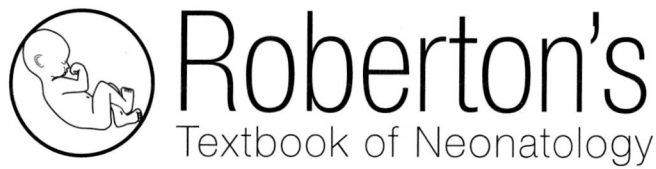

Roberton's
Textbook of Neonatology

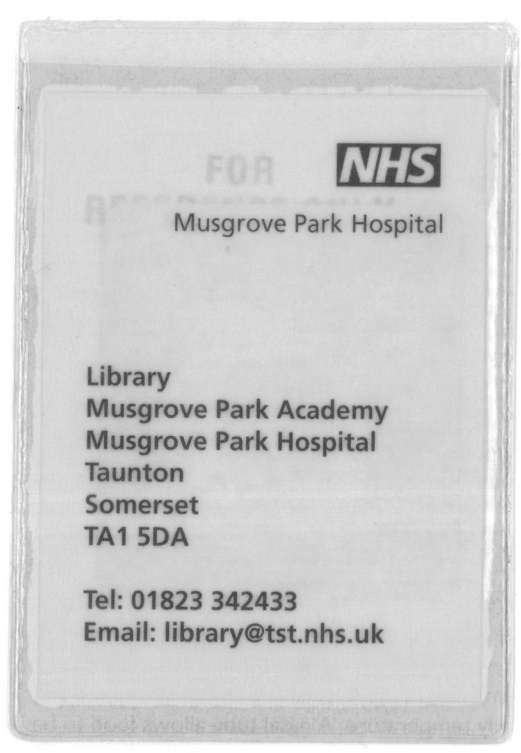

Commissioning Editor: Todd Hummel
Project Development Manager: Hilary Hewitt
Project Manager: Cheryl Brant
Design Manager: Andy Chapman
Illustration Manager: Mick Ruddy
Illustrator: Martin Woodward
Marketing Manager(s) (UK/USA): Catherine Dunningham (UK), Theresa Dudas (US)
Cover illustration: Samuel Ashfield/ Science Photo Library (Caption: Premature baby in an incubator. Babies born before 37 weeks of development require constant monitoring in a contained environment. Their immune system and internal organs are under-developed and they have difficulty maintaining a constant body temperature. A nasal tube allows food to be passed into the stomach.)

Fourth edition

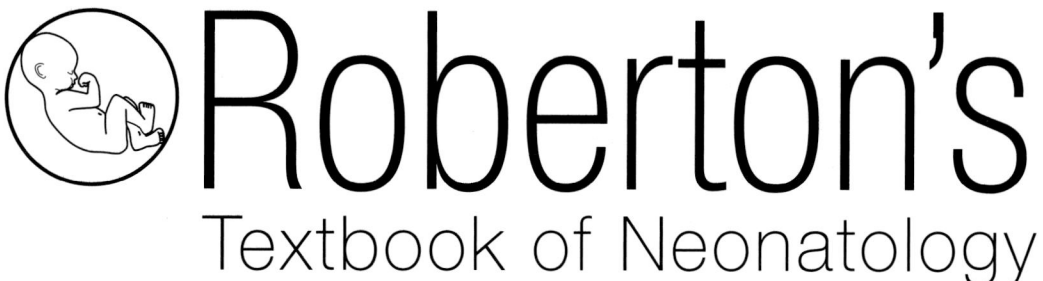

Roberton's
Textbook of Neonatology

EDITED BY

Janet M Rennie MA, MD, FRCP, FRCPCH, DCH
Consultant and Senior Lecturer in Neonatal Medicine
Elizabeth Garrett Anderson Obstetric Hospital,
University College London Hospitals,
London, UK

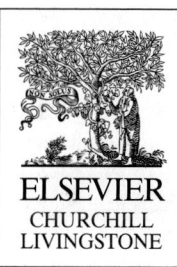

ELSEVIER
CHURCHILL
LIVINGSTONE

ELSEVIER
CHURCHILL
LIVINGSTONE

An imprint of Elsevier Limited

First edition 1986
Second edition 1992
Third edition 1999
Fourth edition 2005

ISBN 0 443 07355 4

British Library Cataloguing in Publication Data
A catalogue record for this book is available from the British Library

Library of Congress Cataloging in Publication Data
A catalog record for this book is available from the Library of Congress

Notice
Medical knowledge is constantly changing. Standard safety precautions must be followed, but as new research and clinical experience broaden our knowledge, changes in treatment and drug therapy may become necessary or appropriate. Readers are advised to check the most current product information provided by the manufacturer of each drug to be administered to verify the recommended dose, the method and duration of administration, and contraindications. It is the responsibility of the practitioner, relying on experience and knowledge of the patient, to determine dosages and the best treatment for each individual patient. Neither the Publisher nor the author assume any liability for any injury and/or damage to persons or property arising from this publication.
The Publisher

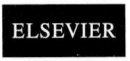 **ELSEVIER** your source for books, journals and multimedia in the health sciences
www.elsevierhealth.com

The Publisher's policy is to use **paper manufactured from sustainable forests**

Printed in China
Last digit is the print number: 9 8 7 6 5 4 3 2 1

Contents

Appendices

Contributors

Jagjit S Ahluwalia MA, MBBCh, DRCOG, DCH, MRCGP, FRCPCH, FRCP
Consultant Neonatologist
Neonatal Intensive Care Unit
Addenbrookes Hospital
Cambridge
UK

Nick Archer MA, FRCP, FRCPCH, DCH
Consultant Paediatric Cardiologist,
    Honorary Clinical
Senior Lecturer
Department of Paediatric Cardiology
John Radcliffe Hospital
Oxford
UK

Ruth M Ayling PhD, MRCP, MRCPath
Consultant Chemical Pathologist,
    Honorary Senior Lecturer
Derriford Combined Laboratory
Derriford Hospital
Plymouth
UK

Philip Baker DM, MRCOG
Professor of Maternal and Fetal Health
St Mary's Hospital
Manchester

Peter G Barth MD, PhD
Emeritus Professor in Paediatric
    Neurology
Department of Paediatric Neurology
Emma Children's Hospital
Academic Medical Center
Amsterdam
The Netherlands

Nick Bishop MBChB, MRCP, MD, FRCPCH
Professor of Paediatric Bone Disease
Academic Unit of Child Health
University of Sheffield
Sheffield
UK

Jeffrey L Brain MS, FRCS
Consultant Neonatal Surgeon
Addenbrookes NHS Trust
Cambridge
UK

Elizabeth Bryan MD, FRCP, FRCPCH
Consultant Paediatrician and Medical
    Consultant to the Multiple Births
    Foundation
Queen Charlotte's and Chelsea Hospital
London
UK

Pamela Cairns MD, MRCP, MRCPCH, DCH
Consultant Neonatologist
Directorate of Children's Services
Neonatal Medicine
Bristol
UK

Andrew J Cant BSc, MD, FRCP, FRCPCH
Consultant in Paediatric Immunology &
    Infectious Diseases
Paediatric Immunology and Infectious
    Diseases Unit
Newcastle General Hospital
Newcastle-upon-Tyne
UK

Fiona Carragher MSc, MRCPath
Principal Biochemist
Department of Clinical Biochemistry
Guy's and St Thomas's Hospital
London
UK

Patrick H T Cartlidge MBChB, DM, FRCP, FRCPCH
Senior Lecturer in Child Health
Department of Child Health
University of Wales College of Medicine
Cardiff
UK

Lord Chan of Oxton MD, FRCPCH, FRCP, FRACP, MFPHM
Visiting Professor in Ethnic Health
University of Liverpool
House of Lords
London
UK

Radha Chari MD, FRCSC
Associate Professor
Department of Obstetrics and
    Gynecology
University of Alberta
Director
Division of Maternal Fetal Medicine
Women's Health Program
Royal Alexandra Hospital
Edmonton
Canada

Adrian K Charles MA, MB, BChir, MD, MRCP, MRCPCH, FRCPath, FRCPA
Paediatric and Perinatal Pathologist
Department of Histopathology
Women's and Children's Pathology
Princess Margaret and King Edward
    Memorial Hospitals
Perth
Australia

Tim Cheetham BSc, MBChB, MD, MRCP, MRCPCH
Senior Lecturer in Paediatric
    Endocrinology
Institute of Child Health
School of Clinical Medical Sciences
University of Newcastle upon Tyne
Royal Victoria Infirmary
Newcastle upon Tyne
UK

Imti Choonara MBChB
Professor in Child Health
Academic Division of Child Health
University of Nottingham
Derbyshire Children's Hospital
Derby
UK

Nicholas M P Clarke ChM, FRCS
Consultant Orthopaedic Surgeon and
   Reader
University Orthopaedics
Southampton General Hospital
Southampton
UK

Sharon Conroy BPharm, MRPharm
Lecturer in Paediatric Clinical Pharmacy
Academic Division of Child Health
University of Nottingham
Derbyshire Children's Hospital
Derby
UK

Christopher J Dare BSc(Hons), BM(Hons),
MRCS(Eng)
Specialist Registrar in Trauma and
   Orthopaedics
University Orthopaedics
Southampton General Hospital
Southampton
UK

Mark Davenport ChM, FRCS(Paed),
FRCS(Eng)
Consultant and Reader in Paediatric
   Surgery
Department of Paediatric Surgery
King's College Hospital
London
UK

Linda S de Vries MD, FRCP
Professor in Neonatal Neurology
Dept of Neonatology
Wilhelmina Children's Hospital
UMC
Utrecht
The Netherlands

Peter Dear MD, FRCP, FRCPCH
Consultant and Senior Lecturer in
   Neonatal Medicine
Neonatal Intensive Care Unit
St James' University Hospital
Leeds
UK

Nestor Demianczuk MD, DES, FRCSC,
ABOG
Professor
Department of Obstetrics and Gynecology
University of Alberta
Royal Alexandra Hospital
Edmonton
Alberta
Canada

Mark Denbow MBBS, MRCOG, PhD
Consultant in Fetal Medicine
Fetal Medicine Unit
St Michael's Hospital
Bristol
UK

D Keith Edmonds FRCOG, FRANZCOG
Consultant Obstetrician & Gynaecologist
Department of Obstetrics & Gynaecology
Queen Charlotte's & Chelsea Hospital
London
UK

Philip Etches MA, MB, FRCP(C), FRCP(Lond),
FAAP, FRCPCH, DCH
Clinical Professor
Department of Paediatrics
University of Alberta
Royal Alexandra Hospital
Edmonton
Canada

David J Evans BM, MRCP(UK), FRCPCH
Consultant Neonatologist
Neonatal Intensive Care Unit
Southmead Hospital
Westbury-on-Trim
Bristol BS10 5NB
UK

Kate Farrer MBChB, FRCPCH, MRCP,
MRCGP, DRCOG, DCH
Consultant Neonatologist
Neonatal Intensive Care Unit
St George's Hospital
London
UK

Mary Fewtrell MD, MA, FRCPCH, DCH
Clinical Scientist and Honorary Senior
   Lecturer
MRC Childhood Nutrition Research
   Centre
Institute of Child Health
London
UK

David Field MBBS(Hons), DCH, FRCPCH,
FRCP(Edin). DM
Professor of Neonatal Medicine
University of Leicester Neonatal Unit
Leicester
UK

Alistair R Fielder FRCS, FRCOphth, FRCP
Professor of Ophthalmology
Department of Visual Neuroscience
Imperial College London
London
UK

Grenville F Fox MBChB, MRCP, FRCPCH
Consultant Neonatologist
Guy's and St Thomas's Hospital
London
UK

Andrew R Gennery MBChB, DCH, MRCP,
MRCPCH, DipMedSci, MD
Senior Lecturer/Honorary Consultant in
   Paediatric Immunology & Bone Marrow
   Transplantation
Paediatric Immunology & Infectious
   Diseases Unit
Newcastle General Hospital
Newcastle-upon-Tyne
UK

Andrew Green PhD, FRCPI, FFPath(RCPI)
Director
National Centre for Medical Genetics;
Professor in Medical Genetics
University College Dublin;
Consultant in Medical Genetics
Our Lady's Hospital and The Children's
   University Hospital
Dublin
Ireland

Anne Greenough MD, FRCP, FRCPCH,
DCH
Professor of Neonatology and Clinical
   Respiratory Physiology
Division of Asthma, Allergy and Lung
   Biology
Guy's, King's and St Thomas' School of
   Medicine
King's College London
London
UK

Nedim Hadzic MD, MSc, FRPCH
Consultant, Honorary Senior Lecturer in
    Paediatric Hepatology
Department of Child Health and Institute
    of Liver Studies
King's College Hospital
London
UK

Simon Hannam MBChB
Children Nationwide Neonatal Unit
King's College Hospital
London
UK

Francoise-Helene D Harlow BSc(Hons),
MRCOG
Consultant Obstetrician and
    Gynaecologist
Norfolk and Norwich University
    Hospital
Norwich
UK

Jane Hawdon MA, MBBS, PhD, MRCP,
FRCPCH
Consultant Neonatologist
Neonatal Unit
Elizabeth Garrett Anderson and
    Obstetrical Hospital
University College London Hospitals
London
UK

Joanna Hawthorne PhD
Senior Research Associate
Centre for Family Research
Cambridge
UK

George Haycock MBBChir, FRCP,
FRCPCH
Professor of Paediatrics
Department of Paediatrics
Eveline Children's Hospital
London
UK

Michael Hird MBBS, MRCP
Consultant in Obstetrics and
    Gynaecology
Royal London Hospital
London
UK

N Kevin Ives MA, MB, BChir, DCH, MRCP,
FRCPCH, MD
Consultant Neonatologist and Honorary
    Senior Clinical Lecturer in Paediatrics
Neonatal Unit
Women's Centre
Oxford
UK

Anthony W Kelsall BSc, MBBCh, FRCPCH,
FRCP
Consultant Neonatologist
Addenbrooke's NHS Trust
Cambridge
UK

Phillipa Kyle MChB, MD, FRCOG,
FRANZCOG
Professor of Obstetrics and Gynaecology
Christchurch School of Medicine and
    Health Sciences
Christchurch
New Zealand

Ian A Laing MA, MD, FRCPE, FRCPCH
Consultant Neonatologist
Neonatal Unit
Simpson Centre for Reproductive Health
Royal Infirmary of Edinburgh
Edinburgh
UK

Victor F Larcher MA, MB, FRCP, FRCPCH
Consultant Paediatrician & Honorary
    Senior Lecturer
Queen Elizabeth Children's Service
Royal London Hospital
London
UK

M A M S Leigh BA
Senior Partner
Hempsons House
London
UK

Malcolm Levene MD, FRCP, FRCPCH,
FMedSci
Professor of Paediatrics
University Department of Paediatrics
Leeds General Infirmary
Leeds
UK

Alan Lucas MD, MA, FRCP, FMedSci
Director/MRC Clinical Professor
MRC Childhood Nutrition Research
    Centre
Institute of Child Health
London
UK

Martin G F Lupton MBBS, MA, MRCOG
Consultant Obstetrician (Locum)
Academic Department of Obstetrics and
    Gynaecology
Chelsea and Westminster Hospital
London
UK

Andrew Lyon MA, MB, FRCP, FRCPCH
Consultant Neonatologist
Neonatal Unit
The Simpson Centre for Reproductive
    Health
Royal Infirmary of Edinburgh
Edinburgh
UK

Alison MacFarlane BA, DipStat, CStat,
FPHM
Professor of Perinatal Health
Department of Midwifery
City University
London
UK

Adnan Manzur MBBS, DCH, FRCPCH
Consultant in Paediatrician
Department of Paediatrics and Neonatal
    Medicine
Imperial College
London
UK

Neil Marlow DM, FRCPCH
Professor of Neonatal Medicine
Academic Division of Child Health
School of Human Development
Nottingham
UK

Hazel E McHaffie PhD, SRN, RM
Deputy Director of Research
Institute of Medical Ethics
Edinburgh
UK

John McIntyre MBChB, BSc, DM, MRCPCH
Senior Lecturer in Child Health
Academic Division of Child Health
University of Nottingham
Derbyshire Children's Hospital
Derby
UK

Eugenio Mercuri FRCPH, MD, PhD
Professor of Paediatric Neurology
Department of Paediatrics and Neonatal
    Medicine
Imperial College
London
UK

Giorgina Mieli-Vergani MD, PhD, FRCP, FRCPH
Alex Mowat Professor of Paediatric
  Hepatology
Paediatric Liver Service
Institute of Liver Studies
King's College Hospital
London
UK

Anthony D Milner MD, FRCP, FRCPCH, DCH
Emeritus Professor of Neonatology
Division of Asthma, Allergy and Lung
  Biology
Guy's, King's and St Thomas' School of
  Medicine
King's College London
London
UK

Neena Modi MBChB, MD, FRCPCH, FRCP, FRCPCH
Clinical Reader in Neonatal Medicine
Department of Paediatrics
Imperial College School of Medicine
London
UK

Gavin Morrison MA, FRCS
Consultant Otolaryngologist
Department of ENT Surgery
Guy's and St Thomas's Hospital
London
UK

Pierre Mouriquand MD, FRCS(Eng), FEBU
Consultant Paediatric Urologist
Department of Paediatric Urology
Hospital Debrousse
Lyon
France

Miranda Mugford BA(Hons), DPhil, HonMFPH
Professor of Health Economics
Institute of Health
University of East Anglia
Norwich
UK

Francesco Muntoni FRCPCH, MD, FMedSci
Professor of Paediatric Neurology
Department of Paediatrics and Neonatal
  Medicine
Imperial College
London
UK

Neil A Murray MD, FRCPH
Senior Lecturer in Neonatal Medicine
Department of Paediatrics and Neonatal
  Medicine
Hammersmith Hospital
London
UK

Simon J Newell MD, FRCPCH, FRCP
Consultant in Neonatal Medicine and
  Paediatric Gastroenterology
Neonatal Unit
St James's University Hospital
Leeds
UK

Eugene Oteng-Ntim MBBS, MRCOG
Consultant Obstetrician
Academic Department of Obstetrics and
  Gynaecology
Guy's and St Thomas' Hospital
London
UK

Roger D Palmer BSc(Hons), MB, BChir, MRCP(UK), MRCPCH
Specialist Registrar in Paediatric Oncology
Addenbrooke's NHS Trust
Cambridge
UK

Michael Patton MA, MSc, MBChB, FRCP, FRCPCH
Professor of Medical Genetics
Department of Medical Genetics
St George's Hospital Medical School
London
UK

David W Pilling MBChB, DCH, DMRD, FRCR, FRCPCH
Consultant Paediatric Radiologist
Department of Radiology
Royal Liverpool Children's Hospital,
  Alder Hey and
Liverpool Women's Hospital
Liverpool
UK

Esther J Posner BSc, MBBS, FRCOphth
Specialist Registrar in Ophthalmology
Western Eye Hospital
London
UK

Janet M Rennie MA, MD, FRCP, FRCPCH, DCH
Consultant and Senior Lecturer in
  Neonatal Medicine
Elizabeth Garrett Anderson Obstetric
  Hospital
University College London Hospitals
London
UK

Sam Richmond MBBS, FRCP, FRCPCH
Consultant Neonatologist
Neonatal Unit
Sunderland Royal Hospital
Sunderland
UK

Rodney Rivers MB, BChir, FRCP, MRCPH, DCH
Reader in Paediatrics
Department of Academic Paediatrics
Imperial College London
London
UK

N C R Roberton MA MB FRCP
Formerly Consultant Paediatrician and
  Neonatologist
Rosie Maternity Hospital
Cambridge
UK

Irene A G Roberts MD, FRCP, FRCPath, DRCOG
Professor of Paediatric Haematology
Department of Haematology
Hammersmith Hospital
Imperial College London
London

Maureen Rogers MBBS, FACD
Head
Department of Dermatology
The Children's Hospital at Westmead
Westmead
Australia

Nicholas Rutter MD, FRCP, FRCPCH
Professor of Paediatric Medicine
University of Nottingham
Academic Division of Child Health
Queen's Medical Centre
Nottingham
UK

Steven M Sale MBChB, FRCA
Fellow in Paediatric Anaesthesia
Bristol Royal Hospital for Children
Bristol
UK

Nicholas M Smith BMedSci(Hons), MBBS,
FRCPath, FRCPA
Paediatric and Perinatal Pathologist
Department of Histopathology
Women's and Children's Pathology
Princess Margaret Hospital for Children
Perth
Australia

Alistair G Smyth BDS, MBBS, FRCS,
FDSRCS
Consultant Cleft, Oral and Maxillofacial
    Surgeon
Northern and Yorkshire Regional Cleft Lip
    and Palate Service
Leeds General Infirmary
Leeds
UK

John A D Spencer MBBS, FRCOG
Consultant Obstetrician and
    Gynaecologist
Northwick Park Hospital
Middlesex
UK

Philip Steer BSc, MBBS, MD, FRCOG
Professor of Obstetrics
Academic Department of Obstetrics and
    Gynaecology
Imperial College Faculty of Medicine
Chelsea and Westminster Hospital
London
UK

Mark D Stringer BSc, MS, FRCS, FRCP,
FRCPCH
Consultant Paediatric Hepatobiliary and
    Reader in Paediatric Surgery
Children's Liver & GI Unit
St James's University Hospital
Leeds
UK

Ian Sugarman FRCS(Edin), FRCS (Paed)
Consultant Paediatric Surgeon
Department of Paediatric Surgery
Leeds General Infirmary
Leeds
UK

Clare Tower MBChB
Wellcome Clinical Research Training
    Fellow
Department of Molecular Medical
    Sciences
University of Nottingham
Queen's Medical Centre
Nottingham
UK

A Michael Weindling BSc, MA, MD, FRCP,
FRCPCH
Professor of Perinatal Medicine
School of Reproductive and
    Developmental Medicine
Liverpool Women's Hospital
Liverpool
UK

Duncan T Wilcox FRCS, MD
Honorary Senior Lecturer
Nephro-Urology Department
Institute of Child Health
London
UK

Denise Williams MB, FRCP, MRCPCH
Consultant Paediatric Oncologist
Department of Paediatrics
Addenbrooke's NHS Trust
Cambridge
UK

Andrew R Wolf MA, MB, BChir, FRCA, MD
Professor of Anaesthesia and Intensive
    Care
University of Bristol
Paediatric Intensive Care Unit
Bristol Royal Children's Hospital
Bristol
UK

James E Wraith MC ChB, FRCPCH
Consultant Paediatrician
Willink Biochemical Genetics Unit
Royal Manchester Children's Hospital
Manchester
UK

Preface

The availability of full text journals on the Web has led many to predicted the demise of the large multi-author textbook, which cannot include the very latest research findings. In my view this prediction will continue to prove fallacious. A good textbook chapter remains the best first step on the pathway to individual learning; it provides background, context and balance for juniors who are working up a topic for the first time, and acts as an *aide-memoire* for experienced consultants who want to check a fact, find a key reference or learn about current management from an expert. A textbook also provides the opportunity to review important areas of practice such as the complications of procedures, standards, epidemiological trends and counselling which are difficult to find covered anywhere in the research literature. With these objects in mind, I have worked with the chapter authors to produce a book which I hope combines solid scientific background information with readable text giving sensible advice, which is readily accessible because it is organized into sections and contains plenty of tables and illustrations. I have made a particular effort to include information on prognosis in this edition because as neonatology has evolved, more is known about the outcome of many conditions and parents and clinicians want access to this information as early as possible.

By the time this book is published it will be almost twenty years since the publication of the first edition. Cliff Roberton, sole editor of the first two editions and my co-editor for the third, has now retired. The book is renamed *Roberton's Textbook of Neonatology* in his honour, and to reflect the enormous contribution that Cliff made to British neonatology. I have taken sole responsibility for the contents and editing of this, the fourth edition, and am accountable for any omissions. Any suggestions for topics to be included in future editions are gratefully received. As ever, I have learned much from reading and re-reading the individual contributions and I am immensely grateful to a large number of people, too many to name individually in the acknowledgement section which follows.

The long cycle of planning, commissioning, writing, reading, checking and rechecking is now at an end. My hope is that all those who use this book will discover something to interest them and find the answers to most of their questions, with a pointer to the right source of further information for their complex queries. Above all, I hope that copies of the book will be found, not in libraries on high dusty shelves, but at the baby's cot-side, where they have become dog-eared and scruffy from everyday use because the content has proved indispensable to those who are striving to deliver high quality neonatal care.

Janet M Rennie
University College London Hospitals
2005

Acknowledgements

The acknowledgement section of a large multi-author textbook such as this inevitably includes mention of partners neglected, holidays missed, and theatre trips abandoned, in addition to the loss of Sunday afternoons with the children. Sadly, all this remains true and as a result I am doubly grateful to the individual chapter authors, who were no doubt aware of the likely cost to their personal lives when they accepted my invitation to contribute. I owe all of them a great deal, and take this opportunity not only to thank them, but to apologise once again to those whose work had to be cut down or altered in order to squeeze the material into one volume. All showed remarkable tolerance in answering queries and accommodating my suggestions, and I hope they are pleased with the result of their labours. Behind them are massed armies of partners, secretaries, and librarians too many to count, but who also deserve praise. Particular thanks of my own are due to the staff of the library at the Royal Society of Medicine in London, who are unfailingly helpful, and produced many obscure references from the basement rolling stacks within days. My secretary Jane Paget has also spent many hours obtaining references and typing in citations to Reference Manager without complaint and with good humour, and I take this opportunity to thank her too.

Hilary Hewitt at Elsevier bore the brunt of the immense amount work involved in getting a project of this size through on time, and she remained cheerful and unflappable throughout, in spite of delivering a baby of her own during the gestation period of the book. It has been a pleasure to work with her. Many others at Elsevier have also made great contributions, particularly Cheryl Brant and Judy Fletcher. The copy editing has been first-class, and the illustrators have managed to produce beautiful figures from many back-of-the envelope sketches.

Last, but by no means least, the person who has borne the largest burden from the impact that editing the book made on my disposable time was of course my husband, Ian Watts. He has been supportive throughout, and to him this book is dedicated, with much love.

Janet M Rennie
University College London Hospitals
2005

Abbreviations

A

α_1AT	Alpha-1-antitrypsin
α_1ATD	Alpha-1-antitrypsin deficiency
α2M	Alpha-2-macroglobulin
a/A ratio	Arterial alveolar ratio (of PaO_2)
AA	Arachidonic acid
A-aDO$_2$	Alveolar–arterial oxygen difference (of PaO_2)
ABR	Auditory brainstem evoked responses
AC	Aplasia cutis
ACE	Angiotensin-converting enzymes
AchR	Acetylcholine receptor
ACT	Activated clotting time
ACTH	Adrenocorticotrophic hormone, corticotrophin
AD	Autosomal dominant
ADA	Adenosine deaminase
ADCC	Antibody-dependent cytotoxicity
ADH	Antidiuretic hormone
ADP	Adenosine diphosphate
ADPKD	Autosomal dominant polycystic kidney disease
AFI	Amniotic fluid index
AFP	Alpha fetoprotein
AGA	Appropriate for gestational age
AGM	Aorto-gonad-mesonephros
AIDS	Aquired immune deficiency syndrome
AIHA	Autoimmune haemolytic anaemia
ALEC	Artificial lung expanding compound (Pumactant)
ALL	Acute lymphoblastic leukaemia
AMH	Antimüllerian hormone
AML	Acute myeloid leukaemia
AMP	Adenosine monophosphate
ANP	Atrial natriuretic peptide
AP	Aorto-pulmonary
APC	Activated protein C
	Antigen-presenting cells
APH	Antepartum haemorrhage
APTT	Activated partial thromboplastin time
AR	Amnioreduction
	Aortic regurgitation
	Autosomal recessive
ARDS	Adult (acute) respiratory distress syndrome
ARM	Artificial rupture of the membranes
ARPKD	Autosomal recessive polycystic kidney disease
ART	Assisted reproductive techniques

AS	Aortic stenosis
ASD	Atrial septal defect
ATP	Adenosine triphosphate
ATS	Anti-tetanus serum
AV	Atrioventricular
AVM	Arteriovenous malformation
AVP	Arginine vasopressin (i.e. ADH)
AVSD	Atrioventricular septal defect

B

BAER	Brainstem accoustic evoked responses
BAL	Bronchoalveolar lavage
BAPM	British Association of Perinatal Medicine (formerly BAPP – British Association of Perinatal Paediatrics)
BASM	Biliary atresia splenic malformation (syndrome)
BBA	Born before arrival
BCG	Bacillus Calmette Guérin
BCSH	British Committee for Standards in Haematology
BMC	Bone mineral content
BMR	Basal metabolic rate
BMT	Bone marrow transplant
BPA	British Paediatric Association
BP	Blood pressure
BPD	Biparietal diameter
	Bronchopulmonary dysplasia
BPSU	British Paediatric Surveillance Unit
BSDL	Bile-salt-dependent lipase
BSEP	Bile salt export pump
BT	Bleeding time

C

CaO$_2$	Arterial oxygen content
CA	Carbonic anhydrase
CAH	Congenital adrenal hyperplasia
cAMP	Cyclic adenosine monophosphate
CBF(V)	Cerebral blood flow (velocity)
CcO$_2$	Capillary oxygen content
CCAM	Congenital cystic adenomatoid malformation
CD	Cluster of differentiation

CDA	Congenital dyserythropoietic anaemia
CDG	Carbohydrate-deficient glycoprotein
CDH	Congenital diaphramatic hernia
	Congenital dislocation of the hip (see DDH, p. 255–6)
CDP	Cytidine choline diphosphate
CEMD	Confidential Enquiry into Maternal Deaths
CESDI	Confidential Enquiry into Stillbirths and Deaths in Infancy
CF	Cystic fibrosis
CFM	Cerebral function monitor
CFTR	Cystic fibrosis transmembrane regulator
CGD	Chronic granulomatous disease
cGMP	Cyclic guanosine monophosphate
CHARGE	Coloboma, heart disease, choanal atresia, retardation, genital and ear anomalies
CHB	Complete heart block
	Congenital heart block
CHD	Congenital heart disease
CHIPA	Chronic in-utero partial asphyxia
CHS	Chediak–Higashi syndrome
CI	Confidence interval
CK	Creatine phosphokinase
CLAPA	Cleft lip and palate association
CLD	Chronic lung disease
CLSE	Calf lung surfactant extract
CM	Capillary malformation
CMD	Congenital muscular dystrophy
CMO	Corticosterone methyloxidase
CMV	Cytomegalovirus
CNEP	Continuous negative external pressure
CNS	Central nervous system
CONS	Coagulase-negative staphylococci
CoA	Co-enzyme A
COP	Colloid osmotic pressure
CP	Cerebral palsy
CPAP	Continuous positive airways pressure
CPC	Choroid plexus cyst
CPD(A)	Citrate phosphate dextrose (adenine)
CPHD	Combined pituitary hormone deficiency
CPR	Cardiopulmonary resuscitation
CPS	Carbamyl phosphate synthetase
CRH	Corticotrophin releasing hormone
CRIB	Clinical risk index for babies
CRP	C-reactive protein
CS	Caesarean section
CSAG	Clinical Standards Advisory Group
CSF	Cerebrospinal fluid
CT	Computed tomography
CTEV	Congenital talipes equinovarus
CTG	Cardiotocogram (cardiotocography)
CvO_2	Mixed venous oxygen content
CVB(S)	Chorionic villus biopsy (sampling)
CVP	Central venous pressure
CVS	Cardiovascular system
	Chorionic villus sampling
CXR	Chest X-ray

D

2:3 DPG	2:3 diphosphoglycerate
DA	Ductus arteriosus
DAT	Direct antiglobulin (Coombs') test
DBA	Diamond–Blackfan anaemia
DBM	Drip/donor breast milk
DC	Dichorionic
DCM	Dilated cardiomyopathy
DCT	Direct Coombs' test
DDAVP	Desmopressin: 1-deamino-8-D-arginine vasopressin
DDH	Developmental dysplasia of the hip
del	deletion
DH	Department of Health
DHA	Docosahexaenoic acid
DHSS	Department of Health and Social Security
DHT	Dihydrotestosterone
DIC	Disseminated intravascular coagulation
DIDMOAD	Diabetes insipidus, diabetes mellitus, optic atrophy, deafness
DILV	Double-inlet left ventricle
DIV	Double-inlet ventricle
DMSA	Dimercaptosuccinic acid
DNA	Deoxyribonucleic acid
DOC	Deoxycorticosterone
DOH	Department of Health
DORV	Double-outlet right ventricle
DOV	Double-outlet ventricle
DPG	Diphosphoglycerate
DPPC	Dipalmitoyl phosphatidyl choline (lecithin)
DQ	Development quotient
DRG	Diagnostic related groups
	Dorsal respiratory group
DTP	Diptheria–tetanus–pertussis
DTPA	Diethylenetriaminepentacetic acid
DVM	Delayed visual maturation
DVT	Deep vein thrombosis
DXA	Dual energy X-ray absorptiometry
DZ	Dizygotic

E

EB	Epidermolysis bullosa
EBF	Exclusive breastfeeding
EBM	Expressed breast milk
EBV	Epstein-Barr virus
EC	European Community
	Ejection click
ECF	Extracellular fluid
ECG	Electrocardiogram
ECM	External cardiac massage
ECMO	Extracorporeal membrane oxygenation
ECV	External cephalic version
EDD	Estimated date of delivery
EDF	End-diastolic flow
EDFV	End-diastolic flow velocity

EDTA	Ethylenediamine tetracetic acid
EEG	Electroencephalogram
EFE	Endocardial fibroelastosis
EFM	Electronic fetal monitoring
EGF	Epithelial/epidermal growth factor
ELBW	Extremely low birthweight (1.0 kg birthweight)
ELISA	Enzyme-linked immunosorbent assay
ELSO	Extracorporeal-like support organisation
EM	Electron microscope
EMG	Electromyogram/electromyography
EMLA	Eutectic mixture of local anaesthetic
ERCP	Endoscopic retrograde cholangiopancreatography
ERG	Electroretinogram
ESPGAN	European Society for Paediatric Gastroenterology and Nutrition
ETT	Endotracheal tube
EVT	Extravillous trophoblast

F

FACS	Fluorescence activated cell sorting
FAITP	Fetal alloimmune thrombocytopenic purpura
FBC	Full blood count
FBM	Fetal breathing movements
FBS	Fetal blood sampling
FCE	Finished consultant episode
FDP	Fibrin degradation products
Fe_{H_2O}	Fractional excretion of water
Fe_{Na}	Fractional excretion of sodium
FEV_1	Forced expiratory volume in one minute
FEVR	Familial exudative vitreoretinopathy
FFP	Fresh frozen plasma
FFTS	Feto-fetal transfusion syndrome
FGR	Fetal growth restriction
FH	Family history
FHR	Fetal heart rate
FIGO	International Federation of Gynaecology & Obstetrics
FIL	Feedback inhibitor of lactation
F_IO_2	Fractional inspired oxygen concentration
FISH	Fluorescent in-situ hybridisation
FOE	Fractional oxygen extraction
FRC	Functional residual capacity
FSE	Fetal scalp electrode
FSH	Follicle-stimulating hormone
FTA-ABS	Fluorescent treponemal antibody absorption test
FUV	Fetal umbilical vein

G

GAD	Glutamic acid decarboxylase
GALT	Gut-associated lymphoid tissue
γGT	Gamma-glutamyl transferase
GABA	Gamma amino butyric acid

G6PD	Glucose-6-phosphate dehydrogenase
GBS	Group B beta-haemolytic streptococcus
G-CSF	Granulocyte colony-stimulating factor
GCT	Germ cell tumours
GDP	Gross domestic product
GFAP	Glial fibrillary acidic protein
GFR	Glomerular filtration rate
GGT	Gamma-glutamyl transpeptidase
GH	Growth hormone
GHRH	Growth hormone releasing hormone
GIFT	Gamete intrafallopian transfer
GI	Gastrointestinal
GIT	Gastrointestinal tract
GM-CSF	Granulocyte–macrophage colony-stimulating factor
GMH-IVH	Germinal matrix/intraventricular haemorrhage
GMP	Guanosine monophosphate
GnRH	Gonadotrophin releasing hormone
GOR	Gastro-oesophageal reflux
GP	General Practitioner
GSD	Glycogen storage disease
GSH	Reduced glutathione
GTP	Guanosine triphosphate
GTT	Glucose tolerance test
GU	Genitourinary
GVHD	Graft-versus-host disease

H

HAA	Hospital activity analysis
HAS	Human albumin solution
HBV	Hepatitis B virus
hCG	Human chorionic gonadotrophin
HCM	Hypertrophic cardiomyopathy
HCV	Hepatitis C virus
HDL	High-density lipoprotein
HDN	Haemolytic disease of the newborn Haemorrhagic disease of the newborn (VKDB)
Hep A, B, C	Hepatitis A, B, C
HELLP	Haemolysis, elevated liver enzymes, low platelets
HES	Hospital episode system
HFFI	High-frequency flow interruption
HFJV	High-frequency jet ventilation
HFOV	High-frequency oscillatory ventilation
HFPPV	High-frequency positive pressure ventilation
HI	Hyperinsulinism in infancy
HIE	Hypoxic ischaemic encephalopathy
HIV	Human immunodeficiency virus
HLA	Human leucocyte antigen
HLH	Haemophogocytic lymphohistiocytosis
HLHS	Hypoplastic left heart syndrome
HMD	Hyaline membrane disease
HMF	Human milk formula
HPA	Hypothalamic-pituitary-adrenal Human platelet antigen

HPI	Haemorrhagic parenchymal infarction
HPP	Hereditary pyropoikilocytosis
HPS	Hypertrophic pyloric stenosis
HPV	Human parvovirus
HRG	Health Resource Groupings
HS	Hereditary spherocytosis
HSV	Herpes simplex virus (I, II)
HVA	Homovanillic acid
HVS	High vaginal swab
Hz	Hertz (cycles/second)

I

IAA	Interrupted aortic arch
ICAM	Intracellular adhesion molecule
ICD	International classification of disease
ICH	Intracranial haemorrhage
ICP	Intracranial pressure
IDA	Iminodiacetic acid
IDM	Infant of the diabetic mother
I:E	Inspiratory to expiratory ratio
IEM	Inborn error of metabolism
IFN	Interferon
IgA, D, G, M	Immunoglobulins A, D, G, and M
IGF	Insulin-like growth factor
IHV	Intrahepatic venous (sampling)
IL	Interleukin
i.m.	Intramuscular
IMF	International Monetary Fund
INO	Inhaled nitric oxide
INR	International normalised ratio
IPL	Intraparenchymal lesion
IPPV	Intermittent positive pressure ventilation
IPT	Intraperitoneal transfusion
IQ	Intelligence quotient
IRT	Immunoreactive trypsin
ITP	Idiopathic/immune thrombocytopenic purpura
IUD	Intrauterine death
IUGR	Intrauterine growth retardation/restriction
i.v.	Intravenous
IVC	Inferior vena cava
IVF	In-vitro fertilisation
IVH	Intraventricular haemorrhage
IVIG	Intravenous immunoglobulin
IVS	Intact ventricular septum
IVT	Intravascular transfusion
IVU	Intravenous urogram

K

KCCT	Kaolin cephalin clotting time
KHE	Kaposiform haemangioendothelioma
KIR	Killer inhibitory receptors
kPa	Kilopascal (= 7.5 mmHg)

L

LA	Laser ablation
LAD	Left axis deviation
LBND	Livebirth with no defects
LBW	Low birthweight (<2.50 kg)
LC	Locus ceruleus
LCAD	Long-chain fatty acyl-CoA dehydrogenase
LCHAD	Long-chain fatty 3-hydroxyacyl-CoA dehydrogenase
LCPUFA	Long-chain polyunsaturated fatty acids
LCT	Long-chain triglyceride
LE	Lupus erythematosus
LGA	Large for gestational age
LH	Luteinising hormone
LLSE	Lower left sternal edge
LM	Lymphatic malformation
LMP	Last menstrual period
LMWH	Low-molecular-weight heparin
LOS	Lower oesophageal sphincter
LP	Lumbar puncture
L:S	Lecithin to sphingomyelin ratio
LSCS	Lower segment caesarean section
LT	Leukotriene
LV	Left ventricle
LVH	Left ventricular hypertrophy
LVOT	Left ventricular outflow tract

M

MACS	Magnetically activated cell sorting
MAD	Multiple acyl-CoA dehydrogenase
MAG-3	Mercaptoacetyl triglycine
MAP	Mean airway pressure
MAPCA	Major aorto-pulmonary communicating arteries
MAS	Meconium aspiration syndrome
MC	Monochorionic
MCA	Middle cerebral artery
MCAD	Medium-chain fatty acyl-CoA dehydrogenase
MCH	Mean corpuscular haemoglobin
MCHC	Mean corpuscular haemoglobin content
MCP	Major cationic protein
MCT	Medium-chain triglycerides
MCUG	Micturating cysto-urethrogram
MCV	Mean corpuscular volume
meg CSF	Megakaryocyte colony-stimulating factor
MHC	Major histocompatibility complex
MIC	Minimum inhibitory concentration
MIF	Migration inhibitory factor
MIP	Macrophage inflammatory protein
MMC	Meningomyelocele
mmHg	Millimetres of mercury
MMR	Mumps, measles and rubella vaccine
MOM	Multiples of the median
MPH	Massive pulmonary haemorrhage

MPI	Milk protein intolerance
MR	Magnetic resonance
	Mitral regurgitation
MRC	Medical Research Council
MRI	Magnetic resonance imaging
mRNA	Messenger ribonucleic acid
MRS	Magnetic resonance spectroscopy
MRSA	Methicillin-resistant *Staphylococcus aureus*
MS	Mitral stenosis
MSH	Melanocyte-stimulating hormone
mt	Mitochondrial
MZ	Monozygotic

N

Naa	*N*-acetyl-aspartate
NADPH	Nicotinamide adenine dinucleotide phosphate
NAITP	Neonatal alloimmune thrombocytopenic purpura
NALD	Neonatal adrenoleucodystrophy
NBAS	Neonatal behavioural assessment scale
NBT	Nitroblue tetrazolium
NCT	National Childbirth Trust
NEC	Necrotising enterocolitis
NG	Nasogastric
NGF	Nerve growth factor
NGT	Nasogastric tube
NH	Neonatal haemochromatosis
NHS	National Health Service
NICHHD	National Institute of Child Health and Human Development
NICU	Neonatal Intensive Care Unit
NIDCAP	Neonatal Individual Developmental Care and Assessment Programme
NIDDM	Non-insulin-dependent diabetes mellitus
NIH	Non-immune hydrops
NIRS	Near infrared spectroscopy
NK	Natural killer (lymphocytes)
NMDA	*N*-methyl-D-aspartate
NMR	Nuclear magnetic resonance
	Neonatal mortality risk
NO	Nitric oxide
NRCT	National Registry of Childhood Tumours
NSAID	Non-steroidal anti-inflammatory drugs
NT	Nuchal translucency
NTD	Neural tube defect

O

17-OHP	17-hydroxyprogesteron
OA	Oesophageal atresia
OC	Obstetric cholestasis
OCT	Ornithine carbamyl transferase
OFC	Occipito-frontal circumference
OI	Osteogenesis imperfecta
ONS	Office of National Statistics

OPCS	Office of Population, Censuses and Surveys
OR	Odds ratio
OTC	Ornithine transcarbamylase

P

PA	Pulmonary artery
PABS	Pulmonary artery branch stenosis
$PaCO_2$	Partial pressure of CO_2 in arterial blood
$PACO_2$	Partial pressure of CO_2 in alveolar gas
PAF	Platelet-activating factor
PAGE	Perfluorocarbon-assisted gas exchange
PAH	Para-amino hippurate
PAI-1	Plasminogen activator inhibitor 1
PAIgG	Antiplatelet autoantibodies
PaO_2	Partial pressure of oxygen in arterial blood
PAO_2	Partial pressure of oxygen in alveolar gas
PAP	Pulmonary artery pressure
PAPP-A	Pregnancy-associated plasma protein A
PAPVC	Partial anomalous pulmonary venous connection
PARP	poly(ADP-ribose) polymerase
PC	Phosphatidylcholine
PCA	Postconceptional age
PCH	Pontocerebellar hypoplasia
PCP	*Pneumocystis carinii* pneumonia
PCr	Phosphocreatine
PCR	Polymerase chain reaction
PCV	Packed cell volume
PDA	Patent ductus arteriosus
PDF	Post-discharge formula
PE	Phosphatidylethanolamine
PEEP	Positive end-expiratory pressure
PET	Pre-eclamptic toxaemia
PF 3	Platelet factor 3
PF 4	Platelet factor 4
PFC	Persistent fetal circulation
	Perfluorocarbon
PFIC	Progressive familial intrahepatic cholestasis
PFK	Phosphofructokinase
PFO	Patent foramen ovale
PG	Phosphatidylglycerol
PGE, F, G, H	Prostaglandins E, F, G and H
PGI_2	Prostacyclin
PGSI	Prostaglandin synthetase inhibitor
pH	Hydrogen ion concentration
PHD	Pituitary hormone deficiency
PHHI	Persistent hyperinsulinaemic hypoglycaemia of infancy (nesidioblastosis)
PHT	Pulmonary hypertension
PHVD	Post-haemorrhagic ventricular dilatation
Pi	Inorganic orthophosphate
PI	Phosphatidylinositol
PIE	Pulmonary interstitial emphysema
PIH	Pregnancy-induced hypertension
PIP	Peak inflating pressure
PIVKA	Protein produced in vitamin K absence

PK	Pyruvate kinase
	Prekallikrein
PKU	Phenylketonuria
PLP	Proteolipid protein
PLV	Partial liquid ventilation
PNET	Primitive neuroectodermal tumour
PNMR	Perinatal mortality rate
PNP	Purine nucleotide phosphorylase
PNW	Postnatal ward
POEMS	Programmable otoacoustic emissions
PSARP	Posterior sagittal anorectoplasty
PP	Pancreatic polypeptide
PPF	Purified plasma fraction
PPHN	Persistent pulmonary hypertension of the newborn
PPROM	Preterm premature rupture of the membranes
PRA	Plasma renin activity
PRISM	Paediatric risk of mortality score
PRL	Prolactin
PROM	Preterm rupture of the membranes
PS	Pulmonary stenosis
	Phosphatidylserine
PSM	Pansystolic murmur
PT	Prothrombin time
PTC	Percutaneous transhepatic cholangiography
PTH	Parathyroid hormone
PTHrP	Parathyroid hormone-related peptide
PTL	Preterm labour
PTM	Preterm milk
PTT	Partial thromboplastin time
PTTK	PTT kaolin
PTV	Patient trigger ventilation
PUBS	Percutaneous umbilical blood sampling
PUFA	Polyunsaturated fatty acids
PUJ	Pyelo/pelvi ureteric junction
PUV	Posterior urethral valves
PVD	Pulmonary vascular disease
PVH	Periventricular haemorrhage
PVL	Periventricular leukomalacia
PVR	Pulmonary vascular resistance

Q

QALY	Quality-adjusted life year
Qs	Proportion of the cardiac output which is shunted
Qt	Total cardiac output
q.v	*Quod vide* = which see

R

RA	Right atrium
RAAS	Renin–angiotensin–aldosterone system
RAH	Right atrial hypertrophy
RBC	Red blood cell
RBP	Retinol-binding protein

RCOG	Royal College of Obstetricians and Gynaecologists
RCPCH	Royal College of Paediatrics and Child Health
RCT	Randomised controlled trial
RDA	Recommended dietary allowance
RDS	Respiratory distress syndrome
REM	Rapid eye movement (sleep)
RF	Risk factor
RFLP	Restriction fragment length polymorphism
RHA	Regional Health Authority
rHuEpo	Recombinant human erythropoietin
RICH	Rapidly involuting congenital haemangioma
RIP	Respiratory inductance plethysmography
	Rest in Peace
RIS	Respiratory insufficiency syndrome
RLF	Retrolental fibroplasia
RNA	Ribonucleic acid
RNCE	Routine neonatal clinical examination
RO	Retinopathy of prematurity
ROC	receiver operating characteristics
RP	Ribosomal protein
RSV	Respiratory syncytial virus
RTH	Resistance to thyroid hormone
RV	Right ventricle
	Residual volume
RVET	Right ventricular ejection time
RVH	Right ventricular hypertrophy
RVOT	Right ventricular outflow tract
Rx	Recipe – prescribe for

S

SAH	s-adenosylhomocysteine
SANDS	Stillbirth and Neonatal Death Society
SaO_2	True arterial haemoglobin oxygen saturation
SB	Stillborn
SBR	Stillbirth rate
SBS	Short bowel syndrome
s.c.	Subcutaneously
SCBU	Special Care Baby Unit
SCID	Severe combined immunodeficiency
SCT	Sacrococcygeal tumour
SD	Standard deviation (of the mean)
SEH	Subependymal haemorrhage
SEP(R)	Somatosensory evoked potential (response)
SF-1	Steroidogenic factor 1
SFD	Small for dates
SGA	Small for gestational age
SH	Sulphydryl
SHO	Senior House Officer
SIADH	Syndrome of inappropriate ADH secretion
SIDS	Sudden infant death syndrome
SIMV	Synchronised intermittent mandatory ventilation
SLE	Systemic lupus erythematosus
SLO	Smith–Lemli–Opitz syndrome
SMA	Spinal muscular atrophy

SMS	Somatostatin
SNAP	Score for neonatal acute physiology
SNHL	Sensorineural hearing loss
SOD	Septo-optic dysplasia
	Superoxide dismutase
SP-A, -B, -C, -D	Surfactant apoproteins A, B, C, D
SPA	Suprapubic aspiration (urine)
	Single photon absorptiometry
sPDA	Symptomatic patent ductus arteriosus
SpO_2	Transcutaneous haemoglobin oxygen saturation (from oximeter)
SpR	Specialist Registrar
SSCA	Single-stranded conformational assay
StAR	Steroidogenic regulatory protein
SVT	Supraventricular tachycardia

T

T_3	Tri-iodothyronine
T_4	Thyroxine
TA	Tufted angioma
TAFI	Thrombin-activated fibrinolysis inhibitor
TA-GVHD	Transfusion-associated graft-versus-host disease
TAM	Transient abnormal myelopoiesis
TAMBA	Twins and multiple births association
TAPVC/D	Total anomalous pulmonary venous connection/drainage
TAR	Thrombocytopenia and absent radius (syndrome)
TB	Tuberculosis
TBG	Thyroxine-binding globulin
$tcPCO_2$	Transcutaneous PCO_2
$tcPO_2$	Transcutaneous PO_2
TCR	T-cell receptor
TCT	Thrombin clotting time
TCU	Transitional care unit
T_E	Expiratory time
TEWL	Transepidermal water loss
TF	Tissue factor
TFPI	Tissue factor pathway inhibitor
TGA	Transposition of the great arteries
TGF	Tissue growth factor
TGV	Thoracic gas volume
THAM	Tris-hydroxymethylaminomethane
T_I	Inspiratory time
TI	Tricuspid incompetence
TINA	Transport of Neonates by Ambulance
TLC	Total lung capacity
TLV	Total liquid ventilation
TMD	Transient myeloproliferative disorder
$TNF\alpha$	Tumour necrosis factor alpha
TOE	Transoesophageal echocardiography
TOF	Tracheo-oesophageal fistula
TORCH	Toxoplasma, rubella, cytomegalovirus, herpes
t-PA	Tissue plasminogen activator
TPFR	Total period fertility rate

TPHA	*Treponema pallidum* haemagglutination assay
TPN	Total parenteral nutrition
TPR	Temperature, pulse and respiration
TPV	Time to peak velocity
TR	Tricuspid regurgitation
TRAP	Twin reversed arterial perfusion
TRH	Thyrotrophin-releasing hormone
tRNA	Transfer RNA
TS	Tuberous sclerosis
TSH	Thyroid-stimulating hormone (thyrotrophin)
TSI	Thyroid-stimulating immunoglobulins
TT	Thrombin time
TTN	Transient tachypnoea of the newborn
TTTS	Twin–twin transfusion syndrome
TXA_2	Thromboxane A2

U

UAC	Umbilical artery catheter
UapH	Umbilical artery pH
UDPGT	Uridine diphosphoglucuronyl transferase
UFH	Unfractionated heparin
UFI	Urine flow impairment
UK	United Kingdom
u-PA	Urokinase-type plasminogen activator
URTI	Upper respiratory tract infection
US	Ultrasound
USA	United States of America
USS	Ultrasound scan
UTI	Urinary tract infection
UVC	Umbilical venous catheter

V

VACTERL	As for VATER with cardiac and limb defects
VATER	Vertebral defects, anal atresia, T-E fistula, radial and renal dysplasia
VC	Vital capacity
VDDR	Vitamin D-dependent rickets
VDRL	Veneral disease research laboratory (test for syphilis)
V_E	Minute volume
VE	Ventricular ectopics
VEGF	Vascular endothelial growth factor
VEP	Visual evoked potential
vi	*Vide infra* (see below in text)
viz	*Videlicet* = namely
VKDB	Vitamin K deficiency bleeding
VLBW	Very low birthweight (<1.50 kg)
VM	Venous malformation
VMA	Vanillylmandelic acid
VRG	Ventral respiratory group
vs	*Vide supra* (see above in text)
VSD	Ventricular septal defect
V_T	Tidal volume
VT	Ventricular tachycardia
VTE	Venous thromboembolism

VUJ	Vesico-ureteric junction
vWD	von Willebrand's disease
vWF	von Willebrand's factor
VZV	varicella zoster virus

W

WBC	White blood cell
	White blood (cell) count
WHO	World Health Organization
WPW	Wolff–Parkinson–White syndrome

X

XLD	X-linked dominant
XLR	X-linked recessive

Z

ZIG	Zoster immune globulin

Section One

Organisation, Delivery and Outcome of Neonatal Care

CHAPTER I

Epidemiology

Alison Macfarlane, Miranda Mugford

Births and birth rates

How birth statistics are compiled

There are three main routes through which data about births are collected. These have been described in considerable detail elsewhere[86,90] but a brief description and update are given here.

The most frequently used source of data on a national scale is civil registration. In the UK parents are required by law to register a birth with the local Registrar of Births, Marriages and Deaths. As well as issuing a certificate, the registrar passes the information to a central office, which compiles both national and local statistics. Scotland, Northern Ireland and the Republic of Ireland each have separate General Register Offices. In 1970, the General Register Office for England and Wales was merged with the Government Social Survey to form the Office of Population Censuses and Surveys. Then, in April 1996, OPCS merged with the Central Statistical Office and the Labour Market Statistics Group of the former Department of Employment to form the Office for National Statistics, which compiles and publishes a wide range of health, social and economic statistics. In 1999, the Office for National Statistics started to undertake a major review of civil registration.[110,111,57] The overall conclusions of this review, which proposed wide-ranging changes to the registration process including the establishment of 'through life records', have yet to be published. Proposals were presented to Parliament in a Draft Regulatory Reform Order in July 2004.[58]

In the UK, the law originally required all fetal deaths after 28 completed weeks of gestation to be registered as stillbirths. This limit was lowered to 24 weeks on 1 October 1992. All live births at any gestation have to be registered. In the Republic of Ireland there was no system for registering stillbirths before 1995 but they have been notified to Directors of Community Care since 1957.

The second method of information collection is through birth notification. In the UK all births have to be notified to the local Director of Public Health under a system introduced in 1907 and made compulsory in 1915. This is usually done by midwives immediately after the birth, and must be done within 36 hours.

The system was devised so that a health visitor could be informed and then call to see the mother and baby. From the 1960s onwards, local and health authorities developed child health computer systems initiated by the birth notification and used to administer vaccination and immunisation programmes and to monitor developmental testing. Since the introduction in England and Wales of the allocation of National Health Service (NHS) numbers for babies at birth in October 2002, the data flows have changed. As the minimum dataset associated with NHS Numbers for Babies is very limited, many maternity units continue to send the fuller dataset used previously in parallel. In Wales, child health systems are being developed so that data from birth notifications can be aggregated nationally and used to produce national maternity and perinatal statistics. In Northern Ireland, each of the four Health and Social Services Boards holds data from child health systems. Perinatal data from these are pooled to produce data for the province as a whole. These are published in reports, *Perinatal information: Northern Ireland*, which are available on paper and on the Northern Ireland NHS intranet. In the Republic of Ireland, a subset of vital statistics data derived from the four-part birth notifications along with data from birth and death registrations is analysed and published centrally by the Central Statistics Office. More detailed perinatal statistics, including clinical and socio-demographic data from the third part of the form, are analysed through the National Perinatal Reporting System and published separately by the Economic and Social Research Institute.

The third route for collecting data about births is through hospital-based systems. Traditionally these have collected data at discharge about hospital inpatient stays. More recently, systems have been developed that gather data about a person's episodes of care within a given trust. NHS commissioners should hold information about care given to their residents wherever this is provided. The ways in which this is done are changing rapidly with the development of information technology systems within the NHS.

In England, information about inpatient stays in NHS hospitals is aggregated nationally through the Hospital Episode Statistics (HES) system. There is a separate Maternity Hospital Episode Statistics system to collect information about women delivering in and babies born in the maternity departments of

NHS hospitals. Maternity HES records include the standard admitted patient record plus a 'maternity tail', with a 'minimum dataset' and 'clinical options'. The items in the minimum datasets were specified by the Steering Group on Health Services Information,[142] chaired by Edith Körner. This was known as the Körner Committee and the datasets it recommended are usually referred to as 'Körner minimum datasets'. The 'clinical options' were set out in publications but were never implemented at a national level.

The Hospital Episode Statistics system started in April 1987 and Maternity HES finally got under way in September 1988, after a delay of 6 months. In the mid-1990s it was still very incomplete. By the financial year 1994–95 the system contained records for only 67% of deliveries in England.[68] This reached 72% in 2002–03 and statistical bulletins containing data from the system are now published annually.[45] Data are still missing for some units, either because they do not have a computer system in their maternity unit or because systems are not linked to other systems in the hospital so the data in them do not reach systems operating at national level.[81] Major changes are imminent, however, with the implementation of the National Care Records Service for individual patient records. It is unclear at the time of writing how this will affect the derivation of statistical records, which have lower priority as a 'secondary use'.

In Wales and Northern Ireland systems similar to Maternity HES were introduced but very few delivery records have data in the 'maternity tail'. Analyses of data about method of delivery and length of stay have been derived from the Patient Episode Database Wales and published in bulletins on paper and on the Statistics Wales web site[104] but, as described above, the dearth of data from 'maternity tails' has led to decisions to use child health systems for collecting more detailed maternity data.

In England data about episodes of care in neonatal intensive care units are collected, along with data about other episodes in paediatric departments, in the main part of HES. Unfortunately, these data are not routinely linked, at national level at least, to the record of the baby's delivery, but the allocation of NHS numbers to babies at birth may make this possible in the future. There is also a lack of consistency in recording levels of special and intensive care in HES and these data are not published routinely.

Scotland has had a maternity information system working nationally since the mid-1970s. Since the mid 1970s, data about mothers have been collected through the SMR2 Maternity Discharge Sheet, and data about babies through the SMR11 record. The system as a whole was known as Core Patient Profile Information in Scottish Hospitals (COPPISH). Some of the data are published annually in *Scottish Health Statistics*, now published electronically on the ISD Scotland web site and others are used for ad hoc analyses. Data from these and other sources have been brought together in a series of publications by ISD and the Scottish Programme for Clinical Effectiveness in Reproductive Health. They include *Births in Scotland 1976–1995*,[75] *Small babies in Scotland*[76] and *Operative vaginal delivery in Scotland: a 20 year overview (with a chapter on multiple pregnancy in Scotland)*.[77] Data from SMR2 are combined with those from the Scottish Perinatal and Infant Mortality Survey and published annually on the ISD web site in the *Scottish Perinatal and Infant Mortality and Morbidity Report*.

In 2003 Scotland started to implement a completely new system, the Scottish Child Health Information Development (SCHID) Project. The first step in this is to implement a web-based Scottish Birth Record and an electronic woman-held record. Scotland is the only country in the UK that makes a concerted attempt to collect data about babies admitted to neonatal units, and the new system will develop this further. The other three countries include them in statistics collected about activity in paediatric departments, but have not so far been able to identify them in separately published data. In England the intention was to code 'levels of care' but this has given rise to problems, which are described later. The Department of Health does publish counts of the numbers of 'well babies' born in NHS hospitals in England but not admitted to neonatal units.

Trends and variations in birth rates

The numbers of live births registered in recent years in each of the four countries of the UK and in the Republic of Ireland are shown in Table 1.1. This shows that in the late 1980s the numbers of births rose everywhere except in the Republic of Ireland, before falling again in the early 1990s. A slight increase in the mid 1990s was followed by a further decline, until there was an upturn in 2002 and 2003. These figures are useful as a measure of the workload of the maternity and paediatric services but shed very little light on the reasons for the increases and decreases. Fluctuations can arise either as a result of changes in the size and age structure of the childbearing population or as a consequence of changes in the birth rate within each age group.

One of the most long-standing measures of birth rate is the general fertility rate. In this the number of live births is expressed as a rate per 1000 women aged 15–44 or, in some cases, 15–49. Figure 1.1 shows the general fertility rate for England and Wales since 1838, the first full year after civil registration began in July 1837. The rates for the mid-19th century are probably an underestimate, as birth registration did not become compulsory in England and Wales until 1874. Shortly after this the fertility rate began to decline, a trend that continued steadily until the 1930s. This was interrupted only by a trough during the First World War and a short-lived peak after the war ended. A similar peak followed the Second World War. After this there was longer-term rise in the 1950s and 1960s, followed by a decline through most of the 1970s. Since the rate reached a minimum in 1977 it has fluctuated, gradually increasing in the late 1980s and decreasing through the 1990s with a slight upturn in 2003.

This overall rate masks changes since 1977 within age groups. Rates for England and Wales are set out in Table 1.2, which shows birth rates among women in their late teens and 20s rising slightly in the late 1980s as the 'bulge' of women born in the mid-1960s entered the childbearing age range[38] and then falling through the 1990s and the early years of the 21st century. In contrast, rates among women in their early 30s rose before levelling off in the mid 1990s, while rates for women in their late 30s and 40s have risen consistently.

These age-specific rates can be summed up in a statistic called the 'total period fertility rate' (TPFR). This is a standardised

Table 1.1 Live births in England, Wales, Scotland and Ireland 1975–2003

Year	England	Wales	England and Wales*	Scotland	Northern Ireland†	Republic of Ireland
1975	568 900	38 030	603 445	67 943	26 130	67 178
1976	550 383	36 883	584 270	64 895	26 361	67 718
1977	536 953	31 765	569 259	62 342	25 437	68 892
1978	562 589	33 308	596 418	64 295	26 239	70 299
1979	601 316	36 174	638 028	68 366	28 178	72 539
1980	618 371	37 357	656 234	68 892	28 582	74 064
1981	598 126	35 842	634 492	69 054	27 166†	72 158
1982	589 711	35 720	625 931	66 196	26 872	70 843
1983	593 255	35 494	629 134	65 078	27 026	67 117
1984	600 573	35 861	636 818	65 106	27 477	64 062
1985	619 301	36 771	656 417	66 676	27 427	62 388
1986	623 609	37 038	661 018	65 812	27 975	61 620
1987	643 330	37 816	681 511	66 241	27 653	58 433
1988	654 363	38 824	693 577	66 212	27 514	54 600
1989	649 357	38 019	687 725	63 480	25 831	52 018
1990	666 920	38 866	706 140	65 973	26 251	53 044
1991	660 806	38 079	699 217	67 024	26 028	52 718
1992	651 784	37 523	689 656	65 789	25 354	51 089
1993	636 461	36 578	673 467	63 337	24 722	49 304
1994	628 956	35 366	664 726	61 656	24 098	48 255
1995	613 257	34 477	648 138	60 051	23 693	48 787
1996	614 188	34 894	649 489	59 296	24 382	50 655
1997	608 202	34 520	643 095	59 440	24 087	52 775
1998	602 111	33 438	635 901	57 319	23 668	53 969
1999	589 468	32 111	621 872	55 147	22 957	53 924
2000	572 826	31 304	604 441	53 076	21 512	54 789
2001	563 744	30 616	594 634	52 527	21 962	57 854
2002	565 709	30 205	596 122	51 270	21 385	60 521§
2003	589 851	31 400	621 469	52 408‡	21 648	61 517§

* Including births in England and Wales to women normally resident outside England and Wales.

† Live birth figures from 1981 are resident births only.

‡ Provisional.

§ Births for Ireland for 2002 and 2003 are year of Registration figures.

Sources: ONS, General Register Offices for Scotland and Northern Ireland; Department of Health, Ireland.

measure that gives the total number of children who would be born to each woman if she experienced the age-specific fertility rates for the year in question throughout her childbearing life. As Table 1.2 shows, the rate for England and Wales rose gradually in the latter half of the 1980s, before falling gradually since then, with a slight rise from 2002. Figure 1.2 shows how TPFRs varied within England and between the countries of Britain and Ireland in 2002. The South West and North East Government Office Regions had the lowest rates, at 1.62, and the West Midlands had the highest at 1.75. Even this was considerably lower than the rates of 1.77 for Northern Ireland and 1.98 for the Republic of Ireland.

These overall rates mask differences within regions and countries. For example, in 2002 in Northern Ireland, the TPFR ranged from 1.50 in Belfast to 2.02 in Dungannon. TPFRs for primary care trusts in England and local areas within Wales can be found in the VS1 tables on CD-ROM. These data are now

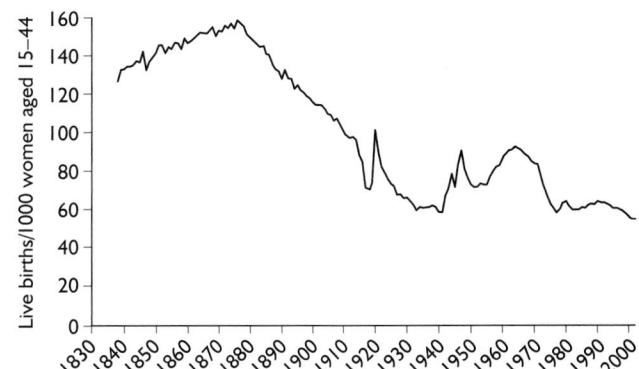

Fig. 1.1 General fertility rate, England and Wales, 1838–2002. Data from General Register Office, OPCS, Office for National Statistics, Birth Statistics, Series FM1.

available only to people who are NHS staff. The country with the lowest TPFR is Scotland, which has been experiencing a major decline in fertility and also a decrease in population in the absence of inward migration.[62]

For planning services it would be useful to have some idea of future trends in births, but these are notoriously difficult to predict. Nevertheless, government statisticians attempt to make such projections, combining analyses of past trends with replies

Table 1.2 Age-specific fertility rates, England and Wales, 1964–2003

Year	Live births, thousands	Live births per 1000 women in age group							
		15–44	Under 20	20–24	25–29	30–34	35–39	40–44	45 and over
1964 (max)	876.0	92.9	42.5	181.6	187.3	107.7	49.8	13.0	0.9
1977 (min)	569.3	58.1	29.4	103.7	117.5	58.6	18.2	4.1	0.3
1979	638.0	63.3	30.3	111.3	131.2	69.0	21.3	4.3	0.4
1984	636.8	59.8	27.4	95.5	126.2	73.6	23.6	4.5	0.4
1985	656.4	61.0	29.5	94.5	127.6	76.4	24.1	4.6	0.4
1986	661.0	60.6	30.1	92.7	124.0	78.1	24.6	4.5	0.4
1987	681.5	62.0	30.9	93.4	125.1	81.3	26.5	4.8	0.4
1988	693.6	63.0	32.4	94.9	123.8	82.7	27.9	4.8	0.4
1989	687.7	62.5	31.9	92.2	120.0	83.7	29.4	4.9	0.3
1990	706.1	64.3	33.3	91.7	122.4	87.3	31.2	5.0	0.3
1991	699.2	63.8	33.1	89.6	119.9	87.0	32.1	5.0	0.3
1992	689.7	63.6	31.7	86.2	117.5	87.3	33.4	5.5	0.3
1993	673.5	62.7	30.9	82.6	114.4	87.3	34.1	5.9	0.3
1994	664.7	62.0	28.9	79.1	112.4	89.3	35.8	6.1	0.3
1995	648.1	60.5	28.5	76.4	108.7	88.2	36.4	6.5	0.3
1996	649.5	60.6	29.7	77.0	106.9	89.7	37.5	6.9	0.3
1997	643.1	60.0	30.3	75.9	104.5	89.8	39.3	7.3	0.3
1998	635.9	59.3	31.3	74.8	101.5	90.7	40.4	7.5	0.3
1999	621.9	57.9	31.1	73.1	98.4	89.7	40.6	7.7	0.4
2000	604.4	56.0	29.5	70.2	94.5	88.1	41.4	8.0	0.4
2001	594.6	54.8	28.1	69.2	91.9	88.2	41.6	8.4	0.5
2002	596.1	54.8	27.1	69.2	91.6	89.9	43.2	8.7	0.5
2003	621.5	56.9	27.0	71.5	95.8	94.9	46.5	9.3	0.5

The rates for women of all ages, under 20, and 45 and over are based upon the female population aged 15–44, 15–19 and 45–49, respectively. All 2001 and 2002 birth rates for England and Wales are based on the revised mid 2001 and mid 2002 population estimates published on 26 September 2003. Birth rates for 2003 are based on the 2002-based population projections for 2003.
Source: ONS Birth Statistics, Series FM1.

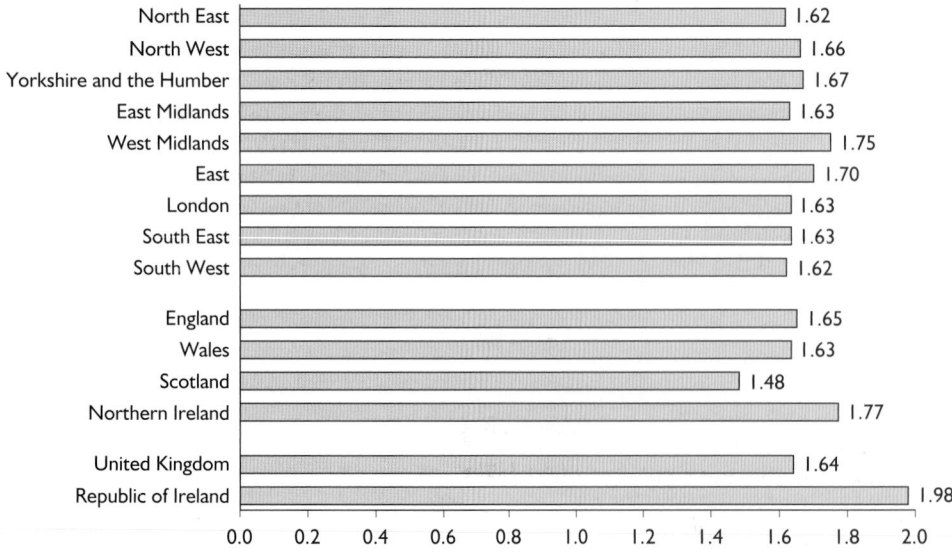

North East	1.62
North West	1.66
Yorkshire and the Humber	1.67
East Midlands	1.63
West Midlands	1.75
East	1.70
London	1.63
South East	1.63
South West	1.62
England	1.65
Wales	1.63
Scotland	1.48
Northern Ireland	1.77
United Kingdom	1.64
Republic of Ireland	1.98

Fig. 1.2 Total period fertility rates, Britain and Ireland, 2002. Data from ONS, Health Statistics Quarterly 19 and CSO Ireland.

to surveys about people's intentions to have children. Population projections for the countries of the UK are produced by the Government Actuary's Department. The 2002-based projections published in 2004 suggest that fertility rates will continue to rise and that the numbers of births in the UK will increase to an average of 709 thousand per year in the 5-year period 2016–2021, before falling again.[38,140]

The incidence of preterm birth and low birthweight

In England and Wales, birthweight data have been collected since the mid-1950s through the birth notification system. From 1953 to 1973, each local authority, and from 1974 to 1986 each health authority, submitted a form to central government giving the numbers of low-weight births to women living in their area. Data from this source have been used in Figure 1.3, which shows that the percentage of liveborn babies weighing 2500 g and less, the original definition of 'low birthweight', remained at a similar level of between 6% and 7% from the mid-1950s to the mid-1980s. The definition of low birthweight was changed in the ninth revision of the International Classification of Diseases[153] to 'under 2500 g'. Babies weighing under 1500 g at birth are now categorised as 'very low birthweight', and those weighing under 1000 g are described as 'extremely low birthweight'.[155]

These birthweight groups are used in Table 1.3 and in the data for more recent years in Figure 1.3. These both show recent trends in the incidence of low birthweight in England and Wales. Although the percentage of liveborn babies weighing under 2500 g has fluctuated since 1983, the general trend was upwards. There was a continuing increase in all groups of babies weighing under 2000 g. Between 1983 and 1988 there was no clear trend in the very small proportion of liveborn babies for whom birthweight was missing, and who are known to include a high proportion of small and immature babies.[4] In the middle of 1989, financial constraints in the OPCS led to a decline in the completeness of recording of birthweight on birth registration

records. Birthweight was missing on up to 4% of records from 1989 to 1994, making the data for these years difficult to interpret. As shown later in Table 1.13, the mortality rate among babies with missing birthweights was well above the overall rate, suggesting that the group included a relatively high proportion of low-birthweight babies. By 1995, the numbers of missing birthweights had declined markedly and the data for 1995 onwards used in Tables 1.3, 1.7, 1.8, 1.9 and 1.13 and Figure 1.3 are much more reliable than those for the preceding years.

The reported incidence of low-weight births in 1995 was well above that for 1988 and rose markedly after 1995, as Figure 1.3 shows. Analyses of birthweight data for both England and Wales and Scotland identified two separate trends, however. Although the percentages of low-weight births had increased during the 1980s, there had also been an increase in the proportion of heavier babies.[14,129,96] From the 1996s onwards in England and Wales, the proportion of heavier babies levelled off.

When OPCS made the arrangements in the 1970s to acquire the information about babies' birthweights from birth notification, it also requested gestational age. For reasons that are long forgotten, access to this was refused by clinical organisations. As a result, until recently in the UK there have been few routinely collected data about gestational age, except in Scotland.[75,89,90] A reported increase in the proportion of preterm births in Scotland can be seen in Figure 1.4 and Table 1.4, which are derived from information in the SMR2 system. Although multiple births have contributed to the rise, preterm singleton births have also increased since the mid 1970s as a proportion of all live births.

The data for both England and Wales and Scotland suggest that there has been an increase in the reported incidence of very small and very preterm babies. Although the rising incidence of multiple birth, discussed later, has made a major contribution to this rise, it is certainly not the only factor. It has been suggested that an increasing tendency to admit smaller and iller babies to neonatal nurseries has also contributed to the rise. By law all live births should be registered but there is a subjective element in distinguishing between a live birth and a miscarriage, particularly if the baby dies very shortly after birth. In the past some of these very tiny babies would have been regarded as miscarriages

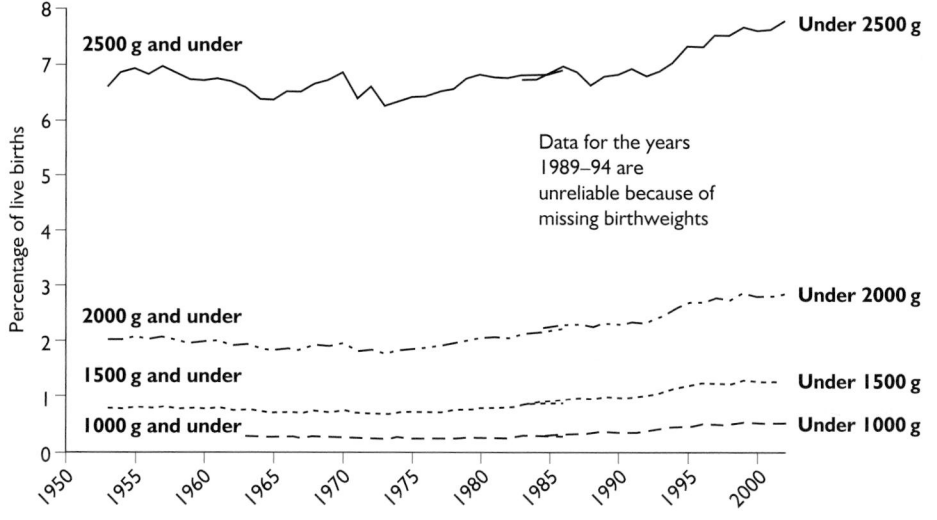

Fig. 1.3 Incidence of low birthweight, England and Wales, 1953–2002. Data from LHS 27/1 low birthweight returns 1953–86 and ONS mortality statistics, Series DH3, 1983–2002. As different definitions were used, the lines are broken.

Table 1.3 Low-birthweight live births, England and Wales, 1983–2002

Year	Total live births	Live births with birthweight	Percentage of live births with stated birthweight				
			Less than 1000 g	Less than 1500 g	1500–1999 g	2000–2499 g	Under 2500 g
1983	629 134	628 269	0.27	0.84	1.26	4.60	6.70
1984	636 818	636 006	0.29	0.87	1.28	4.55	6.70
1985	656 417	655 549	0.29	0.90	1.30	4.61	6.81
1986	661 018	660 394	0.31	0.92	1.35	4.66	6.92
1987	681 511	681 009	0.31	0.96	1.33	4.55	6.83
1988	693 577	692 746	0.32	0.94	1.30	4.36	6.59
1989	687 725	666 612	0.37	0.98	1.32	4.45	6.74
1990	706 140	678 374	0.34	0.96	1.32	4.51	6.79
1991	699 217	673 299	0.34	0.96	1.36	4.57	6.89
1992	689 656	663 689	0.36	1.00	1.30	4.51	6.82
1993	674 467	651 166	0.40	1.03	1.40	4.42	6.85
1994	664 726	646 914	0.44	1.12	1.41	4.44	6.98
1995	648 138	645 641	0.44	1.17	1.50	4.65	7.33
1996	649 485	647 948	0.49	1.22	1.45	4.61	7.28
1997	643 095	641 979	0.47	1.23	1.53	4.69	7.45
1998	635 901	635 116	0.48	1.22	1.50	4.76	7.48
1999	621 872	619 963	0.51	1.29	1.56	4.76	7.61
2000	603 421	602 401	0.50	1.25	1.53	4.81	7.59
2001	594 634	593 753	0.51	1.26	1.52	4.82	7.60
2002	596 122	595 213	0.50	1.25	1.57	4.90	7.72
2003	621 469				1.3		7.17

Source: Office for National Statistics, Mortality statistics, Series DH3.

Table 1.4 Gestational age of live births in Scotland, 1990, 1995, 2002, 2003, as a percentage of all live births

Year	Total	Gestational age, weeks						
		Less than 24	24–27	28–31	32–36	37–41	42+	Not known
All								
1990	63 351	0.0	0.3	0.7	5.3	87.5	5.5	0.6
1995	60 261	0.0	0.3	0.8	5.7	88.2	4.7	0.2
2002	50 592	0.0	0.3	0.8	6.2	89.2	3.4	0.0
2003*	50 157	0.1	0.3	0.9	6.2	89.5	2.9	0.0
Singleton								
1990	61 937	0.0	0.2	0.5	4.6	88.3	5.6	0.7
1995	58 712	0.0	0.2	0.7	4.8	89.2	4.9	0.2
2002	49 060	0.0	0.3	0.6	5.0	90.5	3.5	0.0
2003*	48 650	0.0	0.3	0.7	5.1	90.8	3.0	0.0
Multiple								
1990	1414	0.4	3.6	7.8	35.7	52.3	0.1	0.1
1995	1549	0.6	4.1	5.4	39.3	50.6	–	–
2002	1532	0.3	2.0	7.9	43.7	46.1	–	–
2003*	1507	0.9	2.4	6.3	42.7	47.5	0.1	–

* Provisional.
Source: ISD Scotland.

and would not therefore have been registered as live births. The lowering of the gestational age limit for registering fetal deaths as stillbirths in all countries of the UK in October 1992 may well have reinforced changes in people's perceptions of which events should be registered as live births.

Another factor that may have contributed to the increase in registration is the growing recognition of parents' need to mourn an unsuccessful outcome of pregnancy (Chapter 5). The formalities of registration can sometimes form part of this, together with the process of holding a funeral.

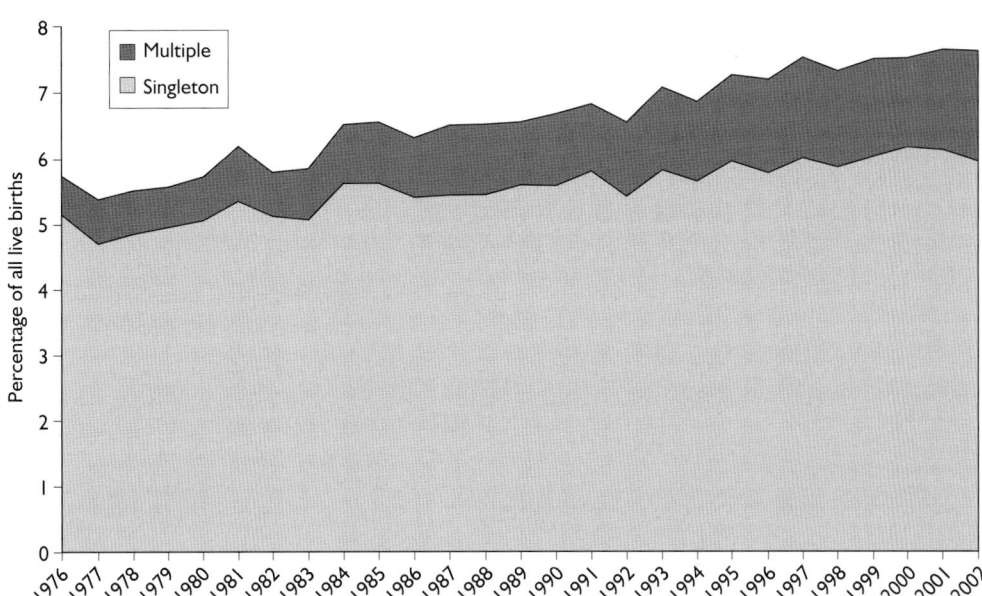

Fig. 1.4 Percentage of live births born before 37 weeks of gestation, by multiplicity, Scotland, 1976–2002. Data from ISD, SMR2.

The incidence of low birthweight varies between different geographical areas and different sectors of the population. Considerable differences were seen in the late 1980s between the countries and parts of countries that took part in the International Collaborative Effort on birthweight, plurality and perinatal and infant mortality.[64] This showed that Norway and Sweden had a much lower incidence of low birthweight than the other countries, whereas England and Wales, Scotland, Israel and the six states of the USA that took part in the study were among the places with the highest reported incidence. Similar differences were seen in the incidences of low birthweight in 1990[97] and for the years around 2000, which are shown in Table 1.5.[24] They are taken from a European study, the PERISTAT perinatal indicator project, which used data collected routinely through the countries' vital statistics systems or medical birth registers.[157] In the EURONATAL study, with data for the mid 1990s and common cutoffs, the differences between countries were not the same as when all births were included.[60,61]

Although the overall incidence of low birthweight in a population tends to be a reflection of the health of that population in general, and of women of childbearing age in particular, at the bottom end of the birthweight range it is affected by the country's criteria for birth registration. In theory this should not affect live births, as in most countries a live birth is registrable regardless of gestational age or birthweight. There are, however, considerable variations in the criteria for the registration of late fetal deaths as stillbirths. This ranges from 12 weeks of gestational age in Japan to 22 weeks in countries that follow World Health Organization (WHO) recommendations, 24 weeks in the countries of the UK, and 28 weeks in Denmark and Sweden.[59,64] In the USA each state has its own registration system, and most use a gestational age of 20 weeks as a criterion for registering fetal deaths.[2] More recent data, for the years around 2000 in European countries participating in the PERISTAT perinatal indictors project and for which data are available, are shown in Figure 1.5.[24]

Inevitably, these wide differences in the gestational age at which fetal deaths are registrable as stillbirths affect decisions about whether a very preterm birth should be regarded as a registrable live birth or as a miscarriage, although the extent to which they do so appears to vary from country to country. In the PERISTAT study, the percentage of live births weighing under 500 g ranged from 0.00% in Denmark and 0.01% in Portugal to 0.06% in the four countries of the UK combined and the French-speaking community of Belgium. Although these differences have a very limited impact on the comparability of statistics about low birthweight, they have a much larger impact on the comparability of mortality statistics.[24] To deal with this problem, the WHO recommends that babies weighing under 500 g or born before 22 completed weeks of gestation are excluded from comparative statistics (ICD10–144).[155] Of the countries participating in the PERISTAT project, Flanders, Spain and the Republic of Ireland followed this recommendation.[93]

A further factor that has to be taken into account is the extent to which data about gestational age and birthweight are missing, either because the information was not recorded initially, or because it was not passed on to population-based data collection systems. This is likely to have affected the trends shown in Figures 1.3 and 1.4, as well as comparisons between countries. Furthermore, where data are almost complete, birthweight is most likely to go unrecorded for babies who die very soon after birth.

Real differences in the low-birthweight rates within countries with the same or similar data collection systems are shown in Table 1.6. In 2002, the incidence of low-weight births in the Government Office regions of England ranged from 6.69% in the South West Region to 8.73% in the West Midlands Region. Each of these regions includes a variety of different populations. Differences between strategic health authorities are wider and the differences between local authority districts in the incidence of low birthweight are wider still. Even though these small babies make up a tiny proportion of all births, they make a considerable contribution to mortality rates. Comparing the countries of the UK, the incidences of low-weight and very-low-weight births in Wales were lower than those for England in 2002, while those for Scotland and Northern Ireland were lower still and the lowest shown in Table 1.6 was in the Republic of Ireland.

Table 1.5 Birthweight distribution of live births in member states participating in the PERISTAT European indicators project

Member state	Coverage if not national	Year and data source	Birthweight g (percentage of live births)							
			Under 500	500–1499	Under 1500	1500–2499	Under 2500	2500–4499	4500 and over	All
Austria		A1-2001	0.03	1.06	1.09	5.54	6.63	92.30	1.08	100.00
Belgium	Flanders	B2-2000	n/a	0.90	0.90	5.66	6.56	92.49	0.95	100.00
Belgium	French community	B3-2000	0.06	1.18	1.24	6.25	7.48	90.77	1.75	100.00
Denmark		DK1-2000	0.04	0.83	0.87	4.11	4.98	90.82	4.20	100.00
Finland		FIN1-2000	0.03	0.73	0.76	3.58	4.34	92.36	3.30	100.00
France	Perinatal survey	F1-1998	0.00	0.78	0.78	5.99	6.77	92.42	0.81	100.00
Germany		D2-1999	0.05	1.05	1.10	5.45	6.54	91.82	1.64	100.00
Greece	Perinatal survey	EL1-1998	0.02	0.96	0.98	6.20	7.19	92.02	0.80	100.00
Ireland		IR1-1999	n/a	0.82	0.82	4.17	4.99	92.10	3.00	100.00
Italy		I1-1998	0.30	0.65	0.91	5.01	5.93	91.46	2.61	100.00
Luxembourg		L2-2000	0.02	0.02	0.04	4.08	4.12	95.09	0.79	100.00
Netherlands		NL1-1999	0.04	0.99	1.04	5.50	6.54	91.15	2.31	100.00
Portugal		P1-1999	0.01	0.95	0.95	6.15	7.10	92.16	0.74	100.00
Spain	Madrid, Valencia, Pais Vasco	EL2-2000	n/a	1.22	1.22	7.32	8.53	91.47	n/a	100.00
Sweden		S1-2000	0.02	0.75	0.77	3.64	4.41	91.33	4.26	100.00
United Kingdom		UK 1,6,7-2000	0.08	1.18	1.24	5.24	6.38	90.63	1.75	100.00

Source: PERISTAT project.[24] See report for descriptions of data sources.[93]

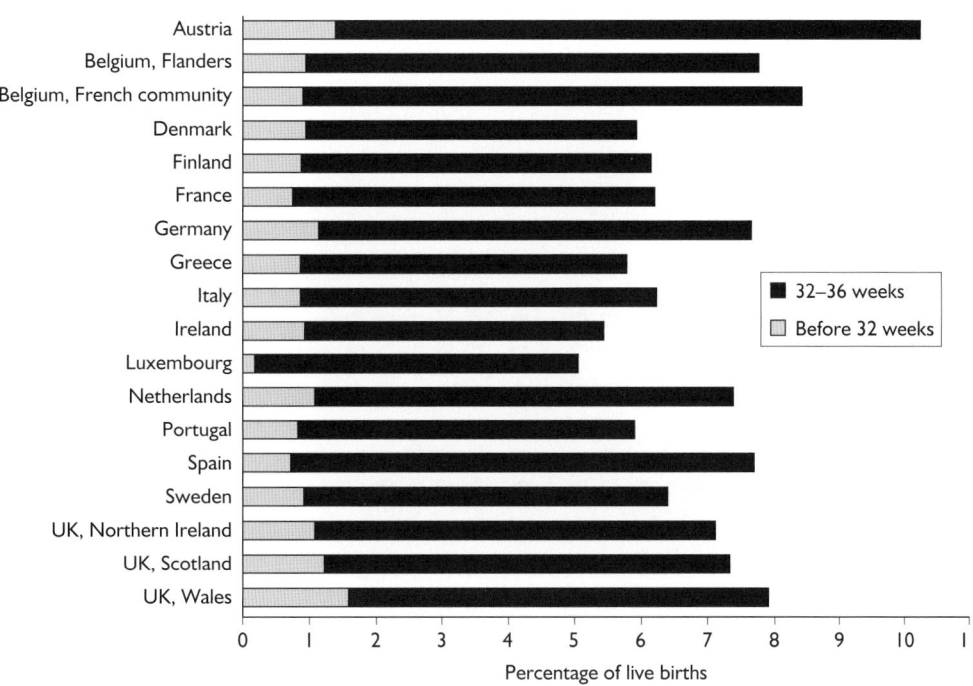

Fig. 1.5 Percentage of live births that were preterm in EU member states participating in the PERISTAT project in years around 2000. Data from PERISTAT project.[24] See report for descriptions of data sources.

Table 1.6 Incidence of low-weight live births in the Government office regions of England, Wales, Scotland and the Irish Republic, 2002

Country or Government office region	Number	Number with stated birthweight	Percentage weighing				
			Under 1000 g	1000–1499 g	1500–1999 g	2000–2499 g	Under 2500 g
North East	26 261	26 251	0.48	0.80	1.73	4.99	8.00
North West	74 588	74 535	0.49	0.76	1.69	5.19	8.14
Yorkshire and the Humber	55 508	55 481	0.52	0.85	1.64	5.27	8.28
East Midlands	45 002	44 965	0.50	0.76	1.62	5.05	7.93
West Midlands	60 985	60 935	0.60	0.90	1.74	5.49	8.73
East	60 120	60 069	0.39	0.64	1.44	4.40	6.88
London	105 042	104 481	0.62	0.78	1.61	5.21	8.22
South East	88 007	87 932	0.43	0.64	1.41	4.38	6.86
South West	49 310	49 288	0.43	0.68	1.35	4.23	6.69
England	564 823	563 937	0.50	0.75	1.57	4.92	7.75
Wales	30 182	30 159	0.46	0.76	1.58	4.59	7.38
Scotland*	50 318	50 312	0.40	0.68	1.53	4.65	7.26
Northern Ireland	21 449	21 447	0.48	0.70	1.31	3.78	6.27
Republic of Ireland	60 521	59 922	0.30	0.50	1.00	3.04	4.84

*Estimated.

Source: ONS VS Tables 2002; Information and Statistics Division, Scottish Health Statistics; Perinatal statistics, Northern Ireland; CSO, Ireland.

Differences between smaller areas are even more marked. In each of the countries of the UK, area deprivation scores have been constructed using data from the census and other data, such as unemployment and crime rates, that can be disaggregated to a local level, to classify small areas. These can be used to group together areas with similar characteristics.

Differences between geographical areas reflect, in their turn, differences in the characteristics of the populations and

differences between groups within the population in the incidence of low birthweight. Table 1.7 shows differences in the incidence of low birthweight when live births are tabulated by the father's social class. The classes used are the eight-class version of the National Statistics Socio-economic classes, which have been used since 2001, superseding the Registrar General's social classes, which were used during the 20th century.[90,136] For babies in each group, and for all birthweights under 2500 g

Table 1.7 Low birthweight by National Statistics Socio-economic Classification of father and registration status for live births, England and Wales, 2002

Social class of father/registration status	Percentage weighing					Percentage of births that were multiple
	Under 1000 g	1000–1499 g	1500–1999 g	2000–2499 g	Under 2500 g	
All	**0.50**	**0.75**	**1.57**	**4.90**	**7.72**	**2.92**
All inside marriage or jointly registered, by National Statistics socio-economic classification of father	0.48	0.74	1.55	4.73	7.51	2.98
1.1 Large employers and higher managerial occupations	0.35	0.54	1.43	3.56	5.88	3.82
1.2 Higher professional occupations	0.46	0.47	1.16	4.09	6.18	2.97
2 Lower managerial and professional occupations	0.38	0.75	1.49	3.88	6.49	3.60
3 Intermediate occupations	0.58	0.71	1.55	3.90	6.74	3.19
4 Small employers and own account workers	0.42	0.78	1.50	4.95	7.65	2.90
5 Lower supervisory and technical occupations	0.35	0.69	1.70	4.84	7.57	2.68
6 Semi-routine occupations	0.67	0.66	1.71	5.83	8.88	2.45
7 Routine occupations	0.69	1.05	1.57	6.00	9.31	2.63
8 Never worked and long-term unemployed	–	–	–	–	–	–
Not classified	0.65	0.96	2.22	5.51	9.34	2.15
All inside marriage	**0.43**	**0.68**	**1.43**	**4.53**	**7.07**	**3.28**
All outside marriage	**0.61**	**0.85**	**1.78**	**5.43**	**8.67**	**2.38**
Joint registration/same address	0.54	0.73	1.62	4.91	7.80	2.51
Joint registration/different address	0.80	1.14	1.98	6.05	9.96	2.17
Sole registration	0.66	0.99	2.14	6.65	10.43	2.15

Source: ONS mortality statistics 2002, Series DH3, No 35.

combined, the table shows clear differences between the higher rates of low birthweight among babies with fathers in routine and semi-routine occupation and the lower rates among babies with fathers in professional and managerial occupations.

Ideally, these data and those in Table 1.6 should be restricted to singleton births because the birthweight distribution for multiple births is different.

Since 1986 mothers have had the option of recording their occupation on their baby's birth certificate but many mothers still do not do so, either because they are not in paid employment or, in the case of the youngest women, because they do not yet have an occupation. For this reason, tabulations by mother's social class are not routinely published.[90,136]

In Scotland, an analysis of births in the years 1980–84 showed a clear social class gradient in the incidence of preterm births at 20–27, 28–31 and 32–36 weeks.[74,84,89] In this case, the gestational ages of babies born within marriage were tabulated according to their father's social class, and births outside marriage were grouped into a single category. An analysis of data for the early 1990s, which extended this to include analyses of low birthweight and preterm birth among births outside marriage by mother's social class, found social class differences in low birthweight but not in preterm birth.[90] More recent analyses are currently under way.

Birthweight distributions are known to differ among ethnic and racial groups.[90,124,132] At the time of writing, ethnic origin is not recorded at birth registration, but it should be recorded in national NHS data collection systems. Although it has been recorded on most hospital notes and on some districts' birth notification forms for some years, the way it was recorded and classified varied widely. In the mid 1990s, it was decided that the definitions used in the 1991 census should be used universally.[107,108] These have now been superseded by the revised classifications used in the 2001 census. In many cases, the data are incomplete and of questionable quality. Although data on birthweight and method of delivery, collected through the Maternity Hospital Episode Statistics, are published annually, black and Asian groups are aggregated in an attempt to overcome problems with data quality.[45]

The 1991 population census was the first in which people were asked to indicate how they described their ethnic origin. The categories used in the question were: White, Black–Caribbean, Black–African, Black–Other, Indian, Pakistani, Bangladeshi, Chinese, and any other ethnic group. People descended from more than one ethnic or racial group were asked to tick the one to which they considered they belonged, or to tick the 'Any other ethnic group' box and describe their ancestry.[118] This classification has been criticised on the grounds that it is more an indicator of skin colour than of cultural and social identity.[1]

After examining the 1991 census data in detail,[32] the Office for National Statistics revised the questions for use in the 2001 census, when slightly different questions were asked in each of the countries of the UK. In England and Wales, specific categories for people of mixed ethnic background were added, along with the terms Black British and Asian British, while Scotland added Black Scottish and Asian Scottish categories. ONS has subsequently revised its categories further in the slight

of subsequent criticisms and the need to take account of national identity within the UK.[112] In addition, in 2001, questions on religion, previously asked only in Northern Ireland, were added in England, Wales and Scotland, where they focussed particularly on religions practised by minority ethnic groups.

The ethnic origins of parents are not recorded at birth and infant death registration in England and Wales but their countries of birth are recorded. Although not a measure of ethnic origin, as many women in some minority ethnic groups having babies in the UK today were themselves born in the UK, country of birth is useful as an approximate measure of migrant status. Despite these limitations, Table 1.8 gives some insight into the differences in the incidence of low birthweight in 2002. As in other years it was highest among babies with mothers born in Pakistan, India and Bangladesh, and nearly as high among babies whose mothers were born in the Caribbean Commonwealth, East Africa and the 'rest of Africa', which essentially means West Africa. In contrast, the incidence of very low birthweight was markedly higher among babies whose mothers were born in the Caribbean Commonwealth and the 'rest of Africa'.[33]

These data illustrate the considerable differences that exist between groups within the population in the incidence of low birthweight and in the distribution of birthweights within the low birthweight range. The association between these and differences in mortality and morbidity will be discussed later but it is important to remember when interpreting the data that being classified as low birthweight does not necessarily imply that the baby had clinical problems, particularly at the upper end of the low-birthweight range. On the other hand, the smaller the baby and the shorter its gestational age, the higher the risk of morbidity.

Multiple births

In England and Wales, multiple births accounted for just under a quarter of live babies born in 2001 weighing under 1500 g, as Table 1.9 shows. After declining for many years, the incidence of multiple births, shown in Figure 1.6, started to increase from the mid-1970s onwards. The increase continued through the 1980s, from 10.1 multiple births per 1000 maternities in 1982 to 11.4 in 1989, 14.1 in 1995 and 15.0 in 2002. There are no data about multiple birth rates for England and Wales for 1981, as multiplicity was not recorded during this year because of industrial action by local registrars of births and deaths.

Multiple birth rates for England and Wales are compared with those for Scotland and Ireland in Table 1.10. Trends in Scotland were similar to those for England and Wales, although rates were slightly lower in Scotland up to the early 1990s. In Northern Ireland the twinning rate was already higher and did not increase in the latter half of the 1980s, but rose considerably in the early 1990s. The rates reached a similar level by the beginning of the 21st century.

The triplet and higher-order birth rates for England and Wales, shown in Figure 1.7, present a rather more dramatic picture than that for multiple births as a whole. After rising slightly during the 1970s, the proportion of triplet and higher-order births more

Table 1.8 Low birthweight by mother's country of birth, England and Wales, 2002

Mother's country of birth	All	All stated	Under 1500 g	1500–1999 g	2000–2499 g	Under 2500 g	Under 1500 g	1500–1999 g	2000–2499 g	Under 2500 g
			Numbers of live births				Percentage of live births with stated birthweight			
All	596 122	595 213	7456	9362	29 139	45 957	1.25	1.57	4.90	7.72
UK	490 711	490 125	5982	7702	23 219	36 903	1.22	1.57	4.74	7.53
Outside the UK	105 411	105 088	1474	1660	5920	9054	1.40	1.58	5.63	8.62
Republic of Ireland	3708	3700	37	41	135	213	1.00	1.11	3.65	5.76
Other European Union	11 449	11 421	108	154	463	725	0.95	1.35	4.05	6.35
Rest of Europe	8142	8103	69	82	263	414	0.85	1.01	3.25	5.11
Australia, Canada and New Zealand	3885	3882	28	43	130	201	0.72	1.11	3.35	5.18
New Commonwealth	54 037	53 873	940	1012	3893	5845	1.74	1.88	7.23	10.85
Bangladesh	8486	8477	115	136	761	1012	1.36	1.60	8.98	11.94
India	7222	7212	120	152	609	881	1.66	2.11	8.44	12.22
Pakistan	15 357	15 336	241	303	1245	1789	1.57	1.98	8.12	11.67
East Africa	3724	3709	66	83	254	403	1.78	2.24	6.85	10.87
Southern Africa	2654	2647	36	32	97	165	1.36	1.21	3.66	6.23
Rest of Africa	8073	8016	226	153	450	829	2.82	1.91	5.61	10.34
Far East	1351	1345	13	16	68	97	0.97	*1.19*	5.06	7.21
Mediterranean	1065	1064	6	19	48	73	0.56	*1.79*	4.51	6.86
Caribbean	3598	3572	87	67	207	361	2.44	1.88	5.80	10.11
Rest of the New Commonwealth	2507	2495	30	51	154	235	1.20	2.04	6.17	9.42
Rest of the world and not stated	24 190	24 109	292	328	1036	1656	1.21	1.36	4.30	6.87

Percentages in italics are based on fewer than 20 births.
Source: ONS mortality statistics 2002, Series DH3, No 35.

Table 1.9 Multiple births as a percentage of all births occurring in 2001, England and Wales

Birthweight (g)	Multiple births as a percentage of		
	Stillbirths	Live births	Infant deaths
Under 1500	12.7	24.1	23.9
1500–1999	9.1	28.7	17.1
2000–2499	3.2	18.1	9.0
Under 2500	10.4	21.2	21.2
2500 and over	1.6	1.4	1.4
All weights	8.6	2.9	14.3

Source: ONS mortality statistics, Series DH3, No 35.

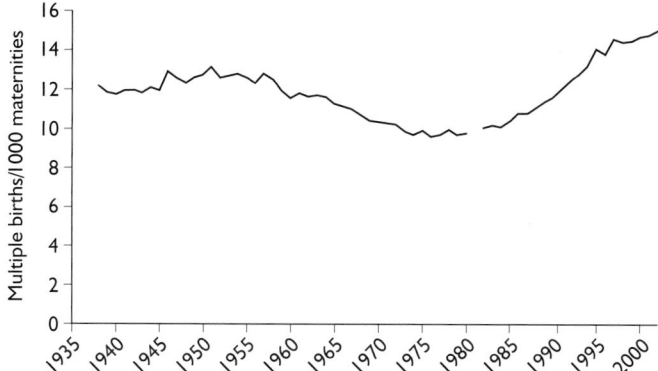

Fig. 1.6 Multiple birth rates, England and Wales, 1938–2002. Data from Office for National Statistics, Birth statistics, Series FM1.

Table 1.10 Multiple birth rates, England and Wales, Scotland and Ireland

	England and Wales	Scotland	Northern Ireland	Republic of Ireland
Twins per 1000 maternities				
1971–75	9.9	10	10.7	12.3
1976–80	9.6	9.4	10.1	11.2
1981–85	10.1[*]	9.9	10.6	10.7
1986–90	10.9	11	10.7	11.5[†]
1991–95	12.6	12.3	12.2	12.4[†]
1996–2000	13.9	13.8	13.8	13.7[†]
2001–02	14.6	14.8	15.0	15.6[‡]
Triplet and higher-order births per 1000 maternities				
1971–75	0.11	0.08	0.08	0.12
1976–80	0.13	0.09	0.14	0.13
1981–85	0.14[*]	0.10	0.12	0.11
1986–90	0.25	0.19	0.14	0.15[†]
1991–95	0.37	0.31	0.31	0.25[†]
1996–2000	0.45	0.36	0.33	0.44[†]
2001–02	0.33	0.25	0.54	0.34[‡]

[*] Excluding 1981.
[†] Based on a revised methodology to take better account of multiple births including stillbirths.
[‡] 2001 only.
Source: ONS; General Register Offices for Scotland and Northern Ireland; Central Statistics Office, Republic of Ireland, *Vital statistics 2001*, Table 2.18.

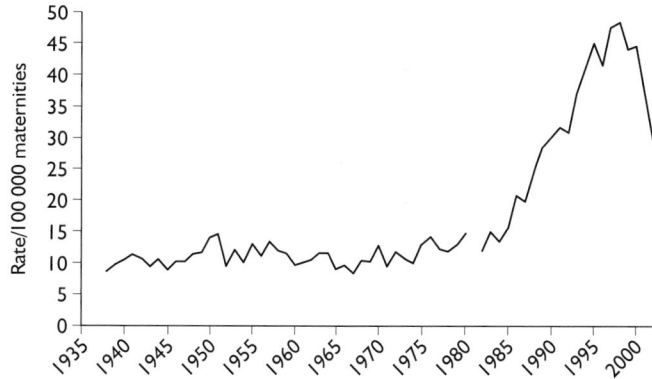

Fig. 1.7 Triplet and higher order births, England and Wales, 1938–2002. Data from Office for National Statistics, Birth statistics, Series FM1.

than doubled during the 1980s, rising from 12.2 per 100 000 maternities in 1982 to 28.6 in 1989. After a slight pause it rose again sharply to 45.0 in 1995. After reaching a peak of 48.3 in 1998, it started to fall, reaching 29.8 in 2002. Rates for Scotland, shown in Table 1.10, followed the same pattern but at a lower level. In Northern Ireland the rate rose in the late 1970s and then remained fairly level, before rising considerably since the 1990s and remaining at a high level. In contrast to this, the rate has started to fall in the Republic of Ireland, where there was a slight rise in the latter half of the 1980s and a bigger rise in the 1990s.

The rising triplet rate was a common feature in most European countries. By 1990, the rates in Belgium and the Netherlands were the highest in Europe, followed by those in West Germany, Italy and France.[97] Despite its reputation for high rates of triplet and higher-order births, Australia's rate for 1994, 35.0 per 100 000 maternities, was no higher than some of these.[6] As Table 1.11 shows, triplet rates were still high in the Netherlands, Belgium, Italy and Germany at the beginning of the 21st century but had fallen in France.[18]

The rise in the incidence of multiple births in general, and triplet and higher-order births in particular, is usually attributed to the increasing use of drugs for the medical management of subfertility and, since the mid-1980s, to techniques for assisted conception. Unfortunately, there are few data available to quantify their contribution over and above the increase that will have occurred spontaneously as a result of the rising age at childbirth.[12] The

National Study of Triplet and Higher-Order Births estimated that 36% of mothers of triplets and 70% of mothers of quadruplet and higher-order births born in the years 1980 and 1982–85 had used drugs for the medical management of subfertility.[16]

The impact of in-vitro fertilisation (IVF) was negligible before 1985 but since then it has become considerable. Statistics produced by the Human Fertilisation and Embryology Authority[71] and its predecessor the Interim Licensing Authority for Human In Vitro Fertilisation and Embryology[78] show a clear association between the rise in triplet and higher-order births from 1985 onwards and

Table 1.11 Multiple birth rates in European member states participating in the PERISTAT project

EU member state	Coverage, if not national	Year	Rate per 1000 maternities		
			Twins	Triplets and higher-order births	All
Austria		2001	14.95	0.42	15.37
Belgium	Flanders	2000	18.04	0.30	18.33
Belgium	French community	2000	13.31	0.55	13.86
Denmark		2000	19.68	0.32	20.00
Finland		2000	15.88	0.16	16.04
France		2000	14.98	0.28	15.26
Germany	Nine Bundeslander	2000	15.82	0.62	16.44
Greece	Perinatal survey	1998	20.05	0.21	20.26
Ireland		1999	13.00	0.52	13.52
Italy		1998	11.73	0.52	12.25
Luxembourg		2000	10.55	0.18	10.72
Netherlands		1999	18.98	0.38	19.37
Portugal		1999	11.07	0.32	11.38
Spain		1999	15.22	0.70	15.92
Sweden		2000	15.99	0.20	16.19
United Kingdom		2000	14.24	0.44	14.69

Source: PERISTAT report.[18] See report for description of data sources.[93]

the increasing use of IVF, gamete intrafallopian transfers (GIFT) and associated procedures.[90] Research commissioned by the Medical Research Council[99] confirmed that multiple births often result from these procedures, as did a survey of triplet and higher-order births undertaken by the British Association of Perinatal Medicine (BAPM) in 1989.[82] A subsequent analysis of data for England and Wales showed rising rates of multiple births on the one hand and of assisted conception and prescriptions for drugs for the medical management of subfertility but was unable to quantify the association as it was based solely on routinely collected data.[47]

Since the mid 1990s, the numbers of NHS prescriptions for the medical management of subfertility has declined but it is unclear whether this is a real decline or simply a shift to the private sector, about which no statistics are collected routinely. The decrease in the triplet rate in Britain follows guidance from the Royal College of Obstetricians and Gynaecologists (RCOG) in 2000 that no more than two embryos should be replaced in IVF procedures involving women under 40.[137] The Human Fertilisation and Embryology Authority included this in its Code of Practice, launched in January 2004.[72] In Australia and New Zealand, multiple pregnancies occurred in 28.1% of GIFT pregnancies and 22.1% of all assisted conception pregnancies in 2000, compared to only 1.6% of all pregnancies in Australia in 2000.[6,40]

Mortality in the first year of life

Trends in mortality rates

The classic indicators of the outcome of pregnancy are stillbirth rates and death rates during the first year of life. These are defined

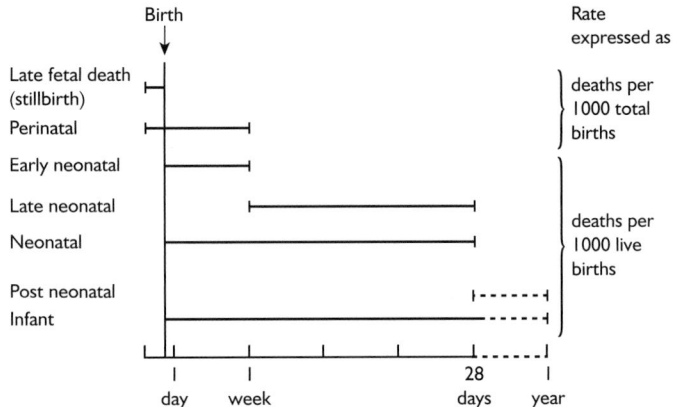

Fig. 1.8 Definitions of stillbirth and infant mortality rates.

in Figure 1.8. Trends since 1905 in neonatal and postneonatal mortality rates for England and Wales are illustrated in Figure 1.9. Although the series of infant mortality rates reaches back to the mid-19th century, the current subdivision of the first year of life into the first month and deaths at ages of at least 1 month but under 1 year started in 1905. The publication of more detailed analyses started at a time when public concern about infant mortality, stemming from the unfitness of many potential recruits for the Boer War, led to a request to the General Register Office for more detailed statistics.[145]

Whereas neonatal mortality rates have decreased relatively steadily during the 20th century, postneonatal mortality, which was initially higher, shows a different pattern. It decreased very rapidly in the first half of the century with the decline in fatality from communicable diseases. It showed signs of levelling off between the mid-1970s and mid-1980s. After virtually halving in the late

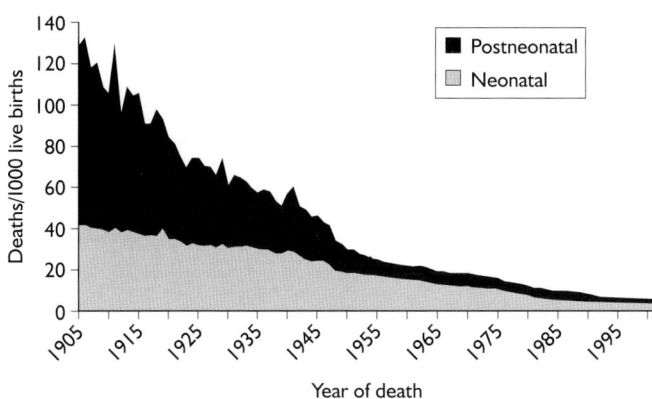

Fig. 1.9 Infant mortality, England and Wales, 1905–2002. Data from Office for National Statistics, Mortality statistics, Series DH3.

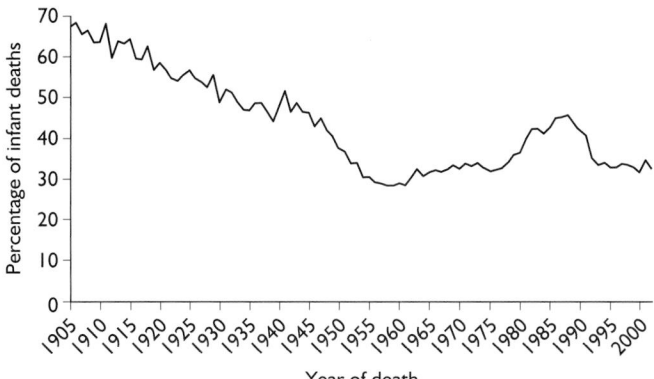

Fig. 1.10 Postneonatal deaths as a percentage of infant deaths, England and Wales, 1905–2002. Data from Office for National Statistics, Mortality Statistics, Series DH3.

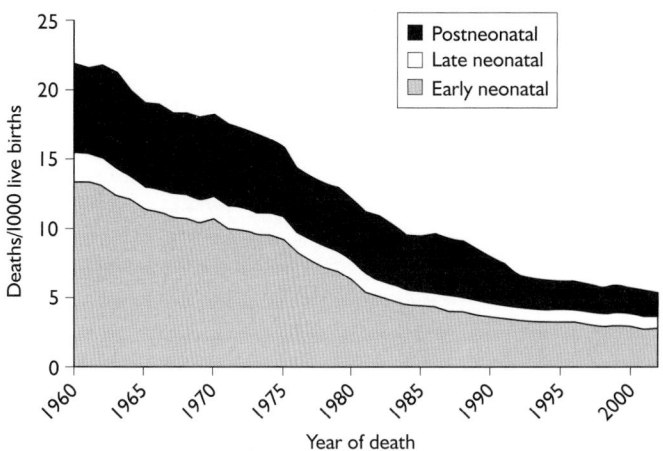

Fig. 1.11 Infant mortality, England and Wales, 1960–2002. Data from OPCS and ONS mortality statistics, Series DH3.

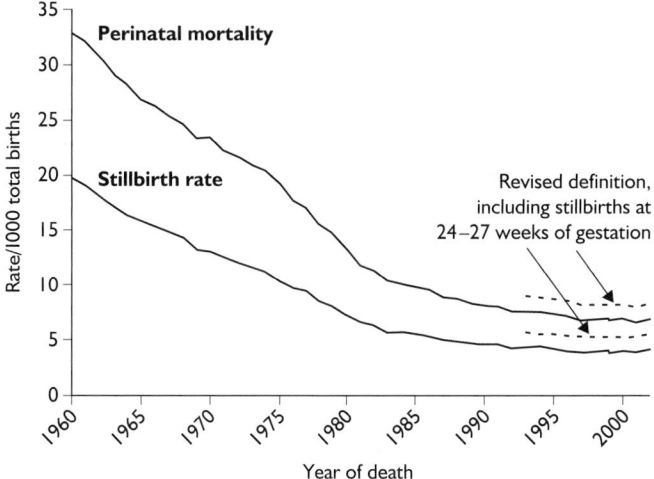

Fig. 1.12 Stillbirth and perinatal mortality rates, England and Wales 1960–2002. Data from Office for National Statistics, Mortality statistics, Series DH3.

1980s and early 1990s, the rate has levelled off again, accounting for about a third of infant deaths, as Figure 1.10 shows.

More recent trends in infant mortality are shown in Figure 1.11, which shows early and late neonatal mortality rates separately. The impact of the change in legislation about stillbirth registration on published stillbirth and perinatal mortality rates is illustrated in Figure 1.12. The published rates, shown with a dotted line from 1992 onwards, showed an apparent increase. Rates from which stillbirths at 24–27 weeks of gestation have been excluded are shown as a continuation of the solid line, and show an apparent halt in the downward trend seen in previous years.

Neonatal, postneonatal and infant mortality rates for England, Wales, Scotland and Ireland in the years since 1970 are shown in Table 1.12. These show continuing small declines in neonatal mortality through the 1990s. As in England and Wales, there was a tendency for the postneonatal mortality rate to level off in the 1980s in each of the other countries, followed by a fall in the late 1980s and early 1990s. The trends in Scotland, Wales and both parts of Ireland are less clear than those in England and Wales, as they are based on smaller numbers of deaths. Similar trends were seen in the regions of England[90,92,126] and in other developed countries.[97] As a whole, however, infant mortality continues to decline in most countries, although it shows some signs of levelling off in the countries with the lowest rates, notably the Nordic countries and Switzerland.[148]

To what extent do trends in infant mortality in the UK reflect changes in the relative size of high-risk groups, and to what extent has mortality fallen within these groups? Figure 1.3 shows no increase in the incidence of low birthweight in England and Wales between the mid-1950s and mid-1980s, but a rise in more recent years. Table 1.3 shows a similar picture but with an increase in the reported incidence of babies in the lowest birthweight groups, who have the highest mortality. It has been suggested that the change in definition of stillbirth may have increased the tendency to register very preterm live births, rather than regarding them as miscarriages.

Within birthweight groups, however, trends in mortality look different. A very marked fall between 1963 and 1986 in mortality in the first week after live birth among babies weighing 2500 g and under, followed by a further fall in the late 1980s, can be seen in Figure 1.13. A different pattern can be seen in Figure 1.14, which shows a more recent and very marked decline from the late 1970s onwards in mortality rates among babies weighing 1000 g and under, and subsequently among babies weighing under 1000 g.

Table 1.12 Neonatal, postneonatal and infant mortality rates since 1970, England and Wales, Scotland and Ireland

	England	Wales	England and Wales	Scotland	Northern Ireland	Irish Republic
Neonatal mortality						
1970	12.3	12.8	12.3	12.8	15.8	12.8
1975	10.7	10.3	10.7	11.8	13.2	12.0
1980	7.6	7.9	7.7	7.8	8.0	6.7
1985	5.3	5.8	5.4	5.5	5.6	5.3
1986	5.2	5.0	5.3	5.2	6.0	5.0
1987	5.0	5.0	5.1	4.7	4.8	4.3
1988	4.9	4.7	4.9	4.5	5.4	5.3
1989	4.7	4.7	4.8	4.7	4.0	4.8
1990	4.6	3.9	4.6	4.4	4.0	4.8
1991	4.3	4.1	4.3	4.4	4.6	5.0
1992	4.3	3.8	4.3	4.6	4.1	4.3
1993	4.2	3.4	4.2	4.0	4.9	4.0
1994	4.0	4.1	4.1	4.0	4.2	4.0
1995	4.2	3.9	4.2	4.0	5.5	4.8
1996	4.1	3.6	4.1	3.9	3.7	4.1
1997	3.9	3.9	3.9	3.2	4.2	3.5
1998	3.8	3.6	3.8	3.6	3.9	4.3
1999	3.9	4.0	3.9	3.3	4.8	4.0
2000	3.9	3.5	3.9	4.0	3.8	4.3
2001	3.6	3.5	3.6	3.8	4.4	4.0
2002	3.6	3.1	3.6	3.2	3.4	3.5
2003	3.6	3.0	3.6	3.4+		3.8
Postneonatal mortality						
1970	5.9	6.4	5.9	6.9	7.1	6.7
1975	5.3	4.2	5.0	5.4	7.2	5.6
1980	4.4	3.5	4.4	4.3	7.6	3.8
1985	3.9	4.0	4.0	3.9	4.0	3.6
1986	4.2	3.9	4.3	3.6	4.2	3.9
1987	4.0	4.5	4.1	3.8	3.8	3.6
1988	4.1	2.9	4.1	3.7	3.6	3.5
1989	3.7	3.3	3.7	4.0	2.9	3.3
1990	3.3	3.0	3.3	3.3	3.5	3.4
1991	3.0	2.4	3.0	2.7	2.8	2.6
1992	2.2	2.2	2.3	2.2	1.9	2.2
1993	2.1	2.1	2.1	2.5	2.1	2.1
1994	2.0	2.2	2.1	2.2	1.9	1.7
1995	2.0	2.0	2.0	2.2	1.6	1.6
1996	2.0	2.0	2.0	2.2	2.0	1.9
1997	2.0	2.0	2.0	2.1	1.4	2.6
1998	1.8	2.0	1.9	2.0	1.7	1.6
1999	1.8	2.1	1.9	1.7	1.6	1.8
2000	1.7	1.8	1.7	1.8	1.2	1.9
2001	1.8	1.9	1.9	1.7	1.6	1.7
2002	1.7	1.6	1.7	2.1	1.2	1.5
2003	1.7	1.1	1.7	1.7+		1.3
Infant mortality						
1970	18.2	18.7	18.2	19.6	22.9	19.5
1975	15.7	14.5	15.7	17.2	20.4	17.5
1980	12.0	11.4	12.0	12.1	15.6	10.3
1985	9.2	9.8	9.4	9.4	9.6	8.8

(Continued)

Table 1.12 (Continued)

	England	**Wales**	**England and Wales**	**Scotland**	**Northern Ireland**	**Irish Republic**
1986	9.5	9.5	9.6	8.8	10.2	8.9
1987	9.1	9.5	9.2	8.5	8.7	7.9
1988	9.1	7.6	9.0	8.2	8.9	8.9
1989	8.4	8.0	8.4	8.7	6.9	8.1
1990	7.9	6.6	7.9	7.7	7.4	8.2
1991	7.3	6.6	7.4	7.1	7.4	7.6
1992	6.5	6.0	6.6	6.8	6.0	6.5
1993	6.3	5.5	6.3	6.5	7.1	6.1
1994	6.1	6.1	6.2	6.2	6.1	5.7
1995	6.1	5.8	6.1	6.2	7.1	6.4
1996	6.1	5.6	6.1	6.2	5.8	6.0
1997	5.9	5.9	5.9	5.3	5.6	6.1
1998	5.6	5.6	5.7	5.6	5.6	5.9
1999	5.7	6.1	5.8	5.0	6.4	5.9
2000	5.6	5.3	5.6	5.7	5.0	6.2
2001	5.4	5.4	5.4	5.5	6.0	5.7
2002	5.3	5.3	4.7	5.3	4.6	5.1
2003	5.3	4.1	5.3	5.1+	5.3	5.1

Figures for Ireland for 2002 and 2003 are year of registration figures.
Source: ONS, General Register Offices for Scotland and Northern Ireland and Central Statistics Office, Ireland.

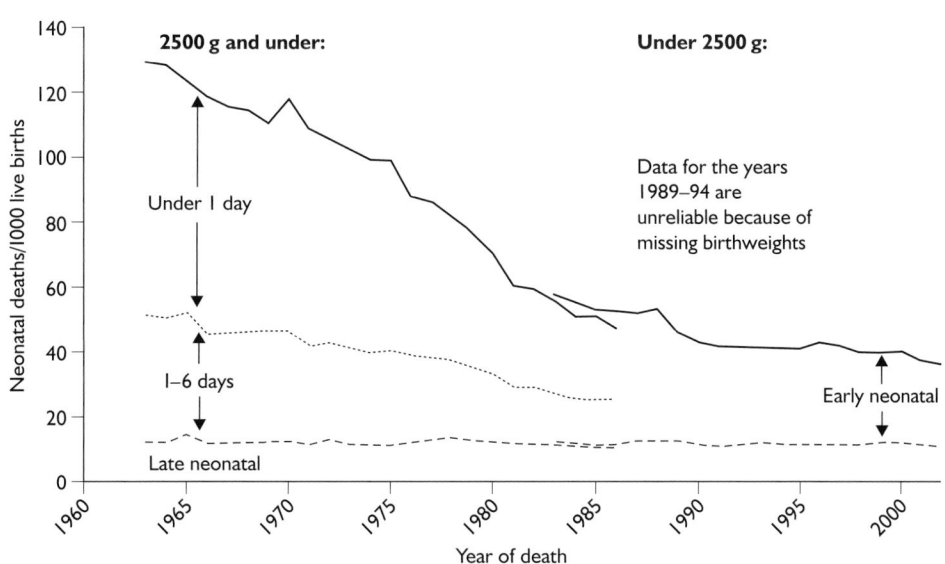

Fig. 1.13 Neonatal mortality among low birthweight babies, England and Wales, 1963–2002. Data from LHS 27/1 low birthweight returns 1963–86 and ONS mortality statistics, Series DH3, 1983–2002. As different definitions were used, the lines are broken.

The fuller data in Table 1.13 show that neonatal mortality continued to fall in England and Wales from the mid-1980s until the early 1990s, but from the mid 1990 onwards the decline appeared to be confined to babies weighing between 1000 g and 2499 g. Trends for the larger babies are far from clear. Table 1.13 also illustrates the impact of the increase in 1989 of the numbers of birth records with missing birthweights. Between 1983 and 1988, when very few birthweights were missing, mortality in this group was very high, suggesting that the babies might not have been weighed because they were very ill or immature. Between 1989 and 1994 mortality in this group was lower than before, but still markedly higher than average. Thus, mortality

in the groups under 2500 g is likely to have been artificially depleted over this period. In 1995, when the proportion of babies with missing birthweights was very much smaller, mortality among them rose, but not to its former level. This means that caution is needed when interpreting the trends in mortality among low-birthweight babies in the late 1980s and early 1990s, shown in Figures 1.13 and 1.14 and Table 1.13.

Table 1.14 shows neonatal mortality rates by birthweight for singleton babies without lethal anomalies born in Scotland over the years 1985–2002. These are tabulated by gestational age in Table 1.15. Neonatal mortality rates tended to decline, although there was considerable fluctuation because of the smaller numbers

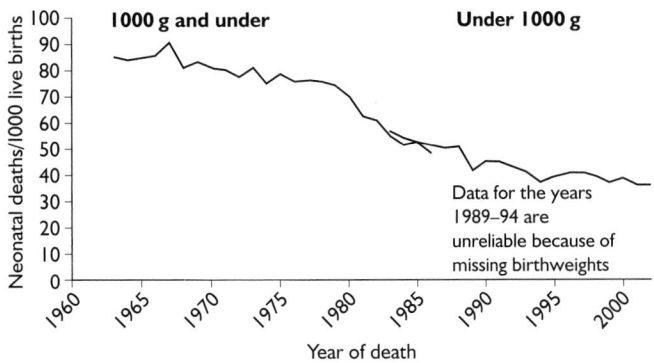

Fig. 1.14 Neonatal mortality among extremely low birthweight babies, England and Wales, 1963–2002. Data from LHS 27/1 low birthweight returns 1963–86 and ONS mortality statistics, Series DH3, 1983–2002. As different definitions were used, the lines are broken.

of babies involved. The exception was babies born between 24 and 27 weeks of gestational age, suggesting that the numbers of babies in this group may have risen with the increasing inclusion of babies with poor survival prospects.

Postneonatal mortality rates for England and Wales, given in Table 1.13, showed no sign of a decline over the years 1983–88, particularly for babies with birthweights under 2500 g. Apart from a possible increase in the 2000–2499 g group, the picture was one of fluctuation, the extent of which is not surprising, given the relatively small numbers of deaths in each group. This was followed by a sharp decline between 1989 and 1992 in all groups, except for babies weighing under 1000 g. This pattern persisted at a slower level from the mid 1990s onwards.

Putting the neonatal and postneonatal mortality rates together to look at infant mortality as a whole, it can be seen that rates tended to decline up until 1985 and then started to level off. After a decline over the period 1989–93, they appeared to level off again before declining very slowly from the late 1990s onwards.

Table 1.13 Neonatal, postneonatal and infant mortality by birthweight, England and Wales, 1985–2001

Year of birth	All weights	Total stated	Under 1000 g	1000–1499 g	Under 1500 g	1500–1999 g	2000–2499 g	Under 2500 g	2500 g and over	Not stated
Neonatal mortality rate per 1000 live births										
1985	5.3	5.1	525.5	134.7	262.0	37.9	12.5	50.3	1.8	156.7
1990	4.4	3.9	444.3	88.4	215.1	25.1	6.4	39.5	1.3	17.3
1995	4.1	4.0	390.1	63.8	187.7	17.5	6.5	37.7	1.4	28.4
1996	4.0	3.9	407.3	59.7	198.0	14.9	5.8	39.9	1.1	50.1
1997	3.9	3.8	404.8	60.2	192.6	17.6	5.6	38.8	1.0	60.9
1998	3.8	3.7	389.1	52.6	185.1	15.4	5.3	36.6	1.0	79.3
1999	3.9	3.8	368.8	55.8	180.6	15.8	4.7	36.8	1.1	36.1
2000	3.8	3.7	383.9	46.5	181.9	16.7	5.3	36.7	1.0	51.0
2001	3.6	3.5	360.6	47.4	173.2	14.2	4.8	34.6	1.0	56.8
Postneonatal mortality rates per 1000 live births										
1985	4.1	4.1	53.1	33.2	39.7	19.8	9.9	15.7	3.2	10.4
1990	3.1	3.1	59.6	31.8	41.7	17.1	7.0	13.9	2.3	3.8
1995	2.0	2.0	62.2	20.4	36.3	9.2	5.1	10.9	1.3	6.3
1996	1.9	1.9	48.9	19.3	31.1	9.1	5.9	10.7	1.2	3.3
1997	1.8	1.8	51.9	18.6	31.4	8.7	4.8	10.0	1.2	4.5
1998	1.9	1.9	58.1	18.3	34.0	7.8	5.1	10.3	1.2	2.4
1999	1.8	1.8	55.9	18.7	33.6	8.7	3.9	9.9	1.1	1.6
2000	1.8	1.8	50.6	16.0	29.9	10.5	4.5	9.9	1.1	2.9
2001	1.7	1.7	57.3	12.7	30.6	8.5	4.5	9.6	1.0	1.1
Infant mortality rates per 1000 live births										
1985	9.4	9.2	578.6	167.9	301.7	57.6	22.4	66.0	5.0	167.1
1990	7.6	7.0	503.9	120.2	256.8	42.2	13.4	53.3	3.6	21.1
1995	6.1	6.0	452.2	84.2	223.9	26.7	11.5	48.6	2.6	34.7
1996	5.9	5.8	456.2	79.0	229.0	24.0	11.7	50.6	2.3	53.3
1997	5.7	5.6	456.7	78.8	224.0	26.3	10.3	48.8	2.1	65.4
1998	5.7	5.6	447.2	71.0	219.1	23.1	10.4	47.0	2.2	81.7
1999	5.6	5.5	424.8	74.6	214.2	24.5	8.6	46.7	2.2	37.7
2000	5.6	5.5	434.5	62.5	211.8	27.2	9.8	46.6	2.2	53.9
2001	5.3	5.2	417.9	60.2	203.9	22.7	9.3	44.2	2.0	57.9

Source: Birth counts, Table A3.5.2 and ONS mortality statistics, Series DH3; for data for individual years for 1983–1994, see Birth counts, Table A3.5.2.[91]

Table 1.14 Birthweight-specific neonatal mortality rates for singleton babies without lethal anomalies, Scotland 1994–2002

	Birthweight (g)					
	Under 1500	**1500–2499**	**2500–3499**	**3500–4499**	**4500 and over**	**Total**
Neonatal deaths without lethal anomalies per 1000 live births						
1994	176.4	3.6	0.6	0.4	–	2.2
1995	175.5	1.8	0.9	0.3	1.9	2.0
1996	200.0	4.1	0.5	0.6	–	2.2
1997	155.3	2.6	0.7	0.5	–	1.9
1998	159.3	4.1	0.9	0.4	0.0	2.0
1999	171.4	2.3	0.6	0.2	0.9	2.0
2000	182.3	5.6	0.9	0.3	1.0	2.7
2001	178.6	2.6	0.8	0.7	1.0	2.3
2002*	145.2	6.1	0.3	0.5	1.0	2.1

* Provisional SMR02.
Source: ISD Scotland, SMR02 and Scottish Perinatal and Infant Mortality and Morbidity Survey.

Table 1.15 Gestation specific neonatal mortality rates for singleton babies without lethal anomalies, Scotland 1985–2002

	Gestational age, weeks					
	Under 24	**24–27**	**28–31**	**32–36**	**37 and over**	**Total**
Neonatal deaths without lethal anomalies per 1000 live births						
1985	*	620.4	114.3	6.7	0.6	3.1
1986	*	491.2	94.9	7.8	0.7	2.6
1987	*	477.3	117.6	7.1	0.7	2.8
1988	*	466.1	49.6	7.6	0.5	2.3
1989	*	448.0	94.3	4.2	0.6	2.5
1990	*	392.2	83.9	6.4	0.6	2.7
1991	*	455.1	73.6	5.8	0.6	2.5
1992	*	425.0	44.6	5.4	0.8	2.6
1993	*	349.4	70.4	4.4	0.6	2.1
1994	*	410.1	40.1	3.6	0.5	2.2
1995	*	420.6	56.0	2.9	0.6	2.0
1996	*	433.3	47.9	4.3	0.5	2.2
1997	*	336.1	30.6	2.1	0.5	1.9
1998	*	313.6	28.0	3.6	0.6	2.0
1999	*	345.9	38.6	2.2	0.4	2.0
2000	*	311.6	57.6	6.0	0.6	2.7
2001	*	308.3	36.8	3.4	0.7	2.3
2002†	*	359.2	33.5	3.1	0.5	2.1

* Rates not calculated as SMR2 data are incomplete.
† Provisional SMR02.
Source: ISD Scotland, *Scottish Perinatal and Infant Mortality and Morbidity Survey*. Data for 1985 to 1993 derived from Birth counts, Table A3.5.5.[91]

There are considerable differences between the countries of Europe in their mortality rates for low- and very-low-birthweight babies. For example, although rates fell during the 1980s in all countries for which birthweight-specific early neonatal mortality rates were available, in 1990 rates for babies born weighing under 1500 g ranged from 175 per 1000 live births in Norway to 297 in Ireland and 398 in Hungary. Although the differences may reflect variations in the criteria for birth registration, the most marked differences are between the countries of eastern and western Europe.[97]

It is usual to present birthweight-specific mortality rates in 500 g groups, and mortality rates for babies born in 2001 in singleton and multiple births are compared in Figure 1.15, but there is considerable variation within these groups, particularly at the bottom end of the scale. A fuller picture could be seen of the 'crossover' of rates in an earlier special analysis in which infant

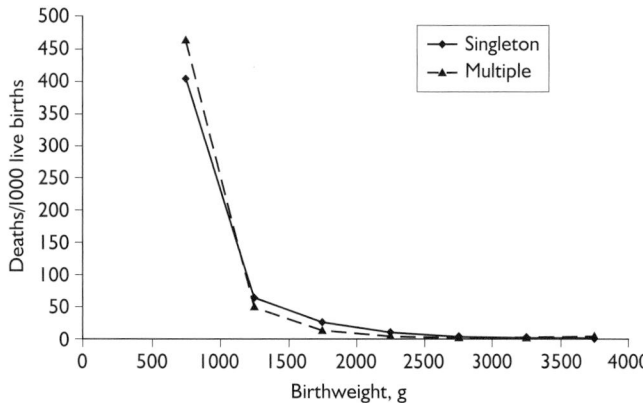

Fig. 1.15 Infant mortality rates for babies from singleton and multiple births born in 2001 in England and Wales. Data from Office for National Statistics, Mortality statistics 2002, Series DH3, Table 26.

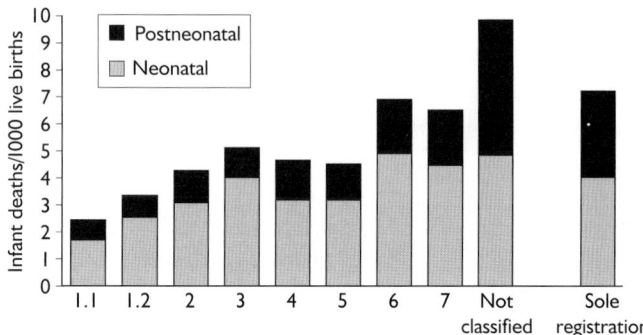

Fig. 1.16 Infant mortality by National Statistics socio-economic Classification of father, England and Wales, births in 2001. Data from Office for National Statistics, Mortality statistics, Series DH3.

mortality rates for the years 1983–87 combined were analysed in 100 g groups.[4] It was necessary to combine 5 years' data to have sufficient numbers of deaths in each group to eliminate the effects of random variation.

Innumerable studies over the years have shown social class gradients in stillbirth and infant mortality rates for the Registrar General's social classes.[46,88,90,95,96,109,116,117] Neonatal and post-neonatal mortality rates for England and Wales, analysed by the National Statistics Socio-economic Class of the baby's father, are shown in Figure 1.16. The analysis includes both births within marriage and those outside marriage registered jointly by both parents, who account for the majority of the rising proportion of births outside marriage. The very high mortality rates among babies registered by the mother on her own are also shown. The data are from the infant-mortality-linked file of ONS.[109]

The most striking feature is that, although there are marked differences between groups, using the new classification does not produce a straightforward gradient. Unlike the Registrar General's classification, which was based on crude assessments of the status of individual occupations, the new classification is based more firmly in sociological theory. In particular, group 4, which consists of people working on their own account, enjoys comparatively low mortality and good health, despite their lack of high status. The explanation advanced is that this results from the amount of autonomy they experience.[135] When the groups are amalgamated to form the three-class version of the classification, as has been done in the revised version of the Department of Health's infant mortality target, this distinction disappears.[136] Another notable feature in Figure 1.16 is the difference between neonatal and postneonatal mortality rates, with the latter showing much wider differences between classes. Deaths attributed to the sudden infant death syndrome show particularly marked social class differences, which contribute substantially to the social class differences in postneonatal mortality.[90]

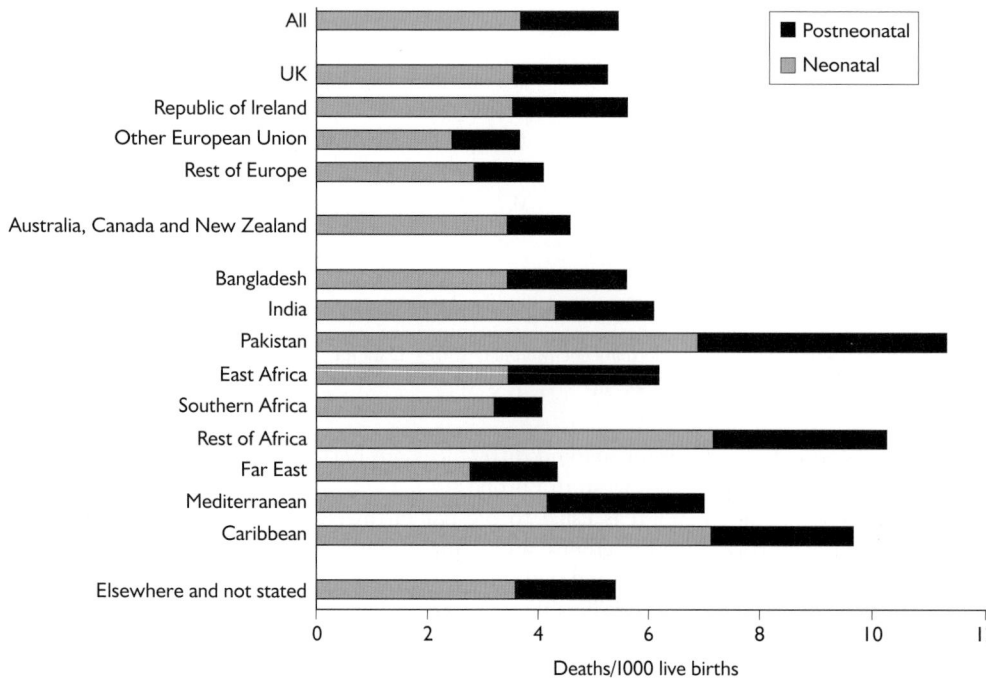

Fig. 1.17 Infant mortality by mother's country of birth, England and Wales, 1999–2002. Data from Office for National Statistics, Mortality statistics, Series DH3.

Neonatal and postneonatal mortality rates for selected mothers' countries of birth are shown in Figure 1.17 and tabulated more fully in Table 1.16. As in other years, mortality rates for babies whose mothers were born in Pakistan are markedly higher than those with mothers born elsewhere in the Indian subcontinent, which are much closer to the overall level. Babies whose mothers came from Pakistan tend to have raised mortality rates associated with congenital anomalies and relatively high mortality rates compared with other groups right across the birthweight range.[9] As in other recent years, mortality rates are also relatively high for babies born to women born in the Caribbean Commonwealth and the largely west African 'rest of Africa'. These groups have high mortality associated with immaturity, which is compatible with their exceptionally high proportions of very-low-birthweight babies.[33]

Multiple births accounted for nearly a quarter of infant deaths of babies born in 2001 weighing under 1500 g at birth and well over a tenth of all infant deaths among babies born in 2001, as Table 1.9 shows. Figure 1.15 gives an indication of how the relationship between mortality rates for singleton and multiple births changes with birthweight within the category below 1500 g. Overall infant mortality rates are higher for multiple than for singleton births. Not surprisingly, mortality is highest among babies born in triplet and higher-order births. This can be seen in Table 1.17, in which infant mortality rates for babies born in multiple births in the years 1975–2001 are compared with those for singletons. Mortality among twins and among triplet and higher-order births fell markedly in the 1970s, then showed no consistent trend in more recent years. Despite year-to-year fluctuations because of the small numbers involved, there was a marked decrease from the early 1990s onwards. No data are available about the extent to which the increasing survival of triplet and higher-order births is associated with morbidity in the survivors. These births create problems not only for the staff of neonatal units but for parents faced with the problems of caring for three or more babies of the same age. These have considerable implications for families and for the health and social services so the downturn in the triplet rate has welcome consequences.[16]

Geographical variations in mortality

Variations from district to district in perinatal and infant mortality rates have received considerable attention from the press and parliament.[69,105] Politicians have sometimes assumed that these variations simply reflect differences in the quality of maternity care. As a result, they have tended to imply that districts and

Table 1.16 Infant mortality by mother's country of birth, England and Wales, 1999–2002 combined

Mother's country of birth	Live births	Neonatal deaths	Postneonatal deaths	Deaths per 1000 live births		
				Neonatal	Postneonatal	Infant
All	**2 417 069**	**8916**	**3230**	**3.7**	**1.7**	**5.0**
UK	2 031 111	7267	2597	3.6	1.7	4.9
England and Wales	1 987 315	7116	2539	3.6	1.6	4.9
Scotland	32 376	114	46	3.5	1.8	4.9
Northern Ireland	10 080	30	11	3.0	1.5	4.1
Elsewhere	1340	7	1	5.2	0.7	6.0
Outside the UK	385 958	1649	633	4.3	2.2	5.9
Irish Republic	16 071	57	27	3.5	2.1	5.2
Other European Union	44 343	109	39	2.5	1.2	3.3
Rest of Europe	28 788	82	28	2.8	1.2	3.8
Australia, Canada and New Zealand	14 746	51	16	3.5	1.1	4.5
New Commonwealth	**197 534**	**1042**	**415**	**5.3**	**2.8**	**7.4**
Bangladesh	31 507	109	46	3.5	2.1	4.9
India	26 967	116	36	4.3	1.8	5.6
Pakistan	56 978	393	180	6.9	4.4	10.1
East Africa	15 587	54	36	3.5	2.7	5.8
Southern Africa	8405	27	4	3.2	0.8	3.7
Rest of Africa	27 743	199	63	7.2	3.1	9.4
Far East	5793	16	8	2.8	1.6	4.1
Mediterranean	4580	19	11	4.1	2.8	6.6
Caribbean	11 900	85	24	7.1	2.5	9.2
Rest of the new Commonwealth	8074	24	7	3.0	1.2	3.8
Rest of the world and not stated	**84 476**	**308**	**108**	**3.6**	**1.8**	**4.9**

Source: ONS mortality statistics, Series DH3.

Table 1.17 Infant mortality rates for singleton and multiple births by year of birth, England and Wales, 1975–2001

Year of birth	Singleton		Twins		Triplets and above	
	Number	**Rate**	**Number**	**Rate**	**Number**	**Rate**
1975	8438	14.3	824	71.8	56	249.3
1976	7459	13.0	665	61.8	42	169.4
1977	7697	12.7	586	55.3	26	133.3
1978	7172	12.2	648	56.9	52	248.8
1979	7395	11.8	621	52.3	41	167.3
1980	7057	11.0	583	47.4	43	154.7
1981	n/a		n/a		n/a	
1982	6089	9.9	496	40.8	19	82.6
1983	5786	9.4	492	39.9	21	75.8
1984	5318	8.5	492	39.6	35	138.9
1985	5642	8.8	504	38.3	25	79.4
1986	5508	8.5	611	44.7	38	92.5
1987	5573	8.4	574	40.6	46	113.0
1988	5384	7.9	593	40.4	52	101.2
1989	5065	7.5	562	37.6	58	98.6
1990	4740	6.9	565	36.1	45	71.9
1991	4168	6.1	531	33.0	67	101.4
1992	3858	5.7	473	28.8	49	77.3
1993	3604	5.5	481	29.6	55	75.1
1994	3444	5.3	494	29.8	51	64.4
1995	3399	5.4	493	28.7	66	77.0
1996	3324	5.3	485	28.6	44	55.1
1997	3213	5.1	409	23.3	55	61.8
1998	3134	5.1	426	24.7	50	56.1
1999	3010	5.0	500	27.2	38	47.7
2000	2951	5.0	392	23.4	44	55.8
2001	2686	4.7	417	24.9	30	47.2

Source: ONS Mortality Statistics, Series DH3.

countries with the highest rates simply have to copy the practices of those with the lowest rates and the problem will be solved almost instantly. As a consequence of this, infant mortality rates and their components have frequently featured over the years in government 'performance indicators' and targets, both as proxy measures of the health of the population and as proxy measures of the quality of health care in an area. Closer inspection of these data shows that these interpretations are oversimplified and that the differences arise from a number of factors.

First, there is the question of which babies to register as births and deaths and which to categorise as miscarriages, which go unrecorded. Decisions about this are likely to reflect cultural, religious and social factors, which may vary from place to place.

Next, it is necessary to consider random variation. Neonatal and infant mortality rates for administrative districts within the UK, such as primary care trusts in England, are now based on such small numbers of events that what appear to be quite large differences from area to area, or from year to year within an area, are actually no larger than would be expected by chance. In the 1980s OPCS published perinatal and infant mortality rates for NHS districts in England and Wales based on 3 years' aggregated data in addition to rates for the most recent year. ONS was forced

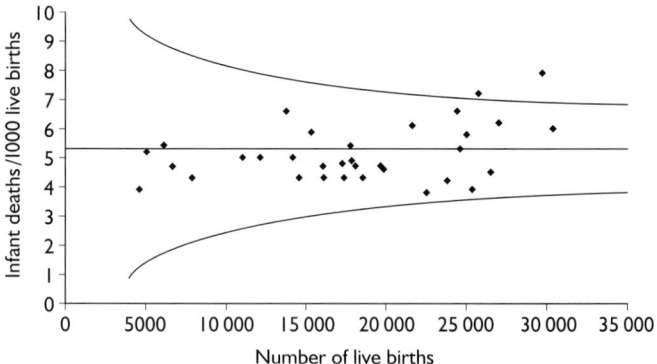

Fig. 1.18 Infant mortality rate by strategic health authority, with 95 per cent confidence intervals for the overall rate based on numbers of live births, England and Wales, 2002.

by the plethora of boundary changes to stop aggregating data in the 1990s. Finally, it has stopped putting data for primary care trusts in the public domain and only NHS staff have access to them.

The data shown in Figure 1.18 are therefore based on data for strategic health authorities for a single year.[113] This shows the

Table 1.18 Neonatal mortality rates in countries participating in the PERISTAT project

Member state	Coverage	Source	Live births	Neonatal deaths (*n*)	Neonatal mortality rate (per 1000 live births)	95% confidence interval	
						Lower	Upper
Austria		A1-2001	75 433	226	3.0	2.6	3.4
Belgium	Flanders	B2-2000	61 844	188	3.0	2.6	3.5
Denmark		DK1-2000	67 084	266	4.0	3.5	4.4
Finland		FIN1-2000	56 541	134	2.4	2.0	2.8
France		F2-2000	774 782	2297	3.0	2.8	3.1
Germany		D2-1999	770 744	2041	2.7	2.5	2.8
Greece	Perinatal survey	EL1-1998	14 277	97	6.8	5.4	8.1
Ireland		IR2-1999	54 242	218	4.0	3.5	4.6
Italy		I-1998	531 650	2031	3.8	3.7	4.0
Luxembourg		L1-2000	5696	11	1.9	0.8	3.1
Netherlands		NL1-1999	200 115	805	4.0	3.7	4.3
Portugal		P1-1999	120 071	407	3.4	3.1	3.7
Spain	Madrid, Valencia, Pais Vasco	E2-2000	85 478	233	2.7	2.4	3.1
Sweden		S1-2000	89 377	203	2.3	2.0	2.6
UK	England and Wales	UK1,8-2000	621 872	2307	3.7	3.6	3.9
UK	Northern Ireland	UK7,10-2000	21 699	78	3.6	2.8	4.4
UK	Scotland	UK6,11-2000	52 115	212	4.1	3.5	4.4

Source: PERISTAT project.[24] See report for descriptions of data sources.[93]

infant mortality rate for each strategic health authority in 2002 plotted against the number of live births to residents in this year. The horizontal line is the rate for England and Wales. The curved lines are its 95% confidence intervals for the relevant numbers of live births. It can be seen that in some of the smaller authorities the rates differed considerably from that for England and Wales, without going outside the 95% confidence interval. In these instances, the difference between the authority's rate and that for England and Wales is no greater than would be expected by chance.

Random variation should also be taken into account when making comparisons between countries, especially when some of them have small populations. Table 1.18 shows neonatal mortality rates for countries participating in the PERISTAT European Perinatal Indicator Project, together with 95% confidence intervals.[24] These show that even the differences between crude mortality rates are by no means as clear cut as is commonly assumed.

Returning to England and Wales, a special analysis for the years 1983–85 found that the districts whose mortality rates fell below the lower 95% confidence limit tended to be those with a high proportion of fathers in professional occupations and a low proportion of mothers born in the 'new Commonwealth' or Pakistan.[15] Most analyses showed a high correlation between perinatal mortality rates and the proportion of low-weight births. This study showed that, when mortality was analysed within birthweight groups, different districts had high and low rates.

These analyses lent support to earlier proposals that birthweight-specific mortality rates were a better proxy measure of the quality of services than crude mortality rates. These had also proposed that multiple births and deaths attributed to congenital malformations should be excluded. Now that, as a result of both decline in natural incidence and the introduction of screening programmes,

mortality attributed to central nervous system anomalies has declined to a much lower level, its inclusion is no longer such a critical factor. In any case, it would be more helpful to use birthweight-specific mortality rates as health service indicators or 'floor targets' than to continue the present practice of using crude rates. It is also a principle to consider when looking at trends over time and differences between countries.

The extent to which differences in the incidence and reporting of low birthweight can affect international comparisons of infant mortality rates is illustrated in Figure 1.19, which is based on data from the PERISTAT European Perinatal Indicator Project referred to earlier. It shows the contribution of preterm and very preterm births to neonatal deaths in the participating countries which had data about gestational age.[24] Because of these differences, the World Health Organization has recommended that babies with gestational ages below 22 weeks and birthweights below 500 g should be excluded from comparisons between countries.[155]

Classification of clinical causes of death

In publications based on death registration, information about causes of death is usually classified to a single 'underlying cause' using the International Classification of Diseases, which is revised approximately every 10 years by the World Health Organization. Since the mid 1990s, the tenth revision (ICD10) has been widely used for most other purposes.[155] The exception is stillbirth and death registration data. Use of ICD10 for this purpose started in

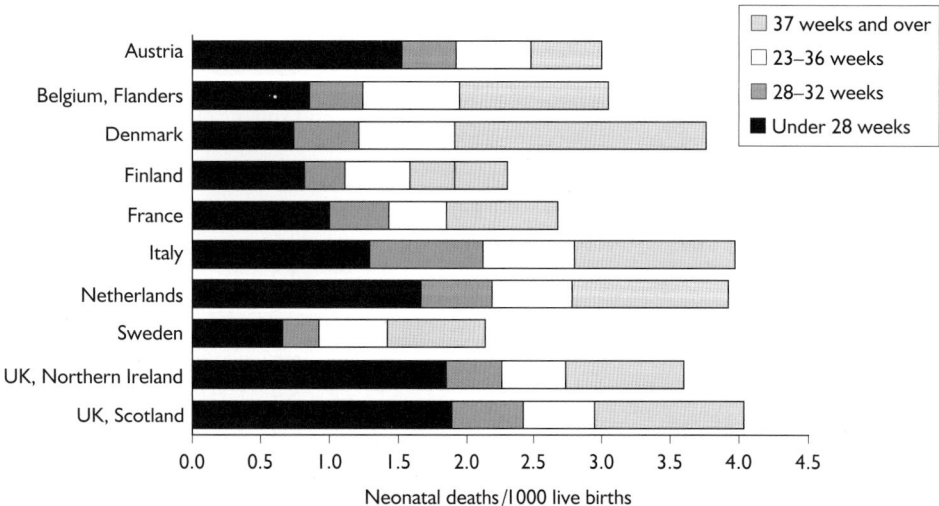

Fig. 1.19 The contribution of preterm births to neonatal mortality in years around 2000 in countries participating in the PERISTAT project. Data from PERISTAT project.[24] See report for descriptions of data sources.[93]

Table 1.19 Stillbirths and infant deaths by ONS cause group, England and Wales, 2002

ONS cause group	Live births	Stillbirths	Neonatal deaths	Postneonatal deaths	Infant deaths	Rate*			
						Stillbirths	Neonatal deaths	Postneonatal deaths	Infant deaths
All causes	596 122	3372	2101	978	3079	5.66	3.52	1.64	5.17
Congenital anomalies		490	538	333	871	0.82	0.90	0.56	1.46
Antepartum infections		25	51	15	66	0.04	0.09	0.03	0.11
Immaturity related conditions		–	1188	186	1374	–	1.99	0.31	2.30
Asphyxia, anoxia or trauma		111	196	9	205	0.19	0.33	0.02	0.34
External conditions		7	11	52	63	0.01	0.02	0.09	0.11
Infections		–	22	120	142		0.04	0.20	0.24
Other specific conditions		210	20	23	43	0.35	0.03	0.04	0.07
Asphyxia, anoxia or trauma		914	–	–	–	1.53	–	–	–
Remaining antepartum deaths		1543	–	–	–	2.59	–	–	–
Sudden infant deaths		–	30	134	164	–	0.05	0.22	0.28
Other conditions		72	45	106	151	0.12	0.08	0.18	0.25

* Stillbirths per 1000 total births and neonatal, postneonatal and infant deaths per 1000 live births.
Source: ONS mortality statistics, Series DH3, 2002 No 35, Table 8.

2000 in Scotland and in 2001 in England, Wales and Northern Ireland. The ICD is designed primarily for use in circumstances in which only limited amounts of clinical information, such as that given on death certificates, is available.

In the perinatal field, other classifications have been developed for use by people with access to the more detailed clinical information found in case notes and pathologists' reports. Perhaps the best known is the classification first developed in Aberdeen in the 1940s by Sir Dugald Baird.[7] This was revised in the early 1980s for use in stillbirth and neonatal mortality surveys in Scotland and the northern region of England, and has separate classifications for conditions in mothers[31] and babies.[65]

A further classification, designed by a pathologist, Jonathan Wigglesworth, is based on externally observable features, supplemented by information from the clinical history.[151] A modified version, produced for the International Collaborative Effort on Birthweight, Plurality, Perinatal and Infant Mortality, was designed for use by people who are further removed from clinical details, and is therefore based on the underlying cause of death coded using the ICD.[30] It also extended the classification to cover conditions associated with death in the postneonatal period. OPCS used this as a basis for a classification it developed for use on the new form of stillbirth and neonatal death certificate introduced in 1986.[5] These certificates have separate spaces to list conditions in the mother, the baby and other factors relating to the death. The system was further developed for classifying stillbirths.[3] Since then, the classification has been used routinely by ONS in its published tabulations of cause of death. It was revised for use with ICD10 and extended to postneonatal mortality rates.[39] It is illustrated in Table 1.19, which shows stillbirth and infant mortality rates for 2002.

Confidential enquiries

As a result of public concern about levels of perinatal and infant mortality in the late 1970s, many special regional and local surveys and enquiries were set up. These varied in their format. Some were largely restricted to reviews of case notes, whereas others involved interviews with bereaved parents. Some took the form of 'confidential enquiries' based on the model of the Confidential Enquiries into Maternal Deaths. Some of these initiatives were for a single year or a limited period.[51] Others, notably those in Scotland and in the former Northern and South East Thames Regions of England, had been in existence for some years.

The rise in infant mortality in England and Wales in 1986 prompted a further enquiry into perinatal, neonatal and infant mortality by the backbench House of Commons Social Services Committee, as it was then called. This recommended 'a targeted programme to reduce perinatal and infant mortality rates, particularly in poorer families where rates are still unnecessarily high'.[69] In addition, it said: 'We recommend that all Regions introduce a regular system of confidential inquiries into all unexplained infant deaths and report to the Department of Health on a regular basis. We also recommend that Regions and the Department of Health set up a system for monitoring the results of such inquiries and making the lessons learned available to all health districts.'[69] In its reply, published in 1989, the government announced that it would be setting up a Confidential Enquiry into Stillbirths and Infant Deaths, and the Chief Medical Officer was setting up a working group to consider what form it might take.[42] Secondly, it acknowledged that many regions already conducted epidemiological surveys of stillbirths and neonatal deaths and it had asked the NHS Management Executive to ensure that all regions were doing them by April 1991. Instead of a targeted programme to reduce infant mortality, it stated that 'Targets need to be set to improve performance'.[42] The Chief Medical Officer's working group reported in 1990.[43] It recommended a national enquiry, with a regional and district reporting structure, into subsets of individual late fetal losses, stillbirths and infant deaths.

The Confidential Enquiry into Stillbirths and Deaths in Infancy (CESDI) was set up in 1992, with a budget of over £2 million per year for England,[67] Wales and Northern Ireland to conduct their own enquiries on the same lines, and the data for all three countries are combined. Scotland has been conducting its own enquiries over a much longer period. As the name suggests, the Enquiry's brief was to collect information on all late fetal losses at 20–23 weeks of gestation and all stillbirths and deaths in the first year of life, and to try to establish ways in which these deaths might be prevented. It was also to establish panels in each former NHS region to perform enquiries into a designated subset of the deaths.

One of its first priorities were 'sudden unexpected deaths in infancy', a category which went wider than the 'sudden infant death syndrome'. These were the focus of its 1994 report and of two papers in the *British Medical Journal* on smoking and sleeping position.[11] These distracted attention from the fuller data published in the CESDI report, which showed that a high proportion of the babies who died were in very deprived circumstances.[36,83,87] CESDI's other early priority was intrapartum-related deaths of normally formed mature babies. These were the subject of confidential enquiries from 1993 to 1995, the initial results of which were published in CESDI's report for 1995.[35-37] In 1996 and 1997 the deaths of a random sample of immature babies were the subject of confidential enquiries. Since then, enquiries have focussed on large babies, babies born at 27 or 28 weeks of pregnancy and the outcome of diabetic pregnancies. After being taken over by the National Institute for Clinical Excellence, which reviewed all the four confidential enquiries, it was merged with the Confidential Enquiry into Maternal Deaths and given a much wider remit as the Confidential Enquiry into Maternal and Child Health. The Enquiry transferred to the National Patient Safety Agency in April 2004.

Morbidity in childhood in relation to circumstances at birth

Although trends in mortality since the mid-1980s are somewhat uncertain, it is clear that over the preceding 20 years there was a dramatic decline in neonatal mortality, particularly among very small and immature babies. This raises the question of whether this fall in mortality has been associated with an increase, a decrease or no change in the rate of morbidity among the survivors.

Although there are a large number of follow-up studies in the medical and education literature, it has been difficult to answer this question. This is because information about long-term morbidity has not been collected in a standardised and comparable way, either in the countries of the UK or in most other countries.

There are few routine sources of information on morbidity available. Because of this, data about morbidity in children who were born with low birthweight or who needed neonatal intensive care for other reasons are available mostly from studies of cohorts of babies cared for in individual hospitals or, occasionally, born to residents in geographically defined populations. Comparisons between these studies and over time is difficult for a number of reasons, which will be outlined.

Routinely collected morbidity data

At present the routinely available sources of information on childhood morbidity in the UK include the censuses and surveys, hospital activity statistics, data from general practice systems, child health computer systems, the BD8 register of people with visual impairments and registers of children with disabilities. A web publication *The health of children and young people*, reviewing data for England and Wales, can be found on the ONS web site.[115]

The General Household Survey, which interviews samples of households in Great Britain, asks people whether they have 'long-standing illness, disability or infirmity' and, if so, whether this restricts their activities in any way. In the case of children, this information is obtained from interviews with parents or other members of the household. In 2002, 5% of boys aged 0–4 years and 3% of girls were reported as having a limiting long-standing illness, compared with 3% and 2%, respectively, in 1975.[114]

For the first time since 1911, the population census taken in 1991 contained a question about health. It was similar but not identical to that in the General Household Survey, and asked whether people had 'any long-term illness, health problem or handicap which limits his/her daily activities or the work he/she can do'.[26,119] In the 2001 census, a question about general health was added. Neither of these two involves clinical examinations or collecting diagnostic data. Since the early 1990s this has been done in a series of health surveys that have been established in each of the four countries of the UK. Since 1995, the Health Survey for England has included children aged 2–15 and from 2002, children under the age of 2 have been surveyed. Data about disability are collected for those aged 10 or over.[130] As only small numbers of children aged 10–15 with a disability are sampled in any given year, it is difficult to draw any firm conclusions about patterns of disability. After an enhanced sample of children was taken in 1997, a special report was published on *The health of young people*.[131]

As has been mentioned earlier, information on inpatient stays in NHS hospitals is collected routinely in all four countries of the UK. This can be used to analyse trends in inpatient and day-case care for particular conditions or in particular specialties. In England, episodes of inpatient care in NHS hospitals, including those in neonatal units, are collected through the Hospital Episode System. The quality and completeness of the diagnostic data vary from district to district, although concerted attempts have been made to improve this. In Wales and Northern Ireland the data are collected through the Patient Episode Database Wales (PEDW) and the Hospital Inpatients System respectively. In Scotland, the SMR1 system deals with general hospital episodes. The SMR11 system, which dealt with neonatal stays, is being superseded by elements of the SCHID project, described above.

In the past, records about successive hospital stays by the same person were not linked, but increasing potential for this now exists. There are now techniques that allow data about babies and children to be linked to data, such as birthweight, from birth records. If records are linked, as has been the case for some years in the Oxford Record Linkage Study, it then becomes possible, for example, to look at the impact of increasing survival of low-birthweight babies on hospital readmission rates in the early years of life.[103] In Scotland, record linkage at a national level is well developed. The other three countries of the UK lag behind, but it is possible to do some linkage locally. The inclusion of NHS numbers on all NHS records increase the potential for record linkage. At the time of writing it is unclear whether the National Care Records Service will be available to provide linked anonymised records for analytical purposes.

Since the mid-1930s visually impaired children and adults living in England and Wales have been able to register with local authorities as 'blind' or 'partially sighted', using a BD8 form. Although the registration system is used primarily for service planning, the new BD8 form introduced in 1990 also has a section that is anonymised and contains some epidemiological data.[53] This is used for monitoring the frequency and causes of blindness in the population, but some visually impaired people are not registered. Cross-checks with other sources suggest that the register is much more complete for people who are blind than for those who are partially sighted. As a result, the reported numbers and rates of visual impairment in England are probably underestimates.[54] Unless there are incentives for earlier reporting of children, it will continue to be difficult to monitor fluctuations in the prevalence of eye conditions such as retinopathy of prematurity.

Under the 1989 Children Act, health authorities, educational authorities and social services are required to cooperate in maintaining registers of children with particular problems or conditions.[41] Such registers, which form a basis for service planning, may be part of the child health information systems held by community trusts, either as free-standing special needs registers[34] or as modules of an integrated computerised system that provides information on all children within an area.[152] The focus of these registers is primarily on service provision but, if appropriately compiled, they could also be used as a source of information on many aspects of health and development in childhood.

A further potential source of information on childhood morbidity in the UK is from the records of general practitioners. Until recently, most data about care given by general practitioners have come from four national surveys of people consulting GPs in sets of volunteer practices. Surveys took place in 1955–56, 1970–71, 1981–82 and 1991–92.[85] As well as background information about patients, diagnostic information was collected about each episode of illness and consultations within it.

Now that most general practices have computer systems, further developments are possible. Data from practices having computer systems provided by VAMP Health Ltd have been pooled for research or monitoring purposes in the General Practice Research Database.[66] More recently, the MIQUEST project has been attempting to aggregate anonymised data from a variety of systems used in general practice.[106] A major problem with all these initiatives is the lack of consistency in the way different practices record clinical and other information. Thus the potential of general practice systems to provide data about health service use and patterns of illness in young children in relation to birthweight and events occurring around the time of birth has yet to be realised.[94]

Special studies to follow children exposed to adverse perinatal events

This section and the following one provide the epidemiological background to the more detailed information and studies reported in Chapter 3, and should be read in conjunction with it.

There are two methods that are commonly used to investigate morbidity in specific groups of children. One is to survey a total population in order to detect impairments and disabilities. This may be done as a 'one-off' cross-sectional point prevalence survey, or alternatively by developing an ongoing register to which children are added when impairments or disabilities are identified. The contribution of the specific group of children to the total pool of impairment in the population can then be estimated and monitored over time.

Population registers of this sort have been set up to list children with particular impairments, such as cerebral palsy, sensorineural deafness and visual impairment.[79] These registers are based on populations defined by residence at the time of birth. Population movement across regional boundaries may result in under-ascertainment, particularly as diagnosis may be delayed in milder cases.

The other method of ascertaining the status of groups of children is to define a cohort or group of children for study and follow them longitudinally to monitor function and health status. This is known as a cohort study. Hundreds of such studies have been done over the past 30 years, but for a number of reasons difficulties are met when trying to interpret them, particularly in making comparisons between them.

First, cohorts for study are defined in differing ways. Most are derived from individual hospitals or units and are therefore subject to selection biases. Populations defined by geographical boundaries are more likely to be free of these biases and to reflect the care given to all babies born to residents in the area. This is the case with the much larger Millennium Cohort, based on a national sample of babies born in 2000 and 2001, but this does not have a clinical focus and children were not recruited to the cohort until they were approximately 10 months old.

Other difficulties in interpretation arise when differing birthweight and gestational age groupings and diagnostic criteria are used. There are, for example, differences in the criteria for including children in diagnostic categories such as small for gestational age or chronic lung disease. Some standardisation is possible by adopting WHO recommendations for grouping birthweight data[155] and, when available, agreed classifications and definitions of neonatal conditions and diseases.

Differences in denominators make it difficult to interpret the numbers and rates of impaired children within a specific cohort. Changes of practice, such as the increasing tendency to register very-low-birthweight births, may alter survival rates independently of any changes in care.[52] Similarly, an increase in the number of children with impairments within a cohort can merely reflect an increased rate of survival with a constant rate of impairment. To improve comparability, the total number of births, the total number of live births, the total number of stillbirths and the number of survivors to hospital discharge within a cohort should all be reported.

A further problem in comparability results from the many different ways in which morbidity and health status may be ascertained and reported. The challenge is to reflect the complexity of the consequences of disease or organ damage in simple descriptive terms. This has often been attempted by considering separate domains or systems, such as neurodevelopmental state, sensory impairment, growth, behavioural attributes and learning abilities, and so on. Alternative measures of health service use, such as hospital admission, primary health care and ancillary services, can be used as a proxy measure of morbidity. These have additional important economic implications. Further measures could include family integrity and social adjustment.

In the past, a clear distinction between the concepts of impairment, disability and handicap, as defined in the International Classification of Impairments, Disabilities and Handicaps,[154] has made a useful basis for describing the effects of disease and illness on children. There have been attempts to standardise systems for describing impairment in children, and these are described in Chapter 3.

Standard descriptions of disability are less easy to define, particularly the allocation of degrees of severity of the disability. Although a number of schemes have been suggested, many studies have an arbitrary categorisation of disability, usually into severe, moderate and mild. This means that pooling and cross-comparison of disability data is not often possible. Further difficulties arise in the presence of multiple system involvement. As part of the surveys of disability done by OPCS in the mid-1980s, objective measures of severity were derived by asking panels of judges to assign relative weightings to different abilities and disabilities, first within one domain and then within several together.[13]

In recent years, particularly with the emergence of international disability movements, this type of classification has been rejected in favour of a social model of disability, where the focus moves from the effects of disease and impairment on the person to society's response to that person. A model has been devised by the British Association for Community Child Health, which retains the traditional concept of disease, impairment and disability but acknowledges the importance of environment in determining disadvantage and loss of social role.[73] A second version of the ICIDH, the International Classification of Functioning, Disability and Health, which takes a more social approach, has now been published.[156]

Another recent advance has been the development of quality of life measures. These focus on relating the impairments present to the quality of life experienced by the child and by the caregivers. Multi-attribute health status descriptions, which were first developed for use in the cancer field, have been adapted. From these, a single value is estimated that reflects the global health-related quality of life for an individual.[139,146] The extent to which these will be used to inform parents confronted with treatment decisions or to inform those allocating limited resources to health care remains to be seen.

Finally, studies differ widely in the ages at which they measure morbidity. Discussions on the 'best' age for follow-up are usually non-productive, as at each age and developmental age the range of abilities and the impact of disabilities differ. Early ascertainment of morbidity allows rapid reporting back to the providers of neonatal intensive care, but the evaluation will inevitably be incomplete or perhaps inaccurate, and will be misleading for parents.[149] Later assessments allow a more detailed and accurate assessment of areas such as learning ability, social skills, language function and school performance, but mean that more children may be lost to follow-up.

Loss to follow-up is a concern if there is a difference in the characteristics of the children who are successfully followed and those who are lost. There is some evidence that in families who are difficult to locate, there is a higher frequency of disability among the children than in families who are easy to find.[150] If this occurs, there will be a selection bias resulting in an underestimate of the rate of disability in the cohort.

Monitoring trends in morbidity among children in relation to factors at birth

Despite their problems, data from the various sources described above can give some insight into trends in morbidity among children in relation to their circumstances at birth. Recent trends are reviewed in Chapter 3. This section discusses some of the epidemiological issues involved.

Cerebral palsy registers rely on multiple and differing sources of ascertainment but all report prevalence rates close to 2 per 1000 liveborn children. For example the data from the 4Child register in the former Oxford Region consistently show that the rate of cerebral palsy is highest among children with the lowest birthweights and the earliest gestational ages. Despite the higher rate of motor deficit associated with immaturity and low birthweight, half of the children on these population registers of cerebral palsy weighed more than 2500 g at birth, as shown in Figure 1.20.[121]

In recent years, the focus of attention has been on the later outcome of babies born before 28 weeks of gestation or weighing less than 1000 g at birth. It is generally agreed that disability rates are highest among the smallest and most preterm babies, so these groups of babies are particularly vulnerable. The numbers of such survivors are small, however, making it difficult to obtain an overall picture of trends in their outcome over time. This has been compounded by the changing perception of viability, a change in registration practice in the presence of transient signs of life, and more aggressive obstetric and neonatal management, which may have led to an increase in the numbers of live births and fewer fetal deaths in these groups. It is therefore useful to have concurrent information on stillbirths and late fetal deaths.

A further problem in assessing changing outcome over time has been the tendency to report the outcome of babies admitted to large regional centres, rather than all babies from a geographical area. Finally, among the studies of geographically defined populations of babies, some are defined by birthweight group and some by gestational age group. There is some evidence that both mortality and morbidity are more closely related to gestational age than birthweight, and information about prognosis by week of gestation is of more value to obstetricians than similar information by birthweight group.[133]

Studies following children into the school years have shown that those who had low birthweights are more likely than average to have learning difficulties, adverse behavioural traits and motor difficulties.[63,120,127] Despite this, it is clear from studies of children of all birthweights that those who had a low birthweight make up a very small proportion of the total number of children who have special educational needs.[80,98]

Finally, babies who were born in the early 1980s and who were very preterm or with a very low birthweight have now reached adulthood. Early behavioural difficulties, such as attention deficit and hyperactivity disorders, may be associated with later adverse psychosocial outcomes in adolescence.[17] Growth patterns and sexual maturity may also have an impact on later psychological and physical health.

The increasing demand for neonatal care

The increase over the last three decades in the proportion of babies that are born alive and that survive the first few days of life has led to a corresponding increase in the numbers requiring the normal level of neonatal care given by mothers, with the support of midwives, health visitors, general practitioners and paediatric staff. There has also been an increase in the numbers of babies likely to need additional care. The likelihood that a baby will need specialist neonatal care is highest among those with the lowest birthweights, and the proportion of babies of low or very low birthweight who survive birth has increased more quickly than the total numbers of live births.

Trends in resources for neonatal care

Between 1976 and 1988, routine health service statistics presented a contradictory picture of neonatal resources. In 1992, the political debate about resources for neonatal care cited data about cots to make the case that the health service resources were being reduced, whereas the increasing number of whole-time equivalent midwives was quoted as evidence of health service expansion. As we show in the following paragraphs, the interpretation of the data was not correct in either case.

Nationally available data about the NHS include numbers of cots in neonatal units and their use, numbers of paediatric medical staff employed by health authorities, and numbers of midwifery and nursing staff working in maternity and neonatal units. So far there is little information about the resources needed from health and social services and families once babies leave neonatal units, although these cannot be assumed to be negligible.[100,125]

Cots for neonatal care

Cots for neonatal care are funded differently depending on the type of care that is expected to be provided: the more intensive the nursing and the more equipment required, the greater the cost of providing the care. As techniques for care change continually,

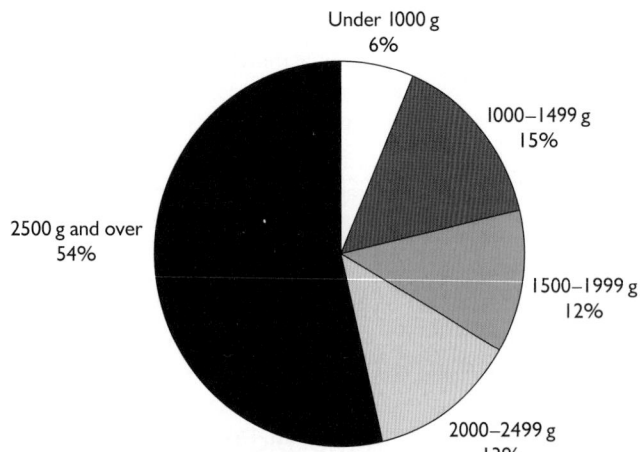

Fig. 1.20 Birthweight distribution of children with cerebral palsy born 1984–97 in the counties of Oxfordshire, Berkshire, Buckinghamshire and Northamptonshire. Data from Oxford Register of Early Childhood Impairments, now known as 4Child.[121]

the definitions of levels of care need to change also, so the relevant professional bodies update these definitions from time to time. A working party set up jointly by the British Paediatric Association and the RCOG published a report in 1978, in which it defined levels of care and the levels of staffing per cot it considered were necessary for each level.[23] These were revised by the BAPM in 1985, 1992 and 1995.[20–22] Whereas details of definitions change at national level, data collected routinely at hospital level count staffed available cots for care of babies and, until the late 1990s, included relatively little additional evidence about the type of cot or level of care provided. Further consultation was taking place at the time of writing about the definition and reporting of services for neonatal care[44] (see also Chapter 2 on recent development in services for neonatal care in the UK).

Data about neonatal cots in England up to 1986 are derived from the SH3 Hospital Return. Numbers of available cots were based on a daily count of staffed available cots in each neonatal unit or special care baby unit (SCBU). Confusion can arise because the numbers of cots counted on the SH3 return were commonly referred to as 'special care cots' and levels of care within the neonatal units were not differentiated. As a result, the total number of cots included those designated for intensive care. The Steering Group on Health Services Information[142] drew on the reports of the professional bodies mentioned above when compiling the definitions of special and intensive care used in the definition of cots for hospital statistics to be collected from 1987 onwards. Such designation is at best artificial, as it is likely that care considered to be intensive often takes place other than in the intensive care area within a special-care nursery. Indeed, in many units such an area may not even be identifiable. Data required to monitor further changes to provision of services within clinical networks are being discussed at the time of writing.[44]

Table 1.20 shows that there has been a fall in the absolute numbers of cots in SCBUs in each of the four countries of the UK. This trend was quoted in newspapers and political campaigns as evidence of cuts in NHS spending, but such an interpretation did not take account of the changing definitions of cots and changing practice in neonatal care over the last three decades. The basis for data collection changed in 1988, and in England the number and use of cots was from that time measured in two different routine systems. Numbers of hospital cots were recorded in the KP70 hospital data system, and the use of cots was derived from the Hospital Episode System, both of which derived data from local health information systems and were administered centrally by the Department of Health. The numbers of cots for neonatal care appeared to have continued to decline until 1990, with a levelling of the numbers and rates per 1000 births after that. Since 1996–97, the numbers of cots for intensive neonatal care have been shown separately.

With increasing concern in the 1970s and 1980s about the separation of babies from their mothers, policies of routine admission to special care for many babies changed. Evidence of this is found in Table 1.20, which shows falling admission rates to SCBUs. The rate fell from a high point of about 20% of births in England in the mid-1970s to just over 10% in 1987. Since 1988 it is no longer the number of admissions but rather the number of 'finished consultant episodes' (FCEs) that is counted. Any baby who is admitted for neonatal care but receives care from different consultants during one admission will be described as receiving more than one FCE during that admission. This can happen if surgery or specialist diagnostic skills are required. Not surprisingly, therefore, numbers of FCEs for babies admitted aged under 28 days and excluding healthy newborns, shown in Table 1.20 for 1989–90 until 1995–96, are

Table 1.20 Cots for neonatal care, England, Wales, Scotland and Northern Ireland, 1980–1988, 1987/88–2002/03

Year	Available cots*		Admissions†		Length of stay‡
	Number	Rate§	Number	Rate§	Average days
England					
1980	3959	6.40	89 277	14.44	8.6
1981	3940	6.59	84 061	14.05	8.9
1982	3902	6.62	76 279	12.93	9.5
1983	3898	6.57	71 184	12.00	10.0
1984	3872	6.45	68 777	11.45	10.5
1985	3756	6.06	68 634	11.08	10.8
1986	3651	5.85	66 725	10.70	11.0
1987	3572	5.55	–	–	–
1987–88	3625	5.63	–	–	–
1988–89	3581	5.47	–	–	–
1989–90	3496	5.38	60 743	9.35	9.6
1990–91	3375	5.06	75 545	11.33	8.7
1991–92	3412	5.16	77 301	11.70	9.4
1992–93	3403	5.22	75 018	11.51	10.0

(Continued)

Table 1.20 (*Continued*)

Year	Available cots*		Admissions†		Length of stay‡ Average days
	Number	**Rate§**	**Number**	**Rate§**	
1993–94	3286	5.04	83 307	13.09	9.9
1994–95	3341	5.25	80 229	12.76	10.6
1995–96	3219	5.12	75 736	12.35	11.1
1996–97	1537	2.50	–	–	–
1997–98	1530	2.52	–	–	–
1998–99	1525	2.53	–	–	–
1999–2000	1534	2.60	–	–	–
2000–01	1517	2.65	–	–	–
2001–02	1543	2.74	–	–	–
2002–03	1551	2.74	–	–	–
2003–04	1491	2.53	–	–	–
Wales					
1980	237	6.34	5359	14.35	8.1
1981	238	6.64	4886	13.63	8.4
1982	236	6.61	4951	13.86	8.4
1983	231	6.51	4386	12.36	8.7
1984	229	6.39	4330	12.07	8.6
1985	223	6.06	4327	11.77	9.4
1986	221	5.97	4097	11.06	10.0
1987	218	5.76	4037	10.68	10.4
1988	219	5.64	3927	10.11	10.6
1987–88	218	5.76	4042	10.69	7.8
1988–89	219	5.64	3892	10.02	7.4
1989–90	219	5.76	4356	11.46	7.6
1990–91	194	4.99	3512	9.04	7.8
1991–92	223	5.86	3796	9.97	7.5
1992–93	210	5.60	3546	9.45	7.5
1993–94	214	5.82	3320	9.08	7.8
1994–95	226	6.40	3215	9.09	13.5
1995–96	208	6.00	3116	9.04	14.5
1996–97	182	5.20	2700	7.74	13.9
1997–98	–	–	–	–	–
1998–99	218	6.51	2917	8.72	15.0
1999–2000	202	6.30	2929	9.12	14.8
2000–01	206	6.57	3012	9.62	13.9
2001–02	202	6.61	2803	9.16	13.8
2002–03	195	6.45	3015	9.98	14.1
Scotland					
1980	626	9.10	20 202	29.3	6.2
1981	621	9.00	19 763	28.6	5.9
1982	619	9.40	17 824	26.9	6.1
1983	608	9.30	16 952	26.0	5.9
1984	597	9.20	15 869	24.4	6.5
1985	580	8.70	15 021	22.5	6.6
1986–87	563	8.50	14 189	21.4	6.8
1987–88	552	8.30	14 500	21.9	6.9
1988–89	543	7.90	12 925	18.5	7.4
1989–90	520	7.80	12 257	18.3	7.8
1990–91	497	7.20	11 597	18.3	8.3
1991–92	477	6.90	10 013	15.2	9.2

(*Continued*)

Table 1.20 (*Continued*)

Year	Available cots*		Admissions[†]		Length of stay Average days
	Number	**Rate**[§]	**Number**	**Rate**[§]	
1992–93	465	6.80	10 020	15.0	8.8
1993–94	448	6.70	9339	14.2	9.1
1994–95	426	6.90	9144	14.4	9.4
1995–96	421	7.00	8619	14.4	9.6
1996–97	404	6.80	8758	14.9	–
1997–98	468	7.20	8220	13.8	7.8
1998–99	420	7.33	–	–	9.2
1999–2000	384	6.96	–	–	10.2
2000–01	380	7.15	–	–	10.3
2001–02	354	6.73	–	–	11.1
2002–03	332	6.47	–	–	10.9
Northern Ireland					
1980	195	6.80	–	–	–
1981	198	7.30	3764	13.80	9.3
1982	–	–	–	–	–
1983	208	7.60	3657	13.40	9.0
1984	218	7.90	3856	13.90	9.1
1985	218	7.90	3667	13.30	9.6
1986	208	7.40	3570	12.70	10.0
1987	–	–	3729	–	9.9
1988–89	176	6.34	3420	12.32	10.3
1989–90	171	6.54	3495	13.40	9.6
1990–91	171	6.45	3608	13.62	9.6
1991–92	170	6.48	3481	13.25	9.7
1992–93	169	6.61	3103	12.13	10.2
1993–94	168	6.74	2870	11.52	10.4
1994–95	166	6.80	2698	11.10	11.1
1995–96	Not available from 1995–96 onwards				

* Neonatal unit and postnatal cots. For England, up to 1986, staffed available cots in SCBU. After 1988, staffed cots available for neonatal care. From 1996–7, average daily number of available and occupied neonatal intensive care beds, line 1 on KH03.
[†] Up to 1986, numbers of babies admitted to SCBU. For England, after 1988, finished consultant episodes for admissions of babies under 28 days of age.
[‡] Mean days of stay/episode.
[§] Rate per 1000 live births.
Source: NHS Executive and DH Statistics Divisions 2&3.

much higher than the previous numbers of admissions to neonatal units. Although this analysis of FCEs is not available for later years, the Department of Health publishes analyses of occupancy (percentage of days an available cot is occupied), which show that, although there was a slight increase in the available cots per 1000 livebirths in the most recent period, the occupancy was constant at about 70%, suggesting that an increasing number of intensive care cot days were being provided.

Falling admission rates between 1980 and 1990 were not accompanied by a significant fall in workload, as those babies who are admitted stay for longer. Table 1.20 also shows that the mean length of stay increased between 1980 and 1986. Data for 1989–90 until 1995–96 show that the mean duration of consultant episodes for babies admitted aged under 28 days has no clear trend, varying between 8.7 and 11.1 days. Data from this source cannot tell us how the casemix has changed, but there is evidence from local surveys done over the period that an increasing proportion of babies admitted received intensive care.[25]

Although data about numbers of intensive care cots have not been routinely collected until recently, national surveys of cot provision have been conducted, and these give some idea of the changes over time, although methods and coverage differ. Table 1.21 summarises data from three of these surveys. In 1980, the Department of Health and Social Security published data from the English NHS regions, which showed that out of a total of 268 consultant units there were 42 with some intensive care

Table 1.21 Neonatal intensive care facilities in England 1980, 1986, 2001 and UK 1989–91

Year and country	England			United Kingdom		
	Nurseries No.	Intensive care cots		Nurseries No.	Intensive care cots	
		No.	Rate per 1000 live births		No.	Rate per 1000 live births
1980	42	173	0.22			
1986	65	341	0.55			
1989				n/a	514	0.66
1990				n/a	549	0.69
1991				257	584	0.74
2001	139	1194	2.12			

Sources: Data for 1980 from Hansard; data for 1986 from BAPM survey of neonatal referrals;[19] data for 1989–90 from BAPM survey;[28] data for 2001 from Department of Health form KH03.

cots, and that the total number of intensive care cots available was 173. By the end of 1986, a national survey of neonatal units[19] found that the number of cots available for intensive care in units where it was regularly practised had increased more than twofold since 1980, with 341 cots in 1986. In the 242 consultant obstetric units in England in 1986, 65 had at least three intensive care cots.

The BAPM survey of transfers for neonatal care was repeated for the years 1989–91 for a report on the access and availability of neonatal intensive care by a working party of the Clinical Standards Advisory Group.[28] Data from this source, which refer to the UK as a whole and are not identified separately for England, are also included in Table 1.21. These show that the rate of intensive care cot provision continued to increase from 0.22 cots per 1000 live births in England in 1980 to 0.74 per 1000 live births in the UK in 1991. A more recent survey in 1999, conducted for the British Association of Perinatal Medicine, was based on a smaller sample of the 37 largest high risk perinatal centres in the UK and also does not provide data about numbers of intensive care cots in all the countries of the UK.[123] Since 1996–97, the KH03 form has listed numbers of intensive cots in England and the nurseries where they are. Although the definitions have changed, it appears that the number of nurseries providing intensive care and the number of cots have fluctuated around a similar level.

Staff for neonatal care

The medical specialty of paediatrics has grown considerably, both in absolute numbers of 'whole-time equivalent' staff and in relation to the numbers of births, as Table 1.22 shows. Data about the division of work between neonatology and other paediatric work are not routinely collected and so it is only possible to comment on the numbers in the specialty of paediatrics as a whole. Data are collected differently from each country's health administration and are not always available on the same basis. Northern Ireland data include community paediatricians and paediatric surgeons in the total figures for paediatrics and paediatric neurology and therefore the totals are not strictly comparable with those from the other countries. The commentary on the data from Northern Ireland also warns that: 'due to coding difficulties within the system, it is impossible to identify paediatric neurology staff working within paediatrics' and that 'it is most probable that all medical staff working within paediatrics are not captured in these figures'.

Recommendations for staffing of neonatal units have been made by successive committees. A report from the Royal College of Physicians[138] made a range of recommendations depending on the size of units and whether they provide a regional referral service. The report concluded that 150 consultant neonatal paediatricians, 120 middle-grade medical staff and about 424 senior house officers would be needed in England and Wales to meet these recommendations. This represented about a third of the whole-time equivalent staff in the paediatric specialties at the time. The numbers of paediatric staff subsequently increased, and so the recommended staffing for neonatal care represented less than a quarter of the 1993 staffing for paediatrics in England and Wales.

The staff numbers are expressed as whole-time equivalents, with each member of staff being counted as the proportion of the full contract hours worked. This avoids the problem of how to count part-time staff, but trends over time can be misleading when nationally agreed hours of work change. It is important to note that changes in the contractual hours of doctors during the last decade will have reduced the total medical time represented by the whole-time equivalent number of staff. Further recommendations for staffing are included in the Report of the DH expert working group.[44]

National data about midwives and nurses can be analysed to indicate how many of them work in neonatal areas. In many maternity units a certain amount of neonatal special care, such as phototherapy, is given in postnatal wards. Because of this blurring of the boundary between different levels of care, it is important to look at the total numbers of maternity unit staff available per birth, as well as the numbers of neonatal unit staff.

The total numbers of qualified hospital nurses and midwives working in the maternity area who were in post on 30 September in each of the years 1982–2003 in England are presented in

Table 1.22 Paediatric medical staff in England, Wales, Scotland and Northern Ireland, 1980–2003

Year	England		Wales		Scotland		Northern Ireland[‡]	
	wte*	Rate[†]	wte*	Rate[†]	wte*	Rate[†]	wte*	Rate[†]
Paediatrics and paediatric neurology								
1982	1745	2.96	110	3.08	214	3.23	–	–
1983	1780	3.00	117	3.30	216	3.32	62	2.27
1984	1821	3.03	119	3.32	217	3.33	66	2.38
1985	1837	2.97	122	3.32	223	3.34	65	2.35
1986	1933	3.10	125	3.37	226	3.43	69	2.45
1987	1994	3.10	–	–	229	3.46	72	2.58
1988	2322	3.55	124	3.19	238	3.59	77	2.77
1989	2222	3.42	135	3.55	246	3.88	77	2.95
1990	2339	3.51	145	3.73	260	3.94	78	2.94
1991	2410	3.65	159	4.18	272	4.06	79	3.01
1992	2559	3.93	160	4.26	267	4.06	94	3.68
1993	2833	4.45	188	5.14	271	4.28	96	3.89
1994	3070	4.88	216	6.11	289	4.69	103	4.28
1995	3892	6.35	228	6.61	321	5.34	126	5.33
1996	3973	6.47	238	6.81	349	5.89	137	5.63
1997	4305	7.08	250	7.23	369	6.21	143	5.93
1998	4487	7.45	260	7.79	374	6.52	154	6.52
1999	4698	7.97	272	8.48	396	7.17	173	7.53
2000	4590	8.01	293	9.35	–	–	174	8.10
2001	4600	8.16	293	9.57	–	–	187	8.53
2002	–	–	311	10.28	–	–	183	8.54
2003	5414	–	–	–	435	8.30	186	–
Paediatric surgery								
1982	–	–	5	0.14	38	0.57	–	–
1983	–	–	5	0.14	36	0.55	11	0.40
1984	–	–	11	0.31	45	0.69	14	0.51
1985	100	0.16	4	0.11	43	0.64	14	0.51
1986	119	0.19	5	0.13	40	0.61	13	0.46
1987	131	0.20	–	–	45	0.68	12	0.43
1988	127	0.19	7	0.18	53	0.80	12	0.43
1989	141	0.22	7	0.18	54	0.85	13	0.50
1990	128	0.19	6	0.15	48	0.73	9	0.34
1991	155	0.23	4	0.11	s	0.49	11	0.42
1992	157	0.24	3	0.08	49	0.74	11	0.43
1993	163	0.26	3	0.08	44	0.69	10	0.40
1994	162	0.26	7	0.20	51	0.83	9	0.37
1995	196	0.32	4	0.12	56	0.93	9	0.38
1996	213	0.35	3	0.09	49	0.83	10	0.41
1997	219	0.36	7	0.20	50	0.84	10	0.41
1998	259	0.43	7	0.21	39	0.67	9	0.37
1999	226	0.38	6	0.19	36	0.65	8	0.34
2000	269	0.47	7	0.22	–	–	4	0.18
2001	261	0.46	8	0.26	–	–	5	0.22
2002	–	–	10	0.33	–	–	5	0.22
2003	247	–	–	–	64	1.23	7	–

*Whole-time equivalent.

[†] Per 1000 live births.

[‡] Figures for Northern Ireland for 1997 onwards are taken from the trust and board human resource management systems. They exclude all agency and bank staff. Bank staff maintain service delivery by covering staff shortfalls and fluctuating workloads. As a consequence their input to the service is difficult to measure. Because of coding difficulties within the system, it is impossible to identify paediatric neurology staff working within paediatrics. Despite the fact that the attached figures are shown by paediatric departments, it is most probable that all medical staff working within paediatrics are not captured in these figures.
Source: NHS Executive and Department of Health, National Assembly for Wales, ISD Scotland, Department of Health, Personal Social Services and Public Safety, Northern Ireland.

Table 1.23. Data are shown only for England, as the other countries of the UK do not provide data in this form. In 1980 changes were made in the nationally agreed hours of work for nursing and midwifery staff in the UK. The change in weekly working hours from 40 to 37.5 had the effect of increasing the whole-time equivalents of part-time staff artificially by 6.7% with no actual increase in available staff. Since 1982 the numbers of whole-time equivalent midwives and nurses has not increased, and the rate per 1000 live births has fallen over the period. This trend is associated with a change in training for nurses under 'Project 2000'. Before 1989 student nurses and midwives were counted as part of the NHS workforce, but students are now supernumerary and are not recorded in staff numbers. In 2003, the rates of provision of midwives and maternity nursing staff per 1000 births in England were near to the lowest rates shown in the two decades.

As staffing always has to be responsive to pressures in different parts of the maternity unit, the subdivision of midwives by place of work should not be seen as a rigid indication of staff available in the neonatal unit or elsewhere. All the same, in England the proportion of qualified midwives working in hospital maternity units who were recorded as neonatal staff increased from under 3% in 1984 to nearly 8% in 1994. This rise must be interpreted with caution, as the numbers in the denominator changed with the fall in numbers of student midwives on the payroll. Table 1.24 shows the numbers and rates per 1000 live births of nursing and midwifery staff in neonatal care, as analysed by the NHS executive from the staff census data. In parallel with the increased numbers of intensive care cots, rates of neonatal nursing and midwifery staff increased from 4 per 1000 live births in 1984 to over 6 per 1000 in 1994. Midwives formed about a third of the neonatal nursing workforce in 1994.

Organisation of neonatal resources

Neonatal workload is to a large extent unpredictable. Fluctuations in workload mean that neonatal units are alternately underoccupied or overstretched, as has been shown in local surveys of neonatal unit activity.[25] In most NHS regions the problem of fluctuating demand is met by transfer of babies between units, so long as all units are not busy at the same time. The organisation and success of such arrangements varies, as was shown in the BAPM surveys of referrals for neonatal medical care.[19,28,123] To formalise these arrangements in local management the Department of Health has recommended the development of clinical networks, and this includes neonatal care.[44] For more information on organisation and transport in neonatal care see Chapters 2 and 13.2.

Relationship between resources for neonatal care and outcomes

It is clear from the above that over the past 30 years there has been a shift of resources towards neonatal intensive care and that this has coincided with a decline in neonatal and infant mortality. At the same time there have been changes in other factors known to be associated with neonatal mortality and other measures of the outcome of pregnancy. Because of the inter-relationship between all of the variables, the relative contribution of care and other factors to the change in mortality and other outcomes is not easy to interpret. Some studies in the USA, Norway, Canada and England found a statistical association between increased amounts of 'care' and lower mortality for some groups of babies after taking account of pre-existing risk factors.[8,27,122,141,143]

Against this apparent trend, a series of papers from Sweden show that perinatal mortality was higher in the maternity hospitals with paediatric departments than in those without, even after taking account of differences in other factors likely to affect mortality.[48,49] Most of the studies quoted here were based on data from the late 1970s, when mortality was higher and resources for neonatal care less widespread.

More recent evidence is less clear. As there are fewer deaths, and as differences between the availability of resources become less pronounced, it becomes more likely that any statistical associations that do exist are masked by chance variation. In a replication[56] of the Norwegian study of access to care at the time of birth, the relationship between mortality and access to care was less strong for babies of different birthweights born between 1979 and 1981 than it had been for those born between 1967 and 1973.

A study in the West Midlands also showed that the inverse association between numbers of paediatricians and neonatal mortality was more marked in the earlier years of the study.[143] This study also illustrated the effect of including outcomes and resources beyond the hospital of birth, that is, where newborn babies are referred between hospitals. When this factor was taken into account, the apparent relationship between paediatric staffing and neonatal mortality almost disappeared.[102]

In a survey of 186 UK neonatal units during 1998 and 1999, the researchers found risk adjusted mortality to be unrelated to either patient volume or staffing levels. However, increasing workload was directly related to higher mortality, although this was not statistically significant at conventional levels.[147] Workload was measured as occupancy as a percentage of maximum capacity, and also as the ratio of nurses to babies.

It is important to take into account not only the quantity of resources but how they are used. Several studies have attempted to adjust outcomes in terms of both mortality and morbidity to take account of predisposing factors, and then to assess the relationship between unexplained differences in outcome and aspects of care provision. With the purpose of such audit of practice in mind, several groups have developed risk scoring methods for admitted babies.[10,128,144] (See also Chapter 2, referring to research on effects of organisation on outcomes of neonatal intensive care.)

The growing evidence from randomised controlled trials of particular aspects of perinatal care makes it clear that the choice of method of care can make a significant difference to mortality and morbidity.[29] In some cases this may mean that more resources are required to improve outcomes, but this is not necessarily the case. For example, giving inexpensive antenatal corticosteroids to women who are at high risk of preterm delivery can reduce the incidence of neonatal respiratory distress syndrome

Table 1.23 Maternity, midwifery and nursing staff in England, 1982–2001

	Midwives*		Nurses working in maternity care[†]	
	wte[‡]	Rate[§]	wte[‡]	Rate[§]
1982	20 250	34.3	10 670	18.1
1983	22 070	37.2	9840	16.6
1984	22 570	37.6	9520	15.9
1985	22 810	36.8	9250	14.9
1986	23 030	36.9	9100	14.6
1987	23 300	36.2	8780	13.7
1988	23 310	35.6	8590	13.1
1989	23 170	35.7	8100	12.5
1990	23 980	36.0	7930	11.9
1991	22 830	34.6	8240	12.5
1992	22 800	35.0	8160	12.5
1993	21 530	33.8	8630	13.6
1994	20 740	33.0	8030	12.8
1995	18 292	29.8	8237	13.6
1996	18 548	30.2	8009	13.2
1997	18 310	30.4	7691	12.8
1998	18 479	31.0	7869	13.2
1999	17 856	30.3	8050	13.7
2000	17 640	30.8	8076	14.1
2001	18 011	31.9	7530	13.4
2002	18 097	32.0	7864	13.9
2003	18 428		8385	

	Nurse consultant	Manager	Reg. sick children nurse	Other 1st level	Other 2nd level		
1998		311	328	3848	442	4929	7869
1999		264	330	4064	405	5063	8050
2000		237	375	4185	339	5136	8076
2001	9	232	480	3604	348	4673	7530
2002	18	274	558	3728	367	4946	7864
2003	31	311	611	4060	317	5330	8385

	Nursery nurse	Nursing assistant/ auxillary	Healthcare assistant	Support worker	
1998	244	3007	928	540	4719
1999	253	2998	996	545	4792
2000	263	2914	1074	530	4781
2001	275	2814	1248	543	4880
2002	289	2903	1294	500	4986
2003	300	3065	1410	575	5351

* Qualified midwives or students on NHS payroll, excludes 'Project 2000' students. Excludes agency staff.
[†] Includes registered, enrolled and unqualified, excludes 'Project 2000' students. Excludes agency staff.
[‡] Whole-time equivalent.
[§] Rate per 1000 live births (after 1997 per 1000 maternities).
Source: NHS Executive and Department of Health Non-medical Staff Census.

Table 1.24 Nurses and midwives in neonatal care in hospital and community health services in England

	1984	1989	1993	1994
No., whole time equivalents*				
Nursing staff, excluding midwives				
Qualified[†]	1040	1740	2160	2170
Unqualified	710	360	370	330
Others	na	10	20	20
Total	1750	2110	2650	2520
Midwives, total	770	1100	1580	1650
Rate per 1000 live births				
Nursing staff, excluding midwives	2.91	3.25	4.16	4.01
Midwives	1.28	1.69	2.48	2.62

* NHS hospital and community health services qualified and unqualified nursing and midwifery staff working in neonatal areas, excluding agency staff and excluding 'Project 2000' students.
[†] Includes seniors 1–5.
Source: NHS Executive Department Stats(W)B Quarry House, Leeds.

and thus the cost of neonatal care.[101] In contrast, other types of care, such as neonatal extracorporeal membrane oxygenation (ECMO) for term babies with severe breathing difficulties, have been shown to reduce mortality and morbidity but can increase the cost of neonatal care.[70] Although the cost of care may be higher overall, benefits are also increased. Research alongside the UK ECMO trial[50,134] shows that the cost of additional healthy survival is comparable to other widely adopted life-extending technologies. Such data can help decisions about prioritising the use of resources, which have to take into account both the costs and the likely benefits.

References

1. Ahmad W I U, Sheldon T 1992 'Race' and statistics. In: Ahmad W I U (eds) The politics of 'race' and health. University of Bradford and Ilkley Community College, Bradford
2. Alberman E, Bergsjo P, Cole S et al 1989 International collaborative effort (ICE) on birthweight, plurality and perinatal and infant mortality. Acta Obstetricia et Gynecologica Scandinavica 68: 5–10
3. Alberman E, Blatchley N, Botting B, Schuman J, Dunn A 1997 Medical causes on stillbirth certificates in England and Wales: distribution and results of hierarchical classification tested by the Office for National Statistics. British Journal of Obstetrics and Gynaecology 104: 1043–1049
4. Alberman E, Botting B 1991 Trends in prevalence and survival of very low birthweight infants, England and Wales: 1983–7. Archives of Disease in Childhood 66: 1304–1308
5. Alberman E, Botting B, Blatchley N, Twidell A 1994 A new hierarchical classification of causes of infant deaths in England and Wales. Archives of Disease in Childhood 70: 403–409
6. Australian Institute of Health and Welfare National Perinatal Statistics Unit 2003 Australia's mothers and babies 2000. Perinatal Statistics Series No 12. AIHW National Perinatal Statistics Unit, Sydney, Australia
7. Baird D, Wyper J F B 1941 High stillbirth and neonatal mortalities. Lancet 2: 657–659
8. Bakketeig L S, Hoffman H J, Sternthal P M 1978 Obstetric service and perinatal mortality in Norway. Acta Obstetricia et Gynecologica Scandinavica 77(Suppl): 3–19
9. Balarajan R, Raleigh V S 1990 Variations in perinatal, neonatal, postneonatal and infant mortality in England and Wales by mother's country of birth, 1982–85. In: Britton M (ed) Mortality and geography: a review in the mid-1980s in England and Wales. Series DS no 9. HMSO, London
10. Bard H 1993 Assessing neonatal risk: CRIB versus SNAP. Lancet 342: 449–450
11. Blair P S, Fleming P J, Bensley D 1996 Smoking and the sudden infant death syndrome: results from 1993–95 case-control study for confidential inquiry into stillbirths and deaths in infancy. British Medical Journal 313: 195–198
12. Blondel B, Macfarlane A 2003 Rising multiple maternity rates and medical management of subfertility: better information is needed. European Journal of Public Health 13: 83–86
13. Bone M, Meltzer H 1989 OPCS survey of disability in Great Britain. Report No 3. HMSO, London
14. Bonelli S R, Raab G M 1997 Why are babies getting heavier? Comparison of Scottish births from 1980 to 1992. British Medical Journal 315: 1205
15. Botting B J, Macfarlane A J 1990 Geographic variations in infant mortality in relation to birthweight 1983–85. In: Britton M (ed) Mortality and geography: a review in the mid-1980s in England and Wales. Series DS no 9. HMSO, London
16. Botting B J, Macfarlane A J, Price F V (eds) 1990 Three, four and more: a study of triplet and higher order births. HMSO, London
17. Botting N, Powls A, Cooke R W I, Marlow N 1997 Attention deficit hyperactivity disorders and other psychiatric outcomes in very low birthweight children at age 12 years. Journal of Child Psychology and Psychiatry 38: 931–941
18. Bréart G, Barros H, Wagener Y, Prati S 2003 Characteristics of the childbearing population in Europe. European Journal of Obstetrics, Gynecology and Reproductive Biology 111: S45–S52
19. British Association of Perinatal Medicine 1989 Referrals for neonatal medical care in the United Kingdom over one year. British Medical Journal 298: 169–172
20. British Association of Perinatal Medicine 1992 Categories of babies requiring neonatal care. British Paediatric Association, London
21. British Association of Perinatal Medicine and Neonatal Nurses Association 1995 Standards for hospitals providing intensive care. BAPM, London
22. British Paediatric Association and British Association for Perinatal Paediatrics 1985 Categories of babies requiring neonatal care. Archives of Disease in Childhood 60: 599–600
23. British Paediatric Association/Royal College of Obstetricians and Gynaecologists Liaison Committee 1978 Recommendations for the improvement of infant care during the perinatal period in the UK. In: Second report from the Social Services Committee, Session 1979–80 HC 663 Vol 2. HMSO, London, pp 256–284
24. Buitendijk S, Zeitlin J, Cuttini M, Langhoff-Roos J, Bottu J 2003 Indicators of fetal and infant health outcomes. European Journal of Obstetrics, Gynecology and Reproductive Biology 111: S66–S77

25. Catterson J 1996 Special care baby units study, 11th report 1995. Public Health Resource Unit, Oxford

26. Charlton J, Wallace M, White I 1994 Long-term illness: results from the 1991 census. Population Trends 75: 18–25

27. Chase H C 1973 A study of risks, medical care and infant mortality. American Journal of Public Health 63(Suppl)

28. Clinical Standards Advisory Group 1993 Neonatal intensive care: access and availability of specialist services HMSO, London

29. Cochrane Library 1997 Issue 1 1997 Update Software, Oxford

30. Cole S K, Hartford R B, Bergsjo P, McCarthy B 1989 International Collaborative Effort (ICE) on birthweight, plurality, perinatal and infant mortality III: A method of grouping underlying causes of infant death to aid international comparisons. Acta Obstetrica Scandinavica 68: 113–117

31. Cole S K, Hey E N, Thomson A M 1986 Classifying perinatal death: an obstetric approach. British Journal of Obstetrics and Gynaecology 93: 1204–1212

32. Coleman D, Salt J (eds) 1996 Ethnicity in the 1991 census, vol 1. Demographic characteristics of ethnic minority populations. HMSO, London

33. Collingwood Bakeo A 2004 Trends in live births by mother in country of birth in England and Wales 1983–2001. Health Statistics Quarterly 23: 25–33

34. Colver A F, Robinson A 1989 Establishing a register of children with special needs. Archives of Disease in Childhood 64: 1200–1203

35. Confidential Enquiry into Stillbirths and Deaths in Infancy 1995 Report, 1 January–31 December 1993. Department of Health, London

36. Confidential Enquiry into Stillbirths and Deaths in Infancy 1996 Third Annual Report, 1 January–31 December 1994. Department of Health, London

37. Confidential Enquiry into Stillbirths and Deaths in Infancy 1997 Fourth Annual Report, 1 January–31 December 1995. Maternal and Child Health Research Consortium, London

38. Craig J 1997 Population review: (9) Summary of issues. Population Trends 88: 5–12

39. Dattani N, Rowan S 2002 Causes of neonatal deaths and stillbirths: a new hierarchical classification in ICD 10. Health Statistics Quarterly 15: 16–22

40. Dean J H, Sullivan E A 2003 Assisted conception in Australia and New Zealand, 2000 and 2001. Assisted conception series no 7. AIHW National Perinatal Statistics Unit, Sydney, Australia

41. Department of Health 1989a An introduction to the Children Act. HMSO, London

42. Department of Health 1989b Perinatal and neonatal mortality. Government reply to the first report from the Social Services Committee, Session 1988–89. Cmd 741. HMSO, London

43. Department of Health 1990 Confidential enquiry into stillbirths and deaths in infancy. Report of a Working Group set up by the Chief Medical Officer. Department of Health, London

44. Department of Health 2003 Report of the DH expert working group on neonatal intensive care services. Available on line at: www.gov.uk/nsf/neonatal.htm

45. Department of Health 2004 NHS maternity statistics, England: 2002–03. Bulletin 2004/10. Department of Health, London

46. Drever F, Whitehead M 1997 Inequalities in health. Series DS No 15. The Stationery Office, London

47. Dunn A, Macfarlane A J 1996 Recent trends in the incidence of multiple births and associated mortality in England and Wales. Archives of Disease in Childhood 75: F10–F19

48. Eksmyr R 1985a Early neonatal deaths in geographically defined populations with different organisation of medical care. Acta Paediatrica Scandinavica 74: 848–854

49. Eksmyr R V 1985b Geographically defined populations with different organisation of medical care. Comparison of perinatal risks. Acta Paediatrica Scandinavica 74: 855–860

50. Elbourne D, Field D, Mugford M 2002 Extracorporeal membrane oxygenation for severe respiratory failure in newborn infants (Cochrane Review). In: The Cochrane Library, Issue 1. Oxford: Update Software

51. Enkin M, Chalmers I 1980 Inquiries into perinatal deaths at area health authority level: a status report winter 1979/80. Community Medicine 2: 219–224

52. Ens-Dokkum M, Johnson A, Schreuder A M et al 1994 Comparison of mortality and rates of cerebral palsy in two populations of very low birthweight infants. Archives of Disease in Childhood 70: F96–F100

53. Evans J R, Wormald R P 1993 Epidemiological functions of BD8 certification. Eye 7: 172–179

54. Evans J, Rooney C, Ashwood F, Dalton N, Wormald R 1996 Blindness and partial sight in England and Wales: April 1990–March 1991. Health Trends 28: 5–12

55. Fleming P J, Blair P S, Bacon C et al 1996 Environment of infants during sleep and risk of the sudden infant death syndrome: results of 1993–95 case-control study for confidential enquiry into stillbirths and deaths in infancy. British Medical Journal 313: 191–195

56. Forbes J F, Larssen K, Bakketeig L S 1987 Access to intensive neonatal care for low birthweight infants: a population study in Norway. Paediatric and Perinatal Epidemiology 1: 33–42

57. General Register Office 2003 Civil registration: delivering vital change. Office for National Statistics, London

58. General Register Office 2004 Proposals to modernise civil registration presented to Parliament. Press release. Office for National Statistics, London

59. Gourbin C, Masuy-Stroobant G 1995 Registration of vital data: are live births and stillbirths comparable all over Europe? Bulletin of the World Health Organization 73: 449–460

60. Graafmans W C, Richardus J H, Borsboom G J J M et al 2002 Birthweight and perinatal mortality and seven western European countries. Epidemiology 13: 569–574

61. Graafmans W C, Richardus J-H, Macfarlane A et al 2001 Comparability of published perinatal mortality rates in Western Europe: the quantitative impact of differences in gestational age and birthweight criteria. British Journal of Obstetrics and Gynaecology 108: 1237–1245

62. Graham E, Boyle P 2003 Low fertility in Scotland: a wider perspective. In: Scotland's population 2002 – the Registrar General's annual review of demographic trends. General Register Office, Edinburgh

63. Hall A, McLeod A, Counsell C, Thomson L, Mutch L 1995 School attainment, cognitive ability and motor function in a total Scottish very-low-birthweight population at eight years: a controlled study. Developmental Medicine and Child Neurology 37: 1037–1050

64. Hartford R B 1990 Definitions, standards, data quality and comparability. Paper given at the International Symposium on perinatal and infant mortality, Bethesda, Maryland, USA, 30 April–2 May

65. Hey E N, Lloyd D J, Wigglesworth J S 1986 Classifying perinatal death: fetal and neonatal factors. British Journal of Obstetrics and Gynaecology 93: 1213–1223

66. Hollowell J 1997 The General Practice Research Database: quality of morbidity data. Population Trends 87: 36–40

67. Horam J 1997 Reply to written question from Audrey Wise. Hansard, 20 March col 811. The Stationery Office, London

68. House of Commons Health Committee 1996 Public expenditure on health and personal social services. HC 698. The Stationery Office, London

69. House of Commons Social Services Committee 1988 Perinatal, neonatal and infant mortality. HC 54. HMSO, London

70. Howard S, Mugford M, Normand C et al 1996 A cost effectiveness analysis of neonatal ECMO using existing evidence. International Journal of Technology Assessment in Health Care 12: 80–92

71. Human Fertilisation and Embryology Authority 1994 Third Annual Report. HFEA, London

72. Human Fertilisation and Embryology Authority 2004 Code of practice, 6th ed. HFEA, London

73. Hutchinson T 1995 The classification of disability. Archives of Disease in Childhood 73: 91–99

74. Information and Statistics Division 1987 Birthweight statistics 1980–84. Information and Statistics Division, Edinburgh

75. Information and Statistics Division 1997 Births in Scotland 1976–1995. Information and Statistics Division, Edinburgh

76. Information and Statistics Division 1998 Small babies in Scotland. Information and Statistics Division, Edinburgh

77. Information and Statistics Division 2003 Operative vaginal delivery in Scotland: a 20 year overview with a chapter on multiple pregnancy in Scotland. Information and Statistics Division, Edinburgh

78. Interim Licensing Authority for Human In Vitro Fertilisation and Embryology 1990 Fifth report. Interim Licensing Authority, London

79. Johnson M A, King R 1989 A regional register of early childhood impairments: a discussion paper. Community Medicine 11: 352–363

80. Kempley S T, Diffley F S, Ruiz G, Lowe D, Evans B G, Gamsu H R 1995 Birth weight and special educational need: effects of an increase in the survival of very low birthweight infants in London. Journal of Epidemiology and Community Health 49: 33–37

81. Kenney N, Macfarlane A 1999 Identifying problems with data collection at a local level: survey of NHS maternity units in England. British Medical Journal 319: 619–622

82. Levene M I, Wild J, Steer P 1992 Higher multiple births and the modern management of infertility in Britain. British Journal of Obstetrics and Gynaecology 99: 607–613

83. Logan S, Spencer N, Blackburn C 1996 Smoking is part of a causal chain (letter). British Medical Journal 313: 1332–1333

84. Lumley J 1997 How important is social class a factor in preterm birth? Commentary. Lancet 49: 1040–1041

85. McCormick A, Fleming D, Charlton J 1995 Morbidity statistics from general practice. Fourth national study 1991–92. Series MB5 no 3. HMSO, London

86. Macfarlane A J 1994 Sources of data. In: Maresh M (ed) Audit in obstetrics and gynaecology. Blackwell, Oxford, pp 18–49

87. Macfarlane A J 1996a Sudden infant death syndrome: more attention should have been paid to socioeconomic factors (letter). British Medical Journal 313: 1332

88. Macfarlane A J 1996b Inégalités en santé des enfants en Europe: une perspective épidémiologique. In: Santé et mortalité des enfants en Europe. Proceedings of the Chaire Quêtelet, 13–15 September 1994. Academia-Bruylant, Louvain-la-Neuve

89. Macfarlane A J, Cole S, Johnson A, Botting B 1988 Epidemiology of birth before 28 weeks of gestation. British Medical Bulletin 44: 861–893

90. Macfarlane A J, Mugford M 2000 Birth counts: statistics of pregnancy and childbirth. Vol 1, Text, 2nd edn. The Stationery Office, London

91. Macfarlane A J, Mugford M, Henderson J, Furtado A, Stevens J, Dunn A 2000 Birth counts: statistics of pregnancy and childbirth. Vol 2, Tables, 2nd edn. The Stationery Office, London

92. Macfarlane A J, Prager K 1990 What is happening to postneonatal mortality? Paper given at International Symposium on perinatal and infant mortality, Bethesda, Maryland, USA 30 April–2 May

93. Macfarlane A, Gissler M, Bolumar F, Rasmussen S 2003 The availability of perinatal health indicators in Europe. European Journal of Obstetrics, Gynecology and Reproductive Biology 111: S15–S32

94. Macfarlane A, Hockley C, Johnson A, McCandlish R, McNiece R 2002 Can the General Practice Research Database be used to monitor the health of babies and their mothers? Health Statistics Quarterly 13: 5–15

95. Macfarlane A, Stafford M, Moser K 2004 Social inequalities. In: Office for National Statistics (ed) The health of children and young people. Office for National Statistics, London

96. Maher J, Macfarlane A 2004 Trends in live births and birthweight by social class and mother's age, 1976–2000. Health Statistics Quarterly 23: 34–43

97. Masuy-Stroobant G 1996 Santé et mortalité infantile en Europe. Victoires d'hier et enjeux de demain. In: Masuy-Stroobant G, Gourbin C, Buekens P (eds) Santé et mortalité des enfants en Europe. Inégalités sociales d'hier et d'aujourd'hui, Chaire Quetelet 1994. Academia-Bruylant, Louvain-la-Neuve

98. Middle C, Johnson A, Alderdice F, Petty T, Macfarlane A J 1996 Birthweight and health and development at the age of 7 years. Child Care, Health and Development 22 1: 55–72

99. MRC Working Party on children conceived by in-vitro fertilisation 1990 Births in Great Britain resulting from assisted conception. British Medical Journal 300: 1229–1233

100. Mugford M 1990 The costs of a multiple birth. In: Botting B J, Macfarlane A J, Price F V (eds) Three four and more: a study of triplet and higher order births. HMSO, London, pp 205–217

101. Mugford M, Piercy J, Chalmers I 1991 Reducing the costs of neonatal care by effective prevention of respiratory distress syndrome. Archives of Disease in Childhood 66: 757–764

102. Mugford M, Szczepura A, Lodwick A, Stilwell J 1988 Factors affecting the outcome of maternity care II. Neonatal outcomes and resources beyond the hospital of birth. Journal of Epidemiology and Community Health 42: 170–175

103. Mutch L M, Ashurst A, Macfarlane A J 1992 Birthweight and hospital admission before the age of two years. Archives of Disease in Childhood 67: 900–904

104. National Assembly for Wales 2004 Maternity statistics: method of delivery 1995–2003. Statistical release 40/2004. National Assembly for Wales, Cardiff

105. National Audit Office Maternity Services 1990 Report by the Controller and Auditor General. HMSO, London

106. National Health Service Executive 1996 Collection of data from general practice: overview. NHS Executive, Leeds

107. National Health Service, Department of Health 1990a Working Paper 11. Framework for information systems: overview. HMSO, London

108. National Health Service, Department of Health 1990b Framework for information systems: the next steps. HMSO, London

109. Office for National Statistics (published annually) Mortality statistics: childhood, infant and perinatal, England and Wales, Series DH3 Office for National Statistics. London

110. Office for National Statistics 1999 Registration: Modernising a vital service: births, marriages and deaths in the 21st century. Office for National Statistics, London

111. Office for National Statistics 2002 Civil registration: vital change: births, marriages and deaths in the 21st century. Cmd 5355. The Stationery Office, London

112. Office for National Statistics 2003a Ethnic group statistics: a guide to the collection and collection of ethnicity data. The Stationery Office, London

113. Office for National Statistics 2003b Infant and perinatal mortality 2002: health areas, England and Wales. Health Statistics Quarterly 19; 70–73

114. Office for National Statistics 2004a Living in Britain. Results from the 2002 General Household Survey. The Stationery Office, London

115. Office for National Statistics 2004b The health of children and young people. Office for National Statistics, London. Available on line at: http://www.statistics.gov.uk/children

116. Office of Population Censuses and Surveys 1978 Occupational mortality 1970–72 England and Wales, decennial supplement. Series DS no 1. HMSO, London

117. Office of Population Censuses and Surveys 1988 Occupational mortality 1979–80, 1982–83 England and Wales, childhood supplement. Series DS no 8. HMSO, London

118. Office of Population Censuses and Surveys and General Register Office, Scotland 1989 Publication of draft census order. Census newsletter No 11. OPCS, London

119. Office of Population Censuses and Surveys, General Register Office, Scotland 1993 1991 Census. Limiting long-term illness: Great Britain. HMSO, London

120. Ornstein M, Ohlsson A, Edmonds J, Asztalos E 1991 Neonatal follow-up of very low birthweight/extremely low birthweight infants to school age: a critical over-view. Acta Paediatrica Scandinavica 80: 741–748

121. Oxford Register of Early Childhood Impairments 2003 Annual report 2002. National Perinatal Epidemiology Unit, Oxford

122. Paneth N, Kiely J L, Wallenstein S, Marcus M, Pakter J, Susser M 1982 Newborn intensive care and neonatal mortality in low birthweight infants. New England Journal of Medicine 307: 149–155

123. Parmanum J, Field D, Rennie J, Steer P on behalf of the British Association of Perinatal Medicine 2000 National census of availability of neonatal intensive care. British Medical Journal 321: 727–729

124. Parsons L, Macfarlane A J, Golding J 1993 Pregnancy, birth and maternity care In: Ahmad WIU (ed) Race and health in contemporary Britain. Open University Press, Buckingham, pp 51–75

125. Petrou S, Mugford M 2000 Predicting the cost of neonatal care. In: Hansen T and McIntosh N, eds. Current topics in Neonatology IV. London, Harcourt Health Sciences, pp 149–174

126. Pharaoh P O D, Macfarlane A J 1982 Recent trends in postneonatal mortality. In: Studies in sudden infant deaths. Studies on Medical and Population Subjects No 45. HMSO, London

127. Pharaoh P O D, Stevenson C J, Cooke R W, Stevenson R C 1994 Clinical and subclinical deficits at 8 years in a geographically defined cohort of low birth-weight infants. Archives of Disease in Childhood 70: 264–270

128. Pollack M M, Ruttiman U E, Getson P R 1988 The pediatric risk of mortality (PRISM) score. Critical Care Medicine 16: 1110–1116

129. Power C 1994 National trends in birth weight: implications for future adult disease. British Medical Journal 308: 1270–1271

130. Prescott-Clarke P, Primatesta P 1997 Health survey for England, 1995. Vol I, Findings. The Stationery Office, London

131. Prescott-Clarke P, Primatesta P (eds) 1998 Health survey for England. The health of young people, '95–97. Vol 1, Findings. The Stationery Office: London

132. Raleigh V S, Balarajan R 1995 The health of infants and children among ethnic minorities. In: Botting B (ed) The health of our children. Series DS no 11. HMSO, London

133. Rennie J M 1996 Perinatal management at the lower margin of viability. Archives of Disease in Childhood 74: F214–F218

134. Roberts T and the ECMO Economics Working Group on behalf of the ECMO Trial Steering Group 1998 Economic evaluation alongside the UK collaborative ECMO trial. British Medical Journal 317: 911–914

135. Rose D, O'Reilly K 1998 The ESRC review of government social classifications. Office for National Statistics and the Economic and Social Research Council, London

136. Rowan S 2003 Implications of changes in the United Kingdom social and occupational classifications in 2001 on infant mortality statistics. Health Statistics Quarterly 17: 33–40

137. Royal College of Obstetricians and Gynaecologists 2000 National evidence-based guidelines. The management on infertility in tertiary care. RCOG, London

138. Royal College of Physicians 1988 Medical care of the newborn in England and Wales. Royal College of Physicians, London

139. Saigal S, Feeny D, Rosenbaum P, Furlong W, Burrows E, Stoskopf B 1996 Self-perceived health status and health-related quality of life of extremely low-birth-weight infants at adolescence. Journal of the American Medical Association 276: 453–459

140. Shaw C 2002-based national projections for the United Kingdom and constituent countries. Population Trends 2004; 115: 6–15

141. Sinclair J C, Torrance G W, Boyle M H, Horwood S P, Saigal S, Sackett D L 1981 Evaluation of neonatal intensive care programs. New England Journal of Medicine 305: 489–494

142. Steering Group on Health Services Information 1985 Supplement to first and fourth reports to the Secretary of State. HMSO, London

143. Stilwell J, Szczepura A, Mugford M 1988 Factors affecting the outcome of maternity care I. Relationship between staffing and perinatal deaths at the hospital of birth. Journal of Epidemiology and Community Health 42: 157–169

144. Tarnow-Mordi W O, Ogston S, Wilkinson A R et al 1990 Predicting death from initial disease severity in very low birthweight infants: a method for comparing the performance of neonatal units. British Medical Journal 300: 1611–1614

145. Tatham J 1907 Letter to the Registrar General. In: 68th report of the Registrar General of Births Marriages and Deaths in England and Wales 1905. Cmd 3279. HMSO, London

146. Tyson J E, Broyles R S 1996 Progress in assessing the long-term outcome of extremely low-birth-weight infants (editorial). Journal of the American Medical Association 276: 492–493

147. UK Neonatal Staffing Study Group 2002 Patient volume, staffing and workload in relation to risk-adjusted outcomes in a random stratified sample of UK neonatal intensive care units: a prospective evaluation. Lancet 359: 99–107

148. UNICEF 2004 Infant mortality country data. Updated May 2004. Available on line at: http://www.childinfo.org/ (accessed June 3 2004)

149. Victorian Infant Collaborative Study Group 1995 Neurosensory outcome at 5 years and extremely low birthweight. Archives of Disease in Childhood 73: F143–F146

150. Wariyar U K, Richmond S 1989 Morbidity and preterm delivery: importance of 100% follow-up (letter). Lancet 1: 387–388

151. Wigglesworth J S 1980 Monitoring perinatal mortality – a pathophysiological approach. Lancet 2: 684–686

152. Woodruffe C, Abra A 1991 A special conditions register. Archives of Disease in Childhood 66: 927–930

153. World Health Organization 1977 Manual of the International statistical classification of diseases, injuries and causes of death, 9th revision. WHO, Geneva

154. World Health Organization 1980 International classification of impairments, disabilities and handicaps. WHO, Geneva

155. World Health Organization 1992 International statistical classification of diseases and related health problems, 10th revision. WHO, Geneva

156. World Health Organization 2001 International Classification of Functioning, Disability and Health. WHO, Geneva

157. Zeitlin J, Wildman K, Bréart G et al 2003 Selecting an indicator set for monitoring and evaluating perinatal health in Europe: criteria, methods and results from the PERISTAT project. European Journal of Obstetrics, Gynecology and Reproductive Biology 111: S5–S14

CHAPTER 2

Organisation and evaluation of perinatal care

Neil Marlow

The great majority of babies require no specialist neonatal care after birth. Only a small proportion of births occur where there is predicted or unpredicted need for neonatal intervention and immediate or continuing neonatal care.

Advances in the understanding and delivery of neonatal care, together with important developments in obstetric practice and fetal medicine, have combined to produce steady improvement in gestation- or birthweight-specific death rates (Chapter 1) and in reducing morbidity in survivors (Chapter 3). However neonatal intensive care remains a low-volume, high-cost area of practice, one which is becoming increasingly technical. Care now involves sicker and more immature babies as good perinatal care, the use of antenatal steroids and postnatal surfactant improve the outlook for the more mature preterm baby.

Pressures on the health services of developed countries make clinical areas such as the neonatal unit difficult to staff with trained and competent personnel. Most health communities have taken steps to concentrate resources into specialist centres while developing excellence in resuscitation practice and short term stabilisation in other units to provide the most effective compromise. Such services require careful clinical governance to ensure their efficacy and effectiveness.

In this chapter the organisation and structure of neonatal services will be discussed in context of current evidence and a system of clinical governance will be outlined. Within the UK this is a time of reflection and reconfiguration of neonatal services. Thus the current and planned scenarios will be discussed.

Organisation of neonatal services

Neonatal Intensive Care (NIC) services have developed differently in different health systems, to some extent depending on the proximity of the children's and maternity services. In some health systems NIC is located within a Children's Hospital, which has advantages for paediatric specialist care but places the postpartum mother at a disadvantage and all children have to be transferred in for care. In other systems NIC has developed alongside maternity services. The degree of centralisation of services has also been driven by external factors, either by financial control, as in the USA, or by population distribution, as in Australia. Many health systems mix these structures according to local geography. The relationship between organisational structures and outcome is highly contentious and not easily amenable to study (see below).

Pressures of health economics have driven most services to concentrate intensive care services in fewer expert centres and to review the structure and function of the other neonatal units (which care for the majority of babies) in terms of their effectiveness at providing a highly expert resuscitation service. One example of this is the development of highly centralised neonatal intensive care in Australia. There are relatively few large population centres in many areas of the continent and as a result the whole country is served by 22 Level 3 (intensive care) nurseries and a highly developed antenatal and neonatal retrieval service has developed. This contrasts with the 171 neonatal units providing intensive care for extremely preterm babies in the UK as part of the EPICure study in 1995. Many European countries have developed neonatal intensive care within Children's Hospitals, and thus all babies needing care are transferred in from often smaller and less expert clinics. Slowly this model is being replaced with a centralised system where expertise can be concentrated in fewer, better-resourced maternity/neonatal centres.

Several classifications or categorisations of neonatal units have been used. Most use the concept that a three-tier service is most efficient, the least intensive category of unit only providing short-term stabilisation prior to transfer, the most intensive carrying out a full range of intensive care activity, and the intermediate tier providing varying degrees of postnatal support depending on local resources.

Such organisation can only function if units work together in a clinical network and if the health commissioners work to ensure that each network has the capacity and resources to provide for the predicted demand. Such a working pattern has major potential advantages in terms of high-throughput NIC units (NICUs) for the maintenance of clinical skills, high occupancy for intensive care cots permitting efficient use of resources and ability to staff the high-intensity areas.

Within the UK, intensive care resources for adults and for children have been incorporated into 'managed clinical networks'. Services are planned based on a geographical population with different ranges of facilities at each centre. The key issue in the success of these services is the central management of resources across several otherwise independent health service units ('Trusts'). The argument for centralisation of paediatric intensive care has been well made[39] and improved early care, triage and outcome can be anticipated through the underpinning of the network with a strong educational and training base. Despite these structures it remains important in any health system that children access the appropriate level of care.[30]

Although arguments similar to these have been accepted in most health-care systems across the world, and within other intensive care disciplines, in the UK NIC has not developed such firm structures and what are in effect intermediate-sized units have provided and continue to provide a range of intensive care facilities. There is a paucity of information as to the relative performance of individual units at different levels and national or regional studies have not provided clarification.[13,44] There has been a reluctance to move to a system that would seem to restrict access to expert care for babies born outside the intensive care centre (as many currently have inadequate intensive care capacity), as this increases the number of transfers, disrupts family life for parents or their relationship with local clinicians, and there is concern over potentially deskilling staff in local units. These concerns are enhanced by the lack of evidence for benefit available to drive change, despite the overwhelming logic of developing network-based care.

Overall the demand for neonatal intensive care has risen (see p. 43). In parallel, the UK has seen increasing public demand for transparency in the delivery of health care, in the wake of several high-profile government reports, and there is a drive to

ensure that care is provided by professionals whose expertise is appropriate to the clinical situation. Recent changes in law are leading a reduction in the traditionally overlong working hours for doctors and there is currently a paucity of nursing and specialist doctors to provide specialist neonatal care. These drivers are fuelling the major proposals for reorganisation in the UK that are currently being considered.

Current provision of neonatal care in the UK

In a survey established by the British Association of Perinatal Medicine in 1994, separate facilities for the care of newborns were identified in 251 maternity units.[32] Of these 211 contributed to a survey of provision. Using then current definitions of levels of care, nearly 60% of units identified three or fewer staffed intensive care cots and no unit had more than 12 intensive care cots. The survey estimated that there were around 800 IC cots, 1100 HD cots and 2200 SC cots across the UK in 1993. Part of the reason for the continuing development of intensive care in this large number of centres was the recommendation of a minimum of 500 intensive care days to maintain skills,[5] considered by many to be much too low to sustain real expertise across the range of staff in a smaller unit, and the 'market forces' approach to the organisation of care, which in turn encouraged hospitals to provide high cost services such as these.

In 1997 the UK Neonatal Staffing Study team obtained responses from all units regarding their care profile in 1995/6.[45] Of the 246 units then active, 76% provided intensive care and 24% special care and stabilisation for transfer to a unit that provided intensive care. The reported activity is shown in Table 2.1. From this it is evident that the median number of intensive care

Table 2.1 Reported unit profiles for UK neonatal units providing neonatal intensive care in 1996

Activity indicators	Median	Range	Response rate (%)
Total no. of admissions	318	48–1020	100
Total no. of cots	18	4–55	100
Total cots for intensive care	4	0*–16	100
No. infants offered respiratory support			
Endotracheal ventilation only	52	10–269	18
All support (includes CPAP)	66	12–310	76
Respiratory support in days			
Endotracheal ventilation only	281	19–2688	18
All support (includes CPAP)	451	13–3324	62
No. VLBW infants admitted	40	2–227	95

*Four units reported and verified that they carried out sustained intensive care despite having no designated intensive care cots.
Source: Tucker J, Tarnow-Mordi W, Gould C, Parry G, Marlow N 1999 UK neonatal intensive care services in 1996. On behalf of the UK Neonatal Staffing Study Collaborative Group. Archives of Disease in Childhood. Fetal and Neonatal Edition 80: F233–F234.

cots in the UK had risen, but that many units had low activity and throughput. The extent to which the changes in market orientation that were a feature of the National Health Service (NHS) at that time contributed to these changes is unknown but there was a lack of concerted planning for regional care at the time in most areas of the country.

That specific surveys are required to estimate the national picture poses a problem. Within the current proposals for reconfiguration of neonatal services, the UK Department of Health (DH) has recognised that collection and collation of data are of critical importance to the allocation of resources and investment is currently under way to address this. To help with this issue, the British Association of Perinatal Medicine (BAPM) has provided definitions of care categories (see below) that can be used to define activity levels across the country[6] and has recommended a dataset for use in units that provide neonatal care[4] so that harmonisation of definitions and reporting strategies can help to resolve these issues (see 'Audit' below).

Classification of neonatal care in the UK

One difficulty in determining the size of the workforce needed to staff a neonatal service is the range of activity and case mix of different services. It is therefore helpful to define a range of categories of care, which may allow the planning of resources.

The DH has supported the classification of neonatal services into three types, which generally follows the model in place in several countries[33] (Table 2.2).

Within any type of neonatal unit, care for an individual baby can be classified by the level of clinical dependency, which should provide a measure of the resources needed to look after that baby. The definitions of these 'categories of care' will differ between health systems. Within the UK there are several contenders, some of which have been developed using formal studies,[34,48] whereas the nationally recommended categories[6] have been developed by professional consensus. Formal studies are under way to evaluate the validity of each. The BAPM and the DH presently recommend that inpatient neonatal care is divided into four categories (Table 2.3).

These levels of care have been tightly defined (Table 2.4) to ensure that there is consistency in definition across the country. The previous definitions, published in 1996,[5] did leave some room for inconsistency. However they themselves were useful in determining the range of cot requirements. The number of intensive care days needed for a particular population will vary depending primarily on the number of low-birthweight babies cared for, as they use up the majority of resources. This in turn is dependent upon the social and environmental mix of the population: within the regions of the south-east of the UK, which includes inner city and rural districts, the cot requirement in each region varied between 1.0 and 1.9 intensive care cots per 1000 births, estimated at the recommended 70% occupancy.

To these categories of care, which are dependency-based, many hospitals have introduced an intermediate category between the neonatal unit and routine postnatal ward, the so-called 'transitional care'. This is primarily aimed at nursing babies who still need 'special care' (e.g. gavage feeding) in an area with their mother and supporting the mother while she provides the majority of care. In different hospitals this is developed and organised differently and there are no formal definitions to facilitate comparisons. Transitional care has an important effect on neonatal unit activity in that special care activity is transferred out to a ward staffed primarily by midwives and thus is not counted in terms of service activity. This may free up staff to increase more intensive activity in the neonatal unit. In addition, it becomes a local responsibility to determine staffing levels for this area and to ensure that adequate support for mothers is available.

Table 2.2 UK categorisation of neonatal units

- Level 1 units provide special care but do not aim to provide any continuing high dependency or intensive care. This term includes units with or without resident medical staff.
- Level 2 units provide high dependency care and some short-term intensive care as agreed within the network. These units will need separate staffing but their resident medical staff may be shared with other paediatric areas.
- Level 3 units provide the whole range of neonatal medical care but not necessarily all specialist services such as cardiology, extracorporeal membrane oxygenation or surgery. These units will have their own separate medical staffing.

Source: British Association of Perinatal Medicine 2001 Standards for hospitals providing intensive and high dependency care. BAPM, London.

Table 2.3 UK definitions of dependency levels

- **Intensive care**. These babies have the most complex problems. This category has been defined by the level of nursing and medical support needed. Babies in this category need one-to-one care by a nurse with a neonatal qualification and the possibility of acute deterioration is such that a competent doctor should be available constantly.
- **High dependency**. These babies have significant dependency and often complex needs but the support required is such that less nursing time is required (one nurse to two babies).
- **Special care**. This description is used for care provided for all other babies who could not reasonably be expected to be looked after at home by their mother.
- **Normal care**. Where the care is provided primarily by the baby's mother (with support from midwives) but where there is no medical indication for the baby to be in hospital.

Source: British Association of Perinatal Medicine 2001 Standards for hospitals providing intensive and high dependency care. BAPM, London.

Table 2.4 An example of a checklist to record daily categories of dependency of care

Level of Care definitions (BAPM 2001)
Please read the list in order and record the level of care that first describes the baby's condition

The following statements refer to the 24 h up to midday and apply to care delivered any time in the past 24 h period (** and in the 24 h following withdrawal)		Intensive care (level 1)	High-dependency care (level 2)	Special care (SC)
** Has the baby been intubated?	Yes →	✓		
Is the baby 4 days old or less AND has received CPAP? (A)	Yes →	✓		
** Is the baby <1000 g AND has received CPAP? (B)	Yes →	✓		
Was the baby <28 w 6 d gestation at birth AND <48 hours old?	Yes →	✓		
Is the baby due for surgery in the next 24 h?	Yes →	✓		
Has the baby had surgery in the past 48 h?	Yes →	✓		
Has the baby had: Exchange transfusion? Peritoneal dialysis? ** Infusion of inotrope, vasodilator or prostaglandin?	Yes →	✓		
Is the baby receiving terminal care or has the baby died?	Yes →	✓		
Has the baby received CPAP (excludes A/B)?	Yes →		✓	
Is the baby <1000 g (excludes A)?	Yes →		✓	
On TPN?	Yes →		✓	
Having convulsions?	Yes →		✓	
In oxygen AND <1500 g?	Yes →		✓	
On treatment for drug withdrawal?	Yes →		✓	
Has the baby had: Indwelling arterial line? Partial exchange transfusion? Tracheostomy care (unless supervised by parent)?	Yes →		✓	
Frequent stimulation for severe apnoea?	Yes →		✓	
Other care in the neonatal unit not covered above?	Yes →			✓

Staffing

Having defined the categories of care, the staffing requirements for a neonatal service can be established. Medical staffing is dependent upon the degree of cross-covering required to run the service and this is in turn dependent on the intensity of care that can effectively be offered.

- For level 1 (or special care) units it is envisaged that no intensive care will take place. Staff will be available in the hospital to attend infrequent emergencies and this cover will be provided as part of an acute paediatric service.
- For level 2 ('high-dependency') units continuous bedside medical support will be required, either by a trainee – senior house officer (SHO) or resident – or by an advanced neonatal nurse practitioner (ANNP), while middle and consultant tier cover is provided as part of the adjacent acute paediatric service.
- For level 3 intensive care services dedicated specialist staff are required with two resident tiers (SHO/ANNP and registrar/consultant) with a supervising consultant available to provide continuity.

In the UK Neonatal Staffing Study, 25% of units providing intensive care in 1996 did not have a consultant with more than 50% time dedicated to neonatal care.[45] This is clearly unsatisfactory given the huge advances in neonatal care over the past 30 years. As workforce directives reduce the working hours available for all staff, the grade and competency of staff providing first-call care must be examined carefully if we are to continue

Table 2.5 Calculation of number of nurses required to staff a neonatal unit (nursing establishment)
(No. of intensive care cots × 1) + (No. of high dependency cots/2) + (No. of special care cots/4) = No. of clinical practice nurses per shift + 1 shift coordinator = Total number of nurses per shift × 5.75 = Establishment in wte

HD = high dependency; IC = intensive care; SC = special care.

to provide high-quality care. In many units this is now contributed to by advanced nurse practitioners, who form an intermediate tier of carers outside the clinical practice nursing teams, because of their expertise and wider responsibilities.

Nurse staffing relates to dependency levels and generally is calculated from an estimated establishment for a particular cot number and configuration. Daily monitoring will confirm the adequacy of this. Nurse staffing is the largest part of the unit budget and thus most vulnerable: in 1996, 79% of units had a ratio of nursing provision to that recommended of less than 1.0 (median 0.84; interquartile range 0.73–0.98) indicating significant underestablishment for the activity that was being carried out, despite taking conservative staffing levels as the norm (1:2 intensive care and 1:4 for all others).[45] This wide variation in the adequacy of local resources to carry out neonatal care is reflected in the findings of other studies[35] and has provided the impetus for the changes proposed in 2003 (see below).

Nurse establishment is usually calculated on the basis that a baby receiving intensive care requires 1:1 nursing, one receiving high dependency requires 1 nurse:2 babies and one requiring special care 1:4 nursing (Table 2.5). In practice, within present resources this is not often achievable and as a minimum 1:2 nursing for intensive care is substituted. These are then minimal requirements and do not include managerial and other specialist roles (advanced practice, family care, practice development), which have evolved within the nursing sphere but require extra resources.

Transfers

Any configuration of neonatal services within a region is dependent upon the availability of both cots and effective patient transport. Transfer of the pregnant woman or her infant is commonplace but within the current service the destination of any transfer cannot be determined with any certainty, as beds are often unavailable at the natural referral centre. Part of the drive to reconfigure services is to remove this lottery.

The relative merits of in-utero and postnatal transfer for care require careful consideration. Studies comparing the results of each all have an inherent bias, as the need for intensive care or ventilation cannot be predicted before birth and postnatal transfer will generally be for ongoing ventilator care, although some babies may die before transfer can be effected. Thus a true study on unselected populations is almost impossible to achieve. None the less, within well centralised systems with often independent transport services, as in the USA[3] and Australia,[38] a more consistent service

can be achieved. Even within the UK there is evidence that babies are not placed at significant risk during a well-planned transfer.[26,27] There are, however, data that suggest that mortality is increased when transfer is requested but unavailable[2] and babies moved between tertiary centres unable to cope with peaks of demand have poorer outcomes.[35] The key to effective transfer is the establishment of proper capacity within a clinical network, to allow planned flows of referrals that can be discussed in early pregnancy with all pregnant women.

One study has evaluated the pattern of 'inappropriate transfers' as a measure of the adequacy of capacity in tertiary units.[35] Inappropriate transfers were defined as those out of a perinatal centre. Over 3 months in 1999, 264 in-utero transfers and 45 postnatal transfers were recorded in 37 such units. Rates of transfer in each region varied from 0.20 to 5.44 per 1000 live births. The risks and outcomes of these transfers were studied in 242 cases.[2] Of in utero transfers, only 61% delivered at the accepting hospital, 12% were moved to a third hospital following delayed delivery and 29% were returned to deliver at their referring hospital. One mother delivered during the journey and nine within 1 hour of arrival. Transfer of mothers and their babies should be a planned process with defined levels of referral and, as far as possible, guaranteed capacity at the natural referral centres.

In-utero transfers

It is important to distinguish the urgency with which mothers are referred for specialist care, usually because of impending prematurity, from more elective transfers for expert assessment of fetal malformation or growth restriction. There must be close liaison between both obstetric and the receiving neonatal team before any decision to move a woman is undertaken. The presence of vaginal bleeding, pre-eclampsia or labour and the obstetric history of the woman must be carefully weighed against the need for transfer. Where urgent transfer can be effected safely this must be the best mode of transfer, as both mother and baby will be cared for in the same centre and separation avoided and the baby will be exposed to minimised postnatal risk. However there is a chance of delivery during the journey and a risk of other unforeseen problems. Not infrequently, women are moved before birth because of a risk of early delivery and do not deliver. This delay in delivery may even then lead to a further transfer.

Postnatal transfers

In most areas of the UK, postnatal transfer services have developed on an ad-hoc basis. Nursing and medical competencies for carrying out safe transfers have not been defined nationally and the mobilisation of a team to carry out a transfer usually results in a senior doctor and nurse being absent from their base units, where they have been integral to care. Postnatal transfer is frequently unavoidable, because there has been no time to arrange in-utero transfer, or because of clinical contraindications, and thus provides an unpredictable drain on staffing in tertiary units. In the past, such transfers were deemed 'flying squads', where a rapid emergency response team travelled rapidly to support the local team in early care scenarios. With improvements in care and expertise at local hospitals it should be possible to effect elective transfers at a time that is clinically appropriate for the baby, although emergencies arising in units without on-site specialist neonatal staff must be planned for and robust arrangements put in place to ensure that these risks are minimised.

The physical environment for transfer, the development of which was as ad hoc as the development of the transport teams, has recently come under scrutiny. Following the Transport of Neonates by Ambulance (TINA) report of 1995[43] and evolving European Union legislation, health and safety issues relating to neonatal transfers and the indemnification arrangements for staff have been clarified and improved. The increasing use of air transport has similarly resulted in the UK Civil Aviation Authority producing and testing to specification equipment for use in such circumstances.

Proposed UK model of neonatal intensive care

The pattern of provision of neonatal care in the UK is currently undergoing change under the influence of the factors listed above. These changes will facilitate a coordinated approach to the provision of care for sick newborn infants and the pattern of care will thus be more predictable than the current situation.

Women and their families expect that pregnancy, delivery and postnatal care will be delivered in one local centre as close as possible to the family home, and this perception is encouraged by health care managers within the NHS hierarchy. Problems arise when problems with either the woman or the fetus develop that cannot be managed by the local services. At present further management is dictated by the availability of obstetric and neonatal resources at the referral centre. Central to the planning of care is the need to pre-warn parents as to what the likely arrangements will be if problems develop, so that families are not faced suddenly by the prospect of their care being transferred to another centre, often at some distance, without warning.

With the introduction of the 'managed clinical network' it should be possible to map out a plan for most eventualities so that a pregnant woman understands the management plan for the anticipated normal pregnancy, what is to happen if a fetal anomaly is discovered, what will happen if very preterm delivery seems likely and what care arrangements are to be made if there is an unanticipated need for neonatal intensive care. Despite the often quoted maxim that pregnant women do not wish to travel for their care, all the evidence points to the woman willingly allowing transfer of care if it is in her baby's best interests.

The detail of the proposals for managed neonatal networks in England is set out in the report of the Department of Health External Working Group[33] and annexes (Fig. 2.1). In essence, neonatal care will be commissioned by the NHS on a regional basis following local discussion to determine the extent of the 'region'. The network should comprise a minimum of 15 000 births per year. A managed network will encompass at least one level 3 NICU with other units of varying expertise. If there is more than one level 3 unit then one will assume a lead role and responsibility for education/practice development and for transport. The

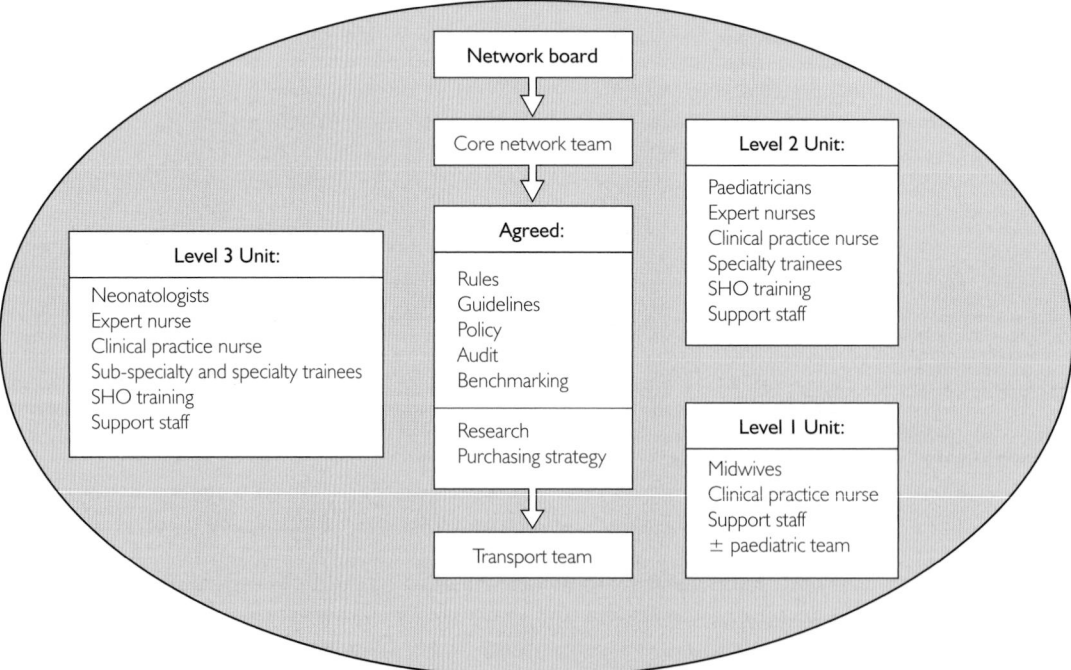

Fig. 2.1 The proposed structure of a managed clinical neonatal network – each network will have different numbers of units at each level and the population covered by each network will be more than 15 000 births. Capacity will be determined by the need to accommodate more than 95% of intensive care activity within the network and for units to function at 70% occupancy. (Expert nurses: specialist nurses in advanced neonatal practice, practice development, family care, transport, etc.; subspecialty trainees: trainee neonatologists; specialty trainees: trainee paediatricians.)

core network team (manager, clinician and nurse) will have responsibility for overseeing the development of the network in terms of policy, guidelines and clinical governance. Within any network there will be agreed rules as to which levels of care are delivered and which babies are cared for in each unit. The planned capacity for the various levels of care in a network will be such that over 95% of activity will be retained within the network.

Relationship of organisation to outcomes

Given the stress placed on the structure to support neonatal care, one would anticipate that structural elements are clearly related to outcomes. Within the UK system this is far from clear. Several attempts to investigate this relationship have been undertaken. The relationship between organisational issues and mortality is the easiest to undertake but, given the decrease in mortality over the past 10 years, death is a relatively rare event and thus small differences in mortality are more difficult to demonstrate. Furthermore, large tertiary units treat a different range of babies from those managed in local services and tend to be overcrowded, with high occupancy rates and more likelihood of understaffing. Smaller units may also transfer out sick babies soon after birth, the mortality being attributed to the receiving unit. The complexity of these issues makes drawing conclusions from comparisons extremely difficult.

Studies of regional outcomes for mixed hospital groups have shown inconsistent effects. In the late 1980s mortality was higher for babies cared for in smaller units in the Trent region of the UK compared to babies cared for in larger units.[16] This longitudinal study was reanalysed in the early 1990s following a NHS reorganisation and then demonstrated no difference in mortality by size of unit.[15] This was ascribed to enhancements in neonatal provision at local hospitals but clearly the relationship is more complex than that.

Scoring systems for neonatal illness provide one way of correcting for case mix, adjustment being made for the illness severity measure when comparing outcomes. The use of such measures is established in paediatric and adult critical care services. In neonatal care the two most frequently used scoring systems are the Score for Neonatal Acute Physiology (SNAP[40]) (plus SNAP-II and SNAPPE-II[41]) and Clinical Risk Index for Babies (CRIB[23]) (and recently CRIB II[37]), although there are others. Care should be taken when using these measures, as they are not an attempt to predict outcome for an individual but a score describing the clinical condition so that some adjustment between outcomes in a population can be made.[22,29] These scores require regular review and updating as techniques and interventions change. For example, a tertiary unit that uses delivery room surfactant or early high-frequency oscillatory ventilation may appear to have low severity of illness scores (based on oxygenation) but similar mortality to other units because the gestational age of the babies cared for is lower. Hence the score itself may partly reflect the care given as much as the underlying characteristics of the baby, i.e. it may itself be an outcome variable for perinatal care.[29]

CRIB originally included data from worst base deficit and highest and lowest inspired oxygen concentrations over the first 12 hours, making it particularly sensitive to changes in early interventions. In contrast, CRIB II uses temperature on admission and maximal base deficit over the first hour as the clinical variables,

The maximum (worst) score for birthweight and gestation is 15, which is obtained for a 22 week male infant in less than 501g birthweight

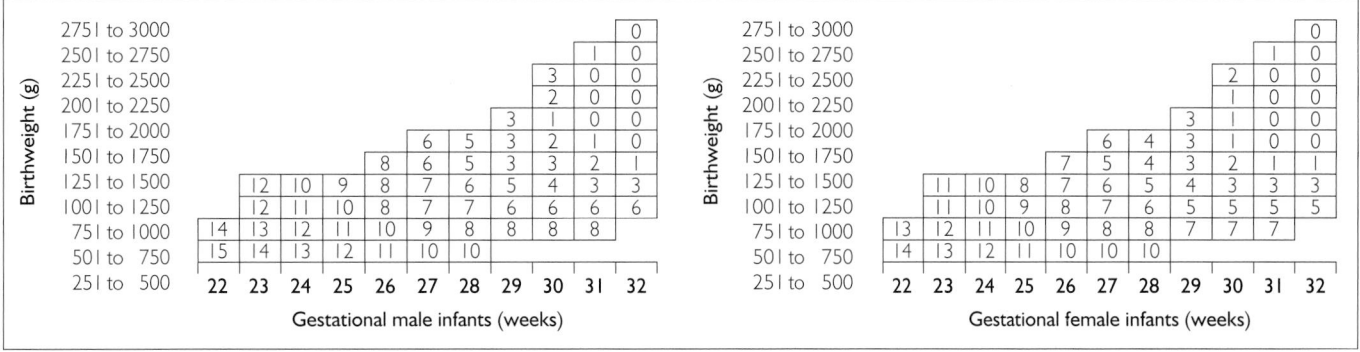

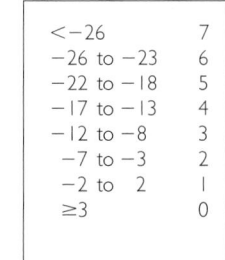

Fig. 2.2 Calculation matrix for the Clinical Risk Index for Babies (CRIB-II). (With permission from Parry G, Tucker J, Tarnow-Mordi W 2003 CRIB II: an update of the clinical risk index for babies score. Lancet 361: 1789–1791.)

which, together with sex, gestational age and birthweight, provide the basis for the score (Fig. 2.2). Using this recently validated model with a high degree of predictive value for mortality (area under the receiver operating characteristics (ROC) curve: 0.92), analysis of the data collected as part of the UK Neonatal Staffing Study, CRIB-II-adjusted mortality did not differ between large and small units in the UK (odds ratio (OR) 1.06; 95% confidence interval (CI) 0.70–1.60).[44]

Nonetheless, corrections for disease severity can provide useful information concerning the relative performance of neonatal services to facilitate the identification of areas for investigation and throw up intriguing questions when applied to cross-national[18,24] or national comparisons.[36] For example, risk-adjusted mortality appears to be significantly higher in Scotland than in England or Australia.[24] The question is raised as to whether this relates to organisation of care, being highly centralised in Australia and devolved in the UK. Caution is required when interpreting these studies as the ethnic, social and demographic profiles of any population may account for more of the variance in outcomes than the perinatal services and the obvious difference, i.e. organisation, may be confounded by population differences. This is emphasised by a further comparison of outcome for babies born at less than 28 weeks of gestation or less than 1000 g birthweight between the Trent region of the UK and Denmark.[18] Births in this group were more prevalent in Trent and, despite a higher use of antenatal steroid, babies had higher CRIB scores, received more mechanical ventilation and were more likely to die compared to the Danish population.

The UK Neonatal Staffing Study randomly selected 54 of 186 units in the UK to study the relationship between throughput, consultant and nurse staffing and outcome as mortality, cerebral damage as detected by ultrasound and nosocomial infection.[44] Data from 13 334 babies were used. High-volume NICUs, treating the sickest babies, had the highest crude mortality but this difference disappeared when risk adjustment was made. However there were important findings relating the risk of dying to the staffing levels on the shift during which a baby was admitted. Babies admitted to a unit working at full capacity were 50% more likely to die than babies admitted to a unit working at 50% capacity (Fig. 2.3). The BAPM has commented that this may be attributable to a number of factors including inadequate staffing and change of case mix as workload increases. It is crucial that staffing levels and expertise are appropriate to the dependency of the babies.

In a further epidemiological study from the USA, there appeared to be an optimal relationship between neonatologist staffing and mortality.[21] The numbers of neonatologists and numbers of cots (expressed in quintiles from the distribution) were related to national statistics of neonatal deaths (in the first 28 days). On average there were 6.2 neonatologists, 33.7 intensive care cots and 17.7 high-dependency cots per 10 000 births. There was lower neonatal mortality where there were 4.8 neonatologists per 10 000 births compared to 2.7 per 10 000 births (OR for death 0.93; 95% CI: 0.88–0.99) but increasing the number above this level did not result in further improvements. Furthermore the availability of neonatal cots was not related to mortality risk and the need for cots (as expressed by the number of babies with birthweight below 1501 g) did not

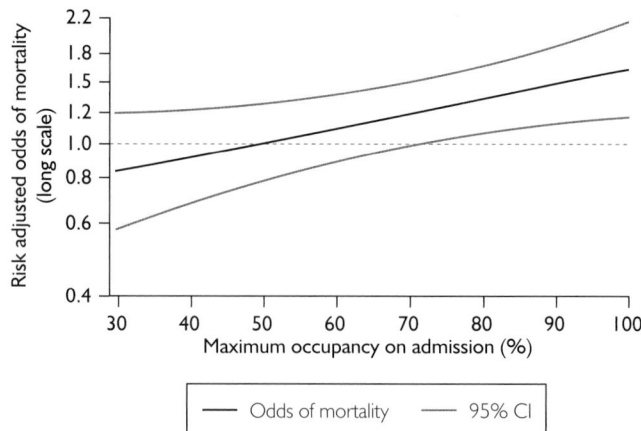

Fig. 2.3 Relationship of risk adjusted odds of mortality and unit occupancy on day of admission. (With permission from Parry G, Tucker J, Tarnow-Mordi W 2003 CRIB II: an update of the clinical risk index for babies score. Lancet 361: 1789–1791.)

relate to cot availability. This must be placed in contrast to the calculated requirement of 10–19 intensive care cots per 10 000 UK births (see above).

The relationship between organisational factors and simple outcome measures is therefore far from clear. In the UK proposals for managed clinical networks it would be incumbent on each network to ascertain and monitor the availability of cots and access for its residents to the service when required, and to benchmark these services against other national data.

Philosophy of care and survival

Mortality at low gestations has improved over the past 20 years such that the great majority of babies born at 26 weeks of gestation or more now survive. Attitudes to babies born at lower gestational ages will therefore have a profound effect on the rates of survival and thus confound comparisons of different services. The extent of the differences brought about by extremes of practice was explored by Lorenz and colleagues,[28] who demonstrated marked differences in survival and prevalence of cerebral palsy in two studies with widely differing approaches to outcome (see Chapter 3, p. 64). In the UK in 1995 the EPICure study group collected information on all livebirths and survivors born at 25 weeks of gestation or less.[11,49] These survival figures are considerably lower than those from, for example, Rhode Island[14] (Fig. 2.4), even allowing for different population sizes. Without a detailed study of the approach to care at these extremely low gestations the reasons for these differences cannot be explored.

Furthermore, it is critical that the denominator data are carefully collected and reported. At extremely low gestations, for example, some babies will fail to respond to resuscitation, whatever the philosophy of care, and the correct denominator is probably the number of fetuses alive at the onset of labour.

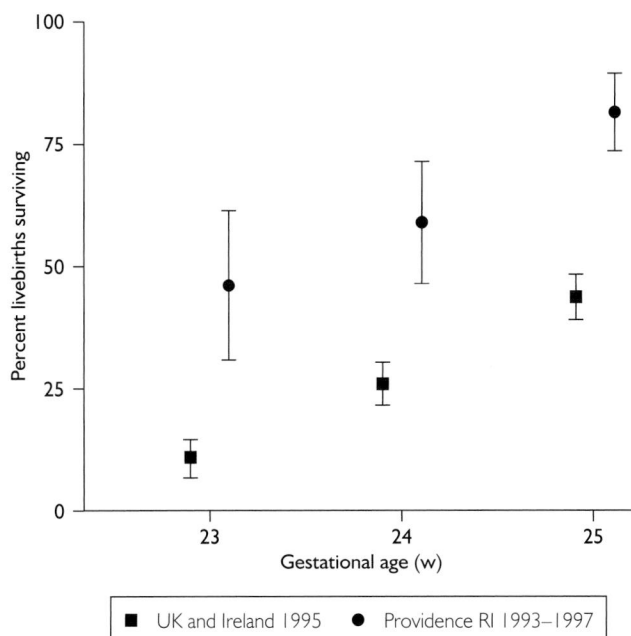

Fig. 2.4 Comparison of mortality following livebirth at 23–25 weeks of gestation in two studies.

Service evaluation

Clinical governance is the framework in which we as professionals assure that our care is accountable to our patients and to our host institutions. There are a range of schemes for this and this section will focus on those applicable to perinatal care under the following headings:

- the clinical governance philosophy;
- clinical audit;
- standards, guidelines and perinatal audit tools;
- benchmarking and evidence based care.

The clinical governance philosophy

Medical audit was promoted in 1989 by the UK government as a means of protecting the interests of patients in the then new health market, but audit and quality assurance were not new developments, particularly in non-medical areas within the NHS. It rapidly became clear that the performance of many services was based upon access and availability, or the personal style directed by consultants, rather than evidence-based practice. The concept was widened to 'clinical audit' involving multidisciplinary teams and achieved some limited success. Neonatal and perinatal care provide prime examples of areas of truly multidisciplinary practice where collaboration must occur across doctors, nurses, midwives and other professional groups for a successful service to evolve.

Clinical audit failed to reach the hearts and minds of clinicians and gradually evolved into the wider concept of clinical

governance in the late 1990s. The most widely used definition of clinical governance is 'a framework through which NHS organisations are accountable for continually improving the quality of their services and safeguarding high standards of care by creating an environment in which excellence in clinical care will flourish'.[42] Thus it is designed to introduce a systematic approach to the delivery of NHS care, in which there is corporate accountability for clinical quality and performance. The essential features of the process are not disputed:

- patient-centred care;
- widely available information about the quality of care;
- reduction in the variations of process, outcomes and access to care;
- reduction in risks and hazards to patients;
- widespread dissemination and adoption of good and research based practice.

The key to the delivery of this process is reliable and comprehensive information about the service, something that has been sadly lacking in the NHS. Indeed, the reforms of the mid-1990s may be likened to an experiment without defined outcome measures.[31] The more recent reforms have increased reporting centrally and hence central control over services,[25] which has exacerbated the difficulties of running acute services with unpredictable workloads. The formation of managed clinical networks (see above) should help to resolve some of these issues.

The clinical audit process

Audit is defined as 'an evaluation (esp. by formal, systematic review) of the effectiveness of the management, working practices, and procedures of a company or other professional body' (Oxford English Dictionary).

The key to the audit process is the setting of standards and the appraisal of the clinical service against those standards. This is often assembled into what is commonly called the audit cycle (Fig. 2.5). Standards may be set nationally, regionally or locally and may evaluate three major aspects of care:

- the structure of the service;
- the process of care;
- the outcome of care or the result of clinical intervention.

The structure of care

This is concerned with the quantity and type of resources and how they are used, for example the number and experience of medical nursing or paramedical staff or the availability of cots. These data are relatively simple to collect and are usually accurate. Standards are produced nationally (see below)[6] and these data can be powerful in the process of bidding for resources. For example, the shortage of neonatal nursing staff was emphasised in the UK Neonatal Staffing Study (Fig. 2.6), which is an example of a national audit of the structure of care.[45]

Audit of structure by itself can only demonstrate potential areas where services may be inadequate and does not form a measure of quality of care until it is matched with patient based

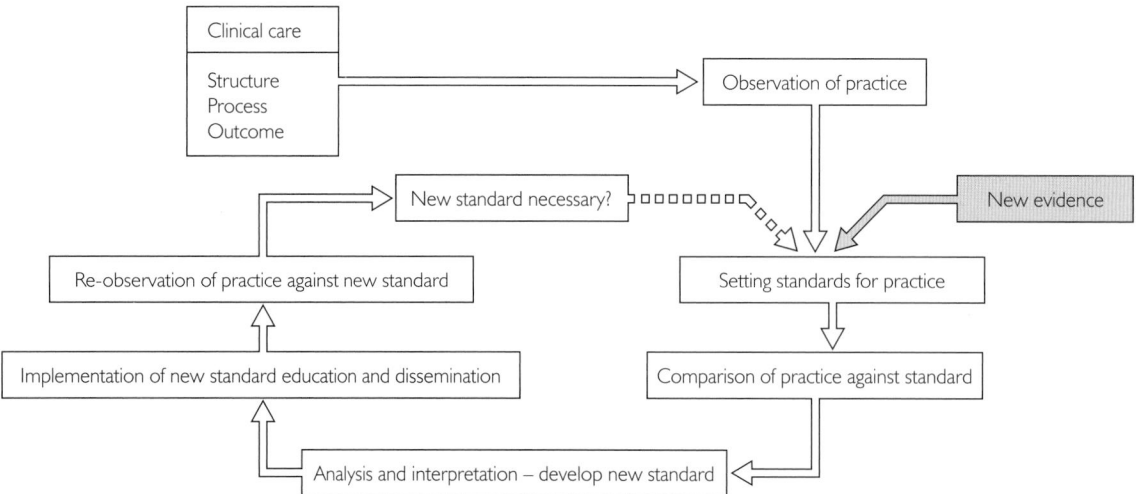

Fig. 2.5 The process of clinical audit. The cycle commences with the observation of practice and the integration of new evidence into the setting of standards and is completed when a new standard is re-evaluated to confirm the effectiveness changes in clinical care.

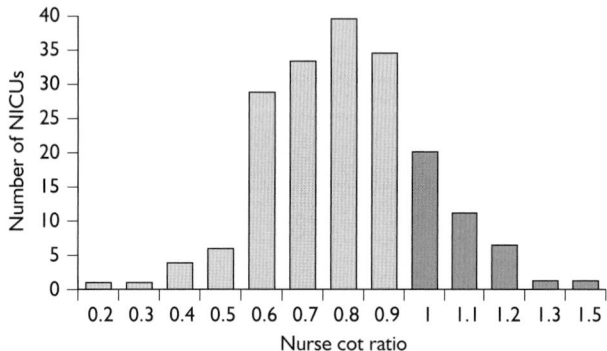

Fig. 2.6 Appropriateness of nursing establishments in all UK neonatal units (actual/recommended numbers of nurses from published standards – lighter bars denote units with lower establishments than required). (With permission from Tucker J, Tarnow-Mordi W, Gould C, Parry G, Marlow N 1999 UK neonatal intensive care services in 1996. On behalf of the UK Neonatal Staffing Study Collaborative Group. Archives of Disease in Childhood. Fetal and Neonatal Edition 80: F233–F234.)

information when it merges with the two other areas of audit. Structural deficiencies may provide one explanation for poor results found during process or outcome audit.

The process of care

This may be considered in three ways:

- the way patients progress through the system – examples would be admission and discharge procedures, the recording of clinical data in the patient notes and the recording of communication with parents;
- the way particular resources are used – examples would be attendance at delivery by appropriate levels of staff, occupancy and case mix studies, the use of transitional care facilities;

- the way particular conditions are managed – examples here relate to particular admission criteria or to diagnostic groups or to interventions; in this area evidence-based practice may be introduced into care via the development of guidelines.

An example of a nationally based audit of the care process is provided by the joint venture between the RCPCH, the BAPM and Royal College of Ophthalmologists. Standards for screening and treatment of retinopathy of prematurity were issued in 1995. Subsequently a nationwide education programme was undertaken followed by an audit of cases registered as requiring treatment. Further audit of the adequacy of cover will be repeated in due course.

The outcome of care

The outcome of care (or the result of interventions) provides the final arbiter of success for a service and includes important mortality and morbidity measures. Outcomes may relate to the child (occurrence of death, complications of treatment or longer-term neurological development), the parent (satisfaction, breastfeeding rates) or the staff (recruitment, retention, levels of competency or ability to perform procedures).

Mortality rates are well defined (Table 2.6) and widely available, and many are collated nationally (Table 2.7, Fig. 2.7) or regionally. Although these data offer the opportunity to set local targets and review local performance, extreme care should be exercised in their interpretation as they may be subject to random variation due to small numbers and systematic variation in methodology of collection. Correction for illness severity has been recommended as a way of avoiding some of these problems (see above).

Choosing outcome measure for specific audit is fraught with difficulty. Outcomes need to be specific, measurable and relevant. For example, babies who receive pulmonary vasodilators to reverse pulmonary hypertension may be audited on their response to treatment, in terms of oxygenation over the period of use and immediately afterwards, but to use duration of ventilation or

Table 2.6 Perinatal definitions

- **Livebirth**. Baby with signs of life observed after complete expulsion from the mother irrespective of the duration of the pregnancy (signs of life include breathing, heart beat, cord pulsation or voluntary movement)
- **Stillbirth (or late fetal death)**. Fetal death prior to complete delivery of a baby born after the 24th week of pregnancy (168 days after the first day of the last menstrual period (LMP)
- **Abortion**. A conceptus born without signs of life before the end of the 24th week of pregnancy (<168 days after LMP)
- **Birthweight**. The first weight of a fetus or newborn baby obtained after birth (preferably within the first hour after birth)
- **Gestational age**. The duration of gestation measured from the first day of the LMP expressed in completed weeks and days (note that gestational age is never rounded up and thus a baby born at 24 weeks and 6 days is usually considered to be of '24 weeks gestational age')
- **Preterm**. Birth at less than 37 weeks of gestation (<259 days after LMP)
- **Term**. From 37 to 42 completed weeks of gestation (259–293 days after LMP)
- **Post-term**. More than 42 weeks (>293 days after LMP)
- **The neonatal period**. The first 28 days after delivery
- **Lethal congenital malformation**. Death primarily due to congenital malformation

Table 2.7 Total births and deaths for England and Wales (2001) by causes of stillbirth, neonatal and infant deaths

ONS cause	Births		Deaths			All infant deaths
	Livebirths	Stillbirths	Early neonatal	Neonatal	Postneonatal	
All causes	594 634	3159	1582	2107	1065	3172
Congenital anomalies	–	446	380	530	361	891
Antepartum infections	–	25	28	66	18	84
Immaturity-related conditions	–	–	975	1216	156	1372
Asphyxia, anoxia or trauma (intrapartum)	–	98	163	199	11	210
External conditions	–	8	4	7	66	73
Infections	–	–	10	23	144	167
Other specific conditions	–	182	9	16	17	33
Asphyxia, anoxia or trauma (antepartum)	–	952	–	–	–	–
Remaining antepartum deaths	–	1383	–	–	–	–
Sudden infant deaths	–	–	1	24	188	212
Other conditions	–	65	12	26	104	130

Source: Office of National Statistics (ONS) – available online at: http://www.statistics.gov.uk

longer-term outcomes (e.g. neurodevelopment) would be inappropriate as many other things determine these outcomes. The only way to determine the effect of vasodilators on these outcomes is within a randomised controlled trial where comparison groups are tightly matched.

Services should regularly monitor quality aspects of care and it is recommended that these are published as an annual report. Ideally these data would be collated on a regional or national basis, and there are excellent examples of this (Fig. 2.8). The minimal content of an annual report has been defined[5] and should also include the monitoring of the rates of disability in defined groups of survivors (see Chapter 3 and Fig. 3.4).

The audit cycle

The audit cycle (Fig. 2.5) comprises a series of processes needed to integrate the results of audit into clinical practice. The identification of topics for audit may be defined within the neonatal team in response to an observation that prompts the initiation of the investigation; the topic may be identified by health commissioners (mortality and disability rates) or regionally/nationally. The American Academy of Pediatrics issues regular statements of policy or guidance, which may form the basis for audit. In the UK the medical Royal Colleges have established audit groups and formulate guidance in specialty. Within neonatology both the Royal College of Paediatrics and Child Health (RCPCH; www.rcpch.ac.uk – Clinical Effectiveness) and the Royal College of Obstetricians and Gynaecologists (RCOG; www.rcog.org.uk – Good Practice) produce guidance of relevance to neonatal practice, but globally within the UK there are few national neonatal guidelines.

Despite a huge investment by the NHS, audit has not won the hearts and minds of many doctors. Part of the reason for this is the failure to understand the importance of a scientific base to the collection, analysis and interpretation of audit data, which is as important in the audit process as it is in research. Appropriate support for audit is often not available locally, in terms of either manpower or expertise, but investment in the clinical governance process has improved the situation greatly over the past 5 years. Correctly supported and executed, audit may make an important contribution to the success of a neonatal service.

Much audit is achieved by examining medical case records. Ideally, prospective data collection should be established as variations in recording information may render the audit data set incomplete. Retrospective audit from case notes should recognise its limitations but it remains an important part of the

process. Problems that occur in retrospective and (to a lesser extent) prospective audit data collection are:

- bias due to poor diagnostic coding;
- bias in record retrieval (difficulty in identifying 'cases' particularly if they have died);
- bias relating to sample size;
- reliability of audit data (e.g. variation in recording or definition between patients and errors in filing of investigation results in notes);
- bias due to missing information;
- inadequate capture of 'non-routine' data to be used in audit;
- case mix and comorbidity;
- inability to assess qualitative aspects of care – timeliness, coordination, empathic components and appropriateness.

A good audit design will address these deficiencies in the planning stage and thereby avoid major errors. It will also include and involve staff from outside the immediate neonatal team who are critical to its success. Once the results are available the critical decision is which of the (any) changes in management that flow from the audit are to be effected. The line of action and responsibility for implementation should be carefully addressed. Financial consequences of audit/changes in practice must be identified and early managerial involvement in implementation is clearly crucial to the success of a project. Medical and nursing education and training for staff in support services must include the development of skills in the audit process.

Finally, the audit cycle is a continuous loop: once an audit is complete and the recommendations are implemented further audit should be planned to ensure the success of these changes.

Benchmarking

A 'benchmark' was originally a surveying mark placed to allow repeated measurements using a levelling staff; it is thus a point of reference, a criterion or touchstone (Oxford English

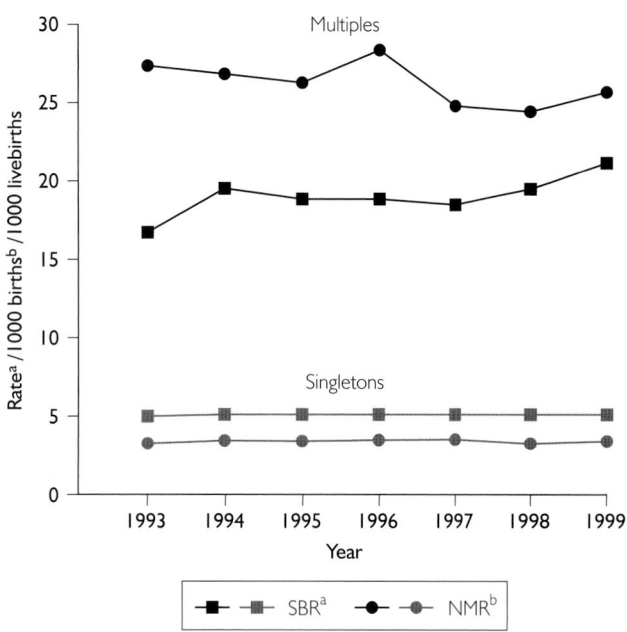

Fig. 2.7 Stillbirth and Neonatal Death rates 1993–1999 for singletons and multiple births: England and Wales (Source: Confidential Enquiry into Stillbirths and Deaths in Infancy. 8th Annual Report. London: Maternal and Child Health Research Consortium; 2001).

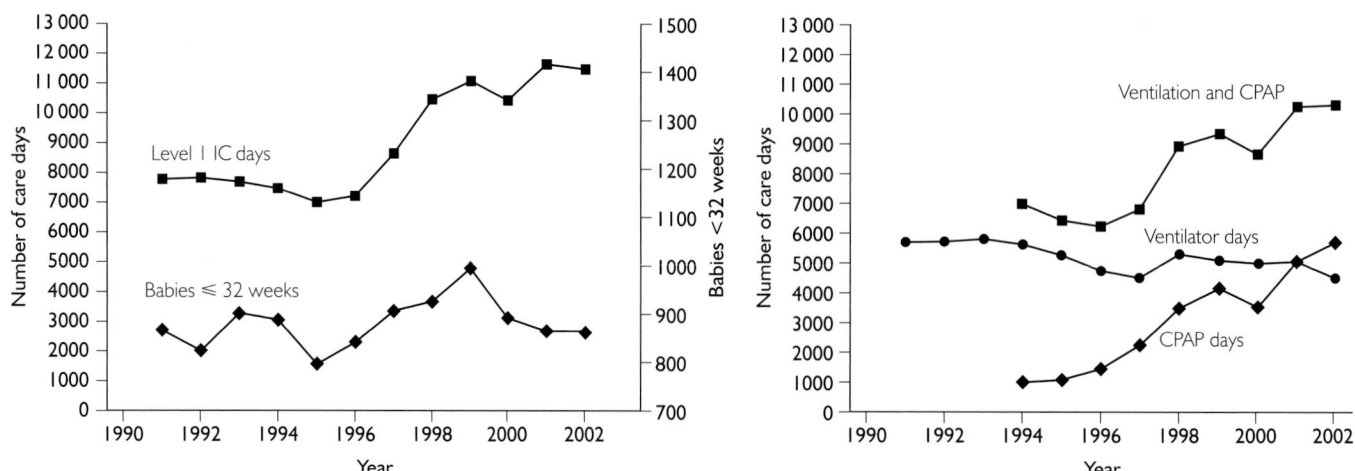

Fig. 2.8 Annual statistics for hospitals contributing to the Trent Neonatal Survey, showing a rise in intensive care activity from 1996, despite consistent numbers of babies born at 32 weeks of gestation or less (left panel), which is due to a rise in the use of continuous positive airway pressure (CPAP) (right panel). Source: Trent Neonatal Survey (with permission).

Dictionary). The process of assessing the structure, process or outcome of a service against an externally derived standards is often termed 'benchmarking', in contrast to audit, which is carried out in response to locally derived standards. In effect they are similar processes carried out to different reference points.

Within the professional neonatal community there are a range of initiatives that are designed to benchmark performance against that of other services, regional/network-based groups (e.g. the Trent Neonatal Survey; the Thames Perinatal Group Accreditation Scheme) or internationally using schemes such as the Vermont Oxford Network (www.vtoxford.org).

Other aspects of clinical governance

Like medical audit, there is a danger that clinical governance will be applied 'top-down' and therefore become irrelevant to many of the staff. Over recent years several hospitals across the UK have encouraged the development of shared governance – a system of encouraging ownership, widening involvement and engagement. With its origins in the USA health community several models have evolved.[7] Although this is often seen as a nursing development 'which seeks to grant nursing staff control over their professional practice and develop and make a genuine contribution to the wider corporate agenda',[20] the principles can and probably should be extended to multidisciplinary teams such as those that work in neonatal care. Retention and recruitment of nursing staff can be materially enhanced by the inclusion of all grades of staff, enhancing acceptance of responsibility for the service, improving communication and respecting time spent in developing the shared governance process. This process demands a fundamental reappraisal of neonatal teams and is not a 'quick-fix' or panacea to aid a failing system.

In a UK health service increasingly driven by elective targets, clinical governance provides a method whereby acute services can ensure that their configuration and resources are not passed by. NHS Trusts have widely accepted a risk-management approach and these need to be stated and addressed or accepted by the corporate structure. Increasingly, neonatal care is being addressed by a range of corporate agenda such as corporate benchmarking, meeting of standards to minimise the risk of litigation and standard pricing. External reviews of service by NHS sponsored bodies, such as the Audit Commission,[1] the Clinical Standards Advisory Group[8,9] and the Department of Health External Review Group[33] have been regularly published over the past 10 years. The effect that these initiatives have on the delivery of neonatal care remains to be seen.

Standards and perinatal audit tools

Standards

Several standards (benchmarks q.v.) have been published against which neonatal services can be appraised in audit of the structure of care. The most important of these in the UK are the *Standards for Hospitals providing Neonatal Intensive and High Dependency Care*. These standards act as a reference point against which resources available may be assessed. The first edition of these standards was published in 1996 and covered staffing, service size and management of neonatal services.[5] Where possible statements were based on published evidence but it was recognised that for many none existed. Detailed recommendations covered the following areas:

- service size;
- medical and nurse staffing;
- support staff;
- equipment;
- audit;
- continuing education within neonatal care.

Following the publication of these standards, it was recognised that intensive care was increasingly directed at the management of a small number of extremely premature infants and particularly sick term infants, for whom increasingly complex care was required. The standards were therefore reviewed, revising in particular the nursing support required for intensive care and the definitions of care categories (intensive, high dependency, special and normal care) and adding a new categorisation of neonatal unit (see above).[6] Whereas the previous standards had been based on pragmatic levels of nursing support, the new standards are in effect aspirational in this area.[33]

Neonatal services are also expected to be evaluated against a range of local professional health organisation standards, such as record-keeping, as are all other hospital-based areas.

Definitions – mortality and morbidity

Conventionally, birthweight is subdivided into low birthweight (LBW: <2501 g), very low birthweight (VLBW: <1501 g) and extremely low birthweight (ELBW: <1001 g). Similar groupings are often used for preterm gestation but there is little agreement as to the definition of very preterm (birth at either <30 weeks or <32 weeks) or extremely preterm (usually birth at ≤25 weeks of gestation). These broad categories are based on risk of death and perinatal complications.

Definition of the causes of perinatal and infant death may help to understand the relationship between specific causes and developments in health care. One such classification is that proposed by Wigglesworth, which has been used to classify deaths over several years as part of the Confidential Enquiry into Stillbirths and Deaths in Infancy (CESDI) (Fig. 2.9). Much of the fall in post-neonatal infant mortality has been due to a reduction in the proportion of deaths ascribed to the sudden infant death syndrome (SIDS) category, initially over the 1980s because of improvements in pathological practice and better diagnosis and then during the 1990s following the observation that prone lying was associated with SIDS,[19,47] alongside intercurrent illness and parental smoking.

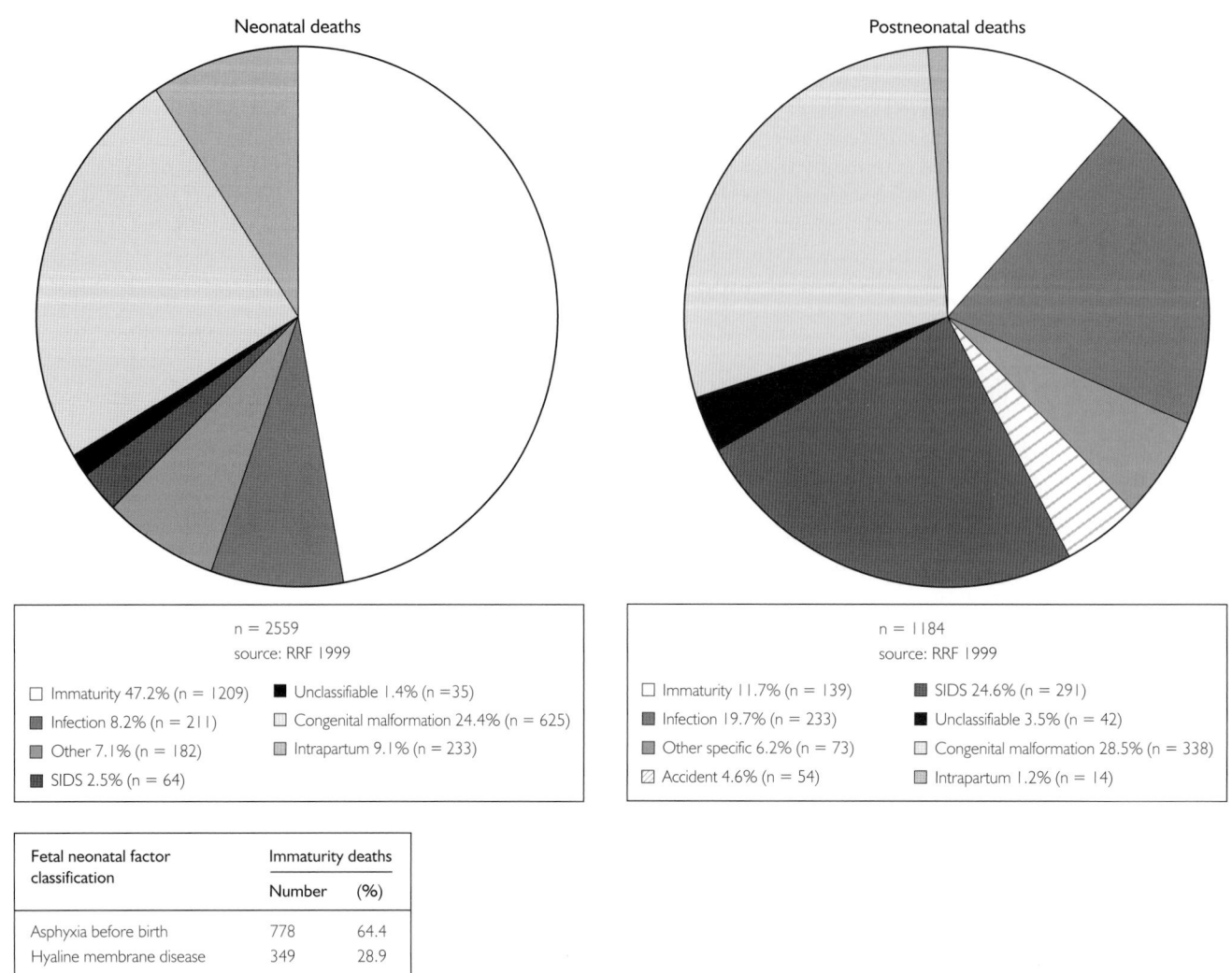

Neonatal deaths

n = 2559
source: RRF 1999

☐ Immaturity 47.2% (n = 1209) ■ Unclassifiable 1.4% (n =35)
■ Infection 8.2% (n = 211) ☐ Congenital malformation 24.4% (n = 625)
■ Other 7.1% (n = 182) ▨ Intrapartum 9.1% (n = 233)
■ SIDS 2.5% (n = 64)

Postneonatal deaths

n = 1184
source: RRF 1999

☐ Immaturity 11.7% (n = 139) ■ SIDS 24.6% (n = 291)
■ Infection 19.7% (n = 233) ■ Unclassifiable 3.5% (n = 42)
■ Other specific 6.2% (n = 73) ☐ Congenital malformation 28.5% (n = 338)
▨ Accident 4.6% (n = 54) ▨ Intrapartum 1.2% (n = 14)

Fetal neonatal factor classification	Immaturity deaths	
	Number	(%)
Asphyxia before birth	778	64.4
Hyaline membrane disease	349	28.9
Intraventricular haemorrhage	39	3.2
Infection	34	2.8
Unclassifiable	9	0.7
Total	1209	100.0

Fig. 2.9 Causes of neonatal and infant deaths in England and Wales using the Wigglesworth classification of deaths (with permission from Confidential Enquiry into Stillbirths and Deaths in Infancy. 8th Annual Report. London: Maternal and Child Health Research Consortium; 2001).

The International Federation of Gynaecology & Obstetrics (FIGO) and the World Health Organization (WHO) have defined datasets to facilitate international comparison of neonatal and perinatal morbidity (Table 2.8). In particular, the definitions and methods of reporting data recommended by FIGO allow correction for major differences in neonatal service provision, presenting the information as totals and then excluding babies with lethal malformations and those of greater than 1000 g birthweight.

Although these classifications are very helpful on an international stage, providing benchmarking for developing health communities, within a highly developed health service mortality and morbidity at borderline gestation and weight have become of equal importance.

Mortality and morbidity rates are critically dependent on the definition of the baseline population and reports of poor outcomes must be clear in their definition for their interpretation and comparison with other reports. For example, a report of outcome for very preterm children will have differing mortality rates if only babies who are admitted for intensive care are considered compared to a report where all liveborn babies are included, as the latter also includes delivery room deaths and the former may include postnatal transfers. It is important to attribute deaths appropriately to the unit or population from which the infant derived and not to the unit to which they were transferred. In the EPICure study livebirth at 20–25 completed weeks of gestation was used and the effect of simply using babies who were admitted for neonatal care is shown in Fig. 2.10.[49] For babies born at or after 26 weeks of gestation rarely die in the delivery room and differences between outcomes based on livebirths or admissions become less important.

Table 2.8 International Federation of Gynecology and Obstetrics (FIGO) recommendations for the international collection of perinatal mortality statistics

Data collection

Collect numbers of births >500 g birthweight, early and late neonatal deaths (<28 days) and identify stillbirths and neonatal deaths with lethal malformations or with birthweight <1000 g

Perinatal statistics

- Lethal malformation rate per 1000 births
- Stillbirth rate (SBR) per 1000 births
- Neonatal mortality rate (NMR) per 1000 livebirths (livebirths dying up to and including 28 days after birth)
- Perinatal mortality rate (PNMR) per 1000 births (stillbirths plus livebirths dying up to and including 7 days after birth)
   Excluding lethal malformations (include all birthweights): SBR; NMR, PNMR
   Excluding lethal malformations and births <1000 g birthweight: SBR; NMR, PNMR
   Excluding births <1000 g birthweight (including lethal malformations): SBR; NMR, PNMR

Table 2.9 WHO international classification of impairments, disabilities and handicaps

- **Impairment**. Any loss or abnormality of psychological, physiological or anatomical structure or function
- **Disability**. Any restriction or lack (resulting from an impairment) of ability to perform an activity in the manner or within the range considered normal for a human being
- **Handicap**. A disadvantage for a given individual, resulting from an impairment or a disability, that limits or prevents the fulfilment of a role that is normal (depending on age, sex and social and cultural factors) for that individual

The definition, use and interpretation of longer-term morbidity data are discussed in Chapter 3. The use of standardised definitions of disability[46] (Tables 3.2 and 3.3 in Chapter 3) enhances the ability to benchmark outcomes in one population against another and are to be encouraged. Current international definitions (Table 2.9) are currently undergoing re-evaluation (see pp. 65–6). Historically these data have been collected in high-risk populations by neonatal teams but ideally this information should be available from routine systems to provide a global picture of impairment using the child health computer system or local disability registers. In such situations it is clear that the majority of impairment and disability in the community occurs in children who were born at or near full term but birthweight- or gestational-age-specific rates of disability increase as birthweight and gestation fall. Attempts to harness parental or non-clinical assessment to improve data collection have not been entirely successful.[17]

Neonatal data recording

Population data

Statutory registration of birth and death provides an opportunity for universal data collection which may be targeted at information gathering or to provide ongoing data for subsequent health care, for instance child health systems. In the UK these have been brought together to provide a comprehensive picture of population variation and trends. Standardisation of data collection is still not achieved across the UK despite initiatives to enhance it. In the smaller population of Scotland the SMR-11 birth data collection form has provided an excellent source of population-based information. The development of the rapid reporting form for perinatal death by the CESDI has facilitated a range of investigations into perinatal death and presently continues as an important source of information (www.cemach.org.uk) (see below).

The year 2003 saw the introduction of a new method for allocating the NHS number at birth, instead of the old system of allocation at registration of the birth up to 6 weeks of age (www.nhsia.nhs.uk/nn4b/pages/overview). This important development will make tracking and tracing of individuals within the health system considerably easier, particularly when babies are transferred between units for complex treatments.

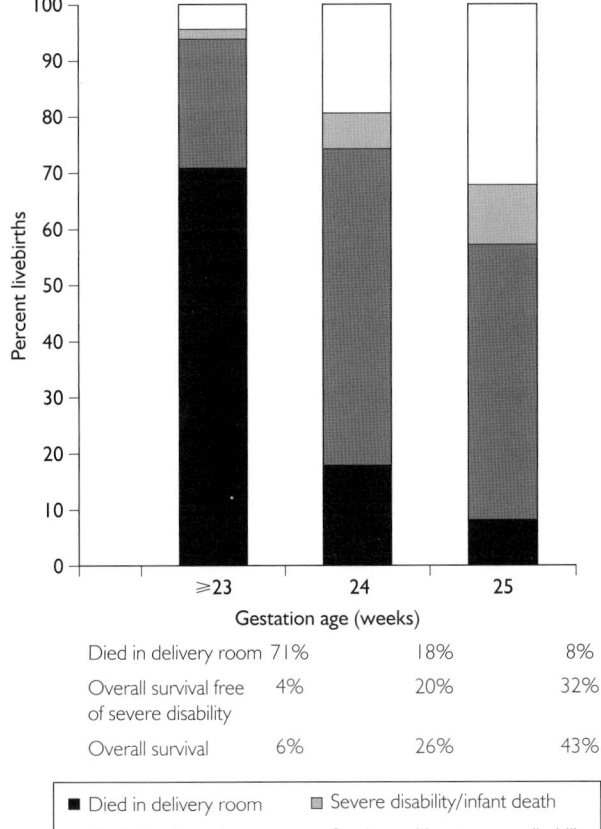

	≥23	24	25
Died in delivery room	71%	18%	8%
Overall survival free of severe disability	4%	20%	32%
Overall survival	6%	26%	43%

- ■ Died in delivery room
- ■ Died after intensive care
- ▨ Severe disability/infant death
- ☐ Survivor without severe disability

Fig. 2.10 Survival and risk of severe disability in the EPICure Study (livebirths in UK and Ireland in 1995) (With permission from Wood N S, Marlow N, Costeloe K, Gibson A T, Wilkinson A R 2000. Neurologic and developmental disability after extremely preterm birth. EPICure Study Group. New England Journal of Medicine 343: 378–384).

Table 2.10 Summary of two recommended minimum datasets to support annual reporting for neonatal intensive care units

Patient-based data	Unit-based data
32 items and eight optional data points*	22 items to describe unit structure/staffing

Patient-based data

32 items and eight optional data points*

1. Name of hospital[†]
2. Mother's NHS number
3. Postcode of mother's residence at birth
4. Planned place of delivery at booking
5. Place of birth
6. Reason for change in place of birth
7. Baby's NHS number
8. Date of birth
9. Time of birth
10. Source of admission to unit
11. Reason for admission to unit
12. Date of admission
13. Date of discharge, transfer or death
14. Discharge or transfer destination
15. Reason for discharge or transfer
16. Birthweight
17. Best estimate of gestation at delivery
18. Plurality
19. Whether post mortem performed
20. Time of death
21. Early neonatal encephalopathy
22. Retinopathy of prematurity examination
23. Retinopathy of prematurity stage
24. Therapy for retinopathy of prematurity
25. Cerebral ultrasound (as per policy)
26. Hearing screening (as per policy)
27. Days of endotracheal ventilation
28. Days of continuous positive airways pressure
29. Number of level 1 intensive care days[‡]
30. Number of level 2 intensive care days[‡]
31. Number of special care days
32. Date of final added oxygen therapy
   - Gender
   - Air leak requiring drainage
   - Worst changes of intraventricular haemorrhage
   - Ventricular size
   - Cystic leukomalacia
   - Highest appropriate percentage inspired O_2
   - Lowest appropriate percentage inspired O_2
   - Worst base excess

Unit-based data

22 items to describe unit structure/staffing

1. Name of hospital[†]
2. Number of livebirths
3. Number of designated intensive care cots
4. Number of designated special care cots

Nursing staff

5. Funded nursing establishment by grade
6. Nursing numbers in post by grade
7. Trained neonatal nursing numbers
8. Number of nurses in training
9. Senior nurse with managerial responsibility
10. Nurse responsible for further education

Medical staff

11. Number of consultants with major involvement in neonatal care
12. Consultant 24-hour cover
13. Resident middle grade 24-hour cover
14. Middle grade cover shared with paediatrics
15. Number of middle grade doctors providing cover
16. Resident SHO 24-hour medical cover
17. Number of professionals contributing to 24-hour resident cover
18. Number of advanced neonatal nurse practitioners
19. Neonatal transport service
20. Babies receiving levels A and B care[§]
21. Babies receiving levels C and D care[§]
22. Transfer in requests refused

*These data points are defined in the dataset and comprise definitions for items that many units will collect, but which do not form part of the minimum dataset.
[†]Variable common to both datasets.
[‡]British Association of Perinatal Medicine/Neonatal Nurses Association definition.
[§]Northern Neonatal Network definitions.
Source: British Association of Perinatal Medicine 1996 The BAPM neonatal dataset. BAPM, London.

High risk groups

In the UK there is no national system for recording outcomes following neonatal intensive care and collating them on a national basis. Many regions do collect such information but there is little attempt to standardise data definitions or reporting between the different systems. The BAPM has defined a data set that would fulfil these requirements (Table 2.10; www.bapm.org/publications.php)[4] so that neonatal services can report data in comparable ways. This data set is currently being re-evaluated

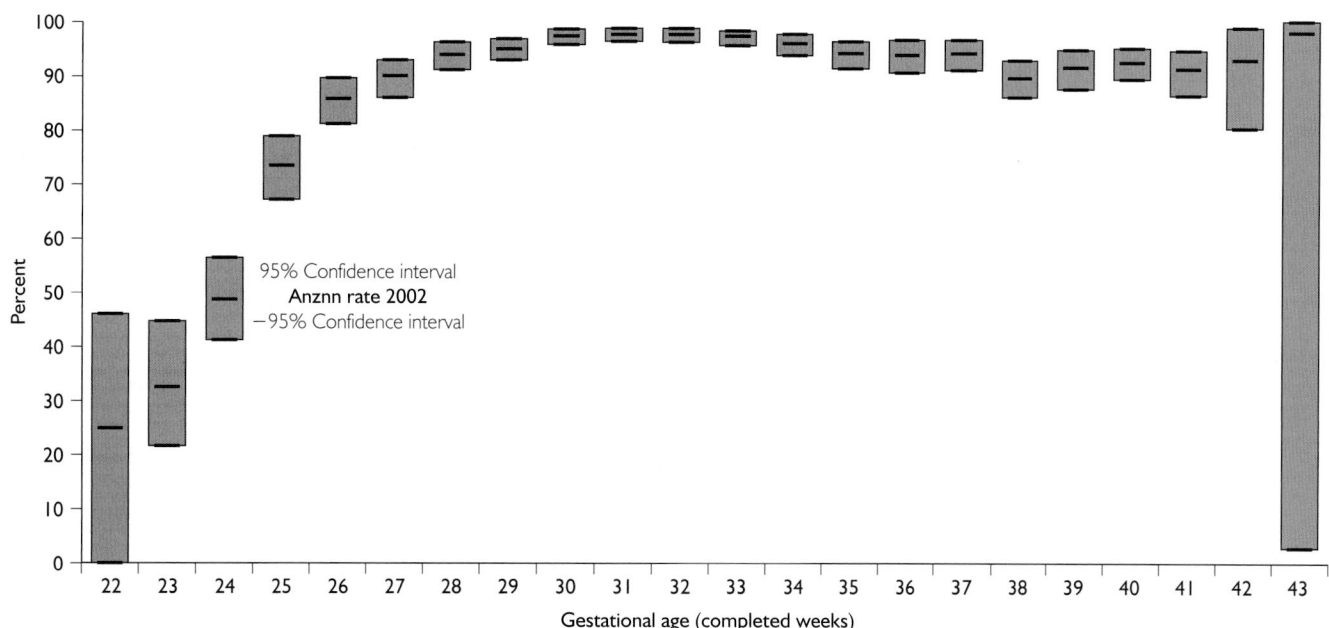

Fig. 2.11 Survival for babies admitted to Neonatal Intensive Care Units in Australia and New Zealand in 2001 with 95% confidence intervals (With permission from Donoghue D, the AZNN Executive 2003 Report of the Australian & New Zealand Neonatal Network 2001. ANZNN, Sydney.).

and developments in central investment in information give hope that this will evolve into a national facility.

As an example of good practice the Australian and New Zealand Neonatal Network have collated information from 22 NICUs from 1994 for babies under 32 weeks of gestation or less than 1500 g birthweight (www.usyd.edu.au/cphsr/anznn). All units are part of a highly developed, regionalised system with centralised care and well organised neonatal retrieval services. In the first report of this collaboration they identified four main objectives:

1. to provide a core dataset that will:
   a. identify trends and variations in mortality and morbidity which warrant further study
   b. enhance the ability to carry out multicentre studies and randomised trials
   c. provide information on neonatal outcomes adjusted for casemix and disease severity to assist with quality improvement;
2. to monitor the use of new technologies
3. to develop and evaluate a risk score for babies in the network
4. to develop and assess clinical indicators for perinatal care through neonatal outcomes.

The most recent report[12] indicates that most of these aims have been met and that the information provides an excellent set of data against which other neonatal services can be benchmarked. The network also acts as a facilitator for a range of academic activity to ensure that care and outcome continue to improve. The critical mass provided by such a collaboration produces narrow confidence intervals for important outcomes (Fig. 2.11).

A further example of international collaboration in this field is the Vermont Oxford Network (www.vtoxford.org). Initially designed to collect and collate patient-based information to facilitate interunit comparisons, it now receives data from over 350 neonatal units worldwide and records information on over 30 000 infants, including datasets from over 50% of NICUs in the USA and 50 units in other countries.

Guidelines and evidence-based care

Perinatal care is one area of modern medicine that has embraced the concept of the randomised controlled trial and thus in many areas it is possible to base care on secure scientific evidence. The collation of these results has allowed a number of statements to be made about good practice in a wide range of areas, brought together in the Cochrane Collaboration. Neonatal reviews are freely available (www.nichd.nih.gov/cochraneneonatal). Not all areas of practice are covered by such reviews, however, and clinical practice must take account of a much broader range of evidence and personal experience. Although national and professional bodies may produce guidance for good practice from time to time (Table 2.10), clear information is required in the context of the working environment and the local development of guidelines is necessary. The establishment of managed clinical networks poses an opportunity for these to be developed on a network basis, reducing the workload for an individual unit and ensuring a more even delivery of quality care.

Guidelines are not mandatory protocols. Care must be individually tailored to the individual's clinical needs and it may thus be necessary to deviate from unit guidelines if it is deemed necessary in a particular situation. However, default management plans are possible for many areas of care and it is primarily in these areas of care that guidelines make a valuable contribution to good practice. When guidelines are drawn up it is helpful to identify audit points and methods of audit so that prospective data collection against the standards set may be made.

The process of integrating scientific evidence into practice has been adopted widely as the practice of 'evidence-based medicine'. A full description of this process is outside the remit of this chapter (www.cebm.net). However, the processes of asking answerable questions, assembling and critically appraising the evidence, acting on the evidence and establishing performance against the evidence are central to the audit/guideline philosophy.

Within a single service it is often difficult to demonstrate benefit from the introduction of evidence-based changes in management. Working together as a local network will clearly bring advantages in terms of population size but using the powerful resources of a large organisation such as the Vermont Oxford Network allows a more rapid introduction of change from a broader range of services.

As part of the NIC/Q2000 scheme the Vermont Oxford Network facilitated a range of service quality improvements in the areas of nosocomial infection, chronic lung disease, postnatal dexamethasone use, prevention of brain haemorrhage and ischaemic brain injury, and family-centred care. This is the first time that such an undertaking has been attempted in the field of clinical care. Each service improvement occurred across a group of neonatal units with variable success. The success of this scheme provides powerful evidence that with a facilitated approach, using common methodology across a network of units, evidence-based changes in practice can be implemented and audited.

In the UK the most effective audit process has been the CESDI, now CEMACH. Registered deaths from 20 weeks of gestation until the end of the first postnatal year are reported centrally. Within this system a series of confidential structured enquiries have been organised, each focussed on a different theme to identify both avoidable factors and good practice in the management of reported cases. Recently this process has been supplemented by the collection of a comparison group of surviving children born at 27 and 28 competed weeks of gestation (Project 27–28). The report from this powerful evaluation of practice has important implications for neonatal practice in the UK.

Conclusions

Within a modern health service, neonatal care makes an important contribution to the health of the population, providing critical care support to babies who are seriously ill and taking evidence-based measures to avoid illness and unnecessary intervention. NIC has developed greatly over the past 30 years with demonstrable improvements in survival and morbidity. Organisation of what are now complex services must be demonstrated to be clinically and financially efficient and clinical care must be transparent and evidence-based. These are challenges that are met though clinical governance and service improvement, as described above. These are now key areas of neonatal practice and central to the delivery of improved outcomes in the future.

References

1. Audit Commission 1993 Children first. HMSO London
2. Bennett C C, Lal M K, Field D J, Wilkinson A R 2002 Maternal morbidity and pregnancy outcome in a cohort of mothers transferred out of perinatal centres during a national census. British Journal of Obstetrics and Gynaecology 109: 663–666
3. Bowen S L 2002 Transport of the mechanically ventilated neonate. Respiratory Care Clinics of North America 8: 67–82
4. British Association of Perinatal Medicine 1996a The BAPM neonatal dataset. BAPM, London
5. British Association of Perinatal Medicine 1996b Standards for hospitals providing neonatal intensive care. BAPM, London
6. British Association of Perinatal Medicine 2001 Standards for hospitals providing intensive and high dependency care. BAPM, London
7. Burnhope C, Edmonstone J 2003 'Feel the fear and do it anyway': the hard business of developing shared governance. Journal of Nursing Management 11: 147–57
8. Clinical Standards Advisory Group 1993 Neonatal intensive care: access to and availability of specialist services. HMSO, London
9. Clinical Standards Advisory Group 1995 Neonatal intensive care: access to and availability of specialist services: Second report to CSAG by a working group. HMSO, London
10. Confidential Enquiry into Stillbirths and Deaths in Infancy 2001 8th Annual Report. Maternal and Child Health Research Consortium: London
11. Costeloe K, Hennessy E, Gibson A T, Marlow N, Wilkinson A R 2000 The EPICure study: outcomes to discharge from hospital for infants born at the threshold of viability. Pediatrics 106: 659–671
12. Donoghue D, the AZNN Executive 2003 Report of the Australian & New Zealand Neonatal Network 2001. ANZNN, Sydney
13. Draper E S, Manktelow B, Field D J, James D 2000 Prediction of survival for preterm births. British Medical Journal 321: 237
14. El-Metwally D, Vohr B, Tucker R 2000 Survival and neonatal morbidity at the limits of viability in the mid 1990s: 22 to 25 weeks. Journal of Pediatrics 137: 616–622
15. Field D, Draper E S 1999 Survival and place of delivery following preterm birth: 1994–96. Archives of Disease in Childhood. Fetal and Neonatal Edition 80: F111–F114
16. Field D, Hodges S, Mason E, Burton P 1991 Survival and place of treatment after premature delivery. Archives of Disease in Childhood 66: 408–10; discussion 410–411
17. Field D, Draper E S, Gompels M J et al 2001 Measuring later health status of high risk infants: randomised comparison of two simple methods of data collection. British Medical Journal 323: 1276–1281
18. Field D, Petersen S, Clarke M, Draper E S 2002 Extreme prematurity in the UK and Denmark: population differences in viability. Archives of Disease in Childhood. Fetal and Neonatal Edition 87: F172–F175
19. Fleming P, Berry J, Gilbert R, Rudd P 1990 Bedding and sleeping position in the sudden infant death syndrome. British Medical Journal 301: 871–872
20. Gavin M, Ash D, Wakefield S, Wroe C 1999 Shared governance: time to consider the cons as well as the pros. Journal of Nursing Management 7: 193–200
21. Goodman D C, Fisher E S, Little G A, Stukel T A, Chang C H, Schoendorf K S 2002 The relation between the availability of neonatal intensive care and neonatal mortality. New England Journal of Medicine 346: 1538–1544
22. Hope P 1995 CRIB, son of Apgar, brother to APACHE. Archives of Disease in Childhood. Fetal and Neonatal Edition 72: F81–F83
23. International Neonatal Network 1993 The CRIB (clinical risk index for babies) score: a tool for assessing initial neonatal risk and comparing performance of neonatal intensive care units. Lancet 342: 193–198
24. International Neonatal Network, Scottish Neonatal Consultants, Nurses Collaborative Study Group 2000 Risk adjusted and population based studies of the outcome for high risk infants in Scotland and Australia. Archives of Disease in Childhood. Fetal and Neonatal Edition 82: F118–F123
25. Klein R 2001 Milburn's vision of a new NHS. Adopting the missionary position. British Medical Journal 322: 1078–1979
26. Leslie A J, Stephenson T J 1997 Audit of neonatal intensive care transport – closing the loop. Acta Paediatrica 86: 1253–1256
27. Leslie A, Stephenson T 2003 Neonatal transfers by advanced neonatal nurse practitioners and paediatric registrars. Archives of Disease in Childhood. Fetal and Neonatal Edition 88: F509–F512
28. Lorenz J M, Paneth N, Jetton J R, den Ouden L, Tyson J E 2001 Comparison of management strategies for extreme prematurity in New Jersey and the Netherlands: outcomes and resource expenditure. Pediatrics 108: 1269–1274

29. Marlow N 2002 Illness severity measures in neonatal intensive care. Acta Paediatrica 91: 367–368

30. Maybloom B, Chapple J, Davidson L L 2002 Admissions for critically ill children: where and why? Intensive and Critical Care Nursing 18: 151–161

31. Maynard A, Bloor K 1996 Introducing a market to the United Kingdom's National Health Service. New England Journal of Medicine 334: 604–608

32. Milligan D W A 1997 Neonatal intensive care provision in the United Kingdom 1992–3. Archives of Disease in Childhood. Fetal and Neonatal Edition 76: F197–F200

33. Neonatal Intensive Care Services Review Group 2003 Neonatal intensive care review – strategy for improvement. Department of Health, London

34. Northern Neonatal Network 1993 Measuring neonatal nursing workload. Archives of Disease in Childhood 68: 539–543

35. Parmanum J, Field D, Rennie J, Steer P 2000 National census of availability of neonatal intensive care. British Association for Perinatal Medicine. British Medical Journal 321: 727–729

36. Parry G J, Gould C R, McCabe C J, Tarnow-Mordi W O 1998 Annual league tables of mortality in neonatal intensive care units: longitudinal study. International Neonatal Network and the Scottish Neonatal Consultants and Nurses Collaborative Study Group. British Medical Journal 316: 1931–1935

37. Parry G, Tucker J, Tarnow-Mordi W 2003 CRIB II: an update of the clinical risk index for babies score. Lancet 361: 1789–1791

38. Rashid A, Bhuta T, Berry A 1999 A regionalised transport service, the way ahead? Archives of Disease in Childhood 80: 488–492

39. Ratcliffe J 1998 Provision of intensive care for children. A geographically integrated service may now be achieved. British Medical Journal 316: 1547–1548

40. Richardson D K, Gray J E, McCormick M C, Workman K, Goldmann D A 1993 Score for neonatal acute physiology: a physiologic severity index for neonatal intensive care. Pediatrics 91: 617–623

41. Richardson D K, Corcoran J D, Escobar G J, Lee S K 2001 SNAP-II and SNAPPE-II: Simplified newborn illness severity and mortality risk scores. Journal of Pediatrics 138: 92–100

42. Scally G, Donaldson L J 1998 The NHS's 50th anniversary. Clinical governance and the drive for quality improvement in the new NHS in England. British Medical Journal 317: 61–65

43. TINA. Transport of Neonates by Ambulance. 1996

44. Tucker J 2002 Patient volume, staffing, and workload in relation to risk-adjusted outcomes in a random stratified sample of UK neonatal intensive care units: a prospective evaluation. Lancet 359: 99–107

45. Tucker J, Tarnow-Mordi W, Gould C, Parry G, Marlow N 1999 UK neonatal intensive care services in 1996. On behalf of the UK Neonatal Staffing Study Collaborative Group. Archives of Disease in Childhood. Fetal and Neonatal Edition 80: F233–F234

46. Ventriculomegaly Trial Group 1995 Disability and perinatal care: report of two working groups. NPEU and Oxford Health Authority, Oxford

47. Wigfield R E, Fleming P J, Berry P J, Rudd P T, Golding J 1992 Can the fall in Avon's sudden infant death rate be explained by changes in sleeping position? British Medical Journal 304: 282–283

48. Williams S, Whelan A, Weindling A, Cooke R 1993 Nursing staff requirements for neonatal intensive care. Archives of Disease in Childhood 68: 534–538

49. Wood N S, Marlow N, Costeloe K, Gibson A T, Wilkinson A R 2000 Neurologic and developmental disability after extremely preterm birth. EPICure Study Group. New England Journal of Medicine 343: 378–384

CHAPTER 3

Outcome following preterm birth

Neil Marlow

Being born prematurely is not a normal outcome for a fetus. For babies born near term this may have relatively few short- or long-term consequences but for babies born particularly early, at 30 weeks gestational age or less, there is a threat to survival and the subsequent quality of life. All organ systems are growing, developing and maturing rapidly over the period when the baby is exposed to fetal and neonatal risk. The interruption to normal fetal development may have significant long-term consequences. It is encouraging that many adults who were born very preterm function well in later life[63,98] but a significant proportion develop disabilities and impairments that are the subject of this chapter.

History

Early neonatal care

Interest in the care of the newborn has waxed and waned through history. The invention that marked the dawn of 'modern' neonatal care was the incubator, first credited to a French obstetrician, Mon Tarnier. The introduction into the Paris Maternité hospital in 1878 facilitated the development of the ideas published by Pierre Budin in his classic monograph entitled *Le Nourissant* (*The Nursling*).[19] Although mainly concerned with inpatient care, there is one surviving photograph of his 'graduates'. Martin Couney, a pupil of Budin, requested a chance to exhibit the new incubators in the World Exposition in Berlin in 1896. Permission granted, he conceived of the idea of a live exhibit with babies, otherwise destined to die, from a local charitable hospital. These *Kinderbrutanstäldter* ('child hatcheries') proved a great success and were soon imitated across the world. Couney himself settled in Cooney Island where his exhibitions became famous; his own daughter was born prematurely and was incubated for 3 months.[145]

Couney's influence led Julius Hess to establish the eight-cot Premature Baby Station at the Sarah Morris Hospital, Chicago. This rapidly expanded and led to the first reliable reports of survival and outcome.[75] No significant deviation from normal term controls was noted in this highly selected population and no effects of birthweight, gestation, sex or maternal illness were found on outcome. Indeed Gesell and Armatruda,[57] using graduates of Couney's summer exhibitions, concluded that 'prematurity does not markedly alter the normal course of mental growth. It neither retards nor accelerates'. However, thinking was soon to change.

Over the next decade the importance of the length of gestation was appreciated and increased morbidity in the smaller survivors was noted, leading to questions about care for these vulnerable babies that persist right through to today. For example, Sheridan observed that improvements in mortality had 'been accompanied by a rising survival of immature, malformed, birth injured and weakly babies'[143] and Drillien warned that improvements in care might lead to increasing numbers of handicapped children in the community.[42]

Care had up to this point been crude, as exemplified by the uncertainty surrounding the use of oxygen,[29] but the 1960s heralded the start of more careful and considered interventions such as early feeding with breast milk and more appropriate respiratory interventions. There were conflicting reports as to trends in outcomes during this time. The first important systematic attempt to review trends in outcome for very-low-birthweight births was published by Ann Stewart and colleagues.[149] They indicated some of the difficulties in comparing reports, often from specialist centres reporting selected groups of infants. They summarised outcome from published reports as death, handicapped or healthy survivor and averaged over adjacent 5-year periods over 32 years. From 1960 mortality was found to have fallen progressively, but in each epoch 6–8% of total livebirths had handicaps. There was no evidence, therefore, of an excess of handicapped children in the community as a result of these improvements in care. The same trends applied equally to the subgroup with a birthweight less than 1000 g.

The contribution of prematurity to disability in the community

The notion that increased survival brought an additional burden of disability into the population remains even today. The concept of a 'gain' in a healthy survivor is set against a 'loss' as a child with disability. Stewart has summarised these studies, as shown in Table 3.1,[147] demonstrating that the gain in terms of healthy

Table 3.1 Estimated 'gains' and 'losses' per 1000 live births in Sweden, Western Australia and England and Wales

Birthweight	Population	Year	'Gains'	'Losses'	Condition
All	Sweden	1971–75	3.8	0.1	Cerebral palsy
<2000 g	Western Australia	1979	101	5	Neurodevelopmental abnormality
<2500 g	England and Wales	1979	33	3.5	Neurodevelopmental abnormality
<1500 g	England and Wales	1979	168	21	Neurodevelopmental abnormality
<1500 g	England and Wales	1981	264	35	Neurodevelopmental abnormality

Adapted from Stewart A 1999 Neurodevelopmental outcome. In: Rennie J M, Roberton N R C (eds) Textbook of neonatology. Churchill Livingstone, Edinburgh, pp 79–100.

survivors far outweighs the increasing burden of disability in the population. Since the early 1980s there has been an explosion of interest in this area and a huge literature base has evolved. Over short periods of time it is clear that trends in disability rates are hard to demonstrate but mortality has continued to decrease as the gestational age at which birth is considered of borderline viability has fallen. This was recognised in the UK by the reduction from 28 weeks to 24 weeks gestational age for the definition of stillbirth in 1992.

Philosophy of care and outcome

The increasing anxiety surrounding the provision of care for the baby of borderline viability has continued and is now directed to babies born before 26 weeks of gestation, such is survival at later gestational age. Survival is in part determined by the attitudes of caregivers, some centres preferring not to offer care at these low gestations in the belief that outcome is likely to be so poor that to attempt intensive care is wrong. Very few studies have attempted to define the results of different models of care. One important study compares the outcome in a heath service with near-universal initiation of intensive care in the USA to selective initiation in the Netherlands; this resulted in 24.1 additional survivors and 7.2 additional cases of cerebral palsy for each 100 live births.[96] Thus the gain and loss account is still in favour of intensive care if cerebral palsy is used as an outcome. Many would argue that cognitive and behavioural impairment is an even more important adverse outcome measure, but the appropriate study has not been done.

It is important that we continue to collect information on the progress of children exposed to neonatal intensive care, as is recommended in UK national standards,[18] not least to provide important information for parents facing an extremely preterm birth and to assist with counselling after birth. Used wisely, they may also be able to provide information as to the adequacy of service provision (Chapter 2).

Reporting outcomes and study design

Data concerning the progress of neonatal intensive care graduates can be used as part of an ongoing audit of outcome or as part of a hypothesis-based research study. Such a study may explore factors that influence development (e.g. social or nutritional factors) or the predictive value of particular observations (e.g. cranial ultrasound appearances). Increasingly, randomised trials of neonatal interventions are including longer-term outcomes (usually for 1–2 years) as secondary or even primary outcomes for a range of neonatal treatments and in economic appraisals of such. In an ideal world these would be collected in an agreed fashion for all children using routine systems, but this is as yet not possible.

Comparing studies in this area is fraught with methodological problems which often preclude comparison of outcome statistics between studies, despite attempts to do so (see below). It is important, therefore, that the data are presented as fully as possible to facilitate comparison year-on-year and between studies. Reports of population outcomes should contain as a minimum:

- information on the birth population:
  - all births or livebirths in a given geographical population
  - numbers of babies admitted for neonatal intensive care
  - details of transfers for care (in and ex utero)
  - survivors to discharge home;
- age at assessment (with range) and correction for prematurity if applied;
- proportion of the population assessed and reasons for non-assessment – a diagram similar to that recommended for randomised trials in the Consort statement (http://www.consort-statement.org/statement.html) is often the clearest way of displaying this;
- measures used to define performance of population (e.g. intelligence test) and definitions of categories used to classify outcome and the numbers with disability in each domain comprising the outcome measure (e.g. cerebral palsy, cognitive function, hearing or visual impairment).

More detailed descriptions of the requirements for such studies have been published.[85,108] This requirement applies less to targeted studies of interventions but nonetheless the discipline of identifying the sample used by reporting the population as suggested above allows much better understanding of the applicability of the results of studies to routine practice.

In 1994, because of a lack of consistency between studies in terms definitions for long-term outcomes, two working groups established by the National Perinatal Epidemiology Unit and Oxford Health Authority developed guidelines for the categorisation of outcome following prematurity.[8] The resulting recommendations allow for consistent reporting of functional outcomes at a corrected age of 2 years (Table 3.2). Two years was

Table 3.2 Disability and prematurity – health status at 2 years: criteria for disability in preterm children

Domain and key questions	Criteria for impairment or disability (criteria for severe disability in bold)
Malformation Does the child have a malformation?	Any anomaly detected at birth or apparent within the first two postnatal years, which is likely to result in death, disfigurement or disability, and which is likely to require medical or surgical treatment (other than a simple cosmetic procedure) **Any malformation which despite physical assistance impairs the performance of daily activities**
Neuromotor function Does the child have any difficulty walking?	Non-fluent gait Abnormal gait reducing mobility **Unable to walk without assistance**
Does the child have any difficulty sitting?	Sits unsupported but unstable Sits supported **Unable to sit**
Does the child have any difficulty with hand use?	Some difficulty feeding with one hand Some difficulty feeding with both hands **Unable to use hands to feed self**
Does the child have any difficulty with head control?	Unstable but no support required **Unable to control head movement without support** **No head control**
Seizures Does the child have seizures?	No treatment required No seizures on treatment Seizures less than 1/month despite treatment **Seizures more than 1/month despite treatment**
Auditory function Does the child have any difficulty hearing?	Hearing impaired, not aided Hearing impaired, corrects with aids **Hearing impaired, uncorrected even with aids**
Communication Is there any difficulty with communication?	Unable to comprehend word/sign out of familiar context **Unable to comprehend word/sign in cued situation** Uses single words only/vocabulary >10 words Vocabulary <10 words **Unable to produce >5 recognisable sounds** **No vocalisation**
Visual function Does the child have any difficulty with vision?	Normal vision with correction Not fully correctable **Blind or sees light only**
Cognitive function Does the child have any learning difficulty?	Developmental quotient 2 to 3 SD below mean **Developmental quotient >3 SD below mean**
Other physical disability Does the child have any other disability? Respiratory	Limited exercise tolerance, no drug treatment Limited exercise tolerance, on drug treatment **Requires continual oxygen therapy** **Requires mechanical ventilation**

(Continued)

Table 3.2 (Continued)

Domain and key questions	Criteria for impairment or disability (criteria for severe disability in bold)
Gastrointestinal	Requires special diet
	Has stoma
	Requires tube feeding
	Requires parenteral nutrition
Renal	Renal impairment; no treatment
	Renal impairment; drug or dietary treatment only
	Requires dialysis
Growth	Height or weight 2 to 3 SD below mean for age
	Height or weight >3 SD below mean for age

From: Anon 1995 Disability and perinatal care: report of two working groups. NPEU and Oxford Health Authority, Oxford.

Table 3.3 Ophthalmic outcomes for low-birthweight (LBW) infants compared to normal birthweight controls

	LBW infants (%)	Comparison (%)	OR (95%CI) for abnormality in LBW group
Birthweight <1750 g assessed at 10–12 years of age[110]	*n* = 254	*n* = 169	
Normal vision (%)	76	93	
Slightly impaired acuity	20	7	4.05 (2.10–7.79)
Moderate impaired acuity	3.5	0	(for any impairment)
Overall morbidity	51	20	4.25 (2.70–6.69)
Birthweight <1501 g assessed at 11–13 years of age[127]	*n* = 137	*n* = 163	
Strabismus	9.5	2.5	4.17 (1.33–13.1)
Abnormal acuity:			
Distance (6 m)	17	8	2.33 (1.13–4.80)
Near (0.6 m)	14	6	2.46 (1.10–5.50)
Spectacles worn	23	13	1.98 (1.08–3.60)
Poor stereopsis	36	15	3.33 (1.91–5.80)
Poor contrast sensitivity	48	19	3.96 (2.36–6.63)

the age at which the panel of interested parties agreed would be most likely to identify serious cerebral palsy with some confidence, bearing in mind the difficulty in interpreting very early assessments. These definitions have good validity when compared to other published criteria[82] with some modification for growth impairment, which is not strictly a severe disability and particularly common among extremely preterm children.[170] The predictive value of these definitions for later disability remains to be elucidated. Alongside the disability data the groups also recommended a minimum data set to allow the identification of each child in UK databases.

The definition of disability at later ages is less well supported by consensus. There are formal definitions of disability available from the World Health Organization (WHO) that should underpin any scheme, but these are currently undergoing re-evaluation (http://www.who.int/health_topics/disabilities/en/) and the detail of categorisation for follow-up is much less clear. The use of different standardised outcome measures (e.g. cognitive, neurological, motor or behavioural domains) will to a large extent depend upon the hypothesis under investigation and attempts to standardise these measures are in truth misguided, excepting that where there are clear internationally accepted definitions (e.g. DSM-IV) these should be reported alongside measures specific to the individual study.

Research evaluations should be focussed on a population base as described above and report data in a standardised fashion.[108] However the research hypothesis will determine the choice and selection of investigation required and the selection of such tests is outside the remit of this chapter. The importance of recruiting contemporary comparison groups is stressed as secular upward drifts in IQ scores are well described[55] and the results of categorisation of children's performance will depend on which reference norms are selected with older measures.[166]

The importance of attempting to examine or at least obtain classifying information on all children in a population as possible has been stressed. There is some evidence that the non-responders may comprise an excess of severely disabled children,[153,168] although there is a paucity of data from other studies to support this. Increasingly the issue of research governance and the necessity to respect parents' privacy means that fewer attempts to contact parents for follow-up investigations are justifiable and research ethics committees are mindful to limit these. Difficulties with contacting parents after some time means that the taking of consent for later research evaluations should be done at the point of original entry into the study and contact maintained with newsletters, birthday cards or similar should help to minimise loss to follow-up.

The development of neonatal networks with consistent data collection will help us better to understand the relationship between our care and outcome (Chapter 2).

Outcome in early infancy

Motor development

Schemes for neurological examination of the newborn, such as those of Amiel-Tison, Dubowitz and Prechtl, are described in Chapter 41.1. Neonatologists must be aware of the different patterns of development over the first year and, where supported by evidence, be prepared to embrace a range of interventions in the nursery and after discharge to optimise a child's development.

Despite the reliance on ultrasound-detected brain lesions for prognosis, clinical assessment of the infant at discharge is of at least equal importance to evaluating the results of cranial imaging. Amiel-Tison and colleagues have described a simple functional examination to be performed at around 40 weeks postmenstrual age. At this age, the very preterm baby is quite different from a newborn term infant, particularly if born at a very low gestational age. Ex-preterm babies are more visually active and demonstrate less flexion and more extensor activity. When the examination is optimal and the results of cranial ultrasound normal, the risk of abnormality at 12 months of age is negligible.[133] The positive predictive value is less useful and many will eventually lose their non-optimal signs early in the first year.

The very preterm baby is hypotonic and weak, with a poorly calcified skeleton. These characteristics impart particular vulnerability to external influences on the development of neurological tone and to skeletal deformations. Nursing postures may lead to changes in head and chest shape if they are not varied and prone positioning will encourage extensor posturing and external hip rotation with shortening of the hip adductors.[4] This may encourage hip dislocation if the child develops spasticity but may easily be avoided using simple postural management.[39] The recent interest in nursing positioning will facilitate normal postural development. Long-term ventilation and chronic lung disease are associated with similar positional issues; neck retraction and truncal extension are features of airway shortening manoeuvres. Irritability associated with these deformities produces a picture that may be attributed to neurological injury, and handling or feeding children with fixed postural deformity is difficult and may lead to difficulties in maternal attachment.

These influences may all modify the trajectory of development. De Groot and colleagues have described a group of ex-preterm infants with discrepancies between active and passive muscle tone that are most obvious in the extensor muscles of the trunk[32] and may also be asymmetric.[33] This usually transient dystonia may be a feature of the developing ex-preterm infant independent of positional changes. De Groot and colleagues argue that these tonal abnormalities lead to delay in unsupported sitting and rotation towards the end of the first year. These have implications for transition between postures and also lead to delay in fine motor development[31] and behavioural changes, through impairment of ability to optimise gross motor and hand function in an otherwise normal child because of truncal fixation.

Transient dystonia was described in preterm children by Drillien[43] as infants with an excess of extensor hypertonicity in the trunk and legs, increased hip adductor tone and delayed supporting reactions. Such changes tend to resolve at around the child's first birthday or over the second year and be initially diagnosed as cerebral palsy. Other more recent studies have evaluated motor development over the first 18 months. Pederson and Markestad[115] studied a geographically based cohort of babies of less than 2000 g birthweight. They categorised 29% as dystonic, 10% as hypotonic and 8% as suspected cerebral palsy. The prevalence of dystonia was 35% in babies under 1000 g, 35% for 1000–1499 g and 21% in babies 1500–1999 g. The peak prevalence of dystonia was at 7 months of age corrected for prematurity. Of children at 18 months of age with suspected cerebral palsy, when examined at 7 months, five had been labelled as suspect cerebral palsy, eight dystonia and one hypotonia. In another study the prevalence of dystonia was 36% of 260 very-low-birthweight (VLBW) infants.[112]

Three studies have indicated long-term outcomes for dystonic infants. In Drillien's original study they were found to have an excess of educational difficulties,[44] in a study of 50 children there was a trend towards more neuromotor difficulties[146] and in a further study dystonic infants had lower cognitive scores and higher disability grades at early school age.[84]

Screening vision and hearing

Screening for retinopathy of prematurity is addressed in Chapter 34, but this cannot form the basis for screening for visual or ocular impairments. Squints and refractive errors are frequently found at follow-up in infancy and each assessment must include adequate examination of visual activity and ocular movements. Refractive errors and subtle disorders of vision such as poor stereognosis and contrast sensitivity are found frequently at longer-term follow-up,[110,116,127] and should be sought in assessments at school age. Table 3.3 shows the outcomes for two recent cohorts detailing the difference from comparative populations. In the recent teenage follow-up of the East Midlands cohort, ophthalmic morbidity was found in 67.8% of children born weighing less than 1000 g, 51.6% of those weighing 1001–1250 g, 44.3% of those weighing 1251–1500 g and 49.5% of those weighing 1501–1750 g compared to 19.5% of their comparison group.[110]

Sensorineural hearing loss is more prevalent in preterm populations, although the aetiology is still obscure and may well be multifactorial.[99] Found in 1–4% of VLBW children, this represents a tenfold increase over unselected populations.[6,25,130] Because of this, most services have developed targeted neonatal screening policies in which prematurity (either as VLBW or birth before 32 weeks gestation) is included in the screened population alongside children with family history of deafness, orofacial anomalies and perinatal central nervous system infection. More recently there has been a move towards universal neonatal hearing screening, predicated on the thesis that early intervention for children with severe or profound hearing loss may improve later language and speech development.[171] Most targeted screening involves automated or manual evoked responses (ABR) which will identify children with significant hearing loss. Universal screening in the USA and most European countries involves testing with automated ABR technology, whereas currently in the UK a 'two-step' approach has been adopted using initial screening with oto-acoustic emissions and automated ABR for failures. Universal screening has a sensitivity of between 80% and 90% and a specificity of above 90%[30] and the median age of detection of severe hearing loss may be as low as 2 months, facilitating early intervention.

Cerebral palsy

The association between spastic diplegia and prematurity was first described in a paper entitled 'Zum Cerablen Diplegien' published in 1896 by Sigmund Freud, during his work as a paediatric neurologist with Charcot in Paris.[2] Thus the increased risk of cerebral palsy following preterm birth has been known for some time and, indeed, cerebral palsy is often considered to be the most common and important disability following preterm birth. In fact this is not the case, as developmental delay and cognitive impairments are by far the commonest disabilities. Nonetheless cerebral palsy remains one of the most important outcomes and in the early 1980s spastic diplegia was used as a marker of the success of perinatal services.[71]

The risk of cerebral palsy is inversely related to gestational age at birth and increased in the presence of intrauterine growth restriction (IUGR), at least among moderately preterm children.[14] As many older studies are birthweight-based the results must be treated with some caution because of the varying proportion of babies born after IUGR (see Chapter 1). The evaluation of secular trends in cerebral palsy must be related to either birthweight or gestation because of the close links. The evolution of birthweight-specific trends in the prevalence of cerebral palsy over the time period of introduction of neonatal intensive care in Mersey, UK have been described.[118] As birthweight-specific survival increased there was an initial rise in the prevalence of cerebral palsy within that birthweight band, followed by a levelling out. This may relate to the increasing survival of children with cerebral palsy who would otherwise have died, up to an equilibrium point. This is in contrast to the pattern described prior to 1980, where there was an initial increase in handicap rates as survival increased followed by a fall as care improved.[149] Cerebral palsy registers can provide excellent population-based data on trends but recent changes in UK data protection law have placed these at some risk.

Population trends have not revealed consistent directions of change in the prevalence of cerebral palsy as a group or in birthweight-specific groupings.[68–72] Figure 3.1 shows a selection of

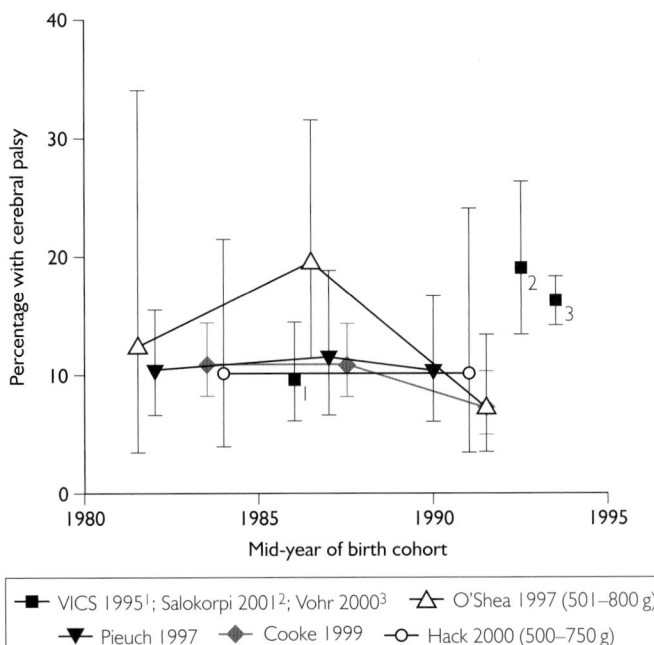

Fig. 3.1 Proportion of children followed up with birthweight below 1000 g who had cerebral palsy (with 95% confidence intervals). (Data from references 6, 26, 66, 111, 121, 137, 159.)

reports of cerebral palsy rates in children born at 1000 g birthweight or less. Age at assessment varied between 18 months and 5 years. Although some studies show significant falls,[26] there are no consistent trends and the more recent reports from Finland[137] and the USA[159] report point estimates for children born in the early 1990s that are higher than previous reports, which may reflect increasing survival at extremely low gestations (25 weeks gestational age or less).[47] The mean prevalence in these studies is 10.4%. Survival and low numbers confound all attempts to compare the prevalence of cerebral palsy by weeks of gestation but eight studies including births from 1982 through to 1995 show a remarkably consistent mean cerebral palsy rate of around 14.7% for babies born at 26 weeks gestational age or less (Fig. 3.2). For births in the UK and Ireland in 1995, 17.7% (95% confidence interval (CI) 13.7–22.6%) children had cerebral palsy at 2.5 years of age.[170] These data hint that rates for 1990s births may be higher than for 1980s births, probably reflecting changes in survival rates.

The distribution of impairment in cerebral palsy is determined by the pattern of brain injury. Diplegia, in which the impairment is more severe caudally, is considered to be the result of damage to the internal capsule as part of periventricular leukomalacia (PVL). This usually symmetrical lesion is commonly observed on magnetic resonance imaging (MRI) scans at follow-up even if no neonatal ultrasound evidence of injury was observed.[21] Diplegia is often associated with relatively mild disability and there is often less severe impairment in other domains compared to other patterns of cerebral palsy. In the EPICure cohort of babies of 25 weeks gestational age or less, only 44%[12/27] children with diplegia had severe disability and thus were likely to have persisting disability at later ages.[170]

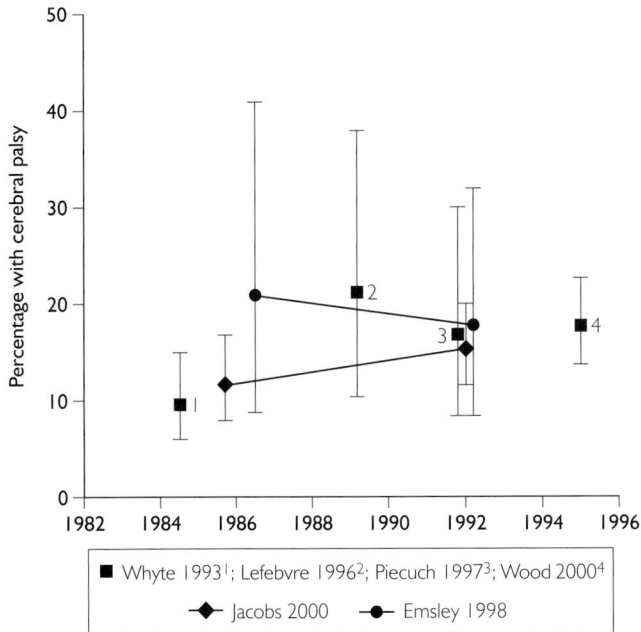

Fig. 3.2 Proportion of children followed up after birth before 26 completed weeks gestational age (with 95% confidence intervals). (Data from references 48, 78, 90, 121, 165, 170.)

Spastic hemiplegia, where the distribution of impairment is the reverse of diplegia and where there is usually significant asymmetry, results from lesions involving the cortex, such as cerebral venous infarction accompanying GMH-IVH. Spastic quadriplegia, where there is four-limb involvement equally distributed in upper and lower limbs, occurs in variable proportions in reports. The distribution of disability in children with diplegia and hemiplegia is not always confined to the legs or to one side of the body and it is a subjective decision as to how to categorise the impairments. This accounts for many of the differences found between different observers. However, the impairment in quadriplegia is more extensive than the other two and the disability is frequently severe (11/12 in the EPICure cohort). Other types of cerebral palsy are found less frequently in very preterm populations.

The timing of diagnosis in follow-up reports is important in determining the prevalence of cerebral palsy: the predictive value of a label of cerebral palsy increases as the child grows up. There is some consensus that the diagnosis of cerebral palsy producing significant disability is usually accurate by the age of 2 years[80] but that before that abnormal patterns of motor development and dystonia or developmental delay may confuse the unwary. In the National Collaborative Perinatal Project cerebral palsy was overdiagnosed at 12 months compared to assessment at 7 years, such that half of the children with the diagnosis at 1 year were free of neurological signs 6 years later.[109] The most common types of cerebral palsy to resolve were categorised as mild and were of the monoparetic, dyskinetic or diplegic types; resolution was more frequent in black infants. However a significant proportion of the children in whom signs had resolved (13% white and 25% blacks) had an IQ of less than 70 at 7 years, emphasising the importance of careful early examination. Despite

the recommendation to wait until 2 years, even at this age there is overdiagnosis[40] and some less severe impairment may not be detectable until early school age.[10]

Developmental progress

Central to the definition of disability in preterm populations is an estimate of the child's developmental level. Clinic assessment using one of the widely available developmental screening tools (e.g. the Denver Developmental Screening Inventory or Schedule of Growing Skills) may indicate normal or very abnormal progress but the diagnostic utility and predictive value are not known; in particular variations in assessment technique may wrongly classify a child if an equivalent DQ of 70 (2 standard deviations (SD) below the mean) is sought as a categorical outcome. Assessment using the Griffiths scales may now be more accurate, using the newly revised scales, which currently extend only to 2 years. The Griffiths scales have the advantage of five subscales, each with clinical relevance.

The more commonly used tool for research evaluation is the Bayley Scales of Infant Development (BSID), now in its second edition. For this it has been extensively revised and the psychometric properties re-evaluated but its predictive value for later intellectual function in preterm populations is not yet well established. This scale produces a mental development index (MDI – to reflect cognitive function) and the psychomotor development index (PDI – more focused on motor function). Many observers simply report the MDI, which is standardised to a mean of 100 and SD of 15 in the general population.

Using the BSID-II, 30% of the EPICure cohort had scores below 70 and 11% scores below 55, representing -2 and -3 SD respectively. Scores were lower in boys but did not vary with gestational age or plurality.[170] Mean scores were MDI: 82 (SD 15) and PDI 83 (SD 16) for those tested but 9.5% of the children assessed failed to complete the BSID-II. Evaluating mean scores of various studies is fraught with difficulty, mainly because exclusions can seriously modify results. It is important to include the whole population in any assessment. Nominal scores can be allocated to children who perform below the lower level of the test range, but the value given should be stated, as even allocating a score of 50 is very different from allocating a score of -4 SD (equivalent to a score of 40), as is often done.

Correction for prematurity is usually applied up to 2 years but may be extended to 3 years for extremely preterm children where the correction still makes around 10% difference, depending on gestational age (Fig. 3.3). This correction is controversial as some prefer to assess against chronological age-related norms, claiming that this more correctly identifies those with developmental problems, but as increasingly preterm children survive this has fallen out of practice. Correcting for prematurity once the child is in the education system, where he is compared to his peers, is unnecessary.

A formal developmental assessment is expensive and time-consuming for service or research purposes, particularly where a categorisation around one figure is required. Increasingly 18–24-month assessments are being used as outcome measures for randomised trials and their inclusion adds very significantly to the

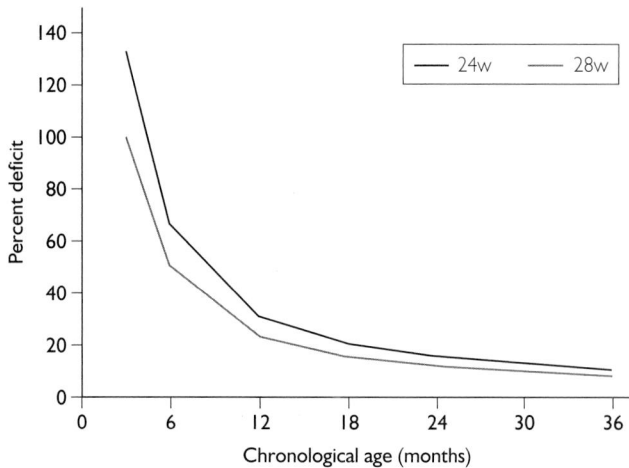

Fig. 3.3 Percent deficit in developmental terms produced by using chronological age rather than corrected age for 24- and 28-week babies.

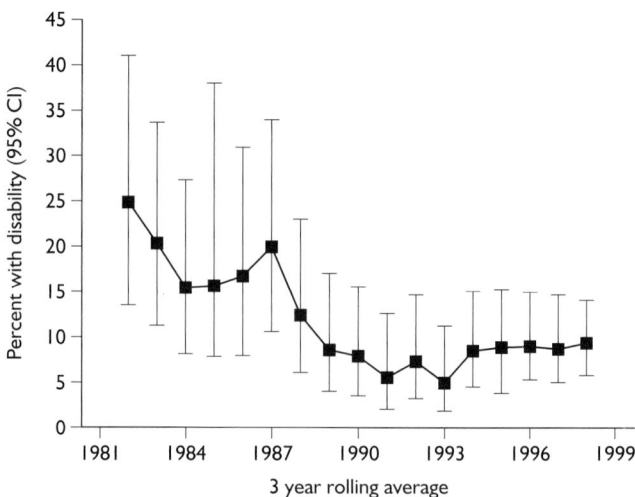

Fig. 3.4 Disability rates among children of less than 1000 g birthweight cared for by the Nottingham Neonatal Service 1981–99 (rolling 3-year averages with 95% confidence intervals shown). From the Nottingham Neonatal Service Passport Scheme, with permission of Dr E Knight Jones.

cost of the project. We have recently validated an adapted parent report questionnaire[139] against the Bayley Scales at 2 years in 64 very preterm children.[81] This has high correlation ($r = 0.68$) and good diagnostic utility (sensitivity 81%; specificity 81%) for a Bayley Scales mental development index of less than 70 and is likely to be as accurate as repeating the developmental assessment with another observer. This may prove a useful tool in the routine follow-up of preterm populations or for use in multicentre trials, where follow-up is important to the evaluation of the safety and efficacy of an intervention but expensive.

There are no particular patterns of developmental impairments associated with prematurity; this reflects the perhaps surprising lack of specific learning impairments at later ages. Behavioural difficulties are particularly difficult to evaluate in infancy but the knowledge that attention deficit hyperactivity disorder (ADHD) is a persistent and constant finding in later studies encourages assessment in infancy. Sadly there are no well respected measures that help to identify children at risk, although direct observation in the clinic does seem to identify a significant proportion of children with inattention and distractibility.[10]

Current follow-up practice

Our present practice in Nottingham is to review children in the neonatal follow-up clinic until 2 years corrected for prematurity who fall into one of three distinct groups – babies of 30 weeks gestation or less, babies with a birthweight of less than 1001 g and babies who have demonstrated neonatal encephalopathy. Follow-up is performed by the attending neonatologist at birth. At 1 and 2 years a health status questionnaire (Table 3.2) is completed and neurological signs are reported. At 2 years we use a parent-report measure, as described above,[81] to quantify developmental status alongside an informal developmental assessment, as this appears as diagnostic as a formal assessment. At 2 years all children in follow-up are referred to their locality community paediatrician who reviews the child through to early school age and is responsible for ensuring that the school is aware of the potential for learning difficulties.

It should be stressed that this is an environment where we have good community-based family support from health visitors, primary care physicians and community paediatric staff. There is also good support from and easy access to advice from dietetics and locality-based physiotherapy and other family support teams for children with special needs. In other health systems alternative arrangements may be necessary.

Although this system is a relatively new development, children had been followed locally since 1981 using a standard follow-up system with referral to a single developmental paediatrician at 12 months of age. Smoothing out year-on-year variation by using 3-year rolling averages, there is a fall in disability rates from 1981 through to the mid 1990s (X_2 (trend): $p < 0.0001$) (Fig. 3.4). Following this, the prevalence of disability in this unit-based population has remained constant at around 9% of babies of less than 1001 g birthweight.

Interventions to improve outcomes for very preterm babies

The knowledge that developmental and cognitive disadvantage are associated with preterm birth has prompted several important efforts to provide developmental or educational therapy. Many of the strategies stem from the early attempts to enhance developmental outcome for children with Down's syndrome. Although referral to early education schemes is commonplace, the evidence that these schemes provide benefit in the long term is wanting.[5,128] Nonetheless these schemes may be essential methods of supporting families who are particularly disadvantaged, in whom there are without doubt impressive short-term gains, particularly in the families of heavier and more mature preterm children,[5] but the evidence for long term benefit in terms of cognitive and learning ability is still lacking.[97]

A formal review of this area is outside the remit of this chapter and the reader is referred to key publications.[62,97,128] The literature is further complicated by a range of short-term neonatal interventions for which methodological issues dominate the interpretation of the results. Well-designed randomised trials of key interventions are required in this area, where subtle effects are particularly sensitive to a range of confounding factors.

School age outcomes

Cognitive function

Despite the early assertions of pioneers in the field, it is clear that prematurity results in significant cognitive disadvantages for surviving populations. This does not mean that all preterm children have learning impairment and will go on to fail at school but that as a group such outcomes occur more frequently. Interpreting the reports of cognitive disadvantage requires close examination of the individual studies and an understanding of the methodology. In particular, the base population must be clearly defined. Several studies have excluded those with severe disability, or those requiring separate special education, in order to concentrate on teasing out the factors that determine outcome in those with less obvious disability.

Bhutta and colleagues have systematically reviewed school age outcomes.[12] They identified 15 case-control studies of VLBW children reporting cognitive data after 5 years of age with attrition rates of less than 30%. They pooled data from 1556 cases and 1720 controls. The weighted mean difference for individual studies when children unable to undertake tests of cognition were excluded ranged from 7.4 to 16.7 IQ points in favour of controls, with an overall weighted mean difference of 10.2 points (95% CI 9–11.5). There was a tendency within the preterm group for scores to be higher with higher birthweight and gestation. There were no differences between US-based and non-US-based studies or between hospital- and population-based data, or with age at assessment.

The relationship between cognitive function and gestation may not be linear as is suggested above. In the Bavarian Longitudinal Study there was no relationship between gestational age and IQ at 33 weeks gestation or more, but a progressive reduction in cognitive scores for each week from 32 to 27 weeks.[167] Similarly, IQ fell with birthweight (in 250 g groups) below 1500 g. In gestational age terms this represents an average deficit of approximately 2.5 IQ points per week below 33 weeks gestational age. This predicts a 20 point deficit for babies of 24 weeks gestation. Considering the EPICure 6-year assessments (Fig. 3.5), which used the same cognitive assessment, confirms this prediction. If IQ is significantly related to gestational age, then interpretation of test scores for birthweight-based cohorts becomes much more difficult.

Cognitive function may also be assessed using school achievement tests, which in essence show very similar relationships between standardised scores as IQ tests.[16] In whichever area a test is applied, there is a significant excess of ex-preterm children who score in the abnormal range. The concept of specific learning

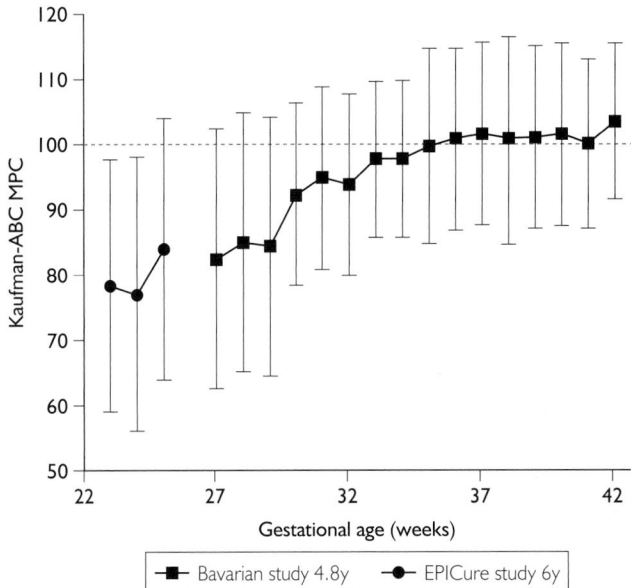

Fig. 3.5 Mean (SD) mental processing composite of the Kaufman-ABC for children in the Bavarian Longitudinal Study (births in 1985)[167] and in the EPICure study (births in 1995).

difficulties has been explored with respect to prematurity. These are usually defined as school achievement in specific areas below that predicted by cognitive assessment. Despite one observation that children of less than 801 g birthweight had an excess of specific learning difficulties,[164] other studies have not replicated this and, indeed, there are no real consistent findings across educational studies to support this, as is our experience.[16,102] In general, the learning difficulties experienced by preterm children are in proportion to their underlying cognitive deficit and the finding of children with intelligence in the normal range but specific functional loss in a particular educational area occurs in a similar frequency to the normal population. As expected, studies indicate a higher proportion of very preterm children with special educational needs, requiring extra support in the classroom, individualised education plans and, where it is practised, education at levels below age-matched peers. This translates into a slight but significant disadvantage in General Certificate of Secondary Education (GCSE) results in VLBW children[119] and to fewer VLBW adults completing higher education.[63]

This cognitive impairment suggests a fundamental underlying problem with brain organisation that may show as disadvantage in multiple areas and may also be related to the adverse behavioural traits described below. Careful, broad educational assessment is indicated for all very preterm children.[11]

Behaviour and psychology

Behavioural assessment is most frequently performed using parent- or teacher-report questionnaires. In the USA and in many European studies the Child Behavior Checklist (CBCL) is used. This is age-banded and provides a way of comparing outcome across different health systems. It is a long questionnaire (over

100 items) and has not been popular in with UK populations. The Strengths and Difficulties Questionnaire has proved more so, providing a shorter, more parent-friendly instrument that has excellent cross-cultural validity. Specific targeted instruments for evaluating attentional disorders, such as the Connors Hyper-activity Scale, are sometimes used.

Bhutta and colleagues also systematically reviewed behavioural measures in 16 studies, comparing 1759 VLBW children and 2629 term controls.[12] Equal numbers of studies reported an excess of externalising and internalising behaviours in preterm children and attentional problems were significantly more common in ten of 15 studies. Formal defined criteria to diagnose ADHD were used in six studies (DSM-III, DSM-III-R, DSM-IV). Relative risks of ADHD for preterm children varied from 1.34 to 4.08 with a pooled risk of 2.64 (95% CI 1.85–3.78). The same caveats concerning birthweight-based research reports hold for these as for cognitive data.

An international comparison of behavioural data between four studies of children below 1001 g birthweight in Canada, Germany, the Netherlands and the USA, tested using parent-report versions of the CBCL, identified that total behavioural scores were more prevalent than in normative or comparison children but that this was only significant in European countries.[76] Subscale scores for social, thought and attentional problems were consistently worse by 0.5–1.2 SD in the extremely-low-birthweight (ELBW) group.

In a detailed neuropsychiatric assessment of 137, 12-year-old VLBW children, ADHD, depression, anxiety and antisocial behaviour were assessed using the Child and Adolescent Psychiatric Assessment parent interview and various parent and child questionnaires.[15] Of the VLBW children, 23% met clinical criteria for ADHD compared to 6% of peers (odds ratio (OR) 4.54, 95% CI 2.1–10). VLBW children were also more likely to have generalised anxiety and more symptoms of depression and the odds ratio for any psychiatric disorder was 3.0 (1.7–5.2).

The high risk of psychiatric disorder, particularly ADHD, thus warrants careful assessment for all very preterm children through school age to provide appropriate intervention and support. Most of the studies cited above used parent-report to detect problems. The use of teacher-report is a valuable way of confirming behaviours at school in direct comparison to peers and should generally be used to support these investigations. The extent to which attention deficit forms one of the basic underlying problems in very preterm children remains to be elucidated.

Motor/neurology

Studies of school-age very preterm children consistently demonstrate poor motor performance in terms of manipulative and gross motor skills. A range of tests can be used but the Movement ABC has been most frequently used to quantify the degree of impairment in this group. In a series of three studies from 6–12 years, persistence of motor difficulties was demonstrated[101,102,124] and these findings have been replicated in many other studies.[83,92] Median scores for the preterm group tend to lie at or outside the 75th percentile for comparison groups. Although a significant disability when in infant school, these

impairments are less intrusive and less obvious as teenagers, where motor skills are less prominent aspects of performance.

An alternative approach is to use detailed standardised or semi-standardised neurological assessments, such as the scheme of Touwen.[154] The detection of 'minor neurological' or 'soft' signs correlates well with the more functional assessments (e.g. the TOMI-r[101]).

The high proportion of children with impaired motor skills/minor neurological abnormalities may be considered the mild end of a spectrum of disability of which cerebral palsy is the extreme expression, and have been labelled as 'borderline' or 'minimal' cerebral palsy.[67] One would predict some correlation with brain injuries but the relationship of either motor skills or minor neurological signs to perinatal events or neonatal ultrasound findings is not clear.[83,92] More recent studies have failed to demonstrate a relationship between function and teenage MRI appearances, despite a high rate of abnormal scan findings.

The motor organisational problems may also be reflected in the high frequency of non-right-handedness and less consistent laterality seen in preterm populations, which show poor correlation with other impaired outcomes or brain injury.[100,125]

Growth and medical outcomes

Despite the concentration on neurological, cognitive and psychological outcomes, it is important not to forget that other aspects of somatic development are frequently disturbed by very preterm birth. VLBW and very preterm children remain smaller throughout childhood than their peers. This is very marked in extremely preterm children, where head growth over the first 3 years remains particularly poor and in whom a slim somatotype persists.[169] Very long-term growth is only rarely reported. In one study, bone age and parental heights of 91 VLBW children were integrated to predict adult height.[126] Heights for the VLBW group were lower than matched comparison children. However, TW2 RUS score was also significantly advanced over chronological age, indicating that final height would also be impaired: 17% were predicted to be below the 3rd percentile and 33% below the 10th percentile as adults.

Respiratory outcomes are discussed in Chapter 27 and other medical outcomes, including auditory and ocular outcomes, in Chapters 41 and 34.

Function and quality of life in surviving ex-preterm children

Although the literature and forgoing discussion are really concerned with the measurement of performance, using narrowly focused cognitive or behavioural assessments, such results are difficult to translate into a comprehensive picture of the function of children within society. To a large extent these integrative aspects of outcome may be more important than focussed measures in determining the progress of a neonatal intensive care survivor through life and the functional definition of outcome at 2 years has been recommended as a means of defining outcomes for comparative work.[80]

Once infancy is past, the development of a child progresses on a variety of planes and functional performance becomes more difficult to register a single summative measure, hence the reliance on 'medical disability' (cerebral palsy, cognitive impairment, sensory loss) as an outcome. The issue of measuring functional outcomes has been recently reviewed by Msall and Tremont.[107] These authors develop the thesis that outcome is assessable in four major domains:

- impairment (disturbance at organ level);
- functional limitations of personal activities (self-care, mobility, communication, social interaction);
- disability in social roles (play, school, work);
- societal limitations (difficulty in participating imposed by social framework).

There are now a range of measures to support such assessments in childhood, each with their own strengths and limitations.[107] Several studies have evaluated functional measures in the preschool years (<6 years).[105,106,114,136] For example, in the survivors of the Cryo-ROP study at 5.5 years, all of less than 1251 g birthweight, 87% had normal functional skills compared to their non-disabled peers and the rates of severe functional disability (<−4 SD of peers) rose from 3.7% of those without retinopathy of prematurity to 26% of those with threshold disease.[104]

Functional status was related to visual status at follow-up; in those with favourable visual status, some disability was found in the domains of self-care (25%), communication (22%), motor (5%) and continence (5%), in contrast to those with poor visual outcomes who had disability in 77%, 66%, 43% and 50% of these domains respectively. Such a picture can demonstrate the vulnerability imposed by medical impairments and help the understanding of those factors that impart protection against disability. In the USA the concept of 'kindergarten-readiness' provides a multidimensional categorisation that can reflect the overall functioning of the child.

Although preschool and school-age children have been frequently studied, a few studies are now starting to evaluate outcome in adolescence and adult life. Hack and colleagues evaluated functional outcomes for a group of teenagers born either weighing less than 750 g, weighing 750–1499 g or at term.[65] For the highest-risk group of ELBW infants as teenagers, two-thirds accessed non-routine educational or medical services, three-quarters used medication, spectacles or other aids to daily living (Fig. 3.6) and 86% demonstrated some functional limitation (Fig. 3.6). The intermediate-birthweight group still had significant functional limitation compared to terms but the differences were less marked. That use of medication and contacts with a doctor did not differ significantly between the three groups

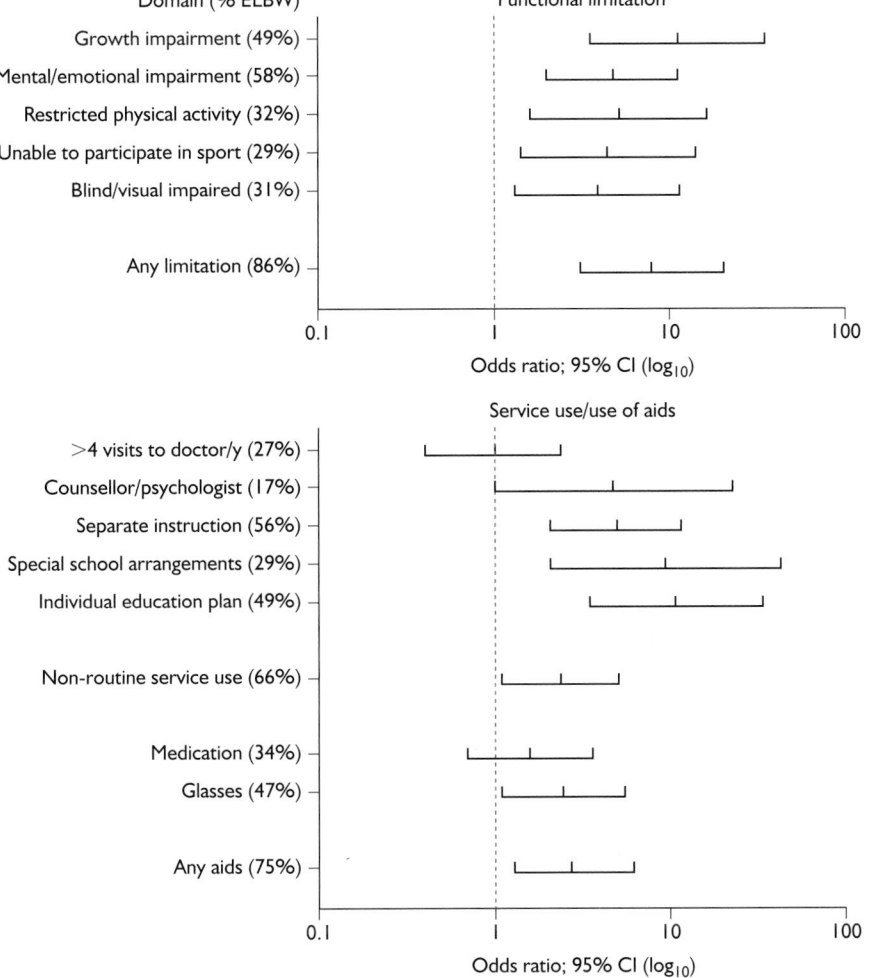

Fig. 3.6 Odds ratio for measures of functional limitation (upper panel) and service/aids use for teenage children of less than 750 g birthweight compared to term comparison children.[65]

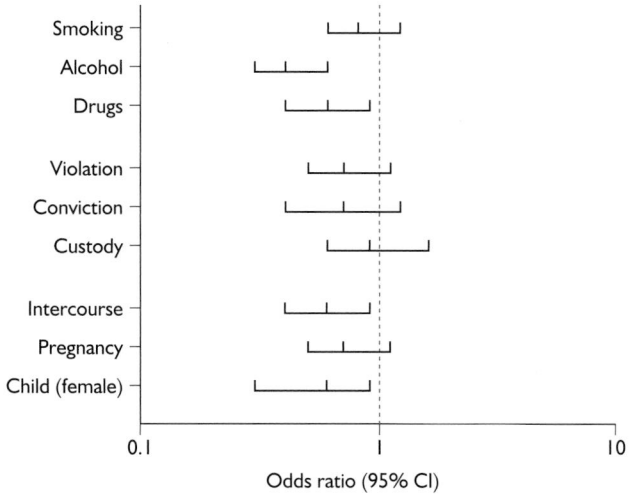

Fig. 3.7 Odds ratio for risk taking behaviours by young adults who were very-low-birthweight compared to normal-birthweight comparison children.[63]

indicates that the needs of these children are generally outside medical practice. Ongoing service provision for this vulnerable group is an important health issue.

The very first reports of outcome in adult life are now starting to appear.[63] Many are the outcomes one might expect from the preceding discussion in terms of lower rates of achievement at school or progression into higher education and higher frequency of low IQ. However, surprisingly, the group of VLBW babies studied by Hack and colleagues were found to engage in less risk-taking behaviour, such as the use of alcohol, tobacco or drugs, and tended to be less likely to come into contact with the law (Fig. 3.7). Whether this represents resilience on the part of the child-cum-adult to engage socially in an appropriate manner or whether this is the end result of the introversion and attentional deficits seen in many of the studies of psychological outcome remains to be determined.[74]

Two groups have explored the quality of life following preterm birth. Using the Health Utilities Index (HUI-2), the health-related quality of life was explored in 141 children of less than 1001 g birthweight at 12–16 years of age.[134] This scale allows quantification of six attributes over a range from 0 (death or the worst outcome) to 1.0 (perfect health). The ELBW children had lower summative index scores than controls (0.87 (SD 0.26) compared to 0.93 (SD 0.11)) over the range of attributes, particularly cognition, sensation, self-care and pain. In contrast, similar proportions scored in the optimal range (scores above 0.95 in 71% and 73% respectively). Despite the excess disability in the ELBW group, a high proportion of ELBW children rated their quality of life similarly to controls. Similarly, self-esteem, measured using the Harter Adolescent Self-Perception Profile, did not differ between ELBW children and controls despite significant differences in academic achievement.[135]

Bjerager and colleagues evaluated quality of life among 18–20-year-old Danish adults born in 1971–4 with a birthweight of less than 1501 g and found no significant differences from controls.[13] This group also evaluated objective and subjective quality of life of 18-year-olds, following birthweights below 1501 g, 1501–2300 g and normal birthweight controls all born in 1980–82.[38] Children with handicap or health problems had lower subjective and objective quality of life scores than other children. Among the remaining children, although subjective scores did not differ between the groups, objective scores for the VLBW group were significantly lower than controls. There appeared to be some improvement in objective scores between the two cohorts but this was less marked in the VLBW group compared to controls.

One can conclude from these two studies that the subjective consideration of quality of life may rise above the objective, performance-driven consideration of impaired function that permeates our description of outcomes. Outcome for young adults who were born very preterm may not be as subjectively bad as is anticipated by the close attention to and concentration on impaired function throughout childhood and the integration of this new generation of survivors into society may be considerably better that anticipated.

Predicting disability in preterm infants

The major determinants of later disability are in essence similar to those predicting perinatal death, often described as part of the continuum of reproductive casualty.[138] Perinatal factors increasing risk of disability include male sex,[88,170] gestational age and birthweight.

The prevalence of disability rises as gestational age and birthweight decrease. The relationship between weight-for-age and disability is much less easy to determine. Tables 3.4 and 3.5 indicate weight- and gestation-based prevalence of disability, respectively, as found in a selection of recent studies. Most queries concern those of extremely low gestation. The prognosis is dependent upon the stage of the process at which the information is to be given. The outcome following live birth at 23 weeks gestation is considerably poorer than the outcome following admission for intensive care, which is poorer than the outcome at 7 days of age. Although it is often stated that individual hospitals should carefully examine their outcomes at these low gestations to use in counselling parents, the confidence with which a statement about outcome is made is low where there are small numbers. For example, in our local population of children born at 30 completed weeks of gestation or less in 1999, the confidence intervals for moderate or severe disability range between 3% and 10% and for those with birthweight below 1001 g between 5% and 18%. EPICure is a population-based outcome study for babies born in the UK and Ireland at 25 completed weeks of gestation or less in 1995.[28,170] Although mortality may have changed since 1995, the order of risk of later disability for a baby remains very similar. These data are displayed in Table 3.5.

The effect of weight-for-gestation is much more difficult to assess. Undoubtedly, fetal growth restriction carries an increased perinatal mortality.[79] At present there is little evidence that intervention with early delivery affects short-term outcomes[9] and it has been possible to construct mortality-based charts

Table 3.4 Details of rates of cerebral palsy in populations defined by birthweight

Author	Area	Birth year	Age (y)	No. studied	Birth-weight (g)	No. seen	IQ < 70 n (%)	Blind n (%)	Deaf n (%)	Severe CP n (%)	Overall n (%)
Lefebvre et al 1988[89]	Montreal, Canada	1976–79	5–9	44	701–1000	44	12 (27)*	0	3 (7)	1 (4)	14 (32)
					1500–1999	114				6 (5)	10 (9)
Forfar et al 1994[56]	Edinburgh, UK	1978–79	1–9	149	1000–1499	32	7 (5)	4 (3)	3 (2)	0	1 (3)
					<1000	3					
					1000–1250	65				1 (33)	1 (33)
Robertson et al 1994[130]	Edmonton, Canada	78–79	1.5–3	82	750–999	15	2 (2)	4 (5)	3 (4)	5 (6)	6 (7)
					500–749	2					
		88–89	1.5–3	197	1000–1250	100	2 (1)	6 (3)	7 (4)	7 (4)	10 (5)
					750–999	70					
					500–749	27					
Doyle 2001[40]	Melbourne, Australia	79–80	14	79	500–999	79	6 (8)	5 (7)	4 (5)	2 (3)	11 (13.9)
Astbury et al 1990[10]	Victoria, Australia	79–81	2	56	≤1000	56	5 (8.9)	1 (2)	2 (4)	2 (4)	5 (8.9)
Anon 1991[6]	Melbourne, Australia	79–80	2	89	≤1000	89	12 (13.5)	6 (6.7)	3 (3.4)	3 (3.4)	24 (27)
		85–87	2	212	≤1000	212	12 (5.7)	9 (4.2)	1 (0.5)	2 (1)	24 (11.4)
O'Shea et al 1997[111]	N. Carolina, USA	79–84	1	24	501–800	24	3 (13)†	2 (8)		3 (13)‡	
		84–89	1	61	501–800	63	12 (20)†	0		12 (19)‡	
		89–94	1	124	501–800	129	8 (7)†	4 (3)		9 (7)‡	
Piecuch et al 1997[121]	San Francisco, USA	79–85	4.6	193	500–999	193	31 (16)§	1 (0.5)	1 (0.5)	19.3 (10)‡	
		86–88	4.6	113	500–999	113	17 (15)§	4 (3.5)	0	9 (8)‡	
		89–91	4.6	136	500–999	136	13 (10)§	0	0	13.6 (10)‡	
Cooke 1999[26]	Liverpool, England	82–85	3	411	<1501	411				45 (10.9)‡	
		86–89	3	387	<1501	387				42 (10.8)‡	
		90–93	3	398	<1501	398				29 (7.3)‡	
Hack et al 1994[64]	Ohio, USA	82–86	6.7	68	<750	68	14 (21)	4 (6)	1 (1.5)	6 (9)‡	
				65	750–1500	65	5 (8)	1 (2)	1 (1.5)	4 (6)‡	
Hack et al 2000[66]	Ohio, USA	82–88	0.7–1.7	49	500–750	49					
		90–92	0.7–1.7	39	500–750	39					
Sauve et al 1998[140]	Alberta, Canada	83–94	3	13	<500	13	8 (61.5)	2 (15.4)	1 (7.6)	2 (15.4)	9 (69)
Dunin-Wasowicz et al 2000[45]	Warsaw, Poland	85–89	7–11	38	<1500	38		2 (5.2)	1 (2.8)	11 (28.9)‡	
		90–94	2–5	51	<1500	51		9 (17.6)	2 (3.9)	18 (35.2)‡	
Salokorpi et al 2001[137]	Finland	91–94	4	142	<1500	142		0		27 (17)‡	
Vohr et al 2000[159]	USA	93–94	1.5–1.9	1151	901–1000	295	86 (31)	3 (1)	20 (7)	45 (15)‡	
					801–900	272	92 (35)	2 (0.7)	24 (9)	42 (15)‡	
					701–800	224	90 (42)	5 (2)	20 (9)	38 (17)‡	
					601–700	202	78 (41)	8 (4)	27 (14)	42 (21)‡	
					501–600	94	42 (45)	1 (1)	10 (11)	16 (17)‡	
					401–500	14	4 (31)	2 (14)	1 (7)	4 (29)‡	
Valkama et al 2000[156]	Oulu, Finland	93–95	1.5	49	<1500	49				5 (10.2)‡	

* DQ < 85; † MDI < 68; ‡ All CP; § IQ < 79.

CP = cerebral palsy.

Table 3.5 Details of rates of disability in populations defined by gestational age

Author	Area	Birth year	Gestation (weeks)	Age at follow-up (years)	Population (n followed/births)	Gestation	n	IQ < 70 n (%)	Blind n (%)	Deaf n (%)	Severe CP n (%)	Overall with any severe disability n (%)
Walker and Patel 1987[160]	Dundee, UK	80-84	26-28	1.5+	24/24	<26	1	0	0	0	0	0
						26-27	5	0	0	0	1 (20)	1 (20)
						28	18	1 (6)	2 (11)	0	2 (11)	5 (28)
Whyte et al 1993[165]	Toronto, Canada	82-87	23-26	1.5	322/322	23	12	1 (8)	2 (17)	0	2 (17)	5 (42)
						24	49	11 (22)	11 (22)	6 (12)	7 (14)	35 (71)
						25	109	18 (17)	4 (4)	0	8 (7)	30 (26)
						26	152	13 (9)	5 (3)	3 (2)	10 (7)	31 (20)
Jacobs et al 2000[78]	Canada	82-87	23-26	1.5-2	239/249	23-26	239	46 (19)	19 (8)	12 (5)	12 (5)	89 (37)
		90-94	23-26	1.5-2	274/305	23-26	274	34 (12)	6 (2)	10 (4)	12 (4)	62 (23)
Emsley et al 1998[48]	Manchester, UK	84-89	23-25	3.3-9.6	24/26	23-25	24	3 (13)	1 (4)	2 (8)	5 (21)	11 (46)
		90-94	23-25	2.2-6.1	40/40	23-25	40	6 (15)	7 (18)	1 (3)	7 (18)	20 (50)
Lefebvre et al 1996[90]	Montreal, Canada	87-92	23-28	1.5	217/254	24	9	3 (33)	1 (11)	1 (11)	0	5 (56)
						25	24	5 (21)	0	0	4 (17)	9 (38)
						26	40	9 (22)	0	0	5 (12)	14 (35)
						27	72	9 (12)	0	0	3 (4)	12 (17)
						28	72	9 (12)	1 (1)	1 (1)	5 (7)	16 (22)
Finnstrom et al 1998[54]	Stockholm, Sweden	90-92	23-27	3	362/369	23-24	29	4 (14)*	16(4)	1†	4 (14)	
						25-26	148	14 (9)*			15 (10)	66 (18)
						≥27	185	6 (3)*			6 (3)	
Piecuch et al 1997[121]	San Francisco, USA	90-94	24-26	1	86/94	24	18	7 (39)	0		2 (11)	
						25	30	9 (30)	1 (3)	2 (2)	6 (20)	35 (41)
						26	38	4 (11)	0		4 (11)	
Doyle 2001[40]	Victoria, Australia	91-92	23-27	5	221/225	23	5	2 (40)‡	4 (1.8)	2 (0.9)	15 (6.8)	65 (29)
						24	21	7 (33)‡				
						25	51	13 (25)‡				
						26	71	17 (24)‡				
						27	77	5 (6)‡				
Wood et al 2000[170]	UK and Ireland	1995	23-25	2.5	283/308	≤23	26	7 (27)	7 (2)	2 (1)	2 (8)	9 (35)
						24	90	17 (19)			11 (12)	31 (34)
						25	167	29 (17)			15 (9)	40 (24)

Key: *Scheffzek category 3-4; †Treacher–Collins syndrome; ‡'major disability'.

which account for weight-for gestation at birth.[41] However, not all babies who are small for gestational age have fetal growth restriction; a significant proportion will be constitutionally small. The risk of cerebral palsy is significantly raised in the face of growth restriction where delivery occurs between 34 and 37 weeks of gestation but any increased risk of cerebral palsy with fetal growth restriction below 34 weeks is lost in the general increased risk following very preterm birth.[14] From cohort studies there is some suggestion that increasing signs of fetal decompensation are associated with poorer cognitive or motor function on testing at school age[93,94,141] but definitive studies are difficult to do when fetal effects of hypoxia on the developing brain are relatively difficult to quantify (see pp. 1129–30).

Prediction of outcome using neonatal cerebral ultrasound

Soon after it was recognised that intraventricular haemorrhage (IVH) was detectable using transfontanellar cranial ultrasound,[23] it was initially thought that disability would be related to the severity of the lesion detected, something that seemed to be deducible from early studies.[152] The technical aspects of the ultrasound examination have improved greatly since these first studies, improving our understanding of the significance of these changes. In particular, the development of higher-frequency transducers (7.5 MHz and higher) has led to better definition of changes in the parenchyma that would not have been identified using 5 MHz sector scanning probes or linear arrays used in earlier studies. There is intense interest in the possibility that the prediction of cerebral palsy may be possible, as this is the outcome that most concerns parents and carers alike. Such information could be of value in determining the balance for continuing intensive care, to set in place early support mechanisms for parents and perhaps even as a basis for early intervention.[161]

The technique of cerebral ultrasound and its interpretation are discussed in Chapters 19 and 41. Although there are many pitfalls in the use and interpretation of ultrasound findings, used with caution it can be a useful prognostic tool for reassurance and early warning.

For ease of description, outcome will be considered in the following categories:

- consistently normal scans;
- germinal matrix–intraventricular haemorrhage (GMH-IVH);
- ventriculomegaly;
- PVL;
- IVH with parenchymal echodensity.

Normal and disabled outcomes are summarised in Table 3.6.

Consistently normal scans

Rennie has reviewed 18 studies, in which births spanned 1979 to 1992, during which time period technology and resolution of images improved.[127] Among these 2290 babies with consistently normal ultrasound findings a disability free outcome occurred in 89% (95% CI 88–90%). Three studies reported data from 1985 onwards with a disability free outcome in 854 of 931 babies (92% (90–93%)) and major 'handicap' in 5% (3–6%). The results of these summary statistics should be treated with caution as the studies were not comparable in terms of populations or of definitions of outcome. Nonetheless, a consistently normal scan carries a risk of serious disability of less than 10% at follow-up.

Germinal matrix–intraventricular haemorrhage

There is general agreement that an uncomplicated subependymal or germinal matrix haemorrhage (GMH) that resolves is not associated with an increased risk of later disability. Among 15 studies including 626 children with isolated GMH, 83% had disability-free outcomes (80–86%) and 13% (10–15%) had major handicap.[129] These data are subject to the same caveats and all reports comprise infants born before the mid-1980s. IVH and GMH are often difficult to distinguish, and it is likely that an uncomplicated IVH that resolves has a similarly good prognosis. One particular caveat is that the large New Jersey study suggested an

Table 3.6 Proportion of children with normal or abnormal outcome defined by neonatal cranial ultrasound findings

Scan classification	No. of studies	No. of babies	Normal outcome (%)	Disabled outcome (%)
Normal scan	3[123,127,163*]	931	92 (90–93)	5 (3–6) (handicap)
Uncomplicated GMH-IVH	7[20,24,86,113,150,151,155]	168	88 (82–92)	7 (4–12) (handicap)
Non progressive ventriculomegaly	10[3,7,24,60,61,87,113,142,148,163]	226		34 (28–40) (handicap)
Ventricles >95th percentile + 4 mm	1[7]	112	10 (5–17)	90 (83–95) (abnormal)
Hydrocephalus with shunt	10[3,17,24,49,51,53,77,95,113,142]	236		59 (53–65) (handicap)
Bilateral cystic PVL	12[24,34,50,52,59,73,103,120,122,132,162,163]	155		88 (82–93) (CP)
Intraparenchymal echodensities >1 cm diameter	1[37]	45	38 (25–52)	62 (48–75) (CP)

CP = cerebral palsy.
* includes only studies with births in 1985 or later.

increase in risk of disabling cerebral palsy in this group to 25% (18–32%; OR 3.5; 1.7–6.9), although the risk following white matter injury (echolucencies or ventricular enlargement) was considerably greater (OR 15; 7.6–31).[123] More recent studies using MRI would suggest that some of this discrepancy relates to unidentified white matter injury (see below).

Ventriculomegaly

The old Papile grading of IVH classed haemorrhages as 'grade III' if an IVH caused distension of the ventricle. However, the terms 'distension' or 'enlargement' are often not tightly defined. Levene has defined percentiles for ventricular size, which demonstrate an increase with postmenstrual age[91] and have been used as definitions for ventriculomegaly (4 mm >95th percentile for postmenstrual age) in studies of management options. Without clear definitions for the assessment of ventricular size, interpretation of data is difficult. Some ventricular enlargement will result from atrophy of the white matter secondary to PVL and is likely to have a different prognosis from transient or progressive ventriculomegaly.

The ventriculomegaly trial provides useful prognostic information. Babies were randomised to expectant versus intermittent tapping when ventricular size progressed beyond 4 mm above the 95th percentile of Levene. Only 11 of 112 were considered normal at 2 years.[7] Ventriculomegaly appears to have worse prognosis in the presence of parenchymal changes or fits.[7] From 10 studies identified by Rennie, there were 226 cases with non-progressive ventriculomegaly, of whom 76 (34%; 28–40%) had major disability at follow-up and in 10 further studies of outcome following shunted hydrocephalus 140/240 babies (59%; 53–65%) had poor outcomes.

Periventricular leukomalacia

The presence of cystic periventricular leukomalacia (cPVL) is the most powerful predictor of cerebral palsy in very preterm children. To a large extent all the forgoing lesions act as proxy indicators for risk of white and grey matter injury, whereas cPVL indicates the end stage of a process where injury has occurred in the white matter. The area and periventricular zone affected by cystic change is, however, of importance in determining prognosis.

The presence of subependymal pseudocysts should be distinguished from that of PVL. Pseudocysts appear as a short string of 'bead-like' cysts lying along the floor of the lateral ventricle or sometimes in the mid zone along the inferolateral margin of the ventricle. They are immediately adjacent to and separated from the ventricle by a thin wall and must not be confused with resolving GMH or with PVL. The cysts of cPVL lie within the white matter and as they develop initially they are separated from the ventricle by a bridge of tissue. Pseudocysts are of no prognostic importance.

Single isolated cysts and cystic changes confined to the frontal zone appear to have better outcome. Although only small numbers have been reported in the literature, most survivors appear to be normal at follow-up.

Cysts that are bilateral and in the occipital zone have a very high risk of later cerebral palsy. In many published reports almost all the cases of cerebral palsy had bilateral occipital cPVL. In 12 studies, 137/155 cases (88% (82–93%)) with bilateral cPVL had cerebral palsy at follow-up. Children with extensive cPVL are also at particular risk of central visual impairment or visuoperceptual problems.[22,46,157]

Cystic change in the intermediate (parietal) zone has a less clear outcome, presumably depending on the degree of injury to the more critical posterior areas; in two studies approximately 50% of babies with frontoparietal or parietal changes developed cerebral palsy compared to none when changes were confined to the frontal zone and all when extended into the occipital zones.[50,59]

In one large study, where cysts were defined as greater than 2 cm diameter, all were associated with cerebral palsy and where the anteroposterior extent of cPVL was more than 2 cm the outlook was particularly poor, all eight cases developing spastic quadriplegia.[132]

Intraventricular haemorrhage with parenchymal echodensity

The early literature confused the occurrence of focal parenchymal haemorrhage and periventricular leukomalacia as 'grade IV' periventricular haemorrhage. In about 10–15% babies with GMH-IVH, unilateral or bilateral parenchymal changes are seen in association with an IVH, which are frequently termed parenchymal extensions and are more common in the extremely preterm infant.[35] These are thought to result from venous infarction[58] due to obstruction to the terminal veins which drain the white matter and lie inferior to the germinal matrix. Careful frequent ultrasound examination allows these to be distinguished from PVL. In the only recent series, 55 of 88 children survived with parenchymal lesions, 45 had lesions more than 1 cm diameter and 38 (69%) did not develop cerebral palsy,[37] which represents a much improved prognosis over older reports of 'grade IV' PVH.

Other lesions in preterm children

There has been debate about the significance of persistent echodensities in the periventricular region, with or without associated GMH-IVH, which do not develop into cystic lesions. De Vries and colleagues have suggested that changes that persist for more than 7 days may be of clinical significance.[36] Several studies have suggested that these appearances may be related to transient neurological abnormalities in infancy or to mild spastic diplegia, and to motor impairments in childhood. Ultrasound is not perhaps the best modality for studying these more subtle changes in brain appearances, as the detection of such lesions is highly machine- and operator-dependent; MRI may be necessary before the significance of these findings becomes clearer.[21,158]

The role of magnetic resonance imaging

MRI is increasingly available for preterm infants during their initial illness. The improved resolution and different imaging modalities provide more detailed information than ultrasound. For example, more cysts are identified using MRI than ultrasound[21,144] and imaging at term-equivalent age allows for better prediction of motor problems by assessing the posterior limb of the internal capsule.[131] Studies to date are difficult to summarise because of small numbers and the range of findings on MRI. Careful studies are required to elucidate the import of more subtle changes on cerebral ultrasound, such as periventricular echodensities that have clear MRI correlates.[158] Quantitative techniques have demonstrated reduced cortical grey matter volume with relatively mild white matter changes, and this reduction was greater in those with ultrasound-identified white matter lesions. Outcome data are awaited for this group.

Studies of late MRI appearances in relation to outcome have not shown good correlation between brain injuries or regional measures of size.[27] However, measures of regional brain volumes in later childhood show significant differences from term controls and, compared to conventional measures of acquired brain injury, hippocampal and caudate nucleus volumes seem to be better associated with subtle measures of outcome, such as cognitive and attentional measures.[1,117]

The pervasive insult provided by preterm birth and subsequent development outside the womb has very significant effects on brain organisation and development that await elucidation.

References

1. Abernethy L J, Palaniappan M, Cooke RW 2002 Quantitative magnetic resonance imaging of the brain in survivors of very low birth weight. Archives of Disease in Childhood 87: 279–283
2. Accardo P J 1982 Freud on diplegia. Commentary and translation. American Journal of Diseases of Children 136: 452–456
3. Allan W C, Riviello J J Jr 1992 Perinatal cerebrovascular disease in the neonate. Parenchymal ischemic lesions in term and preterm infants. Pediatric Clinics of North America 39: 621–650
4. Amiel-Tison C, Grenier A 1986 Neurological assessment in the first year of life. Oxford University Press, Oxford
5. Anon 1990 Enhancing the outcomes of low-birth-weight, premature infants. A multisite, randomized trial. The Infant Health and Development Program. Journal of the American Medical Association 263: 3035–3042
6. Anon 1991 Eight-year outcome in infants with birth weight of 500 to 999 grams: continuing regional study of 1979 and 1980 births. Victorian Infant Collaborative Study Group. Journal of Pediatrics 118: 761–767
7. Anon 1994 Randomised trial of early tapping in neonatal posthaemorrhagic ventricular dilatation: results at 30 months. Ventriculomegaly Trial Group. Archives of Disease in Childhood Fetal and Neonatal Edition 70: F129–F136
8. Anon 1995 Disability and perinatal care: report of two working groups. NPEU and Oxford Health Authority, Oxford
9. Anon 2003 The GRIT Study Group. A randomised trial of timed delivery for the compromised preterm fetus: short term outcomes and Bayesian interpretation. British Journal of Obstetrics and Gynaecology 110: 27–32
10. Astbury J, Orgill A A, Bajuk B, Yu V Y 1990 Neurodevelopmental outcome, growth and health of extremely low-birthweight survivors: how soon can we tell? Developmental Medicine and Child Neurology 32: 582–589
11. Aylward G P 2002 Cognitive and neuropsychological outcomes: more than IQ scores. Mental Retardation and Developmental Disabilities Research Reviews 8: 234–240
12. Bhutta A T, Cleves M A, Casey P H, Cradock M M, Anand K J 2002 Cognitive and behavioral outcomes of school-aged children who were born preterm: a meta-analysis. Journal of the American Medical Association 288: 728–737
13. Bjerager M, Steensberg J, Greisen G 1995 Quality of life among young adults born with very low birthweights. Acta Paediatrica 84: 1339–1343
14. Blair E, Stanley F 1990 Intrauterine growth and spastic cerebral palsy. I. Association with birth weight for gestational age. American Journal of Obstetrics and Gynecology 162: 229–237
15. Botting N, Powls A, Cooke R W, Marlow N 1997 Attention deficit hyperactivity disorders and other psychiatric outcomes in very low birthweight children at 12 years. Journal of Child Psychology and Psychiatry 38: 931–941
16. Botting N, Powls A, Cooke R W, Marlow N 1998 Cognitive and educational outcome of very-low-birthweight children in early adolescence. Developmental Medicine and Child Neurology 40: 652–660
17. Boynton B R, Boynton C A, Merritt T A, Vaucher Y E, James H E, Bejar R F 1986 Ventriculoperitoneal shunts in low birth weight infants with intracranial hemorrhage: neurodevelopmental outcome. Neurosurgery 18: 141–145
18. British Association of Perinatal Medicine 2001 Standards for hospitals providing intensive and high dependency care. BAPM, London: available on line at: www.bapm.org/publications.htm
19. Budin P 1907 The nursling. Caxton Press, London
20. Catto-Smith A G, Yu V Y, Bajuk B, Orgill A A, Astbury J 1985 Effect of neonatal periventricular haemorrhage on neurodevelopmental outcome. Archives of Disease in Childhood 60: 8–11
21. Childs A M, Cornette L, Ramenghi L A et al 2001 Magnetic resonance and cranial ultrasound characteristics of periventricular white matter abnormalities in newborn infants. Clinical Radiology 56: 647–655
22. Cioni G, Fazzi B, Ipata A E, Canapicchi R, van Hof-van Duin J 1996 Correlation between cerebral visual impairment and magnetic resonance imaging in children with neonatal encephalopathy. Developmental Medicine and Child Neurology 38: 120–132
23. Cooke R 1979 Ultrasound examination of neonatal heads. Lancet 2: 38
24. Cooke R W 1987 Early and late cranial ultrasonographic appearances and outcome in very low birthweight infants. Archives of Disease in Childhood 62: 931–937
25. Cooke R W 1993 Annual audit of three year outcome in very low birthweight infants. Archives of Disease in Childhood 69: 295–298
26. Cooke R W 1999 Trends in incidence of cranial ultrasound lesions and cerebral palsy in very low birthweight infants 1982–93. Archives of Disease in Childhood Fetal and Neonatal Edition 80: F115–F117
27. Cooke R W, Abernethy L J 1999 Cranial magnetic resonance imaging and school performance in very low birth weight infants in adolescence. Archives of Disease in Childhood Fetal and Neonatal Edition 81: F116–F121
28. Costeloe K, Hennessy E, Gibson A T, Marlow N, Wilkinson A R 2000 The EPICure study: outcomes to discharge from hospital for infants born at the threshold of viability. Pediatrics 106: 659–671
29. Cross K W 1973 Cost of preventing retrolental fibroplasia? Lancet 2: 954–956
30. Davies A 1997 A critical review of neonatal hearing screening in the detection of congenital hearing impairment. Health Technology Assessment 1: 75
31. De Groot L, de Groot C J, Hopkins B 1997 An instrument to measure independent walking: are there differences between preterm and fullterm infants? Journal of Child Neurology 12: 37–41
32. De Groot L, Hopkins B, Touwen B 1995 Muscle power, sitting unsupported and trunk rotation in pre-term infants. Early Human Development 43: 37–46
33. De Groot L, Hopkins B, Touwen B 1997 Motor asymmetries in preterm infants at 18 weeks corrected age and outcomes at 1 year. Early Human Development 48: 35–46
34. De Vries L S, Connell J A, Dubowitz L M, Oozeer R C, Dubowitz V, Pennock J M 1987 Neurological, electrophysiological and MRI abnormalities in infants with extensive cystic leukomalacia. Neuropediatrics 18: 61–66
35. De Vries L S, Groenendaal F 2002 Neuroimaging in the preterm infant. Mental Retardation and Developmental Disabilities Research Reviews 8: 273–280
36. De Vries L S, Regev R, Pennock J M, Wigglesworth J S, Dubowitz L M 1988 Ultrasound evolution and later outcome of infants with periventricular densities. Early Human Development 16: 225–233
37. De Vries L S, Roelants-van Rijn A M, Rademaker K J, Van Haastert I C, Beek F J, Groenendaal F 2001 Unilateral parenchymal haemorrhagic infarction in the preterm infant. European Journal of Paediatric Neurology 5: 139–149
38. Dinesen S J, Greisen G 2001 Quality of life in young adults with very low birth weight. Archives of Disease in Childhood Fetal and Neonatal Edition 85: F165–F169
39. Downs J A, Edwards A D, McCormick D C, Roth S C, Stewart A L 1991 Effect of intervention on development of hip posture in very preterm babies. Archives of Disease in Childhood 66: 797–801
40. Doyle L W 2001 Outcome at 5 years of age of children 23 to 27 weeks' gestation: refining the prognosis. Pediatrics 108: 134–141
41. Draper E S, Manktelow B, Field D J, James D 1999 Prediction of survival for preterm births by weight and gestational age: retrospective population based study. British Medical Journal 319: 1093–1097
42. Drillien C M 1958 Growth and development of a group of children of very low birthweight. Archives of Disease in Childhood 33: 10–18

43. Drillien C M 1972 Abnormal neurologic signs in the first year of life in low-birthweight infants: possible prognostic significance. Developmental Medicine and Child Neurology 14: 575–584

44. Drillien C M 1980 Low-birthweight Children at Early School-age: a Longitudinal Study. Developmental Medicine and Child Neurology 22: 26–47

45. Dunin-Wasowicz D, Rowecka-Trzebicka K, Milewska-Bobula B et al 2000 Risk factors for cerebral palsy in very-low-birthweight infants in the 1980s and 1990s. Journal of Child Neurology 15: 417–420

46. Eken P, Jansen G H, Groenendaal F, Rademaker K J, de Vries L S 1994 Intracranial lesions in the fullterm infant with hypoxic ischaemic encephalopathy: ultrasound and autopsy correlation. Neuropediatrics 25: 301–307

47. El-Metwally D, Vohr B, Tucker R 2000 Survival and neonatal morbidity at the limits of viability in the mid 1990s: 22 to 25 weeks. Journal of Pediatrics 137: 616–622

48. Emsley H C, Wardle S P, Sims D G, Chiswick M L, D'Souza S W 1998 Increased survival and deteriorating developmental outcome in 23 to 25 week old gestation infants, 1990–4 compared with 1984–9. Archives of Disease in Childhood Fetal and Neonatal Edition 78: F99–F104

49. Etches P C, Ward T F, Bhui P S, Peters K L, Robertson C M 1987 Outcome of shunted posthaemorrhagic hydrocephalus in premature infants. Pediatric Neurology 3: 136–140

50. Fawer C L, Diebold P, Calame A 1987 Periventricular leucomalacia and neurodevelopmental outcome in preterm infants. Archives of Disease in Childhood 62: 30–36

51. Fazzi E, Lanzi G, Gerardo A, Ometto A, Orcesi S, Rondini G 1992 Neurodevelopmental outcome in very-low-birth-weight infants with or without periventricular haemorrhage and/or leucomalacia. Acta Paediatrica 81: 808–811

52. Fazzi E, Orcesi S, Caffi L et al 1994 Neurodevelopmental outcome at 5–7 years in preterm infants with periventricular leukomalacia. Neuropediatrics 25: 134–139

53. Fernell E, Hagberg G, Hagberg B 1990 Infantile hydrocephalus – the impact of enhanced preterm survival. Acta Paediatrica Scandinavica 79: 1080–1086

54. Finnstrom O, Otterblad Olausson P et al 1998 Neurosensory outcome and growth at three years in extremely low birthweight infants: follow-up results from the Swedish national prospective study. Acta Paediatrica 87: 1055–1060

55. Flynn J 1999 Searching for justice, The discovery of IQ gains over time. American Psychologist 54: 5–20

56. Forfar J O, Hume R, McPhail F M et al 1994 Low birthweight: a 10-year outcome study of the continuum of reproductive casualty. Developmental Medicine and Child Neurology 36: 1037–1048

57. Gesell A, Armatruda A 1947 Outcome following prematurity

58. Gould S J, Howard S, Hope P L, Reynolds E O 1987 Periventricular intraparenchymal cerebral haemorrhage in preterm infants: the role of venous infarction. Journal of Pathology 151: 197–202

59. Graham M, Levene M I, Trounce J Q, Rutter N 1987 Prediction of cerebral palsy in very low birthweight infants: prospective ultrasound study. Lancet 2: 593–596

60. Graziani L J, Pasto M, Stanley C et al 1985 Cranial ultrasound and clinical studies in preterm infants. Journal of Pediatrics 106: 269–276

61. Greisen G, Petersen M, Pedersen S A, Baekgaard P 1986 Status at two years in 121 very low birth weight survivors related to neonatal intraventricular haemorrhage and mode of delivery. Acta Paediatrica Scandinavica 75: 24–30

62. Gross R, Spiker D, Haynes C 1997 Helping low birthweight premature babies: the Infant Health and Development Program. Stanford University Press, Palo Alto, CA

63. Hack M, Flannery D J, Schluchter M, Cartar L, Borawski E, Klein N 2002 Outcomes in young adulthood for very-low-birth-weight infants. New England Journal of Medicine 346: 149–157

64. Hack M, Taylor H G, Klein N, Eiben R, Schatschneider C, Mercuri-Minich N 1994 School-age outcomes in children with birth weights under 750 g. New England Journal of Medicine 331: 753–759

65. Hack M, Taylor H G, Klein N, Mercuri-Minich N 2000 Functional limitations and special health care needs of 10- to 14-year-old children weighing less than 750 grams at birth. Pediatrics 106: 554–560

66. Hack M, Wilson-Costello D, Friedman H, Taylor G H, Schluchter M, Fanaroff A A 2000 Neurodevelopment and predictors of outcomes of children with birth weights of less than 1000 g: 1992–1995. Archives of Pediatrics and Adolescent Medicine 154: 725–731

67. Hadders-Algra M, Brogren E, Katz-Salamon M, Forssberg H 1999 Periventricular leucomalacia and preterm birth have different detrimental effects on postural adjustments. Brain 122: 727–740

68. Hagberg B, Hagberg G, Beckung E, Uvebrant P 2001 Changing panorama of cerebral palsy in Sweden. VIII. Prevalence and origin in the birth year period 1991–94. Acta Paediatrica 90: 271–277

69. Hagberg B, Hagberg G, Olow I 1984 The changing panorama of cerebral palsy in Sweden. IV. Epidemiological trends 1959–78. Acta Paediatrica Scandinavica 73: 433–440

70. Hagberg B, Hagberg G, Olow I 1993 The changing panorama of cerebral palsy in Sweden. VI. Prevalence and origin during the birth year period 1983–1986. Acta Paediatrica 82: 387–393

71. Hagberg B, Hagberg G, Olow I, van Wendt L 1996 The changing panorama of cerebral palsy in Sweden. VII. Prevalence and origin in the birth year period 1987–90. Acta Paediatrica 85: 954–960

72. Hagberg B, Hagberg G, Olow I, von Wendt L 1989 The changing panorama of cerebral palsy in Sweden. V. The birth year period 1979–82. Acta Paediatrica Scandinavica 78: 283–290

73. Hansen N B, Kopechek J, Miller R R, Menke J A, Cordero L 1989 Prognostic significance of cystic intracranial lesions in neonates. Journal of Developmental and Behavioral Pediatrics 10: 129–133

74. Harrison H 2002 Outcomes in young adulthood for very-low-birth-weight infants. New England Journal of Medicine 347: 141–143

75. Hess J H, Mohr G J, Bartelme P F 1934 The physical and mental growth of prematurely born children. University of Chicago Press, Chicago

76. Hille E T, den Ouden A L, Saigal S et al 2001 Behavioural problems in children who weigh 1000 g or less at birth in four countries. Lancet 357: 1641–1643

77. Hislop J E, Dubowitz L M, Kaiser A M, Singh M P, Whitelaw A G 1988 Outcome of infants shunted for post-haemorrhagic ventricular dilatation. Developmental Medicine and Child Neurology 30: 451–456

78. Jacobs S E, O'Brien K, Inwood S, Kelly E N, Whyte H E 2000 Outcome of infants 23–26 weeks' gestation pre and post surfactant. Acta Paediatrica 89: 959–965

79. James D K, Parker M J, Smoleniec J S 1992 Comprehensive fetal assessment with three ultrasonographic characteristics. American Journal of Obstetrics and Gynecology 166: 1486–1495

80. Johnson A 1995 Disability and perinatal care. Pediatrics 95: 272–274

81. Johnson S, Marlow N, Wolke D F et al 2004 Validation of a parent report measure of cognitive development for very preterm infants. Developmental Medicine and Child Neurology 46: 389–397

82. Jones H P, Guildea Z E, Stewart J H, Cartlidge P H 2002 The Health Status Questionnaire: achieving concordance with published disability criteria. Archives of Disease in Childhood 86: 15–20

83. Jongmans M, Henderson S, de Vries L, Dubowitz L 1993 Duration of periventricular densities in preterm infants and neurological outcome at 6 years of age. Archives of Disease in Childhood 69: 9–13

84. Khadilkar V, Tudehope D, Burns Y, O'Callaghan M, Mohay H 1993 The long-term neurodevelopmental outcome for very low birthweight (VLBW) infants with 'dystonic' signs at 4 months of age. Journal of Paediatrics and Child Health 29: 415–417

85. Kiely J L, Paneth N 1981 Follow-up studies of low-birthweight infants: suggestions for design, analysis and reporting. Developmental Medicine and Child Neurology 23: 96–100

86. Kitchen W H, Ford G W, Murton L J et al 1985 Mortality and two year outcome of infants of birthweight 500–1500 g: relationship with neonatal cerebral ultrasound data. Australian Paediatric Journal 21: 253–259

87. Kitchen W H, Ford G W, Rickards A L, Doyle L W, Kelly E, Murton L J 1990 Five-year outcome of infants of birthweight 500 to 1500 grams: relationship with neonatal ultrasound data. American Journal of Perinatology 7: 60–65

88. Kraemer S 2000 The fragile male. British Medical Journal 321: 1609–1612

89. Lefebvre F, Bard H, Veilleux A, Martel C 1988 Outcome at school age of children with birthweights of 1000 grams or less. Developmental Medicine and Child Neurology 30: 170–180

90. Lefebvre F, Glorieux J, St-Laurent-Gagnon T 1996 Neonatal survival and disability rate at age 18 months for infants born between 23 and 28 weeks of gestation. American Journal of Obstetrics and Gynecology 174: 833–838

91. Levene M I 1981 Measurement of the growth of the lateral ventricles in preterm infants with real-time ultrasound. Archives of Disease in Childhood 56: 900–904

92. Levene M, Dowling S, Graham M, Fogelman K, Galton M, Phillips M 1992 Impaired motor function (clumsiness) in 5 year old children: correlation with neonatal ultrasound scans. Archives of Disease in Childhood 67: 687–690

93. Ley D, Laurin J, Bjerre I, Marsal K 1996 Abnormal fetal aortic velocity waveform and minor neurological dysfunction at 7 years of age. Ultrasound in Obstetrics and Gynecology 8: 152–159

94. Ley D, Tideman E, Laurin J, Bjerre I, Marsal K 1996 Abnormal fetal aortic velocity waveform and intellectual function at 7 years of age. Ultrasound in Obstetrics and Gynecology 8: 160–165

95. Liechty E A, Gilmor R L, Bryson C Q, Bull M J 1983 Outcome of high-risk neonates with ventriculomegaly. Developmental Medicine and Child Neurology 25: 162–168

96. Lorenz J M, Paneth N, Jetton J R, den Ouden L, Tyson J E 2001 Comparison of management strategies for extreme prematurity in New Jersey and the Netherlands: outcomes and resource expenditure. Pediatrics 108: 1269–1274

97. McCarton C M, Brooks-Gunn J, Wallace I F et al 1997 Results at age 8 years of early intervention for low-birth-weight premature infants. The Infant Health and Development Program. Journal of the American Medical Association 277: 126–132

98. McCormick M C, Richardson D K 2002 Premature infants grow up. New England Journal of Medicine 346: 197–198

99. Marlow E S, Hunt L P, Marlow N 2000 Sensorineural hearing loss and prematurity. Archives of Disease in Childhood Fetal and Neonatal Edition 82: F141–F144

100. Marlow N, Roberts B L, Cooke R W 1989 Laterality and prematurity. Archives of Disease in Childhood 64: 1713–1716

101. Marlow N, Roberts B L, Cooke R W 1989 Motor skills in extremely low birthweight children at the age of 6 years. Archives of Disease in Childhood 64: 839–847

102. Marlow N, Roberts L, Cooke R 1993 Outcome at 8 years for children with birth weights of 1250 g or less. Archives of Disease in Childhood 68: 286–290

103. Monset-Couchard M, de Bethmann O, Radvanyi-Bouvet M F, Papin C, Bordarier C, Relier J P 1988 Neurodevelopmental outcome in cystic periventricular leukomalacia (CPVL) (30 cases). Neuropediatrics 19: 124–131

104. Msall M E, Phelps D L, DiGaudio K M et al 2000 Severity of neonatal retinopathy of prematurity is predictive of neurodevelopmental functional outcome at age 5.5 years. Behalf of the Cryotherapy for Retinopathy of Prematurity Cooperative Group. Pediatrics 106: 998–1005

105. Msall M E, Rogers B T, Buck G M, Mallen S, Catanzaro N L, Duffy L C 1993 Functional status of extremely preterm infants at kindergarten entry. Developmental Medicine and Child Neurology 35: 312–320

106. Msall M E, Tremont M R 2000 Functional outcomes in self-care, mobility, communication, and learning in extremely low-birth weight infants. Clinics in Perinatology 27: 381–401

107. Msall M E, Tremont M R 2002 Measuring functional outcomes after prematurity: developmental impact of very low birth weight and extremely low birth weight status on childhood disability. Mental Retardation and Developmental Disabilities Research Reviews 8: 258–272

108. Mutch L M, Johnson M A, Morley R 1989 Follow up studies: design, organisation, and analysis. Archives of Disease in Childhood 64: 1394–1402

109. Nelson K B, Ellenberg J H 1982 Children who 'outgrew' cerebral palsy. Pediatrics 69: 529–536

110. O'Connor A R, Stephenson T, Johnson A et al 2002 Long-term ophthalmic outcome of low birth weight children with and without retinopathy of prematurity. Pediatrics 109: 12–18

111. O'Shea T M, Klinepeter K L, Goldstein D J, Jackson B W, Dillard R G 1997 Survival and developmental disability in infants with birth weights of 501 to 800 grams, born between 1979 and 1994. Pediatrics 100: 982–986

112. Pallas Alonso C R, de la Cruz Bertolo J, Medina Lopez M C, Orbea Gallardo C, Gomez Castillo E, Simon de las Heras R 2000 [Cerebral palsy and age of sitting and walking in children weighing less than 1500 g at birth]. Anales Espanoles de Pediatria 53: 48–52

113. Palmer P, Dubowitz L M, Levene M I, Dubowitz V 1982 Developmental and neurological progress of preterm infants with intraventricular haemorrhage and ventricular dilatation. Archives of Disease in Childhood 57: 748–753

114. Palta M, Sadek-Badawi M, Evans M, Weinstein M R, McGuinnes G 2000 Functional assessment of a multicenter very-low-birth-weight cohort at age 5 years. Newborn Lung Project. Archives of Pediatrics and Adolescent Medicine 154: 23–30

115. Pederson S J S, Markestad T 2000 Early motor development of premature infants with birthweight less than 2000 grams. Acta Paediatrica 89: 1456–1461

116. Pennefather P M, Clarke M P, Strong N P, Cottrell D G, Fritz S, Tin W 1995 Ocular outcome in children born before 32 weeks gestation. Eye 9(Suppl): 26–30

117. Peterson B S, Vohr B, Staib L H et al 2000 Regional brain volume abnormalities and long-term cognitive outcome in preterm infants. Journal of the American Medical Association 284: 1939–1947

118. Pharoah P O, Platt M J, Cooke T 1996 The changing epidemiology of cerebral palsy. Archives of Disease in Childhood Fetal and Neonatal Edition 75: F169–F173

119. Pharoah P O, Stevenson C J, West C R 2003 General Certificate of Secondary Education performance in very low birthweight infants. Archives of Disease in Childhood 88: 295–298

120. Pidcock F S, Graziani L J, Stanley C, Mitchell D G, Merton D 1990 Neurosonographic features of periventricular echodensities associated with cerebral palsy in preterm infants. Journal of Pediatrics 116: 417–422

121. Piecuch R E, Leonard C H, Cooper B A, Kilpatrick S J, Schlueter M A, Sola A 1997 Outcome of infants born at 24–26 weeks' gestation: II. Neurodevelopmental outcome. Obstet Gynecol 90: 809–814

122. Pierrat V, Eken P, Duquennoy C, Rousseau S, de Vries LS 1993 Prognostic value of early somatosensory evoked potentials in neonates with cystic leukomalacia. Developmental Medicine and Child Neurology 35: 683–690

123. Pinto-Martin J A, Riolo S, Cnaan A, Holzman C, Susser M W, Paneth N 1995 Cranial ultrasound prediction of disabling and nondisabling cerebral palsy at age two in a low birth weight population. Pediatrics 95: 249–254

124. Powls A, Botting N, Cooke R W, Marlow N 1995 Motor impairment in children 12 to 13 years old with a birthweight of less than 1250 g. Archives of Disease in Childhood Fetal and Neonatal Edition 73: F62–F66

125. Powls A, Botting N, Cooke R W, Marlow N 1996 Handedness in very-low-birthweight (VLBW) children at 12 years of age: relation to perinatal and outcome variables. Developmental Medicine and Child Neurology 38: 594–602

126. Powls A, Botting N, Cooke R W, Pilling D, Marlow N 1996 Growth impairment in very low birthweight children at 12 years: correlation with perinatal and outcome variables. Archives of Disease in Childhood Fetal and Neonatal Edition 75: F152–F157

127. Powls A, Botting N, Cooke R W, Stephenson G, Marlow N 1997 Visual impairment in very low birthweight children. Archives of Disease in Childhood Fetal and Neonatal Edition 76: F82–F87

128. Project API 1998 A randomised trial of parental support for families with very preterm children. Archives of Disease in Childhood 79: F4–F11

129. Rennie J M 1997 Neonatal cerebral ultrasound. Cambridge University Press, Cambridge

130. Robertson C, Sauve R S, Christianson H E 1994 Province-based study of neurologic disability among survivors weighing 500 through 1249 grams at birth. Pediatrics 93: 636–640

131. Roelants-van Rijn A M, Groenendaal F, Beek F J, Eken P, van Haastert I C, de Vries L S 2001 Parenchymal brain injury in the preterm infant: comparison of cranial ultrasound, MRI and neurodevelopmental outcome. Neuropediatrics 32: 80–89

132. Rogers B, Msall M, Owens T et al 1994 Cystic periventricular leukomalacia and type of cerebral palsy in preterm infants. Journal of Pediatrics 125: S1–S8

133. Roth S C, Baudin J, McCormick D C et al 1993 Relation between ultrasound appearance of the brain of very preterm infants and neurodevelopmental impairment at eight years. Developmental Medicine and Child Neurology 35: 755–768

134. Saigal S, Feeny D, Rosenbaum P, Furlong W, Burrows E, Stoskopf B 1996 Self-perceived health status and health-related quality of life of extremely low-birth-weight infants at adolescence. Journal of the American Medical Association 276: 453–459

135. Saigal S, Lambert M, Russ C, Hoult L 2002 Self-esteem of adolescents who were born prematurely. Pediatrics 109: 429–433

136. Saigal S, Szatmari P, Rosenbaum P, Campbell D, King S 1990 Intellectual and functional status at school entry of children who weighed 1000 grams or less at birth: a regional perspective of births in the 1980s. Journal of Pediatrics 116: 409–416

137. Salokorpi T, Rautio T, Sajaniemi N, Serenius-Sirve S, Tuomi H, von Wendt L 2001 Neurological development up to the age of four years of extremely low birthweight infants born in Southern Finland in 1991–94. Acta Paediatrica 90: 218–221

138. Sameroff A J, Chandler M J 1975 Reproductive Risk and the Continuum Of Caretaking Causalty. In Horrowitz FD (ed) Review of Child Development Research. Chicago: University of Chicago Press pp 187–244

139. Saudino K, Dale P, Oliver B et al 1998 The validity of parent-based assessment of the cognitive abilities of 2-year-olds. British Journal of Developmental Psychology 16: 349–363

140. Sauve R S, Robertson C, Etches P, Byrne P J, Dayer-Zamora V 1998 Before viability: a geographically based outcome study of infants weighing 500 grams or less at birth. Pediatrics 101: 438–445

141. Scherjon S, Briet J, Oosting H, Kok J 2000 The discrepancy between maturation of visual-evoked potentials and cognitive outcome at five years in very preterm infants with and without hemodynamic signs of fetal brain-sparing. Pediatrics 105: 385–391

142. Shankaran S, Koepke T, Woldt E et al 1989 Outcome after posthemorrhagic ventriculomegaly in comparison with mild hemorrhage without ventriculomegaly. Journal of Pediatrics 114: 109–114

143. Sheridan M D 1962 Infants at risk of handicapping conditions. Monthly Bulletin of the Ministry of Health and Public Health Laboratory Service 238–245

144. Sie L T, van der Knaap M S, Oosting J, de Vries L S, Lafeber H N, Valk J 2000 MR patterns of hypoxic-ischemic brain damage after prenatal, perinatal or postnatal asphyxia. Neuropediatrics 31: 128–136

145. Silverman W A 1979 Incubator-baby side shows (Dr Martin A. Couney). Pediatrics 64: 127–141

146. Sommerfelt K, Pedersen S, Ellertsen B, Markestad T 1996 Transient dystonia in non-handicapped low-birthweight infants and later neurodevelopment. Acta Paediatrica 85: 1445–1449

147. Stewart A 1999 Neurodevelopmental outcome.In: Rennie J M, Roberton N R C (eds) Textbook of neonatology. Churchill Livingstone, Edinburgh, pp 79–100

148. Stewart A L, Reynolds E O, Hope P L et al 1987 Probability of neurodevelopmental disorders estimated from ultrasound appearance of brains of very preterm infants. Developmental Medicine and Child Neurology 29: 3–11

149. Stewart A L, Reynolds E O, Lipscomb A P 1981 Outcome for infants of very low birthweight: survey of world literature. Lancet 1: 1038–1040

150. Szymonowicz W, Yu V Y, Bajuk B, Astbury J 1986 Neurodevelopmental outcome of periventricular haemorrhage and leukomalacia in infants 1250 g or less at birth. Early Human Development 14: 1–7

151. TeKolste K A, Bennett F C, Mack L A 1985 Follow-up of infants receiving cranial ultrasound for intracranial hemorrhage. American Journal of Diseases of Children 139: 299–303

152. Thorburn R J, Lipscomb A P, Stewart A L, Reynolds E O, Hope P L, Pape K E 1981 Prediction of death and major handicap in very preterm infants by brain ultrasound. Lancet 1: 1119–1121

153. Tin W, Fritz S, Wariyar U, Hey E 1998 Outcome of very preterm birth: children reviewed with ease at 2 years differ from those followed up with difficulty. Archives of Disease in Childhood Fetal and Neonatal Edition 79: F83–F87

154. Touwen B C L 1979 The examination of the child with minor neurological dysfunction. Clinics in Developmental Medicine 71. Spastics International Medical Publications, London

155. Tudehope D I, Masel J, Mohay H et al 1989 Neonatal cranial ultrasonography as predictor of 2 year outcome of very low birthweight infants. Australian Paediatric Journal 25: 66–71

156. Valkama AM, Paakko EL, Vainionpaa LK, Lanning FP, Ilkko EA, Koivisto ME. Magnetic resonance imaging at term and neuromotor outcome in preterm infants. Acta Paediatrica 89: 348–55; 2000.

157. Van den Hout B M, Stiers P, Haers M et al 2000 Relation between visual perceptual impairment and neonatal ultrasound diagnosis of haemorrhagic-ischaemic brain lesions in 5-year-old children. Developmental Medicine and Child Neurology 42: 376–386

158. Van Wezel-Meijler G, van der Knaap M S, Sie L T et al 1998 Magnetic resonance imaging of the brain in premature infants during the neonatal period. Normal phenomena and reflection of mild ultrasound abnormalities. Neuropediatrics 29: 89–96

159. Vohr B R, Wright L L, Dusick A M et al 2000 Neurodevelopmental and functional outcomes of extremely low birth weight infants in the National Institute of Child Health and Human Development Neonatal Research Network, 1993–1994. Pediatrics 105: 1216–1226

160. Walker E M, Patel N B 1987 Mortality and morbidity in infants born between 20 and 28 weeks gestation. British Journal of Obstetrics and Gynaecology 94: 670–674

161. Weindling A M, Hallam P, Gregg J, Klenka H, Rosenbloom L, Hutton J L 1996. A randomized controlled trial of early physiotherapy for high-risk infants. Acta Paediatrica 85: 1107–1111

162. Weindling A M, Rochefort M J, Calvert S A, Fok T F, Wilkinson A 1985 Development of cerebral palsy after ultrasonographic detection of periventricular cysts in the newborn. Developmental Medicine and Child Neurology 27: 800–806

163. Weisglas-Kuperus N, Baerts W, Fetter W P, Sauer P J 1992 Neonatal cerebral ultrasound, neonatal neurology and perinatal conditions as predictors of neurodevelopmental outcome in very low birthweight infants. Early Human Development 31: 131–148

164. Whitfield M F, Grunau R V, Holsti L 1997 Extremely premature (≤800 g) schoolchildren: multiple areas of hidden disability. Archives of Disease in Childhood Fetal and Neonatal Edition 77: F85–F90

165. Whyte H E, Fitzhardinge P M, Shennan A T, Lennox K, Smith L, Lacy J 1993 Extreme immaturity: outcome of 568 pregnancies of 23–26 weeks' gestation. Obstet Gynecol 82: 1–7

166. Wolke D, Ratschinski G, Ohrt B, Riegel K 1994 The cognitive outcome of very preterm infants may be poorer than often reported: an empirical investigation of how methodological issues make a big difference. European Journal of Pediatrics 153: 906–915

167. Wolke D, Schulz J, Meyer R 2001 Entwicklungslangzeitfolgen bei ehemaligs, sehr unreifen Frühgeborenen. Monatsschrift für Kinderheilkunde 149: 53–61

168. Wolke D, Sohne B, Ohrt B, Riegel K 1995 Follow-up of preterm children: important to document dropouts. Lancet 345: 447

169. Wood N S, Costeloe K, Gibson A T, Hennessy E, Marlow N, Wilkinson A R 2003 The EPICure Study: growth and associated problems in children born at 25 weeks of gestational age or less. Archives of Disease in Childhood Fetal and Neonatal Edition 88: F492–F500

170. Wood N S, Marlow N, Costeloe K, Gibson A T, Wilkinson A R 2000 Neurologic and developmental disability after extremely preterm birth. EPICure Study Group. New England Journal of Medicine 343: 378–384

171. Yoshinaga-Itano C, Sedey A L, Coulter D K, Mehl A L 1998 Language of early- and later-identified children with hearing loss. Pediatrics 102: 1161–1171

CHAPTER 4

Psychological aspects of neonatal care

Joanna Hawthorne

Babies are born into a social world and are pre-adapted for social life. They have many talents and skills that equip them to be capable social partners, and they start learning about the world immediately. How they are treated from the very beginning can make a difference to their sense of themselves and to their sense of security.

Attachment and social interaction

There is increasing knowledge about the brain of the infant with regard to the development of social relationships. Connections are being formed in the brain from birth, so that the way babies are handled and responded to can improve their future relationships.[25] In fact, Spitz[42] found that babies in orphanages who did not have any social interaction were likely to die. Feeding and changing them was not enough to keep them alive.

Psychologists know that patterns of interaction between the baby and the primary caretaker are set up by three months of age.[54] Difficult experiences during this time can affect the attachment behaviour of the infant. Attachment is defined as the process of forming a relationship, which can take days, weeks or months to develop; the relationship starts in pregnancy. Attachment is affected by the mother's own experience of parenting, and involves making mistakes and repairing them. Children who are securely attached at 12 months and 18 months of age are more cooperative, more empathic, more socially competent, more invested in learning and exploration and more self-confident.[35] It is more appropriate to use the word 'attachment' than 'bonding', which implies an either/or situation, and where the original work was done on animals.[31]

Many studies have shown the difficulties parents face when their baby stays in a neonatal unit. This appears to be mostly due to anxiety about the baby's health, their efforts to parent their baby and the practicalities of visiting, especially if there are other children at home and they live far from the neonatal unit. Murray and Cooper[37] show that the risk of insecure attachment with her infant is increased by 40% if the mother has had a poor relationship with her own mother and a traumatic birth or pregnancy history.

The psychology of parenting

The task of parents is to protect and feed their babies and provide the appropriate environment for them. Parents bring to parenting their own experiences of being parented, which have an impact on their relationship with their baby.[24] If the parents' experiences have been positive, they are more likely to find parenting easier; but if their experiences have been negative, they may have some psychological work to carry out in order to understand how to relate to their child in an appropriate way.[16,44]

Stern[44] describes the support mothers need in their task of mothering. Their primary task is to keep their baby alive, and their primary support people are usually other women who have had babies. The mother's identity becomes reorganised as she takes on a new role.

At the time of birth, families are particularly vulnerable emotionally. Mothers are recovering from labour and delivery and their hormones are changing to allow them to breastfeed and to protect their babies. Winnicott[51] termed this as a state of primary maternal preoccupation, and mothers are likely to be fiercely protective of their babies. Typically, therefore, medical staff would expect to see a mother of a healthy, full-term baby wanting to be close and involved with her baby. The stress on the entire family of having a baby in hospital is well-documented[10,23] and it remains an upsetting and disruptive time for families.

The importance of allowing a parent to feel like a parent when separated from her baby cannot be emphasised enough. The parent can easily be made to feel inferior if health professionals appear to be taking over the parenting role.[29] There can be an effort to 'educate parents' in how to look after their baby in medical settings but this approach can undermine the parent's confidence and create complicated problems around the issues of who the baby belongs to at the vulnerable time of birth.[46] The emphasis may be to teach the mother practical skills, such as bathing the baby and changing nappies. But there is often little support for the emotional side of the relationship, and this may be one factor contributing to low breastfeeding rates. The medical model identifies pathology, so often the emphasis is on the difficulties of the mother–baby couple, rather than on the strengths, or what is functioning well in the relationship.[16]

Respecting and validating parents' observations of their baby can help the parent to feel confident.[17]

It is understandable that roles can be easily confused when a nurse or doctor is providing life-saving support to an ill baby, where the parent feels helpless. As the baby's health improves, and the care is slowly handed over from the medical staff to the parent, there can be some tensions in the parent about her role.[28]

The baby in the neonatal unit – emotional stages parents go through

It is often difficult for staff, who have grown accustomed to the neonatal unit environment, to realise how alien it feels to a parent. The majority of parents, when asked in interviews or questionnaires in the course of research studies, knew little about neonatal intensive care units before their baby was born, or even the fact they existed.[29,39] Therefore, their distress, concern and fear as well as their confusion and anxiety about their baby's survival make it very difficult for them to take in information about their baby, or make decisions.

Parents who have a premature or ill baby commonly suffer a grief reaction.[20] The birth may have come as a shock, as the baby is not the baby they imagined they would have. The baby is tiny, thin, perhaps covered with hair, possibly with eyelids fused shut, and looks far from the ideal of a full-term, chubby baby. Parents may have mixed feelings, as they are happy to have a new baby but feel that it is a loss not to have had a full-term baby.[13] What is more, the parents cannot look after the baby as they would like: the baby needs oxygen, monitoring and feeding, and possibly surgery, and cannot leave the hospital until he is bigger and medically stable. Medicine and supportive machines can help to keep premature and ill babies alive, which means that often these babies are in the neonatal unit for several weeks or months, depending on their medical course and the gestational age at which they were born.

However, parents who have delivered their first live baby after recurrent miscarriages, stillbirths or infertility may react more positively when they finally give birth to a live baby. Their feelings of joy may supersede negative feelings about the baby's condition initially.

Parents of premature or sick babies may be depressed but research studies have shown that some parents may be suffering from post-traumatic stress disorder, which needs entirely different forms of treatment and support.[19]

Because parents are usually in shock when their baby is admitted to a neonatal unit, they may not hear what is being explained to them by the staff. They will need information repeated often, but at their own pace. Often if parents start worrying about the future, they may resist developing a close relationship with the baby, in case the baby dies. They may hesitate to touch or hold their baby for many reasons – the neonatal unit is a very public environment and parents may feel they are being watched. Often parents can feel pressured to perform an interaction with their baby when they are not emotionally ready, and it is important for staff to respect this hesitation. Sometimes, resentment can build

up. Written information can be helpful, but parents may not be able to cope with reading a large amount of information in the early days of their baby's admission to the neonatal unit. Written information needs to be available at the appropriate time for parents and does not take the place of a good relationship between staff and parents and sensitively presented information from the staff.

The next stage of the parents' grief reaction may be guilt, although the stages of grief can be in a different order for each parent, which can lead to misunderstandings and tension between the couple. Parents often feel guilty about giving birth to an ill or premature baby and look for reasons as to why it happened. This guilty stage can be followed by despair, and then anger. Parents can feel despair, as their baby seems to be getting better and then takes a turn for the worse. This period has been described as 'an emotional roller-coaster' and may correspond with the baby's medical course.

The parents' anger can be fuelled by a situation in which they feel they do not have control. They are angry with themselves for giving birth to an ill or premature baby whom they feel they cannot look after properly, and they may take their anger out on the staff, who know their baby intimately. If staff are adequately supported and understand the process of adaptation that parents go through, it improves the staff–parent relationship and helps both parties to work together.[21] Parents build up trust in the staff to look after their baby when they are not there, and parents often become dependent on staff and feel that they and the staff have become a family.

Support for parents while the baby is in the neonatal unit

Most hospitals provide instant photographs of the baby, especially if the mother cannot see her baby immediately, which helps the mother believe she has a baby and dispels any fears she has about the baby's appearance. In some hospitals there is a video-link available between the neonatal unit and the mother's bed, or the hospital or family member may take a video of the baby for the mother to see.

Many studies have shown that, if parents can see, touch and hold their baby in the neonatal unit and be involved in the care of the baby, they feel better and more like a parent.[22,27] Most units have mother and baby rooms where the mother can stay when the baby is in the unit so that she can establish breastfeeding or be near her sick infant. Parents can feel very helpless, anxious and uncomfortable and out of control during their baby's stay, and need to feel cared for themselves in order to provide the best care for their baby.[39,43]

Criteria for admission and discharge are also crucial. Infants with relatively minor problems can be satisfactorily cared for in the general lying-in wards or transitional care wards, where there is more specialised neonatal paediatric nursing and medical support. Transitional care wards where mothers can have their baby beside them are ideal for small babies who need tube-feeding or phototherapy, for instance, without having to be in the special care baby unit.[39,48]

Going home from the neonatal unit

There are many medical, psychological and cultural issues around discharge home for babies who have been premature or ill, and it is worth staff spending time helping to make the appropriate decisions for individual families.[11] While the baby is in the neonatal unit, the parents usually form a close and dependent relationship with the staff. Many parents report feeling angry at this stage, often resenting the perceived tug of war over the baby's care that sometimes seems to take place.[33] Often the baby is medically stable but the feeding and growing is not well-established, and parents find it very difficult to wait for the day the baby can leave the hospital, even though they may understand that the baby's wellbeing is important.

Most hospitals follow up the babies medically and sometimes neurodevelopmentally for 1–2 years. Parents often have many appointments to attend at the hospital but can feel that they need more support emotionally, or for the particular behavioural issues that often arise with babies from neonatal and special care baby units. Babies who were extremely-low-birthweight are well-represented in school populations and have been reported to have more behavioural, social and emotional problems on follow-up.[14,45,36,53] Medical staff need to be aware that behavioural issues should be an important part of follow-up appointments with parents and babies, so an interdisciplinary team may be helpful in addressing the behavioural issues.

Babies from neonatal units may have problems with feeding, sometimes resulting from frequent suctioning and negative aversive experiences with the mouth, and other treatments. Parents can find ongoing feeding problems very distressing and feeding difficulties can become habits if not addressed.[40]

Several studies have discussed the risk of psychological problems with parents and with babies from neonatal units.[52] There are several methods of intervention that have been developed to provide support for parents in neonatal units, in order to minimise the risks of relationship difficulties.

Psychosocial interventions for parents and babies in the neonatal unit

As described earlier, the neonatal unit is a difficult and public place in which to act like a parent and talk to, care for and handle the baby.

While good medical care is paramount and can make a difference to the long-term health of the baby, good psychological care is just as important for these families. There will be individual differences in how each parent, each baby and each member of staff copes with his experiences in a neonatal unit, so a supportive and flexible system needs to be in place in order to address these individual differences.

Some units have interdisciplinary teams to care for the emotional needs of parents. These include counsellors, psychotherapists and psychologists.

However, most units do not provide this kind of support for parents, even though this is increasingly regarded as a necessary part of the system.[21,33] Lewis (personal communication, 1995) reviewed a counselling service in a neonatal unit and found that, if both parents and staff have access to the counsellor, everyone in the unit becomes more open, communicative and supportive. Other therapists have reported that counselling provides parents with help in dealing with the many conflicting feelings that may hamper their parental role, and in coming to terms with their baby's condition and developmental future.[21,33]

Very few neonatal units in the UK employ counsellors or psychotherapists, for parents let alone for staff, but those that do have found them to be helpful. In a few units there are separate counsellors for the parents and the staff. There is evidence that emotional support for staff helps them to cope with the stress of working in a neonatal unit.[21,33]

Staff of all levels can be sensitised to the uniqueness of each parent–baby relationship by role-playing exercises or by teaching sessions with a psychologist or professional who is working with families. Parents and staff alike can be in an emotional state of denial in a neonatal unit, to protect themselves from feeling too much pain. When there is a spokesperson for the baby, staff and parents are often better able to verbalise their feelings, and this in turn helps them take better care of the babies.[21]

Specific interventions have been carried out in neonatal units in recent years. Research has shown that encouraging parents to care for their babies in the neonatal unit helps them to feel better and read their baby's behavioural cues more effectively, supporting contact and development of parental understanding of their baby's needs and strengths.[50] Positive touch and calm holding, Kangaroo care, NIDCAP, NAPI and the Brazelton Neonatal Behavioural Assessment Scale (NBAS), or a shortened version, the Clinical NBAS (CLNBAS), are all ways in which to understand the individual baby's needs, as well as a way of becoming aware of individual differences in temperament, reactivity to stimulation, attentiveness, self-calming, crying, feeding and sleeping behaviours.

The Brazelton assessment, NBAS,[17] is an interactive assessment of newborn behaviour conventionally carried out at or after 37 weeks gestation with term infants or preterm infants who are medically stable. It is designed to facilitate the understanding of the baby's individual ability to habituate to light and sound, regulate state changes (asleep and awake states), self-quiet and respond to visual and auditory stimuli. It takes 20–30 minutes to carry out, preferably between feeds, so that it can be started when the baby is asleep. The assessment can be used as an outcome measure, for example in studies looking at the effects of obstetric analgesia on the baby's behaviour, or as a baseline measure of a baby's behaviour.

The NBAS is currently used as a supportive intervention with parents.[8,18] Fathers who helped perform the assessment on their infants at birth were found to feel closer to them 1 month later.[9] The NBAS provides an opportunity to share with parents the numerous capabilities of their newborn and helps parents to identify the characteristics of the infant that may influence their caregiving. Other work has shown that the NBAS can be particularly useful in helping the emotional relationship between mother and baby. Stern and Bruschweiler-Stern[44] discuss the mother's adjustment to her fetus in pregnancy, and how she imagines the baby she may have. Sometimes the imagined baby is far from the baby she has in reality. The NBAS can help the mother to adjust to the real baby she has delivered.[38] In a study by Widmayer and Field[50] the NBAS was carried out in a group of ex-premature babies. These babies were found to have higher cognitive scores, and the mothers felt more confident with them later.

Keefer[30] has incorporated aspects of the NBAS into the regular paediatric examination of the newborn. The NBAS can be especially helpful with babies of mothers with postnatal depression, babies who have been premature or ill and babies with congenital malformations. This is because the NBAS highlights the positive aspects of the baby's behaviour while also addressing any concerns the mother has about her baby. The Neurobehavioural Assessment of the Preterm Infant (NAPI)[32] assesses the neurobehavioural development of medically stable preterm infants between the ages of 32 weeks gestation and term, and has recently been used with term babies. It is mostly used in research, but can also show parents their baby's skills.

Studies have shown that excessive stimulation such as light, handling and noise, which is non-contingent stimulation in neonatal intensive care units, can be damaging to the baby's efforts to self-regulate.[2,4] Some neonatal units have modified practice in some respects and begun the use of developmental care with premature babies, based on the Neonatal Individualized Developmental Care and Assessment Program (NIDCAP). This was first developed by Als and colleagues,[5] who found that babies who were unable to maintain homeostasis needed physical containment in the fetal position, dimming of lights, protection from loud sounds and less handling. The NIDCAP encourages staff to observe the baby's reaction to stimuli, and then try to reduce the negative aspects of stimuli. This produces a caregiving plan for the infant, so that everyone is helping the baby in the same way. One study found that these babies spent less time on a respirator, less time in oxygen and performed better on developmental tests later.[3] In another study, the baby's physiological stress levels were reduced and weight gain improved using developmental care.[26]

Whitelaw et al[49] and Anderson[6] found that when mothers and fathers hold their preterm infants skin-to-skin ('Kangaroo care') on their chests under protective clothing there was reduced crying, increased breastfeeding, weight gain and early discharge. Both staff and parents need to become sensitive to each infant's cues and signals in order to provide the best possible environment for the baby. Calm holding, light touching[1,12] and 'kangaroo care' are ways to help babies calm and settle that will also help babies learn how to regulate their sleep and awake states.

These kinds of intervention are becoming more frequently used in neonatal units. Because the behaviour of the baby is being closely observed, the baby's voice is being heard. The parents are supported in their efforts to understand and get to know their baby, and the baby's development is optimised.[15] Without these types of intervention, some neonatal units may be neglecting the provision of emotional, behavioural and psychological support for parents and babies. With our increased knowledge of the developing infant brain and the formation of emotional relationships, it is crucial that support is given to parents in understanding their baby in the newborn period.[7]

Support for staff in neonatal units

Staff deal with many conflicting feelings in their work. They often need to deny their sympathetic feelings for the baby in order to inflict pain on him while drawing blood or carrying out other painful procedures. Staff are aware that procedures they carry out can be painful and uncomfortable for babies.[41] A large-scale study of parents' experience in 23 neonatal units in the UK found that: 'the words and actions of nursing and medical staff; the way a unit is run and organised; policies and how these are put into practice all contribute to the parents' sense of wellbeing, confidence and trust'.[39]

While nursing staff themselves emphasise the positive aspects of their role, including high levels of job satisfaction,[39] they nevertheless have a huge emotional task in their everyday relationships with parents. Not only are they attending to the medical needs of the baby but also they usually have the most contact with parents and their concerns.

There is awareness amongst staff that there can be difficulties in communication in the neonatal unit, not only between staff and parents but also between staff and babies. Several strategies can be adopted to minimise these difficulties. Sometimes, parents are encouraged to write notes to the staff, as if from the baby, saying that they like to be handled in a certain way, or that they are wearing their own clothes, for example. Mothers say that they are particularly sensitive to the words used by staff to describe their baby and his behaviour. Negative words and descriptions can be particularly painful to parents, who want their baby to be the best-behaved and most-liked baby in the unit. Both medical and nursing staff need specific training in recognising the changing needs of parents and the complexities of the developing parent–baby relationship. In summary, understanding the concepts of infant mental health will enhance staff's approach to parents.[54]

Bereavement

Recent work has shown that, surrounding the death of a baby, sharing information about the baby's condition and providing parents with the opportunity to be involved in decision making is essential.[34]

In order to support parents best, staff need to form a therapeutic alliance with parents, built on systems theory.[16,43] This means being spontaneous and authentic with parents and understanding how the world of the family is affected by the world of the neonatal unit, which is affected by the world of the staff. Each person, in essence, affects the other. Compassionate and sensitive treatment of parents, showing respect and providing privacy and dignity, should always be the priority. Where units have counsellors trained in bereavement, all members of staff need to work together with them.

There is often a quiet room on a neonatal unit where consultations take place. Parents often refer to this as the 'bad news room' or the 'death room'. It may well have this connotation, but there does need to be such a room in which to talk to parents.

The Child Bereavement Trust[47] has helpful literature available for parents and staff.

Conclusion

Starting life as a baby in a neonatal unit is precarious: Health, development and relationships can be problematic to varying degrees. Medical knowledge in the field of neonatology is expanding, and very sick or small babies survive more frequently. But in order to help babies and parents in the best possible way, great attention must be paid to their behavioural and emotional needs, just as much as to their medical needs. Caring for all aspects of babies' needs will improve their quality of life.

References

1. Adamson-Macedo E N 2002 The psychology of preterm neonates. Mattes Verlag, Germany
2. Als H 1999 Reading the premature infant. In: Goldson E (ed) Nurturing the premature infant. Oxford University Press, Oxford
3. Als H, Lawhon G, Brown E et al 1986 Individualized behavioural and environmental care for the very low birthweight preterm infant at risk for bronchopulmonary dysplasia: neonatal intensive care and development outcome. Pediatrics 78: 1123–1132
4. Als H, Lawhon G, Duffy F H, McAnulty G B, Gibes-Grossman R, Blickman J G 1994 Individualized developmental care for the very low-birthweight preterm infant. Journal of the American Medical Association 272: 853–858
5. Als H, Lester B M, Brazelton T B 1979 Dynamics of the behavioural organization of the premature infant: a theoretical perspective. In: Field T M (ed) Infants born at risk: behaviour and development. S P Medical and Scientific Books, New York
6. Anderson G C 1991 Current knowledge about skin-to-skin (kangaroo) care for preterm infants. Journal of Perinatology 11: 216–226
7. Barnard K E, Morisset C E, Speiker S 2000 Preventive interventions: enhancing parent–infant relationships. In: Zeanah C (ed) Handbook of infant mental health. Guilford Press, New York
8. Beal J A 1986 The Brazelton Neonatal Behavioural Assessment Scale: a tool to enhance parental attachment. Journal of Pediatric Nursing 1: 170–177
9. Beal J A 1989 The effect on father–infant interaction of demonstrating the Neonatal Behavioural Assessment Scale. Birth 16: 18–22
10. Beckwith L, Cohen S E 1978 Preterm birth: hazardous obstetrical and postnatal events as related to caregiver–infant behaviour. Infant Behaviour and Development 1: 403–411
11. Bissell G, Long T 2003 From the neonatal unit to home: how do parents adapt to life at home with their baby? Journal of Neonatal Nursing 91: 7–12
12. Bond C 2002 Positive touch and massage in the neonatal unit: a British approach. Seminars in Neonatology 7: 477–486
13. Boss P 1999 Ambiguous loss. Harvard University Press, Cambridge, Mass.
14. Botting N, Powls A, Cooke R W I, Marlow N 1998 Cognitive and educational outcome of very low birthweight children in early adolescence. Developmental Medicine and Child Neurology 40: 652–660
15. Brazelton T B 1992 Touchpoints: your child's emotional and behavioural development. Perseus Books, Reading, MA
16. Brazelton T B, Cramer B G 1991 The earliest relationship. Karnac Books, London
17. Brazelton T B, Nugent J K 1995 The Neonatal Behavioural Assessment Scale, 3rd edn. MacKeith Press, London
18. Britt G C, Myers B J 1994 The effects of Brazelton intervention: a review. Infant Mental Health Journal 15: 278–292
19. Brockington I 1996 Motherhood and mental health. Oxford University Press, Oxford
20. Caplan G, Mason E A, Kaplan D M 1965 Four studies of crisis in parents of prematures. Communication in Mental Health 1: 149–161
21. Cohen M 2003 Sent before my time – a child psychotherapist's view of life on a neonatal intensive care unit. Karnac, London
22. Davis J A, Richards M P M, Roberton N R C (eds) 1983 Parent–baby attachment in premature infants. Croom Helm, London
23. Divitto, B, Goldberg S 1979 The effects of newborn medical status on early parent–infant relationships. In: Field T M (ed) Infants born at risk: behaviour and development. S P Medical Books, Jamaica, pp. 311–332
24. Fonagy P 2001 Attachment theory and psychoanalysis. Other Press, New York
25. Fox N A, Leavitt L A, Warhol J G 1999 The role of early experience in infant development. Johnson & Johnson Pediatric Institute, Calverton, NY
26. Goldson E 1999 Nurturing the premature infant – developmental interventions in the neonatal intensive care nursery. Oxford University Press, Oxford
27. Hawthorne Amick J 1989 The effect of different routines in a special care baby unit on the mother–infant relationship (Great Britain). In: Nugent J K, Lester B M, Brazelton T B (eds) The cultural context of infancy 1. Ablex, Norwood, NJ
28. Hawthorne J, Alderson P, Killen M, Warren I 2003 Foretelling futures: dilemmas in neonatal neurology. Conference poster: abstract in Journal of Reproductive and Infant Psychology 21, 3253–3254
29. Jacques N C S, Hawthorne Amick J T, Richards M P M 1983 Parents and the support they need. In: Davis J A, Richards M P M, Roberton N R C (eds) Parent–baby attachment in premature infants. Croom Helm, London
30. Keefer C H 1995 The combined physical and behavioral neonatal examination: a parent-centered approach to pediatric care. In: Brazelton T B, Nugent J K (eds) Neonatal Behavioral Assessment Scale, 3rd edn. MacKeith Press, London
31. Klaus N H, Kennell J H, Klaus P H 1995 Bonding. Addison-Wesley, Reading
32. Korner A F, Brown J V, Thom V A, Constantinou J C 1990 Neurobehavioural Assessment of the Preterm Infant (NAPI). Psychological Corporation, New York
33. McFadyen A 1994 Special Care babies and their developing relationships. Routledge, London
34. McHaffie H E 2001 Crucial decisions at the beginning of life; parents' experiences of treatment withdrawal from infants. Radcliffe Medical Press, Oxford
35. Main M, Solomon J 1986 Discovery of an insecure-disorganized/disoriented attachment pattern. In: Brazelton T B, Yogman N W (eds) Affective development in infancy. Ablex, Norwood, NJ
36. Marlow N 1998 Avon Premature Infant Project: a randomised trial of parental support for families with very pre-term children. Archives of Disease in Childhood 79: 4–11
37. Murray L, Cooper P J 1997 The role of infant and maternal factors in postpartum depression, mother–infant interactions, and infant outcomes. In: Murray L, Cooper P J (eds) Postpartum depression and child development. Guilford Press, New York
38. Nugent J K, Brazelton T B 2000 Preventive infant mental health: uses of the Brazelton Scale. In: Osofsky J D, Fitzgerald H E (eds) WAIMH handbook of infant mental health: early intervention, evaluation and assessment: 2. John Wiley, New York
39. Redshaw M E, Harris A, Ingram J C 1996 The Neonatal Unit as a working environment: a survey of neonatal unit nursing. HMSO, London
40. Reilly S M, Skuse D H, Wolke D, Stevenson J 1998 Oral motor dysfunction in children who fail to thrive: organic or non-organic? Developmental Medicine and Child Neurology 41: 115–122
41. Sparshott M 1997 Pain, distress and the newborn baby. Blackwell Science, Oxford
42. Spitz R A 1945 Hospitalism. An inquiry into the genesis of psychiatric conditions in early childhood. Psychoanalytic Study of the Child 1: 53–74
43. Stern D 1995 The motherhood constellation. Basic Books, New York
44. Stern D N, Bruschweiler-Stern 1998 The birth of a mother. Basic Books, New York
45. Stjernqvist K 1992 Extremely low birth weight infants, development, behaviour and impact on the family. Wallin & Dalholm, Lund
46. Strange F 2002 An age of uncertainty: the emotional labour of becoming the parent of a premature baby. Journal of Neonatal Nursing 8: 112–117
47. Thomas J (no date) Supporting parents when their baby dies. Child Bereavement Trust, West Wycombe, Bucks.
48. Whitby C, de Cates C M, Roberton N R C 1983 Neonatal care in the Cambridge unit. In: Davis J A, Richards M P M, Roberton N R C (eds) Parent–baby attachment in premature infants. Croom Helm, London
49. Whitelaw A, Heisterkamp G, Sleath K, Acolet D, Richards M 1988 Skin-to-skin contact for very low birthweight infants and their mothers: a randomized trial of 'kangaroo care'. Archives of Disease in Childhood 63: 1377–1381
50. Widmayer S M, Field T M 1980 Effects of Brazelton demonstrations on early interactions of preterm infants and their teenage mothers. Infant Behavior and Development 3: 78–79
51. Winnicott D W 1988 Babies and their mothers. Free Association Books, London
52. Wolke D 1998 The psychological development of prematurely born children. Archives of Disease in Childhood 78: 567–570
53. Wolke D, Meyer R 1999 Cognitive status, language attainment and pre-reading skills of 6 year old very pre-term children and their peers: The Bavarian Longitudinal Study. Developmental Medicine and Child Neurology 41, 94–109
54. Zeanah C H 2000 Handbook of infant mental health, 2nd edn. Guilford Press, New York

CHAPTER 5

Counselling and support for parents and families

Ian A Laing, Hazel E McHaffie

Introduction

Having a newborn infant ill in a neonatal unit is an extremely stressful experience for parents. The mother is usually suffering from fatigue and physical discomfort from the delivery. Both parents are anxious. Their hopes and dreams are threatened. The future is uncertain, the path unknown. The couple face a strain on their personal and combined resources and cannot know in advance if they will be equal to the challenge.

A principal preoccupation with the parents is the establishment of a relationship with this new member of their family, but conditions are far from ideal. Instead of a 3.5 kg term infant on a postnatal ward, the centre of admiration and congratulations, they have an ill baby, often scrawny, distanced from them by a perspex barrier. Their own feelings of guilt and helplessness are compounded by the fact that there seems to be no role for them; neonatal nurses and doctors are the caregivers; machines and tests replace parental caresses.

If families are to look back on these days and weeks with satisfaction and look forward constructively to the rest of their lives, the professional team must handle them with care. The aim of this chapter is to offer guidance to less experienced clinicians in order to facilitate the best service the circumstances will allow.

No chapter can substitute for personal experience. All junior staff should watch their seniors in action, and take the opportunity to attend counselling sessions where possible. These interactions depend to an extent on an intangible chemistry between parent and professional, and this chemistry is strongly influenced by the personalities of both. But much can be learned from observing closely how the discussions progress, noting the apposite phrase which crystallises a moment, the tactics which deflect anger, the way in which trust is reinforced.

Although the doctor and the parents may differ on many fronts – culture, religious belief, social class, life choices, education, expectations – these differences must not be permitted to create insuperable hurdles. The baby is our patient but he is the parents' child. The decisions should be the right decisions for this family at this point in their lives. The professional's task is to share medical insight and knowledge whilst respecting parental values and beliefs, working with them to make wise choices on behalf of the child.

The relationship with parents

A good working relationship is essential for effective collaboration.

Initial introductions

Courtesy matters. It is polite and helpful, for example, before meeting either or both of the parents, to establish what their names are and how they prefer to be addressed. Similarly the couple need to know their boundaries, and the doctor should introduce himself, and state his role in the team. Shaking hands with both parents at first meeting is symbolic of a future trusting relationship. The overall approach should be one of mutual respect.

Establishing trust

Throughout the exchanges, the doctor should bear in mind the importance of trust. Once lost, it is very hard to regain. And whatever the status or level of experience of the professional, unfounded opinions, unrealistic predictions and false hope undermine confidence.

Before the first interview, the doctor must know any relevant family history, and the details of the pregnancy, labour and delivery. The initial meeting may well take place in the delivery room, with parents who have had only the briefest introduction to their newborn baby. At this stage it is essential to keep things simple. Even for the highly educated, this is no time to be bombarded with complex diagnoses, specialist jargon or intricate pathophysiology. The following example gives basic clear information and may be enough for the first interaction: 'Your baby has come out very early and is very small. His lungs have not yet matured. We have connected him to a ventilator, and he is stable for now. We will tell you much more when you are able to visit the baby unit.'

Questions should be answered honestly. Where doubt exists, professionals should resist the impulse to declare that the baby will be 'fine'. It is much better to reply, 'He's comfortable in his incubator at the moment. But we need to see how he progresses in the next few hours before we can be sure how things will go. We'll keep you informed and I can promise you we won't hide anything from you.'

Roles and responsibilities

In the 21st century, every neonatal unit should have a dedicated counselling room where staff can meet families without fear of interruption. In this room, the parents can be confident that they have the undivided attention of the staff and can have all their concerns addressed. It is a useful rule that doctors should take their cue from the family as to the amount they can absorb or tolerate at a given sitting.

Neonatal units often have written protocols about who should conduct interviews. The consultant holds overall responsibility not only for the child's care but also for the interactions with the family. Junior paediatricians should never be in the position of communicating with families beyond their level of experience. Meetings of a particularly sensitive nature should be conducted by the consultant in the presence of a nurse who is looking after the baby and who has established a rapport with the parents. Although it can be beneficial for junior staff to attend such interviews, it is important to ensure the comfort and privacy of parents is not compromised. And regardless of who is present behind closed doors, the whole team need to know what is said and what decided, in order to facilitate effective teamwork. To that end, full and careful documentation is essential.

A primary task for the consultant is that of assessing the full clinical picture as far as it can be known. Good counselling depends on accurate facts and knowledge of the literature. There will often be areas of uncertainty, but if there have been exhaustive efforts to find out as much as possible, the family will usually respect an honest admission from a senior member of staff of 'I don't know.' A statement such as 'I am confused' does not inspire confidence, but a frank 'There are uncertainties ahead and we can't be sure at this stage how things will go, but we'll continue to discuss everything with you' allows the parent to appreciate the evolving picture. The capacity of the parents to tolerate bad news will vary, but the truth should never be compromised. 'Truth sometimes hurts but deceit hurts more.'[3]

Teamwork

Managing sick infants well is a team effort. A wise doctor will listen to the parents. They have a unique investment in their child and stand in the most privileged position in relation to him. Furthermore, as time goes by, they often become experts in the problems affecting the child. With their focus on the one infant, they not infrequently detect subtle unspecific changes which give rise to unease. Staff should give proper attention to such misgivings. They are often correct.

It is also crucially important to listen to what colleagues say. The nurses are in constant attendance of these babies. The junior doctors see them frequently. Senior colleagues have the benefit of experience. Their instincts and observations may provide insights into both the condition of the baby and the reaction of the parents which are not apparent to a consultant who is present for limited periods of time only. Their voices should be heard and respected.

Consent to treatment

The subject of consent is currently fraught with difficulties in the developed world. Until recent years it was assumed that babies admitted to a neonatal unit brought with them implied consent, which allowed staff to carry out any procedure on the baby without obtaining prior consent. Parents were commonly informed only afterwards. A tension has now arisen, partly stemming from a small number of legal cases in which medical staff strayed beyond ethical boundaries to the clear detriment of the patient. As a result, more and more protocols are being developed demanding that written informed consent be obtained for increasing numbers of procedures, allegedly to protect the child, the parents and the staff. Unfortunately, if genuinely informed consent is to be obtained, each interview between staff and parents must be lengthy in order to do the subject justice. Such interviews erode the time that staff can devote to the child's care, and clearly this could have an adverse effect on prognosis. Should a lumbar puncture be delayed at 0300 hours while parents, already exhausted, are wakened at home and asked to drive to the neonatal unit for an in-depth interview, or should staff be allowed to carry out the procedure and discuss this with the couple during daylight hours? This debate has not yet been resolved.

Nevertheless there are procedures which carry clear risks, and great care should be taken to ensure such procedures are described in detail to the parents by the practitioner designated to carry out the procedure, who must be qualified and trained to do so.

The major decisions

Each neonatal unit should have written guidelines for staff to indicate which procedures require consent to be formally documented. These may include immunisations, transport of an infant from one hospital to another, and operative procedures including laser treatment for retinopathy of prematurity and exchange transfusions.

Consent forms should be readily understood, and inform the signatory of the benefits and risks. National guidelines may be available. However, any such form does not remove the responsibility of the clinician to assess the educational level of the signatory and to ensure that he or she understands the procedure and its implications. Information leaflets describing the procedure and its implications may be a useful adjunct to verbal description, but again they should never be a substitute for the professional interview capturing the essence of what the parents are consenting to and why. Parents should be given a copy of the signed consent form.

The minor decisions

Consent for less invasive procedures with minimal risks is traditionally obtained verbally. Examples include the administration of vitamin K at birth (specifying by which route), immunisations, neonatal screening investigations such as blood sampling to identify phenylketonuria, hypothyroidism, cystic fibrosis and perhaps anonymised testing for human immunodeficiency virus. If it has been decided that written consent is appropriate for all procedures, minor as well as major, the above guidance applies.

Life and death decision-making

Making crucial decisions on behalf of their baby is one of the most difficult experiences parents ever face. Professionals working in neonatal units are understandably anxious about the burden they carry and about the potential for guilt.[8] But recent research has demonstrated that, in reality, parents want to be given the opportunity (though not the obligation) to be active in decision making and they do not appear to suffer adversely as a result.[7]

Of course, they do not do this alone and unsupported. They are dependent on the medical team always for information, often for guidance, and sometimes for a recommendation. A 'guided consensus' is an effective way of handling this process,[4] and it is critical that before withdrawal of neonatal intensive care takes place, the parents as well as the staff are confident that this action is in the child's best interests. Furthermore, the ongoing compassionate support of the team caring for the family is crucial to their ability to cope with this task, and senior staff should be vigilant to ensure that appropriate help is available during each stage of the process. Important elements in this support are good communication, full frank information and, where possible, concrete evidence of a poor prognosis. If each member of the team is to play their part effectively, they too must be adequately supported, and their opinions heard and respected.

In most cases, consensus is reached without dissension. However, if either the family or the staff think that intensive care should continue, then a decision to withdraw would be a gross error of judgement. Usually, parental uncertainty arises from a failure or reluctance to fully comprehend the gravity of the situation. Continued intensive care brings clarity in the fullness of time. The child will either deteriorate or improve, and the decision is then more straightforward.

It is not the intention of this chapter to explore the ethical issues around withdrawal of neonatal intensive care. These have been explored in previous publications.[11,13]

The dying baby

Much has been written recently about the dying baby, and care of the parents.[5,7] There can never be a time when high-quality communication is more important than when a baby is dying. The parents will remember professional sensitivity or insensitivity for the rest of their lives.

In the rare event that a newborn infant collapses and dies without warning, there is little time to build a relationship with the family. The consultant must be summoned and must take control of decision making and communication. Major priorities in these circumstances are that the child should be free of all distress, his or her dignity should be respected, and the family be encouraged to spend the last minutes holding their dying child, free from the encumbrances of intensive care. Such parents should be helped to acknowledge their own unique role, to accept the reality of the short life and death, to create memories, and to be involved with the baby after death.

Much more commonly, babies die in a neonatal unit after some time and following a deliberate reorientation of care to comfort measures. The parents have had time to get to know the staff, and have been closely involved in decision making. Tolerances and preferences as to the exact nature of their own involvement vary, but it is important for clinicians to be aware of the available options and to be non-judgemental of parents.[7]

Managing the dying process

When the parents and staff have agreed that care should be reoriented to comfort measures, then the consultant and a senior nurse should explore with the parents what their wishes may be. They may need guidance as to what options are available, and here senior experienced nursing staff may be especially sensitive. Knowing what they may do – invite close family members and friends to 'say goodbye', organise a baptismal or blessing service, involve siblings, take photographs, collect mementoes, hold and groom the baby, even perhaps take the baby home – enables parents to decide what is right for them and minimises later regret.

The way the death is managed will materially influence parental satisfaction and acceptance of the wisdom of the choices made. Staff should be especially careful in their preparation of parents as to what will or might happen. Protracted deaths, unpleasant sights and sounds, and conflicting advice can all undermine parental confidence and leave families with a burden of guilt and distressing memories.[7] In an individual case, it is difficult to predict, but parents should be reassured that they will be supported by the staff at each stage and that every effort will be made to ensure the baby will slip peacefully into death.

Ensuring freedom from distress is a sensitive issue which has attracted much debate. According to law, any intervention with the purpose of procuring death is illegal, but medication given to alleviate suffering which has the side effect of hastening death is permissible.[12] Comfort may best be assured by the intravenous administration of opiates as necessary, with appropriate reassurance to the parents about the purpose of this analgesia.

Asking for permission to carry out an autopsy is an extremely painful part of this process. With the adverse publicity of recent years, it has become even more sensitive. But where there are unanswered questions about this child or future obstetric risk, it may be the only method of obtaining answers.[1] A principal reason for resisting postmortem examination is the fear of mutilation, and parents may need help to acquire a balance of perspective which will enable them to make appropriate choices.[9]

Memories acquired at this time comfort and sustain parents in the ensuing years.[7] The presence of sensitive staff known to them during the dying process is crucially important if parents are to be maximally involved. Parental reactions vary but will usually include a mixture of anger, denial, numbness and great sadness. Having staff supporting them with whom they have already established a relationship allows them to laugh, or cry, share anecdotes, or express their fears and hostility, without fear of misunderstanding. Although priority must always be given to the parents' needs and privacy, junior staff may learn best from watching the experts at work.

Bereavement

Newly bereaved parents find it difficult to leave behind the support of the team who have known their baby and shared his or her life and death. They have a great need not only to obtain information which enables them to make sense of what has happened, but also to feel that they and their baby were valued and important to the staff.

Parents appreciate staff attending the funeral, contacting them to check they are coping, seeing them to talk about the baby. These things help to avoid a sense of abandonment as well as devastation. Doctors, of course, have many competing demands on their resources and it may not be possible to cultivate an ongoing contact. Commonly it is the nursing staff who provide these signs of caring, often in their own time. But the consultant is the person who is key in the formal bereavement meeting, which takes place 4 to 6 weeks later.[10]

The importance of follow-up cannot be overemphasised. It is crucial in helping the parents to piece together what has happened, accept the reality, and assess their own future obstetric risks. Parents value an unhurried session with the neonatologist and nurse most closely involved with their family, full and frank information, and the opportunity to discuss the implications. The follow-up interview also provides an opportunity for staff to watch and listen to ensure that the couple are mutually supportive and are experiencing a normal grieving process.[10]

Supporting parents

It should be remembered that in these extraordinary and uniquely traumatic circumstances, the usual support systems new parents turn to are inadequate. Parents rely principally on the neonatal team to inform, advise, guide and support them.[6] However, once they have left the neonatal unit, their family and friends are much more in contact with them than are the staff.

There is great potential for such people to compound the pain of bereavement; thus staff should be vigilant to ensure, where possible, that family members are prepared for the task.

Other sources of help exist and should be approached or suggested where appropriate. The staff themselves may seek help in handling difficult situations. A general practitioner, for example, may know the parents intimately, and can often provide information which will help the neonatal-unit staff to understand the family background and its dynamics. Social workers, too, may be able to shed light on what is happening in the family home, and this may be key to parental behaviour in the neonatal unit.

Parents may be directed to alternative forms of support. Religious advisors, other parents who have similar experiences, or self-help groups such as the Stillbirth and Neonatal Death Society, or Compassionate Friends, may all offer solace to certain families, but the difficulty parents sense in approaching strangers when they feel vulnerable and emotional should not be underestimated.

Psychiatric illness is not uncommon in our society and is particularly prevalent among mothers in the early weeks after delivering their infants.[2] Where the mother is separated from her infant during neonatal intensive care, feelings of inadequacy and depression may be exacerbated. A psychiatrist may be invaluable in helping in such a situation.

Conflict

In a well-managed neonatal unit, conflict between staff and families should be rare. Nevertheless, disputes do occasionally occur, and it is the duty of staff to identify why conflict has arisen, and (better) to anticipate and deflect it.

Anticipating trouble

Where emotions run high, there is a constant need for vigilance. Are the parents taking advice from well-meaning but ill-informed members of their family, and should these family members be interviewed too? Is there inter-parental conflict, and should this be acknowledged and sidelined so that both parents, despite their differences, can contribute constructively to their child's care? Is the drug abuse of one or both partners interfering with their ability to make decisions? Should other professionals be brought in to facilitate better control of tempers or hostility so that discussions can be constructive once more?

Averting trouble

Almost always, conflict arises out of uncertainty, parental fatigue, and perceived or actual poor communication. Occasionally a schism can occur on the basis of ethnic or religious differences. Neonatal staff have stressful jobs. They too are only human and personal problems may make them vulnerable. It may be advisable on occasion to allocate another member of staff to a family, where interpersonal tension exists.

In a misguided attempt to cope with all situations, doctors sometimes forget they have allies. Colleagues and peers can be extremely helpful sources of advice. Conflict may diminish simply by bringing in another professional, perhaps of a different gender or ethnic background, perhaps from another city, able to look afresh at the clinical and emotional background out of which tension has emerged. Skilled interpreters may be invaluable in cases where language barriers are the root cause of conflict.

When tension stems from a breakdown of trust, written information may help. A detailed, factual account of the child's illness and prognosis may be taken by parents and discussed with trusted advisors, family and friends. The parents may be encouraged to write down **all** the questions troubling them. Each can then be explored in a follow-up interview. This exchange may also be documented, giving the parents opportunity to consider the situation calmly and in their own time.

Sometimes, parents are helped by having chosen advocates present. Young and inexperienced parents may benefit from their own parents sharing the discussions. A member of a minority religious group may draw strength from a minister or adviser who can explain the parents' stance from a more detached point of view. A sensitive clinician will be aware of special vulnerabilities and needs, and seek to circumvent conflict.

Managing abuse

Staff should be trained in containment of aggression. Occasionally, however, parents may be gratuitously or vindictively verbally abusive. They should be told politely but firmly that this is unacceptable. If the abuse is repeated, senior staff should give serious consideration to excluding the parent(s). If there is any threat of physical violence, security officers should be summoned immediately to have the parent(s) removed, in order to protect the babies, the staff and other visitors to the unit. The consultant will then meet with senior management, social workers, hospital security and the police, to develop a plan which will maximise safety of all those involved, even if it means, in extreme cases, excluding the parents on a permanent basis from the unit.

Dealing with complaints

The consultant takes ultimate responsibility for the care of the baby and family. If a complaint is made, the consultant should be involved in addressing it. It is worth noting that if complaints are not addressed quickly, then they tend to multiply.

A first task is to establish the facts. The responsible team should then meet with the family in a private room where they will be uninterrupted. Listening to the parents is the most important aspect of dealing with such a situation and every effort should be made to adopt an unhurried and sympathetic approach. If the complaint is justified, then staff should be generous in their apology. 'I am sorry we made a mistake. I recognise you are angry. We will do everything to ensure that this does not happen to you or to any other family again.' If the complaint is not justified, then, having listened attentively to the criticisms, the consultant should express regret for the parents' distress but endeavour to give a reasonable and justifiable explanation for any misunderstanding. It may or may not be accepted, but simply being given a fair hearing may well go a long way to satisfying the parents.

Multiple complaints

Multiple complaints usually arise when an initial complaint has not been dealt with immediately. The family should be encouraged to write down each complaint and give the list to the staff beforehand. The consultant and other staff can then explore the justification for each, obtain a full account of the events from those involved, and agree a strategy which promises the best chance of regaining the family's confidence. In this situation, and especially where the complaints are of a serious nature, it is often helpful to have an independent chairperson to reconcile staff and family. Where this person is perceived to be autonomous and impartial, it can be easier to steer clear of personal attack, preserve a proper balance and sense of proportion, and highlight areas of genuine concern.

Special situations

Some situations that are encountered in neonatal units deserve a special mention. Certain types of parents may need special nurturing.

Parents of the acutely collapsed baby

This is often the most demanding of crises. The parents have relaxed, and believe that their child is 'out of the woods'. Suddenly there is an acute deterioration. 'It must be somebody's fault' is a very understandable reaction, but a painful one for dedicated staff to cope with. Immediate answers may not be available. The doctor in charge does not yet know whether the 4-day-old baby has developed an unexpected septicaemia or whether there is a congenital abnormality such as hypoplastic left heart syndrome that has manifested itself now that the ductus has closed. There is a rush to treat infection, and to obtain cardiological advice. The parents may be forgiven for thinking that the staff cannot even identify which organ is triggering the crisis. In such circumstances, honesty is the best policy. The clinician should be very candid but also emphasise the positive aspects of care. 'Your baby, Rosemary, is very ill. We have put her back on the ventilator. There are a number of possible causes and it's important we identify the cause of her problems accurately. At the moment we are treating her for infection. I've asked for a specialist, a cardiologist, to come urgently to the unit so that we can get the best advice available. I am personally taking care of your baby, and as soon as I know the complete answer I will come and discuss our plans with you.'

Parents of the baby with chronic disease

After the whirlwind of delivery, resuscitation, ventilation, replacement surfactant and the roller-coaster of the early days of life, it is very common for a baby to enter a stable phase where there is neither a perceived improvement nor deterioration. This stage can be immensely frustrating for parents. Weeks go by and nothing seems to be happening. Some days the baby looks less good than others. The parents sleep poorly. The staff may also feel discouraged.

Ongoing concern for the parents and good communication are imperative. Parents should never be made to feel they are in the way or troublesome with their frequent questions. Rather, understanding their dilemma can be supportive. 'We know you're having trouble sleeping. Don't hesitate to ring any time in the night just for reassurance. We understand how worrying this stage can be.' Provided it does not encourage false hope, it can be supportive to identify some area of progress and lift the parents' spirits by offering them a different perspective. For example, parents of a child with bronchopulmonary dysplasia may feel discouraged by his ventilator dependency. By saying, 'Yes, your baby is still in 30% oxygen, but look at his excellent growth. With every day that passes, he is making new lung which is no longer being damaged by the ventilator', you are acknowledging the legitimacy of their concerns but giving them encouraging news too.

Long weary days cocooned in a neonatal unit can be depressing. Dedicated parents may need to be given permission to resume a life outside the hospital. Encouraging them to gradually change their visiting patterns may help them to acquire a healthier perspective.

The absent parent

Parents may feel inadequate in the intensive care setting, and may express their fear by staying away. It is the staff's duty to maintain the highest possible standard but this is much harder to achieve without parental collaboration. Every effort should be made to address the cause of their reluctance, to gain their confidence, and, with patience, to draw them into the team. Strategies might include meeting the absent parent on neutral territory; suggesting they bring a supportive friend or relative in too; identifying a specific and positive role for them to play; or cultivating a mutual interest in something outside the unit (e.g. in Edinburgh, the staff have an extensive knowledge of Hibernian Football Club!).

The unsupported teenage mother

Even the most junior members of staff will find themselves caring for mothers and fathers who are several years younger than they are, but their attitude should never be patronising. Though chronologically younger, such parents may be surprisingly mature in experience, outlook and ability to cope. The unsupported teenage mother, however, represents a special challenge. Her abandonment may be temporary or permanent, but efforts should be made to establish the reasons for the schisms. Where the teenager's feelings will not be violated, separate interviews with her own mother may be indicated, in order to befriend her, and to persuade her that both mother and grandmother have an essential role in the child's care and future. If this is inappropriate or fails, then a close friend and/or a social worker should be brought in to support the teenage mother for the important decisions about hers and the baby's future. Patience, gentleness and understanding will all be needed.

The parent who takes control

This is a common situation. It occurs particularly where parents are intelligent, talented and challenging in their own professional lives. They are familiar with Internet searches and soon become 'experts' in their baby's condition, treatment and prognosis. Such parents are used to being in control, and tend to channel their own understandable anxieties into aggression, passive or overt. Staff should be sufficiently resilient to tolerate a mild degree of challenging behaviour, but as soon as it threatens to interfere with the quality of care of the infant, then it must be addressed.

The consultant should meet with staff and listen carefully to the facts, ensuring that they are neither exaggerated nor diminished. Together with another member of staff, he or she should then meet with the parents, and appeal to them to recognise the expertise and professionalism of the staff, and not allow their strong personalities to jeopardise the care the team want to provide for the family. Regaining control is essential to good relationships, and it is a mistake to allow parents to dictate which nurses and doctors they wish to take care of their baby. It may be necessary to set up regular meetings with such a couple to ensure that they are allowing the care of the child to progress unhindered by their anxieties.

The parent with special educational needs

In law, parents have responsibility for their child. Staff have an ethical duty to ensure that the care of the child is equally good no matter the educational attainments of the parents. On rare occasions, however, neonatologists are faced with parents whose educational needs prevent them from understanding what is happening to their child. Sometimes other members of the family may be able to act **in loco parentis**, and it is reassuring to have supportive grandparents who can make rational suggestions in the best interests of the baby. In the absence of such extended family, it may be necessary to contact the Department of Social Work. Doctors' first responsibility is to the child and very occasionally they may be forced to make the child a ward of court, particularly if decisions made by the parents are seen to be against the baby's interests.

The parent who is a healthcare professional

It can be difficult to be the parent of an imperilled infant and also a healthcare professional. Roles and expectations between the two can become confused. Staff should encourage such a person to be a parent first, and expect no more of them than from any other articulate and intelligent mother or father. 'I am going to pretend that you are not a doctor. Indeed, with your permission, I would like to call you Mr Jones while your baby is in the unit', will often produce a smile of relief from the parent.

Preserving your own health

Intensive care is demanding, and neonatal doctors and nurses work extremely hard for the families. We are groomed to succeed, and we feel guilty and inadequate when we do not. Every child's death, every physical deterioration, can feel like failure. It is a mistake to cover up such feelings, and to look for solace in excess.

A healthy way to deal with perceived failure is to discuss troubling cases openly with peers. Reassurance may come from hearing that there was nothing further that could have been done, or a shared sense of sorrow. Some teams favour routine debriefing after any stressful situation. These meetings, if skilfully handled, can be educational, and also beneficial for the corporate as well as individual morale. Maintaining a balance that includes an active life outside the neonatal unit is essential. Whether your interest is in the gym or theatre, climbing mountains or juggling flaming torches, it is essential for the carers to care for themselves if they are to be sufficiently restored to return to the neonatal unit and deal empathically with the next family.

Concluding thoughts

Neonatology combines the rigours of intensive care with the need to communicate openly and in detail with families. Counselling and support for parents cannot adequately be achieved in one meeting and takes great patience and tact. Staff need to be articulate, thoughtful, sensitive and, above all, excellent at listening. It is hoped that this chapter has pointed the way, but excellence in practice is learned from peers, mentors and the families themselves.

References

1. Brodlie M, Laing I A, Keeling J W, McKenzie K J 2002 Ten years of neonatal autopsies in tertiary referral centre: retrospective study. British Medical Journal 324: 761–763
2. Cox J L 1986 Postnatal depression. Churchill Livingstone, Edinburgh
3. Fallowfield L 1997 Truth sometimes hurts, but deceit hurts more. Annals of the New York Academy of Sciences 809: 525–536
4. Laing I A 1989 Withdrawing from invasive neonatal intensive care. In: Mason J K (ed) Paediatric forensic medicine and pathology. Chapman & Hall, London, pp 131–140
5. Laing I A, Halley G 1995 Enough is enough – when to stop neonatal care. Current Paediatrics 5: 53–58
6. McHaffie H E 1992 Social support in the neonatal intensive care unit. Journal of Advanced Nursing 17: 279–287
7. McHaffie H E 2001 Crucial decisions at the beginning of life. Radcliffe Medical Press, Abingdon
8. McHaffie H E, Fowlie P W 1996 Life, death and decisions. Hochland & Hochland, Cheshire
9. McHaffie H E, Fowlie P W, Hume R et al 2001 Consent to autopsy for neonates. Archives of Disease in Childhood. Fetal and Neonatal Edition 85: F4–F7
10. McHaffie H E, Laing I A, Lloyd D J 2001 Follow up care of bereaved parents after treatment withdrawal from newborns. Archives of Disease in Childhood. Fetal and Neonatal Edition 84: F125–F128
11. McHaffie H E, Laing I A, Parker M et al 2001 Deciding for imperilled newborns: medical authority or parental autonomy? Journal of Medical Ethics 27: 104–109
12. Royal College of Paediatrics and Child Health, Ethics Advisory Committee 1997 Withholding and withdrawal of life-saving treatment in children: a framework for practice. Royal College of Paediatrics and Child Health, London
13. Warnock M 1998 An intelligent person's guide to ethics. Gerald Duckworth, London, pp 40–53

Further reading

Gustaitis R, Young E W D 1986 A time to be born, a time to die. Addison-Wesley, Reading, MA
Hindmarch C 2000 On the death of a child. Radcliffe Medical Press, Oxford
Kohner N, Henley A 1995 When a baby dies. The experience of late miscarriage, stillbirth and neonatal death. Pandora Press, London
Kohner N, Leftwich A 1995 Pregnancy loss and the death of a baby: a training pack for professionals. National Extension College, Cambridge
Tschudin V 1997 Counselling for loss and bereavement. Baillière Tindall, London
Warnock M 2002 Making babies. Oxford University Press, Oxford

CHAPTER 6

Ethical and legal aspects of neonatology

PART I

Ethics

Michael Hird, Victor F Larcher

Introduction

As a significant number of deaths occurring in a neonatal unit arise as a consequence of the withholding or withdrawing of life-sustaining treatment,[15] it is important to consider the duties and professional obligations incumbent on those involved in care of the newborn infant, and an ethical framework for this practice is important. We use the term 'life-sustaining treatment' to encompass the use of invasive treatments intended to save or extend the life of an infant who might otherwise die. This includes resuscitation at birth, which may lead to the continuing provision of intensive care, artificial ventilation, other forms of organ support and parenteral nutritional support.

The fundamental principles embodied in the standards governing our approach to these difficult issues can be outlined as follows.

Health professionals must practise in accordance with their duty of care: this includes respecting the autonomy of their patients and acting to restore health, sustain life and prevent illness all to an acceptable and reasonable standard.[2] This is often more simply interpreted as the fact that the child's best interests are considered to be paramount, and this is a tenet found throughout both legal and ethical considerations.

There must be an awareness of the rights of the child as laid out in both the UN Declaration of Human Rights[13] and the UN Convention of the Rights of the Child,[14] where fundamental principles lay down that any decision or action concerning children must have their best interests as a primary consideration. This places a duty on the clinician to respect the life and health of the individual patient by preserving life, restoring health and preventing disease, and to perform these duties to an acceptable standard. Any proposed treatment should confer maximum benefit at the expense of minimal harm with this assessment considering not just clinical factors but also emotional, psychological and social influences affecting both the patient and their family.

A further essential duty is to respect the autonomy of patients. A baby obviously lacks the capacity for self determination, and the primary responsibility for dictating his best interests must be assumed to lie primarily with the parents, whose own concepts are likely to be determined by their own moral framework and cultural and societal mores. This may give rise to conflict, as parental wishes may be at variance with those of the health professionals, whose values may originate from a very different social and economic background. The baby is reliant on his parents and health professionals acting in partnership on his behalf. It is important that this partnership of care incorporates both the parents and the whole health-care team.

Health professionals must undertake to put the interests of the baby above their own. Gorowitz, in defining characteristics associated with a good doctor, said that 'it is important they should understand their own values and motivation well enough to recognise that they can be in conflict with the patient's interests, and also possess the honesty to be truthful about their own fallibility and that of their art'.[4] This is particularly pertinent in situations where continuing efforts to sustain life using the 'sanctity of life' as a guiding principle may represent a breach of professional duty, equal in magnitude to a failure to intervene when it is necessary to do so. Furthermore, it is essential that actions taken or contemplated should be within the framework of the criminal, statute or common law of the country.

Ethical and legal guidance in the UK is available from the Royal College of Paediatrics and Child Health (RCPCH),[12] the British Medical Association[1] and the General Medical Council. None of these, however, will serve to abolish controversy: team members, and indeed parents, may and will have strong views as to the appropriateness of continuing the provision of life-sustaining treatment and time will need to be spent ensuring that there is effective and consistent communication.

Parental demands for continuing life sustaining treatment

Parents may wish intensive care support to be continued when it will neither significantly prolong life nor confer clinical benefit. This may be as a consequence of strongly held parental values or cultural beliefs not shared by the health-care team.

Entitled as they are to make decisions on behalf of their child, it is not axiomatic that parental demands for treatment should be met. Parents need to be helped with sensitivity and compassion to understand the nature and prognosis of their child's illness. Clear and consistent reasons need to be given as to why the clinician's perception is different, and this may require repeated difficult conversations with parents. Communication styles may clash and differences may remain unresolved if time is not spent ascertaining the precise views of the parents.

It is important to emphasise that treatment options are not necessarily all-or-none, particularly for the older neonate. It may be possible to reach a compromise by agreeing to some limited interventions on a therapeutic menu and achieving understanding that overall care is not being withdrawn.

In some uncommon situations, areas of conflict are not resolved and repeated discussions fail to reach a consensus. It may then be necessary to seek judicial review, but if possible all steps should be taken to prevent this.

withhold or withdraw life sustaining treatment could be made (pp. 85–6).

Modern neonatal teams consist of large numbers of professionals with widely differing backgrounds, and it is important that all have a voice. On occasion, evidence of discomfiture may be only subtly exhibited through patterns of behaviour such as a lack of involvement in the case in question or changes in normal posture on ward rounds.[3] An 'in-house' or external second opinion is good practice when withdrawal of care is contemplated.

Guidelines may not alter the final decision relating to withdrawal of intensive care that would otherwise have been made by senior staff. However, their existence does help to clarify the process to all concerned and should help to ensure consistency in discussion with parents. We have been involved in developing multidisciplinary guidelines to help professionals in managing the process of decision making. Included in these is a checklist (Fig. 6.1) which it is hoped will prove helpful.

Withholding or withdrawing life sustaining treatment

Many professionals will instinctively feel that there is a distinction between the withholding and the withdrawal of life-sustaining treatment. Some find it easier not to embark upon a course of action from which they may later have to withdraw. Others find such inactivity difficult. Legally and ethically, however, most authorities would make no such distinction and in many circumstances it may be more appropriate to commence life-sustaining treatment – until for example the prognosis becomes more certain, adequate consultations have been held or the family have come to terms with the situation.

Partnership

Healthcare professionals and parents have a duty to act in partnership and any intervention for a neonate requires valid consent. Parents, confronted with the serious illness of their new baby, may not be able to comprehend the information they are given and its consequences for themselves and their child. A valid consent is one that is sufficiently informed, given by a person able to understand what is involved, and obtained without coercion.[7] It may be difficult to satisfy these conditions in neonatal intensive care. Assimilating information requires time and it is therefore ethical to continue treatment until such criteria are satisfied. However on occasions the baby's clinical condition may change so rapidly that there is no time for informed consent to be obtained.

Guidance

In 1997 the Royal College of Paediatrics and Child Health published an ethical and legal framework within which decisions to

The child's clinical condition
- Are sufficient and adequate medical facts available to make a diagnosis and give accurate prognosis
- Has a potentially treatable condition been excluded
- Is a second medical opinion necessary/desirable
- Is there a need for a psychiatric or psychological assessment of the child
- What are the problems in providing nursing care in the current situation
- What are the views of nursing staff about changing goals for the child
- What are the views of other therapists/professionals involved with the child
- How has dissent in the team been handled
- Is the child able to form a view about what he/she wants
- Has he or she been consulted.

The family
- Is the family's understanding of their child's condition adequate
- What are the family's relevant religious cultural beliefs and values
- Has there been a psycho-social assessment of the family
- What are the family's likely or actual views on changing goals of treatment
- Do the family need the help of an advocate

The decision-making process
- How has uncertainty about the outcome been addressed
- Has there been an ethical review of the case
- Has there been a strategy meeting or psychosocial meeting
- Have Human Rights issues been properly considered
- Is there a proportionate justification for any infringement of Human Rights
- Is there a need for a legal opinion
- Is there a properly formulated care plan
- Has informed consent for this care plan been obtained
- Do the notes adequately reflect the process
- How is the process to be maintained/audited

Fig. 6.1 Checklist for withdrawal of intensive care.

Practical management

Decisions to withhold or withdraw life support or intensive care from infants, whether from birth or following a period of treatment, have to be based on a careful assessment of the infant's clinical condition. While the long-term implications of certain clinical findings such as bilateral intraparenchymal cerebral haemorrhages, diffuse periventricular leukomalacia and severe perinatal asphyxia with grade III hypoxic–ischaemic encephalopathy are relatively well established, the neurodevelopmental outlook in many other situations is often unclear. There is always potential for conflict around such momentous decisions, and the way in which these issues are handled has been shown to have a significant impact on how parents and staff come to terms with the death of the baby. Partnership with parents is an integral part of neonatal care and, while the abiding principle must be that care is directed by the best interests of the baby, this must also try and encompass parental wishes. Honest and effective communication with parents is essential (Chapter 5).

Perinatal management

Involvement in antenatal management where there is threatened preterm labour may be very useful. Good interprofessional communication is important to achieve a consistent management plan.[8] In cases of extreme prematurity, where a decision is being made that resuscitation may not be initiated after birth, parents must be fully aware that their baby may be born alive and remain so for a period of time. The baby may have a definite heartbeat and make weak gasps. In such cases, suitably senior staff should be present to provide support and reassurance to parents and junior staff. The difference between a remote *possibility* of initial survival and the increasing *probability* of survival with increasing gestation needs to be appreciated by the parents if they are to be in a position to make an informed judgement.[5]

The withdrawal process

Good practice dictates that a consensus needs to be achieved without coercion, and frequently this may require repeated discussions with parents, allowing them time to assimilate the information provided and come to terms with events. 'Good medicine' may therefore entail continuing life-sustaining treatment for longer than a purely ethical approach might regard as appropriate.

Cultural and religious beliefs need to be accounted for, with time allowed for baptism or blessing of the child and opportunity offered, within reason, to allow distant family members to visit if desired.

It is necessary to discuss exactly how the withdrawal process is to be managed. Some parents wish their child to be allowed to die spontaneously while still 'on the ventilator'. However, the majority of parents accept the offer of having intensive care support withdrawn and then spending their child's last minutes/hours in the privacy of a parents' room, unfettered by the trappings of technology but always with an awareness of the immediate availability of unit staff. A very small number may wish their child to die at home; this can be achieved, but not without considerable logistical problems.[6]

It is also necessary to be aware of the impact of these events upon parents of other babies on the unit. It is often worthwhile spending time with them to discuss their feelings and at the same time perhaps provide some reassurance as to the progress of their own child. The proviso is that this must be done without compromising the confidentiality of the parents of the baby from whom intensive care support is being withdrawn.

Sedation and paralysis

It is our belief that it is usual, and good practice, for an opiate to be administered prior to withdrawal of ventilatory support, in the normal dose used to provide analgesia or sedation. The intention is to alleviate pain or distress rather than to cause death (although some suppression of respiratory drive is foreseeable and acceptable – so-called doctrine of double effect – and this needs to be both explained and clearly documented). The issue of paralysing agents is more complex. The RCPCH guidelines permit the withdrawal of respiratory support if paralysing agents are concurrently in use but they cannot be initiated just prior to withdrawal. Continuation of paralysing agents during this process may cause discomfort among some members of the team; if they are to be used the members of the team need to be quite clear as to why they are being continued. Some parents and staff will express a wish for drugs to be stopped before withdrawal of intensive care, and this wish should be respected.

After withdrawal of intensive care support

Withdrawal of intensive care on the neonatal unit most commonly involves the cessation of ventilatory support with the expectation that death will usually ensue. On occasions, however, the outcome is less certain and the parents need to be adequately prepared for the possibility that their child may not succumb at once. It is important also to ensure that general supportive and palliative care for both infant *and* parents continues to be provided.

Recently published work by McHaffie et al[11] provides valuable insights into parental perceptions of treatment withdrawal and aspects of subsequent follow-up. It confirmed that parents wish to be involved in both the decision-making and the dying process. One specific area that generated distress was the time taken from the cessation of respiratory support to actual death. A swift demise appeared to confirm to the parents the appropriateness of the decision to withdraw, while delay raised doubts.

After death families must feel at liberty to spend time with their child and may often wish to be involved in bathing them, taking photographs, making hand- and footprints, etc. in accordance with the unit's usual practice and relevant cultural practices.

It is also necessary to notify relevant primary health care professionals, including GPs, community paediatricians, health visitors and midwives, as soon as possible. Units should have appropriate protocols for this. Information needs to be provided about administrative matters relating to certification and funeral arrangements and, while preliminary discussions may on occasions have been held earlier about a post-mortem examination, this will need to be broached and consent sought either at the time or the following day.

Attitudes to post-mortem examination have recently been well explored[9] and the request may be acceded to or declined for a variety of reasons.

Follow-up

This is a very important part of the whole process and significantly assists families in making progress through the normal grieving process. It is clear that contact needs to be made early, possibly within a fortnight, and ideally within 2 months of death. Parents should be able to meet someone they are familiar with and a truthful approach, concern over other family members' welfare and reiteration of details previously relayed to them all help to maintain trust and provide reassurance to the family.[10] Nursing staff in particular are often represented at funerals and may maintain contact for a long time after, and this is much appreciated.

Conclusion

Withholding and withdrawing neonatal intensive care is very much a part of practice in a neonatal unit. Discussions with parents about the possibility of withholding or withdrawing intensive care may have to commence before birth (in extreme preterm labour) and continue through life. It is essential to emphasise that while intensive care may be withdrawn, care to preserve an infant's dignity will not be compromised. It is imperative that there is close senior staff involvement and that all involved strive to manage the process to the best of their abilities.

References

1. British Medical Association 2001 Withholding and withdrawing life-prolonging medical treatment. BMJ Books, London
2. Chantler C, Doyal L 1995 Medical ethics: the duties of care in principle and practice. In: Powers M, Harris N (ed) Clinical negligence. Butterworths, London
3. Chiswick M L 1990 Withdrawal of life support in babies: deceptive signals. Archives of Disease in Childhood 65: 1096–1097
4. Gorowitz S Doctors dilemmas: moral conflicts and medical care. In: Good doctors. ch 12, pp 190–205
5. Halamek L P 2003 Prenatal consultation at the limits of viability. Neoreviews 4: e153–e156
6. Hawdon J M, Williams S, Weindling A M 1994 Withdrawal of neonatal intensive care in the home. Archives of Disease in Childhood; 71: F142–F144
7. Kennedy I, Grubb A 2000 Medical law: text and materials. Butterworths, London
8. Macdonald H and the American Academy of Pediatrics Committee on Fetus and Newborn. 2002 Perinatal care at the threshold of viability. Pediatrics 110: 1024–1027
9. McHaffie H E, Fowlie P W, Hume R, Laing I A, Lloyd D J, Lyon A J 2001 Consent to autopsy for neonates. Archives of Disease in Childhood Fetal and Neonatal Edition 85: F4–F7
10. McHaffie H E, Laing I A, Lloyd D J 2001 Follow up care of bereaved parents after treatment withdrawal from newborns. Archives of Disease in Childhood Fetal and Neonatal Edition 84: F125–F128
11. McHaffie H E, Lyon A J, Fowlie P W 2001 Lingering death after treatment withdrawal in the neonatal intensive care unit. Archives of Disease in Childhood Fetal and Neonatal Edition 85: F8–F12
12. Royal College of Paediatrics and Child Health 1997 Withholding or withdrawing life saving treatment in children: a framework for practice. RCPCH, London
13. United Nations 1948 Declaration of human rights. United Nations, New York
14. United Nations 1989 Convention on rights of the child. United Nations, New York
15. Wall S N, Partridge J C 1997 Death in the intensive care nursery: physician practice of withdrawing and withholding life support. Pediatrics 99: 64–70

PART 2

The law

M A M S Leigh, Janet M Rennie

Introduction

When neonatal medicine emerged as a distinct subspecialty, medical ethics was at a similar stage of infancy. Most decisions were assumed to be matters of 'common sense' and the law was regarded as another country where they did things differently. Today it is accepted that neonatologists have to take profound decisions of public importance, which may be subject to formal analysis in the courts. Decisions taken at the outset of a person's life often have an impact decades later. The baby who is the subject of the decision may be unable to play any part in the discussion today but will as an adult be able to ask pointed questions of his erstwhile clinician. These questions may be very much harder to answer at a time when both the state of the art and the attitudes of society will probably have changed beyond present imagination: the recent organ retention litigation in the UK is a good example of this. In this chapter we will discuss some of these issues and give general advice as to how paediatricians should conduct themselves in those areas of their practice that are likely to bring them into contact with the law.

Clinicians and litigation

Maintaining professional standards

Neonatologists must maintain their skills and the competence of their teams. Remaining 'in good standing' with the Royal College of Paediatrics and Child Health (RCPCH) involves participating in revalidation, appraisal and continuing professional development. Consultants must ensure that the neonatal unit has clear written guidelines and adequate staffing, that the facilities and equipment meet current standards (pp. 48–9) and that outcomes are audited. Accurate, detailed contemporaneous notes must be kept: they are an intrinsic part of good care and the only part that is directly visible when the quality of that care is called into question. Anticipation of possible litigation is not paranoia: it is good medicine to obtain a second opinion in difficult cases. Intemperate remarks about colleagues and hasty judgements about areas that are not within your own competence are poor practice as well as being forensically unwise.

Handling mistakes and complaints

Always be open and honest with the parents but think calmly before you meet them after any adverse event. That a ventilator fails, or an intravenous infusion runs wild, or a nurse makes a drug error is unfortunate but it may not contribute to the baby's eventual problems. Do not make the mistake of thinking that because you are being candid about a complication you should be more hasty than you would be in other circumstances to give a gloomy prognosis. Think carefully about how to treat the baby to minimise any damage and how to break bad news in a way that will reduce parental distress.

If parents complain about your treatment or counselling in an unjustified way, seek the advice and support of senior colleagues, including the Clinical Director and service manager, early on before matters get out of hand.

Appearing in court

Understanding the legal processes outlined in this chapter will help. Sometimes a decision is made not to defend a case even when the staff involved feel that they did nothing wrong and that the adverse outcome was outside their control. There are all sorts of reasons why it is decided not to defend a case in court, and the decision does not necessarily imply that the criticism advanced by the claimant is correct. In this situation, give in gracefully and remember that giving evidence in court is not a pleasant experience for any doctor. However, if it is decided to defend the case, then be prepared to spend time and energy in preparation and in attending court.

In a civil court, remember that the judge is the most important person in the room. Address all your answers to him, not to the barrister who is questioning you. Tell the truth, in simple language, think before you start talking and speak very slowly: this gives the judge time to write down what you are saying and you have time to think carefully about your answer. Do not be afraid of generating silence while you consider your answer. The pace of a courtroom seems very slow to those used to the frenetic activity of intensive care units. Do not engage the opposing barrister in banter, let him needle you or try to score a point at his expense – it is his home territory, not yours; his views are not at issue but your objectivity is. Answer the question after due thought, preferably with a straight 'yes' or 'no' but if you feel you are being forced to answer an inappropriately closed question then do not be afraid to say 'yes, but …' with one concise, crisp sentence. Resist the temptation to embark on a mini-lecture. When you have finished your answer, stop. Do not fall into the temptation to embellish or clarify simply because the cross-examiner waits and looks as if he expects you to do so.

Situations in neonatology with a high risk of litigation

General

Good notekeeping and clear protocols are vital and it is important to keep copies of old protocols when they are updated because they establish the standard of care for that era. Never amend protocols by adding to them in manuscript: always redate and reissue the whole protocol. Do not 'save up' amendments or hesitate to change the protocol simply because the amendment only involves a few words. A protocol you can no longer defend in detail is a hazard to the unit and its patients. Cases are judged by the standards of the day and, in a rapidly advancing field like neonatal medicine, it can be difficult to recall precisely when practice changed. Examples of changes in practice that were sometimes poorly documented and have caused problems in our medico-legal practice were the move to oral vitamin K prophylaxis for vitamin K deficiency bleeding in the autumn of 1992; initiation of surfactant use at around the same time; and the tighter regulation of ventilator settings to avoid hypocarbia in the early to mid 1990s when it was realised that there was a risk of periventricular leukomalacia. The recent recommendations from the Royal College of Obstetricians and Gynaecologists (RCOG) regarding intrapartum antibiotic prophylaxis for group B *Streptococcus* is likely to generate litigation.

The standards of care are those of a reasonably competent practitioner and the courts do not expect that protocols will be changed to reflect every research finding. For a while, there was a fear that protocols would be used to drive litigation in cases where the clinical management had not precisely followed a prescribed guideline. This is not a justification for the lack of a protocol, because in practice claimants usually succeed only when the standard of care is substandard by anybody's definition. Two examples make the point:

■ a preterm baby born after 1982 who required head box oxygen but who had no blood gas measurements taken for 18 hours and then collapsed with terminal respiratory failure and developed a germinal matrix/intraventricular haemorrhage at around the same time;

■ a baby who developed the same lesion (and the same disability) but who was carefully monitored from the start and in whom artificial ventilation was initiated at the appropriate time.

The first child will rightly be entitled to compensation from the hospital; the second will not.

Resuscitation

If a baby develops athetoid cerebral palsy as a result of damage to the basal ganglia after a short period of acute profound hypoxia in the immediate run-up to delivery, the quality and timeliness of the resuscitation will be under intense scrutiny. Minutes matter in this situation and, if the neonatal team arrive late, for whatever reason, the fact should be documented. Common problems are failure to intubate; incorrect endotracheal tube position and failure to use chest compression when appropriate (pp. 232–3). It is not below a reasonable standard of care to intubate the oesophagus but it is substandard care not to recognise it. It may not be below a reasonable standard of care for a junior doctor to be unable to intubate but it will be if he persists in the attempt too long rather than using bag and mask, or fails to call for help. It is substandard care to use a very small size of endotracheal tube in a term baby, or to insert it a very long way.

Example: Baby Z was born at 28 weeks gestation by emergency caesarean section for maternal pre-eclampsia. He weighed a kilo and was resuscitated with intubation and positive pressure ventilation. By 04:50 he was on the neonatal unit, where he extubated himself and was reintubated. He was referred to another hospital for intensive care and this team arrived at 05:20 to find him in very poor condition. His pH was 6.7 with a P_aCO_2 of 22 kPa; a chest X-ray showed that the endotracheal tube was so far in that it abutted the diaphragm on the right side and there was a massive tension pneumothorax, which was drained (Fig. 6.2). Baby Z survived but developed cerebral palsy, and he succeeded in his claim against the original treating hospital. Textbooks such as this one carry information about the correct endotracheal tube size and length (pp. 1256–8), and those who profess the skill of intubation should be aware of the depth to which the tube should be placed and how to assess its position.

A need for resuscitation does not equate to a diagnosis of 'birth asphyxia' and this cannot be stressed too often. Still less does it provide any basis for long-term prognostication. To act on the presumption that it does not discharge a duty of candour: it simply causes needless and unwarranted distress. Use the term 'birth depression', for which there are a number of causes, including hypoxia–ischaemia during labour. Similarly, the term 'flat' is totally imprecise and means different things to different observers. We have seen this term applied to anything from stillborn babies through to babies who responded to blow-by oxygen after a few minutes. Obtain cord pH results and document the baby's early course very carefully, with a narrative about his condition at birth and his response to resuscitation. Remember that babies who recover sufficiently quickly to remain with their mothers are sometimes at the end stage of a prolonged period of 'chronic partial' hypoxic ischaemia and develop seizures at 12–24 hours; it is wise to admit those who require resuscitation

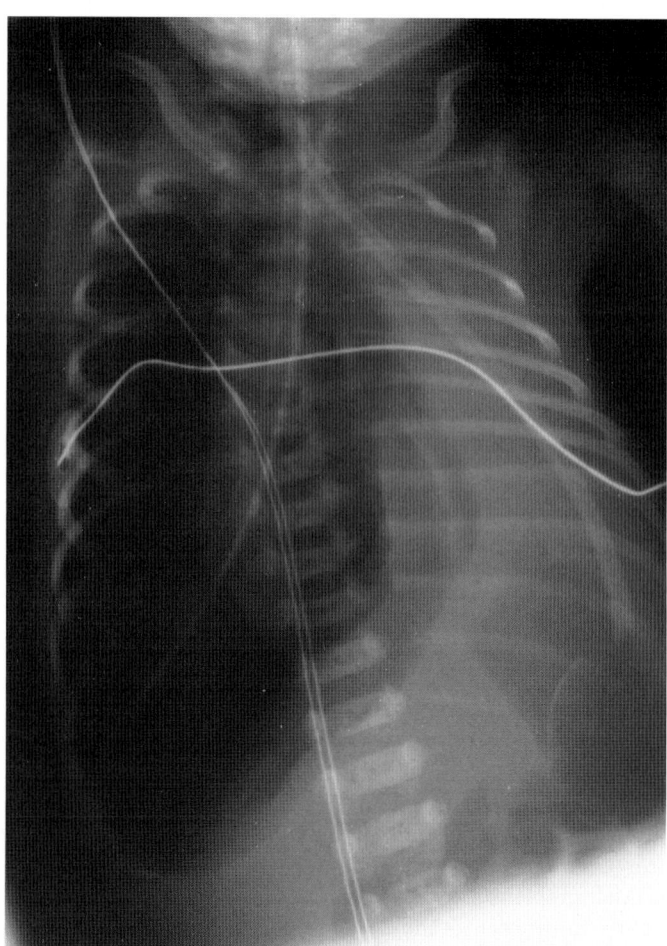

Fig. 6.2 Chest X-ray showing a tension pneumothorax caused by an endotracheal tube that has been inserted too far.

and who also have a cord pH below 7 to avoid a collapse on the postnatal ward.

If resuscitation has to be abandoned, make sure the decision is appropriate, ensure that the baby is not left alone until he has died, and treat the body with dignity at all times. Never, ever leave a baby's body exposed and unattended on the resuscitaire and rush out of the labour ward. Initiating resuscitation in very immature babies generates a great deal of anxiety but, if stopping resuscitation appears to be the appropriate decision, supported by senior input, then fear of litigation should never inhibit clinical judgement.

Example: Baby C was stillborn at term at 04:18 after a period of fetal bradycardia, and resuscitation was initiated by the paediatric senior house officer assisted by the obstetric anaesthetist. Resuscitative efforts continued and the paediatric registrar was called, arriving at 04:40. Documentation was not clear regarding whether or not chest compressions were used from the start, but chest compression and adrenaline (epinephrine) were given when she arrived, at about 04:41. The heart rate returned and the registrar then phoned her consultant for permission to abandon resuscitation; he agreed, not realising that the registrar had only been on the scene for a few minutes. Baby C was given to her grieving parents at 05:00; by 05:20 she was pink, breathing and with a heart rate of 120. C was readmitted to the neonatal unit, where she went on to develop hypoxic–ischaemic encephalopathy. The additional 'hypoxia' time may have made no difference to the outcome, but the quality of the decision making was clearly questionable.

Early neonatal encephalopathy and brain damage

Babies who seize in early neonatal life do not always have hypoxic–ischaemic encephalopathy, even if there was birth depression. However, there is a high risk of sequelae in this situation and the diagnosis should be pursued with vigour. Investigations, including imaging, electroencephalogram (EEG), metabolic screening, lumbar puncture and a search for infection, are mandatory (Ch. 41). Do not prognosticate too early but, if it is appropriate to offer to withdraw care, seek the support of a colleague and warn the parents that the baby might not die.

Current litigation practice in the UK is dominated by claimants with cerebral palsy who ascribe their disability to hypoxia–ischaemia during labour, and a vital plank of their causation argument is their ability to demonstrate early neonatal encephalopathy. There is no specific treatment but the neonatologist must limit any further adverse effects by maintaining blood pressure, glucose levels and blood gases. The notes need to be careful, thorough, non-judgemental and include a daily description of the baby's neurological state. Several suitable systems are published (pp. 57–9). Avoid the temptation to record an absence of change without explaining what has not changed, and make positive factual observations of the child's condition.

Investigation needs to be thorough and appropriate. This is not difficult (Ch. 5) but it is amazing how often there is no arterial and venous cord pH, no head circumference and no description of fontanelle tension, muscle tone, sucking ability or level of alertness in a baby who is being treated with several anticonvulsants and whose nursing notes suggest that he is totally obtunded. It is embarrassing, to say the least, if a diagnosis of congenital cytomegalovirus infection is only established once legal proceedings are well under way.

There is no doubt that asphyxia can cause brain damage, but the majority of babies who suffer asphyxia at birth do not go on to develop brain damage and 90% of cases of cerebral palsy are not attributable to birth asphyxia. Furthermore, fetal distress in labour is sometimes associated with brain damage that has been sustained previously. This means that the association can be difficult to establish and is in part a diagnosis of exclusion. There are various criteria that it has been suggested must be satisfied, but most of these, such as the Template,[9] have proved to be controversial on grounds of dogmatism. We suggest that the following list of features reflects the approach of most experts who advise the courts at the moment.

■ The baby born after 34 weeks must have exhibited severe or moderate neonatal encephalopathy (pp. 1135–6), because this is the stage in the evolution of the disease process in which permanent damage is sustained, and without early neonatal encephalopathy (seizures at less than 24 hours with an abnormal background central nervous system state) it is not probable that brain damage occurred close to the time of birth.

■ The child must suffer from a disability capable of being attributed to birth asphyxia. Traditional thinking held that spastic or athetoid cerebral palsy were the only disabilities in this category, but this has been challenged recently. It appears that, on occasion, learning difficulties can be caused by perinatal hypoxic ischaemia – but in general motor difficulties are paramount.

■ Other more probable diagnoses must be excluded. This necessarily involves a careful and detailed investigation by a wide range of modern modalities, including biochemical tests and magnetic resonance imaging (MRI). Particularly important in this category is the diagnosis of stroke.

■ There must be evidence of significant fetal distress if the fetal heart rate was being monitored at the time when, it is suggested, the damaging hypoxic ischaemia was sustained. Since the vast majority of children tolerate the stresses of labour without sustaining damage, there must be good evidence to pinpoint the insult to this time. Although electronic monitoring is not specific, it is highly sensitive.

■ If it is suggested that profound damage was inflicted at the end of labour, the neonate must exhibit clear evidence of this near-death experience. If the cord blood was sampled the diagnosis of acute profound hypoxic ischaemia in the immediate run-up to delivery becomes difficult to establish if the arterial pH is above 7.0 and the base deficit less than 12, and can usually be excluded if the pH is above 7.1 and the base deficit less than 8. It is always important to consider the arterial as well as the venous cord blood and this is essential in cases of suspected cord occlusion.

■ The Apgar score is not measured to predict outcome, but if the baby scores 2 for circulation at 1 minute it is unlikely that the circulation has recently collapsed, and a 5 minute Apgar score of 6 or above is not usually consistent with a recent acute profound hypoxic–ischaemic injury.

■ It is unlikely that brain damage (particularly of the chronic partial kind) has been sustained without there being damage to at least one other body system, although whether this has been recorded may be a function of how ill the baby was perceived as being at the time.

■ In chronic partial asphyxia leading to cortical watershed damage and spastic cerebral palsy, where the damage has often been inflicted over a period of several hours, the fetus may have had an opportunity to adapt and the picture at birth is more variable. Here the Apgar scores are usually depressed but not necessarily severely so and the requirement for resuscitation is variable. For similar reasons the cord pH is also less informative.

In many of the cases we are asked to assess, the fact that the baby has sustained perinatal hypoxic–ischaemic damage is not in dispute so much as the precise timing of the insult. Where the mother reports a sudden loss of fetal movements a day or two before delivery this may take on a more sinister significance in the light of subsequent events. In all these cases early cerebral imaging, EEG or Doppler studies may be decisive.

Preterm brain injury

Preterm brain injury is usually caused by a complex sequence of interacting factors, which makes establishing causation even more difficult than at term. Further, much preterm brain injury is not preventable at the present state of the art, however meticulous the care. Having said that, if the prematurity was the result of an inappropriate early delivery (for miscalculated dates, say) the child may mount a claim for iatropathic prematurity. Some disabled ex-preterm children born in the mid to late 1990s have mounted successful claims based on the association of hypocarbia with periventricular leukomalacia. The same is true for those whose mothers were not offered antenatal steroids (when appropriate) after about 1994. It remains to be seen whether ex-preterm babies with cerebral palsy who were exposed inappropriately to postnatal steroids (pp. 68–9) will litigate successfully, but this is a good example of the need to keep abreast of the literature. The balance between inducing 'idiopathic' prematurity and avoiding cytokine exposure from chorioamnionitis by delivering the fetus is another example of a situation in which the current state of knowledge is too imprecise to allow a claim to be established based on the link between cytokine exposure and periventricular leukomalacia, but the situation may change.

Adverse outcome after preterm birth is an area where neonatologists need all their skills in communicating with parents as well as treating their patients. The parents of a disabled child understandably seek a reason, and something to blame. If they are kept in touch with their baby's care and given an accurate prognosis and an explanation of any interacting causes as early as possible, they are less likely to ascribe the whole problem to the brief power cut on day 6, or the disconnected ventilator tubing on day 33. Early and full explanations can avoid a long-drawn-out period of attrition, which often ends in disappointment for all concerned. In our experience, it is very unusual to go through a set of notes documenting a neonatal intensive care unit (NICU) stay of several months and find that there were absolutely no problems or errors at all, but it is rarely the case that any deficiency in care can be identified as the cause of an adverse outcome in a very preterm baby. As many studies have shown, there are simply too many hurdles for such babies to surmount for it to be clear which inflicted the lesion that will later prove disastrous.

Jaundice (Ch. 29)

Kernicterus is a preventable disease and although it almost vanished from UK neonatal practice it has now returned with a vengeance. Midwives and others concerned with the management need to be taught that neonatal jaundice can be an emergency. Early discharge policies and the welcome move towards exclusive breastfeeding have produced a new population of vulnerable babies. There is only one way the bilirubin is going in the first few days of life, and that is up.

In our experience the following are especially high-risk groups:

- near-term babies (35–37 weeks) of good weight discharged early;
- babies with haemolytic disease (ABO, glucose-6-phosphate dehydrogenase deficiency, spherocytosis) who develop jaundice early, whether in hospital or at home;
- Afro-Caribbean and oriental babies, in whom clinical detection of jaundice (and transcutaneous bilirubinometry) is unreliable and inaccurate;
- preterm babies with acidosis and/or low albumin levels, or an 'open' blood–brain barrier because of germinal matrix/intraventricular haemorrhage or sepsis, who can develop kernicterus at low levels of bilirubin.

Effective intervention in all such groups requires anticipation as well as reaction.

Example: Baby W was born normally at 07:26 on a Friday in October in the north of England, after a quick and easy labour. He weighed 3.68 kg with a head circumference of 35.5 cm. The baby check was carried out in the hospital during the morning by the family GP, who was providing care, and mother and baby went home soon afterwards. It was the mother's second child. During the pregnancy she had told her carers that her husband had attended the same hospital with a blood disorder, and that he had been told that his red blood cells were a 'different shape to normal'. During the pregnancy he was in fact admitted with a haemolytic crisis and the diagnosis of spherocytosis was conveyed in further letters to the family GP.

On Saturday the community midwife visited at 10 am and noted that W was jaundiced. She advised putting him outside in his pram in the 'sunlight'. By Sunday W was more markedly jaundiced and was feeding less well; again sunlight was advised and the midwife said that a bilirubin estimation would be performed the following day.

On Monday W was irritable and arching his back, and would not feed. His mother took him to the GP, who arranged admission to the hospital, where his bilirubin was found to be 636 micromol/l. An exchange transfusion was done but was too late to prevent kernicterus, which was apparent on the late MRI (see Fig. 29.6). W is disabled by choreoathetoid cerebral palsy, upgaze palsy and deafness.

Hypoglycaemia

This is an area in which far more children attempt litigation than succeed. Most experts consider that as a rule only prolonged periods of symptomatic hypoglycaemia are damaging, and there is now a typical (not pathognomonic) MR pattern described.[5,11,22] (Fig. 6.3) However, this does not mean that there should be complacency about the management of hypoglycaemia (pp. 853–62). Symptomatic hypoglycaemia is an emergency and intravenous treatment is mandatory. For a normal term baby of normal weight whose mother is not diabetic to present with symptomatic hypoglycaemia is unusual, and there should be a high index of suspicion that the underlying diagnosis is hyperinsulinaemia right from the start (pp. 857–8), with the appropriate level of investigation and intervention, and early recourse to expert help.

Like hyperbilirubinaemia, it is now known that the normal healthy breastfed baby is not immune from hypoglycaemic damage due to breast milk insufficiency, albeit the problem is very

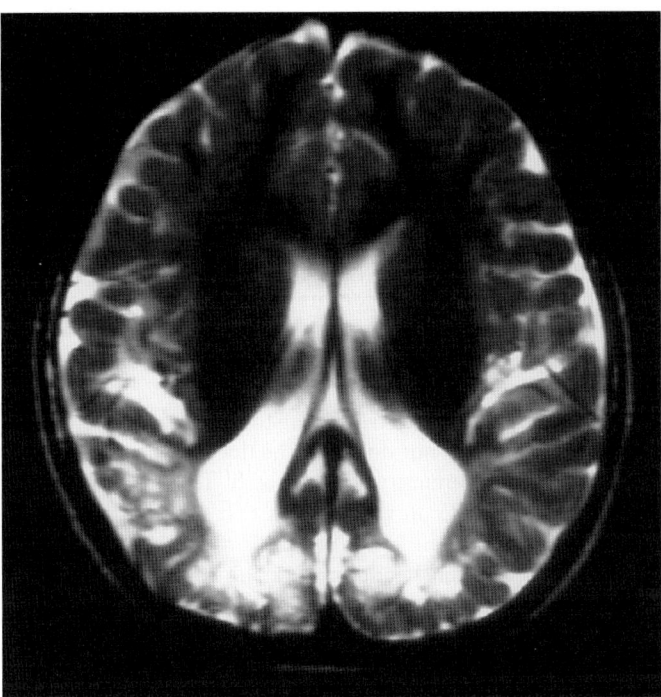

Fig. 6.3 Magnetic resonance image in a case of probable hypoglycaemic brain damage.

rare. Monitoring the adequacy of breastfeeding is difficult, but must be routine midwifery practice (see case history of baby B below). Guidelines regarding the use of supplementary feeds need to be worked out between professionals. Babies who are small for dates or whose mothers have diabetes must have glucose screening using an appropriate method and with reasonable frequency (p. 398).

Example: Baby B was born by elective caesarean section for breech presentation, weighing 2.98 kg. B did not require resuscitation and her Apgar scores were 9_1 and 9_5. She accompanied her mother to the postnatal ward, where she remained well, sucking from the breast seven times over the first night. On the first full day, a Saturday, B sucked three times and was given some boiled water; mother and baby spent a disturbed night. On Sunday the midwife documented that the milk had not yet come in, and by the evening B's mother was upset and tearful; B was taken to the nursery and had one supervised breastfeed in the mid-evening. B was placed in the nursery overnight, and no observations or feeds of any kind were documented. At 06:00 on Monday she was given 10 ml of expressed breast milk with difficulty (because she was 'sleepy'). At 08:00 B collapsed with an unrecordable blood glucose and developed seizures. End stage neuroimaging showed cystic encephalomalacia in the occipitoparietal region, consistent with hypoglycaemic damage (Fig. 6.3).

Retinopathy of prematurity

Children who are blinded from retinopathy of prematurity often litigate, not for poor management of their oxygen therapy but when the screening policy (p. 846) has failed them. This happens in two ways: either the recommended screen does not take place in the critical window of opportunity for treatment, or the screen takes place but the diagnosis is missed. There are clear UK (and international) guidelines for screening, which must be followed; if a planned screening examination cannot take place at the scheduled time (e.g. the baby may be too ill to tolerate the handling or even the dilating drops) the reasons should be carefully documented. The same is true if surgery has to be postponed.

Infectious disease

Neonatal group B streptococcal disease commonly leads to litigation and deviations from standard practice will be harder to defend now that there are guidelines endorsed by the RCOG supporting a 'risk-factor'-based strategy for antenatal prophylaxis. Neonatologists need to work with their obstetric colleagues to devise and implement local guidelines and to think carefully about what should be done, for example, if a baby who should have been exposed to intrapartum prophylaxis is born before her mother receives it (p. 1031).

Neonatal meningitis is hazardous for doctors as well as babies. Although the prognosis of established disease is poor, we see cases in which there is an allegation of delay in investigation or treatment, inadequate dosing, inappropriate antibiotic choice or short duration of treatment. Clinicians must be aware that neonatal meningitis carries a high risk of sequelae and take care to optimise antibiotic and supportive treatment, investigate fully and refer on when appropriate. Increasingly, when a disease has had an adverse outcome, the fact that this was predictable will not of itself prevent those concerned on the patient's behalf from scrutinising the records in retrospect to see whether the management was in fact optimal.

Criticism of failure to diagnose and treat maternal chorioamnionitis is also emerging, reflecting the realisation that cytokines can damage the preoligodendrocytes (pp. 1025–6). However whether there is a real window of opportunity in which such babies can be rescued is yet to be determined; what is clear is that once there are cardiovascular changes the inflammatory cascade is well established and it may already be too late.

'Missed' abnormalities at the neonatal examination

It is difficult for parents to understand that no-one was to blame when their baby, who was checked over and passed fit, collapses with coarctation of the aorta and requires major surgery, or develops amblyopia from a cataract or a limp from developmental dysplasia of the hip. Yet none of these diagnoses are reliably detected by the routine neonatal examination (pp. 249–66). Biochemical screening is reliable but there are sometimes failures in communication that result in a hypothyroid baby starting treatment late. The introduction of screening for medium-chain fatty acyl-CoA dehydrogenase deficiency (pp. 1171–2) in several health regions is welcome but will serve to increase the need for adequate back-up to ensure that affected babies receive appropriate and timely expert advice.

Vitamin K deficiency bleeding

At the moment there is no agreed UK standard regarding the dose, route or frequency of vitamin K prophylaxis for vitamin K deficiency bleeding (p. 298). Parents are offered a choice in many hospitals. Parents who refuse vitamin K for their baby altogether should have their refusal documented. However, sick babies who are admitted to neonatal units should have intramuscular vitamin K. In this instance it does not matter what the mother said before the baby became ill, because by that stage vitamin K is a medically indicated treatment. It is inappropriate to wait for 7 hours for 'consent' in a baby of 32 weeks whose mother required an appendicectomy and who herself was admitted to the intensive care unit ventilated. Any baby can become sick, and if he received oral vitamin K after birth (or no vitamin K) he should be given a further dose intramuscularly, especially if surgery is required.

Scarring and iatropathic problems (p. 92)

The scars of neonatal intensive care are not usually disabling but on occasion extravasation injury can cause tethering around a joint that inhibits movement or is cosmetically disfiguring. Such scarring may be unavoidable but constant vigilance is required to avoid inflicting scars, which will grow with the baby.

Similarly, now that the Department of Health has suggested that there is an increased risk of cardiac tamponade when Silastic long lines are sited in the right atrium (p. 634), neonatologists should only continue to site lines in the heart when there is no alternative. A long line that inadvertently lies in the left ascending lumbar vein can cause permanent paraplegia, via direct extravasation into the subarachnoid space or by causing a vasculitic response with venous congestion in the small veins of the epidural plexus.

Informed consent

General

It is well established in English law that an adult patient with capacity to take a decision can refuse treatment for a good reason, bad reason or no reason at all. The law respects the patient's autonomy and the doctor who operates or treats such a patient without their consent is guilty of an assault.[18] Assault may give rise to a liability to compensate without proof of damage in the civil courts or to a prosecution in the criminal courts, and may be punished by the General Medical Council as professional misconduct. The same legal principles apply to babies save that the operative consent has to be given by someone with parental responsibility.[17] However, parental rights are not beyond the review or control of the court.[17] They derive from the parental duty to look after the child. They exist for the benefit of the child rather than the parent.

Doctors owe a child a duty to care for him in accordance with good medical practice recognised as appropriate by a competent body of professional opinion. This duty is, however, subject to the qualification that, if time permits, they must obtain the consent of the parents before undertaking serious invasive treatment. The parents owe the child a duty to give or withhold consent in the best interests of the child and without regard to their own interests. The court, when exercising the parens patriae jurisdiction, takes over the rights and duties of the parents, although this is not to say that the parents will be excluded from the decision-making process. Nevertheless, in the end the responsibility for the decision whether to give or withhold consent is that of the court alone.

No one can dictate the treatment to be given to the child – neither court, parents nor doctors. The doctors can recommend treatment A in preference to treatment B. They can also refuse to adopt treatment C on the grounds that it is medically contraindicated or for some other reason is a treatment that they could not conscientiously administer. The court, or parents for their part, can refuse to consent to treatment A or B or both, but cannot insist on treatment C. The inevitable and desirable result is that choice of treatment is in some measure a joint decision of the doctors and the court or parents.[18]

Which procedures require written consent?

A consent will be equally valid whether it is given orally or by conduct, as where someone sticks out their arm to receive an injection. Similarly, it does not need to be recorded in writing to provide a defence to a claim of assault. However, when seeking consent a doctor also incurs a duty to explain what is involved in the procedure, to advise of the risks and benefits of the procedure so as to put the parent in a position to take a sensible decision.[21] In order to demonstrate that the parents' rights were respected it is increasingly necessary to record that the proper explanations were given and formalities were complied with. Just as consent to an injection is incomplete without knowing what is in the needle, there is an increasing need to record in detail the explanation that was given. In the past, written consent was only sought for major procedures such as surgery or exchange transfusion. In the future, consent will need to be obtained for many more 'routine' intensive care procedures such as long line insertion or transfusion of blood products. This area has generated much debate and is currently being considered by the British Association of Perinatal Medicine.

Who is able to give consent?

Single mothers

Either parent has the right to consent to the treatment, providing that the parents are married or the father has acquired parental responsibility. If the doctor is on notice that the parents disagree it will be wise either to try to obtain the agreement of the second parent or to suggest that they should go to court to have their differences resolved, but the court stated in one leading case: 'If the parents disagree, one consenting and the other refusing, the doctor will be presented with a professional and ethical dilemma but not with a legal problem because, if he has the consent of one authorised person, the treatment will not without more constitute a trespass or criminal assault.'

Very young mothers

Increasingly common on the NICU is the single mother aged under 16 years. She may be 'Gillick-competent' – able to understand information given to her about her baby and make decisions for herself – but sometimes children are born to mothers so immature that the doctor would be reluctant to accept their consent to treatment of themselves. Nevertheless, only the mother can give a lawful consent to treatment of her child. Often the doctors will be able to involve the grandparents or the biological father in the treatment of the baby, for the same reason that it is good practice to involve the parents of the Gillick-competent child in her own treatment. However it may well be that in such circumstances the hospital will feel that the Social Services Department should be involved because the baby, if not the young mother, is in need of support. Social Services are the lead agency for children in need and may decide to make an application to the court.

Psychiatrically ill mothers

Women with long-standing psychoses sometimes relapse when pregnant or during the puerperium, and women without any previous psychiatric morbidity can become seriously ill for the first time after giving birth. If they are single, this can present major problems for those caring for their baby. The starting point in this situation is with the mother's consultant psychiatrist, in order to establish his perception of her ability to process information and take decisions. On occasion, we have managed withdrawal of care in this situation by involving a team of psychiatrists, social workers, family members and other therapists with a team from the neonatal unit. Where the mother is too ill to give informed consent we have had to involve Social Services or the courts: even here it is good practice to involve the mother as much as possible.

Use of interpreters

Recent National Health Service guidelines have made it clear that the long-established practice of using family members as interpreters is no longer acceptable. The reason for this is that the mother or father may have information that they wish to convey but that they do not want the rest of the family to know – for example a diagnosis of human immunodeficiency virus. Further, there is no way of knowing that family members are translating complex medical information accurately. Using members of staff is also discouraged for the same reason. If parents do not speak English well enough to understand the information that is required for them to give consent, a suitable interpreter must be obtained, booked and paid for from a bank of individuals recognised by the hospital.

There is a scarcity of interpreters in some languages and the full impact and cost of these new recommendations has yet to be appreciated. Three-way telephone consultations may be the only solution in geographically isolated areas where few individuals with language skills are available. Even so, there are problems associated with the everyday informal contact that is essential to effective partnership between the parents and the rest of the team on the neonatal unit, and communication cannot always be confined to the periods when interpreters are available.

Documentation of counselling, and which risks to mention

Neonatologists are under an obligation to ensure that parents understand the nature and purpose of the procedure for which they are seeking consent. This includes making sure that they understand the expected consequences and the risks involved in the procedure. It is less often spelled out that the doctor has an obligation to make clear the consequences and risks of *not* undergoing the procedure. A doctor who negligently deters a patient or parent from consenting to a procedure by giving an exaggerated view of the hazards will incur a potential liability if the parents decide not to allow their baby to undergo the procedure and the baby meets with disaster as a result.

As to what risks should be mentioned, it is sometimes said that there is a 1% rule – that all risks with an incidence of 1% should be mentioned. That may be a useful starting point but it certainly does not describe the risks that need to be mentioned. A much more remote risk of death or disability will usually have to be discussed. The doctor should also take account of how much real choice there is, how much time there is to take the decision and how much information the parents wish to have.

Failing to obtain consent

There are some cases where the parents refuse treatment that the doctor believes is essential in the interests of the child. In those cases the courts can make orders authorising treatment and the doctor must not hesitate to take whatever step is clearly necessary in the interests of the patient. However it is much better to carry the parents with you if possible and conflict resolution can often be achieved by the use of mediation services or family advocates.

Jehovah's Witness parents

An adult Jehovah's Witness is free to refuse a blood transfusion and a doctor who forces an unwilling Jehovah's Witness to accept the treatment will be guilty of an assault. That said, it is important to note that not all Jehovah's Witnesses share the same views; some will accept treatment with some blood products (such as fresh frozen plasma or albumin) and others do choose to accept blood when the alternative is death. It is vital to ascertain the wishes of the individual patient and to help them to stand up to pressure from co-religionists or other family members. Useful guidance on this topic is available from the Association of Anaesthetists' website.

As with any parent, a Jehovah's Witness has the right to take decisions as to what treatment his child should receive. However, if it is plain that the blood needs to be given, the court will make an order that it is lawful to do so, even where both parents object. If the baby's condition is so precarious that death or serious injury is likely to follow unless blood products are immediately given, again it will be lawful to do so even though there is no time to get a court order. In *Re R. (a minor)*[19] the court had to deal with a child suffering from B-cell lymphoblastic leukaemia who was given blood products on admission as an emergency measure without the parents' consent, and the court subsequently approved the administration of blood products in the future. However, it is important to note that the court decided that the medical consultant should not be given a blanket authority to carry out such treatment without further reference to the parents, and that the parents should still be involved as far as possible in the care of their daughter and able to draw attention to treatments alternative to the use of blood products.

In our experience the best approach in this situation is first to think hard about the indication for blood products: Is there an alternative? What is standard and safe practice? Juniors must discuss the situation with a consultant, and consultants may wish to seek the support of another colleague. The reason for the transfusion and the urgency should be carefully explained to the parent (or parents) and an offer made to talk to any religious advisers the family may choose. Many hospitals have panels of on-call volunteer Jehovah's Witness ministers who are prepared to come and help. They can provide invaluable assistance in the counselling and mediation process, and in our experience have largely obviated the need for court applications in recent years. Only if such a reasoned approach fails should a court order be sought, and then only if time allows. Obtaining a court order involves the hospital's solicitors and social workers but when required a court order can usually be obtained within hours.

Emergency situations

In an acute emergency when the parents refuse to consent to treatment that is immediately necessary for the preservation of the life or long-term health of the child, the doctor is empowered to act. The precise basis of this agency of necessity (as it is sometimes called) is unclear, but the doctor's duty is towards the child and if it is clear that the child is about to die because some treatment is immediately necessary and the parents forbid administration of it, the doctor should act in the child's interest.

Parental rights

The relationship with parents

Wherever possible the neonatologist and the parent should form a relationship based on profound mutual trust (pp. 89–90) and close cooperation. The quality of care on the NICU is enhanced if the parent who is to look after the child exclusively in the future is involved as much as possible. Maintaining this relationship requires time and effort, and time can be difficult to find in the hurly-burly of a busy intensive care unit. Continuity can help, and the 'attending' system operated by most neonatal teams may have to be modified to allow parents to form a relationship with one consultant, especially as consultant teams enlarge.[4] On the other hand, many parents find it advantageous to have contact with several consultants, who might put things in different ways – and sharing the emotionally draining load of counselling is valuable if senior staff are to avoid 'burnout'.

Refusal of treatment

Where doctors are confronted with the refusal on the part of a parent to consent to treatment that they consider has a high chance of success, the doctor's responsibility is to the baby. If, after further discussions, the parents are still minded to refuse, the physician can apply to the court for an order. All other avenues need to be explored first. The court has various legal bases on which it can make an order that treatment will be lawful. For example, it can simply determine a single issue as to what would be in the child's interest under section 8 of the Children Act 1989, or it can make the child a ward of court so that all important steps in the child's life have to be sanctioned by the court. Alternatively, under what is called the 'inherent jurisdiction', it can make whatever orders seem appropriate. As Lord Woolf put it, particularly in regard to cases involving children, the last thing the court should be concerned about is whether the right procedure has been used. The important thing is to ensure that the best interests of the child are identified.[16]

The fact that the parents and doctors disagree to such an extent that the court has to resolve the difference of opinion increases the importance of maintaining the doctor–parent relationship. Disagreement with mutual understanding and respect should not entail enmity and the parents usually accept the court's decision and remain the baby's carers.

Unrealistic expectations regarding treatment

Reports of 'miracle survivors' with titles such as 'Neonatal viability: pushing the envelope'[12] have raised parental expectations to the level that a good outcome is assumed for every baby born after 23 weeks gestation. Parents often request that 'everything be done' for their babies, however complex the problem and however overwhelmingly the odds are stacked against success. The most extreme example is probably that of baby K, an anencephalic, whose mother insisted on full intensive care support for over 2 years. Neonatologists need to be careful not to add to these unrealistic expectations or to use the word 'miracle' themselves. The argument used by the doctor who initially resuscitated baby K was that the mother 'needed more time' to adjust to the fact that she could not live. Additional time did not lead to any more acceptance, and baby K's mother continued to believe that a miracle would happen. As Paris puts it, 'if parents are expecting a miracle they have come to the wrong place'.[14]

At the other end of the spectrum are the parents who want a guarantee of success before agreeing to treatment for their child.[13] Things have moved on considerably since the 1963 Johns Hopkins case of a baby with Down's syndrome and duodenal atresia who was 'allowed' to die over an 11-day period, and newborn babies are now recognised to have rights. Few would accede to a parental request for no treatment in this situation today, but the judgement regarding what is a 'reasonable' chance of success does vary between professionals and these differences need to be recognised.

Discontinuation of futile treatment

A decision to withdraw life-sustaining treatment precedes about 30% of deaths in a NICU, and an understanding of the process is an essential part of every consultant neonatologist's training. The best source of guidance is the RCPCH framework for practice of September 1997, and this framework has now been cited with approval by the judiciary on several occasions.

The framework identifies five situations where the decision will be considered; they are:

- the brain-dead child;
- the permanent vegetative state;
- the no-chance situation where disease is so severe that life-sustaining treatment simply delays death without significant alleviation of suffering, rendering medical treatment inappropriate;
- the no-purpose situation where there may be survival with treatment but the degree of impairment will be so great that it is unreasonable to expect the patient to bear it;
- the unbearable situation where the child or family feel that further treatment is more than can be borne.

The detailed guidance given by the RCPCH should be followed. It is vital here to stress the following.

- The withdrawing or withholding of treatment does not imply that a baby will receive no care. The baby remains your patient and you must do your best for him just as much while he is dying.
- It must be noted that there is no significant difference between withholding and withdrawing care as far as the courts are concerned. It is unlawful to take any positive act that will result directly in a person's death, but the withdrawal of treatment in hopeless circumstances is not a positive act.
- The decision should be discussed widely within the clinical team and varying views recorded. If there is substantial dissent or if the parents do not agree, a sensible first course may well be to obtain a second opinion from another clinician with experience of the clinical problem. In the last resort the courts are there to give guidance but, as the RCPCH Framework makes clear, it will in most cases be possible to avoid an application to the court.

Many neonatologists believe that, on occasion, to continue intensive care may be inappropriate and inhumane. Managing this kind of case is challenging and requires a degree of consensus in the treating team. Kant said that 'it is immoral to use one human being as a means rather than as an end in itself'; this implies that inflicting the burden of intensive care on a baby when there is no prospect of success cannot be justified. The problem lies in defining 'no prospect' or 'no chance', because there may be differences of opinion amongst the treating team, or between them and outside experts. When there is unanimity of opinion, the matter can usually be resolved either with or without the intervention of the court.

There are now several documented cases in which the courts have been involved in this situation, both in the USA and the UK. The implication of the decision of the European court in the case of Glass is that doctors should be much more willing to enlist the guidance of the courts at an early stage. We think that in future the courts are likely to be involved in a wider range of these problems than hitherto and that there can be advantages in hospital and parents going to the courts together for guidance at a time when attitudes are less entrenched. The authority of the court can be used as a mediation tool to resolve a shared uncertainty as opposed to an established antagonism. Whatever the decision, it may be easier to implement if both sides have been through this process.

Negligence

Medical negligence consists of a breach of duty of care that causes damage. Claims in the UK are heard in civil (not criminal) courts by a judge sitting alone, who has to find that it is more likely than not that there was a breach of duty and that the claimant's disability was caused by the mistake in question.

Breach of duty

The doctor will be in breach of his duty of care only if he fails to provide a reasonable standard of care. Lord Scarman described the standard which must be achieved by quoting a Scottish judge, who said:

> In the realm of diagnosis and treatment there is ample scope for genuine difference of opinion and one man clearly is not negligent merely because his conclusion differs from that of other professional men … . The true test for establishing negligence in diagnosis or treatment on the part of a doctor is whether he has been guilty of such failure as no doctor of ordinary skill would be guilty of acting with ordinary care.[10]

The principle that the law will respect treatment that accords with a respectable school of thought is known as the Bolam test.[1] It applies whether the doctor is reaching a diagnosis,[10] giving warning of the hazards of treatment[21] or performing a surgical procedure.[23] The court reserves the right to reject an opinion that it believes does not stand up to logical analysis.[2] In the case of care delivered by a team, the law does not require the most junior trainee to have the skills of the consultant. However, it does require the trainee to be competent to perform the tasks allocated to him.[24]

Where a defendant is in breach of his duty of care, the claimant will only be entitled to be compensated for damage caused by that breach of duty. This can cause additional complications; for example, when a senior registrar at a London teaching hospital failed to respond to her bleep to attend a child with croup, the evidence was that it would have made no difference to the exegesis if she had attended, unless she had decided to intubate the child as a precaution against a subsequent attack. The House of Lords held that causation could not be proved if any reasonable senior registrar in her position would have decided not to intubate.[2] If the defendant is guilty of an act of negligence then the court will require that the claimant is put in the position in which he would have been if there had been no negligence, in so far as money can achieve this.

Standards of care

The law holds that doctors are to be judged by the state of their art at the time of treatment. They will not be negligent if they fail to anticipate a hazard that was unknown at the time. This provides a protection for the slower members of the profession, who cannot keep up with the state of their art, provided that they do not fall too far behind. It can be difficult, especially in a case that presents a powerful emotional charge, where the defence that admits that it got it wrong and would do better nowadays cannot be presented as the most impressive face of medicine.

However, because of the problem of limitation, cases sometimes come to court after many years have elapsed. Here the notes are often vestigial by modern standards, or lost. The investigations appear to be sporadic and haphazard. The witnesses are worse: they can rarely remember anything of the facts in issue, even though they may be debating the few hours in which it seems the claimant met with the catastrophe that has blighted his existence. Under the rigours of cross-examination, the paediatrician may be hard pressed to remember the routine practice or treatment policy of 1995 and to describe in coherent terms how it differed from that which was followed in 1985 or 2002.

Limitation

Adult patients of sound mind must issue their writs in respect of personal injuries within 3 years of learning who caused their damage.[7] They do not need to know that the injury was caused by negligence, but they may well be able to argue that only when they knew that their treatment was inadequate did they realise that their injury was not caused by their disease process. The court has a discretion to extend time indefinitely when the interests of justice demand it.[8]

The difficulty for the paediatrician is that time does not run at all against the child under 18, or a patient under a disability. Thus, the survivor of a neonatal disaster has an unfettered right to issue a writ at any time prior to his 21st birthday. If at the age of 18 the young person does not know who or what has caused the damage, time will not start to run until he does. If he never becomes capable of managing his own affairs his 3 years does not start to run until his death. Since individuals with cerebral palsy currently enjoy a life expectancy that sometimes differs only

marginally from the national average, hospitals need to keep neonatal records for a very long time. They are advised to keep all records until the child is aged 26 but records of catastrophic cases should be kept for 80 years. This creates storage problems in the present twilight years of paper records.

Whenever the trial takes place, the court will judge the case on the available evidence. Where a child acquired cerebral palsy because 68 minutes elapsed between the delivery of twins, it seemed that this was in part attributable to a difficulty in finding the registrar because obstetric services were split between two sites. No satisfactory explanation could be provided 17 years after the event. The defendants argued that the judge should be less willing to draw an adverse inference against the defendant, whom delay had deprived of a proper opportunity to rebut the claim. The Court of Appeal concluded:

> our law allows persons under a disability such as Stuart to bring a claim such as this at any time during their lives; indeed their right of action will survive for 3 years after their death. Whoever else may be to blame for the disability Stuart is not. The problem facing the parties and the court as a result of the delay in the present case are far from unique … the delay does not affect the facts which have to be proved, nor the manner of proof. It merely means that both sides will or may be in a position to prove fewer facts. To this extent it may well prejudice both the plaintiff and the defendant …. The court should draw the same inference from those facts as it would if the claim had been promptly made. Likewise, if the facts which have been proved would give rise to a presumption in favour of the plaintiff under the principle of res ipsa loquitor, the court should not decline to apply that principle merely because the claim has been brought after many years.[3]

This case was remarkable in that the court preferred the evidence on causation of a growth expert who did not pretend to be a neonatologist to that of two professors of neonatal medicine and the consultant paediatrician who had originally looked after the baby as a registrar. The claimant had been the donor in twin–twin transfusion syndrome (pp. 151–2), having been delivered at 33 weeks' gestation with a haemoglobin of 9 g/dl where his co-twin had a haemoglobin of 17 g/dl. There was also a weight difference. The claimant's expert was accepted when he told the court that if brain damage had been caused by a chronic twin–twin transfusion syndrome he would have expected it to attack both twins and that an Apgar score of 5 at 5 minutes suggested 'a profound acidosis'.

The timetable of a medical negligence claim

The parents of a child in the UK can consult a specialist solicitor who can obtain government funding for this type of claim. In many other parts of the world the family must find the money to explore the claim or a lawyer willing to accept instructions based on a contingency fee arrangement ('no win no fee').

The lawyer acting for the claimant explores the strength of the claim, by obtaining the hospital records, the results of any risk management investigation and complaints procedure records, and commissioning expert opinion. Then they send a pre-action Letter of Claim, setting out their case in detail.

The defendants have 3 months in which to send a Letter of Response. The defendant's team are instructed by the NHS Litigation Authority in England, who will ultimately meet the claim, and they have a panel of specialist solicitors. The Litigation Authority runs a mutual insurance scheme for NHS bodies, which allows a 'discount' if certain standards are met.

The defendants may have witness statements taken at the time of the incident but with older claims it can be difficult to track down the staff involved. If you are asked to give a witness statement about a case, you will be able to refresh your memory of the case from the notes and a lawyer will help you, but the resulting statement is the evidence that you will give under oath. It is at this point that the inadequacy or inaccuracy of your own notes may come back to haunt you.

If the claimant's team is not persuaded by the letter of response, they will issue formal proceedings and thereafter the action will be controlled by the court. The hospital's team draft and serve a defence, usually based on expert advice. If the case is contested, this is followed by an exchange of expert reports and witness statements, and there may be a meeting of experts to narrow the issues. Over 90% of cases are resolved by agreement at some stage of this process. If the claim succeeds the damages are quantified by teams of experts involving therapists, architects and care providers. Increasingly this is an area where the court tries to save money by using single joint experts. The amount of the settlement includes loss of earnings and costs of care, and so rests heavily on life expectancy. Rather than a lump sum the amount is often paid as a structured settlement, which means that the money is paid out annually to meet the care requirements.

Criminal cases

The doctor enjoys no privileged position under the criminal law of the land and allegations of homicide will be judged by the same rules as apply to the rest of society.

Murder

Murder consists of unlawfully killing a person with the intention of killing or causing grievous bodily harm. It can only be committed by a positive act, unlike manslaughter, which can be committed by omitting to act where there is a duty to do so. There is scope for argument about whether certain events are omissions or positive acts: switching off a ventilator is a positive act whereas ceasing to ventilate may be an omission, depending on the circumstances.

Manslaughter

Medical manslaughter is committed when a doctor causes the death of a patient as a result of an act or omission that amounts to gross negligence. Whether negligence is gross or not is a question of fact for the jury, but the prosecution must first demonstrate a

breach of duty as judged by the Bolam test. The doctor who causes the death of a patient in the course of bona fide treatment without deliberately killing him will not be guilty of any crime if he is acting in accordance with a respectable school of thought.[20]

Where a neonatologist is called and finds a baby weighing 400 g, his first duty is to assess the baby. If he decides not to attempt resuscitation, or to abandon it if the baby does not respond, he cannot be guilty of a crime if a respectable school of thought would have taken the same view, because he will not be guilty of an act of negligence. The case will be judged in all the circumstances, so that a consultant at a major teaching hospital would not be able to rely solely on the fact that a reasonable paediatrician in a peripheral unit with poor facilities would have decided that the case was hopeless. However, the burden will remain on the prosecution throughout to prove, so that the jury is sure, that no respectable neonatologist would have failed to resuscitate that child in those circumstances and that the failure to resuscitate did hasten death. These questions are discussed in a thought-provoking way by Lantos.[6] Furthermore the negligent failure must be gross, so that the jury is sure that the action merits a criminal sanction.

Example: Anthony MacDonald was born on 8 September 1989 at 23 weeks and 4 days gestation with a birth weight of 670 g. The mother presented with a double footling breech, with the feet in the vagina, to a hospital in the USA. Gregory Milleville, a board-certified neonatologist, was present in the delivery room. Anthony was floppy, bruised and bradycardic. After 7–10 minutes of bagging in 100% oxygen the heart rate had not risen above 60, and Dr Milleville wrapped the baby in a blanket and handed him to his parents. About an hour later, he gave a faint cry and the nurse transferred him to the NICU. Dr Milleville placed him on a ventilator. Anthony had a long and stormy course and by the age of 8 he had the skills of a 6–8-month-old baby. The parents pursued a suit against Dr Milleville, claiming that he had violated the requirement for informed consent from the parents by stopping the resuscitation. After a 2-week trial, the jury found that he had no such obligation.[15]

Some very preterm children have been delivered alive as a result of a deliberate procedure to abort the pregnancy following an antenatal diagnosis that there was a substantial risk that the fetus would be born suffering from such abnormalities as would cause it to be born seriously handicapped. Such abortions have been lawful at any stage of gestation in the UK since 1990. The antenatal history does not affect the duty of the neonatologist towards his only patient, the baby. The subsequent death of the baby from the effects of prematurity may or may not ground a prosecution for murder against the obstetrician: legal opinion is divided on the point. However, there is no doubt that, whatever the history in the womb and whatever the parental wishes may be after delivery, the neonatologist must act solely on the basis of what is in the best interests of the child.

Child protection law

Neonatologists need to be aware of the law in this area, particularly with respect to babies under their care whose parents have previous children in care for neglect or who are substance-abusing.

Employment law

Neonatologists are rarely able to confine themselves to treating sick babies. In most cases they have to take on roles as leaders of a multidisciplinary team, trainers of younger doctors, nurses and other colleagues, as well as managers of the vital relationship between the parents and the rest of the clinical team. They need a sophisticated grasp of the expectations of their employers, society and the law in each role. These demands change, sometimes quite rapidly in Western society and expectations also vary from place to place. Doctors will be unable to perform effectively and so fail to achieve the best for their patients if they fail to respond appropriately.

Discrimination

In the UK today the law is comprehensive regarding discrimination on grounds of gender, race, disability, religion and sexual orientation. What would have been considered friendly ward round banter or coffee room gossip only a few years ago is often no longer acceptable. Doctors who seek to exploit their age or clinical seniority to impose their view of what should be tolerated may well cause offence. They could imperil their position as well as the clinical effectiveness of the team while creating financial liabilities for themselves and for their employers.

Paediatrics has a large female workforce and employers and managers have to respond appropriately to the needs of pregnant women and mothers who have legal rights to time off and to work flexibly. Paternity leave is now a legal entitlement. Employees who are adopting children, including those in same-sex relationships, have similar enforceable rights.

Dismissal – the under-performing doctor

The doctor who accepts a role as trainer and supervisor accepts a responsibility to the junior as well as to the patients. The doctor who accepts a role as assessor accepts a less clearly defined responsibility to society and future patients. Assessment of competency remains problematic, but on occasion a neonatal team may be faced with a doctor who appears not to be up to the job.

Such issues should not be evaded. Apparent deficiencies need to be evaluated fairly and communicated clearly. The response should be constructive and remedial. The required improvement should be measurable within agreed time scales where practical.

Dismissal – unacceptable behaviour

Tales of riotous behaviour by junior doctors are legendary, and were formerly almost a rite of passage. Modern employment law takes a dim view of such behaviour, and caution is advised. The use of technology and the increased levels of monitoring of all aspects of employees at work have extended the range of accountability. For example, a doctor was dismissed from his post because he generated a computer image of a young girl's body with the head of the ward sister superimposed upon it. The ward sister was deeply offended by the image and the hospital took disciplinary action against the junior doctor even though he was at the end of his contract. The case ended up at an employment tribunal.

Giving references

When writing references or letters for circulation it is important to remember that a published defamatory statement about a person's character can be libellous. Claims for libel are rare within the current NHS but are not unknown. You owe duties to the subject of the reference, the recipient of the reference, the Service and other patients to exercise reasonable skill and care to ensure the accuracy of all facts included. References need to be accurate, fair and truthful. Where facts are presented accurately they must also be presented in such a way as not to give the reader an unfair overall impression of the subject. Any information provided must not be misleading. However, references do not have to be full and comprehensive. Potential liabilities for discrimination in respect of employees continue to exist in relation to references after the contract has ended.

Acknowledgement

Mr Michael J Ball, employment partner at Halliwells LLP, advised on the section relating to employment law.

References

1. *Bolam* v. *Friern Hospital Management Committee* [1957] 1 WLR 582
2. *Bolitho* v. *City & Hackney Health Authority* [1992] Lloyd's Law Reports Med 1998 26
3. *Bull and Wakeham* v. *Devon Health Authority* [1993] 4 Med LR 117, CA
4. Hack M 2003 Uses of error: continuity of neonatal care. Lancet 361: 1809
5. Kinnala A, Rikkalainen H, Lapinleimu H, Parkkola R, Kormano M, Kero P 1999 Cerebral magnetic resonance imaging and ultrasonography findings after neonatal hypoglycemia. Pediatrics 103: 724–729
6. Lantos J D 2001 The Lazarus case: life and death issues in neonatal intensive care. Johns Hopkins University Press, Baltimore, MD
7. Limitation Act 1980 HMSO, London, section 11
8. Limitation Act 1980 HMSO, London, section 33
9. MacLennan A 1999 A template for defining a causal relation between acute intrapartum events and cerebral palsy: international consensus statement. British Medical Journal 319: 1054–1059
10. *Maynard* v. *West Midlands Regional Health Authority* [1985] 1 All ER 635
11. Murakami Y, Yamashite Y, Matsuishi T, Utsunomiya H, Okudera T, Hashimoto T 1999 Cranial MRI of neurologically impaired children suffering from neonatal hypoglycaemia. Pediatric Radiology 29: 23–27
12. Muraskas J, Bhola M, Tomich P, Thomas D 1998 Neonatal viability: pushing the envelope. Pediatrics 101: 1095
13. Paris J J, Bell A J 1993 Guarantee my child will be 'normal' or stop all treatment. Journal of Perinatology 13: 469–472
14. Paris J J, DeLisser H M, Savani RC 2000 Ending innovative therapy for infants at the margins of viability: case of twins. Journal of Perinatology 4: 251–256
15. Paris J J, Goldsmith J P, Cimperman M 1998 Resuscitation of a micropremie: the case of MacDonald v. Milleville. Journal of Perinatology 18: 302–305
16. *R.* v. *Portsmouth Hospitals NHS Trust, ex parte Glass* [1999] 50 BMLR 269
17. *Re J.* [1990] 3 All ER 930 and [1991] Fam 33
18. *Re J. (a minor)* [1992]
19. *Re R. (a minor)* [1993] 15 BMLR 72
20. *Regina* v. *Adomako* [1995] 1 AC 171
21. *Sidaway* v. *Board of Governors of the Bethlem Royal Hospital and Maudsley Hospital* [1985] AC 871
22. Traill Z, Squier M, Anslow P 1998 Brain imaging in neonatal hypoglycaemia. Archives of Disease in Childhood 79: F145–F147
23. *Whitehouse* v. *Jordan* [1981] 1 All ER 261
24. *Wilsher* v. *Essex Area Health Authority* [1986] 3 All ER 801

CHAPTER 7

Specific problems in developing countries

Lord Chan of Oxton

Introduction

Vast rural areas in the tropics have poorly developed or no obstetric services. Women in those areas tend to be malnourished and during pregnancy continue to do hard manual work. Many babies born to teenage mothers or to grand multiparae continue to be exposed to all the risks of pregnancy attendant on short birth intervals. Tens of millions of pregnant women are exposed to malaria, which is life-threatening to mother and baby and contributes substantially to low birthweight. At parturition, mothers still rely on attendants who lack facilities for simple resuscitation of asphyxiated babies or sterile handling of the umbilical cord and who employ traditional practices injurious to mother and baby.

In urban areas in developing countries, large numbers and many complicated deliveries associated with inadequate antenatal supervision create such pressure of work in the labour ward that little attention is given to the baby after birth. Mothers stay in the maternity ward for hours rather than days and discharge from hospital ends her contact with the service until the next delivery. Neonates needing special care interfere with this delivery-oriented service and are given low priority for medical care and attention.

In the larger cities, where public hospitals are crowded and staff overworked, some mothers have the choice of using private practitioners based in maternity homes, providing obstetric and neonatal care of variable quality. Safe standards of care often depend on the ability of the patient to pay for the services of a consultant obstetrician, trained midwife and a consultant paediatrician.

This unsatisfactory state of affairs has continued during the past two decades, when economic growth of the poorest countries in the 1990s (during the economic boom in Western countries) was slower than in the 1980s. Most of the countries that have slid backwards are in Sub-Saharan Africa and have been savagely hit by acquired immunodeficiency syndrome (AIDS). Fertility and population growth are highest in the poorest countries. Urban growth is fastest among poor populations, where many of the new urban migrants are driven by environmental collapse and economic hardship.

During the closing years of the 20th century, world leaders met regularly in venues in developing countries (Cairo, Rio) to agree on a number of initiatives. They were announced in September 2000 at the United Nations Millennium Summit and endorsed as Millennium Development Goals (MDGs). The eight goals cover: eradication of extreme poverty and hunger; achieving universal primary education; promoting gender equality and empowering women; reducing child mortality; improving maternal health; combating human immunodeficiency virus (HIV)/AIDS, tuberculosis (TB) and malaria; ensuring environmental sustainability; and developing a global partnership for development.[25]

The international community of richer developed countries, G7, has committed itself to an ambitious goal of cutting in half the number of people living in absolute poverty by 2015. But in spite of this agreement to reduce the financial burden of debt in poor countries, debt cancellation has been slow.

Meanwhile, developing countries have been grouped into two categories according to economic and health indicators.[23] The group of least developed countries include most of Sub-Saharan Africa, where infant mortality is around 100 per 1000 live births, adolescent childbearing is common, risk of death in childbirth is worse than 1 in 20, female literacy rate is low, and life expectancy is less than 50 years.

In contrast, rich industrialised countries have infant mortality rates of ≤6 per 1000, risk of death in childbirth is 1 in 4000, female literacy rate is high, and life expectancy is around 77 years.

Between these two groups of rich and poor countries are a number of developing countries with intermediate health indices.

High maternal and infant mortality

Poverty continued to be the biggest single underlying cause of death, disease and suffering in developing countries in the 1990s.

According to World Health Organization (WHO) estimates, maternal mortality remained unchanged at 515 000 women dying every year of the 1990s from pregnancy and childbirth. Maternal mortality was estimated at 400 per 100 000 live births during that decade. The lifetime chance of dying in pregnancy or childbirth was highest in Sub-Saharan Africa (1 in 13) and South

Asia (1 in 54). In industrialised countries, the risk of dying during pregnancy and childbirth was 1 in 4085.

There was a small increase in the percentage of births attended by skilled personnel in 53 countries where maternal mortality is less severe. But in the least developed countries of Sub-Saharan Africa, only 29% of mothers had a skilled attendant at delivery. In 2000, an estimated 53 million women in developing countries gave birth with no professional care whatsoever. Emergency obstetric care supported by UNICEF has reduced the maternal mortality rate in Honduras by almost 40% and is also having dramatic effects in Egypt. Sri Lanka and Malaysia have reduced maternal mortality significantly by making maternity care a priority that guided changes in health services. By looking after pregnant mothers before, during and after delivery, many of the causes of neonatal deaths can be prevented.[24]

Female genital mutilation is outlawed in developed countries but continues to endanger the lives of more than 100 million women in Africa during late pregnancy and labour when surgical intervention is required to allow safe vaginal delivery. Mutilated women living in Britain have presented obstetric problems to maternity teams in NHS hospitals.

Women under 25 years of age in developing countries are becoming infected faster and earlier with HIV/AIDS. In Sub-Saharan Africa, in the 15–24 age group, two females are infected for every male. In the most affected areas, five or six adolescent girls are infected for every boy. During 2002, 14 million children under 15 years had lost one or both parents to AIDS, while in 2000, 2.3 million children became AIDS orphans and nine in 10 of them in Sub-Saharan Africa.[24]

Every year, over 600 000 infants worldwide are infected with HIV from their mothers. The use of antiretroviral prophylaxis such as zidovudine has dramatically reduced mother-to-child transmission of HIV in the world's rich countries. Without intervention, up to 35% of babies are infected, compared with <5% when antiretroviral treatment of mothers and appropriate care are available. Breastfeeding is a major contributing factor to mother-to-child transmission, accounting for one-third of HIV-infected babies when infected mothers are not treated with antiretroviral drugs.[17]

A significant proportion of children born in developing countries are not registered at birth: 71% in Sub-Saharan Africa and 56% in South Asia. In 2000, over 50 million babies were not registered, 41% worldwide.[24]

Two of three deaths in infancy take place during the first month after birth and most of these occur on the first day. An estimated 4 million fetal and another 4 million neonatal deaths occur worldwide annually, 98% in developing countries. Until 1996, almost all programmes to reduce mortality in children under 5 years of age were aimed at tackling deaths from diarrhoea, vaccine-preventable diseases and respiratory infections. This approach met with dramatic success except for neonatal deaths, which now form 40% of all deaths in children aged <5 years. Most of these neonatal deaths can be prevented without the use of complicated techniques or equipment.

Neonatal care in developing countries gained international attention only in 1996, when the WHO Safe Motherhood Programme[20] focused on the main causes of neonatal deaths: birth asphyxia (24%), perinatal infections (32%) and complications of prematurity (24%). Low birthweight (LBW) is an important secondary factor in 40–80% of neonatal deaths according to WHO estimates in 2001.

Subsequently, neonatal care in developing countries received further attention, leading to the Save the Children Fund in the USA publishing *State of the World's Newborns*[21] in September 2001. The report confirmed that improving neonatal health would require:

- improving maternal nutrition, preventing infections such as tetanus by vaccination and malaria by chemoprophylaxis;
- identifying mothers at risk;
- providing skilled attendants for clean deliveries, simple means of resuscitation of the newborn, keeping babies warm and promoting breastfeeding;
- identifying and caring for babies at special risk.

Good survival of neonates can be achieved in poor countries. In Kerala, SE India, where the gross domestic product per person is about US$200, neonatal mortality is 14 per 1000 live births, compared with 50 per 1000 in the wealthier states of Madhya Pradesh and Uttar Pradesh.[6] The key to Kerala's success is the high literacy rate of women: 87% compared with 25% in northern Indian states. It also has basic professional healthcare provided by trained birth attendants, midwives and doctors.[9]

Attempts to improve neonatal care in the 1990s have met with varying success. Training birth attendants to conduct clean deliveries, and in aseptic handling of the umbilical cord by providing them and all pregnant mothers with low-cost WHO-recommended sterile packs containing a sterile razor blade, sterile ligatures and an antiseptic such as gentian violet for the umbilical stump, has been rewarded by an impressive decline in the incidence of neonatal tetanus. By 1999, annual deaths from neonatal tetanus had fallen to 300 000, a saving of half a million lives annually in a decade. This approach to training birth attendants has been adopted in Indonesia since 1993 with success.[30]

More comprehensive care of newborn babies in rural Maharashtra, in NW India, focused on managing sepsis, and this halved neonatal mortality from 55 per 1000 to 25 per 1000 in 3 years. But this model of neonatal care described by Bang et al has not been feasible elsewhere in India because of the high cost of US$5.30 per neonate.[1]

Organising healthcare delivery

In most developing countries, a system of community healthcare is in place in rural settings, comprising health centres aimed at the care of pregnant women and young children. But the effectiveness of this system has been hampered by the variable standard of health workers and the deficiency of basic pharmaceuticals available at the health centres. One initiative piloted in the early 1990s was to charge every user of health centres for the drugs they were prescribed. This payment reduced the number of people who used health centres.

In contrast, most urban towns and cities have no effective system of healthcare provided by local government. The urban drift of people into towns increases the burden on hospitals that are used as primary care clinics by people who are unable to pay for doctors practising in private clinics. Haphazard expansion of slums with neither sanitation nor safe water supply compromises the health of infants and children who commonly suffer from diarrhoea and respiratory illness.

The World Bank in 1993[28] recommended all governments to focus on the poor and expand basic schooling, especially for girls. Government spending on health would be limited to public health measures and essential clinical interventions. Cost-effective public health activities included immunisation, school-based health services, information about family planning and nutrition, programmes to reduce tobacco and alcohol consumption, and AIDS prevention. Essential clinical care in all countries would involve at least prenatal and delivery care, family planning, basic care of the sick child, and simple treatments for TB and sexually transmitted diseases.

This minimum health package recommended by the World Bank could cost as little as US$12 per person annually in low-income countries and reduce the burden of disease by about 25%. Adoption of the package in all developing countries would require a quadrupling of expenditure on public health from US$5 billion in 1993 to US$20 billion annually. Spending on essential clinical services would increase from about US$20 billion to US$40 billion.

Economic stagnation and deflation in the richer industrialised countries over the past decade has made all these recommendations impossible to implement. The economic prospects for the immediate future of developing countries continues to be poor and the above recommendations are impractical. But local examples of successful healthcare systems for mothers and children in developing countries, including some of the poorest, have continued to grow in the 1990s and into this new millennium.

Healthcare has been part of community development in these sustainable schemes of health education, growing fruit and vegetables, rearing fish and chickens, and constructing pit latrines. In 1990, after a decade of the Indonesian government instituting community-based healthcare, primary immunisation coverage was

more than 80%, deaths from diarrhoea decreased, and infant mortality fell to 71 per 1000 live births. By 2001, infant mortality in Indonesia fell to 33 and primary school enrolment/attendance reached 91%.[24] In India and most of Sub-Saharan Africa, successful community-based healthcare initiatives have predominantly been organised by voluntary non-governmental organisations. As a result, the Indian government has encouraged, and continues to encourage, its national health system to work in partnership with their 3000 voluntary charitable health organisations.

The aim of this chapter is to consider specific problems affecting the organisation and delivery of neonatal care in tropical developing countries (Table 7.1) and explore simple effective measures for managing them. Examples of good practice will be described. Attention will also be directed at diseases – including their prevention – that pose a threat to any newborn travelling to the tropics.

Essential newborn care

Neonatal care is essential, not only to reduce mortality and improve the quality of survival by preventing disability, but also to promote positive attitudes to family planning. Parents worldwide show increasing willingness to limit family size as confidence grows in their ability to produce healthy children with a normal life expectancy. In Latin America and the Caribbean, where the mortality rate of children under age 5 years fell from 158 per 1000 live births in 1960 to 47 in 1994, the number of children per mother fell from six in 1950 to three in 1990.

Unsupervised, unskilled, delayed and complicated deliveries that characterise obstetrics in developing countries, and the high frequency of LBW babies, contribute to a high prevalence of birth asphyxia and birth trauma.

Problems associated with perinatal asphyxia emphasise the technological gap between developed and developing countries. Endotracheal intubation and ventilation cannot be applied in health facilities where laryngoscopes and appropriate tubes are not available. Provision of simple mucus extractors and education in their use, together with instruction in bag-and-mask respiration, will do more to lessen the ill effects of birth asphyxia in vast areas of the tropics than will sophisticated technology. India produces a variety of mucus extractors made of plastic and hand-operated bag-and-mask resuscitators for a fraction of the price charged in industrialised countries. This equipment for neonatal resuscitation has been made increasingly available during the past decade in Indian primary health centres where a room is set aside for delivering babies. Mouth-to-mouth respiration can no longer be recommended because of HIV in developing countries. Mouth-to-mask units with a one-way expiratory valve are a safe and appropriate alternative means of resuscitation.

Essential neonatal care for developing countries received a boost when a task force was set up in 1993 by the government of India to train physicians in skills to manage diarrhoea and acute respiratory infections and in neonatal care. The National Neonatology Forum, established by Indian neonatal paediatricians in 1980, launched pilot initiatives in 1994 with their government's Health Ministry in 28 districts across the country.

Table 7.1 Major problems affecting neonates in the tropics

Birth asphyxia and trauma
Low birthweight
Infections
    Hepatitis B, herpes simplex
    Malaria, rubella, syphilis
    Toxoplasmosis, trypanosomiasis
    Tuberculosis, leprosy
    Tetanus
    Ophthalmia – chlamydia, gonococcus
    Amoebiasis
    Strongyloides
    HIV
Jaundice associated with glucose-6-phosphate dehydrogenase
  deficiency
Blood disorders
    Haemorrhagic disease of the newborn
    α-thalassaemia
    Sickle cell anaemia
Urbanisation and the decline in breastfeeding

Table 7.2 Equipment for district neonatal care in India

Primary health centre
Bag resuscitator and mask (1)
Mucus extractor (several)
Weighing scale (1)

First referral centre
Bag resuscitator and mask (2)
Radiant warmer (2)
Weighing scale (2)
Mucus extractor (several)
Oxygen hood (1)
Phototherapy unit (1)

District hospital
Same as for first referral unit, with additional radiant warmer and resuscitation equipment for caesarean section births in the operating theatre

These 'Essential Newborn Care' programmes comprised the establishment of newborn care units with essential equipment (Table 7.2) and appropriate training of doctors and nurses at primary health centres, first-referral units with 10–20 beds attended by a paediatrician and/or obstetrician, and district hospitals. Essential neonatal care includes handwashing facilities, resuscitation of babies who are depressed at birth, provision of warmth, promotion of breastfeeding soon after birth, care of LBW babies, and the identification and appropriate referral of sick neonates. This programme has been extended to scores of districts in India but the impact has yet to be fully assessed.

Low birthweight

The 29th World Health Assembly (1976) defined LBW infants as those weighing <2500 g at birth. The number of LBW babies born in the 1990s remained steady at about 20 million, constituting 16% of all live births worldwide in 1999. The vast majority (>90%) were born in developing countries; of these, 8.1 million took place in India, 1 million in Bangladesh and 1.3 million in Pakistan, accounting for half of the world's LBW babies.

In the past decade, the proportion of LBW babies born in 1999 compared with 1991 fell in industrialised countries from 6% to 4%, in Sub-Saharan Africa from 16% to 14% and in Latin America from 11% to 5%, but rose from 33% to 50% in South Asia.

LBW is a sensitive indicator of socioeconomic development, reflecting the nutritional status and health of mothers and the prospects of survival of newborn infants. Perinatal mortality surveys published in the 1980s confirmed that birthweight and socioeconomic factors are major determinants for neonatal survival in developing countries. In a New Delhi hospital study of 27 794 consecutive singleton births, the perinatal mortality rate dropped from 340 per 1000 births in the 1501–2000 g birthweight group to 46.6 in the group 2001–2500 g; the lowest

mortality rate of 16.7 was in the group 3001–3500 g.[13] Similar findings have been reported from another hospital-based study in Zaria, Nigeria.[14] LBW babies in a hospital in southern Brazil were 17 times more likely to die in the perinatal period than those weighing $\geq$2500 g; babies from the poorest families were three times more likely to die during the perinatal period than those in families with the highest incomes.[4] In this study group, LBW babies comprised 71% of neonatal deaths, and they were 24 times more likely to die in the first month than were normal-weight babies.[3]

Intrauterine growth retardation

In developed countries, the proportion of small-for-gestational age (SGA) infants among babies of LBW ranges from 24% to 45%. In Sub-Saharan Africa, the proportion ranges from 34% in Kenya to 67% in South Africa. The proportion is 58% in Brazil. Much higher frequencies for SGA infants are reported from India: 77–90%. These data were obtained using western centile charts.

However, well-nourished mothers in these countries produce babies of similar weight to their western counterparts, from whom such charts are derived. Although the reliability of some of these estimates is suspect, they emphasise the need to introduce early feeding of LBW babies in developing countries to prevent hypoglycaemia. The low proportion of immature infants among LBW babies in the tropics reduces the need for intensive neonatal care in this group.

The importance of the preponderance of infants with intrauterine growth retardation (IUGR) among LBW babies in developing countries is related to the observation that such infants grow into adults with an increased risk of death from ischaemic heart disease. This association of LBW and heart disease may explain the 45% excess of deaths from cardiovascular disease observed in Bangladeshis, Pakistanis and Indians living in Great Britain. A collaborative study of birthweight and cardiovascular disease in adults from geographical areas in India where migrants to Britain have come showed increased cardiovascular disease and stroke from residents in urban settings but at a lower rate than in their relatives living in Britain.[2]

Factors contributing to LBW births in developing countries are: maternal short stature, teenage pregnancy, short birth interval, maternal anaemia, maternal malnutrition, heavy manual work after mid-pregnancy, smoking and tobacco chewing during pregnancy, and malaria.

Prevention

The best management of LBW births in developing countries would be their prevention by reducing teenage pregnancies, increasing the birth interval using contraception, improving maternal nutrition and treating anaemia, environmental control and prompt treatment of tropical infections, and giving malarial chemoprophylaxis to pregnant women. These measures would promote significant increases in birthweight and break the cycle of growth-retarded female infants becoming stunted adults who will produce growth-retarded babies.

Adolescent childbearing in poor developing countries is associated with pre-eclamptic toxaemia, preterm labour and high frequencies of LBW babies. A substantial reduction in the proportion of babies born within a year of the previous one was identified as an important factor in heavier Pakistani newborns in Birmingham born in 1978 compared with those delivered in 1968.

Food supplementation of pregnant mothers reported increases of birthweight of 25–84 g per 10 000 kcal of maternal energy intake during pregnancy, with mean increases of 135 g occurring with higher intakes. Micronutrient supplements given to women in rural Nepal over 1999–2001 in a randomised controlled trial showed that antenatal folic acid–iron supplements had a modest effect on reducing the risk of LBW. From this trial, 11 women would need to take folic acid–iron supplements, or 12 to take multiple micronutrient supplements, to avert one LBW baby.[8]

Malaria is a contributory cause of LBW and accounts for 25–50% of the attributable risk in primigravidae in malarious areas of Africa. Heavy placental infections with *Plasmodium falciparum* occur more frequently in primiparous indigenous women living in regions of endemic malaria. Infections usually take place during the wet season, when malaria-carrying mosquitoes are abundant. The prevalence rate of placental malaria in tropical Africa is between 20% and 34%. There is abundant evidence that mean birthweights of infants born to women with infected placentae are lower when compared with birthweights of infants born to uninfected mothers. Mean differences, which are consistently in favour of infants born of uninfected placentae, range from 55 to 310 g.[16] Mean birthweights are lower among infants of primiparae than among those of multiparae.

Placental malaria influences birthweight by interfering with placental function and not by direct action of the malarial parasite on the fetus. Garnham, reviewing the morbid histological changes seen in malaria-infected placentae, found it difficult to understand how the fetus could be nourished by an organ showing evidence of such marked pathology which encroaches on and sometimes obliterates the intervillous spaces.[12] Control of malaria in pregnancy through prophylactic antimalarials and using permethrin (insecticide)-impregnated bed nets during the wet season leads to an increase in mean birthweight in malaria-endemic areas and is recommended in antenatal care.

Other tropical diseases also have negative effects on birthweight. Neonates of mothers with leprosy weigh less than those of healthy mothers. IUGR has been observed in babies of mothers with lepromatous leprosy as early as the 16th week of pregnancy. Pregnant women infected with African trypanosomiasis (*T. gambiense* and *T. rhodesiense*) are at high risk of abortion, hydramnios and preterm delivery. In Central and South American countries where Chagas' disease (*T. cruzi*) or American trypanosomiasis is endemic, between 0.5% and 2% of LBW infants under 2000 g have congenital trypanosomiasis. Schistosomiasis can affect the placenta, leading to abortions, preterm delivery and IUGR. Leishmaniasis in pregnancy has been observed to precipitate preterm deliveries. Women with onchocerciasis appear to have a higher-than-expected proportion of LBW babies.

Jaundice

Severe jaundice in newborn infants in the tropics has been a significant public health problem in parts of South East Asia, tropical Africa, the Pacific islands and in some countries bordering the Mediterranean Sea during the last four decades of the 20th century. Neonatal jaundice received high priority at an informal Geneva consultation of senior paediatricians from these regions and WHO officials on the identification of serious diseases affecting child health not covered by WHO programmes in developing countries.[29] The regular use of phototherapy in jaundiced neonates has reduced the need for exchange transfusion with its attendant hazards of using blood that may not have been screened for HIV and hepatitis B.

There appear to be geographical or racial differences in the frequency of severe neonatal jaundice that reflect the interaction of genetic and environmental factors. When compared with European babies, normal-term infants of Chinese and Malay origin tend to have higher maximum bilirubin levels that reach their peak at 4 or 5 days of life.[7] Neonatal jaundice is almost always due to a rise of unconjugated bilirubin in the blood, and it may be difficult to detect in dark-skinned babies. Kernicterus due to the deposition of unconjugated bilirubin in the basal ganglia had been observed as the main cause of death in the first postnatal week in Singapore before a screening programme for glucose-6-phosphate dehydrogenase (G6PD) deficiency was instituted.[27] In the two large cities of Nigeria, Ibadan and Lagos, severe neonatal jaundice continues to be a major cause of admission for infants in the first 2 weeks of life, particularly of those born at home or discharged from hospital within 48 hours of birth. Experience in Ibadan indicates that severe neonatal jaundice is important not only as a cause of cerebral palsy but also in the pathogenesis of deafness and delayed speech.[10]

Causes

The known causes of severe neonatal jaundice in the tropics are different from those found in temperate industrialised countries (Table 7.3). G6PD deficiency is an important cause of neonatal jaundice in South East Asia and West Africa. Haemolysis from factors intrinsic and extrinsic to the red blood cells occurs in neonates with G6PD deficiency. Bacterial infections are frequent in a hot climate without a clean water supply and sanitation. The liver enzyme system for conjugating bilirubin is not functioning

Table 7.3 Common causes of neonatal hyperbilirubinaemia in the tropics

Glucose-6-phosphate dehydrogenase deficiency
Sepsis
Prematurity
Trauma and birth asphyxia
ABO haemolytic disease
Haemolytic agents – naphthalene

optimally in preterm babies. Trauma and asphyxia at birth occur when maternity services are inadequate. Extravasated blood in cephalhaematomata and in bruised tissues is resorbed with the production of bilirubin, which increases the load of unconjugated pigment to be removed by the neonate's liver. Studies in the USA have shown that the incidence of ABO haemolytic disease, based on a positive direct Coomb's test, is increased in black infants.[19] There is some evidence to suggest that the same occurs in African neonates.

In addition, about 20% or 30% of newborn babies with unconjugated bilirubinaemia in tropical countries have none of these causal factors to explain their jaundice. It is probable that environmental factors contribute to neonatal jaundice in the tropics. A report from Papua New Guinea showed the importance of environmental illumination of obstetric wards on the incidence of neonatal jaundice. Architectural modifications to prevent rain blowing into an obstetric ward were made by extending the roof overhangs to a width of several metres so that they excluded most of the daylight. An alarming increase in the incidence of severe neonatal jaundice from 0.5% to 17% was observed after the modifications. Other causes for the increase in neonatal jaundice were excluded.[5] This observation has implications for the design of obstetric wards and neonatal nurseries in the tropics, which should be built with windows facing north–south for coolness, and with roof overhangs limited to a width of 1 m to allow entry of adequate indirect sunlight to reduce neonatal jaundice. The use of natural illumination from indirect sunlight has been found to be of therapeutic value during the day in the tropics; if used with care, it can reduce the need to use phototherapy units during daylight hours.

It has been suggested that the high incidence of severe neonatal jaundice in Nigerian babies could be a result of high exposure to infection and icterogenic drugs and chemicals in their homes.[11,18] Significant exposure to naphthalene, insecticides, mentholated balms and powders, and traditional herbs was found in 65% of families by Familusi & Dawodu.[11] Although the incidence of jaundice did not differ significantly in neonates from households with or without a positive history of exposure, severe jaundice requiring exchange transfusion was significantly more frequent among neonates from families with exposure to naphthalene. Naphthalene can be inhaled or absorbed through the skin of an infant wearing clothes that have been stored in mothballs. It induces haemolysis, fragmentation and Heinz body formation in G6PD-deficient red cells through the oxidising properties of α-naphthol. Even red cells with normal G6PD concentrations undergo haemolysis when exposed to naphthalene.[26] Analysis of high-performance chromatography of some traditional Nigerian remedies for purging neonates of meconium and of mentholated balms has identified naphthalene as an ingredient. Naphthols were found in 6.9% of 625 Nigerian cord blood samples and aflatoxins in 14.6%, indicating perinatal exposure.[15] But there was no significant difference in naphthol or aflatoxin exposure of neonates with and without jaundice. One in three with severe jaundice were G6PD deficient compared with 13.3% of controls (p = 0.009).[22]

Available evidence suggests that neonatal jaundice is common in some tropical communities because of a combination of genetic red cell disorders and exposure of infants to haemolytic environmental agents as a result of traditional practices during the perinatal period.

Protection for newborn travellers to the tropics

Parents with young infants from temperate industrialized countries have become less apprehensive of travelling with them to the tropics. Provided certain measures are taken to protect their health, infants thrive as well in tropical countries as they would in Europe or North America.

Breastfeeding is usually more convenient than bottle-feeding and may be continued into the second year. If the infant is to be bottle-fed, powdered milk should be reconstituted with boiled water, and the milk should not be left to stand unrefrigerated for more than an hour. The same rule applies to liquid milk supplied by manufacturers. Bottles and utensils should be sterilised before use.

Cotton clothing is preferable to clothes made from synthetic fibres because it absorbs perspiration and prevents skin rashes. Although disposable nappies are convenient for travelling, the plastic covers used with them do not allow urine to evaporate and can lead to ammoniacal dermatitis.

Babies should not be exposed to direct tropical light for fear of sunburn. There is also the possibility of long-term dangers of skin cancer. Naked babies lying in the shade for a few hours can become sunburned, particularly on the beach. A bed net impregnated with an insecticide (e.g. permethrin) should be placed over the cot to protect the baby from mosquito bites when asleep during the day and night. Insect repellents may also be used on the skin, care being taken to ensure the baby's skin is not allergic to chemicals used in the repellent.

Immunisation

BCG immunisation is recommended for newborn infants living in cities of developing countries where TB is endemic. The vaccine prevents miliary and meningitic forms of TB. BCG vaccine stored in a refrigerator at 2–8°C should be reconstituted just before use. An intradermal injection of 0.1 ml of the vaccine is introduced into the skin of the left upper arm over the insertion of the left deltoid muscle, and this should produce a weal about 7 mm in diameter. No tuberculin test is necessary before immunisation of a neonate. Between 3 and 6 weeks after the immunisation, a small papule appears at the injection site, indicating the development of delayed hypersensitivity. The papule discharges pus, leaving a shallow ulcer that heals to form a scar. Immunity induced by a successful BCG vaccination provides protection for about 10 years. Immunocompromised infants should not be given this live-attenuated vaccine.

Oral live polio (Sabin) vaccine given in liquid drops is administered to neonates in some developing countries. This method of immunisation is safe and effective and can be recommended to neonates visiting developing countries.

The first dose of diphtheria, pertussis, tetanus and poliomyelitis vaccines is usually administered in the second month of life. Parents should be reminded that two more doses should be given at monthly intervals and that a booster dose is recommended at about 18 months. Measles vaccine or MMR is recommended at 15 months.

Other vaccines, such as cholera, typhoid and yellow fever, are not recommended. Cholera vaccine is not efficient if given in a single dose. Two doses given 4 weeks apart can ensure protection for a maximum of only 6 months. This vaccine if given subcutaneously produces a severe local reaction and pain. The only useful vaccine against *Salmonella typhi* is the live attenuated oral typhoid vaccine administered in an enteric-coated capsule recommended for children over 6 years and for adults. Both cholera and typhoid are diseases that can be avoided if mothers are willing to breastfeed their newborn babies. If they prefer bottle-feeding, then they should be scrupulous in using boiled water for preparing milk and sterilised bottles and teats. Most parents who take their infants abroad live in good accommodation and should be able to take good care of their babies without these vaccines. Yellow fever vaccine is recommended only after 9 months because of the small risk of encephalitis in younger infants.

Meningococcal group C conjugate vaccine provides long-term protection against infection by serogroup C of *Neisseria meningitides* in young children from 2 months of age. It is administered by intramuscular injection. Meningococcal polysaccharide A & C vaccine is effective, but infants respond less well than adults; it is recommended for children over 18 months old.

Pregnant women travelling to the tropics should be given protection against poliomyelitis, using the injectable killed Salk vaccine, and tetanus with two doses of toxoid administered 2 months apart during the third trimester. Yellow fever vaccine may be administered in the third trimester for travellers to endemic regions although it is a live attenuated vaccine. No reliable reports of fetopathy have been recorded with yellow fever vaccination given as recommended here.

Malarial prophylaxis

All newborn infants (including those breastfed) travelling to the tropics should be protected against malaria, a common and life-threatening disease currently endemic in over 100 countries visited by more than 125 million international travellers every year. The malaria parasite Plasmodium is transmitted by various species of Anopheles mosquitoes that bite mainly between sunset and sunrise.

Malaria in pregnant travellers increases the risk of maternal death, miscarriage, stillbirth, LBW and neonatal death. *Plasmodium falciparum* causes the most severe form of malaria and it is endemic in tropical Africa, Asia, the Pacific islands, and Central and South America. In many endemic countries of Central and South America, the Caribbean, Asia and the Mediterranean, the main urban areas are mostly free of malaria transmission. But malaria can occur in urban areas in Africa and India. There is usually less risk of malaria at altitudes above 1500 m, but in favourable climatic conditions (end of the rainy season) it can occur at altitudes up to almost 3000 m. There is no risk of malaria in many tourist destinations in South East Asia, Latin America and the Caribbean.

Prevention and treatment of falciparum malaria are becoming more difficult because *P. falciparum* is increasingly resistant to various antimalarial drugs. Drug resistance has also been reported for *P. vivax*, mainly from Indonesia (Irian Jaya) and Papua New Guinea, with sporadic cases reported from Guyana. The latest advice for travellers can be obtained from the Department of Health's website on *Health Information for Overseas Travel* www.doh.gov.uk/traveladvice/. Details of advice on malaria are also available from the WHO's website on *International travel and health* www.who.int/ith.

Pregnant women and neonates are not encouraged to travel to countries with drug-resistant malaria. But if travel cannot be delayed, the following is recommended. Breastfed as well as bottle-fed babies should be given antimalarial drugs for chemoprophylaxis since they are not protected by the mother's prophylaxis. Dosage schedules should be based on body weight. Chloroquine and proguanil are safe for babies and young children, and mefloquine may be given to infants of more than 5 kg body weight.

The combination of chloroquine, 5 mg/kg body weight weekly, and proguanil, 5 mg/kg daily, will give some protection against *P. falciparum* even in areas where the parasite is resistant to chloroquine, and may alleviate the disease if it occurs despite prophylaxis. Therefore, the possibility of malaria should be considered whenever a child in an endemic area develops a fever. A liquid preparation of chloroquine is available. Proguanil, in either dry or liquid form, is bitter and can be difficult to administer to babies with sensitive tastebuds.

Mefloquine, although effective in areas where falciparum malaria is resistant to chloroquine, is not recommended for neonates. Doxycycline is contraindicated in children below 8 years of age. As a result, the combination of chloroquine and proguanil is the main recommended chemoprophylaxis for neonates in all malaria-endemic countries.

Protection against mosquito bites is essential in addition to malaria chemoprophylaxis. Screening of the bedroom with fine netting will exclude flying insects but allow adequate ventilation. Insecticide-impregnated bed nets are now available that do not require re-impregnation after 6 months or a year. They will repel mosquitoes even when there is a tear and the net is not tucked under the mattress.

Advice should be obtained from specialists in tropical paediatrics if children are likely to live for more than 3 years in a malaria-endemic area. Complications from the long-term continuous use of chloroquine (retinal damage) have to be weighed against the acquisition of immunity from occasional natural infection treated promptly.

References

1. Bang A T, Bang R A, Baitule S B, Reddy M H, Deshmukh M D 1999 Effect of home-based neonatal care and management of sepsis on neonatal mortality: field trial in rural India. Lancet 354: 1955–1961
2. Barker D 1997 Intrauterine programming of coronary heart disease and stroke. Acta Paediatrica Supplement 423: 178–182
3. Barros F C, Victora C G, Vaughan J P, Estanislau H J 1987 Perinatal mortality in southern Brazil: a population based study of 7392 births. Bulletin of the World Health Organization 65: 95–104

4. Barros F C, Victora C G, Vaughan J P, Teixeira A M B, Ashworth A 1987 Infant mortality in southern Brazil; a population based study of causes of death. Archives of Disease in Childhood 62: 487–490

5. Barss P, Comfort K 1985 Ward design and neonatal jaundice in the tropics: report of an epidemic. British Medical Journal 291: 400–401

6. Bhargava S K 2003 Newborn care in India – at the crossroads. Journal of Neonatology 17: 5–13

7. Brown W R, Wong H B 1965 Ethnic group differences in bilirubinemia of Singapore newborns. Bulletin of the Kandang Kerbau Hospital Singapore 4: 35–43

8. Christian P, Khatry S K, Katz J et al 2003 Effects of alternative maternal micronutrient supplements on low birth weight in rural Nepal: double blind randomised community trial. British Medical Journal 326: 571–574

9. Evans I 1995 SAPping maternal health. Lancet 346: 1046

10. Familusi J B, Dawodu A H, Owa J A 1982 Some epidemiological aspects of neonatal hyperbilirubinaemia in Nigeria. In: Fukuyama Y et al (eds) Child neurology. Excerpta Medica, Amsterdam, pp 272–280

11. Familusi J B, Dawodu A H 1985 A survey of neonatal jaundice in association with household drugs and chemicals in Nigeria. Annals of Tropical Paediatrics 5: 219–222

12. Garnham P C C 1938 The placenta in malaria with special reference to reticuloendothelial immunity. Transactions of the Royal Society of Tropical Medicine and Hygiene 32: 13–34

13. Ghosh S, Bhargava S K, Saxena H M K, Sagreiya K 1983 Perinatal mortality – report of a hospital based study. Annals of Tropical Paediatrics 3: 115–119

14. Harrison K A 1985 Childbearing, health and social priorities: a survey of 22,774 consecutive hospital births in Zaria, Northern Nigeria. British Journal of Obstetrics and Gynaecology 92(suppl. 5): 13–22, 61–80, 86–115

15. Maxwell S M, Familusi J B, Sodeinde O, Chan M C K, Hendrickse R G 1994 Detection of naphthols and aflatoxins in Nigerian cord blood. Annals of Tropical Paediatrics 14: 3–5

16. McGregor I A, Wilson M E, Billewicz W Z 1983 Malaria infection of the placenta in the Gambia, West Africa; its incidence and relationship to stillbirth, birthweight and placental weight. Transactions of the Royal Society of Tropical Medicine and Hygiene 77: 232–244

17. McIntyre J, Gray G 2002 What can we do to reduce mother to child transmission of HIV? British Medical Journal 324: 218–221

18. Olowe S A, Ransome-Kuti O 1980 The risk of jaundice in glucose-6-phosphate dehydrogenase deficient babies exposed to menthol. Acta Paediatrica Scandinavica 69: 341–345

19. Peevy K J, Wiseman H J 1978 ABO haemolytic disease of the newborn: evaluation of management and identification of racial and antigenic factors. Pediatrics 61: 475–478

20. Safe Motherhood 1996 Newborn care: getting off to a good start. Safe Motherhood Newsletter 21: 4–8

21. Save the Children Fund 2001 State of the world's newborns. Save the Children Fund, USA

22. Sodeinde O, Chan M C K, Maxwell S M, Familusi J B, Hendrickse R G 1995 Neonatal jaundice, aflatoxins and naphthols: report of a study in Ibadan, Nigeria. Annals of Tropical Paediatrics 15: 107–113

23. UNFPA 2002 State of world population – people, poverty and possibilities. UNFPA, New York

24. UNICEF 2003 The state of the world's children. UNICEF, New York

25. United Nations Millennium Summit 2000 Millennium Development Goals. New York

26. Vales T, Doxiadis S A, Fessas P H 1963 Acute haemolysis due to naphthalene inhalation. Journal of Pediatrics 63: 904–915

27. Wong H B 1966 Singapore kernicterus: a review and the present position. Bulletin of the Kandang Kerbau Hospital Singapore 5: 1–9

28. World Development Report 1993 Investing in health. The World Bank, New York

29. World Health Organization 1985 Serious childhood diseases: priority issues and possible actions at family, community and health centre levels. Report of an informal consultation. WHO MCH/85.3, Geneva

30. World Health Organization 2001 World Health Report. WHO, Geneva

Section Two

Prenatal Life

CHAPTER 8

Basic genetics

Andrew Green

The nature and structure of a gene

Genetics is traditionally defined as the science of biological variation, and has been a scientific discipline for over 100 years. Human genetics makes up a large part of the field of genetics, but the principal laws of genetics are universal and apply equally to all species, including humans. Mendel's studies in the 19th century were originally felt to have no relevance to humans, and it is only in retrospect that their importance can be seen. Many of the principles of genetics were discovered through the study of smaller organisms, such as bacteria, yeast and fruit flies. The basic genetic mechanisms of cell division, development and differentiation happen in the same way in widely divergent species. Therefore, it is impossible to look at human genetics in isolation and there are large amounts of information from lower species which have bearing on human disorders. The study of the genetics of small organisms has had a profound impact on our understanding of human development, and of how human diseases develop. It is likely that such basic science will continue to contribute significantly to the understanding of human genetic disease. In this chapter, I hope to outline the basic elements of genetics, and describe the types of genetic tests now available to help in neonatal diagnosis.

The basic unit of inheritance for any species is the *gene*. The original concept of a gene arose long before the relationship between genes and nucleic acids was ever understood. A gene was considered to be a stable heritable element which conferred a particular property or phenotype on an individual organism. This element was passed on to subsequent generations of a particular species, and the nature of the phenotype varied according to the nature of the gene. The concept of dominant and recessive traits, which will be discussed below, was derived from studies of inheritance patterns, long before the molecular basis of the gene was understood.

A gene can also be considered in another way, as a specific length of deoxyribonucleic acid (DNA) which encodes a particular function, in most cases the synthesis of a protein. This also is a stable heritable unit. Each cell in an organism, regardless of its function, has the entire set of genes for that particular organism, but only a proportion of those genes will be active. DNA is found in the nucleus of every cell of an organism, as a double helix (Fig. 8.1).

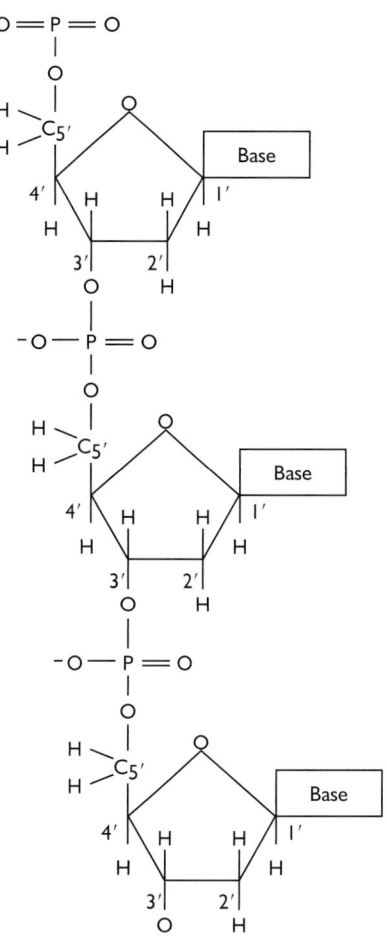

Fig. 8.1 Structure of a DNA chain. The deoxyribose and phosphate residues are linked to form the sugar–phosphate backbone.

Each strand of the double helix has a backbone of alternating phosphate and deoxyribose sugar molecules, with the sugars attached to the 5′ and 3′ hydroxyl groups of the phosphate group. Attached to the sugar molecule, lying within the helix, is one of four nitrogen-containing nucleic acid bases. Two of these bases, adenine (A) and guanine (G), are purines, and two are the smaller pyrimidines cytosine (C) and thymine (T). The A and T bases pair together by hydrogen bonding, and the G and C bases similarly pair by hydrogen bonds (Fig. 8.2). The two strands of the double helix are held together by paired A–T or G–C bases of opposite strands of the double helix. The DNA strand can be read in only one direction, from 5′ (left hand) to 3′ (right hand). The two strands of DNA are complementary to each other, and the sequence of one strand can be predicted from its opposite. If one strand reads 5′-CAGCGTA-3′, then the opposite strand must read 5′-TACGCTG-3′. The double-stranded sequence would then be written as below:

5′-CAGCGTA-3′

3′-GTCGCAT-5′

The simplicity of the double-helix structure allows for several important functions for DNA.

First, huge amounts of information can be stored in the DNA strand. If a molecule of DNA is 1 million bases long, then there are $4^{1\,000\,000}$ possible sequences for that stretch of DNA. A genome is the complete DNA sequence of an organism. In humans, the estimated genome size is 3×10^9 base pairs (bp).

The draft DNA sequence of the entire human genome has been completed, which is a major milestone in human scientific development. It is estimated that the genome has between 30 000 and 40 000 genes. However, despite the DNA sequence being available, the detailed function of many of these genes remains unknown. The next step after the sequencing of the human genome is the understanding of the complexities of all the human genes. The routine practical clinical applications of the knowledge of the human genome is still some way off.

Secondly, the double helix provides a framework for DNA replication. One strand of DNA acts as a template for the synthesis of a new strand. The double helix unwinds, allowing DNA replication enzymes access to the template strand of DNA. The replication system builds a new strand of DNA based on the template. The new double helix formed as a result will contain one original strand and a newly synthesised complementary second strand. This is the basic mechanism of DNA replication in all species.

Thirdly, the double helix provides a basis for repair of damaged DNA. A damaged base can be replaced, knowing its complementary base is present on the opposite strand. Damage to the sugar–phosphate backbone can also be repaired using the opposite strand as a template.

Decoding the information in DNA

About 90% of the DNA in the human genome does not code for any specific property; only about 10% of the genome actually contains coding information in the form of a gene. In simple terms, the genetic code in DNA is transcribed into a molecule called messenger RNA (mRNA). The mRNA is then translated into a protein, which carries out the function encoded by the specific DNA.

A gene has several distinct elements (Fig. 8.3). The major part of the gene is divided into coding regions, called exons, and non-coding regions, called introns. Just before (5′) the first exon, there is a promoter which indicates where transcription of a gene should start. There can be several promoters for one gene, and different promoters can be used according to the tissue in which

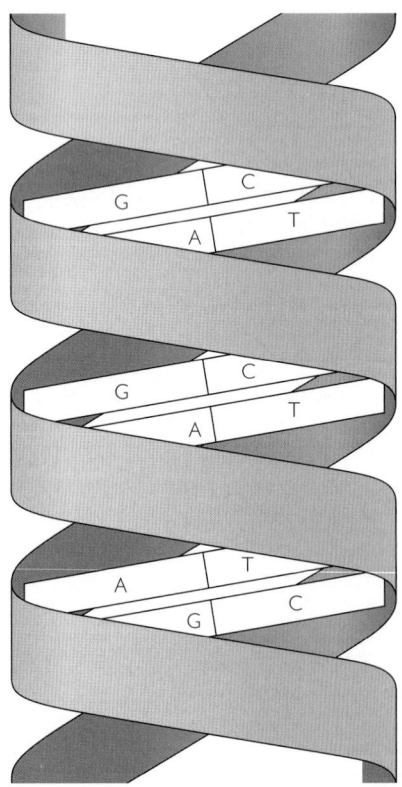

Fig. 8.2 Double helix structure of DNA. The double helix of deoxyribose and phosphate molecules is held together by paired purine and pyrimidine bonds.

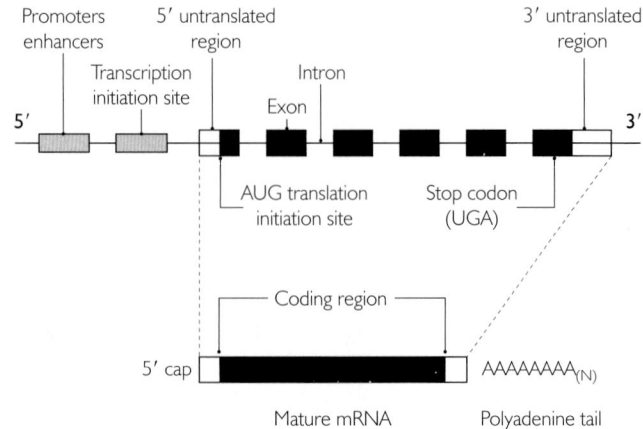

Fig. 8.3 An idealised gene.

the gene is being expressed, in other words the promoter is tissue specific. Further 5' of the promoter there can also be enhancers or suppressors, which can increase or decrease the level of transcription of the gene. Not all of the mRNA will code for protein, as some exons will code for mRNA that does not directly encode protein. These areas, known as untranslated regions, can be either at the start (5') or the end (3') of the mRNA.

To express the DNA code, mRNA is used. There are several different types of RNA, but mRNA is the most important in decoding DNA. There are three differences between RNA and DNA. First, the sugar backbone of RNA contains ribose rather than deoxyribose. Secondly, mRNA exists as a single strand, and remains more unstable. Thirdly, in RNA, the base uracil (U) is used instead of thymine, whereas the other three nucleic acids remain the same.

The DNA code in most genes is expressed as a protein, which is a peptide made of the building blocks of individual amino acids. Each amino acid is coded for by a sequence of three DNA bases, known as a codon. For some amino acids, there is more than one codon (Table 8.1). A long series of DNA codons in a gene will thus code for an entire protein. The mRNA codons coding for amino acids are identical to DNA codons, with the substitution of uracil (U) for thymine (T). There is a tightly controlled mechanism for the generation of protein from a DNA template.

To decode a gene into protein, the DNA is first transcribed into mRNA. A strand (the 'sense' strand) of the DNA double helix is used by the enzyme RNA polymerase to synthesise a complementary strand of mRNA. Transcription of mRNA starts from the 5' end of the first exon of the gene, until the end of the most 3' exon. The intervening introns are initially included, and the first molecule is known as pre-mRNA. The intronic RNA

sequences are spliced out and a 3' polyadenine tail is added, producing mature mRNA. The mature mRNA is then transferred from the nucleus to the ribosome, to be used as a template for the production of protein. The mature mRNA has both 5' and 3' untranslated regions.

Protein synthesis does not begin at the 5' end of the mRNA, but at the first 5' AUG codon, which codes for the amino acid methionine. Protein translation stops at the first truncation codon (usually UGA) thereafter (see Fig. 8.3). In the ribosome, amino acid-specific transfer molecules, called transfer RNAs (tRNAs), bind a free molecule of their specific amino acid. The binding is carried out by an anticodon in the tRNA, which is complementary to the mRNA that codes for that specific amino acid. Using its anticodon, the tRNA binds the specific mRNA codon for its amino acid. By a complex machinery, the amino acid is then added to a growing peptide chain which will eventually form the mature protein (Fig. 8.4). The 5' end of the mRNA

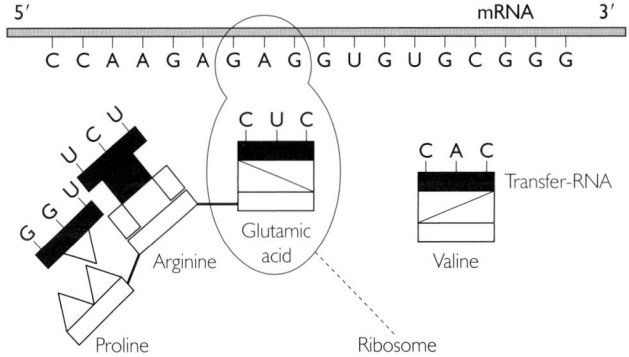

Fig. 8.4 Diagram of protein synthesis from mRNA.

First position	Second position								Third position
	U	Amino acid	C	Amino acid	A	Amino acid	G	Amino acid	
U	UUU	Phe	UCU	Ser	UAU	Tyr	UGU	Cys	U
	UUC	Phe	UCC	Ser	UAC	Tyr	UGC	Cys	C
	UUA	Leu	UCA	Ser	UAA	Stop	UGA	Stop	A
	UUG	Leu	UCG	Ser	UAG	Stop	UGG	Trp	G
C	CUU	Leu	CCU	Pro	CAU	His	CGU	Arg	U
	CUC	Leu	CCC	Pro	CAC	His	CGC	Arg	C
	CUA	Leu	CCA	Pro	CAA	Gln	CGA	Arg	A
	CUG	Leu	CCG	Pro	CAG	Gln	CGG	Arg	G
A	AUU	Ile	ACU	Thr	AAU	Asn	AGU	Ser	U
	AUC	Ile	ACC	Thr	AAC	Asn	AGC	Ser	C
	AUA	Ile	ACA	Thr	AAA	Lys	AGA	Arg	A
	AUG	Met	ACG	Thr	AAG	Lys	AGG	Arg	G
G	GUU	Val	GCU	Ala	GAU	Asp	GGU	Gly	U
	GUC	Val	GCC	Ala	GAC	Asp	GGC	Gly	C
	GUA	Val	GCA	Ala	GAA	Glu	GGA	Gly	A
	GUG	Val	GCG	Ala	GAG	Glu	GGG	Gly	G

Table 8.1 The genetic code

corresponds to the NH$_2$ (amino terminus) of the protein, and the 3′ end of the mRNA corresponds to the COOH (carboxyl terminus) of the protein. Many proteins in higher species are modified after translation by the addition of phosphate or lipid groups.

Chromosomes and cell division

The first coiling of DNA is in the form of the double helix. However, there are subsequent higher orders of coiling and packaging of DNA. The first order gives a loop of about 146 bp in size, wound around a histone protein. The complex is known as a nucleosome. The highest order of coiling of a large DNA molecule, with its associated histones and other proteins, is known as a chromosome.

A chromosome consists of one very long double helix of DNA, containing very many genes in millions of base pairs. Humans are diploid; that is, they have two copies of every chromosome. The normal human chromosome complement is 46, made up of 22 pairs of autosomes (non-sex chromosomes) and two sex chromosomes, either X and Y in a male, or X and X in a female. Each member of a pair of autosomes contains the same genetic information. The pair of X chromosomes in a female will contain the same genetic information, but X and Y chromosomes in a male only have a small number of genes in common. A normal human metaphase karyotype is shown in Figure 8.5.

When cells divide, the genetic content must also be duplicated so that the daughter cells have the correct genetic material. Most cell division occurs as *mitosis*, where one cell divides to give two genetically identical cells. This is the process which allows the formation of a complete human being from one fertilised embryo, and is also the process by which the cells of many organs are constantly renewed. Mitosis is one short period during a carefully programmed cell cycle (Fig. 8.6). After mitosis, the cell may enter a resting phase (G0), or go on to divide again (G1). A cell in G1 will then go on to synthesise new DNA as described above (S phase). There is then a second gap phase (G2), followed by mitosis (M).

Prior to mitosis, the cell can be said to be in *interphase*, during which the chromosomes are very elongated. Just before mitosis, in S phase, the chromosomes are duplicated and begin to

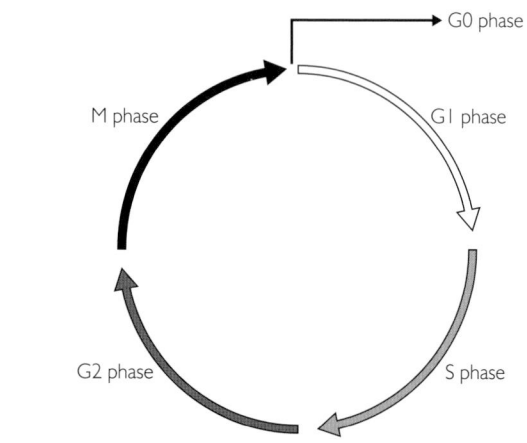

Fig. 8.6 Cell cycle.

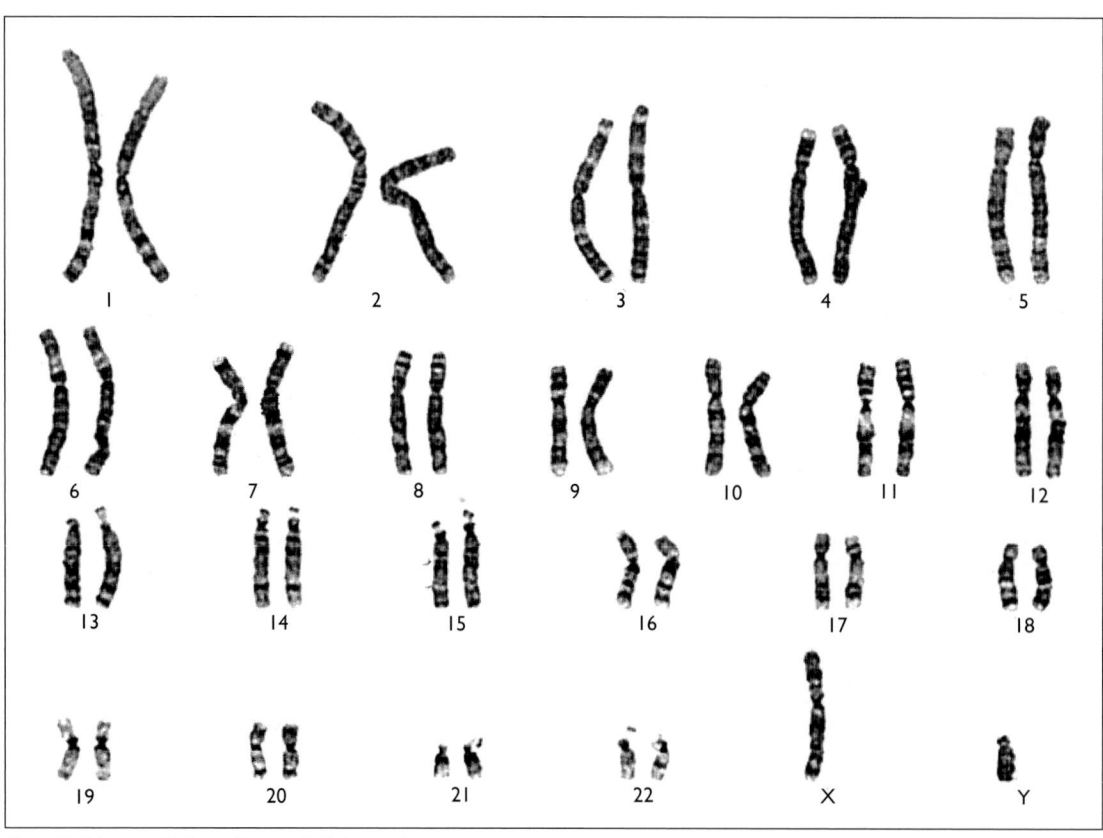

Fig. 8.5 A normal human metaphase karyotype.

Case: Unilabs   Slide: male   Cell: 1   Patient:

condense as two (sister) *chromatids* per chromosome. This condensation phase is known as *prophase*. In the next phase, *metaphase*, the condensed chromatids line up along the plane of the cell, and spindle fibres develop between the centromeres (narrow waist of each chromatid) and the polar centrioles. Standard analysis of human chromosomes is carried out in metaphase. The chromatids separate, starting from each centromere, and pass to the new daughter cell, in the step called *anaphase*. By the *telophase*, the chromatids have reached to opposite poles of the dividing cell, and division completes.

Meiosis is the form of division required to form gametes (sperm or oocyte). Gametes are *haploid*, with only one of each chromosome – 23 in the case of humans. This allows the formation of a new diploid organism from two haploid gametes. Meiosis occurs in two stages, meiosis I and meiosis II. The first phase of meiosis I, prophase I, is similar to that in mitosis, with the appearance of two condensed chromatids which have duplicated. At this stage, crossing over of genetic material from one chromatid to another can occur. It is estimated that one to two crossovers occur per chromosome in each meiosis. This introduces further genetic diversity, ensuring that the inherited chromosomes are different from the chromosomes of the parent. Metaphase I then occurs, where chromatids do not separate but go to the opposite ends of the cell in anaphase I and telophase I. The cells at this stage are still diploid.

The second meiotic division then occurs, where chromatids condense again in prophase II, and line up along the axis of the dividing cell in metaphase II. The chromatids then separate, passing to opposite ends of the cell in anaphase II. The new cells are then haploid, with 23 chromosomes, and the chromatids elongate into thin strands in telophase II.

Chromosome analysis

To examine chromosomes from a patient (a karyotype), dividing cells in culture must be examined. These cells are usually lymphocytes, amniotic fluid cells or fibroblasts. Cells are arrested in the metaphase stage of mitosis, and stained in such a way that the chromosomes are easily visualised. The usual technique used is G-banding (using a Giemsa stain), which gives a characteristic positive and negative banding pattern to each chromosome. Each chromosome has a constriction, called a centromere, dividing the chromosome into a short arm (p) and a long arm (q). Each arm has a number of prominent bands, which can then be subdivided into smaller bands. The gene for the ABO blood group is localised to chromosome 9q34. The gene thus lies in the fourth sub-band from the centromere (q34) of the third band from the centromere (q34) on the long arm (q34) of chromosome 9 (9q34).

Chromosome abnormalities can be broadly classified into abnormalities of chromosome number, or a rearrangement of a normal number of chromosomes. The critical issue in most cases for determining the significance of a chromosome abnormality is whether the abnormality gives rise to an excess or deficiency of the normal diploid state (aneuploidy).

Abnormalities of chromosome number are relatively common, but many are not recognised as they may result in the early loss of a pregnancy. Triploidy (69 chromosomes) and tetraploidy (92 chromosomes) are relatively common causes of early pregnancy loss. Trisomy, the presence of a single extra chromosome (47 chromosomes), is also a common cause of miscarriage. Specific trisomies can give rise to an affected neonate, the commonest being trisomy 21 (Down syndrome), trisomy 13 (Patau syndrome) and trisomy 18 (Edward syndrome). All these trisomies usually occur as a result of autosomal non-dysjunction in meiotic division of the oocyte. In non-dysjunction, the specific chromatids fail to separate, resulting in an extra chromosome in one oocyte and no chromosome in the opposite gamete. A fertilised embryo from the oocyte with an extra chromosome will therefore be trisomic. The fertilised oocyte with an absent chromosome will be monosomic, and be lost as an early miscarriage. Non-dysjunction tends to occur more frequently with increasing maternal age. Non-dysjunction can occur in the male germline, but rarely produces viable offspring.

There are numerous types of chromosome rearrangements, the commonest of which are shown in Figure 8.7. Pericentric and paracentric chromosome inversions are usually balanced, and inherited without any phenotypic effect. Paracentric inversions are usually associated with a low risk of producing a liveborn unbalanced karyotype, but pericentric inversions may carry a higher risk. Insertions, duplications, deletions, isochromosomes and ring chromosomes are all usually aneuploid and associated with significant clinical abnormalities. Reciprocal translocations occur where there is exchange of genetic material from one arm of a chromosome in return for genetic material from a different chromosome. Reciprocal translocations are usually balanced, without any clinical effect, but may carry a risk of having a child with problems due to an unbalanced karyotype.

Another type of translocation is between the acrocentric chromosomes (13–15, 21 and 22), where there is no appreciable coding material on a very small short (p) arm. This is known as a Robertsonian translocation. Robertsonian translocations are one of the commonest human chromosome translocations, and in the balanced form have no clinical effect. A Robertsonian translocation involving chromosomes 14 and 21 is shown in Figure 8.8. Those who carry a Robertsonian translocation involving chromosome 21 may be at significantly higher risk of having a child with Down syndrome as an unbalanced product of the translocation.

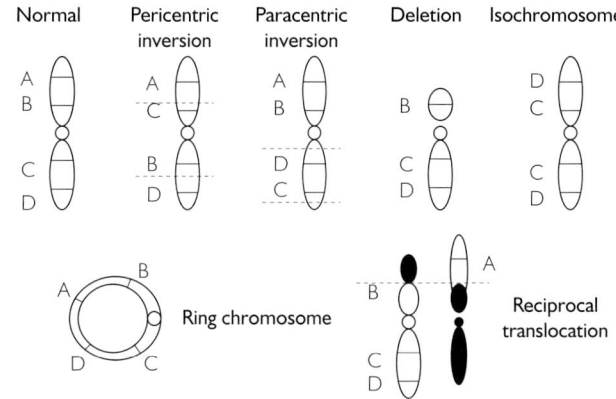

Fig. 8.7 Different types of chromosome anomaly. A–D represent notional chromosomal loci.

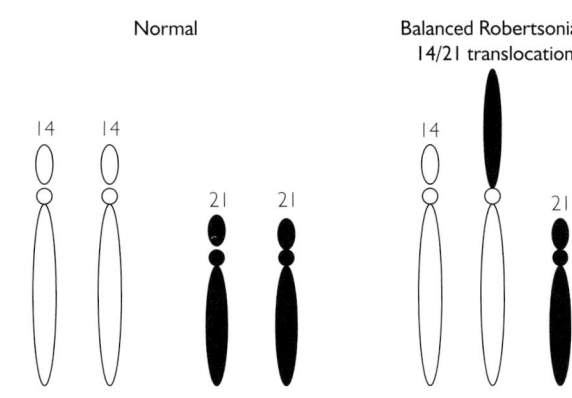

Normal | Balanced Robertsonian 14/21 translocation

Fig. 8.8 Robertsonian translocation.

The same applies to a lesser extent for those carrying a Robertsonian translocation involving chromosome 13, and a subsequent risk of a child with Patau syndrome.

The nomenclature for reporting a chromosome analysis is strict, and needs to be read carefully. A karyotype is reported initially as the number of chromosomes, regardless of whether or not those chromosomes are normal. The sex chromosomes are then described. If there is no further abnormality, the report is then complete. Any further abnormality is added after the sex chromosomes. A normal male karyotype is thus 46,XY. A male with non-dysjunctional Down syndrome will have the karyotype 47,XY,+21, an extra unattached chromosome 21. A male with Down syndrome due to a Robertsonian translocation between chromosomes 14 and 21 will have the karyotype 46,XY,t(14;21), and his carrier mother will have a karyotype 45,XX,t(14;21).

A standard laboratory chromosome analysis will be performed on G-banded chromosomes, which will detect many common and less common chromosome abnormalities, and in most cases no further laboratory work is required. However, recombinant DNA technology has allowed new techniques for chromosome analysis, based on the hybridisation of fluorescently labelled fragments of DNA to the DNA of chromosomes, prepared in a standard fashion, immobilised on a glass slide. The slides can then be visualised by eye using a fluorescent microscope, or indirectly by generating an image of the hybridisation on computer. This technique is known as *FISH*, *f*luorescent *in* s*itu* *h*ybridisation. The information that can be gained from this technique depends on the origin of the fragments of DNA hybridised to the chromosome preparation. Labelled whole chromosome 'paints', consisting of DNA exclusively from one chromosome, are now commercially available. For example, whole chromosome paints can be used to identify the origin of extra chromosomal material which cannot be identified using G-banding techniques. Whole chromosome paints are also helpful in determining the origin of subtle complex translocations. It is also now technically possible to use a chromosome 21 paint on uncultured cells in interphase, to look for trisomy 21. A cell would show three fluorescent nuclear dots, representing three chromosomes 21, as opposed to two in the normal situation.

Fluorescently labelled small DNA fragments, corresponding to 40–50 kb of DNA from a specific chromosomal region, can also be hybridised to metaphase chromosomes. Chromosomal deletions which cannot be detected within the resolution of conventional cytogenetic analysis can be detected by this FISH method. A normal karyotype will give two hybridisation signals, one from the same part of each chromosome. A karyotype containing a submicroscopic chromosomal deletion involving the segment of the chromosome corresponding to the 50 kb DNA fragment will only give one hybridisation signal. An example would be the submicroscopic deletion of chromosome 22q11 which occurs in most cases of the Di George spectrum (see Chapters 28 and 32), which can only be seen by FISH analysis. FISH diagnosis of submicroscopic chromosomal deletions is likely to become available for a variety of specific clinical syndromes.

Patterns of inheritance

Single gene disorders have one of three principal modes of inheritance: autosomal dominant (AD), autosomal recessive (AR) and X-linked recessive (XLR). Other rare forms of inheritance include X-linked dominant (XLD), and mitochondrial disorders, as well as disorders due to abnormalities of genetic imprinting. Disorders caused by inheritance of unstable elements of DNA are now increasingly being recognised (see below).

Autosomal dominant inheritance

AD disorders are characterised by vertical transmission from parent to child, and the hallmark of these conditions is male-to-male transmission of the disease (Fig. 8.9).

Those affected with an AD disorder have a fault in one or other copy of the two genes responsible for that condition. Each child of a person with an AD disorder has a 50:50 chance of inheriting the gene responsible for the condition from its parent. There are many examples of AD disorders, including neurofibromatosis 1 and 2, familial adenomatous polyposis coli, myotonic dystrophy and Huntington's disease. There can often be variability in both *expression* and *penetrance* of AD disorders. For example, neurofibromatosis 1, an AD condition, will almost always manifest in someone who has a neurofibromatosis 1 gene fault. This means that the condition has almost complete *penetrance*. However, different people can manifest the condition in different ways, some showing mild skin lesions and others with severe intracerebral complications. This means that the *expression* of the condition is very variable. In contrast, only 80% of those who have a single gene fault for the rare hereditary form of retinoblastoma will actually develop an eye tumour. The penetrance in this situation is 80%, but the expression of the gene fault is consistent, as manifested by a retinoblastoma.

AD disorders are not commonly seen in neonatal practice. A list of the more frequent conditions is outlined in Table 8.2.

Autosomal recessive inheritance

When a child is diagnosed with an AR disorder, then both copies of a particular gene responsible for the condition are faulty. Both his parents are therefore carriers for that condition, with one

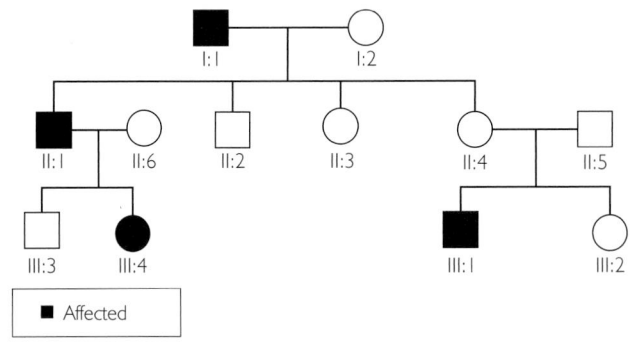

Fig. 8.9 Autosomal dominant inheritance. Note male-to-male transmission and non-penetrance in II:4.

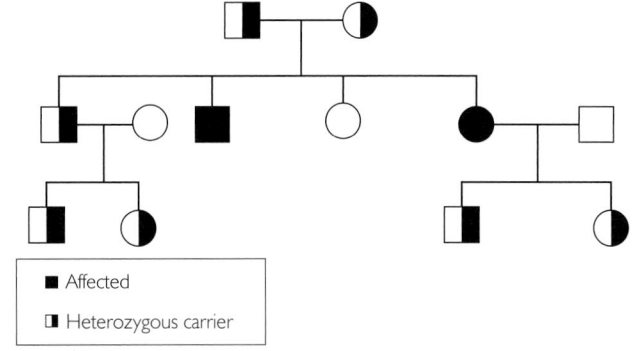

Fig. 8.10 Autosomal recessive inheritance.

Table 8.2 Autosomal dominant disorders in neonatal practice

System affected	Condition
Neurological	Congenital myotonic dystrophy Neurofibromatosis type 1
Ocular	Congenital cataract Retinoblastoma
Haematological	Spherocytosis
Skeletal	Stickler syndrome Craniosynostosis syndromes Achondroplasia Osteogenesis imperfecta
Other	Beckwith–Wiedemann syndrome Noonan syndrome

Table 8.3 Autosomal recessive disorders in neonatal practice

System affected	Condition
Neurological	Spinal muscular atrophy Congenital myopathies
Ocular	Congenital cataract Congenital glaucoma Albinism
Haematological	Thalassaemia Sickle cell anaemia
Skeletal	Short-rib polydactyly syndromes Jeune syndrome
Endocrine	Congenital adrenal hyperplasia
Metabolic	Cystic fibrosis Phenylketonuria Galactosaemia α_1-antitrypsin deficiency

normal and one faulty gene. Two of the child's four grandparents are also carriers, and it is likely that many of the child's relatives are also unknowingly carriers (Fig. 8.10). In most cases, being a carrier for an AR condition has no effect on that person. When both parents are carriers for a fault in the same gene, then there is a 25% chance of each of their children being affected by the condition. The risk of a healthy carrier sibling of having a child with the same condition depends on the chances of that sibling's partner also being a carrier. A child of a person with an AR disorder will automatically be a carrier. The child's chances of being affected will depend upon whether his unaffected parent is a carrier for a fault in the same gene.

AR disorders are commonly encountered in neonatal practice, and the nature of the disorder depends on the population being seen. Each regional population has its own recessive disorder, where the frequency of carriers for that disorder is highest. For instance, cystic fibrosis (CF) is a very common AR disorder in western Europe, whereas sickle cell anaemia is the commonest AR disorder in West Africa. Common examples of AR conditions include CF, sickle cell anaemia, several of the mucopolysaccharidoses, beta-thalassaemia, spinal muscular atrophy and congenital adrenal hyperplasia (Table 8.3). Prenatal diagnosis is available for many of these conditions.

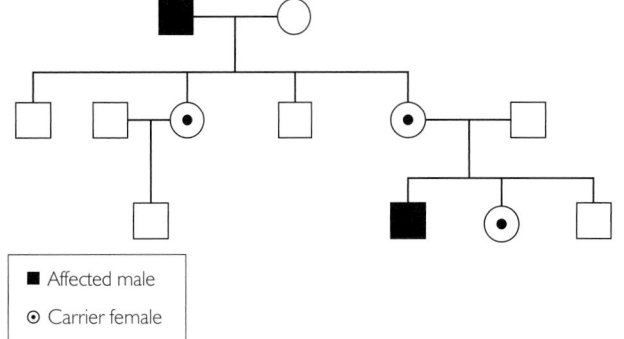

Fig. 8.11 X-linked recessive inheritance.

X-linked recessive inheritance

In XLR inheritance, the condition affects almost exclusively males; females can be carriers (Fig. 8.11). The classic examples of such conditions are haemophilia A and B, Duchenne's and Becker's muscular dystrophy, and Hunter syndrome.

The daughters of a man with an XLR condition are all obligate carriers. The sons of a man with an XLR condition are all normal, as they inherit his Y chromosome and not his X chromosome. When a woman is a carrier of an X-linked condition, each of her sons has a 50:50 chance of being affected and each of her daughters has a 50:50 chance of being a carrier. There can be a relatively high mutation rate for some XLR conditions, and affected boys may not have family history of the condition. About one-third of occurrences of Duchenne's muscular dystrophy are as a result of new mutations. Prenatal diagnosis is available for a wide range of XLR diseases. The more common X-linked disorders in neonatal practice are shown in Table 8.4.

Polygenic inheritance

Many congenital conditions do not have a clear mode of inheritance and can be classed as polygenic or oligogenic, where a disease may arise as a result of the effects of several genes. A good example is cleft lip and palate, which usually occurs in the absence of a family history. However, monozygotic twins have a high concordance for cleft palate, suggesting a genetic influence.

Other forms of inheritance

There are also much rarer forms of inheritance, including XLD, which can be hard to distinguish from AD, except that females will be more mildly affected and there is no male-to-male transmission. An example of an XLD condition is hypophosphataemic rickets.

Mitochondrially inherited diseases show a very unusual pattern of inheritance. Most of the proteins in the mitochondria are encoded for by nuclear genes, but the mitochondria also contain their own small genome of 18 kb, with many copies per cell. The mitochondrial genome replicates independently and far more frequently than the nuclear genome. Several important mitochondrial proteins are encoded by the mitochondrial genome. Mitochondria are only inherited via oocytes, and not sperm. Therefore, when a gene fault is in the mitochondrial genome it will pass exclusively down the female line, but both males and females can be affected. The children of an affected male will not inherit his mitochondrial gene fault. Children with mitochondrial disorders can present with many varied symptoms, including myoclonic seizures, acute acidoses, muscle weakness, deafness or diabetes. A number of mutations or deletions in the mitochondrial genome have been described in patients with a wide variety of conditions, including MELAS (myoclonic epilepsy with lactic acidosis and stroke-like episodes) and MERRF (myoclonic epilepsy with ragged red fibres on muscle biopsy). To complicate matters further, Leber's hereditary ophthalmopathy is a mitochondrially inherited condition with a characteristic mitochondrial mutation, but the expression appears to have an XLR influence.

Some conditions show a phenomenon known as genetic imprinting. An imprinted gene has been marked during meiosis, to indicate the parent from whom it comes. For some genes it appears to be important not only to inherit two copies of that gene, but also to inherit one from each parent. Some genes may be silenced, depending upon which parent has passed on that gene. A good example is the presence of a small deletion of chromosome 15q, which has a different effect depending upon which chromosome 15 is deleted. If the deletion occurs on the chromosome inherited from a child's normal father, the child will develop Prader–Willi syndrome. If the deletion occurs on the chromosome inherited from a child's normal mother, the child will develop a completely different clinical condition, Angelman syndrome. The genes in this area of chromosome 15 are therefore imprinted. In addition, if a child has two maternal copies of chromosome 15 (maternal disomy), but no paternal copy, he or she will also develop Prader–Willi syndrome. Other conditions that show imprinting effects include Russell–Silver syndrome, Beckwith–Wiedemann syndrome, and the rare condition of transient neonatal diabetes mellitus.

A new molecular mechanism for genetic disease has been described, that of inherited unstable triplet repeat expansions. At least nine different conditions are caused by this phenomenon. In one of these conditions, a normal person has a stable number of a repetitive element of three bases of DNA (for example, 20 copies of a CAG repeat) in a particular gene, that gene functions normally, and the children of that person have the same number of repeats in their gene. An affected person has an increased number of repeats (say 100 copies) in that gene, and the affected children of that person have more serious disease, with perhaps 200 repeats in the gene. The molecular genetic findings appear to be the genetic correlate of the phenomenon of anticipation, where a condition appears to worsen from generation to generation. The most extreme example is that of congenital myotonic dystrophy, where a minimally affected mother can have a profoundly affected infant. In this case, there is a small repeat expansion of, say, 150 repeats in the mother, increasing to many hundreds of repeats in her affected infant.

This molecular mechanism is responsible for fragile X syndrome, Huntington's disease, Friedreich's ataxia, several forms of spinocerebellar ataxia, and probably several more conditions.

Table 8.4 X-linked recessive disorders in neonatal practice

System affected	Condition
Neurological	Hunter syndrome
Ocular	Lowe syndrome
	Ocular albinism
Haematological	Glucose-6-phosphate dehydrogenase deficiency
	Haemophilia
Skeletal	Amelogenesis imperfecta
Endocrine	Androgen insensitivity syndrome
Metabolic	Adrenoleukodystrophy
	Fabry's disease
	Lesch–Nyhan syndrome
	Steroid sulphatase deficiency

Molecular genetic analysis for single gene disorders

Laboratory tests for single gene disorders have been available for a considerable time. Haemoglobin electrophoresis for sickle cell anaemia and thalassaemia, and enzyme assays for Tay–Sachs disease, are very effective in resolving clinical issues in individual families. However, an increasing number of specific DNA-based tests can now be used in the diagnosis and prediction of single gene disorders.

The two major techniques used in molecular genetic analysis are the polymerase chain reaction (PCR) and Southern blotting. PCR is a technique which allows amplification of a specific genetic region in large quantities from a small amount of DNA template (Fig. 8.12). The DNA sequence of the region to be amplified must be known, so that synthetic pieces of single-stranded DNA (oligonucleotide primers) corresponding to the region can be designed and manufactured. The oligonucleotide primers are added in great excess to the DNA template, along with a thermostable DNA polymerase, and free nucleotides (A, C, T, G). The mixture is heated up to cause the two strands of template DNA to separate, and then cooled. As the DNA cools, the oligonucleotides bind to the template sequence and are extended by the polymerase. A new copy of the template DNA is thus produced. The cycle is repeated 30–40 times, with an exponential increase in the amount of the target sequence.

DNA generated by PCR can be used in many different ways to detect an abnormality in the sequence. There are numerous techniques which are used to screen PCR products for mutations, such as single-stranded conformational assay, or denaturing gradient gel electrophoresis. In some cases, the complete sequence of the PCR product can be directly determined. Specific PCR assays for mutations have been developed, such as the ARMS test (amplification-resistant mutation system), or the use of a specific DNA restriction enzyme which recognises a known mutant DNA sequence.

Southern blotting is a more protracted procedure involving the digestion of a relatively large amount of DNA by a restriction enzyme. The digested DNA is then electrophoresed through an agarose gel, giving a smear of DNA of different sizes. The DNA is then transferred (blotted) and fixed to a membrane. The fixed DNA is then hybridised to a labelled DNA probe specific for the gene to be analysed, and the specific sizes of DNA to which the probe binds allows determination of the 'genotype' (Fig. 8.13). This test is often superseded by PCR technology.

There are different degrees to which molecular genetic tests can contribute to clinical diagnosis. Some specific molecular genetic tests can be used to detect a known pathogenic DNA mutation and give a diagnosis, even without any knowledge of the patient's clinical status. For instance, the PCR detection of the ΔF508 deletion in both copies of a person's cystic fibrosis (*CFTR*) gene immediately gives a diagnosis of CF. Such direct mutation tests are possible where both the gene responsible for a condition has been isolated and specific pathogenic mutations have been identified. Similarly, a PCR test detects a deletion of exons 7 and 8 in both alleles of a gene called *SMN* on chromosome 5q in almost all children with spinal muscular atrophy. Southern blot analysis of DNA from infants with congenital myotonic dystrophy shows a very large expansion in a triplet repeat DNA sequence in the myotonin kinase gene on chromosome 19, as described earlier.

In other cases, molecular genetic diagnosis can point towards a diagnosis without confirming it. For instance, the presence of a single ΔF508 *CFTR* gene mutation in a child with a history suggestive of CF increases the likelihood of that child being affected.

In some cases, where either a gene is not known or very few gene mutations have been identified in a known gene, gene tracking studies can be performed in a family to predict whether a person in that family is affected. This is known as linkage analysis. Such a study requires careful clinical examination of several family members, to establish whether they are affected or unaffected. When their clinical status is clear, DNA samples are then obtained.

Gene tracking analysis in the family uses the property of normal variations in a gene between different people. Some genetic areas show wide variation between individuals, and a DNA marker from such an area, which can detect many variations, is described as being polymorphic. Each variant of a polymorphic marker is known as an allele. There are now thousands of

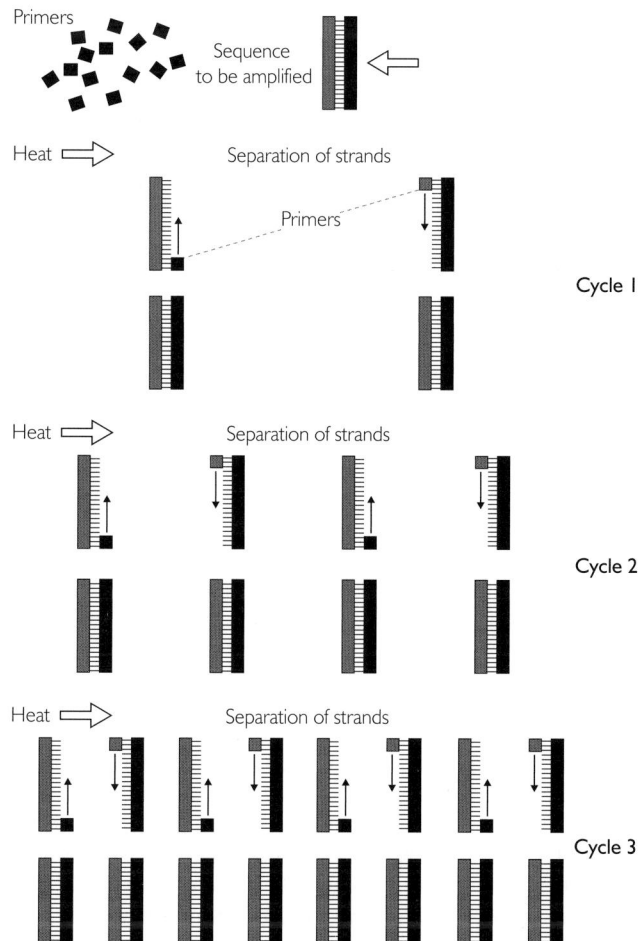

Fig. 8.12 Polymerase chain reaction (PCR).

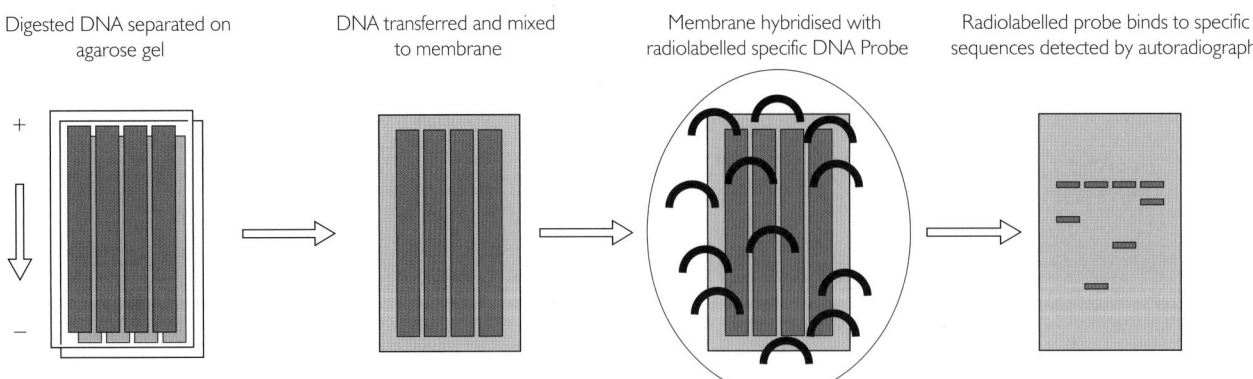

Digested DNA separated on agarose gel | DNA transferred and mixed to membrane | Membrane hybridised with radiolabelled specific DNA Probe | Radiolabelled probe binds to specific sequences detected by autoradiography

Fig. 8.13 Southern blotting and hybridisation.

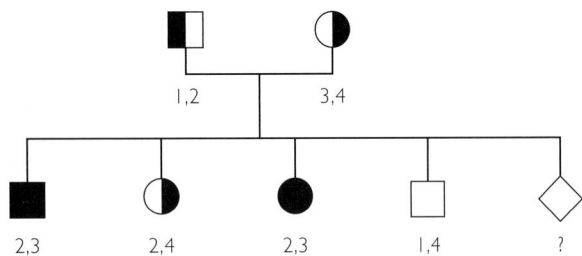

Fig. 8.14 Linkage analysis in an autosomal recessive disorder, using an intragenic polymorphic marker. Alleles 2 and 3 are associated with a gene mutation and can be used to predict the status of another sibling.

polymorphic markers covering most of the human genome, and such markers can be found very close to most known genes. There are several types of polymorphic DNA markers, including those characterised by different numbers of specific DNA-cutting enzymes recognition sites, or restriction fragment length polymorphisms. Other markers detect the variation in number of anonymous elements of repetitive DNA, and are called microsatellites or minisatellites.

If the two alleles of a polymorphic marker can be distinguished, to discriminate between the two copies of that particular chromosome from where the marker comes, then the marker is informative in that individual. Where a gene location is known, but the actual gene has yet to be found, the alleles of informative markers lying either side of the gene will be inherited along with each copy of the gene in question. This can be used to predict a child's clinical status.

If one set of alleles is found in the affected members of the family but not in the unaffected, then the presence or absence of these alleles in the at-risk individual can be used to predict their chances of being affected. An example of linkage analysis for an AR disorder is shown in Figure 8.14. This form of linkage analysis is often used in families with XLR conditions such as Duchenne's muscular dystrophy, to predict whether a woman is a carrier. Such linkage analysis can also be used in prenatal diagnosis.

Because of its nature, linkage analysis is more prone to error than is direct mutation testing. This can be due to difficulties in assessing a person's clinical status, and because of the possibility of recombination between the polymorphic markers. However, with the rapid advances in molecular genetics, many more mutations are being found in many different genes, and linkage analysis is often superseded by direct mutation testing.

A newer development is the ability to immobilise several thousand distinct pieces of DNA on small bits of silicone or glass as ordered microarrays, colloquially known as DNA microchips. This technology can permit thousands of individual DNA analyses very rapidly, and has many potential applications in genetic analysis for inherited disease, and in molecular genetic characterisation of cancers. However, the use of DNA microchips has yet to be applied on a routine basis in genetic diagnosis. There are many other new molecular genetic tests being developed, and it is impossible to cover all such tests in the space available, but it is clear that new genetic tests will alter the clinical management of many infantile conditions.

Further reading

Connor J M, Ferguson-Smith M A 1997 Essential medical genetics. 5th edn. Blackwell Science, Oxford

Lewin B 1994 Genes V. Oxford University Press, Oxford

Online Mendelian Inheritance in Man. A list of genetic disorders and the latest genetic developments for each condition. Website http://www3.ncbi.nlm.nih.gov:80/

Strachan T, Read A P 1996 Human molecular genetics. Bios, Oxford

Watson J D, Hopkins N H, Roberts J W, Steitz J A, Weiner A M 1993 Molecular biology of the gene. 5th edn. Benjamin Cummings, Menlo Park, California

Glossary

3′ distal end of a gene, as indicated by the bond at the third hydroxyl group of the deoxyribose sugar

5′ proximal end of a gene, as indicated by the bond at the fifth hydroxyl group of the deoxyribose sugar

acrocentric a chromosome with effectively only a long arm – chromosomes 13, 14, 15, 21 and 22

allele a genetic variation of a gene or DNA marker

aneuploidy an excess or deficiency of chromosomal material

anticodon an element of transfer RNA which binds a specific amino acid

autosomal dominant inheritance pattern characterised by transmission through several generations, male-to-male transmission, and a 50:50 risk to the children of an affected person

autosomal recessive inheritance pattern characterised by several affected members of the same generation, with carrier parents and a 1:4 recurrence risk where both parents are carriers

base pair unit of double-stranded DNA

centromere element of chromosome involved in chromosome replication, found as a constriction in the chromosome

chromatid condensed chromosome found just before mitosis

codon 3 bp element of DNA encoding an amino acid

diploid a complement of two copies of each chromosome per cell

DNA marker a piece of DNA corresponding to a specific gene or chromosomal segment

enhancers elements of DNA which are involved in increasing gene transcription

exon a part of a gene which is transcribed into mRNA

expression the way in which a gene fault manifests clinically

FISH fluorescent in-situ hybridisation, a powerful technique for studying specific chromosomes or regions of chromosomes

gamete a germ cell – sperm or oocyte

genetic imprinting the marking of a gene according to which parent has passed that gene to the child

haploid a complement of one copy of each chromosome per cell (as in sperm or oocyte)

haplotype a pattern of alleles of DNA markers representing one of the two copies of a chromosomal region

histone a DNA-binding protein important in chromosomal folding

interphase phase of mitosis in which the chromosomes are very elongated

intron the part of a gene between the exons which is not transcribed into mRNA

isochromosome an abnormal chromosome made up of two long or two short arms of a normal chromosome

karyotype an analysis of the chromosome complement of a cell type

linkage analysis the use of polymorphic DNA markers to perform gene tracking studies within a family

meiosis the process of cell division to give haploid germ cells

metaphase phase of mitosis in which the chromosomes are very condensed and easier to analyse

microsatellite marker a DNA marker which detects variation in number of an anonymous small repetitive element of DNA

minisatellite marker a DNA marker which detects variation in number of an anonymous medium repetitive element of DNA

mitosis the normal process of cell division to give two diploid copies of a cell

non-dysjunction a failure of meiosis, giving two copies of a chromosome in one gamete and no copy of a chromosome in the other gamete

nucleosome the combination of a histone and its bound DNA

oligonucleotide primers small lengths of synthetic single-stranded DNA of a specific sequence

paracentric inversion a rearrangement of chromosomal material within one arm of a chromosome

PCR polymerase chain reaction: a method of generating large amounts of specific DNA from a small amount of target sequence

penetrance the number of people known to carry a gene mutation who manifest the condition

pericentric inversion a rearrangement of chromosomal material around the centromere of a chromosome

promoter element of a gene which is necessary to activate gene transcription

prophase phase of the cell cycle where condensation of the chromosomes occurs, just before metaphase

reciprocal translocation exchange of chromosomal segments between different chromosomes

restriction enzyme an enzyme which cuts double-stranded DNA at a specific unique short DNA sequence

restriction fragment length polymorphism a genetic variation between two copies of the same gene, where one gene may have one copy of a restriction enzyme recognition site, and the other two. This variation can be detected using PCR or Southern blotting

ribosome area of the cell where mRNA is converted into protein

ring chromosome an abnormal chromosome where the tips of the long and short arms have fused

Robertsonian translocation a fusion of two acrocentric chromosomes

Southern blotting a process of immobilising DNA to nylon membrane for genetic analysis

suppressor a DNA element which reduces the expression of a gene

telomere the end of a chromosome

telophase the last phase of mitosis

transcription the process of converting DNA into mRNA

translation the production of protein from a DNA sequence

triploidy three of each chromosome, i.e. 69 chromosomes in man

trisomy one extra chromosome, i.e. 47 chromosomes in man

X-linked recessive inheritance characterized by affected males in several generations, and by female carriers

CHAPTER 9

Antenatal diagnosis and fetal medicine

Mark Denbow, Phillipa Kyle

Introduction

Advances continue to be made in the field of prenatal diagnosis and fetal medicine. Improved ultrasound imaging has enhanced the detection of fetal anomaly, and the use of other modalities, such as magnetic resonance imaging (MRI), has allowed further detailed assessment, especially of the central nervous system (CNS).

The drive for early detection of pregnancies at increased risk of aneuploidy continues, with first-trimester combined biochemical and ultrasound assessment now as established practice. Molecular technologies continue to be refined, with the most notable advance being the accurate identification of free fetal deoxyribonucleic acid (DNA) in the maternal circulation, to allow non-invasive determination of fetal Rhesus (Rh) status.

The shift away from invasive procedures to assess fetal well-being continues. Fetal anaemia now is recognised by alterations in middle cerebral artery (MCA) blood flow velocity, and analysis of both the arterial and venous sides of the circulation allows improved accuracy of optimal timing of delivery in cases of fetal growth restriction.

The complications of monochorionic twin pregnancies contribute significantly to the workload of a modern fetal medicine unit. The dilemmas in management in cases of discordant fetal anomaly, and the transfusional complications, including twin-to-twin transfusion syndrome (TTTS), have led to the development of several techniques that enable the relatively safe occlusion of interfetal blood flow.

Fetal surgery continues to be developed. Most units have shifted their emphasis away from open techniques, where maternal complications are common, to endoscopic procedures, with most attention directed towards the repair of neural tube defects (NTDs) and congenital diaphragmatic herniae.

Fetal physiology

Our understanding of fetal physiology has for years been based on indirect sources. Observations in preterm neonates were first assumed to apply to the fetus of comparable gestation, and then extrapolated back to the mid trimester. Non-invasive techniques such as cardiotocography, ultrasound and Doppler have provided information on fetal circulation, growth and behaviour. Amniotic fluid, being largely dependent on fetal urination, has been the traditional source for information about fetal biochemistry and endocrinology.[95] Access to the fetal circulation in the 1980s allowed fetal haematology and biochemistry to be evaluated directly in utero. Knowledge of normal values in the mid-trimester fetus is essential in the prenatal diagnosis of several fetal diseases and forms the basis for more effective treatment of maternal alloimmunisation and better management of growth retardation, and is a prerequisite for other diagnostic and therapeutic approaches in the fetus. The main topics of clinical interest are summarised below, although more detailed listings are available elsewhere.[358]

Haematology

Haemoglobin (Hb), packed cell volume (PCV) and red cell mass increase, while mean corpuscular volume (MCV), reticulocytes and nucleated red blood cells (RBCs) decrease significantly with gestation,[151,263] reflecting the increase in fetal haemopoietic tissue, and the progressive change from hepatic to myeloid erythropoiesis. The normal range for Hb increases from 9–13 g/dl at 17 weeks to 13–18 g/dl at term,[293] and haematocrit from 29–42% at 18 weeks to 35–48% at 30 weeks.[151] The myeloid series does not change with gestation, nor do platelets, which normally exceed $150 \times 10^9/l$. Normal ranges are available for coagulation factors, which are reduced compared with the adult.[260]

Acid–base balance

In normal pregnancies, pH changes with gestational age, and ranges in the umbilical vein from 7.32 to 7.44. On the other hand, PO_2 decreases with gestational age, whereas PCO_2 and bicarbonate rise. The decrease in fetal PO_2 is compensated for by the rise in fetal haemoglobin, so that total oxygen content remains unchanged at 6–7 mmol/l. Normal ranges have been established for both umbilical venous and arterial samples (Fig. 9.1).[296]

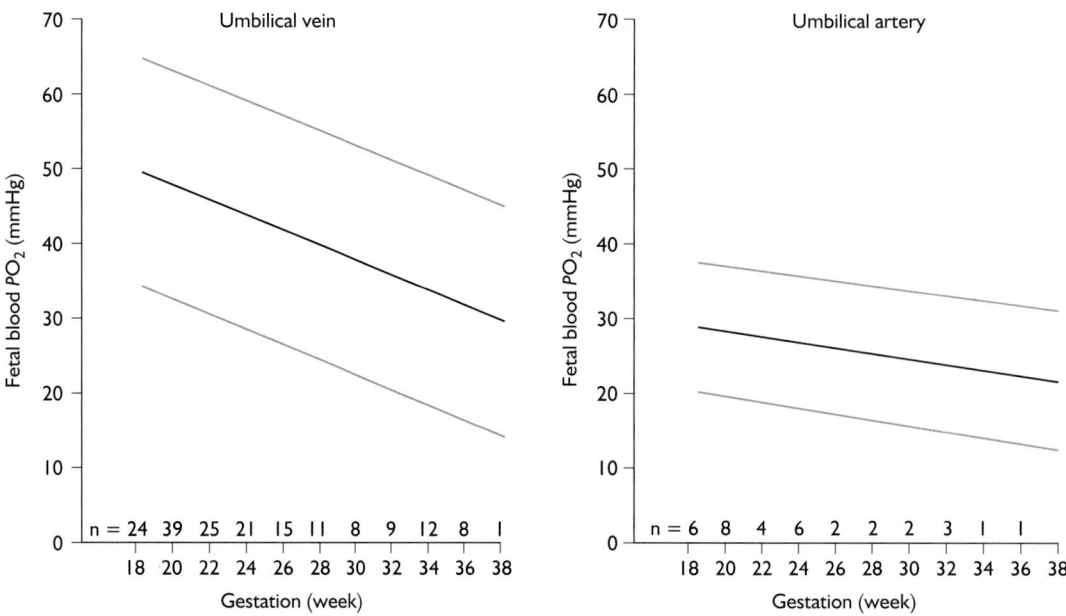

Fig. 9.1 Reference range (mean and 95% data intervals) for PO_2 in umbilical venous and arterial blood throughout gestation. (Reproduced from Nicolaides et al.[296])

Cardiovascular physiology

Mean umbilical venous pressure is 4–5 mmHg between 20 and 33 weeks' gestation.[314] Blood volume has been measured in vivo, on the basis of the change in fetal haematocrit produced by transfusion of a known quantity of red cells. Fetoplacental blood volume rises from 25 ml at 18 weeks to 150 ml at 31 weeks, but during the same interval it decreases when expressed as a function of fetal weight from 117 to 93 ml/kg.[294]

Biochemistry

Reference ranges are available for electrolytes and biochemical indices of renal, hepatic and bone function.[152,267] Fetal sodium and potassium are the same as maternal levels. Fetal glucose levels are lower than in the mother, and their maternofetal gradients have been used as an index of placental transfer.[305] Bilirubin is three times higher in the mid-trimester fetus than in the mother, but albumin levels are considerably lower, with values rising from 16 g/l at 15 weeks to 40 g/l at term.[267]

Renal function

Urea and creatinine levels in utero reflect the excretory function of the placenta and not that of the kidneys. Urinary sodium and phosphate decrease and creatinine increases with gestational age, consistent with progressive maturation of tubular function and an increase in glomerular filtration rate. Potassium and urea, however, do not change, suggesting that the changes in tubular reabsorption occur simultaneously with those in tubular secretion and glomerular filtration. Reference ranges related to gestation are used in the assessment of renal function in fetuses with obstructive uropathies.[303]

Fetal pain

This is a complex area but is of importance with the increasing number of in-utero (and often in-feto) interventions being developed in the field of fetal medicine/surgery. It is clear that the fetus mounts a stress response to painful stimuli from 18 weeks[163,164,402,403] but whether this is perceived as pain is uncertain. Neurons first link the cortex with the rest of the brain at 16 weeks, and their activation might be associated with an unpleasant experience, if not pain itself. By 26 weeks, the system for nociception is present and functioning[224] and it seems likely that the fetus can feel pain from this stage. This evidence leads to the consideration of fetal analgesia for invasive procedures during the second and third trimesters. However, the challenge remains selecting the safest and most effective type and route of analgesic drug without increasing maternal or fetal risks.

Antenatal diagnosis

Ultrasound

Ultrasound is the chief method for detecting structural abnormalities. Since the first report of detection of a fetal anomaly leading to termination of pregnancy,[62] a wide range of major malformations have been detected. With advances in ultrasound imaging, the appearances of an increasing number of minor malformations have now been described, including subtle markers of chromosome abnormalities.

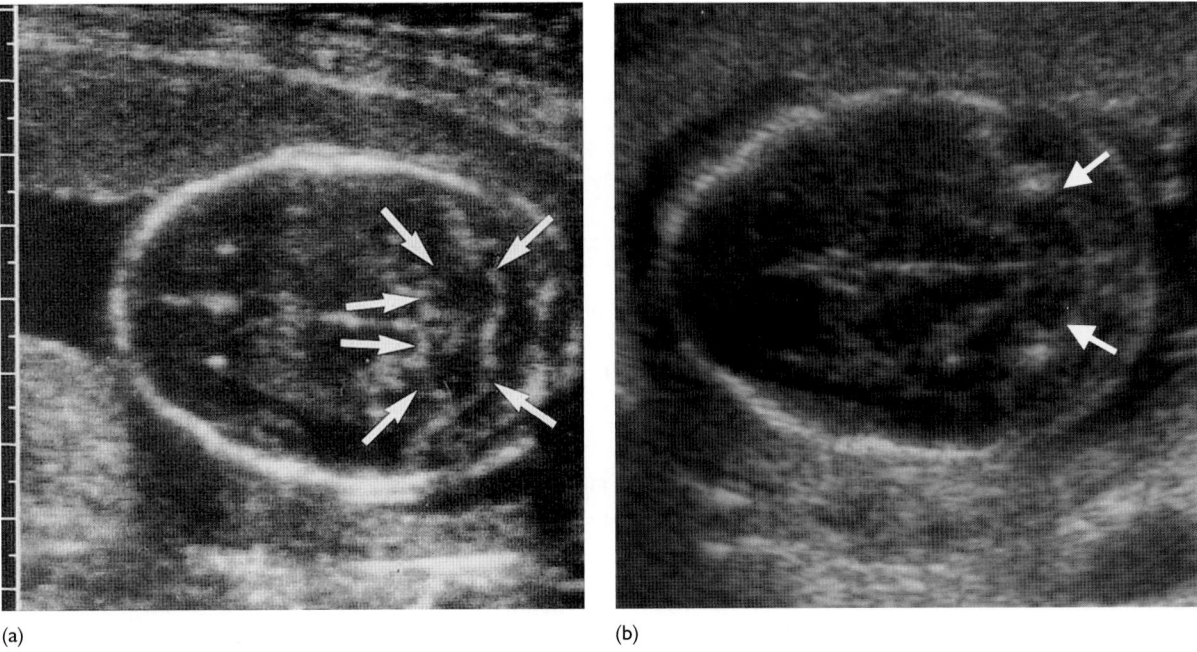

(a)   (b)

Fig. 9.2 (a) The normal dumbbell shape of the cerebellum (arrows) on ultrasound at 18 weeks. (b) Anterior curvature of the cerebellum, the 'banana' sign (arrows) in a fetus of similar gestation with open spina bifida.

The standard of ultrasound achieved in practice has continued to improve dramatically and is available to an increasing proportion of the population. The assignation of 'levels' to various standards of ultrasound was previously used to indicate whether fetal anatomy was examined (level II and beyond), but has fallen into disuse now that visualisation of common fetal structures is within the scope of all those performing obstetric scans.[134]

Routine ultrasound screening is recommended in the UK.[366] This examination is delayed until 18–20 weeks, when cardiac and renal structure becomes discernible. Routine screening detects 60–80% of major and 35% of minor congenital malformations,[78,236,242] in contrast to the 25% detected[193] under the indication-based system favoured in the USA.[280]

Only the main areas of ultrasound diagnoses are summarised below; exhaustive listings are available elsewhere.[364,432]

Neural tube defects

The initial approach to screening for NTDs comprised maternal serum alpha-fetoprotein (AFP) estimation at 16 weeks, with investigation of positive results by amniocentesis for amniotic fluid AFP and acetylcholinesterase. However, only 88% of fetuses with anencephaly, and 79% with myelomeningocoele[411] were so identified. The next advance was to introduce ultrasound at the time of blood collection. The reasons were, first, to exclude twins and death in utero, which raise AFP, and second, the accuracy of AFP screening is increased when dating is based on biparietal diameter[419] although this may be smaller in myelomeningocoele.

The diagnosis of anencephaly is straightforward: the cranial vault cannot be visualised in the standard view for biparietal diameter measurement. Detection of open myelomeningocoele is more complex. Although larger defects may be suggested by gross disruption in vertebral integrity in the longitudinal plane or by soft tissue signs, smaller defects will only be apparent in the horizontal planes of a few localised vertebrae, as subtle splaying in the lateral processes. These views can be difficult, especially if the fetal spine lies against the uterine wall, and in this context screening has been greatly facilitated by two cranial signs found in almost all fetuses with myelomeningocoele. Scalloping of the frontal bones gives the head a lemon-shaped appearance ('lemon' sign), whereas the normally dumbbell-shaped cerebellum appears either absent or banana shaped ('banana' sign, Fig. 9.2).[158,292,335] The latter results from downward herniation of posterior fossa contents, and the former from the subsequent reduction in intracranial volume.

Ultrasound screening using the lemon and banana signs should theoretically detect 96–100% of myelomeningocoele.[61,412] It is important to recognise that ultrasound is both a screening and a diagnostic test, and that small spinal lesions in fetuses with suspicious cranial signs on screening may only be detected on detailed scanning by a very experienced operator. Most centres have dispensed with AFP screening for NTDs, although others have retained it either as a cautious 'belt and braces' approach or as a component of Down syndrome serum screening. With few exceptions, myelomeningocoele is now essentially an ultrasonic diagnosis, although the accuracy of AFP versus ultrasound has not been addressed in comparative trials. In cases of genuine uncertainty, an elevated amniotic fluid concentration of acetylcholinesterase may also be measured to confirm the presence of an NTD.[240]

Other craniospinal malformations

Ventriculomegaly is diagnosed in utero by elevated ratios of various measurements of the lateral ventricle to hemispheric width in the transverse plane[63,146] or enlargement of the atrium of posterior horn of the lateral ventricle.[65] Unless there is progressive or gross dilatation, caution should be exercised in the interpretation of mild ventriculomegaly, especially in the mid trimester. The level of obstruction is determined by examining the third and fourth ventricles and the aqueduct of Sylvius. Hydranencephaly is distinguished from severe hydrocephalus by the absence of midline structures and the lack of a residual cortical rim, but the distinction may be difficult in extreme cases. In holoprosencephaly, the extent of midline ventricular fusion varies with the degree of failure of cleavage of the prosencephalon,[336] and there are often concomitant facial anomalies. The diagnosis of microcephaly should only be made in the presence of serial measurements of head circumference 3–4 standard deviations (SD) below the mean, so as to exclude growth retardation or incorrect dating. The ultrasonic appearances of encephalocoele, and intracranial cysts, tumours and haemorrhage are well described. Agenesis of the corpus callosum, increasingly recognised as separation of the lateral ventricles with upward displacement of the third ventricle, is more difficult to diagnose, and is often detected in association with other CNS abnormalities.[369]

The diagnosis of posterior fossa abnormalities, and most notably the Dandy–Walker malformation, is challenging. The classic appearance is of complete or partial agenesis of the cerebellar vermis with a posterior fossa cyst. However, in one series from a tertiary unit in the UK, the correlation with postmortem was only 43% (6/14) for this abnormality.[68] This has led to evaluation of fetal MRI for complex neurological abnormalities (see below).

Cardiac defects

Following characterisation of the normal ultrasonic appearances of the fetal heart, a wide range of defects have been diagnosed. Inspection of the four-chamber view in a transverse plane during the routine 18-week scan detects approximately 20–40% of severe congenital heart disease.[133,379] This view is abnormal with major defects such as hypoplastic ventricles, atrioventricular canal defects and tricuspid atresia, although minor lesions such as septal defects may be missed. Visualisation of venoatrial and ventriculoarterial connections is more complex, but if it were introduced into routine screening it would theoretically increase the detection rate to greater than 80%.[395] Some cases are missed because of the evolution of the abnormality such that the heart may appear to be normal at the time of screening.

Indications for fetal echocardiography include an abnormal four-chamber view, an affected sibling or parental history, diabetes, exposure to cardiac teratogens, raised nuchal translucency (NT) measurement in an euploid fetus, and monochorionic twin gestations. A high degree of accuracy can then be achieved for diagnosis of major vessel lesions such as pulmonary stenosis, truncus arteriosus, and transposition of the great vessels.[97] Colour flow Doppler facilitates the demonstration of cardiac structure, and M-mode and pulsed wave Doppler provide an index of cardiac function, which is particularly useful in arrhythmias.

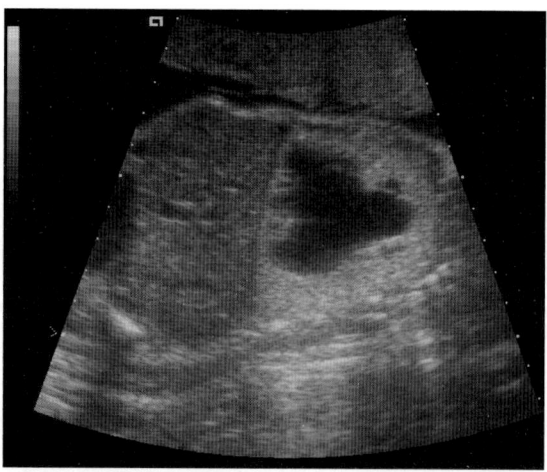

Fig. 9.3 Congenital cystic adenomatous malformation (CCAM) of the lung. A longitudinal view of a large macrocystic CCAM.

Intrathoracic defects (for neonatal surgical management, see Chapter 31)

Most intrathoracic lesions identified prenatally are benign, but their significance is the association with pulmonary hypoplasia. Indirect indices of the severity of compression on the developing lung are the degree of mediastinal shift, the presence of polyhydramnios due to limited swallowing, and hydrops secondary to obstructed venous return. Left-sided diaphragmatic hernias are detected on ultrasound because of displacement of the heart to the right, fluid-filled bowel within the chest, and absence of the stomach intra-abdominally.[75,277] As herniated liver has the same echotexture as the lung, right-sided lesions are more difficult to detect, especially in the absence of polyhydramnios or pleural effusion. Clues include derangement in the normal intra-abdominal course of the gallbladder and intrahepatic vein, although small lesions may go undetected. The appearances of congenital cystic adenomatoid malformation (CCAM) of the lung vary from solitary large cysts to solid echogenic lesions with the worst prognosis (Fig. 9.3).[6,394] The assessment of prognosis is difficult, although in more recent series it appears good, other than in a small minority (6%) in which both mediastinal shift and hydrops are present.[18,360] Some disappear, many get smaller, and only a few stay the same or progress. Diagnosis cannot always be certain antenatally, and differentiation between CCAM, sequestrated lung, tracheal or bronchial atresia, and congenital diaphragmatic hernia may be difficult.[218,243] Mediastinal teratomas have features on ultrasound similar to solid type III or microcystic CCAM lesions.[361]

Gastrointestinal defects (for neonatal surgical management, see Chapter 29)

Oesophageal atresia can be diagnosed when polyhydramnios occurs with non-visualisation of the fetal stomach, although these signs may not be present in the common form associated with tracheo-oesophageal fistula.[131] Duodenal atresia produces polyhydramnios and a characteristic 'double-bubble' appearance (Fig. 9.4), which may not be apparent until the third trimester.[284] Associated anomalies are common in the above two conditions, unlike in

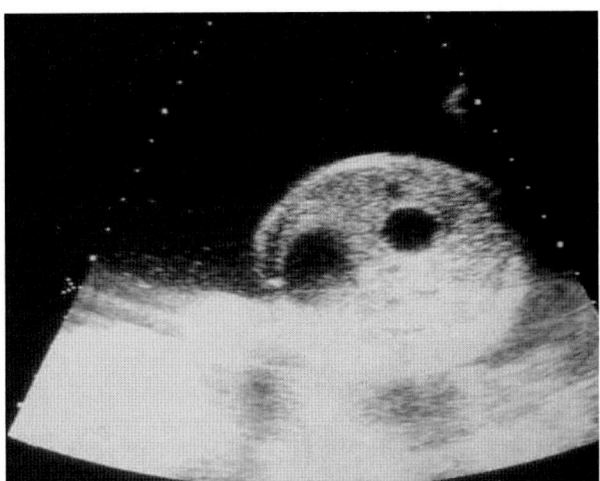

Fig. 9.4 The 'double-bubble' appearance of duodenal atresia.

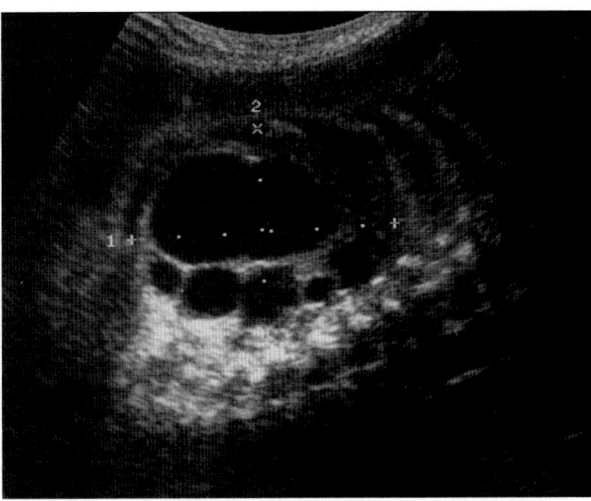

Fig. 9.5 Multicystic kidney disease.

more distal obstructions. Small-bowel obstructions are more likely to be associated with increased amniotic fluid volume than are large-bowel obstructions such as anal atresia, which may go undetected in utero. Peristalsis may be seen[14] and bowel perforations may show up as ascites or, more commonly, hyperechogenicity from meconium peritonitis.[40] Caution must be exercised when gut echogenicity is detected as an isolated finding, as although this may be associated with cystic fibrosis (CF)[274] and aneuploidy, the majority occur in normal fetuses.[130] Meconium peritonitis can also produce pseudocysts, the differential diagnosis of which includes gastrointestinal duplications and choledochal, mesenteric and ovarian cysts.

The distinction of exomphalos from gastroschisis is crucial, given the high incidence of cardiac and chromosomal abnormalities in the former.[165] Exomphalos is characterised on ultrasound by its intimate relation to the umbilical vessels and its covering of omphaloperitoneal membrane. Aneuploidy seems largely confined to fetuses in which the herniated liver is not present within the exomphalos.[28,317] More severe degrees of failure of fusion of the ectomesodermic folds, such as ectopia cordis, ectopia vesicae, pentalogy of Cantrell and the body stalk anomaly, are readily apparent. The incidence of gastroschisis is increasing in the UK, although the underlying reasons have not been determined.[330,398]

Genitourinary defects (for neonatal diagnosis and management, see Chapter 36)

Renal and urinary tract abnormalities are common and comparatively easy to detect, largely because obstructive lesions manifest as cystic spaces, whereas those with poor urine output are characterised by oligohydramnios. Major anomalies such as renal agenesis or low obstructive uropathy will be detected on routine scan at 18–20 weeks, when urine output makes a major contribution to amniotic fluid volume, whereas more minor lesions, such as mild ureteropelvic junction obstruction, may not be obvious until later. As the lack of amniotic fluid in renal agenesis significantly impairs the ultrasound picture, it can be extremely difficult to demonstrate the absence of kidneys in the renal fossae. In these circumstances, referral for confirmation by transvaginal

ultrasound and/or amnioinfusion has been recommended.[143] However, colour flow Doppler imaging of the renal arteries may be adequate to provide the diagnosis: the absence of renal artery colour image confirms no functioning tissue.[378]

Multicystic kidneys are distinguished from hydronephrotic kidneys by their cystic spaces being more peripheral and variable in size, and their stroma more central (Fig. 9.5).[31] The cysts of infantile polycystic kidneys are too small to be resolved by ultrasound, but the kidneys appear enlarged with abnormal echogenicity, associated with oligohydramnios. Occasionally with later-onset infantile polycystic kidney disease the kidneys may appear normal in utero.[362]

The significance of mild pelvicalyceal dilatation remains controversial. Studies show that progressive enlargement, or an anteroposterior diameter of ≥10 mm in the third trimester, is more likely to be associated with pathology.[324] The ultrasound picture in low obstructive uropathy depends on the severity and duration of obstruction. The bladder is variably enlarged and thick walled, and careful scanning reveals dilatation of the upper urethra in those with posterior urethral valves (PUV).[196] Oligohydramnios, upper tract dilatation and hyperechogenic fetal kidneys may also be present.

Skeletal defects (for neonatal diagnosis and management, see Chapter 38)

Isolated malformations detected on routine scanning include kyphoscoliosis, hemivertebrae, limb reduction and shortening, sacral agenesis, polydactyly and flexion deformities. Over 100 distinct skeletal dysplasias are amenable to prenatal diagnosis, both by serial measurement of long bones and by detection of abnormal skeletal shape or mineralisation. Although severe limb shortening, abnormal head or chest shape, or polyhydramnios may alert the sonologist to their presence, determination of the exact type of skeletal dysplasia is difficult in the absence of a previous history, and requires detailed evaluation of hands and feet, thoracic dimensions, face and cranium, and measurement of all the long bones, before consulting comprehensive tables of diagnostic features.[364] Even then, diagnosis may only be made postnatally, when additional investigations such as skeletal X-ray are available. In achondrogenesis, thanatophoric and diastrophic dwarfism, severe limb reduction will be obvious by 18 weeks,[135] whereas in the heterozygous form of achondroplasia this may not be observed until almost the third trimester.[136] If achondroplasia is suspected, amniocentesis can be performed for DNA testing on fibroblasts to detect or exclude the fibroblast growth receptor 3 (FGR-3) mutation known to cause achondroplasia.[42] Abnormal bone shape is a feature of camptomelic and thanatophoric dysplasia, whereas fractures, callus formation and hypomineralisation may be seen in osteogenesis imperfecta types II–IV.[50] Hypomineralisation is also seen in hypophosphatasia and achondrogenesis. Radial aplasia may be associated with trisomy 18, but also with rare genetic syndromes such as Fanconi's anaemia and the thrombocytopenia–absent radius (TAR) syndrome.

Soft tissue abnormalities

Cleft lip, whether isolated or associated with cleft palate, can be detected by imaging the fetal face in coronal and transverse views.[367] Rarer midline clefts are often accompanied by other midline defects, such as holoprosencephaly, ethmocephaly or proboscis. The diagnosis of isolated cleft palate is extremely difficult prenatally.[334] These lesions are usually only detected on detailed scans of patients who have either other abnormalities or an at-risk history. Isolated unilateral clefts are rarely associated with either aneuploidy or genetic syndromes; however, these risks increase with bilateral clefts and the presence of associated anomalies.

Cystic hygromas are readily apparent as multiseptate thin-walled cystic lesions, found most commonly around the dorsolateral region of the neck.[73] As they result from obstruction of the jugulolymphatic channels,[12] hygromas frequently progress in utero to hydrops and fetal demise,[2] although spontaneous resolution is possible.[79] They have a strong association with aneuploidy (50–80%), and therefore karyotyping is advised. Hydrops is obvious as generalised skin oedema with ascites, and in many cases there will also be pericardial and pleural effusions, placentomegaly and polyhydramnios.

Other imaging modalities

Transvaginal ultrasound and MRI

The greater resolution provided by high-frequency transvaginal transducers for structures within their 6–7 cm focal zone is ideal for visualisation of the first-trimester fetus. With experience, the falx, vertebral column, kidneys, bladder, fingers and toes can all be identified by 12 weeks' gestation.[406] This technique can be used at fortnightly intervals from 9–10 weeks in women at high risk. An increasing number of anomalies have now been detected,[3,51] including NTDs, cystic hygromas and skeletal anomalies. Indeed, some workers have proposed early anomaly screening at this gestation.[47] However, caution in diagnosing or excluding anomalies in the first trimester seems prudent; for example, it should be noted that midgut herniation ('exomphalos') is physiological until 11 weeks,[407] and the calvarium may appear normal at 12 weeks in fetuses subsequently shown to be anencephalic.[170]

Transvaginal ultrasound has also been used to assess the uterine cervix during pregnancy for the prediction of preterm labour. While cervical length measurement does appear to be superior to biochemical, microbiological or hormonal methods of screening, the actual length required for intervention, such as cerclage, has yet to be defined in a randomised controlled trial (RCT). However, one group have indicated that in a high-risk population a cut-off of 15 mm is appropriate.[174]

MRI of the fetus was first described in the 1980s. Recently, faster capture times have helped to counter the problems created by fetal movements (Fig. 9.6). Although it has been used to aid the prenatal diagnosis of many conditions, its strength lies in assessing intracranial anatomy, and in particular the posterior fossa. Conditions including agenesis of the corpus callosum and neuronal migration disorders are reliably detected by MRI. Indeed, in one UK series, the ultrasound diagnosis of an intracranial anomaly was modified (but not necessarily refuted) in 71% of cases.[431] It is clear therefore that MRI has a place in prenatal diagnosis, although experience in this form of fetal imaging is still being collected.

Screening strategies for Down syndrome

In the past, standard screening policy was to offer women over the age of 35 years chorionic villus sampling (CVS) or amniocentesis for karyotyping. As only 25–30% of trisomy 21 fetuses are born to 'older' mothers, and as utilisation in this group rarely exceeds 50%, it is hardly surprising that the birth prevalence of Down syndrome fell by only 15% with this strategy.[423] Newer policies, which increase detection rates without increasing the numbers undergoing antenatal karyotyping, have been introduced into practice.

Biochemical

The average maternal serum AFP value in Down pregnancies is 0.7–0.8 multiples of the median.[418] As this association is largely independent of maternal age, the two were then combined to give each woman a specific age- and AFP-adjusted risk.[89] Subsequently, raised human chorionic gonadotrophin (hCG),[41] particularly the free β-hCG subunit, and low unconjugated oestriol[64] levels were found to be associated with trisomy 21. Again, in the absence of any relation to maternal age or each other, their levels and maternal age were next combined using an algorithm to predict fetal risk.[420] The reason for these biochemical changes is not yet understood, but is thought to relate to functional immaturity, producing a delay in the normal gestational rise or fall. Cut-offs of 1:250–1:300 have shown a sensitivity of up to 70%, with a false-positive rate of 5%. The term false positive in this context describes the percentage of the population that would be given a high-risk result if the test were taken up by the entire population. Subsequent refinements using free β-hCG[388] and a prior dating scan,[161] and confining the assay to 15–18 weeks' gestation, have increased the accuracy of the test. There continues to be controversy as to whether the double test (AFP and free β-hCG) is more cost-effective than the triple test (AFP, hCG and oestriol), or indeed the quadruple test (AFP, hCG, oestriol and inhibin), in large cumulative series for each strategy.[216,388,422] Detection rates are greater in older mothers (i.e. over 35 years of age), but this is at the cost of higher false-positive rates.[177]

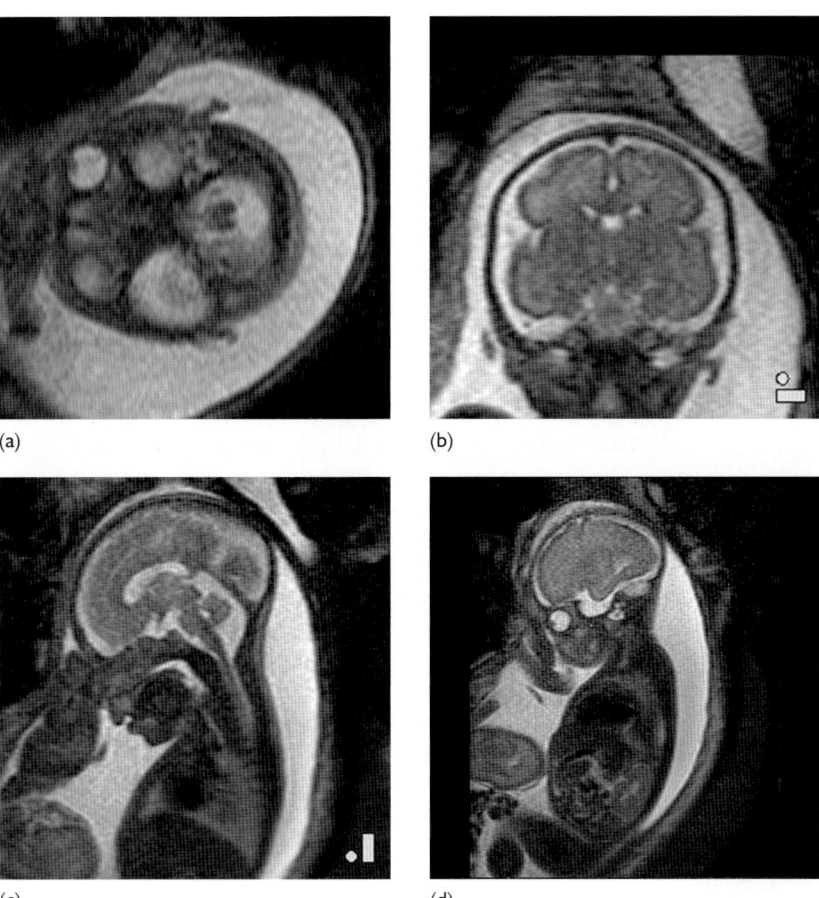

Fig. 9.6 Fetal MRI. Views of the fetal head and brain in a normal midtrimester fetus (a) Transverse, (b) Coronal, and (c), (d) Sagittal.

(a)

(b)

(c)

(d)

As biochemical screening takes place in the mid trimester, it does not allow susceptible women the option of first-trimester CVS for karyotyping. The drive now is to bring screening for aneuploidy into the first and early second trimester, to allow easier termination procedures to be performed. Hopefully, the psychological impact of early diagnosis will be improved by this development.

Ultrasound

There have been major advances in ultrasound screening for aneuploidy. Initially, second-trimester markers were identified in association with various trisomies, including choroid plexus cysts, echogenic bowel, renal pelvic dilatation and increased nuchal thickness. Women carrying fetuses with soft tissue markers of aneuploidy were informed of the increased risk and offered karyotyping. Increasingly, the risks of aneuploidy from these markers are being defined, particularly in relation to maternal age,[384] thus allowing more accurate information to be provided. The interpretation of soft markers is complex. Risk tables now exist, such that risk may be adjusted based on maternal age and single or multiple markers/anomalies, as well as type of marker or anomaly.

The association between increased NT (Fig. 9.7) in the first trimester (10–14 weeks) and aneuploidy has been confirmed in several studies.[229,290,396] The association is with trisomies 21, 18 and 13 in particular. A sensitivity, when related to crown–rump

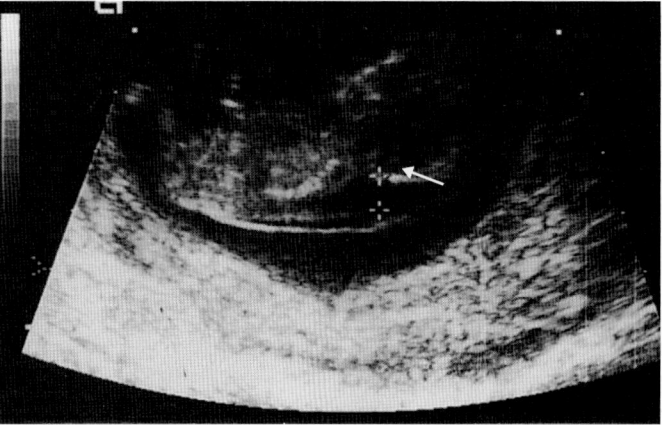

Fig. 9.7 Transabdominal ultrasound view of increased nuchal translucency in a fetus at 11 weeks' gestation.

length and maternal age, of almost 80%, with a false-positive rate of 5%, has been reported by one group in a low-risk population cohort of 96 127.[385]

Anxiety has been raised about the reproducibility of NT measurement.[350] A significant proportion of fetuses so detected miscarry spontaneously rather than continue to term.[37] Indeed, this has led to one group arguing that first-trimester screening tests should detect 8.3% more abnormal fetuses to be compared with methods of second-trimester screening.[112]

Other advantages of early ultrasound for screening include early diagnosis of pregnancy failure, better dating, detection of other abnormalities and, in multiple pregnancy, accurate determination of chorionicity.

Recently, NT measurement has been combined with two first-trimester biochemical markers to improve the efficacy of early screening for trisomy 21. Levels of free β-hCG are increased in the serum of mothers carrying a fetus with Down syndrome, while levels of pregnancy-associated plasma protein A (PAPP-A) are decreased. Combining these two markers with maternal age, the detection rate for trisomy 21 is 60%, with a 5% false-positive rate.[421] Combining this test with NT – the so-called OSCAR test (one-stop clinic for early assessment of fetal risk) – yields a detection rate of 89%.[389]

Finally, those fetuses with an increased NT and normal karyotype are still at risk. A meta-analysis of 16 studies of chromosomally normal fetuses with an increased NT showed that 4% had a cardiac defect,[387] and others have shown that the risk increases with increasing NT measurement.[204] Similarly, this group are at increased risk for having a syndromal defect and poor obstetric outcome. One study has shown that the chance of a livebirth with no defects (LBND) can be stratified according to the first-trimester NT measurement: NT of 3.5–4.4 mm, LBND = 86%; 4.5–5.4 mm, LBND = 77%; 5.5–6.4 mm, LBND = 67%; and >6.4 mm, LBND = 31.[387]

Recently, attention has focused on the relevance of the presence/absence of the fetal nasal bone.[83] In this series from King's College Hospital, the nasal bone was absent in 43 of 59 (73%) trisomy 21 fetuses and in three of 603 (0.5%) chromosomally normal fetuses. The likelihood ratio, therefore, for trisomy 21 was 146 (95% CI, 50–434) for absent nasal bone and 0.27 (0.18–0.40) for nasal bone being present. Subsequent work by the same group[82] has shown in a retrospective series that the integration of nasal bone screening into the OSCAR test would lead to a detection rate of 97%; alternatively, for a false-positive rate of 0.5%, the detection rate is 90.5%. This work needs to be validated by other groups.

Subtle markers of aneuploidy

With advances in ultrasound resolution, many structures not previously visualised, such as the digits, feet and soft tissues of the neck, can now be demonstrated. Accordingly, the minor malformations and abnormal postures characteristic of aneuploid neonates may be seen in utero. Postaxial polydactyly is found more frequently in trisomy 13 than in 18, but ventricular septal defects are common in both.[437] Profile of the trisomy 18 fetus reveals micrognathia and a protuberant upper lip.[24] The hands remain clenched in trisomy 18, with characteristic overlapping of the fingers, and the typical rocker bottom and equinovarus deformity are found in the feet. The sonographic features of trisomy 21 are more elusive. These may include increased nuchal thickness (first or second trimester), mild renal pelvic dilatation, hyperechogenic bowel, brachycephaly, and hypoplasia of the middle phalanx of the fifth finger (clinodactyly).

Choroid plexus cysts (CPCs) are detected in approximately 1% of mid-trimester scans as sonolucent areas within echogenic choroid.[76] Soon after their appearance was described,[81] they were found to be associated with trisomy 18.[157,298] Controversy has centred on whether karyotyping should be offered routinely to all fetuses with CPCs. The size, laterality and shape of the cysts are not helpful in predicting aneuploidy.[269] CPCs are now believed to be benign structures which usually disappear by 22–24 weeks. It has been estimated that the risk of aneuploidy with cysts unassociated with other anomalies lies between 1:350 and 1:500,[27,323] but this takes no account of the *a priori* risk. Current opinion is that if there are isolated CPCs on detailed anomaly scan, the risk of trisomy 18 is increased only marginally (i.e. relative risk 1.5) over that from maternal age alone.[384]

Invasive procedures and prenatal diagnosis

Samples of fetal tissues suitable for karyotyping, biochemical analysis and DNA studies are obtained by CVS and amniocentesis. In many cases the choice of procedure is left to the patient, based on her informed perception of the relative advantages and disadvantages of each. Fetal blood sampling (FBS), a technically more difficult procedure, is performed after 18–20 weeks' gestation, not just for antenatal diagnosis but also for therapy. Each invasive procedure is associated with a small chance of procedure-related loss. In general, therefore, invasive procedures are offered rather than recommended to parents, who, after appropriate counselling, should be given time to consider the various risks of the condition being tested for against those of the procedure.

Amniocentesis

Amniocentesis is the commonest invasive procedure for prenatal diagnosis. Most are done at 14–16 weeks' gestation, when the amniotic cavity contains 150–200 ml of fluid, allowing 15–20 ml to be withdrawn without complication (working rule is x ml withdrawn = x weeks in gestation). A 22G needle is inserted transabdominally and guided to a pool under ultrasound control (Fig. 9.8). Simultaneous ultrasound monitoring reduces the number of dry and bloody taps[99,363] and obviates the rare risk of

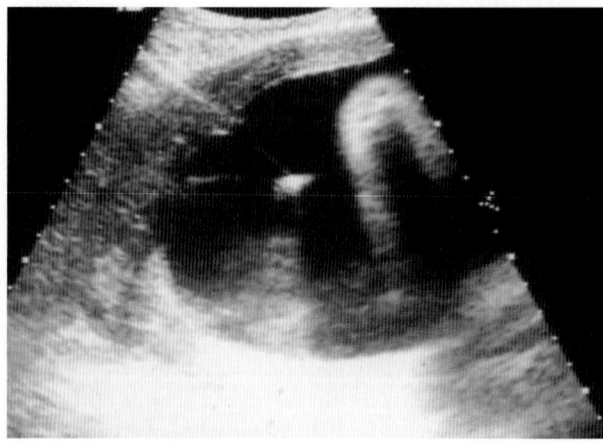

Fig. 9.8 Amniocentesis. The 22G needle is introduced under ultrasound guidance (from top left).

severe fetal trauma. It has thus replaced the older technique of 'semi-blind' insertion following ultrasound identification of a pool. Transplacental insertions have been linked with an increased miscarriage rate[215,397] and should be avoided. Even with an extensive anterior placenta, a small window avoiding the placenta can usually be found.

Patients are quoted a risk of spontaneous miscarriage attributable to the procedure of 1%, based on the results of the only RCT.[397] Of the three major collaborative case–control studies, the Medical Research Council (MRC)[256] reported an increased risk of spontaneous abortion of 1.3%, whereas lower rates were found in the other two.[281,382] As with all invasive procedures, operator experience seems the most important variable, significantly lower miscarriage rates being found for operators with experience of more than 50 procedures.[256,414] The increased risk of respiratory distress identified in the MRC study has not been confirmed,[202] and it is not clear to what extent this was due to prolonged oligohydramnios following amniotic fluid leakage. This issue has not been entirely resolved, given evidence in humans[417] and animals[194] that removal of amniotic fluid on a single occasion may impair respiratory development.

Amniotic fluid contains cells desquamated from fetal skin, gastrointestinal, urogenital and respiratory tracts, and the amnion. In view of their small number, up to 2 weeks' cell culture is required prior to cytogenetic analysis, although with new techniques this period is shortening. A major disadvantage of amniocentesis is that termination of affected fetuses is not performed until well into the mid trimester. Although amniotic fluid can be satisfactorily obtained and cultured at 11–13 weeks,[26,179] the safety of the early procedure has been questioned by a randomised trial showing a greater miscarriage rate than with CVS,[291] and as such is not recommended.

Approximately 0.5% of amniotic cell cultures fail to grow, and maternal cell contamination leads to diagnostic difficulty in <0.2%.[343,405] Level 2 mosaicism (multiple cells with the same abnormality in a single flask) occurs in 0.7% of amniocenteses, and level 3 (multiple cells with the same abnormality in multiple flasks) in 0.2%,[52,199,438] but these are confirmed in the fetus in only 20% and 60% of cases, respectively.

Later in pregnancy, amniocentesis has been used in the management of preterm premature rupture of the membranes (PPROM). However, amniocentesis for bacteriological analysis of amniotic fluid has not attained general usage because of concerns regarding the frequency of low-virulence microorganisms.[141] Amniocentesis is also used for infusing fluid (amnioinfusion) to visualise fetal anatomy in oligohydramnios, and for draining fluid (amnioreduction [AR]) in polyhydramnios secondary to structural problems or TTTS.[143,144]

Recently, fluorescent in-situ hybridisation (FISH) has been introduced to allow rapid detection of trisomy 13, 18 and 21 together with sex chromosome aneuploidies. FISH allows the detection of specific DNA sequences with chromosome-specific painting probes. Uncultured (hence rapid) fetal cells (e.g. amniocytes) are hybridised using DNA-specific probes and the number of signals counted. The technique excludes non-mosaic trisomy but not other aneuploidies. The presence of three signals is consistent with trisomy for that chromosome, but this does not exclude the possibility that the pattern of signals is due to a

structural rearrangement. The probe for chromosome 21 is located in the Down syndrome 'hot-spot' and thus abnormal results are considered reliable. Abnormal results for the probes for chromosomes 13 and 18 should be interpreted with caution, and therefore should not be acted on unless there are clear anomalies on ultrasound consistent with each trisomy.

Chorionic villus sampling

Although obtaining chorionic tissue suitable for cytogenetic and biochemical analysis was first reported more than 30 years ago,[264] CVS was only introduced into clinical practice in the mid-1980s. CVS was originally performed transcervically, but is now commonly performed transabdominally. Not only do operators who perform other transabdominal procedures prefer this, but also it allows samples to be obtained in the second and third trimesters. Furthermore, it may reduce the chance of infection. Safety appears to be better with the transabdominal route (miscarriage rates 1% vs 4%).[207,383] Initially, CVS was performed between 8 and 12 weeks. However, concern was raised following a report of limb reduction defects, some in association with the oromandibular syndrome.[139,140] In all cases, CVS was performed before 66 days' gestation, and by single-needle transabdominal aspiration. Subsequent population and case–control studies have been unable to confirm any link,[156] but theoretically it seems plausible that a procedure which may cause embolism, thrombosis or vasoconstriction at the time of limb bud formation, may lead to such malformations. Thus, it has been recommended that CVS be performed after 10 weeks' gestation.[225,353] In many centres the popularity of CVS declined after these reports, but now, with the potential to test chorionic villi for genetic syndromes together with first-trimester aneuploidy screening, the numbers of CVS performed are again increasing.

Rapid cytogenetic results may be obtained from spontaneous mitoses in direct preparations from the chorionic villus cells[381] or after short-term culture for 12–24 hours. Long-term culture, of up to 2–3 weeks, ensures specimens of sufficient quality for banding studies, but may be complicated by maternal cell contamination and the possibility of culture artefact. Reports of false-negative results on direct analysis[60,116] suggest that long-term culture provides a more accurate reflection of fetal karyotype. Most centres therefore perform both short- and long-term cultures on each specimen. Culture is not needed for most of the enzyme deficiencies underlying inborn errors of metabolism, which can be assayed directly in villi. Villi are also an excellent source of DNA for molecular analysis. Results from CVS are thus available sooner than after amniocentesis, allowing women with abnormal results in the first trimester the option to undergo termination of pregnancy by suction curettage.

The CVS-related fetal loss rate before 28 weeks above the background rate is 1–2% in centres with much experience.[291] One problem with CVS is a 1.0–1.5% incidence of confined placental[48,60,234] or pseudomosaicism,[211] where a discrepancy exists between chorionic and fetal karyotypes, necessitating further investigation by amniocentesis.[262] In most cases, a bizarre aneuploid or polyploid mosaic is identified in the chorion, whereas the fetal karyotype, assessed from skin fibroblasts, is normal. Mosaicism confined to the placenta most likely will not affect the fetal outcome, and this should be suspected when the direct preparation shows a few isolated abnormal cells. In this situation, the cultured cell line result should be awaited, as this will usually be normal as the cells are obtained from the mesenchymal trophoblast and are more representative of the fetus. If the culture still shows mosaicism, then an amniocentesis and a detailed anomaly scan are required. At amniocentesis, fibroblasts are cultured which truly represent the fetus, as they are shed fetal skin cells.

Although DNA analysis for prenatal diagnosis was first used on amniotic cells,[212] it was the application to chorionic villi[320] that precipitated the recent expansion in DNA diagnoses in the first trimester. With the rapid progress that continues in mapping disease-specific gene loci, the list of amenable conditions has increased exponentially, such that advice should be sought with each new request for prenatal diagnosis. The molecular basis of virtually all the common monogenic diseases is now known, and in some cases, such as CF, population screening of prospective parents is a reality.

Direct oligonucleotide probes are suitable for the majority of conditions where the particular point mutation or deletion characterising the disease at the molecular level is known. Examples include sickle cell disease, alpha-thalassaemia and 21-hydroxylase deficiency. In rare cases in which the exact mutation is not yet known, indirect gene tracking is required using a series of informative intra- or extragenic markers around relevant loci, known as restriction fragment length polymorphisms (RFLPs). As this latter approach requires lengthy family studies, including analysis of DNA from a previously affected child, suitability for prenatal diagnosis is best assessed before conception. Recombination is a problem with indirect methods, the exact rate depending on the proximity of the markers used to the disease locus. Genetic heterogeneity and non-paternity are additional sources of error.

Prenatal diagnosis of late-onset autosomal dominant (AD) diseases such as Huntington's chorea and polycystic kidney disease poses counselling difficulties. A currently healthy parent with a 50% risk of having inherited the mutation may request prenatal diagnosis without wishing to know his or her own genetic status.

The polymerase chain reaction (PCR), in which target sequences are exponentially amplified from tiny amounts of DNA, has several implications for prenatal diagnosis. First, results are available more rapidly and can be obtained on amniotic cells without culture. Second, DNA can be obtained for RFLP status from the Guthrie card of a deceased sibling.[434] Third, preimplantation diagnosis after in-vitro fertilisation is now feasible, and in this regard, prenatal diagnosis of human embryos from a single cell biopsied at the eight-cell stage can be performed.[178]

Fetal blood sampling

Early attempts at FBS via placentesis[213] were abandoned because of high fetal mortality and low success rates. Fetoscopy was the first satisfactory method of obtaining pure samples of fetal blood, from either chorionic plate vessels[195] or the umbilical cord.[354] Fetoscopy has now been replaced by the simpler and safer technique of direct ultrasound-guided needling of various fetal vessels. This is done as an outpatient procedure under local anaesthesia

from 17 weeks' gestation. Sedation is rarely necessary. The most common approach, which involves inserting a 20G needle transabdominally into the umbilical vein about 1 cm from the placental cord insertion,[91] yields an adequate sample in 97% of cases.[92] For anterior placentae, the route is transplacental; for posterior, transamniotic. Maternal contamination from inadvertent intervillous sampling is ruled out before removal of the needle by comparing the sample's MCV distribution, determined rapidly on a particle size analyser, to that of the mother.[352] Even at term, fetal MCV, which declines rapidly with gestation, remains significantly higher than that of healthy mothers.[145] The vein is the preferred vessel to sample, being simpler and safer;[424] accidental sampling of the artery can be confirmed by ultrasonic observation of the direction of flow following injection of sterile saline.[302] When there is difficulty approaching the cord insertion because of obesity, oligo- or polyhydramnios, or fetal position, blood may be aspirated from the intrahepatic portion of the fetal umbilical vein.[223,313] Although FBS from the intrahepatic vein is more difficult than at the cord insertion, it obviates the need for laboratory confirmation of its source, and in multiple pregnancies the operator is certain as to which fetus is sampled. Alternative sites of sampling include a free loop of cord and the fetal heart.[15]

FBS was initially developed for the prenatal diagnosis of hereditary disease, particularly the haemoglobinopathies and haemophilias. However, these now are diagnosed by DNA analysis on chorion villi or amniocytes. Standard cytogenetic and DNA studies may be done on fetal blood, and are especially useful when the mother presents too late for amniocentesis or CVS, or when these tests fail. Previously, FBS was used to determine fetal acid–base status, but this now can be inferred from non-invasive Doppler assessment of the fetus.[308] The main indications for FBS are now rapid karyotyping and assessment of potential anaemia or thrombocytopenia.

Determining the loss rate attributable to FBS is difficult, as fetal demise in the weeks after the procedure may instead be due to the underlying high-risk indication. This was clearly demonstrated in one series, which showed increased loss rates in procedures performed on sicker fetuses, i.e. prenatal diagnosis (2%), fetal structural abnormality (6%), assessment of severe fetal growth restriction (FGR, 14%), and hydrops (25%).[255] Daffos et al[92] reported seven losses (1.2%) in 562 continuing pregnancies sampled predominantly for toxoplasmosis, and another group had losses in 0.9% of 469 continuing pregnancies sampled for prenatal diagnosis or karyotyping of minor malformations.[295] Many of these, however, were greater than 21 weeks, and loss rates seem higher earlier in gestation.[43,322] A reported summation of all the published series calculated an overall loss rate in procedures performed in low-risk cases of 2.7%,[162] although others have reported a lower loss rate of 0.9%,[426] and this figure has been corroborated by the USA International Registry.[257] Such results are only achieved after considerable training and experience. Most losses are due to cord haematoma, cord tamponade or haemorrhage, and, unlike losses after CVS or amniocentesis, are apparent at the time of the procedure. In late pregnancy, emergency caesarean section is performed to salvage these infants, although some may be damaged. Intra-amniotic bleeding is observed ultrasonically after 40% of samplings,[92,424] and a histological study of cords within

48 hours of FBS showed that a degree of extravasation occurs in all cases.[208] This bleeding is almost always transient, owing to the abundance of thromboplastins in amniotic fluid.[285]

Skin and muscle biopsy

Prenatal diagnosis of many severe genodermatoses necessitates histological and ultrastructural examination of fetal skin, obtained at 18–22 weeks, initially by fetoscopy[355] but more recently by ultrasound-guided techniques.[16] The usual site chosen is the fetal buttock or leg. Epidermolysis bullosa letalis is characterised by separation of the epidermis from dermis at the lamina lucida on light microscopy, and a paucity of hemidesmosomes on electron microscopy.[355] The prenatal diagnostic features of epidermolysis bullosa dystrophica,[13] epidermolytic hyperkeratosis,[169] harlequin ichthyosis[118] and Sjögren–Larsson syndrome[227] have similarly been described. In oculocutaneous albinism, in which there is a lack of active melanin synthesis in hair bulb melanocytes, the biopsy must be taken from a hair-bearing area such as the scalp.[113] The biopsy site is not detectable at birth, and in a series of 52 skin biopsies there were no procedure-related losses (Rodeck, unpublished observations).

Although DNA analysis is available for the diagnosis of the most common muscular dystrophies, most notably Duchenne muscular dystrophy, there are circumstances when a direct fetal muscle biopsy is required. This is usually when genetic testing has proved inconclusive. The procedure is performed under ultrasound control with the biopsy forceps guided into the outer aspect of the fetal buttock so as to avoid major structures.

Fetal medicine

With the combination of ultrasound and invasive procedures, several conditions can be managed more rationally than in the past, such as congenital malformations, maternal exposure to infectious agents, and FGR. In others, the fetus can be treated; intravascular transfusion has greatly improved the survival of alloimmunised fetuses, making it thus far the best model for fetal therapy.

Management of non-lethal malformations

Table 9.1 lists the risks of chromosomal and other structural malformations associated with common non-lethal congenital malformations. These are considerably higher for anomalies detected in utero than at birth. For example, in the literature the risk of an abnormal karyotype for infants with congenital heart disease is 5–10% and for exomphalos 10%, compared with risks of 32% and 66%, respectively, from antenatal studies.[85,298] Multiple malformations carry a 10 times higher risk of aneuploidy than isolated malformations.[384] The demonstration of any fetal anomaly on ultrasound therefore prompts a detailed search for other abnormalities. Rapid karyotyping by FBS, amniotic fluid FISH

Table 9.1 Reported frequencies of chromosomal and other structural abnormalities in fetuses with malformations detected in utero. The risk of aneuploidy will be lower if the malformation is isolated, and for the softer markers the risk will vary with maternal age

Condition	Aneuploidy (%)	Structural malformations (%)
Hydrocephalus	10–15	30–60
Cystic hygroma	45–80	15–65
Non-immune hydrops	3–15	25
Cleft lip/palate	<1	15–50
Congenital heart disease	25–30	10–20
Diaphragmatic hernia	20–30	17–55
Tracheo-oesophageal fistula	15	50–60
Duodenal atresia	30–35	50–70
Exomphalos	50–65	60–75
Multicystic kidney	5–10	12–40
PUJ obstruction	1–2	20–27
Posterior urethral valves	6–24	25–40
Single umbilical artery	<1	20–45

or transabdominal CVS is offered. This is recommended not only in the mid trimester to allow termination of aneuploid pregnancies, but also in the third trimester, where knowledge of a serious chromosomal defect may alter antenatal and intrapartum management, including mode of delivery. Furthermore, termination of pregnancy after 24 weeks' gestation is legal in the UK if there is a substantial risk that the fetus has an abnormality that would result in the birth of a child with a serious handicap. Karyotyping should also be performed for conditions where the risk of intrauterine death (IUD) is high, such as hydrops, because postmortem autolysis may jeopardise subsequent chromosomal studies and thus future genetic counselling. Indeed, postmortem karyotyping following termination for fetal abnormality has a 27% failure rate, and therefore pre-termination sampling is advised.[228]

The option of termination of pregnancy is offered for severe malformations and support given to those who wish to continue through to delivery despite a poor prognosis. Other malformations are suitable for early postnatal correction, such as certain cardiac defects, duodenal atresia and gastroschisis. Intrauterine surgery may have a role in a few situations, but less so than was originally hoped. The significance of antenatal detection of some conditions, such as PUJ obstruction or multicystic kidney, is not so much the alteration of perinatal management as the initiation of timely investigation and follow-up in infancy.

The worse prognosis for abnormalities diagnosed in utero rather than neonatally largely reflects the increased risks of aneuploidy, multiple malformations and IUD. Whereas cystic hygroma at birth carries an excellent prognosis following surgical correction, the same-named lesion detected in utero leads to survival in less than 5%.[2,231] This high loss rate, which applies equally to euploid fetuses, reflects the frequency of hydrops and hypoxaemia in this condition.[399]

Fetal growth restriction (for more information, see Chapter 10)

The term small for gestational age (SGA) describes both fetuses that are constitutionally small and those with growth restriction (FGR). Approximately 50–70% of fetuses with a birthweight <10th centile are constitutionally small. However, as a group, SGA fetuses are at higher risk of IUD, birth hypoxia, neonatal complications, impaired neurodevelopment, and, according to the Barker hypothesis, potential hypertension and diabetes in later life.

While FGR may be suspected by abdominal palpation and the measurement of the symphyseal–fundal height, the diagnosis is made ultrasonographically, with the abdominal circumference and/or estimated fetal weight <10th centile. Serial measurements are superior to single estimates not only in the prediction of genuine FGR but also in predicting poor outcome.

While ultrasound has assisted in establishing the diagnosis of FGR, the role of Doppler ultrasound has been extensively researched in terms of (i) prediction of risk, and (ii) monitoring affected pregnancies with FGR. The role of uterine artery Doppler analysis in predicting FGR appears to be limited, even in high-risk pregnancies,[74] while screening a low-risk population with umbilical artery Doppler does not reduce perinatal mortality or morbidity.[49] However, monitoring of high-risk pregnancies with umbilical artery Doppler has been shown to reduce perinatal morbidity and mortality.[9,282] In particular, absent end-diastolic flow (EDF) is associated with adverse perinatal outcome.[351] Although acidaemia and hypoxaemia are unlikely in the presence of EDF, 45–80% of fetuses with absent EDF are acidaemic (pH <7.31) and 79–100% hypoxaemic.[288,309]

With knowledge of the fetal compensatory response to hypoxia by redistribution of blood flow, pulsed Doppler investigation of the involved fetal vessels provides more information about fetal condition. Redistribution of blood flow away from the kidneys (leading to oligohydramnios), gut (leading to hyperechogenic bowel) and skin towards the brain, adrenals and heart, can be demonstrated by increased flow velocity within the MCA, and decreased flow velocity within the descending aorta. Alterations in the venous circulatory system may represent an end-stage response with cardiac decompensation, which can be measured at the level of the ductus venosus.[189] Increased pulsatility and reversed velocity at the time of atrial contraction may be found. Decision-making regarding timing of delivery is currently based on combining the results of Doppler studies with growth velocity, amniotic fluid levels and cardiotocography.

The chance of a fetal chromosome abnormality in FGR is as high as 6–16%,[129,295,309] although this risk is based on series of referred patients in which severe FGR, often with oligohydramnios and malformations, was the indication for rapid karyotyping. With severe FGR and no structural malformations, the risk is lower, 2–3%.[384] Clearly, the risk of aneuploidy remains remote in the milder forms of FGR, which complicates 5–10% of all pregnancies in the late third trimester. Karyotyping warrants consideration in severe FGR, when associated with fetal malformations, or in the presence of normal liquor volume or uterine or umbilical Doppler studies.

Red cell alloimmunisation

Despite a dramatic decline in incidence, maternal sensitisation has not disappeared, for a variety of reasons, including antenatal sensitisation, prophylaxis failure and antibodies other than anti-D. Untreated, 45–50% of affected infants will have no or only mild anaemia, and 25–30% will have moderate anaemia posing neonatal problems only. The remaining 20–25% develop hydrops and usually die in utero or neonatally; in half, the hydrops develops prior to 30 weeks.[46] The aim of antenatal management is to identify severely affected fetuses, to correct their anaemia by transfusion, and then deliver them at the optimal time. At each gestational age the risks of invasive monitoring are weighed against those of conservative management and delivery. A suggested algorithm for the management of these cases is outlined in Figure 9.9.

Anti-D prophylaxis

RhD-negative women are at risk of sensitisation from fetomaternal bleeding, not only at delivery but also in other situations, such as external cephalic version and amniocentesis. Although the prevention programme has reduced neonatal deaths attributable to haemolytic disease of the newborn (HDN) from 18.4/100 000 in 1977 to 1.3/100 000 in 1992, there remains a sensitisation rate of around 1.5% among Rh-negative women. Administration of 500 IU of anti-D at 28 and 34 weeks can reduce the risk of immunisation to 0.2%.[88] Anti-D prophylaxis is now recommended by the Royal College of Obstetricians and Gynaecologists[365] and National Institute for Clinical Excellence,[279] with either a dose of 500 IU at 28 and 34 weeks, or a single larger dose early in the third trimester. The rationale for this is that all Rh-negative women are at risk from hidden bleeds.

It is, however, important to note that clinically significant disease can be caused by other red cell alloantibodies such as Rh-c, Kell, Rh-E and Fy^a (Duffy). At present, immunoprophylaxis is not available for non-RhD disease and so immunisation will continue to occur.

Antenatal screening and management of RBC alloimmunisation

Routine serological testing of women is carried out:

- to identify pregnancies at risk of fetal and neonatal alloimmune disease (HDN);
- to identify RhD-negative women who require antenatal anti-D prophylaxis;
- to provide compatible blood swiftly in emergencies.

All women who have no antibodies at 10–16 weeks' gestation should be tested once again between 28 and 36 weeks. Some workers believe that RhD-negative women should have two further tests, one at 28 weeks and one at 34–36 weeks, but sensitisation late in pregnancy is unlikely to result in HDN requiring treatment.

Quantification of the anti-D has simplified interpretation of positive antibody screens. Severe fetal anaemia is not

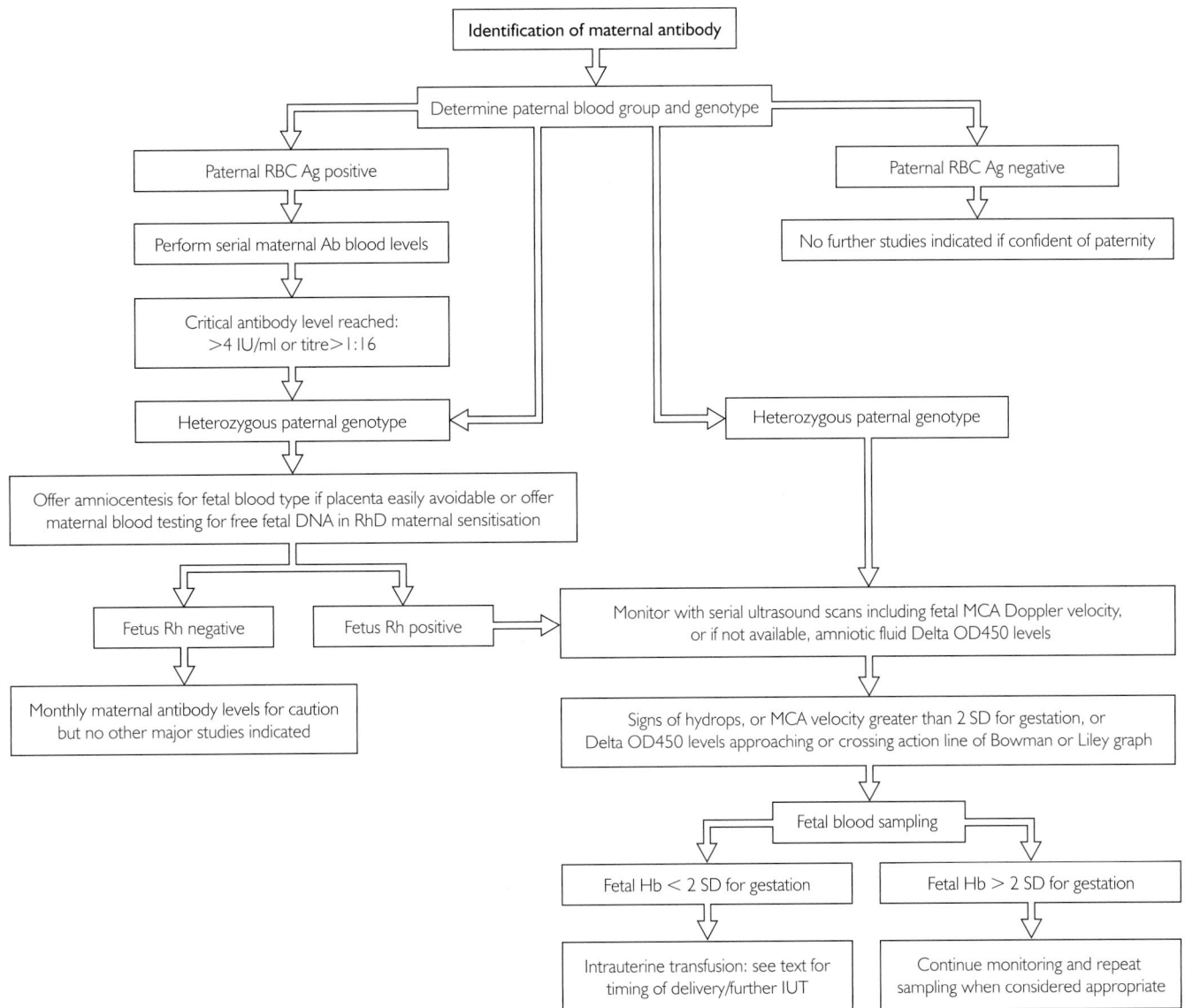

Fig. 9.9 A proposed algorithm for the management of red cell alloimmunisation.

expected <4 IU/ml[44] and is rare (0.25%) <10 IU/ml. Further evaluation therefore is warranted at levels >4 IU/ml. Above this threshold, antibody levels have a limited role as they correlate poorly with the degree of fetal anaemia,[300] although a rising level suggests an increase in severity. Prior to non-invasive methods of assessment, a level >15 IU/ml indicated the need for invasive assessment of fetal anaemia. No such similar cut-off levels apply to anti-c, Kell and Fy[a], and close monitoring is required in these cases, even with low titres.

When the fetus has been shown to be Rh positive, the maternal antibody concentration should be checked every 2–4 weeks. Monitoring is now primarily with assessment of blood velocity in the MCA (see below). Additional ultrasonographic assessments include measurement of placental thickness, umbilical vein diameter, spleen and liver size[77,297,349] or Doppler assessment of velocities in the descending aorta and ductus venosus,[86,287,318,319] although none have been shown to be as reliable as MCA

Dopplers in predicting the degree of anaemia. While the demonstration of fetal ascites indicates severe anaemia (PCV <15%, Hb <4 g/dl) in the mid trimester, ascites only actually develops in two-thirds of fetuses with an Hb <4 g/dl.[300] Anaemia of this degree is not associated with hypoxaemia, but is associated with increased fetal lactate levels suggesting tissue hypoxia.[386] This is unlikely to cause developmental delay, but should be corrected as soon as possible by transfusion.

Determination of paternal zygosity and fetal genotype

Following the identification of antibodies in the maternal circulation, determination of the paternal Rh status is important. Approximately 15% of the UK population are RhD negative, and of the positive fathers, 56% are heterozygous for the D-gene, with a 50% chance of passing this on to the fetus. In cases of proven paternal heterozygosity, fetal antigen status should then be determined. Recent advances, since the identification of the Rh gene in 1991,[84] have allowed fetal antigen status to be determined, firstly from amniotic fluid,[30] and now from maternal blood by identification and analysis of free fetal DNA.[239] The latter has just become available as a clinical service.[138] Concerns of persistence of free fetal DNA from one pregnancy to the next have been largely discounted by the demonstration of its rapid clearance from the maternal circulation soon after birth. Reliability in the case of a RhD-positive fetus appears to be 100% from the data available thus far, as is the demonstration of a RhD-negative male fetus (with detection of the Y chromosome). It is only in the presence of a female RhD-negative fetus (where the chance of analysis of only maternal DNA, i.e. female, is possible) that a confirmatory amniocentesis has been recommended. Fetal blood group typing is also possible from amniocytes using PCR to detect the RhD, c, E and Kell genes.[30,235]

Non-invasive assessment for fetal anaemia

Recent advances in Doppler imaging have resulted in a shift in practice away from early invasive assessment (and hence an avoidance of increased maternal sensitisation). Attention has focused on the Doppler velocimetric assessment of the MCA to predict fetal anaemia (Fig. 9.10). The rationale is that the MCA responds quickly to hypoxaemia owing to the strong dependence of the brain on O_2 and also reflects the hyperdynamic circulation associated with anaemia. Several groups have shown a strong negative correlation between either peak systolic velocity or mean velocity and fetal Hb or haematocrit.[1,251,401] In the largest series, the peak systolic velocity in the MCA predicted moderate or severe anaemia without hydrops in 100% of cases, with a false-positive rate of 12%.[251] The demonstration of increased velocity in the MCA indicates a strong likelihood of fetal anaemia. At this point, invasive testing is indicated. Use of MCA monitoring compared to more traditional methods of monitoring appears to allow the first invasive procedure to be performed later in gestation without compromising fetal wellbeing.[203]

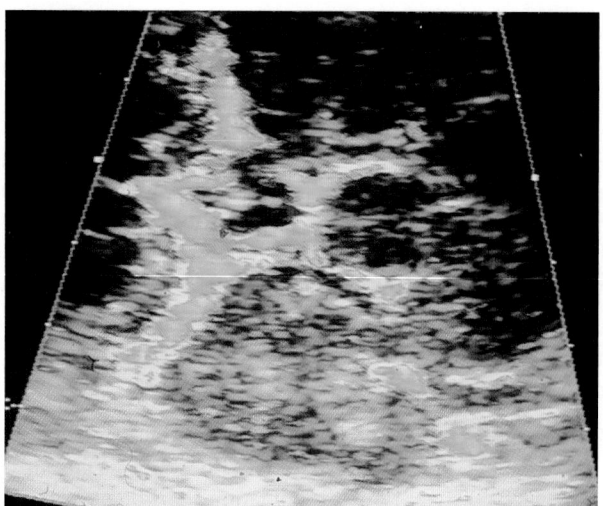

Fig. 9.10 Colour Doppler appearances of the circle of Willis and the middle cerebral arteries.

Fetal blood transfusion

FBS allows direct assessment of fetal PCV and Hb, and permits transfusion to be performed at the same procedure if anaemia is detected. However, as FBS has a loss rate, and provokes fetomaternal haemorrhage and thus increases antibody levels in 70% of procedures in which the placenta is transgressed,[306] it is avoided until MCA Dopplers predict significant anaemia.

Intravascular transfusions (IVTs) were first administered fetoscopically[357] but are now given by ultrasound-guided FBS.[17,32,301] The decision to administer an IVT is based on the PCV or Hb at FBS. Most use an Hb of less than 2 SD for the gestation[288,293] as an indication for transfusion; some use an absolute haematocrit below 30%. The needle tip is kept within the umbilical vein and fresh Rh-negative packed cells compatible with the mother are infused at 10–15 ml/min. The fetal heart rate and flow of infused blood are monitored on ultrasound to guard against inadvertent needle dislodgement and cord tamponade. The volume transfused is determined by consideration of the estimated fetoplacental volume and the fetal and donor PCV[301] or Hb,[293] according to published nomograms. The PCV is rechecked after transfusion, and, if less than the desired 40–45%, a further increment is given.

The timing of the second transfusion should be based on the pre- and post-transfusion fetal Hb from the first transfusion, and from serial MCA Doppler velocities. After the second transfusion, the rate of fall in PCV in the fetus may be determined (when the PCV is estimated to have fallen to 20–25%) and the timing of subsequent transfusions arranged, although these again are often modified by the MCA Doppler velocities. Kleihauer testing of fetal samples indicates that erythropoiesis is usually completely suppressed after two to three transfusions.[307] As the donor blood in the fetal circulation is not susceptible to immune destruction, the rate of fall in PCV declines with increasing transfusions and thus the interval between procedures can be increased. The same principles are used in scheduling delivery between 36 and 38 weeks. Once an intrauterine transfusion has been performed, the timing of delivery will depend on when the last transfusion was performed and how many days it is likely to take for the Hb to fall to a level about 2 SD below the mean. Intrauterine transfusions are not usually performed after 36 weeks. In a woman with no previous history but an antibody level above 4 IU/ml (or 1:16 titre), the delivery can be planned at 37–38 weeks of gestation.

Survival

With serial IVTs, survival rates of 78–95% have been achieved in severely affected fetuses.[301,337] One series has reported that in almost 600 IVTs, intact survival was 98% in those commenced in non-hydropic fetuses at greater than 24 weeks, and 70% in hydropic fetuses less than 24 weeks' gestation.[180] There are few follow-up studies focusing on morbidity, but one published study suggested that when prematurity is removed, long-term morbidity secondary to intrauterine transfusion is low.[200] Therefore, the prognosis is now extremely optimistic. Fetal mortality correlates inversely with gestational age, and operator experience is undoubtedly also of importance.

Fetal thrombocytopenia

Alloimmune thrombocytopenia

Perinatal alloimmune thrombocytopenia complicates 1:5000 births, with intracranial haemorrhage (ICH) affecting 10–20%.[276] Maternal antiplatelet antibodies cross the placenta, in a situation analogous to Rh disease. The consequent fetal thrombocytopenia may be profound, and there have been increasing reports in alloimmune thrombocytopenia of spontaneous ICH in utero, particularly in the third trimester,[102,154,272] but it may occur as early as 18 weeks' gestation. The human platelet-specific antigens are biallelic polymorphisms which involve the platelet surface glycoproteins. Recently, a nomenclature of human platelet antigens (HPAs) has been developed.[416] At present, HPAs 1–5 have been recognised. The genetic basis for these five HPAs has been identified, all involving a single point mutation in the DNA coding for the glycoproteins involved.[435] The most common is HPA 1, which has a high-frequency (85%) or a low-frequency (15%) antigen. Only 2% of women will be homozygous for the low-frequency 'b' allele, and thus at risk for developing antibodies and alloimmunisation. Fortunately, the actual occurrence of alloimmunisation is much rarer than this (0.06%)[39] because the development of antibodies is dependent on the HLA type. HLA-Drw52a and HLA-Dr3 are most commonly associated with the development of HPA 1a antibodies.

Management

The most reliable method of assessing likely disease severity is by inference from previous pregnancies: usually, a current pregnancy will be as severely or more affected than previous pregnancies.[346] This guides when investigation and treatment should begin, which may be as early as 18 weeks' gestation. Percutaneous FBS and estimation of fetal platelet count is the only way to determine whether a fetus is affected.[94]

There are several management options available, and therefore patient care should be tailored dependent on previous history and parental preference.

Fetal platelet transfusions

These are used to cover the samplings and delivery, but may also be employed in a prophylactic manner, with weekly transfusions during the second and third trimesters and delivery once lung maturity is achieved. This prophylactic regimen was favoured in Europe until recently, but is arduous for the mother. In practice, transfusions are usually commenced at 26–28 weeks' gestation to cover the time of greatest risk,[311] although in cases of severe disease the first transfusion may be indicated as early as 20–22 weeks. A normal platelet count does not exclude the diagnosis, and therefore the procedure should be repeated at 28–32 weeks, unless from sampling amniotic fluid or fetal blood the fetal platelet type is found to be compatible.

Intravenous immunoglobulin

Cumulative data suggest that intravenous immunoglobulin (IVIG) is an important treatment option in this condition. Maternal infusion is less invasive and simpler than direct fetal sampling.

However, it is expensive. Reports of maternal IVIG raising the fetal platelet count are variable.[57,315] It may be that the IVIG has a preventative effect on ICH, other than by increasing the fetal platelet count. In a series of 54 women with thrombocytopenic fetuses due to alloimmune thrombocytopenia given IVIG weekly, in whom 10 had a previous infant with ICH, no ICH occurred and yet 20% showed no increase in the platelet count with therapy.[56] Other groups now rely on this treatment solely,[342] or a combination of IVIG and platelet sampling, with the latter's timing and frequency dependent on the previous history, and platelet count.

Conservative

The final option is to follow the fetus regularly by ultrasound and, in countries where late termination is permitted, to offer termination if ICH is found. This approach may be suitable in cases in which there is no severe history and hence the risk of ICH versus a complication from recurrent sampling or transfusion is low. Sampling may be performed prior to delivery to assess whether a transfusion is required to cover this.[214]

There is no clear evidence to demonstrate that one treatment strategy is superior to the others. Although prophylactic platelet transfusions may be the most effective, there is a considerable procedure-related loss secondary to the serial procedures,[428] and therefore this needs to be weighed against the overall risk of ICH with untreated disease. Currently, the balance appears to be swinging to weekly maternal IVIG, with limited FBS, and platelet transfusion if necessary.

Autoimmune thrombocytopenic purpura

Transplacental passage of antibodies in maternal immune thrombocytopenic purpura (ITP) also produces fetal thrombocytopenia, albeit to a lesser degree. The older literature suggested that the 50% of infants with thrombocytopenia had a risk of ICH during vaginal delivery,[192] and accordingly FBS for fetal platelet count determination prior to labour used to be performed in pregnancies complicated by ITP to decide on the mode of delivery.[265,374] More recent studies show a low incidence of severe fetal thrombocytopenia (5–20%) or infant morbidity with maternal ITP,[55,217,425] with no documented cases of antenatal ICH or ICH attributable to mode of delivery even in cases of severe thrombocytopenia. There is no correlation between maternal and fetal platelet counts;[327] the level of platelet-associated antibody does not correlate with fetal thrombocytopenia, but increased levels of free antiplatelet antibody are associated with fetal thrombocytopenia.[53,368] Platelet counts in affected infants may fall following delivery, but generally thrombocytopenia at this stage is not associated with significant morbidity.

Management

Treatment for maternal thrombocytopenia includes steroids, splenectomy (outside pregnancy) and IVIG to raise the platelet count prior to delivery. There is no evidence that these treatments affect fetal platelet count. The investigations required to detect fetal thrombocytopenia in this condition are controversial. The risk of severe fetal thrombocytopenia in a woman presenting with a documented fall in platelet count in pregnancy and no history to suggest ITP is very low,[54,58] and does not justify FBS prior to labour. With a history of chronic ITP, the risk of severe fetal thrombocytopenia ($<50 \times 10^9$/l) is between 5% and 20%, although it is difficult to determine whether mode of delivery affects the outcome. Recommendations have included FBS prior to delivery, and fetal scalp sampling to determine whether caesarean section should be performed. Fetal morbidity appears extremely low in this condition, so that opinion has moved away from fetal intervention unless there has been a strong history of a previous affected child with severe thrombocytopenia.

Congenital infections

Counselling a woman after perinatal exposure to teratogenic infectious agents previously involved quoting empirical risks. Now, direct serological investigation of the fetus and DNA analysis of fetoplacental tissues can be used to determine whether fetal infection has occurred. In rubella this may facilitate continuation of pregnancy, whereas in toxoplasmosis it determines the choice of antimicrobial therapy. FBS has no role in evaluating fetal status in maternal human immunodeficiency virus infection, as the procedure itself could infect the fetus.

Rubella

Prenatal diagnosis of rubella infection is usually indicated following maternal exposure in the early second trimester, or where doubt exists as to whether exposure in the first trimester resulted from primary infection or reinfection. Rubella-specific IgM is detected in fetal serum by radioimmunoassay,[93,273] provided that FBS can be delayed until 21–22 weeks, when the fetal humoral response to infection becomes detectable. Even at 23 weeks occasional false-negative IgMs have been reported.[121] To improve the accuracy of prenatal testing at this late gestation, fetal blood or other tissues are also tested by hybridisation with a cDNA probe to rubella virus.[87] Earlier in pregnancy the same technique can be used on CVS specimens,[404] although concern remains that placental infection may not indicate fetal infection.[10]

Congenital infection leads to the classic rubella triad of cataracts, congenital heart defects (most commonly pulmonary stenosis) and deafness.[173] With advancing gestation, transplacental passage reduces, with congenital infection rates of 50% in the first month falling to just 10% by 3 months.[122] In addition, the severity of the syndrome reduces with advancing gestation.

Cytomegalovirus

The most severe congenital infections are due to primary maternal CMV infection. Primary infection is associated with a 40% transmission rate, although only 10% of those fetuses will develop long-term sequelae, mostly hearing and learning defects.[329] Among the 5–10% who are symptomatic at birth, there will be a neonatal mortality of 30%, with long-term handicap in all survivors. Infection in earlier gestation results in higher transmission and poorer outcome.

Prenatal diagnosis is based on ultrasound findings and the detection of viral particles in the amniotic fluid,[98] or, less commonly, in fetal blood. Specific IgM in fetal sera may also be diagnostic.[230] Ultrasound findings include FGR, ascites or hydrops, intracranial calcification, ventriculomegaly and bowel echogenicity. Nevertheless, 90% of infants with congenital CMV infection remain neurologically and developmentally normal.

If primary CMV with transplacental transmission in pregnancy is confirmed, there is a 5–10% chance of severe clinical disease, and therefore termination of pregnancy should be offered. Recurrent disease carries a much lower risk of handicap, but overall accounts for more affected infants. Attempted treatment of an affected fetus with ganciclovir has been reported with equivocal results,[345] and although there is interest in this therapy, it is unlikely to be introduced until the results of neonatal treatment series are reported.

Toxoplasmosis

Although as pregnancy advances, maternal exposure leads to an increased risk of fetal infection, severity is greatest with exposure in the first trimester, with little chance of severe congenital disease after 20 weeks' gestation. Termination of an infected fetus remains an option, although fetoplacental infection is largely treatable.[109] The aim of fetal testing is to allow optimal transplacental therapy, initially with maternal spiramycin (3 g/day) to prevent transplacental transmission, with the addition of pyrimethamine and sulfadiazine (sulphadiazine) if fetal testing proves positive.[93] These two drugs are directly antiparasitic and have been shown to limit fetal damage. They are not used in the first instance when information about maternal infection is known, but rather only when fetal infection is proven, because of the potential hazards to mother and fetus. The diagnosis of fetal infection is now made with PCR analysis of amniotic fluid, which has replaced the more cumbersome multiple testing that was previously required.[197] If fetal infection is proven, the prognosis is still likely to be good, although vision may be affected later. However, intracranial signs of calcification and/or ventriculomegaly are poor prognostic signs,[35] and termination would be offered.

Parvovirus

Human parvovirus (B19) infection is associated with increased risks of miscarriage, hydrops and IUD,[11] with an overall fetal loss rate of 9% in infected pregnancies.[338] Parvovirus is best identified in fetal blood or other tissues by dot-blot hybridisation, electron microscopy or, most commonly, PCR of B19-specific DNA.[380] The mainstay of diagnosis, however, remains maternal serology in women with appropriate clinical symptoms. Anti-B19 IgM appears in the serum at the onset of illness and remains detectable for up to 3 months. IgG response begins after 7 days and persists, probably to confer lifelong immunity. FBS is not routinely indicated in pregnancies with maternal infection because at least 90% will result in livebirths and parvovirus does not seem to be teratogenic.

It is the profound fetal anaemia secondary to an infective erythroid aplasia that accounts for the significant mortality rate. Following documented maternal infection, close fetal monitoring for signs of anaemia is indicated. Assessment of the MCA velocity for early detection of anaemia may be useful (as with monitoring of fetuses at risk of alloimmunisation) for 12 weeks post exposure, as fetal anaemia may occur 1–11 weeks after maternal infection.[359] FBS and IVT are indicated in the presence of suspected anaemia or hydrops. Hydrops without fetal anaemia has been documented and viral particles have been identified in the fetal myocardium, suggesting that a myocarditis may be contributory. It appears that profoundly anaemic fetuses which are salvaged by transfusion have a good prognosis, although more than one IVT may be necessary on occasion.[331,373]

Tachyarrhythmias

Supraventricular tachycardia (SVT) is the most common fetal tachyarrhythmia, with rates between 200 and 300 beats per minute (bpm). Atrial flutter and fibrillation often run at faster rates. As SVT is often intermittent, treatment is indicated only when SVT is sustained or associated with hydrops.[221] In-utero therapy seems preferable to delivery and neonatal treatment, as the fetus tolerates haemodynamic compromise better in utero, where gas exchange is not hindered by pulmonary oedema. Transplacental treatment by giving the mother digoxin leads to cardioversion in only 25–50% of non-hydropic cases[254,393] and is usually not effective in the presence of hydrops.[155] These poor results partly reflect difficulties in achieving therapeutic maternal levels owing to the increased intravascular volume and glomerular filtration rate of pregnancy.

The addition of second-line drugs, such as flecainide and verapamil, results in improved eventual cardioversion, with over 90% conversion (including fetuses with hydrops) with flecainide in one series.[114] The same group also demonstrated that the fetuses that required second-line therapy in utero, had a significantly more complex postnatal course.

Reports of sudden death in adults with antiarrhythmics such as amiodarone have slowed their incorporation into fetal treatment. Direct fetal intravascular or intraperitoneal therapy may be useful in refractory cases or those with hydrops.[147] Adenosine has recently been reported to cause a chemical cardioversion when injected directly into the fetal circulation, and then sinus rhythm was maintained by transplacental digoxin therapy.[222] This needs to be explored further in cases resistant to initial maternal treatment. Doses required are much higher per kilogram estimated fetal body weight than in the neonate, presumably to allow for transplacental passage into the maternal circulation, and to account for the enhanced fetoplacental blood volume.

Congenital heart block

Complete heart block in the fetus is rare, with a reported incidence of between 1:5000 and 1:20 000. The intrinsic ventricular rate is around 50–65 bpm and the heart usually enlarges and hypertrophies to compensate for the slow rate. Hydrops may occur as congestive heart failure develops.

Congenital heart block (CHB) with a structurally abnormal heart carries a poor prognosis (85% mortality), whereas with a structurally normal heart the prognosis is good.[244] In 1966, the association between isolated CHB and maternal connective tissue disease was first described.[201] Anti-Ro and anti-La (SSA and SSB) antibodies are present in 60–80% of cases, often in mothers with subclinical disease. These antibodies are most frequently found in women with Sjögren's syndrome, or, less often, with systemic lupus erythematosus (SLE). Various therapeutic options based on maternal transplacental therapy are available, although none have shown proven efficacy. These include sympathomimetic agents to increase fetal heart rate and function[175] and maternal dexamethasone to suppress the fetal myocardial inflammation.[38,80] In practice, these are only used with a fetal heart rate <50 bpm, or signs of complication including hydrops.

Abnormalities of amniotic fluid volume

Oligohydramnios

Causes in the mid trimester include urinary tract malformations, PPROM and FGR, and at these gestations survival is less than 25% whatever the cause.[19,258] Conditions with a lethal prognosis, such as renal agenesis and aneuploidies, should be ruled out. Absence of the acoustic window makes inspection of fetal anatomy difficult. Transvaginal ultrasound facilitates visualisation of the renal fossae, as does colour Doppler of the renal arteries.[378] If still equivocal, invasive procedures may be required, including amnioinfusion and/or instillation of fluid into the fetal peritoneal cavity.[312] Amnioinfusion of a warmed physiological solution not only restores the acoustic window, but allows confirmation of PPROM, especially when a dye is added.[143]

As 5–10% of fetuses in pregnancies with severe oligohydramnios will be chromosomally abnormal,[176] rapid karyotyping is carried out at the time of amnioinfusion. In the rare case of a euploid fetus with oligohydramnios, intact membranes and an intact renal tract, there may be a role for serial amnioinfusions in the prevention of lethal pulmonary hypoplasia,[14] which otherwise complicates at least 60% of cases of severe mid-trimester oligohydramnios.[271]

Polyhydramnios

The more severe the polyhydramnios, the more likely that an underlying cause will be found. Using the maximum vertical pocket, mild and severe polyhydramnios have been arbitrarily defined as a deepest pool greater than 8 cm and 15 cm, respectively.[71] The amniotic fluid index (AFI) definitions for mild and severe polyhydramnios are values outside the 97.5th centile for gestation, and an AFI greater than 40 cm, respectively.[270]

Exclusion of maternal diabetes is essential; thereafter, a detailed fetal assessment is mandatory. In one series, 11% of neonates had a structural anomaly (most notably tracheo-oesophageal fistula, oesophageal atresia, duodenal atresia, or conditions that impair fetal swallowing such as arthrogryposis), which increased with increasing severity of the polyhydramnios.[96] If sonographic evaluation was normal, the risk of a major anomaly was just 1% with mild polyhydramnios, but 11% if severe. Aneuploidy was present in 10% of fetuses with sonographic anomalies and in 1% without. Overall the fetal loss rate was 4%, of which 60% had anomalies.

The increased risks of preterm labour and PPROM in polyhydramnios seem mainly confined to those with severe polyhydramnios, i.e. an AFI ⩾40 cm or a deepest pool ⩾15 cm.[67,144] AR has been used with anecdotal success in severe polyhydramnios in order to prolong gestation and relieve maternal discomfort.[132,339] Removal of relatively small volumes of amniotic fluid can restore amniotic pressure to normal,[144] but usually larger volumes are removed to limit the number of procedures that may be required. Nevertheless, removal of volumes greater than 6 l at one time does carry the risk of precipitating abruption and/or preterm labour.[119]

Prostaglandin synthetase inhibitors have been used to reduce amniotic fluid. Indometacin (indomethacin) initially was described at a dose of 75–200 mg/day.[59,248] This acts by reducing fetal urine output[220] and hence amniotic fluid volume.[219] The amniotic cavity and fetal bladder are monitored daily on ultrasound so that the dose can be adjusted to ensure sufficient response without causing oligohydramnios. Concern has arisen about the potential deleterious effects of fetal ductal constriction secondary to indometacin, and therefore monitoring of ductal patency by Doppler has been recommended[266] when exposure is for longer than 1 week. However, the risks of neonatal complications from premature closure of the ductus in utero seem remote, provided therapy is discontinued at 32 weeks. Sulindac, another prostaglandin synthetase inhibitor, has been shown to have less effect on the ductus arteriosus, but still reduces amniotic fluid volume.[66]

Multiple pregnancy

The incidence of twin pregnancies in the UK is 14.4 per 1000 births,[321] an increase of 25% compared with the early 1980s. The incidence is highest in older women (19.1 per 1000 in women aged 35–39 years in 1992), among whom a significant increase occurred owing to assisted reproductive techniques (ART). This relatively small increase in frequency of multiple pregnancy will have a disproportionate effect on perinatal mortality and morbidity. Twin pregnancies have an eight-fold increased risk of cerebral palsy, and triplet pregnancies a 47-fold increase.[333]

Up to a third of twin pregnancies are monozygotic (MZ), of which the majority share a single monochorionic (MC) placenta. For more information about zygosity, see Chapter 23. Perinatal morbidity and mortality in MC twins is three- to five-fold higher than in dichorionic (DC) twins;[22,29,283] furthermore, previable losses are also significantly increased.[375] Much of the increase in risk is due to the presence of vascular anastomoses which are implicated in TTTS, and the co-twin sequelae after IUD of one twin.

Twin–twin transfusion syndrome

TTTS complicates approximately 15% of monochorionic diamniotic (MCDA) twin pregnancies,[376] and accounts for 15–17% of overall perinatal mortality in twins.[391,429] It has classically been attributed to transfusion of blood via placental vascular anastomoses between the two fetal circulations. Vascular anastomoses are present in 96% of MC placentae, and interfetal transfusion is a normal event in the majority of these pregnancies.[106] However, placentae from pregnancies affected by TTTS are characterised

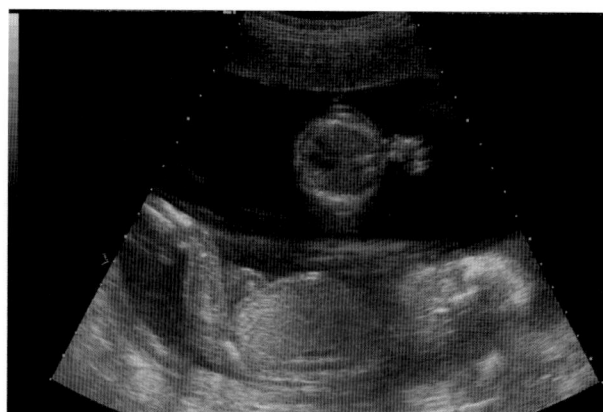

Fig. 9.11 Twin–twin transfusion syndrome. The smaller donor is 'stuck' to the anterior uterine wall, with the larger recipient lying within the polyhydramniotic sac.

by two findings: first, an imbalance in interfetal transfusion is set up by the presence of unidirectional arteriovenous anastomoses, and second, there is an absence of compensatory bidirectional arterio-arterial anastomoses.[105,106,245]

Presentation in the mid trimester has until recently been associated with an 80–100% perinatal loss rate, either from preterm delivery secondary to polyhydramnios, or IUD following severe growth restriction or circulatory overload.[171,429] The majority of cases complicated by TTTS have estimated fetal weight discordance in utero, and differences of <15% are unusual.[142] There is some evidence that the prognosis worsens with an increasing difference in abdominal circumference measurements,[370] cumulatively reflecting the severity of overload/early hydrops in the recipient and growth restriction in the donor.

TTTS presents in the second trimester with discordant amniotic fluid volume (Fig. 9.11).[111] The donor twin becomes oliguric, with consequent oligohydramnios, hence appearing enshrouded within its membrane and finally stuck to the uterine wall. In addition, neither the urinary bladder nor the stomach is usually visible, once anhydramnios is present. The growth velocity of the donor may follow the asymmetrical pattern seen with fetuses affected by FGR. Furthermore, it may also exhibit abnormal umbilical and MCA velocities, with absent/reversed flow in the former, and redistribution in the latter.[190]

The overloaded recipient develops polyuria and severe polyhydramnios. The degree of polyhydramnios cannot be solely explained by the transfusion of blood volume from the donor to the recipient, and there are emerging data implicating alterations in the renin-angiotensin system resulting in the polyhydramnios/oligohydramnios sequence.[246]

Venous Doppler studies in the recipient fetus deteriorate in accordance with the disease process. There may be evidence of pulsatile venous flow, progressing to reverse EDF within the ductus venosus.[191] The development of tricuspid regurgitation indicates worsening of the right-sided cardiac failure. The recipient fetus may develop hydrops, the mechanism of which has been assumed to be volume overload. Doppler studies have shown that severe cases are often associated with venous waveform patterns consistent with raised central venous pressure.[191,347] Typically, recipient fetuses with cardiac dysfunction develop cardiomegaly, tricuspid regurgitation, ventricular hypertrophy and, ultimately, right ventricular outflow tract (RVOT) obstruction.[440]

A number of groups have attempted to 'stage' TTTS in an attempt to rationalise treatment.[341,400] Several prognostic criteria have been used, including arterial and venous Doppler studies, fetal size discordancy, bladder dynamics and amniotic fluid volume. However, sudden unpredictable deterioration in clinical condition can occur, rendering these criteria vulnerable.

Therapeutic options for TTTS

A variety of treatments, including transplacental drug therapy, selective fetocide, AR, laser ablation (LA) of the intertwin placental anastomoses, and intrauterine venesection and exchange transfusion, have been attempted, with varying degrees of success. Current treatment mainly involves the use of AR, LA and selective fetocide, alone or in combination according to disease severity and progression.

Serial amnioreduction

Serial AR remains the simplest of treatment options, with at least one fetus surviving (at 4 weeks postnatal age) in 71% of pregnancies.[252] Although AR aims primarily to control polyhydramnios to allow prolongation of gestation, there is some evidence in TTTS that it may ameliorate fetal condition and the disease process. AR was associated with a 74% median increase in uterine blood flow in one study,[45] while others have demonstrated that fetal MCA pulsatility indices fell acutely with AR in both recipient and donor fetuses.[253]

Until recently, serial aggressive AR was the mainstay of management of this condition. However, because of the high rates of perinatal mortality and morbidity and that no attempt was being made to affect the disease process itself, other techniques have been developed.

Laser ablation

The technique of LA of placental vessels was first developed in animals in 1985[101] and later applied to human pregnancies with TTTS.[100,415] The initial technique involved the photocoagulation of all surface chorionic vessels crossing the interwin septum with a neodymium:yttrium–aluminium–garnet (Nd:YAG) laser. The early results were disappointing, with perinatal survival similar to that of AR.[100,415] The high procedure-related loss rates were attributed to the unnecessary destruction of viable placental tissue using such a non-selective technique.

However, with refinement of the technique and increased operator experience, rates for survival of at least one twin have improved to >75%.[124] Now, most operators perform targeted ablation, with selection and ablation of confirmed anastomoses, while leaving viable placental tissue untouched.

Selective fetocide

Selective fetocide has been suggested to have a role in the management of TTTS by a number of groups. In its favour, the procedure may be performed once the IUD of one of the twins appears imminent, or once all other treatment options have failed. Indeed, this usually allows the parents to feel that the procedure is absolutely necessary to allow even a single twin to be saved. However, this delay may allow some degree of insult to happen to the surviving fetus, before its co-twin is terminated. Either the donor or the recipient fetus may become preterminal, and in order to be a safe and effective procedure, the possibility of acute transfusion of the remaining twin into the terminated twin must be avoided (see below).

Management of TTTS

Most clinicians treat pregnancies complicated by TTTS on a case-by-case basis. First, disease severity is assessed by staging; thereafter, management is contentious. Some groups advocate proceeding to LA in all cases, while others reserve LA for moderate–severe cases and perform AR on milder cases. Selective fetocide is usually only considered in the light of failure of either LA or AR.

Neurological outcome

There are emerging data regarding the longer-term sequelae of TTTS. Cerebral white matter lesions are increased in MC twin pregnancies overall, both with or without TTTS, and this has been attributed to haemodynamic imbalance due to the shared circulation.[22] However, in surviving twins from pregnancies complicated by *severe* TTTS and managed by AR, the incidence of antenatally acquired neurological lesions was found to be 35%, although with the exception of one case, these lesions were relatively subtle, and thus of uncertain long-term significance.[104] Both donors and recipients were shown to be at risk, although the aetiology of the damage is uncertain. It has been speculated that in the recipient the raised haematocrit, and hence potential for intravascular sludging, leads to cortical damage, with the donor's neurological injury secondary to anaemia. However, large differences in fetal Hb concentrations in utero are uncommon.[107] It has been shown that LA, rather than AR, reduces the incidence of cerebral palsy in survivors (4.2% vs 24.4%) because the disease process is largely arrested at the time of treatment;[340] however this has yet to be substantiated in an RCT.

Acute interfetal transfusion

Following the IUD of one of an MC twin pair, there is approximately a 25% incidence of necrotic brain and/or renal lesions (increasing to 50% if the pregnancy was complicated by TTTS) and a similar risk of IUD in the otherwise healthy co-twin.[159,413] The aetiology of this insult appears to be haemodynamic. An imbalance in interfetal transfusion following the death of one twin in utero gives rise to a period of hypotension, potentially resulting in ischaemia, as the initially healthy twin transfuses blood into the dead twin's circulation.[160] The phenomenon of acute interfetal transfusion also has implications in pregnancies where selective fetocide is indicated, e.g. discordant fetal anomaly, TTTS in extremis, and twin reversed arterial perfusion sequence (TRAP).

Selective fetocide ideally should involve an occlusive technique, to prevent any residual possibility of the surviving twin exsanguinating into the non-viable twin's circulation. After initial reports of ultrasound-guided techniques including vascular occlusion with absolute alcohol,[103] histoacryl gel injection[110] or thrombogenic coils,[21] it subsequently became clear that success rates were poor, resulting in co-twin death or damage.[108,310] Now, cord occlusion is performed with bipolar diathermy, with co-twin survival (taking into account pre-existing morbidity) of 76%. It is recommended to perform serial ultrasound or MRI on the surviving twin's brain to exclude evidence of cortical damage.

Multifetal pregnancy reduction and selective fetocide in dichorionic twins

Multifetal pregnancy reduction

This procedure aims to obviate the daunting perinatal mortality in high-order multiple pregnancies (≥ 3) by reducing fetal numbers to a twin or triplet gestation with improved perinatal outcome. In non-reduced higher order (≥ 3 fetuses) pregnancies, approximately one-third will miscarry prior to 24 weeks.[128]

The initial approach, which involved transvaginal aspiration, has been abandoned in view of high loss rates[206] and all are now done by transabdominal injection of KCl into the fetal thorax.[33,125] Most such pregnancies are the result of overzealous use of ovulation induction agents and are therefore usually multizygotic and multichorionic, although not always in twins.[430] The procedure is best delayed until 10–12 weeks, when the risks of abortion and spontaneous regression have subsided and the NT can be measured. The optimal number of fetuses to be left remains controversial, but most centres reduce to twins. The chief risk, that of complete abortion of all fetuses, varies around 4–16% and is influenced by the starting number (triplets 4.5%, quadruplets 8%, quintuplets 11%) and the finishing number after the reduction (ideally two), together with operator experience.[127]

Trichorionic triplets pose the hardest decision in terms of consideration of multifetal pregnancy reduction. One series compared the outcome of reduced trichorionic triplets with that of those managed expectantly.[326] Although the rate of miscarriage in the reduced group was higher (8.3% vs 3.2%), the rate of preterm delivery was considerably lower (9.8% vs 23.1%). Overall, the non-reduced pregnancies had a higher chance of survival (93.3% vs 90.3%) but at the cost of a higher estimated incidence of handicap (1.5% vs 0.6% per fetus).

Selective fetocide

In twin pregnancies discordant for fetal anomaly, selective termination of the affected fetus is an option. Intracardiac KCl injection is the recommended technique,[205] except in MC pregnancies because of the risk of acute interfetal transfusion. In the 20% of cases concordant for fetal sex with a single placental mass on ultrasound, determination of chorionicity will require careful evaluation of the membranous septum. This requires evaluation of the septal thickness and the presence or absence of the lambda sign (Fig. 9.12).[137] A septum that is >2 mm thick and/or contains three to four layers strongly suggests DC placentation,[20,90] although the reproducibility and hence the usefulness of this measurement has been shown to be poor after the first trimester.[390] A combination of all the signs should provide >90% accuracy in chorionicity determination in the second trimester,[371] but 100% accuracy in the first trimester.[69,268] A recent series indicated an overall loss rate of 4% (2.4% in twins, 12.5% in triplets) following selective fetocide,[115] with over 80% of deliveries occurring beyond 32 weeks' gestation. Loss rates are lower if the procedure is performed before 16 weeks.[126]

Fetal stem cell and gene therapy

A large number of haematological and genetic conditions are amenable to bone marrow or stem cell transplantation. The fetus is theoretically the ideal recipient because:

- It is not immunocompetent until the early second trimester at least, so that it would not require the immunosuppressive drugs that have to be used postnatally. Tolerance should therefore be achieved together with long-lasting chimaerism, which is the aim of this therapy;
- Haematopoietic stem cells migrate from the liver to the bone marrow between 12 and 16 weeks of gestation, and therefore a virtual space should be available for the seeding of the graft, obviating the need for marrow ablation with toxic drugs, as in postnatal life.

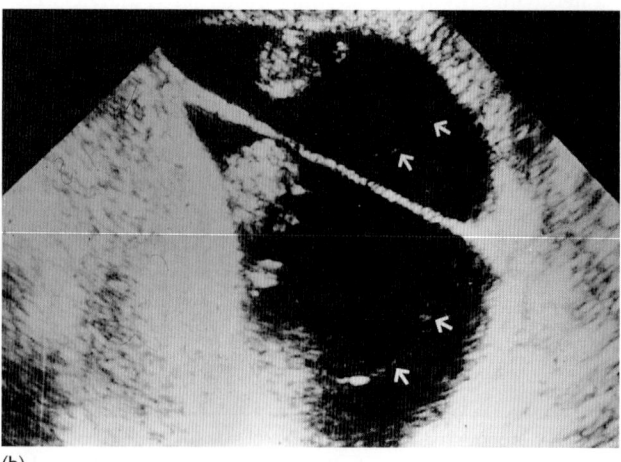

(a) (b)

Fig. 9.12 Transvaginal ultrasound view of first-trimester (a) monochorionic (b) dichorionic twin gestations, showing the amnions and chorions before fusion. (Reproduced from the RCOG Press.)

Success has been achieved in various animal models[377,439] but has been more elusive in the human. The first attempt in the human fetus, using Rh alloimmunisation as a model,[237] showed no evidence of chimaerism. So far, stem cell therapy has only worked in fetuses with immunodeficiency diseases.[150,408]

Appropriate life-threatening disorders may be amenable to fetal gene therapy. In-utero intervention must offer a clear advantage over transplantation or postnatal gene therapy, and can be used only in conditions where there are currently no satisfactory treatments available. An example of such is CF. In-vitro studies where normal and CF airway cells were mixed suggest that only 6–10% of cells expressing normal cystic fibrosis transmembrane regulator (CFTR) are required to correct the ion transport defect in all cells of an epithelial monolayer.[209] Thus, successful gene therapy may require only relatively low-level epithelial airway transduction. The early disease manifestation and poor results from gene therapy treatment of adults with CF has led to research on in-utero treatment in animal models. Submucosal gland progenitors have been identified in the human lung[123] and results of adenoviral-mediated gene transfer to human fetal lung xenografts in vitro are encouraging.[328] More information is awaited in this area.

Fetal surgery

In several congenital malformations, a satisfactory outcome is often achieved with postnatal surgical correction. In some, however, the uncorrected malformation results in progressive organ damage in utero, jeopardising survival. There may be a role in such conditions for in-utero intervention. Initial attempts at fetal surgery took one of two forms: open surgical correction at hysterotomy, or bypassing obstructive lesions by ultrasound-guided insertion of catheter shunts (Fig. 9.13). More recently there has been increasing interest in endoscopic surgical techniques, resulting in lowered maternal morbidity.

These techniques should only be contemplated in centres with expertise, and for conditions in which animal models have demonstrated benefit from correction in utero. Unfortunately, the overall results for open fetal surgery have been disappointing. Despite being limited to a few very specialised centres, the problem of inexorable preterm labour subsequent to surgery has limited the enthusiasm for the approach. If fetal surgery is to be considered in the future, it is essential that chromosomal and other structural malformations first be excluded. Moreover, reliable antenatal predictors are needed when selecting cases for intervention, so that fetal surgery is withheld from those which would otherwise have a satisfactory outcome, and from those in which the pathology is irreversible.

Intrathoracic lesions

Diaphragmatic hernia

The mortality rate from diaphragmatic hernia diagnosed in utero remains high at 75% despite optimal postnatal care.[8,186] The

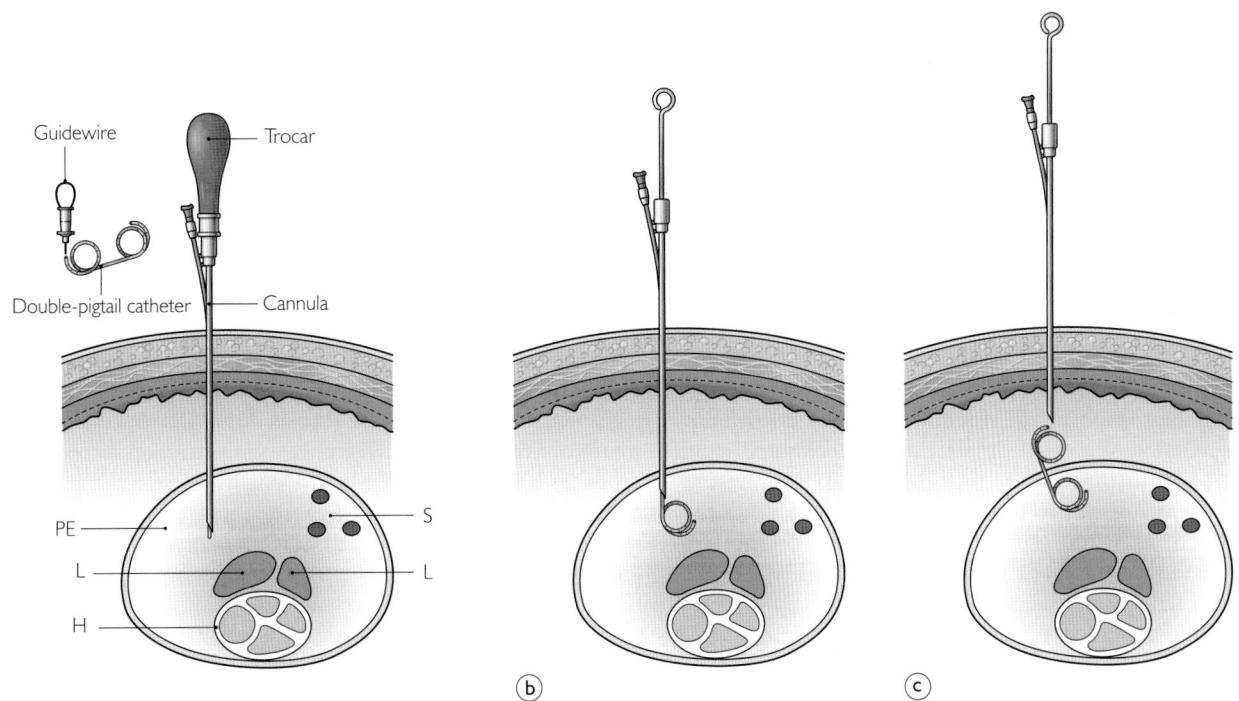

Fig. 9.13 Pleuroamniotic shunting. The trocar (T) and cannula (CA) are inserted transamniotically into the effusion (a). The guidewire (G) is then straightened, the double-pigtail catheter (C) inserted into the cannula, and the wire removed. A short introducer rod then deposits half the catheter within the hemithorax (b). The cannula is then withdrawn into the amniotic cavity, and a long introducer rod is inserted to position the other half of the shunt in the amniotic cavity (c). H, heart; S, spine; L, lungs. (Reproduced from Rodeck et al.[356])

main determinant of outcome is the degree of pulmonary hypoplasia resulting from in-utero lung compression, dependent on the timing and volume of visceral herniation through the diaphragm. Antenatal prediction of neonatal outcome is difficult, but some would say that polyhydramnios, mediastinal shift and a large volume of viscera within the chest are adverse indicators. Studies in an animal model have demonstrated that surgical correction in utero reverses the effects on fetal lung growth and allows survival at birth.[183] The San Francisco group demonstrated in non-human primates the safety and feasibility of fetal surgery,[7] but after a decade of developing appropriate techniques, and operating in the late mid trimester on human fetuses, there have been significant problems. These include difficulty in reducing the herniated liver without kinking the umbilical vein, and the prevention of preterm labour.

An alternative, less invasive corrective approach to diaphragmatic hernia is tracheal ligation. The underlying theory is that preventing drainage of lung liquid will allow the lung to grow (PLUG – plug the lung until it grows), and animal experiments have confirmed this hypothesis.[181,436] Open tracheal ligation, unfortunately, still carries the risk of preterm labour, and may also result in tracheal stenosis. The recent development of endoscopic techniques for insertion of a temporary tracheal plug looks promising[148,182] but much work needs to be done on the optimal timing, duration and method for PLUG before it can be introduced into clinical practice, and the most recent US trial was abandoned.

Fetal hydrothorax

Perinatal mortality in fetal hydrothorax exceeds 50%, and is higher when associated with hydrops than in isolation.[70,348] Compression of the lung during its canalicular phase (17–24 weeks) produces pulmonary hypoplasia, whereas large effusions cause polyhydramnios by impairing swallowing, and hydrops by vena caval obstruction and cardiac compression.[23,332] Chylothorax, the commonest cause in neonates, is diagnosed after alimentation by demonstrating chylomicrons in pleural fluid.[72] The diagnosis may also be made in the fetus by showing high lymphocyte cell counts in aspirated pleural fluid.[25,120]

Ultrasound-guided aspiration of fetal hydrothoraces facilitates neonatal resuscitation if performed immediately prior to delivery.[372] Because the fluid reaccumulates within 6–48 hours,[299,332] long-term drainage is required. This is achieved by a plastic pleuroamniotic shunt, inserted under ultrasound guidance (Fig. 9.13). In three series totalling 34 patients,[241,286,356] resolution was achieved in 17 (50%) patients, 16 (94%) of whom survived, with no respiratory complications. Only two infants survived when hydrops persisted (12%). A single aspiration is performed 1 week beforehand, as the effusion does not always reaccumulate,[23,25] especially with small or unilateral effusions. In fetal hydrothoraces unassociated with other abnormalities, shunting is indicated in the presence of hydrops or polyhydramnios, or if detected in mid trimester. The catheters should be clamped immediately at delivery to prevent a pneumothorax; alternatively, the neonate should be electively intubated and ventilated.

Cystic adenomatoid malformation of the lung (see pp. 584–5)

This rare malformation may result in pulmonary hypoplasia, hydrops and perinatal death in a small percentage of cases.[6] The solid type of lesion is more likely to be associated with a poor prognosis than is the macrocystic lesion, where cysts can be visualised on ultrasound. In the macrocystic type of lesion, long-term drainage of a solitary intrathoracic cyst can be performed, resulting in good outcome at birth.[289] The San Francisco group have also shown that with severe CCAM associated with hydrops, a combination that carries an extremely poor prognosis, open fetal surgical resection by lobectomy offers a good chance of survival. Lobectomy of the massively enlarged pulmonary lobe was performed between 21 and 27 weeks' gestation in eight fetuses, resulting in five survivors.[5] This is therefore one of the conditions where fetal surgery may have a role, although it should only be embarked upon in those cases which otherwise would have an extremely poor outlook.

Obstructive uropathy

Posterior urethral valves (see pp. 947–8)

In fetuses with PUV unassociated with other anomalies, the two main factors determining perinatal outcome are pulmonary hypoplasia and renal dysplasia,[185,278] which seem related to the duration and severity of obstruction. Lack of a urinary contribution to amniotic fluid in the mid trimester leads to pulmonary hypoplasia. Although its pathogenesis is not understood,[304] numerous animal and human studies indicate that lung hypoplasia is a consequence of oligohydramnios. Urethral obstruction has also been considered responsible for renal dysplasia, presumably mediated by raised urinary pressure.[184,226] However, intravesical pressure seems only marginally raised in fetuses with low obstructive uropathies.[316] There is an alternative embryological theory, which suggests that renal dysplasia is not secondary to PUV but results from the same early defect, resulting in abnormal interaction between the urethral bud and the metanephrogenic mesenchyme.[34,392]

As the surgical correction of PUV is relatively simple postnatally, a hypothesis emerged that bypass of the obstruction in utero would minimise renal dysplasia and would restore amniotic fluid, thereby preventing pulmonary hypoplasia and allowing survival at birth.[184] The basis for such intervention was rigorously tested in animals. Urinary obstruction in fetal lambs produces both renal dysplasia and lung hypoplasia,[168,188] whereas early decompression prevents these sequelae.[166,187]

The presence of a normal amniotic fluid volume indicates that lung hypoplasia will not occur, that the obstruction is incomplete, and that the kidneys are producing adequate amounts of urine. Therefore, any benefit from bypass procedures needs to be restricted to those fetuses with severe oligohydramnios, in whom irreversible renal damage has not yet developed. Vesicoamniotic shunting of a fetus with severe renal dysplasia would not only fail to prevent neonatal renal failure, but would also fail to prevent pulmonary hypoplasia if the kidneys in utero were unable to restore amniotic fluid volume. Accordingly, accurate prediction of fetal renal function is important in selecting potential cases for intrauterine surgery. Although renal cysts are visualised in only 44% of dysplastic kidneys, their presence strongly suggests dysplasia.[247] Hyperechogenicity of the renal parenchyma predicts dysplasia with a sensitivity of 73% and a specificity of 80%.[247]

In view of the inaccuracy of ultrasound in predicting renal function, other methods have been sought. Biochemical analysis of fetal urine for the prediction of later renal function has been thought to be useful by some[167,172] but not by others.[427,433] Initially, threshold values to define an isotonic urine with probable poor outcome, $Na^+ > 100$ mEq/l, $Cl^- > 90$ mEq/l and osmolality >210 mmol/l, were used. Refinements have been made by providing normal values for electrolytes (Na^+ and Cl^-) with gestation between 16 and 33 weeks[303] and by serial sampling, which may provide more accurate information.[210] Others have suggested that urinary microproteins may be useful indicators of renal damage, in particular urinary,[238,249,275] and possibly fetal, serum β_2-microglobulin.[36] In present practice a decision whether to shunt or not is based on a combination of urinary electrolytes, β_2-microglobulin, the appearance of the renal tract on ultrasound, and on bladder and liquor volumes.

The standard method of vesicoamniotic shunting is by ultrasound-guided insertion of an indwelling plastic double-pigtail catheter[185,250] as for pleuroamniotic shunting. The results of 73 cases of shunting procedures for low obstructive uropathy reported to the International Registry were not encouraging, with only a 41% perinatal survival rate.[250] However, this included fetuses with pathologies other than PUV, with chromosomal and other abnormalities, and with normal amniotic fluid volume, and 70% of the contributing centres had had experience of only one case. Most of the scepticism about this procedure[117,344] may thus be attributed to poor case selection.

However, more recently, the San Francisco group have published their results of different forms of fetal surgery for obstructive uropathy: techniques included shunt and ureterostomy insertion, LA of the valves and bladder marsupilisation. Of the 14 cases postnatally confirmed to have PUV, the fetal mortality rate was 43%. Chronic renal disease was present in five of the eight survivors, indicating that fetal intervention may not alter postnatal prognosis. Indeed, even favourable fetal urinary electrolyte levels appeared to have no implication postnatally.[198]

It appears, therefore, that inclusion criteria should be rigorously applied to restrict shunting to those few fetuses in which it may be of benefit, i.e. otherwise normal euploid fetuses with sonographically 'normal' kidneys, with severe oligohydramnios and biochemical evidence of adequate renal function.

The long-term outcome following vesicoamniotic shunting is somewhat better when all obstructive uropathies (e.g. prune belly syndrome, urethral atresia, vesicoureteral reflux etc) are considered.[153] At 2-year follow-up of the 62% of fetuses that survived, one-third had undergone renal transplantation for renal failure, with a further 21% having renal impairment; the remaining 43% had normal renal function. Only 50% were acceptably continent at follow-up.

Other surgical conditions

Hydrocephalus (see pp. 1194–6)

Obstruction of the aqueduct of Sylvius causes a rise in cerebrospinal fluid pressure, ventricular enlargement, cortical thinning and irreversible neurological damage. As ventricular shunting in the neonatal period dramatically improves outcome,[233] and as ventriculomegaly may progress in utero, the hypothesis emerged that intrauterine decompression of fetal hydrocephalus would prevent neurological damage. Although initial work in a primate model suggested that in-utero shunting improved survival and outcome,[261] reports to the International Registry[250] demonstrated that in-utero shunting in human fetuses resulted in increased survival of severely handicapped infants, and therefore the technique has been abandoned.

Sacrococcygeal teratoma (see pp. 776, 780, 961)

Congenital sacrococcygeal teratomas are usually benign and in the neonatal period are associated with good outcome after surgical resection. When they are diagnosed in the mid trimester, however, hydrops frequently develops secondary to cardiac failure from arteriovenous shunting, indicating impending fetal demise.[149] One group have reported success with in-utero open surgical resection of the tumour[4] although their previous more problematic experience had suggested that resection must take place before the initiation of end-stage cardiac failure in the fetus and the hydropic placenta leading to the maternal 'mirror syndrome'.[4,232]

Alternative therapies include cytoreduction of the tumour mass by ablative techniques, thereby reducing the venous steal and hence risk of high-output cardiac failure. Several thermocoagulative techniques have been employed with only limited success rates reported.[325]

Neural tube defects (see p. 137)

There is growing experience with in-utero closure of NTDs. An experimental model of spina bifida in the sheep suggests that in-utero correction of the spinal defect can prevent the neurological dysfunction normally seen at birth.[259] Results in humans have been less impressive, although a substantial reduction in shunt-dependent hydrocephalus was demonstrated in one series.[409] It is also clear that in-utero therapy has no benefit with lesions higher in the fetal spine (above L3) and gestations greater than 25 weeks.

Fetal valvuloplasty

There have been several reports of treatment of valve atresia in utero. In one report, two fetuses with complete or almost complete pulmonary atresia and imminent hydrops underwent pulmonary valvuloplasty in utero at mid-gestation.[410] Both children (aged 18 months and 12 months) now have biventricular circulation. As with other fetal surgeries, further research and experience is necessary before this becomes standard practice.

References

1. Abdel-Fattah S A, Soothill P W, Carroll S G, Kyle P M 2002 Middle cerebral artery Doppler for the prediction of fetal anaemia in cases without hydrops: a practical approach. British Journal of Radiology 75: 726–730

2. Abramowicz J S, Warsof S L, Doyle D L, Smith D, Levy D L 1989 Congenital cystic hygroma of the neck diagnosed prenatally: outcome with normal and abnormal karyotype. Prenatal Diagnosis 9: 321–327

3. Achiron R, Achiron A, Yagel S 1993 First trimester transvaginal sonographic diagnosis of Dandy–Walker malformation. Journal of Clinical Ultrasound 21: 62–64

4. Adzick N S, Crombleholme T M, Morgan M A, Quinn T M 1997 A rapidly growing teratoma. Lancet 349: 538

5. Adzick N S, Harrison M R, Flake A W 1993 Fetal surgery for cystic adenomatoid malformation of the lung. Journal of Pediatric Surgery 28: 1–6

6. Adzick N S, Harrison M R, Glick P L et al 1985 Fetal cystic adenomatoid malformation: prenatal diagnosis and natural history. Journal of Pediatric Surgery 20: 483–488

7. Adzick N S, Harrison M R, Glick P L et al 1986 Fetal surgery in the primate. III Maternal outcome after fetal surgery. Journal of Pediatric Surgery 21: 477–480

8. Adzick N S, Harrison M R, Glick P L, Nakayama D K, Manning F A 1985 Diaphragmatic hernia in the fetus: prenatal diagnosis and outcome in 94 cases. Journal of Pediatric Surgery 20: 357–361

9. Alfirevic Z, Neilson J P 1995 Doppler ultrasonography in high-risk pregnancies: systematic review with meta-analysis. American Journal of Obstetrics and Gynecology 172:1379–1387

10. Alford C A, Neva F A, Weller T H 1964 Virologic and serologic studies on human products of conception after maternal rubella. New England Journal of Medicine 271: 1275–1281

11. Anand A, Gray E S, Brown T, Clewley J P, Cohen B J 1987 Human parvovirus infection in pregnancy and hydrops fetalis. New England Journal of Medicine 316: 183–186

12. Andres R L, Brace R A 1990 The development of hydrops fetalis in the ovine fetus after lymphatic ligation or lymphatic excision. American Journal of Obstetrics and Gynecology 162: 1331–1334

13. Anton-Lamprecht I, Jovanovich V, Arnold M L, Rauskolb R, Kern B, Schenck W 1981 Prenatal diagnosis of epidermolysis bullosa dystrophica Hallopeau Siemens with electron microscopy of fetal skin. Lancet ii: 1077–1079

14. Arulkumaran S, Nicolini U, Fisk N M, Rodeck C H 1990 Fetal vesicorectal fistula causing oligohydramnios in the second trimester. British Journal of Obstetrics and Gynaecology 97: 449–451

15. Bang J 1983 Ultrasound guided fetal blood sampling. In: Albertini A, Crosignani P F (eds) Progress in perinatal medicine. Excerpta Medica, Amsterdam, p. 223

16. Bang J 1985 Intrauterine needle diagnosis. In: Holm H A, Kristensen J K (eds) Interventional ultrasound. Munksgaard, Copenhagen, pp 122–128

17. Bang J, Bock J E, Trolle D 1982 Ultrasound guided fetal intravenous transfusion for severe rhesus haemolytic disease. British Medical Journal 284: 373–374

18. Barret J, Chitayat D, Sermer M et al 1995 The prognostic factors in the prenatal diagnosis of the echogenic fetal lung. Prenatal Diagnosis 15: 849–853

19. Barss V A, Benacerraf B R, Frigoletto F D 1984 Second trimester oligohydramnios, a predictor of poor fetal outcome. Obstetrics and Gynecology 64: 608–610

20. Barss V A, Benacerraf B R, Frigoletto F D 1985 Ultrasonographic determination of chorion type in twin gestation. Obstetrics and Gynecology 66: 779–783

21. Bebbington M W, Wilson R D, Machan L, Wittmann B K 1995 Selective feticide in twin transfusion syndrome using ultrasound-guided insertion of thrombogenic coils. Fetal Diagnosis and Therapy 10: 32–36

22. Bejar R, Vigliocco G, Gramajo H et al 1990 Antenatal origin of neurologic damage in newborn infants. American Journal of Obstetrics and Gynecology 162: 1230–1236

23. Benacerraf B R, Frigoletto F D 1985 Mid-trimester fetal thoracocentesis. Journal of Clinical Ultrasound 13: 202–204

24. Benacerraf B R, Frigoletto F D, Greene M F 1986 Abnormal facial features and extremities in human trisomy syndromes: prenatal ultrasound appearances. Radiology 159: 243–246

25. Benacerraf B R, Frigoletto F D, Wilson M 1986 Successful mid-trimester thoracocentesis with analysis of the lymphocyte subpopulation in the pleural effusion. Obstetrics and Gynecology 155: 398–399

26. Benacerraf B R, Greene M F, Saltzman D H et al 1988 Early amniocentesis for prenatal cytogenetic evaluation. Radiology 169: 709–710

27. Benacerraf B R, Harlow B, Frigoletto F D 1990 Are choroid plexus cysts an indication for mid-trimester amniocentesis? American Journal of Obstetrics and Gynecology 162: 1001–1006

28. Benacerraf B R, Saltzman D H, Estroff J A, Frigoletto F D 1990 Abnormal karyotype of fetuses with omphalocele: prediction based on omphalocele contents. Obstetrics and Gynecology 75: 317–319

29. Benirschke K, Kim C 1973 Multiple pregnancy. New England Journal of Medicine 288: 1329–1336.

30. Bennett P R, Kim C L, Colin Y et al 1993 Prenatal determination of fetal RhD type by DNA amplification following chorion villus biopsy or amniocentesis. New England Journal of Medicine 329: 607–610

31. Beretsky L, Lankin D H, Rusoff J H, Phelan L 1984 Sonographic differentiation between the multicystic dysplastic kidney and the uretopelvic junction obstruction in utero using high resolution real time scanners employing digital detection. Journal of Clinical Ultrasound 11: 349–356

32. Berkowitz R L, Chitkara U, Goldberg J D, Wilkins I, Chervenak F A, Lynch L 1986 Intrauterine intravascular transfusion for severe red blood cell iso-immunisation: ultrasound guided percutaneous approach. American Journal of Obstetrics and Gynecology 60: 746–749

33. Berkowitz R L, Lynch L, Chitkara U, Wilkins I A, Mehalek K E, Alvarez E 1988 Selective reduction of multifetal pregnancies in the first trimester. New England Journal of Medicine 318: 1043–1047

34. Berman D J, Maizels M 1982 The role of urinary obstruction in the genesis of renal dysplasia. A model in the chick embryo. Journal of Urology 128: 1091–1096

35. Berrebi A, Kobuch W E, Bessieres M H, Bloom M C, Rolland M, Sarramon M F 1994 Termination of pregnancy for maternal toxoplasmosis. Lancet 355: 36–39

36. Berry S, Lecolier B, Smith R S et al 1995 Predictive value of fetal serum β-microglobulin for neonatal renal function. Lancet 345: 1277–1278

37. Bewley S, Roberts L J, Mackinson A M, Rodeck C H 1995 First trimester nuchal translucency: problems with screening the general population. British Journal of Obstetrics and Gynecology 102: 386–388

38. Bierman F Z, Baxi L, Jaffe I, Driscoll I 1989 Fetal hydrops and congenital complete heart block: response to maternal steroid therapy. Journal of Pediatrics 112: 646–648

39. Blanchette V S, Chen L, Salmon de Freiberg S, Hoghan V A, Trudel E, Decary F 1990 Immunization to the Pl^A1 antigen: results of a prospective study. British Journal of Haematology 74: 209–215

40. Blumenthal D H, Rushovich A M, Williams R K, Rochester D 1982 Prenatal sonographic findings of meconium peritonitis with pathological correlation. Journal of Clinical Ultrasound 10: 350–352

41. Bogart M H, Golbus M S, Sorg N D, Jones O W 1989 Human chorionic gonadotrophin levels in pregnancies with aneuploid fetuses. Prenatal Diagnosis 9: 379–384

42. Bonaventure J, Rousseau F, Legeani-Mallet L, le Merrer M, Munnich A, Maroteaux P 1996 Common mutations in fibroblast growth factor 3 (FGR-3) gene account for achondroplasia, hypochondroplasia, and thanatophoric dwarfism. American Journal of Medical Genetics 63: 148–154

43. Bovicelli L, Orsini L F, Grannum P A T, Pittalis M C, Toffoli C, Dolcini B 1989 A new funipuncture technique: two needle ultrasound and needle biopsy guided procedure. Obstetrics and Gynecology 73: 428–431

44. Bowell P, Wainscoat J S, Peto T E et al 1982 Maternal anti-D concentrations and outcome in rhesus haemolytic disease of the newborn. British Medical Journal 285: 327–329

45. Bower S J, Flack N J, Sepulveda W, Talbert D, Fisk N M 1995 Uterine artery blood flow response to correction of amniotic fluid volume. American Journal of Obstetrics and Gynecology 173: 502–507

46. Bowman J M, Pollack J M 1965 Amniotic fluid spectrophotometry and early delivery in the management of erythroblastosis fetalis. Pediatrics 35: 815–835

47. Braithwaite J M, Armstrong M A, Economides D L 1996 Assessment of fetal anatomy at 12–13 weeks gestation by transabdominal and transvaginal sonography. British Journal of Obstetrics and Gynaecology 103: 82–85

48. Breed A S, Mantingh A, Beekhuis H, Kloosterman M D, Bolscher H T, Anders GJ 1990 The predictive value of cytogenetic diagnosis after CVS: 1500 cases. Prenatal Diagnosis 10: 101–110

49. Bricker L, Neilson J P 2004 Routine Doppler ultrasound in pregnancy (Cochrane Review). In: The Cochrane Library, Issue 2

50. Brons J T J, Wladimiroff J W, Van Der Harten J J et al 1988 Prenatal ultrasonographic diagnosis of osteogenesis imperfecta. American Journal of Obstetrics and Gynecology 159: 176–181

51. Bronshtein M, Blumenfeld I, Kohn J, Blumenfeld Z 1994 Detection of cleft lip by early second-trimester transvaginal sonography. Obstetrics and Gynecology 84: 73–76

52. Bui T H, Iselius L, Lindsten J 1984 European collaborative study on prenatal diagnosis: mosaicism, pseudomosaicism and single abnormal cells in amniotic fluid cell cultures. Prenatal Diagnosis 4: 145–162

53. Burrows R F, Kelton J G 1990 Thrombocytopenia at delivery: a prospective survey of 6715 deliveries. American Journal of Obstetrics and Gynecology 163: 731–734

54. Burrows R F, Kelton J G 1990 Low fetal risks in pregnancies associated with idiopathic thrombocytopenic purpura. American Journal of Obstetrics and Gynecology 163: 1147–1150

55. Burrows R F, Kelton J G 1993 Fetal thrombocytopenia and its relation to maternal thrombocytopenia. New England Journal of Medicine 329: 1463–1466

56. Bussel J B, Berkowitz R L, Lynch L et al 1996 Antenatal management of alloimmune thrombocytopenia with intravenous gamma-globulin: a randomized trial of the addition of low-dose steroid to intravenous gamma-globulin. American Journal of Obstetrics and Gynecology 174: 1414–1423

57. Bussel J B, Berkowitz R L, McFarland J G, Lynch L, Chitkara U 1988 Antenatal treatment of neonatal alloimmune thrombocytopenia. New England Journal of Medicine 319: 1372–1378

58. Bussel J B, McFarland J G, Kaplan C and Working Party 1991 Recommendations for the evaluation and treatment of neonatal autoimmune and alloimmune thrombocytopenia. Thrombosis and Haemostasis 65: 631–634

59. Cabrol D, Landesman R, Muller J, Uzan M, Sureau C, Saxena B B 1987 Treatment of polyhydramnios with prostaglandin synthetase inhibitor (indomethacin). American Journal of Obstetrics and Gynecology 157: 422–426

60. Callen D F, Korban G, Dawson G et al 1988 Extra embryonic/fetal karyotypic discordance during diagnostic chorionic villus sampling. Prenatal Diagnosis 8: 453–460

61. Campbell J, Gilbert W M, Nicolaides K H, Campbell S 1987 Ultrasound screening for spina bifida: cranial and cerebellar signs in a high-risk population. Obstetrics and Gynecology 70: 247–250

62. Campbell S, Johnstone F D, Holt E M et al 1972 Anencephaly: early ultrasonic diagnosis and active management. Lancet ii: 1226–1227

63. Campbell S, Pearce J M 1983 Ultrasound visualization of congenital malformations. British Medical Bulletin 39: 322–331

64. Canick J A, Knight G J, Palomaki G E, Haddow J E, Cuckle H S, Wald N J 1988 Maternal serum unconjugated oestriol as an antenatal screening test for Down's syndrome. British Journal of Obstetrics and Gynaecology 95: 330–333

65. Cardoza J D, Goldstein R B, Filly R A 1988 Exclusion of fetal ventriculomegaly with a single measurement: the width of the lateral ventricular atrium. Radiology 169: 711–714

66. Carlan S J, O'Brien W F, O'Leary T D, Mastrogiannis D 1992 Randomised comparative trial of indomethacin and sulindac for the treatment of refractory preterm labor. Obstetrics and Gynecology 79: 223–228

67. Carlson D E, Platt L D, Medearis A L, Horenstein J 1990 Quantifiable poly-hydramnios: diagnosis and management. Obstetrics and Gynecology 75: 989–993

68. Carroll S G, Porter H, Abdel-Fattah S, Kyle P M, Soothill P W 2000 Correlation of prenatal ultrasound diagnosis and pathologic findings in fetal brain abnormalities. Ultrasound Obstetrics and Gynaecology 16: 149–153

69. Carroll S G, Soothill P W, Abdel-Fattah S, Porter H, Montague I, Kyle P M 2002 Prediction of chorionicity in twin pregnancies at 10–14 weeks of gestation. British Journal of Obstetrics and Gynaecology 109:182–186

70. Castillo R A, Devoe L D, Falls G, Holzman G B, Hadi H A, Fadel H E 1987 Pleural effusions and pulmonary hypoplasia. American Journal of Obstetrics and Gynecology 157: 1252–1255

71. Chamberlain P F, Manning F A, Morrison I, Harman C R, Lange I R 1984 Ultrasound evaluation of AFV. II. The relationship of increased AFV to perinatal outcome. American Journal of Obstetrics and Gynecology 150: 250–254

72. Chernick V, Reed M H 1970 Pneumothorax and chylothorax in the neonatal period. Journal of Pediatrics 76: 624–632

73. Chervenak F A, Isaacson G, Blakemore K J et al 1983 Fetal cystic hygroma. Causes and natural history. New England Journal of Medicine 309: 822–825

74. Chien P F, Arnott N, Gordon A, Owen P, Khan K S 2000 How useful is uterine artery Doppler flow velocimetry in the prediction of pre-eclampsia, intrauterine growth retardation and perinatal death? An overview. British Journal of Obstetrics and Gynaecology 107: 196–208

75. Chinn D H, Filly R A, Callen P W 1983 Congenital diaphragmatic hernia diagnosed prenatally by ultrasound. Radiology 148: 119–123

76. Chitkara U, Cogswell C, Norton K, Wilkins I A, Mehalek K, Berkowitz R L 1988 Choroid plexus cysts in the fetus: a benign anatomic variant or pathological entity? Report of 41 cases and review of the literature. Obstetrics and Gynecology 72: 185–189

77. Chitkara U, Wilkins I, Lynch L, Mehalek K, Berkowitz R L 1988 The role of sonography in assessing severity of fetal anemia in Rh and Kell iso-immunised pregnancies. Obstetrics and Gynecology 71: 393–398

78. Chitty L S, Hunt G H, Moore J, Lobb M O 1991 Effectiveness of routine ultrasonography in detecting fetal structural abnormalities in a low risk population. British Medical Journal 303: 1165–1169

79. Chodirker B N, Harman C R, Greenburg C R 1988 Spontaneous resolution of a cystic hygroma in a fetus with Turner syndrome. Prenatal Diagnosis 8: 291–296

80. Chua S, Ostman-Smith I, Sellers S, Redman C W G 1991 Congenital heart block with hydrops fetalis treated with high-dose dexamethasone: a case report. Journal of Obstetrics and Gynecology and Reproductive Biology 42: 155–158

81. Chudleigh P, Pearce M J, Campbell S 1984 The prenatal diagnosis of transient cysts of the fetal choroid plexus. Prenatal Diagnosis 4: 135–137

82. Cicero S, Bindra R, Rembouskos G, Spencer K, Nicolaides K H 2003 Integrated ultrasound and biochemical screening for trisomy 21 using fetal nuchal translucency, absent fetal nasal bone, free beta-hCG and PAPP-A at 11 to 14 weeks. Prenatal Diagnosis 23: 306–310

83. Cicero S, Curcio P, Papageorghiou A, Sonek J, Nicolaides K 2001 Absence of nasal bone in fetuses with trisomy 21 at 11–14 weeks of gestation: an observational study. Lancet 358: 1665–1667

84. Colin Y, Cherif Zahar B, Le Van Kim C, Raynal V, van Huffel V, Cartron JP 1991 Genetic basis of the RhD positive and RhD negative blood group poly-morphism as determined by Southern analysis. Blood 78: 2747–2752

85. Copel J A, Cullen M, Green J J, Mahoney M J, Hobbins J C, Kleinman C S 1988 The frequency of aneuploidy in prenatally diagnosed congenital heart disease: an indication for fetal karyotyping. American Journal of Obstetrics and Gynecology 158: 409–413

86. Copel J A, Grannum P A, Belanger K, Green J, Hobbins J C 1988 Pulsed Doppler flow–velocity waveforms before and after intrauterine intravascular transfusion for severe erythroblastosis fetalis. American Journal of Obstetrics and Gynecology 158: 768–774

87. Cradock-Watson J E, Miller E, Ridehalgh M K S, Terry G M, Ho-Terry L 1989 Detection of rubella virus in fetal and placental tissues and in the throats of neonates after serologically confirmed rubella in pregnancy. Prenatal Diagnosis 9: 91–96

88. Crowther CA 2003 Anti-D administration in pregnancy for preventing Rhesus alloimmunisation (Cochrane Review). In: The Cochrane Library, Issue 2

89. Cuckle H, Wald N J, Thompson N G 1987 Estimating a woman's risk of having a pregnancy associated with Down's syndrome using her age and maternal serum alpha-fetoprotein level. British Journal of Obstetrics and Gynaecology 94: 387–402

90. D'Alton M E, Dudley D K 1989 The ultrasonographic prediction of chorionicity in twin gestation. American Journal of Obstetrics and Gynecology 160: 557–561

91. Daffos F, Capella-Pavlovsky M, Forestier F 1983 Fetal blood sampling via the umbilical cord using a needle guided by ultrasound. Report of 66 cases. Prenatal Diagnosis 3: 271–277

92. Daffos F, Capella-Pavlovsky M, Forestier F 1985 Fetal blood sampling during pregnancy with use of a needle guided by ultrasound: a study of 606 consecu-tive cases. American Journal of Obstetrics and Gynecology 153: 655–660

93. Daffos F, Forestier F, Capella-Pavlovsky M et al 1988 Prenatal management of 746 pregnancies at risk for congenital toxoplasmosis. New England Journal of Medicine 318: 271–275

94. Daffos F, Forestier F, Kaplan C, Cox W 1988 Prenatal diagnosis and manage-ment of bleeding disorders with fetal blood sampling. American Journal of Obstetrics and Gynecology 158: 939–946

95. Dallaire L, Potier M 1986 Amniotic fluid. In: Milunsky A (ed) Genetic disor-ders and the fetus. Plenum Press, New York, pp 53–67

96. Dashe J S, McIntire D D, Ramus R M, Santos-Ramos R, Twickler D M 2002 Hydramnios: anomaly prevalence and sonographic detection. Obstetrics and Gynecology 100: 134–139

97. Davis G K, Farquhar C M, Allan L D, Crawford D C, Chapman M G 1990 Structural cardiac abnormalities in the fetus: reliability of prenatal diagnosis and outcome. British Journal of Obstetrics and Gynaecology 97: 27–31

98. Davis L E, Tweed G V, Chin T D et al 1971 Intrauterine diagnosis of cytomegalovirus infection: viral recovery from amniocentesis fluid. American Journal of Obstetrics and Gynecology 109: 1217–1219

99. de Crespigny L, Robinson H P 1986 Amniocentesis: a comparison of 'moni-tored' versus 'blind' needle insertion technique. Australian and New Zealand Journal of Obstetrics and Gynecology 26: 124–128

100. de Lia J E, Kuhlmann R S, Harstad T W, Cruikshank D P 1995 Fetoscopic laser ablation of placental vessels in severe previable twin-twin transfusion syndrome. American Journal of Obstetrics and Gynecology 172: 1202–1211

101. de Lia J E, Rogers J G, Dixon J A 1985 Treatment of placental vasculature with a neodymium-yttrium-aluminum-garnet laser via fetoscopy. American Journal of Obstetrics and Gynecology 151: 1126–1127

102. de Vries L, Connell J, Bydder J M et al 1988 Recurrent intracranial haemorrhages in utero in an infant with alloimmune thrombocytopenia. British Journal of Obstetrics and Gynaecology 95: 299–302

103. Denbow M L, Batten M, Kyle P, Fogliani R, Johnson P, Fisk N M 1997 Selective termination of monochorionic twin pregnancy discordant for fetal abnormality. British Journal of Obstetrics and Gynaecology 104: 626–627

104. Denbow M L, Battin M, Cowan F, Azzopardi D, Edwards A, Fisk N 1998 Neonatal cranial ultrasonographic findings in preterm twins complicated by severe feto-fetal transfusion syndrome. American Journal of Obstetrics and Gynecology 178: 479–483

105. Denbow M L, Cox P, Talbert D, Fisk N M 1998 Colour Doppler energy insonation of placental vasculature in monochorionic twins: absent arterio-arterial anastomoses in association with twin-twin transfusion syndrome. British Journal of Obstetrics and Gynaecology 105: 760–765

106. Denbow M L, Cox P, Taylor M, Hammal D, Fisk N M 2000 Placental angioarchitecture in monochorionic twin pregnancies: relationship to fetal growth, feto-fetal transfusion syndrome and pregnancy outcome. American Journal of Obstetrics and Gynecology 182: 417–426

107. Denbow M L, Fogliani R, Kyle P, Letsky E, Nicolini U, Fisk N 1998 Haematological indices at fetal blood sampling in monochorionic pregnancies complicated by feto-fetal transfusion syndrome. Prenatal Diagnosis 18: 941–946

108. Denbow M L, Overton T, Duncan K, Cox P, Fisk N 1999 High failure rate of umbilical vessel occlusion by ultrasound guided injection of absolute alcohol or enbucrilate gel. Prenatal Diagnosis 19: 527–532

109. Desmonts G, Couvreur J 1974 Congenital toxoplasmosis: a prospective study of 378 pregnancies. New England Journal of Medicine 290: 1110–1116

110. Dommergues M, Mandelbrot L, Delezoide A L et al 1995 Twin-to-twin transfusion syndrome: selective feticide by embolization of the hydropic fetus. Fetal Diagnosis and Therapy 10: 26–31

111. Duncan K, Denbow M L, Fisk N 1997 The aetiology and management of twin-twin transfusion syndrome. Prenatal Diagnosis 17: 1227–1236

112. Dunstan F D, Nix A B 1998 Screening for Down's syndrome: the effect of test date on the detection rate. Annals of Clinical Biochemistry 35: 57–61

113. Eady R A J, Gunner D B, Rodeck C H, Garner A 1983 Prenatal diagnosis of oculocutaneous albinism by electron microscopy of fetal skin. Journal of Investigative Dermatology 80: 210–212

114. Ebenroth E S, Cordes T M, Darragh R K 2001 Second-line treatment of fetal supraventricular tachycardia using flecainide acetate. Pediatric Cardiology 22: 483–487

115. Eddelman K, Stone J, Lynch L, Berkowitz R 2002 Selective termination of anomalous fetuses in multifetal pregnancies: two hundred cases at a single center. American Journal of Obstetrics and Gynecology 187: 1168–1172

116. Eichenbaum S Z, Krumins E J, Fortune D W, Duke J 1986 False negative finding on chorionic sampling (letter). Lancet ii: 391

117. Elder J S, Duckett J W, Snyder H M 1987 Intervention for fetal obstructive uropathy: has it been effective? Lancet ii: 1007–1010

118. Elias J, Mazur M, Sabbhaga R, Esterly J, Simpson J L 1980 Prenatal diagnosis of harlequin ichthyosis. Clinical Genetics 17: 275–279

119. Elliot J P, Sawyer S T, Radin T G, Strong R E 1994 Large-volume therapeutic amniocentesis in the treatment of hydramnios. Obstetrics and Gynecology 84: 1025–1027

120. Elser H J, Borutto F, Schneider A, Schneider K 1983 Chylothorax in a twin pregnancy of 34 weeks – sonographically diagnosed. European Journal of Obstetrics, Gynaecology and Reproductive Biology 16: 205–211

121. Enders G, Jonatha W 1987 Prenatal diagnosis of intrauterine rubella. Infection 15: 162–164

122. Enders G, Nickerl-Pacher U, Miller E, Cradock-Watson J E 1988 Outcome of confirmed periconceptual maternal rubella. Lancet 1: 1445–1447

123. Engelhardt J F, Schlossberg H, Yankaskas J R, Dudus L 1995 Progenitor cells of the adult human airway involved in submucosal gland development. Development 121: 2031–2046

124. Eurofetus 2003 Endoscopic access to the fetoplacental unit. www.eurofetus.org

125. Evans M, Fletcher J C, Zador I E, Newton B W, Quigg M H, Struyk C D 1988 Selective first-trimester termination in octuplet and quadruplet pregnancies: clinical and ethical issues. Obstetrics and Gynecology 71: 289–296

126. Evans M I, Goldberg J D, Dommergues M et al 1994 Efficacy of second-trimester selective termination for fetal abnormalities: international collaborative experience among the world's largest centers. American Journal of Obstetrics and Gynecology 171: 90–94

127. Evans M, Krivchenia E, Gelber S, Wapner R 2003 Selective reduction. Clinics in Perinatology 30: 103–111

128. Evans M, Wapner R, Ayoub M, Shalhoub A, Feldman B, Yaron Y 2002 Spontaneous abortions in couples declining multifetal pregnancy reduction. Fetal Diagnosis and Therapy 17: 343–346

129. Eydoux P, Choiset A, Le Porrier N et al 1989 Chromosomal prenatal diagnosis: study of 936 cases of intrauterine abnormalities after ultrasound assessment. Prenatal Diagnosis 9: 255–268

130. Fakhry J, Reiser M, Shapiro L R, Schechter A, Pait L, Glennon A 1986 Increased echogenicity in the lower fetal abdomen: a common normal variant in the second trimester. Journal of Ultrasound in Medicine 5: 489–492

131. Farrant P T 1980 The antenatal diagnosis of oesophageal atresia by ultrasound. British Journal of Radiology 53: 1202–1203

132. Feingold M, Cetrulo C L, Newton E R, Weiss J, Shakr C, Shmoys S 1986 Serial amniocenteses in the treatment of twin-twin transfusion with acute polyhydramnios. Acta Geneticae Medicinae et Gemellologicae 35: 107–113

133. Fermont L, de Geeter B, Aubry M C, Kachener J, Sidi D 1985 A close collaboration between obstetricians and cardiologists allows antenatal detection of severe cardiac malformation by 2D echocardiography. In: Second World Congress of Paediatric Cardiology. Springer-Verlag, New York, p. 10

134. Filly R 1989 Level 1, level 2, level 3 obstetric sonography: I'll see your level and raise you one (letter). Radiology 172: 312

135. Filly R A, Golbus M S 1982 Ultrasonography of the normal and pathological fetal skeleton. Radiology Clinics of North America 20: 311–323

136. Filly R A, Golbus M S, Carey J C, Hall J G 1981 Short-limbed dwarfism: ultrasonic diagnosis by mensuration of the fetal femoral length. Radiology 138: 653–656

137. Finberg H J 1992 The 'twin-peak' sign: reliable evidence of dichorionic twinning. Journal of Ultrasound in Medicine 11: 571–577

138. Finning K M, Martin P G, Soothill P W, Avent N D 2002 Prediction of fetal D status from maternal plasma: introduction of a new noninvasive fetal RHD genotyping service. Transfusion 42: 1079–1085

139. Firth H V, Boyd P A, Chamberlain P F, MacKenzie I Z, Lindenbaum R H, Huson SM 1991 Severe limb abnormalities after chorion villus sampling at 56–66 days gestation. Lancet 337: 762–763

140. Firth H V, Boyd P A, Chamberlain P F, MacKenzie I Z, Morriss-Kay G M, Huson S M 1994 Analysis of limb reduction defects in babies exposed to chorion villus sampling. Lancet 343: 1069–1071

141. Fisk N M 1988 Modifications to selective conservative management in preterm premature rupture of the membranes. Obstetric and Gynecological Survey 43: 328–334

142. Fisk N, Borrell A, Hubinont C, Tannirandorn Y, Nicolini U, Rodeck C 1990 Fetofetal transfusion syndrome: do the neonatal criteria apply in utero? Archives of Diseases in Childhood 65: 657–661

143. Fisk N M, Ronderos-Dumit D, Soliani A, Nicolini U, Vaughan J I, Rodeck C H 1991 Diagnostic and therapeutic transabdominal amnioinfusion in oligohydramnios. Obstetrics and Gynecology 78: 270–278

144. Fisk N M, Tannirandorn Y, Nicolini U, Talbert D G, Rodeck C H 1990 Amniotic pressure in disorders of amniotic fluid volume. Obstetrics and Gynecology 76: 210–214

145. Fisk N M, Tannirandorn Y, Santolaya J, Nicolini U, Letsky E A, Rodeck C H 1989 Fetal macrocytosis in association with chromosomal abnormalities. Obstetrics and Gynecology 74: 611–616

146. Fiske C E, Filly R A, Callen P W 1981 Sonographic measurement of lateral ventricular width in early ventricular dilatation. Journal of Clinical Ultrasound 9: 303–307

147. Flack N J, Zosmer N, Bennett P R, Vaughan J, Fisk N M 1993 Amiodarone given by 3 routes to terminate fetal atrial flutter associated with severe hydrops. Obstetrics and Gynecology 82: 714–716

148. Flake A, Crombleholme T, Johnson M, Howell L, Adzick S 2000 Treatment of severe congenital diaphragmatic hernia by fetal tracheal occlusion: clinical experience with 15 cases. American Journal of Obstetrics and Gynecology 183: 1059–1066

149. Flake A W, Harrison M R, Adzick N S, Laberge J M, Warsof S L 1986 Fetal sacrococcygeal teratoma. Journal of Pediatric Surgery 21: 563–566

150. Flake A W, Roncarolo M G, Puck J M et al 1996 Treatment of X-linked severe combined immunodeficiency by in utero transplantation of paternal bone marrow. New England Journal of Medicine 335: 1806–1810

151. Forestier F, Daffos F, Galacteros F, Bardakjian J, Rainaut M, Beuzard Y 1986 Hematological values of 163 normal fetuses between 18 and 30 weeks of gestation. Pediatric Research 20: 342–346

152. Forestier F, Daffos F, Rainout M, Bruneau M, Trivin F 1987 Blood chemistry of normal human fetuses at mid-trimester of pregnancy. Pediatric Research 21: 579–583

153. Freedman A, Johnson M, Smith C, Gonzalez R, Evans M 1999 Longterm outcome in children after antenatal intervention for obstructive uropathies. Lancet 354: 374–377

154. Friedman J M, Aster R H 1985 Neonatal alloimmune thrombocytopenic purpura and congenital porencephaly in two siblings associated with a 'new' maternal antiplatelet antibody. Blood 65: 1412–1415

155. Frohn-Mulder I, Stewart P, Witsenburg M, Den Hollander N, Wladimiroff J, Hess J 1995 The efficacy of flecainide versus digoxin in the

155. management of fetal supraventricular tachycardia. Prenatal Diagnosis 15: 1297–1302

156. Froster U G, Jackson L 1996 Limb defects and chorionic villus sampling: results from an international registry, 1992–94. Lancet 347: 489–494

157. Furness M E 1987 Choroid plexus cysts and trisomy 18 (letter). Lancet ii: 693

158. Furness M E, Barbary J E, Verco P W 1987 Fetal head shape in spina bifida in the second trimester. Journal of Clinical Ultrasound 15: 451–453

159. Fusi L, Gordon H 1990 Twin pregnancy complicated by single intrauterine death. Problems and outcome with conservative management. British Journal of Obstetrics and Gynaecology 97: 511–516

160. Fusi L, McParland P, Fisk N, Nicolini U, Wigglesworth J 1991 Acute twin-twin transfusion: a possible mechanism for brain-damaged survivors after intrauterine death of a monochorionic twin. Obstetrics and Gynecology 78: 517–520

161. Gardosi J, Mongelli M 1993 Risk assessment adjusted for gestational age in maternal serum screening for Down's syndrome. British Medical Journal 306: 1509–1511

162. Ghidini A, Sepulveda W, Lockwood C, Romero R 1993 Complications of fetal blood sampling. American Journal of Obstetrics and Gynecology 168: 1339–1344

163. Giannakoulopoulos X, Sepulveda W, Kourtis P, Glover V, Fisk N 1994 Fetal plasma cortisol and beta-endorphin response to intrauterine needling. Lancet 344: 77–81

164. Giannakoulopoulos X, Teixeira J, Fisk N, Glover V 1999 Human fetal and maternal noradrenaline responses to invasive procedures. Paediatric Research 45: 494–499

165. Gilbert W M, Nicolaides K H 1987 Fetal omphalocele: associated malformations and chromosomal defects. Obstetrics and Gynecology 70: 633–635

166. Glick P L, Harrison M R, Adzick N S, Noall R A, Villa R L 1984 Correction of congenital hydronephrosis in utero. IV: In utero decompression prevents renal dysplasia. Journal of Pediatric Surgery 19: 649–657

167. Glick P L, Harrison M R, Golbus M S et al 1985 Management of the fetus with congenital hydronephrosis. II: Prognostic criteria and selection for treatment. Journal of Pediatric Surgery 20: 376–387

168. Glick P L, Harrison M R, Noall R A, Villa R L 1983 Correction of congenital hydronephrosis in utero. III: early mid-trimester ureteral obstruction produces renal dysplasia. Journal of Pediatric Surgery 18: 681–687

169. Golbus M S, Sagebiel R W, Filly R A, Gindhart T D, Hall J G 1980 Prenatal diagnosis of bullous ichthyosiform erythroderma (epidermolysis hyperkeratosis) by fetal skin biopsy. New England Journal of Medicine 302: 93–95

170. Goldstein R B, Filly R B, Callen P W 1989 Sonography of anencephaly: pitfalls in early diagnosis. Journal of Clinical Ultrasound 17: 397–402

171. Gonsoulin W, Moise K, Kirshon B, Cotton D, Wheeler J, Carpenter R 1990 Outcome of twin-twin transfusion diagnosed before 28 weeks of gestation. Obstetrics and Gynecology 75: 214–216

172. Grannum P A, Ghidini A, Scioscia A, Copel J A, Romero R, Hobbins J C 1989 Assessment of fetal renal reserve in low level obstructive uropathy. Lancet i: 281–282

173. Gregg N M 1941 Cataract following German measles in the mother. Transactions of the Ophthalmic Society of Australia 3: 34–36

174. Groom K M, Shennan A H, Bennett P R 2002 Ultrasound-indicated cervical cerclage: outcome depends on preoperative cervical length and presence of visible membranes at time of cerclage. American Journal of Obstetrics and Gynaecology 187: 445–449

175. Groves A M, Allan L D, Rosenthal E 1993 Therapeutic use of inotropes in complete heart block in the fetus. British Heart Journal 69: 17 (Abstract)

176. Hackett G A, Nicolaides K H, Campbell S 1987 Doppler ultrasound assessment of fetal and uteroplacental circulations in severe second trimester oligohydramnios. British Journal of Obstetrics and Gynaecology 94: 1074–1077

177. Haddow J E, Palomaki G E, Knight G J, Cunningham G C, Lustig L S, Boyd PA 1994 Reducing the need for amniocentesis in women 35 years of age or older with serum markers for screening. New England Journal of Medicine 330: 1114–1118

178. Handyside A H, Lesko J G, Tarin J J, Winston R M, Hughes M R 1992 Birth of a normal girl after in vitro fertilization and preimplantation diagnostic testing for cystic fibrosis. New England Journal of Medicine 327: 905–909

179. Hanson F W, Zorn E M, Tennant F R, Marianos S, Samuels S 1987 Amniocentesis before 15 weeks gestation: outcome, risks and technical problems. American Journal of Obstetrics and Gynecology 156: 1524–1531

180. Harman C R 1995 Invasive techniques in the management of alloimmune anaemia. In: Harman C R (ed) Invasive fetal testing and treatment. Blackwell Science, Boston, pp 107–192

181. Harrison M R, Adzick N S, Flake A W, Jennings R W 1993 The CDH two-step, a dance of necessity. Journal of Pediatric Surgery 28: 813–816

182. Harrison M, Albanese C, Hawgood S et al 2001 Fetoscopic temporary tracheal occlusion by means of detachable balloon for congenital diaphragmatic hernia. American Journal of Obstetrics and Gynecology 185: 730–733

183. Harrison M R, Bressack M A, Churg A M, de Lorimier A A 1980 Correction of congenital diaphragmatic hernia in utero. II: Simulated correction permits fetal lung growth with survival at birth. Surgery 88: 260–268

184. Harrison M R, Filly R A, Parer J T, Faer M J, Jacobson J B, de Lorimier A A 1981 Management of the fetus with a urinary tract malformation. Journal of the American Medical Association 246: 635–639

185. Harrison M R, Golbus M S, Filly R A et al 1982 Management of the fetus with congenital hydronephrosis. Journal of Pediatric Surgery 17: 728–742

186. Harrison M R, Langer J C, Adzick N S et al 1990 Correction of congenital diaphragmatic hernia in utero. V: Initial clinical experience. Journal of Pediatric Surgery 25: 47–57

187. Harrison M R, Nakayama D K, Noall R, de Lorimier A A 1982 Correction of congenital hydronephrosis in utero. II: Decompression reverses the effects of obstruction on the fetal lung and urinary tract. Journal of Pediatric Surgery 17: 965–974

188. Harrison M R, Ross N A, Noall R, de Lorimier A A 1983 Correction of congenital hydronephrosis in utero. I: The model: fetal urethral obstruction produces hydronephrosis and pulmonary hypoplasia in fetal lambs. Journal of Pediatric Surgery 18: 247–256

189. Hecher K, Campbell S, Doyle P, Harrington K, Nicolaides K 1995 Assessment of fetal compromise by Doppler ultrasound investigation of the fetal circulation. Arterial, intracardiac and venous blood flow studies. Circulation 91: 129–138

190. Hecher K, Ville Y, Nicolaides K 1995 Fetal arterial Doppler studies in twin-twin transfusion syndrome. Journal of Ultrasound in Medicine 14: 101–108

191. Hecher K, Ville Y, Snijders R, Nicolaides K 1995 Doppler studies of the fetal circulation in twin-twin transfusion syndrome. Ultrasound in Obstetrics and Gynecology 5: 318–324

192. Hegde U M 1985 Immune thrombocytopenia in pregnancy and the newborn. British Journal of Obstetrics and Gynaecology 92: 657–659

193. Hegge F N, Franklin R W, Watson P T, Clahoun B C 1989 An evaluation of the time of discovery of fetal malformations by an indication-based system for ordering obstetric ultrasound. Obstetrics and Gynecology 74: 21–24

194. Hislop A, Fairweather D V I, Blackwell R J, Howard S 1984 The effect of amniocentesis and drainage of amniotic fluid on lung development in *Macaca fascicularis*. American Journal of Obstetrics and Gynecology 91: 835–842

195. Hobbins J C, Mahoney M J 1974 In utero diagnosis of haemoglobinopathies: technic for obtaining fetal blood. New England Journal of Medicine 290: 1065–1067

196. Hobbins J C, Romero R, Grannum P, Berkowitz T R L, Cullen M, Mahoney M J 1984 Antenatal diagnosis of renal anomalies with ultrasound. I. Obstructive uropathy. American Journal of Obstetrics and Gynecology 148: 868–877

197. Hohlfield P, Daffos F, Costa J, Thulliez P, Forestier F, Vidaud M 1994 Prenatal diagnosis of congenital toxoplasmosis with a polymerase-chain-reaction test on amniotic fluid. New England Journal of Medicine 331: 695–699

198. Holmes H, Harrison M R, Baskin L S 2001 Fetal surgery for posterior urethral valves: long-term postnatal outcomes. Pediatrics 108: E7

199. Hsu L Y F, Perlis T E 1984 The United States survey on chromosome mosaicism and pseudomosaicism in prenatal diagnosis. Prenatal Diagnosis 4: 97–130

200. Hudon L, Moise K J Jr, Hegemier S E et al 1998 Long-term neurodevelopmental outcome after intrauterine transfusion for the treatment of fetal hemolytic disease. American Journal of Obstetrics and Gynecology 179: 858–863

201. Hull D, Binns B A, Joyce D 1966 Congenital heart block and widespread fibrosis due to maternal lupus erythematosus. Archives of Diseases of Childhood 41: 688–690

202. Hunter A G W 1987 Neonatal lung function following mid-trimester amniocentesis. Prenatal Diagnosis 7: 431–441

203. Hunter A, Denbow M, Bartha J, Abdul-Fattah S, Soothill P, Kyle P 2004 Use of middle cerebral artery Doppler velocities to time invasive procedures in pregnancies affected by Rhesus D alloimmunisation. Submitted for publication

204. Hyett J, Perdu M, Sharland G, Snijders R, Nicolaides K H 1999 Using fetal nuchal translucency to screen for major congenital cardiac defects at 10–14 weeks of gestation: population based cohort study. British Medical Journal 318: 81–85

205. Isada N B, Pryde P G, Johnson M P, Hallak M, Blessed W B, Evans M I 1992 Fetal intracardiac potassium chloride injection to avoid the hopeless resuscitation of an abnormal abortus: I. Clinical issues. Obstetrics and Gynecology 80: 296–299

206. Itskowitz J, Boldes R, Thaler I et al 1989 Transvaginal ultrasonography-guided aspiration of gestational sacs for selective abortion in multiple pregnancy. American Journal of Obstetrics and Gynecology 160: 215–217

207. Jackson L G, Zachary J M, Fowler S E, Desnick R J, Golbus M S, Ledbetter D 1992 A randomized comparison of transcervical and transabdominal chorionic-villus sampling. New England Journal of Medicine 327: 594–598

208. Jauniaux E, Donner C, Simon P, Vanesse M, Hustin J, Rodesch F 1989 Pathological aspects of the umbilical cord after percutaneous umbilical blood sampling. Obstetrics and Gynecology 73: 215–218

209. Johnson L G, Olsen J C, Sarkadi B, Moore K L, Swanstrom R, Boucher R C 1992 Efficiency of gene transfer for restoration of normal airway epithelial function in cystic fibrosis. Nature Genetics 2: 21–25

210. Johnson M P, Bukowski T P, Reitleman C, Isada N B, Pryde P G, Eraus M I 1994 In utero surgical treatment of fetal obstructive uropathy: a new comprehensive approach to identify appropriate candidates for vesicoamniotic shunt therapy. American Journal of Obstetrics and Gynecology 170: 1770–1779

211. Kalousek D K, Dill F J 1983 Chromosomal mosaicism confined to the placenta in human conceptions. Science 221: 665–667

212. Kan Y W, Dozy A M 1978 Antenatal diagnosis of sickle cell anaemia by DNA analysis of amniotic-fluid cells. Lancet ii: 910

213. Kan Y W, Valenti C, Giudotti R, Carnazza V, Rieder R F 1974 Fetal blood sampling in utero. Lancet i: 79–80

214. Kaplan C, Daffos F, Forestier F et al 1988 Management of alloimmune thrombocytopenia: antenatal diagnosis and in utero transfusion of maternal platelets. Blood 72: 340–343

215. Kappel B, Nielsen J, Hansen K B, Mikklesen M, Therkelsen A A J 1987 Spontaneous abortion following mid-trimester amniocentesis. Clinical significance of placental perforation and blood stained amniotic fluid. British Journal of Obstetrics and Gynaecology 94: 50–54

216. Kellner L H, Weiner Z, Weiss R R et al 1995 Triple marker (α-fetoprotein, unconjugated estriol, human chorionic gonadotropin) versus α-fetoprotein plus free-β subunit in second-trimester maternal serum screening for fetal Down syndrome: a prospective comparison study. American Journal of Obstetrics and Gynecology 173: 1306–1309

217. Kelton J G, Inwood M J, Barr R M et al 1982 The prenatal prediction of thrombocytopenia in infants of mothers with clinically diagnosed immune thrombocytopenia. American Journal of Obstetrics and Gynecology 144: 449–454

218. King S J, Pilling D W, Walkinshaw S 1995 Fetal echogenic lung lesions: prenatal ultrasound diagnosis and outcome. Pediatric Radiology 25: 208–210

219. Kirshon B, Mari G, Moise K J 1990 Indomethacin therapy in the treatment of symptomatic polyhydramnios. Obstetrics and Gynecology 75: 202–205

220. Kirshon B, Moise K J, Wasserstrum N, Ou C, Huhta J C 1988 Influence of short term indomethacin therapy on fetal urine output. Obstetrics and Gynecology 72: 51–53

221. Kleinman C S, Copel J A, Weinstein E M, Santulli T V, Hobbins J C 1985 In utero diagnosis and treatment of fetal supraventricular tachycardia. Seminars in Perinatology 9: 113–129

222. Kohl T, Tercanli S, Kececioglu D, Holzgreve W 1995 Direct fetal administration of adenosine for the termination of incessant supraventricular tachycardia. Obstetrics and Gynecology 85: 873–874

223. Koresawa M, Inaba J, Iwasaki H 1987 Fetal blood sampling by liver puncture. Acta Obstetrica et Gynaecologica Japonica 39: 395–399

224. Kostovic I, Rakic P 1990 Developmental history of the transient subplate zone in the visual and somatosensory cortex of the macaque monkey and human brain. J Comp Neurol 297: 441–470

225. Kuliev A M, Modell B, Jackson L et al 1993 Risk evaluation of CVS. Prenatal Diagnosis 13: 197–209

226. Kurth K H, Alleman E R, Schroeder F H 1981 Major and minor complications of posterior urethral valves. Journal of Urology 126: 517–519

227. Kussef B G, Matsouka L Y, Stenn K S, Hobbins J C, Mahoney M J, Hashimoto K 1982 Prenatal diagnosis of Sjögren–Larsson syndrome. Journal of Pediatrics 101: 998–1001

228. Kyle P M, Sepulveda W, Blunt S, Davies G, Cox P M, Fisk N M 1996 High failure rate of postmortem karyotyping after termination for fetal abnormality. Obstetrics and Gynecology 88: 859–862

229. Landwehr J B, Johnson M P, Hume R F, Yaron Y, Sokol R J, Evans M I 1996 Abnormal nuchal findings on screening ultrasonography: aneuploidy stratification on the basis of ultrasonographic anomaly and gestational age at detection. American Journal of Obstetrics and Gynecology 175: 995–999

230. Lange I, Rodeck C H, Morgan-Capner P et al 1982 Prenatal serological diagnosis of intrauterine cytomegalovirus infection. British Medical Journal 284: 1673–1674

231. Langer J C, Fitzgerald P G, Desa D et al 1990 Cervical cystic hygroma in the fetus: clinical spectrum and outcome. Journal of Pediatric Surgery 25: 58–62

232. Langer J C, Harrison M R, Scmidt K G et al 1989 Fetal hydrops and death from sacrococcygeal teratoma: rationale for fetal surgery. American Journal of Obstetrics and Gynecology 160: 1145–1150

233. Laurence K M, Coates S 1962 The natural history of hydrocephalus: detailed analysis of 182 unoperated cases. Archives of Disease in Childhood 37: 345–362

234. Ledbetter D H, Martin A O, Verlinsky Y et al 1990 Cytogenetic results of chorionic villus sampling: high success rate and diagnostic accuracy in the United States collaborative study. American Journal of Obstetrics and Gynecology 162: 495–501

235. Lee S, Bennett P, Overton T, Warwick R, Wu X, Redman C 1996 Prenatal diagnosis of Kell blood group genotypes: KEL1 and KEL2. American Journal of Obstetrics and Gynecology 175: 455–459

236. Levi S, Crouzet P, Schaaps J P et al 1989 Ultrasound screening for fetal malformations. Lancet i: 678

237. Linch D C, Rodeck C H, Nicolaides K H, Jones H M, Brent L 1986 Attempted bone marrow transplantation in a 17 week fetus. Lancet ii: 1453

238. Lipitz S, Ryan G, Samuell C et al 1993 Fetal urine analysis for the assessment of renal function in obstructive uropathy. American Journal of Obstetrics and Gynecology 168: 174–179

239. Lo Y M, Hjelm N M, Fidler C et al 1998 Prenatal diagnosis of fetal RhD status by molecular analysis of maternal plasma. New England Journal of Medicine 339: 1734–1738

240. Loft A G, Hogdall E, Larsen S O, Norgaard-Pedersen B 1993 A comparison of amniotic fluid alpha-fetoprotein and acetylcholinesterase in the prenatal diagnosis of open neural tube defects and anterior abdominal wall defects. Prenatal Diagnosis 13: 93–109

241. Longaker M T, Laberge J, Dansereau J et al 1989 Primary fetal hydrothorax: natural history and management. Journal of Pediatric Surgery 24: 573–576

242. Luck C A 1992 Value of routine ultrasound scanning at 19 weeks: a four-year study of 8894 deliveries. British Medical Journal 304: 1474–1478

243. McCullagh M, MacConnachie I, Garvie D, Dykes E 1994 Accuracy of prenatal diagnosis in congenital cystic adenomatoid malformation. Archives of Disease in Childhood. Fetal and Neonatal Edition 71: F111–F113

244. Machado M V L, Tynan M J, Curry P V L, Allan L D 1988 Fetal complete heart block. British Heart Journal 60: 512–515

245. Machin G, Still K, Lalani T 1996 Correlations of placental vascular anatomy and clinical outcomes in 69 monochorionic twin pregnancies. American Journal of Medical Genetics 61: 229–236

246. Mahieu-Caputo D, Muller F, Joly D et al 2001 Pathogenesis of twin-twin transfusion syndrome: the renin-angiotensin system hypothesis. Fetal Diagnosis and Therapy 16: 241–244

247. Mahoney B S, Filly R A, Callen P W, Hricak H, Golbus M S, Harrison M R 1984 Fetal renal dysplasia: sonographic evaluation. Radiology 152: 143–146

248. Mamopoulos M, Assimakopoulos E, Reece E, Andreou A, Zheng X, Mantelenakis S 1990 Maternal indomethacin therapy in the treatment of polyhydramnios. American Journal of Obstetrics and Gynecology 162: 1225–1229

249. Mandelbrot L, Dumez Y, Muller F, Dommergues M 1991 Prenatal prediction of renal function in fetal obstructive uropathies. Journal of Perinatal Medicine 19: 283–297

250. Manning F A, Harison M R, Rodeck C H and members of the International Fetal Medicine and Surgery Society 1986 Catheter shunts for fetal hydronephrosis and hydrocephalus. New England Journal of Medicine 315: 336–340

251. Mari G, Deter R L, Carpenter R L et al 2000 Noninvasive diagnosis by Doppler ultrasonography of fetal anemia due to maternal red-cell alloimmunization. Collaborative Group for Doppler Assessment of the Blood Velocity in Anemic Fetuses. New England Journal of Medicine 342: 9–14

252. Mari G, Roberts A, Detti L et al 2001 Perinatal morbidity and mortality rates in severe twin-twin transfusion syndrome: results of the International Amnioreduction Registry. American Journal of Obstetrics and Gynecology 185: 708–715

253. Mari G, Wasserstrum N, Kirshon B 1992 Reduction in the middle cerebral artery pulsatility index after decompression of polyhydramnios in twin gestation. American Journal of Perinatology 9: 381–384

254. Maxwell D J, Crawford D C, Curry P V, Tynan M J, Allan L D 1988 Obstetric importance, diagnosis and management of fetal tachycardias. British Medical Journal 297: 107–110

255. Maxwell D, Johnson P, Hurley P, Neales K, Allan L, Knott P 1991 Fetal blood sampling and pregnancy loss in relation to indication. British Journal of Obstetrics and Gynaecology 98: 892–897

256. Medical Research Council Working Party on Amniocentesis 1978 An assessment of the hazards of amniocentesis. British Journal of Obstetrics and Gynaecology 85: suppl. 2

257. Megerian G, Ludomirsky A 1994 Role of cordocentesis in perinatal medicine. Current Opinion in Obstetrics and Gynaecology 6: 30–35

258. Mercer L J, Brown L G 1986 Fetal outcome with oligohydramnios in second trimester. Obstetrics and Gynecology 67: 840–842

259. Meuli M, Meuli-Simmen C, Hutchins G M et al 1995 In utero surgery rescues neurological function at birth in sheep with spina bifida. Nature Medicine 1: 342–347

260. Mibashan R S, Rodeck C H 1984 Haemophilia and other genetic defects of haemostasis. In: Rodeck C H, Nicolaides K H (eds) Prenatal diagnosis. Proceedings of the eleventh study group of the Royal College of Obstetricians and Gynaecologists. RCOG, London, pp 179–194

261. Michejda M, Hodgen G D 1981 In utero diagnosis and treatment of non-human primate fetal skeletal anomalies. I: Hydrocephalus. Journal of the American Medical Association 246: 1093–1097

262. Mikkelsen M, Ayme S 1987 Chromosome findings in chorionic villi. A collaborative study. In: Vogel F, Sperling K (eds) Human genetics: Proceedings of the Seventh International Congress. Springer-Verlag, Berlin, pp 597–606

263. Millar D S, Davis L R, Rodeck C H, Nicolaides K H, Mibashan R S 1985 Normal blood cell values in the early mid-trimester fetus. Prenatal Diagnosis 5: 367–373

264. Mohr J 1968 Foetal genetic diagnosis: development of techniques for early sampling of foetal cells. Acta Pathologica, Microbiologica et Immunologica Scandinavica 73: 73–77

265. Moise K J, Carpenter R J, Cotton D B, Wasserstrum N, Kirshon B, Cano L 1988 Percutaneous umbilical cord blood sampling in the evaluation of fetal platelet counts in pregnant patients with autoimmune thrombocytopenic purpura. Obstetrics and Gynecology 72: 346–350

266. Moise K J, Huhta J C, Sharif D S et al 1988 Indomethacin in the treatment of premature labor. Effects on fetal ductus arteriosus. New England Journal of Medicine 319: 327–331

267. Moniz C F, Nicolaides K H, Bamforth F J, Rodeck C H 1985 Normal ranges for biochemical substances relating to renal, hepatic and bone function in fetal and maternal plasma throughout pregnancy. Journal of Clinical Pathology 38: 468–472

268. Monteagudo A, Timor-Tritsch I E, Sharma S 1994 Early and simple determination of chorionic and amniotic type in multifetal gestations in the first fourteen weeks by high-frequency transvaginal ultrasonography. American Journal of Obstetrics and Gynecology 170: 824–829

269. Montemagno R, Soothill P W, Scarcelli M, Rodeck C H 1995 Disappearance of fetal choroid plexus cysts during the second trimester in cases of chromosomal abnormality. British Journal of Obstetrics and Gynaecology 102: 752–753

270. Moore T R, Cayle J E 1990 The amniotic fluid index in normal human pregnancy. American Journal of Obstetrics and Gynecology 162: 1168–1173

271. Moore T R, Longo J, Leopold G R, Casola G, Gosnik B B 1989 The reliability and predictive value of an amniotic fluid scoring system in severe second trimester oligohydramnios. Obstetrics and Gynecology 73: 739–742

272. Morales W J, Stroup M 1985 Intracranial hemorrhage in utero due to isoimmune neonatal thrombocytopenia. Obstetrics and Gynecology 65: 20S–21S

273. Morgan-Capner P, Rodeck C H, Nicolaides K H, Cradock-Watson J A 1985 Prenatal detection of rubella-specific IgM in fetal sera. Prenatal Diagnosis 5: 21–26

274. Muller F, Aubry M C, Gasser B, Duchatel F, Boue J, Boue A 1985 Prenatal diagnosis of cystic fibrosis. II. Meconium ileus in affected fetuses. Prenatal Diagnosis 5: 109–117

275. Muller F, Dommergues M, Mandelbrot L, Aubry M C, Fekete C, Dumez Y 1993 Fetal urinary biochemistry predicts postnatal renal function in children with bilateral obstructive uropathies. Obstetrics and Gynecology 82: 813–820

276. Muller-Eckhardt C, Grubert A, Weisheit M 1989 348 cases of suspected neonatal alloimmune thrombocytopenia. Lancet i: 363–366

277. Nakayama D K, Harrison M R, Chinn D H et al 1985 Prenatal diagnosis and natural history of the fetus with a congenital diaphragmatic hernia: initial clinical experience. Journal of Pediatric Surgery 20: 118–124

278. Nakayama D K, Harrison M R, de Lorimier A A 1986 Prognosis of posterior urethral valves presenting at birth. Journal of Pediatric Surgery 21: 43–45

279. National Institute for Clinical Excellence 2003 Routine anti-D prophylaxis for rhesus negative women. NICE guideline No. 41. nice.org.uk

280. National Institutes for Health Consensus Development Statement 1984 United States Department of Health and Human Services (NIH publication 84-667), Washington DC

281. National Institutes of Child Health and Human Development 1976 Mid-trimester amniocentesis for prenatal diagnosis. Safety and accuracy. Journal of the American Medical Association 236: 1471–1476

282. Neilson J P, Alfirevic Z 2003 Doppler ultrasound for fetal assessment in high risk pregnancies (Cochrane Review). In: The Cochrane Library, Issue 2

283. Neilson J, Danskin F, Hastie S 1989 Monozygotic twin pregnancy: diagnostic and Doppler ultrasound studies. British Journal of Obstetrics and Gynaecology 96: 1413–1418

284. Nelson L H, Clark C E, Fishburn J I, Urban R B, Penry M F 1982 Value of serial ultrasonography in the in utero detection of duodenal atresia. Obstetrics and Gynecology 59: 657–660

285. Ney J A, Fee S C, Dooley S L, Socol M L, Minogue J 1989 Factors influencing hemostasis after umbilical vein puncture in vitro. American Journal of Obstetrics and Gynecology 160: 424–426

286. Nicolaides K H, Azar G B 1990 Thoraco-amniotic shunting. Fetal Diagnosis and Therapy 5: 153–164

287. Nicolaides K H, Bilardo C M, Campbell S 1990 Prediction of fetal anemia by measurement of the mean blood velocity in the fetal aorta. American Journal of Obstetrics and Gynecology 162: 209–212

288. Nicolaides K H, Bilardo C M, Soothill P W, Campbell S 1988 Absence of end-diastolic frequencies in the umbilical artery: a sign of fetal hypoxia and acidosis. British Medical Journal 297: 1026–1027

289. Nicolaides K H, Blott M, Greenough M 1987 Chronic drainage of fetal pulmonary cyst (letter). Lancet i: 618

290. Nicolaides K H, Brizot M L, Snijders R J M 1994 Fetal nuchal translucency: ultrasound screening for fetal trisomy in the first trimester of pregnancy. British Journal of Obstetrics and Gynaecology 101: 782–786

291. Nicolaides K H, Brizot M, Patel F, Snijders R 1994 Comparison of chorionic villus sampling and amniocentesis for fetal karyotyping at 10–13 weeks gestation. Lancet 344: 435–439

292. Nicolaides K H, Campbell S, Gabbe S G, Giudetti R 1986 Ultrasound screening for spina bifida: cranial and cerebellar signs. Lancet ii: 71–74

293. Nicolaides K H, Clewell W H, Mibashan R S, Soothill P W, Rodeck C H, Campbell S 1988 Fetal haemoglobin measurement in the assessment of red cell isoimmunization. Lancet i: 1073–1075

294. Nicolaides K H, Clewell W H, Rodeck C H 1987 Measurement of human fetoplacental blood volume in erythroblastosis fetalis. American Journal of Obstetrics and Gynecology 157: 50–53

295. Nicolaides K H, Economides D L 1990 Cordocentesis of small-for-gestational age fetuses. In: Chamberlain G (ed) Modern antenatal care of the fetus. Blackwell Science, Oxford, pp 127–149

296. Nicolaides K H, Economides D L, Soothill P W 1989 Blood gases, pH, and lactate in appropriate- and small-for-gestational-age fetuses. American Journal of Obstetrics and Gynecology 161: 996–1001

297. Nicolaides K H, Fontanorosa M, Gabbe S G, Rodeck C H 1988 Failure of ultrasonographic parameters to predict the severity of fetal anemia in rhesus isoimmunisation. American Journal of Obstetrics and Gynecology 158: 920–926

298. Nicolaides K H, Rodeck C H, Gosden C N 1986 Rapid karyotyping in non-lethal malformations. Lancet i: 283–287

299. Nicolaides K H, Rodeck C H, Lange I et al 1985 Fetoscopy in the assessment of unexplained fetal hydrops. British Journal of Obstetrics and Gynaecology 92: 671–679

300. Nicolaides K H, Rodeck C H, Mibashan R S 1985 Obstetric management and diagnosis of haematological disease in the fetus. Clinics in Haematology 14: 775–805

301. Nicolaides K H, Soothill P W, Rodeck C H, Campbell S 1986 Ultrasound guided sampling of umbilical cord and placental blood to assess fetal well-being. Lancet i: 1065–1067

302. Nicolaides K H, Soothill P W, Rodeck C H, Clewell W 1986 Rh disease: intravascular fetal blood transfusion by cordocentesis. Fetal Therapy 1: 185–192

303. Nicolini U, Fisk N M, Rodeck C 1992 Fetal urine biochemistry: an index of renal maturation and dysfunction. British Journal of Obstetrics and Gynaecology 99: 46–50

304. Nicolini U, Fisk N M, Rodeck C H, Talbert D G, Wigglesworth J S 1989 Low amniotic pressure in oligohydramnios – is this the cause of pulmonary hypoplasia? American Journal of Obstetrics and Gynecology 161: 1098–1101

305. Nicolini U, Hubinont C, Santolaya J, Fisk N M, Coe A, Rodeck C H 1989 Maternal–fetal glucose gradient in normal pregnancies and in pregnancies complicated by alloimmunization and fetal growth retardation. American Journal of Obstetrics and Gynecology 161: 924–927

306. Nicolini U, Kochenour N K, Greco P et al 1988 Consequences of fetomaternal haemorrhage after intrauterine transfusion. British Medical Journal 297: 1379–1381

307. Nicolini U, Kochenour N K, Greco P, Letsky E, Rodeck C H 1989 When to perform the next intrauterine transfusion in patients with Rh allo-immunization: combined intravascular and intraperitoneal transfusion allows longer intervals. Fetal Therapy 4: 14–20

308. Nicolini U, Nicolaidis P, Fisk N M et al 1990 Limited role of fetal blood sampling in predicting outcome in intrauterine growth retardation. Lancet ii: 768–772

309. Nicolini U, Nicolaidis P, Fisk N M, Tannirandorn Y, Rodeck C H 1990 Fetal blood sampling from the intrahepatic vein: analysis of safety and clinical experience with 214 procedures. Obstetrics and Gynecology 76: 47–53

310. Nicolini U, Poblete A, Boschetto C, Bonati F, Roberts A 2001 Complicated monochorionic twin pregnancies: experience with bipolar cord coagulation. American Journal of Obstetrics and Gynecology 185: 703–707

311. Nicolini U, Rodeck C H, Kochenour N K et al 1988 In-utero platelet transfusion for alloimmune thrombocytopenia. Lancet ii: 506

312. Nicolini U, Santolaya J, Hubinont C, Fisk N M, Maxwell D, Rodeck C H 1989 Visualization of fetal intra-abdominal organs in second trimester severe oligohydramnios by intraperitoneal infusion. Prenatal Diagnosis 9: 191–194

313. Nicolini U, Santolaya J, Ojo E et al 1988 The fetal intrahepatic vein as an alternative to cord needling for prenatal diagnosis and therapy. Prenatal Diagnosis 8: 665–671

314. Nicolini U, Talbert D G, Fisk N M, Rodeck C H 1989 Pathophysiology of pressure changes during intrauterine transfusion. American Journal of Obstetrics and Gynecology 160: 1139–1145

315. Nicolini U, Tannirandorn Y, Gonzalez P et al 1990 Continuing controversy in alloimmune thrombocytopenia: fetal hyperimmunoglobulinemia fails to prevent thrombocytopenia. American Journal of Obstetrics and Gynecology 163: 1144–1146

316. Nicolini U, Tannirandorn Y, Vaughan J, Fisk N, Nicolaidis P, Rodeck C H 1991 Further predictors of renal dysplasia in fetal obstructive uropathy: bladder pressure and biochemistry of 'fresh urine'. Prenatal Diagnosis 11: 159–166

317. Nyberg D, Fitzsimmons J, Mack L 1989 Chromosomal abnormalities in fetuses with omphalocele: significance of omphalocele contents. Journal of Ultrasound in Medicine 8: 299–308

318. Oepkes D, Brand R, Vandembusschel F P, Meerman R H, Kanhai H H 1994 The use of ultrasonography and Doppler in the prediction of fetal haemolytic anaemia: a multivariate study. British Journal of Obstetrics and Gynaecology 101: 680–684

319. Oepkes D, Vandenbussche F P, Van Bel F, Kanhai H H 1993 Fetal ductus venosus blood flow velocities before and after treatment of red cell alloimmunised pregnancies. Obstetrics and Gynecology 82: 237–241

320. Old J M, Ward R H T, Petrou M et al 1982 First trimester diagnosis of haemoglobinopathies: three cases. Lancet ii: 1413–1416

321. OPCS 1997 Birth Statistics. Review of the Register General on births and patterns of family building in England and Wales. HMSO, London

322. Orlandi F, Damiani G, Jakil C, Lauricella S, Bertolino O, Maggio A 1990 The risks of early cordocentesis (12–21 weeks): analysis of 500 procedures. Prenatal Diagnosis 10: 425–428

323. Ostlere S J, Irving H C, Lilford R J 1989 A prospective study of the incidence and significance of fetal choroid plexus cysts. Prenatal Diagnosis 9: 205–211

324. Ouzounian J G, Castro M A, Fresquez M, Al-Sulyman O M, Kovacs B W 1996 Prognostic significance of antenatally detected fetal pyelectasis. Ultrasound in Obstetrics and Gynecology 7: 424–428

325. Paek B, Jennings R, Harrison M et al 2001 Radiofrequency ablation of human fetal sacrococcygeal teratoma. American Journal of Obstetrics and Gynecology 184: 503–507

326. Papageorghiou A T, Liao A W, Skentou C, Sebire N J, Nicolaides K H 2002 Trichorionic triplet pregnancies at 10–14 weeks: outcome after embryo reduction compared to expectant management. Journal of Maternal Fetal and Neonatal Medicine 11: 307–312

327. Payne S D, Resnik R, Moore T R, Hedriana H L, Kelly T F 1997 Maternal characteristics and risk of severe neonatal thrombocytopenia and intracranial haemorrhage in pregnancies complicated by autoimmune thrombocytopenia. American Journal of Obstetrics and Gynecology 177: 149–155

328. Peault B, Tirouvanziam R, Sombardier M N, Chen S, Perricaudet M, Gaillard D 1994 Gene transfer to human fetal pulmonary tissue developed in immunodeficient SCID mice. Human Gene Therapy 5: 1131–1137

329. Peckham C S, Johnson C, Ades A, Pearl K, Chin K S 1987 Early acquisition of cytomegalovirus infection. Archives of Disease in Childhood 62: 780–785

330. Penman D G, Fisher R M, Noblett H R, Soothill P W 1998 Increase in incidence of gastroschisis in the south west of England in 1995. British Journal of Obstetrics and Gynaecology 105: 328–331

331. Peters M T, Nicolaides K H 1990 Cordocentesis for the diagnosis and treatment of human fetal parvovirus infection. Obstetrics and Gynecology 75: 501–504

332. Petres R E, Redwine F O, Cruickshank D P 1982 Congenital bilateral hydrothorax: antepartum diagnosis and successful intrauterine surgical management. Journal of the American Medical Association 248: 1360–1361

333. Petterson B, Nelson K, Watson L, Stanley F 1993 Twins, triplets, and cerebral palsy in births in Western Australia in the 1980s. British Medical Journal 307: 1239–1243

334. Pilu G, Reece E A, Romero R, Bovicelli L, Hobbins J C 1986 Prenatal diagnosis of craniofacial malformations by ultrasound. American Journal of Obstetrics and Gynecology 155: 45–50

335. Pilu G, Romero R, Reece A, Goldstein I, Hobbins J C, Bovicelli L 1988 Subnormal cerebellum in fetuses with spina bifida. American Journal of Obstetrics and Gynecology 158: 1052–1056

336. Pilu G, Romero R, Rizzo N, Jeanty P, Bovicelli L, Hobbins J C 1987 Criteria for the antenatal diagnosis of holoprosencephaly. American Journal of Perinatology 4: 41–49

337. Poissonier M-H, Brossard Y, Demedeiros N et al 1989 Two hundred intrauterine exchange transfusions in severe blood incompatibilities. American Journal of Obstetrics and Gynecology 161: 709–713

338. Public Health Laboratory Service Working Party on Fifth Disease 1990 Prospective study of human parvovirus B19 infections in pregnancy. British Medical Journal 300: 1166–1170

339. Queenan J T 1970 Recurrent acute polyhydramnios. American Journal of Obstetrics and Gynecology 106: 625–626

340. Quintero R A, Dickinson J E, Morales W J et al 2003 Stage-based treatment of twin-twin transfusion syndrome. American Journal of Obstetrics and Gynecology 188: 1333–1340

341. Quintero R, Morales W, Allen M, Bornick P, Johnson P, Kruger M 1999 Staging of twin-twin transfusion syndrome. Journal of Perinatology 19: 550–555

342. Radder C M, Brand A, Kanhai H H 2001 A less invasive treatment strategy to prevent intracranial hemorrhage in fetal and neonatal alloimmune thrombocytopenia. American Journal of Obstetrics and Gynecology 185: 683–688

343. Reid R S, Sepulveda W, Kyle P M, Davies G 1996 Amniotic fluid culture failure and clinical significance and association with aneuploidy. Obstetrics and Gynecology 87: 588–592

344. Reuss A, Wladimiroff J W, Stewart P A, Scholtmeijer R J 1988 Non-invasive management of fetal obstructive uropathy. Lancet ii: 949–951

345. Revello M G, Percivalle E, Baldanti F 1993 Prenatal treatment of congenital human cytomegalovirus infection by fetal intravascular administration of ganciclovir. Clinical and Diagnostic Virology 1: 61–67

346. Reznikoff-Etievant M F 1988 Management of alloimmune neonatal thrombocytopenia and antenatal thrombocytopenia. Vox Sanguinis 55: 193–201

347. Rizzo G, Arduini D, Romanini C 1994 Cardiac and extracardiac flows in discordant twins. American Journal of Obstetrics and Gynecology 170: 1321–1327

348. Roberts A B, Clarkson N S, Pattison M G, Mok P M 1986 Fetal hydrothorax in the second trimester of pregnancy: successful intrauterine treatment at 24 weeks gestation. Fetal Therapy 1: 203–209

349. Roberts A B, Mitchell J M, Pattison N S 1989 Fetal liver length in normal and isoimmunized pregnancies. American Journal of Obstetrics and Gynecology 161: 42–46

350. Roberts L J, Bewley S, Mackinson A M, Rodeck C H 1995 First trimester fetal nuchal translucency: problems with screening the general population. 1. British Journal of Obstetrics and Gynaecology 102: 381–385

351. Rochelson B, Schulman H, Farmakides G et al 1987 The significance of absent end-diastolic velocity in umbilical artery velocity waveforms. American Journal of Obstetrics and Gynecology 155: 1213–1218

352. Rodeck C H 1980 Fetoscopy guided by real time ultrasound for pure fetal blood samples, fetal skin samples, and examination of the fetus in utero. British Journal of Obstetrics and Gynaecology 87: 449–456

353. Rodeck C H 1993 Fetal development after chorionic villus sampling. Lancet 341: 468–469

354. Rodeck C H, Campbell S 1979 Umbilical cord insertion as a source of pure fetal blood for prenatal diagnosis. Lancet i: 1244–1245

355. Rodeck C H, Eady R A J, Gosden C M 1980 Prenatal diagnosis of epidermolysis bullosa letalis. Lancet i: 949–952

356. Rodeck C H, Fisk N M, Fraser D I, Nicolini U 1988 Long-term in utero drainage of fetal hydrothorax. New England Journal of Medicine 319: 1135–1138

357. Rodeck C H, Holman C A, Karnicki J, Kemp J, Whitmore D N, Austin M A 1981 Direct intravascular fetal blood transfusion by fetoscopy in severe rhesus isoimmunisation. Lancet i: 625–627

358. Rodeck C H, Nicolini U 1988 Physiology of the mid-trimester fetus. British Medical Bulletin 44: 826–849

359. Rodis J, Hovick T J, Quinn D L, Rosengren S S, Tattersall P 1988 Human parvovirus infection in pregnancy. Obstetrics and Gynecology 72: 733–738

360. Roelofsen J, Oostendorp R, Volovics A, Hoogland H 1994 Prenatal diagnosis and fetal outcome of cystic adenomatoid malformation of the lung: case report and historical survey. Ultrasound in Obstetrics and Gynecology 4: 78–82

361. Romero R, Chervenak F A, Kotzen J, Berkowitz R L, Hobbins J C 1982 Antenatal sonographic findings of extralobar pulmonary sequestration. Journal of Ultrasound in Medicine 1: 131–132

362. Romero R, Cullen M, Jeanty P et al 1984 The diagnosis of congenital renal anomalies with ultrasound: II. Infantile polycystic kidney disease. American Journal of Obstetrics and Gynecology 150: 259–262

363. Romero R, Jeanty P, Reece E A et al 1985 Sonographically monitored amniocentesis to decrease intraoperative complications. Obstetrics and Gynecology 65: 426–430

364. Romero R, Pilu G, Pilu G, Jeanty P, Ghidini A, Hobbins J 1988 Prenatal diagnosis of congenital anomalies. Appleton and Lange, Connecticut

365. Royal College of Obstetricians and Gynaecologists 2003 Clinical guidelines: use of anti-D immunoglobulin for Rh prophylaxis. www.rcog.org.uk

366. Royal College of Obstetricians and Gynaecologists Working Party on Routine Ultrasound Examination in Pregnancy 1984 RCOG, London, pp 13–16

367. Salvodelli G, Schmid W, Schinzel A 1982 Prenatal diagnosis of cleft lip and palate by ultrasound. Prenatal Diagnosis 2: 313–317

368. Samuels P, Bussel J B, Braitman L E et al 1990 Estimation of the risk of thrombocytopenia in the offspring of pregnant women with presumed immune thrombocytopenic purpura. New England Journal of Medicine 323: 229–235

369. Sandri F, Pilu G, Cerisoli M, Bovicelli L, Alvisi C, Salvioli G P 1988 Sonographic diagnosis of agenesis of the corpus callosum in the fetus and newborn infant. American Journal of Perinatology 5: 226–231

370. Saunders N, Snijders R, Nicolaides K 1992 Therapeutic amniocentesis in twin-twin transfusion syndrome appearing in the second trimester of pregnancy. American Journal of Obstetrics and Gynecology 166: 820–824

371. Scardo J A, Ellings J M, Newman R B 1995 Prospective determination of chorionicity, amnionicity, and zygosity in twin gestations. American Journal of Obstetrics and Gynecology 173: 1376–1380

372. Schmidt W, Harms E, Wolf D 1985 Successful prenatal treatment of non-immune hydrops fetalis due to congenital chylothorax. British Journal of Obstetrics and Gynaecology 92: 671–679

373. Schwarz T F, Roggendorf M, Hottentrager B et al 1988 Human parvovirus B19 infection in pregnancy. Lancet ii: 566–567

374. Scioscia A L, Grannum P A T, Copel J A, Hobbins J C 1988 The use of percutaneous umbilical blood sampling in immune thrombocytopenic purpura. American Journal of Obstetrics and Gynecology 159: 1066–1068

375. Sebire N, Snijders R, Hughes K, Sepulveda W, Nicolaides K 1997 The hidden mortality of monochorionic twin pregnancies. British Journal of Obstetrics and Gynaecology 104: 1203–1207

376. Sebire N, Souka A, Skentou H, Geerts L, Nicolaides K 2000 Early prediction of severe twin-to-twin transfusion syndrome. Human Reproduction 15: 2008–2010

377. Seller M J, Polani P E 1986 Experimental chimerism in a genetic defect in the house mouse *Mus musculus*. Nature 212: 80–86

378. Sepulveda W, Stagiannis K D, Flack N J, Fisk N M 1995 Prenatal diagnosis of renal agenesis using color flow imaging in severe second-trimester oligohydramnios. American Journal of Obstetrics and Gynecology 173: 1788–1792

379. Sharland G, Allan L 1992 Screening for congenital heart disease prenatally. Results of a 2-year study in the South East Thames Region. British Journal of Obstetrics and Gynaecology 99: 220–225

380. Sheikh A U, Ernest J M, O'Shea M 1992 Long-term outcome in fetal hydrops from parvovirus B19 infection. American Journal of Obstetrics and Gynecology 167: 337–341

381. Simoni G, Brambatti B, Danesino C 1983 Efficient direct chromosome analyses and enzyme determination from chorionic villi samples in the first trimester of pregnancy. Human Genetics 63: 349–357

382. Simpson N E, Dallaire L, Miller J R, Siminovich L, Hamerton J L, Mckeen C 1976 Prenatal diagnosis of genetic disease in Canada: report of a collaborative study. Canadian Medical Association Journal 115: 739–748

383. Smidt-Jensen S, Permin M, Philip J et al 1992 Randomised comparison of amniocentesis and transabdominal and transcervical chorionic villus sampling. Lancet 340: 1238–1244

384. Snijders R J M, Farrias M, von Kaisenberg C, Nicolaides K H 1996 Fetal abnormalities. In: Snijders R J M, Nicolaides K H (eds) Ultrasound markers for fetal chromosomal defects. Parthenon Publishing, London, pp 1–62

385. Snijders R J, Noble P, Sebire N, Souka A, Nicolaides K H 1998 UK multicentre project on assessment of risk of trisomy 21 by maternal age and fetal nuchal translucency thickness at 10–14 weeks gestation. Lancet 352: 343–346

386. Soothill P W, Nicolaides K H, Rodeck C H 1987 The effect of anaemia on fetal acid/base status. British Journal of Obstetrics and Gynaecology 94: 880–883

387. Souka A P, Snijders R J, Novakov A, Soares W, Nicolaides K H 1998 Defects and syndromes in chromosomally normal fetuses with increased nuchal translucency thickness at 10–14 weeks of gestation. Ultrasound in Obstetrics and Gynecology 11: 391–400

388. Spencer K, Carpenter P 1993 Prospective study of prenatal screening for Down's syndrome with free β-HCG. British Medical Journal 307: 764–769

389. Spencer K, Souter V, Tul N, Snijders R, Nicolaides K H 1999 A screening program for trisomy 21 at 10–14 weeks using fetal nuchal translucency, maternal serum free beta-human chorionic gonadotropin and pregnancy-associated plasma protein-A. Ultrasound in Obstetrics and Gynecology 13: 231–237

390. Stagiannis K D, Sepulveda W, Southwell D, Price D, Fisk N M 1995 Ultrasonographic measurement of the dividing membrane during the second and third trimesters: a reproducibility study. American Journal of Obstetrics and Gynecology 173: 1546–1550

391. Steinberg L, Hurley V, Desmedt E, Beischer N 1990 Acute polyhydramnios in twin pregnancies. Australian and New Zealand Journal of Obstetrics and Gynaecology 30: 196–200

392. Stephens F D 1983 Congenital malformations of the urinary tract. Praeger, New York, pp 433–462

393. Stewart P A, Wladimiroff J W 1987 Cardiac tachyarrhythmias in the fetus: diagnosis, treatment and prognosis. Fetal Therapy 2: 7–16

394. Stocker J T, Madewell J E, Drake R M 1977 Congenital cystic adenomatoid malformation of the lung. Classification and morphological spectrum. Human Pathology 8: 155–171

395. Stumpflen I, Stumpflen A, Wimmer M, Bernaschek G 1996 Effect of detailed fetal echocardiography as part of routine prenatal ultrasonographic screening on detection of congenital heart disease. Lancet 348: 854–857

396. Szabo J, Gellen J 1990 Nuchal fluid accumulation in trisomy 21 detected by vaginosonography in the first trimester. Lancet 336: 1133

397. Tabor A, Philip J, Madsen M, Bang J, Obel E B, Norgaard-Oedersen B 1986 Randomised controlled trial of genetic amniocentesis in 4606 low risk women. Lancet i: 1287–1293

398. Tan K H, Kilby M D, Whittle M J, Beattie B R, Booth I W, Botting B J 1996 Congenital anterior abdominal wall defects in England and Wales: retrospective analysis of OPCS data. British Medical Journal 313: 303–306

399. Tannirandorn Y, Nicolini U, Nicolaidis P C, Fisk N M, Arulkumaran S, Rodeck C H 1990 Fetal cystic hygromata: insights gained from fetal blood sampling. Prenatal Diagnosis 10: 189–193

400. Taylor M, Denbow M L, Duncan K, Overton T, Fisk N 2000 Antenatal factors at diagnosis that predict outcome in twin-twin transfusion syndrome. American Journal of Obstetrics and Gynecology 183: 1023–1028

401. Teixeira J M, Duncan K, Letsky E, Fisk N M 2000 Middle cerebral artery peak systolic velocity in the prediction of fetal anemia. Ultrasound in Obstetrics and Gynecology 15: 205–208

402. Teixeira J, Fogliani R, Giannakoulopoulos X, Glover V, Fisk N 1996 Fetal haemodynamic stress response to invasive procedures. Lancet 347: 624

403. Teixeira J, Glover V, Fisk N 1999 Acute cerebral redistribution in response to invasive procedures in the human fetus. American Journal of Obstetrics and Gynecology 181: 1018–1025

404. Terry G M, Ho-Terry L, Warren R C, Rodeck C H, Cohen C H, Rees K R 1986 First trimester prenatal diagnosis of congenital rubella: a laboratory investigation. British Medical Journal 292: 930–933

405. Thirkelsen A J 1979 Cell culture and cytogenetic technique. In: Murken J-D, Stengel-Rutkowski S, Schwinger E N (eds) Prenatal diagnosis (Proceedings of the 3rd European Conference on Prenatal Diagnosis of Genetic Disorders). Ferdinand Enke, Stuttgart, pp 258–270

406. Timor-Tritsch I E, Farine D, Rosen M 1988 A close look at early embryonic development with the high frequency transvaginal transducer. American Journal of Obstetrics and Gynecology 159: 676–681

407. Timor-Tritsch I E, Warren W P, Peisner D B, Pirrone E 1989 First-trimester midgut herniation: a high frequency transvaginal sonographic study. American Journal of Obstetrics and Gynecology 161: 831–833

408. Touraine J L, Raudrant D, Royo C et al 1989 In-utero transplantation of stem cells in bare lymphocyte syndrome. Lancet i: 1382

409. Tulipan N, Sutton L N, Bruner J P, Cohen B M, Johnson M, Adzick N S 2003 The effect of intrauterine myelomeningocoele repair on the incidence of shunt-dependent hydrocephalus. Paediatric Neurosurgery 38: 27–33

410. Tulzer G, Arzt W, Franklin R C, Loughna P V, Mair R, Gardiner H M 2002 Fetal pulmonary valvuloplasty for critical pulmonary stenosis or atresia with intact septum. Lancet 360: 1567–1568

411. UK Collaborative Study on Alpha-Fetoprotein in Relation to Neural Tube Defects 1982 Fourth report. Estimating an individual's chance of having a fetus with open spina bifida and the value of repeat alpha-fetoprotein testing. Journal of Epidemiology and Community Health 36: 87–95

412. Van den Hof M C, Nicolaides K H, Campbell J, Campbell S 1990 Evaluation of the lemon and banana signs in one hundred and thirty fetuses with open spina bifida. American Journal of Obstetrics and Gynecology 162: 322–327

413. van Heteren C, Nijhuis J, Semmekrot B, Mulders L, van den Berg P 1998 Risk for surviving twin after fetal death of co-twin in twin-twin transfusion syndrome. Obstetrics and Gynecology 92: 215–219

414. Verjaal M, Leschot N J 1981 Risk of amniocentesis and laboratory findings in a series of 1500 prenatal diagnoses. Prenatal Diagnosis 1: 173–181

415. Ville Y, Hyett J, Hecher K, Nicolaides K H 1995 Preliminary experience with endoscopic laser surgery for severe twin-twin transfusion syndrome. New England Journal of Medicine 332: 224–227

416. von dem Borne A, Decary F 1990 Nomenclature of platelet-specific antigens. Human Immunology 29: 1–2

417. Vyas H, Milner A D, Hopkin I E 1982 Amniocentesis and fetal lung development. Archives of Disease in Childhood 57: 627–628

418. Wald N J, Cuckle H S 1987 Recent advances in screening for neural tube defects and Down's syndrome. Baillière's Clinical Obstetrics and Gynaecology 1: 649–676

419. Wald N, Cuckle H, Boreham J, Stirrat G 1980 Small biparietal diameter of fetuses with spina bifida: implications for antenatal screening. British Journal of Obstetrics and Gynaecology 87: 219–221

420. Wald N J, Cuckle H S, Densem J W et al 1988 Maternal serum screening for Down's syndrome in early pregnancy. British Medical Journal 297: 883–887

421. Wald N J, George L, Smith D, Densem J W, Petterson K 1996 Serum screening for Down's syndrome between 8 and 14 weeks of pregnancy. International Prenatal Screening Research Group. British Journal of Obstetrics and Gynaecology 103: 407–412

422. Wald N, Huttly W, Hackshaw A 2003 Antenatal screening for Down's syndrome with the quadruple test. Lancet 361: 794–795

423. Walker S, Howard P J 1986 Cytogenetic prenatal diagnosis and its relative effectiveness in the Mersey region and North Wales. Prenatal Diagnosis 6: 13–23

424. Weiner C P 1987 Cordocentesis for diagnostic indications: two years' experience. Obstetrics and Gynecology 70: 664–667

425. Weiner C P 1990 Use of cordocentesis in fetal hemolytic disease and autoimmune thrombocytopenia. American Journal of Obstetrics and Gynecology 162: 1126–1127

426. Weiner C P, Okamura K 1996 Diagnostic fetal blood sampling – technique related losses. Fetal Diagnosis and Therapy 11: 169–175

427. Weiner C P, Williamson R, Bonsib S M et al 1986 In utero bladder diversion – problems with patient selection. Fetal Therapy 1: 196–202

428. Weiner E, Zosmer N, Bajoria R et al 1994 Direct fetal administration of immunoglobulins: another disappointing therapy in alloimmune thrombocytopenia. Fetal Diagnosis and Therapy 9: 159–164

429. Weir P, Ratten G, Beischer N 1979 Acute polyhydramnios – a complication of monozygous twin pregnancy. British Journal of Obstetrics and Gynaecology 86: 849–853

430. Wenstrom K D, Syrop C H, Hammitt D G, Van Voorhis B J 1993 Increased risk of monochorionic twinning associated with assisted reproduction. Fertility and Sterility 60: 510–514

431. Whitby E, Paley M N, Davies N, Sprigg A, Griffiths P D 2001 Ultrafast magnetic resonance imaging of central nervous system abnormalities in utero in the second and third trimester of pregnancy: comparison with ultrasound. British Journal of Obstetrics and Gynaecology 108: 519–526

432. Whittle M J, Connor J M 1994 Prenatal diagnosis in obstetric practice, 2nd edn. Blackwell Science, Oxford

433. Wilkins I A, Chitkara U, Lynch L, Goldberg J D, Mehalek K E, Berkowitz R L 1987 The nonpredictive value of fetal urinary electrolytes: preliminary report of outcomes and correlations with pathological diagnosis. American Journal of Obstetrics and Gynecology 157: 694–698

434. Williams C, Weber L, Williamson R, Hielm M 1988 Guthrie spots for DNA-based carrier testing in cystic fibrosis. Lancet ii: 693

435. Williamson L M, Bruce D, Lubenko A, Chana H J, Ouwehand W H 1992 Molecular biology for platelet alloantigen typing. Transfusion Medicine 2: 225–264

436. Wilson J M, Di Fiore J W, Peters C A 1993 Experimental fetal tracheal ligation prevents the pulmonary hypoplasia associated with fetal nephrectomy: possible application for congenital diaphragmatic hernia. Journal of Pediatric Surgery 28: 1433–1440

437. Wladimiroff J W, Stewart P A, Reuss A, Sachs E S 1989 Cardiac and extracardiac anomalies as indicators for trisomies 13 and 18: a prenatal ultrasound study. Prenatal Diagnosis 9: 515–520

438. Worton R G, Stern R 1987 A Canadian collaborative study of mosaicism in amniotic fluid cell cultures. Prenatal Diagnosis 4: 131–144

439. Zanjani E D, Lim G, McGalve P B et al 1982 Adult haematopoietic cells transplanted to sheep fetuses continue to produce adult globins. Nature 295: 244–246

440. Zosmer N, Bajoria R, Weiner E, Rigby M, Vaughan J, Fisk N 1994 Clinical and echographic features of in utero cardiac dysfunction in the recipient twin in twin-twin transfusion syndrome. British Heart Journal 72: 74–79

Fetal growth, intrauterine growth restriction and small-for-gestational-age babies

Philip Baker, Clare Tower

Introduction

Although infants of small size at birth have been described since the mid 17th century, prematurity was the presumed cause until the 1950s. Even in 1950, the World Health Organization (WHO) considered all infants weighing less than 2500 g as premature.[75] The first report of an 'undernourished full-term infant' was published in 1947,[53] leading to the recognition that some infants less than 2500 g were not premature, but were too small.[76] Subsequent work in the 1960s described increased perinatal morbidity and mortality in infants small for their gestational age, thereby identifying them as a clinically significant group.[6,50] In 1966 the first average growth patterns from 28 weeks were published, documenting reduced growth after 40 weeks' gestation and a reduction in growth with smoking, multiple pregnancies and fetal abnormality (Fig. 10.1).[25,62]

Nomenclature and definition

Intrauterine or fetal growth restriction (IUGR/FGR), rather than growth retardation, is now the preferred terminology, due to adverse associations with the latter. IUGR is defined as an infant that has not reached its growth potential.[46] In other words, growth-restricted babies would have been larger without adverse environmental and/or genetic factors affecting growth. In contrast, small for gestational age (SGA) is a statistical concept based on the distribution of birthweight within a population.[36] Studies have varied in the cut-off for SGA between the 3rd and 10th centile for gestation. However, since birthweight is influenced by constitutional factors such as maternal height, weight, ethnicity, parity and infant sex, some babies less than the 10th centile will be appropriately grown for gestation.[18,70] When no underlying cause has been identified, the term SGA is commonly used.

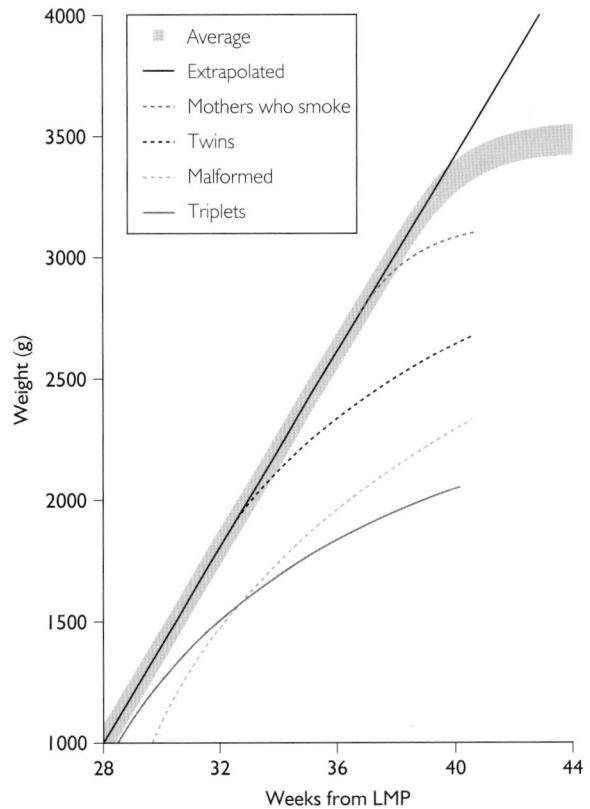

Fig. 10.1 Variation of fetal growth during last trimester of pregnancy. (Adapted from Gruenwald.[25])

Diagnosis

Antenatal diagnosis

The strongest determinant of fetal size is gestational age, hence accurate dating of the pregnancy is vital. There is now growing evidence that ultrasound dating at less than 21–24 weeks is more accurate than dating based on the last menstrual period.[17] However, the majority of units use a combination of certain last menstrual period and ultrasound assessment, only favouring the ultrasound dates if the discrepancy is greater than 7, 10 or 14 days depending on personal preference.

Potentially small fetuses can be clinically identified by measurement of the symphysial–fundal height. After 20 weeks' gestation, the fundal height in centimetres approximates to the number of weeks of gestation, and deviation from this can be used to identify small fetuses. Although a cheap screening tool widely used in antenatal care, it is generally poor at identifying IUGR, due to factors such as subjectivity and maternal build. Sensitivity varies between 60% and 85%, specificity between 80% and 90%, and positive predictive value between 20% and 80%.[69] Therefore, in modern obstetric practice, ultrasound is used to confirm the diagnosis and assess the fetus further.

Ultrasound assessment

It is now generally accepted that measurement of the fetal abdominal circumference is the most sensitive indicator of fetal size (Fig. 10.2).[47] This indicates the nutritional state of the fetus, since it is a measurement of subcutaneous, intra-abdominal and extra-peritoneal fat and liver size.[39] An abdominal circumference of less than the 10th centile on ultrasound scan was found to predict small infants (<10th centile) with an odds ratio (OR) of 13.5 in a low-risk population and 18.4 in a high-risk population.[9] The head circumference should also be measured, although accurate assessments become difficult late in pregnancy due to descent of the fetal head into the pelvis (Fig. 10.3). The combination of head and abdomen measurements can be used to describe the IUGR as *symmetrical*, in which the head and the abdomen are proportionally small, or *asymmetrical*, in which the abdomen is disproportionately small compared with the head.[46] The latter has also been referred to as 'head sparing' and is derived from the assumption that in circumstances of reduced blood supply the fetus diverts blood to 'protect' the head.

It has been suggested that patterns of fetal growth are determined by the timing of any insult. The first 16 weeks of fetal growth represents a period of cellular hyperplasia. From 17 to 32 weeks, there is a period of cellular hypertrophy and hyperplasia, and finally, a phase of (predominantly) hypertrophy follows after 32 weeks. Hence, an insult early in pregnancy, for example a chromosomal abnormality, is believed to produce symmetrical IUGR by reducing overall cell number, whereas an insult later in pregnancy, for example placental insufficiency, produces asymmetrical IUGR. This is undoubtedly a gross oversimplification of

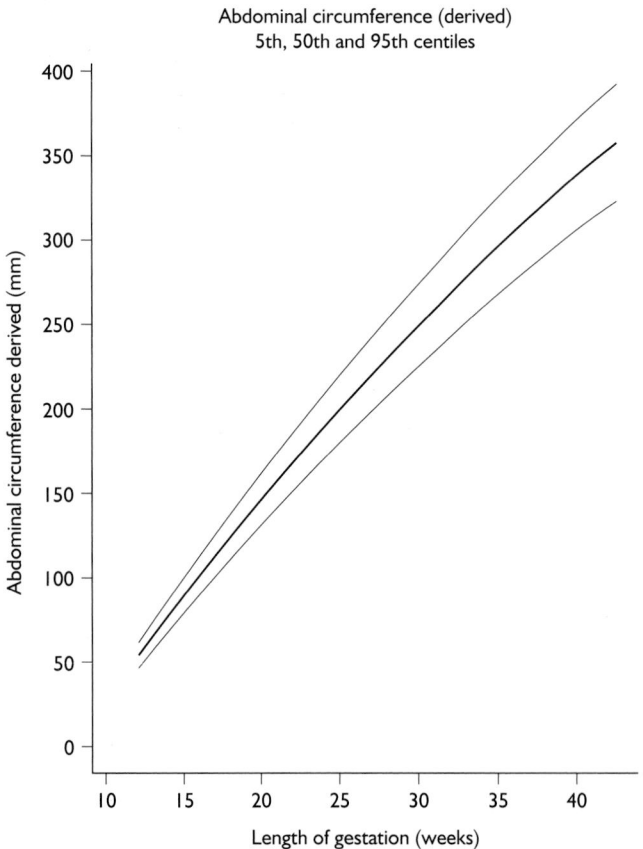

Fig. 10.2 Centile chart for abdominal circumference. (From Chitty L, Altman D G 1993 Charts of fetal size. In: Dewbury K et al (eds) Ultrasound in obstetrics and gynaecology. Churchill Livingstone, Edinburgh.)

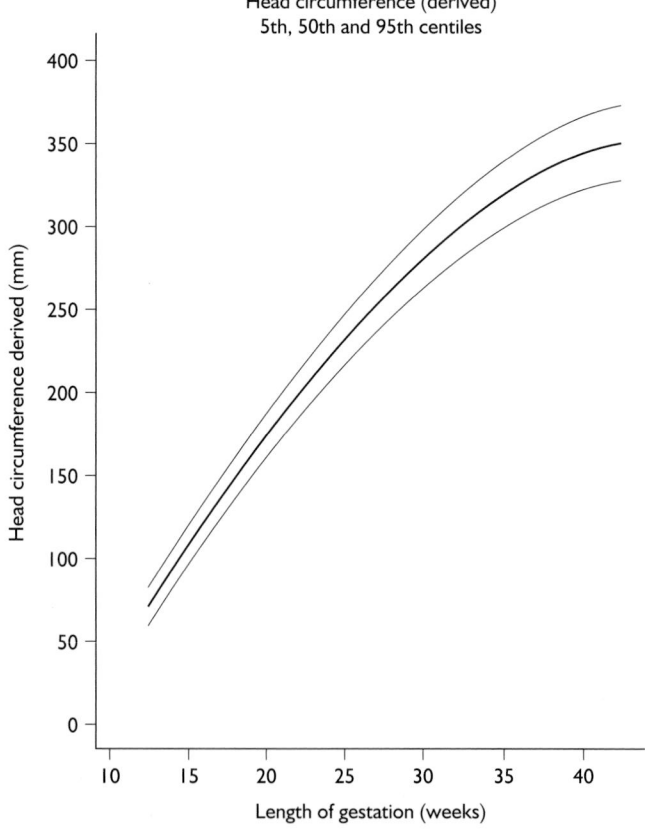

Fig. 10.3 Centile chart for head circumference. (From Chitty L, Altman D G 1993 Charts of fetal size. In: Dewbury K et al (eds) Ultrasound in obstetrics and gynaecology. Churchill Livingstone, Edinburgh.)

the pathophysiology involved, and attempts to correlate these patterns of IUGR with outcome have been conflicting;[12,46] thus, these descriptive terms have limited use as prognostic factors.

Several formulae have been devised to allow estimation of fetal weight from ultrasound measurements. The accuracy of most is ±10%.[69] Although these calculations do not aid significantly in the diagnosis of IUGR, they are helpful in planning delivery and neonatal care (Fig. 10.4). Since growth is a dynamic process, serial measurements every 2–4 weeks should be used to identify any deviation across the centiles.

The diagnosis of IUGR is highly dependent on the centile charts on which the measurements are plotted. Different populations show different characteristics, so, ideally, a chart relevant to the local population should be used. In addition, many of these charts tend to be skewed due to the inclusion or exclusion of certain patient groups. Customised charts are available to take account of factors such as ethnic group but these are rarely practical in a busy antenatal clinic. All these factors contribute to the low predictive ability and high false-positive rate of ultrasound to detect IUGR.

Measurements of fetal size should also be supplemented by assessment of umbilical blood flow and liquor volume as these indicate placental function. Reduced liquor volume (oligohydramnios) is observed on ultrasound in 30% of growth-restricted fetuses.[45] This occurs due to redirection of blood flow away from the fetal kidneys, thus reducing urine output and liquor volume. This is assessed by measuring the maximum pool depth, or more accurately, by adding the pool depth in each four quadrants of

the uterus to produce the amniotic fluid index (AFI). The predictive value of these measurements is not clear, so they are more an adjunct to other elements of the fetal assessment.

Doppler ultrasound can be used to identify changes in the fetal circulation known to be associated with poor placental function. Changes include a reduction in umbilical venous blood flow and increased pulsatility in the umbilical artery and aorta due to increased placental resistance. Reduced pulsatility may be observed in the cerebral arteries, representing reduced resistance and increased flow to this region.

Assessment of blood flow requires knowledge of the vessel diameter, which is difficult for small vessels. Therefore, waveform analysis of the pulsatile flow is utilised. This waveform can be quantified by using the ratio of systolic to diastolic maximum velocity (S/D), the pulsatility index (PI) or the resistance index (RI) (Fig. 10.5).

The PI and RI are more robust than the S/D ratio, therefore are clinically preferable. In normal pregnancy, diastolic flow in the umbilical artery increases as gestation increases, producing a fall in these indices.[28,60]

Umbilical artery (Fig. 10.6)

Increased resistance in the umbilical artery or aorta (increased PI) is associated with low birthweight (LBW), increased risk of operative delivery, increased admission to neonatal units and increased morbidity.[26,27,72] Meta-analyses indicate that the use of Doppler ultrasound to guide clinical decision-making is likely to improve outcomes in pregnancies with suspected growth restriction and pre-eclampsia.[2,55] These meta-analyses found a reduction in perinatal mortality of 38% when Doppler ultrasound was used to guide management. However, late-gestation fetuses (>35 weeks) with IUGR typically have normal umbilical artery Dopplers.[10] Hypoxia is believed to produce peripheral placental angiogenesis that reduces feto-placental (and umbilical) vascular resistance despite compromised uteroplacental blood flow.

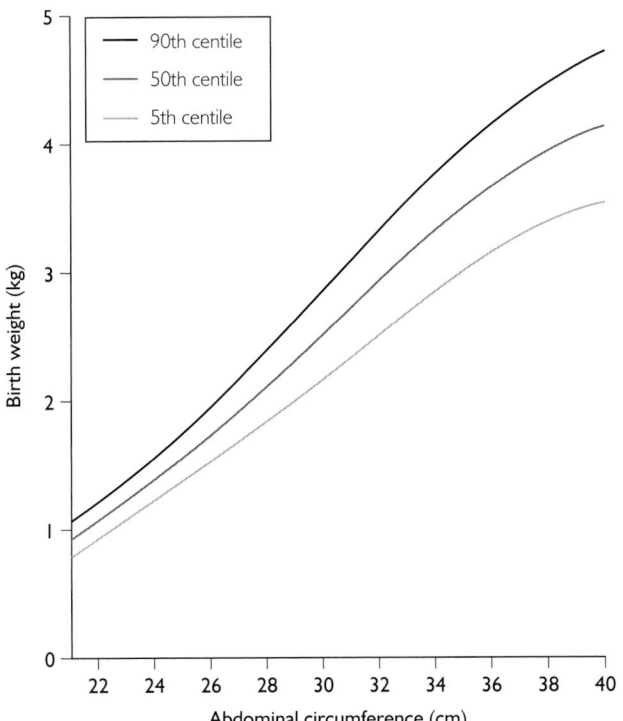

Fig. 10.4 Chart of estimated fetal weight. (From Campbell S, Wilkin D 1975 Ultrasonic measurement of fetal abdomen circumference in the estimation of fetal weight. British Journal of Obstetrics and Gynaecology 82: 689–697.)

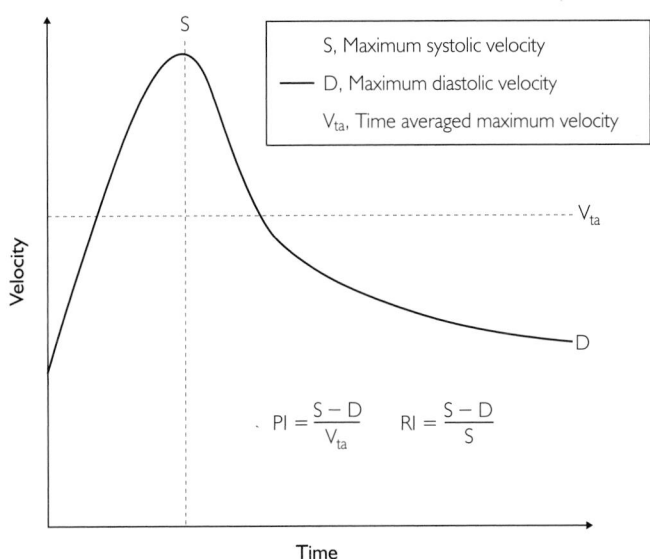

$$PI = \frac{S - D}{V_{ta}} \qquad RI = \frac{S - D}{S}$$

Fig. 10.5 Waveform analysis of pulsatile flow velocity. (Adapted from Kiserud & Marsal.[39])

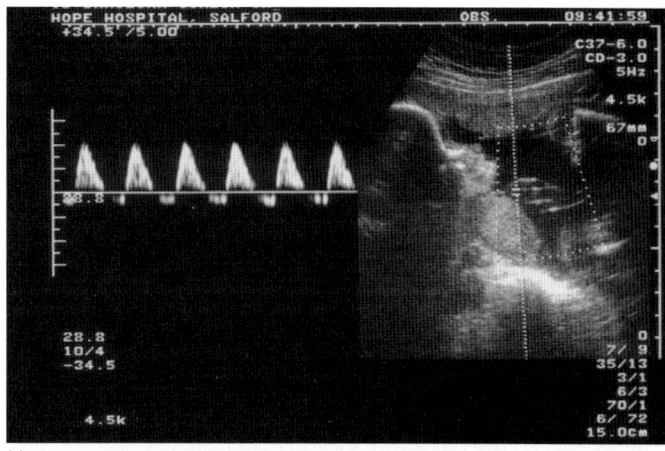

(a)

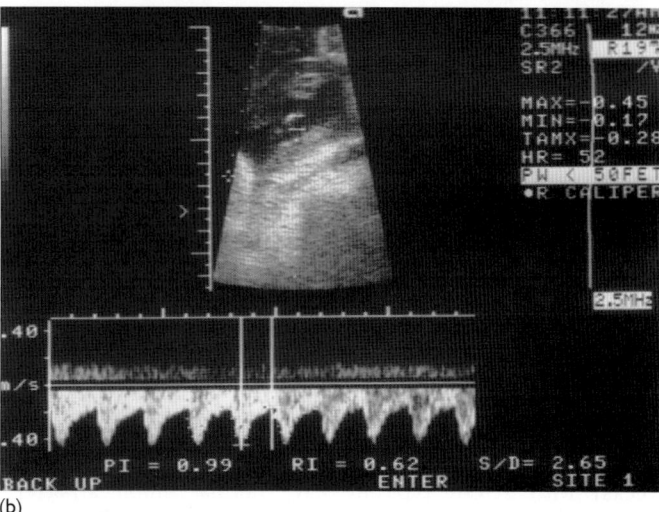

(b)

Fig. 10.6 Umbilical artery Dopplers. (a) Reversed end diastolic flow (EDF) suggesting increased placental resistance. (b) Normal waveform pattern.

Studies have suggested fetal compromise in up to one-third of late-gestation SGA fetuses with normal umbilical Dopplers.[29]

Cerebral circulation

Some growth-restricted fetuses are believed to redistribute blood flow to the brain and therefore demonstrate increased blood flow in cerebral vessels. Doppler ultrasound of vessels such as the middle cerebral artery has been used to assess this. Increased diastolic velocity and, therefore, reduced PI in SGA infants have been associated with abnormal fetal heart rate patterns and increased admission to the neonatal unit.[52]

Uterine artery

Uterine artery Doppler waveforms have been studied to further assess placental function. Abnormal uterine artery blood flow is believed to reflect increased resistance to flow within the placenta earlier in pregnancy than is umbilical artery or middle cerebral artery flow. Therefore, it has been evaluated as a potential screening tool to identify high-risk pregnancy, although it is not yet in widespread use.[66]

Postnatal diagnosis

Birthweight centile alone is ineffective in the postnatal confirmation of IUGR. A long, thin neonate may have a birthweight centile within the normal range but still be malnourished. The ponderal index is an index of body mass and is calculated by (birthweight [g] ÷ crown–heel length [cm]^3) × 100. It is independent of ethnic origin, gender and birth order and is more closely correlated with perinatal morbidity and mortality than birthweight alone.[68]

A further alternative is the gestation-related optimal weight (GROW) centile or the individualised birthweight ratio (IBR) centile.[16,19,70] Both centile calculations incorporate the influence of maternal height, weight, ethnic group, fetal sex and parity and are calculated using computer software available on the Internet. These centiles are a more accurate method of identifying growth-restricted fetuses than birthweight alone. A retrospective study of 31 561 deliveries found that the IBR redefined as normally grown 41% of babies weighing less than the 10th centile.[70] Allowing for these physiological factors also allowed closer correlation with perinatal morbidity.[13]

Causes

SGA and IUGR encompass a wide variety of heterogeneous conditions. Likely causes and associated factors are outlined below (Table 10.1).

Constitutionally small infants

A significant proportion of SGA infants are small but otherwise healthy. An anatomically normal fetus that is symmetrically small with normal liquor volume, normal umbilical Dopplers and normal biophysical profile is most likely to fit into this category. These infants will also maintain their growth velocity and tend not to experience excess morbidity.

Fetal abnormality (Table 10.2)

Chromosomal abnormalities, especially triploidy and trisomy 13, 18 and 21, are associated with IUGR. Commonly, ultrasound abnormalities or markers indicate the diagnosis, although the fetus may be structurally normal. One study from a tertiary referral centre identified karyotypic abnormalities in 19% (89/458) of IUGR fetuses.[65] Aneuploidies can be confirmed or refuted with amniocentesis or chorionic villus sampling. Isolated karyotypic abnormalities within the placenta have also been associated with IUGR.

Almost all structural abnormalities, such as congenital heart disease or neural tube defects, and syndromes such as Russell–Silver are associated with reduced growth.

Infection

Congenital infection is estimated to account for around 5% of cases of IUGR.[59] Direct causal relationships have been demonstrated

Table 10.1 Causes of small-for-gestational-age infants

Fetal factors	Maternal factors	Social/Environmental	Placental
Constitutional	Genetic	Social deprivation	Poor placentation
Chromosomal syndromes	Constitutional	Poor diet	Pre-eclampsia
Malformation	Ill health	Smoking Alcohol Drug misuse	Placental abnormality
Infection	Therapeutic drugs		
Multiple pregnancy	Uterine abnormality		

Table 10.2 Congenital abnormality associated with growth restriction

Type of abnormality	Examples
Chromosomal	Triploidy Trisomy 13 Trisomy 18 Trisomy 21
Cardiac abnormality	Tetralogy of Fallot Atrial septal defect Coarctation Ventricular septal defect
Nervous system	Anencephaly All neural tube defects Hydrocephalus
Renal system	Renal agenesis Bladder exstrophy Urinary tract obstruction Cystic kidneys
Gastrointestinal system	Oesophageal atresia Gastroschisis Cleft lip and palate
Syndromes	Russell–Silver Osteochondrodysplasias, e.g. osteogenesis imperfecta Fanconi Donohue

for cytomegalovirus and rubella, but varicella zoster and human immunodeficiency virus are also possibilities. IUGR is more common if infection occurs early in pregnancy, and the pattern of IUGR is likely (but not exclusively) to be symmetrical. Fetal viral infection has been associated with abnormal placental development and subsequent placental pathology.

Maternal disease

Any serious maternal disease, for example diabetes, asthma, thyrotoxicosis, cardiac and renal disease, can predispose to growth restriction.

Both acquired and inherited thrombophilias have been investigated as predisposing factors for IUGR, as they may increase the risk of thrombotic lesions within the placenta. An increased frequency of the prothrombin mutation and the methylene-tetrahydrofolate reductase mutation in mothers of IUGR infants has been suggested.[43] Antiphospholipid antibodies are an acquired form of thrombophilia and may predispose to an increased risk of growth restriction.[77]

Maternal therapeutic drug administration

Maternal ingestion of beta adrenoreceptor antagonists in the second trimester has been linked to SGA infants, as have anticonvulsants (particularly the hydantoins such as phenytoin), long-term corticosteroids and ciclosporin.

Social and environmental factors

Poor socioeconomic status has long been associated with adverse health problems, and much the same principle applies in pregnancy. A retrospective analysis of obstetric computer databases in the East Midlands used social deprivation scores to investigate the effect of social factors on birthweight.[71] Even allowing for smoking, which has been suggested as the reason for LBW in low socioeconomic groups, those most socially deprived had the lowest-birthweight babies.

Poor diet has also been suggested as a mechanism by which socioeconomic status affects growth. Population studies such as those performed during the Dutch Hunger Winter in 1944 have demonstrated that significant effects were only seen at the extremes of starvation. Even then, the fetus is relatively protected during the first and second trimesters. Anorexic mothers have twice the risk of having an SGA baby, with a similar level of risk being seen in women whose booking body mass index (BMI) is less than 19. Interestingly, high carbohydrate intakes in early pregnancy and low protein intakes in late pregnancy were both associated with a reduction in birthweight.[22]

Tobacco smoking acts in a dose- and gestation-dependent manner to reduce birthweight and increase the risk of IUGR. Therefore, pregnant women who stop smoking by the third trimester are not at increased risk of growth-restricted infants compared with non-smokers.[44] The mechanism by which smoking reduces birthweight is as yet unclear, although it is probably via adverse effects on placental development and blood flow.

Very high alcohol intake (17 units per day in one study[57]) is clearly associated with fetal alcohol syndrome. The diagnostic criteria for fetal alcohol syndrome are growth restriction (weight less than 2 standard deviations below the mean), characteristic facial dysmorphology and neurological damage. The effects of lower alcohol intakes on growth are uncertain, although some prospective studies have shown consumption of three or more units per day is associated with an increased risk of IUGR.[73]

Several recreational drugs of abuse are associated with reduced fetal growth, although the true effect is difficult to assess due to confounding factors. True effects seem likely for opiates, cocaine and amphetamines, but probably not cannabis.[14,30,34,48]

Other environmental influences are known to adversely affect fetal growth, such as living at high altitude. Other less concrete factors suggested include heavy physical activity and living near landfill sites. It is likely that many social factors interact to adversely affect fetal health. A recent retrospective study of social risks in pregnancy, including smoking, alcohol, financial stress and physical violence, found that the OR for delivering an SGA infant increased with the number of risks the mother was exposed to.[1] Although retrospective and based on self-reported risk behaviours, this study highlights the many complex and interacting social factors that may affect pregnancy outcome.

Genetic factors

It has long been recognised that mothers who themselves were small at delivery are at increased risk of delivering a growth-restricted infant.[58] This has been confirmed by later studies, one of which suggested an OR of 3.46 for LBW mothers producing similarly affected infants.[40] Sisters-in-law, who might be expected to experience similar social circumstances, do not exhibit an increased risk.[33] These findings suggest genetic factors, possibly maternal, may be important. A later study also suggested that paternal factors might be important.[51] Despite this epidemiological evidence, there is a paucity of studies suggesting potentially interesting genes. Inherited thrombophilias are among the few investigated to date.[43]

Poor placentation

The human placenta is a villous structure consisting of many branches arising from numerous stem villi. Several changes in the villi have been described in IUGR, including reduced villous density, a reduction in surface area, and fewer loops and coils.[21,32,42] In addition, large plaques of fibrin-like material (similar to acute atheroma) and piling up of trophoblast have been observed.[38] This piling up of trophoblast was subsequently found to represent shedding of apoptotic cells, and increased apoptosis has been described in IUGR placentae.[64]

In addition to the complex branching occurring on the fetal side of the placenta, normal placental development also requires successful trophoblast invasion into the maternal spiral arteries. This trophoblast destroys the muscular and elastic walls of these vessels, producing large flaccid vessels able to meet the growing demands of pregnancy. This is known as physiological change. Placental bed biopsies from pregnancies with IUGR show reduced invasion and physiological change, suggesting a lack of adaptation.[8,63] These vessels also show evidence of atheromatous change. This reduced invasion is believed to produce increased placental resistance to blood flow, and hence the abnormal Doppler waveform patterns. Since similar findings have been described in placentae from pre-eclamptic pregnancy, a common pathogenesis to the two conditions has been suggested. Up to 30% of pregnancies affected by pre-eclampsia are also affected by IUGR.[67]

Other factors

Multiple pregnancies are well documented to be at increased risk of IUGR. Indeed, there is often discordant growth between fetuses. Other important factors include placental abnormalities, such as placental cysts and chorioangiomas, and uterine abnormalities, such as large fibroids or congenital anomalies.

Thus, in summary, using the model espoused by Bobrow & Soothill,[7] SGA fetuses can be categorised according to aetiology into:

1. Normal SGA: no structural anomalies together with normal liquor, normal umbilical artery Doppler waveforms and normal growth velocity.
2. Abnormal SGA: those with structural or genetic abnormalities.
3. FGR: those with impaired placental function identified by abnormal umbilical artery Doppler waveforms and reduced growth velocity.

Implications

SGA (less than the 10th centile) babies have an increased incidence of stillbirth, low Apgar scores, admission to neonatal units, hypoglycaemia, hypothermia, hyperbilirubinaemia and polycythaemia (Table 10.3).[41] There is an increased risk of necrotising enterocolitis, probably due to reduced in-utero blood flow to the bowel. In addition, increased risks of long-term developmental problems have also been described.[49,54] Overall, IUGR confers a 5–10-fold increased risk of both perinatal death and cerebral palsy.[37] There is also a strong association with antepartum stillbirth, in that 60% of 'unexplained' stillbirths were found not to have reached their growth potential when defined by a customised birthweight. Those infants who are preterm as well as SGA are at additional risk.

Table 10.3 Complications associated with small-for-gestational-age infants

Intrapartum	Neonatal	Long term	Adulthood
Abnormal heart rate pattern	Resuscitation	Developmental problems	Fetal origins hypothesis
Acidosis/hypoxia	Low Apgar score	Cerebral palsy	Cardiac disease
Meconium aspiration	Neonatal Unit admission		Diabetes Hypertension
Stillbirth	Hypoglycaemia		Dyslipidaemia
	Hypothermia		
	Polycythaemia		
	Hyperbilirubinaemia		
	Necrotising enterocolitis		
	Coagulopathy		
	Infection		
	Congenital abnormality		

Small size at delivery has also been associated with long-term health problems extending into adulthood. Compilation of detailed infant measurements at birth since the early 20th century in certain areas has allowed the adult health of individuals from these areas to be related to their size at birth. A study based on 16 000 people born in Hertfordshire between 1911 and 1930 found a higher death rate from coronary heart disease among those who weighed less than 2500 g at delivery.[56] A similar study in Sheffield suggested that small size due to growth failure rather than prematurity was responsible for this increased cardiovascular risk.[4] These studies lead to the development of the 'fetal origins', or 'fetal programming', hypothesis, which states that under-nutrition in utero is associated with disproportionate fetal growth and subsequent cardiovascular disease.[5] Similar associations have been described for hypertension, dyslipidaemias and diabetes.[3] However, despite attempts to control for confounding variables such as lifestyle factors and social class, these may have contributed to the differences described.[31]

Prediction

Accurate prediction of those pregnancies destined to be complicated by growth restriction would allow increased vigilance and fetal monitoring, which, in theory, would enable intervention to improve outcomes. Currently, such interventions are limited to avoiding certain risk factors such as smoking, and timely delivery, thereby avoiding the worst sequelae.

History and examination

As outlined above, several risk factors can be identified at booking, such as a BMI under 19 and maternal smoking, which place a pregnancy at high risk of IUGR. In addition, a past history of having an SGA baby increases the risk of recurrence in subsequent pregnancies. Babies born to older mothers are significantly smaller than offspring of younger women, though this effect seems to be largely confined to nulliparous women over 40.

Pregnancy-specific complications are also associated with IUGR. Pre-eclampsia is perhaps the best known, and many of the placental abnormalities are common to both conditions. Retro-placental haemorrhage in the second and third trimesters can impair placental function sufficiently to reduce fetal growth.

Maternal serum screening

Several biochemical markers measured in the maternal serum in the second trimester are associated with reduced growth later in pregnancy. These include α-fetoprotein (AFP), oestriol (E_3), human placental lactogen (HPL) and human chorionic gonadotrophin (hCG). Of these, the most robust is AFP: if the level is 2.5 or more multiples of the median for gestation in the absence of fetal anomaly, there is a 5–10-fold increase in the risk of IUGR.

Ultrasound markers

The best known ultrasonic predictor of subsequent IUGR is abnormal uterine artery Doppler velocimetry; this reflects high impedance levels in the maternal arterial blood supply to the placental unit resulting from deficient trophoblast invasion of the maternal spiral arteries. The abnormalities are apparent as either reduced end-diastolic flow (EDF) or so-called notching of the waveform (Fig. 10.7). Systematic review of 27 studies involving 12 994 women has shown that abnormal uterine artery Doppler flow velocity is associated with a roughly threefold increase in the risk of IUGR, although the diagnostic accuracy of the technique is limited.[11] It would appear that the combination of unexplained elevated maternal AFP and uterine artery Doppler velocimetry is a much more powerful predictor of adverse perinatal outcomes (particularly IUGR).

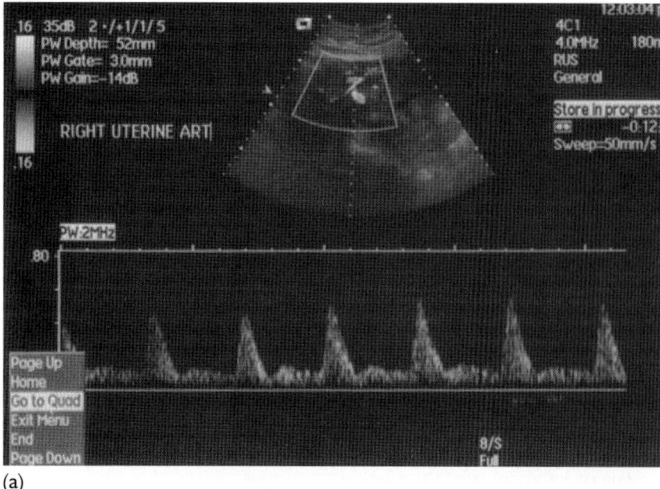

(a)

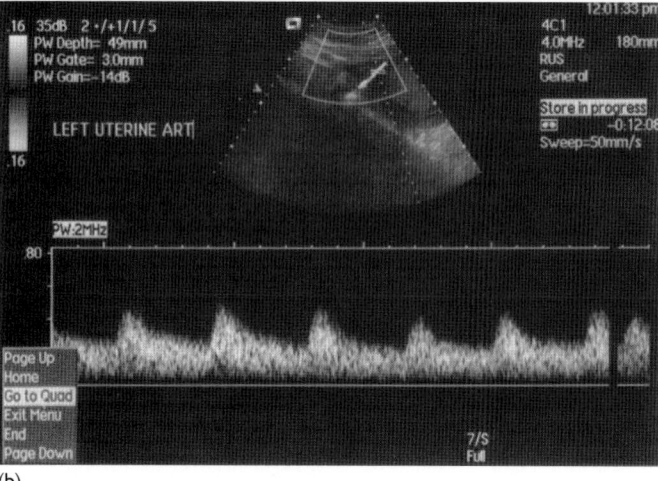

(b)

Fig. 10.7 Uterine artery Dopplers. (a) Increased pulsatility and diastolic notch suggesting increased placental resistance. (b) Normal pattern with high diastolic flow velocity.

Bright or echogenic fetal bowel in the second trimester is associated with an elevated risk of subsequent IUGR. Again, a combination of elevated maternal serum AFP and this ultrasonic marker provides a more precise estimate of the risk of IUGR than either predictor alone.

Scoring systems

Several different scoring systems utilising various risk factors for reduced fetal growth have been devised to better predict women at particular risk of an IUGR baby. All suffer from poor specificity and sensitivity and are therefore of limited clinical usage.

Obstetric management

Obstetric management includes identification of any underlying cause and fetal surveillance. Surveillance consists of regular ultrasound assessment of growth, liquor volume, Doppler assessment

of the fetal circulation, and fetal heart rate monitoring. Since pre-eclampsia occurs in up to 40% of cases of IUGR, maternal surveillance for raised blood pressure, proteinuria and biochemical markers is also important.[35]

Timing of delivery

The only available intervention for growth-restricted pregnancy is delivery. However, there are little available data to assist the timing of such a delivery. Delay may increase the risk of intrauterine hypoxia and adversely affect neurological function,[20] yet premature delivery carries its own risks of neurological impairment.[74] The balance between these factors produces variation in management, and the Growth Restriction Intervention Trial (GRIT) was designed to aid the timing of these deliveries.[23] The entry criteria were singleton or multiple pregnancies between 24 and 36 weeks where the obstetrician was uncertain whether to deliver immediately. Patients were randomised to either deliver immediately (after completion of steroid course) or defer delivery until uncertainty no longer existed. The main outcome measures were infant survival at hospital discharge and paediatric neurodevelopment at 2 years. Initial data have shown that obstetricians were prepared to delay delivery by about 4 days. Although this produced an increased number of stillbirths in the delay group, this was balanced by a similar number of perinatal deaths in the immediate-delivery group.[24] Hence, the 2-year follow-up report is awaited to see if additional guidance will be provided.

Recent guidelines published by the Royal College of Obstetricians and Gynaecologists suggested that where umbilical artery EDF is reversed or absent, admission to hospital for close surveillance and steroids are required.[61] Delivery is advised if any other observation is abnormal (e.g. pathological cardiotocograph). Gestation- and birthweight-specific charts should be used in these circumstances to determine likelihood of survival. If gestation is greater than 34 weeks, delivery should be considered even if other parameters are normal. In cases where EDF is present and other parameters are normal, delivery should be delayed until after 37 weeks.

While the mode of delivery for viable infants less than 35 weeks is likely to be caesarean section following the administration of steroids, the optimal mode of delivery at later gestations is unclear. Careful fetal and cervical assessment is performed prior to considering either induction of labour or caesarean section. Continuous electronic monitoring of the fetal heart rate pattern during labour is indicated due to the increased risk of intrapartum acidaemia. Any suspicious patterns can then be further investigated using fetal blood sampling or, if this is not possible, delivery by caesarean section.

Postnatal examination of the placenta may aid the diagnosis of an underlying cause, and screening the infant for infection or congenital abnormality may be indicated. IUGR with absent or reversed EDF in the umbilical arteries has an overall recurrence risk of 7–20%,[15] hence postnatal counselling is important. Consideration may be given to thrombophilia screening, although it is presently unclear which women may benefit from treatment with low-dose aspirin and low-molecular-weight heparin in subsequent pregnancies.

References

1. Ahluwalia I B, Merritt R, Beck L F, Rogers M 2001 Multiple lifestyle and psychosocial risk and delivery of small for gestational age infants. Obstetrics and Gynecology 97: 649–656

2. Alfirevic Z, Neilson J P 1995 Doppler ultrasonography in high-risk pregnancies: systematic review with meta-analysis. American Journal of Obstetrics and Gynecology 172: 1379–1387

3. Barker D 1995 Fetal origins of coronary heart disease. British Medical Journal 311: 171–174

4. Barker D, Osmond C, Simmonds S, Wield G 1993 The relation of small head circumference and thinness at birth to death from cardiovascular disease. British Medical Journal 306: 422–426

5. Barker D J 1992 Fetal growth and adult disease. British Journal of Obstetrics and Gynaecology 99: 275–276

6. Battaglia F, Lubchenco L 1967 A practical classification of newborn infants by weight and gestational age. Journal of Pediatrics 71: 159–163

7. Bobrow C S, Soothill P W, 1999 Fetal growth velocity: a cautionary tale. Lancet 353: 1460

8. Brosens I, Dixon H, Robertson W 1977 Fetal growth retardation and the arteries of the placental bed. British Journal of Obstetrics and Gynaecology 84: 656–663

9. Chang T, Robson S, Boys R, Spencer J 1992 Prediction of small for gestational age infant: which ultrasonic measurement is best? Obstetrics and Gynecology 80: 1030–1038

10. Chang T, Robson S, Spencer J, Gallivan S 1994 Prediction of perinatal morbidity at term in small fetuses: comparison of fetal growth and Doppler ultrasound. British Journal of Obstetrics and Gynaecology 101: 422–427

11. Chien P, Arnott N, Gordon A et al 2000 How useful is uterine artery Doppler flow velocimetry in the prediction of pre-eclampsia, intrauterine growth restriction and perinatal death? An overview. British Journal of Obstetrics and Gynaecology 107: 196–208

12. Dashe J S, McIntire D D, Lucas M J, Leveno K J 2000 Effects of symmetric and asymmetric fetal growth on pregnancy outcomes. Obstetrics and Gynecology 96: 321–327

13. de Jong C L, Gardosi J, Dekker G A et al 1997 Application of a customised birth weight standard in the assessment of perinatal outcome in a high risk population. British Journal of Obstetrics and Gynaecology 105: 531–535

14. English D, Hulse G, Milne E et al 1997 Maternal cannabis use and birth weight: a meta-analysis. Addiction 92: 1553–1560

15. Farine D, Ryan G, Kelly E N et al 1993 Absent end-diastolic flow velocity waveforms in the umbilical artery – the subsequent pregnancy. American Journal of Obstetrics and Gynecology 168: 637–640

16. Gardosi J 1997 Customized growth curves. Clinical Obstetrics and Gynecology 40: 715–722

17. Gardosi J 1997 Dating of pregnancy; time to forget the last menstrual period. Ultrasound in Obstetrics and Gynecology 9: 367–368

18. Gardosi J, Chang A, Kalyan B et al 1992 Customised antenatal growth charts. Lancet 339: 283–287

19. Gardosi J, Francis A 2000 Software program for the calculation of customised birth weight percentiles. Version 2.0.8. www.wmpi.net/growth/tools.htm

20. Gaudier F, Goldenberg R, Nelson K et al 1994 Acid-base status at birth and subsequent neurosensory impairment in surviving 500 to 1000 gm infants. American Journal of Obstetrics and Gynecology 170: 48–53

21. Giles W, Trudinger B, Baird P 1985 Fetal umbilical artery flow velocity waveforms and placental resistance; pathological correlation. British Journal of Obstetrics and Gynaecology 92: 31–38

22. Godfrey K, Robinson S, Barker D J P et al 1996 Maternal nutrition in early and late pregnancy in relation to placental and fetal growth. British Medical Journal 213: 410–414

23. GRIT Study Group 1996 When do obstetricians recommend delivery for a high-risk preterm growth-retarded fetus? European Journal of Obstetrics and Gynecology and Reproductive Biology 97: 121–126

24. GRIT Study Group 2003 A randomised trial of timed delivery for the compromised preterm fetus: short term outcomes and Bayesian interpretation. British Journal of Obstetrics and Gynaecology 110: 27–32

25. Gruenwald P 1966 Growth of the human fetus. I. Normal growth and its variation. American Journal of Obstetrics and Gynecology 94: 112–121

26. Gudmundsson S, Marsal K 1988 Umbilical and uteroplacental blood flow velocity waveforms in pregnancies with fetal growth retardation. European Journal of Obstetrics and Gynecology and Reproductive Biology 27: 187–196

27. Hackett G, Campbell S, Gamsu H et al 1987 Doppler studies in the growth retarded fetus and prediction of neonatal necrotising enterocolitis, haemorrhage, and neonatal morbidity. British Medical Journal (Clinical Research Edition) 294: 13–16

28. Hendricks S, Sorensen T, Wang K et al 1989 Doppler umbilical artery waveform indices – normal values from fourteen to forty-two weeks. American Journal of Obstetrics and Gynecology 161: 761–765

29. Hershkovitz R, Kingdom J, Geary M, Rodeck C 2000 Fetal cerebral blood flow redistribution in late gestation: identification of compromise in small fetuses with normal umbilical artery Doppler. Ultrasound in Obstetrics and Gynecology 15: 209–212

30. Holzman C, Paneth N 1994 Maternal cocaine use during pregnancy and perinatal outcomes. Epidemiologic Reviews 16: 315–334

31. Huxley R, Neil A, Collins R 2002 Unravelling the fetal origins hypothesis: is there really an inverse association between birthweight and subsequent blood pressure? Lancet 360: 659–665

32. Jackson M R, Walsh A J, Morrow R J et al 1995 Reduced placental villous tree elaboration in small-for-gestational-age pregnancies: relationship with umbilical artery Doppler waveforms. American Journal of Obstetrics and Gynecology 172: 518–525

33. Johnstone F, Inglis L 1974 Familial trends in low birth weight. British Medical Journal 3: 659–661

34. Johnstone F, Raab G, Hamilton B 1996 The effect of human immunodeficiency virus infection and drug use on birth characteristics. Obstetrics and Gynecology 88: 321–326

35. Karsdorp V, van Vugt J, van Geijn H et al 1994 Clinical significance of absent or reversed end diastolic velocity waveforms in umbilical artery. Lancet 344: 1664–1668

36. Kingdom J, Baker P, Blair E 2000 Definitions of intrauterine growth restriction. In: Kingdom J, Baker P (eds) Intrauterine growth restriction. Aetiology and management. Springer-Verlag, London, pp 1–4

37. Kingdom J, Burrell S, Kaufmann P 1997 Pathology and clinical implications of abnormal umbilical artery Doppler waveforms. Ultrasound in Obstetrics and Gynecology 9: 271–286

38. Kingdom J, Huppertz B, Seaward G, Kaufmann P 2000 Development of the placental villous tree and its consequences for fetal growth. European Journal of Obstetrics and Gynecology and Reproductive Biology 92: 35–43

39. Kiserud T, Maršál K 2000 Ultrasound assessment. In: Kingdom J, Baker P (eds) Intrauterine growth restriction. Aetiology and management. Springer-Verlag, London, pp 205–238

40. Klebanoff M, Graubard B, Kessel S, Berendes H 1984 Low birth weight across generations. Journal of the American Medical Association 252: 2423–2427

41. Kramer M, Olivier M, McLean F et al 1990 Impact of intrauterine growth retardation and body proportionality on fetal and neonatal outcome. Pediatrics 86: 707–713

42. Krebs C, Macara L M, Leiser R et al 1996 Intrauterine growth restriction with absent end-diastolic flow velocity in the umbilical artery is associated with maldevelopment of the placental terminal villous tree. American Journal of Obstetrics and Gynecology 175: 1534–1542

43. Kupferminc M J, Eldor A, Steinman N et al 1999 Increased frequency of genetic thrombophilia in women with complications of pregnancy. New England Journal of Medicine 340: 9–13

44. Lieberman E, Gremy I, Lang J, Cohen A 1994 Low birthweight at term and the timing of fetal exposure to maternal smoking. American Journal of Public Health 84: 1127–1131

45. Lin C, Sheikh Z, Lopata R 1990 The association between oligohydramnios and intrauterine growth retardation. Obstetrics and Gynecology 76: 1100–1104

46. Lin C-C, Santolaya-Forgas J 1998 Current concepts of fetal growth restriction: Part I. Causes, classification and pathophysiology. Obstetrics and Gynecology 92: 1044–1055

47. Lin C-C, Santolaya-Forgas J 1999 Current concepts of fetal growth restriction: Part II. Diagnosis and management. Obstetrics and Gynecology 93: 140–146

48. Little B, Snell L, Gilstrap L R 1988 Metamphetamine abuse during pregnancy: outcome and fetal effects. Obstetrics and Gynecology 72: 541–544

49. Low J, Handley-Derry M, Burke S et al 1992 Association of intrauterine growth retardation and learning deficits at 9 to 11 years. American Journal of Obstetrics and Gynecology 167: 1499–1505

50. Lubchenco L, Hansman C, Dressler M, Boyd E 1963 Intrauterine growth as estimated from live birth weight data at 24 to 42 weeks of gestation. Pediatrics 32: 793–800

51. Magnus P, Bakketeig L S, Hoffman H 1997 Birth weight of relatives by maternal tendency to repeat small-for-gestational-age (SGA) births in successive pregnancies. Acta Obstetricia et Gynecologica Scandinavica Supplement 165: 35–38

52. Mari G, Deter R 1992 Middle cerebral artery flow velocity waveforms in normal and small-for-gestational-age fetuses. American Journal of Obstetrics and Gynecology 166: 1262–1270

53. McBurnley R 1947 The undernourished full term infant. A case report. West Journal of Surgical Obstetrics and Gynecology 55: 363–370

54. McCarton C M, Wallace I F, Divon M, Vaughan H G 1996 Cognitive and neurologic development of the premature, small for gestational age infant through age 6: comparison by birth weight and gestational age. Pediatrics 98: 1167–1178

55. Neilson J P, Alfirevic Z 2001 Doppler ultrasound for fetal assessment in high risk pregnancies (Cochrane Review). Cochrane Database for Systematic Reviews (3)

56. Osmond C, Barker D, Winter P et al 1993 Early growth and death from cardiovascular disease in women. British Medical Journal 307: 1519–1524

57. Ouellette E, Rosett H, Rosman N, Weiner L 1977 Adverse effects on offspring of maternal alcohol abuse during pregnancy. New England Journal of Medicine 297: 528–530

58. Ounsted M, Ounsted C 1968 Rate of intrauterine growth. Nature 220: 599–600

59. Pearce M J, Robinson G 1995 Fetal growth and intrauterine growth retardation. In: Chamberlain G (ed) Turnbull's obstetrics, 2nd edition. Churchill Livingstone, Edinburgh, pp 299–312

60. Reed K L 1997 Doppler – the fetal circulation. Clinical Obstetrics and Gynecology 40: 750–754

61. Royal College of Obstetricians and Gynaecologists 2002 The investigation and management of the small-for-gestational-age fetus. Guideline No. 31: 1–16

62. Scott K, Usher R 1966 Fetal malnutrition: its incidence, causes and effects. American Journal of Obstetrics and Gynecology 94: 951–958

63. Sheppard L, Bonnar J 1976 The ultrastructure of the arterial supply of the human placenta in pregnancy complicated by fetal growth retardation. British Journal of Obstetrics and Gynaecology 83: 948–959

64. Smith S C, Baker P N, Symonds E M 1997 Increased placental apoptosis in intrauterine growth restriction. American Journal of Obstetrics and Gynecology 177: 1395–1401

65. Snijders R, Sherrod C, Gosden C, Nicolaides K 1993 Fetal growth retardation: associated malformations and chromosomal abnormalities. American Journal of Obstetrics and Gynecology 168: 547–555

66. Valensise H 1998 Uterine artery Doppler velocimetry as a screening test: where we are and where we go. Ultrasound in Obstetrics and Gynecology 12: 81–83

67. Walker J J 2000 Pre-eclampsia. Lancet 356: 1260–1265

68. Walther F, Ramaekers L 1982 The ponderal index as a measure of the nutritional status at birth and its relation to some aspects of neonatal morbidity. Journal of Perinatal Medicine 10: 42–47

69. Weiner C P 1994 Fetal growth deficiency and its evaluation. In: James D et al (eds) High risk pregnancy. Management options. W B Saunders, London, pp 757–770

70. Wilcox M A, Johnson I R, Maynard P V et al 1993 The individualised birth weight ratio; a more logical outcome measure of pregnancy than birth weight alone. British Journal of Obstetrics and Gynaecology 100: 342–347

71. Wilcox M A, Smith S J, Johnson I R et al 1995 The effect of social deprivation on birth weight, excluding physiological and pathological effects. British Journal of Obstetrics and Gynaecology 102: 918–924

72. Wilson D, Harper A, McClure G et al 1992 Long term predictive value of Doppler studies in high risk fetuses. British Journal of Obstetrics and Gynaecology 99: 575–578

73. Windham G, Fenster L, Hopkins B, Swan S 1995 The association of moderate maternal and paternal alcohol consumption with birth weight and gestational age. Epidemiology 6: 591–597

74. Wood N, Marlow N, Costeloe K et al 2000 Neurologic and developmental disability after extremely preterm birth. EPICure Study Group. New England Journal of Medicine 343: 378–384

75. World Health Organization Expert Group on Prematurity 1950 Final report. WHO, Geneva

76. World Health Organization 1961 Public health aspects of low birth weight. WHO, Geneva

77. Yasuda M, Takakuwa K, Tokunaga A, Tanaka K 1995 Prospective studies of the association between anticardiolipin antibody and outcome of pregnancy. Obstetrics and Gynecology 86: 555–559

Further reading

Kingdom J K, Baker P N 2000 Intrauterine growth restriction: aetiology and management. Springer, London

CHAPTER 11

Maternal illness in pregnancy

Philip Steer, Martin Lupton, Eugene Oteng-Ntim

The most serious outcome of medical complications in pregnancy is death, and the Confidential Enquiry into Maternal Deaths (CEMD)[13] is an important reminder of this. While serious morbidity and death related to pregnancy are relatively rare in the developed world, they are tragically frequent in the developing world, where at least 500 000 women die as a result of pregnancy each year. This chapter considers the most important maternal illnesses in the UK, as reflected in the CEMD.

Thromboembolism associated with pregnancy

Thromboembolic disease is a major cause of maternal mortality in developed countries and a leading cause of maternal death in the UK,[13] accounting for a third of all direct maternal deaths. There is also considerable morbidity associated with thromboembolism, related both to the long-term complications (such as chronic venous insufficiency after deep vein thrombosis [DVT]) and to the side effects of treatment. Thromboembolism has been estimated to complicate 0.6% to 1.2% of pregnancies.[60] The risk of thromboembolism is increased approximately six-fold in pregnancy, due to hormone-induced hypercoagulability, the effects of venous stasis secondary to decreased venous tone, and the mechanical obstruction of the inferior vena cava by the gravid uterus. Other predisposing factors include advanced maternal age, high parity, obesity, bed rest, previous thromboembolism, sickle cell disease, operative delivery, general anaesthesia, and congenital and acquired thrombophilia. The importance of prophylaxis against thromboembolism was highlighted in the CEMD for the tri-ennium 1979–1999.[13] The number of deaths from thromboembolism after caesarean section fell dramatically following the introduction of Royal College guidelines recommending routine thromboprophylaxis. The use of prophylaxis following thrombosis in a previous pregnancy remains controversial, because the reported recurrence rate ranges from a high of 13% to as little as 1%.[40] Moreover, in many published studies the diagnosis was not established objectively, some were retrospective, and those that were prospective had relatively few subjects. However, a recent prospective study[7] reported on 125 pregnant women with a single previous episode of venous thromboembolism (VTE) that had been diagnosed objectively. No heparin was given antenatally but anticoagulant therapy was given for 4 to 6 weeks postpartum. The overall antenatal recurrence rate during pregnancy was 2.4% (95% CI, 0.2–6.9%). There were no episodes of recurrent VTE in the 44 women who did not have an underlying thrombophilia and whose previous VTE had been associated with a non-recurrent risk factor. In contrast, women with an underlying thrombophilia or whose previous VTE was idiopathic (no obvious cause) had an antepartum recurrence rate of 5.9% (95% CI, 1.2–16%). These data suggest that women with a single previous VTE associated with a non-recurrent risk factor and without a thrombophilia do not need routine pharmacological thromboprophylaxis. Nonetheless, given the wide confidence interval and the serious implications of a further VTE, the policy for prophylaxis needs to take into account the views of the woman. In women with underlying thrombophilia, or whose VTE was idiopathic, there is a much stronger case for pharmacological prophylaxis. It is very important that the diagnosis of a suspected DVT or pulmonary embolism in pregnancy is confirmed by an objective test both to avoid unnecessary anticoagulation and because of the implications for future thromboprophylaxis in pregnancy. Non-invasive real-time or duplex ultrasound is the first-line diagnostic tool for DVT in pregnancy. Unfortunately, these ultrasonic methods have limitations, particularly in the investigation of very localised thrombosis in the calf veins, or thrombosis above the inguinal ligament. Venography may be required and should not be withheld because of a negative scan if a VTE is clinically strongly suspected. With adequate shielding of the uterus, the direct radiation dose (and therefore the risk) to the fetus is very small. Chest X-ray, ECG and arterial blood gases should be performed in a pregnant woman with symptoms of a pulmonary embolus, but, if normal, do not completely exclude the diagnosis. Therefore, a perfusion lung scan (ideally with a ventilation scan as well) should also be performed unless the diagnosis is obvious. The isotopes used have a very short half-life and radiation to the fetus is negligible, being about 0.5 Sieverts (50 mrems), which is only a tenth of the maximum gestation exposure recommended in the USA.

Adverse effects of anticoagulation in pregnancy

Heparin is the most widely used anticoagulant in pregnancy because it does not cross the placenta. Furthermore, heparin is not secreted in breast milk and can be used safely during lactation. Heparin, therefore, has no direct adverse effects on the fetus.[5] There are, however, potential risks to the mother from its use. Bleeding may occur, particularly with overdosage during acute therapeutic anticoagulation therapy, and it is important that close monitoring with activated partial thromboplastin time (APTT) for unfractionated heparin (UFH), and anti-Xa assays or heparin levels for low-molecular-weight heparins (LMWHs) is performed. Serious haemorrhage may require reversal of the anticoagulant effect with protamine. However, prophylactic use does not appear to be associated with greater risk of haemorrhage in the antenatal period and can be safely continued even during labour and delivery[31,38,110] although there is a risk of spinal haematoma associated with the insertion of epidural catheters. Most anaesthetists therefore recommend an interval of at least 8 hours from the last heparin injection before such catheters are placed. With modern LMWHs, routine anti-Xa monitoring of prophylactic regimens is not usually necessary.

Heparin-induced thrombocytopenia is a rare but serious side effect. It is an idiosyncratic immune-mediated phenomenon associated with extensive venous thrombosis, which usually occurs between 5 and 15 days after the institution of heparin and may be life-threatening.[76] Thus, the platelet count should be monitored routinely during treatment with heparin, particularly during the first 10 days of use. The risk has been estimated at between 1% and 3% with UFH but is substantially lower with LMWH (1:10 000);[72,118] thus, with LMWHs, monitoring after the first week can probably be as infrequent as once a month.[117]

Heparin-induced osteoporosis is a significant problem with long-term use. The risk to any given individual is difficult to predict because it relates poorly to both dose and duration of therapy. However, an overall 2.2% incidence of osteoporotic fracture has been demonstrated in women taking UFH for a period of over 3 months.[76] LMWHs carry, on the basis of the limited information available, substantially less risk of osteoporosis.[38] The exact mechanism underlying the bone demineralisation is not known.

Although warfarin is not secreted in breast milk in clinically significant amounts, and is safe to use during lactation, it crosses the placenta and is a known teratogen. Warfarin embryopathy (midface hypoplasia, stippled chondral calcification, scoliosis, asplenia, diaphragmatic hernia, short proximal limbs and short phalanges) can occur following exposure to the drug between 6 and 9 weeks' gestation. The incidence of embryopathy has been estimated at between 4% and 5%.[5,80] Warfarin in the second and third trimesters also poses risks to the fetus. Recurrent small intracerebral bleeds can occur, leading to abnormalities such as optic atrophy, microcephaly and mental retardation. The risk is reduced by strict control of maternal anticoagulation (and is smaller if the anticoagulant dose required is less than 5 mg per day). However, fetal intraventricular haemorrhage has been reported even in the presence of low therapeutic INR (international normalised ratio) levels in the mother,[116] probably because of an immature fetal

liver and clotting system. Warfarin should be avoided beyond 36 weeks' gestation because of the excessive haemorrhagic risk to both mother and fetus in the peripartum period.[5,76]

Management of thromboembolism in pregnancy and the puerperium

High-dose subcutaneous LMWH (1 mg/kg b.i.d.) or intravenous UFH is used initially to treat DVT or pulmonary embolism to prevent further, potentially fatal, thromboembolism.[12] Treatment should be started as soon as a provisional diagnosis has been made and should not be delayed until the results of investigations are available. Most treatment guidelines are still based on studies in the non-pregnant population. Two meta-analyses of randomised controlled trials have compared LMWH to UFH in the initial treatment of DVT in non-pregnant subjects.[26,37] LMWH was found to be more effective than UFH, with lower mortality and fewer haemorrhagic complications. LMWH has been used for the initial management of VTE in pregnancy[34,114] and has been recommended in published guidelines.[94] The antenatal use of warfarin in these circumstances is less popular because of the fetal risks. The acute use of thrombolytic agents such as streptokinase are reserved for life-threatening circumstances in pregnancy, because of the possible bleeding complications.

Administration of UFH

Traditionally, intravenous UFH has been the method of choice for heparin administration in acute VTE and may still be preferred in massive pulmonary thromboembolism because of its rapid effect and the extensive experience of its use in this situation. A bolus dose of 5000 units of heparin is injected, followed by an intravenous infusion of between 24 000 and 40 000 units over 24 hours, with the aim of keeping the APTT ratio between 1.5 and 2.5.[56] However, subcutaneous UFH is probably an effective alternative to intravenous administration, and is given as 15 000–20 000 IU, 12 hours apart. This dose will not be expected to alter the APTT ratio, and monitoring can be performed using anti-Xa assays.

Administration of LMWH

In the non-pregnant patient, once-daily administration is recommended for acute treatment of VTE. However, in pregnancy, because of the alteration in the pharmacokinetics, a twice-daily regimen is preferred (enoxaparin 1 mg/kg b.i.d.; dalteparin 100 units/kg b.i.d.). The insertion of an epidural is considered safe in these patients as long as the APTT and platelet count are normal and the administration of UFH was more than 4 hours (or 8 hours for LMWH) prior to insertion. Following delivery, LMWH can be continued or warfarin therapy commenced, for a period of 6 to 12 weeks. Heparin therapy is still required until anticoagulation with warfarin is achieved, which usually takes at least 72 hours (INR 2.0–3.0). The introduction of warfarin in the puerperium reduces maternal exposure to heparin and therefore reduces the risk of osteoporosis. However, following discussion, some women may decide to continue self-injection of heparin in the postnatal period, for simplicity and convenience. Warfarin does not cross into breast milk in any significant quantities, and breastfeeding is not contraindicated.

Thromboprophylaxis in pregnancy

The issue of thromboprophylaxis should preferably be discussed before conception or at least early in pregnancy, so that the associated risks and benefits are fully understood. The timing and duration of prophylaxis will depend on a number of variables, such as the severity of a previous thrombosis, recurrent events, or the presence of a particular risk factor such as thrombophilia. Low-risk patients, such as those with a past history of DVT outside pregnancy and no additional risk factors, may require prophylactic treatment only during delivery and postpartum. High-risk patients, such as women with antithrombin deficiency, will require prophylaxis throughout pregnancy and the puerperium. The management of women who have had pregnancy-associated thromboembolism in the past should include thromboprophylaxis throughout pregnancy and the puerperium. LMWH (e.g. enoxaparin) has been advocated for thromboprophylaxis in pregnancy.[94] The advantages of this type of preparation include once-daily dosage and a possible, although as yet unproven, reduced risk of bleeding, thrombocytopenia and osteoporosis in pregnancy. The disadvantages are higher costs and longer half-life, causing more difficulty if rapid reversal of anticoagulant activity is required. The current recommendation from the CEMD is to offer thromboprophylaxis to all women undergoing caesarean section. A once-daily dose of LMWH should be continued for a period of 5 days or until the patient is mobile and can be discharged from hospital.

An important indication for warfarin during and after pregnancy is the presence of mechanical heart valves; anticoagulation is needed to prevent systemic embolisation. High levels of anticoagulation with warfarin are required long term in these patients outside pregnancy.[57] Low-dose heparin is not adequate to prevent thromboembolism. Transfer to full anticoagulation with heparin should be recommended as soon as the pregnancy test is positive. Warfarin is recommended in the second and third trimesters until approximately 2 weeks prior to anticipated delivery. Heparin is then given until after delivery.

Hypertensive disease in pregnancy

Hypertension complicates between 10% and 15% of all pregnancies. The absolute number of British women dying as a result of the hypertensive diseases of pregnancy has fallen over the last 20 years[13] and now accounts for only 15% of direct maternal deaths. Intracranial haemorrhage is the commonest cause of death associated with hypertension. Unfortunately, the proportion of cases in which there has been substandard care has remained high (80% of cases referred to the CEMD).

There are changes in maternal blood pressure (BP) throughout normal as well as abnormal pregnancy. In normal pregnancy, there are major physiological changes to the mother's cardiovascular system within 3 weeks of conception. There is an increase in heart rate and cardiac output, with a fall in total peripheral resistance. Cardiac output continues to rise until the 24th week of pregnancy, when it has normally increased by approximately 45%. The rise in cardiac output does not keep pace with the fall in systemic vascular resistance, and maternal BP therefore tends to fall during the first and second trimesters, until the 23rd week, when it reaches its nadir. From the 23rd week, the total systemic vascular resistance begins to rise and so maternal BP also rises gradually, the rise becoming more rapid after 34 weeks. The concept of hypertension is imprecise and the thresholds that divide normal from abnormal are fairly arbitrary, with a level at or above 140/90 mmHg being considered abnormal. However, such a fixed threshold probably underestimates hypertension in mid pregnancy and overestimates it at term.

The accurate measurement of BP is critical. Automated BP recording systems can systematically underestimate BP in pre-eclampsia, to a serious degree.[13] The key features of BP measurement in pregnancy are that both K4 and K5 should be measured and annotated, the correct cuff should be selected, and the position of the mother should be consistent.[105] The measurement itself should be to the nearest 2 mmHg.

Women with hypertension in pregnancy can be divided into two groups: those who are hypertensive when they become pregnant (1.5–3% of pregnancies) and those who become hypertensive during pregnancy (7% of pregnancies). Those who become hypertensive during pregnancy can be further subdivided into those who develop pregnancy-induced hypertension (PIH), with no other associated features (PIH is new hypertension in pregnancy appearing after 20 weeks of gestation and resolving after delivery, with a diastolic pressure of at least 90 mmHg on two consecutive occasions measured at least 4 hours apart) and those who develop pre-eclampsia (new hypertension with significant proteinuria [>300 mg/24 h]). There is considerable overlap between the groups, as 25% of women with pre-existing hypertension develop pre-eclampsia at some stage during their pregnancy. The clinical importance of making the correct distinction between the different hypertensive states is that pre-eclampsia is associated with fetal risks (growth restriction, prematurity and death) and maternal risks (cerebrovascular, cardiac, hepatic and renal complications), while PIH and chronic hypertension generally have a far more benign course (mild PIH may even be advantageous for fetal growth).

Chronic hypertension

About 5% of chronic hypertension is known to be secondary to an underlying cause such as renal disease, systemic lupus erythematosus and other rarer diseases such as Cushing's syndrome and Conn's syndrome. Ninety-five per cent of hypertension is primary and has no single identifiable cause. Moderate-to-severe chronic hypertension is defined as a BP of ≥140/90 mmHg at booking or before 20 weeks of pregnancy. Women with essential hypertension tend to be older, parous and are more likely to have a family history of hypertension. In pregnancies where pre-eclampsia does not develop, the risk of a poor outcome (intrauterine growth restriction [IUGR], preterm delivery, maternal renal and vascular problems) is directly proportional to the degree of hypertension and the number of antihypertensives that need to be used to control it. The majority of chronic hypertension is mild or moderate (<160/110 mmHg), and a good outcome can be expected unless pre-eclampsia develops. Antihypertensive medication can sometimes be discontinued in the first and second trimesters because of the fall in BP secondary to the physiological changes of pregnancy. If long-term therapy is required, the most favoured agent is still methyldopa, which has the longest track record of safety in pregnancy. However, it commonly produces side effects such as drowsiness and nightmares, and medications such as calcium channel blockers (e.g. nifedipine or amlodipine) and beta-blockers (e.g. labetolol, atenolol or metoprolol) are increasingly used. There have been some reports of an increase in IUGR with the beta-blockers, so they should be used with caution if there are other risk factors for poor fetal growth. In any case, serial fetal growth monitoring is advisable in all women with hypertension. The early treatment of chronic hypertension does not prevent the later development of pre-eclampsia.[89] The diagnosis of superimposed pre-eclampsia is more difficult in those women with established hypertension, particularly if they already have proteinuria. The development of abnormal liver function tests, clotting disturbances and an increase in plasma urate are useful guides.

Pre-eclampsia

Across the world, pre-eclampsia and eclampsia probably account for up to 50 000 maternal deaths per annum, the vast majority occurring in the developing nations. Pre-eclampsia is a multisystem disorder unique to humans and exclusively associated with pregnancy.[122] It is defined as a syndrome developing after 20 weeks of gestation, characterised by hypertension (a diastolic pressure of at least 90 mmHg on two consecutive occasions at least 4 hours apart) and proteinuria (>300 mg/24 h). The exact cause of pre-eclampsia is still unclear and it remains a 'disease of theories'. All theories agree that the role of the placenta is key, with deficient trophoblastic invasion leading to placental ischaemia, poor placental oxygen transfer with release of oxygen free radicals, and possibly immune maladaptation. The main pathophysiological findings in the mother are widespread vascular endothelial dysfunction with consequent vasoconstriction, haemoconcentration and multi-organ failure.[8]

There is little that can be done to prevent pre-eclampsia. The most recent meta-analysis of the many trials of low-dose aspirin (75 mg/day) suggests a 15% decrease in incidence with its use, but the effect is only of value in women likely to have severe early-onset pre-eclampsia, which is difficult to predict.[30] The trials have however demonstrated the safety of low-dose aspirin in pregnancy. More recently, Shennan et al[101] have proposed that vitamin C and E supplementation (both antioxidants) may be beneficial in the prevention of pre-eclampsia in women at increased risk of the disease; however, this needs to be re-examined by a large-scale clinical trial.

Once pre-eclampsia has developed, it will progress at a variable rate until the fetus and placenta have been delivered. If a women presents at term, labour should be induced to prevent serious deterioration in the maternal and/or fetal condition. At earlier gestations, the antenatal management aims to be conservative in order to prolong pregnancy and improve fetal maturity while attempting to avoid the development of severe maternal complications or fetal compromise. The complaint of symptoms such as headache, visual disturbances, epigastric pain or vomiting, or the presence of proteinuria in a pregnant woman with raised BP, necessitates hospital admission for thorough assessment of the condition and possible delivery. Maternal investigations include blood tests to exclude renal or liver dysfunction, thrombocytopenia and other coagulation disturbances. The assessment of fetal wellbeing should involve growth scans, assessment of liquor volume, and umbilical artery Doppler velocimetry. If delivery appears imminent and the fetus is less than 34 weeks' gestation, antenatal steroids, to improve fetal lung function, must be given whenever possible. Some women with pre-eclampsia have no evidence of fetal compromise while others may have minimal maternal symptoms or signs but significant fetal compromise. The use of antihypertensive agents to control BP should be considered if levels are consistently above 160/100 mmHg. Although control of BP alone will do little or nothing to prevent disease progression, there is an increased risk of stroke, cardiac failure and abruption when hypertension exceeds 170/110 mmHg. By preventing significant rises in BP, antihypertensives may help to prolong the pregnancy for a clinically useful period of fetal development and thus improve neonatal outcome. When the hypertension of pre-eclampsia is masked by treatment, vigilance for the development of other complications must be maintained.

A variety of antihypertensive agents are available which all act by different mechanisms. Methyldopa has a long established and good safety record in pregnancy and is often used for chronic control of BP in pregnant women. Nifedipine SR, amlodipine, atenolol and labetalol are increasingly used as first- and second-line therapies. There is some evidence that β-blockers are associated with fetal growth restriction when used from early in pregnancy, but this does not appear to be a problem when they are prescribed only in the third trimester.[95] Angiotensin-converting enzyme (ACE) inhibitors should not be used in pregnancy as they have an effect on fetal renal function; however, they do not appear to be secreted in the breast milk (in a clinically significant quantity) and some authorities use them for the control of postpartum hypertension. Intravenous hydralazine or labetalol are the mainstay for the acute control of severe hypertension prior to delivery or in the immediate postpartum period. The relationship between maternal BP and fetal compromise is not entirely clear, except that the prolongation of pregnancy usually has benefits for the neonate. Hypotension needs to be avoided, as uteroplacental blood flow can be precarious and sudden falls in BP may lead to fetal compromise.

HELLP syndrome

HELLP syndrome is a particularly aggressive form of pre-eclampsia. Weinstein first used the term in 1982,[119] to describe women whose pre-eclampsia was complicated by haemolysis, elevated liver enzymes and a low platelet count. HELLP syndrome is uncommon, occurring in about 20% of cases of severe pre-eclampsia, with 30% of cases occurring postpartum. Individual features of the HELLP syndrome are seen commonly in severe cases of pre-eclampsia. The importance of recognising the syndrome rests largely on the need to place the woman in a very high-risk category. The occurrence of acute (adult) respiratory distress syndrome in association with HELLP carries a very grave prognosis, with a high maternal mortality.[63] The fetal prognosis includes significant morbidity.

Eclampsia

Eclampsia is uncommon in the UK, occurring in 4.9/10 000 pregnancies,[28] and is three times more likely to occur if the mother is under the age of 19. While the term pre-eclampsia suggests there is a progressive deterioration in the maternal condition to the point of eclampsia, 15–20% of all cases of eclampsia occur without any obvious symptoms and 40% occur before either hypertension or proteinuria is documented. About 40% of cases of eclampsia occur antepartum, 15% intrapartum and 45% postpartum. The pathophysiology of the seizures is uncertain but may involve cerebral vasospasm causing ischaemia, disruption of the blood–brain barrier and cerebral oedema (probably a secondary feature occurring after the seizure). Rarely, cortical blindness can occur.

There is clear evidence that magnesium sulphate should be the drug of choice for the treatment of eclampsia.[29] The 'Magpie' trial demonstrated that the use of magnesium sulphate in pre-eclampsia halves the risk of eclampsia and probably reduces the risk of maternal death. At the dosage given in the trial, there appeared to be no short-term, serious, harmful effects on either the mother or the baby.[61] Unfortunately, 25% of women had some sort of side effect, and this, combined with the fact that there were no maternal deaths in countries with a low perinatal mortality, has meant that there is controversy as to whether in such countries magnesium sulphate should be reserved for those women with severe pre-eclampsia, such as those with HELLP syndrome. The benefits of its use in the developing world are far more obvious.

Heart disease

Heart disease in pregnancy is a worrying condition for the obstetrician as it is one of the leading causes of maternal mortality.[13] In developed countries, the incidence of heart disease in pregnancy has declined over the last 50 years from about 3% to 1%, due to the dramatic reduction in the incidence of rheumatic fever that followed the introduction of penicillin.[57] In contrast, congenital heart disease in pregnancy is increasingly common, owing to the advances in paediatric cardiac surgery and medical therapy that have taken place over the last 30 years, with the result that more affected women are surviving into the reproductive age. In our experience, most of these mothers cope well with the demands of pregnancy provided they are counselled appropriately prior to pregnancy, and care throughout the pregnancy and puerperium is managed by a multidisciplinary team. The risk of a child inheriting polygenic cardiac disease is usually about 3–5%,[92] but recent large studies suggest a risk which varies according to the parent's condition, being 3% in conditions such as tetralogy of Fallot, but as high as 10–18% with atrial septal defect, coarctation of the aorta and aortic stenosis.[9] This is illustrated in Table 11.1. The situation in developing countries is very different, where, due to the continuing high prevalence of rheumatic fever, heart disease is still commonly encountered.

In our preconception and combined obstetric–cardiac clinics, we advise avoidance of pregnancy in women with Eisenmenger's syndrome, primary pulmonary hypertension and inoperable cyanotic heart disease, because of the 30–50% risk of maternal mortality. However, if women choose to go ahead with pregnancy, they are, of course, offered full support. With less severe congenital lesions, the woman and her family must balance the desire for children against the risk of mortality and morbidity. Advice should be given on an individualised basis.

During the antenatal period, the commonest reason for cardiological referral is the detection of a murmur, which proves to be an innocent flow murmur in 90% of cases (such murmurs occur in most pregnant women, due to the 50% increase in cardiac output). The other common presentation is with palpitations, which usually prove to be of no consequence. The majority are due to benign arrhythmias (such as ventricular and atrial unifocal ectopics) that

Table 11.1 Recurrence risk of congenital heart disease (CHD). The prevalence of CHD in offspring of parents with CHD is 3.1%, compared with 1.3% in offspring of parents without CHD. The prevalence may rise to 15% if two affected siblings are born[57]

Cardiac lesion	Risk of recurrence in fetus (%)		
	One sibling affected	Father affected	Mother affected
Aortic stenosis	2	3	17.9
Pulmonic stenosis	2	2	6.5
Marfan's	50	50	50
Ventricular septal defect	3	2	9.5
Atrial septal defect	2.5	1.5	4.6
Patent ductus arteriosus	3	2.5	4.1
Tetralogy of Fallot	2.5	1.5	2.6

require no treatment. Serious dysrhythmias are rare and usually well tolerated. The principles of treatment are no different from those in the non-pregnant, with the exception of some dysrhythmic agents that may be restricted due to insufficient safety data. Adenosine and DC cardioversion can be used safely during pregnancy. Resistant supraventricular tachycardia can be treated with amiodarone. Because of its high iodine content (nearly 40% by weight of each dose), there is a risk of neonatal hypothyroidism. Thus, the drug should be used only when others have failed. It is contraindicated in breastfeeding mothers (p. 419).

Pregnancy in women with artificial heart valves is a major dilemma. Women with advanced valvular disease often need surgical valve replacement. Most cardiologists currently recommend a tissue valve for women wanting to have children, as they avoid the need for anticoagulation. In women with mechanical valves, anticoagulants are essential (see p. 179, the section on thromboprophylaxis).

Peripartum cardiomyopathy is a potentially life-threatening condition that presents during the third trimester or in the puerperium. Treatment is symptomatic and aimed at reducing the risk of both heart failure and thromboembolism.

The main principle of pregnancy management in women with heart disease is very close monitoring. The aim is the early detection of subacute bacterial endocarditis (increase in murmurs, pyrexia), heart failure (audible crackles at the bases of the lungs), valvular dysfunction (new murmurs), and pre-eclampsia. The latter puts a considerable extra strain on the heart and increases risk dramatically; early delivery is usually indicated if it develops. Cardiovascular stress at delivery should be avoided, and this is best achieved by allowing the spontaneous onset of labour, prompt epidural anaesthesia to avoid maternal stress/distress, and an assisted second stage (e.g. ventouse delivery). However, early recourse to caesarean section is necessary if labour is not straightforward or there are obstetric complications.

Neurological disorders in pregnancy

Epilepsy

Approximately 1 in 200 women of childbearing age suffer with epilepsy. Most women with epilepsy have already been diagnosed and need no further investigation, but those with a new onset of fits during pregnancy should be thoroughly investigated and the diagnosis of eclampsia should always be considered. Other causes of fits include cerebral vein thrombosis, thrombotic thrombocytopenic purpura, cerebral infarction, drug and alcohol withdrawal, hypoglycaemia, hyponatraemia, gestational epilepsy and pseudoepilepsy. While the majority (54%) of epileptic women experience no change in the frequency of their fits during their pregnancy, about 30% have an increase in their seizure rate. Putative reasons for this include the pregnancy itself, lack of sleep and decreased serum drug levels due either to poor compliance or to the nausea and vomiting of the first trimester.[99] Serum drug concentrations may also decrease as a result of increased drug metabolism, increased renal clearance and the larger maternal blood volume of pregnancy.[52] While the fetus is

relatively resistant to short episodes of hypoxia and there is no evidence of adverse effects of single seizures on the fetus, status epilepticus has been associated with a 50% risk of fetal loss[36] or handicap. If a woman is fit-free, there is no need to measure the serum anticonvulsant levels. If, however, she is poorly controlled, measurement of serum anticonvulsant levels, at monthly intervals during the pregnancy, can be a useful guide to optimum dosage. If serum levels of anticonvulsant drugs are maintained within the therapeutic range, only 10% of patients will experience an increase in seizure frequency during the pregnancy.[126]

All anticonvulsant drugs marketed up to 1976 have been shown to be teratogenic; it is possible that some of the 'new' anticonvulsants will be shown not to be.[39] Their causation of congenital anomalies appears to be multifactorial, with some degree of genetic involvement, which has not been clearly defined.[50] The risk of congenital malformations is increased in women with epilepsy even if they are not receiving any treatment. If a mother is white, the baseline risk of cleft lip and palate is about 0.1%. When the mother takes phenobarbital (phenobarbitone) – the drug with the strongest association to cleft – there is a threefold increase in the risk[3] but this is still only 0.3%. The underlying risk of malformation for any one drug is about 6–7% (i.e. about two- to threefold the background malformation rate). Unfortunately, the risk rises at least additively with each additional anticonvulsant; thus, it is over 20% if a woman is on three anticonvulsants, and with some combinations the increase in risk is even greater. Theoretically, each anticonvulsant drug can produce specific or distinctive abnormalities. A few of these have been identified:

- **Carbamazepine** – 1% of carbamazepine-exposed infants have spina bifida.[93] There is also an increase in the rate of craniofacial defects and fingernail hypoplasia. There is no evidence of an effect on cognitive function.[100]
- **Phenytoin** has been linked to the 'hydantoin syndrome', in which affected infants suffer with microcephaly, mental retardation, growth deficiency and several other anomalies. However, recent studies have failed to identify an association between phenytoin and either microcephaly or growth deficiency.[79] There is conflicting evidence as to whether phenytoin causes a deterioration in cognitive function,[39] though there is a clear link between phenytoin and congenital heart defects.
- **Sodium valproate** carries a 1–2% risk of neural tube defects (NTDs) occurring in the fetus. It also causes congenital heart defects. Cognitive function is probably affected by valproate, though the size of the effect is uncertain.[39] There is also concern that there may be a link between valproate exposure and autism.[123]
- **Lamotrigine** – the studies of lamotrigine in pregnancy are too small to identify increases in the frequency of all birth defects or even large increases in rare and major defects; however, it appears that there is no increase in the malformation rate when lamotrigine monotherapy is used instead of other antiepileptics.[113]

With the exception of vigabatrin and topiramate, most of the newer antiepileptics do not appear to be teratogenic in animals and nor do they possess the same anti-folate properties as the older antiepileptics.[83] Despite the risk of teratogenicity, it is important to counsel epileptic women who are contemplating pregnancy that uncontrolled seizures are more hazardous to the fetus than are the risks associated with anticonvulsants. The risks of congenital abnormalities may be minimised by maintaining women on the lowest possible dose of drug that keeps them fit-free, and by the use of monovalent rather than polyvalent therapy.[54] Taking two anticonvulsants carries a risk of fetal malformation of approximately 15%, while a combination of valproate, phenytoin and carbamazepine carries a risk of up to 50%. The importance of taking folic acid, 5 mg once per day, both before conception and in the first 3 months of the pregnancy should be emphasised, as the teratogenicity of some of the anticonvulsants may be in part due to their action as folate antagonists.[20] The possibility of withdrawing anticonvulsant therapy in those who have been fit-free for 2 years should also be considered in the pre-pregnancy counselling clinic. Early detailed ultrasound should be offered to all epileptic mothers in order to exclude NTDs.

There is an increased risk of vitamin K deficiency in the neonates of mothers who take anticonvulsants during pregnancy, despite normal maternal clotting factors.[17] To avoid vitamin-K-deficiency bleeding in the newborn (p. 190), vitamin K supplements should be given to the mother in the last few weeks of pregnancy and to the neonate at birth.[68]

There are no particular problems to expect during labour in an epileptic woman, although it is important to ensure that the usual doses of anticonvulsant are not missed. The possibility of fits may be increased because of hyperventilation, exhaustion and lack of sleep. Caesarean section is only indicated for obstetric reasons. If the dose of anticonvulsant has been increased during the pregnancy, a reduction should be made after delivery. None of the anticonvulsants are contraindicated in breastfeeding mothers. Careful contraceptive advice should always be given to epileptic mothers on treatment before they are discharged home.

Stroke

Cerebrovascular disease is a major cause of maternal mortality and morbidity. At least 30% of eclamptic deaths are attributable to cerebral pathology. While strokes are rare in women of childbearing age, with the gradually decreasing maternal mortality rates over the past 20 years they now account for over 10% of the total number of maternal deaths in the UK.[13] Strokes are defined as acute ischaemic or haemorrhagic events causing the onset of focal neurological symptoms.

Ischaemic stroke

Ischaemic strokes may be secondary to arterial occlusion as a result of emboli from distant sources or local thrombosis within the vessel. The incidence of ischaemic stroke is approximately 3–4 cases/100 000 pregnancies per year.[120] This is largely due to the nine-fold increase in risk during the puerperium, with most strokes occurring in the distribution of the carotid and middle cerebral arteries. The hypercoagulable state of pregnancy predisposes the mother to thrombus formation. Potential causes of local arterial abnormalities include atherosclerosis, vasculitis and homocystinuria. Cardiac disease in pregnancy is responsible for a proportion

of embolic strokes. Arrhythmias, infective endocarditis, prosthetic-valve-related emboli and paradoxical embolus may all contribute. Cardiac mural thrombus formation, e.g. in cardiomyopathy or post myocardial infarction, may also give rise to emboli. Haematological disease in pregnancy may also give rise to an increased risk of arterial stroke, e.g. sickle cell anaemia, idiopathic thrombocytopenic purpura and the thrombophilias. Finally, substance abuse is an increasingly frequent cause of ischaemic stroke. Cocaine, amphetamines, heroin and other sympathomimetics are associated with both ischaemic and haemorrhagic strokes.[46]

The management of ischaemic stroke depends on the underlying cause. Neuroimaging techniques such as computed tomography (CT) scanning and magnetic resonance imaging (MRI) are safe in pregnancy with suitable screening of the fetus. Many of the thrombotic and embolic conditions leading to stroke require either prophylactic or therapeutic anticoagulation; however, it is obviously essential to exclude haemorrhagic causes for stroke before anticoagulants are used. In addition, for many of the rarer causes, there is little evidence on risk–benefit ratios, and there are no prospective trials available for guidance. Multidisciplinary management is essential, as is advice from tertiary centres of excellence.

Maternal mortality following cerebral infarction has been reported to be up to 25% of patients.[64] A woman who has had a cerebral ischaemic event which remains unexplained after a thorough evaluation (the aetiology of ischaemic stroke remains elusive in between 20% and 40% of non-pregnant patients, which probably also holds true for pregnant patients)[11] does not appear to be at greater risk of having another ischaemic event during a subsequent pregnancy.

Subarachnoid haemorrhage

The most common causes of intracerebral haemorrhage in pregnancy are arterial aneurysms and arteriovenous malformations (AVMs). The incidence is between 1 and 2 per 10 000, with an overall mortality rate 27–40%.[64] The initial neurological status of the patient following a bleed from an intracranial vascular anomaly correlates well with the risk of death and the neurological prognosis. If there is a profound alteration in consciousness at presentation, mortality rates reach 80–90% and operative mortality is also high (between 25% and 35%). The relative risk of intracerebral haemorrhage is 2.5 during pregnancy and 28.3 during the postpartum period.[48]

It is the suddenness of the onset of the symptoms and the severity of the headache and photophobia which favour the diagnosis of an intracranial bleed over the differential diagnosis of cerebral venous thrombosis, arterial occlusion, eclampsia or meningitis. A CT scan should be performed to confirm the diagnosis. If this is normal but the history is very persuasive, a lumbar puncture may be performed. If an intracerebral haemorrhage is confirmed, then cerebral angiography is required to identify the actual vascular anomaly.

Nimodipine has been shown to reduce posthaemorrhagic vasospasm in aneurysmal bleeding, and therefore lowers the risk of delayed ischaemic neurological deficits and possible death. High-dose steroids may be needed to decrease intracranial oedema. If possible, neurosurgery to excise an AVM or clip an aneurysm should be undertaken during pregnancy, as there is evidence of significant benefits in terms of maternal and fetal mortality.[24] The decision to operate should be made for the same reasons as in the non-pregnant patient, e.g. recurrent haemorrhage (the risk of rebleeding from an AVM in the remainder of pregnancy may be as high as 50%), intractable epilepsy, severe unrelenting headache or cerebrovascular ischaemia secondary to a steal phenomenon. The surgical management of haemorrhage secondary to AVMs is controversial, with no evidence of benefit over non-operative treatment.[24]

The mode of delivery for women with AVMs or aneurysms is still contentious. If the AVM or aneurysm is successfully operated on, vaginal delivery is appropriate. If, however, the lesion is inoperable, then some authorities suggest elective caesarean section[27] while others have argued there is no significant difference in mortality rates following vaginal or caesarean delivery.[24] The risk of recurrent haemorrhage during labour may be reduced by epidural anaesthesia, minimising pushing in the second stage, and by performing an instrumental delivery if required.

Cerebral venous thrombosis

Cerebral venous thrombosis occurs most commonly during the puerperium, particularly in the second to third week postpartum.[104] It has an incidence of 1 per 10 000 deliveries in the developed world, but in the developing world it is the most common cause of stroke, with an incidence of 40–50 per 10 000 deliveries.[27] It is typically associated with infection and dehydration, though there are many other recognised causes. The archetypal presentation is of severe headache, papilloedema and seizures; however, there may also be a focal neurological deficit, aphasia, visual disturbance and the syndrome of 'idiopathic intracranial hypertension'. The diagnosis is best confirmed by CT or MRI. A prospective, randomised case–control study evaluating acute treatment found systemic anticoagulation to be the treatment of choice, even in the presence of intracerebral haemorrhage.[33] Untreated, the mortality is between 20% and 30%.

Multiple sclerosis (MS)

This disease is relatively common, with an incidence of between 0.06% and 0.1%, and it tends to occur during the childbearing years, with a peak incidence at 30 years of age. The cause of MS is unknown and the course is unpredictable. Common symptoms include the acute onset of diplopia, vertigo, gait instability, bladder incontinence, loss of vision and fatigue. The common neuropathological lesion is a plaque, demonstrating myelin loss and gliosis associated with inflammatory infiltrates. During pregnancy, the incidence of new cases of MS falls and the chance of relapse is reduced. This beneficial effect is, however, short term and exacerbation of the condition during the first 6 months postpartum occurs in between 20% and 40% of patients.[16] Spinal and epidural anaesthesia appear to be safe in labour, despite a diagnosis of MS. There is no long-term effect of pregnancy or breastfeeding on the course of MS; however, the children of women with MS have a 30-fold increase in their risk of developing the condition (a risk of 3% as compared with the background rate of 0.1% in the general population).[96]

Psychiatric disease

There is a wide range of psychiatric disease in pregnancy, which the acronym PND (postnatal depression) fails to encompass. Postpartum 'blues' affects between 50% and 70% of women and is a mild, self-limiting condition. It is characterised by symptoms such as weeping, sadness, irritability and anxiety. The symptoms usually peak around the fourth day and resolve by the 10th. In contrast, significant mental illness leading to suicide now accounts for at least 10% of all maternal deaths in the UK.[13] It is probable that this figure represents a significant underestimate, such that psychiatric causes may now be the leading cause of maternal mortality in Britain. This disturbing statistic is made more shocking by the violent nature of the suicides, which include hanging, throat cutting and self-immolation. At other times in women's lives, the most common cause of death by suicide is the ingestion of psychotropic medication.[13]

Postpartum depression

One out of every eight new mothers will have postpartum depression, and if a woman has had a previous episode of postpartum depression, she has a risk of one in four of a recurrence. Of those women who become depressed, between one-third and one-half will suffer from a severe depressive illness, 2% of all new mothers will see a psychiatrist during the first year after delivery, 4 per 1000 will be admitted to a psychiatric hospital, and 2 per 1000 will suffer from a puerperal psychosis.[13] Postpartum depression usually has an insidious onset within the first 3 to 6 months after childbirth. The mother's depressive thoughts typically centre on feelings of inadequacy in the maternal role and concerns for the wellbeing of the infant.[125] The signs and symptoms include increasing sleeplessness, loss of appetite and lack of energy. An assessment of thyroid function should be made and a history taken. If a patient has considered suicide or has thoughts about harming her baby, urgent psychiatric referral should be made and steps taken to ensure the safety of both mother and child. A selective serotonin-reuptake inhibitor is the first-line drug of choice. Given the frequency of postpartum depression, some authorities recommend that all women should be screened after delivery with the Edinburgh Postnatal Depression Scale,[18] which is brief, patient-friendly and reliably detects the presence of postpartum depression (with a score of 10 or more) (Table 11.2).

Diabetes

It is customary to classify women with diabetes in pregnancy into those where the woman had diabetes before conception (i.e. pre-existing diabetes) and those where the condition has developed during the pregnancy. Among the former, the great majority will be insulin-dependent diabetics. The latter will largely have gestational diabetes, where the impairment of glucose tolerance comes on during the pregnancy and resolves following delivery. Thus, the diagnosis of gestational diabetes can

Table 11.2 The Edinburgh Postnatal Depression Score. A score of 12 to 30 triggers a serious response. If the last question scores 3, an urgent response is required

Prompts	Answers	Score
I have been able to laugh and see the funny side of things:	As much as I always could	0
	Not quite so much now	1
	Definitely not so much now	2
	Not at all	3
I have looked forward with enjoyment to things:	As much as I always could	0
	Not quite so much now	1
	Definitely not so much now	2
	Not at all	3
I have blamed myself unnecessarily when things went wrong:	Yes, most of the time	3
	Yes some of the time	2
	Not very often	1
	No never	0
I have been anxious or worried for no good reason:	Yes, most of the time	3
	Yes some of the time	2
	Not very often	1
	No never	0
I have felt scared or panicky for no very good reason:	Yes, most of the time	3
	Yes some of the time	2
	Not very often	1
	No never	0
Things have been getting on top of me:	Yes, most of the time	3
	Yes some of the time	2
	Not very often	1
	No never	0
I have been so unhappy that I have had difficulty sleeping:	Yes, most of the time	3
	Yes some of the time	2
	Not very often	1
	No never	0
I have felt sad or miserable:	Yes, most of the time	3
	Yes some of the time	2
	Not very often	1
	No never	0
I have been so unhappy that I have been crying:	Yes, most of the time	3
	Yes some of the time	2
	Not very often	1
	No never	0
The thought of harming myself has occurred to me:	Yes, most of the time	3
	Yes some of the time	2
	Not very often	1
	No never	0

only be made with certainty once the pregnancy is over and glucose tolerance has returned to normal. There will be some women who happen to be diagnosed for the first time during their pregnancy. The difference between a true gestational diabetic and someone whose glucose impairment will continue in the long term is of little practical importance with respect to management during pregnancy. What matters to the fetus is whether glucose tolerance is normal or not.

Diabetes and the fetus

Congenital anomalies

Despite considerable advances in the management of pregnancy complicated by diabetes, the rate of congenital malformations among babies of women with pre-existing diabetes has not changed in several decades.[90] Overall, the risk is three to five times greater than in the general population and is related directly to the percentage of glycosylated haemoglobin at the time of conception.[109] The mechanism of this teratogenic effect is unknown, but it is related directly or indirectly to impaired glucose tolerance during the period of organogenesis, because the offspring of women with gestational diabetes do not show an excess of congenital abnormalities. It is likely that poor diabetic control later in the pregnancy also has implications for the subsequent wellbeing of the baby. An inverse relationship has been found between the intellectual development of the offspring and ketone and free fatty acid levels in the second and third trimesters.[91]

Spontaneous miscarriage

There appears to be an increased risk of miscarriage among women with pre-existing diabetes. This increased risk is associated with suboptimal diabetic control. Studies from countries such as Norway suggest that this excess pathology can be eliminated by good diabetic control during embryogenesis, which means that good metabolic control must be established before pregnancy.

Intrauterine fetal death

Despite advances in antenatal monitoring, women with poorly controlled diabetes still have an increased incidence of intrauterine fetal death, especially beyond the due date. The underlying mechanism has not been elucidated, but may be related to nocturnal hypoglycaemia.

Perinatal mortality

If deaths from congenital anomalies are excluded, women with well-controlled pre-existing diabetes now have no greater risk of experiencing a perinatal death than do women without diabetes. There is still controversy as to whether gestational diabetes leads to an increased risk of perinatal mortality. Reliable data are surprisingly difficult to obtain, but if there is an increased perinatal mortality, it appears only to be in pregnancies with very poor glucose control.

Neonatal morbidity

In contrast to mortality, neonatal morbidity is still relatively common among the babies of diabetic women. The problems are described in Chapter 22.

Screening for gestational diabetes and impaired glucose tolerance

A condition should not be screened for unless, if diagnosed and treated, health can be improved. Whereas the detection and treatment of overt diabetes is obviously worthwhile, the detection of impaired glucose tolerance in pregnancy remains controversial, apart from its role in identifying women who will be at very high risk of developing diabetes. Screening methods must have high degrees of sensitivity and specificity, and methods such as the use of potential diabetic features, random blood glucose determination and the use of glycosylated haemoglobin do not meet these criteria.

The only screening tests that have acceptable sensitivity and specificity are glucose challenge tests and the use of fasting glucose concentrations. A recent study of both methods[88] showed that for a challenge with a 50 g glucose load, using a cut-off at 1 hour of 7.0 mM resulted in 68% sensitivity and 82% specificity. Using a fasting value of 4.8 mM as a screen resulted in 81% sensitivity and 76% specificity. Although the sensitivity was higher with the fasting method, 30% of the population studied had to undergo a full glucose tolerance test as compared with 14% using the glucose challenge test. The number of tests can be halved by confining the test to women over the age of 25 years, with only a slight reduction in sensitivity. This approach is recommended in the USA, where women under 25 years of age are not usually screened unless they have potential diabetic features.[2] However, until the relevance of gestational impaired glucose tolerance is properly defined, major efforts to implement effective screening practice would not appear to be justified.

If the screening test is abnormal, then the patient should go on to have an oral glucose tolerance test (according to WHO recommendations). The diagnostic criteria are shown in Table 11.3.

Management of diabetic pregnancy

Organisation of care is important and women should preferably be managed in a unit with special interest and expertise in the area. The optimum care of the diabetic pregnancy requires a multidisciplinary approach including not only diabetologists and obstetricians but also dieticians, nurse specialists, neonatologists and ophthalmologists. It is particularly important for women to obtain preconception advice and for the control of the blood sugar to be optimised at that early stage. The aim of treatment is to maintain a normal blood glucose level. Diet and insulin are the key components of diabetic management. Oral hypoglycaemic agents are not widely used in the UK, although in the context of a high incidence of type-2 diabetes (e.g. in the Middle East) they are much more popular. Although there is no consistent evidence that oral hypoglycaemic agents are teratogenic, sulphonylureas cross the placenta and can therefore cause both fetal and neonatal hypoglycaemia.[1]

Diet

The aim is to provide sufficient energy for both mother and fetus, which amounts to 30–35 kcal/kg of non-pregnant ideal body weight. Daily carbohydrate consumption should be in the region of 220–240 g, providing at least 45% of the necessary calorie intake. Detailed and ongoing advice from an experienced dietician is important to the success of dietary management. Diet alone may be sufficient to control gestational diabetes, but if blood glucose exceeds 5.5 mM/l preprandially and 8 mM/l 1 hour postprandially, insulin should be commenced.

Insulin

Women with gestational diabetes who are not controlled by diet alone will need to achieve control using subcutaneous insulin. Increasingly, pen-type syringes are being used to deliver insulin, typically with three doses of short-acting insulin preprandially and one dose of a long-acting insulin at night. However, a woman who is well controlled on a biphasic insulin regimen should not be automatically changed to four times a day. The newer insulin analogues appear very suitable for pregnancy. Continuous subcutaneous insulin infusion appears to offer no advantage to most diabetic pregnant women and should only be used if there is an established continuous subcutaneous insulin service.

Monitoring of glucose

In order to achieve the aim of normoglycaemia throughout the day and night, it is necessary for the diabetic woman to monitor her blood glucose at home, and this would usually be performed between two and six times each day. Well-informed and experienced diabetic patients can then modify their insulin doses themselves. Longer-term control is assessed by measuring glycosylated haemoglobin, which should ideally be in the middle of the normal range.

Labour and the puerperium

Preterm delivery is more common in diabetic pregnancy, and if steroids are given to promote fetal lung maturity, they have a hyperglycaemic effect that usually requires intravenous insulin on a sliding scale to control. The combination of steroids and sympathomimetic drugs (used for tocolysis) requires even larger amounts of insulin for good diabetic control.

The timing of delivery has to be individualized. The woman with well-controlled diabetes, no vascular disease and a normally grown fetus appears to be at no more risk than her non-diabetic counterpart and may be allowed to go to at least the due date.

Table 11.3 Revised WHO criteria for the 75 g oral glucose tolerance test during pregnancy (Adapted from Chelsea and Westminster Hospital Guidelines)		
	Plasma glucose (mmol/l)	
	Fasting	**2 Hours**
Normal	≤5.4	≤7.9
Glucose intolerance	5.5–6.9	8.0–10.9
Gestational diabetes	≥7.0	≥11.0

With a mildly macrosomic fetus, delivery may be contemplated at approximately 37 weeks to try to avoid disproportion and reduce the risk of stillbirth. In a woman with nephropathy, it is often the maternal rather than the fetal condition that determines the timing of delivery.

Insulin requirements fall once labour is established and fall even further once the placenta has been delivered. During labour the most straightforward approach is to use 10% glucose at a constant rate of 1 l every 8 hours with human soluble insulin being given at 1 unit per hour and the dose adjusted according to the hourly blood glucose monitoring. Hyperglycaemia requires more insulin, hypoglycaemia more glucose (the insulin infusion rate should not be reduced below 1 unit per hour as although the blood sugar will then rise, ketoacidosis will occur as the cells will not be able to take up the glucose without sufficient insulin). Once the baby is delivered, the rate of insulin infusion should be reduced (or stopped if the woman has gestational diabetes), with the glucose being continued until the next meal, when pre-pregnancy insulin doses should be commenced. Careful dietary advice is needed in women who are going to breastfeed and they should be alert to the possibility of hypoglycaemia in their baby.

Thyroid disease

Hypothyroidism

Severe hypothyroidism leads to difficulty in conceiving and so is rare in pregnancy. Less severe forms, if untreated, lead to an increased risk of miscarriage and stillbirth through a mechanism which is not understood. It is unusual to diagnose hypothyroidism for the first time during pregnancy, and the majority of women present already on thyroxine (T_4) replacement therapy. Some have suggested that it may be advisable to increase the dose of T_4 as the pregnancy proceeds,[62] but in practice this is rarely judged to be necessary. Nevertheless, even in stable patients it is prudent to check thyroid-stimulating hormone (TSH) levels every trimester.

Thyrotoxicosis

Thyrotoxicosis is the clinical and biochemical state that results from an excess production of, and exposure to, thyroid hormone from any aetiology. It occurs in 0.2% of pregnancies; Graves' disease accounts for 95% of these cases.[32]

Both carbimazole (which is metabolised to methimazole) and propylthiouracil are used in the management of thyrotoxicosis during pregnancy. There are theoretical advantages to using propylthiouracil in that less crosses the placenta than with methimazole, and carbimazole has been associated with cutis aplasia, although the evidence is tenuous. Propylthiouracil also crosses into breast milk in lower quantities than does carbimazole. However, in practice it is doubtful whether there is any material difference between these two drugs, and treatment should be at a dose that maintains the free T_4 at the upper end of the normal range.

It has been reported that in up to 10% of women who have had Graves' disease, TSH receptor-stimulating antibodies cross the placenta and produce a fetal tachycardia (heart rate >160 beats per minute) and a neonatal thyrotoxicosis. Although the levels of these thyroid-stimulating antibodies can be measured in maternal blood, the assays are not readily available and measuring fetal heart rate in at-risk women is likely to be more useful. Treatment of fetal thyrotoxicosis is by increasing the maternal dose of antithyroid drugs until the fetal heart rate is in the normal range. The diagnosis and treatment of neonatal thyrotoxicosis is dealt with elsewhere (pp. 887–8). Although rare, neonatal thyrotoxicosis has a significant mortality, hence early treatment is vital.

Renal disease

A detailed account of this highly specialised subject is beyond the scope of this chapter and the reader should refer to Davison[21] and Williams[121] for recent reviews.

The number of people with end-stage renal disease is growing worldwide, even faster than the rise in the population. It is estimated that for every patient who needs a kidney transplant there are between 20 and 30 who have some degree of renal dysfunction. Diabetes and hypertension are the most common causal pathologies,[44] but whatever the underlying renal pathology, three generalisations can be made about renal disease and pregnancy. The first is that the more severe the disease, the less likely it is that pregnancy will end with a successful outcome. Only 1 in 200 women on long-term dialysis will conceive,[21] with a successful obstetric outcome in between 40% and 50%. The second is that the more severe the renal disease, the higher the likelihood that the pregnancy will result in a permanent deterioration in renal function. The third is that if, in addition to renal impairment, there is hypertension of sufficient severity to require treatment, then the prognosis both for the baby and for maternal renal function is worse than if hypertension were not present. In addition to these general principles the specific renal lesion may influence both the outcome of pregnancy and the subsequent course. Focal glomerulosclerosis, IgA nephropathy and reflux nephropathy, in particular, have been associated with worsening hypertension and renal function during pregnancy. In contrast, chronic glomerulonephritis may run a relatively benign course if hypertension is not present. The level of blood urea is not a particularly good guide to outcome, perhaps because it is a relatively non-toxic transport for nitrogenous waste products. A more useful guide is that, in general, women with serum creatinine (sCr) levels of less than 125 micromol/l have good obstetric outcomes and a good long-term renal prognosis. Those women with moderate (sCr 125–250 micromol/l) or severe (sCr >250 micromol/l) renal insufficiency do less well, with an accelerated deterioration in renal function. When the serum creatinine is greater than 180 micromol/l, it is likely that the risk of severe maternal complications is greater than the probability of a successful obstetric outcome,[41] with a 40–80% risk of developing pre-eclampsia and a 1 in 3 chance of end-stage renal failure within 1 year of delivery.[21] Management of pregnancy is mainly concerned with control of BP and timing of delivery with the aid of detailed maternal and fetal monitoring.

Asymptomatic bacteriuria

The incidence of asymptomatic bacteriuria is in the region of 5%,[78] but varies from 2% to 15%, being highest in those most socioeconomically deprived. *Escherichia coli* is the most commonly isolated pathogen and is present in 80–90% of urinary tract infections (UTIs) and up to 95% of acute pyelonephritis.[15] Between 30% and 50% of women with asymptomatic bacteriuria will develop pyelonephritis.[44] A relationship between asymptomatic bacteriuria, preterm delivery and low birthweight has been proposed,[82] possibly due to the fact that anything that causes inflammation in the mother increases the likelihood of labour (which is itself an inflammatory process, with the release of cytokines and prostaglandins). Some studies have linked untreated UTI in pregnancy with mental retardation and developmental delay in infancy as well as an increase in the rate of intrauterine death,[59] but this remains controversial. The cost-effectiveness of screening for asymptomatic bacteriuria depends on its incidence in any particular population; it is generally thought to be worthwhile if the incidence is 5% or more.

Acute cystitis

Diagnosis is complicated by the fact that most pregnant women experience intermittent frequency and dysuria. UTI is therefore commonly overdiagnosed. In one study of 1040 acute presentations to a labour ward, UTI was suspected in 151 cases but only confirmed on culture in four.[58] The diagnosis is more likely if there is in addition a raised temperature, which should prompt the administration of an appropriate broad-spectrum antibiotic (e.g. amoxicillin [amoxycillin] in non-allergic women). However, in all cases, accurate diagnosis requires urine culture.

Acute pyelonephritis

This occurs in up to 2% of pregnancies and is one of the causes of preterm labour.[19] It is the most common renal complication of pregnancy. The diagnosis is likely if there are symptoms of a UTI together with a high fever, nausea, vomiting and renal angle pain and tenderness. The patient should be admitted to hospital and treated with intravenous broad-spectrum antibiotics.

Renal transplantation and pregnancy

Pregnancy is becoming increasingly common in women who have been the recipients of renal transplants. About 1 in 50 women of childbearing age with renal allografts become pregnant.[21] Approximately 30% of pregnancies do not progress beyond the first trimester and of those pregnancies that do, 5% do not have a live birth. This is due to an increase in the incidence of maternal hypertension, preterm delivery (45–66%) and fetal growth restriction (40%). The prognosis is best when the transplanted kidney comes from a living donor, with no evidence of chronic rejection and the absence of proteinuria. Pregnancy success is also significantly related to the pre-pregnancy SCr level.[121]

Three drugs have been the mainstay of immunosuppressive therapy: prednisolone, ciclosporin A (cyclosporin A; CsA) and azathioprine. Newer agents include tacrolimus and mycophenolate mofetil (MMF). All these drugs cross the placenta, enter the fetal circulation and therefore represent a risk to fetal development.

- **Prednisolone.** There is no evidence that prednisolone is teratogenic in the human. Studies have shown that the number of birth defects observed in a population of women taking prednisolone during pregnancy is no different from that in the normal pregnant population.[6] There is also no persuasive evidence to suggest that prednisolone can affect the fetal or neonatal adrenal gland. This may be because prednisolone is significantly metabolised in the human placenta, with the result that very little reaches the fetus.
- **Azathioprine.** There have been sporadic reports of chromosomal fractures in the gametes of female fetuses exposed in utero to azathioprine, but a cause-and-effect relationship has not yet been established. Azathioprine can cause leukopenia and thrombocytopenia in both the mother and baby. There have been several reports suggesting that azathioprine can cause IUGR, but the relative contributions of drug and underlying disease are difficult to disentangle.
- **CsA.** This drug is not teratogenic in animals. The most recent meta-analysis[4] suggests that CsA is not a major human teratogen, with the overall prevalence of major malformations in the studied population being no different from that reported in the general population. It may, however, be associated with increased rates of preterm delivery.
- **Tacrolimus.** Experience in humans is still fairly limited, though information will become available as this drug is used more widely. Studies suggest that the incidence of malformation is similar to that reported with other immunosupressants.[45]
- **MMF.** Experience in humans is very limited. Case reports[86] have described successful pregnancy outcomes after its use.

In summary, the newborn infants of renal transplant recipients can be affected by the complications of prematurity and the risk of infection. Chromosomal aberrations are a theoretical possibility, but so far the evidence is reassuring. Pregnancy appears to have only a small effect on the medium- to long-term prognosis of the graft and the current view is that the proven benefits of using prednisolone, azathioprine and CsA outweigh their potential for harm, although the balance of benefits and risks may change as more information becomes available.

Haematological disease in pregnancy

Anaemia and pregnancy

Physiological changes

Plasma volume increases progressively throughout pregnancy so that by 36 weeks' gestation it is 50% greater than in the non-pregnant state. Most of the increase occurs by 34 weeks, and the amount of increase is positively correlated with the birthweight of the baby. There is also an increase in the red cell mass; however, the expansion in plasma volume is far greater than the increase in red cell mass, hence the net effect is a fall in haemoglobin concentration, haematocrit and red cell count. Despite this haemodilution, there is usually no change in mean corpuscular volume (MCV) or mean corpuscular haemoglobin concentration (MCHC). Pregnancy causes a two- to three-fold increase in the requirement for iron, and a 10–20-fold increase in folate requirements, to meet the demands of the expanding red cell mass, the fetus and the placenta. The lower limit of normal for haemoglobin concentration in the non-pregnant female is 11.5–12 g/dl. In pregnancy, levels below 10.5 g/dl may be abnormal, although, in certain situations, such as multiple pregnancies, the physiological dilution of haemoglobin may cause even lower concentration of haemoglobin. If there is a haemoglobin level between 9.5 and 11 g/dl with an MCV which is above 84 fl and which has not fallen more than 6 fl during the pregnancy in association with a well-grown fetus, then it probably does not indicate anaemia.[106,107]

Iron-deficiency anaemia

On a global basis, iron-deficiency anaemia is still a leading cause of maternal morbidity and mortality. In developed countries, significant iron-deficiency anaemia is uncommon, although most women are routinely prescribed supplements of iron and folic acid. There is no consensus about the value of giving prophylactic iron to a population which is largely well nourished. Routine administration of iron is cheaper than repeated testing of haemoglobin level, but has the disadvantage that many women experience side effects unnecessarily.

Folate-deficiency anaemia

Folic acid deficiency is the major cause of megaloblastic anaemia in pregnancy; vitamin B12 deficiency is very rare except in developing countries or strict vegans. Folate deficiency is more likely if the woman is taking anticonvulsants drugs or she suffers from haematological conditions such as haemolytic anaemia and thalassaemia. Diagnosis of folate deficiency should be confirmed by the measurement of serum and red cell folate levels (it should be noted that the normal range in pregnancy is lower than in non-pregnant women). All women planning pregnancy are now advised to take 400 microgram/day of folate periconceptionally, to lower the risk of NTDs and other fetal abnormalities, and this reduces the risk of folate deficiency still further. In addition, women who have had a previous fetus with an NTD and women taking anticonvulsants or sulfasalazine (sulphasalazine) are advised to take 5 mg folate periconceptionally.

Malignant disease and pregnancy

As the trend for delaying pregnancy into the later reproductive years continues, the frequency of pregnancy complicated by malignancy will probably increase. At present, cancer complicates

Table 11.4 Incidence of malignant disease in pregnancy (Adapted from Pavlidis[85] and Smith et al[103])

Tumour type	Incidence
Breast cancer	1:5000
Cervical cancer	1.2:10 000
Lymphoma	1:20 000
Melanoma	1:10 000
Leukaemia	1:75 000
Ovarian cancer	1:20 000
Colorectal cancer	1:50 000–100 000

between 1 in 1000 and 1 in 1500 pregnancies.[70] This is still relatively rare, given that cancer is the leading cause of death for women of reproductive age living in the developed world, with 1 in 52 developing an invasive malignancy before the age of 39 years. The most common malignancies associated with pregnancy include cervical cancer, breast cancer, melanoma and haematological cancers (Table 11.4). While the diagnosis, evaluation and treatment of pregnant women with cancer is essentially the same as for the non-pregnant, there is one obvious but crucial difference. How will treatment of maternal disease affect fetal survival and normal development? Treatments such as chemotherapy and radiotherapy clearly represent a risk to the developing fetus; however, this risk is modulated by a variety of factors including gestational age, treatment modality and treatment dose. Cancer per se rarely represents a significant risk to the fetus, and, counterintuitively, continuation of pregnancy has not been associated with accelerated tumour growth or deterioration in maternal prognosis for most malignancies. Thus, elective termination of pregnancy rarely offers a therapeutic advantage to the mother.[85]

Cervical cancer

While the incidence of cervical cancer has declined over recent years, it is still the most common malignancy diagnosed in pregnancy (1.6–10.6 cases per 10 000 pregnancies).[124] Because they are examined more frequently, pregnant women are three times more likely than non-pregnant women to have their disease diagnosed early (stage I disease).[127] Diagnosis can be made by colposcopy and colposcopic biopsy in any trimester. Since the majority of disease is diagnosed at an early stage, treatment can usually be delayed until a viable fetus can be delivered. Cervical cancer does not of itself adversely affect pregnancy and there is no difference in survival between pregnant and non-pregnant women matched for age, stage and year of diagnosis.[127] There is no reported difference in survival between women who deliver vaginally and those delivered by caesarean section. A significant proportion (up to 50%) of pre-invasive disease diagnosed in pregnancy disappears following birth, possibly because of physical changes in the cervix associated with delivery.

Breast cancer

The incidence of breast cancer during pregnancy is approximately 1 in 5000. There is no difference in survival between pregnant and non-pregnant women whose disease is matched for stage.[84] Unfortunately, pregnant women tend to present at a later stage in the disease process, with between 53% and 74% already having lymph node involvement at diagnosis. Ultrasound with fine-needle aspiration is the most sensitive investigation (with a sensitivity of 93%).[42] Modified radical mastectomy has usually been the treatment of choice for stage I and stage II breast cancer, although 'lumpectomy' has recently been reported as giving equivalent results in non-pregnant women.[35] Radiotherapy is usually delayed until after delivery of the fetus, though adjuvant chemotherapy can be given after the first trimester, following discussion with the mother. If breast cancer is treated, future pregnancy does not confer a worse prognosis on the mother. As most disease recurrence occurs within 3 years, some authorities advise delaying future conception until after this.

Malignant melanoma

Melanoma accounts for about 8% of all malignant tumours arising during pregnancy (incidence approximately 1:10 000).[103] The diagnosis of melanoma is made by histological assessment of the excised tumour. Site and depth are key factors in the prognosis, but pregnancy has no effect on survival. Therefore, women with adequate surgical excision should be encouraged to continue with their pregnancy. Unfortunately, however, malignant melanoma can spread to the fetus or placenta, and accounts for 30% of the reported cases of this type of metastasis.

Liver disease

Hepatic dysfunction is an important complication of pre-eclampsia. Apart from this, liver disease in pregnancy is relatively uncommon. However, there are two forms of liver disease specific to pregnancy that pose a risk to the mother and/or baby, intrahepatic cholestasis and acute fatty liver.

Intrahepatic cholestasis of pregnancy

Obstetric cholestasis (OC) is very irritating (literally; it causes severe itching) but carries little risk for the mother (with the exception of a small increase in the postpartum haemorrhage rate). It does, however, pose an important threat to the fetus. Sixty per cent of pregnancies complicated by OC end prematurely (both because of the early onset of spontaneous labour and because of induction of labour). A third are complicated by 'fetal distress' (the nature of which is often not simply hypoxia – see later) and up to 2% are associated with intrauterine death.[51] OC has a geographically variable prevalence, affecting between 0.1% and 1.5% of pregnancies in Europe (the incidence being higher in the Nordic countries) and 9.2–15.6% of pregnancies in South American countries such as Bolivia and Chile.[65]

The aetiology of the condition is not understood, but it appears to have both genetic and environmental components. It seems at least in part to be induced by high levels of oestrogen,

as symptoms may recur if an affected woman subsequently uses combined oral contraception. The hallmark of the condition is 'itch' with generalised pruritus, most notably of the palms and soles, causing great discomfort to the mother. Jaundice is uncommon (even though OC is the second most common cause of jaundice in pregnancy, the first being viral hepatitis),[69] although liver function tests are commonly abnormal. There is a rise in the transaminases in 60% of patients, raised bilirubin in 25% and raised serum bile acids in the vast majority (although not all).[65]

Badly affected women should be offered ursodeoxycholic acid (URSO) to relieve their pruritus. URSO makes the bile acids more hydrophilic and thus aids their excretion. It is not licensed for administration in pregnancy; however, there are no reports of teratogenesis associated with its use. Why the fetus is affected is not known, but it has been suggested that if the placenta has similar difficulty with bile acid transport as the maternal liver (perhaps by inheriting the same defect), then bile acid levels in the fetus will rise to dangerously high levels. Certainly, bile acids have been shown to cause asystole in cardiomyocytes in culture. If this theoretical model is correct, it is possible that URSO may also protect the fetus, but this has not yet been established.

Because almost all of the sudden intrauterine deaths occur after 36 weeks' gestation, it has become usual to induce labour at 37 weeks. Whether the resulting increase in problems associated with early delivery (especially respiratory distress syndrome) are justified by the decreased risk of stillbirth has not yet been established and prospective trials are needed. There is a marked increase in the incidence of meconium staining of the amniotic fluid, both before and during labour. The reasons for this are not known; they do not appear simply to be hypoxia. In a pregnancy complicated by OC, antepartum vitamin K should be given to the mother to reduce the risk of bleeding which occurs secondary to hepatic dysfunction. The symptoms usually resolve within a few days of delivery.

Acute fatty liver of pregnancy

This is an extremely rare condition, unique to pregnancy. Presentation is typically in the third trimester, with nausea and anorexia. There is often hypertension and proteinuria and the condition is associated with pre-eclampsia, multiple pregnancy and maternal obesity. It is also more common when the fetus is male (ratio 3:1). Transaminases are elevated as is alkaline phosphatase (above the normal upper limit for pregnancy), but the biochemical findings that generally distinguish acute fatty liver from pre-eclampsia are a much higher elevation of uric acid and marked hypoglycaemia. Jaundice is a late feature of the disease. MRI or CT scanning may help in the diagnosis. Although liver biopsy is diagnostic (showing microvesicles of fat in the hepatocytes), it is risky in a pregnant woman, especially if her clotting is abnormal. Precise diagnosis is less important than prompt delivery, which is usually mandated by deteriorating maternal condition. The woman's condition must be stabilised by general supportive measures including controlling hypertension and correcting hypoglycaemia and (as far as possible) deficiencies in clotting factors. The baby should then be delivered without delay. Acute fatty liver of pregnancy carries a maternal mortality of 10–20% and a perinatal mortality of 20–30%, but once the baby is born, improvement usually begins. If the mother survives (sometimes even liver transplantation is necessary), then full recovery is the rule.

Hepatitis

Infection with hepatitis viruses A, B, C and D produces a clinical picture in the pregnant woman very similar to that outside pregnancy. Management of vertical transmission of hepatitis A, B and C to the neonate is described elsewhere. Hepatitis E differs in that this usually mild disease carries a significant risk of maternal death, for reasons that are not understood. The high mortality makes it difficult to judge the frequency of vertical transmission, but one report suggests that this is very high.[47]

Respiratory disease

The pregnant woman is susceptible to a variety of respiratory complications and for unknown reasons up to 75% of women experience a subjective feeling of breathlessness at some time during pregnancy. This can lead, particularly in the third trimester, to diagnostic confusion.[77]

Pneumonia

The prevalence of pneumonia in pregnancy is between 0.4% and 1%,[111] the same as in non-pregnant women. With appropriate management, maternal mortality is no longer significantly increased,[23] though preterm labour remains a risk.

Cystic fibrosis

Cystic fibrosis (CF) is an autosomal recessive disorder arising from a defect on chromosome 7. The prevalence of the abnormal gene is about 4% in many white populations, with an incidence of homozygous CF of 1 in 2500 live births.[25] The median survival of women with this condition has changed from the early teens to the fourth decade over the last 50 years. Thus, women with CF are increasingly surviving into the reproductive age. The ability of the mother to carry the pregnancy to term appears to be primarily related to her pre-pregnancy lung function, although severe underweight is also an important risk factor. If the mother is generally fit, there is little evidence to suggest that the fetus will be affected by the mother's CF, though there is an increased risk of preterm delivery.[81] Patients with a low FEV_1 (<50%) should be managed in tertiary centres by a multidisciplinary team, as this level of pulmonary dysfunction carries a significant risk of maternal mortality from respiratory failure.

Asthma

The most commonly encountered respiratory disease in pregnancy is asthma, which affects 3% of the childbearing population.[55]

The prevalence is increasing.[10] There is no consistent effect of pregnancy on asthma, with some individuals showing improvement, some deteriorating, and some experiencing no change in symptoms. Poor control may reflect a variety of issues, including the woman's reluctance to take medication when pregnant because of (incorrect) fears of harmful drug effects on her unborn child, or because of incorrect advice from healthcare professionals.[67] The occurrence of nocturnal dyspnoea is the earliest symptom of inadequate control. Regular use of inhaled steroids should be encouraged as they are effective and pose no risk to the fetus. Regular use of beta sympathomimetics should be discouraged as they are associated with an increased long-term risk of sudden death. Oral steroids can be used safely if needed (see above).

The effect of asthma on pregnancy

In general, when asthma is severe, requiring chronic steroid therapy, there appears to be an increase in maternal and fetal morbidity, particularly if symptom control is poor.[115] Some studies have reported an unexplained increase in the incidence of preterm delivery in this group of women,[87] though other prospective studies have not confirmed this.[108] There are also studies suggesting a higher risk of pre-eclampsia, caesarean section and growth restriction[97] in women with asthma, but, once again, other studies have failed to confirm this.[108] The overall pregnancy outcome for women with well-managed asthma is comparable to that in the general population,[98] and asthmatic women can be reassured that with optimal disease control the outcome of their pregnancy will probably be normal.

The management of asthma in pregnancy

The management of asthma in pregnancy is essentially the same as in a non-pregnant woman. The avoidance of allergens and rapid control of infective exacerbations of disease are necessary. The guidelines of the National Asthma Campaign[71] recommend a stepwise approach to care, with particular emphasis on the prevention of attacks with the early introduction of steroids, rather than acute symptom control with regularly inhaled bronchodilators. Inhaled steroids are preferable to oral treatment because of the reduced incidence of maternal side effects. However, oral prednisolone or prednisone should not be withheld from a pregnant patient if required to treat severe asthma. There is no evidence of any teratogenic effects with the conventional drugs used to treat asthma, including β-agonists, oral or inhaled steroids, sodium cromoglycate and theophyllines. The theoretical risk of suppression of the fetal hypothalamo-pituitary-adrenal axis by maternal steroid therapy has not been substantiated in clinical practice. Beta-agonists do not delay the onset or slow the progress of normal labour.[102] Women who have received chronic steroid therapy for their asthma should be prescribed intramuscular hydrocortisone during labour. Regional anaesthesia is preferable to general anaesthesia because of the increased risks of atelectasis and postoperative chest infection following intubation.

Women who suffer with asthma should be encouraged to breastfeed, as there is some evidence that it may help to prevent atopic problems in their offspring.[43] None of the drugs used in the management of asthma (except tetracycline and iodides) are contraindicated in breastfeeding. The 4% background risk of a child developing asthma is increased approximately two- to threefold if one parent has asthma, particularly if he or she is atopic.

Hyperemesis gravidarum

Vomiting is a very common symptom of pregnancy, with over 50% of women reporting at least one episode by 16 weeks' gestation.[49] Hyperemesis gravidarum occurs when persistent vomiting in early pregnancy results in dehydration, ketosis and weight loss. Hospital admission is often required for intravenous hydration and electrolyte replacement. Most cases will then improve with no subsequent problems, but in some women the symptoms are intractable, necessitating frequent stays in hospital, and an increase in maternal and fetal complications is observed. The mechanisms underlying hyperemesis gravidarum remain unclear. A variety of agents have been linked to the pathogenesis of the disorder. These include hormones such as human chorionic gonadotrophin (hCG), free T_4, progesterone, oestrogen and cortisol, and immunological factors such as complement.[53] Mechanical factors such as delayed gastric emptying and lower oesophageal pressures, and psychological problems, are some of the other contributors.

Mild vomiting in pregnancy is appropriately regarded as a benign condition and, in fact, has been associated with a lower fetal loss rate and less likelihood of delivering preterm compared with pregnancies in which no vomiting occurs.[49] However, women with severe hyperemesis gravidarum associated with altered biochemistry and significant weight loss deliver growth-restricted infants, and hence increased fetal surveillance is mandatory. Severe hyperemesis gravidarum is potentially dangerous for the mother as well as the fetus, with three maternal deaths being reported between 1991 and 1993.[22] Complications include Mallory–Weiss oesophageal tears, Mendelson syndrome, retinal haemorrhage, thromboembolism and abnormal liver function. Raised transaminase levels usually return to normal when maternal nutrition improves. Neurological problems can include Wernicke's encephalopathy attributed to vitamin B_1 or thiamine deficiency, central pontine myelosis, possibly due to overzealous correction of severe hyponatraemia, peripheral neuropathies and muscle wasting or weakness. The psychological morbidity associated with hyperemesis gravidarum can also be severe, and considerable upset to family life may occur, especially if repeated hospital admission is required.

Management

A variety of medical disorders must be excluded when a woman presents with severe vomiting in pregnancy. Initially, an ultrasound scan should be performed to exclude multiple pregnancy and the presence of hydatidiform mole, in which the very high hCG levels may precipitate hyperemesis. A UTI should be considered, as should gastroenteritis, pancreatitis, gallstones and peptic ulcer disease. Endocrine disorders such as overt thyrotoxicosis, diabetic ketoacidosis and Addison's disease are included in the differential diagnosis, as well as vomiting secondary to drugs such as routine iron supplements.

The principles of treatment include appropriate parenteral fluid and electrolyte replacement such as Hartmann's solution or normal saline (0.9%). Oral or intravenous thiamine supplements should be prescribed in women with persistent vomiting. Antiemetics are of limited value (although they may have a placebo effect, they can also cause drowsiness) but should not be withheld if the mother requests them, as none of the commonly prescribed drugs, including phenothiazines, cyclizine and dopamine antagonists, have been found to be teratogenic in human studies.[66] The treatment of gastritis or oesophageal reflux with a histamine receptor antagonist such as ranitidine, the proton pump inhibitor omeprazole, or antacids may be beneficial in some cases. More recently, the use of corticosteroids to treat severe hyperemesis has been reported. Small uncontrolled studies have noted a dramatic rapid improvement in symptoms after oral prednisolone (40–60 mg daily) or intravenous hydrocortisone (50–100 mg b.i.d.).[73,74,112] A recent multicentre, randomised, double-blind, placebo-controlled study demonstrated a beneficial effect of steroids on appetite, weight gain and well-being and suggested that steroids may lead to improvement of nausea, vomiting and oral fluid intake and reduce the duration of dependence on intravenous fluids.[75] A larger study will be needed to determine whether these findings are attributable to chance. Although steroids are known to be safe for the fetus in the short term, there remains some caution regarding maternal side effects, as long-term steroid therapy may occasionally be required to control symptoms throughout pregnancy, and increases in the incidence of adult hypertension and diabetes are a long-term hazard for the fetus.

In patients with very severe weight loss and malnutrition, total parenteral nutrition may be needed.[14] Finally, it is important to provide constant psychological support and encouragement for the woman and her family.

Acknowledgements

This chapter draws heavily from the equivalent chapter in the previous edition of this textbook and the contribution of the earlier authors is gratefully acknowledged. It has, however, been substantially revised and updated.

References

1. Adam P A, King K, Schwartz, R 1968 Model for the investigation of intractable hypoglycemia: insulin-glucose interrelationships during steady state infusions. Pediatrics 41: 91–105
2. American Diabetes Association 1999 American Diabetes Association: clinical practice recommendations 1999. Diabetes Care 22(suppl. 1): S1–S114
3. Arpino C, Brescianini S, Robert E et al 2000 Teratogenic effects of antiepileptic drugs: use of an International Database on Malformations and Drug Exposure (MADRE). Epilepsia 41: 1436–1443

4. Bar Oz B, Hackman R, Einarson T, Koren G 2001 Pregnancy outcome after cyclosporine therapy during pregnancy: a meta-analysis. Transplantation 71: 1051–1055

5. Bates S M, Ginsberg J S 1997 Anticoagulants in pregnancy: fetal effects. Baillières Clinical Obstetrics and Gynaecology 11: 479–488

6. Briggs G G, Freeman R K, Yaffe S J 1994 Drugs in pregnancy and lactation. Williams & Wilkins, Baltimore

7. Brill-Edwards P, Ginsberg J S, Gent M et al 2000 Safety of withholding heparin in pregnant women with a history of venous thromboembolism. Recurrence of Clot in This Pregnancy Study Group. New England Journal of Medicine 343: 1439–1444

8. Broughton P F, Rubin P C 1994 Pre-eclampsia – the 'disease of theories'. British Medical Bulletin 50: 381–396

9. Burn J, Brennan P, Little J et al 1998 Recurrence risks in offspring of adults with major heart defects: results from first cohort of British collaborative study. Lancet 351: 311–316

10. Burney P G, Chinn S, Rona R J 1990 Has the prevalence of asthma increased in children? Evidence from the national study of health and growth 1973–86. British Medical Journal 300: 1306–1310

11. Carhaupoma J, Tomlinson M, Levine S 2000 Neuromuscular diseases. In: James D K, Steer P J (eds) High risk pregnancy. W B Saunders, London, pp 803–837

12. Carson J L, Kelley M A, Duff A et al 1992 The clinical course of pulmonary embolism. New England Journal of Medicine 326: 1240–1245

13. CEMD 2001 Why mothers die 1997–1999: The Confidential Enquiries into Maternal Deaths in the United Kingdom. RCOG Press, London

14. Charlin V, Borghesi L, Hasbun J, Von Mulenbrock R, Moreno MI 1993 Parenteral nutrition in hyperemesis gravidarum. Nutrition 9: 29–32

15. Connolly A, Thorp J M 1999 Urinary tract infections in pregnancy. Urologic Clinics of North America 26: 779–787

16. Cook S D, Troiano R, Bansil S 1993 Multiple sclerosis and pregnancy. In: Devinski C, Feldman E, Hainline B (eds) Neurological complications of pregnancy. Raven Press, New York, pp 83–85

17. Cornelissen M, Steegers-Theunissen R, Kollee L et al 1993 Increased incidence of neonatal vitamin K deficiency resulting from maternal anticonvulsant therapy. American Journal of Obstetrics and Gynecology 168(3 Pt 1): 923–928

18. Cox J L, Holden J M, Sagovsky R 1987 Detection of postnatal depression. Development of the 10-item Edinburgh Postnatal Depression Scale. British Journal of Psychiatry 150: 782–786

19. Cunningham F G, Lucas M J 1994 Urinary tract infections complicating pregnancy. Baillières Clinical Obstetrics and Gynaecology 8: 353–373

20. Dansky L V, Rosenblatt D S, Andermann E 1992 Mechanisms of teratogenesis: folic acid and antiepileptic therapy. Neurology 42(suppl. 5): 32–42

21. Davison J M 2001 Renal disorders in pregnancy. Current Opinion in Obstetrics and Gynaecology 13: 109–114

22. Department of Health 1996 Report on Confidential Enquiries into Maternal Deaths in the United Kingdom 1991–1993. RCOG Press, London

23. de Swiet M 1995 Diseases of the respiratory system. In: De Swiet M (ed) Medical disorders in obstetric practice. Blackwell Science, Oxford, pp 1–33

24. Dias M S, Sekhar L N 1990 Intracranial hemorrhage from aneurysms and arteriovenous malformations during pregnancy and the puerperium. Neurosurgery 27: 855–865

25. Dodge J A, Morison S, Lewis P A et al 1997 Incidence, population, and survival of cystic fibrosis in the UK, 1968–95. UK Cystic Fibrosis Survey Management Committee. Archives of Disease in Childhood 77: 493–496

26. Dolovich L R, Ginsberg J S, Douketis J D, Holbrook A M, Cheah G 2000 A meta-analysis comparing low-molecular-weight heparins with unfractionated heparin in the treatment of venous thromboembolism: examining some unanswered questions regarding location of treatment, product type, and dosing frequency. Archives of Internal Medicine 160: 181–188

27. Donaldson J 1995 Neurological disorders. In: de Swiet M (ed) Medical disorders in obstetric practice. Blackwell Science, Oxford

28. Douglas K A, Redman C W 1994 Eclampsia in the United Kingdom. British Medical Journal 309: 1395–1400

29. Duley L, Henderson-Smart D J 2002 Drugs for treatment of very high blood pressure during pregnancy (Cochrane Review). Cochrane Database of Systematic Reviews (4): CD001449

30. Duley L, Henderson-Smart D, Knight M, King J 2001 Antiplatelet drugs for prevention of pre-eclampsia and its consequences: systematic review. British Medical Journal 322: 329–333

31. Dulitzki M, Pauzner R, Langevitz P, Pras M, Many A, Schiff E 1996 Low-molecular-weight heparin during pregnancy and delivery: preliminary experience with 41 pregnancies. Obstetrics and Gynecology 87: 380–383

32. Ecker J L, Musci T J 1997 Treatment of thyroid disease in pregnancy. Obstetric and Gynecology Clinics of North America 24: 575–589

33. Einhaupl K M, Villringer A, Meister W et al 1991 Heparin treatment in sinus venous thrombosis. Lancet 338: 597–600

34. Ellison J, Walker I D, Greer I A 2000 Antenatal use of enoxaparin for prevention and treatment of thromboembolism in pregnancy. BJOG 107: 1116–1121

35. Fisher B, Jeong J H, Anderson S, Bryant J, Fisher E R, Wolmark N 2002 Twenty-five-year follow-up of a randomized trial comparing radical mastectomy, total mastectomy, and total mastectomy followed by irradiation. New England Journal of Medicine 347: 567–575

36. Gaily E, Kantola-Sorsa E, Granstrom M L 1990 Specific cognitive dysfunction in children with epileptic mothers. Development Medicine and Child Neurology 32: 403–414

37. Gould M K, Dembitzer A D, Doyle R L, Hastie T J, Garber A M 1999 Low-molecular-weight heparins compared with unfractionated heparin for treatment of acute deep venous thrombosis. A meta-analysis of randomized, controlled trials. Annals of Internal Medicine 130: 800–809

38. Greer I A, Thomson A J 2001 Management of venous thromboembolism in pregnancy. Ballieres Best Practice and Research. Clinical Obstetrics and Gynaecology 15: 583–603

39. Holmes L B 2002 The teratogenicity of anticonvulsant drugs: a progress report. Journal of Medical Genetics 39: 245–247

40. Howell R, Fidler J, Letsky E, de Swiet M 1983 The risks of antenatal subcutaneous heparin prophylaxis: a controlled trial. British Journal of Obstetrics and Gynaecology 90: 1124–1128

41. Imbasciati E, Pardi G, Capetta P et al 1986 Pregnancy in women with chronic renal failure. American Journal of Nephrology 6: 193–198

42. Ishida T, Yokoe T, Kasumi F et al 1992 Clinicopathologic characteristics and prognosis of breast cancer patients associated with pregnancy and lactation: analysis of case-control study in Japan. Japanese Journal of Cancer Research 83: 1143–1149

43. Jellife D, Jellife E 2003 'Breast is best': modern meanings. New England Journal of Medicine 297: 912–915

44. Jones C A, McQuillan G M, Kusek J W et al 1998 Serum creatinine levels in the US population: Third National Health and Nutrition Examination Survey. American Journal of Kidney Diseases 32: 992–999

45. Kainz A, Harabacz I, Cowlrick I S, Gadgil S, Hagiwara D 2000 Analysis of 100 pregnancy outcomes in women treated systemically with tacrolimus. Transplant International 13(suppl. 1): S299–S300

46. Kaku D A, Lowenstein D H 1990 Emergence of recreational drug abuse as a major risk factor for stroke in young adults. Annals of Internal Medicine 113: 821–827

47. Khuroo M S, Kamili S, Jameel S 1995 Vertical transmission of hepatitis E virus. Lancet 345: 1025–1026

48. Kittner S J, Stern B J, Feeser B R et al 1996 Pregnancy and the risk of stroke. New England Journal of Medicine 335: 768–774

49. Klebanoff M A, Koslowe P A, Kaslow R, Rhoads G G 1985 Epidemiology of vomiting in early pregnancy. Obstetrics and Gynecology 66: 612–616

50. Koch S, Losche G, Jager-Roman E et al 1992 Major and minor birth malformations and antiepileptic drugs. Neurology 42(suppl. 5): 83–88

51. Lammert F, Marschall H U, Glantz A, Matern S 2000 Intrahepatic cholestasis of pregnancy: molecular pathogenesis, diagnosis and management. Journal of Hepatology 33: 1012–1021

52. Leppik I, Rask C 1989 Pharmacokinetics of antiepileptic drugs during pregnancy. Seminars in Neurology 8: 240–246

53. Leylek O A, Toyaksi M, Erselcan T, Dokmetas S 1999 Immunologic and biochemical factors in hyperemesis gravidarum with or without hyperthyroxinemia. Gynecologic and Obstetric Investigation 47: 229–234

54. Lindhout D 1992 Pharmacogenetics and drug interactions: role in antiepileptic-drug-induced teratogenesis. Neurology 42(suppl. 5): 43–47

55. Littlejohns P, Ebrahim S, Anderson R 1989 Prevalence and diagnosis of chronic respiratory symptoms in adults. British Medical Journal 298: 1556–1560

56. Lowe G D 1997 Treatment of venous thrombo-embolism. Baillières Clinical Obstetrics and Gynaecology 11: 511–521

57. Lupton M, Oteng-Ntim E, Ayida G, Steer P J 2002 Cardiac disease in pregnancy. Current Opinion in Obstetrics and Gynecology 14: 137–143

58. MacDermott R I 1994 The interpretation of midstream urine microscopy and culture results in women who present acutely to the labour ward. British Journal of Obstetrics and Gynaecology 101: 712–713

59. McDermott S, Callaghan W, Swejbka L 2000 Urinary tract infections during pregnancy and mental retardation and developmenal delay. Obstetrics and Gynecology 96: 113–119

60. Macklon N S, Greer I A 1996 Venous thromboembolic disease in obstetrics and gynaecology: the Scottish experience. Scottish Medical Journal 41: 83–86

61. Magpie Trial Co-ordinators Group 2002 Do women with pre-eclampsia, and their babies, benefit from magnesium sulphate? The Magpie Trial: a randomised placebo-controlled trial. Lancet 359: 1877–1890

62. Mandel S J, Larsen P R, Seely E W, Brent G A 1990 Increased need for thyroxine during pregnancy in women with primary hypothyroidism. New England Journal of Medicine 323: 91–96

63. Martin J N Jr, Perry K G Jr, Miles J F Jr et al 1993 The interrelationship of eclampsia, HELLP syndrome, and prematurity: cofactors for significant maternal and perinatal risk. British Journal of Obstetrics and Gynaecology 100: 1095–1100

64. Mas J, Lamy C 1998 Stroke in pregnancy and the puerperium Journal of Neurology 245: 305–313

65. Milkiewicz P, Elias E, Williamson C, Weaver J 2002 Obstetric cholestasis. British Medical Journal 324: 123–124

66. Milkovich L, van der Berg B J 1977 Effects of antenatal exposure to anorectic drugs. American Journal of Obstetrics and Gynecology 129: 637–642

67. Moore-Gillon, J 1994 Asthma in pregnancy. British Journal of Obstetrics and Gynaecology 101: 658–660

68. Moslet U, Hansen E S 1992 A review of vitamin K, epilepsy and pregnancy. Acta Neurologica Scandinavica 85: 39–43

69. Mullally B A, Hansen W F 2002 Intrahepatic cholestasis of pregnancy: review of the literature. Obstetrical and Gynecological Survey 57: 47–52

70. Munkarah A, Morris R 2000 Malignant disease in pregnancy. In: James D K, Steer P J, Weiner C P, Gonik B (eds) High risk pregnancy, management options. W B Saunders, London, pp 945–959

71. National Asthma Campaign 1997 The management of chronic asthma in adults and school children. Thorax 52(suppl. 1): S11

72. Nelson-Piercy C 1994 Low molecular weight heparin for obstetric thrombo-prophylaxis. British Journal of Obstetrics and Gynaecology 101: 6–8

73. Nelson-Piercy C, de Swiet M 1994 Corticosteroids for the treatment of hyperemesis gravidarum. British Journal of Obstetrics and Gynaecology 101: 1013–1015

74. Nelson-Piercy C, de Swiet M 1995 Complications and the use of corticosteroids for the treatment of hyperemesis gravidarum. British Journal of Obstetrics and Gynaecology 102: 507–509

75. Nelson-Piercy C, Fayers P, de Swiet M 2001 Randomised, double-blind, placebo-controlled trial of corticosteroids for the treatment of hyperemesis gravidarum. BJOG 108: 9–15

76. Nelson-Piercy C, Letsky E A, de Swiet M 1997 Low-molecular-weight heparin for obstetric thromboprophylaxis: experience of sixty-nine pregnancies in sixty-one women at high risk. American Journal of Obstetrics and Gynecology 176: 1062–1068

77. Nelson-Piercy C, Williamson C 2001 Medical disorders in pregnancy. In: Chamberlain G, Steer P J (eds) Turnbull's obstetrics. Churchill Livingstone, Edinburgh, pp 275–299

78. Norden C W, Kass E H 1968 Bacteriuria of pregnancy – a critical appraisal. Annual Review of Medicine 19: 431–470

79. Nulman I, Scolnik D, Chitayat D, Farkas L D, Koren G 1997 Findings in children exposed in utero to phenytoin and carbamazepine monotherapy: independent effects of epilepsy and medications. American Journal of Medical Genetics 68: 18–24

80. Oakley C M 1995 Anticoagulation and pregnancy. European Heart Journal 16: 1317–1319

81. Odergraad I, Stray-Pederson B 2002 Maternal and fetal morbidity in pregnancies of Norwegian and Swedish women with cystic fibrosis. Acta Obstetricia et Gynecologica Scandinavica 81: 698–705

82. Ovalle A, Levancini M 2001 Urinary tract infections in pregnancy. Current Opinion in Urology 11: 55–59

83. Palmieri C, Canger R 2002 Teratogenic potential of the newer antiepileptic drugs: what is known and how should this influence prescribing? CNS Drugs 16: 755–764

84. Parente J T, Amsel M, Lerner R, Chinea F 1988 Breast cancer associated with pregnancy. Obstetrics and Gynecology 71: 861–864

85. Pavlidis N A 2002 Coexistence of pregnancy and malignancy. The Oncologist 7: 279–287

86. Pergola P E, Kancharla A, Riley D J 2001 Kidney transplantation during the first trimester of pregnancy: immunosuppression with mycophenolate mofetil, tacrolimus, and prednisone. Transplantation 71: 994–997

87. Perlow J H, Montgomery D, Morgan M A, Towers C V, Porto M 1992 Severity of asthma and perinatal outcome. American Journal of Obstetrics and Gynecology 167: 963–967

88. Perucchini D, Fischer U, Spinas G A, Huch R, Huch A, Lehmann R 1999 Using fasting plasma glucose concentrations to screen for gestational diabetes mellitus: prospective population based study. British Medical Journal 319: 812–815

89. Redman C W 1976 Fetal outcome in trial of antihypertensive treatment in pregnancy. Lancet 2: 753–756

90. Reece E A, Homko C J 2000 Why do diabetic women deliver malformed infants? Clinical Obstetrics and Gynecology 43: 32–45

91. Rizzo T, Metzger B E , Burns W J, Burns K 1991 Correlation between antepartum maternal metabolism and intelligence of offspring. New England Journal of Medicine 325: 9111–9116

92. Romano-Zelekha O, Hirsh R, Blieden L, Green M, Shohat T 2001 The risk for congenital heart defects in offspring of individuals with congenital heart defects. Clinical Genetics 59: 325–329

93. Rosa F W 1991 Spina bifida in infants of women treated with carbamazepine during pregnancy. New England Journal of Medicine 324: 674–677

94. Royal College of Obstetricians and Gynaecologists 2001 RCOG Guideline No 28. Thromboembolic disease in pregnancy and the puerperium: acute management. RCOG, London

95. Rubin P C, Butters L, Clark D M et al 1983 Placebo-controlled trial of atenolol in treatment of pregnancy-associated hypertension. Lancet 1: 431–434

96. Sadovnick A D 1984 Empiric recurrence risks for use in the genetic counselling of multiple sclerosis patients. American Journal of Medical Genetics 17: 713–714

97. Schatz M, Zeiger R S, Hoffman C P 1990 Intrauterine growth is related to gestational pulmonary function in pregnant asthmatic women. Kaiser-Permanente Asthma and Pregnancy Study Group. Chest 98: 389–392

98. Schatz M, Zeiger R S, Hoffman C P et al 1995 Perinatal outcomes in the pregnancies of asthmatic women: a prospective controlled analysis. American Journal of Respiratory and Critical Care Medicine 151: 1170–1174

99. Schmidt D, Canger R, Avanzini G et al 1983 Change of seizure frequency in pregnant epileptic women. Journal of Neurology, Neurosurgery and Psychiatry 46: 751–755

100. Scolnik D, Nulman I, Rovet J et al 1994 Neurodevelopment of children exposed in utero to phenytoin and carbamazepine monotherapy. Journal of the American Medical Association 271: 767–770

101. Shennan A H, Poston L, Chappell L C, Seed P T 2001 Prevention of pre-eclampsia. Lancet 357: 1534

102. Sims C D, Chamberlain G V, de Swiet M 1976 Lung function tests in bronchial asthma during and after pregnancy. British Journal of Obstetrics and Gynaecology 83: 434–437

103. Smith L, Danielsen B, Allen M, Cress R 2003 Cancer associated with obstetric delivery: results of linkage with the California cancer registry. American Journal of Obstetrics and Gynecology 189: 1128–1135

104. Srinivasan K 1983 Cerebral venous and arterial thrombosis in pregnancy and puerperium. A study of 135 patients. Angiology 34: 731–746

105. Steer P J 1999 The definition of pre-eclampsia. British Journal of Obstetrics and Gynaecology 106: 753–755

106. Steer P J 2000 Maternal hemoglobin concentration and birth weight. American Journal of Clinical Nutrition 71(suppl.): 1285S–1287S

107. Steer P, Alam M A, Wadsworth J, Welch A 1995 Relation between maternal haemoglobin concentration and birth weight in different ethnic groups. British Medical Journal 310: 489–491

108. Stenius-Aarniala B, Piirila P, Teramo K 1988 Asthma and pregnancy: a prospective study of 198 pregnancies. Thorax 43: 12–18

109. Stiete H, Stiete S, Jahrig D, Briese V, Willich S N 1995 [Risk groups of newborn infants of diabetic mothers in relation to their somatic outcome and maternal diabetic metabolic status in pregnancy.] Zeitschrift fur Geburtshilfe und Neonatologie 199: 156–162

110. Sturridge F, de Swiet M, Letsky E 1994 The use of low molecular weight heparin for thromboprophylaxis in pregnancy. British Journal of Obstetrics and Gynaecology 101: 69–71

111. Susanti I, Edmundo R 2001 Respiratory complications of pregnancy. Obstetrical and Gynecological Survey 57: 39–46

112. Taylor R 1996 Successful management of hyperemesis gravidarum using steroid therapy. Quarterly Journal of Medicine 89: 103–107

113. Tennis P, Eldridge R R 2002 Preliminary results on pregnancy outcomes in women using lamotrigine. Epilepsia 43: 1161–1167

114. Thomson A J, Walker I D, Greer I A 1998 Low-molecular-weight heparin for immediate management of thromboembolic disease in pregnancy. Lancet 352: 1904

115. Turner E S, Greenberger P A, Patterson R 1980 Management of the pregnant asthmatic patient. Annals of Internal Medicine 93: 905–918

116. Ville Y, Jenkins E, Shearer M J et al 1993 Fetal intraventricular haemorrhage and maternal warfarin. Lancet 341: 1211

117. Warkentin T E 2002 Platelet count monitoring and laboratory testing for heparin-induced thrombocytopenia. Archives of Pathology and Laboratory Medicine 126: 1415–1423

118. Warkentin T E, Levine M N, Hirsh J et al 1995 Heparin-induced thrombocytopenia in patients treated with low-molecular-weight heparin or unfractionated heparin. New England Journal of Medicine 332: 1330–1335

119. Weinstein L 1982 Syndrome of hemolysis, elevated liver enzymes, and low platelet count: a severe consequence of hypertension in pregnancy. American Journal of Obstetrics and Gynecology 142: 159–167

120. Wiebers D O 1985 Ischemic cerebrovascular complications of pregnancy. Archives of Neurology 42: 1106–1113

121. Williams D J 2001 Renal disease and fluid balance in pregnancy. Current Obstetrics and Gynaecology 11: 146–152

122. Williams D J, de Swiet M 1997 The pathophysiology of pre-eclampsia. Intensive Care Medicine 23: 620–629

123. Williams P G, Hersh J H 1997 A male with fetal valproate syndrome and autism. Developmental Medicine and Child Neurology 39: 632–634

124. Wingo P A, Tong T, Bolden S 1995 Cancer statistics, 1995. CA: A Cancer Journal for Clinicians 45: 8–30

125. Wisner K L, Parry B L, Piontek C M 2002 Clinical practice. Postpartum depression. New England Journal of Medicine 347: 194–199

126. Yerby M S, Devinsky O 1994 Epilepsy and pregnancy. Advances in Neurology 64: 45–63

127. Zemlickis D, Lishner M, Degendorfer P, Panzarella T, Sutcliffe S B, Koren G 1991 Maternal and fetal outcome after invasive cervical cancer in pregnancy. Journal of Clinical Oncology 9: 1956–1961

CHAPTER 12

Obstetrics for the neonatologist

Francoise-Helene D Harlow, John A D Spencer

Introduction

Obstetrics is an ever-evolving specialty. In the earlier part of the last century efforts were concentrated on reducing maternal mortality. The results have been dramatic even in recent years. Between 1973/75 and 1988/90 the UK maternal mortality rate fell by 54%, from nine to four maternal deaths per million women aged 15–44.[28–30] During the 1960s to 1980s the focus widened to the fetus. Cardiotocographic (CTG) monitoring and fetal scalp blood sampling were introduced in an attempt to decrease perinatal mortality. Early studies[63] showed that the introduction of continuous fetal heart rate (FHR) monitoring was associated with a reduction in the incidence of intrapartum stillbirths in complicated labours. Consequently, the number of fetal monitors for use during labour in Great Britain increased by nearly 90% between 1977 and 1984.[123] However, subsequent analysis of pooled results[92,118] showed that continuous monitoring had no overall effect on perinatal mortality but did significantly reduce the incidence of neonatal seizures. Despite this apparent advantage, follow-up of the largest study in Dublin[79] showed that the incidence of cerebral palsy was similar in both groups at 4 years of age, and only 22% of children with cerebral palsy had shown signs of birth asphyxia.[45] This study, however, recruited only uncomplicated pregnancies (with a normal volume of clear liquor) in whom the incidence of intrapartum stillbirth was already as low as 0.4 per 1000. Indeed, it seems increasingly likely that perinatal mortality and morbidity has reached its nadir in uncomplicated pregnancies in which placental function is considered normal at the onset of labour.

The focus of obstetric care is, therefore, changing once again. Identification of complicated pregnancies and abnormal placental function is increasingly the aim of modern obstetric management. This is reflected in the recent recommendations for the provision of maternity services.[27] This encourages midwives to manage the majority of low-risk pregnancies, with medical involvement concentrated on cases identified as being at increased risk of complications, or which subsequently deviate from the expected norm.

The aim of this chapter is to outline the intrapartum assessment of fetal wellbeing in the structurally and chromosomally normal fetus. However, the wellbeing of the fetus *prior* to labour or elective delivery is the key to the fetus's ability to tolerate intrapartum stresses. Antenatal assessment of fetal wellbeing is therefore of paramount importance and is covered in detail in other chapters of this book. Antenatal placental function, which determines fetal growth velocity and the liquor volume, is routinely assessed clinically with symphysis–fundal height measurements. Serial growth scans, Doppler studies and cardiotocography are then used selectively when indicated. Pregnancies at increased risk of placental compromise, for example multiple pregnancies or in women who have had previous growth-restricted fetuses, are routinely followed with serial ultrasound scans. Fetuses with poor growth velocities, oligohydramnios, abnormal Doppler studies or abnormal cardiotocographs are less likely to tolerate the stresses of labour, since placental blood flow is compromised with each uterine contraction/tightening. Thus placental reserve at the onset of labour is of critical importance.

Currently, intrapartum assessment of fetal wellbeing determined by placental function is the best available predictor of neonatal outcome. Common complications and management strategies will also be covered in this chapter. Clearly, this account cannot be exhaustive: the intention is to concentrate on aspects of obstetric care of relevance to the neonatologist. Suggestions for further reading and other sources of information are included at the end of the chapter.

Intrapartum assessment and management

This section begins by discussing the mechanism of normal labour and methods of correcting slow progress. It then goes on to describe the fetal response to labour and ways of assessing intrapartum fetal wellbeing. Finally it covers methods of delivery: this is the time at which the neonatologist often becomes involved for the first time. We hope to have demonstrated, however, that the antenatal and intrapartum course leading up to this point should also be of interest to the attending paediatrician.

The mechanism of labour

Recognition of the onset of labour determines all subsequent management objectives.

Diagnosis of labour

A diagnosis of labour is made when regular painful uterine activity effects a change in the cervix. Pain, however, is a subjective experience and is always important to the mother, especially when it is bad enough for her to ask for analgesia. Regularity – an objective observation – is usually accepted when contractions occur more frequently than once every 5 minutes. When regular contractions are considered painful by the mother the question of 'confirming' the diagnosis of labour is appropriate. If the cervix is 3 or more centimetres dilated then labour is usually diagnosed with certainty. If the cervix is less dilated, this is when conservative and active approaches differ in subsequent management.

Early graphical descriptions of labour[38] indicated that 'early' labour (defined as cervical dilatation of less than 3 cm) could last many hours. This led to the idea that there is a slow, or latent, phase of labour, followed by a faster, or active, phase. With a conservative approach, when the cervix is less than 3 cm dilated the woman would be told that she was not yet in 'established labour'. Usually a further examination is performed 4 hours later. 'Early' labour, however, may last for many hours and can lead to maternal exhaustion and reduced fetal reserve.

The philosophy of 'active management' of labour,[95] however, challenges the idea that prolonged labour is a normal and an inevitable consequence if women present 'early' in labour and have yet to get through the latent phase. In the National Maternity Hospital, Dublin, 98% of first labours deliver within 12 hours of the diagnosis of labour. Early and accurate diagnosis of labour is one key feature of the management. Effacement or dilatation of the cervix (by 1 cm), a 'show' and ruptured membranes are all features that are used to 'confirm' the onset of labour in such circumstances. The problem with this approach is that it inevitably leads to a rather low threshold for intervention such as oxytocin infusion.

Progress in labour

Once labour has been diagnosed then progress is expected within certain time limits. Regular examinations of the cervix are made, at least every 4 hours with conservative management and every 1–2 hours with active management, so that the rate of dilatation can be plotted against time. The use of a composite graphical record of progress in labour, described as a 'partogram', was first reported from Africa.[99] This was soon complemented by a nomogram of expected progress.[116] The most widespread expectation for progress in labour is a rate of at least 1 cm cervical dilatation per hour, which derives from the slowest 10% of women reported by Philpott.[99] With conservative management this expectation begins after the cervix has reached 3 cm dilatation; with active management it begins when labour is diagnosed. Interventions to augment progress are more frequent in active management. However, with active management there is a reduction by almost 50%

in the likelihood of a caesarean section due to dystocia, i.e. ineffective uterine activity.[77] Nonetheless, many midwives, some obstetricians and pregnant women see active management of labour as unnecessary 'medical' intervention and prefer the conservative approach.

Management of the second stage of labour has undergone a change in recent years, particularly since the more widespread use of regional analgesia with epidurals. Once the cervix is fully dilated, progress is defined as descent of the presenting part through the birth canal. This is often judged by hourly vaginal examinations. As the fetus exerts pressure on the pelvic floor (levator ani muscles), the mother feels increasing rectal pressure and an irresistible urge to push. In multiparous women this sensation can occur before full dilatation is reached, and active pushing is then usually discouraged to prevent the cervix from becoming oedematous.

In the absence of an epidural, the usual limits of duration for pushing are 60–90 minutes for first labours and 30–60 minutes for multiparous women. These recommendations have some support, in that fetal hypoxia and acidaemia increase progressively during the second stage.[58] However, in recent years, with the increasing use of epidural analgesia, more time in the second stage before pushing has been shown to improve the chance of vaginal delivery[64] without a major deterioration in fetal pH.[83] Nevertheless, the need for operative assistance remains significantly increased[57] and many consider one additional hour sufficient to minimise this possibility.

Interventions during labour

There are two interventions designed to improve the rate of progress during spontaneous labour, amniotomy and intravenous infusion of oxytocin. Both can also be used to induce labour.

Rupture of the membranes

One of the aspects of active management is the use of amniotomy within 2 hours if cervical dilatation is not evident following the diagnosis of labour.[95] However, routine rupture of the membranes to prevent slow progress in labour has been criticised. A large collaborative study[12] showed that membranes ruptured spontaneously in only 66% of women before the second stage. Earlier amniotomy significantly shortened the duration of labour but was associated with a higher incidence of caput formation and moulding of the fetal head. In addition, there was an increased incidence of early uniform FHR decelerations and a significantly lower median umbilical artery pH at birth (albeit still within the normal range). These findings can be explained on the basis of increased uterine activity, greater head compression and cord compression. A more recent study[115] has suggested that the effect of amniotomy on the fetus is a balance between the adverse effects of augmentation and the benefits of reduced duration of labour.

Effects of oxytocin

Augmentation of spontaneous labour by oxytocin infusion aims to achieve optimal uterine activity with a maximum contraction frequency of once every 2 minutes. Uterine perfusion decreases during contractions, resulting in a decrease in blood flow to the intervillous space.[6] As long as the relaxation periods between contractions remain adequate, and sustained uterine tonus is avoided, fetal bradycardia is not seen[14] and fetal cerebral oxygenation remains unaffected.[97] Nevertheless, in clinical practice the use of oxytocin is associated with an increased incidence of FHR decelerations.[107]

Intrapartum fetal assessment

The fetus responds to many aspects of labour and its management. Monitoring of fetal wellbeing requires an understanding of placental function and, in particular, knowledge of the influence of pregnancy complications and labour on maternal-fetal gas exchange. During labour, observations are made on the amount and colour of the amniotic fluid, but the mainstay of fetal monitoring is the recording, either intermittently or continuously, of the FHR. Optimal interpretation of some changes requires fetal blood sampling (FBS) to determine the fetal acid–base level.

Amniotic fluid volume

A normal volume of amniotic fluid offers some degree of protection against the many effects of uterine contractions. The volume of the intervillous space is maintained and is not compressed against the fetus, and the umbilical cord is also less likely to be compressed. Oligohydramnios present before postdates labour is a predictor for intrapartum fetal distress.[25] Therefore, continuous FHR monitoring is advocated and decelerations are more readily interpreted as an indication of clinically important fetal hypoxia. Likewise, reduced liquor volume in early labour, for instance subsequent to amniotomy, is associated with an increased chance of subsequent FHR decelerations.[103] Infusion of saline into the amniotic cavity during labour has been shown to decrease the incidence of FHR decelerations and may reduce the likelihood of caesarean section being considered necessary.

Meconium

The passage of meconium into the amniotic fluid during labour (fresh meconium) is one of the traditional indicators of fetal distress, and is associated with increased perinatal morbidity and mortality.[9] However, meconium-stained amniotic fluid before labour (old meconium) is found increasingly after 37 weeks' gestation, occurring in 15–20% of pregnancies reaching 41 weeks. It is often found at the time of caesarean section after prolonged labour in the absence of other evidence of fetal distress, yet it is rarely seen in situations of acute fetal distress, such as placental abruption and cord prolapse. The mechanism by which the fetal bowel is stimulated to pass meconium is unclear.

Meconium is sterile but its importance lies in the risk of neonatal meconium aspiration syndrome. This only occurs in about 1% of cases with meconium present. It is now believed that meconium aspiration can occur in utero prior to delivery. The precise aetiology remains obscure, although associated fetal distress predisposes to perinatal morbidity if meconium is present. The current view is that fetal hypoxia and acidaemia lead to an increase in fetal gasping and deep breathing movements respectively. These are the breathing movements that cause inhalation of amniotic fluid, with meconium if present. Meconium aspiration is more common if the meconium is thick rather than thin.[105] Oligohydramnios leads to the meconium remaining thick and undiluted, and may be an important determinant of any subsequent fetal distress in such circumstances. The passage of prelabour meconium may represent a previous transient fetal stimulation, possibly hypoxic, although infection and thyrotoxicosis are rare causes.

Thus, meconium remains an indication for continuous monitoring of the FHR during labour, and the presence of meconium lowers the threshold for making a diagnosis of fetal distress if FHR abnormalities occur.

Fetal heart rate monitoring

The value of continuous electronic FHR monitoring (EFM) during labour remains controversial. Randomised trials have suggested that continuous EFM confers no outcome advantage over intermittent auscultation for normal, uncomplicated labours.[79] However, this may be a reflection of the rather simplistic interpretation advocated by early enthusiasts.[56] Simple 'pattern recognition' of changes in the FHR has not been shown to be helpful, and it has since been realised that the FHR is a sophisticated reflection of fetal adaptation to changes in the intrauterine environment. The CTG must therefore be interpreted in the context of the clinical picture. The future of FHR monitoring requires further understanding and acceptance of a more physiological approach to interpretation.[113]

Despite its apparently limited value, EFM is still in widespread use. Continuous monitoring is considered mandatory in high-risk cases, e.g. in the presence of meconium or when there is recognised intrauterine growth restriction (IUGR). It is therefore important that the attending paediatrician has a basic understanding of the implications of normal and abnormal FHR records.

Fetal heart rate records are usually assessed with respect to four main features.[104]

- **Baseline rate**. This is the mean rate in beats per minute determined over a 5–10-minute interval, when stable in the absence of accelerations and decelerations.
- **Baseline variability**. This refers to oscillations of the recorded baseline FHR (previously described as long-term variability). Both amplitude and frequency may be important.
- **Accelerations**. An acceleration is a transient rise in the FHR of at least 15 beats/minute, which lasts for more than 15 seconds. If the rate remains raised then this may be considered a tachycardia.
- **Decelerations**. A deceleration is a transient fall in the FHR. The commonly accepted classification of decelerations will be discussed later.

Normal intrapartum fetal heart rate patterns

The normal baseline FHR lies between 110 and 160 beats/minute at term (Fig. 12.1). During periods of fetal activity, baseline variability is usually greater than 5 beats/minute (and less than 25 beats/minute) and there should be two or more accelerations in a 20-minute period. It has been known for some time that

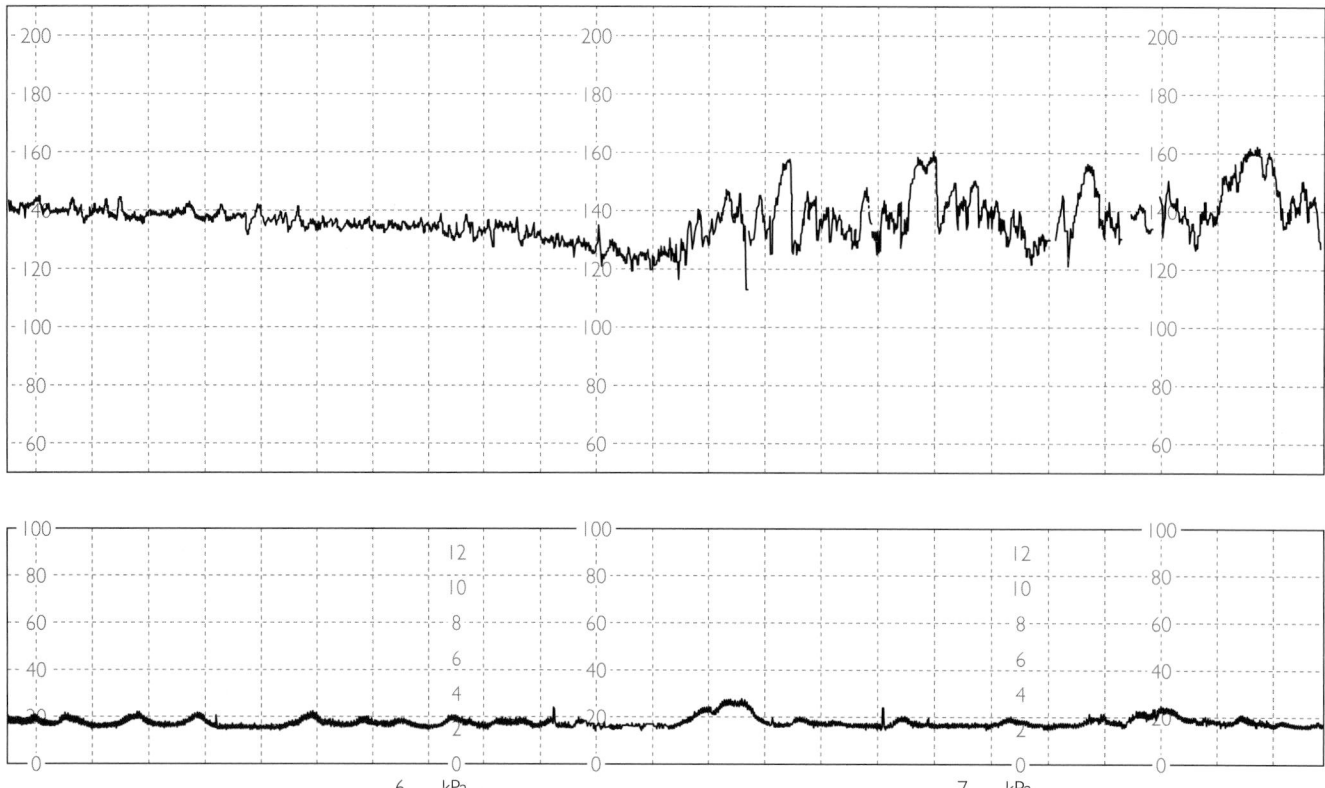

Fig. 12.1 Normal rest activity cycling in a term fetus. The baseline fetal heart rate is 130–140 beats/minute. In the first part of the trace the baseline variability is approximately 5 beats/minute, there are no accelerations and no decelerations (rest cycle). In the latter part of the trace the baseline variability is 10–15 beats/minute, there are plenty of accelerations and no decelerations (active cycle).

acceleration is the only pattern not related to fetal acidaemia.[4] Recent interest in fetal stimulation has confirmed the absence of fetal acidaemia associated with a fetal response in the form of a FHR acceleration.[111] However, the absence of accelerations does not necessarily imply acidaemia: only about 2% will have a pH on a fetal blood sample taken in labour of less than 7.25.[4]

It was not until the 1980s that the influence of the fetal rest–activity behavioural cycle on intrapartum baseline FHR variability became widely recognised.[110] Episodes of low variability, often less than 5 beats/minute, are associated with the quiet fetal behavioural state and an absence of movement-related FHR accelerations. Such physiological episodes do not usually last more than 45 minutes. Further tests of fetal wellbeing are appropriate after this, as it may signify a previously unrecognised chronic placental problem. The typical FHR appearance of normal cyclical fetal behaviour is illustrated in Fig. 12.1.

Fetal heart rate decelerations (of any type) are not part of the normal CTG appearance in term fetuses. Early decelerations (synchronous with the contraction) are common, especially in the second stage of labour (Fig. 12.2) and are usually well tolerated. They are probably caused by a vagal reflex as a response to mild transient hypoxia as the mother bears down with contractions. Provided all the other aspects of the CTG are normal and the liquor is clear, early decelerations can be well tolerated by a healthy fetus.

The interpretation of the FHR pattern of the preterm fetus in labour is similar to that of its term counterpart.[124] However, there are some subtle differences in the FHR pattern. The baseline rate is commonly faster and the variability is often rather less.

Accelerations occur less frequently and are less marked. The differentiation between quiet and active sleep patterns may not be evident until 32 weeks' gestation. Small brief (<20 s) decelerations are often seen and are not considered significant.

Abnormalities of the fetal heart rate pattern

The significance of an abnormal pattern is much more difficult to judge. In general, the more of the four basic aspects of the FHR (baseline rate, baseline variability, accelerations, decelerations) that are abnormal, the more likely the fetus is to be acidaemic. The role of the obstetrician is to seek a cause for the FHR abnormalities, as management will be influenced by the presumed aetiology. For example, repetitive early decelerations in a woman who has progressed from 2 to 10 cm dilation in half an hour will be considered much less sinister than a similar trace in a patient who is thought to have ruptured her previous caesarean section scar. Clearly, the management of these two situations will be quite different. For this reason it is difficult to give a comprehensive yet basic guide to CTG abnormalities in labour.

Abnormalities of the baseline FHR

Acute rises in FHR in labour probably reflect an increase in catecholamine secretion and indicate an early adaptive response to fetal hypoxia before the development of fetal acidaemia. Although chorioamnionitis should always be suspected, recent studies have shown that epidural analgesia is a benign cause of maternal fever and associated fetal tachycardia.[78] β-mimetic tocolytic therapy frequently causes a maternal tachycardia and leads to a

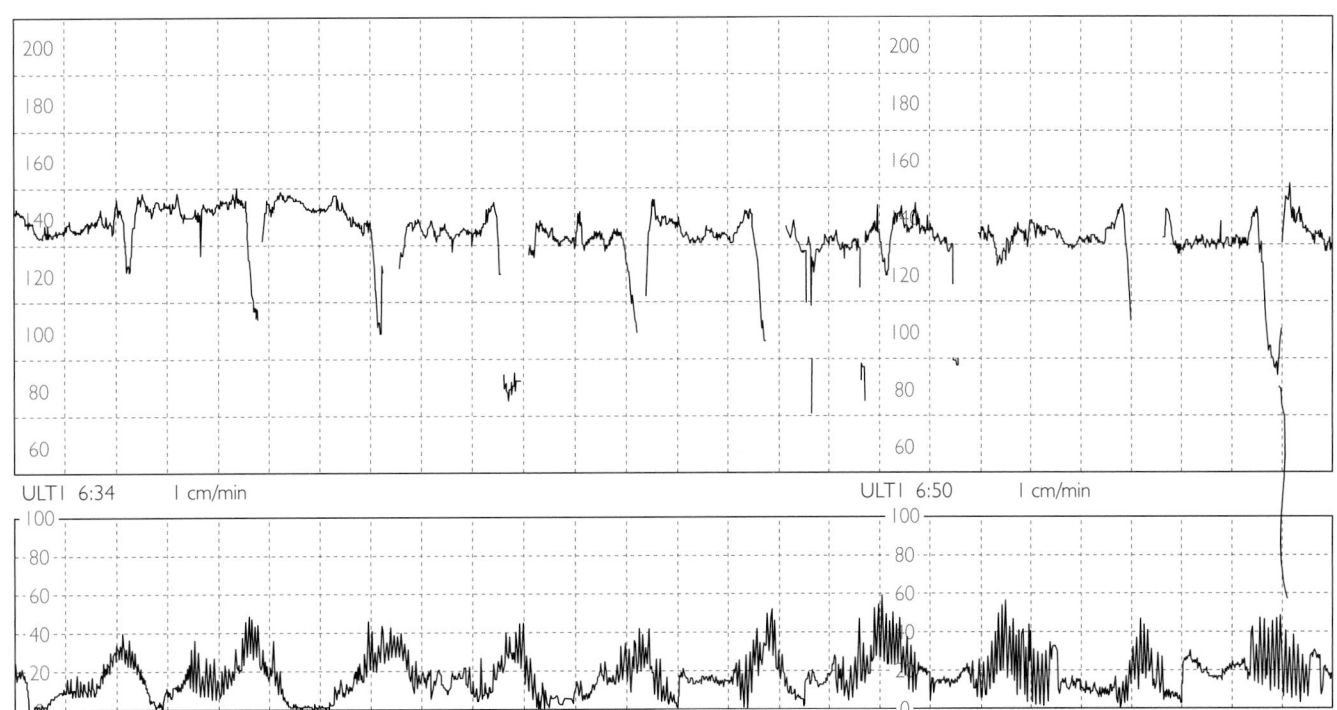

Fig. 12.2 Early decelerations in the second stage of labour. The 'spikes' in uterine activity represent the maternal effort of pushing.

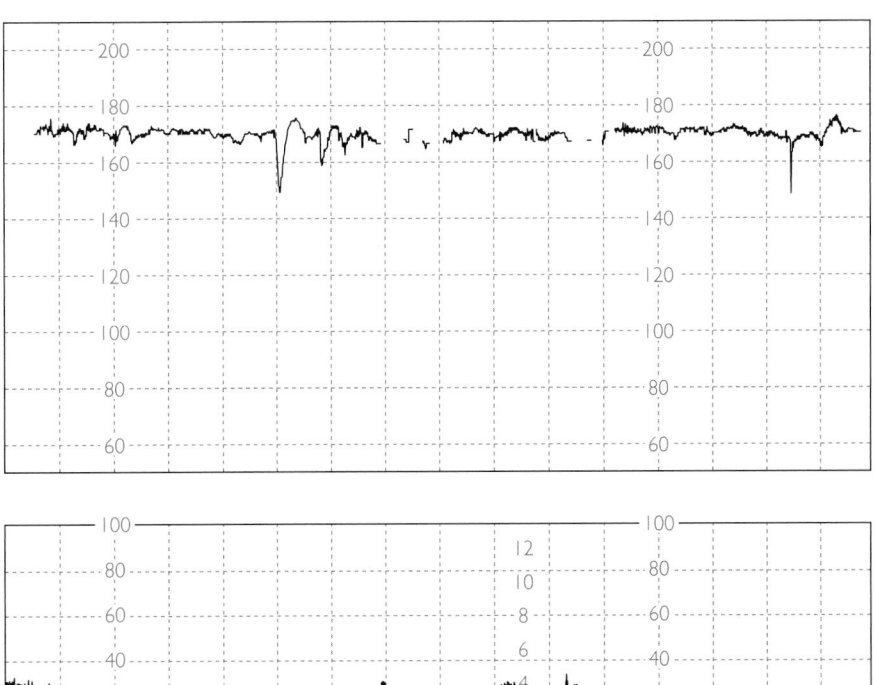

Fig. 12.3 This is a complicated fetal tachycardia (baseline 170 beats/minute, reduced variability and loss of accelerations). The mother had an unexplained pyrexia and was only 1 cm dilated, so a caesarean section was performed. The baby had normal cord gases but a group B streptococcal septicaemia.

benign fetal tachycardia. Rarely a fetal tachyarrhythmia may be recognised for the first time in labour. Fetal tachycardia above 180 beats/minute has traditionally been regarded as a sign of fetal distress. Even in high-risk pregnancies, however, it is not particularly predictive of fetal acidaemia. If found in association with other abnormal FHR patterns the prognosis significantly worsens (Figs 12.3–12.5). Fetal blood sampling or delivery then become more important.

Fetal bradycardia can also be benign. A persistent baseline FHR between 100 and 110 beats/minute can be seen normally in some postdates pregnancies and in patients on beta-blockers. Acute bradycardias below 100 beats/minute can occur in a number

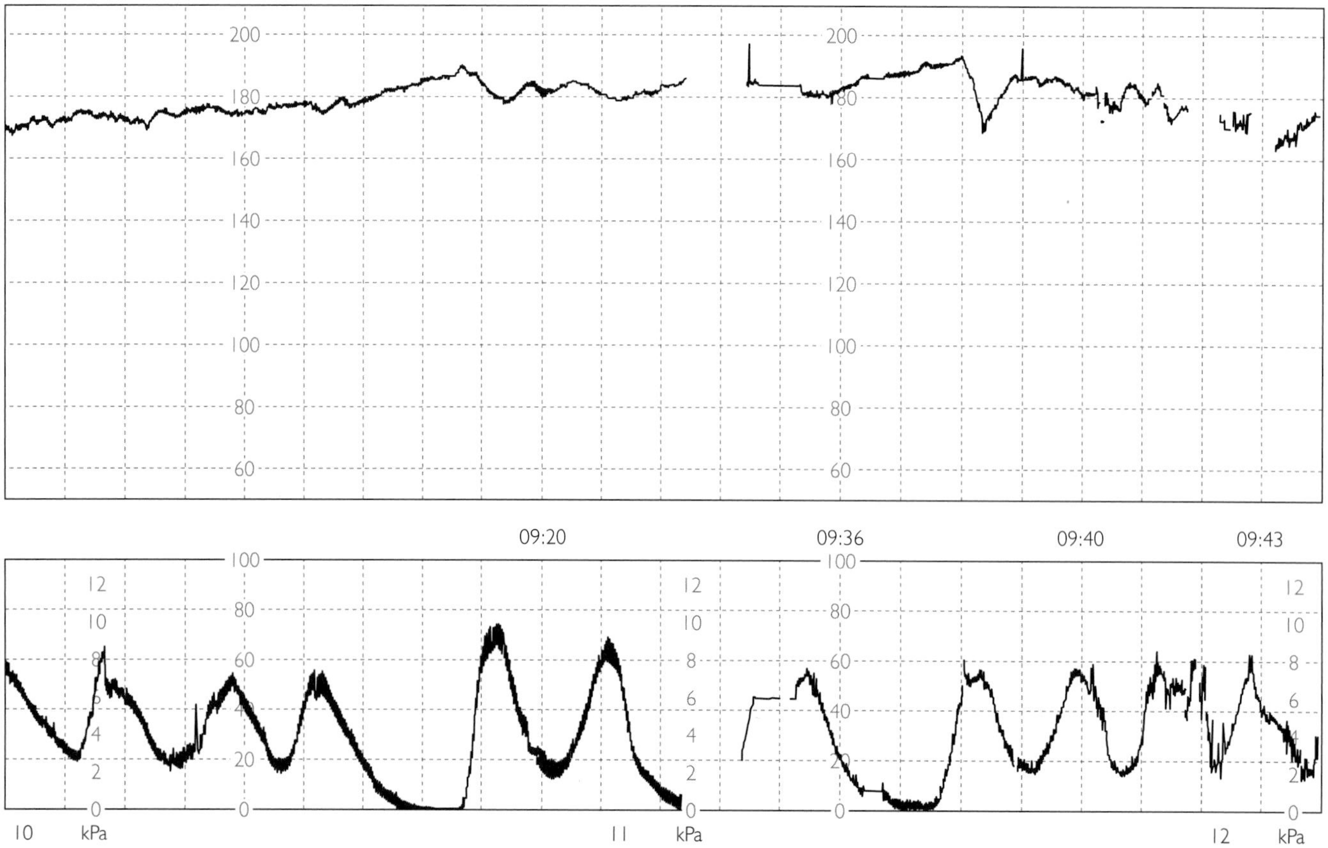

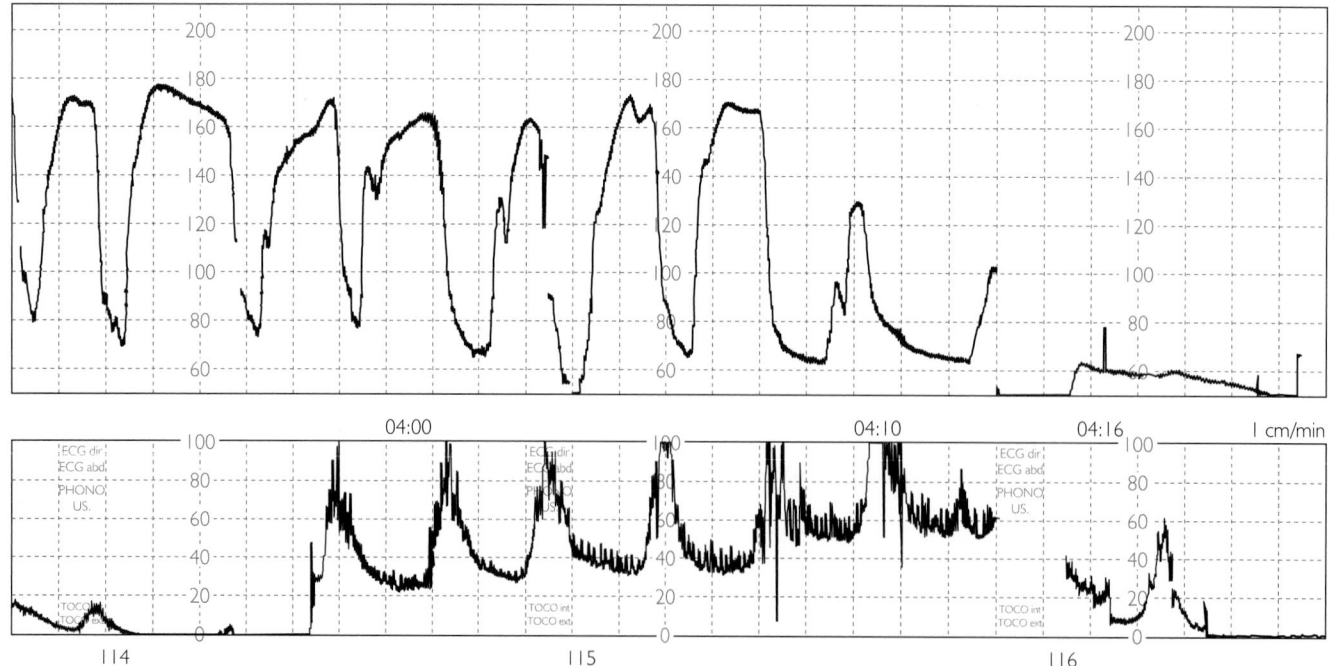

Fig. 12.4 This is a complicated fetal tachycardia with a rising baseline (170–190 beats/minute), almost absent variability and at least one early deceleration. An immediate ventouse delivery was performed. The baby was mildly acidotic at birth but made a full recovery.

Fig. 12.5 This is a complicated fetal tachycardia with no baseline variability and late decelerations. A terminal bradycardia occurred prior to caesarean section. The arterial cord pH was 6.7 and there was thick meconium. The birthweight was 2.1 kg. The baby had a severe hypoxic–ischaemic encephalopathy and ultimately died.

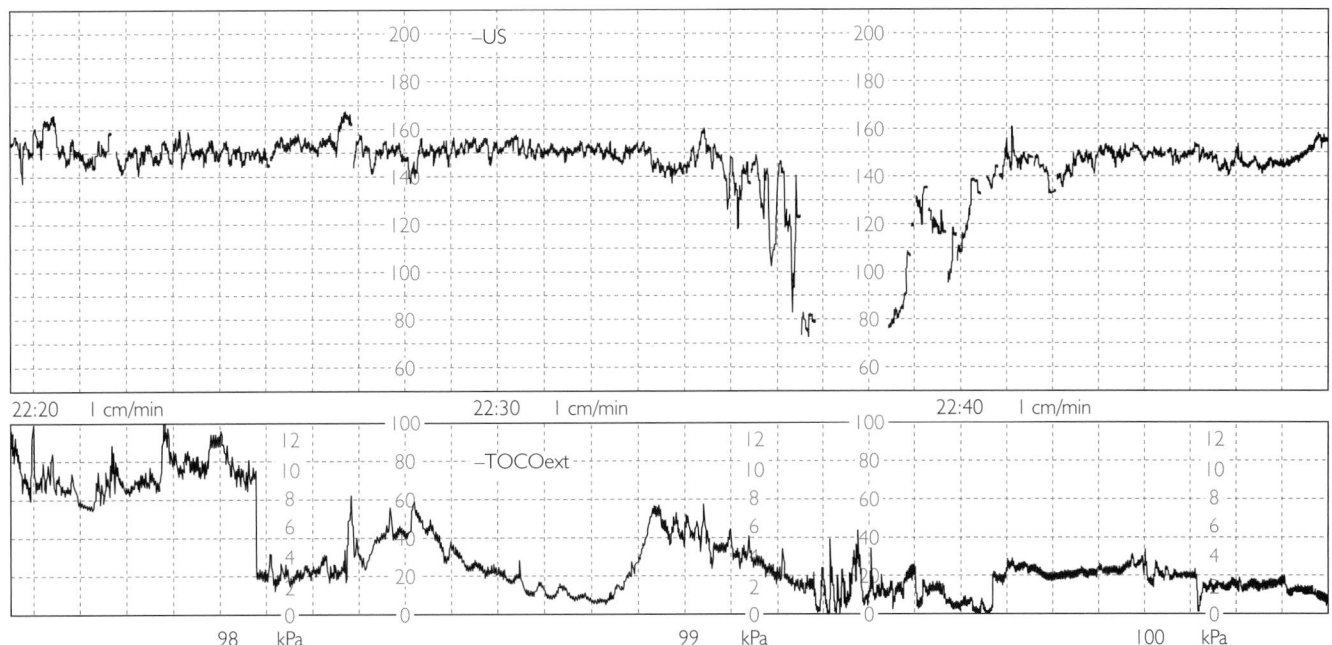

Fig. 12.6 This is an acute fetal bradycardia in an otherwise normal cardiotocograph. The mother was being induced with prostaglandins and had a prolonged tightening prior to the bradycardia. She was also lying flat on her back. Merely moving her into a left lateral position, thus alleviating any element of aortocaval compression, caused the cardiotocograph to return entirely to normal and no further intervention was necessary.

of situations, including vaginal examination, suddenly reaching full dilatation and after epidural top-ups (even in the absence of maternal hypotension). An acute fall in FHR indicates an acute interruption of oxygen delivery, secondary to either maternal hypotension/aortocaval compression or umbilical cord compression (Fig. 12.6). Acidaemia develops within 10–15 minutes and may continue to progress unless the situation is corrected. If the bradycardia fails to recover once appropriate treatment has been instigated, immediate delivery is necessary. However, if the baseline FHR returns to normal and there are no other abnormal FHR features, conservative management is appropriate. If there is no obvious explanation for a recovered bradycardia then FBS should be performed to assess fetal reserve in case there is previously unrecognised chronic placental insufficiency.

Again, fetal bradycardia in association with other abnormalities of the FHR is more sinister. The worst combination of FHR abnormalities described has been progressive bradycardia associated with absent FHR variability, which is regarded as a terminal response of a dying fetus[11,48] (Fig. 12.5).

Abnormalities of the baseline variability
The significance of reduced baseline variability has already been discussed. Excessive variation (>25 beats/minute) is an early adaptive response to fetal hypoxia, and in isolation it has not been found to be particularly predictive of fetal acidaemia.[4] Commonly, however, abnormalities of the baseline variability are seen in conjunction with other FHR abnormalities. In such cases further tests of fetal wellbeing are appropriate.

Presence of decelerations
In general, decelerations should be considered transient bradycardias. FHR decelerations related to uterine contractions certainly represent interruption of maternal-fetal oxygen transfer. In a healthy fetus the most likely mechanism is chemoreceptor stimulation,[47] resulting in a vagal nerve response. Fetal acidaemia only occurs after a considerable reduction in fetal oxygen delivery.[61] Thus, FHR decelerations have a low predictive value for fetal acidaemia, particularly in the absence of associated complications or risk factors.

For example, epidural analgesia is recognised to have an association with late FHR decelerations: however, the outcome appears to be similar (in terms of mean umbilical artery pH and Apgar scores) to cases in which regional analgesia was not employed. Thus, FHR decelerations in this setting are probably more a reflection of adjustments of fetal cardiovascular control rather than an indication of the development of fetal acidaemia.[112] In contrast, however, late FHR decelerations may be the first signs of unrecognised placental insufficiency and may be associated with a faster rate of development of acidaemia.[112] Again we return to the point that CTG interpretation is only one aspect of the emerging clinical picture. The obstetrician needs to work out why the fetus is mounting a response in the form of FHR decelerations. All decelerations indicate hypoxia, but acidaemia will be present in less than 50% of cases.

Various classifications of FHR decelerations have been proposed. The most widely used in the UK is early, variable and late.

■ **Early decelerations**. These are decelerations in which the trough of the decrease in the FHR is synchronous with the peak of the uterine contraction and does not fall below 90 beats/minute (Fig. 12.2). They are not particularly common. In the first stage of labour they are frequently secondary to treatable causes – supine hypotension, epidural analgesia, fetal manipulation, etc. Correction of the apparent cause will allow the FHR to return to the baseline and the prognosis is unaffected. Of the three types of deceleration, early ones are

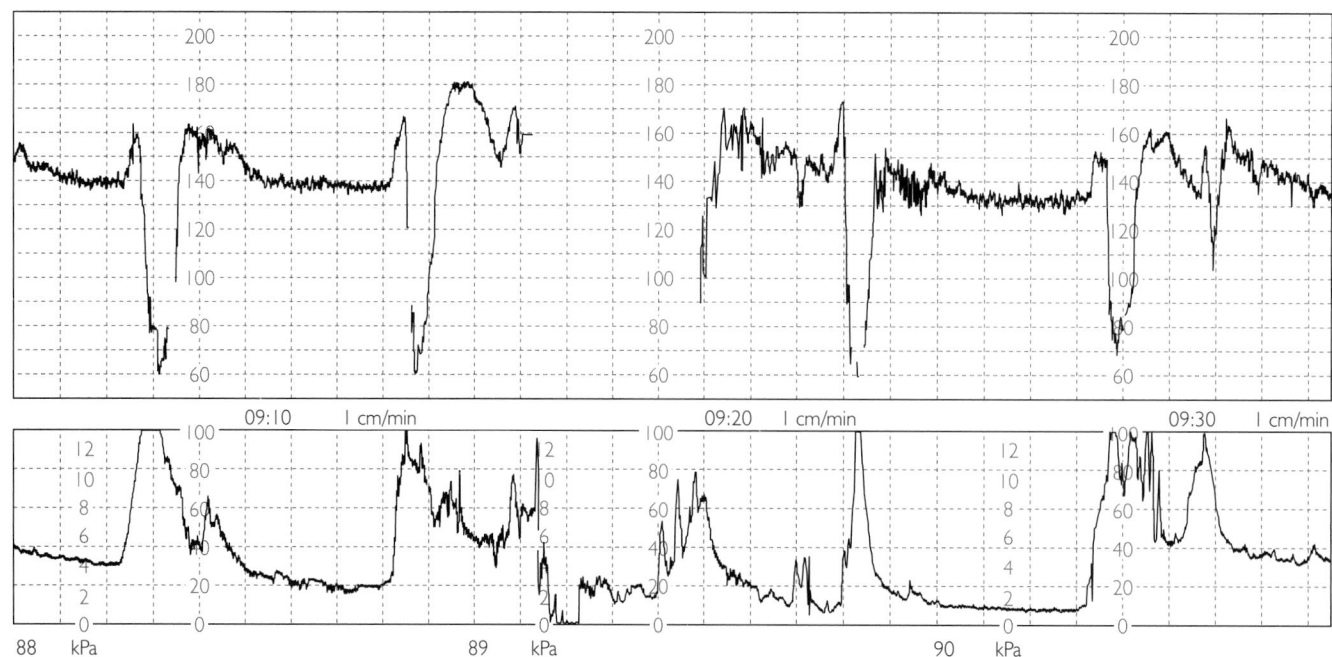

Fig. 12.7 These are typical M-shaped, variable decelerations secondary to cord compression. They are 'early' in timing but deep, and 'shouldered' by transient increases in fetal heart rate. Since the cardiotocograph was otherwise normal, the mother was allowed to continue pushing. She had a normal vaginal delivery of a healthy baby half an hour later.

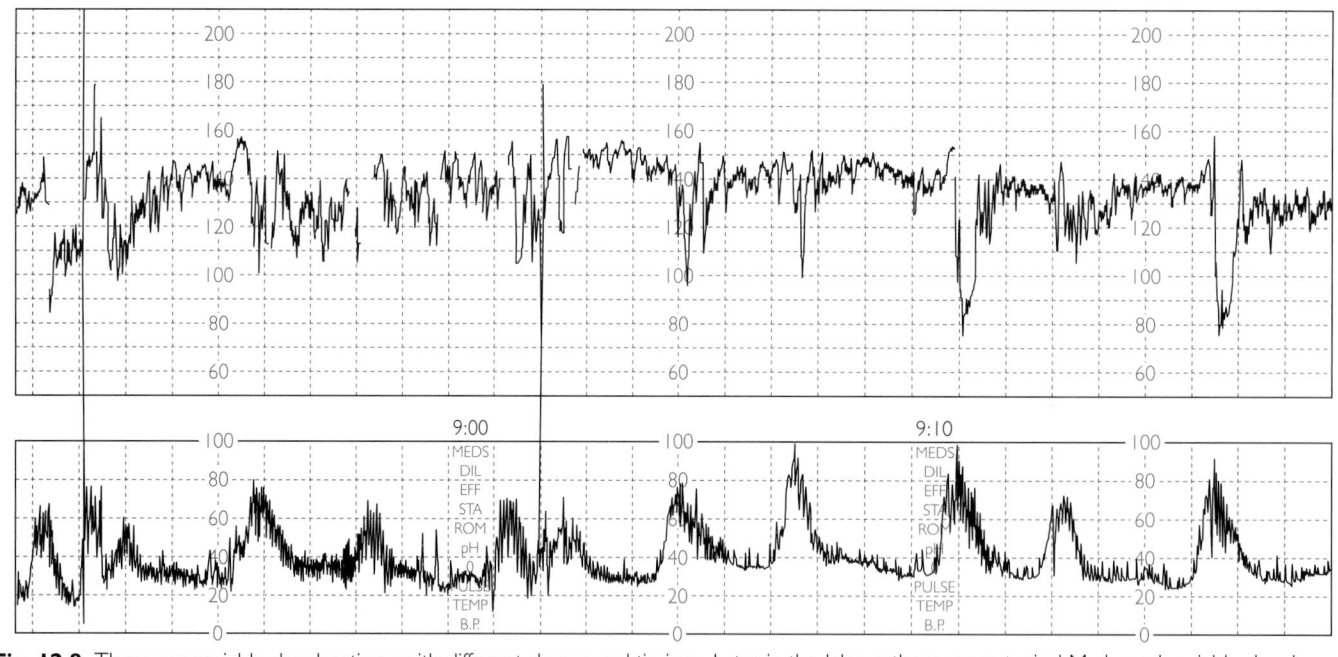

Fig. 12.8 These are variable decelerations with different shapes and timings. Later in the labour there were typical M-shaped variable decelerations in an otherwise normal cardiotocograph. The baby was born in good condition with the cord round his neck.

the most benign. If the early decelerations persist or there are other abnormalities of the FHR, FBS may become indicated.

■ **Variable decelerations**. A clear, concise definition of variable decelerations is difficult to find. They are either early in timing (synchronous with the peak of the contraction) but fall below 90 beats/minute, or they are variable in their shape and timing (Figs 12.7–12.9). Variable decelerations usually represent fetal

responses to umbilical cord compression. FBS or delivery (in the second stage of labour) are often performed, although the fetal prognosis is usually not affected unless the variable decelerations are 'atypical' or associated with other FHR abnormalities.

■ **Late decelerations**. These are decelerations in which the trough of the decrease in the FHR occurs after the peak of the uterine contraction (Figs 12.5, 12.10–12.12). They are more likely to be

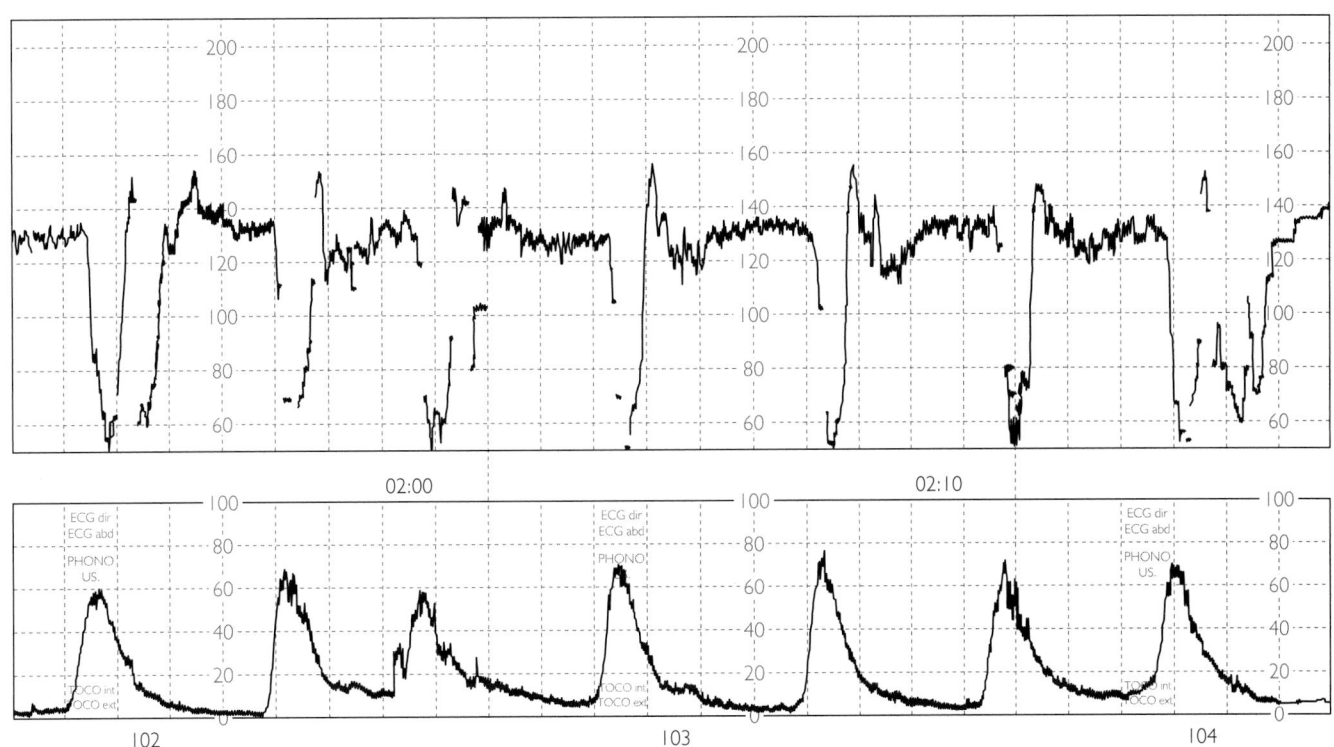

Fig. 12.9 These are atypical variable decelerations. The first and last decelerations are 'biphasic' with a 'late' component, making this a 'pathological' cardiotocograph by National Institute for Clinical Excellence criteria. Unfortunately, fetal blood sampling/delivery was not performed. The later cardiotocograph is shown in Fig. 12.5.

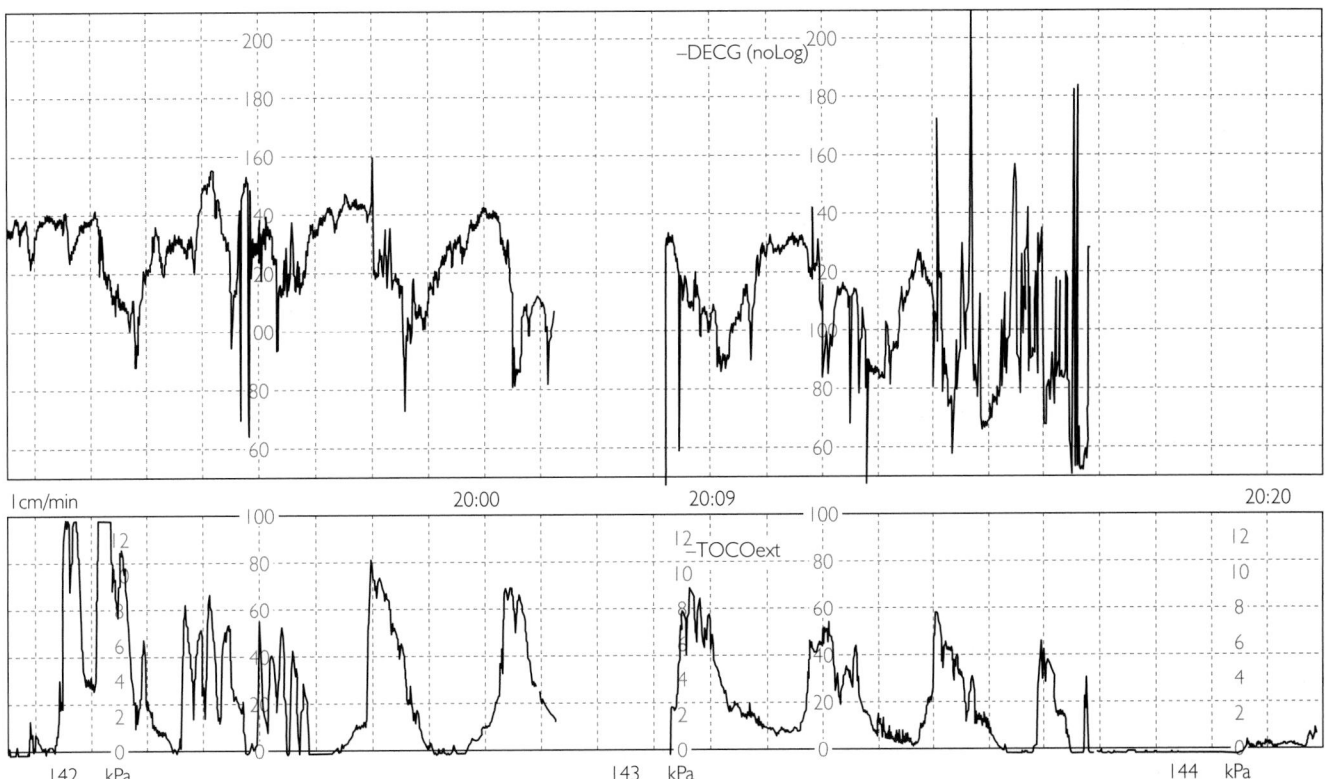

Fig. 12.10 There are persistent late decelerations and the baseline is gradually falling. Spontaneous vaginal delivery was imminent and no intervention was therefore required. A 3.8 kg baby was born in good condition.

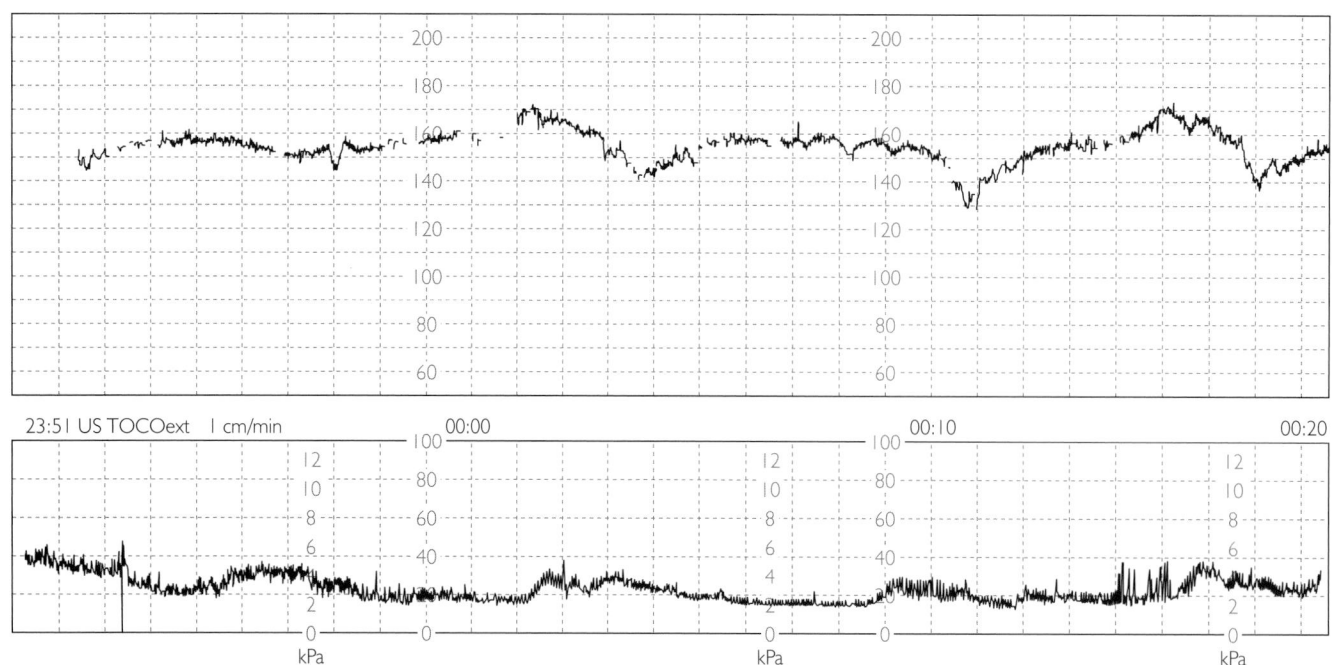

Fig. 12.11 These are late decelerations with reduced baseline variability. The mother had constant abdominal pain and vaginal bleeding. At caesarean section there was evidence of an abruption and the arterial cord pH was 6.9. The baby subsequently did well.

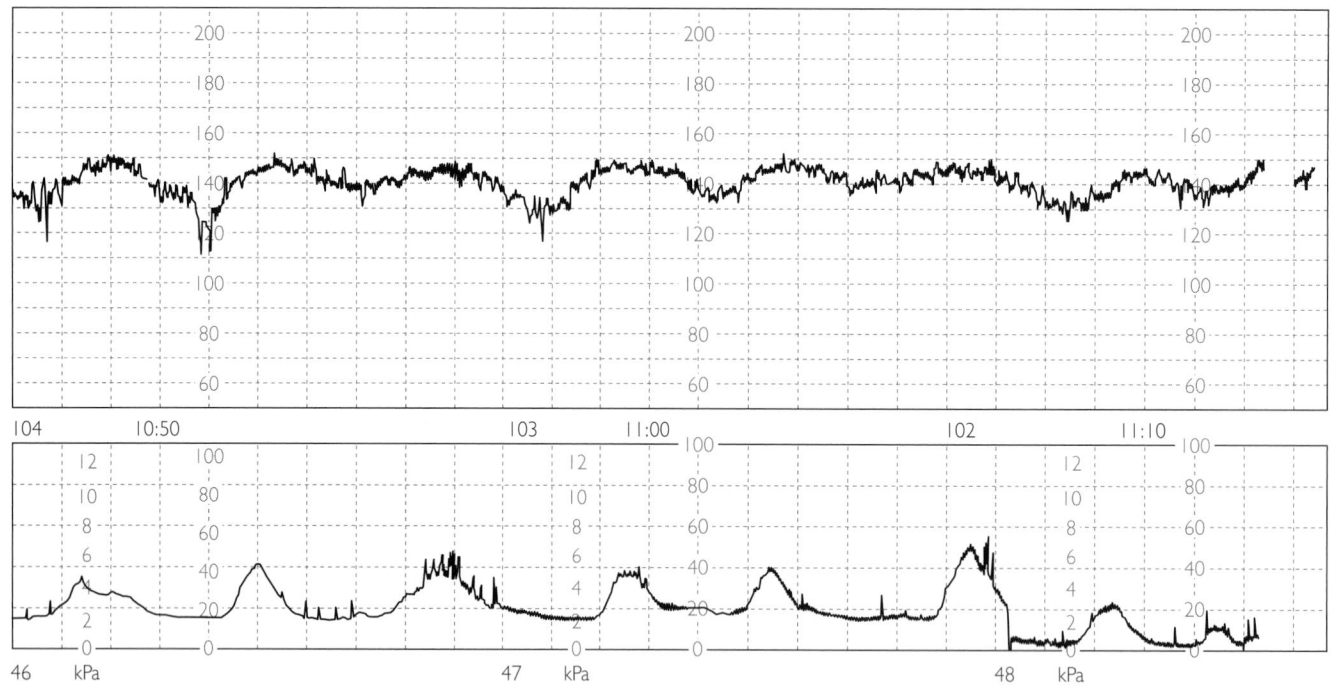

Fig. 12.12 There are persistent shallow, late decelerations. The baseline rate is 150 beats/minute. This cardiotocograph was not acted upon and 2 hours later there was a terminal bradycardia and the baby was delivered stillborn.

associated with fetal acidaemia than other forms of deceleration[4] but the correlation is still poor. Late decelerations, particularly in the setting of other FHR abnormalities, suggest fetal hypoxia secondary to uteroplacental insufficiency. The characteristic changes associated with the progressive effects of chronic placental failure include loss of accelerations (associated with a decrease in fetal movements), a reduced baseline variability and

the onset of recurrent decelerations[69] (Figs 12.5, 12.12, 12.13). There is a significantly higher incidence of metabolic acidosis at delivery[18,122] but if delivery is effected prior to such ominous CTG patterns then fetal decompensation into acidaemia is prevented.[71] FBS or delivery is therefore advisable.

From the review of FHR patterns it is clear that no single abnormal pattern reliably predicts fetal outcome. Comprehensive

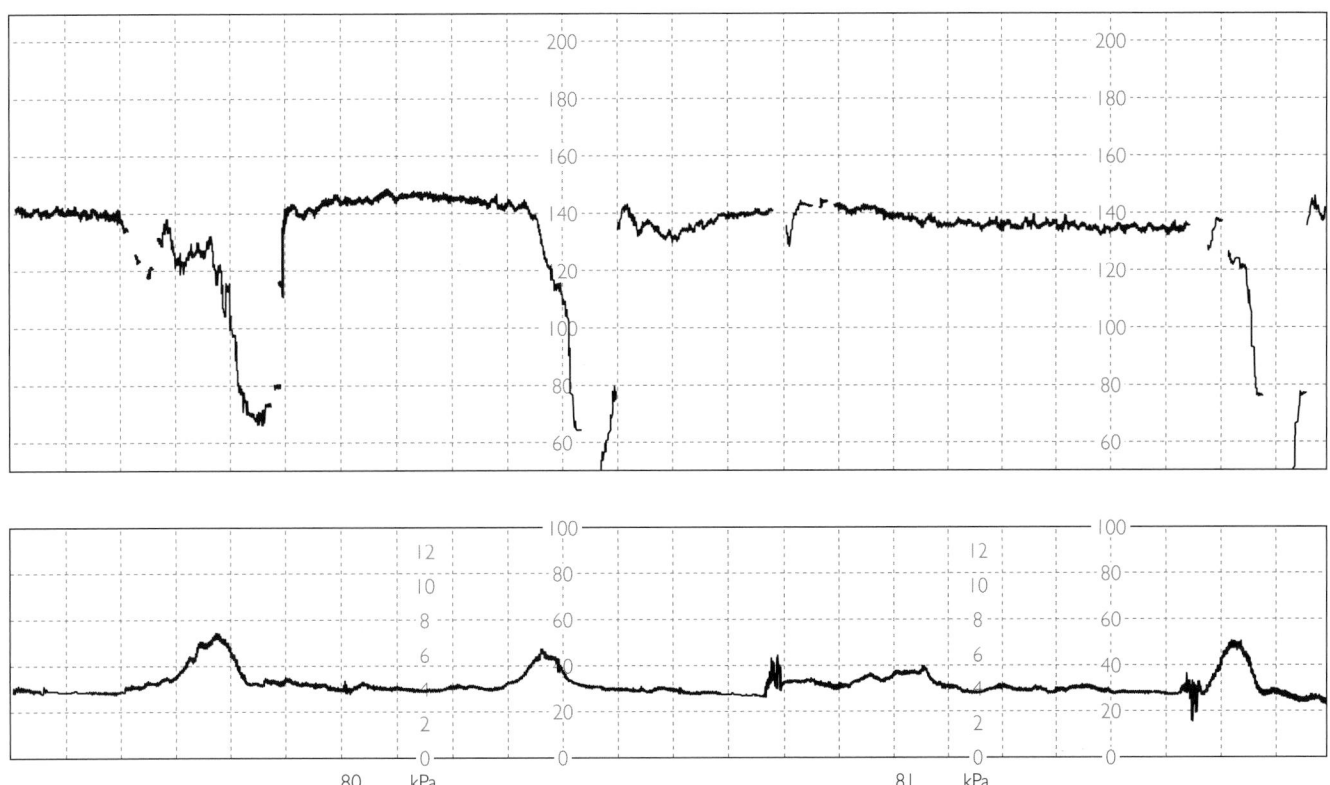

Fig. 12.13 There are late decelerations with reduced baseline variability. The mother had not experienced any fetal movements the preceding day. She was only in early labour and fetal blood sampling was not possible. At caesarean section there was thick meconium and the infant weighed 2.4 kg. The cord pH was normal and the baby did well.

evaluation of all the FHR characteristics previously mentioned is essential. This information must then be integrated into the clinical scenario before decisions can be made on management. Of most importance is the influence of pre-labour placental insufficiency on fetal tolerance to interruptions in oxygen delivery during labour. Acidaemia develops more rapidly in cases of IUGR.

Sinusoidal and pseudosinusoidal fetal heart rate patterns
The classical CTG pattern in severe fetal anaemia (whatever the cause) is described as 'sinusoidal' (Fig. 12.14). This is a preterminal pattern which is *rarely* seen. Six rigid criteria must be fulfilled to make the diagnosis:[84]

- a stable baseline FHR of 120–160 beats/minute, with regular oscillations;
- an amplitude of 5–15 beats/minute;
- a frequency of 2–5 cycles/minute;
- absent short-term variability;
- no areas of normal FHR variability or reactivity.

Pseudosinusoidal FHR patterns (vaguely defined as undulatory waveforms), in contrast, are common and usually innocuous. They are strongly associated with the use of pethidine and epidural analgesia and are also seen with fetal sucking movements. Such patterns will generally improve with time. There have been only occasional reports of major pseudosinusoidal FHR patterns (with amplitudes greater than 24 beats/minute) in association with preterminal fetal anaemia.[91]

Guidelines

Recently the Clinical Effectiveness Support Unit of the Royal College of Obstetricians and Gynaecologists (RCOG) has produced evidence-based guidelines on the use and interpretation of cardiotocography in intrapartum fetal surveillance.[106] They have categorised FHR features into 'reassuring', 'non-reassuring' and 'abnormal' groups (Table 12.1). This enables categorisation of the cardiotocograph trace as 'normal', 'suspicious' or 'pathological' (Table 12.2). 'Suspicious' traces can be managed conservatively but 'pathological' traces demand FBS or delivery.

Fetal scalp blood sampling

This was first described by Saling in Germany in 1962. Later it was suggested that FBS could be deferred until an 'abnormal pattern' was seen on the FHR record.[4] Even then, most cases had a low risk of being associated with fetal acidaemia (always less than 50%). Moreover, clinical trials have clearly indicated that there is an increased risk of caesarean section if cardiotocography is used alone without FBS. This has led the RCOG to recommend that electronic monitoring should not be used without facilities for FBS.[113]

A number of indications for FBS have already been mentioned. If the pH is 7.2 or less, immediate delivery is indicated, providing the FBS was performed for a good reason and at the

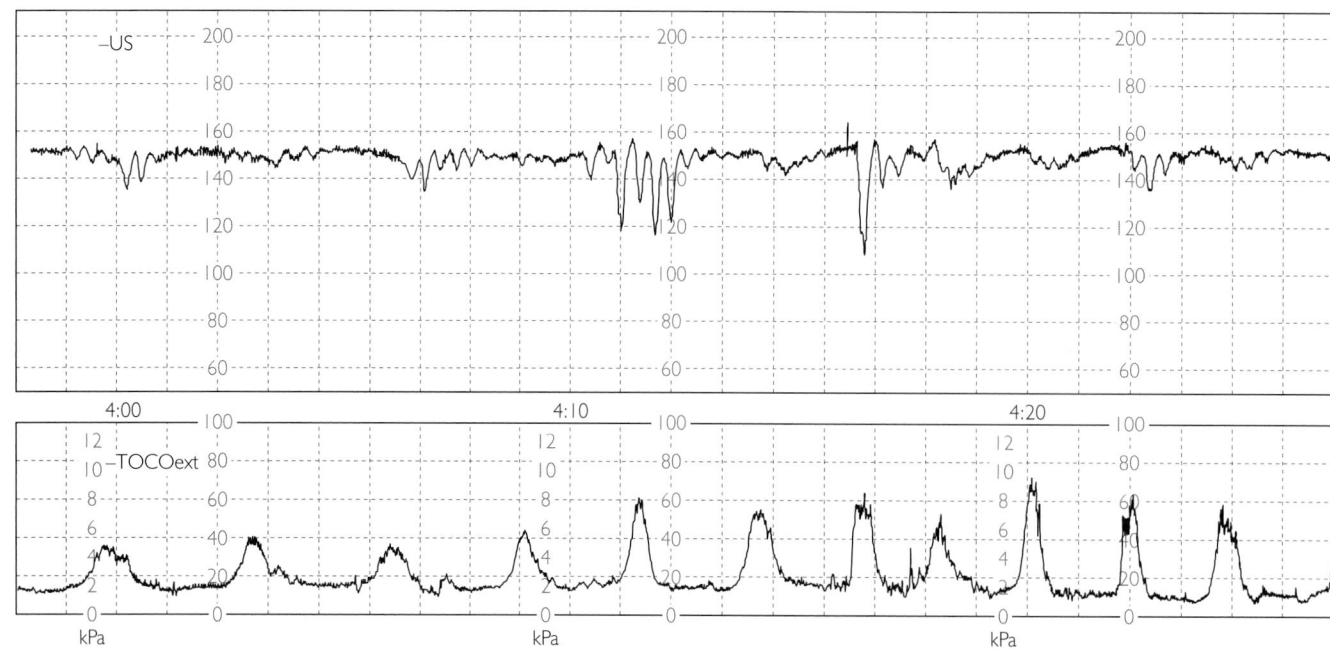

Fig. 12.14 A sinusoidal cardiotocograph in a case of feto-maternal haemorrhage. The infant had a haemoglobin of 8 g/dl at birth.

Table 12.1 National Institute of Clinical Excellence categorisation of fetal heart rate features

Feature	Baseline (bpm)	Variability (bpm)	Decelerations	Acceleration
Reassuring	110–160	≥5	None	Present
Non-reassuring	100–109 or 161–180	<5 for ≥40 but <90 min	Early or Variable or 1 × prolonged (<3 min)	
Abnormal	<100 or >180 or Sinusoidal (≥10 min)	<5 for ≥90 min	Atypical variable or Late 1 × prolonged (>3 min)	

The absence of accelerations in an otherwise normal CTG is of uncertain significance.

Table 12.2 National Institute of Clinical Excellence categorisation of fetal heart rate traces

Category	Definition
Normal	A cardiotocogram where *all four* features fall into the reassuring category
Suspicious	A cardiotocogram whose features fall into *one* of the non-reassuring categories (the remainder of features being reassuring)
Pathological	A cardiotocogram whose features fall into *two or more* non-reassuring categories or *one or more* abnormal categories

correct time. If the FBS pH is more than 7.2, it is usually appropriate to continue with the labour and repeat the sample 1 hour later, unless the situation deteriorates in the meantime, necessitating earlier intervention. The rate of fall of the fetal scalp pH is as important as each absolute value. This must be integrated into the clinical picture. For example, a rapidly falling pH (still above 7.2) in a woman who is soon going to be deliverable vaginally may be acceptable. In contrast, the same fetal scalp pH profile in

Table 12.3 Normal values for umbilical cord blood gas data (in term fetuses with Apgar scores ≥7 at 5 min)[52]

	Mean	Standard deviation	2.5th percentile
UApH	7.26	0.07	7.10
UAPCO$_2$ (mmHg)	53	10	35
UAPO$_2$ (mmHg)	17	6	6
UA BE (mEq/l)	−4	3	−11
UVpH	7.34	0.06	7.20
UVPCO$_2$ (mmHg)	41	7	28
UVPO$_2$ (mmHg)	29	7	16
UV BE (mEq/l)	−3	3	−8

BE = base excess; UA = umbilical artery; UV = umbilical vein.

a labour that is progressing slowly and is complicated by thick meconium is probably an indication for caesarean section.

Fetal pH falls more rapidly during pushing in the second stage.[58,113] The pH may decrease as fast as 0.1 units per 10 minutes during a prolonged bradycardia, and rapid delivery is essential to prevent acidaemia at birth.[65]

Umbilical cord blood sampling

Measurement of pH and blood gas values in blood from the umbilical cord immediately after delivery is an invaluable guide to the interaction between labour and the fetus. Umbilical venous blood values give an indication of the effects of placental gas transfer and correction of buffered arterial metabolic acids. Oxygen saturation and pH values are higher in venous blood, which is the best representation of cerebral blood oxygen content. Umbilical arterial blood gas analysis has shown that the fetal response to labour is a varying degree of acidaemia in the blood supplying the lower body.[113] The range of fetal adaptation to labour is wide. In a study[52] of over 15 000 term newborns with 5-minute Apgar scores of 7 or more, the median umbilical artery pH (UApH) was 7.26, with a 2.5th percentile value of 7.1. The normal values for umbilical blood gas data are shown in Table 12.3. Arterial and venous cord pH are likely to be significantly different if there is an element of cord compression, hence the importance of taking paired cord blood samples. The normal range defines the 'physiological acidaemia' of the normal, vigorous newborn. Indeed, umbilical artery pH values above 7.05 in term infants show no significant association with low Apgar scores[42] or adverse neurodevelopmental outcome.[35] Correction of such severe acidaemia after birth by healthy babies is rapid and correlates with a low P_aCO_2 at 1 hour of age.[114]

The distribution of UApH values in preterm infants (<32 weeks' gestation) is skewed, with a median value of 7.25 (range 6.78–7.49) and mean (SD) of 7.23.[0.15] There is a trend towards more infants having low UApH at lower gestations. After adjustment for other risk factors in preterm infants the UApH is not significantly associated with outcomes of neonatal death, cerebral palsy and developmental quotient at 1 year. Nonetheless, UApH measurement does provide useful information for the paediatrician attending the delivery.

Delivering the infant

This section covers delivery of both preterm and term infants. Common indications for specific modes of delivery, the medical interventions that may be used to effect delivery and the potential complications affecting the newborn infant will be discussed.

Term infants

The majority of term infants will deliver spontaneously with the assistance of a midwife. In England and Wales the spontaneous vaginal delivery rate in 2000/01 was estimated at 67%.[119] While operative vaginal delivery rates have remained constant at approximately 11%, caesarean section rates are increasing.[119] The national caesarean section rate in England and Wales was 21.5% in 2000/01[119] compared to 10.4% in 1985.[80] The current national caesarean section rate is comparable to that in the USA and Italy.[121]

The indications for caesarean section, instrumental delivery and induction of labour in term infants will now be outlined, with particular reference to possible fetal complications. The management of breech presentations and multiple pregnancies will be discussed separately.

Caesarean section delivery

The indications for an elective caesarean section are various. In the recent national audit,[119] 37% of the total caesarean section rate in England and Wales was for elective cases. The most frequently cited primary indications reported by clinicians are previous caesarean section and breech presentation.[119] This agrees with studies in other countries.[90,121] Elective caesarean section by maternal request is an increasing phenomenon but still only accounts for a small proportion of operative deliveries.[119] There are a few 'absolute' indications for elective caesarean section, for instance major placenta praevia or abnormal lie, where the baby cannot be safely delivered vaginally. If placental integrity has to be breached in order to reach the baby there is a risk of fetal anaemia. More commonly, situations arise in which planned caesarean section is strongly recommended, for example breech presentations. In maternal HIV infection there is evidence that caesarean section delivery offers a considerable degree of protection for the baby from vertical transmission[93] and this is the usual mode of delivery in the developed world. Similarly, symptomatic primary genital herpes simplex infection at term (a rare occurrence) is an indication for delivery by caesarean section. Recurrent disease is now known to carry a low risk for the fetus[100] and caesarean section is only contemplated if there are active lesions in labour and the membranes have been ruptured for less than 4 hours at the time of presentation at the hospital.

It is widely assumed that elective caesarean section ensures good condition at birth, and certainly the incidence of seizures in babies born by elective caesarean section is very low, but this is not always the case. Maternal hypotension due to regional anaesthesia, with or without aortocaval compression, can reduce placental perfusion and lead to acute fetal hypoxia.[72] There is also an increased incidence of fetal respiratory complications, such as transient tachypnoea of the newborn and hyaline membrane disease in the absence of the normal 'stress' of labour. The risk of neonatal respiratory morbidity is related to the gestational age at which the elective caesarean section is performed.[87] For this reason, elective caesarean sections should usually be planned for 39 weeks gestation.

Emergency caesarean section (performed in labour) may be indicated either for fetal distress or failure to progress in labour. The urgency of the procedure will be determined by the presumed aetiology and severity of the problem. This information is usually available to the attending paediatrician. In cases of placental abruption with evidence of fetal distress, the data suggest that the perinatal outcome is significantly improved by early caesarean section rather than attempted vaginal delivery.[96] Significant fetal bleeding[43] and transient neonatal coagulopathies[46] have been reported. The main risk to the fetus, however, is from hypoxia-ischaemia.

Instrumental vaginal delivery

This is usually indicated for fetal distress, delay in the second stage of labour or maternal exhaustion. Occasionally 'elective' instrumental delivery is recommended, for example in some women with congenital or acquired cardiac abnormalities, when the systemic effects of active pushing may be deleterious to the mother. Instrumental vaginal delivery can be effected in most cases using either obstetric forceps or the vacuum extractor (ventouse). The trend is towards increased use of the ventouse, as recent studies[62,117] have suggested that maternal trauma and long-term morbidity are less than with forceps. Overall, the incidence of fetal complications is the same using either instrument; however, the nature of potential injuries varies according to the method used. Cephalhaematoma, subgaleal haemorrhage (p. 1126) and superficial scalp trauma are significantly more likely with vacuum extraction, and one study has suggested an association with retinal haemorrhage.[33] Forceps, however, more commonly cause craniofacial injuries such as bruising, linear skull fractures, tentorial tears and facial nerve palsies. There is no significant difference in the number of jaundiced babies requiring phototherapy when forceps are compared with ventouse. Several long-term studies of term infants delivered by ventouse have shown no increase in mental retardation or cerebral palsy, nor any differences from infants delivered by forceps.[10,13] It must be stressed, however, that serious fetal injury is rare nowadays since heroic 'high' instrumental deliveries (using forceps or vacuum extraction) are no longer performed: caesarean section is the preferred mode for a potentially difficult delivery. Instrumental delivery is more likely to be associated with shoulder dystocia, although this can occur with spontaneous vaginal delivery.

Shoulder dystocia

Shoulder dystocia occurs in approximately 1% of total births. It is an obstetric emergency in which acute fetal hypoxia rapidly develops. The principal risk factor is fetal macrosomia, albeit the majority of cases occur in infants weighing less than 4500 g.[44] Additional risk factors include maternal diabetes mellitus, a history of previous shoulder dystocia, prolonged labour and delay in the second stage of labour. Unfortunately, at present there is no reliable method for antenatal prediction of shoulder dystocia. Ultrasound estimations of fetal weight are subject to greater errors in larger babies. Even in cases of suspected macrosomia, routine delivery by caesarean section is not recommended. Indeed, abdominal delivery does not always circumvent the problem as 'shoulder dystocia' can also occur with delivery through a uterine incision.

A number of manoeuvres can be employed to expedite delivery of the shoulders and all obstetricians and midwives should have regular training in 'shoulder dystocia drills'. Occasionally, deliberate fracture of the baby's clavicles is necessary. Excessive traction on the fetal neck can result in brachial plexus injuries (almost always Erb's palsy), the majority of which recover spontaneously. Although the incidence of Erb's palsy (p. 984) is increased in cases of shoulder dystocia, it is important to remember that a substantial proportion of cases of Erb's palsy are unrelated to birth trauma. Often the more serious consequence of shoulder dystocia is severe fetal hypoxia due to delay in delivery of the infant's body.

Induction of labour

The commonest indication for induction of labour is prolonged pregnancy. This term denotes a pregnancy that has gone beyond 42 weeks from the date of the first day of the last menstrual period.[40] In places where women book in the first trimester and dating scans are performed, the incidence of prolonged pregnancy is less than 5%.[34,60] Though small, there is an increased risk of perinatal mortality after 42 weeks.[3,23] This is largely accounted for by an increased incidence of uteroplacental insufficiency and oligohydramnios. There is also an increased perinatal morbidity in prolonged pregnancies due to hypoxia, shoulder dystocia and birth injuries,[3] even when delivery is spontaneous rather than instrumental. A policy of offering routine induction of labour after 41 weeks reduces perinatal mortality without increasing the caesarean section rate. It is therefore usual to offer women induction of labour between 8 and 14 days after their expected date of delivery.[89] If this is declined, an ultrasound scan should be performed to assess the amniotic fluid volume and fetal size. If there is oligohydramnios or IUGR, induction of labour while the fetus is healthy should be strongly advocated. If the scan is reassuring, it is customary to commence regular (at least twice weekly) CTG monitoring after 42 weeks. Provided there is prompt intervention when CTG abnormalities occur, the perinatal outcome in prolonged pregnancies is improved by such monitoring.[31,32]

Induction of labour may be indicated prior to 41 weeks gestation for a variety of indications. The general principle governing such decisions is that delivery of the pregnancy will be of benefit to the health of the fetus or the mother or both. So, for example, induction may be merited on the basis of uncompromised fetal IUGR or maternal pre-eclampsia alone, or in cases of mild pre-eclampsia with associated IUGR.

There are several methods available for inducing labour. Artificial rupture of the membranes and oxytocin stimulation have already been discussed. The most commonly used alternative method, which is particularly suited to women with 'unfavourable' cervices, is the vaginal administration of prostaglandin (PG)E$_2$ gels or pessaries. The 'favourability' of the cervix for induction of labour can be assessed by vaginal examination of the cervix and determination of the Bishop score. Four parameters of the cervix are assessed – the dilation, length and consistency, the position of the cervical os, and the station of the presenting part of the fetus. A score of up to 2 is allocated for each parameter and the total score calculated. A Bishop score of 7 or more is generally considered to be 'favourable' and artificial rupture of the membranes is often possible.

The potential fetal complication of vaginal administration of PGE$_2$ gel/pessary is fetal distress secondary to uterine hyperstimulation. Hyperstimulation is iatrogenic and describes an inappropriate myometrial reaction to exogenous oxytocics, either because of myometrial hypersensitivity or drug overdosage. Hyperstimulation can result in a prolonged elevation of resting intrauterine pressure (hypertonus) or contractions occurring too frequently (tachysystole; ≥ 6 contractions in 10 min). In either case, the fetus does not have long enough to recover from the acute hypoxic stress of the uterine activity and CTG abnormalities (usually late decelerations) ensue. One of the reasons misoprostol, a much cheaper and easier to store PGE$_1$ analogue, is not routinely used in the UK to induce labour is because the incidence of hyperstimulation with the current treatment regimens is higher than with PGE$_2$.

Breech presentation

The management of term breech presentations has, until recently, been the subject of intense controversy. Many of the earlier studies performed to assess the mortality and morbidity of the fetus undergoing vaginal breech delivery were poor. They were mostly retrospective reviews of practice and often simply compared babies delivered vaginally by the breech with those presenting head first.[22] One of the fundamental shifts in opinion over the last 10–15 years has been the realisation that breech presentation itself may well be a bad prognostic feature.[59] In addition, there is a well recognised association with fetal abnormality.[19,73] Vaginal breech delivery carries the risk of cord compression/prolapse and extended arms at delivery, as well as difficult delivery of the aftercoming head. This risk may be approximately 1–2%.[20,41]

The controversy over the mode of delivery of term breech presentations was finally clarified with the publication of the Term Breech Trial in 2000.[49] This was a randomised trial to compare a policy of planned caesarean section with a policy of planned vaginal birth for selected breech-presentation pregnancies. It was conducted in 121 centres in 26 countries and enrolled 2088 women with singleton, flexed or extended, breech fetuses. The primary outcomes were perinatal mortality, neonatal mortality and serious neonatal morbidity, and analysis was by intention to treat. All three primary outcomes were significantly lower for the planned caesarean section group than for the planned vaginal birth group (relative risk 0.33, 95% confidence interval 0.19–0.56) and serious maternal complications were similar between the groups. Consequently, most clinicians in the UK now recommend elective caesarean section for term breech singletons. Some vaginal breech deliveries will inevitably still be conducted, for instance undiagnosed breeches recognised in the second stage of labour, or as a result of informed maternal choice. The challenge for clinicians now is how to maintain and teach vaginal breech delivery skills when these deliveries occur so infrequently.

The alternative management strategy for the breech fetus at term is to attempt to convert the presentation to cephalic by external manipulation prior to labour (external cephalic version, ECV). There is good evidence that ECV for breeches at term can reduce non-cephalic births by nearly 60%[54] and routine tocolysis appears to reduce the failure rate of the procedure.[55] Nonetheless, even in the Term Breech Study,[49] nearly 80% of participants had not had an attempt at ECV. It has been argued[108] that ECV should be offered universally in all obstetric units as an alternative to planned caesarean section for term breech presentations. ECV does carry small risks to the fetus of bradycardia[101] and fetomaternal haemorrhage.[1]

Multiple pregnancy

The optimal mode of delivery in multiple pregnancies is also controversial. Elective caesarean section is frequently performed for triplets and higher-order multiples,[21,76] although no randomised studies are available to support this in preference to vaginal delivery. The planned mode of delivery of twins will be influenced by their presentations. The most common is vertex–vertex, and most obstetricians would currently advise vaginal delivery.[15,17,102] When the first twin presents as a breech, delivery by caesarean section is often recommended.[17] This has a limited evidence base but, subsequent to the Term Breech Trial in singletons,[49] many clinicians are extrapolating the data to apply to multiple pregnancies. For twins presenting as first twin vertex–second twin non-vertex, opinion is currently divided as to the optimal mode of delivery. Some would perform an elective caesarean section, believing that this reduces the neonatal mortality and morbidity of the second twin. Others would advocate that, with careful fetal monitoring and recourse to caesarean section if necessary, the risks to the second twin can be minimised. Vaginal delivery of the second, non-vertex, twin can be effected by external cephalic version or internal podalic version (grasping the feet and converting the lie to longitudinal) followed by breech extraction.

Clearly there are unresolved issues with respect to the optimal mode of delivery of twin gestations. Recently it has been suggested that second twins born at term are at substantially higher risk than first twins of death due to complications of vaginal delivery,[109] irrespective of the presentation of the second twin. However, this was a retrospective cohort study whose results may have been influenced by the potential biases and limitations of such study designs. In an attempt to clarify the situation, the group who carried out the Term Breech Trial[49] are currently setting up the 'Term Twin Trial'. This will have an identical design to its predecessor. Hopefully it will provide a definitive answer to the optimal mode of delivery of term twins.

Other high-risk situations for the fetus

Cord prolapse resulting in fetal bradycardia can lead to rapid development of fetal acidaemia. The obstetric management is to expedite delivery. Meanwhile, the cord should be replaced in the warm environment of the mother's vagina to minimise cord spasm and the presenting part should be lifted out of the pelvis to minimise cord compression. Provided the fetus was in good condition prior to the cord prolapse and the baby is then delivered quickly, the neonate should respond rapidly to resuscitation.

Ruptured uterus is another obstetric emergency in which fetal compromise can rapidly develop. It typically occurs in multiparous women, especially in those with a uterine scar or with uterine stimulation, for instance with oxytocin. The classical clinical symptoms and signs are severe pain (which will 'break through' epidural analgesia), cessation of contractions, intrapartum bleeding and haematuria. Early warning signs are often seen on the cardiotocograph. It is for this reason that continuous electronic fetal monitoring is recommended in women labouring after a previous caesarean section. Again the fetal outcome from this acute hypoxic insult will be determined by the speed of delivery and the fetal condition prior to uterine rupture.

Finally, in the rare event of maternal cardiac/respiratory arrest, fetal delivery is often expedited to assist with maternal resuscitation. The physical effects of a third-trimester uterus on lung expansion and aortocaval compression can make maternal resuscitation especially difficult. If the maternal condition is not dramatically improved after 5 minutes of intensive resuscitation, rapid fetal delivery is recommended. Both the maternal and fetal outcomes are often poor nonetheless. The potential causes for a maternal cardiorespiratory arrest are numerous, for example amniotic fluid embolism, pulmonary embolism, myocardial infarction, massive cerebrovascular event, hypovolaemia.

Preterm infants

Term is defined as 37 completed weeks of gestation. The mode of delivery of preterm infants will be influenced by the gestational age, the fetal and maternal condition and whether the mother is already in spontaneous preterm labour. It is therefore difficult to make generalisations, and decisions need to be taken on an individual basis after discussion with the parents. The optimal management of breech presentations and multiple pregnancies preterm is less well established than in the term setting. Unfortunately, the incidence of breech presentation is higher preterm,[50] when it is usually the chance lie of a mobile fetus in a relatively large volume of amniotic fluid. Multiple pregnancies are at increased risk of almost every pregnancy complication, including preterm labour and delivery.

The antenatal diagnosis of chronic uteroplacental insufficiency and its importance has already been mentioned. If the fetus shows sign of compromise antenatally (i.e. abnormal CTGs on a background of abnormal Doppler studies), delivery should be effected by caesarean section almost irrespective of the gestation. Such fetuses are unlikely to be able to compensate for the acute hypoxic stress of reduced placental perfusion with each uterine contraction for prolonged periods. If, however, the CTGs remain normal antenatally the management will be much more dependent on the gestational age. In the preterm situation, expectant management with daily CTGs, weekly scans to assess liquor volume

and perform Doppler studies, and fortnightly fetal size measurements to assess growth are preferable to delivery, as the risks of prematurity are appreciable. The aim is to quantify the rate of progression of the chronic placental problem. Rapid deterioration or abnormal CTGs should prompt delivery by caesarean section. Alternatively, if the fetus remains uncompromised, induction of labour at 38 weeks' gestation can be planned.

There may be an underlying cause for the IUGR. Maternal pre-eclampsia, particularly if it is severe and of early onset, often causes chronic uteroplacental insufficiency. Recurrent episodes of minor antepartum haemorrhage due to placenta praevia can lead to IUGR.[120] The main risk to the neonate, however, is from preterm delivery. This is not surprising, as a low-lying placenta is more common in earlier pregnancy, and with formation of the lower uterine segment in the third trimester an apparent change in placental position is frequently seen.[16] Preterm placental abruption requiring delivery is also associated with growth restriction in a substantial proportion of cases.[53] The fetal effects of a placental abruption depend on the degree of placental separation and the condition of the placenta prior to the acute event. In addition, the maternal condition in any of these situations can be the principal indication for preterm delivery even when the fetus appears healthy.

Caesarean section delivery for a very preterm infant may involve 'non-lower-segment' uterine incisions, which are more susceptible to rupture in subsequent pregnancies. FBS is usually avoided because of the increased risk of serious fetal trauma. For the same reason, vacuum extraction is not used below 34 weeks gestation. Elective forceps delivery with episiotomy for preterm infants presenting by the vertex (previously thought to protect the fetal head), has not been shown to be of benefit,[67] and hence is normally only performed for standard obstetric reasons.

Preterm labour

There are a number of predisposing causes for preterm labour but often an underlying aetiology is not identifiable. Preterm prelabour rupture of the membranes (PPROM), chorioamnionitis, polyhydramnios and antepartum haemorrhage are common pathologies leading to preterm labour. Antepartum haemorrhage has already been briefly discussed. Polyhydramnios may be related to maternal diabetes, since fetal polyuria occurs in response to exposure to abnormally high glucose concentrations. This may also cause fetal macrosomia with its attendant increased risks of shoulder dystocia.[85] Fetal abnormalities, for example fetal central nervous system and gastrointestinal tract problems, which cause impaired fetal swallowing, and fetal hydrops can also result in polyhydramnios. The abnormally increased intra-amniotic pressure caused by the polyhydramnios is, in itself, a predisposing factor for PPROM.

Preterm prelabour rupture of the membranes

Preterm prelabour rupture of the membranes is diagnosed on the basis of maternal history, liquor visualisation and clinical or ultrasound evidence of oligohydramnios. Again, the cause of PPROM is relevant to both the obstetrician and the neonatologist. Common aetiologies include polyhydramnios, chorioamnionitis, invasive testing (e.g. amniocentesis), maternal urinary tract infection and cervical incompetence. Underlying causes should be treated where possible. The management thereafter is usually conservative unless there is deterioration in the fetomaternal condition. The risks of prematurity are greater than those of the most common complication, chorioamnionitis.[68] Unfortunately, this is difficult to detect clinically in its early stages and conclusive tests are not currently available. Cord prolapse and placental abruption can also occur.

Chorioamnionitis can be caused by a variety of vaginal pathogens. Once the membranes have ruptured, the passage of organisms into the amniotic cavity is facilitated. Group B *Streptococcus* is of particular concern since it can result in serious neonatal morbidity as well as being a prominent cause of preterm labour. Intrapartum antibiotics (even in the 'term labour' setting) have been shown to significantly decrease neonatal colonisation, sepsis and death.[8,30,86] The problem is deciding which women should be treated. Studies have shown that transient and intermittent carriage is common[2] and that antenatal screening is a poor predictor of the intrapartum state.[7] Unfortunately, a rapid assay is not available. Bacterial vaginosis as a possible causal factor in preterm labour is also being investigated.[51]

Thus it is evident that infection is a particularly important factor in both PPROM and preterm labour. This finally led to the design of a large, randomised multicentre trial known as ORACLE (overview of the role of antibiotics in curtailing labour and early delivery).[70,71] ORACLE I[70] included only women with PPROM and showed that maternal administration of oral erythromycin is associated with a range of health benefits for the neonate including delayed delivery and decreased respiratory, cerebral and infective morbidity. Co-amoxiclav, the other study agent, could not be routinely recommended because of its association with necrotising enterocolitis. Consequently, oral erythromycin is now routinely given to women with PPROM. ORACLE II[71] however, which included women in threatened preterm labour without evidence of PPROM, showed no evidence of benefit from prophylactic antibiotic use. Hence antibiotics should not be routinely prescribed for women in spontaneous preterm labour without evidence of clinical infection.

Preterm labour is a frequently overdiagnosed entity, as cervical change in the presence of uterine contractions is necessary to fulfil the criteria for diagnosis. Indeed, in recent years interest has focused on methods of distinguishing those women in threatened preterm labour who will go on to deliver preterm from those whose contractions will settle spontaneously. This would enable treatment to be targeted at the correct patients. Initial studies on fetal fibronectin detection in cervicovaginal secretions were promising.[39,88] More recent work,[74,82] however, has shown that the fetal fibronectin test has relatively poor positive predictive values for preterm delivery (36–50%) but good negative predictive values (91–98%). It has been suggested that fetal fibronectin is released in cases of subclinical chorioamnionitis. Thus, the role of fetal fibronectin testing is yet to be fully established and it is not currently in routine use.

Tocolytic therapy in threatened preterm delivery

Immediate delivery in cases of preterm labour is occasionally indicated for fetal or maternal reasons (e.g. placental abruption). Sometimes the woman is allowed to continue labouring irrespective of the gestational age, as the risks of continued intrauterine existence outweigh the disadvantages of prematurity (e.g. obvious chorioamnionitis). However, in the majority of cases the management is dependent on the gestational age. Previously, long-term tocolytic therapy was widely used. It has since become appreciated that tocolytics can have serious adverse effects and that only in certain situations is there a potential benefit. The neonatal morbidity following delivery between 34 and 37 weeks is unchanged whether or not attempts to arrest labour are successful,[36] and there is now no justification for tocolysis after 34 weeks. However, tocolytics do have a role between 25 and 34 weeks' gestation. Overall, the data of the 15 studies considered by Keirse et al[67] demonstrate that beta-sympathomimetic drug therapy results in a lower incidence of preterm birth. The real value of tocolysis, however, is to enable sufficient time to enhance fetal lung maturity by the concomitant use of maternal corticosteroid therapy.

Antenatal steroid therapy in threatened preterm labour

Maternally administered corticosteroids have been in use since 1972[75] and have been extensively evaluated in the preterm labour setting. Data from 12 controlled trials reviewed by Crowley et al[26] demonstrated that corticosteroids reduce the occurrence of hyaline membrane disease overall, and this reduction in respiratory morbidity was also associated with reductions in the risk of germinal matrix/intraventricular haemorrhage (GMH-IVH), necrotising enterocolitis and neonatal death. A recent meta-analysis of all the randomised trials of antenatal corticosteroid therapy has confirmed these benefits.[24] Initial studies showed no clear evidence of short- or long-term adverse effects on the mother or infant. This led to their elective use in many other settings in which preterm delivery is anticipated, for instance. severe IUGR. The effects of steroids used for this purpose, however, have not been fully established. Indeed, the practice of weekly steroid therapy in higher-order multiple pregnancies has no scientific basis. Steroids are also frequently used outside the gestational age range for which they were originally clinically evaluated (28–34 weeks).

Worryingly, the evidence is now accumulating that antenatal steroids may have long-term deleterious effects on the infant.[66] There are growing concerns, based on animal and some human data, that repeated antenatal doses could lead to a decrease in birthweight, a decrease in fetal brain and other organ size, and abnormal neuronal development. Previous investigations have been hampered by non-standardisation in the type of glucocorticoid, route of delivery, timing of administration and number of treatment courses. There does appear to be a dose-related effect in terms of potential adverse outcomes.

Currently, therefore, obstetricians should be minimising antenatal steroid treatments to a single course with repeated dosing only if there is an imminent risk of preterm delivery. This is the recommendation of the recently updated RCOG guideline on the subject.[98] The previous common practice of giving weekly injections of steroids starting at fetal viability and continuing into the third trimester is to be discouraged.

When tocolytic therapy is indicated, it should be continued if possible for 48 hours to try to maximise the effects of steroids. A variety of tocolytics are available, some of which have fetal side-effects relevant to the neonatologist. Beta-sympathomimetic agents (e.g. ritodrine and salbutamol) cross the placenta and may cause fetal tachycardia and occasionally other adverse fetal cardiac effects, which may be significant in an already compromised fetus.[37,67]

Maternal hyperglycaemia can result in troublesome neonatal hypoglycaemia, but long-term ill effects have not been recognised.

Prostaglandin synthesis inhibitors (e.g. indomethacin), on the other hand, can have more serious neonatal consequences. The predominant problems are premature closure or constriction of the ductus arteriosus and reduced fetal urinary output, leading to oligohydramnios. Necrotising enterocolitis, ileal perforation and neonatal GMH-IVH have also been reported.[81,94] Consequently, indomethacin is now used infrequently and selective cyclooxygenase (COX) II inhibitors are being studied. Atosiban, an oxytocin antagonist, is being increasingly used as a tocolytic in spite of its cost, because of its apparent efficacy in the absence of maternal side effects. No neonatal complications have been recognised. All neonatologists will be aware, however, that tocolysis does not necessarily delay preterm delivery as intended.

Conclusion

The fetus spends many months in utero sustained by its placental 'lifeline'. Although many abrupt changes occur at the time of delivery, the baby's ability to adapt to extrauterine existence is inevitably influenced by antecedent events. It is of fundamental importance, therefore, that neonatologists in training gain some insight into our current understanding of fetal pathophysiology and its assessment and management. This chapter has covered the major areas of interest, but some issues remain unresolved.

References

1. Alexander L, Newton J 1969 Acute renal failure after attempted external cephalic version. Journal of Obstetrics and Gynaecology of the British Commonwealth 76: 711–712
2. Anthony B F, Okada D M, Hobel C J 1978 Epidemiology of group B streptococcus: longitudinal observations during pregnancy. Journal of Infectious Diseases 137: 524–530
3. Bakketeig L, Bergsjo P 1989 Post-term pregnancy: magnitude of the problem. In: Chalmers I, Enkin M, Keirse M J N C (eds) Effective care in pregnancy and childbirth I. Oxford University Press, Oxford, pp 765–775
4. Beard R W, Filshie G M, Knight C A, Roberts G M 1971 The significance of the changes in the continuous fetal heart rate in the first stage of labour. Journal of Obstetrics and Gynaecology of the British Commonwealth 78: 865–881
5. Beeby P J, Elliott E J, Henderson-Smart D J, Rieger I D 1994 Predictive value of umbilical artery pH in preterm infants. Archives of Disease in Childhood 71: F93–F96
6. Borell U, Fernström I, Ohlson L, Wiqvist N 1965 Influence of uterine contractions on the uteroplacental blood flow at term. American Journal of Obstetrics and Gynecology 93: 44–57
7. Boyer K M, Gadzalla C A, Kelly P D, Burd L I, Gotoff S P 1983 Selective intrapartum chemoprophylaxis of neonatal group B streptococcal early-onset disease. II Predictive value of prenatal cultures. Journal of Infectious Diseases 148: 802–809
8. Boyer K M, Gotoff S P 1986 Prevention of early-onset neonatal group B streptococcal disease with selective intrapartum chemoprophylaxis. New England Journal of Medicine 314: 1665–1669
9. Boylan P C 1991 Liquor assessment: meconium and oligohydramnios. In: Spencer J A D (ed) Fetal monitoring. Oxford University Press, Oxford, pp 133–137
10. Byre I, Dahlia K 1974 The long term development of children delivered by vacuum extraction. Developmental Medicine and Childhood Neurology 16: 378–381
11. Caldeyro-Barcia R, Mendez-Bauer C, Poseiro J J et al 1966 Control of human fetal heart rate during labor. In: Cassels D E (ed) The heart and circulation in the newborn and infant. Grune & Stratton, New York, pp 7–36
12. Caldeyro-Barcia R, Schwarcz R, Belizan J M et al 1974 Adverse perinatal effects of early amniotomy during labor. In: Gluck L (ed) Modern perinatal medicine. Mosby Yearbook, Chicago, pp 431–439
13. Carmody F, Grant A, Mutch M, Vacca A, Chalmers I 1986 Follow up of babies delivered in a randomized comparison of vacuum extraction and forceps delivery. Acta Obstetricia et Gynaecologica Scandinavica 65: 763–766
14. Cerevka J, Scheffs J S, Vasicka A 1970 Shape of uterine contractions (intra-amniotic pressure) and corresponding fetal heart rate. 1 Spontaneous and oxytocin induced labours. Obstetrics and Gynecology 35: 695–703
15. Cetrulo C L 1986 The controversy of mode of delivery in twins: the intrapartum management of twin gestation. Seminars in Perinatology 10: 39–40
16. Chapman M G, Furness E T, Jones W R, Sheat J H 1989 Significance of the location of placenta site in early pregnancy. British Journal of Obstetrics and Gynaecology 86: 846–848
17. Chervenak F A, Johnson R E, Youcha S, Hobbins J C, Berkowitz R L 1985 Intrapartum management of twin gestation. Obstetrics and Gynecology 65: 119–124
18. Chew F T, Drew J H, Oats J N, Riley S F, Beischer N A 1985 Nonstressed antepartum cardiotocography in patients undergoing elective Cesarean Section – fetal outcome. American Journal of Obstetrics and Gynecology 151: 318–321
19. Collea J V, Rabin S C, Weghorst G R et al 1978 The randomised management of term frank breech presentation: vaginal delivery versus caesarean section. American Journal of Obstetrics and Gynecology 134: 186
20. Collea J V, Chien C, Quilligan E J 1980 The randomised management of term frank breech presentation: a study of 208 cases. American Journal of Obstetrics and Gynecology 137: 233–239
21. Collins M S, Bleyl J A 1990 Seventy one quadruplet pregnancies: management and outcome. American Journal of Obstetrics and Gynecology 162: 1384–1392
22. Confino E, Gleicher N, Elrad H, Ismajovich B, David M P 1985 The breech dilemma: a review. Obstetrics and Gynecology Survey 40: 330–337
23. Crowley P 1989 Post-term pregnancy: induction or surveillance? In: Chalmers I, Enkin M, Keirse M J N C (eds) Effective care in pregnancy and childbirth I. Oxford University Press, Oxford, pp 776–791
24. Crowley P 2004 Prophylactic steroids for preterm birth. In: Cochrane database of systematic reviews (complete reviews), issue 1. DOI 10.1002/14651858.CD000065. Update Software, Oxford
25. Crowley P, O'Herlihy C, Boylan P 1984 The value of ultrasound measurement of amniotic fluid volume in the management of prolonged pregnancies. British Journal of Obstetrics and Gynaecology 91: 444–448
26. Crowley P, Chalmers I, Keirse M J N C 1990 The effects of corticosteroid administration before preterm delivery: an overview of the evidence from controlled trials. British Journal of Obstetrics and Gynaecology 97: 11–17
27. Department of Health 1993 Changing childbirth: Parts I and II. HMSO, London
28. Department of Health and Social Security 1994 Report on confidential enquiries into maternal deaths in the United Kingdom 1988–1990. HMSO, London.
29. Royal College of Obstetrics and Gynaecology 2001 Why mothers die 1997–1999. The Confidential Enquiries into Maternal deaths in the United Kingdom. RCOG Press, London
30. Easmon C S F, Hastings M J G, Deeley J, Bloxham B, Rivers R P A, Marwood R 1983 The effect of intrapartum chemoprophylaxis on the vertical transmission of group B streptococci. British Journal of Obstetrics and Gynaecology 90: 633–635
31. Eden R D, Gergely R Z, Schifrin B S, Wade M A 1982 Comparison of antepartum testing schemes for the management of postdate pregnancy. American Journal of Obstetrics and Gynecology 144: 683–692
32. Eden R D, Seifert L S, Kodack L D, Trofatter K F, Killam A P, Gall S A 1988 A modified biophysical profile for antenatal fetal surveillance. Obstetrics and Gynecology 71: 365–369
33. Ehlers N, Jensen I K, Hansen K B 1974 Retinal haemorrhages in the newborn – a comparison of delivery by forceps and by vacuum extractor. Acta Ophthalmologica 52: 73–82
34. Eik-Nes S H, Okland O, Aure J C, Ulstein M 1984 Ultrasound screening in pregnancy: a randomised controlled trial. Lancet 1: 1347
35. Fee S C, Malee K, Deddish R, Minogue J P, Socol M L 1990 Severe acidosis and subsequent neurological status. American Journal of Obstetrics and Gynecology 162: 802–806
36. Fox J F, McCaul R W, Martin W E, Roberts W E, McLaughlin B, Morrison J C 1992 Neonatal morbidity between 34–37 weeks gestation. American Journal of Obstetrics and Gynecology 166: 360–363

37. Friedman D M, Blackstone J, Hoskins I 1992 Adverse fetal cardiac effects of oral ritodrine tocolysis. 12th Annual SPO Meeting No. 17. American Journal of Obstetrics and Gynecology 166: 326

38. Friedman E A 1954 The graphic analysis of labor. American Journal of Obstetrics and Gynecology 68: 1568–1575

39. Garite T J 1991 Oncofetal fibronectin in cervico-vaginal secretions is highly predictive of preterm delivery. American Journal of Obstetrics and Gynecology 164: 259–260

40. Gibb D 1984 Prolonged pregnancy. In: Studd J W W (ed) The management of labour. Blackwell Scientific, Oxford, pp 108–122

41. Gimovsky M L, Petrie R H 1989 The intrapartum management of the breech presentation. Clinics in Perinatology 16: 976–986

42. Goldaber K G, Gilstrap L C, Leveno K J, Dax J S, McIntire D D 1991 Pathologic fetal acidemia. Obstetrics and Gynecology 78: 1103–1107

43. Golditch I A, Boyce N E 1970 Management of abruptio placenta. Journal of the American Medical Association 212: 288–293

44. Gonen R, Spiegel D, Abend M 1996 Is macrosomia predictable, and are shoulder dystocia and birth trauma preventable? Obstetrics and Gynecology 88: 526–529

45. Grant A, O'Brien N, Joy M T, Hennessy E, MacDonald D 1989 Cerebral palsy among children born during the Dublin randomised trial of intrapartum monitoring. Lancet 2: 1233–1235

46. Green J R 1989 Placenta abnormalities: placenta praevia and abruptio placentae. In: Creasy R K, Resnik R (eds) Maternal-fetal medicine: principles and practice. W B Saunders, Philadelphia

47. Guissani D A, Spencer J A D, Moore P J, Bennet L, Hanson M A 1993 Afferent and efferent components of the cardiovascular reflex responses to acute hypoxia in term fetal sheep. Journal of Physiology 461: 431–449

48. Hammacher K 1969 The clinical significance of cardiotokography. In: Huntingford P J, Hueter K A, Saling E (eds) Perinatal medicine. Georg Thieme, Stuttgart, pp 80–85

49. Hannah ME, Hannah WJ, Hewson SA, Hodnett ED, Saigal S, William AR 2000 Planned caesarean section versus planned vaginal birth for breech presentation at term: a randomised multicentre trial. Term Breech Trial Collaborative Group. Lancet 356: 1375–1383

50. Haughey M J 1985 Fetal position during pregnancy. American Journal of Obstetrics and Gynecology 153: 885–886

51. Hay P E, Lamont R F, Taylor-Robinson D, Morgan D J, Ison C, Pearson J 1994 Abnormal bacterial colonisation of the lower genital tract as a marker for subsequent preterm delivery and late miscarriage. British Medical Journal 308: 295–298

52. Helwig J T, Parer J T, Kilpatrick S J, Laros R K 1996 Umbilical cord blood acid-base state: What is normal? American Journal of Obstetrics and Gynecology 174: 1807–1814

53. Hibbard B M, Jeffcoate T N A 1966 Abruptio placentae. Obstetrics and Gynecology 27: 155–167

54. Hofmeyr GJ 2000 External cephalic version for breech presentation at term. Cochrane Database of Systematic Reviews 2: CD000184

55. Hofmeyr GJ 2002 Interventions to help ECV for breech presentations at term. Cochrane Database of Systematic Reviews 2: CD000184

56. Hon E H 1968 An atlas of fetal heart rate patterns. Harty Press, Newhaven

57. Hoult I J, MacLennan A H, Carrie L E S 1977 Lumbar epidural analgesia in labour: relation to fetal malposition and instrumental delivery. British Medical Journal 1: 14–16

58. Humphrey M D, Chang A, Wood E C, Morgan S, Hounslow D 1974 A decrease in fetal pH during the second stage of labour, when conducted in the dorsal position. Journal of Obstetrics and Gynaecology of the British Commonwealth 81: 600–602

59. Hytten F 1982 Breech presentation: Is it a bad omen? British Journal of Obstetrics and Gynaecology 60: 417–420

60. Ingemarsson I, Heden L 1989 Cervical score and onset of spontaneous labor in prolonged pregnancy dated by second-trimester ultrasonic scan. Obstetrics and Gynecology 74: 102–105

61. Itskovitz J, Goetzman B W, Rudolf A M 1982 The mechanism of late deceleration of the heart rate and its relationship to oxygenation in normoxemic and chronically hypoxemic fetal lambs. American Journal of Obstetrics and Gynecology 142: 66–73

62. Johanson R B 1994 Vacuum extraction versus forceps delivery. In: Cochrane database of systematic reviews: pregnancy and childbirth module No 03256. Update Software, Oxford

63. Johnstone F D, Campbell D M, Hughes G J 1978 Has continuous intrapartum monitoring made any impact on fetal outcome? Lancet 1: 1298–1300

64. Kadar N, Cruddas M, Campbell S 1986 Estimating the probability of spontaneous delivery conditional on time spent in the second stage. British Journal of Obstetrics and Gynaecology 93: 568–576

65. Katz M, Shani N, Meizner I, Insler V 1982 Is end-stage deceleration of the fetal heart ominous? British Journal of Obstetrics and Gynaecology 89: 186–189

66. Kay HH, Bird IM, Coe CL, Dudley DJ 2000 Antenatal steroid treatment and adverse fetal effects: What is the evidence? Journal of the Society for Gynecologic Investigation 7: 269–278

67. Keirse M J N C, Grant A, King J F 1989 Preterm labour. In: Chalmers I, Enkin M, Keirse M I N C (eds) Effective care in pregnancy and childbirth I. Oxford University Press, Oxford, pp 694–745

68. Keirse M J N C, Ohlsson A, Treffers P E, Kanhai H H H 1989 Prelabour rupture of the membranes preterm. In: Chalmers I, Enkin M, Keirse M J N C (eds) Effective care in pregnancy and childbirth I. Oxford University Press, Oxford pp 666–692

69. Keirse M J N C, Trimbos J B 1980 Assessment of antepartum cardiotocograms in high risk pregnancy. British Journal of Obstetrics and Gynaecology 87: 261–269

70. Kenyon S L, Taylor D J, Tarnow-Mordi W 2001 Broad spectrum antibiotics for preterm, prelabour rupture of fetal membranes: the ORACLE I randomised trial. ORACLE Collaborative Group Lancet 375: 979–988

71. Kenyon S L, Taylor D J, Tarnow-Mordi W 2001 Broad spectrum antibiotics for spontaneous preterm labour: the ORACLE II randomised trial. ORACLE Collaborative Group Lancet 375: 989–994

72. Kinsella S M, Spencer J A D 1995 Maternal and fetal cardiovascular effects of epidural analgesia during labour. Contemporary Reviews in Obstetrics and Gynaecology 7: 145–150

73. Lamont R F, Dunlop P D M, Crowley P et al 1983 Spontaneous preterm labour and delivery at under 34 weeks gestation. British Medical Journal 286: 454–457

74. Leeson S C, Maresh M J A, Martindale E A et al 1996 Detection of fetal fibronectin as a predictor of preterm delivery in high risk asymptomatic pregnancies. British Journal of Obstetrics and Gynaecology 103: 48–53

75. Liggins G C, Howie R N 1972 A controlled trial of antepartum glucocorticoid treatment for prevention of the respiratory distress syndrome in premature infants. Pediatrics 50: 515–517

76. Lipitz S, Reichman B, Panet G et al 1989 The improving outcome of triplet pregnancies. American Journal of Obstetrics and Gynecology 161: 1279–1284

77. Lopez-Zeno J A, Peaceman A M, Adashek J A, Socol M L 1992 A controlled trial of a program for the active management of labor. New England Journal of Medicine 326: 450–454

78. Macaulay J H, Randall N R, Bond K, Steer P J 1992 Continuous monitoring of fetal temperature by noninvasive probe and its relationship to maternal temperature, fetal heart rate, and cord arterial oxygen and pH. Obstetrics and Gynecology 79: 469–474

79. MacDonald D, Grant A, Sheridan-Pereira M, Boylan P, Chalmers I 1985 The Dublin randomised controlled trial of intrapartum fetal heart-rate monitoring. American Journal of Obstetrics and Gynecology 152: 524–539

80. MacFarlane A, Mugford M, Henderson J, Furtado A, Stevens J, Dunn A 2000 Obstetric intervention rates by mothers age and parity, NHS hospital births, England and Wales, 1967,1975, 1980, England, 1980, 1985, 1994/5. Birth Counts: Statistics of Pregnancy and Childbirth. The Stationery Office, London, pp 535–536

81. Major C A, Lewis D F, Harding J A, Porto M A, Garite T J 1994 Tocolysis with indomethacin increases the incidence of necrotizing enterocolitis in the low-birth-weight neonate. American Journal of Obstetrics and Gynecology 170: 102–106

82. Malak T M, Sizmur F, Bell S C, Taylor D J 1996 Fetal fibronectin in cervicovaginal secretions as a predictor of preterm birth. British Journal of Obstetrics and Gynaecology 103: 648–653

83. Maresh M, Choong K-H, Beard R W 1983 Delayed pushing with lumbar epidural analgesia in labour. British Journal of Obstetrics and Gynaecology 90: 623–627

84. Modanlou H D, Freeman R K 1982 Sinusoidal fetal heart rate pattern: its definition and clinical significance. American Journal of Obstetrics and Gynecology 142: 1033–1038

85. Modanlou H D, Komatsu G 1982 Large for gestational neonates: anthropometric reason for shoulder dystocia. Obstetrics and Gynecology 60: 417–423

86. Morales W J, Lim D V, Walsh A F 1986 Prevention of neonatal group B streptococcal sepsis by the use of a rapid screening test and selective intrapartum chemoprophylaxis. American Journal of Obstetrics and Gynecology 155: 979–983

87. Morrison J J, Rennie J M, Milton P J 1995 Neonatal respiratory morbidity and mode of delivery at term: influence of timing of elective caesarean section. British Journal of Obstetrics and Gynaecology 102: 101–106

88. Nageotte M P, Hollenback K A, Vanderwahl B A, Hutch K M 1992 Circulating cellular fibronectin in the prediction of preterm labor. American Journal of Obstetrics and Gynecology 166: 270–273

89. National Institute for Clinical Excellence 2001 Induction of labour. Clinical Guideline D London

90. National Institutes of Health Consensus Development Conference 1980 Cesarean Childbirth. NIH Consensus Statement Online

91. Neesham D E, Umstad M P, Cincotta R B, Johnston D L, McGrath G M 1993 Pseudosinusoidal fetal heart rate pattern and fetal anaemia: case report and review. Australian and New Zealand Journal of Obstetrics and Gynaecology 33: 386–388

92. Thaker S B, Stroup D, Chang M 2004 Continuous electronic heart rate monitoring for fetal assessment during labor. In: The Cochrane database of systematic reviews (complete reviews), issue 1. DOI 10.1002/14651858.CD000063 93. Update Software, Oxford

93. Newell M L 1994 Caesarean section and risk of vertical transmission of HIV I infection. Lancet 343: 1464–1467

94. Norton M E, Merrill J, Cooper B A B, Kuller J A, Clyman R I 1993 Neonatal complications after the administration of indomethacin for preterm labor. New England Journal of Medicine 329: 1602–1607

95. O'Driscoll K, Foley M, MacDonald D 1984 Active management of labor as an alternative to cesarean section for dystocia. Obstetrics and Gynecology 63: 485–490

96. Okonofua F E, Olatubosun O A 1985 Caesarean versus vaginal delivery in abruptio placentae associated with live fetuses. International Journal of Gynaecology and Obstetrics 23: 471–474

97. Peebles D M, Spencer J A D, Edwards A D et al 1993 Relation between frequency of uterine contractions and human fetal cerebral oxygen saturation studied during labour by near infrared spectroscopy. British Journal of Obstetrics and Gynaecology 101: 44–48

98. Penney G C, Cameron M J 2004 Antenatal corticosteroids to prevent respiratory distress syndrome RCOG Press Guideline no. 7

99. Philpott R H 1972 Graphic records in labour. British Medical Journal 4: 163–165

100. Prober C G, Sullender W M, Yasukawa L L, Au D S, Yeager A S, Arvin A M 1987 Low risk of herpes simplex virus infections in neonates exposed to the virus at the time of vaginal delivery by mothers with recurrent genital herpes simplex virus infections. New England Journal of Medicine 316: 240–244

101. Rabinovici J, Barhai G, Reichman B, Serr D M, Mashinach S 1988 Internal podalic version with unruptured membranes for the second twin in transverse lie. Obstetrics and Gynecology 71: 428–430

102. Rayburn W F, Lavin J P, Miodovnik M, Varner M W 1984 Multiple gestation: twin interval between delivery of the first and second twins. Obstetrics and Gynecology 63: 502–506

103. Robson S C, Crawford R A, Spencer J A D, Lee A 1992 Intrapartum amniotic fluid index and its relationship to fetal distress. American Journal of Obstetrics and Gynecology 166: 78–82

104. Rooth G, Hutch A, Hutch R, 1987 Guidelines for the use of fetal monitoring. International Journal of Gynaecology and Obstetrics 25: 159–167

105. Rossi E M, Philipson E H, Williams T G, Kalhan S C 1989 Meconium aspiration syndrome: intrapartum and neonatal attributes. American Journal of Obstetrics and Gynecology 161: 1106–1110

106. Royal College of Obstetrics and Gynaecology, Clinical Effectiveness Support Unit 2001 The use of electronic fetal monitoring: The use and interpretation of cardiotocography in intrapartum fetal surveillance. Evidence-based Clinical Guideline Number 8. RCOG, London

107. Schwarcz R L, Belizan J M, Cifuentes J R, Cuadro J C, Marques M B, Caldeyro-Barcia R 1974 Fetal and maternal monitoring in spontaneous labors and in elective inductions. American Journal of Obstetrics and Gynecology 120: 356–362

108. Shennan A, Bewley S 2001 How to manage term breech deliveries. British Medical Journal 323: 244–245

109. Smith G C S, Pell J P, Dobbie R 2002 Birth order, gestational age, and risk of delivery related perinatal death in twins: retrospective cohort study. British Medical Journal 325: 1004–1006

110. Spencer J A D, Johnson P 1986 Fetal heart rate variability changes and fetal behavioural cycles during labour. British Journal of Obstetrics and Gynaecology 93: 314–321

111. Spencer J A D 1991 Predictive value of a fetal heart rate acceleration at the time of fetal blood sampling in labour. Journal of Perinatal Medicine 19: 207–215

112. Spencer J A D, Koutsoukis M, Lee A 1991 Fetal heart rate and neonatal condition related to epidural analgesia in women reaching the second stage of labour. European Journal of Obstetrics, Gynecology and Reproductive Biology 41: 173–178

113. Spencer J A D 1993 Fetal response to labour. In: Spencer J A D, Ward H R T (eds) Intrapartum fetal surveillance. Royal College of Obstetricians and Gynaecologists, London, pp 17–33

114. Spencer J A D, Robson S C, Farkas A 1993 Spontaneous recovery after severe metabolic acidaemia at birth. Early Human Development 32: 103–111

115. Stewart P, Kennedy J H, Calder A A 1982 Spontaneous labour: when should the membranes be ruptured? British Journal of Obstetrics and Gynaecology 89: 39–43

116. Studd J 1973 Partograms and nomograms of cervical dilatation in management of primigravid labour. British Medical Journal 4: 451–455

117. Sultan A H, Kamm M A, Bartram C I, Hudson C N 1994 Perineal damage at delivery. Contemporary Reviews in Obstetrics and Gynaecology 6: 18–24

118. Thacker S B 1989 Effectiveness and safety of intrapartum fetal monitoring. In: Spencer J A D (ed) Fetal monitoring. Castle House Publications, Tunbridge Wells, pp 211–217

119. Thomas J, Paranjothy S 2001 Royal College of Obstetricians and Gynaecologists, Clinical Effectiveness Support Unit. The National Sentinal Caesarean Section Audit Report. RCOG Press, London

120. Varma T R 1973 Fetal growth and placental function in patients with placenta praevia. Journal of Obstetrics and Gynaecology of the British Commonwealth 80: 311–315

121. Ventura S J, Martin J A, Curtin S C, Menacker F, Hamilton B E 2001 Births: final data for 1999. National Vital Statistics Report 49. HMSO, London, pp 1–74

122. Visser G H A, Redman C W G, Huisjes H J, Turnbull A C 1980 Nonstressed antepartum heart-rate monitoring: implications of decelerations after spontaneous contractions. American Journal of Obstetrics and Gynecology 138: 429–435

123. Wheble A M, Gillmer M D G, Spencer J A D, Sykes G S 1989 Changes in fetal monitoring practice in the UK. British Journal of Obstetrics and Gynaecology 96: 1140–1147

124. Zanini B, Paul R H, Huey J R 1980 Intrapartum fetal heart rate: correlation with scalp pH in the preterm fetus. American Journal of Obstetrics and Gynecology 136: 43–47

Further reading/sources of further information

Enkin M, Keirse M J N C, Neilson J et al 2000 Guide to effective care in pregnancy and childbirth, 3rd edn. Oxford University Press, Oxford

James D K, Steer P J, Weiner C P, Gonik B 1999 High risk pregnancy – management options, 2nd edn. W B Saunders, London

Spencer J A D (ed) 1991 Fetal monitoring – physiology and techniques of antenatal and intrapartum assessment, 2nd edn. Oxford Medical Publications, Oxford

www.cochrane.org/reviews

www.rcog.org.uk/guidelines

Section Three

Care Around Birth

CHAPTER 13

Care around birth

PART 1

Resuscitation of the newborn

Anthony D Milner

Being born is stressful, particularly if it is by vaginal delivery. During normal labour there is transient fetal hypoxia during each uterine contraction,[5,133] which results in the fetus becoming more acidaemic as the labour progresses. These changes have been followed by serial fetal scalp samples during the first and second stages of labour (Table 13.1).[12,131] Hormones associated with a stress response and biochemical markers of asphyxia (Table 13.2) are released by the fetus: in general, the greater the stress and trauma of the labour the higher the level of hormones released. Yet despite enduring this process for several hours, most newborn infants are pink, vigorous and breathing regularly by 1–2 minutes of age.

Unfortunately, not all babies make the transition to an extrauterine environment without help. In these babies the action that is taken in the next few minutes can mean the difference between death, survival with cerebral palsy or neurologically intact survival. In no other area of medicine are the benefits of prompt and correct action more rewarding and more immediate.

Over the last 10 years there have been several national and international protocol statements providing guidance on provision of neonatal resuscitation culminating in the recommendations of the European Resuscitation Council (2000)[53] and the Pediatric Working Party of the International Liaison Committee on Resuscitation.[98,120] These provide consensus statements drawn up by experts but, as there have been surprisingly few controlled trials in this important area, many of the recommendations are based at best on physiological studies and often just on 'best practice.'

Table 13.2 Markers of hypoxia/stress in the neonate as a result of 'normal labour'

- Catecholamines[76,156]
- Arginine vasopressin[146,167]
- Renin[141]
- Angiotensin[117]
- Endothelin I[95]
- Cortisol[17,145]
  - Thyroid activity[17]
  - PaO_2[1]
- Hypoxanthine[140]
- Endorphins[2]
- Plasma creatine kinase-BB[56]

Table 13.1 Changes in fetal blood gases in normal human labour (the standard deviation is given in parentheses)

	Stage of labour					
	Cervix 0–2 cm dilated	Cervix 3–5 cm dilated	Cervix 6 cm to fully dilated	FD(c)	FD(p)	Umbilical artery
pH	7.29 (0.05)	7.30 (0.05)	7.29 (0.02)	7.28 (0.05)	7.23 (0.06)	7.23 (0.05)
BD (mmol/l)	−5.5 (2.4)	−5 (2.2)	−6.3 (2.1)	−6.7 (2.1)	−9.1 (3.5)	−7.4 (2.7)
PCO_2 (mmHg)	44 (6)	42 (6)	42 (6)	40 (5.5)	44 (9)	52 (10.5)
PO_2 (mmHg)		23.7 (5.7)*			21.5 (4.3)†	17.2 (6.0)

* Level taken some time during the first stage. † Level taken some time during second stage.
BD, base deficit; FD(c), full dilatation/head in mid-cavity; FD(p), full dilatation/head on perineum.
Samples collected by fetal scalp sample except for cord arterial blood gas measurements.
Data of Beard and Morris[12] for pH, PCO_2 and base deficit, and of Paterson et al[131] for PO_2.

Causes of delayed onset of regular respiration

A frequent misconception is that delayed onset of respiration at birth is always the result of intrapartum asphyxia, but many additional factors can delay the onset of respiration after delivery (Table 13.3). Several of these may be present in a single baby, yet each one needs to be recognised as quickly as possible and properly treated. In general, asphyxia and the conditions listed in Table 13.3 either prevent the onset of spontaneous respiration or cause a serious reduction in the baby's respiratory efforts. The baby who breathes vigorously but remains cyanosed, or the baby who fails to make any respiratory effort despite the absence of asphyxia, will be considered separately at the end of this chapter, under the heading of babies who fail to respond to resuscitation (pp. 234–7).

It is increasingly recognised[62,130] that perinatal asphyxia is a relatively rare cause of permanent central nervous system (CNS) damage (p. 224). Nevertheless, intrapartum asphyxia is the cause of some cases of perinatally acquired brain damage. If a baby does not breathe after delivery, his PaO_2 falls immediately to close to zero and he rapidly becomes acidotic, that is, he develops the biochemical stigmata of asphyxia (pp. 224–5), which can also cause brain damage or aggravate pre-existing CNS injury.

Acute asphyxia

The animal model for acute neonatal asphyxia[44] has been used to explain the physiological changes in the infant who is not breathing immediately after delivery, and provides the theoretical basis for the management of his resuscitation. It will therefore be described in detail.

Acute postnatal asphyxia is induced in newborn animals by delivering them in good condition by caesarean section and then preventing them from breathing by immediately sealing their heads in a bag of saline. A very characteristic sequence of events

then takes place (Fig. 13.1). After a few shallow breaths which, owing to the nature of the experiment, cannot result in any gas exchange, the animal stops 'breathing'. This early period of apnoea, so-called primary apnoea, may last for up to 10 minutes. However, after 1–2 minutes in primary apnoea the animal usually starts to gasp: the gasps occur with increasing frequency and vigour but then decreasing until the animal literally reaches the last gasp. The heart rate falls rapidly after the onset of asphyxia, plateaus or may rise slightly in primary apnoea and early in the phase of gasping, then begins to slow. Cardiac activity continues

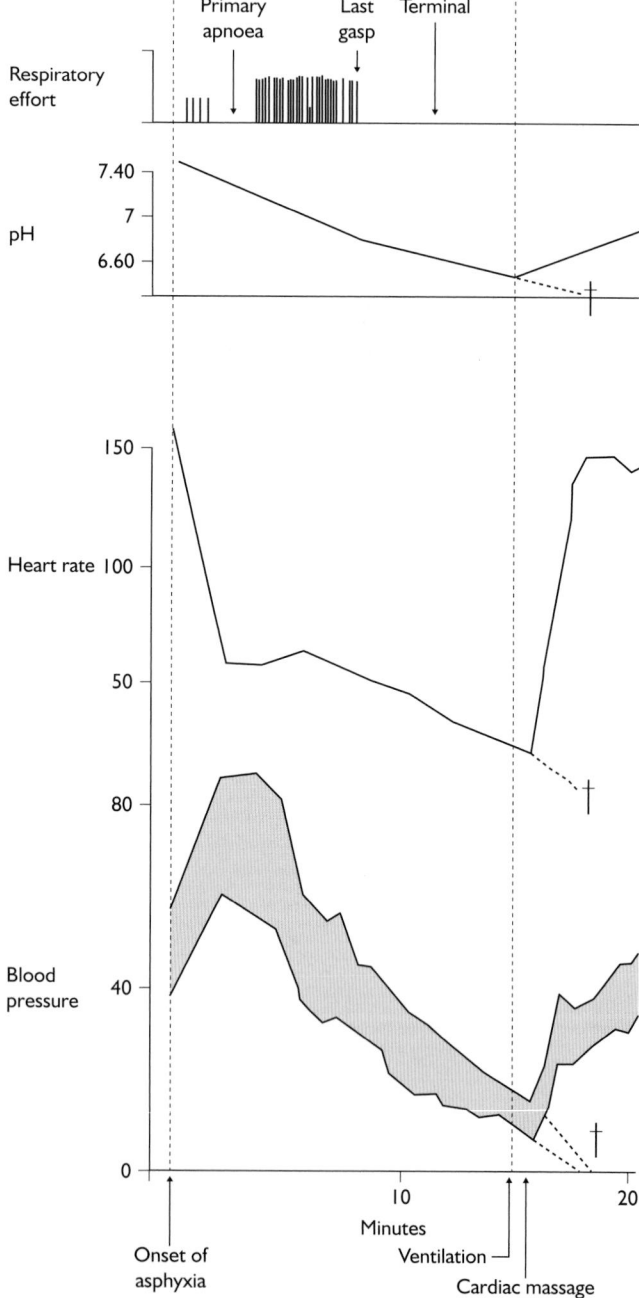

Fig. 13.1 Physiological changes during asphyxia and resuscitation of a newborn animal. (Adapted from Dawes G S, Jacobson H N, Mott J C, Shelley H J, Stafford A 1963 Treatment of asphyxia in newborn lambs and monkeys. Journal of Physiology 169: 167–184.)

Table 13.3 Factors other than asphyxia that may delay the onset of respiration after delivery

- Central nervous system injury or abnormality present prior to labour
- Drugs depressing the central nervous system
- Maternal hypocapnia
- Trauma, especially to the central nervous system
- Prematurity, in particular surfactant-deficient, stiff lungs
- Sepsis, especially group B streptococci
- Muscle weakness due to prematurity or primary muscle disease
- Anaemia, hypovolaemia
- Congenital malformations
  - Obstructing the airway or preventing lung expansion
  - Neurological, impairing respiratory control

for 10 minutes or more after the last gasp. The period between the last gasp and cardiac arrest is known as secondary or terminal apnoea. The changes in blood pressure parallel those in heart rate. A severe mixed acidaemia develops. By the end of terminal apnoea the $PaCO_2$ may exceed 13.5 kPa (100 mmHg), the $[H^+]$ is usually greater than 300 nmol/l (pH <6.5), and the PaO_2 is zero. The serum potassium rises to 15 mmol/l or more.

The neonatal primate is capable of surviving at least 20 minutes of complete oxygen deprivation, but in the latter part of this period brain damage is occurring. Survival is due to the existence of large stores of glycogen in the brain, liver and myocardium, which can produce energy by anaerobic glycolysis during asphyxia,[163] and also to the ability of neonatal brain tissues to metabolise fuels such as lactate and ketones.[61,160,181] Reduction in the stores of glycogen for any reason, such as growth retardation (pp. 116–17) or preceding partial asphyxia (see below), will reduce the fetus's ability to withstand an acute asphyxial insult.

Brain damage has been described in monkeys sacrificed towards the end of the phase of gasping, but as many human neonates clinically assessed to be in terminal apnoea when resuscitated survive without neurological sequelae (see below), it seems probable that brain damage following acute asphyxia is not inevitable unless it is severe, prolonged, or was superimposed on preceding chronic partial asphyxia (see below).

The response to removing the bag of saline from the animal's head during the above experiment (Fig. 13.1) depends on the stage of asphyxia reached. If the animal is in primary apnoea it will remain apnoeic until the pH falls to a level which will provoke gasping, or until external stimuli have the same effect. As it will then inhale air or oxygen the animal's condition rapidly improves and the gasps soon change into regular respiration. If the animal is already making respiratory movements or gasping when the bag is removed, and air or oxygen enters its lungs, a regular respiratory pattern rapidly develops; if the bag is removed in terminal apnoea respiration will not occur. To resuscitate such an animal positive-pressure ventilation must be used, and if the heart rate is very slow (or is absent) external cardiac massage will be necessary.

Giving intravenous glucose and bicarbonate throughout the above experiment to combat the acidaemia and hypoglycaemia resulting from consumption of all the glycogen stores during asphyxia prolongs the survival of the animal. If these agents are given during resuscitation by positive-pressure ventilation they will improve the cardiac output, expedite the onset of spontaneous respiration[4] and thereby minimise the likelihood of subsequent brain damage.[45]

This model is of limited value, as acute total asphyxia is rare in the human neonate; human mothers are not usually anaesthetised for long periods prior to delivery and cord occlusion is not total. Further, there may be other complications such as the presence of heavy sedation or prematurity (see below), the primary apnoea may be prolonged[30] or the gasping efforts may be too weak to establish alveolar ventilation. Still, severe intrapartum terminal profound asphyxia will result in the delivery of an infant with a $[H^+]$ concentration above 100 nmol/l (pH <7.0) who is limp, bradycardic and in terminal apnoea (see above).

The experiments on acute animal asphyxia have provided several other important pieces of information that help us to understand the behaviour and treatment of the human infant who is asphyxiated or apnoeic immediately after delivery. These include the following.

- The onset of gasping and therefore regular respiration can be expedited in primary apnoea by peripheral stimuli, including rubbing the baby with a warm towel, blowing cold gases over the baby's face or giving an intramuscular injection.
- Drugs administered to the mother, including all commonly used sedatives and analgesics, pass to the fetus and may prolong primary apnoea to such an extent that the acidaemia becomes severe and the phase of gasping may never occur. However, they also slow down the accumulation of carbon dioxide and lactic acid.
- A baby born in terminal apnoea will never establish spontaneous respiration unless he is actively resuscitated by intubation and intermittent positive pressure ventilation (IPPV). This crucial fact is the prime reason why, when confronted by an infant who is apnoeic at 2–3 minutes of age, there should be absolutely no delay in establishing effective ventilation.

In infants resuscitated from terminal apnoea the time from the onset of artificial ventilation to either the first gasp or regular respiration is proportional to the severity of the asphyxia before ventilation was started (Fig. 13.2).[4] If artificial ventilation was started before the pH was depressed too far, the infant may be

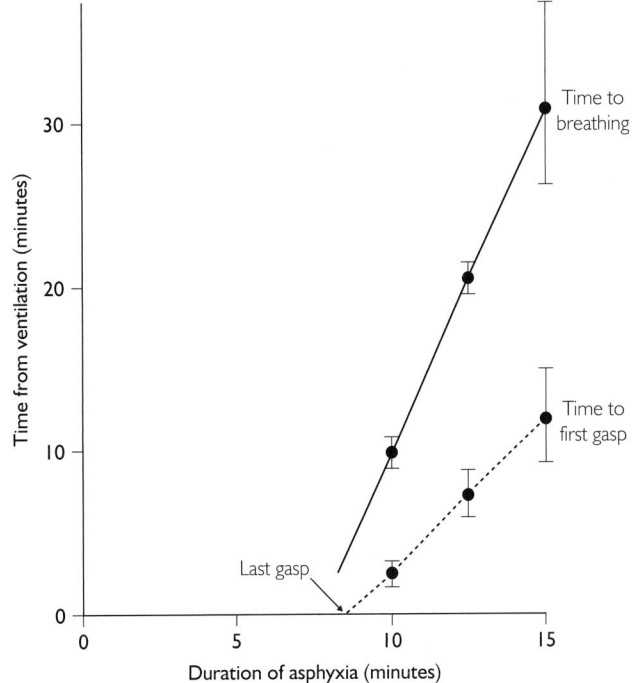

Fig. 13.2 Time from beginning positive-pressure ventilation with oxygen until the first gasp – and until the establishment of regular breathing – in nearly newly delivered Rhesus monkeys asphyxiated for 10, 12.5 or 15 minutes at 30°C. The vertical bars indicate the standard errors of the means in each group of five or six monkeys. (With permission from Adamsons K, Behrman R, Dawes G S, James L S, Koford C 1964 Resuscitation by positive pressure ventilation and tris-hydroxymethylaminomethane of Rhesus monkeys asphyxiated at birth. Journal of Pediatrics 65: 807–818.)

expected to gasp (a Head's paradoxical reflex[77]) and start regular respiration after 3–4 minutes of IPPV, whereas if resuscitation was started well into terminal apnoea when the $[H^+]$ was probably greater than 150 nmol/l (pH <6.8), gasping may be delayed for 20 minutes and regular respiration for over half an hour. Therefore, those infants who have not started to breathe spontaneously 4–5 minutes after starting IPPV should, in the absence of other causes of neonatal respiratory depression, be assumed to have a very low pH.

Chronic in-utero 'prolonged partial' asphyxia

Episodes of acute total asphyxia creating sudden total fetal anoxia as described above are relatively rare in clinical practice. More common are events that lead to the gradual development of fetal hypoxia, acidaemia and chronic partial asphyxia (Ch. 41). This can occur before or during labour. For example, some hours or even days before delivery a fetus may suffer a hypoxic/asphyxial insult that is not severe enough to kill him but that can cause neurological damage.[122,171] By the time the mother of such a baby goes into labour, he may have made a complete biochemical recovery and have normal blood gases.[166] As the baby has not suffered intrapartum asphyxia he may well show no signs of respiratory depression at birth, have a good Apgar score and establish regular breathing without any apparent problems.

In a different set of animal experiments from those described above, pregnant monkeys were given an excess of halothane to render them hypotensive, and their fetus thereby hypoxic and acidaemic, for periods of 4–6 hours. The animals were then delivered of newborns with widespread cortical, midbrain and cerebellar damage.[25] In clinical practice this 'chronic partial' hypoxic ischaemia can occur if labour is augmented or if there are additional problems, such as maternal supine hypotension. Pathological causes of chronic partial hypoxic ischaemia in clinical practice include excessive use of oxytocic drugs, the effect of labour on a growth-retarded fetus who already has reduced umbilical blood flow,[79] which falls even further during the normal uterine contractions of labour, or recurrent episodes of umbilical cord occlusion caused by entanglement around a fetal part or compression of the cord between the presenting part and the pelvis.

During such episodes the fetal blood pressure is normal or high to start with, and although the heart rate is commonly sustained there may be a bradycardia; the cardiac output is diverted primarily to the placenta, adrenals, brain and myocardium.[20,21,148] The fetal PO_2 and pH fall, and energy is produced by anaerobic metabolism of glycogen and glucose to lactate. Because the PCO_2 also rises, a combined metabolic and respiratory acidaemia develops. These changes may resolve rapidly if normal uteroplacental function is restored and the asphyxia is transient or treated.[132] However, if the heart rate and blood pressure fall the vital organs will eventually become ischaemic[20,148] and brain damage occurs. The pattern of damage seen after chronic partial intrauterine hypoxic ischaemia is that of global neuronal loss, (so-called selective neuronal necrosis[184]) and the brain also characteristically shows damage in the watershed areas between the arteries supplying the cerebral cortex, with parasagittal cerebral injury (p. 1133).[184] These ischaemic lesions correspond to those seen in the experimental animal model of partial asphyxia described by Brann and Myers.[25]

If episodes of partial asphyxia have been short-lived the fetus is unlikely to be seriously damaged; if delivered promptly, although his respiration may be depressed immediately after delivery and he may be acidaemic with a poor Apgar score, he usually responds quickly to resuscitation and is unlikely to suffer sequelae.

Sequelae are, however, more likely to occur if chronic partial hypoxic ischaemia has been severe or prolonged.[25] If such asphyxia persists up to the time of delivery it can culminate in a short period of profound asphyxia, following which the baby will be born in very poor condition, with a low Apgar score. If cord blood gas analysis is carried out he will have a marked metabolic, and in some cases respiratory, acidaemia with an $[H^+]$ of more than 100 nmol/l (pH <7.0). However, how much brain damage has been sustained can only be assessed by his clinical condition in the next 12–24 hours, and by whether or not he develops hypoxic ischaemic encephalopathy (HIE; pp. 1128–48). Animal evidence also suggests that permanent neurological damage can occur on occasion with prolonged recurrent partial in-utero asphyxia without the fetal pH falling. This is presumably because, during transient episodes of asphyxia, if the blood pressure is not adequately sustained, cerebral oxygen delivery to watershed areas may fall below critical levels, despite the fact that at the same time there is not sufficient generalised oxygen lack to result in widespread anaerobic glycolysis, lactic acidaemia and a fall in pH. Despite the absence of systemic acidosis in these experiments, it is interesting that there were marked fetal heart rate changes during each episode of asphyxia.[38]

Finally, it is probably quite common for a fetus to recover from, or be resuscitated from, in-utero asphyxia, and even for his acid–base status to recover in the presence of persisting hypoxia.[162,188] In such cases the fetus with a reasonable pH may make a satisfactory transition to extrauterine life (i.e. have a reasonable Apgar score), yet have suffered in-utero asphyxia with damage to his central nervous system, which will manifest as HIE in the neonatal period. Similar in-utero recovery can also occur after a single, acute, brain-damaging asphyxial insult.[111] This potential for 'in-utero resuscitation' is yet another reason for the poor association between Apgar scores, cord blood gases and subsequent neurological disorders, and also explains why some babies who develop severe HIE cause few resuscitation problems in the labour ward.[59,86,91,136,151]

Although the various types of asphyxial insult described above do in their own right cause neuronal death at the time, there are now extensive data to show that a large amount of the long-term damage to the brain of babies who develop HIE is the result of the secondary energy failure that occurs postnatally, which is described in detail in Chapter 41, Part 4.

The fact that prenatal asphyxia can evolve in these many different ways in the hours and days before and after delivery has important clinical and medicolegal implications, of which the three most important are:

- most babies who have signs of fetal distress, a low Apgar score or acidaemia on cord blood gas analysis are normal in the neonatal period and on follow-up;

- intrauterine problems days or weeks before labour can cause severe long-term neurological defects, yet the baby may show few if any neurological abnormalities in the neonatal period;
- in the absence of clinically apparent HIE in the neonatal period it is highly unlikely that intrapartum events are responsible for neurological sequelae.

Pre-existing brain disease

Case reports in the past established that babies who had suffered a severe insult some time before labour could show fetal distress, develop neurological signs including encephalopathy in the neonatal period, and end up with cerebral palsy. A study from Oxford[64] showed that babies who died following a labour characterised by marked cardiotocographic (CTG) abnormalities had pathological changes in their brain that were old and must have antedated labour. Thus brain damage developing before labour can cause fetal distress in labour, a low Apgar score and neonatal death. A case control study in Western Australia found no evidence of intrapartum hypoxic ischaemia in over 70% of babies with early neonatal encephalopathy.[11] Rarely, congenital malformations of the brain (see below[26]) or congenital myopathies may also result in a baby being born with poor Apgar scores not due to perinatal asphyxia, and some babies with diagnoses such as Smith–Lemli–Opitz syndrome (p. 890), other inborn errors of metabolism or chromosomal malformations can develop early encephalopathy.[55]

Depression of the respiratory centre

Pharmacological

Almost all the drugs used as analgesics, sedatives or general anaesthetics during labour can cross the placenta and, in theory, depress the neonatal respiratory centre. However, respiratory depression from drugs is likely to be important only in premature babies or those who have also suffered some degree of intrapartum asphyxia. A drug-exposed full-term baby with an $[H^+]$ less than 55 nmol/l (pH >7.25) will probably establish regular respiration unless the level of drug in the plasma is very high. If, however, respiration is depressed, as in animal experiments, this will take the form of prolongation of primary apnoea and unless artifical ventilation is established the neonate will become progressively hypoxic and acidaemic, with all that this entails. Although sedative drugs do prolong survival in experimental asphyxia, this effect must never lull the paediatrician into believing that resuscitation is less urgent in the infant who is apnoeic because of drug depression than in the one who is apnoeic through asphyxia.

Hypocapnia

The maternal $PaCO_2$ may be reduced in women who are using one of the breathing techniques associated with 'natural' childbirth or an inhalational analgesic such as Entonox. The hyperventilation may be involuntary during a general anaesthetic if there is exuberant bag squeezing by the anaesthetist. The fetal $PaCO_2$ is in equilibrium with that of the mother, and a fetus born with a $PaCO_2$ less than 4 kPa (30 mmHg) lacks the carbon dioxide drive to ventilation and may remain apnoeic until his $PaCO_2$ rises sufficiently to stimulate the respiratory centre.[118] Maternal hypocapnia may also reduce placental blood flow and thereby cause fetal hypoxia and acidaemia.[116,102]

Trauma

In babies born in poor condition at birth after a traumatic forceps or breech extraction it is difficult to separate the effects of trauma from the fetal asphyxia, which often coexists. Trauma alone is now very rare with improvements in obstetric practice[41] but may, for example, cause subdural haemorrhage (pp. 1122–3) in a baby who is in good condition at birth but who deteriorates during the first 12–24 hours as the haematoma increases in volume. It is important to remember that subdural haemorrhage may occur after a spontaneous vaginal delivery.[74]

Endorphin levels are higher in the cord blood of infants exposed to the physical stresses of vaginal delivery[2] and, as these substances may depress neonatal ventilation,[81] it follows that trauma can indirectly depress the central nervous system. Recent research showing that the excitatory neurotransmitters responsible for the secondary energy failure of HIE are also released after traumatic delivery[93] may provide a unifying mechanism for the interrelationship between birth trauma, birth asphyxia and subsequent neurological injury.

A rare traumatic cause of delayed onset of respiration at birth is injury or transection of the spinal cord in the cervical region. Depending on the level of the injury, both the intercostal muscles and the diaphragm will be paralysed and apnoea will result. Formerly common following extended breech presentations,[187] this type of injury now seems to be limited to babies delivered by rotational forceps.[110]

Anaemia

The infant who is severely anaemic may be in high-output heart failure. He lacks haemoglobin to deliver oxygen to the tissues and this will make him more susceptible to asphyxia. Without haemoglobin he lacks one of the body's major buffers and may therefore be more acidaemic.[168] As a result he may be in very poor condition at delivery and may not only breathe inadequately but respond poorly to resuscitation. Although severely asphyxiated infants are pale, coexisting anaemia must always be considered in a pale infant responding poorly to resuscitation.

The two most likely causes of severe anaemia at birth are Rhesus incompatibility and fetal haemorrhage. The delivery of a baby with Rhesus disease is usually expected; unexpected severe anaemia at birth is usually due to feto-maternal haemorrhage although on occasion there can be bleeding from a vasa praevia or hypovolaemia due to a feto-placental blood loss when there is a very tight nuchal cord.[180] In addition to the normal resuscitation routines, such infants require urgent transfusion (pp. 764–8).

Sepsis

Babies suffering from severe intrapartum infection, both preterm and at term, classically due to *Listeria*[23] or group B streptococci,[108,134] can be born with very poor Apgar scores, although they are not asphyxiated. They are critically ill at the time of birth, with hypotension and septicaemia (i.e. a positive blood culture). Although the outlook for these babies is grave, the condition must be diagnosed and vigorous anti-infection therapy commenced (pp. 1026–8), in addition to the management of their initial apnoea.

Subsequent effects of asphyxia (acute or chronic) on body systems

The metabolism of all cells, including those in the central nervous system, is inhibited by a profound acidaemia, and myocardial performance and cardiac output fall as the $[H^+]$ rises above 80 nmol/l (pH <7.10).[15,49] Exposure to an $[H^+]$ above 65 nmol/l (pH <7.25) inhibits surfactant synthesis (p. 481), predisposing to respiratory distress syndrome (RDS) in premature infants (see below). These changes in organ function can be the result of asphyxia occurring before delivery, or of asphyxia secondary to inadequate resuscitation and care in the first few minutes of life in babies who were not asphyxiated at the moment of delivery, or both.

Central nervous system

The most serious impact of asphyxia is on the brain, not only because, by depressing the vital centres in the brain, it results in respiratory depression at birth, but also because asphyxia in term babies leading to HIE is a cause of perinatal brain damage and subsequent neurological handicap (p. 1144).

Cardiovascular system

Heart failure often follows severe birth asphyxia[28] (p. 624). Myers[119] noted that it could be one of the aetiological factors contributing to hypoxic ischaemic encephalopathy, probably by reducing cerebral blood flow at a time when this is pressure-passive. The main cause of the heart failure is hypoxic and hypotensive myocardial ischaemia and necrosis,[29] with cardiac dilatation, stretching of the tricuspid valve ring and tricuspid incompetence. It may be aggravated by hypoglycaemia,[7] constriction of the placental vascular bed in response to asphyxia and hypoxia,[124] or changes in circulating blood volume.[180]

Lung effects

Pulmonary blood flow falls during fetal asphyxia but once the asphyxia is withdrawn there is a reactive hyperaemia,[47] which causes fluid transudation and oedema in the tissues damaged by asphyxia. Preterm newborn animals delivered shortly after such an experiment develop pulmonary oedema and histological changes similar to those seen in human infants with RDS.[43] Intrapartum asphyxia increases the incidence of RDS in short-gestation infants[104,174] (p. 474). The postasphyxial pulmonary oedema causes desquamation of the cells lining the terminal air spaces, which is one of the earliest histological changes seen in the lungs of human neonates dying from RDS,[67] the protein-rich oedema fluid inhibits surfactant,[92] the persisting acidaemia inhibits surfactant synthesis[112] and the defective ventilatory excursion of the asphyxiated infant reduces the release on to the alveolar surface of whatever surfactant he does possess.[191] This is discussed in detail on page 484.

Asphyxiated term infants may gasp for a period after delivery. Alternatively they may be tachypnoeic, driven by the metabolic acidaemia (p. 222), or they may have apnoeic pauses.[152] Severe asphyxia also causes severe lung disease in term babies by a mechanism analogous to acute RDS (pp. 474–5).

Evidence for the role of postnatal asphyxia in causing RDS comes from Drew,[50] who showed that efficient postnatal resuscitation of low-birthweight infants could reduce the severity of, and mortality from, RDS, presumably by preventing the deleterious effects of underventilation and acidaemia.

In term infants massive pulmonary haemorrhage (pp. 512–15) is a rare pulmonary sequel of severe asphyxia.[54] Not only are the lungs damaged by the asphyxia but myocardial ischaemia coupled with fluid overload during resuscitation may result in left ventricular failure.

Renal effects

Whenever a neonate develops severe hypoxia or hypotension kidney damage may result. After birth asphyxia, proteinuria is common,[115] as is haematuria, and in severe cases renal failure develops (pp. 935–40). Myoglobinuria leading to acute tubular necrosis and renal failure can also occur.[101] Some authors have linked severe renal damage with severe neurological disease[137] but the same group, and others, now report that renal damage is common in HIE and does not predict outcome.[161]

Temperature homoeostasis

Severely asphyxiated babies, particularly very-low-birthweight (VLBW) ones, are likely to get cold because it can be difficult to prevent heat loss during resuscitation in the labour ward. In addition, hypoxia is known to depress the thermogenic response to cold (Chapter 27)[157] and even in mildly asphyxiated babies the oxygen consumption is below normal in the first few hours.[155] Sedative drugs given intra partum to the mother may also depress thermogenesis and result in a cold baby (p. 270).

Other organ systems

Intrapartum and postnatal asphyxia reduce gut motility in the neonatal period, causing feed intolerance,[16] and probably predispose the neonate to necrotising enterocolitis.[150] They may also cause hypoglycaemia,[78] hypocalcaemia[178] and hyperammonaemia.[71] The pituitary gland may be affected. Inappropriate antidiuretic hormone production and hyponatraemia are common during the first few days in severely asphyxiated infants, and growth hormone deficiency presenting later in childhood is more common in infants who were breech deliveries.[40] The liver may be damaged and become necrotic,[164] and liver enzymes are raised, although the increased incidence of neonatal jaundice following asphyxia is more likely to be the result of bruising than of hepatic dysfunction.[31,63] Clotting factor deficiencies in asphyxiated infants are not reversed by vitamin K[80] and are usually the result of disseminated intravascular coagulation.[37]

Requirement for resuscitation

Gupta and Tizard[77] reported in 1967 that 5.7% of all deliveries were apnoeic at 1 minute of age and that a quarter of these needed intubation in the delivery room. In the 1970 perinatal mortality survey, Chamberlain et al[35] reported that 4.7% of infants took more than 3 minutes to establish sustained respiration, and half of these required intubation. Milner and Vyas[113] reported that 2.1% of all newborn babies required intubation and IPPV. One study revealed that intubation rates may vary considerably, from 2% to 10% in units in the same area in Scotland.[94] More recently, Palme-Kilander[128] found that only one in 100 babies born in Sweden needed active resuscitation and, unlike previous experience, only 20% of these (0.2% of the total) went on to need intubation and IPPV. There is also evidence that the need for intubation is falling in the UK, from 2.4% in 1993 to 1.2% in 1997, apparently related to improvements in obstetric and midwifery care.[6]

Gupta and Tizard[77] estimated that 70% of infants requiring resuscitation were born in predictably high-risk situations, and similar figures are given by Primhak et al[144] and Palme-Kilander.[128] For this reason skilled staff should attend the complicated deliveries listed in Table 13.4. The reasons for attending

in the presence of meconium-stained liquor (p. 199) or prematurity (pp. 236–7) are explained in detail elsewhere. Intubation is often needed in babies born by caesarean section (6.2%) and by breech (8%).[113] Although a case can be made for not attending non-rotational forceps without fetal distress,[75] or elective repeat caesarean section;[142,73] quality perinatal care with rapid effective resuscitation still requires skilled personnel to attend up to 40% of all deliveries.[144] Furthermore, 30% of babies who need active resuscitation are delivered after an apparently normal labour in which there has been no evidence of fetal compromise.[77,144] Low et al[106] showed that careful assessment of antenatal risk factors failed to identify half of all babies with a base deficit of more than 12 mmol/l at birth. These data are compelling reasons for ensuring that someone capable of resuscitating a newborn baby, be it a midwife, a general practitioner, a paediatrician or an anaesthetist, is present or available within 2–3 minutes at every delivery.

Assessment of the baby after delivery

It is essential that the baby's condition is evaluated as quickly after delivery as possible. The response to resuscitation should be recorded as a narrative in the baby's notes, the account ending only when the baby is pink, breathing normally and active, or is at least pink and stable and connected if necessary to a ventilator. Although the Apgar Score (Table 13.5) has traditionally been used to assess the condition of the baby at birth and the 5-minute score remains a useful marker of asphyxia,[33] the need for intervention depends on just three of the five components: heart rate, colour and respiratory activity.

Babies who require resuscitation fall into four main groups:

- those who are apnoeic or make feeble and inadequate respiratory efforts, are cyanosed but have a heart rate above 100/min and are well perfused;

Table 13.4 Perinatal complications requiring a paediatrician's presence at delivery

- Caesarean section
- Forceps
- Breech
- Ventouse (vacuum extraction)
- Malpresentations
- Multiple pregnancy
- Meconium staining
- Gestation <36 weeks
- Fetal distress
- Known fetal complications
  - Rhesus disease
  - Congenital malformation

Table 13.5 The Apgar score

Clinical feature	Score		
	0	1	2
Heart rate	0	≤100	>100
Respiration	Absent	Gasping or irregular	Regular or crying lustily
Muscle tone	Limp	Diminished, or normal with no movements	Normal with active movements
Response to pharyngeal catheter	Nil	Grimace	Cough
Colour of trunk	White or blue	Pink with blue extremities	Pink

- those who make no respiratory effort at all and are often bradycardic and pale;
- a third and uncommon group that remain cyanosed despite vigorous respiratory efforts
- the very small group in which neonatal apnoea is due to primary disorders in the muscles or the central nervous system.

Labour ward management of resuscitation

Preparation

All delivery suites should be equipped to deal with advanced resuscitation (see below) and, since blind drug or fluid therapy is no longer acceptable, this should include facilities for assessing whether the three most serious complications of asphyxia – acidaemia, hypotension and hypoglycaemia – are present. Furthermore, as the labour ward resuscitation trolley is not the ideal site for complex resuscitation, modern maternity hospitals should be designed so that the delivery suite and the neonatal unit are adjacent to each other, so that the critically ill baby can be referred quickly to the neonatal intensive care unit (NICU) for treatment once he is pink and has an adequate heart rate. Under most circumstances (see below) treatment with drugs or volume expansion can and should wait until the baby is in the NICU and appropriate investigations have been carried out.

Equipment

Most neonatal resuscitation is now carried out on purpose-built resuscitation trolleys (Fig. 13.3), the essential components of which are:

- an adequate shelf on which to lay the infant. This should be at a comfortable height for the resuscitator, be tiltable and permit partial extension of the infant's neck. However, in general babies should lie flat[113] and there is no need to extend the neck during intubation (see below);
- a supply of oxygen for the face mask, bag and mask, T piece or endotracheal tube, capable of giving a flow of 5 l/min (see below);
- a mask for giving oxygen to the cyanosed but breathing baby;
- a suction tube with soft suction catheters sizes French gauge (FG) 8 and 10 to clear the airway, and FG2/3 to suck through the endotracheal tube (ETT). The suction should not exceed 200 mmHg and for routine use should be set at 100 mmHg (136 cmH$_2$O) to prevent damage to the oropharyngeal mucosa. Because of the risk of infection from the neonate, mouth-held mucus extractors should not be used;
- an overhead radiant heat source and sides to the resuscitation shelf to minimise the radiant and convective heat loss respectively;
- an accurate clock with the ability to measure time in seconds, as time passes very quickly in any emergency procedure.

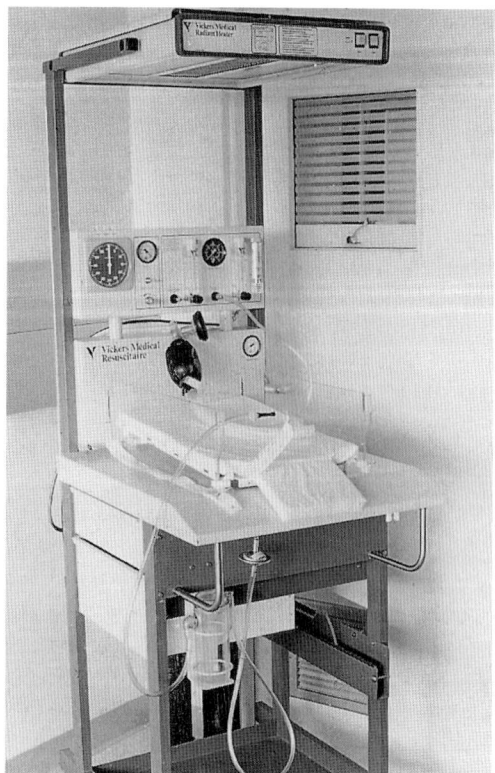

Fig. 13.3 Resuscitation trolley with overhead heater, large clock, adequate resuscitation area and appropriate storage space.

Oxygen supply

Whichever method of administering oxygen is used, the gas *must* be passed through a pressure-limiting device terminating in a variable-pressure blow-off valve, which should normally be set at 30 cmH$_2$O. Babies must never, ever be ventilated with a gas supply that is obtained directly from the medical gas supply of the hospital. This is at a dangerously high pressure and babies have died from massive air leak as a result.

Although the current international recommendations are that, if available, 100% oxygen should be used for resuscitating babies at birth, there is increasing evidence that this may not be optimal as the use of oxygen is associated with the generation of excessive levels of oxygen free radicals.[153] Studies on animals (particularly piglets) have shown that air is as effective as oxygen in resuscitation from acute asphyxia.[149] Although there were no apparent histological differences between those receiving oxygen and those receiving air, the air group had better neurological function after resuscitation.[173] Randomised studies on babies requiring resuscitation at birth have shown that, for most babies, air is as effective as 100% oxygen,[147,154,183] although in these studies the option remained for babies receiving air to be changed to 100% oxygen if cyanosis persisted. Babies resuscitated with oxygen had evidence of oxidative stress persisting for 1 month[182] and oxygen administration was associated with a delay in the onset of spontaneous breathing.[154]

It is likely that as a result of further studies the recommendation to use 100% oxygen will be replaced either by air as a first-line option or by a compromise, perhaps 30% oxygen.

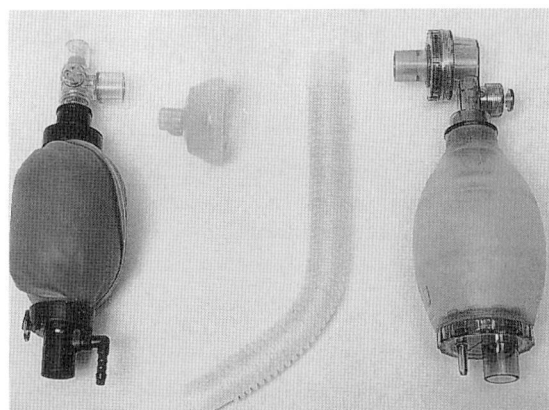

Fig. 13.4 Bag and mask systems appropriate for neonatal resuscitation. Ambu bag on the left; Paediatric Laerdal on the right. The hose should be connected to act as a reservoir if high oxygen concentrations are required.

However, it should be remembered that, when using bag and mask systems without an attached oxygen reservoir (Fig. 13.4) at 5 litres of oxygen per minute the baby receives only about 40% oxygen, while if the reservoir is attached this increases to 60–70%.[83]

Trolley equipment

The equipment on the trolley must include:

- a bag and mask system for artificial ventilation. The easiest masks to use are those with a pneumatic rim to obtain a tight face seal connected to a self-inflating bag. The mask must be detachable from the bag unit and replaceable with a connector for an endotracheal tube. Several bag and mask systems are commercially available (Fig. 13.4), but the Ambu bag and Paediatric Laerdal systems with soft face masks are preferable (see below). They must be squeezed gently;
- T piece face mask system. A good alternative is simply to occlude a T piece connected to a face mask and to the gas supply via a pressure-limiting device[88] but this has the disadvantage that unless the resuscitaire is adapted, pure oxygen will be given. A T connector connected to the ETT is also an effective alternative to using a bag and mask system attached to the ETT in those babies for whom intubation is indicated, but has the same drawback of giving virtually pure oxygen. T-piece systems have many advantages, however: they are easy to sterilise and assemble, and they make it easier to monitor the inflation pressure and give a long inflation time, which is important to establish a functional residual capacity (FRC; see below);
- laryngeal masks, as these have been used successfully for neonatal resuscitation.[27,57,66] This device is passed blind, requires less training and is particularly useful when the baby has an abnormal upper airway;
- a selection of baby-sized oropharyngeal airways (sizes **00** and **000**);
- at least two laryngoscopes (as one may fail at the crucial moment); which blade to have on the laryngoscope is a matter

of individual preference but generally speaking a straight-bladed one of the Wisconsin, Magill or Oxford Infant types is best. Disposable neonatal laryngoscopes are now available and have proved entirely suitable in our hands, circumventing the problems created by damage and loss in the autoclave;
- a selection of endotracheal tubes (2.5, 3.0 and 3.5 mm) and appropriate connectors from them to the resuscitation bag. In general, oral tubes are easier to insert in emergencies, but if the practice of the unit is to use nasal endotracheal tubes for long-term ventilation a supply of these may be left on the trolley for use in appropriate cases;
- endotracheal tube introducers;
- Magill forceps for nasal endotracheal tubes;
- nasogastric tubes type FG 6 and 8 for emptying the stomach, particularly in meconium-affected babies;
- disposable gloves;
- a selection of syringes, needles, specimen bottles and intravenous cannulae;
- adhesive tape of a type that will not damage very fragile preterm skin;
- cord clamps and ties;
- a large pair of scissors;
- a stethoscope;
- equipment for emergency cannulation of the umbilical vessels, (pp. 1240–7) together with equipment for draining a pneumothorax (pp. 490–1);
- intraosseous needles;
- BM/Dextrostix;
- electrocardiographic monitor;
- an oximeter;
- a Dinamap blood pressure recorder.

The only drugs required on the trolley are:

- sodium bicarbonate (4.2% or 8.4%), 10 ml ampoules;
- adrenaline (epinephrine), (1:10 000) 2 ml ampoules;
- Physiological saline (for umbilical catheters), 1 ml ampoules;
- 10% dextrose, 10 ml ampoules;
- Naloxone 0.4 mg/ml, 2 ml ampoules;
- Vitamin K, 1 mg ampoules.

A supply of 1000 U/ml heparin for anticoagulation of syringes used in blood gas analysis should be kept in the labour ward refrigerator. There should be ready access to fresh O-negative blood for emergency transfusion.

Equipment checks on arrival in the labour ward

- Is the gas supply to the resuscitation trolley turned on and working? Is the pressure blow-off valve set at 30 cmH₂O?
- Is the clock working and set to zero?
- Is the suction working at a pressure of 100 mmHg and is a soft suction catheter attached?
- Is the laryngoscope available, clean and working?
- Are appropriately sized endotracheal tubes available, together with matching connectors and T pieces?
- Is the bag and mask unit there, and easily attached to an endotracheal tube connector?

- Is the thermal environment appropriate? Is the resuscitation unit heater switched on? Is the labour ward warm enough? If necessary go round and close windows and doors and turn off fans – when a sick preterm infant is expected his thermal environment takes priority over that of the obstetrician, the delivery ward staff and the parents. The room temperature should be 20°C for a full-term infant, and least 23°C if a preterm baby is expected.
- Are there some warmed dry towels to wrap the baby in during resuscitation, and bonnets for preterm babies?

Personnel

If twins, a VLBW infant or one requiring complex resuscitation, such as known hydrops or exomphalos, are anticipated, ensure that adequate staff are present: at least two neonatologists plus adequate nursing support are needed.

History

In an ideal world a paediatrician would attend all deliveries that are likely to produce an infant requiring resuscitation, having been fully briefed by the obstetrician about the mother's social, medical and obstetric history and having been introduced to the mother and her partner before delivery in order to inform them about the possible course of events. However, the reality is that in many situations much of this history has to be obtained while resuscitation is under way and the neonatologist has not had time to form a relationship with the baby's parents or to appraise himself of their views and expectations.

If possible, the following information should always be readily available for the paediatrician:

- maternal age, parity, occupation and marital status;
- father's age and occupation;
- gestational age;
- reasons for preterm delivery;
- fetal growth during this pregnancy;
- the results of any diagnostic amniocentesis or ultrasound assessment that has been carried out;
- illnesses in this pregnancy, e.g. diabetes, tuberculosis, malaria, rubella, human immunodeficiency virus (HIV);
- complications of this pregnancy, e.g. toxaemia, abruption;
- important drugs taken during this pregnancy, e.g. anticonvulsants, anticoagulants;
- previous perinatal morbidity and mortality, e.g. stillbirths, neonatal deaths or infants admitted to a NICU;
- health of the surviving infants, e.g. cerebral palsy, chromosome abnormalities or hereditary disease such as haemophilia or muscular dystrophy;
- maternal health during labour, e.g. temperature, evidence of infection;
- course of labour, e.g. induction, duration of first and second stages, indications for intervention by forceps, caesarean section, CTG changes, fetal blood gases;
- drugs administered during labour, e.g. uterine stimulants, steroids, antibiotics, opiates, tocolytics.

Initial care of the baby after delivery

Start the clock on the resuscitation trolley the moment the baby is free from the mother's body (not when the cord is clamped). As soon as the baby (usually enclosed in a wet and bloody theatre towel) is placed on the trolley, note his age (usually 30–40 seconds), and assess his heart rate, respiration, colour and tone. To check the heart rate it is essential to listen to the chest with a stethoscope: do not rely on feeling the umbilical arterial pulsation in the cord, as all you feel is your own heartbeat pounding away in your fingertips. Traditional advice has been to dry the infant as soon as you receive him, discard the wet towel and cover him with prewarmed dry towels to minimise heat loss (p. 221). Some units are reporting better thermal control is achieved when the wet (usually preterm) baby is placed directly into a freezer bag closed at the neck, into which holes are cut for access. The stethoscope is applied over the plastic bag.

The first Apgar score (p. 225) should then be awarded, at 1 minute of age. Even more important in the baby who does not breathe adequately is to begin to assess the cause of his poor transition to postnatal life by using the subscore components and the baby's reaction to the initial resuscitation (see above).

Care of the infant after the initial assessment

On the basis of the initial assessment, by 60–90 seconds of age most babies fall into one of the following five groups:

- fit, healthy, crying or breathing regularly (90–95%);
- blue and apnoeic, or not breathing too well; the pulse rate is more than 100/min; probably in primary apnoea or in the phase of gasping (5–6%);
- obvious terminal apnoea, pale, limp and apnoeic, heart rate less than 100 (0.2–0.5%);
- dead but resuscitable (less than 0.1%);
- remaining cyanosed despite vigorous and effective ventilation.

Fit and healthy

Leave this baby alone: do not suck him out, as this may damage the pharyngeal mucosa and is a powerful vagal stimulus that may trigger a reflex bradycardia. Enthusiastic sucking is based on the frequently held misconception that what is coming out of the baby's mouth is inhaled amniotic fluid. It is not: it is fetal pulmonary fluid that has been in the lungs prior to birth, and it will do no harm if it stays there a few moments longer or is swallowed. Upper airway suction is indicated if there is blood or other extraneous material. Laryngoscopy and tracheal toilet are no longer recommended for meconium aspiration if the baby is not asphyxiated and is making vigorous breathing movements as this tends to increase rather than reduce subsequent morbidity.[189]

Table 13.6 Efficacy of neonatal bag and mask systems in resuscitation[58]

System	Inflation pressure achieved (cmH$_2$O)	Expiratory volume (ml)*
Neonatal Laerdal	20.2	5.5
Paediatric Laerdal	26.9	10.4
Penlon	19.2	8.3
Ambu baby	30.3	15.4

* This volume gives a measure of the likely tidal gas exchange.

This lusty, breathing infant should be dried and wrapped in a warm blanket to minimise heat loss, his umbilical cord securely clamped or tied, given a dose of vitamin K and given to his mother, who, if she is intending to breastfeed, should be encouraged to put him to the breast. In the first hour a baby is awake and alert, and this period is very important in establishing a close attachment between mother and baby (Ch. 20). Suckling at this time is also important in establishing long-term and successful lactation (pp. 377–8). There is absolutely no need to bathe the infant immediately: it does not harm him to be covered in vernix or have some blood in his hair, whereas bathing in the labour ward can rapidly reduce a healthy baby's body temperature to less than 35°C.

Apnoeic or breathing inadequately, but with a good heart rate and tone (presumed primary apnoea)

Most of these babies respond to peripheral stimuli, such as rubbing with a warmed towel or flicking their toes (see above), or by giving oxygen by face mask. If this fails to stimulate the baby to commence breathing within 30–60 seconds,[128] basic resuscitation will be required.

Face mask resuscitation

This should be the first line of resuscitation in all babies who make a poor transition to extrauterine life. All staff involved in neonatal resuscitation should be trained to carry out face mask resuscitation effectively. It is essential to have a tight seal where the mask is applied to the baby's face; to ensure an adequate airway the baby's neck should be slightly extended with his jaw held forward (an oropharyngeal airway may help). It is a common mistake either to overextend or overflex the neck: both these manoeuvres obstruct the airway at pharyngeal and laryngeal level.

Studies have shown that a soft-rimmed mask with a small dead space, such as the Bennett or Laerdal, is the easiest to use and gives the best face seal.[127]

Positive pressure inflation can then be provided using either a bag and mask or a T piece and mask device.

Bag and mask devices
There are a variety of self inflating resuscitation bags available on the market including Laerdal and Ambu. Physiological studies

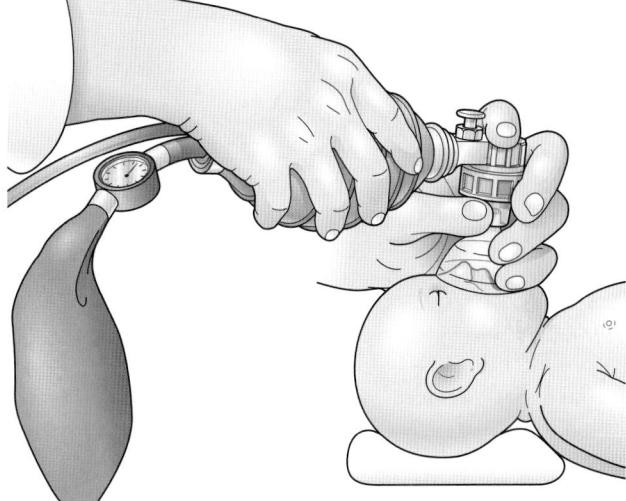

Fig. 13.5 Positive pressure ventilation using a bag and mask system. (With permission from Bossaert L L 1998 European Resuscitation Council Guidelines for Resuscitation. Elsevier, London, p. 108.)

have shown that those with bag volumes of 500 ml (Fig. 13.4) achieve the best respiratory exchange[58] (Table 13.6). Smaller bags, for instance that of the infant Laerdal device, generate too low an inflation pressure for too short an inflation time to overcome the viscosity of the airway fluid and are not suitable for neonatal resuscitation.

In routine use, connecting to 5 l/min oxygen provides 40% oxygen, rising to 60–70% if the reservoir hose is used.

The mask is held over the baby's nose and mouth with one hand, achieving an airtight seal. The bag is then squeezed between the thumb and fingers of the other hand, 30–60 times per minute (Fig. 13.5). These devices all have pressure-limited 'pop-off' valves set to limit the inflation pressure to between 20 and 30 cmH$_2$O, although higher inflation pressures can be achieved if the valve is overridden with the tip of a finger. Despite their relatively poor performance,[58] it is clear from personal experience and the literature[129] that most babies requiring active intervention respond well to bag and mask resuscitation at birth. This is because most such babies are in primary apnoea, and the bag and mask system either augments their own spontaneous respiration when it occurs, or provokes a Head's reflex and thus spontaneous lung aeration.[129]

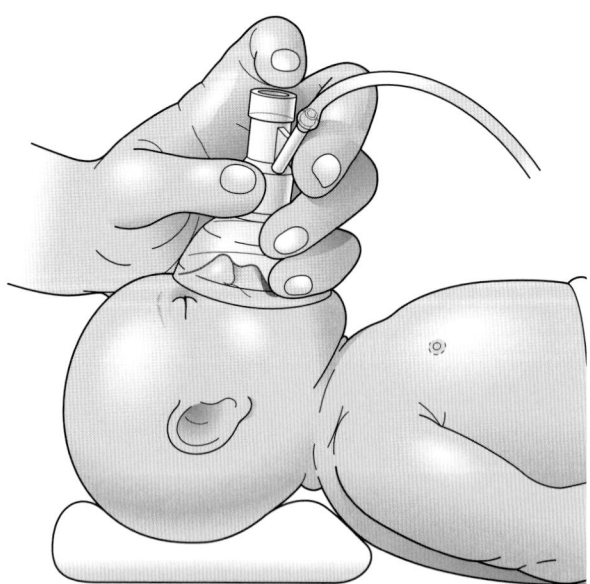

Fig. 13.6 Positive pressure ventilation via endotracheal tube and T piece. (With permission from Bossaert L L 1998 European Resuscitation Council Guidelines for Resuscitation. Elsevier, London, p. 108.)

T piece face mask devices

An alternative which is gaining popularity[6] is to attach a T piece to the face mask. One of the ports is connected to a gas supply (oxygen or air) by a tube that incorporates a pressure limiting device set to 20–30 cmH$_2$O. As already stated, medical gas or air must only ever be given to a baby if it is first passed through a suitable pressure-limiting device. A baby must never be ventilated via a T piece supplied with oxygen from a source meant for adult patients, which is at dangerously high pressure. The face mask is held in place over the baby's mouth and nose, using the thumb and middle finger, while the index finger occludes the remaining free port intermittently (Fig. 13.6). For the first inflation, the pressure is maintained for 2–3 seconds to aid lung expansion, and then at 30 breaths per minute, allowing 0.5–1 second for each subsequent inflation. These devices, which are available commercially (e.g. NeoPuff, Tom Thumb) require less skill than the bag and mask system, leave one of the operator's hands free and in a physiological study produced more effective tidal exchange.[88]

The large majority of babies will respond rapidly to mask resuscitation. A few will remain apnoeic and require intubation and IPPV (see below).

Apnoeic, pale and with heart rates of less than 100/minute (presumed terminal apnoea)

About 0.2–0.5% of all deliveries result in a baby in this poor condition, and such babies represent about 5–10% of all infants apnoeic at 2 minutes of age. Although these babies are likely to have severe asphyxia and will probably not breathe spontaneously unless resuscitated by intubation and positive-pressure

ventilation, it is worth giving face mask resuscitation for 5–10 seconds, as some will respond. If there is no response and the heart rate remains below 100/minute, advanced resuscitation must be commenced without delay. The longer intubation is delayed, the more profound the biochemical and physiological abnormalities and the greater the likelihood of permanent brain damage (Fig. 13.7).

Intubation and intermittent positive-pressure ventilation

In a recent study about one in 500 term neonates did not respond to bag and mask ventilation;[128] this is very close to the estimated incidence of babies born in terminal apnoea. For babies who do not respond to bag and mask resuscitation by 2–3 minutes of age, it is essential to progress at once to endotracheal intubation and IPPV. Intubation should be commenced earlier in those who are bradycardiac (heart rate less than 100/min despite face mask resuscitation) or who have no chest movement or air entry with a bag and mask system.

Intubation

To intubate a baby (pp. 1256–8), lay him with his head in the same plane as his body or only slightly extended; using the left hand, insert the laryngoscope into his mouth. For those who are left-handed, it is possible to buy special laryngoscopes that can be held in the right hand, but this can lead to confusion in the labour suite. With the tip of the blade in the vallecula, pull the epiglottis forward and thus reveal the vocal cords. The view of the larynx is improved if an assistant presses lightly on the cricoid cartilage. Alternatively use the fifth finger of the hand holding the laryngoscope to press down. The tip of the endotracheal tube is then advanced to enter the larynx.

Ideally a shouldered oral endotracheal tube should be used for resuscitation, as the shoulder makes it less likely that the tube will be pushed in too far. Straight endotracheal tubes are difficult to pass without the use of an introducer. If this is used inappropriately (i.e. with its tip extending beyond the end of the endotracheal tube), perforation of the pharynx, trachea or oesophagus may occur, leading to pneumomediastinum and mediastinitis.[65,176,158,48] The operator must hold the tube firmly in place with the finger and thumb of one hand.

Insert either a 3.0 or 3.5 mm internal diameter tube. The former can be inserted into all but the smallest preterm infant (<1.00 kg birthweight), and the latter should be used in full-term infants. A 2.5 mm tube has a high internal resistance[123] and is often pushed in too far (see below). These tubes should only be used if it is not possible to insert a larger one.

Laryngeal mask

Laryngeal masks provide an alternative to tracheal intubation in babies at birth.[57] These are passed blind, without the need for a laryngoscope, and so require less expertise. They are particularly useful in babies with congenital abnormalities of the upper airway, in whom visualisation of the vocal cords can be extremely difficult.[177]

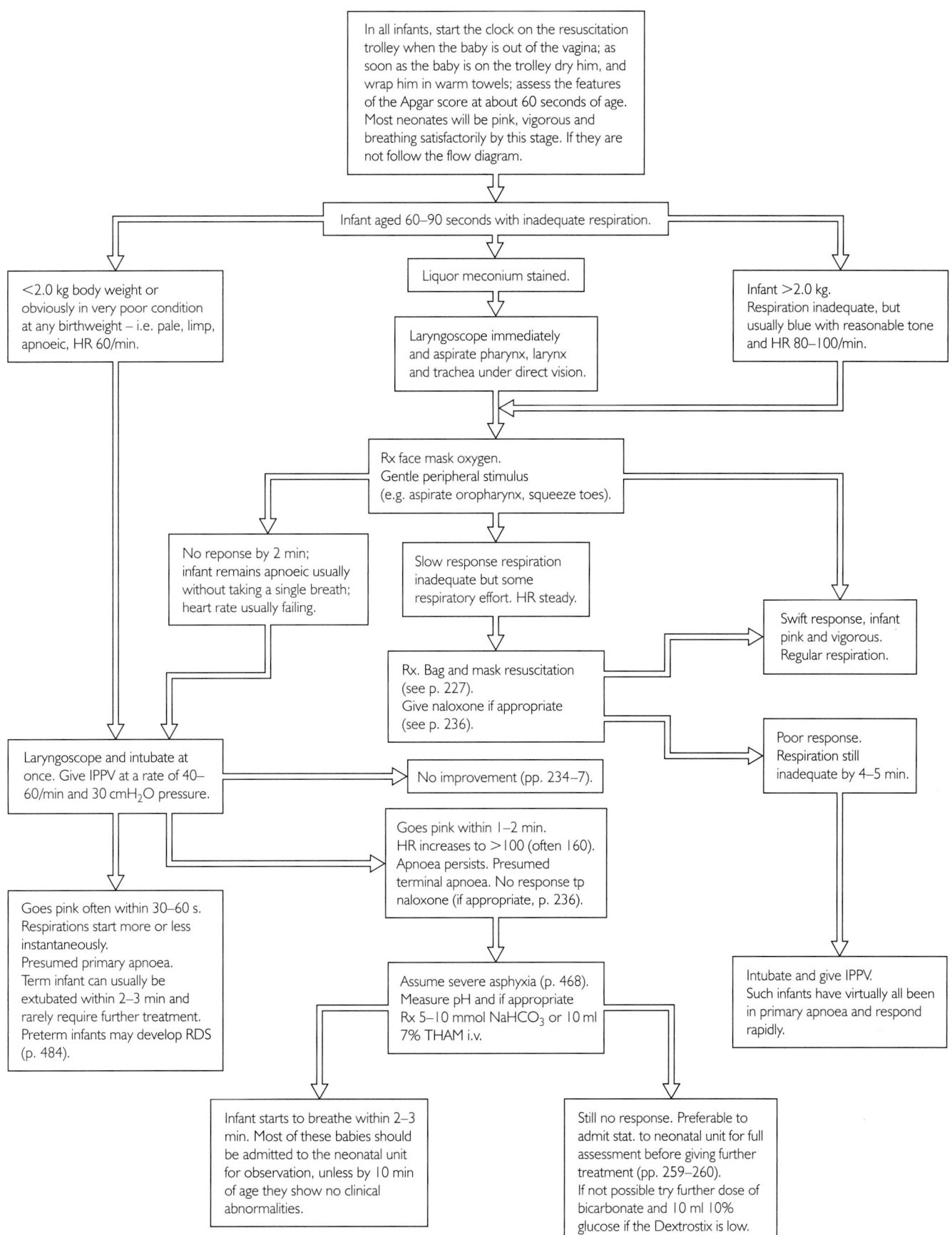

Fig. 13.7 Flow diagram for resuscitation of the newborn.

Intermittent positive pressure ventilation

Connect the tube to a bag system or to a T connector and ventilate the baby, ensuring both by observation of the chest (not the abdomen) and direct auscultation over both lung fields that the lungs are being ventilated.

Physiological studies have shown, perhaps surprisingly, that even IPPV down an endotracheal tube achieves poorer ventilation than the baby's own spontaneous respirations and rarely leads to the formation of a gaseous reservoir, the FRC, with the first few inflations[113] (Table 13.7). To achieve the optimal gas exchange, and at the same time establish an FRC, it is necessary to use a long inflation time. This is best achieved using a T connector to the ETT and occluding the expiratory limb for 2–3 seconds for the first breath (Table 13.7)[22] at an inflation pressure of 30 cmH$_2$O. Subsequently, use an inspiratory time of 1 second and ventilate at an overall rate of 30–40/min. Occasionally, in neonates with severe underlying lung disease, such as early-onset RDS, or with severe meconium aspiration or diaphragmatic hernia, higher pressures and rates may be needed, and the resuscitation trolley should be designed in such a way that these alterations can be made rapidly and safely.

Alternatively, a self inflating bag can be attached to the endotracheal tube. This has the disadvantage that it is very difficult to achieve inflation times in excess of 1 second unless the pressure-limiting valve is occluded. This device is usually used at higher rates (40–60/min).

The vast majority of infants in primary apnoea who require resuscitation by IPPV usually respond at once and will start to breathe very quickly, often gasping in response to lung inflation (Head's reflex), and then become pink. Such infants can usually be extubated within a further 2–3 minutes, rarely require further medical care and can normally be transferred from the labour ward to the postnatal ward with their mothers.

Babies in terminal apnoea will take longer to respond, usually becoming pink before commencing to make respiratory efforts. Some will remain bradycardic and require external cardiac massage and drug therapy before recovering from cyanosis.

Chest compression

Chest compression must be given to any baby who has a heart rate that remains below 60/min despite adequate positive pressure ventilation.

This must be given properly. Unfortunately many authoritative sources give the wrong advice, namely to depress the sternum with two fingers. Several studies[42,177] have shown that this is ineffective. The baby must be held as shown in Fig. 13.8, with the fingers along the thoracolumbar spine and both thumbs placed over the lower sternum.[139,39] The sternum should be firmly depressed at a rate of 120/min, with sufficient vigour to depress the sternum by 2–3 cm in a term baby, allowing one lung inflation for each three chest compressions.[99] The force required can be learned by practising during resuscitation of babies who have suffered cardiac arrest postnatally and have indwelling arterial cannulae connected to a pressure transducer. At best, chest compression achieves a blood pressure of around 20% of normal

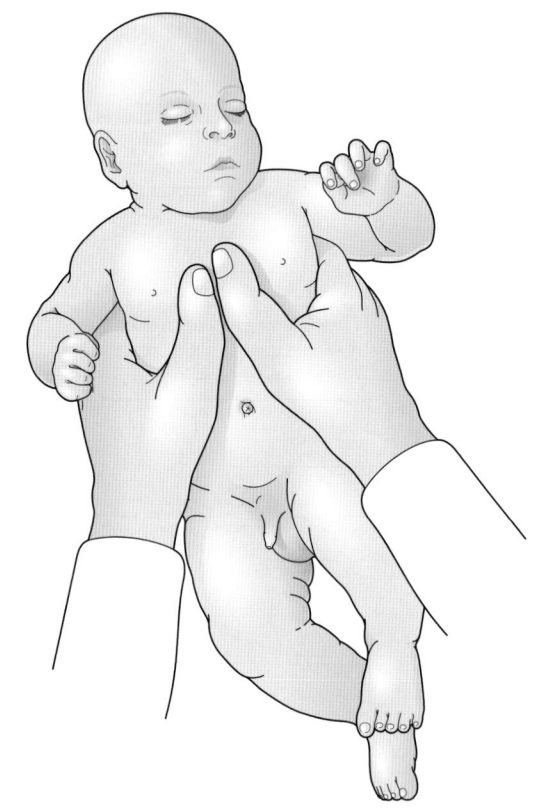

Fig. 13.8 Technique of chest compression for cardiopulmonary resuscitation.

Table 13.7 Tidal exchange and functional residual capacity established in term neonates

	Spontaneous breath	**1 s inflation of IPPV**	**2–5 s inflation of IPPV**
Inspiratory/inflation pressure (cmH$_2$O)	33 (6.1–103)	30	30
Tidal exchange (ml)	40.3 (2.7–90)	18.6 (0–62.5)	33.6 (16.9–70)
FRC (ml)	18.7 (2.7–40)	7.5 (0–15.5)	15.9 (11.7–23.2)

Tidal exchange and functional residual capacity (FRC) established in term neonates taking a first spontaneous breath, and in the first inflation of those resuscitated with a 1 s and 2–5 s inflation time down an endotracheal tube. Mean values are given with range in parentheses.[114]

and is not a substitute for an adequate circulation. Chest compression should be continued until the heart rate is in excess of 100/min or until a decision is made to discontinue resuscitation.

Further therapy

Drugs have a small and controversial role in resuscitation and will be ineffective in the absence of adequate lung ventilation.

Adrenaline (epinephrine)

This drug has a place in the resuscitation of the baby who remains bradycardic with a heart rate of less than 60/min despite a minimum of 30 seconds of ventilation and external cardiac massage,[121] although the outcome in babies in whom it is used is extremely poor.[165] Initially it can be given intratracheally.[103] The recommended initial dose is 0.01 mg/kg (0.1 ml/kg of a 1/10 000 solution). There are claims that adequate plasma levels are only achieved if much higher doses are given when the endotracheal route is used (0.25 ml 1/1000 adrenaline/kg; 250 micrograms/kg).[156] If the bradycardia persists, sodium bicarbonate should be given and then the adrenaline (epinephrine) repeated at a dose of 0.3 mg/kg (0.3 ml/kg of a 1/10 000 solution) either again down the endotracheal tube or via the vascular route used for the administration of the sodium bicarbonate. This cycle of bicarbonate/adrenaline (epinephrine) can be repeated up three times. It is however, important to stress that there have been no randomised controlled trials examining the efficacy of adrenaline (epinephrine) in the resuscitation of the asphyxiated newborn baby.[194]

Sodium bicarbonate

There is a continuing debate[82,90,121,190] about the place of intravenous bicarbonate in neonatal resuscitation. There are theoretical arguments that intravenous bicarbonate reduces the pH of the cerebrospinal fluid, that it results in a worse outcome from cardiac arrest in animals and adults, the latter often with ventricular fibrillation,[9,193] and that it induces hypercapnia.[125,190] Counter arguments can be mounted; namely that bicarbonate speeds the return of respiration,[4] increases tissue sensitivity to catecholamines[143] and in fact raises the intracellular pH of animal brains.[87,159] In practice, it can produce rapid improvement in the clinical condition of severely acidotic pale apnoeic and peripherally shut down babies.

The current recommendation is that, if a neonate has not responded to adrenaline (epinephrine), or external cardiac massage despite adequate IPPV and has persisting bradycardia, he should be given sodium bicarbonate.[99,138]

The optimal route for the administration of sodium bicarbonate is via the umbilical vein. It is dangerous to inject drugs directly into the umbilical vein, as this may:

- swill an umbilical vein clot into the systemic circulation;
- result in the drug not reaching the systemic circulation when using small-volume infusions (e.g. naloxone, adrenaline (epinephrine));
- traumatise the umbilical artery, causing haemorrhage and making subsequent arterial catheterisation difficult;

- go directly into the umbilical artery, causing spasm and ischaemia in the distribution of the iliac vessels (pp. 1242–6);
- go down a patent urachus and into the bladder.

For these reasons an umbilical venous catheter should be inserted (pp. 1246–7) and there should be appropriate provision for doing this on all resuscitation trolleys.

The recommended dose of sodium bicarbonate is 1–2 mmol/kg (2–4 ml of a 4.2% sodium bicarbonate solution), given over at least 2 minutes to reduce adverse effects from the hypertonicity of the solution. Ideally any subsequent doses should be given after arterial blood measurements of the acid–base status of the baby.

Alternatively the sodium bicarbonate and additional doses of adrenaline (epinephrine) can be given after inserting an intraosseous needle. This is both faster and easier than umbilical vein catheterisation,[52,3] although whether it is as effective is unknown. Certainly, intraosseous needles suitable for use in neonates should be immediately available in the labour suite.

Born with absent or inaudible heart beat

If the obstetrician is certain that the fetal heart was heard up to 10 minutes prior to delivery it is always worth attempting to resuscitate the fresh stillbirth, i.e. the neonate with an Apgar score of 0.

Some such infants respond very quickly and dramatically to conventional cardiopulmonary resuscitation and are vigorous and active by 5–10 minutes of age. These were either not stillbirths (i.e. had very quiet and slow heart sounds not detected by the paediatrician) or had undergone a sudden acute asphyxial stimulus that caused cardiac arrest just before delivery, without previous prolonged myocardium and brain-damaging asphyxia.

When confronted with a fresh stillbirth always send for help, as at any cardiac arrest more than one pair of expert hands is needed urgently.

Give five inflations using a face mask system and then proceed to intubation, ventilation and external cardiac massage without delay.

The baby will require either an umbilical catheter or intraosseous needle and probably at least one cycle of adrenaline (epinephrine) and bicarbonate. Oximetry and electrocardiographic monitoring are helpful in the management of these babies and if available should be commenced after the initial phase of resuscitation has been completed.

Other drugs, including atropine, calcium and analeptics, are ineffective, are no longer recommended[190] and should not be given.

If by 15 minutes of age the Apgar score is still 0, and in particular if the oximeter or electrocardiography shows persisting asystole without effective peripheral oxygenation from electrocardiographic monitoring and IPPV, then resuscitation should be withdrawn, as neurologically intact survival is no longer possible.[96] Check for signs such as skin slippage or cloudy corneas (Ch. 14) in case the CTG was artefactual and in fact the baby had died some hours earlier. For the baby who makes no respiratory effort at all by 25–30 minutes but is pink and well perfused, the outlook is also very poor. Such babies, however, should be transferred to the NICU for full evaluation, in particular to exclude non-asphyxial causes of failure to breathe, which may have genetic implications (see below).

Special situations

The infant who does not respond to intermittent positive pressure ventilation and resuscitation

Three main categories of baby behave in this way:

- the baby who clinically is assessed as asphyxiated but, despite the procedures outlined in this chapter, is still cyanosed and often bradycardic at 5–10 minutes of age;
- the baby who is vigorous and active, makes good respiratory efforts, yet fails to go pink – this strongly suggests an unasphyxiated baby with a serious malformation in his respiratory tract (Ch. 27) or cardiovascular system (Ch. 28), or persistent pulmonary hypertension with right-to-left shunting of blood through the patent foramen ovale and patent ductus arteriosus (Ch. 28);
- the baby born apnoeic or with very feeble respiratory efforts and no evidence of intrapartum complication who requires positive pressure ventilation and promptly goes pink with a good heart rate but who remains hypotonic and with inadequate or absent respiration – this strongly suggests suppression of the respiratory centre, a primary neurological or myopathic disorder, or cerebral injury in late pregnancy but before labour.

The baby who remains cyanosed and bradycardic

There are four main reasons for this state of affairs:

- there is some technical error in the resuscitation procedure;
- the baby has developed a pneumothorax;
- there is some congenital structural abnormality that prevents oxygenation;
- the infant is very ill with serious underlying lung disease (pp. 637–43).

Technical error

In babies whose external appearance is normal, by far and away the most common reason for a poor response to resuscitation is a technical error. It is therefore essential to check as quickly as possible for the following errors.

- The endotracheal tube is in the wrong place, either in the oesophagus or down one main stem bronchus, or even in some more distant part of the bronchial tree. This is very likely to occur if too small a tube is used or if the tube is not 'shouldered'. It is very easy to be misled by chest movement and breath sounds over the chest. The baby's chest may move if IPPV is applied to his stomach, and the conducted sounds of gas going in and out of the stomach may trap the unwary into thinking that it is going in and out of the lungs. Exactly the

Table 13.8 Expiratory volume achieved with first three breaths using bag and mask ventilation or endotracheal tubes

	Expiratory volume (ml)		
	Breath 1	**Breath 2**	**Breath 3**
Bag and mask	3.0	4.7	3.9
ETT and IPPV	14.3	10.5	17.0

All babies were ventilated at pressures of approximately 30 cmH$_2$O. The expiratory volume gives a close estimate of the tidal exchange.[114]

same problems can occur if only one lung or a section of it is being ventilated. If in doubt, check by auscultation that gas is not going into the abdomen and that air really does enter both sides of the chest equally. Relaryngoscope the baby to confirm that the endotracheal tube is in the larynx.

- An inadequate inflation pressure (usually set to 30 cmH$_2$O) is being applied. The blow-off valve on the resuscitation trolley may become inadvertently set at a low pressure. Inadequate inflation is particularly common when using bag and mask ventilation, particularly with the small-volume self-inflating bags (Table 13.8).
- Too small an endotracheal tube is being used – a common mistake. The 2.5 mm diameter tubes have a high internal resistance, allow a big air leak and are very easily pushed in too far, so that they lodge well down the bronchial tree. This not only results in very poor ventilation and oxygenation but carries the risk of rupturing the lobe that is being ventilated, causing a pneumothorax.
- The oxygen supply has been disconnected. If in doubt about the integrity of the oxygen supply use mouth to tube ventilation.

As soon as these errors are recognised and remedied, the infant will rapidly pink up and become vigorous and active.

Pneumothorax

This should always be considered in any infant who responds poorly to resuscitation. Of all the medical conditions compromising the response to resuscitation this is not only the easiest to treat but is also the one in which successful treatment is most likely to result in a dramatic clinical improvement. A pneumothorax can occur spontaneously or as a result of some technical error during resuscitation (see above).

The clinical clues suggesting a pneumothorax are:

- a deviated mediastinum;
- a hyperresonant hemithorax;
- a distended abdomen;
- decreased air entry;
- odd vascular changes, e.g. pale lower half and cyanosed upper half.

There is rarely time to confirm the diagnosis radiologically, but a fibreoptic light source may help (p. 488).

In an infant who is deteriorating rapidly despite other resuscitative efforts, and in whom a pneumothorax is suspected clinically, insert a wide-bore needle into the second intercostal space in the midclavicular line. If you are wrong, surprisingly little harm is done: if you are right there will be a gratifying hiss of escaping air, the infant's condition will rapidly improve, and a chest drain can then be inserted (pp. 1259–60).

Severe illness affecting response to resuscitation
Some neonatal lung diseases may prevent adequate oxygenation of the neonate during and after resuscitation: obvious diagnostic clues are usually present.

Meconium aspiration (pp. 502–8)
The history will be obvious, and an integral part of the resuscitation of such infants is efficient and meticulous bronchial toilet. These babies have often suffered intrapartum asphyxia as well and may be delivered in terminal apnoea; appropriate treatment for this is also necessary. However, if the baby remains very difficult to ventilate and oxygenate, and his lungs 'feel' stiff and there is poor pulmonary expansion, one option available is to attempt further bronchopulmonary lavage. The only other short-term available treatment is raising the oxygen concentration, inflation pressures and ventilator rate until the baby turns pink.

Congenital pneumonia (p. 1042)
Does the maternal history suggest systemic or genital infection? If it does, there is nothing that can be done in the short term other than increasing the oxygen, pressure and rate of ventilation, plus correcting acidaemia, hypoglycaemia and hypotension. In addition, the investigations and treatment appropriate for sepsis must be initiated as soon as possible.

Hypovolaemia
Excessive blood loss, for example as a result of placenta praevia or ruptured vasa praevia, will result in hypovolaemia with pallor, poor pulse volume and, if sufficiently severe, persisting bradycardia. Very occasionally, an extremely tight nuchal cord can produce the same effect.[180] Under these conditions, give 10–20 ml/kg of crystalloid intravenously or intraosseously over 10–15 minutes. Albumin is no longer recommended.[120] This can be repeated if necessary. If the hypovolaemia was obviously due to catastrophic blood loss, transfusions of O-negative blood should then be given.

Severe congenital structural abnormalities of the respiratory tract affecting ventilation
As a result of routine antenatal anomaly scanning, the large majority of these conditions will have already been identified. There will, however, be some mothers who have had no antenatal care, or have arrived just before delivery from developing countries with poor scanning facilities.

Although babies with the rare disorders listed in Table 13.9 may behave like asphyxiated babies and breathe poorly after delivery, more often and more characteristically they cry and have vigorous respiratory efforts (because they are not asphyxiated) but fail to go pink because of their underlying lung or

Table 13.9 Malformations causing persistent cyanosis or dyspnoea after delivery

Upper respiratory tract
- Choanal atresia (p. 604)
- Pierre Robin's syndrome (p. 622)
- Laryngeal and tracheal malformations
  - Atresia
  - Webs
  - Luminal tumours
  - Clefts (pp. 609–10)

Lung
- Pulmonary hypoplasia
  - Potter's syndrome (p. 940)
  - Prolonged membrane rupture (p. 198)
  - Idiopathic
- Pleural effusions with or without hydrops (pp. 516–19)
- Congenital cystic adenomatoid malformation (pp. 584–5)
- Congenital lobar emphysema (pp. 589–90)
- Pulmonary lymphangiectasia (p. 557)

Extrapulmonary
- Diaphragmatic hernia (pp. 594–603)
- Diaphragmatic eventration
- Intrathoracic space-occupying tumours
- Gross abdominal distension splinting the diaphragm
  - Tumours
  - Hepatosplenomegaly
  - Ascites
  - Dilated renal tract
- Small chest
  - Asphyxiating thoracic dystrophy
  - Thanatophoric dwarfism

airway disorder. This pattern is so characteristic that when seen it should alert the physician to seek structural malformations, of which the commonest is lung hypoplasia accompanying diaphragmatic hernia.

Initially many of the babies are not asphyxiated, but the underlying malformation results in defective oxygenation and inadequate ventilation and the infant may rapidly develop the biochemical changes of asphyxia with secondary depression of ventilation.

Infants with laryngeal and tracheal malformations are usually not resuscitable unless someone with extreme presence of mind not only recognises the problem but can also perform an emergency tracheostomy (pp. 614–16).

Infants with lung hypoplasia may have an instantly recognisable malformation such as thanatophoric dwarfism (pp. 777, 794, 926) or Potter's syndrome (p. 940), in which case active resuscitation can be withdrawn. In others, urgent transport to the NICU and X-ray is essential to establish the presence of potentially treatable conditions such as diaphragmatic hernia (pp. 594–603), pleural effusion (pp. 516–19) adenomatoid malformation (pp. 584–5), Pierre Robin's syndrome (pp. 582–4) or choanal atresia (p. 604).

Persisting apnoea with hypotonia but good cardiovascular response

This can, of course, be due to severe terminal apnoea (see above) but, if there is nothing in the maternal history to suggest this, the most likely cause is respiratory suppression from opiates given to the mother within a few hours of delivery. If this is suspected, give naloxone.

Naloxone

Naloxone is a pure antagonist of exogenous and endogenous opioids. Because of the surge of endorphins perinatally, naloxone was tried as a general treatment for apnoea at birth but this proved unsuccessful.[36] It is not without hazard, and its use in animals may increase the severity of asphyxial brain damage,[192] perhaps by causing a surge in catecholamines.[126] Care should be taken in administering naloxone to the newborn of narcotic addicts, as this may precipitate an acute withdrawal episode.[70]

Whatever the mechanism, the effects of intravenous naloxone are complex and potentially dangerous. It must therefore only be used if the mother of an apnoeic infant has received opiate analgesics in the 4–6 hours before delivery. Furthermore, it must only be given after respiration has been established, by IPPV if necessary, and the baby has become pink. Never give naloxone to an apnoeic unventilated infant, although if a baby is pink but breathing irregularly it is perfectly safe to give intramuscular naloxone while watching the baby carefully until the drug begins to work and respiration becomes regular. A dose of 0.1 mg/kg (0.25 ml/kg of the adult strength solution) should be given intramuscularly or intravenously[8] and may be repeated if necessary. Neonatal Narcan should no longer be used and should not be stocked on resuscitation trolleys.

If the diagnosis is correct, a response will be seen within a few minutes. If there is no response, other diagnoses need to be considered. These include some structural disorder of the CNS or a primary neuromuscular disease (Table 13.10).

The many, individually rare, conditions that present in this way are reviewed by Brazy et al.[26]

Meconium aspiration syndrome

The management of the condition is discussed in detail elsewhere (pp. 502–8).

As already stated (p. 221), tracheal toilet is not indicated for babies born through meconium-stained amniotic fluid who remain vigorous, as a large multicenter study has shown that this does not reduce subsequent morbidity.[189] However, if the meconium-stained baby has depressed respiration, reduced muscle tone and a heart rate of less than 100/min, tracheal suctioning should be carried out under laryngoscopic vision. Suction should be limited to 3 seconds using a wide-bore catheter or endotracheal tube. This manoeuvre can be repeated if meconium is aspirated and the heart rate remains above 60/min.[121]

Babies with congenital diaphragmatic hernias

These are also covered in detail elsewhere (pp. 594–603).

Table 13.10 Neurological causes of persisting hypoventilation and failure to respond to resuscitation

- Structural central nervous system malformations
- Severe antenatal brain damage (p.225)
- Fractured cervical spine with cord damage (p. 259)
- Dystrophia myotonica (p. 510)
- Congenital myopathies (pp. 1183–5)
- Werdnig–Hoffmann disease (p. 1182)
- Brain tumour
- Degenerative brain disorders (pp. 1169–77)
- Ondine's curse (central hypoventilation syndrome)

From Brazy J E, Kinney H C, Oakes W J 1987 Central nervous system structural lesions causing apnea at birth. Journal of Pediatrics 111: 163–175.

It is now rare for the diagnosis of diaphragmatic hernia not to be made antenatally. All except those with small defects and little pulmonary hypoplasia are likely to need intubation and IPPV. Face mask resuscitation is contraindicated as this may distend the intestinal contents within the thoracic cavity, reducing further the ability for the lungs to expand. If there is significant pulmonary hypoplasia, inflation pressures of up to 40 cmH$_2$O may be required.

Prematurity

It is well recognised that the Apgar score is often low in premature babies[34] (Fig. 13.9) and that active resuscitation is frequently required[10] (Table 13.4). The score is a poor indicator of asphyxia in this group and correlates much better with gestation.[34,72,107,135] However, Goldenberg et al[72] did show that those preterm neonates who are asphyxiated (low pH) are more likely to have a low Apgar score. It is also clear that, whatever the cause of the low Apgar score in preterm babies, the score is a good marker of the neonate who is more likely to suffer sequelae or to die.[13,14,69,109] Against this background it is interesting to note that the antenatal administration of dexamethasone to induce lung maturity (p. 341) is associated with a higher Apgar score in treated preterm babies.[68]

The decision of whether to electively intubate a VLBW infant for resuscitation in the labour ward is bound up with the controversies about the prophylactic administration of surfactant (p. 475). The much quoted study by Drew[50] who found that the mortality in babies born at less than 30 weeks gestation was reduced from 49% to 23% is not helpful, as only 3% of the 96 control babies in the selective group were intubated and resuscitated. The current recommendation is that there is no need to intubate all babies born prematurely but that if the baby fails to cry by 15 seconds or establish regular respiration by 30 seconds, face mask resuscitation should be commenced and intubation carried out if the baby has not achieved satisfactory respiratory exchange by a further 30 seconds.[53]

Apart from the risk of pneumothorax, the term infant is unlikely to suffer damage from the inflation pressures currently recommended. There are increasing anxieties that these same

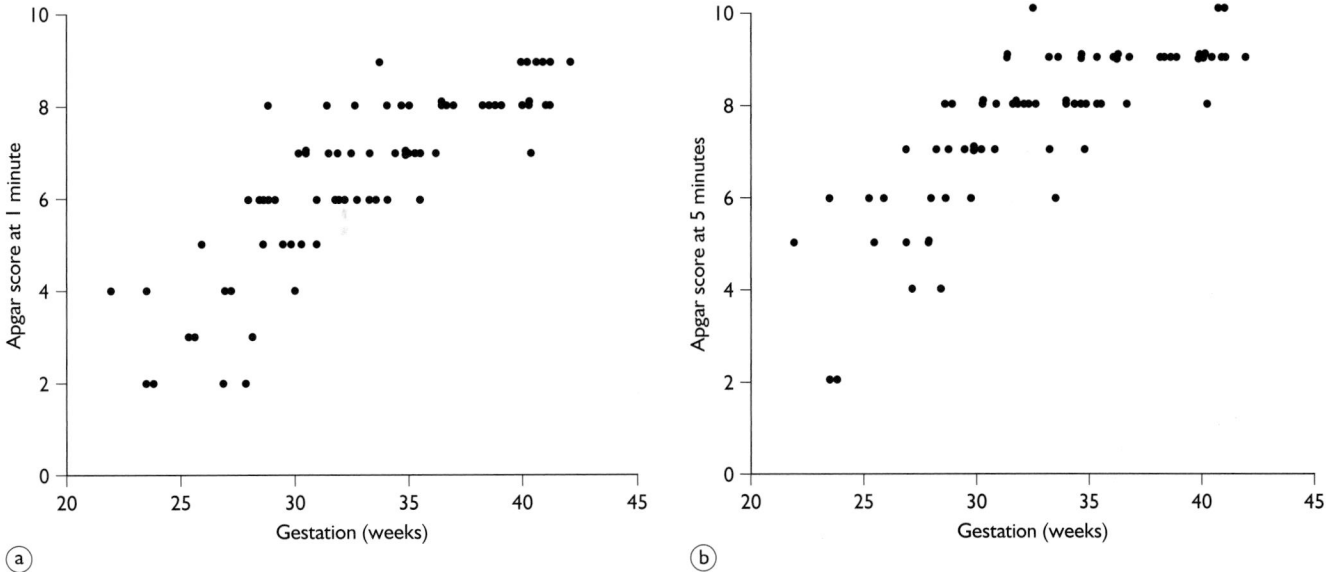

Fig. 13.9 Scattergram of 1-minute (a) and 5-minute (b) Apgar scores plotted against gestation. (With permission from Catlin E A, Carpenter M W, Brann B S et al 1986 The Apgar score revisited: influence of gestational age. Journal of Pediatrics 109: 865–868.)

pressures may cause lung damage in the very immature baby and increase the risk of chronic lung disease (pp. 554–73) so that there is doubt about how these babies should be resuscitated.

Physiological studies[89] have shown that inflation pressures of 25–30 cmH$_2$O rarely produce inflation volumes greater than twice the anatomical dead space during the initial phases of resuscitation, a minimum required for effective alveolar ventilation. However, in another study, all preterm infants who were born and required resuscitation over a period of a year were initially exposed to inflation pressures limited to 16 cmH$_2$O. This pressure could be increased if there was no apparent chest wall movement. Using this protocol, no infant received more than 32 cmH$_2$O, with a mean of 23 cmH$_2$O.[85]

Resuscitation studies on immature animals have produced worrying results. Bjorklund and colleagues[19] found that six inflations of 60 cmH$_2$O, lasting for 5 seconds each resulted in stiffer lungs over the subsequent 4 hours and worse lung histology in preterm lambs than in controls. Five sustained lung inflations of 8, 16 and 32 ml/kg produced a dose-dependent degree of lung damage, but even 8 ml resulted in reduced lung compliance compared to non-intubated controls.[18] This volume is less than the 10 ml/kg achieved on the first breath by term babies commencing to breathe spontaneously.[185] Studies on animal models have shown that the lung damage is avoided even when high inflation pressures are used if lung expansion is prevented using rubber bands[51,84,32] or plaster cast[84] around the chest wall, indicating that it is excessive volume change rather than pressure that is responsible for the lung damage – i.e. volutrauma not barotrauma.

It is not clear what inflation pressures and volumes are safe for the surfactant-deficient preterm infant. It may be that even limiting lung inflation to the minimum necessary to permit adequate gaseous exchange will result in damage in some very immature infants.

Current recommendations on resuscitation of preterm infants

Relatively low pressures (15–20 cmH$_2$O) should be used initially, and should be sustained for approximately 3 seconds but increased as necessary if there is no apparent chest wall movement.

Continuous positive airway pressure

An alternative approach, providing continuous positive airway pressure (CPAP) administered by nasal cannula at the time of delivery, has been explored in very immature infants.[105] A CPAP of 20–25 cmH$_2$O was applied for 15–20 seconds, followed by a CPAP level of 4–6 cmH$_2$O. This was associated with a reduction in the need for intubation and IPPV from 84% to 40%, compared to historical controls. There was also a significant reduction in the incidence of severe intraventricular haemorrhage, bronchopulmonary dysplasia and time spent in hospital. This approach needs further investigation.

Devices are now available (e.g. Neopuff) that permit PEEP to be provided during the phase of active resuscitation and CPAP once the infant begins to breathe spontaneously. This may be of benefit as CPAP will help in the establishment of the FRC. Failure to establish an FRC during the early stages of resuscitation has been shown to be related to more severe RDS and lower rates of survival.[179]

Resuscitating at the limit of viability

Although the results of external cardiac massage have been very poor in extremely-low-birthweight babies, Finer and colleagues[60] found that, of 13 babies born weighing less than 750 g who required cardiopulmonary resuscitation, ten survived and six of seven assessed after infancy had normal neurological outcomes, indicating that very preterm babies can be saved.

The current recommendation is that babies born at a gestation of less than 23 weeks should not be resuscitated, although there are situations in which, despite appropriate counselling, parents will pressurise the paediatrician to taking active steps[24,99] Many units will not commence resuscitation in babies born in very poor condition, with bradycardia, at 23 and 24 weeks gestation. There is, however, an ongoing debate about whether there is a place for drug therapy, including adrenaline (epinephrine) for babies born at less than 26 weeks gestation, as the outcome is so poor. If there is any doubt about the gestation of the baby, resuscitation should be commenced and advice on whether to continue should be sought from a senior colleague.

Cord blood gas analysis

In the heat of the moment in the labour ward this is usually the only other piece of information available to help diagnose the cause of a neonate's failure to breathe. It is the most satisfactory way of assessing whether or not asphyxia, rather than one of the other conditions listed in Table 13.3, is present.[175] Ideally, at all deliveries samples should be collected from both the umbilical artery and vein in a section of the cord double-clamped immediately after delivery.[97] In normal deliveries the umbilical arterial pH is lower than that of the umbilical vein (Table 13.11).[186] In the presence of cord compression the umbilical vein samples may still be normal and give a false impression of the fetal health, whereas the arterial sample, which is fetal blood, may show severe acidaemia. These blood gas data can be available within minutes and can then be extremely useful in guiding the management of the baby's subsequent resuscitation.

Other measurements

Analysing blood for biochemical indicators of asphyxia, such as lactate, hypoxanthine or creatine kinase, may be useful as a research tool in assessing the management and outcome of antepartum events but is of no value in the care of the baby in the labour ward, or in the first 60 minutes of life. An important part of the early assessment of the baby who responds slowly to

Table 13.11 Mean pH and base deficit of infants with different Apgar scores[172]

	1 min Apgar score								
	1	2	3	4	5	6	7	8	9
No. of infants	5	12	17	11	22	30	62	147	589
Mean pH	7.17	7.12	7.10	7.22	7.18	7.17	7.19	7.20	7.21
SD	0.5	0.13	0.13	0.10	0.08	0.09	0.08	0.07	0.08
Mean BD	10.6	11.8	11.5	7.8	9.6	10.6	8.8	8.4	7.9
SD	4.0	5.9	6.3	5.5	4.3	3.2	4.1	3.7	3.6

BD = base deficit (mEq/l); SD = standard deviation.

resuscitation is to measure his blood glucose (p. 1302) and blood pressure (pp. 1293–4).

Continuing therapy following resuscitation

The infant who has established regular respiration

Unless an infant assessed as being in terminal apnoea responds very rapidly to resuscitation and is pink, vigorous and neurologically normal by 8–10 minutes of age, he should be admitted to the NICU. On admission, as well as carefully examining him and measuring his blood pressure, his packed cell volume, blood glucose and blood gases should be measured. A chest X-ray is indicated if there is any evidence of cardiorespiratory distress. In most term babies these investigations are usually normal, no further treatment is required and, apart from looking slightly wide-eyed and overalert for a few hours (i.e. grade I HIE p. 1136), they make a very rapid recovery. Hypoglycaemia (glucose <1.5 mmol/l) should always be corrected but base deficits of 10–20 mmol/l usually correct spontaneously and rapidly[169] and there is no need to give otherwise asymptomatic acidaemic term babies intravenous bicarbonate or tris-hydroxymethylaminomethane (THAM).

These babies can usually be transferred to their mothers on the postnatal ward by 24–36 hours of age.

If a preterm infant suffers this degree of asphyxia he will almost certainly develop RDS and his subsequent management is described fully on pages 479–84. The treatment of the minority of term babies who develop grade I–III hypoxic ischaemic encephalopathy with multiorgan involvement is described on page 1136.

The infant who does not start to breathe

If an infant has become pink with a good cardiac output, yet by 20 minutes of age has made no spontaneous respiratory effort despite adequate oxygenation and appropriate treatment with bicarbonate, glucose and naloxone, further therapy should be delayed until further blood gas analysis, blood glucose measurements and a chest X-ray have been carried out. If these show some persisting abnormality, appropriate therapy can be given, but if they are normal yet apnoea persists this is very suggestive of either profound neurological problems, with a grave prognosis, or, particularly if the evidence for asphyxia is minimal, some underlying neurological disorder (see below).

Despite controlling blood gases and biochemistry and achieving satisfactory cardiac, pulmonary and renal function, the occasional baby who has suffered from severe asphyxia may develop severe intractable cerebral oedema and may never establish spontaneous respiration. The prognosis for such babies is grim.[96,170] After making absolutely sure that the apnoea does not represent drug depression or an inherited neurological defect, and after discussion with the parents, it is appropriate to discontinue life-support procedures in a way and at a time that allows the parents to be with and to hold their baby.

References

1. Aarnoudse M D, Huisjes H J, Gordon H, Oeseburg B, Zijlstra W G 1985 Fetal subcutaneous scalp PO_2 and abnormal heart rate during labour. American Journal of Obstetrics and Gynecology 153: 565–566

2. Abboud T K 1988 Maternal and fetal endorphins: effects of pregnancy and labour. Archives of Disease in Childhood 63: 707–709

3. Abe K K, Blum G T, Yamamoto L G 2000 Intraosseous is faster and easier than umbilical venous catheterization in newborn emergency vascular access models. American Journal of Emergency Medicine 18: 126–129

4. Adamsons K, Behrman R, Dawes G S, James L S, Koford C 1964 Resuscitation by positive pressure ventilation and tris-hydroxymethylaminomethane of Rhesus monkeys asphyxiated at birth. Journal of Pediatrics 65: 807–818

5. Aldrich C J, D'Antona D, Wyatt J S et al 1994 Fetal cerebral oxygenation measured by near-infra red spectroscopy shortly before birth and acid base status at birth. Obstetrics and Gynecology 84: 861–866

6. Allwood A C, Madar R J, Baumer J H, Readdy L, Wright D 2003 Changes in resuscitation practice at birth. Archives of Disease in Childhood Fetal and Neonatal Edition 88: F375–F379

7. Amatayakul O, Cumming G R, Haworth J C 1970 Association of hypoglycaemia with cardiac enlargement and heart failure in newborn infants. Archives of Disease in Childhood 45: 717–720

8. American Academy of Pediatrics 1990 Naloxone dosage and route of administration for infants and children: addendum to emergency procedures for infants and children. Pediatrics 86: 484–485

9. Arieff A I, Leach W, Park R, Lazarowitz V C 1982 Systemic effects of $NaHCO_3$ in experimental lactic acidosis in dogs. American Journal of Physiology 242: F586–591

10. Ayoubi J M, Audibert F, Boithias C et al 2002 Perinatal factors affecting survival and survival without disability of extreme premature infants at two years of age. European Journal of Obstetrics, Gynecology, and Reproductive Biology 105: 124–131

11. Badawi N, Kurinczuk J J, Keogh J M et al 1998 Intrapartum risk factors for newborn encephalopathy: the Western Australia case control study. British Medical Journal 317: 1554–1558

12. Beard R W, Morris E D 1965 Foetal and maternal acid base balance during normal labour. Journal of Obstetrics and Gynaecology of the British Commonwealth 72: 496–503

13. Beeby P J, Elliott E J, Henderson-Smart D et al 1994 Predictive value of umbilical artery pH in preterm infants. Archives of Disease in Childhood 71: F93–F96

14. Behnke M, Carter R L, Hardt N S, Eyler F D, Cruz A C, Resnick M B 1987 The relationship of Apgar scores, gestational age and birthweight to survival of low birthweight infants. American Journal of Perinatology 4: 121–124

15. Beierholm E A, Grantham N, O'Keefe D D, Laver M B, Daggett W M 1975 Effects of acid – base changes, hypoxia and catecholamines on ventricular performance. American Journal of Physiology 228: 1555–1561

16. Berseth C L, McCoy H H 1992 Birth asphyxia alters neonatal intestinal mobility in term neonates. Pediatrics 90: 669–673

17. Bird J A, Spencer J A D, Mould T, Symonds M E 1996 Endocrine and metabolic adaptation following caesarean section or vaginal delivery. Archives of Disease in Childhood 74: F132–F134

18. Bjorklund L J, Curstedt T, Ingimarsson J 1996 Lung injury caused by neonatal resuscitation of immature lambs – relation to volume of lung inflation. Pediatric Research 39: 362A

19. Bjorklund L J, Ingimarsson J, Curstedt T et al 1997 Manual ventilation with a few large breaths at birth compromises the therapeutic effect of subsequent surfactant replacement in immature lambs. Pediatric Research 42: 348–355

20. Block B S, Schlafer D H, Wentworth R A, Kreitzer L A, Nathanielsz P W 1990 Intrauterine asphyxia and the breakdown of the physiologic circulatory compensation in fetal sheep. American Journal of Obstetrics and Gynecology 162: 1325–1331

21. Bocking A D, Gagnon R, White S E, Homan J, Milne K M, Richardson B S 1988 Circulatory responses to prolonged hypoxemia in fetal sheep. American Journal of Obstetrics and Gynecology 159: 1418–1424

22. Boon A W, Milner A D, Hopkin I E 1979 Lung expansion, tidal exchange and formation of the functional residual capacity during resuscitation of asphyxiated neonates. Journal of Pediatrics 95: 1031–1036

23. Boucher M, Yonekura M L 1986 Perinatal listeriosis (early onset): correlation of antenatal manifestations and neonatal outcome. Obstetrics and Gynecology 68: 593–597

24. Boyle R J, McIntosh N 2001 Ethical considerations in neonatal resuscitation: clinical and research issues. Seminars in Neonatology 6: 261–269

25. Brann A W, Myers R E 1975 Central nervous system findings in the newborn monkey following severe in utero partial asphyxia. Neurology 25: 327–330

26. Brazy J E, Kinney H C, Oakes W J 1987 Central nervous system structural lesions causing apnea at birth. Journal of Pediatrics 111: 163–175

27. Brimacombe J, Gandini D 1995 Resuscitation of neonates with the laryngeal mask airway. A caution. Pediatrics 95: 453–454

28. Burnard E D, James L S 1961 Failure of the heart after undue asphyxia at birth. Pediatrics 28: 545–565

29. Cabal L A, Devaskar U, Siassi B, Hodgman J E, Emmanouilides G 1980 Cardiogenic shock associated with perinatal asphyxia in term infants. Journal of Pediatrics 96: 705–710

30. Campbell A G M, Milligan J E, Talner J S 1968 The effect of pretreatment with phenobarbital, meperidine or hyperbaric oxygen on the response to anoxia and resuscitation in newborn rabbits. Journal of Pediatrics 72: 518–527

31. Campbell N, Harvey D R, Norman A P 1975 Increased frequency of neonatal jaundice in a maternity hospital. British Medical Journal 2: 548–552

32. Carlton D P, Cummings J J, Scheerer R G, Poulain F R, Bland R D 1990 Lung overexpansion increases pulmonary microvascular protein permeability in young lambs. Journal of Applied Physiology 69: 577–583

33. Carter B S, Haverkamp A D, Merenstein G B 1993 The definition of acute perinatal asphyxia. Clinics in Perinatology 20: 287–304

34. Catlin E A, Carpenter M W, Brann B S et al 1986 The Apgar score revisited: influence of gestational age. Journal of Pediatrics 109: 865–868

35. Chamberlain R, Chamberlain G, Howlett B, Claireaux A 1975 British births 1970, vol. I. The first week of life. Heinemann, London, ch 4

36. Chernick V, Manfreda J, DeBooy V, Davi M, Rigatto H, Seshia M 1988 Clinical trial of naloxone in birth asphyxia. Journal of Pediatrics 113: 519–525

37. Chessells J M, Wigglesworth J S 1971 Coagulation studies in severe birth asphyxia. Archives of Disease in Childhood 46: 253–256

38. Clapp J F III, Peress N S, Wesley M, Mann L I 1988 Brain damage after intermittent partial cord occlusion in the chronically instrumented fetal lamb. American Journal of Obstetrics and Gynecology 159: 504–509

39. Clements F, McGowan J 2000 Finger position for chest compressions in cardiac arrest in infants. Resuscitation 44: 43–46

40. Craft W H, Underwood L E, Van Wyk J J 1980 High incidence of perinatal insult in children with idiopathic hypopituitarism. Journal of Pediatrics 96: 397–402

41. Cyr R M, Usher R H, McLean F H 1984 Changing patterns of birth asphyxia and trauma over 20 years. American Journal of Obstetrics and Gynecology 148: 490–498

42. David R 1988 Closed chest cardiac massage in the newborn infant. Pediatrics 81: 552–554

43. Davis J A, Stafford A 1964 Respiratory distress in newborn rabbits. Biologia Neonatorum 7: 129–140

44. Dawes G S 1968 Fetal and neonatal physiology. Year Book, Chicago, pp 141–159

45. Dawes G S, Hibbard E, Windle W F 1964 The effect of alkali and glucose infusion on permanent brain damage in rhesus monkeys asphyxiated at birth. Journal of Pediatrics 65: 801–806

46. Dawes G S, Jacobson H N, Mott J C, Shelley H J, Stafford A 1963 Treatment of asphyxia in newborn lambs and monkeys. Journal of Physiology 169: 167–184

47. Dawes G S, Mott J C 1962 The vascular tone of the foetal lung. Journal of Physiology 164: 465–477

48. Devine S T, Rosenberg H K, Kumar L S, Bhandari V 2002 Esophageal perforation in the premature newborn: case report and review of the literature. Connecticut Medicine 66: 131–135

49. Downing S E, Talner N S, Gardner T H 1966 Influences of hypoxemia and acidemia on left ventricular function. American Journal of Physiology 210: 1327–1334

50. Drew J H 1982 Immediate intubation at birth of the very-low-birth-weight infant. American Journal of Diseases of Children 136: 207–210

51. Dreyfuss D, Soler P, Basset G, Saumon G 1988 High inflation pressure pulmonary edema. Respective effects of high airway pressure, high tidal volume, and positive end-expiratory pressure. American Review of Respiratory Disease 137: 1159–1164

52. Ellemunter H, Simma B, Trawoger R, Maurer H 1999 Intraosseous lines in preterm and full term neonates. Archives of Disease in Childhood Fetal and Neonatal Edition 80: F74–F75

53. European Resuscitation Council 2000 Part II: Neonatal resuscitation. Resuscitation 46: 401–416

54. Fedrick J, Butler N R 1971 Certain causes of neonatal death. iv. Massive pulmonary haemorrhage. Biology of the Neonate 18: 243–262

55. Felix J F, Badawi N, Kurinczuk J, Bower C, Keogh J M, Pemberton P J 2000 Birth defects in children with newborn encephalopathy. Developmental Medicine and Child Neurology 42: 803–808

56. Fernandez, F, Verdu A, Queso J, Perez-Higueras A 1987 Serum CPK-BB Isoenzyme in the assessment of brain damage in asphyctic term infants. Acta Paediatrica Scandinavica 76: 914–918

57. Fernandez-Jurado M I, Fernandez-Baena M 2002 Use of laryngeal mask airway for prolonged ventilatory support in a preterm newborn. Paediatric Anaesthesia 12: 369–370

58. Field D, Milner A D, Hopkin I E 1986 Efficacy of manual resuscitation at birth. Archives of Disease in Childhood 61: 300–302

59. Finer N N, Robertson C M, Richards R T et al 1981 Hypoxic ischaemic encephalopathy in term neonates. Perinatal factors and outcome. Journal of Pediatrics 98: 112–117

60. Finer N N, Tarin T, Vaucher Y E, Barrington K, Bejar R 1999 Intact survival in extremely low birth weight infants after delivery room resuscitation. Pediatrics 104: e40

61. Fisher D J, Heyman M A, Rudolph A M 1981 Myocardial consumption of oxygen and carbohydrates in newborn sheep. Pediatric Research 15: 843–846

62. Freeman J M, Nelson K B 1988 Intrapartum asphyxia and cerebral palsy. Pediatrics 82: 240–249

63. Friedman E A, Sachtleben M R 1976 Neonatal jaundice in association with oxytocin stimulation of labour and operative delivery. British Medical Journal 1: 198–199

64. Gaffney G, Squier M V, Johnson A et al 1994 Clinical associations of prenatal ischaemic white matter injury. Archives of Disease in Childhood 70: F101–F106

65. Galvis A G, Kelley C F 1979 Hypopharynx perforation during infant's resuscitation. Journal of the American Medical Association 242: 1526–1527

66. Gandini D, Brimacombe J 2003 Laryngeal mask airway for ventilatory support over a 4-day period in a neonate with Pierre Robin sequence. Paediatric Anaesthesia 13: 181–182

67. Gandy G M, Jacobson W, Gairdner D 1970 Hyaline membrane disease. I. Cellular changes. Archives of Disease in Childhood 45: 289–295

68. Gardner M O, Goldenberg R L, Gaudier F L et al 1995 Predicting low Apgar scores of infants weighing less than 1000 grams: the effect of corticosteroids. Obstetrics and Gynecology 85: 170–174

69. Gaudier F L, Goldenberg R L, Nelson K. G et al 1996 Infant's acid–base status at birth and Apgar scores on survival in 500–1000 g infants. Obstetrics and Gynecology 87: 175–180

70. Gibbs J, Newson T, Williams J, Davidson D C 1989 Naloxone hazard in infants of opioid abusers. Lancet 2: 159–160

71. Goldberg R N, Cabal L A, Sinatra F R, Plajstek C E, Hodgman J E 1979 Hyperammonemia associated with perinatal asphyxia. Pediatrics 64: 336–341

72. Goldenberg R L, Huddleston J F, Nelson K G 1984 Apgar scores and umbilical pH in preterm newborn infants. American Journal of Obstetrics and Gynecology 149: 651–654

73. Gonzalez F, Juliano S 2002 Is pediatric attendance necessary for all cesarean sections? Journal of the American Osteopathic Association 102: 127–129

74. Govaert P 1993 Cranial haemorrhage in the term newborn infant. Cambridge University Press, Cambridge, pp 52–57

75. Gray L C, Grant H W 1984 Should a paediatrician be present at non-rotational forceps deliveries? British Journal of Obstetrics and Gynaecology 91: 899–900

76. Greenough A, Lagercranz H, Pool J, Dahlin I 1987 Plasma catecholamine levels in preterm infants. Acta Paediatrica Scandinavica 76: 54–59

77. Gupta J M, Tizard J P M 1967 The sequence of events in neonatal apnoea. Lancet 2: 55–59

78. Gutberlet R L, Cornblath M 1976 Neonatal hypoglycemia revisited 1975. Pediatrics 58: 10–17

79. Hackett G A, Campbell S, Gamsu H, Cohen-Overbeek T, Pearce J M F 1987 Doppler studies in the growth retarded fetus and prediction of neonatal necrotising enterocolitis, haemorrhage and neonatal morbidity. British Medical Journal 294: 13–16

80. Hambleton G, Appleyard W J 1973 Controlled trial of fresh frozen plasma in asphyxiated low birthweight infants. Archives of Disease in Childhood 48: 31–35

81. Hazinski T A, Grunstein M M, Schlueter M A, Tooley W H 1981 Effect of naloxone on ventilation in newborn rabbits. Journal of Applied Physiology 50: 713–717

82. Hein H A 1993 The use of sodium bicarbonate in neonatal resuscitation: help or harm. Pediatrics 91: 496–497

83. Hermansen M C, Prior M M 1993. Oxygen concentrations from self inflating resuscitation bags. American Journal of Perinatology 10: 79–80

84. Hernandez L A, Peevy K J, Moise A A, Parker J C 1989 Chest wall restriction limits high airway pressure-induced lung injury in young rabbits. Journal of Applied Physiology 66: 2364–2368

85. Hird M F, Greenough A, Gamsu H R 1991 Inflating pressures for effective resuscitation of preterm infants. Early Human Development 26: 69–72

86. Holden K R, Mellits E D, Freeman J M 1982 Neonatal seizures. 1. Correlation of prenatal and perinatal events with outcomes. Pediatrics 70: 165–176

87. Hope P L, Cady E B, Delpy D T et al 1988 Brain metabolism and intracellular pH during ischaemia: effects of systemic glucose and bicarbonate administration studied by ^{31}P and ^{1}H nuclear magnetic resonance spectroscopy in vivo in the lamb. Journal of Neurochemistry 50: 1394–1402

88. Hoskyns E W, Milner A D, Hopkin I E 1987 A simple method of face mask resuscitation at birth. Archives of Disease in Childhood 62: 376–378

89. Hoskyns E W, Milner A D, Boon A W, Vyas H, Hopkin I E 1987 Endotracheal resuscitation of preterm infants at birth. Archives of Disease in Childhood 62: 663–666

90. Howell J H 1987 Sodium bicarbonate in the perinatal setting revisited. Clinics in Perinatology 14: 807–816

91. Hull J, Dodd K L 1992 Falling incidence of hypoxic ischaemic encephalopathy in term infants. British Journal of Obstetrics and Gynaecology 99: 386–391

92. Ikegami M, Jacobs H, Jobe A 1983 Surfactant function in respiratory distress syndrome. Journal of Pediatrics 102: 443–447

93. Ikonomidou C, Qin Y, Labruyere J, Kirby C, Olney J W 1996 Prevention of trauma induced degeneration in infant rat-brain. Pediatric Research 39: 1020–1027

94. Information and Statistical Division, SHCSA 1992 Hospital and Health Board Comparisons in Obstetrics: 57

95. Isozaki-Fukuda Y, Kojima T, Hirata Y et al 1991 Plasma immunoreactive endothelin 1 concentration in human fetal blood: its relation to asphyxia. Pediatric Research 30: 244–247

96. Jain L, Ferre C, Vidyasagar D et al 1991 Cardiopulmonary resuscitation of apparently stillborn infants: survival and long term outcome. Journal of Pediatrics 118: 778–782

97. Johnson J W C, Ricards D S, Wagaman R A 1990 The case for routine umbilical acid–base studies at delivery. American Journal of Obstetrics and Gynecology 162: 621–625

98. Kattwinkel J, Niermeyer S, Nadkarni V et al 1999 Resuscitation of the newly born infant: an advisory statement from the Pediatric Working Group of the International Liaison Committee on Resuscitation. Resuscitation 40: 71–88

99. Kattwinkel J, Niermeyer S, Nadkarni V et al 2001 An advisory statement from the Pediatric Working Group of the International Liaison Committee on Resuscitation. Middle East Journal of Anesthesiology 16: 315–351

100. Khare S K 1977 Neurohypophyseal dysfunction following perinatal asphyxia. Journal of Pediatrics 90: 628–629

101. Kojima T, Kobayashi T, Matsuzaki S, Iwase S, Kobayashi Y 1985 Effects of perinatal asphyxia and myoglobinuria on development of acute neonatal renal failure. Archives of Disease in Childhood 60: 908–912

102. Levinson G, Shnider S M, Delorimier A A, Steffenson J L 1974 Effects of maternal hyperventilation on uterine blood flow and fetal oxygenation and acid base status. Anesthesiology 40:340–347

103. Lindemann R 1984 Resuscitation of the newborn: endotracheal administration of adrenaline. Acta Paediatrica Scandinavica 73: 210–212

104. Linderkamp O, Versmold H T, Fendel H, Riegel K P, Betke K 1978 Association of neonatal respiratory distress with birth asphyxia and deficiency of red cell mass in premature infants. European Journal of Pediatrics 129: 167–173

105. Lindner W, Vossbeck S, Hummler H, Pohlandt F 1999 Delivery room management of extremely low birth weight infants: spontaneous breathing or intubation? Pediatrics 103: 961–967

106. Low J A, Panagiotopoulos C, Derrick E J 1995 Newborn complications after intrapartum asphyxia with metabolic acidosis in the preterm fetus. American Journal of Obstetrics and Gynecology 172: 805–810

107. Luthy D A, Shy K K, Strickland D et al 1987 State of infants at birth and risk for adverse neonatal events and long term sequelae. A study in low birthweight infants. American Journal of Obstetrics and Gynecology 157: 676–679

108. Maberry M C, Ramin S M, Gilstrap L C, Leveno K L, Dax J S 1990 Intrapartum asphyxia in pregnancies complicated by intra-amniotic infection. Obstetrics and Gynecology 76: 351–354

109. McDonald H M, Mulligan J C, Allen A C, Taylor P M 1980 Neonatal asphyxia. I. Relationship of obstetric and neonatal complications to neonatal mortality in 38 405 consecutive deliveries. Journal of Pediatrics 96: 898–902

110. MacKinnon J A, Perlman M, Kirpalani H et al 1993 Spinal cord injury at birth. Diagnostic and prognostic data in 22 patients. Journal of Pediatrics 122: 431–437

111. Mallard E C, Gunn A J, Williams C E et al 1992 Transient umbilical cord occlusion causes hippocampal damage in the fetal sheep. American Journal of Obstetrics and Gynecology 167: 1423–1430

112. Merritt T A, Farrell P M 1976 Diminished pulmonary lecithin synthesis in acidosis. Experimental findings as related to the respiratory distress syndrome. Pediatrics 57: 32–40

113. Milner A D, Vyas M 1985 Resuscitation of the newborn. In: Milner A D, Martin R J (eds) Neonatal and pediatric respiratory medicine. Butterworth, London, p 16

114. Milner A D, Vyas H, Hopkin I E 1984 Efficacy of face mask resuscitation at birth. British Medical Journal 289: 1563–1565

115. Miltényi M, Pohlandt F, Boka G, Kun E 1981 Tubular proteinuria after perinatal hypoxia. Acta Paediatrica Scandinavica 70: 399–403

116. Motoyama E K, Rivard G, Acheson F, Cook C D 1966 Adverse effects of maternal hyperventilation on the fetus. Lancet 2: 286–288

117. Mott J C 1975 The place of the renin-angiotensin system before and after birth. British Medical Bulletin 31: 44–50

118. Moya F, Morishima H O, Schnider S M, James L S 1965 Influence of maternal hyperventilation on the newborn infant. American Journal of Obstetrics and Gynecology 91: 76–84

119. Myers R E 1972 Two patterns of perinatal brain damage and their conditions of occurrence. American Journal of Obstetrics and Gynecology 112: 246–276

120. Niermeyer S, Kattwinkel J, Van Reempts P et al 2000 International Guidelines for Neonatal Resuscitation: an excerpt from the Guidelines 2000 for Cardiopulmonary Resuscitation and Emergency Cardiovascular Care: International Consensus on Science. Contributors and Reviewers for the Neonatal Resuscitation Guidelines. Pediatrics 106: e29

121. Niermeyer S, Van Reempts P, Kattwinkel J et al 2001 Resuscitation of newborns. Annals of Emergency Medicine 37(4 Suppl): S110–S125

122. Nijhuis J G, Kruyt N, Van Wijck J A M 1988 Fetal brain death. Two case reports. British Journal of Obstetrics and Gynaecology 95: 197–200

123. Oca M J, Becker M A, Dechert R E, Donn S M et al 2002 Relationship of neonatal endotracheal tube size and airway resistance. Respiratory Care 47: 994–997

124. Oh W, Omori K, Emmanouilides G, Phelps D L 1975 Placenta to lamb fetus transfusion in utero during acute hypoxia. American Journal of Obstetrics and Gynecology 122: 316–322

125. Ostrea E M, O'Dell G B 1972 The influence of bicarbonate administration on blood pH in a closed system: clinical implications. Journal of Pediatrics 80: 671–680

126. Padbury J F, Agata Y, Polk D H, Wang D L, Callegari C C 1987 Neonatal adaptation: naloxone increases the catecholamine surge at birth. Pediatric Research 21: 590–593

127. Palme C, Nystrom B, Tunell R 1985 An evaluation of the efficiency of face masks in the resuscitation of newborn infants. Lancet 2: 207–210

128. Palme-Kilander C 1992 Methods of resuscitation in low Apgar score newborn infants – a national survey. Acta Paediatrica 81: 739–744

129. Palme-Kilander C, Tunell R 1993 Pulmonary gas exchange during face mask ventilation immediately after birth. Archives of Disease in Childhood 68: 11–16

130. Paneth N, Stark R I 1983 Cerebral palsy and mental retardation in relation to indicators of perinatal asphyxia. American Journal of Obstetrics and Gynecology 147: 960–966

131. Paterson P J, Dunstan M K, Trickey N R A, Beard R W 1970 A biochemical comparison of the mature and post-mature fetus and newborn infant. Journal of Obstetrics and Gynaecology of the British Commonwealth 77: 390–397

132. Patriarco M S, Viechnicki B M, Hutchinson T A, Klasko S K, Yeh S-Y 1987 A study on intrauterine fetal resuscitation with terbutaline. American Journal of Obstetrics and Gynecology 157: 384–387

133. Peebles D M, Spencer J A D, Edwards A D et al 1994 Relation between frequency of uterine contractions and human fetal cerebral oxygen saturation studied during labour by near infrared spectroscopy. British Journal of Obstetrics and Gynaecology 101: 44–48

134. Peevy K J, Chalhub E G 1983 Occult group B streptococcal infection: an important cause of intrauterine asphyxia. American Journal of Obstetrics and Gynecology 146: 989–990

135. Perkins R P, Papile L A 1985 The very low birthweight infant: incidence and significance of low Apgar scores, 'asphyxia' and morbidity. American Journal of Perinatology 2: 108–113

136. Perlman J M, Risser R M 1996 Can asphyxiated infants at risk for neonatal seizures be rapidly identified by current high risk markers. Pediatrics 97: 456–462

137. Perlman J M, Tack E D 1988 Renal injury in the asphyxiated newborn infant: relationship to neurologic outcome. Journal of Pediatrics 113: 875–879

138. Phillips B, Zideman D, Wyllie J, Richmond S, van Reempts P; European Resuscitation Council 2001 European Resuscitation Council Guidelines 2000 for newly born life support. A statement from the Paediatric Life Support Working Group and approved by the Executive Committee of the European Resuscitation Council. Resuscitation 48: 235–239

139. Phillips G W L, Zideman D A 1986 Relation of infant heart to sternum: its significance in cardiopulmonary resuscitation. Lancet 2: 1024–1025

140. Pietz J, Guttenberg N, Gluck L 1988 Hypoxanthine: a marker of asphyxia. Obstetrics and Gynecology 72: 762–766

141. Pohjavuori M 1983 Obstetric determinants of plasma vasopressin concentrations and renin activity at birth. Journal of Pediatrics 103: 966–968

142. Press S, Tellechea C, Pregen S 1985 Caesarean delivery of full term infants: identification of those at high risk for requiring resuscitation. Journal of Pediatrics 106: 477–479

143. Preziosi M P, Roig J C, Hargrove N et al 1993 Metabolic acidaemia with hypoxia attenuates the haemodynamic responses to epinephrine during resuscitation in lambs. Critical Care Medicine 21: 1901–1907

144. Primhak R A, Herber S M, Whincup G, Milner R D G 1984 Which deliveries require paediatricians in attendance? British Medical Journal 289: 16–18

145. Procianoy R S, Cecin S K G 1985 The influence of labour and delivery on preterm fetal and renal function. Acta Paediatrica Scandinavica 74: 400–404

146. Puolakka J, Kauppila A, Tuimala R, Jouppila R, Vuori J 1983 The effect of parturition on umbilical blood plasma levels of norepinephrine. Obstetrics and Gynecology 61: 19–21

147. Ramji S, Ahuja S, Thirupuram S, Rootwelt T, Rooth G, Saugstad O D 1993 Resuscitation of asphyxic newborn infants with room air or 100% oxygen. Pediatric Research 34: 809–812

148. Richardson B S 1989 Fetal adaptive responses to asphyxia. Clinics in Perinatology 16: 595–611

149. Rootwelt T, Loberg E M, Moen A, Oyasaeter S, Saugstad O D 1992 Hypoxemia and reoxygenation with 21% or 100% oxygen in newborn pigs: changes in blood pressure, base deficit, and hypoxanthine and brain morphology. Pediatric Research 32: 107–113

150. Ryder R W, Shelton J D, Guinan M E, The Committee on Necrotising Enterocolitis 1980 Necrotising enterocolitis. A prospective multicenter investigation. American Journal of Epidemiology 112: 113–124

151. Sarnat H B, Sarnat M S 1976 Neonatal encephalopathy following fetal distress. Archives of Neurology 33: 696–705

152. Sasidharan P 1992 Breathing pattern abnormalities in full term asphyxiated newborn infants. Archives of Disease in Childhood 67: 440–442

153. Saugstad O D 2001 Resuscitation of newborn infants with room air or oxygen. Seminars in Neonatology 6: 233–239

154. Saugstad O D, Rootwelt T, Aalen O 1998 Resuscitation of asphyxiated newborn infants with room air or oxygen: an international controlled trial: the Resair 2 study. Pediatrics 102: e1

155. Schubring C 1986 Temperature regulation in healthy and resuscitated newborns immediately after birth. Journal of Perinatal Medicine 14: 27–33

156. Schwab K O, von Stockhausen H B 1994 Plasma catecholamines after endotracheal administration of adrenaline during postnatal resuscitation. Archives of Disease in Childhood 70: F213–F217

157. Scopes J W, Ahmed I 1966 Minimal rates of oxygen consumption in sick and premature newborn infants. Archives of Disease in Childhood 41: 407–416

158. Seefelder C, Elango S, Rosbe K W, Jennings R W 2001 Oesophageal perforation presenting as oesophageal atresia in a premature neonate following difficult intubation. Paediatric Anaesthesia 11: 112–118

159. Sessler D, Mills P, Gregory G et al 1987 Effects of bicarbonate on arterial and brain intracellular pH in neonatal rabbits recovering from hypoxic lactic acidosis. Journal of Pediatrics 111: 817–823

160. Settergren G, Lindblad B S, Persson B 1976 Cerebral blood flow and exchange of oxygen, glucose, ketone bodies, lactate, pyruvate and amino acids in infants. Acta Paediatrica Scandinavica 65: 343–353

161. Shah P, Rophagen S, Beyene J, Perlman M 2004 Multiorgan dysfunction in infants with post asphyxial hypoxic ischaemic encephalopathy. Archives of Disease in Childhood 89: F152–F155

162. Shekarloo A, Mendez-Bauer C, Cook V, Freese U 1989 Terbutaline (intravenous bolus) for the treatment of acute intrapartum fetal distress. American Journal of Obstetrics and Gynecology 160: 615–618

163. Shelley H J 1961 Glycogen reserves and their changes at birth and in anoxia. British Medical Bulletin 17: 137–143

164. Shiraki K 1970 Hepatic cell necrosis in the newborn. American Journal of Diseases of Children 119: 395–400

165. Sims D G, Heal C A, Bartle S M 1994 Use of adrenaline and atropine in neonatal resuscitation. Archives of Disease in Childhood 70: F3–F10

166. Skillman C A, Plessinger M A, Woods J R, Clark K E 1985 Effect of graded reductions in uteroplacental blood flow in the fetal lamb. American Journal of Physiology 249: H1098–H1105

167. Smith A, Prakash P, Nesbitt J et al 1990 The vasopressin response to severe birth asphyxia. Early Human Development 22: 119–129

168. Soothill P W, Nicolaides K H, Rodeck C H 1987 Effect of anaemia on fetal acid–base status. British Journal of Obstetrics and Gynaecology 94: 880–883

169. Spencer J A D, Robson S C, Farakas A 1993 Spontaneous recovery after severe metabolic acidaemia at birth. Early Human Development 32: 103–112

170. Steiner H, Neligan G 1975 Perinatal cardiac arrest: quality of survivors. Archives of Disease in Childhood 50: 696–702

171. Stoddard R A, Clark S L, Minton S D 1988 In utero ischaemic injury: sonographic diagnosis and medicolegal implications. American Journal of Obstetrics and Gynecology 159: 23–25

172. Sykes G S, Molloy P M, Johnson P et al 1982 Do Apgar scores indicate asphyxia? Lancet 2: 494–496

173. Temesvari P, Karg E, Bodi I et al 2001 Impaired early neurologic outcome in newborn piglets reoxygenated with 100% oxygen compared with room air after pneumothorax-induced asphyxia. Pediatric Research 49: 812–819

174. Thibeault D W, Hobel C J 1974 The interrelationship of the foam stability test, immaturity and intrapartum complications in the respiratory distress syndrome. American Journal of Obstetrics and Gynecology 118: 56–61

175. Thorp J A, Sampson J E, Parisi V M, Creasy R K 1989 Routine umbilical cord blood gas determinations. American Journal of Obstetrics and Gynecology 161: 600–605

176. Topsis J, Kinas H Y, Kandall S R 1989 Esophageal perforation – a complication of neonatal resuscitation. Anesthesia and Analgesia 69: 532–534

177. Trawoger R, Mann C, Mortl, Riha K 1999 Use of laryngeal masks in the resuscitation of a neonate with difficult airway. Archives of Disease in Childhood Fetal and Neonatal Edition 81: F160

178. Tsang R C, Chen I, Hayes W, Atkinson W, Atherton H, Edwards N 1974 Neonatal hypocalcaemia in infants with birth asphyxia. Journal of Pediatrics 84: 428–433

179. Upton C J, Milner A D 1991 Endotracheal resuscitation of neonates using a rebreathing bag. Archives of Disease in Childhood 66: 39–42

180. Van Haesbrouck P, Vanneste K, Pretere C et al 1987 Tight nuchal cord and neonatal hypovolaemic shock. Archives of Disease in Childhood 62: 1276–1277

181. Vannucci R C 1992 Perinatal brain metabolism. In: Polin R A, Fox W W (eds) Fetal and neonatal physiology. W B Saunders, Philadelphia, pp 1510–1519

182. Vento M, Asensi M, Sastre J, Garcia-Sala F, Pallardo F V, Vina J 2001 Resuscitation with room air instead of 100% oxygen prevents oxidative stress in moderately asphyxiated term neonates. Pediatrics 107: 642–647

183. Vento M, Asensi M, Sastre J, Garcia-Sala F, Vina J 2001 Six years of experience with the use of room air for the resuscitation of asphyxiated newly born term infants. Biology of the Neonate 79: 261–267

184. Volpe J J 1995 Neurology of the newborn. W B Saunders, Philadelphia, pp 279–313

185. Vyas H, Field D, Milner A D, Hopkin I E 1986 Determinants of the first inspiratory volume and functional residual capacity at birth. Pediatric Pulmonology 2: 189–193

186. Westgate J, Garibaldi J M, Greene K R 1994 Umbilical cord blood gas analysis at delivery: a time for quality data. British Journal of Obstetrics and Gynaecology 101: 1054–1063

187. Westgren M, Grundsell H, Ingemarsson I, Muhlow A, Svenningsen N W 1981 Hyperextension of the fetal head in breech presentation. A study with long term follow-up. British Journal of Obstetrics and Gynaecology 88: 101–104

188. Wilkenning R B, Doyle D W, Meschia G 1993 Fetal pH improvement after 24 hours of severe non-lethal hypoxia. Biology of the Neonate 63: 129–132

189. Wiswell T E, Gannon C M, Jacob J et al 2000 Delivery room management of the apparently vigorous meconium-stained neonate: Results of the multicenter, international collaborative trial. Pediatrics 105: 1–7

190. Wyckoff M H, Perlman J, Niermeyer S 2001 Medications during resuscitation – what is the evidence? Seminars in Neonatology 6: 251–259

191. Wyszogrodski I, Kyei-Aboagye K, Taeusch H W, Avery M E 1975 Surfactant inactivation by hyperventilation: conservation by end expiratory pressure. Journal of Applied Physiology 38: 461–466

192. Young R S K, Hessert T R, Pritchard G A, Yagel S K 1984 Naloxone exacerbates hypoxic-ischaemic brain injury in the neonatal rat. American Journal of Obstetrics and Gynecology 150: 52–56

193. Zaritsky A 1995 Bicarbonate in cardiac arrest: the good, the bad and the puzzling. Critical Care Medicine 23: 429–430

194. Ziino A J, Davies M W, Davis P G 2003 Epinephrine for the resuscitation of apparently stillborn or extremely bradycardic newborn infants. Cochrane Database of Systematic Reviews 2: CD003849

PART 2

Neonatal transport

David Field

Introduction

Throughout the developed world there are no countries in which all newborns have immediate access to neonatal care. As a result every country has a need to transfer some babies for medical reasons. On many occasions this need can be anticipated (e.g. a mother in preterm labour at 28 weeks gestation) and an in-utero transfer can take place. While it is generally accepted that this approach has many advantages it is important to stress that it is not risk-free. A full discussion of in-utero transfer is beyond the remit of this chapter and can be found elsewhere.[16]

There are many circumstances in which a baby will need access to neonatal care not available at the point of delivery and these vary around the world. For example:

- to receive neonatal intensive care when either this is not available locally or the in-house facilities are full;

- to undergo an investigation or procedure not available on site (in countries where separate maternity services exist transfer may be needed even for basic interventions such as phototherapy);

- to return to a local hospital after a period of treatment elsewhere.

Therefore, depending on the organisational structure of neonatal and maternity care in a particular country and its geography, the numbers of babies requiring transfer and the nature of the service provided will vary enormously. For example in France a large number of babies are born in maternity hospitals away from neonatal services and hence a significant number of transfers involve mature babies, but typically they are moved by road. In parts of Australia similar problems exist but the long distances mean that air transport is the only practical option.[1] In contrast, within the UK few transfers occur without the need for intensive care at least being anticipated, but the majority of transfers take place by road in under 1 hour. A more detailed description of these practical differences can be found elsewhere.[12]

These inherent differences are clearly major influences on how a country or region chooses to organise neonatal transport services. The two most common models are (1) as a separate organisation and (2) as part of a neonatal intensive care service. The latter was certainly the norm in the UK throughout the 1970s, 1980s and 1990s. In other parts of the world (e.g. Australia and the USA), transport developed with a separate, more specialist identity.[11,14] Although the transport teams were often linked physically with a neonatal unit there were separate staffing and administrative arrangements. This allowed transport services to focus on their core activity, with benefits in terms of the quality of the service provided. Those transport services whose staffing was completely separate were also able to undertake transfers without jeopardising the cover available to babies already in the neonatal unit. The advantages of a stand-alone specialist service are slowly being accepted worldwide.

Whatever the choice of organisational model the basic principles set out below should not be compromised.

Basic principles

The organisation

The most respected transport services around the world aim to facilitate the whole process of moving a baby, for whatever reason. Once the referring hospital asks for help the transport service takes responsibility for moving and placing the baby appropriately. Clearly these aims can be achieved in a variety of ways but the following are particularly helpful:

- a single telephone contact point manned 24 hours a day 365 days a year;
- a conference call facility to permit senior staff at the referring hospital to be able to speak directly to senior staff at the potential receiving unit;
- up to date information about cot availability in potential receiving units.

Whether the transport service is a stand-alone organisation or part of another service there must be a director to provide clinical leadership. One or more technicians are essential to ensure that appropriate equipment is purchased and maintained. Training and clinical governance must also be the responsibility of named individuals.

Personnel and training

Retrieval teams around the world are based in a variety of staffing models. Both nurses and doctors can undertake this role provided they have the necessary knowledge and skills. The transport service should, as part of a process of induction, ensure that all staff undertaking transfers are adequately prepared. Important areas to cover include the following.

- **Understanding the local perinatal service.** Staff must appreciate the catchment area they cover – how far away is unit 'x', what

staffing does it have, how long does it take to get there by road? Similarly, if transport vehicles are supplied by a different organisation, procedures for ordering a vehicle must be clear.
- **Equipment orientation.** Staff should not only be familiar with the normal use of the transport incubator and its associated equipment but also be capable of basic troubleshooting. Familiarity with any communication system is particularly important where long-distance transfers are undertaken.
- **Local policies and procedures.** Since neonatal transport is performed by a team, many organisations adopt a didactic approach to all elements of basic care (e.g. vascular access), processes for accepting a transfer request, team make-up and individual roles. These must be taught and knowledge assessed before any new staff member actually undertakes transfers unsupported.
- **Clinical skills.** All team members should be taught and then be able to demonstrate all basic clinical skills in 'scenario training' before undertaking transfers unsupported.
- **Special skills.** Where transport services regularly use air transport, personnel should be trained on those particular aircraft. This should include not only how to load and fix the equipment but safety training – for example how to escape from a helicopter ditched in the sea. An appreciation of how altitude affects the patient's physiology and the functioning of equipment is also vital.
- **'Buddying' of new members of staff with seniors** during the first few transfers allows them to familiarise themselves with processes and procedures while gaining confidence.

With regard to ongoing training, one of the most important aspects is a careful debriefing. This allows any problems, whether clinical, procedural or mechanical, to be dealt with. Actions that follow debriefing might include more training for an individual or modification to a piece of equipment.[2,8,9]

Vehicles

Teams undertaking transport should plan to have appropriate vehicles available (i.e. reflecting their catchment area). If journey times by road are likely to regularly exceed 2 hours, air transport should be considered.

Road vehicles (not always traditional ambulances) should:

- be easy to load;
- be able to secure safely the equipment and staff;
- provide forward-facing seats for staff (reduces motion sickness);
- provide sufficient space to permit staff to work on the baby if required;
- provide oxygen and electrical supplies for the transport incubator during the journey;
- permit continuing communication with referring and receiving hospitals during the transfer.

Some transport services deal with these points by having a dedicated vehicle. Clearly, this has advantages in terms of optimising the transport environment but, unless the number of transports performed is very high, is a costly approach. Problems also arise if the vehicle breaks down or is unavailable during a routine service. For those relying on a local ambulance or vehicle supplier it is vital to know their response times and the type of vehicle they will be able to supply.[10]

Fixed wing aircraft allow transport over much greater distances. However, loading can be a major problem and space available during the journey may be very limited. Strict regulations ensure that equipment used during the transfer does not interfere with the aircraft system. The same problems relate to helicopter transfers. Here limited payload, space and noise are particular problems.

Medical equipment

The most demanding type of neonatal transfer occurs when a baby is being moved to receive intensive care or some other specialist intervention such as extracorporeal membrane oxygenation. Here it is necessary to reproduce, as closely as possible, the facilities of the base intensive care unit. 'Transport incubator systems' are intended to provide these facilities but there are serious practical considerations that limit what can actually be supplied.[5]

- **Weight**. Moving the transport incubator system to the transport vehicle and safely loading and securing it, without breaking health and safety rules, limits the total weight. In the European Union this weight limit has been set at 140 kg. Where helicopters or fixed-wing aircraft are to be used, physical size is also a consideration.
- **Suitability for use in the transport setting**. Equipment used during transport is often bumped, subjected to vibration and exposed to extremes of temperature. Therefore, equipment used during transport should be capable of withstanding, and working normally in, these adverse circumstances. Conversely the equipment (including the vehicle) should be designed to minimise the baby's exposure to excessive noise and mechanical vibration.[3,13]
- **Gas and power supplies**. Most intensive care equipment requires an electricity supply, which, during transport, must come from the reserve battery of the transport incubator system or the transport vehicle. Transport equipment must therefore be efficient in its use of power if it is not to jeopardise the functioning of other equipment or of the vehicle itself. Similarly gas supplies, other than air, must be carried and hence ventilators that require high volumes of gas in order to function are best avoided in the transport environment.

Despite these caveats the transport incubator system must be capable of supplying the following.

- **An incubator**. Although it would be desirable to provide both temperature regulation and humidity for the smallest babies, the latter is not practical. Fluid and evaporative heat loses are best controlled by placing the baby in a plastic bag.
- **A ventilator**. An efficient ventilator capable of working in the transport environment is more important than a machine capable of working in a large variety of modes.
- **A cardiorespiratory monitor** (including invasive blood pressure).
- An adequate number of **infusion pumps**.
- **Drugs**.

- A full range of **consumables**. (These last two items are often carried separately from the transport incubator system.)
- **Gas supplies**. There should be sufficient gas for the whole journey, even after allowing for some delays, carried between the vehicle and the transport incubator system. In case the vehicle fails, the transport incubator systems alone should be capable of working alone for at least 1 hour.
- **Power supply** – see comments under 'Gas supplies' above.

A variety of other equipment can be carried in special circumstances, e.g. nitric oxide, or a portable blood gas analyser where local geography means long-distance transfers are regularly undertaken.

Safety

Neonatal transport places both the patient and staff at increased risk (Fig. 13.10). There are numerous examples of fatalities during transfers from around the world. Solutions to some of the risks involved are not yet available (e.g. a safe restraining device for babies in the transport incubator). However other risks can be reduced by careful planning, training and common sense.

- Arrangements for loading and unloading of the transport incubator system should minimise the need for staff actually to lift the device. The equipment should not be used in a way that would put it at risk of falling, e.g. from a narrow loading ramp.
- All equipment must be properly restrained while the vehicle is in motion. Proper restraint means that the restraining device and the anchorage points both on the equipment and the vehicle must be carefully chosen and tested.[4]
- Seats for staff must face forward and seat belts must be worn.
- Staff involved in air transport must be familiar with evacuation procedures and, if appropriate, have access to life jackets. In some circumstances staff should wear survival suits during the transfer.
- Staff using air transport should be familiar with 'flight decision making', i.e. the process by which a pilot will decide whether it is or is not safe to fly.

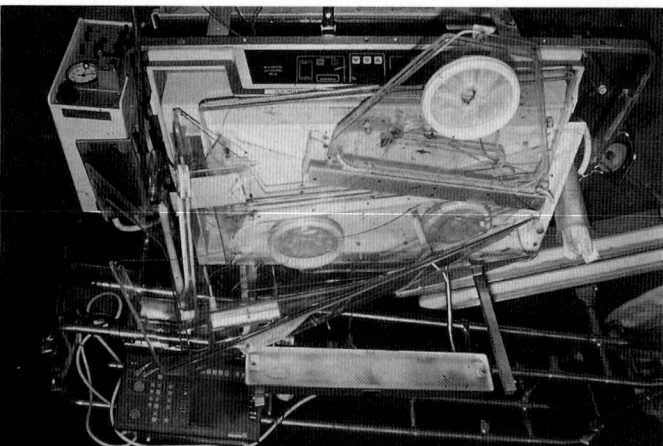

Fig. 13.10 Damage done to a transport incubator by a road traffic accident.

The medical aspects of neonatal transport for intensive care

Although many aspects of routine neonatal care apply during all types of transfer it is during the transfer of infants for intensive or specialist care (e.g. cardiac) that special considerations and attention to detail become particularly important.[2,15] Some of the important points to be considered in relation to any urgent transfer are outlined below:

- First contact: The initial discussion to arrange the transfer should be between senior clinicians. Where the receiving hospital and the transport service are separate organisations, ideally this should take the form of a conference call during which the baby's current condition and most appropriate future management can be discussed by all relevant parties. One result of this discussion should be advice to the referring hospital about the baby's management prior to transfer. The manner of this exchange is also vital in building a relationship between all those involved in the baby's care and avoiding any sense of condescension. Since it is not always possible to involve experienced individuals, many services use a checklist of points to be covered and information to be noted at the first contact.
- Routine checks should have been carried out on the transport equipment but it is important to double-check any items of particular relevance after the baby has been referred. For example, the baby may have a chest drain in place and hence portable valves are essential. In addition some items of equipment (e.g. for nitric oxide administration) may not be routinely carried and will need to be added.[7] As a general rule it is a mistake to assume that the referring hospital will be able to supply any item of equipment for use during the journey back, as it may be incompatible or conflict with some other aspect of the transport incubator system.
- When the transport team arrive at the referring hospital they should take time to get a careful handover. The whole team should promote a philosophy of team work with staff at the referring unit.
- The baby must be stabilised. The aim of this process should be to ensure that nothing unexpected happens on the return journey. The most difficult decision often relates to the airway and whether the baby should be intubated and ventilated for the journey. While this is certainly not mandatory it is sensible to take this course if there is any doubt about the baby's ability to maintain an airway and or keep breathing. If necessary, delay any return journey until after the circulation has been improved by the use of volume and or inotropes. Metabolic instability, particularly hypoglycaemia, should also be dealt with.
- Ensure that there is time to speak to parents about the baby's condition and pass on contact information for the new unit. It is essential that parents have a chance to see the baby before departure.
- Moving the baby from the intensive care cot into the transport incubator requires great skill. Lines must be protected, appropriate new infusions prepared, the transport ventilator adjusted, etc. so that everything is ready in the transport incubator system to receive the baby. This move must take place very smoothly if the baby is to avoid heat loss. This risk can be reduced if the transport incubator is positioned temporarily under a radiant heater.
- Continue monitoring the baby during the journey back. If there are concerns about the baby's condition during the journey, ideally the vehicle should be stopped while any problems are dealt with. This is unlikely to be possible in the case of air transport.
- Because neonatal transfer services move babies with a variety of problems, it is important for teams to have clear guidelines for the management of specialist 'high-risk' situations – for example, babies with gastroschisis, tracheo-oesophageal atresia and all either undiagnosed or known duct-dependent cardiac lesions.

Audit and understanding outcomes

Because only small numbers of individuals are involved in any one neonatal transfer it is important that the process is the subject of careful audit. This should involve all types of transfer, not just those for intensive care. This is best achieved by the team completing a form that documents various aspects of the transfer. The broad areas that should be covered include:

- personnel involved;
- times, e.g. initial call received, time that the team left to retrieve the baby, time of arrival in referring unit;
- problems with availability or use of the transport vehicle;
- equipment problems;
- clinical problems encountered;
- physiological parameters of the baby, e.g. temperature on leaving the referring unit and on arrival back, change in blood gases.

These data alone allow both the performance of the service and that of individual team members to be monitored. Where any kind of adverse incident occurs a more detailed debriefing can be helpful in identifying whether the problem can be avoided in the future and act as a learning exercise for the whole transport service.

The later outcome of babies has been the subject of a number of publications in the past. These appeared to demonstrate an adverse outcome for babies involved in urgent postnatal transfers compared to babies whose entire course was within a tertiary neonatal unit. It has become clear more recently that this type of comparison is not 'fair', as babies chosen for urgent postnatal transfer represent a selected group with disease that is significantly more severe than that of infants of a similar gestation not involved in any kind of transfer.

For an individual transport service it is important to monitor the outcome (at the very least survival corrected for disease severity) of the babies it transfers. However, at the present time there is no evidence that postnatal transfer per se has an adverse effect on the babies' chances of survival.[6]

References

1. American Academy of Pediatrics 1993 Taskforce on Interhospital Transport. Guidelines for air and ground transport of neonatal and paediatric patients. AAP, Elk Grove Village, IL

2. Berry A B 1999 Training and organisation of retrieval. Seminars in Neonatology 4: 253–263

3. Campbell A N, Lightstone A D, Smith J M, Kirpalani H, Perlman M 1984 Mechanical vibration and sound levels experienced in neonatal transport. American Journal of Disease in Childhood 138: 967–970

4. CEN TC 239 2001 Rescue systems – transportation of incubators. Part 1: Interface conditions. European Committee for Standardization, Brussels, EN 13976-1.2003

5. CEN TC 239 2001 Rescue systems – transportation of incubators. Part 2: System requirements. European Committee for Standardization, Brussels, EN 13976-2.2003

6. Field D, Draper E S 1999 Survival and place of delivery 1994–96. Archives of Disease in Childhood 80: F111–F114

7. Kinsella J P, Griebel J, Schmidt J M, Abman S H 2002 Use of inhaled nitric oxide during interhospital transport of newborns with hypoxemic respiratory failure. Pediatrics 109: 158–161

8. Leslie A 1994 Formation of a neonatal transport team. Paediatric Nursing 6: 18–22

9. Leslie A, Bose C 1999 Nurse-led neonatal transport. Seminars in Neonatology 4: 265–271

10. Little J W 1999 Ambulance transport for the newborn. Seminars in Neonatology 4: 247–251

11. Rashid A, Bhuta T, Berry A 1999 A regionalised transport service: the way ahead? Archives of Disease in Childhood 80: 488–492

12. Roy R N D, Langford S, Charbenaud J-L et al 1999 Neonatal transport around the world. Seminars in Neonatology 4: 219–235

13. Shenai J P, Johnson G E, Varney R V 1981 Mechanical vibration in neonatal transport. Pediatrics 68: 55–57

14. Shenai J P, Major C W, Gaylord M S et al 1991 A successful decade of regionalized perinatal care in Tennessee: the neonatal experience. Journal of Perinatology 11: 137–143

15. Skeoch C H, Booth P 1999 Medical care during transport. Seminars in Neonatology 4: 281–287

16. Steer P 1999 Maternal transfer. Seminars in Neonatology 4: 237–240

Section Four

General Neonatal Care

CHAPTER 14

Examination of the newborn

Janet M Rennie

Introduction

A thorough physical examination of every neonate is accepted as good practice and forms a core item of the child health surveillance programme in many countries.[33] There is no nationally agreed standard for the conduct of the examination, although the Royal College of General Practitioners in the UK – under the auspices of the National Institute for Clinical Excellence (NICE) – is developing guidelines for routine postnatal care, due in 2006.

The aims of the routine newborn examination are:

- to review any problems arising or suspected from antenatal screening, family history or the events of labour;
- to acertain whether or not the family have any worries about the baby and to try to address them;
- to initiate appropriate treatment and follow up where indicated (e.g. hepatitis vaccination, phototherapy for jaundice, special teat for cleft palate);
- to screen for specific target conditions, including developmental dysplasia of the hip (DDH), cataract and congenital heart disease (CHD);
- to diagnose congenital malformations and common neonatal problems, and give advice about management;
- to detect the occasional baby who is obviously ill and requires urgent treatment;
- to collect baseline information about weight and head circumference, and to check that the baby has passed urine and meconium;
- to identify parents who may have problems in caring for their baby due to substance abuse, mental health problems, learning difficulties or very poor housing and to alert the appropriate professional groups;
- to begin to provide health education advice, e.g. regarding breastfeeding, cot death prevention, safe transport in cars.

For some babies, early diagnosis may make all the difference to their subsequent health; examples are congenital cataract and urethral valves. For others, reassurance about minor deviations from normal (birthmarks, syndactyly of the toes, extra digits) is all that is required. The slightest variation from what the family consider to be normal may produce the most intense distress and anxiety at a stage when the mother is emotionally very labile.

The yield of abnormal findings is surprisingly high, with up to 20% of healthy newborns being found to have one minor anomaly.[1] Most of these are of no importance, although the number of such abnormalities matters (Table 14.1). Only 0.5% of babies have

Table 14.1 Common minor neonatal abnormalities and their importance

Abnormalities that do not matter when isolated. Three or more such abnormalities do matter
Folded-over ears
Hyperextensibility of thumbs
Syndactly of the 2nd and 3rd toes
Single palmar crease
Polydactyly, especially if familial
Umbilical hernia, especially in Afro-Caribbean babies
Single umbilical artery
Hydrocoele
5th finger clinodactly
Simple dimple just above the natal cleft (see text for definition)
Undescended testes
Single café-au-lait spot
Single ash-leaf macule
Third fontanelle (5% of babies)
Capillary or strawberry haemangioma
Accessory nipples
Abnormalities that might matter even when they are isolated
Ear pits and tags
More than three café-au-lait spots in a Caucasian baby, more than five in black African babies
Multiple haemangiomatas, or strawberry haemangiomas in specific places (e.g. ophthalmic division of the trigeminal nerve in Sturge–Weber, or in the midline over the spine)
Oedema of the feet – think of Turner's syndrome
Asymmetric crying facies
Microcephaly
Macrocephaly
Micrognathia
Midline skin defects over the spine other than simple dimples
Scrotal swelling/discoloration (think of torsion of the testes)

three such anomalies, and the risk of an accompanying major malformation then rises from 3% (with one minor anomaly) to 20%. Unfortunately, the examination performs poorly as a screen for several important conditions such as DDH, cataract, and CHD.

Who should examine the baby?

Babies should be examined by a trained practitioner who has the time to talk and listen to the mother. In the past, all neonatal examinations were carried out by paediatricians, usually junior paediatricians with some specific basic training. Generations of paediatric residents have learnt the range of normality by performing large numbers of 'baby checks', and they have the advantage of a full medical training and a direct chain of referral. Recently, advanced neonatal nurse practitioners (ANNPs) and trained midwives have begun to undertake the examination, and mothers are usually very satisfied with the service they provide.[47,80] In the randomised trial conducted in South East England,[80] mothers whose baby was examined by a midwife were more satisfied than the group whose baby was examined by a paediatric senior house officer (SHO), although the general level of satisfaction was very high. The reason why the midwives' examination was preferred was that there was more provision of health education advice (related to feeding, sleeping and skin care). Once this was controlled for, the differences in satisfaction disappeared. The midwives took 5 minutes longer, on average, to conduct the examination than the SHOs. Randomisation only took place during the working day, and half of all babies born during the study period were excluded from randomisation because of problems such as maternal disease, low birthweight (LBW), operative delivery or a need for resuscitation at birth.

When should babies be examined?

Besides the routine check immediately after delivery, every newborn infant deserves at least one full examination before discharge home. For many years it was customary for a second examination to be carried out, but the value of this has been shown to be limited and a single examination is now the norm.[28,54] The timing for the full examination is probably not crucial, and the optimum time for a single examination has yet to be determined.

Examination in the delivery room

All babies should be checked soon after birth; this will generally be done by the midwife following uncomplicated full-term labour, but if the paediatrician has been called to the delivery, he should make a quick appraisal of the infant after any necessary resuscitation. This examination is usually confined to checking that the infant looks well and that there are no major abnormalities requiring immediate attention or explanation to the parents, such as hare lip/cleft palate, spina bifida, anal atresia or ambiguous genitalia. This is a most sensitive and important time for parents and they should be given the opportunity to be left alone with their baby as soon as possible.

Full routine examination

Mothers meticulously inspect their own babies; hence, one of the most important functions of the examination is to answer any questions that the mother may raise. It follows that the examination should, if possible, always be done in her presence. The following general format is recommended:

1. Check the maternal medical, obstetric and social history from the notes, the mother and the nursing staff.
2. Introduce yourself to the mother with an explanation about what you are doing.
3. Fully examine the baby.
4. Give advice and information, arrange follow-up and provide reassurance where appropriate. When giving advice, remember that the neonatal examination is not a perfect screening tool.

History and background knowledge

Before approaching the mother and infant, read the baby notes to obtain basic information about the mother's previous obstetric and medical history as well as the type of delivery and the baby's condition at birth; note also the birthweight, gestational age and sex. If there are complicated medical or social problems, it is helpful to discuss them with the nursing staff beforehand and also to check the mother's notes for details.

It is useful to have a mental checklist of relevant background information to obtain before starting the examination. This should include:

- The baby's sex.
- The baby's birthweight and reputed gestational age and whether these are mutually compatible.
- The mother's age and social background.
- Is there any chronic maternal disease? If so, what treatment is the mother receiving?
- Is there a history of recreational drug and/or alcohol use; is the mother a smoker?
- Is there any possibly relevant family history?
- The outcome and dates of any previous pregnancies.
- Was the pregnancy normal? Were there any complications?
- What were the results of pregnancy screening tests, e.g. 19-week ultrasound scan?
- Were any special diagnostic procedures, e.g. amniocentesis, performed?
- Was there any discrepancy between the mother's dates and those derived by the obstetrician from clinical ultrasound assessments?
- Were there any signs of fetal distress?
- What drugs and/or anaesthesia were given during labour?
- How was the infant delivered?

- What was his condition at birth (e.g. Apgar scores at 1 and 5 minutes)?
- Was any resuscitation needed?
- How long before sustained respiration was established?
- Was the baby in the neonatal unit? If so, why?

Introductions and general 'gestalt' inspection

The doctor should introduce himself and say what he has come for. To ask the baby's name and record it helps to establish a good relationship. Because so many early worries are concerned with feeding, one should always enquire what method the mother is using and whether she is happy with it. Routine weighing and feed charts have been abandoned in most UK maternity units, but the incidence of readmission with hypernatraemic dehydration due to breast-milk insufficiency is rising.[45] All babies lose weight after birth; 2–3% each day to a maximum of around 10% (p. 343), but it is rare for a baby to lose more weight than this, or to remain more than 10% below birthweight after the 5th day.[82] If there is a current weight, then a quick calculation of weight lost or gained since birth should be made.

Enquire about the health of any previous children. There may have been previous stillbirths, infant deaths or adverse outcomes about which the mother may be extremely anxious. The paediatrician should also review and confirm any relevant items of background information gleaned from the notes. Always ask the mother whether she has any specific worries, when she is expecting to be discharged and what support she has at home. Knowledge of the father's and mother's occupation provide useful background information. By means of these preliminary pleasantries one can usually quickly establish a relationship and can gauge the level at which to discuss any problems. During these introductory minutes, the examiner can try to make the mother and her partner (if present) feel like individuals, and can also do two other very important things:

- observe the mother's attitude to her baby, and whether she is confident and happy or tense and withdrawn;
- observe the baby, noting colour, facies, breathing pattern, posture and movements.

An enormous amount can be learned by these simple observations while continuing to chat to the mother. For recording purposes, it is useful to have a checklist printed or stamped in the baby's notes to serve as an aide memoire. The examination must be dated and signed. The experienced observer uses 'gestalt' to assess the importance of minor dysmorphic features (Table 14.1), subtle signs of illness, or atypical behaviour patterns.

Formal examination

The baby must be undressed down to the nappy for most of the examination time; it is impossible to examine a baby properly when clothed. Most parts of the examination can be performed in any behavioural state, and the order in which this is done is largely a matter of personal preference, but working from top to toe down the front and vice versa up the back is as good as any other. Full advantage should be taken of any quiet or sleeping periods to feel the anterior fontanelle, look at the eyes, auscultate the heart and palpate the abdomen. It is wise to leave the hips until nearly the end of the examination, even though this item is arguably one of the most important items on the agenda and must be done with the infant quiet and relaxed, because the Ortolani/Barlow test often does make the baby cry. Throughout the whole examination, one is at first consciously, later almost subconsciously, observing such things as posture, muscle tone, movements and reaction to stimuli so that finally there is very little need for a formal evaluation of the central nervous system (CNS) unless suspicious signs have come to light. A suggested order for the examination is given below: details of what one is looking for are given in the section on Systematic Review.

Order of examination

1. Remove the baby's clothes except the nappy.
2. Feel the anterior fontanelle for tension (leave until later if the baby is crying!).
3. Look at the face for colour or any peculiarities.
4. Listen to the heart and estimate heart rate and respiratory rate. The lungs can also be auscultated but this is seldom informative.
5. Palpate the abdomen.
6. Return to the head and examine scalp and skull and measure head circumference and record it, together with the weight.
7. Examine the eyes, ears, nose and mouth.
8. Examine the neck, including the clavicles.
9. Examine the arms, hands, legs and feet.
10. Remove the nappy.
11. Feel for the femoral pulses.
12. Examine the genitalia and anus.
13. Turn the baby to the prone position and examine the back and spine, and assess tone.
14. Return the infant to the supine position and evaluate the CNS.
15. Examine the hips.
16. Make sure you have not omitted anything and check you have paid attention to any concerns expressed by the mother.

Systematic review

Skin

During the general examination, the colour and texture of the skin should be noted, as well as any birthmarks or rashes. Birthmarks are common in babies, and most are vascular or pigmentary lesions.[35] Many are normal variants, but some are of great importance. Sturge–Weber syndrome (p. 830) occurs in 10% of those who have a port-wine stain involving the ophthalmic division of the trigeminal nerve, for example.

The frequency of café-au-lait spots varies tremendously and it is common to see one spot, although more than three are rare. Some have recommended that any Caucasian baby with more than three such spots, and any African baby with more than five, be followed for the development of multisystem disease.[46] Many other skin lesions are described in Chapter 33, and some excellent illustrated textbooks are available.[19]

Skin colour

Healthy warm Caucasian babies should be reddish pink all over after the first few hours of life, but they can be covered with white cheesy vernix; this can also be stained a golden yellow in post-maturity or appear greenish if meconium has been passed before birth.

Cyanosis

Cyanosis is usually discernible when arterial blood is 80% saturated, but the ability to detect cyanosis varies between individuals and with different lighting conditions. Cyanosis can be difficult to evaluate in an infant who is very pale (anaemic or peripherally shut down) or racially pigmented. Plethoric infants (central packed-cell volume >65%) can appear cyanosed because they have more than 5 g of reduced haemoglobin per 100 ml even when adequately oxygenated. Peripheral cyanosis of the hands and feet and circumoral cyanosis (acrocyanosis) is common during the first 48 hours. It is essential to ascertain that cyanosis is not central by noting whether or not the tongue is blue. Traumatic cyanosis or bruising of the presenting part, sometimes associated with petechiae, is also quite common, particularly over the face if there has been a nuchal cord. If there is any doubt, check arterial oxygen saturation with a pulse oximeter. Babies with confirmed central cyanosis should be admitted to the neonatal unit and investigated urgently, beginning with a blood gas estimation and a chest X-ray (CXR) and proceeding to an early echocardiogram if there is no evidence of respiratory disease.

Cyanosis during crying early in postnatal life may be quite normal as a result of transient elevation of pulmonary vascular resistance with right-to-left shunting, but cyanotic attacks should always be taken seriously.

Pallor

Mature babies appear paler than preterm ones, because of their relatively thick skin. Generalised pallor may indicate anaemia, peripheral shutdown with shock, or both. The capillary filling time can be estimated by pressing on the skin and should not be longer than 3 seconds if the skin is warm.

Jaundice

This is discussed in detail elsewhere (Chapter 29, Part 1) but is often detected first during the routine newborn examination. Icterus appearing in the first 24 hours requires urgent investigation and treatment and should at once evoke the response 'What is the mother's Rh and ABO group? Were there any antibodies and are there any other signs of congenital infection?'

Jaundice appearing between 2 and 4 days is extremely common, with 65% of normal full-term infants acquiring a serum bilirubin of over 80 micromol/l, the level at which jaundice is visible in white-skinned babies. The peak level, reached on the third or fourth day, is around 220 micromol/l. Jaundice in preterm (including near-term) babies requires very careful evaluation, and if any jaundiced baby is ill in any way (unduly lethargic, feeding poorly, vomiting, or has an unstable temperature), infection – or worse, bilirubin encephalopathy (p. 665) – must be excluded. The level of bilirubin is hard to judge by eye, so if in doubt it must be measured. This is particularly important in Afro-Caribbean, Oriental and Asian babies, in whom clinical assessment of jaundice is fraught with hazard. Jaundice stains the skin in a cephalo-caudal direction, so that any jaundice extending to the umbilicus in a term infant is likely to correspond to a bilirubin level of over 200 micromol/l. Healthy term infants are not immune from kernicterus but levels of bilirubin above 500 micromol/l are probably required to produce it (Chapter 29, Part 1).

Sadly, kernicterus has returned: more than 80% of the cases reported to the US registry were born after 1990. Audit showed that common factors were lack of professional concern about jaundice, inadequate breastfeeding and a failure to recognise that the near-term baby (35–37 weeks) is particularly susceptible. A third of the cases in the registry had glucose-6-phosphate dehydrogenase (G6PD) deficiency (p. 747), meaning that special attention must to be paid to male babies who are of Afro-Caribbean, Greek, Italian or southeast Asian origin.[39] Most babies are now at home when bilirubin levels are peaking, hence parents, midwives and general practitioners require education and training in the assessment of neonatal jaundice (p. 669). In the USA, the parent support group Parents of Infants and Children with Kernicterus[59] is campaigning for all babies to have their bilirubin measured before discharge, but the predictive ability of this test as a screen is not yet fully established.[3]

Skin texture

Note whether the skin is peeling (common in post-term infants), nice and firm (normal) or very loose (intrauterine growth retardation or dehydration). Oedema is uncommon in full-term infants and should always raise the question of hypoalbuminaemia. Pedal oedema and a low hairline should make the examiner think of Turner's syndrome in a baby girl (p. 249).

Skin rashes

These are very common in newborn babies. Flat lesions are described as macular (by definition, macules are <1 cm, but the term is not always used this way). Raised lesions are described as papular when they are up to 1 cm in size and nodular up to 2 cm. Raised lesions filled with clear fluid are vesicular (<1 cm) or bullous (>1 cm). When raised lesions contain purulent fluid, they are termed pustular. Diagnosis of a petechial rash, which does not blanch on pressure, should prompt a platelet count. Milia are tiny cream papules, which are inclusion cysts containing trapped keratinised stratum corneum, and which usually resolve without treatment.

The most frequent skin disorder of newborn infants is erythema toxicum neonatorum (toxic erythema: p. 819). There is an eosinophilic infiltrate into the dermis and there can be an associated eosinophilia in the blood. The rash usually starts between

24 and 48 hours of age and resolves by the 5th day. Transient neonatal pustular melanosis (p. 819) is extremely common in Afro-Caribbean babies, and is a similar reaction to erythema toxicum although the lesions are present from birth. These pustules contain neutrophils. The pustules fade into hyperpigmented brown macules resembling lentils (lentigines) which last for several months before themselves fading. Miliaria rubra, or prickly heat, is common in hot humid climates. The rash usually occurs mainly on the head and upper trunk.

Head and skull

Babies' heads can be considerably distorted and moulded during labour and delivery; there may be a marked caput succedaneum (oedema caused by pressure over the presenting part) which subsides in 2–3 days, or the soft skull bones can be greatly moulded. Either or both of these factors can produce bizarre head shapes which persist for the first few days and sometimes longer. It is important to distinguish deformation – the result of impact from mechanical forces on normal tissue – from malformation. Up to 20% of babies show effects of intrauterine constraint.[31] Babies who have been in the breech presentation for a long time in utero often have a 'breech head' with a prominent occipital shelf.[17]

Feel the anterior fontanelle for its tension and size: it can measure up to 3 × 3 cm at its widest points, though the size is very variable. Fullness may indicate raised intracranial pressure (cerebral oedema, hydrocephalus or meningitis). The posterior fontanelle is often open at this age but is usually only fingertip size, with only 3% more than 2 cm in diameter. Examine the cranial sutures for any undue separation, which is abnormal. Over-riding of the bones of the vault is common in the first 48 hours, but ridging at the suture lines, as opposed to the 'step-up' feel of over-riding, implies craniosynostosis (premature fusion of the sutures). The sagittal suture is the most commonly affected. Craniosynostosis occurs in about 0.4 per 1000 births and may require a neurosurgical procedure for cosmetic correction (p. 1201), or to allow brain growth if several sutures are fused.[38] Limb defects, particularly syndactyly, are the most common associated malformations and it may be worth asking the parents if they have fused toes.

Palpate the skull bones: small areas of craniotabes caused by pressure from the maternal pelvis occur in 2% of normal newborns and are of no significance.[32] Cephalhaematomata – collections of blood between the periosteum and the skull bones – are felt as softish bumps over the affected bone, most commonly the parietal, and do not extend across the suture lines. Explain their benign nature to the mother and add that they may take 6 weeks or more to subside. A boggy swelling crossing a suture line is more sinister and can indicate subgaleal haemorrhage (p. 1126). There may be a chignon from the use of a vacuum extractor. Neonatal skull fractures are rare. Elevation of the 'ping-pong' ball type of fracture where the bone is depressed but not fractured can be achieved with the application of a vacuum extractor. Linear skull fractures usually require no treatment but should be followed with a repeat X-ray, because if the dura has been torn, a 'growing' fracture can develop.[69,72]

Inspect the scalp for any injury such as forceps marks or lacerations from scalp electrodes, fetal blood sampling or instrumental delivery. Look also for any bald patches or naevi over the scalp. A small defect of the scalp – cutis aplasia–can be confused with the scar of a scalp clip electrode. Cutis aplasia (p. 832) is a serious congenital abnormality with a risk of infection and bleeding from the underlying dural venous sinuses, and may be a clue to an underlying diagnosis such as Adams–Oliver syndrome.

Measure the occipitofrontal head circumference (OFC) at its maximum and ensure that it falls within the normal range (approximately 33–37 cm at term). Compare the measurement with any pre-existing measurements: rapid enlargement of the head after birth with boggy swelling crossing the suture lines is due to the rare and dangerous condition of subgaleal haemorrhage (p. 1126). There is a strong association with ventouse delivery. If the head is unduly small (below the 2nd centile), consider dysmorphic syndromes, congenital infections or isolated microcephaly. If the head is unduly large from the beginning, consider familial megalencephaly or hydrocephalus. A large head in the presence of widely separated sutures or a full fontanelle requires immediate ultrasound evaluation. Remember that moulding of the skull can lead to an erroneous OFC measurement which returns to normal once the moulding has subsided.

Face

Most babies' faces are unremarkable, apart from perhaps resembling one or other parent. Occasionally, however, the facial appearance is the first clue to an underlying disorder such as Down's syndrome. The bloated cherubic face of infants born to mothers with diabetes is also characteristic (Chapter 22). If unusual facial features are seen, this should prompt a particularly diligent search for other dysmorphic manifestations, but if the baby is asymptomatic and otherwise normal, the appearance may well be familial and a glance at the parents may confirm this.

There is a difference between facial palsy and asymmetric crying facies. The latter is often due to congenital absence of the depressor anguli oris muscle (DAOM); these babies can wrinkle their foreheads and close their eyes, in contrast to babies with a facial nerve palsy. The incidence of absent DAOM is about 0.6–0.8% of the population, and there is an association with CHD.[49]

Ears

Look at the general shape, size and position of the ears and feel the cartilage. Low-set ears are those in which the top of the pinna falls below a line drawn from the outer canthus of the eye at right angles to the facial profile (Fig. 14.1). Abnormally small or large floppy ears are characteristic of several syndromes. Overfolding of the helix can result from fetal constraint, and in mild cases resolves without treatment over the first weeks of life. Taping and splinting has now been shown to be remarkably successful even in cases which would previously have required surgery.[10] Note any preauricular pits, skin tags or accessory auricles. Otoscopic examination does not usually form part of the routine examination.

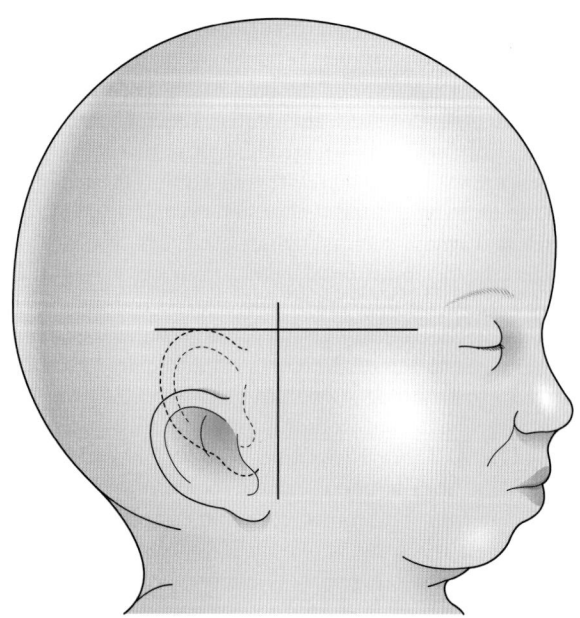

Fig. 14.1 In normal ears (dotted line) the top of the helix lies on a line drawn at right angles to the facial profile from the outer canthus of the eye. Low-set ears (solid line) are those in which the helix is set below the line.

Prevalence of isolated ear tags is 1.7 per 1000, with bilateral tags in 6%.[1] Ear pits and tags can be autosomal dominant, but it is important to assess hearing in these babies. Routine renal ultrasonography is probably unnecessary if ear pits or tags are isolated.[44]

Hearing screening

Congenital bilateral hearing impairment affects about 1:1000 babies, and early aiding is associated with better language, communication, mental health and employment prospects. Much congenital deafness is now known to be genetic, with recessive mutations at the connexin locus accounting for many cases.[55] Universal hearing screening in the neonatal period is feasible and is currently available in the US but not in Europe. Successful screening has been achieved in large studies using transient evoked oto-acoustic emissions with automated threshold brainstem evoked responses in those who fail the initial screen,[79] although arguments still rage about the effectiveness.[70] Most neonatal units in the UK are currently using targeted screening, limiting testing to babies with a family history of congenital deafness, craniofacial abnormalities, significant jaundice or a diagnosis of perinatal infection. Many units test all babies who are ill enough to require admission.

Nose

Inspect the nose for its general shape and width of the bridge. If it appears abnormally wide, measure the distance between the inner canthi: this should not exceed about 2.5 cm in the term infant. The nose can appear quite squashed as a result of intrauterine compression. Occasionally, the septal cartilage is dislocated, and this can be recognised by deviation of the columella. Compression of the tip of the nose causes collapse and increased deviation of the nostrils in this condition, which requires treatment by an ENT surgeon. Flaring of the alae nasi is not normal and its presence indicates some respiratory illness. Babies are obligate nose breathers and hence complete nasal obstruction (diagnosed by failure to mist a mirror) causes intense respiratory distress, which requires immediate investigation. Snuffly noses are quite common, but providing the babies can breathe normally during feeding, serious problems are rarely present; if in doubt, ensure that both nares are patent by passing a fine catheter through each nostril. The mother should be reassured that the symptom will disappear as the baby (and his nose) grows bigger.

Eyes

The eyes should always be inspected for any gross abnormality, noting their size, dimensions and slant; check for any strabismus or nystagmus. A third of newborns have an intermittent exotropia, but esotropia is not normal. Congenital cataract is the commonest form of preventable childhood blindness and evaluating the red reflex is an essential part of the neonatal examination (see below), although it is not feasible to perform full fundoscopy on every baby. Fundoscopy should of course be attempted if there is any question of abnormality. A mydriatic may be needed, and if there is any doubt, the opinion of an ophthalmologist should be sought. Normally, the optic disc appears pale and the temporal side of the retina is less well vascularised than the nasal. Isolated retinal haemorrhages may be seen and have no significance.

Look for (and ask about) any discharge from the eyes. A slight mucoid discharge ('sticky eye') is very common in the first 2 days after birth, but later is likely to be due to failure of canalisation of the nasolacrimal duct. A membranous obstruction in this structure persists in 70% of neonates, but resolves spontaneously by 3 months of age in 70% and by a year in 96%.[84] After a year, probing may be required; earlier in life, simple cleaning of crusts is the best treatment. Referral is not required, but beware photophobia or conjunctivitis which suggest another diagnosis. Occasionally, congenital obstruction of the nasolacrimal duct combines with an obstruction to retrograde flow to produce a dacrocystocoele; a tense blue–grey swelling just beneath the medial canthus. These often become infected and an early ophthalmic opinion should be obtained. A frankly purulent discharge, particularly if accompanied by redness and swelling of the eyelids, should always be taken seriously and demands bacterial investigation and treatment (pp. 841–2). Subconjunctival haemorrhages are very common after birth (analogous to petechiae in the skin) and are harmless, although the mother may need reassurance. The sclerae provide a guide to jaundice, particularly in Afro-Caribbean or Asian babies.

Iris

The iris is normally blue or grey in the newborn. Look for colobomata (keyhole-shaped pupil): if present, there could also be a defect in the retina, and this should prompt a search for other congenital malformations. Babies with aniridia often have a poor visual outcome.

Cornea

Check that the cornea does not appear abnormally large, especially if the baby has prominent eyes. The corneal diameter is normally about 10 mm, and if this is greater than 13 mm (particularly if the cornea is also hazy) the baby might have congenital glaucoma (pp. 839–40). The cornea should be bright and clear; corneal opacities deserve referral to an ophthalmologist as they can be due to herpetic ulceration, posterior corneal defects, endothelial dystrophies or abnormal metabolic infiltrations. Corneal haze after a forceps delivery usually resolves.

Cataracts can be occasionally seen with the naked eye using a bright light shone tangentially. The lens should always be examined through an ophthalmoscope held 6–8 inches from the eye. If the lens is clear, you should be able to see a red retinal reflex. If there is any doubt, an ophthalmological opinion must be sought urgently, as the baby may have a congenital cataract. The best results are obtained after early treatment, before there is any chance of stimulus-deprivation amblyopia (p. 836). A dull red reflex can also be secondary to congenital melanoma or cytomegaloviral retinitis. Unfortunately, the neonatal screen performs poorly in the detection of cataract: 83/235 (35%) of cases diagnosed in the UK between 1995 and 1996 were detected at the newborn screen, with a further 30 cases being uncovered at the 6-week check.[64] As yet, no better strategy has been proposed. Babies in whom cataract is diagnosed must be investigated for the cause (p. 795).

Mouth

Note if the mouth is of normal size or if there is micrognathia. Observe any asymmetry of the corners of the mouth and the nasolabial folds.

Inspection of the inside of the mouth is best done either while the baby is crying lustily or by making him open it (pressing down on the chin sometimes does the trick). It is better not to use a tongue depressor. One should ensure that the palate is intact by seeing it directly; palpation is not enough. It is embarrassing, to say the least, to have missed a cleft in the soft palate which later turns up as a feeding problem or nasal regurgitation.

Minor variations of normal which may be seen include: Epstein's pearls (white patches of microkeratosis akin to milia on the palate or gums, usually at the junction between the hard and soft palate); natal teeth (which are rare in Caucasian populations but are usually best removed, especially if loose); short frenulum or 'tongue tie' (which virtually never needs treatment, p. 381); and bluish swellings (ranulae) on the floor of the mouth which are mucus retention cysts and need no treatment.

Neck

The infant has a relatively short neck, which should be inspected for general shape and symmetry, palpated for any lumps or swellings, and tested for its full range of movements.

A webbed neck may suggest Turner syndrome (pp. 895–6). A very short webbed neck with or without torticollis may indicate underlying abnormalities of the cervical spine (Klippel–Feil syndrome, p. 981). Redundant skin posteriorly is one of the characteristics of Down's syndrome (pp. 785–6).

Cystic hygromas are soft fluctuant swellings, usually arising in the posterior triangle, which transilluminate readily. Sternomastoid 'tumours' are lesions in the sternomastoid muscle caused by haemorrhage or ischaemia resulting in secondary fibrosis.

The clavicles should be palpated for fractures, especially if there is any suggestion of an Erb's palsy, if delivery was a difficult breech extraction, or if there was shoulder dystocia.

Chest and cardiorespiratory system

In spite of advances in antenatal scanning, most CHD is still unsuspected before birth, and babies still present with cyanosis, shock or a murmur. Unfortunately, the neonatal examination performs no better in the detection of CHD or DDH than it does for cataract. Even in the best hands, the neonatal check fails to detect over half of all babies who are subsequently found to have significant heart disease.[2,47,81] A large retrospective study of all births in the northern region of the UK revealed 1590 babies with CHD diagnosed by the age of 1 year from a cohort of 300 102 births.[81] As many as 33% presented with signs before the newborn examination was carried out (five died); of the remaining 1061 babies, the examination revealed an abnormality in just under half. Even when an abnormality was suspected, the usual arrangement for discharge with a 6-week paediatric follow-up was shown to be too late for some; a further nine babies died between discharge and 6 weeks. The main causes of death were hypoplastic left heart, interruption of the aortic arch, and coarctation of the aorta. One of the implications of this study is that a baby with suspected heart disease should be referred for an early definitive cardiological opinion. This has major resource implications in the UK, where paediatric cardiologists are few and far between. Certain groups of babies are at high risk of CHD, including those with Down's syndrome (40–50% have heart defects).

Start by inspecting the chest. Breast swelling is quite normal at this age and a few drops of 'witches' milk' may be expressed from them. These changes are of no significance unless there is obvious inflammation, but the mother may need reassurance.

Many deductions about the cardiorespiratory state can also be made by simple inspection. As well as noting the infant's colour – the single best clue to overall function – observe the respiratory rate and other signs of respiratory distress, such as retractions and grunting. If there is any doubt about the presence of cyanosis, check with a pulse oximeter. Several groups have now suggested that pulse oximetry should be added to the neonatal examination in order to improve the yield of detection of CHD.[42,65,66] About 5% of babies had a postductal oxygen saturation <95% at more than 2 hours of age, but only 1% of babies had a low result when it was checked twice; 10% of these had cardiac disease.[66] As yet, the cost-effectiveness and feasibility of adding pulse oximetry to the routine 'baby check' is not established and it cannot be recommended as routine practice. The pulse oximetry test missed coarctation, still a common cause of unexpected collapse after discharge.[42,66]

The respiratory rate is normally 40–60 breaths/min. A baby whose respiratory rate is persistently above 55 breaths/min needs very careful evaluation and continued observation, because this is unusual. Remember that all infants, particularly preterm ones, can have pauses of 5–10 seconds interspersed with periods of regular breathing (periodic breathing, p. 575). True apnoeic attacks (pp. 573–7) last longer than this and are extremely rare in the full-term neonate. Observe the respiratory pattern. When the infant is quiet, there should be no flaring of the alae nasi, no grunting and no retractions. On crying, some babies, especially if premature, may exhibit mild sternal or subcostal retraction.

The lungs can be auscultated at the same time as the heart, but by and large this is an unrewarding exercise if there are no respiratory symptoms.

Palpate the precordium for any thrills or a pronounced ventricular heave. The point of maximal impulse is usually found in the left fourth intercostal space inside the midclavicular line. Percussion of an asymptomatic infant's chest is a waste of time.

Check the peripheral pulses: a persistent ductus arteriosus with a significant left-to-right shunt produces a bounding quality. Always palpate the femoral pulses: if they are absent or difficult to feel, suspect coarctation. Four-limb blood pressure may help by confirming a differential between the upper and lower limbs; however, normal newborns can have a difference of up to 20 ± 3.5 mmHg.[62] A difference of 20 mmHg or more suggests coarctation (pp. 649–50).

Innocent heart murmurs

An innocent murmur is one that does not signify cardiac disease. Approximately 60% of normal newborns have a systolic murmur at the age of 2 hours,[9] but the incidence falls to around 1% by the time the routine neonatal examination is performed.[2,24] Murmur is not the only sign of significant heart disease, and currently the neonatal examination detects only about a half of all babies who eventually present in the neonatal period with significant problems. Ainsworth et al[2] found a high incidence of problems when a murmur was present, but all those who care for the newborn must be aware that the absence of a murmur does not guarantee a normal heart, and vice versa. It is possible to make a positive diagnosis of an innocent murmur using clinical skills alone,[24] and the following features were emphasised in a study from Oxford:[4]

- grade 1–2/6 murmur at the left sternal edge;
- no clicks on auscultation;
- normal pulses;
- otherwise normal clinical examination.

When a positive diagnosis of an innocent murmur was made in this way, no babies with cardiac disease were identified with subsequent echocardiography. About 23% of those who were offered echocardiography had significant cardiac disease.[24]

The usual origin of an innocent murmur is the acute angle at the pulmonary artery bifurcation; a few cases have patent ductus arteriosus or tricuspid regurgitation which resolves rapidly. McCrindle and his colleagues[51] suggested six features to help non-cardiologists identify significant murmurs:

- pansystolic;
- grade 3/6 or more;
- best heard in the upper left sternal border;
- harsh quality;
- abnormal second heart sound;
- early or mid systolic click.

Clinical examination was correct 98% of the time when similar criteria were applied to childhood murmurs, albeit by paediatric cardiologists.[51,74] Clinical evaluation without laboratory tests was equally effective in the hands of general paediatricians in Denmark.[34] ECG and CXR have traditionally been used to assist in the classification of murmurs as innocent, but the clinical diagnosis is rarely changed by ECG[57,74] or CXR,[57,77] and these tests should be abandoned for this purpose. An examination by an experienced colleague is a better aid to the identification of genuinely innocent murmurs. I agree with Hall & Elliman[33] that the widespread availability of echocardiography now means that this investigation, with the accompanying expert consultation, should be offered early to babies whose neonatal murmur cannot confidently be classified as innocent.

Mention of 'heart murmurs' produces intense anxiety, and talking about 'holes in the heart' is guaranteed to produce a flood of tears; now that it is clear that many are due to pulmonary vessel 'kinking' **in a normal heart**, this is perhaps a less disturbing explanation. You can reassure the parents that 80–90% of murmurs found in the neonatal period will disappear during the first year, most of them within the first 3 months, and that if this is the case, the baby will be discharged from outpatients. A practical guide to the action to be taken when a murmur is discovered is given in Table 14.2.

Abdomen

Inspection

Simple observation may yield quite a lot of information. Abdominal distension is easily appreciated, and because of the poorly developed abdominal musculature and scanty subcutaneous fat, the intra-abdominal organs can sometimes be seen, particularly the bowel in premature infants. Look for any discharge or reddening of the skin around the umbilicus, which is a common source of infection. The state of the cord stump will depend on the age of the baby, but the cord usually separates by 2 weeks and a delay of longer than 30 days should be investigated (pp. 369–70). Shortly after birth the three vessels are easily seen. A single umbilical artery is present in 0.3% of newborns, and there is an association with renal abnormalities, which were found in 7% of cases in one series.[8] A single umbilical artery in a baby with any other problem justifies further investigation of the renal tract. There is no need to investigate for isolated single umbilical artery in a well baby with no other problem.

Further investigation of the renal tract will also be required for infants who were found to have abnormalities on prenatal

Table 14.2 Action to be taken when a heart murmur is heard

Is there peripheral circulatory collapse?	If so, immediate investigation is required
Is there central cyanosis?	Confirm with pulse oximeter. Urgent investigation
Is there any evidence of heart failure? (tachycardia, tachypnoea, enlarged liver)	If so, immediate investigation is required
Can the femoral pulses be felt easily?	If not, check four-limb blood pressure
Are there any dysmorphic features?	If so, investigation should be done
Is the murmur grade 1–2/6, systolic, not harsh, heard at the left sternal edge only in a well baby with normal pulses?	The murmur is innocent. If the baby is less than 48 hours old and remaining in hospital, listen again before discharge as the murmur may have gone. If mother and baby are about to go home, tell the parents the diagnosis and arrange follow-up at 3–4 weeks. Some units offer echocardiography to these infants
Is the murmur grade 3+ or more, running into diastole, or pansystolic, or is there a click, abnormal second heart sound or femoral pulses which are difficult to feel?	This murmur may be pathological. Even if the baby is well, ask a more senior colleague to listen. Watch the baby for signs of heart failure. Arrange echocardiography with the accompanying expert opinion as soon as possible. Carry out pulse oximetry, a chest X-ray and ECG as a baseline and to assist in differential diagnosis

ultrasonography. Vesicoureteric reflux is now known to be a familial disease; 30% of infants screened because of a positive family history were found to have the condition.[73] In future this may emerge as a further important part of neonatal screening. A thick cord with profuse jelly is characteristic of infants of diabetic mothers and a thin one is often seen in small-for-dates babies. Green discoloration indicates the passage of meconium before birth. The stump becomes dark and shrivelled and separates at about 10–14 days, longer if antibiotic prophylaxis is used. Persistent discharge should make one think of a patent urachus (p. 233). Note if there is an umbilical hernia and reassure the mother that no treatment is indicated. Record the time of first passage of meconium and urine.

Palpation

It is essential for your hands to be warm and for the infant to be quiet and relaxed; if necessary, have him suck on a dummy or a clean finger. Remember that a baby with a full stomach may well regurgitate milk if you press too hard, often to the distress of the mother who may have just spent a lot of time feeding and then cleaning up the baby!

Palpate the abdominal musculature; there is frequently a diastasis of the recti. Feel for the liver edge, which can be up to 2 cm below the right costal margin in normal infants. The kidneys are usually palpable with patience, and some observers have even gone so far as to state that failure to feel them indicates their absence. It is, however, probably much more important to detect any abnormally large renal masses. The spleen can often be 'tipped', but if more than 1 cm is palpable, investigation is needed. Feel for an enlarged bladder; if present, try to express it and observe the urinary stream. Auscultation need not form part of the routine abdominal examination unless there is reason to suspect gastrointestinal abnormality (distension, bile-stained vomit, failure to pass meconium, or bloody stools).

Genitalia

Male

Inspect the penis for length (normally about 3 cm); occasionally, a penis looks deceptively short, but palpation will usually disclose a respectable organ buried in suprapubic fat. True micropenis is rare but is an important sign of congenital hypopituitarism (pp. 870–1). Check the position of the urethral meatus, and if it is abnormally situated, describe the hypospadias as glandular, coronal, mid-shaft or perineal; also inspect the shaft of the penis for curvature and compress it at its base to stimulate an erection, which may reveal a latent chordee. Glandular hypospadias without chordee usually needs no treatment, but in more severe degrees of hypospadias the baby will need corrective surgery at some time before school age. All cases should have the benefit of specialist advice and the parents must be told not to circumcise the baby, because the foreskin will be essential for the future repair.

Always ask about the urinary stream in boys. A poor stream may be present if there is meatal stenosis with hypospadias; constant dribbling of urine is nearly always abnormal and may indicate urethral valves.

Examine the scrotum for rugosity and feel for the testes, although the size of the scrotum is not a good guide to the position of the testes in the newborn. At full term, both testes should be palpable, even if retractile. Six per cent of male babies have at least one testis which is undescended at birth (more in VLBW babies); after 3 months of age, further natural descent is unlikely. If one or both testes are undescended at the neonatal examination, a follow-up appointment should be made, but if the testis is not descended by 3 months, the baby should be referred for surgical review. A bluish black discoloration of the scrotum suggests testicular torsion, especially now that very few baby boys acquire bruising of their genitalia during a vaginal breech delivery. Neonatal testicular torsion occurs some time before birth in almost all cases, and in this situation the testis is hard and not tender.[14] Urgent referral to a paediatric surgeon is indicated because, although the testis is usually already infarcted, most recommend that the contralateral testis is fixed.

Hydroceles can occur in the newborn period, but usually resolve spontaneously and do not require treatment. Examine the groins for indirect inguinal herniae; these are not uncommon, particularly in preterm infants, and can usually be reduced easily. If present, the mother should be warned about the symptoms and signs of incarceration/strangulation and an urgent surgical appointment organised so that early surgery can be arranged.

Female

Inspect the vulva – the clitoris and labia minora are relatively prominent in preterm infants, but at full term the labia majora should cover the labia minora although the clitoris may still appear relatively large. There is often a white mucoid vaginal discharge which is occasionally bloodstained; this is normal and the mother should be reassured accordingly. Small hymenal skin tags or mucoid cysts which resolve spontaneously may occur around the vaginal opening. Inguinal herniae are rare in the female and their presence should raise the question of other abnormalities in the genital tract. For further advice, see Chapter 39.

At this stage in the examination, check the position of the anus and anal tone. A 'wink' can be produced by gently touching the anal margin.

Spine

With the baby prone, inspect the back for any obvious curvature and look for any midline abnormality over the spine and base of skull, such as a swelling, dimple, hairy patch or naevus. Any of these may indicate an underlying abnormality of the vertebral column or spinal cord; occult spinal dysraphism is the most common spinal axis malformation by far, and early detection should prevent upper urinary tract deterioration, infection, and permanent damage to the nervous system.

Simple sacrococcygeal pits are common and harmless; in a study from St George's Hospital, London, no infant in a series of 75 with sacral dimple or pit alone was found to have a spinal abnormality.[26] The problem lies in defining the 'simple dimple' or 'simple pit', because any midline lesion other than those in or just above the natal cleft should be investigated. Similarly, any lesion at any level with a fatty pad, hairy patch or an area of atretic skin deserves further investigation. One helpful definition was given by Kriss & Desai.[43] These authors carefully evaluated 207 neonates with 216 dorsal cutaneous stigmata who were born in their hospital between 1993 and 1996 (the 207 were 4.8% of the births). All 207 (but not all babies) had ultrasound of the spine. Magnetic resonance imaging (MRI) was performed only if the ultrasound was abnormal. Of the 160 with 'simple' dimples – defined as being less than 2.5 cm from the anus, less than 5 mm wide, and with a midline placement and no other cutaneous stigmata – no baby had spinal dysraphism. Sixteen of the other babies were found to have abnormalities. Ultrasound was used to assess the position of the conus of the spinal cord (around L1–2 in the

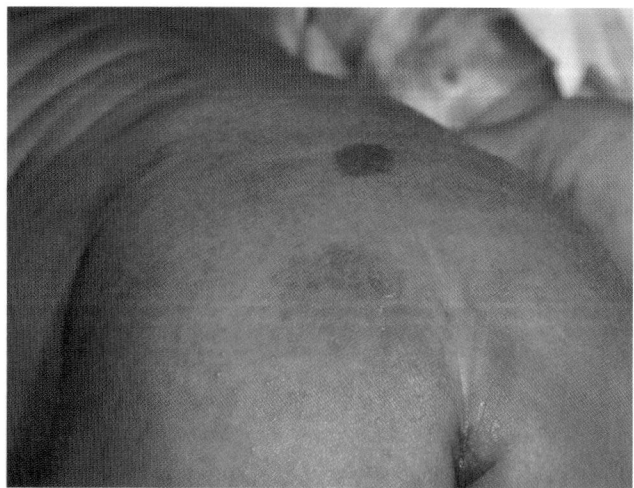

Fig. 14.2 A simple dimple above the anus, with an erythematous macule in the midline over the spine at a higher level.

newborn, below L3 abnormal[36]), the mobility of the nerve roots, and the presence of an intrathecal mass. Fig. 14.2 shows an example of a 'simple dimple' but with an associated midline erythematous macule, which is a trigger for investigation. Kriss & Desai[43] did not attempt to assess the incidence of spinal lesions in the babies without cutaneous markers; 50–80% of late-presenting cases with spinal dysraphism have a cutaneous marker.

Ultrasound is not the gold standard, and the radiological expertise is not always available; in groups at very high risk, MRI is indicated.[52] Both MRI and ultrasound are better than plain radiographs.

See page 1191 for more information on spinal cord diastematomyelia and midline abnormalities. See *http://www.btinternet. com/~tetheredcordresources/personal_story.htm* for a description of the lifelong consequences of cord tethering arising from spinal dysraphism. Always examine the back in the midline if at follow-up a baby has a limp, foot abnormalities, bladder or bowel problems, or scoliosis.

Upper limbs

Inspect the arms for shape, posture, symmetry and size. In normal upper limbs, the fingertips reach to mid-thigh when the arms are abducted to the body. Examine the hand for any flexion deformities of the fingers and inspect the palms for the arrangement of creases. Although about 45% of individuals with Down's syndrome have single transverse palmar creases, this finding occurs unilaterally in 4% and bilaterally in 1% of the Caucasian population and is a normal phenotypic variant in the Chinese population (16.8%). Polydactyly (hands and feet) is sometimes a familial trait, but look carefully for any other dysmorphic features. All digital remnants should be removed surgically. Previously some were tied off with black silk and left to separate by dry gangrene, but this left a stump which produced an unsightly lump or a painful neuroma in many cases.

Observe spontaneous arm movements: stroking the hand or forearm is sometimes necessary to elicit active motion in the shoulder, elbow, wrist and hand. Test passive movements for muscle tone and range of motion. Owing to intrauterine restriction of space and activity, the newborn may lack some elbow extension. Lack of active movement and pain on passive manoeuvres suggests a fracture or infection, whereas in brachial plexus or cervical spine injury passive motion is not restricted. A brachial plexus lesion is revealed by lack of movement in the arm; initially the arm is flaccid. After 48 hours, an upper palsy can be distinguished from a complete palsy. In an upper root palsy (C5, 6, sometimes C7) the arm is internally rotated and pronated, and there is no active abduction or elbow flexion (Erb's palsy, the waiter's tip position). The incidence of brachial plexus palsy remains around 1.6–2.9 per 1000,[63] although a recent UK study reported a lower incidence of 0.4 per 1000.[22] In a complete palsy of upper and lower roots, the arm is flail; there may be a ptosis and a Horner's syndrome due to damage to the stellate ganglion adjacent to C8 and T1. Phrenic palsy should be considered in these cases. The hand may become clawed (Klumpke's paralysis). Whilst the prognosis of brachial plexus lesions is generally good, with most series reporting a recovery rate of 75–95%, this may be over-optimistic: over half the babies in the UK series still had signs at 6 months.[22] The results of surgical repair have improved markedly since the early days, and babies who have no recovery in biceps function by 3 months should be referred to a specialist.[27]

Lower limbs

Inspect the legs and feet for posture, symmetry, general size and shape, as well as for any obvious deformities. Observe spontaneous or stimulated active movements and test the range of passive movements.

The midpoint of the newborn baby's length is just above the umbilicus (cf. the symphysis pubis in the adult). Asymmetry in leg girth or length suggests one of the limb reduction defects (p. 806). Some restriction of joint motion is usual, secondary to limitation of intrauterine space. Babies who were vertex presentations usually have fully flexed hips and knees, but in those who were extended breech presentations, the knees may remain fully extended for a few days, so that the feet are somewhere near the mouth. The knees may lack up to 30° of full extension in the neonate. The tibiae are often laterally bowed and internally rotated. The feet should be inspected for their general configuration. They may provide confirmatory evidence of dysmorphic syndromes, such as the 'rocker bottom' shape and short hallux in Edward's syndrome. A convex 'rocker bottom' sole and a rigid foot may also indicate congenital vertical talus which will require surgery.[75] Puffy feet and hypoplastic nails are characteristic of Turner syndrome.

The feet and ankles may be found in many positions, most of which are related to intrauterine moulding (especially if there has been oligohydramnios); much more rarely, there is an underlying neurological deficit. A calcaneovalgus position of the foot is almost invariably due to fetal position in utero and will correct in time, with or without simple manipulation. If there is an equinovarus position, without using undue force an attempt should be made to overcorrect it by abduction and dorsiflexion of the foot

and ankle so that the little toe touches the outside of the leg. If this manoeuvre is successful, no treatment is indicated, but deformities that cannot be so corrected (true talipes equinovarus) require urgent orthopaedic attention (pp. 972–3). Simple metatarsus adductus (i.e. inturning of the forefoot) is not uncommon, 90% of cases resolving with no treatment.

Over-riding toes are common; syndactyly is often familial; neither usually needs treatment. It is most important to explain the nature and natural history of these minor deformities to the parents.

Hips

Screening for congenital dislocation of the hip was introduced into the UK in 1966 and remains one of the most important items in the newborn examination. This condition is now termed developmental dysplasia of the hip (DDH) (pp. 967–71). The incidence of DDH is around 1–2 per 1000 births, whereas the incidence of unstable hips is around 10 per 1000 births. Expert management of DDH diagnosed in the neonatal period can be expected to produce a normal hip, while treatment initiated after the first year of life is usually followed by a worse result, even after surgical treatment. Up to a quarter of adult hip osteoarthritis requiring surgery may be associated with DDH.[50] Sadly, despite initial confidence in the ability of the Ortolani and Barlow tests to detect DDH, the number of cases diagnosed late (0.2 per 1000) has not reduced and may even have increased.[71] The number of babies who require surgery for DDH has not much changed since the 1960s, at 0.78 per 1000 births.[29] This study showed that 70% of cases were not detected by the current neonatal screening examination, and it has even been suggested that enthusiastic or repeated clinical examination may provoke harm.[53]

The Standing Medical Advisory Committee[76] recommended three clinical screening examinations for the newborn in order to detect DDH. These were to be conducted at less than 24 hours of age, at discharge from the maternity hospital, and at 6 weeks. Several studies, including that of Glazener et al,[28] have shown that two clinical examinations in the newborn period does not improve the yield for detection of DDH, and very few UK maternity units currently offer two hip checks. There are as yet no specific UK Government guidelines regarding ultrasonographic screening. The UK National Screening Committee (founded in 1996: www.nsc.nhs.uk) recommends that an ultrasound be performed in babies with an abnormal clinical examination, but considers that the position for those with risk factors alone has yet to be evaluated. DDH is commoner following breech presentation, in females, if there is oligohydramnios, and in those with a positive family history.[11] In spite of the recommendations of the UK Screening Committee, the use of 'selective' ultrasound for babies with risk factors, in addition to ultrasound for those with a suspect clinical examination, is widespread practice in the UK at present. The reasons for this include concern that clinical examination in the hands of an inexperienced examiner performs little better than no screen at all, with a detection rate of around 35%.[13] A check by an experienced examiner or universal ultrasound screening was followed by a good result in 76–80%,

Table 14.3 Screening strategy for using ultrasound in the detection of developmental dysplasia of the hip

- Breech presentation (whether delivered by caesarean section or vaginally), particularly with extended knees
- Family history of dysplastic hip
- Any deformity suggesting intrauterine compression (e.g. torticollis), or oligohydramnios
- Any abnormality of the lower limb
- Clicky hip on clinical examination, or one with restricted abduction
- If sufficient manpower available, consider firstborn females

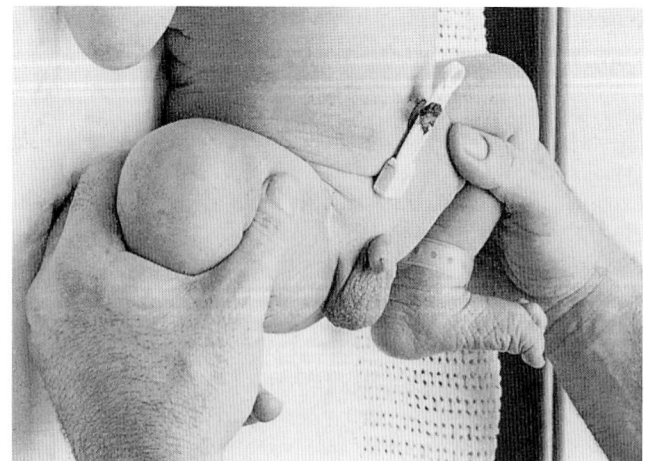

Fig. 14.3 Ortolani test.

with 'selective' ultrasound achieving around 60% detection rate in this modelling study.[13]

Ultrasound can detect clinically stable but anatomically abnormal hips, and show normality in clinically suspect hips.[30] Wholesale ultrasound screening is labour-intensive, produces a high number of false positive results with a concomitant high early treatment rate, is expensive, and is probably not the solution for the UK at present.[20] A study in Norway showed that universal screening was of marginal benefit.[68] Nevertheless, several large European programmes are in place, and in the UK the Coventry results are impressive.[18]

In my view, the best current strategy is to use selective ultrasound (that is, ultrasound based on risk factors; Table 14.3) together with clinical neonatal examination. The choice of risk factors depends on the local population and availability of ultrasound time; for example, screening all breech infants (approximately 4% of births) yields 22% of the cases of DDH, whereas adding firstborn females (approximately 18% of births) would uncover a further 29% of cases, bringing the total yield to 51%, at a 'cost' of screening 23% of all births (breech and/or firstborn females).[83] The risk factors in Table 14.3 should also be used to identify infants who need to be examined again at 6 weeks of age with extra care.

The cornerstone of the screening strategy for DDH remains a careful history and clinical examination. The Ortolani/Barlow manoeuvres must be performed in every newborn. Details follow, although these tests are hard to describe in words and are much better taught by demonstration. A teaching aid, the 'baby hippy' is also available, although rarely used. The timing of the examination is crucial: most unstable hips that are detected by clinical examination (or ultrasound) during the first day are false positive findings. There is a therapeutic dilemma between splinting all unstable hips immediately, risking avascular necrosis in otherwise normal hips, and delaying treatment, risking a falsely reassuring second examination[12] and a poor result. Avascular necrosis is the main disadvantage arising from 'overtreatment' of babies with unstable hips demonstrated with ultrasound who will not go on to develop a dislocation.[13]

Procedure

The infant should be lying supine on a flat firm surface, with the legs relaxed, pacified if necessary by sucking on a dummy or finger. The examination may well make the baby cry and interpretation is difficult if the thigh muscles are actively contracting.

First, straighten out the legs and look for any obvious inequality in length, and then carry out Ortolani's test.[58] This manoeuvre is designed to return a dislocated femoral head to the acetabulum. Fully flex the knees and flex the hips to a right angle. Place the middle finger of each hand over the greater trochanters, thumbs over the internal aspect of the thighs, and palms over the knees. Then, simultaneously, pull the leg away from the pelvis and slowly abduct and externally rotate the hips, pressing forwards and medially with the middle fingers (Fig. 14.3). A previously dislocated hip is indicated by a definite 'clunk' as the displaced femoral head slips forward into the acetabulum, rather like engaging the gear lever of a car. This is a quite different sensation from a ligamentous 'click', which is more common but may still be of significance.[40] It does, however, take some experience to tell the difference, the clue being whether there is any sensation of movement. In almost all normal babies it is possible to fully abduct the hips so that the knees almost touch the couch. Inability to do so may indicate a dislocated hip that cannot be reduced and is an indication for an ultrasound scan (Table 14.3).

The next stage of the examination is to do Barlow's test.[7] This test is designed to 'dislocate' an unstable hip that is in joint. Some hips are 'loose' but cannot be completely dislocated using this clinical test. Hold the hips and knees as before. With the hips at about 70° abduction, test each hip in turn by pressing forwards and medially (i.e. towards the symphysis pubis) with the finger. Normally no movement is felt, but if the hip is dislocated, the femur is felt to move, again with a 'clunk' as it slips into the acetabulum. The reverse procedure is then performed by pressing backwards and laterally with the thumb. Normally there is again no movement, but a dislocatable hip will 'clunk' out of the acetabulum and will return there when the pressure is released.

Following the examination and ultrasound screening for high-risk groups, it should be possible to classify the hip(s) into one of the following categories:

- normal;
- a stable hip with acetabular dysplasia on ultrasound (found because of positive family history, etc.);
- a clinically unstable ('loose') hip with acetabular dysplasia on ultrasound;

- a dislocatable hip (one that can be pushed out of the acetabulum and back again) – Barlow positive;
- a reducible dislocated hip – Ortolani positive;
- an irreducible dislocated hip (this may easily be missed);
- a dislocatable or dislocated hip secondary to another problem e.g. CNS disease.

For further information on the management of these types of DDH, see Chapter 38.

Neurological

Although much has been written about the neurological assessment of the neonate, formal testing is seldom needed during routine examination of the newborn. More detail is contained in Chapter 41. Enough screening information can usually be gleaned from talking to the mother and from carefully watching, handling and listening to the baby throughout the examination.

The following general observations can act as a screening test, although one must take into account both gestational age (considered in more detail elsewhere) and postnatal age. The infant may be neurologically very labile during the first few days, and the most meaningful results are obtained only after this time. For a more comprehensive neurological assessment of both preterm and full-term neonates, see Dubowitz & Dubowitz.[16]

Behavioural state

Healthy term infants should move between behavioural states, spending most time in quiet and active sleep.

Posture

The undisturbed normal neonate lies predominantly in a flexed position with no lateral preference (Fig. 14.4). When prone, the knees are often tucked under the abdomen. The fists are clenched and the thumbs are intermittently furled. With the head in the midline, the limbs are roughly symmetrical. Remember, however, that the presentation at birth can influence posture for several days.

Spontaneous motor activity

Normal infants move their limbs in an alternating fashion. Many babies may appear jittery. The prevalence of jittering was 44% in a sample of almost 1000 infants in Boston examined between 8 and 72 hours of age.[60] Half were jittery solely when crying and the remainder were jittery during several behavioural states. How to distinguish jittering from fits is discussed in Chapter 41.

Muscle tone and strength

This is tested by:

1. Assessing resistance to passive movements.
2. Pull-to-sit manoeuvre (Fig. 14.5) Pull the baby up from the supine position by his wrists. In term infants there should be some elbow flexion and the head should come up almost in line with the body. When held sitting, the head should remain erect for 2–3 seconds. The palmar grasp reflex may be tested at the same time.

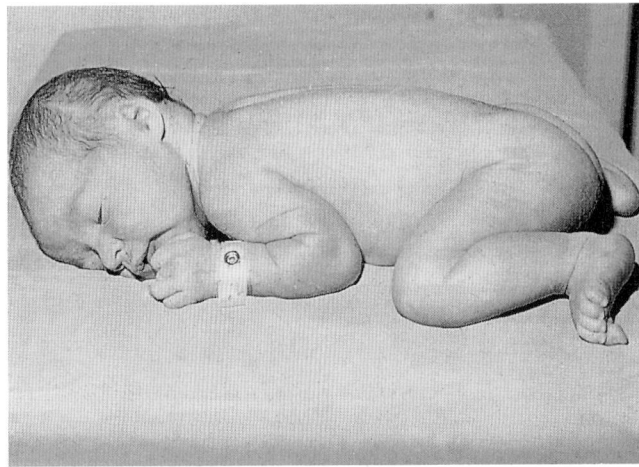

Fig. 14.4 Posture in prone position.

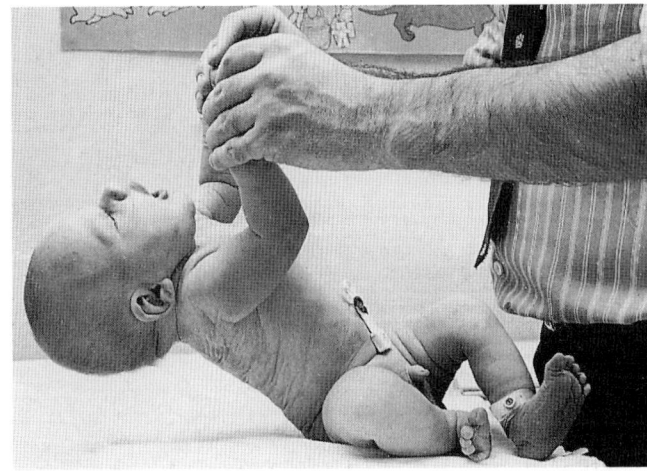

Fig. 14.5 Pull-to-sit manoeuvre. Note flexion of elbows and slight flexion of neck as the infant is pulled up by his wrists.

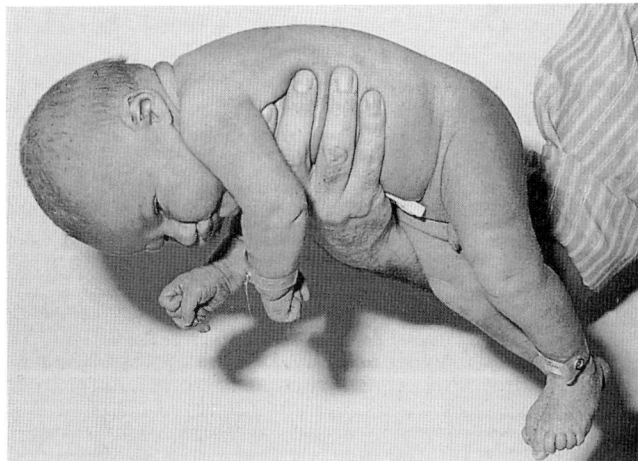

Fig. 14.6 Ventral suspension. Note the flexed arms and the head lying almost on a plane with the body.

3. Ventral suspension (Fig. 14.6). Hold the baby in the air with a hand under the chest – he should be able to hold his head in line with his body for a few seconds and he should be able to flex his limbs against gravity.

Other general observations

Crying will almost certainly be noted at some time during the examination. Pay particular attention if it is either high-pitched or very weak, or if the infant is reported to cry excessively.

Feeding and sucking patterns will be obvious from the history.

The eyes have already been discussed – they should lie in the mid-position in the orbit and move in a conjugate fashion; note any constant deviation, persistent strabismus and nystagmus.

Suspicious neurological signs

With practice and experience, one is soon able to judge from the history and handling of an infant during the examination whether he is behaving normally. The purpose of such a screening procedure is to pick out those infants who merit more detailed study and follow-up. The features that should arouse suspicion and which need careful follow-up are:

- persistent failure to suck properly;
- a high-pitched cry;
- extreme irritability or 'starey-eyed' appearance;
- abnormal posturing, e.g. opisthotonus, excessive fisting, constantly fisted thumbs;
- generalised persistent hypertonia;
- 'frog' posture or generalised hypotonia; paucity of spontaneous movements, including facial expressions;
- asymmetric movements;
- a history of convulsions;
- midline lesions over the spine.

Feeding assessment: screening for breast-milk insufficiency

Complete failure of lactogenesis is very rare. Secondary lactation insufficiency is more common and occurs in about 10% of women; risk factors include flat or inverted nipples, breast engorgement and sore nipples, leading to problems latching on, with the consequence that insufficiently frequent nursing leads to a reduction in the milk supply. Although the assessment of breastfeeding is primarily a midwifery task, it is important that feeding is established before the baby goes home. Breast-milk insufficiency is the underlying reason for many readmissions for jaundice, and there has been a resurgence in hypernatraemic dehydration. It is no longer standard practice in the UK to weigh babies daily, or as part of the discharge examination, although the American Academy of Pediatrics do support weighing. Laing & Wong have called for the re-introduction of weighing, but so far there have been few moves in this direction in spite of a general murmur of support from the paediatric community.[45]

Biochemical screening

The list of conditions which can be identified by screening a blood sample in the newborn period grows longer every year (Chapter 43), and various pressure groups have campaigned for the introduction of tests for maple syrup urine disease, congenital adrenal hyperplasia, galactosaemia, biotinidase deficiency and familial hyperlipidaemia, for example. Screening for cystic fibrosis is to be introduced into England (and probably Scotland) in the near future, following a Government decision in July 2001.[21,56] Tandem mass spectrometry enables the measurement of many compounds on dried blood spots. As a result, screening for medium-chain acyl CoA dehydrogenase (MCAD) deficiency and glutaric aciduria type I has been suggested; both of these inborn errors of metabolism are easily treatable, with early intervention offering the potential to prevent death and neurological disability. MCAD deficiency is as common as phenylketonuria, and the results of an evaluation of screening are awaited. The UK Health Technology assessment programme recommended that screening for these disorders be given a high priority in the 1990s, but many clinicians in this field remain disillusioned and frustrated by the lack of progress since then.[48]

Health education

The normal newborn examination represents an opportunity to provide advice about well-baby care. Information is contained in the parent-held child health records, but a selection of leaflets on the following topics should be available, and the examining doctor needs to be prepared to give advice on a range of topics, including those following. Women who reported receiving healthcare advice were more satisfied with the consultation about their newborn than those who were not offered such advice.[80] Mothers appreciated advice on topics such as jaundice, skin care, sleeping, and stool and nappy care.

- **Jaundice** – kernicterus is a preventable disease, and its resurgence has been a distressing feature of the otherwise welcome early-discharge policy. Jaundice is the most common reason for readmission to the maternity unit. Leaflets should be available informing parents of the importance of deepening jaundice, particularly in babies who become sleepy and develop an unusual cry. Health professionals need education that abnormal neurological signs in a very jaundiced baby are an emergency, and that babies of certain ethnic groups are at higher risk because of the chance of G6PD deficiency.[59]
- **Cot death prevention**[25] – babies should sleep alone, on their backs; parents should not smoke; infant bedrooms should be kept at a comfortable temperature of about 18°C and babies should be kept warm but not overclothed. There may be local initiatives in place for Care of the Next Infant (CONI) – next siblings of infants who died of cot death.
- **Prevention of haemorrhagic disease of the newborn** – if the parents choose oral vitamin K and the baby is to be breastfed, further oral doses of vitamin K are needed (p. 372). Local policies may vary as to which babies are not considered suitable for oral vitamin K prophylaxis, i.e. require intramuscular treatment because they are at high risk of vitamin K deficiency bleeding. Examples include preterm babies, babies whose mothers are taking antituberculous or anticonvulsant drugs, and babies with evidence of liver disease.
- **Breastfeeding promotion** – the hospital should try to become a 'baby friendly' environment. The simple rules that have

been shown to help promote breastfeeding (Chapter 16) should be followed. A breastfeeding counsellor should be on hand to provide advice and suitable literature.

- **Sleeping** – advice on sleeping position, co-sleeping and bedding ties in with cot death prevention. Parents may welcome suggestions regarding websites or books with information about sleep routines, crying babies, and colic.
- **Hearing screening** – until universal hearing screening is introduced, parents should be given advice on signs which suggest that a baby might not be hearing properly, such as failing to startle to loud sounds, failing to turn to sound or quieten when spoken to (especially singing or 'motherese'), and failing to make tuneful babble.
- **Nutrition advice** – advice on weaning (no cow's milk until a year, to avoid iron deficiency) can begin in the maternity hospital.
- **Hygiene advice** – need for and methods of sterilising bottles, dummies, etc.; nappy care.
- **Sibling management** – many parents request literature on dealing with rivalry.
- **Screening for those in need of immediate vaccination** – this mainly refers to hepatitis and TB vaccination. For information, see Chapter 29, Part 2.
- **HIV-positive mothers** – treatment of babies should begin immediately for the best results. In the UK, HIV-positive mothers are advised against breastfeeding.
- **Advice on handling** – how to deal with crying babies – no shaking.
- **Safe transport in cars** – the newborn period is a good time to give advice on the purchase of safe types of car seat and to encourage their use.
- **Maternal depression** – those working in a maternity hospital should be aware of the maternal depression scales and how to administer them. Literature informing mothers about this common and important problem and where to get help could help prevent tragedy. Screening for depression is not advocated at present.

Gestational age

The most reliable basis for assigning gestational age is an early obstetric ultrasound, and when this agrees with the mother's menstrual dates this gives the best assessment. An evaluation of the neonatal methods of estimating gestational age revealed that even the best were only half as accurate as those based on obstetric ultrasound at 15–19 weeks of gestation.[78] The clinical methods had 95% confidence intervals of 17 days, whereas the obstetric ultrasound had 95% confidence intervals of less than 7 days. Any maturity estimation based on ultrasound obtained only during the second half of pregnancy is unreliable, and information from uterine size, date of quickening, etc. is valueless from the neonatal point of view.

The criteria used for estimating gestational age after birth may be divided into those that are based on physical maturation and those that are dependent on development of the nervous system. Many complex scoring systems have been devised.

Some criteria are more valuable than others, and little is lost by using only a few items.[41,61] The physical items proved more robust than the items assessing tone and posture in the evaluation of Wariyar et al, and a retrospective assessment based on when the infant acquired the ability to suck and swallow reliably (34–35 weeks) was surprisingly accurate, providing the infant was not oxygen dependent.[78] Direct ophthalmoscopy can be used to visualise the lens, although the cornea is usually too opaque for this to be possible in very preterm babies (whose eyelids may also be fused). After about 27 weeks, a grading system can be applied to the vessels of the lens: these cover the entire anterior surface between 27 and 28 weeks, reach only to the middle of the lens by 31–32 weeks, and are at the periphery by 33–34 weeks.[37] This method of assessment is not much used because it requires dilatation of the pupil and is only applicable at less than 48 hours of age.

Physical characteristics

The physical signs that are most valuable in the assessment of gestational age are ear firmness, breast and genital development, creases on the soles of the feet, and hair development. Tone and posture are also valuable (see next section).

The skin of the very immature infant (<27 weeks) appears dark red in colour because it is so thin and fragile; it gradually thickens and by full term is starting to desquamate. Blood vessels may at first be prominent and later disappear. Very fine lanugo hair is present initially and gradually vanishes by full term. The nails may reach the fingertips by 32 weeks but extend beyond them at term. Plantar skin creases are absent in immature infants but start to appear at around 32 weeks and gradually increase to cover the heel by full term. Plantar skin creases are only useful if they are evaluated in the first few hours. The ears (pinnae) are flat in very preterm babies, in whom they have no cartilage and remain in bizarre shapes after folding. From about 33 weeks, some cartilage can be felt, the pinna starts incurving and recoils after folding, so that at term the ear is firm and fully shaped with immediate recoil. The breasts of the very immature infant are non-existent, even the nipple being barely visible. A breast nodule is palpable by about 36 weeks. In the male, the testes descend to the inguinal canal after about 29 weeks but may not be fully in the scrotum until term, the latter becoming progressively more rugose during this time. The immature female has a prominent clitoris with relatively small, widely separated labia majora. By full term, both labia minora and clitoris are covered by the larger labia majora.

Various attempts have been made to quantify some of these changes by using scoring systems. Farr et al[23] used a system of 34 points derived from 11 criteria; Dubowitz et al[15] used the same physical criteria with a total of 35 points. Parkin et al[61] produced a much simpler scheme with 13 points derived from only four of the above criteria. This simple system proved as accurate as the Dubowitz or expanded Ballard[5,6] score if half scores were allotted.[78] The new Ballard score[5] (Fig. 14.7) is valid for very preterm infants, although the accuracy in this group has been questioned.

Neuromuscular Maturity

	−1	0	1	2	3	4	5
Posture							
Square window (wrist)	>90°	90°	60°	45°	35°	0°	
Arm recoil		180°	140°–180°	110°–140°	90°–110°	<90°	
Popliteal angle	180°	160°	140°	120°	100°	90°	<90°
Scarf sign							
Heal to ear							

Physical Maturity

								Maturity rating	
Skin	Sticky friable transparent	Gelatinous red, translucent	Smooth pink, visable veins	Superficial peeling and/or rash. few veins	Cracking pale areas rare veins	Parchment deep cracking no vessels	Leathery cracked wrinkled	Score	Weeks
Lanugo	None	Sparse	Abundant	Thinning	Bald areas	Mostly bald		−10	20
								−5	22
Planter surface	Heel–toe 40–50mm: −1 <40mm: −2	>50 mm no crease	faint red marks	Anterior transverse crease only	Creases ant. 2/3	Creases over entire sole		0	24
								5	26
								10	28
Breast	Imperceptible	Barely perceptible	Flat areola no bud	Stippled areola 1–2 mm bud	Raised areola 3–4 mm bud	Full areola 5–10 mm bud		15	30
								20	32
Eye/ear	Lids fused loosely: −1 tightly: −2	Lids open pinna flat stays folded	Sl. curved pinna; soft; slow recoil	Well-curved pinna; soft but ready recoil	Formed and firm instant recoil	Thick cartilage ear stiff		25	34
								30	36
Genitals male	Scrotum flat, smooth	Scrotum empty faint rugae	Testes in upper canal rare rugae	Testes decending few rugae	Testes down good rugae	Testes pendulous deep rugae		35	38
								40	40
Genitals female	Clitoris prominent labia flat	Prominent clitoris small labia minora	Prominent clitoris enlarging minora	Majora and minora equally prominent	Majora large minora small	Majora cover clitoris and minora		45	42
								50	44

Fig. 14.7 The new Ballard score. (From Ballard et al.[5])

Neurological criteria

The development of some reflexes and a gradual increase in muscle tone combined with changes in the range of passive joint movements with advancing gestation provide much information about maturity. Some of these items have been semi-quantified into scoring systems for use in conjunction with physical characteristics.

The appearance times of four reflexes as described by Robinson[67] are probably most useful for premature infants <34 weeks. The items are not scored, but their presence or absence should give a reasonable idea of whether a given LBW infant is compatible with his reputed gestational age. To these can be added the ability to suck/swallow reliably at 34–35 weeks of gestation. The five reflexes are thus as follows:

- Pupil reaction to light – this appears between 29 and 31 weeks, and is reliable after 32 weeks. The response can be extremely difficult to see in a tiny baby; one method is to look at the eye through the magnifying lens of an otoscope head, which is used as the light source.
- Glabellar tap – a blink in response to a tap on the glabella appears between 32 and 34 weeks.
- Traction response – flexion of the neck or arms when the baby is pulled up by the wrists from the supine position – appears between 33 and 36 weeks.
- Neck righting – the trunk follows the head when the neck is passively rotated in either direction from the supine – appears between 34 and 37 weeks.
- Ability to suck/swallow reliably – this matures with remarkable consistency between 34 and 35 weeks and allows the infant to bottle feed, providing he is not oxygen dependent.

The postnatal development of these reflexes can be used sequentially after birth so that an estimate of gestational age may be arrived at retrospectively.

Combination of the Robinson neurological assessment for infants <34 weeks' gestation and the Parkin modification of the Farr score for infants >32–34 weeks' gestation is usually all that is required to assess a neonate's gestation. However, the more complex scheme of Dubowitz et al[15] is widely used, though it is doubtful if it adds to the accuracy of the simple schemes.

The Dubowitz/Ballard scores are based on a combination of physical criteria and others that are largely dependent on the assessment of muscle tone. The very immature infant is extremely floppy, with very little flexor tone in the neck, trunk or limbs. As gestation advances, he gradually adopts a flexed posture and muscle tone increases, together with an ability to move against gravity.

Muscle tone can be assessed and graded by:

- observing the infant's posture in the supine position;
- assessing the head lag in response to traction on the wrists (pull-to-sit manoeuvre);
- observation in ventral suspension;
- manipulating the arms (scarf sign) and legs (heel-to-ear manoeuvre and popliteal angle);
- observing the flexion responses of the limbs following passive extension (arm and leg recoil);
- estimating the angles to which the wrist and ankle can be passively flexed (square window and ankle dorsiflexion). N.B. This test is not one of muscle tone since a greater degree of flexion can be obtained in the more mature infant; it must therefore represent an increase in the mobility of the joints concerned.

These items (35 points derived from 10 criteria) have been meticulously scored. The total score so obtained is added to that derived from the Farr and Dubowitz physical criteria. The gestational age is then estimated using a graph.

References

1. Adam M, Hudgins L 2003 The importance of minor anomalies in the evaluation of the newborn. NeoReviews 4: e99
2. Ainsworth S B, Wyllie J P, Wren C 1999 Prevalence and clinical significance of cardiac murmurs in neonates. Archives of Disease in Childhood. Fetal and Neonatal Edition 80: F43–F45
3. Alpay F, Sarici U, Tosuncuk D, Serdar M A, Inanc N, Gokcay E 2000 The value of first day bilirubin measurement in predicting the development of significant hyperbilirubinaemia in healthy term newborns. Pediatrics 106: e16
4. Arlettaz R, Archer L N J, Wilkinson A R 1998 Natural history of innocent heart murmurs in newborn babies: controlled echocardiographic study. Archives of Disease in Childhood. Fetal and Neonatal Edition 78: F166–F170
5. Ballard J L, Khoury J C, Wedig K, Wang L, Eilers-Walsman B L, Lipp J R 1991 New Ballard score, expanded to include extremely premature infants. Journal of Pediatrics 119: 417–423
6. Ballard J L, Novak K K, Driver M A 1979 A simplified score of fetal maturation of newly born infants. Journal of Pediatrics 95: 769–774
7. Barlow T G 1962 Early diagnosis and treatment of congenital dislocation of the hip. Journal of Bone and Joint Surgery (British Volume) 44: B292–B301
8. Bourke W G, Clarke T A, Mathews T G, O'Halpin D O, Donoghue V B 1993 Isolated single umbilical artery – the case for screening. Archives of Disease in Childhood 68: 600–601
9. Brando M, Rowe R D 1961 Auscultation of the heart in the early neonatal period. American Journal of Diseases of Children 101: 575–586
10. Brown F E, Cohen L B, Addante R R, Graham J M Jr 1986 Correction of congenital auricular deformities by splinting in the neonatal period. Pediatrics 78: 406–441
11. Chan A, McCaul K A, Cundy P J, Haan E A, Byron-Scott R 1997 Perinatal risk factors for developmental dysplasia of the hip. Archives of Disease in Childhood. Fetal and Neonatal Edition 76: F94–F100
12. Clarke N M P 1992 Diagnosing congenital dislocation of the hip. British Medical Journal 305: 435–436
13. Dezateux C, Brown J, Arthur R, Karnon J, Parnaby A 2003 Performance, treatment pathways, and effects of alternative policy options for screening for developmental dysplasia of the hip in the United Kingdom. Archives of Disease in Childhood 88: 753–759
14. Driver C P, Losty P D 1998 Neonatal testicular torsion. British Journal of Urology 82: 855–858
15. Dubowitz L M S, Dubowitz V, Goldberg C 1970 Clinical assessment of gestational age in the newborn infant. Journal of Pediatrics 77: 1–10
16. Dubowitz L, Dubowitz V 1981 The neurological assessment of the preterm and fullterm newborn infant. Clinics in Developmental Medicine No 79. SIMP/Heinemann, London
17. Dunn P M 1976 Congenital postural deformities. British Medical Bulletin 32: 71–76
18. Eastwood D M 2003 Neonatal hip screening. Lancet 361: 595–597
19. Eichenfield L F, Frieden I J, Esterly N B 2001 Textbook of neonatal dermatology. W B Saunders, Philadelphia
20. Elbourne D, Dezateux C, Arthur R et al 2002 Ultrasonography in the diagnosis and management of developmental hip dysplasia (hip trial): clinical and economic results of a multicentre randomised controlled trial. Lancet 360: 2009–2018
21. Elliman D, Dezateux C, Bedford H E 2002 Newborn and childhood screening programmes: criteria, evidence and current policy. Archives of Disease in Childhood 87: 6–9
22. Evans-Jones G, Kay S P J, Weindling A M et al 2003 Congenital brachial palsy: incidence, causes and outcome in the UK and Republic of Ireland. Archives of Disease in Childhood. Fetal and Neonatal Edition 88: F185–F189
23. Farr V, Kerridge D F, Mitchell R G 1966 The value of some external characteristics in the assessment of gestational age. Developmental Medicine and Child Neurology 8: 657–660
24. Farrer K F M, Rennie J M 2003 Neonatal murmurs: are senior house officers good enough? Archives of Disease in Childhood. Fetal and Neonatal Edition 88: F147–F151
25. Foundation for the Study of Infant Deaths 2004 Available on www.sids.org.uk
26. Gibson P, Britton J, Hall D M B, Rowland Hill C 1995 Lumbosacral skin markers and identification of occult spinal dysraphism in neonates. Acta Paediatrica Scandinavica 84: 208–209
27. Gilbert A, Brockman R, Carlioz H 1991 Surgical treatment of brachial plexus palsy. Clinical Orthopaedics and Related Research 264: 39–47

28. Glazener C M A, Ramsay C R, Campbell M K et al 1999 Neonatal examination and screening trial (NEST): a randomised, controlled, switchback trial of alternative policies for low risk infants. British Medical Journal 318: 627–632

29. Godward S, Dezeteux C 1998 Surgery for congenital dislocation of the hip as a measure of outcome of screening. Lancet 351: 1149–1152

30. Graf R, Wilson B 1995 Sonography of the infant hip and its therapeutic implications. Chapman & Hall, Weinheim

31. Graham J M Jr 1994 When is it best to be born? A morphological perspective – craniofacial deformation. In: Amiel-Tison C, Stewart A (eds) The newborn infant: one brain for life. INSERM, Paris, pp 23–38

32. Graham J M Jr, Smith D W 1979 Parietal craniotabes in the neonate: its origin and significance. Journal of Pediatrics 95: 114–116

33. Hall D M B, Elliman D (eds) 2003 Health for all children, 4th edn. Oxford University Press, Oxford. Text available from: http://www.health-for-all-children.co.uk

34. Hansen L K, Birkebaek N H, Oxhoj H 1995 Initial evaluation of children with heart murmurs by the non-specialised paediatricians. European Journal of Pediatrics 154: 15–17

35. Hernandez J A, Morelli J G 2003 Birthmarks of potential medical significance. NeoReviews 4: e263

36. Hill C A, Gibson P J 1995 Ultrasound determination of the normal location of the conus medullaris in neonates. American Journal of Neuroradiology 16: 469–472

37. Hittner H M, Hirsch N J, Rudolph A J 1977 Assessment of gestational age by examination of the anterior vascular capsule of the lens. Journal of Pediatrics 91: 455–458

38. Hunter A G W, Rudd N L 1977 Craniosynostosis. II. Coronal synostosis: its familial characteristics and associated clinical findings in 109 patients lacking bilateral polysyndactyly or syndactyly. Teratology 15: 301–309

39. Johnson L H, Bhutani V K, Brown A K 2002 System based approach to management of neonatal jaundice and prevention of kernicterus. Journal of Pediatrics 140: 396–403

40. Jones D A 1989 Importance of the clicking hip in screening for congenital dislocation of the hip. Lancet 1: 599–601

41. Klimek R, Klimek M, Rzepecka-Weglarz B 2000 A new score for postnatal clinical assessment of fetal maturity in newborn infants. International Journal of Gynecology and Obstetrics 71: 101–105

42. Koppel R I, Druschel C M, Carter T et al 2003 Effectiveness of pulse oximetry screening for congenital heart disease in asymptomatic newborns. Pediatrics 111: 451–455

43. Kriss V M, Desai N S 1998 Occult spinal dysraphism in neonates: assessment of high risk cutaneous stigmata on sonography. American Journal of Radiology 171: 1687–1693

44. Kugelman A, Tubi A, Bader D, Chemo M, Dabbah H 2002 Pre-auricular tags and pits in the newborn: the role of renal ultrasonography. Journal of Pediatrics 141: 388–391

45. Laing I A, Wong C M 2002 Hypernatraemia in the first few days: is the incidence rising? Archives of Disease in Childhood. Fetal and Neonatal Edition 87: F158–F161

46. Landau M, Krafchik B R 1999 The diagnostic value of café-au-lait macules. Journal of the American Academy of Dermatology 40: 877–890

47. Lee T W R, Skelton R E, Skene C 2001 Routine neonatal examination: effectiveness of trainee paediatrician compared with advanced neonatal nurse practitioner. Archives of Disease in Childhood. Fetal and Neonatal Edition 85: F100–F104

48. Leonard J V, Dezateux C 2002 Screening for inherited metabolic disease in newborn infants using tandem mass spectrometry. British Medical Journal 324: 4–5

49. Lin D S, Huang F Y, Lin S P et al 1997 Frequency of associated anomalies in congenital hypoplasia of depressor anguli oris muscle: a study of 50 patients. American Journal of Medical Genetics 71: 215–218

50. Lloyd-Roberts G C 1955 Osteoarthritis of the hip: a study of clinical pathology. Journal of Bone and Joint Surgery (British Volume) 37: 8–47

51. McCrindle B W, Shaffer K M, Kan J S, Zahka K G, Rowe S A, Kidd L 1996 Cardinal clinical signs in the differentiation of heart murmurs in children. Archives of Paediatric and Adolescent Medicine 150: 169–174

52. Medina L S, Crone K, Kuntz K M 2001 Newborns with suspected occult spinal dysraphism: a cost effectiveness analysis of diagnostic strategies. Pediatrics 108: e101

53. Moore F H 1989 Examining infants' hips – can it do harm? Journal of Bone and Joint Surgery (British Volume) 71: 4–5

54. Moss G D, Cartlidge P H T, Speidel B D, Chambers T L 1991 Routine examination in the newborn period. British Medical Journal 302: 878–879

55. Nance W E 2003 The genetics of deafness. Mental Retardation and Developmental Disability Research Reviews 9: 109–119

56. National electronic Library for Screening 2004 Available on *www.nelh.nhs.uk/screening/vbls.html*

57. Newburger J W, Rosenthal A, Williams R G, Fellows K, Miettinen O S 1983 Noninvasive tests in the initial evaluation of heart murmurs in children. New England Journal of Medicine 308: 61–64

58. Ortolani M 1937 Un segno poco noto e sua importanza per la diagnosi precoce di prelussazione congenita dell'anca. Pediatrica (Napoli) 45: 129–136

59. Parents of Infants and Children with Kernicterus 2004 Available on www.pickonline.org

60. Parker S, Zuckerman B, Bauchner H, Frank D, Vinci R, Cabral H 1990 Jitteriness in full term neonates: prevalence and correlates. Pediatrics 85: 17–23

61. Parkin J M, Hey E N, Clowes J S 1976 Rapid assessment of gestational age at birth. Archives of Disease in Childhood 51: 259–263

62. Piazza S F, Chandra M, Harper R G, Sia C G, McVicar M, Huang H 1985 Upper- vs lower-systolic blood pressure in full-term normal newborn. American Journal of Diseases of Children 139: 797–799

63. Pondaag W, Malessy M J A, Thomeer R T W M 2004 Natural history of obstetric brachial plexus palsy: a systematic review. Developmental Medicine and Child Neurology 46: 138–144

64. Rahi J S, Dezateux C 1999 National cross sectional study of detection of congenital and infantile cataract in the United Kingdom: role of childhood screening and surveillance. British Medical Journal 318: 362–365

65. Reich J D, Miller S, Brogdon B et al 2003 The use of pulse oximetry to detect congenital heart disease. Journal of Pediatrics 142: 268–272

66. Richmond S, Reay G, Abu Harb M 2002 Routine pulse oximetry in the asymptomatic newborn. Archives of Disease in Childhood. Fetal and Neonatal Edition 87: F83–F88

67. Robinson R J 1966 Assessment of gestational age by neurological examination. Archives of Disease in Childhood 41: 437–447

68. Rosendahl K, Markestad T, Lie R T 1994 Ultrasound screening for developmental dysplasia of the hip in the neonate: the effect on treatment rate and prevalence of late cases. Pediatrics 94: 47–52

69. Rothman L, Rose J S, Laster D W, Quaker R, Tenner M 1976 The spectrum of growing skull fracture. Pediatrics 57: 26–31

70. Russ S A, Rickards F, Poulakis Z, Barker M, Saunders K, Wake M 2002 Six year effectiveness of a population based two tier infant hearing screening programme. Archives of Diseases in Childhood. 86: 245–250

71. Sanfridson J, Redland-Johnell I, Uden A 1991 Why is congenital dislocation of the hip still missed? Analysis of 96,891 infants screened in Malmo, 1956–1987. Acta Orthopaedica Scandinavica 62: 87–91

72. Scarfo G B, Mariotti A, Tomaccini D, Palma L 1989 Growing skull fracture. Childs Nervous System 5: 163–167

73. Scott J E S, Swallow V, Coulthard M G, Lambert H J, Lee R E J 1997 Screening newborn babies for familial ureteric reflux. Lancet 350: 396–400

74. Smythe J F, Teixeira O H, Vlad P, Demers P P, Feldman W 1990 Initial evaluation of heart murmurs: are laboratory tests necessary? Pediatrics 86: 497–500

75. Staheli L T 1993 Shoes and common lower limb problems. In: David T J (ed) Recent Advances in Paediatrics Vol 11. Churchill Livingstone, Edinburgh, pp 161–173

76. Standing Medical Advisory Committee 1986 Screening for detection of congenital dislocation of the hip in infants. DHSS, London. Full text obtainable from: http://www.steps-charity.org.uk/forms/SMAC_booklet.pdf

77. Temmerman A M, Mooyaart E L, Taverne P P 1991 The value of the routine chest roentenogram in the cardiological evaluation of infants and children: a prospective study. European Journal of Pediatrics 150: 623–636

78. Wariyar U, Tin W, Hey E 1997 Gestational assessment assessed. Archives of Disease in Childhood. Fetal and Neonatal Edition 77: F216–F220

79. Wessex Universal Neonatal Hearing Screening Trial Group 1998 Controlled trial of universal neonatal screening for early identification of permanent childhood hearing impairment. Lancet 352: 1957–1964

80. Wolke D, Dave S, Hayes J, Rownsend J, Tomlin M 2002 Routine examination of the newborn and maternal satisfaction: a randomised controlled trial. Archives of Disease in Childhood. Fetal and Neonatal Edition 86: F155–F160

81. Wren C, Richmond S, Donaldson L 1999 Presentation of congenital heart disease in infancy: implications for routine examination. Archives of Disease in Childhood. Fetal and Neonatal Edition 80: F49–F53

82. Wright C M, Parkinson K N 2004 Postnatal weight loss in term infants: what is 'normal' and do growth charts allow for it? Archives of Disease in Childhood. Fetal and Neonatal Edition 89: F254–F257

83. Yiv B C, Saidin R, Cundy P J et al 1997 Developmental dysplasia of the hip in South Australia in 1991: prevalence and risk factors. Journal of Paediatrics and Child Health 33: 151–156

84. Young J D H, MacEwen C J 1997 Managing congenital lacrimal obstruction in general practice. British Medical Journal 315: 293–296

CHAPTER 15

Temperature control and disorders

Nicholas Rutter

Children and adults can control their body temperature over a wide range of ambient conditions. They achieve this by making physiological or behavioural adjustments that affect the rate at which they produce or lose heat. The newborn baby is similarly homoeothermic but there are differences, mainly of degree, which make it more difficult for him to maintain a constant body temperature. A low bodyweight to surface area ratio means that heat production is low relative to heat loss. The physiological and behavioural responses to a warm or cold environment are less well developed than in older babies or children. The part played by the mother in the thermoregulation of newborn animals is vital, maternal body heat being used to warm the young as before delivery. However, routine care of the preterm newborn human often demands that the baby is removed from the mother, stripped naked and nursed in dry, draughty surroundings, conditions which may produce severe thermal stress.

An appropriate thermal environment with maintenance of a normal body temperature is important to the newborn, particularly if ill or small. Several studies in the past have shown that if such babies are allowed to become cold, their chances of survival are considerably reduced, their incidence of illness is increased and their rate of growth is diminished. Although these studies were made when mortality rates were high and the babies were severely cold stressed, the implication is that cold stress is harmful and should be avoided. To these important reasons for choosing a baby's thermal environment carefully should be added thermal comfort, a concept that is well defined in children and adults. There is no reason to suppose that babies do not feel uncomfortably cold or hot because their neurological development is too immature for them to express their feelings.

Those who care for newborn babies take responsibility for selecting an appropriate physical environment. This is not instinctive, and thought needs to be given to those factors that determine the thermal environment, so that suitable conditions can be provided. Obsessive attention to detail, particularly in the management of the preterm baby, is important.

Physical, physiological and behavioural aspects of thermoregulation

Heat balance

The law of conservation of energy demands that under equilibrium conditions, heat losses balance heat production. If production exceeds loss, the body temperature rises until a new equilibrium is reached; if losses exceed production, body temperature falls.

$$\text{Heat production} = \text{heat loss by convection} + \text{radiation} + \text{evaporation}$$

The amount of heat that a newborn baby loses by conduction is small and can be ignored.

Heat production

The newborn baby produces heat by metabolic activity in all body tissues. Basal metabolic rate is difficult to measure since the newborn is rarely awake, quiet and starved, but resting levels can be measured. The resting metabolic rate (usually measured indirectly as the resting oxygen consumption) describes the metabolism of a baby who is lying still, asleep, more than an hour after the previous feed, and in neutral thermal surroundings (for definition, see later). Under these conditions, the heat production of a healthy term newborn baby is similar to that of an adult when expressed per unit weight, but almost half that of an adult when expressed per unit surface area. As it is surface area that determines a subject's heat loss, this relatively low heat production per unit area explains why the newborn requires a much warmer environment than an adult. Resting metabolic rate is similar in term and preterm babies when expressed per unit weight, but considerably lower in preterm babies when expressed per unit surface area (Fig. 15.1). Preterm babies thus

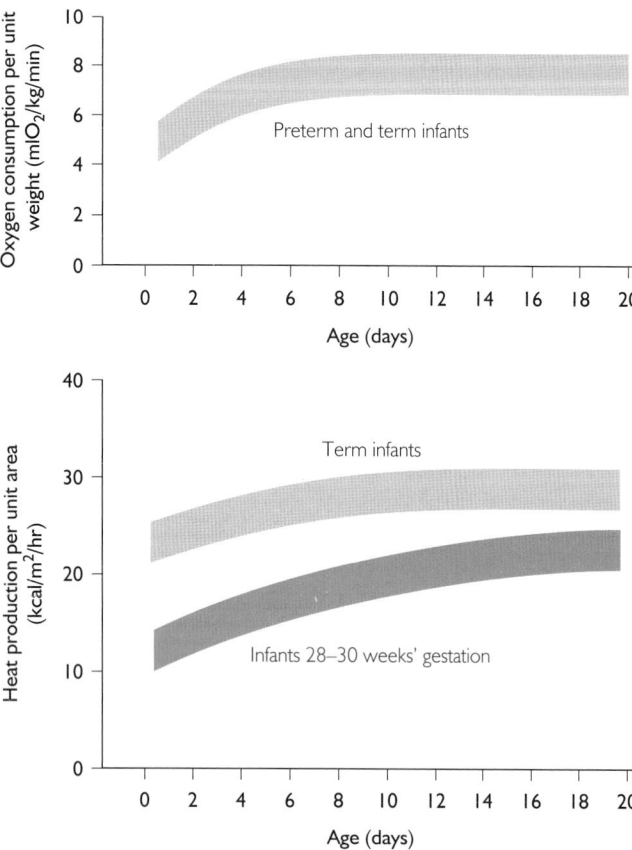

Fig. 15.1 Resting metabolic rate in the newborn period when expressed per unit weight (upper) and per unit surface area (lower). The ranges shown are the mean values ± 1 standard deviation. (Derived from data of Hey.[29])

Table 15.1 Factors affecting a newborn infant's heat production

Heat production increased	Heat production decreased
Awake	In deep sleep
Active	Ill infants especially with asphyxia or hypoxia
After food	Fasting
Rapid growth	Malnutrition
Neonatal thyrotoxicosis	Hypothyroidism
Cardiac left-to-right shunt	Cyanotic congenital heart disease
Drugs, e.g. theophylline, caffeine	Drugs, e.g. chlorpromazine

require higher ambient temperatures than term babies.[34] Resting metabolic rate rises in the immediate newborn period.[29,37] The maximum rate of approximately 50 kcal/m²/h is reached by the age of 3–6 months, and thereafter remains constant through childhood into adult life. Many factors influence a baby's heat production (Table 15.1). It is higher in rapid eye movement sleep than deep sleep, suggesting that the brain is metabolically highly active. The newborn baby is also able to increase heat

production in response to cold stress (see below). There is considerable individual variation, particularly in small babies.

Heat loss

Convection

Heat is lost by convection from the exposed surface of the baby to the surrounding air, and is determined largely by the difference in temperature between the two. If the ambient temperature exceeds the surface temperature of the baby, heat will be gained by convection. Convective heat loss also depends on the air speed. If it is rapid, the insulating effect of still air close to the baby's surface is lost (forced convection) and convective heat loss increases. Convection is a major source of heat loss when newborn babies are exposed in cool, draughty rooms.

Radiation

Heat is lost by radiation from the exposed surface of the baby to the surrounding surfaces that directly overlook the baby. This is proportional to the difference between these surface temperatures but independent of the temperature and speed of the intervening air. It is an important channel of heat loss when babies are exposed naked in a delivery room or a single-walled incubator, but a source of heat gain when a baby is nursed under a radiant warmer.

Evaporation of water

As water evaporates from the baby, heat is lost (each millilitre of water that evaporates removes 560 calories of heat). Under normal conditions, in a term baby, evaporative heat loss amounts to about a quarter of the resting heat production.[33] About a quarter of this loss is by evaporation of water from the respiratory tract, the remainder occurring by passive diffusion of water through the epidermis (transepidermal water loss [TEWL]). Evaporative heat loss is nevertheless not important in term babies, except at delivery, when the skin is wet with amniotic fluid. Mature babies have the ability to increase evaporative heat loss in response to a warm environment by sweating.[26,33]

Preterm babies, however, have high evaporative heat losses. Their insensible water loss is high compared with term babies, particularly in the most immature in the early neonatal period.[16,52] This is the result of a high TEWL, which is up to six times higher per unit surface area in a newborn baby of 26 weeks' gestation than in a term baby (Fig. 15.2).[22,24,56] The high TEWL occurs because the immature baby's skin has a thin, poorly keratinized stratum corneum that offers little resistance to the diffusion of water. Postnatal existence rapidly hastens the development of an effective epidermal barrier, so that by about 2 to 3 weeks of age even the most immature baby has a TEWL approaching that of a term baby. The high TEWL of preterm babies is further increased by adhesive trauma to the skin.[27]

Evaporative heat loss is increased in the newborn by exposure to radiant energy. Use of a radiant warmer increases evaporative

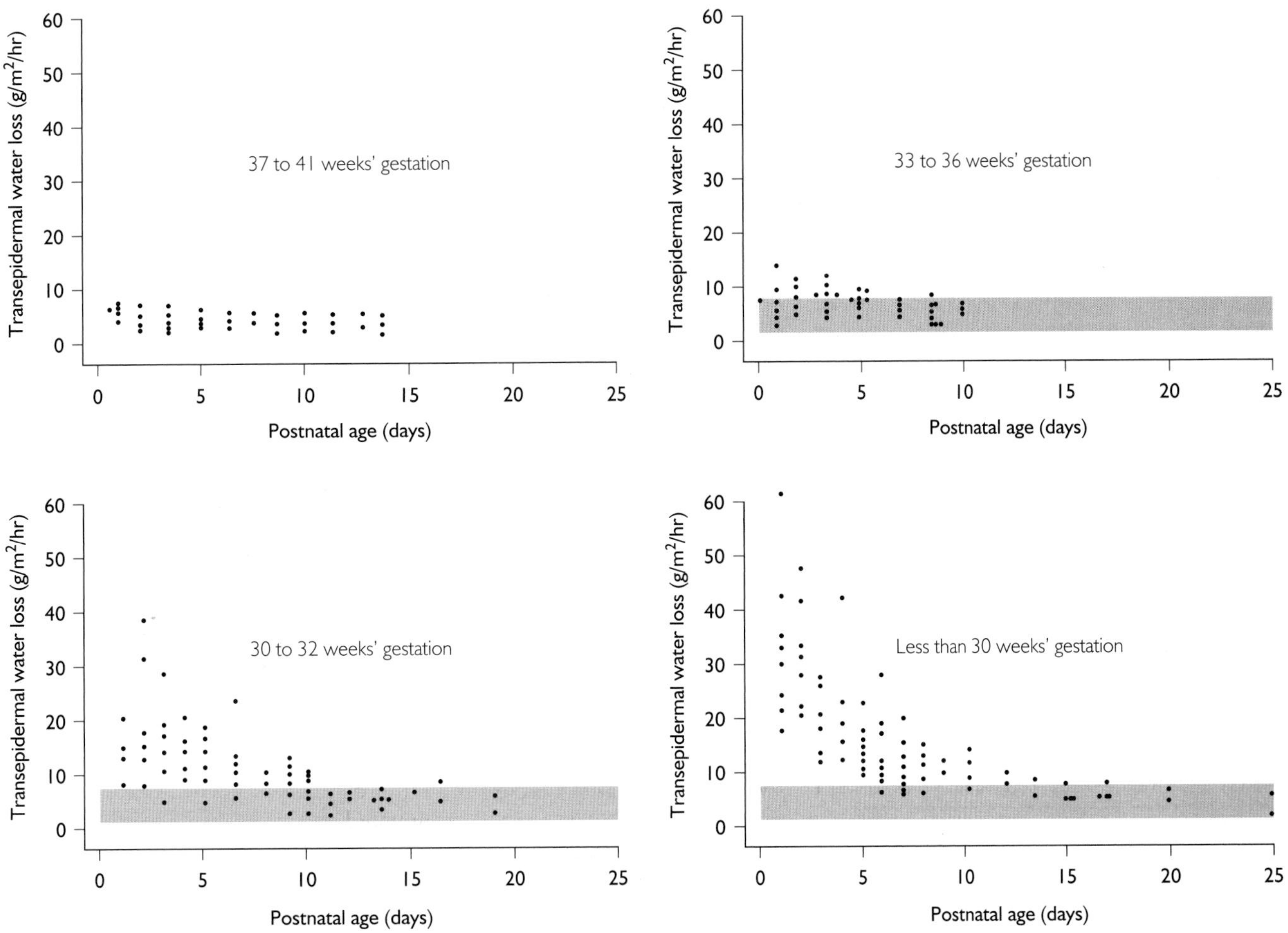

Fig. 15.2 Transepidermal water loss from the abdomen of newborn infants, showing the separate influences of gestation and postnatal age. The shaded area is the range of water loss in term infants for comparison. (From data of Harpin & Rutter.[27])

heat loss by a factor of about 0.5–2.0 and phototherapy by 0.4–2.0. The two together are additive. This is probably caused by the higher surface temperatures, greater air speeds and lower humidity when babies are exposed to radiant energy, physical factors that increase evaporative heat loss. When these are allowed for, radiant warmers[41] and phototherapy[42] have little direct effect in increasing TEWL.

The high evaporative heat losses of babies of less than 30 weeks' gestation in the first week or so of life make their clinical management difficult. If nursed in dry incubators, they readily become hypothermic; and if nursed under radiant warmers, difficulties in management of fluid balance arise. Reduction of this high evaporative loss is necessary and can be achieved in a number of ways:

- by increasing the ambient humidity – evaporative heat loss decreases linearly as humidity rises (Fig. 15.3), so that losses at high humidity are very low;[22,33,61]
- by protecting the baby from draughts – for example, an incubator with low air speeds can be used,[51,69] or the baby can be nursed under a perspex shield closed at one end;[16]
- by attempting to waterproof the baby – plastic bubble blankets or clear plastic film draped over the preterm baby will

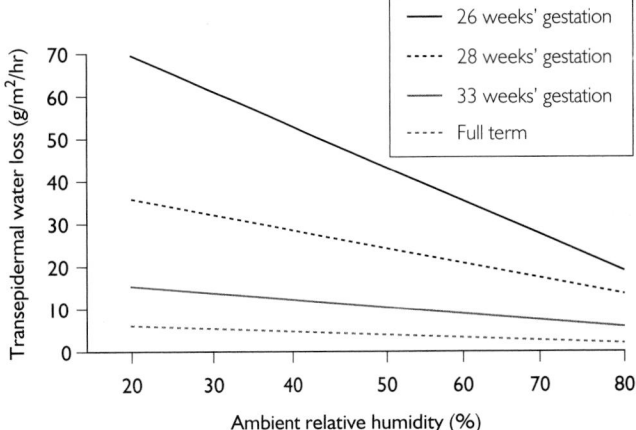

Fig. 15.3 The effect of ambient relative humidity on transepidermal water loss. It is most marked in the immature infant with a very high water loss. (Derived from Hammarlund & Sedin.[22])

reduce insensible water loss by 75%.[45] Topical application of an emollient grease (soft paraffin, Aquaphor™) may reduce TEWL in preterm babies by 50% although it confers no overall benefit in terms of survival or morbidity. A similar reduction in

TEWL can be achieved by using a semi-permeable polyurethane membrane as an artificial skin.[43,63]

Response to a cold environment

As the environmental temperature falls, the newborn baby makes physiological and behavioural responses to maintain a constant deep-body temperature. These are initiated by hypothalamic and cutaneous temperature receptors.

Physiological

The baby can increase heat production in response to cold stress without any increase in physical activity (shivering does not occur in the newborn). Non-shivering thermogenesis results from the metabolic activity of a specialised organ of heat production, brown adipose tissue. This distinctive fat is found superficially (especially between the scapulae) and deep within the body (especially along the aorta) of the newborn baby. In response to cold, catecholamines are released which act directly on brown adipose tissue, uncoupling oxidative phosphorylation and releasing energy as heat. A newborn baby can more than double his or her rate of heat production in this way.[29] Non-shivering thermogenesis is impaired in all newborn babies in the first 12 hours, in ill babies especially following asphyxia or with hypoxia, and after maternal sedative administration, especially diazepam. Peripheral vasoconstriction also occurs in response to cold, diverting blood from the baby's surface to the core. This is well developed in term babies but limited in very immature babies in the immediate neonatal period.

Behavioural

Whereas a child or adult will wake up and become restless when cold, the newborn baby may continue to sleep. Cold babies, however, do tend to be more active, sleep less and adopt a flexed posture in an attempt to increase heat production and decrease heat loss. These responses are also seen in preterm babies.

Response to a warm environment

As the environmental temperature rises, the newborn baby attempts to prevent a rise in body temperature.

Physiological

Sweating in response to a warm environment occurs in term babies from birth.[26,33] The amount of water lost by sweating per unit area of skin is considerably lower than that lost by a heat-acclimatized adult, although the density of sweat glands is greater in the newborn. The amount of sweat produced by each gland is therefore much lower in the newborn than in the adult. Sweating in the newborn is most marked on the forehead, temple and occiput, but occurs everywhere except the palms and the soles (which only sweat in response to emotional stress).

It provides some measure of defence against overheating. In congenital hypohidrotic ectodermal dysplasia, in which sweating is impaired, the newborn baby is particularly susceptible to heat stress. Sweating is absent in babies below 36 weeks' gestation at birth but usually appears by about 2 weeks of age. It occurs at fewer sites and is less marked than in term babies, providing poor defence against overheating. Babies born to mothers who have abused opiates during pregnancy have a well-developed ability to sweat, even if born prematurely. Vasodilatation in response to heat occurs in term and preterm babies, so that the skin of an overheated baby is warm and red.[25]

Behavioural

As the environmental temperature increases, newborn babies become less active, sleep more and lie in an extended, sunbathing posture. Preterm babies also make these responses.[25,55]

Body temperature and thermal neutrality

There is a zone of environmental temperature within which a baby's heat production is at a minimum, the body temperature is normal, and there is no sweating. Fine thermoregulation is maintained by changes in skin blood flow, posture and activity.[31] This is termed the thermoneutral range (Fig. 15.4). Babies are best nursed at an environmental temperature close to this range, probably around the lower end, since this is more comfortable for children and adults.[30] The width and the absolute values of this neutral thermal range depend on the baby's resting heat production and insulation. In the term baby nursed naked, the range is wider and lower than in the preterm baby who has a low metabolic rate and poor tissue insulation. Clothing and wrapping babies greatly widens and lowers the neutral thermal range.[36] Thus, for a term baby in the first week, the range is about 32–33.5°C when nursed naked, and 24–27°C when clothed. For a preterm baby of 30 weeks' gestation weighing 1.5 kg, the range is about 34–35°C when nursed naked and 28–30°C when clothed.

Body temperature falls when a baby can no longer increase heat production in response to a cool environment, and rises when sweating is insufficient as a means of heat loss. Between these extremes, a normal body temperature is maintained. Clearly, a baby with a normal body temperature can be sweating or be markedly cold stressed, so body temperature is an insensitive guide to the suitability of the thermal environment. Doctors and nurses commonly assume that if a baby has a normal body temperature the ambient temperature conditions must be satisfactory. In doing so, they fail to distinguish between being cold and feeling cold. A careful observer can recognise that a baby is feeling cold before he actually becomes cold, by assessing the baby's posture, activity, skin colour and peripheral skin temperature. However, the very-low-birthweight (VLBW) baby is an exception. A baby of less than 1 kg has such a low heat production per surface area, limited metabolic response to cold, and poor tissue insulation that he appears poikilothermic (body temperature drifts up and down with the ambient temperature).

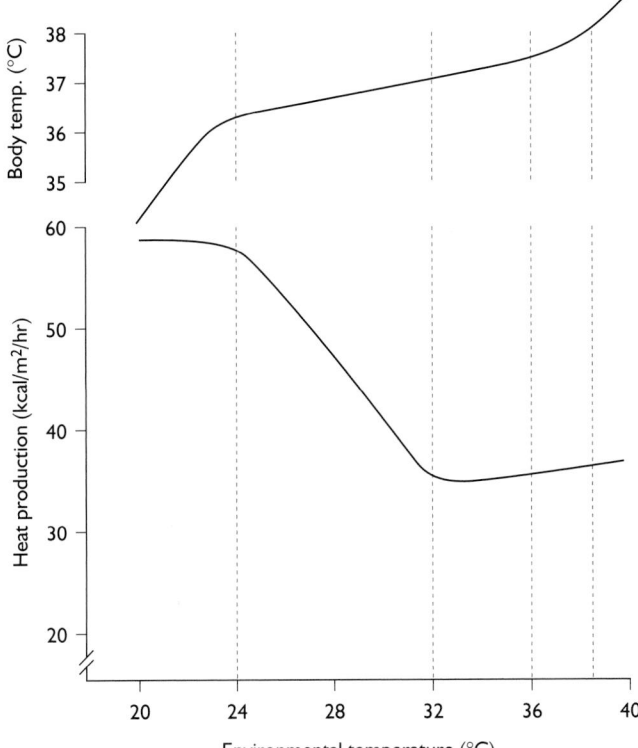

Fig. 15.4 The effect of environmental temperature on heat production and body temperature of a 1.9 kg infant of 34 weeks' gestation, nursed naked in surroundings of uniform temperature and moderate humidity. Between 32°C and 36°C, heat production is minimal, there is no sweating, and body temperature is normal (neutral thermal range). When the environmental temperature exceeds 36°C, the infant sweats, and above 38°C, the body temperature rises rapidly. Below 32°C, heat production increases by non-shivering thermogenesis, but below 24°C, heat production has reached its maximum and body temperature rapidly falls.

Measurement of body temperature in such a baby is a convenient and reliable guide to the suitability of the thermal environment.

Measurement of temperature

Some measurement of core or surface temperature is useful in the newborn as a guide to the suitability of the thermal environment and in the detection of illness. The relative insensitivity of body temperature as a guide to the thermal environment of the mature neonate has been mentioned, but it is useful in VLBW babies in the early neonatal period when they behave as if they were poikilothermic. In larger healthy babies, considerable thermal stress is needed to raise or lower body temperature outside the normal range. Surface temperature measurements change readily, but normal values are less well defined and the measuring devices themselves alter temperature, so that a composite measurement influenced by both environmental and skin

temperature is recorded. Rectal, axillary and between skin and mattress temperatures correlate well with core temperature as recorded by an electronic thermometer inserted 5 cm beyond the anus.[47]

Rectal temperature

This can be measured using a flexible thermocouple or thermistor inserted 5 cm from the anal margin. There is little increase in temperature if the probe is inserted more deeply, but there is a considerable gradient in the first 5 cm, most of which occurs in the first 3 cm. A flexible probe can be left in situ for continuous monitoring but is easily pushed out by the straining baby. The mercury-in-glass thermometer is still used: it should be lubricated with soft paraffin and inserted in a downwards and backwards direction (at an angle of 30° to the horizontal) to a depth of 3 cm from the anal margin (2 cm in a preterm baby).[70] Shallower insertion gives a falsely low recording because blood from the surface of the legs may return via venous plexuses around the anus. Most equilibration has occurred by a minute after insertion. The dangers of using a glass thermometer for rectal temperature measurement are haemorrhage and perforation of the rectum, which are particularly likely to occur if the baby is struggling. Rectal temperature measurement is contraindicated in necrotising enterocolitis.

Because of the small risk associated with rectal temperature measurement, axillary measurement is preferred. This is the current recommendation of the American Academy of Pediatrics. However, a single rectal temperature measurement in all newborn babies soon after delivery is an effective screening test for imperforate anus. The normal range in babies is 36.5–37.5°C regardless of weight or gestation.

Axillary temperature

This is usually measured by an electronic thermometer with the probe placed firmly in the roof of the axilla and the baby's upper arm held against the side of the chest wall. It is safe. The normal range in babies of all weights and gestation is 35.6–37.3°C. On average, it is about 0.5°C lower than rectal temperature, but the difference in an individual baby is unpredictable.

Skin temperature

A thermocouple or thermistor lightly taped to the baby's skin can be left for repeated or continuous measurements. The upper abdomen is a convenient site, as changes with environmental temperature are not as great as at a peripheral site and the skin is conveniently flat. The normal range depends on the tissue insulation and therefore on the baby's size. In term babies, the range is 35.5–36.5°C; in a preterm baby, 36.2–37.2°C. The baby below 1 kg birthweight has an abdominal skin temperature close to the rectal or axillary temperature. If the temperature probe is placed between the baby's back and the underlying mattress and then allowed to equilibrate, the final measured temperature is similar to core, rectal or axillary measurements.[47]

Practical management of the thermal environment

At delivery

The rectal temperature of the newborn baby at delivery averages 37.8°C (range 37–39°C), about 1°C higher than the maternal temperature. The placenta is an efficient heat exchanger in pregnancy, removing the heat produced by the fetus, but this is impaired during labour. The baby's body temperature falls immediately after delivery and can easily reach subnormal levels if steps are not taken to conserve heat. Heat losses in a newly born baby are very high.[23] Most delivery rooms and operating theatres are comfortable for clothed adults but cold for exposed babies. Heat losses by convection and radiation are high, and evaporative heat losses from the wet skin far exceed the baby's metabolic heat production. Furthermore, the ability of the baby to increase his or her metabolic rate immediately after birth is impaired, particularly in the presence of birth asphyxia or maternal sedation. As ever, the VLBW baby is at greater risk of cold stress because of an unfavourable weight to surface area ratio. The body temperature of an exposed 1 kg baby can fall by 1°C every 5 minutes.

There is no evidence that a marked fall in body temperature is an advantage to the baby. Preterm babies who become cold at delivery have a greater chance of dying, particularly of hyaline membrane disease. Cold stress is associated with acidosis and hypoxia,[18] factors which impair surfactant production in the preterm newborn. It is difficult to separate the effects of cold itself from the effects of birth asphyxia, hypoxia and the need for resuscitation (which in turn cause a fall in body temperature). However, the poor outcome of preterm babies who become cold after delivery justifies strenuous efforts to keep them warm. By contrast, the healthy term baby is less susceptible to cold stress at delivery and more resistant to the effects. Acidosis and hypoxia may occur, but transient grunting is the usually the only clinical effect. With care, this can be prevented without separating mother and baby.

The ideal temperature of a delivery room or operating theatre is about 25°C, comfortable for the mother and her attendants and for the baby. The baby should be dried at once and then given to the mother. Direct physical contact between the mother and the baby is a mode of thermoregulation much used in the animal world and is most effective when there are no intervening clothes or blankets. Unless the room temperature is in excess of 25°C or there is supplementary heating, the exposed parts of the baby should be dry and covered. Weighing, cleaning, bathing, care of the umbilical cord and the fixing of name-bands not only interrupt contact between the mother and her baby, but also cause cold stress and are best postponed. Resuscitation should be carried out after the baby has been dried. Supplementary heat is essential during resuscitation and can conveniently be provided with a fixed-output radiant heat source above the baby. The exposed trunk and legs of a baby born by breech delivery should be dried and wrapped before the head is delivered.

The delivery room or operating theatre is always too cold for a VLBW baby. The baby should be thoroughly dried, wrapped, resuscitated and removed to a warmer environment as soon as possible. Wrapping the baby in a polyethylene film straight away without prior drying, until after transfer to a warmer or an incubator, has been shown to be an effective way of avoiding a fall in body temperature in the immediate postnatal period.[64]

Nursing care of the newborn baby

A newborn baby when dressed, wrapped, placed in a cot and nursed in a warm room is in a neutral thermal environment (see above). Heat production is at a minimum and energy intake is therefore available for growth. Mothers prefer to see their babies dressed rather than naked, and the clothed newborn seems more contented. A naked baby is poorly insulated and heat losses are high even in a warm room. Clothing more than doubles the insulation, and bedding (a sheet and two blankets) further increases it, so that the resistance to heat loss of a clothed, wrapped baby is three times greater than that of a naked one (Table 15.2).[32,35] The head is a large part of the total surface area of the newborn baby and has a higher surface temperature because of the brain's high rate of metabolism. A woollen bonnet is an effective method of increasing thermal insulation, and is especially useful in low-birthweight (LBW) babies, who have relatively larger heads and whose trunk may need to be exposed.

The following recommendations are made for nursing healthy babies in the newborn period:[30]

- 2–2.5 kg: clothed, with bedding, in a room temperature of about 24°C;
- 1.5–2 kg: clothed, with a bonnet and bedding, in a room temperature of about 26°C;
- <1.5 kg: clothed, with a bonnet, in an incubator temperature of about 30–32°C.

Babies weighing more than about 1.80 kg are commonly nursed in an environment 1–2°C cooler than this. They will have a minor and clinically unimportant increase in oxygen consumption as a result. Large term babies who are wrapped and covered with a sheet and blanket have a wide neutral thermal range and can tolerate cooler environments with little increase in metabolic rate. A newborn baby should be nursed clothed, even in an incubator, unless exposure is necessary for observation or access. Skin-to-skin contact between mother and baby is an effective and safe method of keeping a healthy preterm baby warm.

Incubator care

A closed incubator provides a baby with a high ambient temperature whilst allowing attendants to work at a lower, more comfortable temperature. Most incubators work by forced convection: air is heated and then circulated by a fan within the

Table 15.2 Resistance to heat loss (insulation) in an infant weighing 2.5 kg lying on a foam mattress in a cool, draught-free room. Insulation is measured in clo units (1 clo unit = $0.155\,°C\,m^2\,W^{-1}$ or $0.18\,°C\,m^2\,kcal^{-1}$) (Reproduced from Hey[32])

Resistance due to	Completely naked	Wearing bonnet, wrapped in one sheet	Fully clothed under blankets, in a cot
One flannelette sheet and two blankets around a clothed baby	–	–	0.61
One flannelette swaddling sheet around an unclothed baby	–	0.81	–
Thick gauze bonnet over head	–	0.22	0.22
Vest, napkin and long nightdress	–	–	1.25
Boundary layer of still air around the skin	0.78	0.78	0.78
Body tissues (when vasoconstricted)	0.29	0.29	0.29
Total resistance	1.07	2.10	3.15

canopy of the incubator at an air speed of about 20 cm/s. There are two means of controlling the heater output:

- **Air mode.** The air temperature is set to a desired level and maintained by thermostat. The heater output is proportional to the difference between the set temperature and the actual temperature. If the incubator air temperature is just below the set temperature, the heater output will be low; if it is substantially below the set temperature, the heater will be on full power. This means that fluctuations in air temperature due to cycling of the thermostat are small.

- **Servo mode.** The heater output is controlled by the baby's skin temperature. A temperature probe is taped to the skin, preferably the upper abdomen, and the heater cycles to keep the skin temperature at that site constant. In practice, air temperature fluctuations are greater in servo mode than air mode, especially when the baby is handled (Fig. 15.5).

Air mode is probably satisfactory for nursing most newborn babies.[8] Servo mode has the disadvantages of wide fluctuations in air temperature,[15] particularly during nursing procedures, of providing an inappropriately low ambient temperature when the baby is febrile, and of lack of control when a baby with very high insensible water loss is nursed in a dry incubator.[6] The probe may become detached, resulting in an inappropriate air temperature. A naked baby in an incubator loses heat predominantly by radiation, less by convection and evaporation (Fig. 15.6). Heat loss by radiation can be reduced by covering or clothing the baby, often impractical, or by use of a double-walled incubator.[46] In practice, the radiant losses can be compensated by a higher air temperature setting. Incubators are useful for nursing small babies who can be clothed but need a very warm ambient temperature, and for naked or sick babies who need to be observed and who need intervention. They allow added oxygen and humidity to be given. Nursing and medical procedures disrupt the environmental temperature control, resulting in temperature instability.[50]

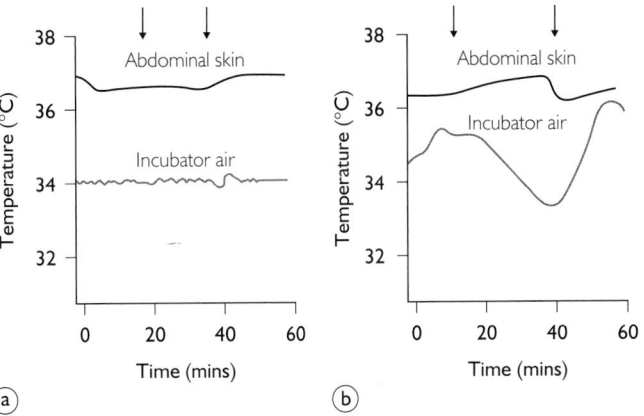

Fig. 15.5 Fluctuations in incubator air temperature when used (a) in air mode and (b) in servo mode. In air mode, the set temperature (air) is 34°C, and in servo mode, the set temperature (skin) is 36.3°C. Handling for brief spells for routine nursing procedures is indicated (↓).

Temperature settings depend on whether the baby is clothed or naked, on the weight and the postnatal age. The values shown in Table 15.3 are estimated to provide an environmental temperature at the lower end of the neutral thermal range under conditions of low air speed (below 10 cm/s), moderate relative humidity (50%), and where the temperature of the inner wall is the same as the air temperature. When used in the servo mode, the required set skin temperatures are the same as those recommended for babies nursed under radiant warmers (Table 15.4).

There is a complex relationship between the water content of the air (absolute humidity), the water content of the air expressed as a percentage of the maximum possible water content (relative humidity), and air temperature.[30] Room air at 20°C in the British Isles has a relative humidity of about 50%. In a warm neonatal intensive care unit at 30°C the same room air is only about 30% saturated, whereas in an unhumidified

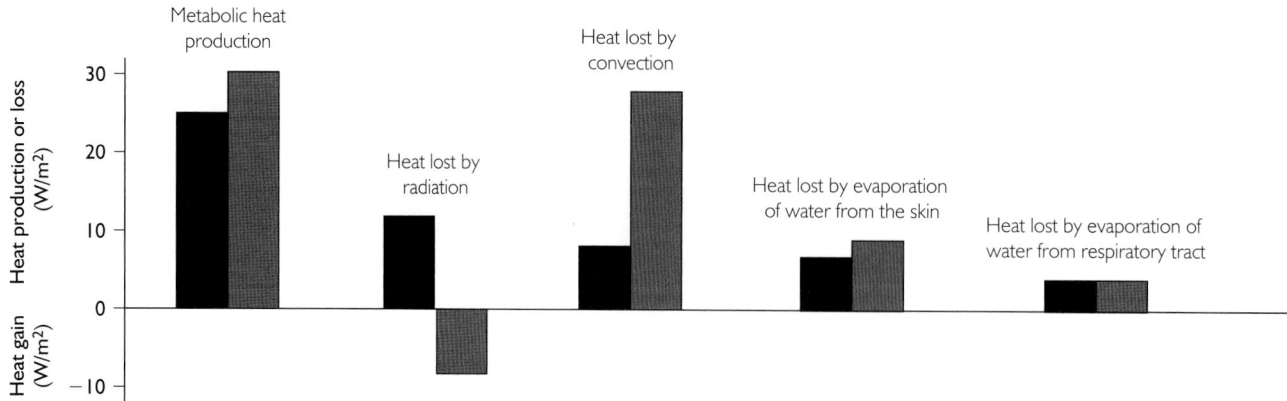

Fig. 15.6 Heat production, losses and gains of 11 preterm infants (mean birthweight 1.58 kg, gestation 32 weeks, age 7 days) nursed naked in an incubator (black bars) and under a radiant warmer (grey bars) in presumed neutral thermal conditions. (Redrawn from Wheldon & Rutter.[67])

Table 15.3 Average incubator air temperatures needed to provide a suitable thermal environment for naked, healthy infants (From Hey[31])

Birthweight (kg)	Environmental temperature			
	35°C	34°C	33°C	32°C
1.0–1.5	For 10 days	After 10 days	After 3 weeks	After 5 weeks
1.5–2.0		For 10 days	After 10 days	After 4 weeks
2.0–2.5		For 2 days	After 2 days	After 3 weeks
>2.5			For 2 days	After 2 days

Note:

- In a single-walled incubator, the environmental temperature needs to be increased by 1°C for every 7°C difference between room and incubator temperature.
- Very-low-birthweight infants (<1 kg) need higher air temperatures and a humidified incubator in the first week.[59,66]
- The values are averages but there is considerable individual variation.

incubator at 37°C the relative humidity may be as low as 25%. A baby of less than 30 weeks' gestation, a day or so old, nursed in an unhumidified incubator, may have an evaporative heat loss that exceeds metabolic heat production (Fig. 15.7). The baby may therefore remain cold, even in an air temperature of 37°C. Humidification is an effective way of reducing this evaporative heat loss and maintaining a normal body temperature (Fig. 15.8). Its routine use is recommended in incubator-nursed babies below 30 weeks' gestation in the first week of life.[28] Modern incubator humidifiers provide good humidity control: the maximum setting should be used, producing a relative humidity of 80–90% at the maximum air temperature. Humidification itself is probably of no advantage to the more mature baby. The disadvantages of humidification are condensation of moisture on the inner wall of the incubator ('rain-out') and infection. Condensation can be reduced by use of a high room temperature or a double-walled incubator. Risk of infection has perhaps been exaggerated. Alternative methods of reducing high evaporative heat losses, such as plastic covering or an emollient ointment, are less effective (see earlier).

Table 15.4 Suggested abdominal skin temperature settings for infants nursed under radiant warmers or in servo-mode incubators

Weight (kg)	Abdominal skin temperature (°C)
<1.0	36.9
1.0–1.5	36.7
1.5–2.0	36.5
2.0–2.5	36.3
>2.5	36.0

Incubators are generally safe. Overheating of the baby is rare unless the incubator is subjected to an additional source of heat such as direct sunlight. Cold stress is more common than heat stress. The perspex canopy provides a welcome barrier between the ill baby and his or her attendant, except when access is necessary for practical procedures, but parents often dislike this barrier and are relieved when their baby is transferred to a cot.

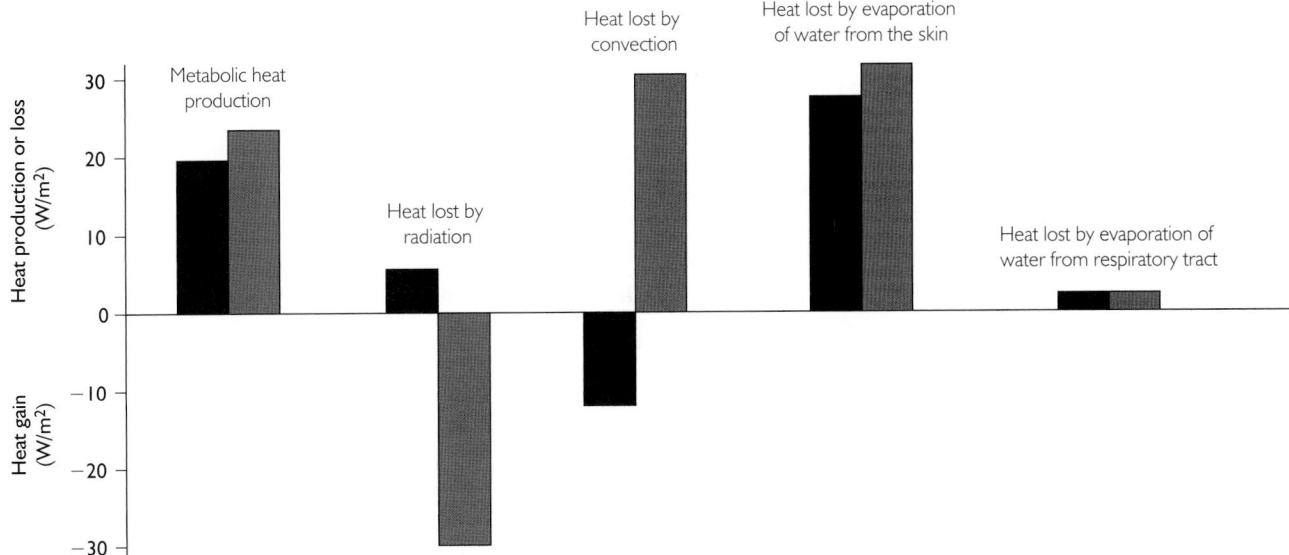

Fig. 15.7 Heat production, losses and gains of an infant of 28 weeks' gestation, birthweight 1.08 kg, on the third day. When nursed naked in a dry incubator (black bars), air temperature 37.7°C, rectal temperature fell to 36.4°C. This is because her high skin evaporative heat loss exceeded the metabolic heat production. When nursed under a radiant warmer (grey bars), set to provide a skin temperature of 36.8°C, rectal temperature rapidly rose to 36.8°C because of the high radiant heat gain. (Redrawn from Wheldon & Rutter.[67])

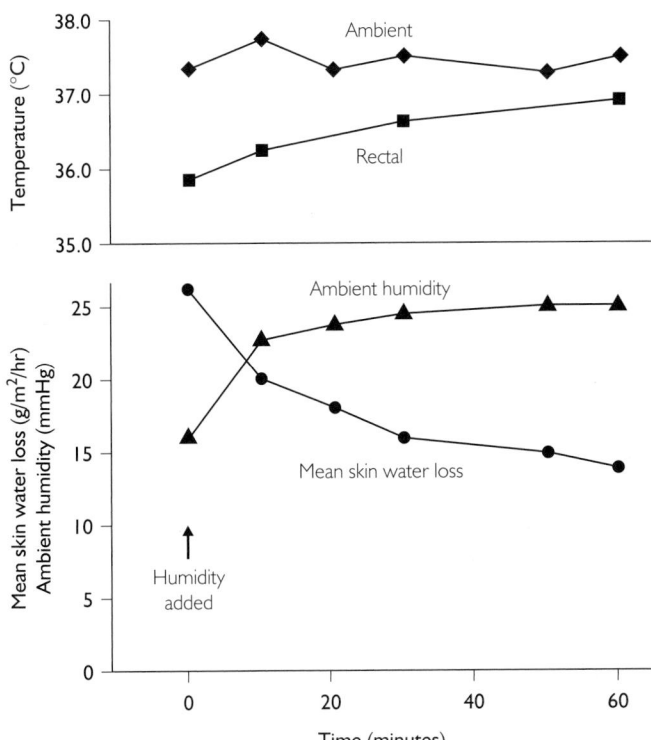

Fig. 15.8 The effect of humidifying an incubator. The baby (30 weeks' gestation, 1 day old) has a rectal temperature of 35.8°C in spite of an incubator temperature of 37.3°C. When humidity is added, skin water loss falls and the rectal temperature steadily increases to 37.0°C.

Care under radiant warmers

This is an alternative device for nursing naked babies who need to be observed closely. The baby lies on an open cradle over which is suspended a heat source emitting radiant energy in the frequency spectrum 700–300 000 nm. The heater is placed approximately 90 cm from the baby's surface and the maximum output does not usually exceed 500 W/m,[2] being controlled in a proportional way by the baby's skin temperature. A thermistor is lightly taped to the upper abdomen and the desired temperature selected. The recommended set temperatures depend on the baby's size (see Table 15.4). Fixed-output low-power heaters are only suitable for keeping babies warm during brief procedures such as resuscitation.

The thermal environment is obviously different from that provided by an incubator.[3,67] The baby is exposed to cool, dry, draughty air and a markedly fluctuating radiant heat source (Fig. 15.9). Heat loss by convection is therefore high, but heat is gained by radiation (see Fig. 15.6). Several studies have shown that babies nursed under radiant warmers have higher resting levels of oxygen consumption than those nursed in incubators: the increase is about 10–20%. Evaporative heat loss is consistently higher in babies nursed under radiant warmers and is due to an increase in water loss from the skin rather than from the respiratory tract.[67] The increase varies from 25% to 150%. Surface temperature distribution is more uneven in babies nursed under radiant warmers: the peripheries are cooler than in babies nursed in incubators with the same mean skin temperature. Skin and limb blood flow is increased by 50% and there is a small (5%) increase in cardiac output caused by an increase in heart rate. Radiant warmers therefore produce a fluctuating, asymmetrical thermal environment compared to the constant even temperature provided by an incubator. No study has shown that either method is superior to the other in terms of the mortality, morbidity and growth of babies nursed in them.[17] Radiant warmers are, however, potentially more dangerous than incubators. Overheating from probe detachment or interference can occur quickly, so the baby's surface or core temperature

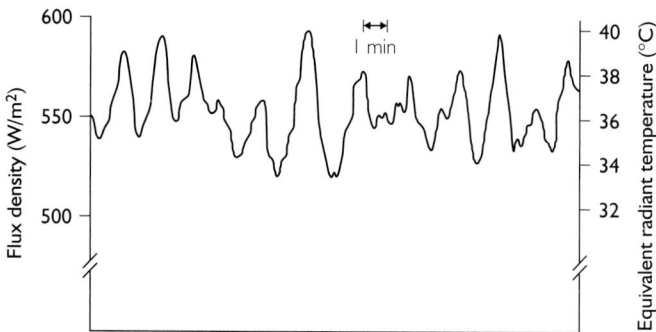

Fig. 15.9 Typical recording of radiant flux density incident on the upper abdomen of an infant nursed under a radiant warmer. The infant is 32 weeks' gestation, birthweight 1.42 kg, age 9 days: the room temperature is 28.5°C. The estimated mean radiant temperature is shown on the right-hand axis. Fluctuations are due to cycling of the servo-control system. (Redrawn from Wheldon & Rutter.[67])

needs continuous independent monitoring. The increased evaporative water loss may result in hypernatraemic dehydration[38] or, if overenthusiastically replaced, in an increased incidence of patent ductus arteriosus. The baby's fluid intake needs to be carefully assessed. Insensible water loss can be reduced in babies under radiant warmers by covering them with a rigid perspex box.[9,68] This impairs the radiant heat exchange between baby and warmer, producing a thermal environment with features of a warmer and an incubator. A more acceptable measure is to cover the baby in a clear plastic film.[4,5] This results in lower oxygen consumption and less demand for radiant heat.[2]

The advantages of using a radiant warmer are threefold: it is the most effective way of keeping a very small baby warm (see Fig. 15.7), particularly in the first 24 hours after delivery when considerable handling is necessary;[49] it is the quickest way of rewarming a cold baby; and it allows easy access for practical procedures.

The heated water-filled mattress

This was developed to provide an alternative method of keeping small babies warm, suitable for use in developing countries. Compared with the incubator or radiant warmer, it is cheap, simple, readily acceptable to mothers and babies, and is not dependent on a continuous supply of electricity. The mattress is a polyvinyl bag filled with 10 l of water and heated by a foil pad. This has a high thermal capacity and will therefore continue to provide warmth after the power source is interrupted. The water temperature is thermostatically controlled and can be regulated from 35°C to 38°C. Preterm babies can be safely nursed in a cot on a heated water-filled mattress if they are stable and do not have to be undressed for observation.[58] Temperature control, metabolic rate and weight gain compare favourably with similar babies nursed in incubators. The heated water-filled mattress is an excellent method for rewarming hypothermic preterm infants, being safer than and superior to an incubator.[57] Preterm babies nursed on a water-filled mattress suffer less cold stress and may grow better than those nursed in a warm room.[19]

Thermal environment during transport

Transporting a small sick baby from one hospital to another for intensive care is a considerable challenge. Such babies are often cold to start with, their heat losses are great and their heat production is small. Furthermore, the environmental temperature during transport may be very low, sometimes below 0°C. Transport incubators are generally less satisfactory in terms of performance than nursing incubators. The essentials of keeping a small sick baby warm during transport are:

- to reduce the high radiant heat losses which occur if the baby is nursed naked – this can be achieved by covering the baby or by use of a double walled incubator;
- to reduce the high evaporative heat loss – the baby should be covered in a plastic film or bubble blanket;
- to observe the baby by remote means – heart rate, respiratory rate, temperature and transcutaneous oxygen tension or saturation can be measured without touching the baby;
- to maintain a high air temperature – in babies of 1 kg or below, the required air temperature will be close to 37°C.

A portable incubator with double walls or with a radiant heat source in the wall will substantially reduce a baby's heat loss in very cold environments. Added humidity greatly assists maintenance of a normal body temperature in the very immature baby.

Surgery

The newborn baby undergoing surgery is at particular risk of cold stress. The operating theatre air and wall temperatures are often low and the room is draughty. The baby is usually starved and drugged, so that his or her response to cold stress is blunted. Furthermore, exposed organs lose water, and therefore heat, by evaporation.

Cold stress can be minimised by the following measures:

- the air temperature in the theatre should be raised to 28–30°C;
- the baby should be well insulated before being taken to theatre: this is effectively achieved by wrapping the limbs, trunk and scalp with cotton-wool lagging;
- the area of the baby exposed for surgery should be kept to a minimum;
- some supplementary source of heat should be provided: an electric warming pad below, or a radiant heater above the baby can be used.

Disorders of temperature control

The baby with a low body temperature (below 36°C rectal)

Mild degrees of hypothermia are common, particularly following delivery. More severe hypothermia (below 34°C rectal) is less common and usually due to overwhelming cold stress. In hospital, it is typically seen in small, sick preterm babies in the early neonatal period, when they are nursed in incubators and handled frequently. Use of a polyethylene bag to cover the newly born preterm baby in the delivery room has been shown to reduce early hypothermia.[64] The use of a radiant warmer also avoids this early hypothermia.[49] Outside hospital, accidental hypothermia is liable to occur when a baby is born unexpectedly or when the birth is concealed. Hypothermia may occur in the first few weeks of life, particularly if the baby is nursed in an unheated room and the outside temperature drops below freezing on a cold winter night. Infection (particularly pneumonia and septicaemia), serious congenital abnormality (particularly cyanotic heart disease or severe cardiac failure) and low birthweight are predisposing factors. Malnutrition also predisposes to hypothermia, by reducing tissue insulation and the metabolic response to cold. Rapid screening for hypothermia is feasible using a simple chemical strip to record axillary or abdominal skin temperature.[40]

Babies with moderate or severe hypothermia are lethargic, feed poorly, have a weak cry and reduced movements. Peripheral oedema is common and areas of sclerema may occur in severe cases. Marked facial erythema may give a false impression of a healthy baby, but the skin always feels strikingly cold. The diagnosis will be made when rectal temperature is measured with a low-reading thermometer, but will be missed if the usual clinical thermometer with a minimum reading of 35°C is used. In very severe cases (rectal temperature below 28°C), the baby may appear virtually dead, with profound cardiorespiratory depression. There are anecdotal reports of such babies being left for dead but eventually making a full recovery.

There is limited information available about the safest and most effective method of rewarming cold babies. Very slow rewarming over several days has been advocated, particularly in babies with chronic cold exposure who have developed cold injury. Increasingly, though, it appears that it is safe to rewarm cold babies more rapidly, at a rate of 1–2°C/h. In an incubator, this can be achieved using the maximum air temperature setting, or by setting the air temperature to a level which is 1–2°C higher than body temperature, and increasing it in a stepwise fashion until the baby is warm. Radiant warmers are effective in treating hypothermic babies, using a set skin temperature of 37°C.[39] Sarman et al[57] found that a heated water-filled mattress was superior to an incubator in rewarming 53 hypothermic preterm babies. Skin-to-skin contact has also been shown to be a safe and effective method of rewarming.[12]

Complications may occur during rewarming. If rapid rewarming of the baby's surface diverts blood from the core, hypotension can result. It has been suggested that use of a plasma expander during rewarming may improve survival.[60] Hypoglycaemia should be looked for and prevented by a slow intravenous infusion of 10% dextrose. Care should be taken in interpreting blood gas results, as pH is temperature dependent. It rises by 0.016 pH units for every 1°C fall in temperature, so that blood with a pH of 6.94 at 37°C will have a pH of 7.10 at 27°C. Because pH is always measured at 37°C, it is easy to overestimate and therefore overtreat a metabolic acidosis in a hypothermic baby. Abdominal distension is common and necrotising enterocolitis may occur. Feeding should not start until a normal body temperature has

been achieved. Haemorrhagic pulmonary oedema is a sinister sign and a common autopsy finding in babies who die from hypothermia. The reported mortality rate in severe hypothermia is 20–50%, but this includes babies with congenital abnormalities or serious infection that contributed to the hypothermia. Most survivors develop normally.

If the cause of the hypothermia is obvious, as for example in a small baby born unattended at home or a baby abandoned in the cold, further investigation is not necessary as a routine. If, however, a young baby is admitted to hospital and found to be hypothermic, with a recent history of being unwell, then an infective cause should be looked for. A full infection screen, including a chest X-ray and a lumbar puncture, will be necessary. Respiratory syncytial virus infection, especially pneumonia or bronchiolitis, is particularly associated with hypothermia in very young babies. If accidental cold exposure and infection have been eliminated as the cause, hypothyroidism should be considered.

The baby with a raised body temperature (above 38°C rectal)

There are two explanations for a raised body temperature: the baby may have an increased set-point temperature or may be overheated. In a study of a large number of term babies, a raised body temperature was found in 1% in the early neonatal period.[65] Of these, 10% had a bacterial infection and 90% were overheated. Babies with a raised set-point temperature behave as if they are cold. Heat production is increased, probably by non-shivering thermogenesis, and heat loss is reduced by cutaneous vasoconstriction. An increase in set-point temperature is a common finding in an infected newborn, although this is a less reliable and less marked sign than in older babies and children with infection. Of 371 babies aged up to 30 days, the rates of serious bacterial infection were 4.4% for those with a rectal temperature of 38.1–39.0°C, 7.6% for the range 39.1–39.9°C, and 18% above 39.9°C, but only 6% of febrile babies had a temperature in the latter range.[11] An increased set-point temperature is also seen in babies with a serious congenital abnormality of the brain, especially hydranencephaly, encephalocoele, holoprosencephaly and trisomy 13, and following severe birth asphyxia, where it is a poor prognostic sign. Such babies have an instability of thermoregulation as a result of hypothalamic damage.[13] Overheating is the commonest cause of a raised temperature and almost always the cause of hyperpyrexia (above 41°C rectal). It is common in restless, active babies and in overwrapped babies left in a warm room. It is also seen in a baby born to a pyrexial mother, regardless of whether the baby is infected. A baby's temperature at birth reflects maternal temperature and is usually about 0.5°C higher. Epidural anaesthesia is commonly associated with an elevated maternal temperature. The baby is therefore likely to have a raised temperature and to be investigated for sepsis.[44]

Hyperpyrexia is rare in the newborn and usually results from mechanical or electrical failure of a warming device. An incubator in direct sunlight behaves like a greenhouse: short-wave radiation passes directly through the perspex canopy and long-wave radiation heats the perspex, which in turn radiates to the

Table 15.5 Differences between a healthy infant who is overheated and a febrile infant with a raised set-point

Overheated infant	Febrile infant
High rectal temperature	High rectal temperature
Warm hands and feet	Cool hands and feet
Abdominal exceeds hand skin temperature by less than 2°C	Abdominal exceeds hand skin temperature by more than 3°C
Pink skin	Pale skin
Extended posture	Lethargic
Healthy appearance	Looks unwell

baby. Serious overheating may occur if the servo probe becomes detached from a baby under a powerful radiant warmer. In early infancy, overheating occurs with excessive wrapping, during heatwaves and when babies are left in closed cars exposed to sunlight. A mild fever of abrupt onset and short duration on the third or fourth day of life is described in babies who are otherwise well and show no signs of infection. It corresponds with the nadir of early neonatal weight loss, and, as the latter is the result of extracellular fluid loss, it is sometimes referred to as dehydration fever.

Mild overheating is not dangerous. It may be associated with an increase in apnoea of prematurity,[7,53] although this is over-emphasised. An increased set-point temperature is possibly beneficial to a baby with an infection. However, hyperpyrexia from overheating is dangerous. Shock, protracted fits, diarrhoea, disseminated intravascular coagulation, and renal and hepatic failure occur in overheated babies,[1] but the few who have died from overheating in the newborn period have done so suddenly, without prior symptoms. Sudden death in infancy has been linked with overheating,[21] and is described in families with a history of malignant hyperpyrexia[14] and hypohidrotic ectodermal dysplasia.[10]

The distinction between an overheated baby and one with an increased set-point temperature is important.[25,54] The overheated baby needs a cooler environment, not a series of painful investigations to find an infective cause for the 'fever'. There are several important differences (Table 15.5). A history of symptoms of infection and an immediate assessment of the thermal environment are important. A useful physical sign is the degree of difference in skin temperature between the abdomen and the hand: the abdomen is always warmer than the hand; in the overheated baby the difference is less than 2°C (often less than 1°C), but in the infected baby it usually exceeds 3.5°C. The same applies to the difference between the rectal temperature and the sole temperature.[48]

Therapeutic hypothermia

Hypothermia has been successfully used in conjuction with cardiopulmonary bypass in babies undergoing open-heart surgery, to extend the time of surgery. Body temperature is lowered rapidly by surface cooling to about 28°C – rewarming is also rapid and appears to be well tolerated. Recently, hypothermia has been explored as a method of cerebral protection in newborn babies who have been subjected to acute asphyxial brain injury during labour.[20] Two methods have been suggested: mild whole body hypothermia (to 34–35°C) by surface cooling of the trunk, and local cooling of the head using a water-cooled cap. The effectiveness of this intervention has yet to be shown, but it appears to be well tolerated.[62]

References

1. Bacon C, Scott D, Jones P 1979 Heat stroke in well-wrapped infants. Lancet i: 422–425
2. Baumgart S 1984 Reduction of oxygen consumption, insensible water loss and radiant heat demand with use of a plastic blanket for low birthweight infants under radiant warmers. Journal of Pediatrics 100: 787–790
3. Baumgart S 1985 Partitioning of heat losses and gains in premature newborn infants under radiant warmers. Pediatrics 75: 89–99
4. Baumgart S, Engle W D, Fox W W, Polin R A 1981 Effect of heat shielding on convective and evaporative heat losses and on radiant heat transfer in the premature infant. Journal of Pediatrics 99: 948–956
5. Baumgart S, Fox W W, Polin R A 1982 Physiologic implications of two different heat shields for infants under radiant warmers. Journal of Pediatrics 100: 787–790
6. Belgaumkar T K, Scott K E 1975 Effects of low humidity on small premature infants in servocontrol incubators. I. Decrease in rectal temperature. Biology of the Neonate 26: 337–347
7. Belgaumkar T K, Scott K E 1975 Effects of low humidity on small premature infants in servocontrol incubators. II. Increased severity of apnoea. Biology of the Neonate 26: 348–352
8. Bell E F, Rios G R 1983 Air versus skin temperature servocontrol of infant incubators. Journal of Pediatrics 103: 954–959
9. Bell E F, Weinstein M R, Oh W 1980 Heat balance in premature infants: comparative effect of convectively incubated and radiant warmer, with and without plastic heat shield. Journal of Pediatrics 96: 460–465
10. Bernstein R, Hatchuel I, Jenkins T 1980 Hypohidrotic ectodermal dysplasia and sudden infant death syndrome. Lancet ii: 1024
11. Bonadio W A, Romine K, Gyuro J 1990 Relationship of fever magnitude to rate of serious bacterial infections in neonates. Journal of Pediatrics 116: 733–735
12. Christensson K, Bhat G J, Amadi B C, Eriksson B, Hojer B 1998 Randomised study of skin-to-skin versus incubator care for rewarming low-risk hypothermic neonates. Lancet 352: 1115
13. Cross K W, Hey E N, Kennaird D L, Lewis S R, Urich H 1971 Lack of temperature control in infants with abnormalities of the central nervous system. Archives of Disease in Childhood 46: 437–443
14. Denborough M A, Galloway G J, Hopkinson K C 1982 Malignant hyperpyrexia and sudden infant death. Lancet ii: 1068–1069
15. Ducker D A, Lyon A J, Ross Russell R, Bass C A, McIntosh N 1985 Incubator temperature control: effects on the very low birthweight infant. Archives of Disease in Childhood 60: 902–907
16. Fanaroff A A, Wald M, Gruber H S, Klaus M H 1972 Insensible water loss in low birth weight infants. Pediatrics 50: 236–245
17. Flenady V J, Woodgate P G 2000 Radiant warmers versus incubators for regulating body temperature in newborn infants (Cochrane Review). Cochrane Database of Systematic Reviews (2): CD000435
18. Gandy G M, Adamsons K, Cunningham N, Silverman W A, James L S 1964 Thermal environment and acid-base homeostasis in human infants during the first few hours of life. Journal of Clinical Investigation 43: 751–758
19. Greenabate C, Tafari N, Rao M R, Yu K F, Clemens J D 1994 Comparison of heated water-filled mattress and space-heated room with infant incubator in providing warmth to low birthweight newborns. International Journal of Epidemiology 23: 1226–1233
20. Gunn A J, Bennet K 2002 Cerebral hypothermia in the management of hypoxic-ischemic encephalopathy. NeoReviews 3: 116–122
21. Guntheroth W G, Spiers P S 2001 Thermal stress in sudden infant death: is there an ambiguity with the rebreathing hypothesis? Pediatrics 107: 693–698
22. Hammarlund K, Sedin G 1979 Transepidermal water loss in newborn infants. III. Relation to gestational age. Acta Paediatrica Scandinavica 68: 795–801

23. Hammarlund K, Nilsson G E, Oberg P A, Sedin G 1980 Transepidermal water loss in newborn infants. V. Evaporation from the skin and heat exchange during the first hours of life. Acta Paediatrica Scandinavica 69: 385–392

24. Hammarlund K, Sedin G, Stromberg B 1983 Transepidermal water loss in newborn infants. VIII. Relation to gestational age and postnatal age in appropriate and small for gestational age infants. Acta Paediatrica Scandinavica 72: 721–728

25. Harpin V A, Chellapah G, Rutter N 1983 The responses of the newborn infant to overheating. Biology of the Neonate 44: 65–75

26. Harpin V A, Rutter N 1982 Sweating in preterm babies. Journal of Pediatrics 100: 614–618

27. Harpin V A, Rutter N 1983 Barrier properties of the newborn infant's skin. Journal of Pediatrics 102: 419–425

28. Harpin V A, Rutter N 1985 Humidification of incubators. Archives of Disease in Childhood 60: 219–224

29. Hey E N 1969 The relation between environmental temperature and oxygen consumption in the new-born baby. Journal of Physiology 200: 589–603

30. Hey E N 1971 The care of babies in incubators. In: Gairdner D, Hull D (eds) Recent advances in paediatrics, 4th edn. J & A Churchill, London, pp 171–216

31. Hey E N 1975 Thermal neutrality. British Medical Bulletin 31: 69–74

32. Hey E N 1983 Temperature regulation in sick infants. In: Tinker J, Rapin M (eds) Care of the critically ill patient. Springer, Berlin, pp 1013–1029

33. Hey E N, Katz G 1969 Evaporative water loss in the new-born baby. Journal of Physiology 200: 605–619

34. Hey E N, Katz G 1970 The optimum thermal environment for naked babies. Archives of Disease in Childhood 45: 328–334

35. Hey E N, Katz G, O'Connell B 1970 The total thermal insulation of the newborn baby. Journal of Physiology 207: 683–698

36. Hey E N, O'Connell B 1970 Oxygen consumption and heat balance in the cot-nursed baby. Archives of Disease in Childhood 45: 335–343

37. Hill J R, Rahimtulla K A 1965 Heat balance and the metabolic rate of new-born babies in relation to environmental temperature, and the effect of age and of weight on basal metabolic rate. Journal of Physiology 280: 239–265

38. Jones R W A, Rochefort M J, Baum J D 1976 Increased insensible water loss in newborn infants nursed under radiant heaters. British Medical Journal ii: 1347–1350

39. Kaplan M, Eidelman A I 1984 Improved prognosis in severely hypothermic newborn infants treated by rapid rewarming. Journal of Pediatrics 105: 470–474

40. Kennedy N, Gondwe L, Morley D C 2000 Temperature monitoring with ThermoSpots in Malawi. Lancet 355: 1364

41. Kjartansson S, Arsan S, Hammarlund K, Sjors G, Sedin G 1995 Water loss from the skin of term and preterm infants nursed under a radiant heater. Pediatric Research 37: 233–238

42. Kjartansson S, Hammarlund K, Sedin G 1992 Insensible water loss from the skin during phototherapy in term and preterm infants. Acta Paediatrica 81: 764–768

43. Knauth A, Gordin M, McNelis W, Baumgart S 1989 Semipermeable polyurethane membrane as an artificial skin for the premature neonate. Pediatrics 83: 945–950

44. Lieberman E, Lang J M, Frigoletto F, Richardson D K, Ringer S A, Cohen A 1997 Epidural analgesia, intrapartum fever and neonatal sepsis evaluation. Pediatrics 99: 415–419

45. Marks K H, Friedman Z, Maisels M J 1977 A simple device for reducing insensible water loss in low birth weight babies. Pediatrics 60: 223–226

46. Marks K H, Lee C, Bolan C D, Maisels M J 1981 Oxygen consumption and temperature control of premature infants in a double-wall incubator. Pediatrics 68: 93–98

47. Mayfield S R, Bhatia J, Nakamura K T, Rios G R, Bell E F 1984 Temperature measurement in term and preterm infants. Journal of Pediatrics 104: 271–275

48. Messaritakis J, Anagnostakis D, Laskari H, Katerelos C 1990 Rectal-skin temperature difference in septicaemic newborn infants. Archives of Disease in Childhood 65: 380–382

49. Meyer M P, Payton M J, Salmon A, Hutchinson C, de Klerk A 2001 A clinical comparison of radiant warmer and incubator care for preterm infants from birth to 1800 grams. Pediatrics 108: 395–401

50. Mok Q, Bass C A, Ducker D A, McIntosh N 1991 Temperature instability during nursing procedures in preterm neonates. Archives of Disease in Childhood 66: 783–786

51. Okken A, Blijam C, Franz W, Bohn E 1982 Effects of forced convection of heated air on insensible water loss and heat loss in preterm infants in incubators. Journal of Pediatrics 101: 108–112

52. Okken A, Jonxis J H P, Rispens P, Zijlstra W G 1979 Insensible water loss and metabolic growth rate in low birth weight newborn babies. Pediatric Research 13: 1072–1075

53. Perlstein P H, Edwards N K, Sutherland J M 1970 Apnoea in premature infants and incubator air temperature changes. New England Journal of Medicine 282: 461–466

54. Pomerance J J, Brand R J, Meredith J L 1981 Differentiating environmental from disease-related fevers in the term newborn. Pediatrics 67: 485–487

55. Rutter N, Hull D 1979 Response of term babies to a warm environment. Archives of Disease in Childhood 54: 178–183

56. Rutter N, Hull D 1979 Water loss from the skin of term and preterm babies. Archives of Disease in Childhood 54: 858–868

57. Sarman I, Can G, Tunell R 1989 Rewarming preterm infants on a heated, water filled mattress. Archives of Disease in Childhood 64: 687–692

58. Sarman I, Tunell R 1989 Providing warmth for preterm babies by a heated, water filled mattress. Archives of Disease in Childhood 64: 29–33

59. Sauer P J J, Dane H J, Visser H K 1984 New standards for neutral thermal environment of healthy very low birthweight infants in week one of life. Archives of Disease in Childhood 59: 18–22

60. Tafari N, Gentz J 1974 Aspects of rewarming newborn infants with severe accidental hypothermia. Acta Paediatrica Scandinavica 63: 595–600

61. Thompson M H, Stothers J K, McLellan N J 1984 Weight and water loss in the neonate in natural and forced convection. Archives of Disease in Childhood 59: 951–956

62. Thoreson M, Whitelaw A 2000 Cardiovascular changes during mild therapeutic hypothermia and rewarming in infants with hypoxic-ischemic encephalopathy. Pediatrics 106: 92–99

63. Vernon H J, Lane A T, Wischerath L J, Davis J M, Menegus M A 1990 Semipermeable dressing and transepidermal water loss in premature infants. Pediatrics 86: 357–362

64. Vohra S, Frent G, Campbell V, Abbott M, Whyte R 1999 Effect of polyethylene occlusive skin wrapping on heat loss in very low birth weight infants at delivery: a randomized trial. Journal of Pediatrics 134: 547–551

65. Voora S, Srinivasan G, Lilien L D, Yeh T F, Pildes R S 1982 Fever in full-term newborns in the first four days of life. Pediatrics 69: 40–44

66. Wheldon A E, Hull D 1983 Incubation of very immature infants. Archives of Disease in Childhood 58: 504–508

67. Wheldon A E, Rutter N 1982 The heat balance of small babies nursed in incubators and under radiant warmers. Early Human Development 6: 131–143

68. Yeh T F, Amma P, Lilien L D et al 1979 Reduction of insensible water loss in premature infants under the radiant warmer. Journal of Pediatrics 94: 651–653

69. Yeh R F, Voora S, Lilien L D, Matwynschyn J, Srinivasan G, Pildes R S 1980 Oxygen consumption and insensible water loss in premature infants in single-space vs double-walled incubators. Journal of Pediatrics 97: 967–997

70. Young D G 1965 'Spontaneous' rupture of the rectum. Proceedings of the Royal Society of Medicine 58: 615–616

CHAPTER 16

Infant feeding

PART I

Nutritional physiology: dietary requirements of term and preterm infants

Mary Fewtrell, Alan Lucas

New perspectives in neonatal nutrition

Since the first edition of this textbook there have been major conceptual changes in neonatal nutrition. Previously, the main objective in feeding infants was meeting nutritional needs, preventing nutritional deficiencies and promoting growth. However, increasing evidence shows that early nutrition has biological effects on the individual with important implications for later health. Thus, the way infants are fed may influence clinical course and prognosis. For instance, in preterm infants, early nutrition may influence propensity to life-threatening diseases such as necrotising enterocolitis (NEC)[85] and systemic sepsis, and, in the long term, have a major impact on cognitive function[88] and disease risk in later life – notably cardiovascular disease.[132]

Until recently, early nutritional practice was underpinned largely by observational or physiological studies, or by small clinical trials designed to test for the effects of specific products on nutritional status, growth and tolerance. Our new understanding of the importance of early nutrition has emerged with the application of the pharmaceutical trial model to nutritional interventions. Formal randomised trials have now produced an evidence-base for nutritional practice, rooted in short-term and, importantly, long-term efficacy and safety testing.

Nutritional programming

The concept that there are sensitive periods in early life when insults or stimuli may have long-term or lifetime effects is known as 'programming',[80] and has been recognised for over a century.

The evidence that nutrition could operate as a programming agent was first shown in animals 40 years ago.[94] Animal studies have shown that nutrition during critical periods in early life can programme outcomes such as changes in metabolism, endocrine function, gut function, size, body fatness, blood pressure, insulin resistance, blood lipids, learning, behaviour and longevity.[81] Over the past decade, the long-term findings from large-scale randomised intervention studies in human infants have been emerging. These studies show that human infants, like other species, are programmed by early diet to a major degree. Early diet can have long-term effects on blood pressure,[132] insulin resistance,[135] blood lipids,[133] tendency to obesity,[134] bone health,[47] atopy,[84] cognitive function[88] and brain structure. The effect sizes are large; in the case of cardiovascular risk factors (blood pressure, blood lipids, insulin resistance), the programming effects of early nutrition are greater than non-pharmacological interventions in adult life, such as exercise and weight loss. These new findings must now be factored into the design of modern nutritional practices and are considered further in the following sections.

Nutrition during fetal life

An understanding of fetal nutritional physiology is vital to clinical practice. From analysis of 'reference fetuses' of different gestational ages, it is possible to calculate daily fetal nutrient accretion rates[49,154,162] and to use these as a basis for studying postnatal nutrition and its disorders. For example, the intrauterine accretion of calcium and phosphorus is substantially higher than that which can be supplied by a standard formula or mature breast milk to premature infants.

Several other nutrients are laid down late in gestation, so that the preterm infant has low body stores. One example is body fat. By mid-gestation, body fat content is less than 1% of body weight; at 28 weeks, 3.5%; at 34 weeks, 7.8%; and at term, 15%. During the last month of intrauterine life, the fetus lays down about 7 g of fat per day.[154]

Carbohydrate stores are also laid down relatively late. Shelley[128] estimated liver glycogen to be about 1 g/100 g of tissue at 31 weeks and 4 g/100 g at term. Widdowson[154] calculated total body carbohydrate to be 9 g at 33 weeks and 34 g at term. These data have been used to calculate the ability of infants of different gestations to withstand starvation and maintain glucose homoeostasis after birth.

Total body water falls progressively from over 95% of body weight in the first trimester to around 75% at term[54] and continues to fall throughout infancy.

Lipid-soluble vitamins are transferred across the placenta by simple or facilitated diffusion,[93,107] hence fetal blood concentrations of such vitamins correlate well with those in the mother, with the exception of vitamin E – for which fetal blood levels are around 30% of maternal values.[99] These vitamins accumulate in fetal tissues throughout pregnancy. Blood concentrations, and perhaps body stores, are reduced in preterm infants and those of poorly nourished mothers. Water-soluble vitamins are transported against concentration gradients, mostly by active transport: fetal blood levels of vitamins B_1, B_2, B_6, B_{12}, folate and vitamin C are two- to fourfold higher than those in maternal blood. Preterm babies and babies of undernourished mothers have lower blood levels of water-soluble vitamins at birth.[8]

'Biological clock' of fetal development

Intermediary metabolism

Throughout fetal life there is a progressively changing picture of enzymatic differentiation.[62] Certain enzymes of amino acid metabolism develop late, including those concerned with the synthesis of cysteine from methionine, taurine from cysteine, and tyrosine from phenylalanine, with degradation of tyrosine[112] and production of urea.[15] As a result, low-birthweight (LBW) infants might be expected to have increased dietary requirements for certain amino acids (such as cysteine and taurine; p. 326) and be at risk for possibly deleterious accumulation of others (such as phenylalanine, tyrosine and methionine; pp. 326–7).

Key enzymes in gluconeogenic pathways (e.g. phosphoenolpyruvate carboxykinase) may not develop until near or even just after term delivery.[62] A constant transplacental glucose infusion renders gluconeogenesis relatively unimportant in utero, and the fetal liver is more concerned with the storage of glucose as glycogen; phosphorylase and glucose 6-phosphatase ensure immediate glucose release after birth and defer the need for gluconeogenesis until around 24–48 hours of age; in contrast, the preterm neonate, born with low stores of liver glycogen[154] and reduced gluconeogenic ability, is at risk of hypoglycaemia (pp. 853–62).

Gastrointestinal tract

See Chapter 31.

Adaptations to extrauterine nutrition

Adaptation to feeding after birth involves major postnatal changes in gut structure and function and in intermediary metabolism. Although the fetal intestine is structurally mature by 25 weeks' gestation and capable of digesting and absorbing milk feeds, motor activity develops more slowly, and may limit the tolerance to enteral feeds.

Postnatally, enteral feeding appears to play a key part in triggering gut development. Studies on piglets and rats show marked structural and functional changes in the gastrointestinal (GI) tract and its adnexae following feeding – changes not seen in unfed animals. These effects are not confined to the gut: for example, enteral feeding may cause increased responsiveness to glucose by pancreatic β cells. Enteral feeding is not a new experience for the newborn infant: by the end of pregnancy, the fetus is swallowing about 500 ml of amniotic fluid daily, providing up to 3 g of protein,[54] a similar fluid intake and about 25–50% of the protein intake of the breastfed infant at term. Enteral feeding in utero contributes to fetal nutrition and may help to prepare the gut for extrauterine feeding.

The following factors are important in regulating the adaptation of the intestine to extrauterine nutrition:

- **Endocrine secretion**. Corticosteroids and thyroxine are critical triggers for gut development.[78] Adrenalectomy, hypophysectomy and thyroidectomy in animals delay gut maturation, whereas administration of glucocorticoids or thyroxine prior to delivery causes elongation of microvilli, increases the activities of the brush-border enzymes sucrase, enteropeptidase and alkaline phosphatase, and induces pancreatic enzyme secretion postnatally.

- **Intraluminal factors**. These may be endogenous (secreted by the GI tract) or exogenous (dietary nutrients), and act either directly on the cells of the GI tract, or indirectly via effects on hormone secretion. For example, in neonatal rats, enteral feeding with sucrose increases intestinal sucrase and isomaltase, whereas lactose increases gut lactase,[78] a finding consistent with the observed tolerance of preterm infants to lactose despite the late development of lactase in infants born at term. Surges in plasma levels of gut hormones can be induced by small, nutritionally insignificant volumes of milk, leading to the concept of minimal enteral feeding, where small volumes of milk are used to promote intestinal maturation and adaptation even when the infant is too sick to tolerate full enteral nutrition. Minimal enteral feeding has been demonstrated to produce more ordered patterns of gut motility,[12] more rapid gut transit times,[95] and results in improved growth, greater energy intakes, fewer episodes of culture-confirmed sepsis, reduced requirements for supplemental oxygen, and earlier tolerance of enteral feeds, with reduced requirements for parenteral nutrition.[96] However, although intraluminal factors undoubtedly influence GI development, they do not provide the sole trigger for ontogenetic changes, as normal maturational patterns of enzymes may occur in surgically bypassed segments of gut.[143]

- **Breast-milk hormones and growth factors** (Chapter 16, Part 2, p. 309). A large number of substances present in human milk have been demonstrated to play a role in regulating the adaptive changes that accompany the transition to enteral feeding. These include bombesin, somatostatin, epidermal growth factor, IGF-1 and IGF-2, and nucleotides. In many cases these substances undergo only limited degradation in the stomach and appear to retain bioactivity in the intestine. Although they may not be essential for survival, the higher incidence of GI disease in infants fed formula raise the possibility that these compounds may contribute to the protective effect of human milk.
- **Bacteria.** Studies on the GI flora of infants fed human milk or formula suggest that the indigenous microflora are an important factor in GI development and function, altering the activities of various enzymes.[140]

Biological consequences of depriving babies of enteral feeds after birth

Exclusive intravenous feeding in rats results in decreased weight of the small intestine, pancreas and oxyntic area of the stomach, associated with a significant reduction in small-intestinal DNA and a dramatic reduction in antral gastrin content; in contrast, animal studies have shown that other organs not directly concerned with nutrition, such as spleen and testes, remain unaffected,[71] and Heird[65] has demonstrated intestinal mucosal atrophy during parenteral nutrition, with concomitant reduction in brush-border enzyme activities. These effects may be related to the very low concentrations of circulating gut hormones found in human infants deprived of enteral feeding.

Although after short periods of parenteral nutrition in neonates tolerance to enteral feeds usually increases rapidly (in the absence of structural anomaly of the gut), it remains to be established whether prolonged avoidance of enteral feeding could deprive the neonate of critical signals for gut development.

Non-nutritional consequences of enteral feeding

When a neonate is fed, dynamic alterations occur in splanchnic blood flow, with a significant increase in velocity, which is 35% greater in formula-fed term infants than in breastfed infants. Fasting velocities are also higher in formula-fed infants.[32] In preterm infants, there is a significant correlation between the increase in mean superior mesenteric artery (SMA) blood flow seen after a test feed and subsequent early tolerance of enteral feeds.[42] Preterm infants fed hourly have higher preprandial blood flow in the SMA, with no significant postprandial change, whereas those fed 3 hourly show lower preprandial blood flow and significant postprandial hyperaemia, with a longer latency and smaller amplitude after expressed breast milk than after preterm formula.[77]

These findings suggest that both the frequency and composition of feeds influence splanchnic blood flow in preterm infants. Changes may also occur in pulmonary function, with decreased tidal volume, minute ventilation and compliance in very-low-birthweight (VLBW) infants randomised to intermittent versus continuous feeds.[14]

Individual nutrients: physiology and dietary needs of term and preterm infants

Calculation of the nutrient requirements for term infants has traditionally been based on the composition of breast milk. However, the precise dietary intake of breastfed babies is unknown, and there is ongoing uncertainty over what should be regarded as an ideal pattern of growth during infancy, with data from animals and now humans increasingly suggesting that accelerated early growth may be associated with adverse effects on later health. Thus, appropriate dietary goals continue to be disputed. The EC Directive on Infant Formulae[31] recommendations for the nutrient content of the diet of formula-fed babies are shown in Table 16.1. All infant-formula manufacturers in the UK are required by law to comply with these, under the Infant Formula and Follow-On Formula Regulations[68] of 1995 and 1997.

LBW babies are not a homogeneous population: their requirements and tolerance of individual nutrients are influenced by gestation, postnatal age and concomitant illness. Nevertheless, there is some international consensus on the advisable intakes for each nutrient. This field was comprehensively reviewed by the Committee on Nutrition of the European Society for Paediatric Gastroenterology and Nutrition,[41] and most recently by a panel of international experts,[142] who considered separately the needs of infants above or below 1000 g; a summary of the recommendations by this panel for intakes of individual nutrients is shown in Table 16.2. The scientific and clinical basis for current recommendations for the desirable nutrient intakes in preterm infants is illustrated below.

Proteins and amino acids

The protein intake per kilogram bodyweight for the human infant is greater than for adults. In mammals, the protein content of milk correlates highly with postnatal growth rate. Nine amino acids are considered essential in human nutrition: arginine, lysine, leucine, isoleucine, valine, methionine, phenylalanine, threonine and tryptophan. However, because of the late development of certain enzymes of amino acid metabolism, the newborn infant may have a temporarily increased requirement for cysteine and histidine, and perhaps for taurine (see below).

Digestion and absorption

Luminal hydrolysis results in the breakdown of most large molecular weight proteins into peptides and amino acids. Most peptides are then hydrolysed by peptidases on the microvillus

Table 16.1 Composition of mature human milk and nutritional guidelines for the composition of artificial feeds for full-term infants per 100 ml (EC Directive Guidelines, 1991[31])

	Mean values for pooled samples of expressed mature human milk	Guidelines for infant formulas	
		Minimum	Maximum
Energy			
kJ	293	250	315
kcal	70	60	75
Protein (g)	1.3		
Casein dominant			
Infant formula		1.35	2.25
Whey dominant			
Infant formula		1.08	2.25
Lactose (g)	7	2.1	NS
Total carbohydrate (g)		4.2	10.5
Fat (g)	4.2	2.0	4.9
Vitamins (μg)			
A	60	36	135
D	0.01	0.6	1.9
E*	0.35	0.3	NS
K	0.21	2.4	NS
Thiamin	16	24	NS
Riboflavin	30	36	NS
Nicotinic acid	230	150	NS
Pyridoxine	6	21	NS
B_{12}	0.01	0.06	NS
Folic acid	5.2	2.4	NS
Biotin	0.76	0.9	NS
C	3.8	4.8	NS
Minerals			
Sodium (mg)	15	12	45
Potassium (mg)	60	36	109
Chloride (mg)	43	30	94
Calcium (mg)	35	30	NS
Phosphorus (mg)	15	15	67.5
Magnesium (mg)	2.3	3.0	11.25
Iron (μg)	76	600	1500
Iodine (μg)	7	3.0	NS
Zinc (mg)	0.295	0.45	1.8
Copper (μg)	39	12	60

*mg(TE) – tocopherol equivalents. NS, not specified.

membrane prior to transport through the membrane, but some are absorbed intact. Although pepsin secretion is lower in preterm than term infants at birth, it is unaffected by the type of diet.[63] The activity of brush-border peptidases is also low in preterm infants at birth, but increases rapidly.

Protein requirements for term babies

These are discussed further on page 303. The EC Directive guidelines[31] recommend that formulas containing unmodified cow's milk protein should contain 1.35–2.25 g of protein per 100 ml of reconstituted feed, whereas if the casein/whey ratio is adjusted to be closer to human milk (2:3), a minimum of 1.1 g of protein per 100 ml of feed is suggested. This implies that cow's milk whey has a higher biological value for human infants than cow's milk casein, but this has never been proven. As growth velocity falls during infancy, there is a progressively decreased need for protein intake per kilogram of bodyweight.

Estimating the protein requirements for the preterm baby

That the rapid growth in preterm babies might greatly increase the need for dietary protein has been appreciated for over 40 years.

Table 16.2 Recommended intakes of individual nutrients for (formula-fed) stable/growing preterm infants (International Consensus Recommendation, Tsang et al 1993[142])

	<1000 g			>1000 g		
	Per kg per day SI units	Per kg per day mass units	Per 100 kcal mass units	Per kg per day SI units	Per kg per day mass units	Per 100 kcal mass units
Energy						
kcal	110–120	110–120	100	110–120	110–120	100
kJ	460–502	460–502	419	460–502	460–502	419
Protein (g)	3.6–3.8	3.6–3.8	3.0–3.16	3.0–3.6	3.0–3.6	2.5–3.0
Fat (g)						
Linoleic	4–15% cal	4–15% cal	0.44–1.7 g	4–15% cal	4–15% cal	0.44–1.7 g
Linolenic	1–4% cal	1–4% cal	0.11–0.44 g	1–4% cal	1–4% cal	0.11–0.44 g
C18:2/C18:3	⩾5	⩾5	⩾5	⩾5	⩾5	⩾5
Carbohydrate (g)						
Lactose	3.8–11.4	3.8–11.4	3.16–9.5	3.8–11.8	3.8–11.8	3.16–9.8
Oligomers	0–8.4	0–8.4	0–7.0	0–8.4	0–8.4	0–7.0
Sodium (mmol/mg)	2–3	46–69	38–58	2–3	46–69	1.66–2.5
Potassium (mmol/mg)	2–3	78–120	65–100	2–3	78–120	1.66–2.5
Chloride (mmol/mg)	2–3	70–105	59–89	2–3	70–105	1.66–2.5
Calcium (mmol/mg)	2–3	120–230	100–192	2–3	120–230	1.66–2.5
Phosphorus (mmol/mg)	1.94–4.52	60–140	50–117	1.94–4.52	60–140	1.61–3.77
Magnesium (mmol/mg)	0.33–0.63	7.9–15	6.6–12.5	0.33–0.63	7.9–15	0.275–0.53
Iron (μmol/mg)	36	2	1.67	36	2	30
Zinc (μmol/μg)	15	1000	833	15	1000	12.7
Copper (μmol/μg)	1.9–2.4	120–150	100–125	1.9–2.4	120–150	1.6–2.0
Selenium (nmol/μg)	16–38	1.3–3.0	1.08–1.25	16–38	1.3–3.0	14–32
Manganese (nmol/μg)	136	7.5	6.3	136	7.5	115
Iodine (nmol/μg)	236–472	30–60	25–50	236–472	30–60	197–394
Vitamin A (IU)	700–1500	700–1500	583–1250	700–1500	700–1500	583–1250
Vitamin D (IU)	150–400*	150–400	125–333	150–400*	150–400	125–333
Vitamin E (IU)	6–12+	6–12	5–10	6–12+	6–12	5–10
Vitamin K (nmol/μg)	18–22	8–10	6.66–8.33	18–22	8–10	15–18.5
Vitamin C (mmol/mg)	102–136	18–24	15.20	102–136	18–24	85–114
Thiamin (μmol/μg)	0.53–0.71	180–240	150–200	0.53–0.71	180–240	0.45–0.59
Riboflavin (μmol/μg)	0.66–0.96	250–360	200–300	0.66–0.96	250–360	0.53–0.8
Pyridoxine (μmol/μg)	0.73–1.02	150–210	125–175	0.73–1.02	150–210	0.61–0.85
Niacin (mmol/mg)	30–39	3.6–4.8	3–4	30–39	3.6–4.8	25–33
B12 (nmol/μg)	0.22	0.3	0.25	0.22	0.3	0.18
Folate (nmol/μg)	56–113	25–50	21–42	56–113	25–50	48–95
Taurine (μmol/mg)	36–72	4.5–9.0	3.75–7.5	36–72	4.5–9.0	30–60
Carnitine (μmol/mg)	~18	~2.9	~2.4	~18	~2.9	~15
Inositol (mmol/mg)	0.18–0.45	32–81	27–67.5	0.18–0.45	32–81	0.15–0.375
Choline (μmol/mg)	138–270	14.4–28	12–23.4	138–270	14.4–28	115–225

*aim for 400 IU per day.
+max = 25 IU.

The principles used to assess protein needs serve as a model for the investigation of requirements for other nutrients.

Relation of protein intake to growth

Weight gain and linear growth are the traditional measures of nutritional status. Gordon et al[60] demonstrated in 1947 that preterm infants gained weight more rapidly on high protein-containing formulas than on human milk, and Davidson et al[37] showed that weight gain was greater in preterm infants fed a formula supplying 4 g/kg/24 h rather than 2 g/kg/24 h. High intakes of protein may also result in an increase in linear growth and a greater rate of increase in head circumference.[17,87]

A factorial approach

Protein requirements may be derived using a combination of values for body composition[163] and for nitrogen retention, obtained from balance studies. The results from a number of such studies show that protein gain increases linearly with intakes between approximately 2 g/kg/24 h and 4 g/kg/24 h.[98] These calculations involve making assumptions about desirable postnatal growth performance, but the results emphasise that, in order to achieve the accretion of nitrogen at the same rate as seen in utero during the third trimester, the preterm infant requires substantially greater intakes of protein than would be obtained by a term infant fed on breast milk.

In a sick infant in whom a temporary period of reduced nutritional intake is necessary, it is important at least to prevent catabolism. Theoretically, a protein intake of 0.5 g/kg/24 h will result in a reduction of protein turnover to the point of equilibrium (that is, zero gain and zero loss), and from a pragmatic point of view this should be the minimum acceptable daily intake. However, nutritional restriction for medical reasons must be weighed against the long-term consequences of suboptimal nutrition (see below).

Assessment of protein undernutrition

A low concentration of plasma protein is a traditional index of protein malnutrition. Preterm infants fed on human milk (banked or own mother's) may develop hypoproteinaemia after the second month of postnatal life, and this is prevented by protein supplementation.[118] By using traditional nitrogen balance studies, the protein deposition in new tissue can be estimated. In one such study of infants fed on a preterm formula providing 3.6 g protein per kilogram per day, the percentage of protein in new tissue (12.8%) was within the range described in utero (11–14%); in contrast, those fed on mature donor breast milk, providing around 2.2 g protein per kilogram per day, had only 8.7% protein in new tissue, suggesting a low protein content in lean body mass, as seen in experimental malnutrition.[117]

Assessment of protein 'overload'

The Committee of Nutrition of the American Academy of Pediatrics[2] stated in 1977 that 'The optimal diet for the low-birthweight infant may be defined as one that supports a rate of growth approximating that of the third trimester of intrauterine life, without imposing stress on the developing metabolic and excretory system.' Although the first part of this statement could be disputed, the second part is a matter of general agreement. Schultz et al[125] showed that compared with a breastfed control group of infants receiving 2.0 g protein per kilogram per day, a formula-fed group receiving 4.4 g protein per kilogram per day demonstrated azotaemia, a lower blood glucose, hyperaminoacidaemia (especially phenylalanine) and metabolic acidosis, and regained birthweight more slowly. However, balance and stable isotope studies[160] have emphasised that the amount of energy absorbed is critical for the rate of protein synthesis. If energy intake is low, high protein intakes cannot be utilised and the infant's metabolic machinery is stressed; in contrast, diets with high available energy and large protein intakes, of at least 4 g/kg/24 h, result in increased nitrogen retention and growth, without

metabolic strain. For this reason, it is conventional to express protein (and indeed other nutrient requirements) in relation to energy intake (Table 16.2) as well as in absolute terms.

Long-term outcome studies

Most important is whether early protein intake could have long-term consequences, either adverse or beneficial. Using an experimental approach, Goldman et al[59] studied 304 infants below 2000 g who had been randomised to 2% or 4% protein diets, providing, respectively, 3.0–3.6 g and 6.0–7.2 g protein per kilogram per day. Infants below 1300 g in the high protein intake group had a markedly higher incidence of low IQs (below 90) by Stanford–Binet score at 5 years of age. The incidence of strabismus in infants below 1700 g fed on a high protein intake was also increased. It has been suggested that transient hyperaminoacidaemia (especially tyrosine) on high protein intakes might have been responsible for these adverse outcomes, but currently the explanation is uncertain. Indeed, in a more recent study, Lucas et al[82] looked at a group of preterm infants who had elevated plasma phenylalanine levels during the neonatal period, associated with the use of intravenous Vamin 9. Despite phenylalanine levels in the range reported to produce long-term cognitive deficits in infants with phenylketonuria, neurodevelopmental testing at 18 months post-term showed no difference between infants who had neonatal hyperphenylalaninaemia and those who did not. This study also noted that infants who developed hyperphenylalaninaemia had typically received total parenteral nutrition (TPN) with a low energy:protein ratio, emphasising the importance of considering protein and energy intakes together.

On the positive side, there is evidence suggesting that long-term outcome may be improved by meeting the increased protein requirements of certain groups of infants, for example those born prematurely. Preterm infants randomised to receive a preterm formula containing 2 g/100 ml protein showed both better short-term growth than those fed a standard term formula containing 1.45 g/100 ml[87] and improved neurodevelopment 7.5–8 years later.[88]

Protein quality

Whey proteins have a lower concentration of aromatic amino acids (tyrosine and phenylalanine) than are found in caseins; the studies by Goldman[59] were performed with high-casein formulas (like cow's milk), but most modern formulas are whey predominant, reducing the possibility of hypertyrosinaemia and hyperphenylalaninaemia.[112] Whey is also a good source of cysteine, a potentially essential amino acid in the newborn period (see above). However, a high whey intake is associated with plasma threonine concentrations which are three times those of the infant fed breast milk. In fact, plasma threonine (and other amino acid) concentrations are higher in the fetus than they are postnatally,[7] raising the possibility that high values in babies born preterm are not necessarily toxic.

Amino acid composition

Breastfed infants have higher plasma and urine taurine concentrations and a higher rate of synthesis of bile acids than those fed on formula; the latter may partially explain the better fat absorption of infants fed human milk rather than formulas.[56,151] Rhesus monkeys fed a taurine-deficient formula for the first 6 or 12 months of life show abnormal retinal structure, although the abnormalities show some degree of spontaneous regression by 12 months even when the animals remain on the deficient diet.[67] A randomised trial of taurine supplementation in formula-fed preterm infants[145] showed no effect on growth, behaviour or electroretinograms, but some evidence of more rapid auditory maturation in the supplemented group at the equivalent of term (as assessed by brainstem-evoked response). More recently, we have shown that preterm infants with the highest plasma taurine concentrations during the neonatal period have better numeracy skills during adolescence and better development of the related parietal cortical grey matter (Wharton, unpublished). Thus, it seems prudent to add taurine to LBW formulas to achieve concentrations similar to those of breast milk.

Glutamine is used as a fuel by the small intestine and as a precursor for the synthesis of purine and pyrimidine bases. Numerous studies in animals and adult humans have demonstrated that it has beneficial effects on the GI tract, including the maintenance of structure and function during parenteral nutrition. These findings have led to the suggestion that glutamine may be particularly important for the stressed preterm infant. A systematic review that included data from three small randomised trials of glutamine supplementation in preterm infants concluded that they showed no evidence of a beneficial effect of supplementation, but that a larger randomised trial was required.[144] More recently, Vaughn[148] reported the results of a large (n = 649) multicentre randomised trial of enteral glutamine supplementation (0.3 g/kg/day) versus sterile water for the first 28 days in infants with birthweights between 500 g and 1250 g. There was no significant difference between groups in culture-proven sepsis or suspected sepsis, although supplemented neonates had less GI dysfunction.

Arginine is a precursor for the synthesis of nitric oxide, which in turn is important as a regulator of vascular perfusion. Plasma arginine concentrations have been found to be inversely related to the severity of respiratory distress syndrome, and low concentrations have been reported in infants who develop NEC. A recent randomised trial of arginine supplementation (1.5 mmol/kg/day, given either enterally or parenterally) versus placebo in preterm infants found a significantly reduced incidence of NEC in supplemented infants.[3]

Fat

Digestion and absorption[63]

Fat provides about half the energy for infants fed human milk, and its digestion commences in the stomach, catalysed by lingual lipase[51] and gastric lipase. Gastric lipolysis is quantitatively greater in the infant than in the adult, and the output and activity of lipases in the preterm infant are equal to those of adults maintained on a high-fat diet. Although gastric function and the production of lipase are unaffected by infant diet, the extent of fat digestion is greater in babies fed human milk (25%) than formula

(14%), probably because of the structural differences between triglyceride in human milk fat globules and that in formula fat particles. Both lingual and gastric lipases are able to penetrate the milk fat globule membrane and digest triglyceride without disrupting its structure. The contribution of pancreatic lipases is relatively lower in infants than in adults. However, the bile salt-dependent lipase (BSDL) present in human milk may contribute significantly to fat digestion. BSDL is present in high quantities even in the milk of mothers who deliver prematurely, and its concentration is independent of milk volume. Unlike gastric and pancreatic lipases, BSDL shows no positional or fatty acid specificity and is able to produce free fatty acids which are more easily absorbed than mono- or diglycerides at the low bile-salt concentration seen in newborn infants.

The products of fat digestion are absorbed, resynthesised as triglycerides and secreted mainly into the lymphatic system as chylomicrons, and thence into the blood via the great veins. The foregoing applies to long-chain triglycerides, which are best absorbed if they are unsaturated. In contrast, medium-chain triglycerides (MCTs; 8–10 carbon atoms to the chain) are handled quite differently: their digestion is largely independent of bile salts; they are well absorbed, hydrolysed or intact, and pass to the liver via the portal system. Faecal fat excretion in newborn infants is greater in infants fed on cow's milk than in those fed on human milk or vegetable fats.

Most modern formulas contain a mixture of animal and vegetable oils, adjusted to mimic the pattern of fatty acid saturation and chain lengths found in breast milk. When compared with human milk, such fat mixtures have a reduced content of fatty acids esterified to glycerol in the 2 position and an increase in those esterified in the 1 and 3 positions. The latter undergo hydrolysis in the gut, releasing palmitic acid, which is poorly absorbed and tends to form calcium soaps; this may be partly responsible for the harder stools seen in formula-fed infants, and could influence calcium absorption. Studies using a modified fat blend ('Betapol') containing a high proportion of fatty acids esterified in the 2 position to mimic that found in human milk[111] showed increased calcium absorption (measured by stable isotope) and fat absorption in term[24,48] and preterm[23,91] infants. In term infants, the use of a formula containing Betapol for the first 3 months of life was also associated with reduced stool soap fatty acids and softer stools, together with an increase in whole body bone mass, suggesting that increased calcium absorption resulted in measurable biological effects.[72] Whether the effect on skeletal mass persists is unknown.

An alternative strategy for reducing stool fatty acid soap formation is to reduce the palmitate content of infant formulas to much lower levels than are found in breast milk. This approach has recently been shown to result in increased whole body bone mass, presumably due to improved fat, and therefore calcium, absorption.[75]

Fat requirements

Because there are clinical and physiological ceilings on the amount of dietary energy that it is desirable to supply as carbohydrate or protein, a minimum of around 30% of dietary energy needs to be supplied as fat. Linoleic and α-linolenic acids are essential fatty acids for the development of the brain and for prostaglandin synthesis. Essential fatty acid deficiency is also associated with skin lesions and retarded growth.

Two other dietary factors are important for lipid metabolism. Carnitine[108,153] plays a key role by facilitating transport of long-chain fatty acids across the mitochondrial membrane prior to their oxidation. Carnitine deficiency during the neonatal period has been reported in infants who experience intrapartum hypoxia and acidosis.[11] Preterm and small-for-gestational age (SGA) infants may have impaired endogenous carnitine synthesis, and if carnitine intake is deficient (as in TPN) plasma and tissue concentrations fall. Nevertheless, whether such infants are put at clinical risk from a low-carnitine diet is uncertain. A recent randomised trial found that preterm infants who received supplemental carnitine in parenteral nutrition did not demonstrate any reduction in apnoea of prematurity, ventilatory requirements or need for supplemental oxygen therapy compared with those who received placebo.[105] A study of formula-fed term SGA infants randomly assigned a carnitine supplement or placebo showed no significant effect of supplementation on growth up to 1 year of age (Lucas et al, unpublished). Standard formulas usually contain similar concentrations of carnitine to those in breast milk, but some preterm formulas have additional carnitine.

Choline[64,153] is required for phospholipid and acetylcholine synthesis. About half the choline requirement is derived from the diet. Human and cow's milk-based diets provide a sufficient intake.

Inositol, a six-carbon cyclic polyalcohol sugar, is a component of membrane phospholipids, and compounds containing inositol are important in signal transduction. Breast milk, particularly colostrum, contains high concentrations, whereas the levels in infant formulas are lower and intravenous feeding solutions have none. At present, it is recommended that all preterm infants receive supplementation based upon the level of inositol in human milk. A systematic review of four randomised controlled trials (RCTs) of inositol supplementation in preterm infants concluded that supplementation results in a statistically significant and clinically important reduction in the risk of chronic lung disease, retinopathy of prematurity (stage 4 or needing therapy) and death.[66] The authors suggest a multicentre RCT of appropriate size is required to confirm these findings.

Essential fatty acid requirements

Two groups of long-chain polyunsaturated fatty acids (LCPUFA; i.e. polyunsaturated fatty acids with greater than 18-carbon chain length) have received increasing interest in recent years: these are homologues of linoleic acid of the n-6 series (dihomo-gammalinolenic acid, arachidonic acid [AA]) and of α-linolenic acid of the n-3 series (eicosapentanoic acid, docosahexaenoic acid [DHA]). The LCPUFA are synthesised from the precursor essential fatty acids by a process of chain elongation and desaturation (Fig. 16.1). They are found in high concentrations in the phospholipids of cell membranes, notably in the central nervous system.[103] In addition, AA, dihomogammalinolenic acid and eicosapentanoic acid are precursors for eicosanoids – important modulators and mediators of a variety of essential biological processes.

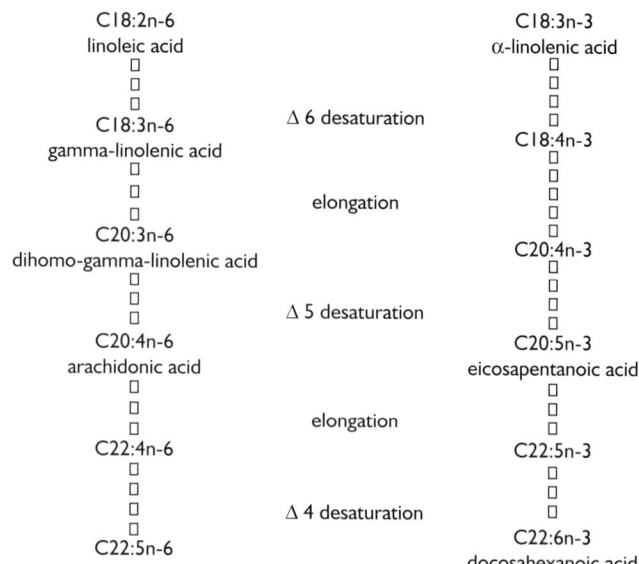

Fig. 16.1 Major steps in the formation of long chain polyunsaturated fatty acids (LPCs) from the C:18 essential fatty acids. Unsaturated fatty acids contain at least one double bond between adjacent carbon atoms: the number of double bonds is represented by 1n, 2n, 3n, etc. LPCs are further classified by the position of the first double bond from the methyl or omega end of the hydrocarbon chain, represented as -3, -6, -9 or ω-3, ω-6, ω-9. Linoleic acid (C18:2n-6) thus has a chain length of 18 carbons with two double bonds, the first of which is at the sixth carbon atom from the omega end.

Rapid accumulation of LCPUFA in the brain, particularly DHA, occurs from the third trimester to 18 months postpartum.[28] Human milk contains both the precursor essential fatty acids *and* adequate LCPUFA for structural lipid accretion,[27] but infant formulas traditionally contained only the parent essential fatty acids, the assumption being that the infant could synthesise LCPUFA from these. However, term and preterm infants fed on formulas which contain minimal LCPUFA have been shown to have lower red cell LCPUFA, and lower LCPUFA in the phospholipids of the cerebral cortex and subcutaneous tissues than infants fed breast milk.[21,43,44,92] Largely on the basis of the biochemical data supporting the view that preterm infants may have a reduced ability to synthesise LCPUFA from the parent essential fatty acids, ESPGAN[41] recommended that formulas for LBW infants should be enriched with metabolites of both linoleic and linolenic acids, approximating the levels typical of human milk. However, whether the biochemical LCPUFA deficiency in formula-fed infants has clinical relevance in terms of long-term growth or neurodevelopment remains controversial, despite several RCTs. At present, although there is clear evidence that supplementing infant formulas with LCPUFA results in *biochemical* improvement, there are less published data demonstrating lasting *clinical* benefits (see below).

LCPUFA and clinical outcome in preterm infants
The suggestion that LCPUFA might have a beneficial effect on neurodevelopment in preterm infants gained support from the

finding that those fed human milk have better developmental outcome than those fed unsupplemented formulas.[89] However, such comparisons are obviously confounded by socioeconomic factors, and there are many other differences between breast milk and formula which might explain the differences in outcome. Systematic reviews[123,131] have concluded that LCPUFA supplementation results in more rapid visual maturation, which is transient, but that there is no convincing evidence of cognitive benefit. Since the Simmer review was last updated, two studies have reported some evidence for a beneficial effect of LCPUFA supplementation on neurodevelopment. Clandinin et al[29] have recently reported, in abstract form, the results of a study in which preterm infants fed formula supplemented with LCPUFA up to 1 year post-term had significantly higher Bayley developmental scores at 18 months than infants fed unsupplemented formula. Finally, our own randomised trial demonstrated a positive effect of LCPUFA supplementation on Bayley Mental Developmental Index (MDI) at 18 months post-term in boys.[45]

It is important to appreciate that to date, follow up has only been reported up to 2 years post-term, using tests of global development. It is possible that LCUFA supplementation results in more subtle effects on areas of development that may only be detected using more specific tests at a later age.

LCPUFA and clinical outcome in term infants

The situation regarding the need for LCPUFA supplementation of term infant formulas is controversial. Simmer concluded that there is little evidence from randomised trials to support the hypothesis that LCPUFA supplementation confers a benefit for visual or general development,[130] and that, whilst a beneficial effect on information processing is possible, larger studies conducted over longer periods are required to conclude that LCPUFA supplementation provides a benefit when compared with standard formula. Recently, Forsyth et al[50] published results of a 6-year follow-up of infants from a randomised trial of LCPUFA supplementation, showing that supplemented infants had lower blood pressure during childhood. These findings raise the possibility that LCPUFA supplementation might have effects beyond those on neurodevelopment.

Safety and LCPFA supplementation

A further important consideration is whether the addition of selected LCPUFAs is safe in both preterm and term infants. It seems unlikely that either DHA or AA is inherently harmful, since they are present in human milk. However, various strategies have been used to supplement formula with LCPUFA, and they have not been without problems. There is a fine balance between the relative amounts of linoleic and linolenic acids and their longer-chain products, with inhibition of linoleic acid desaturation by long-chain n-3 fatty acids, and competition between AA and eicosapentanoic acid for incorporation into membrane lipids. Early attempts at LCPUFA supplementation using fish oils alone as a source of DHA actually resulted in a growth disadvantage,[20,22,120] possibly due to a reduction in AA formation. However, two recent studies using a balanced combined

addition of DHA with AA, have also found reduced linear growth in LCPUFA-supplemented infants up to 12 months[147] and 18 months[46] post-term. In contrast, two trials have shown significant benefits of LCPUFA-supplemented formulas for growth in preterm infants.[29,69]

The optimum sources of LCPUFA require further investigation. Indeed, it seems probable that the inconsistent findings in randomised trials relate more to the different strategies used to add LCPUFA to the formula rather than to the actual LCPUFA themselves. LCPUFA may be sourced from fish oils, egg lipids or single-cell organisms. Each supplementation strategy may lead to alterations, not only in the desired LCPUFA, but also to other fatty acids and nutrients, including the addition of 'unphysiological' fatty acids not found in breast milk. For this reason, in future it may be important to evaluate LCPUFA-supplemented formulas on an individual basis rather than grouping them all together in meta-analyses.

Term babies

The EC Directive guidelines[31] recommend that the fat content of infant formulas should lie between 2.0 g and 4.9 g per 100 ml of feed.

Preterm babies

The main problem with dietary fat in preterm infants is the increased tendency to steatorrhoea. Reduced fat absorption in LBW infants relates to:[115]

- reduced pancreatic lipase and carboxylic ester hydrolase activity;
- reduced bile acid pool size and secretion rate: the duodenal bile acid concentration may well be below the critical level for micelle formation;
- possible reduction in activity or excretion of lingual lipase.

Fat absorption from fresh breast milk is approximately 90%, but the observed range is enormous. Williamson et al[156] found that fat absorption from expressed breast milk fell to 55% in VLBW infants fed pasteurised milk, and to around 45% when the milk was boiled. These data may reflect loss of the bile salt-stimulated lipase found in human milk due to heat treatment.

A controversial issue is the addition of large quantities of MCTs to specially designed preterm infant formulas, largely because such babies absorb palmitic acid (n-16) poorly. The MCT content of human milk is low (less than 2% total fatty acids), whereas modern preterm formulas may contain up to 40% of the fat in this form. MCTs may spare dietary nitrogen and enhance calcium and magnesium absorption.[139] However, recent studies have failed to show improved energy or nitrogen balance, or better weight gain, in preterm infants fed MCTs. Indeed, Okatmoto et al[106] showed that although better fat absorption occurred with a high-MCT diet, the infants had a higher incidence of abdominal distension, loose stools, vomiting and increased gastric aspirates. The availability of newer fat blends such as Betapol may present an alternative solution in the future.

Carbohydrate

Physiology[73]

The carbohydrate in human milk is almost entirely lactose, which provides 40% of ingested energy. Other carbohydrates, e.g. sucrose and maltodextrins, may be hydrolysed efficiently by active brush-border sucrase, maltase and isomaltase, even in preterm infants, and starch or glucose polymers can be digested by salivary and pancreatic amylase, by amylase present in human milk, and by intestinal mucosal hydrolases.

Dietary lactose undergoes one of two processes: hydrolysis into glucose and galactose by the intestinal brush-border lactase, followed by absorption of glucose and galactose, or fermentation in the colon, with production of various gases and short-chain fatty acids.[6] The latter may be important in the nutrition and function of the intestine and colon. For example, short-chain fatty acids administered into the colon have been shown to stimulate intestinal growth following gut resection in animal models, and prevent mucosal atrophy after resection and TPN. There is controversy over the possible role of lactose fermentation in the development of NEC. However, although there are some experimental data linking excessive carbohydrate fermentation in the small intestine with an inflammatory condition resembling NEC, there is little evidence that *colonic* lactose fermentation is a primary factor.

Galactose and glucose are absorbed by the same carrier mechanism, and more than 90% reaches the portal vein. Most galactose is removed by the liver on first pass, and appears to be preferentially used for glycogen synthesis rather than conversion to glucose.

There is currently intense interest in the probiotic role of oligosaccharides in human milk. Probiotics are defined as non-digestible food ingredients that selectively stimulate the growth and/or activity of one or more bacteria in the colon, and therefore benefit the host. Human milk contains hundreds, if not thousands, of oligosaccharides. These are thought to promote the bifidogenic-dominant colonic microflora observed in breast-fed infants, which in turn protect the infant from enteropathogenic bacteria. Cow's milk formulas traditionally contain no oligosaccharides. However, a recent randomised trial in term infants reported significantly higher proportions of bifidobacteria in the stools of infants fed a formula containing synthetic oligosaccharides than in those fed standard formula.[124]

Term infants' requirements

The EC Directive recommendation[31] for carbohydrate intake is that it should be between 4.2 g and 10.5 g per 100 ml of reconstituted feed, and that the lactose content should be above 2.1 g/100 ml (Table 16.1). Other carbohydrate sources that are used (successfully) in modern formulas are maltodextrin and amylose. Although sucrose is well digested by human infants, it renders formulas significantly 'sweeter' than human milk: it is not incorporated in formulas used in the UK, but is present in certain soy-based formulas in the USA.

Preterm infants' requirements

It is difficult to infer from physiological studies which carbohydrate is optimal for LBW infants. Lactose enhances gut absorption of calcium and magnesium and may encourage a favourable gut flora;[19] excessive intakes may result in diarrhoea and metabolic acidosis,[6] yet in practice a high lactose intake in preterm infants is usually well tolerated.

One approach in the design of preterm formulas is to use lactose as the principal carbohydrate source, but to replace a proportion of the carbohydrate with glucose polymers in order to prevent excess osmolality (see Table 16.2 for recommended intakes).

There has been interest in the provision of lower-carbohydrate high-fat formulas to preterm infants with chronic lung disease; the aim of the reduced carbohydrate is to lower the respiratory quotient and thereby reduce carbon dioxide production. Such formulas have been demonstrated to support adequate growth while reducing arterial carbon dioxide levels, but their role remains to be defined.[109]

Energy

The fundamental energy (E) equation is:

$$E_{intake} = E_{stored} + E_{expended} + E_{excreted} \qquad \text{Eqn. (1)}$$

Energy expended may be subdivided further:

$$E_{expended} = E_{BMR} + E_{activity} + E_{synthesis} + E_{thermoreg} \qquad \text{Eqn. (2)}$$

where E_{stored} is the energy deposited during growth, E_{BMR} is the basal energy requirement, $E_{activity}$ is the additional cost of muscular activity, $E_{synthesis}$ is the metabolic cost of growing (excluding energy actually stored in new tissue) and $E_{thermoreg}$ is the energy cost of maintaining body temperature.

Traditionally, the tools used to derive these values have been energy balances and indirect calorimetry (energy expenditure calculated from oxygen consumption and carbon dioxide production) performed under different experimental conditions during rest. More recently, the 'doubly labelled water method' has been used to measure total energy expenditure over periods of several days. (The method depends on monitoring the differential disappearance from the body of two stable isotopes, ^{18}O and deuterium, both administered orally as labelled water.)

There has been dispute over which conversion factors should be used for either human or cow's milk to derive the metabolisable energy content (the gross energy of the food from bomb calorimetry minus the energy lost in the stools and urine) from macronutrient concentrations. Although not entirely appropriate to the milk-fed neonate, the conventional Atwater conversion factors derived by Southgate and Durnin[136] are commonly used (Table 16.3).

Term infants' requirements

The EC Directive guidelines[31] recommend that formula should contain similar energy contents to those reported in human milk,

Table 16.3 Conventional Atwater conversion factors

	kcal/g	kJ/g
Carbohydrate (expressed as monosaccharide or lactose monohydrate)	3.75	16
Protein (total N × 6.38)	4	17
Fat	9	37

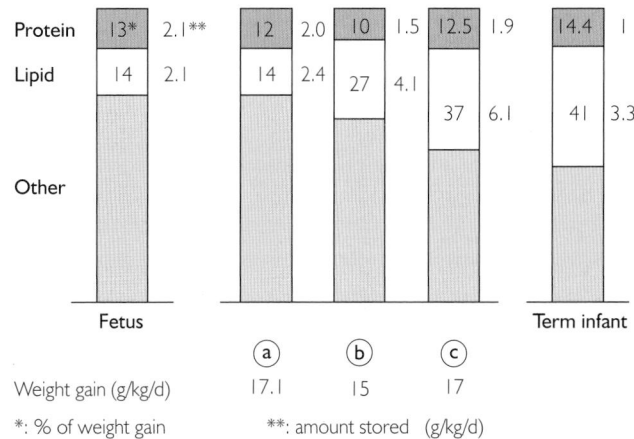

Fig. 16.2 Weight gain composition of the fetus (32–36 weeks) and of the term infant (0–4 months), compared with that of preterm infants fed different diets. (a) Protein-supplemented pooled human milk. (b) Pooled human milk. (c) Preterm formula. Figures represent the percentage of weight gain as protein or fat.

i.e. 60–75 kcal/100 ml of reconstituted feed. However, from studies employing the doubly labelled water method, Lucas et al[86] suggested that infants fed on human milk may receive lower energy intakes than those commonly reported and those employed in modern formulas – they obtained a value of 58 kcal/100 ml at 3 months; this may explain why modern formula-fed term infants grow faster than their breastfed counterparts.

Term SGA infants have been reported to have energy expenditures 5–10% higher than infants who are appropriate for gestational age (AGA), and may therefore benefit from increased energy to promote catch-up growth. In one study, a high-energy formula resulted in a marginal increase in weight gain and head growth.[16] However, it is likely that both extra energy and protein are required simultaneously (see p. 303).

Preterm infants' requirements

The energy requirements for preterm infants cannot be calculated without some consideration of the desired composition of weight gain, as the deposition of different types of tissue incurs different energy costs. For example, 9 kcal are stored in each gram of fat, compared with 4 kcal per gram of protein. Thus, a weight gain high in fat will require more energy to be stored than one high in protein. As previously mentioned (p. 290), the ratio of energy to protein is important in determining the relative amount of lean tissue versus fat which is deposited. These considerations are not just theoretical, as the different diets used for preterm infants do result in variations in the composition of tissue deposited (Fig. 16.2). At present it is not known whether it is best to aim for a weight gain with 15% fat (as in the fetus) or nearer 40% fat (as in a term infant), and unless this can be shown to have implications for future health, one might argue that it is academic. The results to date have been conflicting: DeGamarra[39] and Cooper[33] both found no differences in growth at 2 or 3 years of age in preterm infants who had shown wide differences in adiposity as infants. However, Agras et al[1] reported that greater adiposity at birth was a predictor of greater fatness at 6 years of age. In our own randomised trial of diet in preterm infants we found major differences in growth rates between diet groups during the neonatal period, but no differences in either growth[47] or body fatness[46a] between diet groups at follow-up between 8 and 12 years of age.

All the components of the energy equation have been either measured or estimated in preterm infants, in order to calculate the optimal energy intake. The daily energy cost of activity is around 10 kcal/kg; the cost of thermogenesis, 10 kcal/kg/24 h (depending on thermal environment); and, at growth rates

of 15 g/kg/24 h, the cost of tissue synthesis is about 10–20 kcal/kg.[113,153] The remaining component of energy expenditure, basal metabolic rate (BMR), cannot be measured in preterm infants as it requires at least a 12-hour fast. However, total energy expenditure, which includes all four of these components, has been measured over 5 days with both the doubly labelled water method and indirect calorimetry in four preterm infants[116] growing at a mean rate of 15 g/kg/24 h, and was 58 kcal/kg/24 h (range 57–60). Other studies making measurements over 24-hour periods have produced similar figures, in the range 50 to 70 kcal/kg/24 h. If these figures are entered into Equation (2):

$$E_{expended} = E_{BMR} + E_{activity} + E_{synthesis} + E_{thermoreg}$$
$$57\text{--}70 \qquad ? \qquad 10 \qquad 10\text{--}20 \qquad 10$$

a value for BMR of between 17 and 40 g/kg/24 h^{-1} is obtained.

In order to estimate energy requirements, it is necessary to consider both energy stored and energy excreted. In the study by Roberts et al,[116] energy stored was 59 kcal/kg/24 h (which is about twice the figure for in utero energy deposition and substantially higher than ideal estimates for preterm infants, owing to the increased fat deposition seen postnatally). Energy losses in the stools have been estimated to be around 10–30 kcal/kg bodyweight, but massive losses may occur (well in excess of 50% of intake) in sick babies with an immature gut. If these figures are entered into Equation (1):

$$E_{intake} = E_{stored} + E_{expended} + E_{excreted}$$
$$59 \qquad 57\text{--}70 \qquad 10\text{--}30$$

the required intake would be between 126 and 159 kcal/kg/24 h. This is in the middle of the range recommended by ESPGAN of 110–165 kcal/kg/24 h, and slightly above the 120 kcal/kg/24 h recommended by the recent international panel of experts for the stable preterm infant.

For logistic reasons, very few data are available on the specific energy requirements of sick (as opposed to stable) preterm infants; the techniques used to estimate energy expenditure are not easily applied in such cases. There are no definite data showing an advantage from increasing the energy intake above that recommended for stable preterm infants, and in practice the challenge is usually to provide the desired intake in the face of fluid restriction or feed intolerance associated with the prevailing illness. There are some data on infants with chronic lung disease demonstrating an increase in energy expenditure of 15–30%, particularly in those who are failing to thrive.[38,76,152,159] However, the poor growth in these infants may more often reflect suboptimal nutrient intake, since in most studies energy intakes fail to reach the estimated requirements for stable preterm infants, let alone those who might have higher requirements.[157]

Water (Chapter 36, Part 1)

Water is a major nutrient (for review, see Wharton[153]). However, the quantity deposited in growth (around 10 ml/kg/24 h by preterm infants, for instance) is minute compared with water turnover. Clearly, in sick babies it would be impossible to allow nutrient intakes to vary in parallel with water requirement, and water must be treated as an 'independent variable'.

Nucleotides[161]

There has been increasing interest over the last decade in the role of nucleotides in infant nutrition. Breast milk contains at least 13 different nucleotides, accounting for 5% of non-protein nitrogen.[70] Cow's milk has lower levels and a different nucleotide profile. Nucleotides are important in cell-mediated immunity, and it has been suggested that they are one of the anti-infective agents in breast milk, responsible for the lower levels of infection reported in breastfed infants. There is good evidence for the role of dietary nucleotides in animals (for example, enhancing T-cell function,[119] and improving intestinal growth and maturation in weaning rats.[146]

A variety of short-term effects have been reported for nucleotide-supplemented formulas in infants, including an alteration in the bowel flora following supplementation, with a predominance of lactobacilli as seen in the breastfed infant,[57] although this latter finding could not be reproduced by Balmer et al.[9] Pickering et al[110] found a significantly higher *Haemophilus influenzae* type b polysaccharide antibody concentration at 7 and 12 months of age, and a significantly higher diphtheria antibody concentration at 7 months in infants fed a nucleotide-supplemented formula compared with those fed a control formula. No differences were found in growth or serum immunoglobulin levels. Navarro et al[100] reported that preterm infants fed nucleotide-supplemented formula during the first 3 months of life had higher plasma IgM and IgA concentrations than infants fed unsupplemented formula. Dietary nucleotides may also modulate lipid metabolism, increasing serum lipoprotein concentrations[122] predominantly due to an increase in apolipoprotein content.

There is little available evidence on the effect of nucleotide supplementation on clinical outcome in infants. A non-randomised trial of infants living in poor socioeconomic circumstances in Chile found a reduced incidence of diarrhoea in those who received nucleotide-supplemented formulas compared with unsupplemented formulas.[18] At least 13 studies have shown that nucleotide-supplemented formulas have no effect on physical growth in healthy AGA infants.[25] However, one randomised trial demonstrated positive effects on growth during the first 6 months of life in term SGA infants.[34] This effect was not associated with altered patterns of illness, and it was postulated that it might reflect trophic effects of nucleotides on the GI tract.

Macrominerals (Tables 16.1, 16.2, 16.4)

Sodium, potassium and chloride

Calculation of desirable intakes of sodium, potassium and chloride requires a knowledge of renal function (Chapter 36, Part 1).

Term infants' requirements
Two factors have had an important bearing on recommendations for dietary sodium intake in young infants. First, the concern that high salt intake might result in dangerous hypernatraemia at times of excessive water loss (e.g. diarrhoea), and secondly, the now unconvincing evidence that early salt intake might predispose to later high blood pressure.

Preterm infants' requirements
Sodium.
Major adjustments in body sodium occur in the neonatal period: massive renal losses of up to 10 mmol/kg/24h or more can occur in the first week and may be independent of intake. It is impossible accurately to predict sodium needs in the early neonatal period, and in very small and sick infants, regardless of diet, plasma sodium should be monitored and hyponatraemia of <133 mmol/l – and certainly <130 mmol/l – should be corrected.

Preterm breast milk has a higher sodium content (≥10–20 mmol/l during the early weeks of lactation) than mature donor milk (about ≤6 mmol/l). Hyponatraemia has been noted in preterm infants fed human milk; it is more severe in those fed donor milk. Intakes from donor milk and preterm milk, providing around 1 and 2 mmol/kg/24 h, respectively, during the first month, are often inadequate, and Aperia et al[4] have recommended 3 mmol/kg/24 h.

The high sodium content of modern preterm formulas is usually only required in the early neonatal period. After that, the excess sodium needs to be excreted. However, in a large randomised study,[90] preterm neonates fed on a formula providing 3.6 mmol/l did not have an increased risk of hypernatraemia, compared with those fed standard formula or breast milk (providing under half the sodium intake), and 13–16 years later did not show any elevation in blood pressure.[132]

Potassium and chloride.
In general, human milk and the available adapted formulas provide adequate potassium and chloride to meet intrauterine accretion rates of 0.9 and 0.7 mmol/kg/24h, respectively.[153]

Table 16.4 Digestion, physiological role and deficiency states of calcium, phosphorus and magnesium

	Digestion	Physiological role	Deficiency states
Calcium	Absorption by both passive and active transport: Ca, Mg-ATPase facilitates uptake into the mucosal cells, where a calcium-binding protein is induced by vitamin D. 20–60% retention, according to diet (better with human milk) but increased by vitamin D and parathormone and reduced by complexing with dietary fat, phosphate and phytates. Part bound, e.g. to protein, part free in plasma	Bones are major stores. Also required for cell membrane function, neuromuscular activity, clotting and a wide variety of cellular functions	Tetany, bone demineralisation, arrhythmias, paralytic ileus, fits
Phosphorus	70–95% absorption, increased by vitamin D, reduced by insoluble intraluminal complex formation, e.g. with phytate or if excessive calcium salts added. Commonly elevated in plasma in neonatal period in cow's milk formula-fed term infants; nadir in preterm infants at 1–2 weeks	Bone mineralization, ATP, DNA, RNA, phospholipids and many other biological roles	Rickets is rare in full term newborns. Phosphate deficiency syndrome may arise, particularly in infants fed by total parenteral nutrition: listlessness, poor feeding, rapid shallow breathing, muscle weakness, impaired oxygen release from haemoglobin, bone disease, nephrocalcinosis
Magnesium	Some transport mechanisms may be shared with calcium: absorption increased by vitamin D and parathormone and decreased by steatorrhoea and phytates. High fetal plasma levels, which may fall after birth	Stored in bone. Important intracellular cation, muscle contraction, cofactor for carbohydrate, protein and energy metabolism	Weakness, poor feeding, failure to thrive, paralytic ileus, calcium-resistant tetany, fits, apnoea

Calcium and phosphorus (Table 16.4)

Term infants

Calcium is less well absorbed from cow's milk than from human milk. However, in spite of the high levels of calcium and phosphorus in cow's milk, the relatively higher phosphorus intake has in the past resulted in hyperphosphataemia, hypocalcaemia with convulsions (see below), and other complications such as dental hypoplasia.[138] Moreover, the high phosphorus content in unmodified cow's milk may also induce hypomagnesaemia, and, in some cases of neonatal tetany, convulsions can be alleviated only by administration of magnesium.[30] Current recommendations for calcium and phosphorus are shown in Table 16.1.

Preterm infants' requirements

Considerable attention has been focused on the calcium and phosphorus requirements of LBW infants,[153] stimulated by the high incidence of metabolic bone disease seen in this population (Chapter 35, Part 4).

Magnesium

The recommended intake for term infants is given in Table 16.1, and the physiology outlined in Table 16.4. Body magnesium content, largely in bone, rises rapidly in the third trimester, so that preterm infants are born with low reserves.[36] In preterm infants, net magnesium absorption in the first week is about 50% and is largely independent of vitamin D. Magnesium deficiency may

impair calcium homoeostasis. Atkinson et al[5] showed that infants fed on preterm milk (2.5–3.0 mg magnesium per 100 ml) failed to retain this element at intrauterine accretion rates, and showed evidence of falling reserves; in contrast, a formula-fed group receiving two to three times more magnesium retained it at a somewhat greater rate than in utero. In infants fed human milk, dietary supplementation with phosphorus improves magnesium retention by reducing urine losses.[74]

Iron

Term infants

Iron stores at birth are influenced by gestation, birthweight and the extent of the placental transfusion at delivery. Healthy breastfed infants absorb iron well from human milk and usually maintain normal iron stores during the first 4–6 months (p. 307). However, the bioavailability of iron in cow's milk (especially) and cow's milk formulas is much less than in human milk. The EC Directive[31] recommended that formulas used from birth should, if iron is added, contain 0.5–1.5 mg/100 kcal, and follow-on milks should contain 1–2 mg/100 kcal (Table 16.1). The recommended daily intake in infancy is 6 mg, but in the USA 10–15 mg/day is recommended.

Preterm infants' requirements

A 1.0 kg fetus contains 64 mg iron,[155] and this increases subsequently in utero at a rate of 1.8 mg/kg/24 h. About 25% of iron is stored in the liver as ferritin, and most of the rest is present in haemoglobin. After birth, therefore, a 1.0 kg infant only has sufficient iron to synthesise about 18.0 g of haemoglobin (3.4 mg iron per gram haemoglobin), and since the iron content of human milk is 40 micrograms per 100 ml or less (providing 80 micrograms/kg/24 h fed at 200 ml/kg/24 h), preterm infants fed human milk will eventually develop an iron-deficiency anaemia without supplementation.

Iron stores usually remain adequate during the first 6–8 weeks, and iron supplementation at this stage has no influence on anaemia of prematurity. By 12 weeks, iron stores become depleted in unsupplemented infants, and iron-deficiency anaemia develops.[61] Intakes of 2.0–3.0 mg/kg/24 h have been shown by several groups to prevent such anaemia.

It is recommended that preterm infants receive a supplement of no more than 2.5 mg/kg/24 h of iron, starting between 6 and 8 weeks of age and continuing until 12 months, or until full mixed feeding provides an adequate iron intake. A recent trial of high (20.7 mg/l) versus normal (13.4 mg/l) iron formulas in preterm infants found no difference in weight gain nor development at 12 months post-term.[52]

Recently there has been increasing interest in the use of recombinant human erythropoietin (r-HuEPO) in preterm infants to reduce the requirement for blood transfusion. Studies have demonstrated[126] that infants treated with r-HuEPO require higher amounts of iron – up to 6 mg/kg/24 h – and that this should be initiated at the same time as the r-HuEPO.

Trace metals

Summaries of the physiological roles and the consequences of deficiency are shown in Table 16.5, and recommended intakes for term infants in Table 16.1.

Table 16.5 Trace metals

	Physiology	Deficiency states
Iodine	Well absorbed, concentrated in thyroid gland, incorporated in thyroxine and tri-iodothyronine. Excess is excreted in urine	Endemic goitre in areas where human milk is deficient; soy formulas are iodine-deficient and are usually supplemented
Zinc	Present in a large number of metalloenzymes, including alkaline phosphatase and carbonic anhydrase. Required for insulin activity. Absorption partly by active transport. Bioavailability influenced by diet: poor absorption from diets of plant origin. Nadir in plasma zinc at around 2–3 months. Infants fed by total parenteral nutrition and those with gut disease are especially liable to clinical deficiency	Acrodermatitis syndrome. Delayed diagnosis if signs mistaken for 'nappy rash' of another aetiology. (NB May be inherited as a rare autosomal recessive disorder). Also mild deficiency in infancy, or later, may be associated with reduced growth, loss of appetite, impaired taste acuity and perhaps pica. Impaired immune responses, poor wound healing
Copper	Copper-containing enzymes include cytochrome oxidase, tyrosinase and uricase; required for iron utilization, myelinization and connective tissue formation. Absorption: stomach and small intestine. Stored in liver and muscle, attached to caeruloplasmin	See text
Manganese	Role: found in mitochondria, required for carbohydrate metabolism; actively absorbed in duodenum. Transport protein: transmanganin, a specific β-globulin. Excretion is largely biliary	No deficiency state described in human infants
Chromium	Role: potentiates insulin-induced glucose uptake. Poorly absorbed. Transported by transferring. Body stores: low	In one study, diabetic glucose tolerance tests were corrected in infants with kwashiorkor
Fluoride	Enters bone and teeth, increasing their hardness. Supplementation is not recommended currently during the first 6 months	Dental caries. Excess: fluorosis, including rotting of teeth
Molybdenum	Present in xanthine oxidase. Active transfer across the placenta	No deficiency disease clearly recognised in human infants
Selenium	Role: antioxidant – cofactor for vitamin E	Deficiency not defined in neonates but described in children and adults living in the Keshan province of China: generalised myopathy with cardiac failure and haemolytic anaemia. Possibly occurs in preterm infants on unsupplemented long-term parenteral nutrition
Cobalt	Cobalt is a component of vitamin B_{12} and may not be needed independently of B_{12} requirement	

Zinc

Zinc has been found in over 70 metalloproteins, mostly enzymes, including both DNA and RNA polymerase; it plays a critical role in cell replication and growth.[127,153]

Zinc accumulates in the fetus during the last trimester at around 250 micrograms/kg/24 h. The amount of zinc provided by 200 ml of human milk per kilogram per day falls from 1650 micrograms on the first day of lactation to 160 micrograms after 4 months. Therefore, human milk collected during the early (but not later) months of lactation theoretically provides enough zinc to meet 'in utero' accretion rates. Zinc in banked donor milk should be adequate, although Goes et al[58] reported that redistribution and alterations in the zinc-binding pattern during processing in human milk banks with an increase in the fat fraction and decrease in the whey fraction might reduce zinc bioavailability. Dauncey et al[36] found that preterm infants fed human milk did not achieve positive zinc balance until after 40 days of age.

Zinc deficiency has been described as a late sequel (2–4 months) of preterm birth.[114] These infants develop a syndrome very similar to acrodermatitis enteropathica, with growth arrest, irritability, anorexia, alopecia, diarrhoea, vesiculopustular lesions of the hands and feet, and the characteristic perioral, facial and perineal dermatitis; plasma zinc levels, though not necessarily helpful, are usually <35 micrograms/100 ml (5.4 mmol/l) (normal >70 micrograms/100 ml). Infants respond rapidly to oral zinc sulphate (providing 1.0–3.5 mg zinc per day).

Although there is some evidence that plasma zinc levels are lower in healthy formula-fed term infants than breastfed ones,[79] this does not appear to be reflected in any differences in growth; indeed, in another study,[121] zinc supplementation of formula had no effect on growth velocity. However, the situation may be different in more vulnerable groups. For example, a randomised study in preterm infants fed either a zinc-supplemented or a placebo-supplemented term formula for 6 months from the time at which they attained 1.8 kg, showed higher plasma zinc levels, significantly greater linear growth velocity and higher maximum motor development scores in the supplemented group.[53] More recently, a randomised study of zinc supplementation in formula-fed SGA infants in Chile showed greater catch-up growth over the first 6 months of life in the supplemented group.[26]

The EC Directive guidelines[31] recommend a zinc concentration of 300–750 micrograms/100 ml formula for term infants, and the International Consensus Committee[142] recommended 490 micrograms/100 ml of formula for preterm infants. The value of zinc supplementation for the long-term growth and development of infants born preterm or SGA requires further study.

Copper

Copper accumulates in the fetus during the last trimester at about 50 micrograms/kg/24 h; 200 ml per kilogram per day of human milk provides about 60–80 micrograms/kg/24 h. Nevertheless, Dauncey et al[36] found that preterm infants fed human milk were in negative balance during the first 12 days of life, and one out of six infants were still in negative balance at 40 days.[127,153]

Several cases of copper deficiency have been described in infants born prematurely and fed on cow's milk-based formulas or copper-free parenteral nutrition solutions.[127] The features of copper deficiency include psychomotor retardation, hypotonia, pallor and hypopigmentation, hepatosplenomegaly, X-ray changes of osteoporosis, blurring and cupping of metaphyses with subperiosteal new bone formation and fractures, and sideroblastic anaemia resistant to iron therapy. Neutropenia may also be present and the bone marrow shows vacuolated erythroid and myeloid cells, with iron deposition in the vacuoles. Several of these features are liable to develop when plasma copper falls below 20 mg/100 ml and caeruloplasmin below 5 mg/100 ml. Treatment with copper 0.6–0.8 mg/kg/24 h, given as 1% copper sulphate solution, is effective. There is no evidence that human milk-fed preterm infants require additional copper.

Iodine

Iodine is found almost entirely in the thyroid, where it is incorporated into thyroglobulin and thyroid hormones. It is possible that a syndrome of transient hypothyroidism, seen in preterm infants, could be due to lack of iodine in iodine-deficient areas.[40] The iodine content of breast milk is affected by maternal diet[101] but is usually sufficient. The EC Directive guidelines[31] suggest a minimum of 8 micrograms per 100 ml of formula.

Other trace minerals

Manganese, selenium, chromium and molybdenum are all essential elements, but no definite deficiency states have been described in preterm infants fed human milk or cow's milk-based formulas;[153] quantitative recommendations cannot be made on strong grounds. Manganese is found in very large unphysiological quantities in some formulas (especially soy-based ones), with values up to 100–1000 times those in human milk. It is not known whether these intakes are toxic, but there seems no basis for giving more than 5 micrograms per 100 ml of formula (human milk contains around 0.5–2.5 micrograms/100 ml).

Aluminium

Aluminium is not a nutrient – it has not been found in any metalloprotein, yet it has been added to drinking water (as a clarifying agent); it contaminates artificial formulas, especially soy formulas, which may contain 100 times the aluminium level of breast milk, and is present in high concentrations in some components of intravenous feeding solutions, notably calcium and phosphorus preparations.[97] In patients on renal dialysis, with limited ability to excrete aluminium, toxicity is well described, with dementia, anaemia and bone disease. Preterm infants have immature kidney function and their intake of aluminium from parenteral nutrition solutions – and to a lesser extent from formulas – may be much higher than from breast milk. A randomised trial[13] in 227 preterm infants who received standard versus low aluminium parenteral nutrition solution showed significant deficits in neurodevelopment at 18 months post-term of the order of a one developmental quotient point loss for each day of standard TPN received. Further follow-up of this cohort is planned. Neonatal units should discuss with their pharmacy how to minimise the aluminium content of their TPN solutions.

Vitamins

Clinical vitamin deficiency is rare in the neonatal period. Vitamin deficiency can occur in certain circumstances; these include maternal vitamin depletion, with reduced placental transport and low vitamin concentrations in breast milk, unsupplemented formulas, TPN, the use of unconventional non-milk-based diets, parasitic infestation, neonatal gut and biliary disease, and prematurity.

Optimal intake levels for many vitamins have not been determined in human infants. Broadly, vitamin intakes from breast milk have been taken as a guide (Table 16.1), but excess supplementation in formulas is usually employed in order to compensate for losses during preparation and storage and lower bioavailability. There is no clear evidence showing detrimental effects of excess vitamin supplementation, except for vitamins A and D, though it has been suggested that excessive vitamin E intake may interfere with wound healing and iron 'status'.

The physiological roles of vitamins and clinical consequences of deficiency are summarised in Table 16.6.

Table 16.6 Vitamins: physiology and diseases caused by deficiency (or excess)

	Physiology	Deficiency (or excess)
Vitamin A	Retinyl esters are the main contributor to Vitamin A activity in milk, though both cow's and human milk contain the retinal precursor beta-carotene. Partly emulsified by bile salts, partly hydrolysed by lipase and re-esterified to retinyl palmitate in gut mucosa. One-sixth of dietary carotene is converted into active vitamin A. Stored in liver. Secreted by liver into the bloodstream in association with retinal-binding protein: secretion of vitamin A is tightly regulated like that of a hormone. Required for the synthesis of rhodopsin and other retinal pigments: important for the development of epithelial cells (and therefore the maintenance of epithelial membranes). Degraded by light	Xerophthalmia, susceptibility to infection, keratinization of mucous membranes, blindness. Excess, e.g. 18 000 IU/day or above: raised intracranial pressure, dry skin, loss of hair, brittle bones, irritability
Vitamin E	Placental transfer low. Liver stores may be low. Iron may interfere with absorption and activity. Polyunsaturated fatty acids increase E requirement. Role: antioxidant, prevents oxidation of unsaturated fats thereby increasing stability of cell membranes	Clinical disease states poorly defined. Reduces postnatal red cell haemolysis
Vitamin D	Absorptive mechanisms not fully investigated in human infant: bile salts may be required – absorbed into lymphatic system. Stored in adipose tissue and muscle with small amounts in skin and liver. Sunlight-induced synthesis in the skin from 7-dehydrocholesterol will be minimal in many neonates; active metabolites are 25- and 1,25-hydroxyvitamin D (25-OHD and 1,25-$(OH)_2$D): these act as steroid hormones. Principal role: the enhancement of calcium and phosphate absorption from gut and renal conservation of these elements. Also important for the normal mineralization of bones and teeth	Rickets, tetany. Maternal vitamin D deficiency may rarely result in neonatal rickets. Very small amounts of vitamin D in breast milk – occasionally insufficient, especially if light exposure minimal. Excess: intakes of over 4000 IU/day may result in hypercalcaemia. At intakes greater than 10 000 IU/kg per day: ectopic calcification, failure to thrive
Vitamin K	Emulsified by bile salts. Synthesis by gut flora is much debated. Stores in liver are relatively small. Maternal deficiency predisposes to neonatal deficiency. Role: manufacture of clotting factors (including II, VII, IX and X) and bone metabolism	Haemorrhagic disease of newborn. Excess: haemolytic anaemia can be caused by the water-soluble analogue
Thiamine (B$_1$)	Role: coenzyme in many enzyme systems: pathways involving acetyl CoA	Anorexia, irritability, fatigue, oedema, heart failure, constipation, peripheral neuropathy
Riboflavin (B$_2$)	Component of flavoenzymes: involved in electron transport processes, e.g. in energy metabolism, fatty acid oxidation. Degraded by light	Cheilosis, angular stomatitis, impaired fatty acid oxidation and iron economy
Niacin	Part of NAD–NADP system of Krebs cycle; involved in protein and fat synthesis. Dietary tryptophan will supply niacin: 60 mg tryptophan = 1 mg niacin	Diarrhoea, dermatitis, neurological disturbance

(Continued)

Table 16.6 (*Continued*)

	Physiology	Deficiency (or excess)
Pyridoxine (B$_6$)	Role: modification of functional groups, especially in amino acid metabolism (decarboxylation, transamination, oxidation, desulphurylation)	Convulsion, dermatitis, weakness, anaemia
Vitamin B$_{12}$	Coenzyme for methionine synthesis and indirectly for DNA synthesis, folic acid metabolism, conversion of methylmalonic to succinic acid	Pernicious anaemia, central nervous system damage
Folic acid	Role: enzyme systems taking part in one-carbon transfers in DNA, RNA, methionine and serine synthesis, needed for histidine utilization. Synthesized by gut flora	Megaloblastic anaemia, retarded growth, gastrointestinal disturbance
Pantothenic acid	Roles: part of coenzyme A system, involved in energy and fat metabolism. Synthesized by gut flora	No dietary deficiency state described in man
Biotin	Role: carboxylation reactions, especially concerned with fatty acid synthesis. Produced by gut flora	Possibly skin rashes
Vitamin C	Water-soluble. Absorbed in upper intestine. Not stored: excess excreted in urine. Maternal deficiency may result in neonatal deficiency. Intake from unsupplemented pasteurized cow's milk is minimal. Role: involved in collagen synthesis and in several aspects of amino acid metabolism: protects against hypertyrosinaemia and hyperphenylalaninaemia in newborn period; promotes conversion of folic acid to folinic acid, catecholamine synthesis, carnitine synthesis, iron absorption	Biochemical deficiency may arise in newborn period – overt scurvy rare below 3 months of age

Term infants

Current recommended levels for formula-fed infants are shown in Table 16.1.

Preterm infants' requirements (Table 16.2)

Preterm infants may have special needs for some vitamins because:

- they are born with low body stores, especially of the fat-soluble vitamins which normally accumulate during the third trimester;
- they may have reduced absorptive capacities for some vitamins (e.g. vitamin E);
- they might benefit from 'pharmacological doses' of certain vitamins, e.g. vitamin E.

A brief account follows, summarising information about vitamins of particular importance.[141,153]

Vitamin A

Vitamin A is required for the synthesis of retinal pigments and for the development and maintenance of epithelial membranes. The active form, retinol, is transported in plasma, bound to retinol-binding protein (RBP). Synthesis of RBP usually occurs late in gestation, and plasma retinol and RBP concentrations are lower in preterm than in term infants.[129] RBP also has a lower level of saturation in premature neonates. These data suggest that preterm infants have low body stores of vitamin A and are therefore at risk of deficiency. Low vitamin A status has been associated with an increased risk of chronic lung disease.

In view of these observations, vitamin A supplementation of human milk-fed preterm infants seems wise (see below). Vitamin A can be obtained from the diet in two forms: pre-formed vitamin A (largely retinol) and carotenoids (chiefly β-carotene). Although β-carotene is potentially a good, non-toxic source of vitamin A, its use in preterm infants is relatively unexplored. Vitamin A is light degraded: 70% can be lost from human milk during a 3-hour enteral infusion into an infant under phototherapy lighting.[10] Care must be taken to ensure that the principal source of vitamin A given to preterm infants is not light exposed.

Several studies have been performed to assess whether large doses of vitamin A can reduce the incidence of chronic lung disease (Chapter 27, part 3). Meta-analysis of these studies suggests that regular intramuscular doses of vitamin A are associated with a reduction in oxygen requirement at 36 weeks' gestation.[35] However, a more recent study using large (5000 IU per day) oral doses of vitamin A failed to find any benefit.[150] Darlow[35] suggested that the benefits, safety and acceptability of delivering vitamin A in an intravenous emulsion compared with repeated intramuscular injections should be assessed in future.

Vitamin D

The term 'vitamin D' is often used to refer to both vitamin D$_2$, originating from the plant sterol ergosterol, and vitamin D$_3$, the natural vitamin synthesised in the skin from 7-dehydrocholesterol. Vitamin D$_2$ (or D$_3$) is converted to 25-hydroxyvitamin D (25-OHD, calcidiol) in the liver, and thence into the active metabolite

1,25-dihydroxyvitamin D (1,25-$(OH)_2$D, calcitriol) in the kidney. A major function of 1,25-$(OH)_2$D is to increase calcium and phosphorus absorption from the intestine, but it also conserves these two elements by its action on the kidney.

Preterm infants may have greater requirements for vitamin D than infants born at term; they have lower stores at birth and greater demands for skeletal mineralisation, and although the vitamin D pathway is intact, it may not be fully developed at very low gestation. The dose normally recommended for full-term infants, 400 IU per day, is probably well in excess of requirements for normal babies. However, in preterm infants, doses of up to 800–2000 IU per day have been given. Although these high doses have been shown to increase calcium absorption, vitamin D is no substitute for calcium and phosphorus supplementation in the prevention of bone disease (Chapter 35, Part 4). If intake of these minerals is adequate, there seems no justification in giving more than 400–600 IU vitamin D per day. The use of 1,25-OHD rather than vitamin D may seem logical, as in very small preterm infants absorption of vitamin D may be impaired by a small bile-salt pool size and fat malabsorption. Nevertheless, the use of such active metabolites of vitamin D, and especially the more potent ones (for example 1α-OHD), is experimental and potentially dangerous.

Vitamin E

Increased intakes of vitamin E, which is a powerful antioxidant, may be required to prevent haemolytic anaemia in preterm infants, especially those receiving a diet rich in PUFA or iron. (Polyunsaturated lipids in cell membranes are liable to oxidative damage, which may be enhanced by iron.) There has been much interest in the use of pharmacological doses of vitamin E in preterm infants, but current evidence suggests that it is of no proven benefit in preventing or treating clinically significant retinopathy of prematurity (Chapter 34), and has no role in bronchopulmonary dysplasia (Chapter 27, Part 3) or in the prevention of intraventricular haemorrhage (Chapter 41, Part 3). Against giving high (pharmacological) doses of vitamin E is its potential toxicity; local reactions may occur at the site of intramuscular injection, and high plasma levels have been associated with sepsis and NEC in preterm infants.

Vitamin E requirements must be related to the amount of PUFA in the diet. Human milk contains adequate vitamin E in relation to its PUFA content. Additional supplements are of dubious benefit, but 5 mg/24 h is safe if the objective is to attempt to reduce anaemia. The better-absorbed water-soluble form should be used. High pharmacological doses (25–100 mg/24 h) require concomitant monitoring of plasma levels, which should not exceed 4 mg/100 ml.

Vitamin K

Despite recent controversy over the optimum route for administration and the dose required, vitamin K should be given routinely to all newborn babies as a prophylaxis against vitamin K-deficiency bleeding (VKDB). When given orally to breastfed infants, repeat doses are required at around 1 and 6 weeks, to avoid the risk of intracranial bleeding from late VKDB. A Danish group reported that 12-weekly oral doses are completely effective, even in infants

with liver disease.[102] However, von Kries[149] reported that not all cases of late-onset VKDB were prevented by three doses of oral vitamin K. The situation in sick term or preterm babies is not controversial: all such infants should receive 0.5–1.0 mg of vitamin K parenterally on the first day.

Folic acid

Folic acid dosages for preterm infants vary considerably. Gandy and Jacobson[55] showed benefit from high-dose folic acid supplementation on the growth of erythroblastotic infants. In a large randomised study, Stevens et al[137] were unable to demonstrate differences in growth between LBW infants given either a supplement of 100 micrograms of folic acid per day (from 3 weeks to 12 months) or a formula containing only 3.5 micrograms folic acid per 100 ml (similar to human milk), and no infant became anaemic. More recently, however, Worthington-White et al[158] showed that formula-fed preterm infants who received supplemental folate for the first 6 months (100 micrograms/24 h) had higher serum folate concentrations and a significantly reduced fall in haemoglobin over the study period. An intake of at least 100 micrograms/24 h seems prudent for all LBW infants until 40 weeks postconceptional age.

Vitamin C and pyridoxal phosphate (B_6)

Vitamin C has been shown to prevent hypertyrosinaemia and hyperphenylalaninaemia in LBW infants, especially those on high protein intakes. In view of this and the low vitamin C levels of unsupplemented preterm infants, a supplement is recommended (see below).

Supplementary B_6 might also be expected to improve protein utilisation, in view of its role as a cofactor in amino acid metabolic pathways.

Riboflavin (B_2)

The requirement of preterm infants for riboflavin is currently under review. Most human milk-fed preterm infants develop biochemical evidence of riboflavin deficiency if they have received no supplement after the first week.[83] This problem is compounded by the massive destruction of riboflavin by light when milk is handled in neonatal units. Early biochemical riboflavin deficiency has been shown to be prevented using a preterm formula containing 180 micrograms of riboflavin per 100 ml, or by using a riboflavin-containing multivitamin preparation.[83]

References

1. Agras W S, Kraemer H C, Berkowitz R I, Hommer L D 1990 Influence of early feeding style on adiposity at 6 years of age. Journal of Pediatrics 116: 805–809
2. American Academy of Pediatrics Committee on Nutrition 1977 Nutritional needs of low-birth-weight infants. Pediatrics 60: 519–530
3. Amin H J, Zamora S A, McMillan D D et al 2002 Arginine supplementation prevents necrotizing enterocolitis in the premature infant. Journal of Pediatrics 140: 425–431
4. Aperia A, Broberger O, Zetterstrom R 1982 Implications of limitation of renal function for the nutrition of low birthweight infants. Acta Paediatrica Scandinavica Supplement 296: 49–52

5. Atkinson S A, Radde I C, Anderson G H 1983 Macromineral balances in premature infants fed their own mother's milk or formula. Journal of Pediatrics 102: 96–106

6. Aurichio S, Rubino A, Murset G 1965 Intestinal glycosidase activities in the human embryo, fetus and newborn. Pediatrics 35: 944–954

7. Aynsley-Green A 1985 Metabolic and endocrine interrelations in the human fetus and neonate. American Journal of Clinical Nutrition 41: 399–418

8. Baker H, Frank O, Thompson A D et al 1975 Vitamin profile of 174 mothers and newborn at parturition. American Journal of Clinical Nutrition 28: 59–65

9. Balmer S E, Hanvey L S, Wharton B A 1994 Diet and faecal flora in the newborn: nucleotides. Archives of Disease in Childhood. Fetal and Neonatal Edition 70: F137–F140

10. Bates C J, Liu D-S, Fuller N J, Lucas A 1985 Susceptibility of riboflavin and vitamin A in breast milk to photodegradation and its implications for the use of banked breast milk in infant feeding. Acta Paediatrica Scandinavica 74: 40–44

11. Bayes R, Campoy C, Goicoechea A et al 2001 Role of intrapartum hypoxia in carnitine nutritional status during the early neonatal period. Early Human Development 65: S103–S110

12. Berseth C L, Nordyke C 1993 Enteral nutrients promote postnatal maturation of intestinal motor activity in preterm infants. American Journal of Physiology 264: 1046–1051

13. Bishop N J, Morley R, Day J P, Lucas A 1997 Aluminium neurotoxicity in preterm infants receiving intravenous-feeding solutions. New England Journal of Medicine 336: 1557–1561

14. Blondheim O, Abbasi S, Fox W W, Bhutani V K 1993 Effect of enteral gavage feeding rate on pulmonary functions of very low birth weight infants. Journal of Pediatrics 122: 751–755

15. Boehm G, Muller D M Beyreiss K, Raiha N C 1988 Evidence for functional immaturity of the ornithine-urea cycle in very-low-birth-weight infants. Biology of the Neonate 54: 121–125

16. Brooke O G, Kinzey J M 1985 High energy feeding in small for gestation neonates. Archives of Disease in Childhood 60: 42–46

17. Brooke O G, Wood C, Barley J 1982 Energy balance, nitrogen balance and growth in preterm infants fed expressed breast milk, a premature infant formula and two low-solute adapted formulae. Archives of Disease in Childhood 57: 898–904

18. Brunser O, Espinoza J, Araya M, Cruchet S, Gil A 1994 Effect of dietary nucleotide supplementation on diarrhoeal disease in infants. Acta Paediatrica 83: 188–191

19. Bullen C L, Willis A T 1971 Resistance of the breast fed infant to gastroenteritis. British Medical Journal iii: 338–343

20. Carlson S E, Cooke R J, Werkman S H, Tolley E A 1992 First year growth of preterm infants fed standard compared to marine oil (fish oil) supplemented formula. Lipids 27: 901–907

21. Carlson S E, Rhodes P G, Ferguson M G 1986 Docosahexaenoic acid status of preterm infants at birth and following feeding with milk or formula. American Journal of Clinical Nutrition 44: 798–804

22. Carlson S E, Werkman S H, Tolley E A 1996 The effect of long chain n-3 fatty acid supplementation on visual acuity and growth of preterm infants with and without bronchopulmonary dysplasia. American Journal of Clinical Nutrition 63: 687–697

23. Carnielli V P, Luijendijk I H T, van Goudoever J B et al 1995 Feeding premature newborn infants palmitic acid in amounts and sterioisomeric position similar to that of human milk: effects on fat and mineral balance. American Journal of Clinical Nutrition 61: 1037–1042

24. Carnielli V P, Luijendijk I H T, van Goudoever J B et al 1996 Structural position and amount of palmitic acid in infant formula: effects on fat, fatty acid and mineral balance. Journal of Pediatric Gastroenterology and Nutrition 23: 553–560

25. Carver J D, Walker W A 1995 The role of nucleotides in human nutrition. Journal of Nutritional Biochemistry 6: 58–72

26. Castillo-Duran C, Rodriguez A, Venegas G, Alvarez P, Icaza G 1995 Zinc supplementation and growth of infants born small for gestational age. Journal of Pediatrics 127: 206–211

27. Clandinin M T, Chappell J E, Heim T, Swyer P R, Chance G W 1981 Fatty acid utilization in perinatal de novo synthesis of tissues. Early Human Development 5: 355–366

28. Clandinin M T, Chappell J E, Leong S, Heim T, Swyer P R, Chance G W 1980 Extrauterine fatty acid accretion in infant brain: implications for fatty acid requirements. Early Human Development 4: 131–138

29. Clandinin M, VanAerde J, Antonson D et al 2002 Formulas with docosa-hexaenoic acid (DHA) and arachidonic acid (AA) promote better growth and development scores in very-low-birth-weight infants. Pediatric Research 51: 187A–188A

30. Cockburn F, Brown J K, Belton N R, Forfar J O 1973 Neonatal convulsions associated with primary disturbance of calcium, phosphorus and magnesium. Archives of Disease in Childhood 48: 99–103

31. Commission Directive on Infant Formulae and Follow-on Formula (91/321/EC) 1996 O.J.No. L 175/35

32. Coombs R C, Morgan M E, Durbin G M, Booth I W, McNeish A S 1992 Doppler assessment of human neonatal gut blood flow velocities: postnatal adaptation and response to feeds. Journal of Pediatric Gastroenterology and Nutrition 15: 6–12

33. Cooper P A, Rothberg A, Davies V A, Horn J, Vogelman L 1989 Three-year growth and developmental follow-up of very low birth weight infants fed own mother's milk, a premature formula, or one of two standard formulas. Journal of Paediatric Gastroenterology and Nutrition 8: 348–354

34. Cosgrove M, Davies D P, Jenkins H R 1996 Nucleotide supplementation and the growth of term small for gestational age infants. Archives of Disease in Childhood. Fetal and Neonatal Edition 74: F122–F125

35. Darlow B A, Graham P J 2000 Vitamin A supplementation for preventing morbidity and mortality in very low birth weight infants (Cochrane Review). Cochrane Database of Systematic Reviews (2): CD000501

36. Dauncey M J, Shaw J C, Urman J 1977 The absorption and retention of magnesium, zinc and copper by low birthweight infants fed pasteurized human breast milk. Pediatric Research 11: 1033–1039

37. Davidson M, Levine S, Bauer C, Dann M 1967 Feeding studies in low birthweight infants. Journal of Pediatrics 70: 695–713

38. De Gamarra E 1992 Energy expenditure in premature newborns with bronchopulmonary dysplasia. Biology of the Neonate 61: 337–344

39. De Gamarra M E, Schutz Y, Catzeflis C et al 1987 Composition of weight gain during the neonatal period and longitudinal growth follow-up in premature babies. Biology of the Neonate 52: 181–187

40. Delange F, Bourdoux P, Ketelbant-Balasse P, Van Humskerken A, Glinoer D, Ermans A M 1983 Transient primary hypothyroidism in the newborn. In: Dussault J H, Walker P (eds) Congenital hypothyroidism. Marcel Dekker, New York, pp 275–301

41. ESPGAN 1987 Nutrition and feeding of preterm infants. Committee on Nutrition of the Preterm Infant, European Society of Paediatric Gastroenterology and Nutrition. Acta Paediatrica Scandinavica Supplement 336: 1–14

42. Fang S, Kempley S T, Gamsu H R 2001 Prediction of early tolerance to enteral feeding in preterm infants by measurement of superior mesenteric artery blood flow velocity. Archives of Disease in Childhood. Fetal and Neonatal Edition 85: F42–F45

43. Farquharson J, Cockburn F, Patrick W A, Jamieson E C, Logan R W 1992 Infant cerebral cortex phospholipid fatty acid composition and diet. Lancet 340: 810–813

44. Farquharson J, Jamieson E C, Abbasi K A, Patrick W J A, Logan R W, Cockburn F 1995 Effect of diet on the fatty acid composition of the major phospholipids of infant cerebral cortex. Archives of Disease in Childhood 72: 198–203

45. Fewtrell M S, Abbott R A, Kennedy K et al 2004 Randomized, double-blind trial of long-chain polyunsaturated fatty acid supplementation with fish oil and borage oil in preterm infants. Journal of Pediatrics 111: 471–479

46a. Fewtrell M S, Lucas A, Cole T J et al 2004 Prematurity and reduced body fatness at 8–12 y of age. American Journal of Clinical Nutrition 80: 436–440

46. Fewtrell M S, Morley R, Abbott R A et al 2002 Double-blind randomized trial of long-chain polyunsaturated fatty acid supplementation in formula fed to preterm infants. Pediatrics 110: 73–82

47. Fewtrell M S, Prentice A, Jones S C et al 1999 Bone mineralization and turnover in preterm infants at 8–12 years of age: the effect of early diet. Journal of Bone and Mineral Research 14: 810–820

48. Filer I J, Mattson F, Fomon S J 1969 Triacylglycerol configuration and fat absorption by the human infant. Journal of Nutrition 99: 293–298

49. Fomon S J, Kaschke F, Ziegler E E, Nelson S E 1982 Body composition of reference children from birth to age 10 years. American Journal of Clinical Nutrition 35: 1169–1175

50. Forsyth J S, Willatts P, Agostoni C, Bissenden J, Casaer P, Boehm G 2003 Long chain polyunsaturated fatty acid supplementation in infant formula and blood pressure in later childhood: follow up of a randomized controlled trial. British Medical Journal 326: 953

51. Fredrikzon B, Hernell O, Blackberg L 1982 Lingual lipase: role in lipid digestion in infants with low birthweight and/or pancreatic insufficiency. Acta Paediatrica Scandinavica Supplement 296: 75–80

52. Friel J K, Andrews W I, Aziz K, Kwa P G, Lepage G, L'Abbe M R 2001 A randomized trial of two levels of iron supplementation and developmental outcome in low birth weight infants. Journal of Pediatrics 139: 254–260

53. Friel J K, Andrews W L, Matthew J D et al 1993 Zinc supplementation in very low birth weight infants. Journal of Pediatric Gastroenterology and Nutrition 17: 97–104

54. Friis-Hansen B 1982 Body water metabolism in early infancy. Acta Paediatrica Scandinavica Supplement 296: 44–48

55. Gandy G M, Jacobson W 1977 Influence of folic acid on birth-weight and growth of the erythroblastotic infant. Archives of Disease in Childhood 52: 7–15, 16–21

56. Gaull G E, Rassin D K, Raiha N C R, Heinonen K 1977 Milk protein quantity and quality in low-birth-infants. III. Effects on sulfur amino acids in plasma and urine. Journal of Pediatrics 90: 348–355

57. Gil A, Corral E, Martinez A et al 1986 Effects of the addition of dietary nucleotides to an adapted milk formula on the microbial pattern of faeces in term newborn infants. Journal of Clinical Nutrition and Gastroenterology 1: 127–131

58. Goes H C, Torres A G, Donangelo C M, Trugo N M 2002 Nutrient composition of banked human milk in Brazil and influence of processing on zinc distribution in milk fractions. Nutrition 18: 590–594

59. Goldman H I, Goldman J S, Kaufman I 1974 Late effects of early dietary protein intake on low birthweight infants. Journal of Pediatrics 84: 764–769

60. Gordon H, Levine S, McNamara H 1947 Feeding of premature infants. American Journal of Diseases of Children 73: 442–452

61. Graham G C, Placko R P, Moralls E, Acevedo G, Cordaus A 1970 Dietary protein quality in infants and children. American Journal of Diseases of Children 120: 419–423

62. Greengard O 1977 Enzymic differentiation of human liver: comparison with the rat model. Pediatric Research 11: 669–676

63. Hamosh M 1996 Digestion in the newborn. Clinics in Perinatology 23: 191–210

64. Hanin I, Schuberth J 1974 Labelling of acetylcholine in the brain of mice fed on a diet containing deuterium labelled choline. Journal of Neurochemistry 23: 819–824

65. Heird W C 1977 Effects of total parenteral alimentation on intestinal function. In: Sunshine P (ed) Gastrointestinal function and neonatal nutrition. Ross Laboratories, Columbus, Ohio, p. 16

66. Howlett A, Ohlsson A 2000 Inositol for respiratory distress syndrome in preterm infants (Cochrane Review). Cochrane Database of Systematic Reviews (4): CD000366

67. Imaki H, Jacobson S G, Kemp C M, Knighton R W, Neuringer M, Sturman J 1993 Retinal morphology and visual pigment levels in 6- and 12-month-old rhesus monkeys fed a taurine-free human infant formula. Journal of Neuroscience Research 36: 290–304

68. Infant formula and follow-on formula regulations 1995 Statutory Instrument No. 77. HMSO, London

69. Innis S M, Adamkin D H, Hall R T et al 2002 Docosahexaenoic acid and arachidonic acid enhance growth with no adverse effects in preterm infants fed formula. Journal of Pediatrics 140:547–554

70. Janas L M, Picciano M F 1982 The nucleotide profile of human milk. Pediatric Research 16: 659–662

71. Johnson L R, Copeland E, Dudrick S J, Lichtenberger L M, Castro G A 1975 Structural and hormonal alterations in the gastrointestinal tract of parenterally fed rats. Gastroenterology 68: 1177–1183

72. Kennedy K, Fewtrell M S, Morley R, Quinlan P T, Wells J C K, Lucas A 1999 Double-blind randomised trial of a synthetic triglyceride (betapol) in formula fed term infants: effects on stool biochemistry, stool characteristics and bone mineralisation. American Journal of Clinical Nutrition 70: 920–927

73. Kien C L 1996 Digestion, absorption and fermentation of carbohydrates in the newborn. Clinics in Perinatology 23: 211–228

74. Koo W K K, Tsang R C 1993 In: Tsang R C, Lucas A, Uauy R, Zlotkin S (eds) Nutritional needs of the preterm infant. Scientific basis and practical guidelines. Caduceus Medical Publishers, New York, pp 135–156

75. Koo W W, Hammami M, Margeson D P, Nwaesei C, Montalto M B, Lasekan J B 2003 Reduced bone mineralization in infants fed palm olein-containing formula: a randomized, double-blinded, prospective trial. Pediatrics 111: 1017–1023

76. Kurzner S I, Garg M, Bautista D B, Sargent C W, Bowman C M, Keens T G 1988 Growth failure in infants with bronchopulmonary dysplasia. Nutrition and elevated resting metabolic expenditure. Pediatrics 81: 379–384

77. Lane A J, Coombs R C, Evans D H, Levin R J 1998 Effect of feed interval and feed type on splanchnic haemodynamics. Archives of Disease in Childhood. Fetal and Neonatal Edition 79: F49–F53

78. Lebenthal E, Lee P C, Heitlinger L E 1983 Impact of development of the gastrointestinal tract on infant feeding. Journal of Pediatrics 102: 1–9

79. Lombeck I, Fuchs A 1994 Zinc and copper in infants fed breast-milk or different formula. European Journal of Pediatrics 153: 770–776

80. Lucas A 1991 Programming by early nutrition in man. Ciba Foundation Symposium 156: 38–50

81. Lucas A 1994 Role of nutritional programming in determining adult morbidity. Archives of Disease in Childhood 71: 288–290

82. Lucas A, Baker B A, Morley R 1993 Hyperphenylalaninaemia and outcome in intravenously fed preterm neonates. Archives of Disease in Childhood 68: 579–583

83. Lucas A, Bates C 1984 Transient riboflavin depletion in preterm infants. Archives of Disease in Childhood 59: 837–841

84. Lucas A, Brooke O G, Morley R, Cole T J, Bamford M F 1990 Early diet of preterm infants and development of allergic or atopic disease: randomised prospective study. British Medical Journal 300: 837–840

85. Lucas A, Cole T J 1990 Breast milk and neonatal necrotising enterocolitis. Lancet 336: 1519–1523

86. Lucas A, Ewing E, Roberts S B, Coward W A 1987 How much energy does the breast-fed infant consume and expend? British Medical Journal 295: 75–77

87. Lucas A, Gore S M, Cole T J et al 1984 A multicentre trial on the feeding of low birthweight infants: effects of diet on early growth. Archives of Disease in Childhood 59: 722–730

88. Lucas A, Morley R, Cole T J 1998 Randomised trial of early diet in preterm babies and later intelligence quotient. British Medical Journal 317: 1481–1487

89. Lucas A, Morley R, Cole T J, Lister G, Leeson-Payne C 1992 Breast milk and subsequent intelligence quotient in children born preterm. Lancet 339: 261–264

90. Lucas A, Morley R, Hudson G J et al 1988 Early sodium intake and later blood pressure in preterm infants. Archives of Disease in Childhood 63: 656–657

91. Lucas A, Quinlan P, Abrams S, Ryan S, Meah S, Lucas P J 1997 Randomized controlled trial of a synthetic triacylglycerol milk formula for preterm infants. Archives of Disease in Childhood. Fetal and Neonatal Edition 77: F178–F184

92. Makrides M, Neumann M A, Byard R W, Simmer K, Gibson R A 1994 Fatty acid composition of brain, retina and erythrocytes in breast- and formula-fed infants. American Journal of Clinical Nutrition 60: 189–194

93. Malone J L 1975 Vitamin passage across the placenta. Clinics in Perinatology 2: 295–307

94. McCance R 1962 Food, growth, and time. Lancet 2: 271–272

95. McClure R J, Newell S J 1999 Randomised controlled trial of trophic feeding and gut motility. Archives of Disease in Childhood. Fetal and Neonatal Edition 80: F54–F58

96. McClure R J, Newell S J 2000 Randomised controlled study of clinical outcome following trophic feeding. Archives of Disease in Childhood. Fetal and Neonatal Edition 82: F29–F33

97. McGraw M, Bishop N, Jamieson R et al 1986 Aluminium content of milk formula and intravenous fluids used in infants. Lancet i: 157

98. Micheli J-L, Schutz Y 1993 In: Tsang R C, Lucas A, Uauy R, Zlotkin S (eds) Nutritional needs of the preterm infant. Scientific basis and practical guidelines. Caduceus Medical Publishers, New York, pp 31–32

99. Mino M, Nishino H 1973 Fetal and maternal relationship in serum vitamin E level. Journal of Nutritional Science and Vitaminology 19: 475–482

100. Navarro J, Maldonada J, Narbona E et al 1999 Influence of dietary nucleotides on plasma immunoglobulin levels and lymphocyte subsets of preterm infants. Biofactors 10: 67–76

101. Nohr S B, Laurberg P, Borlum K-G et al 1994 Iodine status in neonates in Denmark: regional variations and dependency on maternal iodine supplementation. Acta Paediatrica 83: 578–582

102. Norgaard-Hansen K, Ebbesen F 1996 Neonatal vitamin K prophylaxis in Denmark: three years' experience with oral administration during the first three months of life compared with one oral administration at birth. Acta Paediatrica 85: 1137–1139

103. O'Brien J S, Fillerup D L, Mead J F 1964 Quantification and fatty acid and fatty aldehyde composition of ethanolamine, choline, and serine glycerophosphatides in human cerebral grey and white matter. Journal of Lipid Research 5: 329–338

104. O'Connor D, Hall R, Adamkin D et al 2001 Growth and development in preterm infants fed long-chain polyunsaturated fatty acids: a prospective, randomized controlled trial. Pediatrics 108: 359–371

105. O'Donnell J, Finer N N, Rich W, Barshop B A, Barrington K J 2002 Role of L-carnitine in apnea of prematurity: a randomized, controlled trial. Pediatrics 109: 622–626

106. Okatmoto G, Muttard C R, Sucker C L, Hierd W C 1982 Use of medium chain triglycerides in feeding the low birthweight infant. American Journal of Diseases of Children 136: 428–431

107. Orzalesi M 1987 Vitamins and premature infants. Biology of the Neonate 52 (suppl. 1): 97–112

108. Penn D, Schmidt-Sommerfeld E, Pascu F 1981 Decreased tissue carnitine concentrations in newborn infants receiving total parenteral nutrition. Journal of Pediatrics 98: 976–978

109. Pereira G R, Baumgart S, Bennett M J et al 1994 Use of high-fat formula for premature infants with bronchopulmonary dysplasia: metabolic, pulmonary, and nutritional studies. Journal of Pediatrics 124: 605–611

110. Pickering L K, Granoff D M, Erickson J R et al 1998 Modulation of the immune system by human milk and infant formula containing nucleotides. Pediatrics 101: 242–249

111. Quinlan P, Moore S 1993 Modification of triglycerides by lipases: process technology and its application to the production of nutritionally improved fats. Inform 4: 580–585

112. Raiha N C R 1981 Perinatal development of some enzymes of amino acid metabolism in the liver. In: Davis J A, Dobbing J (eds) Scientific foundations of pediatrics. Heinemann, London, pp 129–138

113. Reichman B L, Chessex P, Putet G et al 1982 Partition of energy metabolism and energy cost of growth in the very low-birthweight infant. Pediatrics 69: 443–451

114. Reifen R M, Zlotkin S 1993 In: Tsang R C, Lucas A, Uauy R, Zlotkin S (eds) Nutritional needs of the preterm infant. Scientific basis and practical guidelines. Caduceus Medical Publishers, New York, p. 198

115. Rey J, Schuri Z L, Amedee-Manesme O 1982 Fat absorption in low birthweight infants. Acta Paediatrica Scandinavica Supplement 296: 81–84

116. Roberts S B, Coward W A, Schlingenseipen K-H, Nohria V, Lucas A 1986 Comparison of doubly labelled water method with calorimetry and a nutrient balance study for assessing energy expenditure, water intake and metabolizable energy intake in preterm infants. American Journal of Clinical Nutrition 44: 315–322

117. Roberts S B, Lucas A 1985 The effects of two extremes of dietary intake on body composition in preterm infants. Early Human Development 12: 301–307

118. Ronnholm K A R, Sipila I, Siimes M A 1982 Human milk protein supplementation for the prevention of hypoproteinemia without metabolic imbalance in breast milk fed very low birthweight infants. Journal of Pediatrics 101: 243–247

119. Rudolph F B, Kulkarni A D 1984 Involvement of dietary nucleotides in T lymphocyte function. Advances in Experimental Medicine and Biology 165: 175–178

120. Ryan A S, Montalto M B, Groh-Wargo S et al 1999 Effect of DHA-containing formula on growth of preterm infants to 59 weeks postmenstrual age. American Journal of Human Biology 11: 457–467

121. Salmenpera L, Perheentupa J, Pakerinen P, Siimes M A 1994 Zinc supplementation of infant formula. American Journal of Clinical Nutrition 59: 985–989

122. Sanchez-Pozo A, Morillas J, Molto L, Robles R, Gil A 1994 Dietary nucleotides influence lipoprotein metabolism in newborn infants. Pediatric Research 35: 112–116

123. SanGiovanni J P, Parra-Cabrera S, Colditz G A, Berkey C S, Dwyer J T 2000 Meta-analysis of dietary essential fatty acids and long-chain polyunsaturated fatty acids as they relate to visual resolution acuity in healthy preterm infants. Pediatrics 105: 1292–1298

124. Schmelzle H, Wirth S, Skopnik H et al 2003 Randomized double-blind study of the nutritional efficacy and bifidogenicity of a new infant formula containing partially hydrolyzed protein, a high beta-palmitic acid level, and nondigestible oligosaccharides. Journal of Pediatric Gastroenterology and Nutrition 36: 343–351

125. Schultz K, Soltesz G, Mestyan J 1980 The metabolic consequences of human milk and formula feeding in premature infants. Acta Paediatrica Scandinavica 69: 647–652

126. Shannon K 1995 Recombinant human erythropoetin in neonatal anaemia. Clinics in Perinatology 22: 627–640

127. Shaw J C L 1982 Trace metal requirements of preterm infants. Acta Paediatrica Scandinavica Supplement 296: 93–100

128. Shelley H J 1964 Carbohydrate reserves in the newborn infant. British Medical Journal i: 273–275

129. Shenai J P, Chytil F, Jhaveri A, Stahlman M T 1981 Plasma vitamin A and retinol binding protein in premature and term neonates. Journal of Pediatrics 99: 302–305

130. Simmer K 2001 Longchain polyunsaturated fatty acid supplementation in term infants (Cochrane Review). Cochrane Database of Systematic Reviews (4): 000376

131. Simmer K, Patole S 2004 Longchain polyunsaturated fatty acid supplementation in preterm infants (Cochrane Review). In: The Cochrane Library, Issue 3. John Wiley & Sons, Chichester

132. Singhal A, Cole T J, Lucas A 2001 Early nutrition in preterm infants and later blood pressure: two cohorts after randomised trials. Lancet 357: 413–419

133. Singhal A, Cole T, Fewtrell M, Lucas A 2004 Breast milk feeding and the lipoprotein profile in adolescents born preterm. Lancet (In press)

134. Singhal A, Farooqi I S, O'Rahilly S, Cole T J, Fewtrell M, Lucas A 2002 Early nutrition and leptin concentrations in later life. American Journal of Clinical Nutrition 75: 993–999

135. Singhal A, Fewtrell M, Cole T J, Lucas A 2003 Low nutrient intake and early growth for later insulin resistance in adolescents born preterm. Lancet 361: 1089–1097

136. Southgate D A T, Durnin J V G A 1970 Calorie conversion factors. An experimental reassessment of the factors used in the calculation of the energy values of human diets. British Journal of Nutrition 24: 517–535

137. Stevens D, Burman D, Strelling K, Morris A 1979 Folic acid supplementation in low birthweight infants. Pediatrics 64: 333–335

138. Stimmler L, Snodgrass G J A I, Jaffe E 1973 Enamel hypoplasia of the teeth associated with neonatal tetany. Lancet i: 1085–1086

139. Tantibhedyangkul P, Hashim S A 1978 Medium chain triglyceride feeding in premature infants: effects on calcium and magnesium absorption. Pediatrics 61: 537–545

140. Thomson A B R, Keelen M 1986 The development of the small intestine. Canadian Journal of Physiology and Pharmacology 64: 13–29

141. Tsang R E 1985 Vitamin and mineral requirements in preterm infants. Marcel Dekker, New York

142. Tsang R C, Lucas A, Uauy R, Zlotkin S (eds) 1993 Nutritional needs of the preterm infant. Scientific basis and practical guidelines. Caduceus Medical Publishers, New York, pp 288–289

143. Tsuboi K K, Kwon L K, Ford W D A et al 1986 Delayed ontological development in the bypassed ileum of the infant rat. Gastroenterology 80: 1550–1556

144. Tubman T R, Thompson S W 2001 Glutamine supplementation for preventing morbidity in preterm infants (Cochrane Review). Cochrane Database of Systematic Reviews (4): CD001457

145. Tyson J E, Lasky R, Flood D, Mize C, Picone T, Paule C L 1989 Randomized trial of taurine supplementation for infants ≤1300 gram birth weight: effect on auditory brainstem-evoked responses. Pediatrics 83: 406–415

146. Uauy R, Stringel G 1988 Effect of dietary nucleotides on growth and maturation of the developing gut in the rat. Pediatric Research 23: 494A

147. Vanderhoof J, Gross S, Hegyi T 2000 A multicenter long-term safety and efficacy trial of preterm formula supplemented with long-chain polyunsaturated fatty acids. Journal of Pediatric Gastroenterolgy and Nutrition 30: 121–127

148. Vaughn P, Thomas P, Clark R, Neu J 2003 Enteral glutamine supplementation and morbidity in low birth weight infants. Journal of Pediatrics 142: 662–668

149. von Kries R, Hachmeister A, Gobel U 1999 Can 3 oral 2mg doses of vitamin K effectively prevent late vitamin K deficiency bleeding? European Journal of Pediatrics 158: S183–S186

150. Wardle S P, Hughes A, Chen S, Shaw N J 2001 Randomised controlled trial of oral vitamin A supplementation in preterm infants to prevent chronic lung disease. Archives of Disease in Childhood. Fetal and Neonatal Edition 84: F9–F13

151. Watkins J B, Jarvenpaa A-L, Szczepanik-Van Leeuwen P et al 1983 Feeding the low-birth-weight infant. V. Effects of human milk taurine and cholesterol on bile acid kinetics. Gastroenterology 85: 793–800

152. Weinstein M R, Oh W 1981 Oxygen consumption in infants with bronchopulmonary dysplasia. Journal of Pediatrics 99: 958–961

153. Wharton B A 1987 Nutrition and feeding of preterm infants. Blackwell Scientific, Oxford

154. Widdowson E M 1981 Nutrition. In: Davis J A, Dobbing J (eds) Scientific foundations of pediatrics, 2nd edn. Heinemann, London, pp 41–43

155. Widdowson E M, Dickerson J W T 1964 Chemical composition of the body. In: Comar C L, Bronner F (eds) Mineral metabolism Vol. II, Part A. Academic Press, New York, pp 1–247

156. Williamson S, Finucane E, Elliott J, Gamsu H R 1978 Effect of heat treatment of human milk on absorption of nitrogen, fat, sodium, calcium and phosphorus by preterm infants. Archives of Disease in Childhood 53: 555–563

157. Wilson D C, McClure G, Halliday H L, Reid M M, Dodge J A 1991 Nutrition and bronchopulmonary dysplasia. Archives of Disease in Childhood 66: 37–38

158. Worthington-White D A, Behnke M, Gross S 1994 Preterm infants require additional folate to reduce the severity of the anemia of prematurity. American Journal of Clinical Nutrition 60: 930–935

159. Yeh T F, McClenan D A, Ajayi O A, Pildes R S 1989 Metabolic rate and energy balance in infants with bronchopulmonary dysplasia. Journal of Pediatrics 114: 448–451

160. Young V R 1981 Protein-energy interrelationships in the newborn: a brief consideration of some basic aspects. In: Lebenthal E (ed) Textbook of gastroenterology and nutrition in infancy Vol. 1. Raven Press, New York, pp 257–263

161. Yu V Y R 2002 Scientific rationale and benefits of nucleotide supplementation of infant formula. Journal of Paediatrics and Child Health 38: 543–549

162. Ziegler E E 1986 Protein requirements of preterm infants. In: Fomon S J, Heird W C (eds) Energy and protein needs during infancy. Academic Press, Orlando

163. Ziegler E E, Biga R L, Fomon S J 1981 Nutritional requirements of the premature infant. In: Suskind RM (ed) Textbook of pediatric nutrition. Raven Press, New York, pp 29–39

PART 2

Feeding the full-term baby

Mary Fewtrell, Alan Lucas

Breastfeeding

Breastfeeding is a complex physiological event: indeed, the term itself could be regarded as a misnomer, since 'feeding' is only one of several physiological processes that occur when a newborn infant is put to the breast. These processes can be summarised as follows:

- provision of nutrients;
- provision of immunological and antimicrobial protection;
- induction of adaptive events that equip the infant for extrauterine nutrition;
- the passage of non-nutritive factors (other than antimicrobial ones) from mother to infant, e.g. breast milk hormones and growth factors;
- provision of digestive enzymes, e.g. milk lipases;
- effects on the mother, e.g. contraceptive role;
- facilitation of mother–infant bonding;
- 'programming' effects on long-term health.

Nutritive aspects of human milk

Human milk does not have a constant composition, and significant changes take place during the course of lactation, diurnally and during each feed. Uncertainty over the precise dietary intake of breastfed infants poses a major problem for nutritional science. In Tables 16.7 and 16.8, the composition of average mature human milk is tabulated[15] together with the composition of unmodified cow's milk.

Protein

The protein content of milks of mammalian species appears to be related to the postnatal growth rate of the infant.[6] Human infants have especially slow postnatal growth rates compared with many other mammals, and the protein content of human milk is correspondingly very low. Previously, the protein content of mature human milk may have been overestimated, because of its high content of non-protein nitrogen: a realistic figure is 1.0 g/100 ml compared with 3.5 g/100 ml in cow's milk.

The two main classes of protein in milk are whey and casein. Human milk is whey predominant (around 60% of total protein), though the casein content is still debated. Cow's milk, however, is casein predominant, with only 20% whey. In human whey, α-lactalbumin is the dominant protein, followed by lactoferrin. In contrast, the major whey protein in cow's milk is β-lactoglobulin, which is absent from human milk and may be antigenic when fed to human infants. α-Lactalbumin is present in

cow's milk, but lactoferrin occurs in only small amounts. Whey proteins have a high nutritive value for human infants: their essential amino acid content is high. Some work has suggested that infants fed on modified whey-predominant formulas retain more nitrogen and grow faster than those fed on unmodified (casein-predominant) formulas, but this is debatable and formulas marketed in the USA are often casein predominant. Caseins may precipitate at low pH, forming a 'curd' in the infant's stomach, and this has led to the widespread belief that casein-dominant formulas may be more satisfying for hungry infants. Human milk casein yields a softer, more flocculent curd than cow's milk casein.

Human milk has a cysteine content about twice that of cow's milk and a methionine/cysteine ratio content that is seven times less than cow's milk. In view of the late development of cystathionase (which converts methionine to cystine), cysteine may be an essential amino acid in the newborn, and it has been suggested that the high cysteine content of human milk is biologically advantageous. In addition, the relatively low content of tyrosine and phenylalanine in human milk may be related to the newborn infant's limited capacity to metabolise them.

The non-protein nitrogen content in human milk is unusually high: about 25% of the total, compared with 6% in cow's milk. It consists of free amino acids, urea, creatinine, creatine, uric acid and ammonia. Clearly, free amino acids must be included with protein from a nutritional point of view; it is unknown whether other non-protein nitrogen fractions have nutritional value.[9] The free amino acids in human milk include taurine, which is present in significantly higher amounts than in cow's milk. During early lactation, milk protein content is much higher than in mature milk (Fig. 16.3). The falling protein content could represent an adaptation to the infant's decreasing protein requirements, or simply reflect the maturation of the mammary gland.

Energy

Published values for the energy content of breast milk (obtained unphysiologically as expressed breast milk) of around 70 kcal/100 ml have been challenged. Using the doubly labelled water method, which avoids milk sampling, Lucas et al[48] suggest that a figure close to 60 kcal per 100 ml is realistic. Most formulas have significantly higher energy contents than this (see below).

Fat

The fat content of milk from different mothers is very variable, and in an individual usually increases during early lactation (1–2 weeks) and later declines. (Indeed, with the exception of lactose and lysozyme, most breast milk nutrients, including minerals and vitamins, decline after the first 2–3 months of lactation.)

Table 16.7 Nutrient content of baby milks available in the UK (per 100 ml)

Composition per 100 ml	Mature human milk		Demineralised whey-based formulas					Modified milk formulas			
	DHSS[a]	Macy et al[b]	Aptamil First with Milupan** (M)	Premium** (C&G)	Farley's First Milk (FHP)**	SMA Gold** (Wyeth)	HiPP Organic Infant Milk	Aptamil Extra** with Milupan (M) (FHP)	Plus** (C&G) (Wyeth)	Farley's** Second Milk	SMA White**
Macronutrients											
Protein* (g)	1.34	1.45	1.40	1.40	1.45	1.5	1.6	1.6	1.7	1.7	1.6
Casein (%)	–	32	40	40	40	40	40	80	77	80	80
Whey (%)	–	68	60	60	60	60	60	20	23	20	20
Fat (g)	4.2	3.8	3.6	3.5	3.82	3.6	3.3	3.2	3.4	2.9	3.6
LCPUFA	+	+	+	+	+	+	–	+	–	–	–
Carbohydrate+											
Lactose (g)	7.0	7.0	7.3	7.4	6.96	7.2	7.9	8.1	7.2	2.8	7.0
Maltodextrin (g)	–	–	–	–	–	–	–	–	5.5	–	–
Total (g)	7.0	–	7.3	7.5	6.96	7.2	7.9	8.3	7.3	8.3	7.0
Energy											
kcal	70	68	67	67	68	67	68	68	67	66	67
kJ	293	285	280	280	284	280	284	285	280	277	280
Minerals (mg)											
Calcium	35	33	45	52	39	46	65	70	80	61	56
Chloride	43	43	46	43	45	43	41	47	53	55	55
Magnesium	2.8	4.0	5	5.0	5.2	6.4	7.0	5.9	5.4	6.0	5.3
Phosphorus	15	15	28	26.0	27	33	38	47	45	48	44
Potassium	60	55	70	64	57	70	65	80	82	86	80
Sodium	15	15	17	19	17	18	20	29	21	25	22
Trace elements (µg)											
Copper	39	40	50	40	42	33	17	30	40	40	33
Iodine	76	150	10	10	4.5	10	8.1	9.3	10	10	10
Iron	76	150	700	500	690	800	700	700	500	660	800
Manganese	ND	0.7	8.4	7.4	3.4	5	NS	10	10	3.3	10
Zinc	295	530	500	500	340	600	500	600	500	330	600
Potential renal solute load^ (mosmol/l)	88	91	94	93	93	97	NS	110	113	116	110

(Continued)

Table 16.7 (Continued)

Composition per 100 ml	Mature human milk		Demineralised whey-based formulas					Modified milk formulas			
	DHSS[a]	Macy et al[b]	Aptamil First with Milupan** (M)	Premium** (C&G)	Farley's First Milk (FHP)**	SMA Gold** (Wyeth)	HiPP Organic Infant Milk	Aptamil Extra** with Milupan (M) (FHP)	Plus** (C&G) (Wyeth)	Farley's** Second Milk	SMA White**
Vitamins											
A retinol (µg)	60	53	67	65	100	78	73	59	65	97	75
B_1 thiamin (µg)	16	16	50	40	42	100	59	40	40	39	100
B_2 riboflavin (µg)	31	42.6	100	110	55	150	73	60	110	53	150
B_6 pyridoxine (µg)	6	11	50	40	35	60	59	50	40	33	60
B_{12} (µg)	0.01	trace	0.3	0.2	0.14	0.2	0.14	0.3	0.2	0.13	0.2
Biotin (µg)	0.76	0.4	1.4	1.7	1.0	2.0	1.5	1.3	1.5	1.0	2.0
Folic acid (µg)	5.2	0.18	13.0	11	3.4	8.0	4.9	11.0	11.0	3.3	8.0
Niacin (µg)	230	172	700	760	690	900	0.96	800	750	660	900
C ascorbic acid (mg)	3.8	4.3	8.0	8.2	6.9	9.0	8.6	9.0	8.0	6.6	9.0
SD cholecalciferol (µg)	0.01	0.01	1.0	1.4	1.0	1.1	0.9	1.0	1.4	1.0	1.1
ED-x-tocopherol (mg)	0.35	0.56	1.2	1.3	0.48	0.74	0.41	1.1	1.1	0.46	0.74
K phytomenadione (µg)	ND	1.7	4.0	5.1	2.7	6.7	4.1	3.8	5.0	2.6	6.7
Others											
Nucleotides	+	+	–	–	–	+	–	–	–	–	+

* total nitrogen × 6.38.
+ figures declared as disaccharide.
# liquid formulation – sodium 34, chloride 67.
^ method of Ziegler & Fomon (1971):[79] calculated values.

M, Milupa.

C&G, Cow & Gate Nutricia.

[a] DHSS Reports on Health and Social Subjects Nos 12(1977), 18(1980), 20(1983).
[b] Macy, Kelly and Sloan (1953) and Mettler (1976).
** manufacturer's information.
NS, not stated.
FHP, Farley Health Products.

Table 16.8 Nutrient content of follow-on baby milks available in the UK (per 100 ml)

Composition per 100 ml	Follow-on milks					
	Cow's milk	Step-up** (C&G)	Farley's Follow-on milk** (FHP)	SMA progress** (Wyeth)	Milupa Forward	HiPP Organic Follow-on milk
Macronutrients						
Protein* (g)	3.4	1.8	2.1	2.2	2.1	2.1
Casein (%)	77[a]	80	80	80	–	55
Whey (%)	23[a]	20	20	20	–	45
Fat (g)	3.9	3.4	3.1	3.0	3.3	3.5
Saturated (%)	63.2[a]	36	50	45	–	37
Unsaturated (%)	36.6[a]	64	50	55	–	63
Carbohydrate+ (g)						
Lactose	4.6	7.8	5.3	7.8	7.0	7.2
Maltodextrin	–	–	2.7	–		
Amylose	–	–	–	–		
Glucose	–	–	–	–		
Total	4.6	8.0	8.0	7.8	9.0	7.2
Energy						
kcal	67	70	68	67	74	69
kJ	280	290	285	281	311	285
Minerals (mg)						
Calcium	124	88	72	90	87	99.2
Chloride	98	55	68	62	71	68.8
Magnesium	12	7	7.8	8.0	9.0	10.3
Phosphorus	98	51	55	62	62	68.9
Potassium	155	87	91	107	127	133
Sodium	52	27	31	33	30	36.5
Trace elements (μg)						
Copper	20	50	41	60	70	20.5
Iodine	ND	11	11	12	12.4	10
Iron	50	1300	1200	1300	1200	1200
Manganese	ND	10	4.0	4.3	10	NS
Zinc	360	900	400	900	600	700
Potential renal solute load ^ (mosmol/l)	225	122	140	150	149	NS
Vitamins						
A retinol (μg)	40	65	80	75	62	72.9
B_1 thiamin (μg)	40	40	40	100	50	60
B_2 riboflavin (μg)	200	120	150	150	160	270
B_6 pyridoxine (μg)	40	40	40	60	50	30
B_{12} cyanocobalamin (μg)	0.3	0.16	0.15	0.2	0.2	0.3
Biotin (μg)	2.1	1.6	3.0	2.0	1.0	2.5
Folic acid (μg)	5	11	7.0	8.0	11	–
Niacin (μg)	80	830	650	900	1200	–
C ascorbic acid (mg)	1.5	8	10	14	9.0	8.6
SD cholecalciferol (μg)	0.02	1.9	1.1	1.5	1.0	0.9
ED-X-tocopherol (mg)	0.09	1.1	0.48	0.74	0.6	0.4
K phytomenadione (μg)	ND	5.0	2.7	6.7	3.1	1.0

* total nitrogen × 6.38.
+ figures declared as disaccharide.
# liquid formulation – sodium 34, chloride 67.
^ method of Ziegler & Fomon (1971):[79] calculated values.
M, Milupa.
C&G, Cow & Gate Nutricia.

[a] DHSS Reports on Health and Social Subjects Nos 12(1977), 18(1980), 20(1983).
[b] Macy, Kelly and Sloan (1953) and Mettler (1976).
** manufacturer's information.
NS, not stated.
FHP, Farley Health Products.

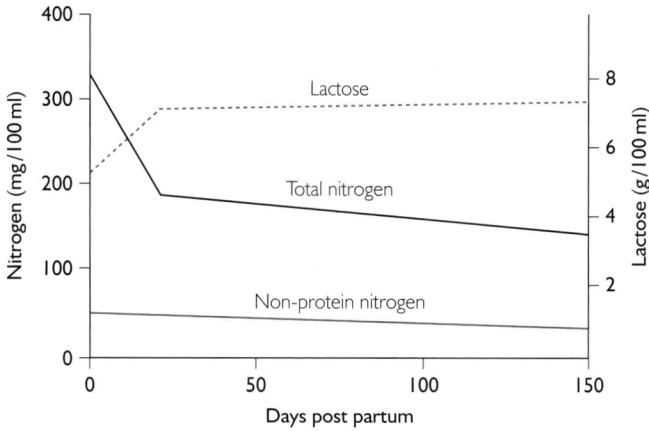

Fig. 16.3 Concentration of lactose, total nitrogen and non-protein nitrogen in human milk during the course of lactation. (After George & Lebenthal[23].)

Table 16.9 Fatty acid composition of mature human and cow's milk lipids (%, w/w)

Fatty acid	Human milk	Cow's milk
4:0	–	3.0
6:0	Trace	1.6
8:0	Trace	1.3
10:0	1.3	3.0
12:0	3.1	3.1
14:0	5.1	14.2
15:0	0.4	1.3
16:0	20.2	49.9
16:1	5.7	3.7
18:0	5.9	5.7
18:1	46.4	16.7
18:2	13.0	1.6
18:3	1.4	1.8

The fat concentration rises markedly during a feed, from around 2.1 g/100 ml to 4.1 g/100 ml.[49]

Cow's milk and human milk have similar fat contents and most of the lipid is triglyceride (98%); the principal difference is the pattern of fatty acids (Table 16.9). Human milk fatty acid profiles are, however, markedly influenced by diet. Vegetarians, for instance, consume more long-chain fatty acids than those on a mixed diet. Human milk has a higher proportion of unsaturated fatty acids than cow's milk and a greater concentration of the essential fatty acids. Unlike cow's milk, long-chain fatty acids in human milk are esterified to glycerol predominantly in the 1 position, which improves their absorption.

Breast milk lipids occur as globules ranging in size from 1 micron to 10 microns, emulsified in the aqueous phase of milk.[35] These globules consist of non-polar core lipids (such as triglycerides and cholesterol esters) covered with bipolar materials (including protein and phospholipids) which constitute the milk lipid globule membrane. The latter prevents the globules from coalescing and presents a large surface area for the action of lipolytic enzymes.

Carbohydrate

Lactose is present in higher concentrations in human milk (7 g/100 ml) than in cow's milk (4.7 g/100 ml). Lactose enhances calcium absorption from the gut, promotes the growth of lactobacilli, and may help to create a favourable gut flora that protects against gastroenteritis.

Minerals

All major minerals are present in higher concentrations in cow's milk than in human milk (see Table 16.7); with the higher protein content of cow's milk, they account for its high renal solute load. The amount of sodium in cow's milk is regarded as excessive for the human infant. However, early human milk has a high sodium content which may be 10 times that seen in mature milk. The raised phosphate/calcium ratio in cow's milk has been implicated in neonatal hypocalcaemia (see below).

Trace metals

The major trace metal concentrations in mature human and cow's milk are shown in Table 16.8. Zinc concentrations in mature human milk are rather less than those in cow's milk, whereas the reverse is the case for copper; cow's milk has a substantially greater magnesium content. Copper, iron and zinc are present in higher concentrations in human colostrum than in later milk. However, the comparison of levels of trace nutrients in different milks is of less relevance than the bioavailability of these elements. There is good bioavailability of iron and other minerals from human milk. In cow's milk, iron and zinc are less available, the latter being bound to high-molecular-weight fractions.

Vitamins

In the west, vitamin deficiencies are generally rare in fully breastfed infants when the mother is well nourished. Vitamins K and D, however, require special consideration.

Vitamin K

Levels are low in breast milk (0.4–2.8 micrograms/ml), though they are higher in colostrum (0.8–4.8 micrograms/ml). In contrast, non-supplemented formulas usually contain around 6–11 micrograms/ml and supplemented formulas up to 100 micrograms/ml. Parenteral prophylaxis at birth with 1 mg vitamin K is effective against vitamin K-deficiency bleeding (p. 372). There is still debate about a suitable oral regimen (p. 372).

Vitamin D

The need for vitamin D supplementation is controversial. In the human infant, cholecalciferol (vitamin D) is derived mainly from the skin, synthesised from 7-dehydrocholesterol under the influence of sunlight. Breast milk provides only about 10 IU of vitamin D daily in winter and 20 IU daily in the summer, and water-soluble vitamin D is present only in trace amounts that have negligible activity.[26] Healthy, exclusively breastfed infants have adequate bone mineralisation in the first 16 weeks of life[61] and maintain satisfactory serum levels of 25-hydroxycholecalciferol for at least 6 months,[7] suggesting that vitamin D supplements during this period are unnecessary. However, rickets has been reported in association with prolonged breastfeeding.[55] Over the past 2 years there have also been reports of an increase in the incidence of rickets in children of South East Asian origin living in the UK, particularly those living in the North. Although the Committee on Medical Aspects of Food Policy (COMA) recommended that all infants receive 280–340 IU of vitamin D daily, either in a multivitamin preparation or in infant formula, and that Asian children should continue vitamin D supplements until 5 years of age, this does not appear to happen in practice, and there have been calls for a renewed campaign to raise awareness.[66]

Multivitamins

It has been recommended that in the UK children receive daily vitamin A (200 mg), vitamin C (200 mg) and vitamin D (7 mg) as a combined preparation (available under the Welfare Food Scheme; five-drop dosage) from 6 months to 5 years.[17] However, many professionals give multivitamins from 1 month to babies receiving breast milk. This is also supported,[17] especially when there is doubt about the mother's dietary status.

Iron

The breastfed infant's requirement for supplemental iron is controversial. The low levels of iron in breast milk (compared with those in supplemented modern formulas) are very well absorbed (around 80%, compared with about 4–6% from fortified formulas). Nevertheless, a small proportion of breastfed infants have lower iron stores at 6 months, and a greater proportion appear deficient at 9 months or later, than those fed iron-supplemented formula.[22,32,62] The recent UK Government advice to exclusively breastfeed for 6 months may have an effect on iron status.

Iron-deficiency anaemia is common in infancy and childhood. Although often asymptomatic, iron deficiency may be associated with adverse effects on cognitive outcome, although it remains uncertain whether the poor development of iron-deficient infants is due to poor social background or iron deficiency or a combination of the two factors.[25] In the toddler age group, the prevalence of iron deficiency varies with socioeconomic background and ethnic group. The 1995 National Diet and Nutrition Survey[27] reported that 12% of 2-year-olds had a haemoglobin (Hb) concentration below 11.0 g/dl. A more recent survey, involving 1057 2-year-olds with Asian parents living in England, reported Hb <11.0 g/dl in 29% of Pakistani, 25% of Bangladeshi and 20% of Indian children.[41]

This is a major community health concern. In bottle-fed infants, continued use of iron- and vitamin C-fortified formulas during infancy is effective in preventing iron-deficiency anaemia,[72] but in babies receiving breast milk plus weaning foods beyond 6 months, good nutritional advice is required. Iron from iron-fortified cereals may not be well absorbed. Haem iron, preferably from red meat, is ideal, though often not consumed in sufficient quantities. Other meats and vitamin C will enhance iron absorption from a meal. However, if there is any doubt about the sufficiency of iron intake, it may be prudent to give supplemental iron drops;[13] careful instruction is required on the danger to the child and other siblings of accidental iron overdosage. Because iron stores are proportional to body mass at birth, babies who are small for gestational age may become iron-depleted well before 6 months.

Fluoride

Fluoride is not a nutrient, although epidemiological studies show its role in preventing dental caries. It has both systemic and topical actions. Systemically it acts on the teeth prior to eruption, being built into the structure of the enamel and making it resistant to decay. It also limits enamel demineralisation. Fluoride also acts topically by promoting remineralisation, possibly through antibacterial effects. The relative roles of systemic versus topical fluoride are still being debated. In areas where the water supply is fluoridated (fluoride ion >0.3 ppm), infants consuming reconstituted formulas will have adequate intake, but in breastfed babies intake will inevitably be low. The British Dental Association[18] and the American Academy of Pediatrics[1] have recommended that an intake of 0.25 mg of fluoride should be achieved from 2 weeks to 2 years of age (available as drops), but emphasise the dangers (fluorosis) of exceeding this dosage from all sources combined. When water becomes the principal part of the breastfed infant's fluid intake, supplementation is no longer required if the water supply is fluoridated.

Adequacy of breast milk as the sole diet for healthy term babies

Maternal breast milk production rises to a peak in the third and fourth months after delivery, providing a mean of around 750–850 ml/24 h (more in boys than girls). The majority of exclusively breastfed babies consume between 500 ml and 1200 ml per 24 h.[57] By the end of this period, at intakes of 150 ml/kg the infant would consume 1.5 g/kg/24 h of protein and 85–105 kcal/kg/24 h (according to which values for milk energy are accepted: see Lucas et al[48]). Beyond this age, protein and energy intakes per kilogram body weight will fall as the infant grows, and eventually, without the introduction of weaning foods, breast milk alone will no longer meet the infant's needs. The point at which this occurs is variable and difficult to define, even for populations. The recommended dietary allowance (RDA) for protein, usually set near 2 g/kg/24 h for infancy, has an in-built safety margin, and it is now recognised that the RDA for energy (e.g. 116 kcal/kg/24 h at 3 months) is unrealistically high compared with the much lower intakes of breastfed babies growing and developing normally.

The traditional approach to assessing the adequacy of the diet is to monitor growth and watch for centile crossing. However, healthy breastfed babies being fed in accordance with present-day practices do not grow according to the accepted international National Center for Health Statistics (NCHS) growth standard, which was based largely on formula-fed infants. Data from several countries[76] show a marked secular trend in growth performance with the recent resurgence of breastfeeding. Typically, in the first 3 months the breastfed baby gains weight and length at a relatively fast rate, so that the centiles are above the NCHS values. However, beyond 4 months there is a progressive deceleration of growth, a process which persists throughout infancy, despite the introduction of weaning foods. At least three studies have now reported that breastfed infants remain leaner during infancy and childhood, with a lower risk of obesity.[3,14,75] Whether these data should be treated as indicating that breast milk is an inadequate source of nutrition beyond 4 months (on average), or rather that new standards are required to accommodate the growth pattern of breastfed babies, is a matter of considerable debate. The latest British growth standards may go some way towards addressing this issue; the data covering the newborn period and infancy are based on a representative sample of infants including both breast and bottle feeders from the Cambridge area.[20] Indeed, data for the breastfed infants are now available as a separate growth chart.[11] The World Health organization (WHO) is currently developing growth charts from breastfed infants from five countries. These are expected to be available in 2005.

A systematic review on the optimal duration of exclusive breastfeeding (EBF) was commissioned recently by WHO, primarily to assess the effects on growth and health of EBF for 6 months versus 3–4 months, with mixed breastfeeding (with complementary foods) thereafter.[38] Sixteen studies meeting the specified inclusion criteria for the review were included; seven from developing counties and nine from developed countries. With the exception of two randomised trials conducted in Honduras, all studies were observational. The conclusions were as follows:

- Infants with EBF for 6 months show no evidence of weight or length deficits compared to those with EBF until 3–4 months, although larger sample sizes would be required to rule out small increases in the risk of undernutrition.

- Infants with suboptimal iron stores at birth who receive EBF for 6 months without iron supplementation may be at risk of inadequate iron stores during infancy. This is more likely to occur in a developing country.

- Infants with EBF until 6 months have a significantly reduced incidence of one or more episodes of gastrointestinal (GI) infection during the first year. This finding is based primarily on an observational analysis of data from a large randomised trial of a breastfeeding promotion intervention in Belarus.[37] Because of its healthcare system and clean water supply, Belarus is regarded as a 'developed' country in the context of infection risk. The incidence of GI infection during the first year was 7.4% (213/2862) in infants with EBF to 3–4 months, compared with 5.0% (31/621) in those with EBF to 6 months (odds ratio [OR] 0.61, 95% confidence interval [CI] 0.41–0.93). However, the difference in the proportion of infants hospitalised with GI infection did not differ significantly between groups (2.2% vs 1.8%, OR 0.75, 95% CI 0.38–1.04).

The authors of the review concluded that 'the available evidence demonstrates no apparent risks in recommending, as public health policy, EBF for the first 6 months of life in both developing and developed country settings.' Interestingly, a second systematic review on the same topic came to different conclusions. Lanigan et al[40] used different selection criteria, and included 33 studies in their review. They concluded that there is a lack of clear evidence to either support or refute the existing (i.e. 4–6 month) recommendation for the age of introduction of complementary foods to the breast milk- or formula-fed infant.

Both reviews commented on the generally poor standard of evidence available on which to base recommendations, and the Kramer review specifically called for large randomised trials 'to rule out small adverse effects on growth and to confirm the reported health benefits of EBF for 6 months'.

The UK Department of Health has recently altered the advice for England and Wales in line with WHO recommendations, and suggested that mothers should exclusively breastfeed for the first 6 months before introducing solids. More recently, the advice to delay the introduction of solids until 6 months has been extended to formula-fed infants. However, regardless of the deliberations of health professionals, breastfed babies themselves may play an important part in influencing the time of weaning.

Antibacterial aspects of human milk[24,45]

Grulee's studies in Chicago in the 1930s, based on a 9-month period of supervised follow-up of 20 061 babies, provided convincing evidence of the anti-infective advantages of breastfeeding in the pre-antibiotic era.[28] With overall improvements in public health and obstetric and paediatric care in western countries, these major differences in infection rates have diminished dramatically, though much less so in developing countries. In western society, an increased morbidity (but not mortality) due to infection in bottle-fed babies is supported by recent evidence,[34] even when account has been taken of class differences in feeding preferences, but the major clinical importance of the protective properties of breast milk relates to infants in the developing world.

It is now apparent that, as well as reducing infection risk during the period of breastfeeding, human milk has a protective effect against diarrhoea, respiratory tract infections and otitis media well beyond this period.[31]

Immunoglobulins

The principal immunoglobulin in milk, secretory IgA, is present in the highest concentrations in the first few days postpartum. There is little evidence that absorption of the relatively low concentrations of IgG in human milk occurs. Secretory IgA is relatively resistant to low pH and proteolytic enzymes, and can be recovered from the stools of breastfed infants. It is likely that its protective effects are confined to the gut and perhaps to the respiratory tract. A wide variety of antibodies against viruses and bacteria and their toxins have been described in human milk, but their actions within the gut are not fully understood.

Other antimicrobial factors

Although all complement components have been demonstrated in human milk, their relatively low concentration, and the observation that heating milk up to 56°C for 30 minutes does not decrease its bacteriostatic action against *E. coli*, has cast doubt on the anti-infective role of milk complement. Human milk is one of the richest sources of lysozyme, which is present in about

3000 times the concentration reported in cow's milk. In vitro, it acts with IgA to lyse *E. coli* and some salmonellae, but its role in vivo is not established.

The iron-binding protein lactoferrin may deprive gut organisms of free iron as a growth factor, and has been shown to be bacteriostatic and bacteriocidal in vitro, although its protective role in vivo is uncertain. Lactoferrin increases markedly in milk during lactation, and has received recent attention as a possible growth factor.

Other factors present in human milk, for example oligonucleotides and glycoconjugates, may act as receptors and divert pathogens or toxins away from binding to the infant's pharynx or gut. Breast milk also contains nucleotides, which may promote cell-mediated immunity (see pp. 994–6).

Nutritive aspects of antimicrobial factors

Previously it was believed that antimicrobial proteins, including IgA and lactoferrin, which comprise a significant proportion (30–40%) of milk protein, were not available for nutrition. Prentice et al[59] have challenged this view, suggesting that the great majority of these proteins are digested: by 6 weeks, only 1% of lactoferrin and 17% of secretory IgA is detected in the stools, and 95% of total dietary protein could be regarded as nutritionally available.

Effects on gut flora

Breastfeeding promotes the growth of harmless lactobacilli (bifidobacteria) in the infant's gut, compared to the higher numbers of *E. coli* in formula-fed infants; this has been partly attributed to the presence of a growth factor ('bifidus factor') in human milk. More recent work suggests that factors that influence postnatal colonisation of the gut are more complex; one group has observed that, whereas Nigerian breastfed infants showed the expected predominance of bifidobacteria in their gut, UK infants, whether breastfed or bottle-fed, had a predominance of *E. coli* and *Bacteroides* spp. in their gut flora.[67]

Cells in milk

Human milk is populated with macrophages, polymorphonuclear leukocytes, and T and B lymphocytes; it has been calculated that the breastfed infant ingests as many viable leukocytes each day as he has circulating at any one time. The B lymphocytes contain cell lines that have synthesised IgA in the breast, but whether these cells survive for long enough in the infant's gut to carry out any further useful biological role is unknown. There is evidence that T cells in milk may transfer tuberculin sensitivity from mother to infant,[64] presumably mediated through lymphokines, which might have been secreted before the infant ingested the milk. There is no evidence that T lymphocytes are transferred across the gut in humans or participate in 'graft versus host' disease. However, cells transferred from mother to infant may induce tolerance of maternal HLA status; previously breastfed infants who receive a renal allograft from their mother have less organ rejection.[19]

Table 16.10 Hormones reported in breast milk

Steroids	Prolactin
Thyroxine	Erythropoietin
Gonadotriophins	Melatonin
Luteinizing hormone-releasing hormone	Epidermal growth factor
Thyropin-releasing hormone	Prostaglandins
Thyroid-stimulating hormone	Calcitonin
Adrenocorticotrophic hormone	

Breast milk cells might protect against necrotising enterocolitis (NEC), though this is disputed. In a neonatal rat model, a disease resembling NEC, induced by hypoxia and an enteral challenge with *Klebsiella*, could be prevented by fresh breast milk.[58] Whatever the mechanism, NEC is less common in preterm infants fed breast milk than in those fed formula.[47]

Breast milk hormones

Possible 'messenger' substances in human milk

In recent years a wide variety of hormones and growth factors have been described in human milk.[63] A selection of these are listed in Table 16.10. In animals, such factors may be absorbed from the gut, and data from preterm human neonates suggest that epidermal growth factor crosses the gut wall into the circulation.[21] It is an important question whether or not the lactating mother, in addition to providing nutrients and anti-infective factors, might also exert some control over neonatal metabolism and development through the mediation of 'chemical messengers' and trophic factor secreted into her milk.

Enzymes in human milk[29]

The bile salt-stimulated lipase in human milk may play a significant part in intestinal lipolysis. Its presence may partly account for improved fat absorption from human milk compared with cow's milk, and for the observation that pasteurisation results in lower fat absorption from breast milk in preterm infants.[77] Bile salt-stimulated lipase also has esterase activity, which may assist the digestion of breast milk retinyl esters.

Several other enzymes have been described in human milk. Breast milk amylase is identical in structure to the salivary enzyme, and probably compensates for the relatively slow postnatal development of the latter. Several proteases are also present, including trypsin, elastase and plasmin. However, it is doubtful whether they play an important role in the neonatal period because of the high antiprotease activity of human milk.

Other factors in breast milk

Babies may consume from breast milk a variety of substances which have no physiological value to them. Maternal medications are discussed in Chapter 11. Addictive drugs cause increasing concern. Some evidence suggests a need for caution over the regular use of alcohol by breastfeeding mothers: Little et al[43] initially showed that one unit of alcohol or more each day for the first 3 months was associated with reduced motor development scores in the infant at 1 year. However, in a more recent study of 915 infants from the ALSPAC cohort, alcohol use during lactation was not associated with a deficit in motor skills at 18 months.[44]

Pesticide residues are officially monitored. Organohalogens such as dioxins and polychlorinated biphenyls (PCBs) in breast milk are of current concern. These lipophilic chemicals are excreted in breast milk in 10–50 times the concentration in cow's milk or formulas, frequently exceeding accepted safety limits for cow's milk.[4] They accumulate in fat over long periods, and some are highly toxic to skin, liver, and immune and nervous systems. They are also suspected carcinogens. Studies in infants to date have suggested that prenatal exposure to these substances may be associated with decreased psychomotor function, abnormal thyroid function tests (decreased T_3 and T_4 with elevated TSH), and effects on immune status. However, despite relatively high levels of PCBs in breast milk, reflected in a threefold level of plasma PCBs in children at 2.5 years of age compared with formula-fed infants, no significant negative effects on outcome have been found. Indeed, a recent study of Dutch infants followed up to 6 years of age suggested that breastfeeding itself counteracts the adverse developmental effects of dioxins and PCBs.[8]

Human immunodeficiency virus and other viruses in breast milk[46]

Human immunodeficiency virus (HIV) has been found in breast milk in HIV-positive mothers, and there is now good evidence that transmission to the breastfed baby occurs in 14–16% of cases (pp. 1073–4). Whether HIV-positive mothers or those at high risk should avoid breastfeeding has evoked heated debate; in developing countries, there may be no satisfactory alternative, and research is underway to determine strategies for minimising virus transmission by either reducing plasma viral load or preventing subclinical mastitis. However, in many countries, including the UK, it is recommended that such mothers do not breastfeed.

Both hepatitis B virus (HBV) and hepatitis C virus (HCV) may be found in the breast milk of seropositive mothers,[10,74] and transmission to the infant has been reported.[74] However, most evidence suggests that breast milk is an uncommon route of infection.[5,10,39,54] Mothers who wish to donate breast milk are now routinely screened for HBV, HCV and HIV, and excluded if positive.

Cytomegalovirus is found in the milk of between 32% and 96% of seropositive mothers when polymerase chain reaction is used,[30] and breastfed babies of seropositive mothers show a higher rate of seropositivity at 1 year of age (70%) than those who are bottle fed (30%).[53] This does not generally pose a problem for healthy term babies, but may do in those born preterm (see p. 1016).

Maternal aspects of breastfeeding

Advice and assistance

The practical management of breastfeeding is outlined on pages 378–9. The UK Baby Friendly Initiative, under the umbrella of UNICEF, was set up in 1994 and aims to increase the incidence and duration of breastfeeding. More information about the Baby Friendly Initiative, and aspects of breastfeeding the normal term baby, is given in Chapter 20.

Artificial feeding for the normal term infant

General considerations

The purpose of artificial feeding is to provide a satisfactory food for infants in situations where a substitute for breast milk is required. The 'ideal' artificial diet should:

- meet the nutrient needs of healthy infants;
- be well tolerated without inducing metabolic stress or biochemical disturbance;
- not result in short- or long-term morbidity.

Until recent years, the artificial milks failed to meet any of these criteria – sometimes with serious consequences. Modern formulas come much closer to attaining these goals (Table 16.8).

Recommended dietary allowances for formula-fed infants

From a teleological point of view, breast milk should be the nutritional standard for formula-fed infants. Many of the current RDAs are based on the concentrations of nutrients in human milk. However, in constructing a formula from non-human milk components, account must be taken of (a) the bioavailability, (b) the digestibility and (c) the biological value of the nutrients, all of which may differ from those in human milk.

Milk volume

Based on human lactational studies, fluid intakes of around 150 ml/kg/24 h are satisfactory for the first 3–4 months in formula-fed infants. However, this is only an approximate guideline: healthy infants fed on formula ad libitum (as with breastfed infants) will show considerable variations in intake in association with normal growth.

Artificial formula

Unmodified cow's milk

'Doorstep' milk should not be used for infants in the first 12 months.[13] Problems that may be encountered with cow's milk, or unmodified cow's milk formulas, include hyperosmolar dehydration associated with high renal solute load, hypocalcaemic fits associated with phosphate overload, casein curd obstruction, vitamin deficiency (e.g. rickets, scurvy) and iron-deficiency anaemia. These problems are rarely seen in infants fed modern formulas. Skimmed and semi-skimmed milk should not be used because of their low energy and vitamin A contents. Indeed, the DHSS[17] recommends that fully skimmed milk should not be given before the age of 5 years.

Goat's milk

Goat's milk is not suitable for infant feeding because of its high solute load and low vitamin content. It is particularly deficient in folate, and severe megaloblastic anaemia may result if goat's milk is the sole feed.

Modern cow's milk-based formulas

Modern milk formulas have been extensively modified from their predecessors in their protein, lipid, electrolyte and trace nutrient composition. Table 16.7 shows the composition of the standard infant formulas available in Britain, and Table 16.8 the composition of follow-on formulas. There is no information on whether or not the more recent finer degrees of modification have resulted in significant benefits, but it seems reasonable on empirical grounds to manufacture products resembling human milk as closely as possible. The need for further 'humanisation' of infant formulas is still actively under investigation. Topical issues include the possibility of lowering total protein content to, say, $1.2–1.4\,g/100\,ml$ (cf. $1.5\,g/100\,ml$ currently; Table 16.7); the addition of sources of very-long-chain lipids (C20 or greater) in view of their importance in the brain; and the addition of further factors found in human milk, including nucleotides (p. 292) and oligosaccharides.

Soya formulas

The problems encountered with earlier soya-based formulas have been largely overcome; formulas are now supplemented with methionine, taurine and carnitine, and contain adequate minerals to allow for losses due to phytate binding in the gut. They are able to support normal growth and bone mineralisation when used as the sole diet.[33,52] However, some issues remain unresolved. Soya beans have a high aluminium content, but it is not known whether this has any clinical relevance. More recently, attention has been drawn to the potentially large amounts of plant oestrogen (phytoestrogen) that may be ingested by infants who are fully fed on soya formulas: studies have shown that infants fed soya formula have plasma concentrations of phytoestrogens hundreds of times higher than those fed breast milk or cow's milk formula.[56,65] However, a follow-up study of adults who had received either soya formula or cow's milk formula in infancy found no evidence of long-term effects of early soya exposure on either general or reproductive health.[73]

Although many infants receive soya formulas because of suspected cow's milk allergy, it should be recognised that soya protein is itself potentially allergenic. Double-blind placebo-controlled challenges with soya milk in infants with proven allergy to cow's milk protein have suggested that around 5% of these infants are also intolerant of soya protein.[12]

Practical aspects of formula feeding

Detailed instructions for the reconstitution of artificial feeds and the hygienic use of feeding utensils can be obtained from manufacturers, but the following points need emphasising.

1. The safety of modern infant formulas is highly dependent on:
   - correct reconstitution of feeds, with accurate use of the scoops provided by manufacturers;
   - attention to sterility.

   A recent systematic review concluded that errors in the reconstitution of infant formulas are widespread, with a tendency to overconcentrate, although underconcentration also occurred. This review also highlighted the range of different scoop sizes produced by manufacturers.[60]

2. Infant formulas may be provided in 'ready to feed' liquid form (commonly used by hospitals for convenience, and now gaining popularity in the community) or as powder (less expensive and most commonly used by parents). When powdered milk is used, the water added deserves attention:
   - Water which has passed though a water softener will have an increased sodium content and should not be used.[17]
   - Although water should be boiled before addition to powder formulas, repeated or prolonged boiling may raise the sodium content in the water to an undesirable extent.[17]
   - Environmental contaminants, e.g. nitrates, lead, aluminium and agrochemicals,[17] continue to be a topic of public interest. High nitrate concentrations in the water supply have been associated with rare cases of methaemoglobinaemia (current recommended nitrate levels in water are $<50\,mg/l$).[17] Lead is still found in tap water in some pre-1976 houses with lead pipes. Soft water is particularly plumbosolvent. The 1993 WHO guidelines for the quality of drinking water recommended that the lead concentration of water used to make up formula feeds should not exceed 10 micrograms/l (48.3 nmol/l).[78]
   - The poor microbiological standards of drinking water that may be found in developing countries, among other factors, makes formula feeding highly undesirable in this situation.
   - It is the duty of the water authority to provide a safe water supply that fulfils international guidelines on chemical composition. Nevertheless, consumers have frequently wished to 'play safe'. Bottled water should be the same standard as water from the public supply, but some marketed waters are unsuitable for infants; for example, 'natural mineral water' may contain unacceptable levels of carbon dioxide, sodium, nitrate and fluoride.[17] Some water-filter manufacturers do not recommend their product for preparing water for babies, because silver may leach from the filter.

Breast versus bottle

The relevant question for the medical profession is whether or not there are clinical grounds for wishing to influence parental choice. In the developing world, the evidence that breastfeeding has a major influence on infant mortality and morbidity is well established and the case for medical intervention is strong. In the developed world, the situation is rather different: in spite of considerable speculation on the benefits of breastfeeding, it has been harder to prove major detrimental effects of bottle-feeding. Comparisons between breast- and bottle-fed infants are almost exclusively epidemiological, and as it is not possible to randomise infants to one feeding regimen or another, it is difficult to be certain that observed differences are not due to social class, social circumstances or other factors, rather than to the selection of diet per se. Such confounding has made it difficult to evaluate published data on the differences between breast- and bottle-fed babies in their subsequent health and development. It has been supposed by many authors that mother–infant interaction would be favourably affected by breastfeeding; however, in his review, Levy[42] argued that there was no evidence to suggest that breast- and bottle-fed infants differed in this respect, and concluded that bottle-feeding per se could not be held responsible for disturbance in the mother–infant relationship in infancy or later. Levy also pointed out that during the early months the infant is not capable of clearly deciding that the bottle is not part of the mother's body, and that if a bottle is offered with love, warmth and sensitivity, there is no evidence that the infant's chances of normal psychological development are impaired. A variety of emotional benefits to the mother have been put forward for breastfeeding, but these may cease to be benefits if the mother has set her mind against feeding her baby this way.

Evidence is accumulating to suggest breastfeeding has health benefits, both short and long term. More recently, data supporting the benefits of breastfeeding have been obtained from trials using a randomised, experimental design. The Promotion of Breastfeeding Intervention Trial (PROBIT),[36] a cluster-randomised study conducted in Belarus, involved more than 17 000 mother and term-infant pairs. Clinics were assigned either to standard practice or to an intervention modelled on the UNICEF Baby Friendly Initiative, designed to increase the incidence and exclusivity of breastfeeding. Although individual infants were not randomly assigned to diet, the intervention resulted in significantly higher breastfeeding rates and duration of EBF, and infants from this group had a significantly lower risk of developing both gastroenteritis and eczema during the first year of life. Further follow-up of this cohort is underway and should provide valuable data on the longer-term effects of breastfeeding.

Some of the most persuasive evidence for the benefits of breast milk has come from a large randomised trial of diet during the neonatal period in preterm infants. Those who received human milk, whether mother's own or banked, were significantly less likely to develop NEC or systemic infection, and showed better feed tolerance. More recently, longer-term benefits have become apparent. The use of human milk was associated with lower blood pressure,[68] reduced insulin resistance,[71] and a more favourable plasma lipid profile during adolescence.[69]

Epidemiological data have linked breastfeeding with a variety of benefits, including, in the short term, reduced gastroenteritis, otitis media and atopy (at least in infants with a positive family history). In the longer term, there is persuasive evidence that breastfeeding is associated with:

- Lower blood pressure.
- A more favourable plasma lipid profile.

- A lower risk of childhood obesity.[3,70,75]
- Improved cognitive development – meta-analyses of studies examining the effect of feeding on later cognitive development have suggested that, even after adjusting for appropriate confounding factors, breastfeeding is associated with significantly higher scores for cognitive development, and that the developmental benefits increase with the duration of breastfeeding. Differences are larger for low birthweight infants (mean advantage 5.18 points) than for normal birthweight infants (mean advantage 2.66 points).[2]
- Reduced risk of atopy, at least in infants with a positive family history.

The data presented suggest that there is sufficient evidence of clinical benefit to promote breastfeeding as the 'ideal' for term infants in developed countries. To help achieve this goal, better health education (starting at school) is required in order to promote a culture in which breastfeeding is regarded as the normal way to feed infants (see above).

References

1. American Academy of Pediatrics Committee on Nutrition 1986 In: Forbes G B (ed) AAP Pediatric nutrition handbook, pp 170–173
2. Anderson J W, Johnstone B M, Remley D T 1999 Breastfeeding and cognitive development: a meta-analysis. American Journal of Clinical Nutrition 70: 525–535
3. Armstrong J, Reilly J J; Child Information Team 2002 Breastfeeding and lowering the risk of childhood obesity. Lancet 359: 2003–2004
4. Astrup-Jensen A 1988 Environmental and occupational chemicals. In: Bennett P N (ed) Drugs and human lactation. Elsevier, Amsterdam, pp 551–573
5. Beasley R P, Stevens C E, Shiao I S, Meng H C 1975 Evidence against breastfeeding as a mechanism for vertical transmission of hepatitis B. Lancet 2: 740–741
6. Bernhart F W 1961 Correlation between growth-rate of the suckling of various species and the percentage of total calories from protein in the milk. Nature 191: 358–360
7. Birkbeck J A, Scott H F 1980 25-Hydroxycholecalciferol serum levels in breastfed infants. Archives of Disease in Childhood 55: 691–695
8. Boersma E R, Lanting C I 2000 Environmental exposure to polychlorinated biphenyls (PCBs) and dioxins. Consequences for longterm neurological and cognitive development of the child. Advances in Experimental Medicine and Biology 478: 271–287
9. Carlson S E 1985 Human milk non-protein nitrogen: occurrence and possible functions. Advances in Pediatrics 32: 43–70
10. Chaudary R K 1983 Perinatal transmission of hepatitis B virus. Canadian Medical Association Journal 128: 664–666
11. Cole T J, Paul A A, Whitehead R G 2002 Weight reference charts for British long-term breastfed infants. Acta Paediatrica 91: 1296–1300
12. Dean T P, Adler B R, Ruge F, Warner J O 1993 In vitro allergenicity of cow's milk substitutes. Clinical and Experimental Allergy 23: 205–210
13. Department of Health 1994 Weaning and the weaning diet. Report on Health and Social Subjects No. 45. HMSO, London
14. Dewey K G, Heinig M J, Nommsen L A, Peerson J M, Lonnerdal B 1991 Growth of breast-fed and formula-fed infants from 0–18 months: the DARLING study. Pediatrics 89: 1035–1041
15. DHSS 1977 The composition of mature human milk. Report on Health and Social Subjects No. 12. HMSO, London
16. DHSS 1980 Artificial feeds for the young infant: Report on Health and Social Subjects No. 18. Report of the Committee on Medical Aspects of Food Policy. HMSO, London
17. DHSS 1988 Present day practice in infant feeding, third report. Report on Health and Social Subjects No. 32. HMSO, London
18. Dowell T B, Joyston-Bechal S 1981 Fluoride supplements – age related dosage. British Dental Journal 150: 273–275
19. Flores H C, Cromwell J W, Leventhal J R, Najarian J S, Matas A J 1993 Does previous breast feeding affect maternal donor renal allograft outcome? A single-institution experience. Transplantation Proceedings 25: 212

20. Freeman J V, Cole T J, Chinn S, Jones P R M, White E M, Preece M A 1995 Cross-sectional stature and weight reference curves for the UK. Archives of Disease in Childhood 73: 17–24

21. Gale S M, Read L C, George-Nascimento C, Wallace J C, Ballard F J 1989 Is dietary epidermal growth factor absorbed by premature human infants. Biology of the Neonate 55: 104–110

22. Garry P, Owen G M, Hooper E M, Gilbert B A 1981 Iron absorption from human milk and formula with and without iron supplementation. Pediatric Research 15: 822–828

23. George D E, Lebenthal E 1981 Human breast milk in comparison with cow's milk. In: Lebenthal E (ed) Textbook of gastroenterology and nutrition in infancy. Raven Press, New York, pp 295–320

24. Goldman A S, Thorpe L W, Goldblum R M, Hanson L A 1986 Review article. Anti-inflammatory properties of human milk. Acta Paediatrica 75: 689–695

25. Grantham-McGregor S, Ani C 2001 A review of studies on the effect of iron deficiency on cognitive development in children. Journal of Nutrition 131: 649S–668S

26. Greer F R, Reeve L E, Chesney R W, DeLuca H F 1982 Water-soluble vitamin D in human milk: a myth. Pediatrics 69: 238

27. Gregory J, Collins D L, Davies P S W, Clark P L, Hughes J M 1995 National Diet and Nutrition Survey: children aged 1½–4½ years. Volume I: Report of the Diet and Nutrition Survey. HMSO, London

28. Grulee C G, Sanford H N, Herron P H 1935 Breast and artificial feeding. Journal of the American Medical Association 104: 1986–1988

29. Hamosh M 1996 Digestion in the newborn. Clinics in Perinatology 23: 191–210

30. Hamprecht K, Maschmann J, Vochem M, Dietz K, Speer C P, Jahn G 2001 Epidemiology of transmission of cytomegalovirus from mother to preterm infant by breastfeeding. Lancet 357: 513–518

31. Hanson L A 1998 Breastfeeding provides passive and likely long-lasting active immunity. Annals of Allergy, Asthma, and Immunology 81: 523–533

32. Haschke F, Vanura H, Male C et al 1993 Iron nutrition and growth of breast- and formula-fed infants during the first 9 months of life. Journal of Pediatric Gastroenterology and Nutrition 16: 151–156

33. Hillman L S 1990 Mineral and vitamin D adequacy in infants fed human milk or formula between 6 and 12 months of age. Journal of Pediatrics 117: S134–S142

34. Howie P W, Forsyth J S, Ogston S A, Clark A, Florey C D 1990 Protective effect of breast feeding against infection. British Medical Journal 300: 11–16

35. Jensen R G 1996 The lipids in human milk. Progress in Lipid Research 35: 53–92

36. Kramer M, Chalmers B, Hodnett E et al 2001 Promotion of breastfeeding intervention trial (PROBIT): a randomized trial in the Republic of Belarus. Journal of the American Medical Association 285: 413–420

37. Kramer M S, Guo T, Platt R W et al 2003 Infant growth and health outcomes associated with 3 compared with 6 mo of exclusive breastfeeding. American Journal of Clinical Nutrition 78: 291–295

38. Kramer M S, Kakuma R 2002 Optimal duration of exclusive breastfeeding (Cochrane Review). Cochrane Database of Systematic Reviews (1): CD003517

39. Kurauchi O, Furui T, Itakura A et al 1993 Studies on transmission of hepatitis C virus from mother-to-child in the perinatal period. Archives of Gynecology and Obstetrics 253: 121–126

40. Lanigan J A, Bishop J A, Kimber A C, Morgan J B 2001 Systematic review concerning the age of introduction of complementary foods to the healthy full-term infant. European Journal of Clinical Nutrition 55: 309–320

41. Lawson M S, Thomas M, Hardiman A 1998 Iron status of Asian children aged 2 years living in England. Archives of Disease in Childhood 78: 420–426

42. Levy R 1981 Mother-infant relations in the feeding situation. In: Lebenthal E (ed) Textbook of gastroenterology and nutrition in infancy. Raven Press, New York, pp 633–645

43. Little R E, Anderson K W, Ervin C H, Worthington-Roberts B, Clarren S K 1989 Maternal alcohol use during breast-feeding and infant mental and motor development at one year. New England Journal of Medicine 321: 425–430

44. Little R E, Northstone K, Golding J; ALSPAC Study Team 2002 Alcohol, breastfeeding and development at 18 months. Pediatrics 109: E72–2

45. Lucas A 1983 Human milk and infant feeding. In: Boyd R, Battaglia F C (eds) Perinatal medicine. Butterworths, London, pp 172–200

46. Lucas A 1988 Aids and human milk banking. In: Hudson C N, Sharp F (eds) Proceedings of 19th RCOG Study Group: Aids in obstetrics and gynaecology. Royal College of Obstetricians and Gynaecologists, London, pp 271–281

47. Lucas A, Cole T J 1990 Breast milk and neonatal necrotising enterocolitis. Lancet 336: 1519–1523

48. Lucas A, Ewing G, Roberts S B, Coward W A 1987 How much energy does the breast fed baby consume and expend? British Medical Journal 295: 75–77

49. Lucas A, Lucas P J, Baum J D 1980 The Nipple Shield Sampling System: a device for measuring the dietary intake of breast fed infants. Early Human Development 4: 365–372

50. Macy I G, Kelly H J, Sloan R E 1953 The composition of milks. National Academy of Science, National Research Council, Washington DC, Publication 254

51. Mettler A E 1976 Infant milk powder feeds compared on a common basis. Postgraduate Medical Journal 52(suppl 8): 3–20

52. Mimouni F, Campaigne B, Neylan M, Tsang R C 1993 Bone mineralisation in the first year of life in infants fed human milk, cow-milk formula or soy-based formula. Journal of Pediatrics 122: 348

53. Minamishima I, Ueda K, Minematsu T et al 1994 Role of breast milk in acquisition of cytomegalovirus infection. Microbiology and Immunology 38: 549–552

54. Moriya T, Sasaki F, Mizui M et al 1995 Transmission of hepatitis C virus from mothers to infants: its frequency and risk factors revisited. Biomedicine and Pharmacotherapy 49: 59–64

55. Mughal M Z, Salama H, Greenaway T et al 1999 Florid rickets associated with prolonged breast feeding without vitamin D supplementation. British Medical Journal 318: 39–40

56. Oehlschlager S, Fewtrell M, Barnes K, Damant A, Smith R, Hanley B 1999 Levels of the soya isoflavones genistein and daidzein in blood and urine of infants fed soya formula, cow's milk formula, and breast milk. Archives of Disease in Childhood 80(suppl 1): A23

57. Paul A A, Black A E, Evans J, Cole T J, Whitehead R G 1985 Breastmilk intake and growth in infants from two to ten months. Journal of Human Nutrition and Dietetics 1: 437–450

58. Pitt J, Barlow B, Heird W C 1977 Protection against experimental necrotizing enterocolitis by maternal milk. I. Role of milk leucocytes. Pediatric Research 11: 906–909

59. Prentice A, Ewing G, Roberts S B et al 1987 The nutrition role of breast-milk IgA and lactoferrin. Acta Paediatrica Scandinavica 76: 592–598

60. Renfrew M, Ansell P, Macleod K L 2003 Formula feed preparation: helping reduce the risks; a systematic review. Archives of Disease in Childhood 88: 855–858

61. Roberts C C, Chan G M, Follard D, Rayburn C, Jackson R 1981 Adequate bone mineralization in breast fed infants. Journal of Pediatrics 99: 192–196

62. Saarinen U M, Siimes M A 1979 Iron absorption from breast milk, cow's milk and iron supplemented formula. Pediatric Research 13: 143–147

63. Sack J 1980 Hormones in milk. In: Firer S, Eidelman A I (eds) Human milk, its biological and social value. Excerpta Medica, Amsterdam, pp 56–61

64. Schlesinger J J, Covelli H D 1977 Evidence for transmission of lymphocyte responses to tuberculin by breast-feeding. Lancet 2: 529–532

65. Setchell K D, Zimmer-Nechemias L, Cai J, Heubi J E 1997 Exposure of infants to phyto-oestrogens from soy-based infant formula. Lancet 350: 23–27

66. Shaw N J, Pal B R 2002 Vitamin D deficiency in UK Asian families: activating a new concern. Archives of Disease in Childhood 86: 147–149

67. Simhon A, Douglas J R, Drasar B S, Soothill J F 1982 Effect of feeding on infants' faecal flora. Archives of Disease in Childhood 57: 54–58

68. Singhal A, Cole T J, Lucas A 2001 Early nutrition in preterm infants and later blood pressure: two cohorts after randomised trials. Lancet 357: 413–419

69. Singhal A, Cole T, Fewtrell M, Lucas A 2004 Breast milk feeding and the lipoprotein profile in adolescents born preterm. Lancet 363: 1571–1578

70. Singhal A, Farooqi I S, O'Rahilly S, Cole T J, Fewtrell M, Lucas A 2002 Early nutrition and leptin concentrations in later life. American Journal of Clinical Nutrition 75: 993–999

71. Singhal A, Fewtrell M, Cole T J, Lucas A 2003 Low nutrient intake and early growth for later insulin resistance in adolescents born preterm. Lancet 361: 1089–1097

72. Stekel A 1984 Prevention of iron deficiency. In: Stekel A (ed) Iron nutrition in infancy and childhood. Raven Press, New York, pp 179–192

73. Strom B L, Schinnar R, Ziegler E E et al 2001 Exposure to soy-based formula in infancy and endocrinological and reproductive outcomes in young adulthood. Journal of the American Medical Association 286: 2402–2403

74. Uehara S, Abe Y, Saito T et al 1993 The incidence of vertical transmission of hepatitis C virus. Tohoku Journal of Experimental Medicine 171: 195–202

75. von Kries R, Koletzko B, Sauerwald T et al 1999 Breastfeeding and obesity: cross sectional study. British Medical Journal 319: 147–150

76. Whitehead R G, Paul A A, Cole T J 1989 Diet and the growth of healthy infants. Journal of Human Nutrition and Dietetics 2: 73–84

77. Williamson S, Finucane E, Elliott J, Gamsu H R 1978 Effect of heat treatment of human milk on absorption of nitrogen, fat, sodium, calcium and phosphorus by preterm infants. Archives of Disease in Childhood 53: 555–563

78. World Health Organization 1993 Guidelines for drinking-water quality. Vol 1. Recommendations. WHO, Geneva

79. Ziegler E E, Fomon S J 1971 Fluid intake, renal solute load and water balance in infancy. Journal of Pediatrics 78: 561–568

PART 3

Feeding low-birthweight infants

Alan Lucas, Mary Fewtrell

General considerations

The principal matters to be decided when planning enteral feeding in low-birthweight (LBW) infants are which diet, which route of administration and what feeding schedule should be selected. Valuable short-term studies have been performed on preterm infant feeding, but only recently have data become available on the longer-term effects of early nutrition for later health and development. Information of this nature is critical in order to assess the value of current practice.

Choice of diet

A wide range of diets have been used for feeding LBW infants, including the following:

- Human milk:
  - mother's own: 'preterm milk';
  - banked donor milk (expressed breast milk or drip breast milk);
  - fortified human milk;
  - human milk formulas (separated and reconstituted human milk).
- 'Term' infant formulas:
  - cow's milk based;
  - soya based.
- Special 'preterm' infant formulas.
- Parenteral feeding (Chapter 17):
  - partial;
  - total.

Human milk

There is now major interest in human milk for feeding LBW infants, and the practice of encouraging mothers to provide milk for their own preterm infants has become widespread. The value of breast milk in neonatal intensive care needs critical appraisal.

Nutritional considerations

Unmodified human milk may not always meet the theoretical requirements of LBW infants for several nutrients, including:

- protein (especially when 'mature' donor milk is used, p. 316);
- energy (especially donor 'drip breast milk', p. 316);
- sodium (pp. 284, 303);
- calcium, phosphorus and magnesium (pp. 284, 303);
- trace elements, e.g. iron, zinc and copper (pp. 284, 303);
- certain vitamins (e.g. B_2, B_6, folic acid, C, D, E and K, pp. 284, 304, 306–7).

However, human milk does have theoretical nutritional advantages compared with formulas, including the composition and easier absorption of its fats (p. 306), and the bioavailability of certain trace metals (p. 294). Formulas designed to meet the calculated nutrient needs of preterm infants result, inevitably, in a greater renal solute load imposed on the infant (p. 303) than that seen with human milk.

Infection and necrotising enterocolitis

Information on the protective advantages in the west of human milk used for feeding LBW infants is very scanty. However, in the developing world, where infection rates are high, the anti-infective role of human milk assumes much greater importance.[69]

In a large study, with formal dietary assignments, Lucas and Cole[47] showed that babies fed exclusively on formula had six times more confirmed necrotising enterocolitis (NEC) than infants fed exclusively on breast milk (fresh or pasteurised), and three times the NEC rate of those fed formula in conjunction with breast milk. The authors suggested that using either raw maternal milk or pasteurised donor milk in the early diet of preterm infants might prevent about 500 cases of NEC each year in the UK.

Allergy

There is a theoretical possibility that feeding the preterm infant with cow's milk proteins at a time when gut permeability may be increased[73] could raise the chance of later cow's milk allergy. Indeed, Lucas et al[56] showed that preterm neonates rapidly developed latent sensitisation to cow's milk. At the 18-month follow-up of a randomised trial of early nutrition, Lucas et al[46] found no overall difference in allergic reactions between infants fed formula or donor breast milk, but in the subgroup of infants with atopy in one or more first-degree relatives, early formula feeding was associated with twice the incidence of subsequent allergic reactions compared with those in the exclusively human milk-fed group (for eczema the respective incidences were 41% and 16%).

Gastrointestinal 'tolerance'

Gastrointestinal 'tolerance' of human milk is greater than that of formulas. Cavell[11] has shown that human milk passes through

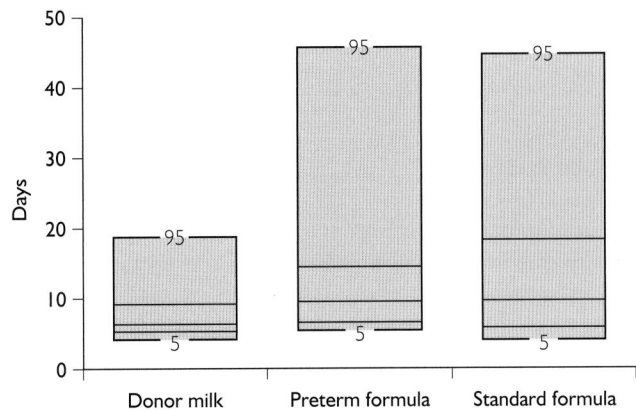

Fig. 16.4 Days to attain full enteral feeds according to diet in over 300 preterm infants under 1850 g birthweight. Data are represented in centiles; the horizontal lines in the data bar for each diet represent, from bottom to top, the 5th, 25th, 50th, 75th and 95th centiles for the number of postnatal days to reach an enteral intake of 150 mg/kg/24 h

the stomach faster than formula in preterm infants, and this observation is compatible with our own finding of increased vomiting and a higher residual intragastric volume in preterm infants fed either standard or special formulas. As a result, it may take substantially longer to establish full enteral feeding in infants fed formulas; in a five-centre study, 95% of infants fed breast milk were on full feeds by 18 days, whereas the 95th centile for formula-fed babies was more than 40 days, owing to a proportion of infants in whom it was difficult to achieve feed tolerance (Fig. 16.4).[52] These data have implications for the design of feeding regimens (see below).

Developmental scores

Preterm babies fed on their own mother's milk have been shown to have higher developmental scores at 18 months and higher IQs at 7.5–8 years than those fed on other diets, even after adjusting for a range of demographic, social and clinical factors that might confound this comparison.[61,66] Whether these findings reflect a failure to adjust for further (unknown) confounding factors, or whether fresh human milk has a beneficial effect on development, is an important question for investigation. The latter explanation is favoured by the observation that infants fed banked breast milk had higher developmental scores at 18 months than those fed term formulas, despite the lower macronutrient content of banked breast milk.[60]

Long-term cardiovascular health

A recent follow-up of adolescents born preterm and randomised to banked breast milk or preterm formula during the neonatal period has shown significantly lower blood pressure and a more favourable lipid profile in those who received human milk.[75,76] Children randomised to receive human milk had lower LDL-cholesterol to HDL-cholesterol ratios, lower apolipoprotein-B to apolipoprotein-A-1 ratios and lower CRP concentrations (a measure of the inflammatory process associated with atherosclerosis) than those who received preterm infant formula during the neonatal period.[76] There was a dose–response effect between each of these outcome measures and the proportion of human milk in the neonatal diet. Breast milk-fed children had an LDL/HDL cholesterol ratio that was 14% lower than formula-fed children, an effect size very similar to the 10–16% benefit in this ratio associated with breastfeeding reported in subjects born at term.[25,72] The 10% lowering of LDL-cholesterol observed with the use of human milk in this cohort would be estimated, in an adult population, to reduce the incidence of cardiovascular disease by 25% and mortality by 13–14%. A 10% lowering of LDL-cholesterol is also greater than that typically seen with dietary interventions in adults. Children who had received human milk also had significantly lower mean blood pressure than those who received preterm infant formula (81.9 [SD 7.8] mmHg vs 86.1 [6.5] mmHg).[75] The effect was seen whether fresh mother's milk or banked donor breast milk was used. Moreover, there was a dose-response effect – blood pressure at follow-up decreased as the proportion of human milk received during the neonatal period increased. The average effect size seen in this study is larger than that produced by any non-pharmacological method of reducing blood pressure during adult life (weight loss, exercise, diet). Moreover, this magnitude of reduction in blood pressure in an adult population would be expected to reduce the prevalence of hypertension by 17%, the risk of cardiovascular disease by 6%, and the risk of strokes and transient ischaemic attacks by 15%.

Interestingly, children who received human milk also had evidence of both lower insulin resistance[78] (Singhal, unpublished) and better arterial distensibility (an early marker of vascular disease) than children from the preterm formula group. These effects seemed to be mediated by growth predominantly during the first 2 weeks of postnatal life, and raise the hypothesis that promoting growth early in the neonatal period may not be optimal for certain aspects of longer-term cardiovascular health.

Types of breast milk

The composition of breast milk depends on its source, the mode of its collection and on the postnatal and postconceptional age of the donor; it can be further modified by its subsequent treatment.

Preterm milk

The milk of mothers who have delivered preterm infants – so-called preterm milk (PTM) – has a different composition from that of mothers delivered at term. PTM has a higher concentration of total nitrogen,[1] protein nitrogen, sodium, chloride, magnesium and iron,[44] copper and zinc,[3] with a raised IgA content in early lactation.[35] The reasons for these differences remain speculative but may relate to the low volume often produced by PTM donors.[53]

PTM is thus more suitable than term donor milk for feeding preterm infants, particularly in view of its higher concentration of protein. However, protein intakes from PTM are very variable, and by the second month of PTM production protein concentrations often fall to values at which theoretical needs would be met only by very high volume intakes. PTM may be given raw to the mother's own infant, in which case antimicrobial components will remain intact. Neither microbiological examination nor pasteurisation is necessary in this situation, provided that the collected milk is refrigerated adequately and fed to the infant within 48 hours, or at most 72 hours, or if it is frozen.

Many mothers who elect at the outset to provide milk for their own infants either totally or partially fail to do so. In over 600 mother's milk-fed infants from several centres studied between 1982 and 1985, maternal milk comprised less than 50% of total enteral intake. In a further study between 1988 and 1990, this figure had fallen below 40%. Factors contributing to lack of success in producing sufficient PTM include physical separation of mother and child, inadequate support, the inherent difficulty of maintaining the milk supply by manual or mechanical expression, lack of motivation, and – not least – poor advice. The difficulties faced by mothers trying to provide milk for their preterm infant must not be underestimated. They may need to express milk for a period of weeks in the absence of significant suckling stimulus and in the presence of a great deal of stress, a potent inhibitor of the milk ejection reflex. Despite the fact that an increasing proportion of mothers are now attempting to express breast milk, there has been relatively little research on ways to improve milk yield or composition. Simple measures have been shown to improve milk volume. These include increasing the frequency of expression.[15] Mothers need to be advised to express their milk at least as often as they would normally nurse a baby, that is, around six to eight times a day as a minimum. Other measures that may be effective include kangaroo care or skin-to-skin contact,[39] relaxation tapes,[26] and avoidance of smoking.[38] The type of breast pump and mode of expression may also be important. Jones et al[40] showed that the use of breast massage prior to pumping, and the use of simultaneous as opposed to sequential pumping both increased milk volumes in mothers using the Ameda electric breast pump, and that there was an additive effect of massage and simultaneous pumping. Recently, there has been some interest in the design of more physiological breast pumps – that is, using alternative strategies to simple suction which is inherently unphysiological in human lactation. A randomised trial comparing the use of a standard hospital electric breast pump with a novel manual pump designed to use compression stimuli as well as suction to extract milk found that the pumps showed similar efficacy in everyday clinical practice, and the manual pump received higher ratings for a number of consumer characteristics than did the electric pump.[28]

Expressed donor milk

Expressed donor milk can be foremilk or hindmilk, obtained either before or after the donor's own infant has fed from the breast; these two types of milk will have, respectively, lower or higher fat and energy contents than milk received by the breastfed infant. Mature donor milk will have a lower protein, sodium, zinc and copper content than that of milk produced in early lactation.

Drip breast milk

This is the milk that drips spontaneously from the contralateral breast during feeding in a proportion of lactating mothers – about 20% produce significant quantities. It can be collected during feeding into a presterilised glass or plastic shell worn over the contralateral nipple and areola. Drip breast milk has a similar composition to foremilk, with a low fat and energy content (often around 50 kcal/100 ml in pooled milk). Fat concentration and energy value correlate positively with the volume of drip breast milk obtained, and negatively with the postnatal stage of the donor. Pools of donor breast milk may have energy contents as low as 45 kcal/100 ml, compared with around 65 kcal/100 ml in mature expressed breast milk.[33,51]

Fortified human milk

One solution to overcome the nutrient deficits in human milk for the preterm infant is to add a milk fortifier containing protein, energy, macrominerals, trace minerals and a comprehensive range of vitamins. Several are now commercially available (Table 16.11), usually in the form of a powder which is added to a fixed volume of milk. However, the addition of nutrients to a complex biological medium such as milk poses theoretical problems. In particular, breast milk varies greatly in composition, and the addition of a fixed supplement may result in some infants exceeding the upper recommended limit for certain nutrients while others remain below desirable intake levels. Fortification may also influence nutrient availability or alter the biological properties of human milk.

A review for the Cochrane collaboration, last updated in 1999, concluded that the use of multinutrient fortifiers is associated with short-term improvements in weight gain, linear growth and head growth, but that there is currently no evidence of long-term benefit, and insufficient evidence to be reassured that there are no deleterious effects.[43] In a study of 275 infants randomised to receive either a breast-milk fortifier or control supplement containing only vitamins and phosphate, there was no significant difference in neurodevelopmental outcome at 18 months of age.[49] This study included infants who received preterm formula if insufficient breast milk was available. In the short term, the fortifier was well tolerated, and there was an increased growth rate in infants who received more than 50% of their intake as breast milk. However, the study also produced findings of potential concern: infants who received the fortifier had a significant increase in the incidence of infection (proven plus suspected), and a trend towards an increase in the incidence of NEC (a much larger study would be needed to detect such an effect as significant). It remains to be established whether overall outcome in infants fed fortified breast milk is better than that in infants fed a preterm formula when both diets provide similar nutrient intakes.

Table 16.11 Major nutrient composition of breast milk fortifiers available in the UK (amounts given are what would be added to 100 ml of human milk)

	Cow & Gate Nutriprem	Milupa Eoprotein	Mead Johnson Enfamil	SMA Breast Milk Fortifier
Energy				
kJ	44	65	58	64
kcal	10	15	14	15
Protein (g)	0.7	0.8	0.7	1.0
Carbohydrate (g)	2.0	3.0	2.73	2.4
Fat (g)	nil	0	0.05	0.16
Sodium (mg)	6.0	10	7.0	18
Potassium (mg)	4.0	8	45	27
Calcium (mg)	60	65	90	90
Phosphorus (mg)	40	45	45	45
Magnesium (mg)	6.0	6.0	1.0	3.0
Vitamin A (μg)	130	130	234	270
Vitamin D (μg)	5.0	5.0	6.5	7.6
Vitamin E (mg)	2.6	2.6	2.3	3.0
Vitamin K (μg)	6.3	6.3	9.1	11.0

(Manufacturers' data.)

Although further research is required, the concept of human milk fortification, of both mother's own and donor milk, is promising and offers the potential benefits of human milk (discussed above) while avoiding the problem of nutrient deficits. It is unlikely that further trials evaluating fortification versus no supplementation will be performed, and further research is likely to be directed towards comparing different fortifier preparations, evaluating both short- and long-term outcomes, and developing practical methods for dealing with the variability in nutrient content of expressed milk. At present, we would suggest that human milk should be fortified if the infant's weight gain is unsatisfactory.

Human milk formula

This involves the addition of human milk protein and fat preparations (together with additional minerals) to whole human milk.[55] Rohnholm et al[74] have demonstrated that breast milk fortification with human milk protein improves growth and prevents hypoproteinaemia. However, the manufacture of human milk formula requires a large supply of donor milk and is impractical for most neonatal units.

Human milk banking

Units wishing to set up a human milk bank should consult the DHSS report[20] on the collection and storage of human milk, and the more recent review by Balmer and Wharton.[4] It is important to appreciate that once milk has been collected, bacterially decontaminated, stored, frozen and thawed, pasteurised, exposed to light, aliquoted and instilled into feeding apparatus, it may have undergone qualitative alterations that render it significantly different from milk obtained by an infant during normal suckling.[32] Freezing, thawing and heat treatment damage antimicrobial factors in milk and denature milk lipase; milk cells seldom survive the banking process. Evans et al[24] showed that accurate pasteurisation for 30 minutes at 62.5°C destroyed 24% of the lysozyme, 57% of the lactoferrin, 34% of the IgG, but little IgA (though loss of biological activity of IgA was not assessed), whereas after treatment at 73°C (as might occur with inaccurate pasteurisation), only minimal quantities of these constituents remained intact. Heating milk may also reduce the vitamin C content. In addition, pasteurisation may reduce fat absorption, perhaps by damaging milk lipase. The optimal time and temperature required to destroy bacteria reliably and preserve antimicrobial properties is under investigation: Wills et al[81] suggest that short-time, low-temperature pasteurisation (56°C for 15 minutes) is effective, but milk should always be checked bacteriologically after pasteurisation and before banking, although it does not require further checks after thawing. Some workers have argued that banked milk could be given raw, but others are concerned about bacteriological safety,[6] since the milk may contain potential pathogens, such as β-haemolytic streptococci. Light exposure of breast milk results, within 3 hours, in a 50% reduction in riboflavin content and 70% loss of vitamin A.[5]

Screening of breast milk donors for human immunodeficiency virus (HIV), hepatitis B virus and hepatitis C virus is now advised. The risk of acquiring HIV from donor breast milk is unknown (see above), but there have been no reported cases of preterm infants infected in this way. Published evidence suggests that pasteurisation destroys HIV,[22] although some virologists continue to have doubts about this. Pasteurisers should be frequently calibrated to ensure their temperature-control settings remain in the effective range (60–66°C).

'Term' infant formulas

For many years, formulas designed for full-term infants were used to feed LBW infants. Such formulas (see Table 16.7) contain around 1.5 g of protein/100 ml and 65–70 kcal/100 ml. Fed at 180–200 ml/kg, they provide only 2.7–3.0 g of protein/kg/24 h – below the limit recommended by the International Consensus Committee (see Table 16.2). Sodium, calcium and phosphorus intakes, together with those of several trace nutrients, do not meet the calculated needs of LBW infants. Data from a large multicentre trial show that infants fed standard formulas grow more slowly in the short term than those fed 'preterm' formulas, and have substantially lower motor and mental development scores at 18 months and lower IQs at 7.5–8 years.[57,59] In our view, standard formulas have no place in the future management of preterm infants under 2 kg bodyweight, and preterm formulas should be used in their place. Soya formula should not be used for feeding LBW infants.

Special preterm infant formulas

In recent years, a variety of formulas have been designed to meet the theoretical nutrient needs of LBW infants (see Part 1). These formulas (see Table 16.12) vary significantly in their detailed composition, and continue to evolve.

The potential of preterm formulas for inducing 'metabolic strain' (e.g. renal solute and protein overload) is greater than with other available diets, particularly in very small and sick infants. However, clinical trials have shown that such formulas may carry a number of short-term advantages over unsupplemented human milk: they promote faster weight, length and head circumference gain (see below), reduce hospital stay, and reduce the incidence of hyponatraemia, bone disease of prematurity, hypophosphataemia, hyperbilirubinaemia and some vitamin deficiencies.[8,34,45] More importantly, at follow-up, infants previously fed preterm formulas are advantaged over those fed standard 'term' formula in linear growth,[45] developmental scores and IQ.[58,59]

Diets for preterm infants: overview

In summary, recent evidence suggests that human milk has an important place in neonatal intensive care. Many infants tolerate human milk better than formula, and enteral feeds can be established faster, reducing the requirement for parenteral nutrition (with its known hazards: see Chapter 17). The use of breast milk is likely to be associated with a reduction in the incidence of NEC and systemic infection, and it is associated with improved cognitive outcome, lower blood pressure and more favourable plasma lipid profile during childhood and adolescence. In addition, the slower initial growth rates seen in infants receiving human milk may be beneficial for later insulin resistance and arterial distensibility. However, in the preterm population, the risks and benefits of promoting growth must be balanced; poor early growth may have adverse consequences for short-term survival and for later cognitive development and bone health, whereas promoting growth (particularly during very early postnatal life) may be bad for later cardiovascular risk. On balance, in this group of infants current data support the promotion of growth, since the later cardiovascular outcome of infants who grow well is no worse than that of infants born at term.

Our recommendation is to use breast milk, preferably the mother's own, but donor milk if it is not available, to establish enteral feeds (up to 150 ml/kg) in infants of 28 weeks' gestation or less and in infants who have had prolonged intravenous feeding (when the gut may be atrophic) or prolonged respiratory disease. When mothers do not provide breast milk, preterm formula should be used as a sole diet from after birth in larger, well babies and after the establishment of human milk feeds in smaller or ill babies. If no breast milk is available, either maternal or banked, preterm formula should be cautiously introduced. Although term formula is sometimes used to establish enteral feeds in infants who appear not to tolerate preterm formula, there is no scientific evidence to support this; a large randomised study of diet in preterm infants found no difference in the amount of vomiting, the time to tolerate full enteral feeds, or the incidence of NEC between infants receiving term formula versus preterm formula as their sole diet (Lucas et al, unpublished data). If term formula *is* used in this situation, it should be replaced by preterm formula as soon as possible. Preterm formula may also be used as a supplement when mothers elect to provide their milk but do not have sufficient for the infant's requirements. Breast milk should be supplemented with phosphorus as a minimum to prevent metabolic bone disease. A multi-nutrient breast milk fortifier may be added if growth is unsatisfactory once the infant is tolerating full enteral feeds with breast milk.

However, preterm infants are not a homogeneous population, and with the survival of extremely low birthweight (ELBW) babies any single diet is now unlikely to be optimal from birth to discharge. For instance, from the calculations of Ziegler et al,[82] a baby of 800–1200 g requires 15% more protein than one between 1200 g and 1800 g. Furthermore, certain groups of babies appear more vulnerable than others to the effects of suboptimal nutrition. Lucas et al showed that small-for-gestational-age (SGA) preterm babies and males particularly were disadvantaged in terms of developmental scores in infancy if they were fed on mature pasteurised milk or standard term formula rather than a nutrient-enriched preterm formula.[58,59] Further work is required to explore how diets can be tailored to individual patients' needs.

Route of administration of feeds

Infants less than 34 weeks' gestation seldom have adequately developed reflexes to suck, so that feeding has to be intragastric, transpyloric or intravenous (Chapter 17). Short-term partial parenteral nutrition, accompanied by gradually increasing enteral feeding, often needs to be employed in immature infants.

Table 16.12 Nutrient content of low-birthweight formulas available in the UK (per 100 ml)

Composition per 100 ml	Mature human milk		Pre-Aptamil with Milupan~** (M)	Nutriprem 1 LBW** (C&G)	Osterprem (FHP)**	SMA LBW** (Wyeth)
	DHSS[a]	Macy et al[b]				
Macronutrients						
Protein* (g)	1.34	1.45	2.4	2.4	2.0	2.0
Fat (g)	4.2	3.8	4.4	4.4	4.6	4.4
Saturated (%)	50.1	52	79	43.4	42.3	49
Unsaturated (%)	48.5	48	21	56.6	57.7	51
LCP	+	+	+	+	+	+
Carbohydrate+ (g)						
Lactose	7.0	7.0	6.0	6.0	6.0	4.3
Maltodextrin	−	−		1.65	4.3	
Total	7.0	7.0	7.9	7.9	7.65	8.6
Energy						
kcal	70	68	80	80	80	82
kJ	293	285	335	335	335	343
Minerals (mg)						
Calcium	35	33	100	100	110	80
Chloride	43	43	48	48	60	60
Magnesium	2.8	4.0	10	10	5.0	8
Phosphorus	15	15	50	50	63	43
Potassium	60	55	80	80	72	85
Sodium	15	15	41	41	42	35
Trace elements (μg)						
Copper	39	40	80	80	96	83
Iodine	7	7	14	25	8	10
Iron	76	150	90	900	40	800
Manganese	ND	0.7	5.0	10	3.0	10
Zinc	295	530	700	700	880	800
Potential renal solute load ^ (mosmol/l)	88	91	148	148	134	129
Vitamins						
A retinol (μg)	60	53	108	227	100	90
B₁ thiamin (μg)	16	16	140	140	95	120
B₂ riboflavin (μg)	31	42.6	200	200	180	200
B₆ pyridoxine (μg)	6	11	120	120	100	72
B₁₂ cyanocobalamin (μg)	0.01	trace	0.2	0.2	0.2	0.3
Biotin (μg)	0.76	0.4	3.0	3.0	2.0	2.4
Folic acid (μg)	5.2	0.18	48	48	50	48
Niacin (μg)	230	172	300	3000	1000	1320
C ascorbic acid (mg)	3.8	4.3	16	16	28	11
SD cholecalciferol (μg)	0.01	0.01	2.4	5.0	2.4	1.5
ED-X-tocopherol (mg)	0.35	0.56	3.0	3.0	10	1.2
K phytomenadione (μg)	ND	1.7	6.6	6.6	7.0	8.0
Other (mg)						
Carnitine	ND	ND	2.0	2.0	1.0	2.6
Choline	ND	9	10	10	5.6	15
Inositol	ND	39	30	30	3.2	4.5
Taurine	4.8	ND	5.5	5.5	5.1	4.7

* total nitrogen × 6.38.
+ figures declared as disaccharide.
\# liquid formulation – sodium 34, chloride 67.
^ method of Ziegler & Fomon (1971):[83] calculated values.
~ Milupan is a lipid mixture containing LCPUFA.

[a] DHSS Reports on Health and Social Subjects.[18,19,21]
[b] Macy et al[63] and Mettler.[64]
** manufacturer's information.
NS, not stated.
LCPUFA, long chain polyunsaturated fatty acids: + added, − not added.

Intragastric feeding

Nasogastric or orogastric gavage feeding is the most commonly practised method of enteral feeding for preterm infants. An important pitfall to remember when giving human milk by tube is that significant loss of energy may occur from the adherence of fat to the feeding vessels.[7] This process may be accentuated by the change in physical characteristics of the fat induced by freezing for long periods. In addition, when a syringe pump is used to infuse human milk continuously the syringe should be positioned *below* the infant, otherwise the fat rises up the connecting tube towards the syringe and may never be received by the infant.

Transpyloric feeding

Transpyloric feeding (into the duodenum or jejunum) has been widely used in the past. There is no convincing evidence that it improves feed tolerance and growth, or reduces aspiration, and a meta-analysis of studies comparing transpyloric with intragastric feeds found that the mortality rate was 15% higher in the transpyloric group.[79] Thus, current evidence does not support the routine use of this method.

Feeding schedules

Large, well, preterm infants

It is neither possible nor desirable to adhere to rigid feeding policies for LBW infants: gastointestinal 'tolerance' of enteral feeding is very variable and concomitant illness may impose additional constraints, and therefore feeding must be managed on an individual basis.

The following guidelines are suggested for infants less than 1500 g birthweight. Feeding, by nasogastric tube if necessary, should start early to prevent hypoglycaemia, at about 2 hours of age. A commonly employed schedule for increasing feed volumes is to give, on the first four successive days, 60, 90, 120 and 150 ml/kg/24 h, and for infants on diets requiring greater feed volumes than this, to make further daily increments to 180 ml/kg/24 h by day 10, and 200 ml/kg/24 h by day 14. There are few data on the rate at which bolus feeds should be instilled down a tube: most units favour gravity feeding over 10–20 minutes, rather than by injection from a syringe.

Most infants weighing more than 1500 g will tolerate 3-hourly feeds; smaller infants will need to be fed every 1–2 hours. Initially, the nasogastric tube should be aspirated at least 4- to 6-hourly, just before a feed. If the volume of aspirate is small, e.g. up to 10% of the accumulated feed intake since the previous aspiration, it may be replaced without altering the feed schedule; if it is significantly more than this, it is advisable to reduce the feed intake accordingly, especially in infants showing increased abdominal girth. In infants who develop increasing abdominal distension, constipation or very loose stools, with or without blood in the stools, enteral feeds should be stopped temporarily and NEC

(pp. 694–703) considered. If feed volumes need to be reduced below the required total fluid for more than a few hours, an intravenous infusion must be considered.

Sick and very immature preterm infants

In infants who are sick or very immature it is both undesirable and often impossible to commence full enteral feeds after birth, and an intravenous infusion must be commenced. There are theoretical and clinical trial data to support the idea of using small, subnutritional quantities of enteral food in babies who will not tolerate full feeds (see pp. 282–3).[65] In extremely immature infants (<27 weeks), however, even minimal enteral feeds may not be tolerated initially. A recent Cochrane review[42] comparing early versus delayed initiation of enteral feeds for parenterally fed LBW infants concluded that there was a lack of evidence on which to base practice. The timing of introduction of enteral feeds in preterm infants with severe intrauterine growth retardation, particularly when accompanied by absent or reversed end-diastolic blood flow, remains particularly controversial. Such infants may be at greater risk of NEC if they are fed, but they may also benefit more from the effects of minimal enteral feeding, in terms of adapting to enteral feeds. At present the best approach may be to attempt minimal enteral feeding as soon as possible with human milk.

In newborn infants who are receiving either minimal or no enteral nutrition, the immediate aim of the intravenous infusion is to meet the infant's needs for water and electrolyte homoeostasis (pp. 335–54) and to prevent hypoglycaemia: the decision about when to add nutrients other than glucose to the infusion will depend on the patient's age, birthweight, the severity of his illness, and how well he tolerates enteral feeds. The consequences of early deprivation of nutrients have received inadequate attention, but the calculated nutritional reserves of an infant weighing 1000 g would last for only 4–5 days in the unfed state. It is important to attend to early intravenous intake in such babies (Chapter 17) while enteral feeds are being established.

A systematic review comparing rapid versus slow rate of advancement of enteral feeds for parenterally fed LBW infants[41] concluded that there was some evidence that more rapid rates were associated with a shorter time to regain birthweight and to achieve full feeds. However, the authors also concluded that there were insufficient data regarding the safety of rapid advancement of feeds, and a particular lack of data in ELBW infants. When enteral feeding is commenced in very immature or sick infants, it may be advisable to use either a continuous infusion pump suitable for accurately administering volumes to the nearest 0.5 ml/h or less, or slowly infused hourly boluses. Subsequent increments in feed frequency are a matter for clinical judgement, together with careful monitoring of enteral tolerance.

Recording the daily intakes of each diet received by the infant, as opposed to that prescribed, is important, as the two may be significantly different; if the desired intake cannot be achieved, consideration should be given to altering the type of feed or route of administration. The commonest cause of growth failure in preterm infants is poor nutrient intake. Protein intake is as important as energy intake, and the addition of energy alone to the diet will not promote satisfactory growth if protein intake is also deficient.

Psychosocial aspects

Practical involvement of parents in infant feeding during the period when suckling is not possible has considerable psychological benefits. Parents (under supervision) may be encouraged to measure out and give nasogastric tube feeds. Mothers who wish ultimately to breastfeed may start to put their infant to the breast from an early stage, even at 1000 g provided the infant is well. Randomised studies looking at the effects of non-nutritive sucking during the administration of tube-feeds have not shown consistent beneficial effects on growth or gastrointestinal function, although it may reduce hospital stay by up to 6 days.[79]

The difficulties encountered by mothers trying to express their own breast milk for their preterm infants are discussed on page 316.

Post-discharge nutrition[27]

Preterm infants frequently leave hospital severely growth retarded and fulfilling the criteria for 'failure to thrive', yet until recently little attention has been paid to their subsequent nutrition. In our cohort of 926 preterm infants, 77% were below the 10th centile for weight at the time of hospital discharge, and the percentages remaining below this centile at 9 months, 18 months and 7.5–8 years were 38%, 34% and 19%, respectively. The figures were even higher for those infants weighing less than 1000 g at birth: 98%, 69%, 58% and 26%, respectively.[67]

The small size of preterm infants at discharge is likely to be associated with deficits of a variety of nutrients, including calcium, phosphorus, iron, zinc and copper. A recent study of nutrient intakes in hospitalised preterm infants found cumulative energy and protein deficits of 406 kcal/kg and 14 g/kg at 1 week and 813 kcal/kg and 23 g/kg at 6 weeks of age in infants less than 31 weeks' gestation.[23] Such deficits would inevitably increase in infants fed term formula or unsupplemented breast milk after discharge.

Four main dietary options are available for use in preterm infants after hospital discharge:

- human milk;
- term infant formula;
- preterm infant formula;
- nutrient-enriched post-discharge formula (PDF).

Formula-feeding post discharge

A study of formula-fed preterm infants after discharge from hospital demonstrated that, when fed ad libitum, these infants frequently consume volumes far in excess of those usually recommended by paediatricians: 16% took more than 350 ml/kg/24 h, 50% consumed more than 165 kcal/kg/24 h, and 35% more than 4 g/kg/24 h of protein.[54] Cooke[13] studied 129 preterm infants randomised to receive preterm formula or term formula up to 6 months post term. Boys (but not girls) fed preterm formula after discharge showed significantly greater weight and length gain and larger head circumference by

6 months post term than those fed term formula throughout. At 18 months post term, boys previously fed preterm formula were, on average, 1 kg heavier, 1 cm longer and had 1 cm greater head circumference than those fed term formula.[12] Body composition measurements made using dual X-ray absorptiometry (DXA) suggested that the additional weight gain was composed predominantly of lean tissue rather than fat.[14] There were no significant differences in neurodevelopment measured using the Bayley Scales of Infant Development at 18 months.

The use of preterm formula after hospital discharge is associated with growth benefits, particularly in boys. However, infants fed on demand may consume high volumes of preterm formula, and this could result in potentially toxic intakes of certain nutrients such as vitamin D.[68] Such considerations, together with the desire to promote catch-up growth and replenishment of nutrient stores after discharge, led to the development of special 'post-discharge' formulas. These formulas were designed such that all nutrient levels are within the range set for a standard term formula, although towards the upper end of this range for a number of nutrients (Table 16.13). Compared with a term formula, PDFs have higher protein content to promote catch-up growth, accompanied by a modest increase in energy to allow utilisation of the additional protein, additional calcium and phosphorus to permit adequate bone mineralisation, and additional zinc, trace elements and vitamins to support the projected increase in growth rates.

A large randomised trial[50] involving 284 preterm infants randomised to either term formula or PDF for the first 9 months post term, found that, 9 months post term, PDF-fed infants were significantly heavier (mean difference 370 g) and longer (1.1 cm) than infants fed term formula, and the length difference persisted to 18 months post term. Differences between diet groups were significantly greater in boys, who had a length advantage of 1.5 cm at 18 months if they received PDF. There was no evidence the PDF had made infants fat; their mean weight centile was still below the 50th centile and skin-fold thicknesses were not increased. Head circumference and developmental outcome at 9 or 18 months did not differ significantly between groups.

Three other studies have compared term formula and PDF fed up to 12 months post term. Carver et al[10] reported that PDF-fed infants were significantly heavier at 1 and 2 months post term and longer at 3 months. There were particular benefits in infants with birthweights less than 1250 g and in boys; male infants with a birthweight <1250 g who were fed PDF were longer at 6 months, weighed more at 12 months, and had greater head circumference up to 12 months post term. Atkinson et al[2] found significantly greater weight in PDF-fed infants but no difference in length or head circumference. Finally, Brunton et al[9] compared term formula and PDF in 60 preterm infants with bronchopulmonary dysplasia. Those fed PDF had higher nitrogen, mineral and zinc retention and, by 3 months post term, attained significantly greater length, greater radial bone mineral content and greater lean mass than infants fed term formula.

Breastfeeding post discharge

Breast milk is strongly promoted as the optimum diet for preterm infants in hospital in view of its proven benefits. However, it is not

Table 16.13 Nutrient content of post-discharge formulas available in the UK (per 100 ml)

Composition per 100 ml	Post-discharge formulas	
	Nutriprem 2** (C&G)	**Farley's Premcare****
Macronutrients		
Protein* (g)	2.0	1.85
Casein (%)	40	40
Whey (%)	60	60
Fat (g)	4.1	3.96
LCP	+	+
Carbohydrate+ (g)		
Lactose	5.9	6.2
Total	7.4	7.24
Energy		
kcal	75	72
kJ	310	301
Minerals (mg)		
Calcium	94	70
Chloride	46	45
Magnesium	6.7	5.2
Phosphorus	50	35
Potassium	77	78
Sodium	26	22
Trace elements (µg)		
Copper	60	57
Iodine	20	4.5
Iron	1200	650
Manganese	10	5
Zinc	710	600
Potential renal solute load ^ (mosmol/l)	124	NS
Vitamins		
A retinol (µg)	99	100
B$_1$ thiamin (µg)	90	95
B$_2$ riboflavin (µg)	110	100
B$_6$ pyridoxine (µg)	80	80
B$_{12}$ cyanocobalamin (µg)	0.28	0.2
Biotin (µg)	3	1.1
Folic acid (µg)	20	25
Niacin (µg)	1.7	1000
C ascorbic acid (mg)	16	15
SD cholecalciferol (µg)	1.6	1.3
ED-X-tocopherol (mg)	1.9	1.5
K phytomenadione (µg)	5.9	6.0
Others		
Choline (mg)	32	
Inositol (mg)	29	
Taurine (mg)	4.9	
Osmolality (mOsmol/kg)	290	

* total nitrogen $\times$ 6.38.
+ figures declared as disaccharide.
# liquid formulation – sodium 34, chloride 67.
^ method of Ziegler & Fomon (1971):[83] calculated values.
** manufacturer's information.

clear whether unsupplemented breast milk meets the nutritional requirements of preterm infants after discharge. Whilst the number of mothers providing breast milk for their infant for at least part of the hospital stay has increased, the proportion of these mothers fully breastfeeding their infant after discharge is still relatively small – around 20% in a recent American study.[31] However, a greater proportion of infants receive some breast milk, along with an infant formula, for at least the first few weeks after discharge.

A number of studies have reported slower growth rates and lower bone mass in human milk-fed infants, at least in the short term. Lucas et al[50] studied 65 preterm infants who were breastfed (but allowed up to 2 oz of formula daily) for at least 6 weeks after discharge. Although similar in size to formula-fed infants at discharge, by 6 weeks post term breastfed infants were significantly lighter and shorter than formula-fed infants (on average 513 g lighter and 1.6 cm shorter than infants fed PDF). Deficits persisted up to 9 months post term, by which time all the breastfed infants were receiving term formula and solids. Collectively, these data suggest that preterm infants who are breastfed after discharge grow more slowly and have lower bone mass than formula-fed infants. Whether the differences persist or indeed have any consequences for later outcome is currently under investigation.

Introduction of solid foods

There are no published data to guide either the optimal timing of weaning or the nature of solid foods for preterm infants. The 1994 Department of Health (DOH) report recommended that 'a reasonable compromise may need to be adopted such that weaning can be advised when the infant weighs at least 5 kg, has lost the extrusion reflex and is able to eat from a spoon'.[16] However, the 5 kg guideline could mean that the most preterm infants growing below the 3rd centile could be 10 months old before they reach this weight, and well beyond sensitive periods for texture and taste.

The age of introduction of solids and the nature of the diet could have consequences in both the short and longer term. The introduction of solids is likely to result in a reduction in milk intake. If the quality of solid food is poor, this may result in a reduction in overall nutrient density that could compromise growth. In a recent observational study of weaning practices in preterm infants from three Surrey hospitals, solids were introduced at a mean chronological age of 17 weeks, and a mean post-term age of 11.5 weeks.[70] Twenty-one per cent of infants were weaned before the suggested DOH guideline of 5 kg. The same investigators randomised preterm infants to either current weaning practice, or to a 'new solid food strategy', which recommended the early onset of weaning (from 13 weeks chronological age) and the use of foods with a higher energy, protein, iron and zinc content. The intervention group achieved increased protein and energy intake and better iron status by 6 months post term, and had improved linear growth velocity at 12 months.[30]

On a more practical level, preterm infants are at risk of developing feeding difficulties that may have a significant impact on their post-discharge nutrition and growth. Infants who require prolonged respiratory support, have delayed introduction and establishment of oral feeds, or who develop chronic lung disease[63] are particularly vulnerable, and are more likely to have feeding problems, especially cough and vomit during feeds, throughout the first year of life.[37] Early intervention in such infants, before oral feeding is introduced, may help minimise the potential for aversion to oral feeding and maximise the development of oro-motor skills.

The term growth-retarded infant

Growth-retarded term infants are known to be at risk of continued growth failure[71,80] as well as learning and behavioural problems.[36] However, until recently, relatively little attention has been paid to the nutritional management of such infants.

de Rooy and Hawdon[17] studied metabolic adaptation in 65 SGA infants with birthweights below the 2nd centile over the first week of life, in relation to their mode of feeding. Exclusively breastfed infants showed a significantly greater production of ketone bodies, with no increase in the incidence of hypoglycaemia, suggesting better metabolic adaptation. Ketone body production was lowest in formula-fed infants and intermediate in partially breastfed infants. These data strongly support breastfeeding in healthy term SGA infants, although adequate maternal support is clearly required to achieve this.

Most data suggest that catch-up growth in SGA infants, if it occurs, is largely completed during the first 9 months of life. It is not clear at present why a minority of growth-retarded infants fail to catch up, and to what extent this reflects their genetic potential. However, the possibility that catch-up growth might be influenced by early nutrition warrants investigation as a potential mechanism for influencing long-term morbidity.

In a recent trial,[29] term SGA infants randomised to a nutrient-enriched PDF during the first 9 months showed increased gains in length and head circumference up to 18 months – 9 months beyond the period of nutritional intervention – compared with infants fed standard term formula. There were no significant differences between groups in developmental outcome at 18 months. A reference group of breastfed term SGA infants showed more gradual catch-up growth than the PDF-fed infants, but attained the same size by 18 months, and had higher developmental scores. These findings suggest that nutritional manipulation of growth patterns in term SGA infants is possible. However, more recently a six year follow-up of this cohort has shown higher blood pressure in those fed and the nutrient-enriched formula with no persisting benefits for size (Singhal, unpublished). Data have also emerged from a number of other studies suggesting that early growth acceleration (generally defined as upward centile crossing for weight) may have adverse consequences, increasing the risk of later insulin resistance and higher blood pressure. Thus, the short-term benefits of promoting catch-up in growth-restricted infants must be weighed against potential adverse consequences for later health, and decisions made on an individual basis. The balance of risks and benefits of promoting early growth is likely to vary depending on the environment (for example, developing versus developed world settings). Available data suggest that breastfeeding should be encouraged as the optimal source of nutrition for these infants, since it produces more gradual catch-up growth, with better developmental outcome.

References

1. Atkinson S A, Bryan M H, Anderson G H 1978 Human milk: difference in nitrogen concentration in milk from mothers of term and premature infants. Journal of Pediatrics 93: 67–69
2. Atkinson S A, Randall-Simpson J, Chang M, Bosco P 1999 Randomized trial of feeding nutrient-enriched vs standard formula to premature infants during the first year of life. Pediatric Research 45: 276A
3. Atmmo T, Omololu A 1982 Trace element content of breast milk of mothers of preterm infants in Nigeria. Early Human Development 6: 309–313
4. Balmer S E, Wharton B A 1992 Human milk banking at Sorrento Maternity Hospital, Birmingham. Archives of Disease in Childhood 67: 556–559
5. Bates C J, Lui D S, Fuller N J, Lucas A 1985 Susceptibility of riboflavin and vitamin A in breast milk to photodegradation, and its implications for the use of banked breast milk in infant feeding. Acta Paediatrica Scandinavica 74: 40–44
6. Baum J D 1979 Raw breast milk for babies in neonatal units. Lancet ii: 898
7. Brooke O G, Barley J 1978 Loss of energy during continuous infusions of breast milk. Archives of Disease in Childhood 53: 344–345
8. Brooke O G, Wood C, Barley J 1982 Energy balance, nitrogen balance and growth in preterm infants fed expressed breast milk, a premature infant formula and two low-solute adapted formulae. Archives of Disease in Childhood 57: 898–904
9. Brunton J A, Saigal S, Atkinson S A 1998 Growth and body composition in infants with bronchopulmonary dysplasia up to 3 months corrected age: randomized trial of a high-energy nutrient-enriched formula fed after hospital discharge. Journal of Pediatrics 133: 340–345
10. Carver J D, Wu P Y, Hall R T et al 2001 Growth of preterm infants fed nutrient-enriched or term formula after hospital discharge. Pediatrics 107: 683–689
11. Cavell B 1982 Reservoir and emptying function of the stomach of the premature infant. Acta Paediatrica Scandinavica Supplement 296: 60–61
12. Cooke R J, Embleton N D, Griffin I J, Wells J C, McCormick K P 2001 Feeding preterm infants after hospital discharge: growth and development at 18 months of age. Pediatric Research 49: 719–722
13. Cooke R J, Griffin I J, McCormick K et al 1998 Feeding preterm infants after hospital discharge: effect of dietary manipulation on nutrient intake and growth. Pediatric Research 43: 355–360
14. Cooke R J, McCormick K, Griffin I J et al 1999 Feeding preterm infants after hospital discharge: effect of diet on body composition. Pediatric Research 46: 461–464
15. de Carvalho M, Anderson D M, Giangreco A, Pittard W B 3rd 1985 Frequency of milk expression and milk production by mothers of non-nursing premature neonates. American Journal of Diseases of Children 139: 483–485
16. Department of Health 1994 Weaning and the weaning diet. Report on Health and Social Subjects No. 45. London, HMSO
17. de Rooy L, Hawdon J 2002 Nutritional factors that affect the postnatal metabolic adaptation of full-term small- and large-for-gestational-age infants. Pediatrics 109: E42
18. DHHS 1977 The composition of mature human milk. Report on Health and Social Subjects No. 12. HMSO, London
19. DHSS 1980 Artificial feeds for the young infant. Report on Health and Social Subjects No. 12. Report of the Committee on Medical Aspects of Food Policy. HMSO, London
20. DHSS 1981 The collection and storage of human milk. Report on Health and Social Subjects No. 22. HMSO, London
21. DHSS 1983 Present day practice in infant feeding. Report on Health and Social Subjects No. 20. HMSO, London
22. Eglin R-P, Wilkinson A R 1987 HIV infection and pasteurisation of breast milk. Lancet i: 1093
23. Embleton N, Pang N, Cooke R J 2001 Postnatal malnutrition and growth retardation: an inevitable problem in preterm infants? Pediatrics 107: 270–273
24. Evans T J, Ryley J C, Neale L M 1978 Effects of storage and heat on antimicrobial proteins in human milk. Archives of Disease in Childhood 53: 239–241
25. Fall C H D, Barker D J P, Osmond C, Winter P D, Clark P M S, Hales C N 1992 Relation of infant feeding to adult serum cholesterol concentration and death from ischaemic heart disease. British Medical Journal 304: 801–805
26. Feher S D, Berger L R, Johnson J D, Wilde J B 1989 Increasing breast milk production for premature infants with a relaxation/imagery audiotape. Pediatrics 83: 57–60
27. Fewtrell M S 2003 Growth and nutrition after discharge. Seminars in Perinatology 8: 169–176
28. Fewtrell M S, Lucas P, Collier S, Singhal A, Ahluwalia J S, Lucas A 2001 Randomized trial comparing the efficacy of a novel manual breast pump with a

standard electric breast pump in mothers who delivered preterm infants. Pediatrics 107: 1291–1297

29. Fewtrell M S, Morley R, Abbott R A et al 2001 Catch-up growth in small for gestational age term infants: a randomized trial. American Journal of Clinical Nutrition 74: 516–523

30. Foote K D, Marriott L D, Bishop J A, Kimber A C, Morgan J B 2001 Preterm infants post-discharge growth in length improves with a novel nutritional strategy. Early Human Development 63: 59–60

31. Furman L, Minich N M, Hack M 1998 Breastfeeding of very low birth weight infants. Journal of Human Lactation 14: 29–34

32. Garza C, Johnson C A, Nichols B L 1982 Effects of methods of collection and storage on nutrients in human milk. Early Human Development 6: 295–303

33. Gibbs J A H, Fisher C, Bhattacharya S, Goddard P, Baum J D 1978 Drip breast milk: its composition, collection and pasteurisation. Early Human Development 1: 227–245

34. Gross S J 1983 Growth and biochemical response of preterm infants fed human milk or modified infant formula. New England Journal of Medicine 308: 237–241

35. Gross S J, Buckley R H, Wakil S S, McAllister D C, David R J, Faix R G 1981 Elevated IgA concentration in milk produced by mothers delivered of preterm infants. Journal of Pediatrics 99: 389–393

36. Hadders-Algra M, Touwen B C L 1990 Body measurements, neurological and behavioural development in six-year-old children born preterm and/or small-for-gestational age. Early Human Development 22: 1–13

37. Hawdon J M, Beauregard N, Slattery J, Kennedy G 2000 Identification of neonates at risk of developing feeding problems in infancy. Developmental Medicine and Child Neurology 42: 235–239

38. Hopkinson J M, Schanler R J, Fraley J K, Garza C 1992 Milk production by mothers of premature infants: influence of cigarette smoking. Pediatrics 90: 934–938

39. Hurst N M, Valentine C J, Renfro L, Burns P, Ferlic L 1997 Skin-to-skin holding in the neonatal intensive care unit influences maternal milk volume. Journal of Perinatology 17: 213–217

40. Jones E, Dimmock P W, Spencer S A 2001 A randomised controlled trial to compare methods of milk expression after preterm delivery. Archives of Disease in Childhood. Fetal and Neonatal Edition 85: F91–F95

41. Kennedy K A, Tyson J E, Chamnanvanakij S 2000 Rapid versus slow rate of advancement of feedings for promoting growth and preventing necrotizing enterocolitis in parenterally fed low-birth-weight infants (Cochrane Review). Cochrane Database of Systematic Reviews (2): CD001241

42. Kennedy K A, Tyson J E, Chamnanvanakij S 2000 Early versus delayed initiation of progressive enteral feedings for parenterally fed low birth weight or preterm infants (Cochrane Review). Cochrane Database of Systematic Reviews (2): CD001970

43. Kuschel C A, Harding J E 2000 Multicomponent fortified human milk for promoting growth in preterm infants (Cochrane Review). Cochrane Database of Systematic Reviews (2): CD000343

44. Lemons J A, Moyle L, Hall D, Summons M 1982 Differences in the composition of preterm and term human milk during early lactation. Pediatric Research 16: 113–117

45. Lucas A, Brooke O G, Barker B A, Bishop N, Morley R 1989 High alkaline phosphatase activity and growth in preterm neonates. Archives of Disease in Childhood 64: 902–909

46. Lucas A, Brooke O G, Morley R, Cole T J, Bamford M F 1990 A randomised prospective study of early diet and later allergic or atopic disease. British Medical Journal 300: 837–840

47. Lucas A, Cole T J 1990 Breast milk and neonatal necrotising enterocolitis. Lancet 336: 1519–1523

48. Lucas A, Fewtrell M S, Davies P S W et al 1997 Breastfeeding and catch-up growth in infants born small for gestational age. Acta Paediatrica 86: 564–569

49. Lucas A, Fewtrell M S, Morley R et al 1996 Randomized outcome trial of human milk fortification in preterm infants. American Journal of Clinical Nutrition 64: 142–151

50. Lucas A, Fewtrell M S, Morley R et al 2001 Randomized trial of nutrient enriched formula versus standard formula for post-discharge preterm infants. Pediatrics 108: 703–711

51. Lucas A, Gibbs J A H, Baum J D 1978 The biology of drip breast milk. Early Human Development 2: 351–361

52. Lucas A, Gore S M, Cole T J et al 1984 Multicentre trial on feeding low birthweight infants: effect of diet on early growth. Archives of Disease in Childhood 59: 722–730

53. Lucas A, Hudson G 1984 Preterm milk as a source of protein for low birthweight infants. Archives of Disease in Childhood 59: 831–836

54. Lucas A, King F J, Bishop N J 1992 Postdischarge formula consumption in infants born preterm. Archives of Disease in Childhood 67: 691–692

55. Lucas A, Lucas P J, Chavin S L, Lyster R L J, Baum D 1980 Human milk formula. Early Human Development 4: 15–21

56. Lucas A, McLaughlan P, Coombs R R A 1984 Latent anaphylactic sensitisation of infants of low birthweight to cow's milk proteins. British Medical Journal 289: 1254–1256

57. Lucas A, Morley R, Cole T J 1998 Randomised trial of early diet in preterm babies and later intelligence quotient. British Medical Journal 317: 1481–1487

58. Lucas A, Morley R, Cole T J et al 1989 Early diet in preterm babies and developmental status in infancy. Archives of Disease in Childhood 64: 1570–1578

59. Lucas A, Morley R, Cole T J et al 1990 Early diet in preterm babies and developmental status at 18 months. Lancet 335: 1477–1481

60. Lucas A, Morley R, Cole T J, Gore S M 1994 A randomised multicentre study of human milk versus formula and later development in preterm infants. Archives of Disease in Childhood. Fetal and Neonatal Edition 70: F141–F146

61. Lucas A, Morley R, Cole T J, Lister G, Leeson-Payne C 1992 Breast milk and subsequent intelligence quotient in children born preterm. Lancet 339: 261–264

62. Macy I G, Kelly H J, Sloan H E 1983 The composition of milks. National Academy of Science, National Research Council, Publication 254, Washington DC

63. Martin M, Shaw N J 1997 Feeding problems in infants and young children with chronic lung disease. Journal of Human Nutrition and Dietetics 10: 271–275

64. Mettler A E 1976 Infant milk powder feeds compared on a common basis. Postgraduate Medical Journal 52(suppl. 8): 3–20

65. McClure R J, Newell S J 2000 Randomised controlled study of clinical outcome following trophic feeding. Archives of Disease in Childhood. Fetal and Neonatal Edition 82: F29–F33

66. Morley R, Cole T J, Lucas P J et al 1988 Mothers' choice to provide breast milk and developmental outcome. Archives of Disease in Childhood 63: 1382–1385

67. Morley R, Lucas A 2000 Randomized diet in the neonatal period and growth performance until 7.5–8 y of age in preterm children. American Journal of Clinical Nutrition 71: 822–828

68. Nako Y, Fukushima N, Tomomasa T, Nagashima K 1993 Hypervitaminosis D after prolonged feeding with a premature formula. Pediatrics 92: 862–863

69. Narayanan I, Prakash K, Gujral V V 1982 The value of human milk in the prevention of infection in the high risk low birthweight infant. Journal of Pediatrics 99: 496–498

70. Norris F J, Williams C M, Larkin M, Hampton S M, Morgan J B 2002 Factors affecting the introduction of complementary feeding in the preterm infant. European Journal of Clinical Nutrition 56: 448–454

71. Ounsted M K, Moar V A, Scott A 1984 Children of deviant birthweight at the age of seven years: health, handicap, size and developmental status. Early Human Development 9: 323–340

72. Plancoulaine S, Charles M A, Lafay L et al 2000 Infant-feeding patterns are related to blood cholesterol concentration in prepubertal children aged 5–11y: the Fleurbaix-Laventie Ville Sante study. European Journal of Clinical Nutrition 54: 114–119

73. Roberton D M, Paganelli R, Dinwiddie R, Levinski R J 1982 Milk antigen absorption in the neonate. Archives of Disease in Childhood 57: 369–372

74. Rohnholm K A R, Sipila I, Siimes M A 1982 Human milk protein supplementation for the prevention of hypoproteinaemia without metabolic imbalance in breast milk fed very low birthweight infants. Journal of Pediatrics 101: 243–247

75. Singhal A, Cole T J, Lucas A 2001 Early nutrition in preterm infants and later blood pressure: two cohorts after randomised trials. Lancet 357: 413–419

76. Singhal A, Cole T, Fewtrell M, Lucas A 2004 Breast milk feeding and the lipoprotein profile in adolescents born preterm. Lancet (In press)

77. Singhal A, Farooqi I S, O'Rahilly S, Cole T J, Fewtrell M, Lucas A 2002 Early nutrition and leptin concentrations in later life. American Journal of Clinical Nutrition 75: 993–999

78. Singhal A, Fewtrell M, Cole T J, Lucas A 2003 Low nutrient intake and early growth for later insulin resistance in adolescents born preterm. Lancet 361: 1089–1097

79. Steer P, Lucas A, Sinclair J C 1992 Feeding the low birth-weight infant. In: Sinclair J C, Bracken M B (eds) Effective care of the newborn infant. Oxford University Press, New York, pp 94–160

80. Walther F J 1988 Growth and development of term disproportionate small-for-gestational-age infants at the age of 7 years. Early Human Development 18: 1–11

81. Wills M E, Han V E M, Harris D A, Baum J D 1982 Short time low temperature pasteurisation of human milk. Early Human Development 7: 71–80

82. Ziegler E E, Biga R L, Fomon S J 1981 Nutritional requirements of the premature infant. In: Suskind R M (ed) Textbook of pediatric nutrition. Raven Press, New York, pp 29–39

83. Ziegler E E, Fomon S J 1971 Fluid intake, renal solute load and water balance in infancy. Journal of Pediatrics 78: 561–568

CHAPTER 17

Parenteral nutrition

Pamela Cairns

The fetus is nourished parenterally during pregnancy via the placenta. This is abruptly discontinued at birth and the vast majority of babies then make a successful transition to enteral feeding. Parenteral nutrition is indicated in the infant for whom feeding via the enteral route is impossible, inadequate or hazardous, because of malformation, disease or immaturity. It is used in infants with major anomalies such as intestinal atresia or omphalocoele, necrotising enterocolitis (NEC) or protracted diarrhoea. Babies with congenital anomalies of the gut will require parenteral support perioperatively until normal gut function has returned. In babies with NEC or a chylothorax, resting the gastrointestinal (GI) tract for a prolonged period may be curative. Parenteral nutrition is also used in extremely preterm babies prior to enteral feeding or to supplement milk feeds which can then be increased slowly while continuing to satisfy nutritional requirements. Some preterm infants have ineffective gut motility leading to feed intolerance. Sepsis and various commonly used drugs such as morphine may also adversely affect gut motility. Many very preterm babies require prolonged parenteral support.

As with any treatment, parenteral nutrition is only justified if the benefits outweigh the hazards (Table 17.1). As the safety of the technique depends on available resources and expertise, indications for parenteral nutrition necessarily vary between centres. Centres without facilities for intensive medical and nursing care and frequent biochemical monitoring using microtechniques must transfer babies requiring parenteral nutrition to appropriately equipped units.

Benefits

The long-term impact of inadequate nutrition during the neonatal period is now becoming clearer. The third trimester is a critical period for neuronal development. Work in the rodent model has demonstrated permanent impairment in dendritic arborisation and axonal myelination if early nutrition is inadequate.[41] Clinical trials of enteral nutrition in preterm human infants have suggested that nutrition during the same period may impact on long-term neurodevelopmental outcome.[80]

Randomised controlled trials (RCTs) have shown that infants on total[51,137] and supplemental[6,24] parenteral nutrition have significantly earlier and faster weight gain compared with those fed conventionally. Weight gain consistently at a rate above intrauterine growth rate can be achieved after 2 weeks of age for those born at 29 weeks' gestation.[47] It has been shown that total body water and extracellular fluid volume do not increase during parenteral nutrition but rather remain unchanged or decrease in spite of weight gain, thus supporting the hypothesis that the weight gain is due to tissue accretion rather than fluid retention.[33,102]

Apart from achieving nutritional adequacy and satisfactory postnatal growth, parenteral nutrition may also reduce the morbidity and mortality from specific diseases. Early introduction and excessive increases in oral feeding in preterm or sick infants increase the risk of aspiration pneumonia, cardiorespiratory disturbances and NEC. Parenteral nutrition, which allows the cautious and gradual establishment of oral feeding, is likely to minimise these risks in preterm or sick infants. A meta-analysis of the two RCTs of total parenteral nutrition (TPN)[52,137] showed that the incidence of NEC was significantly reduced with parenteral nutrition.[58] The increased use and earlier initiation of parenteral nutrition have been associated with better tolerance of enteral

Table 17.1 Risks associated with TPN

Metabolic
- Hyperglycaemia
- Hyperchloraemic acidosis
- Metabolic bone disease of prematurity
- Abnormal aminogram
- Hyperlipidaemia

Line-related (p. 330)
- Infection
- Atrial or superior venocaval thrombus
- Pleural effusions
- Pericardial tamponade
- Tissue necrosis from extravasation injury

General
- Cholestasis
- Gut mucosal atrophy

feeds and a shorter convalescent period in preterm infants requiring prolonged assisted ventilation.[86]

Composition of infusates

Fluids (fluid balance is also covered in Chapter 18)

The maturity of the infant, the type of incubator used, and the methods employed to curtail water loss will determine parenteral fluid requirements. Preterm infants adapt poorly to inadequate or excessive fluid intake compared with term infants. They have increased amounts of extracellular fluid, their kidneys have a poorer concentrating and diluting ability (pp. 932–4), they have a larger surface area in relation to weight, and their insensible water loss through the skin, especially in the first week, is significantly higher (p. 268). Increased fluid loss occurs when the infant is placed under radiant warmers or phototherapy.[15] Fluid requirements are decreased with the use of double-walled incubators,[135] heat shields or plastic blankets[11] and high ambient humidity.[54]

A review of the evidence for restricted versus liberal early fluid intake indicated that a restricted approach significantly reduced the risks of patent ductus arteriosus, NEC and death.[14] It would therefore seem sensible to carefully restrict the water intake to premature babies initially, while avoiding significant dehydration. If extremely preterm infants are nursed in maximally humidifed incubators, their fluid requirement should be no greater than that of more mature infants, that is, 60–80 ml/kg/day increasing to 100–120 ml/kg/day in the second week. On the other hand, if measures to reduce insensible water loss are not taken, fluid requirements for some extremely preterm infants could be in excess of 150 ml/kg/day. Serial assessment of hydration status is mandatory. The hydration status and fluid prescription should be reviewed no less than 12 hourly in the first week of life, assessing weight loss, urine output, and serum urea and electrolytes.

Energy

The estimation of energy requirement takes into account the components of total heat production (basal metabolic rate, physical activity, specific dynamic action of food, thermoregulatory heat production) and the energy cost of growth. In preterm infants, the basal metabolic rate is about 40 kcal/kg/day.[110] The energy cost of activity is 4 kcal/kg/day with minimal handling[110] and the specific dynamic action of parenteral nutrition is 13% of the basal heat production or 10% of the calories infused.[113] If an infant is nursed in a thermoneutral environment, an input of 50 kcal/kg/day is sufficient to match ongoing expenditure but it does not meet additional requirements of growth.[57]

Growth failure will result unless additional energy is provided. The energy cost of gaining 1 g of new tissue is 5 kcal.[110] To achieve the equivalent of third-trimester intrauterine weight gain of 14–15 g/kg/day, an additional 70 kcal/kg/day is required.

Parenterally fed infants, compared with those enterally fed, begin to grow at a lower energy intake because of smaller faecal energy losses and reduced energy expenditure. Nevertheless, the goal energy intake for a rapidly growing preterm infant is theoretically about 120 kcal/kg/day, or even higher in long-term ventilated infants with chronic lung disease (CLD), whose energy requirements are increased by 25–30%.[132]

Protein

The goal of supplying protein to the neonate is to achieve nitrogen retention at in-utero rates without causing metabolic disturbance. In sick preterm infants, it is inadvisable to attempt to meet their energy needs immediately after birth with intravenous glucose as the sole energy source.[43] Randomised clinical trials in sick, preterm infants showed that an intake of 1.5 g/kg/day of amino acids from the day of birth resulted in a nitrogen retention rate of 9 mmol/kg/day and improved protein synthesis.[111] In contrast, the control group had a negative nitrogen balance of about 10 mmol/kg/day, equivalent to a daily loss of 3% of the body's protein in the first 3 days after birth before amino acids were commenced. The energy intake should be at least 40–50 kcal/kg/day when amino acids are introduced, because with lower energy intakes, more of the infused amino acids are oxidised to meet endogenous energy needs and less remain for tissue synthesis. Energy from non-protein sources is essential for optimal nitrogen economy in parenteral nutrition. Zlotkin et al[140] found that when energy intakes of more that 70 kcal/kg/day were given to preterm infants, the major determinant of nitrogen retention was the protein intake. At least 25 non-protein calories are needed for each gram of protein added to the solution. Whether this non-protein energy is derived from glucose or fat makes no difference to the nitrogen-sparing effect (see below).

Parenteral protein requirements, as determined by a variety of methods, are in the range of 2.0–2.5 g/kg/day for term infants and 2.7–3.5 g/kg/day for preterm infants.[75] The intrauterine nitrogen accretion rate for a fetus is 24 mmol/kg/day at 24–36 weeks' gestation. The parenteral nitrogen required to achieve retention equal to the fetal accretion rate depends on a number of factors such as energy intake derived from glucose and fat, the quality of infused amino acids, vitamin and mineral co-factors, and the patient's clinical status. Crystalline amino acids in the form of L-stereoisomers are the preferred nitrogen source in parenteral nutrition as they have a high bioavailability, resulting in a nitrogen retention of over 70% of the amount infused.[29,60] A parenteral nitrogen intake of 32 mmol/kg/day (equivalent to 3.3 g/kg/day of amino acids) can result in duplication of intrauterine nitrogen accretion rates. RCTs have shown that a parenteral intake of 4 g/kg/day, as compared with 2–3 g/kg/day, resulted in higher nitrogen retention, net protein synthesis and weight gain.[37,140]

Preterm infants require not only more amino acids than term infants but also qualitatively different amino acids. Cysteine, taurine, tyrosine and histidine have been considered as conditionally essential amino acids in preterm infants.[73] Conversion of methionine to cysteine and taurine, and conversion of phenylalanine to tyrosine, are affected by enzyme immaturity. However, the addition of cysteine[81] and taurine[127] to parenteral nutrition solutions in preterm infants did not improve nitrogen retention or weight gain. Taurine is important in the conjugation of bile acids, although humans can also conjugate bile acids with glycine. Some investigators consider that the addition of taurine to TPN reduces the incidence of cholestasis.[59] Comparison of amino acid solutions based on the composition of egg protein and breast milk has shown that the latter results in a lower risk of high plasma phenylalanine levels but a higher risk of low tyrosine levels.[83,104] No adverse neurodevelopmental outcome has been observed after hyperphenylalaninaemia induced by parenteral nutrition.[77] If adequate non-protein energy is provided, the risk of hyperphenylalaninaemia is reduced (intravenous energy intake of greater than 34 kcal/g protein). Amino acid solutions designed for paediatric patients have been shown to result in a more favourable plasma aminogram, higher nitrogen retention and better weight gain in preterm infants.[61] Amino acid solutions have also been designed using the engineering technique of optimisation, in which the composition is derived from calculations based on a large body of plasma amino acid data from patients who have received a variety of parenteral amino acid solutions. Studies have shown that preterm infants tolerate these 'designer' amino acid solutions well.[65]

Babies who are considered to be unlikely to tolerate full enteral feeds within the first week of life should be commenced on amino acid solution as soon as is practical. The use of 'standard bags' allows parenteral nutrition to be started at times when technical help for sterile manufacture is unavailable. Parenteral nutrition should be started with 1–1.5 g/kg/day amino acids (using a paediatric or neonatal formulation). Adequate non-protein energy should be provided. If this is not tolerated due to fluid restriction or hyperglycaemia, then the quantity of amino acids should be reduced accordingly. The protein content of the infusion should be increased stepwise by 1 g/kg/day to a total of 3.5 g/kg/day. In the absence of renal disease, a metabolic acidosis or rising urea is unlikely to be due to the infant's intravenous protein intake, and other causes should be sought. An elevated urea in the absence of an elevated creatinine may reflect underhydration. If other causes have been excluded, the amino acid intake should be reduced to 2.5 g/kg/day.

Carbohydrate

The goal of carbohydrate provision for the neonate is to maintain euglycaemia and promote optimal growth and body composition.

The consensus interpretation of the neurophysiological and neurodevelopmental outcome data is currently that neonatal blood glucose concentration should be maintained above 2.6 mmol/l (p. 852).[70,79] Parenteral glucose can reduce endogenous protein catabolism of preterm infants by about 80%.[7] The risks of hyperglycaemia and glycosuria increase with decreasing gestation and birthweight.[76]

The rate of endogenous glucose metabolism in well, fasting neonates has been estimated to be 4–6 mg/kg/min.[36] Some premature infants will require more than this to maintain a satisfactory blood glucose. Glucose infusions should be commenced at 4 mg/kg/min (e.g. 10% dextrose at 60 ml/kg/day will provide an infusion rate of 4 mg/kg/min) and increased as required. If more

than 80 ml/kg/day of fluid intake is prescribed in extremely preterm infants below 1000 g birthweight, it is advisable to use 5% dextrose to avoid hyperglycaemia. If a concentration of more than 12.5% dextrose is required, this should be given centrally due to the risks of subcutaneous tissue infiltration. Since glucose tolerance improves with increasing postnatal age,[136] the glucose infusion rate can usually be progressively increased to 18–20 g/kg/day (12–14 mg/kg/min) in the second week after birth, if tolerated.

If hyperglycaemia (serum glucose of over 8 mmol/l with glycosuria) occurs, the baby should be carefully assessed. Hyperglycaemia occurring in a previously metabolically stable baby may be the first sign of infection. Immature infants may have limited tolerance of intravenous glucose even when infused at physiological rates. Hyperglycaemia during glucose infusion appears to be due primarily to persistent endogenous hepatic glucose production secondary to an insensitivity of hepatocytes to insulin.[34,101] Insulin can be infused in infants who remain hyperglycaemic at a glucose infusion rate of 8 g/kg/day (6 mg/kg/min),[92] commencing at 0.05 units/kg/h.[19] An RCT in infants of below 1000 g birthweight with glucose intolerance has shown that insulin therapy improves glucose intake and weight gain.[30]

Lipid

The goals of providing fat to neonates are to prevent fatty acid deficiency, facilitate provision of lipid-soluble vitamins and promote optimal growth and body composition.

Nitrogen-sparing effects of carbohydrate and fat are similar in parenterally fed infants, although lipid has the benefit of being calorie dense.[99,131] Abnormal plasma fatty acid patterns have been noted within 2–3 days of lipid-free alimentation, with a deficiency state in 10 days.[74] Essential fatty acid deficiency can be prevented by as little as 0.5 g/kg/day of Intralipid,[74] a fat emulsion derived from soybean oil containing 54% linoleic acid and 8% linolenic acid. Fat emulsions containing equal proportions of long- and medium-chain triglycerides (LCT/MCT) have been used in infants,[114] and one study showed greater nitrogen retention with LCT/MCT than with LCT emulsions.[128]

Lipid utilisation is limited and often unpredicatable in preterm and in small-for-gestational-age infants, due to deficient cellular uptake and utilisation of free fatty acids rather than to low lipoprotein lipase activity.[112] Although heparin releases endothelial-bound lipoprotein lipase and hepatic lipase in the circulation,[139] it does not improve fat clearance in infants.[124] Carnitine plays an important role in the oxidation of fatty acids by facilitating their transport across mitochondrial membranes. Preterm infants fed parenterally with carnitine-free solutions develop low blood and tissue carnitine concentrations because of their small carnitine depots and limited capacity for carnitine biosynthesis. Carnitine supplementation, however, does not improve growth or lipid tolerance and is not recommended.[27]

There have been a number of concerns over the early use of lipid; however, RCTs have established the benefits and safety of parenteral fat commenced on the day of birth.[26,45,122] One RCT reported significantly prolonged oxygen and ventilatory therapy in infants commenced on parenteral fat on day 3 compared with controls.[52] In subsequent studies, oxygenation and pulmonary haemodynamics in preterm infants with severe respiratory distress syndrome were not adversely affected when parenteral fat was infused at a dose of 1–4 g/kg/day[1,22,45] but deteriorated when the infusion rate exceeded an equivalent of 6–7 g/kg/day.[94] An association between parenteral fat administration and coagulase-negative staphylococcal bacteraemia in infants has been found[44] but there is no evidence that it impairs immune function in infants.[40,62,125,130] An increase in circulating free fatty acid levels can theoretically compete with bilirubin for binding to albumin. However, fat emulsion is also capable of binding unconjugated bilirubin[126] and infusions of 2–4 g/kg/day have been found to have no effect on total or unbound serum bilirubin.[23,124] At levels of free fatty acids, bilirubin and albumin usually occurring in this population, significant displacement does not occur.[2] A transient increase in blood glucose occurs with parenteral fat infusion, owing to altered glucose utilisation.[138] Currently available parenteral fat emulsions do not contain long-chain polyunsaturated fatty acids of the n-6 and n-3 family which might be important for neurodevelopment. Infants are incapable of synthesising these fatty acids and prolonged parenteral nutrition may result in a deficiency which is of potential importance. Free radicals generated when Intralipid undergoes peroxidation could be potentially damaging to preterm infants.[100] Phototherapy-induced formation of triglyceride hydroperoxides can be prevented by covering the Intralipid with aluminium foil, although this has largely fallen out of fashion.[89]

Lipid tolerance can be improved by using a continual infusion over 24 hours and by using 20% rather than 10% concentration. Two RCTs have shown that a continuous fat infusion regimen is better than an intermittent regimen, as reflected by less fluctuation in serum levels and a lower incidence of clinical and metabolic complications.[21,68] Compared with 10% Intralipid, 20% Intralipid has a lower phospholipid/triglyceride ratio and liposomal content, and RCTs have shown that the 20% emulsion results in lower plasma triglyceride, cholesterol and phospholipid concentrations.[55,56]

A 20% lipid emulsion should be started at 1 g/kg/24 h and increased daily by 1 g/kg to 3 g/kg/24 h as tolerated.[63] The lipid is run into the parenteral nutrition solution through a Y connection placed near to the baby. Plasma triglyceride levels should be monitored, as plasma turbidity assessed by visual inspection or nephelometry does not reliably predict serum concentration.[116] If the baby has poor growth but is tolerating lipids, the total dose can be increased to 3.5 g/kg/day. When triglyceride levels exceed 1.7 mmol/l, it is necessary to reduce or interrupt fat infusion until normal values are regained.[31] The lipid infusion should be reduced or interrupted for 24–48 hours during acute sepsis, because of reduced fat oxidation rate.[93]

Lipaemia may interfere with biochemical tests, leading to spurious conjugated hyperbilirubinaemia, hypercalcaemia and hyponatraemia. This is less of a problem with modern analysers but should be borne in mind in the interpretation of unexpected results.

Minerals and trace elements

Early hypernatraemia in preterm infants is caused mainly by their high insensible water loss (p. 268), while early hyponatraemia is caused mainly by arginine vasopressin release associated with periventricular haemorrhage, pneumothorax or hyaline membrane disease.[109] Late hyponatraemia in preterm infants is due to limited tubular sodium reabsorption.[3] No sodium should be added until postnatal natriuresis has occurred (pp. 336, 338). Thereafter, 3–5 mmol/kg/day is recommended, to prevent late hyponatraemia, and further increased if the infant is receiving furosemide (frusemide) for CLD or has significant ongoing renal losses. Although a potassium intake of 1–2 mmol/kg/day is required for the growing preterm infant, it should be withheld in the first 3 days after birth in those who are extremely preterm, because they are at risk of developing non-oliguric hyperkalaemia from immature distal tubular function.[25,50] Hypochloraemic alkalosis is prevented by a chloride intake of 2 mmol/kg/day. Chloride intakes in excess of 6 mmol/kg/day are inadvisable because of the risk of hyperchloraemic metabolic acidosis.[49] This can be explained by the physicochemical model. The electroneutrality of plasma is maintained by the charge buffers H^+ and OH^-. If the concentration of negatively charged chloride increases, then the concentration of positively charged hydrogen is increased to balance it. This results in a fall in pH. Hyperchloraemic acidosis can be avoided by replacing part of the sodium chloride load with sodium acetate.[91]

Parenteral administration of calcium at 1 mmol/kg/day from birth can reduce early neonatal hypocalcaemia in preterm infants.[115] Requirements calculated to match intrauterine accretion rates in a rapidly growing preterm infant are, however, higher than that used to maintain short-term homeostasis. Parenteral nutrition solutions should contain 1.3–1.5 mmol/100 ml of calcium and phosphorus (molar ratio of 1:1 or a ratio of 1.3:1 by weight) and 0.2–0.3 mmol/100 ml of magnesium, administered with a fluid intake of 120–150 ml/kg/day.[48] These recommendations are described per unit volume to prevent administration of high concentrations of calcium and phosphorus, resulting in precipitation of these minerals when fluid intake is restricted. Factors that affect solubility of calcium and phosphorus are discussed below (see 'Preparation'). High intakes of calcium and phosphorus should only be given through a central venous line.

Table 17.2 summarises the recommendations on parenteral minerals and trace elements for preterm infants based on guidelines published by the American Society for Clinical Nutrition.[48] If parenteral nutrition is supplemental or is limited to 4 weeks, only zinc needs to be added to the infusate. Other trace elements are required if TPN continues for over 1 month. The risk of zinc deficiency is increased with excessive GI fluid losses, as is the risk of copper deficiency when there are losses of copper-containing biliary secretion. Both copper and manganese supplementation should be withheld when cholestasis is present. Because selenium and chromium are excreted mainly through the kidneys, less should be given when renal function is impaired. Since destruction of erythrocytes postnatally provides the infant with 18 micromol/kg/day of iron, iron supplementation is unnecessary, especially if the infant is receiving repeated top-up blood transfusions. Molybdenum and fluoride supplements are recommended only with long-term (3–6 months) TPN. The aluminium content of parenteral nutrition infusates may be up to 1 micromol/dl as a result of aluminium contamination of the components used, such as calcium gluconate, which can contribute up to 80% of the total aluminium load. As it has been suggested that

Table 17.2 Recommendations for intravenous minerals and trace elements in preterm infants (amount per kilogram per day)

Sodium	3–5 mmol	(70–120 mg)
Chloride	3–5 mmol	(110–180 mg)
Potassium	1–2 mmol	(40–80 mg)
Calcium*	1.5–2.2 mmol	(60–90 mg)
Phosphorus*	1.5–2.2 mmol	(50–70 mg)
Magnesium	0.3–0.4 mmol	(7–10 mg)
Zinc	6–8 micromols	(400–500 micrograms)
Copper	0.3–0.6 micromols	(20–40 micrograms)
Selenium	13–25 nmol	(1–2 micrograms)
Manganese	18–180 nmol	(1–10 micrograms)
Iodine	8 nmol	(1 microgram)
Chromium	4–8 nmol	(0.2–0.4 micrograms)
Molybdenum	2–10 nmol	(0.2–1 micrograms)

*Based on a 120–150 ml/kg/day fluid intake of a solution which contains 1.3–1.5 mmol/dl of calcium and phosphorus (molar ratio 1:1) equivalent to 50–60 mg/dl of calcium and 40–45 mg/dl of phosphorus (weight ratio 1.3:1).

Table 17.3 Composition of Multivitamin Infusion Paediatric (amount per 5 ml vial)

Vitamin A	0.7 mg
Vitamin D	10 micrograms
Vitamin E	7 mg
Vitamin K	0.2 mg
Vitamin C	80 mg
Vitamin B$_1$	1.2 mg
Vitamin B$_2$	1.4 mg
Vitamin B$_6$	1 mg
Nicotinamide	17 mg
Panthenol	5 mg
Biotin	20 micrograms
Folic acid	140 micrograms
Vitamin B$_{12}$	1 microgram

this will adversely affect neurodevelopment, aluminium contamination should be reduced as far as possible.[20,85]

Vitamins

The ideal parenteral vitamin preparation for use in infants is not yet available. One multivitamin infusion (M. V. I. Paediatric) is designed for paediatric use (Table 17.3). Term infants on this daily dose maintain serum vitamin levels within acceptable ranges.[84] Preterm infants should be given 40% of the standard dose (2 ml) per kilogram bodyweight, with a maximum not to exceed the term infant's dose of 5 ml, even though this dose results in low serum levels of vitamin A.[46] About 80% of vitamin A and 30% of vitamins D and E are lost during administration owing to adherence to tubing and photodegradation, especially during phototherapy.[46,120] By adding the vitamin preparation into the fat emulsion instead of the amino acid–glucose mixture, vitamin losses can be reduced and the risk of deficiency minimised.[9,35]

Techniques

All preparations should be carried out under strict aseptic conditions using a laminar flow hood and terminal filtration with a 0.22-micron filter prior to delivery to the ward.

The solubility of calcium and phosphorus depends on other components within the infusate and the order in which they are mixed. Because of the low solubility product of these minerals, the one-bag system (amino acid, glucose and fat mixed into a single bag) is unable to deliver adequate amounts to prevent osteopenia and rickets in extremely preterm infants. The higher amino acid concentrations recommended for use in preterm infants do help to enhance their solubility by decreasing the pH of the solution. Phosphorus should be added before calcium to avoid the high concentrations of phosphorus causing immediate precipitation with calcium. Precipitation with phosphates is more likely with calcium chloride than with the gluconate salt. Glycerophosphates may allow greater delivery of calcium and phosphorus because they are stable in solution and have equivalent retention rates to standard salts.[53,107]

Administration

An infusion pump is required to maintain a constant rate of delivering the parenteral nutrition solution. A 0.22-micron bacterial filter is commonly used if terminal filtration is not carried out in the pharmacy. Distal to the filter, a second infusion pump delivers the fat emulsion close to the intravascular catheter. It is important to minimise mixing of the fat emulsion with calcium and heparin as this increases the risks of formation of calcium–phosphorus crystals and flocculation of Intralipid due to the destabilising effect of divalent cations.[108] Peripheral veins can be repeatedly cannulated using short 22- or 24-gauge catheters. When central venous catheters are used, the distal tip of the catheter is placed in the superior or inferior vena cava outside the right atrium (pp. 1249–52). Percutaneous central venous catheterisation[28,87,88] is preferred over the surgical cutdown approach,[118] although the Broviac catheter, which requires a cutdown, has also been used successfully, even in infants below 1000 g birthweight.[90,133] The addition of heparin (1 unit/ml) to the infusate further reduces significantly the incidence of phlebitis and thrombosis of both peripheral[5] and central venous catheters.[10] However, concern remains about the effect of heparin on the stability of calcium and lipid, as the addition of heparin to the amino acid mixture risks flocculation of lipid occurring at the Y site where the solutions mix. Many pharmacies therefore prefer not to add heparin to parenteral nutrition. Infusion of lipid emulsions is known to prolong survival times of peripheral venous lines.[97,98] Parenteral nutrition has been administered routinely

Table 17.4 Monitoring during parenteral nutrition

- Daily bodyweight and weekly body length and head circumference
- Initially during grading up of parenteral nutrients or during periods of metabolic instability:
  - Strict fluid balance
  - 6- to 12-hourly urine/blood glucose
  - Daily plasma sodium, potassium, calcium, urea and acid–base
  - Twice-weekly triglycerides
- When on full parenteral nutrition and during metabolic steady state:
  - Strict fluid balance
  - 12- to 24-hourly urine/blood glucose
  - Once/twice-weekly plasma sodium, potassium, calcium, urea and acid–base
- Plasma magnesium, phosphorus, alkaline phosphatase, albumin, transaminases, triglycerides and bilirubin (total and conjugated) weekly
- Plasma amino acids and ammonia not usually routinely monitored
- Trace elements should be monitored monthly
- Screening for infection or coagulation defects as indicated

Table 17.5 Precautions taken to minimise the risk of sepsis

- Preparation of individual aliquots of parenteral nutrition solutions in the pharmacy
- Manipulations carried out in the ward to be avoided
- Silastic catheters instead of polyethylene/polyvinyl catheters to be used
- Central venous catheters must be placed under strict aseptic conditions
- Skin exit site for catheter placed in area which can be meticulously cleansed
- Proper care of the site and all the connectors and tubings essential
- The TPN line should not be broken for the administration of drugs

through umbilical arterial catheters in infants who require arterial access for blood gas and blood pressure monitoring in the first 2 weeks after birth. This has been found to be comparable to central venous catheters in efficacy and safety.[67] The umbilical venous catheter has also been compared favourably with the use of peripheral veins in delivering parenteral nutrition.[95]

The importance of careful monitoring of the baby receiving TPN cannot be overemphasised (Table 17.4).

Hazards

Infections and technical complications

Infants on parenteral nutrition have an increased risk of bacterial sepsis caused by *Staphylococcus epidermidis* or *S. aureus*[13] and fungal sepsis caused by *Candida*.[134] The prevalence of catheter-related sepsis in infants ranges from 8% to 45%, with staff training playing a key role in its prevention.[105] The risk of polymicrobial bacteraemia is increased by manipulations of the parenteral infusate at the bedside.[42,66] Precautions which should be taken to minimise the risk of sepsis are listed in Table 17.5.

Uncommon but serious complications of central venous catheterisation include superior or inferior vena cava obstruction, cardiac arrhythmia or tamponade, intracardiac thrombi, pleural effusion or chylothorax, pulmonary embolism, Budd–Chiari syndrome, and hydrocephalus secondary to jugular venous thrombosis. The success or failure of parenteral nutrition is obviously a function of careful technique. While many of these technical problems can be avoided with peripheral vein infusion, this has

the risks of excessive handling of the infant, diminished delivery of nutrition due to 'down time', localised necrosis tissue ulceration and subcutaneous calcium depositions.

Metabolic complications

The risks of abnormal plasma aminograms, hyperammonaemia, hyperchloraemic metabolic acidosis, metabolic bone disease and trace element deficiencies are minimised with the careful choice of amino acid solutions and appropriate additives to the infusate. Cholestatic jaundice occurs in 10–40% of infants on parenteral nutrition; it is very uncommon in those who receive it for less than 2 weeks, but 80% of those who require TPN for more than 2 months develop cholestasis.[12] Likely mechanisms include immaturity of the hepatobiliary system,[82] prolonged fasting,[106] impaired bile secretion and bile salt formation,[121] coexisting sepsis,[71] and underlying medical conditions associated with hypoxia or GI conditions requiring surgery.[16] In the vast majority, cholestasis resolves when enteral feeding is initiated, but progression to biliary cirrhosis[96] and liver failure[103] can occur. Discontinuing the TPN for 1–2 weeks may allow significant recovery; phenobarbital (phenobarbitone) therapy[123] and surgical biliary irrigation[32] have also been used successfully.

In view of the potential metabolic complications, parenteral lipids should be used with caution in infants with fulminating sepsis or NEC, prior to adequate clinical stabilisation with antibiotic therapy. Amino acids and electrolyte solutions should be monitored with great care in infants with severely impaired renal function. The total nitrogen intake may be limited, but should not be discontinued completely, as this will result in catabolism.

Transition to enteral nutrition

In spite of the adequacy of parenteral nutrition in meeting nutritional requirements for postnatal growth, enteral feeding itself is vital for adaptation to extrauterine nutrition through its trophic effects on the GI tract and its physiological effects on GI exocrine and endocrine secretion and motility.[78] Milk feeds result in surges of secretion, glucagon, gastrin and motilin, all of which have trophic effects and mediate GI secretion and motility. Parenterally fed young animals demonstrate not only a failure of growth of the stomach, small intestine and pancreas compared with those enterally fed, but also decreased disaccharidase activity in the atrophic proximal small intestine mucosa.[47] It has been shown in human infants that enteral feeding is necessary for normal gastric acid secretion.[64] Enteral feeding is associated with increases in blood gastrin and motilin levels[117] and intestinal motor activity.[18] Amino acid nitrogen flux, protein synthesis and breakdown are significantly higher during enteral than parenteral nutrition, reflecting the rapid growth and development of the gut in the enterally fed infant.[37] Glucagon, in addition to its role in GI motility, stimulates bile flow.[8] Infants on TPN with no enteral intake secrete extremely dilute bile, a finding which may explain some of the adverse hepatobiliary changes associated with TPN.[4] Those who are parenterally fed also have significantly fewer immunoglobulin-containing intestinal plasma cells than those who are enterally fed.[69]

The early introduction of milk feeds prescribed even in subnutritional quantities is therefore beneficial for growth, development and maintenance of normal structure and function in the GI and hepatobiliary systems.[17] Early introduction of enteral feeding is associated with a lower prevalence of severe feeding intolerance[72] and nosocomial infection.[129] RCTs have compared the effects of early (2–7 days) versus late (9–18 days) enteral feeding, both groups initially receiving the majority of their energy intake by the parenteral route.[39,119] Infants who received early low-volume enteral feeding had improved feeding tolerance, reached full enteral nutrition faster and had less indirect hyperbilirubinaemia, cholestatic jaundice and osteopenia of prematurity.

Conclusion

Parenteral nutrition, despite the many unanswered questions, represents a major breakthrough in the ability to provide adequate nutrition and to achieve normal growth in many preterm or sick infants who cannot tolerate or utilise enteral nutrients for long periods. Because of its potential complications, which can only be kept at an acceptable level by obsessional attention to detail, parenteral nutrition should be used only in neonatal units where there are appropriate facilities and staff. Parenteral nutrition is life-saving in many instances of neonatal GI failure and is an essential facet of modern neonatal intensive care.

References

1. Adamkin D H, Gelke K N, Wilkerson S A 1985 Clinical and laboratory observations: influence of intravenous fat therapy on tracheal effluent phospholipids and oxygenation in severe respiratory distress syndrome. Journal of Pediatrics 106: 122–124
2. Adamkin D H, Radmacher P G, Klingbeil R L 1992 Use of intravenous lipid and hyperbilirubinemia in the first week. Journal of Pediatric Gastroenterology and Nutrition 14: 135–139
3. Al-Dahhan J, Haycock G B, Chantler C, Stimmler L 1983 Sodium homeostasis in mature and immature neonates. I. Renal aspects. Archives of Disease in Childhood 58: 335–342
4. Al-Rabeeah A, Thurston O G, Walker K 1986 Effect of total parenteral nutrition on biliary lipids in neonates. Canadian Journal of Surgery 29: 289–291
5. Alpan G, Eyal F, Springer C, Glick B, Goder K, Armon J 1984 Heparinization of alimentation solutions administered through peripheral veins in premature infants: a controlled study. Pediatrics 74: 374–378
6. Anderson T L, Muttart C R, Bieber M A, Nicholson J F, Heird W C 1979 A controlled trial of glucose versus amino acids in premature infants. Journal of Pediatrics 94: 947–951
7. Auld P A M, Bhagananda P, Mehta S 1966 The influence of an early caloric intake with I-V glucose on catabolism of premature infants. Pediatrics 37: 592–596
8. Aynsley-Green A 1983 Plasma hormone concentrations during enteral and parenteral nutrition in the human newborn. Journal of Pediatric Gastroenterology and Nutrition 2: 108–112
9. Baeckert P A, Greene H L, Fritz I, Oelberg D G, Adcock E W 1988 Vitamin concentrations in very low birth weight infants given vitamins intravenously in a lipid emulsion: measurement of vitamins A, D and E and riboflavin. Journal of Pediatrics 113: 1057–1063
10. Bailey M J 1979 Reduction of catheter-associated sepsis in parenteral nutrition using low-dose intravenous heparin. British Medical Journal i: 1671–1673
11. Baumgart S, Engle W D, Fox W W, Polin R A 1981 Effect of heat shielding on convective and evaporative heat loss and on radiant heat transfer in the premature infant. Journal of Pediatrics 99: 948–956
12. Beale E F, Nelson R M, Bucciarelli R L, Donnelly W H, Eitzman D V 1979 Intrahepatic cholestasis associated with parenteral nutrition in premature infants. Pediatrics 64: 342–347
13. Beganovic N, Verloove-Vanhorick S P, Brand R, Ruys J H 1988 Total parenteral nutrition and sepsis. Archives of Disease in Childhood 63: 66–69
14. Bell E F, Acarregui M J 2001 Restricted versus liberal water intake for preventing morbidity and mortality in preterm infants (Cochrane Review). Cochrane Database of Systematic Reviews (3): CD000503
15. Bell E F, Neidich G A, Cashore W J, Oh W 1979 Combined effect of radiant warmer and phototherapy on insensible water loss in low-birth-weight infants. Journal of Pediatrics 94: 810–813
16. Bell R L, Ferry G D, Smith E O et al 1986 Total parenteral nutrition related cholestasis in infants. Journal of Parenteral and Enteral Nutrition 10: 356–359
17. Berseth C L 1995 Minimal enteral feedings. Clinics in Perinatology 22: 195–204
18. Berseth C L, Nordyke C 1993 Enteral nutrients promote postnatal maturation of intestinal motor activity in preterm infants. American Journal of Physiology 264: G1046–G1051
19. Binder N D, Raschko R K, Benda G I, Reynolds J W 1989 Insulin infusion with parenteral nutrition in extremely low birthweight infants with hyperglycemia. Journal of Pediatrics 114: 273–280
20. Bishop N J, Morley R, Day J P, Lucas A 1997 Aluminum neurotoxicity in preterm infants receiving intravenous-feeding solutions. New England Journal of Medicine 336: 1557–1561
21. Brans Y W, Andrew D S, Carrillo D W, Dutton E P, Menchaca E M, Puleo-Schappke B A 1988 Tolerance of fat emulsions in very low birth weight neonates. American Journal of Diseases of Children 142: 145–152
22. Brans Y W, Dutton E B, Andrew D S, Menchaca E M, West D L 1986 Fat emulsion tolerance in very low birth weight neonates: effect on diffusion of oxygen in the lungs and on blood pH. Pediatrics 78: 79–84
23. Brans Y W, Ritter D A, Kenny J D, Andrew D S, Dutton E B, Carillo D W 1987 Influence of intravenous fat emulsion on serum bilirubin in very low birthweight infants. Archives of Disease in Childhood 62: 156–160
24. Brans Y W, Sumners J E, Dweck H S, Cassady G 1974 Feeding the low birth weight infant: orally or parenterally? Preliminary results of a comparative study. Pediatrics 54: 15–22
25. Brion L P, Schwartz G J, Campbell D, Fleischman A R 1989 Early hyperkalaemia in very low birthweight infants in the absence of oliguria. Archives of Disease in Childhood 64: 270–282
26. Brownlee K G, Kelly E J, Ng P C, Kendall-Smith S C, Dear P R 1993 Early or late parenteral nutrition for the sick preterm infant? Archives of Disease in Childhood 69: 281–283
27. Cairns P A, Stalker D J 2000 Carnitine supplementation of parenterally fed neonates (Cochrane Review). Cochrane Database of Systematic Reviews (4): CD000950
28. Chathas M K, Paton J B, Fisher D E 1990 Percutaneous central venous catheterization. American Journal of Diseases of Children 144: 1246–1250
29. Chessex P, Zebiche H, Pineault M, Lopage D, Dallaire L 1985 Effect of aminoacid composition of parenteral solutions on nitrogen retention and metabolic response in very low birth weight infants. Journal of Pediatrics 106: 111–117
30. Collins J W Jr, Hoppe M, Brown K, Edidin D V, Padbury J, Ogata E S 1991 A controlled trial of insulin infusion and parenteral nutrition in extremely low birth weight infants with glucose intolerance. Journal of Pediatrics 118: 921–927

31. Cooke R J, Yeh Y, Gibson D, Debo D, Bell G L 1987 Soybean oil emulsion administration during parenteral nutrition in the preterm infant: effect on essential fatty acid, lipid and glucose metabolism. Journal of Pediatrics 111: 767–773

32. Cooper A, Ross A J III, O'Neil J A, Bishop H C, Templeton J M, Ziegler M M 1985 Resolution of intractable cholestasis associated with total parenteral nutrition following biliary irrigation. Journal of Pediatric Surgery 20: 772–774

33. Coran A G, Drongowski R A, Wesley J R 1984 Changes in total body water and extracellular fluid volume in infants receiving total parenteral nutrition. Journal of Pediatric Surgery 19: 771–776

34. Cowett R M, Anderson G E, Maguire C A, Oh W 1988 Ontogeny of glucose homeostasis in low birth weight infants. Journal of Pediatrics 112: 462–465

35. Dahl G B, Svensson L, Kinnander N J G, Zander M, Berstrom U K 1994 Stability of vitamins in soybean oil fat emulsion under conditions simulating intravenous feeding of neonates and children. Journal of Parenteral and Enteral Nutrition 18: 234–239

36. Denne S C 1998 Carbohydrate requirements. In: Polin R A, Fox W W (eds) Fetal and neonatal physiology, 2nd edn. WB Saunders, Philadelphia, pp 325–327

37. Duffy B, Pencharz P 1986 The effect of feeding route (IV or oral) on the protein metabolism of the neonate. American Journal of Clinical Nutrition 43: 108–111

38. Duffy B, Pencharz P 1986 The effects of surgery on the nitrogen metabolism of parenterally fed human neonates. Pediatric Research 20: 32–35

39. Dunn L, Hulman S, Weiner J, Kliegman R 1988 Beneficial effects of early hypocaloric enteral feeding on neonatal gastrointestinal function: preliminary report of a randomized trial. Journal of Pediatrics 112: 622–629

40. English D, Roloff J S, Lukens J N, Parker P, Greene H L, Ghishan F K 1981 Intravenous lipid emulsions and human neutrophil function. Journal of Pediatrics 99: 913–916

41. Escobar C, Salas M 1995 Dendritic branching of claustral neurons in neonatally undernourished rats. Biology of the Neonate 68: 47–54

42. Fleer A, Senders R C, Visser M R et al 1983 Septicemia due to coagulase-negative staphylococci in a neonatal intensive care unit: clinical and bacteriological features and contaminated parenteral fluids as a source of sepsis. Pediatric Infectious Disease 2: 426–431

43. Forsyth J S, Crighton A 1995 Low birthweight infants and total parenteral nutrition immediately after birth. I. Energy expenditure and respiratory quotient of ventilated and non-ventilated infants. Archives of Disease in Childhood. Fetal and Neonatal Edition 73: F4–F7

44. Freeman J, Goldman D A, Smith N E, Sidebottom D G, Epstein M F, Platt R 1990 Association of intravenous lipid emulsion and coagulase-negative staphylococcal bacteremia in neonatal intensive care units. New England Journal of Medicine 323: 301–308

45. Gilbertson N, Kovar I Z, Cox D J, Crowe L, Palmer N T 1991 Introduction of intravenous lipid administration on the first day of life in the low birth weight neonate. Journal of Pediatrics 119: 615–623

46. Gilles J, Jones G, Pencharz P 1983 Delivery of vitamins A, D and E in parenteral nutrition solutions. Journal of Parenteral and Enteral Nutrition 7: 11–14

47. Goldstein R M, Hebiguchi T, Luk G D et al 1985 The effects of total parenteral nutrition on gastrointestinal growth and development. Journal of Pediatric Surgery 20: 785–791

48. Greene H L, Hambidge K M, Schanler R, Tsang R C 1988 Guidelines for the use of vitamins, trace elements, calcium, magnesium and phosphorus in infants and children receiving total parenteral nutrition: report of the Subcommittee on Pediatric Parenteral Nutrition Requirements from the Committee on Clinical Practice Issues of the American Society for Clinical Nutrition. American Journal of Clinical Nutrition 48: 1324–1342

49. Groh-Wargo S, Ciaccia A, Moore J 1988 Neonatal metabolic acidosis: effect of chloride from normal saline flushes. Journal of Parenteral and Enteral Nutrition 12: 159–161

50. Gruskay J, Costarino A T, Polin R A, Baumgart S 1988 Nonoliguric hyperkalemia in the premature infant weighing less than 1000 grams. Journal of Pediatrics 113: 381–386

51. Gunn T, Reaman G, Outerbridge E W, Cole E 1978 Peripheral total parenteral nutrition for premature infants with the respiratory distress syndrome: a controlled study. Journal of Pediatrics 92: 608–613

52. Hammerman C, Aramburo M J 1988 Decreased lipid intake reduces morbidity in sick premature neonates. Journal of Pediatrics 113: 1083–1088

53. Hanning R M, Atkinson S A, Whyte R K 1991 Efficacy of calcium glycerophosphate vs conventional mineral salts for total parenteral nutrition in low-birth-weight infants: a randomized clinical trial. American Journal of Clinical Nutrition 54: 903–908

54. Harpin V A, Rutter N 1985 Humidification of incubators. Archives of Disease in Childhood 60: 219–224

55. Haumont D, Deckelbaum R J, Richelle M et al 1989 Plasma lipid and plasma lipoprotein concentrations in low birth weight infants given parenteral nutrition with twenty or ten percent lipid emulsion. Journal of Pediatrics 115: 787–793

56. Haumont D, Richelle M, Deckelbaum R J, Coussaert E, Carpentier Y A 1992 Effect of liposomal content of lipid emulsions on plasma lipid concentrations in low birth weight infants receiving parenteral nutrition. Journal of Pediatrics 121: 759–763

57. Heimler R, Doumas B T, Jendrzejczak B M, Nemeth P B, Hoffman R G, Nelin L D 1993 Relationship between nutrition, weight change, and fluid compartments in preterm infants during the first week of life. Journal of Pediatrics 122: 110–114

58. Heird W C 1992 Parenteral feeding. In: Sinclair J C, Bracken M B (eds) Effective care of the newborn infant. Oxford University Press, Oxford, pp 141–160

59. Heird W C, Dell R B, Helms R A et al 1987 Amino acid mixture designed to maintain normal plasma amino acid patterns in infants and children requiring parenteral nutrition. Pediatrics 80: 401–408

60. Heird W C, Hay W, Helms R A, Storm M C, Kashyap S, Dell R B 1988 Pediatric parenteral amino acid mixture in low birth weight infants. Pediatrics 81: 41–50

61. Helms R A, Herrod H G, Burckart G J, Christensen M L 1983 E-rosette formation, total T-cells, and lymphocyte transformation in infants receiving intravenous safflower oil emulsion. Journal of Parenteral and Enteral Nutrition 7: 541–545

62. Helms R A, Christensen M L, Mauer E C, Storm M C 1987 Comparison of a pediatric versus standard amino acid formulation in preterm neonates requiring parenteral nutrition. Journal of Pediatrics 110: 466–470

63. Hilliard J L, Shannon D L, Hunter M A, Brans Y W 1983 Plasma lipid levels in preterm neonates receiving parenteral nutrition. Archives of Disease in Childhood 58: 29–33

64. Hyman P E, Feldman E J, Ament M E, Bryne W J, Euler A R 1983 Effect of enteral feeding on the maintenance of gastric acid secretory function. Gastroenterology 84: 341–345

65. Imura K, Okada A, Fukui Y et al 1988 Clinical studies on a newly devised amino acid solution for neonates. Journal of Parenteral and Enteral Nutrition 12: 496–504

66. Jarvis W R, Highsmith A K, Allen J R, Haley R W 1983 Polymicrobial bacteremia associated with lipid emulsion in a neonatal intensive care unit. Pediatric Infectious Disease 2: 203–208

67. Kanarek K S, Kuznicki M B, Blair R C 1991 Infusion of total parenteral nutrition via the umbilical artery. Journal of Parenteral and Enteral Nutrition 15: 71–74

68. Kao L C, Cheng M H, Warburton D 1984 Triglycerides, free fatty acids, free fatty acids/albumin molar ratio, and cholesterol levels in serum of neonates receiving long-term lipid infusions: controlled trial of continuous and intermittent regimes. Journal of Pediatrics 104: 429–435

69. Knox W F 1986 Restricted feeding and human intestinal plasma cell development. Archives of Disease in Childhood 61: 744–749

70. Koh T H H G, Aynsley-Green A, Tarbit M, Eyre J A 1988 Neural dysfunction during hypoglycaemia. Archives of Disease in Childhood 63: 1353–1358

71. Kubota A, Okada A, Nezu R, Kamata S, Imura K, Takagi Y 1988 Hyperbilirubinemia in neonates associated with total parenteral nutrition. Journal of Parenteral and Enteral Nutrition 12: 602–606

72. LaGamma E F, Ostertag S G, Birenbaum H 1985 Failure of delayed oral feedings to prevent necrotizing enterocolitis. American Journal of Diseases of Children 139: 385–389

73. Laidlaw S A, Kopple J D 1987 Newer concepts of the indispensable amino acids. American Journal of Clinical Nutrition 46: 593–605

74. Lee E J, Simmer K, Gibson R A 1993 Essential fatty acid deficiency in parenterally fed preterm infants. Journal of Paediatrics and Child Health 29: 51–55

75. Lemons J A, Neal P, Ernst J 1986 Nitrogen sources for parenteral nutrition in the newborn infant. Clinics in Perinatology 13: 91–109

76. Louik C, Mitchell A A, Epstein M F, Shapiro S 1985 Risk factors for neonatal hyperglycemia associated with 10% dextrose infusion. American Journal of Diseases of Children 139: 783–786

77. Lucas A, Baker B A, Morley R M 1993 Hyperphenylalaninaemia and outcome in intravenously fed preterm infants. Archives of Disease in Childhood 68: 579–583

78. Lucas A, Bloom S R, Aynsley-Green A 1983 Metabolic and endocrine effects of depriving preterm infants of enteral nutrition. Acta Paediatrica Scandinavica 72: 245–249

79. Lucas A, Morley R, Cole T J 1988 Adverse neurodevelopmental outcome of moderate neonatal hypoglycaemia. British Medical Journal 297: 1304–1308

80. Lucas A, Morley R, Cole T J 1998 Randomised trial of early diet in preterm babies and later intelligence quotient. British Medical Journal 317: 1481–1487

81. Malloy M H, Rassin D K, Richardson C J 1984 Total parenteral nutrition in sick preterm infants: effects of cysteine supplementation with nitrogen intakes of 240 and 400 mg/kg/day. Journal of Pediatric Gastroenterology and Nutrition 3: 239–244

82. Merritt R J 1986 Cholestasis associated with total parenteral nutrition. Journal of Pediatric Gastroenterology and Nutrition 5: 9–22

83. Mitton S G, Burston D, Brueton M J, Kovar I Z 1993 Plasma amino acid profiles in preterm infants receiving Vamin 9 glucose or Vamin Infant. Early Human Development 32: 71–78

84. Moore M C, Greene H L, Phillips B et al 1986 Evaluation of a pediatric multiple vitamin preparation for total parenteral nutrition in infants and children. Pediatrics 77: 530–538

85. Moreno A, Dominguez C, Ballabriga A 1994 Aluminium in the neonate related to parenteral nutrition. Acta Paediatrica 83: 25–29

86. Moyer-Mileur L, Chan G M 1986 Nutritional support of very low birth weight infants requiring prolonged assisted ventilation. American Journal of Diseases of Children 140: 929–932

87. Nakamura K T, Sato Y, Erenberg A 1990 Evaluation of a percutaneously placed 27-gauge central venous catheter in neonates weighing < 1200 grams. Journal of Parenteral and Enteral Nutrition 14: 295–299

88. Neubauer A P 1995 Percutaneous central i.v. access in the neonate: experience with 535 silastic catheters. Acta Paediatrica 84: 756–760

89. Neuzil J, Darlow B A, Inder T E, Sluis K B, Winterbourn C C, Stocker R 1995 Oxidation of parenteral lipid emulsion by ambient and phototherapy lights: potential toxicity of routine parenteral feeding. Journal of Pediatrics 126: 785–790

90. Ogata E S, Schulman S, Raffensperger J, Luck S, Rusnak M 1984 Caval catheterisation in the intensive care nursery: a useful means for providing parenteral nutrition to the extremely low birthweight infant. Journal of Pediatric Surgery 19: 258–262

91. Olunfunmi P, Ryan S, Matthew L, Cheung K, Lunn J 1997 Randomised controlled trial of acetate in preterm neonates receiving parenteral nutrition. Archives of Disease in Childhood. Fetal and Neonatal Edition 77: F12–F15

92. Ostertag S G, Jovanovic L, Lewis B, Auld P A M 1986 Insulin pump therapy in the very low birth weight infant. Pediatrics 78: 625–630

93. Park W, Paust H, Brosicke H, Knoblack G, Helge H 1986 Impaired fat utilization in parenterally fed low birth weight infants suffering from sepsis. Journal of Parenteral and Enteral Nutrition 10: 627–630

94. Pereira G R, Fox W W, Stanley C A, Baker L, Schwartz J G 1980 Decreased oxygenation and hyperlipemia during intravenous fat infusions in premature infants. Pediatrics 66: 26–30

95. Pereira G R, Lim B K, Ing C, Medeiros H F 1992 Umbilical vs peripheral vein catheterization for parenteral nutrition in sick premature neonates. Yonsei Medical Journal 33: 224–231

96. Pereira G R, Sherman M S, DiGiacomo J, Zieler M, Roth K, Jacobowski D 1981 Hyperalimentation induced cholestasis. American Journal of Diseases of Children 135: 842–845

97. Phelps S J, Cochran E B 1989 Peripheral venous line infiltration in infants receiving 10% dextrose, 10% dextrose/amino acids, or 10% dextrose/amino acids/fat emulsion. Journal of Parenteral and Enteral Nutrition 13: 628–632

98. Phelps S J, Helms R A 1987 Risk factors affecting infiltration of peripheral venous lines in infants. Journal of Pediatrics 111: 384–389

99. Pineault M, Chessex P, Bisaillon S, Brisson G 1988 Total parenteral nutrition in the newborn: impact of the quality of infused energy on nitrogen metabolism. American Journal of Clinical Nutrition 47: 298–304

100. Pitkanen O, Hallman M, Anderson S 1991 Generation of free radicals in lipid emulsion used in parenteral nutrition. Pediatric Research 29: 56–59

101. Pollak A, Cowett R M, Schwartz R, Oh W 1978 Glucose disposal in low birth weight infants during steady state hyperglycemia: effects of exogenous insulin administration. Pediatrics 61: 546–549

102. Polley T Z, Benner J W, Rhodin A, Weintraub W H, Coran A G 1979 Changes in total body water in infants receiving total intravenous nutrition. Journal of Surgical Research 26: 555–559

103. Postuma R, Trevenen C L 1979 Liver disease in infants receiving total parenteral nutrition. Pediatrics 63: 110–115

104. Puntis J W, Ball P A, Preece M A, Green A, Brown G A, Booth I W 1989 Egg and breast milk based nitrogen sources compared. Archives of Disease in Childhood 64: 1472–1477

105. Puntis J W, Holden C E, Smallman S, Finkel Y, George R H, Booth I W 1991 Staff training: a key factor in reducing intravascular catheter sepsis. Archives of Disease in Childhood 66: 335–337

106. Rager R, Finegold M J 1975 Cholestasis in immature newborn infants: is parenteral alimentation responsible? Journal of Pediatrics 86: 264–269

107. Raupp P, von Kries R, Pfahl H, Manz F 1991 Glycero- vs glucose phosphate in parenteral nutrition of premature infants: a comparative in vitro evaluation of calcium/phosphorus compatibility. Journal of Parenteral and Enteral Nutrition 15: 469–473

108. Raupp P, von Kries R, Schmidt E, Pfahl H, Gunther O 1988 Incompatibility between fat emulsion and calcium plus heparin in parenteral nutrition of premature babies. Lancet I: 700

109. Rees L, Shaw J C L, Brook C G D, Forsling M L 1984 Hyponatraemia in the first week of life in preterm infants. II Sodium and water balance. Archives of Disease in Childhood 59: 423–429

110. Reichman B L, Chessex P, Putet G et al 1982 Partition of energy metabolism and energy cost of growth in the very low birth weight infant. Pediatrics 69: 446–451

111. Rivera A Jr, Bell E F, Bier D M 1993 Effect of intravenous amino acids on protein metabolism of preterm infants during the first three days of life. Pediatric Research 33: 106–111

112. Rovamo L M, Nikkila E A, Raivio K O 1988 Lipoprotein lipase, hepatic lipase, and carnitine in premature infants. Archives of Disease in Childhood 63: 140–147

113. Rubecz I, Mestyan J 1973 Energy metabolism and intravenous nutrition of premature infants. Biology of the Neonate 23: 45–58

114. Rubin M, Harell D, Naor N et al 1991 Lipid infusion with different triglyceride cores (long-chain vs medium-chain/long-chain triglycerides): effect on plasma lipids and bilirubin binding in premature infants. Journal of Parenteral and Enteral Nutrition 15: 642–646

115. Salle B L, David L, Chopard J P, Grafmeyer D C, Renaud H 1977 Prevention of early neonatal hypocalcemia in low birth weight infants with continuous calcium infusion: effect on serum calcium, phosphorus, magnesium, and circulating immunoactive parathyroid hormone and calcitonin. Pediatric Research 11: 1180–1185

116. Schreiner R L, Glick M R, Nordschow C D, Gresham E L 1979 An evaluation of methods to monitor infants receiving intravenous lipids. Journal of Pediatrics 94: 197–200

117. Shulman D I, Kanarek K 1993 Gastrin, motilin, insulin, and insulin-like growth factor-I concentrations in very low birth weight infants receiving enteral or parenteral nutrition. Journal of Parenteral and Enteral Nutrition 17: 130–133

118. Shulman R J, Pokorny W J, Martin C G, Petitt R, Baldaia L, Roney D 1986 Comparison of percutaneous and surgical placement of central venous catheters in neonates. Journal of Pediatric Surgery 21: 348–350

119. Slagle T A, Gross S J 1988 Effect of early low-volume enteral substrate on subsequent feeding tolerance in very low birth weight infants. Journal of Pediatrics 13: 526–531

120. Smith J L, Canham J E, Wells P A 1988 Effect of phototherapy light, sodium bisulfite, and pH on vitamin stability in total parenteral nutrition and mixtures. Journal of Parenteral and Enteral Nutrition 12: 394–402

121. Sondheimer J M, Bryan H, Andrews W, Forster G G 1978 Cholestatic tendencies in premature infants on and off parenteral nutrition. Pediatrics 62: 984–989

122. Sosenko I R S, Rodriguez-Pierce M, Bancalari E 1993 Effect of early initiation of intravenous lipid administration on the incidence and severity of chronic lung disease in premature infants. Journal of Pediatrics 123: 975–982

123. South M, King A 1987 Parenteral nutrition associated cholestasis: recovery following phenobarbitone. Journal of Parenteral and Enteral Nutrition 11: 208–209

124. Spear M L, Stahl G E, Hamosh M, McNelis W G, Richardson L L, Spence V 1988 Effect of heparin dose and infusion rate on lipid clearance and bilirubin binding in premature infants receiving intravenous fat emulsions. Journal of Pediatrics 112: 94–98

125. Strunk R C, Murrow B W, Thilo E, Kunke K S, Johnson E G 1985 Normal macrophage function in infants receiving Intralipid by low-dose intermittent administration. Journal of Pediatrics 106: 640–645

126. Thaler M M, Wennberg R P 1977 Influence of intravenous nutrients on bilirubin transport. II Emulsified lipid solutions. Pediatric Research 11: 167–171

127. Thornton L, Griffin E 1991 Evaluation of a taurine containing amino acid solution in parenteral nutrition. Archives of Disease in Childhood 66: 21–25

128. Uhlemann M, Plath C, Heine W et al 1989 MCT fat emulsions enhance efficacy of whole-body protein metabolism in very small preterm neonates. Clinical Nutrition 8: 84

129. Unger A, Goetzman B W, Chan C, Lyons A B, Miller M F 1986 Nutritional practices and outcome of extremely premature infants. American Journal of Diseases of Children 140: 1027–1033

130. Usmani S S, Harper R G, Usmani S F 1988 Effect of a lipid emulsion (Intralipid) on polymorphonuclear leukocyte functions in the neonate. Journal of Pediatrics 113: 132–136

131. Van Aerde J E, Sauer P J, Pencharz P B, Smith J M, Heim T, Swyer P R 1994 Metabolic consequences of increasing energy intake by adding lipid to parenteral nutrition in full-term infants. American Journal of Clinical Nutrition 59: 659–662

132. Wahlig T M, Georgieff M K 1995 The effects of illness on neonatal metabolism and nutritional management. Clinics in Perinatology 22: 77–96

133. Warner B W, Gorgone P, Schilling S, Farell M, Ghory M J 1987 Multiple purpose central venous access in infants less than 1000 grams. Journal of Pediatric Surgery 22: 820–822

134. Weese-Mayer D E, Fondriest D W, Brouilette R T, Shulman S T 1987 Risk factors associated with candidemia in the neonatal intensive care unit: a case control study. Pediatric Infectious Disease Journal 6: 190–196

135. Yeh T F, Voora S, Lilien L D, Matwynshyn J, Srinivasan G, Pildes R S 1980 Oxygen consumption and insensible water loss in premature infants in single-versus double-walled incubators. Journal of Pediatrics 97: 967–971

136. Yu V Y H, James B E, Hendry P G, MacMahon R A 1979 Glucose tolerance in very low birthweight infants. Australian Paediatric Journal 15: 147–151

137. Yu V Y H, James B, Hendry P, MacMahon R A 1979 Total parenteral nutrition in very low birthweight infants: a controlled trial. Archives of Disease in Childhood 54: 653–661

138. Yunis K A, Oh W, Kalhan S, Cowett R M 1992 Glucose kinetics following administration of an intravenous fat emulsion to low birth weight neonates. American Journal of Physiology 263: E844–E849

139. Zaidan H, Dhanireddy R, Hamosh M, Bengtsson-Olivecrona G, Hamosh P 1985 Lipid clearing in premature infants during continuous heparin infusion: role of circulating lipases. Pediatric Research 19: 23–25

140. Zlotkin S H, Bryan M H, Anderson G H 1981 Intravenous nitrogen and energy intakes required to duplicate in utero nitrogen accretion in prematurely born human infants. Journal of Pediatrics 99: 115–120

Appendix

How to write a TPN prescription

There are two approaches to the provision of neonatal TPN. The first is to use standard bags – that is, bags containing the desired quantity of amino acids, dextrose and electrolytes for a preterm infant receiving 150 ml/kg/day TPN. Therefore the nutrients are increased proportionately as the fluid volume is increased over the first week. These have the advantage of cost and convenience and are suitable for the majority of preterm infants. Those with high electrolyte requirements, a significant volume of non-nutritional infusates or prolonged fluid restriction, benefit from individualised prescriptions. Some units use individualised prescriptions for all their patients for this reason.

The actual method of prescribing TPN also varies widely across units. The precise volume and concentrations of amino acid, dextrose and electrolyte solutions may be calculated in the NICU or in the pharmacy, with or without the aid of a computer program. In St Michael's Hospital, Bristol, we prescribe the desired quantity of nutrients for each individual baby and the calculations are carried out in the pharmacy. It is important to be familiar with the exact process in each hospital as 15% dextrose in one hospital may refer to an overall concentration of 15% while in another it may mean that 15% dextrose has been added to the solution, resulting in a significantly more dilute product.

General guidelines

- Decide total daily fluid intake for baby.
- Subtract all other intravenous infusion volumes (such as arterial line fluid or inotropes).
- Order TPN for the remaining volume. As the enteral input increases, the intravenous protein, lipid and carbohydrate intake will reduce proportionately.
- When calculating the desired sodium intake, remember to take into consideration any saline or sodium bicarbonate infusions.

Protein

- Start early (within the first 24 hours if possible for all preterm infants).
- Start at 1 g/kg/day.
- Use a neonatal formulation.
- Increase by 1 g/kg/day to a total of 3.5 g/kg/day.
- Use with caution in babies with renal impairment (may need restriction to 2.5 g/kg/day) or with suspected inborn errors of metabolism (stop while investigations awaited).

Dextrose

- Prescribe as mg/kg/min starting at 6 mg/kg/min.
- Increase by daily increments of 2 mg/kg/min if tolerated.
- If using a peripheral cannula, note that the maximum overall dextrose concentration of the solution should be 12.5%.

Lipid

- Start at 1 g/kg/day on day 1 of TPN. Use 20% emulsion.
- Increase by 0.5 g/kg/day to a maximum of 3.5 g/kg/day.
- Check triglyceride levels after a 4-hour lipid-free period twice weekly.
- Use with caution in babies with acute sepsis (temporary lipid intolerance), labile pulmonary hypertension (altered prostaglandin synthesis) or severe jaundice (fatty acid displacement of bilirubin from albumin).

Electrolytes and minerals

- Add sodium when the plasma sodium starts to fall, and titrate. The usual maintenance dose is a total of 2–4 mmol/kg/day. Allow for sodium content of other infusions. Once sodium intake is greater than 3 mmol/kg/day, use sodium acetate.
- Start potassium at 1–2 mmol/kg/day on day 3 and titrate.
- Start calcium and phosphate at 1–1.5 mmol/kg/day on day 1. Discuss with pharmacist if higher concentrations desired.
- Start magnesium at 0.2 mmol/kg/day and titrate.
- Add maintenance trace elements, such as Pedi trace (Fresenius Kabi) 1 ml/kg/day.

Vitamins

- Add water-soluble vitamins to amino acid solution from day 1, such as Solvito N (Fresenius Kabi) 1 ml/kg/day.
- Add fat-soluble vitamins to lipid emulsions from day 1, such as Vitlipid N Infant (Fresenius Kabi) 4 ml/kg/day to a maximum of 10 ml.

CHAPTER 18

Fluid and electrolyte balance

Neena Modi

Introduction

The management of fluid balance in neonates differs from that in other age groups in several important respects. Neonatal physiology is not static. The immediate postnatal period is a time during which the transition from the fluid, intrauterine environment to the gaseous, postnatal environment must be successfully made. Developmental changes continue after delivery and are particularly relevant in very immature infants. Postnatal adaptation of extra-renal systems affect fluid balance and the influences of illness and medication may be superimposed upon this. Disturbances in electrolyte and water balance are not uncommon in newborn infants and this chapter will approach the regulation of fluid balance and its management from the perspective of the clinician.

Renal and extra-renal determinants of sodium, water and acid–base balance

Sodium balance

In adults, approximately 80–90% of filtered sodium is reabsorbed in the proximal tubule (Fig. 18.1)[34] and in the thick ascending limb of the loop of Henlé. Unabsorbed sodium passes into the distal tubule and collecting duct. Here, sodium is absorbed in exchange for potassium and hydrogen ions. Distal tubular sodium reabsorption is regulated via the renin–angiotensin–aldosterone system (RAAS). In neonates, a smaller proportion of filtered sodium is absorbed in the proximal tubule and a correspondingly larger proportion delivered distally.

The sodium retention that characterises growth is due to the influence of very high RAAS activity.[134] In contrast to the term neonate, the preterm neonate has a reduced capacity to retain sodium. Poor sodium retention is due to impaired reabsorption

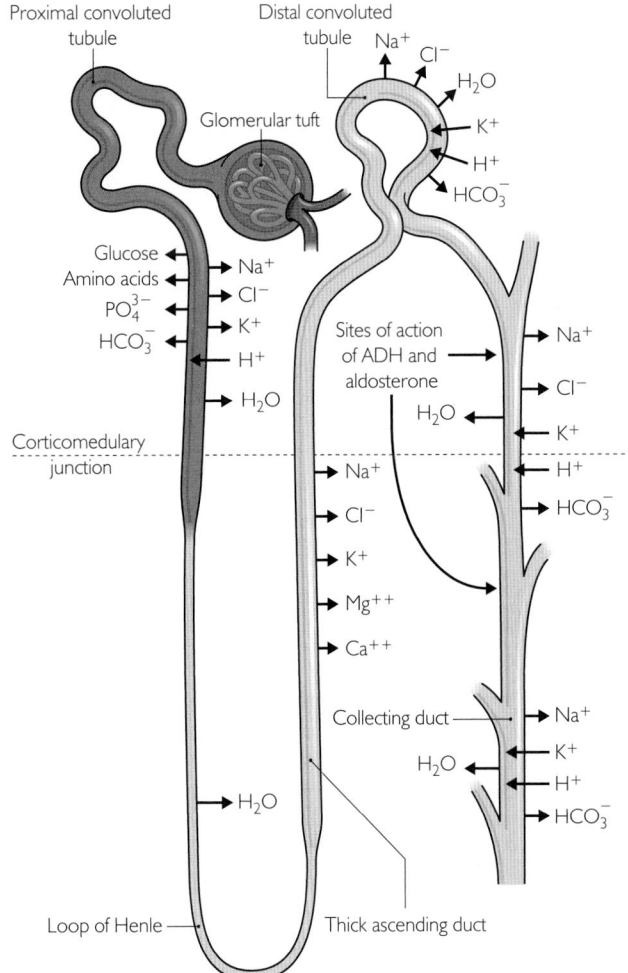

Fig. 18.1 Excretion of water and electrolytes. Water is reabsorbed in the proximal tubule together with glucose, amino acids, phosphate, sodium and bicarbonate, and from the distal nephron under the influence of AVP and the hypertonic medulla. In the distal tubule, sodium is reabsorbed under the influence of aldosterone with associated excretion of potassium and hydrogen ions. (Adapted from Cumming & Swainson.[34])

at the proximal tubule, resulting in a higher distal sodium delivery, and to limited aldosterone responsiveness at the distal tubule.[139] Intestinal absorption is also limited.[2] Both preterm and full-term neonates have a limited capacity to excrete a sodium load. This is not due to a low glomerular filtration rate (GFR), because filtration, in even the most immature neonate, greatly exceeds the amount that is ultimately retained, but because acute sodium loading results in only a blunted fall in RAAS activity and a limited natriuretic response.[38] Overall, homeostasis is dependent on the regulation of tubular reabsorption, a process that in turn is dependent upon the stage of developmental maturation.

Tubular epithelial cells are bound by an apical membrane that faces the tubular lumen, and a basolateral membrane that lines the lateral and basal intercellular space and faces the peritubular capillaries. The lipid bilayer of the cell membrane is poorly permeable and solutes cross the membrane via transporters. These are specialised proteins inserted into the cell membrane. Their regulation is complex and involves hormones, intracellular signalling systems, protein phosphorylation, and endo- and exocytosis, each of which in turn undergoes developmental regulation. Na^+/K^+-ATPase is the enzyme responsible for active sodium transport in all eukaryotic cells. There are many forms of Na^+/K^+-ATPase, each encoded by specific groups of Na^+/K^+ ATPase genes. In renal tubular cells, Na^+/K^+-ATPase, present on the basolateral membrane, creates an electrochemical gradient which is the energy source for the co-transport, involving specific transporter proteins, of Na^+ and glucose, and Na^+ and amino acids, and the countertransport of Na^+ and H^+ across the luminal membrane.[73] The long-term regulation of sodium balance is brought about by changes in the abundance of sodium transporters. During ontogenesis, there are tissue-specific patterns of increase in activity accompanied by an increase in Na^+/K^+-ATPase mRNA.[107] Antenatal glucocorticoid treatment increases the abundance of Na^+/K^+-ATPase in both lungs and kidney and enhances the maturation of renal tubular transport.

The postnatal enhancement in sodium conservation is brought about by the increasing responsiveness of the distal tubule to aldosterone[1,138] and by an increase in the abundance of Na^+/K^+-ATPase and transporter proteins.[67,70] The ability to excrete a sodium load also matures during development. An increase or decrease in activity of renal Na^+/K^+-ATPase is the final common pathway for the short-term regulation of natriuresis.[6] Downregulatory factors, which cause natriuresis, include atrial natriuretic peptide (ANP), dopamine and diuretics. Noradrenaline is an upregulatory factor, which results in sodium retention. The peptide regulatory factors bind to cell membrane receptors and exert their effects via a cascade of intracellular messengers. Developmental maturation of these intracellular signalling systems fine-tunes the regulation of sodium balance.[40,51,77,93,135] Clinical observations offer some substantiation of these in-vitro studies. ANP stimulates membrane-bound guanylate cyclase, which leads to an increase in the intracellular second messenger, cyclic guanosine monophosphate (cGMP), generated from endogenous guanosine triphosphate. cGMP interacts with specific protein kinases which in turn catalyse the phosphorylation of several protein substrates and finally leads to a biological effect such as inhibition of sodium reabsorption. In a study of preterm babies,[93] the ratio of urinary cGMP to ANP was found to increase exponentially in the first 3 days after birth and then to reach a plateau. The ratio of sodium excretion to cGMP continued to increase over the 10 days of the study. This suggests a postnatal maturation in the ANP/cGMP/sodium excretion cascade and thus an increasing postnatal ability to excrete sodium.

Renal water handling

As nutrition can be provided to babies only in liquid form, a high fluid intake is mandatory and an infant must have a high urine flow in order to maintain water balance. A high urine flow rate is achieved by a much greater fractional excretion of glomerular filtrate (Fe_{H_2O}). In newborn babies, decreased hydrostatic and osmotic forces across the peritubular space result in decreased proximal tubular reabsorption of filtered water. A greater proportion of water is therefore delivered distally as compared with in older subjects. In the distal nephron, water reabsorption is regulated by the antidiuretic hormone (ADH), arginine vasopressin (AVP). The ADH-dependent increase in water permeability is brought about by the insertion of water channels, the acquaporins, from an intracellular vesicular reservoir into the apical membranes of cells of the collecting ducts,[36] allowing the movement of water across the tubular membrane in response to the high concentration of the medullary interstitium. Not all acquaporin (AQP) isoforms are expressed in the human kidney and there are differences in expression during development, but fetal animals and preterm babies are sensitive to ADH.[43] The regulation of collecting-duct water permeability by vasopressin is mediated by *AQP2* expression. Humans with mutations in the *AQP2* gene have nephrogenic diabetes insipidus.[35]

The capacity to concentrate urine develops progressively during postnatal life. In neonates, maximum urine osmolality is about half that of older subjects. This difference is due to shorter loops of Henlé, reduced tonicity of the medullary interstitium as urea concentrations are low because of the highly anabolic state of the rapidly growing infant, and reduced expression of *AQP2*. Higher urine concentrations, however, can be produced under conditions of severe dehydration stress and in response to antenatal glucocorticoid therapy.[155]

Preterm babies are able to achieve similar minimal urine osmolalities to adults and diluting ability is unlikely to limit water excretion. The peak urine flow of mature infants given a water load is the same as that of adults when expressed per unit body water.[90] Coulthard & Hey[33] have also challenged the view that newborns have a limited capacity for water excretion. They showed that healthy preterm babies are able to adjust water excretion appropriately from the second day after birth, when their daily intakes were varied between 95 and 200 ml/kg, sodium intake remaining constant. The Fe_{H_2O} increased from a mean of 7.4% to 13.1% of the filtered volume with the higher intake. A similarly high Fe_{H_2O} in adults would result in a daily urine volume of over 20 litres. It is of note that there was no concomitant increase in the loss of sodium in the urine, an observation that refutes the widely held view that babies are unable to sustain a high urine flow without an inevitable increase in the loss of sodium.

Acid–base balance

The normal pH range of extracellular fluid is 7.35 to 7.45, corresponding to an H^+ concentration of 35–45 mEq/l. The regulation of acid–base balance involves, in order of speed of response, body buffers, respiratory function and renal function. In the proximal tubular cells, carbon dioxide, derived from cellular metabolism or diffusion from the tubular lumen, combines with water to form carbonic acid. This dissociates to H^+ and HCO_3^-. The H^+ is actively pumped into the tubular lumen and combines with filtered bicarbonate to form carbonic acid, which dissociates to water and CO_2. The CO_2 then diffuses back into the tubular cell to repeat the cycle. The net effect is that for each hydrogen ion excreted, one bicarbonate ion is retained, so that bicarbonate reserves are continuously regenerated.

$$CO_2 + H_2O \leftrightarrow H_2CO_3 \leftrightarrow H^+ + HCO_3^-$$

In mature subjects, bicarbonate is regenerated by this process to maintain a plasma concentration of about 25 mmol/l, but preterm babies have a lower threshold.[24] Hydrogen ions are excreted all along the nephron and combine with other bases, chiefly phosphate and ammonia, in the tubular fluid, when bicarbonate reabsorption is complete. In health, renal excretion is the only route for acid loss. Acid gain may arise from respiratory or metabolic disorders.

Acidosis

Acidosis may be respiratory, metabolic or mixed. In respiratory failure, carbon dioxide retention shifts the above equation to the right, with an increase in carbonic acid. Renal compensation is accomplished over a period of several days, by an increase in hydrogen ion excretion and bicarbonate regeneration. Blood gas analysis will reveal a compensated respiratory acidosis, with a high PCO_2, raised bicarbonate and a normal pH (Fig. 18.2).[53]

A metabolic acidosis is due to an increase in acid or a decrease in base. The most common cause for metabolic acidosis in neonatal intensive care is tissue hypoxia leading to lactic acidosis. Metabolic acidosis occurs with sepsis, renal failure, amino acid intolerance during parenteral nutrition, and in inborn errors of metabolism. Hyperchloraemia may occur with some parenteral nutrition formulations and should be considered in the investigation of metabolic acidosis. Chloride is predominantly an extracellular anion and the normal serum level is 90–110 mmol/l. Partly replacing chloride with acetate in parenteral nutrition reduces the risk of hyperchloraemic metabolic acidosis.[110]

In an otherwise normal subject, a fall in pH will stimulate hyperventilation, shift the carbonic acid equation to the left, and increase CO_2 elimination. The features of a compensated metabolic acidosis are a low bicarbonate, low PCO_2 and normal pH. Infants with both respiratory disease and a metabolic acidosis will show a mixed picture, with a high PCO_2, low bicarbonate and low pH. Renal tubular acidosis is discussed in Chapter 36.

Alkalosis

A metabolic alkalosis is caused by gain of base, as in the injudicious use of sodium bicarbonate, or loss of acid. Gastric acid loss

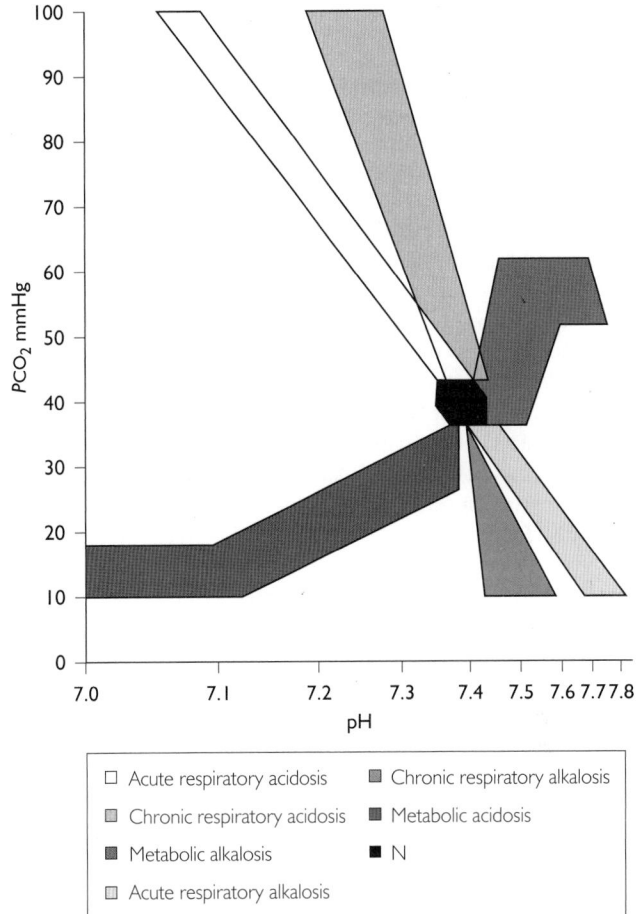

Fig. 18.2 Interpretation of changes in acid–base balance. (Adapted from Golberger.[53])

Table 18.1 Causes of metabolic alkalosis

Gastric loss	Vomiting, pyloric stenosis, high intestinal obstruction, continuous aspiration of gastric fluid
Excessive bicarbonate administration	Diuretic therapy, inadequate intake
Hypokalaemia	Diuretic therapy, diarrhoea
Hypochloraemia	
Adrenal hypersecretion	
Barrter's syndrome	

may occur in high intestinal obstruction. In the distal tubule and collecting duct, sodium is reabsorbed in exchange for either potassium or hydrogen ions, under the influence of aldosterone. If intracellular H^+ is low, potassium is preferentially lost, and vice versa. This explains the association between alkalosis and hypokalaemia. A metabolic alkalosis is often seen in chronic diuretic therapy. Causes of metabolic alkalosis are shown in Table 18.1. A respiratory alkalosis results from hyperventilation. The commonest cause in the neonatal unit is iatrogenic and occurs during assisted ventilation. Hyperventilation may also be seen in neurologically damaged infants and in rare conditions such as Leigh's disease and Joubert's disease.

Postnatal alterations in body water distribution

The size of the extracellular compartment decreases steadily throughout life, from around 65% of bodyweight at 26 weeks' gestation, to 40% at term and 20% by the age of 10 years (Fig. 18.3).[49,50] Superimposed on this gradual reduction, a more abrupt contraction of the extracellular compartment occurs shortly after birth[12,14,69,126,127,131] due to loss of interstitial fluid. This accounts, at least in part, for early postnatal weight loss. The onset of extracellular fluid loss is closely related to cardiopulmonary adaptation. Loss of extracellular fluid occurs rapidly in healthy babies but may be delayed in babies with respiratory distress syndrome (RDS).[98] Several studies now suggest that the contraction of the extracellular compartment is triggered by ANP released in response to increased atrial stretch as pulmonary vascular pressure falls[22,79,120,145] and left atrial venous return increases. The intravascular compartment may also be acutely expanded during birth by the reabsorption of lung liquid and the effect of a variable placental transfusion. As the timing of the diuresis/natriuresis is a consequence of the fall in pulmonary vascular pressure, it is not surprising that attempts to improve the course of RDS with diuretics have not shown benefit.[25]

A corollary of the isotonic loss of extracellular fluid is that net water and sodium balance in the first days after birth is negative (Fig. 18.4).[128] This is borne out by the observation that in newborn babies an increase in the intake of sodium leads to an increase in sodium excretion[82,114,127] until contraction of the extracellular compartment occurs. Sodium balance then becomes positive, commensurate with the need for growth. However, preterm babies have a limited, though variable, capacity to excrete a sodium load, so that, despite increasing excretion in response to an increase in intake, sodium retention occurs readily.[22,32] If there is concurrent restriction in the intake of water, these babies readily become hypernatraemic. This was demonstrated in a study by Shaffer & Meade[127] in which babies between 25 and 31 weeks' gestation were randomised to receive a sodium intake of 3 mmol/kg/day or 1 mmol/kg/day. The intake of water was restricted to 75 ml/kg/day on the first day, increasing by 10 ml/kg/day until day 5. In the former group, 50% became hypernatraemic, compared with 20% in the latter.

If a more liberal intake of water accompanies the intake of sodium, extracellular tonicity is maintained but the extracellular compartment expands. This is shown by weight gain at a time when weight loss is to be expected. In the majority of babies, this cumulative positive balance is subsequently lost, so that the normal postnatal change in body water distribution occurs but is delayed.[22] However, delayed loss of extracellular fluid increases the risk of later morbidity (vide infra). Exogenous surfactant administration has modified the natural history of RDS, but in the pre-surfactant era, it was well recognised that a diuresis/natriuresis[98] occurred at the time of improving respiratory function.

Insensible water loss

Insensible water loss occurs through the respiratory tract, in stool and across the skin. Stool water loss is small and usually less than

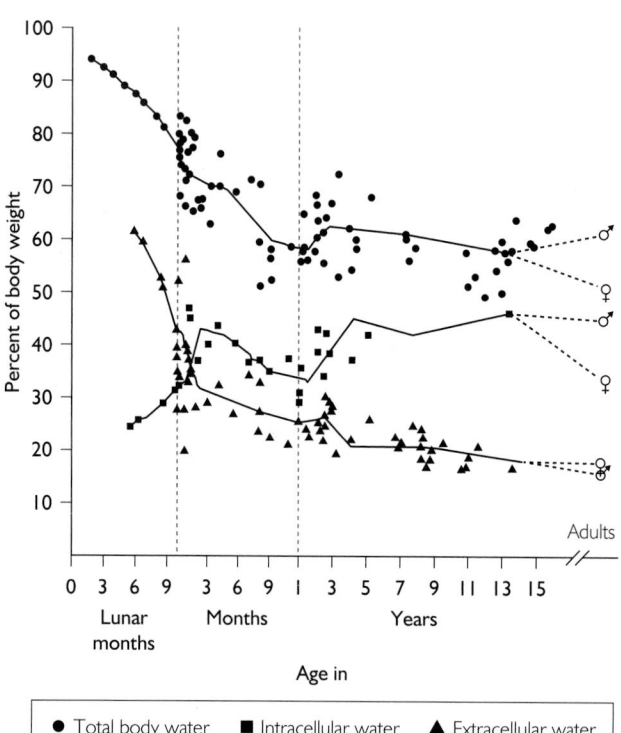

Fig. 18.3 Body water compartments as percentages of bodyweight from early fetal life to adult life. (Adapted from Friis-Hansen.[49])

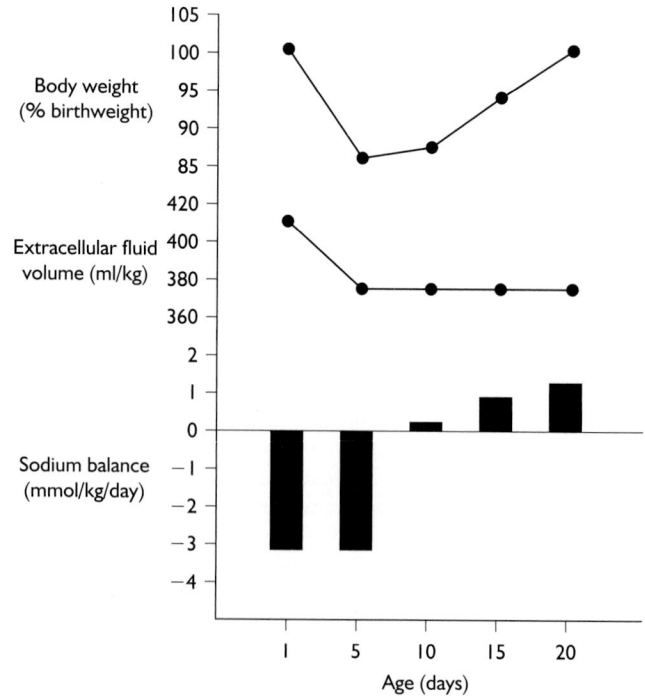

Fig. 18.4 Postnatal changes in bodyweight, extracellular volume and sodium balance. (Adapted from Shaffer & Weismann.[128])

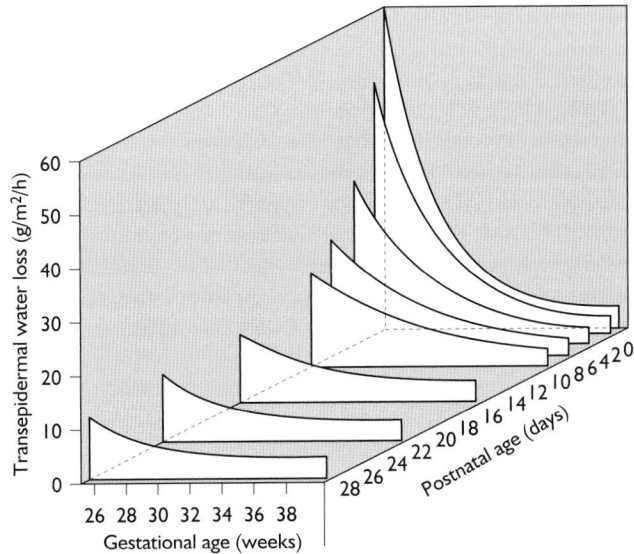

Fig. 18.5 Transepidermal water loss in relation to gestational age at birth at different postnatal ages in appropriate-for-gestational-age infants. (Adapted from Sedin et al.[124])

Table 18.2 Factors influencing insensible water loss

Increased loss	Lower gestational age
	Lower postnatal age
	Denuded/broken skin
	Increased skin temperature
	Activity
	Increased environmental temperature
	Radiant heat sources
	Radiant warmers
	Phototherapy units
	Draughts
	Crying
Decreased loss	Clothing
	High ambient humidity
	High humidity microenvironment
	Body box
	Plastic blanket
	Good skin care
	Topical ointment
	Humidification of inspired gases

5 ml/kg/24 h in the first days after birth, but losses from the respiratory tract may be high if inspired gases are not adequately humidified. The upper respiratory tract both warms and humidifies inspired gases, and full saturation (44 mg/l) is achieved by mid trachea. If the upper respiratory tract is bypassed with an endotracheal tube, respiratory water loss must be reduced by adequate humidification of inspired gases. Care must be taken when selecting humidifiers for use with neonatal ventilators, ensuring that this level of saturation is achieved within the operating temperature range.

Transepidermal water loss may be considerable in preterm babies and reflects both skin immaturity and the large surface area to weight ratio. In this population, the skin is an important determinant of water balance during the first days after birth. Sodium is not lost through the skin, because babies born below 36 weeks' gestation do not sweat, though this develops within the first 2 weeks after birth.[61]

The stratum corneum of the skin consists of overlapping, dead, epidermal cells that have been filled with keratin, a fibrous protein. This layer is the barrier to water loss. Although keratinisation begins at around 18 weeks' gestation, the fetal epidermis is still very thin at 26 weeks and the stratum corneum barely visible. During the last trimester, the epidermis and stratum corneum thicken and keratinisation becomes more marked.[45] Skin maturation, unlike the maturation of renal function, is accelerated by birth, and transepidermal loss falls exponentially with increasing gestational and postnatal age (Fig. 18.5).[57–59,124] After 32 weeks' gestation, water loss through the skin is low and has fallen to around 12 ml/kg/day.[122] Transepidermal loss is also influenced by ambient humidity, skin integrity, environmental and skin temperature, airspeed and radiant heat sources, including phototherapy (Table 18.2). Radiant heat sources can increase transepidermal water loss by a factor of up to 0.5–2.[122] Epidermal maturation is not accelerated by antenatal steroid therapy.[72]

In immature babies, the highest transepidermal losses occur during the first days after birth (Table 18.3). In the most vulnerable group, below 28 weeks' gestation, water lost through the skin may exceed urine volume, without adequate measures to decrease losses, when nursed naked under a radiant warmer. Each millilitre of water that evaporates from the skin is accompanied by the loss of 560 calories of heat, and so it is also difficult to keep a baby with a high transepidermal water loss warm. A high ambient humidity reduces transepidermal water loss and this effect is most marked in the most immature infants (Fig. 18.6). A decrease in ambient humidity from 60% to 20% will increase water lost through the skin by 100% in infants below 26 weeks'

Table 18.3 Transepidermal water loss at an ambient humidity of 50% (mean ± SD)[59]

Gestational age (weeks)	Postnatal age (days)					
	n	0–1	3	7	14	21	28
25–27	9	129 ± 39	71 ± 9	43 ± 9	32 ± 10	28 ± 10	24 ± 10
28–30	13	42 ± 13	32 ± 9	24 ± 7	18 ± 6	15 ± 6	15 ± 6
31–36	22	12 ± 5	12 ± 4	12 ± 4	9 ± 3	8 ± 2	7 ± 1
37–41	24	7 ± 2	6 ± 1	6 ± 1	6 ± 1	6 ± 0	7 ± 1

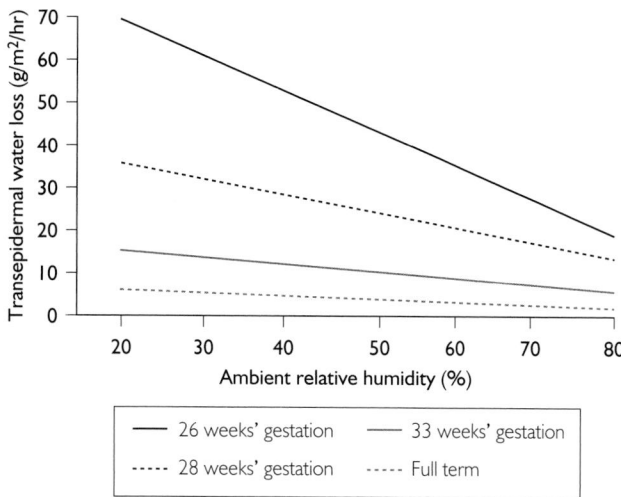

Fig. 18.6 The effect of ambient relative humidity on transepidermal water loss (based on the data of Hammarlund & Sedin[57]). (From Rutter.[122])

gestation.[57] Takahashi et al[140] showed that insensible water loss in infants weighing less than 1000 g is reduced to less than 40 ml/kg/day if ambient humidity is above 90%. Humidification is easier with an incubator, but a high humidity microenvironment well above 60% may be maintained immediately around a baby nursed under a radiant warmer by using bubblewrap or other plastic sheeting and a humidified body box. Draughts should be eliminated. Stripping of the stratum corneum and deeper abrasions of the skin can be reduced by using non-abrasive tape such as micropore, neonatal electrodes, and skin protectants, prior to affixing urine bags and transcutaneous oxygen electrodes.[27,46] Water-impermeable barriers, such as soft paraffin, or topical ointments reduce transepidermal water loss[109,150] but have only entered into use to a limited extent. An adequate provision of fluid is also necessary, using a system that allows the glucose delivery rate to be altered independently of fluid volume in order to avoid hyperglycaemia.[5]

The extent to which transepidermal water loss is reduced, hypernatraemic dehydration and hyperglycaemia avoided, and temperature stability maintained, may be regarded as an index of the overall quality of nursing and medical care and are useful measures for longitudinal audit.

Appropriate and inappropriate antidiuretic hormone secretion

The release of ADH (AVP) is stimulated by a rise in osmolality and by baroreceptors located in the heart and great vessels. ADH has two principal actions: it increases the reabsorption of water and it is a potent vasoconstrictor, contributing to the maintenance of blood pressure (BP). The pressor effect of ADH appears to be one of the mediators through which central arterial BP is maintained, and both hypovolaemia and hypotension will result in a rise in circulating ADH.[39] Under experimental conditions, a rise in ADH occurs when intravascular volume falls

by about 10%.[39] Little is known of setting of baroreceptor responses in the human preterm newborn, though Rees et al[113] described a doubling of urinary AVP after blood loss of the order of 10% in a 26-week, 800 g infant.

It has been suggested that the syndrome of inappropriate ADH secretion (SIADH) occurs frequently in the newborn.[113] Certainly, raised ADH levels and hyponatraemia are common in acutely ill infants. However, the maintenance of central BP overrides the defence of tonicity. This was clearly demonstrated in experiments on human volunteers in whom progressive salt depletion was induced by a salt-free diet and vigorous sweating[89] but water intake was unrestricted. Whole body sodium depletion was initially accompanied by isotonic contraction of the extracellular compartment and rapid weight loss. With increasing depletion of the intravascular compartment, baroreceptor-stimulated ADH-induced water reabsorption slowed down the rate of weight loss but at the cost of a fall in plasma osmolality. In such a situation, the release of ADH is not inappropriate for volume status. Evidence suggests that this effect underlies the impaired water excretion seen in ill infants. In a large prospective study, Gerigk et al[52] found that although plasma osmolality was lower in acutely ill infants and children, compared with a control group, both ADH and plasma renin activity (PRA) were raised, indicating activation of the RAAS. The intravenous infusion of isotonic saline resulted in a better reduction in ADH and PRA when compared with hypotonic saline and oral fluid. This suggests that ADH was appropriately elevated as a consequence of a reduced intravascular volume.

The recognition of an inadequate intravascular volume can be difficult. In the study by Gerigk et al[52] described above, only a third of infants and children had overt signs of dehydration. Newborn babies are at particular risk of intravascular volume depletion[151] from immediate cord clamping, which may lead to a reduction in blood volume by as much as 50% when compared with late clamping,[85] and subsequently from frequent blood sampling. As the normal range for BP in the newborn is wide and BP correlates poorly with blood volume,[9,13] BP measurements cannot be relied upon to detect hypovolaemia. Careful attention should be paid to assessment of the circulation using central venous pressure monitoring,[132] capillary-refill time, the core–peripheral temperature difference and Doppler echocardiographic assessments.[44,111] The core–peripheral temperature difference correlates with circulating AVP.[82]

Postoperatively, a low serum sodium concentration is usually a result of unrecognised intravascular volume depletion and continuing provision of salt-poor fluid, with ADH-driven water retention. The appropriate management of postoperative fluid balance includes circulatory support and the relative restriction of salt-poor fluid together with the adequate use of salt-containing fluid.[74] Normal saline, not colloid, is now considered the preferred fluid.[133] Once water retention and hyponatraemia have occurred, water restriction is necessary to correct the hyponatraemia safely. True inappropriate ADH secretion is probably rare in the newborn.[66] This diagnosis should be made only in accordance with the classic criteria of Bartter and Schwartz,[11] when hyponatraemia exists with normovolaemia, normal BP, normal renal and cardiac function, evidence of continuing sodium excretion, and urine that is not maximally dilute. In the newborn,

SIADH has been described in acute brain injury and central nervous system infection and following maternal substance abuse.[154]

In pathological circumstances such as heart or liver failure, hypotension occurs together with an expanded extracellular compartment and there is whole body sodium excess despite hyponatraemia. Myocardial dysfunction, whether arising from ischaemia, metabolic acidosis, immaturity or other cause, is increasingly recognised during neonatal intensive care and may contribute to impaired water excretion. Hyponatraemia is also commonly observed in infants with chronic lung disease (CLD), often with clinical signs suggestive of an expanded extracellular compartment. Whole body sodium may be depleted by chronic diuretic therapy but levels of ADH are raised and free water clearance reduced.[68] It is possible that in this situation abnormal transmural pressure gradients lead to effective central hypotension, increased AVP release and impaired water excretion. During acute episodes of respiratory failure associated with air trapping, a decrease in central venous return, pulmonary blood flow and left atrial filling will lead to a similar situation.[112] However, the aetiology of disordered salt and water balance in CLD is inadequately understood. Pulmonary hypertension, initially reversible, is an almost invariable accompaniment of CLD, and fluid retention may be attributable to cor pulmonale, though cardiac performance may be impaired by other factors such as dexamethasone therapy.[23,60]

Pharmacological influences on fluid balance

Indometacin (indomethacin)

Indometacin is a prostaglandin synthetase inhibitor that is commonly used to facilitate the closure of a symptomatic patent ductus arteriosus (PDA). It is also administered antenatally as a tocolytic, and to reduce liquor volume in polyhydramnios. In older subjects it is known to reduce sodium excretion and urine flow by enhancing tubular reabsorption, but in addition to this there have been anxieties that it may lower GFR in preterm infants. This difference may reflect the dependence of these subjects on renal prostaglandins to maintain an adequate renal blood flow in the face of high RAAS activity; a parallel can be seen in a study in dogs, where indometacin was shown to induce a fall in GFR only when RAAS activity was increased by sodium depletion.[106] Conversely, there is also evidence to suggest that inhibition of prostaglandin synthesis has no effect on renal blood flow.[7] Walker et al[149] studying the chronically catheterised fetal sheep, describe the amelioration of the oliguric response to indometacin in the presence of an AVP V2-receptor antagonist. They speculate that indometacin stimulates the release of AVP, resulting in oliguria.

A temporary reduction of sodium and water excretion is described in all reports of babies given indometacin for duct closure. In the early days of its use, salt and water retention and dilutional hyponatraemia were a common occurrence. The simultaneous administration of 1 mg/kg of furosemide (frusemide) has been shown to eliminate the renal side effects of 0.3 mg/kg indometacin without reducing its efficacy in duct closure.[156]

In a randomised controlled trial, similar claims for concurrent dopamine therapy were found to be unsubstantiated.[47] If indometacin is to be used in a dose of 0.2 mg/kg, 12 hourly, it is appropriate to restrict sodium and water intake by approximately 30% and monitor fluid balance carefully. Smaller doses of 0.1 mg/kg, 24 hourly, as suggested by Rennie & Cooke[116] are less likely to result in adverse renal effects. Ibuprofen is entering into use as an alternative to indometacin, though oligohydramnios and neonatal renal failure have been described after maternal exposure to ibuprofen.[16,75]

Steroids

The synthetic glucocorticoids dexamethasone and betamethasone are widely used in perinatal medicine, antenatally to promote fetal lung maturation and postnatally in the management of CLD. These drugs have a number of potent actions on several organ systems. They are gene transducers as well as having direct effects at the level of the cell membrane. They increase β_2 receptor density, antioxidant levels and the density of Na^+/K^+-ATPase, affect a variety of cytokines and growth factors, enhance surfactant production, increase clearance of lung liquid, and suppress inducible nitric oxide synthase. Glucocorticoids are also catabolic agents. A temporary inhibition in growth is well documented during therapy and this often results in a rise in blood urea.

The abundance of Na^+/K^+-ATPase is regulated by glucocorticoids[28] in an age-dependent manner.[29] In rats, betamethasone will increase Na^+/K^+-ATPase mRNA in the kidney during infancy, but not during fetal life, nor in adults. In contrast, lung tissue Na^+/K^+-ATPase is maximally induced by glucocorticoids during the perinatal period. The inference is that glucocorticoids interact with other transcriptional factors, expressed in an age-dependent fashion, to activate the genes for Na^+/K^+-ATPase so that different tissues have different periods of sensitivity to glucocorticoid regulation. Glucocorticoids enhance renal tubular regulation of sodium balance, potentiate ANP stimulation of cGMP production,[64] and enhance the maturation of renal acidification.[15] In addition to the well-known effects on the lungs, antenatal exposure to dexamethasone accelerates the maturation of renal function in human preterm newborns[4] and induces both Na^+/K^+-ATPase and Na^+ channels in lung epithelial cells, thus facilitating the clearance of lung liquid.[104] This may underlie the seemingly paradoxical effect of glucocorticoids in triggering a diuresis in the fluid-retaining baby with CLD.[55,123]

Inotropic agents

Dopamine and dobutamine are now frequently used in neonatal intensive care to support BP and cardiac output, and also for their purported renal effects at low dose. In addition to cardiovascular effects which influence renal function, dopamine has direct renal actions, inhibiting renal Na^+/K^+-ATPase and Na^+H^+ exchanger activity and attenuating the actions of aldosterone and AVP.[125] The cellular signalling system that transduces the signal from activated dopamine receptors to inhibit renal Na^+/K^+-ATPase undergoes developmental regulation.[51]

Three randomised clinical studies[56,78,119] comparing the efficacy of dopamine and dobutamine all showed that dopamine is more effective at raising and maintaining BP than dobutamine. However, in only one of these studies was left ventricular output measured as well and this showed that dopamine did not increase cardiac output in contrast to dobutamine, which produced a mean increase in left ventricular output of 21%.[119] Seri et al[125] showed that dopamine at a dose of 2 micrograms/kg/min induced maximal diuresis and natriuresis in sick preterm neonates if systemic BP was within the normal range. An increase to 4 micrograms/kg/min resulted in a further increase in BP, but no change in urine output and sodium excretion. As dopamine raises BP through its vasoconstrictor actions, renal perfusion may in fact be impaired at higher doses.

Three trials to determine whether dopamine therapy may prevent indometacin-mediated deterioration in renal function in the preterm newborn infant have been included in a Cochrane review. Though dopamine improved urine output, there was no evidence of effect on serum creatinine or the incidence of oliguria.[10]

Low-dose dopamine has commonly been administered to critically ill adult patients with evidence of renal dysfunction, because, in healthy volunteers, low-dose dopamine increases renal blood flow and induces natriuresis and diuresis. Renal ischaemia is the commonest cause of acute renal failure in this patient group and the hope has been that low-dose dopamine, by increasing renal blood flow, might help preserve renal cellular oxygenation, GFR and urine output. However, dopamine is also a proximal-tubular diuretic, so it increases the presentation and reabsorption of chloride by the ascending limb of the loop of Henlé, an effect that may increase medullary oxygen consumption and exacerbate medullary ischaemia. In a recent large randomised trial in critically ill adult patients, low-dose dopamine (2 micrograms/kg/min) did not protect against renal dysfunction.[20] To date, there is only limited evidence that low-dose dopamine (3–5 micrograms/kg/min) improves urine output in very immature infants.[41]

Clinical implications of postnatal and developmental changes

The first days after birth

The principles that govern the management of sodium and water balance during the period of postnatal adaptation differ from those that govern subsequent management. Early fluid management, during the period of postnatal adaptation, should permit an isotonic contraction of the extracellular compartment and a brief period of negative sodium and water balance. Extracellular water overload increases the risks and severity of respiratory illness in the newborn,[62,100,117,129,130] and weight gain in the first days after birth, in babies with RDS, is associated with an increased risk of developing CLD.[147]

Routine sodium administration in parenteral fluid will promote the retention of extracellular fluid, including pulmonary interstitial fluid, and in infants requiring intensive care, should be avoided until the physiological postnatal diuresis/natriuresis[22,98] is underway. If this point is indeterminate, sodium administration should be deferred until postnatal weight loss has occurred.[12,131,143] There is no 'correct' figure for postnatal weight loss, as hydration at birth is variable[142] and birthweight does not correlate closely with extracellular water volume.[126] The baby with RDS may be regarded as a model of delayed postnatal maturation in whom the postnatal diuresis is delayed. In contrast, in the healthy preterm baby, postnatal cardiopulmonary adaptation occurs over the same rapid timescale as in a full-term baby.

The immediate administration of 'maintenance' sodium in parenteral fluid is unnecessary and adversely affects respiratory outcome. Costarino et al[32] first provided some evidence for this approach in a blind trial comparing sodium restriction in the first 5 days after birth with sodium administration of 3–4 mmol/kg/day from birth. Water was prescribed independently. Extracellular volume was not measured, nor were the babies weighed in this study, but sodium balance was positive in the sodium-supplemented group on the first day after birth and this group had a significantly higher incidence of bronchopulmonary dysplasia (BPD). Antenatal glucocorticoid therapy induces maturation of sodium excretion and confers partial protection against the adverse consequences of early sodium administration. However, even in infants exposed to antenatal steroids, early sodium administration increases the risk of adverse respiratory outcome. This was shown by Hartnoll et al[62] in a blinded, randomised controlled trial in which infants born at 25–30 weeks' gestation received a parenteral sodium intake of 4 mmol/kg/day either from the first day after birth or when a weight loss of 6% had occurred. Extracellular fluid volume was measured at birth and on day 14. A significant reduction in extracellular fluid volume was observed in the group who received the delayed intake of sodium, in contrast to the early-intake group, in whom no reduction was seen. By the end of the first week, 35% of babies in the delayed-intake group and 8.7% of the early-intake group, and by 28 days after birth, 40% of the delayed-intake group compared with 18% of the early-intake group, no longer required additional oxygen. There was no difference between the groups in the rate of reduction in pulmonary artery pressure,[63] suggesting that the poorer respiratory outcome in the early-intake group was not attributable to delayed cardiopulmonary adaptation but rather to persistent expansion of the extracellular compartment and delayed clearance of pulmonary interstitial fluid.

Water should be provided in an intake sufficient to allow the excretion of a relatively small initial renal solute load[157] and to maintain tonicity in the face of initially high, but rapidly falling, transepidermal losses. In very immature babies, the principal determinant of water requirement in the first days after birth is the magnitude of insensible water loss, and every effort should be made to reduce this to a minimum. Although negative water balance is the physiological norm during this period, the provision of sodium-free fluid, and hence compromise in the extent to which nutrition can be delivered, does not have to be restricted in order to achieve this. Although babies who are hypoxaemic and hypovolaemic may have reduced glomerular filtration, this is not the case for infants with stable clinical parameters.[97] Observations of the effects of positive airway pressure in newborn animals with normal lungs should not be extrapolated to babies with non-compliant lungs. In the former, but not the latter, high inflation pressures will be transmitted to the intrathoracic contents, affecting venous return and altering intrarenal blood flow[101] and glomerular filtration.[48] As discussed above, ADH-driven water retention is a more common cause of impaired water excretion than is renal diluting capacity.

Early postnatal weight loss reflects both the loss of body water and the loss or gain of body solids. As nutritional support for sick preterm babies improves, it is likely that early postnatal weight loss will be diminished, though body water will still be lost to the same extent. This was shown in a study comparing healthy preterm babies with a group with RDS, during the first week after birth. Both groups lost an identical amount of body water, namely 10% of the total body water content at birth. However, the healthy babies lost a maximum of 5.9% of birthweight, in contrast to 8.6% in the RDS group. This was because, although both groups gained in body solids during the period of weight loss, the healthy babies, who received a higher energy intake, gained solids to a significantly greater extent (Fig. 18.7).[143]

Neonatal paediatricians have long been concerned about 'excessive fluid intake'. Associations have been described between high fluid intakes and increased risk of symptomatic PDA,[19,136] necrotising enterocolitis (NEC)[18] and BPD.[26,32,76,141,147] Though an expanded intravascular compartment might exacerbate left-to-right shunting through a PDA, Reller et al[115] found no benefit from a reduced fluid intake in preterm infants. It is also plausible that interstitial oedema is implicated in the pathogenesis of NEC and BPD. On the basis of a systematic review of four randomised trials,[19,87,141,148] only one of which found a significant reduction in the subsequent diagnosis of a PDA and no overall difference in BPD, Bell & Accaregui[17] recommend 'careful restriction' of fluid intake. Though the aim of this systematic review was to examine the effects of differences in water intake, sodium intake was not controlled in these studies, so that increased 'fluid' meant an increased intake of both sodium and water. A large body of evidence suggests that it is the increased intake of sodium and resulting expansion of the extracellular compartment, and not an 'excessive' intake of water, that is responsible for the increase in morbidity.

The growing infant

Growth is of paramount importance in the newborn baby. Once the phase of immediate postnatal adaptation is over, the management of fluid and electrolyte balance must be tailored to the demands of growth. It is questionable whether stepwise increments in parenteral nutrition are necessary once postnatal weight loss has been achieved, since healthy preterm babies are capable of excreting large volumes of water.[33,97] Enteral feeds may be commenced concurrently.

Sodium is a permissive factor for growth, and a deficiency inhibits DNA synthesis in the most immature cells.[108] Chronic limitation of intake is associated not only with extracellular volume contraction and poor weight gain, but also with poor skeletal and tissue growth[30,65,67,152] and adverse neurodevelopmental outcome.[65] Human milk will provide a daily sodium intake of about 1 mmol/kg bodyweight, which, if retained, is sufficient

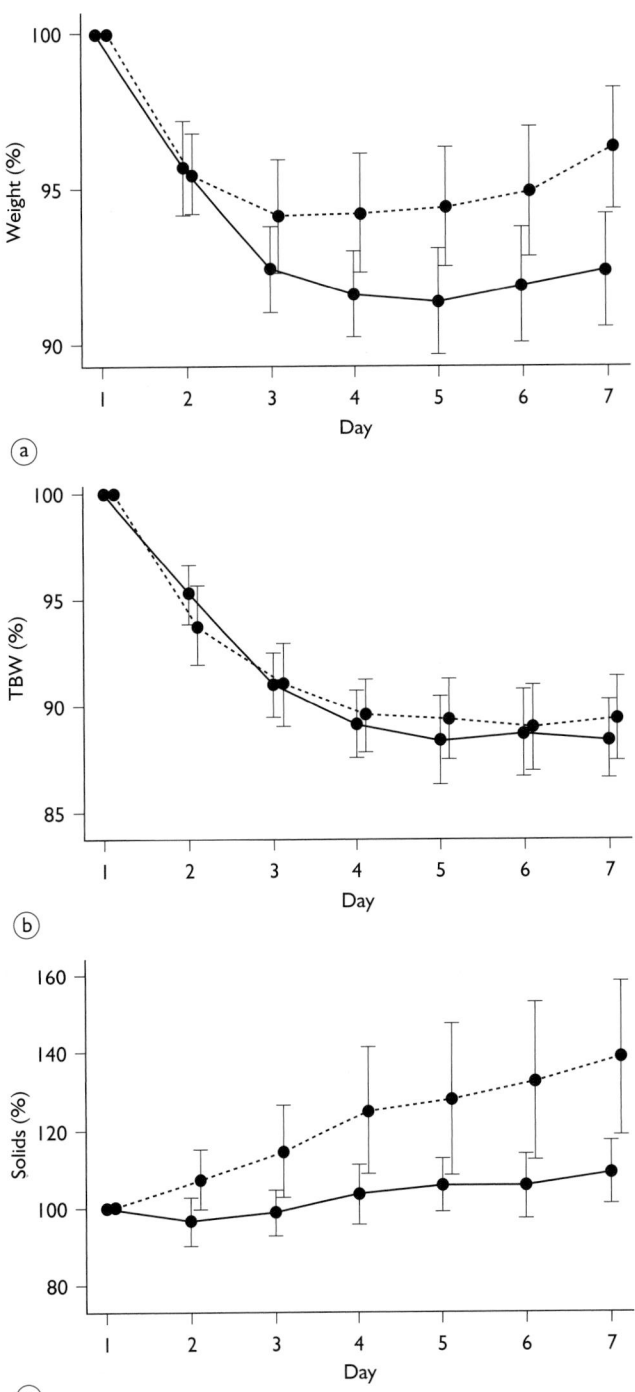

Fig. 18.7 Weight, total body water and body solids during the first week after birth in healthy preterm babies (dotted line) and babies with respiratory distress syndrome (solid line). Values (mean ± 95% CI) are expressed as a percentage of the value at birth. (Adapted from Tang et al.[143])

for normal growth. The full-term baby is able to do so virtually completely, by both renal tubular and intestinal reabsorption. However, extremely immature babies require a sodium intake of at least 4 mmol/kg/day, or more if, for example, they are on treatment with xanthines or other diuretics, in order to ensure the retention of 1 mmol/kg/day.[67] In babies below 36 weeks' gestation, commence full sodium administration at 4 mmol/kg/day once 5% weight loss has been achieved.

If preterm babies are fed unsupplemented or unfortified breast milk, chronic sodium depletion will be revealed in the first instance by poor weight gain. Sodium administration at 4 mmol/kg/day should continue until around 32–34 weeks postmenstrual age, by which time maturation of sodium conservation should have occurred.[3,118] It is not known whether continued administration at this dose beyond this postmenstrual age is harmful and might, for example, increase the risk of later hypertension.

Constructing a fluid prescription

Didactic recommendations for fluid prescriptions are inappropriate, given variations in gestational age, ambient humidity, nursing practices and clinical condition. With an understanding of the principles involved, it is a straightforward matter to construct an initial prescription when a newborn baby is admitted to an intensive care unit. First make a judgement of the likely magnitude of insensible water loss, taking into account sources of radiant heat, ambient humidity, humidification of inspired gases, respiratory rate, and gestational and postnatal age, using the information presented in Figures 18.5 and 18.6 and Tables 18.2 and 18.3. A rational *initial* intravenous volume prescription would be the sum of an allowance for urinary water of 30–60 ml/kg/day PLUS estimated insensible water loss (Table 18.4).[96] Glucose delivery should commence at around 7 mg/kg/min. For example, insensible water loss in an infant below 1000 g birthweight, during the first week after birth, will be of the order of 40 ml/kg/day when ambient humidity exceeds 90%,[140] but around 100 ml/kg/day in 40% humidity. The initial volume necessary might therefore be anything from 70 to 160 ml/kg/day. If insensible water losses are predicted to be high, for example during the period immediately after delivery when the baby is under a radiant warmer as lines are being inserted and the baby is being stabilised, start with a high intake but reduce this once a stable high-humidity microenvironment is established. As neither transepidermal water loss, the integrity of renal function nor the timing of the postnatal natriuresis/diuresis can be predicted precisely, the adequacy of the estimate must be assessed within 6–8 hours.

It is important to ensure that blood glucose levels remain stable. The use of a single solution containing a fixed concentration of glucose will obviously increase the chances of hypoglycaemia or hyperglycaemia if the volume of fluid administered cannot be altered independently. The use of 5% and 50% glucose solutions delivered through a Y connection allows both the glucose delivery rate and the volume infused to be readily altered independently.[5] For example, a 10% solution will provide a glucose delivery rate of 4.8 mg/kg/min at 70 ml/kg/24 h and 9.7 mg/kg/min at 140 ml/kg/24 h. A constant glucose delivery rate of, for example, 7 mg/kg/min, could be achieved by the infusion of 5% glucose at 2.3 ml/kg/h with 50% glucose at 0.6 ml/kg/h (for a total of 70 ml/kg/24 h) or 5% glucose at 5.5 ml/kg/h with 50% glucose at 0.3 ml/kg/h (for 140 ml/kg/24 h). If the blood glucose rises, the glucose delivery rate may be reduced to 5 mg/kg/min without altering the total volume infused, by altering the proportion of 5% and 50% glucose to 2.6 ml/kg/h and 0.3 ml/kg/h or 5.8 ml/kg/h and 0 ml/kg/h, to deliver 70 ml/kg/24 h or 140 ml/kg/24 h respectively.

The aims of fluid management in preterm infants with RDS are outlined in Table 18.5. The principles underlying the management of fluid balance in other common situations in neonatal intensive care are outlined in Table 18.6.

Monitoring fluid balance

Fluid balance should be monitored meticulously in sick newborn babies requiring intensive care. All too often, a failure to detect a problem in its early stages leads to a potentially reversible situation becoming irreversible. Good monitoring is the responsibility of both medical and nursing staff. The serum sodium, potassium and creatinine should be assessed regularly, urine output carefully measured and the baby weighed daily (Table 18.7). As concentrations at birth reflect maternal concentrations, a baseline measure of serum creatinine, sodium and potassium

Table 18.4 Estimated starting intravenous intake, at an ambient humidity of 50% [A]

Gestational age (weeks)	Birthweight (kg)	Approximate[124] transepidermal water loss (ml/kg/24 h)	Allowance for urine output (ml/kg/24 h)	Estimated intake range (ml/kg/24 h)	Suggested starting[Y] volume (ml/kg/24 h)
<27	<1.0	120	30–60	150–180	150*[A]
27–30	1.0–1.5	40	30–60	70–100	90
31–36	1.5–2.5	15	30–60	45–75	60
>36	>2.5	10	30–60	40–70	60

* The most immature infants are particularly at risk of renal impairment, and a cautious approach, commencing at the lower end of the estimated requirement, is recommended.

[A] At higher ambient humidities, transepidermal water losses will be reduced and requirements will be lower.

[Y] Once sustained weight loss of at least 5% is achieved, proceed to the intravenous volume necessary to support nutritional goals without stepwise increments.

Table 18.5 Aims of fluid balance management in preterm babies with respiratory distress syndrome

Reduce insensible water loss to a minimum	Provide high humidity via incubator or deliver to microenvironment; use bubblewrap, plastic blanket or body box; meticulous skin care; draught elimination
Facilitate early postnatal loss of extracellular interstitial fluid	Reduce the early intake of sodium to a minimum
Maintain glucose homeostasis	Use a volume-independent, variable glucose delivery system
Optimise nutritional support	Early provision of parenteral and minimal enteral nutrition
Maintain renal perfusion	Monitor blood pressure, core–peripheral temperature gap, capillary refill time, urine output, cardiac performance and central venous pressure; use volume and inotropic support as necessary

should be obtained on admission in order to be able to interpret subsequent levels. Nursing charts should be designed so that hourly intake and output volumes can be recorded clearly. Satisfactory management is marked by a urine flow rate of at least 0.5–1 ml/kg/h on the first day, rising to 2–3 ml/kg/h thereafter, daily weight loss of the order of 1–2%, followed by weight gain of the order of 14–16 g/kg/day once an adequate nutritional intake has been achieved, a steady fall in serum creatinine, and electrolyte concentrations within the normal range (Table 18.7).

Serum creatinine

Creatinine is derived from the turnover of phosphocreatine in muscle and is excreted in the urine. At steady state, creatinine excretion is an indirect measure of muscle mass. In everyday clinical practice, the serum creatinine is used as an index of GFR. The serum creatinine at birth is a reflection of the maternal concentration. Subsequently this changes at a rate based on the balance between creatinine production rate, dependent on muscle mass,[99] and clearance rate, dependent on GFR, which in turn varies with postconceptional age (Fig. 18.8). The wide range of values seen for serum creatinine against postnatal age is

Table 18.6 Common clinical problems in fluid balance management

Respiratory distress syndrome	Starting infusion volume dependent on magnitude of anticipated insensible water loss. Delay intravenous sodium administration until after the postnatal diuresis/natriuresis has commenced and steady weight loss is underway
Patent ductus arteriosus	Fluid restriction is inappropriate unless there is evidence of heart failure as this will compromise nutrition. Indometacin toxicity is exacerbated by dehydration
Severe birth asphyxia at term	Anticipate possibility of renal failure. Initially restrict salt-free intake to 20–30ml/kg/day until renal function can be assessed. Optimise renal perfusion. Central vascular access may be necessary for infusion of hypertonic dextrose
Chronic lung disease	Avoid prolonged periods of fluid restriction as poor nutrition will worsen prognosis. If diuretics are necessary, be wary of chronic sodium depletion that will further compromise growth
Necrotising enterocolitis	Third-space fluid losses may be considerable and the interpretation of an acute change in body weight is difficult. Profound intravascular volume depletion may be present without weight loss
Postoperative	Reduce salt-poor fluid by 30%. Unrecognised hypovolaemia is common and may contribute to postoperative hyponatraemia if there is inadequate support with salt-containing fluid

Table 18.7 Monitoring fluid balance in intensive care

Weight	Daily	Steady initial loss of 1–2% daily; maximum weight loss variable but usually in the range of 5–10%; weight gain should have commenced by 7–10 days
Urine output	Continuously	Review 4–8 hourly; should exceed 0.5 ml/kg/h on day 1 in extremely preterm infants; thereafter, >2–3 ml/kg/h in all infants; <1 ml/kg/h requires investigation of renal impairment
Serum sodium	Daily or twice daily	132–144 mmol/l
Serum potassium	Daily or twice daily	3.8–5.7 mmol/l; spurious elevation due to haemolysis common
Serum creatinine	Daily	Should see steady decline after birth

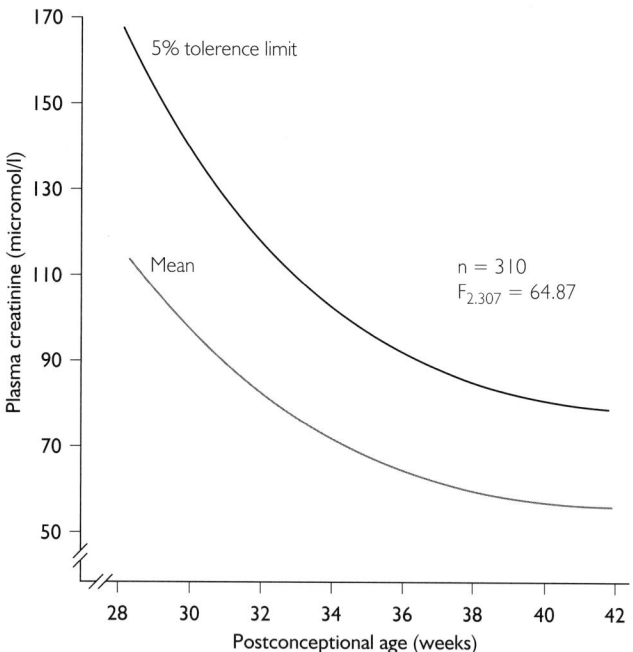

Fig. 18.8 Normal ranges for plasma creatinine by postconceptional age. (Adapted from Trompeter et al.[144])

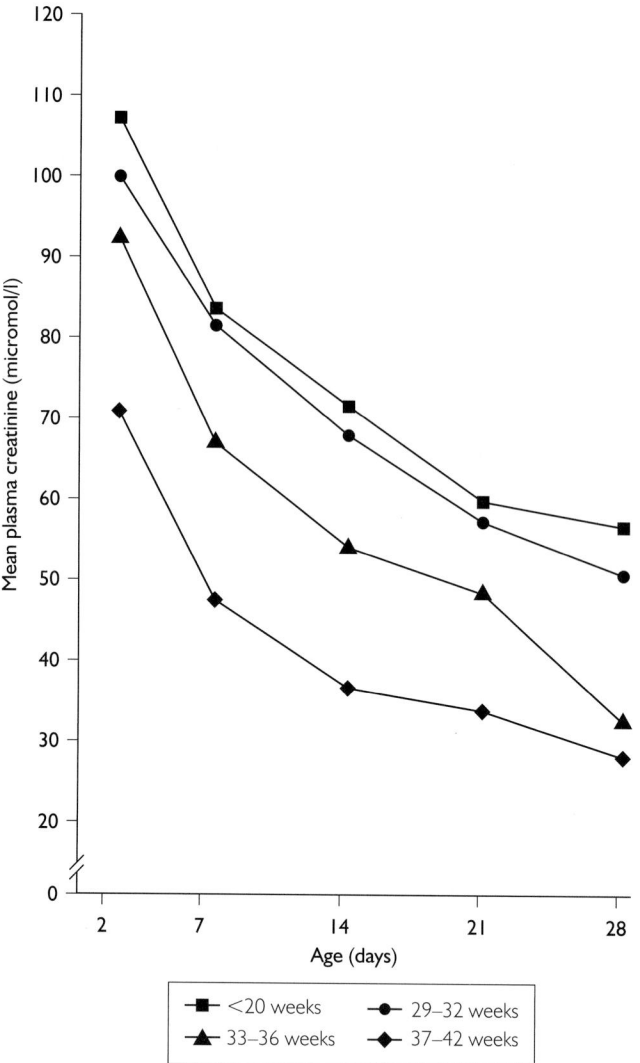

Fig. 18.9 Relationship between plasma creatinine and postnatal age in different gestational age groups. (Adapted from Rudd et al.[121])

due predominantly to the large variation that exists in weight for postconceptional age.

In the first weeks after birth, serum creatinine falls, initially exponentially as the maternally derived creatinine load is excreted, then more gradually.[121] A single measure of serum creatinine provides no more than a crude estimate of renal function and observing the change over days is of more help. A useful clinical pointer to renal insufficiency is a failure to see the expected postnatal decline in serum creatinine (Fig. 18.9). In the neonate, a sustained rise in serum creatinine or a failure to fall, is indicative of a reduced GFR. The blood urea is of little value in the assessment of renal function in the newborn as it is influenced by numerous non-renal factors. For example, an elevated blood urea may result from sequestered blood in the gastrointestinal tract (GIT) or be due to catabolism during treatment with dexamethasone, despite normal renal function.

Alterations in body weight

The importance of accurate, daily weighing as part of the assessment of fluid balance in babies requiring intensive care cannot be overemphasised. Isotonic expansion of the extracellular compartment can, and frequently does, occur in the preterm neonate. This will be missed if changes in bodyweight are not considered in conjunction with serum electrolytes. If a newborn baby gains weight in the first days after birth at a time when weight loss would be anticipated and the serum sodium concentration is normal, isotonic expansion of the extracellular compartment has occurred and sodium balance in these babies is positive, at a time when it should be negative.[22]

Conversely, poor growth, in the face of an adequate energy intake, may reflect chronic sodium depletion and this may occur with a normal or low-normal serum sodium concentration. Electronic scales, accurate to at least 5 g, are required. The net weight should be documented, taking into account the weights of attachments, as these may vary substantially from day to day for babies in intensive care. There are preliminary indications that bioelectrical impedance analysis may be helpful in the longitudinal assessment of body water compartments in neonates and may be particularly useful when clinical instability of the baby precludes weighing.[146]

Urinary indices

The fraction of filtered sodium excreted (Fe_{Na}) and urinary sodium concentration rise transiently during the postnatal natriuresis and then fall with postnatal age. Values for the former, in babies between 25–34 weeks' gestation, in the first week after birth, often exceed 5%. The median urinary sodium concentration is around 80 mmol/l. The fractional sodium excretion is often

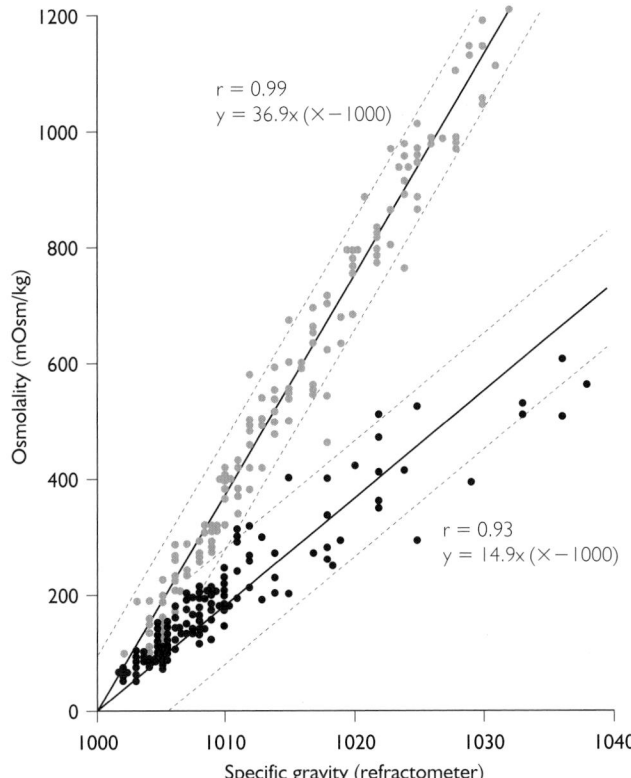

Fig. 18.10 Relationship between specific gravity and urinary osmolality in newborn infants (●) and older children (●). Dotted lines show 95% prediction limits for individual observations. (Adapted from Benitez et al.[21])

Table 18.8 Protein excretion in the newborn[37]

Gestational age (weeks)	Number of subjects	Protein excretion (mg/m²/24h)	
		Mean	Range
<28	5	21	4.8–31
30	12	50	0–226
32	15	56	0–125
34	15	60	0–314
36	17	30	0–110
40	26	31	0–146

Dark brown or red urine usually suggests haematuria, but may be caused by bile pigments, haemoglobin, rifampicin, porphyrins or urates. Urine microscopy is necessary to detect red blood cells, leukocytes and casts. Red blood cell casts imply renal parenchymal pathology. Haematuria may occur in renovascular disease, cortical and tubular necrosis, neoplasia, obstructive uropathy, coagulopathy, nephritis and infection. A clean catch or suprapubic aspirate of urine should contain less than five white blood cells.[86] Leukocyturia is most often caused by infection, but pyrexia or any inflammatory process may also be responsible. Newborns normally excrete small amounts of protein (Table 18.8).[37] The heaviest proteinuria is seen in congenital nephrotic syndrome.

Urine flow rate

As neonates do not empty their bladders completely on voiding and as 7% fail to void during the first 24 hours after birth, external urine collections of short duration may be inaccurate. Urine can easily be collected into adhesive urine bags in boys, but with more difficulty in girls. Self-adhesive urine bags in a wide variety of different sizes and designs are now commercially available. In order to protect the skin and prevent breakdown, it is important to 'prep' the skin first and to use a suitable medical adhesive if necessary. Repeated application, because of poor adhesion, rapidly leads to excoriation of the delicate skin around the groin. Many urine bags are designed for once-only use and cannot be emptied through an integral port. If so, ensure that urine can be aspirated without having to remove the bag, by inserting a soft feeding tube into the bag before application. Collection into pre-weighed nappies or cotton wool balls is widely practised, but can be misleading, as evaporation, leading to volume loss and increased osmolality, may be appreciable.[153] Catheterisation is a practicable option even in the tiniest of babies.

Given a diluting and concentrating capacity that extends from 50 to 600 mOsm/kg and a daily renal solute load of approximately 10–15 mOsm/kg,[158] the maximum and minimum urine flow rates that preterm infants can achieve are 300 and 25 ml/kg/24 h, respectively. The latter value, which represents the minimum urine flow rate beyond which solute retention would result, approximates to 1 ml/kg/h and is the justification

used in the evaluation of the oliguric infant and is discussed further below. 'Spot' urinary sodium concentrations bear no relationship to daily sodium balance and are of little use in determining the cause of hyponatraemia.

Well, preterm infants are able to achieve a minimum urine osmolality of around 50 mOsm/kg,[33,158] and infants with RDS, around 90 mOsm/kg.[94] Maximum osmolality is of the order of 600–800 mOsm/kg, though higher values exceeding 1000 mOsm/kg are occasionally seen. A urine osmolality that lies between 200 and 400 mOsm/kg usually suggests that fluid intake is satisfactory. However, as immature babies in the first days after birth may have even more limited concentrating abilities, these infants may become dehydrated while continuing to pass urine of low osmolality. Specific gravity is often measured in place of osmolality as it can easily be performed on the ward. The presence of glucose or protein (both often found in samples from sick preterm babies) will, however, falsely elevate the specific gravity. In addition, the relationship between specific gravity, as measured with a refractometer, and osmolality differs between the newborn and older children, so that in the newborn, an osmolality of 400 is indicative of a specific gravity anywhere between 1020 and 1030 (Fig. 18.10).[21] Reagent strip test measurement of urinary specific gravity is unsatisfactory.[54]

Dipstick urinalysis may be used as a screening test for proteinuria, haematuria and glycosuria. Bilirubin causes dark-yellow to brown discoloration and suggests a conjugated hyperbilirubinaemia.

for the use of this figure as a clinical indication of renal failure. Extremely immature infants have considerably smaller solute loads on the first day after birth, and in these infants it may be more appropriate to regard a urine flow rate of less than 0.5 ml/kg/h on day 1 and 1 ml/kg/h thereafter, as abnormal. Leake et al[83] showed that babies between 28 and 34 weeks' gestation could increase urine flow rate to a mean of 12 ml/kg/h during acute increases in infusion rates to 250 ml/kg/day. Extremely immature preterm babies, in whom minimum urine osmolality is of the order of 90 mOsm/kg, will be able to achieve a urine flow rate of around 7 ml/kg/h.[33]

Common clinical problems

Disorders of sodium concentration

Changes in the serum sodium concentration reflect both sodium and water balance. In hypernatraemic states there is an absolute or relative deficit of water in relation to body sodium. Conversely, in hyponatraemia, there is relative or absolute excess of body water. In both hypernatraemia and hyponatraemia, total body sodium may be increased, decreased or unchanged. Common situations in which hyponatraemia occurs in the neonate are listed in Table 18.9. It is a reasonable assumption that hyponatraemia and hypernatraemia contribute to neurological morbidity in sick newborn babies, though quantification of the effect, particularly in preterm babies, is difficult. Brain cell volume is affected by acute changes in extracellular tonicity. The regulation of cell volume following cell swelling or shrinkage in response to changes in extracellular tonicity is brought about by the accumulation or loss of inorganic ions and organic solutes. Compensatory changes in electrolyte content occur rapidly, so that during acute exposure to hypertonicity, there is a rapid movement of electrolytes into the cell, in favour of water retention. Adaptation to chronic hyperosmolar states occurs by increasing the concentration of intracellular organic osmolytes.[137] These include polyols (sorbitol, myo-inositol), certain amino acids (taurine, alanine, proline) and methylamines (betaine, glycerylphosphorylcholine).

Loss of organic osmolytes occurs more slowly than movement of electrolytes. Thus, if chronic hyperosmolality is corrected rapidly, the influx of water into the cell continues, resulting in cell swelling and cerebral oedema. Cell swelling can lead to occlusion of blood flow, hypoxia and release of cytoxic neuroexcitatory amino acids. Conversely, an acute fall in serum sodium concentration will first lead to the movement of water into cells and the development of intracellular oedema and brain swelling. Over a period of time, the concentration of intracellular osmolytes decreases, so as to favour the movement of water out of the cell. If extracellular hypotonicity is then corrected rapidly, the continued movement of water out of the cell will result in brain shrinkage.

Although the time-scale over which the human brain adapts to alterations in tonicity by increasing or decreasing intracellular organic osmolytes is not clearly established, a chronic imbalance in tonicity should be corrected slowly over at least 48–72 hours. The

Table 18.9 Causes of hyponatraemia in neonates

Primary water excess
Excess intake
    To mother: large intrapartum infusion of sodium-free fluid
    To baby: excessive intravenous intake
Impaired excretion
    Intrinsic renal failure
    Indometacin
    Appropriate or inappropriate ADH secretion
    Adrenocortical failure

Primary sodium depletion
Insufficient intake
    Maternal laxative or diuretic abuse
    Use of non-sodium-supplemented donor breast milk for preterm babies
Excessive loss
    Renal
        Diuretics including xanthines
        Tubular dysfunction
            Pyelonephritis
            Nephrotoxic agents
            Obstructive uropathies
    Endocrine
        Salt-losing forms of congenital adrenal hyperplasia
        Hypoaldosteronism
    Gastrointestinal
        External
            Vomiting
            Ileostomy/colostomy loss
        Sequestered
            Ileus
            Obstruction
            Necrotising enterocolitis
    Central nervous system
        Following repeated drainage of CSF in posthaemorrhagic hydrocephalus
        Cerebral salt wasting

Mixed
Water excess and sodium depletion
    Sodium and water depletion treated with continued infusion of sodium-free fluid
    Chronic lung disease treated with long-term diuretic therapy
Water excess disproportionate to whole body sodium excess
    Congestive cardiac failure
    Liver failure
    Nephrotic syndrome

management of acute imbalance may be quicker. If hypernatraemia has developed rapidly, over a period of hours, reducing the serum sodium by 1 mmol/l/h appears safe. If hypernatraemia develops slowly, over a period of days, the rate of reduction in serum sodium should not exceed 0.5 mmol/l/h.

Proton magnetic resonance spectroscopy provides a non-invasive direct means to quantify the organic osmolyte response to disturbances in osmolality. Lee et al[84] reported a 44% increase in cerebral osmolyte content in a child with chronic hypernatraemia (serum Na 195 mmol/l) that returned to normal 36 days after start of therapy. We have found a normal cerebral myo-inositol 8 days after the start of therapy in a term neonate in whom hypernatraemia (serum Na 173 mmol/l) developed over a period of 8 days (unpublished data).

The key to establishing the cause of hyponatraemia or hypernatraemia, developing after birth, is to assess the change in body-weight in conjunction with the clinical context. Hyponatraemia with weight loss or inadequate weight gain suggests sodium depletion. Hyponatraemia with inappropriate weight gain suggests water excess (Table 18.9). Hypernatraemia with weight loss suggests dehydration; hypernatraemia with weight gain, sodium and water overload. Hyponatraemia due to water excess responds to water restriction but should not detract from treatment of the underlying cause. Hyponatraemia due to sodium deficit requires an increase in sodium intake, but once body stores have been replenished, this should be reduced to maintenance requirements.

Hypernatraemia

In extremely preterm babies, hypernatraemia occurring in the first few days of postnatal life is usually due to excessive transepidermal water loss, possibly compounded by excessive sodium administration. As this is a situation in which hypernatraemia may escalate rapidly, it should be treated promptly by increasing the volume of infused fluid, avoidance of an excessive sodium intake and redoubling efforts to reduce insensible water loss.

Hypernatraemia arising in otherwise healthy, breastfed, full-term neonates is also well described. The incidence has been variably reported because of differences in methods of ascertainment. Oddie et al[105] in a large population-based survey describe an occurrence of 7.1/10 000 breastfed infants. Laing & Wong[81] report an occurrence of 14.4/10 000 infants in a single large centre, and Manganaro et al[88] 276/10 000 breastfed hospital admissions. Some authors cite the finding of a high urinary sodium concentration in the infant and a high breast milk sodium concentration as evidence that the condition is due to an excessive sodium intake.[8] However, the condition is more likely due to a failure of breastfeeding and dehydration. Neville et al[103] have shown that breast milk sodium is inversely related to breast milk volume. The concentration of sodium in breast milk has been used as an index of lactogenesis.[102] In a study involving 130 nursing mothers, 95.4% of mothers with a normal initial breast milk sodium concentration were breastfeeding successfully at 1 month whereas only 55% of those with a high breast milk sodium concentration were successful despite intervention with support and counselling. The longer the breast milk sodium concentration remained elevated, the lower the success rate. The highest breast milk sodium seen in this study was 134 mmol/l on the eighth day. The term neonate who has had an inadequate intake of breast milk is both dehydrated and sodium depleted. As the total volume of milk ingested is severely reduced, total sodium intake is not elevated. Volume depletion, by stimulating the RAAS, would normally reduce the urinary loss of sodium. The explanation for the seemingly paradoxical occurrence of a high urinary sodium concentration is that severe dehydration initiates a compensatory natriuresis in many mammalian species, including man, and is a homeostatic response that serves to protect against hypernatraemia and hyperosmolality.[91] This dehydration-induced natriuresis is a physiological response that occurs even in the sodium-restricted state and appears to be mediated by osmoreceptor-stimulated oxytocin release.[71] In addition to the need to avoid rehydration with hypo-osmolar salt-poor fluid, this sodium deficit also needs replenishing. Evidence of circulatory collapse or compromise should be treated with a resuscitation volume of 20–30 ml/kg of normal saline administered over 30–60 minutes. Enteral feeds should be continued except where a specific contraindication exists. The remainder of the deficit may be replaced intravenously, initially as normal saline and subsequently half-normal saline with dextrose,[81] aiming to reduce the serum sodium at a rate not exceeding 12 mmol/l/day.

Hyponatraemia

The serum sodium concentration at birth reflects the maternal value. Often, a low serum sodium at birth suggests that the mother has received a large volume of salt-poor intravenous fluid during labour, resulting in an excess transfer of water to the baby. Labour ward policies should avoid the use of fixed-concentration solutions for intrapartum drug administration, as under these circumstances an increase in dose will result in increasing infusion volumes. Newborn hyponatraemia has also been described following maternal diuretic and laxative abuse and in pre-eclampsia.

In the first few days after birth, prior to the postnatal diuresis/natriuresis and in the absence of substantial sodium intake, hyponatraemia is almost invariably dilutional, due to excessive water retention or administration and not to sodium depletion. Chronic sodium loss will first be accompanied by extracellular volume contraction, poor weight gain and a normal serum sodium concentration. Hyponatraemia will only ensue as a late sign. Donor breast milk contains variable but inadequate quantities of sodium. Breast milk from mothers delivering preterm contains larger amounts, but this is not sustained and even in these babies supplementation is necessary from the third to fourth week. Many babies receive xanthines to treat apnoea of prematurity. These are weak diuretics, but chronic use will predispose to sodium depletion. Potent agents such as furosemide (frusemide) may cause large sodium losses. An acute fall in serum sodium usually reflects impaired water excretion but may occur following a single dose of furosemide (frusemide) or with sudden gastrointestinal loss, as in NEC. Sodium loss may occur from the GIT as visible external loss, as in vomiting or as ileostomy or colostomy losses, or as sequestered loss, as with an ileus or obstruction. In the latter case, there will be no weight loss. Renal tubular loss of sodium may arise in acute pyelonephritis and following relief of obstructive uropathy. Endocrine causes of hyponatraemia are discussed in Chapter 35 Part 2. The diagnostic approach in suspected inappropriate ADH secretion is discussed above.

Hyperkalaemia and hypokalaemia

Potassium is the principal intracellular cation and is important for the maintenance of intracellular fluid volume. Total body potassium is approximately 46 mmol/kg, a value that is similar in babies and adults. Unrecognised negative potassium balance may be relatively common in neonates receiving intensive care. It is all too easy to mask a falling serum potassium if blood samples are slightly haemolysed. Engle & Arant[42] found that newborns with RDS had a mean cumulative negative potassium balance of approximately 4 mmol/kg by day 4. This represents approximately 10% of total body potassium. Preterm neonates should receive a potassium intake of 2 mmol/kg/day, commencing within 48 hours of birth if urine output is satisfactory and there are no concerns about renal function. A high potassium level may be reported if there has been difficulty in obtaining the blood sample or a delay in processing it, as potassium is released from damaged cells. True hyperkalaemia occurs in the context of extensive tissue damage, such as following extensive bruising, shock and ischaemia, and in renal failure. The management of hyperkalaemia is discussed in Chapter 36.

Causes of potassium depletion are shown in Table 18.10. Hypokalaemia may result from gastrointestinal or urinary loss. Most gastrointestinal disorders are also associated with sodium loss and the resulting increase in circulating aldosterone exacerbates potassium loss. Hypokalaemia is usually accompanied by a metabolic alkalosis.

Oligoanuria

Oligoanuria is the commonest presenting sign of renal impairment in the neonatal intensive care unit. It was formerly most often seen in the context of severe respiratory disease, but, with improvements in the management of this condition, perinatal asphyxia, sepsis, NEC and major surgery have emerged as the four most common predisposing causes. Other clinical settings in which it may occur include intrapartum blood loss, as in acute feto-maternal or feto-fetal haemorrhage. This may not be immediately obvious, unlike serious neonatal haemorrhage.

The spectrum of renal injury following hypoxic-ischaemic injury extends from mild tubular dysfunction to acute tubular necrosis or irreversible cortical necrosis. Acute retention of urine is also often seen in this situation. Myoglobinuria following rhabdomyolysis, and haemoglobinuria due to intravascular haemolysis, may affect renal function.[80]

Dehydration resulting from failure to replace high insensible water losses readily occurs in extremely preterm infants. Fluid may be lost acutely into the GIT, as in acute obstruction and NEC. Myocardial compromise, following asphyxia, in heart failure, in complex congenital heart disease or following cardiac surgery, will lead initially to decreased renal perfusion. Pharmacological agents may lead to catastrophic hypotension. Tolazoline, an alpha agonist, is occasionally employed for its pulmonary vasodilator actions. It is also a systemic vasodilator, and systemic hypotension, leading to renal failure, is a serious side effect of therapy. Acute falls in BP have also been described following the use of fentanyl and the angiotensin-converting enzyme (ACE) inhibitors. Antenatal exposure to ACE inhibitors may lead to renal impairment in the newborn.[92]

Hydration and the adequacy of the circulation require careful and continuous assessment in neonatal intensive care. Failure to accurately monitor urine output will delay recognition and increase the risk of pre-renal impairment progressing to intrinsic renal failure. It is important to exclude congenital abnormalities of the kidneys such as dysplasia and infantile-type polycystic disease, and to diagnose renal venous thrombosis or treatable obstructive lesions such as posterior urethral values.

Investigation and management of oligoanuria

The management of the newborn should always include anticipation of likely problems. The probability of renal impairment is high in severely asphyxiated full-term babies and initial fluid intake should be restricted to 20–30 ml/kg/day until the situation is clear (Table 18.6). This will not result in dehydration as it is considerably more than the transepidermal insensible loss of full-term babies, which is around 12 ml/kg/day. Hypoglycaemia may be a problem at low infusion volumes, and hypertonic dextrose, infused centrally, may be necessary. The circulation should be carefully supported bearing in mind that myocardial compromise may also be present and that these babies are at risk of pulmonary haemorrhage. Maintenance sodium administration should be avoided. Urinary retention will require catheterisation.

Careful monitoring of urine output should commence immediately on admission. If the urine flow rate falls abruptly in a previously stable infant, or drops below 1 ml/kg/h in the first few days after birth, immediate investigation is mandatory. First consider the clinical context and whether the problem is likely to be pre-renal, renal or post-renal. Pre-renal failure as a consequence of renal hypoperfusion may occur with hypovolaemia

Table 18.10 Causes of potassium depletion

- Inadequate intake

- Gastrointestinal loss
  Aspiration of gastrointestinal contents
  Vomiting
  Pyloric stenosis
  Ileus
  Ileostomy loss
  Diarrhoea

- Renal loss
  With metabolic alkalosis
  Excessive base administration
  Furosemide and other loop diuretics
  Congenital chloride diarrhoea
  Hyperaldosteronism
  Bartter's syndrome
  Cushing's syndrome
  With metabolic acidosis
  Renal tubular acidosis
  Diuresis during recovery from acute renal failure

or dehydration. The possibility of pre-renal failure should be addressed as a matter of urgency, as it is reversible, but will rapidly lead to established renal failure if untreated. A diagnosis of post-renal failure from an obstructed renal tract can be easily identified using ultrasound.

It has been suggested that the best indicator to distinguish pre-renal from established renal failure, in the oliguric neonate, is the fractional excretion of sodium (Fe_{Na}). This is readily calculated from the sodium and creatinine concentrations of serum (S) and a spot urine (U) sample:

$$Fe_{Na}\% = (U/S) \text{ sodium} \times (S/U) \text{ creatinine} \times 100$$

If tubular function is intact and sodium reabsorption continues, the infant is in oliguric pre-renal failure and the Fe_{Na} will be less than 3%. Once tubular necrosis has occurred, the Fe_{Na} is usually above 10%. Pre-renal oliguria demands urgent attention to renal perfusion, whereas a high Fe_{Na} suggests established renal failure and the equally urgent need for restriction of fluid intake. Unfortunately, the Fe_{Na} and other indices such as the renal failure index (U sodium $\times$ S/U creatinine) have poor sensitivity and specificity.[95] In extremely immature infants, values for Fe_{Na} in pre-renal and renal failure overlap. The urinary sodium concentration cannot be interpreted clearly if furosemide (frusemide) has already been used, nor is delaying further action until urinary sodium and creatinine estimations have been obtained, acceptable.

Impaired renal perfusion as a cause of oligoanuria is more likely if other evidence of circulatory compromise exists. If the clinical assessment is equivocal, a fluid challenge is an appropriate approach. Administer normal saline, 10–20 ml/kg, followed by furosemide (frusemide). A note of caution should be sounded here: in the critically ill neonate with severe respiratory failure, impaired renal perfusion may be unresponsive to volume replacement and the risk of exacerbating respiratory function through the injudicious use of large intravenous volumes is substantial. A urine flow rate of 0.5 ml/kg/h is acceptable on the first day after birth in such infants and attention should be directed towards improving renal perfusion through optimal respiratory and cardiovascular support. If there are signs of extracellular volume overload, with weight gain or weight retention, or the infant appears frankly oedematous, a fluid challenge may well worsen the situation, and inotropic support of cardiac output with dobutamine, 10–20 micrograms/kg/min, should be considered. The role of low-dose dopamine is discussed above. Furosemide (frusemide) increases the flow of tubular fluid, but also stimulates prostaglandin release and reduces renal metabolic requirements by inhibiting the sodium pump. Although doses of 1–3 mg/kg have been recommended, a higher dose of 4–5 mg/kg is probably more appropriate, as furosemide (frusemide) exerts its effects on the loop of Henlé only after glomerular filtration, and high plasma levels are necessary when the GFR is low.[97] However, because the half-life of furosemide (frusemide) clearance is almost 24 hours in healthy preterm infants who are not in renal failure,[31] clearance will almost certainly be several days in babies remaining in renal failure, and there is no rationale for repeating the dose; this would only lead to accumulation and the risks of ototoxicity, interstitial nephritis and possibly persistence of ductal patency.

If a volume challenge does not produce a prompt diuresis, fluid intake should immediately be reduced to no more than insensible water loss plus urine output. Further management is that of established renal failure (Chapter 36 Part 1).

References

1. Al-Dahhan J, Haycock G B, Chantler C, Stimmler L 1983 Sodium homeostasis in term and preterm neonates. I. Renal aspects. Archives of Disease in Childhood 58: 335–343
2. Al-Dahhan J, Haycock G B, Chantler C, Stimmler L 1983 Sodium homeostasis in term and preterm neonates. II. Gastrointestinal aspects. Archives of Disease in Childhood 58: 343–345
3. Al-Dahhan J, Haycock G B, Nichol B, Chantler C, Stimmler L 1984 Sodium homeostasis in term and preterm neonates. III. Effect of salt supplementation. Archives of Disease in Childhood 59: 945–950
4. Al-Dahhan J, Stimmler L, Chantler C, Haycock G B 1987 The effect of antenatal dexamethasone administration on glomerular filtration rate and renal sodium excretion in premature infants. Pediatric Nephrology 1: 131–135
5. Al-Rubeyi B, Murray N, Modi N 1994 A variable dextrose delivery system for use in neonatal intensive care. Archives of Disease in Childhood. Fetal and Neonatal Edition 70: F79
6. Aperia A, Holtback U, Syren M L, Svensson L B, Fryckstedt J, Greengard P 1994 Activation/deactivation of renal Na^+, K^+-ATPase: a final common pathway for regulation of natriuresis. FASEB Journal 8: 436–439
7. Arnold-Aldea S A, Auslender R A, Parer J T 1991 The effect of the inhibition of prostaglandin synthesis on renal blood flow in fetal sheep. American Journal of Obstetrics and Gynecology 165: 185–190
8. Bajpai A, Aggarwal R, Deorari A K, Paul V K 2002 Neonatal hypernatremia due to high breast milk sodium. Indian Pediatrics 39: 193–196
9. Barr P A, Bailey P E, Sumners J, Cassady G 1977 Relation between arterial blood pressure and blood volume and effect of infused albumin in sick preterm infants. Pediatrics 60: 282–289
10. Barrington K, Brion L P 2002 Dopamine versus no treatment to prevent renal dysfunction in indomethacin-treated preterm newborn infants (Cochrane Review). Cochrane Database of Systematic Reviews (3): CD003213
11. Bartter F C, Schwartz W B 1967 The syndrome of inappropriate secretion of antidiuretic hormone. American Journal of Medicine 42: 790–806
12. Bauer K, Bovermann G, Roithmaier A, Gotz M, Proiss A, Versmold H 1991 Body composition, nutrition and fluid balance during the first two weeks of life in preterm neonates weighing less than 1500 g. Journal of Pediatrics 118: 615–620
13. Bauer K, Linderkamp O, Versmold H T 1993 Systolic blood pressure and blood volume in preterm infants. Archives of Disease in Childhood 69: 521–522
14. Bauer K, Versmold H 1989 Postnatal weight loss in preterm neonates less than 1500 g is isotonic dehydration of the extracellular volume. Acta Paediatrica Scandinavica Supplement 360: 37–42
15. Baum M, Quigley R 1993 Glucocorticoids stimulate rabbit proximal convoluted tubule acidification. Journal of Clinical Investigation 91: 110–114
16. Bavoux F 1992 [Fetal toxicity of non-steroidal anti-inflammatory agents]. Presse Médicale 21: 1909–1912 (in French)
17. Bell E F, Acarregui M J 2001 Restricted versus liberal water intake for preventing morbidity and mortality in preterm infants (Cochrane Review). Cochrane Database of Systematic Reviews (3): CD000503
18. Bell E F, Warburton D, Stonestreet B, Oh W 1979 High volume fluid intake predisposes premature infants to necrotising enterocolitis. Lancet ii: 90
19. Bell E F, Warburton D, Stonestreet B, Oh W 1980 Effect of fluid administration on the development of symptomatic patent ductus arteriosus and congestive heart failure in premature infants. New England Journal of Medicine 302: 598–604
20. Bellomo R, Chapman M, Finfer S, Hickling K, Myburgh J 2000 Low-dose dopamine in patients with early renal dysfunction: a placebo-controlled randomised trial. Australian and New Zealand Intensive Care Society (ANZICS) Clinical Trials Group. Lancet 356: 2139–2143
21. Benitez O A, Benitez M, Stijnen T, Boot W, Berger H M 1986 Inaccuracy in neonatal measurement of urine concentration with a refractometer. Journal of Pediatrics 108: 613–616
22. Bétrémieux P, Modi N, Hartnoll G, Midgley J 1995 Longitudinal changes in extracellular fluid volume, sodium excretion and atrial natriuretic peptide, in preterm neonates with hyaline membrane disease. Early Human Development 41: 221–222
23. Brand P L, van Lingen R A, Brus F, Talsma M D, Elzenga N J 1993 Hypertrophic obstructive cardiomyopathy as a side effect of dexamethasone treatment for bronchopulmonary dysplasia. Acta Paediatrica 82: 614–617

24. Brewer E D 1992 Urinary acidification. In: Polin RA, Fox WW (eds) Fetal and neonatal physiology. WB Saunders, Philadelphia, pp 1657–1660

25. Brion L P, Soll R F 2001 Diuretics for respiratory distress syndrome in preterm infants (Cochrane Review). Cochrane Database of Systematic Reviews (2): CD001454

26. Brown E R, Stark A, Sosneko I, Lawson E E, Avery M E 1978 Bronchopulmonary dysplasia: possible relationship to pulmonary oedema. Journal of Pediatrics 92: 982–984

27. Cartlidge P H T, Rutter N 1987 Karaya gum ECG electrodes for the preterm infant. Archives of Disease in Childhood 62: 1281–1282

28. Celsi G, Nishi A, Akusjärvi G, Aperia A 1991 Abundance of Na^+, K^+-ATPase mRNA is regulated by glucocorticoid hormones in infant rat kidneys. American Journal of Physiology 260: F192–F197

29. Celsi G, Wang Z M, Akusjarvi G, Aperia A 1993 Sensitive periods for glucocorticoid regulation of Na^+, K^+-ATPase mRNA in the developing lung and kidney. Pediatric Research 33: 5–9

30. Chance G W, Radde I C, Willis D M, Roy R N, Park E, Ackerman J 1977 Postnatal growth of infants of <1.3 kg birth weight; effects of metabolic acidosis, of caloric intake and of calcium, sodium and phosphate supplementation. Journal of Pediatrics 91: 787–793

31. Chevalier R L, Campbell F, Brenbridge A N A G 1984 Prognostic factors in neonatal acute renal failure. Pediatrics 74: 265–272

32. Costarino A T, Gruskay J A, Corcoran L, Pollin R A, Baumgart S 1992 Sodium restriction versus daily maintenance replacement in very low birth weight premature neonates: a randomised, blind therapeutic trial. Journal of Pediatrics 120: 99–106

33. Coulthard M G, Hey E N 1985 Effect of varying water intake on renal function in healthy preterm babies. Archives of Disease in Childhood 60: 614–620

34. Cumming A D, Swainson C P 1995 Disturbances in water, electrolyte and acid-base balance In: Edwards C R W, Bouchier I A D, Haslett C, Chilvers E R (eds) Davidson's principles and practice of medicine. Churchill Livingston, Edinburgh, p. 587

35. Deen P M, Knoers N V 1998 Vasopressin type-2 receptor and aquaporin-2 water channels mutants in nephrogenic diabetes insipidus. American Journal of the Medical Sciences 316: 300–309

36. Deen P M, Verdijk M A, Knoers N V et al 1994 Requirement of human renal water channel aquaporin-2 for vasopressin dependent concentration of urine. Science 264: 92–95

37. De Luna M B, Hallet W H 1967 Urinary protein excretion in healthy infants, children and adults. Proceedings of the American Society of Nephrology 16: 16

38. Drukker A, Goldsmith D I, Spitzer A, Edelmann C M, Blaufox M D 1980 The renin angiotensin system in newborn dogs: developmental patterns and response to acute saline loading. Pediatric Research 14: 304–307

39. Dunn F L, Brennan T J, Neelson A E, Robertson G L 1976 The role of blood osmolality and volume in regulating vasopressin secretion by the rat. Journal of Clinical Investigation 52: 3212–3219

40. Ekblad H, Aperia A, Larsson S H 1992 Intracellular pH regulation in cultured renal proximal tubule cells in different stages of maturation. American Journal of Physiology 263: F716–F721

41. Emery E F, Greenough A 1993 Efficacy of low dose dopamine infusion. Acta Paediatrica 82: 430–432

42. Engle W D, Arant B S 1984 Urinary potassium excretion in the critically ill neonate. Pediatrics 74: 259–64

43. Ervin M G 1988 Perinatal fluid and electrolyte regulation: role of arginine vasopressin. Seminars in Perinatology 12: 134–142

44. Evans N 2003 Volume expansion during neonatal intensive care: do we know what we're doing? Seminars in Neonatology 8: 315–323

45. Evans N J, Rutter N 1986 Development of the epidermis in the newborn. Biology of the Neonate 49: 74–80

46. Evans N J, Rutter N 1986 Reduction of skin damage from transcutaneous oxygen electrodes using a spray-on dressing. Archives of Disease in Childhood 61: 881–884

47. Fajardo C A, Whyte R K, Steele B T 1992 Effect of dopamine on failure of indomethacin to close the patent ductus arteriosus. Journal of Pediatrics 121: 771–775

48. Fewell J E, Norton J B 1980 Continuous positive airway pressure impairs renal function in newborn goats. Pediatric Research 14: 1132–1134

49. Friis-Hansen B 1961 Body water compartments in children: changes during growth and related changes in body composition. Pediatrics 28: 169–181

50. Friis-Hansen B 1983 Water distribution in the fetus and newborn infant. Acta Paediatrica Scandinavica Supplement 305: 7–11

51. Fukuda Y, Bertorelli A, Aperia A 1991 Ontogeny of the regulation of Na^+, K^+-ATPase activity in the renal proximal tubular cell. Pediatric Research 30: 131–134

52. Gerigk M, Gnehm HE, Rascher W 1996 Arginine vasopressin and renin in acutely ill children: implications for fluid therapy. Acta Paediatrica 85: 550–553

53. Golberger E 1986 A primer of water, electrolyte and acid-base disorders, 7th edn. Lea & Febinger, Philadelphia, p. 55

54. Gouyon J B, Houchan N 1993 Assessment of urine specific gravity by reagent strip test in newborn infants. Pediatric Nephrology 7: 77–78

55. Greenough A, Chan V, Emery E F, Gamsu H R 1993 Respiratory status and diuresis following treatment with dexamethasone. Early Human Development 32: 87–91

56. Greenough A, Emery E F 1993 Randomised trial comparing dopamine and dobutamine in preterm infants. European Journal of Pediatrics 152: 925–927

57. Hammarlund K, Sedin G 1979 Transepidermal loss in newborn infants. III. Relation to gestational age. Acta Paediatrica Scandinavica 68: 795–801

58. Hammarlund K, Sedin G, Stromberg B 1982 Transepidermal water loss in newborn infants. VII. Relation to postnatal age in very preterm and full term appropriate for gestational age infants. Acta Paediatrica Scandinavica 71: 369–374

59. Hammarlund K, Sedin G, Stromberg B 1983 Transepidermal water loss in the newborn. VIII. Relation to gestational age and postnatal age in appropriate and small for gestational age infants. Acta Paediatrica Scandinavica 72: 721–728

60. Haney I, Lachance C, van Doesburg N H, Fouron J C 1995 Reversible steroid induced hypertrophic cardiomyopathy with left ventricular outflow tract obstruction in two newborns. American Journal of Perinatology 12: 271–274

61. Harpin V A, Rutter N 1982 Sweating in preterm babies. Journal of Pediatrics 100: 614–619

62. Hartnoll G, Bétrémieux P, Modi N 2000 Randomised controlled trial of postnatal sodium supplementation on body composition in 25–30 week gestation infants. Archives of Disease in Childhood. Fetal and Neonatal Edition 82: F24–F28

63. Hartnoll G, Modi N, Bétrémieux P 2001 Randomised controlled trial of postnatal sodium supplementation in 25–30 week gestational age infants: effects on cardiopulmonary adaptation. Archives of Disease in Childhood. Fetal and Neonatal Edition 85: F29–32

64. Hayamizu S, Kanda K, Ohmori S, Murata Y, Seo H 1994 Glucocorticoids potentiate the action of atrial natriuretic polypeptide in adrenalectomized rats. Endocrinology 135: 2459–2464

65. Haycock G B 1993 The influence of sodium on growth in infancy. Pediatric Nephrology 7: 871–875

66. Haycock G B 1995 The syndrome of inappropriate secretion of antidiuretic hormone. Pediatric Nephrology 9: 375–381

67. Haycock G B, Aperia A 1991 Salt and the newborn kidney. Pediatric Nephrology 5: 65–70

68. Hazinski T A, Blalock W A, Engelhardt B 1988 Control of water balance in infants with bronchopulmonary dysplasia: role of endogenous vasopressin. Pediatric Research 23: 86–88

69. Heimler R, Doumas B T, Jendrzejczak B M, Nemeth P B, Hoffman R G, Nelin L D 1993 Relationship between nutrition, weight change and fluid compartments in preterm infants during the first week of life. Journal of Pediatrics 122: 110–114

70. Herin P, Aperia A 1994 Neonatal kidney, fluids and electrolytes. Current Opinion in Pediatrics 6: 154–157

71. Huang W, Lee S L, Arnason S S, Sjoquist M 1996 Dehydration natriuresis in male rats is mediated by oxytocin. American Journal of Physiology 270: R427–R433

72. Jain A, Rutter N, Cartlidge P H 2000 Influence of antenatal steroids and sex on maturation of the epidermal barrier in the preterm infant. Archives of Disease in Childhood. Fetal and Neonatal Edition 83: F112–F116

73. Jörgensen P L 1986 Structure, function and regulation of Na, K-ATPase in the kidney. Kidney International 29: 10–20

74. Judd B A, Haycock G B, Dalton N, Chantler C 1987 Hyponatraemia in premature babies and following surgery in older children. Acta Paediatric Scandinavica 76: 385–393

75. Kaplan B S, Restaino I, Raval D S, Gottlieb R P, Bernstein 1994 Renal failure in the neonate associated with in utero exposure to non-steroidal anti-inflammatory agents. Pediatric Nephrology 8: 700–704

76. Kavvadia V, Greenough A, Dimitriou G, Hooper R 2000 Randomised trial of fluid restriction in ventilated very low birthweight infants. Archives of Disease in Childhood 83: F91–F96

77. Kinoshita S, Jose P A, Felder R A 1989 Ontogeny of the dopamine 1 receptor in rat renal proximal convoluted tubule. Pediatric Research 25: 68A

78. Klarr J M, Faix R G, Pryce C J, Bhatt-Mehta V 1994 Randomised blind trial of dopamine versus dobutamine for treatment of hypotension in preterm infants with respiratory distress syndrome. Journal of Pediatrics 125: 117–122

79. Kojima T, Hirata Y, Fukuda Y, Iwase S, Koboyashi Y 1987 Plasma atrial natriuretic peptide and spontaneous diuresis in sick neonates. Archives of Disease in Childhood 62: 667–670

80. Kojima T, Kobayashi T, Matsuzaki S, Iwase S, Kobayashi Y 1985 Effects of perinatal asphyxia and myoglobinuria on development of acute neonatal renal failure. Archives of Disease in Childhood 60: 908–912

81. Laing I A, Wong C M 2002 Hypernatraemia in the first few days: is the incidence rising? Archives of Disease in Childhood. Fetal and Neonatal Edition 87: F158–F162

82. Lambert H J, Coulthard M G, Palmer J M, Baylis P H, Matthews J N S 1990 Control of sodium and water balance in the preterm neonate. Pediatric Nephrology 4: C53

83. Leake R D, Zakauddin S, Trygstad C W, Fu P, Oh W 1976 The effect of large volume intravenous fluid infusion on neonatal renal function. Journal of Pediatrics 89: 968–972

84. Lee J H, Arcinue E, Ross B D 1994 Brief report: organic osmolytes in the brain of an infant with hypernatremia. New England Journal of Medicine 331: 439–442

85. Linderkamp O, Nelle M, Kraus M, Zilow E P 1992 The effect of early and late cord-clamping on blood viscosity and other hemorheological parameters in full-term neonates. Acta Paediatrica 81: 745–750

86. Littlewood J M 1971 White cells and bacteria in voided urine of healthy newborns. Archives of Disease in Childhood 56: 167–172

87. Lorenz J M, Kleinman L I, Kotagal U R, Reller M D 1982 Water balance in very low birth weight infants: relation to water and sodium intake and effect on outcome. Journal of Pediatrics 101: 423–432

88. Manganaro R, Mami C, Marrone T, Marseglia L, Gemelli M 2001 Incidence of dehydration and hypernatremia in exclusively breast-fed infants. Journal of Pediatrics 139: 673–675

89. McCance R A 1936 Experimental sodium chloride deficiency in man. Proceedings of the Royal Society of London (Biology) 119: 245–268

90. McCance R A, Naylor N J B, Widdowson E M 1954 The response of infants to a large dose of water. Archives of Disease in Childhood 29: 104–109

91. McKinley M J, Evered M D, Mathai M L 2000 Renal Na excretion in dehydrated and rehydrated adrenalectomized sheep maintained with aldosterone. American Journal of Physiology. Regulatory, Integrative and Comparative Physiology 279: R17–R24

92. Mehta N, Modi N 1989 ACE inhibitors in pregnancy. Lancet ii: 96

93. Midgley J P, Modi N, Littleton P, Carter N, Royston P, Smith A 1992 Atrial natriuretic peptide, cyclic guanosine monophosphate and sodium excretion during postnatal adaptation in male infants below 34 weeks gestation with severe respiratory distress syndrome. Early Human Development 28: 145–154

94. Modi N 1988 Development of renal function. British Medical Bulletin 44: 935–956

95. Modi N 1989 Treatment of renal failure in neonates. Archives of Disease in Childhood 64: 630

96. Modi N 1997 Management of postnatal disorders of fluid balance. In: Brace R (ed) Fetus and neonate volume IV – Body fluids and kidney. Cambridge University Press, Cambridge, pp 299–322

97. Modi N, Coulthard M 1999 Renal function. In: Levitt G, Harvey D, Cooke RWI (eds) Practical perinatal care – the baby under 1000 g. Butterworth Heinemann, Oxford, pp 199–211

98. Modi N, Hutton J L 1990 The influence of postnatal respiratory adaptation on sodium handling in preterm neonates. Early Human Development 21: 11–20

99. Modi N, Hutton J L 1990 Urinary creatinine excretion and estimation of muscle mass in infants of 25–34 weeks gestation. Acta Paediatrica Scandinavica 79: 1156–1162

100. Mohan P, Rojas J, Davidson K K et al 1984 Pulmonary air leak associated with neonatal hyponatraemia in premature infants. Journal of Pediatrics 105: 153–157

101. Moore E S, Galvez M B, Paton J B, Fisher D E, Behrman R E 1974 Effects of positive pressure ventilation on intrarenal blood flow in infant primates. Pediatric Research 8: 792–796

102. Morton J A 1994 The clinical usefulness of breast milk sodium in the assessment of lactogenesis. Pediatrics 93: 802–806

103. Neville M C, Keller R, Seacat J et al 1988 Studies in human lactation: milk volume in lactating women during the onset of lactation and full lactation. American Journal of Clinical Nutrition 48: 1375–1386

104. O'Brodovich H, Canessa C, Ueda J, Rafii B, Rossier BC, Edelson J 1993 Expression of the epithelial Na$^+$ channel in the developing rat lung. American Journal of Physiology 265: C491–C496

105. Oddie S, Richmond S, Coulthard M 2001 Hypernatraemic dehydration and breast feeding: a population study. Archives of Disease in Childhood 85: 318–320

106. Oliver J A, Pinto J, Sciacca R R, Cannon P J 1980 Increased renal secretion of norepinephrine and prostaglandin E$_2$ during sodium depletion in the dog. Journal of Clinical Investigation 66: 748–756

107. Orlowski J, Lingrel J B 1988 Tissue-specific and developmental regulation of rat Na,K-ATPase catalytic α isoform and β subunit mRNAs. Journal of Biological Chemistry 263: 10436–10442

108. Ostlund E V, Eklof A C, Aperia A 1993 Salt deficient diet and early weaning inhibit DNA synthesis in immature rat proximal tubular cells. Pediatric Nephrology 7: 41–44

109. Pabst R C, Starr K P, Qaiyumi S, Schwalbe R S, Gewolb I H 1999 The effect of application of aquaphor on skin condition, fluid requirements and bacterial colonisation in very low birth weight infants. Journal of Perinatology 19: 278–283

110. Peters O, Ryan S, Matthew, Cheng K, Lunn J 1997 Randomised controlled trial of acetate in preterm neonates receiving parenteral nutrition. Archives of Disease in Childhood. Fetal and Neonatal Edition 77: F12–F15

111. Pladys P, Bétrémieux P, Lefrancois C, Schleich J M, Gourmelon N, Le Marec B 1994 [Doppler echocardiography in the evaluation of volume expansion effects in newborn infants]. Archives of Pediatrics 1: 470–476 (in French)

112. Rao M, Eid N, Herrod L, Parekh A, Steiner P 1986 Antidiuretic response in children with bronchopulmonary dysplasia during episodes of acute respiratory distress. American Journal of Diseases in Childhood 140: 825–828

113. Rees L, Brook C D G, Shaw J C L, Forsling M L 1984 Hyponatraemia in the first week of life in preterm infants. I. Arginine vasopressin secretion. Archives of Disease in Childhood 59: 414–422

114. Rees L, Shaw J C L, Brook C D G, Forsling M L 1984 Hyponatraemia in the first week of life. II. Sodium and water balance. Archives of Disease in Childhood 59: 423–429

115. Reller M D, Lorenz J M, Kotagal U R, Meyer R, Kaplan S 1985 Hemodynamic significant PDA: an echocardiographic and clinical assessment of incidence, natural history and outcome in very low birth weight infants maintained in negative fluid balance. Pediatric Cardiology 6: 17–24

116. Rennie J, Cooke R W I 1991 Prolonged low dose indomethacin for persistent ductus arteriosus of prematurity. Archives of Disease in Childhood 66: 55–58

117. Rojas J, Mohan P, Davidson K K 1984 Increased extracellular water volume associated with hyponatremia at birth in premature infants. Journal of Pediatrics 105: 158–161

118. Roy R N, Chance G W, Radde I C, Hill D E, Willis D M, Sheepers J 1976 Late hyponatremia in very low birthweight infants (<1.3 kg). Pediatric Research 10: 526–531

119. Rozé J C, Tohier C, Maingueneau C, Lefèvre M, Mouzard A 1993 Response to dobutamine and dopamine in the hypotensive, very preterm infant. Archives of Disease in Childhood 69: 59–63

120. Rozycki J H, Baumgart S 1991 Atrial natriuretic factor and postnatal diuresis in respiratory distress syndrome. Archives of Disease in Childhood 66: 43–47

121. Rudd P T, Hughes E A, Placzek M M, Hodes D T 1983 Reference ranges for plasma creatinine during the first month of life. Archives of Disease in Childhood 58: 212–215

122. Rutter N 1989 The hazards of an immature skin. In: Harvey D R H, Cooke R W I, Levitt G A (eds) The baby under 1000g. Butterworth, London, p 99

123. Schrod L, Frauendienst-Egger G, Forgber I, von Stockhausen H B 1991 [Dexamethasone in the treatment of bronchopulmonary dysplasia]. Pneumologie 45: 892–896 (in German)

124. Sedin G, Hammarlund K, Nilsson G E, Strömberg B, Oberg P 1985 Measurements of transepidermal water loss in newborn infants. Clinics in Perinatology 12: 79–99

125. Seri I, Rudas G, Bors Z, Kanyicska B, Tulassay T 1993 Effects of low dose dopamine infusion on cardiovascular and renal functions, cerebral blood flow and plasma catecholamine levels in sick, preterm neonates. Pediatric Research 34: 742–749

126. Shaffer S G, Bradt S K, Hall R T 1986 Postnatal changes in total body water and extracellular volume in the preterm infant with respiratory distress syndrome. Journal of Pediatrics 109: 509–514

127. Shaffer S G, Meade V M 1989 Sodium balance and extracellular volume regulation in very low birth weight infants. Journal of Pediatrics 115: 285–290

128. Shaffer S G, Weismann D N 1992 Fluid requirements in the preterm infant. Clinics in Perinatology 19: 233–250

129. Singhi S C, Chookang E 1984 Maternal fluid overload during labour, transplacental hyponatraemia and risk of transient neonatal tachypnoea in term infants. Archives of Disease in Childhood 59: 1155–1158

130. Singhi S C, Chookang E, Hall J S, Kalghatgi S 1985 Iatrogenic neonatal and maternal hyponatraemia following oxytocin and aqueous glucose infusion during labour. British Journal of Obstetrics and Gynaecology 92: 356–363

131. Singhi S C, Sood V, Bhakoo N K, Ganguly N K, Kaur A 1995 Composition of postnatal weight loss and subsequent weight gain in preterm infants. Indian Journal of Medical Research 101: 157–162

132. Skinner J R, Milligan D W A, Hunter S, Hey E 1992 Central venous pressure in the ventilated neonate. Archives of Disease in Childhood 67: 374–377

133. So K W, Fok T F, Ng P C, Wong W W, Cheung K L 1997 Randomised controlled trial of colloid or crystalloid in hypotensive preterm infants. Archives of Disease in Childhood. Fetal and Neonatal Edition 76: F43–F46

134. Spitzer A 1982 The role of the kidney in sodium homeostasis during maturation. Kidney International 21: 539–545

135. Sposi N M, Bottero L, Cossu G, Russo G, Testa U, Peschle C 1989 Expression of protein kinase C genes during ontogenic development of the central nervous system. Molecular and Cellular Biology 9: 2284–2288

136. Stevenson J G 1977 Fluid administration in the association of patent ductus arteriosus complicating respiratory distress syndrome. Journal of Pediatrics 90: 257–261

137. Strange K 1993 Maintenance of cell volume in the central nervous system. Pediatric Nephrology 7: 689–697

138. Sulyok E, Nemeth M, Tenyi I et al 1979 Postnatal development of renin-angiotensin-aldosterone system, RAAS, in relation to electrolyte balance in premature infants. Pediatric Research 13: 817–820

139. Sulyok E, Varga F, Gyory E, Jobst K, Csaba I F 1979 Postnatal development of renal sodium handling in premature infants. Journal of Pediatrics 95: 787–792

140. Takahashi N, Hoshi J, Nishida H 1994 Water balance, electrolytes and acid base balance in extremely premature infants. Acta Paediatrica Japonica 36: 250–252

141. Tammela O K, Koivisto M E 1992 Fluid restriction for preventing bronchopulmonary dysplasia? Reduced fluid intake during the first weeks of life improves the outcome of low-birth-weight infants. Acta Paediatrica 81: 207–212

142. Tang W, Modi N, Clark P 1994 Dilution kinetics of H_2^{18} for the measurement of total body water in preterm babies in the first week after birth. Archives of Disease in Childhood 69: 28–31

143. Tang W, Ridout D, Modi N 1997 Influence of respiratory distress syndrome on body composition after preterm birth. Archives of Disease in Childhood. Fetal and Neonatal Edition 77: F28–F31

144. Trompeter R S, Al-Dahhan J, Haycock G B, Chik G, Chantler C 1983 Normal values for plasma creatinine concentration related to maturity in normal term and preterm infants. International Journal of Pediatric Nephrology 4: 145–148

145. Tulassay T, Seri I, Rascher W 1987 Atrial natriuretic peptide and extracellular volume control after birth. Acta Paediatrica Scandinavica 76: 444–446

146. Uthaya S, Tang W, Doré CJ, Modi N Clinical utility of bioelectrical impedance analysis for the estimation of total body water during neonatal intensive care. (Submitted)

147. Van Marter L J, Leviton A, Allred E N, Pagano M, Kuban K C 1990 Hydration during the first days of life and the risk of bronchopulmonary dysplasia in low birth weight infants. Journal of Pediatrics 116: 942–949

148. von Stockhausen H B, Struve M 1980 [Effects of highly varying parenteral fluid intakes in premature and newborn infants during the first three days of life]. Klinische Padiatrie 192: 539–546 (in German)

149. Walker M P R, Moore T R, Brace R A 1994 Indomethacin and arginine vasopressin interaction in the fetal kidney: a mechanism of oliguria. American Journal of Obstetrics and Gynecology 171: 1234–1241

150. Wananukul S, Praisumanna P 2002 Clear topical ointment decreases transepidermal water loss in jaundiced infants receiving phototherapy. Journal of the Medical Association of Thailand 85: 102–106

151. Wardrop C A, Holland B M 1995 The roles and vital importance of placental blood to the newborn infant. Journal of Perinatal Medicine 23: 139–143

152. Wassner S J 1991 The effect of sodium repletion on growth and protein turnover in sodium depleted rats. Pediatric Nephrology 5: 501–504

153. Williams P R, Kanarek K S 1982 Urine evaporative loss and effects on specific gravity and osmolality. Journal of Pediatrics 100: 626–628

154. Winrow A P, Kovar I Z, Jani B R, Gatzoulis M 1992 Early hyponatraemia and neonatal drug withdrawal. Acta Paediatrica 81: 847–848

155. Yasui M, Marples D, Belusa R et al 1996 Development of urinary concentrating capacity: role of aquaporin-2. American Journal of Physiology 271: F461–F468

156. Yeh T F, Wilks A, Singh J, Betkerur M, Lilien L, Pildes R S 1982 Furosemide prevents the renal side effects of indomethacin therapy in premature infants with patent ductus arteriosus. Journal of Pediatrics 101: 433–437

157. Ziegler E, Fomon S J 1971 Fluid intake, renal solute load and water balance in infancy. Journal of Pediatrics 78: 561–568

158. Ziegler M D, Ryu J E 1976 Renal solute load and diet in growing premature infants. Journal of Pediatrics 89: 609–611

CHAPTER 19

Intensive care monitoring and data handling

Andrew Lyon

Introduction

Successful care of the newborn depends on understanding the pathophysiology of the conditions affecting the baby. To follow changes in clinical condition, and the effects of treatment, it is essential that we are able to monitor the progress of the baby.

There are a plethora of devices to help with monitoring. Many are well established and of accepted benefit, e.g. heart rate, while others are still to be shown to have an impact on clinical care, e.g. Cerebral Function Monitors. There is debate about which method gives the best information, e.g. transcutaneous PO_2 versus saturation, and also about when invasive monitoring, such as intra-arterial blood pressure (BP), should be used.

If information is collected from monitors it must be interpreted and then acted upon. This requires not only a knowledge of the underlying physiology, but also at least a basic understanding of how the monitors work. In particular it is important to know the limitations of the devices and the circumstances in which they become unreliable.

Electrical safety

With the large number of devices attached to babies, electrical safety is of paramount importance and all equipment must conform to strict regulations.

The Medical Device Regulations of 1994 (SI 1999/3017) state that all equipment placed on the market within the European Community must comply with the essential requirements of the European Union Directive on medical devices. In essence this means that devices must carry a CE-mark as a sign of conformity. This includes assurance that the device meets the general requirements for safety of medical electrical equipment laid down in IEC 601-1. This also applies to any equipment used for research and there must be no possibility that the baby could act as an earth.

Units must have an agreed policy for the purchase and maintenance of all equipment, as well as for staff support and training. This must be done in consultation with a Department of Medical Physics and be supported by an adequate budget.[15]

Mobile phones can interfere with monitoring systems and should not be used in hospitals and particularly within intensive care areas.

Cardiovascular monitoring

Heart rate and ECG

The electrodes used to obtain the ECG should be placed lateral enough on the chest to minimise any shadow on X-ray. Correct positioning is important if these leads are used also to produce a respiratory trace by impedance changes.

The displayed ECG is not of diagnostic quality and a full 12-lead ECG must be requested if an arrythmia is suspected (pp. 651–7).

Changes in the ECG pattern can indicate conditions such as hyperkalaemia and myocardial ischaemia. A reduction in size of the complexes may be an early sign of pulmonary air leak or cardiac tamponade.[45]

Heart rate can be derived and displayed from the ECG. With many multiparameter monitors, the heart rate can also be obtained from the BP trace, removing the need to stick electrodes onto fragile skin. Access to the ECG signal does have the advantage that it is possible to check artefacts such as 'double counting' of the QRS and T waves resulting in an artificially high heart rate.

Tachycardia is associated with haemorrhage, hypovolaemia or inadequate analgesia. Bradycardia in the ventilated infant is often a sign of blocked endotracheal tube, while in the self-breathing baby it is usually an indicator of apnoeic episodes.

Echocardiography

Echocardiography is used for the assessment of structural heart defects as well as helping to detect, and determine management of, the patent ductus arteriosus. It can also help in the assessment of ventricular function following asphyxia and in chronic lung disease. Although echocardiography may help guide in the use of volume replacement or inotrope support in a baby with hypotension, there is, as yet, no evidence that its routine use in monitoring the newborn baby has any impact on long-term outcome.

Perfusion

Tissue survival depends on both oxygenation and the blood flow (perfusion) through the capillary bed. Monitoring tissue perfusion is important for early recognition of circulatory failure and in assessing response to therapy.

Blood pressure

Perfusion is dependent on the systemic BP. Normal values in the neonate are shown in Appendix 4.

BP can be monitored directly with transducers attached to arterial lines. These need calibrating to zero and changes in position of the transducer relative to the heart may alter the reading. The calibration and position should be checked if there has been a sudden change in BP. Visual display of the waveform is important in assessing reliability, as damping of the arterial trace affects systolic and diastolic BP. Mean pressure remains more reliable but even this can become unreliable when the trace is damped.[20]

Non-invasive oscillometric methods significantly overestimate BP at the lower end and are poor at detecting hypotension. They should not be used to verify low readings from arterial lines. Mean BP is taken as the point where the oscillations in the cuff are maximum and, although related to the true mean BP, this value will differ from that obtained from an intra-arterial line.[25]

Hypotension occurs when compensatory mechanisms can no longer sustain the BP. Such decompensation should be avoided and what is needed is a reliable method of assessing tissue perfusion before any change in BP.

Skin perfusion

In low-flow states, blood supply in the skin is reduced to protect perfusion of vital organs. Skin blood flow is used as a marker of overall perfusion but it is also affected by the thermal environment.[32]

Capillary refill time correlates poorly with hypovolaemia in adults.[8] Normal values for neonates, nursed in different thermal environments, have been published,[74] and, in general, the skin reperfuses in less than 3 seconds. Capillary refill is better estimated on the skin of the forehead or chest rather than the toes, but the value of its routine determination is debatable.

Decreasing skin blood flow results in a widening of the central–peripheral temperature gap. This can indicate hypovolaemia, or a decrease in venous return, before the BP falls.[39] Delay is establishing vasomotor tone makes these changes an unreliable measure of tissue perfusion in the very-low-birthweight infant immediately after birth. In the absence of other indicators of hypovolaemia, such as a rising heart rate, a widening temperature gap is more likely to be due to cold stress.[41]

Central venous pressure (CVP)

CVP can be measured with an umbilical venous catheter in the right atrium. Close attention to maintaining the position of the transducer relative to the heart is essential, and the monitor must be calibrated to zero frequently. There is little information on the use of CVP in the newborn baby. A value of zero in the ventilated neonate is usually associated with other signs of hypovolaemia.[68]

Lactate

Measurement of lactate can be incorporated into blood gas or glucose analysers. Accumulation of lactate, implying increasing anaerobic metabolism, occurs in sepsis and with a reduction in tissue perfusion. There is poor correlation with arterial pH and, in the absence of a raised lactate, a metabolic acidosis is unlikely to be due to hypoperfusion. Values above 3 mmol/l soon after birth are abnormal and serial measurements can provide important prognostic information in ill, ventilated neonates.[23]

Lactate levels are elevated following asphyxia. Levels below 5 mmol/l, at 30 minutes of age, have been followed by a good outcome, while those above 9 mmol/l have been associated with moderate or severe encephalopathy.[22]

Persistently high lactate levels, above 10–15 mmol/l, suggest an inborn error of metabolism (pp. 907–21).

Other measures of perfusion

Change in urine output, monitored using pre-weighed nappies or cotton wool balls, is an insensitive marker of tissue perfusion, with volumes decreasing only after a fall in BP. Normal urine output is discussed on pages 336, 373.

Venous oxygen tension or saturation, measured in blood taken from a catheter passed through the foramen ovale into the left atrium, may be a better indicator of oxygen delivery but is not in routine use.[52] Near-infrared spectroscopy (NIRS)[83] and gastric intramucosal pH measured by tonometry[16] are techniques not yet applicable to everyday clinical use. Using echocardiography to measure flow in the superior vena cava gives a better reflection of cerebral blood flow than does cerebral artery Doppler measures or mean BP.[27]

Respiratory system monitoring

Respiration

Respiration monitors are used routinely to detect apnoea. They add little extra benefit to the monitoring of the ventilated baby, where more useful information is obtained from the ventilator.

There are several methods used for respiratory monitoring and these are discussed in Chapter 27.

The relationship between apnoea, bradycardia and desaturation is complex. In the majority of episodes, apnoea or hypoventilation is the initiating event, causing a fall in oxygen saturation, which in turn triggers a reflex bradycardia.[4]

Apnoea monitors alone have been shown to miss significant episodes of both apnoea and bradycardia.[70] In the absence of monitors that measure airflow, mixed or obstructive apnoea will only be identified by the accompanying bradycardia and desaturation.

An apnoea monitor should be attached to all spontaneously breathing babies who either have apnoeic attacks, or respiratory disease likely to be complicated by apnoea. However, if there are true concerns, then respiratory monitoring should always include a measure of heart rate and oxygen saturation.

Oxygen

A knowledge of the partial pressure of oxygen in arterial blood (PaO_2) is essential in intensive care. This can be measured intermittently, by arterial puncture or sampling from an indwelling catheter, or continuously, by use of an intravascular transducer. The frequency of sampling depends on the clinical condition of the baby and on the reliability placed on values obtained from continuous oxygen monitors.

Arterial puncture

This is painful, and crying alters the PaO_2.[24] A patent ductus arteriosus may result in a higher PaO_2 in the right arm and head/neck compared with other areas of the body.

Capillary and venous samples

Results from arterialised capillary samples can be misleading if the baby is poorly perfused or the blood not free flowing. They should not be used in the assessment of the acutely ill baby. Capillary samples underestimate PaO_2 significantly and should never be used to assess oxygenation.[44] They do not accurately predict arterial values in neonates[18] but can be useful for monitoring trends in PCO_2 and acid–base state in the stable baby.

Venous blood is of no use in the estimation of arterial PO_2 but may be an acceptable alternative to capillary samples for following trends in PCO_2 and acid–base state,[42] although the evidence in the literature is very limited. Venous samples should not be used in the assessment of the acutely ill baby.

Indwelling arterial lines

Indwelling arterial lines allow repeated sampling without disturbing the infant and can be used for continuous BP monitoring. Further information on the techniques used to insert arterial lines, and their complications, can be found in Chapter 28.

Umbilical artery catheter (UAC)

The tip of the UAC is positioned in the descending aorta (pp. 1240–1). High catheters (above the diaphragm) have fewer complications (Chapter 44) than those positioned low (just above the aortic bifurcation), and can remain in situ for longer.[9] Low-dose heparin (1 unit/ml) added to the infusion fluid reduces the risk of catheter blockage.[10]

To help position the catheter, many reference charts have been produced,[62,64] but an X-ray is needed to confirm the site of the tip (pp. 1240–1).

Peripheral artery catheters

The radial or posterior tibial arteries are commonly used, but the ulnar, dorsalis pedis and axillary arteries are alternatives (p. 1247–9). The brachial and femoral arteries should be avoided.

Complications are rare, but vasospasm and thrombus formation can cause major problems, even when collateral circulations are intact.

Total occlusion of the artery may persist after the catheter is removed. For this reason, the ulnar artery should not be used if the radial artery in that hand has been cannulated previously.

Low-dose heparin must be added to the infusion, the limb observed closely, and the catheter removed at the first sign of impaired perfusion.

Continuous intravascular blood gas monitoring

With intermittent sampling, major fluctuations in condition may be difficult to follow. Increasing the frequency of sampling introduces significant blood loss in small infants.

Continuous intravascular PaO_2 monitoring is possible.[30] Although reliable, the accuracy of these electrodes deteriorates with time, due to fibrin deposition. An intravascular catheter which measures PO_2, PCO_2, pH and temperature continuously, has been developed (Neotrend – Diametrics Medical Ltd, High Wycombe, UK). There can be difficulties with insertion, but they work well giving continuous blood gas data.[47]

Transcutaneous monitoring

These probes contain a heater that arterialises the blood in the skin. Oxygen diffuses through a membrane into the electrode, where it is reduced, setting up an electric current, the size of which is related to the partial pressure. This is displayed as the transcutaneous PO_2 (TcO_2).

Calibration takes several minutes and, once sited, the electrode takes around 15 minutes to equilibrate. The heat from the probe will burn the skin if not moved every 2–4 hours.[31,56] The combination of resiting and recalibration can mean that the sensor is not recording on the baby for substantial periods of time.

Falsely low readings are obtained if the probe is placed over poorly perfused skin, e.g. a bony surface,[76] if the infant lies on the electrode, or if there is poor peripheral circulation.[81] Falsely high readings occur when there is poor contact with the skin, allowing air to get under the electrode.

There is a larger difference between TcO_2 and PaO_2 in older infants,[57] but within infants the ratio between TcO_2 and PaO_2 remains constant. Although absolute values may not be accurate, the trend in TcO_2 can still give useful information.

The sensitivity and specificity of transcutaneous monitors at detecting hypoxia (PaO_2 <6.6 kPa) have been estimated at 85% and 97%, respectively. For hyperoxia (PaO_2 >13.3 kPa), the sensitivity is 87% and specificity 89%. This means that the monitors will miss approximately 15% of both hypoxic and hyperoxic events, defined by these limits.[57]

Target values for TcO_2 depend on maturity, severity of illness and underlying diagnosis. It is common practice in preterm infants to aim for TcO_2 between 6 and 10 kPa.

Saturation monitoring

Pulse oximetry is now the predominant method of oxygen monitoring. It is based on the principle that oxygenated haemoglobin absorbs light in the infrared region of the spectrum (850–1000 nm) while deoxygenated haemoglobin absorbs light in the visible red band (600–750 nm). The ratio of the light absorbed at two different wavelengths correlates with the proportions of oxygenated and deoxygenated haemoglobin in the tissues. The oximeter detects pulsation, which ensures that it is measuring only light absorbed by the haemoglobin in the blood vessels.

Pulse oximeters are easy to use, require no calibration and give immediate information. They are prone to artifact, and users must be aware of the many problems that can result in incorrect readings.

Strong ambient light and light bypassing the tissues cause an optical shunt, which is a common cause of artifact. Poor perfusion will affect the function of the oximeter, with most needing a pulse pressure of >20 mmHg[28,48] or a systolic BP >30 mmHg.[66]

Tight tape around the probe can affect the signal by impairing arterial pulsation, and can cause scarring and deformation of the hand or foot.

On the same infant, two oximeters may give different readings.[33] Some display 'functional' saturation and others 'fractional' saturation. The latter allows for levels of carboxyhaemoglobin and methaemoglobin, and is, in general, 2% lower.

Movement artifact is common and often makes interpretation of readings difficult, as well as being the most common cause of false alarms. It is important to check that the light plethysmography waveform shows a good-quality signal.[57] Another method of validation is to compare the pulse rate measured by the oximeter with that from an ECG monitor.[58] The readings are reliable only when the two heart rates are the same. In practice this usually means that the rates are within 5–10 beats of each other.

Figure 19.1 shows a typical trace with both heart rates. There is initially a period of poor agreement between the rates, and the dips in the saturation are caused by artifact. There then follows a period of good agreement, with reliable saturation readings.

Recent developments in pulse oximetry have reduced the false-alarm rates. In particular, instruments using the Masimo Signal extraction technology have been shown to identify true desaturations and bradycardias at least as reliably as a conventional oximeter[12] but with 93% fewer false alarms.[14]

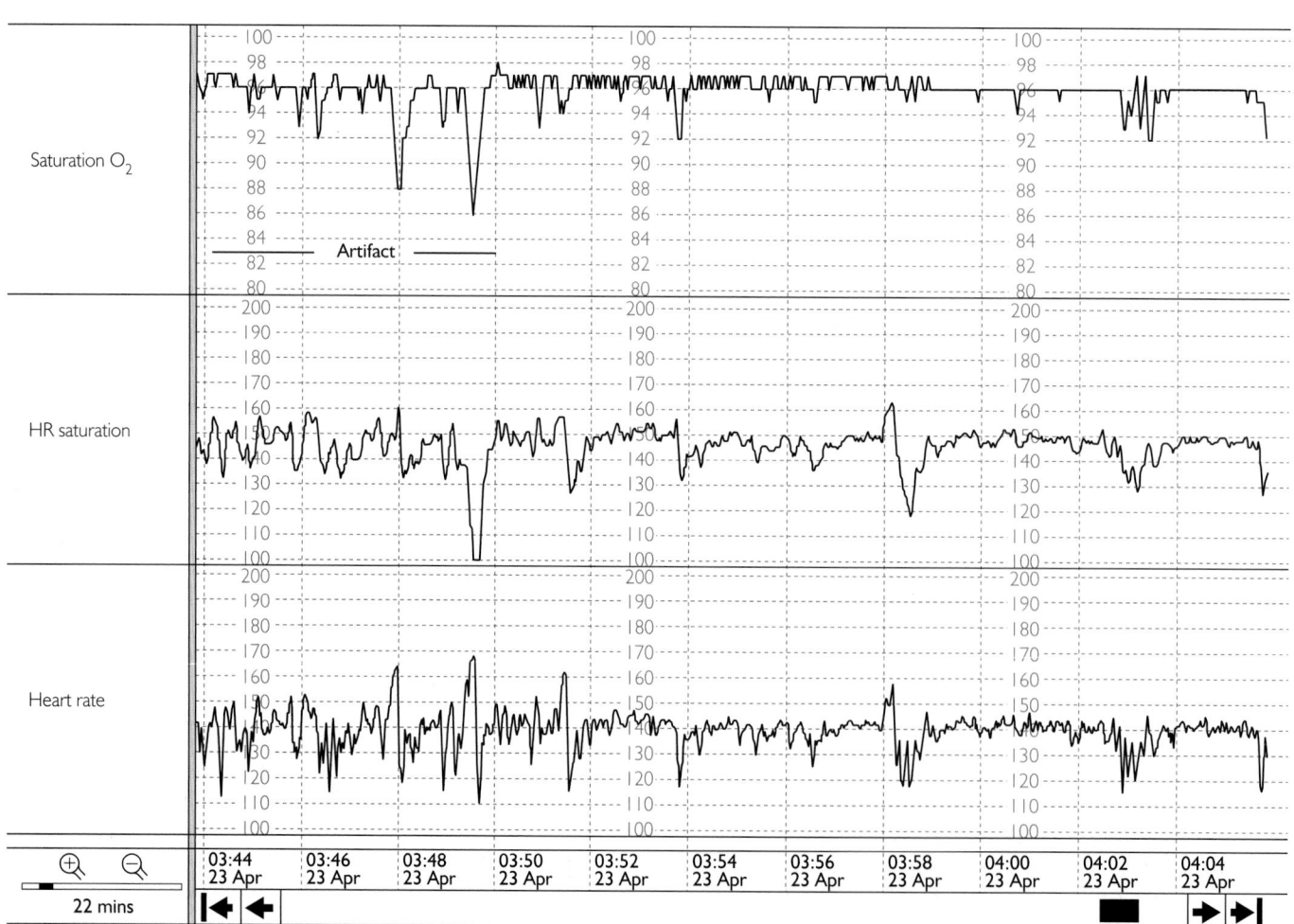

Fig. 19.1 Artifact on oxygen saturation recording shown by lack of agreement of heart rate traces.

Detection of hypoxia

Oximeters use 'look up' tables based on data from healthy adults to convert light absorption to saturation. Low levels have been derived by extrapolation from higher values and as a consequence these monitors underestimate the true degree of hypoxaemia. Sensitivity and specificity for the detection of hypoxaemia have been estimated at 92% and 97%, respectively.[57]

Hyperoxia

The shape of the haemoglobin dissociation curve means that oximeters have a low sensitivity to hyperoxia, with small shifts in saturation reflecting large changes in PO_2. With an upper alarm limit set at 95%, newer instruments detect hyperoxia (>10.6 kPa) with a sensitivity of around 95% but a specificity of only 26–45%. Lowering the alarm limits improves the sensitivity but decreases the specificity even further.[13]

Normal values for oxygen saturation

A functional saturation below 95%, obtained repeatedly while the infant is breathing regularly, should be regarded as abnormal, irrespective of age. Occasional falls in saturation below 80% are probably normal during the first 6 months of life.[55] However, there are no data that tell us at what baseline saturation level intervention should be considered or how often, or for how long, and to what nadir, saturation may be allowed to fall. We know a lot about saturation monitoring in normal babies but remain uncertain about how to apply this technology to infants with respiratory disease.

It is difficult to recommend limits for oxygen saturation in babies with lung disease. Applying data from normal babies may increase their exposure to inspired oxygen, which in itself may be damaging,[2,65,78] while low saturations in infants have been associated with acute life-threatening events.[37] Many recommend that oxygen therapy be considered when baseline saturation is less than 93%.[54] The safe upper limit is uncertain but recent outcome data suggest around 95%. In clinical practice it is impossible to set such tight limits without there being an unacceptable number of false alarms. Infants in hospital are commonly allowed lower saturations, but, if being discharged home in oxygen, they should be maintained with a saturation above 93%.[54]

Carbon dioxide

The partial pressure of carbon dioxide (PCO_2) is important in determining the adequacy of alveolar ventilation and interpreting the acid–base balance. PCO_2 is affected by crying, which commonly occurs during intermittent sampling. Capillary samples are useful for monitoring stable infants with chronic respiratory problems, but care must be exercised in their interpretation.[18] Venous samples may be an acceptable alternative when monitoring trends in PCO_2, but the literature is limited and even greater care should be taken in interpreting the values obtained. The new generation of multiparameter intravascular sensors (Neotrend) include continuous PCO_2 monitoring.

Transcutaneous CO_2 monitoring

Transcutaneous CO_2 (TcCO_2) is commonly combined with oxygen monitoring in the same probe. Most TcCO_2 electrodes work by measuring the change in pH of an electrolyte solution, separated from the skin by a hydrophobic membrane, which is permeable to carbon dioxide but not to hydrogen ions.

TcCO_2 is in general 27% higher than the corresponding arterial measurement, due partly to local tissue production of carbon dioxide as well as to the heating coefficient of blood. The electrodes need calibration against a known concentration of carbon dioxide every 4 hours. This can take 10 minutes, adding to the time that the probe is not in use monitoring the baby.

Over a 4-hour period, there is an upward drift in the TcCO_2 but overall there remains a good correlation between transcutaneous and arterial CO_2, making it a useful trend monitor. Repeated blood gas estimations are still required, but changes in TcCO_2 can give early warning of developing problems, such as a blocking endotracheal tube (Fig. 19.2). In transport, TcCO_2 monitoring has resulted in babies arriving with lower ventilator pressures and better blood gases.[51]

There are no data on normal values for TcCO_2. Experience with these monitors has been that each baby has an individual relationship between arterial and TcCO_2. These probes are more useful as a means of following trends than as a measurement of true arterial PCO_2.

End-tidal CO_2 monitoring

Capnography measures the concentration of CO_2 in exhaled gas and has been used extensively in patients under general anaesthesia and in adult intensive care. Small tidal volumes, rapid respiratory rates and inhomogeneous alveolar ventilation/perfusion in neonates with lung disease have limited the use in the newborn.[34] TcCO_2 monitoring provides a more accurate estimation of $PaCO_2$.[79]

The problem of inhomogeneous lung disease has been diminished by replacement surfactant. Studies using newer mainstream monitors, with low dead-space and resistance, have shown capnography to have some place in monitoring trends in carbon dioxide.[63] It may be useful in recognising oesophageal intubation.[60]

Acid–base balance

The pH, bicarbonate and base-excess are important in the assessment of respiratory status. The multiparameter UAC (Neotrend) records pH continuously and can also derive bicarbonate and base-excess. Capillary samples can be used to monitor changes in acid–base state in the stable baby. The usefulness of venous samples in such situations is uncertain.

Continuous on-line respiratory function monitoring

This is now available on most ventilators. Data are presented as numerical values, time-based waveforms of flow, volume and

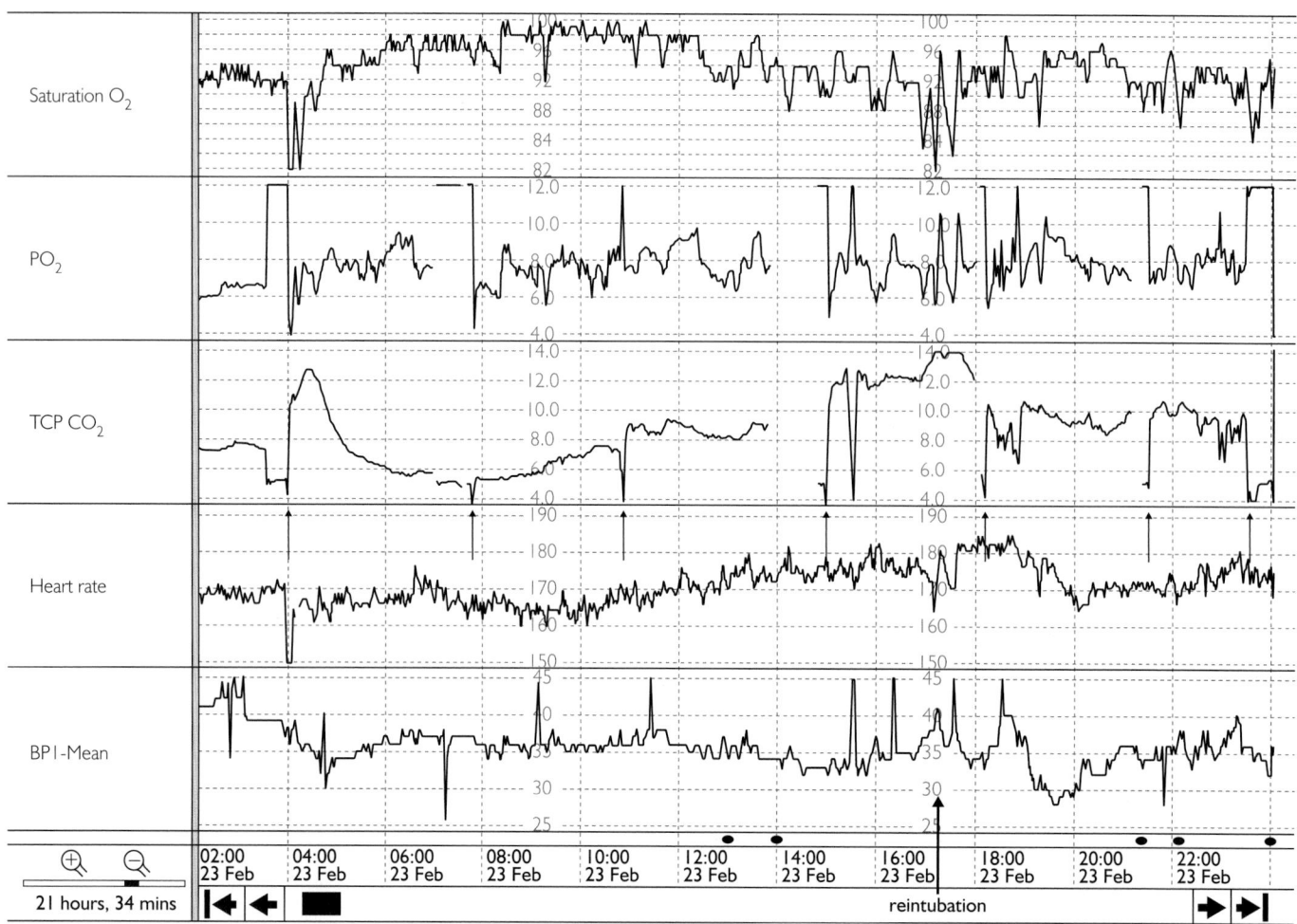

Fig. 19.2 Trend graphs of infant showing rise in transcutaneous CO_2 for several hours before blocked tube diagnosed. Black arrows show times when probe was off baby for recalibration.

airway pressures, and flow/volume and pressure/volume loops. The interpretation of this information requires a knowledge of how the data are obtained as well as an understanding of the underlying pathophysiology.

These monitors have been shown to reduce mortality in adults with acute respiratory distress syndrome.[3] In infants, their use has reduced ventilator time[72] and short-term morbidity,[61] although as yet there is little evidence that overall outcome is improved. Further critical evaluation is required, as not all the information used in adult trials can be obtained reliably in newborn infants.

A flow sensor, usually a hot-wire anemometer, needs to be connected directly to the endotracheal tube and this adds 1 ml to the respiratory dead-space. In the smallest infants this could necessitate increased minute ventilation to maintain CO_2 elimination.[73] Data from different devices may not be comparable. Changes in gas composition affect the measurements. Pure oxygen is 12% more viscous than room air, so reducing the fraction of inspired oxygen (FiO_2) may result in an apparent increase in tidal volume.[82]

Functional residual capacity

Measurements of tidal volume and functional residual capacity (FRC) can be used to avoid high end-inspiratory and low end-expiratory lung volumes. FRC varies considerably over the course of an illness and can change rapidly with treatments such as surfactant or high-frequency oscillatory ventilation. There is presently no readily applicable method for repeated measurements of FRC that would be suitable for routine clinical use. FRC is inferred from the chest X-ray appearances and the FiO_2 required to achieve adequate oxygenation, although the relationship between the radiographic and measured lung volumes is inconsistent.[77]

Leaks

There is generally some leak around the un-cuffed endotracheal tubes used in newborn infants. Bernstein et al[11] report a mean leak size of around 15%. A leak makes some of the derived data, such as compliance and resistance, unreliable and also complicates the interpretation of loops and waveforms. Most of the leak occurs in inspiration and is calculated as inspired minus expired volume, expressed as a percentage of the inspired volume. The displayed expired tidal volume has usually taken leak into account and further correction is not needed.

The size of leak only becomes important if there is a problem with ventilation. Flow-triggered ventilators are susceptible to autocycling in the presence of an airway leak, the rate of auto-cycling being proportional to the size of the leak.[11]

Tidal volume

A healthy, spontaneously breathing term infant with no lung disease has a tidal volume of around 7–9 ml/kg bodyweight.[1] The ventilated infant with respiratory disease has fewer functional airspaces, and there may be regional inhomogeneity of pressure volume characteristics within the lungs. 'Normal' tidal volumes may therefore expose parts of the lungs to excess end-inspiratory volume. Because of this, target tidal volumes are generally set around the 4–6 ml/kg range, depending on the CO_2 elimination. When there is pulmonary hypoplasia, target tidal volumes may need to be lowered as the inspiratory capacity of the lungs per unit bodyweight will be less than normal.

Some devices display tidal volume breath by breath, others give a rolling average. Spontaneous breaths are generally smaller than ventilator breaths, so if averaging is used it will not give a true impression of the ventilator tidal volumes, if there is significant spontaneous breathing. Displayed values are not weight corrected.

Minute ventilation

A rolling average of expired minute ventilation can be calculated and subdivided into the relative proportions attributable to ventilator and spontaneous breaths. Whether this is any more useful than looking at tidal volumes is unclear. There is no evidence that measuring minute ventilation is any more useful than monitoring transcutaneous PCO_2.

Compliance and resistance

There are a variety of methods for deriving these data from continuous dynamic pressure volume traces, but they are unlikely to be useful in everyday clinical practice. The values are affected by lung volume at the time of measurement and are unreliable if inappropriately short inspiratory or expiratory times are used. They are made inaccurate by leaks around the endotracheal tube. The variable nature of infant–ventilator interactions complicate their interpretation in real-time.

The C20:C ratio is a derived index of lung overdistension which compares the compliance during the last 20% of inflation with that of the whole breath.[29] This index is unreliable in newborn infants because it requires a ventilator which generates a slow rise in inflation pressure, or a constant flow of gas into the lungs during inflation, and little or no air leak,[49] conditions seldom met in neonatal ventilation.

Waveforms

Simultaneous time-based traces of flow, volume and pressure are the most commonly used graphical representation of respiratory function and provide the most readily interpretable information. The scaling of the graphs is important. Autoscaling should be used with caution, as changes in the size of the waveforms, due

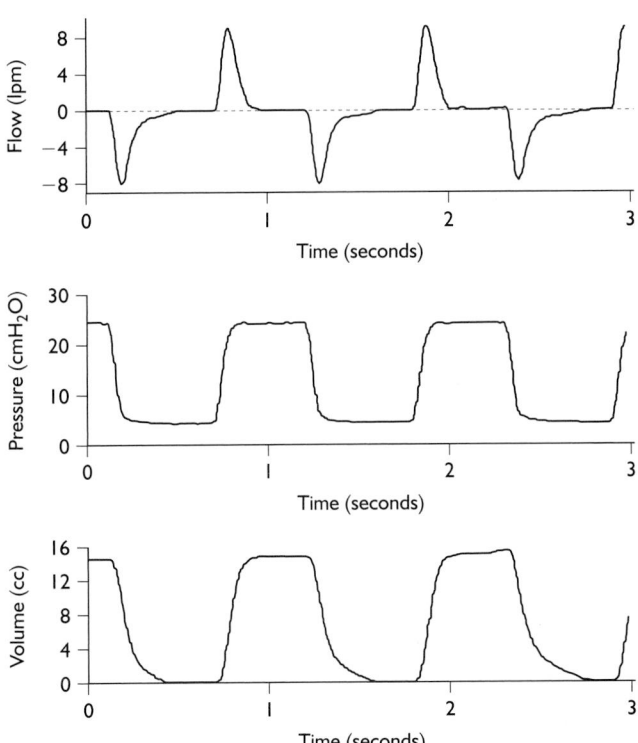

Fig. 19.3 Simultaneous time-based waveforms of flow, pressure and volume from a ventilated infant.

to variation in respiratory function, may be obscured by the system re-drawing them on a new scale.

The time-based waveforms help in determining appropriate inspiratory and expiratory times. Figure 19.3 shows simultaneous traces of flow, volume and pressure over time from a ventilated infant. With the onset of inflation, pressure rises to a peak and is maintained at this level for the duration of inspiration. As the pressure has risen, gas flows into the lungs and inspiratory flow (shown above the line) rises rapidly to a peak before falling to zero. No further volume passes into the lungs for the remainder of the set inspiratory time. The volume trace rises rapidly to a peak and then plateaus, with the inspired tidal volume held in the lungs until the onset of expiration. If there is an air leak around the endotracheal tube, the volume plateau is not horizontal but slopes upward from left to right (Fig. 19.4). The gradient of the slope reflects the size of the leak. Under these circumstances, the flow trace does not return to zero but continues at a low level after the initial rapid rise and fall (Fig. 19.4). In the case of a very large leak, or when the endotracheal tube has slipped out of the trachea, the volume trace continues to rise steeply until it goes off the screen and the flow remains high throughout inspiration. Under these circumstances, little or no expiratory flow is seen at the onset of expiration.

At the onset of expiration, the pressure in the ventilator circuit falls to the set positive end-expiratory pressure (PEEP) level. Gas flows out of the lungs and expiratory flow (conventionally displayed below the baseline) accelerates to a peak and then falls to zero (Fig. 19.3). The volume trace falls from the inspiratory volume peak to zero. If there is an air leak around

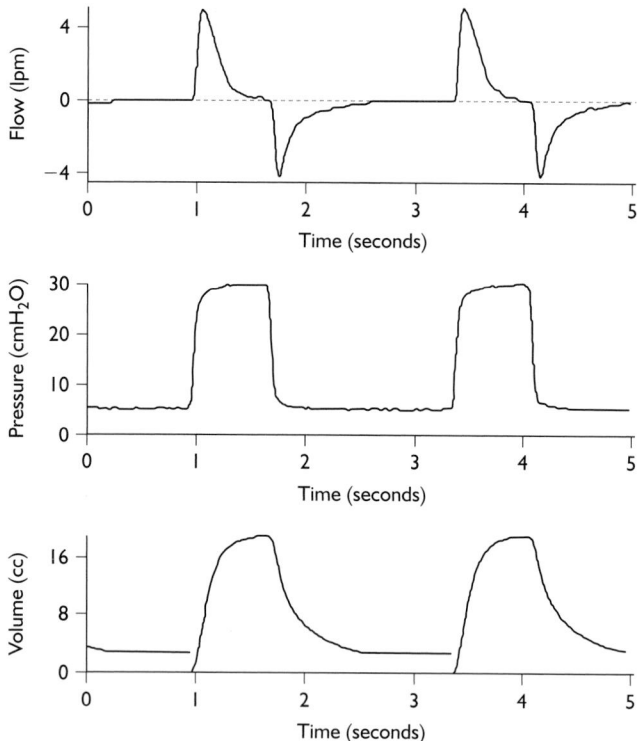

Fig. 19.4 Time-based waveforms from an infant with a modest leak around the endotracheal tube.

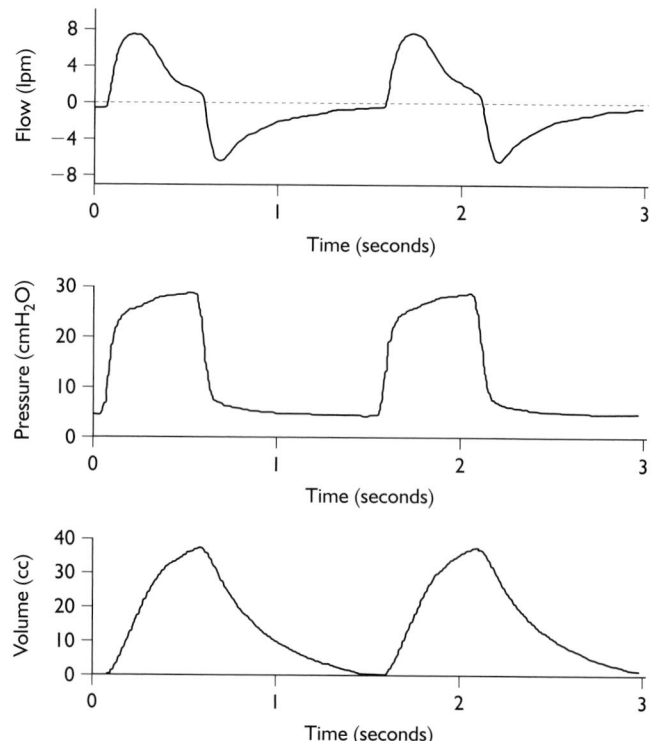

Fig. 19.5 Simultaneous waveforms from an infant with a long expiratory phase. After 1 second in expiration, expiratory flow has not quite reached zero before the onset of the next inspiration.

the endotracheal tube, the volume trace does not return to zero because the gas that leaked around the tube in inspiration cannot be exhaled (Fig. 19.4). Monitoring devices are usually set to re-zero the volume baseline at the onset of the next inspiratory flow. If the next inflation begins before the expiratory flow has returned to zero, gas is trapped in the lungs. This phenomenon is called occult or inadvertent PEEP.[67] It will impair gas exchange and occasionally may be life-threatening.[71] Inspection of the expired flow waveform allows the clinician to ensure that expiratory flow has returned to zero before the onset of the next inflation and prevent this complication. In Figure 19.5, expiratory flow has not quite returned to zero when the next inflation arrives, despite an expiration time of around 1 second.

With an obstructing endotracheal tube, the height of the peak flow on the inspiratory and expiratory flow waveforms lessens, and the width of the expiratory flow pattern broadens because the increase in airway resistance makes gas movements take longer.

Excessive rain-out of humidity in the tubing can partially obstruct the bias flow in the circuit. This causes fluctuations in airway pressure, resulting in small flow oscillations at the airway, which are seen in the flow baseline at times when there should be no flow. They can result in autocycling of the ventilator, and the presence of an oscillating flow baseline should prompt inspection of the circuit for trapped water.

Loops

Pressure/volume and flow/volume are the commonest displayed loops. They are distorted by infant–ventilator interactions. If the screen is watched in real time, breaths that are relatively free from interaction can be identified when the infant is settled. Pressure/volume loops can be inspected to determine the critical opening pressure of the airspaces and the upper inflection point where the slope of the pressure/volume relationship begins to flatten because of overdistension. This has been used in adults to facilitate less damaging ventilation strategies.[59] However, in order to plot the progressive change in lung volume that occurs for a given change in pressure, the pressure has to rise slowly enough to allow changes in volume to keep pace. Pressure-limited neonatal ventilators generate relatively square pressure waves with a rapid rise to peak inspiratory pressure and an equally rapid fall to the PEEP level in expiration. This means that the changes in lung volume during inspiration are mostly plotted against the peak inspiratory pressure and during expiration against the end pressure, giving the loops a rectangular appearance which bears little relationship to the underlying pressure/volume characteristics of the lung (Fig. 19.6). Significant leaks around the endotracheal tube make interpretation even more difficult.

Inspection of flow/volume loops can give information about airway resistance. If resistance is increased, flow is slower. This can be observed from the time-based waveforms without the need to look at flow/volume loops. If there are secretions in the endotracheal tube, the expiratory limb of the loop can show a saw-tooth pattern, indicating the need for endotracheal suction.[38]

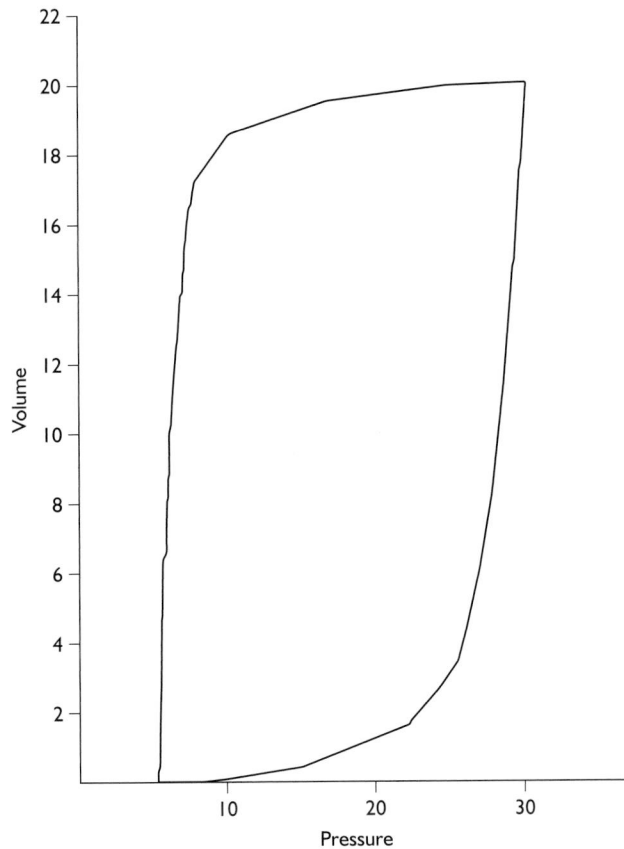

Fig. 19.6 Pressure/volume loop from an infant on pressure-limited ventilation.

Neurological system monitoring

Compared with the respiratory and cardiovascular systems, there is little available for continuous neurological monitoring. Examination of the nervous system is often intermittent and assessment subjective. It is more difficult when sedative drugs and neuromuscular paralysis agents are given.

EEG and cerebral function monitors

Continuous EEG recording is now feasible and clinically useful. EEG is the best method for detecting seizure activity. Changes in the background give important prognostic information following hypoxic-ischaemic injury (Chapter 41).

Interpretation of the full EEG can be difficult and techniques to simplify the data have been introduced. Amplitude-integrated EEG (aEEG) monitoring, using the Cerebral Function Monitor (CFM), is produced from a single EEG lead. Two electrodes are attached to the scalp. Although adhesive is often used, more reliable recordings over long periods of time are obtained using needle electrodes placed under the skin. The CFM has been shown to be effective in monitoring cerebroelectrical background activity in sick neonates[36] and in detection of subclincal seizures.[35] It has a predictive value in the first hours of life following asphyxial injury.[5]

Although aEEG can be used for long periods, it must be remembered that it is a simplified method for monitoring electrocortical background activity and has limitations. Its simplicity is an advantage but can result in difficulties in interpreting whether a pattern represents seizure or other activity. A least one standard EEG should be recorded in monitored infants.

Cerebral ultrasound

Ultrasound offers an easy method of imaging the neonatal brain. Repeated scans allow progress to be monitored and give prognostic information. Abnormalities that persist are more likely to be genuine, and most conditions evolve over time, allowing more certain diagnosis. Ultrasound changes must be interpreted with care and its use is covered in pages 77–8.

Intracranial pressure monitoring

Indirect measurements of intracranial pressure taken across the anterior fontanelle have been found to be unreliable and inaccurate. Invasive intracranial pressure monitoring may have its place in specialist units, but has not been shown to improve outcome in the baby with neonatal encephalopathy secondary to a hypoxic-ischaemic insult.

Near-infrared spectroscopy

NIRS is capable of providing information on cerebral haemoglobin oxygen saturation, cerebral blood volume, cerebral blood flow, cerebral oxygen delivery, cerebral venous saturation and cerebral oxygen availability-utilisation. Although giving useful information on cerebral haemodynamics, this technique remains mainly a research tool and has not yet become established in everyday clinical care.

Temperature monitoring

Measuring central temperature is important. The rectum should not be used as there is a significant risk of damage to the mucosa. Rectal temperature is unreliable and is affected by the depth of insertion of the thermometer, whether the baby has just passed a stool and by the temperature of the blood returning from the lower limbs.

The temperature of the skin over the liver or in the axilla reflects central temperature. A more accurate measurement can be obtained by placing the probe between the scapulae and a non-conducting mattress. No tape is needed on the skin since the baby lies on the probe, holding it in place. This so-called zero heat flux temperature has been shown to be very close to the central temperature.[26]

The measure of a single temperature tells us how well the baby is maintaining that temperature but nothing about how

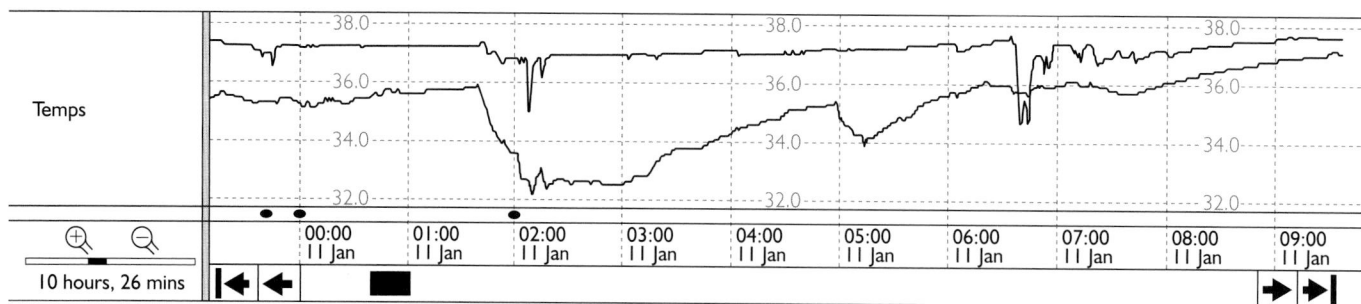

Fig. 19.7 Trend in central (top trace) and peripheral (bottom trace) temperatures, showing widening of the gap during handling, with slow recovery after the procedure.

much energy is being used to achieve thermal balance. The continuous measurement and display of a central (abdominal, axilla or zero heat flux) and a peripheral (foot) temperature detects cold stress. Figure 19.7 shows an increasing temperature gap during a procedure. The baby is exposed to cold stress, but if the central temperature alone was being measured, then this would not have been apparent. Central measures of temperature vary, but the baby is usually between 36.8°C and 37.3°C with a central–peripheral temperature gap of around 1°C.

A high central temperature, particularly if unstable, along with a wide central–peripheral gap is seen in septic babies.[46]

Monitoring the sick baby

What needs to be monitored will always depend on the clinical condition of the baby. The sick or unstable baby, and this includes the preterm ventilated newborn, should, wherever possible, have continuous intra-arterial BP monitoring, as hypotension is an important factor in poor outcome. Continuous measurement and display of dual temperatures gives useful information on thermal balance and perfusion.

The monitoring of oxygen, carbon dioxide and acid–base state is essential in intensive care. It is vital to have a method of continuous oxygen monitoring, although there will still be a need for intermittent blood sampling – usually 4–6 hourly, but this may be more frequent if there are repeated changes in ventilation or the clinical condition dictates.

There is debate about the best method of continuous oxygen monitoring. Further research is needed before any definite recommendation can be made about whether saturation or PO_2 should be used. Despite the lack of comparative literature, saturation is now the most widely used method, but this is subject to artifact and can underestimate both hypoxia and hyperoxia. Saturation monitors are easy to use but the information they produce is often more difficult to interpret than many inexperienced users think. Indwelling arterial probes and transcutaneous monitors measure PO_2 but in both it can be difficult to maintain reliable readings in the baby. Transcutaneous monitors give very useful information on the trend in PCO_2.

Whatever method is used to monitor blood gases, users must have a good understanding of how the values are obtained and the pitfalls in their interpretation.

Clinical and laboratory monitoring

Infection

Infection is an important cause of morbidity and mortality. Babies must be screened whenever there is a clinical indication of suspected sepsis. The screen should include culture of blood, cerebrospinal fluid, urine, secretions and swabs, although which are needed in each case will depend on the clinical picture and the policy of the individual unit.

The coagulase-negative staphylococcus is commonly grown in cultures and the differentiation of infection from colonisation can be difficult. In all situations, the result of cultures must be interpreted in the light of the clinical features and other supportive laboratory tests, particularly differential white count, platelet count and C-reactive protein. There are many studies looking at the best predictors of infection in the neonate but none have come up with any method that has acceptable values for sensitivity and specificity.

In the ventilated baby there is debate about the usefulness of routine culture of endotracheal aspirates. Some studies have shown a close association[40] between organisms isolated in the trachea and those grown from blood cultures, while other have not.[69]

A knowledge of the organisms colonising the respiratory tract can be useful if there is a clinical deterioration or change in other laboratory markers of infection. They give a guide to antibiotic choice until further culture results are available. A Gram stain of the secretions showing increasing white cell count may be indicative of infection rather than colonisation.

Fluid balance

Input/output charts should be used to help assess fluid balance, but it is important to measure all fluids given to the baby, including drugs and flushes for catheters.[50]

Allowance must be made for evaporative fluid losses unless the baby is nursed in high humidity. Respiratory fluid losses can be high if there is inadequate humidification of the ventilator gases.

Urine output can be assessed by using pre-weighed nappies or cotton wool balls, but these must be weighed as soon as possible after voiding, to avoid evaporative loss.[17]

Fluid shifts in the baby are reflected in weight changes, but it is difficult in clinical practice to get good reproducible measurements, even when using within-incubator scales.

In the first days of life, changes in plasma sodium reflect hydration, with hyponatraemia being due to fluid overload and hypernatraemia to dehydration. Analysers now measure sodium along with the blood gases. Several measurements of plasma sodium throughout the day, along with the input/output chart, gives a good estimate of fluid balance in the sick neonate.

Biochemistry

As well as repeated estimations of plasma sodium, to help assess fluid balance, other electrolytes, glucose, creatinine, bilirubin, and calcium should be measured once daily, and more often if clinically indicated. Laboratory methods are discussed in Chapter 43 and normal values are given in Appendix 6. If parenteral nutrition is being used, then appropriate biochemical monitoring is needed (Chapter 17).

Haematology

Blood losses from sampling should be recorded and the sick ventilated baby must have a haemoglobin and/or haematocrit measured at least daily. Deciding on the optimum time for transfusion with red cells is difficult and there are no good data in the literature to help. Individual units need to develop their own guidelines.

Thrombocytopenia is often seen in sepsis, particularly if there is a consumptive coagulopathy or where central intravenous lines have been infected with coagulase-negative staphylococci. In ill babies, the platelet count, clotting studies and fibrinogen should be monitored regularly. Heparin in arterial lines can contaminate the samples for clotting studies and care must be taken in the interpretation of the results.

Daily total white counts, and the differential, can give an indication of developing sepsis. Absolute values are very varied, but changes, either up or down, can be indicative of infection.

Flow charts and plotting results on graphs are useful as they show trends in biochemical and haematological data.

Point-of-care testing

Point-of-care (near-patient) testing is expanding with the development of highly accurate instruments.

Blood gas analysers on the nursery are a mandatory part of the equipment of any intensive care unit. Glucose should always be measured using whole blood glucose analysers such as the Yellow Springs; cotside stick methods (Dextrostix, BM-glycaemie, or reflostix) are no longer considered sufficiently accurate for neonatal use (p. 1219).

New generations of analysers allow the measurement of a whole range of parameters without sending blood to the laboratory. Each unit must determine which bedside tests are indicated based on an analysis of test accuracy, clinical importance and cost–benefit ratio. There are major issues about maintenance of appropriate standards and quality control that also need to be addressed.

X-ray monitoring (Chapters 29 and 44)

Although routine radiographs have been shown to be safe and not expose the extremely-low-birthweight infant to any excessive radiation risk,[75] the use of X-rays should be limited and determined by clinical need.

The chest X-ray is vital in the initial assessment of all babies with respiratory disease. Further X-rays, throughout the course of the respiratory illness, should be done as clinically indicated.

Abdominal X-rays help in the diagnosis of necrotising enterocolitis (NEC) and in detecting intestinal perforation. There is debate in how often these X-rays should be repeated in infants with NEC.

There are many other indications for X-rays, including to check the position of endotracheal tubes and the tips of central arterial and venous lines.

Intravenous pumps

All pumps used to deliver intravenous fluids must have in-line pressure alarms. These detect occlusion in the line distal to the pump. Many have adjustable limits and can be set to detect small changes in pressure, which could give an early warning of fluid extravasation into the tissues.

Unfortunately there is no evidence that any of the currently marketed infusion devices are capable of predicting or detecting infiltration in any patient population. Pressure changes caused by patient movement are far greater than those found in the early stages of fluid extravasation.[53]

Close observation of the infusion site at regular intervals, stopping the infusion at the first sign of swelling or redness, is all that is available to detect fluid extravasation and hopefully prevent or minimise subsequent tissue damage. Scarring from tissue infiltration is now a common cause of complaint and litigation. It is important that all units have a policy for the observation of intravenous infusions and that there is a record of the sites being observed at least hourly.

Data handling

Technical advances have increased the amount and complexity of data from monitors, but 'more' is not necessarily 'better'. For example, although there are theoretical reasons why the large number of parameters available from ventilator monitors should be helpful, there is, for many, little evidence that in routine clinical care they make any difference. Inexperienced doctors and nurses, who may be responsible for much of the day-to-day care, are faced with increasingly complex, and potentially useless, information, before they have even grasped the basic principles. There is a serious danger of 'data overload'. An increasing multitude of alarms, often indicating minor technical problems only, result in the 'crying wolf' situation, with staff less likely to react appropriately to correct alarms.[80] There is a need to assess critically what is essential for the care of the baby, and the introduction of new monitoring parameters should be resisted without assessment of their usefulness by rigorous clinical trials.

Monitoring is not just about reading values from machines. It is the ability to integrate a whole range of data, including observation of the 'whole' baby, into meaningful information. 'Experience' and 'gut feeling' are really recognition of patterns, although the process may occur subconsciously. Experienced nursing staff are an essential part of the monitoring of the baby and they often raise concerns about potential problems. However, even the most experienced clinical staff are slow at recognising developing problems even when the patterns, on retrospective review, have been obvious for some time.[6]

Continuous trend monitoring

Monitors and blood tests give information on the condition of the baby at a single moment. Displaying data as a continuous graph allows trends to be visualised, hopefully facilitating detection of abnormalities and allowing earlier intervention. The typical patterns in the trends of central–peripheral temperature differences shown in Figure 19.7 are a good example.

Plotted trends can show that a parameter is changing significantly, even before the values are outside the set alarm ranges. They may also make it clearer which readings are due to artifact.

Figure 19.2 shows the high PCO_2 associated with a blocked endotracheal tube, necessitating an emergency reintubation. Although the clinical deterioration was sudden, it can be seen that the PCO_2 had been rising slowly for several hours. Earlier assessment may well have avoided the subsequent collapse. Trend monitoring of $TcCO_2$ may also facilitate earlier diagnosis of pulmonary air leak.[43]

A randomised controlled trial of trend monitoring in neonatal intensive care failed to show that it improved outcome.[19] Data overload, an inability to ascertain which data were important, a failure to include enough relevant information, or simply that staff were ignorant of the patterns that existed may be the reasons why trend monitoring did not make any difference to outcome. Also, it is often the change in a number of parameters that is important and it can be difficult to visualise these all at once. Computers can be used to recognise complex trends and what is needed are computerised decision support systems if the full potential of continuous trend data is to be recognised.[7] In such systems, artifact detection and removal remains a challenge but this has been shown to be feasible.[21]

References

1. [Anonymous] 1993 Respiratory mechanics in infants: physiologic evaluation in health and disease. American Thoracic Society/European Respiratory Society. American Review of Respiratory Disease 147: 474–496
2. [Anonymous] 2000 Supplemental Therapeutic Oxygen for Prethreshold Retinopathy Of Prematurity (STOP-ROP), a randomized, controlled trial. I: Primary outcomes. Pediatrics 105: 295–310
3. [Anonymous] 2000 Ventilation with lower tidal volumes as compared with traditional tidal volumes for acute lung injury and the acute respiratory distress syndrome. The Acute Respiratory Distress Syndrome Network. New England Journal of Medicine 342: 1301–1308
4. Adams J A, Zabaleta I A, Sackner M A 1997 Hypoxemic events in spontaneously breathing premature infants: etiologic basis. Pediatric Research 42: 463–471
5. al Naqeeb N, Edwards A D, Cowan F M et al 1999 Assessment of neonatal encephalopathy by amplitude-integrated electroencephalography. Pediatrics 103: 1263–1271
6. Alberdi E, Becher J-C, Gilhooly K et al 2001 Expertise and the interpretation of computerised physiological data: implications for the design of computerised physiological monitoring in neonatal intensive care. International Journal of Human Computer Studies 55: 191–216
7. Alberdi E, Gilhooly K, Hunter J et al 2000 Computerisation and decision making in neonatal intensive care: a cognitive engineering investigation. Journal of Clinical Monitoring 16: 85–94
8. Baraff L J 1993 Capillary refill time: is it a useful clinical sign? Pediatrics 92: 723–724
9. Barrington K J 2000 Umbilical artery catheters in the newborn: effects of position of the catheter tip (Cochrane Review). Cochrane Database of Systematic Reviews (2): CD000505
10. Barrington K J 2000 Umbilical artery catheters in the newborn: effects of heparin (Cochrane Review). Cochrane Database of Systematic Reviews (2): CD000507
11. Bernstein G, Knodel E, Heldt G P 1995 Airway leak size and autocycling of three flow-triggered ventilators. Critical Care Medicine 23: 1739–1744
12. Bohnhorst B, Peter C S, Poets C F 2000 Pulse oximeters' reliability in detecting hypoxemia and bradycardia: comparison between a conventional and two new generation oximeters. Critical Care Medicine 28: 1565–1568
13. Bohnhorst B, Peter C S, Poets C F 2002 Detection of hyperoxaemia in neonates: data from three new pulse oximeters. Archives of Disease in Childhood. Fetal and Neonatal Edition 87: F217–F219
14. Bohnhorst B, Poets C F 1998 Major reduction in alarm frequency with a new pulse oximeter. Intensive Care Medicine 24: 277–278
15. British Association of Perinatal Medicine 2001 Standards for hospitals providing neonatal intensive and high dependency care, 2nd edition.
16. Campbell M E, Costeloe K L 2001 Measuring intramucosal pH in very low birthweight infants. Pediatric Research 50: 398–404
17. Cooke R J, Werkman S, Watson D 1989 Urine output measurements in premature infants. Pediatrics 83: 116–118
18. Courtney S E, Weber K R, Breakie L A et al 1990 Capillary blood gases in the neonate. A reassessment and review of the literature. American Journal of Diseases of Children 144: 168–172
19. Cunningham S, Deere S, Symon A et al 1998 A randomized, controlled trial of computerized physiologic trend monitoring in an intensive care unit. Critical Care Medicine 26: 2053–2060
20. Cunningham S, Symon A G, McIntosh N 1994 Changes in mean blood pressure caused by damping of the arterial pressure waveform. Early Human Development 36: 27–30
21. Cunningham S, Symon A G, McIntosh N 1994 The practical management of artifact in computerised physiological data. International Journal of Clinical Monitoring and Computing 11: 211–216
22. Da Silva S, Hennebert N, Denis R, Wayenberg J-L 2000 Clinical value of a single postnatal lactate measurement after intrapartum asphyxia. Acta Paediatrica 89: 320–323
23. Deshpande S A, Ward Platt M P 1997 Association between blood lactate and acid-base status and mortality in ventilated babies. Archives of Disease in Childhood. Fetal and Neonatal Edition 76: F15–F20
24. Dinwiddie R, Patel B D, Kumar S P et al 1979 The effects of crying on arterial oxygen tension in infants recovering from respiratory distress. Critical Care Medicine 7: 50–53
25. Diprose G K, Evans D H, Archer L N J, Levene M I 1986 Dinamap fails to detect hypotension in very low birth weight infants. Archives of Disease in Childhood 61: 771–773
26. Dollberg S, Xi Y, Donnelly M M 1993 A noninvasive transcutaneous alternative to rectal thermometry for continuous measurement of core temperature in the piglet. Pediatric Research 34: 512–517
27. Evans N, Klucklow M, Simmons M et al 2002 Which to measure, systemic or organ blood flow? Middle cerebral artery and superior vena cava flow in very preterm infants. Archives of Disease in Childhood. Fetal and Neonatal Edition 87: F181–F184
28. Falconer R J, Robinson B J 1990 Comparison of pulse oximeters: accuracy at low arterial pressure in volunteers. British Journal of Anaesthetics 65: 552–557

29. Fisher J B, Mammel M C, Coleman J M et al 1988 Identifying lung overdistension during mechanical ventilation by using volume-pressure loops. Pediatric Pulmonology 5: 10–14

30. Goddard P, Keith I, Marcovitch H et al 1974 Use of a continuously recording intravascular oxygen electrode in the newborn. Archives of Disease in Childhood 49: 853–860

31. Golden S M 1981 Skin craters – a complication of transcutaneous oxygen monitoring. Pediatrics 67: 514–516

32. Gorelick M H, Shaw K N, Baker M D 1993 Effect of ambient temperature on capillary refill in healthy children. Pediatrics 92: 699–702

33. Grieve S H, McIntosh N, Laing I A 1997 Comparison of two different pulse oximeters in monitoring preterm infants. Critical Care Medicine 25: 2051–2054

34. Hand I L, Shepard E K, Krauss A N et al 1989 Discrepancies between transcutaneous and end-tidal carbon dioxide monitoring in the critically ill neonate with respiratory distress syndrome. Critical Care Medicine 17: 556–559

35. Hellstrom-Westas L, Rosen I, Svenningsen N W 1985 Silent seizures in sick infants in early life. Acta Paediatrica Scandinavica 74: 741–748

36. Hellstrom-Westas L, Rosen I, Svenningsen N W 1990 Cerebral complications detected by EEG-monitoring during neonatal intensive care. Acta Paediatrica Supplement 360: 83–86

37. Iles R, Edmunds A T 1996 Prediction of early outcome in resolving chronic lung disease of prematurity after discharge from hospital. Archives of Disease in Childhood 74: 304–308

38. Jubran A, Tobin M J 1994 Use of flow-volume curves in detecting secretions in ventilator-dependent patients. American Journal of Respiratory and Critical Care Medicine 150: 766–769

39. Lambert H J, Baylis P H, Coulthard M G 1998 Central-peripheral temperature difference, blood pressure, and arginine vasopressin in preterm neonates undergoing volume expansion. Archives of Disease in Childhood. Fetal and Neonatal Edition 78: F43–F45

40. Lau Y L, Hey E N 1991 Sensitivity and specificity of daily tracheal aspirate cultures in providing organisms causing bacteremia in ventilated neonates. Pediatric Infectious Disease Journal 10: 290–294

41. Lyon A J, Pikaar M E, Badger P et al 1997 Temperature control in very low birthweight infants during the first five days of life. Archives of Disease in Childhood. Fetal and Neonatal Edition 76: F47–F50

42. McGillivray D, Ducharme F M, Carron Y, Mattimoe C, Treherne S 1999 Clinical decision making based on venous versus capillary blood gas values in the well-perfused child. Annals of Emergency Medicine 34: 58–63

43. McIntosh N, Becher J-C, Cunningham S et al 2000 Clinical diagnosis of pneumothorax is late: use of trend data and decision support might allow preclinical detection. Pediatric Research 48: 408–415

44. McLain B I, Evans J, Dear P R 1988 Comparison of capillary and arterial blood gas measurements in neonates. Archives of Disease in Childhood 63: 743–747

45. Merenstein G B, Dougherty K, Lewis A 1972 Early detection of pneumothorax by oscilloscope monitor in the newborn infant. Journal of Pediatrics 80: 98–101

46. Messaritakis J, Anagnostakis D, Laskari H et al 1990 Rectal-skin temperature difference in septicaemic newborn infants. Archives of Disease in Childhood 65: 380–382

47. Morgan C, Newell S J, Ducker D A et al 1999 Continuous neonatal blood gas monitoring using a multiparameter intra-arterial sensor. Archives of Disease in Childhood. Fetal and Neonatal Edition 80: F93–F98

48. Morris R W, Nairn M, Torda T A 1989 A comparison of fifteen pulse oximeters. Part I: A clinical comparison; Part II: A test of performance under conditions of poor perfusion. Anaesthesia and Intensive Care 17: 62–73

49. Neve V, de la Roque E D, Leclerc F et al 2000 Ventilator-induced overdistension in children: dynamic versus low-flow inflation volume-pressure curves. American Journal of Respiratory and Critical Care Medicine 162: 139–147

50. Noble-Jamieson C M, Kuzmin P, Airede K I 1986 Hidden sources of fluid and sodium intake in ill newborn infants. Archives of Disease in Childhood 61: 695–696

51. O'Connor T A, Grueber R 1998 Transcutaneous measurement of carbon dioxide tension during long-distance transport of neonates receiving mechanical ventilation. Journal of Perinatology 18: 189–192

52. O'Connor T A, Hart R T 1994 Mixed venous oxygenation in critically ill neonates. Critical Care Medicine 22: 343–346

53. Phelps S J, Tolley E A, Cochran E B 1990 Inability of inline pressure monitoring to predict or detect infiltration of peripheral intravenous catheters in infants. Clinical Pharmacy 9: 286–292

54. Poets C F 1998 When do infants need additional inspired oxygen? A review of the current literature. Pediatric Pulmonology 26: 424–428

55. Poets C F 1999 Assessing oxygenation in healthy infants. Journal of Pediatrics 135: 541–543

56. Poets C F, Samuels M P, Noyes J P et al 1991 Home monitoring of transcutaneous oxygen tension in the early detection of hypoxaemia in infants and young children. Archives of Disease in Childhood 66: 676–682

57. Poets C F, Southall D P 1994 Noninvasive monitoring of oxygenation in infants and children: practical considerations and areas of concern. Pediatrics 93: 737–746

58. Poets C F, Stebbens V A 1997 Detection of movement artifact in recorded pulse oximeter saturation. European Journal of Pediatrics 156: 808–811

59. Ranieri V M, Suter P M, Tortorella C et al 1999 Effect of mechanical ventilation on inflammatory mediators in patients with acute respiratory distress syndrome: a randomized controlled trial. Journal of the American Medical Association 282: 54–61

60. Roberts W A, Maniscalco W M, Cohen A R et al 1995 The use of capnography for recognition of esophageal intubation in the neonatal intensive care unit. Pediatric Pulmonology 19: 262–268

61. Rosen W C, Mammel M C, Fisher J B et al 1993 The effects of bedside pulmonary mechanics testing during infant mechanical ventilation: a retrospective analysis. Pediatric Pulmonology 16: 147–152

62. Rosenfeld W, Biagtan J, Schaeffer H et al 1980 A new graph for insertion of umbilical artery catheters. Journal of Pediatrics 96: 735–737

63. Rozycki H J, Sysyn G D, Marshall M K et al 1998 Mainstream end-tidal carbon dioxide monitoring in the neonatal intensive care unit. Pediatrics 101: 648–653

64. Rubin B K, McRobert E, O'Neill M B 1986 An alternate technique to determine umbilical arterial catheter length. Clinical Pediatrics 25: 407–408

65. Saugstad O D 2001 Update on oxygen radical disease in neonatology. Current Opinion in Obstetrics and Gynecology 13: 147–153

66. Severinghaus J W, Spellman M J J 1990 Pulse oximeter failure thresholds in hypotension and vasoconstriction. Anesthesiology 73: 532–537

67. Simbruner G 1986 Inadvertent positive end-expiratory pressure in mechanically ventilated newborn infants: detection and effect on lung mechanics and gas exchange. Journal of Pediatrics 108: 589–595

68. Skinner J R, Milligan D W A, Hunter S et al 1992 Central venous pressure in the ventilated neonate. Archives of Disease in Childhood 67: 374–377

69. Slagel T A, Bifano E M, Wolf J W et al 1989 Routine endotracheal cultures for the prediction of sepsis in ventilated babies. Archives of Disease in Childhood 64: 34–38

70. Southall D P, Levitt G A, Richards J M et al 1983 Undetected episodes of prolonged apnea and severe bradycardia in preterm infants. Pediatrics 72: 541–551

71. Stenson B J, Glover R M, Wilkie R A et al 1995 Life-threatening inadvertent positive end-expiratory pressure. American Journal of Perinatology 12: 336–338

72. Stenson B J, Glover R M, Wilkie R A et al 1998 Randomised controlled trial of respiratory system compliance measurements in mechanically ventilated neonates. Archives of Disease in Childhood. Fetal and Neonatal Edition 78: F15–F19

73. Stokes G M, Milner A D, Wilson A J et al 1986 Ventilatory response to increased dead spaces in the first week of life. Pediatric Pulmonology 2: 89–93

74. Strozik K S, Pieper C H, Roller J 1997 Capillary refilling time in newborn babies: normal values. Archives of Disease in Childhood 67: 374–377

75. Sutton P M, Arthur R J, Taylor C et al 1998 Ionising radiation from diagnostic x rays in very low birthweight babies. Archives of Disease in Childhood. Fetal and Neonatal Edition 78: F227–F229

76. Takiwaki H, Nakanishi H, Shono Y et al 1991 The influence of cutaneous factors on the transcutaneous pO2 and pCO2 at various body sites. British Journal of Dermatology 125: 243–247

77. Thome U, Topfer A, Schaller P et al 1998 Comparison of lung volume measurements by antero-posterior chest X-ray and the SF6 washout technique in mechanically ventilated infants. Pediatric Pulmonology 26: 265–272

78. Tin W, Milligan D W, Pennefather P et al 2001 Pulse oximetry, severe retinopathy, and outcome at one year in babies of less than 28 weeks gestation. Archives of Disease in Childhood. Fetal and Neonatal Edition 84: F106–F110

79. Tobias J D, Meyer D J 1997 Noninvasive monitoring of carbon dioxide during respiratory failure in toddlers and infants: end-tidal versus transcutaneous carbon dioxide. Anesthesia and Analgesia 85: 55–58

80. Tsien C L, Facklet J 1997 Poor prognosis for existing monitors in the intensive care unit. Critical Care Medicine 25: 614–619

81. Vyas H, Helms P, Cheriyan G 1988 Transcutaneous oxygen monitoring beyond the neonatal period. Critical Care Medicine 16: 844–847

82. Yeh M P, Adams T D, Gardner R M et al 1984 Effect of O2, N2, and CO2 composition on nonlinearity of Fleisch pneumotachograph characteristics. Journal of Applied Physiology 56: 1423–1425

83. Yoxall C W, Weindling A M 1996 The measurement of peripheral venous oxyhaemoglobin saturation in newborn infants by near infrared spectroscopy with venous occlusion. Pediatric Research 39: 1103–1106

CHAPTER 20

Care of the normal term newborn baby

Patrick H T Cartlidge

Normal healthy term newborn babies who remain in the maternity hospital for a few days after birth are most appropriately cared for by their mothers, supervised by midwives. Neonatologists are rarely involved, but clear protocols and guidelines need to be put in place to detect the rare baby who develops a problem such as symptomatic hypoglycaemia, marked jaundice, sepsis, or hypernatraemic dehydration due to breast milk insufficiency. Many routine procedures are required, feeding has to be established, and every baby needs to be examined carefully. Minor problems are common and often cause considerable parental anxiety, but they are rarely of clinical importance.

The information in this chapter aims to guide those who are responsible for well, term newborns, highlighting common problems and areas where local protocols may need to be developed. Further useful information can be found elsewhere in this book, and in other texts.[81]

Anticipatory care

Many babies are normal at birth yet their mother had a medical complication of pregnancy such as pre-eclampsia, or a chronic illness such as asthma or diabetes (Table 20.1). The condition itself may have an effect on the newborn, as may the drugs required for treatment. However, with the exception of the important examples marked by an asterisk in Table 20.1, most maternal illnesses have no serious effects on the baby, who will be normal at birth, will stay normal thereafter, and should be cared for alongside the mother. Nevertheless, it is essential to be aware of all these illnesses so that appropriate and prompt action can be taken to prevent unnecessary sequelae, such as severe jaundice in babies with a family history of hereditary spherocytosis. Fetal medicine has had a dramatic impact in this area, providing prior warning of such diverse problems as ambiguous genitalia, cardiac disease and intrathoracic masses.

The effects of drugs passing to the fetus transplacentally and to the neonate in breast milk are discussed fully in Chapter 24.

Care immediately after birth

Neonatal resuscitation (Chapter 13, Part 1)

Umbilical cord clamping

Umbilical blood flow decreases rapidly after delivery to less than 20% of the fetal value by 40 to 60 seconds of age.[30,60,105] There is little evidence to support the need to rush immediately to clamp the cord if uterine contraction is not artificially induced, since there are few, if any, risks associated with delayed clamping.[65] However, there is a theoretical risk of a large placental transfusion and polycythaemia if cord clamping is delayed after a uterine stimulant (Syntometrine) has been used, and so in these circumstances the cord should be clamped promptly.

It is essential that there is a foolproof routine for clamping or ligating the umbilical cord in the labour ward, otherwise a fatal neonatal haemorrhage can ensue. Either two ligatures or one of the commercially available cord clamps should be used.

Umbilical cord care

Correct umbilical care during the first week significantly reduces the incidence of infection, not only in the neonate but also in the mother.[19,31] Necrotic Wharton's jelly is readily colonised by organisms from the environment, which may spread to cause skin, conjunctival or systemic infection in the baby, or mastitis in the mother.

Umbilical cord colonisation and infection can be reduced by using topical antibiotics.[8,28] Yet, in developed countries, there is no evidence that topical antibiotics or antiseptics reduce systemic infection, and moreover they both delay cord separation.[106] Thus, simply keeping the cord clean is a reasonable and safe mode of care.[106] This advice is not applicable in countries with a high incidence of serious bacterial infection in babies, or harmful cord care traditions. In these situations, various techniques

Table 20.1 Maternal illness: effect on the baby and neonatal management

Maternal illness	Effect on baby	Neonatal management
Cardiovascular disease		
Ischaemic heart disease	–	–
Rheumatic heart disease	–	–
Congenital heart disease		
■ acyanotic	Increased risk of congenital heart disease	Echocardiogram
■ cyanotic	IUGR	Echocardiogram
	Increased risk of congenital heart disease	
Hypertension	IUGR, may need to be delivered preterm	Check blood pressure if unwell
	Neonatal hypotension from drug therapy	
Respiratory disease		
Asthma	IUGR if severe	No neonatal intervention proven to
	Increased incidence of asthma	reduce the risk of asthma
Chronic bronchitis	IUGR	–
Cystic fibrosis	–	No hazard from maternal lung pathogens
		Breastfeeding is safe
Endocrine and metabolic disease		
Diabetes*	Infant of a diabetic mother (Chapter 22)	Needs careful neonatal evaluation*
Thyrotoxicosis*	Neonatal thyrotoxicosis (pp. 877–8)	Needs careful neonatal evaluation
Hyperparathyroidism	Neonatal hypocalcaemia (pp. 883–5)	Monitor serum calcium during first 7 days
Other endocrine disease,	–	–
e.g. Addison's disease,		
hypothyroidism		
Phenylketonuria*	Impaired development and microcephaly	Nothing can be done in the neonatal period
	Congenital heart disease	
Gastrointestinal disease		
Coeliac disease	–	–
Crohn's disease	Prematurity or IUGR if severe	–
Ulcerative colitis	Prematurity or IUGR if severe	–
Peptic ulceration	–	–
Stomas, colostomy etc.	–	–
Renal disease		
Chronic renal disease	IUGR	Depends on aetiology and inheritance risk
(nephrotic, renal failure etc.)	Some forms of renal disease are hereditary,	
	e.g. polycystic disease, Alport's syndrome	
Urinary infection	IUGR	Usually none
		Investigate if mother has vescico-
		ureteric reflux
Neurological disease		
Epilepsy: effect of anticonvulsants	Teratogenic drug effects, but rare with	Give i.m. vitamin K because risk
	common anticonvulsants (pp. 1114–17)	of haemorrhagic disease increased
	Sedation from maternal drugs	Monitor
	Occasional withdrawal symptoms	Monitor
	Sedation from maternal drugs in	Monitor, breastfeeding rarely
	breast milk (rare)	interrupted
Dystrophia myotonica*	Infant affected (usually more severely)	See page 510
	May be seriously ill in respiratory failure	
Myasthenia*	Neonatal myasthenia (p. 1185)	Monitor, usually no problems
Degenerative disease		
■ multiple sclerosis	–	–
■ motor neurone disease	–	–

(Continued)

Table 20.1 (Continued)

Maternal illness	Effect on baby	Neonatal management
Infection in the mother		
Pyrexia of unknown origin	–	Monitor for infection
Recognisable acute infection	Usually nil	See page 1016
	Risk greatest for viral infections (pp. 1053–61)	
Chronic maternal infection and carrier state*	Can be serious, e.g. HIV, tuberculosis	See Chapter 11
Allergic disorders		
Hayfever, eczema etc.	Inherited atopic tendency	Avoid early allergen exposure (e.g. cow's milk), particularly if mother has severe atopic disease
Haematological disorders		
Anaemia (iron, folate deficiency)	–	–
Autoimmune haemolytic anaemia	IgG transmitted to fetus causing haemolysis	Monitor for jaundice and anaemia
Haemoglobinopathies	Neonatal problems uncommon since most are β-chain defects (p. 377)	–
Hereditary spherocytosis	Neonatal haemolysis and jaundice in the 50% of infants affected	Monitor for jaundice and anaemia
Idiopathic thrombocytopenic purpura	Fetal haemorrhage can occur but is rare	Check platelet count and observe for bleeding; may need treating (pp. 149–50)
	Neonatal haemorrhage also rare	
Glucose-6-phosphate dehydrogenase deficiency	Neonatal jaundice	Monitor for jaundice and sepsis
	Increased risk of infection (p. 671)	
Autoimmune disease		
Systemic lupus erythematosus*	Congenital heart block	Cardiac pacing if heart block (pp. 655–7)
		No treatment if heart rate normal
Psychiatric disorders		
Drug dependency	IUGR	Monitor and treat drug withdrawal (Chapter 26)
	Drug withdrawal	
	Drug effects (occasionally)	
Malignant disease		
Ongoing malignancy	May need preterm delivery	–
Previously treated malignancy	Reduced fertility but no neonatal effects except IUGR after Wilms tumour	–
Miscellaneous		
Abdominal trauma	Rare	–
Malnutrition	IUGR (p. 510)	–
Smoking	IUGR	–
	Increased respiratory morbidity and sudden infant death syndrome in infancy	

* Maternal illnesses that may seriously affect the baby.
IUGR, intrauterine growth retardation.

may be used to prevent infection, such as the use of a hexachlorophene-containing powder. Spraying the umbilical cord with an antibiotic powder gives even better protection, a lower incidence of subsequent topical and superficial staphylococcal infections, and is safe.[8,28]

Prevention of eye infection

In many countries, it is routine to instil one drop of 0.5–1.0% silver nitrate into each eye immediately after delivery, to prevent gonococcal ophthalmia. The technique is effective, reduces the incidence of other types of conjunctivitis, and is largely free from side effects,[10] though some studies have reported a chemical conjunctivitis in up to 90% of recipients.[71] A 2.5% solution of povidone-iodine has been shown to be more effective[45] and protects against chlamydial conjunctivitis, which is otherwise more difficult to prevent even with the use of erythromycin ointment. Whether or not prophylaxis is justified depends on the incidence and severity of neonatal conjunctivitis in the local population; it is not used in the UK.

Vitamin K

Haemorrhagic disease of the newborn is potentially fatal. It exists in an early and late form, and is primarily a risk in breastfed babies and those with liver disease.[3] Indeed, it may be the presenting feature of liver disease. The condition can be prevented by giving 1 mg of vitamin K intramuscularly (i.m.) after delivery to all babies.[62] However, a paper from Bristol that suggested an increased risk of leukaemia in later childhood generated considerable anxiety about this practice.[33] Many subsequent studies from different parts of the world – Sweden,[27] USA,[50] Denmark,[73] Germany[92] and UK[6] – have failed to confirm the Bristol findings.

Various oral regimens have been used, either to avoid giving injections or, more recently, to avoid the putative risk of malignancy. From these studies it is clear that a single oral dose at birth does not prevent the risk of haemorrhagic disease, particularly the late-onset disease,[38] which in one series was 13 times more common following oral vitamin K than after i.m. vitamin K prophylaxis.[62] Repeated doses of oral vitamin K have been suggested as an alternative to a single dose of the i.m. vitamin K. Current practice continues to vary widely in Britain,[9] but the following regimen is advised by the Royal College of Paediatrics and Child Health:[83]

- i.m. Konakion – a single 1 mg dose at or soon after birth, *or*
- oral Konakion MM Paediatric – 2 mg at birth and at 4–7 days for all babies, and a third dose at 1 month of age for breastfed babies.

Infants at increased risk of haemorrhagic disease because of maternal liver disease, or maternal anticonvulsant or anti-tuberculosis drugs, should receive i.m. or i.v. Konakion.[83] In addition, there remains a concern that the oral regimen may not prevent late haemorrhagic disease, particularly in breastfed babies. This is only in part because of the failure to administer a complete course.[93] This concern can be ameliorated by giving an oral dose of 2 mg at birth followed by 1 mg weekly for 3 months.[38]

Thermal care (Chapter 15)

The risk of developing hypothermia is greatest immediately after delivery. It is not uncommon for the body temperature of a normal full-term baby to drop to 35–35.5°C by 15–30 minutes of age because of slipshod thermal care. The adverse effects of more severe hypothermia are detailed on pages 276–7 and include hypoglycaemia, acidosis, pulmonary hypertension and impaired surfactant production.

The best way to prevent hypothermia is to remember the underlying mechanisms of heat exchange: evaporation, conduction, convection and radiation. Evaporative heat loss, even of babies born into a water pool, is almost eliminated by prompt drying. Conductive heat loss is lessened by pre-warming the towels and any other equipment that will be in contact with the baby. Convective heat loss is ameliorated by having a warm and draught-free delivery room and covering the baby. All doors and windows should be closed, air circulation systems likely to cool the baby should be turned off (or the baby placed away from the air vent), and the room temperature should be at least 20°C. Radiant heat is lost from the exposed skin of the baby to any surrounding surfaces that directly overlook the infant, and is proportional to the difference in temperature between these surfaces and to the distance between the surfaces. Thus, particularly in winter, walls and windows 'feel' cold even when not directly touched. This problem is readily overcome by avoiding leaving the baby exposed and staying away from cold (external) windows and walls. Radiant heaters and heated blankets achieve a reversal of some of these processes and can allow the infant to gain heat.

Many mothers wish to have early skin–skin contact with their baby and this should be encouraged. Because the baby will be naked, it is sensible to increase the temperature of the room to a level comfortable for a naked and resting person (23–25°C), and/or use an overhead heat source. The baby should be dry and covered with a warm towel or sheet, and draughts should be avoided. These are all wise precautions that do not distract from the intensely personal experience. Babies cared for like this maintain their body temperature, cry less, have better blood glucose control and base-excess values than do cot-nursed babies.[14] They are also more likely to establish successful long-term lactation.[80]

Bathing babies shortly after birth is a fairly certain way of causing neonatal hypothermia and should be avoided.[40] Most blood, meconium and vernix is quickly and effectively removed during the initial drying in warm towels, and thereafter any surplus can be wiped clear with a tissue.

Measurement

Babies should be weighed shortly after birth for social as well as medical reasons. The head circumference is often measured at this stage although it is often inaccurate due to the presence of a caput succedaneum or moulding; it is more appropriately done as part of the routine clinical examination. There is no evidence that routine length measurement is useful, but if performed it must be done properly with an infant stadiometer, taking care to have the baby properly extended. Stretching a tape-measure alongside a supine or upside down baby is inaccurate and a waste of time.

Labelling and security

In hospital, as opposed to home confinements, it is essential to attach a nametag to the baby immediately after delivery to prevent ghastly incidents of confused identity. There seems to be little benefit, however, from the more complex procedure of footprinting the baby.[88] Recent abductions of babies from postnatal wards in the UK have led to the introduction of additional security measures in many hospitals.

Bonding

The scientific basis of early mother–child interaction is outlined in detail in Chapter 4. In simple practical terms, both parents should be left alone with their baby immediately after birth, when babies are particularly bright-eyed and attractive. Putting the baby to the breast early is one of the most important determinants of successful lactation[14,84] and, by releasing oxytocin, promotes uterine contraction, the milk-ejection reflex, and complex maternal behavioural responses.[90] Moreover, even simple skin contact at this stage has been shown to stimulate release of maternal oxytocin and prolactin and aid the first breastfeed.[23,24,80]

The normal neonate

Cardiorespiratory function

The normal term infant has a pulse rate of 120–160/min and a blood pressure of 50–55/30 to 80/50 mmHg (p. 623). Occasional ectopic beats are quite common. The respiratory rate should be less than 60/min and is usually 35–45/min. During REM sleep, breathing is often irregular, with pauses of 3–5 seconds, but more prolonged apnoeic spells should never be accepted as normal. In non-REM sleep, breathing is very regular and shallow.

Temperature

The term baby maintains a core temperature very accurately around 37°C, so that any departure from this always requires careful evaluation, in particular to exclude sepsis. For the healthy clothed term baby who is in a cot, keeping the room at a temperature of 20–22°C is adequate. If the room temperature falls below 20°C, the baby should be covered with one or two blankets and may need to wear a bonnet. It is very important, however, to avoid overheating by lying the baby by a radiator, in direct sunlight, overwrapping, or putting an external heat source inside the cot.

Weight changes

All babies should be weighed shortly after birth. Thereafter there is usually little point in re-weighing until the third or fourth day. Normal infants lose up to 10% of birthweight during this time, primarily as a result of extracellular water loss. The fourth-day weight is the only readily available check that breastfeeding is progressing satisfactorily (see below). Many babies who are discharged early are not weighed at this time, but a re-evaluation of the practice has recently been suggested, and seems sensible.[55]

Weight loss in the first few days averages 4–7% and should not exceed 10% of the birthweight. It should always be assessed in relative terms, even though it means that a 4500 g baby may lose up to 450 g. In general, breastfed babies lose more weight (5–10%) than bottle-fed ones (2–6%),[57] but this difference may be less if the baby breastfeeds more frequently.[7] From 1 week of age, the normal baby should gain weight at 20–30 g/day until the age of 6 months.[82]

Urine output and staining of nappies

Many babies pass urine immediately after birth, and then, particularly if breastfed with a poor fluid intake, may pass very little urine in the next 24–36 hours. Thereafter they pass 40–60 ml of urine/kg/24 h. It is exceptionally unusual for any illness to present in an otherwise normal baby with just anuria or oliguria. Pink staining of the nappy is commonly due to harmless urate crystals.

Bowel activity

Many babies open their bowels in the first 2 minutes, and usually regularly thereafter. Initially babies pass meconium, a dark-greenish substance composed of intestinal secretions, bile (including bilirubin), swallowed amniotic debris and the remains of desquamated intestinal mucosal cells.[39] By 2–3 days, 'changing' stools, a mixture of meconium and more normal stools, are passed. Once feeding is established, breastfed babies pass very soft mustard-yellow stools, often with every feed. Their stools are acid (pH <6).[51] Bottle-fed babies pass a less acid (pH 6–7.5), firmer and paler stool, only once or twice a day. The bacterial flora in the stools is described on page 290.

Neurological activity

The neurological capabilities of the neonate are outlined on pages 1096–7. Newborn babies can see, and prefer a face to 'scrambled' shapes, they can hear and smell, and within the first few days and weeks of life they learn to recognise their mother by these senses.[61,89,91]

In the neonatal period, babies have irregular sleep–waking cycles. In the first few days they spend up to 18 hours asleep, with 50–60% of the sleep being REM.[86] They wake to feed or when uncomfortable, usually because the nappy is wet or soiled, but the sleep–wake pattern gradually becomes more regular.[75] Circadian rhythmicity is detectable in heart rate and body temperature by 1 month of age.[32]

Postnatal care

Routine observation

At about 4 hours after birth, it is desirable to make a check of general wellbeing and to measure the baby's temperature, pulse and respiration. In hospital, this is often conveniently done on admission to the postnatal ward. In this situation, the baby's identity should also be verified, the security of the cord clamp confirmed, and a check made to establish that vitamin K has been given. There is no need routinely to check the blood pressure, haematocrit or blood glucose.[4] Thereafter, temperature, pulse and respiration should be recorded if the baby becomes unwell. Temperature instability, tachycardia and tachypnoea are important signs of neonatal sepsis (pp. 1017–28).[68]

Rooming-in

The standard management should be that the mother has her baby with her in a cot beside her bed throughout the 24 hours (rooming-in). This is advantageous from the point of view of preventing cross-infection and it also promotes successful breastfeeding. This practice also facilitates the mother's desire to learn how to recognise, respond and manage every demand and need of her baby. If the mother is ill or exhausted, or if she requests it, help may be needed to settle her baby, although in many hospitals there is no longer a ward nursery.

Sleeping position

The risk of sudden infant death syndrome (SIDS) is reduced if babies are placed to lie on their back (Fig. 20.1). Side sleeping is not as safe and sleeping on the front is associated with the highest risk. Occasionally, babies are placed to sleep on their front for medical reasons, but this is the exception. The risk of SIDS is also reduced by the avoidance of cigarette smoking during pregnancy, avoiding exposure of the baby to cigarette smoking after birth, and by precautions to avoid overheating.

Prevention of infection on a postnatal ward

Handwashing and gowns

The major risk to the normal baby is from organisms carried by the medical and nursing staff, who must be meticulous in washing their hands before they touch any baby (Fig. 20.2). The extended family should do the same. The parents (particularly mother) and baby quickly share commensal organisms, but even so, good hygiene is important. Gowns are not required for staff or family.[11]

Baby washing

If the cross-infection techniques are good, and the baby rooms-in, so that he is colonised from the mother, all that is required is a wash with any of the commercial baby soaps. If there is an outbreak of skin infection, then chlorhexidine washing can be instituted. The use of hexachlorophene to wash babies should be avoided because it can be toxic.[58]

Nursing routine

The nursing routines designed to prevent transmission of infection from staff to baby or from baby to baby are outlined on pages 1015–16.

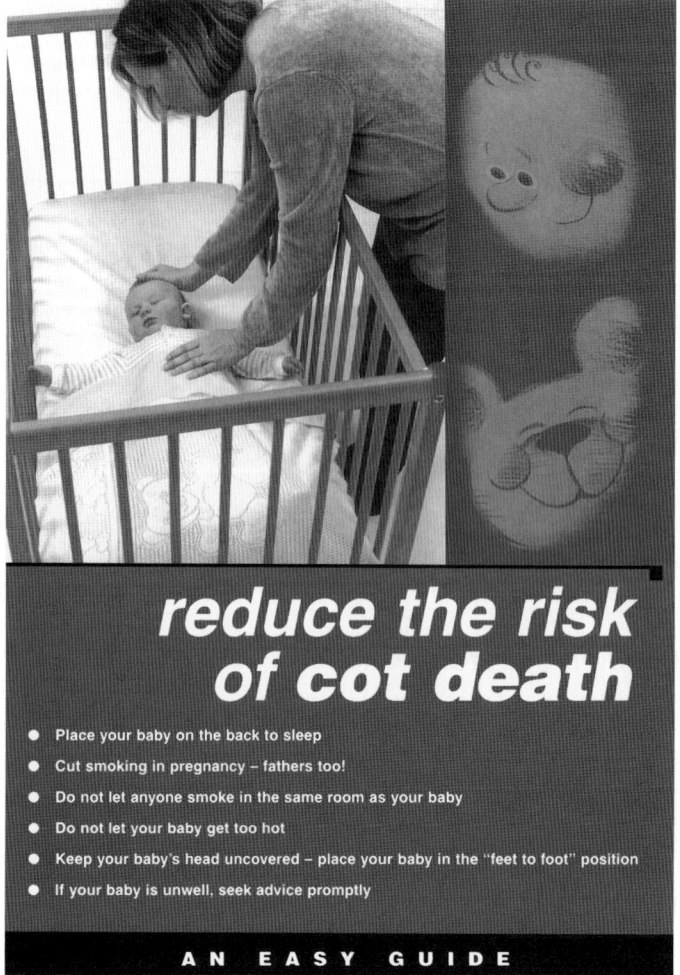

Fig. 20.1 Leaflet with advice on reducing the risk of sudden infant death syndrome. (Courtesy of the Department of Health.)

reduce the risk of cot death

- Place your baby on the back to sleep
- Cut smoking in pregnancy – fathers too!
- Do not let anyone smoke in the same room as your baby
- Do not let your baby get too hot
- Keep your baby's head uncovered – place your baby in the "feet to foot" position
- If your baby is unwell, seek advice promptly

AN EASY GUIDE

Visitors

Healthy visitors are not an infectious hazard, and the number allowed should be decided on a commonsense basis. There are no medical reasons why grandparents, fathers and siblings should not be allowed free access to the new family member.

Cord care

The early care of the cord with simple cleaning is described above. A 'healthy' cord is dry. The cord usually drops off naturally within 2 weeks, but this may be delayed if antibiotics or antiseptics are applied.[106]

Skin care

No special skin care is given other than to protect the perianal area and genitalia with a barrier cream at each nappy change.

Well-baby care

The hazards of hypothermia lessen once the baby has adapted to extrauterine life, and so it is not necessary to delay washing beyond the second or third day of life. At this time the mother can

The steps to effective hand hygiene

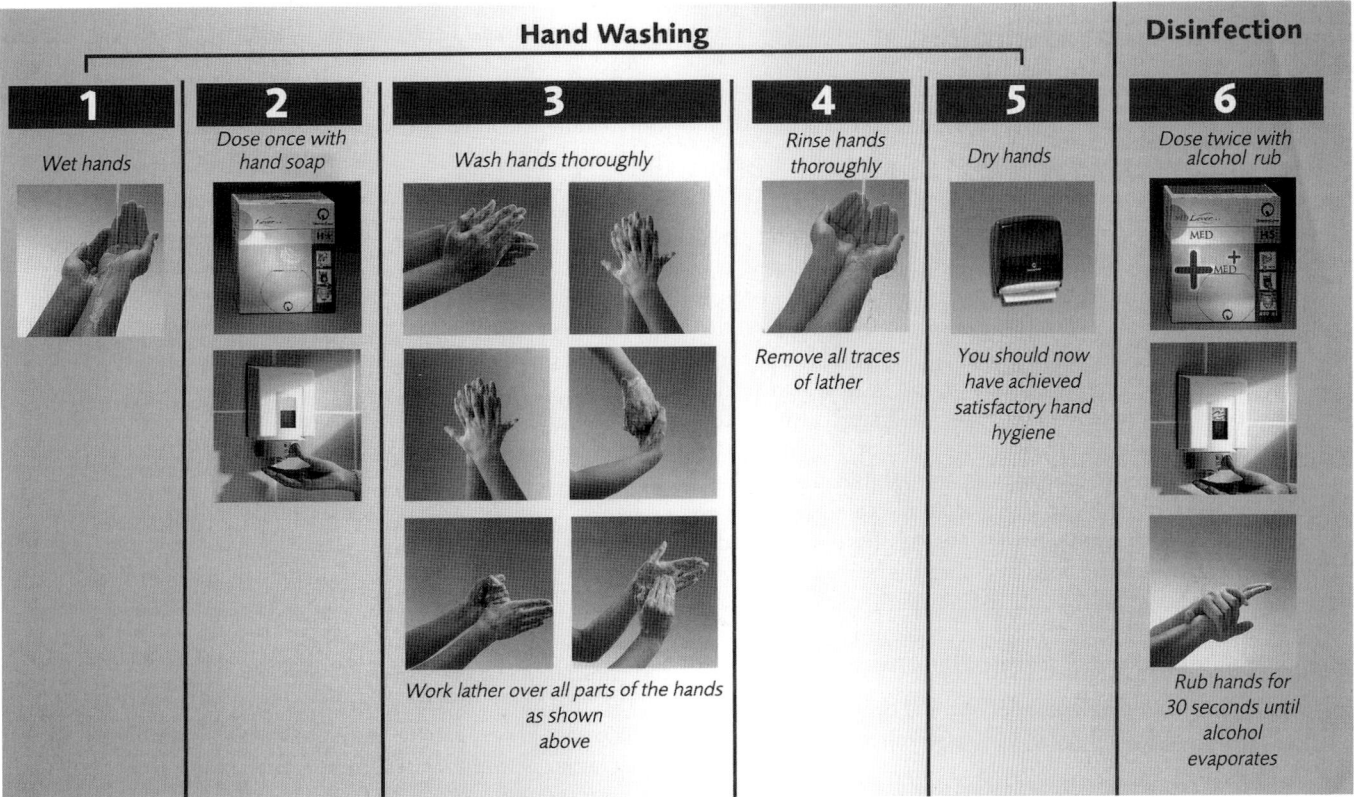

Fig. 20.2 Poster to promote effective handwashing and hygiene. (Courtesy of DiverseyLever Ltd.)

participate fully. This first wash can be just 'topping and tailing', that is, washing the face and hair and cleaning up the groin and perineum. For primiparae, this first bath may need to be a supervised or even a demonstrated affair. It is a good opportunity to reinforce any advice given at parent-craft classes that the parents attended.

The foreskin

At birth the foreskin is adherent to the surface of the glans penis, and is not meant to be retractile. Indeed, the foreskin remains non-retractile in most boys until about 2 years of age. Forcible retraction during infancy tears the prepuce and may cause scarring and a phimosis in later life. There is some evidence that urinary tract infections are less common in circumcised boys,[18,85] but this is not sufficient justification for routine neonatal circumcision.[102] Parents who elect to have their son circumcised usually do so for cultural or religious reasons. The operation should always be performed by a trained anaesthetic and surgical team.

Immunisations

Poliomyelitis

In areas of the developing world where poliomyelitis is endemic, there is a case for immunising the neonate with oral polio vaccine, since there is a good antibody response in neonates given the vaccine at 7 days.[47] In developed countries, routine polio vaccination is commenced at 2–3 months of age.

Hepatitis B

In the UK, vaccination is offered to infants of mothers who are seropositive for at least one of the hepatitis B antigens, although there is some local variation in practice. At birth, at-risk babies should receive 2 ml (200 microlitres) of the hepatitis B immunoglobulin and a first dose of one of the hepatitis B vaccines, ideally within the first 12 hours of life. Repeat doses of vaccine should be given at 1 and 6 months of age.[25]

The American Academy of Pediatrics recommends universal immunisation of all neonates against hepatitis B,[2] and there is much to commend this approach where hepatitis B is endemic.

Tuberculosis

In communities where the prevalence of tuberculosis is high, BCG should be given in early infancy. In the UK, this includes babies born into ethnic groups with a high incidence of close contact with a sputum-positive case (see also Table 20.1). The conversion rate to Mantoux positivity is nearly 100%.[74] It is estimated that this gives 60–80% protection against childhood tuberculosis, with perhaps even greater protection against meningitis.[15,16]

In the developed world, BCG should not be given to the baby of an HIV-positive woman, but HIV screening is not justified in countries where universal neonatal BCG immunisation is practised.[72]

Routine neonatal clinical examination

Timing and personnel

All newborn babies should be examined carefully at least once in the first few days.[70] The examination should be carried out by someone experienced in neonatal care, not so much because of what might otherwise be missed clinically, but because the examiner must know how to interpret a finding which is commonly trivial but which might be sinister, and how to answer the plethora of questions about all aspects of well-baby care that the parents are likely to ask.

It is essential for those carrying out the examination to have a clear understanding of what they are trying to achieve. They must remember that the midwives will usually have recognised a cleft palate or Down syndrome, and that the parents will have been over their new baby with a fine-tooth comb and will already have detected most visible abnormalities. There are, therefore, four main functions to the examination:

1. Detectings serious problems which would otherwise not have been detected and which merit early assessment and treatment.

Table 20.2 Minor abnormalities and normal variations that may cause parental anxiety

Skin lesions
  'stork bite'
  milia
  erythema toxicum
  strawberry naevi (rarely present at birth)
  cutis marmorata
  miliaria
  mongolian patches
  innocent pigmented naevi
  epithelial pearls in the mouth
Cephalhaematoma
Subconjunctival haemorrhage
Peripheral and traumatic cyanosis
Tongue-tie
Diastasis recti
Protuberant xiphisternum
Hydrocoeles
Sacral dimple
Umbilical anomalies, e.g. hernia
Physiological jaundice
Snuffles
Talipes calcaneovalgus
Vulval mucosal tag
Breast enlargement

Basically there are only three common ones: congenital heart disease, developmental dysplasia of the hip, and visual defects.

2. Checking for many very rare but serious conditions, e.g. the enlarged bladder of posterior urethral valves, the posterior abdominal mass of a congenital tumour, or a dermal sinus leading to the theca.
3. Noting and explaining to the parents the multitude of normal variations and minor anomalies that may be present (Table 20.2).
4. Health promotion: give advice on nutrition, reducing the risk of SIDS, parental smoking, transport in cars, etc. It also gives the parents a chance to ask about any aspects of the health-care of their baby.

Medically, the ideal time to carry out the examination is towards the end of the first week, since by that time transient abnormalities present on the first day, such as murmurs and slightly unstable hips, will have resolved. By implication, therefore, a first-day examination is primarily for the reassurance of the parents, and if it is decided to offer such a service in a maternity unit, it should be designed with this in mind. However, with the increasing trend towards early discharge, this examination may be the only opportunity for a professional paediatrician to check the baby, and this opportunity must be taken.

The examination has a low specificity and low sensitivity, so findings must be interpreted with caution.[70] On the one hand, the clinician has to be careful not to over-interpret signs found on the first day in such a way that the infant is subjected to unnecessary investigations and treatment, and the parents to unnecessary anxiety. On the other hand, most congenital heart disease is not detected at this examination and false reassurance should be avoided.[1] The details of the examination are given in Chapter 14.

Gestational-age assessment

Gestational age is most accurately calculated using early antenatal ultrasound data and the menstrual history. If these are unreliable or unavailable, gestational age can be determined using the examination and assessment as outlined in Chapter 14. Knowledge of whether a baby is preterm and/or small for dates, may alter management of an infant less than 2800 g, and so it is important to know such a baby's gestational age. In contrast, a detailed assessment of gestational age rarely influences the management of the asymptomatic infant over 2800 g, and in practice it is not required.

Biochemical screening

Currently, all newborn babies in the UK are screened for phenylketonuria (PKU) and hypothyroidism. In addition, galactosaemia, cystic fibrosis (CF), haemoglobinopathies and various aminoacidopathies are screened for in some parts of the country (p. 377).

Phenylketonuria

At 5–9 days of age, all babies have a heel-prick blood sample analysed for phenylalanine: a raised level may indicate PKU. The baby should only be tested if his or her milk intake is normal. The blood is collected onto an absorbent card, taking care to fill each of the circles with blood. Approximately 1:2000 of all infants are positive on screening, about five times more than the prevalence of the disease (1:10 000). Those with positive tests are recalled and their plasma phenylalanine re-measured to determine whether or not they have PKU. If PKU or a variant is confirmed by a second raised phenylalanine level, the baby should be referred to a specialist centre for full investigation and ongoing care.

Hypothyroidism

Using another of the blood spots, a radioimmunoassay is done for thyroid-stimulating hormone (TSH): those with a high TSH are then recalled for further evaluation. This is required in about 0.2–0.3% of all infants tested. The incidence of hypothyroidism detected in this way is about 1:3500 (p. 874). All infants identified should be treated as quickly as possible. The diagnosis of hypothyroidism can be confirmed later, and the precise aetiology defined (p. 875).

Other metabolic errors

The screening for these is described on pages 914–15.

Cystic fibrosis

Blood spots from the neonatal screening blood card can be analysed for immunoreactive trypsin (IRT), which is markedly raised in most neonates with CF (incidence 1:2000). The test is very specific, with a recall rate of only 0.5% and very few false-positive or false-negative results. The accuracy of the screening can be improved if positive IRT tests are combined with polymerase chain reaction analysis for the ΔF508 genotype in CF.[35,100] Screening for CF is not yet universally practised in the UK, although preliminary studies show a definite benefit.[20,54,96]

Haemoglobinopathies

In areas of the UK where there are significant numbers of babies of ethnic groups known to be at high risk of sickle cell disease or thalassaemia (e.g. South East London), neonatal screening is offered.

Hearing screening

Currently, neonatal hearing screening is performed only for high-risk infants. Universal neonatal hearing screening has been accepted as a priority in the UK and is likely to be introduced very soon. More information about methods of hearing screening can be found on pages 254, 263, 377.

Feeding the normal term baby

Human milk is undoubtedly the preferred food for term infants, and every effort should be made to encourage a mother to breast-feed. In the developing world, breastfeeding dramatically improves survival and so bottle-feeding should be avoided if at all possible. Indeed, promoting breastfeeding is one of the main World Health Organization strategies for reducing infant mortality. However, it should be acknowledged that in developed countries, the evidence for the superiority of breast milk relative to modified cow's milk formula is weak, and so it is unjustifiable to pressurise a woman into breastfeeding. Schemes that give mothers accurate, evidence-based information about breastfeeding to enable informed choice of feeding method (such as the UNICEF Baby Friendly Initiative) demonstrate improvements in breastfeeding rates.[52,87]

Breastfeeding

Despite numerous initiatives, through UNICEF, the Department of Health and the Royal College of Midwives, only 66% of mothers in the UK initiate breastfeeding, and at 6 weeks of age, only 42% of babies are still breastfed.[37] These figures have not improved significantly over the last few years.[98]

Preparation

In the UK at least, breastfeeding is a learned skill not an instinctive behaviour, and it should not be assumed to occur easily for all women. Ideally, breastfeeding education should start in the antenatal period, with advice on what constitutes normal breastfeeding behaviour. Practical help should be available in the immediate postnatal period to assist in the proper initiation of lactation (Table 20.3).

Lactation

Following the expulsion of the placenta, the anterior pituitary gland releases large amounts of prolactin, a hormone essential for

Table 20.3 Hospital policies intended to promote breastfeeding
Antenatal education
Baby put to breast as soon after birth as possible
Establish rooming-in
Feed at least 8 times per day, up to 12 times if necessary
Do not have specific duration of feeds at the breast
Finish the first breast, going to the second if hungry
No supplementary/complementary feeds
No dummies
No discharge gift packs
Regular assessment of the mother's breasts

lactation. Frequent breastfeeds in the early postnatal period stimulate the development of prolactin receptors in the mammary gland. It is thought that breast milk output is related more to the number of prolactin receptors than to levels in the blood.[22] It seems likely that the more the receptors are sensitised in the early postpartum period, the more abundant will be the milk production. In contrast, delayed suckling results in reduced levels of prolactin and thus less prolactin receptors stimulated. When the baby suckles, nerve impulses are sent from the breast to the posterior pituitary and oxytocin is released. Oxytocin causes the myoepithelial cells to contract and milk is squeezed from the alveoli towards the nipple and into the mouth of the suckling infant. This is the milk-ejection reflex or let-down reflex. At first an unconditional reflex, it quickly becomes conditional and readily inhibited by anxiety and pain.

Initially, lactation is hormonally driven, and colostrum will be produced whether or not suckling takes place. Colostrum is thick, viscous and small in volume, with intakes of 4–14 ml each feed. Over the next 48 to 96 hours, milk production increases markedly[22] and the volumes produced start to be governed by suckling and milk removal, activities that are essential for the continuation of lactation.[76] After 1 to 2 weeks, on average 700–800 ml per day of milk is produced, with a wide range from 450 to 1200 ml. At the end of each feed, about 100 ml of milk is left in the breasts.[26] Babies seem able to judge their own intake such that they grow normally, so an assessment of intake should only be attempted if weight gain is unsatisfactory.

Milk is produced for as long as it is removed from the breast. The rate of milk secretion may differ between breasts if the duration or frequency of suckling is not equal. This suggests autocrine regulation of milk secretion by the production of a local factor within each breast that controls lactation. This factor has been identified and is termed the feedback inhibitor of lactation (FIL).[77,101]

Attachment and positioning

Correct attachment and positioning are of fundamental importance to successful breastfeeding, so the mother should be taught these skills at the first feed. Correct technique ensures effective milk drainage and a satiated (briefly) infant,[103] thereby minimising problems such as sore and cracked nipples, breast engorgement and mastitis. The baby will feed frequently until the milk supply is abundant. If incorrectly positioned, the stimulus for an increase in yield will be compromised, FIL will remain in the breast, and lactation will decrease. Resulting breast pain or anxiety about sufficiency of milk supply will inhibit the milk-ejection reflex, a demoralising experience for the mother.

With the baby positioned for breastfeeding, the head and body must be in alignment, with baby well supported in a position that is sustainable for mother and baby and brought in close to the mother's body. Correct attachment is vital for the lips to form a seal with the breast. The mouth is open wide against the breast and the tongue protrudes beyond the lower gum. The baby's nose is aimed toward the nipple to facilitate extension of the lower jaw (Fig. 20.3). The baby is attached with the nipple adjacent to the junction of the hard and soft palate in the roof of the mouth. A significant amount of breast is drawn into the mouth, enabling the baby's jaw and tongue to compress and strip

or milk the lactiferous sinuses. The nipple only forms one third of the 'teat' in baby's mouth; the rest is breast tissue.

The appearance of a correctly attached baby is shown in Figure 20.4. The baby's head is slightly extended and both nostrils are clear of the breast. The mouth is wide open and lips flanged backwards. The chin must be touching the breast. If the areola is visible, more should be seen above than below the mouth, indicating that the nipple is in the roof of the mouth. A correctly attached baby makes long deep sucks with pauses.

Frequency and duration

The optimum time to initiate breastfeeding is shortly after delivery, ideally during the period of skin contact, since for the first

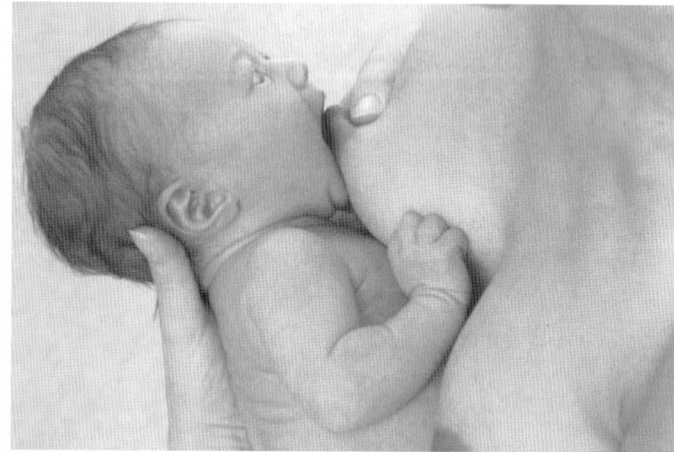

Fig. 20.3 Positioning for breastfeeding. The head and body must be in alignment, with baby well supported in a position that is sustainable for mother and baby and brought in close to the mother's body. The mouth is open wide against the breast and the tongue protrudes beyond the lower gum. The baby's nose is aimed toward the nipple to facilitate extension of the lower jaw. (With permission from Mother & Baby Picture Library/Ruth Jenkinson.)

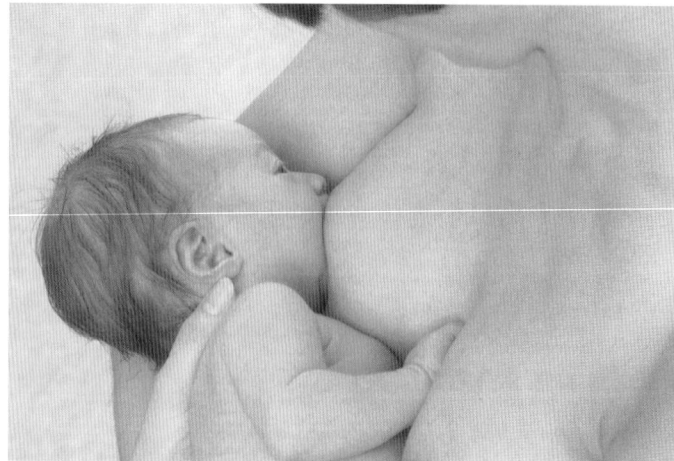

Fig. 20.4 A correctly attached baby. (With permission from Mother & Baby Picture Library/Ruth Jenkinson.)

2 hours of life babies are usually alert and the sucking reflex intense.[5] It is important not to miss this phase since thereafter babies enter a deep sleep before periods of wakefulness ensue, which are accompanied by the desire for frequent short feeds. Healthy infants may feed 10 or more times a day in the first few days and this should not be limited.[13,22] At this time, when only colostrum is being produced, the baby should suckle both breasts during a feed. The duration of each feed is variable; in general, the endpoint is when the baby loses interest in sucking or the breast is empty, usually 7–10 minutes.

After the first few days, most breastfed babies will gradually settle into a 2–3-hourly feeding pattern. Most of the milk will come in the first 4–6 minutes, although many babies will continue to suck intermittently thereafter for comfort. At this time there is some evidence to show that prolonged feeding at one breast, ensuring that it is empty, reduces complications.[29] Also, the fat content of breast milk increases during the feed, and so it is important not to limit the length of time a baby suckles.[104] After this breast is empty, if the baby has gone to sleep, then the feed is over; however, if he is still hungry, some milk should be given from the other breast. To ensure that one breast at a time is completely emptied, the mother should alternate which breast she offers first.

Complementary and supplementary feeds

Complementary feeds are those offered after a baby has breast-fed. Supplementary feeds are those that replace the entire breastfeed. They may be given from a bottle, cup or syringe and can consist of mother's expressed milk or modified cow's milk formula. The decision to give such feeds to a breastfeeding baby is a major one, since it frequently inhibits the establishment of successful breastfeeding.[12,53,67] Probably the only genuine justifications for complementary or supplementary feeds are hypoglycaemia and dehydration with a weight loss more than 10% of birthweight. Whatever the reason for using complementary or supplementary feeds, the mother should, if at all possible, continue to express milk on a regular basis until breastfeeding is established. Topping up with water or a glucose solution is a major cause of lactation failure and should be avoided.

Monitoring breastfeeding

Whilst breastfeeding is being established, it is wise to monitor the frequency of feeds and weight changes. If weight gain is poor or persistent weight loss occurs (pp. 307–9), examine the baby carefully for signs of ill health and take a urine sample to exclude infection (p. 1218). If these are normal, the problem is almost certainly a poor intake; in such babies, urine output is low and hypernatraemia is common. The only way to confirm a poor intake is by test weighing, but caution is needed since the technique is inaccurate unless it is done very carefully, and in particular it may underestimate low intakes.[99] Test weighing must be a last resort, and only in infants in whom failure to gain weight is becoming a serious problem. The anxiety provoked in a mother by the procedure can inhibit lactation[23] and may therefore make things worse.

Bottle-feeding

Starting feeds

There are many modified cow's milk formulae available and they are very similar to each other; which to use is down to parental choice. Tables of composition of currently available formula milks compared with breast milk can be found in Chapter 16. The first feed should be offered at about 4 hours of age. If the baby falls asleep, there is no need to do anything, since a term neonate is designed on the assumption that he will be breastfed and receive few calories during the first 24–48 hours. Thereafter, the baby is fed on demand, which in most cases is about every 4 hours, less frequent than most breastfed babies. As with breastfed neonates, there is no justification for offering water or a glucose solution.

Technique of feeding

The baby should be swaddled and held closely and comfortably to the mother so that she can hold the bottle with her free hand. Touching the baby's mouth or lips with the teat will usually evoke the rooting reflex. The mouth will open, the teat can be popped in, and he will begin to suck. The sucking mechanism is different from breastfeeding[59] since there is not the equivalent of the milk-ejection reflex, so that in addition to compressing the teat with the gums and squeezing milk into the mouth as in breastfeeding, the baby has to generate a vacuum in his or her mouth to suck the milk out of the bottle. The amount obtained per suck can be altered by varying the size of the hole in the teat, but, in general, large holes should be used only in babies with sucking problems.

Temperature

Traditionally, bottle milk is warmed to body temperature before feeding, but there is no need to do this. Babies take room-temperature milk perfectly satisfactorily.

Frequency of feeds

Demand feeding should be the norm, and bottle-fed babies usually settle into a 3–4-hourly schedule, taking about six feeds per day.

Volume of feeds

Healthy term infants should be demand fed and allowed to take what they want. Most babies take the volumes outlined in Table 20.4 and settle down to an intake of 150–180 ml/kg/24 h.

Table 20.4 Volumes of modified cow's milk to feed to normal full-term babies

Day 1	60 ml/kg
Day 2	90 ml/kg
Day 3	120 ml/kg
Days 4–6	150 ml/kg
Days 7–10	180 ml/kg

As with breastfed babies, if weight gain is satisfactory, a relaxed attitude should be adopted towards individual variation.

Feeding problems

Feeding problems must be sorted out with the mother and baby together. Feeding problems are emphatically not an indication for transferring an otherwise normal baby to a neonatal intensive care unit.

Maternal symptoms

For obvious reasons, these are limited to the breastfeeding mother.

Nipple problems (Table 20.5)

Correct positioning and attachment of the baby is the key to preventing and treating sore nipples. If the nipples do become sore, the mother should be encouraged to persevere, while being meticulous with her feeding technique, in the justified expectation that things will rapidly improve within 2–3 days. Covering the sore nipple with a shield may be helpful, but should be managed carefully and the baby weaned off the nipple shield as soon as possible. If feeding is too painful, or if a fissure develops which is not healing, then there may be no alternative but to abandon feeding from that breast until it has healed, but the baby can continue to feed from the other breast. The affected breast must be emptied 3–4 hourly by hand expression or with a breast pump, and the milk can be fed to the baby by cup, spoon or bottle, according to the wishes of the mother.

An inflamed nipple can be treated with a moist wound-healing agent such as Gelonet, or with Vaseline, which is gently removed with a tissue before the baby feeds. There is no evidence to support the use of other topical agents.

Breast engorgement

When the milk first comes in, the breasts may become full very quickly, which can make it difficult for the baby to attach to the breast as the nipple and areola are tense and hard. If this occurs, before each feed the mother can hand express a little (20–30 ml) milk to slacken her breasts sufficiently for the baby to attach satisfactorily. In most cases engorgement is transient and the milk supply settles down to meet demand within the first week or two. If it does not, a small amount of milk may always need to be expressed before the start of a feed. True engorgement occurs if the baby is incorrectly attached and therefore unable to drain the breast efficiently, or if feeding time is restricted. These aspects must be corrected to relieve the engorgement and to prevent the action of feedback inhibitor of lactin (FIL), which will inhibit milk supply.

The discomfort caused by engorgement may merit analgesia. In some women the engorgement results in extravasation of milk into a segment of the breast tissue itself. The mother may then become pyrexial, the breast red and tender, and a mass may be palpable in one lobule. This is the condition known as mastitis. The treatment is to give analgesics and regularly empty the breast every 4 hours. However, since manual expression is extremely painful, a breast pump is essential.

Breast abscess

This is usually secondary to mastitis, but can result from superficial staphylococcal infection if the cord care has been poor (pp. 369–70). The mother is febrile and toxic, with an acutely tender inflamed breast lobule. She needs antibiotics, antipyretics and analgesics. Lactation and breastfeeding can usually continue, but it may be painful or difficult to feed. The milk will remain clean unless the abscess ruptures into the ductal system. If surgery is necessary to drain the abscess, the breast should be manually drained of milk frequently, to maintain the milk supply until feeding can resume. Rarely does lactation need to be suppressed.

Inadequate milk production

In most cases, the mother's perception that she is not producing enough milk is incorrect.[41] However, if poor intake is documented (see above), the first thing to do is to increase the frequency of sucking (or expressing) to 2–3 hourly,[22] and to ensure that the baby is correctly positioned and attached to the breast in order to drain milk effectively. If this does not increase milk production, metoclopramide or domperidone, drugs that increase prolactin production, can be tried.[49]

If the baby is still not gaining weight, the mother should start complementary feeds (pp. 379, 382). There are many ways of giving complementary feeds, and currently popular is the nursing supplementer, which enables the baby to take extra milk while sucking at the breast. This is achieved by means of a fine-bore tube which is taped to the mother's breast and leads into the baby's mouth. The baby thus sucks on the tube and the breast at the same time. The use of complementary feeds is, however, often the beginning of a downhill course that may lead to lactation failure and the cessation of breastfeeding.

Too much milk

Milk may come out of the contralateral breast when the baby is sucking, it may drip out of both breasts between feeds, and/or the woman may have persistent problems with engorgement. Leaking milk can be absorbed with pads, and breast engorgement can be treated by emptying some milk before the start of a feed. In general, these problems settle down with the passage of time, as, physiologically, milk production is linked to consumption.

Table 20.5 Factors contributing to sore nipples
Poor baby position at feeding
Sucking the nipple rather than the areola
Licking the nipple pre/post feeding
Poor hygiene – dried milk left on the nipple after a feed
Friction from clothing
Chemical irritation – soap, tincture of benzoin

Taste

Babies appear to be able to distinguish different flavours in milk, as they take less if the milk contains lactic acid after vigorous maternal exercise[95] or it contains alcohol;[63] they take more if it contains garlic.[64]

Suppression of lactation

In most women, in the absence of sucking, prolactin secretion rapidly declines and the milk production stops, with very little breast discomfort or engorgement. Bromocriptine is no longer available for the suppression of lactation,[79] and so for women with discomfort, simple analgesia and breast support is indicated.

Breast cancer

For most women, breastfeeding does not influence the subsequent development of breast cancer.[66,94] There is, however, some evidence that prolonged lactation is protective.[17] If breast cancer is diagnosed late in pregnancy or after delivery, immediate maternal treatment is imperative and this prohibits breastfeeding.

Breast abnormalities

Women with unilateral absence of a breast or who have had a mastectomy can try to feed from their single breast, since in principle the challenge is no different to that faced by women with twins. Rare women, despite apparently normal breasts, fail to lactate, presumably owing to end-organ insensitivity to the hormonal stimuli.

Women who have had augmentation mammoplasty can breastfeed, as the augmentation procedure is carried out behind the glandular tissue, which is left undamaged by the procedure. However, in general such women are less likely to be successful breastfeeders.[43] Recently, anxiety has been expressed about whether the increased incidence of immune-mediated rheumatic disease in such women could be transmitted to babies in breast milk.[56] However, an overview of the literature suggests that there is no contraindication to breastfeeding.[48] Women who have had reduction mammoplasty are unlikely to breastfeed since the procedure disconnects the areola from the underlying structures.

Baby symptoms

Feeding problems are common. Typical symptoms include poor feeding, crying, poor weight gain, and vomiting.

Poor feeding

Babies feed at variable intervals and durations, and if a baby is gaining weight normally, he is getting enough nutrition regardless of his habit. The time to be concerned is if feeding lasts for only 2–3 minutes, if weight gain is poor, or if a baby deviates from a previously recognised pattern of feeding. The first thing to do is to ensure that the baby has a normal oro-pharynx and is not ill. The examination should be focused on the detection of a cleft palate (clefts of the soft palate are unfortunately often missed by routine neonatal examinations), thrush or the very rare occurrence of significant tongue-tie. Also assess for signs of respiratory distress, congenital heart disease, infection, a dysmorphic syndrome (e.g. Down syndrome) or a primary neuromuscular disorder. Check for hypoglycaemia as a consequence of a poor intake. Investigations will depend on the clinical circumstances.

If all these are normal but the baby still feeds poorly, the commonest causes are:

1. Preterm
2. The aftermath of a difficult delivery, e.g. vacuum extraction
3. Sedation from intrapartum or antenatal drug therapy (e.g. maternal pethidine)
4. Sedation from drugs in the breast milk.

The identification of a large-for-dates preterm infant will depend on an assessment of gestational age if obstetric data are uncertain. Such a baby may remain sleepy with poor feeding for some time, and tube feeding with expressed breast milk or a chosen formula is often necessary. In groups 2 and 3, the baby will improve spontaneously within 24–48 hours. If a narcotic analgesic was given during the intrapartum period, the baby may be reluctant to feed, and a dose of naloxone should reverse the sedative effect. It may be necessary to give the baby one or two tube feeds of expressed breast milk or a chosen formula in the interim. Prolonged sedation from drugs in breast milk is very unusual, and is rarely a contraindication to breastfeeding. If babies continue to be floppy and feed poorly, consider investigations along the lines suggested for hypotonia (p. 236).

Tongue-tie (ankyloglossia)

The evidence that tongue-tie is a common cause of neonatal feeding problems is weak. The practice of snipping the frenulum without anaesthetic is cruel.

Crying

Persistent crying in the neonate is usually due to hunger. There are many other causes for babies crying, notably pain. If the diagnosis is hunger, the appropriate treatment is milk, even if the baby was fed only 2 hours previously. If the crying baby shows no enthusiasm for feeding and is clean and dry, then he probably just needs a cuddle; skin contact can be particularly comforting. If this does not work, one must exclude occult but painful conditions such as otitis media, urinary tract infection, intussusception, bone and joint sepsis, and incarcerated hernia. It is commonly believed that crying in a baby is due to wind, but this should be assumed only when other causes have been excluded. Infantile colic is discussed below.

Wind

The bottle-fed baby will usually swallow some air with a feed. This may be because the hole in the teat is too small to let milk into the mouth as quickly as a hungry baby wishes, and so he sucks air around the teat. A large hole may also result in air swallowing because the milk comes into the mouth too rapidly and the baby splutters. Poor parental feeding technique may allow the level of the milk in the teat to go below the hole in the teat, or the baby may continue to suck on an empty teat and swallow air. The breastfed baby should swallow less air during a feed. Air swallowing is most common in the first 2 weeks whilst supply and demand are being established. With insufficient milk, the baby may suck in air; with an abundance of milk, the baby may splutter at an over-vigorous milk-ejection reflex.

Regardless of the type of feed, afterwards it is traditional to sit the baby upright in the hope that the stomach gas bubble will lie underneath the oesophageal hiatus and then, by rubbing or patting the back, the bubble will be induced to burst upwards – very satisfying for all. 'Winding' the baby in this way is supposed to prevent excess gas being propelled through the infant's small intestine, where, by analogy with older patients, it is believed to cause abdominal pain and/or infantile colic. This may not be evidence based but it has a long tradition and appears harmless. Nevertheless, it should be considered the cause of crying only once an alternative explanation has been excluded.

Colic

Infantile colic can occur in the late neonatal period. Its aetiology remains a mystery, although food and lactose intolerance in the mother and baby have been investigated, with equivocal results.[44,46,69] Stressful psychosocial factors may play a part.[78] The treatment includes reassurance about the benign nature of the symptoms. Massage of the abdomen, and patting the baby's back whilst he lies prone with the abdomen supported, appear to help, as do antispasmodic drugs.[97] Feeding technique should be checked, but giving up breastfeeding or changing the type of milk in bottle-fed babies is not justified without a clearly defined reason.

Poor weight gain/persisting hunger

Bottle-fed babies receive ad-libitum calories and fluid in measurable quantities, so this problem is much more common in breastfed infants, who, if denied adequate liquid and/or calories, will present with poor weight gain, persistent crying or both. If no other cause for these features is found, inadequate intake can be documented by careful test weighing. Checking the serum electrolytes may uncover hypernatraemic dehydration. If, despite implementing all the tricks outlined above to improve milk intake, the breastfed baby still fails to thrive, there comes a time when some extra source of liquid and/or calories is indicated. This time has come when:

- there is persistent failure to settle a crying fractious breastfed baby over a short period of time;
- the initial weight loss exceeds 10–12%;
- there is dehydration, hypoglycaemia, hypernatraemia or severe jaundice (see pp. 661–78);
- there is no weight gain by 6–7 days of age;
- there are sore nipples or engorgement, only one breast is being used, and the baby is hungry;
- the mother is demoralised by a crying baby – calming the baby and offering help to correct poor positioning and attachment, with expression of milk, which can be given by cup, spoon or bottle, may transform the situation and allow normal lactation to be established.

One of the purported advantages of breastfeeding is a reduction in the incidence of cow's milk protein allergy.[42] There is the possibility that this syndrome may be induced even by one or two cow's milk formula feeds in the neonatal period. However, the evidence for this is weak, and the giving of glucose solution when breast milk is insufficient has little to recommend it. Moreover, there is no evidence that this practice decreases atopic disease in general.[36]

Complementary and supplementary feeds

One may be forced into trying complementary and/or supplementary feeds in term babies with feeding problems, although the use of such feeds can make matters worse and cause lactation to fail completely. It may be, however, that the use of such feeds is the first objective marker of lactation that, for some reason or another, is inevitably going to prove inadequate.[34]

Dehydration fever

If a baby in the first week of life develops a fever, two likely and important causes are infection (pp. 1011–75) and overheating due to some defect in the environmental control (pp. 277–8). If these are excluded in a febrile baby who appears well but has an inadequate intake and has lost 10% or more of his birthweight, he may be suffering from dehydration. This can be confirmed clinically, and by measuring the plasma osmolality, which in dehydration fever will usually exceed 310 mOsmol/l.[21] Such a baby drinks clear fluids (or bottle milk) avidly, whereupon his temperature falls and he gains weight.

Gastroenterological symptoms

Vomiting (pp. 693–4), diarrhoea (p. 694), abdominal distension (p. 698) and jaundice (pp. 661–78) all require evaluation in their own right: they are rarely due to feeding problems, although jaundice is frequently associated with breastfeeding (pp. 664–5).

Acknowledgement

I would like to acknowledge the help and advice of Grace Thomas in writing the infant feeding section.

References

1. Abu-Harb M, Hey E, Wren C 1994 Death in infancy from unrecognised congenital heart disease. Archives of Disease in Childhood 71: 3–7
2. American Academy of Pediatrics 1992 Universal hepatitis B immunization. Pediatrics 89: 795–800
3. American Academy of Pediatrics 1993 Controversies concerning vitamin K and the newborn. Pediatrics 91: 1001–1003
4. American Academy of Pediatrics 1993 Routine evaluation of blood pressure, hematocrit and glucose in newborns. Pediatrics 92: 474–476
5. Anderson G C 1982 Development of sucking in term infants from birth to four hours postbirth. Research in Nursing and Health 5: 21–27
6. Ansell P, Bull D, Roman E 1996 Childhood leukaemia and intramuscular vitamin K: findings from a case-control study. British Medical Journal 313: 204–205

7. Avoa A, Fischer P R 1990 The influence of prenatal instruction about breast feeding on neonatal weight loss. Pediatrics 86: 313–315

8. Barrett F F, Mason F O, Flemming D 1979 The effect of three cord care regimens on bacterial colonization of normal newborn infants. Journal of Pediatrics 94: 796–799

9. Barton J S, Tripp J H, McNinch A W 1995 Neonatal vitamin K prophylaxis in the British Isles: current practice and trends. British Medical Journal 310: 632–633

10. Bell T A, Grayson T J, Krohn M A et al 1993 Randomized trial of silver nitrate, erythromycin and no eye prophylaxis for the prevention of conjunctivitis among newborns not at risk for gonococcal ophthalmitis. Pediatrics 92: 755–760

11. Birenbaum H J, Glorioso L, Rosenberger C et al 1990 Gowning on a postpartum ward fails to decrease colonization in the newborn infant. American Journal of Diseases of Children 144: 1031–1033

12. Blomquist H K, Jonsbo F, Serenius F, Persson L A 1994 Supplementary feeding in the maternity ward shortens the duration of breast feeding. Acta Paediatrica 83: 1122–1126

13. Cable T A, Rothenberger L A 1984 Breast feeding behavioral patterns among La Leche League mothers. A descriptive study. Pediatrics 73: 830–835

14. Christensson K, Siles C, Moreno L 1992 Temperature, metabolic adaptation and crying in healthy full term newborns cared for skin to skin or in a cot. Acta Paediatrica 81: 488–493

15. Clarke A, Rudd P 1992 Neonatal BCG immunization. Archives of Disease in Childhood 67: 473–474

16. Colditz G A, Berkey C S, Mosteller F et al 1995 The efficacy of Bacillus Calmette-Guerin vaccination of newborns and infants in the prevention of tuberculosis: meta-analysis of the published literature. Pediatrics 96: 29–35

17. Collaborative Group on Hormonal Factors in Breast Cancer 2002 Breast cancer and breastfeeding: collaborative reanalysis of individual data from 47 epidemiological studies in 30 countries, including 50,302 women with breast cancer and 96,973 women without the disease. Lancet 360: 187–195

18. Craig J C, Knight J F, Sureshkumar P et al 1996 Effect of circumcision on the incidence of urinary tract infection in pre-school boys. Journal of Pediatrics 128: 23–27

19. Cushing A H 1985 Omphalitis: a review. Pediatric Infectious Disease 4: 282–285

20. Dankert-Roelse J E, Te Meerman G J, Martijn A, Ten Kate L P, Knol K 1989 Survival and clinical outcome in patients with cystic fibrosis, with or without neonatal screening. Journal of Pediatrics 114: 362–367

21. Davis J A, Harvey D R, Stevens J F 1966 Osmolality as a measure of dehydration in the neonatal period. Archives of Disease in Childhood 41: 448–450

22. De Carvalho M, Robertson S, Friedman A, Klaus M 1983 Effect of frequent breastfeeding on early milk production and infant weight gain. Pediatrics 72: 307–311

23. De Chateau P, Holmberg H, Jakobsson K, Winberg J 1977 A study of factors promoting and inhibiting lactation. Developmental Medicine and Child Neurology 19: 575–584

24. De Chateau P, Wilberg B 1977 Long-term effect on mother-infant behaviour of extra contact during the first hour postpartum. Acta Paediatrica Scandinavica 66: 145–151

25. Delage G, Remy-Prince S, Ducic S, Pierri E, Montplaisir S 1988 Combined passive-active immunization against the hepatitis B virus of 132 newborns of chronic carrier mothers: long term results. Pediatric Infectious Disease Journal 7: 769–776

26. Dewey K G, Heinig M J, Nonunsen L A, Lonnerdal B 1991 Maternal versus infant factors related to breast milk intake and a residual milk volume: the DARLING Study. Pediatrics 87: 829–837

27. Ekelund H, Finnstrom O, Gunnarskog J, Kallen B, Larsson Y 1993 Administration of vitamin K to newborn infants and childhood cancer. British Medical Journal 307: 89–91

28. Elias-Jones A C 1986 Triple antibiotic spray application to umbilical cord. Early Human Development 13: 299–302

29. Evans K, Evans R, Simmer K 1995 Effect of the method of breast feeding on breast engorgement, mastitis and infantile colic. Acta Paediatrica 84: 849–852

30. Gill R W, Trudinger B J, Garrett W J, Kossoff G, Warren P S 1981 Fetal umbilical venous flow measured in utero by pulsed Doppler and B-mode ultrasound. I: Normal pregnancies. American Journal of Obstetrics and Gynecology 139: 720

31. Gillespie W A, Simpson K, Tozer R C 1958 Staphylococcal infection in a maternity hospital: epidemiology and control. Lancet ii: 1075–1080

32. Glotzbach S F, Edgar D, Boeddiker M, Ariagno R L 1994 Biological rhythmicity in normal infants during the first 3 months of life. Pediatrics 94: 482–488

33. Golding J, Greenwood R, Birmingham K, Mott M 1992 Childhood cancer, intramuscular vitamin K and pethidine given during labour. British Medical Journal 305: 341–346

34. Gray-Donald K, Kramer M S, Munday S, Leduc D G 1985 Effect of formula supplementation in the hospital on the duration of breast feeding: a controlled clinical trial. Pediatrics 75: 514–518

35. Green M R, Weaver L T, Heeley A F et al 1993 Cystic fibrosis identified by neonatal screening: incidence, genotype and early natural history. Archives of Disease in Childhood 68: 464–467

36. Gustafsson D, Lowhagen T, Andersson K 1992 Risk of developing atopic disease after early feeding with cow's milk based formula. Archives of Disease in Childhood 67: 1008–1010

37. Hamlyn B, Brooker S, Oleinikova K, Wands S 2002 Infant feeding 2000. The Stationery Office, London

38. Hanson K N, Ebbesen F 1996 Neonatal vitamin K prophylaxis in Denmark: three years experience with oral administration during the first 3 months of life compared with one oral administration at birth. Acta Paediatrica 85: 1137–1139

39. Harries J T 1978 Meconium in health and disease. British Medical Bulletin 34: 75–78

40. Henningsson A, Nystrom B, Tunnell R 1981 Bathing or washing babies after birth. Lancet ii: 1401–1403

41. Hillervik-Lindquist C, Hofvander Y, Sjolin S 1991 Studies on perceived breast milk insufficiency. Acta Paediatrica Scandinavica 80: 297–303

42. Host A, Husby S, Osterballe O 1988 A prospective study of cows milk allergy in exclusively breast fed infants. Acta Paediatrica Scandinavica 77: 663–670

43. Hurst N M 1996 Lactation after augmentation mammoplasty. Obstetrics and Gynecology 87: 30–34

44. Illingworth R S 1985 Infantile colic revisited. Archives of Disease in Childhood 60: 981–985

45. Isenberg S J, Apt L, Wood M 1995 A controlled trial of povidone iodine as prophylaxis against ophthalmia neonatorum. New England Journal of Medicine 332: 562–566

46. Jakobsson I, Linberg T 1983 Cow's milk proteins cause infantile colic in breast fed infants: a double blind crossover study. Pediatrics 71: 268–271

47. John T J 1984 Immune response of neonates to oral poliomyelitis vaccine. British Medical Journal 289: 881

48. Jordan M E, Blum R W M 1996 Should breast feeding by women with silicone implants be recommended? Archives of Pediatrics and Adolescent Medicine 150: 880–888

49. Kauppila A, Kivinen S, Ylikorkala D 1981 Metoclopramide increases prolactin release and milk secretion in puerperium with stimulating the secretion of thyrotropin and thyroid hormones. Journal of Clinical Endocrinology and Metabolism 52: 436–439

50. Klebanoff M A, Read J S, Mills J L, Shiono P H 1993 The risk of childhood cancer after neonatal exposure to vitamin K. New England Journal of Medicine 329: 905–908

51. Kleessem B, Bunke H, Tovar K et al 1995 Influence of two infant formulas and human milk on the development of the fecal flora in newborn infants. Acta Paediatrica 84: 1347–1356

52. Kramer M S, Chalmers B, Hodnett E D et al 2001 Promotion of breastfeeding intervention trial (PROBIT). Journal of the American Medical Association 285: 413–420

53. Kurinij N, Shiono P H 1991 Early formula supplementation of breast feeding. Pediatrics 88: 745–750

54. Kuzemko J A 1986 Screening, early neonatal diagnosis and prenatal diagnosis. Journal of the Royal Society of Medicine 79(suppl. 12): 2–5

55. Laing I A, Wong C M 2002 Hypernatraemia in the first few days: is the incidence rising? Archives of Disease in Childhood 87: 158–162

56. Levine J J, Lin H-C, Rowley M et al 1996 Lack of autoantibody expression in children born to mothers with silicone breast implants. Pediatrics 97: 243–245

57. Maisels M J, Gifford K, Antle C E, Leib G R 1988 Jaundice in the healthy newborn: new approach to an old problem. Pediatrics 81: 505–511

58. Martin-Bouyer G, Lebreton R, Toga M, Stolley P D, Lockhart J 1982 Outbreak of hexachlorophene poisoning in France. Lancet 1: 91

59. Mathew O P 1991 Science of bottle feeding. Journal of Pediatrics 119: 511–519

60. McCallum W D 1977 Thermodilution measurement of human umbilical blood flow at delivery. American Journal of Obstetrics and Gynecology 127: 491

61. McFarlane J A, Smith D M, Garrow D H 1978 The relationship between mother and neonate. In: Kitzinger S, Davis J A (eds) The place of birth. Oxford University Press, Oxford, pp 185–200

62. McNinch A W, Tripp J H 1991 Haemorrhagic disease of the newborn in the British Isles: 2 year prospective study. British Medical Journal 303: 1105–1109

63. Mennella J A, Beauchamp G K 1991 The transfer of alcohol to human milk. New England Journal of Medicine 325: 981–985

64. Mennella J A, Beauchamp G K 1993 The effects of repeated exposure to garlic flavoured milk on the nursling's behaviour. Pediatric Research 34: 805–808

65. Mercer J S 2001 Current best evidence: a review of the literature on umbilical cord clamping. Journal of Midwifery and Women's Health 46: 402–414

66. Michaels K B, Willett W C, Rosner B A et al 1996 Prospective assessment of breast feeding and breast cancer among 89887 women. Lancet 347: 431–436

67. Michaelsen K F, Larsen P S, Thomsen B L, Samuelson G 1994 The Copenhagen cohort study on infant nutrition and growth: duration of breast feeding and influencing factors. Acta Paediatrica 83: 565–571

68. Mifsud A, Seal D, Wall R, Valman B 1988 Reduced neonatal mortality from infection after introduction of respiratory monitoring. British Medical Journal 296: 17–18

69. Moore D J, Robb T A, Davidson G P 1988 Breath hydrogen response to milk containing lactose in colicky and non-colicky infants. Journal of Pediatrics 113: 979–984

70. Moss G D, Cartlidge P H T, Speidel B D, Chambers T L 1991 Routine examination in the neonatal period. British Medical Journal 302: 878–879

71. Nishida H, Risenberg H M 1975 Silver nitrate ophthalmic solution and chemical conjunctivitis. Pediatrics 56: 368–373

72. O'Brien K L, Ruff A J, Louise M A et al 1995 Bacillus Calmette-Guerin complications in children born to HIV-1 infected women, with a review of the literature. Pediatrics 95: 414–418

73. Olsen J H, Hertz H, Blinkenberg K, Verder H 1994 Vitamin K regimens and incidence of childhood cancer in Denmark. British Medical Journal 308: 895–896

74. Ormerod L P, Garnett J M 1988 Tuberculin response after neonatal BCG vaccination. Archives of Disease in Childhood 63: 1491–1492

75. Parmelee A H 1961 Sleep patterns in infancy. Acta Paediatrica Scandinavica 50: 160–170

76. Prentice A, Addey C V P, Wilde C J 1989 Evidence for local feedback control of human milk secretion Biochemical Society Transactions 17: 122

77. Prentice A, Wilde J 1989 Evidence for local feedback control of human milk secretion. Biochemical Society Transactions 17: 489–492

78. Rautava P, Helenius H, Lehtonen L 1993 Psychosocial predisposing factors for infantile colic. British Medical Journal 307: 600–604

79. Rayburn W F 1996 Clinical commentary: the bromocriptine (Partodel) controversy and recommendations for lactation suppression. American Journal of Perinatology 13: 69–71

80. Righard L, Alade M O 1990 Effect of delivery room routines on success of first breastfeed. Lancet 336: 1105–1107

81. Roberton N R C 1996 A manual of normal neonatal care, 2nd edn. Edward Arnold, London

82. Roche A F, Guo S, Moore W M 1989 Weight and recumbent length from 1–12 months of age: reference data for 1 month increments. American Journal of Clinical Nutrition 49: 599–607

83. Royal College of Paediatrics and Child Health 1999 Medicines for children. RCPCH, London

84. Salariya E M, Easton P M, Cater J I 1978 Duration of breast feeding after early initiation of frequent feeding. Lancet ii: 1141–1143

85. Schoen E J 1993 Circumcision updated – indicated? Pediatrics 92: 860–861

86. Schulte F J 1981 Developmental neurophysiology. In Davis J A, Dobbing J (eds) Scientific foundation of paediatrics, 2nd edn. Heinemann, London, pp 785–829

87. Tappin D M, Mackenzie J M, Brown A J et al 2001 Breastfeeding rates are increasing in Scotland. Health Bulletin 59: 102–113

88. Thompson J E, Clark D A, Salisbury B, Cahill J 1981 Footprinting the newborn infant: not cost effective. Journal of Pediatrics 99: 797–798

89. Trevarthen C, Murray L, Hubley P 1981 Psychology of infants. In: Davis J A, Dobbing J (eds) Scientific foundation of paediatrics, 2nd edn. Heinemann, London, pp 211–274

90. Unvas-Moberg K, Eriksson M 1996 Breast feeding: physiological endocrine and behavioural adaptations caused by oxytocin and local neurogenic activity in the nipple and mammary gland. Acta Paediatrica 85: 525–530

91. Varendi H, Porter R H, Winberg J 1994 Does the newborn baby find the nipple by smell? Lancet 344: 989–990

92. Von Kries R, Gobel U, Hachmeister A, Kaletsch U, Michaelis J 1996 Vitamin K and childhood cancer: a population based case-control study in Lower Saxony, Germany. British Medical Journal 313: 199–203

93. Von Kries R, Hachmeister A, Gobel U 1995 Repeated oral vitamin K prophylaxis in West Germany: acceptance and efficacy. British Medical Journal 310: 1097–1098

94. Vorherr H 1979 Pregnancy and lactation in relation to breast cancer risk. Seminars in Perinatology 3: 299–311

95. Wallace J P, Inbar G, Emsthausen K 1992 Infant acceptance of post exercise breast milk. Pediatrics 89: 1245–1247

96. Weaver L T, Green M R, Nicholson K et al 1994 Prognosis in cystic fibrosis treated with continuous flucloxacillin from the neonatal period. Archives of Disease in Childhood 70: 84–89

97. Weissbluth M D, Christoffel K K, Todd-Davis A 1984 Treatment of infantile colic with dicyclomine hydrochloride. Journal of Pediatrics 104: 951–955

98. White A, Freeth S, O'Brien M 1992 Infant feeding 1990. Office for Population Censuses and Surveys, London

99. Whitfield M F, Kay R, Stevens S 1981 Validity of routine clinical test weighing as a measure of the intake of a breast fed infant. Archives of Disease in Childhood 56: 919–921

100. Wilcken B, Wiley V, Sherry G et al 1995 Neonatal screening for cystic fibrosis: a comparison of two strategies for case detection in 1.2 million babies. Journal of Pediatrics 127: 965–970

101. Wilde C J, Addey C V P, Boddy L M et al 1995 Autocrine regulation of milk secretion by a protein in milk. Biochemical Journal 305: 51

102. Winberg J, Bollgren I, Gothefors L et al 1989 The prepuce: a mistake of nature. Lancet i: 598–599

103. Woolridge M W 1986 The 'anatomy' of infant sucking. Midwifery 2: 164–171

104. Woolridge M W, Fisher C 1988 Colic, 'overfeeding' and symptoms of lactose malabsorption in the breast-fed baby: a possible artifact of feed management? Lancet 2: 382–384

105. Yao A C, Lind J 1974 Blood flow in the umbilical vessels during the third stage of labour. Biology of the Neonate 25: 186

106. Zupan J, Garner P 2000 Topical umbilical cord care at birth (Cochrane Review). Cochrane Database of Systematic Reviews (2): CD001057

CHAPTER 21

Transitional care and the convalescing NICU graduate

Kate Farrer

Introduction

This chapter focuses on the care of babies who are suitable for transitional care, together with the care of well, convalescing, neonatal intensive care unit (NICU) graduates.

Admission criteria to the NICU varies between units. Birthweight has traditionally been one criteria, and many neonatal units admit all babies with a birthweight below 1.7 kg. Although babies weighing 1.7–2 kg have been shown to be at greater risk of complications during the neonatal period, for those who are asymptomatic at birth, there is no evidence that caring for them on a postnatal ward with their mother causes any harm so long as certain basic monitoring procedures can be undertaken.[19,28] NICU admission criteria should thus be:

- illness;
- birthweight and gestation – locally agreed criteria.

The weight and gestation should be selected locally following consultation between NICU and postnatal ward staff, and reflect the weight and gestation that the postnatal ward staff feel able to supervise. Typically, babies less than 32–34 weeks' gestation or below 1.7 kg will require NICU admission. Babies develop a sucking reflex at around 32 weeks but usually cannot sustain regular sucking feeds until 35 weeks. The necessity for tube feeding is often the dominant factor in babies who require transitional care unit (TCU) care.

Transitional care units

During the 1970s, TCUs, also called intermediate care units, were developed. Often sited on postnatal wards, they cared for babies who were well enough to stay with their mothers but who required a greater level of supervision than other well babies. Unfortunately, in recent years the availability of TCUs has declined, mainly due to a lack of appropriately trained nursing or midwifery staff. However, they remain popular with staff and patients (Table 21.1).[28,68] A TCU isolation room is particularly useful for the care of big babies with infectious disorders, which in themselves might not be a serious problem but which would pose a major risk of cross-infection if they were in a routine postnatal ward or in the neonatal unit, e.g. gonococcal ophthalmia, MRSA colonisation.

There is evidence that caring for appropriately selected babies on the TCU decreases the risks of mother–child separation (Chapter 20) and decreases the risk of nosocomial infection.[16,38,41] Babies separated from their mother at birth, display separation distress calls which cease at reunion,[24] and separation from the mother on the first night may increase the risk of allergy in later life.[53]

Equipment for transitional care

In addition to appropriately skilled nursing staff and regular neonatal medical input, TCUs should be maintained at a stable temperature at all times. Necessary equipment includes radiant

Table 21.1 Patients in TCUs

LBW and IUGR babies
Convalescent NICU graduates, e.g. completing course of antibiotics
Infants of drug-abusing, diabetic or thyrotoxic mothers
Babies with specific feeding difficulties
  – cleft lip or palate
  – requiring tube feeds (⩾2 hourly)
Babies requiring phototherapy
Babies requiring close observation
  – potential to develop meconium aspiration
  – at risk of hypoxic-ischaemic encephalopathy with poor cord gas but well following delivery
Twins and triplets of appropriate weight and gestation
Isolation for babies posing infection risk (ideal if isolation cubicle available), e.g. gonococcal ophthalmia

overhead heaters, phototherapy units, blood glucose monitoring equipment, breast pumps and electronic scales. There must be a fully equipped resuscitation area with piped oxygen, air and suction. The usual strict precautions to minimise nosocomial infection should apply (pp. 1033–4); each baby should have his or her own equipment, e.g. stethoscope, cotton wool and alcohol for hand rubbing.

Routine care of babies on a TCU

Labour ward care for these babies is identical to that described for term babies (Chapter 20); for small babies, there should be particular emphasis on temperature control (see below). Routines, including clinical examination, cord care, screening, weighing, family visiting and administration of vitamin K, are as for term babies – remembering that all low-birthweight (LBW) babies should have intramuscular vitamin K (p. 372).

Observations

Small and preterm babies have greater risk of developing illnesses in the neonatal period[19] than mature well-grown babies, thus temperature, pulse and respiratory rate (TPR) should be recorded on admission and 4–6-hourly for 24–48 hours. Daily observations thereafter are acceptable. Deviation from the normal range for TPR should prompt admission to the NICU. Normal range for pulse is 120–160 bpm and for respiration is 40–60/min. Apnoea monitoring is inappropriate in the TCU and should necessitate admission to the NICU.

Temperature control

The term baby maintains a core temperature very accurately around 37°C. Small babies, with a larger surface area to body mass ratio than term babies, are prone to hypothermia. If the baby is in an ambient temperature below 22–23°C, he may be using the thermoregulatory mechanisms described in Chapter 15, which will place a metabolic demand on him.[6]

If a small baby has a temperature of 36.0°C or less on admission to the TCU, examine him and check that he is otherwise well. Check he is dry, then fully clothe him, including a hat, before swaddling him in a sheet and blankets. Extra heat can be provided by placing him under a radiant heater or by using a heated water mattress. If, despite adequate warming attempts, the baby remains hypothermic, or if a baby who has been a TCU resident for some time develops hypothermia, he requires admission to the NICU and evaluation to exclude sepsis.

Weight

Like term babies, preterm and LBW babies lose up to 10% of their body weight in the first 4–5 days, and then gain weight at 10–15 g/kg/day. It may take 6–10 days before the 32-week gestation, or 1.5–1.8 kg, baby shows steady weight gain.

Infection

Babies born at 32–35 weeks have 'physiological immunodeficiency' (p. 996). They are born before the transplacental transfer of maternal immunoglobulin is complete, and lymphocyte function is not fully developed. Babies nursed in TCUs are susceptible to infection and strict nosocomial precautions should apply. If the baby has been delivered after premature rupture of the membranes, or other antenatal risk factors for neonatal infection are present (e.g. maternal factors including ill health, offensive lochia or liquor, and abnormal white cell count and C-reactive protein [CRP]), then the baby requires a full infection screen plus antibiotic treatment pending results (p. 1014). Symptoms suggesting infection should be meticulously assessed. In fact, babies are less exposed to nosocomial infection in the TCU than in the NICU, and infection rarely develops.[16,19,38]

Skin

Adhesive tape is the primary cause of skin breakdown in LBW babies.[48] Tape should be thoughtfully applied and its use minimised.

Jaundice

Preterm babies and those with intrauterine growth retardation/restriction (IUGR) are at greater risk of jaundice, particularly if they are not feeding well or have been polycythaemic. If jaundice appears, the bilirubin level must be checked and phototherapy instituted at bilirubin levels appropriate for gestation (pp. 672–3). When assessing whether a jaundiced baby is safe for discharge, many variables have to be taken into account, e.g. age, gestation, weight gain/loss, feeding, bilirubin trend, rate of rise/fall, and time since cessation of phototherapy. The bilirubin level should be checked for rebound 6 hours after ceasing phototherapy and sometimes again after 12 hours, depending on the cause of the jaundice. The bilirubin level usually plateaus by day 5 in the term baby and day 6–7 in the preterm baby.

Small-for-dates babies

All babies weighing below the 10th centile have traditionally been regarded as small for dates (SFD), although, in reality, babies with birthweights between the 3rd and 10th centile rarely pose a problem if clinically well and feeding adequately. Modern antenatal care should distinguish genuine IUGR from the normal small baby. IUGR babies (pp. 116–17) require close observation for such problems as hypoglycaemia (pp. 853–62) and polycythaemia (p. 751) and are discussed in greater detail in Chapter 10.

Hypoglycaemia (also see pp. 853–62)

The definition and pathophysiology of hypoglycaemia is discussed in Chapter 35. Preterm and IUGR babies are more likely to develop hypoglycaemia than term or appropriate-for-gestation-age babies even if they are feeding well. The fear of hypoglycaemia was the main reason that for many years these babies were always admitted to the NICU and separated from their mothers. However, for the healthy LBW and IUGR babies, the techniques for monitoring for hypoglycaemia, and appropriate prophylaxis to prevent hypoglycaemia by adequate feeding, can be administered safely on the TCU.

The blood glucose level at which adverse sequelae might arise is uncertain. IUGR babies have low glycogen stores and have a poor ketone body response to hypoglycaemia; if the caloric intake is poor, then the baby is at risk of falling to a level of hypoglycemia where, if this level is maintained, adverse neurological sequelae can occur. The risk is greatest in the first 48 hours of life, hence the importance of accurate monitoring in this group. Ideally, monitoring should be done with a whole blood glucometer because it is now realised that reagent sticks are insufficiently reliable for this important task. Hypoglycaemia diagnosed on the ward using a glucometer should always be confirmed with a laboratory glucose level. Consideration should be given to further investigation with insulin levels. Attempts should be made to keep the blood glucose above 2.5 mmol/l; this minimises the risk of developing severe hypoglycaemia (<1.0 mmol/l). There is no evidence that transient low levels of glucose which are not associated with signs cause any adverse long-term sequelae.

Hypoglycaemia – monitoring, prevention and treatment

For those at risk, feeds should be started as soon as possible after birth. The mother should be encouraged to put the baby to the breast in the labour ward. In general, within the first 24 hours, every endeavour should be made to keep the blood glucose >2.0 mmol/l and thereafter above 2.5 mmol/l. Blood glucose monitoring should start at 4 hours of age (earlier if IUGR) and then every 4 hours until two consecutive levels are above 2.5 mmol/l, then daily until 72 hours. Monitoring should recommence if feeding is reduced or the baby is unwell. If there is difficulty keeping the blood glucose level more than 2.0 mmol/l, an extra feed should be given by cup, bottle or tube. If the level remains low, or the baby had clinical signs or will not tolerate further feeds, then he should be admitted to the NICU.

Feeding the baby on the TCU

Breastfeeding

If the mother intends to breastfeed, if possible, the baby should go to the breast in the labour ward. Subsequently, regular breast-feeds help to stimulate colostrum and establish lactation. Preterm and LBW babies may need complementary feeds by bottle, cup or tube until effective suckling feeds and weight gain are achieved. These babies should be monitored for hypoglycaemia (pp. 858–9) for at least the first 48 hours and again if the feeding is poor.

Bottle-feeding

If bottle-feeding is the desired, or required, method of feeding, ideally the baby should be demand fed, initially aiming for a 3-hourly schedule, extending towards a 4-hourly schedule and six feeds per day. If most of the required volume is taken (Table 21.2) and the baby is not hypoglycaemic, no further 'top-up' feed is necessary. One of the advantages of bottle-feeding is that the exact volume of feed is known; if the baby is not taking enough and if there are problems with his weight, hypoglycaemia or jaundice, he should be topped up 3-hourly using a nasogastric tube. Formula feeding is further discussed on pages 379–80.

Tube feeding

Indications

The decision to feed via a nasogastric or orogastric tube is usually based on several factors, including:

- the baby's gestation at birth;
- the number of times a baby wakes for a feed – too often or too few;
- how well he suckles during a feed;
- the volume taken;
- the amount of weight lost, or the paucity of weight gain;
- blood glucose levels.

The most common indication for tube feeding is the preterm or LBW baby who, in the first 48 hours of life, is prone to hypoglycaemia and yet unable to effectively suck the required amount of milk from the breast or bottle. He may require tube feeds for an unpredictable length of time. Tube feeds can be given on a TCU if they are not required more frequently than every 2 hours.

Technique

Oral tubes are marginally easier to pass and do not have the disadvantage that they partially obstruct the nasal airway. However, if more than an occasional tube feed is likely to be necessary, an indwelling 4FG nasogastric feeding tube should be inserted, as these remain in place more reliably than orogastric tubes.

Table 21.2 Volumes of milk to feed to normal 1.60–2.50 kg preterm and small neonates

Day	Volume (ml/kg/24 h)
1	60
2	90
3	120
4	150
7–10	180–200

Breast- and bottle-feeding are both still possible with an indwelling nasogastric tube, and this spares the baby the discomfort of repeated tube passage. The position of the tube should be confirmed by aspirating acid gastric contents or by auscultation over the stomach while blowing 5 ml of air down the tube. The tube should be aspirated before the start of each feed. This is not only essential to confirm that the tube is still in the stomach, but identifies those babies who are not tolerating oral feeds and have milk pooling in their stomach.

To give a tube feed under the influence of gravity the appropriate volume of milk should be allowed to run from an open syringe (without the plunger). The plunger should never be used other than to overcome the surface tension of bubbles in the tube at the start of a feed. The milk should flow freely, usually over a period of 5–20 minutes, depending on the volume.

Volume and frequency

In general, in preterm and SGA babies the volume given (Table 21.2) should be divided into a 3-hourly feeding schedule. Two-hourly feeds can be given on a TCU for a day or two, but usually these babies and any needing hourly tube feeds are transferred to the NICU.

If the tube feed is complementing a bottle feed, the deficit should be made up. If the tube feed is complementing a breast-feed, in the first few days when only colostrum is likely to have been taken, the full volume should be given (Table 21.2). Thereafter, a smaller proportion can be given based on clinical assessment, the blood glucose, the weight gain and the hydration of the baby.

Complications of tube feeding

Complications from tube feeding include pharyngeal, oesophageal, gastric and duodenal perforation with pneumomediastinum and peritonitis.[10,64] Soft silicone tubes have been passed into the bronchus.[45] Gastric perforation can occur spontaneously in the neonatal period, possibly secondary to gut ischaemia around the time of delivery,[8] thus it is possible that in at least some of the reported cases the tube merely passed through a hole that was already there. Gastro-oesophageal reflux has been shown to be almost universal in tube-fed preterm infants, increasing the risk of aspiration pneumonia.[55]

Cup feeding

This technique has grown in popularity without clear evidence of benefit. Avoidance of 'nipple confusion' and increased rates of establishing breastfeeding have been postulated as reasons for advocating cup feeding. Cup feeding involves swaddling the baby and sitting him in an upright position. The rim of a cup half full of milk is then gently placed on the baby's lower lip, directing the rim towards the corners of the upper lip, tipping the milk to touch the baby's lip as he swallows it. The current evidence from small studies suggests physiological stability; the volume and length of feed do not differ between cup- and bottle-feeding babies.[39] Other authors conclude cup feeding takes longer, with increased spillage but reduced desaturations and a higher incidence of breastfeeding at 3 months.[32,51,62] Appropriate circumstances in which to consider cup feeding are maternal ill-health and the baby with cleft lip or palate.

Finger feeding

Finger feeding involves attaching a feeding tube to the side of a finger which is then inserted into the mouth in order to stimulate sucking. The tube is attached to an open syringe containing breast milk and thus theoretically associates the sucking reflex with the taste of breast milk. This technique is useful to assess the ability to suck and swallow, but, as it involves the same sucking movements and technique as bottle-feeding, it should be used with caution if breastfeeding is the desired outcome.

Non-nutritive sucking

The sucking reflex develops from 28 weeks, with effective suck, coordinated with breathing and swallowing, developing from 32 weeks. Non-nutritive sucking, using a pacifier or finger during tube feeding, may help develop or maintain an effective sucking mechanism and maintain association between enteral feeding and sucking in babies unable to orally feed, e.g. babies with bulbar palsies.[72]

Care of the intensive-care graduate

Babies who have required neonatal intensive care usually have a phase when they are asymptomatic but are still not ready for discharge. Satisfactory feeding and growth, maintenance of temperature at ambient room temperature, and maintenance of adequate oxygen saturation levels without supplementary oxygen all need to be achieved before discharge. A small number of NICU graduates with chronic lung disease (CLD) will be discharged still needing supplementary oxygen (p. 563).

Convalescing NICU graduates in general remain well but routines should be in place to detect any new problems. Serious complications of prematurity, such as CLD (pp. 554–73), retinopathy of prematurity (ROP; pp. 843–7) and post-haemorrhagic ventricular dilatation (PHVD; pp. 1157–9) are dealt with elsewhere in this book.

Emotional, developmental and environmental needs

The emotional and psychological needs of the baby and his family continue to be important and are addressed in Chapter 4. Developmental programmes such as the newborn individualised developmental care and assessment programme (NIDCAP) are increasingly popular, despite conflicting evidence of benefit. Many small studies show some developmental programmes may have positive benefits, but larger randomised controlled trials (RCTs) with longer follow-up are required.[40,58] Numerous small, often poorly designed, studies from developing countries demonstrate the potential positive benefits of kangaroo care (KC) in term and preterm babies. KC, the practice of nursing the baby skin-to-skin in his mother's cleavage, improves temperature stability[23] and gaseous exchange in preterm babies[37] and, in term babies, improves weight gain and decreases nosocomial infection. KC is associated with a greater sense of maternal competence and less parental dissatisfaction but there is no effect on mortality and overall there is insufficient evidence to recommend its routine use in LBW babies.[25] Non-nutritive sucking, as preterm infants learn to establish oral feeding, has been shown to have some clinical benefit, including decreased length of hospital stay.[72]

Natural fetal posture is that of increasing flexion towards term. Historically, practices in the NICU tended to discourage this, allowing the hypotonic preterm infant to lie extended with a frog-like posture. This has adverse effects on later posture and neuromotor development;[33] thus, current practices focus on flexed positioning and body containment manoeuvres. Rest periods,[73] massage[35] and swaddling[54] may all have a role.

Noise levels should be minimised[57] and staff need to be aware that their conversation is the greatest contributor to the din.[61] Appropriate music has been shown to be soothing to the term, but not preterm, baby.[18,42] Circadian rhythms of temperature and sleep appear to develop as a function of gestational age,[52] independently of cycled light exposure.[14] However, other studies show that establishing light–dark circadian cycles may have some benefit,[49] as exposure to bright lights is associated with adverse events.[67] Overall it would seem appropriate to seek to adopt a less 'chaotic, non-circadian environmental approach' in the modern neonatal nursery.[52]

Routine surveillance

The NICU graduate usually has a full examination once or twice a week. The routine should include the details in Figure 21.1. Each week, full blood and reticulocyte count, and electrolyte

Routine 1-week examination

Age (days)		CGA	
Weight		Head circumference	
Current problems			
Medication			
Feeding			
CVS			
Murmurs		Pulses	
Respiratory system			
Abdomen		Genitalia	
CNS		Eyes	
Skin			
Other findings			

Fig. 21.1 Routine 1 week examination.

and alkaline phosphatase levels should be assessed. The baby's bodyweight and head circumference should be plotted weekly on an appropriate chart to ensure normal progression.

New clinical findings which might arise during this time include herniae, anaemia, metabolic bone disease, murmurs, poor weight gain and cavernous haemangiomas.

Weight gain

The standard rules of neonatal weight gain apply. Babies should gain weight at 15 g/kg/24 h. The baby may feed voraciously, particularly towards the end of his convalescent phase in the neonatal unit. If allowed, many will take more than 180–200 ml/kg/24 h, and will gain weight at a faster rate. This sort of catch-up growth is frequently seen once the baby goes home and the parents are much less rigid than the nursing staff, feeding volumes of up to 300 ml/kg/24 h.[47] At this time the baby may develop some peripheral, rather firm, oedema. This can cause concern. However, if the baby is otherwise well and with no evidence of heart failure or any condition likely to cause peripheral oedema, the condition is benign and requires no treatment. There is no need to reduce feeds, and in particular there is no need to prescribe diuretics in the vain hope of removing this oedema.

Poor weight gain (Table 21.3)

The commonest cause of poor weight gain is inadequate caloric intake. Intake should be increased to a volume of 180–200 ml/kg/day of breast milk if tolerated. If weight gain remains poor, then supplementation should be directed towards the nutritional state of the infant and appropriate supplements of carbohydrate-, protein- or calorie-enriched formula will help improve weight gain (pp. 318–19). CLD, anaemia, and hyponatraemia in the breastfed baby[4] also cause poor weight gain. If, despite adequate calorie, sodium and nutrient intake, weight gain remains poor, other causes of failure to thrive should be considered (Table 21.3).

Murmurs

During this period, a heart murmur may be noted for the first time. Murmurs associated with heart failure, cyanosis or decreased femoral pulses need prompt investigation. Murmurs from the pulmonary vessels may be noted as a soft ejection systolic murmur maximal in the pulmonary area, radiating to the axillae. This benign murmur arises as blood flows across the pulmonary valve or at the bifurcation of the pulmonary arteries. It does not require further investigation, and resolves as the baby grows.[5]

Head size and shape

Weekly occipito-frontal circumference (OFC) measurement is crucial. Accelerated growth might imply PHVD (pp. 1157–9) and slow growth may indicate cerebral atrophy (p. 1150). Preterm babies have a tendency to develop a long thin dolichocephalic head shape. This is due to the effect of gravity on the soft

Table 21.3 Causes of poor weight gain

Inadequate caloric intake
  Expressed breast milk
  Vomiting
  Low-volume feeds (e.g. because of tachypnoea)

Insufficient supply of essentials other than energy
  Sodium deficiency
  Anaemia (inadequate oxygen-carrying capacity)

Increased energy expenditure
  Sepsis
    Urinary tract infection
  Bronchopulmonary dysplasia
  Hyperactivity
    thyrotoxicosis
    cerebral irritability
    seizures
    drug withdrawal
  Drug therapy
    diuretic
    theophylline
  Cold stress
    bathing, handling, inadequate clothing (supply bonnets)
  Misery
    no non-nutritive sucking
    discomfort from sheets (lambswool better)

Excessive nutrient losses
  Gastro-oesophageal reflux
  Hypertrophic pyloric stenosis
  Necrotising enterocolitis
  Gastroenteritis
  Protein–energy malnutrition
  Milk lactose and protein intolerance
  Congenital enteropathies
  Short bowel syndrome

skull bones whilst the relatively immobile baby lies predominantly on his side.[21] As geometrically the most efficient way of containing a given volume is within a sphere, if the baby's brain growth is normal but is contained in an elliptical skull, the OFC may appear larger than anticipated for the baby's gestation. The skeletal abnormality can be minimised by nursing techniques in the early neonatal period that support the skull, such as an O-ring,[21] but even without intervention the head shape normalises spontaneously.[63]

Herniae and testes

Inguinal hernias occur in 11% of babies under 1500 g and 17% under 1000 g; they are more likely to occur in males and in babies with CLD.[44] Hernias ideally need repair prior to the baby's discharge. The timing of surgery is a matter of clinical judgement. Repairing large hernias in babies with severe CLD can result in serious deterioration; other babies with CLD may have improved respiratory status and handling following repair.[34] There is no need to rush into surgery for 'cosmetic' reasons.

Delay in testicular decent in male babies with extremely low birthweight (ELBW) is common. No specific treatment is indicated, but if the testes are still not descended by the time of discharge, appropriate follow-up should be arranged with a paediatric surgeon.

Umbilical hernias are common especially in Down syndrome, Afro-Caribbean babies and those with CLD. They invariably resolve but may become large, and if still present at 1 year of age, referral should be made to a paediatric surgeon.

Retinopathy of prematurity

All babies less than 32 weeks' gestation and below 1.50 kg birthweight who received additional oxygen should be examined on a weekly or fortnightly basis for the development of ROP (pp. 843–7). For extremely preterm babies, this screening should start at 32 weeks' corrected gestational age (CGA). The examination can destabilise the sick baby and care should be taken when giving a mydriatic with systemic side effects (e.g. bradycardia and arrhythmias).

Biochemical abnormalities

Weekly electrolytes, calcium, phosphorus and alkaline phosphatase should be measured. Abnormalities such as metabolic bone disease and hyponatraemia can occur particularly in breast-fed babies, as mature breast milk lacks adequate amounts of sodium and phosphate for the needs of the preterm baby (p. 314). Hyponatraemia is common due to a combination of a low sodium intake and the relatively high fractional excretion of sodium (p. 292). Sodium supplements should be given; some babies need up to 10 mmol/kg/24 h.

ELBW babies are also at risk of metabolic bone disease (Chapter 35, Part 4). This manifests biochemically as hypophosphataemia, a rise in alkaline phosphatase, and occasionally, in severe cases, hypercalcaemia. This condition should be prevented by appropriate use of supplements in breastfed babies (pp. 316–17).

Anaemia of prematurity

The surviving very-low-birthweight (VLBW) baby becomes anaemic, with a haemoglobin nadir at 6–8 weeks of age of 7–9 g/dl. The aetiology of the condition is multifactorial (p. 749). It is contributed to by iatrogenic blood loss at a time when the rapidly expanding intravascular volume of the growing baby may outstrip the bone marrow's capacity to produce sufficient red cells. Deficiency of haematinics such as iron and folate may play a small part, but vitamin E has no role.[76] Most babies with anaemia of prematurity and a low reticulocyte count have low levels of plasma erythropoietin (p. 750). The therapeutic use of erythropoietin is discussed in detail on page 750.

If the baby is well, the haemoglobin may fall as low as 7 g/dl without the need for transfusion; particularly reassuring is a good reticulocyte count (3–10%). If symptoms of anaemia such as poor feeding, lethargy or congestive heart failure[1] occur, the simplest form of treatment is a 10–15 ml/kg transfusion of packed red cells.

Data reporting the effects of transfusion on apnoea are conflicting. Some authors conclude that transfusion decreases the frequency of apnoea.[70] However, others suggest that transfusion has little effect on apnoea but tachycardia and tachypnoea may be significantly improved.[75]

Eosinophilia

VLBW babies may have a marked eosinophilia (1×10^9/l) by the age of 3–4 weeks. This often follows an episode of proven sepsis,[50] but is otherwise a benign finding and should not trigger the neonatologist into a hunt for causes for eosinophilia such as parasitic infection.[71]

Feeding the convalescent premature baby

It is now clear that many advantages result from the early introduction of minimal enteral feeding to VLBW babies even while they are still very ill (pp. 282–3). Full enteral nutrition is achieved sooner and the complications of long-term total parenteral nutrition reduced (p. 330). By the time the baby is convalescent from his acute neonatal illness, he will usually be tolerating hourly feeds at a total daily volume of 180–200 ml/kg.

A large body of experience shows that, when introducing feeds, breast milk is better tolerated than formula (pp. 314–15). Non-nutritive sucking using a pacifier during tube feeding may have benefits[72] and help train the baby in the techniques of sucking. Once a baby is 30–32 weeks' gestation, so long as he is well enough, he can be put to the mother's breast if she intends to breastfeed him.[12] It is unlikely that significant amounts of milk will be ingested in this way, but it can dramatically improve the mother's morale.

Continuous and bolus feeds have advantages and disadvantages.[26,65] There may be less feed intolerance with 3-hourly bolus feeds[65] but overall there is little evidence from RCTs to support the superiority of either method.[59] Nasojejunal tube feeds are rarely used as they have a high incidence of complications (p. 510), and the percentage of ingested calories absorbed is less as the gastric intraluminal phase of digestion is bypassed.

Once the baby is 33–34 weeks' gestation he should make a reasonable attempt at sucking feeds from the bottle or the breast, and by 35 weeks most neurologically normal convalescent ex-premature babies should be able to suckle feed satisfactorily. For those mothers who have maintained their lactation by expression, every attempt should be made to encourage the baby to go to the breast, and if possible to have the mother rooming-in on the NICU.

Nutritional supplements

Vitamin D

The convalescent ex-premature infant should be given vitamin D supplementation, 400 units daily, with appropriate phosphate supplements, to reduce the risk of metabolic bone disease (p. 923).

Folic acid

Preterm babies who are not folic acid supplemented may become folate deficient and develop megaloblastic anaemia.[69] Most NICUs give 100 micrograms of folic acid daily until term CGA or until discharge.

Iron

VLBW babies are born before most of the body's stores of iron are laid down in the third trimester of pregnancy. Early iron supplements have made no significant difference to the severity of the anaemia of prematurity (p. 750) although concomitant treatment with erythropoietin can result in a better response to iron (p. 750).

Iron, particularly parenteral, has been associated with increased risk of infection.[9] The surviving ELBW baby may have received multiple blood transfusions and thus doses of intravenous iron; he is likely to have greatly elevated ferritin levels. Thus, iron supplements can be delayed. Many units wait until the baby is at least 6 weeks old, or shortly before discharge, before starting supplements such as sodium iron EDTA 5.5 mg daily.

Discharging small babies

Whether it is the 32–36-week asymptomatic baby on a TCU, a normal small term baby, or the long-term NICU survivor, many factors need to be considered when preparing a baby for discharge. Traditionally there has been a focus on the need to attain a particular weight, e.g. 1.7 or 1.8 kg, prior to discharge. The advent of neonatal community nurses has made such rules more flexible and successful discharge at 1.5 kg and below has been achieved.[17] Current practices should focus on careful multidisciplinary assessment of the baby, the parents and the home environment before discharge can take place. The recommendations of the American Academy of Pediatrics[2] should be achieved:

- a sustained pattern of weight gain rather than a specific achieved weight;
- physiological stability with the ability to suckle feed and maintain normal body temperature in an open environment;
- parental involvement and preparation prior to discharge;
- home support post discharge;
- frequent outpatient follow-up to ensure adequate weight gain and to monitor development.

Evidence to support the exact timing of discharge for NICU graduates who have had prolonged oxygen requirements or recurrent apnoeas is lacking. Adequate oxygen saturations at all times, including feeding, should be demonstrated for at least a week prior to discharge, with no apnoeas for at least 5 days. The management of the baby with CLD still needing oxygen is discussed on page 563.

Prior to discharge, each baby should have a complete neonatal examination, including visualisation of the normal red light reflex and examination of the hips to assess stability (pp. 259–61); unnecessary repeated hip examination is not advised as this can predispose to the development of dysplasia.[3] Hearing (p. 254) and ROP (p. 846) checks should be performed for those who qualify, and follow-up arranged if indicated.

Advice to parents

Information giving, parent information leaflets and useful website addresses can help parent understanding and preparation prior to discharge.[74] Discharge advice to parents should include recommendations for the baby to sleep on his back in a cigarette-free environment and not to be overwrapped.[36] Parents are advised not to sleep in the same bed as the baby especially if they smoke, have recently drunk alcohol, are very tired or are taking drugs which make them sleepy. A baby under 8 weeks old sharing a bed with his parents has a twofold risk of sudden infant death syndrome (SIDS) if the parents are non-smokers and 11-fold if the parents smoke.[20] Babies should not sleep on a sofa with adults, as they have a 50-fold increased risk of SIDS.[13] The baby's cot should probably be in the parents' bedroom until 6 months of age.[36] Teaching parents resuscitation procedures can help alleviate anxiety and increase parental confidence[43] but there is no evidence that this reduces post-discharge mortality or morbidity.

Immunisations

Premature babies should be vaccinated according to the recommended schedule without correction for prematurity.[29,30] There is evidence that this results in good antibody response to diptheria–tetanus–pertussis (DTP), haemophilus and poliomyelitis.[11,27] However, hepatitis B[46] and BCG[66] immunisations may be less effective in preterm babies, but should be given where appropriate. Although no case of vaccine-transmitted polio has been reported within an NICU, there is a risk from using oral polio virus vaccine,[56] thus inactivated polio vaccine is recommended for those babies in whom discharge is not imminent.[22] In addition, influenza vaccine should be given to NICU graduates who are discharged during the winter months. Babies with CLD, especially those going home in oxygen, should receive palivizumab respiratory syncytial virus prophylaxis during their first winter. Babies who have CLD or had a prolonged oxygen requirement should receive conjugate pneumococcal vaccine.[31]

Apnoea has been reported in up to 30% of babies born at less than 31 weeks' gestation, following immmunisation at 2 months of age with whole cell DTP and Hib.[15] Most life-threatening events occur soon after the vaccination, so that appropriate monitoring for 48 hours post immunisation is recommended. Minor adverse events are also more common in preterm babies;[15] these are not serious but can be distressing for parents. Warning parents about possible adverse events can help to alleviate parental anxiety. Minor adverse events include low-grade fever (2–3%), soreness at the injection site (5–15%) and malaise. Vaccination also causes a rise in CRP.[7]

There are very few contraindications to immunising these babies. However, if a baby has recently been extubated, vaccination may precipitate reintubation. A period of respiratory stability is recommended before vaccination. There is little information regarding the immunological response to vaccination of preterm babies who have received steroids for CLD or upper airway obstruction. Previously, routine practice was to wait for 6–12 weeks post steroid course; there is no evidence to support the need for this, and vaccinations can be given as soon as post-steroid stability has been achieved. Acquired neurological disease in the neonatal period is not a contraindication to vaccination, even to the pertussis component of the vaccine. It is particularly important that babies with CLD receive the pertussis component, as pertussis superimposed on lung disease can be a devastating illness.

Feeding

For the larger preterm baby and the normal SGA baby discharged from a TCU who is not breastfeeding, formula feeds, appropriate for their postconceptional age, should be used (pp. 318, 319). Post-discharge nutrition and follow-on formulas for the NICU graduate are discussed in Chapter 16.

Post-discharge care

Monitors

Preterm infants have 8–10 times the risk of SIDS compared with low-risk term babies.[36] There is no evidence that home apnoea alarms reduce the incidence of SIDS or acute life-threatening events and it is possible that many cardiorespiratory events are missed by standard monitors. Although preterm babies are more likely than term babies to have adverse cardiorespiratory events until 43 weeks' CGA, there is no evidence that these events are precursors to SIDS, and after 43 weeks' CGA, the frequency of cardiorespiratory events in preterm babies is the same as for healthy term babies.[60]

Vitamin and iron supplements

The NICU graduate should receive iron and vitamin D supplementation from the time of discharge until he is at least 6 months old. For the preterm TCU graduate, similar supplementation should be given if he is breastfed, but, as all formulae are now supplemented, it is doubtful whether additional vitamins and iron are required for bottle-fed babies. SGA graduates from the TCU do not in general require supplements.

Follow-up

A baby discharged from the TCU who had an uncomplicated course does not need hospital follow-up, except if there was

Table 21.4 Criteria for follow-up of NICU graduates

≤32 weeks' gestation
≤1.50 kg birthweight
Neonatal encephalopathy
Seizures
Meningitis
Septicaemia
Necrotising enterocolitis
Significant hyperbilirubinaemia (including those requiring exchange transfusion)
Intracranial lesion on ultrasound scan
Persisting murmurs
Persisting structural abnormalities, e.g. hernia, vesicoureteric reflux, undescended testicles
Babies with CLD at discharge
Babies with social problems, e.g. narcotic abstinence syndrome
Infants of HIV-positive mothers

significant IUGR. The routine child health surveillance system is adequate for the needs of these babies.

Most NICU graduates require follow-up, but it is important to be selective (Table 21.4). Careful multidisciplinary follow-up is necessary for babies with complex actual, or potential, problems so that motor delay, spasticity and poor weight gain are detected and managed promptly. Long-term follow-up of very sick or preterm babies, with accurate data collection, can help consolidate epidemiological information about outcome for this group.

References

1. Alvarson D C 1995 The physiologic impact of anemia in the neonate. Clinics in Perinatology 22: 609–625
2. American Academy of Pediatrics 1998 Hospital discharge of the high-risk neonate – proposed guidelines. Pediatrics 102: 411–417
3. American Academy of Pediatrics 2000 Clinical practice guideline: early detection of developmental dysplasia of the hip. Pediatrics 105: 896–905
4. Arant B S 1993 Sodium chloride and potassium. In: Tsang R C, Lucas A, Uauy R, Zlotkin S (eds) Nutritional needs of the preterm infant. Williams & Wilkins, Baltimore, pp 157–175
5. Arlettaz R, Archer N, Wilkinson A R 2001 Closure of the ductus arteriosus and development of pulmonary branch stenosis in babies of less than 32 weeks gestation. Archives of Disease in Childhood. Fetal and Neonatal Edition 85: F197–F200
6. Azaz Y, Fleming P J, Levine M et al 1992 The relationship between environmental temperature, metabolic rate, and evaporative water loss in infants from birth to three months. Pediatric Research 32: 417–423
7. Balkundi D R, Nycyk J A, Cooke R W I 1994 Immunization and C reactive protein in infants on neonatal intensive care units. Archives of Disease in Childhood. Fetal and Neonatal Edition 71: F149
8. Bayatpour M, Bernard L, McCune F et al 1979 Spontaneous gastric rupture in the newborn. American Journal of Surgery 137: 267–269
9. Beecroft D M O, Dix M R, Farmer K 1977 Intramuscular iron-dextran and susceptibility of neonates to bacterial infections. Archives of Disease in Childhood 52: 778–781
10. Bell M J 1985 Perforation of the gastrointestinal tract and peritonitis in the neonate. Surgery, Gynecology and Obstetrics 160: 20–26
11. Bernbaum J C, Daft A, Anolik R et al 1985 Response of preterm infants to diphtheria-tetanus-pertussis immunizations. Journal of Pediatrics 107: 184–188
12. Bier J A B, Ferguson A, Anderson L et al 1993 Breast feeding of very low birth-weight infants. Journal of Pediatrics 123: 773–778
13. Blair B, Fleming P, Smith I 1999 Babies sleeping with parents: case control study of factors influencing the risk of the sudden infant death syndrome. British Medical Journal 319:1457–1462
14. Boo N Y, Chee S C, Rohana J 2002 Randomised controlled study on the effects of different durations of light exposure on weight gain by preterm infants in a neonatal intensive care unit. Acta Paediatrica Scandinavica 91: 674–679
15. Botham S J, Isaacs D 1997 Incidence of apnoea and bradycardia in preterm infants following DTPw and Hib immunization: a prospective study. Journal of Paediatrics and Child Health 33: 418–421
16. Boxall A, Orme R L E, Cruickshank J G 1982 Shared care and infection in a special care baby unit. Nursing Times 78: 1848–1850
17. Bromley P 2000 Transitional care: let's think again. Journal of Neonatal Nursing 6: 60–64
18. Burke M, Walsh J, Oehler J et al 1995 Music therapy following suctioning. Neonatal Network 14: 41–49
19. Campbell D M, Gandy G M, Roberton N R C 1983 Which babies need admission to special care baby units? In: Davis J A, Richards M P M, Roberton N R C (eds) Parent–baby attachment in premature infants. Croom Helm, London, pp 67–85
20. Carpenter R G, Irgens L M, Blair P et al 2004 Sudden unexplained infant death in 20 regions in Europe: case control study. Lancet 363: 185–191
21. Cartlidge P H T, Rutter N 1988 Reduction of head flattening in preterm infants. Archives of Disease in Childhood 63: 755–757
22. Cherry J D 1995 Enteroviruses. In: Remington J S, Klein J O (eds) Infectious diseases of the fetus and newborn infant, 4th edn. W B Saunders, Philadelphia, pp 404–446
23. Christensson K, Bhat G J, Amadi B C et al 1998 Randomised study of skin-to-skin versus incubator care for re-warming low-risk hypothermic neonates. Lancet 352: 1115
24. Christensson K, Cabrera T, Christensson E et al 1995 Separation distress call in the human neonate in the absence of maternal contact. Acta Paediatrica 84: 468–473
25. Conde-Agudelo A, Diaz-Rossello J L, Belizan J M 2003 Kangaroo mother care to reduce morbidity and mortality in low birth weight infants (Cochrane Review). Cochrane Database of Systematic Reviews (2): CD002771
26. Cooke R J, Embleton N D 2000 Feeding issues in preterm infants. Archives of Disease in Childhood. Fetal and Neonatal Edition 83: F215–F218
27. D'Angio C T, Maniscalco W M, Pichichero M E 1995 Immunologic response of extremely premature infants to tetanus, haemophilus influenzae and polio immunization. Pediatrics 96: 18–22
28. Dear P R F, McClain B I 1987 Establishment of an intermediate care ward for babies and mothers. Archives of Disease in Childhood 62: 597–600
29. Department of Health 1996 The immunisation schedule. In: Salisbury D, Begg N (eds) Immunisation against infectious disease 1996 – 'The Green Book'. DoH, London, pp 45–47
30. Department of Health 1999 Start of the new meningococcal C conjugate vaccine immunisation programme. PL/CMO/99/4
31. Department of Health 2002 Update on immunisation issues. PL/CMO/2002/4
32. Dowling D, Meirer P, DiFiore J et al 2002 Cup-feeding for preterm infants: mechanics and safety. Journal of Human Lactation 18: 13–20
33. Downs J A, Edwards A D, McCormick D C et al 1991 Effect of intervention on development of hip posture in very preterm babies. Archives of Disease in Childhood 66: 797–801
34. Emberton M, Patel L, Zideman D A et al 1996 Early repair of inguinal hernia in preterm infants with oxygen dependent bronchopulmonary dysplasia. Acta Paediatrica 85: 96–99
35. Field T 2002 Massage therapy. Medical Clinics of North America 86: 163–171
36. Fleming P J, Blair P S, Bacon C et al 1996 Environment of infants during sleep and risk for SIDS: results of 1993-1995 case control study for CESDI. British Medical Journal 313: 191–195
37. Fohe K, Kropf S, Avenarius S 2000 Skin-to-skin contact improves gas exchange in premature infants. Journal of Perinatology 5: 311–315
38. Goldman D A, Leclair J, Malone A 1978 Bacterial colonization of neonates admitted to an intensive care environment. Journal of Pediatrics 63: 288–293
39. Howard C, De Blieck E, Ten Hoopen C et al 1999 Physiologic stability of newborns during cup- and bottle-feeding. Pediatrics 104(5 suppl.): 1204–1207
40. Jacobs S E, Sokol J, Ohlsson A 2002 The newborn individualised developmental care and assessment programme is not supported by meta-analyses of the data. Journal of Pediatrics 140: 699–706
41. Jarvis W R 1987 Epidemiology of nosocomial infections in pediatric patients. Pediatric Infectious Disease Journal 6: 344–351
42. Kaminski J, Hall W 1996 The effect of soothing music on neonatal behavioural states in the hospital newborn nursery. Neonatal Network 15: 45–54
43. Komelasky A L, Bond B S 1993 The effect of teaching two forms of learning reinforcement on parental retention of CPR skills. Pediatric Nursing 19: 96–98

44. Kumar V H, Clive J, Rosenbrantz T S et al 2002 Inguinal hernia in preterm infants (⩽32-week gestation). Pediatric Surgery International 18: 147–152

45. Laing I A, Lang M A, Callaghan O et al 1986 Nasogastric compared with nasoduodenal feeding in low birthweight infants. Archives of Disease in Childhood 61: 138–141

46. Lau Y-L, Tam A Y C, Ng K W et al 1992 Response of preterm infants to hepatitis B vaccine. Journal of Pediatrics 121: 962–965

47. Lucas A, King F, Bishop N R 1992 Post-discharge formula consumption in infants born preterm. Archives of Disease in Childhood 67: 691–692

48. Lund C, Osbourne J, Kuller J et al 2001 Neonatal skin care: clinical outcomes of the AWHONN/NANN evidence-based clinical practice guideline. Journal of Obstetric, Gynaecology and Neonatal Nursing 30: 41

49. Mann N P, Haddow R, Stokes L et al 1986 Effect of night and day on preterm infants in a newborn nursery: randomised trial. British Medical Journal 293: 1265–1267

50. Manoura A, Hatzidaki E, Karakaki E 2002 Eosinophilia in sick neonates. Haematologica 32: 31–37

51. Marinelli K, Burke G, Dodd V 2001 A comparison of the safety of cupfeedings and bottlefeedings in premature infants whose mothers intend to breastfeed. Journal of Perinatology 21: 350–355

52. Mirmiran M, Ariagno R L 2000 Influence of light in the NICU on the development of circadian rhythms in preterm infants. Seminars in Perinatology 24: 247–257

53. Montgomery S M, Wakefield A J, Morris D L et al 2000 The initial care of newborn infants and subsequent hayfever. Allergy 55: 916–922

54. Neu M, Browne J 1997 Infant physiologic and behavioural organisation during swaddled versus unswaddled weighing. Journal of Perinatology 17: 193–198

55. Newell S J, Booth I W, Morgan M E I et al 1989 Gastro-oesophageal reflux in preterm infants. Archives of Disease in Childhood 64: 780–786

56. Paz J A, Vallada M G, Marques S N 2000 Vaccine-associated paralytic poliomyelitis: a case report of domiciliary transmission. Revista do Hospital das Clínicas 55: 101–104

57. Philbin M, Robertson A, Hall J 1999 Recommended permissible noise criteria for occupied, newly constructed or renovated hospital nurseries. Journal of Perinatology 19: 559–563

58. Pinelli J, Symington A 2003 Developmental care for promoting development and preventing morbidity in preterm infants (Cochrane Review). Cochrane Database of Systematic Reviews (4): CD001814

59. Premji S, Chessell L 2003 Continuous nasogastric milk feeding versus intermittent bolus milk feeding for premature infants less than 1500 grams. (Cochrane Review). Cochrane Database of Systematic Reviews (1): CD001819

60. Rangasamy R, Corwin M, Hunt C et al 2001 Cardiorespiratory events recorded on home monitors; comparison of healthy infants with those at increased risk for SIDS. Journal of the American Medical Association 285: 2199–2207

61. Robertson A, Cooper-Peel C, Vos P 1999 Sound transmission into incubators in the NICU. Journal of Perinatology 19: 494–497

62. Rocha N, Martinez F, Jorge S 2002 Cup or bottle for preterm infants: effects on oxygen saturation, weight gain and breastfeeding. Journal of Human Lactation 18: 132–138

63. Rutter N, Hinchcliffe W, Cartlidge P H T 1993 Do preterm infants always have flattened heads? Archives of Disease in Childhood 68: 606–607

64. Sands T, Glasson M, Berry A 1989 Hazards of nasogastric tube insertion in the newborn infant. Lancet ii: 680

65. Scahnler R J, Schulman R J, Lau C et al 1999 Feeding strategies for premature infants: randomised trial of gastrointestinal priming and tube-feeding methods. Pediatrics 103: 434–439

66. Sedaghatian M R, Kardouni K 1993 Tuberculin reponse in preterm infants after BCG vaccination at birth. Archives of Disease in Childhood. Fetal and Neonatal Edition 69: F309–F311

67. Shiroiwa Y, Kamiya Y, Uchibori S et al 1986 Activity, cardiac and respiratory responses of blindfold preterm infants in a neonatal intensive care unit. Early Human Development 14: 259–265

68. Simpson D 2000 Transitional care for neonates. The Practising Midwife 3: 13–15

69. Strelling M K, Blackledge D G, Goodall H B 1979 Diagnosis and management of folate deficiency in low birthweight infants. Archives of Disease in Childhood 54: 271–277

70. Stute H, Greiner B, Linderkamp O 1995 Effect of blood transfusion on cardiorespiratory abnormalities in preterm infants. Archives of Disease in Childhood. Fetal and Neonatal Edition 72: F194–F196

71. Sullivan S E, Calhoun D A 2000 Eosinophilia in the neonatal intensive care unit. Clinics in Perinatology 27: 603–622

72. Symington A, Pinelli J 2001 Non-nutritive sucking for promoting physiologic stability and nutrition in preterm infants (Cochrane Review). Cochrane Database of Systematic Reviews (3): CD001071

73. Torres C, Holditch-Davis D, O'Hale A et al 1997 Effect of standard rest periods on apnoea and weight gain on preterm infants. Neonatal Network 16: 35–43

74. Vanderberg K 1999 What to tell parents about the developmental needs of their baby at discharge. Neonatal Network 18: 57–59

75. Westkamp E, Soditt V, Adrian S et al 2002 Blood transfusion in anemic infants with apnea of prematurity. Biology of the Neonate 82: 228–232

76. Zipursky A 1984 Vitamin E deficiency anemia in newborn infants. Clinics in Perinatology 11: 393–402

CHAPTER 22

The infant of a diabetic mother

Jane Hawdon

Diabetes may complicate the pregnancy of a woman with established diabetes or one who develops transient or permanent diabetes during pregnancy. The fertility and wellbeing of diabetic women dramatically improved with the availability of insulin, but a high perinatal mortality rate of 20–25% persisted until the 1960s. In the last three decades, perinatal mortality rates have fallen and rates below 3% have been achieved in some centres.[20,41,81] However, in some regions, for example Northern England, high perinatal mortality rates, four to six times baseline, persist.[16,37]

Especially when there is good pre-conceptional care and maternal diabetic control, infants of diabetic mothers (IDMs) who do not have congenital malformations may be expected to have an uncomplicated neonatal course and should be managed as any other healthy term baby. For example, few UK units now insist on routine attendance of paediatricians at the delivery or routine admission to a neonatal unit, unless complications are expected. However, the pregnancy in established or gestational diabetes may be complicated by one or more of a wide variety of problems in the fetus and in the newborn. Adequate antenatal screening and assessment should indicate the pregnancies at greatest risk so that an antenatal plan may be made.

Before discussing the aetiology and management of the fetal and neonatal complications of maternal diabetes, it is appropriate to be reminded of Farquhar's[29] vivid and classic description of infants of poorly controlled diabetic mothers:

> They emerge at least alive from within the fiery metabolic furnace of diabetes mellitus, but they resemble one another so closely that they might well be related. They are plump, sleek, liberally coated with vernix caseosa, full-faced and plethoric. During their first two or more extrauterine hours they lie on their backs, bloated and flushed, their legs flexed and abducted, their lightly closed hands on each side of the head, the abdomen prominent and their respiration sighing. They convey a distinct impression of having such a surfeit of both food and fluid pressed upon them by an insistent hostess that they desire only peace so that they may recover from their excesses.

Congenital anomalies

Despite major improvements in the care of diabetic pregnancies, there has been little overall change in the incidence of congenital malformations.[16,62,80] Congenital anomalies in the offspring of a diabetic woman occur with a frequency up to 10 times that observed in the general population. The problem has become even more compelling as the perinatal mortality has fallen, because malformations now account for a large proportion of perinatal losses and have replaced respiratory distress syndrome (RDS) as the leading cause of death in IDMs.[1,16,20,23]

The cause of diabetic embryopathy is not fully understood. Genetic factors (diabetes-related genes) are unlikely to play a role, as the incidence of birth defects is not increased in the newborn infants of diabetic fathers.[17] It is likely that congenital anomalies are related to the diabetic intrauterine environment during the period of organogenesis, before the seventh week of gestation.[54] Therefore, most malformations take place before the pregnancy is recognised and the intensified diabetes treatment is initiated. This supports the recommendation that good diabetic control before conception is mandatory.

The teratogenic effect of hyperglycaemia has been suggested by human studies,[60] and has been confirmed in animal studies.[31] However, animal studies have demonstrated additional factors such as hyperketonaemia[40,82] increased levels of somatomedin-inhibiting factors[83] and decreased myoinositol concentration in the neuroectoderm.[92]

Insulin cannot be teratogenic, because the human placenta is impermeable to insulin at early gestation[4] and fetal pancreatic β cells are not present before the 10th week.[48] However, disturbances in the secretion of relaxin, an insulin homologue, have been suggested to be potentially teratogenic.[28]

Finally, hypoglycaemia can also be embryotoxic in experimental animals,[13] but data from human studies are reassuring.[60]

Although IDMs are at risk for a wide variety of malformations, one syndrome seems to be particularly strongly associated with diabetes, with a relative risk of 212 compared with non-diabetics.[18] The syndrome of caudal regression is a condition in which agenesis or hypoplasia of the femora occurs in conjunction with agenesis of the lower vertebrae (sacral agenesis).[67] Other anomalies over-represented in IDMs are anencephaly, meningomyelocele, holoprosencephaly,[7] vertebral dysplasia, congenital heart disease, ventricular septal defect, transposition of the great vessels and small left colon syndrome.[75]

It is clear that efforts to prevent birth defects should start before conception, with contraceptive advice offered so that every pregnancy can be planned in advance with optimum periconceptual metabolic control. Some reports suggest that early first-trimester improvement in glycaemic control,[27,32] combined with prenatal diagnosis of anomalies using serum α-fetoprotein determinations and ultrasound scanning,[61] could reduce the impact of congenital anomalies.

Macrosomia and smallness for gestational age

Macrosomia and organomegaly attributed to fetal hyperinsulinaemia are well-known characteristics of many diabetic pregnancies. Glucose crosses the placenta by facilitated diffusion, therefore maternal hyperglycaemia imposes a carbohydrate surplus on the fetus. The fetus responds with increased secretion of insulin. Because insulin is an anabolic hormone, the fetal hyperinsulinaemia stimulates protein, lipid and glycogen synthesis to cause macrosomia. Although this classic maternal hyperglycaemia–fetal hyperinsulinism theory of Pedersen[69] is widely accepted, the metabolic and endocrine disturbances are much more complex. For example, free amino acids also have a stimulatory effect on

the development of the β cell, and the anabolic actions of insulin, in utero at least, could in part be mediated through the insulin-induced release of insulin-like growth factors.[24,55] In addition, birthweight is positively correlated with maternal concentrations of triglycerides and free fatty acids.[44,45]

Rates of macrosomia vary between centres – for example, from only 8% with birthweights above the 90th centile in an Italian study of strict maternal diabetic control[81] to 35% with birthweights above the 95th centile in the Northern Region in the UK.[37] The relationship between overall maternal diabetes control and macrosomia is not close,[10] in that some infants may still be born with macrosomia after a pregnancy in which maternal blood glucose levels were apparently well controlled. The reason for this may include the fact that glucose level is not the only parameter describing optimal diabetic control in pregnancy. However, some studies suggest that optimal management of diabetic pregnancies may reduce the incidence of macrosomia.[39,52]

The striking physical appearance (Fig. 22.1) of these infants has already been described. Much of the increased mass is fat.[99] The organomegaly is selective: the liver and heart are often enlarged and skeletal length is increased in proportion to weight, but the brain size is not increased relative to gestational age and so the head may appear disproportionately small.[64]

The clinical significance of macrosomia is the risk of the complications of delivery of a large infant, such as shoulder dystocia, obstructed labour and perinatal asphyxia.[3,57] In one study,[3] 30% of IDMs with a birthweight above 4000 g who were delivered vaginally developed shoulder dystocia, with frequent complications such as fractures and brachial plexus palsy.

Maternal diabetic vascular disease leading to placental insufficiency can impair fetal growth, so some of the infants will be born small for gestational age (SGA).[19] Overzealous diabetic control and maternal hypoglycaemia may have the same result.[47] The SGA IDM appears to be at even greater risk of adverse outcome, especially neurodevelopmental sequelae,[74] because the perinatal problems of the IDM are compounded by those of intrauterine malnutrition (Chapter 10).

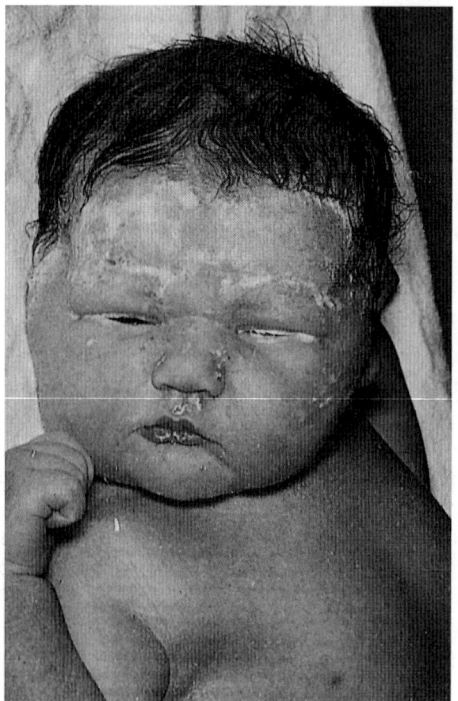

Fig. 22.1 An infant born to a poorly controlled diabetic mother. There is increased adiposity and facial plethora, together with respiratory distress.

Respiratory complications

Although the incidence of RDS was previously reported to be five to six times higher in IDMs than in the normal population, this incidence is falling in line with improved maternal diabetic control and prevention of preterm delivery.[34] IDMs may have typical RDS despite a normal lecithin–sphingomyelin ratio in the amniotic fluid. This may be because RDS is secondary to the retarded maturation of the pulmonary surfactant system (p. 469), including surfactant proteins,[15,33,65] rather than simply to the reduced production of phospholipids. Animal studies have demonstrated that insulin inhibits cortisol-induced lecithin synthesis by pneumocytes,[87] probably by inhibiting the production of fibroblast-pneumocyte factor, which promotes phosphatidylcholine synthesis. It has also been demonstrated that butyrate inhibits the transcription of mRNA for surfactant proteins.[73]

IDMs are also at increased risk for transient tachypnoea of the newborn (TTN)[34] or respiratory distress associated with cardiac abnormalities. Finally, many diabetic women are delivered before term and/or by caesarean section, and the contribution of these factors to increased respiratory morbidity from RDS or TTN must be considered.[63] The management of these respiratory complications, should they occur, should be according to each unit's standard policy.

Hypocalcaemia and hypomagnesaemia

Neonatal hypocalcaemia has been reported in up to 50% of IDMs,[58,93] and both its incidence and severity appear to be related to the degree of maternal diabetes control.[25,93] Hypocalcaemia is usually associated with hyperphosphataemia and occasionally with hypomagnesaemia. The aetiology is not entirely clear, but neonatal hypoparathyroidism has been demonstrated and may in part be secondary to maternal magnesium loss.[25,50,59] Birth asphyxia may also exacerbate hypocalcaemia.

None of the studies that report hypocalcaemia have commented on whether an isolated biochemical finding is of clinical significance. Usually no clinical signs are seen and no treatment is necessary. However, in the presence of clinical signs of hypocalcaemia and hypomagnesaemia, the deficits should be corrected as described elsewhere in this book (p. 882).

Hyperviscosity, polycythaemia, jaundice

IDMs have an increased risk of being polycythaemic and developing the neonatal hyperviscosity syndrome.[58]

Normoblastaemia and extensive extramedullary erythropoiesis in the IDM were observed as early as 1944,[53] and the aetiology of the increased erythropoiesis has since been described.[76] Elevated umbilical plasma erythropoietin concentrations have been found in IDMs, and these correlated directly with plasma insulin levels in both IDMs and controls.[100] The raised erythropoietin levels are thought to be secondary to relative cellular hypoxia, which is the result of insulin-induced high glucose uptake and high metabolic rates. A more direct effect of insulin was shown in another study,[71] in which insulin stimulated growth in culture of late erythroid progenitors in cord blood from premature, term and IDM infants.

Lysis of this red cell load contributes to the prolonged unconjugated hyperbilirubinaemia often found in IDMs.[70] There may also be functional immaturity of hepatic enzymes.[91]

Renal vein thrombosis and thrombosis in other vessels, which has been reported to occur with increased frequency in IDMs, is probably related to polycythaemia and hyperviscosity.[5]

Polycythaemia and hyperbilirubinaemia should be managed as described in Chapter 30 and Chapter 29, Part 1, respectively.

Hypertrophic cardiomyopathy

Cardiac enlargement and hypertrophy in IDMs was reported as early as 1944.[53] The condition has now been studied more extensively.[94] Improved echocardiographic techniques have shown a generalised myocardial hypertrophy with a disproportionate thickening of the septum.[49,77] Symptomatic infants generally have severe hypertrophy and the hypertrophied septal muscles may bulge into the left ventricle, thereby narrowing the left ventricular outflow tract (Fig. 22.2). The condition may cause fetal or neonatal death.[51,84] The cardiomyopathy may be related to maternal diabetes control[49,77] and to fetal and neonatal hyperinsulinaemia.[11]

If clinical signs occur, the presentation is usually within the first weeks of postnatal life with cardiorespiratory distress and congestive heart failure. Systolic ejection murmurs can be heard in most affected infants, and chest radiography reveals cardiomegaly.[98] The majority of the infants need supportive care only. If congestive heart failure develops, propranolol is recommended.[98] Digitalis and other positive inotropic agents are generally contraindicated because they increase systolic contraction and may exacerbate the outflow tract obstruction.[98]

The hypertrophic cardiomyopathy of the IDM is transient. Resolution of the signs can be expected in 2–4 weeks, and the septal hypertrophy regresses within 2–12 months (see also p. 645).[77,98]

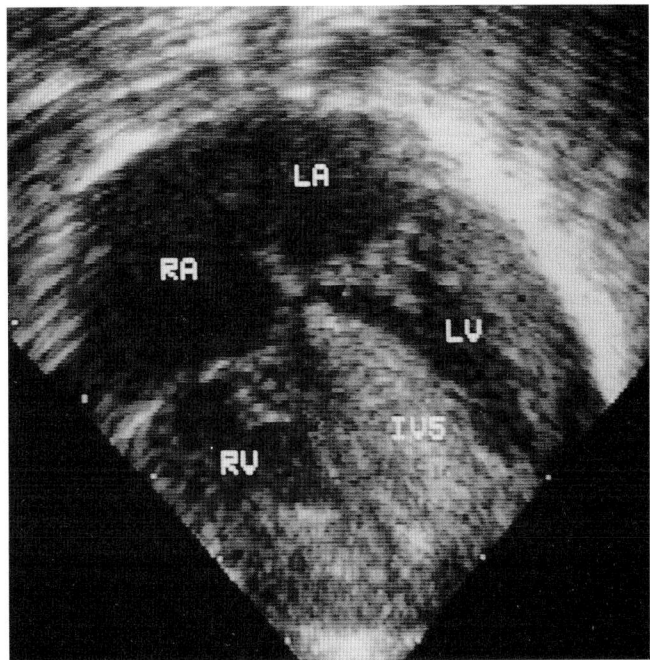

Fig. 22.2 Echocardiographic image of a four-chamber view of a neonatal heart, demonstrating hypertrophy of the intraventricular septum (IVS) secondary to fetal hyperinsulinism. RA, right atrium; LA, left atrium; RV, right ventricle; LV, left ventricle.

Hypoglycaemia
(see also Chapter 35, Part I)

Most IDMs have transient (1–4 hours postnatally) asymptomatic hypoglycaemia before a spontaneous increase in blood glucose level occurs, a pattern also seen in newborn babies of non-diabetic mothers.[46] Others have a more prolonged period of severe symptomatic hypoglycaemia, and a minority develop late hypoglycaemia after an initial benign course. However, all regain normal blood glucose control within the first few days after birth. Recent data have shown that plasma insulin levels fall to normal within 12–24 hours of birth in all infants except those whose mothers' diabetes was poorly controlled.[35] For the full definition and symptoms of hypoglycaemia, see pages 854–5.

IDMs may have hyperinsulinism at birth owing to increased placental transfer of glucose and other nutrients stimulating increased insulin secretion (see above).[8] The pancreas shows hyperplasia and hypertrophy of the islets of Langerhans[14,53] without evidence of pancreatic pathology. An increase of the glucagon and pancreatic polypeptide cell fractions in the pancreas has also been shown by immunocytochemical methods,[56] and a counterregulatory hormone response has been demonstrated which may curtail the period of hypoglycaemia.[12,38] However, it has been reported that some infants fail to develop the normal increase in plasma glucagon at 2–4 hours of age.[9]

The effect of hyperinsulinism on the liver has been confirmed using stable isotope methods,[42] which demonstrated decreased glucose production. If raised insulin levels persist beyond the first postnatal day, other metabolic fuels may be affected. For example, in theory, plasma free fatty acid and blood ketone body concentrations may be lower than in normal term infants, although clinical studies have not confirmed this.[68] Plasma amino acid concentrations are less affected than in organic hyperinsulinism secondary to congenital pancreatic disorders (pp. 857–8). The characteristic low blood levels of branched-chain amino acids are not an invariable finding,[88,95] possibly because of other transient disturbances in postnatal metabolic adaptation, including the effects of concurrent asphyxia or hypoxia.

In relation to management, a blood glucose level should be obtained from the mother (or cord) at delivery and from the infant 3–4-hourly, before feeds, for 6–12 hours after birth. Frequency and duration of monitoring will depend upon antenatal diabetic control and maternal blood glucose concentration – when control has been poor and maternal or cord blood glucose levels high, monitoring should be more intensive. Blood glucose screening may be discontinued when at least two consecutive pre-feed blood glucose levels are satisfactory and the baby remains well (Chapter 21). It should be noted that test strip reagents are inaccurate, especially at high packed cell volume.[22] Therefore, in polycythaemic infants it is important to use accurate methods, and if test strips are to be used, measure the plasma and not the whole blood concentration of glucose.

Hypoglycaemia may usually be prevented by giving enteral feeds with milk within 1–2 hours after delivery, as it has been shown that a feed of 10 ml/kg human milk can cause an increase of blood glucose in the order of 1 mmol/l at this time.[6]

Breastfeeding should be encouraged, with additional breast milk or formula supplementation as indicated by clinical signs and blood glucose levels. There is evidence in other groups of babies that excessive formula supplementation may impair counterregulatory responses, so volumes of formula should be kept to the minimum required.[26] However, for some infants, daily feed volumes of at least 100 ml/kg may be required to maintain normoglycaemia.

Sick infants unable to tolerate enteral feeding, or those who remain hypoglycaemic despite full enteral feeds, should receive an intravenous infusion of glucose at an initial rate of 5 mg/kg/min (3 ml/kg/hour of 10% dextrose) but increasing rapidly if indicated by repeat blood glucose monitoring. Some hyperinsulinaemic babies require glucose infusions in excess of 10 mg/kg/min, but glucose should not be administered at rates higher than that required to maintain normoglycaemia, in order to avoid continued stimulation of insulin secretion. If enteral feeds have been tolerated, these should not be reduced when intravenous glucose is commenced. Neurological signs of hypoglycaemia in any infant warrant immediate correction by a bolus injection of 200–400 mg/kg glucose followed by glucose infusion or increased rate of glucose infusion, the rate being adjusted as necessary to maintain normoglycaemia. In other circumstances, boluses should be avoided, as increased insulin secretion and rebound hypoglycaemia will result.

Cortisol (5 mg/kg) has been recommended by others to be given intravenously or intramuscularly at 12-hour intervals. A single injection of glucagon (0.03–0.1 mg/kg), which has a temporary hyperglycaemic effect by releasing glucose from glycogen stores, is a useful measure in the event of delay in siting intravenous lines.

Intravenous glucose should be weaned gradually, as indicated by blood glucose monitoring. Reactive hypoglycaemia may occur if the glucose infusion is decreased too quickly.

Outcome

According to some studies, infants of poorly controlled diabetic mothers are at greater risk of brain damage, poor psychomotor development, subtle neurological abnormalities ('minimal brain dysfunction', hyperactivity) and EEG changes. There are a number of risk factors – birth trauma, placental dysfunction, hypoxia-ischaemia, episodes of maternal ketosis or hypoglycaemia during pregnancy (p. 186), neonatal hypoglycaemia.[36,78,89] As these are all interdependent variables, it is impossible to determine which is the most important factor. For example, both neonatal hypoglycaemia and adverse neurodevelopmental outcome are associated with aberrant antenatal metabolic control.[66,86,90] Studies of well-controlled diabetes in pregnancy show a favourable neurodevelopmental outcome.[72,79,85]

Although many studies have shown that, on follow-up, the majority of children of diabetic mothers have normal weight-for-height and normal height-for-age, in some cases, poor antenatal diabetic control and the presence of neonatal macrosomia increase the risk of obesity in later life.[2,21,86,96]

The risk of insulin-dependent diabetes developing by the age of 20 years in the offspring of diabetic women is at least seven times that for non-diabetic parents, and later impaired glucose tolerance is associated with aberrant maternal diabetic control.[72,86] Interestingly, this is only one-third of the risk reported for the offspring of fathers with insulin-dependent diabetes,[97] and this is possibly because of a lower rate of *DR4* allele transmission from mothers or an effect of programming by the intrauterine environment.[30]

Careful medical and obstetric care to achieve strict glycaemic control throughout pregnancy, in combination with appropriate neonatal care, greatly reduces the risk of the many complications discussed in this chapter. Perinatal mortality for IDMs is now less than 3% in most major centres, and the vast majority of infants of strictly controlled euglycaemic mothers are of normal size and post-natal metabolic adaptation is normal.[12,43] Therefore it is important to avoid iatrogenic problems such as needless separation of mothers and babies or practices which impede successful breastfeeding.

References

1. [Anonymous] 1988 Congenital abnormalities in infants of diabetic mothers. Lancet i: 1313–1315

2. [Anonymous] 1990 Hyperinsulinaemia and macrosomia. New England Journal of Medicine 323: 340–342

3. Acker D B, Sachs B P, Friedman E A 1985 Risk factors for shoulder dystocia. Obstetrics and Gynecology 66: 762–768

4. Adam P A J, Teramo K, Raiha N, Gitlin D, Schwartz R 1969 Human fetal insulin metabolism early in gestation. Response to acute elevation of the fetal glucose concentration and placental transfer of human insulin. Diabetes 18: 403–416

5. Avery M E, Oppenheimer E H, Gordon H H 1957 Renal vein thrombosis in newborn infants of diabetic mothers. New England Journal of Medicine 256: 1134–1138

6. Aynsley-Green A, Soltesz G 1985 Hypoglycaemia in infancy and childhood. Current Reviews in Paediatrics 1: 54–58

7. Barr M, Hanson J W, Currey K et al 1983 Holoprosencephaly in infants of diabetic mothers. Journal of Pediatrics 102: 565–568

8. Block M B, Pildes R S, Mossabhoy N A, Steiner D F, Rubenstein A 1974 C-peptide immunoreactivity: a new method for studying infants of insulin-treated diabetic mothers. Pediatrics 53: 923–928

9. Bloom S R, Johnston D F 1972 Failure of glucagon release in infants of diabetic mothers. British Medical Journal iv: 453–454

10. Bradley R J, Nicolaides K H, Brudenell J M 1988 Are all infants of diabetic mothers 'macrosomic'? British Medical Journal 297: 1583–1584

11. Breitweser J A, Meyer R A, Sperling M A, Tsang R C, Kaplan S 1980 Cardiac septal hypertrophy in hyperinsulinaemic infants. Journal of Pediatrics 96: 535–539

12. Broberger U, Hansson U, Largercrantz H, Persson B 1984 Sympathoadrenal activity and metabolic adjustment during the first 12 hours after birth in infants of diabetic mothers. Acta Paediatrica Scandinavica 73: 620–625

13. Buchanan T A, Schemmer J K, Freinkel N 1986 Embryotoxic effects of brief maternal insulin hypoglycaemia during organogenesis in the rat. Journal of Clinical Investigation 78: 643–649

14. Cardell B S 1953 Hypertrophy and hyperplasia of the pancreatic islets in newborn infants. Pathology 66: 335–341

15. Carlson K S, Smith B T, Post M 1984 Insulin acts on the fibroblast to inhibit glucocorticoid stimulation of lung maturation. Journal of Applied Physiology 57: 1577–1579

16. Casson I F, Clarke C A, Howard C V et al 1997 Outcomes of pregnancy in insulin dependent diabetic women: results of a five year population cohort study. British Medical Journal 315: 275–278

17. Comess L J, Bennett P H, Man M B et al 1969 Congenital anomalies and diabetes in the Pima Indians of Arizona. Diabetes 18: 471–477

18. Coombs C A, Kitzmuiller J C 1991 Spontaneous abortion and congenital malformation in diabetes. Clinical Obstetrics and Gynecology 5: 315–331

19. Cordero L, Landon M B 1993 Infant of the diabetic mother. Clinics in Perinatology 20: 635–648

20. Coustan D R 1988 Pregnancy in diabetic women. New England Journal of Medicine 319: 1663–1665

21. Cummins M, Norrish M 1980 Follow-up of children of diabetic mothers. Archives of Disease in Childhood 55: 259–264

22. Dacombe C M, Dalton R G, Goldie D F, Osborne J P 1981 Effect of packed cell volume on blood glucose estimations. Archives of Disease in Childhood 56: 789–791

23. Damm P, Molsted-Pedersen L 1989 Significant decrease in congenital malformations in newborn infants of an unselected population of diabetic mothers. American Journal of Obstetrics and Gynecology 161: 1163–1167

24. Delmis J, Drazaneic A, Ivanisevic M, Suchanek E 1992 Glucose, insulin, HGH and IGF-I levels in maternal serum, amniotic fluid and umbilical venous serum: a comparison between late normal pregnancy and pregnancies complicated with diabetes and fetal growth retardation. Journal of Perinatal Medicine 20: 47–56

25. Demaini S, Mimouni F, Tsang R C, Khoury J, Hertzberg V 1994 Impact of metabolic control of diabetes during pregnancy on neonatal hypocalcaemia: a randomized study. Obstetrics and Gynecology 83: 918–922

26. de Rooy L J, Hawdon J M 2002 Nutritional factors that affect the postnatal metabolic adaptation of full-term small- and large-for-gestational-age infants. Pediatrics 109: E42

27. Diabetes Control and Complications Trial Research Group 1993 The effect of intensive treatment of diabetes on the development and progression of long term complications in insulin dependent diabetes mellitus. New England Journal of Medicine 329: 977–986

28. Edwards J R G, Newall D R 1988 Relaxin as an aetiological factor in diabetic embryopathy. Lancet i: 1428–1430

29. Farquhar J W 1959 The child of a diabetic woman. Archives of Disease in Childhood 34: 76–96

30. Field L L 1988 Insulin-dependent diabetes mellitus: a model for the study of multifactorial disorders. American Journal of Human Genetics 43: 793–798

31. Freinkel N 1988 Diabetic embryopathy and fuel-mediated organ teratogenesis: lessons from animal models. Hormone and Metabolic Research 20: 463–475

32. Fuhrmann K, Reicher H, Semmler K, Fisher F, Fisher M, Glockner E 1983 Prevention of congenital malformations in infants of insulin-dependent diabetic mothers. Diabetes Care 6: 213–223

33. Gewolb I H 1993 High glucose causes delayed fetal lung maturation in vitro. Experimental Lung Research 19: 619–630

34. Hanson U, Persson B 1993 Outcome of pregnancies complicated by type I insulin dependent diabetes in Sweden: acute pregnancy complications, neonatal mortality and morbidity. American Journal of Perinatology 10: 330–333

35. Hawdon J M, Aynsley-Green A 1996 Neonatal complications, including hypo-glycaemia. In: Dornhorst A, Hadden D (eds) Diabetes and pregnancy: an international approach to diagnosis and management. Wiley, Chichester, pp 303–318

36. Haworth J C, McRae K N, Dilling L A 1976 Prognosis of infants of diabetic mothers in relation to neonatal hypoglycaemia. Developmental Medicine and Child Neurology 18: 471–479

37. Hawthorne G, Robson S, Ryall E A, Sen D, Roberts S H, Ward Platt M P 1997 Prospective population based survey of outcome of pregnancy in diabetic women: results of the Northern Diabetic Pregnancy Audit, 1994. British Medical Journal 315: 279–281

38. Hertel J, Kuhl C 1986 Metabolic adaptation during the neonatal period in infants of diabetic mothers. Acta Endocrinologica 277(suppl.): 136–140

39. Hod M, Rabinerson D, Kaplan B et al 1996 Perinatal complications following gestational diabetes mellitus how 'sweet' is ill? Acta Obstetricia et Gynecologica Scandinavica 75: 809–815

40. Horton W E Jr, Sadler T W 1983 Effects of maternal diabetes on early embryogenesis: alterations in morphogenesis produced by ketone body, beta-hydroxybutrate. Diabetes 32: 610–616

41. Hunter D J S 1992 Diabetes in pregnancy. In: Chalmers I, Enkin M, Keirse M J N C (eds) Effective care in pregnancy and childbirth. Oxford University Press, Oxford, pp 579–594

42. Kalhan S C, Savin S M, Adam P A F 1977 Attenuated glucose production rate in newborn infants of insulin dependent diabetic mothers. New England Journal of Medicine 296: 375–376

43. King C K, Tserng K, Kalhan S C 1982 Regulation of glucose production in newborn infants of diabetic mothers. Pediatric Research 16: 608–612

44. Knopp R H, Magee M S, Walden C E, Bonet B, Benedetti T J 1992 Prediction of infant birth weight by GDM screening tests. Importance of plasma triglyceride. Diabetes Care 15: 1605–1613

45. Knopp R H, Warth M R, Charles D et al 1986 Lipoprotein metabolism in pregnancy, fat transport to the fetus, and the effects of diabetes. Biology of the Neonate 50: 297–317

46. Komrower G M 1954 Blood sugar levels in babies born of diabetic mothers. Archives of Disease in Childhood 25: 28–33

47. Langer O, Levy J, Brustman C 1989 Glycemic control in gestational diabetes mellitus – how tight is tight enough: small for gestational age versus large for gestational age? American Journal of Obstetrics and Gynecology 161: 646–653

48. Like A, Orci L 1972 Embryogenesis of the human pancreatic islets. A light and electron microscopic study. Diabetes 21: 511–534

49. Mace S, Hirschfeld S S, Riggs T, Fanaroff A A, Merkatz I R 1979 Echocardiographic abnormalities in infants of diabetic mothers. Journal of Pediatrics 95: 1013–1019

50. Martinez M E, Catalan P, Lisbona A et al 1994 Serum osteocalcin concentrations in diabetic pregnant women and their newborns. Hormone and Metabolic Research 26: 338–342

51. McMahon J N, Berry P J, Joffe H S 1990 Fatal hypertrophic cardiomyopathy in an infant of a diabetic mother. Pediatric Cardiology 11: 211–212

52. Mello G, Parretti E, Mecacci F et al 2000 What degree of maternal metabolic control in women with type 2 diabetes is associated with normal body size and proportions in full term infants? Diabetes Care 23: 1494–1498

53. Miller H C, Johnson R D, Durlacher S H 1944 A comparison of newborn infants with erythroblastosis fetalis with those born to diabetic mothers. Journal of Pediatrics 24: 603–615

54. Mills J L, Baker L, Goldman A S 1979 Malformations in infants of diabetic mothers occur before the seventh gestational week. Diabetes 28: 292–293

55. Milner R D G 1988 Endocrine control of fetal growth. In: Linblad B S (ed) Perinatal nutrition. Academic Press, New York, pp 45–62

56. Milner R D G, Wirdham P K, Tsanakas J 1981 Quantitative morphology of B, A, D and PP cells in infants of diabetic mothers. Diabetes 30: 271–274

57. Mimouni F, Miodovnik M, Siddiqi T A, Khoury J, Tsang R C 1988 Perinatal asphyxia in infants of insulin-dependent diabetic mothers. Journal of Pediatrics 113: 345–353

58. Mimouni F, Tsang R C, Hertzberg V S, Miodovnik M 1986 Polycythemia, hypomagnesemia and hypocalcemia in infants of diabetic mothers. American Journal of Diseases of Children 140: 798–800

59. Mimouni F, Tsang R C, Hertzberg V S, Neumann V, Ellis K 1989 Parathyroid hormone and calcitriol changes in normal and insulin dependent diabetic pregnancies. Obstetrics and Gynecology 74: 49–54

60. Miodovnik M, Mimouni F, Dignan P S J et al 1988 Major malformations in infants of IDDM women. Vasculopathy and early first-trimester poor glycemic control. Diabetes Care 11: 713–718

61. Molsted-Pedersen L, Pedersen J F 1985 Congenital malformations in diabetic pregnancies. Acta Paediatrica Scandinavica Supplement 320: 79–84

62. Molsted-Pedersen L, Tygstrup I, Pedersen J 1964 Congenital malformations in newborn infants of diabetic women. Lancet i: 1124–1126

63. Morrison J J, Rennie J M, Milton P J D 1995 Neonatal respiratory morbidity and timing of elective caesarean section at term. British Journal of Obstetrics and Gynaecology 102: 101–106

64. Naeye R L 1965 Infants of diabetic mothers: a quantitive, morphologic study. Pediatrics 35: 980–988

65. Nogee L, McMahan M, Whitsett J A 1988 Hyaline membrane disease and surfactant protein, SAP-35, in diabetes in pregnancy. American Journal of Perinatology 5: 374–377

66. Ornoy A, Ratzon N, Greenbaum C, Wolf A, Dulitzky M 2001 School-age children born to diabetic mothers and to mothers with gestational diabetes exhibit a high rate of inattention and fine gross motor impairment. Journal of Paediatric Endocrinology and Metabolism 14(suppl. 1): 681–689

67. Passarge E, Lenz W 1966 Syndrome of caudal regression in infants of diabetic mothers: observation of further cases. Pediatrics 37: 672–675

68. Patel D, Kalhan S 1992 Glycerol metabolism and triglyceride-fatty acid cycling in the human newborn: effect of maternal diabetes and intrauterine growth retardation. Pediatric Research 31: 52–58

69. Pedersen J 1954 Weight and length at birth of infants of diabetic mothers. Acta Endocrinologica 16: 330–341

70. Peevy K J, Landaw S A, Gross S J 1980 Hyperbilirubinemia in infants of diabetic mothers. Pediatrics 66: 417–419

71. Perrine S P, Greene M F, Lee P D K, Cohen R A, Faller D V 1986 Insulin stimulates cord blood erythroid progenitor growth: evidence for an aetiological role in neonatal polycythaemia. British Journal of Haematology 64: 503–511

72. Persson B, Gentz J 1984 Follow-up of children of insulin-dependent and gestational diabetic mothers. Neuropsychological outcome. Acta Paediatrica Scandinavica 73: 343–358

73. Peterec S M, Nichols K V, Dynia D W, Wilson C M, Cross I 1994 Butyrate modulates surfactant protein mRNA in fetal rat lung by altering mRNA transcription and stability. American Journal of Physiology 267: L9–L15

74. Petersen M B, Pedersen S A, Greisen G, Pedersen J F, Molsted-Pedersen L 1998 Early growth delay in diabetic pregnancy: relation to psychomotor development at age 4. British Medical Journal 296: 598–600

75. Philippart A J, Reed O J, Georgeson K E 1975 Neonatal small left colon syndrome: intramural not intraluminal obstruction. Journal of Pediatric Surgery 10: 733–739

76. Phillips A F, Dubin J W, Malty P J, Raye J R 1982 Antenatal hypoxaemia and hyperinsulinaemia in the chronically hyperglycaemic fetal lamb. Pediatric Research 16: 653–658

77. Reller M D, Kaplan S 1988 Hypertrophic cardiomyopathy in infants of diabetic mothers: an update. American Journal of Perinatology 5: 353–358

78. Rizzo T A, Dooley S L, Metzger B E, Cho N H, Ogata E S, Silverman B L 1995 Prenatal and perinatal influences on longterm psychomotor development in offspring of diabetic mothers. American Journal of Obstetrics and Gynecology 173: 1753–1758

79. Rizzo T A, Ogata E S, Dolley S L, Metzger B E, Cho N H 1994 Perinatal complications and cognitive development in 2 to 5-year-old children of diabetic mothers. American Journal of Obstetrics and Gynecology 171: 706–713

80. Roberts A B, Pattison N S 1990 Pregnancy in women with diabetes mellitus, twenty years experience: 1968-1987. New Zealand Medical Journal 103: 211–213

81. Roversi G D, Garguilo M, Nicolini U et al 1979 A new approach to the treatment of diabetic pregnant women. American Journal of Obstetrics and Gynecology 135: 567–576

82. Sadler T W, Hunter II E S, Wynn R E, Phillips L S 1989 Evidence for multifactorial origin of diabetes-induced embryopathies. Diabetes 38: 70–74

83. Sadler T W, Phillips L S, Balkan W, Goldstein S 1986 Somatostatin inhibitors from diabetic rat serum after birth and development of mouse embryos in culture. Diabetes 35: 861–865

84. Sardesai M G, Gray A A, McGrath M M, Ford S E 2001 Fatal hypertrophic cardiomyopathy in the fetus of a woman with diabetes. Obstetrics and Gynecology 98: 925–927

85. Sells C J, Robinson N M, Brown Z, Knopp R H 1994 Longterm developmental follow up of infants of diabetic mothers. Journal of Pediatrics 125: S9–S17

86. Silverman B L, Rizzo T A, Cho N H, Metzger B E 1998 Long-term effects of the intrauterine environment. The Northwestern University Diabetes in Pregnancy Center. Diabetes Care 21(suppl. 2): B142–B149

87. Smith B T, Giroud C J P, Robert M, Avery M E 1975 Insulin antagonism of cortisol action on lecithin synthesis by cultured fetal lung cells. Journal of Pediatrics 87: 953–955

88. Soltész G, Schultz K, Mestyan G, Horvath M 1978 Blood glucose and plasma free amino acid concentrations in infants of diabetic mothers. Pediatrics 61: 77–82

89. Stenninger E, Flink R, Eriksson B, Sahlen C 1998 Long-term neurological dysfunction and neonatal hypoglycaemia after diabetic pregnancy. Archives of Disease in Childhood. Fetal and Neonatal Edition 79: F174–F179

90. Stenninger E, Schollin J, Aman J 1997 Early postnatal hypoglycaemia in newborn infants of diabetic mothers. Acta Paediatrica 86: 1374–1376

91. Stevenson D K, Ostrander C R, Hopper A O, Cohen R S, Johnson J D 1981 Pulmonary excretion of carbon monoxide as an index of bilirubin production. II a. Evidence for possible delayed clearance of bilirubin in infants of diabetic mothers. Journal of Pediatrics 98: 822–824

92. Sussman I, Matschinsky F M 1988 Diabetes affects sorbitol and myoinositol levels of neuroectodermal tissue during embryogenesis in rats. Diabetes 37: 974–981

93. Tsang R C, Kleinman L I, Sutherland J M, Light J 1972 Hypocalcaemia in infants of diabetic mothers: studies in calcium, phosphorus and magnesium metabolism and parathormone responsiveness. Journal of Pediatrics 80: 384–395

94. Veille J-C, Sivakoff M, Hanson R, Fanaroff A A 1992 Interventricular septal thickness in fetuses of diabetic mothers. Obstetrics and Gynecology 79: 51–54

95. Vejtorp M, Pedersen F, Klebbe F G, Lund E 1977 Low concentration of plasma amino acids in newborn babies of diabetic mothers. Acta Paediatrica Scandinavica 66: 53–58

96. Vohr B R, Lipsitt L P, Oh W 1980 Somatic growth of children of diabetic mothers with reference to birth size. Journal of Pediatrics 97: 196–199

97. Warram J H, Krolewski A S, Gottlieb M S, Kahn C R 1984 Differences in risk of insulin dependent diabetes in offspring of diabetic mothers and diabetic fathers. New England Journal of Medicine 311: 149–152

98. Way G L, Wolfe R R, Eshaghpour E, Bender R L, Jafe R B, Ruttenberg H D 1979 The natural history of hypertrophic cardiomyopathy in infants of diabetic mothers. Journal of Pediatrics 95: 1020–1026

99. Whitelaw A 1977 Subcutaneous fat in newborn infants of diabetic mothers: an indication of quality of diabetic control. Lancet i: 15–18

100. Widness J A, Susa J B, Garcia J F et al 1981 Increased erythropoiesis and elevated erythropoietin in infants born to diabetic mothers and in hyperinsulinemic rhesus fetuses. Journal of Clinical Investigation 67: 637–642

CHAPTER 23

Multiple births

Elizabeth Bryan

As multiple births are increasingly large contributors to the preterm and low-birthweight population, a special chapter on multiple births is justified by the disproportionate number of problems they present for the neonatologist.

Twinning rates

Estimates of the incidence of twins are hampered by the unknown number of abortions and early fetal deaths that occur in multiple pregnancies. Ultrasound studies in early pregnancy frequently reveal the death and later reabsorption of one fetus in the first trimester – the vanishing twin syndrome.[50,72] Thus the prevalence of twins at a certain time is all that can be accurately estimated.

Furthermore, some multiple births may not be recorded if a pair, one stillborn and one liveborn, are delivered before 24 weeks' gestation. The stillborn would be registered as an abortion and the liveborn would thus appear in the records as a single birth.

Following a fall in the multiple birth rate, the incidence has been steadily increasing in all developed countries since the early 1980s.[43,47] In England and Wales it has risen from 9.0/1000 births in 1980 to 14.8/1000 in 2001 (Fig. 23.1). The incidence of triplets rose much faster still until 1998, quadrupling in 15 years. It has now started to decline again[69] (Fig. 23.2).

The increase in multiple births is largely due to the widespread use of poorly monitored ovulation induction and to multiple embryo transfer in the treatment of subfertility[55] but is also due to the rise in average maternal age.[47] The most recent figures from the UK's Human Fertilisation and Embryology Authority reported 26.7% of multiple births following in-vitro fertilisation, of which 1.7% were triplets. With donor insemination, 6.7% were multiple births.[41]

Dizygotic (DZ), and therefore overall, twinning rates vary greatly in different parts of the world. In general, black Africans have the highest rates; the Far-Eastern, mongolian, races the lowest; the rates for Asian Indians and Caucasians lie between these. The prevalence of monozygotic (MZ) twin births had been constant worldwide at 3.5/1000 maternities until recently. A small increase in the MZ twinning rate has been noted since the 1980s.[2]

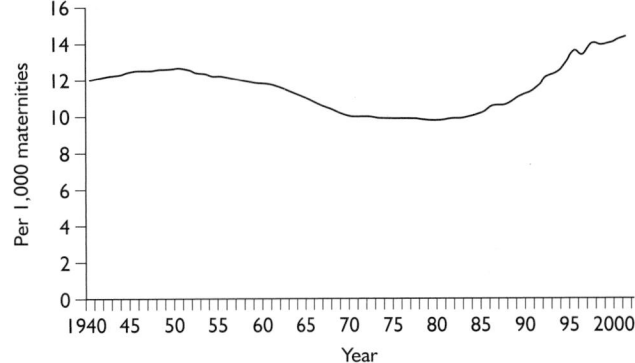

Fig. 23.1 Twinning rate in England and Wales 1940–2001.

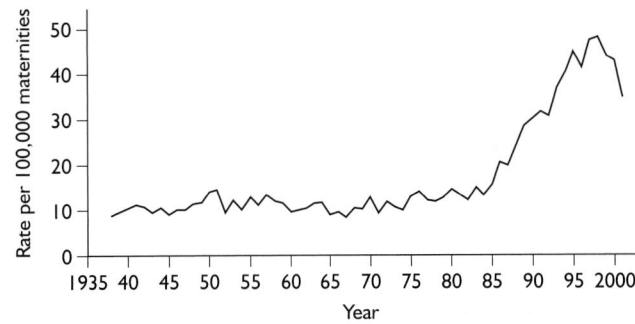

Fig. 23.2 Triplet rate in England and Wales 1938–2001.

Types of twins

Dizygotic twins arise when two ova are released and fertilised in one menstrual cycle, whereas MZ twins arise when one ova is fertilised and the resulting zygote divides into two. The ratio of MZ to DZ twins varies in different populations. In the UK approximately two-thirds are DZ, so in all, about one-third of the pairs will be of unlike sex, one-third both girls, and one-third both boys.

There are no known factors affecting the rate of MZ twinning, although MZ splitting appears to be 6–12 times more common following ovulation stimulation, whether or not fertilisation took place in vitro.[10,25] There also appear to be some extremely

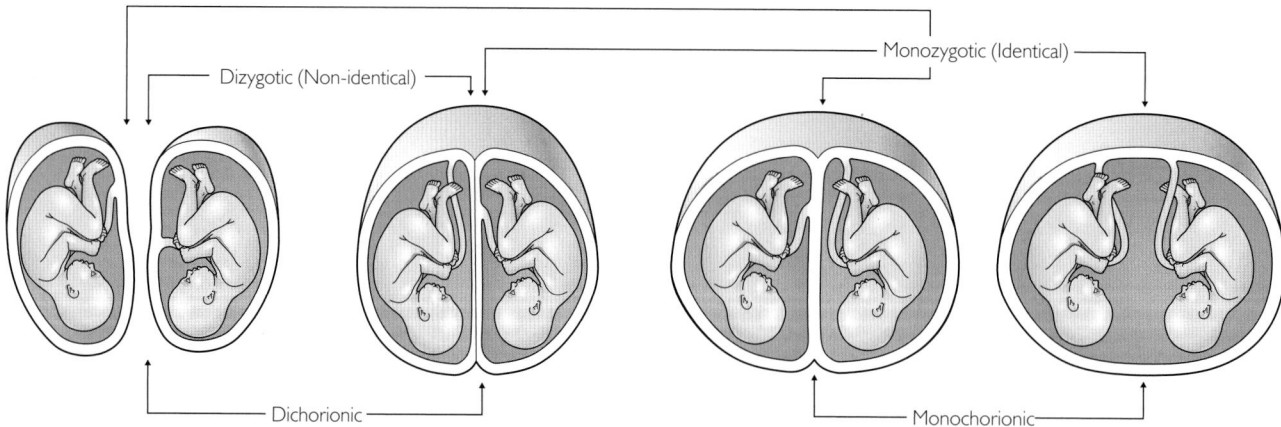

Fig. 23.3 Relationship between zygosity and chorionicity. (With permission from Multiple Births Foundation 1997 Are they identical? Zygosity determination for twins, triplets and more. MBF, London.)

rare examples of MZ twinning occurring as an autosomal dominant.[78] DZ twinning is known to be affected by a number of factors in addition to race, many of which appear to be related to differing maternal gonadotrophin levels. There are definite maternal genetic determinants but there is still uncertainty about paternal ones, if any. The rates are known to increase with maternal age, height, parity and frequency of intercourse.[57] Many other factors have been suggested but most are as yet unconfirmed.

Determination of zygosity

Zygosity determination should be part of the routine care of multiple pregnancies. Information on zygosity is of importance not only for epidemiological, genetic, obstetric and paediatric reasons but also because of the difference in prognosis between MZ and DZ sets.[29] Furthermore, the parents themselves usually want to know about it, not least because their chances of having multiple births in future pregnancies will vary according to the zygosity. Too often, however, the zygosity is not considered during the pregnancy or even after birth so that invaluable information from the placenta is lost and blood samples become harder to collect.

The zygosity of approximately half of Caucasian twins can be determined during the pregnancy and confirmed at birth either because the infants are of different sex and therefore DZ or because ultrasonography reveals a monochorionic placenta, thus conclusively demonstrating monozygosity. Very, very rarely DZ twins can have a monochorionic placenta.[80] In MZ twins whose zygote division occurs within the first 4 days or so of fertilisation, the resulting two placental discs (separate or fused) and therefore two chorions (Fig. 23.3) are indistinguishable from those of DZ twins. Nevertheless, many parents are still mistakenly told that their children are DZ on the evidence of a dichorionic placenta.

Like-sex DZ twins can only be distinguished reliably from the one-third of MZ twins who have dichorionic placentas by DNA analysis. The minisatellite probe test is a highly reliable tool[39] requiring only small quantities of blood or other tissues. Tests are

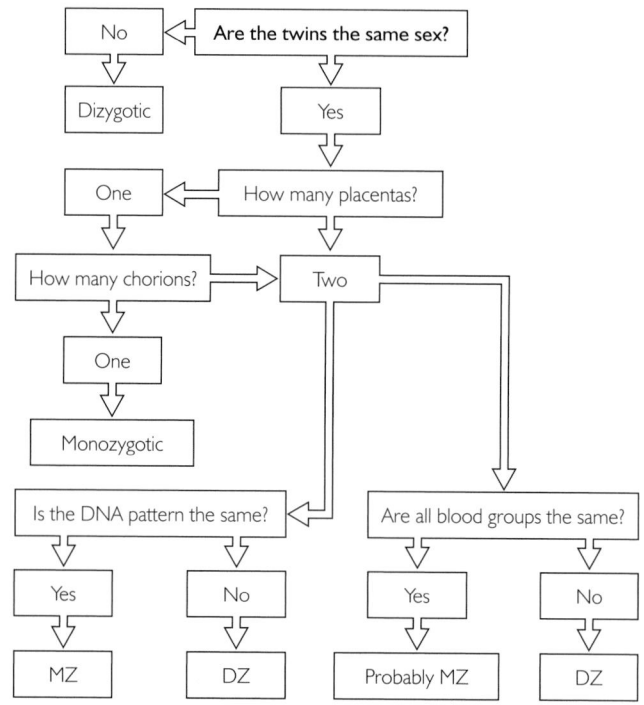

Fig. 23.4 Flow chart for determining zygosity.

most practically done on placental samples at delivery or on cheek swabs taken from infants or children. Cord blood is frequently used but great care is required to avoid contamination with maternal blood. Blood groups or other genetic markers such as red cell enzymes, serum proteins and tissue enzymes (in particular from the placenta) have all been used for determining zygosity but DNA analysis has now become the standard method. The steps to determine zygosity in newborn twins are shown in Fig. 23.4.[66]

Fetal growth

The growth and development of the twin fetus is affected not only by the same intrauterine factors as the singleton fetus but by the interaction with the second fetus. At best it must compete for nutrition. At worst it may be severely, even lethally, damaged by the co-twin.[14]

Intrauterine growth rates differ between singletons and twins from about 26 weeks, with the divergences then increasing with increasing gestational age.[1,35,54,64] As with singletons, primiparous pairs grow more slowly than multiparous.[54] The typical pattern of intrauterine growth of twins is similar to that of a growth-retarded singleton in that the weight falls disproportionately more than the occipitofrontal circumference. Birthweight and OFC centile charts for English twins are now available.[17] Some 52% of twins and 92% of triplets are of low birthweight (<2500 g) compared with 6% of singletons, and as many as 10% of twins and 32% of triplets are of very low birthweight (VLBW; <1500 g).[9] Indeed, twins and triplets contributed at least 35% of the VLBW infants in a recent population-based study.[9] The average weight of a newborn twin is about 800 g less than a singleton[54] but if allowance is made for differences in gestational age the discrepancy is reduced to 500 g. Opposite-sex twins tend to be heavier than like-sex twins[54] and boys than girls in both like- and opposite-sex pairs.[54] Dichorionic twins tend to be heavier than monochorionic[4] but DZ twins are heavier than both di- and monochorionic MZ twins.[22]

Intrapair discordance

Discordant growth refers to interfetal differences in birthweight between the large and small infant, expressed as a percentage of the large twin's weight: its defining value varies from 10–25% in different reports. Birthweight discordance may be due to the different sites of implantation of the two placentas or of the umbilical cords, but the commonest cause of large discrepancies in fetal growth is probably haemodynamic imbalance in the chronic form of twin–twin transfusion syndrome (TTTS; Fig. 23.5). Discordant size during the first half of gestation is likely to be associated with an intrinsic factor such as a malformation.[87]

Twin–twin transfusion in monochorionic pregnancies[86]

All monochorionic placentas have vascular anastomoses between the two fetal circulations: intertwin transfusion is therefore a normal event. It is only when this transfusion becomes unbalanced that problems arise.

Acute TTTS results from an acute haemodynamic imbalance across the superficial arterioarterial or venovenous anastomoses. It most commonly occurs during labour and may cause severe hypovolaemia in one twin and hypervolaemia in the other. An acute haemodynamic imbalance may also occur following the intrauterine death of one twin (see p. 405).

Chronic TTTS results from a haemodynamic imbalance in the parenchymatous arteriovenous network and there is a conspicuous absence of superficial anastomoses.[6] It complicates, to a varying degree, up to a third of monochorionic pregnancies and is the cause of up to 20% of perinatal mortality in twins. In the past,

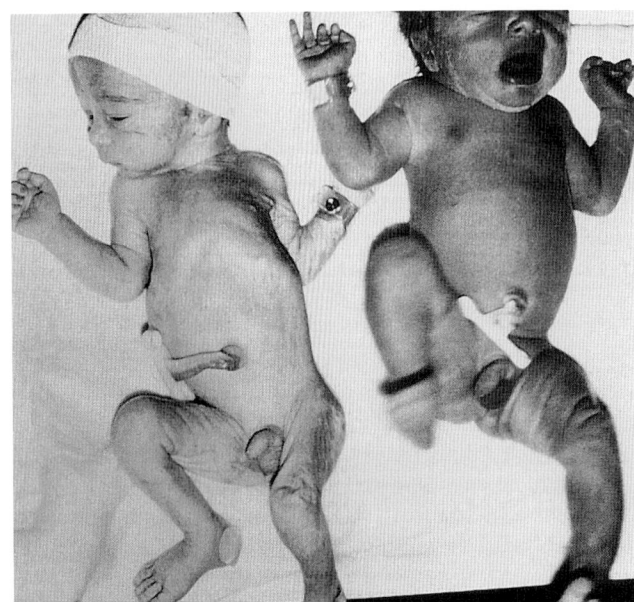

Fig. 23.5 The fetofetal transfusion syndrome, showing intrauterine growth retardation and pallor of the donor (weight 1.6 kg, haemoglobin (Hb) 7.9 g/100 ml) and plethora of the recipient (weight 2.7 kg, Hb 21 g/100 ml).

the diagnosis was made on the neonatal criteria of an intrapair cord blood haemoglobin difference of 5 g/l and birthweight discrepancy. It is now recognised that, in the more severe cases, presenting in the second trimester, these differences are usually absent and the main problems for the recipient fetus are severe polyhydramnios, cardiac hypertrophy, tricuspid regurgitation, venous overload and hydrops and, for the donor, oligohydramnios sometimes resulting in a 'stuck' twin.[86] Changes in the renin–angiotensin system in response to hypovolaemia in the donor fetus may play a key role in the development of the syndrome.[59]

In the newborn, the recipient twin is characteristically heavier and polycythaemic and faces the complications of high blood viscosity, such as cardiac failure, hyperbilirubinaemia and intravascular thromboses, whereas the donor shows signs of intrauterine growth retardation, anaemia and hypoproteinaemia. Renal failure and/or renal tubular dysgenesis due to chronic renal hypoperfusion in utero may also occur.[48] When anaemia is the presenting feature, care must be taken to distinguish from other causes of anaemia such as fetomaternal haemorrhage.

Prenatal treatment has included repeated amniocenteses, laser ablation of anastomoses, amniotic septostomy, selective feticide and transfusion of the donor with exsanguination of the recipient,[86] with amnioreduction resulting in higher survival rates than laser ablation in the less severe cases, whereas laser ablation appears to be more successful than amnioreduction in the most severe.

Postnatally, the treatment of the polycythaemic or anaemic twin is similar to singletons with the same problems (Ch. 30). In addition, the recipient may have short- and long-term cardiovascular problems.[46] Right ventricular outflow obstruction may become severe enough to require valvotomy in infancy.

There is a relatively high risk of brain damage, often due to periventricular leukomalacia, in TTTS whether or not the donor twin dies, although the risk is undoubtedly increased when there is intrauterine death of one twin.

The Australian and New Zealand TTTS registry logged 112 cases between 1995 and 1998. Fully 27% of all the babies had abnormal cranial ultrasound scans, with 10% developing periventricular leukomalacia.[26] Cincotta et al[20] reported periventricular leukomalacia in 17% of TTTS babies in a series of 17 pregnancies, of which five had intrauterine death of one twin. The International Amnioreduction Registry reported on outcomes of 223 twin sets with TTTS diagnosed before 28 weeks gestation and treated by aggressive amniodrainage between 1990 and 1998.[61] The likelihood of cranial ultrasound scan abnormalities increased with the haemoglobin difference between the twins; 24% of the recipients and 25% of the donors had major abnormalities. Haverkamp et al[37] describe a higher incidence of periventricular leukomalacia in the recipient twin (5/19) than the donor (0/21). Only 18/40 twins afflicted with TTTS during intrauterine life in this series were completely normal at neurodevelopmental follow-up.

Monoamniotic twins

Monoamniotic (MA) twins arise in MZ twins when the splitting of the single zygote is delayed until the end of the second week after fertilisation. Monoamnionicity can be established after 6 weeks by the presence of a single yolk sac and the lack of an intertwin septum. Monoamniotic twins account for approximately 1% of MZ twin pregnancies. Earlier studies have reported perinatal mortality rates as high as 30–70%[3] but in cases diagnosed during the second trimester the mortality rate is probably much lower – about 10%. Nevertheless, monoamniotic twins represent a serious and shared challenge to obstetricians and neonatologists in balancing the risk of intrauterine death against the complications associated with preterm delivery. The primary cause of fetal death is cord compression as a result of cord entanglement.

There have been no randomised trials on the management of monoamniotic pregnancies but a review of the literature[3] and personal communications reveal various empirical protocols employed to reduce the risk of cord compression. (It is unlikely that cord entanglement per se can be prevented as it not uncommonly occurs during the first trimester.) Protocols include planned caesarean delivery, with or without prophylactic corticosteroids, at a certain gestation (30–34 weeks). Some centres recommend continuous monitoring in hospital from 25 weeks. Recently, efforts to reduce amniotic fluid volume, and therefore fetal movements and the associated risk of compression of entangled cords, have been attempted by medical treatments such as sulindac or indometacin (indomethacin). Superficial vascular anastomoses are common in MA pregnancies[5] and TTTS is rare.

Congenital anomalies

In most, though not all, studies a higher prevalence of anomalies has been found among multiple births as compared with singletons.[53] Factors that may cause this apparent variation include the gestational criterion used for defining stillbirth, the range of anomalies studied, opportunities for and thoroughness of examination, twinship itself, maternal age and zygosity distribution.

The increase is limited to MZ twins.[21] Concordance rates vary considerably by type of anomaly but in general discordance is more common even among MZ twins.[53] The less favourable environment of a monochorial placentation accounts for some, but not all, of the increase seen in MZ.[21,62]

Congenital anomalies in twins pose additional dilemmas. Not only may some conditions be treated antenatally but the possibility of selective feticide, when one twin has an irremediable anomaly, provides a new and difficult choice for both obstetricians and parents.[13]

Anomalies unique to multiple conception

Anomalies unique to the twinning process include conjoined twinning, fetus in fetu, acardia and fetus papyraceus.

Conjoined twinning

Conjoined twins occurs in approximately 1/50 000 pregnancies.[90] They are a form of MZ twinning in which the division of the zygote is incomplete. The increased incidence of additional unrelated malformations suggests that conjoined twinning may be associated with a fundamental disturbance of embryogenesis.[28]

There are no known predisposing factors to conjoined twinning but it is more common in females.[7,63,90] There is an increased frequency among triplet sets[76] and in parts of Africa.[90] Seasonal clustering has also been reported.[63]

The site and extent of the fusion is highly variable. Thoracopagus is the commonest form and accounts for about 70% of cases.[28,75]

Inevitably ethical dilemmas arise with conjoined twins, particularly when surgical separation means that the life of one is likely to be at the expense of the other.[73]

Twin reversed arterial perfusion

Twin reversed arterial perfusion (TRAP), previously known as acardia or chorioangiopagus parasiticus, occurs in about 1/30 000–35 000 deliveries.[34] It varies in its manifestations from a mass of amorphous tissues to an incomplete but otherwise well-formed fetus. An imbalance in the interfetal circulation resulting in atrophy of the heart or a primary failure of cardiac development have both been suggested as the aetiological mechanisms.

As survival of the acardiac fetus is dependent on a shared circulation with the (usually normal) co-twin, TRAP occurs only in monochorionic, and therefore MZ, pregnancies. However, in one instance, a triploid twin acardiac with a 70 XXX + 15 karyotype was delivered with a co-twin with a normal male karyotype and a monochorionic placenta.[8] This sex discordance may be due to polar body twinning.

The male:female ratio in TRAP twins is lower than in twins in general.[45] The mean maternal age is high[31] consistent with the finding that some acardiacs are trisomic.[77]

Relatively little attention has been paid to the pump twin. They appear to have a surprisingly high incidence of malformations[76] but, even when potentially normal, these babies have a high mortality rate of up to 50%, usually as a result of the combination of intrauterine cardiac failure and prematurity.[84] The size of the acardiac twin relative to the pump twin appears to strongly influence the perinatal outcome, with a significantly higher rate of prematurity and therefore mortality among those with a higher birthweight ratio.[65] Their perinatal management should be greatly improved now that the problems can be foreseen by routine ultrasonic examination. Intrauterine treatment can be given for cardiac failure, and amniocentesis or indometacin (indomethacin) for polyhydramnios. Recently, various methods, including embolisation and laser coagulation, have been used to cause feticide of the acardiac twin.

Death of one fetus

The possible dangers of an intrauterine death to a surviving monochorionic twin are now well recognised. Many types of anomalies have been reported in the surviving twin[53] and the nature of these anomalies probably depends on the stage of gestation at which the co-twin dies.[40] Review of pooled data on 53 cases suggests that disruptions of the central nervous system are the most common complication (72%), followed by the gastro-intestinal system (19%), kidneys (15%) and lungs (8%).[82] Cardiac malformations have also been reported,[23] as have cases of aplasia cutis.[60] These diverse lesions are probably all the result of a damaging, if not lethal, hypoxic episode resulting from the severe transient hypotension that may occur as the vascular resistance falls in the dying fetus.[32]

Chromosomal anomalies

These are usually discordant in DZ twins and, surprisingly, also occasionally in MZ.[74] The twins are then known as heterokary-otypes and it is assumed that the maldistribution of chromosomes occurred at about the same time as the twinning process. Heterokaryotypes XY/XO are the explanation for the occasional pair of MZ twins of different sexes.[74]

Klinefelter's syndrome appears to be more common in twins and in their relatives.[79] There also appears to be an increased incidence of Turner's syndrome in twins[19] and of twinning among the (normal) family members of patients with Turner's syndrome.[67] Carothers et al[19] suggest that there may be a postzygotic mechanism common to twinning and X chromosome loss. Genotypic discordance in MZ twins may be caused by a variety of mechanisms.[36,58] X inactivation is likely to be the cause of some cases of discordancy for genetic disorders such as Duchenne's muscular dystrophy in MZ twins.

Some anomalies, such as oesophageal atresia[85] and some cardiac malformations,[18] occur more commonly in twins. Cardiac malformations are usually discordant in MZ twins, suggesting that the malformation develops as a result of some process peculiar to MZ twins. The TTTS syndrome is responsible for some cardiac anomalies in recipient twins (see pp. 152–3) but it has also been suggested that a disturbance in laterality may be the cause in others.[18]

The teratogenic effects of both drugs and intrauterine infections may have intrapair differences in expression.[16] This may be because of a difference in fetal susceptibility. In other instances where the teratogenic effect of the drug is sharply limited, as in the case of thalidomide, the discordance could be due to the insult acting at the very beginning or end of the sensitive period. As DZ twins can be conceived several days apart, one embryo may be a few days retarded or accelerated in development and therefore escape unscathed.

Perinatal mortality

Perinatal mortality data for multiple births can be misleading. If a multiple birth occurs before 24 weeks gestation and includes both live births and dead fetuses, the fetal deaths are not registrable. Thus some very preterm multiples will be registered as singleton (or lower-order multiples). The reverse may also occur. If a dead fetus, including a fetus papyraceus, is delivered with a live birth after 24 weeks it should be registered as a stillbirth even if the intrauterine death occurred many weeks previously.

Although there has been a somewhat greater fall in perinatal mortality rates in twins than in singletons in recent years[71] and even more in triplets,[44,56] a striking difference remains. The perinatal mortality rate is over four times higher in twins and four to nine times higher in triplets. The main contributor to the high perinatal death toll in multiples is prematurity and for this reason twins have a relatively higher neonatal than intrauterine mortality compared to singletons. Nevertheless, the stillbirth rate in twins is three times that of singletons, with TTTS being a significant contributor to this. Following the fetal death of one MZ twin, the co-twin has a 20-fold risk of intrauterine death, as well as twice the chance of dying in the neonatal period.[88]

When adjusted for birthweight, however, twins fare better than singletons in the low-birthweight groups between 1000 and 2500 g.[27,71,88] This is presumably because of the greater gestational age of twins at any given weight. Only above 2500 g does the mortality rate become higher in twins.

Most, but not all, studies have shown the second-born baby to be at higher risk of death and morbidity. Boys fare worse than girls, regardless of zygosity. The highest perinatal mortality rate occurs in male–male pairs and in unlike-sex pairs the male is at a significant disadvantage. The mortality rate is higher in MZ than in DZ twins and a recent study showed that this increase is limited to monochorionic pairs.[55] The TTTS accounts for many of these; cord complications in monoamniotic twins and the higher incidence of lethal malformations such as acardia are further contributors to the death toll in monochorionic twins.

Twins conceived as a result of infertility treatment tend to be delivered earlier and to be of lower birthweight than spontaneously conceived twins[49] and babies from these pregnancies have a higher perinatal mortality rate than the spontaneously conceived.[42] The explanation is uncertain but the cause of the parental subfertility may be a contributory factor.

Perinatal bereavement

Parents who lose one twin face particular problems.[15,52] They have to experience the joy of a new baby and the tragedy of bereavement simultaneously. Because they still have a live infant their loss is usually greatly underestimated, if it is acknowledged at all.

The parents are too often discouraged from talking about their dead baby. Yet concentration on the healthy baby to the exclusion of the stillbirth or neonatal death may encourage the mother to idealise the dead child (her angel baby) and hence alienate her from the survivor, especially if the surviving twin is difficult to handle because of illness or disturbed behaviour.

The pride involved in expecting twins is enormous, and failure is therefore deeply felt. Mothers inevitably feel shame and often some guilt. This guilt may be increased by any implication from friends or medical staff that the death was all for the best, even if logically this may seem so. Twinship is also important to the survivor and this continues into adulthood. This has implications for the care of the surviving twin and his parents from birth onwards.[89]

Some parents have difficulty in distinguishing the two babies in their own minds. Some may feel that the dead one never existed – a fantasy baby. Substantive mementos, such as photographs or even an ultrasound scan showing the two babies together, can help to clear the emotional confusion. Naming the dead baby not only helps to distinguish the babies but later makes it much easier to talk to the survivor (who should always be told) about his twin.

Blood or placental samples should always be taken for zygosity determination. Even if one baby dies, parents usually want to know whether or not their twins were identical. The zygosity may also be important for reliable genetic counselling about congenital anomalies and the chances of further twin conceptions.

Where both babies are born alive but one baby is likely to die, the family should be encouraged to spend extra time with this one so that precious memories can be created and the parents may later find comfort in knowing that they gave this baby as much love and care as they could. A photograph of the two babies (together with their parents if they so wish) should be taken as quickly as possible.

If a twin is born dead before 24 completed weeks of the pregnancy (a miscarriage) and a sibling is liveborn, the legal paradox and ambiguity add to the parents' difficulties.

Most, if not all, mothers continue to think of their surviving child as a twin even if the other baby was stillborn. Many parents welcome the opportunity to reminisce about their lost baby, particularly with the medical staff, who may be the only people who knew him. Many years later they still appreciate an enquiry about their feelings towards the dead baby and any concerns about the survivor's feelings about his dead twin.

An increasing number of parents are likely to face bereavement through choosing to lose a malformed twin fetus through selective feticide. Their grief can be powerful but may be delayed until the delivery of the healthy baby. It is important that the fetus is respected and its loss recognised.[13]

Parents' responses to the loss of normal fetuses in a multifetal pregnancy reduction vary.[12] Some are just relieved to have two (or one) healthy babies. Others will value support in coping with their guilt and grief over the death of one or more potentially healthy children. Some will not wish the subject to be mentioned, especially if they have not told their family.

Social

Parents of multiples need particular understanding. Few are prepared for the emotional as well as practical and financial stresses involved in caring for more than one baby at once.[11,33,81,83] They are often faced not only with the problem of caring for and relating to two babies at once but two babies each of whom is more difficult because of the prematurity, low birthweight and other neonatal problems already described. Furthermore, many twins will be separated from their mother on intensive care neonatal wards. It may be particularly difficult for the mother if the two babies are on different wards; she may well forget the baby in a distant incubator.

If one baby is much more demanding, mothers may feel guilty that they are unable to give their twins equal attention. They should be reassured that sometimes that baby may need more attention.

A mother's relationship with her babies will be further impeded if she finds it difficult to tell them apart. The babies should always be clearly identifiable and called by their names. The cot should be made recognisable at a distance so that the parents can start relating to the particular baby as they approach. Similarly, parents should be encouraged to dress the babies differently from the start despite pressure from friends and relatives. Twin names such as Joy and Jay or Robert and Roberta are also best avoided if the children's individuality is to be respected.

The long-term effects of early mother–twin relationships have yet to be established. Mothers of preterm twins have been found to show fewer initiatives and responses to their babies than mothers of preterm singletons and to be less responsive to both positive signals and to crying. They also had less physical contact with and talked less to them. At 18 months, the cognitive development of the twins was less advanced than that of the single-born controls and maternal behaviour in the newborn period was predictive of the level of development of the children at 18 months.[70]

One twin may be ready to go home before the other, but most units now try to discharge the babies together, otherwise the baby left behind may suffer in his relationship with his mother. Moreover, it has been shown that earlier discharge from hospital is the most important factor affecting the self-esteem of a school-age twin.[38] If discharge together is not practicable, because one baby needs a much longer stay, parents should be encouraged and helped to visit the remaining baby. Facilities for the healthy child to attend with the parents must always be provided.

Feeding

It is enormously important for a mother of twins to establish the easiest and most satisfactory feeding routine for both herself and her babies as soon as possible.[51] For far too many, the feeding of their twins is remembered as a period of frustration, exhaustion and failure. Many who planned to breastfeed have been bitterly disappointed.

For some, the advantages of bottlefeeding so that others can feed their babies outweigh other considerations. But any mother who would like to breastfeed should be given every encouragement and practical help. Most mothers can fully breastfeed two babies but they will need informed prenatal preparation,[30,51] including demonstrations by mothers, as well as a lot of help during the neonatal period. No mother should be expected to feed her newborn twins simultaneously without an attendant.

Whether the babies are fed together or separately is entirely up to the mother's preference and practicality. There have been no studies that compare milk production in the two methods. Many find it easier to feed separately initially until breastfeeding is well established.

Co-bedding

Many parents now choose to co-bed their twins in the neonatal period and early months. Preliminary studies suggest that the babies may have more settled sleep and more synchronous waking.[68] In preterm twins, more rapid weight gain and earlier discharge from hospital has been reported.[24] A recent study found that there was no significant increase in core temperature or lowering of oxygen saturation in co-bedded infants (Ball et al, personal communication). There is currently no evidence of an increase in sudden infant death syndrome in co-bedded twins and there is anecdotal evidence that such physical contact with each other can reduce the frequency of apnoeic episodes in some preterm pairs. Furthermore, babies in one cot have the advantage of being more likely to remain longer in the parents' bedroom.

References

1. Alexander G R, Kogan M, Martin J, Papiernik E 1998 What are the fetal growth patterns of singletons, twins and triplets in the United States? Clinical Obstetrics and Gynecology 41: 114–125
2. Allen G, Parisi P 1990 Trends in monozygotic and dizygotic twinning rates by maternal age and parity. Further analysis of Italian data, 1949–1985, and rediscussion of US data, 1964–1985. Acta Geneticae Medicae et Gemellologiae 39: 317–328
3. Allen V M, Windrim R, Barrett J, Ohlsson A 2001 Management of monoamniotic twin pregnancies: a case series and systematic review of the literature. British Journal of Obstetrics and Gynaecology 108: 931–936
4. Ananth C V, Vintzileos A M, Shen-Schwarz S, Smulian J C, Lai W L 1998 Standards of birthweight in twin gestations stratified by placental chorionicity. Obstetrics and Gynecology 91: 917–924
5. Bajoria R 1998. Abundant vascular anastomoses in monoamniotic versus diamniotic monochorionic placentas. American Journal of Obstetrics and Gynaecology 179: 788–793
6. Bajoria R, Wigglesworth J, Fisk N 1995 Angioarchitecture of monochorionic placentas in relation to the twin twin transfusion syndrome. American Journal of Obstetrics and Gynecology 172: 856–863
7. Benirschke K, Kim C K 1973 Multiple pregnancy. New England Journal of Medicine 288: 1329–1336
8. Bieber F R, Nance W E, Morton C C et al 1981 Genetic studies of an acardiac monster: evidence of polar body twinning in man. Science 214: 775–777
9. Blickstein I 2002 Normal and abnormal growth in multiples. Seminars in Neonatology 7: 177–185
10. Blickstein I, Jones C, Keith L G 2003 Zygotic splitting rates following single embryo transfers in in-vitro fertilization. New England Journal of Medicine 348: 2366–2367
11. Botting B J, Macfarlane A J, Price F V (eds) 1990 Three four and more. A study of triplets and higher order births. HMSO, London
12. Bryan E 2002 Loss in higher multiple pregnancy and multifetal pregnancy reduction. Twin Research 5: 169–174
13. Bryan E 2004 Problems surrounding selective feticide. In: Abramsky L, Chapple J (eds) Prenatal diagnosis. The human side. London, Chapman & Hall
14. Bryan E M 1986 The intrauterine hazards of twins. Archives of Disease in Childhood 61: 1044–1045
15. Bryan E M 1995 Perinatal bereavement after the loss of a twin. In: Ward H, Whittle M (eds) Multiple pregnancy. RCOG Press, London, ch 19, pp 186–195
16. Bryan E M, Little J, Burn J 1987 Congenital anomalies in twins. Baillière's Clinical Obstetrics and Gynaecology 1: 697–721
17. Buckler J M H, Green M 1994 Birth weight and head circumference standards for English twins. Archives of Disease in Childhood 71: 516–521
18. Burn J, Corney G 1984 Congenital heart defects and twinning. Acta Geneticae Medicae et Gemellologiae 33: 61–69
19. Carothers A D, Frackiewicz A, deMey R et al 1980 A collaborative study of the aetiology of Turner syndrome. Annals of Human Genetics 43: 355–368
20. Cincotta R B, Gray P H, Phythian G, Rogers Y M, Chan F Y 2000 Long term outcome of twin – twin transfusion syndrome. Archives of Disease in Childhood. 83: F171–F176.
21. Corney G, MacGillivray I, Campbell D M, Thompson B, Little J 1983 Congenital anomalies in twins in Aberdeen and North-East Scotland. Acta Geneticae Medicae et Gemellologiae 28: 353–360
22. Corney G, Robson E B, Strong S J 1972 The effects of zygosity on the birthweight of twins. Annals of Human Genetics 36: 45–59
23. Daw E 1983 Fetus papyraceus – 11 cases. Postgraduate Medical Journal 59: 598–600
24. DellaPorta K, Aforismo D, Butler-O'Hara M 1998. Co-bedding of twins in the neonatal intensive care unit. Pediatric Nursing 24: 529–531
25. Derom R, Derom C, Vlietinck R. 2000 The risk of monozygotic twinning. In: Blickstein I, Keith L G.(eds) Iatrogenic multiple pregnancy. London, Parthenon Press, ch 2, pp 9–19.
26. Dickinson J E, Evans S F 2000. Obstetric and perinatal outcomes from the Australian and New Zealand twin – twin transfusion syndrome registry. American Journal of Obstetrics and Gynecology 182, 706–712.
27. Dunn A, Macfarlane A 1996 Recent trends in the incidence of multiple births and associated mortality in England and Wales. Archives of Disease in Childhood 75: F10–F19
28. Edmonds D E, Layde P M 1982 Conjoined twins in the United States 1970–1977. Teratology 25: 301–308
29. Fisk N, Bryan E 1993 Routine prenatal determination of chorionicity in multiple gestation: a plea to the obstetrician. British Journal of Obstetrics and Gynaecology 100: 975–977
30. Flidel-Rimon O, Shinwell E S 2002 Breast-feeding multiples. Seminars in Neonatology 7: 231–239
31. Frutiger P 1969 Zum Problem der Akardie. Acta Anatomica (Basle) 74: 505–531
32. Fusi L, McParland P, Fisk N, Nicolini U, Wigglesworth J. 1991 Acute twin–twin transfusion: a possible mechanism for brain-damaged survivors after intrauterine death of a monochorionic twins. Obstetrics and Gynecology 78: 517–520
33. Garel M, Salobir C, Blondel B 1997 Psychological consequences of having triplets: a 4-year follow-up study. Fertility and Sterility 67: 1162–1165
34. Gillim D L, Hendricks C H 1953 Holoacardius: review of the literature and a case report. Obstetrics and Gynecology 2: 647–653
35. Gliniania S V, Skjaerven R, Magnus P 2000 Birthweight percentiles by gestation age in multiple births – a population-based study of Norwegian twins and triplets. Acta Obstetricia et Gynecologica Scandinavica 79: 450–458
36. Gringras P, Chen W 2001 Mechanisms for differences in monozygous twins. Early Human Development 64: 105–117

37. Haverkamp F, Lex C, Hanisch C, Fahnenstich H, Zerres K 2001 Neurodevelopmental risks in twin-to-twin transfusion syndrome: preliminary findings. European Journal of Paediatric Neurology 5: 221–227

38. Hay D A, O'Brien P J 1987 Early influences on the school social adjustment of twins. Acta Geneticae Medicae Gemellologiae 36: 239–248

39. Hill A V S, Jeffreys A J 1985 Use of minisatellite DNA probes for determination of twin zygosity at birth. Lancet 2: 1394–1395

40. Hoyme H E, Higginbottom M C, Jones K L 1981 Vascular etiology of disruptive structural defects in monozygotic twins. Pediatrics 67: 288–291

41. Human Fertilisation and Embryology Authority 2002 The HFEA patients guide to infertility and IVF and the patients guide for DI. London HFEA

42. Hurst Y, Lancaster P 2001 Assisted conception in Australia and New Zealand 1999 and 2000 (Assisted Conception Series no 6). AIHW, Sydney

43. Imaizumi Y 1997 Trends of twinning rates in ten countries, 1972–1996. Acta Geneticae Medicae Gemellologiae 46: 209–218

44. Imaizumi Y 2003 Perinatal mortality in triplet births in Japan: time trends and factors influencing mortality. Twin Research 6: 1–6

45. James W H 1978 A note on the epidemiology of acardiac monsters. Teratology 16: 211–216

46. Karatza A A, Wolfenden J L, Taylor M J O, Wee L, Fisk N M, Gardiner H M 2002 The influence of twin–twin transfusion syndrome on fetal cardiovascular structure and function: prospective study of 136 monochorionic twins. Heart 88: 271–277

47. Kiely J L, Kiely M 2001 Epidemiological trends in multiple births in the United States, 1971–1998. Twin Research 3: 131–133

48. Kriegsmann J, Coerdt W, Kommoss F, Beetz R, Hallermann C, Muntefering H 2000 Renal tubular dysgenesis (RTD) – an important cause of the oligohydramnion-sequence. Report of 3 cases and review of the literature. Pathology, Research and Practice 196: 861–865

49. Lambalk C B, van Hooff M 2001 Natural versus induced twinning and pregnancy outcome: a Dutch nationwide survey of primiparous dizygotic twin deliveries. Fertility and Sterility 75: 731–736

50. Landy H J, Weiner S, Corson S L, Batzer F R, Bolognese R J 1986 The 'vanishing twin': ultrasonic assessment of fetal disappearance in the first trimester. American Journal of Obstetrics and Gynecology 155: 14–19

51. Leonard L G 2003 Breastfeeding rights of multiple birth families and guidelines for health professionals. Twin Research 6: 34–45

52. Lewis E, Bryan E M 1988 Management of perinatal loss of a twin. British Medical Journal 297: 1321–1323

53. Little J, Bryan E M 1988 Congenital anomalies in twins. In: MacGillivray I, Campbell D, Thompson B (eds) Twinning and twins. John Wiley, Chichester, pp 207–240

54. Liu Y C, Blair E 2002 Predicted birthweight for singletons and twins. Twin Research 5: 529–537

55. Loos R, Derom C, Vlietinck R, Derom R 1998 The East Flanders Prospective Twin Survey (Belgium): a population-based register. Twin Research 1: 167–175

56. MacFarlane A, Mogford M 2000 Characteristics of babies. In: Macfarlane A, Mogford M (eds) Birth counts. The Stationery Office, London, ch 6, pp 165–189

57. MacGillivray I, Samphier M, Little J 1988 Factors affecting twinning. In: MacGillivray I, Campbell D M, Thompson B (eds) Twinning and twins. John Wiley, Chichester, pp 67–93

58. Machin G A 1996 Some causes of genotypic and phenotypic discordance in monozygotic twin pairs. American Journal of Medical Genetics 61: 216–228

59. Mahieu-Caputo D, Muller F, Joly D et al 2001 Pathogenesis of twin–twin transfusion syndrome: the rennin – angiotensin system hypothesis. Fetal Diagnosis and Therapy 16: 241–244

60. Mannino F L, Jones K L, Benirschke K 1977 Congenital skin defects and fetus papyraceus. Journal of Pediatrics 91: 559–564

61. Mari G, Roberts A, Detti L et al 2001 Perinatal morbidity and mortality rates in severe twin–twin transfusion syndrome: results of the international amnioreduction registry. American Journal of Obstetrics and Gynecology 185: 708–715

62. Melnick M, Myrianthopoulos N C 1979 The effects of chorion type on normal and abnormal developmental variation in monozygous twins. American Journal of Medical Genetics 4: 147–156

63. Milham S 1966 Symmetrical conjoined twins: an analysis of the birth records of 22 sets. Journal of Pediatrics 69: 643–647

64. Min S J, Luke B, Gillespie B et al 2000 Birthweight references for twins. American Journal of Obstetrics and Gynecology 182: 1250–1257

65. Moore T R, Gale S, Benirschke K 1990 Perinatal outcome of forty-nine pregnancies complicated by acardiac twinning. American Journal of Obstetrics and Gynecology 163: 907–912

66. Multiple Births Foundation 1997 Are they identical? Zygosity determination for twins, triplets and more. MBF, London

67. Nielsen J, Dahl G 1976 Twins in the sibships and parental sibships of women with Turner's syndrome. Clinical Genetics 10: 93–96

68. Nyqvist K H, Lutes L M 1998 Co-bedding twins: a developmentally supportive care strategy. Journal of Obstetrics and Gynecology Neonatal Nursing 27: 450–456

69. Office of National Statistics 2001 Series DH3 no 32. ONS, London

70. Ostfeld B M, Smith R H, Hiatt M, Hegyi T 2000 Maternal behaviour toward premature twins: implications for development. Twin Research 3: 234–241

71. Parker J D, Schoendorf K C, Kiely J K 2001 A comparison of recent trends in infant mortality among twins and singletons. Paediatrics and Perinatal Epidemiology 15: 12–18

72. Pharoah P O D, Anand D, Platt M J, Briscoe L 2001 Epidemiology of the vanishing twins. Twin Research 4: 202

73. Reijal A-L R, Nazer H M, Abu-Osba Y K, Rifai A, Ahmed S 1992 Conjoined twins: medical, surgical and ethical challenges. Australia and New Zealand Journal of Surgery 62: 287–291

74. Riekhof P L, Horton W A, Harris D J, Schimke R N 1972 Monozygotic twins with the Turner syndrome. American Journal of Obstetrics and Gynecology 112: 59–61

75. Rudolph A J, Michaels J P, Nichols B L 1967 Obstetric management of conjoined twins. In: Bergsme D (ed) Conjoined twins. D Birth Defects Original Article Series III. National Foundation March of Dimes, New York

76. Schinzel A A G L, Smith D W, Miller J R 1979 Monozygotic twinning and structural defects. Journal of Pediatrics 95: 921–930

77. Scott J M, Ferguson-Smith M A 1973 Heterokaryotypic monozygotic twins and the acardiac monster. Journal of Obstetrics and Gynaecology of the British Commonwealth 80: 52–59

78. Segreti W D, Winter P M, Nance W E 1979 Familial studies of monozygotic twinning. In: Nance W E, Allens G, Parisi P (eds) Twin research. Biology and epidemiology. Allan R Liss, New York, pp 55–60

79. Soltan H C 1968 Genetic characteristics of families of XO and XXY patients, including evidence of source of X chromosomes in 7 aneuploid patients. Journal of Medical Genetics 5: 173–180

80. Souter V L, Kapur T P, Nyholt D R et al 2003 A report of dizygous monochorionic twins. New England Journal of Medicine 349: 154–158

81. Spillman J R 1992 A study of maternity provision in the UK in response to the needs of families who have a multiple birth. Acta Geneticae Medicae et Gemellologiae 41: 353–364

82. Szymonowicz W, Preston H, Yu V Y H 1986 The surviving monozygotic twin. Archives of Disease in Childhood 61: 454–458

83. Taylor E M, Emery J L 1988 Maternal stress, family and health care of twins. Children and Society 4: 351–366

84. Van Allen M I, Smith D W, Shepard T H 1983 Twin reversed arterial perfusion (TRAP) sequence: a study of 14 twin pregnancies with acardius. Seminars in Perinatology 7: 285–293

85. Van Staey M, De Bie S, Matton M T, De Roose J 1984 Familial congenital esophageal atresia. Personal case report and review of the literature. Human Genetics 66: 260–266

86. Wee L Y, Fisk N M 2002 The twin–twin transfusion syndrome. Seminars in Neonatology 7: 187–202

87. Weissman A, Achiron R, Lipitz S, Blickstein I, Mashiach S 1994 The first trimester growth-discordant twin: an ominous prenatal finding. Obstetrics and Gynecology 84: 110–11470

88. West C R, Adi Y, Pharoah P O D 1999 Fetal and infant death in mono- and di-zygotic twins in England and Wales 1982–91. Archives of Disease in Childhood Neonatal and Fetal Edition 80: F217–F220

89. Woodward J 1998 The lone twin. Understanding twin bereavement and loss. Free Association Books, London

90. Zake E Z N 1984 Case reports of 16 sets of conjoined twins from a Uganda hospital. Acta Geneticae Medicae Gemellologiae 33: 75–80

Further reading

Bryan E, Denton J, Hallett F 2001 Guidelines for professionals: multiple births and their impact on families. Multiple Births Foundation, London

CHAPTER 24

Pharmacology

Imti Choonara, John McIntyre, Sharon Conroy

Introduction

Medicines have made a significant contribution to reducing both mortality and morbidity in neonates. The benefits of antibiotics, analgesics, surfactant and anticonvulsants are discussed in detail in other sections of this textbook.

The practising neonatologist does not need to be an expert in clinical pharmacology. There are, however, advantages in understanding some basic facts regarding how neonates handle medicines and some of the practical problems associated with the administration of medicines to neonates of different weights and gestation.

History of drug toxicity in neonates

Some of the most important examples of drug toxicity in humans have occurred in newborn infants or the developing fetus. These cases illustrate the difference between neonates and adults in relation to drug absorption, distribution, metabolism and toxicity, as well as formulation issues (Table 24.1).

Table 24.1 Important examples of drug toxicity in the neonate

Year	Drug/Compound	Toxicity	Mechanism
1886	Aniline dye	Methaemoglobinaemia	Percutaneous absorption
1956	Sulphisoxazole	Kernicterus	Bilirubin displacement from plasma proteins
1959	Chloramphenicol	Grey baby syndrome	Impaired metabolism
1961	Thalidomide	Phocomelia	Fetal production of teratogenic metabolite
1982	Sodium chloride/water	Alcohol poisoning	Formulation
1984	Vitamin E	Coagulopathy, hepatic and renal failure	Formulation?
1998	Cisapride	Arrhythmia	Drug interaction

Percutaneous toxicity

One of the earliest recognised drug toxicities in humans was methaemoglobinaemia, due to the effects of aniline dye, which was reported in 1886! The dye had been used to stamp the name of the institution (Marylebone Workhouse) on nappies for newborn babies. Ten newborn infants developed cyanosis after percutaneous absorption of the dye. Several months later another outbreak was observed and the connection to the dye was noted.[11] Subsequently there have been other cases of newborn infants developing cyanosis following percutaneous absorption of aniline dye.

The absorption of compounds is enhanced by prolonged contact of a wet nappy with the perineum. The greater surface area to weight ratio of newborn infants in comparison to children and adults results in greater relative exposure of topical medicines/chemicals. Also the relative increase in the water content of the dermis and the thinner stratum corneum facilitates transcutaneous diffusion of small molecules. There have been other examples of percutaneous toxicity occurring in the newborn infant, including neurotoxicity in association with hexachlorophane and hypothyroidism following the use of topical iodine.[11]

Protein binding and sulphonamides

In 1956, Silverman and colleagues reported a difference in mortality rate and kernicterus among premature infants who received two different antibiotic regimens.[11] Neonates who received a combination of penicillin and sulphisoxazole had a significantly higher mortality than those who received oxytetracycline. It was almost 10 years before laboratory studies showed that the sulphonamide had displaced bilirubin from albumin by nature of its higher binding affinity. This marked increase in the free bilirubin concentration resulted in ill preterm neonates developing kernicterus. The mean plasma concentrations of total bilirubin were the same in both treatment groups and also in the babies who developed kernicterus. This unfortunate adverse drug reaction shows the importance of considering protein binding of drugs in the neonate. This is especially so in sick preterm infants where there are high plasma concentrations of bilirubin together with an impaired capacity to metabolise and excrete bilirubin due to the reduced activity of glucuronosyltransferase.

Impaired metabolism and chloramphenicol

In 1959, the grey baby syndrome was reported in association with the use of the antibiotic chloramphenicol. Newborn infants developed abdominal distension, vomiting, cyanosis, cardiovascular collapse, irregular respiration and eventually death.[11] The following year, pharmacokinetic studies showed that neonates were unable to metabolise chloramphenicol to the same extent as children and adults. This was due to impaired glucuronidation of chloramphenicol, and a halving of the dose of chloramphenicol prevented the development of the grey baby syndrome. Recognition of the limited capacity for drug metabolism in the neonate has led to more appropriate dosage regimens for other medicines.

Thalidomide and teratogenicity

Only 2 years after the death of several newborn infants in association with the use of chloramphenicol, a short letter to *The Lancet* reported the possible association between the administration of thalidomide, given as an antiemetic or sedative during pregnancy, and multiple congenital abnormalities in the newborn infant, in particular phocomelia.[43] Thalidomide was an exceptionally safe antiemetic when studied in healthy adult volunteers. Animal studies involving thalidomide in pregnant rats initially showed no evidence of teratogenicity. Careful retrospective analysis showed that the effect of thalidomide on the human fetus was time-specific (Table 24.2). Subsequent studies in rats showed that the species was sensitive but only at 12 days gestation. It is important to remember the difference between the human fetus and animal models and to be aware of the potential teratogenic effect of medicines that are otherwise exceptionally safe.

Thalidomide itself is not teratogenic. It is the metabolites of thalidomide, in particular the monocarboxylic and dicarboxylic

metabolites, that are teratogenic. These metabolites, however, do not cross over from maternal plasma into the fetus. Thalidomide itself crosses over into the fetus and is then metabolised to produce the toxic metabolites.[4] It is unfortunate that the fetus with limited capacity to metabolise medicines can, in this case, metabolise the drug with the subsequent formation of a potent teratogen.

Formulation problems

In the early 1980s there were two major tragedies involving premature infants that were thought to be related to the constituents of the medicinal products rather than the actual drug itself. Ten preterm infants who were receiving mechanical ventilation developed central nervous system depression with associated hypotonia, apnoea and seizures.[22] This was followed by a severe metabolic acidosis and multi-organ failure and was described as the gasping syndrome. These infants all had umbilical arterial catheters and were receiving multiple injections of heparinised bacteriostatic sodium chloride, used for flushing the catheters, and also medications reconstituted with bacteriostatic water. Both the sodium chloride and the water contained 0.9% benzylalcohol. The infants who died had significant levels of benzylalcohol in their serum.

The unit that described this inadvertent poisoning stopped using bacteriostatic saline and water and subsequently no further cases of the gasping syndrome were noted. The healthy adult can tolerate up to 30 ml of 0.9% benzylalcohol as a single dose (approximately 0.5 ml/kg). The newborn infants who developed the gasping syndrome were receiving between 20 and 50 times this amount on a daily basis.

In 1983, an intravenous (i.v.) form of vitamin E was marketed as a prevention for the retinopathy of prematurity. Seven months later, E-ferol was withdrawn from the market following the deaths of 38 infants who had received the drug.[48] The affected infants showed signs of hepatic, renal and haematopoietic toxicity. The exact mechanism of the toxicity is still not understood but it has been postulated that the emulsifiers used to solubilise vitamin E may have been responsible.

Cisapride and drug interactions

Cisapride has been used extensively in children and neonates for gastro-oesophageal reflux.[5] Serious cardiac arrhythmias, in particular ventricular tachycardia and fibrillation, have been reported in patients taking cisapride. Sudden death has been described, both in adults and in neonates. The efficacy of cisapride in the neonate is dealt with elsewhere within this textbook. The metabolism of cisapride is dependent upon CYP3A4 enzyme activity, which is reduced in the neonatal period and in particular in the preterm neonate. The risk of sudden death is considerably increased by the administration of medicines that inhibit CYP3A4, e.g. erythromycin.

Clinicians cannot be expected to remember all potentially significant drug interactions but they need to be aware that cisapride must not be prescribed alongside CYP3A4-inhibiting drugs such as erythromycin, clarithromycin, fluconazole, itraconazole

Table 24.2 Time course of thalidomide teratogenicity in humans

Days gestation on exposure	Effect
21–22	Absence of external ears and paralysis of central nerves
24–27	Phocomelia of arms
26–29	Phocomelia of legs
34–36	Hypoplastic thumbs and anorectal stenosis

or ketoconazole. More importantly, they need to be aware of the risk of drug interactions and ensure the involvement of paediatric/neonatal pharmacists in neonatal intensive care units (NICUs).

Licensing

The Medicines Act of 1968 requires that all medicines manufactured or marketed in the UK have been authorised by the Licensing Authority, the Medicines Control Agency. The aim is to ensure that medicines are examined for efficacy, safety and quality. The Medicines Act was introduced as a response to significant cases of drug toxicity that occurred in the late 1950s and early 1960s. Two of these involved the developing fetus (thalidomide) and the newborn infant (chloramphenicol). It is ironic that legislation that was introduced to protect all humans has failed to protect those who are at the greatest risk, i.e. newborn infants. This is despite the fact that tragedies in the newborn infant precipitated the legislation.

Unlicensed and off-label use

Unlicensed medicines involve modifications to a licensed medicine (e.g. tablets that are crushed and prepared into suspensions), using chemicals as medicines, the manufacture of formulations under a 'specials' licence and using medicines licensed in other countries. A particular problem in neonates and children is the off-label use of medicines. This includes the use of licensed medicines: at doses outside that stated in the product licence; for different indications; outside the licensed age range; and by an alternative route, e.g. the use of an i.v. formulation orally. Examples of off-label drug prescriptions in the newborn infant are given in Table 24.3.

In a UK study, over 50% of drug prescriptions on an NICU were off-label and 90% of babies received a drug that was either unlicensed or used in an off-label way.[12] Ten per cent of drug prescriptions were unlicensed. Studies in an NICU in the Netherlands showed a higher percentage of unlicensed use (62%) and this was associated with the preparation of specific formulations in the hospital pharmacy.[37] Such results do not imply that current prescribing is inappropriate but reflect the lack of scientific evidence and appropriate formulations for drug therapy in the neonate.

Table 24.3 Examples of off-label drug use

Off-label for	Example
Dose	Gentamicin
Age	Morphine
Route	Sodium chloride
Indication	Albumin

Risk

One purpose of the licensing system is to reduce the risk to patients of unexpected side effects. In children there is a greater risk associated with the use of unlicensed and off-label medicines.[54] This is not to say that clinicians should restrict themselves solely to the use of licensed products. However, the newborn infant deserves the same high standards in drug treatment expected by adults. This can only be achieved by the careful scientific study of clinically needed medicines in newborn infants in a controlled setting. Such clinical trials would not only provide evidence of efficacy but also dramatically reduce the number of deaths associated with the use of new medicines in a non-controlled manner. If there are deaths in a clinical trial, the investigators and regulatory authorities have a responsibility to review the reasons for any deaths at an early stage and to consider whether the experimental drug may be responsible.

Furthermore, licensing should provide appropriate formulations. Many ampoules of off-label drugs contain amounts such that 10-fold errors can occur with the use of a single vial, e.g. morphine.

Legislative changes

There have been major changes in legislation in the USA, where the 1997 Food and Drug Administration's Modernization Act (FDAMA) has resulted in an increase in clinical trials in children.[53] The FDAMA provides a substantial financial incentive for the pharmaceutical industry to study medicines in paediatric patients. The 1998 FDA Pediatric Rule obliges the pharmaceutical industry to consider whether a new drug would be of benefit to children or not. These legislative changes have resulted in significant numbers of clinical trials in children, but unfortunately has only had a minor impact on increasing clinical trials in neonates. Current legislation in the USA aims to improve this situation.

In Europe, discussions are taking place within the European Commission and Parliament regarding children and medicines. Legislation is likely to provide a similar financial incentive, in the form of a patent life extension, to encourage the pharmaceutical industry to study appropriate medicines in newborn infants. It is essential that any clinical trials in neonates relate to medicines that are likely to be of significant clinical benefit to neonates and are not simply studied to increase the considerable profits that can be obtained by such a patent extension.[36] Health professionals have a responsibility to ensure that neonates are beneficiaries of clinical trials.

Drug handling

Large variations in gestation, size and disease states, combined with rapid maturational changes, make optimising drug therapy in the neonatal period more challenging than at any other time. This section focuses on what the body might do to drugs, using specific examples relevant to clinical practice to illustrate key principles. An overview of the major components involved in drug handling is given in Figure 24.1.

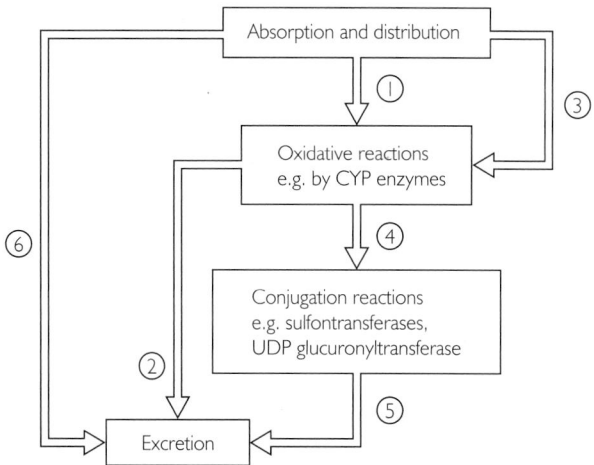

Fig. 24.1 Biotransformation of drugs. 1, Transformation of hydrophobic compounds to more soluble compounds by adding a functional group (oxygen, sulphur or carbon). The cytochrome P450 is the largest group of these enzymes. 2, Direct excretion via bile or urine. 3,4, The substrates are conjugated to increase their water solubility and excretion. 5, Excretion of the conjugated compound. 6, Some drugs are excreted unchanged in the urine or bile. (Adapted from de Wildt et al.[20])

Absorption

Many drugs in neonatal practice are administered i.v. and bypass the need for absorption. However, for drugs administered extravascularly, absorption is an important process, as the body compartment the drug is delivered to is usually separated from the intended site of action. Absorption characteristics are relevant to drugs given orally, intramuscularly, rectally or transcutaneously. In practice, oral administration is the only one commonly used, as the variability from the other sites is usually too great for predictable drug therapy.

Clinical implications

Absorption from the gastrointestinal tract will depend on the physicochemical properties of the drug and individual patient factors[8] and may be significantly different in newborns compared with older children and adults. Table 24.4 summarises the major factors likely to influence gastrointestinal absorption.

Gastric acid secretion can be extremely variable. In the immediate newborn period, gastric pH may be neutral. With increasing maturity and postnatal age, there is a decrease in intragastric pH.[38] There is a rapid fall within hours to between 1.5 and 3.5 in preterm and term infants. However, other factors such as feeds make it difficult to consistently maintain an acid pH in the neonatal period.

The gastric emptying time will affect the absorption time profile. Gut motility is influenced by gestational age, postnatal age and the type of feeding used.[9,49,58] Another variable that alters absorption is the colonisation of the gastrointestinal tract with microflora. This is influenced by maternal flora, type of feed and antibiotic use. The metabolic capacity of microflora may influence absorption of drugs, but the clinical importance of this is far from clear.

Table 24.4 Factors affecting drug absorption

Drug properties
Molecular weight
Lipid solubility
Degree of ionisation
Drug release characteristics
Drug-induced alterations in gut motility

Patient characteristics
Surface area available for absorption
pH of stomach and duodenum
Gastric emptying rate
Gastrointestinal microflora
Enzyme activity in gut wall
Gastrointestinal blood flow

Examples

The potential implications of varying gastric pH are that some acid-labile drugs, such as oral penicillin, may have enhanced absorption during a relative hypochlorhydric phase. Acidic drugs, such as phenobarbital, may have reduced absorption, due to their increased degree of ionisation in the more neutral environment.

Nevertheless, some drugs are given orally with good effect. Caffeine to treat apnoea of prematurity is often administered by an oral route, and effective, therapeutic concentrations of caffeine are achieved rapidly.[23]

Key message

Absorption of drugs given by the extravascular route will depend on the physiochemical properties of the drug and patient characteristics. Extreme variability in patient characteristics means extrapolating bioavailability data from adult studies is flawed. Theoretical considerations give little insight into the practical realities of how a drug will be absorbed in the newborn period. Furthermore, other issues such as administration difficulties, losses due to vomiting and spillage may be far more important determinants of drug effect than absorption characteristics. Oral administration cannot guarantee predictable drug delivery in the critical situation.

Drug distribution

In an optimum drug dosage regimen, a desired target concentration is achieved. This requires consideration of the distribution volume of the drug, usually referred to as the apparent volume of distribution (Vd). This is not a real physiological volume but relates the amount of drug in the body to the blood concentration. The distribution of the drug depends on:

- the size of the body water and fat compartments;
- protein-binding capacity;
- haemodynamic factors such as cardiac output and regional blood flow.

Clinical implications

The age-related changes in body compartments and protein binding are particularly relevant in the neonatal period (see also, fluid and electrolyte balance [pp. 335–54] and neonatal renal disease [pp. 935–40]). In adults, the total body water is 50–55% of bodyweight. In an extremely premature infant, total body water comprises approximately 92% of bodyweight and body fat comprises less than 1%. At term, the total body water is around 75% of bodyweight and the total amount of fat has increased to around 15%. The intracellular volume increases from 25% bodyweight in the preterm infant to around 33% at term. Selecting a drug dose is made more difficult by rapid postnatal changes. There is a rapid contraction in the extracellular volume shortly after birth, with interstitial fluid loss.[28]

For water-soluble and highly protein-bound drugs, the differences in body composition tend to result in Vd that are greater in newborns, especially preterms. Therefore, at equal doses per bodyweight, peak concentrations in blood will be lower (although mean concentration at steady state is unaffected by Vd). For drugs distributed mainly in the extracellular fluid space, the dose required on a milligram per kilogram basis would be significantly greater, because of the larger extracellular fluid compartment. However, for highly lipophilic drugs, very premature infants may have a reduced Vd.

Examples

Aminoglycosides, such as gentamicin, bind minimally to proteins and are mainly distributed in body water. Therefore, with increasing prematurity, the Vd is likely to be greater and would be a rationale for using a higher loading dose. The available data supports this. For gentamicin, the Vd range in preterm infants is 0.35–0.75 l/kg,[50,60] whereas values in older children merge with accepted adult values of 0.25–0.32 l/kg.[39]

By contrast, benzodiazepines are lipophilic and highly protein bound. The median Vd of midazolam in preterm neonates is 1.1 l/kg, which is similar to that seen in children or adults.[18] Recommended loading doses per bodyweight are similar in neonates and children.

Protein binding

The pharmacological effect of a drug is related to the unbound fraction in the blood. The degree of binding to plasma proteins is a major factor in determining drug distribution. The age-related quantitative and qualitative changes in plasma proteins are crucial to the likely clinical effects. Acidic and neutral drugs are largely bound to albumin, whereas basic drugs bind to albumin, α1-acid glycoprotein and lipoprotein.[8]

Clinical implications

With increasing prematurity, the total plasma protein and plasma albumin are lower[46] and the binding affinity less. The consequence is increased concentrations of unbound drug. Protein binding is also affected by endogenous substances, most notably bilirubin. Because of competitive binding, increased bilirubin levels may displace and therefore increase the free drug levels. Conversely,

Table 24.5 Protein binding of drugs

Drug	% bound to protein	Potential problem
Aspirin	95	Yes
Caffeine	25	No
Diazepam	75–90	Possible
Digoxin	16–30	No
Furosemide (frusemide)	95	Yes
Indometacin (indomethacin)	95	Yes
Penicillin	65	No
Phenobarbital (phenobarbitone)	20–35	No
Phenytoin	90	Yes
Theophylline	35–55	No

Table 24.6 Clinical relevance of protein binding

Potency of displacing property	Drug/Drug group
Very strong	X-ray contrast media
Moderate to strong	Indometacin (indomethacin) and other NSAIDs
Weak	Furosemide (frusemide)
Unlikely to displace	Antibiotics, antihistamines, opiates

certain drugs may displace bilirubin from albumin binding sites and so increase the risk of bilirubin toxicity. In practice, it is only when plasma protein binding is high (90% or more) that clinically important displacement of bilirubin will occur. Table 24.5 shows examples of where this may happen.

The in-vitro binding studies alert us to potential risks of drugs displacing bilirubin. The affinity for albumin binding by bilirubin exceeds the affinity for most drugs and the actual clinical risk is likely to be very small. Table 24.6 shows some areas of clinical relevance.

Examples

Phenytoin is a relatively insoluble weak acid that is extensively bound to plasma protein (around 90%). Developmental changes in protein binding would suggest a greater unbound fraction in the blood with increasing prematurity. Furthermore, clinically important displacement by bilirubin and from fluctuations in blood pH may also occur. In practice, predicting drug levels and therapeutic effect is fraught with difficulty, and, given the narrow therapeutic index, drug monitoring is required.

Key message

The neonate has a very different body composition and protein binding capacity. Rapid changes occur in the context of a unique set of circumstances for each individual, altering the Vd and protein binding. Predicting drug levels, both blood and tissue, is difficult, and standard pharmacokinetic data from adults are of little practical help.

Biotransformation

The process of removing the drug from the body is called clearance, and the total body clearance is a summation of all the clearance mechanisms involved. There are a number of pathways that can lead to the elimination of drugs from the body (see Fig. 24.1) but the two principal mechanisms in the newborn are the hepatic and renal pathways. The ontogeny of these clearance mechanisms is crucial to the pharmacological response of the newborn.[1]

For many drugs, elimination requires a chemical alteration of the drug molecule: biotransformation. Most drugs are lipophilic and a transformation to more water-soluble metabolites is a key step. Biotransformation reactions are conventionally grouped into two main types, phase 1 and phase 2 reactions. Phase 1 reactions, by adding or revealing a functional group (oxygen, sulphur or carbon), make a compound more water soluble. This may then be directly excreted or act as a substrate for the phase 2 reaction.

The primary organ for drug biotransformation is the liver, where a variety of enzymes are involved in modifying both endogenous and exogenous substances. Other organs such as the kidney, gut, lung and skin may also have some biotransforming capacity. These are probably of little clinical relevance.

Phase 1 reactions

Phase 1 reactions include oxidation, reduction, hydrolysis and hydroxylation reactions. Most of these are carried out by the hepatic cytochrome P-450 (CYP) oxidase system, involving haem-containing proteins. Recent reviews have addressed the nomenclature and clinical relevance to paediatrics.[1,20,29] The nomenclature for CYP uses a three-tier classification based on the genes: the family (at least 40% homology, e.g. CYP3), a subfamily (highly related genes, e.g. CYP3A) and the individual gene (e.g. CYP3A4). The isoforms of the 3A subfamily (CYP3A4, CYP3A5, CYP3A7) account for the majority of drug-metabolising enzymes. They are responsible for metabolism of about 50% of drugs.[1] Other enzymes involved in drug metabolism are shown in Table 24.7. The activity of most of these enzymes is significantly reduced in the neonate. The neonate compensates for reduced activity in the major pathways by utilising alternative pathways. Enzyme activity may increase rapidly after birth (CYP2D and CYP2E1) or slowly during infancy (CYP1A2).

Phase 2 reactions

In these reactions, excretion of the drug is enhanced by conjugation of endogenous molecules to drug substrate. The important reactions in the newborn are glucuronidation, sulphation, acetylation, glutathione conjugation, methylation and amino acid conjugation. Compared with phase 1 enzymes, the ontogeny of these phase 2 reactions is less well established.

Clinical implications

The rapidly changing balance of different phase 1 enzymes explains many of the noticeable differences in drug clearance during the newborn period. Each enzyme has an independent developmental pattern. Fetal CYP enzymes such as CYP3A7 decline rapidly

Table 24.7 Major cytochromes involved in drug metabolism

CYP	Activity in neonates	Drug substrates of the enzyme	Drug inhibitors of the enzyme
1A2	↓	Caffeine Theophylline	Amiodarone Cimetidine
2C9	↓	Ibuprofen Phenytoin	Amiodarone Fluconazole
2C19	↓	Diazepam	Cimetidine Indometacin (indomethacin)
2D6	↓?	Codeine Metoclopramide	Amiodarone Cimetidine Ranitidine
2E1	↓	Paracetamol	
3A4/7	↓ (3A4) ↑ (3A7)	Cisapride Erythromycin Fentanyl Lidocaine Midazolam	Amiodarone Cimetidine Ciprofloxacin Erythromycin

after birth and activities of neonatal ones such as CYP3A4 rise within a few weeks of birth and continue to do so in the first year.[20]

The clinical implications for changes in phase 2 enzymes are likely to be important because of their role in many of the reactions required for homeostasis, but ontogeny is less well described. However, there is evidence of unique maturational profiles relevant to clinical practice.

Glucuronidation is probably the most common pathway but is most deficient in the immediate neonatal period, and other conjugation pathways, such as sulphation, have to compensate. Methylation reactions are often insignificant in adults but may have a prominent role in the neonate. However, as a recent review of the glucuronosyl transferase (UGT) isoforms indicated, clinically useful generalisations are hard to make.[19]

Examples

Midazolam clearance reflects hepatic CYP3A, and in adults, clearance correlates with hepatic CYP3A4/5 activity. As the ontogeny of CYP3 activity would predict, plasma clearance is reduced in the newborn period, particularly the preterm infant. Pharmacokinetic studies show clearance rates of 1.8 ml/min/kg in preterm/term infants[18,34] compared with 3 ml/min/kg in infants, 9.2 ml/min/kg in children and 10 ml/min/kg in adults.[17]

CYP2C9 is primarily responsible for phenytoin biotransformation. The delay in appearance of active CYP2C9 activity could well explain the prolonged half-life in preterm infants of 75 hours, that rapidly declines in term infants to 20 hours and continues to decline in the first weeks of age to 8 hours.[42]

Theophylline is a CYP1A2 substrate. Clearance is low in the first few days after birth. CYP1A2 activity increases over the first 6 months of life. The clearance and metabolite pattern reaches

Table 24.8 Clearance and dose for paracetamol

Postconceptional age (weeks)	Clearance (ml/min/kg)	Suggested dose (mg/kg/day)
30	1.33	25
34	2.33	45
40	3.50	60
60	4.50	90

adult values by 55 weeks of age and is related mainly to post-conceptional age.

Paracetamol is metabolised in the liver by capacity-limited pathways of glucuronidation and sulphation (phase 2 reactions). These combined account for 82% and 68% of paracetamol metabolites excreted in the urine in adults and children, respectively. There are significant changes in the elimination pathway with increasing maturity. The sulphation pathway is relatively well developed compared to glucuronidation in the fetal/early neonatal period, as demonstrated by a low glucuronide to sulphate ratio in the preterm infant (0.1–0.2).[59] This changes over time to 0.3, 0.75, 1.6 and 1.8 in the term infant, young child, adolescent and adult, respectively.[41,44] The clearance increases with postconceptional age and therefore dose regimens that achieve a target concentration must be adapted accordingly (Table 24.8).[2]

Morphine is conjugated in the liver to morphine-3-glucuronide (M3G) and morphine-6-glucuronide (M6G). The analgesic properties are thought to come from morphine and M6G. Glucuronidation of morphine is reduced in premature infants and morphine clearance in the neonate (range 0.8 to 7.8 ml/min/kg) closely correlates with increasing postconceptional age.[51] As would be predicted, clearance in children (25 ml/min/kg) is considerably greater.[10]

Excretion

Most drugs or their metabolites are ultimately eliminated from the body via the kidney. Renal excretion depends on glomerular filtration, tubular reabsorption and tubular secretion. The dynamics of this system change with advancing maturity and postnatal age (see Chapter 36).

The elimination half-life ($t_{1/2}$) describes the disappearance of a drug from the blood and is the time taken for the concentration of a drug to fall by one half. It is helpful in determining drug dose intervals. Many drugs follow first-order kinetics and are eliminated by the kidneys in proportion to the glomerular filtration rate (GFR). Knowledge of the $t_{1/2}$ for the drug will then allow dose adjustment when renal function is impaired, a common problem in the neonatal period.

Clinical implications

The amount of drug filtered by the glomerulus depends on its functional capacity and the blood flow. The amount of drug–protein binding is also a determinant, as the amount of drug filtered is inversely related to the degree of protein binding.

During fetal life, GFR is low. It rises with increasing gestational age but is constant when corrected for fetal bodyweight. At birth, the GFR in preterm infants is 0.6–0.8 ml/min and in term infants 2–4 ml/min (pp. 929–30).[55–57] Increases in cardiac output, changes in vascular resistance that increase renal blood flow, and increased permeability of the glomerular membrane result in significant increases in GFR in the first few days of life. These changes occur in both term and preterm infants. The implication for many drugs in the immediate newborn period, particularly for preterm infants, is a longer $t_{1/2}$ and extended dosing interval. However, this then changes during the first week of life. Changes in serum creatinine after the first 48 hours of life may give an approximate measure of the newborn's GFR.[21]

Tubular reabsorption and secretory function may be functionally immature in the neonate. The rate of maturation is slower than for GFR. This is an additional modulator in renal elimination to consider for some drugs, such as penicillins, where tubular secretion is the main mechanism of excretion. Furthermore, concomitant drugs that alter renal function or maturation, such as indometacin (indomethacin), can also profoundly alter excretion.[56]

Examples

Vancomycin is eliminated by glomerular filtration and therefore gestational and postnatal age would be expected to affect the pharmacokinetics. The elimination $t_{1/2}$ in neonates ranges from 3.5 to 10 hours and there is a positive correlation with serum creatinine.[35] Dosage schedules based on bodyweight and serum creatinine have been shown to be clinically useful.[25] However, neonates rarely receive vancomycin in the first week of life when renal function is most likely to be impaired and a dosing regimen based on weight alone can be effective.[16] Furthermore, exposure to antenatal corticosteroids diminishes the gestational age-dependent difference in the renal excretion of antibiotics.[56]

Ceftazidime is also predominantly eliminated through glomerular filtration. With increasing gestational age and GFR, clearance increases and $t_{1/2}$ decreases; dosage recommendations should be based on gestational age and GFR.[57]

Key message

Renal function is crucial to clearance of a drug from the serum and elimination from the body. Gestational age and postnatal age are important determinants of renal function. Dosing schedules that allow for this are required, to achieve a therapeutic drug concentration.

Drug prescribing and administration

Safe and accurate drug prescribing and administration in the neonatal patient can present complex challenges. The risks involved can be minimised by applying common sense to prescribing practice. There is no point in prescribing doses based on bodyweight such that it is impractical to measure the dose from the drug formulations available. Additionally, this may increase the risk of medication errors. It is difficult to accurately measure volumes less than 0.05 ml even with a 1 ml syringe. This applies to both i.v. and oral drug therapy.

Prescribing protocols should be agreed by medical, pharmacy and nursing staff which include rounding up or down of doses to an acceptable number of whole numbers or decimal places, depending on the drug and the preparations available for administration.

Oral or nasogastric route of administration

The oral route of administration is an option for some drugs in a neonatal patient who is well enough to tolerate milk feeds. Absorption may be unreliable and unpredictable, however, due to changes in gastric emptying time or the lack of gastric acid production (see above). Liquid formulations of medicines are necessary for oral or nasogastric administration. They should not be mixed with milk or other feeds as interactions can occur with the feed, rendering the drug unavailable. Also the feed may not be completed and therefore all the dose will not be administered. Drugs may create an unpleasant taste in the milk, which may discourage the baby from feeding.

Certain liquid medicines contain excipients that have been added to enhance flavour and acceptability of the formulation, or to improve solubility of the drug or to stabilise the final product. These may be inappropriate for administration to a neonate. Examples include a commercially available preparation of phenobarbital elixir containing 38% alcohol (phenobarbital elixir BP) that is not recommended for the neonatal patient.

Liquid medicines should always be measured in an oral syringe in order to ensure accurate measurement. Hypodermic syringes should never be used for oral or nasogastric administration as they may result in inadvertent i.v. administration. This has been reported with nystatin oral suspension, digoxin oral liquid, crushed baclofen tablets suspended in water, paracetamol oral suspension and potassium chloride oral liquid.[13,14] Children were involved in several of these incidents and fortunately suffered no apparent harm. However, this has resulted in deaths in adult patients.[14] Hospitals should introduce and implement policies whereby oral medicines must be measured in dedicated oral syringes which are not compatible with i.v. access devices. Many liquid medicines can be administered down a nasogastric tube when necessary, provided that adequate care is taken to prevent blockage of the tube. All doses should be flushed through using sterile water. Ancillary connectors are available to allow oral syringes to be connected to nasogastric and gastrostomy tubes, avoiding the need to use i.v. syringes in these situations.

Topical

The skin of a neonate, especially if premature, offers an immature protective barrier to substances applied topically, particularly in the first week of life. The skin is well hydrated due to the high total body and extracellular fluid content in a newborn baby, and offers a large surface area for absorption in proportion to bodyweight. This has resulted in instances of drug toxicity (see

above). However, this route of absorption has also been exploited for therapeutic effect with drugs such as theophylline and caffeine for the treatment and prevention of neonatal apnoea.[6] This route of drug delivery may overcome the problems of oral or i.v. therapy but further work is necessary to develop reliable drug delivery systems.

Intravenous administration

Commercially available preparations are often in forms suitable for the administration of adult doses, not paediatric and neonatal doses. Many drugs need to be diluted before they can be given i.v. in neonates. Inappropriate excipients may be present; for example, phenobarbital elixir BP injection contains 80–90% w/v propylene glycol, which can cause hyperosmolality unless diluted. Injections presented as dry powders in vials for reconstitution are likely to have a displacement volume, which must be taken into account if the correct dose is to be drawn from the vial. An example is benzylpenicillin injection, where the powder in the injection vial occupies 0.4 ml when dissolved; hence, 4.6 ml should be added to the vial to give a concentration of 600 mg in 5 ml. This can make a significant difference when reconstituting a vial, from which a small proportion must be taken for the neonatal dose.

The hub of a syringe contains a 'dead space' that may be more than 0.1 ml.[40] Because of this, care must be taken in drawing up drugs requiring dilution. If the active drug is drawn up first, followed by the diluent, the syringe will contain around 0.1 ml extra of the concentrated drug solution. This may be clinically significant. It is therefore safer to draw up some of the diluent first into the syringe, add the required amount of drug solution from another syringe, and follow with the rest of the diluent to the required final volume.

If drugs are being given as a bolus into an i.v. infusion line, then they should be given at an access point as close to the patient as possible. If the infusion is running, then it is not normally necessary to flush the drug through with an extra bolus of a compatible solution, other than a small amount to clear the drug from the point of access. More than this is likely to result in the baby receiving significant volumes of extra fluid. In fluid-restricted babies, these flush volumes should be taken into account. Many drugs contain considerable amounts of sodium or potassium, e.g. benzylpenicillin injection contains 1.68 mmol of sodium per 600 mg vial. This needs to be considered in babies undergoing strict fluid balance and electrolyte monitoring, or babies with unexplained electrolyte disturbances.

With drugs required to reach the patient quickly, e.g. adenosine for supraventricular tachycardia (SVT), a flush will be needed to deliver the drug to the patient in the required timeframe. Otherwise it may take some time before the drug reaches the patient, especially if the infusion rate is low. Similarly with drugs undergoing monitoring, such as aminoglycoside antibiotics, it is important that the time the drug is delivered to the patient is known for results to be interpretable; hence a flush is advisable.

Central venous access should be used for irritant or inotropic drugs, and for administration of medicines over long periods of time. Aseptic technique is essential when using this route of administration. All i.v. drugs should be given slowly either as an infusion or as a bolus over 3–5 minutes (except for adrenaline in a cardiac arrest [p. 1276] and adenosine for SVT [pp. 151, 1276]).

Compatibilities of i.v. fluids must be known before drugs/fluids are allowed to mix together in i.v. circuits, if precipitation and formation of particles is to be avoided. These may be obvious – for example, flucloxacillin and gentamicin form a dense white precipitate when they come into contact with each other, which is likely to be sufficient to block a cannula. However, other interactions may be less obvious, but still result in emboli formation, with potentially serious complications in the baby. If in doubt, contact the pharmacist for information or advice on alternative methods of drug delivery.

If, due to lack of alternative access, a bolus drug must be given down a line delivering a continuous infusion, it is advisable to 'sandwich' the drug between bolus doses of a fluid known to be compatible with both drugs involved. Care must be taken not to bolus either the flush or the drug too quickly, as the baby is then likely to receive an unintended bolus of the main infusion drug, which for drugs such as morphine, midazolam, dopamine and dobutamine is undesirable (Table 24.9).

Entry sites should be carefully observed for signs of thrombophlebitis or 'tissuing'. They should not be bandaged in a manner that obscures a good view of the tissues surrounding the point of cannula entry. Extravasation of drugs can result in pain, oedema, irritation and even necrosis leading to permanent scarring (p. 92). Advice should be sought as to measures to minimise damage caused by extravasated drugs (pp. 1253–4). Guidelines should be available locally to deal with extravasation.

Use of in-line filters should be considered. Some of the available products are now appropriate for neonatal use as they are of low volume and therefore do not require large flush volumes to push drugs through them. Some of the available products have 0.2-micron filters and are capable of removing air, particulate matter, microbial contaminants and endotoxins, thus protecting the baby from the risk of emboli, thrombophlebitis and infection. Intravenous infusion lines may be left up for up to 96 hours when certain filters are included in the circuit. This saves nursing time and money from changing of infusion sets on a 24-, 48- or 72-hourly basis, as is the policy in most NICUs.[7]

Intramuscular

The intramuscular (i.m.) route of administration should be avoided if possible, as it is a painful route of administration, especially in the neonate who has very little muscle mass. It is also an unreliable route of drug administration, as absorption from the i.m. site can be slow and erratic. This is due to poor blood supply to the site, reduced muscular contractions and vasomotor instability which can result in an exaggerated vasoconstriction reflex, further reducing blood flow to the site.[6] The i.m. route should never be used if there is a bleeding problem, e.g. thrombocytopenia or in a patient on anticoagulants.

Rectal

This can be a useful route of administration for some drugs if the oral and i.v. routes are not available, though, in the neonate, absorption may be less complete and slower than if drugs are given orally or i.v.. Suppositories containing appropriate neonatal doses, however, are not always available. Suppositories are often cut in half or quarters. The drug content is not necessarily distributed evenly through the suppository and therefore the actual dose administered may differ from that intended. Consequently, this is a practice that should not be encouraged.

Drug interactions

Serious drug interactions are fortunately uncommon. They are preventable by the involvement of clinical pharmacists in reviewing drug prescription charts. Some of the major types of drug interactions and their mechanism are described below (Table 24.10).

Pharmacodynamic interactions

These occur when drugs given together have similar or antagonistic pharmacological effects or side effects. Such interactions are usually predictable from a knowledge of the pharmacology of both drugs and may be caused by competition at receptor sites or occur when both drugs act on the same physiological system.

Table 24.9 Administration of intravenous drugs

Administer the drug at an access point close to the patient
Be aware of the fluid volume and/or electrolytes administered with the drug and flush solutions
Give slowly over 3–5 minutes or as an infusion
Be aware of the danger of bolus and flushes into infusions containing maintenance drugs
Ensure that drugs and fluids are compatible before allowing them to mix together

Table 24.10 Major drug interactions

Drugs	Type of interaction	Effect
Midazolam + Morphine	Pharmacodynamic	Increased sedation
Indometacin (indomethacin) + Gentamicin	Renal excretion reduced	Increased risk of nephrotoxicity
Erythromycin + Cisapride	Enzyme inhibition	Decreased metabolism of cisapride → ↑ risk of toxicity
Erythromycin + Midazolam	Enzyme inhibition	Decreased metabolism of midazolam → ↑ sedation

An example is the co-prescribing of drugs with sedative side effects, many of which affect cerebral and respiratory function. When morphine and midazolam are administered together to provide analgesia and sedation for ventilation, the two drugs interact. Their similar adverse effect profile causes increased sedation (in this case the desired effect) and respiratory depression. However, they can be given safely together, provided that adequate monitoring of the patient is assured, appropriate respiratory support is available, and dose adjustment is performed in relation to the clinical response of the patient.

Pharmacokinetic interactions

If the administration of one drug changes the absorption, distribution, metabolism or excretion of another drug, resulting in increased or decreased amount of drug becoming available to produce an effect, then this is a pharmacokinetic interaction. They can be divided into several types.

Drug absorption interactions

The rate of absorption of a drug, or the total amount finally absorbed, may be altered by such an interaction. Delayed absorption is unlikely to be a major clinical problem, unless the drug involved requires a high peak plasma concentration to be rapidly achieved, e.g. a sedative or an analgesic agent. However, if the interaction results in a reduction in the total amount of drug absorbed, the result may actually be ineffective therapy.

An example is the concomitant administration of oral theophylline and erythromycin, resulting in sub-therapeutic levels of erythromycin with consequent lack of efficacy. The mechanism is unknown.

Protein-binding alterations

Most drugs are bound loosely to plasma proteins. Drugs can displace each other from such protein binding sites, and the displaced drug will therefore be available for effect or toxicity in its free form in the plasma. This is only likely to be significant if the drug is normally extensively protein bound, i.e. to an extent greater than 90%, and is not normally widely distributed throughout the body. In most patients, such displacement interactions rarely produce more than a short-lived effect. However, for the neonate with reduced renal and hepatic excretion, it may be relevant in a small number of drugs.

Enzyme induction

Many drugs are metabolised in the liver. Induction of the hepatic microsomal enzyme system by one drug may increase the rate of metabolism of another drug. This may result in lowered plasma concentrations of the second drug and potentially a reduced effect.

An example is the increase in the metabolism of corticosteroids such as dexamethasone by phenobarbital. This results in a reduction of the steroid plasma concentration and consequently reduced clinical effectiveness. The steroid dose will need to be increased to produce the desired clinical response.

Discontinuation of a drug known to induce hepatic enzymes may result in increased serum concentrations of a second drug, with toxicity as a result. Care must therefore be taken when discontinuing enzyme-inducing agents, as dose reduction of interacting drugs may be necessary. Phenobarbital, phenytoin, carbamazepine and rifampicin are examples of important enzyme-inducing agents.

Enzyme inhibition

Drugs that inhibit hepatic microsomal enzymes may result in reduced metabolism of other drugs and therefore raised serum concentrations, with potential for increased effect and toxicity. These are usually the most dangerous type of drug interactions. Erythromycin, cimetidine, ciprofloxacin and fluconazole are examples of common enzyme inhibitors.

An important example is the use of erythromycin and midazolam together. Erythromycin inhibits the metabolism of midazolam, resulting in markedly increased plasma midazolam concentrations with accompanying profound sedation.[31] Dose reductions are necessary to avoid toxicity and may need to be of the order of 50–75%.

Cimetidine inhibits the metabolism of phenytoin, with a resulting increase in plasma concentrations of the anticonvulsant and the potential for toxicity. Metronidazole may also have the same effect on phenytoin levels in some patients. It is necessary to monitor the phenytoin levels carefully and make careful dose adjustments as needed.

Ciprofloxacin inhibits the metabolism of caffeine/theophylline and again may predispose to toxicity.[47]

Renal excretion

Many drugs are renally excreted through glomerular filtration and active tubular secretion. Some drugs are actively transported across the kidney tubules and competition for such active transport mechanisms may occur. This can result in delayed excretion of competing drugs. Similarly, the concomitant administration of indometacin and aminoglycoside antibiotics, such as gentamicin, may result in drug toxicity. Indometacin reduces glomerular filtration in the kidney, the main route of elimination for these antibiotics. This may result in retention of the antibiotic, with consequential high levels and the potential for both renal toxicity and ototoxicity.

Drug therapy for the fetus

Improved diagnostic methods during pregnancy have led to the development of drug interventions for fetal disorders diagnosed in utero.

Corticosteroid administration in preterm labour

An example frequently seen is the use of corticosteroid therapy in mothers threatening preterm labour. The Cochrane review by

Crowley, in 2002, of trials using corticosteroid drugs for women expected to deliver prematurely, showed administration between 48 hours and 7 days pre-delivery significantly reduced respiratory distress syndrome and its sequelae.[15] Weekly courses do not confer a benefit over a single course.[27]

Antiarrhythmic agents in fetal tachycardia

Intrauterine development of sustained fetal tachycardia and congestive heart failure is a life-threatening condition requiring urgent treatment. Treatment of the fetal arrhythmias by giving drugs to the mother can be successful (p. 780). Drugs used include digoxin, quinidine, verapamil, flecainide, propafenone, propranolol, procainamide, amiodarone and sotalol. This wide range of drugs suggests that the search for optimal therapy of this condition is still ongoing. Digoxin and flecainide have been the most commonly used agents, but sotalol may also be a valuable treatment option in some circumstances.[45]

Antiretroviral therapy to prevent vertical transmission of HIV

There is an increasing prevalence of women infected with HIV and they now account for almost half the annual incidence of infections. Most of these women are of childbearing age and it has been estimated that they transmit the infection to their babies at a rate of around 1500 cases per day.[3]

In the developed world, the administration of intensive and complex regimens combining antepartum, intrapartum and postpartum administration of antiretroviral therapy together with prudent use of caesarian section can reduce transmission of infection from mother to baby to 0–2.8% (pp. 1073–4).[26] Zidovudine has been the drug used in most of the studies. Nevirapine and lamivudine have also been studied.[3]

Unfortunately, neither expensive and complicated drug therapy nor avoidance of breastfeeding are likely to be practical in many parts of the world where the rates of HIV infection are at their highest. Work is ongoing to evaluate the benefit of simpler, cheaper and more practical methods of drug delivery in these areas.

Endocrine disorders

Other conditions such as congenital adrenal hyperplasia and fetal thyroid disorders have also been treated by maternal administration of drugs. This field of therapeutics is an exciting and developing area, which requires more research in the future.

Drugs in breast milk

Breastfeeding has significant advantages for both the infant and mother (pp. 302–10 and 377–9). It is associated with a significant reduction in both morbidity and mortality in the infant and is therefore to be encouraged.

Risk of drug toxicity in breastfed infants

The risk of an adverse drug reaction following breastfeeding by a mother taking medicines is small. A prospective study of over 800 infants who were being breastfed by women taking regular medicines detected no major adverse drug reactions.[33] Just over 10% of mothers reported a minor adverse drug reaction in the infant (diarrhoea, drowsiness or irritability were the most frequent). This important study emphasises the safety of breastfeeding in mothers requiring medicines.

There are, however, certain groups of medicines where breastfeeding is contraindicated (Table 24.11). It is important to recognise that a woman who is receiving these medicines may be less likely to conceive or breastfeed and it is rare for breastfeeding to be absolutely contraindicated.

More frequent is the larger group of medicines where a potential problem may arise during breastfeeding. Most adverse events reported following breastfeeding relate to isolated case reports.[33] It is important to be aware that certain medicines may cause a problem.[30] If any of the medicines listed in Table 24.12 are prescribed to a breastfeeding mother, it is advisable to discuss management with the local paediatric clinical pharmacist or the local drug information centre for a risk/benefit assessment. Alternative medicines may be available in some cases (see website run by the UK Midlands Medicines Information *www.ukmicentral.nhs.uk/ drugpreg/guide.htm*). Other approaches involve administration of the medicine immediately after the mother has breastfed an infant. Caffeine is only likely to be a problem if the mother is having a large daily intake. In the majority of cases, breastfeeding should be encouraged, even when the mother requires a medicine.

Table 24.11 Drugs contraindicated in breastfeeding mothers

Cytotoxics
Ergotamine
Immunosuppressants
Lithium
Phenindione

Table 24.12 Drugs that may cause problems during breastfeeding

Group	Drugs
Anticonvulsants	Ethosuximide, phenobarbital (phenobarbitone), primidone
Antidepressants	Doxepin, fluoxetine
Antibiotics	Chloramphenicol, metronidazole
Anxiolytics	Alprazolam, diazepam
Antihypertensives	Acebutolol, atenolol, nadolol, sotalol
Antiarrhythmics	Amiodarone
Bronchodilators	Theophylline
Radioisotopes	–
Non-medicinal	Alcohol, coffee

Therapeutic drug monitoring

Therapeutic drug monitoring (TDM) has been defined as 'the measurement of drug concentrations in biologic fluids to assess whether they correlate with the patient's clinical condition and whether the dosage or dosage intervals need to be changed'.[52] The purpose is to optimise the management of patients receiving drug therapy for the treatment or prevention of disease.

For TDM to aid in drug therapy, the following criteria must be satisfied:[52]

■ Clinically interpretable correlation between serum drug concentration and pharmacodynamic effect.
■ Narrow margin (therapeutic index) between serum concentrations causing toxic effects and those producing therapeutic effect.
■ Serum concentration produced by a given dose is unpredictable due to inter- and intra-patient pharmacokinetic differences.
■ Pharmacodynamic effects of the drug are not easily measurable.
■ A rapid and reliable method for drug serum concentration analysis must be available.

Certain drugs used in the neonate should be monitored using serum concentrations in order to ensure that the doses being administered are both safe and therapeutically effective.

An example is phenobarbital for neonatal seizures. The therapeutic drug concentration is in the range 15–40 mg/l. Below this range, the drug is likely to be ineffective; above it, toxic effects are more likely. It is, however, important to treat the patient and not purely a serum concentration: if the patient has a level of 8 mg/l yet is seizure-free, then a dose increase may not be indicated.

Another example for which TDM is important is phenytoin. As the capacity of the neonate to metabolise phenytoin nears saturation, small dose increments result in disproportionate increases in plasma concentrations. Saturation of metabolism can occur with therapeutic doses and safe dose adjustment is difficult and must be done with caution.

Blood sampling

The timing of blood sampling for analysis is very important. It is desirable for steady state to be reached before levels are meaningful, unless, of course, toxicity is suspected before this time. It takes the order of three to four half-lives of the drug to reach steady state. For a drug such as phenobarbital that has a $t_{1/2}$ of around 2–4 days in the neonate, steady state will not be achieved until after 1–2 weeks of treatment. Steady state can be achieved much more quickly using a loading dose and therefore it is then appropriate to check levels earlier. A further complicating factor in neonates is the rapidly changing pharmacokinetic capacity of these patients. The significant improvements in renal and hepatic elimination mechanisms after birth may mean steady state is never achieved for drugs given in the neonatal period.

Many drugs need to have blood sampled at specific times in relation to the dosing schedule (Table 24.13). These times need to be accurate for the results to be interpretable and dose

Table 24.13 Neonatal drugs that require monitoring

Drug	When to sample	Therapeutic range
Amikacin	Pre-dose (trough): just prior to next dose	Trough level 2–5 mg/l
	Post-dose (peak): 1 hour after an i.v. dose	Peak level 15–30 mg/l
Digoxin	At least 6 hours after dose	0.8–2.2 micrograms/l
Gentamicin/ Tobramycin	Pre-dose (trough): just prior to next dose	Trough level <2 mg/l
	Post-dose (peak): 1 hour after an i.v. dose	Peak level 5–10 mg/l
Phenobarbital (phenobarbitone)	Immediately prior to next dose	15–40 mg/l
Phenytoin	Immediately prior to next dose	10–20 mg/l
Vancomycin	Pre-dose (trough): immediately prior to next dose	Trough level 5–10 mg/l
	Post-dose (peak): 1 hour after completion of infusion	Peak level 25–40 mg/l*

* There is controversy regarding the value of measuring peak levels of vancomycin, as there is no evidence that transiently high peak levels cause toxicity

adjustment to be made safely. Neonatal pharmacists will usually be able to help with advice regarding sampling and dose adjustment.

Therapeutic ranges

Recommended therapeutic ranges for drugs are usually based on adult pharmacokinetic and pharmacodynamic data. Little is known on whether the same reference ranges should be applied to children and even less regarding neonates. Hospital laboratories tend to quote the same reference ranges irrespective of the age of the patient. This leads to the assumption that patients of all ages respond in the same way to similar blood levels. This is unlikely to be the case, as receptor numbers and sensitivities may be different, and the actual drug concentration reaching the receptor sites in patients of different ages is also likely to vary, due to altered pharmacokinetic handling. The therapeutic range for phenobarbital has been shown to be higher in the neonate than in older children and adults.[24]

Furthermore, neonates have reduced levels of plasma proteins, and those plasma proteins have a reduced affinity and capacity to bind drugs. This means that drugs which are normally highly protein bound will be less so in the neonate, resulting in a higher free – and, therefore, active – fraction of drug. Levels are usually reported in terms of total concentration, hence the same level in a neonate and an adult may produce very different effects in terms of efficacy and toxicity.

Difficulties in relation to TDM in the neonate also occur with the presence of interfering endogenous compounds that may not be present in adult patients. Digoxin-like immunoreactive substances may be present in neonates. These cross-react with many digoxin assay methods, falsely elevating total serum drug concentrations.[24,52] It is possible that other compounds interfering with other drug assays may be found in the future.

Despite these current deficiencies in information relevant to the neonate, TDM is still recommended for the drugs in Table 24.13, but with a keen awareness of the patient's clinical response.

References

1. Alcorn J, McNamara P J 2002 Ontogeny of hepatic and renal systemic clearance pathways in infants: part 1. Clinical Pharmacokinetics 41: 959–998
2. Anderson B J, van Lingen R A, Hansen T G et al 2002 Acetaminophen developmental pharmacokinetics in premature neonates and infants: a pooled population analysis. Anesthesiology 96: 1336–1345
3. Andiman W A 2002 Transmission of HIV-1 from mother to infant. Current Opinion in Pediatrics 14: 78–85
4. Aranda J V, Stern L 1983 Clinical aspects of developmental pharmacology and toxicology. Pharmacology and Therapeutics 20: 1–51
5. Augood C, Gilbert R, Logan S et al 2002 Cisapride treatment for gastro-oesophageal reflux in children (Cochrane Review). Cochrane Database of Systematic Reviews (3): CD002300
6. Barrett D A, Rutter N 1994 Transdermal delivery and the premature neonate. Critical Reviews in Therapeutic Drug Carrier Systems 11: 1–30
7. Bennion D, Martin K 1991 In-line filtration. Paediatric Nursing 3: 20–21
8. Besunder J B, Reed MD, Blumer J L 1988 Principles of drug biodisposition in the neonate. A critical evaluation of the pharmacokinetic-pharmacodynamic interface (part 1). Clinical Pharmacokinetics 14: 189–216
9. Cavell B 1979 Gastric emptying in preterm infants. Acta Paediatrica Scandinavica 68: 725–730
10. Choonara I A, McKay P, Hain R et al 1989 Morphine metabolism in children. British Journal of Clinical Pharmacology 28: 599–604
11. Choonara I, Rieder M J 2002 Drug toxicity and adverse drug reactions in children – a brief historical review. Paediatric and Perinatal Drug Therapy 5: 12–18
12. Conroy S, McIntyre J, Choonara I 1999 Unlicensed and off label drug use in neonates. Archives of Disease in Childhood. Fetal and Neonatal Edition 80: F142–F145
13. Cousins D, Upton D 1997 Increased funding can cut risk. Pharmacy in Practice 7: 597–598
14. Cousins D, Upton D 1998 Inappropriate syringe use leads to fatalities. Pharmacy in Practice 8: 209–210
15. Crowley P 2002 Prophylactic corticosteroids for preterm birth (Cochrane Review). In: The Cochrane Library, Issue 3. Update Software, Oxford
16. de Hoog, Schoemaker R C, Mouton J W et al 2000 Vancomycin population pharmacokinetics in neonates. Clinical Pharmacology and Therapeutics 67: 360–367
17. de Wildt S N, Johnson T N, Choonara I 2003 The effect of age on drug metabolism. Paediatric and Perinatal Drug Therapy 5: 101–106
18. de Wildt S N, Kearns G L, Hop W C et al 2001 Pharmacokinetics and metabolism of intravenous midazolam in preterm infants. Clinical Pharmacology and Therapeutics 70: 525–531
19. de Wildt S N, Kearns G L, Leeder J S et al 1999 Glucuronidation in humans. Pharmacogenetic and developmental aspects. Clinical Pharmacokinetics 36: 439–452
20. de Wildt S N, Kearns G L, Leeder J S et al 1999 Cytochrome P450 3A: ontogeny and drug disposition. Clinical Pharmacokinetics 37: 485–505
21. Drukker A, Guignard J P 2002 Renal aspects of the term and preterm infant: a selective update. Current Opinion in Pediatrics 14: 175–182
22. Gershanik J, Boecler B, Ensley H et al 1982 The gasping syndrome and benzyl alcohol poisoning. New England Journal of Medicine 307:1384–1388
23. Giacoia G P, Jungbluth G L, Jusko W J 1989 Effect of formula feeding on oral absorption of caffeine in premature infants. Developmental Pharmacology and Therapeutics 12: 205–210
24. Gilman J 1990 Therapeutic drug monitoring in the neonatal and paediatric age group: problems and clinical phamacokinetic implications. Clinical Pharmacokinetics 19: 1–10
25. Grimsley C, Thomson A H 1999 Pharmacokinetics and dose requirements of vancomycin in neonates. Archives of Disease in Childhood. Fetal and Neonatal Edition 81: F221–F227
26. Grosch-Wörner I, Schäfer A, Obladen M et al 2000 An effective and safe protocol involving zidovudine and caesarean section to reduce vertical transmission of HIV-1 infection. AIDS 14: 2903–2911
27. Guinn D A, Atkinson M W, Sullivan L et al 2001. Single vs weekly courses of antenatal corticosteroids for women at risk of preterm delivery: a randomised controlled trial. Journal of the American Medical Association 286: 1581–1587
28. Hartnoll G, Betremieux P, Modi N 2000 Body water content of extremely preterm infants at birth. Archives of Disease in Childhood. Fetal and Neonatal Edition 83: F56–F59
29. Hines R N, McCarver D G 2002 The ontogeny of human drug-metabolizing enzymes: phase I oxidative enzymes. Journal of Pharmacology and Experimental Therapeutics 300: 355–360
30. Howard C R, Lawrence R A 2001 Xenobiotics and breastfeeding. Pediatric Clinics of North America 48: 485–504
31. Hughes J, Gill A, Leach H J et al 1994 A prospective study of the adverse effects of midazolam on withdrawal in critically ill children. Acta Paediatrica 83: 1194–1199
32. Ito S 2000 Drug therapy for breast-feeding women. New England Journal of Medicine 343: 118–126
33. Ito S, Blajchman A, Stephenson M et al 1993 Prospective follow-up of adverse reactions in breast-fed infants exposed to maternal medication. American Journal of Obstetrics and Gynaecology 168: 1393–1399
34. Jacqz-Aigrain E, Wood C, Robieux I 1990 Pharmacokinetics of midazolam in critically ill neonates. European Journal of Clinical Pharmacology 39: 191–192
35. James A, Koren G, Milliken J et al 1987 Vancomycin pharmacokinetics and dose recommendations for preterm infants. Antimicrobial Agents and Chemotherapy 31: 52–54
36. Jong G W, van den Anker J, Choonara I 2001 FDAMA's written request list: medicines for children. Lancet 357: 398
37. Jong G W, Vulto A G, de Hoog M et al 2001 A survey of the use of off-label and unlicensed drugs in a Dutch children's hospital. Pediatrics 108: 1089–1093
38. Kelly E J, Newell S J, Brownlee K G et al 1993 Gastric acid secretion in preterm infants. Early Human Development 35: 215–220
39. Kelman A W, Thomson A H, Whiting B et al 1984 Estimation of gentamicin clearance and volume of distribution in neonates and young children. British Journal of Clinical Pharmacology 18: 685–692
40. Koren G 1997 Therapeutic drug monitoring principles in the neonate. Clinical Chemistry 43: 222–227
41. Levy G, Khanna N N, Soda D M et al 1975 Pharmacokinetics of acetaminophen in the human neonate: formation of acetaminophen glucuronide and sulfate in relation to plasma bilirubin concentration and D-glucaric acid excretion. Pediatrics 55: 818–825
42. Loughnan P M, Greenwald A, Purton W W et al 1977 Pharmacokinetic observations of phenytoin disposition in the newborn and young infant. Archives of Disease in Childhood 52: 302–309
43. McBride W G 1961 Thalidomide and congenital abnormalities. Lancet ii: 1358
44. Miller R P, Roberts R J, Fischer L J 1976 Acetaminophen elimination kinetics in neonates, children and adults. Clinical Pharmacology and Therapeutics 19: 284–294
45. Oudijk M A, Michon M M, Kleinman C S et al 2000. Sotalol in the treatment of fetal dysrhythmias. Circulation 101: 2721–2726
46. Pacifici G M, Viani A, Taddeucci-Brunelli G et al 1986 Effects of development, ageing, and renal and hepatic insufficiency as well as hemodialysis on the plasma concentrations of albumin and alpha 1-acid glycoprotein: implications for binding of drugs. Therapeutic Drug Monitoring 8: 259–263
47. Parker A C, Preston T, Heaf D et al 1994 Inhibition of caffeine metabolism by ciprofloxacin in children with cystic fibrosis as measured by the caffeine breath test. British Journal of Clinical Pharmacology 38: 573–576
48. Phelps D L 1984 E-Ferol: What happened and what now? Pediatrics 74: 1114–1116

49. Riezzo G, Indrio F, Montagna O et al 2001 Gastric electrical activity and gastric emptying in preterm newborns fed standard and hydrolysate formulas. Journal of Pediatric Gastroenterology and Nutrition 33: 290–295

50. Rocha M J, Almeida A M, Afonso E et al 2000 The kinetic profile of gentamicin in premature neonates. Journal of Pharmacy and Pharmacology 52: 1091–1097

51. Saarenmaa E, Neuvonen P J, Rosenberg P et al 2000 Morphine clearance and effects in newborn infants in relation to gestational age. Clinical Pharmacology and Therapeutics 68: 160–166

52. Soldin O P, Soldin S J 2002 Review: therapeutic drug monitoring in pediatrics. Therapeutic Drug Monitoring 24: 1–8

53. Spielberg S P 2000 Paediatric therapeutics in the USA and internationally: an unparalleled opportunity. Paediatric and Perinatal Drug Therapy 4: 71–74

54. Turner S, Nunn A J, Fielding K et al 1999 Adverse drug reactions to unlicensed and off-label drugs on paediatric wards: a prospective study. Acta Paediatrica 88: 965–968

55. van den Anker J N 1996 Pharmacokinetics and renal function in preterm infants. Acta Paediatrica 85: 1393–1399

56. van den Anker J N, Hop W C, de Groot R et al 1994 Effects of prenatal exposure to betamethasone and indomethacin on the glomerular filtration rate in the preterm infant. Pediatric Research 36: 578–581

57. van den Anker J N, Hop W C, Schoemaker R C et al 1995 Ceftazidime pharmacokinetics in preterm infants: effect of postnatal age and postnatal exposure to indomethacin. British Journal of Clinical Pharmacology 40: 439–443

58. van den Driessche M, Peeters K, Marien P et al 1999 Gastric emptying in formula-fed and breast-fed infants measured with the 13C-octanoic acid breath test. Journal of Pediatric Gastroenterology and Nutrition 29: 46–51

59. van Lingen R A, Deinum J T, Quak J M et al 1999 Pharmacokinetics and metabolism of rectally administered paracetamol in preterm neonates. Archives of Disease in Children. Fetal and Neonatal Edition 80: F59–F63

60. Vervelde M L, Rademaker C M, Krediet T G et al 1999 Population pharmacokinetics of gentamicin in preterm neonates: evaluation of a once daily dosage regimen. Therapeutic Drug Monitoring 21: 514–519

CHAPTER 25

Analgesia

Steven M Sale, Andrew R Wolf

Introduction

Pain has been described as 'an unpleasant sensory and emotional experience which is usually associated with tissue damage or described in terms of such damage'. While neonates have a broadly similar type of response to painful stimuli as the adult, the presence or absence of pain as a conscious event can never be proven. Infants and neonates have only a limited ability to communicate compared with adults, and their responses can be inconsistent or absent.[66] Little can be inferred on the actual experience of pain or the attendant emotions, if any, relating to it in the neonate. Much depends on the nature of self awareness, consciousness and the development of 'self' in fetal life.[39,63,91] Given the impossible task of making judgements on the nature of pain perception in the fetus and neonate, the term nociception (the anatomical and physiological system of pain sensation) has been felt to be more appropriate.

Despite increasing interest in provision of analgesia in neonates, a recent survey of Canadian practice showed that procedural pain still remains poorly treated.[53] Moreover, this is not a small problem: neonates, particularly those who are unwell, are subjected to a large number of nociceptive stimuli, a total of 500 invasive procedures being recorded in a single neonate during a single hospital stay.[16]

Nociception in the infant

Nociceptive pathways develop early in gestation: as early as 6 weeks' gestation, dorsal horn cells in the spinal cord have formed synapses with the developing sensory neurons.[74] These sensory neurons grow peripherally to reach the skin of the limbs by 11 weeks, the rest of the trunk by 15 weeks and the remaining cutaneous and mucosal surfaces by 20 weeks.[48,99] At full term, the density of nociceptive nerve endings in the newborn skin is at least as great as that of the adult.[38] Further organisation of the laminar structure of the cells in the dorsal horn (Rexed's laminae) and their synapses, together with the appearance of specific neurotransmitter vesicles, begins at 13 weeks and is completed by 30 weeks.[83]

By this time, nerve tracts associated with nociception are fully myelinated up to the thalamic level.[37] Synaptic connections of the thalamocortical tracts occur at 24 weeks' gestation,[57] and myelination of the nociceptive thalamocortical radiations are complete by 37 weeks.[37] Other nociceptive tracts may not be fully myelinated until much later,[7] but lack of myelination does not imply lack of function. Synaptic connections of C fibres do not appear functionally mature until the third trimester, but noxious stimuli can still be transmitted via A-β fibres.[31] Descending inhibitory tracts, which act via inputs into spinal cord cells to suppress the transmission of noxious stimuli, are also not fully functional at term. The lack of descending inhibition from higher centres will tend to increase afferent nociceptive transmission in the spinal cord.

Few neurophysiological or cytochemical studies have been attempted in the human infant. Positron emission tomography has shown that glucose utilisation – and, by inference, cerebral metabolism – is maximal in sensory areas of the neonatal brain[22] and that auditory and visual evoked potentials have developed by 30 weeks' gestation.[45] These data, along with EEG data,[96] imply a very complex level of integration and maturity within the cerebral cortex by this time. Somatosensory evoked responses (SERs) are present from 28 weeks' gestation, although the latency is long, due to slow peripheral and central transmission.

While nociceptive connections remain immature in the preterm neonate, the larger receptive fields, the immaturity of the descending inhibitory pathways, and the ability of non-C fibres to transmit nociceptive inputs into the dorsal horn facilitated by subthreshold C-fibre effects give the impression of an underdamped, poorly discriminative system with a potential for much exaggerated responses. This is born out in Fitzgerald's observations on the cutaneous withdrawal reflex[11,32] and other studies which have shown that newborn reactions to painful stimuli can be diffuse, unlocalised or sometimes completely absent.[66] This failure to respond consistently to a standard noxious stimulus can confound attempts to quantify pain using behavioural measurement.

Effects of nociception

The initial effects of nociception can be categorised under physiological responses, stress responses and behavioural responses.

Haemodynamic responses to noxious stimuli occur as early as 18 weeks' gestation in the human fetus.[95] Neonates undergoing awake nasotracheal intubation have a rise in mean arterial pressure of 57%, with a similar rise in intracranial pressure, during the procedure.[55] Age-related differences in cardiovascular responses to noxious stimuli have been reported.[80] In a study on lumbar puncture in preterm infants, the younger babies (<32 weeks' gestational age) showed the greatest rise in blood pressure during the handling phase rather than during the actual procedure. This was in contrast to the older babies, who displayed maximum response during the procedure itself. Other physiological responses that have been investigated in the context of nociception are R-to-R interval and frequency analysis on ECG,[81] transcutaneous oxygen tension, ventilatory patterns and sweating.

Hormonal responses to noxious stimuli can also be identified in the human fetus and the response obtunded by opioids.[30] Neonatal stress responses to surgery appear to be greater in magnitude and shorter lived than in older infants[5,75] and the subsequent nitrogen loss appears to be greater in the younger age groups. Inadequate suppression of these responses during major surgery affects postoperative recovery,[9] but it remains unclear if complete elimination of the responses is desirable either. Some measure of stress response during surgery can be achieved by real-time analysis of blood sugar, provided glucose-containing solutions are avoided.[103]

Preterm infants exhibit hypersensitivity and postinjury hyperalgesia, similar to adults, following heel lancing, which can be prevented by the application of local anaesthetic.[32] There is also evidence that early tissue injury can cause hyperinnervation (increased branching of nociceptive nerve endings), which persists and may lead to hyperalgesia and allodynia.[24]

The impression that emerges is that even the very preterm infant has complex interneuronal connections capable of integrated responses to tactile or nociceptive input. They have inconsistent responses to external stimuli, which may reflect the late functional connections of sensory afferents (particularly C fibres) within the spinal cord. However, the combination of larger receptive fields, recruitment of non-nociceptive afferents and reduced inhibitory controls results in 'underdamped' responses (long lasting, exaggerated and poorly localised) once afferent stimuli have achieved central activation above a threshold level. Inconsistency of response may reflect the profound effects that conscious state[42] and other external responses[44] have on behaviour.

Secondary effects of nociception

Neonates who experience repeated noxious stimuli can show both short-term hypersensitivity[32] and longer-term persistence of immature pain responses.[54] At 18 months they have been reported to respond less than normal infants to everyday painful experiences,[43] and at 4–5 years show increased somatisation (an inappropriate expression of psychosocial distress as physical symptomatology). Awake circumcision without analgesia causes irritability, reduced attentiveness and poor orientation that can last longer than the expected duration of pain,[28] and 3–6 months later these babies have exaggerated responses to painful stimuli compared with a matched group who have not been circumcised.[92]

Comforting strategies that reduce the stress of interventional procedures in preterm infants are associated with improved developmental and clinical outcomes.[2] The results of the multicentre NOPAIN trial provide compelling evidence for the benefits of providing analgesia to ventilated neonates. A low-dose morphine infusion was found to reduce the incidence of neurological complications (intraventricular haemorrhage and periventricular leukomalacia) in ventilated infants when compared with midazolam or dextrose.[6] However, liberal use of opioids may also alter longer-term responses to painful stimuli. Early opioid exposure appears to increase subsequent responses to painful stimuli.[70] It has even been claimed that early exposure to opioids may be associated with self-destructive behaviour in adolescence.[51]

Measurement of pain/nociception in the neonate

Most of the early studies on infant pain measurement were based on a single noxious stimulus such as heel prick (procedural pain) and were primarily developed for research purposes. This was a useful model because it provided a relatively consistent stimulus from which to identify and grade responses. However, the behavioural tools derived from studies on procedural pain have limited applicability to other situations such as postoperative pain and the discomfort from prolonged immobility in the neonatal intensive care unit. There are few validated tools for prolonged pain or discomfort, they require training to increase reliability and are labour intensive with a low degree of clinical utility. In the Bristol Royal Hospital for Children we use a modified observational pain scale that is simple to use, requires minimal training and is feasible in a clinical setting (Table 25.1). Tools available are either unidimensional – using behavioural responses to pain – or multidimensional – using a combination of behavioural, physiological and contextual indicators. Behavioural indicators are more specific than physiological changes in all age groups. Many of these tools are developed from validated techniques used in older children and infants, such as the Children's Hospital of Eastern Ontario Scale (CHEOPS).

Unidimensional measures

The Neonatal Facial Coding System (NFCS), developed by Grunau and Craig,[42] has been extensively studied and validated for procedural pain in both preterm and term infants. It uses a variety of facial actions discussed above (Fig. 25.1). The EDIN scale (Échelle Douleur Inconfort Nouveau-Né, neonatal pain and discomfort scale) is a recently developed scale that has been validated for prolonged pain in preterm infants, using five behavioural indicators (facial activity, body movement, sleep, contact quality with carers and consolability).[27] Other behavioural tools described include:

- Maximally Discriminative Facial Coding System (MAX),[50] which uses facial expressions to identify 10 emotions, one of which is pain;

Table 25.1 Modified observational pain scale

Agitation	Facial expression	Movement	Ventilation
2 = Major	2 = Grimace/nasal flare	2 = Flexed/tense	2 = Fighting ventilator
1 = Responds to comforting	1 = Movement	1 = Appropriate	1 = Comfortable
0 = No movement	0 = No movement	0 = No movement	0 = Apnoea

A modified observational pain scale used on the Paediatric Intensive Care unit in the Bristol Royal Hospital for Children. Hourly observations are recorded. A total score of 2 or less implies oversedation, 3–5 is ideal, and 6 or more implies undersedation.

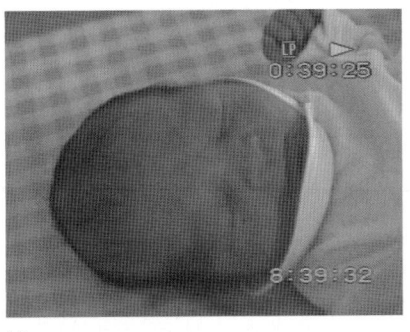

(a)

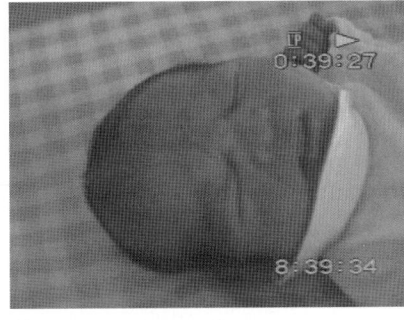

(b)

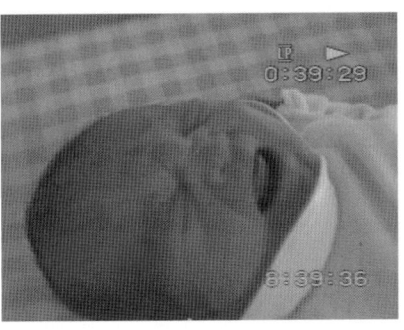

(c)

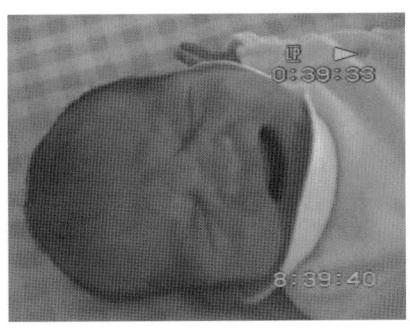

(d)

Fig. 25.1 Stills from video footage showing an infant 1 second before and 1, 3 and 7 seconds after venepuncture (a, b, c and d, respectively). Some of the consistent facial actions to a painful stimulus (as described by the Neonatal Facial Coding System) can be identified – brow bulge, eye squeeze, nasolabial furrow, lip opening, vertical and horizontal stretching of the mouth, and taut tongue.

- Mills Infant/Toddler Pain Index (MITPI);[1]
- Clinical Scoring System (CSS),[17] which was developed to assess postoperative pain in infants;
- Infant Body Coding System (IBCS),[26] which was developed by Craig to assess body activity and has been used in conjuction with the NFCS;
- Behavioural Pain Score (BPS),[79] which was adapted from the CHEOPS to evaluate response to opioids in preterm and full-term infants;
- Liverpool Infant Distress Score (LIDS),[47] which scores eight behavioural characteristics to identify postoperative pain in infants.

Multidimensional measures

The COMFORT scale was developed for use on the paediatric intensive care unit, to be used from newborns to adolescents.[4] It was intended to measure distress associated with anxiety and fear, as well as pain. Eight indicators were found, including mean arterial blood pressure, heart rate, muscle tone, alertness, agitation, respiratory behaviour, physical movement and facial tension. The Premature Infant Pain Profile (PIPP), which uses behavioural (brow bulge, eye squeeze and nasolabial furrow), physiological (heart rate and oxygen saturation) and contextual (gestational age and behaviour state) indicators, is also clinically useful.[87] Other validated tools include the Neonatal Infant Pain Scale (NIPS)[61] and CRIES,[58] which was developed for postoperative pain. In the paralysed neonate, behavioural tools cannot be employed and physiological measures such as cardiovascular responses to handling have to be used.

Pharmacological considerations

Classically, neonates are regarded as highly susceptible to opioid drugs both in terms of pharmacodynamics (physiological effects of the drug on the body) and pharmacokinetics (how the body handles the drug). However, the limited studies available have shown that there is a large individual variability in this population, associated with maturity, previous exposure to drugs and organ function. Individual drug effects from dosing regimens are therefore poorly predictive and can only be described in general terms.

Pharmacodynamics

Opioid receptors change both in numbers and in type during development, and in the rat this is associated with a large change in sensitivity.[77] It has been suggested from human studies which have compared plasma concentrations of opioid drugs that human neonates could be relatively resistant to the ventilatory effects of opioids, and that the sensitivity observed after opioid administration is due to selective distribution of the drug to the brain after administration. Lipid-soluble drugs, such as fentanyl, are preferentially redistributed into the neonatal brain after a bolus injection and attain high initial peak concentrations at the effect site (biophase). In contrast, elimination of the drug from biophase is slow because of the limitations on peripheral uptake and drug elimination. Fat-soluble opioids such as fentanyl will therefore have a more rapid onset of effect, greater potency and slower offset than can be predicted by simply analysing pharmacokinetic data. Delivery of morphine into biophase may also be enhanced in the neonate and young infant due to immaturity of the blood–brain barrier.[59]

Pharmacokinetics

Neonates have a high percentage of body water and less fat than older infants. Consequently, relatively large loading doses of water-soluble drugs such as morphine may need to be given over the first few hours of an infusion to achieve adequate plasma concentrations and effect. Subsequent drug elimination in the 'drug naïve' neonate is delayed due to immaturity of hepatic and renal function. Therefore, once steady state has been achieved, infusion rates need to be reduced substantially to prevent accumulation.

A fourfold reduction in the elimination half-life of morphine takes place in the first few years of life, with mean values of 7.2 hours below 1 month, compared with 1.7 hours in adults.[71] This is due primarily to the prolonged clearance of the drug. Other similar data also demonstrated the large individual variability between subjects, particularly in the neonate. The mean elimination half-life in the newborn was measured to be 13.9 hours, with a standard deviation of 6.4 hours.[76] Pharmacokinetic data for fentanyl show a similar pattern, with even greater variability in the premature infant.[23,35,56] Hepatic clearance of fentanyl may be drastically reduced in neonates undergoing intra-abdominal surgery or those with raised intra-abdominal pressure.[56] This has been attributed to the effects of raised intra-abdominal pressure on liver blood flow.[68] The implications for infants undergoing abdominal surgery are clear: some infants will have a sustained effect from doses of opioid that would normally be expected to have a limited duration of action.

Clinical analgesia

Opioids and paracetamol remain the most commonly used analgesics but there is increasing use of ketamine (an NMDA antagonist), clonidine (α_2 agonist), local anaesthetics and other non-steroidal anti-inflammatory drugs (NSAIDs).

Opioids

Morphine, fentanyl and codeine are the most commonly used opioids in the UK. All can cause ventilatory depression, urinary retention and decreased intestinal motility leading to delayed feeding after abdominal surgery.

Morphine remains the historical gold standard with which other analgesics are compared. Morphine has both slower onset and offset than fentanyl after a single dose, but after long-term infusion this effect is reversed due to the shorter terminal elimination half-life of morphine. In the ventilated neonate, an intravenous loading dose (50–150 micrograms/kg) is required to achieve effective analgesia, followed by an infusion rate between 5 and 20 micrograms/kg/h. However, as tolerance develops, the infusion rate may need to be further increased. 'Nurse-controlled analgesia' (NCA) is a useful technique for control of infant pain. The patient receives a background morphine infusion (2.5–10 micrograms/kg/h) topped up at appropriate intervals by 'nurse-controlled' doses (varying from about 2.5 to 10 micrograms/kg) according to formal pain assessment.

Morphine should be used with caution in the spontaneously breathing postoperative neonate. Loading doses of 10–50 micrograms/kg morphine can be given by slow infusion over 15 minutes in conjunction with sedation scores at 5-minute intervals. Once the desired level of comfort has been achieved, the infusion is discontinued, even if the full dose has not been delivered. Additional doses are then given in the same fashion according to regular documented pain scores, thereby maintaining a therapeutic level on an individual titrated basis. NCA can also be used with a low background morphine infusion (1–5 micrograms/kg/h). All infants under 6 months receiving opioids need to stay in a high-dependency unit for continual monitoring with direct observation, pulse oximetry and ventilatory monitoring.

Fentanyl provides intense analgesia and relative cardiovascular stability. At high doses (10–150 micrograms/kg as a single injection), it can control pulmonary hypertension.[46] These doses are well above analgesic doses (0.5–10 micrograms/kg). Fahnenstich and colleagues observed chest wall rigidity in eight out of 89 neonates following relatively small doses of 3–5 micrograms/kg fentanyl; all cases responded quickly to either naloxone or neuromuscular blockade.[29] The high lipid solubility of fentanyl and increased skin permeability of the preterm neonate makes the transdermal route of administration feasible and this is currently being evaluated. Transtracheal fentanyl provides rapid absorption in rabbits but awaits clinical trials in humans.[49]

Codeine has, reputedly, a lower incidence of opioid-related side effects. It has been advocated for use in neonatal practice at a dose of 1 mg/kg, by the oral, intramuscular or rectal route. Single dose administration appears safe, but with repeated doses, unwanted side effects do occur.[82] Codeine is metabolised to morphine, but there is considerable variability, and in a small genetic subgroup of 'poor metabolisers' (9% in UK, 30% in Hong Kong Chinese) codeine has virtually no analgesic effect.[102] This large inter-patient variability necessitates caution when using codeine long term in neonates.

Tolerance and withdrawal

While initial doses of opioid infusions needed for analgesia and sedation are low, the dose requirements increase rapidly. Neonates undergoing extracorporeal membrane oxygenation require five times the initial opioid infusion rate by day 6 to achieve the same level of sedation, due to a combination of enhanced elimination[14] and true tolerance.[41] The use of long-term infusions of morphine for sedation alone is debatable: it is better to reserve analgesic drugs for pain relief or use low-dose infusions of morphine in conjunction with other long-acting sedatives such as chloral hydrate or promethazine.

Opioid antagonists (naloxone 4–10 micrograms/kg) easily reverse opioid side effects but must be used with caution in neonates receiving opioid infusions, as acute antagonism may trigger a syndrome of withdrawal. Withdrawal is characterised by an excitation of the central nervous system, the gastrointestinal system and the autonomic nervous system.[90] Opioid abstinence syndrome can occur after 48 hours of morphine infusion but is more usually observed after 4 to 5 days. Management includes the use of a reducing opioid regimen (with morphine or methadone), α_2 antagonists (clonidine 3–5 micrograms/kg 8–12 hourly) and benzodiazepines for anxiolysis. Weaning schedules can last weeks. Preventative methods include the judicious use of opioids combined with formal comfort scores to optimise the rate of opioid withdrawal.

Non-opioids

Paracetamol (acetaminophen) is primarily metabolised by glucuronidation in older children but by sulphation in neonates.[100] Once the main metabolic pathways are saturated, paracetamol is oxidated by the cytochrome P450 system to a reactive intermediary compound which is bound to glutathione, but can react with hepatocyte macromolecules in the absence of glutathione. Neonates may have some protection from the hepatic toxicity effects of paracetamol by having greater glutathione stores and slower oxidative metabolism.[97] Paracetamol is a widely accepted treatment for moderate pain in neonates. Current data suggest that its short-term use in term and preterm neonates is safe and efficacious.[8] It has additive effects when combined with opioids, thereby allowing lower doses and subsequently lower incidence of side effects.[72] Loading doses of paracetamol are similar for premature and term neonates (25 mg/kg orally or 35 mg/kg by triglyceride suppository). Subsequent maintenance regimens must be tailored to the maturity of the infant. Anderson et al[10] found that adequate plasma concentrations can be achieved by an oral dose of 25 mg/kg/day in premature neonates at 30 weeks' post-conception, 45 mg/kg/day at 34 weeks' gestation, 60 mg/kg/day at term, and 90 mg/kg/day at 6 months of age. Rectal doses must be increased by a third the oral dose to account for the decreased absorption by this route. These regimens may cause hepatotoxicity in some individuals if used for longer than 2–3 days. An intravenous pro-drug is now available (propacetamol) which liberates half the mass of paracetamol. Autret et al[15] found that with neonates aged less than 10 days, a 15 mg/kg dose of propacetamol 6 hourly (i.e. 30 mg/kg/day paracetamol) resulted in sufficient antipyretic plasma levels; however, double this dose was required for older infants. More trials are needed to establish the safety of propacetamol.

NSAIDs have antipyretic and anti-inflammatory properties with no respiratory depressant or sedative side effects. As with paracetamol, they have an opioid-sparing effect in older children. Concern over potentially serious side effects has limited NSAID use for analgesia. Current knowledge of their neonatal effect results almost entirely from their use in the treatment of patent ductus arteriosus (PDA). Side effects of indometacin (indomethacin) include oliguria from decreased renal perfusion, necrotising enterocolitis and gut perforation from decreased splanchnic perfusion,[86] and gastrointestinal bleeding from reduced platelet function. Decreased cerebral blood flow may have a preventative effect on intraventricular haemorrhage in preterm neonates.[73] Ibuprofen has been used as an oral analgesic in term neonates and has a lower incidence of side effects than indometacin when used for treatment of PDAs.[101] It should be used with caution in jaundiced patients as it may displace bilirubin from albumin, and, at a dose of 5–10 mg/kg, ibuprofen need only be repeated every 12–24 hours, as its half-life is prolonged compared with in adults.[12]

Recently there has been a resurgence of interest in ketamine and clonidine. Ketamine is a centrally acting NMDA receptor antagonist and potent analgesic. It has been used with proven efficacy and safety for the anaesthesia of neonates for some years. It can be given intravenously (0.5–2 mg/kg), rectally (3–8 mg/kg), intramuscularly (2–5 mg/kg) and via the neuro-axial route.[78] It has the advantage of promoting cardiovascular stability, especially in hypovolaemic patients; it maintains respiratory drive and is a bronchodilator. It increases salivation and respiratory secretions and is usually given with an anticholinergic agent (e.g. atropine 10 micrograms/kg i.v.) and is often combined with midazolam (e.g. 25 micrograms/kg) to provide procedural analgesia and sedation. Intravenous doses of 2 mg and intramuscular doses of 3 mg/kg have been found to induce sedation in 45 seconds and 4 minutes, respectively.[25] S(+) ketamine, one of the two enantiomers of ketamine, has an analgesic potency threefold that of the racemic ketamine and may prove to have fewer side effects. It has been used effectively in caudal anaesthesia[65] but further clinical trials are needed to evaluate its parenteral use in neonates.

Clonidine is an α_2 agonist that is commonly used via the caudal route (1–2 micrograms/kg) in combination with local anaesthetic drugs. It provides dose-dependent analgesia following oral and intravenous administration. It has the advantage of having less respiratory depression than opioids, although there are case reports of postoperative apnoea in term and preterm infants.[20,21] Oral doses of up to 4 micrograms/kg 8 hourly have been used in the treatment of neonatal opioid withdrawal.[90]

Pure sedative drugs have an adjuvant role in the treatment of neonatal pain. In combination with analgesics, they may reduce anxiety and stress by promoting sleep. Of the benzodiazepines, lorazepam (20–100 micrograms/kg) has a longer duration, resulting in a smoother sedative effect.[69] Benzodiazepines have an additive effect on the respiratory depression of opioids. Chloral hydrate, promethazine and triclofos sodium are other popular sedative drugs.

Local anaesthetics

The use of local and regional anaesthesia/analgesic techniques has a significant, albeit specialised, role in the treatment of neonatal pain (see Table 25.2). High-dose opioid techniques may be beneficial to the sick neonate by suppressing nociceptive processing and the neural-humoral responses to pain, but are complicated by respiratory depression. Conversely, regional analgesia has been shown to be as effective as morphine infusions without causing sedation or ventilatory depression,[13,104] leading to faster recovery times. There are many recent studies to suggest that in experienced hands regional anaesthesia/analgesia is safe and easy with few side effects.[36,67,89,98] Local anaesthetics can block nociceptive transmission at various sites – topically and by local infiltration to the skin, regionally by nerve blocks or neuro-axially via the caudal, lumbar or thoracic epidural route. Single-shot administration can provide up to 12 hours of analgesia or indwelling catheters can be used for local anaesthetic infusions or repeat bolus.

Newborns are at a higher risk for local anaesthetic toxicity, which had previously led to concern over the use of local anaesthetics in this age group. Lower α_1-acid glycoprotein levels[62] and reduced clearance of amide local anaesthetics results in potentially higher plasma levels, which can cause seizures and cardiovascular collapse.[19] This is further exacerbated by acidosis, hypoxia, hypercapnia, hyponatraemia and hyperkalaemia – many

Table 25.2 Analgesic doses

	Population	Dose	Notes
Morphine	Ventilated neonate	50–150 micrograms/kg i.v.	Loading dose
		5–20 micrograms/kg/h i.v.	Infusion
		2.5–10 micrograms/kg i.v.	NCA (bolus every 30 min)
		2.5–10 micrograms/kg/h i.v.	NCA (background infusion)
	Unventilated neonate	10–50 micrograms/kg i.v.	Slow loading dose
Fentanyl	For ventilated neonates only	0.5–10 micrograms/kg i.v.	
Alfentanil	For ventilated neonates only	5–10 micrograms/kg i.v.	Loading dose
		0.5–1 micrograms/kg/h i.v.	Infusion
Codeine		1 mg/kg p.o./p.r.	
Paracetamol	All ages	25 mg/kg p.o., 35 mg/kg p.r.	Loading dose
	30 weeks' PCA	25 mg/kg p.o., 30 mg/kg p.r.	Maximum daily dose
	34 weeks' PCA	45 mg/kg p.o., 60 mg/kg p.r.	Maximum daily dose
	40 weeks' PCA	60 mg/kg p.o., 80 mg/kg p.r.	Maximum daily dose
	60 weeks' PCA	90 mg/kg p.o., 120 mg/kg p.r.	Maximum daily dose
Propacetamol	Term neonates <10 days	60 mg/kg i.v.	Maximum daily dose
	Term neonates >10 days	120 mg/kg i.v.	Maximum daily dose
Ibuprofen		5–10 mg/kg p.o.	Every 12–24 hours
Ketamine		0.5–2 mg/kg i.v.*, 3–8 mg/kg p.r.	Co-administration with an anticholinergic advised due to increased respiratory secretions
Clonidine		2–4 micrograms/kg p.o.	For opioid withdrawal
Lorazepam		20–100 micrograms/kg i.v.	
Chloral hydrate/ Triclofos sodium		30–50 mg/kg p.o./p.r.	
Promethazine		0.5 mg/kg i.v./p.o.	

Doses of commonly used analgesic and sedative drugs. These dosing regimens are guides only and care must be taken as there is considerable variation in effect.
* 2 mg/kg ketamine is an anaesthetic dose and may cause apnoea.
NCA, nurse-controlled analgesia; PCA, postconceptional age.

of which the neonate is at a greater risk for developing. Care should be taken when calculating the safe maximum doses of lidocaine (lignocaine; 3 mg/kg) and bupivicaine (2 mg/kg bolus). Epidural infusions of bupivicaine (0.2 mg/kg/h, 1.25 mg/ml) can be given safely for up to 48 hours, but Larsson et al found a significant number of neonates had a still rising plasma bupivicaine level at 48 hours,[60] suggesting that accumulation may occur with prolonged epidural infusions.

Eutectic mixture of local anaesthetics (EMLA) contains 2.5% lidocaine (lignocaine) and 2.5% prilocaine. Prilocaine has a metabolite, o-toluidine, which can cause methaemoglobinaemia. Taddio et al, in a meta-analysis of 11 trials, showed the incidence of clinically relevant methaemoglobinaemia to be zero,[93] allaying previous concerns over the use of EMLA in those under 3 months. However, the risk of significant methaemoglobinaemia increases if excess doses are used too frequently and if other methaemoglobin-inducers are used. Tetracaine (amethocaine) is an alternative topical anaesthetic that is being increasingly used in the UK. Further studies are needed to establish its safety for the newborn, but early work suggests it to be a safe and effective anaesthetic for venepuncture.[52] Both EMLA and tetracaine (amethocaine) gel (Ametop) have been found to be not particularly effective for heel-lancing pain. Venepuncture by an experienced practitioner causes less pain than heel lancing and should

Table 25.3 A suggested plan for provision of analgesia in the neonatal unit for various common scenarios

A. Postoperative analgesia

Non-ventilated baby	1. Determine opioid history e.g. loading dose in theatre or long-term administration 2. Inadequate analgesia 10–50 micrograms/kg i.v. morphine* bolus over 15 minutes with formal pain/comfort scoring at 5-minute intervals until analgesia is optimal 3. Analgesia maintenance 0–20 micrograms/kg/h i.v. morphine* 4. Regular paracetamol (caution after 48 hours – see text) 5. Transfer to enteral analgesics, e.g. codeine, as soon as possible
Ventilated baby	1. Inadequate analgesia 50–150 micrograms/kg i.v. morphine* bolus as required 2. Analgesia maintenance 0–40 micrograms/kg/h i.v. morphine* 3. Regular paracetamol (caution after 48 hours – see text) 4. Fentanyl* with critically ill babies (conveys haemodynamic stability) 0.5–10 micrograms/kg i.v. bolus if analgesia inadequate 2.5–10 micrograms/kg/h for i.v. maintenance

B. Background sedation

Ventilated baby	1. Opioid infusion Critically ill baby use fentanyl* 2.5–10 micrograms/kg/h i.v. Otherwise morphine* 0–20 micrograms/kg/h 2. Optimise opioid infusion with pain/comfort scoring Limit dose to reduce tolerance (kinetic and dynamic) Ensure adequate analgesia to avoid stress response 3. Consider secondary agents to reduce opioid requirements Sedatives e.g. Triclofos or lorazepam Clonidine 4. Non-pharmacological strategies (see text)

C. Procedural analgesia

e.g. venepuncture or chest-drain insertion	1. Use local anaesthesia where possible; first establish appropriate safe dose for patient, then consider: Local infiltration EMLA (allow skin contact of at least 60 minutes) Ametop (allow skin contact of 45 minutes) 2. Non-pharmacological strategies (see text) 3. Consider single i.v. opioid bolus

* Infants receiving opioid infusions must be fully monitored with regular formal pain/comfort scoring in a high dependency or intensive care unit.

be the method of choice.[85] Neonatal circumcision, which is still performed without anaesthesia in parts of the world, has been shown to have long-term effects on pain perception 6 months after the procedure.[92] In a recent Cochrane review, EMLA was found to attenuate the physiological effects of pain following circumcision.[94] However, the authors concluded that while EMLA was more effective than placebo and should be used in place of nothing, there are more effective analgesic methods, such as penile dorsal nerve blocks and ring blocks, which need further evaluation. Initial reports suggest dorsal nerve blocks to be safe, with a low incidence of complications.[33]

Environmental and behavioural interventions

There is a growing body of evidence that environmental, behavioural and non-pharmacological strategies can reduce the behavioural and physiological indicators of pain and stress in the newborn. These principles are encompassed in the concept of developmental care which leads to improved neuro-behavioural organisation, lower morbidity and earlier discharge.[2,3] Minimising painful procedures to those absolutely necessary and clustering them together can reduce the frequency of noxious stimuli. Other techniques thought to be beneficial include decreasing handling, reducing ambient noise and light, and establishing day – night cycles.[34]

Behavioural strategies useful in reducing pain scores during painful procedures include gentle sensory stimulation of the visual, tactile,[40] auditory[64] and taste senses. Oral sucrose and sweet compounds are safe and effective at reducing pain scores during invasive procedures. There is a dose-dependent effect from 5% to 50%, but the optimal dose is not known.[88] Bellieni et al combined oral 10% glucose, non-nutritive sucking and multisensorial stimulation into a process of 'sensorial saturation'. They found that this was more effective at reducing pain scores than any of these techniques alone.[18] Proprioceptive, vestibular and thermal stimulation occurs through swaddling, rocking and maintaining a flexed position (facilitated tucking).[34] The use of melatonin is still in the research domain but it may prove useful to regulate the circadian rhythm.[84] An overview of general strategy is shown in Table 25.3.

References

1. Abu-Saad H H, Bours G J, Stevens B et al 1998 Assessment of pain in the neonate. Seminars in Perinatology 22: 402–416
2. Als H, Lawhon G, Brown E et al 1986 Individualized behavioral and environmental care for the very low birth weight preterm infant at high risk for bronchopulmonary dysplasia: neonatal intensive care unit and developmental outcome. Pediatrics 78: 1123–1132
3. Als H, Lawhon G, Duffy F H et al 1994 Individualized developmental care for the very low-birth-weight preterm infant. Medical and neurofunctional effects. Journal of the American Medical Association 272: 853–858
4. Ambuel B, Hamlett K W, Marx C M et al 1992 Assessing distress in pediatric intensive care environments: the COMFORT scale. Journal of Pediatric Psychology 17: 95–109
5. Anand K J 1990 Neonatal stress responses to anesthesia and surgery. Clinics in Perinatology 17: 207–214
6. Anand K J, Barton B A, McIntosh N et al 1999 Analgesia and sedation in preterm neonates who require ventilatory support: results from the NOPAIN trial.

Neonatal Outcome and Prolonged Analgesia in Neonates. Archives of Pediatrics and Adolescent Medicine 153: 331–338
7. Anand K J, Carr D B 1989 The neuroanatomy, neurophysiology, and neurochemistry of pain, stress, and analgesia in newborns and children. Pediatric Clinics of North America 36: 795–822
8. Anand K J, Menon G, Narsinghani U et al 2000 Systemic analgesic therapy. In: Anand, K J, Stevens B, McGrath P (eds) Pain in neonates. Elsevier, Amsterdam, pp 159–188
9. Anand K J, Sippell W G, Aynsley-Green A 1987 Randomised trial of fentanyl anaesthesia in preterm babies undergoing surgery: effects on the stress response. Lancet 1: 62–66
10. Anderson B J, van Lingen R A, Hansen T G et al 2002 Acetaminophen developmental pharmacokinetics in premature neonates and infants: a pooled population analysis. Anesthesiology 96: 1336–1345
11. Andrews K, Fitzgerald M 1994 The cutaneous withdrawal reflex in human neonates: sensitization, receptive fields, and the effects of contralateral stimulation. Pain 56: 95–101
12. Aranda J V, Varvarigou A, Beharry K et al 1997 Pharmacokinetics and protein binding of intravenous ibuprofen in the premature newborn infant. Acta Paediatrica 86: 289–293
13. Armitage E N 1988 Is there a place for regional anesthesia in pediatrics? – Yes! Acta Anaesthesiologica Belgica 39: 191–195
14. Arnold J H, Truog R D, Scavone J M et al 1991 Changes in the pharmacodynamic response to fentanyl in neonates during continuous infusion. Journal of Pediatrics 119: 639–643
15. Autret E, Dutertre J P, Breteau M et al 1993 Pharmacokinetics of paracetamol in the neonate and infant after administration of propacetamol chlorhydrate. Developmental Pharmacology and Therapeutics 20: 129–134
16. Barker D P, Rutter N 1995 Exposure to invasive procedures in neonatal intensive care unit admissions. Archives of Disease in Childhood. Fetal and Neonatal Edition 72: F47–F48
17. Barrier G, Attia J, Mayer M N et al 1989 Measurement of post-operative pain and narcotic administration in infants using a new clinical scoring system. Intensive Care Medicine 15(suppl. 1): S37–S39
18. Bellieni C V, Buonocore G, Nenci A et al 2001 Sensorial saturation: an effective analgesic tool for heel-prick in preterm infants: a prospective randomized trial. Biology of the Neonate 80: 15–18
19. Berde C B 1993 Toxicity of local anesthetics in infants and children. Journal of Pediatrics 122(5 Pt 2): S14–S20
20. Bouchut J C, Dubois R, Godard J 2001 Clonidine in preterm-infant caudal anesthesia may be responsible for postoperative apnea. Regional Anesthesia and Pain Medicine 26: 83–85
21. Breschan C, Krumpholz R, Likar R et al 1999 Can a dose of 2 microg.kg^{-1} caudal clonidine cause respiratory depression in neonates? Paediatric Anaesthesia 9: 81–83
22. Chugani H T, Phelps M E 1986 Maturational changes in cerebral function in infants determined by 18-FDG positron emission tomography. Science 231: 840–844
23. Collins C, Koren G, Crean P et al 1985 Fentanyl pharmacokinetics and hemodynamic effects in preterm infants during ligation of patent ductus arteriosus. Anesthesia and Analgesia 64: 1078–1080
24. Constantinou J, Reynolds M L, Woolf C J et al 1994 Nerve growth factor levels in developing rat skin: upregulation following skin wounding. Neuroreport 5: 2281–2284
25. Cotsen M R, Donaldson J S, Uejima T et al 1997 Efficacy of ketamine hydrochloride sedation in children for interventional radiologic procedures. American Journal of Roentgenology 169: 1019–1022
26. Craig K D, McMahon R J, Morison J D et al 1984 Developmental changes in infant pain expression during immunization injections. Social Science and Medicine 19: 1331–1337
27. Debillon T, Zupan V, Ravault N et al 2001 Development and initial validation of the EDIN scale, a new tool for assessing prolonged pain in preterm infants. Archives of Disease in Children. Fetal and Neonatal Edition 85: F36–F41
28. Dixon S, Snyder J, Holve R et al 1984 Behavioral effects of circumcision with and without anesthesia. Journal of Developmental and Behavioral Pediatrics 5: 246–250
29. Fahnenstich H, Steffan J, Kau N et al 2000 Fentanyl-induced chest wall rigidity and laryngospasm in preterm and term infants. Critical Care Medicine 28: 836–839
30. Fisk N M, Gitau R, Teixeira J M et al 2001 Effect of direct fetal opioid analgesia on fetal hormonal and hemodynamic stress response to intrauterine needling. Anesthesiology 95: 828–835
31. Fitzgerald M, Butcher T, Shortland P 1994 Developmental changes in the laminar termination of A fibre cutaneous sensory afferents in the rat spinal cord dorsal horn. Journal of Comparative Neurology 348: 225–233

32. Fitzgerald M, Millard C, McIntosh N 1989 Cutaneous hypersensitivity following peripheral tissue damage in newborn infants and its reversal with topical anaesthesia. Pain 39: 31–36

33. Fontaine P, Dittberner D, Scheltema K 1994 The safety of dorsal penile nerve block for neonatal circumcision. Journal of Family Practice 39: 243–248

34. Franck L S, Lawhon G 1998 Environmental and behavioral strategies to prevent and manage neonatal pain. Seminars in Perinatology 22: 434–443

35. Gauntlett I S, Fisher D M, Hertzka R E et al 1988 Pharmacokinetics of fentanyl in neonatal humans and lambs: effects of age. Anesthesiology 69: 683–687

36. Giaufre E, Dalens B, Gombert A 1996 Epidemiology and morbidity of regional anesthesia in children: a one-year prospective survey of the French-Language Society of Pediatric Anesthesiologists. Anesthesia and Analgesia 83: 904–912

37. Gilles F J, Shankle W, Dooling E C 1983 Myelinated tracts: growth patterns. In: Gilles F J, Leviton A, Dooling E C (eds) The developing human brain: growth and epidemiologic neuropathy. John Wright, Boston, pp 117–183

38. Gleiss J, Stuttgen G 1970 Morphologic and functional development of the skin. In: Stave U (ed) Physiology of the perinatal period. Appleton-Century-Crofts, New York, pp 889–906

39. Glover V, Fisk N 1996 We don't know; better to err on the safe side from midgestation. British Medical Journal (Clinical Research Ed.) 313: 796

40. Gray L, Watt L, Blass E M 2000 Skin-to-skin contact is analgesic in healthy newborns. Pediatrics 105: 14

41. Greeley W J, Debruijn N P 1998 Changes in sufentanil pharmacokinetics within the neonatal period. Anesthesia and Analgesia 67: 86–90

42. Grunau R V, Craig K D 1987 Pain expression in neonates: facial action and cry. Pain 28: 395–410

43. Grunau R V, Whitfield M F, Petrie J H 1994 Pain sensitivity and temperament in extremely low-birth-weight premature toddlers and preterm and full-term controls. Pain 58: 341–346

44. Haouari N, Wood C, Griffiths G et al 1995 The analgesic effect of sucrose in full term infants: a randomised controlled trial. British Medical Journal 310: 1498–1500

45. Henderson-Smart D J, Pettigrew A G, Campbell D J 1983 Clinical apnea and brain-stem neural function in preterm neonates. New England Journal of Medicine 308: 353–357

46. Hickey P R 1985 Blunting of the stress response in the pulmonary circulation of infants with fentanyl. Anesthesia and Analgesia 64: 1137–1141

47. Horgan M, Choonara I 1996 Measuring pain in neonates: an objective score. Paediatric Nursing 8: 24–27

48. Humphrey T 1964 Some correlations between the appearance of human fetal reflexes and the development of the nervous system. Progress in Brain Research 4: 93–135

49. Irazuzta J E, Ahmed U, Gancayco A et al 1996 Intratracheal administration of fentanyl: pharmacokinetics and local tissue effects. Intensive Care Medicine 22: 129–133

50. Izard C E, Huebner R R, Risser D et al 1980 The young infant's ability to produce discrete emotion expressions. Developmental Psychology 16: 132–140

51. Jacobson B, Eklund G, Hamberger L et al 1987 Perinatal origin of adult self-destructive behaviour. Acta Psychiatrica Scandinavica 76: 364–371

52. Jain A, Rutter N 2000 Does topical amethocaine gel reduce the pain of venepuncture in newborn infants? A randomised double blind controlled trial. Archives of Disease in Childhood, Fetal and Neonatal Edition 83: F207–F210

53. Johnston C C, Collinge J M, Henderson S J et al 1997 A cross-sectional survey of pain and pharmacological analgesia in Canadian neonatal intensive care units. Clinical Journal of Pain 13: 308–312

54. Johnston C C, Stevens B J 1996 Experience in a neonatal intensive care unit affects pain response. Pediatrics 98: 925–930

55. Kelly M A, Finer N H 1984 Nasotracheal intubation in the neonate: physiological responses and the effects of atropine and pancuronium. Journal of Pediatrics 105: 303–309

56. Koehntop D E, Rodman J H, Brundage D M et al 1986 Pharmacokinetics of fentanyl in neonates. Anesthesia and Analgesia 65: 227–232

57. Kostovic I, Rakie P 1984 Development of prestriate visual projections in the monkey and human fetal cerebrum revealed by transient cholinesterase staining. Journal of Neuroscience 4: 25–42

58. Krechel S W, Bildner J 1995 CRIES: a new neonatal postoperative pain measurement score. Initial testing of validity and reliability. Paediatric Anaesthesia 5: 53–61

59. Kupfererberg H J, Way E L 1963 Pharmacologic basis for increased sensitivity of the newborn rat to morphine. Journal of Pharmacology and Experimental Therapeutics 141: 105–112

60. Larsson B A, Lonnqvist P A, Olsson G L 1997 Plasma concentrations of bupivacaine in neonates after continuous epidural infusion. Anesthesia and Analgesia 84: 501–505

61. Lawrence J, Alcock D, McGrath P et al 1993 The development of a tool to assess neonatal pain. Neonatal Network Journal of Neonatal Nursing 12: 59–66

62. Lerman J, Strong H A, LeDez K M et al 1989 Effects of age on the serum concentration of alpha 1-acid glycoprotein and the binding of lidocaine in pediatric patients. Clinical Pharmacology and Therapeutics 46: 219–225

63. Lloyd-Thomas A R, Fitzgerald M 1996 Reflex responses do not necessarily signify pain. British Medical Journal (Clinical Research Ed.) 313: 797–798

64. Locsin R G 1981 The effect of music on the pain of selected post-operative patients. Journal of Advanced Nursing 6: 19–25

65. Marhofer P, Krenn C G, Plochl W et al 2000 S(+)-ketamine for caudal block in paediatric anaesthesia. British Journal of Anaesthesia 84: 341–345

66. Marshall R E, Stratton W C, Moore J A et al 1980 Circumcision. 1. Effects upon newborn behavior. Infant Behavior and Development 3: 1–9

67. Martinez-Telleria A, Cano Serrano M E, Martinez-Telleria M J et al 1997 [Analysis of regional anesthetic efficacy in pediatric postoperative pain.] Cirugia Pediatrica 10: 18–20

68. Masey S A, Koehler R C, Buck J R et al 1985 Effect of abdominal distention on central and regional hemodynamics in neonatal lambs. Pediatric Research 19: 1244–1249

69. McDermott C A, Kowalczyk A L, Schnitzler E R et al 1992 Pharmacokinetics of lorazepam in critically ill neonates with seizures. Journal of Pediatrics 120: 479–483

70. McRae M E, Rourke D A, Imperial-Perez F A et al 1997 Development of a research-based standard for assessment, intervention, and evaluation of pain after neonatal and pediatric cardiac surgery. Pediatric Nursing 23: 263–271

71. McRorie T I, Lynn A M, Nespeca M K et al 1992 The maturation of morphine clearance and metabolism. American Journal of Diseases of Children 146: 972–976

72. Menon G, Anand K J, McIntosh N 1998 Practical approach to analgesia and sedation in the neonatal intensive care unit. Seminars in Perinatology 22: 417–424

73. Ment L R, Vohr B, Oh W et al 1996 Neurodevelopmental outcome at 36 months' corrected age of preterm infants in the Multicenter Indomethacin Intraventricular Hemorrhage Prevention Trial. Pediatrics 98(4 Pt 1): 714–718

74. Okado N 1981 Onset of synapse formation in the human spinal cord. Journal of Comparative Neurology 201: 211–219

75. Okur H, Kucukaydin M, Ustdal K M 1995 The endocrine and metabolic response to surgical stress in the neonate. Journal of Pediatric Surgery 30: 626–630

76. Olkkolo K T, Maunuksela E L, Korpela R et al 1988 Kinetics and dynamics of postoperative morphine in children. Clinical Pharmacology and Therapeutics 44: 123–136

77. Pasternak G W, Zhang A Z, Tecoff L 1980 Developmental differences between high and low affinity opioid binding sites: their relationship to analgesia and ventilatory depression. Life Sciences 27: 1185–1190

78. Pellier I, Monrigal J P, Le Moine P et al 1999 Use of intravenous ketamine-midazolam association for pain procedures in children with cancer. A prospective study. Paediatric Anaesthesia 9: 61–68

79. Pokela M L 1994 Pain relief can reduce hypoxemia in distressed neonates during routine treatment procedures. Pediatrics 93: 379–383

80. Porter F L, Blackwell M, Miller J P 1991 Differences in developmental blood pressure regulation during lumbar puncture in newborns. Pediatric Research 29: 230

81. Porter F L, Porges S W, Marshall R E 1988 Newborn pain cries and vagal tone: parallel changes in response to circumcision. Child Development 59: 495–505

82. Reisime T, Pasternak G 1996 Opioid analgesics and antagonists. In: Hardman J G, Limbird L E, Mounoff P B et al (eds) Goodman and Gilman's: The pharmacological basis of therapeutics. McGraw-Hill, New York, pp 521–555

83. Rizvi T A, Wadhwa S, Mehra R D et al 1986 Ultrastructure of marginal zone during prenatal development of human spinal cord. Experimental Brain Research 64: 483–490

84. Seron-Ferre M, Torres-Farfan C, Forcelledo M L et al 2001 The development of circadian rhythms in the fetus and neonate. Seminars in Perinatology 25: 363–370

85. Shah V, Ohlsson A 2001 Venepuncture versus heal lance for blood sampling in term neonates (Cochrane Review). Cochrane Database of Systematic Reviews (2): CD0001452

86. Shorter N A, Liu J Y, Mooney D P et al 1999 Indomethacin-associated bowel perforations: a study of possible risk factors. Journal of Pediatric Surgery 34: 442–444

87. Stevens B, Johnston C, Petryshen P et al 1996 Premature Infant Pain Profile: development and initial validation. Clinical Journal of Pain 12: 13–22

88. Stevens B, Ohlsson A 2001 Sucrose for analgesia in newborn infants undergoing painful procedures (Cochrane Review). Cochrane Database of Systematic Reviews (4): CD001069

89. Strafford M A, Wilder R T, Berde C B 1995 The risk of infection from epidural analgesia in children: a review of 1620 cases. Anesthesia and Analgesia 80: 234–238

90. Suresh S, Anand K J 1998 Opioid tolerance in neonates: mechanisms, diagnosis, assessment, and management. Seminars in Perinatology 22: 425–433

91. Szawarski Z 1996 Probably no pain in the absence of self. British Medical Journal (Clinical Research Ed.) 313: 796–797

92. Taddio A, Katz J, Ilersich A L et al 1997 Effects of neonatal circumcision on pain response during subsequent routine vaccination. Lancet 349: 599–603

93. Taddio A, Ohlsson A, Einarson T R et al 1998 A systematic review of lidocaine-prilocaine cream (EMLA) in the treatment of acute pain in neonates. Pediatrics 101: E1

94. Taddio A, Ohlsson K, Ohlsson A 2000 Lidocaine-prilocaine cream for analgesia during circumcision in newborn boys. Cochrane Database of Systematic Reviews (2): CD000496

95. Teixeira J, Fogliani R 1996 Fetal haemodynamic stress response to invasive procedures. Lancet 347: 524

96. Torres F, Anderson C 1985 The normal EEG of the human newborn. Journal of Clinical Neurophysiology 2: 89–103

97. Truog R, Anand K J 1989 Management of pain in the postoperative neonate. Clinics in Perinatology 16: 61–78

98. Uguralp S, Mutus M, Koroglu A et al 2002 Regional anesthesia is a good alternative to general anesthesia in pediatric surgery: experience in 1,554 children. Journal of Pediatric Surgery 37: 610–613

99. Valman H B, Pearson J F 1980 What the fetus feels. British Medical Journal (Clinical Research Ed.) 280: 233–234

100. van Lingen R A, Deinum J T, Quak J M et al 1999 Pharmacokinetics and metabolism of rectally administered paracetamol in preterm neonates. Archives of Disease in Childhood. Fetal and Neonatal Edition 80: F59–F63

101. Van Overmeire B, Smets K, Lecoutere D et al 2000 A comparison of ibuprofen and indomethacin for closure of patent ductus arteriosus. New England Journal of Medicine 343: 674–681

102. Williams D G, Hatch D J, Howard R F 2001 Codeine phosphate in paediatric medicine. British Journal of Anaesthesia 86: 413–421

103. Wolf A R, Doyle E, Thomas E 1998 Modifying infant stress responses to major surgery: spinal vs extradural vs opioid analgesia. Paediatric Anaesthesia 8: 305–311

104. Wolf A R, Hughes D 1993 Pain relief for infants undergoing abdominal surgery: comparison of infusions of i.v. morphine and extradural bupivacaine. British Journal of Anaesthesia 70: 10–16

CHAPTER 26

The baby of a substance-abusing mother

Rodney Rivers

The spread of illicit drug use from the developed to many of the developing countries is resulting in a worldwide increase in drug abuse. A survey carried out in 1995 revealed a concerning level of involvement by the young. In the annual report (2001) on the UK drug situation to the European Monitoring Commission on dangerous drugs, among people aged 16–29, 25% had reported using drugs in the previous year with over 500 000 of 16–24 year olds using class A drugs in the year 2000. Regional differences are apparent, with relatively greater use of ecstasy, diazepam and cocaine in Scotland.[19] In the USA it is believed that about 3% of the 4.1 million drug-abusing women of childbearing age in the 1995 and 1996 survey continue drug use during pregnancy.

Because of associated polydrug use, including alcohol, the attribution of a causal relationship between fetal drug exposure and a neonatal outcome measure becomes difficult; self-reporting in pregnancy is also unreliable. Attribution of long-term outcome measures to fetal drug exposure becomes even more problematic because of the difficulty of controlling for complications arising in pregnancy, including abruptio placenta, poor health, squalid accommodation, unemployment and poverty on a background of unsatisfactory relationships, periods of imprisonment and social instability. Malnutrition, chronic pelvic infection, human immunodeficiency virus (HIV) and hepatitis B, C and D may further contribute to an inability of a mother to provide appropriate child care. Finally, the selection of positive associations rather than negative ones for publication influences the readership's perception of the effects of drugs on the fetus and child.[42] Can one ever be certain that so-called normal controls have not been exposed to any 'recreational' drugs during pregnancy? Use of neuroactive drugs in pregnancy may result in a withdrawal syndrome in the newborn consequent upon the deprivation following birth. The hallmark of neonatal withdrawal, as highlighted by Volpe, is the dramatic movement disorder, jitteriness.[83] Drugs used by substance-abusing women that have been associated with neonatal withdrawal syndromes are listed in Table 26.1 and those associated with withdrawal seizures in Table 26.2.

Table 26.1 Drugs described as being associated with a neonatal withdrawal syndrome

Drug	Time of onset of withdrawal
Heroin	0–96 hours – peak 12–24 hours
Methadone	12 to >72 hours – peak 24–48 hours (can be up to 7 days)
Barbiturates	
Shorter-acting	0–24 hours
Longer-acting	≥7 days
Diazepam	2–6 hours
Chlordiazepoxide	3 weeks
Tricyclic antidepressants	0–12 hours
Propoxyphene	<24 hours
Pentazocine	<24 hours
Codeine	<24 hours
Dihydrocodeine (DF 118)	<48 hours
Alcohol	<24 hours
OxyContin	<24 hours

Table 26.2 Neonatal seizures following passive addiction

- Opiates
- Opioids
- Barbiturates – shorter-acting
- Tricyclic antidepressants
- Propoxyphene
- Alcohol

Narcotics

Opiates

Heroin has high lipid and membrane solubility and is hydrolysed to morphine. Morphine itself, the component of the opium poppy with most analgesic activity, is principally metabolised to 3- and 6-morphine glucuronides (M3G, M6G) and to codeine. Following morphine dosing, the ratio of M3G to M6G is similar in the plasma of newborns and older children. However, since M3G is larger and more polar than morphine, placental transfer of fetally formed metabolite to the maternal circulation is likely to be restricted and fetal accumulation will occur.[58] M6G has some 37 times the analgesic effect of morphine sulphate but M3G has excitatory effects. In the newborn, although M3G excitation may be blocked by receptor occupancy by morphine,[35] as the morphine level falls, M3G becomes a potential cause of seizures.[59] This may partly explain why morphine is the drug of choice in heroin abstinence withdrawal seizures.[85]

Chronic opiate exposure

Chronic opiate exposure in animals[68] and primates[24] results in changes in the cells of the major noradrenergic nucleus of the brain stem, the locus ceruleus (LC). Upregulation of cyclic adenosine monophosphate (cAMP), protein phosphorylation and enhanced nuclear c-*fos* proto-oncogene expression[29] result in alterations in neuronal metabolism and excitability.[53] Increased sensitivity at postsynaptic and beta-adrenergic receptors innervated by the LC in thalamus, hypothalamus, spinal cord and cerebral cortex is reported.

Opiate withdrawal

On withdrawal or inhibition by an opiate antagonist, increased LC neurone firing causes adrenaline (epinephrine) depletion at 48–72 hours in the dog[26] and is associated with hypertension, a fall in heart rate, pH and PaO_2, and with defaecation in the fetal sheep.[8] In human pregnancy, raised levels of adrenaline (epinephrine) from the fetal adrenal and of noradrenaline (norepinephrine) from fetal sympathetic nervous system activation have been found in amniotic fluid during maternal opiate withdrawal, these changes being reversed by increasing the maternal methadone dosage.[91] The increased firing of LC neurones in the rat is paralleled by the behavioural signs of withdrawal[68] and the syndrome, deriving from LC neuronal representation throughout the neuraxis, can be suppressed by the action of the α_2-agonist clonidine.[1]

Opiates in pregnancy

The problems posed by narcotic use in pregnancy have been outlined.[32] The aim must be to reduce fetal exposure to fluctuating drug levels and repeated episodes of 'withdrawal' by replacing heroin, with its short half-life, by a cross-tolerant synthetic drug such as methadone or buprenorphine.[36] Randomised trials of methadone maintenance programs have been shown to reduce heroin use, mortality and criminality[84] and in pregnancy to result in higher mean birthweights and larger head circumferences. Taken orally, methadone has high bioavailability and a long half-life (20–30 hours), being metabolised in the liver. However, the higher the fetal plasma level is at birth the more rapid the initial fall and the more severe the neonatal withdrawal.[14] In a study in which babies were grouped by severity of withdrawal, the plasma half-life of methadone was 16 hours in the severe group and 23 hours in the mild withdrawing group; signs of withdrawal did not develop while methadone levels were above 0.06 micrograms/ml.[72]

Maternal dose at delivery does not always correlate with withdrawal severity,[15,72] although in general the lower the maternal methadone intake the lower the incidence and severity of the neonatal withdrawal. Although a maternal intake of less than 20 mg/day may be sought to achieve a better outcome and a shorter period of neonatal hospital supervision, there is always concern that illicit drugs may be utilised to counter the effects of the dose reduction.[47,63,77] Some success has been achieved with discontinuation of methadone in pregnancy[46] but this must always be balanced against the risk of a resumption of illicit drug use and fetal instability with signs of withdrawal including fetal hyperactivity, tachycardia on cardiotocography and stillbirth.

The neonate

Infants born to mothers abusing heroin tend to be of low birthweight and to demonstrate a withdrawal syndrome.[28] Some 50% will be less than 2500 g at birth and 45–70% are below the 10th percentile for gestational age. The intrauterine growth retardation is frequently symmetrical, implying a disturbance of brain growth with as many as 40% having head circumference measurements of below the 10th percentile; causation, as indicated above, is likely to be multifactorial.[83] In a comparison of methadone versus high-dose buprenorphine in pregnancy, high-dose buprenorphine was associated with a lower preterm delivery rate and a shorter time to peak neonatal withdrawal score than methadone.[44] Withdrawal may also be shorter following buprenorphine exposure.

Pregnancy-related substitution programmes

The success of antenatally directed drug substitution programmes using methadone and, more recently, buprenorphine, have been consistently reported.[10] The incidence of low birthweight and of severe neonatal withdrawal have been reduced and improved parenting has also been reported.[51] Continuation of care via a special postnatal follow-up clinic has enabled babies to be discharged on medication rather than having to remain in hospital until weaned off therapy.[56] The consistent approach that such clinics can provide is exemplified by the experience at the Wirral Hospital on Merseyside, where in 1996 a prioritised, sequential reduction and elimination of alcohol, cocaine, benzodiazepines and heroin with methadone substitution led to a reduction in the need for admission to the neonatal unit of the babies of abusing mothers for neonatal withdrawal management from 50% to 15% by 1997 (J L Robertson, personal communication, 1998).

Substitution programmes in the UK may account for much of methadone usage. Babies born to mothers on methadone may be below 2500 g at birth (10–35%), up to 40% being small for gestational age. The neonatal withdrawal syndrome can be particularly severe and occurs in 60–95%.[38,83] A correlation between methadone dosage at delivery, withdrawal severity, length of stay and duration of treatment has been reported,[48] although previous workers found no correlation between the severity of withdrawal and maternal dose.[28] Withdrawal signs occur later (day 2 and 3) than with heroin, with some only becoming severe by 10–14 days. Delayed withdrawal may relate to maternal use of benzodiazepines or other drugs.[78] Duration of withdrawal is longer and seizures more frequent with methadone than with heroin, occurring in 8% of one series (ten of 127) at a mean age of onset of 10 days. Electroencephalographic paroxysmal activity may precede or accompany observed seizures[31] and nutritive sucking can be profoundly affected.[43] With intervention, hyperphagia and excessive weight gain have been observed, apparently unrelated to withdrawal severity or maternal drug dosage.[49]

Opiate withdrawal syndrome

This occurs in 60–90% of babies in reported series although it is highly probable that many mildly affected infants go unrecognised. Clinically evident withdrawal is more likely in the term than the preterm infant.[15] Both in rats and humans, it would seem that the gestationally related behavioural repertoire may affect the apparent incidence of withdrawal (Table 26.3).[37] The absence of withdrawal behaviour should not lead to the assumption that a preterm infant does not undergo withdrawal, as evidenced by the findings during fetal withdrawal.[91]

Initial signs relate to central nervous system disturbance and are dominated by a very stimulus-sensitive, rhythmic tremulousness, which is stopped by the passive flexion of the part involved. In contrast to seizures, as emphasised by Volpe,[83] these movements are not accompanied by clonic jerks or abnormalities of gaze or eye deviation. Excessive alertness, agitation, activity and hypertonia become evident, with frantic sucking of fingers and hands. This is in contrast to the reduced level of consciousness associated with the jitteriness of hypoxic ischaemic injury, of hypoglycaemia and of polycythaemia. In spite of the sucking behaviour, coordination of sucking and swallowing is disorganised, regurgitation and vomiting are common and diarrhoea may develop by day 4–6. Seizures occur in some 2–11% of cases[31,40] but may relate to accompanying conditions or even to treatment (e.g. chlorpromazine). Their occurrence demands full investigation. Abnormal electroencephalograms without overt seizures have been reported in over 30%.[80] In the preterm baby, it has been thought that withdrawal is more likely to be manifested by higher scores for tremor, high-pitched cry, tachypnoea and poor feeding with less sleep disturbance, fever, diarrhoea, hypertonia and hyperreflexia than in term infants. It has therefore been suggested that they might benefit from the application of a different withdrawal scoring system. Extrapolating from the fetal evidence, the development of hypertension might be an indication of withdrawal.

Differential diagnosis

Withdrawal signs are non-specific; infections, metabolic and electrolyte derangements and focal central nervous system pathology

Table 26.3 Neonatal heroin withdrawal syndrome

	Moderate (%)	Severe (%)	Convulsions (%)
Term	50	16	7.3
Preterm	21	0	2.9

Severity of withdrawal in relation to gestational age in 178 infants. (From Doberczak et al 1991.[15])

must be sought and polycythaemia excluded. Infection with syphilis, gonorrhoea or chlamydia may become manifest. Vigilance is required if other diagnoses are not to be missed.

Management

When opiate use is revealed, the constellation of withdrawal signs in the baby is readily recognised (Table 26.4). The appearance of this range of signs in a young infant should always alert carers to the possibility of drug withdrawal as a cause, even in the face of maternal denial. Analysis of both urine and meconium may reveal evidence of in-utero drug exposure.[61] The lack of controlled trials and of comparisons between former treatments and the currently favoured morphine or methadone is recognised.[79]

Several scoring systems have been developed, although all are open to the problems of observer subjectivity. Their use does, however, introduce a degree of objectivity, thereby helping to determine when pharmacological intervention is required, as well as providing a basis for increasing or reducing the dosage of the drug being administered. In the USA, more reliance is placed on supportive treatment. A detailed appraisal of the various drugs that have been used has been published by the Committee on Drugs of the American Academy of Pediatrics, together with recommendations.[52] Whether it is appropriate to delay treatment when signs of brain excitation are evident, as is implied in the recommendations, can be questioned in the light of published research on the deleterious effects of brain excitation on neurodevelopment, neuronal migration and synapse formation.

On the basis that the central nervous system excitation is the most undesirable feature of withdrawal and that signs of this precede the appearance of autonomic sequelae, a scoring system was developed[70] that is weighted towards the central neurologically based signs, treatment being commenced with a score of 6 or more on two successive occasions, 2–4 hours apart (Fig. 26.1). The importance of investigating for alternative explanations of the observed abnormalities cannot be overemphasised.

Several scoring systems of varying complexity exist. They aim to reduce interobserver score variability by utilising grading systems. One such scoring system, modified from that of Finnegan

Table 26.4 Signs of opiate withdrawal

Central nervous system	Gastrointestinal	Other
Jitteriness	Regurgitation	Snuffles
Irritability	Vomiting	Sneezing
Shrill cry	Diarrhoea	Salivation
Hyperactivity		Tachypnoea
Hypertonia		Yawning
Increased wakefulness		Hiccoughs
Excessive sucking		Sweating
Poor feeding		Fever/temperature
Exaggerated Moro		instability
reflex		Poor weight gain
Seizures		

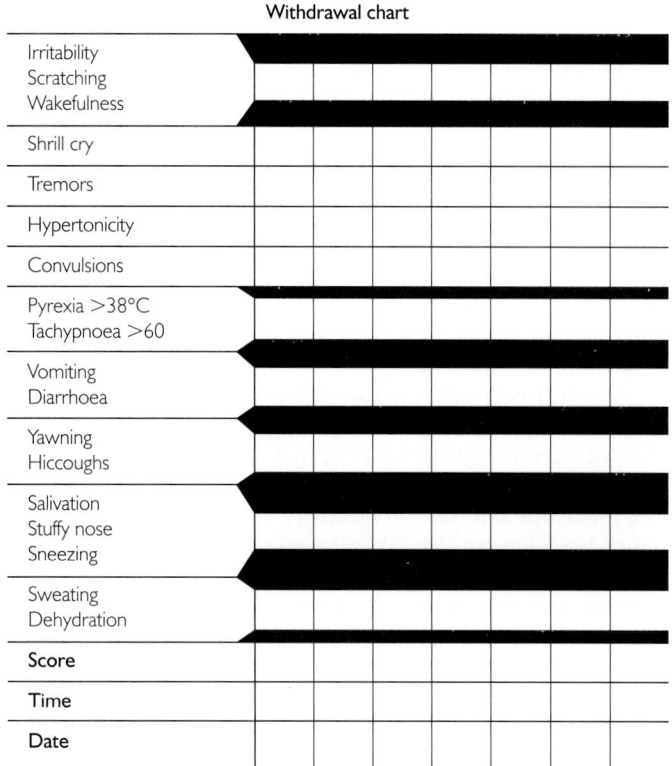

Withdrawal chart

Irritability Scratching Wakefulness								
Shrill cry								
Tremors								
Hypertonicity								
Convulsions								
Pyrexia >38°C Tachypnoea >60								
Vomiting Diarrhoea								
Yawning Hiccoughs								
Salivation Stuffy nose Sneezing								
Sweating Dehydration								
Score								
Time								
Date								

Fig. 26.1 Severity of drug withdrawal score chart based on clinical observations. Each square at the time a baby is assessed may receive a score of 0 or 1. Only one item in any of the groups of items needs to be present for a score of 1 to be awarded. The maximum total score at a given time is therefore 10. Scores are recorded 2–4-hourly.

and having the benefit of relative simplicity, grades certain observations – e.g. 'Sleeps <1 or <2 or <3 hours after feeds' scoring 1, 2 or 3 – and distinguishes tremors when disturbed from those occurring when undisturbed. Together with other items, treatment is commenced with scores of 8 or above on three occasions each 4 hours apart.[73]

The accuracy with which scoring charts are completed is likely to be dependent on many factors including staff training and staff:mother ratios on postnatal wards, where scoring for withdrawal is usually initiated. A case can be made for simplicity on postnatal wards to ensure that staff become alerted to a baby needing closer supervision and possible intervention while perhaps using a more discriminating score chart on the neonatal unit if staff numbers and training levels in the use of the system permit. In the final analysis, scoring systems are inherently subjective and staff need training in their use. Comparisons of the simultaneous use of different scoring systems in relation to frequency of therapeutic intervention and outcome are not available.

General care of the infant

These babies are at risk of meconium aspiration and the consequences of preterm delivery and poor intrauterine growth in addition to withdrawal itself.[62] At delivery, naloxone is contraindicated: it has provoked withdrawal seizures in a neonate who responded

Table 26.5 Seizure outcome by year in neonates requiring drug therapy for opiate withdrawal

Year	Number of cases	Withdrawal therapy	Seizures (cases)	Seizure therapy
1987	10	C	1	Mo
1988	9	C	3	≠C
			2	Mo
1989	8	C	1	Mo
1990	2	C	0	–
1991	7	C	2	D
1992	2	C	1	Mo
1993	4	C	2	Mo
1994	6	C: 2	2	Mo
		Me: 3	0	–
		Mo: 1	0	–
1995	4	Me	0	–
1996–2002	>20	Me	0	–

Of 44 treated with chlorpromazine, 14 developed seizures.
C = chlorpromazine; Mo = morphine; Me = methadone; D = diazepam.

to morphine.[22a] Since studies on the efficacy of stimulus-reduction have shown little beneficial effect on withdrawal,[69] appropriate drug therapy, hydration and provision of nutrients are the cornerstones of management. Additional considerations are the provision of antenatal and postnatal therapy to reduce HIV acquisition, when a mother is infected, and hepatitis B protection.

Drug treatment of withdrawal

The introduction of an opiate when signs of significant central neurological disturbance develop will usually prevent the emergence of the later signs described above. Although the four most used drugs in treatment have been paregoric, phenobarbital (phenobarbitone), diazepam and chlorpromazine,[9] these have been superseded either by the use of the intravenous formulation of methadone, given orally,[32] or by the use of oral morphine. Methadone prevents withdrawal seizures, unlike phenobarbital (phenobarbitone) and diazepam, which ironically were often ineffectual.

Although in practice there may be little to choose between oral methadone and oral morphine, the reasons for replacing the formerly used drugs with the preferred methadone include less predictable or undesirable pharmacokinetics (variable absorption – oral morphine, delayed excretion – diazepam and chlorpromazine) and depression of feeding and production of oversedation (phenobarbital (phenobarbitone), diazepam, chlorpromazine). There is an increased seizure risk with chlorpromazine and potential side effects from other components in the formulations used including alcohol, benzoic acid (interference with albumin/bilirubin binding), phenol, sodium bisulfite (anaphylaxis in older patients) and propylene glycol (hyperosmolality in the newborn).

One unit's experience of the occurrence of seizures in term babies on chlorpromazine therapy for opiate withdrawal is shown in Table 26.5. Since converting from chlorpromazine to methadone in 1993, term babies have been treated for opiate withdrawal with methadone under the author's supervision and no opiate withdrawal-related seizures have been encountered. In the period 1987–1993 all babies with seizures on chlorpromazine who were treated with morphine had immediate cessation of seizures; control of seizures with diazepam was less satisfactory. It is noteworthy that, at the time of seizure occurrences, other signs of withdrawal were minimal.

Treatment regimen

A proposed algorithm is shown in Fig. 26.2. With repeated withdrawal scores of 6 and above, oral methadone is commenced at 6-hourly intervals until control is achieved (score 5 or less), commencing at 0.1 mg/kg/dose orally and increasing stepwise every 6 hours by 0.05 mg/kg. With control, the total administered over the preceding 24 hours is divided twice daily for the succeeding 24 hours (doses at noon and midnight) and, providing control remains satisfactory (score <5), dose reductions are made by 20% each day until 0.05 mg/dose has been reached. Dose reduction has then often to be lessened to 0.005 mg/day if excessive agitation is to be avoided. On cessation of treatment, the baby is observed for any significant relapse (continuous score >5) for a further 48 hours. Administering a dose twice daily rather than once daily appears to reduce undesirable oversedation as well as preventing the emergence of agitation before the next dose is due.

Seizures would be best treated by a single dose of parenteral methadone (0.25 mg/kg) or morphine (0.15 mg/kg) followed by maintenance therapy but have not been observed with the above regimen. A failure of opiate to control seizures could result from other drug withdrawal (e.g. barbiturates, alcohol) or other causes, and uncontrolled seizures should be further investigated and treated with phenobarbital (phenobarbitone). Monitoring for apnoea should be maintained in the early stages of stabilisation.

These recommendations are based on the observation that a score of 6 achieved as a 'one-off' may sometimes be recorded on a single occasion only and such babies may go on to avoid drug treatment altogether. However, two scores of 6 or a rising score of more than 6 is indicative of severe withdrawal. Recordings of withdrawal status tend to be made more frequently during obvious withdrawal because these babies are not easily ignored; to ensure that a score of 6 is not a 'one-off,' further assessment 2–4 hours later is recommended before commencing drug treatment.

Because of the sequential nature of the development of signs of withdrawal, a baby scoring 6 or more on sequential occasions would inevitably be manifesting significant neurobehavioural disturbance. A reduction in treatment dosage should not be commenced until withdrawal is under control (score <5).

Dosing at 12 midnight and 12 noon allows adjustments in dosage to be made on the morning ward round against the knowledge of the withdrawal scores following previous dose reduction or dose increase instigated at noon the day before.

The specialised follow-up clinic reported from Australia enabled discharge on continuing treatment to be achieved. Only very gradual withdrawal of oral morphine was practised so that the duration of morphine exposure was significantly longer than during a previous period of hospital care (60 versus 17 days, $p = 0.0001$).[56]

Withdrawal score/monitoring	Intervention
≤5 ↓	Normal newborn care Low stimulation environment No drug intervention
≥6 × 2, 2–4 hours apart ↓	Commence oral methadone
≥6 on 2–4 hourly assessments	Stepwise ↑ in methadone dosage every 6 hours
↓ ≤5 × 2 on 2–4 hourly assessments	Stabilise dosage giving the total of the previous 24 hours as a divided dose, twice daily, at noon and 12 midnight. Giving this regime for 48 hours
↓ <5	Commence reducing dosage every 24 hours by 20% each day
↓ ≥6 × 2, 2–4 hours apart	Increase dosage to that given before the last dose reduction
↓ ≥6 × 2, 2–4 hours apart	Increase dosage further
↓ <5	Recommence reducing dose on a daily basis
↓ <5	If dose reduction has been difficult, when dose is 0.05 mg/dose twice daily, reduce by 0.005 mg/day in order to avoid excessive agitation, until cessation of treatment
↓ <5	Observe 48 hours following discontinuation of treatment
↓ ≥6 × 2, 2–4 hours apart	Recommence at 0.005 mg/kg twice daily Consider possibility of benzo withdrawal
↓ <5	Reduce dosage as above (0.005 mg/day) Observe 48 hours following discontinuation of treatment

Fig. 26.2 Oral methadone regimen for opiate/methadone withdrawal.

Outcome

If withdrawal is recognised for what it is, babies should no longer die from it. In one of the more dramatic case descriptions,[65] a woman with two normal children, who had acquired the 'opium habit' having been prescribed opium to prevent a miscarriage in her third pregnancy, went on to have 15 neonatal deaths, all occurring within 3 days of birth from opiate withdrawal. Only with her 18th pregnancy was the baby prescribed paregoric to protect the infant from the 'shock' of withdrawal. The baby survived.

Among more recent reports of neonatal death, the mortality does not appear to be necessarily related to withdrawal.[22,23,63,88] A subacute withdrawal syndrome is recognised, which, if it occurs after discharge home, may tax the parents to the limits of their tolerance; this is especially likely if the baby fails to sleep, is difficult to feed or makes apparently excessive demands for milk, suffering severe colic and vomiting. In some, these features may persist for several months and a small dose of diazepam may be prescribed with benefit, initially under supervision following re-hospitalisation. Frequent home visiting by a designated health visitor can ensure that late withdrawal is recognised and appropriately managed.

Postnatal growth has been reported to show some catch-up, but persistent weight retardation at 12 months has been shown to correlate with methadone dosage in the pregnancy.[81] Prenatal and infancy nurse home visit programmes have been shown to reduce the number of observed hazards for children in the home, to result in fewer injuries and to reduce visits to the emergency department in socially deprived families[57] but not convincingly in homes of drug abusing mothers.

Breastfeeding

This is not usually recommended for mothers on heroin, as high peak blood levels are reflected in breast milk heroin concentrations. However, mothers on methadone, codeine or morphine, when appropriately prescribed, may be recommended to take their medication after completion of a breastfeed. Undetectable or only very low plasma levels of methadone have been found in the babies of mothers whose doses of methadone are between 20 and 80 mg/24 hours, these plasma levels reflecting a mean methadone milk:plasma ratio of 0.44; they are quite insufficient to prevent the neonatal withdrawal syndrome.[87] Breastfeeding is therefore not contraindicated. The poor initial weight gain associated with withdrawal, possibly deriving from increased neonatal energy expenditure, may be improved by calorie supplementation. Hyperphagia[49] may result in the need for top-up formula feeds.

Discharging home on medication

A favourable report on the experience derived from a multidisciplinary follow-up clinic set up to follow up babies discharged after stabilisation on oral morphine has been published from Australia.[56] In a retrospective study comparing a group of 17 early discharges with a historic control group of 60, the duration of hospital stay was reduced from a mean of 7.8 days to 5.4 days ($p < 0.01$). Follow-up was achieved in all but one case. The success of such a policy would depend on many factors, including the motivation and mobility of the population under study.

Sudden infant death syndrome

A number of studies have reported an increased risk of this, particularly following moderate or severe withdrawal.[39] It may be difficult to differentiate true sudden infant death syndrome from babies dying from neglect relative to their needs or from unrecognised infections.

Neurodevelopment

In spite of recently reviewed animal studies pointing to disordered neuronal and glial proliferation following in-utero opiate exposure,[83] published human follow-up studies, with all their methodological difficulties,[27] suggest that by 2 years of age and at school entry age there may be no delay.[86] However, intrauterine growth retardation, toxic compounds in street drug preparations, alcohol exposure, postnatal undernutrition and lack of social stimulation may all have additional subtle effects on the final intellectual performance and social integration of surviving infants.

Cocaine

Effects

Cocaine use in pregnancy has become a major concern.[30] The effects on the fetus and neonate have been extensively discussed,[82] although the scientific validity of some of the reported associations has been questioned because of inadequate recruitment of controls.[50] Causal relationships can be difficult to prove[54,67] but, from the increasing body of available data, it seems probable that disruption of brain architecture and possibly of long-term functioning could result from human fetal exposure. Disentangling the interrelationships between the biologic and social factors remains a target for future research.[74,89]

The extent of cocaine usage in the UK during pregnancy remains unknown. The unreliability of interviewing techniques and of maternal urine testing (positive only for 24 hours following administration)[90] mitigate against the acquisition of firm data both on the number of fetuses being exposed and on the severity of individual exposure. Neonatally derived urine is positive for cocaine between 12 and 24 hours from the time of last fetal exposure, with the metabolite benzoylecgonine being detectable for up to 7 days.[60] Although results of screening by analysis of meconium have been reported,[61] if it is exposure to high concentrations that poses most risk, mere detection will not help to predict outcome. Hair analysis can be informative on duration of exposure.[4] Reduced activity of plasma cholinesterase in the fetus and during infancy delays the metabolism of cocaine.[76]

Cocaine as water-soluble cocaine hydrochloride is taken by nasal insufflation, by mouth or intravenously; following alkali extraction, as heat-stable cocaine alkaloid (crack), it is inhaled as vapour on heating. Cocaine's pharmacological effects arise from blockading catecholamine, dopamine and tryptophan uptake, leading to prolonged sympathetic nervous stimulation with hypertension and vasoconstriction. Reduced serotonin synthesis may explain the alterations in sleep–wake cycling and reduced sleep requirements of affected babies.[21] A plasma catecholamine precursor and cerebrospinal fluid catecholamine levels[51] are raised in cocaine-exposed newborns. Some of the described clinical associations

Table 26.6 Effects of cocaine on fetus and newborn

Observation	Putative mechanisms
Uterine stimulation	1. Catecholamines
Placental abruption	2. Direct effect on myometrium
Preterm birth	
Fetal hypoxia, death	3. Catecholamine-induced vasoconstriction of materno-fetal unit
Intrauterine growth retardation	
Low birthweight	4. Increased fetal metabolic rate
Intermittent hypoxia	1
Diminished head circumference for gestation	3 & 4 above Impaired neuronal proliferation, migration and differentiation
Abnormalities of central nervous system development	
Intraventricular and parenchymal haemorrhage/infarction	Disturbed autoregulation Hypertensive episodes Ischaemic, vasoconstrictive episodes
Meconium staining of liquor	Sympathetic activation
Necrotising enterocolitis	Sympathetic activation
Limb reduction defects	Vasoconstrictive episodes
Gut atresias	
Myocardial ischaemia	

of cocaine use in pregnancy and their possible mechanisms are shown in Table 26.6. Confounding effects of other drugs, alcohol exposure and smoking are difficult to determine. Morphological changes in neuronal differentiation have been found in adult rats exposed to cocaine in utero,[25] and exaggeration of the deleterious effects of hypoxia by the presence of cocaine is reported.[75]

Cocaine may be present at birth or may be derived postnatally in breast milk[7] or from a nipple if topically applied as an analgesic.[5] Although the excessive sympathetic pathway activity of opiate withdrawal occurs as the opiate levels decline, with cocaine, maximal sympathetic activity is seen at around its peak level. Abnormal sleep patterns are noted, with tremors and hypertonia being particularly prominent together with long dull–alert periods of poor visual responsiveness but with the eyes open.[60]

Seizures caused by cocaine are well recognised in adults and have been seen in exposed toddlers and infants.[3,71] Abnormalities of the electroencephalogram have been recorded.[16] Increased anterior cerebral artery blood flow consistent with the vasoconstrictive effects of the drug have been reported.[41] Persisting hypertension was found in one small study.[33] The problems of small studies and confounding variables occur repeatedly in the literature. Although cocaine withdrawal is recognised in adults and can be induced in rats, it has been difficult to disentangle neonatal cocaine effects from possible withdrawal. Until recently, studies have generally not observed behavioural patterns different from those in control term newborns.[20] In a carefully designed multicentre study comparing central nervous system and autonomic manifestations in control babies with babies following fetal exposure to cocaine,

or to cocaine plus opiates, jitteriness was seen in 14.6% and irritability in 12.2% of cocaine-only-exposed babies (controls 5.9% and 5.8% respectively.)[2] The period of observation however was short and later manifestations of the exposure would not have been detected. A dose effect on neurobehavioral performance has also been reported.

Management

Usually no intervention is required; since breast feeding shortly after crack use can cause seizures,[7] it would seem prudent to discourage breast feeding in known crack users.

Outcome

Variable increases in sudden infant death syndrome with an overall risk of 8.5/1000 have been calculated from available reports; these reports have, however, been challenged.[50] Impaired respiratory and arousal responses have been cited as being of possible relevance;[11] heart rate variability is also increased.[69]

As regards the more global effects of cocaine on the fetal brain, a correlation between small head size, cocaine exposure and developmental scores has been reported,[7] although many of the cases were lost to follow-up. If the establishment of interneuronal connections is dependent on grouped repetitious patterns of neuronal stimulation,[18] then attention span, social stimulation and the child's own directed motivation will all have an impact upon brain development. Deficits leading to impulsiveness, deviant behaviour and inability to respond to normal educative techniques will only be discernible by appropriate longitudinal long-term testing. Poorer novelty preference performance in follow up to 13 months has been demonstrated.[34]

The best hope for any fetus must be preceding, population-based, school-age and preconceptual education concerning the wide-ranging potential effects of cocaine, together with comprehensive prenatal and postnatal support programs.

Other drugs of addiction

Many drug-exposed infants must escape detection because of the mildness and non-specificity of withdrawal signs, early discharge from hospital and slow elimination of many sedative/hypnotic/anxiolytic drugs. Most withdrawal signs are similar in content to those of opiate withdrawal, although there are exceptions.

Short-acting barbiturates are associated with withdrawal seizures following jitteriness and hyperactivity while **longer-acting barbiturates** cause a withdrawal syndrome with an onset of up to 14 days that may last for months.[13]

Alcohol exposure is associated with physical stigmata in one-third of infants together with profound neurodevelopmental sequelae. Withdrawal occurs early, usually between 3 and 12 hours after delivery and is associated with hyperactivity, irritability and excessive crying; poor sucking, a disturbed sleeping pattern, tremors and seizures have also been reported.[55,66] Seizures in the first 12 hours of life are a particular feature of alcohol and tricyclic withdrawal following the development of tremulousness; seizures of either origin are best controlled with phenobarbital (phenobarbitone).

Benzodiazepines can be associated with neonatal hypotonicity and poor feeding[64] and can be responsible for a withdrawal syndrome occurring beyond 10 days of age that can be mistaken for a relapse of opiate withdrawal during weaning from opiates postnatally.

Marijuana has not been consistently shown to be associated with neonatal or developmental abnormalities.[12]

Newer drugs of abuse

OxyContin, a long-acting oxycodone, has been reported as causing neonatal withdrawal and is potentially important since it is not detected by routine enzymatic screening for opiates. A drug that is increasingly being used as a recreational drug in Europe is **gamma-hydroxybutyrate** – a form of Ecstasy – and its analogues. Chronic abuse and withdrawal are well recognised in adults;[17] paediatricians should therefore be aware of a possible neonatal withdrawal counterpart. Agitation and tremors are features described and management with benzodiazepines is recommended in adults. Withdrawal can be prolonged.

Those caring for neonates have therefore to maintain awareness of new trends in drug usage if they are to prevent withdrawal from going unrecognised or from being inappropriately investigated and managed.

Polydrug exposure

This may increase the complexity of the observed withdrawal and its management, with the combination of opiate and cocaine being reported as giving rise to a more severe withdrawal than opiates alone.[2]

Additional management issues

A plan of management applicable to the UK support agencies is shown in Fig. 26.3. This involves an antenatal planning meeting for all agencies involved in the care of the mother and baby, followed by postnatal monitoring in a transitional care facility on a postnatal ward for up to 5 days in known cocaine exposure and for up to 14 days with moderate- to high-dose methadone usage. Cranial ultrasound examinations are obtained and other focal lesions sought as indicated. A further planning meeting is held prior to discharge. Discharge would not be undertaken if there is evidence of infant abuse or neglect or if there is serious conflict or violence between the parents.

Drug treatment, if required, is initiated on the special care baby unit and, unless going into foster care, babies are currently only

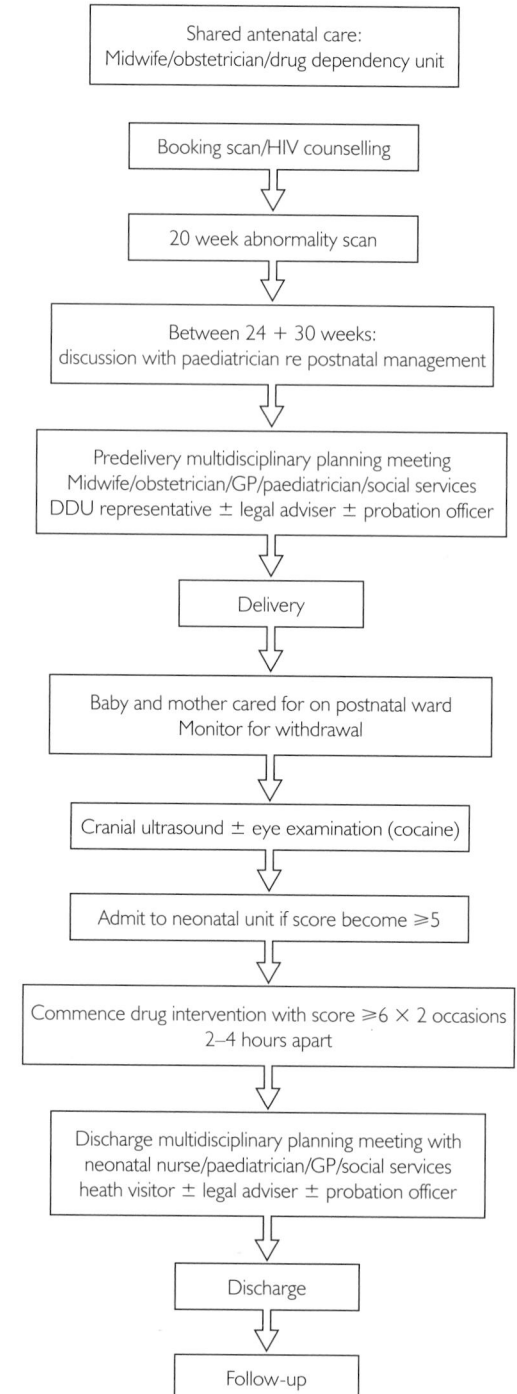

Fig. 26.3 Antenatal and postpartum plan.

rarely transferred home on continuing withdrawal treatment. Some mothers will spend a period under supervision in a mother and baby home but, once at home, their health visitor and social worker are the principal sources of surveillance, in addition to paediatric follow-up. Facilitating parental involvement when their baby provides little positive behavioural return for their efforts is an essential part of the nursing support from birth onwards.

The disorganised social lifestyle and variable involvement in criminality to fund a continuing habit create a conflict of interests with the need of a developing child for social interaction and care. These children are often very demanding and may have disorganised sleep patterns for months. The inability to separate biological from social causes of impaired growth and developmental achievements does nothing to allay the fear that these children are often exposed to persistent disadvantage. A follow-up of 85 babies at 2–13 years after discharge following treatment for opiate withdrawal after birth at a London teaching hospital between 1968 and 1983 revealed that only 25% were living with both parents, 20% were with their mother and 12% were with their father. A further 36% were with relatives, had been adopted, fostered or were in other placements. Six parents and four children had died (M J H Williams and S Cavanagh, personal communication 1986). A not dissimilar experience has been reported from France.[45] Not infrequently, well-intentioned plans for providing family support have to be reversed and the children taken into care to avoid abuse or neglect.

References

1. Aghajanian G K 1978 Tolerance of locus coeruleus neurons to morphine and suppression of withdrawal in response to clonidine. Nature 276: 186–188
2. Bada H S, Bauer C R, Shankaran S et al 2002 Central and autonomic system signs with in utero drug exposure. Archives of Disease in Childhood Fetal and Neonatal Edition 87: F106–F112
3. Bateman D A, Heagarty M C 1989 Passive freebase cocaine ('crack') inhalation by infants and toddlers. American Journal of Diseases of Children 143: 25–27
4. Callahan C M, Grant T M, Phipps P et al 1992 Measurement of gestational cocaine exposure: sensitivity of infants' hair, meconium and urine. Journal of Pediatrics 120: 763–768
5. Chaney N E, Franke J, Wadlington W B 1988 Cocaine convulsions in a breast-feeding baby. Journal of Pediatrics 112: 134–135
6. Chasnoff I J, Griffith D R, Freier C et al 1992 Cocaine/polydrug use in pregnancy: two year follow up. Pediatrics 89: 284–289
7. Chasnoff I J, Lewis D E, Squires L 1987 Cocaine intoxication in a breast-fed infant. Pediatrics 80: 836–838
8. Cohen M S, Rudolph A M, Melmon K L 1980 Antagonism of morphine by naloxone in pregnant ewes and fetal lambs. Developmental Pharmacology and Therapeutics 1: 58–69
9. Committee on Drugs 1983 Neonatal drug withdrawal. Pediatrics 72: 895–902
10. Connaughton J F, Reeser D, Schut J et al 1977 Perinatal addiction. Outcome and management. American Journal of Obstetrics and Gynecology 129: 679–686
11. Davidson Ward S L, Bautista D, Chan L et al 1990 Sudden infant death syndrome in infants of substance-abusing mothers. Journal of Pediatrics 117: 876–881
12. Day M L, Richardson G A 1991 Prenatal marijuana use: epidemiology, methodologic issues, and infant outcome. Clinics in Perinatology 18: 77–91
13. Desmond M M, Schwanecke R R, Wilson G S et al 1972 Maternal barbiturate utilization and neonatal withdrawal symptomatology. Journal of Pediatrics 80: 192–197
14. Doberczak T M, Kandall S R, Friedmann P 1993 Relationships between maternal methadone dosage, maternal–neonatal methadone levels, and neonatal withdrawal. Obstetrics and Gynecology 81: 936–940
15. Doberczak T M, Kandall S R, Wilets I 1991 Neonatal opiate abstinence syndrome in term and preterm infants. Journal of Pediatrics 118: 933–937
16. Doberczak T, Shonzer S, Senie R et al 1988 Neonatal neurologic and EEG effects of intrauterine cocaine exposure. Journal of Pediatrics 113: 354–359
17. Doyon S 2001 The many faces of ecstasy. Current Opinion in Pediatrics 13: 170–176
18. Edelman G M 1987 Neural Darwinism. The theory of neuronal group selection. Basic Books, New York, p 308–330
19. European Drugs Monitoring Centre 2001 Annual report on the state of the Drugs problem in the European Union. European Monitoring Centre on Drugs and Drug Addiction, Lisbon. Available on line at: http://www.emcdda.org
20. Eyler F D, Behnke M, Garvan C W et al 2001 Newborn evaluations of toxicity and withdrawal related to prenatal cocaine exposure. Neurotoxicology and Teratology 23: 399–411
21. Farrar H C, Kearns G L 1989 Cocaine: clinical pharmacology and toxicology. Journal of Pediatrics 115: 665–675
22. Fricker H S, Segal S 1978 Narcotic addiction, pregnancy, and the newborn. American Journal of Diseases of Children 132: 360–366
22a. Gibbs J, Newson T, Williams J et al 1989 Naloxone hazard in infant of opioid abuser. Lancet 2: 159–160
23. Goodfriend M J, Shey I A, Milton D K 1956 The effects of maternal narcotic addiction on the newborn. American Journal of Obstetrics and Gynecology 71: 29–36
24. Grant S J, Huang Y H, Redmond D E Jr 1988 Behaviour of monkeys during opiate withdrawal and locus coeruleus stimulation. Pharmacol Biochem Behav 30: 13–19
25. Gressens P, Kosofsky B E, Evrard P 1992 Cocaine-induced disturbances of corticogenesis in the developing murine brain. Neuroscience Letters 140: 113–116
26. Gunne L-M 1962 Catecholamine metabolism in morphine withdrawal in the dog. Nature 195: 815–816
27. Hans S L, Marcus J, Jeremy R J et al 1984 Neurobehavioural development of children exposed in utero to opioid drugs. In: Yanai J (ed) Neurobehavioural teratology. Elsevier Science, Amsterdam, pp 245–273
28. Harper R G, Solish G I, Purow H M et al 1974 The effect of a methadone treatment program upon pregnant heroin addicts and their newborn infants. Pediatrics 54: 300–305
29. Hayward M D, Duman R S, Nestler E J 1990 Induction of the c-*fos* proto-oncogene during opiate withdrawal in the locus coeruleus and other brain regions of the rat brain. Brain Research 525: 256–266
30. Heagarty M C 1990 Crack cocaine. A new danger for children. American Journal of Diseases of Children 144: 756–757
31. Herzlinger R A, Kandall S R, Vaughan H G J. 1977 Neonatal seizures associated with narcotic withdrawal. Journal of Pediatrics 91: 638–641
32. Hoegerman G, Schnoll S 1991 Narcotic use in pregnancy. Clinics in Perinatology 18: 51–76
33. Horn P T 1992 Persisting hypertension after prenatal cocaine exposure. Journal of Pediatrics 121: 288–291
34. Jacobson S W, Jacobson J L, Sokol R J 1996 New evidence for neurobehavioural effects of in utero cocaine exposure. Journal of Pediatrics 129: 581–590
35. Jacquet Y F, Klee W A, Rice K C et al 1977 Stereospecific and nonstereospecific effects of + and − morphine: Evidence for a new class of receptors? Science 198: 842–845
36. Jernite M, Viville B, Escande B et al 1999 Buprenorphine and pregnancy. Analysis of 24 cases. Archives de Pediatrie 6: 1179–1185
37. Jones K L, Barr G A 1995 Ontogeny of morphine withdrawal in the rat. Behavioural Neuroscience 109: 1189–1198
38. Kandall S R, Albin S, Gartner L M et al 1977 The narcotic-dependent mother: fetal and neonatal consequences. Early Human Development 1/2: 159–169
39. Kandall S R, Gaines J, Habel L et al 1993 Relationship of maternal substance abuse to subsequent sudden infant death syndrome in offspring. Journal of Pediatrics 123: 120–126
40. Kandall S R, Gartner L M 1974 Late presentations of drug withdrawal symptoms in newborns. American Journal of Diseases of Children 127: 58–61
41. King T A, Perlman J M, Laptook A R et al 1995 Neurologic manifestations of in utero cocaine exposure in near-term and term infants. Pediatrics 96: 259–264
42. Koran G, Graham K, Shear H et al 1989 Bias against the null hypothesis: The reproductive hazards of cocaine. Lancet 2: 1440–1442
43. Kron R E, Litt M, Phoenix M D et al 1976 Neonatal narcotic abstinence: effect of pharmacotherapeutic agents and maternal drug usage on nutritive sucking behaviour. Journal of Pediatrics 88: 637–641
44. Lejeune C, Aubisson S, Simmat-Durand L et al 2001 Withdrawal syndromes of newborns of pregnant drug abusers maintained under methadone or high dose buprenorphine: 246 cases. Annales de Medicine Interne (Paris) 152(Suppl 7): 21–27
45. Lejeune C, Ropert J C, Montamat S et al 1997 Medical-social outcome of 59 infants born to addicted mothers. Journal de Gynecologie, Obstetrique et Biologie de la Reproduction (Paris) 26: 395–404
46. Maas U, Kattner E, Weingart J B et al 1990 Infrequent neonatal opiate withdrawal following maternal methadone detoxification during pregnancy. Journal of Perinatal Medicine 18: 111–118
47. Madden J D, Chappel J N, Zuspan F et al 1997 Observation and treatment of non-narcotic withdrawal. American Journal of Obstetrics and Gynecology 127: 199–201
48. Malpas T J, Darlow B A, Lennox R et al 1995 Maternal methadone dosage and neonatal withdrawal. Australian and New Zealand Journal of Obstetrics and Gynecology 35: 175–177
49. Martinez A, Kastner B, Taeusch H W 1999 Hyperphagia in neonates withdrawing from methadone. Archives of Disease in Childhood Fetal and Neonatal Edition 80: F178–F182

50. Mayes L C, Granger R H, Bornstein M H 1992 The problem of prenatal cocaine exposure. A rush to judgment. Journal of the American Medical Association 267: 406–408

51. Needlman R, Zuckerman B S, Anderson G et al 1993 CSF monoamine precursors and metabolites in human neonates following in utero cocaine exposure. Pediatrics 92: 55–60

52. American Academy of Pediatrics Committee on Drugs 1998 Neonatal drug withdrawal policy statement. Pediatrics 101: 1079–1088

53. Nestler E J 1992 Molecular mechanisms of drug addiction. Journal of Neuroscience 12: 2439–2450

54. Newspiel D R 1992 Cocaine-associated abnormalities may not be causally related. American Journal of Diseases of Children 146: 278–279

55. Nichols M M 1967 Acute alcohol withdrawal syndrome in a newborn. American Journal of Diseases of Children 113: 714–715

56. Oei J, Feller J M, Lui K 2001 Coordinated outpatient care of the narcotic-dependent infant. Journal of Pediatrics and Child Health 37: 266–270

57. Olds D L, Henderson C R Jr, Kitzman H 1994 Does prenatal and infancy nurse home visitation have enduring effects on qualities of parental caregiving and child health at 25 and 50 months of life. Pediatrics 93: 89–98

58. Olsen G D, Gasser S R, Sommer K M et al 1987 Placental permeability for morphine 3-glucuronide. In: Xth International Congress of Pharmacology Proceedings, Sydney, Australia

59. Olsen G D, Sommer K M, Wheeler P L et al 1988 Accumulation and clearance of morphine 3-β-D glucuronide in fetal lambs. Journal of Pharmacology and Experimental Therapeutics 247: 576–584

60. Oro A S, Dixon S D 1987 Perinatal cocaine and methamphetamine exposure: maternal and neonatal correlates. Journal of Pediatrics 111: 571–578

61. Ostrea E M, Brady M J, Parks P M et al 1989 Drug screening of meconium in infants of drug-dependent mothers: an alternative to urine testing. Journal of Pediatrics 115: 474–477

62. Ostrea E M, Chavez C J 1979 Perinatal problems (excluding neonatal withdrawal) in maternal drug addiction: a study of 830 cases. Journal of Pediatrics 94: 292–295

63. Ostrea E M, Chavez C J, Strauss M E 1976 A study of factors that influence the severity of neonatal narcotic withdrawal. Journal of Pediatrics 88: 642–645

64. Perault M C, Favreliere S, Minet P et al 2000 Benzodiazepines and pregnancy. Therapie 55: 587–595

65. Petty G E 1913 Narcotic drug disease and allied ailments. J A Davies, Tennessee

66. Pierog S, Chandavasu O, Wexler I 1977 Withdrawal symptoms in infants with fetal alcohol syndrome. Journal of Pediatrics 90: 630–633

67. Potter S, Klein J, Valiante G et al 1994 Maternal cocaine use without evidence of fetal exposure. Journal of Pediatrics 125: 652–654

68. Rasmussen K, Beitner-Johnson D B, Krystal J H et al 1990 Opiate withdrawal and the rat locus coeruleus: behavioural, electrophysiological and biochemical correlates. Journal of Neuroscience 10: 2308–2317

69. Regalado M G, Schechtman V L, Del Angel A P et al 1996 Cardiac and respiratory patterns during sleep in cocaine-exposed neonates. Early Human Development 44: 187–200

70. Rivers R P A 1986 Neonatal opiate withdrawal. Archives of Disease in Childhood 61: 1236–1239

71. Rivkin M, Gilmore H E 1989 Generalised seizures in an infant due to environmentally acquired cocaine. Pediatrics 84: 1100–1102

72. Rosen T S, Pippenger C E 1976 Pharmacologic observations on the neonatal withdrawal syndrome. Journal of Pediatrics 88: 1044–1048

73. Royal Prince Alfred Hospital 1998 Department of Neonatal Medicine Protocol Book: Drug withdrawal score. Available on line at: http://www.cs.nsw.gov.au/rpa/ neonatal/newprot/score.htm

74. Singer L T, Yamashita T S, Hawkins S et al 1994 Increased incidence of intraventricular hemorrhage and developmental delay in cocaine-exposed very low birthweight infants. Journal of Pediatrics 124: 765–771

75. Spraggins Y R, Seidler F J, Slotkin T A 1994 Cocaine exacerbates hypoxia-induced cell damage in the developing brain: effects on ornithine decarboxylase activity and protein synthesis. Biology of the Neonate 66: 254–266

76. Stewart D J, Inaba T, Lucassen M 1979 Cocaine metabolism: cocaine and norcocaine hydrolysis by liver and serum esterases. Clinical Pharmacology and Therapeutics 25: 464–468

77. Strauss M E, Andresko M, Stryker J C et al 1976 Relationship of neonatal withdrawal to maternal methadone dose. The American Journal of Drug and Alcohol Abuse 3: 339–345

78. Sutton L R, Hinderliter S A 1990 Diazepam abuse in pregnant women on methadone maintenance. Implications for the neonate. Clinical Pediatrics (Philadelphia) 29: 108–111

79. Theis J G W, Selby P, Ikizler Y et al 1997 Current management of the neonatal abstinence syndrome: a critical analysis of the evidence. Biology of the Neonate 71: 345–356

80. Van Baar A L, Fleury P, Soepatmi S et al 1989 Neonatal behaviour after drug-dependent pregnancy. Archives of Disease in Childhood 64: 235–240

81. Vance J C, Chant D C, Tudehope D I et al 1997 Infants born to narcotic dependent mothers: physical growth patterns in the first 12 months of life. Journal of Paediatrics and Child Health 33: 504–508

82. Volpe J J 1992 Effect of cocaine use on the fetus. New England Journal of Medicine 327: 399–407

83. Volpe J J 2001 Teratogenic effects of drugs and passive addiction. In: Neurology of the newborn, 4th edn. WB Saunders, Philadelphia, pp 859–898

84. Ward J, Mattick R P, Hall W 1992 Key issues in methadone maintenance treatment. Univ of New South Wales Press, Sydney

85. Wijburg F A, de Kleine M J K, Fleury P et al 1991 Morphine as an anti-epileptic drug in neonatal abstinence syndrome. Acta Paediatrica Scandinavica 80: 875–877

86. Wilson G S, Desmond M M, Wait R B 1981 Follow-up of methadone-treated and untreated narcotic dependent women and their infants: health, developmental, and social implications. Journal of Pediatrics 98: 716–722

87. Wojnar-Horton R E, Kristensen J H, Yapp P et al 1997 Methadone distribution and excretion into breast milk of clients in a methadone maintenance programme. British Journal of Clinical Pharmacology 44: 543–547

88. Zelson C, Rubio E, Wasserman E 1971 Neonatal narcotic addiction: 10 year observation. Pediatrics 48:178–189

89. Zuckerman B, Frank D A 1994 Prenatal cocaine exposure: 9 years later. Journal of Pediatrics 124: 731–733

90. Zuckerman B, Frank D A, Hingson R et al 1989 Effects of maternal marijuana and cocaine use on fetal growth. New England Journal of medicine. 320: 762–768

91. Zuspan F P, Gumpel J A, Mejia-Zelaya A et al 1975 Fetal stress from methadone withdrawal. American Journal of Obstetrics and Gynecology 122: 43–47

Section Five

Disorders of the Newborn

CHAPTER 27

Pulmonary disease of the newborn

PART 1

Physiology
Anne Greenough, Anthony D Milner

Introduction

Intensive care is required to support newborn infants who have been born with a respiratory system which cannot provide adequate spontaneous ventilation, usually because of immature birth, or who have failed to adapt to an extrauterine existence (as evidenced by their need for resuscitation at birth, their delayed lung fluid clearance or development of persistent pulmonary hypertension). This chapter, therefore, reviews the growth of the respiratory system before and after birth, the mechanisms responsible for the production and clearance of lung fluid, how the healthy infant achieves an expanded air-filled lung, the fetal and postnatal development of respiratory control, and the development and function of surfactant and the surfactant proteins.

Morphological development of the lung

The human fetal lung originates in the 3-week-old embryo as a ventral diverticulum that arises from the caudal end of the laryngotracheal groove of the foregut. The commitment of the foregut endoderm cell to form the lung bud is dependent on the transcription factor, hepatocyte nuclear factor 3-beta.[4] There are four major stages of lung development based on its microscopic appearance: embryonic, 3–6 weeks; pseudoglandular, 6–17 weeks; canalicular, 17–26 weeks and alveolar, 27 weeks to term. The nerves of the lung develop from neural crest cells and migrate via the vagus nerve to the future trachea and lung; there is then progressive extension of the nerve supply.[213] The bronchial tree is developed by the 16th week of gestation. Gli proteins are essential for lung branching morphogenesis.[167] During the canalicular stage of development, there is continued branching of respiratory bronchioles, vascularisation of the terminal tubules and thinning of the airway epithelium. Arteries and veins develop alongside the respiratory airways. Airway branching and pulmonary vasculogenesis involve reciprocal epithelial–mesenchyme interactions mediated by growth factors, possibly with interplay from physical stimuli.[233] Towards the end of this stage (24 weeks), pulmonary gas exchange becomes theoretically possible. By 20 to 22 weeks of gestation, both type I and type II pneumocytes can be identified. Type I cells are flattened and form over 90% of the gas-exchanging surface of the mature lung. The cuboidal type II cells have a secretory function, and from 24 weeks, osmiophilic lamellar bodies containing surfactant can be identified. From 24 weeks to term, further terminal branching occurs, with the development of saccules, which become the alveolar ducts. Although alveoli begin to appear as shallow indentations at about 32 weeks of gestation, most alveolar development occurs post term.

The lung grows postnatally mainly by an increase in alveolar number, and by 4 years of age, the adult number of alveoli is present.[220] The subsequent increase in lung volume and surface area is due to an increase in alveolar size. In the first 5 years, there is little elastin in the alveolar walls, which only extends around the alveolar walls by 18 years;[147] the early 'relative' deficiency of elastin may facilitate the increase in size of the alveoli in the growing lung. There is a two- to threefold increase in diameter and length of airways between birth and adulthood.[104] The amount of bronchial smooth muscle relative to airway size increases between birth and adulthood, the increase in the first weeks after birth being particularly rapid.

Factors influencing lung growth and development

Abnormal lung growth can be the result of inadequate space, or reduction in either fetal breathing or amniotic fluid volume. The time of onset of the insult determines which structures are affected. Prior to 16 weeks of gestation, branching of the airways is impaired permanently, which will also reduce the potential for the number of alveoli. An insult occurring later affects the number of alveoli. Space restriction can be due to an abnormality extrinsic to the lung, for example congenital diaphragmatic hernia, pleural effusion or asphyxiating thoracic dystrophy, or intrinsic to the lung, for example cystic adenomatoid malformation. Other factors influencing lung growth and development include malnutrition, particularly vitamin A deficiency,[153,154] maternal smoking[160] and glucocorticoid administration.[25]

Fetal breathing movements

Phrenic nerve or cervical cord resections which abolish fetal breathing movements (FBMs) are associated with arrest of lung growth. Fetal breathing is dependent on normal diaphragmatic function, and pulmonary hypoplasia in newborns occurs with generalised neuromuscular disorders, isolated phrenic nerve agenesis and diaphragmatic amyoplasia. During periods of FBM, rhythmical contractions of the diaphragm retard the loss of lung liquid and help to maintain lung expansion when the upper airway resistance is reduced;[108] this may be the mechanism by which FBMs preserve lung growth.

Fetal lung liquid

In fetal life the lung is filled with liquid, increasing from 4–6 ml/kg bodyweight at mid-gestation to about 20 ml/kg near term. The hourly rate of production is initially 2 ml/kg, increasing to 5 ml/kg at term. Fetal lung liquid contributes one-third to one-half to the daily turnover of amniotic fluid. Compared with either amniotic fluid or plasma, lung liquid has a high chloride, but low bicarbonate and protein concentration. The dominant force mediating lung liquid secretion is the secondary active transport of chloride ions from the interstitial space into the lung lumen (Fig. 27.1).[175] Sodium ions and water follow passively down electrical and osmotic gradients. The volume of fetal lung liquid is principally regulated by the resistance to lung liquid efflux through the upper airway and by the presence of diaphragmatic activity associated with FBMs.[108] A pressure in the lumen of the lung approximately 1 cm of water greater than that in the amniotic cavity is generated, which is essential for lung growth. The presence of lung liquid is important for normal lung development; chronic drainage results in pulmonary hypoplasia,[62] and lung fluid restriction in the embryonic rat lung affects growth but not airway branching.[212] Tracheal ligation increases fetal intrathoracic pressure and causes lung hyperplasia; this experimentally can reverse the pulmonary hypoplasia associated with oligohydramnios and congenital diaphragmatic hernia.[53,91] There is, however, concern that although tracheal ligation results in increased cell proliferation and normal-sized lungs, it may be associated with decreased surfactant production[24] and altered alveolar structure.[43]

During labour and delivery, the concentration of adrenaline increases, and, as a consequence, lung liquid secretion ceases and resorption begins. Fetal lung liquid absorption is via activation or opening of sodium channels on the apical surface of the pulmonary epithelium.[110] Thyroid hormone and cortisol are necessary for

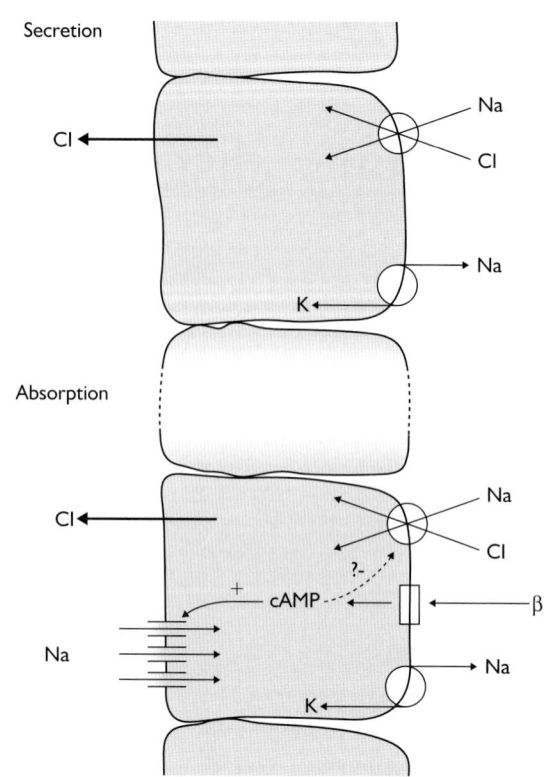

Fig. 27.1 Schematic model to explain the secretory and absorptive states of the lung. Na^+/K^+-ATPase (K ⊸ Na) generates a gradient for Na^+ which enters the intracellular space across the basolateral membrane linked to Cl^- (≢). β (▯) receptor; (Na, ⊗) sodium channel in apical membrane; cAMP, cyclic AMP. (Reproduced from Walters & Ramsden.[231])

maturation of the normal response of the fetal lung to ephinephrine.[9] Exposure to postnatal oxygen tensions increases sodium transport across the pulmonary epithelium.[190]

Amniotic fluid volume

Pulmonary hypoplasia is associated with oligohydramnios following prolonged rupture of the membranes, or chronic drainage following amniocentesis. It appears to be due to the increased efflux of lung liquid from the intrapulmonary space and is not the result of external compression of the fetal thorax squeezing out lung liquid, as the amniotic fluid pressure under such circumstances is at or below the normal range.[169] Prolonged oligohydramnios is associated with a decrease in lung liquid volume and a reduction in both the rate of lung liquid secretion and tracheal fluid flow rate.[52]

Pulmonary circulation

The pulmonary blood vessels and lymphatics develop from the mesenchyme of the splanchnic mesoderm of the foregut; this surrounds the lung buds as they push out from the laryngeal floor.

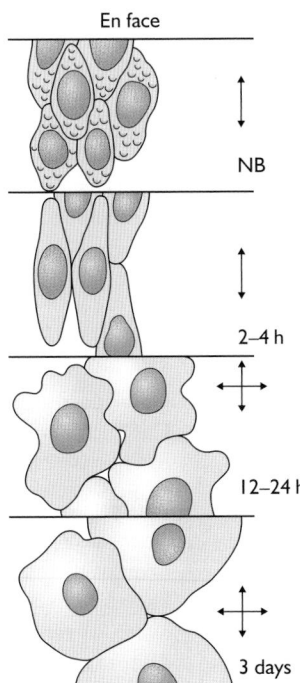

Fig. 27.2 Illustration of en face shape changes – the spreading of endothelial cells from birth to 3 days. (Reproduced from Haworth.[96])

Adjacent blood vessels fuse to form a rudimentary vasculature. The vascular plexus within each lung bud becomes supported by paired segmental arteries, which arise from the dorsal aorta. At 32 days of gestation, the sixth branchial arches appear, which give off the pulmonary arteries, hence the segmental arteries cease to supply the lung. By 50 days of fetal age, the adult blood supply pattern is achieved. Occasionally, an early segmental artery persists, captured within a lobe or lung segment (see sequestered lobe p. 588).[96] There is progressive dichotomous branching of the pulmonary arteries during lung growth; 70% of the preacinar arteries are formed between the 10th and 14th week of gestation. Additional branching in the canalicular phase and in the last trimester around the developing saccules greatly increases the vascular supply to the area of gas exchange.

During fetal as compared with adult life, the arterial walls contain a greater proportion of smooth muscle. Postnatally, there is rapid thinning – in the first 2 weeks, due to distension, and over the next year, due to a slow reduction in the number of muscle fibres.[105] If such remodelling does not occur, the pulmonary vascular resistance (PVR) remains high, leading to persistent pulmonary hypertension (pp. 496–502). Abnormal remodelling alters the pulmonary vascular reactivity and the response to pharmacological agents. Normal postnatal development can be divided into three overlapping phases.[83,96] Stage one starts from birth and lasts for about 4 days, and represents adaptation to extrauterine life. The vessel walls become thinner.[97] Initially, the endothelial cells are squat, have a low surface to volume ratio and have many surface projections, but within 5 minutes after birth, the endothelial cells become thinner with less cell-to-cell contact; fewer projections are evident as their surface membrane material is donated to allow the cells to spread rapidly (Fig. 27.2). During stage two, when the cells have taken up their

definitive position, they deposit connective tissue and fix the wall structure. In stage three, there is growth of the pulmonary vasculature, which lasts until adulthood. At birth, almost the entire pulmonary vasculature is innervated. The majority of nerves contain the vasoconstrictor neuropeptides tyrosine and tyrosine hydroxylase.[96] Both nerve density and the immunoreactive expression of the neurotransmitters increase particularly rapidly in the first 2 weeks.[239]

Cardiorespiratory adaptation at birth

Aeration of the lungs at birth

In fetal life, the respiratory system is fluid filled. The replacement of lung liquid by air is largely accomplished within a few minutes of birth. Lung liquid production ceases during labour and this effect is mediated by catecholamines[230] and arginine vasopressin.[109] Some liquid is squeezed out under the high vaginal pressure during the second stage of delivery,[126] while the majority is absorbed into the pulmonary lymphatics and capillaries.[215] The transpulmonary pressure, which inflates the lungs, displaces liquid from the terminal respiratory units into the perivascular spaces. Air entry into the lung displaces liquid and reduces the hydraulic pressure in the pulmonary circulation, increasing blood flow. This increases the effective vascular surface area for fluid exchange, facilitating water absorption into the pulmonary vascular bed.

Stimulus for the first breath

Fetal breathing activity ceases during labour. Following birth, one of the most important stimuli to the onset of breathing is cooling. Audiovisual, proprioceptive and touch stimuli recruit central neurons and increase central arousal.[38,92] Hypoxia mediated by central chemoreceptors is important, but peripheral chemoreceptor activity is not critical to the onset of respiration (pp. 452–4).

The median time for the onset of respiratory activity is 10 seconds.[229] A high negative pressure is required to overcome the high flow resistance and inertia of liquid in the airways, as well as the surface tension at the air–liquid interface.[126] Both Karlberg et al[126] and Milner & Saunders[161] recorded inspiratory pressures during the first breath of greater than 20 cmH$_2$O, but not in all infants. Subsequently, using a dual pressure tip transducer, Vyas et al[228] demonstrated that pressures of greater than 20 cmH$_2$O were the norm. Expiration is also active for the first few breaths, with pressures ranging from 18 to 115 cmH$_2$O; this may aid the distribution of ventilation and facilitate further fluid clearance from the lungs.

Changes in lung mechanics after birth

There is a fall in airways resistance and rise in functional residual capacity (FRC), which is most rapid in the first 2 hours. Compliance, however, progressively increases over the 24-hour period as lung liquid is gradually absorbed. The changes in lung mechanics occur at a slower rate following elective caesarean section, when there is a delay in lung fluid absorption.

Circulatory changes at birth

In the fetus, only about 12% of the right ventricular output enters the pulmonary circulation,[66] because of the high PVR, the presence of a patent ductus arteriosus and the low-resistance placental component of the systemic circulation. At birth, clamping of the umbilical cord and removal of the placenta from the circulation reduces venous return through the inferior vena cava to the right atrium. The foramen ovale closes because of the resultant lower right atrial pressure and the increase in left atrial pressure that occurs with the increased pulmonary venous return. The loss of the umbilical venous return also means diminished flow through the ductus venosus and passive closure occurs usually within 3 to 7 days after birth.

PVR falls rapidly in the first minutes after birth, then more gradually over the next days and weeks of life. This fall in PVR, which is associated with a structural reorganisation and thinning of the vessel walls, allows for an eightfold increase in pulmonary blood flow. There are several mechanisms responsible for the fall in PVR. Lung aeration results in opening up the pulmonary capillary bed, acute lowering of PVR and an increase in pulmonary blood flow. This is due to both a mechanical effect and oxygenated blood passing through the pulmonary circulation. In fetal lambs, mechanical expansion of the lungs with a non-oxygenated gas caused a decrease in PVR and a fourfold increase in pulmonary blood flow; a further increase resulted when oxygen was used as the ventilatory gas.[221] Inflation of the lungs also stimulates pulmonary stretch receptors, which leads to reflex vasodilation of the pulmonary vascular bed. Mechanical expansion additionally creates surface forces at the gas–liquid interface within the alveoli, which physically expand small blood vessels and decrease perivascular pressure.[232]

Prostaglandins and endothelial-derived products (endothelin-1 [ET-1] and nitric oxide [NO]) are important in regulating fetal and transitional pulmonary vascular tone (Table 27.1).[207,253] The fetal PVR is high because of the low oxygen tension and PGI_2 and NO levels, and the presence of vasoconstrictor substances such as ET-1. PGI_2 production increases soon after birth and falls 2–5 hours later. Its production and release is related to pulmonary tissue stretch. PGI_2 participates in the reduction of PVR accompanying ventilation, but is not essential for maintaining low PVR once it has been established.[143] NO is produced by the vascular endothelial cells, by the effects of NO synthase on L-arginine, forming citrulline and NO. The NO then diffuses into the smooth muscle cells, stimulating guanylate cyclase and increasing guanosine monophosphate (GMP) production and resulting in smooth muscle relaxation. Pharmacological NO blockade inhibits endothelium-dependent pulmonary vasodilation and attenuates the rise in pulmonary blood flow after birth. Increased fetal oxygen tension augments endogenous NO release. The vasodilator effects of exogenous PGI_2 are blocked by NO synthase inhibitors, which suggests that NO modulates PGI_2 activity.[252] Decreased production of endogenous vasoconstrictors, such as thromboxane and ET-1, may also participate in the decrease in

Table 27.1 Factors that modulate pulmonary vascular resistance (PVR) in the near-term and term transitional and neonatal pulmonary circulation (From Kinsella & Abman.[128])

Lowers PVR	Increases PVR
Endogenous mediators and mechanisms	*Endogenous mediators and mechanisms*
Oxygen	Hypoxia
Nitric oxide	Acidosis
PGI_2, E_2, D_2	Endothelin-1
Adenosine, ATP, magnesium	Leukotrienes
Bradykinin	Thromboxanes
Atrial natriuretic factor	Platelet activating factor
Alkalosis	Ca^{++} channel activation
K^+ channel activation	α-adrenergic stimulation
Histamine	$PGF_{2\alpha}$
Vagal nerve stimulation	
Acetylcholine	*Mechanical factors*
β-adrenergic stimulation	Overinflation or underinflation
	Excessive muscularisation,
Mechanical factors	vascular remodeling
Lung inflation	Altered mechanical properties of
Vascular cell structural	smooth muscle
changes	Pulmonary hypoplasia
Interstitial fluid and	Alveolar capillary dysplasia
pressure changes	Pulmonary thromboemboli
Shear stress	Main pulmonary artery distention
	Ventricular dysfunction,
	venous hypertension

PVR at birth. In healthy infants, the majority of measurable changes in cardiopulmonary haemodynamics occur by 8 hours, although some degree of right-to-left ductal shunting may be found up to 12 hours after birth.[232] In most infants the ductus has closed or is closing by 24 hours of age, but there is a significant delay in ductal closure in infants with respiratory failure and pulmonary hypertension. During early neonatal life, the pulmonary circulation remains unstable, and in certain disease states, particularly those associated with asphyxia or chronic hypoxia, the PVR increases or remains at the high fetal levels – persistent pulmonary hypertension (pp. 496–502).

Postnatal function

The airways

The nasal portion of the airway is supported by its larger bony and smaller cartilaginous portions. Nasal resistance to airflow, which comprises approximately one-third of the total pulmonary resistance, is determined by the physical dimensions in a given individual, which are related to ethnic origin,[172] and the state of the mucous membranes lining the airway. The prime function of the nose is to act as an entry port for respiration, humidifying and warming inspired gas and trapping extraneous particles.

Infants are not necessarily obligate nose breathers and full-term infants can establish oral breathing in the presence of nasal occlusion.[197] The pharyngeal portion of the airway is very compliant. In the absence of active muscle contraction, there is apposition of the soft palate and tongue against the posterior pharyngeal wall, which is accentuated by neck flexion and negative pressures during inspiration, leading to collapse and obstruction of the airway. This is usually prevented by the splinting and dilating actions of pharyngeal muscles. In the fetus and newborn infant, there is increased flexibility of the epiglottis and the hyoid, thyroid and cricoid cartilages. In term infants, the region is stabilised by a fat-laden superficial fascia which covers the neck and face; this is absent in the premature infant, as fat accumulation occurs in the last third of gestation.

Chemoreceptors in the larynx serve to prevent the entry of foreign material by triggering reflex apnoea. Changes in laryngeal diameter modulate airway resistance, and lung volume can be maintained by expiratory adduction of the vocal cords.[58] Laryngeal resistance can be varied by active abduction of the vocal cords during inspiration and by passive as well as active adduction during expiration. Inspiratory abduction and expiratory adduction of the vocal cords occur during fetal breathing movements.[42]

The trachea and main bronchi are supported by cartilaginous rings; nevertheless, smooth muscle contraction can cause narrowing and markedly increase resistance, at least in the adult. In the newborn, the small airways are more compliant than in the adult and expiratory collapse tends to lead to air trapping.

The thorax

In the newborn, compared with the adult, the thorax is round rather then dorsoventrally flattened and the rib orientation is horizontal rather than caudal, thus the expansion potential of the thorax is limited. The neonatal thoracic cage has relatively soft and flexible bony elements, which makes the chest wall subject to collapse during increased inspiratory efforts and the lungs rather collapsed at rest. To compensate, the infant attempts to elevate his lung volume at end expiration by a rapid breathing rate, a short expiratory time, intercostal activity and grunting (expiratory laryngeal adduction). Grunting disappears in rapid eye movement (REM) sleep.[89] Instability of end-expiratory lung volume, particularly in the premature neonate, may explain fluctuations in arterial oxygen levels.[5]

The respiratory muscles (Fig. 27.3)

The main inspiratory muscle is the diaphragm, a dome-shaped muscle attached to the ribs. Diaphragmatic contraction results in the abdominal contents moving downwards, increasing the vertical dimension of the thoracic cavity. If the dome's descent is impeded by abdominal pressure, then the lower ribs are pulled up. This increases the ribcage diameter by virtue of the linkages between ribs provided by the intercostal muscles and by the articulations of the ribs that lead to the 'pump and bucket handle

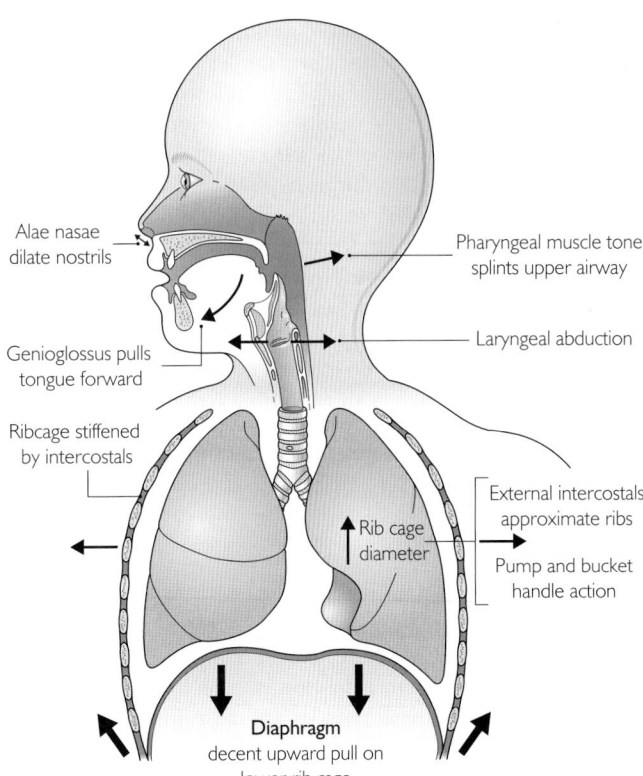

Alae nasae dilate nostrils

Pharyngeal muscle tone splints upper airway

Genioglossus pulls tongue forward

Laryngeal abduction

Ribcage stiffened by intercostals

Rib cage diameter

External intercostals approximate ribs

Pump and bucket handle action

Diaphragm decent upward pull on lower rib cage

Fig. 27.3 Diagrammatic representation of the respiratory pump showing the various muscles and actions that make up inspiration. Although the diaphragm is the main muscle, many others act to optimise its function by opening the airways and splinting the floppy ribcage.

action'. The configurations of the adult and neonatal diaphragm differ, the latter being relatively flat following birth, the dome shape developing with the physical growth of the thorax and internal organs.[50] There is an exaggerated asymmetrical movement of the newborn diaphragm during respiration. These differences mean the diaphragm is less efficient in the neonate than in the adult. The number of skeletal muscle fibres in the diaphragm is, however, fixed at the time of birth and the subsequent increase in muscle weight is due to hypertrophy. The diaphragm consists of type I fibres, which are oxidative with a slow twitch and fatigue-resistant, type IIa fibres, which are oxidative-glycolytic with a fast twitch but also fatigue-resistant, and type IIb fibres, which are glycolytic with a fast twitch and are fatiguable.[246] The proportion of type I fibres is low at birth and increases until 6 months of age; there is an associated increase in type IIb, but a decrease in type IIa fibres. Type IIc fibres, which are present at birth, disappear completely by 6 months.[155] This means that at birth the diaphragm has a relatively high percentage of oxidative fibres (type I, IIa and IIc) which are fatigue-resistant. The proportion of type I fibres, however, may be low in the preterm infant, putting him at risk of diaphragmatic muscle fatigue. Optimal function of the diaphragm is dependent on ribcage stability and adequate abdominal muscle tone. This is particularly important when the system is loaded, as with stiff lungs or obstructed airways.

The internal and external intercostal muscles are components of the chest wall. Their actions are similar and depend on the volume of the ribcage: elevating the ribs at low lung volumes, but lowering them at high lung volumes.[45] The intercostal muscles also maintain the stability of the chest wall during inspiration and limit volume reduction during expiration. This tonic activity is abolished in REM sleep, resulting in destabilisation and distortion of the chest wall and asynchronous movements of the abdomen and ribcage.[42] These problems particularly compromise the premature newborn, because of his soft thoracic skeleton. During REM sleep, such infants rely on diaphragmatic activity to compensate for the inefficiency of the chest wall and thus diaphragmatic fatigue can result in a reduction in tidal volume and much of the increased diaphragmatic work being dissipated in 'sucking in ribs instead of air'.[23] Abdominal muscle tone may also be important in stabilising the ribcage in REM sleep.

Upper airway muscles

Patency of the upper airway is dependent on the upper airway muscles and the diaphragm. The genioglossus, geniohyoid, sternohyoid, sternothyroid and parohyoid muscles are most important in maintaining the patency of the oropharynx. There is active contraction of the laryngeal muscles, particularly in early expiration, and there is relatively late relaxation of the inspiratory muscles. That activity reduces the flow rate and is modified by carbon dioxide levels, high levels resulting in a reduced resistance to flow. If the FRC is reduced, the above muscle activity is increased, such that the airway is almost completely occluded in expiration and gas has to be forced out by contraction of the abdominal muscles, producing a grunt.

Gas exchange in the neonatal lung

At rest, oxygen consumption in the newborn (7 ml/min/kg) is approximately twice that of adults. Minute ventilation is proportionally increased and is achieved largely by an increased breathing rate. This increased rate presumably results from the constraints on increasing tidal volume imposed by the relatively stiff lungs and unstable ribcage. The disadvantage is that this increases the amount of dead-space ventilation, although this is minimised by the relatively low volume of the proximal airways.[165] In addition, overventilation or underperfusion of some lung units contributes to the wasted ventilation. The contribution of ventilation–perfusion mismatch, as estimated from the arterial–alveolar differences for oxygen (a-ADO$_2$) is most marked in preterm infants in the first hours after birth.

A major difference between the blood gases of newborn and older infants is the lower PaO_2 in relation to the inspired oxygen tension. This is largely because of right-to-left shunting of blood either through areas of the lung with very low ventilation–perfusion ratios or, less commonly, through persisting fetal vascular channels (foramen ovale and ductus arteriosus). Estimates of the total shunt in healthy infants are 24% of the cardiac output in the first hour after birth and 10% at 1 week of age. Shunting through fetal vascular channels is important immediately after birth in immature infants or in sick infants with raised PVR. The low PaO_2 due to right-to-left shunting (through cardiac shunts and perfused but non-ventilated lung units) cannot be overcome by administering 100% oxygen, because the blood that is being ventilated soon becomes fully saturated and increasing the oxygen tension adds little further oxygen. On the other hand, carbon dioxide accumulation from partial right-to-left shunting can be compensated for by increased ventilation of functioning lung units. Thus, provided respiratory efforts are maintained, $PaCO_2$ will be normal or even low, despite right-to-left shunting.

Gas transport in the blood[47]

Oxygen

Haemoglobin increases the oxygen transport capacity of the blood 70-fold over that of plasma. As a consequence, the majority of oxygen in whole blood is transported as oxyhaemoglobin (HbO$_2$) and only a small proportion dissolved in solution. The haemoglobin concentration is regulated by a renal sensing mechanism, which operates to maintain a balance between the oxygen supply and requirement of the renal tissues. A decrease in concentration or arterial oxygen saturation of haemoglobin or an increase in haemoglobin affinity for oxygen increases erythropoietin production. Haemoglobin is a tetramer; each of the four subunits contains a haem moiety (porphyrin and one atom of ferrous iron) attached to a polypeptide (globin) chain. The four iron atoms can each combine with an oxygen molecule; they remain in the ferrous state, that is, the reaction is oxygenation rather than oxidation. In adult haemoglobin, the four globin chains are predominantly $\alpha_2\beta_2$ (HbA), whereas in the fetus they are $\alpha_2\gamma_2$ (HbF). The quarternary structure of haemoglobin determines its affinity for oxygen: uptake of oxygen by haemoglobin results in a change of position of the haem moieties, facilitating further oxygen binding. The result is that the oxygen–haemoglobin dissociation curve (the relationship of the percentage oxygen saturation of haemoglobin to the PO_2) has a characteristic sigmoid shape (Appendix 9). The oxygen–haemoglobin disssociation curve is affected by the pH, temperature and concentration of 2,3-diphosphoglycerate (2,3-DPG). A rise in temperature or fall in pH (Bohr shift) shifts the curve to the right, which means that a higher PO_2 is required for haemoglobin to bind to a given amount of oxygen. This is quantified as the P$_{50}$, the PO_2 at which the haemoglobin is half saturated with oxygen. The higher the P$_{50}$, the lower the affinity of haemoglobin for oxygen. 2,3-DPG is formed from a product of glycolysis and thus its concentration falls when the pH is low. 2,3-DPG binds preferentially to the β chains of deoxygenated haemoglobin. An increase in 2,3-DPG causes more oxygen to be liberated, that is, the oxygen dissociation curve is shifted to the right.

The fetus and newborn

Compared with in the adult, fetal red blood cells (RBCs) are larger, have a shorter half-life and differ in ultrastructure

(p. 740). They also differ with regard to their mechanical, osmotic, thermal and acidic fragility, and contain haemoglobin (HbF) which is less easily denatured in alkaline or acidic solutions than is adult haemoglobin. The γ chains of HbF have the same number of amino acids as the β chains, but differ in sequence by 39 amino acids. The γ chains of HbF have poorer binding to 2,3-DPG. The effect of 2,3-DPG on the P_{50} of fetal haemoglobin is approximately 40% of the effect on the P_{50} of adult haemoglobin (Appendix 9). The oxygen tension of fetal blood is one-fifth to one-quarter that of the adult, but the fetal arterial blood oxygen content and oxyhaemoglobin saturation are similar to those of the adult. This results from the high oxygen-carrying capacity and the increased oxygen affinity of HbF. The latter facilitates the movement of oxygen from mother to fetus. Oxygen delivery to the fetal tissues is sustained because the steep fetal oxygen dissociation curve means that a small decrease in oxygen tension results in a major change in oxyhaemoglobin saturation and unloading of oxygen.

In the term newborn, 70–80% of the haemoglobin is HbF: in preterm babies, about 90% of haemoglobin is HbF (pp. 740, 741). Neither birth, intrauterine hypoxia nor haemolytic disease of the newborn causes a change in the proportions of HbA and HbF at any given gestational age. Near term, however, the demand for accelerated erythropoeisis leads preferentially to synthesis of HbA. During the first year, HbF decreases from 70% to less than 2% of the total haemoglobin.

The high oxygen affinity of HbF has disadvantages in postnatal life. In particular, the low P_{50} decreases the driving potential for oxygen diffusion, limiting the rate at which oxygen can be unloaded.[2] The oxygen consumption of the newborn at minimal activity, even in a thermally neutral environment, increases by 100–150% in the first few days. To meet these demands, the baby's blood oxygen affinity decreases rapidly over the first 5 days and then more gradually, reaching adult values by 6 months.[48] During the first 5 days, the 2,3-DPG levels rise to above those found in the adult; this decreases blood oxygen affinity by lowering intercellular pH. Prematurely born babies have a lower 2,3-DPG content, lower P_{50} and higher fetal haemoglobin concentration. They have a smaller oxygen unloading capacity and do not catch up until 3 months of age.[80]

Carbon dioxide

Carbon dioxide is 20 times more soluble in water than is oxygen. Carbon dioxide is carried in the blood by three mechanisms: the majority as bicarbonate (85%), but also dissolved and in combination with proteins as carbamino compounds. Bicarbonate is formed very rapidly in RBCs, because of the presence of carbonic anhydrase, which catalyses the first part of the following reaction:

$$CO_2 + H_2O \rightarrow H_2CO_3 \rightarrow HCO_3^- + H^+$$

Ionic dissociation of H_2CO_3 is fast. HCO_3^- then diffuses out of the RBC down a concentration gradient, but H^+ cannot follow and binds to haemoglobin. This is facilitated in the presence of reduced haemoglobin, which is a weaker acid than oxyhaemoglobin, and thus deoxygenation of the blood increases its ability to carry carbon dioxide (the Haldane effect). To maintain electrical neutrality, as HCO_3^- diffuses out, Cl^- diffuses into the RBC (the chloride shift). These events increase the osmolar content of the RBC, thus the packed cell volume is higher on the venous than on the arterial side of the circulation. Carbon dioxide also combines with the N terminals of amino acids of proteins, particularly haemoglobin, to form carbamino compounds:

$$CO_2 + R_2 + NH_2 \rightarrow RNHCOO^- + H^+$$

The newborn's blood has a greater carbon dioxide transport capacity. This is because of the high haemoglobin level. In addition, carbon dioxide competes with 2,3-DPG for the haemoglobin binding site, and since 2,3-DPG binds less avidly with HbF than with adult haemoglobin, more carbon dioxide can be taken up. RBC carbonic anhydrase levels, however, are 25% lower in the neonate and even more so in those born prematurely.[130]

Regulation of breathing

The rhythmic transition from the inspiratory to the expiratory phase of the respiratory cycle is ordered by a centrally generated respiratory rhythm, which consists of three neural phases:[21]

- inspiration, corresponding to inspiratory muscle contraction;
- phase one expiration, corresponding to post inspiration or passive expiration, when inspiratory muscles cease to progressively contract;
- phase two expiration, corresponding to active exhalation with expiratory muscle contraction.

Respiratory 'centre'

The respiratory rhythm (described above) is generated by a loose complex of respiratory neurons, which lie within the ventrolateral region of the brainstem. The respiratory rhythm generator also produces sighs and gasps. A variety of models of the central respiratory rhythm generator have been proposed, but a common assumption is that chemical neurotransmission is required to mediate the synaptic interactions which play a role in generation of transmission and expression of the respiratory rhythm.[21] The hybrid pacemaker – network model incorporates a critical neuronal kernel of a network of excitatory neurons with pacemaker properties, which are located in the pre-Botzinger complex of the ventrolateral medulla. The kernel is embedded in a larger network that interacts with it via inhibitory synaptic connections, which provide the dynamic control required for the evolution of the complete pattern of inspiratory and expiratory network activity.[211] As rhythm is generated, it is ultimately synaptically transmitted to spinal motor neurons and cranial pre-motor neurons; the latter control the activity of airway muscles.[21] Afferents from the forebrain, hypothalamus, central and peripheral chemoreceptors, muscles, joints and pain receptors are integrated into the 'centre'. The number of intersynaptic connections reaches a peak towards the end of fetal life.

Neurotransmitters

Excitatory

The excitatory neurotransmitters include glutamate, which excites NMDA and non-NMDA receptors; the latter are involved in generating and transmitting respiratory rhythms to spinal and cranial respiratory neurons.[68] The transmission of inspiratory drive is further fine tuned by presynaptic glutaminergic modulation at the level of the spinal cord. Serotonin (5HT) has diverse effects on respiratory neuronal activity, but the most consistent effect is to restore a normal breathing pattern in metabolic states such as hypoxia or ischaemia which cause apneustic breathing.[140] Substance P is largely excitatory. It may stimulate respiration by effects within the primary medullary respiratory network;[249] there may also be endogenous release from projections from the caudal raphe nuclei to the inspiratory neurons.[107] Around birth there is elevation of noradrenergic activity, leading to activation of the locus coeruleus, which may be important for the forebrain drive of breathing.[138] Cooling stimulates noradrenaline turnover and is important for stimulating breathing at birth; the stimulatory effect on breathing of cooling, however, is not mediated by a noradrenergic mechanism.[73]

Inhibitory

Both GABA and glycine are essential for generating respiratory rhythm in the primary network. These inhibitory amino acids provide phasic waves of inhibitory postsynaptic potentials which are received by the medullary respiratory neurons during their silent periods.[192] GABA and glycine are released by late and post-inspiratory neurons to turn off inspiratory neurons and so facilitate the transition from inspiration to expiration. Deficiency of glycinergic inhibition in knockout mice results in a slower frequency of breathing.[150] Synaptic inputs from peripheral sensory receptors and brain regions outside the primary medullary respiratory network input affect the full expression of the respiratory rhythm.[61] Phasic transition is modulated by two sources of synaptic inputs from outside the primary network: the slowly adapting pulmonary stretch receptors and pontine neurons. Suppression of either of these inputs prolongs inspiration (apneusis). Opioids (endorphins and exogenous drugs) decrease respiration by peripheral[17] and central actions; the latter are due to a decrease in spontaneous respiratory unit activity and suppression of recurrent excitation by glutaminergic inputs within the primary respiratory network.[49] There may be endogenous endorphinergic tonic inhibition of breathing in the neonate, which vanishes after the neonatal period.[137] Adenosine is ubiquitously formed in the body and has both central and peripheral effects. When administered centrally, it depresses ventilation; this effect is most pronounced in young full-term and preterm models. If adenosine is given systemically, however, it stimulates breathing, probably by stimulating peripheral chemoreceptors; this effect may be more important in the adult. Adenosine antagonists (theophylline and caffeine) stimulate breathing and also block, but not in humans, hypoxia-induced respiratory depression.[203] In a rat model, theophylline administration reversed the adenosine-induced age-dependent reduction in respiratory frequency.[101]

Adenosine may mediate the secondary apnoea seen after birth asphyxia; removal of an inhibitory substance might explain why it is often necessary to artificially ventilate an infant for a period that is two- to threefold longer than the duration of asphyxia.[159] PGE_2 inhibits fetal breathing movements, and prostaglandin inhibitors, such as indometacin (indomethacin), stimulate FBM. Plasma concentrations of PGE_2 decrease at birth and it has been suggested this may be important for the onset of respiration. In the neonate, PGE_1 and PGE_2 depress ventilation. A significant correlation has been found between the occurrence of central apnoeas and the PGE-M concentration in urine of preterm babies.[106]

Chemoreceptors

Both central and peripheral chemoreceptors are involved in modification of respiratory activity in response to changes in blood gases. The central chemoreceptors are situated near the ventral surface of the medulla and respond to changes in carbon dioxide/pH and oxygen supply. The peripheral chemoreceptors are situated at the bifurcation of the common carotid arteries (carotid bodies) and in the aortic bodies above and below the aortic arch, the former being more important in man.

In the fetus, the arterial chemoreceptors are active in utero, but have reduced sensitivity. They are virtually silenced when the arterial PO_2 rises at birth.[18] Resetting of the carotid chemoreceptors to hypoxia then occurs. This is probably triggered by the rise in blood oxygen levels. The resetting of the chemoreceptors to hypoxia is essentially complete within 24 to 48 hours of birth[26] and may be due to a change in dopamine levels. Dopamine inhibits chemoreceptor discharge in both the newborn and adult. If rat pups are delivered into a hypoxic environment (12%), they maintain both their low sensitivity to hypoxia, with persistence of the immature inhibitory response to hypoxia,[59] and a high dopamine turnover.[102] In the lamb, hyperoxia induced by mechanical ventilation of the fetus for a few days before birth causes premature resetting.[19]

At birth, blood gas measurements indicate that there should be a powerful chemoreceptor drive to breathe. The carotid chemoreceptors, however, do not appear to be essential for the initiation of air breathing and are probably quickly silenced by the rise in the PaO_2 that occurs. The relative inactivity of the chemoreceptors during this period is indicated by the reduced immediate ventilatory responses to hypoxia and hyperoxia in humans and an inability to detect chemoreceptor afferent activity in the lamb carotid sinus nerve. Presumably other drives maintain breathing efforts at this time.

Although the peripheral chemoreceptors are not essential for initiation of respiration, they are important in the development of breathing control, as their denervation increases the neonatal mortality of newborn animals.[57] Carotid and aortic chemoreceptor denervation in newborn piglets, however, demonstrated that there are other sites of residual chemosensitivity.[206] The carotid chemoreceptor responses to both oxygen and carbon dioxide are weak in the newborn and increase during postnatal development.[27,149] The mechanisms of carotid body maturation are unknown, but are unlikely to be due to changes in dopamine secretion, which takes place over days rather than weeks.[102]

Responses to changes in oxygen tension (Fig. 27.4)

The fetus

Fetuses respond to hypoxia with a suppression of ventilation, which is most marked in growth-retarded fetuses;[14] the hypoxic suppression of ventilation is mediated by the lateral part of the lower pons. The hypoxic respiratory depression in a rat model is emphasised after in-utero exposure to caffeine and this coincides with an increased Fos expression pattern in the area postrema and nucleus raphe obscurus.[20] In response to hypoxia there are also cardiovascular reflexes; these include bradycardia and redistribution of the circulation to favour the heart, brain and adrenals,[176] which minimise oxygen consumption and conserve oxygen supplies for vital organs. Hyperoxia stimulates continuous fetal breathing.

The newborn

The newborn's response to hypoxia in the perinatal period is a biphasic response: a transient increase in minute ventilation followed by a decrease to or below baseline levels. The initial increase in ventilation is probably due to activation of peripheral chemoreceptors, as it is abolished by carotid sinus nerve section. The subsequent reduction in ventilation may result from a fall in $PaCO_2$ following the initial hyperventilation and may be due to a depression of central respiratory neurons.[196] It may also be explained by the suppressant effect of hypoxia in the fetal state persisting into the neonatal period. The biphasic response to hypoxia disappears at 12 to 14 days and the adult pattern is then seen, that is, stimulation without depression (Fig. 27.4). Very immature infants respond to hypoxia in a similar fashion to fetuses, that is, with apnoea. This inhibition of breathing is at a suprapontine level. More mature preterm infants have an initial increase (but less than in term infants) and then a more dramatic fall in ventilation in response to hypoxia.[194] In non-REM sleep, the decrease in ventilation is the predominating response. The response to hypoxia is also modified by the temperature of the environment in which the infant is nursed; transient hyperventilation on exposure to 12% O_2 is not seen if the infant is in a cold rather than a warm environment.[30]

A hyperoxic gas causes a temporary suppression of breathing; this is attributed to the withdrawal of peripheral chemoreceptor drive. During the first few days, the reduction in ventilation with 100% oxygen is less, consistent with inactivity of the carotid afferents during this resetting period. After a few minutes of hyperoxia, ventilation increases to above control levels. In adults, a similar but less marked hyperventilation has been attributed to hyperoxic cerebral vasoconstriction, which leads to increased brain tissue carbon dioxide. The response to hyperoxia is slower in more immature infants. Prolonged exposure to supplemental oxygen also reduces the response to hyperoxia.

Response to carbon dioxide/acidosis

The fetus

Fetal breathing can be detected as early as 14 weeks of gestation in the human. The amount of time the fetus spends breathing increases with advancing gestational age. Initially, fetal breathing was thought to depend only on behavioural reflexes, as it was only observed during REM sleep. It is now known that fetal breathing is modified by chemical stimuli; the fetus responds to an increase in $PaCO_2$ with an increase in breathing, both elevated frequency and diaphragmatic activity. It is probably that the hydrogen ion concentration, rather than carbon dioxide per se, is the major stimulus to respiratory activity, although there is some evidence that carbon dioxide may have an effect independent of pH.[158] During non-REM sleep, however, only very high $PaCO_2$ levels (>100 mmHg) can initiate breathing activity.[196] Hypoxia inhibits fetal breathing. Lesions in the ventrolateral pons eliminate the hypoxic inhibition of breathing and are associated with a lower threshold for carbon dioxide drive-augmented breathing through all states.[121] Fetal breathing is also suppressed during labour.

The newborn

Inhalation of CO_2 increases ventilation in the newborn in both REM and quiet sleep. The slope of minute ventilation versus $PaCO_2$ levels in the newborn is similar to that of adults, but the response is shifted to the left because of lower resting carbon dioxide levels.[23,193] The tidal volume component of the ventilatory response assumes greater importance with postnatal development. The percentage of inhaled CO_2 influences the pattern of breathing. A low percentage of CO_2 (<2%) primarily stimulates an increase in tidal volume,[122] whereas a higher percentage provokes an increase in respiratory frequency and tidal volume.[163] Periodic breathing is abolished with a small increase in inhaled CO_2.[122] Sleep state also influences the response to carbon dioxide, both in adults[181] and in the newborn.[23] In term infants, the slope of ventilatory response is less during active than quiet

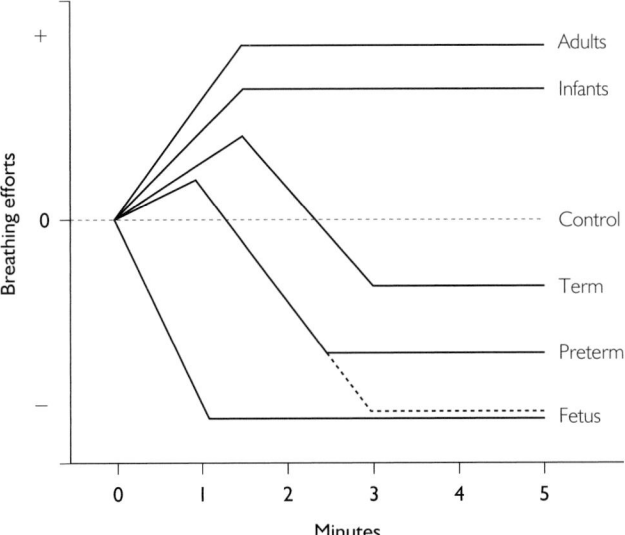

Fig. 27.4 Diagrammatic representation of the age-related responses to hypoxia, induced by breathing hypoxic gases for 5 minutes (solid bar). Breathing efforts assessed by diaphragmatic EMG in the fetus and by ventilatory responses in others. Dashed interrupted line indicates that apnoea may occur in preterm infants, resembling a fetal response. (Reproduced from Henderson-Smart.[99])

sleep (Fig. 27.5). This may be due to mechanical instability associated with ribcage distortion in active sleep, since the diaphragmatic response is intact. In preterm infants,[195] the slope of the ventilatory response is less, but increases with postnatal growth. As diaphragm EMG responses to CO_2 inhalation are also reduced in the preterm infant, this is probably due to the immaturity of the central chemoreceptors rather than mechanical differences in the respiratory pump.[193]

Respiratory reflexes

The Hering–Breuer reflexes

Hering & Breuer[100] described three respiratory reflexes. The Hering–Breuer inflation reflex is stimulated by lung inflation and results in cessation of respiratory activity. This reflex is generated by stretch receptors within the airway and has an afferent pathway lying within the vagi. In the newborn, the reflex produces a pattern of rapid, shallow tidal breathing and operates within the tidal volume range. The reflex is active from FRC and is maximal after an inspiration of approximately 4 ml/kg above FRC.[93] In older subjects, the reflex prevents excessive volume exchange and can only be stimulated if the inflating volume is increased above a critical threshold.[35,77] In the first 4 to 6 weeks after birth, there does not appear to be any change in the reflex,[31] but its strength then declines over the first year.[188] The reflex is increased in infants with non-compliant lungs and by administration of theophylline, but not caffeine.[141] The influence of maturity at birth on the strength of the reflex is controversial.[31,65,129] Hypoxia in adults, but not newborns, has been shown to reduce the strength, but the reflex response to lung inflations can be greater during hypoxic hyperthermia than normoxia, which may be of importance in the pathophysiology of apneas.[156]

The Hering–Breuer expiratory reflex is stimulated if inhalation is prolonged. The active expiration seen in infants ventilated at slow rates and long inflation times may be a manifestation of this reflex.[76]

In animal models, the Hering–Breuer deflation reflex is evidenced by a prolonged inspiration generated in response to deflating the lung rapidly, either by attaching the endotracheal tube to a suction source or creating a pneumothorax, or following an unusually vigorous expiratory effort which takes the lung below its end-expiratory level. This response does occur in the newborn[151] and may have a role in maintaining the FRC. The strength of the reflex is increased if rapid lung volume reduction is commenced at FRC rather than end inspiration.[88]

Head's paradoxical reflex

Head[98] noted that if vagal conduction was blocked, rapid inflation, instead of producing apnoea, resulted in a stronger and more pronounced diaphragmatic contraction; this was named Head's paradoxical reflex. It has subsequently been termed the inspiratory augmenting reflex or provoked augmented inspiration and is the underlying mechanism of the first breath and sighing. This reflex improves compliance and reopens partially collapsed airways. It has an important role in promoting lung expansion during resuscitation. Its frequency is increased by low compliance, hypercapnia and hypoxia.[33]

The intercostal phrenic inhibitory reflex

Rapid chest wall distortion results in a shortening of inspiratory efforts. This reflex response is inhibited by an increase in FRC or applying continuous positive airway pressure (CPAP); the mechanism may be improved chest wall stability.[152]

Irritant reflexes

Subepithelial chemoreceptors in the trachea, bronchi and bronchioles detect insults to the epithelial surfaces; thus, inhalation of toxic gases causes a change in frequency and depth of respiration. The response is less in REM sleep and in the premature infant,[63] who has a smaller number of small myelinated vagal fibres and poorly developed receptors.

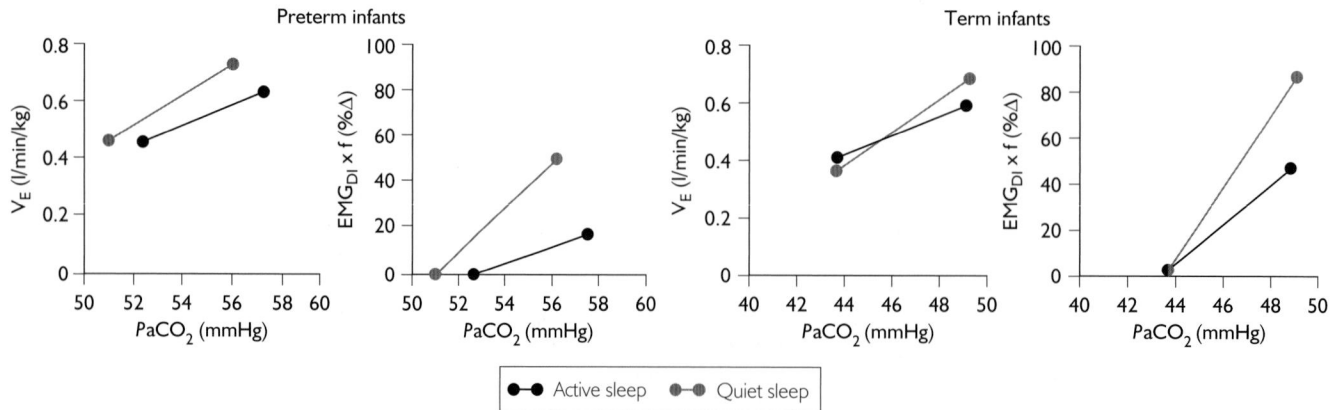

Fig. 27.5 The ventilatory response to CO_2 re-breathing in neonates. Note that (A) preterm and (B) term infants showed a decreased response to CO_2 in 'phasic' REM sleep as compared with quiet sleep. The vertical axis on the figures on the right is a measure of EMG activity multiplied by the change in respiratory rate. (Reproduced from Rigatto.[194])

Upper airway reflexes

Breathing is stimulated by cold via the trigeminal afferents of the facial skin, whereas irritant stimuli to the nasal mucosa cause inhibition of breathing and cardiovascular reflex responses resembling those in diving mammals. The latter response is enhanced under anaesthesia and in the newborn,[234] when cortical dampening of the responses is reduced. Vigorous suctioning of the nasopharynx can stimulate apnoea and bradycardia via these reflexes.[39]

The laryngeal chemoreceptors defend the lower airway from inhalation. Introduction of water into the interarytenoid notch induces apnoea.[182] In active sleep, laryngeal stimulation is more likely to induce apnoea and less likely to cause arousal.[181] This is of potential clinical significance since gastro-oesophageal reflux is more common during active sleep.[114] There may be 'chemically selective' responses, as apnoea is more common if water rather than saline is used,[44] but differences in response to species-specific and other milks has not been demonstrated in man.

Lung mechanics (Table 27.2)

Lung volumes

The tidal volume is the amount of gas entering or leaving the lung with each breath. Minute volume is calculated by multiplying the tidal volume by the respiratory rate over one minute. The volume exchanged following a maximum inspiratory and expiratory effort is called the vital capacity and in the infant can be measured during crying (crying vital capacity), or more accurately by pressurising a face mask to 20–25 cmH$_2$O and then inflating a rigid walled jacket with pressures of 40–60 cmH$_2$O.[224] The residual volume (RV) remains after a maximum expiratory effort; RV plus vital capacity gives the total lung capacity. At end expiration, the volume of gas remaining in the lung is referred to as the FRC and can be estimated by rebreathing an inert gas, such as helium. Only areas of the lung in communication with the airways will be measured by such a method. Alternatively, the patient can be placed in a body plethysmograph and the thoracic gas volume (TGV) estimated by applying Boyle's law during airway occlusion; TGV is FRC plus trapped gas. The dead space is the part of the respiratory system which does not take part in ventilation and is made up of the anatomical dead space (the conducting airways) and the physiological dead space, which includes non-functioning alveoli. Alveolar ventilation can be estimated from the tidal volume minus the dead space. In infants with respiratory distress, particularly transient tachypnoea of the newborn, the respiratory rate is increased and the tidal volume may be decreased. In respiratory distress syndrome (RDS) and pneumonia, the FRC is low (p. 447) and the physiological dead space increased.

Compliance

Compliance is a measure of the distensibility of the lungs and chest wall, the change in volume per unit pressure. Dynamic compliance is assessed during tidal breathing by measurement of

Table 27.2 The tidal flow and volume were measured by a Type 00 Fleisch pneumotachograph, and intrathoracic pressure with a 4 cm oesophageal balloon. Babies supine and in quiet sleep. Dead space eliminated by a bias flow of air. Data of Milner and Marsh reproduced with their permission.

Measurements	No of infants studied	Mean	Standard deviation	Range
Tidal volume (ml/g)	266	4.8	1.0	2.9–7.9
Respiratory rate (bpm)	266	50.9	13.1	25–104
Minute volume (ml/min/kg)	266	232	3.6	78–444
Dynamic compliance (ml/cmH$_2$O/kg)	266	1.72	0.5	0.9–3.7
Total pulmonary resistance (cmH$_2$O/l/s)	266	42.5	1.6	3.1–171
Work of breathing (G.cm)	266	11.9	7.4	1.1–52.6
Expiratory time (s)	291	0.57	0.17	0.27–1.28
Inspiratory time (s)	291	0.51	0.10	0.28–0.87
Time to maximum expiratory flow/total expiratory time (s)	291	0.51	0.12	0.18–0.83
Static compliance (ml/cmH$_2$O)	299	3.70	1.45	2.0–14.8
Respiratory system resistance (cmH$_2$O/l/s)	299	63.4	16.6	34.9–153.3
Time constant of respiratory system (s)	299	0.24	0.10	0.08–1.1
Thoracic gas volume (ml/kg)	271	29.8	6.2	14.5–45.6

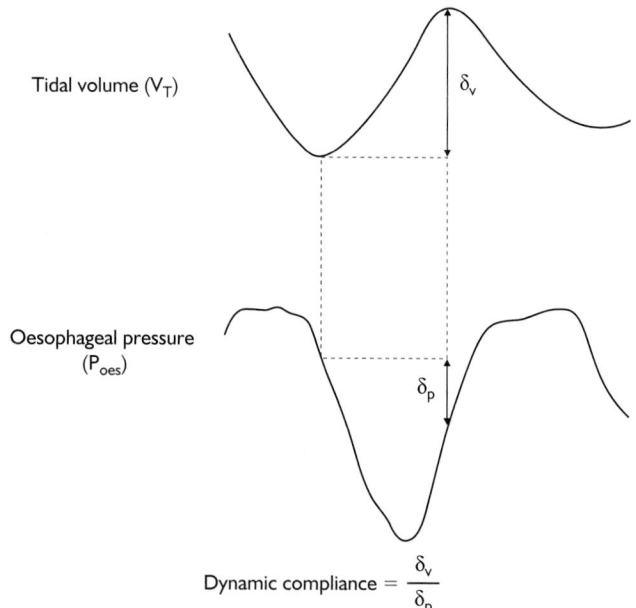

$$\text{Dynamic compliance} = \frac{\delta_v}{\delta_p}$$

Fig. 27.6 Volume and oesophageal pressure traces during spontaneous breathing. The dynamic compliance is calculated by dividing the tidal volume (δ_v) by the pressure gradient between the beginning and end of inspiration (δ_p). (Reproduced from Greenough et al.[78])

the change in volume (usually using the integrated signal of a flow-measuring device, a pneumotachograph) divided by the change in pleural pressure (which under certain conditions is similar to the change in oesophageal pressure) between points of zero airflow (Fig. 27.6). In situations with a rapid respiratory rate and chest wall distortion, dynamic compliance measurements can be inaccurate. Dynamic compliance is measured in ventilated infants by relating the volume change from a positive pressure inflation to the pressure drop (that is, PIP–PEEP), providing that the infant is not making spontaneous respiratory efforts, as these might interfere with volume delivery during inflation.

Static compliance requires the measurement of changes in lung volume over a larger range than the tidal volume or an assumption has to be made that the end-expiratory transpulmonary pressure represents a static value, which is unlikely to be true in infants with lung disease.[208] Static compliance is usually measured in spontaneously breathing infants using an occlusion technique, which relies on occlusion during inspiration causing a transient inhibition of breathing by stimulation of the Hering–Breuer reflex. The airway pressure during the occlusion is related to the volume above end expiration at which the occlusion was made. This technique requires temporary cessation of breathing, which may be difficult to provoke in an infant with a rapid respiratory rate or a weak Hering–Breuer reflex. Static compliance measurements assess the compliance of both the lung and chest wall. In the newborn, the chest wall compliance is very high, so, essentially, dynamic and static compliance values are similar. Compliance is reduced in infants with RDS.

Resistance

Resistance is a measure of the pressure necessary to generate airflow. Airway resistance can be assessed in a body plethysmograph,

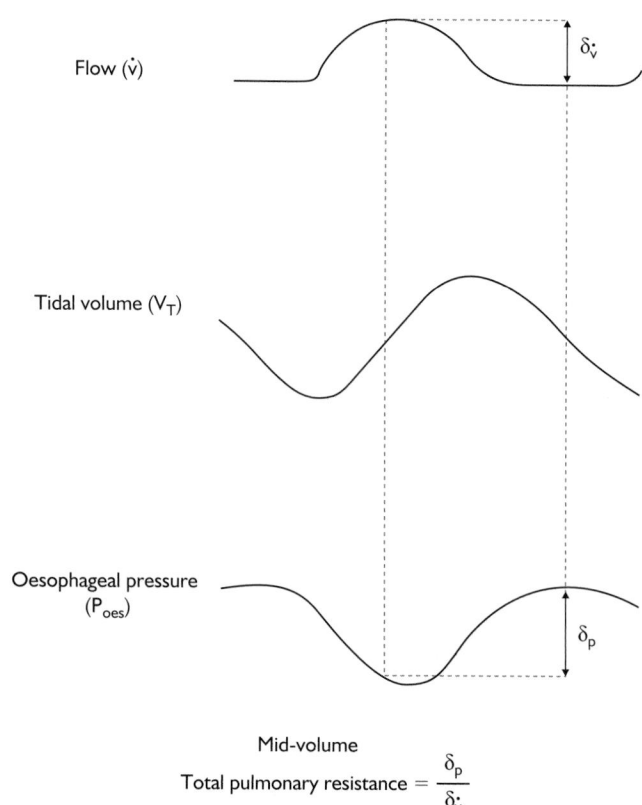

$$\text{Total pulmonary resistance} = \frac{\delta_p}{\delta_{\dot{v}}}$$

Mid-volume

Fig. 27.7 Flow, volume and pressure traces during tidal breathing. The total pulmonary resistance is calculated by dividing the pressure gradient between mid-inspiration and mid-expiration (δ_p) by the simultaneous flow difference (δ_v). (Reproduced from Greenough et al.[78])

but after the first week the infant will usually require sedation and this technique is not applicable to oxygen-dependent patients. Pulmonary resistance (Fig. 27.7), however, can be measured on the NICU, using an oesophageal balloon and pneumotachograph; the pressure difference corresponding to the flow change between points of equal lung volume is measured. Resistance is increased in infants with meconium aspiration syndrome and, at follow-up, in those who required neonatal ventilation.[251] Resistance can also be calculated from the volume and flow traces obtained after the release of the occlusion discussed above. The time constant, the time for 63% of the volume to leave the lungs, can be measured; thus, the resistance can be calculated, as the time constant equals the product of the compliance and the resistance.[144]

Surfactant

Origins of surfactant

Alveolar type II cells

Alveolar type II cells produce surfactant (Fig. 27.8).[185] They are compact cuboidal cells, occurring most often at the corners of the air spaces. They cover about 2% of the alveolar surface and account for about 15% of the cell numbers. They differentiate

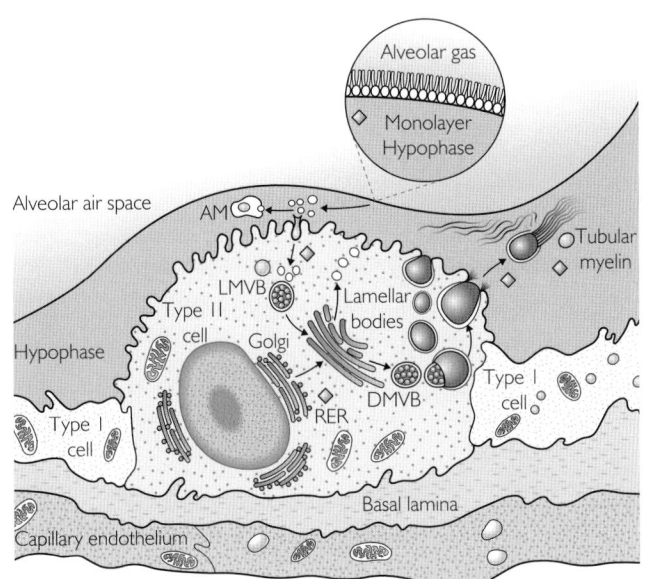

Fig. 27.8 An alveolar type II cell showing two surfactant release mechanisms: lamellar bodies and the constitutive release of surfactant protein A. Surfactant is shown being both phagocytosed by an alveolar macrophage (AM) and being taken back into the cell and being reutilised. The inset shows a monolayer, which, in the gel phase, is able to withstand very large lateral forces, literally splinting open the alveolus. RER, rough endoplasmic reticulum; LMVB, light multivesicular body; DVMB, dense multivesicular body. ◇ indicate the possible sites of damage in ARDS; these include the synthesis, release and reuptake of surfactant, and the formation of tubular myelin and of the monomolecular layer. (Reproduced from Nicholas et al.[168])

from the columnar epithelium during the canalicular phase of development (p. 445), but are not prominent until about 24 weeks' gestation, when they can be identified by their osmiophilic lamellar inclusion bodies.[136] The biosynthesis of surfactant phosphatidylcholine occurs in the endoplasmic reticulum of the type II cell. The phospholipid then moves via intracellular pathways towards the lamellar bodies, for secretion into the alveolus. The characteristic feature of the alveolar type II cell is the lamellar body, storage granules of surfactant.[85]

Lamellar bodies

A mature lamellar body is about 1.5 microns in diameter. They consist of a limiting membrane surrounding about 20 to 70 close-packed phospholipid bilayers, or lamellae, each with a width of 66 Å, arranged in a hemisphere. The ends of these lamellae abut onto a baseplate, which is probably an extension of the limiting membrane. In the centre is a matrix core of proteinaceous material.[216,217] Lamellar bodies, isolated from lung tissue by density gradient centrifugation, contain surfactant lipids and the surfactant proteins A, B and C (SP-A, SP-B, SP-C).

The lamellar bodies unravel to tubular myelin, a lattice of parallel lipid bilayers approximately 6.0 nm thick with a regular spacing of approximately 50 nm. It is highly surface active, containing phospholipids and surfactant proteins in the presence of calcium. SP-A is more abundant in tubular myelin than in lamellar bodies and is probably an important organiser of tubular myelin. There is direct transition from the tubular myelin to the surface film, with absorption of a mixture of saturated and unsaturated phospholipids. The surface film is then refined by selective squeeze out of the unsaturated phospholipids;[177] thus it consists almost entirely of dipalmitoyl phosphatidylcholine (DPPC) at expiration to FRC. During this cycling, small vesicular forms of surfactant are generated; these have poor surfactant activity and are mainly taken up by type II cells, although some are degraded by macrophages or lost from the airways. The loss of surfactant into the airways is proportional to the rate and depth of respiration and can be greatly reduced by addition of CPAP during mechanical ventilation.[248] Surfactant lost in this way is swallowed or, in the case of the fetus, finds its way into the amniotic fluid.

Recycling of surfactant

Surfactant may be degraded locally in the alveoli and small airways, the breakdown products being absorbed and recycled by the alveolar cells (Fig. 27.9). More than 90% of the phosphatidylcholine on the alveolar surface is reprocessed; this conserves surfactant components as well as reactivating them to regenerate surfactant. The turnover time is approximately 10 hours.[214] The contribution, therefore, to the alveolar surfactant pool from de novo synthesis is modest. The molecules seem to be taken up by the type II cell intact rather than broken down into their component parts. The surface of the type II cell facing the alveolus is covered with microvilli and lectin receptors. Aerosolised DPPC and lectins can rapidly enter type II cells and become associated with multivesicular bodies and subsequently lamellar bodies.[244] These clearance pathways are much less active in the developing lung, with a longer turnover time for surfactant phosphatidylcholine. In the preterm ventilated lamb, the turnover time is approximately 13 hours, reprocessing the alveolar surfactant with little catabolic activity.[118] In the adult, large amounts of surfactant phospholipid can be cleared in a dose-dependent fashion. The system is not overwhelmed by an exogenous dose 40 times greater than the size of the endogenous pool.

There is negative feedback regulation of surfactant production mediated by SP-A binding to type II cells.[222] Surfactant secretion is controlled by stretch receptors and stimulated by gas entering the lung, causing alveolar distension.[202] Other factors controlling secretion[200] include β-adrenergic receptors on alveolar type II cells, which increase in number towards the end of gestation.

Composition

Surfactant is a complex mixture of substances including phospholipids, neutral lipids and proteins.

Phosphatidylcholine and phosphatidylglycerol

Lipids are the major constituent of surfactant and the most important are phosphatidylcholine (PC) and phosphatidylglycerol (PG), representing 70–80% and 5–10% of the lipids,

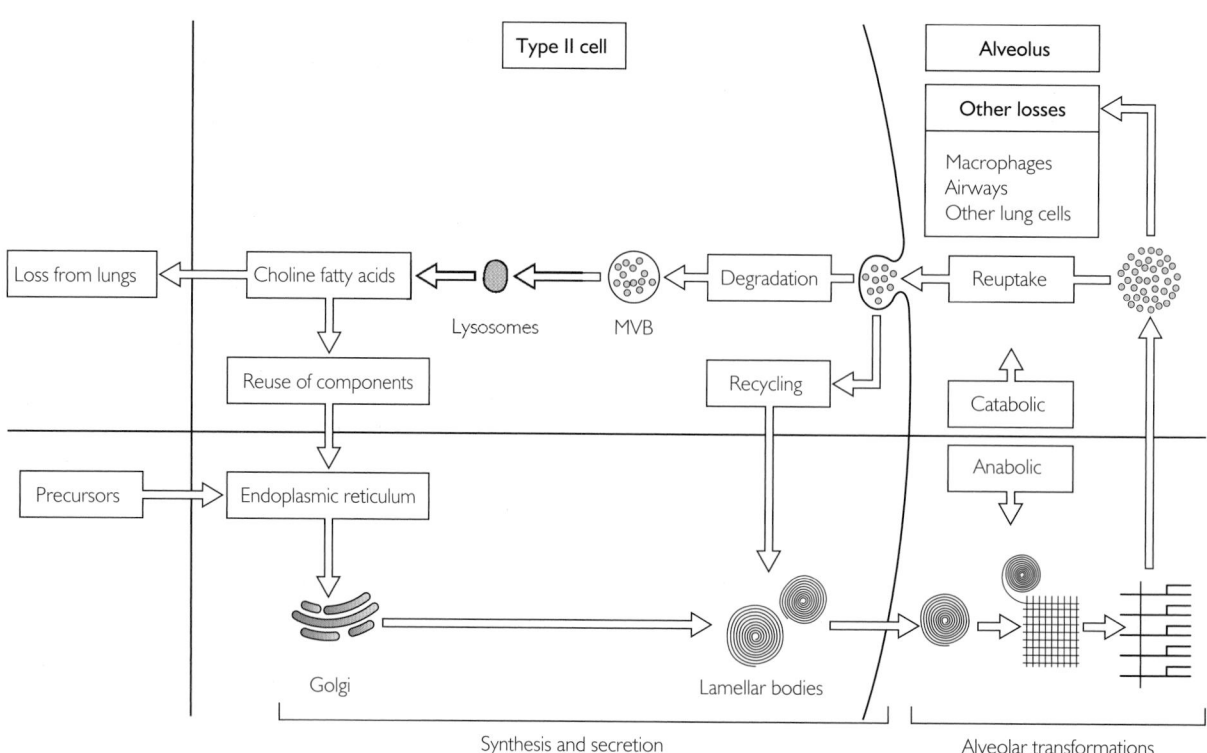

Fig. 27.9 Illustration of surfactant metabolism based on the saturated phosphatidylcholine component of surfactant. The anabolic pathway for synthesis and secretion links with alveolar transformations of the lamellar surfactant to tubular myelin and the monolayer. Catabolic pathways for phospholipid vesicles are minor pathways in the newborn lung but active in the adult lung. The majority of the surfactant is taken back into type II cells for recycling during the newborn period. (Reproduced from Jobe & Ikegami.[115])

respectively. Another 10% of the lipids is made up of phosphatidylinositol (PI), phosphatidylserine (PS) and phosphatidylethanolamine (PE). Approximately 60% of the PC has both fatty acids saturated (i.e. disaturated) and, as the primary saturated fatty acid is palmitic acid, the major compound in surfactant is DPPC. The palmitic acid residues are non-polar and hydrophobic and orient towards the air, whereas the PC is polar and hydrophilic and associates with the liquid phase.[111] The shape and orientation of the DPPC means that it generates a stable monolayer and is able to maintain low surface pressures: during expiration the molecules become very closely packed, as the palmitoyl moieties lack the C=C bonds that produce the kinks in the acyl chains.[247] DPPC is relatively rigid at body temperature and cannot adsorb to a surface,[74] its phase transition (melt) being approximately at 41°C. At body temperature, DPPC cannot move rapidly enough to maintain a surface monolayer during the respiratory cycle and a 'spreading' agent such as PG is required for normal surfactant function.

PC is synthesised in the endoplasmic reticulum of the type II pneumocytes. There is an increase in surfactant production towards the end of gestation. From 27 to 31 days (term) in rabbits, there is a 10-fold increase in surfactant; during a similar time period, PC increases from 30% to 70% of the total phospholipids, whereas sphingomyelin decreases from 40% to 10%. This change is due to increased synthesis, whereas after birth there is increased secretion. In surfactant from human term and preterm infants, the fractional concentrations of not only

PC16:0/16:0 (DPPC), but also palmitoylmyristoyl PC (PC16:0/14:0) and palmitoylpalmitoleoyl PC (PC16:0/16:1) increase with maturation;[16] in animal models, the concentrations of the latter phospholipids correlate significantly with respiratory rate. The proportions of the acidic phospholipids PG and PI change with lung development. Initially PI is the primary acidic phospholipid, but with increasing maturation is replaced by PG. Patients with RDS have low levels of DPPC and absent PG.[84] In poorly controlled diabetic pregnancies, the fetuses have low levels of PG even near term. If RDS progresses to chronic lung disease, the appearance of PG is delayed; PI also predominated with acute lung injury.[116]

Other lipids

About 10% of the total lipids in surfactant are neutral lipids. These are cholesterol, triacylglycerols and free fatty acids.[183] They appear to be an integral part of the surfactant in lamellar bodies and on the alveolar surface. Cholesterol alters the fluidity and organisation of lipid-rich membranes. Sphingomyelin represents less than 2% of surfactant lipid, and glycolipids and carbohydrates a very small fraction of the surfactant mass. The amount of sphingomyelin, a minor component of surfactant, remains unchanged through gestation and thus the change in the amount of DPPC or lecithin can be assessed by comparing it to the amount of sphingomyelin. Thus, lung maturity can be assessed by measurement of the ratio of lecithin to sphingomyelin, the L:S ratio (p. 556).

Surfactant proteins

Four surfactant-associated proteins – SP-A, SP-B, SP-C and SP-D – have been identified and comprise 5–10% of surfactant by weight.[56]

Surfactant protein A

SP-A is composed of approximately 248 amino acids.[15] It is a large glycoprotein belonging to the calcium-dependent collectin family of proteins. It comprises approximately 5% of surfactant by weight. There is considerable heterogeneity in its structure because of extensive post-translational modification. The human gene is located on chromosome 10; gene expression occurs exclusively in type II pneumocytes,[22] which appear to be the main site of synthesis.[245] Lamellar bodies are enriched with SP-A compared with lung homogenates.[176]

Synthesis of SP-A increases after 28 weeks of gestation.[12] Antibodies to this protein, however, are present in lung tissue at gestations as early as 16 weeks.[7] SP-A is developmentally regulated and induced in vivo by corticosteroids and thyrotrophin-releasing hormone (TRH).[111] SP-A synthesis is enhanced by cAMP, beta-adrenergic agents and epidermal growth factor (EGF). Dexamethasone increases the level of SP-A.[180,241,242] Insulin inhibits the accumulation of SP-A and SP-B mRNA, but has no effect on SP-C mRNA in vitro.[46] Insulin inhibits both SP-A and SP-B gene expression in vitro, and the levels of SP-A in the amniotic fluid of pregnancies complicated by diabetes mellitus are lower than in controls. In the mature lung, SP-A is expressed predominately in type II cells and Clara cells, but there is some expression in tracheal glands.

SP-A binds to and confers calcium-dependent aggregation on surfactant phospholipids.[94] SP-A has an essential role in determining the structure of tubular myelin, and the stability and rapidity of spreading and recycling of phospholipids.[225,240] It regulates the synthesis and secretion of phospholipids, and enhances their uptake by type II cells by binding to specific high-affinity receptors on the apical surface of the type II cells. SP-A partially inhibits surfactant secretion from type II cells[55] and may prevent the accumulation of surfactant on the alveolar surface. Its major contribution towards surface activity is to enhance the effects of SP-B and/or SP-C.[95] SP-A and SP-D form part of the innate host defence against infection. As collectins, they can target carbohydrate structures on invading microorganisms, particularly bacteria, resulting in agglutination and enhanced clearance.[82] SP-A binds endotoxin and a wide range of Gram-positive and Gram-negative organisms, promoting phagocytosis and killing of microorganisms by alveolar macrophages. It acts also as an opsonin for the phagocytosis of viruses, such as herpes simplex, influenza A and respiratory syncytial virus (RSV). SP-A increases NO production by macrophages to promote pathogen killing.[116] Knockout of the SP-A gene makes mice unable to form tubular myelin[131] and results in increased susceptibility to infection.[145] A low concentration of SP-A in lavage fluid in premature baboons has been correlated with a high infection index, based on histopathology, microbiological cultures and clinical indications of sepsis.[6] SP-A polymorphisms have been associated with severe RSV infection[146] and an increased risk of bronchopulmonary dysplasia.[236]

Surfactant protein B

The active 79 amino acid SP-B peptide (molecular weight [MW] 7500–9000) is produced by the proteolytic cleavage of pro SP-B, a 25 000–33 000 MW precursor protein.[41] SP-B comprises 1–2% of surfactant by weight.[235] The active SP-B peptide contains highly positively charged amino acids that form an amphipathic helix with the hydrophilic amino acid residues positioned near the phospholipid head groups at the membrane surface.[240] It is composed of two identical polypeptide chains, held together by a disulphide bond.[120] SP-B is encoded by a single copy gene located on chromosome 2.[60] The mRNA for SP-B is detectable in human fetal lung tissue as early as 12–14 weeks of gestation, localised in the epithelial cells of bronchi and bronchioles. After 25 weeks it is localised in the type II cells. Glucocorticoids increase expression of SP-B in fetal lung. Expression is restricted to type II pneumocytes and Clara cells. The active SP-B peptide is stored in lamellar bodies and secreted with phospholipids into the airway lumen.

SP-B is required for the formation of tubular myelin and increases the spreading of surfactant phospholipids onto an air–water interface.[32] SP-B disrupts phospholipid vesicles and alters the ordering and packing of the PC molecules. SP-B combined with lipid mixtures constitutes most of the surface activity of natural surfactant in vitro and increases lung compliance in vivo; SP-C and SP-B together are even more effective. SP-C and SP-B both stimulate lipid uptake in isolated cells. SP-B can also protect the pulmonary surfactant film from inactivation by serum proteins.[67]

Absence of SP-B influences the composition of pulmonary surfactants. It is associated with absence or markedly decreased PG and an additional aberrant SP-C peptide.[227] DPPC synthesis is preserved in SP-B deficiency but SP-C cannot be processed to its active peptide and no secretion of normal surfactant occurs.[13] In SP-B knockout mice, both lamellar bodies and tubular myelin structures are absent. SP-B deficiency, with complete absence of SP-B, is an autosomal recessively inherited disorder.[3] SP-B deficiency causes hypoxaemic respiratory failure and leads to lethal respiratory failure within the first year of life and is refractory to mechanical ventilation, surfactant therapy, glucocorticoids and extracorporeal membrane oxygenation.[34,87] It can present as a congenital form of alveolar proteinosis, but not all cases have this feature; pulmonary hypertension is a prominent clinical finding. Lung transplanation is currently the only successful intervention. High-frequency oscillatory ventilation and neuromuscular blockade may optimise oxygenation in SP-B-deficient infants awaiting lung transplantation, but such data are from the retrospective examination of only five infants' records.[127] SP-B deficiency can be demonstrated by the absence of SP-B in amniotic fluid or airway samples.[116] The most frequent mutation is a 121ins2 frame shift mutation; the gene frequency of this mutation is one per 1000–3000.[37]

Partial deficiencies of SP-B with less severe clinical courses have now been reported.[219] Glucocorticoid treatment may increase SP-B expression in infants with mutations that result in a low expression of SP-B.[8] SP-A and SP-B genetic variants have been identified as risk or protection factors for RDS.[64,81] SP-B polymorphisms are important determinants for RDS and may explain differences between black and white subjects, as well as between males and females, regarding the risk for RDS.[64]

Surfactant protein C

This hydrophobic protein has an MW of 3000–6000 depending on the separation system used. It comprises 1–2% of surfactant by weight.[119] The mRNA for SP-C is present from early lung morphogenesis at the distal tips of the branching airways,[238] but subsequently SP-C expression occurs only in the type II cells. The SP-C gene is located on chromosome 8.[72] SP-C contains 35 amino acids and is likely to be a transmembranous peptide. It has a hydrophobic valine-rich region, which may be required for its function. SP-C can impart surface-like properties to phospholipids.[133,191] Concentrations as low as 1% can dramatically enhance surface adsorption and spreading of phospholipids in vitro. It may play a role in enhancing the reuptake of phospholipids. Surprisingly, SP-C knockout mice have normal respiratory function and lung development;[71] it is possible that SP-B replaces SP-C. In humans, however, SP-C deficiency has been associated with an interstitial lung disease.[170]

Surfactant protein D

SP-D has an MW of 46 000 and is produced by type II and bronchiolar epithelial cells. Its expression increases with advancing gestation in association with differentiation of terminal airway cells;[40] SP-D production begins in the bronchiolar and terminal epithelium from about 21 weeks of gestation.[162] SP-D expression is widely distributed in epithelial cells in the body; in the lung, SP-D expression occurs in the type II cells, Clara cells and other airway cells and glands. Glucocorticoids increase SP-D expression. SP-D does not have significant surfactant-like activities when mixed with phospholipids. It is, however, involved in the immune function of the lung,[135] binding to a variety of complex carbohydrates and glycolipids and may have a role in host defence functions in the lung by interacting with the surfaces of bacteria and other microorganisms.[240] An SP-D polymorphism has been associated with severe RSV infection.[139] SP-D alters SP-A-dependent inhibition of surfactant secretion.[1] SP-D knockout produces alveolar accumulation of lipids and proteins.[132]

Synthesis

Phosphatidylcholine synthesis

PC is produced by the cytidine diphosphate (CDP) choline pathway (Fig. 27.10).[198] Choline is taken up by the cell by facilitated transport and is then phosphorylated by choline kinase to phosphocholine, which in turn is converted to CDP choline (the rate-limiting step), which is then transferred to diacylglycerol to give PC. This produces molecules containing one saturated fatty acid, palmitic acid, and one unsaturated fatty acid, usually oleic acid. This molecule is then remodelled by deacylation to lysophosphatidylcholine, followed by reacylation with a palmitic acid derived from either palmitoyl CoA or a second molecule of lysophosphatidylcholine[11] to give DPPC. It has been suggested that only 50% of the DPPC is synthesised directly from saturated diacylglycerols as precursors[184] and the rest by remodelling. Two remodelling mechanisms exist; both involve deacylation of de-novo synthesised 1-saturated-2-unsaturated PC to acyl-2-lysophosphatidylcholine. The latter is then either reacylated by reaction with a saturated acyl CoA or transacylated in a reaction involving two molecules of lysophosphatidylcholine.[199] Only the former mechanism is quantitatively important. Cholinephosphate

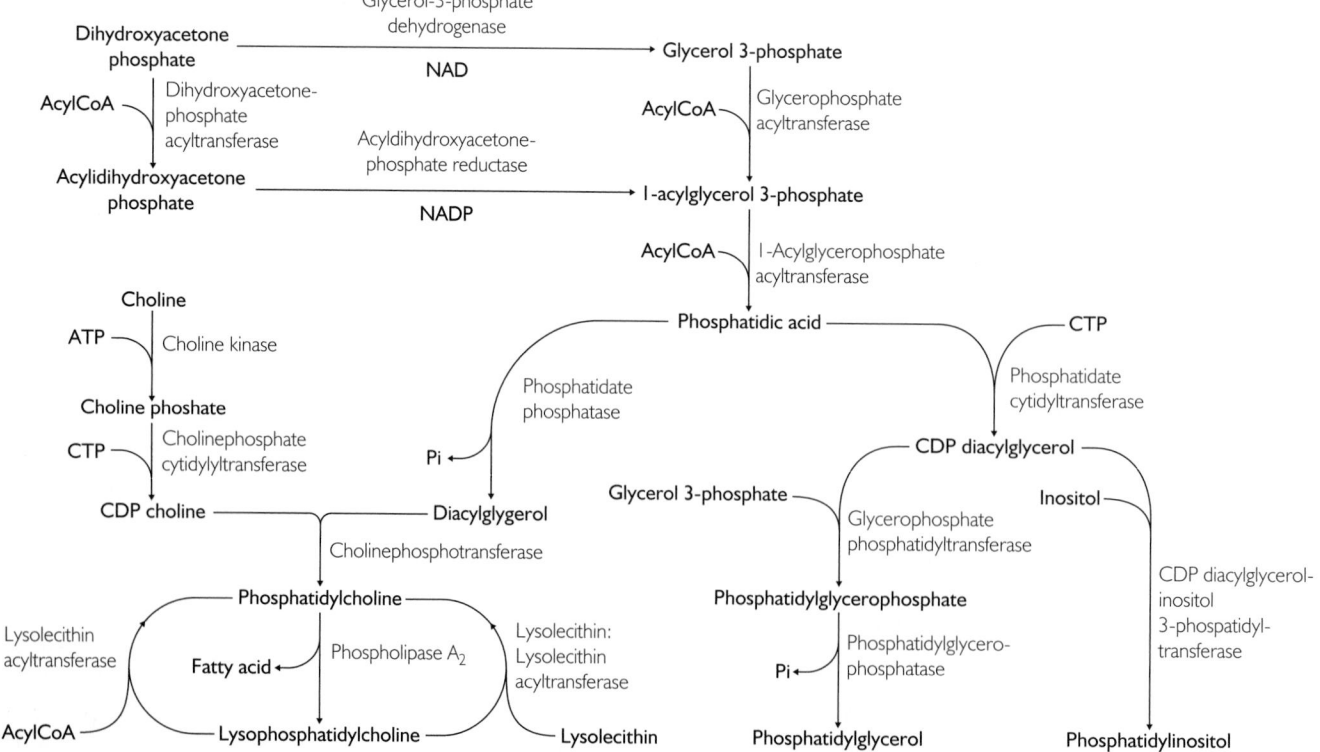

Fig. 27.10 Pathways in the biosynthesis of phosphatidylcholine, phosphatidylglycerol and phosphatidylinositol. (Reproduced from Rooney.[198])

cytidylyltransferase (CT), which catalyses phosphocholine to CDP choline, is essentially inactive without lipids; CT activity is activated during fetal lung development and after corticosteroid administration. Several other hormones, including thyroid hormones and insulin, and EGF influence this sequence of events. PC synthesis via the methylation of PE is of minor importance, except in conditions of choline deficiency.[250]

Phosphatidylglycerol synthesis

PG is synthesised together with the other acidic phospholipids, PI and PS, from CDP-diacylglycerol, which is in turn derived from phosphatidic acid (Fig. 27.10).

Factors affecting surfactant maturation

Glucocorticoids

Endogenous cortisol is an important physiological stimulus to fetal lung maturation. In the fetal sheep, there is a marked increase in plasma cortisol concentration at the end of gestation and this is associated with an increase in DPPC in lung tissue and lung lavage fluid.[53] Administration of betamethasone to pregnant rabbits results in an increase in the total amount of phospholipid, as well as an increase in the percentage in PC of the total phospholipids.[201] Cortisol induces fetal lung fibroblasts to produce fibroblast pneumocyte factor, which then stimulates surfactant production by the fetal type II pneumocytes.[209] In animal experiments, glucocorticoids increase lung aeration, decrease the surface tension of the lung extract and increase synthesis of both surfactant phospholipids and proteins.[125] In preterm infants, antenatal treatment with dexamethasone increases the surface activity of surfactant isolated from airway specimens and the ratio of SP-A to PC, but not in offspring of mothers with severe hypertension.[125] Dexamethasone increases pulmonary surfactant secretion through an enhancement of β_2-adrenoreceptor gene expression.[113] In a primary culture of rat alveolar cells, while dexamethasone had no effect on the basal secretion rate of PC, it augmented both the PC secretion and the cAMP formation increased by terbutaline, and increased the mRNA expression of β_2 receptors in type II cells.[113]

Beta-adrenergic drugs

Beta-adrenergic drugs stimulate adenylcyclase and inhibit phosphodiesterases, thereby increasing the amount of intracellular cAMP, which in turn increases the production[142] and secretion of surfactant. cAMP stimulates the synthesis of disaturated phospholipids and SP-A; in addition, it mediates the effect of a number of hormones. Terbutaline, a β-adrenergic agonist, can stimulate the secretion of PC from undifferentiated type II cells.[134] The pattern of response, however, was different from that seen in differentiated cells, suggesting that the developmental secretion of surfactant is complex and probably involves both excitatory and inhibitory mechanisms that develop at different stages.[134] Stimulation of the β_2-agonist system (using either a long-acting β_2 agonist, formeterol, or agents which elevate intracellular cAMP), however, may not augment postnatal function significantly above that noted for single-dose betamethasone therapy.[117]

Thyroid hormones

Thyroxine (T_4) increases surfactant production and lung maturation. Infants who develop RDS have lower cord blood levels of T_4 compared with those who do not. T_4 does not easily cross the placenta, but triiodothyronine (T_3) given to pregnant rats is associated with an increase in T_3 in the fetal serum. T_3 increases the type II cell receptors' response to fibroblast pneumocyte factor, which is necessary for appropriate surfactant production. TRH, unlike T_4 and T_3, readily crosses the placenta; it increases the amount of surfactant phospholipid. The effects of TRH are not entirely mediated by thyroid hormone. TRH stimulates prolactin production and functions as a neurotransmitter in the central nervous system.

Prolactin

Prolactin levels are lower in infants who develop RDS compared with those who do not and also are lower in immature versus mature infants and males versus females.[51] The effect of prolactin both in vivo and in cultured lung systems, however, is variable and the role of prolactin in surfactant production regulation remains speculative.

Epidermal growth factor

EGF may be important in the development of the pulmonary epithelium. Infusion of this substance into lambs prevents the development of hyaline membrane disease[29] and increases lung distensibility. There is a reduced amount of SP-A in the offspring of rats with EGF autoantibodies.[187] Muellerian inhibiting substance inhibits lung maturation by blocking phosphorylation of EGF receptors;[28] this may be an explanation for the higher incidence of RDS in males. In non-human primate fetuses delivered at 78% of term, in-utero treatment with EGF resulted in higher SP-A levels and L:S ratios in treated compared to untreated fetuses.[75]

Fibroblast pneumocyte factor

Alveolar cells need the presence of fibroblasts and their pneumocyte factor to produce surfactant.[210] Glucocorticoids act on the fetal lung fibroblasts to induce the production of fibroblast pneumocyte factor, which in turn stimulates rapid surfactant synthesis by the alveolar type II cell.

Insulin

Insulin delays the maturation of alveolar type II cells and decreases the proportion of saturated PC.[79] In addition, infants of diabetic mothers have delayed appearance of PG.[174] Hyperglycaemia also plays a role in the delay in lung maturation seen in these babies.[69] Insulin inhibits SP-A gene expression.[157]

Testosterone

Premature male infants are more prone to RDS than are similarly immature female infants.[179] Male lungs are approximately 1 week more immature as determined by the disaturated PC content. These differences may be due to inhibition of surfactant production in males by androgens;[223] lipid concentration in the lung appears to be at least partly directly or indirectly regulated by androgens.[173] In addition, androgens delay lung maturation through their action on lung fibroblasts.[186]

Surfactant physical properties and functions

Surfactant prevents atelectasis and thus reduces the work of breathing. This is achieved by reduction of surface tension and by surfactant becoming a 'solid' monolayer, promoting stability of the alveoli, in expiration. Surfactant also prevents the transudation of fluid: in conditions of high surface tension, fluid is sucked into the alveolar spaces from the capillaries.

The presence of an insoluble surface film capable of maintaining a very low surface tension (or high surface pressure) in the air spaces was first inferred by Pattle.[178] A small bubble will normally diminish in size and disappear; the smaller it becomes, the more rapidly its diameter decreases. This follows from the relationship described by the Laplace equation

$$P = 2\gamma/r$$

where P = internal pressure, γ = surface tension and r = radius, that is, that the pressure difference across the bubble's wall is given by twice the tension in the wall divided by the radius. Thus, in the presence of a high surface tension and small radius, the high pressure difference causes gas to diffuse from the bubble into the surrounding liquid. In the lung, however, the presence of an insoluble surface film means that the surface tension is reduced as the radius decreases. The contribution of surface tension to the pressure volume behaviour of the lung was demonstrated by von Neergaard,[226] who showed that lungs inflated with saline have a higher compliance than if filled with air. Saline abolishes the surface tension forces, which are an important component of the static recoil force of the lung.

Surfactant lowers surface tension by forming an insoluble surface film. This opposes the surface tension of the underlying liquid by exerting surface pressure. The surface properties of surfactant result from its composition, that is, molecules with both a hydrophobic and hydrophilic chain. When forming a film on water, the polar group is attracted to the water, whereas the non-polar group is turned towards the gas phase. DPPC is a symmetrical molecule and the two straight hydrophobic fatty acid chains allow close packing of the monolayer. Compression of such a monolayer results in it being changed from a liquid to a condensed gel or solid state;[36,164] this is because the transition temperature of the refined mixture rises to above 37°C, so that in vivo the refined monolayer may be solid.[36] In RDS, the PC is relatively unsaturated and of lower quantity than in the mature species. This means an unstable monolayer is formed on compression in expiration, which buckles and does not reduce surface tension effectively. Even when the monolayer has been refined,

there is so little DPPC available the alveoli are of small size. Thus, infants with RDS have a low FRC and an increased work of breathing.

Inhibition of surface activity of surfactant by proteins

The alveolar surfactant system may be altered by an inhibitory effect of proteins leaked from the intravascular or interstitial space, due to an increased permeability of the capillary endothelial and/or alveolar–epithelial barrier.[205] In RDS, the alveolar capillary membrane permeability is increased, and the hyaline membranes are a massive aggregation of fibrin. In addition, proteinaceous material may be inhaled, for example as in meconium aspiration syndrome. There is a marked rank order of potency of proteins in interfering with surfactant function – fibrinmonomer > fibrinogen > albumin > elastin > IgG > IgM – such that fibrin has 50 times greater effectiveness than albumin. Once the proteins are present in the surface monolayer, they inhibit the ability of the compressed surfactant to lower surface tension. The leakage of protein onto the alveolar surface, at least in premature rabbits, can be inhibited by surfactant treatment and treatment with antenatal steroids or TRH.[112] In other conditions, such as meconium aspiration syndrome, the inhibitory effect of the proteins can be overcome by increasing the dose of surfactant. Exogenous surfactants differ with regard to their inhibition by proteins; calf lung surfactant extract and Alveofact are only moderately inhibited by fibrinogen.[204] KL_4 surfactant, which has a synthetic peptide in lieu of SP-B, resists inhibition to serum proteins more than a natural surfactant (beractant).[148]

Assessment of surfactant maturity

The fluid which is secreted by the fetal lung moves out into the amniotic fluid, carrying surfactant with it. As the lung matures, so the composition of the surfactant in the amniotic fluid changes. The proportion of surfactant (lecithin) in the amniotic fluid can be compared with that of sphingomyelin (L:S ratio). An L:S ratio greater than 2.0 is usually associated with lung maturity and in 95% of cases will predict the absence of RDS. A mature L:S ratio, however, can be associated with RDS in the infants of diabetic mothers or those with rhesus disease; in these cases, the abnormality is deficiency of PG rather than a lack of DPPC. Relating the amniotic fluid surfactant to the albumin level provides a more reliable predictor of the absence of RDS in infants of diabetic mothers than assessing the amount of DPPC.[218] Unfortunately, an L:S ratio less than 2.0 predicts RDS with an accuracy of only 54%.[86] The lower the L:S ratio, the more likely the baby is to develop RDS: 21% of babies with an L:S ratio of 1.5 to 2.0 being affected, compared to 80% with an L:S ratio below 1.5.

The L:S ratio cannot necessarily be predicted by the fetal gestational age, as accelerated maturation can be seen in small-for-dates babies, whereas delayed maturation is associated with lung hypoplasia, mild diabetes, very small twins[171] and occasionally is familial.[86] Abnormal L:S ratios occur when the specimen is contaminated with blood, meconium or vaginal secretions. The predictive value of L:S ratios depends on amniotic fluid being sampled within 3 days of delivery. Once the patient is in labour, the amniotic fluid L:S ratio is increased compared with that obtained at elective caesarean section.

Identification of PG in the amniotic fluid is helpful, as babies with PG rarely develop RDS. A combination of a low L:S ratio with absence of PG from amniotic fluid samples obtained within 3 days of delivery is a better predictor of the duration of respiratory support than is either gestational age or birthweight, but only in pregnancies not complicated by premature rupture of the membranes.[90] In diabetic pregnancies, the presence of PG correlated to an L:S ratio of $\geqslant 3.0$ and a lamellar body count of at least 50 000.[70]

The L:S ratio can also be assessed in fluid from the pharynx[10,103,237] or stomach.[166] This can give retrospective demonstration that a baby had mature lungs at birth or provide further documentation on the course of a baby's illness.[124]

Alternative methods which correlate highly to the L:S ratio are available; these include fluorescence polarisation[189] and assessment of lamellar body concentration. Such tests are less labour intensive and have a turnaround time of 1 hour.[54] Meta-analysis of six studies demonstrated that the lamellar body count performed slightly better than the L:S ratio in the prediction of RDS; in addition, the test can be performed more quickly and is less expensive.[243]

The level of serum SP-A in the first 24 hours has been shown to increase with advancing gestational age and differs significantly between infants with and without RDS.[123] SP-A can also be measured in cord blood using an enzyme-linked immunosorbent assay system, so has been suggested to be a useful serum marker to predict the development of RDS.[123] Tests of surfactant maturity, however, are now rarely employed, as many clinicians have the policy of giving exogenous surfactant very soon after birth to all infants born below a certain gestational age, because of the proven efficacy of prophylactic surfactant administration.

References

1. Akino T, Shiratori M, Tsuzuki A et al 1991 Native form of surfactant protein D (SP-D) which lipids are associated with, affects the activity of SP-A on type II cells. American Review of Respiratory Disease 143: A316

2. Altura B M, Chand N 1981 Bradykinin-induced relaxation of renal and pulmonary arteries is dependent upon intact endothelial cell. British Journal of Pharmacology 74: 10–11

3. Andersen C, Ramsay J A, Nogee L M et al 2000 Recurrent familial neonatal deaths: hereditary surfactant protein B deficiency. American Journal of Perinatology 17: 219–224

4. Ang S L, Rossan J 1994 HNF-3beta is essential for node and notocord development in mouse development. Cell 78: 561–574

5. Asonye U O, Vidyasagar D 1981 Clinical applications of continuous transcutaneous PO_2 monitoring. In: Lauersen N H, Hochberg H M (eds) Clinical perinatal biochemical monitoring. Williams & Wilkins, Baltimore, pp 205–219

6. Awasthi S, Coalson J J, Yoder B A, Crouch E, King R J 2001 Deficiencies in lung surfactant proteins A and D are associated with lung infection in very premature neonatal baboons. American Journal of Respiratory and Critical Care Medicine 163: 389–397

7. Ballard P L, Hawgood S, Liley H 1986 Regulation of pulmonary surfactant apoprotein SP 28-36 gene in fetal human lung. Proceedings of the National Academy of Sciences of the United States of America 83: 9527–9531

8. Ballard P L, Nogee L M, Beers M F et al 1995 Partial deficiency of surfactant protein B in an infant with chronic lung disease. Pediatrics 96: 1046–1052

9. Barker P M, Walters D V, Markiewicz M et al 1991 Development of the lung liquid reabsorptive mechanism in fetal sheep: synergism of triiodothyronine and hydrocortisone. Journal of Physiology 433: 435–449

10. Barr P A, Jenkins P A, Baum J D 1975 L/S ratio in hypopharyngeal aspirate of newborn infants. Archives of Disease in Childhood 50: 856–861

11. Batenburg J J 1982 The phosphatidylcholine-lysophosphatidylcholine cycle. In: Farrell P M (ed) Lung development: biological and clinical perspectives. Academic Press, New York, p. 36

12. Batenburg J J, Hallman M 1990 Developmental biochemistry of alveoli. In: Scarpelli E M (ed) Pulmonary physiology: fetus, newborn, child and adolescent. Lea & Febiger, Philadelphia, pp 106–139

13. Beers M F, Hamvas A, Moxley M A et al 2000 Pulmonary surfactant metabolism in infants lacking surfactant B. American Journal of Respiratory Cell and Molecular Biology 22: 380–391

14. Bekedam D J, Visser G H A 1985 Effects of hypoxemic events on breathing, body movements and heart rate variation: a study in growth retarded human fetuses. American Journal of Obstetrics and Gynecology 153: 52–56

15. Benson B, Hawgood S, Schilling J et al 1985 Structure of canine pulmonary surfactant apoprotein: cDNA and complete amino acid sequence. Proceedings of the National Academy of Sciences of the United States of America 82: 6379–6383

16. Bernhard W, Hoffman S, Dombrowsky H et al 2001 Phosphatidylcholine molecular species in lung surfactant: composition in relation to respiratory rate and lung development. American Journal of Respiratory Cell and Molecular Biology 25: 725–731

17. Bianchi A L, Denavit-Saubie M, Champagnat J 1995 Central control of breathing in mammals: neuronal circuitry, membrane properties, and neurotransmitters. Physiological Reviews 75: 1–45

18. Blanco C E, Dawes G S, Hanson M A et al 1984 The response to hypoxia of arterial chemoreceptors in fetal sheep and newborn lambs. Journal of Physiology 351: 25–37

19. Blanco C E, Hanson M A, McCooke H B et al 1987 Studies of chemoreceptor resetting after hyperoxic ventilation of the fetus in utero. In: Ribero J A, Pallot D J (eds) Chemoreceptors in respiratory control. Croom Helm, London, pp 221–227

20. Bodineau L F, Cayetanot F, Sadani-Makki F et al 2003 Consequences of in utero caffeine exposure on respiratory output in normoxic and hypoxic conditions and related changes of Fos expression: a study on brainstem-spinal cord preparations isolated from newborn rats. Pediatric Research 53: 266–273

21. Bonham A C 1995 Neurotransmitters in the CNS control of breathing. Respiration Physiology 101: 219–230

22. Bruns G S, H, Veldman G M, Latt S A et al 1987 The 35 kd pulmonary surfactant associated protein is encoded on chromosome 10. Human Genetics 76: 58–62

23. Bryan A C, Bowes G, Maloney J E 1986 Control of breathing during sleep. In: Cherniack N S, Widdicombe J G (eds) Handbook of physiology – the respiratory system. American Physiological Society, Bethesda, pp 529–579

24. Bullard K M, Sonne J, Hawgood S et al 1997 Tracheal ligation increases cell proliferation but decreases surfactant protein in fetal murine lungs in vitro. Journal of Pediatric Surgery 32: 207–213

25. Burri P H, Hislop A A 1998 Structural considerations. European Respiratory Journal 12(suppl. 27): 59s–65s

26. Calder N A, Williams B A, Kumar P et al 1994 The respiratory response of healthy term infants to breath-by-breath alternations in inspired oxygen at two postnatal ages. Pediatric Research 35: 321–324

27. Carroll J L, Bamford O S, Fitzgerald R S 1993 Postnatal maturation of carotid chemoreceptor responses to O_2 and CO_2 in the cat. Journal of Applied Physiology 75: 2383–2391

28. Catlin E A, Uitvlugt N D, Donahoe P K et al 1991 Muellerian inhibiting substance blocks epidermal growth factor receptor phosphorylation in fetal rat lung membranes. Metabolism 40: 1178–1184

29. Catterton W Z, Escobedo M B, Sexson W R et al 1979 Effect of epidermal growth factor on lung maturation in fetal rabbits. Pediatric Research 13: 104–110

30. Ceruti E 1966 Chemoreceptor reflexes in the newborn infant: effect of cooling on the response to hypoxia. Pediatrics 37: 556–564

31. Chan V, Greenough A 1992 Lung function and the Hering Breuer reflex in the neonatal period. Early Human Development 28: 111–118

32. Chang R, Nir S, Poulain FR 1998 Analysis of binding and membrane destabilisation of phospholipid membranes by surfactant apoprotein B. Biochemica et Biophysica Acta 1371: 254–264

33. Cherniack N S, von Euler C, Glogowska M et al 1981 Characteristics and rate of occurrence of spontaneous and provoked augmented breaths. Acta Paediatrica Scandinavica 111: 349–360

34. Chetcuti P A J, Ball R J 1995 Surfactant aproprotein B deficiency. Archives of Disease in Childhood. Fetal and Neonatal Edition 73: F125–F127

35. Clark F J, von Euler C 1972 On the regulation of depth and rate of breathing. Journal of Physiology 222: 267–295

36. Clements J A 1977 Functions of the alveolar lining layer. American Review of Respiratory Disease 115: 67–71

37. Cole F S, Hamvas A, Rubenstein P et al 2000 Population based estimates of surfactant protein B deficiency. Pediatrics 105: 538–541

38. Condorelli S, Scarpelli E M 1975 Somatic-respiratory reflex and onset of regular breathing movements in the lamb foetus in utero. Pediatric Research 9: 879–884

39. Cordero L, Hon E 1971 Neonatal bradycardia following nasopharyngeal stimulation. Journal of Pediatrics 78: 441–447

40. Crouch E, Rust K, Marinecheck W et al 1991 Developmental expression of pulmonary surfactant protein D (SP-D). American Journal of Respiratory Cell and Molecular Biology 5: 13–18

41. Curstedt T, Johansson J, Barros-Soderling J 1988 Low molecular mass surfactant protein type 1. The primary structure of hydrophobic 8-Kda polypeptide with eight half cysteine residues. European Journal of Biochemistry 172: 521–525

42. Curzi-Dascalova L 1978 Thoraco-abdominal respiratory correlations in infants: constancy and variability in different sleep states. Early Human Development 2: 25–38

43. Davey M G, Hooper S B, Cock M L, Harding R 2001 Stimulation of lung growth in fetuses with lung hypoplasia leads to altered postnatal lung structure in sheep. Pediatric Pulmonology 32: 267–276

44. Davies A M, Koenig J S, Thach B T 1988 Upper airway chemoreflex responses to saline and water in preterm infants. Journal of Applied Physiology 64: 1412–1420

45. De Troyer A, Kelly S, Macklem P T et al 1985 Mechanics of intercostal space and actions of external and internal intercostal muscles. Journal of Clinical Investigation 75: 850–857

46. Dekowski S A, Snyder J M 1992 Insulin regulation of messenger ribonucleic acid for the surfactant associated proteins in human fetal lung in vitro. Endocrinology 131: 669–676

47. Deli009-Papadopoulos M, DiGiacomo J E 1992 Oxygen transport and delivery. In: Polin R A, Fox W W (eds) Fetal and neonatal physiology. W B Saunders, Philadelphia, pp 801–813

48. Deli009-Papadopoulos M, Roncevic N P, Oski F A 1971 Postnatal changes in oxygen transport of term, premature and sick infants: the role of red cell 2,3-diphosphoglycerate and adult hemoglobin. Pediatric Research 5: 235–245

49. Denavit-Saubié M, Champagnat J, Zieglgaensberger W 1978 Effects of opiates and methionine-enkephalin on pontine and bulbar respiratory neurones of the cat. Brain Research 155: 55–67

50. Devlieger H 1987 The chest wall in the preterm infant. MD Thesis. Universite Catholique de Louvain, Louvain, pp 136–140

51. Dhanireddy R, Smith Y F, Hamosh M et al 1983 Respiratory distress syndrome in the newborn: relationship to serum prolactin, thyroxine and sex. Biology of the Neonate 43: 9–15

52. Dickinson K A, Harding R 1987 Decline in lung liquid volume and secretion and tracheal flow rate in lambs. Journal of Applied Physiology 62: 24–38

53. DiFiore J W, Wilson J M 1994 Lung development. Seminars in Pediatric Surgery 3: 221–232

54. Dilena B A, Ku F, Doyle I et al 1997 Six alternative methods to the lecithin/sphingomyelin ratio in amniotic fluid for assessing fetal lung maturity. Annals of Clinical Biochemistry 34: 106–108

55. Dobbs D L, Wright J R, Hawgood S et al 1987 Pulmonary surfactant and its components inhibit secretion of phosphatidylcholine from cultured rat alveolar type II cells. Proceedings of the National Academy of Sciences of the United States of America 84: 1010–1014

56. Dobbs L G 1989 Pulmonary surfactant. Annual Review of Medicine 40: 431–446

57. Donnelly D F, Haddad G G 1990 Prolonged apnea and impaired survival in piglets after sinus and aortic nerve section. Journal of Applied Physiology 68: 1048–1052

58. Duara S 1992 Structure and function of the upper airway in neonates. In: Polin R A, Fox W W (eds) Fetal and neonatal physiology. W B Saunders, Philadelphia, pp 823–828

59. Eden G J, Hanson M A 1987 Effects of chronic hypoxia on chemoreceptor function in the newborn. In: Ribero J A, Pallot D J (eds) Chemoreceptors in respiratory control. Croom Helm, London, pp 369–377

60. Emrie P A, Jones C, Hofmann T 1988 The coding sequence for the human 18 000 dalton hydrophobic pulmonary surfactant protein is located on chromosome 2 and identifies a restriction fragment length polymorphism. Somatic and Cellular Molecular Genetics 14: 105–110

61. Feldman J L 1986 Neurophysiology of breathing in mammals. In: Bloom F E (ed) Handbook of physiology, Section 1: The nervous system, Vol. IV: Intrinsic regulatory systems of the brain. American Physiological Society, Bethesda, pp 463–524

62. Fewell J E, Hislop A A, Kitterman J A et al 1983 Effect of tracheostomy on lung development in fetal lambs. Journal of Applied Physiology 55: 1103–1108

63. Fleming P J, Bryan A C, Bryan M H 1978 Functional immaturity of pulmonary irritant receptors and apnea in newborn preterm infants. Pediatrics 61: 515–518

64. Floros J, Fan R, Diangelo S, Guo X, Wer J, Luo J 2001 Surfactant protein B associations and interactions with SP-A in white and black subjects with respiratory distress syndrome. Pediatrics International 43: 567–576

65. Frantz I D, Alder S M, Abroms I F et al 1976 Respiratory response to airway occlusion in infants: sleep state and maturation. Journal of Applied Physiology 41: 634–635

66. Friedman A H, Fahey J T 1993 The transition from fetal to neonatal circulation: normal responses and implications for infants with heart disease. Seminars in Perinatology 17: 106–121

67. Friedrich W, Schmalisch G, Stevens P A, Wauer R R 2000 Surfactant protein SP-B counteracts inhibition of pulmonary surfactant by serum proteins. European Journal of Medical Research 5: 277–282

68. Funk G D, Smith J C, Feldman J J 1993 Generation and transmission of respiratory oscillations in medullary slices: role of excitatory amino acids. Journal of Neurophysiology 70: 1497–1515

69. Gewolb I H, Rooney S A, Barrett C 1985 Delayed pulmonary maturation in the fetus of the streptozotocin-diabetic rat. Experimental Lung Research 8: 141–151

70. Ghidini A, Spong CY, Goodwin K, Pezzullo J C 2002 Optimal thresholds of the lecithin/sphingomyelin ratio and lamellar body count for the prediction of the presence of phosphatidylglycerol in diabetic women. Journal of Maternal-Fetal & Neonatal Medicine 12: 95–98

71. Glasser S W, Burhans M S, Korfhagen T R et al 2001 Altered stability of pulmonary surfactant in SP-C deficient mice. Proceedings of the National Academy of Sciences of the United States of America 98: 6366–6371

72. Glasser S W, Korfhagen T R, Perne C M 1988 Two genes encoding human pulmonary surfactant proteolipid SPL (pVal). Journal of Biological Chemistry 263: 10326–10331

73. Gluckman P D, Gunn T R, Johnston B M 1983 The effect of cooling on breathing and shivering unanaesthetized fetal lambs in utero. Journal of Physiology 343: 495–506

74. Goerke J 1998 Pulmonary surfactant: functions and molecular composition. Biochimica et Biophysica Acta 1408: 79–89

75. Goetzman B W, Read L C, Plopper C G et al 1994 Prenatal exposure to epidermal growth factor attenuates respiratory distress syndrome in rhesus infants. Pediatric Research 35: 30–36

76. Greenough A 1988 The premature infant's respiratory response to mechanical ventilation. Early Human Development 17: 1–5

77. Greenough A, Pool J 1991 Hering Breuer reflex in young asthmatic children. Pediatric Pulmonology 11: 345–349

78. Greenough A, Roberton N R C, Milner A D 1995 Neonatal respiratory disorders. Edward Arnold, London, p. 105

79. Gross I, Smith G J, Wilson C M et al 1980 The influence of hormones on the biochemical development of fetal rat lung in organ culture: II insulin. Pediatric Research 14: 834–838

80. Guyton A C 1971 Regulation of cardiac output. Anaesthesiology 29: 314–326

81. Haataja R, Ramet M, Marttila R, Hallman M 2000 Surfactant proteins A and B as interactive genetic determinants of neonatal respiratory distress syndrome. Human Molecular Genetics 9: 1751–1760

82. Hakansson K, Reid K B M 2000 Collectin structure: a review. Protein Science 9: 1607–1617

83. Hall S M, Haworth S G 1986 Conducting pulmonary arteries structural adaptation to extrauterine life. Cardiovascular Research 21: 208–216

84. Hallman M, Feldman B H, Kirkpatrick E et al 1977 Absence of phosphatidylglycerol (PG) in RDS in the newborn. Pediatric Research 11: 714–720

85. Hallman M, Miyai K, Wagner R M 1976 Isolated lamellar bodies from rat lung; correlated ultrastructural and biochemical studies. Laboratory Investigation 35: 79–86

86. Hallman M, Teramo K, Kankaanpaa K et al 1980 Prevention of respiratory distress syndrome: current view of lung maturity studies. Annals of Clinical Research 12: 36–44

87. Hamvas A, Nogee L M, deMello D E et al 1995 Pathophysiology and treatment of surfactant protein-B deficiency. Biology of the Neonate 67(suppl. 1): 18–32

88. Hannam S, Ingram D M, Rabe-Hesketh S, Milner A D 2001 Characterisation of the Hering Breuer deflation reflex in the human neonate. Respiration Physiology 124: 51–64

89. Harding R 1986 The upper respiratory tract in perinatal life. In: Johnston B M, Gluckman P D (eds) Reproductive and perinatal medicine. Respiratory control and lung development in the fetus and newborn. Perinatology Press, Ithaca, pp 331–376

90. Harper M A, Lorentz W B 1993 Immature lecithin:sphingomyelin ratios and neonatal respiratory course. American Journal of Obstetrics and Gynecology 168: 495–498

91. Harrison M R, Adzick N S, Flake A W et al 1996 Correction of congenital diaphramgatic hernia in utero VIII: Response of the hypoplastic lung to tracheal occlusion. Journal of Pediatric Surgery 31: 1339–1348

92. Hasan S J, Rigaux A 1992 Effect of bilateral vagotomy on oxygenation, arousal and healthy movements in fetal sheep. Journal of Applied Physiology 73: 1402–1412

93. Hassan A, Gossage J, Ingram D et al 2001 Volume of activation of the Hering Breuer inflation reflex in the newborn infant. Journal of Applied Physiology 90: 763–769

94. Hawgood S, Benson B J, Hamilton R L 1985 Effects of surfactant associated protein and calcium ions on the structure and surface activity of lung surfactant lipids. Biochemistry 24: 185–190

95. Hawgood S, Benson B J, Schilling J et al 1987 Nucleotide and amino-acid sequences of pulmonary surfactant SP18 and evidence for cooperation between SP18 and SP28-36 in surfactant lipid adsorption. Proceedings of the National Academy of Sciences of the United States of America 84: 66–70

96. Haworth S G 1992 Development of the pulmonary circulation. In: Polin R A, Fox W W (eds) Fetal and neonatal physiology. W B Saunders, Philadelphia, pp 671–682

97. Haworth S G, Hall S M, Chew M et al 1987 Thinning of fetal pulmonary arterial wall and postnatal remodelling: ultrastructural studies on the respiratory unit arteries of the pig. Virchows Archiv. A, Pathological Anatomy and Histopathology 411: 161–171

98. Head H 1889 On the regulation of respiration. Journal of Physiology 10: 1–70

99. Henderson-Smart D J 1983 Regulation of breathing in the perinatal period. In: Saunders N A, Sulivan C E (eds) Sleeping and breathing: lung biology in health and disease. Marcel Dekker, New York

100. Hering E, Breuer J 1868 Die selbsteurung der Amnung durch den nevus vagus sitzber. Sitzungsbericht der Kaiserlichen Akademie der Wissenschaften in Wien 57: 672–677

101. Herlenius E, Aden U, Tang L Q, Lagercrantz H 2002 Perinatal respiratory control and its modulation by adenosine and caffeine in the rat. Pediatric Research 51: 4–12

102. Hertzberg T, Hellstrom S, Holgert H et al 1992 Ventilatory response to hyperoxia in newborn rats born in hypoxia – possible relationship to carotid body dopamine. Journal of Physiology 456: 645–654

103. Hill C M 1976 The determination of the fatty acid profile of lecithin from human amniotic fluid and the pharyngeal aspirate of the newborn. Journal of Physiology 257: 15–17P

104. Hislop A, Haworth S G 1989 Airway size and structure in the normal fetal and infant lung and the effect of premature delivery and artificial ventilation. American Review of Respiratory Disease 140: 1717–1726

105. Hislop A, Reid L 1981 Growth and development of the respiratory system. Anatomical development. In: Davis J A, Dobbing J (eds) Scientific foundations of paediatrics. Heinemann, London, pp 390–432

106. Hoch B, Bernhard M 2000 Central apnoea and endogenous prostaglandins in neonates. Acta Paediatrica 89: 1364–1368

107. Holtman J R J, Speck D F 1994 Substance P immunoreactive projections to the ventral respiratory group in the rat. Peptides 15: 803–805

108. Hooper S B, Harding R 1995 Fetal lung liquid: a major determinant of the growth and functional development of the fetal lung. Clinical and Experimental Pharmacology and Physiology 22: 235–247

109. Hooper S B, Wallace M J, Harding R 1993 Amiloride blocks the inhibition of fetal lung liquid secretion caused by AVP but not by asphyxia. Journal of Applied Physiology 74: 111–115

110. Hummler E, Barker P, Gatzy J et al 1996 Early death due to defective neonatal lung fluid clearance in alpha-EnaC-deficient mice. Nature Genetics 12: 325–328

111. Ikegami M, Jobe A H 1993 Surfactant metabolism. Seminars in Perinatology 17: 233–240

112. Ikegami M, Jobe A, Pettenazzo A et al 1987 Effects of maternal treatment with corticosteroids, T₃, TRH and their combinations on lung function of ventilated preterm rabbits with and without surfactant treatments. American Review of Respiratory Disease 136: 892–898

113. Isohama Y, Kumanda Y, Tanaka K, Kai H, Takahama M, Miyata T 1997 Dexamethasone increases beta 2-adrenoreceptor-regulated phosphatidylcholine secretion in rat alveolar type II cells. Japanese Journal of Pharmacology 73: 163–169

114. Jeffery H E, Reid I, Rahilly P et al 1980 Gastro-esophageal reflux in "near-miss" sudden infant death infants in active but not quiet sleep. Sleep 3: 393–399

115. Jobe A H, Ikegami M 1993 Surfactant metabolism. Clinics in Perinatology 20: 683–696

116. Jobe A H, Ikegami M 2001 Biology of surfactant. Clinics in Perinatology 28: 655–669

117. Jobe A H, Ikegami M, Padbury J et al 1997 Combined effects of fetal lamb beta agonist stimulation and glucocorticoids on lung function of preterm lambs. Biology of the Neonate 72: 305–310

118. Jobe A, Ikegami M, Seidner S R et al 1989 Surfactant phosphatidylcholine metabolism and surfactant function in preterm ventilated lambs. American Review of Respiratory Disease 139: 352–359

119. Johansson J 1998 Structure and properties of surfactant protein C. Biochimica et Biophysica Acta 1408: 161–171

120. Johansson J, Curstedt 1997 Molecular structures and interactions of pulmonary surfactant. European Journal of Biochemistry 244: 675–693

121. Johnston B M, Bennet L, Gluckman P D 1989 In: Gluckman P D, Johnston B M, Nathanielsz P W (eds) Research in perinatal medicine, Vol. VIII Advances in fetal physiology. Perinatology Press, Ithaca, pp 77–193

122. Kalapesi Z, Durand M, Leahy F N et al 1981 Effect of periodic or regular respiratory pattern on the ventilatory response to low inhaled CO2 in preterm infants during sleep. American Review of Respiratory Disease 123: 8–11

123. Kaneko K, Shimizu H, Arakawa H, Ogawa Y 2001 Pulmonary surfactant protein A in sera for assessing neonatal lung maturation. Early Human Development 62: 11–21

124. Kanto W P, Borer R C, Barr M et al 1976 Tracheal aspirate lecithin:sphingomyelin ratios as predictors of recovery from respiratory distress syndrome. Journal of Pediatrics 89: 612–616

125. Kari M A, Akino T, Hallman M 1995 Prenatal dexamethasone and exogenous surfactant therapy: surface activity and surfactant components in airway specimens. Pediatric Research 38: 678–684

126. Karlberg P, Cherry R B, Escardo F E et al 1962 Respiratory studies in newborn infants II. Pulmonary mechanics of breathing in the first minutes of life, including the onset of respiration. Acta Paediatrica Scandinavica 51: 121–136

127. King E L, Shackelford G D, Hamvas A 2001 High-frequency oscillation and paralysis stabilize surfactant protein-B-deficient infants. Journal of Perinatology 21: 421–425

128. Kinsella J P, Abman S H 1995 Recent developments in the pathophysiology and treatment of persistent pulmonary hypertension of the newborn. Journal of Pediatrics 126: 853–864

129. Kirkpatrick S M L, Olinsky A, Bryan M H et al 1976 Effect of premature delivery on the maturation of the Hering-Breuer inspiratory inhibitor reflex in human infants. Journal of Pediatrics 88: 1011–1014

130. Kleinmann L I, Petering H G, Sutherland J M 1967 Blood carbonic anhydrase activity and zinc concentration in infants with respiratory distress syndrome. New England Journal of Medicine 227: 1157–1161

131. Korfhagen T R, Bruno M D, Ross G G et al 1996 Altered surfactant function and structure in SP-A gene targeted mice. Proceedings of the National Academy of Sciences of the United States of America 93: 9594–9599

132. Korfhagen T R, Sheftelyevich V, Burhans MS et al 1998 Surfactant protein D regulates surfactant phospholipid homeostasis in vivo. Journal of Biological Chemistry 273: 28438–28443

133. Kraemer A, Wintergalen A, Sieber M, Galla H J, Amrein M, Guckenberger R 2000 Distribution of surfactant-associated protein C within a lung surfactant model film investigated by near field optical microscopy. Biophysical Journal 78: 458–465

134. Kresch M J, Lima D M, Lu H 1996 Developmental regulation of phospholipid secretion by fetal type II pneumocytes. Biochimica et Biophysica Acta 1299: 39–46

135. Kuan S F, Rust K, Crouch E 1992 Interactions of surfactant protein D with bacterial lipopolysaccharides. Surfactant protein D is an Escherichia coli-binding protein in bronchoalveolar lavage. Journal of Clinical Investigation 90: 97–106

136. Kuhn C 1982 The cytology of the lung: ultrastructure of the respiratory epithelium and extracellular lining layers. In: Farrell P M (ed) Lung development: biological and clinical perspectives. Academic Press, New York, p 27

137. Lagercrantz H 1987 Neuromodulators and respiratory control in the infant. Clinics in Perinatology 14: 683–695

138. Lagercrantz H, Pequignot J M, Hertzberg T et al 1994 Birth-related changes of expression and turnover of some neuroactive agents and respiratory control. Biology of the Neonate 65: 145–148

139. Lahti M, Lofgren J, Marttila R et al 2002 Surfactant protein D gene polymorphism associated with severe respiratory syncytial virus infection. Pediatric Research 51: 696–699

140. Lalley P M, Bischoff A M, Richter D W 1994 Serotonin 1-alpha-receptor activation suppresses respiratory apneusis in the cat. Neuroscience Letters 172: 59–62

141. Laubscher B, Greenough A 1998 Comparative effects of theophylline and caffeine on respiratory function of preterm infants. Early Human Development 50: 185–192

142. Lawson E E, Brown E R, Torday J S et al 1978 The effect of epinephrine on tracheal fluid flow and surfactant flux in fetal sheep. American Review of Respiratory Disease 118: 1023–1026

143. Leffler C W, Hessler J R, Green R S 1984 The onset of breathing at birth stimulates pulmonary vascular prostacyclin synthesis. Pediatric Research 18: 938–942

144. Lesouef P N, England S J, Bryan A C 1984 Passive respiratory mechanics in newborns and children. American Review of Respiratory Disease 129: 552–556

145. LeVine A M, Bruno M D, Huelsman K M, Ross G F, Whitsett J A, Korfhagen T R 1997 Surfactant protein A-deficient mice are susceptible to group B streptococcal infection. Journal of Immunology 158: 4336–4340

146. Lofgren J, Ramet M 2002 Association between surfactant protein A gene locus and severe respiratory syncytial virus infection in infants. Journal of Infectious Diseases 185: 283–289

147. Loosli C G, Potter E L 1959 Pre and postnatal development of the respiratory portion of the human lung. American Review of Respiratory Disease 80: 5–20

148. Manalo E, Merritt T A, Kheiter A et al 1996 Comparative effects of some serum components and proteolytic products of fibrinogen on surface tension-lowering abilities of beractant and a synthetic peptide containing surfactant KL$_4$. Pediatric Research 39: 947–952

149. Marchal F, Bairam A, Haouzi P et al 1992 Carotid chemoreceptor response to natural stimuli in the newborn kitten. Respiration Physiology 87: 183–193

150. Markstahler U E, Kremer E, Kimmina S, Becker K, Richter D W 2002 Effects of functional knock-out alpha 1 glycine-receptors on breathing movements in oscillator mice. Respiratory Physiology & Neurobiology 130: 33–42

151. Marsh M, Fox G, Hoskyns E W et al 1994 The Hering Breuer deflationary reflex in the newborn infant. Pediatric Pulmonology 18: 163–169

152. Martin R J, Nearman H S, Katona P G et al 1977 The effect of a low continuous positive airway pressure on the reflex control of respiration in the preterm infant. Journal of Pediatrics 90: 976–981

153. Massaro G D, Massaro D 1996 Formation of pulmonary alveoli and gas exchange surface area: quantitation and regulation. Annual Review of Physiology 58: 73–92

154. Massaro G D, Massaro D 2000 Retinoic acid treatment partially rescues failed septation in rats and in mice. American Journal of Physiology 278: L955–L960

155. Mayock D E, Hall J, Watchko J F et al 1987 Diaphragmatic muscle fiber type development in swine. Pediatric Research 22: 449–454

156. Merazzi D, Mortola J P 1999 Hering Breuer reflex in conscious newborn rats: effects of changes in ambient temperature during hypoxia. Journal of Applied Physiology 87: 1656–1661

157. Miakotina O L, Goss K L, Snyder J M 2002 Insulin utilises the PI 3-kinase pathway to inhibit SP-A gene expression in lung epithelial cells. Respiratory Research 3: 27

158. Millhorn D E, Eldridge F L 1986 Role of ventrolateral medulla in regulation of respiratory and cardiovascular systems. Journal of Applied Physiology 61: 1249–1263

159. Millhorn D E, Eldridge F L, Kiley J P et al 1984 Prolonged inhibition of respiration following acute hypoxia in glomectomized cats. Respiration Physiology 57: 331–340

160. Milner A D, Marsh M J, Ingram D M et al 1999 Effects of smoking in pregnancy on neonatal lung function. Archives of Disease in Childhood. Fetal and Neonatal Edition 80: F8–F14

161. Milner A D, Saunders R A 1977 Pressure and volume changes during the first breath of human neonates. Archives of Disease in Childhood 52: 918–924

162. Mori K, Kurihara N, Hayashida S, Tanaka M, Ikeda K 2002 The intrauterine expression of surfactant protein D in terminal airways of human fetuses compared with surfactant protein A. European Journal of Pediatrics 161: 431–434

163. Moriette G, van Reempts P, Moore M et al 1985 The effect of rebreathing CO$_2$ on ventilation and diaphragmatic electromyography in newborn infants. Respiration Physiology 62: 387–397

164. Morley C J, Bangham A D 1981 Physical properties of surfactant under compression. In: Wichert V (ed) Progress in respiratory research 15. Clinical importance of surfactant defects. Karger, Basle, p. 188

165. Mortola J P 1983 Some functional mechanical implications of the structural design of the respiratory system in newborn mammals. American Review of Respiratory Disease 128: S69–S72

166. Motoyama E K, Namba Y, Rooney S A 1976 Phosphatidylcholine content and fatty acid composition of tracheal and gastric liquids from premature and full term newborn infants. Clinica Chimica Acta 70: 449–454

167. Motoyoma J, Liu J, Mo R et al 1998 Essential function of Gli2 and Gli3 in the formation of the lung, trachea and oesophagus. Nature Genetics 20: 54–57

168. Nicholas T E, Doyle I R, Bersten A D 1997 Surfactant replacement therapy in ARDS: white knight or noise in the system? Thorax 52: 195–197

169. Nicolini U, Fisk N M, Talbert D G et al 1989 Intrauterine manometry: technique and application to fetal pathology. Prenatal Diagnosis 9: 243–254

170. Nogee L M, Wert S E, Proffitt S A et al 2000 Allelic heterogeneity in hereditary SP-B deficiency. American Journal of Respiratory and Critical Care Medicine 161: 973–981

171. Obladen M, Gluck L 1977 RDS and tracheal phospholipid composition in twins: independent of gestational age. Journal of Pediatrics 90: 799–802

172. Ohki M, Naito K, Cole P 1991 Dimensions and resistances of the human nose: racial differences. Laryngoscope 101: 276–278

173. Ojeda M S, Gomez N, Giminez M S 1997 Androgen regulation of lung lipids in the male rat. Lipids 32: 57–62

174. Ojomo E O, Coustan D R 1990 Absence of evidence of pulmonary maturity at amniocentesis in term infants of diabetic mothers. American Journal of Obstetrics and Gynecology 163: 954–957

175. Olver R E, Strang L B 1974 Ion fluxes across the pulmonary epithelium and the secretion of lung liquid in the foetal lamb. Journal of Physiology 241: 327–357

176. O'Reilly M A, Nogee L, Whitsett J A 1988 Requirement of the collagenous domain for carbohydrate processing and secretion of surfactant protein of Mr = 35 000. Biochimica et Biophysica Acta 969: 176–184

177. Pastrana-Rios B, Flach C R, Brauner J W, Mautone A J, Mendelsohn R 1994 A direct test of the "squeeze-out" hypothesis of lung surfactant function. Biochemistry 33: 5121–5127

178. Pattle R E 1955 Properties, function and origin of the alveolar lining layer. Nature 175: 1125–1126

179. Perelman R H, Palta M, Kirby R et al 1986 Discordance between male and female deaths due to the respiratory distress syndrome. Pediatrics 78: 238–244

180. Phelps D S, Church S, Kourembanas S 1987 Increases in the 35 kDa surfactant associated protein and its mRNA following in vivo dexamethasone treatment in fetal and neonatal rats. Electrophoresis 8: 235–238

181. Phillipson E A, Bowes G 1986 Control of breathing during sleep. In: Cherniack N S, Widdicombe J G (eds) Handbook of physiology – the respiratory system. American Physiological Society, Bethesda, pp 649–690

182. Pickens D L, Schefft G L, Thach B T 1989 Pharyngeal fluid clearance and aspiration preventive mechanisms in sleeping infants. Journal of Applied Physiology 66: 1164–1171

183. Post M, Batenburg J, Schuurmans E et al 1982 Lamellar bodies isolated from adult human lung tissue. Experimental Lung Research 3: 17–28

184. Post M, Schuurmans E A, Batenberg J J et al 1983 Mechanisms involved in the synthesis of disaturated phosphatidylcholine by alveolar type II cells isolated from adult rat lung. Biochimica et Biophysica Acta 750: 68–77

185. Post M, van Golde L M G 1988 Metabolic and developmental aspects of the pulmonary surfactant system. Biochimica et Biophysica Acta 947: 249–286

186. Provost P R, Blomquist C H, Drolet R, Flamand N, Tremblay Y 2002 Androgen inactivation in human lung fibroblasts: variations in levels of 17 beta-hydroxysteroid dehydrogenase type 2 and 5 alpha-reductase activity compatible with androgen inactivation. Journal of Clinical Endocrinology and Metabolism 87: 3883–3892

187. Raaberg L, Nexo E, Jorgensen P E et al 1995 Fetal effects of epidermal growth factor deficiency induced in rats by autoantibodies against epidermal growth factor. Pediatric Research 37: 175–181

188. Rabbette P S, Dezateux C A, Fletcher M E et al 1991 The Hering Breuer reflex declines during the first year of life. European Respiratory Journal 4: 533S

189. Ragosch V, Juergens S, Lorenz U et al 1992 Prediction of RDS by amniotic fluid analysis: a comparison of the prognostic value of traditional and recent methods. Journal of Perinatal Medicine 20: 351–360

190. Ramminger S J, Baines D L, Olver R E, Wilson S M 2000 The effects of PO$_2$ upon transepithelial ion transport in fetal rat distal lung epithelial cells. Journal of Physiology 524: 539–547

191. Revak S D, Merritt T A, Degryse E et al 1988 Use of human surfactant low molecular weight apoproteins in the reconstitution of surfactant biological activity. Journal of Clinical Investigation 81: 826–833

192. Richter D W, Ballanyi K, Schwarzacher S 1992 Mechanisms of respiratory rhythm generation. Current Opinion in Neurobiology 2: 788–793

193. Rigatto H 1984 Control of ventilation in the newborn. Annual Review of Physiology 46: 661–674

194. Rigatto H 1992 Control of breathing in fetal life and onset and control of breathing in the neonate. In: Polin R A, Fox W W (eds) Fetal and neonatal physiology. W B Saunders, Philadelphia, pp 790–801

195. Rigatto H, Kwiat Kouski K A, Hansan S U et al 1991 The ventilatory response to endogenous CO2 in preterm infants. American Review of Respiratory Disease 143: 101–104

196. Rigatto H, Lee D, Davi M et al 1988 Effect of increased arterial PaCO$_2$ on fetal breathing and behavior in sheep. Journal of Applied Physiology 64: 982–987

197. Rodenstein D O, Perlmutter N, Stanescu D C 1985 Infants are not obligatory nasal breathers. American Review of Respiratory Disease 131: 343–347

198. Rooney S A 1985 The surfactant system and lung phospholipid biochemistry. American Review of Respiratory Disease 131: 439–460

199. Rooney S A 1992 Regulation of surfactant-associated phospholipid synthesis and secretion. In: Polin R A, Fox W W (eds) Fetal and neonatal physiology. W B Saunders, Philadelphia, pp 971–985

200. Rooney S A 2001 Regulation of surfactant secretion. Comparative Biochemistry and Physiology 129: 233–243

201. Rooney S A, Gobran L I, Marino P A et al 1979 Effects of betamethasone on phospholipid content, composition and biosynthesis in fetal rabbit lung. Biochimica et Biophysica Acta 572: 64–76

202. Rooney S A, Gobran L I, Wai-Lee T S 1977 Stimulation of surfactant production by oxytocin-induced labour in the rabbit. Journal of Clinical Investigation 60: 754–759

203. Runold M, Lagercrantz H, Prabhakar M R et al 1989 Role of adenosine in hypoxic ventilatory depression. Journal of Applied Physiology 67: 541–546

204. Seeger W, Grube C, Gunther A et al 1993 Surfactant inhibition by plasma proteins: differential sensitivity of various surfactant preparations. European Respiratory Journal 6: 971–977

205. Seeger W, Stohr G, Neuhof H 1985 Surfactant inhibitory plasma-derived proteins. In: Walters D V, Strang L B, Geubelle F (eds) Physiology of the fetal and neonatal lung. Kluwer Academic Press, Lancaster, pp 225–240

206. Serra A, Brozoski D, Hodges M, et al 2002 Effects of carotid and aortic chemoreceptor denervation in newborn piglets. Journal of Applied Physiology 92: 893–900

207. Shaul P W 1995 Nitric oxide in the developing lung. Advances in Pediatrics 42: 367–414

208. Silverman M 1983 Respiratory function testing in infancy and childhood. In: Laszlo G, Sudlow M F (eds) Measurement in clinical respiratory physiology. Academic Press, London, pp 293–328

209. Smith B T 1978 Fibroblast pneumocyte factor: intercellular mediator of glucocorticoid effect on fetal lung. In: Stern L (ed) Neonatal intensive care. Mason, New York, pp 25–32

210. Smith B T 1979 Lung maturation in the fetal rat: acceleration by injection of fibroblast pneumocyte factor. Science 204: 1094–1095

211. Smith J C, Butera R J, Koshiya N, Del Negro C, Wilson C G, Johnson S M 2000 Respiratory rhythm generation in neonatal and adult mammals: the hybrid pacemaker-network model. Respiration Physiology 122: 131–147

212. Souza P, O'Brodovich H, Post M 1995 Lung fluid restriction affects growth but not airway branching of embryonic rat lung. International Journal of Developmental Biology 39: 629–637

213. Sparrow M P, Weichselbaum M, McCray P B 1999 Development of the innervation and airway smooth muscle in human fetal lung. American Journal of Respiratory Cell and Molecular Biology 20: 550–560

214. Stevens P A, Wright J R, Clements J A 1989 Surfactant secretion and clearance in the newborn. Journal of Applied Physiology 67: 1595–1605

215. Strang L B 1977 Neonatal respiration. Blackwell Scientific, Oxford

216. Stratton C J 1976 The high resolution ultrastructure of the periodicity and architecture of the lipid-retained and extracted lung multilamellar body laminations. Tissue and Cell 8: 713–728

217. Stratton C J 1976 The three dimensional aspect of mammalian lung lamellar bodies. Tissue and Cell 8: 693–712

218. Tanasijevic M K, Winkelman J W, Wybenga D R et al 1996 Prediction of fetal lung maturity in infants of diabetic mothers using the FLM S/A and disaturated phosphatidylcholine tests. American Journal of Clinical Pathology 105: 17–22

219. Thompson M W 2001 Surfactant protein B deficiency: insights into surfactant function from clinical surfactant protein deficiency. American Journal of the Medical Sciences 321: 26–32

220. Thurlbeck W M 1982 Postnatal human lung growth. Thorax 37: 564–571

221. Tietel D F, Iwamoto H S, Rudolph A M 1987 Effects of birth related events on central blood flow patterns. Pediatric Research 22: 557–566

222. Tino M J, Wright J R 1998 Interactions of surfactant protein A with epithelial cells and phagocytes. Biochimica et Biophysica Acta 1408: 241–263

223. Torday J S 1985 Dihydrotesterone inhibits fibroblast pneumocyte factor-mediated synthesis of saturated phosphatidylcholine by fetal rat lung cells. Biochimica et Biophysica Acta 835: 23–28

224. Turner D J, Stick S M, Lesouef K L, Sly P D, Lesouef P N 1995 A new technique to generate and assess forced expiration from raised lung volume in infants. American Journal of Respiratory and Critical Care Medicine 151: 1441–1450

225. Veldhuizen R A W, Yao L-J, Hearn S A et al 1996 Surfactant-associated protein A is important for maintaining surfactant large-aggregate forms during surface-area cycling. Biochemical Journal 313: 835–840

226. von Neergaard K 1929 Neue auffassungen uber einen grundbegriff der Atemmechanik. Die Retraktionskraft der Lunge abhaengig von der Oberflaechenspannung in den Alveolen. Zeitschrift fur die Gesamte Experimentelle Medizin 66: 373–394

227. Vorbroker D K, Profitt S A, Nogee L M et al 1995 Aberrant processing of surfactant protein C in hereditary SP-B deficiency. American Journal of Physiology 268: L647–L656

228. Vyas H, Field D, Hopkin I E et al 1986 Determinants of the first inspiratory volume and functional residual capacity at birth. Pediatric Pulmonology 2: 189–193

229. Vyas H, Milner A D, Hopkin I E 1981 Comparison of intrathoracic pressure and volume changes during the spontaneous onset of respiration in babies born by caesarean section and by vaginal delivery. Journal of Pediatrics 99: 787–791

230. Walters D V, Olver R E 1978 The role of catecholamines in lung liquid absorption at birth. Pediatric Research 12: 239–242

231. Walters D V, Ramsden C A 1985 The secretion and absorption of fetal lung liquid. In: Walters D V, Strang L B, Geubelle F (eds) Physiology of the fetal and neonatal lung. Kluwer Academic Press, Lancaster, pp 61–74

232. Walther F J, Benders M J, Leighton J O 1993 Early changes in the neonatal circulatory transition. Journal of Pediatrics 123: 625–632

233. Warburton D, Zhao J, Berberich M A, Bernfield M 1999 Molecular embryology of the lung: then, now and in the future. American Journal of Physiology 276: L697–L704

234. Wealthall S R 1975 Factors resulting in a failure to interrupt apnea. In: Bosma J F, Showacre J (eds) Development of upper respiratory anatomy and function. US Government Printing Office, Washington DC, pp 212–225

235. Weaver T E 1998 Synthesis, processing and secretion of surfactant proteins B and C. Biochimica et Biophysica Acta 1408: 173–179

236. Weber B, Borkhardt A 2000 Polymorphisms of surfactant protein A genes and the risk of bronchopulmonary dysplasia in preterm infants. Turkish Journal of Pediatrics 41: 181–185

237. Weller P H, Jenkins P A, Gupta J et al 1976 Pharyngeal lecithin:sphingomyelin ratio in newborn infants. Lancet i: 12–14

238. Wert S E, Glasser S W, Korfhagen T R et al 1993 Transcriptional elements from the human SP-C gene direct expression in the primordial respiratory epithelium of transgenic mice. Developmental Biology 156: 426–443

239. Wharton J, Haworth S G, Polak J M 1988 Postnatal development of the innervation and paraganglia in the porcine pulmonary arterial bed. Journal of Pathology 154: 19–27

240. Whitsett J A, Nogee L M, Weaver T E et al 1995 Human surfactant protein B: structure, function, regulation and genetic disease. Physiological Reviews 75: 749–757

241. Whitsett J A, Pilot T, Clark J C et al 1987 Induction of surfactant protein in fetal lung: effects of cAMP and dexamethasone on SAP-35 RNA and synthesis. Journal of Biological Chemistry 262: 5256–5261

242. Whitsett J A, Weaver T E, Lieberman M A et al 1987 Differential effects of epidermal growth factor and transforming growth factor beta and synthesis of Mr = 35 000 surfactant associated proteins in fetal lung. Journal of Biological Chemistry 262: 7908–7913

243. Wijnberger L D, Huisjes A J, Voorbij H A, Franx A, Bruinse H W, Mol B W 2001 The accuracy of lamellar body count and lecithin/sphingomyelin ratio in the prediction of neonatal respiratory distress syndrome: a meta-analysis. BJOG 108: 583–588

244. Williams M C 1987 Vesicles within vesicles: what role do multivesicular bodies play in alveolar type II cells? American Review of Respiratory Disease 135: 744–746

245. Williams M C, Benson B J 1981 Immunocytochemical localization and identification of the major surfactant protein in adult rat lung. Journal of Histochemistry and Cytochemistry 29: 291–305

246. Woodrum D 1992 Respiratory muscles. In: Polin R A, Fox W W (eds) Fetal and neonatal physiology. W B Saunders, Philadelphia, pp 829–841

247. Wright J R, Clements J A 1987 Metabolism and turnover of lung surfactant. American Review of Respiratory Disease 135: 426–444

248. Wyszogrodski I, Kyei-Aboagye K, Taeusch H W J 1975 Surfactant inactivation by hyperventilation: conservation by end expiratory pressure. Journal of Applied Physiology 38: 461–466

249. Yamamoto M, Lagercrantz H, von Euler C 1981 Effects of substance P and TRH on ventilation and pattern of breathing in newborn rabbits. Acta Physiologica Scandinavica 113: 541–543

250. Yost R W, Chander A, Dodia C et al 1986 Stimulation of the methylation pathway for phosphatidylcholine synthesis in rat lungs by choline deficiency. Biochimica et Biophysica Acta 875: 122–125

251. Yüksel B, Greenough A 1992 Neonatal respiratory support and lung function abnormalities at follow-up. Respiratory Medicine 86: 97–100

252. Zenge J P, Rairigh R L, Grover T R et al 2001 NO and prostaglandins modulate the pulmonary vascular response to hemodynamic stress in the late gestation fetus. American Journal of Physiology. Lung Cellular and Molecular Physiology 281: 1157–1163

253. Ziegler J W, Ivy D D, Kinsella J P et al 1995 The role of nitric oxide, endothelin and prostaglandins in the transition of the pulmonary circulation. Clinics in Perinatology 22: 387–403

PART 2

Acute respiratory disease

Anne Greenough, Anthony D Milner

Respiratory problems are the commonest cause both of admission to a neonatal unit and of requirement for mechanical ventilation.

Respiratory distress syndrome

Respiratory distress syndrome (RDS), in non-intubated babies who have not received exogenous surfactant therapy, is characterised clinically by a respiratory rate >60/min, dyspnoea (intercostal, subcostal indrawing, sternal retraction) with a predominantly diaphragmatic breathing pattern and a characteristic expiratory grunt or moan, all presenting within 4 to 6 hours of delivery. Oxygen administration is required to prevent cyanosis, and there is a reticulogranular chest X-ray (CXR) appearance as a result of widespread atelectasis. Nowadays, this classical presentation is unusual, as very prematurely born babies are intubated and given surfactant within the first few hours after birth. The diagnosis in such babies then is based on their premature birth and CXR appearance. Pathophysiologically, the condition is characterised by non-compliant (stiff) lungs, which contain less surfactant than normal and become atelectatic at end-expiration. Histologically, hyaline membranes occur, lining the terminal airways. These membranes give the condition its alternative name, hyaline membrane disease (HMD), which, to be semantically correct, should be used only in the presence of histological confirmation (that is at autopsy); thus, the term RDS is preferred.

Incidence

Prior to routine use of either antenatal corticosteroids or postnatal surfactant, the prevalence of lung disease in newborn babies was reported to be between 2% and 3% in Europe[276,430] and, in 1986–1987, 1.72% of liveborn babies developed RDS in the USA.[54] In the modern era of neonatal intensive care, approximately 1% of infants develop RDS.[765]

Aetiology

RDS results from immaturity of the lungs, particularly the surfactant-synthesising systems. Various factors contribute to the immaturity and others interact with it to increase or decrease the incidence of the disorder.

Predisposing factors

Prematurity

The risk of RDS is inversely proportional to gestational age; 50% of babies less than 30 weeks of gestational age, as compared with 2% of those between 35 and 36 weeks, developing RDS.[765] RDS is almost invariable in infants <28 weeks' gestation, but it does remain a significant problem up to 34 weeks' gestation.[563] The maturation of surfactant synthesis is a mirror image of the incidence of RDS at different gestations. Some of the dyspnoea and hypoxaemia in very preterm babies is due to their immature lung structure, with increased connective tissue and poorly developed alveoli. Other factors make the preterm neonate inherently susceptible to RDS. Their lung epithelia are more leaky than those of a baby born at term, increasing the likelihood of protein passing onto the alveolar surface, where it will inhibit surfactant function (see below). They are more prone to asphyxia, hypoxia, hypotension and hypothermia, all of which are likely to impair surfactant synthesis or increase alveolar capillary leakiness.

Gender

Boys are much more likely to develop RDS than girls, with a male to female ratio of 1.7:1, and are more likely to die from the disease.[270] In male fetuses, the delayed maturation of the lecithin-to-sphingomyelin (L:S) ratio and late appearance of phosphatidylglycerol (PG)[284] are androgen induced.[528,881]

Race

Black babies have a lower incidence of RDS, 60–70% of that of white babies of the same gestational age.[445] This is evident even in very immature babies, only 40% of African infants <32 weeks' gestational age developing RDS, compared with 75% of Caucasian infants.[488] No black baby with an L:S ratio >1.2 developed RDS, but white babies did develop the disease at those low ratios.[742] Allelic variation in the surfactant protein A gene has been reported between American whites and Nigerian blacks.[745]

Caesarean section

Caesarean section carried out before the mother went into labour was reported to increase the risk of her baby developing RDS,[272,894,895] although this was not a consistent finding.[854] That is in keeping with the findings that surfactant is released into the airways[112] and the pharyngeal L:S ratio is higher in babies born by caesarean section with, rather than without, labour.[939] Data from infants born at gestations above 32 to 34 weeks confirm the association of caesarean section before labour with both RDS and transient tachypnoea of the newborn (TTN; pp. 485–6).[23,158,641] The timing of the caesarean section is also important; the need for mechanical ventilation being 120 times greater after elective caesarean section at 37 to 38 weeks as compared with 39 to 41 weeks.[598]

Birth depression

Babies who are depressed at birth have been reported to be at increased risk of RDS.[871] The incidence of RDS in babies less than 32 weeks of gestation was 54% in those with an Apgar <4 compared with 42% in babies with Apgars >4 (p < 0.005).[57] During fetal asphyxia, lung perfusion falls, resulting in ischaemic damage to pulmonary capillaries. When the fetus recovers from the acute asphyxia, pulmonary hyperperfusion occurs, and if delivery occurs shortly afterwards, a protein-rich fluid leaks out of the damaged pulmonary capillaries.[470] This leakage of proteins inhibits surfactant activity on the alveolar surface.[449] The protein leak can be prevented by exogenous surfactant,[453] but in babies who respond poorly to surfactant administration, this benefit is probably overwhelmed by a large alveolar protein leak.[307,523] The surfactant protein A (p. 459) is of specific benefit in minimising the inhibitory effect of protein on either endogenous or exogenous surfactant.[975] One of the beneficial effects of antenatal steroids (pp. 473–4) may be that they reduce this capillary leakiness.[450] The association between asphyxia and RDS is also influenced by the fact that hypoxia and acidaemia predispose to pulmonary hypertension and hypoperfusion with a right-to-left shunt (p. 450) and reduce surfactant synthesis by inhibiting synthetic enzymes. RDS following birth depression blends into a spectrum with acute respiratory distress syndrome (ARDS; pp. 468–85).

Maternal diabetes

Fetuses of diabetic mothers have abnormal surfactant synthesis, in particular a delay in the appearance of PG.[677] Insulin delays the maturation of alveolar type II cells and decreases the proportion of saturated phosphatidylcholine in the surfactant.[374] There are decreased levels of surfactant protein (SP)-A in amniotic fluid from diabetic pregnancies as compared with fluid from non-diabetic women.[486,826] In cultured human lung tissue, insulin inhibits accumulation of SP-A and its mRNA during culture.[213,826] The incidence of RDS in infants of diabetic mothers (IDM) was also increased by elective caesarean section before labour at 36–37 weeks. Improvements in maternal diabetic control during pregnancy have now facilitated delay in delivery until the 39th–40th week of gestation and RDS now occurs in less than 1% of patients,[517] even though in some the surfactant pattern at amniocentesis remains immature.[677]

Hypothyroidism

Thyroid activity is important in the prenatal development of the surfactant system (pp. 461, 484). Preterm babies who develop RDS have lower levels of thyroid hormones in their cord blood than do controls.[182,220] The postnatal nadir in serum thyroxine concentration seen in preterm infants is very low in neonates with RDS.[917] Although most term babies with congenital hypothyroidism detected by screening do not have RDS, some cases do occur.[157]

Genetic predisposition

Families in which several relatively mature babies have developed RDS have been reported. At preterm gestations, if a woman has one baby with RDS, the relative risk of RDS in a subsequent low-birthweight (LBW) baby may be increased threefold.[651] SP-B deficiency (p. 459) results in lethal respiratory failure,[665] which in some has been associated with histopathological features of congenital alveolar proteinosis.[664] This abnormality has now been described in families[32,33,664,665] and the inheritance is autosomal recessive. Partial deficiency of SP-B, which may be compatible with survival, has now been reported.[160] Polymorphisms in intron 4 of the SP-B gene have been found to independently modify the course of RDS, as indicated by the frequency of severe RDS and the occurrence of chronic lung disease (CLD).[602] Specific alleles of the SP-A and SP-B genes associate interactively with susceptibility to RDS, and dominant mutations of SP-C associate with CLD.[389]

Twins

The second twin is more likely to develop RDS,[381,671] although this is not a consistent finding and others have reported no difference between twins and singletons.[950] There is similarity of L:S ratios in twins, which is greater in monozygotic than dizygotic pairs.[236,559]

Hypothermia

Surfactant function is defective in cold babies[332] and the concomitant hypoxia and acidaemia impair surfactant synthesis.[626] In addition, below 34°C, even in the presence of adequate amounts of PG, dipalmitoyl phosphatidylcholine (DPPC) cannot spread to form an adequately functioning monolayer. Hypothermia in animals induces pulmonary hypertension and a fall in PaO_2;[945] similar mechanisms may occur in neonates. Coagulation disorders are more common in hypothermic infants.

Nutrition

In animal studies, maternal malnutrition compromises fetal surfactant synthesis as well as lung growth.[549,569] Postnatally, although calorie deprivation does not appear to be important,[269] specific deficiencies of fatty acids or inositol may be relevant.[304,387] Inositol supplementation in babies with RDS improves outcome,[388] reducing the risk of CLD or death, and severe retinopathy of prematurity (ROP).[442]

Intrauterine growth retardation

An appropriately grown infant of 28 weeks' gestational age is much more likely to develop severe RDS than a growth-retarded 32-week-gestation infant of similar birthweight.[711] Severely growth-retarded infants, however, have a higher incidence of RDS and it is more severe.[711,874]

Haemolytic disease of the newborn (HDN)

The development of pulmonary maturity may be delayed in severely affected HDN infants with or without hydrops.[724,937] A possible mechanism is the increased levels of insulin due to beta-islet cell hypertrophy, as occurs in IDM (p. 398). The presence of heart failure with proteinaceous pulmonary oedema fluid aggravates any pre-existing surfactant deficiency due to prematurity.

Time of cord clamping

Preterm neonates who had undergone early cord clamping and had a low red cell mass, particularly when combined with some degree of birth depression, were more prone to develop

RDS.[255,572,896] As a consequence, it was recommended that following preterm delivery the cord should not be clamped until 1–1½ minutes after delivery.[896] A small prospective study of babies less than 33 weeks' gestation showed that a 30-second delay in cord clamping had no effect on mortality, but that the late-clamped babies were easier to ventilate in the first few days and required fewer blood transfusions.[512]

Factors with equivocal effects on the incidence of RDS

Maternal hypertension
Some have reported a higher incidence of RDS in preterm infants of hypertensive mothers,[884,957] perhaps due to delivery by caesarean section pre-labour. In contrast, no effect of pre-eclampsia with or without growth retardation was demonstrated on the results of lung maturity tests, neonatal morbidity including RDS, or mortality.[303,784] In another study, RDS occurred in 15% of infants of mothers with hypertensive pre-eclampsia but in 38% of non-hypertensive controls of similar weight and gestation.[800]

Prolonged rupture of membranes
There is no consensus regarding the impact of prolonged rupture of membranes.[383,957] An apparent benefit may be explained by greater use of antenatal steroids in pregnancies affected by such.[875]

Factors reducing the incidence of RDS (see prevention of RDS, pp. 472–5)

Maternal addiction
Maternal narcotic addiction, smoking[566] and alcohol ingestion[456] all reduce the incidence of RDS. Heroin can mature the surfactant synthesising systems. The effect of cocaine is unclear,[59,397] although in animal models it induces surfactant synthesis.[834]

Pathology

The initial histological finding[310] in non-surfactant-treated infants with RDS is alveolar epithelial cell necrosis, which develops within half an hour of birth. The epithelial cells become detached from the basement membrane and small patches of hyaline membranes form on the denuded areas. At the same time, there is diffuse interstitial oedema. The lymphatics are dilated by the delayed clearance of fetal lung fluid and the capillaries next to the membranes have a sludged appearance. There are very few osmiophilic granules in the type II cells (p. 445), which in places contain vacuoles, suggesting that all the lamellar bodies have been discharged. In the early stages, all these changes are rather patchy, but, by 24 hours, more extensive generalised membrane formation in the transitional ducts and respiratory bronchioles occurs. Hyaline membranes line the overdistended terminal and respiratory bronchioles (Fig. 27.11), particularly where the airways branch, and may extend into the putative alveolar ducts. The most distal component of the respiratory unit, the terminal sacs, although collapsed are not lined by membranes. The hyaline membranes are eosinophilic on staining with haematoxylin and

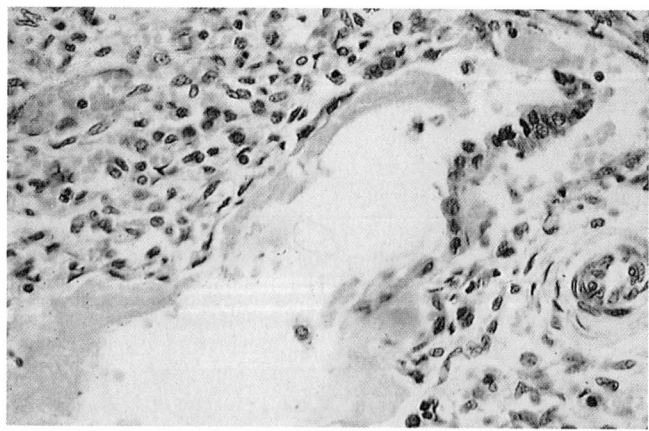

Fig. 27.11 Histology of respiratory distress syndrome, showing pink-staining hyaline membranes lining a terminal bronchiole with surrounding atelectasis.

eosin, and contain nuclear debris from necrotic pneumocytes. Occasionally, when the infant has hyperbilirubinaemia, the membranes are yellow, reflecting the presence of unconjugated bilirubin. The hyaline membranes are formed by coagulation of plasma proteins, which have leaked onto the lung surface through damaged capillaries and epithelial cells; the fibrillary component of the membranes is derived from exuded fibrin. After 24 hours, a few inflammatory cells appear within the airway lumen; macrophages are usually the most prominent cell, although some polymorphs may also be present. Ingestion of the membrane by macrophages takes place over the next 2 or 3 days as the membrane separates. Macrophages are also present beneath the membrane within the interstitium, which is usually oedematous and where there may be a mild fibroblastic response. Epithelial regeneration is detectable after 48 hours, usually beneath the separating membranes. Cuboidal cells from the unaffected transitional ducts become large and mitotic; they flatten out and spread beneath the hyaline membranes. Other cells produce lamellar bodies. Many of these reparative cells form abnormally thick epithelial squames and, with damaged capillaries, can present a considerable barrier to efficient gas exchange. During this stage of repair, surfactant can be detected in increasing quantities on the alveolar surface.[310] By 7 days of age, the hyaline membranes will have disappeared in an infant with uncomplicated RDS. In ventilated babies, however, the healing process is markedly altered and delayed. There is a hyperplastic healing process, with massive shedding of bronchiolar epithelial cells and type II pneumocytes. Hyaline membranes remain prominent. The terminal airways may be plugged with secretions and there is progressive scarring and fibrosis of the alveoli and airways, leading to the picture of CLD (pp. 554–73).

Pathophysiology

Lung function

The lungs are non-compliant, approximately 0.3–0.5 ml/cmH_2O/kg, when the disease is at its worst[75,242] (Table 27.3). As

Table 27.3 Values for lung mechanics in respiratory distress syndrome (from various sources quoted in text)

Tidal volume (V_T)	4–6 ml/kg
Minute volume (V_E)	250–400 ml/kg/min
Alveolar ventilation (V_A)	50–90 ml/kg/min
Physiological dead space (V_D/V_T)	60–75%
Functional residual capacity (FRC)	3–20 ml/kg
Crying vital capacity	20–30 ml
Dynamic compliance (C_L)	0.0003–0.0005 l/cmH$_2$O/kg
Inspiratory resistance ($R_{aw\ Insp}$)	55–95 cmH$_2$O/l/s
Expiratory resistance ($R_{aw\ Exp}$)	140–200 cmH$_2$O/l/s
Work of breathing	800–3000 g.cm/min/kg

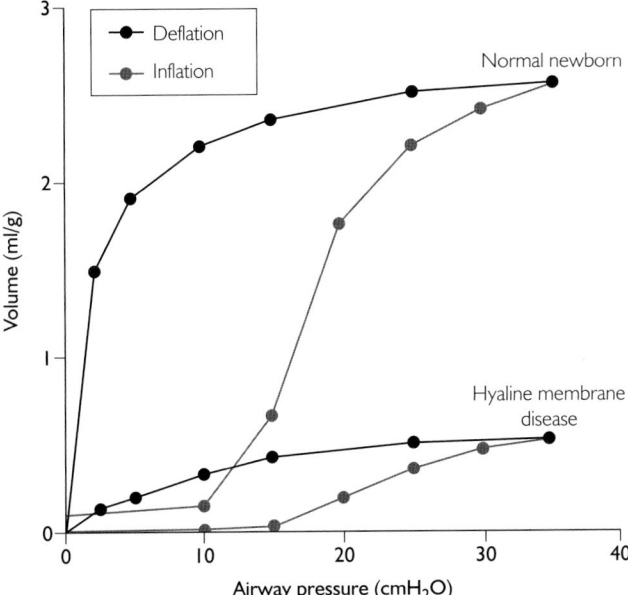

Fig. 27.12 Pressure–volume loops in excised lungs of neonates dying with and without hyaline membrane disease (HMD). In HMD, the deflation curve closely follows the inflation curve and little air is retained at zero pressure. In normal lungs, much more air is retained on the deflation limb of the loop (the phenomenon of hysteresis). (Reproduced from Gribetz et al.[368])

surfactant begins to appear, the compliance improves and has usually returned to values of 1–2 ml/cmH$_2$O/kg[165,628] by 6 to 7 days of age. In severe disease, the functional residual capacity (FRC) may be as low as 3 ml/kg,[221] whereas the FRC is at a normal level of 25–30 ml/kg in recovering babies.[743] Babies with RDS have a low tidal volume and a large physiological dead space. Minute ventilation, however, may be increased by an elevated respiratory rate in an attempt to sustain alveolar ventilation, but this is usually unsuccessful, resulting in alveolar underventilation and carbon dioxide retention. Pressure–volume loops on lungs excised at post mortem from babies dying of HMD have a characteristic pattern (Fig. 27.12). During inflation, the volume change for a given increase in pressure is very small, and during deflation, the change in volume follows a track almost similar to

that seen during inflation, whereas in the normal lung, air is retained until low pressures are reached (hysteresis). As the pressure drops to zero, very little or no air is retained within the surfactant-less alveoli, corresponding to the very small FRC measured in vivo. Inspiratory resistance is usually normal in RDS,[165,431] but expiratory resistance is increased, probably as a result of the closure of the airway prior to the expiratory grunt.[852] It is also increased by the presence of an endotracheal tube (ETT).[248] An inevitable sequel of the abnormal lung mechanics is that the work of breathing is increased in neonates with RDS to twice that seen in those without RDS.[432,588]

The time constant gives a measure of the time available for gas to leave the lung during expiration, which is normally accepted to take three time constants. The time constant is the compliance (l/cmH$_2$O) multiplied by the airways resistance (in cmH$_2$O/l/s). It is very short in neonates with severe RDS:

$$\underset{\text{(compliance)}}{0.001\,\text{l/cmH}_2\text{O}} \times \underset{\text{(resistance)}}{100\,\text{cmH}_2\text{O/l/s}} = \underset{\text{(time constant)}}{0.1\text{s}}$$

In babies with less stiff lungs, however, the time constant will be longer, and if the baby breathes rapidly (at 80/min), this will result in gas being retained in his lungs when the next inspiration starts.[852] Clinical studies[424,837] have shown the respiratory rate of infants with RDS to be about 80–90/min, with an average inspiratory time of 0.25–0.35 seconds. This pattern of respiration may be adopted so that the neonate retains gas within his lungs and some level of FRC is maintained.

A characteristic feature of RDS is the expiratory grunt. This is the result of the baby attempting to sustain an FRC by delaying the escape of air from his lungs during expiration. They try to do this in two ways: firstly, during expiration, the diaphragm continues to contract, trying to delay or brake the reduction in thoracic volume and thus retain gas within the alveoli;[198] secondly, by contracting the constrictor muscles of the larynx, an attempt is made to close the upper airway as in the Valsalva manoeuvre. Since the abdominal muscles contract at the same time as the laryngeal muscles relax, there is an explosive exhalation of air, which is the characteristic 'grunt'. Bypassing this laryngeal component of expiratory braking by putting an ETT through the cords results in a fall in the PaO_2 in babies with RDS.[399]

Surfactant

The preterm baby is born with poor reserves of surfactant (pp. 462–3). Most babies, however, have some present in the first few hours after birth.[740] The deterioration seen in babies with non-surfactant-treated RDS is due in part to the disappearance of these small quantities of surfactant, compounded by fatigue as the neonate struggles to sustain ventilation in stiff, surfactant-deficient lungs. The disappearance of surfactant is primarily due to the inhibitory effect of proteins on surfactant (see above),[451] which leak onto the alveolar surface in the early oedematous stage of lung damage. The deleterious effect of hypoxia and acidaemia on surfactant synthesis (p. 481) may also play a part, but patency of the ductus is not relevant.[14] The levels of surfactant proteins are also low in the first few hours in babies with RDS and rise as the babies recover. The lungs remain non-compliant and atelectatic until surfactant begins to reappear from 36 to 48 hours of age, as demonstrated by measurement of L:S ratios of pharyngeal aspirates.[480]

Pulmonary hypertension

Pulmonary artery pressure (PAP) remains high throughout the first week and even longer in some cases of RDS.[261,819] The more severe the RDS, the higher the PAP, which may remain close to systemic levels in fatal cases (Fig. 27.13).[926] At least during systole, PAP can be higher than systemic pressure, at which time there is likely to be right-to-left ductal shunting. In diastole, the systemic pressure is likely to be higher than the pulmonary pressure and the overall effect is bidirectional ductal shunting, and this is frequently detected echocardiographically in RDS.[260,261,819]

Mechanisms of hypoxia: right-to-left shunt with ventilation–perfusion imbalance

Hypoxaemia in RDS is due to a large right-left shunt.[855,930] There are four main sites of right–left shunts:

1. Obligatory shunts present due to drainage of the veins of the myocardium directly into the left side of the heart and anastomoses between the bronchial and pulmonary circulation. These are small and of no haemodynamic or clinical significance.

2. Shunting through the foramen ovale occurs if right atrial pressure is higher than left atrial pressure. Interatrial right–left shunting is rare in neonates with RDS.[262,842]

3. Shunting through a patent ductus arteriosus (PDA): the ductus arteriosus is patent in most babies with RDS during the first 48–72 hours.[245,744] If the PAP exceeds the aortic pressure, there will be a significant right–left shunt. Right–left shunts at ductal level are common in persistent pulmonary hypertension of the newborn (PPHN; p. 450) but in uncomplicated RDS are small and constitute <10% of the total right-left shunt.[792] Right-to-left ductal shunting means that blood taken from an umbilical artery catheter (UAC) can have a much lower PaO_2 than blood passing up the carotid arteries to the eyes (p. 480). Colour Doppler studies in babies with RDS have demonstrated that intravascular shunting at ductal or foramen ovale level is relatively unusual and the shunts through these channels are predominantly bidirectional or left–right in the first few days after birth. This has little effect on blood gas values, but increases the cardiac output and the load on the right ventricle.[260,262,792]

4. The true intrapulmonary right–left shunt, when pulmonary capillary blood passes through the lung without coming into contact with a ventilated alveolus.

The combination of 1 to 4 is the true right-to-left shunt. There is another right-to-left shunt, which contributes to the total shunt or venous admixture seen in babies with RDS, and it is the result of pulmonary blood flow passing partially ventilated alveoli, ventilation–perfusion imbalance. This large component of the right–left shunt in RDS can be eliminated, by giving the baby 100% oxygen to breathe for 15 minutes (the hyperoxia or nitrogen washout test). This eliminates shunting resulting from partially oxygenated alveoli, and a shunt calculated at the end of a period breathing 100% oxygen is the true shunt outlined above. In most babies with RDS, the majority of the right-to-left shunt is the fourth component of the true shunt plus this ventilation–perfusion imbalance.

Carbon dioxide retention

The increased $PaCO_2$ in RDS is due to hypoventilation secondary to atelectasis, decreased tidal volume and increased dead space. Ventilation is also non-homogeneous, so whereas end-tidal $PACO_2$ is a good measure of $PaCO_2$ in patients with normal lungs, in babies with RDS there is a risk that measurement of $PACO_2$ will seriously underestimate $PaCO_2$.[531] Since the mixed venous PCO_2 (normally 6.13 kPa, 46 mmHg) is usually only a fraction of a kilopascal above arterial or alveolar PCO_2 (normally 5.33 kPa, 40 mmHg), the right–left shunt has to be enormous before the admixture of venous blood significantly contributes to hypercapnia in RDS.

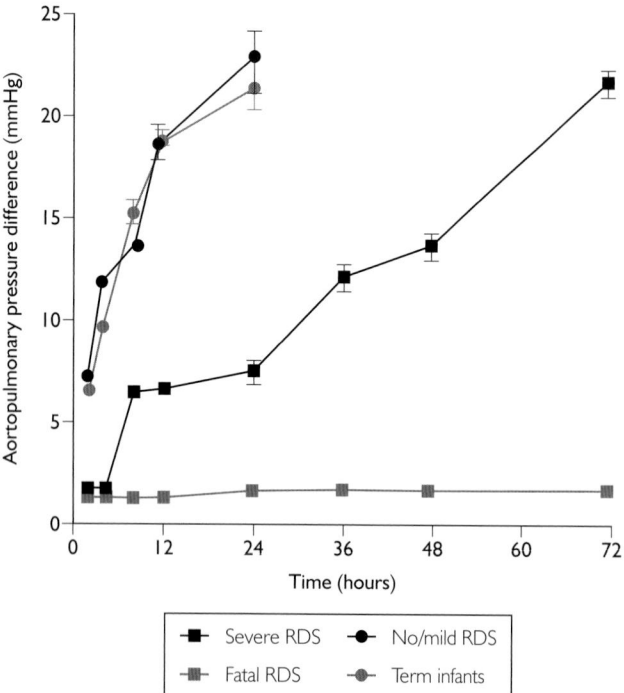

Fig. 27.13 Aortopulmonary pressure differences (mmHg, mean ± SEM) from 2 hours until 24 hours of age in term and premature neonates with no or mild respiratory distress syndrome (RDS) and until 72 hours of age in premature neonates with severe or fatal RDS. (Reproduced from Walther et al.[926])

Prevention of respiratory distress syndrome

Prevention of prematurity

Premature birth is associated with social deprivation: it has been suggested that the incidence of prematurity could be reduced by manipulation of economic variables,[690] but, in general, the results are not convincing.[807,914] Tocolytic drugs to prevent preterm labour have proved disappointing,[510,556] prolonging pregnancy for not more than 48 hours.[497] Genital tract infection is associated with preterm labour, and in women with preterm rupture of the membranes (PROM) there is evidence that treatment with antibiotics reduces the prematurity rate.[335]

Antenatal steroid therapy

Not all steroids cross the placenta; cortisol is largely inactivated, but degradation is resisted by synthetic steroids such as betamethasone and dexamethasone. Antenatal administration of dexamethasone or betamethasone to pregnant women in preterm labour significantly reduces the incidence of RDS (odds ratio [OR] 0.63; 95% confidence interval [CI] 0.44, 0.82) and neonatal death (OR 0.60; 95% CI 0.48, 0.75). Several other serious complications of prematurity, including germinal matrix/intraventricular haemorrhage (GMH/IVH: OR 0.48; 95% CI 0.32, 0.72) and necrotising enterocolitis (NEC: OR 0.58; 95% CI 0.32, 1.09), are also reduced.[180,929] No long-term adverse effects have been demonstrated from a single course of antenatal corticosteroids.[219]

The effects of antenatal steroids (Table 27.4) include inducing the enzymes for surfactant synthesis and the genes for the production of the surfactant proteins A, B, C and D,[623] and improving the quality of the surfactant produced.[890] Glucocorticoids, such as dexamethasone, can cause substantial stimulation of SP-B gene expression to two to three times adult levels in fetal lung explants.[64] They mature the non-surfactant-producing tissues of the lung;[107,540] the septa become longer, thinner and less cellular, with larger air spaces and increased numbers of alveolar divisions.

Table 27.4 Some benefits of antenatal steroids

Improved Apgar scores	Gardner et al[313]
Maturation of lung structure	Bunton & Plopper[107]
	Lanteri et al[540]
Initiation of surfactant protein synthesis	Mendelson et al[623]
Improved NO-mediated pulmonary venous relaxation	Zhou et al[983]
Reduced pulmonary capillary leakiness	Ikegami et al[450]
Interaction with postnatal exogenous surfactant therapy	p. 461
Increased resistance to high oxygen exposure	Frank[294]
Better blood pressure in early neonatal period	Moise et al[633]
Higher neonatal white cell counts	Barak et al[40]
Less patent ductus arteriosus	Ward,[929] Eronen et al[259]
Less GMH-IVH	Crowley,[180] Garland et al[316]
Less NEC	Ward[929]

Timing of treatment

Results from randomised trials have demonstrated that the benefit is maximal in babies delivered between 24 and 168 hours of starting the maternal therapy.[180] A smaller but useful benefit is also seen in women receiving less than 24 hours of therapy. In a retrospective study,[791] however, one dose given 4 to 24 hours prior to delivery appeared to be as effective as two or more doses given 24 hours to 7 days before delivery.

Number of courses

There are doubts about the safety of multiple courses of corticosteroids,[301,452] which at this time cannot be recommended as routine treatment. Repeated courses of therapy may suppress the maternal and fetal hypothalamic-pituitary-adrenal axis,[35] as well as increasing the risk of maternal hyperglycaemia and infection. Neonatal Cushing's syndrome has been reported after repeated antenatal courses of steroids.[95] Conversely, steroids may depress the neonatal adrenal gland when used in conventional doses.[482] Evidence from eight randomised controlled trials in animal models highlighted that, although repeated doses of antenatal corticosteroids have beneficial effects in terms of lung function, they may have adverse effects on brain function and fetal growth.[5]

Gestational age

In the original study by Liggins & Howie,[568] the greatest benefit was seen at gestations of 30–34 weeks, with a much smaller although statistically significant benefit below 30 weeks. Crowley's meta-analysis[180] demonstrated a benefit in neonates less than 31 weeks, but evidence for benefit in babies of less than 28 weeks is less strong.[241,314]

Preterm rupture of membranes

Although there has been concern that in PROM, antenatal steroids may increase risk of infection, with appropriate clinical surveillance, this was not a problem in the studies reviewed by Crowley;[180] indeed, a beneficial effect was demonstrated.

Maternal hypertension

Liggins & Howie[568] reported that steroid-treated hypertensive women had a significantly increased stillbirth rate and perinatal mortality; as a consequence, such women were excluded from trials.[180] Clinical experience and observational studies, however, suggest that steroids can be used safely in this situation.[539]

Diabetes

In the past, glucocorticoids were avoided in diabetic pregnancies because of their potential for causing hyperglycaemia; however, they should be given, as the insulin regimen can be altered during the brief period of hyperglycaemia. Steroids switch on the surfactant protein-synthesising systems in experimental diabetic rats.[631]

Twins

Multiple pregnancies have often been excluded from trials of antenatal corticosteroids, but twins represent 28% of cohorts of prematurely born babies.

General effects

As well as the specific benefits for RDS outlined above, antenatal steroids appear to have a generally beneficial effect in preterm infants (Table 27.4). Some of these are as a consequence of reducing the incidence and severity of RDS, whereas others represent the maturing effect of steroids on many body systems. The interaction with the benefits of postnatal exogenous surfactant therapy is of particular importance (pp. 483–4). Follow-up of steroid-treated babies shows no excess of handicap compared with controls.[240,587]

Guidelines for antenatal steroid usage

Guidelines have been produced by the Royal College of Obstetricians and Gynaecologists,[762] the British Association of Perinatal Medicine, and the National Institutes for Health of the USA.[663] Their recommendations include:

- Antenatal treatment with corticosteroids should be considered for all women at risk of preterm labour between 24 and 36 weeks. Treatment should consist of two doses of betamethasone given intramuscularly 24 hours apart or four doses of dexamethasone given 12 hours apart. Betamethasone, however, is now preferred, as in an observational study[48] it was associated with a lower risk of periventricular leukomalacia (PVL).
- Treatment for less than 24 hours is associated with significant improvement in outcome; thus, corticosteroids should be given unless immediate delivery is anticipated.
- In the absence of chorioamnionitis, antenatal corticosteroids are recommended in pregnancies complicated by preterm premature rupture of the membranes.
- Unless there is evidence that corticosteroids will have an adverse effect on the mother, they are also recommended in other complicated pregnancies.

Thyroid preparations

Thyroid hormones are involved in the induction of surfactant synthesis.[34,337] There are reports of apparent success with intra-amniotic therapy,[758] as thyroid hormones and thyroid-stimulating hormone (TSH) do not cross the placenta, but most workers have studied the administration of thyrotrophin-releasing hormone (TRH) to the mother, usually in combination with dexamethasone. There is a consistent synergism between TRH and steroids in animal studies.[635,717] The results of an initial study in humans[636] were also promising. Subsequently, a prospective study showed a significant reduction in RDS,[522] but in another study, only the incidence of CLD in survivors was significantly reduced.[36] The ACTOBAT study,[4] however, showed no benefit from TRH administration, and, although the dose of TRH was half that used in the earlier studies, the TRH group suffered increased morbidity, as they delivered at significantly earlier gestations. Meta-analysis of the results of 11 trials, which included 4500 women, has demonstrated that prenatal administration of TRH in addition to corticosteroids did not reduce the risk of neonatal respiratory distress or bronchopulmonary dysplasia (BPD). Indeed, the data showed there were adverse effects: an increase in requirement for ventilation and more likelihood of having a low Apgar score at 5 minutes.[181] Antenatally administered TRH can also produce transient suppression of the pituitary–thyroid axis and transient complications in the mother, including nausea, vomiting and increased blood pressure (BP).[373]

Other antenatal drugs

Various drugs have been used in animal experiments to mature the surfactant synthetic pathways. These include opiates,[331] aminophylline[485] and ambroxol.[752] Benefit from ambroxol has been reported,[932] but this is not a consistent finding.[190] Some[967] but not all[273] animal experiments suggest that antenatal beta-mimetics may improve neonatal lung function. Their effect in the human neonate appears to be small,[541] although, in a randomised controlled trial[252] infants whose mothers had received an infusion of terbutaline prior to elective delivery had significantly better lung function.

Prevention of intrapartum asphyxia

Asphyxia worsens RDS and predisposes to pulmonary haemorrhage. If asphyxia is absent and the preterm neonate is presenting by the vertex, there is no need to proceed to caesarean section on a routine basis,[7] but if fetal distress develops, delivery by caesarean section should be considered even at early gestations.

Prevention of postnatal asphyxia

It is important to prevent postnatal hypoxic damage to lung capillaries and minimise the risk of haemorrhagic pulmonary oedema, by rapidly establishing normal blood gases and normal pulmonary perfusion and ensuring maximum surfactant release from the type II pneumocytes by adequate expansion of the lungs. Inadequate ventilation leads to poor surfactant release, resulting in hypoxia and acidaemia, leading to a vicious cycle (Fig. 27.14). As a consequence, it had been argued that unless a baby of <30 weeks' gestation is in excellent condition at 30 seconds of age and crying and vigorous, he should be actively resuscitated by intubation and intermittent positive pressure ventilation (IPPV). The studies[243,755] that demonstrated such an approach reduced morbidity and mortality from RDS were performed before the modern era of neonatal intensive care and a less aggressive approach; using continuous positive airways pressure (CPAP) rather than IPPV is now preferred in some centers (pp. 520–1). Prevention of asphyxia, however, remains important, and appropriate resuscitation may require endotracheal intubation.[571]

Avoiding drug depression

Many drugs given to the mother in preterm labour – including opiate analgesics, anaesthetic agents, benzodiazepines, and the drugs used to control fulminating eclampsia, such as magnesium sulphate – can cause marked hypotonia and respiratory depression. In general, as well as using the specific opiate antagonist naloxone (except in infants of drug-addicted mothers, in whom naloxone will precipitate drug withdrawal signs), affected babies

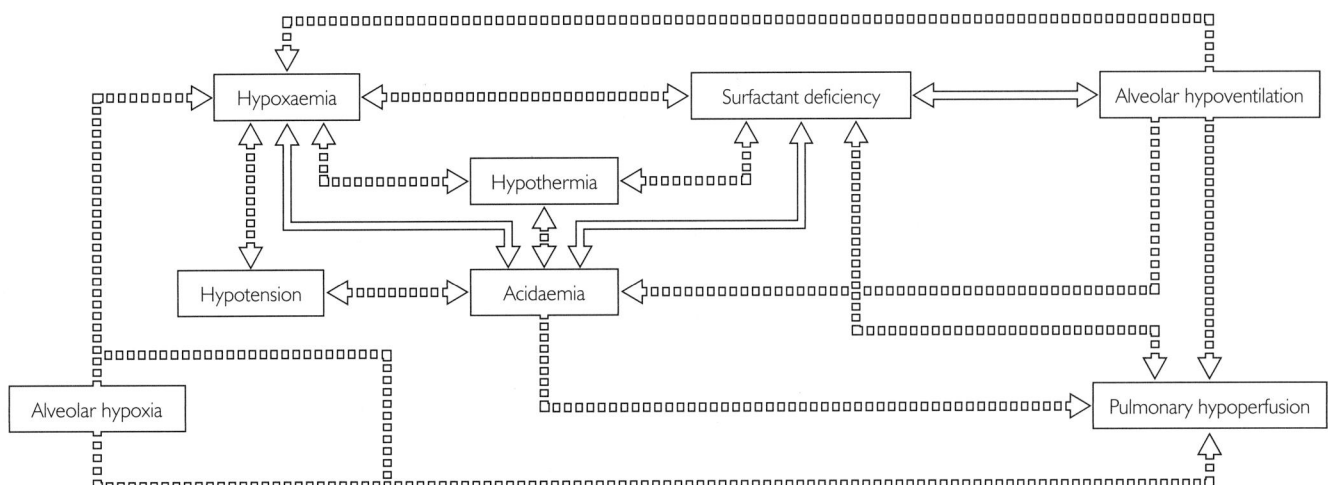

Fig. 27.14 Interrelationship of factors affecting surfactant and other components of lung function; solid lines indicate major effects. (Reproduced from Roberton.[750])

may require ventilation from birth until the drugs are excreted or metabolised.

Avoidance of maternal fluid overload

Excessive fluid administration to the mother in labour may result in neonatal hyponatraemia,[867] which may predispose to pneumothorax if the baby develops RDS.[632]

Prophylactic surfactant

A large number of studies have been carried out assessing the impact of prophylactic surfactant, i.e. administering surfactant within the first few minutes after birth. Many varieties of surfactant have been used (Table 27.5). Meta-analyses of the results have been performed,[827,829–831,833] demonstrating positive effects of both synthetic and natural surfactants. Prophylactic use of natural surfactant results in a significant reduction in pneumothorax (OR 0.35; 95% CI 0.26, 0.49), mortality (OR 0.60; 95% CI 0.44, 0.83), and the combined outcome of mortality and CLD (OR 0.84; 95% CI 0.75, 0.93) but not CLD alone (OR 0.93; 95% CI 0.80, 1.07).[829]

All trials of surfactant therapy have shown a reduction in oxygen requirements and the ventilator pressures required. Problems with the measurement techniques resulted in confusion regarding the effect of surfactant on compliance, as the early improvements may not be detected by dynamic compliance measurements.[498] Surfactant also results in elevation of lung volume,[173] in association with increased oxygenation.[230] Meta-analyses of the results of trials comparing administering surfactant prophylactically or selectively, or early versus late have demonstrated prophylactic/early administration is more effective. Prophylactic versus selective surfactant administration has been associated with a significant reduction in neonatal mortality (OR 0.61; 95% CI 0.28, 0.77), CLD/death (OR 0.85; 95% CI 0.76, 0.95) and pneumothorax (OR 0.54; 95% CI 0.42, 0.84);[833] early versus late revealed a reduction in neonatal mortality (OR 0.87; 95% CI 0.77, 0.99) and pneumothorax (OR 0.70; 95% CI 0.58, 0.82).[972]

Table 27.5 Surfactants which have been used in clinical studies		
Type of surfactant	**Animal source**	**Composition (or additives if animal derived)**
Animal lung wash:		
Surfactant TA	Cow	DPPC, palmitic acid triglyceride
Survanta	Cow	Similar to surfactant TA
Infasurf (CLSE)	Cow	
Curosurf	Pig	
Alveofact SF-RI 1	Cow	
Human surfactant:	Liquor amnii	
Artificial surfactant:		
Belfast		DPPC + HDL
ALEC (Pumactant)		70% DPPC, 30% PG
Exosurf		DPPC + tyloxapol and hexadecanol
Surfactant KL$_4$	Cow	Synthetic SP-B analogue made of lysine + leucine

Clinical features of respiratory distress syndrome

The diagnostic criteria for RDS were laid down before use of prophylactic surfactant. These comprised: a respiratory rate above 60/min; grunting expiration; indrawing of the sternum, intercostal spaces and lower ribs during inspiration; and cyanosis without added oxygen.[766]

Natural history

The disease is present within the first 4 hours after birth. In the absence of treatment with exogenous surfactant, over the next

24–36 hours the baby tires, his dyspnoea worsens and he becomes oedematous. As surfactant synthesis commences, the severity of the disease begins to abate from 36–48 hours of age, and this is associated with a spontaneous diuresis.[491]

Respiratory signs

The more mature baby with RDS may breathe at a fast respiratory rate, exceeding 100/min. This faster rate is more efficient in terms of work of breathing. Some babies may alternate a breathing pattern of shallow tachypnoea up to 100–120/min with one in which they breathe comparatively slowly (40–60/min) with marked recession and grunting. The slow-breathing baby often has episodes of apnoea, and this is a sign that respiration is beginning to fail.[198] In addition to tachypnoea, there is marked intercostal and sternal recession, and flaring of the alae nasi. The main respiratory muscle is the diaphragm. In the presence of a compliant ribcage, diaphragmatic contraction results in a marked seesaw pattern to respiration, with the chest moving inwards and the abdomen moving outwards during inspiration, and vice versa on expiration. On auscultation there is a reduction in air entry. An expiratory grunt is a feature of most forms of neonatal respiratory disease, and is an attempt by the baby to sustain his FRC (p. 360). In uncomplicated RDS, these clinical features gradually return to normal by 7 days at the latest.

Cardiovascular signs

The heart rate in mild to moderate cases of RDS is 140–160/min and shows normal variability. In infants with severe RDS, the heart rate tends to be slower (120/min) with little beat-to-beat variation. The heart sounds are normal. Murmurs are not normally present; if heard in the first 24–48 hours, they suggest congenital heart disease or ischaemic myocardial injury and require further investigation. A murmur appearing after 3–4 days is usually due to a PDA. Heart failure is not a feature of RDS; if present, it suggests cardiac disease.

Neonates with RDS are often hypotensive and this is associated with a worse prognosis.[390] Hypotension is less common in babies who receive antenatal steroids.[633] There are many causes for the hypotension, including hypoxia and acidaemia depressing the myocardium and reducing cardiac output, a low blood volume, and high pressure ventilation compromising venous return and reducing cardiac output. Hypotension predisposes to acidaemia, which increases pulmonary vascular resistance, GMH/IVH (pp. 1150–9), renal failure (p. 484) and NEC (pp. 694–703). It is essential, therefore, to measure the BP and to correct hypotension as soon as possible.

Central nervous system

The preterm baby even without RDS is hypotonic, inactive and lies in the frog position, spending most of his day asleep. Abnormal neurological signs are often subtle (pp. 71–2), but if present they are ominous, suggesting development of a GMH/IVH.

Abdominal examination

Examination of the abdomen is usually unremarkable; the liver, spleen and kidneys are often palpable but are rarely significantly enlarged. Hepatosplenomegaly suggests heart failure or sepsis and should be dealt with accordingly, and an easily felt liver in a baby with severe respiratory failure suggests a right tension pneumothorax (p. 484).

Most babies with severe RDS have an ileus,[246] and do not pass meconium. Improvement in their general condition is often heralded by the appearance of bowel sounds and the passage of meconium, although gastric emptying may still be delayed. Jaundice is not uncommon; phototherapy and exchange transfusion are indicated in preterm infants at much lower bilirubin levels than in the full-term neonate (pp. 674, 675).

Differential diagnosis (Table 27.6)

The differential diagnosis in the first 6 hours can usually be made on the basis of the history (including the gestation), the clinical examination, the blood gases and the CXR. It is impossible, however, to exclude infection as the cause of the baby's symptoms. Furthermore, infection with group B streptococci (GBS; *Streptococcus agalactiae*) can coexist with RDS.[461] As a consequence, it is important to treat all infants presenting with respiratory distress with antibiotics until the results of cultures are available. Primary PPHN (pp. 496–502) can be differentiated by the absence of significant parenchymal lung disease and the relevant echocardiographic findings. Infants with RDS, however, may also have marked pulmonary hypertension[926] and it is useful to identify these infants, as they can benefit from pulmonary vasodilator therapy. Such infants are likely to have an oxygen requirement that is out of proportion to their CXR appearance and a poor response to surfactant therapy. Respiratory distress presenting after 4–6 hours of age in an infant who has been adequately observed is usually due to pneumonia or heart failure secondary to heart disease. Other conditions such as aspiration and inhalation of the feed, some malformations and, occasionally, a small pneumothorax can present after 6 hours of age, but these are less common.

Investigations

Haematological

There are no unique haematological findings in RDS. The haemoglobin will vary with the local practice for cord clamping.[968] Anaemia may develop later due to GMH/IVH (pp. 1150–9) or iatrogenic losses (p. 1238). Results of measurements of the coagulation system are often prolonged due to prematurity in infants with RDS, although disseminated intravascular coagulation (DIC) is rare. The presence of a coagulopathy can be due to complications such as birth asphyxia, septicaemia or a GMH/IVH.[140,612] Infants who have suffered intrauterine growth retardation are also at increased risk of coagulation abnormalities.[398] The white blood count is normal for the baby's birthweight and gestation.[610] Thrombocytopenia is not a feature of RDS unless there is DIC (pp. 759–60) or the baby is ventilated.[37]

Biochemical

The plasma electrolyte pattern is usually normal, although marked early hyponatraemia can be seen if the mother has been

Table 27.6 Differential diagnosis of dyspnoea in the neonate

Condition	Gestational age	History	Examination[a]	Gases[b]	Presentation[c] <6h	Presentation[c] >6h	Chest radiograph	Comments
Respiratory distress syndrome	Prem				+++	N	Diagnostic but see pp. 220–2	Working diagnosis in all preterm neonates unless chest radiograph suggests alternative. Always consider infection (p. 479)
Transient tachypnoea	FT >prem[d]	Often CS delivery	Mild hypoxaemia needing 40% O_2		+++	R	Diagnostic but see p. 486	Commonest cause of breathlessness in term babies. By definition, a mild disease (pp. 1011–75)
Meconium aspiration	FT[e]	Meconium-stained liquor at resuscitation. Post-maturity	Meconium-stained baby. Meconium in larynx		+++	N	Streaky	Diagnosis obvious on history. Infection may coexist
Pneumothorax or pneumomediastinum	FT >prem	May be excessive resuscitation at birth			++	R[f]	Diagnostic	
Massive pulmonary haemorrhage	Prem >FT	Asphyxia or other cause of heart failure, bleeding tendency. Use of artificial surfactant	Crepitations; usually marked pallor. Blood up larynx or in endotracheal tube. PDA after presentation		+	+++	Unhelpful; usually a white-out	Diagnosis based on clinical findings
After severe asphyxia	FT[g]	Severe asphyxia Low Apgar May be helpful	Other features of asphyxia (pp. 485–6) Rarely differentiates this from other causes of dyspnoea	Marked metabolic acidaemia	++	N	Unhelpful	Tachypnoea driven by acidaemia
Infection (pneumonia)	Any			Often severe acidaemia and easy to reduce CO_2 without increasing PaO_2	++	+++	Unhelpful in most cases though may show patchy changes	Impossible to exclude in any baby (pp. 1020–1). This is the working diagnosis in the absence of specific chest radiograph findings in neonates >6 hours old with respiratory disease. WBC.CRP may be helpful (p. 485)
Congenital malformations	FT >prem	Usually normal delivery. May have been detected on antenatal ultrasound	Rarely helpful	May be profound hypoxaemia with raised CO_2	+++	+	Virtually always diagnostic	Diaphragmatic hernia, cysts effusions, agenesis all present this way. TOF should not present this way (pp. 715–17)

(Continued)

Table 27.6 (Continued)

Condition	Gestational age	History	Examination[a]	Gases[b]	Presentation[c] <6 h	Presentation[c] >6 h	Chest radiograph	Comments
Congenital heart disease	FT >prem		Murmurs, heart size, signs of heart failure	CO_2 normal or reduced. In cyanotic CHD PaO_2 rarely >6–7 kPa even in oxygen with IPPV	R	+++	May be helpful or diagnostic	The alternative common diagnosis in infants presenting after 6 hours and particularly after 24 hours of age. ECG and echocardiogram usually diagnostic. Virtually always rapidly fatal
Pulmonary hypoplasia	Any	Prolonged rupture of membranes	Potter's features (p. 604). No kidneys palpable, amnion nodosum. Dwarf (p. 790)	Profound hypoxaemia and hypercapnia	+++	N	Diagnostic; very small lungs	
Persistent pulmonary hypertension	FT >prem	May have had mild asphyxia	May hear soft murmur of TI	Gases like cyanotic CHD, i.e. marked hypoxaemia with normal or reduced CO_2	+++	+	Usually normal or nearly so	Can be difficult to exclude cyanotic CHD unless echocardiogram available
Inhalation of feed	Any	Obvious			R	+++	Unhelpful	Should not happen in well-run units. Normal term babies rarely inhale, so always seek alternative diagnosis, especially infection
Inborn errors of metabolism	FT >prem	May be positive FH or history of unexplained NND in the past	No evidence of lung disease. Tachypnoea driven by acidaemia	Severe metabolic acidaemia, normal PaO_2; low $PaCO_2$	R	+++	Often normal	Diagnosis based on blood changes plus ketonaemia in many cases (p. 777)
Primary neurological or muscle disease	FT >prem	May be positive FH or history of unexplained NND or infant death. Polyhydramnios may occur	Marked hypotonia. Areflexia, odd face, deformities. No evidence of lung disease	Gases normal (unless apnoeic)	++	++	Often normal	Usually easy to identify as a group
Upper airway obstruction	FT >prem	May be typical in choanal atresia (p. 395)	Stridor present. Problems resolve on intubation. Laryngoscopy be diagnostic	Gases normal when intubated; CO_2 may be raised beforehand	++	++	Often normal	

a Mentioning features other than cardinal features of respiratory disease (pp. 468–554).
b Most conditions cause hypoxaemia and hypercarbia; only if the blood gas patterns differ from this is it noted here.
c Frequency of presentation graded + to +++; N = never, R = rarely.
d Full term greater than premature. This means that the condition can occur at any gestation, but since full-term babies are more common than preterm ones, there are more cases in full-term neonates.
e If preterm, consider listeria.
f Usually as a complication of pre-existing severe lung disease, especially HMD.
g Severely asphyxiated premature babies will get RDS.

overloaded with fluid during labour.[867] The plasma calcium is frequently low (1.5–1.7 mmol/l) in the first 48–72 hours in ill LBW babies. Although infants of very low birthweight (VLBW) are prone to hypoglycaemia, when sick they are also susceptible to hyperglycaemia (pp. 863–4). Infection should be considered in a baby with hyperglycaemia. Babies with RDS may have impaired renal function, with a reduced glomerular filtration rate and renal plasma flow and a correspondingly raised urea and creatinine;[377] they are also poor at excreting hydrogen ions.[10] Fluid restriction has been advocated to improve lung function, but no such effect was seen in a randomised trial.[491]

Serum albumin levels are often below 25–30 g/l in preterm infants[120] and are lower in the cord blood of babies who develop RDS than in controls.[78] The albumin may remain below 25 g/l for days or even weeks in critically ill babies; this is the result of albumin leaking into the subcutaneous tissues, poor protein intake and impaired albumin synthesis. Administration of albumin, however, does not improve lung function[346] and may increase the risk of CLD development;[231] hence it should be avoided. Total complement levels are normal,[124] but anaphylotoxins are released if complications or RDS occur, such as pneumothorax or GMH/IVH.[258]

Blood gas measurements

Hypoxaemia occurs and can be used to assess the severity of the lung disease (p. 532). A mixed metabolic and respiratory acidaemia is found in most cases of RDS, with the $PaCO_2$ being raised in all but the mildest cases; indeed, the absence of hypercapnia or the presence of a low $PaCO_2$ should suggest a diagnosis other than RDS in a dyspnoeic neonate (pp. 472, 516).

Hormone levels

Cortisol levels of ill 26-week babies are lower than those of healthy preterm babies; they remain low for several days after birth and are further depressed by prenatal therapy with dexamethasone.[482] Levels of TSH, T4 and T3, although initially normal in cord blood,[519] drop below normal during the first week.[297]

Echocardiography

Echocardiographic studies in neonates with RDS confirm the presence of a PDA in most cases (p. 636), but are otherwise normal in the absence of PPHN or severe depression of myocardial function. Doppler echocardiography is used to investigate the degree of pulmonary hypertension (pp. 498–9).

Measurement of surfactant status

These have limited applicability, as apparently typical RDS can develop in the presence of L:S ratios greater than 2.0, even when PG is present[942] and surfactant-deficient RDS and congenital pneumonia due, in particular, to GBS can coexist. In addition, although assessment of surfactant proteins can be used to determine pulmonary maturity, the tests are expensive and time-consuming. There may, however, be a role for rapid early assessments of neonatal surfactant levels,[72,143] if supplies of surfactant are limited.

Chest X-ray

The CXR appearance contributes to the establishment of the diagnosis. In addition, thymic (Fig. 27.15), cardiac and skeletal abnormalities can be identified and the positions of ETTs and indwelling cannulae checked. Classically, in RDS the CXR shows diffuse, fine granular opacification in both lung fields with an air bronchogram where the air-filled bronchi stand out against the atelectatic lungs. In reality, the appearance can be very variable, from a slight granularity to lungs that are so opaque that it is impossible to distinguish between the lung field and the cardiac silhouette. A 'whiteout' on a 1-hour X-ray, however, may be due to retained fetal lung fluid; by 4 hours of age, presumably as a result of clearance of the liquid, the CXR appearance may show marked improvement. The CXR appearance also depends on the phase of the respiratory cycle, the appearance being much worse on an expiratory rather than an inspiratory one. Positive pressure support with both CPAP and IPPV can improve the CXR appearance in a baby who had marked X-ray changes while breathing spontaneously; surfactant treatment has the same effect.[251] As a consequence, the appearance of a CXR taken in the first few hours is a poor guide to both prognosis[481] and the response to exogenous surfactant therapy.[229]

Treatment

Initial care

Transportation from the labour ward to the NICU

It is essential to ensure that there is no deterioration in a baby's lung disease during transfer. All VLBW neonates who require intubation for resuscitation should be ventilated in the transport incubator. Ventilator settings during transport are based on the oxygen saturation and the clinical assessment of the baby, in particular whether there is adequate chest wall expansion. Practice

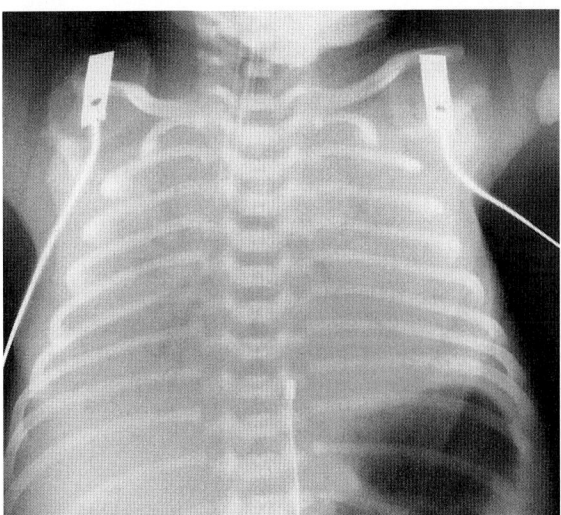

Fig. 27.15 Severe respiratory distress syndrome. The lungs are totally opaque and cannot be separated from the heart border because of widespread atelectasis. An air bronchogram can be seen in the right lung.

differs regarding whether babies who have been intubated to be given surfactant should be extubated onto nasal CPAP (nCPAP) or remain intubated for transfer and until assessment can take place on the NICU. Others do not intubate infants routinely in the labour ward, but use nCPAP and transfer the babies using that method of respiratory support.

Initial management in the NICU

As soon as the baby arrives in the NICU, he must be put into an incubator prewarmed to 35–36°C or placed under a radiant heater. In the next 30–60 minutes, the following procedures should be carried out in all neonates with RDS:

- Weigh the infant.
- Examine carefully.
- Measure the head circumference to facilitate diagnosis of the rare infant with a subgaleal haemorrhage and subsequently rapidly enlarging head circumference (p. 1126).
- Connect to ECG and respiration monitors (pp. 624–7).
- Measure the baby's temperature.
- Insert a UAC (or, failing that, a peripheral arterial cannula) and measure PaO_2, $PaCO_2$ and pH.
- Measure the BP using a continuously recording device once an arterial cannula is in situ, and Dinamap if no cannula is in place.
- Treat abnormalities of blood gases (p. 474), and BP (p. 481).
- Draw blood for haemoglobin and white cell count. Cross-match all ill neonates, as most eventually need transfusion.
- Take a set of cultures, including a blood culture; a lumbar puncture is not required for all infants (p. 1263). A blood sample for culture can be taken from the UAC during the sterile insertion routine.
- Send blood for electrolyte measurement; this establishes a baseline and identifies early abnormalities due to problems with maternal fluid balance.
- Measure coagulation in ill and bruised babies and those less than 30 weeks' gestation.
- Insert a peripheral cannula for the administration of antibiotics.
- In critically ill infants or those with extremely low birthweight (ELBW), insert an umbilical or central venous catheter.
- Obtain a CXR, preferably after inserting the UAC.
- Give surfactant, if it has not been given prophylactically in the labour ward (pp. 483–4).
- Update the parents.

In relatively mature infants with apparently mild lung disease, a peripheral arterial sample is advisable prior to inserting the UAC. If this confirms that the disease is only mild, arterial cannulation is not required, although an i.v. catheter should be inserted for antibiotics and parenteral fluids.

General management of the baby with RDS

Minimal handling

If hypoxic babies are disturbed and handled, their respiration may become very irregular or stop altogether, their right–left shunt increases, and their PaO_2 falls rapidly. Major disturbances, such as sucking out an ETT, performing a lumbar puncture or taking a CXR, can cause catastrophic falls in PaO_2. The 'minimal

handling' maxim dominates the whole approach to managing all sick babies with RDS.

Physiotherapy

In the first 24 to 48 hours, secretions are not a problem unless infection develops. As a consequence, chest physiotherapy and routine suctioning of the ETT are contraindicated.

Temperature control

The baby's thermal environment should be controlled and if babies are exposed during any procedure, they should be under a radiant heat source, with as much of their surface as possible covered in order to minimise heat losses.

Blood gas management

Abnormalities of PaO_2, $PaCO_2$ and acid–base metabolism are characteristic of RDS, and keeping them within a reasonably normal range is the single most important component of the treatment. The detailed management of oxygen administration, CPAP and IPPV are covered on pages 520–4.

PaO_2

The PaO_2 drawn from a UAC distal to the ductus should be maintained in the range 7–10 kPa (50–75 mmHg).

$PaCO_2$

The $PaCO_2$ in a normal newborn baby is in the range 4.6–5.4 kPa (35–40 mmHg). Cerebral blood flow increases about 30% with each 1 kPa increase in $PaCO_2$, but a degree of permissive hypercarbia has been associated with a reduced incidence of CLD.[316] Higher $PaCO_2$ levels in more mature neonates with RDS and in <1.50 kg infants more than a week old who are being weaned off IPPV are acceptable, providing the baby is clinically stable with satisfactory pH and base excess levels. Hypocapnia ($PaCO_2$ <3.3 kPa) should be avoided because of its role in the genesis of PVL (pp. 1159–64) and CLD (pp. 554–73). A rapidly rising $PaCO_2$ is a sign of impending respiratory failure, usually associated with a fall in pH, and therefore indicates that the baby should be intubated and ventilated irrespective of his postnatal age. More gradual changes, or a stable high $PaCO_2$ with an acceptable pH (>7.25), can be managed conservatively, particularly when the baby is not in the acute phase of illness.

pH

Metabolic alkalaemia is rare, is almost always iatrogenic as a result of excessive i.v. bicarbonate use, and requires no therapy. Respiratory alkalaemia is usually due to excessive use of ventilator pressures or a deliberate attempt to dilate the pulmonary vasculature in PPHN (pp. 496–502).

Acidaemia is common in neonates with RDS. It is always essential to establish whether the acidaemia is respiratory, with a raised $PaCO_2$, or metabolic, with a normal $PaCO_2$ and a negative base excess, or a combination of a metabolic and respiratory acidosis, which is more usual. The commonest cause of a metabolic acidaemia in a baby with RDS is a raised lactate from anaerobic metabolism. This in turn can be secondary to hypoxaemia, hypotension, anaemia, infection, sepsis or strenuous respiratory muscle activity. When a metabolic acidaemia does develop, it is essential to identify the cause, so direct treatment can be instituted – for example, oxygen for hypoxia, antibiotics for infection, transfusion for anaemia and hypotension, or IPPV for exhaustion.

Acidaemia inhibits surfactant synthesis (p. 224) and increases pulmonary vascular resistance.[768] Once the pH falls below 7.15, other physiological functions such as myocardial contractility[60] and diaphragmatic activity[441] begin to deteriorate. The sick neonate has difficulty in excreting an acid load.[10] Ill VLBW neonates should have their pH kept >7.25 at all times. If the pH is <7.25 with a base deficit >10 mmol/l, intravenous alkali therapy is appropriate, if other therapies are not immediately successful. Inappropriately large or fast infusions of base to correct metabolic acidaemia, however, may cause hypernatraemia or cerebral haemorrhage.[440] Two alkalis have been used in neonatal therapy, sodium bicarbonate and trishydroxymethyl-laminomethane (THAM). Both are effective. The theoretical risk that following infusion of bicarbonate the cerebrospinal fluid might become even more acidotic does not seem to apply to the neonate.[438,795] THAM administration does not give a sodium load or increase the $PaCO_2$ and is preferable to bicarbonate if the neonate has a high $PaCO_2$ but apnoea may result[746] and thus THAM should only be given to ventilated neonates. The dose of base to be given is calculated as:

$$\text{Dose (mmol)} = \text{base deficit (mmol/l)} \times \text{body weight (kg)} \times 0.4$$

The rate of infusion should never exceed 0.5 mmol/min. Seven per cent THAM solution contains approximately 0.5 mmol/ml of base.

Blood pressure

All neonates suffering from RDS must have their BP monitored regularly (p. 623). It is important to determine whether a baby is hypotensive because he is anaemic. In general, the first transfusion should be 15 ml/kg given by infusion over 10–15 minutes if the hypotension is severe in the first hours after birth; thereafter, transfusions of blood or albumin are better given more slowly, at a rate guided by the condition of the neonate, his clinical response and the BP rise during the transfusion. Transfusions should also be given to babies who are not hypotensive but have features suggesting hypovolaemia, such as poor capillary filling, peripheral vasoconstriction and a falling pH, coupled with the record of large volumes of blood having been removed for analysis. There is, however, no place for routine plasma expanders soon after delivery.[667] If the neonate's haemoglobin is not low, saline should be given rather than albumin, because the response to albumin is small and rarely sustained[76,254] and it has adverse effects (p. 235). If the hypotensive neonate is severely hypoxic or acidaemic, his cardiac function may be impaired and he will tolerate volume expansion badly, in which case dopamine is the preferred treatment.[328] Dopamine should also be used in those in whom volume expansion has failed to increase BP; trials have shown it to be more effective than dobutamine.[253,518] The actions of dopamine are complex.[793] At 0.5–2.0 microgram/kg/min, dopaminergic actions dilate renal, mesenteric and coronary arteries; from 2 to 10 microgram/kg/min, myocardial contractility is increased directly by both α and β receptor-mediated actions and also by the release of noradrenaline from cardiac adrenergic nerves. At doses above 10–15 microgram/kg/min, dopamine begins to show α-adrenergic activity and is a vasoconstrictor of all vascular beds. Initially, therefore, 2–4 microgram/kg/min should be given,[794] increasing the dosage until the BP is acceptable.

If plasma volume expansion plus dopamine does not reverse hypotension, other agents can be tried:

- Dobutamine. This is an isoprenaline analogue with a primarily β-adrenergic inotropic effect on the myocardium, with little peripheral vascular effect, and no specific effect on the renal vascular bed.
- Isoprenaline. This beta-mimetic drug has a chronotropic and inotropic effect and is therefore of greatest benefit if hypotension is accompanied by bradycardia. It is not useful in shock because of its peripheral vasodilator effects.
- Adrenaline. This increases BP by peripheral vasoconstriction plus increased myocardial contractility. Its vasoconstrictor effects on the renal vasculature are clearly undesirable.
- Dopexamine hydrochloride. This is a synthetic catecholamine with predominant β2-adrenergic and dopaminergic activity. In low doses (2–4 microgram/kg/min) it can improve BP and urine output,[494] but at higher doses it drops systemic vascular resistance.
- Hydrocortisone 1–2 mg may be successful.[408]

Maintenance of haemoglobin

There are many reasons for a preterm neonate being anaemic (pp. 743, 748–9). There may have been an intrapartum haemorrhage, defective placental transfusion, or a twin–twin or fetomaternal haemorrhage. Blood loss after birth is iatrogenic, but a sudden drop in the haematocrit/haemoglobin level in a baby with RDS suggests the development of a GMH-IVH (pp. 1123–4). Ill neonates, in particular those who are premature, tolerate haemoglobin levels <13 g/dl (PCV <40%) poorly.[856] This is presumably because of the increase in cardiac output required to meet the oxygen demands of the tissues when there is reduced blood oxygen-carrying capacity. One policy, therefore, is to transfuse all ill neonates when their haemoglobin has fallen below 13 g/dl (PCV 40%).[465] Blood for transfusion should be from a cytomegalovirus-negative donor and be partially packed to a haemoglobin level appropriate for a premature baby (PCV 40–45%), but it does not need to be fresh blood, as the adverse metabolic features of 2- to 3-week-old donor blood are of no clinical significance when given as a 15 ml/kg transfusion over 30–120 minutes. The blood should be irradiated to avoid the risk of graft-versus-host disease (p. 1002). If the baby has a clinically important patent ductus, he should receive furosemide (frusemide) 1.0 mg/kg during the transfusion; otherwise, there is no need to give diuretic cover. Transfusions may need to be given several times a week during the acute phase of the illness and should be continued for as long as the baby is ventilated or has CLD requiring more than 30–40% oxygen (pp. 559–60). With modern transfusion practice, donor exposure can be reduced to a minimum (pp. 764–8).

Coagulation abnormalities

Routine administration of fresh frozen plasma (FFP) soon after birth is of no benefit,[667] but it is important to check for coagulation disorders, as these may be of sufficient magnitude to require treatment, particularly in a baby who is small for gestational age (SGA).[398]

If an overt coagulation disturbance occurs, such as DIC or thrombocytopenia, this should be treated by appropriate factor replacement (p. 761), but it is also essential to control and reverse the underlying problem, such as hypoxaemia or sepsis, which caused the coagulopathy in the first place. Exchange transfusion has no place in the routine management of RDS but may be indicated in the presence of DIC or sepsis.

Fluid and electrolyte balance

Renal function is often impaired in RDS (p. 485). Urine production may be no more than 1.0–1.5 ml/kg/h, close to the definition of oliguric renal failure (1 ml/kg/h) (pp. 350–1); however, peripheral oedema is usually due to leaky capillaries.

Antidiuretic hormone (ADH) levels are raised in babies with RDS, particularly when they are very ill[734] or after they develop a pneumothorax.[695,951] Babies who develop CLD have particularly raised ADH levels in the first few days after birth.[492] Plasma levels of atrial natriuretic peptide (ANP) are also high in the first few days in babies with RDS.[798] There is a complex inter-relationship between ANP levels, ductal shunting with atrial distention in RDS, and the postnatal natriuresis that appears to be an integral part of the recovery phase of RDS (pp. 336, 338).[476] The increased capillary permeability in RDS (p. 498) results in fluid loss into all tissues, including the lungs, and this is worse when pancuronium is given (p. 531). If fluid and sodium balance are inadequately controlled, the risks of PDA (p. 484), NEC (p. 345), CLD (pp. 882–3) and probably GMH-IVH are increased.

Infants with RDS should start on 40–60 ml/kg/24 h of a 10% dextrose solution. The fluid intake subsequently should be guided by the electrolyte levels and the change in the baby's weight. The ill neonate loses about 1–3% of bodyweight per day;[797] a greater loss may indicate dehydration, whereas a static or increase in weight suggests too much fluid has been given.

Appropriate supplements of electrolytes can be given in the light of the serum electrolyte analyses. Sodium and potassium do not usually need to be added to the fluid intake for the first 36–48 hours, though the frequent presence of hypocalcaemia in such babies (p. 882) means that calcium should usually be given (p. 861).

Glucose infusion rates in excess of 6 mg/kg/min (p. 316; approximately 85 ml of 10% dextrose per kilogram per 24 hours) are likely to cause hyperglycaemia, glycosuria and an osmotic diuresis. If more than 80–100 ml/kg/24 h of fluid is necessary, it is essential to monitor the blood glucose regularly and change to 5% dextrose infusions if the blood glucose exceeds 7–8 mmol/l and/or there is glycosuria.

Characteristically, a diuresis occurs around the time the baby's lung function improves.[491] Once this happens, previous constraints on the fluid balance to 40–60 ml/kg/24 h need to be relaxed to prevent dehydration, haemoconcentration and jaundice.

Albumin

Hypoalbuminaemia, with a low colloid osmotic pressure predisposing to tissue oedema, is common in RDS. Infusions of albumin, however, do not improve respiratory function;[346] indeed, they may impair it[491] and increase the risk of CLD.[231]

Nutrition in RDS

Since the protein and caloric reserves of the VLBW neonate are small, it is essential that some form of nutrition, including protein, is given as soon after birth as possible. Neonates with severe respiratory illness may have an ileus and delayed gastric emptying; bowel sounds are absent, and meconium is not passed. Enteral feeding initially may not be feasible in some ventilated babies <1.5 kg or some larger sick neonates. Parenteral nutrition, initially amino acids and glucose, should be given, progressing to full TPN, including intravenous fat, until an adequate enteral intake of protein and calories has been achieved. There are anxieties regarding the use of intralipid in neonates with severe lung disease, in whom it may cause a fall in PaO_2 by increasing pulmonary vascular resistance.[719] In addition, preterm neonates given intralipid have been reported to be supplementary oxygen- and ventilator-dependent longer than controls, and more developed BPD.[392,836] Intralipid also predisposes the VLBW baby to *Staphylococcus epidermidis* sepsis. Pulmonary lipid emboli are more common in, but not exclusively limited to, neonates receiving intravenous fat.[812] Therefore, if lipid is to be used during the first week in ventilated neonates, the dose should not exceed 3 g/kg/24 h, or 2 g/kg/24 h if there is evidence of sepsis.

Milk in the stomach may compromise ventilation, increase the work of breathing,[409] lower the PaO_2 and even cause apnoea. In spontaneously breathing babies, respiratory problems may be aggravated by the presence of a nasogastric tube obliterating one half of the upper airway.[363] Neither gastro-oesophageal reflux (GOR), NEC, nor the physiological changes mentioned, however, appear to be a major problem in VLBW neonates,[658,659] even in those who are ventilated and with an indwelling UAC, provided that milk (ideally breast milk) is only given to babies in whom it is clear that bowel activity is present. Furthermore, there are powerful reasons for attempting to introduce enteral feeds as soon as possible. The prolonged absence of enteral feeding compromises gut growth, the development of enzymes and normal peristaltic activity, and limits early weight gain, with the implication that may have for long-term neurological development. The sooner enteral feeding is attempted in VLBW neonates, the sooner full enteral feeding is established.[583,883] Thus, once bowel sounds are present in a ventilated neonate who is appropriately grown and has passed meconium, irrespective of whether or not there is an indwelling UAC,[883] enteral feeding should be started, using if possible the mother's milk (pp. 330–1).

Initially, small volumes (0.5–1.0 ml every hour or every other hour)[70] should be given to preterm infants. The stomach should be aspirated through a nasogastric tube every 4–6 hours to confirm that the milk is passing through the pylorus, and if it is not and there is abdominal distension, then the feeding should be discontinued for 24–48 hours before trying again. Once tolerated, the amount given can be steadily increased to the appropriate volume for the neonate's postnatal age and weight (p. 379).

Drug therapy in RDS

Antibiotics

It is impossible to differentiate severe early-onset septicaemia from RDS, and both conditions may coexist. Without antibiotic treatment, early-onset septicaemia can be fatal within hours (pp. 1028–33). For this reason, all dyspnoeic newborn babies, irrespective of their gestation or CXR appearance, should have appropriate bacterial cultures taken and be treated with antibiotics from the earliest signs of respiratory illness. Penicillin and gentamicin are appropriate therapy as they act synergistically against GBS and are also effective against many of the other organisms that cause early-onset septicaemia and pneumonia. In babies with RDS who are stable or who are improving, antibiotics should be stopped when negative culture results are notified at 48–72 hours.

Diuretics
The oliguria, peripheral and pulmonary oedema of early RDS, and the fact that a spontaneous diuresis is associated with improvement in respiratory status, prompted several trials of the use of diuretics in preterm infants with RDS. No long-term benefits have been described; thus, diuretics should be reserved for infants who are oliguric and have obvious signs of fluid retention and deteriorating lung function. The response to a dose of 1 mg/kg furosemide (frusemide) should be evaluated. If a diuresis does not result, a combination of furosemide (frusemide) and dopamine may be effective.[886]

Vitamins
Vitamin K should be given to all neonates (p. 298).

Pulmonary vasodilators
Pulmonary hypertension should be suspected in infants whose hypoxia is more severe than would be anticipated from their CXR appearance. Affected infants can benefit from pulmonary vasodilators, with an improvement in oxygenation, but all have side-effects (pp. 500–1). Randomised trials have not demonstrated any long-term benefits in administering inhaled nitric oxide (iNO) to prematurely born infants (pp. 500–1).[293,515,655,858]

Analgesia/sedation
Appropriate analgesia/sedation should be given to ventilated infants (Chapter 25) and analgesia should be administered prior to a painful procedure being undertaken. Sedation is contraindicated in infants with RDS who are breathing spontaneously.

Methylxanthines
Methylxanthines are of proven benefit in apnoea of prematurity (p. 578) and in weaning babies less than 30 days old from IPPV (pp. 533–4). In spontaneously breathing babies with RDS, apnoeic attacks are usually a sign of impending ventilatory exhaustion[198] and are then an indication for IPPV rather than administration of a methylxanthine.

Indometacin (indomethacin)
The use of indometacin (indomethacin) in preventing or treating a patent ductus is discussed in detail on page 484.

Surfactant therapy
Surfactant given as 'rescue' therapy improves the outcome in babies with established RDS, resulting in a reduction in pneumothorax, mortality and the combined outcome of mortality and BPD. Surfactant administration also is associated with a reduction in oxygen requirement, intensity of ventilation and an improvement in blood gases.

Method of administration   The surfactant preparation is delivered over a period of a few seconds down an ETT via an injection device at the ETT connector. The surfactant usually disseminates homogenously,[200] particularly if large rather than small doses are used.[905] As might be expected, deposition is influenced by gravity, with dependent parts of the lung receiving more of the dose.[98] There seems, however, to be no benefit from manoeuvres aimed at trying to improve the distribution to different lobes.[985]

Mechanism of action   Exogenous surfactants work in two ways. Firstly, by coating the alveolar surface, they improve lung volume and thus pulmonary perfusion and oxygenation. Lung histology improves.[709] A fall in PAP and a rise in pulmonary blood flow and left-to-right ductal shunting have been reported in most studies[391,792] but not all.[83] The second effect of exogenous surfactant administration is that it is incorporated into the type II cells and can provide substrate for, or even stimulate, surfactant production.[673,709]

Size and number of doses   Early studies[527] suggested that at least 100 mg/kg of whichever surfactant was used should be given. Subsequent studies have confirmed that small doses are less effective, e.g. 2.5 ml/kg Exosurf compared with 5 ml/kg[69] and 50 mg/kg Alveofact compared with 100 mg/kg,[341] but that larger doses, e.g. 200 mg/kg tds Curosurf compared with 100 mg/kg tds,[386] conferred no extra benefit.

Although beneficial effects, both clinically and physiologically, are seen after a single dose of surfactant, usually in the range of 100 mg/kg,[168,211] most studies show that better results are obtained with more than one dose. The Osiris trial,[684] however, showed no benefit of three to four doses of Exosurf compared with two doses. Meta-analysis has demonstrated that multiple doses give a better outcome than a single dose, with a significant reduction in the pneumothorax rate (relative risk [RR] 0.51; 95% CI 0.30, 0.88).[828]

Variation in individual response   Not all babies respond to surfactant; factors that lead to an unsatisfactory response include the presence of a PDA, cardiogenic shock or PPHN, and airleaks, which in some cases will lead to protein leaking onto the alveolar surface, impairing surfactant function.[307,523] Failure to respond to surfactant marks out a group of babies with a poorer prognosis.[394,534,818]

Different types of surfactant   Natural surfactants, as they more closely mimic the 'physiological' mixture of lipids and proteins (SP-B and SP-C), have a more rapid effect on oxygenation than do older synthetic surfactants. Meta-analysis of randomised trials comparing natural and synthetic surfactants demonstrated that the natural surfactant was associated with a significant reduction in mortality (RR 0.87; 95% CI 0.76, 0.98) and pneumothorax (RR 0.63; 95% CI 0.53, 0.75).[831] A synthetic surfactant containing a polypeptide KL4 composed of lysine and leucine, which mimics the effects of SP-B, however, has been produced.[156] It appears to be as resistant as natural surfactants to the inhibitory effects of proteins on the alveolar surface.[606] Attempts are also being made to produce SP-C analogues.[471]

Prophylactic versus selective/rescue therapy   Administering surfactant prophylactically compared to selectively or as rescue therapy is associated with a lower mortality and has other advantages. Early surfactant replacement with extubation to nCPAP, as compared with later, selective surfactant replacement and continued mechanical ventilation, was associated with a reduced need for mechanical ventilation, although an increased utilisation of exogenous surfactant replacement therapy.[849] In addition, early compared with delayed dosing with surfactant followed by high-frequency oscillatory ventilation (HFOV) facilitated and accelerated early stabilisation during the acute phase of RDS.[712]

Side effects   During the administration of the surfactant, there may be transient hypoxaemia and bradycardia.[567] There were initial anxieties that, following surfactant instillation, there was either a fall[177] or a rise in cerebral blood flow velocity[901,904] and even an increase in GMH-IVH.[164] Systemic hypotension and a transient flattening of the EEG were also reported.[177,410] More detailed studies have shown little more than a transient perturbation in cerebral haemodynamics, without evidence of cerebral ischaemia, if care is taken with the surfactant instillation[61,250,585] and the pooled data show either no effect or even a slight reduction in the incidence of GMH-IVH following surfactant administration.

Swamping alveolar macrophages with instilled surfactant could, in theory, increase the baby's susceptibility to infection;[786] no clinical evidence has, however, been found for such an association. Anxiety has been expressed that immune responses to exogenous surfactant proteins instilled into the lung would cause short- or long-term problems, but none have been reported. Surprisingly, antibodies to surfactant proteins have been found in both surfactant- and placebo-treated infants.[142]

Massive pulmonary haemorrhage (MPH), particularly in ELBW neonates, has been noted following surfactant administration. This was increased (doubled) with the use of a synthetic surfactant (Exosurf).[727,851]

Follow-up studies have not demonstrated any additional neurological deficits in surfactant-treated survivors,[577,640] nor any increase in severe ROP.[870] Surfactant-treated infants may have improved long-term lung function compared with untreated controls.[1,979]

Monitoring

The general principles of monitoring the ill preterm neonate are laid out in Chapter 19.

Complications

Many of the complications are dealt with in detail elsewhere and only the briefest of outlines will be given here.

Airleaks, pneumothorax, pulmonary interstitial emphysema (pp. 487–96)

In the past, some form of airleak was reported in about 5% of babies with RDS who were breathing spontaneously; the incidence doubled with CPAP and rose to as high as 35–40% in babies treated with IPPV plus positive end-expiratory pressure (PEEP) and inspiratory times exceeding 1 second. Nowadays, with use of 'synchronous' IPPV (pp. 521–4) and surfactant (p. 475), the overall incidence of airleaks is between 5% and 10% in ventilated infants.

Patent ductus arteriosus

The incidence of symptomatic PDA is increased by fluid overload.[62] A clinically significant ductus in a ventilated preterm baby aged 5–7 days presents as signs of heart failure and a loud precordial murmur filling systole, frequently extending into diastole. The oxygen and ventilatory requirements increase and affected babies may develop MPH (pp. 512–15). At this stage, fluids should be restricted and treatment given to effect closure, unless there are contraindications. If the first course is unsuccessful, then a second one can be given; in such cases, a prolonged course, 0.1 mg/kg daily for 6 days, might be more successful.[736] Meta-analyses of studies of prophylactic indometacin (indomethacin) given on the first day would suggest that this is beneficial, as its administration was associated with a significant reduction in symptomatic PDA, although no effect on neonatal mortality.[288] Given the beneficial effect of indometacin (indomethacin) also on the incidence of GMH-IVH and MPH as well as PDA, there is a case for prophylactic therapy in babies <28 weeks' gestational age with a high incidence of these complications.[155]

Ligation is used only in neonates who have not responded to conservative management. The size of the neonate should not be a deterrent to surgery, since it is in the ELBW infant <1.00 kg in whom the ductus does not respond to indometacin (indomethacin) that successful weaning from the ventilator will not take place until the duct is ligated.

Germinal layer/intraventricular haemorrhage (Chapter 41, Part 5)

The development of a large GMH-IVH is usually associated with clinical deterioration characterised by anaemia, increased ventilatory requirements, and neurological signs, which can be subtle (p. 1155). In many cases, smaller GMH-IVHs are asymptomatic and detected only on routine ultrasound. Many aspects of the management of respiratory failure in the neonate are directed towards preventing GMH-IVHs, for example avoiding procedures which might provoke surges in cerebral blood flow (p. 1154) and correcting coagulation disturbances (p. 756–60).

Chronic lung disease

This has now become the single most important complication of RDS in terms of morbidity, duration of therapy and cost. CLD also occurs in infants who initially had mild or even no respiratory distress.[39] It is described in detail in Chapter 27, Part 3.

Renal failure

One of the purposes of attempting early correction and maintenance of BP, using dopamine to preserve renal perfusion and paying meticulous attention to the fluid balance in babies with RDS, is to sustain renal function. In some cases this is not successful, and in others an acute episode of collapse, such as may occur with bilateral tension pneumothoraces, results in acute tubular necrosis (p. 936). If renal failure develops, it should be treated as outlined on pages 937–40. If biochemical control cannot be achieved, then either peritoneal dialysis or haemofiltration[174] may be used. Haemofiltration avoids the major problem with peritoneal dialysis, which is that the intraperitoneal fluid splints the diaphragm and makes oxygenation difficult in ventilated neonates

Outcome

Survival

Death from RDS in a baby weighing more than 1.5 kg is exceptionally rare and the overall mortality from the condition has now been reduced to between 5% and 10%.

Sequelae

Readmission to a general paediatric ward within the first year after discharge from the neonatal unit is common[637,650] and prematurely born infants continue to have a high incidence of readmission throughout childhood.[589] Amongst VLBW infants, infants with birthweight <750 g and gestational age <28 weeks require the greatest number of admissions and longest duration of stay. In the first year, the duration of stay is inversely related to birthweight.[977] Readmissions are particularly likely in infants who developed BPD and subsequently suffered an RSV infection;[348] other causes of readmission include sequelae of surgery in NEC, failure to thrive, and repair of an inguinal hernia, which is very common in males weighing <1.00 kg at birth.

Respiratory

The most important respiratory sequel of RDS is CLD (Chapter 27, part 3). Airway problems secondary to prolonged intubation may also occur (pp. 1257–8). After discharge, babies who have survived RDS in the neonatal period are more likely to have respiratory illness, particularly in the first year of life, than are infants born at term or prematurely without respiratory problems. Preterm babies have function abnormalities at follow-up; an increased airways resistance and air trapping. These sequelae are more common in neonates who required prolonged ventilation[976] and they are particularly severe in those who developed BPD (pp. 554–6).

Long-term neurological sequelae (pp. 71–2)

VLBW neonates who have been ventilated for RDS have a higher incidence of neurological sequelae than do control infants. Infants born at less than 26 weeks' gestational age have a particularly poor prognosis.[172]

Transient tachypnoea of the newborn

Incidence

This is between 4[765] and 5.7[641] per 1000 infants delivered between 37 and 42 weeks of gestation. TTN does occur in prematurely born infants, although coexisting problems such as RDS may mask the presentation; an incidence of 10 per 1000 has been reported,[191] which is higher than in term infants.

Aetiology

TTN is due to a delay in fetal lung fluid clearance.[27] It is more common in infants who are born by caesarean section without labour.[641] In such infants who develop TTN, noradrenaline levels are lower than in those delivered following labour.[354] In the absence of labour, anticipatory lung fluid clearance will not have occurred (p. 446).[925]

The relative risk for respiratory distress after birth by caesarean section without labour has been reported to be 1.74 if delivery occurs at 37 rather than 38 weeks of gestation.[641] Similarly, TTN and RDS were found to be more common in twins delivered by caesarean section if this was performed prior to 38 weeks of gestation.[137] Others,[563] however, have suggested that respiratory morbidity may only be increased by delivery by caesarean section if this occurs prior to the 36th week of gestation.

Respiratory distress after elective caesarean section in babies born at term may be due to surfactant deficiency per se,[598] but surfactant deficiency may also be important in the pathogenesis of TTN.[464] Other risk factors for TTN include male sex[191,933] and a family history of asthma.[217,782,783] The proposed mechanism for the association of TTN and maternal asthma is that infants of asthmatic mothers have a genetic predisposition to β-adrenergic hyporesponsiveness.[783]

Presentation

The classical presentation is isolated tachypnoea with respiratory rates up to 100–120/min. The infants rarely grunt, which is a sign indicating atelectasis. Retraction, indicating non-compliant lungs, is minimal. The chest may be barrel shaped as a result of hyperinflation, and the liver and spleen are palpable because of downward displacement of the diaphragm. Peripheral oedema is often present, and affected babies lose weight more slowly than controls.[731] On auscultation, there may be added moist sounds, similar to those heard in heart failure. Tachycardia is common, but the BP is usually normal. TTN usually settles within 24 hours, but may persist for several days. Some infants with TTN have been reported to require high concentrations of supplementary oxygen,[385] even 100% oxygen for several days[104] or IPPV;[885] whether such patients had TTN is arguable.

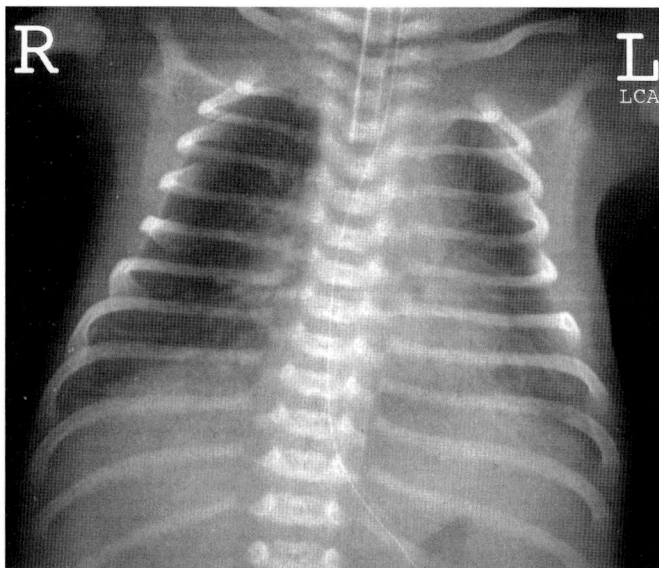

Fig. 27.16 Transient tachypnoea of the newborn. There is fluid in the right horizontal fissure and pulmonary venous congestion.

Investigations

Affected infants usually have a mild hypoxia; a marked respiratory or metabolic acidosis is unusual, and, if present, makes a review of the diagnosis mandatory. The CXR shows hyperinflation, prominent perihilar vascular markings, oedema of the interlobar septae, and fluid present in the fissures[191] (Fig. 27.16). The prominent perihilar streaking is due to engorgement of the periarterial lymphatics, which participate in the clearance of lung fluid; fluid may also be present in the costophrenic angles. The CXR usually clears by the next day, although complete resolution may take 3–7 days. Infants with TTN have a reduced tidal volume, but a raised minute volume due to the increased respiratory rate. Compliance is reduced; airways resistance and FRC raised.[778]

Interleukin-6, but not C-reactive protein, levels at the onset of symptoms in newborns evaluated for sepsis in the perinatal period differentiated between those infants who had TTN and those who had proven or suspected sepsis.[477]

Differential diagnosis

A rapid respiratory rate may be due to cerebral irritation from subarachnoid blood or perinatal hypoxic ischaemia (p. 455), but these infants are distinguished by their history and the presence of a respiratory alkalaemia. The CXR appearance of TTN may be mimicked by heart failure. If the heart failure is due to asphyxia, there will be a positive history and the heart will usually be enlarged; if it is due to congenital heart disease, a murmur may be present. It is not possible to differentiate TTN from early-onset sepsis (pp. 1028–33) and this needs to be considered when planning the initial treatment.

Prevention

Continuous infusion of terbutaline given to mothers prior to elective caesarean section was associated with improved lung function,[252] but the mothers who received terbutaline had significantly higher levels of bleeding.

Treatment

Most infants with TTN require no form of respiratory support other than added oxygen, and rarely require an inspired oxygen concentration greater than 40% or support for more than 3 days. Intravenous penicillin and gentamicin should be administered until infection has been excluded (pp. 1019–26). Hydration should be maintained with intravenous glucose electrolyte solutions, and nasogastric tube feeds withheld until the respiratory rate settles. Diuretics are of no proven benefit.[564,952] In a randomised trial, although infants who were given oral furosemide (frusemide), 2 mg/kg followed by 1 mg/kg 12 hours later, lost more weight than the placebo group, there were no significant differences between the two groups with regard to duration of tachypnoea or hospitalisation, or the severity of symptoms.[564]

Monitoring

The standard monitoring outlined on pages 577–8 should be applied. A UAC should be inserted if the baby has a persisting requirement for more than 40% oxygen.

Complications

These are rare, though airleaks may occur, particularly if the baby has required CPAP or IPPV.

Prognosis

The condition is self-limiting, although the symptoms may last throughout the perinatal period. There is debate whether babies who have had TTN are more likely to wheeze at follow-up.[783,809]

Minimal respiratory disease

This entity is usually defined as transient respiratory signs persisting for a mean of only 4 hours.[430]

Aetiology

Some babies are hypothermic, with a temperature of less than 35°C. Surfactant function is temperature-dependent[332] and the babies often improve within an hour or two when their temperature returns to normal. Some babies have a moderately low pH at 7.20–7.25, and this may transiently compromise surfactant synthesis.[626] In other babies, the tachypnoea may be the result of mild intrapartum asphyxia with or without minor degrees of aspiration of meconium or amniotic squames. In most cases, the condition probably represents the very mild end of the spectrum of delayed clearance of lung liquid, which in the more marked form is diagnosed as TTN.

Clinical features

The baby, near or at term, presents within the first 2–3 hours, commonly after being transferred to the postnatal ward with his mother. The infant usually have an expiratory grunt or moan, which may be quite loud; there is mild sternal or intercostal recession, and a respiratory rate of up to 80–100/min. Cyanosis, if present, is relieved by putting the infant in 25–30% oxygen. There are no added sounds in the chest, and the rest of the clinical examination is normal.

Differential diagnosis

This is always a retrospective one, made once the baby has recovered and shows no signs of infection or more serious pulmonary disease. The major anxiety when the baby first presents is whether he has early-onset sepsis (pp. 1028–33). The only presenting feature in some infants with mild pulmonary hypoplasia can be tachypnoea;[8] such cases, however, can be distinguished by the persistence of the tachypnoea, small volume lungs on CXR, and abnormal lung function tests.

Investigations

It is advisable to check the infant's blood gas, take a CXR to exclude other diagnoses, and send off a blood count and culture. Hypoglycaemia should be excluded, particularly if the baby is an IDM or is small for dates. The blood gas analyses will usually show mild hypoxaemia in air (PaO_2 6–8 kPa, 45–60 mmHg), which rapidly becomes normal in 25–30% oxygen; $PaCO_2$ and the pH will usually be normal or show a mild metabolic acidaemia, with a pH of 7.20–7.25 and a base deficit of 10 mmol/l. The haemoglobin and white cell count will be normal. The CXR, particularly if taken within 1–2 hours of birth, often shows some streakiness or a rather non-specific haziness, both of which probably represent delayed clearing of the fetal lung liquid.

Treatment

Antibiotics should be given to all infants with respiratory distress, as infection cannot be excluded until the results of the cultures are available at 48 hours after birth.

Prognosis

The prognosis is excellent. Most babies are asymptomatic and in room air by 12 hours of age.

Pulmonary airleaks

Pneumothorax and pulmonary interstitial emphysema (PIE) are the most common forms of airleaks in the newborn; pneumomediastinum, pneumopericardium and pneumoperitoneum also occur. Rarely, multiple airleaks may be complicated by subcutaneous emphysema and systemic air embolism.

Pathophysiology

Pulmonary airleaks occur when there is uneven alveolar ventilation, air trapping and high transpulmonary pressure swings, the final common pathway being alveolar overdistension and rupture. Uneven ventilation is compounded by a lack of redistribution of pressure through the alveolar connecting channels (the pores of Kohn), which are reduced in number in the immature lung.[594] The rupture is thought to occur at the alveolar bases, in apposition to blood vessels. The gas tracks along the sheaths of pulmonary blood vessels to the mediastinum, where it accumulates in the roots of the lungs; air may then rupture into the pleura, mediastinum, pericardium or extrathoracic areas. The existence of PIE supports this hypothesis, as, after alveolar rupture, gas is trapped in the parenchyma by the extensive connective tissue matrix and increased interstitial water in the preterm lung. This prevents decompression into the mediastinum, thereby splinting the lung and compressing the blood vessels. An alternative hypothesis is that interstitial air directly enters the pleural cavity after rupture of a subpleural bleb.[713]

Pneumothorax

Incidence

An early study,[844] which involved X-raying the chest of all newborns, demonstrated that 1% had airleaks, although only 10% of those with airleaks were symptomatic. The incidence was reported to be higher if there was associated lung disease or the neonate was receiving assisted ventilation; 4% of infants with lung disease developed airleaks, compared with 16% on CPAP and 34% of those being ventilated.[597] In the last decade, however, the incidence of pneumothorax has decreased dramatically in response to use of surfactant therapy (p. 475), pancuronium (p. 489) and fast ventilator rates (pp. 526–8). Nowadays, most units report airleak rates of 5–10% in ventilated babies.

Aetiology

Spontaneous pneumothoraces may occur immediately after birth due to the high transpulmonary pressure swings generated by the newborn during their first breaths[918] or because of active resuscitation (pp. 219–42). Familial spontaneous pneumothoraces occurring in neonates are very rare.[256] Pneumothorax is usually a complication of respiratory disease, for example RDS or meconium aspiration syndrome (MAS), and congenital malformations, in which there is uneven ventilation, alveolar overdistension and air trapping, made worse in many cases by IPPV. Pneumothorax may occasionally result from direct injury to the lung by causes other than mechanical ventilation, for example direct perforation by suction catheters or introducers passed through the ETT[20,910] or by central venous catheter placement.[308]

Components of ventilatory support have been incriminated in increasing the incidence of airleak. These include addition of PEEP of 3–8 cmH$_2$O,[66] but the data were not from a randomised study. A prolonged inflation time was also noted to be a risk factor,[721] perhaps because of provocation of active expiration against the ventilator.[345] The higher (50% vs 16%) incidence of airleak with an inspiratory:expiratory (I:E) ratio of $\geq$1.0:1 compared with an I:E ratio of $\leq$0.7:1[866] might also be explained by a similar mechanism. High peak inspiratory pressures[349,675] and mean airway pressures (MAPs) increased the incidence of airleaks.[868] Airleaks occur in babies who have started to exhale while the ventilator is still trying to inflate their lungs (active expiratory reflex).[358]

Clinical features

Small pneumothoraces may be asymptomatic, but, when a large pneumothorax develops, all of the clinical features of respiratory distress may be present. In addition, with very large or tension pneumothoraces, the infant's overall condition usually deteriorates, often dramatically, with pallor, shock and deterioration in oxygenation. An increased resonance on percussion may be detected, and there is a decrease in air entry on the affected side. A tension pneumothorax will result in a shift of the mediastinum and the position of the cardiac impulse; there is also abdominal distension due to displacement of the diaphragm and, with a right-sided pneumothorax, downward displacement of the liver. At the time of a pneumothorax, there is a marked increase in cerebral blood flow velocity, which correlates closely with the systemic haemodynamic changes.[421] Pneumothorax causes and aggravates haemorrhage into the germinal layer and ventricles of preterm infants. Increased levels of AVP may also occur, resulting in fluid retention (p. 482).

Diagnosis

Continuous monitoring of the heart rate, BP and $PaCO_2$ will give warning of the baby's deterioration. Transillumination with an intense beam from a fibreoptic light is of considerable help in the preterm baby with a thin chest wall: abnormal air collections cause increased transmission of light on the involved side;[533] however, PIE can give a similar appearance. The CXR remains the gold standard for diagnosing pneumothorax and should be done unless the infant's clinical condition makes emergency drainage mandatory. The diagnosis of a pneumothorax on the CXR is usually obvious, but rarely the appearance of either lobar emphysema or cystic adenomatoid malformation of the lung

may resemble a pneumothorax.[565] A small pneumothorax may only be recognised by a difference in radiolucency between the two lung fields (Fig. 27.17). A large pneumothorax will be associated with absent lung markings and a collapsed lung on the ipsilateral side (Fig. 27.18). A tension pneumothorax will be demonstrated by eversion of the diaphragm, bulging intercostal spaces, and mediastinal shift (Fig. 27.19).

Ill, ventilated infants are usually nursed in the supine position and intrapleural air rises to lie retrosternally. Retrosternal air

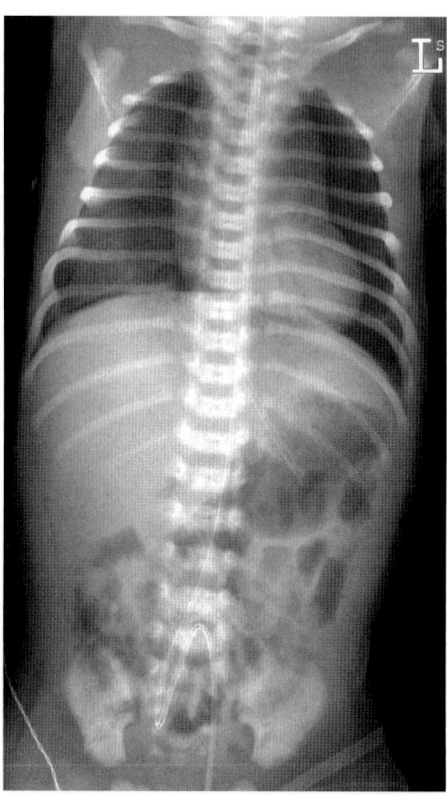

Fig. 27.17 Bilateral pneumothoraces. Note bulging at the intercostals' margins. The difference in the translucency of the two sides indicates that there is more free air on the left.

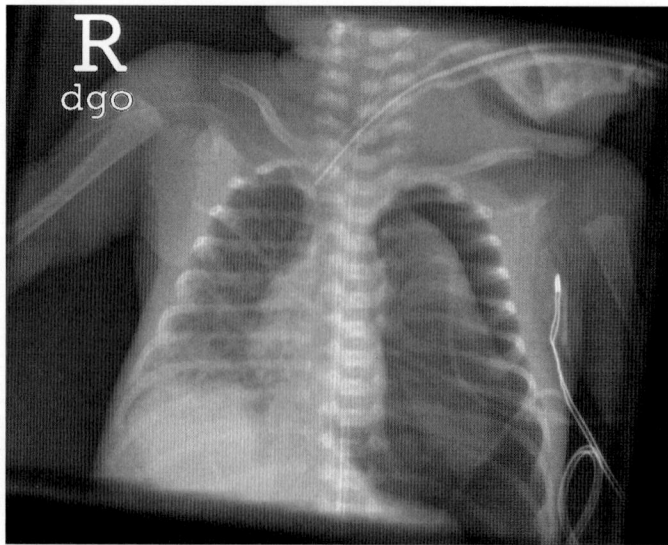

Fig. 27.18 Large left-sided tension pneumothorax. Note that the non-compliant lung has only partially collapsed.

is best demonstrated by a horizontal-beam, lateral-view CXR (Fig. 27.20), which is also useful in demonstrating the position of the chest-drain tip (see below, Fig. 27.21).

Prevention

The risk of pneumothorax can be reduced by administering surfactant (p. 475), by using the minimum ventilator pressure required (pp. 523–4), and by abolishing the baby's active expiratory efforts.

Paralysis/sedation

Breathing out of phase with the ventilator during IPPV increases the incidence of pneumothorax (see above). Routine paralysis of all ventilated babies, however, is no better at preventing pneumothorax than is synchronised ventilation.[802] Pancuronium

should be given selectively, only to infants with an active expiratory pattern (see above), if pneumothoraces are to be prevented.[167,360] Active expiration may be difficult to detect clinically at slow rates; however, if a neonate's oxygenation fails to improve and obvious respiratory efforts continue as the ventilator rate is increased to 60–80/min, this identifies the majority of neonates with a persisting active respiratory pattern who are likely to benefit from paralysis.[351] Infants who receive neuromuscular blocking agents, such as pancuronium, require higher peak pressures when the first dose is given, to maintain oxygenation, and ventilator rates should be reduced to ≤60/min to avoid gas trapping.[425]

If 'paralysis' is required for a prolonged period, infants become oedematous, and this is only partially responsive to fluid restriction. Consequently, many clinicians now prefer to avoid use of neuromuscular blocking agents and administer analgesics and/or sedatives to try and suppress respiratory activity, but also

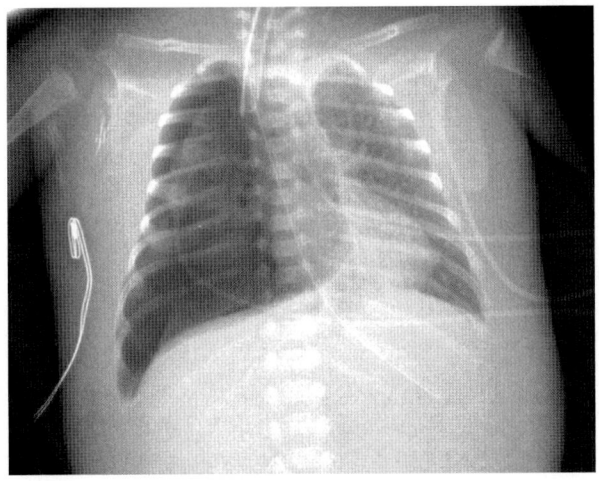

Fig. 27.19 Large right-sided tension pneumothorax with bulging over the midline and compression of the left lung.

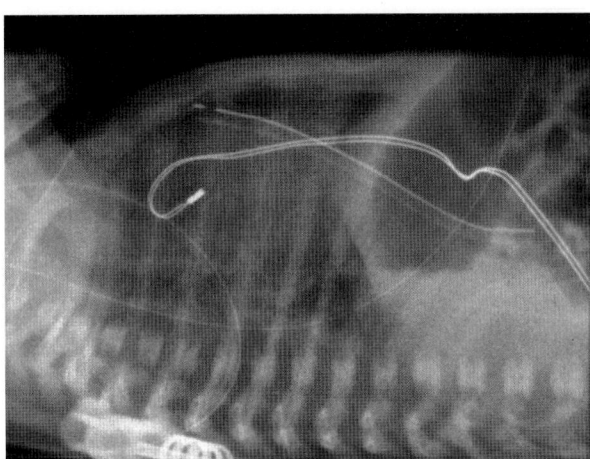

Fig. 27.21 Lateral chest X-ray demonstrating a correctly anteriorly placed tip of a chest drain.

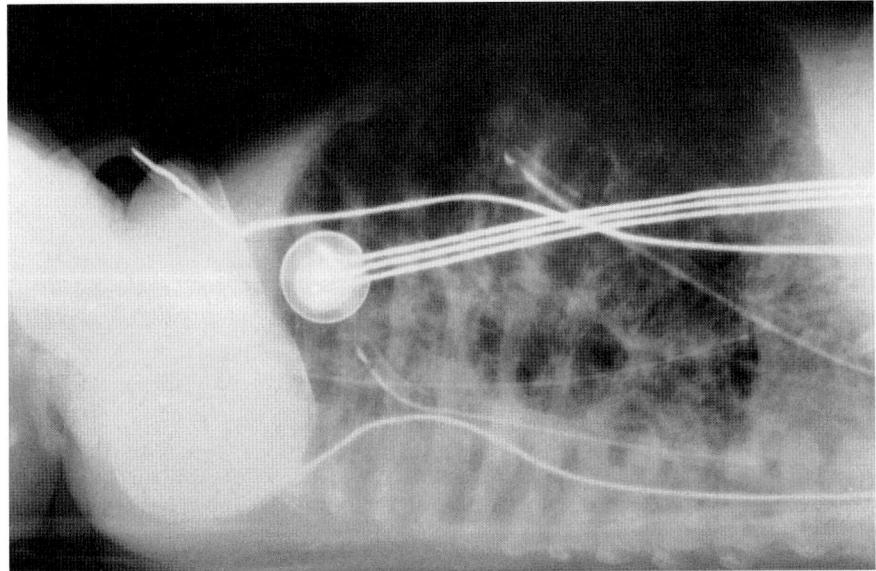

Fig. 27.20 Lateral chest X-ray with anterior collection of air. Only one chest drain is positioned to lie anteriorly; the other tip lies posteriorly and the pneumothorax has been inadequately drained.

to minimise any discomfort felt by a ventilated baby. Stress hormone levels have been demonstrated to be significantly related to the severity of illness and to fall with sedation.[42] It has been suggested that pre-emptive analgesia might reduce the incidence of poor neurological outcome in preterm infants who require ventilatory support.[18] Administration of analgesics and/or sedatives, although having benefits, has not been demonstrated in randomised trials to reduce the pneumothorax rate[537] and they too have side effects. For example, in a randomised trial,[683] fentanyl administration was associated with a reduction in stress markers, but no improvements in long-term outcome. Fentanyl can cause muscle rigidity and precipitate movement disorders, and withdrawal symptoms can occur. Plasma fentanyl clearance increases with maturity; thus, gestational age should be taken into account when prescribing fentanyl.[773] Naloxone is an effective antidote to fentanyl. Morphine, compared with placebo, also significantly reduced adrenaline concentrations in ventilated neonates, but did not influence the occurrence of airleak.[725] Morphine does not appear to be associated with adverse effects on intelligence, motor function or behaviour at follow-up,[593] but should be used with caution in prematurely born infants, because of its low clearance, which correlates with gestational age.[772] Diamorphine may be preferable to morphine: in a randomised trial,[960] both agents reduced the stress response to ventilation, but diamorphine had a more rapid onset of sedation and did not have morphine's hypotensive tendency. Midazolam is sedative in ventilated babies,[463] but it does not influence the course of RDS and in high doses it causes respiratory suppression, hypotension and reduced cerebral blood flow. Long-term use can result in accumulation, and an encephalopathic illness has been described. Midazolam is reversed by flumazenil. Midazolam is not as effective a sedative as chloral,[666] but chloral can cause gastric irritation and its metabolite is hepatotoxic.

Modes of ventilation

High-frequency positive pressure ventilation

Ventilating babies at rates of ≥60/min rather than at 30–40/min reduced the incidence of airleaks.[81,407] Those data were subsequently confirmed by the results of two multicentre, randomised studies.[672,715] Meta-analysis of the results of the randomised trials[356] demonstrated that the risk for airleak at the faster compared with the slower rate was significantly reduced (RR 0.69; 95% CI 0.51, 0.93). The most likely explanation for the reduction in airleak at the faster frequency was that spontaneous respiration synchronises with the ventilator at fast rates,[359] whereas infants actively expire at slow rates. There have, however, been no randomised trials comparing different ventilator rates in infants routinely exposed to antenatal steroids and postnatal surfactant; whether fast rates are more effective than slow rates in preventing pneumothoraces in such a population remains unknown.

Patient-triggered ventilation

Comparison with historical controls suggested that patient-triggered ventilation (PTV) might reduce the incidence of pneumothorax. Meta-analysis of the results of six randomised trials, however, has not confirmed that effect (RR for airleak 1.03; 95% CI 0.80, 1.34).[356] During pressure support ventilation (PSV), both the initiation and termination of ventilator inflation are determined by the infant's respiratory efforts. Studies have demonstrated that PSV reduces the rate of asynchrony (p. 525), but whether this form of ventilation will reduce the incidence of pneumothorax remains untested.

High-frequency oscillation

Meta-analysis of the results of randomised trials has demonstrated that high-frequency oscillation (HFO) does not reduce the incidence of pneumothorax in preterm infants. Indeed, if a high-volume strategy is used, it has been suggested that HFO may even increase the pneumothorax rate (RR 1.19; 95% CI 1.03, 1.38).[411] In infants born at term, in a randomised trial,[420] use of HFO was associated with a reduction in the incidence of pneumothorax, but this was at the expense of an increase in intracerebral haemorrhage.

Treatment

Asymptomatic pneumothoraces need no treatment, other than careful observation of the infant. In term infants with mild symptoms, a pneumothorax may respond to increasing the inspired oxygen concentration to 100%, which will favour resorption of the extra-alveolar gas; this strategy should not be used in prematurely born infants at risk of ROP.

A pneumothorax must always be drained using a chest drain in symptomatic and/or ventilated babies and those with tension pneumothoraces. If the infant is in extremis, and there is no time for formal insertion of a chest drain, emergency drainage of a pneumothorax can be done by needle aspiration. A butterfly needle (18 G) should be used. This is then attached to a three-way tap, which is held under water in a small sterile container. The needle is inserted through the skin in the second intercostal space anteriorly, and then the skin and needle moved sideways before advancing the needle through the underlying muscle; this reduces the likelihood of leaving an open needle track for entry of air once the needle has been removed. Care must be taken not to remove too much air by needle aspiration, as the needle might then tear the expanding lung. Following emergency drainage, a chest tube should be inserted (pp. 1259–60).

Insertion of a chest tube (10–14 FG) should be under local anaesthesia and by blunt dissection through either the second intercostal space just lateral to the mid-clavicular line or the sixth space in the mid-axillary line. The tip of the chest tube should lie retrosternally to achieve the most effective drainage (Fig. 27.22). A retrospective review of 149 cases of chest drain placement[12] revealed that inserting the chest drain through the anterior chest wall achieved retrosternal positioning in 85% of occasions compared with only 47% inserted through the lateral chest wall. The lateral site, however, is preferred for cosmetic reasons, as any resultant scar is less obvious. If the lateral site is chosen, to maximise the likelihood of retrosternal placement of the drain tip, the infant should be turned so that the affected side is uppermost and the drain inserted aiming anteriorly. The drain should be positioned with the trocar removed and the infant very temporarily disconnected from the ventilator, as this reduces the risk of inserting the drain into the lung. This complication should be suspected if there is continuous drainage of air or the

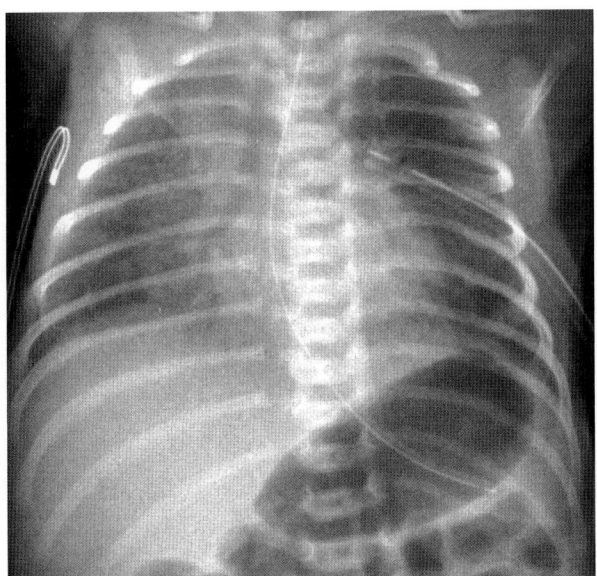

Fig. 27.22 Anteroposterior chest X-ray of the infant in Fig. 27.21, demonstrating the pneumothorax has been adequately drained.

pneumothorax persists. Retrosternal placement of the chest tube tip should be confirmed by CXR (p. 1260); a second drain is only infrequently required to ensure complete drainage if the first drain has been appropriately sited. Complications of malpositioned tubes include traumatisation of the thoracic duct resulting in a chylothorax, cardiac tamponade due to a haemorrhagic pericardial effusion, and phrenic nerve injury; the latter complication is more likely if the drainage tube is positioned deep in the chest.[946] Once inserted, the tube should be connected to an underwater seal drain with suction of 5–10 cmH$_2$O. Heimlich valves are useful during transport, but can become blocked and so fail to operate if left in situ for any length of time. Once a chest drain has been inserted, it should be left in situ for at least 72–96 hours, or for 24 hours after it is no longer bubbling. The chest tube should then be clamped for a further 24 hours and only removed if no pleural air accumulates. Pneumothoraces persisting for an average of 10 days may respond to fibrin glue, but this treatment has been reported to have significant risks.[779]

After drainage of an uncomplicated pneumothorax, a baby not on IPPV usually improves rapidly. In a ventilated, very prematurely born baby, a pneumothorax often precipitates a serious deterioration in his condition, with the development of a large intracerebral bleed.

Bronchopleural fistula

A large tear in the pleural surface of the lung, a bronchopleural fistula, may not close with conventional tube drainage of the pneumothorax. Alternative strategies are surgical closure at thoracotomy,[371] selective bronchial intubation (see below),[13,969] or instillation of fibrin glue into the pleural space.[67]

Prognosis

The mortality, though not the incidence, varies with birthweight and is in general double that of babies who have RDS but no airleak. If a parenchymal haemorrhage occurs in association with a pneumothorax (pp. 487–91), this has a detrimental effect on the neurological outcome.

Pulmonary interstitial emphysema

Aetiology

Pulmonary interstitial emphysema is gas trapped within the perivascular sheaths of the lung. In the surfactant-deficient lung of the preterm infant,[713] rupture of the small airways occurs distal to the termination of their fascial sheath, and air dissects into the interstitium. PIE occurs mainly in neonates with RDS,[113] but has been noted, though much less frequently, in aspiration syndromes and sepsis. PIE is associated with positive pressure ventilation, high peak inspiratory pressures and malpositioned ETTs.[349,400] It has rarely been described in spontaneously breathing infants.[218] PIE may be lobar in distribution, but more commonly involves both lungs. It frequently occurs with either a pneumothorax or pneumomediastinum.

Incidence

There is an inverse relationship between the incidence of PIE and birthweight.[400] The new ventilatory strategies and the use of surfactant have considerably reduced the incidence of PIE.

Pathophysiology

In infants with PIE, the trapped gas reduces pulmonary perfusion by compressing the vessels and interfering with ventilation. As a result, there is profound hypoxaemia combined with carbon dioxide retention.

Presentation

PIE virtually always presents radiologically – that is, it is found on the CXR of a severely ill neonate carried out either on a routine basis or because his condition was deteriorating.

Diagnosis

Transillumination of the chest with diffuse PIE will give the same appearance as a large pneumothorax. The CXR, however, is diagnostic, demonstrating hyperinflation and a characteristic cystic appearance, which may be diffuse, multiple, small, non-confluent, cystic radiolucencies (Figs 27.23 & 27.24), which may be unilateral (Fig. 27.25); at a later stage, large bullae may appear (Fig. 27.26). The appearance may be confused with lobar emphysema or with cystic adenomatoid malformation of the lung.

Treatment

Affected babies usually have severe RDS and/or sepsis; their ventilator management is particularly difficult. For both generalised and localised disease, ventilator pressures should be kept at the minimum compatible with acceptable gases (PaO_2 >6–7 kPa [45–52 mmHg], pH >7.25), and the baby paralysed to minimise

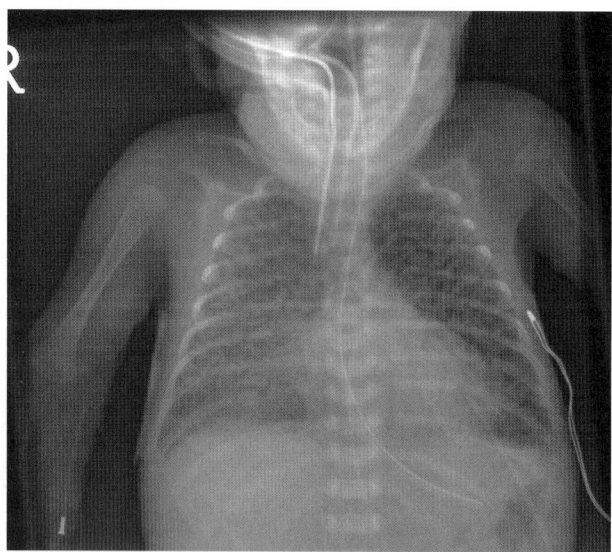

Fig. 27.23 Bilateral pulmonary interstitial emphysema.

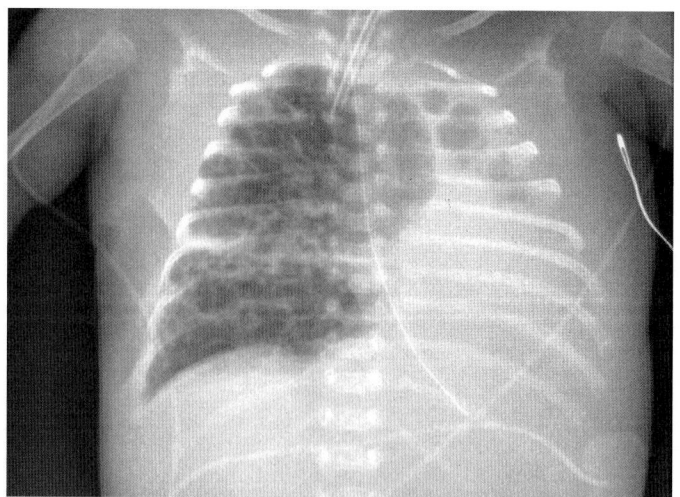

Fig. 27.25 Severe pulmonary interstitial emphysema of the right lung with mediastinal shift and compression of the left lung.

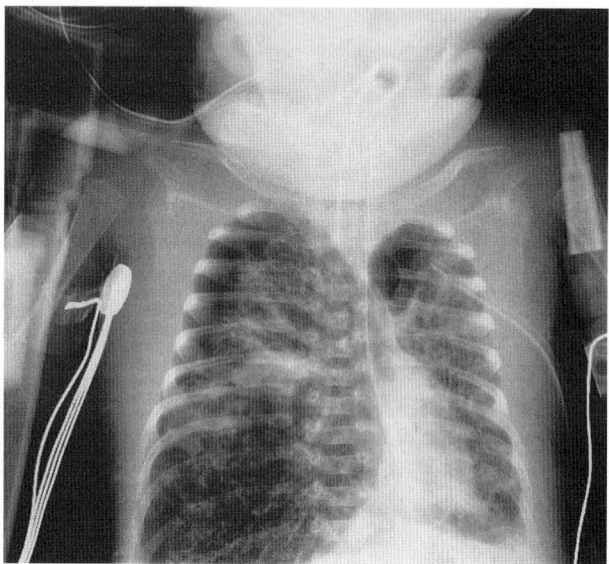

Fig. 27.24 Gross pulmonary interstitial emphysema (PIE) of right lung with overdistension and downward displacement of diaphragm and moderately severe PIE of left lung.

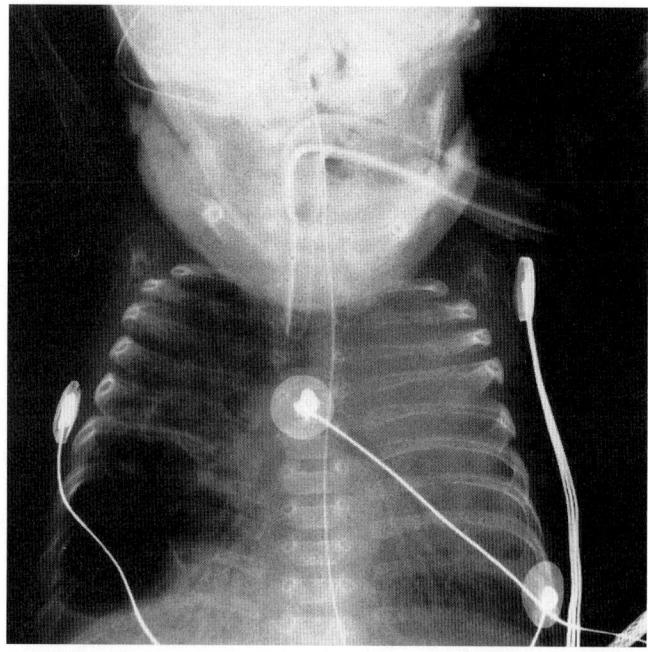

Fig. 27.26 Pulmonary interstitial emphysema of the right lung with gross cystic changes in the right middle lobe compressing the right lower lobe and left lung.

the risk of extension of the airleaks. Withdrawal of PEEP may result in disappearance of the PIE.[557]

Generalised PIE may respond to increasing the ventilator rate to 100–120/min.[660] Using such rates, the number of babies who progress to pneumothorax may be reduced, but without any other advantage. Indeed, in one series,[349] the severity of the PIE increased, possibly because of the absence of a pneumothorax decompressing the interstitial emphysema. Transfer from conventional ventilators to high-frequency jet ventilation (HFJV),[90,716] high-frequency flow interruption[300] or oscillation[149] has improved oxygenation in some infants with severe respiratory failure due to PIE, but a randomised controlled trial failed to show that HFO had benefit in PIE.[420] HFJV has been reported in a randomised

trial to be more successful support than rapid-rate conventional ventilation;[503] survival and the incidence of BPD, GMH-IVH, PDA, airway obstruction and airleak, however, were similar in the two groups. Treatment with continuous negative pressure and intermittent mandatory ventilation was reported to improve oxygenation in a small study.[187] The results of a retrospective review of a case series suggested that a 3-day course of dexamethasone (0.5 mg/kg/day) might reduce ventilatory requirements in infants with PIE.[283]

If the lungs do not decompress in response to different ventilator strategies, linear pleurotomies have been carried out to

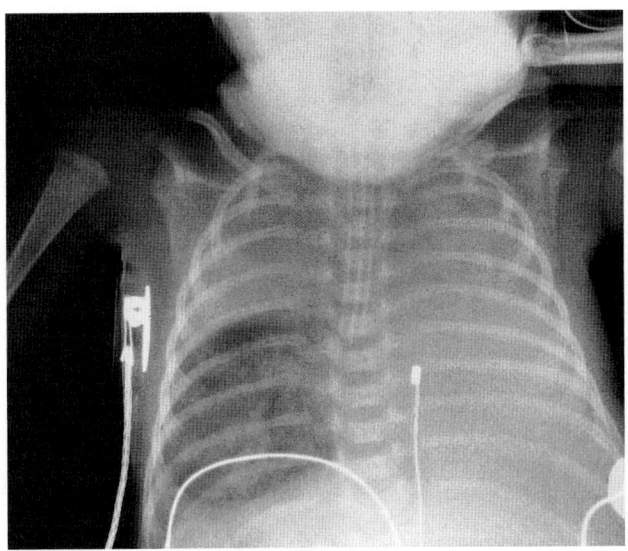

Fig. 27.27 Endotracheal tube inserted into right main bronchus with resultant collapse of left lung and right upper lobe.

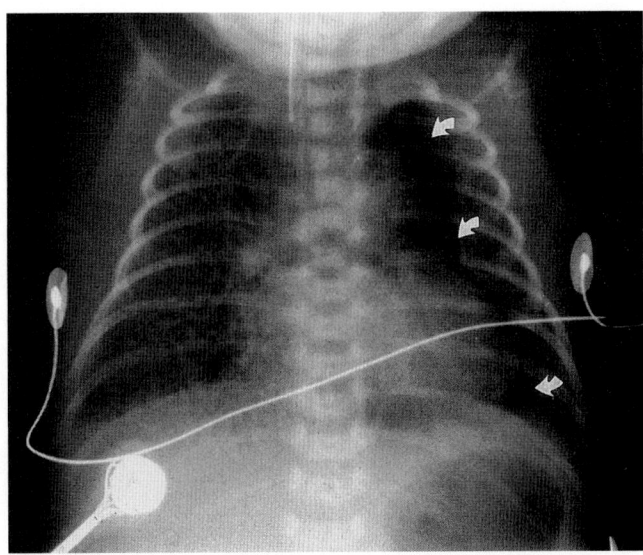

Fig. 27.28 Left-sided pneumomediastinum (between the arrows and the heart border).

create an artificial pneumothorax. This can be done by scarification of the lung using either a 21 G needle inserted through the chest wall[630] or puncturing multiple blebs at thoracotomy.[982]

The conservative ventilatory management outlined above for generalised PIE should also be tried for localised disease and is often successful.[580] In addition, in localised PIE, placing the infant with his hyperinflated lung dependent in the lateral decubitus position at all times can result in partial or complete atelectasis of the desired segments.[159,863] In this position, the upper 'good' lung receives a greater proportion of the ventilation,[405] the affected dependent lung being underventilated and hence decompressing. Selective bronchial intubation may also be useful. As soon as the affected lung is bypassed, it becomes atelectactic (Fig. 27.27); if selective intubation is maintained for 24–48 hours, when the affected lung is reventilated the PIE does not usually recur.[13,100,126] This technique is more useful if the left lung is affected, as selective intubation of the right main bronchus is easier to perform. It may be necessary to support the infant on HFOV to maintain adequate blood gases during selective intubation.[737] When using selective intubation of the right main bronchus, cutting an additional side hole in the ETT has been suggested to reduce the problem of right upper lobe collapse.[595] Selective obstruction of one main bronchus has also been achieved by inserting a handmade latex oesophageal balloon under bronchoscopic control.[618] If selective bronchial intubation fails, insertion of a pneumothorax tube directly into the blebs[747] or carrying out multiple linear pleurotomies as in generalised disease[982] might be considered. The collections may persist and compress the adjacent normal lung parenchyma, causing a sudden deterioration in the infant's condition. Resection of the affected area may be required to alleviate the respiratory distress.

Prognosis

The incidence of CLD is greatly increased following diffuse PIE (pp. 554–73),[843,974] and radiologically the changes of PIE may merge imperceptibly into those of BPD. The mortality from diffuse PIE is high, but studies reporting outcome generally predate routine use of antenatal steroids and postnatal surfactant.[349,400,639]

Pneumomediastinum

Pneumomediastinum occurs in approximately 2.5 per 1000 livebirths, in babies where there is gas trapping associated with RDS, pneumonia, MAS and mechanical ventilation.

Presentation

The infant with an isolated pneumomediastinum may be asymptomatic or have mild respiratory distress; it only rarely causes severe symptoms. The sternum may appear bowed and the heart sounds muffled. Mediastinal shift rarely occurs. Air may track up into the soft tissues of the neck, but this is uncommon. Pneumomediastinum often coexists with multiple airleaks, including PIE and pneumothorax, in severely ill, ventilated babies (Fig. 27.28).

Diagnosis

This is made on the CXR (Fig. 27.28), as a halo of air adjacent to the borders of the heart, and on lateral view it produces marked retrosternal hyperlucency. The mediastinal gas may elevate the thymus away from the pericardium, resulting in a cresentic configuration resembling a spinnaker sail.[642]

Treatment

An isolated pneumomediastinum is often asymptomatic and in general requires no treatment. It is very difficult to drain a pneumomediastinum, as the gas is collected in multiple independent lobules. Relatively successful attempts have been made, however,

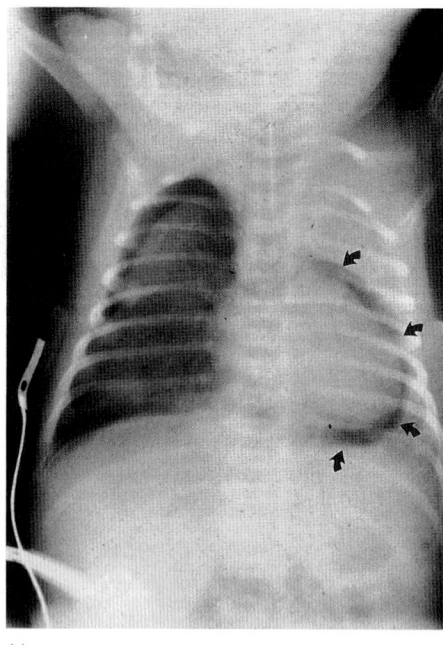
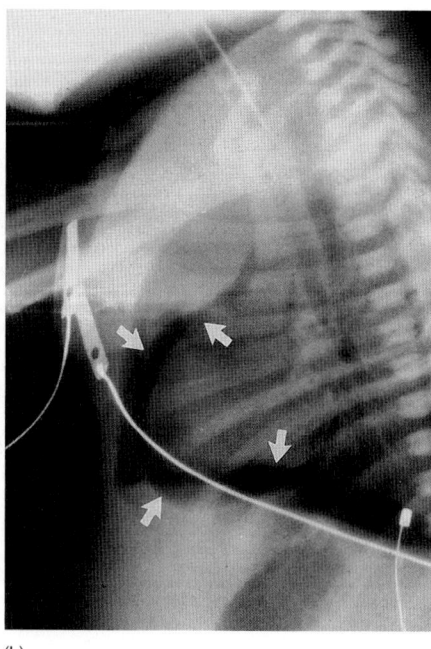

(a) (b)

Fig. 27.29 Pneumopericardium: (a) anteroposterior view; (b) lateral view. There is also a right pneumothorax.

with multiple needling and tube drainage.[869] In term infants, use of a high inspired oxygen concentration will be associated with resorption of the extra-alveolar air, but this should not be attempted in preterm infants at risk from ROP (pp. 843–7).

Pneumopericardium

A pneumopericardium is rarely asymptomatic and usually causes cardiac tamponade with sudden hypotension, bradycardia and cyanosis. The heart sounds are muffled, but a friction rub is rarely audible. The signs may be confused with those of a tension pneumothorax, but the CXR is diagnostic (Fig. 27.29). It is usually accompanied by other major airleaks such as pneumomediastinum, widespread PIE or tension pneumothorax.

Aetiology

Pneumopericardium may rarely occur spontaneously[458] or in babies supported by CPAP,[406] but the majority of cases occur in ventilated, prematurely born babies. Its frequent association with PIE and pneumomediastinum suggests that the gas enters the pericardium through a defect in the pericardial sac, probably at the pericardial reflection near the ostia of the pulmonary veins.

Diagnosis

The CXR demonstrates gas completely surrounding the heart (Fig. 27.29), outlining the base of the great vessels and contained within the pericardium. Gas can be seen inferior to the diaphragmatic surface of the heart, differentiating this abnormality from a pneumomediastinum in which the mediastinal gas is limited inferiorly by the attachment of the mediastinal pleura to the central tendon of the diaphragm. In a haemodynamically significant pneumopericardium, the transverse diameter of the heart is significantly reduced.

Treatment

A conservative approach can be adopted for small asymptomatic lesions. All symptomatic pneumopericardia should be drained immediately by direct pericardial tap via the subxiphoid route. The BP should be monitored continuously, and the tap repeated if bradycardia or hypotension recurs. Catheter drainage may be necessary if the pericardial air reaccumulates.

Prognosis

The mortality for symptomatic pneumopericardium is between 80% and 90%[436] and many survivors have neurological sequelae.

Pneumoperitoneum

This may result from perforation of the gut, but may also be caused by air dissecting from the chest through the diaphragmatic foramina into the peritoneum[24] (Fig. 27.30), particularly in ventilated babies who already have a pneumothorax and a pneumomediastinum. In some cases, the gas localises in the connective tissue on the posterior wall of the abdomen, a pneumoretroperitoneum.[484]

Diagnosis

If the pneumoperitoneum is large, the diagnosis can be made from the anteroposterior X-ray (Fig. 27.31). For smaller leaks, a horizontal-beam lateral or right lateral X-ray is required (Fig. 27.32). Rupture of the bowel, usually due to NEC, can generally be excluded by the absence of a history of gastrointestinal disease, in particular bloody stools or intestinal obstruction, and a normal gut gas pattern on erect abdominal X-ray. If there is still doubt, differentiating a pneumoperitoneum caused by transdiaphragmatic air dissection from one due to perforated bowel can

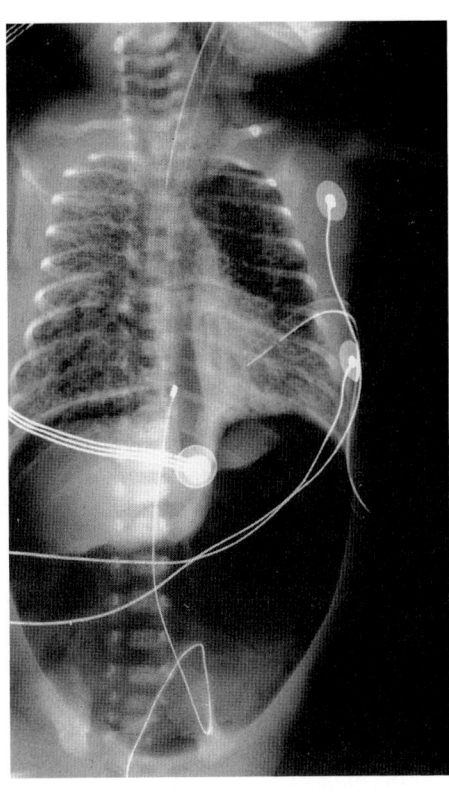

Fig. 27.30 Pneumoperitoneum associated with gross pulmonary interstitial emphysema.

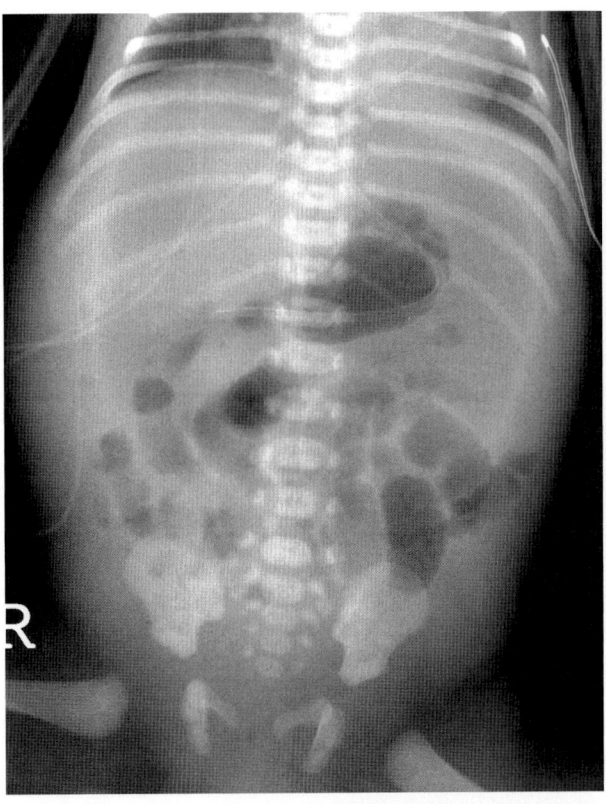

(a)

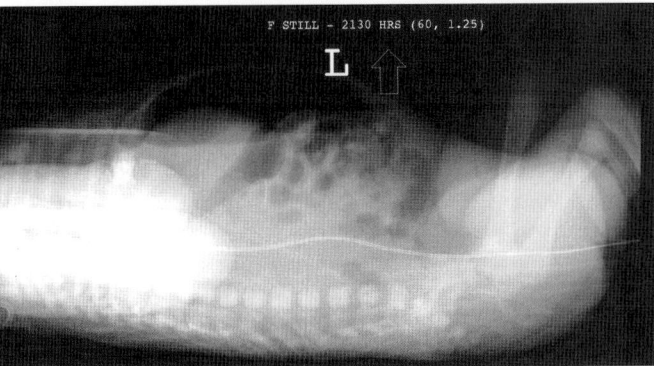

(b)

Fig. 27.31 Pneumoperitoneum due to gastrointestinal perforation. (a) Anteroposterior view shows classic 'football' sign. (b) The lateral X-ray of the same infant shows a large collection of free air above the liver.

be made by measuring the PO_2 of aspirated intraperitoneal gas.[907] In ventilator-induced pneumoperitoneum, the intraperitoneal PO_2 is very high, reflecting PAO_2, whereas the PO_2 of a surgical pneumoperitoneum is similar to that of room air or lower.

Treatment

If the abdomen is not under sufficient tension to cause respiratory embarassment, then no treatment is necessary. If there is tension, the peritoneum should be drained either by needle aspiration or by inserting a drainage tube.

Systemic air embolism

This is a rare complication of IPPV. Affected infants are usually premature, have severe pulmonary insufficiency necessitating very high ventilator pressures ($>40\,cmH_2O$) and the majority (94%) have other airleaks.[550] This condition has, however, been reported in infants supported by CPAP.[959] It is associated with a sudden and catastrophic deterioration in the baby's condition, with either pallor or cyanosis, hypotension and bizarre ECG irregularities.

Pathogenesis

Gas embolism results from alveolar–capillary or bronchovenous fistulae, which have been demonstrated by barium studies at autopsy.[93] Such communications are more likely to occur in airleak syndromes, but may also follow trauma to the lung. Laceration of lung tissue favours reversal of the intrabronchial pressure–pulmonary venous pressure gradient, thereby increasing the risk of pulmonary vascular air embolism.

Diagnosis

On the CXR, gas can be seen in the systemic and pulmonary arteries and veins (Fig. 27.33). Gas can be withdrawn from the umbilical venous or arterial catheters, and this has been observed in over half the reported cases.

Treatment

Early withdrawal of air from the UAC may be of benefit, particularly if the leak is small or has been introduced through an intravascular line.

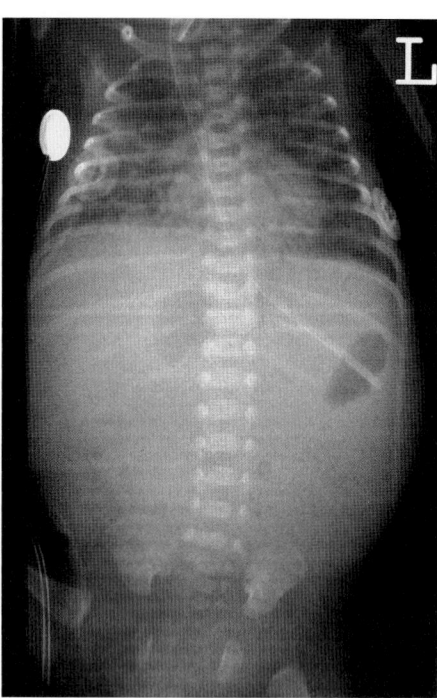

Fig. 27.32 Pneumoperitoneum indicated on the anteroposterior view by a small amount of non-anatomical air to the right of the vertebral column.

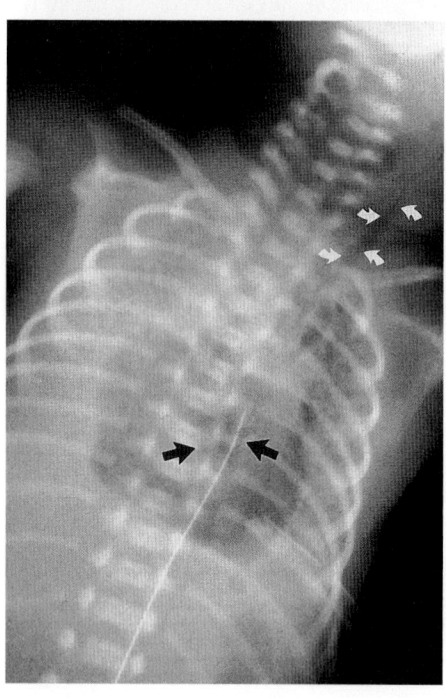

Fig. 27.33 Postmortem X-ray of a baby who died from systemic air embolism. Gas can be seen (black arrows) within the heart and in the great vessels in the neck (white arrows).

Prognosis

This condition is usually fatal.[550]

Subcutaneous emphysema

This condition, with air tracking into the neck or other subcutaneous tissues, is usually associated with a pneumomediastinum. It requires no treatment. A localised subcutaneous collection of air under tension – a bronchocutaneous fistula – has been described.[30]

Persistent pulmonary hypertension of the newborn

The dominant pathophysiological feature of PPHN is a high PAP. This condition has been called persistent fetal circulation (PFC), but this term should be avoided, as one of the characteristic features of the fetal circulation, the high-flow, low-resistance circuit through the placenta, is missing.

Definition and classification

The PFC syndrome was first used by Gersony et al[324] to describe babies who had a structurally normal heart, but large right-to-left shunts at atrial and ductal levels secondary to pulmonary hypertension. It is now understood that PPHN is the common endpoint of several different pathophysiological mechanisms. PPHN is present when an infant with an echocardiographically confirmed structurally normal heart has:

- severe hypoxaemia, usually a $PaO_2 < 5$–$6\,kPa$ (37.5–45 mmHg) in an F_IO_2 of 1.0 and IPPV if necessary;
- mild lung disease, but the hypoxaemia is disproportionately severe for the radiological, clinical and acid–base abnormalities;
- evidence of a right-to-left ductal shunt (usually a PaO_2 in the distal aortic [UAC] blood 1–2 kPa [7.5–15 mmHg] lower than simultaneous preductal [right radial artery] PaO_2 estimation); in the absence of a ductal shunt, a large shunt may be demonstrated echocardiographically at the foramen ovale.[899]

There are a number of distinct syndromes which can result in a baby developing PPHN:

- **Primary PPHN, or PPHN in the presence of mild neonatal lung disease.** Those with primary disease are the babies originally described by Gersony et al[324] who are profoundly hypoxic but have no clinical or autopsy evidence of lung disease. This entity merges into PPHN in babies who have disproportionately severe hypoxaemia from what appears clinically, radiologically and on $PaCO_2$ measurements to be mild parenchymal lung disease. There is now considerable evidence to suggest that this entity is due to excessive muscularisation of the pulmonary arterial system starting in the antenatal period (see below), perhaps aggravated by intrapartum asphyxia[733] and iatrogenic overventilation in the early stages of mild respiratory disease.[739]
- **PPHN secondary to severe intrapartum asphyxia.** In these babies, hypoxia and acidaemia, both of which are powerful pulmonary artery constrictors[586] and are present in severe asphyxia, prevent the normal postnatal changes in circulation. The tendency to PPHN may be increased in such neonates by similar structural changes in the vasculature to those outlined above, and the large right–left shunt may be aggravated by systemic hypotension secondary to post-asphyxial myocardial damage.[111]

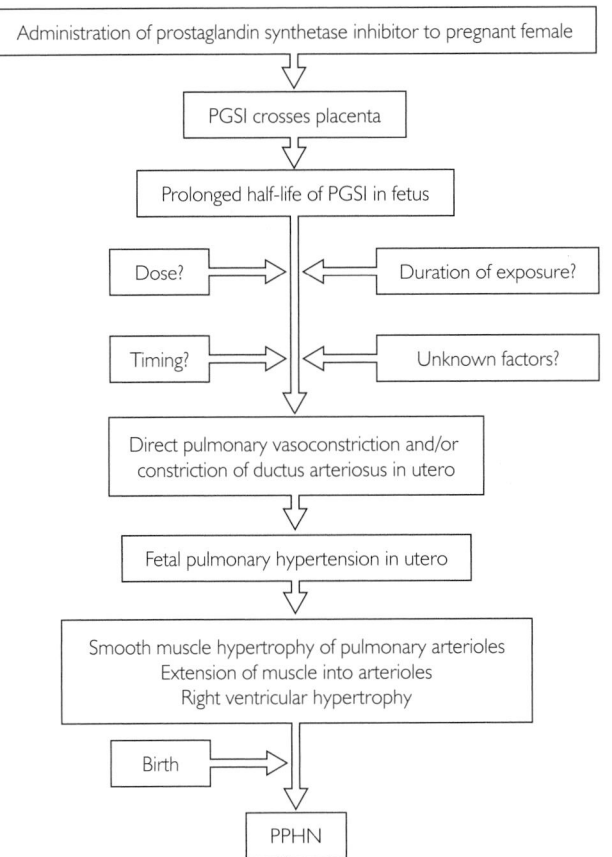

Fig. 27.34 Mechanism of drug-induced persistent pulmonary hypertension of the newborn. (Reproduced from Turner & Levin.[887])

- **PPHN secondary to infection.** This particularly severe form of the disease, characteristically associated with GBS sepsis, is probably due to the release of vasoactive substances.
- **PPHN secondary to pulmonary hypoplasia.** This is characteristic of neonates with diaphragmatic hernia, and is due to the abnormal development and reduced cross-sectional area of the pulmonary vasculature.[322]
- **PPHN secondary to drug therapy.** This has been reported after the use of prostaglandin synthetase inhibitors (PGSI) before delivery. One survey demonstrated that mothers of inborn term babies with PPHN were 9.6 times more likely to have taken aspirin in pregnancy and 17.5 times more likely to have taken other PGSI drugs.[903] These drugs, either by a direct effect on the pulmonary vasculature or by closing the fetal ductus, cause fetal pulmonary hypertension which persists postnatally.[561,887] It is probably the result of changes in the pulmonary arterial musculature similar to those reported in primary PPHN[560] (Fig. 27.34). Administration of ibuprofen, a cyclo-oxygenase inhibitor, in the first 6 hours after birth has been associated with the development of pulmonary hypertension.[342]
- **PPHN secondary to alveolar capillary dysplasia.** Several reports have appeared of babies with clinical PPHN in whom, at post mortem, there appeared to be misalignment of the pulmonary vessels and poor apposition of the vessels to the alveoli.[125] This condition is fatal and does not respond to extracorporeal membrane oxygenation (ECMO).[139]

- **PPHN secondary to congenital heart disease.** Conditions that obstruct the venous outflow from the lungs or cause myocardial failure can cause pulmonary hypertension and/or marked right–left shunting with hypoxaemia. They are considered in detail in Chapter 28.
- **Iatrogenic PPHN secondary to overventilation** (p. 531).

Pathophysiology

The pathognomonic feature of this condition is the presence of pulmonary hypertension, producing right–left shunts at the level of the ductus arteriosus and the foramen ovale.[244,820] The comparatively small difference between pre- and postductal PaO_2 levels, rarely greater than 2–3 kPa (15–21 mmHg), however, suggests that only a small component of the shunt occurs at duct level and the majority is through the foramen ovale.[899] The pulmonary artery pressure is at or above systemic levels. Skinner et al[820] have shown that a marked reduction in left ventricular function is the most significant marker of severe disease.

Abnormal pulmonary vasculature

Infants with PPHN have abnormal pulmonary vascular reactivity, structure and/or growth. In post-mortem studies on babies with PPHN, virtually all secondary to meconium inhalation, the muscularity of the pulmonary arteries is markedly increased.[648,649] Not only is the amount of muscle in the vessel wall increased, but also the muscle extends into vessels surrounding the alveoli, whereas in the normal baby muscular pulmonary arteries rarely extend past the terminal bronchiole. The exact intrauterine events that increase pulmonary vascular reactivity and impair structure are poorly understood. Impaired vascular epidermal growth factor (VEGF) signalling, however, can cause fetal pulmonary hypertension with structural remodelling, right ventricular hypertrophy and impaired pulmonary vasodilation in experimental models.[376] Chronic intrauterine pulmonary hypertension can markedly decrease lung VEGF expression; selective inhibition of VEGF mimics the structural and physiological changes of experimental PPHN.[376] Babies with PPHN have lower blood VEGF levels than controls.[542] Postnatally, sustained pulmonary hypertension rapidly accelerates pulmonary vascular injury, with aggressive smooth muscle proliferation and remodelling. Initially the effects of hypertension are at least partially offset by release of endogenous vasodilators, but this may not be sustained.[2]

Vasoactive agents

NO is a potent pulmonary vasodilator, active in the transition of the circulation at birth (p. 448). A significant rise in pulmonary blood flow at birth is related to the acute release of NO; vasodilation occurs through cGMP kinase-mediated stimulation of K^+ channels.[171] Other vasodilator products, including PGI_2, also modulate changes in pulmonary vascular tone at birth. NO modulates PGI_2 activity in the perinatal lung.[981] Adenosine release may also contribute to the fall in pulmonary vascular resistance; this may be through enhanced production of NO.[526]

Endothelin-1 (ET-1) is a potent pulmonary vasoconstrictor; the plasma level is raised in neonates with hypoxia[530] and severe PPHN.[535,760] Increased circulating levels of ET-1 mediate in part GBS-induced pulmonary hypertension.[653] Raised levels of the constrictor leukotrienes LTC4 and LTD4 have been found in the blood of some, but not all, neonates with PPHN when compared with ventilated neonates without this complication; the levels fall with successful therapy.[237,393,532,846] In the PPHN accompanying sepsis due to GBS or other organisms,[326,801,921] including viruses,[878] there is initial severe arterial spasm followed by increased vascular permeability and an increased lung fluid content and lymph flow.[705,756,777] In these babies it is thought that thromboxane A[2][326,393,769] is responsible and that it has its effect without affecting the morphometry of the pulmonary vasculature.[41] In animal models, PPHN, but not the haematological features of GBS sepsis, can be prevented by treatment with drugs which inhibit thromboxane A$_2$ synthesis, such as indometacin (indomethacin),[769] and can be reversed by intravenous infusion of the vasodilator prostaglandin PGE$_2$ and by isoprenaline.[96,179] The increased capillary permeability in sepsis-induced PPHN appears to be due to the action of bacterial endotoxins sequestering white cells in the lungs,[757,777] where they release vasoactive agents such as tumour necrosis factor. There is also an additional effect of thromboxane A$_2$ since, as with the short-term effects on the pulmonary vasculature, long-term effects can be mitigated by the use of indometacin (indomethacin).

Vascular hypoplasia

The PPHN of diaphragmatic hernia and other conditions associated with pulmonary hypoplasia is due to a reduction in the number of intralobar arteries and their increased muscularity.[321]

Blood gas changes/asphyxia

A fall in pH causes pulmonary vasoconstriction in experimental animals,[767,768] and hypoxia is a potent vasoconstrictor.[586] Neonatal pulmonary vasculature is extremely sensitive to changes in pH, PaO_2 and $PaCO_2$.[123] Therefore, perinatal and postnatal hypoxaemia and metabolic or respiratory acidaemia can cause marked pulmonary arterial spasm, pulmonary hypertension, a large right–left shunt and PPHN, particularly in babies with prenatal pulmonary arterial muscular hypertrophy.

Polycythaemia

A rise in haematocrit in experimental animals causes pulmonary hypertension. The factors involved, however, are not clear, since a rise in pulmonary vascular resistance is not seen if fetal blood as opposed to adult blood is used to raise the haematocrit[287] and polycythaemia is not a consistent feature of neonates with PPHN.[290]

Mode of delivery

PPHN can follow inappropriately preterm caesarean section.

Heredity

Familial cases have been reported.

Clinical features

In babies with primary PPHN, the presentation is often subtle and may mimic that of cyanotic congenital heart disease. Babies with primary PPHN virtually always present within 12 hours of birth, and very rarely after 24 hours. In PPHN which is secondary to pre-existing lung disease, the clinical features will be those of GBS sepsis (pp. 1029–32), RDS (pp. 468–85) or MAS (pp. 502–8), together with the cyanosis of severe PPHN. Secondary effects from the hypoxia, such as acidaemia and hypotension, may be present. The age at diagnosis still depends on the underlying problem and its severity. In GBS infection (p. 1029), severe asphyxia (p. 224) and congenital diaphragmatic hernia (CDH; pp. 594–603), PPHN will appear within 6 hours of birth in a critically ill neonate.

The baby remains cyanosed even when high oxygen concentrations are administered by IPPV. Respiratory distress, however, is often mild. The respiratory rate is usually increased to 60–100/min, the higher rates being seen in term babies. Retraction is mild, and grunting rare. The air entry is normal and there are rarely added sounds. The heart rate is normal or slightly increased. All pulses, including the femorals, are normal. The first heart sound is normal, but the second is commonly single and loud because of the rise in PAP. There is a right parasternal heave, and a soft systolic murmur may be heard, signifying tricuspid incompetence or, occasionally, mitral incompetence. Heart failure is not usually present, but the infant may be hypotensive. Examination of the abdomen, genitourinary system and the CNS are usually normal in the absence of predisposing factors such as sepsis or asphyxia.

Differential diagnosis (pp. 637–8)

Cyanotic congenital heart disease, which presents in the first 12 hours, is usually a severe form, with heart failure, distinctive murmurs and obvious changes on the CXR and ECG. In PPHN, however, the CXR and ECG are often within the normal limits, and the findings on examination of the cardiovascular system are comparatively subtle (see above).

Echocardiography will establish the normal cardiac anatomy in PPHN. The response to ventilation with 100% oxygen may differentiate PPHN from cyanotic congenital heart disease.[290] In the former, the PaO_2 will usually increase to >13 kPa (100 mmHg), whereas in cyanotic heart disease it will not rise above 5–6 kPa (37.5–45 mmHg). Not all neonates with PPHN, especially those with sepsis and CDH, however, respond in this way.

Investigations

Haematological and biochemical

There are no specific haematological abnormalities in babies with PPHN, but thrombocytopenia has been reported in severe cases.[790] The thrombocytopenia may be a manifestation of abnormal prostaglandin activation.

Blood gases

In both primary and secondary PPHN, maximal PaO_2 values of 6 kPa (45 mmHg) are characteristic, often with a difference of at least 1–2 kPa (7.5–15 mmHg) between preductal and postductal PaO_2 (p. 497). At diagnosis there may be a metabolic acidaemia, but respiratory acidaemia, by definition, is unusual. Metabolic acidaemia can be controlled by an initial infusion of base, followed by BP support and maintaining the haematocrit above 40%. A resistant acidosis is a feature of either the terminal stages of PPHN or some other underlying problem – in particular, overwhelming sepsis.

Chest X-ray

In secondary PPHN, the X-ray will be that of the underlying lung disease, although, by definition, the appearance will be less severe than anticipated for the severity of the hypoxaemia. In primary PPHN, the CXR changes are often minimal; there may be a mild non-specific increase in lung markings, but little else is noted.

Electrocardiogram

Various ECG changes have been reported in neonates with PPHN. The ECG may be normal, or more typically shows changes of right axis deviation, right atrial enlargement and right ventricular hypertrophy and overload.[413] In babies who develop PPHN following severe asphyxia, the ECG may show the changes of subendocardial ischaemia (p. 506).

Echocardiography

This is the single most useful investigation in establishing the diagnosis. Firstly, and most importantly, it will exclude the various forms of cyanotic congenital heart disease by showing a normal cardiac anatomy. Secondly, pulmonary hypertension, right-to-left shunting at the ductal and foramen ovale level and ventricular function can be assessed.[820]

Bacteriology

PPHN can be secondary to sepsis; thus it is important that the infant is screened for infection, including routine swabs and blood cultures (p. 1019).

Treatment

The treatment of PPHN can be divided into two components: that of the hypoxaemia and PPHN, and that of the coexisting lung disease, which is covered elsewhere.

Minimal handling

It is important to adhere to the 'minimal handling' maxim (p. 480). Slight disturbance, for example turning the baby or taking his temperature, may precipitate severe hypoxaemia, and major interventions such as ETT suctioning or physiotherapy can have devastating effects. Monitoring must therefore be continuous and interference with the baby reduced to an absolute minimum. ETT suctioning should be carried out only when essential to maintain ETT patency; chest physiotherapy is contraindicated.

Blood pressure and blood volume

The size of the right–left shunt is in part dependent on the systemic BP (see above); thus, in babies born at term, the systemic BP should be maintained at a mean of at least 40 mmHg, with a systolic of 50 mmHg. Aggressive therapy should be used to achieve an appropriate systemic BP, including volume challenges and, particularly, administration of inotropes. The haemoglobin level should be kept greater than 13 g/dl (PCV 40%) in order to maximise oxygen transport to the tissues. If polycythaemia (central PCV >70–75%) is present, the existence of PPHN is one of the situations in which a dilutional exchange transfusion is justified.

Coagulation disorders

If present, these should be corrected by appropriate factor replacement.

Fluid and electrolyte balance

Electrolyte abnormalities and hypoglycaemia must be corrected and pH and base deficit kept within normal limits by use of THAM or bicarbonate as appropriate. Urine output must be carefully monitored.

Antibiotics

Broad-spectrum antibiotic cover should be given to all these babies.

Nutrition

Enteral feeding should be avoided; as a consequence, infants who are still ventilator-dependent on day 3 or 4 should be started on intravenous nutrition.

Respiratory support

Once a baby's PaO_2 falls below 5–6 kPa (37–45 mmHg) in 70% oxygen, he should be ventilated. If IPPV is needed, initial settings should be at rates of 60–80/min, an I:E ratio of 1:1.2, a PEEP of 3 cmH$_2$O, and sufficient peak pressure to achieve a $PaCO_2$ of not greater than 4.8–5.5 kPa (35–40 mmHg) and a pH >7.30. The inspired oxygen concentration should be increased as necessary to achieve a PaO_2 of at least 8–9 kPa (56–63 mmHg). For the full-term baby prone to fight the ventilator, neuromuscular blocking agents should be used, and in this situation there are theoretical reasons for preferring D-tubocurarine to pancuronium.[448]

PPHN unresponsive to conservative treatment

Hyperventilation

This was described first by Peckham & Fox.[696] Reduction of the $PaCO_2$ to 2.5–3.5 kPa (19–26 mmHg) and elevation of the pH to 7.55–7.60 resulted in a rise in PaO_2. Hyperventilation is no longer advocated, because a $PaCO_2$ of 2.5–3.5 kPa (19–26 mmHg) results in a 50% reduction of cerebral blood flow, which could cause cerebral ischaemia. Although in babies born at term no long-term adverse sequaelae have been described,[102] hypocapnia in preterm babies has been linked to PVL,[370,454] and marked hypocapnia (<2.5 kPa, [19 mmHg]) may reduce cardiac output.[122] Hyperventilation, via barotrauma, may also result in airleaks[289] and CLD.[55,290] Persisting hypocapnic alkalaemia markedly increases hypoxic reactivity of the pulmonary vasculature, thus tending to perpetuate the pathophysiology of PPHN.[340]

High-frequency oscillation: jet ventilation

Anecdotally, these forms of respiratory support have been associated with improvements in oxygenation,[524,840,909] but, although many babies have been so treated, the data are uncontrolled.

ECMO

ECMO is an effective rescue therapy for infants with PPHN[891] (see pp. 528–9).

Vasodilator drugs

Tolazoline, prostacyclin and magnesium sulphate were widely used until the advent of NO. Other drugs have been reported to be beneficial. Diltiazem, a calcium channel antagonist, has reduced right ventricular pressure in neonates with PPHN.[457] In animal models of pulmonary hypertension, sildenafil (a phosphodiesterase-5 inhibitor) has been demonstrated to be more effective than iNO in the treatment of pulmonary hypertension.[803]

Tolazoline

Tolazoline is no longer the drug of choice for PPHN, although historically it was the most commonly used drug. Between 25% and 50% of babies with primary PPHN or PPHN secondary to RDS or MAS respond to this agent, but the effects on the systemic circulation are at least as great as those on the pulmonary vasculature, and side effects, including significant hypotension, are common. Other side effects have been reported and include renal failure and gastrointestinal haemorrhage.[928] Side effects may be minimised by a dilute, slow infusion,[669] but we strongly recommend that iNO be considered first if a baby is sick enough to require consideration for tolazoline therapy.

Prostacyclin

This agent in doses of 5–40 ng/kg/min is an effective pulmonary vasodilator, but has a wide list of side effects.[701] The same comments apply regarding consideration of iNO as for tolazoline.

Endotracheal administration of tolazoline[184] or prostacyclin[500] can cause selective vasodilation. Inhalation of prostacyclin in animals and babies has been shown to be at least as effective as the parenteral preparation, with fewer side effects, and to cause an equivalent response to iNO.[77,984] High doses of aerosolised PGI_2, however, could spill over into the systemic circulation, and thus the magnitude of the dose administered is critical if this therapy is to be a selective pulmonary vasodilator.

Magnesium sulphate

As a loading dose of 200 mg/kg followed by an infusion of 20–100 mg/kg/h, it is effective,[879,963] but less so and with more side effects than iNO.[771] During magnesium therapy, levels must be carefully monitored, as hypermagnesmia can cause sedation, muscle relaxation, hyporeflexia, and calcium and potassium disturbances.

Inhaled nitric oxide (p. 563)

NO is a vasodilator substance that relaxes vascular smooth muscle. It is synthesised in the endothelial cells from L-arginine and oxygen.[249] Neonates who suffer from PPHN may have low levels of arginine,[916] but this is not a universal finding.[493] NO diffuses into the smooth muscle cells, where it activates guanylate cyclase to increase 3,5 GMP and hence produces relaxation of the smooth muscles. When NO is inhaled, it diffuses across the alveolar capillary membrane and activates guanylate cyclase in the pulmonary arteriolar smooth muscle. The resulting increase in cGMP causes smooth muscle relaxation. NO then binds rapidly to haemoglobin; once bound, it is inactivated and therefore produces no systemic effects.

Clinical studies Since the preliminary studies of Kinsella et al[514] and Roberts et al,[751] there have been many reports of the benefit of NO in PPHN. The efficacy of iNO is improved if combined with a strategy to improve lung volume.[513,944] Even in patients with moderate PPHN, iNO can increase arterial oxygenation and reduce the amount of ventilatory support required.[774] Not all term babies, however, respond, a poor response being seen in those with severe parenchymal disease, systemic hypotension and myocardial dysfunction, as well as in those with structural pulmonary abnormalities, for example infants with pulmonary hypoplasia and dysplasia, who can develop a sustained dependence on iNO.[334] A poor response to iNO is predictive of a poor outcome.

In term-born babies, meta-analysis of the results of eight randomised trials demonstrated that use of iNO was associated with an improvement in oxygenation and a reduction in the combined outcome of death or need for ECMO; the effect was due to a reduction in the need for ECMO.[278] The combined intervention of iNO and HFOV has been demonstrated to be more successful than use of iNO or HFOV alone in rescuing infants at or near term with severe respiratory failure.[515] No significant long-term benefits of iNO have been demonstrated in babies with CDH. No excess of adverse neurodevelopmental outcomes have been demonstrated in babies exposed to iNO in randomised trials;[657] babies with CDH, however, have a higher incidence of sensorineural hearing loss.[656]

Randomised trials have failed to demonstrate that iNO has any significant long-term benefits for preterm babies, with no significant differences in mortality.[293,516,858] A shorter duration of ventilation, however, was noted in one trial.[516]

iNO delivery   Studies in term infants have demonstrated that levels of 5 ppm are equally as effective as higher doses,[195,961] but lower doses (2 ppm) are not;[170] indeed, initial treatment with a subtherapeutic dose of iNO may diminish the clinical response to higher doses and have adverse sequealae.[170] We therefore use 5 ppm of iNO in term infants and then wean as rapidly as possible (see below). In preterm infants, higher doses (up to 40 ppm) may be needed to improve oxygenation,[544] but have not been shown to improve long-term outcome.

NO has a very short duration of action; thus, rebound vasoconstriction and hypoxaemia can result if the NO is suddenly withdrawn. Therefore, to prevent sudden withdrawal of NO during routine nursing procedures, in-line suction devices are recommended to prevent interrupting the circuit and handbagging circuits should contain an additional iNO source. It is important to wean iNO as soon as oxygenation has improved and the baby stabilised, otherwise tolerance may occur. During weaning from iNO, the level should be gradually reduced; decreasing to 1 ppm minimises the deterioration in oxygenation.[196] Increasing the inspired oxygen concentration by 10–20% immediately prior to cessation of iNO may also be helpful. Scavenging is not necessary in a well-ventilated environment (8–12 air changes per hour), but, even so, environmental checks are recommended to reassure staff accidental macrocontamination has not occurred. It is important to exclude congenital heart disease in neonates being considered for iNO and thus facilities for echocardiography should be readily available.

Infants at or near term with hypoxic respiratory failure (an oxygenation index of at least 25) should be considered for iNO, but only after their lung volume has been optimised and their cardiovascular status stabilised. Neonates who are hypoxaemic secondary to congenital heart disease, right ventricular-dependent circulation, severe left ventricular dysfunction, duct-dependent circulation or methaemoglobinaemia should not be given iNO. There is currently insufficient evidence to recommend routine use of iNO in prematurely born babies or in term babies with CDH.

Side effects   NO should be administered only if continuous NO and nitrogen dioxide (NO_2) monitoring are available and there is immediate access to methaemoglobin analysis.[973] NO reacts rapidly with O_2 to form NO_2, which is toxic to the lung. The nitrosylhaemoglobin produced by NO binding to haemoglobin is rapidly converted to methaemoglobin, which is then reduced by methaemoglobin reductase in erythrocytes. Unfortunately, immature infants and those of certain ethnic groups have low levels of methaemoglobin reductase. Particularly in VLBW babies with RDS,[645] care needs to be taken that NO_2 is not being formed,[629] and that the baby is not developing methaemoglobinaemia.[513,924] These problems are more likely if high concentrations of NO[6] are used for prolonged periods in high inspired oxygen concentrations.[629] Inhaled NO administration has been associated with an increased bleeding time.[323] Although no excess of intracranial haemorrhage (ICH) in preterm infants has been described in randomised trials (p. 1129), it seems prudent to avoid iNO therapy in babies with a low platelet count or a bleeding diathesis, until these have been treated.

Inhaled ethyl nitrite gas
Inhaled O-nitrosoethanol gas (ENO) administered to seven babies with PPHN produced sustained improvements in oxygenation, without adverse effects.[644]

PPHN associated with sepsis

Infants who have PPHN secondary to sepsis are difficult to treat. The presence of sepsis and its complications, such as hypotension, hypoglycaemia and coagulation disturbances, makes most of the therapies for PPHN either impossible or very difficult to use. This is particularly a problem if there is oliguric renal failure, which limits the baby's ability to deal with the volume of the intravenous infusions of base, albumin, glucose, coagulation factors and inotropes that are necessary. Frequently, severely affected babies are hypocapnic and alkalaemic, yet despite aggressive ventilation this rarely achieves pulmonary vasodilatation and a rise in PaO_2. Vasodilator drugs, even in the presence of an adequate blood volume and systemic BP support with dopamine and/or dobutamine, virtually always cause profound hypotension in babies who are already tending to hypotension, and thus vasodilators are probably contraindicated in septic babies. The small amount of animal data using NO suggests that this is likely to be of only marginal benefit if used early in the illness, as the endogenous system becomes maximally stimulated trying to relieve the pulmonary hypertension caused by the infection.[325] For all these reasons, the clinician is left with little alternative than using the most vigorous therapy for neonatal sepsis (pp. 1017–28) in the hope that the situation will gradually improve. ECMO has been used successfully in some affected term babies.

Monitoring babies with PPHN

This has to be meticulous and continuous. Particular care must be taken to observe minimal-handling routines, as disturbing these babies can result in severe treatment-resistant hypoxaemia. Meticulous continuous PaO_2 monitoring is essential. An indwelling continuously recording PaO_2 cannula should be placed in the aorta, but the umbilical artery PaO_2 measurements should be supplemented by a measure of the preductal PaO_2, using either a right radial artery catheter or a transcutaneous monitor placed on the right upper chest. Pre- (right hand) and postductal (either foot) SpO_2 measurements give useful additional information.

Weaning the baby with PPHN off therapy

Once the neonate has acceptable blood gases (a term neonate has a PaO_2 of 16 kPa [120 mmHg] and a pH >7.55–7.60) and has been stable at these readings for 4 hours, weaning can begin. This should be done cautiously as, for some days afterwards, a fall in pulmonary artery pressure and a decrease in the right–left shunt can result in the pulmonary arteries once more going into spasm, perhaps due to the sensitising effects of alkalaemia.[340] The ventilator pressure should be reduced to <30 cmH$_2$O first, and then the rate of infusion of the vasodilator drugs reduced. In PPHN, the ventilator pressures should never be reduced by more than 1–2 cmH$_2$O increments, and the oxygen concentration by no more than 3–5%.

Complications

If a pneumothorax occurs, it must be drained; the hypoxaemia caused by a pneumothorax may so aggravate the pulmonary arterial vasocontriction that it pushes the baby into irreversible hypoxaemia, hypotension and bradycardia. PIE is particularly difficult to manage, as reduction in ventilator pressure will almost inevitably result in a rise in $PaCO_2$ and a reduction in pH and PaO_2, with worsening of the PPHN. The preterm baby with PPHN who is severely hypoxaemic, acidotic and/or hypotensive is at risk of brain injury, particularly if hypocapnia is used as treatment.

Natural history and prognosis

This varies with the aetiology, but is in general unpredictable. Many neonates respond promptly to treatment and the resulting mortality is low, in the 10–20% range, with most of the deaths being due to complications of prematurity or the neurological sequelae of severe birth asphyxia. For those requiring ECMO with primary PPHN or PPHN complicating RDS or MAS, survival figures of 80–90% are reported (p. 485). In babies with GBS sepsis, the mortality rate ranges from 10% to 50% (p. 1031). Most of the babies die either from irreversible hypoxia secondary to the PPHN or from myocardial failure as bacterial toxins cause arrhythmias or profound hypotension. The results in diaphragmatic hernia are given on page 599.

Sequelae

Once the pulmonary arteries relax and the lungs are perfused, the normal progression of postnatal cardiopulmonary adaptation should take place, and the baby can be expected to make a complete recovery. Whether or not sequelae occur in survivors depends on whether the intensity of respiratory support caused CLD, and whether any neurological damage resulted from severe hypoxia.

Meconium aspiration syndrome

MAS results from the inhalation of meconium before, during or immediately after delivery.

Incidence

In Europe the incidence is between 1:1000 and 1:5000, whereas in North America, rates of 2–5:1000 have been reported. Five per cent of babies born through meconium-stained liquor develop MAS.[154]

Aetiology

Meconium inhalation

To develop MAS, an infant must pass meconium, inhale it, and the inhaled material must damage the lungs. All these factors are inextricably interlinked with the presence of fetal asphyxia (see below, pp. 506–7).

Passage of meconium

An overall prevalence of 8–22% is quoted.[154,366,729] Meconium aspiration is a disease of term or post-term babies. Meconium staining of the liquor occurs in 5% or less of preterm pregnancies,[620] when it suggests chorioamnionitis,[620] but the prevalence increases to 10% or more after 38 weeks, reaching 22% in patients at a gestational age of 42 weeks, and 44% in babies who deliver 1 to 2 weeks later. Meconium staining is reported in association with in-utero infections.[759]

The fetal passage of meconium may be due to a vagal reflex, but more convincing are the data showing that motilin, which is produced mainly by the jejunum and stimulates peristalsis, is very low in preterm infants and non-asphyxiated term infants, but is raised in asphyxiated term babies who pass meconium intrapartum.[600]

Inhalation of meconium

During normal fetal breathing activity there is net movement of fluid out of the lung,[205] which will normally prevent meconium inhalation. Meconium inhalation, however, can occur before the onset of labour, as meconium has been found in the lungs of stillborn babies[101] and in babies who die in the early neonatal period, who could not have inhaled meconium intrapartum.[110,609,860] Prolonged severe fetal hypoxia can stimulate fetal breathing, to the extent that amniotic fluid is inhaled,[437] and fetal gasping movements also draw intra-amniotic material into the alveoli.[84,608] Perinatally, meconium inhalation can occur if the baby breathes or gasps with his mouth, pharynx or larynx full of meconium-stained liquor. This may occur late in the second stage of labour, particularly if there is a severe mixed acidaemia with a fetal pH <7.0,[729] when the raised $PaCO_2$ may have provoked intrapartum gasping. Postnatally, any meconium in the upper airway potentially can cause MAS. If meconium is inhaled, development of severe MAS depends in part on whether there is coexisting asphyxia,[415,487] although respiratory disease can develop when cord blood gases are normal.[729]

Effect of meconium on the lungs

Meconium is a sticky material composed of inspissated fetal intestinal secretions. When inhaled, it probably has at least four interacting deleterious effects on a neonatal lung (Fig. 27.35):

- It creates a ball valve mechanism in the airways whereby air can be sucked in past the plug but cannot be exhaled. This increases airways resistance, mainly in expiration, causing gas trapping, lung overdistension and pneumothorax.
- It acts as a chemical irritant. Inflammatory cells and mediators are released, which affect vessel contractility, lead to capillary

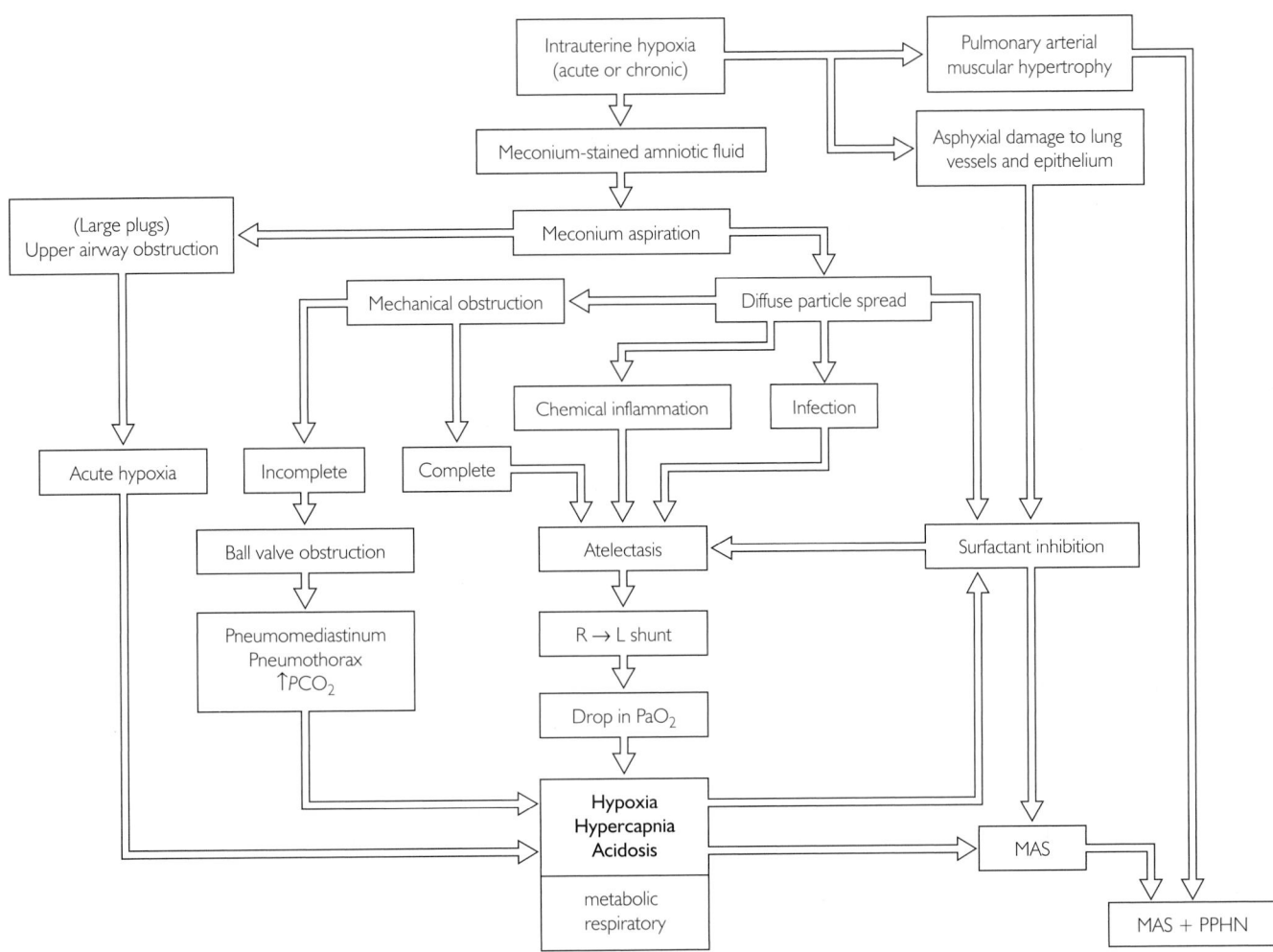

Fig. 27.35 Aetiology of meconium aspiration syndrome and its associated clinical syndromes.

leakage, and injure the lung parenchyma. The cytokines cause airway and alveolar epithelial necrosis.[980] Cell injury and apoptosis may also result from the high concentrations of phospholipase A2 found in meconium.[435] Thus, 24 to 48 hours after inhalation there is an exudative and inflammatory pneumonitis with alveolar collapse and cellular necrosis.

■ The organic nature of inhaled material, although initially sterile, may predispose the baby to pulmonary infection, particularly with *Escherichia coli*. Meconium may inhibit phagocytosis and the neutrophil oxidative burst,[148] hence bacteria can grow in meconium-stained amniotic fluid. Meconium staining of the liquor may be a marker of chorioamnionitis, predisposing the baby to congenital pneumonia,[620,935] and meconium inhibits polymorph function.[148]

■ Meconium inhibits surfactant function and production;[145,193,643] the inhibition is in a concentration-dependent manner.[859] The water/methanol-soluble phase (bilirubin and proteins) and, particularly, the chloroform-soluble phase (free fatty acids, triglycerides and cholesterol) of meconium inhibit surfactant.[859] In addition, phospholipase A2 degrades surfactant[785] and lysophosphatidylcholine can inhibit surfactant secretion.[375] Meconium alters the morphological ultrastructure of surfactant and hence decreases its surface tension-lowering ability.[29]

These four factors combine to cause the severe airway and alveolar disease which is more likely to occur if there is coexisting asphyxial lung damage.[475,487,729]

Effect on pulmonary vasculature

A rise in pulmonary artery pressure occurs in all babies with hypoxia and acidaemia (p. 475). Meconium in the lung increases pulmonary artery pressure, even if the blood gases are normal.[889] The inflammatory response (see above) results in release of vasoactive substances, which cause vasoconstriction; in addition, there may be maldevelopment of the pulmonary vessels secondary to chronic hypoxia (p. 453). MAS is the commonest respiratory disorder associated with PPHN.

Pathology

The pleura may be normal or petechial haemorrhages may be present on the lung surfaces due to acute hypoxaemia, particularly if death has occurred rapidly after birth. The lungs may be greenish yellow in colour. The cut surface can show congestion and haemorrhage, and meconium can be expressed from the cut ends of the smaller bronchi. The pathognomonic histological feature is the presence of amniotic squames, together with meconium in the terminal airways. Meconium itself appears as a granular eosinophilic material, often containing small yellow 'meconium bodies'. Aspirated material will stimulate a macrophage reaction, but, in the absence of an infective process, acute inflammation with neutrophils is not a feature. In addition to the meconium, hyaline membranes are frequently present. There may also be non-specific changes of an asphyxial insult to the lung, which include interstitial oedema and haemorrhage. The changes of PPHN (pp. 496–502) may be seen in the pulmonary vascular tree. Infants who die of MAS will have been ventilated at high pressures and rates and thus the histological changes merge into those of BPD. In babies with MAS who die early in the neonatal period, severe asphyxial damage may be seen in other organs, in particular the brain, kidney and myocardium.

Prevention

Antenatal

An inverse relationship has been found between amniotic fluid volume and fetal heart rate decelerations, a possible mechanism being either cord or head compression. Amnioinfusion, by maintenance of amniotic fluid volume during labour, aims to stop this problem occurring and hence reduce the likelihood of MAS.[185] It also dilutes any meconium. Amnioinfusion using 1000 ml of saline 6-hourly until delivery was associated with better Apgar scores, less meconium below the cords and a lower rate of caesarean section,[936] and, in a randomised trial[857] involving women with oligohydramios, amnioinfusion starting in the latent phase of labour reduced meconium passage and operative deliveries for fetal distress. The results of a meta-analysis[433] suggested that amnioinfusion, particularly in settings of limited perinatal survelliance, would improve perinatal outcome, with a significant reduction in MAS, HIE and neonatal ventilation or ICU admission. Retrospective studies, however, have not always demonstrated positive effects[897,936] and there are adverse outcomes of amnioinfusion, which include an increased incidence of cord prolapse, infection and requirement for instrumental delivery; in addition, the duration of labour may be prolonged.[857]

Suppression of fetal breathing movements by maternal narcotic administration, although successful in a baboon model,[82] did not reduce the incidence of MAS in two clinical series.[110,239]

Intrapartum/postpartum

Mode and timing of delivery

MAS is frequently reported to be higher in infants born by caesarean section rather than vaginal delivery; caesarean sections are usually performed on infants with fetal distress, a risk factor for MAS, and hence this may explain the association. The incidence of MAS, however, was significantly higher in infants of women with singleton pregnancies complicated by thick-consistency meconium-stained liquor who were randomised to undergo elective caesarean section (11/35) rather than spontaneous vaginal delivery (4/35).[627]

A prospective study[971] demonstrated that reduction in post-term delivery was the most important factor in reducing MAS.

Airway suctioning

Although it is clear that some meconium can be inhaled pre-labour, it is assumed that the majority of cases of MAS arise due to inhalation of meconium postnatally or during fetal gasping during the last few minutes of the second stage of labour. In uncontrolled studies, meticulous clearing of the airway at delivery was reported to reduce the incidence of MAS.[119,366,877] The results of several subsequent studies, however, suggested that routine suctioning through the cords or intubation with endotracheal toilet was not justified, as the manoeuvres not only failed to reduce the incidence of MAS but also were associated with increased morbidity.[266,267,570] Randomised trials have now been reported which have addressed whether intrapartum intubation and tracheal suctioning are necessary. No significant differences in the incidence of MAS or in other major outcomes were demonstrated between babies randomised to receive either naso- or oropharyngeal suctioning prior to delivery of the shoulders or no suctioning.[898] Similarly, no significant differences were demonstrated in the incidence of MAS or other respiratory complications between apparently vigorous infants who were randomised to intubation and tracheal suctioning or routine delivery room care.[953] In addition, meta-analysis of the results of four randomised trials which included vigorous term meconium-stained babies[384] did not demonstrate significant benefit with regard to mortality, MAS or HIE from routine endotracheal intubation at birth as compared with routine resuscitation including oropharyngeal suction. The event rates for the outcomes, however, were low, thus making reliable estimates of treatment effect impossible. Nevertheless, on the evidence to date, intubation and suctioning should be restricted to newborns who are depressed – that is, they have a heart rate of less than 100 beats per minute, poor respiratory effort and poor tone. It is important that an experienced paediatrician attends such deliveries. As soon as possible after delivery, affected babies should be handed to the paediatrician, who should gently insert a laryngoscope and carefully clear the upper airway of any meconium-stained material present. If no meconium is seen below the cords, it is not worth proceeding.[570] If, however, meconium is seen, direct tracheal suction is indicated. Studies in kittens have demonstrated that inhaled meconium stayed in the trachea and major bronchial divisions for several minutes after the onset of respiration and was, therefore, still in a site from which it could be aspirated.[702]

IPPV

The indications for resuscitation by IPPV (pp. 521–4) are not affected by the presence of meconium, other than it is always important to clear as much meconium from the airway as possible before applying positive pressure ventilation.

Compression of the neonatal thorax

This is not recommended, as it seems unlikely to prevent gasping, which has a large diaphragmatic component, and compression of the thorax can actually stimulate respiratory efforts.

Bronchial lavage

Instilling water or saline into the lower respiratory tract is controversial; an increase in wet lung has been noted following this procedure[119] and repeated bronchial lavage can do harm. Once on IPPV, tracheal suction with saline lavage, however, resulted in a 35% improvement in airway resistance.[58]

Postnatal gastric aspiration

Many clinicians routinely aspirate the stomach of a baby who has inhaled meconium at delivery, assuming the baby will have also swallowed meconium and gastric aspiration will prevent subsequent meconium inhalation following vomiting or reflux. Routine gastric lavage prior to feeding, however, did not decrease the incidence of MAS in babies born through meconium-stained liquor.[652]

Clinical signs

The baby is usually mature, or post mature, with long fingernails and a dry skin which soon starts to flake. The skin, nails and umbilical cord are often stained greenish yellow. The baby is not usually febrile, unless secondarily infected. Peripheral oedema is not a feature, and if present, suggests either renal damage with renal failure (pp. 935–40) or iatrogenic fluid overload.

Respiratory

The baby has tachypnoea, which may exceed 120/min. Intercostal and subcostal recession occur and there is use of accessory muscles and flaring of the nostrils. An expiratory grunt may be heard. The meconium in the airways causes widespread sticky crepitations and occasional rhonchi, air trapping and an overdistended chest with an increased anteroposterior diameter. The baby may remain symptomatic for only 24 hours or be very dyspnoeic for 7–10 days before recovery. In patients who required ventilation, the respiratory disease has usually abated to a resting tachypnoea of 50–70/min in room air by 14 days of age.

Cardiovascular

In the absence of asphyxial damage to the myocardium, there are no specific cardiovascular features of MAS. Hypotension suggests myocardial damage, as do signs of congestive heart failure. In uncomplicated MAS, the heart rate tends to be around 110–125/min, and the BP is maintained within the normal range. If PPHN (pp. 496–502) develops, S2 may remain single, and there may be the murmur of tricuspid incompetence (p. 498).

Abdominal examination

The liver and spleen are often palpable because of downward displacement of the diaphragm caused by air trapping. In a severely affected infant, bowel sounds may be absent, with delayed passage of meconium. The kidneys are not usually palpable, but there may be urinary retention and bladder distension in babies with severe neurological problems or those who receive pancuronium.

Central nervous system

Depending on the severity of the coexisting neurological insult, the baby may behave normally or show any of the neurological features of birth depression, ranging from the over-alert stage I hypoxic-ischaemic encephalopathy (HIE) to the flaccid, unresponsive, ventilated baby in stage III (p. 469). Convulsions may occur.

Differential diagnosis

Apparently faeculent liquor may be due to yellow–green bilious vomiting secondary to upper gastrointestinal tract obstruction.[965] It is important to exclude concurrent illness, especially infection and PPHN.

Pathophysiology

The respiratory failure and hypoxaemia in babies with MAS are due to stiff lungs, marked ventilation–perfusion imbalance and pulmonary hypertension precipitating extrapulmonary right–left shunts. Babies with MAS have a reduced compliance and tidal volume, and an increased airways resistance, but the tachypnoea increases the minute volume to twice normal.[38] In the early stages of the disease, when the airways are plugged by meconium, there is a marked ventilation–perfusion abnormality, which lessens as the lungs recover. In those who develop PPHN, the pulmonary artery pressure will be higher than the systemic, with right–left shunting through the ductus arteriosus and/or the foramen ovale.

Investigations

Haematological

The haemoglobin is normal, but the nucleated red blood cell[238] and the white cell[610,625] counts are often raised. White cell function is reduced.[148] Thrombocytopenia occurs in neonates with meconium aspiration who have PPHN,[790] are ventilated,[37] or develop DIC secondary to severe asphyxia (pp. 759–60).

Biochemical

There are no characteristic biochemical features of MAS. If coexisting asphyxia is severe, there may be inappropriate ADH production and hyponatraemia (pp. 340–1). Renal failure secondary to acute tubular necrosis may cause hyperkalaemia and a raised urea. Hypocalcaemia may also occur, as in any critically ill neonate (pp. 882–3).

Blood gases

Hypoxia is common, but in mature infants with mild–moderate disease and an efficient respiratory pump (p. 1309), ventilation is not a problem, and the $PaCO_2$ may even be low, normal or only slightly raised. A $PaCO_2$ >8 kPa (60 mmHg) is unusual and is seen only in patients with severe lung disease who eventually need ventilation.

Changes in pH initially reflect the metabolic acidaemia of intrapartum asphyxia; mature babies commonly correct their acidaemia spontaneously from pH levels in the 7.10 to 7.15 range and base deficit values of 10 to 15 mmol/l.[839] After the first hour or two, persisting metabolic acidaemia indicates an underlying problem such as sepsis, hypotension and/or renal failure, which should be sought and remedied.

Urine analysis

Unless renal failure supervenes, the urinary output is normal (p. 373). Many babies with MAS, although not in overt renal failure, have a raised urinary β2-microglobulin, indicating they have incurred some renal damage.[161] The urine may be greenish-brown in colour as a result of the absorption of meconium pigments across the pulmonary epithelium and their excretion in the urine.[212]

ECG, echocardiography

In uncomplicated MAS, the ECG and echocardiogram will be normal. If there has been severe intrapartum asphyxia, there may be ECG changes suggesting subendocardial ischaemia, and the echocardiogram will show reduced cardiac contractility. In those with PPHN, echocardiography demonstrates right-to-left shunting at ductal and atrial levels and a jet of tricuspid insufficiency, indicating raised right ventricular pressures.

Chest X-ray

The common early changes are widespread patchy infiltration and, in 20–30% of the patients, small pleural effusions. Overexpansion is also common in the early stage. In mild–moderate cases, the changes resolve within 48 hours. In severe cases, as the disease progresses, by 72 hours of age with or without ventilation the appearance is often changed to that of diffuse and homogeneous opacification of both lung fields, as a result of a pneumonitis and interstitial oedema secondary to the irritant effect of the inhaled meconium (Fig. 27.36). These changes gradually resolve over the next week, but in severe cases the X-ray may still be abnormal at 14 days, and may merge into the pattern seen in BPD, although this is uncommon. Airleaks, in particular pneumothorax and pneumomediastinum, are very common in MAS (p. 508).

Microbiology

All babies suffering from MAS should have an infection screen as soon as possible after admission to the NICU. This is the only way to establish the coexistence of sepsis and, since antibiotics will be used in virtually all cases (p. 507), provides the essential baseline information upon which further antibiotic therapy can be planned.

Monitoring

There is a temptation to under-monitor full-term babies with MAS because, despite marked tachypnoea and a very abnormal CXR appearance, they often look surprisingly pink and vigorous.

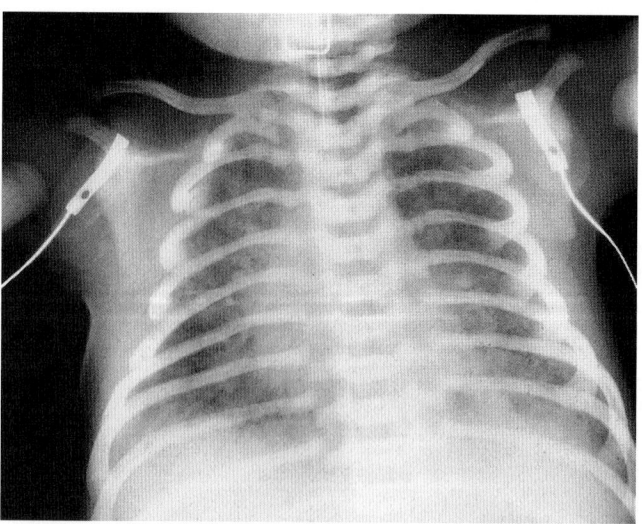

Fig. 27.36 Severe confluent pneumonitis in meconium aspiration syndrome.

This temptation should be resisted, not only because of the importance of early detection of blood gas abnormalities, electrolyte disturbance or hypotension before secondary effects develop, but also because the baby with MAS has a major risk of sudden deterioration due to a tension pneumothorax.

Treatment

There is no specific treatment for MAS. The aim is to support the baby until alveolar macrophages clear the debris and lung function returns to normal.

Respiratory failure

The relative efficiency of the respiratory pump in mature babies will enable them to control their $PaCO_2$, unless the disease is severe or their respiration depressed by the neurological effects of asphyxia. Since these mature babies are not susceptible to ROP, the prime concern is preventing hypoxaemia.

Oxygen therapy

Many babies with MAS can be managed by giving an appropriate concentration, up to 80–90%, of warmed humidified oxygen into a headbox. The oxygen saturation should be maintained at 95%, or the PaO_2 greater than 10 kPa, during the acute stage of the illness. In many mild cases, oxygen therapy at 40% or less for 24–48 hours is all that is required and their PaO_2 in room air is normal by 48 hours of age.

Acid–base homeostasis

Carbon dioxide retention is only a problem in severe cases. A $PaCO_2$ of 7.5–8 kPa (55–60 mmHg) is acceptable, providing the pH is sustained above 7.25. Intubation and ventilation are indicated if the $PaCO_2$ rises above 8 kPa (60 mmHg), particularly in the presence of a PaO_2 <6 kPa (45 mmHg) early in the disease.

The first blood gas analysis taken after birth may show a marked metabolic acidaemia. Provided that the baby is otherwise stable, with a normal PaO_2 and $PaCO_2$ and is passing urine, base deficits of 10 to 15 can be left to correct spontaneously (p. 481). The acidaemia should be corrected, however, if the base deficit is greater than 15 or the pH below 7.10.

In babies who show features of HIE, more rigid control of the blood gases is required (pp. 1135–6); hypoxia, hypercapnia and acidaemia are all undesirable. This indication for intubation and ventilation takes priority over the more conservative management of the blood gases outlined for babies with uncomplicated lung disease.

CPAP

CPAP at pressures of 4–7 cmH$_2$O can improve oxygenation, but it is likely to increase the risk of pneumothorax. In addition, use of nasal prongs in term neonates usually makes them irritable and restless, with a fall in PaO_2.

IPPV

Babies with MAS can be very difficult to ventilate; a long expiratory time and a low level of PEEP are theoretically best in MAS; elevation of PEEP can improve oxygenation, but increases the risk of pneumothorax. Administration of a neuromuscular blocking agent is virtually always required. When the blood gases start to improve, weaning can usually be rapid. Once the infant is in ≤50–60% oxygen and peak pressures of 20 cmH$_2$O, neuromuscular blockade can be stopped. We then prefer to transfer infants to PTV and wean by reduction in peak pressures, extubating infants into headbox oxygen without a period on CPAP.

High-frequency ventilation

HFJV used with surfactant, but not alone, has been reported to improve oxygenation in MAS.[199] A retrospective review, however, reported no significant difference in the outcome of infants with MAS supported by HFJV.[51] HFOV, particularly when used with NO, improved oxygenation and outcome in infants with PPHN and MAS.[515]

ECMO

In a randomised trial, ECMO improved survival of MAS infants with an oxygenation index >40 by 50%.[891] Approximately 94% of babies with MAS who are managed with ECMO survive; this does not appear to be at an increased risk of disability or adverse neurological outcome.[892]

Liquid ventilation

The results of liquid ventilation in animal models[317,678] suggest this could be an advantageous method of respiratory support in babies with MAS.

Pulmonary vasodilators

Drugs used to treat pulmonary hypertension can be effective in babies with MAS.[279,333,514,850,879] Inhaled NO improves oxygenation and decreases the need for ECMO,[151,655] but in those trials no other significant differences in major outcomes were noted. Inhaled NO has been reported to improve oxygenation in ventilated infants, who were not exposed to hyperventilation or induced alkalosis.[379] Results from animal models suggest that the phophodiesterase-5 inhibitor sildenafil may be at least as effective as iNO.[803]

Surfactant

Exogenous surfactant therapy has been used with anecdotal success.[25,507] In a randomised prospective study, babies who received surfactant within 6 hours of birth, had fewer airleaks, were on IPPV and oxygen for a shorter period and were much less likely to require ECMO.[277] The maximum effect on oxygenation was after three doses or more, suggesting that larger doses are required in MAS. Once on ECMO, the use of surfactant speeds recovery and the rate of weaning from ECMO.[581] In a randomised trial, up to four doses of surfactant reduced the need for ECMO in term infants with respiratory failure, half of whom had MAS;[582] however, there were no other significant differences in outcome. Meta-analysis of the results of the two randomised trials[277,582] demonstrated that surfactant administration reduced the risk of requiring ECMO (RR 0.64; 95% CI 0.46, 0.91), but not mortality.[832]

Lavage with surfactant may be a particularly effective method of improving gas exchange by washing out meconium and the products of inflammation,[676] as well as diluting the meconium. Multiple small-volume dilute surfactant lavages have been reported to improve oxygenation.[538] In a randomised trial, lavage with the protein-containing synthetic surfactant Surfaxin (KL-4 surfactant) improved lung function.[955] Results from in-vitro studies have suggested that that surfactant, compared with commercially available surfactants (Survanta, Alveofact and Curosurf), better resists meconium inhibition.[417]

Antibiotics

The presence of organic and potentially infected material in the liquor and in the lung may predispose to pneumonia; there are some data from animals to support this view.[103,285,935] After taking cultures, but not necessarily doing a lumbar puncture, neonates diagnosed as suffering from MAS should be put on broad-spectrum antibiotics, penicillin and gentamicin. The antibiotics should be discontinued when the culture results are known to be negative or after 7 days, when the baby is in the convalescent stage of the illness and requiring less than 30–40% oxygen.

Blood volume and blood pressure

Anaemia is not usually a problem in babies with MAS immediately after delivery; however, during subsequent management, if the haemoglobin falls below 13 g/dl or the PCV below 40%, the baby should be transfused. BP control is essential in all neonates with MAS, aiming to keep the pressure within the normal range (pp. 1293–4). Hypotension is usually only a problem in babies who have suffered severe intrapartum asphyxia with coexisting myocardial injury or after vasodilators (p. 356). If hypotension occurs, it is managed in the usual way with volume expansion and/or inotropes, depending on the neonate's myocardial and renal function (p. 481).

Physiotherapy

In neonates with mild to moderate disease who are not ventilated and require less than 60% inspired oxygen concentration, chest physiotherapy is rarely necessary. In the severely affected baby who is intubated and paralysed, chest percussion and ETT suction may be helpful, but should be continued only as long as this produces significant amounts of greenish material, and abandoned if the neonate becomes irritable, restless and hypoxaemic.

Steroids

In an animal model, although steroids reduced respiratory symptoms due to MAS, the mortality rate was higher.[299] In a randomised trial involving 35 infants,[970] steroid treatment in the first 6 hours after birth resulted in no significant differences in the duration of ventilation or survival and the steroid-treated group experienced an increased time to wean. In a subsequent small trial,[962] major outcomes (mortality and CLD) were not influenced by steroid therapy. More recently, steroid administration resulted in more rapid improvement in ventilated infants with MAS and PPHN.[188] Further studies are required to determine if steroid administration influences long-term outcomes.

Fluid and electrolyte balance

In uncomplicated MAS, this is rarely a problem, and standard fluid therapy, starting with 40 ml/kg/24 h on the first day and increasing thereafter, can be used. When MAS has been accompanied by severe birth asphyxia, fluid restriction to 40 ml/kg/24 h at least is indicated until urine output improves. The initial fluid given should be 10% dextrose, with electrolytes added only after 24–48 hours. If asphyxia has occurred, blood glucose levels should be carefully monitored and hypoglycaemia treated promptly.

Complications

Babies with MAS may suffer from HIE (pp. 1128–48) and renal failure (pp. 935–40). These are dealt with elsewhere.

Pneumothorax, airleaks

Pneumomediastinum, pneumopericardium and pneumoperitoneum can all occur; approximately 50% of ventilated MAS babies suffer some form of airleak, but PIE is unusual. Pneumothoraces may be both bilateral and under tension, and commonly cause acute deterioration in the baby's condition.

Persistent pulmonary hypertension

This is a common complication of severe MAS, and, on histological and clinical grounds, it appears to be particularly frequent in fatal cases.[956]

Bronchopulmonary dysplasia

This is a rare complication of MAS,[619] although it may occur in any baby who survives after long-term high-pressure IPPV.

Mortality

Mortality rates are between 4% and 12%.[154] The majority of deaths are from respiratory failure, PPHN or airleaks,[956] but some die from the associated neurological or renal sequelae of severe asphyxia.

Morbidity

Neurological

The neurological sequelae in these babies are those of the coexisting HIE (p. 1144).

Pulmonary

MAS predisposes to long-term respiratory morbidity.[592,862,978] At school age, although the majority of neonates who survived MAS were completely asymptomatic, 30–40% had problems with asthma and less than half had completely normal lung function tests.[592,862] Other data[529] also suggest that meconium aspiration predisposes to increased bronchial hyperreactivity. Yuksel et al[978] demonstrated that lung function abnormalities at follow-up relate to the severity of MAS. In addition, at 6 to 9 years of age, evidence of residual airways disease was seen in patients who had moderate to severe MAS,[169] whereas 12 children who had had mild MAS had normal lung function.[848]

Aspiration of amniotic fluid

Post-mortem studies of stillbirths have revealed that amniotic squames can be inhaled by the fetus in utero, presumably as a result of 'terminal' gasping activity preceding intrauterine death.[941] The importance of less severe manifestations of this entity, in the absence of meconium staining of the amniotic fluid, is speculative, but it is clear that there is a postnatal lung disease attributed to the inhalation of non-meconium-stained amniotic squames.[781]

Aspiration of fluid at delivery

Aspiration of blood can result in early-onset respiratory distress and a radiographic appearance of aspiration syndrome.[339] It occurs during birth by caesarean section or a vaginal birth complicated by *abruptio placenta*.

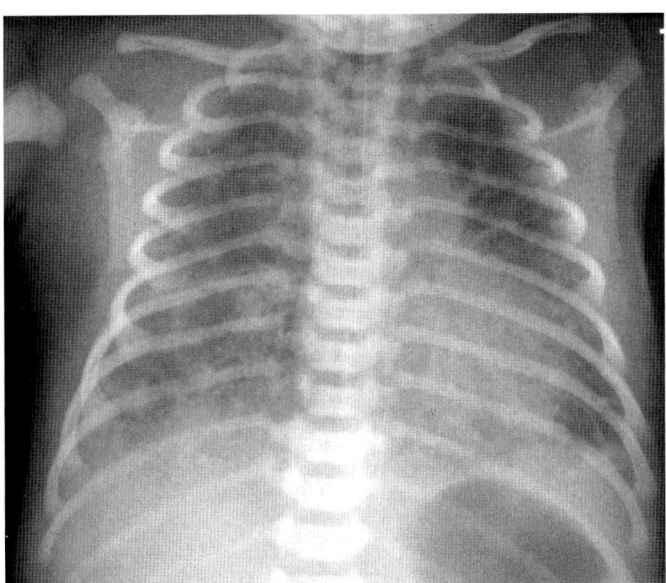

Fig. 27.37 Bilateral changes due to aspiration of pool fluid at an underwater birth.

Aspiration of 'pool' fluid during a water birth may also cause respiratory distress (Fig. 27.37).

Other aspiration syndromes (Table 27.7)

In the neonatal period, aspiration can occur due to malfunction of coordination of sucking, swallowing and breathing.

Swallowing incoordination

Pathophysiology

The anatomical structure of the pharynx and larynx protects the airway from inhalation[584] and there are defensive reflexes. The presence of any material in the pharynx initiates swallowing and reflex breath-holding.[949] If the airway remains threatened, additional reflexes, including more prolonged apnoea, choking, laryngospasm and coughing, are provoked.[197,707] These mechanisms provide a less effective shield over the airway in the neonatal period than they do in older children and adults. During sucking, the term neonate may have a reduction in ventilation,[15] PaO_2 and heart rate,[616] progressing to apnoea in some.[378,459,617,845] This may be because of poor breathing/swallowing coordination or additional problems such as velopalatine insufficiency with reflux into the nasopharynx.[714]

The preterm neonate has greater problems, including immature sucking/swallowing coordination,[808] which may be overwhelmed by oral feeding, and a high incidence of GOR.[658] If there has been brain damage, the neurological control of swallowing may be compromised. The preterm infant can protect his

Table 27.7 Types of aspiration syndrome in the newborn

1. Sucking/swallowing incoordination
   a. Prematurity
   b. Secondary to structural malformation or neurological disorders
     cleft palate, Pierre-Robin syndrome
     tracheo-oesophageal fistula, laryngeal cleft
     hypoxic-ischaemic encephalopathy
   c. Syndromes with poor sucking, e.g. Prader-Willi

2. Syndromes attributed to gastro-oesophageal reflux
   a. In babies on IPPV – right upper lobe collapse
   b. Wilson-Mikity syndrome
   c. Apnoeic attacks

3. Massive regurgitation and inhalation of a feed

airway as well as an infant born at term can, but these frequent challenges mean that its integrity may eventually be breached[459] and inhalation of stomach contents results. Even if the defence mechanisms are effective in preventing intrapulmonary inhalation, significant symptoms, especially apnoea,[613,658] may still result.

Coordinating sucking, swallowing and breathing becomes more difficult at all gestations if the neonate is sedated, for example by the transplacental passage of opiates, or if he is tachypnoeic with RDS or TTN.[876]

Other common causes of breathing/swallowing incoordination in both preterm and term babies are structural malformations in the upper airway or gastrointestinal tract, or neurological problems interfering with normal swallowing. Biochemical problems such as hypoglycaemia or hyponatraemia may occasionally have the same effect. Most causes of dysphagia and sucking/swallowing incoordination are extremely rare and usually present with the primary disorder rather than with dysphagia.

Clinical features

The commonest manifestation of swallowing/breathing incoordination in the term baby is choking, spluttering and becoming transiently apnoeic and blue during a feed. The baby thereafter usually remains asymptomatic. Many of these babies are at the extreme end of the normal spectrum of the response to feeding.[616] More serious examples are seen in babies who have brain damage or have problems such as cleft palate. In these, even saliva may continually collect in the pharynx and the baby will be 'mucousy'. In severe cases, babies have saliva dribbling from their mouths, and may cough and splutter when trying to clear their airways: cyanosis and bradycardia can occur.[378,459] Persisting retention of secretions in the pharynx and larynx, in addition to causing noisy breathing and upper respiratory tract symptoms, may result in tachypnoea and retraction, and, on auscultation, widespread conducted sounds are heard. Affected babies can have reflex apnoea caused by the presence of foreign materials in the larynx.[44]

Table 27.8 Dysphagia in the newborn. (Modified from Illingworth[455])

Gross anatomical defects

Palate	Cleft palate, submucous cleft
Tongue	Macroglossia, cysts, tumours, lymphangioma, ankyloglossia superior
Nose	Choanal atresia
Mandible	Micrognathia, Pierre-Robin syndrome
Temporomandibular joint	Ankylosis (congenital or infective), hypoplasia
Pharynx	Cyst, diverticulum, tumour
Larynx	Cleft, cyst
Oesophagus	Atresia, stenosis, short oesophagus, web, diverticulum, duplication, lung buds, tracheo-oesophageal fistula
Thorax	Vascular rings

Neuromuscular incoordination

Delayed maturation	Prematurity, normal variant
Cerebral palsy	All types
Brain damage	Post-asphyxial, postinfection (prenatal or postnatal)
Abnormalities of the cranial nerve nuclei and their tracts	Bulbar and suprabulbar palsy Moebius syndrome Pharyngeal, cricopharyngeal incoordination (idiopathic, secondary to brain damage)

Congenital laryngeal stridor

Myopathies	Myotonic dystrophy, myasthenia gravis
Hypotonia from any cause	Brain damage, Werdnig–Hoffman syndrome
Infections	Tetanus, polio, stomatitis, oesophagitis

Investigation and differential diagnosis

On the basis of the history and clinical examination, it should be possible to distinguish babies who have had a single or at most two to three episodes due to immature mechanisms being overwhelmed, from those with GOR or a chronic neurological or structural problem (Table 27.8). The clinical presentation of oesophageal atresia, with maternal polyhydramnios, followed by the baby having major problems with his secretions in the first 2–3 hours, is sufficiently classical that it should not be missed. Other babies may have covert GOR, or may be refluxing into the nasopharynx during a feed, with subsequent reflex apnoea.[714] Appropriate oesophageal pH[506,658] or contrast studies will demonstrate the abnormality.

Treatment

If no clinical abnormality is found (which is usually the case) in a term baby who has been admitted to the neonatal unit following such an episode on the postnatal ward, breast- or bottle-feeding can be continued under careful supervision, proceeding to further investigation only if choking persists. In convalescent LBW neonates, or those with recognised neurological or structural problems, all that is usually necessary in the absence of signs of aspiration pneumonia is to omit one or two feeds, before carefully restarting them, by nasogastric tube if necessary.

Babies with a tracheo-oesophageal fistula or laryngeal cleft should have surgical repair as soon as possible (pp. 715–7). Problems associated with palatal defects may be considerably improved by the use of a palatal prosthesis (p. 714). In babies with Pierre-Robin syndrome, laryngomalacia or other surgical problems in which there is not only tongue/palate incoordination but also a structural predisposition to inhalation, and, in addition, no prospect of immediate surgical correction, the airways should be meticulously suctioned and the baby nursed prone. It may, however, occasionally be necessary to resort to tracheostomy in order to protect the lungs.

A small group of babies, typically those with severe neurological damage secondary to HIE or with a primary problem such as dystrophia myotonica, may have prolonged difficulties. Frequent suctioning of the mouth and pharynx will be required and it may help to keep the babies lying prone or semi-prone, allowing their mouth to empty by gravity. Persistence of problems is an ominous prognostic feature; despite suctioning and positioning and meticulous nursing care, inhalation of secretions will eventually result, progressing to aspiration pneumonia, which is a common terminal event in such cases.

Gastro-oesophageal reflux (p. 704)

This has been recognised with increasing frequency in the neonate (pp. 510–11) and may occur in association with a hiatus hernia. Newell et al[658] found an overall incidence of 85% in babies <1.50 kg, but, unlike Goodwin et al,[338] found the incidence to be much lower during IPPV.[659] GOR is still present in many ex-prematures at the time of discharge,[613] but less so than in term babies of the same postconceptional age (PCA);[469] the clinical relevance of these data are speculative. GOR should be suspected in neonates with apparently inexplicable and recurrent respiratory problems, especially if there is recurrent apnoea unresponsive to theophylline,[658] a history suggesting reflux or recurrent vomiting, or right upper lobe collapse or consolidation on X-ray. To confirm the diagnosis, the demonstration of fat-laden macrophages in the tracheobronchial secretions is of value[661,670] combined with radiological or pH probe demonstration of reflux.[443,658,680]

Treatment

If episodes of apnoea or recurrent pulmonary disease in a neonate are attributed to reflux, small frequent feeds or continuous milk infusion are advocated; nasojejunal feeds or thickened feeds may also be beneficial.[658] Lying a baby prone, as well as improving the blood gases (p. 1309), can reduce the amount of reflux.[681] Antacids should be given if there is evidence of oesophagitis. Cisapride is no longer prescribed, because of the reports of toxicity and apparent lack of efficacy. Consequently, if the above measures fail, some clinicians prescribe another prokinetic agent, domperidone. Whether neonates benefit from any form of medical therapy for reflux has been questioned[443] and, therefore, fundoplication is recommended if problems from GOR persist. In our experience, this is rarely necessary, except in babies with chronic severe reflux and CLD.

Aspiration pneumonia

This may occur following one of the episodes of sucking/swallowing incoordination or reflux described above and is most likely to occur in babies with neurological defects or structural malformations. It may be covert due to reflux, or can follow an episode of massive regurgitation and vomiting, which is virtually limited to ill and convalescent babies of all gestations on the NICU. The baby, often still tube-fed, is found covered in vomit, and is usually cyanosed, apnoeic or gasping, and bradycardic.

Prevention

Most cases of aspiration pneumonia can and should be prevented by prompt clinical recognition and appropriate management of the disorders in which they are likely to occur (Table 27.7) and by careful attention to the feeding technique. This includes:

- not feeding babies (other than trophic feeds, pp. 330–1, 697) with respiratory distress, until their condition has stabilised, they have bowel sounds and have passed meconium;
- careful use of tube feeding in preterm babies (pp. 387–8), those recovering from respiratory distress, and those with HIE or structural malformations; progress to bottle/breast-feeding should occur when the baby has no biochemical or haematological problems, is tolerating nasogastric tube feeding well, has no problems with secretions and is showing spontaneous sucking activity on the tube or on a dummy;
- aspirating the indwelling nasogastric tube every 4–6 hours to ensure that milk, even with minimal enteral feeds, has not pooled in the stomach, posing the threat of regurgitation;
- avoiding all enteral feeds (tube or oral) for at least 12 hours after extubation (pp. 607–8).

Pathophysiology

The foreign material aspirated into the airway can have three effects: physical obstruction, chemical irritation and promotion of infection. The major problem is the irritant potential of the inhaled fluid. All fluids, including water, are damaging, but gastric contents are particularly damaging because of their acidic pH.[464] In the first few days after birth, the pH of a neonate's stomach contents can be 2.5 or less if the infant is unfed[26] or fed only clear fluids with no buffering capacity. Inhaled curd is particulate, and can obstruct airways, leading to lung collapse and/or consolidation, and may predispose to infection.

Clinical findings

In babies with sucking–swallowing incoordination, the features of their primary diagnosis will be present (Table 27.8). In addition, if such infants have chronic pooling of secretions in their upper airway, they will be mucousy with rattling, noisy respiration, often coupled with respiratory distress due to obstruction of the airway by secretions. Widespread conducted sounds, therefore, are often heard on auscultation of the chest.

After a massive regurgitation or vomit which triggers an episode of apnoea, cyanosis and bradycardia, but which has been promptly and efficiently dealt with (see below), many neonates show no abnormal physical signs 10–15 minutes later. In these babies and those with more chronic problems, the clinical features suggesting that inhalation pneumonia has actually occurred are the non-specific ones of respiratory distress (pp. 643–8). In a neonate with pre-existing lung disease, respiratory function deteriorates. In both, crepitations and rhonchi may be heard on auscultation.

Investigations

In the baby who rapidly reverts to normal and shows no signs of respiratory compromise 15–30 minutes after the episode, it is still advisable to do a CXR. A new area of consolidation, particularly in the right upper lobe, is very suggestive of inhalation, but more generalised and non-specific changes may occur. In either the chronic situation or following a single severe episode, if the baby has the signs of respiratory disease he should be investigated for infection (pp. 1018–26). Measuring the electrolytes, blood sugar and calcium is indicated in all babies, and may identify a cause of a convulsion.

Treatment

The vomiting episode
When the baby is found, his mouth, nose and pharynx should be quickly and effectively sucked out. If the infant has become cyanosed, oxygen should be given by mask. Most babies respond briskly at this stage, and no further treatment is required other than the evaluation outlined above. If the baby does not respond promptly, the airway should be cleared using a laryngoscope, and inhaled material aspirated under direct vision. This should always be done if the episode is so severe that the baby remains apnoeic or intubation is required for resuscitation.

General management
Oxygen
Sufficient oxygen should be given to keep the PaO_2 in the normal range. If the aspiration has been severe, or it complicates pre-existing lung disease in a small preterm baby, the episode may trigger apnoea or cause such severe pneumonitis that the baby will require IPPV.

Physiotherapy
If there are copious secretions following inhalation, or if the CXR shows an area of consolidation, then 4-hourly physiotherapy should be given to encourage drainage from the affected region. The baby should also be nursed in the position that optimises drainage from the affected lobe.

Feeding

In most babies it is wise to stop oral feeds for 24–48 hours after an episode of aspiration/inhalation. In the preterm neonate, recourse to intravenous feeding may be necessary. In the term baby, once the tachypnoea has settled, oral feeding can be restarted unless there is some chronic problem, in which case a period of nasogastric feeds will need to be used.

Antibiotics

Until the cultures are negative, it is impossible to be sure that the whole episode was not triggered by infection. As a consequence, broad-spectrum antibiotic cover should be given, usually flucloxacillin and an aminoglycoside (p. 1041). Antibiotics should be continued for at least 5–7 days or until the baby is clinically much improved if there are marked CXR changes or the neonate required IPPV, even if the cultures are negative.

Morbidity and mortality of aspiration pneumonia

This is completely dependent on the underlying pathology, since the lung disease following inhalation on its own is rarely, if ever, fatal. Babies with persistent failure to suck or swallow secretions after severe birth asphyxia and those with congenital neurological problems have a guarded prognosis on the basis of their underlying defects. Most babies with a structural defect do well with appropriate surgery, but there remains an appreciable mortality with laryngotracheo-oesophageal cleft (p. 717) or Pierre-Robin syndrome (pp. 714, 800). For the baby whose problems are due to immaturity, the outlook is excellent, since it can be anticipated that the lung disease will respond to the therapy outlined, although some infants may develop BPD and have a prolonged convalescence.

Pulmonary haemorrhage

This condition is better named haemorrhagic pulmonary oedema and is a form of fulminant lung oedema with leakage of red cells and capillary filtrate into the lungs.[853] It must be clearly differentiated from the common occurrence of a small amount of blood-stained material aspirated from the ETT of a ventilated baby as a result of trauma. Pulmonary haemorrhage occurs most commonly in babies weighing <1500 g, who often have a PDA[315] and have been treated with surfactant.

Incidence

The incidence of pulmonary haemorrhage in infants with a birth-weight less than 1500 g, treated with surfactant, was reported to be 11.9%.[688]

Aetiology

MPH represents the extreme end of the spectrum of pulmonary oedema in the neonate. This has four main causes[79] (Table 27.9), which all increase fluid leak into the pulmonary interstitium and thus elevate pulmonary lymphatic flow. Although intra-alveolar fluid may appear at an early stage of interstitial oedema,[825] pulmonary oedema usually occurs as lung interstitial fluid rises and fluid leaks into the alveoli because the alveolar epithelium either has been damaged or becomes leaky due to distension by the interstitial fluid. The first change is a rise in pulmonary capillary pressure; this causes an increase in interstitial fluid, which eventually leaks into the alveoli through holes in the epithelium. Initially these holes are large enough to allow passage of molecules such as albumin, but small enough to retain molecules such as IgG, IgM, and fibrinogen, and the majority of red cells. As the changes become more marked, the holes in the endothelium and epithelium increase in size and larger molecules leak through. In most cases, the amount of blood lost is small and the haematocrit of the lung effluent is less than 10%. MPH can occur following severe birth depression and in infants with hydrops due to rhesus haemolytic disease, left heart failure, congenital heart disease, sepsis, hypothermia, fluid overload, oxygen toxicity and haemostatic failure. Infants who are SGA are more likely to suffer a pulmonary haemorrhage,[207] the association being independent of other factors.[281] In addition, the neonate with severe RDS on IPPV in a high oxygen concentration and with heart failure secondary to a large pulmonary blood flow from a PDA may suffer an MPH.[315] Preterm infants with echocardiographic evidence of a large left-to-right shunt across a PDA and a high pulmonary blood flow also had a high incidence of MPH.[264] MPH can also

Table 27.9 Causes of pulmonary oedema in the neonate. (Reproduced with permission from Bland[79])

Increased pulmonary microvascular pressure	Reduced intravascular oncotic pressure	Reduced lymphatic drainage	Increased microvascular permeability
Heart failure	Prematurity	PIE	Sepsis
Hypoxia	Hydrops	Pulmonary fibrosis	Endotoxaemia
Transfusions	Fluid overload	Raised CVP	Emboli
Intravenous fat	Hypoproteinaemia		Oxygen toxicity
Increased pulmonary blood flow	loss in gut		
Pulmonary hyperplasia	loss from kidneys		
	malnutrition		

occur as a complication of exogenous surfactant replacement therapy, perhaps by increasing pulmonary blood flow as PaO_2 rises. Administration of the artificial surfactant Exosurf (pp. 483, 484) increased the incidence of MPH.[575,902] Meta-analysis of the results of 29 trials[727] demonstrated an association of MPH with synthetic, but not natural, surfactant use. The risk of MPH associated with prophylactic and rescue surfactant therapy has been addressed in two Cochrane reviews. Rescue surfactant therapy was not demonstrated to have a significant effect on MPH,[833] but prophylactic surfactant increased the risk (RR 3.28; 95% CI 1.5, 9.2).[830] MPH is seen in babies with DIC, albeit rarely, but does not usually occur in babies with thrombocytopenia, haemorrhagic disease of the newborn or haemophilia. Following the marked clinical deterioration with an MPH, however, it is not uncommon for secondary DIC to develop.[162]

Pathology

The changes present in the lungs are dependent on the stage of the illness reached by the time of death. In deaths before 48 hours of age and in stillbirths, interstitial haemorrhage is common, but in deaths after 48 hours and following surfactant administration,[691] intra-alveolar bleeding dominates the clinical picture. The lungs are solid at post mortem and usually a deep reddish-purple colour; they are gasless and sink in water. Their pressure/volume characteristics will be those of low compliance, surfactant-less lungs (p. 471). Hyaline membranes will often be present, since MPH frequently complicates primary RDS. As in RDS, there will be necrosis and desquamation of the alveolar lining cells. In cases which come to autopsy more than 48 hours after the haemorrhage, and particularly if the neonate survives for several days on IPPV, usually in a high oxygen concentration and at high pressures, the changes merge into those seen in severe CLD (pp. 554–73).

Clinical features

The two striking clinical features of MPH are a sudden deterioration and usually the simultaneous appearance of copious bloody secretions from the baby's airway – either up the ETT or from the larynx and mouth in a non-intubated infant. The baby usually is hypotensive, pale and frequently limp and unresponsive, although term babies may occasionally be active and restless secondary to hypoxaemia, and 'fight' the ventilator. Occasionally, collapse antedates the overt haemorrhage by an hour or two, and rarely the baby looks surprisingly well despite the production of copious bloodstained pulmonary oedema.

Cardiac

As the condition is commonly secondary to heart failure, the infant may have a tachycardia greater than 160/min and the murmur of a PDA is frequently heard.[315] Other signs of heart failure, including hepatosplenomegaly and a triple rhythm, can occur. The presence of peripheral oedema may indicate heart failure, hydrops, hypoalbuminaemia or fluid overload. Hypotension is virtually always present, because of a combination of blood and fluid loss, heart failure, and coexisting hypoxaemia and acidaemia.

Respiratory

Infants are dyspnoeic and cyanotic and auscultation of the chest reveals widespread crepitations with reduction in air entry.

Differential diagnosis

Small amounts of blood coming up the ETT are usually due to trauma. A few babies may deteriorate clinically without apparent cause for an hour or two before the haemorrhage develops, but once copious bloodstained fluid appears from the airway, the diagnosis is self-evident. The underlying cause, however, should be established, since this will influence subsequent treatment.

Investigations

Haematological

Although the haematocrit of the oedema fluid is usually <10%, considerable quantities of blood may be lost, and the haemoglobin may fall to 10 g/dl or even lower. There are no specific white cell changes in MPH. Cole et al[162] found that coagulation disturbances were not a regular feature of their patients prior to the haemorrhage, but DIC is not uncommon afterwards.

Biochemical

Affected preterm babies usually have the same problems as those with severe RDS. In particular, hypoglycaemia, hypocalcaemia, hypoalbuminaemia and renal failure should be sought and remedied.

Chest X-ray

The CXR in the baby who has had a large MPH shows a virtual 'whiteout' (Fig. 27.38) with just an air bronchogram visible. This appearance is indistinguishable from severe surfactant deficiency and may be a reflection of the secondary surfactant deficiency that occurs following pulmonary haemorrhage. As the condition improves on IPPV, the changes may clear or merge into those of BPD. Rarely, a lobar pattern of consolidation is found, suggesting that the haemorrhage has just occurred in part of the lung.

Bacteriology

The haemorrhage may be precipitated by sepsis. For this reason, an infection screen must always be taken immediately after the event. The baby's condition, however, will usually preclude performing a lumbar puncture (p. 1263).

Blood gases

All components of arterial blood gas analysis deteriorate rapidly after the bleed. Hypoxia is severe, the $PaCO_2$ may increase to

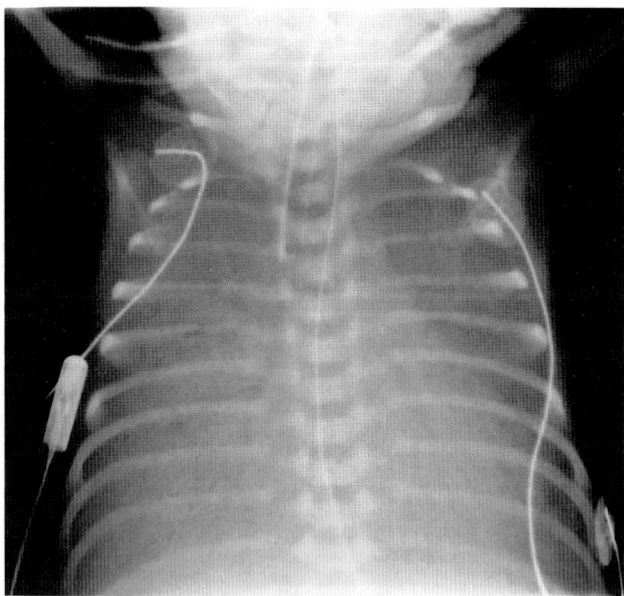

Fig. 27.38 Widespread homogeneous opacification of the lungs in a baby with massive pulmonary haemorrhage. (Reproduced from Greenough et al.[357])

10 kPa (75 mmHg) or more and there is usually a marked metabolic acidosis with a base deficit of at least 10 mmol/l. The combined respiratory and metabolic acidaemia may result in a pH of 7.10 or less.

Monitoring

The blood gases should be meticulously supervised in preterm babies susceptible to ROP. Clotting studies should be done daily until they normalise. A daily CXR should be taken because of the high ventilator pressures that are frequently required, and the potential complications.

Treatment

Particular attention must be paid to maintaining the BP with blood transfusion, progressing to inotropes as necessary (p. 499). The severe acidaemia should be corrected with intravenous base if IPPV and correction of the hypoxia and hypotension do not promptly return the pH and base deficit to an acceptable level. Underlying disorders must be treated. Heart failure due to anaemia in, for example, haemolytic disease, should be treated by exchange transfusion with packed cells, aiming for a haemoglobin of 13–14 g/dl. Asphyxial myocardial damage may need inotrope support (see below), and sepsis should be treated as outlined on pages 1026–8.

Control of pulmonary oedema and heart failure

Fluid balance
Fluid input should be restricted to 60–80 ml/kg/24 h, particularly if there is a coexisting patent ductus. The BP can be sustained by judicious infusion of blood, but mainly by the use of inotropes.

Diuretics
These babies have left ventricular failure and pulmonary oedema. Furosemide (frusemide; 1 mg/kg) should be given as soon as possible after the haemorrhage and repeated as necessary, to treat fluid overload.

IPPV
All babies with MPH should be intubated and ventilated. They usually have severe lung disease, and peak inflating pressures above 30 cmH$_2$O may be necessary. For this reason (p. 521), and since mature babies in particular become very restless, neuromuscular blockade and sedation should be used routinely until the haemorrhage is controlled. During IPPV, a high PEEP (up to 6–7 cmH$_2$O) is employed. Although in experimental studies this does not reduce the total lung water, it redistributes it back into the interstitial space, improving oxygenation and ventilation–perfusion balance.[603,694]

Surfactant
Paradoxically, although surfactant may precipitate MPH (p. 582), after stabilising the baby on IPPV after the haemorrhage, a single dose of surfactant has been suggested to improve oxygenation.[687]

Patent ductus arteriosus
PDA is common in preterm neonates who develop MPH; use of prophylactic indometacin (indomethacin) may reduce both complications.[155] While the baby is critically ill, the use of indometacin (indomethacin) or equivalent is contraindicated, but this should be reconsidered 24–48 hours later, once the coagulopathy is controlled and the hypoxia and acid–base disorders corrected.

Physiotherapy/suction
In the first few hours after the haemorrhage, there may be copious bloody secretions. Suction is required every 10–15 minutes in extreme cases, as there is a significant risk of the secretions clotting and blocking the airway or ETT. Physiotherapy, however, is not of proven value, and as these neonates are extremely fragile, it should not be used as a routine in the early stages, instead relying on adequate humidification to keep the secretions sufficiently liquid that they can be sucked up the ETT.

Coagulopathy
The features of DIC are frequently present. Transfusion of platelets, however, is rarely required, but infusions of FFP are indicated and are usually successful in promptly correcting the clotting deficiencies. After the first 24–48 hours when the baby has become stable on IPPV, the acid–base disturbances have been corrected and septicaemia (if present) treated, the coagulation problems usually remit and further factor replacement is not usually necessary.

Antibiotics
Sepsis is a recognised cause of MPH; thus, antibiotics should be started after taking cultures. If the baby is already receiving

antibiotics, it is sensible to broaden the spectrum to cover infection by staphylococci and *Pseudomonas* species.

Complications

These babies are susceptible to all the major complications of respiratory failure. High-pressure ventilation predisposes them to airleaks, and BPD is a common sequel.[688] At the time of their sudden collapse, they are susceptible to neurological damage and GMH/IVH (p. 1123); the occurrence of cerebral bleeds may be doubled in babies who suffer pulmonary haemorrhage.[281] The occurrence of seizures is increased in infants with pulmonary haemorrhage.[880]

Mortality

For many years this was regarded as a universally fatal condition.[315] In the modern era of intensive care, survival is improved; but affected infants are the sickest and most immature and their mortality rate is of the order of 38%.[688]

Asphyxial lung disease/acute respiratory distress syndrome

Many lung diseases may be the sequel of intrapartum asphyxia in the neonate, including meconium aspiration (pp. 502–8), persistent pulmonary hypertension (pp. 496–502) and MPH (pp. 512–15). Once these clear-cut clinical conditions have been excluded, intrapartum asphyxia or severe lung injury may result in severe respiratory distress, acute respiratory distress syndrome (ARDS).

Aetiology

ARDS results from lung injury from a number of causes. These include asphyxia, shock, sepsis, MAS and DIC.

Pathophysiology

Asphyxia damages pulmonary blood vessels, making them leaky, and this, plus the pulmonary oedema secondary to heart failure occurring as a result of asphyxial damage to the myocardium,[105,109,927] may compromise surfactant function (pp. 491–3). Severe metabolic acidaemia can also depress myocardial contractility, again leading to heart failure, pulmonary oedema and tachypnoea.[60,931] If the leak of protein-rich fluid onto the alveoli becomes large enough, ARDS develops, with epithelial degeneration, surfactant inhibition, interstitital cellular infiltration, pulmonary hypertension and eventually alveolar fibrosis.[763]

Metabolic acidaemia stimulates hyperventilation.[467] In the neonate, the chemoreceptors are sensitive to pH;[654,922] the increase in respiration is more likely to be due to stimulation of peripheral chemoreceptors than medullary centres.[108]

Damage to the CNS may stimulate tachypnoea by two mechanisms. Firstly, the neural control of respiration may be damaged, resulting in hyperventilation. This is well recognised in older patients.[553] Neurologically damaged babies may hyperventilate to $PaCO_2$ levels of 2.5–3.0 kPa (19–23 mmHg) in the first few days after birth. Secondly, neurogenic pulmonary oedema may occur following any rise in intracranial pressure (ICP) or brain injury. It is primarily due to an increased pulmonary vascular permeability leading to interstitial pulmonary oedema, hypoxia and tachypnoea.[163,614] The mechanism is probably active in the newborn, and explains, for example, the sudden deterioration in respiratory function following a GMH/IVH, but may also be of importance in babies with HIE or subdural haemorrhage following birth asphyxia.

Asphyxia caused by cord occlusion may trap blood in the placenta, causing fetal anaemia,[804,908] and acute fetal haemorrhage from ruptured vasa praevia or following a large fetomaternal haemorrhage will result in the birth of a baby who is anaemic, shocked and acidotic.[732] Chronic fetal anaemia due to rhesus disease or fetomaternal haemorrhage also produces babies with acidaemia, anaemia and tachypnoea.[704] The lowered buffering capacity of blood with a low haemoglobin will also potentiate the effect of metabolic acidaemia on respiration (see above).

Clinical features

Some babies who suffer intrapartum asphyxia remain tachypnoeic for 24–48 hours after delivery;[871] less commonly, severe lung disease, ARDS,[265] occurs.

Infants with ARDS are severely hypoxaemia. This is primarily a disease of term babies, who, within the first hour or two, usually present with tachypnoea of 100/min or more, rather than with retraction and grunting, although in some babies the clinical picture may be dominated by the neurological sequelae of asphyxia, and apnoea may occur.[871] The baby may be tachycardic and hypotensive with a triple rhythm, or have the systolic murmurs of tricuspid or mitral incompetence;[105,282] if there has been severe myocardial damage, other signs of heart failure, crepitations and hepatomegaly may be found.[111]

Differential diagnosis

This is a diagnosis of exclusion in the neonate who has suffered intrapartum asphyxia. The CXR excludes complications such as pneumothorax, and does not show the features of 'wet lung' seen in transient tachypnoea. Excluding sepsis, as always, is important, as GBS infection may masquerade as asphyxia.[697]

Investigations

The blood gases should be measured on an arterial sample; babies with ARDS are severely hypoxaemic. Respiration is stimulated by the metabolic acidaemia (base deficit >20 mmol/l, with a corresponding low pH), damage to the CNS or by lung receptors stimulated by pulmonary oedema; the $PaCO_2$ is usually <4 kPa (30 mmHg). Hypoglycaemia is common after asphyxia, as is DIC (pp. 759–60); both should be remedied promptly if found.

A CXR is essential and will demonstrate diffuse pulmonary infiltrates. In severe cases there will be a 'whiteout' as in severe RDS.

Evidence of myocardial damage should be sought by performing an echocardiograph to assess ventricular function and an ECG should be obtained. If myocardial damage is present, much greater care has to be taken regarding use of bolus infusions. The ECG may show changes of ST-segment depression and T-wave inversion if there is severe asphyxia,[111,796] but in lesser degrees of asphyxia there may only be slight flattening of the T-wave.[468] The level of the myocardial isoenzyme of creatine kinase may be raised.[722]

Monitoring

A UAC is the preferred site for monitoring blood gases and BP. Affected babies are peripherally shut down, making clinical assessment of oxygenation impossible and arterial puncture difficult; frequent samples may be needed until the pH returns to normal.

Management

Surfactant administration can improve oxygenation in ARDS. It is most effective if given early and in larger doses than in RDS.[674] In adults and children with ARDS, prone positioning has been shown to improve oxygenation.[183]

Blood gases

The baby should receive sufficient warmed humidified oxygen to keep his PaO_2 above 8 kPa (60 mmHg). Prolonged high-pressure ventilation similar to that used for neonatal RDS (pp. 480–1) may be necessary.[265] A high level of PEEP should be used to try and restore the FRC to more normal values; this will also increase the MAP level and hence oxygenation. An excessive amount of PEEP, however, will impair gas exchange by causing alveolar overdistension. High-volume strategy HFO can also improve oxygenation,[327] particularly in those patients who had a positive response to PEEP elevation (pp. 522). HFJV has also been used with anecdotal success.[703] Inhaled NO has been used in patients with ARDS to improve oxygenation.[216]

Metabolic acidaemia

Term neonates can recover spontaneously and quickly from pH levels of 7.10–7.15 and base deficits of >15 mmol/l.[192,839,864] For this reason, immediately after delivery, expectant treatment of uncomplicated metabolic acidaemia is justified if the pH is above 7.10, but an arterial gas should be checked 30–60 minutes later to ensure that spontaneous correction is taking place. If the pH is below this value, or the infant has heart failure attributed to acidaemia, then the pH should be corrected to 7.30–7.40 using the standard formula (p. 1315).

Hypotension and heart failure

These are two of the most serious complications of severe asphyxia, as they are associated with secondary ischaemic injury to the CNS, myocardium (endocardial ischaemia), kidneys (renal failure) and intestine (NEC). They must, therefore, be corrected urgently. The general approach to hypotension outlined on pages 530–1 should be followed, taking great care with fluid balance if the myocardium is compromised. In general, the fluid intake should initially be restricted to 40 ml/kg/24 h. If heart failure is present, furosemide (frusemide) should be given. IPPV with PEEP helps to control pulmonary oedema.

Anaemia

A haemoglobin <13 g/dl (PCV <40%) is an indication for transfusion in asphyxial lung disease. If there is coexisting myocardial asphyxial injury, the transfusion should be given slowly and carefully with a diuretic. In such a situation, if the haemoglobin level is <8–9 g/dl, the safest way of increasing it is with a single-volume exchange transfusion using packed red blood cells.

Hypoxic-ischaemic encephalopathy

The management of this is outlined in detail on pages 1128–48. If there is severe HIE, it is essential to prevent blood gas abnormalities (p. 1309).

Antibiotics

After collecting the appropriate samples for culture, including blood culture, broad-spectrum antibiotics, usually penicillin plus an aminoglycoside (pp. 1037–9), should be administered. Aminoglycoside levels must be carefully monitored, as these infants are at risk of renal dysfunction.

Prognosis

The mortality of ARDS is high,[703] particularly in those infants who develop secondary infection or do not respond to elevation of their PEEP level. Airleaks and infection are commonly seen in infant with ARDS.

Pleural effusions

Isolated

These are uncommon in the neonatal period. The incidence of primary fetal hydrothorax is estimated at one case per 15 000 pregnancies.[578]

Aetiology

Pleural effusions diagnosed antenatally are frequently associated with chromosomal or congenital abnormalities.[662] Intrauterine (cytomegalovirus, toxoplasmosis, rubella, adenovirus), perinatal (GBS and *Staphylococcus*) and postnatal (*Staphylococcus*) infection can all result in pleural effusions. Isolated effusions are usually a chylothorax (pp. 518–19). Approximately 9% of infants with MAS have pleural effusions; rarer associations are TTN, PPHN, heart failure and congenital myotonic dystrophy. Right-sided diaphragmatic hernia can be associated with a hydrothorax, which results from a fluid-filled peritoneal sac in the right side of the chest.[938] An effusion will develop following repair of CDH (pp. 596–8). Trauma, for example by direct erosion of the inferior vena cava by a TPN catheter into the pleural space, can result in a pleural effusion.[554] A unilateral hydrothorax may also occur if a central venous catheter migrates into the pulmonary vasculature.[599] Pleural effusions are usually part of a generalised oedematous state (hydrops fetalis); an isolated fetal pleural effusion can progress to generalised hydrops.

Clinical signs

Infants with large effusions are frequently difficult to resuscitate as, antenatally, the pleural effusion may have prevented normal lung growth. In infants with underlying pulmonary hypoplasia, there will be a reduced pulmonary vascular bed and the babies will have PPHN. On examination, the trachea and mediastinum will be shifted to the contralateral side and the ipsilateral lung dull to percussion with absent breath sounds. Small effusions may be asymptomatic and diagnosed incidentally on a chest radiograph.

Diagnosis

Antenatally, pleural effusions are detected by ultrasonography and should be suspected in fetuses whose mothers have polyhydramnios.[708] Postnatally, on the CXR there may be a 'whiteout' on the affected site (Figs 27.39 & 27.40), but if the pleural effusion is small, it is important to remember that fluid will collect in the most dependent parts of the chest, around the lateral chest wall or the diaphragm (Figs 27.41 & 27.42).

Differential diagnosis

At birth, the presentation of a large effusion is similar to that of CDH (p. 596), but there are no bowel sounds in the chest. The CXR appearance may be confused with an eventration or atelectasis.

Treatment

Antenatally, pleural effusions are drained either intermittently by thoracocentesis[700] or continuously by a thoracoamniotic shunt.[87] Indications for antenatal drainage include the development of hydrops, and mediastinal shift with unilateral effusions. At birth, infants with large pleural effusions require active resuscitation by intubation and positive pressure ventilation.[708] Thoracocentesis

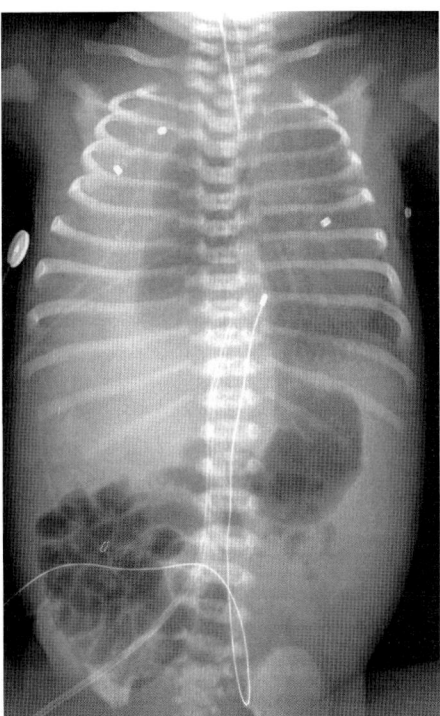

Fig. 27.39 Chest X-ray demonstrates a right pleural effusion. Antenatally, the infant was hydropic with bilateral pleural effusions; pigtail catheters were inserted bilaterally (with successful drainage on the right) and are still in situ, shown by the two radio-opaque dots on each side of the chest.

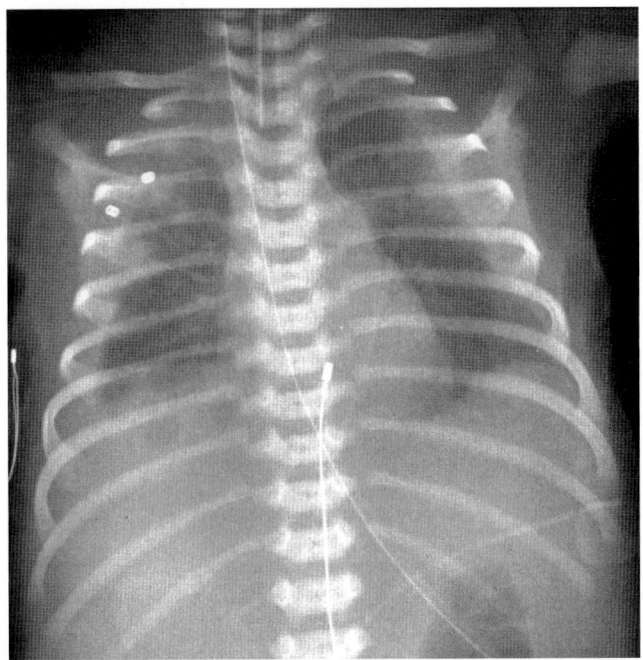

Fig. 27.40 Bilateral pleural effusions. Note the presence of a pigtailed catheter on the right side of the chest, which was placed antenatally.

may also be required to achieve effective ventilation and this may also be necessary later in the postnatal period. To perform a thoracocentesis, the infant should be turned onto the contralateral side and a 21 G butterfly needle attached to a syringe inserted via a Z-track 1 cm above the vertebral column in between the fifth and sixth or sixth and seventh ribs. Unless the infant is very oedematous, fluid can be easily obtained with the needle tip only 0.5 cm below the skin surface. Aspirated fluid should always be sent for

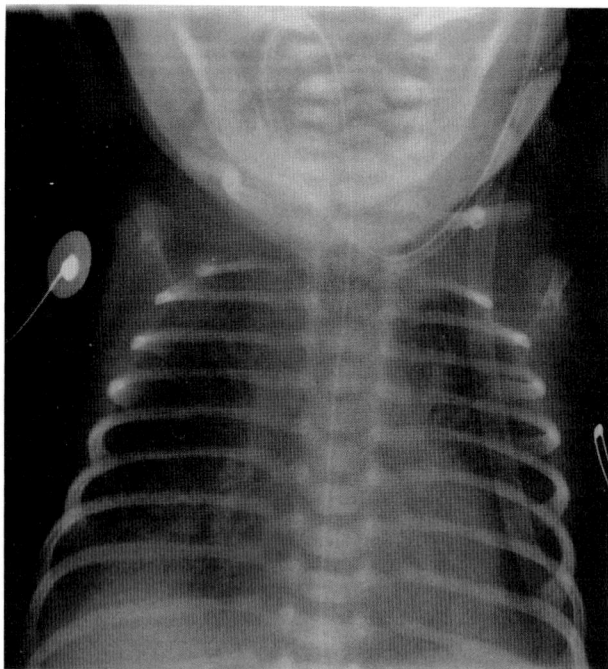

Fig. 27.41 Small pleural effusion. Chest X-ray in erect position: note obliteration of the right hemidiaphragm. (Reproduced from Greenough et al.[357])

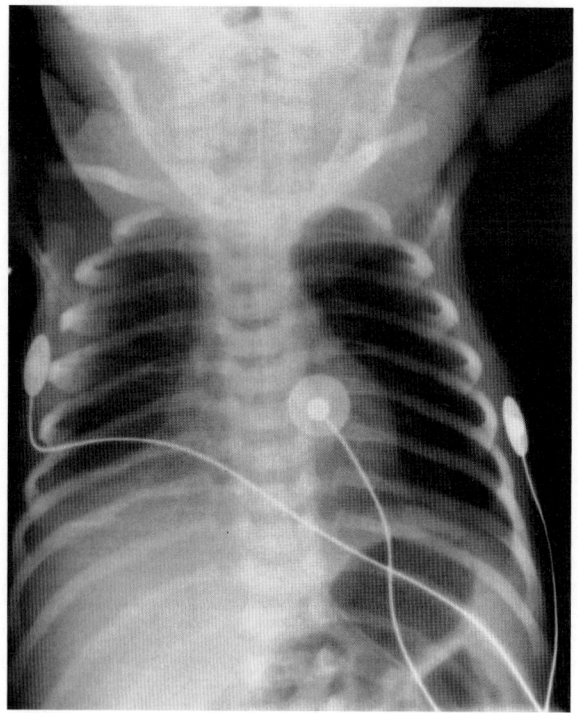

Fig. 27.42 Small pleural effusion. Supine X-ray showing a rim of fluid. (Reproduced from Greenough et al.[357])

cytology to determine the lymphocyte count, and for biochemical and microbiological analysis. If the effusion is due to infection, the fluid will have a high protein content, with neutrophils present, and organisms may be isolated. The fluid should also be sent for

cytological examination, a high lymphocyte count indicating a chylothorax. If a chest tube is used to drain a pleural effusion, it is important to ensure the tip does not abut the mediastinum, as this increases the risk of phrenic nerve injury.[946]

Prognosis

Antenatally diagnosed pleural effusions, particularly if present prior to 32 weeks of gestation, have a mortality rate as high as 55%.[382] Bilateral fetal pleural effusions are frequently associated with pulmonary hypoplasia. Postnatally, effusions persisting for more than 3 days increase the risk of chronic oxygen dependency.[576]

Chylothorax

Incidence

One in 10 000 deliveries and one in 2000 neonatal intensive care admissions were reported to have a chylothorax.[900]

Aetiology

Chylothorax may occur spontaneously or be associated with lymphoedema due to congenitally abnormal lymph vessels in conditions such as Turner's or Noonan's syndrome or congenital lymphangiectasia. In the latter condition, there is diffuse dilatation of the interlobular and subpleural lymphatics. A congenital abnormality in the lymphatic system at the level of the thoracic duct below or above the fifth thoracic vertebrae leads to a right- or left-sided chylothorax.[900] It can be associated with foregut malformations and extralobar sequestration. Rarely, trauma to the thoracic duct at delivery by hyperexpansion of the spinal column in association with increased venous pressure during birth results in a chylothorax, but more commonly it is a complication of certain types of cardiac surgery (repair of coarctation of the aorta or ligation of a PDA) or repair of a congenital posterolateral diaphragmatic hernia.[624] Another iatrogenic cause is superior vena caval (SVC) obstruction in patients who have had venous catheterisation for TPN.[17]

Clinical signs

Unusually, chylothoraces result in hydrops, due to impairment of venous return by cardiac and vena caval compression and/or loss of protein into the pleural space. In 50% of cases, chylothoraces present in the first week with symptoms as described under isolated pleural effusion. Typically, the lesion is right-sided. Chronic chylothorax may be associated with hypovolaemia, hypoalbuminaemia, hyponatraemia and weight loss. Such patients are immunocompromised due to loss of lymphocytes and humoral antibodies.

Diagnosis

In an unfed infant, the fluid obtained at thoracocentesis is clear, yellow and contains large numbers of lymphocytes (20 to 50 per high-power field). Lipoprotein electrophoresis demonstrates a high triglyceride and a low cholesterol level. Once the infant is milk-fed, the fluid will become chylous, clearing once a medium-chain triglyceride (MCT) formula is introduced. Chylothorax associated with SVC obstruction should be suspected in infants with swelling of the face, neck and upper extremities; ultrasonography will confirm the presence of fluid in the chest and the position of the catheter tip. Doppler ultrasonography will identify the SVC obstruction.

Treatment

Chylothoraces may need to be drained antenatally (see above). Postnatally, many cases respond to a single thoracocentesis, as this results in lung expansion tamponading the defect and preventing further pleural fluid formation. If the fluid reaccumulates, drainage is required and the baby should be fed with a milk containing fat only in the form of MCTs. In the gut, long-chain fatty acids pass into the lymph as chylomicrons after being re-esterified to triglycerides, before entering the venous network, whereas medium-chain fatty acids pass directly into the portal venous blood. Pregestemil or Pepti junior can be tried, but a semi-elemental milk may be required and should be continued for at least 2 weeks after the effusion has disappeared.[99,401,723] Rarely, in non-responsive cases, TPN should be used. Pleural abrasion, ligation of the thoracic duct and pleurodesis are possible options for those chylothoraces that fail to respond to medical management.[19,723]

Prognosis

This condition usually resolves, but the mortality rate has been suggested to be as high as 60% for bilateral chylothoraces.[117]

Haemothorax

Aetiology

Trauma with damage to the arteries alongside the ribs from misplacement of a chest drain to drain a pneumothorax is the commonest cause of a neonatal haemothorax; it can also occur at thoracic surgery. Rare causes include clotting abnormalities,[344] penetration of the fetal thorax at amniocentesis,[3] spontaneous rupture of a PDA, and arteriovenous malformations.

Diagnosis

The CXR will demonstrate a 'whiteout', and a radioisotope lung scan can identify an underlying arteriovenous fistula.

Treatment

Resuscitation by urgent transfusion of blood and clotting factors may be required. Surgical intervention should be considered if a large blood vessel has been traumatised.

Management of neonatal respiratory failure

Oxygen therapy

Supplementary oxygen therapy

In mild–moderate respiratory disease, all that is usually required to keep the baby's PaO_2 at 8–12 kPa (60–90 mmHg) (p. 1309) is the administration of warmed humidified supplementary oxygen. Additional support by CPAP or IPPV is indicated only if a satisfactory PaO_2 cannot be achieved in 60–80% oxygen in a headbox, or at lower inspired oxygen concentrations if there are other features of respiratory failure. To avoid sudden changes in the inspired oxygen concentration, the oxygen should be given into a perspex box placed over the baby's head and shoulders (headbox). The concentration of oxygen administered should be measured by an analyser placed near the baby's mouth. This form of therapy is frequently sufficient for preterm babies more than 30 weeks of gestational age with RDS, all babies with minimal respiratory disease and most with TTN (pp. 485–6). The occasional mature baby with RDS and most cases of meconium aspiration can also be managed with headbox oxygen, even though they may require concentrations of up to 80% for 72 hours or more, providing they do not develop other signs of respiratory failure.

Nasal cannula-administered oxygen

In babies requiring prolonged oxygen therapy for BPD, administration of oxygen by nasal cannula allows the baby to be picked up and cuddled and bottle- or breastfed. It is, however, difficult to assess the concentration of oxygen administered to such babies. Purpose-built double cannulae or an 8 FG feeding catheter cut to length and inserted 2–3 cm into one nostril can be used. Correct fixation of the catheter to the nostril is important to prevent restricting the flow rate, accidental displacement and excessive advancement of the catheter, which has been associated with gastric rupture.[144]

Percutaneous oxygen

Oxygen can be absorbed through the thin skin of VLBW babies. The average rise in PaO_2 when the babies were transferred from ambient air to 95% oxygen was 1.2 kPa (9 mmHg).[121]

Oxygen toxicity

Oxygen is toxic to tissues because it forms free radicals, such as superoxide (O_2^-) and hydroxyl (OH^-).[499] The neonate is exposed to complex physiological and pharmacological stresses from these agents.[780,824] The effect of oxygen on the lung is complex. If adults are exposed to even a few hours of pure oxygen, they develop a tracheitis and reduced tracheal mucus velocity. After about 16–24 hours, they experience chest discomfort and cough. Dyspnoea develops after a further 24–48 hours.[460]

During the first 24 hours, there is a significant alveolar-capillary leak of protein.[204] If pure oxygen exposure is continued for 3–4 days, animals develop a fatal lung disease with oedematous alveolar walls, interstitial haemorrhage, atelectasis,[146] and type II cell hyperplasia.[209] Surfactant is depleted in the early stages of oxygen exposure, with a reduction in both DPPC and PG,[511] and the levels continue to fall after the animal is removed from 100% oxygen.[214,434] Another deleterious effect of breathing pure oxygen is that all the nitrogen is washed out of the alveoli; as oxygen is much more rapidly taken up by pulmonary capillary blood than is nitrogen, this predisposes to atelectasis. Pulmonary alveolar macrophage function is significantly reduced in animals by exposure to more than 80% oxygen for at least 3 days.[806]

Exposure of the neonatal lung to a high inspired oxygen concentration in the presence of lung disease also causes damage, probably because the oxygen free radicals interact with lung cell lipids. Neonates, however, seem to be more resistant to pulmonary oxygen toxicity than are adults.[146] This resistance is dependent on the presence in the tissues of antioxidant enzymes such as superoxide dismutase, catalase and glutathione peroxidase. In the term lung, the cells, including type II pneumocytes, are able rapidly to switch on antioxidant enzymes after birth,[295,495] an effect that may be stimulated by epidermal growth factor,[720] but this is less efficient in the preterm lung.[296,496,579] The level of antioxidant enzymes and the resistance of the lung to hyperoxia are increased at term by prenatal maternal and postnatal treatment with dexamethasone.[201,294] In preterm animals, the postnatal increase in enzymes and oxygen resistance may be absent.[496,835] Administration of surfactant protects against oxygen toxicity.[444,706]

Although 100% oxygen clearly damages the lungs, the danger of lower oxygen concentrations to the human neonate is much less clear. In adult humans, oxygen concentrations less than 60% rarely do harm, and exposure to between 50% and 90% resulted in limited damage.[520] In mature rabbits, exposure to 60% oxygen for 3 weeks caused alveolar interstitial oedema but increased surfactant production.[434] Rats kept in 60% oxygen for 2 weeks had small lungs with parenchymal thickening.[395] Studies in neonatal baboons suggest that exposure to a high oxygen concentration even without IPPV is damaging.[214]

Administration of 100% oxygen to babies is never justified, as, with large shunts (p. 450), the increase in PaO_2 achieved by increasing from 90% oxygen to 100% oxygen is trivial and is not worth the risks of both oxygen toxicity to the lung and the atelectasis that results from nitrogen washout.

Assisted ventilation in the newborn

Continuous positive airways pressure

CPAP is a positive distending pressure applied continuously. The aim of CPAP is to hold the alveoli and airways open and prevent them collapsing during expiration. The major benefit of CPAP is that it stabilises the ribcage, reducing chest wall distortion during inspiration, and consequently increases the efficiency of the diaphragm.[799] It regularises the respiratory rate, which usually falls because of stimulation of the Hering–Breuer reflex, and

results in an increase in inspiratory time and tidal volume. There is an increase in the FRC in proportion to the level of applied pressure; some alveoli, however, will be overdistended, resulting in a fall in dynamic compliance.[634] If too small a diameter tube is used to administer the CPAP, the work of breathing may increase as a result of the increased effort required to overcome the resistance of the tube.[545]

CPAP techniques

CPAP was initially given through an ETT,[367] but, in an attempt to avoid the hazards of intubation, many other devices have been used, including Gregory's original headbox, face chambers and negative-pressure chambers. These devices have mostly been abandoned, and CPAP is now given by facemask or, more usually, nasal prongs. Facemask CPAP has a high complication rate[365] and is thus not recommended. The mask must be applied firmly to the face to prevent gas leaks and maintain the pressure, and this can distort the baby's face; furthermore, the apparatus holding the mask in place must be strapped tightly around the back of the head, which can distort its shape. In early series, pressure necrosis and even GMH/IVH or cerebellar haemorrhage were reported.[689] It is difficult to use a nasogastric tube with facemask CPAP because this breaks the seal; yet, without this tube, the stomach cannot be easily aspirated and gaseous abdominal distension results. The presence of the facemask also makes it difficult to tend to the baby's mouth and nose. CPAP can be delivered using an underwater seal;[208] if the bubbling is vigorous, the baby experiences vibration of his chest at frequencies similar to those experienced during HFOV (pp. 526–8). In a small randomised trial of infants ready for extubation, gas exchange was maintained despite a significant reduction in minute volume during 'bubble' CPAP, suggesting that the chest vibrations may have contributed to gas exchange.

CPAP is usually delivered to the baby through either a pair of tubes inserted into both nostrils, or a single tube into one nostril. A prong, cut down from a soft, 3.0 mm, blue-line Portex ETT, is inserted 1 cm into one nostril and connected to a lightweight T-piece circuit attached to a standard neonatal ventilator in CPAP mode. In this way, the gas-mixing, pressure-measuring and humidification facilities of the ventilator circuit can be used. The tube is kept in place by a soft cord tied around it and fastened to both cheeks by lightweight sticky tape. An alternative device, described by Benveniste et al,[65] applies a jet of gas near to the exit of the curved attachment for the prongs in a way that mimics the actions of an expiratory valve and thus applies CPAP. This device has been widely used in the Scandinavian studies of CPAP in RDS.[462,478]

The method of nCPAP delivery used influences outcome. For example, there is a variation in the resistance to flow with the different nCPAP devices; the resistance is lowest in devices with short double prongs. That finding may explain why meta-analysis of the results of two studies demonstrated that short binasal prongs were more effective at preventing reintubation than were single nasal or nasopharyngeal prongs.[210] Variable flow nCPAP is associated with better lung recruitment than is either continuous flow nCPAP via nasal prongs or continuous flow nCPAP via modified nasal cannulae.[175] The work of breathing is also lower with variable flow CPAP.[686] These beneficial effects may be due to gas entrainment by the high-velocity jet flows; lung overdistension, however, may occur in infants with mild disease if CPAP levels greater than 6 cmH$_2$O are used with variable flow CPAP.

CPAP settings

In relatively mature infants with acute RDS who have not received treatment with surfactant, CPAP pressures of 5–8 cmH$_2$O may be required; however, in immature infants in the recovery stage of their illness who have more compliant lungs, levels in excess of 2–3 cmH$_2$O may not be tolerated. It is important not to use too high a CPAP level, as this will cause lung overdistension, resulting in impairment of ventilation and carbon dioxide retention. The CPAP and F$_1$O$_2$ levels are adjusted on the basis of blood gas analyses. If the neonate still has unsatisfactory oxygenation in 50–60% oxygen, he should be intubated and ventilated.

Hazards of CPAP

Traumatic injuries to the nose and face from the prong(s) can occur,[754] and, although these can be minimised by good nursing technique, they are not completely avoidable. More serious complications are pneumothorax and GMH/IVH. Airleaks do occur in infants supported by CPAP.[206,380] Indeed, in a non-randomised study,[601] pneumothoraces developed more often in infants supported by nCPAP than in those supported by synchronised intermittent mandatory ventilation (SIMV). Nasal CPAP, then, should never be used in units without facilities for both the rapid recognition and drainage of a tension pneumothorax and the subsequent use of IPPV.

Clinical studies

When first introduced, CPAP was applied to babies requiring 50–60% oxygen to keep their PaO_2 >8 kPa (60 mmHg). With increased familiarity, the technique was used earlier in babies with RDS, often when they needed no more than 35–40% oxygen to maintain an acceptable PaO_2. Used in this way, it improved blood gases and seemed to cause more rapid recovery.[11,49,92,247,367] In early randomised controlled trials, however, the benefits of CPAP seemed to be small[748] and problems were experienced, and the results of prospective trials of CPAP in babies with relatively mild lung disease suggested that treated babies did less well than controls.[396,402] Nevertheless, early CPAP is now used in many centres in preference to early intubation and IPPV.[28,330,462,478,571] In non-randomised trials, its use has been associated with a reduction in the requirement for mechanical ventilation and in the incidence of BPD. Use of early CPAP has also been associated with a reduction in the duration of ventilation in a randomised trial,[873] but whether such an approach influences neurodevelopmental outcome requires testing.[208] If early CPAP is used, the baby should be temporarily intubated so that surfactant can be given,[913] which should be administered early rather than late.[912] It is also important to remember that use of nCPAP requires meticulous attention to the airway, and frequent suctioning may be necessary. Rigorous training is required for success; the correct size prongs should be used and the neonate's neck properly positioned.[208]

CPAP is frequently used during the recovery stage of RDS to support neonates following extubation from the ventilator

(pp. 607–8).[233] It is helpful in the management of infants with recurrent apnoeic attacks (Chapter 27, part 4); nCPAP dilates the upper airway, which may explain its selective beneficial effects on mixed and obstructive apnoea.[311] CPAP is also sometimes useful in upper airways obstruction due to Pierre–Robin syndrome or congenital laryngeal stridor, when nasopharyngeal CPAP may be preferable, with the tip of the nasal cannula passing through the posterior choanae into the upper pharynx.[404]

Nasal-delivered ventilatory modes

Experience of ventilatory modes delivered by nasal prongs is limited and there have been no large randomised trials to determine whether these techniques offer long-term advantages for neonates. Nasal prong-delivered IPPV appears to augment the beneficial effects of nCPAP in prematurely born infants with apnoea;[555] there are, however, case reports of gastrointestinal perforation with this mode of respiratory support. In two small trials, delivery of SIMV compared with CPAP via nasal prongs was associated with a lower incidence of respiratory failure[302] and reintubation.[43] HFOV has been delivered by nasal prongs and resulted in a reduction in carbon dioxide levels in some infants with a moderate respiratory acidosis on nCPAP.[906]

Continuous negative expanding pressure

This is an alternative way of providing distending pressure in which the infant's body is placed in a negative pressure box from which the head protrudes and continuous negative external pressure (CNEP) in the range −4 to −10 cmH$_2$O is applied.[776] In patients already ventilated, the peak and positive end-expiratory pressures are reduced by the level of negative pressure applied.

Early studies[685] demonstrated CNEP was associated with improvements in oxygenation, the best results being experienced in infants with severe RDS. In addition, respiratory rate decreased and, in infants with stiff lungs, compliance improved on CNEP.[312] In a randomised trial,[775] use of CNEP (−4 to −6 cmH$_2$O) was associated with a lower duration of oxygen therapy (18.3 vs 33.6 days), but there were trends towards an increase in mortality and cranial ultrasound abnormalities in the CNEP group. CNEP in combination with intermittent mandatory ventilation, in anecdotal series, has been demonstrated to improve oxygenation in infants with PPHN,[813] PIE[186] and BPD.[776]

Early attempts at CNEP were poorly tolerated, particularly in ELBW infants, because of difficulties in securing the infant and hypothermia. These problems have been overcome by specially designed neck seals[776] and providing a circulation of warm air. CNEP can, however, overdistend the lung and impair lung function in infants with CLD. The considerable technical challenges have meant that CNEP is not widely used in the UK.

Intermittent positive pressure ventilation

Indications

There are two absolute indications for starting IPPV:

- sudden collapse with apnoea, bradycardia and failure to establish satisfactory ventilation after a short period of bag-and-mask ventilation;

- failure to establish adequate spontaneous ventilation in the labour ward after prompt and active resuscitation (pp. 230, 232).

The relative indications for intubation and IPPV apply to babies who are breathing spontaneously but are clinically, or on the basis of blood gas results, showing signs of impending respiratory failure. These indications vary with the gestational and postnatal age of the baby, the nature of the underlying disease, and whether the major feature of the respiratory failure is carbon dioxide retention, hypoxaemia or recurrent apnoeic spells.

Most babies in impending respiratory failure fall into one of three clearly separate groups, which require different plans of action:

- VLBW neonates <28 weeks' gestation and <1.00 kg. These babies are usually ventilated from the time of resuscitation in the labour ward (p. 236). This also applies to many babies between 28 and 32 weeks' gestation weighing 1.0–1.5 kg. A small number of these infants establish adequate regular respiration after birth but subsequently develop signs of RDS. To prevent sudden collapse with its attendant complications (p. 468) and to give surfactant (p. 475), these babies should be ventilated once they need more than 40% oxygen on CPAP to keep their PaO_2 >7–8 kPa (52–60 mmHg) or have a $PaCO_2$ >6–6.5 kPa (45–50 mmHg) with a pH <7.25.
- Babies 1.50–2.25 kg at 32–35 weeks' gestation, usually with RDS. Nasal CPAP may be sufficient support for infants whose $PaCO_2$ exceeds 6.5–7.0 kPa (50–52 mmHg) but who maintain their pH >7.25 and have an oxygen requirement of less than 60%. If, however, CPAP does not result in a prompt improvement, such babies should be ventilated.
- Mature babies >2.25–2.50 kg and >36–37 weeks' gestation. These babies have a comparatively rigid ribcage and well-developed respiratory muscles, so can sustain vigorous respiratory efforts and tachypnoea >100–120/min for some days. They also tolerate CPAP badly, becoming distressed and irritable when the device is attached. They can be left in headbox oxygen at ≤80% for several days, intervening with intubation and IPPV only if the $PaCO_2$ exceeds 8–9 kPa (60–67 mmHg), the PaO_2 is <6 kPa (45 mmHg) in 80–90% oxygen, or a metabolic acidaemia or hypotension are developing, which do not respond to increasing the inspired oxygen concentration, plasma expansion or infusion of base.

Other indications for IPPV in the neonatal period include:

- PPHN. For the neonate with primary PPHN or pulmonary hypertension secondary to mild lung disease, intubation and tight control of the $PaCO_2$ can be beneficial (p. 498).
- Severe early-onset sepsis (pp. 1028–33). The incidence of apnoea and pulmonary hypertension is high in this group of babies who present within 6–12 hours of delivery.
- MPH.
- Diaphragmatic hernia. These babies should be ventilated and paralysed from birth (pp. 594–603).
- HIE. Although hyperventilation to prevent cerebral oedema by keeping the $PaCO_2$ in the 3.0–3.5 kPa (22–25 mmHg) range (pp. 1140–1) is no longer justified, the $PaCO_2$ in such babies should not be allowed to rise above 6 kPa (45 mmHg). Sedation from anticonvulsant drugs often requires ventilation.

- Apnoea. The small preterm baby with recurrent apnoea, which is not controlled by methylxanthines or CPAP, requires IPPV (pp. 573, 574).

Techniques of IPPV and ventilator settings

Pressure-limited, time-controlled ventilation

A continuous flow of gas is delivered which distends the lung for a preset inflation time to a predetermined pressure. During expiration, the ventilator gas flow continues to deliver PEEP if required. Gas enters the lungs during the inspiratory time; the amount entering is determined by the set peak pressure and the gas flow rate. The latter should always be large enough to ensure that the preset peak pressure can be reached during the available inflation time. At a fast flow, the lungs are distended more quickly, and the peak pressure is reached sooner, thereby creating a relatively square-wave inspiratory gas flow. When the desired pressure has been reached, the pressure-limiting valve opens and prevents any further rise. The longer the inflation time, the longer the lungs are held distended at this pressure. The higher the pressure is set, depending on the compliance of the lungs, the larger the volume of gas which enters the lungs, though this is limited in non-compliant lungs by the size of the leak around the ETT.

Peak inflating pressures: When starting a baby on IPPV, the peak inflating pressure should be adjusted to ensure adequate, but not excessive, chest wall expansion; in practice this usually equates to a delivered volume of approximately 6 ml/kg.[221] Sufficient pressure must be used to achieve acceptable blood gases. Since high pressures are likely to cause a pneumothorax (pp. 487–91) or lead to BPD (pp. 554–66), the lowest possible peak pressure compatible with normal blood gases should be employed. In general, the starting pressures for a baby with respiratory distress should be about 16–18 cmH$_2$O. The peak pressure is then adjusted according to the blood gas results, which should be determined within 15 minutes of commencing mechanical ventilation. Underventilation produces a high $PaCO_2$ and a low PaO_2, and overventilation a low $PaCO_2$ and sometimes an excessively high PaO_2.

Positive end-expiratory pressure: This acts like CPAP to hold the peripheral airways open during expiration. PEEP should always be used during ventilation, as it conserves surfactant on the alveolar surface, except in severe PIE or certain cases of over-inflation.[966] If too high a PEEP level is applied, particularly if combined with a short expiratory time, the lung cannot deflate properly. This causes hyperinflation, a reduced tidal volume and compromised gas exchange, and the $PaCO_2$ rises[799] accompanied by a fall in PaO_2. Early studies demonstrated that a PEEP of about 5 cmH$_2$O, rather than no PEEP or much higher levels, improved oxygenation;[414,622] the mechanism was via an increase in MAP. More recent studies have suggested that babies with acute RDS or apnoea do not require more than 3 cmH$_2$O of PEEP;[274,347] however, in babies who have severe RDS even after surfactant, increasing PEEP up to 5 cmH$_2$O may result in a useful increase in lung volume.[189] Infants ventilated beyond the first week without cystic CLD have improved oxygenation at 6 cmH$_2$O.[347]

Mean airway pressure: There is a good correlation between the MAP level and oxygenation,[91,414] such that PaO_2 may be improved by increasing the inspiratory time, the level of PEEP or the peak inflating pressure, all three manoeuvres elevating MAP. Elevation of the PEEP level is the most effective method of increasing lung volume and hence oxygenation. At a critical level, determined by the infant's lung function, further elevation of the MAP level can impair oxygenation. The MAP level can be calculated from various formulae, but they assume a square-wave inflating pressure and therefore overestimate the MAP. Such calculations are now rarely necessary as the MAP level is displayed on virtually all the currently available ventilators.

Ventilator rates: Historically, babies with RDS were ventilated at a ventilator rate that matched their respiratory rate, about 80–100/min, but this resulted in a high incidence of BPD.[741] Studies[89,414,738] then showed that if an I:E ratio of 1:2 was used, the PaO_2 was higher at ventilator rates of 30/min compared with 80/min. At a rate of 30/min, the PaO_2 was found to be higher if the inspiratory time was longer than the expiratory time (a reverse I:E ratio) and 5 cmH$_2$O of PEEP was employed. Those data were restricted to neonates with severe RDS. Nevertheless, by the late 1970s, ventilator rates of 20–40/min with long inspiratory times were being widely used in infants with all types of lung disease, with an incidence of pneumothorax and other forms of airleak of 35–40% (pp. 487–96). Subsequently, faster rates were preferred. Heicher et al[407] found that they could ventilate babies at 60/min with inspiratory times of 0.5 seconds at lower peak inspiratory pressures and with better blood gases and fewer pneumothoraces than when rates of 30/min and inspiratory times of 1 second were used. Subsequently, Greenough et al[362] showed that when babies with RDS were kept at the same MAP, rates of 120/min produced an improvement in PaO_2 compared with rates of 30 and 60/min (Fig. 27.43). This improvement resulted from the neonates breathing in synchrony with the ventilator. By increasing the ventilator rate to 75–100/min, most neonates were induced to breathe in synchrony[359,837] and thus had better blood gases,[362] but whether synchrony decreased the pneumothorax rate was not investigated. In paralysed infants, however, it was important to reduce the ventilator rate to 60/min or less, to reduce the likelihood of gas trapping.[425]

Inspiratory and expiratory times, inspiratory–expiratory ratios: In the 1970s' studies, when rates of 20–40/min were being used, inspiratory to expiratory ratios of 2:1 or even 3:1 were applied, giving inspiratory times as long as 1.5 seconds. This increased the MAP and improved oxygenation, but the reverse I:E ratio, with a concomitant prolongation of the inflation time, was one of the factors which correlated with the high pneumothorax rate.[721,866] Subsequently, the average inspiratory and expiratory times in ventilated babies with RDS were demonstrated to be 0.31 seconds (SD 0.06 s) and 0.42 seconds (SD 0.13 s), respectively,[838] i.e. an I:E ratio of approximately 1:1.3. Employment of such a ratio with an appropriate rate for gestational age[353] resulted in many babies with RDS breathing in synchrony with the ventilator, with an attendant improvement in oxygenation. Similar studies have not been undertaken in very immature infants with mild

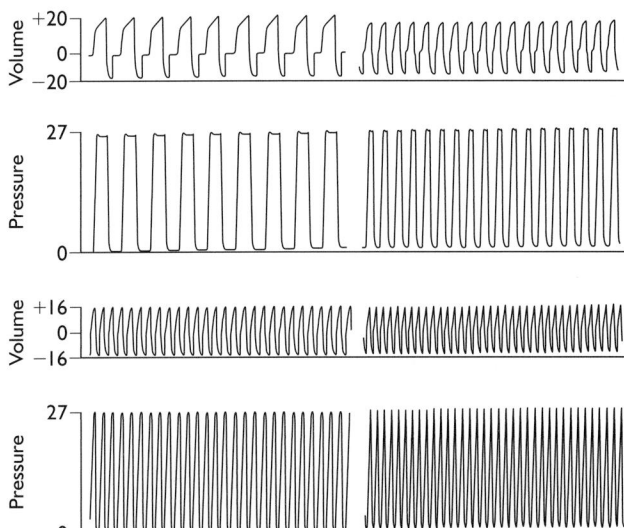

Fig. 27.43 Changes in airway pressure waveform and delivered volume as frequency increases. In each of the four recordings, the upper trace is the volume trace (inflation upwards, deflation downwards) and the lower trace is the airway pressure recording. A Sechrist ventilator was used: flow 10/min; peak pressure 30 cmH$_2$O; PEEP 3 cmH$_2$O; I:E 1:1. The ventilator rates are: upper right 30/min; upper left 60/min; lower right 90/min; lower left 120/min.

lung disease who have received both antenatal steroids and postnatal surfactant therapy; but it is likely that such infants, if they have vigorous respiratory efforts, would be best ventilated with a physiological I:E ratio (i.e. a longer expiratory to inspiratory time) and a rate similar to their spontaneous respiratory frequency.

An I:E ratio of 1:1 results in best gas exchange for babies ventilated beyond the first week after birth.[131] Increasing the ventilator rate above 60/min offers no advantage in such babies.

Problems with pressure-limited ventilators

The ventilators currently available may fail to maintain tidal volume at fast rates (>80–100/min) and short inflation times. This results from a failure to achieve the peak inflating pressure, to maintain a positive pressure plateau and/or the development of inadvertent PEEP.[221] The resultant reduction in minute volume and MAP results in a fall in PaO_2 and a rise in $PaCO_2$, which can be overcome only by increasing the gas flow to make the waveform more square or by increasing the peak inflating pressure.

Ventilator settings with pressure-limited ventilators (Table 27.10)

Babies with abnormal lungs
Initially guided by the baby's colour and chest expansion, the following initial ventilator settings are appropriate, providing the chest wall moves adequately, until the result of blood gas analyses are available (Table 27.11).

Pressure:	16–18/3 cmH$_2$O
Rate:	60/min
Inspiratory time:	0.3–0.4 s
Oxygen concentration:	60–80%

Table 27.10 Adjustments to conventional ventilation according to disease

Respiratory disease	Ventilatory settings
RDS	Low PEEP
	Rates 60–80/min
MAS	Low PEEP
	Long expiratory time
Pulmonary hypoplasia	Low PEEP
Pulmonary airleak	Minimise PIP
Pulmonary haemorrhage	High PEEP
Pulmonary oedema	Long inspiratory times

Table 27.11 Adjustments to ventilator settings on the basis of blood gas changes

Low PaO_2	High $PaCO_2$	Increase peak pressure, which will also increase mean airway pressure: in spontaneously breathing babies ↑ rates may also work.
Low PaO_2	Normal $PaCO_2$	↑ F_IO_2; ↑MAP but maintain PIP (i.e. ↑ PEEP or ↑ T_I)
Low PaO_2	Low $PaCO_2$	Consider alternative diagnosis, e.g. PPHN, sepsis, overventilation. ↑ F_IO_2; ↑ MAP; use vasodilators.
PaO_2 normal	High $PaCO_2$	↓ PEEP, ↑ rate; keep MAP constant.
PaO_2 normal	Low $PaCO_2$	↓ rate: maintain MAP.
PaO_2 high	$PaCO_2$ high	Rare: check for mechanical problems, e.g. blocked tube, ↓ PEEP, ↓ T_I: ↑ rate ↓ F_IO_2
PaO_2 high	$PaCO_2$ normal	↓ MAP (usually ↓ PIP): ↓ F_IO_2
PaO_2 high	$PaCO_2$ low	↓ pressure, ↓ rate, ↓ F_IO_2 (see text)
PaO_2 normal	$PaCO_2$ normal	Sit tight! Unless plan to wean.

Babies with normal lungs

For babies with primary neurological or myopathic problems, e.g. congenital myopathy (pp. 1183–5), fractured cervical spine (p. 259), severe neurological depression due to birth asphyxia (pp. 224–5), drugs (p. 576), or preterm babies with recurrent apnoea (pp. 573–7), the initial ventilator settings should be:

Pressure:	15/3 cmH$_2$O
Rate:	20–30/min
Inspiratory time:	0.35–0.40 s
Oxygen concentration:	21–30%

Volume-set, time-limited ventilation

These ventilators deliver a predetermined tidal volume, irrespective of the pressure necessary to achieve that volume. The volume delivered is detemined by the inflation time, flow, pressure limit, and patient compliance and resistance.

Randomised trials of volume-controlled ventilation (VCV) have suggested that it has advantages over pressure-controlled ventilation. VCV was associated with less hypotension and severe intracerebral haemorrhage in one trial[710] and a shorter duration of ventilation in another.[816]

The main problem with volume ventilation is that not all the tidal volume is delivered to the baby's lungs, as with the onset of inflation, the pressure rises, compressing the gas in the ventilator circuit as well as in the baby. Furthermore, unless cuffed ETTs are used, as the pressure rises, there is a variable leak of gas around the ETT. As a consequence, the volume required to ventilate the baby cannot be calculated with accuracy.

Patient-triggered ventilation

PTV is a mode in which the patient's inspiratory efforts 'trigger' positive pressure inflations.

Assist/control and synchronous intermittent mandatory ventilation

The initial triggered ventilation modes used in the 1980s were assist/control (A/C) or synchronous intermittent positive pressure ventilation (SIPPV), during which all of the infant's respiratory efforts could trigger positive pressure inflations, and SIMV, during which the maximum number of breaths that could be triggered was determined by the preset SIMV rate.

Early attempts at A/C or SIMV were with modified conventional ventilators. Devices were developed to detect inspiratory activity in a variety of ways, including changes in abdominal expansion by a body movement sensor (Graseby capsule),[621] oesophageal pressure,[350] airflow,[361] airway pressure[423] and impedance.[915] If a critical change in inspiratory activity was detected by any of these methods, the inspiratory control was triggered. The subsequently produced purpose-built ventilators have trigger sensors with improved function compared with the early devices. The function of the triggering systems can be evaluated by their susceptibility to autotrigger, their sensitivity (the number of the baby's inspiratory efforts that are detected) and their trigger delay or response time (the delay between the sensor being activated and the ventilator inflating the baby). Auto-triggering occurs if there is excessive condensation in the ventilator circuit, which can cause changes in flow or pressure, and if there is a large leak around the ETT, when there will be detectable flows in expiration. There have been many studies comparing triggering devices, but the majority have been performed on relatively mature infants with RDS. A further limitation is that different triggering systems have been compared with different ventilators and thus it is not possible to determine if the results seen are explained by differences in the function of the ventilators, triggering systems or both. Use of a single ventilator type has allowed comparison of an airflow and airway pressure trigger and demonstrated that the former functioned better in very immature infants.[226] All triggering systems, however, perform less well in very immature infants.

During A/C or SIMV, it is important to limit the ventilator inflation time, otherwise it may extend into the spontaneous expiration of the baby, resulting in asynchrony or even active expiration.[423] In addition, a prolonged inflation time has been shown to reduce the triggering rate by stimulation of the Hering–Breuer reflex.[893] If, however, the inflation time is too short (<0.2 s), the volume delivered by the ventilator is compromised.[223,275] The optimum inflation time, therefore, appears to between 0.2 and 0.4 seconds.

Clinical studies

A/C or SIMV, compared with conventional ventilation, in a series of physiological studies were associated with a lower rate of asynchrony,[68] higher tidal volume and improved blood gases;[153] additional advantages were reduced fluctuations of both BP[446] and cerebral blood flow velocity.[343] Those findings would suggest that triggered ventilation might reduce the incidence of BPD or severe ICH. Meta-analysis[348] of the results of six randomised trials, however, demonstrated that the only advantage of A/C or SIMV was a significantly shorter duration of ventilation, the incidences of BPD, severe ICH and airleaks and the mortality rate being similar. No significant excess of adverse effects were demonstrated,[356] but in the largest trial,[50] a greater proportion of infants departed from their randomised mode on the A/C arm and there was a trend for more of the immature infants supported by A/C to have airleaks. In that trial,[50] however, a variety of ventilators were used, which may have influenced the outcome;[223] in addition, an airway pressure trigger, which performs less well than an airflow trigger in very immature infants,[226] was used for the majority of babies in the A/C arm. Nevertheless, on current evidence, use of A/C or SIMV cannot be recommended for infants with RDS. A/C, however, is useful in infants recovering from RDS; in a randomised trial it was shown to significantly shorten the duration of weaning.[127]

There have been no randomised comparisons of A/C and SIMV in RDS, but the results of three randomised trials suggest that A/C rather than SIMV is the more efficacious weaning mode.[128,130,228] Weaning involving reducing the SIMV rate below 20/min, compared with reduction in the peak inflating pressures during A/C, was associated with a significantly longer duration of weaning (pp. 532–5).

Pressure support ventilation

During PSV, the patient's inspiratory effort triggers the onset of a positive pressure inflation and the end of the spontaneous inspiration dictates the termination of the inflation. PSV has been demonstrated[235] to reduce the asynchrony rate; it is important to determine whether this translates into a lower incidence of airleak.

Volume guarantee (VG)

In this mode, the peak inflating pressure is servo-controlled so that a preset volume is delivered during triggered ventilation (A/C, SIMV, PSV). Adequate gas exchange can be achieved at lower MAPs when VG is instituted,[138] probably because the baby makes a greater contribution to minute ventilation.[416] It seems likely that use of VG may be particularly advantageous during weaning.

Proportional assist ventilation (PAV)

During PAV, the applied ventilator pressure is servo-controlled throughout each respiratory cycle, based on a continuous input from the patient, such that the baby controls the timing, depth and airflow contour of the entire ventilator breath. In addition, negative ventilator resistance and elastance can be applied (unloading), to relieve the resistive and elastic work of breathing, respectively. The clinician sets the level of unloading and this enhances the effect of respiratory muscle effort.

During PAV, it is essential that there is adequate backup ventilation should the baby develop hypoventilation or apnoea. Other possible adverse effects include excessive resistive and elastic unloading, which result, respectively, in resonant oscillations and runaway ventilator pressures.[788] It is also important to avoid using PAV with a major leak around the ETT, as the leak-flow mimics inspiration and hence may cause the ventilator to repeatedly deliver inflations to the set upper pressure limit.

Clinical studies

In preterm infants, PAV compared with A/C and IMV, in a short-term physiological study,[787] allowed adequate gas exchange at lower MAPs. It is important to determine if PAV offers long-term advantages over other modes of ventilation in appropriately designed trials.

High-frequency jet ventilation

HFJV is a modification of the technique initially developed to provide respiratory support during bronchoscopy. Frequencies between 60 and 600/min may be used. During HFJV, a high-pressure source delivers gas in short bursts down a small-bore injector cannula, the tip of the cannula usually lying within the ETT, pointing towards the lung.[306] The bursts of gas entrain additional gas from areas surrounding the jet cannula down the ETT; expiration is passive. In most studies, rates of 100–200/min have been used. In an animal model,[934] a relatively narrow range of inspiratory and expiratory times was demonstrated to provide optimum HFJV. A significantly higher airway pressure gradient is necessary to maintain a constant tidal volume if the inspiratory time is shortened, and reduction in expiratory time below 170 ms results in air trapping. Most jet ventilators operate like constant-flow time-cycled ventilators, and the pressure waveform is typically triangular, although pressure servo-controlled jet ventilators are available and produce a square pressure waveform. Keszler & Durand[504] have described jet ventilators in detail. On HFJV, the PEEP is increased to optimise lung volume and a background IMV rate of 2–5/min employed to open up the alveoli on inspiration.[504] During weaning, it is also important to maintain lung volume; thus, as with HFO, the F_1O_2 is reduced before the MAP.

Clinical studies

HFJV has been used as a rescue mode of support to improve blood gas tensions in infants with respiratory failure unresponsive to conventional ventilation;[716] adequate blood gas tensions were achieved with lower peak inflation pressures.[115] It was also used with good results in babies with airleaks, in particular bronchopleural fistulae,[90,336] PPHN[114] and diaphragmatic hernia.[90] The results of randomised trials, however, have been conflicting. In a small trial of 42 infants, no improvement in outcome with HFJV was demonstrated,[116] and in another study,[257] although oxygenation improved in infants with PPHN, no long-term benefits were ascribed to HFJV use. Keszler et al reported two positive trials:[503,505] HFJV use was associated in the first[503] with more rapid resolution of PIE, and in the second[505] with a reduction in the incidence of BPD at 36 weeks and need for home oxygen. Another trial,[954] however, was halted for safety reasons, as infants exposed to HFJV as opposed to conventional mechanical ventilation (CMV) had higher rates of severe ICH (41% vs 22%) and PVL (31% vs 6%). Nevertheless, meta-analysis of three trials demonstrated that HFJV use was associated with a significant reduction in BPD, but a non-significant trend towards an increase in PVL.[71]

Complications

HFJV use has been associated with a high incidence of necrotising tracheobronchitis,[604] an ischaemic lesion resulting from intraluminal tracheal pressure compromising mucosal and submucosal blood flow. In HFJV, the lesions range from moderate erythema of the airway to severe necrotising tracheobronchitis with total tracheal obstruction.[90] The high mean pressure and near-constant intraluminal pressure may be important factors in the pathogenesis of this problem.[215] Not all workers find a high incidence, perhaps because of meticulous humidification,[116] but others have reported that HFJV causes more tracheal damage than IPPV[591,679] and that the longer the technique is applied, the more likely that necrotising tracheobronchitis will develop.[90,292]

High-frequency flow interrupters

High-frequency flow interrupters (HFFIs) deliver small volumes of gas at high frequencies. A high-pressure gas source fed into a CPAP circuit immediately opposite the ETT connector is interupted. These devices can be used at frequencies of up to 20 Hz (1200/min).

Clinical studies

HFFI use has been associated with improvements in blood gases in babies with PIE, and radiological resolution of the PIE.[300,320] No long-term benefits of HFFI have been reported from randomised trials.[178,693]

Complications

Unlike HFOV (see below), neither HFJV nor HFFI incorporates an active expiratory phase and thus gas trapping may be experienced, particularly at fast frequencies. Tracheal necrosis has been experienced with HFFI.

High-frequency oscillatory ventilation

During HFOV, frequencies between 180 and 3000/min (3–50 Hz) may be used; however, in practice, frequencies of 10–15 Hz are most commonly employed. Unlike other forms of respiratory

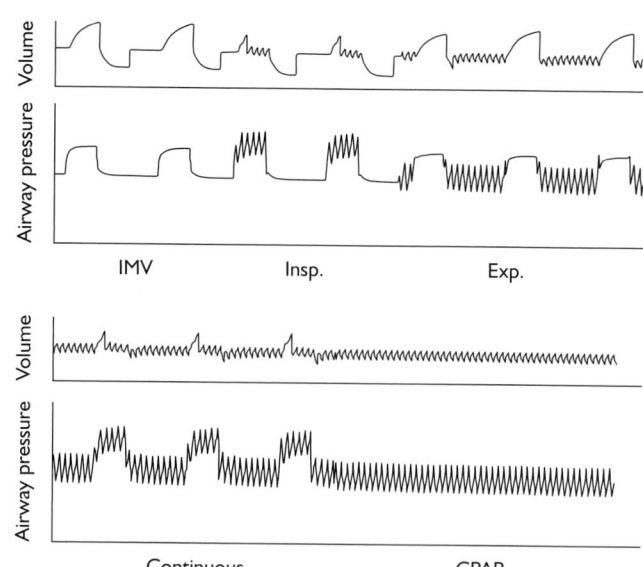

Fig. 27.44 High-frequency oscillatory ventilation with conventional ventilation. The upper trace demonstrates intermittent mandatory ventilation (IMV), then a combination of IMV plus oscillation on the positive pressure plateau (Insp.) and on the right-hand part of the trace IMV plus oscillation on the expiratory pressure (Exp.). The lower two traces demonstrate oscillation throughout the ventilation cycle (continuous) and on top of constant mean airway pressure (CPAP). (Reproduced from Laubscher et al.[543])

support, there is an active expiratory phase as well as an active inspiratory phase; this means that gas trapping is unlikely, even though very fast frequencies are employed. During HFOV, a volume generator feeds into a CPAP circuit close to the patient. The generator can be a piston, bellows or a loudspeaker driven by a generator and audio amplifier. Continuous flow is necessary to add fresh gas to the circuit and remove expired gas. HFOV may also be given at the same time as conventional ventilation[646] (Fig. 27.44), but there are no data to suggest such an approach has long-term benefit. HFOV can also be applied externally by means of a thoracoabdominal chamber connected to a vacuum source and a high-frequency oscillator.[403]

During HFOV, two volume strategies have been pursued: a low-volume strategy, in which MAP is limited with the aim of preventing damage due to barotrauma, and a high-volume strategy, in which MAP is elevated to promote optimum alveolar expansion and hence improve oxygenation. Comparison of the two strategies in animal models demonstrated that the high-volume strategy is less damaging to the lungs.[590] Volume delivery during HFOV is proportional to the product of the frequency and the square of the oscillatory amplitude.[823] Early studies suggested that HFOV provided a tidal exchange considerably less than the baby's anatomical dead space.[306] It was suggested that gas exchange occurred additionally by mechanisms distinct from those operating during conventional ventilation; these included bulk flow by convection, convective mixing between lung units (Pendelluft) and augmented diffusion.[136] It has more recently been demonstrated that infants are oscillated at a tidal volume similar to their anatomical dead space.[232]

Management during HFOV

Oxygenation is influenced by the inspired oxygen concentration and the MAP, the latter controlling lung volume. If a high-volume strategy is used as a rescue support, then the infants should be transferred to HFOV at a MAP 2 cmH$_2$O higher than that on CMV.[129] The MAP is then gradually increased to optimise oxygenation. Infants with severe respiratory failure on conventional ventilation often have very low lung volumes and an increase in MAP on HFOV of up to 10 cmH$_2$O may be necessary to maximise oxygenation.[222] The optimum MAP and the change in MAP necessary to optimise oxygenation are dependent on the severity of the infant's lung disease and his lung volume. If too high a level of MAP is used, this will result in lung overdistension and deterioration in blood gases. It is thus important to increase the MAP in incremental stages, leaving sufficient time at each step for the lung volume to equilibrate; this usually happens within 10 minutes, but may take up to 20 minutes.[872] Continuous monitoring of oxygenation should be employed; in an infant with atelectasis this will demonstrate an improvement in oxygenation when the MAP is increased. The MAP should then only be further increased once the monitoring demonstrates no further change in oxygenation, i.e. the lung volume has stabilised; such an approach will minimise the risk of overdistension.

Carbon dioxide elimination is dependent on the delivered volume, which is influenced primarily by the oscillatory amplitude but also by the frequency and I:E ratio. On commencing HFOV, the oscillatory amplitude is increased until chest wall vibration is apparent, and then adjusted as needed to correct hypocapnia or hypercapnia. If an oscillator capable of delivering a constant volume is employed, oscillating at the resonant frequency of the respiratory system in RDS (between 12 and 24 Hz, 720–1440/min) is associated with an increased volume delivery to the infant.[439] The resonant frequency of the respiratory system in preterm infants with RDS remains remarkably constant in the early stages of their illness, despite large changes in static compliance.[551] Unfortunately, this does not apply to the majority of commercially available oscillators, whose performance is impaired at increased frequencies.[543] Thus, altering the frequency from 10 to 15 Hz using such oscillators has very little impact on carbon dioxide elimination.[132] Reducing the frequency below 10 Hz, particularly with the Sensor Medics oscillator, however, results in a greater volume delivery[543] and thus this manoeuvre can be very useful to improve carbon dioxide elimination in a mature infant with severe respiratory failure. Increasing the I:E ratio from 1:2 to 1:1 on the Sensor Medics increases the delivered volume and hence carbon dioxide elimination[234] and has not been associated with gas trapping in infants with respiratory failure.[9]

HFOV in animals suppresses spontaneous respiration; although this in part is explained by changes in blood gas tensions, this effect also appears to be related to stimulation of pulmonary mechanoreceptors; vagal fibres are stimulated continuously and to a greater extent during HFOV than with static lung inflation.[605] In humans, however, spontaneous respiration is reduced, but not usually inhibited;[133] however, this rarely interferes with the effectiveness of respiratory support.[133,419] Hence, we do not recommend routine neuromuscular blockade for infants supported by HFOV.

Early versus selective, delayed surfactant administration resulted in a better outcome for infants supported by high-volume strategy HFOV.[712] In a randomised trial involving 43 infants, a smaller proportion of infants given early rather than delayed surfactant suffered the combined outcome of death or supplementary oxygen requirement at 36 weeks' PCA (29% vs 64%) or had had an ICH (43% vs 82%).[712]

Clinical studies

There have been many anecdotal reports of benefit using HFOV[611] in babies with severe RDS,[134] hypoplastic lungs, pneumonia, PPHN,[94] PIE[149] and diaphragmatic hernia.[483] Use of HFOV enabled blood gas tensions to be maintained, with a lowering of MAP and resolution of PIE,[149] and may be applied only to the affected side if selective intubation is employed.[737] Severe lobar emphysema may resolve on HFOV if a low-volume strategy is pursued.[525] HFOV, however, is not a successful form of rescue respiratory support in all babies. Failure to improve oxygenation after 6 hours of treatment identifies those babies most likely to die[134,692] or survive with disability.[141]

There have been two randomised trials of HFOV in infants with severe respiratory failure. In term-born infants,[150] HFOV was a more effective rescue support than CMV, but there were no significant differences in the requirement for ECMO or duration of ventilator or oxygen dependency between the two groups. In preterm infants,[420] use of HFOV was associated with a significant reduction in new pulmonary airleak (RR 0.73, 95% CI 0.55–0.96), but a significant increase in ICH (RR 1.77, 95% CI 1.06–2.96).

There have now been at least ten randomised prophylactic trials in which infants have been randomised to receive HFOV or CMV in the first 24 hours after birth. The trials have differed with respect to administration of antenatal corticosteroids and postnatal surfactant, and the types of oscillator and conventional ventilator used. Meta-analysis of the results of those trials[411] has demonstrated that HFOV had no significant effect on mortality, but was associated with a modest reduction in BPD in survivors at term (number needed to treat [NNT] 17).

Complications

In an initial prospective randomised study,[419] prophylactic use of HFOV in infants of birthweight between 750 g and 2000 g with respiratory failure due to RDS, pneumonia or PPHN was associated, worryingly, with a significant increase in the incidence of complicated GMH-IVH. The study design, however, has been criticised, as, in particular, a low-volume strategy was pursued. In a more recently reported trial,[638] even though a high-volume strategy was used, a trend towards an increase in severe ICH was also noted, although this did not reach statistical significance when adjusted for differences in pregnancy-related hypertension rates between the two groups. Meta-analysis of the results of ten prophylactic studies,[411] however, did not find a statistically significant effect overall on short-term neurological abnormality and no significant excess of ICH or PVL was noted in the HFOV arm of the largest trial to date which only included very immature infants.[473]

During HFOV, very effective carbon dioxide elimination can be achieved. Rapid, large changes in carbon dioxide tensions can occur and are associated with changes in cerebral blood flow velocity.[489] In a case–control study,[224] rescue HFOV was associated with worse neurodevelopmental status at 2 years; this adverse outcome was commoner in very immature babies and could not be predicted by their initial response to HFOV.

Extracorporeal membrane oxygenation

ECMO, a form of cardiopulmonary bypass, provides a method of gas exchange in patients with respiratory failure without resorting to damaging patterns of ventilatory support and allows the lungs a chance to recover. ECMO has been used as a method of respiratory support in newborns suffering from RDS, MAS, sepsis, primary PPHN, congenital heart disease and diaphragmatic hernia. Introduction of the new techniques of respiratory support for term infants has been associated with a reduction in the number of infants being referred for ECMO.[422] A greater proportion of infants now receive HFOV, iNO and/or surfactant prior to being referred for ECMO. Delay in the institution of ECMO in infants with severe MAS, however, has been associated with longer post-ECMO ventilation and a higher mortality rate.[329] Delay in referral may reflect an inappropriately pessimistic view of the survival rate of MAS infants supported by ECMO.[923] Early discussion with an ECMO centre is advocated to ensure appropriate timing of referral and it has been recommended that ECMO be thought of as an extension of conventional treatment in severe MAS, rather than as a last resort.[203]

Criteria for instituting ECMO
These have included:[22,45,56,574]

- severe but reversible cardiac or pulmonary disease unresponsive to optimal ventilation and pharmacological therapy; there should be no ventilator-induced damage or CLD and the baby must have had less than 10 days of aggressive IPPV;
- estimated mortality risk greater than 80%; an oxygen index (OI, MAP $\times F_1O_2/PaO_2$ postductal $\times$ 100) greater than 40, historically had been associated with >90% mortality, but in the UK ECMO trial,[891,892] an OI >40 was associated with a 41% mortality rate;
- birthweight >2.0 kg;
- gestational age greater than 34 weeks;
- no bleeding disorder;
- absence of prolonged perinatal hypoxic ischaemia predicted to produce brain damage;
- no chromosomal or congenital abnormality incompatible with quality of life.

Technique
Cannulation for ECMO is either venoarterial (VA) or venovenous (VV).[21] Venous blood is usually drained from the right jugular vein; oxygen is then added and carbon dioxide removed by the membrane lung; oxygenated blood is then returned to the patient. For VA bypass, the right common carotid artery and right internal jugular vein are used. Approximately 80% cardiopulmonary bypass is achieved and the level of respiratory support can be reduced, limiting further barotrauma. In VV bypass, oxygenated blood is returned via the right femoral vein or umbilical vein and the carotid artery spared. VV ECMO can also be undertaken through a double-lumen catheter. A disadvantage of VV ECMO is that cardiopulmonary bypass is not attained and thus the infant must have good myocardial function. There have been no head-to-head trials comparing VA and VV ECMO, but data from the ELSO registry suggest that mortality may be lower with VV ECMO (8.5% vs 16.2%).[319]

Total respiratory support is provided by an extracorporeal blood flow of approximately 100 ml/kg/min, increasing up to 120 ml/kg/min.[45,574] To allow the lung to rest, during VA ECMO, inspired oxygen concentrations of 21–40% and ventilator rates of 10–20/min at pressures of 16–20 cmH$_2$O are used. In both VA and VV ECMO, venous blood is pumped to an oxygenator, which has blood and gas compartments separated by a semipermeable membrane, where diffusion of oxygen and carbon dioxide occurs. Oxygen transfer is controlled by the membrane's surface area, pump flow and the degree of saturation of the venous blood. Carbon dioxide elimination is adjusted by altering the flow rate. Infants are heparinised to achieve whole-blood activated clotting times (ACT) two to three times normal (an ACT of 160–200 s). Haematocrit and platelet count are maintained with transfusion of saline-washed, packed red blood cells and platelet concentrates as necessary.

When the baby starts to improve, as indicated by improving oxygenation, the ECMO circuit flow is gradually reduced to 50 ml/min. When stable vital signs, adequate urine output and acceptable arterial blood gases are achieved on this minimal flow for 4–5 hours, the ECMO cannulae are clamped, and the baby excluded from the ECMO circuit, which can be restarted if necessary.

Results
An initial randomised controlled study[46] was analysed by a statistical method called 'play the winner'. In that study, although ECMO was associated with a significant improvement in survival rate, only one of the 12 infants entered into the study was randomised to conventional therapy. O'Rourke et al[682] abandoned their prospective trial when four out of ten conventionally treated babies had died, compared with none of nine treated with ECMO (p = 0.054). A multicentre UK trial involving 185 infants was then performed and demonstrated that, compared with CMV, ECMO reduced mortality by 50% in infants with PPHN or MAS.[891]

More than 18 000 neonates have been reported to the ELSO registry as receiving ECMO, with survival rates of 86% in infants with respiratory disorders and 56% in infants with cardiac disorders. Survival rates are highest in infants with MAS (90%), are only 50% in CDH infants but are 76% in CLD infants[418] (Table 27.12).

Complications
Local vascular complications occur, including haemorrhage, vessel thrombosis and problems with wound healing. The babies can suffer from anaemia and thrombocytopenia as the result of consumption of blood products at the oxygenator's membrane surface. Mechanical problems occur in up to 20% of patients.

Table 27.12 Survival related to disease of the first 7647 infants reported to the ELSO registry. (From Kanto[479] with permission)

Diagnosis	Survival rate
Meconium aspiration syndrome	93
Severe respiratory distress syndrome	83
Persistent pulmonary hypertension of the newborn	83
Sepsis	77
Congenital diaphragmatic hernia	59

Sequelae

The results of anecdotal follow-up studies need to be interpreted with caution, as the infants were extremely ill prior to receiving ECMO and their original illness may be at least partially responsible for any chronic morbidity. Follow-up at 1 year of infants entered into the UK multicentre randomised trial did not demonstrate any excess of severe disability. At 4 years of age, one in four survivors had evidence of impairment with or without disability; the ECMO group had higher survival rates.[63]

There have been few studies reported on the long-term respiratory status of ECMO survivors. Short et al[810] found a 15% prevalence of BPD, the risk factors being culture-proven streptococcal sepsis and late placement (7–8 days of age) on ECMO. Other risk factors for BPD are lung hypoplasia and failure to respond to a trial of HFOV.[789] Comparison of non-randomised infants suggested that conventionally treated patients, compared with those supported by ECMO with similar illness severity, have a higher rate of BPD.[924] Examination at 1 year of 77 infants from the UK randomised trial demonstrated that the ECMO-treated infants had slightly better lung function, with higher inspiratory conductance and $V_{max}FRC$.[53]

Liquid ventilation

Liquid ventilation[147] is performed using perfluorocarbons (PFCs), which have a low surface tension (25% of that of water) and a high solubility for respiratory gases, particularly oxygen. PFCs contain carbon and fluorine bonds, which are extremely strong, making them pharmacologically and chemically inert; in addition, they are radio-opaque.

Liquid ventilation may be total (TLV), in which the PFC is pre-oxygenated and warmed as it is circulated to fill the lungs to the expected FRC.[426] The PFC is then moved backwards and forwards at a relatively slow rate and high tidal volume because of the high viscosity of PFC.[426] TLV requires different circuitry than used in current clinical practice. Partial liquid ventilation (PLV) or perfluorocarbon-associated gas exchange (PAGE) has been used to support patients. During PLV, PFC again fills the lungs to FRC, but the patient is then gas ventilated 'on top'. If no further PFC is given, the PFC in the lung simply evaporates away. Throughout the period of PLV, usually less than 7 days, the PFC is topped up via a side port in the ETT so that a meniscus remains visible there.[428,546]

In animal models, liquid, as compared with gas, ventilation has been demonstrated to reduce ventilation–perfusion mismatch and improve compliance and oxygenation.[888] It also appears to be a less damaging form of respiratory support, particularly in very immature animals.[426,958] It is compatible both with NO[943] and surfactant.[548] Indeed, it appears to have several advantages over surfactant therapy, as it is not inactivated by proteins and has better spreading capability.[548]

Clinical studies

Experience to date is limited to small series, the majority of patients receiving PLV while on ECMO. Under such circumstances, in adults,[428] children and neonates,[364,372,546] PLV has been demonstrated to improve oxygenation and compliance. PLV has also improved oxygenation in premature infants with severe respiratory failure.[547] It has been suggested that PLV can enhance pulmonary function[718] and that lung growth can apparently be induced by distension of the lung with perfluorocarbon in neonates with CDH.[427] In a small randomised trial, however, no statistically significant differences in the number of ventilator-free days or survival rate were found between CDH infants supported by ECMO who did or did not additionally receive PLV.[427]

Care of babies on ventilators

Intubation

The technique of intubating babies and the choice of tubes is described on pages 1256–8. Intubating small, sick babies can be difficult, babies becoming hypoxaemic, acidaemic and bradycardic during the procedure. During intubation, stress hormones are released,[552,811] BP and ICP rise,[728] and this, together with the blood gas changes, predisposes the neonate to GMH/IVH (pp. 1150–9).[305,501,615] For this reason, it was recommended[501] that intubation should only be carried out once the infant had received pancuronium and atropine, as this mitigated the adverse physiological changes. Atropine abolishes the bradycardia and muscle relaxants attenuate the rise in ICP. In addition, use of suxamethonium, a rapidly acting muscle relaxant, shortens the duration of intubation and hence reduces the duration of hypoxaemia that commonly occurs during intubation. Suxamethonium should, however, be given with a vagolytic drug to pre-empt the potential profound bradycardia that can occur with its administration. Sedation analgesia should also be administered with the muscle relaxant. Morphine commonly has been used, often on its own,[940] but fentanyl and alfentanil have a more rapid onset and shorter duration of action. Fentanyl can cause chest wall rigidity, but this resolves promptly with administration of suxamethonium and can be minimised by slow bolus administration.

Type of endotracheal tube

Straight or shouldered, but not cuffed, ETTs are used in neonates. Shouldered tubes, because of their greater width at the mouth, may be easier to fix, but there is no evidence from randomised trials that either type of tube is associated with a lower incidence of subglottic stenosis. Nevertheless, care should be taken to ensure that the shouldered part of the tube does not impact onto the cricoid ring, as this could lead to pressure necrosis in the subglottic region; this can be avoided by checking on the CXR that the position of the tip of the tube is at or above the level of the clavicles. It should be remembered, however, that neck position affects the position of the tip of the ETT; the tube tip moves caudally with neck flexion and cephaladly with extension.[761] An advantage of using a shouldered (Coles) tube is that its resistance is approximately 50% lower than that of a straight tube with the same internal diameter as the narrow part of the shouldered tube;[607] the resistance of the ETT adds to the inspiratory work of breathing.

It is important to use an appropriate-sized tube. If too small a tube is used, suctioning becomes difficult. In addition, if there is a large leak around the tube, high peak inflating pressures cannot be achieved. Tube size also influences the inspiratory and expiratory resistance; the calculated mean difference in expiratory resistance between tubes of 2.5 mm and 3.5 mm internal diameter was 93 cmH$_2$O.[271] Shortening an ETT to an appropriate length also reduces its resistance.

Changing an oral ETT used for labour ward resuscitation to a nasal ETT on a routine basis is not necessary. There is no evidence that nasal tubes are superior to oral tubes for routine use.[596] Nasal ETTs can be easily fixed at the nose, which might reduce laryngeal trauma, but ulceration and excoriation of the nostrils can occur. Oral tubes are generally thought to be easier to insert, but infants may suck on an oral ETT and at follow-up, high palatal arches, pressure-induced grooves and even clefts in the palate have been described.

Humidification

Inadequate warming and humidification of inspired gases will cool the baby and lead to dehydration of the bronchial secretions with airway plugging and obstruction of the ETT. The gas from the ventilator should reach the ETT adequately warmed and humidified. The British Standards Institution[97] recommend that the minimal accepted humidity is 33 mgH$_2$O per litre inspired gas, which is 75% of that obtained during normal breathing.

Fixation

Many techniques for immobilising ETTs have been described; these include purpose-made devices such as a flange sewn to the ETT and then tied to either side of a bonnet or simply using adhesive tape stuck around the tube and then to the infant's face. It is important to use a system which minimises accidental extubation and avoids causing cosmetic deformity (p. 1259).

Suctioning

Suctioning can cause bradycardia, hypoxia, bacteraemia and pneumothorax, and an increase in cerebral blood flow and ICP but a fall in cerebral oxygenation,[647,699,814,822,865] though these effects are less in the paralysed baby.[268] The technique of ETT suction must allow oxygen administration throughout the procedure, and if the baby becomes bradycardic or the tcPO$_2$, continuous PaO_2 monitoring or oximetry demonstrates the oxygenation to have fallen below 6 kPa or the SpO$_2$ below 80%, suction should be discontinued and the infant reconnected to the ventilator.

Inserting the suction catheter until a resistance is felt (when the catheter hits the carina) should be avoided (p. 504). The suction tube should only be inserted far enough to reach just beyond the tip of the ETT.[31]

As a prelude to suction, a small amount of water or saline is often put down the ETT. Both of these may damage the lungs and/or the surfactant system,[536] particularly if the fluid is not adequately warmed.[472] If some form of lubrication is deemed essential to enable the suction catheter to pass down the ETT, the smallest amount of fluid necessary, probably 0.3–0.5 ml, should be used.

Endotracheal suctioning during the acute respiratory illness should be minimised and tailored to the need of the individual neonate. There is no evidence that suctioning is needed more often than every 12 hours in the routine care of babies ventilated for RDS.[948]

Complications of intubation

The mucosa of the larynx and trachea shows deciliation, necrosis and desquamation within hours of intubation[318,474] and metaplastic change in the trachea occurs.[730] Nevertheless, remarkably few long-term sequelae are seen. Many neonates have some hoarseness and/or mild stridor, but only in the 24–48 hours after extubation, and although tracheomegaly can occur after prolonged intubation,[74] it seems to cause little functional problem. Serious damage to the larynx and trachea, such as granulomata or subglottic stenosis or cysts, is uncommon. These sequelae occur in babies who have had prolonged and/or repeated intubations[805] and can be minimised by meticulous attention to ETT immobilisation and by skilled and judicious timing of extubation.

Tracheostomy

Once a tracheostomy is placed in a neonate, they often become very tracheostomy-dependent and thus difficult to decannulate; consequently, a 'routine' change to a tracheostomy is contraindicated. Since ETTs can be used for 3–4 months or more if indicated in neonates, resort to tracheostomy is only necessary when attempts to extubate a baby have been persistently thwarted by laryngeal or tracheal problems.

Prevention of infection

All infants who are commenced on ventilation should receive antibiotics. If, after 48 hours, there are no ongoing signs of infection and the cultures are negative, consideration should be given to stopping the antibiotics.

Maintenance of blood volume and blood pressure

Anaemia commonly compounds the problem of hypotension and ventilated babies should have their haemoglobin kept above 13–14 g/dl (PCV >40%).[465] In ventilated babies with RDS, Skinner et al[821] found that CVP ranged from 0 to 12 mmHg, but that when it fell to the 0–3 mmHg range, the babies showed clinical evidence of hypovolaemia. Although not studied by Skinner et al,[821] by analogy with adult studies,[726] one would anticipate that such babies would respond to volume expansion.

A cause of hypotension in ventilated neonates is a reduction in cardiac output secondary to IPPV and PEEP. High-pressure IPPV, particularly when accompanied by high levels of PEEP, can compromise cardiac output by reducing venous return, obstructing the pulmonary vasculature and increasing right ventricular overload and thus the right ventricular volume, which in turn squashes the left ventricular cavity, reducing left ventricular output and splinting the heart and pericardium between overinflated lungs. The output from both ventricles is lowest in the sickest babies, MAP being an important variable in reducing cardiac output.[263] Iatrogenic pulmonary hypertension causing profound hypoxia can be caused by overventilation, which can also obstruct the bronchial circulation.[920] Particularly when PIE is present, the CXR in such babies shows that the heart is squashed and markedly reduced in volume. Problems with hypotension and a low cardiac output can usually be overcome by transfusion; however, if the problem is left ventricular compression, this can be improved only if it is possible to reduce the ventilator pressure.

Cerebral blood flow

IPPV also influences the cerebral circulation in various ways and thus may influence the incidence of GMH/IVH and PVL. Ventilated VLBW babies have a highly variable cerebral blood flow velocity, which can be reduced by the use of pancuronium[698] or by adequate volume replacement.[735] Hyperventilation resulting in hypocarbia reduces cerebral blood flow and should be avoided in preterm babies, as it increases the risk of PVL (pp. 1159–64).

Paralysing babies during ventilation

Administration of neuromuscular blocking agents can reduce the incidence of airleaks if given to preterm babies who are actively expiring against the ventilator.[360] Such agents, however, do have adverse effects (p. 1282). In babies with active respiration, albeit out of phase with ventilator inflation, abolition of spontaneous respiratory activity is associated with a fall in PaO_2 and a rise in $PaCO_2$;[769] following pancuronium or morphine administration, lung function may deteriorate, with a fall in compliance and FRC and a rise in airways resistance, leading to a fall in oxygenation.[73] This deterioration in oxygenation can usually be overcome by increasing the peak inspiratory pressure by 4–6 cmH$_2$O immediately prior to giving the first dose of pancuronium. The use of a neuromuscular blocker results in neonates being ventilated for a longer period of time and developing moderate oedema,[353] although this is not associated with a fall in plasma volume.[106] Prolonged use has been suggested to cause contractures or muscle atrophy,[770,817] but this can be avoided by appropriate passive physiotherapy.

Paralysis should also be considered for:

- the mature term baby with MAS, PPHN or GBS sepsis who is chronically restless, hypoxic and impossible to maintain in synchrony with the ventilator, despite sedation and rate and inspiratory time manipulation; infants with CDH should all be paralysed from birth (pp. 554–73);
- any neonate, irrespective of gestation, who shows the 'active expiratory reflex' pattern and in whom this is not abolished by synchronous ventilation and sedation;
- any neonate who develops severe PIE and infants who remain restless despite sedation following drainage of a pneumothorax.

Pancuronium is the most commonly used drug in this situation, given at intervals to suppress all respiratory activity, as it has fewer side effects than curare. Strict attention to fluid balance is mandatory, as fluid retention during paralysis is common. The excretion of pancuronium in the neonate with kidney and liver problems is variable and this agent interacts with other drugs, in particular the aminoglycosides;[668] in consequence, very high plasma levels and prolonged paralysis may occur with infusions of the drug. This may worsen pulmonary mechanics.[73] Hence, infusions should be avoided and the drug given by boluses as required, although this does not necessarily avoid all the side effects. Vecuronium and atracurium have been used as alternatives, particularly as the latter's metabolism is independent of renal activity. Variations in sensitivity of the neuromuscular junction in neonates, however, means that the inital dose of veuronium given should be small (10–20 microgram) and, as the duration of action and recovery time is longer in babies, maintenance doses should also be low.

Analgesia/sedation (Chapter 25)

Neonates in pain show stress reactions and being ventilated may be unpleasant and painful. For this reason, ventilated babies should receive some form of analgesic with or without a sedative (p. 483).

Physiotherapy in ventilated neonates

Problems with retained sticky secretions or ETT blockage are rare in the first 3–4 days of IPPV if adequate humidification of the ventilator gases is undertaken. Chest physiotherapy on ventilated babies with RDS may cause serious hypoxia and release of stress hormones;[369] physiotherapy is, therefore, not warranted as a routine.[291,814,948] Frequent endotracheal suction and/or regular chest physiotherapy may be needed, however, in babies with:

- pneumonia and increased secretions (pp. 1042–4);
- meconium aspiration (pp. 502–8);
- MPH (pp. 512–15);
- bronchorrhoea as CLD develops (p. 1044).

Posture

The position of ventilated neonates should be changed 2- to 3-hourly from the back to the right and then the left side, to aid movement of airway secretions. The prone position (except in babies with UACs) with the baby's head turned to one side should also be used, since this will facilitate drainage of secretions and improvement of blood gases.[225,919] The neonate with severe PIE should lie on the affected side, since this hastens the disappearance of interstitial gas (pp. 491–3).

Deterioration on IPPV

Not all babies who are stable on IPPV remain so: their condition may, and often does, worsen, and this can be a sudden collapse or a gradual deterioration.

Sudden collapse

Sudden spontaneous episodes of hypoxaemia are not uncommon in ventilated preterm babies. These may be due to episodes of active exhalation[86] and usually Arespond to short-term increases in F_1O_2 or pressure; infants who continue to actively expire should be paralysed (pp. 489–90). More prolonged deterioration is usually due to one of three things: a blocked or displaced ETT, an acute airleak, usually a pneumothorax, or the sudden development of a large GMH/IVH (pp. 1152–9). If the third possibility is not present, prompt and efficient management of the other two are essential to prevent it developing. Firstly it is important to establish that the ETT is in situ and patent by observing whether there is adequate chest wall excursion and auscultating the chest. Use of a portable, battery-operated capnometer, which detects exhaled carbon, may facilitate detection of extubation[861] by demonstrating the absence of intermittent changes in carbon dioxide in time with ventilation. The development of a pneumothorax, by either transillumination or CXR, must then be excluded; if the infant's condition is critical, emergency chest aspiration should be considered (pp. 1258–60).

Gradual deterioration

The respiratory condition of infants with RDS who have not received surfactant will worsen over the first 24–48 hours. Other reasons for a ventilated baby to gradually deteriorate include the development of pneumonia, a GMH/IVH, anaemia, hypotension, an airleak or pulmonary oedema. In addition, partial blockage of the ETT and progression to BPD will be associated with worsening blood gases.

The severely hypoxic neonate

Hypoxia with normocapnia or hypocapnia

In the absence of severe lung disease and in infants with mild RDS or MAS, the blood gas abnormalities should be managed as outlined for PPHN. In infants with severe lung disease who remain severely hypoxic (PaO_2 <5 kPa in 95% oxygen) despite treatment of coexisting problems, the options are to increase the level of ventilatory support, use vasodilator drugs (pp. 481–2) and, in an infant born at or near term, consider use of ECMO (pp. 528–9). The MAP should be increased because, by causing an improvement in lung volume, this can increase oxygenation. MAP can be increased by elevating either the peak inflating pressure or PEEP level or by prolonging the inflation time (with a reversed I:E ratio); the most effective manoeuvre, however, is to increase the PEEP level. Infants who are actively expiring against the ventilator and/or are receiving a peak inflating pressure .25 cmH$_2$O should be paralysed. If these manoeuvres fail and the infant has an adequate BP (pp. 1293–4), pulmonary vasodilator drugs (pp. 500–1) should be given.

It is essential to check that the baby has not been overventilated to such an extent that the MAP is compromising pulmonary artery perfusion and causing iatrogenic PPHN. The diagnostic clues are a low PaO_2 and a very low $PaCO_2$, often less than 3–3.5 kPa (23–26 mmHg), a raised pH (>7.45–7.50) and a CXR showing dark overexpanded lungs. A similar situation may be seen with inadvertent PEEP in older babies with BPD and an increased airways resistance; reducing the ventilator rate and hence increasing the expiratory time will dramatically improve ventilation.[847]

Profound hypoxaemia with carbon dioxide retention

If severe hypoxaemia is combined with hypercapnia, particularly if this is >7–8 kPa (52–60 mmHg), and technical problems with the ventilator circuit and tube have been excluded, the ventilator pressure and/or rate should be increased. If very high inflation pressures (35 cmH$_2$O) are being used, in a neonate who is clinically stable with an acceptable BP, less than perfect blood gases can be tolerated, provided that the PaO_2 is >5.5–6.0 kPa (41–45 mmHg), the $PaCO_2$ <8 kPa (60 mmHg) and the pH >7.25.

Weaning

It is important to wean an infant from mechanical ventilation and extubate as soon as possible, as complications of IPPV such as infection, BPD and airleak are related to the duration of IPPV. There are, however, dangers in trying to get a baby off IPPV too quickly, particularly in the very preterm baby in whom too rapid a weaning process may result in a recurrence of severe atelectasis (Fig. 27.45) and the need for more intensive ventilator support than before.

Once satisfactory blood gases have been achieved (PaO_2 8–12 kPa [60–90 mmHg], $PaCO_2$ <5.5–6.5 kPa [40–50 mmHg], pH >7.25) and the baby has been stable at these levels for 6 hours, weaning should begin. When weaning, the most damaging modality of ventilation should be reduced first, i.e. the peak inspiratory pressure, as this is a factor in the aetiology of pneumothorax and BPD (pp. 478–9, 554–6). After reducing the peak pressures down to 25 cmH$_2$O and the inspired oxygen concentration to less than 60%, if the PaO_2 is >8–9 kPa (60–70 mmHg) and the $PaCO_2$ is well controlled or if there is a respiratory alkalaemia, the oxygen concentration and peak pressures can then be reduced simultaneously. In general, the settings should be reduced in small increments; 5–10% for oxygen and 2–3 cmH$_2$O for peak inspiratory pressure; too rapid or too large changes can result in the baby becoming hypercapnic and/or hypoxic. After each change, it is important to check the blood gases within 30–60 minutes to ensure that they are still satisfactory. If the blood gases are acceptable (PaO_2 >8 kPa [60 mmHg], pH >7.25) and the baby is breathing spontaneously, the settings should be reduced every 4–6 hours.

Pancuronium should not be discontinued until problems due to airleaks (severe PIE or pneumothorax) have been controlled, and the ventilator settings have been reduced to 22–25 cmH$_2$O and 50–60% oxygen.

Once the baby is making spontaneous respiratory efforts and the peak pressures have been reduced to 14–18/3 cmH$_2$O (depending on the size of the baby), the ventilator rate can also be reduced, but to a minimum of 20/min (see below) in steps of 5–10/min, in the expectation that the baby's spontaneous efforts will contribute more to the minute ventilation as the rate is reduced. During this phase, the inflation time should be <0.5 seconds as, compared with using a longer inflation time, this results in a faster weaning process.[352] Others prefer to maintain the ventilator rate at 60/min and reduce the peak inflating pressure to very low levels (8–10 cmH$_2$O), as, theoretically, using such an approach, the baby may stay synchronous for longer. As the baby recovers from RDS, however, his lungs will become

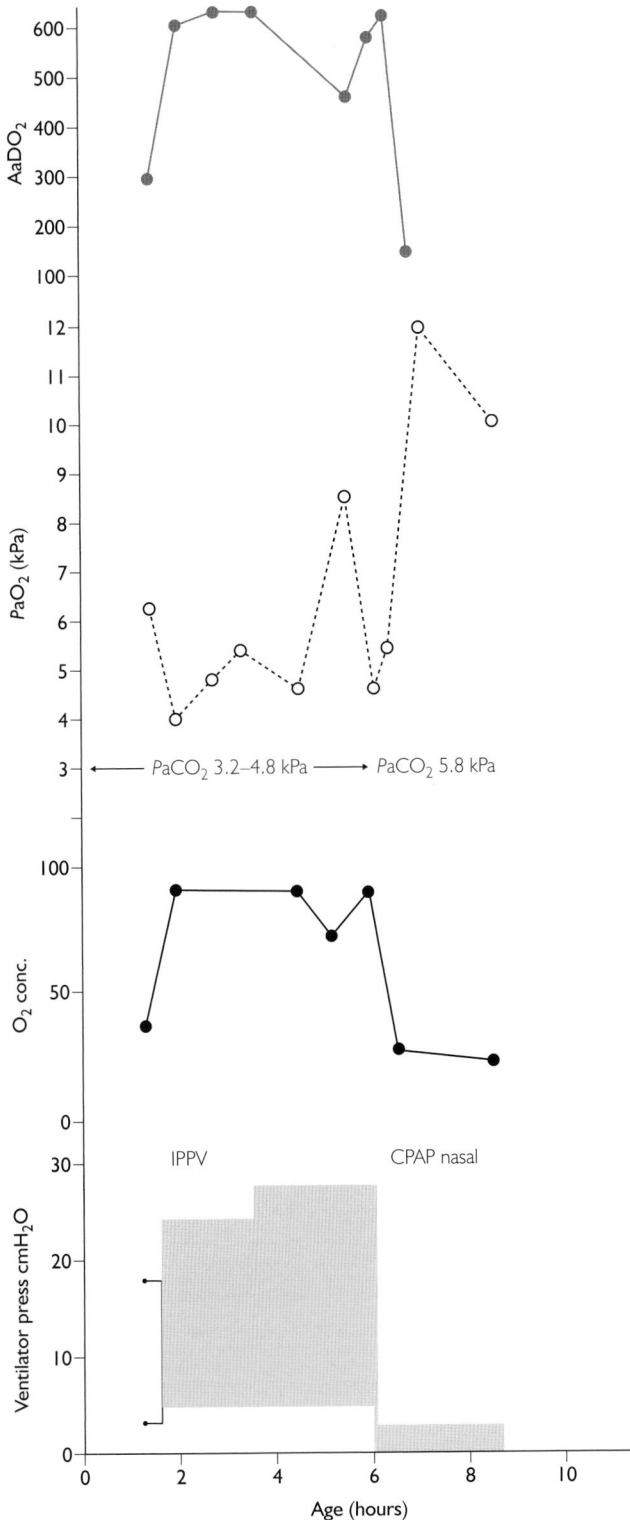

Fig. 27.45 Iatrogenic persistent pulmonary hypertension of the newborn in a 29-week 1.28-kg neonate initially assessed to have severe respiratory distress syndrome and ventilated as shown in 80–95% oxygen. The chest X-ray showed dark, well-expanded lungs. At 6 hours of age, the infant was switched from IPPV 28/5 cmH₂O in 95% oxygen to nCPAP in 30% oxygen, with dramatic improvement in oxygenation. AaDO₂ = Alveolar–arterial oxygen difference. (Reproduced from Roberton.[749])

more compliant and his spontaneous respiratory rate may decrease. A more effective method of weaning than reducing rate is to transfer the infant to A/C and reduce the inflating pressures to 10–14 cmH₂O, depending on the size of the infant, before considering extubation. This approach has been shown to significantly shorten the duration of weaning.[127] If SIMV rather than A/C is used during the weaning process, it is important not to reduce the SIMV rate below 20/min. Reducing the ventilator rate below 20/min, regardless of whether a patient-triggered mode is used, increases the work of breathing.[764] Other triggered modes, for example PSV with or without VG (p. 525), can be used to wean babies; whether these modes are more effective than A/C requires investigation in appropriately designed randomised trials.

Once the neonate is in 30% oxygen and the peak inflating pressures further reduced to 10–16 cmH₂O, the baby will usually be ready to extubate. Some prefer to extubate babies only after they have been able to maintain their blood gases on endotracheal CPAP (etCPAP). The period on etCPAP should, however, be limited to an hour or less,[509] as breathing through a narrow ETT increases the work of breathing (p. 530), so the baby can tire easily. Indeed, in randomised trials, direct extubation from a low IMV rate rather than after a period of etCPAP was associated with an increased chance of successful extubation.[202]

Infants with a birthweight less than 1.0 kg should be extubated onto nCPAP rather than directly into supplementary oxygen delivered into a headbox. Randomised trials have demonstrated that use of nCPAP post extubation reduces the need for increased respiratory support.[233] If nCPAP is used, after 48 to 72 hours the baby should then be nursed in a headbox in the same inspired oxygen concentration, nCPAP being restarted if the baby develops apnoeas of signs or increasing respiratory distress. Others, in contrast, prefer to time-cycle babies on and off CPAP, with increasingly longer periods off CPAP on successive days if tolerated; that method, however, has not been shown to have any advantages over taking them directly off the nCPAP.[753] Particularly in very preterm babies, nCPAP may be required for several days or weeks to prevent recurrent apnoeic attacks (pp. 573–7).

In babies >1.50 kg birthweight, weaning can often be rapid, over a period of 12 to 24 hours, with no need for prolonged periods on nCPAP. Conversely, in neonates <1.00 kg birthweight, the later stages of weaning may take weeks (see below). Infants older than a week of age may benefit from extubation onto higher levels of CPAP than preterm infants less than a week of age (6 rather than 3 cmH₂O).[127]

In babies <1.5 kg and <32 weeks' gestational age, aminophylline or oral theophylline (5 mg/kg/24 h) or caffeine citrate (5 mg/kg/24 h) should be administered at least 12 hours prior to extubation. In prospective controlled trials, administration of methylxanthines has been demonstrated to shorten the duration of weaning.[412] Theophylline, however, has side effects, including tachycardia, vomiting, diuresis and hyperglycaemia; these are dose related, hence it is important to monitor levels carefully. Theophylline also increases energy expenditure and augmented carbohydrate utilisation, which could be detrimental to growth.[118] A further disadvantage is that theophylline has to be given three times a day. Caffeine, then, is the weaning agent of choice, as it is administered once daily, has a lower toxicity level and fewer side effects and in a randomised trial[815] was demonstrated to be equally effective as theophylline. Doxapram has been used in infants who appear resistant to methylxanthines, but even in low dose may cause elevation of BP and result in high plasma levels of doxopram;[447] thus, we do not recommend its use.

Weaning problems

After any step in weaning, the baby may deteriorate or the blood gases at the new setting may be unacceptable. One finding which is common in VLBW neonates and which suggests that the weaning procedure is not progressing smoothly is the development over 6 to 12 hours of a metabolic acidaemia, a sign that the work of breathing at the new ventilator setting is excessive. In this situation, after ensuring that the baby has not suffered some unrelated adverse event such as a blocked ETT or a pneumothorax, all that is usually required is to revert to the previous ventilator setting. In some babies, however, following the deterioration, much more vigorous ventilation may be necessary for 24 to 48 hours before the weaning process can once more be resumed.

Extubation

Extubation carries the risk of severe hypoxia leading to GMH/IVH, inhalation of gastric contents and the need for reintubation, with a possibility of laryngeal trauma. It is essential, therefore, only to attempt extubation with the baby in the best possible condition, including normal electrolytes, a haemoglobin >13 g/dl and normal acid–base status. Feeding should be discontinued 6 to 12 hours before extubation and not restarted for a further 12 hours, so that the risks of regurgitation and inhalation of milk are reduced to a minimum.

After extubation, the neonate often has considerable difficulty clearing his secretions as airway ciliary function has been compromised by the damage caused by the ETT. The inspired oxygen must, therefore, be humidified and warmed. Regular physiotherapy and oropharyngeal suction should be started,[280] as always, applied in such a way that it does not cause deterioration in the baby's blood gases or result in apnoea and bradycardia. In general, both physiotherapy and suction should be used 3- to 4-hourly, adapting the frequency on the basis of clinical findings or the CXR (see below). Nursing recently extubated babies in the prone position results in better blood gases.[573]

Prediction of successful extubation

The results of lung mechanics measurements have been used to predict extubation outcome. A spontaneously generated minute volume at least 50% of the mechanically generated minute ventilation has been noted to predict readiness for extubation.[947] In another study,[490] however, a low lung volume (FRC <26 ml/kg) was more predictive of extubation failure (need for reintubation) than compliance, tidal volume or respiratory rate results, but only if the lung volumes post- rather than pre-extubation were considered. Extubation failure occurs if the respiratory load is greater than the respiratory muscle strength; a low gestational age, however, was more predictive of extubation failure in very immature infants than were the results of compliance measurements to assess respiratory load or inspiratory pressures generated against an occlusion to assess respiratory muscle strength.[227]

Extubation problems

Stridor

Minor degrees of stridor are not uncommon and usually only last for an hour or two or at most 24 hours. If persistent, the infant may benefit from high-pressure nasopharyngeal CPAP (pp. 520–1), using pressures up to 6–8 to 10 cmH$_2$O; whether or not this will work can only be assessed on a trial-and-error basis. Nebulised adrenaline can also be administered. If the stridor is marked and unresponsive with severe respiratory distress and there is progressive deterioration of the blood gases, there is no alternative but to reintubate. In such patients, the ETT should be left in place with the baby on minimal ventilation for at least 2 to 3 days before a further attempt at extubation is made after pretreating the baby with dexamethasone (0.5 mg/kg) for 24 hours and continuing the drug for 24 to 48 hours after extubation.[176] The management of the baby in whom this does not work and in whom some more serious laryngeal damage has occurred is outlined on page 608.

Lobar collapse

Despite careful physiotherapy and suction post extubation (p. 607), up to 20% of neonates develop collapse consolidation of one lung or just one lobe, particularly the right upper, because of plugging of the bronchi with secretions[964] (Fig. 27.46). This complication seems to be more common after nasal intubation.[841] It may cause such severe deterioration that reintubation and IPPV are necessary, but in other infants may be virtually asymptomatic. The milder cases can be treated by vigorous physiotherapy. Occasionally it is worth sucking out the airway of more severely affected neonates under direct vision at laryngoscopy. By turning the head away from the affected lung, the suction catheter can usually be directed into the appropriate main stem bronchus.

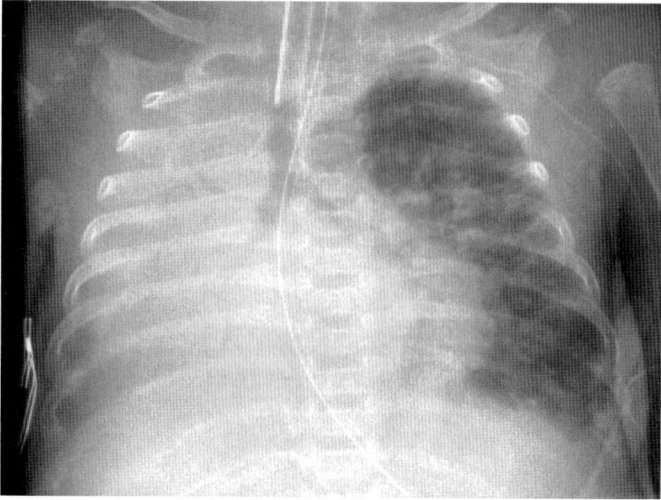

Fig. 27.46 Atelectasis of the right lung. The infant required reintubation and ventilation prior to the chest radiograph because of poor blood gases post extubation.

In order to detect areas of asymptomatic collapse, particularly in the right upper lobe, before they progress to total lung collapse, neonates should be X-rayed within 24 hours after extubation and whenever there is any deterioration in their clinical condition or blood gases. The development of significant intercostal/subcostal retractions and an increase in the inspired oxygen concentration of at least 7% has been suggested to be a sensitive indicator of radiological deterioration.[286]

Recurrent failure to wean or extubate

Repeated unsuccessful attempts to extubate a neonate over a period of a week is usually only a problem in ELBW neonates whose weight is not increasing and in whom the repeated episodes of extubation and deterioration make adequate nutrition even more difficult to achieve. Rarely it is due to laryngeal damage. Poor lung function is not usually responsible.[911] Affected infants should be reintubated and restarted on IPPV at the minimal settings necessary to achieve normal blood gases and kept there until they are in a better condition and gaining weight consistently. Repeated failure to wean a neonate off IPPV is very suggestive of a neurological problem, either secondary to GMH/IVH or some primary muscular or neurological disorder, including, particularly in term babies, the congenital hypoventilation syndrome (Ondine's curse).

References

1. Abbasi S, Bhutani V K, Gerdes J S 1993 Long term pulmonary consequences of respiratory distress syndrome in preterm infants treated with exogenous surfactant. Journal of Pediatrics 122: 446–452

2. Abman S H, Ivy D, Ziegler J W, Kinsella J P 1996 Mechanisms of abnormal vasoreactivity in persistent pulmonary hypertension of the newborn infant. Journal of Perinatology 16: S18–S23

3. Achiron R, Zakut H 1986 Fetal haemothorax complicating amniocentesis. Acta Obstetrica Gynaecologica Scandinavica 65: 869–870

4. ACTOBAT Study Group 1995 Australian collaborative trial of antenatal thyrotropin releasing hormone (ACTOBAT) for prevention of neonatal respiratory disease. Lancet 345: 877–882

5. Aghajafari F, Murphy K, Matthews S, Ohlsson A, Anankwah K, Hannah M 2002 Repeated doses of antenatal corticosteroids in animals: a systematic review. American Journal of Obstetrics and Gynecology 186: 843–849

6. Ahluwalia J S, Kelsall A W R, Raine J et al 1994 Safety of inhaled nitric oxide in premature neonates. Acta Paediatrica 83: 347–348

7. Ahn M O, Cha K Y, Phelan J P 1992 The low birthweight infant: is there a preferred route of delivery? Clinics in Perinatology 19: 411–423

8. Aiton N R, Fox G R, Hannam S, Stern C M M, Milner A D 1996 Pulmonary hypoplasia presenting as persistent tachypnoea in the first few months of life. British Medical Journal 312: 1149–1151

9. Alexander J, Blowes R, Ingram D, Milner A D 1993 Determination of the resonant frequency of the respiratory system during high frequency oscillatory ventilation. Early Human Development 35: 234

10. Allen A C, Usher R H 1971 Renal acid excretion in infants with respiratory distress syndrome. Pediatric Research 5: 345–355

11. Allen L P, Reynolds E O R, Rivers R P A, LeSouef P N, Wimberley P D 1977 Controlled trial of continuous positive airway pressure given by face mask for hyaline membrane disease. Archives of Disease in Childhood 52: 373–378

12. Allen R W, Jung A L, Lester P D 1981 Effectiveness of chest tube evacuation of pneumothorax in neonates. Journal of Pediatrics 99: 629–634

13. Al-Nishi N, Dyer D, Sharief N, Al-Alaiyan S 1994 Selective bronchial occlusion for treatment of bullous interstitial emphysema and bronchopleural fistula. Journal of Pediatric Surgery 29: 1545–1547

14. Alpan G, Mauray F, Clyman R I 1989 Effect of patent ductus arteriosus on water accumulation and protein permeability in the lungs of mechanically ventilated premature lambs. Pediatric Research 26: 570–575

15. Al-Sayed L, Schrank W, Thach B T 1994 Ventilatory sparing strategies and swallowing pattern during bottle feeding in human infants. Journal of Applied Physiology 77: 78–83

16. Aly H Z 2001 Nasal prongs continuous positive airway pressure: a simple yet powerful tool. Pediatrics 108: 759–761

17. Amodio J, Abramson S, Berdon W et al 1987 Iatrogenic causes of large pleural fluid collections in the premature infant: ultrasonic and radiographic findings. Pediatric Radiology 17: 104–108

18. Anand K J S, McIntosh N, Lagercrantz H et al 1999 Analgesia and sedation in preterm infants who require ventilatory support. Results from the NOPAIN Trial. Archives of Pediatric Adolescent Medicine 153: 331–338

19. Andersen E A, Hertel J, Pedersen S A, Sorensen J R 1984 Congenital chylothorax: management by ligature of the thoracic duct. Scandinavian Journal of Thoracic and Cardiovascular Surgery 18: 193–194

20. Anderson K D, Chandra R 1976 Pneumothorax secondary to perforation of segmental bronchi by suction catheters. Journal of Pediatric Surgery 11: 687–693

21. Andrews A F, Klein M D, Tommasian J M 1983 Venovenous ECMO in neonates with respiratory failure. Journal of Pediatric Surgery 18: 339–346

22. Andrews A F, Roloff D, Bartlett R H 1984 Use of extracorporeal membrane oxygenation in persistent pulmonary hypertension of the newborn. Clinics in Perinatology 11: 729–735

23. Annibale D J, Hulsey T C, Wagner C L et al 1995 Comparative neonatal morbidity of abdominal and vaginal deliveries after uncomplicated pregnancies. Archives of Pediatrics and Adolescent Medicine 149: 862–867

24. Aranda J V, Stern L, Dunbar J S 1972 Pneumothorax with pneumoperitoneum in a newborn infant. American Journal of Diseases of Children 123: 163–166

25. Auten R L, Notter R H, Kendis J W, Southgate W M 1991 Surfactant treatment of full term newborns with respiratory failure. Pediatrics 87: 101–107

26. Avery G B, Randolph J G, Weaver T 1966 Gastric acidity in the first day of life. Pediatrics 37: 1005–1007

27. Avery M E, Gatewood O B, Brumley G 1966 Transient tachypnea of the newborn. American Journal of Diseases of Children 111: 380–385

28. Avery M E, Tooley W H, Keller J B et al 1987 Is chronic lung disease in low birthweight infants preventable? A survey of eight centers. Pediatrics 79: 26–30

29. Bae C W, Takahasi A, Chida S, Sasaki M 1998 Morphology and function of pulmonary surfactant inhibited by meconium. Pediatric Research 44:187

30. Baildam E M, Dady I M, Chiswick M L 1993 Bronchocutaneous fistula associated with mechanical ventilation. Archives of Disease in Childhood 69: 525–526

31. Bailey C, Kattwinkel J, Teja K, Buckley T 1988 Shallow versus deep endotracheal suctioning in young rabbits: pathological effects on the tracheal and bronchial wall. Pediatrics 82: 746–751

32. Ball R, Chetcuti P, Beverley D 1995 Fatal familial surfactant protein B deficiency (letter). Archives of Disease in Childhood. Fetal and Neonatal Edition 73: F53

33. Ball R, Chetcuti P, Primhak R 1995 Clinical aspects of familal surfactant protein B deficiency (abstract). Biology of the Neonate 67(suppl. 1): 81

34. Ballard P L 1984 Combined hormonal treatment and lung maturation. Seminars in Perinatology 8: 283–292

35. Ballard P L, Gluckman P D, Liggins G C, Kaplan S L, Grumbach M M 1980 Steroid and growth hormone levels in premature infants after prenatal betamethasone therapy to prevent respiratory distress syndrome. Pediatric Research 14: 122–127

36. Ballard R A, Ballard P L, Creasy R K et al 1992 Respiratory disease in very-low-birthweight infants after prenatal thyrotropin-releasing hormone and glucocorticoids. TRH Study Group. Lancet 339: 510–515

37. Ballin A, Koren G, Kohelet D et al 1987 Reduction in platelet counts induced by mechanical ventilation in newborn infants. Journal of Pediatrics 111: 445–449

38. Bancalari E, Berlin J A 1978 Meconium aspiration and other asphyxial disorders. Clinics in Perinatology 5: 317–334

39. Bancalari E, del Morval T 2001 Bronchopulmonary dysplasia and surfactant. Biology of the Neonate 80(suppl. 1): 7–13

40. Barak M, Cohen A, Herschikowitz S 1992 Total leukocyte and neutrophil count changes associated with antenatal betamethasone administration in premature infants. Acta Paediatrica 81: 760–763

41. Barefield E S, Hicks T P, Phillips J B 1994 Thromboxane and pulmonary morphometry in the development of the pulmonary hypertensive response to group B streptococcus. Critical Care Medicine 22: 506–514

42. Barker D P, Rutter N 1996 Stress, severity of illness, and outcome in ventilated preterm infants. Archives of Disease in Childhood. Fetal and Neonatal Edition 75: F187–F190

43. Barrington K J, Bull D, Finer K N 2001 Randomized trial of nasal synchronized intermittent mandatory ventilation compared with continuous positive airway

pressure after extubation of very low birth weight infants. Pediatrics 107: 638–641

44. Bartlett D 1985 Ventilatory and protective mechanisms of the infant larynx. American Review of Respiratory Disease 131(suppl.): 49–50

45. Bartlett R H, Andrews A F, Toomasian J M, Haiduc N J, Gazzaniga A B 1982 ECMO for newborn respiratory failure, 45 cases. Surgery 92: 425–433

46. Bartlett R H, Roloff D W, Cornell R G, Andrews A F, Dillon P W, Zwishenberger J B 1985 Extracorporeal membrane oxygenation in neonatal respiratory failure. A prospective randomized study. Pediatrics 76: 479–487

47. Bartmann P, Bamberger U, Pohlandt F, Gortner L 1992 Immunogenicity and immunomodulatory activity of bovine surfactant (SF-RI 1). Acta Paediatrica 81: 383–388

48. Baud O, Foix-L'Helias L, Kaminski M et al 1999 Antenatal glucocorticoid treatment and cystic periventricular leukomalacia in very premature infants. New England Journal of Medicine 341:1190–1196

49. Baum J D, Roberton N R C 1974 Distending pressure in infants with respiratory distress syndrome. Archives of Disease in Childhood 49: 771–781

50. Baumer J H 2000 International randomized controlled trial of patient triggered ventilation in neonatal respiratory distress syndrome. Archives of Disease in Childhood. Fetal and Neonatal Edition 82: F5–F10

51. Baumgart S, Hirsch R B, Butler S Z, Coburn C E, Spitzer A R 1992 Diagnosis related criteria in the consideration of extracorporeal membrane oxygenation in neonates previously breathed with high frequency jet ventilation. Pediatrics 89: 491–494

52. Beard R W, Morris E D 1965 Foetal and maternal acid-base balance during normal labour. Journal of Obstetrics and Gynaecology of the British Commonwealth 72: 496–506

53. Beardsmore C, Dundas I, Poole K et al 2000 Respiratory function in survivors of the United Kingdom Extra Corporeal Membrane Oxygenation Trial. American Journal of Respiratory and Critical Care Medicine 161: 1129–1135

54. Becerra J E, Rowley D L, Atrash H K 1992 Case fatality rates associated with conditions originating in the perinatal period: United States 1986 through 1987. Pediatrics 89: 1256–1259

55. Beck R 1985 Chronic lung disease following hypocapnic alkalosis for persistent pulmonary hypertension. Journal of Pediatrics 106: 527–528

56. Beck R, Anderson K D, Pearson G D, Cronin J, Miller M K, Short B L 1986 Criteria for extracorporeal membrane oxygenation in a population of infants with persistent pulmonary hypertension of the newborn. Journal of Pediatric Surgery 21: 297–302

57. Beeby P J, Elliott E J, Henderson-Smart D J, Rieger I D 1994 Predictive value of umbilical artery pH in preterm infants. Archives of Disease in Childhood. Fetal and Neonatal Edition 71: F93–F96

58. Beeram M R, Dhanireddy R 1992 Effects of saline instillation during tracheal suction on lung mechanics in newborn infants. Journal of Perinatology 12: 120–123

59. Beeram M R, Young M, Abedin M 1995 Effect of maternal illicit drug use on the mortality of very low birth weight infants. Journal of Perinatology 15: 456–460

60. Beierholm E A, Grantham N, O' Keefe D D, Laver M B, Daggett W M 1975 Effects of acid-base changes, hypoxia and catecholamines on ventricular performance. American Journal of Physiology 228: 1555–1561

61. Bell A H, Skov L, Lundstrom K E, Saugstad O D, Griesen G 1994 Cerebral blood flow and plasma hypoxanthine in relation to surfactant treatment. Acta Paediatrica 83: 910–914

62. Bell E F, Warburton D, Stonestreet B S, Oh W 1980 Effect of fluid administration on the development of symptomatic patent ductus arteriosus and congestive heart failure in premature infants. New England Journal of Medicine 303: 598–604

63. Bennett C C, Johnson A, Field D J et al 2001 UK collaborative randomised trial of neonatal extracorporeal membrane oxygenation: follow-up to age 4 years. Lancet 357: 1094–1096

64. Benson B J 1993 Genetically engineered human pulmonary surfactant. Clinics in Perinatology 20: 791–811

65. Benveniste D, Berg O, Pederson J E P 1976 A technique for delivery of continuous positive pressure to the neonate. Journal of Pediatrics 88: 1015–1019

66. Berg T J, Pagtakhan T D, Reed M H et al 1975 Bronchopulmonary dysplasia and lung rupture in hyaline membrane disease: influence of continuous distending pressure. Pediatrics 55: 51–53

67. Berger J T, Gilhooly J 1993 Fibrin glue treatment of persistent pneumothorax in a premature infant. Journal of Pediatrics 122: 958–960

68. Bernstein G, Cleary J P, Heldt G P et al 1993 Response time and reliability of three neonatal patient triggered ventilators. American Review of Respiratory Disease 148: 358–364

69. Berry D D, Pramanik A K, Philips J B 3rd et al 1994 Comparison of the effect of three doses of a synthetic surfactant on the alveolar-arterial oxygen gradient in infants weighing > or = 1250 grams with respiratory distress syndrome. American Exosurf Neonatal Study Group II. Journal of Pediatrics 124: 294–301

70. Berseth C L 1995 Minimal enteral feedings. Clinics in Perinatology 22: 195–205

71. Bhuta T, Henderson-Smart D J 2000 Elective high frequency jet ventilation versus conventional ventilation for respiratory distress syndrome in preterm infants (Cochrane Review). Cochrane Database of Systematic Reviews (2): CD000328

72. Bhuta T, Kent-Biggs J, Jeffrey H E 1997 Prediction of surfactant dysfunction in term infants by click test. Pediatric Pulmonology 23: 287–291

73. Bhutani V K, Abbasi S, Silvieri E M 1988 Continuous skeletal muscle paralysis: effect on neonatal pulmonary mechanics. Pediatrics 81: 419–422

74. Bhutani V K, Ritchie W G, Shaffer T H 1986 Acquired tracheomegaly in very preterm neonates. American Journal of Diseases of Children 140: 449–452

75. Bhutani V K, Sivieri E M, Abbasi S, Shaffer T H 1988 Evaluation of neonatal pulmonary mechanics and energetics. Pediatric Pulmonology 4: 150–158

76. Bignall S, Bailey P C, Bass C A et al 1989 The cardiovascular and oncotic effects of albumin infusion in premature infants. Early Human Development 20: 191–201

77. Bindl L, Fahnenstich H, Peukert U 1994 Aerosolized prostacyclin for pulmonary hypertension in neonates. Archives of Disease in Childhood. Fetal and Neonatal Edition 71: F214–F216

78. Bland R D 1972 Cord blood total protein level as a screening aid for the idiopathic respiratory distress syndrome. New England Journal of Medicine 287: 9–13

79. Bland R D 1982 Edema formation in the newborn lung. Clinics in Perinatology 9: 593–611

80. Bland R D 1992 Formation of fetal liquid and its removal near birth. In: Polin R A, Fox W W (eds) Fetal and neonatal physiology. W B Saunders, Philadelphia, pp. 782–789

81. Bland R D, Kim M H, Light M J, Woodson J L 1980 High frequency ventilation in severe hyaline membrane disease: an alternative therapy. Critical Care Medicine 8: 275–280

82. Block M R, Kallenberger D A, Kern J D, Nerveux D 1981 In utero meconium aspiration by the baboon fetus. Obstetrics and Gynecology 57: 37–40

83. Bloom M C, Roques-Gineste M, Fries F, Lelong-Tissier M C 1995 Pulmonary haemodynamics after surfactant replacement in severe neonatal respiratory distress syndrome. Archives of Disease in Childhood. Fetal and Neonatal Edition 73: F95–F98

84. Boddy K, Dawes G S 1975 Fetal breathing. British Medical Bulletin 31: 3–7

85. Bodmer B, Benjamin A, McLean F, Usher R H 1986 Has the use of cesarean section reduced the risks of pregnancy in the preterm breech presentation? American Journal of Obstetrics and Gynecology 154: 244–250

86. Bolivar J M, Gerhardt T, Gonzalez A et al 1995 Mechanism for episodes of hypoxemia in preterm infants undergoing mechanical ventilation. Journal of Pediatrics 127: 767–773

87. Booth P, Nicolaides K H, Greenough A, Gamsu H R 1987 Pleuroamniotic shunting for fetal chylothorax. Early Human Development 15: 365–367

88. Boros S J, Bing D R, Mammel M C, Hagen E, Gordon M J 1984 Using conventional infant ventilators at unconventional rates. Pediatrics 74: 487–492

89. Boros S J, Campbell K 1980 A comparison of the effects of high frequency–low tidal volume and low frequency–high tidal volume mechanical ventilation. Journal of Pediatrics 97: 108–112

90. Boros S J, Mammel M C, Coleman J M et al 1985 Neonatal high frequency jet ventilation: four years' experience. Pediatrics 75: 657–663

91. Boros S J, Matalon S, Ewald R, Leonard A, Hunt C 1977 The effect of independent variations in inspiratory:expiratory ratio and expiratory pressure during mechanical ventilation in hyaline membrane disease. The significance of mean airway pressure. Journal of Pediatrics 91: 794–798

92. Boros S J, Reynolds J W 1975 Hyaline membrane disease treated with early nasal end expiratory pressure: one year's experience. Pediatrics 56: 218–223

93. Bowen F W, Chandra R, Avery G B 1973 Pulmonary interstitial emphysema with gas embolism in hyaline membrane disease. American Journal of Diseases of Children 126: 117–118

94. Boynton B R, Mannino F L, Davis R F, Kopotic R J, Friedrichsen G 1984 Combined high-frequency oscillatory ventilation and intermittent mandatory ventilation in critically ill neonates. Journal of Pediatrics 105: 297–302

95. Bradley B S, Kumar S P, Mehta P N, Ezhuthachan S G 1994 Neonatal cushingoid syndrome resulting from serial courses of antenatal betamethasone. American Journal of Obstetrics and Gynecology 83: 869–872

96. Brigham K L, Serafin W, Zadoff A, Blair I, Meyrick B, Oates J A 1988 Prostaglandin E_2 attenuation of sheep lung responses to endotoxin. Journal of Applied Physiology 64: 2568–2574

97. British Standards Institution 1970 Specifications for humidifiers for use with breathing machines. BS4494. London

98. Broadbent R, Fox T F, Dolovich M et al 1995 Chest position and pulmonary deposition of surfactant in surfactant depleted rabbits. Archives of Disease in Childhood. Fetal and Neonatal Edition 72: F84–F89

99. Brodman R F, Zarelson T M, Schiebler G L 1974 Treatment of congenital chylothorax. Journal of Pediatrics 85: 516–520

100. Brooks J G, Bustamente S A, Koops B L 1977 Selective bronchial intubation for the treatment of severe localised pulmonary interstitial emphysema in newborn infants. Journal of Pediatrics 91: 648–652

101. Brown B L, Gleicher N 1981 Intrauterine meconium aspiration. Obstetrics and Gynecology 57: 26–29

102. Bruce D A 1984 Effects of hyperventilation on cerebral blood flow and metabolism. Clinics in Perinatology 11: 673–680

103. Bryan C S 1967 Enhancement of bacterial infection by meconium. Johns Hopkins Medical Journal 121: 9–16

104. Bucciarelli R L, Egan E A, Gressner I H, Eitzman D V 1976 Persistence of fetal cardiopulmonary circulation. Manifestation of transient tachypnea of the newborn. Pediatrics 58: 192–197

105. Bucciarelli R L, Nelson R M, Egan E A et al 1977 Transient tricuspid insufficiency of the newborn. A form of myocardial dysfunction in stressed newborns. Pediatrics 59: 330–337

106. Buckner P S, Todd D A, Lui K, John E 1991 Effect of short-term muscle relaxation on neonatal plasma volume. Critical Care Medicine 19: 1357–1361

107. Bunton T E, Plopper C G 1984 Triamcinolone induced structural alterations in the development of the lung of the fetal rhesus Macaque. American Journal of Obstetrics and Gynecology 148: 203–215

108. Bureau M A, Begin R, Berthiaume Y 1979 Central chemical regulation of respiration in term newborn. Journal of Applied Physiology 47: 1212–1217

109. Burnard E D, James L S 1961 Failure of the heart after undue asphyxia at birth. Pediatrics 28: 545–565

110. Byrne D L, Gau G 1987 In utero meconium aspiration: an unpreventable cause of neonatal death. British Journal of Obstetrics and Gynaecology 94: 813–814

111. Cabal L A, Devaskar U, Siassi B, Hodgman J E, Emmanouilides G 1980 Cardiogenic shock associated with perinatal asphyxia in preterm infants. Journal of Pediatrics 96: 705–710

112. Callen P, Goldsworthy S, Graves I, Harvey D, Mellows H, Parkinson C 1979 Mode of delivery and the lecithin/sphingomyelin ratio. British Journal of Obstetrics and Gynaecology 86: 965–968

113. Campbell R E 1970 Intrapulmonary interstitial emphysema. A complication of hyaline membrane disease. American Journal of Radiology 110: 449–456

114. Carlo W A, Beoglos A, Chatburn R L, Walsh M C, Martin R J 1989 High frequency jet ventilation in neonatal pulmonary hypertension. American Journal of Diseases of Children 143: 233–238

115. Carlo W A, Chatburn R L, Martin R J 1984 Decrease in airway pressure during high frequency jet ventilation versus conventional ventilation in infants with respiratory distress syndrome. Journal of Pediatrics 104: 101–107

116. Carlo W A, Chatburn R L, Martin R J 1987 Randomized trial of high frequency jet ventilation in respiratory distress syndrome. Journal of Pediatrics 110: 275–278

117. Carmant L, Le Guennec J-C 1989 Congenital chylothorax and persistent pulmonary hypertension of the newborn. Acta Paediatrica Scandinavica 78: 789–792

118. Carnielli V P, Verlato G, Benini F et al 2000 Metabolic and respiratory effects of theophylline in the preterm infant. Archives of Disease in Childhood. Fetal and Neonatal Edition 83: F39–F43

119. Carson B S, Losey R W, Bowes W W, Simmons M A 1976 Combined obstetric and pediatric approach to prevent meconium aspiration syndrome. American Journal of Obstetrics and Gynecology 126: 712–715

120. Cartlidge P H T, Rutter N 1986 Serum albumin concentrations and oedema in the newborn. Archives of Disease in Childhood 61: 657–660

121. Cartlidge P H T, Rutter N 1988 Percutaneous oxygen delivery to the preterm infant. Lancet i: 315–317

122. Cartwright D, Gregory G A, Lou H, Heyman M A 1984 The effect of hypocarbia on the cardiovascular system of puppies. Pediatric Research 18: 685–690

123. Cassin S, Dawes G S, Mott J C, Ross B B, Strang L B 1964 The vascular resistance of the fetal and newly ventilated lung of the lamb. Journal of Physiology 171: 61–79

124. Cat R, Rosario N A, Taborda de Messias I 1993 Evaluation of complement activation in premature newborn infants with hyaline membrane disease. European Journal of Pediatrics 152: 205–208

125. Cater G, Thibeault D W, Beatty E C et al 1989 Misalignment of lung vessels and alveolar capillary dysplasia: a cause of persistent pulmonary hypertension. Journal of Pediatrics 114: 293–300

126. Chan V, Greenough A 1992 Severe localized pulmonary interstitial emphysema – decompression by selective bronchial intubation. Journal of Perinatal Medicine 20: 313–316

127. Chan V, Greenough A 1993 Randomized trial of methods of extubation in acute and chronic respiratory distress. Archives of Disease in Childhood 68: 570–572

128. Chan V, Greenough A 1993 Randomised controlled trial of weaning by patient triggered ventilation or conventional ventilation. European Journal of Pediatrics 152: 51–54

129. Chan V, Greenough A 1993 Determinants of oxygenation during high frequency oscillation. European Journal of Pediatrics 152: 350–353

130. Chan V, Greenough A 1994 Comparison of weaning by patient triggered ventilation or synchronous intermittent mandatory ventilation in preterm infants. Acta Paediatrica 83: 335–337

131. Chan V, Greenough A 1994 Inspiratory and expiratory times for infants ventilator-dependent beyond the first week of life. Acta Paediatrica 83: 1022–1024

132. Chan V, Greenough A 1994 The effect of frequency on carbon dioxide levels during high frequency oscillation. Journal of Perinatal Medicine 22: 103–106

133. Chan V, Greenough A, Dimitriou G 1995 High frequency oscillation, respiratory activity and changes in blood gases. Early Human Development 40: 87–94

134. Chan V, Greenough A, Gamsu H R 1994 High frequency oscillation for preterm infants with severe respiratory failure. Archives of Disease in Childhood. Fetal and Neonatal Edition 70: F44–F46

135. Chan V, Greenough A, Hird M F 1991 Comparison of different rates of artificial ventilation for preterm infants ventilated beyond the first week of life. Early Human Development 26: 177–183

136. Chang H K 1984 Mechanisms of gas transport during ventilation by high frequency oscillation. Journal of Applied Physiology 56: 553–563

137. Chasen S T, Madden A, Chervenak F A 1999 Cesarian delivery of twins and neonatal respiratory disorders. American Journal of Obstetrics and Gynecology 181: 1052–1056

138. Cheema I U, Ahluwara J S 2001 Feasibility of tidal volume guided ventilation in newborn infants: a randomized crossover trial using the volume guarantee modality. Pediatrics 107: 1323–1328

139. Chelliah B P, Brown D, Cohen M, Talleyrand A J, Shen-Schwarz S 1995 Alveolar capillary dysplasia – a cause of persistent pulmonary hypertension unresponsive to a second course of extracorporeal membrane oxygenation. Pediatrics 96: 1159–1161

140. Chessels J M, Wigglesworth J S 1972 Coagulation studies in preterm infants with respiratory distress and intracranial haemorrhage. Archives of Disease in Childhood 47: 564–570

141. Cheung P Y, Prasertsom W, Finer N N, Robertson C M T 1997 Rescue high frequency oscillatory ventilation for preterm infants: neurodevelopmental outcome and its prediction. Biology of the Neonate 71: 282–291

142. Chida S, Phelps D S, Soll R F, Taeusch H W 1991 Surfactant proteins and anti-surfactant antibodies in sera from infants with respiratory distress syndrome with and without surfactant treatment. Pediatrics 88: 84–89

143. Chida S, Tujiwara T, Konishi M et al 1993 Stable microbubble test for predicting the risk of respiratory distress syndrome. European Journal of Pediatrics 152: 152–156

144. Cigada M, Gavazzi A, Assi E, Luccarelli M 2001 Gastric rupture after nasopharyngeal oxygen administration. Intensive Care Medicine 27: 939

145. Clark D A, Nieman G F, Thompson J E, Paskanik A M, Rokhar J E, Bredenberg C E 1987 Surfactant displacement by meconium free fatty acids: an alternative explanation for atelectasis in meconium aspiration syndrome. Journal of Pediatrics 110: 765–770

146. Clark J M, Lambertsen C J 1971 Pulmonary oxygen toxicity. Pharmacology Review 23: 37–133

147. Clark L C, Gollan F 1966 Survival of mammals breathing organic liquids equilibrated with oxygen at atmospheric pressure. Science 152: 1756

148. Clark P, Duff P 1995 Inhibition of neutrophil oxidative burst and phagocytosis by meconium. American Journal of Obstetrics and Gynecology 173: 1301–1305

149. Clark R H, Gerstmann D R, Null D N et al 1986 Pulmonary interstitial emphysema treated by high frequency oscillatory ventilation. Critical Care Medicine 14: 926–930

150. Clark R H, Gertsman D R, Null D M, deLemos R A 1992 Prospective randomized comparison of high frequency oscillatory and conventional ventilation in respiratory distress syndrome. Pediatrics 89: 5–12

151. Clark R H, Kueser T J, Walker M W et al 2000 Low-dose nitric oxide therapy for persistent pulmonary hypertension of the newborn. Clinical Inhaled Nitric Oxide Research Group. New England Journal of Medicine 342: 469–474

152. Clark R H, Yoder B A, Sell M S 1994 Prospective randomized comparisons of high frequency oscillation and conventional ventilation in candidates for extracorporeal membrane oxygenation. Journal of Pediatrics 124: 447–454

153. Cleary J P, Bernstein G, Mannino F L, Heldt G P 1995 Improved oxygenation during synchronized intermittent mandatory ventilation in neonates with respiratory distress syndrome: a randomized crossover study. Journal of Pediatrics 126: 407–411

154. Cleary J M, Wiswell T E 1998 Meconium-stained amniotic fluid and the meconium aspiration syndrome: an update. Pediatric Clinics of North America 45: 511–529

155. Clyman R I 1996 Recommendations for the postnatal use of indomethacin: an analysis of four separate treatment strategies. Journal of Pediatrics 128: 601–607

156. Cochrane C G, Revak D S, Merritt T A et al 1996 The efficacy and safety of KL4 surfactant in preterm infants with respiratory distress syndrome. American Journal of Respiratory and Critical Care Medicine 153: 404–410

157. Cohen G R, Thorp J, Yeast J D, Meyer B A, O'Kell R, Macy C 1991 A markedly immature lecithin:sphingomyelin ratio at term and congenital hypothyroidism. American Journal of Diseases of Children 145: 1227–1228

158. Cohen M, Carson B S 1985 Respiratory morbidity benefit of awaiting onset of labour after elective cesarean section. Obstetrics and Gynecology 65: 818–824

159. Cohen R S, Smith D W, Stevenson D K, Moskowitz P S, Graham C B 1984 Lateral decubitus position as therapy for persistent pulmonary interstitial emphysema in neonates: a preliminary report. Journal of Pediatrics 104: 441–443

160. Cole F S, Hamvas A, Rubenstein P et al 2000 Population based estimates of surfactant protein deficiency. Pediatrics 105: 538–541

161. Cole J W, Portman R J, Lim Y, Perlman J M, Robson A M 1985 Urinary β_2-microglobulin in full term newborns: evidence for proximal tubular dysfunction in infants with meconium stained amniotic fluid. Pediatrics 76: 958–964

162. Cole V A, Normand I C S, Reynolds E O R et al 1973 Pathogenesis of hemorrhagic pulmonary edema and massive pulmonary hemorrhage in the newborn. Pediatrics 51: 175–187

163. Colice G L, Matthay M A, Bass E, Matthay R A 1984 Neurogenic pulmonary edema. American Review of Respiratory Disease 130: 941–948

164. Collaborative European Multicentre Study Group 1991 Factors influencing the clinical response to surfactant replacement therapy in babies with severe respiratory distress syndrome. European Journal of Pediatrics 150: 433–439

165. Cook C D, Sutherland J M, Segal S et al 1957 Studies of respiratory physiology in the newborn infant. III. Measurements of the mechanics of respiration. Journal of Clinical Investigation 36: 440–448

166. Cooke R W I, Gribbin B, Gunning A J, Pickering D 1978 Ligation of patent ductus arteriosus in the very low birthweight newborn infant. Archives of Disease in Childhood 53: 271–275

167. Cooke R W I, Rennie J M 1984 Pancuronium and pneumothorax. Lancet i: 286–287

168. Corbet A, Bucciarelli R, Goldman S, Mammel M, Wold D, Long W 1991 Decreased mortality rate among small premature infants treated at birth with a single dose of synthetic surfactant. A multicenter controlled trial. Journal of Pediatrics 118: 277–284

169. Cordier M P, Gaultier C L, Boule M 1984 Infants with meconium aspiration syndrome: follow-up study (abstract). American Review of Respiratory Disease 129: 218

170. Cornfield D N, Maynard R C, de-Regnier R-A O et al 1999 Randomized controlled trial of low dose inhaled nitric oxide in the treatment of term and near term infants with respiratory failure and pulmonary hypertension. Pediatrics 104: 1089–1094

171. Cornfield D N, Reeve H L, Tolarova S et al 1996 Oxygen causes fetal pulmonary vasodilation through activation of a calcium-dependent potassium channel. Proceedings of the National Academy of Sciences of the the United States of America 93: 8089–8094

172. Costelo K, Hennessey E, Gibson A T et al 2000 The Epicure Study: outcomes to discharge from hospital for infants born at the threshold of viability. Pediatrics 106: 659–671

173. Cotton R B, Olsson T, Law A B et al 1993 The physiological effects of surfactant treatment on gas exchange in newborn premature infants with hyaline membrane disease. Pediatric Research 34: 495–501

174. Coulthard M G, Sharp J 1995 Haemodialysis and ultrafiltration in babies weighing under 1000 g. Archives of Disease in Childhood. Fetal and Neonatal Edition 73: F162–F165

175. Courtney S E, Pyon K H, Saslow J G et al 2001 Lung recruitment and breathing pattern during variable versus continuous positive airway pressure in premature infants: an evaluation of three devices. Pediatrics 107: 304–308

176. Couser R J, Ferrara T B, Falde B et al 1992 Effectiveness of dexamethasone in preventing extubation failure in preterm infants at increased risk for airway edema. Journal of Pediatrics 121: 591–596

177. Cowan F, Whitelaw A, Wertheim D, Silverman M 1991 Cerebral blood flow velocity changes after rapid administration of surfactant. Archives of Disease in Childhood 66: 1105–1109

178. Craft A P, Bhandari V, Finer N N 2003 The sy-fi study: a randomized prospective trial of synchronized intermittent mandatory ventilation versus a high-frequency flow interrupter technique in infants less than 1000 g. Journal of Perinatology 23: 14–19

179. Crowley M R, Fineman J R, Soier S J 1991 Effect of vasoactive drugs on thromboxane A_2 mimetic-induced pulmonary hypertension in newborn lambs. Pediatric Research 29: 167–172

180. Crowley P A 1995 Antenatal corticosteroid therapy. A meta-analysis of the randomized trials 1972–1994. American Journal of Obstetrics and Gynecology 173: 322–335

181. Crowther C A, Alfirevic Z, Haslam R R 2000 Prenatal thyrotropin-releasing hormone for preterm birth (Cochrane Review). Cochrane Database of Systematic Reviews (2): CD000019

182. Cuestas R A, Lindall A, Engel R R 1976 Low thyroid hormones and respiratory distress syndrome of the newborn. New England Journal of Medicine 295: 297–302

183. Curley M A, Thompson J E, Arnold J H 2000 The effects of early and repeated positioning in paediatric patients with acute lung injury. Chest 118: 156–163

184. Curtis J, O'Nell J T, Pettett G 1993 Endotracheal administration of tolazoline in hypoxia induced pulmonary hypertension. Pediatrics 92: 403–408

185. Cusick W, Smulian J C, Vintzileos A M 1995 Intrapartum use of fetal heart rate monitoring, contraction monitoring, and amnioinfusion. Clinics in Perinatology 22: 875–906

186. Cvetnic W G, Cunningham M D, Sills J H, Gluck L 1990 Reintroduction of continuous negative pressure ventilation in neonates: two years experience. Pediatric Pulmonology 8: 245–253

187. Cvetnic W G, Waffarn F, Martin J M 1989 Continuous negative pressure and intermittent mandatory ventilation in the management of pulmonary interstitial emphysema. Journal of Perinatology 9: 26–32

188. Da Costa D E, Nair A K, Pai M G, Al Khusarby S M 2001 Steroids in full term infants with respiratory failure and pulmonary hypertension due to meconium aspiration syndrome. European Journal of Pediatrics 138: 113–115

189. da Silva W J, Abbasi S, Pereira G, Bhutani V K 1994 Role of positive end expiratory pressure changes on functional residual capacity in surfactant treated preterm infants. Pediatric Pulmonology 18: 89–92

190. Dani C, Grella P V, Lazzarin L, Rubaltelli F F 1997 Antenatal ambroxol treatment does not prevent the respiratory distress syndrome in premature infants. European Journal of Pediatrics 156: 392–393

191. Dani C, Reali M F, Bertini G et al 1999 Risk factors for the development of respiratory distress syndrome and transient tachypnoea in newborn infants. Italian Group of Neonatal Pneumology. European Respiratory Journal 14: 155–159

192. Daniel S S, Adamsons K, James L S 1966 Lactate and pyruvate as an index of prenatal oxygen deprivation. Pediatrics 37: 942–953

193. Dargaville P A, South M, McDougall P N 2001 Surfactant and surfactant inhibitors in meconium aspiration syndrome. Journal of Pediatrics 138: 113–115

194. Davey A M, Becker J D, Davis J M 1993 Meconium aspiration syndrome: physiological and inflammatory changes in newborn piglet model. Pediatric Pulmonology 16: 101–108

195. Davidson D, Barefield E S, Kattwinkel J et al 1998 Inhaled nitric oxide for the early treatment of persistent pulmonary hypertension of the term newborn: a randomized double-masked, placebo-controlled, dose-response multicenter study. The I-NO/PPHN Study Group. Pediatrics 101: 325–334

196. Davidson D, Barefield E S, Kattwinkel J et al 1999 Safety of withdrawing inhaled nitric oxide therapy in persistent pulmonary hypertension of the newborn. Pediatrics 104: 231–236

197. Davies A M, Koenig J S, Thach B T 1989 Characteristics of upper airway chemoreflex prolonged apnea in human infants. American Review of Respiratory Disease 139: 668–673

198. Davis G M, Bureau M A 1987 Pulmonary and chest wall mechanics in the control of respiration in the newborn. Clinics in Perinatology 14: 551–579

199. Davis J M, Richter S E, Kendig J W, Notter R H 1992 High frequency jet ventilation and surfactant treatment of newborns with severe respiratory failure. Pediatric Pulmonology 13: 108–112

200. Davis J M, Russ G A, Metlay L, Dickerson B, Greenspan B S 1992 Short-term distribution kinetics of intratracheally administered exogenous lung surfactant. Pediatric Research 31: 445–450

201. Davis J M, Whitin J 1992 Prophylactic effects of dexamethasone in lung injury caused by hyperoxia and hyperventilation. Journal of Applied Physiology 72: 1320–1325

202. Davis P G, Henderson-Smart D J 2001 Extubation from low rate intermittent positive airways pressure versus extubation after a trial of endotracheal continuous positive airways pressure in intubated preterm infants (Cochrane Review). Cochrane Database of Systematic Reviews (4): CD0001078

203. Davis P J, Skekerdemian L S 2001 Meconium aspiration syndrome and extracorporeal membrane oxygenation. Archives of Disease in Childhood. Fetal and Neonatal Edition 84: F1–F3

204. Davis W B, Rennard S I, Bitterman P B, Crystal R G 1983 Early reversible changes in human alveolar structures induced by hyperoxia. New England Journal of Medicine 309: 878–883

205. Dawes G S, Fox H E, LeDuc B M, Liggins G C, Richards R T 1972 Respiratory movements and rapid eye movement in the fetal lamb. Journal of Physiology 220: 119–143

206. De Bie H M, van Toledo-Eppinga L, Verbeke J I, van Elburg R M 2002 Neonatal pneumatocele as a complication of nasal continuous positive airway pressure. Archives of Disease in Childhood. Fetal and Neonatal Edition 86: F202–F203

207. De Carolis M P, Romagnoli C, Cafforio C et al 1998 Pulmonary haemorrhage in infants with gestational age of less than 30 weeks. European Journal of Pediatrics 157: 1037–1038

208. De Klerk A M, de Klerck R K 2001 Use of continuous positive airway pressure in preterm infants: comments and experience from New Zealand. Pediatrics 108: 761–763

209. De Los Santos R, Seidenfeld J J, Anzueto A et al 1987 One hundred percent oxygen lung injury in adult baboons. American Review of Respiratory Disease 136: 657–661

210. De Paoli A G, Morley C J, Davis P G, Lau R, Hingeley E 2002 In vitro comparison of nasal continuous positive airway pressure devices for neonates. Archive of Disease in Childhood. Fetal and Neonatal Edition 87: F42–F45

211. de Winter J P, Merth I T, van Bel F, Egberts J, Brand R, Quanjer P H 1994 Changes in respiratory system mechanics in ventilated lungs of preterm infants with two different schedules of treatment. Pediatric Research 35: 541–549

212. Dehan M, Francoual J, Lindenbaum A 1978 Diagnosis of meconium aspiration by spectrophotometric analysis of urine. Archives of Disease in Childhood 53: 74–76

213. Dekowski S A, Snyder J M 1992 Insulin regulation of messenger ribonucleic acid for the surfactant-associated protein in human fetal lung in vitro. Endocrinology 131: 669–676

214. DeLemos R A, Coalson J J, Gerstmann D R, Kuehl T J, Null D M 1987 Oxygen toxicity in the premature baboon with hyaline membrane disease. American Review of Respiratory Disease 136: 677–682

215. DeLemos R A, Gerstmann D R, Clark R H, Guajardo A, Null D M 1987 High frequency ventilation – the relationship between the ventilator design and clinical strategy in the treatment of hyaline membrane disease and its complications: a brief review. Pediatric Pulmonology 3: 370–372

216. Demirakca S, Dortsch J, Knotlie C et al 1996 Inhaled nitric oxide in neonatal and paediatric acute respiratory distress syndrome: dose response, prolonged inhalation and weaning. Critical Care Medicine 24: 1913–1919

217. Demissie K, Marcella S W, Breckenridge M B, Rhoads G G 1998 Maternal asthma and transient tachypnea of the newborn. Pediatrics 102: 84–90

218. Dembinski J, Herep A, Kan N, Knopfle G, Bartmann P 2002 CT imaging of pulmonary lobar interstitial emphysema in spontaneously breathing preterm infant. American Journal of Perinatology 19: 285–290

219. Dessens A B, Smolders-de Haas H, Koppe J G 2000 Twenty-year follow-up of antenatal corticosteroid treatment. Pediatrics 105: E77

220. Dhanireddy R, Smith Y F, Hamosh M et al 1983 Respiratory distress syndrome in the newborn: relationship to serum prolactin, thyroxine and sex. Biology of the Neonate 43: 9–15

221. Dimitriou G, Greenough A 1995 Volume delivery during positive pressure inflation – relationship to spontaneous tidal volume of neonates. Early Human Development 41: 61–68

222. Dimitriou G, Greenough A 1995 Measurement of lung volume and optimization of oxygenation during high frequency oscillation. Archives of Disease in Childhood. Fetal and Neonatal Edition 72: F180–F183

223. Dimitriou G, Greenough A 2000 Performance of neonatal ventilators. British Journal of Intensive Care 10: 186–188

224. Dimitriou G, Greenough A, Broomfield D et al 2002 Rescue high frequency oscillation and predictors of adverse neurodevelopmental outcome in preterm infants. Early Human Development 66: 133–141

225. Dimitriou G, Greenough A, Castling D, Kavvadia V 1996 A comparison of supine and prone positioning in oxygen-dependent and convalescent premature infants. British Journal of Intensive Care 6: 254–259

226. Dimitriou G, Greenough A, Cherian S et al 2001 Comparison of airway pressure and airflow triggering systems using a single type of neonatal ventilator. Acta Paediatrica 90: 445–447

227. Dimitriou G, Greenough A, Endo A et al 2002 Prediction of extubation failure in preterm infants. Archives of Disease in Childhood. Fetal and Neonatal Edition 86: F32–F35

228. Dimitriou G, Greenough A, Giffin F, Chan V 1995 Synchronous intermittent mandatory ventilation modes versus patient triggered ventilation during weaning. Archives of Disease in Childhood. Fetal and Neonatal Edition 72: F188–F190

229. Dimitriou G, Greenough A, Giffin F J, Karani J 1995 The appearance of early chest radiographs and the response to surfactant replacement therapy. British Journal of Radiology 68: 1177–1180

230. Dimitriou G, Greenough A, Kavadia V 1997 Changes in lung volume, compliance and oxygenation in the first 48 hours of life in infants given surfactant. Journal of Perinatal Medicine 25: 49–54

231. Dimitriou G, Greenough A, Kavvadia V 2002 Fluid restriction, colloid infusion and chronic lung disease development in very low birth weight infants. Neonatal Intensive Care 15: 13–18

232. Dimitriou G, Greenough A, Kavvadia V et al 1998 Volume delivery during high frequency oscillation. Archives of Disease in Childhood. Fetal and Neonatal Edition 78: F148–F150

233. Dimitriou G, Greenough A, Kavvadia V et al 2000 Elective use of nasal continuous positive airways pressure following extubation of preterm infants. European Journal of Pediatrics 159: 434–439

234. Dimitriou G, Greenough A, Kavvadia V, Milner A D 1999 Comparison of two inspiratory:expiratory ratios during high frequency oscillation. European Journal of Pediatrics 158: 796–799

235. Dimitriou G, Greenough A, Lubscher B et al 1998 Comparison of airway pressure triggered and airflow triggered ventilation in very immature infants. Acta Paediatrica 87: 1256–1260

236. Dobbie H G, Whittle M J, Wilson A I, Whitfield C R 1983 Amniotic fluid phospholipid profile in multiple pregnancy and the effect of zygosity. British Journal of Obstetrics and Gynaecology 90: 1001–1006

237. Dobyns E L, Wescott J Y, Kennaugh J M, Ross M N, Stenmark K R 1994 Eicosanoids decrease with successful extracorporeal membrane oxygenation therapy in neonatal pulmonary hypertension. American Journal of Respiratory and Critical Care Medicine 149: 873–880

238. Dollberg S, Livny S, Mordecheyev N, Mimouni F B 2001 Nucleated red blood cell counts in meconium aspiration syndrome. Obstetrics and Gynecology 97: 593–596

239. Dooley S L, Pesavento D J, Depp R et al 1985 Meconium below vocal chords at delivery; correlation with intrapartum events. American Journal of Obstetrics and Gynecology 153: 761–770

240. Doyle L W, Kitchen W H, Ford G W, Rickards A L, Kelly E A 1989 Antenatal steroid therapy and 5 year outcome of extremely low birthweight infants. Obstetrics and Gynecology 73: 743–746

241. Doyle L W, Kitchen W H, Ford G W, Rickards A L, Lissenden J V, Ryan M M 1986 Effects of antenatal steroid therapy on mortality and morbidity in very low birthweight infants. Journal of Pediatrics 108: 287–292

242. Dreizzen E, Migdal M, Praud J P et al 1988 Passive compliance of total respiratory system in preterm newborn infants with respiratory distress syndrome. Journal of Pediatrics 112: 778–781

243. Drew J H 1982 Immediate intubation at birth of the very low birthweight infant. American Journal of Diseases of Children 136: 207–210

244. Duara S, Fox W W 1986 Persistent pulmonary hypertension of the neonate. In: Thibeault D W, Gregory G A (eds) Neonatal pulmonary care, 2nd edn. Appleton Century Crofts, Norwalk, CT, pp. 461–481

245. Dudell G G, Gersony W M 1984 Patent ductus arteriosus in neonates with severe respiratory disease. Journal of Pediatrics 104: 915–920

246. Dunn P M 1963 Intestinal obstruction in the newborn with special reference to transient functional ileus associated with respiratory distress syndrome. Archives of Disease in Childhood 38: 459–467

247. Durbin G M, Hunter N J, McIntosh N, Reynolds E O R, Wimberley P D 1976 Controlled trial of continuous inflating pressure for hyaline membrane disease. Archives of Disease in Childhood 51: 163–169

248. Edberg K E, Sandberg K, Silberberg A 1991 Lung volumes, gas mixing and mechanics of breathing in mechanically ventilated very low birth weight infants with idiopathic respiratory distress syndrome. Pediatric Research 30: 496–500

249. Edwards A D 1995 The pharmacology of inhaled nitric oxide. Archives of Disease in Childhood. Fetal and Neonatal Edition 72: F127–F130

250. Edwards A D, McCormick D C, Roth S C et al 1992 Cerebral hemodynamic effects of treatment with modified natural surfactant investigated by near infrared spectroscopy. Pediatric Research 32: 532–536

251. Edwards D K, Hilton S V W, Merritt T A, Hallman M, Mannino F, Boynton B R 1985 Respiratory distress syndrome treated with human surfactant. Radiographic findings. Radiology 157: 329–334

252. Eisler G, Hjertberg R, Lagercrantz H 1999 Randomised controlled trial of effect of terbutaline before elective caesarian section on postnatal respiration and glucose homeostasis. Archives of Disease in Childhood. Fetal and Neonatal Edition 80: F88–F92

253. Emery E F, Greenough A 1993 Randomized trial of two inotropes in preterm infants. European Journal of Pediatrics 152: 1–3

254. Emery E F, Greenough A, Gamsu H R 1992 Randomized controlled trial of colloid infusions in hypotensive preterm infants. Archives of Disease in Childhood 67: 1185–1188

255. Emmanouilides G C, Moss A J 1971 Respiratory distress in the newborn. Effects of cord clamping before and after onset of respiration. Biology of the Neonate 18: 363–368

256. Engdahl M S, Gershan W M 1998 Familial spontaneous pneumothorax in neonates. Pediatric Pulmonology 25: 398–400

257. Engle W D, Yoder M C, Andreoli S P et al 1997 Controlled prospective randomised comparison of high frequency jet ventilation and conventional ventilation in neonates with respiratory failure and persistent pulmonary hypertension. Journal of Perinatology 17: 3–9

258. Enskog A, Bengtsson A, Bengtson J P, Heideman M, Andreasson S, Larsson L 1996 Complement anaphylatoxin C3a and C5a formation in premature children with respiratory distress. European Journal of Pediatrics 155: 41–45

259. Eronen M, Kari A, Pesonen E, Hallman M 1993 The effect of antenatal dexamethasone administration on the fetal and neonatal ductus arteriosus. American Journal of Diseases of Children 147: 187–192

260. Evans N J, Archer L N J 1991 Doppler measurement of pulmonary artery pressure and extrapulmonary shunting in the acute phase of hyaline membrane disease. Archives of Disease in Childhood 66: 6–11

261. Evans N J, Archer L N J 1991 Doppler assessment of pulmonary artery pressure during recovery from hyaline membrane disease. Archives of Disease in Childhood 66: 802–804

262. Evans N J, Iyer P 1994 Incompetence of the foramen ovale in preterm infants supported by mechanical ventilation. Journal of Pediatrics 125: 786–792

263. Evans N, Kluckow M 1996 Early determinants of right and left ventricular output in ventilated preterm infants. Archives of Disease in Childhood. Fetal and Neonatal Edition 74: F88–F94

264. Evans N, Kluckow M 1999 High pulmonary blood flow and pulmonary hemorrhage. Pediatric Research 45: 195a

265. Faix R G, Viscardi R M, Dipietro M A, Nicks J J 1989 Adult respiratory distress syndrome in full term newborns. Pediatrics 83: 171–176

266. Falciglia H S 1988 Failure to prevent meconium aspiration syndrome. Obstetrics and Gynecology 71: 249–253

267. Falciglia H S, Henderschott C, Potter P et al 1992 Does DeLee suction at the perineum prevent meconium aspiration syndrome? American Journal of Obstetrics and Gynecology 167: 1243–1249

268. Fanconi S, Duc G 1987 Intratracheal suction in sick preterm infants: prevention of intracranial hypertension and cerebral hypoperfusion by muscle paralysis. Pediatrics 79: 538–543

269. Farrell P M 1986 Nutrition and infant lung function. Pediatric Pulmonology 2: 44–59

270. Farrell P M, Avery M E 1975 State of the art. HMD. American Review of Respiratory Disease 111: 657–688

271. Farstad T, Bratlid D 1991 Effect of endotracheal tube size and ventilator settings on the mechanics of a test system during intermittent flow ventilation. Pediatric Pulmonology 11: 15–21

272. Fedrick J, Butler N R 1970 Certain causes of neonatal death. I. Hyaline membranes. Biology of the Neonate 15: 229–255

273. Fiascone J M, Hu L-M, Vreeland P N 1992 Terbutaline does not improve lung function in preterm infants. American Journal of Obstetrics and Gynecology 167: 847–853

274. Field D, Milner A, Hopkin I E 1985 Effects of positive end expiratory pressure during ventilation of the preterm infant. Archives of Disease in Childhood 60: 843–847

275. Field D J, Milner A D, Hopkin I 1985 Inspiratory time and tidal volume during high frequency positive pressure ventilation. Archives of Disease in Childhood 60: 259–261

276. Field D J, Milner A D, Hopkin I E, Madeley R J 1987 Changing patterns in neonatal respiratory disease. Pediatric Pulmonology 3: 231–235

277. Findlay R D, Taeusch H W, Walther F J 1996 Surfactant replacement therapy for meconium aspiration syndrome. Pediatrics 97: 48–52

278. Finer N N, Barrington K J 1999 Nitric oxide for respiratory failure in infants born at or near term (Cochrane Review). Cochrane Database of Systematic Reviews (4): CD000399

279. Finer N N, Etches P C, Kamstra B, Tierney A J, Peliowski A, Ryan C A 1994 Inhaled nitric oxide in infants referred for extracorporeal membrane oxygenation: dose response. Journal of Pediatrics 124: 302–308

280. Finer N N, Moriartey R R, Boyd J, Phillips H J, Stewart A R, Ulan O 1979 Post-extubation atelectasis: a retrospective review and prospective controlled study. Journal of Pediatrics 94: 110–113

281. Finlay E R, Subhedar N V 2000 Pulmonary haemorrhage in preterm infants. European Journal of Pediatrics 159: 870–871

282. Finley J P, Howwman-Giles R B, Gilday D L, Bloom K R, Rowe R D 1979 Transient myocardial ischemia of the newborn infant demonstrated by thallium myocardial imaging. Journal of Pediatrics 94: 263–270

283. Fitzgerald D, Willis D, Usher R, Outerbridge E, Davis G M 1998 Dexamethasone for pulmonary interstitial emphysema in preterm infants. Biology of the Neonate 73: 34–39

284. Fleisher B, Kulovich M V, Hallman M, Gluck L 1985 Lung profile: sex difference in normal pregnancy. Obstetrics and Gynecology 66: 327–330

285. Florman A L, Teubner D 1969 Enhancement of bacterial growth in amniotic fluid by meconium. Journal of Pediatrics 74: 111–114

286. Fok T F, Kew J, Loftus W K et al 1998 Clinical predictors of post-extubation radiological changes of the chest in newborn infants. Acta Paediatrica 87: 88–92

287. Fouron J C, Bard H, Riopel L, deMuylder X, van Ameringer M-R, Urfer F 1985 Circulatory changes in newborn lambs with experimental polycythemia: comparison between fetal and adult type blood. Pediatrics 75: 1054–1060

288. Fowlie P W 1996 Prophylactic indomethacin: systemic review and meta-analysis. Archives of Disease in Childhood. Fetal and Neonatal Edition 74: F81–F87

289. Fox W W 1982 Mechanical ventilation in the management of persistent pulmonary hypertension of the neonate (PPHN). 83rd Ross Conference on Pediatric Research: Cardiovascular Sequelae of Asphyxia in the Newborn. Ross Laboratories, Columbus, OH, p. 102

290. Fox W W, Duara S 1983 Persistent pulmonary hypertension in the neonate. Diagnosis and management. Journal of Pediatrics 103: 505–514

291. Fox W W, Schwartz J G, Shaffer T H 1978 Pulmonary physiotherapy in neonates: physiologic changes and respiratory management. Journal of Pediatrics 92: 977–981

292. Fox W W, Spiker A R, Musci M 1984 Tracheal secretion impaction during hyperventilation for persistent pulmonary hypertension of the neonate (abstract). Pediatric Research 18: 323

293. Franco-Belgium Collaborative NO Trial Group 1999 Early compared with delayed inhaled nitric oxide in moderately hypoxaemic neonates with respiratory failure: a randomised controlled trial. Lancet 354: 1066–1071

294. Frank L 1992 Prenatal dexamethasone treatment improves survival of newborn rats during prolonged high oxygen exposure. Pediatric Research 32: 215–221

295. Frank L, Bucher J R, Roberts R J 1978 Oxygen toxicity in neonatal and adult animals of various species. Journal of Applied Physiology 45: 699–704

296. Frank L, Sosenko I R S 1991 Failure of premature rabbits to increase antioxidant enzymes during hyperoxic exposure: increased susceptibility to pulmonary oxygen toxicity compared with term rabbits. Pediatric Research 29: 292–296

297. Franklin R C, Purdie G L, O'Grady C M 1986 Neonatal thyroid function: prematurity, prenatal steroids and respiratory distress syndrome. Archives of Disease in Childhood 61: 589–592

298. Frantz I D, Close R H 1985 Elevated lung volume and alveolar pressure during jet ventilation of rabbits. American Review of Respiratory Disease 131: 134–138

299. Frantz I D, Wang N S, Thach B T 1975 Experimental meconium aspiration: effects of glucocorticoid treatment. Journal of Pediatrics 86: 434–441

300. Frantz I D, Werthammer J, Stark A R 1983 High frequency ventilation in premature infants with lung disease: adequate gas exchange at low tracheal pressure. Pediatrics 71: 483–488

301. French N P, Hagan R, Evans S F et al 1999 Repeated antenatal corticosteroids: size at birth and subsequent development. American Journal of Obstetrics and Gynecology 180: 114–121

302. Friedlich P, Lecart C, Posen R, Ramicone E, Chan L, Ramanathan R 1999 A randomised trial of nasopharyngeal-synchronised intermittent mandatory ventilation versus nasopharyngeal continuous positive airway pressure in very low birthweight infants after extubation. Journal of Perinatology 191: 413–418

303. Friedman S A, Schiff E, Kao L, Sibai B M 1995 Neonatal outcome after preterm delivery for pre-eclampsia. American Journal of Obstetrics and Gynecology 172: 1785–1792

304. Friedman Z, Rosenberg A 1979 Abnormal lung surfactant related to essential fatty acid deficiency in a neonate. Pediatrics 63: 855–859

305. Friesen R H, Honda A T, Thieme R E 1987 Changes in anterior fontanelle pressure in preterm neonates during tracheal intubation. Anesthesia and Analgesia 66: 874–878

306. Froese A B, Bryan A C 1987 High frequency ventilation. American Review of Respiratory Disease 135: 1363–1374

307. Fuchimukai T, Fujiwara T, Takahishi A, Enhorning G 1987 Artificial pulmonary surfactant inhibited by proteins. Journal of Applied Physiology 62: 429–437

308. Gabwell C E, Salzberg A M, Sonnino R E, Haynes J H 2000 Potentially lethal complications of central venous catheter placement. Journal of Pediatric Surgery 35: 709–713

309. Gage J E, Taeusch H W, Treves S, Caldicott W 1981 Suctioning of upper airway meconium in newborn infants. Journal of the American Medical Association 246: 2590–2592

310. Gandy G, Jacobson W, Gairdner D 1970 Hyaline membrane disease. I. Cellular changes. Archives of Disease in Childhood 45: 289–310

311. Gaon P, Lee S, Hannam S et al 1999 Assessment of effect of nasal continuous positive pressure on laryngeal opening using fibreoptic laryngoscopy. Archives of Disease in Childhood. Fetal and Neonatal Edition 80: F230–F232

312. Gappa M, Costeloe K, Southall D P, Rabbette P S, Stocks J 1994 Effect of continuous negative extrathoracic pressure on respiratory mechanics and timing in infants recovering from neonatal respiratory distress syndrome. Pediatric Research 36: 364–372

313. Gardner M O, Goldenberg R L, Gaudier F L, Dubard M B, Nelson K G, Hauth J C 1995 Predicting low Apgar scores of infants weighing less than 1000 grams: the effect of corticosteroids. Obstetrics and Gynecology 85: 170–174

314. Garite J J, Rumney P J, Briggs G G et al 1992 A randomized placebo-controlled trial of betamethasone for the prevention of respiratory distress syndrome at 24–28 weeks' gestation. American Journal of Obstetrics and Gynecology 166: 646–651

315. Garland J, Buck R, Weinberg M 1994 Pulmonary hemorrhage risk in infants with a clinically diagnosed patent ductus arteriosus. A retrospective cohort study. Pediatrics 94: 719–723

316. Garland J, Buck R K, Allred E N et al 1995 Hypocarbia before surfactant therapy appears to increase bronchopulmonary dysplasia risk in infants with respiratory distress syndrome. Archives of Pediatrics and Adolescent Medicine 149: 617–622

317. Gastiasoro-Cuesta E, Alvarez-Diaz F J Arnaiz-Renedo A et al 2001 The cardiovascular effects of partial liquid ventilation in newborn lambs after experimental meconium aspiration. Pediatric Critical Care Medicine 2: 334–339

318. Gau G S, Ryder T A, Mobberley M A 1987 Iatrogenic epithelial change caused by endotracheal intubation of neonates. Early Human Development 15: 221–229

319. Gauger P G, Hirschl R B, Delosh T N et al 1995 A matched pairs analysis of venoarterial and venovenous extracorporeal life support in neonatal respiratory failure. ASAIO Journal 41: M573–M579

320. Gaylor M S, Quissell B J, Lair M E 1987 High frequency ventilation in the treatment of infants weighing less than 1500 grams with pulmonary interstitial emphysema. Pediatrics 79: 915–921

321. Geggel R L, Murphy J D, Langleben D, Crone R K, Vacanti J P, Reid L M 1985 Congenital diaphragmatic hernia: arterial structural changes and persistent pulmonary hypertension after surgical repair. Journal of Pediatrics 107: 457–464

322. Geggel R L, Reid L M 1984 The structural basis for persistent pulmonary hypertension of the newborn. Clinics in Perinatology 11: 525–549

323. George T N, Johnson K J, Bates J N et al 1998 The effect of inhaled nitric oxide therapy on bleeding time and platelet aggregation in neonates. Journal of Pediatrics 132: 731–734

324. Gersony W M, Duc G V, Sinclair J C 1969 'PFC' syndrome (abstract). Circulation 40(suppl. III): 87

325. Gibson R L, Berger J I, Redding G J, Standaert T A, Mayock D E, Truog W E 1994 Effect of nitric oxide synthase inhibition during group B streptococcal sepsis in neonatal piglets. Pediatric Research 36: 776–783

326. Gibson R L, Truog W E, Redding G J 1988 Thromboxane associated pulmonary hypertension during three types of Gram positive bacteremia in piglets. Pediatric Research 23: 553–556

327. Giffin F, Greenough A 1994 ARDS type disease in children: modern respiratory management. Intensive Care Britain, 3rd edn. Greycoat Publishing, London, pp. 28–31

328. Gill A B, Weindling A M 1993 Randomized controlled trial of plasma protein fraction versus dopamine in hypotensive very low birthweight infants. Archives of Disease in Childhood 69: 284–287

329. Gill B S, Neville H L, Khan A M et al 2002 Delayed institution of extracorporeal membrane oxygenation is associated with increased mortality rate and prolonged hospital stay. Journal of Pediatric Surgery 37: 7–10

330. Gitterman M K, Fusch C, Gitterman A R et al 1997 Early nasal continuous positive airway pressure treatment reduces the need for intubation in very low birthweight infants. European Journal of Pediatrics 156: 384–388

331. Glass L, Rajegowda B D, Evans H E 1971 Absence of respiratory distress syndrome in premature infants of heroin addicted mothers. Lancet i: 685–686

332. Gluck L, Kulovich M V, Eidelman A I, Cordero L, Khazin A F 1972 Biochemical development of surfactant activity in mammalian lung. IV. Pulmonary lecithin synthesis in the human fetus and newborn and etiology of the respiratory distress syndrome. Pediatric Research 6: 81–99

333. Goetzman B W, Sunshine P, Johnson J D et al 1976 Neonatal hypoxia and pulmonary vasospasm: response to tolazoline. Journal of Pediatrics 89: 617–621

334. Goldman A P, Tasker R C, Haworth S G, Sigston P E, Macrae D J 1996 Four patterns of response to inhaled nitric oxide for persistent pulmonary hypertension of the newborn. Pediatrics 98: 708–713

335. Gomez R, Ghezzi F, Romero R, Munoz H, Tolosa J E, Rojas I 1995 Premature labor and intra-amniotic infection. Clinical aspects and role of the cytokines in diagnosis and pathophysiology. Clinics in Perinatology 22: 281–342

336. Gonzales F, Harris T, Black P et al 1987 Decreased gas flow through pneumothoraces in neonates receiving high frequency jet ventilation versus conventional ventilation. Pediatrics 110: 464–466

337. Gonzales L W, Ballard P L, Ertsey R, Williams M C 1986 Glucocorticoids and thyroid hormones stimulate biochemical and morphological differentiation of human fetal lung in organ culture. Journal of Clinical Endocrinology and Metabolism 62: 678–691

338. Goodwin S R, Graves S A, Haberkern C M 1985 Aspiration in intubated premature infants. Pediatrics 75: 85–88

339. Gordon E, South M, McDougall P N et al 2003 Blood aspiration syndrome as a cause of respiratory distress in the newborn infant. Journal of Pediatrics 142: 200–202

340. Gordon J B, Martinez F R, Keller P A, Tod M L, Madden J A 1993 Differing effects of acute and prolonged alkalosis on hypoxic pulmonary vasoconstriction. American Review of Respiratory Disease 148: 1651–1656

341. Gortner L, Pohlandt F, Bartmann P et al 1994 High dose versus low dose bovine surfactant treatment in very premature infants. Acta Paediatrica 83: 135–141

342. Gournay V, Savagner C, Thiriez G et al 2002 Pulmonary hypertension after ibuprofen prophylaxis in very preterm infants. Lancet 359: 1486–1488

343. Govindaswami B, Heldt G P, Bernstein G, Beyar R 1993 Reduction in cerebral blood flow velocity (CBFV) variability in infants <1500 g during synchronized ventilation (SIMV) (abstract). Pediatric Research 33: 1258

344. Grausz J P, Harvey D R 1967 Neonatal haemothorax: a report of two cases. Archives of Disease in Childhood 42: 675–676

345. Greenough A 1988 The premature infant's respiratory response to mechanical ventilation. Early Human Development 9: 1–5

346. Greenough A 1998 Use and misuse of albumin infusions in neonatal care. European Journal of Pediatrics 157: 699–702

347. Greenough A, Chan V, Hird M F 1992 Positive end expiratory pressure in acute and chronic neonatal respiratory distress. Archives of Disease in Childhood 67: 320–323

348. Greenough A, Cox S, Alexander et al 2001 Health care utilisation of infants with chronic lung disease, related to hospitalisation for RSV infection. Archives of Disease in Childhood 85: 463–468

349. Greenough A, Dixon A D, Roberton N R C 1984 Pulmonary interstitial emphysema. Archives of Disease in Childhood 59: 1046–1051

350. Greenough A, Greenall F 1988 Patient triggered ventilation in premature neonates. Archives of Disease in Childhood 63: 77–78

351. Greenough A, Greenall F 1988 Observation of spontaneous respiratory interaction with artificial ventilation. Archives of Disease in Childhood 63: 168–171

352. Greenough A, Greenall F, Gamsu H R 1987 Inspiratory times when weaning from mechanical ventilation. Archives of Disease in Childhood 62: 1269–1270

353. Greenough A, Greenall F, Gamsu H R 1987 Synchronous respiration – which ventilator rate is best? Acta Paediatrica Scandinavica 76: 713–718

354. Greenough A, Lagercrantz H 1992 Catecholamine abnormalities in transient tachypnoea of the premature newborn. Journal of Perinatal Medicine 20: 223–226

355. Greenough A, Milner A D 1987 High frequency ventilation in the neonatal period. European Journal of Pediatrics 146: 446–449

356. Greenough A, Milner A D, Dimitriou G 2001 Synchronised ventilation (Cochrane Review). Cochrane Database of Systematic Reviews (1): CD000456

357. Greenough A, Milner A D, Roberton N R C 1996 Neonatal respiratory disorders. Edward Arnold, London

358. Greenough A, Morley C J, Davis J A 1983 The interaction of spontaneous respiration with artificial ventilation in preterm babies. Journal of Pediatrics 103: 769–773

359. Greenough A, Morley C J, Pool J 1986 Fighting the ventilator: are fast rates an effective alternative to paralysis? Early Human Development 13: 189–194

360. Greenough A, Morley C J, Wood S, Davis J A 1984 Pancuronium prevents pneumothoraces in ventilated premature babies who actively expire against positive pressure ventilation. Lancet i: 1–3

361. Greenough A, Pool J 1988 Neonatal patient triggered ventilation. Archives of Disease in Childhood 63: 394–397

362. Greenough A, Pool J, Greenall F, Morley C J, Gamsu H 1987 Comparison of different rates of artificial ventilation in premature neonates with respiratory distress syndrome. Acta Paediatrica Scandinavica 76: 706–712

363. Greenspan J S, Wolfson M R, Holt W J, Shaffer T H 1990 Neonatal gastric intubation: differential respiratory effects between nasogastric and orogastric tubes. Pediatric Pulmonology 8: 254–258

364. Greenspan J S, Wolfson M R, Rubenstein D et al 1997 Partial liquid ventilation of human preterm neonates. Journal of Pediatrics 117:106–111

365. Gregory G A 1986 Devices for applying continuous positive airway pressure. In: Thibeault D W, Gregory G A (eds) Neonatal pulmonary care, 2nd edn. Appleton Century Crofts, Norwalk CT, pp. 307–320

366. Gregory G A, Gooding C A, Phibbs R H, Tooley W H 1974 Meconium aspiration in infants: a prospective study. Journal of Pediatrics 85: 848–852

367. Gregory G A, Kitterman J A, Phibbs R H, Tooley W H, Hamilton W K 1971 Treatment of idiopathic respiratory distress syndrome with continuous positive pressure. New England Journal of Medicine 284: 1333–1340

368. Gribetz I, Frank N R, Avery M E 1959 Static volume pressure relations of excised lungs of infants with hyaline membrane disease; newborn and stillborn infants. Journal of Clinical Investigation 38: 2168–2175

369. Griesen G, Frederiksen P S, Hertel J, Christensen N J 1985 Catecholamine response to chest physiotherapy and endotracheal suctioning in preterm infants. Acta Paediatrica Scandinavica 74: 525–529

370. Griesen G, Munck H, Lou H 1987 Severe hypocarbia in preterm infants and neurodevelopmental deficit. Acta Paediatrica Scandinavica 76: 401–404

371. Grosfeld J, Lemons J, Ballantine T V, Schreiner R L 1980 Emergency thoracotomy for acquired bronchopleural fistula in the premature infant with respiratory distress. Journal of Pediatric Surgery 15: 416–421

372. Gross G W, Greenspan J S, Fox W W, Rubenstein D, Wolfson M R, Shaffer T H 1995 Use of liquid ventilation with perflubron during extracorporeal membrane oxygenation: chest radiographic appearances. Pediatric Radiology 194: 717–720

373. Gross I, Moya F R 2001 Is there a role for antenatal TRH therapy for the prevention of neonatal lung disease? Seminars in Perinatology 25: 406–416

374. Gross I, Smith G J, Wilson C M et al 1980 The influence of hormones on the biochemical development of the fetal rat lung in organ culture. Pediatric Research 14: 834–838

375. Grossman G, Tashiro K, Kobayaski T et al 1999 Experimental neonatal respiratory failure induced by lysophosphatidyl choline: effect of surfactant treatment. Journal of Applied Physiology 86: 633–640

376. Grover T R, Parker T A, Zenge J P, Markham N E, Kinsella J P, Abman S H 2003 Intrauterine hypertension decreases lung VEGF expression and VEGF inhibition causes pulmonary hypertension in the ovine fetus. American Journal of Physiology. Lung Cellular and Molecular Physiology 284: L508–L517

377. Guignard J-P, Torrado A, Mazouni S M, Gautier E 1976 Renal function in respiratory distress syndrome. Journal of Pediatrics 88: 845–850

378. Guilleminault C, Coons S 1984 Apnea and bradycardia during feeding in infants weighing >2000 gm. Journal of Pediatrics 104: 932–935

379. Gupta A S, Rastogi S, Sahni R et al 2002 Inhaled nitric oxide and gentle ventilation in the treatment of pulmonary hypertension of the newborn – a single-center, 5-year experience. Journal of Perinatology 22: 435–441

380. Gurakan B, Tarcan A, Arda I S, Coskun M 2002 Persistent pulmonary interstitial emphysema in an unventilated neonate. Pediatric Pulmonology 34: 409–411

381. Hacking D, Warkins A, Fraser S et al 2001 Respiratory distress syndrome and birth order in premature twins. Archives of Disease in Childhood. Fetal and Neonatal Edition 84: F117–F121

382. Hagay Z, Reece A, Roberts A, Hobbins J C 1993 Isolated fetal pleural effusion: a prenatal management dilemma. Obstetrics and Gynecology 81: 147–152

383. Hallak M, Bottoms S F 1993 Accelerated pulmonary maturation from preterm premature rupture of membranes: a myth. American Journal of Obstetrics and Gynecology 169: 1045–1049

384. Halliday H L 2000 Endotracheal intubation at birth for preventing morbidity stained infants born at term (Cochrane Review). Cochrane Database of Systematic Reviews (2): CD000500

385. Halliday H L, McClure G, Reid M McC 1981 Transient tachypnoea of the newborn: two distinct clinical entities? Archives of Disease in Childhood 56: 322–325

386. Halliday H L, Tarnow-Mordi W O, Corcoran J D, Paterson C C 1993 Multicentre randomized trial comparing high and low dose surfactant regimens for the treatment of respiratory distress syndrome (Curosurf 4 trial). Archives of Disease in Childhood 69: 276–280

387. Hallman M, Arjomaa P, Hoppu K 1987 Inositol supplementation in respiratory distress syndrome: relationship between serum concentration, renal excretion and lung effluent phospholipids. Journal of Pediatrics 110: 604–610

388. Hallman M, Bry K, Hoppu K, Lappi M, Pohjavuori M 1992 Inositol supplementation in premature infants with respiratory distress syndrome. New England Journal of Medicine 326: 1233–1239

389. Hallman M, Haataja K 2003 Genetic influences and neonatal lung disease. Seminars in Neonatalogy 8: 19–27

390. Hallman M, Merritt T A, Bry K, Berry C 1993 Association between neonatal care practices and efficacy of exogenous human surfactant: results of a bi-center randomized trial. Pediatrics 91: 552–560

391. Hamdan A H, Shaw N J 1995 Changes in pulmonary artery pressure in infants with respiratory distress syndrome following treatment with Exosurf. Archives of Disease in Childhood. Fetal and Neonatal Edition 72: F176–F179

392. Hammerman C, Aramburo M J 1988 Decreased lipid intake reduces morbidity in sick premature neonates. Journal of Pediatrics 113: 1083–1088

393. Hammerman C, Lass N, Strates E, Komar K, Bui K-C 1987 Prostanoids in neonates with persistent pulmonary hypertension. Journal of Pediatrics 110: 470–472

394. Hamvas A, Devine T, Cole F S 1993 Surfactant therapy failure identifies infants at risk for pulmonary mortality. American Journal of Diseases of Children 147: 665–668

395. Han R N N, Buch S, Tseu I et al 1996 Changes in structure, mechanics and insulin-like growth factor related gene expression in the lungs of newborn rats exposed to air or 60% oxygen. Pediatric Research 39: 921–929

396. Han V K M, Beverly D W, Clarson C et al 1987 Randomized controlled trial of very early continuous distending pressure in the management of preterm infants. Early Human Development 15: 21–32

397. Hanlon-Lundberg K, Williams M, Rhim T, Covert R F, Mittendorf R, Holt J A 1996 Accelerated fetal lung maturity profiles and maternal cocaine exposure. Obstetrics and Gynecology 87: 128–132

398. Hannam S, Lees C, Edwards R J, Greenough A 2003 Neonatal coagulopathy in preterm, small-for-gestational-age infants. Biology of the Neonate 83: 177–181

399. Harrison V C, Heese H deV, Klein M 1968 The significance of grunting in hyaline membrane disease. Pediatrics 41: 549–559

400. Hart S M, McNair M, Gamsu H R, Price J F 1983 Pulmonary interstitial emphysema in very low birthweight infants. Archives of Disease in Childhood 58: 612–615

401. Hashim S A, Roholt H B, Babayan V K, Van Itallie T B 1964 Treatment of chyluria and chylothorax with medium chain triglyceride. New England Journal of Medicine 270: 756–761

402. Hauer A C, Rosegger H, Haas J, Haxhija E Q 1996 Reaction of term newborns with prolonged postnatal dyspnoea to early oxygen, mask CPAP and volume expansion: a prospective randomized clinical trial. European Journal of Pediatrics 155: 805–810

403. Hayek Z, Peliowski A, Ryan C A, Jones R, Finer N N 1986 External high frequency oscillation in cats. Experience in the normal lung and after saline lung lavage. American Review of Respiratory Disease 133: 630–634

404. Heaf D P, Helms P J, Dinwiddie R 1982 Nasopharyngeal airways in Pierre Robin syndrome. Journal of Pediatrics 100: 698–703

405. Heaf D P, Helms P, Gordon I, Turner H M 1983 Postural effects on gas exchange in infants. New England Journal of Medicine 308: 1505–1508

406. Heckman M, Linder W, Pohlandt F 1998 Tension pneumopericardium in a preterm infant without mechanical ventilation; a rare cause of cardiac arrest. Acta Paediatrica 87: 346–348

407. Heicher D A, Kasting D S, Richards J R 1981 Prospective clinical comparison of two methods of mechanical ventilation of neonates: rapid rate and short inspiratory time versus slow rate and long inspiratory time. Journal of Pediatrics 98: 957–961

408. Helbock H J, Insoft R M, Conte F A 1993 Glucocorticoid responsive hypotension in extremely low birthweight newborns. Pediatrics 92: 715–717

409. Heldt G P 1988 The effect of gavage feeding on the mechanics of the lung, chest wall and diaphragm in preterm infants. Pediatric Research 24: 55–58

410. Hellstrom-Westas L, Bell A H, Skov L, Greisen G, Svenningsen N W 1992 Cerebro-electrical depression following surfactant treatment in preterm neonates. Pediatrics 89: 643–647

411. Henderson-Smart D J, Bhuta T, Cools F et al 2003 Elective high frequency oscillatory ventilation versus conventional ventilation for acute pulmonary dysfunction in preterm infants (Cochrane Review). Cochrane Database of Systematic Reviews (1): CD000104

412. Henderson-Smart D J, Davis P J 2003 Prophylactic methylxanthines for extubation in preterm infants (Cochrane Review). Cochrane Database of Systematic Reviews (1): CD000139

413. Henry G W 1984 Non-invasive assessment of cardiac function and pulmonary hypertension in persistent pulmonary hypertension of the newborn. Clinics in Perinatology 11: 627–640

414. Herman S, Reynolds E O R 1973 Methods for improving oxygenation in infants mechanically ventilated for severe HMD. Archives of Disease in Childhood 48: 612–617

415. Hernandez C, Little B B, Dax J S, Gilstrap L C, Rosenfeld C R 1993 Prediction of the severity of meconium aspiration syndrome. American Journal of Obstetrics and Gynecology 169: 61–70

416. Herrera C M, Gerhardt T, Claure N et al 2002 Effects of volume guaranteed synchronized intermittent mandatory ventilation in preterm infants recovering from respiratory failure. Pediatrics 110: 529–533

417. Herting G, Rauprick P, Stitchenother G et al 2001 Resistance of different surfactant preparations to inactivation by meconium. Pediatric Research 50: 44–49

418. Hibbs A, Evans J R, Gerdes M et al 2001 Outcome of infants with bronchopulmonary dysplasia who receive extracorporeal membrane oxygenation therapy. Journal of Pediatric Surgery 36: 1479–1484

419. HIFI Study Group 1989 High-frequency oscillatory ventilation compared with conventional mechanical ventilation in the treatment of respiratory failure in preterm infants. New England Journal of Medicine 320: 88–93

420. HiFO Study Group 1993 Randomized study of high-frequency oscillatory ventilation in infants with severe respiratory distress syndrome. Journal of Pediatrics 122: 609–619

421. Hill A, Perlman J M, Volpe J J 1982 Relationship of pneumothorax to occurrence of intraventricular hemorrhage in the premature newborn. Pediatrics 69: 144–149

422. Hintz S R, Suttner D M, Sheehan A M et al 2000 Decreased use of neonatal extracorporeal membrane oxygenation (ECMO): how new treatment modalities have affected ECMO utilization. Pediatrics 106: 1339–1343

423. Hird M F, Greenough 1990 Causes of failure of neonatal patient triggered ventilation. Early Human Development 23: 101–108

424. Hird M F, Greenough A 1991 Inflation time in mechanical ventilation of preterm neonates. European Journal of Pediatrics 150: 440–443

425. Hird M, Greenough A, Gamsu H R 1990 Gas trapping during high frequency positive pressure ventilation using conventional ventilators. Early Human Development 22: 51–56

426. Hirschl R B, Merz S I, Montoya J P et al 1995 Development and application of a simplified liquid ventilator. Critical Care Medicine 23: 157–163

427. Hirschl R B, Philip W F, Glick V 2003 A prospective randomized trial of perfluorocarbon-induced lung growth in newborns with congenital diaphragmatic hernia. Journal of Pediatric Surgery 38: 283–289

428. Hirschl R B, Pranikoff T, Gauger P, Schreiner R J, Dechert R, Bartlett R H 1995 Liquid ventilation in adults, children and full term neonates. Lancet 346: 1201–1202

429. Hirschl R B, Tooley R, Parent A C, Johnson K, Bartlett R H 1995 Improvement of gas exchange pulmonary function and lung injury with partial liquid ventilation. Chest 108: 500–508

430. Hjalmarson O 1981 Epidemiology and classification of acute neonatal respiratory disorders. Acta Paediatrica Scandinavica 70: 773–783

431. Hjalmarson O, Olsson T 1974 Mechanical and ventilatory parameters in healthy and diseased newborn infants. Acta Paediatrica Scandinavica Supplement 247: 26–48

432. Hjalmarson O, Olsson T 1974 Work of breathing. Acta Paediatrica Scandinavica Supplement 247: 49–60

433. Hofmeyer G J 2002 Amnioinfusion for meconium stained liquid in labour (Cochrane Review). Cochrane Database of Systematic Reviews (1): CD000014

434. Holm B A, Notter R H, Leary J F, Matalon S 1987 Alveolar epithelial changes in rabbits after a 21 day exposure to 60% oxygen. Journal of Applied Physiology 62: 2230–2236

435. Holopainen R L, Aho H, Laine D J et al 1999 Human meconium has high phospholipase A2 activity and induces cell injury and apoptosis in piglet lungs. Pediatric Research 46: 626–632

436. Hook B, Hack M, Morrison S, Borawski-Clark E, Newman N S, Fanaroff A 1995 Pneumopericardium in very low birthweight infants. Journal of Perinatology 15: 27–31

437. Hooper S B, Harding R 1990 Changes in lung liquid dynamics induced by prolonged fetal hypoxemia. Journal of Applied Physiology 69: 127–135

438. Hope P L, Cady E B, Delpy D T, Ives N K, Gardner R M, Reynolds E O R 1988 Brain metabolism and intracellular pH during ischaemia: effects of systemic glucose and bicarbonate administration studied by ^{31}P and ^{1}H nuclear magnetic resonance spectroscopy in vivo in the lamb. Journal of Neurochemistry 50: 1394–1402

439. Hoskyns E N, Milner A D, Hopkin I E 1991 Combined conventional ventilation with high frequency oscillation in neonates. European Journal of Pediatrics 150: 357–361

440. Howell J H 1987 Sodium bicarbonate in the perinatal setting – revisited. Clinics in Perinatology 14: 807–816

441. Howell S, Fitzgerald R S, Roussos C 1985 Effects of uncompensated and compensated metabolic acidosis on canine diaphragms. Journal of Applied Physiology 59: 1376–1382

442. Howlett A, Ohlsson A 2003 Inositol for respiratory distress syndrome in preterm infants (Cochrane Review). Cochrane Database of Systematic Reviews (4): CD000366

443. Hrabovsky E E, Mullett M D 1986 Gastroesophageal reflux and the premature infant. Journal of Pediatric Surgery 21: 583–587

444. Huang Y-C T, Sane A C, Simonson S G 1995 Artificial surfactant attenuates hyperoxic lung injury in primates. I: Physiology and biochemistry. Journal of Applied Physiology 78: 1816–1822

445. Hulsey T C, Alexander G R, Robillard P Y, Annibale D J, Keenan A 1993 Hyaline membrane disease: the role of ethnicity and maternal risk characteristics. American Journal of Obstetrics and Gynecology 168: 572–576

446. Hummler H, Gerhardt T, Claure N, Everett R, Bancalari E 1994 Influence of patient triggered ventilation (PTV) on ventilation and blood pressure fluctuations in neonates. Pediatric Research 35: 338A

447. Huon C, Rey E, Mussat P, Parat S, Moriette G 1998 Low-dose doxapram for treatment of apnoea following early weaning in very low birthweight infants: a randomized, double-blind study. Acta Paediatrica 87: 1180–1184

448. Hutchinson A A, Yu V Y H 1980 Curare in the treatment of pulmonary hypertension as it occurs in the idiopathic respiratory distress syndrome. Australian Journal of Paediatrics 16: 94–100

449. Ikegami M 1994 Surfactant inactivation. In: Boynton B R, Carlo W A, Jobe A H (eds) New therapies for neonatal respiratory failure. Cambridge University Press, Cambridge, pp. 36–48

450. Ikegami M, Berry D, Elkady T, Pettenazzo A, Seidner S, Jobe A 1987 Corticosteroids and surfactant change lung function and protein leaks in the lungs of ventilated premature rabbits. Journal of Clinical Investigation 79: 1371–1378

451. Ikegami M, Jacobs H, Jobe A 1983 Surfactant function in respiratory distress syndrome. Journal of Pediatrics 102: 443–447

452. Ikegami M, Jobe A H, Newnham J, Polk D H, Willet K E, Sly P 1997 Repetitive prenatal glucocorticoids improve lung function and decrease growth in preterm lambs. American Journal of Respiratory and Critical Care Medicine 156: 178–184

453. Ikegami M, Jobe A H, Tabor B L, Rider E D, Lewis J F 1992 Lung albumin recovery in surfactant treated preterm ventilated lambs. American Review of Respiratory Disease 145: 1005–1008

454. Ikonen R S, Janas M O, Koivikko M J et al 1992 Hyperbilirubinaemia, hypocarbia and periventricular leukomalacia in preterm infants: relationship to cerebral palsy. Acta Paediatrica 81: 802–809

455. Illingworth R S 1969 Sucking and swallowing difficulties in infancy. Diagnostic problems of dysphagia. Archives of Disease in Childhood 44: 655–665

456. Ioffe S, Chernick V 1987 Maternal alcohol ingestion and the incidence of respiratory distress syndrome. American Journal of Obstetrics and Gynecology 156: 1231–1235

457. Islam S, Masiakos P, Schnitzer J J et al 1999 Diltiazem reduces pulmonary arterial pressures in recurrent pulmonary hypertension associated with pulmonary hypoplasia. Journal of Pediatric Surgery 34: 712–714

458. Itani M H, Mikati M A 1998 Early onset neonatal spontaneous pneumopericardium. Lebanese Medical Journal 46: 165–167

459. Itani Y, Fujioka M, Nishimura G, Nitsu N, Oono T 1988 Upper GI examination in older premature infants with persistent apnea: correlation with simultaneous cardiorespiratory monitoring. Pediatric Radiology 18: 464–467

460. Jackson R M 1985 Pulmonary oxygen toxicity. Chest 88: 900–905

461. Jacob J, Edwards D, Gluck L 1980 Early onset sepsis and pneumonia observed as respiratory distress syndrome. American Journal of Diseases of Children 134: 766–768

462. Jacobsen T, Gronvall J, Petersen S, Andersen G E 1993 Minitouch treatment of very low birthweight infants. Acta Paediatrica 82: 934–938

463. Jacqz-Aigrain E, Daoud P, Burtin P et al 1994 Placebo-controlled trial of midazolam sedation in mechanically ventilated newborn babies. Lancet 334: 640–650

464. James D K, Chiswick M L, Harkes A et al 1984 Non-specificity of surfactant deficiency in neonatal respiratory disorders. British Medical Journal (Clinical Research Ed) 288: 1635–1638

465. James L, Greenough A, Naik S 1997 The effect of blood transfusion on oxygenation in premature ventilated neonates. European Journal of Pediatrics 156: 139–141

466. James L, Jardin F, Farcot J C et al 1981 Influence of positive end expiratory pressure on left ventricular performance. New England Journal of Medicine 304: 387–392

467. Javaheri S, Herrera L, Kazemi H 1979 Ventilatory drive in acute metabolic acidosis. Journal of Applied Physiology 45: 913–918

468. Jedeikin R, Primhak A, Shennan A T, Swyer P R, Rowe R D 1983 Serial electrocardiographic changes in healthy and stressed neonates. Archives of Disease in Childhood 58: 605–611

469. Jeffery H E, Page M 1995 Developmental inactivation of gastro-oesophageal reflux in preterm infants. Acta Paediatrica 84: 245–250

470. Jeffries A L, Coates G, O'Brodovich H 1984 Pulmonary epithelial permeability in hyaline membrane disease. New England Journal of Medicine 311: 1075–1080

471. Johansson J, Curstedt T, Robertson B 1996 Synthetic protein analogues in artificial surfactants. Acta Paediatrica 85: 642–646

472. John E, Ermocilla R, Golden J, Cash R, McDevitt M, Cassady G 1980 Effects of gas temperature and particulate water on rabbit lung during ventilation. Pediatric Research 14: 1186–1191

473. Johnson A H, Peacock J C, Greenough A et al for the United Kingdom Oscillation Study Group 2002 High frequency oscillation ventilation for the prevention of chronic lung disease of prematurity. New England Journal of Medicine 347: 633–642

474. Joshi V V, Mandavia S G, Stern L, Wigglesworth F W 1972 Acute lesions induced by endotracheal intubation. American Journal of Diseases of Children 124: 646–649

475. Jovanovic R, Nguyen H T 1989 Experimental meconium aspiration in guinea pigs. Obstetrics and Gynecology 73: 652–656

476. Kääpä P, Seppänen M, Kero P, Ekblad H, Arjamaa O, Vuolteenaho O 1995 Haemodynamic control of atrial natriuretic peptide plasma levels in neonatal respiratory distress syndrome. American Journal of Perinatology 12: 235–239

477. Kallman J, Ekholm L, Eriksson M, Malmstrom B, Schollin J 1999 Contribution of interleukin-6 in distinguishing between mild respiratory distress and neonatal sepsis in the newborn infant. Acta Paediatrica 88: 880–884

478. Kamper J, Wulff K, Larsen C, Lindeqvist S 1993 Early treatment with nasal continuous positive airway pressure in very low birthweight infants. Acta Paediatrica 82: 193–197

479. Kanto W P 1994 A decade of experience with neonatal extracorporeal membrane oxygenation. Journal of Pediatrics 124: 335–347

480. Kanto W P, Borer R C, Barr M, Roloff D W 1976 Tracheal aspirate lecithin-sphingomyelin ratios as predictors of recovery from respiratory distress syndrome. Journal of Pediatrics 89: 612–616

481. Kanto W P, Kuhns L P, Borer R C, Roloff D W 1978 Failure of serial chest radiographs to predict recovery from respiratory distress syndrome. American Journal of Obstetrics and Gynecology 131: 757–760

482. Kari M A, Raivio K O, Stenman U H, Voutilainen R 1996 Serum cortisol, dehydroepiandrosterone sulphate and steroid-binding globulins in preterm neonates: effect of gestational age and dexamethasone therapy. Pediatric Research 40: 319–324

483. Karl S R, Ballantine T V N, Schnides M T 1983 High frequency ventilation at rates of 375–1800 cycles/minute in 4 neonates with congenital diaphragmatic hernia. Journal of Pediatric Surgery 18: 822–828

484. Karlowicz M G 1994 Pneumoretroperitoneum and perirenal air associated with tension pneumothorax. American Journal of Perinatology 11: 63–64

485. Karotkin E H, Kido M, Cashore W J et al 1976 Acceleration of fetal lung maturation by aminophylline in fetal rabbits. Pediatric Research 10: 722–724

486. Katyal S L, Amenta J S, Singh G, Silverman J A 1984 Deficient lung surfactant apoproteins in amniotic fluid with mature phospholipid profile from diabetic pregnancies. American Journal of Obstetrics and Gynecology 184: 48

487. Katz V L, Bowes W A 1992 Meconium aspiration syndrome: reflections on a murky subject. American Journal of Obstetrics and Gynecology 166: 171–183

488. Kavvadia V, Greenough A 1998 Influence of ethnic origin on respiratory distress syndrome in very premature infants. Archives of Disease in Childhood. Fetal and Neonatal Edition 78: F25–F28

489. Kavvadia V, Greenough A, Boylan G et al 2001 Effect of a high volume strategy high frequency oscillation on cerebral haemodynamics. European Journal of Pediatrics 160: 140–141

490. Kavvadia V, Greenough A, Dimitriou G 2000 Prediction of extubation failure in preterm neonates. European Journal of Pediatrics 159: 227–231

491. Kavvadia V, Greenough A, Dimitriou G, Forsling M 1998 Comparison of respiratory function and fluid balance in very low birthweight infants given artificial or natural surfactant or no surfactant. Journal of Perinatal Medicine 26: 469–474

492. Kavvadia V, Greenough A, Dimitriou G, Forsling M L 2000 A comparison of arginine vasopressin levels and fluid balance in the perinatal period in infants who did and did not develop chronic oxygen dependency. Biology of the Neonate 78: 86–91

493. Kavvadia V, Greenough A, Lilley J et al 1999 Plasma arginine levels and the response to inhaled nitric oxide in neonates. Biology of the Neonate 76: 340–347

494. Kawczynski P, Piotrowski A 1996 Circulatory and diuretic effects of dopexamine infusion in low birthweight infants with respiratory failure. Intensive Care Medicine 22: 65–70

495. Keeney S E, Cress S E, Brocon S E, Bidani A 1992 The effect of hyperoxic exposure on antioxidant enzyme activities of the alveolar type II cells in neonatal and adult rats. Pediatric Research 31: 441–444

496. Keeney S E, Mathews M J, Rassin D K 1993 Antioxidant enzyme responses to hyperoxia in preterm and term rats after prenatal dexamethasone administration. Pediatric Research 33: 177–180

497. Keirse M J N C 1995 Betamimetic tocolytics in preterm labour. In: Enkin M N, Kierse M J N C, Renfrew M J, Neilson J P, Crowther C (eds) Pregnancy and childbirth module of the Cochrane Collaboration; Issue 2. Update Software, Oxford

498. Kelly E, Bryan H, Possmayer F, Findova H, Bryan C 1993 Compliance of the respiratory system in newborns pre and post surfactant replacement therapy. Pediatric Pulmonology 15: 225–230

499. Kelly F J, Lubec G 1995 Hyperoxic injury of immature guinea pig lung is mediated by hydroxyl radicals. Pediatric Research 38: 286–291

500. Kelly L K, Porta N F, Goodman D M, Carroll C L, Steinhorn R H 2002 Inhaled prostacyclin for term infants with persistent pulmonary hypertension refractory to inhaled nitric oxide. Journal of Pediatrics 141: 830–832

501. Kelly M A, Finer N N 1984 Nasotracheal intubation in the neonate: physiologic responses and effects of atropine and pancuronium. Journal of Pediatrics 105: 303–309

502. Keszler M, Carbone M T, Cox C, Schumacher R E 1992 Severe respiratory failure after elective repeat cesarean delivery: a potentially preventable condition leading to extracorporeal membrane oxygenation. Pediatrics 89: 670–672

503. Keszler M, Donn S M, Bucciarelli R L et al 1991 Multicenter controlled trial comparing high frequency jet ventilation and conventional mechanical ventilation in patients with pulmonary interstitial emphysema. Journal of Pediatrics 119: 85–93

504. Keszler M, Durand D J 2001 Neonatal high-frequency ventilation. Past, present and future. Clinics in Perinatology 28: 579–607

505. Keszler M, Modanlou H D, Brudno S et al 1997 Multicenter controlled clinical trial of high frequency jet ventilation in preterm infants with uncomplicated respiratory distress syndrome. Pediatrics 120: 107–113

506. Khalaf M N, Porat R, Brodsky N L, Bhandart V 2001 Clinical correlations in infants in the neonatal intensive care unit with varying severity of gastroesophageal reflux. Journal of Gastroenterology and Nutrition 32: 45–49

507. Khammash H, Perlman M, Wojtulewicz J, Dunn M 1993 Surfactant therapy in full term neonates with severe respiratory failure. Pediatrics 92: 135–139

508. Kiely J L 1991 Mode of delivery and neonatal death in 17 587 infants presenting by the breech. British Journal of Obstetrics and Gynaecology 98: 898–904

509. Kim E H, Boutwell W C 1987 Successful direct extubation of very low birthweight infants from low intermittent mandatory ventilation rate. Pediatrics 80: 409–414

510. King J F, Grant A, Keirse M J N C, Chalmers I 1988 Betamimetics in preterm labour: an overview of the randomised controlled trials. British Journal of Obstetrics and Gynaecology 95: 211–222

511. King R J, Coalson J J, Seidenfeld J, Anzueto A R, Smith D B, Peters J I 1989 Oxygen and pneumonia induced lung injury. II. Properties of surfactant. Journal of Applied Physiology 67: 357–365

512. Kinmond S, Aitchison T C, Holland B M, Jones J G, Turner T L, Wardrop C A 1993 Umbilical cord clamping and preterm infants: a randomized trial. British Medical Journal 306: 172–175

513. Kinsella J P, Abman S H 1995 Recent developments in the pathophysiology and treatment of persistent pulmonary hypertension of the newborn. Journal of Pediatrics 126: 853–864

514. Kinsella J P, Neish S R, Shaffer E, Abman S H 1992 Low dose inhalational nitric oxide in persistent pulmonary hypertension of the newborn. Lancet 340: 819–820

515. Kinsella J P, Truog W E, Walsh W F et al 1997 Randomised multicentre trial of inhaled nitric oxide and high frequency oscillatory ventilation in severe persistent pulmonary hypertension of the newborn. Journal of Pediatrics 131: 55–62

516. Kinsella J P, Walsh W F, Bose C L et al 1999 Inhaled nitric oxide in premature neonates with severe hypoxaemic respiratory failure: a controlled trial. Lancet 354: 1061–1065

517. Kjos S L, Walter F J, Montorom M, Paul R H, Diaz F, Stabiler M 1990 Prevalence and etiology of respiratory distress in infants of diabetic mothers: predictive value of lung maturation tests. American Journal of Obstetrics and Gynecology 163: 898–903

518. Klarr J M, Faix R G, Pryce C J E, Bhatt-Mehta V 1994 Randomized trial of dopamine versus dobutamine for treatment of hypotension in preterm infants with respiratory distress syndrome. Journal of Pediatrics 125: 117–122

519. Klein A H, Foley B, Foley T P, MacDonald H M, Fisher D A 1981 Thyroid function studies in cord blood from premature infants with and without RDS. Journal of Pediatrics 98: 818–820

520. Klein J 1990 Normobaric pulmonary oxygen toxicity. Anesthesia and Analgesia 70: 195–207

521. Klein M D, Whittlesey G C 1994 Extracorporeal membrane oxygenation. Pediatric Clinics of North America. 41: 365–384

522. Knight D B, Liggins G C, Wealthall S R 1994 A randomized controlled trial of antepartum thyrotropin releasing hormone and betamethasone in the prevention of respiratory disease in preterm infants. American Journal of Obstetrics and Gynecology 171: 11–16

523. Kobayashi T, Nitta K, Ganzuka M, Inui S, Grossmann G, Robertson B 1991 Inactivation of exogenous surfactant by pulmonary edema fluid. Pediatric Research 29: 353–356

524. Kohelet D, Perlman M, Kirpalani H, Hanna G, Koren G 1988 High frequency oscillation in the rescue of infants with persistent pulmonary hypertension. Critical Care Medicine 16: 510–516

525. Kohlhauser C, Popow C, Helbich T, Hermon M, Weninger M, Herold C J 1995 Successful treatment of severe neonatal lobar emphysema by high frequency oscillatory ventilation. Pediatric Pulmonology 19: 52–55

526. Konduri G G, Mital S 2000 Adenosine and ATP cause NO-dependent pulmonary vasodilation in fetal lambs. Biology of the Neonate 78: 220–229

527. Konishi M, Fujiwara T, Takeuki Y et al 1988 Surfactant replacement therapy in neonatal respiratory distress syndrome. European Journal of Pediatrics 144: 20–25

528. Kotas R V, Avery M E 1971 Accelerated appearance of pulmonary surfactant in the fetal rabbit. Journal of Applied Physiology 30: 358–361

529. Koumbourlis A C, Mutich R L, Motoyama E S 1995 Contribution of airway hyperresponsiveness to lower airway obstruction after extracorporeal membrane oxygenation for meconium aspiration syndrome. Critical Care Medicine 23: 749–754

530. Kourembanas S, Marsden P A, McQuillan L P, Fuller D V 1991 Hypoxia induces endothelin gene expression and secretion in cultured human endothelium. Journal of Clinical Investigation 88: 1054–1057

531. Krauss A N, Auld P A M 1969 Ventilation perfusion abnormalities in the premature infant: triple gradient. Pediatric Research 3: 255–264

532. Kühl P G, Cotton R B, Schweer H, Seyberth H 1989 Endogenous formation of prostanoids in neonates with persistent pulmonary hypertension. Archives of Disease in Childhood 64: 949–952

533. Kuhns L R, Bednarek F J, Wyman M L, Roloff D W, Borer R C 1975 Diagnosis of pneumothorax or pneumomediastinum in the neonate by transillumination. Pediatrics 56: 355–360

534. Kuint J, Reichman B, Neumann L, Shinwell E S 1994 Prognostic response of the immediate response to surfactant. Archives of Disease in Childhood. Fetal and Neonatal Edition 71: F170–F173

535. Kumar P, Kazzi N J, Shankaran S 1996 Plasma immunoreactive endothelin-1 concentrations in infants with persistent pulmonary hypertension of the newborn. American Journal of Perinatology 13: 335–341

536. Lachman B 1987 Combination of saline instillation with artificial ventilation damages bronchial surfactant. Lancet i: 1375

537. Lago P, Benini F, Agosto C, Zacchello F 1998 Randomised controlled trial of low dose fentanyl infusion in preterm infants with hyaline membrane disease. Archives of Disease in Childhood 79: 194–197

538. Lam B C, Yeung C Y 1999 Surfactant lavage for meconium aspiration syndrome: a pilot study. Pediatrics 103: 1014–1018

539. Lamont R F, Dunlop P D M, Levene M I, Elder M G 1983 Use of glucocorticoids in pregnancies complicated by severe hypertension and proteinuria. British Journal of Obstetrics and Gynaecology 90: 199–202

540. Lanteri C J, Willet K E, Kano S et al 1994 Time course in lung mechanics following fetal steroid treatment. American Journal of Respiratory and Critical Care Medicine 150: 759–765

541. Laros R K, Kitterman J A, Heilbron D C 1991 Outcome of very low birthweight infants exposed to beta sympathomimetics in utero. American Journal of Obstetrics and Gynecology 164: 1657–1665

542. Lassus P, Turanlati M, Heikkala P et al 2001 Pulmonary vascular endothelial growth factor and Ftt-1 in fetuses in acute and chronic lug disease and in PPHN. American Journal of Respiratory and Critical Care Medicine 164:1961–1967

543. Laubscher B, Greenough A, Costeloe K 1996 Performance of four neonatal high frequency oscillators. British Journal of Intensive Care 6: 148–152

544. Laubscher B, Greenough A, Devane S P 1997 Response to nitric oxide: influence of gestational age. European Journal of Pediatrics 156: 639–642

545. Le Souef P, England S J, Bryan A C 1984 Total resistance of the respiratory system in preterm infants with and without an endotracheal tube. Journal of Pediatrics 104: 108–111

546. Leach C L, Greenspan J S, Rubenstin S D et al 1995 Partial liquid ventilation with Liquivent: a pilot and safety and efficacy study in premature newborns with severe respiratory distress syndrome (abstract). Pediatric Research 37: 220

547. Leach C L, Greenspan J S, Rubenstein S D et al 1996 Partial liquid ventilation with perfluorocarbon in premature infants with severe respiratory distress syndrome. New England Journal of Medicine 335: 761–767

548. Leach C L, Holm B, Morin F C et al 1995 Partial liquid ventilation in premature lambs with respiratory distress syndrome: efficacy and compatibility with exogenous surfactant. Journal of Pediatrics 126: 412–420

549. Lechner A J, Winson D C, Bauman J E 1986 Lung mechanics, cellularity and surfactant after prenatal starvation in guinea pigs. Journal of Applied Physiology 60: 1610–1614

550. Lee S K, Tanswell A K 1989 Pulmonary vascular air embolism in the newborn. Archives of Disease in Childhood 64: 507–510

551. Lee S, Milner A D 2000 Resonance frequency in respiratory distress syndrome. Archives of Disease in Childhood. Fetal and Neonatal Edition 83: F203–F206

552. Lehtinen A-M, Hovorka J, Widholm O 1984 Modification of aspects of the endocrine response to tracheal intubation by lignocaine, halothane and thiopentone. British Journal of Anaesthesia 56: 239–246

553. Leigh R J, Shaw D A 1976 Rapid regular respiration in unconscious patients. Archives of Neurology 33: 356–361

554. Leipala J A, Petaja J, Fellman V 2001 Perforation complications of percutaneous central venous catheters in very low birthweight infants. Journal of Paediatrics and Child Health 37: 168–171

555. Lemyre B, Davis P G, de Paoli A G 2002 Nasal intermittent positive pressure ventilation (NIPPV) versus nasal continuous positive airway pressue (NCPAP) for apnea of prematurity (Cochrane Review). Cochrane Database of Systematic Reviews (1): CD002272

556. Leonardi M R, Hankins G D V 1992 What's new in tocolytics. Clinics in Perinatology 19: 367–384

557. Leonidas J C, Hall R T, Rhodes P G 1975 Conservative management of unilateral pulmonary interstitial emphysema under tension. Journal of Pediatrics 87: 776–778

558. Leslie G I, Gallery E D M, Arnold J D, Nicholson E 1991 Hyaline membrane disease and early neonatal aldosterone metabolism in infants of less than 33 weeks gestation. Acta Paediatrica Scandinavica 80: 628–633

559. Leveno K J, Quirk J G, Whalley P J, Herbert W N P, Trubey R 1984 Fetal lung maturation in twin gestations. American Journal of Obstetrics and Gynecology 148: 405–411

560. Levin D L, Fixler D E, Morriss F C, Tyson J 1978 Morphologic analysis of the pulmonary vascular bed in infants exposed in utero to prostaglandin synthetase inhibitors. Journal of Pediatrics 92: 478–483

561. Levin D L, Mills L J, Parkey M, Garriott J, Campbell W 1979 Constriction of the fetal ductus arteriosus after administration of indomethacin to the pregnant ewe. Journal of Pediatrics 94: 647–650

562. Levin D L, Weinberg A G, Perkin R M 1983 Pulmonary microthrombi syndrome in newborn infants with unresponsive persistent pulmonary hypertension. Journal of Pediatrics 102: 299–303

563. Lewis D F, Futayyeh S, Towers C V, Asrat T, Edwards M S, Brooks G G 1996 Preterm delivery from 34 to 37 weeks of gestation: is respiratory distress syndrome a problem? American Journal of Obstetrics and Gynecology 174: 525–528

564. Lewis V, Whitelaw A 2002 Furosemide for transient tachypnoea of the newborn (Cochrane Review). Cochrane Database of Systematic Reviews (1): CD000366

565. Liang J S, Lu F L, Tang J R, Yang K 2000 Congenital diaphragmatic hernia misdiagnosed as pneumothorax in a newborn. Taiwan Erch Koi Hseh Hui Tsa Chih 41: 221–223

566. Lieberman E, Torday J, Barbieri R, Cohen A, Van Vunakis H, Weiss S T 1992 Association of intrauterine cigarette smoke exposure with indices of fetal lung maturation. Obstetrics and Gynecology 79: 564–570

567. Liechty E A, Donovan E, Purohit D et al 1991 Reduction of neonatal mortality after multiple doses of bovine surfactant in low birthweight neonates with respiratory distress syndrome. Pediatrics 88: 19–28

568. Liggins G C, Howie R N 1972 A controlled trial of antepartum glucocorticoid treatment for prevention of the respiratory distress syndrome in premature infants. Pediatrics 50: 515–525

569. Lin Y, Lechner A J 1991 Surfactant content and type II cell development in fetal guinea pig lungs during prenatal starvation. Pediatric Research 29: 288–291

570. Linder N, Aranda J V, Tsur M et al 1988 Need for endotracheal intubation and suction in meconium stained neonates. Journal of Pediatrics 112: 613–615

571. Linder W, Vossbeck S, Hummler H et al 1999 Delivery room management of extremely low birthweight infants: spontaneous breathing or intubation? Pediatrics 103: 961–967

572. Linderkamp O, Versmold H T, Fendel H, Riegel K P, Betke K 1978 Association of neonatal respiratory distress with birth asphyxia and deficiency of red cell mass in premature infants. European Journal of Pediatrics 129: 167–173

573. Lioy J, Manginello F P 1988 A comparison of prone and supine positioning in the immediate post-extubation period of neonates. Journal of Pediatrics 112: 982–984

574. Loe E A, Graves E D, Ochsner J L, Falterman K W, Arensman R M 1985 ECMO for newborn respiratory failure. Journal of Pediatric Surgery 20: 684–688

575. Long W, Corbet A, Allen A et al 1992 Retrospective search for bleeding diathesis among premature newborn infants with pulmonary hemorrhage after synthetic surfactant treatment. Journal of Pediatrics 120: S45–S48

576. Long W A, Lawson E E, Harned H S, Kraybill E N 1984 Pleural effusion in the first days of life. American Journal of Perinatology 1: 190–194

577. Long W, Zucker J A, Kraybill E N 1995 Symposium in synthetic surfactant. II. Health and developmental outcomes at one year. Journal of Pediatrics 126: S1–S80

578. Longaker M T, Laberge J M, Dansereau J et al 1989 Primary fetal hydrothorax: natural history and management. Journal of Pediatric Surgery 24: 573–576

579. Loo C K, Smith G J, Lykke A W J 1989 Effects of hyperoxia on surfactant morphology and cell viability in organotypic cultures of fetal rat lungs. Experimental Lung Research 15: 597–617

580. Lopez J B, Campbell R E, Bishop H C 1977 Clinical note: non-operative resolution of prolonged localized intrapulmonary interstitial emphysema associated with hyaline membrane disease. Journal of Pediatrics 91: 653–654

581. Lotze A, Knight G R, Martin G R 1993 Improved pulmonary outcome after exogenous surfactant for respiratory failure in term infants requiring extracorporeal membrane oxygenation. Journal of Pediatrics 121: 261–268

582. Lotze A, Mitchell B R, Short B L et al 1998 Multicenter study of surfactant (Beractant) use in the treatment of term infants with severe respiratory failure. Journal of Pediatrics 132: 40–47

583. Lucas A, Bloom S R, Aynsley-Green A 1986 Gut hormones and minimal enteral feeding. Acta Paediatrica Scandinavica 75: 719–723

584. Lund W S 1976 Deglutition. In: Hinchcliffe R, Harrison D (eds) Scientific foundations of ortolaryngology. Heinemann, London, pp. 591–598

585. Lundstrom K E, Greisen G 1996 Changes in EEG, systemic circulation and blood gas parameters following two or six aliquots of porcine surfactant. Acta Paediatrica 85: 708–712

586. Lyrene R K, Philips J B 1984 Control of pulmonary vascular resistance in the fetus and newborn. Clinics in Perinatology 11: 551–564

587. MacArthur B A, Howie R N, Dezcete J A, Elkins J 1981 Cognitive and psychosocial development of 4-year-old children whose mothers were treated antenatally with betamethasone. Pediatrics 68: 638–643

588. McCann E M, Goldman S L, Brady J P 1987 Pulmonary function in the sick newborn infant. Pediatric Research 21: 313–325

589. McCormick M D, Workman Daniels K, Grooks Gunn J et al 1993 Hospitalization of very low birthweight children at school age. Journal of Pediatrics 122: 360–365

590. McCulloch P R, Fokert P G, Froese A B 1988 Lung volume maintenance prevents lung injury during high frequency oscillatory ventilation in surfactant deficient rabbits. American Review of Respiratory Disease 137: 1185–1192

591. McEvoy R D, Davies N J, Hedenstierna G, Hartman M T, Spragg R G, Wagner P D 1982 Lung mucociliary transport during high frequency ventilation. American Review of Respiratory Disease 126: 452–456

592. MacFarlane P I, Heaf D P 1988 Pulmonary function in children after neonatal meconium aspiration syndrome. Archives of Disease in Childhood 63: 368–372

593. MacGregor R, Evans D, Sugden D, Gaussen T, Levene M 1998 Outcome at 5–6 years of prematurely born children who received morphine as neonates. Archives of Disease in Childhood. Fetal and Neonatal Edition 79: F40–F43

594. Macklin C C 1936 Alveolar pores and their significance in the human lung. Archives of Pathology 21: 202–210

595. MacMahon P, Fleming P J, Thearle M J, Speidel B D 1982 An improved selective bronchial intubation technique for managing severe localized interstitial emphysema. Acta Paediatrica Scandinavica 71: 151–153

596. McMillan D D, Rademaker A W, Buchan K A, Reid A, Machin G, Sauve R S 1986 Benefits of orotracheal and nasotracheal intubation in neonates requiring ventilatory assistance. Pediatrics 7: 39–44

597. Madansky D L, Lawson E E, Chernick V, Taeusch H W 1979 Pneumothorax and other forms of pulmonary air leak in the newborn. American Review of Respiratory Disease 120: 729–737

598. Madar J, Richmond S, Hey E 1999 Surfactant deficient respiratory distress after elective delivery at 'term'. Acta Paediatrica 88: 1244–1248

599. Madhavi P, Jameson R, Robinson M J 2000 Unilateral pleural effusion complicating central venous catheterisation. Archives of Disease in Childhood. Fetal and Neonatal Edition 82: F248–F249

600. Mahmoud E L, Benirschke K, Vaucher Y E, Poitras P 1988 Motilin levels in term neonates who have passed meconium prior to birth. Journal of Paediatric Gastroenterology and Nutrition 7: 95–99

601. Makhoul I R, Smolkin T, Sujov P 2002 Pneumothorax and nasal continuous positive airway pressure ventilation in premature neonates: a note of caution. ASAIO Journal 48: 476–479

602. Makri V, Hospes B, Stoll-Becker S, Borkhardt A, Gortner L 2002 Polymorphisms of surfactant protein B encoding gene: modifiers of the course of neonatal respiratory distress. European Journal of Pediatrics 161: 604–608

603. Malo J, Ali J, Wood L D H 1984 How does positive end expiratory pressure reduce intrapulmonary shunt in canine pulmonary edema? Journal of Applied Physiology 57: 1002–1010

604. Mammel M C, Boros S J 1987 Airway damage and mechanical ventilation. Pediatric Pulmonology 3: 443–447

605. Man G C W, Man S F P, Kappagoda C T 1983 Effects of high frequency oscillatory ventilation on vagal and phrenic nerve activity. Journal of Applied Physiology 54: 502–507

606. Manalo E, Merritt T A, Kheiter A, Amirkhanian J, Cochrane C 1996 Comparative effects of some serum components and proteolytic products of fibrinogen in surface tension-lowering abilities of Beractant and a synthetic peptide containing surfactant KL4. Pediatric Research 39: 947–952

607. Manczur T, Greenough A, Nicholson G P et al 1999 Resistance of pediatric and neonatal endotracheal tubes – influence of flow, rate, size and shape. Critical Care Medicine 28: 1595–1598

608. Manning F A, Martin C B, Murata Y, Miyaki K, Danzier G 1979 Breathing movements before death in the primate fetus. American Journal of Obstetrics and Gynecology 135: 71–76

609. Manning F A, Schreiber F A, Turkel S B 1978 Fatal meconium aspiration 'in utero'. A case report. American Journal of Obstetrics and Gynecology 132: 111–113

610. Manroe B L, Weinberg A G, Rosenfield C R, Browne R 1979 The neonatal blood count in health and disease. I. Reference value for neutrophil cells. Journal of Pediatrics 95: 89–98

611. Marchak B E, Thompson W K, Duffty P 1981 Treatment of RDS by high frequency oscillatory ventilator. A preliminary report. Journal of Pediatrics 99: 287–292

612. Margolis C Z, Orzalesi M M, Schwartz A D 1973 Disseminated intravascular coagulation in the respiratory distress syndrome. American Journal of Diseases of Children 125: 324–326

613. Marino A J, Assing E, Carbone M T, Hiatt I M, Hegyi T, Graff M 1995 The incidence of gastroesophageal reflux in preterm infants. Journal of Perinatology 15: 369–371

614. Maron M B 1987 Analysis of airway fluid protein concentration in neurogenic pulmonary edema. Journal of Applied Physiology 62: 470–476

615. Marshall T A, Deeder R, Pai S, Berkowitz G P, Austin T L 1984 Physiological changes associated with endotracheal intubation in preterm infants. Critical Care Medicine 12: 501–503

616. Mathew O P 1991 The science of bottle feeding. Journal of Pediatrics 119: 511–519

617. Mathew O P, Clark M L, Pronske M L, Luna-Solarzano H G, Peterson M D 1985 Breathing pattern and ventilation during oral feeding in term newborn infants. Journal of Pediatrics 106: 810–813

618. Mathew O P, Thach B T 1980 Selective bronchial obstruction for treatment of bullous interstitial emphysema. Journal of Pediatrics 96: 475–477

619. Mayes L, Perkett E, Stahlman M T 1983 Severe bronchopulmonary dysplasia: a retrospective review. Acta Paediatrica Scandinavica 72: 225–229

620. Mazor M, Furman B, Wiznitzer A, Hipps R 1995 Maternal and perinatal outcome of patients with preterm labour and meconium stained amniotic fluid. Obstetrics and Gynecology 86: 830–833

621. Mehta A, Callan K, Bright B M, Stacey T E 1986 Patient triggered ventilation in the newborn. Lancet ii: 706–712

622. Memon A, Dave R, Branca P A, Atkinson G W, Kagen J J 1979 Improved method of gas exchange in HMD (abstract). American Review of Respiratory Disease 119(suppl.): 275

623. Mendelson C R, Alcorn J L, Gao E 1993 The pulmonary surfactant protein genes and their regulation in fetal lung. Seminars in Perinatology 17: 223–232

624. Mercer S 1986 Factors involved in chylothorax following repair of congenital posterolateral diaphragmatic hernia. Journal of Pediatric Surgery 21: 9–11

625. Merlob P, Amir J, Zaizov R, Reisner S H 1980 The differential leukocyte count in full term newborn infants with meconium aspiration and neonatal asphyxia. Acta Paediatrica Scandinavica 69: 779–780

626. Merritt T A, Farrell P M 1976 Diminished pulmonary lecithin synthesis in acidosis: experimental findings as related to the RDS. Pediatrics 57: 32–40

627. Meydanli M M, Dilbaz B, Caliskan E et al 2001 Risk factors for meconium aspiration syndrome in infants born through thick meconium. International Journal of Obstetrics and Gynaecology 72: 9–18

628. Migdal M, Dreizzen E, Praud J P et al 1987 Compliance of the total respiratory system in healthy preterm and fulterm newborns. Pediatric Pulmonology 3: 214–218

629. Miller O I, Celermajer D S, Deanfield J E, Macrae D J 1994 Guidelines for the safe administration of inhaled nitric oxide. Archives of Disease in Childhood. Fetal and neonatal Edition 70: F47–F49

630. Milligan D W A, Issler H, Massam M, Reynolds E O R 1984 Treatment of neonatal pulmonary interstitial emphysema by lung puncture. Lancet i: 1010–1011

631. Moglia B B, Phelps D S 1996 Changes in surfactant protein A mRNA levels in a rat model of insulin-treated diabetic pregnancy. Pediatric Research 39: 241–247

632. Mohan P, Rojas J, Davidson K et al 1984 Pulmonary air leak associated with neonatal hyponatremia in premature infants. Journal of Pediatrics 105: 153–157

633. Moise A A, Wearden M E, Kozinetz C A, Gest A L, Welty S E, Hansen T N 1995 Antenatal steroids are associated with less need for blood pressure support in extremely premature infants. Pediatrics 95: 845–850

634. Moomjian A S, Schwartz J G, Shutack J-G, Rooklin A R, Shaffer T H, Fox W W 1981 Use of external expiratory resistance in intubated neonates to increase lung volume. Archives of Disease in Childhood 56: 869–873

635. Moraga F A, Riquelme R A, Lopez A A, Moya F R, Llanos A J 1994 Maternal administration of glucocorticoid and thyrotropin-releasing hormone enhances fetal lung maturation in undisturbed preterm lambs. American Journal of Obstetrics and Gynecology 171: 729–734

636. Morales W J, O'Brien W F, Angell J L, Knuppel R A, Sawai S 1989 Fetal lung maturation: the combined use of corticosteroids and thyrotropin-releasing hormone. Obstetrics and Gynecology 73: 111–116

637. Morgan M E I 1985 Late morbidity of very low birthweight infants. British Medical Journal 29: 171–173

638. Moriette G, Pars- Uado J, Walt H et al 2001 Prospective randomized multicenter comparison of high frequency oscillatory ventilation and conventional ventilation in preterm infants less than 30 weeks with respiratory distress syndrome. Pediatrics 107: 365–372

639. Morisot C, Kacet N, Bouchez M C et al 1990 Risk factors for fatal pulmonary interstitial emphysema in neonates. European Journal of Pediatrics 149: 493–495

640. Morley C J, Morley R 1990 Follow-up of premature babies treated with artificial surfactant (ALEC). Archives of Disease in Childhood 65: 667–669

641. Morrison J J, Rennie J M, Milton P J 1995 Neonatal respiratory morbidity and mode of delivery at term: influence of timing of elective caesarean section. British Journal of Obstetrics and Gynaecology 102: 101–106

642. Moseley J E 1960 Loculated pneumomediastinum in the newborn. A thymic 'spinnaker' sign. Radiology 75: 788–790

643. Moses D, Holm B A, Spitale P, Liu M Y, Enhorning G 1991 Inhibition of pulmonary surfactant function by meconium. American Journal of Obstetrics and Gynecology 164: 477–481

644. Moya M P, Gow A J, Califf R M, Goldberg R N, Stamler J S 2002 Inhaled ethyl nitrite gas for persistent pulmonary hypertension of the newborn. Lancet 360: 141–143

645. Mupanemunda R H, Edwards A D 1995 Treatment of newborn infants with inhaled nitric oxide. Archives of Disease in Childhood. Fetal and Neonatal Edition 72: F131–F134

646. Murthy B V, Petros A J 1996 High-frequency oscillatory ventilation combined with intermittent mandatory ventilation in critically ill neonates and infants. Acta Anaesthesiologica Scandinavica 40: 679–683

647. Murdoch D R, Darlow B A 1984 Handling during neonatal intensive care. Archives of Disease in Childhood 59: 957–961

648. Murphy J D, Rabinowitz M, Goldstein J D, Reid L M 1981 Structural basis of persistent pulmonary hypertension of the newborn infant. Journal of Pediatrics 98: 962–967

649. Murphy J D, Vawter G F, Reid L M 1984 Pulmonary vascular disease in fatal meconium aspiration. Journal of Pediatrics 104: 758–762

650. Mutch L, Newdick M, Lodwick A, Chalmers I 1986 Secular changes in re-hospitalization of very low birthweight infants. Pediatrics 78: 164–171

651. Nagourney B A, Kramer M S, Klebanoff M A, Usher R H 1996 Recurrent respiratory distress syndrome in successive preterm pregnancies. Journal of Pediatrics 129: 591–596

652. Narchi H, Kulaylat N 1999 Is gastric lavage needed in neonates with meconium-stained amniotic fluid? European Journal of Pediatrics 158: 315–317

653. Navarrete C T, Devia C, Lessa A C et al 2003 The role of endothelin converting enzyme inhibition during group B streptococcus-induced pulmonary hypertension in newborn piglets. Pediatric Research 54: 387–392

654. Nelson N M 1976 Respiration and circulation after birth. In: Smith C A, Nelson N M (eds) The physiology of the newborn infant, 4th edn. Charles C Thomas, Springfield, IL, pp. 210–214

655. Neonatal Inhaled Nitric Oxide Study Group 1997 Inhaled nitric oxide in full term and nearly full term infants with hypoxic respiratory failure. New England Journal of Medicine 336: 597–603

656. Neonatal Inhaled Nitric Oxide Study Group (NINOS) 1997 Inhaled nitric oxide and hypoxic respiratory failure in infants with congenital diaphragmatic hernia. Pediatrics 1999: 838–845

657. Neonatal Inhaled Nitric Oxide Study Group (NINOS) 2000 Inhaled nitric oxide in term and near term infants: neurodevelopmental follow-up of the Neonatal Inhaled Nitric Oxide Study Group (NINOS). Journal of Pediatrics 136: 611–617

658. Newell S J, Booth I W, Morgan M E I et al 1989 Gastro-oesophageal reflux in preterm infants. Archives of Disease in Childhood 64: 780–786

659. Newell S J, Morgan M E I, Durbin G M, Booth I W, McNeish A S 1989 Does mechanical ventilation precipitate gastro-oesophageal reflux during enteral feeding? Archives of Disease in Childhood 64: 1352–1355

660. Ng K P K, Easa D 1979 Management of interstitial emphysema by high frequency low positive pressure hand ventilation in the neonate. Journal of Pediatrics 95: 117–118

661. Nicholson B G 1997 A test for recurrent aspiration in children. Pediatric Pulmonology 3: 65–69

662. Nicolaides K H, Azar G B 1990 Thoracoamniotic shunting. Fetal Diagnosis and Therapy 5: 153–164

663. NIH Consensus Panel Development 1995 Effect of corticosteroids on fetal maturation and perinatal outcomes. Journal of the American Medical Association 273: 413–418

664. Nogee L, de Mello D, Dehner L, Colten H 1993 Pulmonary surfactant protein B deficiency in congenital pulmonary alveolar proteinosis. New England Journal of Medicine 328: 406–410

665. Nogee L, Garnier G, Singer L et al 1994 A mutation in the surfactant protein B gene responsible for fatal neonatal respiratory disease in multiple kindreds. Journal of Clinical Investigation 93: 1860–1863

666. Northern Neonatal Network 2000 Neonatal Formulary. BMJ Books, London

667. NNNI Trial Group (Northern Neonatal Nursing Initiative) 1996 A randomized trial comparing the effect of prophylactic intravenous fresh frozen plasma, gelatin or glucose on early mortality and morbidity in preterm babies. European Journal of Pediatrics 155: 580–588

668. Nugent S K, Laravuso R, Rogers M C 1979 Pharmacology and use of muscle relaxants in infants and children. Journal of Pediatrics 94: 481–487

669. Nuntnarumit P, Korones S B, Yang W, Bada H S 2002 Efficacy and safety of tolazoline for treatment of severe hypoxemia in extremely preterm infants. Pediatrics 109: 852–856

670. Nussbaum E, Maggi J C, Mathis R, Galant S P 1987 Association of lipid laden alveolar macrophages and gastroesophageal reflux in children. Journal of Pediatrics 110: 190–194

671. Obladen M, Gluck L 1977 RDS and tracheal phospholipid composition in twins: independent of gestational age. Journal of Pediatrics 90: 799–802

672. Octave Study Group 1991 Multicentre randomised controlled trial of high against low frequency positive pressure ventilation. Oxford Region Controlled Trial of Artificial Ventilation. Archives of Disease in Childhood 66: 770–775

673. Oetomo S B, Lewis J, Ikegami M, Jobe A H 1990 Surfactant treatments alter endogenous surfactant metabolism in rabbit lungs. Journal of Applied Physiology 68: 1590–1596

674. Ogawa Y, Shimizu H, Ikatura Y et al 1999 Functional pulmonary surfactant deficiency and neonatal respiratory disorders. Pediatric Pulmonology 18: 175–177

675. Oh W, Stern L 1977 Diseases of the respiratory system. In: Behrman R E (ed) Neonatal and perinatal medicine: disease of the fetus and infant. C V Mosby, St Louis, p. 558

676. Ohama Y, Itakura Y, Koyama N, Eguchi H, Ogawa Y 1994 Effect of surfactant lavage in a rabbit model of meconium aspiration syndrome. Acta Paediatrica Japonica 36: 236–238

677. Ojomo E O, Coustan D R 1990 Absence of evidence of pulmonary maturity at amniocentesis in term infants of diabetic mothers. American Journal of Obstetrics and Gynecology 163: 954–957

678. Onasanya B I, Rais-Bahrami K, Rivera O, Seale W R, Short B L 2001 The use of intratracheal pulmonary ventilation and partial liquid ventilation in newborn piglets with meconium aspiration syndrome. Pediatric Critical Care Medicine 2: 69–73

679. Ophoven J P, Mammel M C, Gardon M J 1984 Tracheobronchial histopathology associated with high frequency ventilation. Critical Care Medicine 12: 829–832

680. Orenstein S R, Orenstein D M 1988 Gastroesophageal reflux and respiratory disease in children. Journal of Pediatrics 112: 847–858

681. Orenstein S R, Whitington P F 1983 Positioning for prevention of infant gastroesophageal reflux. Journal of Pediatrics 103: 534–537

682. O'Rourke P P, Crone R K, Vacanti J P et al 1989 Extracorporeal membrane oxygenation and conventional medical therapy in neonates with persistent pulmonary hypertension of the newborn: a prospective randomized study. Pediatrics 84: 957–963

683. Orsini A G, Leef K H, Costarino A, Dettorre M D, Stefana J L 1996 Routine use of fentanyl infusions for pain and stress reduction in infants with respiratory distress syndrome. Journal of Pediatrics 129: 140–145

684. Osiris Collaborative Group 1992 Early versus delayed neonatal administration of a synthetic surfactant – the judgement of Osiris. Lancet ii: 1363–1369

685. Outerbridge E 1979 The negative pressure ventilator. In: Thibeault G W, Gregory G A (eds) Neonatal pulmonary care. Addison-Wesley, CA, pp. 168–177

686. Pandit P B, Courtney S E, Pyon K H et al 2001 Work of breathing during constant- and variable-flow nasal continuous positive airway pressure in preterm neonates. Pediatrics 108: 682–685

687. Pandit P B, Dunn M S, Colucci E A 1995 Surfactant therapy in neonates with respiratory deterioration due to pulmonary hemorrhage. Pediatrics 95: 32–36

688. Pandit B P, O'Brien K, Aztalos E et al 1999 Outcome following pulmonary haemorrhage in infants dying after surfactant therapy. Journal of Pediatrics 124: 621–626

689. Pape K E, Armstrong D L, Fitzhardinge P M 1976 Central nervous system pathology associated with mask ventilation in the very low birthweight infant: a new etiology for intracerebellar hemorrhages. Pediatrics 58: 473–483

690. Papiernik E, Bouyer J, Dreyfus J et al 1985 Prevention of preterm births: a perinatal study in Hagenau, France. Pediatrics 76: 154–158

691. Pappin A, Shenker N, Hack M, Redline R W 1994 Extensive intraalveolar pulmonary hemorrhage in infants dying after surfactant therapy. Journal of Pediatrics 124: 621–626

692. Paranka M S, Clark R H, Yoder B A, Null D M 1995 Predictors of failure of high frequency oscillatory ventilation in term infants with severe respiratory failure. Pediatrics 95: 400–404

693. Pardou A, Vermeylen D, Muller M F, Determmerman D 1993 High frequency ventilation and conventional mechanical ventilation in newborn babies with respiratory distress syndrome: a prospective randomized trial. Intensive Care Medicine 19: 406–410

694. Pare P D, Warriner B, Baile E M, Hogg J C 1983 Reduction of pulmonary extravascular water with positive end expiratory pressure in canine pulmonary edema. American Review of Respiratory Disease 127: 590–593

695. Paxson C L, Stoerner J W, Denson S E, Adcock E W, Morriss F H 1977 Syndrome of inappropriate antidiuretic hormone secretion in neonates with pneumothorax or atelectasis. Journal of Pediatrics 91: 459–463

696. Peckham G J, Fox W W 1978 Physiologic factors affecting pulmonary artery pressure in infants with persistent pulmonary hypertension. Journal of Pediatrics 93: 1005–1010

697. Peevy K J, Chalhub E G 1983 Occult group B streptococcal infection: an important cause of intrauterine asphyxia. American Journal of Obstetrics and Gynecology 146: 989–990

698. Perlman J M, Goodman S, Kreusser K L, Volpe J J 1985 Reduction in intraventricular hemorrhage by elimination of fluctuating cerebral blood flow velocity in preterm infants with respiratory distress syndrome. New England Journal of Medicine 312: 1352–1357

699. Perlman J M, Volpe J J 1983 Suctioning in the preterm infant: effects on cerebral blood flow velocity, intracranial pressure and arterial blood pressure. Pediatrics 72: 329–334

700. Petres R E, Redwine F O, Cruikshank D P 1982 Congenital bilateral chylothorax: antepartum diagnosis and successful intrauterine surgical management. Journal of the American Medical Association 248: 1360–1365

701. Petros A J 1995 Epoprostenol (prostacyclin) for the treatment of pulmonary hypertension. BPA Medicines Standing Committee, London

702. Pfenninger E, Dick W, Brecht-Krauss D, Bitter F, Hofmann H, Bowdler I 1984 Investigation of intrapartum clearance of the upper airway in the presence of meconium contaminated amniotic fluid using an animal model. Journal of Perinatal Medicine 12: 57–68

703. Pfenninger J, Tschappler M, Wagner B P et al 1991 The paradox of the adult respiratory distress syndrome in neonates. Pediatric Pulmonology 10: 18–24

704. Phibbs R H, Johnson P, Kitterman J A, Gregory G A, Tooley W H 1972 Cardiorespiratory status of erythroblastotic infants. Pediatrics 49: 5–14

705. Philips J B III, Lyrene R K, Godoy G et al 1988 Hemodynamic responses of chronically instrumented piglets to bolus injections of group B streptococcus. Pediatric Research 23: 81–85

706. Piantadosi C A, Fracicia P J, Duhaylongsod F G et al 1995 Artificial surfactant attenuates hyperoxic lung injury in primates. II: Morphometric analysis. Journal of Applied Physiology 78: 1823–1831

707. Pickens D L, Scheft G, Thach B T 1988 Prolonged apnea associated with upper airway protective reflexes in apnea of prematurity. American Review of Respiratory Disease 137: 113–118

708. Pijpers L, Reuss A, Stewart P A, Wladimiroff J W 1989 Non-invasive management of isolated bilateral fetal hydrothorax. American Journal of Obstetrics and Gynecology 161: 330–332

709. Pinkerton K E, Lewis J E, Rider E D et al 1994 Lung parenchyma and type II cell morphometrics: effect of surfactant treatment on preterm ventilated lamb lungs. Journal of Applied Physiology 77: 1953–1960

710. Piotrowski A, Sobala W, Kawczynski P 1997 Patient initiated, pressure regulated volume controlled ventilation compared with intermittent mandatory ventilation in neonates: a prospective randomised study. Intensive Care Medicine 23: 975–981

711. Piper J M, Xenakis E M-J, McFarland M 1996 Do growth retarded premature infants have different rates of perinatal morbidity and mortality than appropriately grown premature infants? Obstetrics and Gynecology 87: 169–174

712. Plavka R, Kopecky P, Sebron V et al 2002 Early versus delayed surfactant administration in extremely premature neonates with respiratory distress syndrome ventilated by high-frequency oscillatory ventilation. Intensive Care Medicine 28:1483–1490

713. Plenat F, Vert P, Didier F, Andre M 1978 Pulmonary interstitial emphysema. Clinics in Perinatology 5: 351–375

714. Plexico D T, Loughlin G M 1981 Nasopharyngeal reflux and neonatal apnea. American Journal of Diseases of Children 135: 793–794

715. Pohlandt F, Sayle H, Schroeder H et al 1992 Decreased incidence of extra-alveolar air leakage or death prior to air leakage in high versus low rate positive pressure ventilation: results of a seven centre randomized trial in preterm infants. European Journal of Pediatrics 151: 904–909

716. Pokora T, Bing D, Mammel M, Boros S 1983 Neonatal high frequency jet ventilation. Pediatrics 72: 27–32

717. Polk D H, Ikegami M, Jobe A H et al 1995 Postnatal lung function in preterm lambs: effects of a single exposure to betamethasone and thyroid hormones. American Journal of Obstetrics and Gynecology 172: 872–881

718. Pranikoff T, Gauger P G, Hirschl R B 1996 Partial liquid ventilation in newborn patients with congenital diaphragmatic hernia. Journal of Pediatric Surgery 31: 613–618

719. Prasertsom W, Phillipos E Z, van Aerde J E, Robertson M 1996 Pulmonary vascular resistance during lipid infusion in neonates. Archives of Disease in Childhood. Fetal and Neonatal Edition 74: F95–F98

720. Price L T, Chen Y, Frank L 1993 Epidermal growth factor increases antioxidant enzyme and surfactant system development during hyperoxia and protects fetal rat lungs in vitro from hyperoxic toxicity. Pediatric Research 34: 577–585

721. Primhak R A 1983 Factors associated with pulmonary airleak in premature infants receiving mechanical ventilation. Journal of Pediatrics 102: 764–767

722. Primhak R A, Jedeikin R, Ellis G et al 1985 Myocardial ischaemia in asphyxia neonatorum. Acta Paediatrica Scandinavica 74: 595–600

723. Puntis J W L, Roberts K D, Handy D 1987 How should chlyothorax be managed? Archives of Disease in Childhood 62: 593–596

724. Quinlan R W, Buhi W C, Cruz A C 1984 Fetal pulmonary maturity in isoimmunized pregnancies. American Journal of Obstetrics and Gynecology 148: 787–789

725. Quinn M W, Wild J, Dean H G et al 1993 Randomized double-blind controlled trial of effect of morphine on catecholamine concentrations in ventilated preterm babies. Lancet 342: 324–327

726. Qvist J, Pontoppidan H, Wilson R S et al 1975 Hemodynamic responses to mechanical ventilation with PEEP: the effect of hypervolemia. Anesthesiology 42: 45–55

727. Raju T N K, Langenberg P 1993 Pulmonary hemorrhage and exogenous surfactant therapy: a meta-analysis. Journal of Pediatrics 123: 603–610

728. Raju T N K, Vidyasagar D, Torres C, Grundy D, Bennett E J 1980 Intracranial pressure during intubation and anesthesia in infants. Journal of Pediatrics 96: 860–862

729. Ramin K D, Leveno K J, Kelly M A, Carmody T J 1996 Amniotic fluid meconium: a fetal environmental hazard. Obstetrics and Gynecology 87: 181–184

730. Rasche R F H, Kuhns L P 1972 Histopathologic changes in airway mucosa of infants after endotracheal intubation. Pediatrics 50: 632–637

731. Rawlings J S, Smith F R, Wiswell T E 1984 Transient tachypnea of the newborn. An analysis of neonatal and obstetric risk factors. American Journal of Diseases of Children 138: 869–871

732. Raye J R, Gutberlet R L, Stahlman M 1970 Symptomatic posthemorrhagic anemia in the newborn. Pediatric Clinics of North America 17: 402–413

733. Reece E A, Moya F, Yakigi R, Holford T, Duncan C, Ehrenkranz R A 1987 Persistent pulmonary hypertension: assessment of perinatal risk factors. Obstetrics and Gynecology 70: 696–700

734. Rees L, Forsling M L, Brook C D G 1980 Vasopressin concentrations in the neonatal period. Clinical Endocrinology 12: 357–362

735. Rennie J M 1989 Cerebral blood flow velocity variability after cardiovascular support in premature babies. Archives of Disease in Childhood 64: 897–901

736. Rennie J M, Cooke R W 1991 Prolonged low dose indomethacin for the persistent ductus arteriosus of prematurity. Archives of Disease in Childhood 66: 55–58

737. Rettwitz-Volk W, Schloesser R, von Loewenich V 1993 One-sided high frequency oscillating ventilation in the treatment of unilateral pulmonary emphysema. Acta Paediatrica 82: 190–192

738. Reynolds E O R 1971 Effects of alterations in mechanical ventilation settings on pulmonary gas exchange in hyaline membrane disease Archives of Disease in Childhood 46: 152–159

739. Reynolds E O R 1994 Commentator on: Carlo WA, Greenough A, Chatburn R L. Advances on conventional mechanical ventilation. In: Boynton B R, Carlo W A, Jobe A H (eds) New therapies for neonatal respiratory failure. Cambridge University Press, Cambridge, p. 138

740. Reynolds E O R, Roberton N R C, Wigglesworth J S 1968 Hyaline membrane disease, respiratory distress and surfactant deficiency. Pediatrics 42: 758–768

741. Reynolds E O R, Taghizadeh A 1974 Improved prognosis of infants mechanically ventilated for hyaline membrane disease. Archives of Disease in Childhood 49: 505–515

742. Richardson D K, Torday J S 1994 Racial differences in predictive value of the lecithin/sphingomyelin ratio. American Journal of Obstetrics and Gynecology 170: 1273–1278

743. Richardson P, Bowes C L, Carlstrom J R 1986 The functional residual capacity of infants with respiratory distress syndrome. Acta Paediatrica Scandinavica 75: 267–271

744. Rigby M L, Pickering D, Wilkinson A 1984 Cross sectional echocardiography in determining persistent patency of the ductus arteriosus in preterm infants. Archives of Disease in Childhood 59: 341–345

745. Rishi A, Hatzis D, McAlmon F, Floros J 1992 An allelic variant of the 6A gene for surfactant protein A. American Journal of Physiology 262: 2566–2573

746. Roberton N R C 1970 Apnoea after THAM administration in the newborn. Archives of Disease in Childhood 45: 206–214

747. Roberton N R C 1976 Treatment of cystic ventilator lung disease. Proceedings of the Royal Society of Medicine 69: 344–347

748. Roberton N R C 1976 CPAP or not CPAP? Archives of Disease in Childhood 51: 161–162

749. Robertson N R C 1985 Persistent fetal circulation. Chairman's summary. In: Clinch J, Matthews T (eds) Perinatal medicine. MTP Press, Lancaster, pp. 199–200

750. Roberton N R C 1992 A manual of neonatal intensive care, 3rd edn. Edward Arnold, London pp. 128–129

751. Roberts J D, Polaner D M, Lang P, Zapol W M 1992 Inhaled nitric oxide in persistent pulmonary hypertension of the newborn. Lancet 340: 818–819

752. Robertson B 1981 Neonatal pulmonary mechanics and morphology after experimental therapeutic regimes. In: Scarpelli E M, Cosmi E V (eds) Reviews in perinatal medicine, Vol. 4. Raven Press, New York, pp. 337–379

753. Robertson N J, Hamilton P A 1998 Randomised trial of elective continuous positive airway pressure (CPAP) compared with rescue CPAP after extubation Archives of Disease in Childhood. Fetal and Neonatal Edition 79: F58–F60

754. Robertson N J, McCarthy L S, Hamilton P A, Moss A L 1996 Nasal deformities resulting from flow driver continuous positive airway pressure. Archives of Disease in Childhood. Fetal and Neonatal Edition 75: F209–212

755. Robson E, Hey E 1982 Resuscitation of preterm babies at birth reduces the risk of death from hyaline membrane disease. Archives of Disease in Childhood 57: 184–186

756. Rojas J, Larsson L E, Hellerqvist C G, Brigham K L, Gray M E, Stahlman M T 1983 Pulmonary hemodynamic and ultrastructural changes associated with group B streptococcal toxemia in adult sheep and newborn lambs. Pediatric Research 70: 1002–1008

757. Rojas J, Stahlman M 1984 The effects of group B streptoccocus and other organisms on the pulmonary vasculature. Clinics in Perinatology 11: 591–599

758. Romaguera J, Ramirez M, Adamsons K 1993 Intra-amniotic thyroxine to accelerate fetal maturation. Seminars in Perinatology 17: 260–266

759. Romero R, Hanaoka S, Mazor M et al 1991 Meconium-stained amniotic fluid: a risk factor for microbial invasion of the amniotic cavity. American Journal of Obstetrics and Gynecology 164: 859–862

760. Rosenberg A A, Kennaugh J, Koppenhafer S L, Loomis M, Chatfield B A, Abman S H 1993 Elevated immunoreactive endothelin I levels in newborn infants with persistent pulmonary hypertension. Journal of Pediatrics 123: 109–114

761. Rost J R, Frush D P, Auten R L 1999 Effect of neck position on endotracheal tube location in low birthweight infants. Pediatric Pulmonology 27: 199–202

762. Royal College of Obstetricians and Gynaecologists 1996 Antenatal corticosteroids to prevent respiratory distress syndrome. www.rcog.org.uk/guidelines/corticosteroids

763. Royall J A, Levin D L 1988 Adult respiratory distress syndrome in pediatric patients. I. Clinical aspects, pathophysiology, pathology and mechanisms of lung injury. Journal of Pediatrics 112: 169–180

764. Roze J C, Liet J M, Gournay V et al 1997 Oxygen cost of breathing and weaning process in newborn infants. European Respiratory Journal 10: 2583–2585

765. Rubatelli F F, Bonale L, Tangucci M et al 1998 Epidemiology of neonatal acute respiratory disorders. Biology of the Neonate 74: 7–15

766. Rudolph A J, Smith C A 1960 Idiopathic respiratory distress syndrome of the newborn. Journal of Pediatrics 57: 905–921

767. Rudolph A M 1977 Fetal and neonatal pulmonary circulation. American Review of Respiratory Disease 115(suppl.): 11–18

768. Rudolph A M, Yuan S 1966 Response of the pulmonary vasculature to hypoxia and hydrogen ion changes. Journal of Clinical Investigation 45: 399–411

769. Runkle B, Goldberg R N, Streitfeld M M et 1984 Cardiovascular changes in group B streptococcal sepsis in the piglet: response to indomethacin and the relationship to prostacyclin and thromboxane A_2. Pediatric Research 18: 874–878

770. Rutledge M, Hawkins E, Langston C 1986 Skeletal muscle atrophy induced in infants by chronic pancuronium treatment. Journal of Pediatrics 109: 883–886

771. Ryan C A, Finer N N, Barrington K J 1994 Effects of magnesium sulphate and nitric oxide in pulmonary hypertension induced by hypoxia in newborn piglets. Archives of Disease in Childhood. Fetal and Neonatal Edition 71: F151–F155

772. Saarenmaa E, Neuvonen P J, Fellman V 2000 Gestational age and birthweight effects on plasma clearance of fentanyl in newborn infants. Journal of Pediatrics 136: 767–770

773. Saarenmaa E, Neuvonen P J, Rosenberg B, Fellman V 2000 Morphine clearance and effects in newborn infants in relation to gestational age. Clinical Pharmacology and Therapeutics 68: 160–166

774. Sadiq H F, Mantych G, Benawra R S, Devaskar U P, Hocker J R 2003 Inhaled nitric oxide in the treatment of moderate persistent pulmonary hypertension of the newborn: a randomized controlled multicenter trial. Journal of Perinatology 23: 98–103

775. Samuels M P, Raine J, Wright T et al 1996 Continuous negative extrathoracic pressure in neonatal respiratory failure. Pediatrics 98: 1154–1160

776. Samuels M P, Southall D P 1989 Negative extrathoracic pressure in treatment of respiratory failure in infants and young children. British Medical Journal 299: 1253–1257

777. Sandberg K, Engelhardt B, Hellerqvist C, Sundell H 1987 Pulmonary response to group B streptococcal toxin in young lambs. Journal of Applied Physiology 63: 2024–2030

778. Sandberg K, Sjoqvist B A, Hjalmarson O, Olsson T 1987 Lung function in newborn infants with tachypnea of unknown cause. Pediatric Research 22: 581–586

779. Sarkar S, Hussain N, Herson V 2003 Fibrin glue for persistent pneumothroax in neonates. Journal of Perinatology 23: 82–84

780. Saugstad O D 1996 Mechanisms of tissue injury by oxygen radicals: implications for neonatal disease. Acta Paediatrica 85: 1–4

781. Schaffer A J, Avery M E 1977 Aspiration pneumonia. In: Schaffer A J, Avery M E (eds) Disease of the newborn, 3rd edn. W B Saunders, Philadelphia, pp. 116–126

782. Schatz M 1999 Asthma and pregnancy. Lancet 350: 1202–1204

783. Schatz M, Zeiger R S, Hoffman C P, Saunders B S, Harden K M, Forsythe A B 1991 Increased transient tachypnea of the newborn in infants of asthmatic mothers. American Journal of Diseases of Children 145: 156–158

784. Schiff E, Friedman S A, Mercer B M, Sibai B M 1993 Fetal lung maturity is not accelerated in pre-eclamptic pregnancies. American Journal of Obstetrics and Gynecology 169: 1096–1101

785. Schrama A J, de Beaufort A J, Sukul Y R M et al 2001 Phospholipase A₂ is present in meconium and inhibits the activity of pulmonary surfactant: an in vitro study. Acta Paediatrica 90: 412–416

786. Schrod L, Hornemann F, von Stockhausen H B 1996 Chemiluminescence activity of phagocytes from tracheal aspirates of premature infants after surfactant therapy. Acta Paediatrica 85: 719–723

787. Schulze A, Gerhardt T, Musante G et al 1999 Proportional assist ventilation in low birthweight infants with acute respiratory disease. A comparison to assist/ control and conventional mechanical ventilation. Journal of Pediatrics 135: 339–344

788. Schulze A, Rich W, Schellenberg L et al 1998 Effects of different gain settings during assisted mechanical ventilation using respiratory unloading in rabbits. Pediatric Research 44: 132–138

789. Schwendeman C A, Clark R H, Yoder B A, Null D M, Gertsmann D R, De Lemos R A 1992 Frequency of chronic lung disease in infants with severe respiratory failure treated with high frequency ventilation and/or extracorporeal membrane oxygenation. Critical Care Medicine 20: 372–377

790. Segal M L, Goetzman B W, Schick J B 1980 Thrombocytopenia and pulmonary hypertension in the perinatal aspiration syndrome. Journal of Pediatrics 96: 727–730

791. Sen S, Reghu A, Ferguson S D 2002 Efficacy of a single dose of antenatal steroid in surfactant-treated babies under 31 weeks' gestation. Journal of Maternal-Fetal and Neonatal Medicine 12: 298–303

792. Seppänen M P, Kääpä P O, Kero P O, Saraste M 1994 Doppler derived systolicpulmonary artery pressure in acute neonatal respiratory distress syndrome. Pediatrics 93: 769–773

793. Seri I 1995 Cardiovascular, renal and endocrine actions of dopamine in neonates and children. Journal of Pediatrics 126: 333–344

794. Seri I, Rudas G, Bors Z, Kanyicska B, Tulassay T 1993 Effects of low dose dopamine infusion on cardiovascular and renal functions, cerebral blood flow and plasma catecholamine levels in sick preterm neonates. Pediatric Research 34: 742–749

795. Sessler D, Mills P, Gregory G, Litt L, James T 1987 Effects of bicarbonate on arterial and brain intracellular pH in neonatal rabbits recovering from hypoxic lactic acidosis. Journal of Pediatrics 111: 817–823

796. Setzer E, Ermocilla R, Tonkin I, John E, Sansa M, Cassady G 1980 Papillary muscle necrosis in a neonatal autopsy population. Incidence and associated clinical manifestations. Journal of Pediatrics 96: 289–294

797. Shaffer S G, Bradt S K, Hall R T 1986 Postnatal changes in total body water and extracellular volume in the preterm infant with respiratory distress syndrome. Journal of Pediatrics 109: 509–514

798. Shaffer S G, Geer P G, Goetz K L 1986 Elevated atrial natriuretic factor in neonates with respiratory distress syndrome. Journal of Pediatrics 109: 1028–1033

799. Shaffer T H, Koen P A, Moskowitz G D, Ferguson J D, Delivoria-Papadopoulos M 1978 Positive end expiratory pressure: effects on lung mechanics of premature lambs. Biology of the Neonate 34: 1–10

800. Shah D M, Shenai J P, Vaughn W K 1995 Neonatal outcome of mothers with pre-eclampsia. Journal of Perinatology 15: 264–267

801. Shankran S, Farooki Z Q, Desai R 1982 Hemolytic streptococcal infection appearing as persistent fetal circulation. American Journal of Diseases of Children 136: 725–727

802. Shaw N J, Cooke R W I, Gill A B, Shaw N J, Saaed M 1993 Randomised trial of routine versus selective paralysis during ventilation for neonatal respiratory distress syndrome. Archives of Disease in Childhood 69: 479–482

803. Shekerdemian L S, Ravn H B, Penny D J 2002 Intravenous sildenafil lowers pulmonary vascular resistance in a model of neonatal pulmonary hypertension. American Journal of Respiratory and Critical Care Medicine 165: 1098–1102

804. Shepherd A J, Richardson C J, Brown J P 1985 Nuchal cord as a cause of neonatal anemia. American Journal of Diseases of Children 139: 71–73

805. Sherman J M, Lowitt S, Stephenson C, Ironson G 1986 Factors influencing aquired subglottic stenosis in infants. Journal of Pediatrics 109: 322–327

806. Sherman M P, Evans M J, Campbell L A 1988 Prevention of pulmonary alveolar macrophage proliferation in newborn rabbits by hyperoxia. Journal of Pediatrics 112: 782–786

807. Shiono P H, Klebanoff M A 1993 A review of risk scoring for premature birth. Clinics in Perinatology 20: 107–125

808. Shivpuri C R, Martin R J, Carlo W A, Fanaroff A S 1983 Decreased ventilation in preterm infants during oral feeding. Journal of Pediatrics 103: 285–289

809. Shohat M, Levy G, Levy I et al 1989 Transient tachypnoea of the newborn and asthma. Archives of Disease in Childhood 64: 277–279

810. Short B L, Miller M K, Anderson K D 1987 Extracorporeal membrane oxygenation in the management of respiratory failure in the newborn. Clinics in Perinatology 14: 737–748

811. Shribman A J, Smith G, Achola K J 1987 Cardiovascular and catecholamine responses to laryngoscopy with and without intubation. British Journal of Anaesthesia 59: 295–299

812. Shulman R J, Langston C, Schanler R J 1987 Pulmonary vascular lipid deposition after administration of intravenous fat to infants. Pediatrics 79: 99–102

813. Sills J H, Cvetnic W G, Pretz J 1989 Continuous negative pressure in the treatment of infants with pulmonary hypertension and respiratory failure. Journal of Perinatology 9: 43–48

814. Simbruner G, Coradello H, Foder M, Havelec L, Lubec G, Pollak A 1981 Effects of tracheal suction on oxygenation, circulation and lung mechanics in newborn infants. Archives of Disease in Childhood 54: 326–330

815. Sims M E, Rangasamy R, Lee S et al 1989 Comparative evaluation of caffeine and theophylline for weaning premature infants from the ventilator. American Journal of Perinatology 6: 72–75

816. Sinha S A, Donn S M, Gavey J, McCarthy M 1997 Randomised trial of volume controlled versus time cycled, pressure limited ventilation in preterm infants with respiratory distress syndrome. Archives of Disease in Childhood. Fetal and Neonatal Edition 77: F202–F205

817. Sinha S K, Levene M I 1984 Pancuronium bromide induced joint contractions in the newborn. Archives of Disease in Childhood 59: 73–75

818. Skelton R, Jeffery H E 1996 Factors affecting the neonatal response to artificial surfactant. Journal of Paediatrics and Child Health 32: 236–241

819. Skinner J R, Boys R J, Hunter S, Hey E N 1992 Pulmonary and systemic arterial pressure in hyaline membrane disease. Archives of Disease in Childhood 67: 366–373

820. Skinner J R, Hunter S, Hey E N 1996 Haemodynamic features at presentation in persistent pulmonary hypertension of the newborn and outcome. Archives of Disease in Childhood. Fetal and Neonatal Edition 74: F26–F32

821. Skinner J R, Milligan D W A, Hunter S, Hey E N 1992 Central venous pressure in the ventilated neonate. Archives of Disease in Childhood 67: 374–377

822. Skov L, Ryding J, Pryds D, Greisen G 1992 Changes in cerebral oxygenation and cerebral blood volume during endotracheal suctioning in ventilated neonates. Acta Paediatrica 81: 389–393

823. Slutsky A S, Brown R, Lehr J et al 1981 High frequency ventilation: a promising new approach to mechanical ventilation. Medical Instrumentation 15: 228–233

824. Smith C V, Hansen T N, Martin N E et al 1993 Oxidant stress responses in premature infants during exposure to hyperoxia. Pediatric Research 34: 360–365

825. Snashall P D 1980 Pulmonary oedema. British Journal of Diseases of the Chest 74: 2–22

826. Snyder J M, Mendelson C R 1987 Insulin inhibits the accumulation of the major lung surfactant apoprotein in human fetal lung explants maintained in vitro. Endocrinology 120: 1250–1257

827. Soll R F 1996 Appropriate surfactant usage. European Journal of Pediatrics 155: S8–S13

828. Soll R F 2000 Multiple versus single dose natural surfactant extract for severe neonatal respiratory distress syndrome (Cochrane Review). Cochrane Database of Systematic Reviews (2): CD000141

829. Soll R F 2000 Prophylactic natural surfactant extract for preventing mortality and morbidity in preterm infants (Cochrane Review). Cochrane Database of Systematic Reviews (2): CD000511

830. Soll R F 2000 Prophylactic synthetic surfactant for preventing mortality and morbidity in preterm infants (Cochrane Review). Cochrane Database of Systematic Reviews (2): CD001079

831. Soll R F, Blanco F 2001 Natural surfactant extract versus synthetic surfactant for neonatal respiratory distress syndrome (Cochrane Review). Cochrane Database of Systematic Reviews (2): CD000144

832. Soll R F, Dargaville P 2002 Surfactant for meconium aspiration syndrome in full term infants (Cochrane Review). Cochrane Database of Systematic Reviews (2): CD002054

833. Soll R F, Morley C J 2001 Prophylactic versus selective use of surfactant for preventing morbidity and mortality in preterm infants (Cochrane Review). Cochrane Database of Systematic Reviews (2): CD000510

834. Sosenko I R 1993 Antenatal cocaine exposure produces accelerated surfactant maturation without stimulation of antioxidant enzyme development in the late gestation rat. Pediatric Research 33: 327–331

835. Sosenko I R S, Chen Y, Price L, Frank L 1995 Failure of premature rabbits to increase lung antioxidant enzyme activities after hyperoxic exposure: antioxidant enzyme gene expression and pharmacologic intervention with endotoxin and dexamethasone. Pediatric Research 37: 469–475

836. Sosenko I R S, Rodriguez-Pierce M, Bancalari E 1993 Effect of early initiation of intravenous lipid administration on the incidence and severity of chronic lung disease in premature infants. Journal of Pediatrics 123: 975–982

837. South M, Morley C J 1986 Synchronous mechanical ventilation of the neonate. Archives of Disease in Childhood 61: 1190–1195

838. South M, Morley C J 1986 Spontaneous respiratory timing in intubated neonates with RDS (abstract). Early Human Development 14: 147–148

839. Spencer J A D, Robson S C, Farkas A 1993 Spontaneous recovery after severe metabolic acidaemia at birth. Early Human Development 32: 103–112

840. Spitzer A R, Davis J, Clarke W T, Bernbaum J, Fox W W 1988 Pulmonary hypertension and persistent fetal circulation in the newborn. Clinics in Perinatology 15: 389–413

841. Spitzer A R, Fox W W 1982 Post-extubation atelectasis – the role of oral versus nasal endotracheal tubes. Journal of Pediatrics 100: 806–811

842. Stahlman M, Blankenship W J, Shepard F M, Gray J, Young W C, Malan A F 1972 Circulatory studies in clinical hyaline membrane disease. Biology of the Neonate 20: 300–320

843. Stahlman M T, Cheatham W, Gray M E 1979 The role of air dissection in bronchopulmonary dysplasia. Journal of Pediatrics 95: 878–885

844. Steele R W, Metz J R, Bass J W, DuBois J J 1971 Pneumothorax and pneumomediastinum in the newborn. Radiology 98: 629–632

845. Steinschneider A, Weinstein S L, Diamond E 1982 The sudden infant death syndrome and apnea/obstruction during neonatal sleep and feeding. Pediatrics 70: 858–863

846. Stenmark K R, James S L, Voelkel N F, Toews W H, Reeves J T, Murphy R C 1983 Leukotriene C_4 and D_4 in neonates with hypoxia and pulmonary hypertension. New England Journal of Medicine 309: 77–80

847. Stenson B J, Glover R M, Wilkie R A et al 1995 Life-threatening inadvertent positive end expiratory pressure. American Journal of Perinatology 12: 336–338

848. Stevens J C, Eigen H, Wysomierski D 1988 Absence of long term pulmonary sequelae after mild meconium aspiration syndrome. Pediatric Pulmonology 5: 74–81

849. Stevens T P, Blennow M, Soll R F 2002 Early surfactant administration with brief ventilation versus selective surfactant and continued mechanical ventilation for preterm infants with or at risk for RDS (Cochrane Review). Cochrane Database of Systematic Reviews (2): CD003063

850. Stevenson D K, Kasting D S, Darnall R A et al 1979 Refractory hypoxemia associated with neonatal pulmonary disease. Journal of Pediatrics 95: 595–599

851. Stevenson D, Walther F, Long W et al 1992 Controlled trial of a single dose of synthetic surfactant at birth in premature infants weighing 500–699 grams. Journal of Pediatrics 120: S3–S12

852. Strang L B (ed) 1977 Neonatal respiration. Blackwell Scientific, Oxford, p. 207

853. Strang L B 1977 Haemorrhagic lung oedema and massive pulmonary haemorrhage. In: Strang L B (ed) Neonatal respiration. Blackwell Scientific, Oxford, p. 259

854. Strang L B, Anderson G S, Platt J W 1957 Neonatal death and selective caesarean section. Lancet i: 954–956

855. Strang L B, McLeish M H 1961 Ventilatory failure and right-to-left shunt in newborn infants with respiratory distress. Pediatrics 28: 17–27

856. Strauss R G 1995 Red blood cell transfusion practices in the neonate. Clinics in Perinatology 22: 641–655

857. Strong T H, Hetzler G, Sarno A P, Paul R H 1990 Prophylactic intrapartum amnioinfusion: a randomized clinical trial. American Journal of Obstetrics and Gynecology 162: 1370–1375

858. Subhedar N V, Ryan S W, Shaw N J 1997 Open randomised controlled trial of nitric oxide and early dexamethasone in high risk preterm infants Archives of Disease in Childhood. Fetal and Neonatal Edition 77: F185–F190

859. Sun B, Curstedt T, Robertson B 1993 Surfactant inhibition in experimental meconium aspiration. Acta Paediatrica 82: 182–189

860. Sunoo C, Kosasa T S, Hale R W 1989 Meconium aspiration syndrome without evidence of fetal distress in early labour before elective caesarean delivery. Obstetrics and Gynecology 73: 707–709

861. Sutherland P D, Quinn M 1993 Nellcor Stat Cap differentiates oesophageal from tracheal intubation. Archives of Disease in Childhood. Fetal and Neonatal Edition 73: F184–F186

862. Swaminathan S, Quinn J, Stabile M W, Bader D, Platzker A C G, Keens T G 1989 Long term pulmonary sequelae of meconium aspiration syndrome. Journal of Pediatrics 114: 356–361

863. Swingle H M, Eggert L D, Bucciarelli R L 1984 New approach to management of unilateral tension pulmonary interstitial emphysema in premature infants. Pediatrics 74: 354–357

864. Sykes G S, Molloy P M, Johnson P et al 1982 Do Apgar scores indicate asphyxia? Lancet i: 494–496

865. Tarnow-Mordi W 1991 Is routine endotracheal suction justified? Archives of Disease in Childhood 66: 374–375

866. Tarnow-Mordi W O, Narang A, Wilkinson A R 1985 Lack of association of barotrauma and airleak in hyaline membrane disease. Archives of Disease in Childhood 60: 555–560

867. Tarnow-Mordi W O, Shaw J C L, Liu D, Gardner D A, Flynn F V 1981 Iatrogenic hyponatraemia of the newborn due to maternal fluid overload – a prospective study. British Medical Journal 283: 639–642

868. Tarnow-Mordi W O, Wilkinson A R 1985 Inspiratory: expiratory ratio and pulmonary interstitial emphysema. Archives of Disease in Childhood 60: 496–497

869. Taylor J, Dibbins A, Sobel D B 1993 Neonatal pneumomediastinum: indications for and complications of treatment. Critical Care Medicine 21: 296–298

870. Termote J U M, Schalij-Delfos N E, Wittebol-Post D et al 1994 Surfactant replacement therapy: a new risk factor in developing retinopathy of prematurity? European Journal of Pediatrics 153: 113–116

871. Thibeault D W, Hall F K, Sheehan M B, Hall R T 1984 Postasphyxial lung disease in newborn infants with severe perinatal acidosis. American Journal of Obstetrics and Gynecology 150: 393–399

872. Thome U, Toepfer A, Schaller P, Pohlandt F 1998 Effect of mean airway pressure on lung volume during high-frequency oscillatory ventilation of preterm infants. American Journal of Respiratory and Critical Care Medicine 157:1213–1218

873. Thompson M A 2002 Early nasal continuous positive airways pressure (nCPAP) with prophylactic surfactant for neonates at risk for RDS; the IFDAS multicentre randomised trial. Archives of Disease in Childhood 86(suppl): A7

874. Thompson P J, Greenough A, Gamsu H R, Nicolaides K H 1992 Ventilatory requirements for respiratory distress syndrome in small for gestational age infants. European Journal of Pediatrics 151: 528–531

875. Thompson P J, Greenough A 1993 Steroid usage in pregnancies complicated by premature rupture of the membranes. Journal of Perinatal Medicine 21: 219–224

876. Timms B J M, Di Fiore J M, Martin R J, Miller M J 1993 Increased respiratory drive as an inhibitor of oral feeding of preterm infants. Journal of Pediatrics 123: 127–131

877. Ting P, Brady J P 1975 Tracheal suction in meconium aspiration. American Journal of Obstetrics and Gynecology 122: 767–770

878. Toce S S, Keenan W J 1988 Congenital echovirus 11 pneumonia with pulmonary hypertension. Pediatric Infectious Disease 7: 360–361

879. Tolsa J F, Cotting J, Sekarski N, Payot M, Micheli J L, Calame A 1995 Magnesium sulphate as an alternative and safe treatment for severe persistent pulmonary hypertension of the newborn. Archives of Disease in Childhood. Fetal and Neonatal Edition 72: F184–F187

880. Tomaszcwska M, Stork E K, Friedman H G et al 1998 Pulmonary haemorrhage in VLBW (<1.5 kg) infants: correlates of death and neonatal and neurodevelopmental outcomes. Pediatric Research 43: 230A

881. Torday J 1992 Cellular timing of fetal lung development. Seminars in Perinatology 16: 130–139

882. Towne B H, Lott I T, Hicks D A, Healey T 1985 Long term follow-up of infants and children treated with extracorporeal membrane oxygenation (ECMO) – a preliminary report. Journal of Pediatric Surgery 20: 410–414

883. Troche B, Harvey-Wilkes K, Engle W D et al 1995 Early minimal feedings promote growth in critically ill premature infants. Biology of the Neonate 67: 172–181

884. Tubman T R J, Rollins M D, Patterson C C et al 1990 Increased incidence of respiratory distress syndrome in babies of hypertensive mothers. Archives of Disease in Childhood 66: 52–54

885. Tudehope D I, Smyth M H 1979 Is transient tachypnoea of the newborn always a benign condition? Australian Paediatric Journal 15: 160–165

886. Tulassay T, Seri I 1986 Acute oliguria in preterm infants with hyaline membrane disease. Interaction of dopamine and frusemide. Acta Paediatrica Scandinavica 75: 420–424

887. Turner G R, Levin D L 1984 Prostaglandin synthesis inhibition in persistent pulmonary hypertension of the newborn. Clinics in Perinatology 11: 581–589

888. Tütüncü A S, Faithfull N S, Lachmann B 1993 Comparison of ventilatory support with intratracheal perfluorocarbon administration and conventional mechanical ventilation in animals with acute respiratory failure. American Review of Respiratory Disease 148: 785–792

889. Tyler D C, Murphy J, Cheney F W 1978 Mechanical and chemical damage to lung tissue caused by meconium aspiration. Pediatrics 62: 454–459

890. Ueda T, Ikegami M, Polk D 1995 Effects of fetal corticosteroid treatment on postnatal surfactant function in preterm lambs. Journal of Applied Physiology 79: 846–851

891. UK Collaborative ECMO Trial Group 1996 UK collaborative randomised trial of neonatal extracorporeal membrane oxygenation. Lancet 348: 75–82

892. UK Collaborative ECMO Group 1998 UK collaborative ECMO trial; follow up to 1 year of age. Pediatrics 101: E1

893. Upton C J, Milner A D, Stokes G M 1990 The effect of changes in inspiratory time on neonatal triggered ventilation. European Journal of Pediatrics 149: 668–670

894. Usher R H, Allen A C, McLean F H 1971 Risk of respiratory distress syndrome related to gestational age, route of delivery and maternal diabetes. American Journal of Obstetrics and Gynecology 111: 826–832

895. Usher R H, McLean F, Maughan G B 1964 Respiratory distress syndrome in infants delivered by caesarean section. American Journal of Obstetrics and Gynecology 88: 806–815

896. Usher R H, Saigal S, O'Neill A, Surainder Y, Chua L-B 1975 Estimation of RBC volume in premature infants with and without respiratory distress syndrome. Biology of the Neonate 26: 241–248

897. Usta I M, Mercer B M, Aswad N K, Sibai B M 1995 The impact of a policy of amnioinfusion for meconium stained amniotic fluid. Obstetrics and Gynecology 85: 237–241

898. Vain N, Sozylд E, Prudent L et al 2002 Oro-and nasopharyngeal suction of meconium stained neonates before delivery of their shoulders does not prevent meconium aspiration syndrome: results of the international, multicenter, randomized controlled trial. Pediatric Research 51: 379A

899. Valdes-Cruz L M, Dudell G G, Ferrara A 1981 Utility of M-mode echocardiography for early identification of infants with persistent pulmonary hypertension of the newborn. Pediatrics 68: 515–525

900. Van Aerde J, Campbell A, Smyth J et al 1984 Spontaneous chylothorax in newborns. American Journal of Diseases of Children 138: 961–964

901. van Bel F, de Winter P J, Wijnands H B, van de Bor M, Egberts J 1992 Cerebral and aortic blood flow velocity patterns in preterm infants receiving prophylactic surfactant treatment. Acta Paediatrica 81: 504–510

902. van Houten J, Long W, Mullett M 1992 Pulmonary haemorrhage in premature infants after treatment with synthetic surfactant. An autopsy evaluation. Journal of Pediatrics 120: S40–S44

903. van Marter L J, Leviton A, Allred E N et al 1996 Persistent pulmonary hypertension of the newborn and smoking and aspirin and nonsteroidal antiinflammatory drug consumption during pregnancy. Pediatrics 97: 658–663

904. van de Bor M, Ma E J, Walther F J 1991 Cerebral blood flow velocity after surfactant instillation in preterm infants. Journal of Pediatrics 118: 285–287

905. van der Bleek J, Plötz F B, van Overbeek F M et al 1993 Distribution of exogenous surfactant in rabbits with severe respiratory failure: the effect of volume. Pediatric Research 34: 154–158

906. Van der Hoeven M, Brouwer E, Blanco C E 1998 Nasal high frequency ventilation in infants with moderate respiratory insufficiency. Archives of Disease in Childhood. Fetal and Neonatal Edition 79: F61–F63

907. Vanhaesebrouck P, Leroy J G, Depraeter C, Parijs M, Thiery M 1989 Simple test to distinguish between surgical and non-surgical pneumoperi-toneum in ventilated neonates. Archives of Disease in Childhood 64: 48–49

908. Vanhaesebrouck P, Vanneste K, de Praeter C, van Trapper Y, Thiery M 1987 Tight nuchal cord and neonatal hypovolaemic shock. Archives of Disease in Childhood 62: 1276–1277

909. Varnholt V, Lasch P, Suske G, Kachel W, Brands W 1992 High frequency oscillatory ventilation and extracorporeal membrane oxygenation in severe persistent pulmonary hypertension of the newborn. European Journal of Pediatrics 151: 769–774

910. Vaughan R S, Menke J A, Giacoia G P 1978 Pneumothorax: a complication of endotracheal tube suctioning. Journal of Pediatrics 92: 633–635

911. Veness-Meeham K A, Richter S, Davis J M 1990 Pulmonary function testing prior to extubation in infants with respiratory distress syndrome. Pediatric Pulmonology 9: 2–6

912. Verder H, Albertsen P, Ebbesen F et al 1999 Nasal continuous positive airway pressure and early surfactant therapy for respiratory distress syndrome in newborns of less than 30 weeks gestation. Pediatrics 103: E24

913. Verder H, Robertson B, Greisen G et al 1994 Surfactant therapy and nasal continuous positive airway pressure for newborns with respiratory distress syndrome. New England Journal of Medicine 331: 1051–1055

914. Villar J, Farnot U, Barros F, Victora C, Langer A, Belizan J M 1992 A randomized trial of psychosocial support during high risk pregnancies. New England Journal of Medicine 237: 1266–1271

915. Vishveshwara N, Freeman B, Peck M, Calwag N, Shock S, Rajani K B 1991 Patient triggered synchronized ventilation of newborns: report of a preliminary study and three years' experience. Journal of Perinatology 11: 347–354

916. Vosatka R J, Kashjap S, Trifiletti R R 1994 Arginine deficiency accompanies persistent pulmonary hypertension of the newborn. Biology of the Neonate 66: 65–70

917. Vulsma T, Kok J H 1996 Prematurity-associated neurologic and developmental abnormalities and neonatal thyroid function. New England Journal of Medicine 334: 857–858

918. Vyas H, Field D, Hopkin I E, Milner A D 1986 Determinants of the first inspiratory volume and functional residual capacity at birth. Pediatric Pulmonology 2: 189–193

919. Wagaman M J, Shutack J G, Moomjian A S, Schwartz J G, Shaffer T H, Fox W W 1979 Improved oxygenation and lung compliance with prone positioning of the neonates. Journal of Pediatrics 94: 789–791

920. Wagner E M, Mitzner W A, Bleecker E R 1987 Effects of airway volume on bronchial blood flow. Journal of Applied Physiology 62: 561–566

921. Waites K B, Grouse D T, Philips J B, Canupp K C, Castle G H 1989 Ureaplasmal pneumonia and sepsis associated with persistent pulmonary hypertension of the newborn. Pediatrics 83: 79–85

922. Walker D W 1984 Peripheral and central chemoreceptors in the fetus and newborn. Annual Review of Physiology 46: 687–703

923. Walker G M, Coutts J A, Skeoch C, Davis C F 2003 Paediatrician's perception of the use of extracorporeal membrane oxygenation to treat meconium aspiration syndrome. Archives of Disease in Childhood. Fetal and Neonatal Edition 88: F70–F71

924. Walsh-Sukys M C 1993 Persistent pulmonary hypertension of the newborn. Clinics in Perinatology 20: 127–143

925. Walters D V, Olver R E 1978 The role of catecholamines in lung liquid absorption at birth. Pediatric Research 12: 239–242

926. Walther F J, Benders M J, Leighton J O 1992 Persistent pulmonary hypertension in premature neonates with severe respiratory distress syndrome. Pediatrics 90: 899–904

927. Walther F J, Siassi B, Ramadan N A, Wu P Y K 1985 Cardiac output in newborn infants with transient myocardial dysfunction. Journal of Pediatrics 107: 781–785

928. Ward R M 1984 Pharmacology of tolazoline. Clinics in Perinatology 11: 703–713

929. Ward R M 1994 Pharmacologic enhancement of fetal lung maturation. Clinics in Perinatology 21: 523–542

930. Warley M A, Gairdner D 1962 Respiratory distress syndrome of the newborn – principles of treatment. Archives of Disease in Childhood 37: 455–465

931. Watters T A, Weydland M F, Parmley W W et al 1987 Factors influencing myocardial response to metabolic acidosis in isolated rat hearts. American Journal of Physiology 253: H1261–H1270

932. Wauer R R, Schmalisch G, Bohme B, Arand J, Lehmann D 1992 Randomized double blind trial of ambroxol for the treatment of respiratory distress syndrome. European Journal of Pediatrics 151: 357–363

933. Webb R D, Shaw R J 2001 Respiratory distress in heavier versus lighter twins. Journal of Pediatric Medicine 29: 60–63

934. Weisberger S A, Carlo W A, Chatburn R L, Fouke J M, Martin R J 1986 Effect of varying inspiratory and expiratory times during high-frequency jet ventilation. Journal of Pediatrics 108: 596–600

935. Wen T S, Eiriksen N L, Blanco J D, Graham J M, Oshiro B T, Prieto J A 1993 Association of clinical intra-amniotic infection and meconium. American Journal of Perinatology 10: 438–440

936. Wenstrom K D, Parsons M T 1989 The prevention of meconium aspiration in labour using amnioinfusion. Obstetrics and Gynecology 73: 647–651

937. Whitfield C R, Chan W H, Sproule W B, Stewart A D 1972 Amniotic fluid lecithin-sphingomyelin ratio and fetal lung development. British Medical Journal ii: 85–86

938. Whittle M J, Gilmore D H, McNay M B et al 1989 Diaphragmatic hernia presenting in utero as a unilateral hydrothorax. Perinatal Diagnosis 9: 115–118

939. Whittle M J, Hill C M 1980 Relationship between amniotic lecithin-sphingomyelin ratio, fetal cord blood cortisol levels and duration of induced labour. British Journal of Obstetrics and Gynaecology 87: 38–42

940. Whyte S, Birrell G, Wyllie J 2000 Premedication before intubation in UK neonatal units. Archives of Disease in Childhood. Fetal and Neonatal Edition 82: F38–F41

941. Wigglesworth J S 1984 Perinatal pathology. W B Saunders, Philadelphia, pp. 106–107

942. Wigton T R, Tamura R K, Wickstrom E, Atkins V, Deddish R, Socol M L 1993 Neonatal morbidity after preterm delivery in the presence of documented lung maturity. American Journal of Obstetrics and Gynecology 169: 951–955

943. Wilcox D T, Glick P L, Karamanoukian H L, Leach C, Morin F C, Fuhrman B P 1995 Perfluorocarbon-associated gas exchange improves pulmonary mechanics, oxygenation, ventilation, and allows nitric oxide delivery in the hypoplastic lung congenital diaphragmatic hernia lamb model. Critical Care Medicine 23: 1858–1863

944. Wilcox D T, Glick P L, Karamanoukian H L, Morin F C, Fuhrman B P, Leach C L 1994 Perfluorocarbon associated gas exchange (PAGE) and nitric oxide in the lamb congenital diaphragmatic hernia model. Pediatric Research 35: 260A

945. Will D H, McMurtry I F, Reeves J T, Grover R F 1978 Cold induced pulmonary hypertension in cattle. Journal of Applied Physiology 45: 469–473

946. Williams O, Greenough A, Mustafa N, Houghton S, Rafferty G R 2003 Extubation failure due to phrenic nerve injury. Archives of Disease in Childhood. Fetal and Neonatal Edition 88: F72–F73

947. Wilson B J, Becker M A, Linton M E et al 1998 Spontaneous minute ventilation predicts readiness for extubation in mechanically ventilated infants. Journal of Perinatology 18: 436–439

948. Wilson G, Hughes G, Rennie J, Morley C 1991 Evaluation of two endotracheal suction regimes in babies ventilated for respiratory distress syndrome. Early Human Development 25: 87–90

949. Wilson S L, Thach B T, Brouilette R T, Abu-Osba Y K 1981 Coordination of breathing and swallowing in human infants. Journal of Applied Physiology 50: 851–858

950. Winn H N, Romero R, Roberts A, Liu H, Hobbins J C 1992 Comparison of fetal lung maturation in preterm singleton and twin pregnancies. American Journal of Perinatology 9: 326–328

951. Wiriyathian S, Rosenfield C R, Arant B S, Porter J C, Faucher D J, Engle W D 1986 Urinary arginine-vasopressin in the neonatal period. Pediatric Research 20: 103–108

952. Wiswell M T, Rawlings J S, Smith F R, Goo E D 1985 Effects of frusemide on the clinical course of transient tachypnoea of the newborn. Pediatrics 75: 908–910

953. Wiswell T E, Gannon C M, Jacob J et al 2000 Delivery room management of the apparently vigorous meconium stained neonate: results of the multicenter international collaborative trial. Pediatrics 105: 1–7

954. Wiswell T E, Graziani L J, Kornhauser M S et al 1996 High-frequency jet ventilation in the early management of respiratory distress syndrome is associated with a greater risk for adverse outcomes. Pediatrics 98: 1035–1043

955. Wiswell T E, Knight G R, Finer N N et al 2002 A multicenter, randomized controlled trial comparing surfaxin (lucinactant) lavage with standard care for treatment of meconium aspiration syndrome (MAS). Pediatrics 109: 1081–1087

956. Wiswell T E, Tuggle J M, Turner B S 1990 Meconium aspiration syndrome: have we made a difference? Pediatrics 85: 715–721

957. Wolf E J, Vintzileos A M, Rosenkrantz T S, Rodis J F, Salafia C M, Pezzullo J G 1993 Do survival and morbidity of very low birthweight infants vary according to the primary pregnancy complication that results in preterm delivery? American Journal of Obstetrics and Gynecology 169: 1233–1239

958. Wolfson M R, Greenspan J S, Deoras K S, Rubenstein S D, Shaffer T H 1992 Comparison of gas and liquid ventilation: clinical, physiological and histological correlates. Journal of Applied Physiology 72: 1024–1031

959. Wong W, Tok T F, Ng P C et al 1997 Vascular air embolism: a rare complication of nasal CPAP. Journal of Paediatrics and Child Health 33: 444–445

960. Wood C M, Rushforth J A, Hartley R, Dean H, Wild J, Levene M 1998 Randomised double blind trial of morphine versus diamorphine for sedation

of preterm infants. Archives of Disease in Childhood. Fetal and Neonatal Edition 79: F34–F39

961. Wood K S, McCaffery M J, Donovan J C et al 1999 The effect of nitric oxide concentration on outcome in infants with persistent hypertension of the newborn. Biology of the Neonate 75: 215–224

962. Wu J M, Yeh T F, Wang J Y et al 1999 The role of pulmonary inflammation in the development of pulmonary hypertension in the newborn with meconium aspiration syndrome (MAS). Pediatric Pulmonology Supplement 18: 205–208

963. Wu T J, Teng R J, Yau K I T 1995 Persistent pulmonary hypertension of the newborn treated with magnesium sulphate in premature neonates. Pediatrics 96: 472–474

964. Wyman M L, Kuhns L R 1977 Lobar opacification of the lung after tracheal extubation in neonates. Journal of Pediatrics 91: 109–112

965. Wynn R J, Schreiner R L 1979 Spurious elevation of amniotic fluid bilirubin in acute hydramnios with fetal intestinal obstruction. American Journal of Obstetrics and Gynecology 134: 105–106

966. Wyszogrodski J, Kyei-Aboagye N, Taeusch H W Jr 1975 Surfactant inactivation by hyperventilation: conservation by end-expiratory pressure. Journal of Applied Physiology 38: 461–466

967. Wyszogrodski J, Taeusch H W Jr, Avery M E 1974 Isoxuprine induced alterations of pulmonary pressure volume relationship in premature rabbits. American Journal of Obstetrics and Gynecology 119: 1107–1111

968. Yao A C, Lind J 1974 Placental transfusion. American Journal of Diseases of Children 127: 128–141

969. Yeh T, Pildes R, Salem M 1978 Treatment of persistent tension pneumothorax in a neonate by selective bronchial intubation. Anesthesiology 49: 37–38

970. Yeh T F, Srinivasan G, Harris V, Pildes R S 1977 Hydrocortisone therapy in meconium aspiration syndrome: a controlled trial. Journal of Pediatrics 90: 140–143

971. Yoder B A, Kirsch E A, Barth W H, Gordon M C 2002 Changing obstetric practices associated with decreasing incidence of meconium aspiration syndrome. Obstetrics and Gynecology 99: 731–739

972. Yost C C, Soll R F 2000 Early versus delayed slective surfactant treatment for neonatal respiratory distress syndrome (Cochrane Review). Cochrane Database of Systematic Reviews (2): CD001456

973. Young J D, Dyar O J 1996 Delivery and monitoring of inhaled nitric oxide. Intensive Care Medicine 22: 77–86

974. Yu V Y K, Orgill A A, Lim S B, Bajuk B, Astbury J 1983 Bronchopulmonary dysplasia in very low birthweight infants. Australian Paediatric Journal 19: 233–236

975. Yukitake K, Brown C L, Schlueter M A 1995 Surfactant apoprotein A modifies the inhibitory effect of plasma proteins on surfactant activity in vivo. Pediatric Research 37: 21–25

976. Yuksel B, Greenough A 1992 Neonatal respiratory support and lung function abnormalities at follow-up. Respiratory Medicine 86: 97–100

977. Yuksel B, Greenough A 1994 Birth weight and hospital readmission of infants born prematurely. Archives of Pediatrics and Adolescent Medicine 148: 384–388

978. Yuksel B, Greenough A, Gamsu H R 1993 Neonatal meconium aspiration syndrome and respiratory morbidity during infancy. Pediatric Pulmonology 16: 358–361

979. Yuksel B, Greenough A, Gamsu H R 1993 Respiratory function at follow-up after neonatal surfactant replacement therapy. Respiratory Medicine 87: 217–221

980. Zagariya A, Bhat R, Uhal B, Novale S, Freidine M, Vidyasagar D 2000 Cell death and lung cell histology in meconium aspirated newborn rabbit lung. European Journal of Pediatrics 59: 819–826

981. Zenge J P, Rairigh R L, Grover T R et al 2001 NO and prostaglandins modulate the pulmonary vascular response to hemodynamic stress in the late gestation fetus. American Journal of Respiratory Cell and Molecular Biology 281: 1157–1163

982. Zerella J T, Trump D S 1987 Surgical management of neonatal interstitial emphysema. Journal of Pediatric Surgery 22: 34–37

983. Zhou H, Gao Y, Raj J U 1996 Antenatal betamethasone therapy augments nitric oxide mediated relaxation of preterm ovine pulmonary veins. Journal of Applied Physiology 80: 390–396

984. Zobel G, Dacar D, Rodl S, Friehs I 1995 Inhaled nitric oxide versus inhaled prostacyclin and intravenous versus inhaled prostacyclin in acute respiratory failure in pulmonary hypertension in piglets. Pediatric Research 38: 198–204

985. Zola E M, Gunkel J H, Chan R K et al 1993 Comparison of three dosing procedures for administration of bovine surfactant to neonates with respiratory distress syndrome. Journal of Pediatrics 122: 453–459

PART 3

Chronic lung disease
Anne Greenough, Anthony D Milner

Chronic lung disease (CLD) has been used as the diagnosis for all babies who are oxygen dependent beyond 28 days of age with an abnormal chest X-ray (CXR) appearance. It is possible, however, on the basis of the clinical course and/or CXR appearance, to identify distinct forms of 'CLD', such as Wilson–Mikity syndrome or bronchopulmonary dysplasia (BPD). It had been suggested[86] that the diagnosis of BPD should be restricted to babies with severe CLD, whose CXR appearance fulfilled the Northway criteria.[179] The consensus of an NIH-sponsored workshop, however, was to use the term BPD rather than CLD as the 'umbrella' term for all oxygen-dependent babies, as it better distinguished the neonatal lung process from the chronic lung illnesses seen in later life.[125] As a consequence, the term BPD will be used according to the NIH consensus in this chapter and distinctive forms of 'CLD' described subsequently.

Bronchopulmonary dysplasia

The four stages of BPD were originally based on a sequence of CXR changes.[179] In the present population of babies, particularly those born at very early gestations, those stages do not occur consistently. Indeed, babies may develop BPD even though they had mild or absent initial respiratory distress.[41] As a consequence, simpler diagnostic criteria for BPD have been used, including a requirement for supplementary oxygen and an abnormal CXR appearance at more than 28 days after birth.[116] It was then argued that oxygen dependency beyond 36 weeks' postconceptional age (PCA) was a better definition than oxygen dependency at 28 days, as it correlated more closely with continuing morbidity after discharge.[230] A subsequent study,[140] however, demonstrated that oxygen dependency at 28 days rather than at 36 weeks' PCA more accurately predicted chronic respiratory morbidity at preschool age. Others[186] have suggested that the CXR appearance is more predictive than oxygen dependency at either 30 days or 36 weeks' PCA. At an NIH-sponsored workshop, a more extensive definition was proposed. Babies were considered to have BPD if they had been oxygen dependent for at least 28 days, but were then classified as suffering from mild, moderate or severe BPD according to their respiratory support requirement at a later date. It was recommended that immature babies (less than 32 weeks of gestational age) be assessed at 36 weeks' PCA or at discharge home, whichever came first. They were diagnosed as having mild BPD if at that time they were breathing air, moderate BPD if they required less than 30% supplementary oxygen, and severe BPD if they needed more than 30% oxygen and/or positive pressure ventilation or nasal continuous positive airways pressure (CPAP).

It was recommended that infants born at 32 weeks of gestation or greater be assessed at 56 days postnatal age or discharge home, whichever came first, and at that time the severity of their BPD be graded, as for the more immature babies, according to their respiratory support requirement.[125]

Incidence

The incidence of BPD in very-low-birthweight (VLBW) babies has been reported to vary from 15% to 50%. This is partially explained by differences in the proportions of very immature babies in the populations considered, as the incidence of BPD is inversely related to gestational age. Another factor that influences the incidence of BPD is the criteria for the use of supplementary oxygen. A survey of members of the Vermont Oxford Network highlighted that pulse oximetry saturation thresholds varied from <84% to <96%, with only 41% of the respondents using the same criteria (<90%).[69] Others have argued that the differences in BPD rates between institutions might be the result of the different ventilatory strategies they employed (p. 559). A reduction in the incidence of BPD from 1980 to 1990 seen in a UK study[48] was ascribed to use of lower maximum peak inspiratory pressures and oxygen concentrations. In anecdotal series, use of CPAP has been associated with low BPD rates (pp. 520–1). In some centres, the number of BPD infants is increasing. A survey of a geographically defined population in the Trent Health Region demonstrated that the incidence of BPD had increased from 25% in 1987 to 42% in 1997 when defined as oxygen dependency at 28 days and from 11% to 29% over the same time period when defined as oxygen dependency at 36 weeks' PCA. It was noted that this increase was associated with a greater number of babies of less than 33 weeks' gestational age being admitted to the neonatal units.[155] The increase in the number of cases of BPD has also been suggested to be due to the improved survival of very immature babies.[192]

Aetiology (Fig. 27.47)

BPD commonly occurs in prematurely born babies who have had respiratory distress syndrome (RDS), but also occurs in immature infants who had no initial lung disease.[41] Babies born at term may also develop BPD,[13,207] particularly if they suffer severe initial lung disease, as evidenced by a requirement for extracorporeal membrane oxygenation (ECMO).[143]

Many factors increase the risk of BPD development, including those listed below.

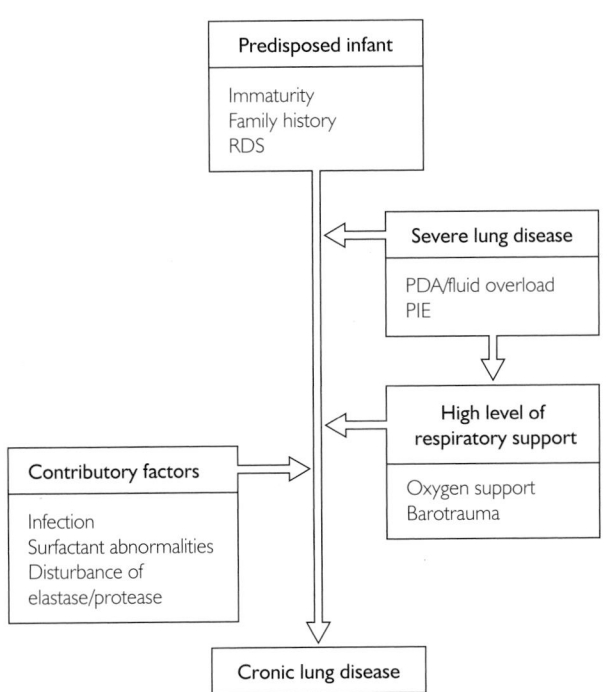

Fig. 27.47 Aetiological associations of BPD. (Redrawn from Greenough et al.[97])

Oxygen toxicity

Northway et al[179] originally ascribed BPD to oxygen toxicity, as the chronic phase was invariably associated with high oxygen concentrations for more than 150 hours. Prolonged exposure to high oxygen concentrations has complex biochemical, microscopic and gross anatomical effects on lung tissues.[26,51,73] Oxygen toxicity is caused by the increased production of cytotoxic oxygen free radicals, which overwhelm the antioxidant defences. Prematurely born infants are particularly vulnerable; they have incomplete development of their pulmonary antioxidant enzyme systems and low levels of antioxidants such as vitamins C and E.

Baro- or volutrauma

BPD was first reported in babies who received oxygen concentrations of less than 60%, when used in association with CPAP[257] or mechanical ventilation.[13] Intermittent positive pressure ventilation (IPPV) seemed particularly damaging if peak inflating pressures above 35 cmH$_2$O were used.[17,251] Baro- or volutrauma was further incriminated by the demonstration of an inverse relationship between hypocarbia and BPD development.[81,147] Infants with $PaCO_2$ levels $\leqslant$29 mmHg before surfactant therapy had an odds ratio of 5.6 for developing BPD as compared with babies who had a $PaCO_2$ of at least 40 mmHg.[81] Volutrauma may occur at resuscitation if rapid lung expansion is attempted. Prematurely born lambs given six manual inflations of 35–40 ml/kg, compared with those not 'bagged' at birth, had poorer lung function at 4 hours of age, as indicated by lower inspiratory capacities.[22] Use of high tidal volumes at resuscitation can also compromise the response to surfactant therapy in preterm lambs.[263]

Immaturity

There is an inverse relationship between the incidence of BPD and gestational age. Agents prolonging pregnancy, however, may not reduce BPD. Antenatal administration of indometacin (indomethacin) significantly prolonged the gestation of women who threatened with preterm labour between 24 and 34 weeks. There was, however, an increased BPD rate, particularly in babies delivering within 120 hours of their mothers starting treatment.[72] Administration of indometacin (indomethacin) may have delayed development of lamellar bodies and surfactant components.[72]

Patent ductus arteriosus and fluid balance

The association of patent ductus arteriosus (PDA) and an increased risk of BPD has frequently been reported. The effect is potentiated by infection, particularly if temporally related.[84] Prophylactic use of low-dose indometacin (indomethacin), initiated in the first 24 hours after birth, however, did not significantly reduce the incidence of BPD, even though it decreased the incidence of symptomatic PDA.[50,75] Fluid overload may explain the association of PDA and BPD, as it causes congestive heart failure and hence deterioration in lung function. A retrospective review[261] demonstrated that BPD babies, compared with controls, had received greater quantities of total, crystalloid and colloid fluids in the perinatal period. Multivariate assessment of the traditional risk factors for BPD in babies with birthweight less than 1200 g also highlighted that oxygen dependency was associated with high fluid intake, as well as with PDA and ventilator pressure at 96 hours.[185] Babies destined to develop BPD may handle fluids differently from 'controls'. The spontaneous diuresis that occurs in the first days after birth in babies who have had respiratory distress, happens at a significantly older age in BPD babies.[63,241] In addition, babies who subsequently develop BPD experience less weight loss or even weight gain during the perinatal period; this is in association with significantly raised arginine vasopressin (AVP) levels.[138] This may reflect that the babies had more severe initial lung disease: mechanical ventilation, pneumothorax and infection are all risk factors for raised AVP levels. Elevated vasopressin levels have also been noted in BPD babies aged 1 to 4 months.[115]

Air leak

Pulmonary interstitial emphysema (PIE) has been associated with a high incidence of BPD.[45,168] Respiratory function is compromised by air dissection into false air spaces, which creates a large dead space for ventilation; these spaces then increase in size with time and compress lung tissue.[242]

Infection

Antenatal

Chorioamnionitis may predispose to BPD. In one series,[267] 63% of babies with BPD but only 21% of babies without BPD had exposure to chorioamnionitis. BPD is increased in babies who have been exposed to high levels of tumour necrosis factor-alpha (TNFα) in amniotic fluid.[118]

Postnatal

BPD is twice as common in babies who develop postnatal infection with cytomegalovirus than in non-infected babies.[221] Review of 17 studies demonstrated that the relative risk (RR) for BPD development in babies colonised with *Ureaplasma urealyticum* was 1.72 (95% CI 1.5–1.96).[265] The effect may be greatest in babies with a birthweight less than 1250 g[264] and in those who did not receive surfactant.[265] Only those with persistent colonisation (which accounted for 45% of *U. urealyticum*-positive VLBW babies in one series) might be at increased risk of BPD.[36]

Surfactant abnormalities

BPD has been associated with persisting surfactant abnormalities.[180] The lecithin:sphingomyelin ratio increased slowly in BPD babies[110] and phosphatidylglycerol was noted to appear several months later in BPD babies who died rather than survived. Proliferative changes in BPD may reduce the number of type II cells, explaining the above findings. Abnormalities related to surfactant proteins, particularly SP-A, have also been associated with BPD.[249] In addition, deficiency of SP-A mRNA expression persisted following RDS in a model of chronic lung injury.[43] SP-A is important in blocking the surfactant-inactivating effects of serum proteins during oedema formation (p. 459).

Predisposition to BPD

The role of a family history of asthma is controversial.[37,175] Babies unable to secrete adequate amounts of cortisol in settings of increased stress injury may be at risk of continuing lung injury. At the end of the first week, babies who subsequently developed BPD had significantly lower cortisol secretion in response to ACTH than babies who recovered without BPD.[269]

Clinical presentation

The majority of babies with BPD are born very prematurely and at 2 to 3 months of age remain dyspnoeic and require oxygen supplementation. Some may have had minimal or no initial respiratory distress, but then deteriorate and become chronically oxygen dependent. A minority, who have severe BPD, are oedematous and have signs of right heart failure. In addition, they have retractions and other abnormalities related to a chronic increased work of breathing, such as a Harrison's sulcus. These patients, despite increasing postnatal age, frequently fail to thrive and are at high risk of deterioration related to recurrent respiratory infections. Cor pulmonale develops in those who are chronically hypoxaemic. Copious endotracheal secretions, persistent atelectasis, lobar hyperinflation, aspiration and abnormalities of the trachea and/or bronchus are common. Bronchoscopy reveals tracheomalacia and/or bronchomalacia.[162] Large airway collapse can be seen on the CXR as thinning or tapering of the

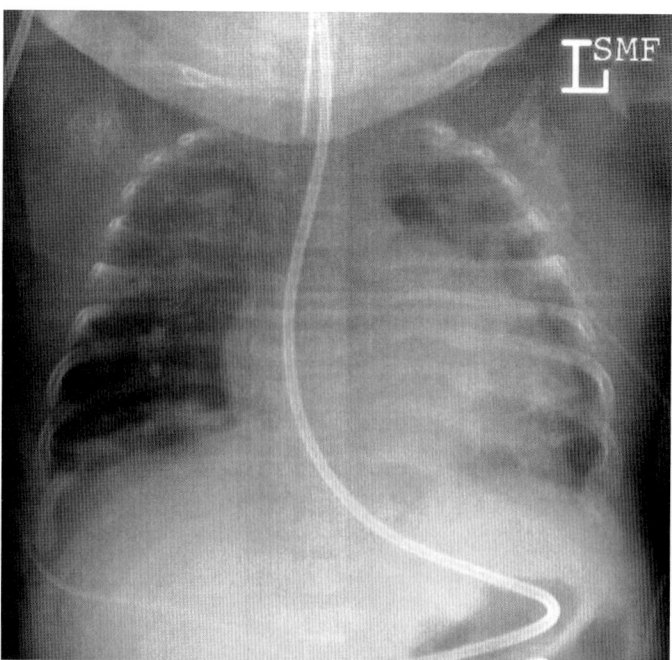

Fig. 27.48 Chest radiograph of a baby with BPD and rib fractures due to metabolic bone disease.

airways, or demonstrated by cine-computed tomography (cine-CT).[154] Tracheo- and bronchomalacia usually improve as the infant grows, but in severe cases surgery may be necessary. Increasing oxygen requirements, hypoxic and hypercapnic episodes in association with radiological changes of fixed lobar emphysema or recurrent atelectasis may be associated with tracheobronchial stenosis. In some affected patients, endoscopy and balloon dilation may be successful.[19] Extubation may be complicated by inspiratory stridor secondary to tracheal scarring (p. 534).

Feeding difficulties and aspiration are common, due to bulbar dysfunction or gastro-oesophageal reflux. Parenteral nutrition may be needed, although excessive infusions of lipid solutions may compromise pulmonary function[56] and have been implicated in increasing the risk of BPD.[47,238] Growth failure is common. Osteopenia has been reported as a complication of BPD,[243] although no difference was found in the degree of mineralisation of BPD and gestational age-matched control babies in one series.[214] Nevertheless, fractures can occur due to severe metabolic bone disease in BPD babies (Fig. 27.48).

Imaging

Northway et al[179] described four distinct radiographic appearances:

Stage 1: Radiographically indistinguishable from severe RDS (1–3 days);
Stage 2: Marked radio-opacity of the lungs (4–10 days);
Stage 3: Clearing of the radio-opacity into a cystic, bubbly pattern (10–20 days) (Fig. 27.49);

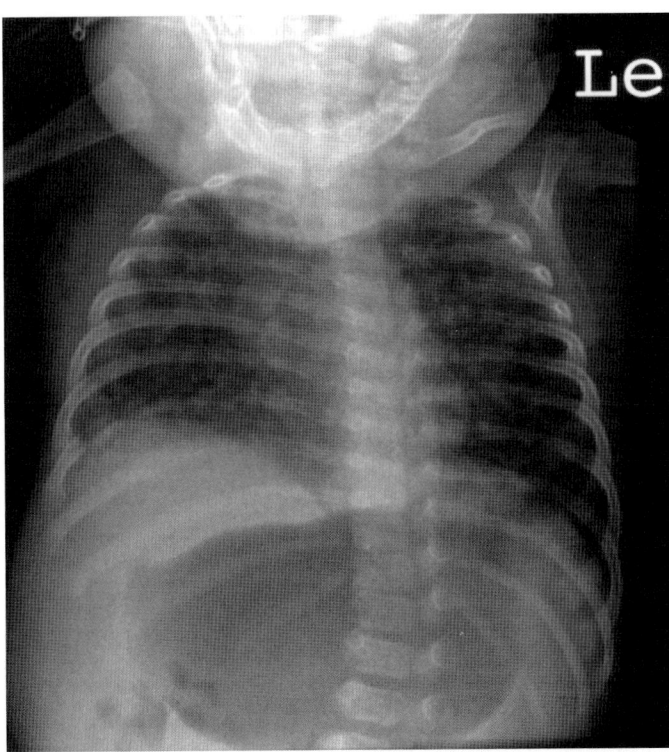

Fig. 27.49 Stage 3 BPD with widespread cystic abnormalities.

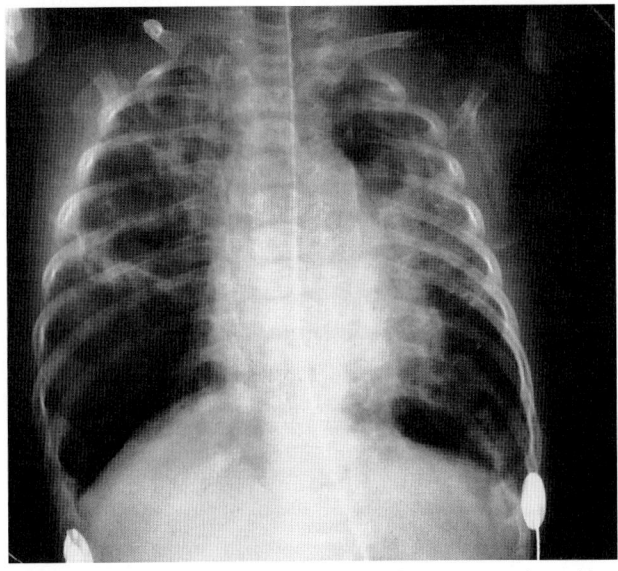

Fig. 27.50 Late stage 4 BPD with gross cystic overexpansion with compression of the mediastinum.

Stage 4: Hyperexpansion, streaks of abnormal density and areas of emphysema with variable cardiomegaly (from 1 month) (Fig. 27.50).

Hyde et al[122] suggested that babies with BPD who have an abnormal CXR appearance on the 28th day after birth can be divided into two groups, those with homogeneous or patchy ill-defined opacification in the lungs without coarse reticulation being classified as having type I disease and those with classical coarse reticulation and streaky densities interspersed with small cystic translucencies as having type II disease. Resolution occurred in babies with type I disease, whereas type II disease always followed PIE and had a poorer prognosis.

A variety of scoring systems to quantify the CXR appearance abnormalities have been developed. One system scored the volume of the lungs, the degree of hyperinflation, and the presence and severity of interstitial changes and cysts.[282] Using that scoring system, it was possible from the appearance of the CXR at 1 month to predict the most severe lung function abnormalities at 6 months of age.[282] It was noted that the babies with the highest CXR scores and lung function abnormalities were those who had cystic elements and/or interstitial changes. As a consequence, a simplified CXR score was subsequently developed, in which only the lung volume and the presence of interstitial shadows and cysts were scored.[94] The CXR appearance so assessed differed significantly between babies who were and were not oxygen dependent at 36 weeks' PCA[90] and those who were and were not symptomatic in the first 6 months.[255]

In older babies with BPD, CT scans, rather than CXR, give more detailed information. Common findings on CT scan of such patients are multifocal areas of hyperaeration, linear and triangular subpleural opacities, but not bronchiectasis.[183]

Pathology

In babies who develop 'traditional' BPD, there is progression from the initial exudative stage of diffuse alveolar damage in RDS to a regenerative and fibroproliferative reparative stage. This can be divided into three phases: an early reparative stage, a subacute proliferative stage and a chronic fibroproliferative stage.[8] In early BPD, the lungs have a grossly abnormal appearance, being firm, heavy and darker than normal; the surface is irregular, with emphysematous areas alternating with areas of collapse. Histological examination demonstrates areas of emphysema, which may coalesce into larger cystic areas, surrounded by areas of atelectasis. Florid obliterative bronchiolitis occurs, particularly if high peak inflating pressures have been used,[251] and results in occlusion of the airway lumen and distal pulmonary collapse. In older babies, airway injury is marked by smooth-muscle hypertrophy, squamous metaplasia of the respiratory epithelium and glandular hyperplasia[156] and fibrosis alternating with areas of emphysema. Hypertrophy of the pulmonary arterial smooth muscle in the media and adventitial fibrous tissue is increased.[117] Later, normal conducting bronchi may be found, with marked uniform expansion of distal air spaces with little or no interstitial fibrosis. In longstanding, healed BPD, seen in babies aged between 2 and 40 months, there is alveolar septal fibrosis, cardiomegaly and evidence of pulmonary hypertensive vascular disease.[246]

The pathology of BPD is now very heterogeneous, influenced by the age at death and severity of the initial illness and can include a combination of airway, interstitial and blood vessel abnormalities.[260] Babies with a predominantly bronchiolar pattern rather than interstitial damage usually have had more severe acute lung disease, required a greater degree of ventilatory support and died at a younger age.[260] There are few reports describing the pathology of 'new' BPD: they highlight dilated distal gas exchange structures, decreased alveolarisation, minimal small airway injury and less prominent inflammation and fibrosis.[71] Similarly, in ventilated and oxygen-exposed preterm baboons and lambs, the major abnormalities are dilated alveolar ducts and decreased alveolarisation[44] and a decreased total internal lung surface area.[43] As a consequence, it has been proposed that the 'new' BPD is not primarily the injury/repair paradigm of traditional BPD, but rather a maldevelopment sequence resulting from interference/interruption of normal developmental signalling for terminal maturation and alveolarisation of the lungs of very preterm infants.[126]

Cytology of tracheal aspirates

Neutrophils are present in 90% of aspirates from days 1 to 4, but are present on days 11 to 15 only in babies who go on to develop BPD (p. 554). Initially, in babies developing 'traditional' BPD, there is evidence of a destructive process with sloughed epithelial cells and fragments of hyaline membrane. This is replaced by regenerative changes with metaplastic epithelial cells and histiocytes and followed by a transitional stage with evidence of epithelial recovery, but with dysplastic and metaplastic cells still present.[55] In the most severe stage, histiocytes plus sheets of cells showing squamous metaplasia and dysplasia are present. The speed of progression from one stage to another is dependent on the oxygen dose, which is the product of oxygen concentration and hours of exposure.[210] Surfactant replacement therapy can modify the progression of the cytological changes.[161]

Pathophysiology

Babies with RDS, compared with healthy subjects, have an excess of neutrophils and alveolar macrophages in their lung effluent. Barotrauma and oxygen toxicity induce an inflammatory reaction, which persists in babies who develop BPD; 95% of 11- to 15-day-old babies with BPD have neutrophils in their aspirates. The activated neutrophils mediate endothelial cytotoxicity and inhibit phosphatidylcholine synthesis.[284] During the acute phase of lung injury, a host response is initiated.[182] Pro-inflammatory cytokines (interleukin [IL]-1β, IL-6)[144] and soluble intercellular adhesion molecule (ICAM-1) are demonstrated in the lung lavage from day 1, reaching a peak in the second week. IL-1β activity also increases during the first week, inducing the release of inflammatory mediators, activating inflammatory cells and upregulating adhesion molecules on endothelial cells. There is release of chemokines, including the α-chemokine IL-8, which induces neutrophil chemotaxis, and the β-chemokine macrophage inflammatory protein (MIP)-1-α, which is chemotactic for monocytes and macrophages. High concentrations of MIP-1-α have been associated with the later development of fibrosis.[170] The anti-inflammatory cytokine IL-10 partly regulates the production of TNFα, IL-6 and IL-8. Sequential bronchoalveolar lavage (BAL) samples over the first 96 hours demonstrated that IL-10 mRNA was absent, possibly predisposing to chronic lung inflammation.[130]

Mediator release from the neutrophils may increase airway hyperreactivity, as the BAL fluid contains elevated levels of lipid mediators, including leukotrienes,[101,163] which cause bronchoconstriction, vasoconstriction, oedema, neutrophil chemotaxis and mucus production in the lung. Leukotriene B4 (LTB4), the anaphylatoxin C5a and IL-8 have been detected in the BAL fluid of BPD infants.[100] Urinary leukotriene levels are high at 28 days[58] and remain elevated in BPD babies as compared with in healthy controls, even when studied at 6 months of age.[46] In addition to LTC4, which is a potent bronchoconstrictor, eicosanoids and platelet-activating factor (PAF), potent lipid mediators with known injurious effects on the lung,[245] are also found in large quantities in the tracheobronchial effluent of babies who subsequently develop BPD. Levels of endothelin-1, a potent vasoconstrictor and bronchoconstrictor peptide, are also elevated in the first days after birth in tracheal aspirates of babies who develop BPD.[176] C5a and IL-8, via activation of neutrophils and breakdown of pulmonary vascular endothelium and/or inducing PAF production, may contribute to the persistently abnormal lung permeability in early BPD.[102] The increase in vascular permeability leads to movement of macrocytes, then neutrophils, and subsequently monocytes and lymphocytes, into the interstitial and alveolar spaces.[182] The activated neutrophils release elastase,[160] with higher elastase activity in the tracheal lavage of BPD babies than in that of similarly aged controls.[266] Free elastase activity in tracheal aspirate fluid has also been associated with an increased risk of PIE.[240] There are also raised levels of collegenase and phospholipase A2.[111] The protease–antiprotease imbalance is further contributed to by inactivation of α-1-antiprotease by oxidative modification, and hence can be modified by α-1-antitrypsin administration. The latter resulted in prevention of the reduced lung compliance observed in untreated hyperoxia-exposed neonatal rats.[142]

There are increased concentrations of the soluble form of ICAM-1, a glycoprotein that allows cell-to-cell contact, in the tracheal aspirates of babies with early BPD.[141] Levels of soluble E-selectin, another cell adhesion molecule, are also increased in the perinatal period in babies developing BPD.[202] Direct contact between activated cells leads to further production of proinflammatory cytokines and other mediators. The inflammatory infiltrate is associated with striking loss of endothelial, basement membrane and interstitial sulphated glycoaminoglycans (GAGs).[169] GAGs are important in restricting albumin and ion flux, inhibiting fibrosis in fetal animals and controlling cellular proliferation and differentiation.

TNFα activity increases late,[10] the highest levels occurring between days 14 and 28. TNFα and IL-6 induce fibroblast and collagen production and cause pulmonary fibrosis in animal models. TNFα is a potent inducer of IL-6 expression by inflammatory and structural cells, and IL-6 inhibits release of TNFα by macrophages, forming a negative feedback loop. Therefore, it was proposed that early elevated IL-6 might be a response to severe lung injury and an early marker of BPD, whereas TNFα may contribute to the chronic inflammation.[10]

Differential diagnosis of BPD

Viral pneumonia, aspiration problems and lung infections associated particularly with immune deficiency can usually be differentiated from BPD on the history. The changes in the CXR appearance due to either total anomalous pulmonary venous return or pulmonary lymphangiectasia are present from birth.

Management

General

The aim is to keep the baby free from infection, while gradually weaning him off the ventilator and into progressively lower concentrations of oxygen. It is important to ensure that older babies have a comprehensive care plan, which includes attention to appropriate auditory, tactile and visual experiences and the opportunity to suckle. The provision of sleep–wake rhythms is also important. Parental support is essential through these prolonged admissions. Home oxygen therapy allows early discharge, except in those babies who require intermittent positive pressure support or are failing to gain weight. Babies who remain chronically ventilator dependent should be transferred to a ward more suited to deal with older infants.

Ventilator management

The peak inspiratory pressures and inspired oxygen concentrations should be kept at the minimum compatible with achieving a PaO_2 of 6.7–9.3 kPa (50–70 mmHg) and oxygen saturations of at least 92% (pp. 358–9). In infants with evidence of pulmonary hypertension, the oxygen saturation level should be maintained at least at 95%. Ventilator rates over 60 bpm using a conventional ventilator offer no advantage to babies developing BPD.[40] After the first week, increasing the positive end-expiratory pressure (PEEP) level to 6 cmH₂O can improve oxygenation without adversely affecting CO_2 elimination,[89] but this strategy may not be successful in babies with severe cystic BPD. Carbon dioxide levels can be allowed to rise, provided that there is no evidence of a respiratory acidosis (pH < 7.25). Sedation should be kept to the minimum, as the aim is to promote the infant's respiratory efforts so that he can become independent of the ventilator. Certain babies, despite appropriate respiratory support, suddenly become grey, pale, sweaty and cyanosed, frequently associated with poor chest wall expansion (BPD spells). The babies are difficult to ventilate by bag and mask and may take many minutes to resuscitate. These episodes seem to occur in agitated babies. Simultaneous measurements of tidal flow, airway and oesophageal pressure and oxygen saturation demonstrated that the hypoxaemic episodes were preceded by an active exhalation and a decrease in end expiratory lung volume, which could lead to small airway closure and the development of intrapulmonary shunts.[25] Sedation can help to reduce the number of episodes, but if they are very frequent and troublesome it may be necessary to paralyse affected babies.

Anecdotally, patient-triggered ventilation has been used with success, but BPD babies may not generate sufficient flow or pressure to exceed the critical trigger level (pp. 524–5). High-volume strategy, high-frequency oscillation (HFO) can improve oxygenation in babies who deteriorate acutely, but may cause overexpansion in those who have cystic BPD.

Babies with BPD may require prolonged ventilation. Chronic use of either an oral or nasal endotracheal tube can result in cosmetic defects (p. 1259). Tracheostomy avoids those problems and eases nursing of an increasingly active infant. Tracheostomies, however, may be difficult to close in this population; thus, their use should be restricted to babies who remain fully ventilated after 3 months of age.

Weaning

Frequent attempts should be made to wean the baby from the ventilator. During weaning, a rise in $PaCO_2$ should be ignored, unless the pH falls below 7.25. Methylxanthines may be useful to hasten weaning, but have been of proven value only in babies less than 1 month old (p. 562). Corticosteroids facilitate extubation,[106] but their short-term beneficial effects have to be weighed against possible long-term adverse effects (p. 562). Extubation initially should be attempted after a short period (not more than 1 hour) on endotracheal CPAP, to ensure that the infant has adequate respiratory drive. Nasal CPAP may be poorly tolerated in relatively mature babies,[38] but is useful for those who have acquired tracheobronchomalacia.[188] If nasal CPAP is required for prolonged periods, it is important that an appropriate method of fixation is used (p. 1257). Reintubation and ventilation should be avoided, unless the baby suffers frequent troublesome or a major apnoea, severe metabolic acidosis indicating respiratory fatigue or a marked deterioration in blood gases. Physiotherapy and increasing the inspired oxygen concentration should be the first-line treatment for worsening blood gases, which will usually be due to atelectasis associated with secretions.

Oxygen therapy and monitoring

Administration of supplementary oxygen via nasal cannulae has advantages regarding ease of nursing care, but the exact oxygen concentration is difficult to monitor and, as a consequence, this mode of delivery should not be used in immature babies at risk of retinopathy.

Transcutaneous oxygen monitoring significantly underestimates arterial PO_2 in babies with BPD.[112,208] Oxygen saturation monitoring is preferred, as, over a wide range of PaO_2, $PaCO_2$, pH, heart rate, blood pressure, haematocrit and fetal haemoglobin levels, a close correlation between pulse oximeter values and arterial SaO_2 at saturations greater than 78% has been demonstrated.[201,236] Chronic intermittent hypoxia may result in increased pulmonary vascular resistance, pulmonary hypertension and right heart failure, and in non-randomised studies, administering supplementary oxygen to keep the oxygen saturation at ≥92% has been associated with a better growth rate and a reduction in hospital admissions. Aiming for higher saturations in the majority of babies with BPD, however, may be not only unnecessary but also harmful. In a trial examining the efficacy and safety of supplemental therapeutic oxygen for babies with pre-threshold retinopathy of prematurity, those maintained at saturations of 96% to 99% rather than 89% to 94% had an increased risk of adverse pulmonary events, including pneumonia and/or exacerbations of BPD.[248] Our policy is for babies with

BPD who are more than 1 month of age to have an echocardiograph to determine whether they have pulmonary hypertension; if detected, then their oxygen saturations are maintained at ≥95%; if pulmonary hypertension is not present, then the oxygen saturation is maintained at 92%.

Cardiovascular status

Approximately one-quarter of babies with BPD develop pulmonary hypertension. This can be indicated clinically by a single heart sound and the murmur of tricuspid regurgitation. An enlarged liver may simply reflect hyperexpanded lungs. Although cardiac catheterisation of babies with BPD is not routinely indicated, it can be used to assess the responsiveness of the pulmonary vascular bed to changes in the oxygen tension.[2] If the pulmonary artery pressure falls with a rise in oxygenation, continuous oxygen therapy by nasal cannula should be used. Pulmonary hypertension may also be detected non-invasively by echocardiography.

Systemic hypertension is common in BPD babies and can appear after discharge. Hypertension may result from renal damage following prolonged umbilical artery catheter usage or nephrocalcinosis due to chronic diuretic therapy. In addition, certain medications, including corticosteroids,[91] elevate the blood pressure. Although the hypertension is frequently transient and responds to antihypertensive medication,[70] it can result in left ventricular hypertrophy or cerebrovascular accident.

Infection

Chest infections occur frequently in babies with BPD[278] and should be treated promptly with physiotherapy, antibiotics or antiviral therapy, as appropriate. The respiratory tract of a baby with BPD is frequently colonised with potentially pathogenic bacteria and it is important to differentiate this from true infection. If there is a deterioration in respiratory status or radiological appearance (Fig. 27.51), endotracheal or nasopharyngeal secretions should be cultured. In addition, nasopharyngeal secretions should be sent for immunofluorescence screening for respiratory syncytial virus (RSV), adenovirus and influenza. If such infections are identified and other causes of a respiratory deterioration have been excluded (for example a PDA, Fig. 27.52) treatment with ribavirin should be considered.[83]

Routine immunisations, but a killed polio vaccine, should be given once BPD babies reach 2 months of age, even though they remain on the NICU. Immunisation against influenza should also be considered, especially for babies receiving home oxygen therapy. Immunoprophylaxis with Palivizumab against RSV should be given for babies discharged home on supplementary oxygen and considered for other BPD babies, particularly if they are less than 6 months of age at the start of the RSV season.[159]

Haematology

Babies who require an inspired oxygen concentration of greater than 30% should have regular packed cell volume (PCV) estimations and a transfusion (15 ml/kg) given if their PCV falls below 40%. Once respiratory support is no longer required, it is sufficient to check the haemoglobin level on a weekly basis and to transfuse only those babies who have symptomatic anaemia with a poor reticulocyte response.

Fluid and electrolytes

Excessive fluid intake should be avoided. Babies with severe BPD usually will not tolerate more than 150 ml/kg/24 h. If their weight gain is greater than 20 g/kg/24 h on such a regimen, this may indicate heart failure and regular diuretics should be considered. If chronic diuretic therapy is given, acid–base balance,

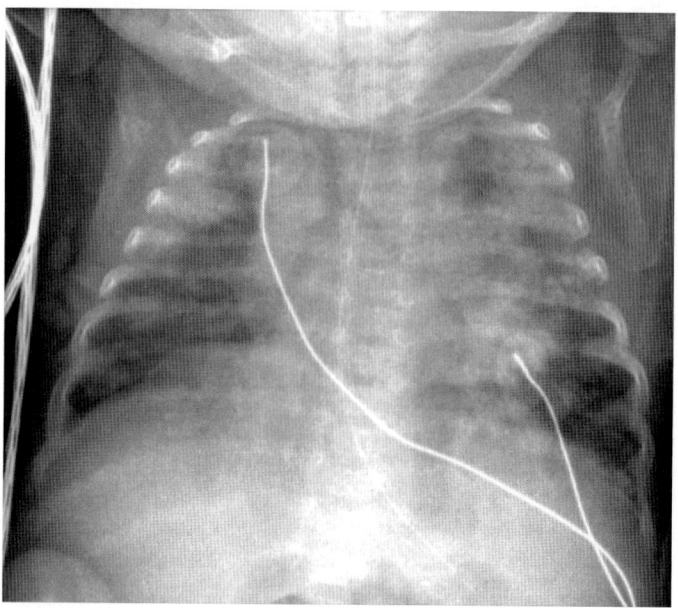

Fig. 27.51 Deterioration due to *Staphylococcus epidermidis* infection; note the left upper lobe consolidation. The baby has metabolic bone disease.

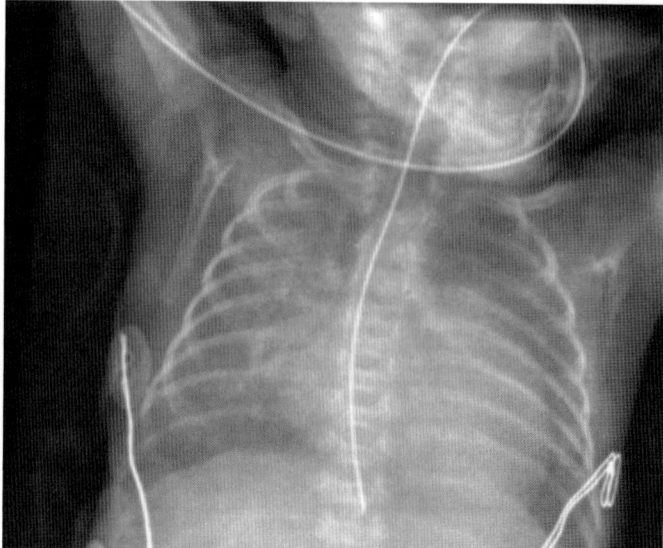

Fig. 27.52 Deterioration in a BPD infant due to symptomatic patent ductus arteriosus. Note the enlarged heart and pulmonary oedema. The nasogastric tube is poorly positioned.

chloride and calcium levels must be carefully monitored and appropriate supplements administered if these become abnormal. Regular renal ultrasounds should be performed to check for the development of nephrocalcinosis.

Nutrition

Babies with BPD requires a calorie intake approximately 20% to 40% greater than age-matched infants without respiratory embarrassment. Energy requirements above 150 kcal/kg are rare and usually associated with malabsorption.[206] Prolonged periods of total parenteral nutrition (TPN) should be avoided because of the adverse effects, particularly of intralipid on the lungs,[200] and may be impractical because of limited venous access. Large-volume enterally administered feeds are poorly tolerated and restriction to 120 ml/kg/day, using either a concentrated feed or calorie supplementation, is preferable. A milk fortifier should be used if the infant is receiving human milk. If a preterm formula is being given, this should be continued until the infant reaches approximately 3.0 kg. If those options fail to provide adequate calories for growth, because of fluid restriction or high calorie needs, then addition of modular components such as carbohydrate or fat or both can be used to concentrate the formula to 30 kcal/oz. Fats are available as long-chain (LCT) or medium-chain triglycerides (MCT). The standard supplemental dose is 1.0 or 0.5 ml/oz of formula, respectively. LCT is available as a fat emulsion (4.5 kcal/ml), whereas MCT is not emulsified (8.3 kcal/ml). MCT must be mixed thoroughly and added just prior to a bolus feed or it will separate out and adhere to the tubing. To avoid the risk of ketosis, fat should not provide more than 60% of the total calories. Fat can slow gastric emptying, so is contraindicated in patients with reflux. Carbohydrate is available as readily digestible glucose polymers (powder 4–5 kcal/g or liquid 2 kcal/ml). A typical supplement is 1 g of powder or 1–2 ml of liquid per ounce of formula. It is usually well tolerated, but occasionally can cause loose stools.[24]

Administration of a nutrient-enriched formula (higher intake of protein, calcium, phosphorus and zinc), rather than a standard formula, can achieve greater linear growth, radial bone mineral content and lean mass.[31] The early provision of adequate protein/caloric support and specific antioxidant-related nutrients is also important to try and limit the immature lung's susceptibility to oxygen-induced damage.[76] Early lipid provision, especially in the form of polysaturated fatty acids (PUFAs), may reduce endogenous CO_2 production, improving the bioavailability of fat-soluble vitamins and providing an alternative means of augmenting antioxidant defence.[76] High-fat compared with high-carbohydrate formula feeds result in similar adequate growth in babies with BPD, but lower carbon dioxide production.[195] Survival in more than 95% oxygen was greater in rats given a high PUFA diet.[237] Unfortunately, BPD babies may have limited fat absorption,[24] with low duodenal lipase activity and a high faecal fat excretion rate. This may be due to the longer duration of TPN to which BPD babies are exposed. Compared with enteral feeding, TPN is associated with lower stimulation of postnatal development of the liver and pancreas and decreased secretion of enterohormones, as well as choleostasis.

Babies with BPD can suffer from aspiration and gastro-oesophageal reflux. This can be difficult to manage, but a fundoplication is rarely required. The osmolality should be checked if thickeners are used with a concentrated feed. Other feeding problems are common and include tiring on feeding and vomiting. Oral hypersensitivity can occur and results from repeated negative stimuli to the oral area and lack of development of appropriate feeding behaviour.

Drug therapy

Diuretics

Administration of furosemide (frusemide) can acutely increase lung compliance and reduce airway resistance,[136,171] facilitating a reduction in ventilator requirements[153] and transient improvements in blood gases in both ventilated and non-ventilated babies.[134,136] Systematic review of studies, however, demonstrated that in preterm babies less than 3 weeks of age with BPD, furosemide (frusemide) administration had either inconsistent or no detectable effects.[28] In babies older than 3 weeks, a single dose of 1 mg/kg of furosemide (frusemide) improved lung compliance and airway resistance for 1 hour. Chronic administration of furosemide (frusemide) also improved both oxygenation and lung compliance, but the positive effects were limited to the duration of the treatment. Prolonged therapy with hydrochlorothiazide and spironolactone had been suggested to be useful in hypertensive, BPD babies[1] and to improve the outcome of babies with severe BPD.[4] Unfortunately, those results were not confirmed in a randomised trial;[132] administration of spironolactone and chlorothiazide to oxygen-dependent BPD babies improved pulmonary function and reduced the fractional inspired oxygen requirement, but did not result in any long-term benefits.

Diuretics have many side effects. Furosemide (frusemide) increases the urinary excretion of sodium, chloride and potassium and consequently may cause hypochloraemia, hyponatraemia and hypokalaemia, in addition to hypocalcaemia.[153] It may also cause a metabolic alkalosis,[60] and compensatory hypoventilation and hypercarbia have been described.[114] Other side effects include secondary hyperparathyroidism, rickets and ototoxicity.[215] In adults, the ototoxicity of furosemide (frusemide) is related to its plasma concentration and there is a synergistic effect with aminoglycosides. Chronic diuretic therapy may cause hypercalcuria, renal calcification and nephrolithiasis.[121] Nephrocalcinosis is commonest in the most immature babies and those receiving the longest course of therapy or given furosemide (frusemide) by the intravenous route.[232] Other risk factors for nephrocalcinosis include a family history, fluid restriction, TPN or methylxanthine administration, and renal candidiasis. Nephrocalcinosis is associated with urinary tract infection and haematuria and, at follow-up, chronic glomerular and tubular dysfunction.

Aerosolised furosemide (frusemide) has been given to babies with or developing BPD,[148] the rationale being that lung mechanics in patients with lung oedema might be improved by diuresis-independent lung fluid reabsorption and/or there may be alleviation of reactive airway disease, as occurs in adults and children. Systematic review of results of studies in which a single dose of aerosolised furosemide (frusemide) was given demonstrated significant improvement in tidal volume after 1 and 2 hours, but no improvement in compliance or resistance at either time point.[28] A dose of 1 mg/kg appears more effective than lower doses.[204]

Methylxanthines

Intravenous aminophylline therapy can improve lung function and hasten weaning from the ventilator in babies with BPD, but only in those less than 30 days old.[209] The lack of response in the older age group might be explained by extensive pulmonary fibrosis resulting in irreversible airways obstruction. Oral theophylline can improve lung function in BPD babies, the addition of a diuretic being synergistic.[131]

Bronchodilator therapy

Inhaled bronchodilator can reduce airways resistance in babies with BPD at term[135,166,273] and improve pulmonary resistance, dynamic compliance, tidal volume and transcutaneous blood gases when administered to ventilated babies with BPD at approximately 1 month of age.[33] Salbutamol administration results in a dose-related improvement in lung mechanics in ventilator-dependent babies, beneficial effects of 200 micrograms of salbutamol lasting 3 hours.[61] Inhaled ipratropium bromide gives similar short-term improvements.[273] Synergism occurs between ipratropium bromide and salbutamol in improving respiratory mechanics in ventilated babies for up to 1 to 2 hours after administration.[30] No synergy, however, was shown between metaproterenol and atropine, and with both treatments lung function returned to baseline values within 3 hours.[133] There are no randomised trials with long-term outcomes in which treatment with bronchodilator had been initiated before discharge from the neonatal unit.[173]

After discharge, inhaled bronchodilators administered via a spacer device can improve lung function and reduce symptoms in wheezy VLBW survivors.[277,283] Nebulised bronchodilator, however, may cause a deterioration in lung function, as evidenced by an increase in airways resistance;[281] this can be avoided by administering the bronchodilator by inhaler and spacer device.[277] Although individual BPD babies may benefit from bronchodilator administration, routine treatment is not warranted in stable patients. In such patients with a corrected age of 1 year, neither salbutamol nor ipatropium bromide resulted in a significant reduction in pulmonary resistance.[59]

Disodium cromoglycate

Disodium cromoglycate both has an anti-inflammatory effect and reduces non-specific bronchial hyperreactivity; its use has been associated with a clinical improvement and a reduction in the inspired oxygen concentration and ventilator pressures.[244] At follow-up, disodium cromoglycate can reduce symptoms and bronchodilator usage in VLBW infants.[279]

Corticosteroids

Steroids have a number of beneficial actions, including stabilising membranes and reducing pulmonary oedema, enhancing surfactant synthesis, suppressing collagen synthesis, and reducing bronchospasm and inflammation in small airways and leukotriene production. Dexamethasone given to ventilated babies reduces the pulmonary inflammatory response, microvascular permeability and release of inflammatory mediators and neutrophil influx into the airways.[101]

Systematic reviews of the results of randomised trials investigating the efficacy of systemic corticosteroids have demonstrated

that the timing of administration influences the impact of treatment. Commenced in the first 96 hours after birth, corticosteroids reduce the risk of BPD at both 28 days and 36 weeks' PCA, lower the risk of PDA and pulmonary airleak and promote earlier extubation.[107] Corticosteroids given in the second week after birth, however, not only significantly reduce BPD at 28 days and 36 weeks' PCA but also lower mortality at 28 days.[20] If corticosteroids are started after 3 weeks of age, the positive effects are a significant reduction in BPD at 36 weeks' PCA and a reduction in failure to extubate by 28 days, need for late rescue dexamethasone and home oxygen therapy.[106]

The results of one randomised trial demonstrated that giving corticosteroids for 6 weeks compared with a shorter course or no steroids was associated with a reduction in oxygen dependency and improved neurodevelopmental outcome; few infants, however, were included in the follow-up.[54] Others[7] found no difference in long-term outcome between babies randomised to a 6-week course of dexamethasone and those who received a 3-day pulsed course. A sensitivity analysis of randomised trials in which corticosteroid therapy was commenced in the first 2 weeks after birth demonstrated that similar effects could be achieved if dexamethasone was given at a dose of 0.5 mg/kg/day for 7 to 14 days or for higher doses or longer courses.[20] The efficacy of shorter courses (3 days or less) has also been examined. Combining such a course with 18 days of inhaled therapy did not improve outcome.[145] Repeating the course[29] or commencing it in the first 48 hours after birth[80] is more efficacious, but the latter regimen has been associated with an increase in intestinal perforation.[80] Recent studies have focused on determining the efficacy of low-dose dexamethasone. Comparable improvements in lung function were seen in infants given 0.2 mg/kg/day for 3 days then 0.1 mg/kg/day for 4 days and those given 0.5 mg/kg/day for 3 days, 0.25 mg/kg/day for 3 days and 0.1 mg/kg for a seventh day.[65]

Numerous side effects of steroid therapy have been reported. These include pneumothorax, sepsis, necrotising enterocolitis (NEC), hyperglycaemia, hypertension, periventricular densities and leukomalacia, diabetic ketoacidosis, hypertrophic cardiomyopathy and greater weight loss.[105,123,177,199,203,205,239] A similar incidence and pattern of septicaemia in babies given steroids or not so treated has been documented,[174] but nosocomial infection may be more likely to occur in babies in whom treatment is commenced at 2 rather than 4 weeks of age.[190] In addition, dexamethasone use prior to 14 days of age has been associated with an increased risk of candidal sepsis.[194] It is important, therefore, to exclude sepsis before embarking on steroid therapy, but a policy of prophylactic antibiotics or antifungal agents to run concurrently is not evidence based. Dexamethasone can cause secondary adrenal suppression at the hypothalmic–pituitary level.[52]

The possible long-term effects of corticosteroids are of concern. In animal models, corticosteroids significantly impair cell multiplication in the lung and central nervous system. Dexamethasone given to rats at a critical period after birth (4 to 14 days) resulted in increased lung volumes, enlarged air spaces and reduced alveolar surface area and total DNA content. After the drug was withdrawn, the trend towards precocious puberty was reversed, but late sequelae were described, that is, emphysematous lungs with larger and fewer air spaces.[258] In animal models, decreased brain weight and DNA content have also been reported, with a delay in cortical dendritic branching and disrupted postnatal glial cell formation. Follow-up of babies entered into early trials did not suggest that dexamethasone increased neurological problems, but the sample sizes were small, comparison was made with historical controls or the discriminatory power of the study was reduced because up to 40% of the controls also received corticosteroids. Follow-up of babies entered into more recently reported studies has demonstrated that the risk of cerebral palsy and adverse neurodevelopmental outcome is increased following dexamethasone administration.[184,231] The risk may be related to the timing of administration: adverse neurological outcome was significantly more common if dexamethasone was commenced in the first 96 hours after birth, but if started after 3 weeks, the increase in cerebral palsy was only of borderline significance. Spastic diplegia appears to be the most common form of cerebral palsy following dexamethasone administration.

To avoid the side effects of systemically administered steroids, this therapy has been given by inhalation. Side effects are indeed less common[108] and include tongue hypertrophy which resolves after cessation of treatment,[150] but this mode of administration is less efficacious. Inhaled compared with systemic administration of corticosteroids results in a slower onset of action and a smaller magnitude of effect.[62,99] Review of randomised trials assessing the efficacy of inhaled steroid therapy initiated in the first 2 weeks after birth demonstrated no statistically significant effects on BPD at 28 days or 36 weeks' PCA or on mortality.[224] There was, however, a reduction in requirement for rescue systemic steroids.

Surfactant

Surfactant dysfunction may persist and contribute to the continuing respiratory support required by neonates with BPD (p. 556). In a pilot study, a single dose of a natural surfactant reduced the inspired oxygen concentration requirement in babies aged between 7 and 30 days.[187]

Inhaled nitric oxide

Inhaled nitric oxide (iNO) may be useful in infants with or developing BPD to reduce their oxygenation index, but the magnitude of response can be variable and the optimum dose ranges from 6 to 60 ppm.[151] In early BPD (infants aged from 10 to 30 days), however, iNO administered at a dose of 20 ppm or less was associated with improvements in oxygenation without inducing changes in markers of inflammatory or oxidative injury.[42] A positive response to iNO in babies with severe BPD has been associated with an improved outcome in a non-randomised study;[12] four of 11 babies who responded were ultimately weaned off mechanical ventilation, whereas all five non-respondents either died or continued to require mechanical ventilation.

Recommendations regarding drug therapy

A single dose of furosemide (frusemide) should be given to treat acute fluid overload, and regular chlorothiazide and spironolactone should be administered to infants who have signs of incipient right heart failure or are poorly tolerant of a modest fluid

volume regimen (120 ml/kg/day). Caffeine, commenced to facilitate extubation, should be continued while infants are at risk of apnoeic episodes, but stopped if symptomatic gastro-oesophageal reflux develops. On the NICU, bronchodilators are rarely necessary and should be administered only to those BPD infants who have symptomatic wheeze. We consider corticosteroids only for infants who are at least 2 weeks of age and have severe lung disease, remaining ventilator dependent and in high oxygen concentrations. Systemic corticosteroids are prescribed for 3 days and only continued, for a further 6 days in a reducing dose, if there has been an obvious clinical response (i.e. a significant reduction in respiratory support requirements). It is possible that much smaller doses than previously used are efficacious; research is required to determine if there is a dosage regimen with a positive risk–benefit ratio. We do not use inhaled steroids on the NICU, except for BPD babies who have troublesome symptomatic wheeze. Other drug therapies discussed above are used only on an individual basis or in the context of a randomised trial.

Home respiratory support

Home oxygen therapy should be considered for babies who have no medical problem other than their increased inspired oxygen requirement. Some parents, however, will also cope with tube feeding their baby. Supplementary oxygen can be delivered via either a single feeding catheter inserted into one nostril or twin nasal cannulae. Oxygen concentrators should be used, unless the baby requires only low amounts of oxygen. Small portable oxygen cylinders should also be provided, whichever system is used, as they are necessary for transporting the baby. At regular intervals, the babies should be seen at home or in hospital and their progress and weight checked. Their oxygen saturation needs to be monitored preferably for at least 24-hour periods, if not continuously. The oxygen saturation should be maintained above 92% to ensure appropriate weight gain;[103] others have recommended a minimum SaO_2 of 95%.[120,198] Weaning from supplementary oxygen should be gradual; if the inspired oxygen concentration is abruptly reduced, resulting in hypoxaemia, this can lead to worsening pulmonary hypertension[254] and an increased incidence of apnoea, which responds to improving arterial oxygen saturation.[223] It is essential to ensure patients maintain their oxygen saturation levels at all times; desaturation occurs particularly after feeding[234] and lower oxygen saturation levels are frequently recorded when the baby is asleep. For the first month after oxygen is no longer needed, parents should keep the equipment at home in case of increased oxygen need associated with even minor respiratory infections. Home oxygen facilitates earlier discharge from the neonatal unit and corresponding financial savings.[196] It is important, however, to be aware that some infants may require months or even years of home oxygen.[93]

Only a very small number of babies with BPD have been discharged on home ventilation.[74] The babies must have a tracheostomy. Home ventilation requires an enormous investment in equipment, community services and education for parents.[189] In one series,[222] the average duration of home ventilation was 365 days.

Prophylaxis

Antenatal therapy

Corticosteroid treatment given to women at high risk of preterm delivery reduces the incidence of neonatal death and RDS by approximately 50%,[53] but, even in combination with postnatal surfactant, fails to favourably impact on the incidence of BPD.[127] The positive effects of thyrotrophin-releasing hormone seen in early studies[11] have not been confirmed in large randomised trials.[3]

Fluid management

Promotion of an early diuresis with a diuretic[220] or an albumin infusion[92] does not significantly improve perinatal respiratory status, and fluid restriction in the first weeks after birth does not reduce BPD,[139,252] although early studies demonstrated that fluid restriction reduced the incidence of NEC and PDA.[15,152] Limiting colloid administration and avoiding early sodium supplementation might, however, reduce the incidence of BPD. Inverse relationships between the amount of colloid received and perinatal lung function[137] and the risk of BPD development[63] have been demonstrated. A lower rate of BPD was noted in infants in whom sodium supplementation was not given in the first 3 to 5 days compared with those receiving daily maintenance sodium.[49] In addition, in a randomised trial, withholding sodium supplementation until there was evidence of weight loss equalling 6% of birthweight, rather than giving routine maintenance, was associated with a reduction in the proportion of babies who required supplementary oxygen at 7 days.[113]

Vitamin E

The toxic effects of oxygen upon the lung are enhanced by vitamin E deficiency and prevented by vitamin E treatment.[253] Healthy term and premature babies have mean plasma vitamin E levels of less than 0.25 mg/dl in the first 24 hours after birth;[167] a level of less than 0.5 mg/dl indicates vitamin E inadequacy in adults. Daily vitamin E administration to infants requiring an inspired oxygen concentration of greater than 40% was associated with a reduction in the number of babies with a CXR appearance compatible with BPD.[68] The results of randomised trials,[67,216] however, failed to demonstrate that vitamin E administration reduced the incidence of BPD. It may be that too low a dosage was used, but the incidence of culture-proven neonatal sepsis and NEC was significantly higher in infants maintained at pharmacological levels of vitamin E for 8 days or more compared with those placebo treated. Vitamin E decreases the oxygen-dependent intracellular killing ability of neutrophils, resulting in a decreased resistance to infection in preterm babies.[129] Thus, higher doses of vitamin E are not recommended in this context.

Vitamin A

Vitamin A supplementation influences the normal differentiation of regenerating airways. VLBW infants are frequently deficient in vitamin A because of deprivation of transplacental acquisition. In addition, parenteral administration of vitamin A is inefficient[39] because of photodegradation and absorption of the vitamin to the intravenous tubing. VLBW neonates with BPD may have suboptimal plasma concentrations of vitamin A for extended periods.[228] In a randomised study,[229] vitamin A (retinyl palmitate 2000 IU), given by the intramuscular route on postnatal day 4 and every other day thereafter for a total of 14 injections over 28 days to oxygen-dependent babies resulted in significantly higher mean plasma concentrations of vitamin A and a reduction in BPD and the need for supplementary oxygen, mechanical ventilation and intensive care. The results of subsequent trials have been conflicting,[193,227,259] but meta-analysis of the results of seven randomised trials[57] highlighted that vitamin A supplementation reduced death or oxygen requirement at 1 month of age (RR 0.93, 95% CI 0.88–0.99) and oxygen requirement at 36 weeks' PCA (RR 0.87, 95% CI 0.77–0.99). The optimal dosage, mode and duration of administration of vitamin A in VLBW babies, however, needs further investigation.[124] Vitamin A administration must be carefully monitored if side effects, such as non-specific neurological signs secondary to raised intracranial pressure caused by toxic levels, are to be avoided.

Superoxide dismutase

Superoxide dismutase (SOD) is a naturally occurring intracellular enzyme which converts the toxic superoxide radical into the potentially less toxic hydrogen peroxide. Pretreatment of rats with SOD prevents toxic changes in lung macrophages[233] and damage to lung cells[23] when exposed to hyperoxia. Human neonates are deficient in SOD.[212,276] The efficacy of prophylactic SOD has been tested in two randomised trials;[250] no favourable effect on oxygen dependency at 28 days or 36 weeks' PCA was noted. In one study,[211] however, treated babies, compared with those who received placebo, had a lower frequency of respiratory problems after discharge (RR 0.30, 95% CI 0.11–0.87). Toxicity has not been reported, but antioxidant therapy may affect the bactericidal activity of polymorphonuclear cells.

Allopurinol

Allopurinol is a synthetic competitive inhibitor of xanthine oxidase and a free-radical scavenger. Enteral administration of 20 mg/ml for 7 days, in a randomised placebo-controlled trial, however, failed to significantly reduce the incidence of BPD.[213]

Surfactant

Exogenous surfactant replacement therapy, although significantly reducing the combined outcome of BPD and death, does not reduce the incidence of BPD alone (p. 563).

Inositol

Inositol supplementation (80 mg/kg) during the first 5 days after birth improved survival without BPD from 55% to 71%.[109]

Bronchodilators

Prophylaxis with salbutamol, started in the first 2 weeks after birth, was not associated with a significant reduction in the duration of ventilatory support, incidence of BPD or mortality, in a randomised trial.[173]

Cromolyn sodium

Cromolyn sodium inhibits neutrophil activation and neutrophil chemotaxis and thus can modulate the inflammatory process in the lung.[172] In randomised trials,[268] however, prophylactic cromolyn sodium failed to significantly reduce the incidence of BPD or any other clinically important outcome.

Ambroxol

Ambroxol given over the first 5 days has been associated with a 50% reduction in the incidence of BPD, without adverse effect.[270]

Respiratory support

Avoidance of 'aggressive' respiratory support may be associated with a reduction in BPD. Avery et al[9] reported an eight-centre comparison and highlighted that the lowest incidence of BPD was in the institution using CPAP (5 cmH$_2$O via nasal prongs) soon after birth, in preference to intubation and mechanical ventilation. Other management policies differed between the eight centres examined and as the babies were not randomised, it cannot be confidently concluded that the use of CPAP alone explained the lower BPD incidence. Others have also reported that the incidence of BPD appears to be lower in institutions in which a smaller proportion of patients are intubated and mechanically ventilated.[197] Minimal ventilation (partial pressure of carbon dioxide >52 mmHg) compared with routine ventilation (partial pressure of oxygen <48 mmHg) in a randomised trial involving 220 babies, however, was not associated with a significant reduction in the incidence of death or BPD.[34]

Meta-analysis of the results of randomised trials has demonstrated that patient-triggered ventilation does not reduce the incidence of BPD.[96] Certain trials have demonstrated that high-volume strategy, HFO was associated with a lower rate of BPD. Such a favourable outcome, however, was not seen in a trial in which 797 very immature babies (23 to 28 weeks of gestation) were randomised to HFO or conventional ventilation in the first hour after birth.[128]

Nitric oxide

Three randomised trials assessing the efficacy of iNO have included prematurely born babies; none have demonstrated that iNO results in a significant reduction in BPD.[14]

Tri-iodothyronine (T$_3$)

In a randomised, placebo-controlled trial, administration of T$_3$ and hydrocortisone for 7 days after birth to infants of less than 30 weeks' gestation was not associated with a reduction in BPD.[21]

Prognosis

Mortality

Predischarge mortality is usually caused by intercurrent infection, cor pulmonale or respiratory failure. Predictors of death in hospital include male gender and length of ventilatory support and supplementary oxygen.[226] Sudden infant death syndrome (SIDS) was reported to be higher in babies with BPD,[271] but this has not been subsequently confirmed.[85,219]

Morbidity

BPD infants require a median of two (range 0–20) re-hospitalisations in the first 2 years.[88] Preterm babies with BPD are twice as likely to be hospitalised in the first 2 years than are preterm babies without BPD.[104] Re-hospitalisations are significantly more common in BPD babies requiring supplementary oxygen at home[87] and those that develop RSV infections.[88] A higher number of days of re-hospitalisations for respiratory causes has also been noted in BPD babies oxygen dependent beyond 36 weeks' PCA, compared with those oxygen dependent only beyond 28 days or less than 28 days.[64]

Morbidity relating to growth

The average weight and height at term of babies with severe BPD is frequently at or below the third centile; growth failure being partially the result of increased metabolic demands from increased work of breathing.[149] Growth accelerates as respiratory symptoms improve. At school age, children who had had BPD did not have poorer growth than controls.[262]

Central nervous system morbidity

Delays in development have been reported to be common,[178] with poor developmental outcome correlating positively with prolonged hospitalisation and requirement for oxygen in babies with severe BPD.[157,225] Developmental delay was reported to be commoner in BPD babies oxygen dependent beyond 36 weeks' PCA than in those oxygen dependent only beyond 28 days or less.[98] Requirement for mechanical ventilatory support of more than 50 days had been associated with a poor prognosis, with no intact survivors in one series.[272] More recently, ventilation for longer than 28 days has been associated with intact survival, but not in VLBW babies with evidence of significant brain injury.[256]

Pulmonary morbidity

Prospective follow-up of inborn VLBW babies[95] revealed approximately twice as much wheezing amongst BPD survivors as in term babies from the same geographical area. Pulmonary function abnormalities in the first year after birth in BPD babies include a high airways resistance, low dynamic pulmonary compliance, reduced functional residual capacity (FRC), abnormal gas exchange (hypercarbia, low oxygen saturation), elevated minute volume and lower gas mixing index. The most consistent finding in BPD has been increased pulmonary or airway resistance.[165,181,247,280] Lung function usually improves with age.[82,165,275] Nevertheless, pulmonary function tests may still be abnormal, with reduced exercise tolerance, in school-age children.[235] Affected children had a positive methacholine challenge test, indicating bronchial hyperreactivity, and a positive response to bronchodilator therapy. Andreasson et al[6] reported airways obstruction in 10 out of 11 8-year-olds with BPD, but in only nine out of 24 controls who just had RDS; hyperinflation was more common and FRC significantly higher in the children with BPD. At approximately 8 years of age, 'BPD' children may still have exercise intolerance,[164,191] even if pulmonary function at rest is only slightly impaired.[217]

Numerous chronic complications may be seen on the CXR of BPD infants at follow-up,[66] including cor pulmonale, right ventricular hypertrophy and enlargement of the main pulmonary artery, reflecting pulmonary hypertension. Atelectasis and subsegmental or segmental collapse may occur, frequently affecting the left lower lobe. Rickets, due to dietary or parenteral nutritional deficiency of calcium and vitamin D or to the calciuric effect of furosemide (frusemide), may manifest by rib fractures together with generalised demineralisation and metaphyseal fraying, widening and cupping. The CXR abnormalities of severe BPD may persist for some years.[158] Most patients, however, remain either radiologically stable or show a trend towards improvement. High-resolution CT scanning demonstrated that adult survivors of 'traditional' BPD, compared with similar aged young adults, had multifocal areas of reduced attenuation and perfusion, bronchial thickening and decreased bronchus-to-pulmonary artery diameter ratios.[119]

Cardiovascular morbidity

Cardiac catheterisation of survivors of severe BPD revealed persisting elevation of pulmonary artery pressure and a high pulmonary vascular resistance, cardiac index and intrapulmonary shunt fraction.[18] Pulmonary hypertension can be detected noninvasively by Doppler echocardiographic demonstration of tricuspid regurgitation or estimation of the pulmonary systolic time interval. Such measurements can be used to identify a response to elevation of the inspired oxygen concentration.[16] Systemic hypertension is also common in babies with severe BPD, affecting 13% of 87 patients who required home oxygen therapy. In the survivors, however, it resolved prior to weaning from supplementary oxygen.[5]

Other forms of chronic lung disease

It is not uncommon for very prematurely born babies who have had no acute respiratory illness to develop chronic pulmonary problems. In the past, affected babies would have been described as suffering from conditions such as respiratory insufficiency syndrome (RIS).[35] Nowadays, these babies are simply described as having BPD. Nevertheless, certain diagnoses are still used for babies who have a distinctive clinical presentation and/or CXR appearances; as a consequence, these are described below.

Chronic pulmonary insufficiency of prematurity

Chronic pulmonary insufficiency of prematurity (CPIP) is diagnosed in very immature babies who have made at least a partial recovery from RDS but then go on to develop apnoea and have increasing oxygen requirements. Many would now describe these babies as having a mild form of BPD. The babies have low lung volumes and it is useful to consider the diagnosis of CPIP, as it reminds the clinician that affected babies respond well to CPAP (see below).

Diagnosis

The CXR demonstrates small-volume lungs with hazy lung fields (Fig. 27.53).

Management

The babies frequently require supplementary oxygen, and CPAP is useful to treat worsening hypoxaemia and apnoea. Caffeine administration can be helpful, but antibiotics are only necessary to treat secondary infection.

Prognosis

The babies have slowly progressive atelectasis, hypoxaemia and hypercarbia, but recovery is usually complete by 6 weeks of age.

Wilson–Mikity syndrome

Prematurely born babies, classically who have had no respiratory problems in the first week after birth, are affected. The diagnosis is made when progressive respiratory failure develops during the second week, in association with diffuse small bilateral cystic translucencies on the CXR.[274] The babies have intrapulmonary shunting and maldistribution of ventilation and perfusion;[146] pulmonary hypertension can be detected at cardiac catheterisation. There appears to be geographical variations in

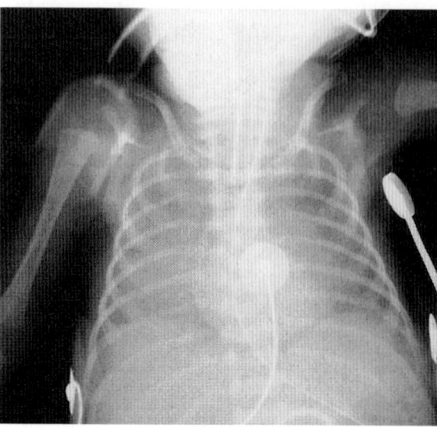

Fig. 27.53 Chronic pulmonary insufficiency of prematurity; note the small-volume, hazy lung fields.

the incidence of this condition; for example, it is rarely diagnosed in the UK but is more common in Japan.

Clinical signs

There is an insidious onset of tachypnoea and cyanosis, and dyspnoea, especially on effort. The infant frequently has an overexpanded chest, wheezing and coughing.

Aetiology

The syndrome usually occurs in babies of less than 32 weeks' gestational age;[32] it thus may represent a functional and anatomical immaturity of the airways.[218] Intrauterine infection may also be responsible, as babies with Wilson–Mikity syndrome have been found to have high plasma immunoglobulin M (IgM) levels on the first day after birth.[78] In addition, the mothers of affected babies have been noted to have a high incidence of chorioamnionitis, in association with a raised cord blood IgM.[79] Babies with a condition resembling Wilson–Mikity syndrome have been reported to have increased leukocyte elastase in tracheal aspirates at birth, indicating antenatal leukocyte migration to the lungs.[77]

Diagnosis

A diffuse fine reticular pattern infiltrating both lung fields, interspersed with areas of emphysematous cysts, is seen on the CXR of affected babies (Fig. 27.54). The changes initially, unlike in BPD, are more marked in the upper zones. As the disease progresses, the cysts coalesce and marked hyperinflation is a prominent feature.

Prognosis

Symptoms may persist for many months and respiratory infections are common during infancy. Abnormal lung function, suggesting persistent small airway damage, has been found in survivors even at 8 to 10 years of age, but usually the pulmonary disease resolves. Death may occur due to cardiac failure, respiratory failure or infection.

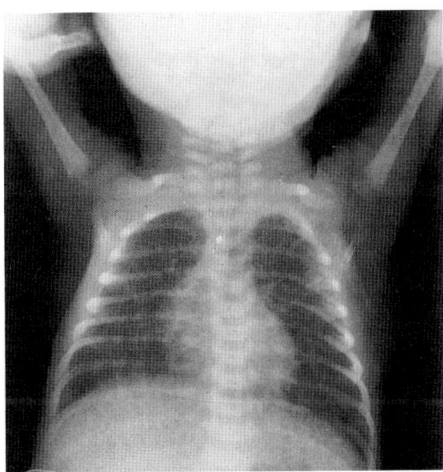

Fig. 27.54
Wilson–Mikity syndrome.

References

1. Abman S H, Accurso F J, Koops B L 1984 Experience with home oxygen in the management of infants with bronchopulmonary dysplasia. Clinical Pediatrics (Philadelphia) 23: 471–476
2. Abman S H, Wolfe R R, Accurso F J et al 1985 Pulmonary vascular response to oxygen in infants with severe bronchopulmonary dysplasia. Pediatrics 75: 80–84
3. ACTOBAT Study Group 1995 Australian collaborative trial of antenatal thyrotropin releasing hormone (ACTOBAT) for prevention of neonatal respiratory disease. Lancet 345: 877–882
4. Albersheim S G, Solimano A J, Sharma A K et al 1989 Randomized double blind controlled trial of long term diuretic therapy for bronchopulmonary dysplasia. Journal of Pediatrics 115: 615–620
5. Anderson A H, Warady B A, Daily D K et al 1993 Systemic hypertension in infants with severe bronchopulmonary dysplasia: associated clinical factors. American Journal of Perinatology 10: 190–193
6. Andreasson B, Lindstrom M, Mortensson W et al 1989 Lung function eight years after neonatal ventilation. Archives of Disease in Childhood 64: 108–113
7. Armstrong D L, Penrice J, Bloomfield F H, Knight D B, Dezoete J A, Harding J E 2002 Follow up of a randomised trial of two different courses of dexamethasone for preterm infants at risk of chronic lung disease. Archives of Disease in Childhood. Fetal and Neonatal Edition 86: F102–F107
8. Askin F 1991 Respiratory tract disorders in the fetus and neonate. In: Wigglesworth J S, Singer D B (eds) Textbook of fetal and perinatal pathology. Blackwell Scientific, Oxford, pp. 643–688
9. Avery M E, Tooley W H, Keller J B et al 1987 Is chronic lung disease in low birth weight infants preventable? A survey of eight centers. Pediatrics 79: 26–30
10. Bacchi A, Viscardi R M, Tacrak V et al 1994 Increased activity of interleukin-6 but not tumour necrosis factor-alpha in lung lavage of premature infants is associated with the development of bronchopulmonary dysplasia. Pediatric Research 36: 244–252
11. Ballard R A, Ballard P L, Creasy R K et al 1992 Respiratory disease in very low birthweight infants after prenatal thyrotropin-releasing hormone and glucocorticoids. Lancet 339: 510–515
12. Banks B A, Seri I, Ischiropoulos H et al 1999 Changes in oxygenation with inhaled nitric oxide in severe bronchopulmonary dysplasia. Pediatrics 103: 610–618
13. Barnes N D, Glover W J, Hull D et al 1969 Effects of prolonged positive pressure ventilation in infancy. Lancet ii: 1096–1099
14. Barrington K J, Finer N N 2001 Inhaled nitric oxide for respiratory failure in preterm infants (Cochrane Review). Cochrane Database of Systematic Reviews (3): CD000509
15. Bell E F, Warburton D, Stonestreet B et al 1980 Effect of fluid administration on the development of symptomatic patent ductus arteriosus and congestive heart failure in premature infants. New England Journal of Medicine 302: 598–604
16. Benatar A, Clarke J, Silverman M 1995 Pulmonary hypertension in infants with chronic lung disease: non-invasive evaluation and short term effect of oxygen treatment. Archives of Disease in Childhood. Fetal and Neonatal Edition 72: F14–F19
17. Berg T J, Pagtakhan T D, Reed M H et al 1975 Bronchopulmonary dysplasia and lung rupture in hyaline membrane disease: influence of continuous distending pressure. Pediatrics 55: 51–53
18. Berman W, Yabek S M, Dillon T et al 1982 Evaluation of infants with bronchopulmonary dysplasia using cardiac catheterization. Pediatrics 70: 708–712
19. Betremieux P, Treguier C, Pladys P et al 1995 Tracheobronchography and balloon dilatation in acquired neonatal tracheal stenosis. Archives of Disease in Childhood. Fetal and Neonatal Edition 72: F3–F7
20. Bhuta T, Ohlsson A 1998 Systematic review and meta-analysis of early postnatal dexamethasone for prevention of chronic lung disease. Archives of Disease in Childhood. Fetal and Neonatal Edition 79: F26–F33
21. Biswas S, Buffery J, Enoch H et al 2003 Pulmonary effects of triiodothyronine (T_3) and hydrocortisone (HC) supplementation in preterm infants less than 30 weeks gestation: THORN trial – thyroid hormone replacement in neonates Pediatric Research 53: 48–57
22. Bjorklund L L, Ingimarsson J, Curstedt T et al 1997 Manual ventilation with a few large breaths at birth compromises the therapeutic effect of subsequent surfactant replacement in immature lambs. Pediatric Research 42: 348–355
23. Block E R, Fisher A B 1977 Protection of hyperoxic induced depression of pulmonary serotonin by pre-treatment with superoxide dismutase. American Review of Respiratory Disease 116: 441–446

24. Boehm G, Bierbach U, Moro G et al 1996 Limited fat digestion in infants with bronchopulmonary dysplasia. Journal of Pediatric Gastroenterology and Nutrition 22: 161–166

25. Bolivar J M, Gerhardt T, Gonzalez A et al 1995 Mechanisms for episodes of hypoxemia in preterm infants undergoing mechanical ventilation. Journal of Pediatrics 127: 767–773

26. Bonikos D S, Benson K G, Northway W H J 1976 Oxygen toxicity in the newborn. The effect of chronic continuous 100 per cent oxygen exposure on the lung of newborn mice. American Journal of Pathology 85: 623–650

27. Brion L P, Primhak R A 2002 Intravenous or enteral loop diuretics for preterm infants with (or developing) chronic lung disease (Cochrane Review). In: The Cochrane Library, Issue 4. Update Software, Oxford

28. Brion L P, Primhak R A, Yong W 2002 Aerosolized diuretics for preterm infants with (or developing) chronic lung disease (Cochrane Review). In: The Cochrane Library, Issue 4. Update Software, Oxford

29. Brozanski B S, Jones J G, Gilmour C H et al 1995 Effect of pulse dexamethasone therapy on the incidence and severity of chronic lung disease in the very low birthweight infant. Journal of Pediatrics 126: 769–776

30. Brundage K L, Mohsini K G, Froese A B et al 1990 Bronchodilator response to ipratropium bromide in infants with bronchopulmonary dysplasia. American Review of Respiratory Disease 142: 1137–1142

31. Brunton J A, Saigal S, Atkinson S A 1998 Growth and body composition in infants with bronchopulmonary dysplasia up to 3 months corrected age: a randomized trial of a high-energy nutrient enriched formula fed after hospital discharge. Journal of Pediatrics 133: 340–345

32. Burnard E D 1966 The pulmonary syndrome of Wilson and Mikity and respiratory function in very small premature infants. Pediatric Clinics of North America 13: 999–1016

33. Cabal L A, Larrazabal C, Ramanathan R et al 1987 Effects of metaproterenol on pulmonary mechanics, oxygenation and ventilation in infants with chronic lung disease. Journal of Pediatrics 110: 116–119

34. Carlo W A, Stark A R, Wright L L et al 2002 Minimal ventilation to prevent bronchopulmonary dysplasia in extremely-low-birth-weight infants. Journal of Pediatrics 141: 370–374

35. Carlsson J, Svenningsen N W 1975 Respiratory insufficiency syndrome (RIS) in preterm infants with gestational age of 32 weeks and less. Acta Paediatrica Scandinavica 64: 813–821

36. Castro-Alcaraz S, Greenberg E M et al 2002 Patterns of colonisation with *Ureaplasma urealyticum* during neonatal intensive care unit hospitalisations of very low birthweight infants and the development of chronic lung disease. Pediatrics 110: e45

37. Chan K N, Noble-Jamieson C M, Elliman A et al 1988 Airway responsiveness in low birthweight children and their mothers. Archives of Disease in Childhood 63: 905–910

38. Chan V, Greenough A 1993 Randomized trial of methods of extubation in acute and chronic respiratory distress. Archives of Disease in Childhood 68: 570–572

39. Chan V, Greenough A, Cheeseman P et al 1993 Vitamin A levels and feeding practice of neonates with and without chronic lung disease. Journal of Perinatal Medicine 21: 205–210

40. Chan V, Greenough A, Hird M F 1991 Comparison of different rates of artificial ventilation for preterm infants ventilated beyond the first week of life. Early Human Development 26: 177–183

41. Charafeddine L, D'Angio C T, Phelps D L 1999 Atypical chronic lung disease patterns in neonates. Pediatrics 103: 759–765

42. Clark P L, Ekekezie I I, Kaftan H A, Castor C A, Truog W E 2002 Safety and efficacy of nitric oxide in chronic lung disease. Archives of Disease in Childhood. Fetal and Neonatal Edition 86: F41–F45

43. Coalson J J, King R J, Yang F et al 1995 SP-A deficiency in primate model of bronchopulmonary dysplasia with infection. In situ mRNA and immunostains. American Journal of Respiratory and Critical Care Medicine 151: 854–866

44. Coalson J J, Winter V V, Gertsmann D R et al 1992 Pathophysiologic, morphometric and biochemical studies of the premature baboon with bronchopulmonary dysplasia. American Review of Respiratory Disease 145: 872–881

45. Cochran D P, Pilling D W, Shaw N J 1994 The relationship of pulmonary interstitial emphysema to subsequent type of chronic lung disease. British Journal of Radiology 76: 1155–1157

46. Cook A J, Yuksel B, Sampson A P et al 1996 Cysteinyl leukotriene involvement in chronic lung disease in premature infants. European Respiratory Journal 9: 1907–1912

47. Cooke R 1991 Factors associated with chronic lung disease in preterm infants. Archives of Disease in Childhood 66: 776–779

48. Corcoran J D, Patterson C C, Thomas P S et al 1993 Reduction in the risk of bronchopulmonary dysplasia from 1980–1990: results of a multi-variate logistic regression analysis. European Journal of Pediatrics 152: 677–681

49. Costarino A T J, Gruskay J A, Corcoran L et al 1992 Sodium restriction versus daily maintenance replacement in very low birth weight premature neonates: a randomized, blind therapeutic trial. Journal of Pediatrics 120: 99–106

50. Couser R J, Ferrara B, Wright G B et al 1996 Prophylactic indomethacin therapy in the first 24 hours of life for the prevention of patent ductus arteriosus in preterm infants treated prophylactically in the delivery room. Journal of Pediatrics 128: 631–637

51. Crapo J D, Peters-Golden M, Marsh-Salin J et al 1978 Pathologic changes in the lungs of oxygen-adapted rats. A morphometric analysis. Laboratory Investigation 39: 640–653

52. Cronin C M G, Dean H, MacDonald N T et al 1993 Basal and post-ACTH cortisol levels in preterm infants following treatment with dexamethasone. Clinical and Investigative Medicine 16: 8–14

53. Crowley P, Chalmers I, Keirse M 1990 The effects of corticosteroid administration before preterm delivery: an overview of the evidence from controlled trials. British Journal of Obstetrics and Gynaecology 97: 11–25

54. Cummings J J, D'Eugenio D B, Gross S J 1989 A controlled trial of dexamethasone in preterm infants at high risk for bronchopulmonary dysplasia. New England Journal of Medicine 320: 1505–1510

55. D'Ablang G, Bernard B, Zahavov I et al 1975 Neonatal pulmonary cytology and bronchopulmonary dysplasia. Acta Cytologica 19: 21–27

56. Dahms B B, Halpin T C 1980 Pulmonary arterial lipid deposit in infants receiving intravenous lipid infusion. Pediatrics 97: 800–805

57. Darlow B A, Graham P J 2002 Vitamin A supplementation for preventing morbidity and mortality in very low birthweight infants (Cochrane Review). In: The Cochrane Library, Issue 4. Update Software, Oxford

58. Davidson D, Drafta D, Wilkens B A 1995 Elevated urinary leukotriene E4 in chronic lung disease of extreme prematurity. American Journal of Respiratory and Critical Care Medicine 151: 841–845

59. De Boeck K, Smith J, van Lierde S et al 1998 Response to bronchodilators in clinically stable 1-year-old patients with bronchopulmonary dysplasia. European Journal of Pediatrics 157: 75–79

60. De Rubertis F R, Michelis M F, Beck N et al 1970 Complications of diuretic therapy: severe alkalosis and syndrome resembling inappropriate secretion of anti-diuretic hormone. Metabolism 19: 709–719

61. Denjean A, Gulmaraes H, Migdal M et al 1992 Dose-related bronchodilator response to aerosolized salbutamol (albuterol) in ventilator-dependent premature infants. Journal of Pediatrics 120: 974–979

62. Dimitriou G, Greenough A, Giffin F J et al 1997 Inhaled versus systemic steroids in chronic oxygen dependency in preterm infants. European Journal of Pediatrics 156: 51–55

63. Dimitriou G, Greenough A, Kavvadia K 2004 Fluid retention, colloid infusion and chronic lung disease development in very low birthweight infants. Neonatal Intensive Care (in press)

64. Duff A L, Pomeranz E S, Gelber L E et al 1993 Risk factors for acute wheezing in infants and children: viruses, passive smoke and IgE antibodies to inhalant allergens. Pediatrics 92: 535–540

65. Durand M, Mendoza M E, Tantivit P, Kugelman A, McEvoy C 2002 A randomised trial of moderately early low-dose dexamethasone therapy in very low birth weight infants: dynamic pulmonary mechanics, oxygenation and ventilation. Paediatrics 109: 262–268

66. Edwards D K 1979 Radiographic aspects of bronchopulmonary dysplasia. Journal of Pediatrics 95: 823–829

67. Ehrenkranz R A, Ablow R C, Warshaw J B 1979 Prevention of bronchopulmonary dysplasia with vitamin E administration during the acute stages of respiratory distress syndrome. Journal of Pediatrics 95: 873–878

68. Ehrenkranz R A, Bonta B W, Ablow R C et al 1978 Amelioration of bronchopulmonary dysplasia following vitamin E administration. A preliminary report. New England Journal of Medicine 299: 564–568

69. Ellsbury D L, Acarregui M J, McGuiness G A, Klein J M 2002 Variability in the use of supplemental oxygen for bronchopulmonary dysplasia. Journal of Pediatrics 140: 247–249

70. Emery E F, Greenough A 1992 Effect of dexamethasone on blood pressure: relationship to postnatal age. European Journal of Pediatrics 151: 364–366

71. Erickson A M, de la Monte S M, Moore G W et al 1987 The progression of morphologic changes in bronchopulmonary dysplasia. American Journal of Pathology 127: 474–484

72. Eronen M, Pesonen E, Kurki T et al 1994 Increased incidence of bronchopulmonary dysplasia after antenatal administration of indomethacin to prevent preterm labor. Journal of Pediatrics 124: 782–788

73. Escobedo M B, Gonzalez A 1982 A baboon model of bronchopulmonary dysplasia. Experimental and Molecular Pathology 37: 323–334

74. Fauroux B, Sardet A, Foret D 1995 Home treatment for chronic respiratory failure in children: a prospective study. European Respiratory Journal 8: 2062–2066

75. Fowlie P W 1996 Prophylactic indomethacin: systematic review and meta-analysis. Archives of Disease in Childhood. Fetal and Neonatal Edition 74: F81–F87

76. Frank L 1992 Antioxidants, nutrition and bronchopulmonary dysplasia. Clinics in Perinatology 19: 541–561

77. Fujimura M, Kitajima H, Nakayama M 1993 Increased leukocyte elastase of the tracheal aspirate at birth and neonatal pulmonary emphysema. Pediatrics 92: 564–569

78. Fujimura M, Takeuchi T, Ando M et al 1983 Elevated immunoglobulin M levels in low birthweight neonates with chronic respiratory insufficiency. Early Human Development 9: 27–32

79. Fujimura M, Takeuchi T, Kitajima H et al 1989 Chorioamnionitis and serum IgM in Wilson-Mikity syndrome. Archives of Disease in Childhood 64: 1379–1383

80. Garland J S, Alex C P, Pauly T H et al 1999 A three-day course of dexamethasone therapy to prevent chronic lung disease in ventilated neonates: a randomized trial. Pediatrics 104: 91–99

81. Garland J S, Buck R K, Allred E N et al 1995 Hypocarbia before surfactant therapy appears to increase bronchopulmonary dysplasia risk in infants with respiratory distress syndrome. Archives of Pediatrics and Adolescent Medicine 149: 617–622

82. Gerhardt T, Hehre D, Feller R et al 1987 Serial determination of pulmonary function in infants with chronic lung disease. Journal of Pediatrics 110: 448–456

83. Giffin F, Greenough A, Yuksel B 1995 Antiviral therapy in neonatal chronic lung disease. Early Human Development 42: 97–109

84. Gonzalez A, Sosenko I R S, Chandar J et al 1996 Influence of infection on patent ductus arteriosus and chronic lung disease in premature infants weighing 1000 g or less. Journal of Pediatrics 128: 470–478

85. Gray P H, Rogers Y 1994 Are infants with bronchopulmonary dysplasia at risk for sudden infant death syndrome? Pediatrics 93: 774–777

86. Greenough A 1990 Personal practice. Bronchopulmonary dysplasia. Early diagnosis, prophylaxis and treatment. Archives of Disease in Childhood 65: 1082–1088

87. Greenough A, Alexander J, Burgess S et al 2001 Home oxygen status on rehospitalisation and primary care requirements of chronic lung disease infants. Archives of Disease in Childhood 86: 40–43

88. Greenough A, Boorman J, Alexander J et al 2001 Health care utilisation of CLD infants related to hospitalisation for RSV infection. Archives of Disease in Childhood 85: 463–468

89. Greenough A, Chan V, Hird M F 1992 Positive end expiratory pressure in acute and chronic neonatal respiratory distress. Archives of Disease in Childhood 67: 320–323

90. Greenough A, Dimitriou G, Johnson A H et al 2000 The chest radiograph appearances of very premature infants at 36 weeks post conceptional age. British Journal of Radiology 73: 366–369

91. Greenough A, Emery E F, Gamsu H R 1992 Dexamethasone and hypertension in chronic lung disease of preterm infants. European Journal of Pediatrics 152: 134–135

92. Greenough A, Emery E F, Hird M F et al 1993 Randomized controlled trial of albumin infusion in ill preterm infants. European Journal of Pediatrics 152: 157–159

93. Greenough A, Hird M F, Gamsu H R 1991 Home oxygen therapy following neonatal intensive care. Early Human Development 26: 29–35

94. Greenough A, Kavvadia K, Johnson A H et al 1999 A simple chest radiograph score to predict chronic lung disease in prematurely born infants. British Journal of Radiology 72: 530–533

95. Greenough A, Maconochie I, Yüksel B 1990 Recurrent respiratory symptoms in the first year of life following preterm delivery. Journal of Perinatal Medicine 18: 489–494

96. Greenough A, Milner A D, Dimitriou G 2001 Synchronized mechanical ventilation for respiratory support in newborn infants (Cochrane Review). In: The Cochrane Library, Issue 1. Update Software, Oxford

97. Greenough A, Milner A D, Roberton N R C 1995 Neonatal respiratory disorders. Edward Arnold, London, p. 396

98. Gregoire M-C, Lefebvre F, Glorieux J 1998 Health and developmental outcomes at 18 months in very preterm infants with bronchopulmonary dysplasia. Pediatrics 101: 856–860

99. Groneck P, Goetze-Speer B, Speer C P 1999 Effects of inhaled beclomethasone compared to systemic dexamethasone on lung inflammation in preterm infants at risk of chronic lung disease. Pediatric Pulmonology 27: 383–387

100. Groneck P, Goetze-Speer B, Oppermann M et al 1994 Association of pulmonary inflammation and increased microvascular permeability during the development of bronchopulmonary dysplasia: a sequential analysis of inflammatory mediators in respiratory fluids of high risk preterm neonates. Pediatrics 93: 712–718

101. Groneck P, Reuss D, Goetze-Speer B et al 1993 Effects of dexamethasone on chemotactic activity and inflammatory mediators in tracheobronchial aspirates of preterm infants at risk for chronic lung disease. Journal of Pediatrics 122: 938–944

102. Groneck P, Speer C P 1995 Inflammatory mediators and bronchopulmonary dysplasia. Archives of Disease in Childhood. Fetal and Neonatal Edition 73: F1–F3

103. Groothuis J R, Rosenberg A A 1987 Home oxygen promotes weight gain in infants with bronchopulmonary dysplasia. American Journal of Diseases of Children 141: 992–995

104. Gross S J, Iannuzzi D M, Kveselis D A et al 1999 Effect of preterm birth on pulmonary function at school age: a prospective controlled study. Journal of Pediatrics 133: 188–192

105. Gunn T, Reece E R, Metrakos K et al 1981 Depressed T cells following neonatal steroid treatment. Pediatrics 67: 61–67

106. Halliday H, Ehrenkranz R A 2001 Delayed (>3 weeks) postnatal corticosteroids for chronic lung disease in preterm infants (Cochrane Review). In: The Cochrane Library, Issue 2. Update Software, Oxford

107. Halliday H, Ehrenkranz R A 2001 Early postnatal (<96 hours) corticosteroids for preventing chronic lung disease in preterm infants (Cochrane Review). In: The Cochrane Library, Issue 2. Update Software, Oxford

108. Halliday H L, Patterson C C, Halahakoon C W N L et al 2001 A multicenter, randomized open study of early corticosteroid treatment (OSECT) in preterm infants with respiratory illness: comparison of early and late treatment and of dexamethasone and inhaled budesonide. Pediatrics 107: 232–240

109. Hallman M, Bry K, Hoppu K et al 1992 Inositol supplementation in premature infants with respiratory distress syndrome. New England Journal of Medicine 326: 1233–1239

110. Hallman M, Pitkainen O, Rauvala H et al 1987 Glycolipid accumulation in lung effluent in bronchopulmonary dysplasia. Pediatric Research 21: 454A

111. Hallman M, Spragg R G, Harrell J H et al 1982 Evidence of lung surfactant abnormality in respiratory failure. Journal of Clinical Investigation 70: 673–683

112. Hamilton P A, Whitehead M D, Reynolds E O R 1985 Underestimation of arterial oxygen tension by transcutaneous electrode with increasing age in infants. Archives of Disease in Childhood 60: 1162–1165

113. Hartnoll G, Betremieux P, Modi N 2000 Randomised controlled trial of postnatal sodium supplementation on oxygen dependency and body weight in 25–30 week gestational age infants. Archives of Disease in Childhood. Fetal and Neonatal Edition 82: F19–F23

114. Hazinski T A 1985 Furosemide decreases ventilation in young rabbits. Journal of Pediatrics 106: 81–85

115. Hazinski T A, Blalock W A, Engelhardt B 1988 Control of water balance in infants with bronchopulmonary dysplasia: role of endogenous vasopressin. Pediatric Research 23: 86–88

116. HIFI Study Group 1989 High-frequency oscillatory ventilation compared with conventional mechanical ventilation in the treatment of respiratory failure in preterm infants. New England Journal of Medicine 320: 88–93

117. Hislop A A, Haworth S G 1990 Pulmonary vascular damage and the development of cor pulmonale following hyaline membrane disease. Pediatric Pulmonology 9: 152–156

118. Hitti J, Krohn M A, Patton D L et al 1997 Amniotic fluid tumor necrosis factor-α and the risk of respiratory distress syndrome among preterm infants. American Journal of Obstetrics and Gynecology 177: 50–56

119. Howling S J, Northway W H, Hansell D M et al 2000 Pulmonary sequelae of bronchopulmonary dysplasia survivors: high-resolution CT findings. American Journal of Roentgenology 174: 1323–1326

120. Hudak B B, Allen M C, Hudak M L et al 1989 Home oxygen therapy for chronic lung disease in extremely low birthweight infants. American Journal of Diseases of Children 143: 357–360

121. Hufnagle K G, Khan S N, Penn D et al 1982 Renal calcification: a complication of long term frusemide therapy in premature infants. Pediatrics 70: 360–363

122. Hyde I, English E R, Williams J A 1989 The changing pattern of chronic lung disease of prematurity. Archives of Disease in Childhood 64: 448–451

123. Israel B A, Sherman F S, Guthrie R D 1993 Hypertrophic cardiomyopathy associated with dexamethasone therapy for chronic lung disease in preterm infants. American Journal of Perinatology 10: 307–310

124. Italian Collaborative Group on Preterm Delivery (ICGPD) 1993 Supplementation and plasma levels of vitamin A in premature newborns at risk for chronic lung disease. Developmental Pharmacology and Therapy 20: 144–151

125. Jobe A H, Bancalari E 2001 Bronchopulmonary dysplasia. NICHD-NHLBI-ORD Workshop. American Journal of Respiratory and Critical Care Medicine 163: 1723–1729

126. Jobe A H, Ikegami M 1998 Mechanisms initiating lung injury in the preterm. Early Human Development 53: 81–94

127. Jobe A H, Michell B R, Gunkel J H 1993 Beneficial effects of the combined use of prenatal corticosteroids and postnatal surfactant on preterm infants. American Journal of Obstetrics and Gynecology 168: 508–513

128. Johnson A H, Peacock J L, Greenough A et al 2002 High frequency oscillatory ventilation for the prevention of chronic lung disease of prematurity. New England Journal of Medicine 347: 633–642

129. Johnson L, Bowen F W J, Abbasi S et al 1985 Relationship of prolonged pharmacologic serum levels of vitamin E to the incidence of sepsis and necrotizing enterocolitis in infants with birthweight <1500 g or less. Pediatrics 75: 619–638

130. Jones C A, Cayabyab R G, Kwong K Y C et al 1996 Undetectable interleukin (IL)-10 and persistent IL-8 expression early in hyaline membrane disease: a possible developmental basis for the predisposition to chronic lung inflammation in preterm newborns. Pediatric Research 39: 966–975

131. Kao L C, Durand D J, Dhillias B L et al 1987 Oral theophylline and diuretics improve pulmonary mechanics in infants with bronchopulmonary dysplasia. Journal of Pediatrics 111: 439–444

132. Kao L C, Durand D J, McCrea R C et al 1994 Randomized trial of long-term diuretic therapy for infants with oxygen-dependent bronchopulmonary dysplasia. Journal of Pediatrics 124: 772–781

133. Kao L C, Durand D J, Nickerson B G 1989 Effects of inhaled metaproterenol and atropine on the pulmonary mechanics of infants with bronchopulmonary dysplasia. Pediatric Pulmonology 6: 74–80

134. Kao L C, Warburton D, Cheng M H et al 1984 Effect of oral diuretics on pulmonary mechanics in infants with chronic bronchopulmonary dysplasia: results of a double-blind crossover sequential trial. Pediatrics 74: 37–44

135. Kao L C, Warburton D, Platzker A C G et al 1984 Effect of isoproterenol inhalation on airways resistance in chronic bronchopulmonary dysplasia. Pediatrics 73: 509–514

136. Kao L C, Warburton D, Sargent C W et al 1983 Furosemide acutely decreases airway resistance in chronic bronchopulmonary dysplasia. Journal of Pediatrics 103: 624–629

137. Kavvadia V, Greenough A, Dimitriou G et al 1999 Comparison of the effect of two fluid input regimes on perinatal lung function in ventilated infants of very low birthweight. European Journal of Pediatrics 158: 917–922

138. Kavvadia V, Greenough A, Dimitriou G et al 2000 A comparison of arginine vasopressin levels and fluid balance in the perinatal period in infants who did and did not develop chronic oxygen dependency. Biology of the Neonate 78: 86–91

139. Kavvadia V, Greenough A, Dimitriou G et al 2000 Randomized trial of fluid restriction in ventilated very low birthweight infants. Archives of Disease in Childhood. Fetal and Neonatal Edition 83: F91–F96

140. Kinali M, Greenough A, Dimitriou G, Yuksel B 1999 Chronic respiratory morbidity following premature delivery – prediction of prolonged respiratory support requirement. European Journal of Pediatrics 158: 493–496

141. Kojima T, Sasai M, Kobayashi Y 1993 Increased soluble ICAM-1 in tracheal aspirates of infants with bronchopulmonary dysplasia. Lancet 342: 1023–1024

142. Koppel R, Han R N N, Cox D et al 1994 Alpha-1-antitrypsin protects neonatal rats from pulmonary vascular and parenchymal effects of oxygen toxicity. Pediatric Research 36: 763–770

143. Kornhauser M S, Cullen J A, Baumgart S et al 1994 Risk factors for bronchopulmonary dysplasia after extracorporeal membrane oxygenation. Archives of Pediatrics and Adolescent Medicine 148: 820–825

144. Kotecha S, Wilson L, Wangoo A et al 1996 Increase in interleukin (IL)-1β and IL-6 in bronchoalveolar lavage fluid obtained from infants with chronic lung disease of prematurity. Pediatric Research 40: 250–256

145. Kovacs L, Davis G M, Faucher D et al 1998 Efficacy of sequential early systemic and inhaled corticosteroid therapy in the prevention of chronic lung disease of prematurity. Acta Paediatrica 87: 792–798

146. Krauss A N, Levin A R, Grossman H et al 1970 Physiologic studies on infants with Wilson-Mikity syndrome. Journal of Pediatrics 77: 27–36

147. Kraybill E N, Runyan D K, Bose C L et al 1989 Risk factors for chronic lung disease in infants with birth weights of 751 to 1000 grams. Journal of Pediatrics 115: 115–120

148. Kugelman A, Durand M, Garg M 1997 Pulmonary effect of inhaled furosemide in ventilated infants with severe bronchopulmonary dysplasia. Pediatrics 99: 71–75

149. Kurzner S I, Garg M, Bautista D B et al 1988 Growth failure in bronchopulmonary dysplasia: elevated metabolic rates and pulmonary mechanics. Journal of Pediatrics 112: 73–80

150. Linder N, Kuint J, German B et al 1995 Hypertrophy of the tongue associated with inhaled corticosteroid therapy in premature infants. Journal of Pediatrics 127: 651–653

151. Lonnqvist P A, Jonsson B, Winberg P et al 1995 Inhaled nitric oxide in infants with developing or established chronic lung disease. Acta Paediatrica 84: 1188–1192

152. Lorenz J M, Kleinman L I, Kotagal U R et al 1982 Water balance in very low birthweight infants: relationship to water and sodium intake and effect on outcome. Journal of Pediatrics 101: 423–432

153. McCann E M, Lewis K, Demin D D et al 1985 Controlled trial of furosemide therapy in infants with chronic lung disease. Journal of Pediatrics 106: 957–962

154. McCubbin M, Frey E E, Wagener J S et al 1989 Large airway collapse in bronchopulmonary dysplasia. Journal of Pediatrics 114: 304–307

155. Manktelow B N, Draper E S, Annamalai S et al 2001 Factors affecting the incidence of chronic lung disease of prematurity in 1987,1992 and 1997. Archives of Disease in Childhood. Fetal and Neonatal Edition 85: F33–F35

156. Margraf L R, Tomashefski J F, Bruce M C et al 1991 Morphometric analysis of the lung in bronchopulmonary dysplasia. American Review of Respiratory Disease 143: 391–400

157. Markestad T, Fitzhardinge P M 1981 Growth and development in children recovering from bronchopulmonary dysplasia. Journal of Pediatrics 98: 597–602

158. Mayes L, Perkett E, Stahlman M T 1983 Severe bronchopulmonary dysplasia: a retrospective review. Acta Paediatrica Scandinavica 72: 225–229

159. Meissner C D, Welliver R C, Chartrand S A et al 1996 Prevention of respiratory syncytial virus infection in high risk infants: consensus opinion on the role of immunoprophylaxis with respiratory syncytial virus hyperimmune globulin. Pediatric Infectious Disease Journal 15: 1059–1068

160. Merritt T A, Cochrane C G, Holcomb K et al 1983 Elastase and alpha-1 protease inhibitor activity in tracheal aspirates during RDS: the role of inflammation and pathogenesis of bronchopulmonary dysplasia. Journal of Clinical Investigation 72: 656–666

161. Merritt T A, Hallman M, Holcomb K 1986 Human surfactant treatment of severe respiratory distress: pulmonary effluent indicators of lung inflammation. Journal of Pediatrics 108: 741–748

162. Miller R W, Woo P, Kellman R K et al 1987 Tracheobronchial abnormalities in infants with bronchopulmonary dysplasia. Journal of Pediatrics 111: 779–782

163. Mirro R, Armstead W, Leffler C 1990 Increased airway leukotriene levels in infants with severe bronchopulmonary dysplasia. American Journal of Diseases of Children 144: 160–161

164. Mitchell S H, Teague W G, Robinson A 1998 Reduced gas transfer at rest and during exercise in school-age survivors of bronchopulmonary dysplasia. American Journal of Respiratory and Critical Care Medicine 157: 1406–1412

165. Morray J P, Fox W W, Kettrick R G et al 1982 Improvement in lung mechanics as a function of age in the infant with severe bronchopulmonary dysplasia. Pediatric Research 16: 290–294

166. Motoyama E K, Fort M D, Klesh K W et al 1987 Early onset of airway reactivity in premature infants with bronchopulmonary dysplasia. American Review of Respiratory Disease 136: 50–57

167. Moyer W J 1950 Vitamin E levels in term and premature newborn infants. Pediatrics 6: 893–896

168. Moylan F M B, Walker A M, Kramer S S et al 1978 Alveolar rupture as an independent predictor of bronchopulmonary dysplasia. Critical Care Medicine 6: 10–13

169. Murch S H, Costeloe K, Klein N J et al 1996 Mucosal tumour necrosis factor-α production and extensive disruption of sulfated glycosaminoglycans begin within hours of birth in neonatal respiratory distress syndrome. Pediatric Research 40: 484–489

170. Murch S H, Costeloe K, Klein N J et al 1996 Early production of macrophage inflammatory protein-1-alpha occurs in respiratory distress syndrome and is associated with poor outcome. Pediatric Research 40: 490–497

171. Najak Z D, Harris E M, Lazzara A et al 1983 Pulmonary effects of furosemide in preterm infants with lung disease. Journal of Pediatrics 102: 758–763

172. Ng G Y, Ohlsson A 2002 Cromolyn sodium for the prevention of chronic lung disease in preterm infants (Cochrane Review). In: The Cochrane Library, Issue 4. Update Software, Oxford

173. Ng GY, Da S, Ohlsson A 2001 Bronchodilators for the prevention and treatment of chronic lung disease in preterm infants (Cochrane Review). Cochrane Database of Systematic Reviews (3): CD003214

174. Ng P C, Thomson M A, Dear P R F 1990 Dexamethasone and infection in preterm babies: a controlled study. Archives of Disease in Childhood 65: 54–56

175. Nickerson B G, Taussig L M 1980 Family history of asthma in infants with bronchopulmonary dysplasia. Pediatrics 65: 1140–1144

176. Niu J O, Munshi U K, Siddiq M M, Parton L A 1998 Early increase in endothelin-1 in tracheal aspirates: correlation with bronchopulmonary dysplasia Journal of Pediatrics 132: 965–970

177. Noble-Jamieson C M, Regev R, Silverman M 1989 Dexamethasone in neonatal chronic lung disease: pulmonary effects and intracranial complications. European Journal of Pediatrics 148: 365–367

178. Northway W H 1979 Observations on bronchopulmonary dysplasia. Journal of Pediatrics 95: 815–818

179. Northway W H J, Rosan R C, Porter D Y 1967 Pulmonary disease following respiratory therapy of hyaline membrane disease: bronchopulmonary dysplasia. New England Journal of Medicine 276: 357–368

180. Obladen M 1988 Alterations in surfactant composition. In: Merritt A, Northway W H, Boynton B R (eds) Bronchopulmonary dysplasia. Blackwell Scientific, Boston, pp. 131–141

181. O'Brodovich H M, Mellins R B 1985 Bronchopulmonary dysplasia. Unresolved neonatal acute lung injury. American Review of Respiratory Disease 132: 694–709

182. Odezmir A, Brown M A, Morgan W J 1997 Markers and mediators of inflammation in neonatal lung disease Pediatric Pulmonology 23: 292–306

183. Oppenheim C, Marmou-Mani T, Sayegh N et al 1994 Bronchopulmonary dysplasia: value of CT in identifying pulmonary sequelae. American Journal of Roentgenology 163: 169–172

184. O'Shea T M, Kothadia J M, Klinepeter K L et al 1999 Randomized placebo-controlled trial of a 42-day tapering course of dexamethasone to reduce the duration of ventilator dependency in very low birth weight infants: outcome of study participants at 1-year adjusted age. Pediatrics 104: 15–21

185. Palta M, Gabbert D, Weinstein M R, Peters M E 1991 Multivariate assessment of traditional risk factors for chronic lung disease in very low birth weight neonates. The Newborn Lung Project. Journal of Pediatrics 119: 285–292

186. Palta M, Sadek M, Barnet J H et al 1998 Evaluation of criteria for chronic lung disease in surviving very low birthweight infants. Journal of Pediatrics 132: 57–63

187. Pandit P B, Dunn M S, Kelly E N et al 1995 Surfactant replacement in neonates with early chronic lung disease. Pediatrics 95: 851–854

188. Panitch H B, Allen J L, Alpert B E et al 1994 Effects of CPAP on lung mechanics in infants with acquired tracheobronchomalacia. American Journal of Respiratory and Critical Care Medicine 150: 1341–1346

189. Panitch H B, Downes J J, Kennedy J S et al 1996 Guidelines for home care of children with chronic respiratory insufficiency. Pediatric Pulmonology 21: 52–56

190. Papile L-A, Tyson J E, Stoll B J et al 1998 A multicenter trial of two dexamethasone regimens in ventilator-dependent premature infants. New England Journal of Medicine 338: 1112–1118

191. Parat S, Moriette G, Delaperche M-F et al 1995 Long term pulmonary functional outcome of bronchopulmonary dysplasia and premature birth. Pediatric Pulmonology 20: 289–296

192. Parker R A, Lindstrom D P, Cotton R B 1992 Improved survival accounts for most, but not all, of the increase in bronchopulmonary dysplasia. Pediatrics 90: 663–668

193. Pearson E, Bose C, Snidow T et al 1992 Trial of vitamin A supplementation in very low birth weight infants at risk for bronchopulmonary dysplasia. Journal of Pediatrics 121: 420–427

194. Pera A, Byun A, Gribar S, Schwartz R, Kumar D, Parimi P 2002 Dexamethasone therapy and Candida sepsis in neonates less than 1250 grams. Journal of Perinatology 22: 204–208

195. Pereira G R, Baumgart S, Bennett M J et al 1994 Use of high fat formula for premature infants with bronchopulmonary dysplasia: metabolic, pulmonary and nutritional studies. Journal of Pediatrics 124: 605–611

196. Pinney M A, Cotton E K 1976 Home management of bronchopulmonary dysplasia. Pediatrics 58: 856–859

197. Poets C F, Sens B 1996 Changes in intubation rates and outcome of very low birth weight infants: a population-based study. Pediatrics 98: 24–27

198. Poets C F, Wilken M, Seidenberg J et al 1993 Reliability of a pulse oximeter in the detection of hyperoxemia. Journal of Pediatrics 122: 87–90

199. Pomerance J J, Puri A P 1980 Treatment of neonatal bronchopulmonary dysplasia with steroids. Pediatric Research 14: 649A

200. Prasertsom W, Phillipos E Z, van Aerde J E et al 1996 Pulmonary vascular resistance during lipid infusion in neonates. Archives of Disease in Childhood. Fetal and Neonatal Edition 74: F95–F98

201. Ramanathan R, Durand M, Larrazabal C 1987 Pulse oximetry in very low birth weight infants with acute and chronic lung disease. Pediatrics 79: 612–617

202. Ramsay P L, O'Brien Smith E, Hegemier S, Welty S E 1998 Early markers for the development of bronchopulmonary dysplasia: soluble E-selectin and ICAM-1. Pediatrics 102: 927–932

203. Rastogi A, Akintorin S M, Bez M L et al 1996 A controlled trial of dexamethasone to prevent bronchopulmonary dysplasia in surfactant-treated infants. Pediatrics 98: 204–210

204. Rastogi A, Luayon M, Ajayi O A et al 1994 Nebulized furosemide in infants with bronchopulmonary dysplasia. Journal of Pediatrics 125: 976–979

205. Regev R, DeVries L S, Noble-Jamieson C M et al 1987 Dexamethasone and increased intracranial echogenicity. Lancet i: 632–633

206. Reimers K J, Carlson S J, Lombard K A 1992 Nutritional management of infants with bronchopulmonary dysplasia. Nutrition in Clinical Practice 7: 127–132

207. Rhodes P G, Hall R T, Leonidas J C 1975 Chronic pulmonary disease in neonates with assisted ventilation. Pediatrics 55: 788–795

208. Rome E S, Stork E K, Carlo W A 1984 Limitations of transcutaneous PO$_2$ and PCO$_2$ monitoring in infants with bronchopulmonary dysplasia. Pediatrics 74: 217–220

209. Rooklin A R, Moomjian A S, Shutack J G et al 1979 Theophylline therapy in bronchopulmonary dysplasia. Journal of Pediatrics 95: 882–888

210. Rosan R C 1975 Hyaline membrane disease and a related spectrum of neonatal pneumopathies. Perspectives in Pediatric Pathology 2: 15–60

211. Rosenfeld W, Evans H, Concepcion L et al 1984 Prevention of bronchopulmonary dysplasia by administration of bovine superoxide dismutase in preterm infants with respiratory distress syndrome. Journal of Pediatrics 105: 781–785

212. Rosenfeld W, Sadhev S, Zabalera I et al 1986 Measurement of superoxide dismutase in neonates utilizing polyclonal antibodies. Pediatric Research 20: 209A

213. Russell G A B, Cooke R W I 1995 Randomised controlled trial of allopurinol prophylaxis in very preterm infants. Archives of Disease in Childhood. Fetal and Neonatal Edition 73: F27–F31

214. Ryan S, Congdon P J, Horsman A et al 1987 Bone mineral content in bronchopulmonary dysplasia. Archives of Disease in Childhood 62: 889–894

215. Rybak L P 1982 Pathophysiology of frusemide toxicity. Journal of Otolaryngology 11: 127–133

216. Saldanha R L, Cepeda E E, Poland R L 1982 The effect of vitamin E prophylaxis on the incidence and severity of bronchopulmonary dysplasia. Journal of Pediatrics 101: 89–93

217. Santuz P, Baraldi E, Zaramella P et al 1995 Factors limiting exercise performance in long term survivors of bronchopulmonary dysplasia. American Journal of Respiratory and Critical Care Medicine 152: 1284–1289

218. Saunders R A, Milner A D, Hopkin I E 1978 Longitudinal studies of infants with the Wilson-Mikity syndrome. Biology of the Neonate 33: 90–99

219. Sauve R S, Singhal N 1985 Long term morbidity of infants with bronchopulmonary dysplasia. Pediatrics 76: 725–733

220. Savage M O, Wilkinson A R, Baum J D et al 1975 Frusemide in respiratory distress syndrome. Archives of Disease in Childhood 50: 709–713

221. Sawyer M H, Edwards D K, Spector S A 1987 Cytomegalovirus infection and bronchopulmoary dysplasia in premature infants. American Journal of Diseases of Children 141: 303–305

222. Schreiner M S, Donar M E, Kettrick R G 1987 Pediatric home mechanical ventilation. Pediatric Clinics of North America 34: 47–60

223. Sekar K C, Duke J C 1991 Sleep apnea and hypoxemia in recently weaned premature infants with and without bronchopulmonary dysplasia. Pediatric Pulmonology 10: 112–116

224. Shah V, Ohlsson A, Halliday H L, Dunn M S 2000 Early administration of inhaled corticosteroids for preventing chronic lung disease in ventilated very low birth weight preterm neonates (Cochrane Review). Cochrane Database of Systematic Reviews (2): CD001969

225. Shankaran S, Szego E, Eizert D et al 1984 Severe bronchopulmonary dysplasia: predictors of survival and outcome. Chest 86: 607–610

226. Shaw N J, Ruggins N, Cooke R W I 1993 Infants with chronic lung disease: predictors of mortality at Day 28. Journal of Perinatology 13: 464–467

227. Shenai J P 1999 Vitamin A supplementation in very low birth weight neonates: rationale and evidence. Pediatrics 104: 1369–1374

228. Shenai J P, Chytil F, Stahlman M T 1985 Vitamin A status of neonates with bronchopulmonary dysplasia. Pediatric Research 19: 185–188

229. Shenai J P, Kennedy K A, Chytil F et al 1987 Clinical trial of vitamin A supplementation in infants susceptible to bronchopulmonary dysplasia. Journal of Pediatrics 111: 269–277

230. Shennan A T, Dunn M S, Ohlsson A et al 1988 Abnormal pulmonary outcomes in premature infants: prediction from oxygen requirement in the neonatal period. Pediatrics 82: 527–532

231. Shinwell E S, Karplus M, Reich D et al 2000 Early postnatal dexamethasone treatment and increased incidence of cerebral palsy. Archives of Disease in Childhood. Fetal and Neonatal Edition 83: F177–F181

232. Short A, Cooke R W I 1991 The incidence of renal calcification in preterm infants. Archives of Disease in Childhood 66: 412–417

233. Simon L 1980 Protection against toxic effect of sustained hyperoxia on lung macrophages by superoxide dismutase. Clinical Research 28: 432A

234. Singer L, Martin R J, Hawkins S W et al 1992 Oxygen desaturation complicates feeding in infants with bronchopulmonary dysplasia after discharge. Pediatrics 90: 380–384

235. Smyth J A, Tabachnik E, Duncan W J et al 1981 Pulmonary function and bronchial hyperreactivity in long-term survivors of bronchopulmonary dysplasia. Pediatrics 68: 336–340

236. Solimano A J, Smyth J A, Mann T K et al 1986 Pulse oximetry advantages in infants with bronchopulmonary dysplasia. Pediatrics 78: 844–849

237. Sosenko I R S, Frank L 1991 Oxidants and antioxidants. In: Cherniak N, Mellins R B (eds) Basic mechanisms of paediatric respiratory disease: cellular and integrative. B C Decker, Philadelphia, p. 315

238. Sosenko I R S, Rodriguez-Pierce M, Bancalari E 1993 Effects of early initiation of intravenous lipid administration on the incidence and severity of chronic lung disease in premature infants. Journal of Pediatrics 123: 975–982

239. Spear M L, Reeves G, Pearlman S A 1993 Diabetic ketoacidosis after steroid administration for bronchopulmonary dysplasia: a case report. Journal of Perinatology 13: 232–234

240. Speer C P, Ruess D, Harms K et al 1993 Neutrophil elastase and acute pulmonary damage in neonates with severe respiratory distress syndrome. Pediatrics 91: 794–799

241. Spitzer A R, Fox W W, Delivoria-Papadopoulos M 1981 Maximum diuresis – a factor in predicting recovery from respiratory distress syndrome and the development of bronchopulmonary dysplasia. Journal of Pediatrics 98: 476–479

242. Stahlman M T, Cheatham W, Gray M E 1979 The role of air dissection in bronchopulmonary dysplasia. Journal of Pediatrics 95: 878–885

243. Steichen J J, Gratton T L, Tsang R C 1980 Osteopenia of prematurity: the cause and possible treatment. Journal of Pediatrics 96: 528–534

244. Stenmark K R, Eyzaguine M, Remigio L et al 1985 Recovery of platelet activating factor and leukotrienes from infants with severe bronchopulmonary dysplasia: clinical improvement with cromolyn treatment. American Review of Respiratory Disease 131: 236A

245. Stenmark K R, Eyzaguirre M, Westcott J Y et al 1987 Potential role of eicosanoids and PAF in the pathophysiology of bronchopulmonary dysplasia. American Review of Respiratory Disease 136: 770–772

246. Stocker J T 1986 Pathologic features of long standing "healed" bronchopulmonary dysplasia: a study of 28 3- to 40-month old infants. Human Pathology 17: 943–961

247. Stocks J, Godfrey S, Reynolds E O R 1978 Airway resistance in infants after various treatments for hyaline membrane disease: special emphasis on prolonged high levels of inspired oxygen. Pediatrics 61: 178–183

248. STOP-ROP Multicenter Study Group 2000 Supplemental Therapeutic Oxygen for Prethreshold Retinopathy Of Prematurity (STOP-ROP), a randomized, controlled trial. I: Primary outcomes. Pediatrics 105: 295–310

249. Strayer D S, Merritt T A, Lwebuga-Mukasa J et al 1986 Surfactant–antisurfactant immune complexes in infants with respiratory distress syndrome. American Journal of Pathology 122: 353–362

250. Suresh G K, Soll R F 2002 Superoxide dismutase for preventing chronic lung disease in mechanically ventilated preterm infants (Cochrane Review). In: The Cochrane Library, Issue 4. Update Software, Oxford

251. Taghizadeh A, Reynolds E O R 1976 Pathogenesis of bronchopulmonary dysplasia following hyaline membrane disease. American Journal of Pathology 82: 241–264

252. Tammela O K T, Lanning F P, Koivisto M E 1992 The relationship of fluid restriction during the first month of life to the occurrence and severity of bronchopulmonary dysplasia in low birthweight infants: a 1-year radiological follow-up. European Journal of Pediatrics 151: 367–371

253. Taylor D W 1956 The effects of vitamin E and of methylene blue on the manifestations of oxygen poisoning in the rat. Journal of Physiology 131: 200–210

254. Teague W G, Pian M S, Heldt G P et al 1988 An acute reduction in the fraction of inspired oxygen increases airway constriction in infants with chronic lung disease. American Review of Respiratory Disease 137: 861–865

255. Thomas M, Greenough A, Johnson A et al 2003 Frequent wheeze at follow-up of very preterm infants: which factors are predictive? Archives of Disease in Childhood. Fetal and Neonatal Edition 88: F329–F332

256. Thomas M, Greenough A, Morton M 2003 Prolonged ventilation and intact survival in very low birth weight infants. European Journal of Pediatrics 162: 65–67

257. Tooley W 1979 Epidemiology of bronchopulmonary dysplasia. Journal of Pediatrics 95: 851–858

258. Tschanz S A, Damke B M, Burri P H 1995 Influence of postnatally administered glucocorticoids on rat lung growth. Biology of the Neonate 68: 229–245

259. Tyson J E, Wright L L, Oh W et al 1999 Vitamin A supplementation for extremely-low-birth-weight infants. National Institute of Child Health and Human Development Neonatal Research Network 340: 1962–1968

260. van Lierde S, Cornelis A, Devlieger H et al 1991 Different patterns of pulmonary sequelae after hyaline membrane disease: heterogeneity of bronchopulmonary dysplasia. Biology of the Neonate 60: 152–162

261. van Marter L J, Leviton A, Allred E N et al 1990 Hydration during the first days of life and the risk of bronchopulmonary dysplasia in low birth weight infants. Journal of Pediatrics 116: 942–949

262. Vrlenich L A, Bozynski M E A, Shyr Y et al 1995 The effect of bronchopulmonary dysplasia on growth at school age. Pediatrics 95: 855–859

263. Wada K, Jobe A H, Ikegami M 1997 Tidal volume effects on surfactant treatment responses with the initiation of ventilation in preterm lambs. Journal of Applied Physiology 83: 1054–1061

264. Wang E E L, Cassell G H, Sanchez P J et al 1993 *Ureaplasma urealyticum* and chronic lung disease of prematurity: critical appraisal of the literature on causation. Clinical Infectious Diseases 17: S112–S116

265. Wang E E, Ohlasson A, Kellner J D 1995 Association of *Ureaplasma urealyticum* colonization with chronic lung disease of prematurity: result of meta-analysis. Journal of Pediatrics 127: 640–644

266. Watterberg K L, Carmichael D F, Gerdes J S et al 1994 Secretory leukocyte protease inhibitor and lung inflammation in developing bronchopulmonary dysplasia. Journal of Pediatrics 125: 264–269

267. Watterberg K L, Demers L M, Scott S M et al 1996 Chorioamnionitis and early lung inflammation in infants in whom bronchopulmonary dysplasia develops. Pediatrics 97: 210–215

268. Watterberg K L, Murphy S 1993 Failure of cromolyn sodium to reduce the incidence of bronchopulmonary dysplasia: a pilot study. The Neonatal Cromolyn Study Group. Pediatrics 91: 803–806

269. Watterberg K L, Scott S M 1995 Evidence of early adrenal insufficiency in babies who develop bronchopulmonary dysplasia. Pediatrics 95: 120–125

270. Wauer R R, Schmatisch G, Bohne B et al 1992 Randomized double blind trial of ambroxol in the treament of respiratory distress syndrome. European Journal of Pediatrics 151: 357–363

271. Werthammer J, Brown E R, Neff R K et al 1982 Sudden infant death syndrome in infants with bronchopulmonary dysplasia. Pediatrics 69: 301–304

272. Wheater M, Rennie J M 1994 Poor prognosis after prolonged ventilation for bronchopulmonary dysplasia. Archives of Disease in Childhood. Fetal and Neonatal Edition 71: F210–F211

273. Wilkie R A, Bryan M H 1987 Effect of bronchodilators on airway resistance in ventilator-dependent neonates with chronic lung disease. Journal of Pediatrics 111: 278–282

274. Wilson M G, Mikity V G 1960 A new form of respiratory disease in premature infants. American Journal of Diseases of Children 99: 489–499

275. Wong Y C, Beardsmore C S, Silverman M 1982 Pulmonary sequelae of neonatal respiratory distress in very low birthweight infants: a clinical and physiological study. Archives of Disease in Childhood 57: 418–424

276. Yoshioka T, Sugive A, Shimaola T 1979 Superoxide dismutase activity in the maternal and cord blood. Biology of the Neonate 36: 173–180

277. Yüksel B, Greenough A 1991 Ipratropium bromide for symptomatic preterm infants. European Journal of Pediatrics 150: 854–857

278. Yüksel B, Greenough A 1992 Acute deteriorations in neonatal chronic lung disease. European Journal of Pediatrics 151: 697–700

279. Yuksel B, Greenough A 1992 Inhaled sodium cromoglycate for preterm infants with respiratory symptoms at follow-up. Respiratory Medicine 86: 131–134

280. Yüksel B, Greenough A, Green S 1991 Lung function abnormalities at six months of age after neonatal intensive care. Archives of Disease in Childhood 66: 472–476

281. Yüksel B, Greenough A, Green S 1991 Paradoxical response to nebulized ipratropium bromide in preterm infants asymptomatic at follow-up. Respiratory Medicine 85: 189–194

282. Yüksel B, Greenough A, Karani J et al 1991 Chest radiograph scoring system for use in preterm infants. British Journal of Radiology 64: 1015–1018

283. Yüksel B, Greenough A, Maconochie I 1990 Effective bronchodilator therapy by a simple spacer device for wheezy premature infants in the first two years of life. Archives of Disease in Childhood 65: 782–785

284. Zimmerman J J 1995 Bronchoalveolar inflammatory pathophysiology of bronchopulmonary dysplasia. Clinics in Perinatology 22: 429–456

PART 4

Apnoea and bradycardia

Simon Hannam

Introduction

Apnoea is a commonly encountered phenomenon on the neonatal unit, particularly in preterm babies. Episodes of cessation of breathing can lead to hypoxaemia and bradycardia requiring resuscitation. As there are many different causes of apnoea, the treatment of the condition depends on the results of investigation into, and diagnosis of, the underlying pathology.

Definition

The American Academy of Pediatrics defines apnoea as a pause in breathing of greater than 20 seconds or one of less than 20 seconds and associated with bradycardia and/or cyanosis.[3] A wide range of apnoea durations have been studied, varying from 2[33] to ≥15 seconds.[6,43] In practice, though, most apnoea alarms on neonatal units are set up to detect those apnoeas lasting for greater than 20 seconds. Apnoea must be distinguished from periodic breathing (see below) which is common in preterm infants and where there are bursts of respiratory activity separated with apnoeic pauses lasting at least 3 seconds.[32]

Incidence of clinical apnoea

There is an inverse correlation between the frequency of apnoea and gestational age. Apnoea occurs in over 80% of babies born at less than 30 weeks' gestation, about 50% of those born at 30–31 weeks', 14% born at 32–33 weeks' and 7% born at 34–35 weeks'.[38]

Types of apnoea

There are three types of apnoea: central, obstructive and mixed. In central apnoea, there is a cessation of both respiratory effort and nasal airflow (Fig. 27.55a). With obstructive apnoea, nasal airflow ceases as the infant makes increasing respiratory effort in an attempt to overcome partial or total upper airway obstruction (Fig. 27.55b). The third type of apnoea is described as mixed and has both central and obstructive components. During central apnoeas, upper airway obstruction can occur, as reflected by the loss of cardiac artefact in the airflow trace (Fig. 27.55a).[66] Recently, a reclassification of apnoea has been proposed using the presence or absence of amplified cardiac airflow artefact in the respiratory airflow trace to define whether an apnoea is central or obstructive.[53] Central apnoeas are those with the cardiac artefact present, obstructive where it is absent, and mixed where the artefact is absent during part of the apnoea.[54] The distribution of apnoea type has been demonstrated to vary with the length of apnoea in preterm infants.[13] Butcher-Peuch et al[13] analysed 1520 episodes of apnoea of over 10 seconds duration. With increasing length of apnoea, the proportion of central apnoea decreased from 69% to 29%, whilst that of mixed apnoeas increased from 20% to 60%. Pure obstructive apnoeas in preterm babies make up between 6% and 10% of the total number of apnoeas.[26,99]

Mechanisms of apnoea

Central apnoea

Signals for the involuntary control of breathing which maintain rhythmic ventilation originate in the brainstem in the area of the medulla oblongata (p. 451). Input into the respiratory centre arises from three primary sources: chemoreceptors, mechanoreceptors of the lung and upper airway, and input from the cerebral cortex. Delayed maturation of any of these sites could potentially result in apnoea.

Brainstem generator

There is evidence for the immaturity of the brainstem generator in the aetiology of apnoea of prematurity. Brainstem conduction times, as detected by auditory evoked responses, shorten with increasing gestational age.[40] Infants experiencing apnoea had longer brainstem conduction times compared with those of equivalent gestational age without apnoea.

Chemoreceptors (see also pp. 452–4)

Central chemoreceptors that detect changes in CO_2 and pH in the arterial blood are located in the brainstem.[35] Preterm babies who are having apnoeas demonstrate a depressed ventilatory

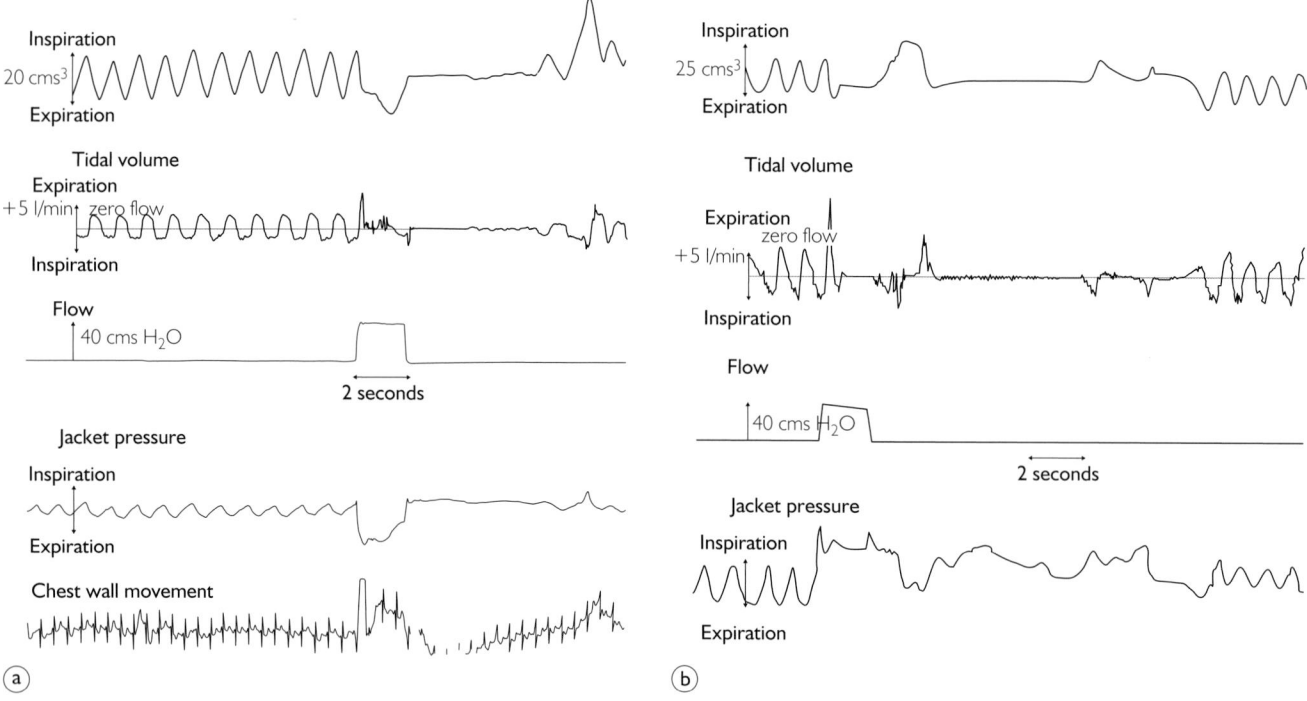

Fig. 27.55 (a) Apnoea in a preterm infant following lung deflation using an inflatable jacket. Note that there is cessation of breathing movements, initially with a closed upper airway, which then opens, as reflected by the appearance of cardiac artefact in the airflow tracing. (b) Obstructive apnoea following lung deflation in a preterm infant. Note that chest wall movements continue in the absence of airflow.

response to CO_2 compared with those not having apnoeas.[29] As there were no differences in the respiratory mechanics or oxygenation between the two groups, this reduced response to CO_2 was attributed to decreased response of chemoreceptors located in the respiratory centre. These findings have been contradicted in a study investigating the response of preterm babies breathing through added dead space, where it was not possible to demonstrate a deficit in central respiratory control in infants experiencing apnoeas.[100]

Peripheral chemoreceptors are located outside the brainstem in the carotid bodies near the bifurcation of the common carotid arteries. Afferent information from the chemoreceptors is transmitted via the glossopharyngeal nerve. The principal role of these receptors is to detect hypoxaemia. In babies, hypoxia elicits an excitatory response with an augmentation of respiratory effort. Preterm and newborn babies exhibit a biphasic response to hypoxia,[60] with an increase in ventilation followed by an inhibition of breathing. In preterm babies, this inhibitory response to hypoxia can extend into the second month of life, when apnoeas can still be a significant problem.

Mechanoreceptors in the lungs and upper airways provide input into the respiratory centre. Functional immaturity in the reflexes transmitted via the vagus nerve has been demonstrated. The Hering–Breuer inflation reflex (p. 454), where inspiration is terminated and expiration promoted, has been shown to be significantly reduced in preterm babies experiencing apnoea.[30] The Hering–Breuer deflation reflex (p. 454), which terminates expiration and promotes inspiration, has also been demonstrated to be immature in preterm babies having apnoeas.[27,33]

Obstructive apnoea

Using the new classification of apnoea, many apnoeas previously described as being central are in fact obstructive or mixed in nature. Mechanisms leading to obstructed breaths include instability of the upper airway in preterm infants, asynchrony of the musculature of the upper airway and diaphragm, pathological changes in the upper airway, and central nervous system (CNS) pathologies. Obstruction of the upper airway may be a result of decreased tone in preterm infants, leading to collapse and obstruction of the upper airway.[45] Using an ultrafine fibreoptic scope, the site of upper airway obstruction in preterm babies has been shown to be at the laryngeal level.[82] It is not clear whether airway closure is a reflection of hypoxia associated with apnoea, whether it is due to asynchrony between the alae nasi and diaphragm sucking in the upper airway[14] or whether it is due to passive airway narrowing due to reduced tone. Spontaneous neck flexion can also lead to obstruction in healthy preterm babies[96] as well as in situations where there are anatomical abnormalities of the upper airway, such as Pierre-Robin sequence and Down syndrome. Obstructive apnoeas are also more common in infants who have had intraventricular haemorrhages, possibly as a result of decreased tone in the upper airway.[13]

Mixed apnoea

With mixed apnoea, most apnoeas commence with central apnoea followed by airway occlusion.[45] Narrowing of the airway occurs about 1 second into a central apnoea.[54] This appears to be due to the loss of tone of the muscles of the upper airway. Clearly, this could then lead to the development of airway obstruction and evolve into a mixed apnoea. All apnoeas persisting for more than 20 seconds fall into the category of mixed apnoea.[99] Obstructing the airway can also lead to central apnoea. Upton et al[101] investigated the response of preterm infants to airway obstruction. There was an increased frequency of central apnoea following relief of the obstruction, raising the possibility that obstruction itself might have a role in the development of the central apnoea.[101] Apnoea may represent an immaturity of the multiple mechanisms that determine the rate and depth of respiration.[106] A relationship between cycle time and length of apnoeic episodes has been demonstrated reflecting a 'hunting' form of ventilation whereby respiration was first stimulated then suppressed. The fact that short respiratory pauses, periodic breathing and prolonged apnoeas all occur at the nadir of spontaneous breathing cycles[105] supports the idea of a common aetiology of apnoea. In the light of recent studies, it appears that central, mixed and obstructive apnoeas are part of a spectrum of apnoea rather than forming distinct entities and that all may have a common underlying mechanism.[73]

Factors involved in apnoea

Most apnoeic episodes in preterm babies are in infants who are otherwise healthy. These are called primary apnoeas, can be attributed to prematurity and are a diagnosis of exclusion. There are many conditions that cause or accentuate apnoea (Table 27.13). It is therefore essential to investigate infants appropriately, with a high index of clinical suspicion, when apnoeas suddenly appear in a previously well baby.

Periodic breathing, sleep state and diaphragmatic fatigue

Periodic breathing can be defined as bursts of respiratory activity of 20 seconds or less, separated by central apnoeic pauses lasting from 3 to 10 seconds.[32] Periodic breathing is present in almost all preterm babies, but is relatively uncommon in term babies.[31] The aetiology of periodic breathing remains obscure, although the finding that it is absent until 48 hours of age suggests that inactivity of peripheral chemoreceptors at this time might play a role.[6] There is disagreement as to whether periodic breathing is a benign or harmful phenomenon. Desaturation during periodic breathing has been reported,[79,80] although whether this is of long-term significance is unclear. Previous research suggested that periodic breathing was not linked to prolonged apnoea in preterm babies.[6] Recent studies have contradicted this finding and have proposed a causal link between periodic breathing and prolonged apnoea.[2,80] In both term and preterm babies, periodic breathing and apnoeas are more common in rapid eye movement (REM) sleep than in non-REM sleep.[88] It has been suggested that the reason for this may be chest wall distortion stimulating the costophrenic inhibitory reflex,[49] despite this distortion being

Table 27.13 Conditions exacerbating or causing apnoea in the neonatal period

Hypoxia
Central nervous system
   Primary apnoea of prematurity
   Intracranial haemorrhage
   Seizures
   Drugs
      Sedatives, narcotics
      Post anaesthesia
      Prostaglandin E_2

Sepsis
   Necrotising enterocolitis
   Meningitis
   Bronchiolitis

Metabolic abnormalities
   Hypoglycaemia
   Hyponatraemia
   Hypocalcaemia
   Inborn errors of metabolism

Environmental
   Hyperthermia
   Hypothermia

Upper airway obstruction
   Choanal atresia
   Micrognathia (Pierre Robin sequence)
   Macroglossia
   Hypotonia of Down syndrome

Circulatory
   Patent ductus arteriosus
   Heart failure
   Anaemia

Vasovagal reflex
   Siting of nasogastric tube
   Upper airway suctioning

Immunisation

present both in REM and non-REM sleep.[20] An alternative mechanism has been suggested in a study demonstrating that arterial oxygen levels were significantly lower in REM compared with quiet sleep.[62] Chest wall distortion might also have a role in the aetiology of apnoea by increasing the work of breathing and causing diaphragmatic fatigue.[37] This is supported by the finding that EMG studies of the diaphragm demonstrated fatigue in preterm infants having apnoeas.[59]

Hypoxia

As discussed previously, hypoxia tends to lead to respiratory depression in very immature babies. It therefore follows that any condition causing respiratory or neurological problems that lead to hypoxia can cause or accentuate apnoea in these babies. It has been demonstrated that preterm babies, with increasing levels of inspired oxygen, have decreasing apnoea frequency.[108]

Infection

Apnoea is more likely to occur in an infected baby. The mechanism by which infection causes apnoea is unclear, although there might be resetting of the afferent inputs to the respiratory centre. This would especially be the case in infections involving the lung parenchyma, with afferent input from lung mechanoreceptors being altered. Apnoeas are common in babies who are developing necrotising enterocolitis. As well as abdominal distension splinting the chest wall, inflammatory mediators might have an effect on vagal afferent input.[63] Preterm infants infected with respiratory syncytial virus (RSV) are particularly prone to develop apnoea.[16] In support of inflammatory mediators having a role in the aetiology of apnoea, interleukin-1β levels in pharyngeal secretions of RSV-infected infants have been demonstrated to correlate with apnoea.[57]

Central nervous system disorders

Trauma, germinal matrix/intraventricular haemorrhage (GMH-IVH) and meningitis are all associated with apnoea. Apnoea can also be a result of seizure activity.[107] Apnoea can be associated with the Arnold–Chiari malformation. The rare condition of congenital central alveolar hypoventilation syndrome (Ondine's curse) is thought to be due to an abnormality of the neural crest cells involved in respiration. Babies with this condition have absent ventilation sensitivity to hypoxia and hypercarbia even when they are awake. Their breathing pattern is normal when they are awake, but they become cyanosed when asleep. Prolonged respiratory support is required.

Environmental temperature

Preterm infants respond to an increase in environmental temperature beyond the thermoneutral range with a rise in apnoea frequency and periodic respiration.[71] The mechanism for this is unclear.

Gastro-oesophageal reflux

Upper airway chemoreceptors may have a role in the development of apnoea. Instillation of saline into the airway of a sleeping infant induces apnoea, swallowing and arousal.[95] These responses could be relevant when considering the role of gastro-oesophageal reflux (GOR) as a cause of apnoea. The association between GOR and apnoea of prematurity has been difficult to prove and recent studies have failed to demonstrate a temporal relationship between episodes of reflux and apnoea.[72] In support of this finding, treatment of GOR has not been shown to reduce the frequency of apnoea of prematurity.[48]

Apnoea and bottle feeding

Some infants, especially those with chronic lung disease, become hypoxaemic during and after bottle feeds.[81] It has not been possible to demonstrate an increased frequency of apnoea when comparing bottle, milk boluses via nasogastric tube, and continuous tube feeds.[74]

Anaemia

If low levels of haemoglobin predispose infants to apnoea, blood transfusion should reduce the incidence of apnoea. A reduction in the incidence of apnoea following transfusion has been reported.[47] Other groups have not seen this response,[109] and doubt remains regarding the efficacy of using transfusions to treat symptomatic apnoea.

Anaesthesia

Following a general anaesthetic, preterm infants are at risk of developing apnoea.[52] This problem worsens in preterm infants of increasing immaturity.[17] As a result, postoperative monitoring in a high-dependency cot is essential for all preterm babies who are recovering from surgery, until they are at least a month post-term equivalent postnatal age.

Patent ductus arteriosus

Infants who develop pulmonary oedema as a consequence of a patent ductus arteriosus are at risk of apnoea. Stimulation of pulmonary C fibres occurs in response to pulmonary oedema,[85] possibly leading to apnoea in a vagally mediated response.

Immunisation

Apnoea in preterm infants following immunisation with DPT has been reported.[83] For this reason, infants receiving immunisations on neonatal units need to be carefully monitored in the period following administration of vaccines.

Drugs

Analgesics such as morphine can depress neonatal respiration.

Bradycardia

As with apnoea, varying definitions of bradycardia in the preterm infant have been used by investigators. A fall in heart rate to less than 100 beats per minute in a preterm infant for over 5 seconds is generally considered to constitute a bradycardia.[23]

Alternatively, a fall in heart rate of more than 30% below baseline has been used as the criteria for bradycardia.[39,76] Whatever method of calculating a bradycardia is employed, a crucial factor to take into consideration is whether or not a bradycardia is clinically significant. Brief falls in heart rate unaccompanied by apnoea or desaturation are unlikely to be of importance. Bradycardias are more common in apnoeas of longer duration.[39]

A series of complex physiological interactions leads to the scenario of apnoea, bradycardia and desaturation.[61] In the majority of cases, there is an apnoea or period of hypoventilation closely followed by a fall in oxygen saturation and then bradycardia.[1] Initially it was thought that this bradycardia was the direct result of myocardial hypoxia. It is now clear that the bradycardia occurs too early in apnoea to be due to this effect.[104] The evidence therefore supports the concept that the bradycardia following apnoea and desaturation is a reflex response. Analysis of the sequence of events leading to bradycardia in preterm infants has demonstrated that almost all the bradycardias commence after the onset of apnoea and after the onset of the fall in oxygen saturation.[76] This would support the theory that the bradycardia occurs via the carotid chemoreceptors. It appears that the combination of apnoea and hypoxaemia has a synergistic effect on the stimulation of arterial chemoreceptors in causing bradycardia[4] rather than hypoxaemia per se. Upper airway closure may also have a role in the development of the bradycardia, perhaps due to the lack of stimulation of a pulmonary inflation reflex.[102] This has been shown by the heart rate not recovering in mixed apnoea until airflow had been restored.[39] A different scenario exists whereby bradycardia occurs simultaneously with apnoea. This presumably represents a vagally mediated, rather than hypoxic, response. It has been proposed that enhanced vagal tone might have a role in predisposing preterm infants to apnoeas and bradycardias.[63] The diving reflex could be the reflex pathway for this type of bradycardia.[18] This reflex can be initiated by immersing the face in ice-cold water, which causes stimulation of the trigeminal nerve[87] and results in apnoea, bradycardia and peripheral vasoconstriction. This dramatic reflex can be harnessed clinically to terminate episodes of supraventricular tachycardia (pp. 652–4). Support for this was provided by Storrs,[94] who used venous occlusion plethysmography to demonstrate that peripheral blood flow was diverted to central organs during bradycardia. This has been contradicted by studies showing a reduction in cerebral blood flow during bradycardia.[70]

Monitoring

Monitoring is essential in babies who have conditions that predispose them to having apnoea. This includes all infants of less than 35 weeks of gestation and those more mature infants with other serious illnesses. There is some controversy as to the type of monitoring that is most appropriate in such babies. Based on the current evidence, we use a combination of a pressure-sensitive apnoea mattress, heart rate monitoring and oxygen saturation monitoring in our special-care nursery.

Cardiorespiratory monitoring (Chapter 19)

Due to the close association between bradycardia and apnoea, all babies who are at risk of apnoea should have monitoring of heart rate as well as respiratory effort. This can be achieved using standard ECG monitors using three electrodes, two of which can be in common with impedance equipment. There can be problems with false alarms due to either detachment of one of the electrodes or body movement. The heart rate signal from a pulse oximeter is even more prone to false alarms.

There are several devices available that monitor the movement of the chest or abdominal wall. Techniques for assessing chest wall movement include: air-filled apnoea mattresses,[56] pressure-sensitive devices which lie under the infant,[89] pressure-sensitive capsules attached to the abdominal wall,[103] and sensors that detect changes in abdominal circumference (impedance monitor and respiratory inductance plethysmography [RIP]). The first three types of devices are bedevilled by problems with false positive alarms, which increase the stress placed on nursing staff and parents. Also, none are able to discriminate between obstructive/mixed apnoea and central apnoea. For this to be possible, a means of measuring nasal airflow, such as a nasal thermistor[22] or an end-tidal CO_2 monitor, need to be used. Impedance monitoring involves measuring the current that passes between two low-voltage electrodes placed on opposite sides of the chest. As the infant inspires, there is an increase in the air/tissue ration and the voltage falls. This system does have the disadvantage of picking up changes in cardiac output during an apnoea and preventing the triggering of the alarm.[91] RIP consists of lightweight bands placed around the chest and the abdomen. Within the bands are coils of copper wire that act as a one-turn transducer. As the cross-sectional area of the chest and abdomen vary with respiration, so does the inductance of the bands. These variations can then be displayed. Paradoxical movements of the chest and abdomen, where the chest and abdomen move out of phase, can be used to accurately diagnose obstructive apnoea. Transthoracic impedance measurements cannot be used for this purpose.[12]

Oxygenation

Babies who are receiving oxygen treatment must have the concentration measured, and their response to oxygen treatment must be assessed (pp. 357–9). This may be achieved using either direct blood gas estimations (pp. 479, 480–1), transcutaneous (tc) oxygen measurements (pp. 357–8) or pulse oximetry (p. 358). Pulse oximeters are easy to site, although care has to be taken not to attach the device too tightly. There is a faster response time than with $tcPO_2$ measurements, with the oximeter signal averaged over 3 to 5 seconds.[34] The monitors are susceptible to both movement artefact and poor cardiac output, which can lead to false alarms. Pulse oximetry is of additional value as preterm infants can have episodes of profound desaturation in the absence of apnoea or bradycardia.[75] In our view, a pulse oximeter is probably the most helpful single device to use when monitoring for apnoea on the neonatal unit. A combination of a cardiorespiratory monitor and pulse oximeter should be used in infants who are having symptomatic apnoeas.[98]

Investigation of apnoea

Investigating a preterm baby who is developing apnoea depends to a great extent on the overall clinical picture. Most apnoea in preterm babies will be related to immaturity and be primary apnoea. This is, however, a diagnosis of exclusion and apnoea can herald the onset of serious disease. Therefore, the following investigations should be considered: infection screen (including lumbar puncture and urinalysis), serum glucose, serum calcium, haemoglobin, chest X-ray, cranial ultrasound scan, arterial blood gas and viral screen (especially RSV). If the apnoeas remain resistant despite treatment, the presence of a convulsive disorder should be considered and an EEG obtained.

Treatment of apnoea of prematurity

Once a preterm baby has been investigated and appropriately treated for conditions aggravating apnoea, other therapies to decrease the frequency of apnoea need to be initiated.

Treatment of individual episodes of apnoea

Most babies respond to conservative treatment of an apnoea. Once an apnoea or bradycardic episode has been detected, usually by a monitor alarming, the baby needs to be assessed urgently. Many of these episodes are self-limiting and no action needs to be taken. If the baby is still apnoeic or bradycardic when examined, a gentle stimulus such as flicking the foot may be sufficient to restore breathing. If it is suspected that the baby might have aspirated a feed, the head should be gently extended and gentle suctioning of the upper airway should be attempted. If, despite these interventions, the baby remains apnoeic or the heart rate is not restored, the baby should be ventilated using either a bag and mask or a mask and T-piece using the baby's usual F_IO_2. This resuscitation should never be done using 100% oxygen, due to the risk of retinopathy of prematurity (ROP) with hyperoxaemia. Careful monitoring of the baby's oxygen saturations should be maintained throughout. Occasionally, intubation is required despite these manoeuvres.

Pharmacotherapy

Methylxanthines (caffeine and aminophylline/theophylline) form the mainstay of the treatment of apnoea of prematurity. The exact mechanism by which these drugs exert their effect is not known. It is thought that their respiratory stimulant effect might partly be due to phosphodiesterase inhibition.[44] Methylxanthines also increase the strength of diaphragmatic contractility.[5] In babies who are not being fed, a loading dose of intravenous aminophylline

followed by maintenance can be administered. Theophylline can be used in babies receiving oral fluids. Due to the variability of the half-life of theophylline, the narrow therapeutic window and the potential toxic side effects of theophylline in preterm infants, blood levels need to be monitored closely. Theophylline is methylated to form caffeine in preterm babies and it may be necessary to monitor levels of both methylxanthines in order to assess the total drug load.[11] The most commonly encountered side effect of theophylline is tachycardia. Less frequent side effects include seizures, abdominal distension, vomiting, diarrhoea, jitteriness and worsening of GOR. There have not been large-scale, randomised controlled trials (RCTs) investigating the efficacy of theophylline in the treatment of apnoea of prematurity. The only double-blind, RCT was carried out in 31 babies experiencing symptomatic apnoea and demonstrated that there was a significant short-term reduction in apnoea in infants treated with theophylline compared with placebo.[69] Aminophylline, when given prophylatically to ventilated preterm babies, has been shown to reduce the frequency of apnoea.[7] Many units are now using caffeine as their first-line therapy instead of theophylline. This is partly due to caffeine having a wider therapeutic range with fewer toxic side effects, although significant tachycardia can still be a problem. Routine blood levels are not required, providing the infant shows a satisfactory response to treatment. In a recent double-blind RCT, caffeine treatment was associated with a significant reduction in apnoeas in preterm infants experiencing symptomatic apnoea.[25] Prophylactic treatment of asymptomatic preterm infants with caffeine, however, does not reduce the incidence of apnoea.[41] In summary, although caffeine treatment of apnoea has a similar clinical response rate to theophylline, there are certain therapeutic advantages to using caffeine.[84,93]

Doxapram, which acts as a non-specific stimulant of the CNS, has been used as a second-line treatment in preterm babies who failed to respond to aminophylline.[8] Side effects include abdominal distension, irritability, jitteriness, vomiting, increased blood pressure, and feed intolerance. There is no evidence to support its use as a first-line agent in the treatment of apnoea of prematurity above methylxanthines in current-day practice.[42]

Ventilation

If, despite treatment with methylxanthines, an infant continues to have frequent apnoeas, continuous positive airways pressure (CPAP) needs to be considered. CPAP reduces the incidence of apnoea by around 50%.[92] The effect of CPAP is selective – it reduces the incidence of mixed or obstructive apnoea but has no effect on central apnoeas.[64] It is possible that CPAP exerts its effect through mechanically splinting the upper airway.[65] On direct visualisation of the upper airway, CPAP has been demonstrated to significantly dilate the laryngeal opening.[28] Nasal intermittent positive pressure ventilation shows promise as a treatment of apnoea of prematurity.[55] Occasionally, apnoeas are resistant to treatment and the infant has to be intubated and ventilated. In these infants, the lowest possible oxygen concentration and ventilatory pressures need to be used, as they are often relatively easy to ventilate.

Other therapeutic options

A variety of kinaesthetic stimulations to prevent apnoeas in preterm infants have been employed. These range from rocking beds to oscillating mattresses. There is little evidence that these methods are of any therapeutic value.[67] Other measures, such as changing the position from supine to prone,[36,51] altering environmental temperature[71] and correcting hypoxia,[108] can decrease the incidence of apnoea.

Stopping treatment, predischarge monitoring and discharge home

Babies who have had apnoeas treated with methylxanthines tend to have had treatment discontinued by 35 weeks' postconceptional age (PCA).[24] Despite this, significant apnoeas can persist up to 43 weeks' PCA.[24,78] Most neonatalogists agree that after stopping methylxanthines, babies who have experienced problematic apnoea of prematurity should have an event-free period of 5–7 days before discharge from the neonatal unit.[19] On the neonatal unit, preterm babies are usually nursed in the prone position to improve oxygenation and reduce apnoea frequency.[36] Due to the increased risk of sudden infant death syndrome (SIDS) in the prone position, babies should spend a period of a week or more in the supine position prior to discharge, unless there are other factors that preclude this being done.[9]

Home monitoring

Preterm infants are at an increased risk of SIDS.[68] It has been recommended that preterm infants who are experiencing symptomatic apnoeas should be discharged on home cardiorespiratory monitors,[58] although there is no evidence that those who have had troublesome apnoea on the neonatal unit are at additional risk of SIDS. Most home cardiorespiratory monitors are unable to detect episodes of obstructive apnoea, due to their reliance on transthoracic impedance measurements. Obstructive apnoeas were the most commonly observed event detected in a recent series investigating the role of home monitoring in preterm infants.[78] However, even these apnoeas did not seem to be precursors to SIDS. At present, therefore, there seems little justification for using home monitoring in preterm infants.

Advice regarding SIDS and acute life-threatening events

Prospective cardiorespiratory monitoring carried out on preterm infants did not identify prolonged apnoea as a risk factor for SIDS.[90] Despite this, prior to discharge of their baby from the neonatal unit, parents need to be advised of the measures that can be taken to reduce the risk of SIDS. These include sleeping in the supine position, avoiding hyperthermia, stopping smoking[68] and not co-sleeping.[10] Following discharge, a baby can occasionally experience an acute life-threatening event (ALTE). An ALTE is said to have occurred when a baby has been found apnoeic, with a change in colour (cyanosis or pallor) and tone (limpness or stiffness), and has required mouth-to-mouth resuscitation or vigorous stimulation. Ex-preterm babies are at increased risk of experiencing an ALTE.[78] For this reason, parents need to be taught basic infant life support prior to their baby being discharged.

Prognosis

It has been difficult to prove that apnoeic episodes have a deleterious effect on neurological development. This is due to the presence of many confounding variables that might affect neurological outcome following intensive care on a neonatal unit. Some studies have found that apnoeas have an adverse effect on neurological development,[13,15,46] whilst others have not been able to demonstrate this association.[50,97] A higher incidence of ROP has been reported in preterm infants who have had troublesome apnoea.[77] The National Institutes of Health Consensus Development Conference on Infantile Apnea in 1986[58] concluded that there was no evidence that primary apnoea of prematurity was associated with problems in long-term development. There have, however, been concerns raised about the long-term safety of methylxanthine usage.[86] Some of the evidence is contradictory, with both the incidence of cerebral palsy and IQ scoring being higher at 14 years of age in children who had received theophylline treatment as a preterm infant.[21]

References

1. Adams J A, Zabaleta I A, Sackner M A 1997 Hypoxemic events in spontaneously breathing premature infants: etiologic basis. Pediatric Research 42: 463–471
2. Al-Saedi S A, Lemke R P, Haider A Z, Cates D B, Kwiatkowski K, Rigatto H 1997 Prolonged apnea in the preterm infant is not a random event. American Journal of Perinatology 14: 195–200
3. American Academy of Pediatrics Taskforce on Prolonged Apnea 1978 Prolonged apnea. Pediatrics 61: 651–652
4. Angell-James J E, Daly M de B 1969 Cardiovascular responses in pnoeic asphyxia: role of arterial chemoreceptors and the modification of their effects by a pulmonary vagal inflation reflex. Journal of Physiology 201: 87–104
5. Aubier M, De Troyer A, Sampson M, Macklem P T, Roussos C 1981 Aminophylline improves diaphragmatic contractility. New England Journal of Medicine 305: 249–252
6. Barrington K J, Finer N N 1990 Periodic breathing and apnea in preterm infants. Pediatric Research 27: 118–121
7. Barrington K J, Finer N N 1993 A randomized, controlled trial of aminophylline in ventilatory weaning of premature infants. Critical Care Medicine 21: 846–850
8. Barrington K J, Finer N N, Peters K L, Barton J 1986 Physiologic effects of doxapram in idiopathic apnea of prematurity. Journal of Pediatrics 108: 124–129
9. Bhat R Y, Leipala J A, Rafferty G F, Hannam S, Greenough A 2003 Survey of sleeping position recommendations for prematurely born infants on neonatal intensive care unit discharge. European Journal of Pediatrics 162: 426–427

10. Blair P S, Fleming P J, Smith I J et al 1999 Babies sleeping with parents: case-control study of factors influencing the risk of the sudden infant death syndrome. CESDI SUDI Research Group. British Medical Journal 319: 1457–1461

11. Bory C, Baltassat P, Porthault M, Bethenod M, Frederich A, Aranda J V 1979 Metabolism of theophylline to caffeine in premature newborn infants. Journal of Pediatrics 94: 988–993

12. Brouillette R T, Morrow A S, Weese-Mayer D E, Hunt C E 1987 Comparison of respiratory inductive plethysmography and thoracic impedance for apnea monitoring. Journal of Pediatrics 111: 377–383

13. Butcher-Puech M C, Henderson-Smart D J, Holley D, Lacey J L, Edwards D A 1985 Relation between apnoea duration and type and neurological status of preterm infants. Archives of Disease in Childhood 60: 953–958

14. Carlo W A, Martin R J, Bruce E N, Strohl K P, Fanaroff A A 1983 Alae nasi activation (nasal flaring) decreases nasal resistance in preterm infants. Pediatrics 72: 338–343

15. Cheung P Y, Barrington K J, Finer N N, Robertson C M 1999 Early childhood neurodevelopment in very low birth weight infants with predischarge apnea. Pediatric Pulmonology 27: 14–20

16. Church N R, Anas N G, Hall C B, Brooks J G 1984 Respiratory syncytial virus-related apnea in infants. Demographics and outcome. American Journal of Diseases of Children 138: 247–250

17. Cote C J, Zaslavsky A, Downes J J et al 1995 Postoperative apnea in former preterm infants after inguinal herniorrhaphy. A combined analysis. Anesthesiology 82 :809–822

18. Daly M D B 1986 Handbook of physiology: the respiratory system, vol. II. American Physiological Society, Bethesda, pp. 529–579

19. Darnall R A, Kattwinkel J, Nattie C, Robinson M 1997 Margin of safety for discharge after apnea in preterm infants. Pediatrics 100: 795–801

20. Davi M, Sankaran K, Maccallum M, Cates D, Rigatto H 1979 Effect of sleep state on chest distortion and on the ventilatory response to CO_2 in neonates. Pediatric Research 13: 982–986

21. Davis P G, Doyle L W, Rickards A L et al 2000 Methylxanthines and senso-rineural outcome at 14 years in children <1501 g birthweight. Journal of Paediatrics and Child Health 36: 47–50

22. Dransfield D A, Fox W W 1980 A noninvasive method for recording central and obstructive apnea with bradycardia in infants. Critical Care Medicine 8: 663–666

23. Dransfield D A, Spitzer A R, Fox W W 1983 Episodic airway obstruction in premature infants. American Journal of Diseases of Children 137: 441–443

24. Eichenwald E C, Aina A, Stark A R 1997 Apnea frequently persists beyond term gestation in infants delivered at 24 to 28 weeks. Pediatrics 100: 354–359

25. Erenberg A, Leff R D, Haack D G, Mosdell K W, Hicks G M, Wynne B A 2000 Caffeine citrate for the treatment of apnea of prematurity: a double-blind, placebo-controlled study. Pharmacotherapy 20: 644–652

26. Finer N N, Barrington K J, Hayes B J, Hugh A 1992 Obstructive, mixed, and central apnea in the neonate: physiologic correlates. Journal of Pediatrics 121: 943–950

27. Fleming P J, Bryan A C, Bryan M H 1978 Functional immaturity of pulmonary irritant receptors and apnea in newborn preterm infants. Pediatrics 61: 515–518

28. Gaon P, Lee S, Hannam S, Ingram D, Milner A D 1999 Assessment of effect of nasal continuous positive pressure on laryngeal opening using fibre optic laryngoscopy. Archives of Disease in Childhood. Fetal and Neonatal Edition 80: F230–F232

29. Gerhardt T, Bancalari E 1984 Apnea of prematurity: I. Lung function and regulation of breathing. Pediatrics 74: 58–62

30. Gerhardt T, Bancalari E 1984 Apnea of prematurity: II. Respiratory reflexes. Pediatrics 74: 63–66

31. Glotzbach S F, Ariagno R L 1992 Periodic breathing. In: Beckerman R C, Broillette R T, Hunt C E (eds) Respiratory control disorders in infants and children. Lippincott Williams & Wilkins, Baltimore, pp. 142–160

32. Glotzbach S F, Tansey P A, Baldwin R B, Ariagno R L 1989 Periodic breathing cycle duration in preterm infants. Pediatric Research 25: 258–261

33. Hannam S, Ingram D M, Milner A D 1998 A possible role for the Hering-Breuer deflation reflex in apnea of prematurity. Journal of Pediatrics 132: 35–39

34. Hay W W, Brockway J M, Eyzaguirre M 1989 Neonatal pulse oximetry: accuracy and reliability. Pediatrics 83: 717–722

35. Heeringa J, Berkenbosch A, de Goede J, Olievier C N 1979 Relative contribution of central and peripheral chemoreceptors to the ventilatory response to CO_2 during hyperoxia. Respiration Physiology 37: 365–379

36. Heimler R, Langlois J, Hodel D J, Nelin L D, Sasidharan P 1992 Effect of positioning on the breathing pattern of preterm infants. Archives of Disease in Childhood 67: 312–314

37. Heldt G P 1988 Development of stability of the respiratory system in preterm infants. Journal of Applied Physiology 65: 441–444

38. Henderson-Smart D J 1981 The effect of gestational age on the incidence and duration of recurrent apnoea in newborn babies. Australian Paediatrics Journal 17: 273–276

39. Henderson-Smart D J, Butcher-Puech M C, Edwards D A 1986 Incidence and mechanism of bradycardia during apnoea in preterm infants. Archives of Disease in Childhood 61: 227–232

40. Henderson-Smart D J, Pettigrew A G, Campbell D J 1983 Clinical apnea and brain-stem neural function in preterm infants. New England Journal of Medicine 308: 353–357

41. Henderson-Smart D J, Steer P A 2002 Prophylactic methylxanthine for prevention of apnea in preterm infants (Cochrane Review). In: The Cochrane Library, Issue 4. Update Software, Oxford

42. Henderson-Smart D J, Steer P 2002 Doxapram versus methylxanthine for apnea in preterm infants (Cochrane Review). In: The Cochrane Library, Issue 4. Update Software, Oxford

43. Hodgman J E, Gonzalez F, Hoppenbrouwers T, Cabal L A 1990 Apnea, transient episodes of bradycardia, and periodic breathing in preterm infants. American Journal of Diseases of Children 144: 54–57

44. Howell L L 1993 Comparative effects of caffeine and selective phosphodiesterase inhibitors on respiration and behavior in rhesus monkeys. Journal of Pharmacology and Experimental Therapeutics 266: 894–903

45. Idiong N, Lemke R P, Lin Y J, Kwiatkowski K, Cates D B, Rigatto H 1998 Airway closure during mixed apneas in preterm infants: is respiratory effort necessary? Journal of Pediatrics 133: 509–512

46. Jones R A, Lukeman D 1982 Apnoea of immaturity. 2. Mortality and handicap. Archives of Disease in Childhood 57: 766–768

47. Joshi A, Gerhardt T, Shandloff P, Bancalari E 1987 Blood transfusion effect on the respiratory pattern of preterm infants. Pediatrics 80: 79–84

48. Kimball A L, Carlton D P 2001 Gastroesophageal reflux medications in the treatment of apnea in premature infants. Journal of Pediatrics 138: 355–360

49. Knill R, Bryan A C 1976 An intercostal-phrenic inhibitory reflex in human newborn infants. Journal of Applied Physiology 40: 352–356

50. Koons A H, Mojica N, Jadeja N, Ostfeld B, Hiatt M, Hegyi T 1993 Neuro-developmental outcome of infants with apnea of infancy. American Journal of Perinatology 10: 208–211

51. Kurlak L O, Ruggins N R, Stephenson T J 1994 Effect of nursing position on incidence, type, and duration of clinically significant apnoea in preterm infants. Archives of Disease in Childhood. Fetal and Neonatal Edition 71: F16–F19

52. Kurth C D, Spitzer A R, Broennle A M, Downes J J 1987 Postoperative apnea in preterm infants. Anesthesiology 66: 483–488

53. Lemke R P, Al-Saedi S A, Alvaro R E et al 1996 Use of a magnified cardiac airflow oscillation to classify neonatal apnea. American Journal of Respiratory and Critical Care Medicine 154: 1537–1542

54. Lemke R P, Idiong N, Al-Saedi S, Kwiatkowski K, Cates D B, Rigatto H 1998 Evidence of a critical period of airway instability during central apneas in preterm infants. American Journal of Respiratory and Critical Care Medicine 157: 470–474

55. Lemyre B, Davis P G, de Paoli A G 2002 Nasal intermittent positive pressure ventilation (NIPPV) versus nasal continuous positive airway pressure (NCPAP) for apnea of prematurity (Cochrane Review). In: The Cochrane Library, Issue 4. Update Software, Oxford

56. Lewin J E 1969 An apnoea-alarm mattress. Lancet 2: 667–668

57. Lindgren C, Grogaard J 1996 Reflex apnoea response and inflammatory mediators in infants with respiratory tract infection. Acta Paediatrica 85: 798–803

58. Little G A, Ballard R A, Brooks J R et al 1987 National Institutes of Health Consensus Development Conference on Infantile Apnea and Home Monitoring, Sept 29 to Oct 1, 1986. Pediatrics 79: 292–299

59. Lopes J M, Muller N L, Bryan M H, Bryan A C 1981 Synergistic behavior of inspiratory muscles after diaphragmatic fatigue in the newborn. Journal of Applied Physiology 51: 547–551

60. Martin R J, DiFiore J M, Jana L et al 1998 Persistence of the biphasic ventilatory response to hypoxia in preterm infants. Journal of Pediatrics 132: 960–964

61. Martin R J, Fanaroff A A 1998 Neonatal apnea, bradycardia, or desaturation: does it matter? Journal of Pediatrics 132: 758–759

62. Martin R J, Okken A, Rubin D 1979 Arterial oxygen tension during active and quiet sleep in the normal neonate. Journal of Pediatrics 94: 271–274

63. Mathew O P 2003 Apnea, bradycardia and desaturation. In: Mathew O P (ed) Respiratory control and disorders in the newborn. Marcel Dekker, New York, pp. 273–293

64. Miller M J, Carlo W A, Martin R J 1985 Continuous positive airway pressure selectively reduces obstructive apnea in preterm infants. Journal of Pediatrics 106: 91–94

65. Miller M J, DiFiore J M, Strohl K P, Martin R J 1990 Effects of nasal CPAP on supraglottic and total pulmonary resistance in preterm infants. Journal of Applied Physiology 68: 141–146

66. Milner A D, Boon A W, Saunders R A, Hopkin I E 1980 Upper airway obstruction and apnoea in preterm babies. Archives of Disease in Childhood 55: 22–25

67. Osborn D A, Henderson-Smart D J 2002 Kinesthetic stimulation for treating apnea in preterm infants (Cochrane Review). In: The Cochrane Library, Issue 4. Update Software, Oxford

68. Oyen N, Markestad T, Skaerven R et al 1997 Combined effects of sleeping position and prenatal risk factors in sudden infant death syndrome: the Nordic Epidemiological SIDS Study. Pediatrics 100: 613–621

69. Peliowski A, Finer N N 1990 A blinded, randomized, placebo-controlled trial to compare theophylline and doxapram for the treatment of apnea of prematurity. Journal of Pediatrics 116: 648–653

70. Perlman J M, Volpe J J 1985 Episodes of apnea and bradycardia in the preterm newborn: impact on cerebral circulation. Pediatrics 76: 333–338

71. Perlstein P H, Edwards N K, Sutherland J M 1970 Apnea in premature infants and incubator-air-temperature changes. New England Journal of Medicine 282: 461–466

72. Peter C S, Sprodowski N, Bohnhorst B, Silny J, Poets C F 2002 Gastroesophageal reflux and apnea of prematurity: no temporal relationship. Pediatrics 109: 8–11

73. Poets C F 2003 Pathophysiology of apnea of prematurity. In: Mathew O P (ed) Respiratory control and disorders in the newborn. Marcel Dekker, New York, pp. 295–316

74. Poets C F, Langner M U, Bohnhorst B 1997 Effects of bottle feeding and two different methods of gavage feeding on oxygenation and breathing patterns in preterm infants. Acta Paediatrica 86: 419–423

75. Poets C F, Stebbens V A, Richard D, Southall D P 1995 Prolonged episodes of hypoxemia in preterm infants undetected by cardiorespiratory monitors. Pediatrics 95: 860–863

76. Poets C F, Stebbens V A, Samuels M P, Southall D P 1993 The relationship between bradycardia, apnea, and hypoxemia in preterm infants. Pediatric Research 34: 144–147

77. Purohit D M, Ellison R C, Zierler S, Miettinen O S, Nadas A S 1985 Risk factors for retrolental fibroplasia: experience with 3,025 premature infants. National Collaborative Study on Patent Ductus Arteriosus in Premature Infants. Pediatrics 76: 339–344

78. Ramanathan R, Corwin M J, Hunt C E et al for the Collaborative Home Infant Monitoring Evaluation (CHIME) Study Group 2001 Cardiorespiratory events recorded on home monitors: comparison of healthy infants with those at increased risk for SIDS. Journal of the American Medical Association 285: 2199–2207

79. Razi N M, Delauter M, Pandit PB 2002 Periodic breathing and oxygen saturation in preterm infants at discharge. Journal of Perinatology 22:442–444

80. Rigatto H 2003 Periodic breathing. In: Mathew O P (ed) Respiratory control and disorders in the newborn. Marcel Dekker, New York, pp. 237–272

81. Rosen C L, Glaze D G, Frost J D 1984 Hypoxemia associated with feeding in the preterm infant and full-term neonate. American Journal of Diseases of Children 138: 623–628

82. Ruggins N R, Milner A D 1991 Site of upper airway obstruction in preterm infants with problematical apnoea. Archives of Disease in Childhood 66: 787–792

83. Sanchez P J, Laptook A R, Fisher L, Sumner J, Risser R C, Perlman J M 1997 Apnea after immunization of preterm infants. Journal of Pediatrics 130: 746–751

84. Scanlon J E, Chin K C, Morgan M E, Durbin G M, Hale K A, Brown S S 1992 Caffeine or theophylline for neonatal apnoea? Archives of Disease in Childhood 67: 425–428

85. Schertel E R, Adams L, Schneider D A, Smith K S, Green J F 1986 Rapid shallow breathing evoked by capsaicin from isolated pulmonary circulation. Journal of Applied Physiology 61: 1237–1240

86. Schmidt B 1999 Methylxanthine therapy in premature infants: sound practice, disaster, or fruitless byway? Journal of Pediatrics 135: 526–528

87. Scholander P F 1963 The master switch of life. Scientific American 209: 92–106

88. Schulte F J, Busse C, Eichhorn W 1977 Rapid eye movement sleep, motoneurone inhibition, and apneic spells in preterm infants. Pediatric Research 11: 709–713

89. Smith J E, Scopes J W 1972 A new apnoea alarm for babies. Lancet 2: 545–546

90. Southall D P, Richards J M, de Swiet M et al for the Multicentre Prospective Study into the Sudden Infant Death Syndrome 1983 Identification of infants destined to die unexpectedly during infancy: evaluation of predictive importance of prolonged apnoea and disorders of cardiac rhythm or conduction. British Medical Journal (Clinical Research Ed.) 286:1092–1096

91. Southall D P, Richards J M, Lau K C, Shinebourne E A 1980 An explanation for failure of impedance apnoea alarm systems. Archives of Disease in Childhood 55: 63–65

92. Speidel B D, Dunn P M 1976 Use of nasal continuous positive airway pressure to treat severe recurrent apnoea in very preterm infants. Lancet 2: 658–660

93. Steer P A, Henderson-Smart D J 2002 Caffeine versus theophylline for apnea in preterm infants (Cochrane Review). In: The Cochrane Library, Issue 4. Update Software, Oxford

94. Storrs C N 1977 Cardiovascular effects of apnoea in preterm infants. Archives of Disease in Childhood 52: 534–540

95. Thach B T 1992 Neuromuscular control of the upper airway. In: Beckerman R C, Broillette R T, Hunt C E (eds) Respiratory control disorders in infants and children. Lippincott Williams & Wilkins, Baltimore, pp. 47–61

96. Thach B T, Stark A R 1979 Spontaneous neck flexion and airway obstruction during apneic spells in preterm infants. Journal of Pediatrics 94: 275–281

97. Tudehope D I, Rogers Y M, Burns Y R, Mohay H, O'Callaghan M J 1986 Apnoea in very low birthweight infants: outcome at 2 years. Australian Paediatrics Journal 22: 131–134

98. Upton C J, Milner A D, Stokes G M 1991 Apnoea, bradycardia, and oxygen saturation in preterm infants. Archives of Disease in Childhood 66: 381–385

99. Upton C J, Milner A D, Stokes G M 1992 Upper airway patency during apnoea of prematurity. Archives of Disease in Childhood 67: 419–424

100. Upton C J, Milner A D, Stokes G M 1992 Response to tube breathing in preterm infants with apnea. Pediatric Pulmonology 12: 23–28

101. Upton C J, Milner A D, Stokes G M 1992 Response to external obstruction in preterm infants with apnea. Pediatric Pulmonology 14: 233–238

102. Upton C J, Milner A D, Stokes G M 1992 Episodic bradycardia in preterm infants. Archives of Disease in Childhood 67: 831–834

103. Valman H B, Wright B M, Lawrence C 1983 Measurement of respiratory rate in the newborn. British Medical Journal (Clinical Research Ed.) 4;286: 1783–1784

104. Vyas H, Milner A D, Hopkin I E 1981 Relationship between apnoea and bradycardia in preterm infants. Acta Paediatrica Scandinavica 70: 785–790

105. Waggener T B, Frantz I D, Cohlan B A, Stark A R 1989 Mixed and obstructive apneas are related to ventilatory oscillations in premature infants. Journal of Applied Physiology 66: 2818–2826

106. Waggener T B, Stark A R, Cohlan B A, Frantz I D 1984 Apnea duration is related to ventilatory oscillation characteristics in newborn infants. Journal of Applied Physiology 57: 536–544

107. Watanabe K, Hakamada S, Kuroyanagi M, Yamazaki T, Takeuchi T 1983 Electroencephalographic study of intraventricular hemorrhage in the preterm newborn. Neuropediatrics 14: 225–230

108. Weintraub Z, Alvaro R, Kwiatkowski K, Cates D, Rigatto H 1992 Effects of inhaled oxygen (up to 40%) on periodic breathing and apnea in preterm infants. Journal of Applied Physiology 72: 116–120

109. Westkamp E, Soditt V, Adrian S, Bohnhorst B, Groneck P, Poets C F 2002 Blood transfusion in anemic infants with apnea of prematurity. Biology of the Neonate 82: 228–232

PART 5

Malformations of the lower respiratory tract
Grenville F Fox

Pulmonary agenesis

Bilateral pulmonary agenesis is an extremely rare abnormality and is obviously not compatible with postnatal life. It has been described in association with anencephaly and other congenital anomalies.[127]

Unilateral pulmonary agenesis also occurs in association with other congenital anomalies, including congenital heart disease (CHD), oesophageal atresia, and vertebral and facial anomalies.[81,120] Antenatal ultrasound diagnosis has been reported,[101] although most cases present with respiratory distress in the early neonatal period. Others may present with recurrent respiratory symptoms in early childhood or be discovered incidentally.[146]

Diagnosis is usually confirmed on a chest X-ray (CXR), which shows absence of aeration on the affected side, with marked mediastinal shift and herniation of the unaffected lung, which often shows compensatory hyperinflation.

Management is supportive only, with treatment of other congenital malformations if possible. Mortality rate is high and often depends on coexisting CHD.

Pulmonary hypoplasia

Primary pulmonary hypoplasia

In this rare form of pulmonary hypoplasia, there is no apparent underlying cause. Familial cases have been described,[33] although the disorder is usually sporadic. Acinar dysplasia has been found in some cases of primary pulmonary hypoplasia, with abnormal development occurring distal to the bronchi. There are no alveoli and the terminal bronchioles have multiple cystic branches lined by bronchial epithelium, equivalent to failure of lung development beyond the pseudoglandular phase.[136]

Secondary pulmonary hypoplasia

A normal-sized thoracic cavity, normal amniotic fluid volume and normal fetal breathing movements are all required for optimal lung growth in utero. Causes of secondary pulmonary hypoplasia can include intrathoracic space-occupying lesions, small chest syndromes, oligohydramnios, congenital neuromuscular disorders and other causes, according to aetiology (Table 27.14).

Reduction in intrathoracic space

Conditions that restrict thoracic volume are frequently associated with pulmonary hypoplasia. Of these, congenital diaphragmatic hernia (CDH) has been extensively researched, and histological studies show that there is decreased bronchial and vascular branching with reduced alveolar number.[42]

Reduction in fetal breathing movements

Pulmonary hypoplasia is associated with a number of congenital neuromuscular diseases. There is a reduction in bronchial branching,

Table 27.14 Causes of secondary pulmonary hypoplasia

Pathophysiology	Condition/aetiology
Reduction in intrathoracic space	Congenital diaphragmatic hernia[7] Congenital cystic adenomatoid malformation[121] Congenital lung cysts Pleural effusions[24] Small chest syndromes (see Table 27.15)
Reduction in fetal breathing movements	Congenital myotonic dystrophy[158] Spinal muscular atrophy[106] Phrenic nerve agenesis[61] Cervical spinal cord lesions[135]
Reduction in amniotic fluid volume	Fetal renal abnormalities Bilateral renal agenesis (Potter syndrome)[126] Multicystic dysplastic kidneys[112] Polycystic kidney disease[76,112] Obstructive uropathy[70] Renal tubular dysgenesis[83,112] Prolonged premature rupture of membranes[11] Uteroplacental insufficiency Amniocentesis
Other	Rhesus disease[26] Trisomies (21[31] and 18) Maternal drugs Angiotensin-converting enzyme inhibitors[66] Sodium valproate[75] Anterior abdominal wall defects[150]

suggesting that lung growth and development is affected before the 16th week of fetal life. Fetal breathing movements are frequently seen with ultrasound scanning (USS) several weeks prior to this, and the amplitude of pressure changes during breaths has been shown to be an important determinant of normal lung growth.[90]

Reduction in amniotic fluid volume

Oligohydramnios from any cause can result in pulmonary hypoplasia, particularly if it develops at less than 26 weeks of pregnancy (Table 27.14). Attempting to restore normal amniotic fluid volume by amnioinfusion is associated with less pulmonary hypoplasia, confirming that adequate amniotic fluid volume is necessary for normal lung growth.[110]

Post-mortem examination shows that in pulmonary hypoplasia caused by renal disease there is a reduction in bronchial branching, indicating maldevelopment prior to 16 weeks of fetal life. There is also a decreased alveolar number and size, suggesting continuing maldevelopment after this.[71]

Premature rupture of membranes prior to 26 weeks' gestation is associated with pulmonary hypoplasia in approximately 23% of cases.[16] The gestational age at the time of membrane rupture and duration of rupture (longer than 14 days) with severe oligohydramnios were found to be independent risk factors for pulmonary hypoplasia in one series.[79] Fetal breathing, fetal movements, and thoracic circumference to abdominal circumference ratios were not predictive. Premature rupture of membranes at less than 25 weeks' gestation and for more than 14 days duration with severe oligohydramnios predicted a neonatal mortality due to pulmonary hypoplasia of greater than 90%.

Although not associated with severe pulmonary hypoplasia, amniocentesis in the first and second trimester may affect lung growth, leading to an increased incidence of respiratory problems and reduced lung volume and function in newborn infants.[1,151,159]

The mechanism for decreased lung growth due to oligohydramnios is uncertain and several mechanisms have been suggested, including thoracic compression,[110] reduced fetal breathing movements[3] and reduced stretching of the developing respiratory tract by fluid.

Clinical features

Bilateral pulmonary hypoplasia varies in severity from a neonate who cannot be resuscitated, through to those who have mild symptoms of respiratory distress which resolve over the first few weeks of life without intervention.[5]

Severe bilateral pulmonary hypoplasia is frequently complicated by pneumothorax and persistent pulmonary hypertension of the newborn (PPHN). When neuromuscular disease such as congenital myotonic dystrophy is present, there may be a history of reduced fetal movements and polyhydramnios due to poor fetal swallowing. There is profoundly decreased muscle tone, myopathic facies and talipes equinovarus is common. The ribs are often hypoplastic and this is associated with a poor prognosis.[49] Respiratory function is further compromised by diaphragmatic hypoplasia. Congenital myotonic dystrophy is usually inherited in

an autosomal dominant pattern via the mother, who is only mildly affected and often undiagnosed until presentation of her more severely affected baby or due to a history of previous stillbirth or neonatal death (pp. 1180–1). The molecular basis of the condition is an expansion in the number of trinucleotide repeats at chromosome 19q13.3.[18] This increases in subsequent generations, accounting for the worsening clinical severity – a phenomenon known as genetic anticipation.

Severe oligohydramnios due to renal disease or early, chronic leakage of amniotic fluid often causes severe pulmonary hypoplasia, resulting in early neonatal death. Affected neonates may be small for gestational age, have limb contractures and typical 'Potter's' facies with abnormal ears, flattened nose and epicanthic folds. The hands and feet are often 'spade like'.

Diagnosis

Antenatal ultrasound may identify factors associated with pulmonary hypoplasia such as CDH and other causes of reduced intrathoracic space, bilateral renal anomalies and oligohydramnios or features of congenital neuromuscular disease. Antenatal three-dimensional ultrasonography and Doppler blood flow velocities of pulmonary arteries have been used to estimate fetal lung volume.[86,165]

Severe bilateral pulmonary hypoplasia presents immediately after birth. Affected neonates are difficult to resuscitate, requiring high-pressure positive pressure ventilation with FiO_2 1.0. Despite this and other extensive interventions, death is likely within minutes of birth. The antenatal history and USS may have identified renal disease, oligohydramnios or other features suggestive of the underlying conditions listed in Table 27.14. The CXR shows small-volume lungs with a bell-shaped chest. Lung volumes can be estimated by measuring functional residual capacity using gas dilution or plethysmographic techniques.[5,151,152]

Management

Antenatal

Antenatal diagnosis of conditions leading to pulmonary hypoplasia is often possible as early as the second trimester. This may provide an opportunity for antenatal fetal intervention in some cases. If polyhydramnios is present, drainage may prolong the pregnancy and reduce the risk and consequences of preterm birth.

Drainage of large fluid-filled congenital cystic adenomatoid malformations (CCAMs), bronchogenic cysts or hydrothoraces with a pigtail intercostal catheter used to create a thoracoamniotic shunt has been shown to be associated with resolution of hydrops and may allow normal subsequent lung growth.[91,152]

Tracheal plugging or occlusion by clipping has been attempted in a small number of human fetuses with CDH (Chapter 27, part 6).[67] This promotes lung growth by preventing egress of fluid produced within the lungs. Outcomes so far have been variable, but less complications and better survival may be possible by fetoscopic insertion of a detachable balloon for tracheal occlusion,[68] although the USA trial has been curtailed early because no benefit was found.[69]

Amnioinfusion for such cases may reduce neonatal mortality due to pulmonary hypoplasia[110,157] but evidence from randomised controlled trials is lacking.

Fetal bladder catheterisation has been carried out successfully in a number of cases of obstructive uropathy diagnosed prior to 24 weeks' gestation, thus avoiding pulmonary hypoplasia, due to resolution of severe oligohydramnios.[144]

Postnatal

The degree of respiratory support required for infants with bilateral pulmonary hypoplasia depends on the severity of underdevelopment of the lungs. In many cases, particularly when there has been anhydramnios or severe oligohydramnios noted from early in the second trimester with other severe congenital anomalies such as bilateral cystic dysplastic kidneys, it may be appropriate to consider withholding or withdrawing ongoing intensive respiratory support. In cases of mild bilateral pulmonary hypoplasia, no respiratory support may be required and close monitoring is recommended over a period of several weeks or months while the lungs grow to a normal size.[5]

Many babies with bilateral pulmonary hypoplasia may require prolonged mechanical ventilation. Ventilatory requirements may be high, particularly initially. Following prolonged rupture of membranes in the second trimester, some infants may require very high-pressure ventilation initially, but recover rapidly over the first 24 hours of life to enable complete weaning from any respiratory support within a few days. This has been attributed to severe atelectasis due to oligohydramnios and referred to as 'dry lung syndrome'.[95] The lung growth in these cases is likely to be normal, but initial CXR appearance and antenatal history may suggest pulmonary hypoplasia.[92]

Due to the increased risk of infection following prolonged rupture of membranes, broad-spectrum antibiotics should be given following appropriate investigations.

Pulmonary hypertension is a common problem. Inhaled nitric oxide (iNO), high-frequency oscillation, calcium antagonists and extracorporeal membrane oxygenation (ECMO) have been advocated, with successful outcome in a small number of cases.[56,74] At 34 weeks, preterm delivery is low risk and may avoid joint contractures.[16]

Prognosis

Survival with bilateral pulmonary hypoplasia is dependent on the degree of lung underdevelopment and other associated anomalies. In one recently published series, survival was 40%, 92% and 100% following rupture of membranes at 14–19 weeks, 20–25 weeks and 26–28 weeks, respectively.[47] Pulmonary hypoplasia accounted for 78% of deaths. Other studies have found that gestational age at the time of membrane rupture, the latency period until birth and the amniotic fluid volume are independent factors which predict the risk of pulmonary hypoplasia and neonatal mortality.[16,164]

Resolution of symptoms due to mild-to-moderate pulmonary hypoplasia may take weeks to months.[5] Long-term ventilatory support may be required for those with more severe problems,

with resolution likely to occur with growth, and good nutrition therefore essential. Lung volume measurements using several different techniques in infants with a number of different underlying diagnoses have suggested that normal lung size is likely by 6 years of age in the vast majority who survive the early neonatal period.[5,27,149]

Small chest syndromes

Table 27.15 shows conditions that have congenital chest wall abnormalities leading to respiratory symptoms in the neonatal period. The ribs are usually short and many are associated with vertebral anomalies resulting in kyphoscoliosis, which may further reduce thoracic volume. Pulmonary hypoplasia may also occur in some of these conditions, but lung growth and development has been documented as being normal in many cases.[163]

Antenatal diagnosis using USS is able to detect many of these conditions before 24 weeks' gestation. In one series, accuracy of diagnosis was only 65%, but prediction of mortality had 100% sensitivity and specificity.[124]

Signs of respiratory distress may develop early in many of these conditions. The thorax often appears bell-shaped and the abdomen large. CXR shows the same, with short horizontal ribs as well as apparent cardiomegaly and clear lung fields. Close examination of the vertebrae and other bones on a skeletal survey, along with detailed family history, may help establish the underlying diagnosis.

Four subtypes of short rib–polydactyly syndromes have been described (Saldino–Noonan, Majewski, Verma–Naumoff and Beemer–Langer syndromes), but these, along with asphyxiating thoracic dystrophy and Ellis van Creveld syndrome, are likely to represent a continuous spectrum.[100] Further advances in molecular genetics may provide further evidence to support this.

In many of these conditions, mechanical ventilation is often required immediately after birth and for a variable time, depending on the underlying diagnosis. Prognosis is often poor, but those surviving the first year may have a good long-term outlook.[117] Surgical reconstruction of the chest wall with bone grafts or synthetic prostheses has been described in cases of asphyxiating thoracic dystrophy and other similar conditions,[154] with good long-term outcome being reported if this is limited to milder cases able to survive to 1 year of age before surgery is contemplated.[39]

Congenital cystic adenomatoid malformation

CCAM is a rare condition, predominantly affecting the lower lobes of the lungs. Unilateral CCAM is more common, with the left lung being affected more commonly than the right.[137] Bilateral cases have also been reported.[14,137] The affected areas of the lung consist of a mass of cysts lined by bronchial or cuboidal epithelium, which may contain cystic and adenomatoid portions with intervening normal lung tissue. Stocker et al described three

Table 27.15 Congenital chest wall abnormalities causing neonatal respiratory symptoms

Condition	Inheritance/genetics	Clinical features	Prognosis
Asphyxiating thoracic dystrophy (Jeune's syndrome)	Autosomal recessive – mutation chromosome 15q13	Short ribs, bell-shaped chest, +/− short limbs, hypoplastic iliac wings, renal abnormalities	Variable severity ranging from mild neonatal respiratory distress and long-term survival, to early severe respiratory failure and death
Chondroectodermal dysplasia (Ellis van Creveld syndrome)	Autosomal recessive – mutation chromosome 4p16	Short ribs, polydactyly (medial), congenital heart disease, cleft lip and palate, hypoplastic nails	Neonatal respiratory distress with good outcome
Short rib–polydactyly syndromes	Autosomal recessive	Short ribs, polydactyly, vertebral and pelvic defects, short limbs, congenital heart disease, renal, genital and intestinal abnormalities	Severe neonatal respiratory failure with early death
Achondroplasia	Autosomal dominant (80% new mutations)	Small chest, short limbs, macrocephaly with frontal bossing	Mild neonatal respiratory distress, upper airway obstruction and apnoea, mild hypotonia. Good prognosis
Achondrogenesis	Autosomal recessive	Type 1 (Parenti–Fraccaro syndrome) – short limbs, large head, small barrel-shaped chest with thin ribs with fractures, unossified vertebral bodies Type 2 (Langer–Saldino syndrome) – short limbs and ribs with more ossification of skull and vertebral bodies	Stillborn or die in early neonatal period
Thanatophoric dysplasia	Sporadic – fibroblast growth factor receptor 3 gene mutation	Very short limbs with 'telephone handle' femurs; very small, pear-shaped chest; clover-leaf skull; occasional other congenital anomalies (congenital heart disease, hydronephrosis, imperforate anus, hydrocephalus)	Severe neonatal respiratory failure usually leading to death within hours. Some may survive several weeks[119]
Camptomelic dysplasia	Autosomal recessive	Short limbs, bowed long bones, narrow thorax, occasionally with 11 ribs. May have female phenotype with male karyotype, hydrocephalus and hypoplasia of larynx and tracheal rings	Usually severe neonatal respiratory failure and early death within weeks. Survival to 17 years noted in one case[140]
Osteogenesis imperfecta	Type II – usually autosomal recessive, but may be dominant. Mutation in type I procollagen genes	Severe deformity of the chest wall and limbs due to mutiple, healed in-utero fractures; soft skull, thin skin	Approximately 50% stillborn. Others usually die immediately after birth. Antenatal diagnosis by ultrasound scan[107] or chorionic villus biopsy possible[78]
	Type III – autosomal recessive. Mutation in type I collagen genes	As above but less severe	Mild respiratory problems may occur in the neonatal period. Chest wall deformity is often progressive, resulting in death later in childhood in many cases

(Continued)

Table 27.15 (Continued)

Condition	Inheritance/genetics	Clinical features	Prognosis
Hypophosphatasia (perinatal form)	Autosomal recessive – mutation in tissue non-specific alkaline phosphatase gene found in some cases[57]	Poorly mineralised bones with multiple pathological fractures, short ribs and long bones, hypercalcaemia, low alkaline phosphatase	Death from respiratory failure in early neonatal period. Antenatal diagnosis possible by alkaline phosphatase assay from chorionic villus biopsy
Cleidocranial dysostosis	Autosomal dominant	Hypoplasia of clavicle, short ribs, delayed closure of anterior fontanelle and delayed eruption of teeth	Variable degree of neonatal respiratory distress may occur
Spondyloepiphyseal dysplasias	Autosomal dominant	Delayed ossification of vertebrae with kyphoscoliosis, small chest and cleft palate	May present with neonatal respiratory distress
Spondylothoracic dysostoses	Autosomal recessive	Vertebral anomalies resulting in severe chest wall deformity due to crowding of the ribs	Severe neonatal respiratory distress resulting in death within first few months[78]
Spondylocostal dysostoses	Autosomal recessive or dominant	Vertebral and rib abnormalities resulting in some chest wall abnormality	Autosomal recessive type more likely to present with severe neonatal respiratory distress. Dominant form may present with mild symptoms only[78]

pathological variations of CCAM.[142] Type 1 is the most common of these, accounting for approximately 50% of cases. It consists of multiple, thin-walled cysts lined with pseudostratified epithelium, which may contain mucus-secreting glands. The cysts are large and may be confused with congenital lobar emphysema. Type 2 CCAM accounts for approximately 40% of cases and consists of multiple, smaller cysts (less than 1–2 cm diameter), which are lined by ciliated cuboidal or columnar epithelium without glandular tissue. Type 3 lesions are rarer (less than 10% of CCAMs) and relatively solid lesions, which have very small cysts lined with ciliated cuboidal epithelium. Subsequently, a fourth type has been described which has acinar-alveolar epithelium, rather than the bronchiolar epithelium found in types 1, 2, and 3 CCAM.[108] This suggests that there are two subtypes of CCAM arising at different stages of the branching morphogenesis of lung development. The first arises at the pseudoglandular stage (types 1, 2 and 3), whilst type 4 lesions arise at the saccular stage. A simpler classification describing microcystic (cysts <5 mm) and macrocystic (cysts >5 mm) lesions has been suggested and also has prognostic value.[153]

The aetiology of CCAM remains obscure, although it has been suggested that it is the result of dysregulation of lung epithelial cell turnover, with both increased cell proliferation and decreased apoptosis.[22] Glial cell-derived neurotropic factor (GDNF) is a growth factor involved in the development of fetal lung and other organs, and increased expression of this has been found in the epithelial cells of CCAM tissue compared with normal lung.[50] Platelet-derived growth factor-BB (PDGF-BB)

stimulates normal lung growth and is maximal during the cannalicular stage. Increased levels of PDGF-BB have been found in rapidly growing CCAMs which were associated with hydrops.[89]

The incidence of CCAM has been estimated at 1 in 25 000–30 000 pregnancies. Males and females are equally affected and there are no recognised patterns of inheritance. Trisomy 18 has been noted in a very small number of cases.[85] Associated congenital anomalies occur in approximately 20% of cases.[142] Other congenital malformations of the lung such as bronchogenic cysts and pulmonary sequestration may also coexist.[21,96]

Clinical features

The majority of cases of CCAM are diagnosed by antenatal USS. After the initial diagnosis, approximately 40% of lesions partially or completely regress as the pregnancy progresses,[10,46,60,137,155] a third of these initially increasing in size.[85] Hydrops occurs in approximately 30% of cases[35,46,97] and polyhydramnios is also common. Echocardiographic studies suggest that raised central venous pressure due to vascular compression is the likely cause of hydrops, whereas polyhydramnios may be due to oesophageal compression leading to reduced swallowing. In-utero death may occur in up to 25% of cases, with polyhydramnios, hydrops, marked mediastinal shift and type 3 CCAM being associated with this and postnatal death.[12,20,84,111] Preterm birth appears to be more common, ranging from 0% to 50%.[46,105,153] This wide variation may reflect differing approaches to antenatal intervention.

Postnatal presentation is variable and ranges from absence of symptoms in up to 50% of cases,[111] to severe respiratory distress requiring artificial ventilation and other forms of respiratory support. Tachypnoea, cyanosis with oxygen requirement and carbon dioxide retention are common features. Pneumothorax[55] and PPHN[129] have also been noted in association with CCAM in the early neonatal period. Late presentation in children and adults, most commonly with recurrent lower respiratory tract infection, is now unusual, due to widespread routine antenatal USS.[93] However, some recently reported cases presenting from infancy to adulthood describe lung abscess,[37] pneumothorax,[88] haemoptysis,[28] and incidental finding on a CXR.[8]

A number of case reports suggest an association between CCAM and various intrathoracic neoplasms. Bronchoalveolar carcinoma has developed both in children as young as 11 years old as well as in adult patients.[62] Pulmonary rhabdomyosarcoma has also been reported in a number of cases,[122] the youngest being 13 months old. Bronchopulmonary blastoma may develop from CCAM and has been found after initial surgical resection.[123]

Diagnosis

Antenatal USS may detect CCAM as early as 16 weeks' gestation, when the lesions appear as a hyperechogenic mass in microcystic lesions or as larger cysts.[153] Ultrasound estimation of the volume of CCAM has been used to predict the development of hydrops,[35] and Doppler blood flow waveforms of fetal pulmonary arteries have been found to accurately predict pulmonary hypoplasia.[51] More recently, fetal magnetic resonance imaging (MRI) has been evaluated and may be useful in distinguishing between CCAM and other anomalies such as CDH.[72]

Initial postnatal imaging with plain CXR usually shows a cystic, solid or mixed lesion in the affected lobes, depending on the underlying type of CCAM. Mediastinal shift is common. Further evaluation with computed tomography (CT) scanning may be helpful to distinguish between CCAM and CDH or in small lesions that are difficult to visualise on a CXR, as well as to accurately depict anatomical location.[80] Colour flow Doppler studies may be useful to exclude systemic arterial blood supply that has been noted in some cases of CCAM, although this may not be apparent until found during surgical resection.[21]

Management

Termination of pregnancy may be considered in pregnancies with poor prognostic features such as bilateral CCAM, early hydrops or associated severe congenital anomalies.[60,85,153] Amniotic fluid reduction by amniocentesis may reduce the risk of preterm birth, although there is no direct evidence supporting this in cases of CCAM. If there is marked mediastinal shift associated with large fluid-filled cysts, thoracoamniotic shunting has led to high survival rates[2,35] but such intervention is indicated only if there is polyhydramnios or hydrops.[44] For massive multicystic or predominantly solid CCAM associated with hydrops, fetal lobectomy may provide an alternative therapeutic option. This was performed in 13 cases between 21 and 29 weeks' gestation, resulting in eight healthy survivors at 1 to 7 years' follow-up.[2]

Early postnatal surgical resection with lobectomy or segmentectomy is required in symptomatic cases. Mediastinal shift, pulmonary hypoplasia and pulmonary hypertension may be problematic in the initial postnatal period and high-frequency oscillatory ventilation (HFOV),[160] iNO,[14] selective intubation of the contralateral lung[23] and ECMO[114] have been used to stabilise infants with CCAM perioperatively. The risk of recurrent infection and malignant change suggests that surgery should also be considered in asymptomatic cases, and this is our current clinical practice.

Prognosis

Poor prognostic indicators include hydrops, polyhydramnios, mediastinal shift, microcystic disease, early antenatal diagnosis, presence of other congenital malformations, and preterm birth.[105,153] Recurrence rates in partially resected CCAM are low.[102]

Congenital lung cysts

Congenital lung cysts may be extrapulmonary (mostly arising from bronchi or trachea) or intrapulmonary (mostly arising from alveoli). They are usually single, confined to one lung and are not associated with cystic changes in other organs. The commonest site is in the carinal region, but they may occur at the periphery of the lung, below the diaphragm or in the mediastinum.[98]

Signs of respiratory distress due to congenital lung cysts are extremely unusual in the neonatal period, with only 10% diagnosed at this stage, a further 14% during the first year and over 50% in adults, many being discovered incidentally by routine CXR.[131] Symptoms and timing of presentation depend on the size and site of congenital lung cysts.

Diagnosis is usually from CXR appearance. CT, MRI or USS may be useful in differentiating large congenital lung cysts from CCAM and congenital lobar emphysema.

Surgical resection is recommended for all congenital lung cysts. More recently, thoracoscopic surgical techniques have been described for these lesions.[134]

Pulmonary sequestration

Pulmonary sequestration is a congenital abnormality consisting of intrathoracic or intra-abdominal lung tissue with arterial blood supply from the thoracic or abdominal aorta. There is usually no connection to the tracheobronchial tree. Traditionally, classification has been according to the position of the lesion, as intra- or extralobular, with intralobular lesions lying adjacent to normal lung tissue within the pleura and extralobular lesions being within their own pleura. Subsequently, a classification based on the airway connection, the arterial supply, venous drainage and lung parenchyma has been advocated.[29]

It was initially suggested that pulmonary sequestrations are likely to arise due to an accessory lung diverticulum from the primitive foregut, with extralobular lesions being more distal. A further explanation of aetiology is that of the haphazard branching theory, in which there are abnormal connections or malinosculations between the primitive foregut and aortic-pulmonary arch system.[87]

Pathophysiology

Intralobular pulmonary sequestrations usually consist of a mass of airless alveoli, which may have a cystic appearance. They are usually left sided and involve the lower zone in 85% of cases.[161] Arterial supply is directly from the aorta in most cases, with venous drainage into a pulmonary vein. Extralobular lesions may be intrathoracic or abdominal, and venous drainage is into systemic veins, usually the vena cava or azygous veins.[52] One variation involves sequestration in the right lung with resultant right lung hypoplasia, with infradiaphragmatic venous drainage to the vena cava from the sequestered lobe and surrounding otherwise normal lung. This is known as Scimitar syndrome, due to the characteristic appearance of the CXR and angiogram.[53]

Clinical features

Antenatal diagnosis may be by USS, showing an echogenic intrathoracic or intra-abdominal mass. Polyhydramnios is common and fetal pleural effusions and hydrops may also occur. More recently, fetal MRI has been used to obtain further detail.[41]

Intralobular lesions may lead to symptoms of respiratory distress in the neonatal period due to compression of adjacent normal lung or heart failure due to a large arteriovenous shunt. However, approximately 80% of babies remain symptom-free but present later in childhood or adulthood with infection, pleural effusion or haemoptysis. The diagnosis may be made on CXR as an incidental finding. Scimitar syndrome can present in the neonatal period with massive haemorrhage from the affected lung.[6]

Other congenital malformations are rarely found in intralobular pulmonary sequestration. However, in two recently described series, more than 50% of pulmonary sequestrations were associated with type 2 CCAM.[17,30] These differed from those without CCAM, with earlier presentation, usually within the first 3 months of life.

Extralobular pulmonary sequestration often remains asymptomatic and is usually found incidentally. Other congenital malformations such as CDH and CHD occur in nearly 60% of cases.[138]

Diagnosis

CXR shows pulmonary sequestration as a radiodensity, usually in the posteromedial part of the left lung. Doppler ultrasonography, spiral CT scanning or MR angiography may be used to determine arterial supply and venous drainage,[65] although aortography remains the definitive investigation for this.

Management

Antenatal drainage of polyhydramnios and insertion of thoraco-abdominal shunts for associated hydrothorax may improve outcome after antenatal presentation of pulmonary sequestration.[91]

Early surgical resection by segmentectomy or lobectomy for intralobar sequestrations, and sequestrectomy for extralobar sequestrations, have generally been recommended in order to alleviate a mass effect in large lesions and prevent other possible short-term complications such as haemorrhage and heart failure, as well as avoiding later infection.[15,64,156] Successful minimally invasive surgery using thoracoscopy or laparoscopy has also been described.[38,103]

Embolisation of the feeding artery using a coil placed via a vascular catheter has been reported recently, with a high rate of success and minimal complications.[36]

Prognosis

Antenatal regression and resolution of pulmonary sequestration may occur in approximately 50% of cases.[15,91] Polyhydramnios and hydrops are likely to be associated with a worse outcome. Postnatal regression has also been described but appears to occur less frequently.[54]

Surgical resection in the neonatal period or later generally leads to excellent results, with favourable long-term outcome.[64,91] Metaplasia or neoplastic change has not been noted from histological examination of resected pulmonary sequestrations.

Congenital pulmonary lymphangiectasis

Congenital pulmonary lymphangiectasis (CPL) is a rare condition in which there is cystic dilatation of the pulmonary lymphatics with obstruction to their drainage. It is usually bilateral and associated with severe respiratory failure, although unilateral and localised lesions have been described.[130] It is more common in males and may be associated with other abnormalities of the lymphatics. Noonan et al described three groups of patients with CPL:[116]

- CPL associated with generalised lymphangiectasis. Presentation is often antenatal with hydrops. Generalised lymphangiectasis develops with malabsorption and hemihypertrophy.
- CPL associated with CHD. Total anomalous venous drainage, hypoplastic left heart, pulmonary stenosis, and atrial and ventricular septal defects have all been described in association with CPL.
- CPL as a primary developmental defect of the lung. This may occur in Noonan's, Turner's and Down's syndrome.

Pathophysiology

CPL may arise due to failure of fusion of embryonic lymphatic channels, which initially develop as spaces within the lung bud.

It has also been suggested that it may be part of a generalised developmental anomaly of lymphatics, rather than an intrinsic lung defect. Lymphatic obstruction results in large, firm and heavy lungs which are poorly expanded.

Clinical features

Presentation is usually antenatal, with hydrops or severe respiratory distress in a term infant. Exogenous surfactant therapy may lead to temporary resolution of respiratory failure.

Diagnosis

In generalised bilateral CPL, lung fields usually have a ground-glass appearance on CXR, but are usually well inflated or even overinflated, and have prominent interstitial lymphatics radiating from the hilar areas. Chylous pleural infusions may be present. The diagnosis is only confirmed by lung biopsy.

Localised lesions may present with a cystic mass, which appears similar to a cystic adenomatoid malformation on antenatal USS or postnatal CXR.[130]

Management

Surgical excision may be possible for localised CPL.[130] Bilateral disease presenting with severe respiratory failure has a poor prognosis.

Pulmonary alveolar proteinosis (congenital alveolar proteinosis)

Pulmonary alveolar proteinosis (PAP) is a rare condition characterised by accumulation of lipoproteinaceous material in the alveolar space, which impedes gas exchange. Presentation is usually in older children and adults; babies can develop severe respiratory failure. Familial recurrence has been reported, suggesting autosomal recessive inheritance in some cases.[13]

Pathology

The lipoproteinaceous material found distending the alveoli stains positive for periodic acid-Schiff and represents surfactant, which accumulates due to defective alveolar macrophage function. Changes are usually generalised in the neonatal form of the disease, although a focal distribution has also been noted.[104] Histological evidence from some reported cases of PAP has suggested that the underlying aetiology is a congenital deficiency of surfactant protein B (SP-B).[115] Several mutations in the SP-B gene have been described, with the 121ins2 mutation occurring in approximately two-thirds of cases.[40]

Clinical features and diagnosis

Presentation is usually with severe, prolonged respiratory failure in a term infant. The CXR appearance is suggestive of surfactant deficiency, with diffuse ground-glass opacification of the lung fields. CT also shows generalised opacification, with prominent interlobular septa.[113]

Diagnosis is confirmed by demonstration of decreased or absent SP-B by enzyme-linked immunosorbent assay (ELISA) in aspirates obtained by alveolar lavage or immunostaining of lung tissue from biopsy.[13]

Management

Ventilatory support is required from birth in congenital alveolar proteinosis. Temporary improvement may result from alveolar lavage and exogenous surfactant therapy, but the condition is usually fatal within a few weeks of birth.[13] Long-term survival has only been reported after lung transplantation.[73]

Congenital lobar emphysema

This is a rare condition in which the affected lobe is hyperinflated. The incidence in babies has been estimated as 1 in 90 000, although it may present in older children and adults.[34,99] Congenital lobar emphysema is more common in males[77] and familial cases have been described, but with no common pattern of inheritance.[132,147] CHD occurs in 10–15% of cases.[77]

Pathophysiology

The hyperinflated lobe or lobes occur due to a 'ball-valve' mechanism for which a number of aetiologies have been implicated. These include defects in bronchial cartilage, resulting in bronchomalacia,[45] partial large airway obstruction due to excessive mucus or inflammatory exudates[148] and extraluminal compression of large airways by bronchogenic cysts[58] or aberrant blood vessels.[128]

The affected lobe or lobes are distended and pale in colour, with absent ventilation and perfusion. Compression resulting in atelectasis of unaffected lobes occurs, along with mediastinal shift.

Clinical features

Presentation in the early neonatal period, with signs of respiratory distress, occurs in 50–60% of cases. Most late presentations occur within the first 6 months, most commonly with recurrent lower respiratory tract infection.[77] On examination, the affected side may be hyperinflated, with reduced breath sounds, an increased percussion note and expiratory wheeze.

In recently published case series, the left upper lobe was affected in 65% of cases, the right middle lobe in 24% and the right upper lobe in 11%.[43,77,139,145] One case series suggested that symptoms were worse when congenital lobar emphysema occurred in either upper lobe.[145]

Diagnosis

Antenatal diagnosis with USS and MRI has been reported in very few cases.[9,118] Like other congenital lung lesions diagnosed on antenatal USS, some appear to decrease in size or even disappear altogether as the pregnancy progresses, but signs may still occur soon after birth.

Postnatally, most cases of congenital lobar emphysema can be diagnosed by a plain CXR, which typically shows hyperinflation of the affected lobe, mediastinal shift and compression of other parts of both lungs. Delayed resorption of lung fluid is commonly seen within the affected lobe as increased opacity within the affected lobe. Ventilation perfusion scintigraphy, showing decreased ventilation and perfusion, and CT scans may also aid diagnosis.[77,141] Echocardiography is necessary to exclude CHD, and barium swallow, bronchoscopy and cardiac catheterisation with angiography may be required to exclude a vascular ring.[133]

Management

Most cases of congenital lobar emphysema presenting in the neonatal period require surgical lobectomy. Mild cases presenting later can usually be managed conservatively.[77] Successful treatment with flexible bronchoscopy[125] and selective bronchial intubation has also been described in a small number of cases.[59]

Ciliary abnormalities

Primary ciliary dyskinesia, also known as the immotile cilia syndrome, is an autosomal recessive condition with an incidence of approximately 1 in 15 000.

Pathophysiology

Ciliary dyskinesia occurs most commonly due to absence of the dynein arms on the outer microtubular doublets.[4] Other abnormalities of cilial ultrastructure, recognised by electron microscopy, have also been described, along with cilial aplasia.[48,143] Patients with typical symptoms and decreased ciliary beat frequency but normal cilial ultrastructure have also been described.[63]

Clinical features

Ciliary dysfunction leads to poor clearance of respiratory tract secretions, which predisposes cases to recurrent upper and lower respiratory tract infections, sinusitis and otitis media. Bronchiectasis may develop by mid to late childhood or during adult life as a result of chronic respiratory infection. The incidence of dextrocardia and situs inversus (Kartagener's syndrome)

varies from 50% to 67% in large case series.[32,109] Male infertility also occurs, due to reduction of sperm motility.

Presentation in the neonatal period occurs in more than two-thirds of cases and may be with otherwise unexplained persistent signs of respiratory distress, pneumonia or mucoid nasal secretions.[19,162] Diagnosis may also be suspected in cases of dextrocardia or with a positive family history.

Diagnosis

A superficial brush biopsy sample of epithelial cells from the nasopharynx can be examined under light microscopy to assess cilial function. An electronic counting device or photometric methods can be used to measure ciliary beat frequency, which is reduced in primary ciliary dyskinesia. Electron microscopic examination is used to assess specific structural defects of cilia.

Management

Antibiotics for respiratory tract and other infections and chest physiotherapy may delay the onset of bronchiectasis. Surgical treatment for bronchiectasis is not normally required but lobectomy and successful lung transplantation have been reported in the most severe cases.[94] Successful intracytoplasmic sperm injection and in-vitro fertilisation has been described in male patients.[25]

Prognosis

Bronchiectasis occurs in approximately one-third of cases by late childhood, but the severity is variable and prognosis is usually better than with cystic fibrosis or other causes of childhood bronchiectasis. Life expectancy can be normal but depends on the severity of bronchiectasis.[82]

References

1. [Anonymous] 1978 An assessment of the hazards of amniocentesis. Report to the Medical Research Council by their Working Party on Amniocentesis. British Journal of Obstetrics and Gynaecology 85(suppl. 2): 1–41
2. Adzick N S, Harrison M R, Crombleholme T M et al 1998 Fetal lung lesions: management and outcome. American Journal of Obstetrics and Gynecology 179: 884–889
3. Adzick N S, Harrison M R, Glick P L et al 1984 Experimental pulmonary hypoplasia and oligohydramnios; relative contributions of lung fluid and fetal breathing movements. Journal of Pediatric Surgery 19: 658–665
4. Afzelius B A 1976 A human syndrome caused by immotile cilia. Science 193: 317–319
5. Aiton N R, Fox G F, Hannam S et al 1996 Pulmonary hypoplasia presenting as persistent tachypnoea in the first few months of life. British Medical Journal 312: 1149–1150
6. Alivizatos P, Cheatle T, de Leval M et al 1985 Pulmonary sequestration complicated by anomalies of pulmonary venous return. Journal of Pediatric Surgery 20: 76–99
7. Areechon W, Reid L 1963 Hypoplasia of lung with congenital diaphragmatic hernia. British Medical Journal i: 230–233

8. Avitabile A M, Greco M A, Hulnick D H et al 1984 Congenital cystic adenomatoid malformation of the lung in adults. American Journal of Surgical Pathology 8: 193–202

9. Babu R, Kyle P, Spicer R D 2001 Prenatal sonographic features of congenital lobar emphysema. Fetal Diagnosis and Therapy 16: 200–202

10. Bagolan P, Nahom A, Giorlandino C et al 1999 Cystic adenomatoid malformation of the lung: clinical evolution and management. European Journal of Pediatrics 158: 879–882

11. Bain A D, Smith I I, Gauld I K 1964 Newborn born after prolonged leakage of liquor amnii. British Medical Journal ii: 598–599

12. Bale P M 1979 Congenital cystic malformation of the lung. A form of congenital bronchiolar ("adenomatoid") malformation. American Journal of Clinical Pathology 71: 411–420

13. Ball R, Chetcuti P A, Beverley D 1995 Fatal familial surfactant protein B deficiency. Archives of Disease in Childhood. Fetal and Neonatal Edition 73: F53

14. Banerjea M C, Wirbelauer J, Adam P et al 2002 Bilateral cystic adenomatoid lung malformation type III – a rare differential diagnosis of pulmonary hypertension in neonates. Journal of Perinatal Medicine 30: 429–436

15. Becmeur F, Horta-Geraud P, Donato L et al 1998 Pulmonary sequestrations: prenatal ultrasound diagnosis, treatment and outcome. Journal of Pediatric Surgery 33: 492–496

16. Blott M, Greenough A 1988 Neonatal outcome after prolonged rupture of the membranes starting in the second trimester. Archives of Disease in Childhood 63: 1146–1150

17. Bratu I, Flageole H, Chen M F et al 2001 The multiple facets of pulmonary sequestration. Journal of Pediatric Surgery 36: 784–790

18. Brook J D, McCurrach M E, Harley H G et al 1992 Molecular basis of myotonic dystrophy: expansion of a trinucleotide (CTG) repeat at the 3' end of a transcript encoding a protein kinase family member. Cell 68: 799–808

19. Buchdahl R M, Reiser J, Ingram D et al 1988 Ciliary abnormalities in respiratory disease. Archives of Disease in Childhood 63: 238–243

20. Budorick N E, Pretorius D H, Leopold G R et al 1992 Spontaneous improvement of intrathoracic masses diagnosed in utero. Journal of Ultrasound in Medicine 11: 653–662

21. Cass D L, Crombleholme T M, Howell L J et al 1997 Cystic lung lesions with systemic arterial blood supply: a hybrid of congenital cystic adenomatoid malformation and bronchopulmonary sequestration. Journal of Pediatric Surgery 32: 986–990

22. Cass D L, Quinn T M, Yang E Y et al 1998 Increased cell proliferation and decreased apoptosis characterize congenital cystic adenomatoid malformation of the lung. Journal of Pediatric Surgery 33: 1043–1046

23. Castillo F, Lucaya J, Tokashiki N et al 1994 Selective intubation in a case of cystic adenomatoid malformation. Archives of Disease in Childhood. Fetal and Neonatal Edition 70: F70–F71

24. Castillo R A, Devoe L D, Falls G et al 1987 Pleural effusions and pulmonary hypoplasia. American Journal of Obstetrics and Gynecology 157: 1252–1255

25. Cayan S, Conaghan J, Schriock E D et al 2001 Birth after intracytoplasmic sperm injection with use of testicular sperm from men with Kartagener/immotile cilia syndrome. Fertility and Sterility 76: 612–614

26. Chamberlain D, Hislop A, Hey E et al 1977 Pulmonary hypoplasia in babies with severe rhesus isoimmunisation: a quantitive study. Journal of Pathology 122: 43–52

27. Chatrath R R, el Shafie M, Jones R S 1971 Fate of hypoplastic lungs after repair of congenital diaphragmatic hernia. Archives of Disease in Childhood 46: 633–635

28. Chen K T 1985 Congenital cystic adenomatoid malformation of the lung and pulmonary tumorlets in an adult. Journal of Surgical Oncology 30: 106–108

29. Clements B S, Warner J O 1987 Pulmonary sequestration and related congenital bronchopulmonary-vascular malformations: nomenclature and classification based on anatomical and embryological considerations. Thorax 42: 401–408

30. Conran R M, Stocker J T 1999 Extralobular sequestration with frequently associated cystic adenomatoid malformation, type 2: report of 50 cases. Pediatric and Developmental Pathology 2: 454–463

31. Cooney T P, Thurlbeck W M 1982 Pulmonary hypoplasia in Down's syndrome. New England Journal of Medicine. 307: 1170–1173

32. Coren M E, Meeks M, Morrison I et al 2002 Primary ciliary dyskinesia: age at diagnosis and symptom history. Acta Paediatrica 91: 667–669

33. Cregg N, Casey W 1997 Primary congenital pulmonary hypoplasia – a genetic component to aetiology. Paediatric Anaesthesia 7: 329–333

34. Critchley P S, Forrester-Wood C P, Ridley P D 1995 Adult congenital lobar emphysema in pregnancy. Thorax 50: 909–910

35. Crombleholme T M, Coleman B, Hedrick H et al 2002 Cystic adenomatoid malformation volume ratio predicts outcome in prenatally diagnosed cystic adenomatoid malformation of the lung. Journal of Pediatric Surgery 37: 331–338

36. Curros F, Chigot V, Emond S et al 2000 Role of embolization in the treatment of bronchopulmonary sequestration. Pediatric Radiology 30: 769–773

37. Dahabreh J, Zisis C, Vassiliou M et al 2000 Congenital cystic adenomatoid malformation in an adult presenting as lung abscess. European Journal of Cardio-thoracic Surgery 18: 720–723

38. Danielson P D, Sherman N J 2001 Laparoscopic removal of an abdominal extralobar pulmonary sequestration. Journal of Pediatric Surgery 36: 1653–1655

39. Davis J T, Heistein J B, Castile R G et al 2001 Lateral thoracic expansion for Jeune's syndrome: midterm results. Annals of Thoracic Surgery 72: 872–877

40. de Mello D E, Lin Z 2001 Pulmonary alveolar proteinosis: a review. Pediatric Pathology and Molecular Medicine 20: 413–432

41. Dhingsa R, Coakley F V, Albanese C T et al 2003 Prenatal sonography and MR imaging of pulmonary sequestration. American Journal of Roentgenology 180: 433–437

42. Dibbins A W, Weiner E S 1974 Mortality from neonatal diaphragmatic hernia. Journal of Pediatric Surgery 9: 653–662

43. Dogan R, Demircin M, Sarigul A et al 1997 Surgical management of congenital lobar emphysema. Turkish Journal of Pediatrics 39: 35–44

44. Dommergues M, Louis-Sylvestre C, Mandelbrot L et al 1997 Congenital adenomatoid malformation of the lung: is active fetal therapy indicated? American Journal of Obstetrics and Gynecology 177: 953–958

45. Doull I J, Connett G J, Warner J O 1996 Bronchoscopic appearances of congenital lobar emphysema. Pediatric Pulmonology 21: 195–197

46. Duncombe G J, Dichinson J E, Kikiros C S 2002 Prenatal diagnosis and management of congenital cystic adenomatoid malformation of the lung. American Journal of Obstetrics and Gynecology 187: 950–954

47. Farooqi A, Holmgren P A, Engberg S et al 1998 Survival and 2-year outcome with expectant management of second-trimester rupture of membranes. Obstetrics and Gynecology 92: 895–901

48. Fonzi L, Lungarella G, Palatresi R 1982 Lack of kinocilia in the nasal mucosa in the immotile cilia syndrome. European Journal of Respiratory Disease 63: 558–563

49. Fried K, Pajewski M, Mundel G et al 1975 Thin ribs in neonatal myotonic dystrophy. Clinical Genetics 7: 417–420

50. Fromont-Hankard G, Philippe-Chomette P, Delezoide A L et al 2002 Glial cell-derived neurotropic factor expression in normal human lung and congenital cystic adenomatoid malformation. Archives of Pathology and Laboratory Medicine 126: 432–436

51. Fuke S, Kanzaki T, Mu J et al 2003 Antenatal prediction of pulmonary hypoplasia by acceleration time/ejection time ratio of fetal pulmonary arteries by Doppler blood flow velocimetry. American Journal of Obstetrics and Gynecology 188: 228–233

52. Gamillscheg A, Beitzke A, Smolle-Juttner F M et al 1996 Extralobular sequestration with unusual arterial supply and venous drainage. Pediatric Cardiology 17: 57–59

53. Gao Y A, Burrows P E, Benson L N et al 1993 Scimitar syndrome in infancy. Journal of the American College of Cardiology 22: 873–882

54. Garcia-Pena P, Lucaya J, Hendry G M et al 1998 Spontaneous involution of pulmonary sequestration in children: a report of two cases and review of the literature. Pediatric Radiology 28: 266–270

55. Gardikis S, Didilis V, Polychronidis A et al 2002 Spontaneous pneumothorax resulting from congenital cystic adenomatoid malformation in a pre-term infant: case report and literature review. European Journal of Pediatric Surgery 12: 195–198

56. Geary C, Whitsett J 2002 Inhaled nitric oxide for oligohydramnios-induced pulmonary hypoplasia: a report of two cases and review of the literature. Journal of Perinatology 22: 82–85

57. Gehring B, Mornet E, Plath H et al 1999 Perinatal hypophosphatasia: diagnosis and detection of heterozygote carriers within the family. Clinical Genetics 56: 313–317

58. Gerami S, Richardson R, Harrington B et al 1969 Obstructive emphysema due to mediastinal bronchogenic cysts in infancy. Case report and brief review of literature. Journal of Thoracic and Cardiovascular Surgery 58: 432–436

59. Glenski J A, Thibeault D W, Hall F K et al 1986 Selective bronchial intubation in infants with lobar emphysema: indications, complications, and long-term outcome. American Journal of Perinatology 3: 199–204

60. Golaszewski T, Bettelheim D, Eppel W et al 1998 Cystic adenomatoid malformation of the lung: prenatal diagnosis, prognostic factors and fetal outcome. Gynecologic and Obstetric Investigation 46: 241–246

61. Goldstein J D, Reid L M 1980 Pulmonary hypoplasia resulting from phrenic nerve agenesis and diaphragmatic amyoplasia. Journal of Pediatrics 97: 282–287

62. Granata C, Gambini C, Balducci T et al 1998 Bronchioalveolar carcinoma arising in congenital cystic adenomatoid malformation in a child: a case report and review on malignancies originating in congenital cystic adenomatoid malformation. Pediatric Pulmonology 25: 62–66

63. Greenstone M A, Dewar A, Cole P J 1983 Ciliary dyskinesia with normal ultrastructure. Thorax 38: 875–876

64. Halkic N, Cuenoud P F, Corthesy M E et al 1998 Pulmonary sequestration: a review of 26 cases. European Journal of Cardio-thoracic Surgery 14: 127–133

65. Hang J D, Guo Q Y, Chen C X et al 1996 Imaging approach to the diagnosis of pulmonary sequestration. Acta Radiologica 37: 883–888

66. Hanssens M, Keirse M J, Vankelecom F et al 1991 Fetal and neonatal effects of treatment with angiotensin-converting enzyme inhibitors in pregnancy. Obstetrics and Gynecology 78: 128–135

67. Harrison M R, Adzick N S, Flake A W et al 1996 Correction of congenital diaphragmatic hernia in utero. VIII: Response of the hypoplastic lung to tracheal occlusion. Journal of Pediatric Surgery 31: 1339–1348

68. Harrison M R, Albanese C T, Hawgood S B et al 2001 Fetoscopic temporary tracheal occlusion by means of detachable balloon for congenital diaphragmatic hernia. American Journal of Obstetrics and Gynecology 185: 730–733

69. Harrison M R, Keller R L , Hawgood S B et al 2003 A randomized trial of fetal endoscopic tracheal occlusion for severe fetal congenital diaphragmatic hernia New England Journal of Medicine 349: 1916–1924

70. Harrison M R, Ross N, Noall R et al 1983 Correction of congenital hydronephrosis in utero. I. The model: fetal urethral obstruction produces hydronephrosis and pulmonary hypoplasia in lambs. Journal of Pediatric Surgery 18: 247–256

71. Hislop A, Hey E, Reid L 1979 The lungs in congenital bilateral renal agenesis and dysplasia. Archives of Disease in Childhood 54: 32–38

72. Hubbard A M, Adzick N S, Crombleholme T M et al 1999 Congenital chest lesions: diagnosis and characterization with prenatal MR imaging. Radiology 212: 43–48

73. Huddleston C B, Bloch J B, Sweet S C et al 2002 Lung transplantation in children. Annals of Surgery 236: 270–276

74. Islam S, Masiakos P, Schnitzer J J et al 1999 Diltiazem reduces pulmonary arterial pressures in recurrent pulmonary hypertension associated with pulmonary hypoplasia. Journal of Pediatric Surgery 34: 712–714

75. Janas M S, Arroe M, Hansen S H et al 1998 Lung hypoplasia – a possible teratogenic effect of valproate. Case report. APMIS: Acta Pathologica, Microbiologica, et Immunologica Scandinavica 106: 300–304

76. Kaariainen H, Koskimies O, Norio R 1988 Dominant and recessive polycystic kidney disease in children: evaluation of clinical features and laboratory data. Pediatric Nephrology 2: 296–302

77. Karnak I, Senocak M E, Ciftci A O et al 1999 Congenital lobar emphysema: diagnostic and therapeutic considerations. Journal of Pediatric Surgery 34: 1347–1351

78. Karnes P S, Day D, Berry S A et al 1991 Jarcho-Levin syndrome: four new cases and classification of subtypes. American Journal of Medical Genetics 40: 264–270

79. Kilbride H W, Yeast J, Thibeault D W 1996 Defining limits of survival: lethal pulmonary hypoplasia after midtrimester premature rupture of membranes. American Journal of Obstetrics and Gynecology 175: 675–681

80. Kim W S, Lee K S, Kim I O et al 1997 Congenital cystic adenomatoid malformation of the lung: CT-pathologic correlation. American Journal of Roentgenology 168: 47–53

81. Knowles S, Thomas R M, Lindenbaum R H et al 1988 Pulmonary agenesis as part of the VACTERL sequence. Archives of Disease in Childhood 63: 723–726

82. Kollberg H, Mossberg B, Afzelius B et al 1978 Cystic fibrosis compared with the immotile-cilia syndrome. A study of mucociliary clearance, ciliary ultrastructure, clinical picture and ventilatory function. Scandinavian Journal of Respiratory Disease 59: 297–306

83. Kriegsmann J, Coerdt W, Kommoss F et al 2000 Renal tubular dysgenesis (RTD) – an important cause of the oligohydramnion-sequence. Report of 3 cases and review of the literature. Pathology, Research and Practice 196: 861–865

84. Kuller J A, Yankowitz J, Goldberg J D et al 1992 Outcome of antenatally diagnosed cystic adenomatoid malformations. American Journal of Obstetrics and Gynecology 167: 1038–1041

85. Laberge J M, Flageole H, Pugash D et al 2001 Outcome of prenatally diagnosed congenital cystic adenomatoid lung malformation: a Canadian experience. Fetal Diagnosis and Therapy 16: 178–186

86. Lee A, Kratochwil A, Stumpflen I et al 1996 Fetal lung volume determination by three-dimensional ultrasonography. American Journal of Obstetrics and Gynecology 175: 588–592

87. Lee M L, Tsao L Y, Chaou W T et al 2002 Revisit on congenital bronchopulmonary vascular malformations: a haphazard branching theory of malinosculations and its clinical classification and implication. Pediatric Pulmonology 33: 1–11

88. Lejeune C, Deschildre A, Thumerelle C et al 1999 [Pneumothorax revealing cystic adenomatoid malformation of the lung in a 13 year old child.] Archives de Pediatrie 6: 863–866 (in French)

89. Liechty K W, Crombleholme T M, Quinn T M et al 1999 Elevated platelet-derived growth factor-B in congenital cystic adenomatoid malformations requiring fetal resection. Journal of Pediatric Surgery 34: 805–809

90. Liggins G C, Vilos G A, Campos G A et al 1981 The effect of bilateral thoracoplasty on lung development in fetal sheep. Journal of Developmental Physiology 3: 275–282

91. Lopoo J B, Goldstein R B, Lipshutz G S et al 1999 Fetal pulmonary sequestration: a favourable congenital lung lesion. Obstetrics and Gynaecology 94: 567–571

92. Losa M, Kind C 1998 Dry lung syndrome: complete airway collapse mimicking pulmonary hypoplasia? European Journal of Pediatrics 157: 935–938

93. Lujan M, Bosque M, Mirapeix R M 2002 Late-onset congenital cystic adenomatoid malformation of the lung. Embryology, clinical symptomatology, diagnostic procedures, therapeutic approach and clinical follow-up. Respiration 69: 148–155

94. Macchiarini P, Chapelier A, Vouhe P et al 1994 Double lung transplantation in situs inversus with Kartagener's syndrome. Journal of Thoracic and Cardiovascular Surgery 108: 86–91

95. McIntosh N 1988 Dry lung syndrome after oligohydramnios Archives of Disease in Childhood 63: 190–193

96. MacKenzie T C, Guttenberg M E, Nisenbaum H L et al 2001 A fetal lung lesion consisting of bronchogenic cyst, bronchopulmonary sequestration and congenital cystic adenomatoid malformation: the missing link? Fetal Diagnosis and Therapy 16: 193–195

97. Mahle W T, Rychik J, Tian Z Y et al 2000 Echocardiographic evaluation of the fetus with congenital cystic adenomatoid malformation. Ultrasound in Obstetrics and Gynecology 16: 620–624

98. Maier H C 1948 Bronchogenic cysts of mediastinum. Annals of Surgery 127: 476–502

99. Man D W, Hamdy M H, Hendry G M et al 1983 Congenital lobar emphysema: problems in diagnosis and management. Archives of Disease in Childhood 58: 709–712

100. Martinez-Frias M L, Bermejo E, Urioste M et al 1993 Lethal short rib-polydactyly syndromes: further evidence for their overlapping in a continuous spectrum. Journal of Medical Genetics 30: 937–941

101. Maymon R, Schneider D, Hegesh J et al 2001 Antenatal sonographic findings of right pulmonary agenesis with ipsilateral microtia: a possible new laterality association. Prenatal Diagnosis 21: 125–128

102. Mentzer S J, Filler R M, Phillips J 1992 Limited pulmonary resections for congenital cystic adenomatoid malformation of the lung. Journal of Pediatric Surgery 27: 1410–1413

103. Mezzetti M, Dell'Agnola C A, Bedoni M et al 1996 Video-assisted thoracoscopic resection of pulmonary sequestration in an infant. Annals of Thoracic Surgery 61: 1836–1837

104. Mildenberger E, de Mello D E, Lin Z et al 2001 Focal congenital alveolar proteinosis associated with abnormal surfactant protein B messenger RNA. Chest 119: 645–647

105. Miller K E, Corteville J E, Langer J C 1996 Congenital cystic adenomatoid malformation in the fetus: natural history and predictors of outcome. Journal of Pediatric Surgery 31: 805–808

106. Moerman P, Fryns J P, Goddeeris P et al 1983 Multiple ankyloses, facial anomalies, and pulmonary hypoplasia associated with severe antenatal spinal muscular atrophy. Journal of Pediatrics 103: 238–241

107. Morin L R, Herlicoviez M, Loisel J C et al 1991 Prenatal diagnosis of lethal osteogenesis imperfecta in twin pregnancy. Clinical Genetics 39: 467–470

108. Morotti R A, Cangiarella J, Gutierrez M C et al 1999 Congenital cystic adenomatoid malformation of the lung (CCAM): evaluation of the cellular components. Human Pathology 30: 618–625

109. Nadel H R, Stringer D A, Levinson H et al 1985 The immotile cilia syndrome: radiological manifestations. Radiology 154: 651–655

110. Nakayama D K, Glick P L, Harrison M R et al 1983 Experimental pulmonary hypoplasia due to oligohydramnios and its reversal by relieving thoracic compression. Journal of Pediatric Surgery 18: 347–353

111. Neilson I R, Russo P, Laberge J M et al 1991 Congenital adenomatoid malformation of the lung: current management and prognosis. Journal of Pediatric Surgery 26: 975–980

112. Newbould M J, Lendon M, Barson A J 1994 Oligohydramnios sequence: the spectrum of renal malformations. British Journal of Obstetrics and Gynaecology 101: 598–604

113. Newman B, Kuhn J P, Kramer S S et al 2001 Congenital surfactant protein B deficiency – emphasis on imaging. Pediatric Radiology 31: 327–331

114. Njinimbam C G, Hebra A, Kicklighter S D et al 1999 Persistent pulmonary hypertension in a neonate with cystic adenomatoid malformation of the lung following lobectomy: survival with prolonged extracorporeal membrane oxygenation therapy. Journal of Perinatology 19: 64–67

115. Nogee L M, de Mello D E, Dehner L P et al 1993 Brief report: deficiency of pulmonary surfactant protein B in congenital alveolar proteinosis. New England Journal of Medicine 328: 406–410

116. Noonan J A, Walters L R, Reeves J T 1970 Congenital pulmonary lymphangiectasis. American Journal of Diseases of Children 120: 314–319

117. Oberklaid F, Danks D M, Mayne V et al 1977 Asphyxiating thoracic dysplasia. Clinical, radiological and pathological information on 10 patients. Archives of Disease in Childhood 52: 758–765

118. Olutoye O O, Coleman B G, Hubbard A M et al 2000 Prenatal diagnosis and management of congenital lobar emphysema. Journal of Pediatric Surgery 35: 792–795

119. O'Malley B P, Parker R, Saphyakhajon P et al 1972 Thanatophoric dwarfism. Journal of the Canadian Association of Radiologists 23: 62–68

120. Osborne J, Masel J, McCredie J 1989 A spectrum of skeletal anomalies associated with pulmonary agenesis: possible neural crest injuries. Pediatric Radiology 19: 425–432

121. Ostor A G, Fortune D W 1978 Congenital cystic adenomatoid malformation of the lung. American Journal of Clinical Pathology 70: 595–604

122. Ozcan C, Celik A, Ural Z et al 2001 Primary pulmonary rhabdomyosarcoma arising within cystic adenomatoid malformation: a case report and review of the literature. Journal of Pediatric Surgery 36: 1062–1065

123. Papagiannopoulos K A, Sheppard M, Bush A P et al 2001 Pleuropulmonary blastoma: is prophylactic resection of congenital lung cysts effective? Annals of Thoracic Surgery 72: 604–605

124. Parilla B V, Leeth E A, Kambich M P et al 2003 Antenatal detection of skeletal dysplasias. Journal of Ultrasound in Medicine 22: 255–258

125. Phillipos E Z, Libsekal K 1998 Flexible bronchoscopy in the management of congenital lobar emphysema in the neonate. Canadian Respiratory Journal 5: 219–221

126. Potter E L 1946 Bilateral renal agenesis. Journal of Pediatrics 29: 68–76

127. Potter E L 1952 Pulmonary pathology of the fetus and the newborn. In: Advances in pediatrics, Vol. IV. Year Book Medical Publishers, Chicago

128. Raynor A C, Capp M P, Sealy W C 1967 Lobar emphysema of infancy: diagnosis, treatment and etiological aspects. Annals of Thoracic Surgery 4: 374–385

129. Rescorla F J, West K W, Vane D W et al 1990 Pulmonary hypertension in neonatal cystic lung disease: survival following lobectomy and ECMO in two cases. Journal of Pediatric Surgery 25: 1054–1056

130. Rettwitz-Volk W, Schlosser R, Ahrens P et al 1999 Congenital unilobar pulmonary lymphangiectasis. Pediatric Pulmonology 27: 290–292

131. Ribet M E, Copin M C, Gosselin B H 1996 Bronchogenic cysts of the lung. Annals of Thoracic Surgery 61: 1636–1640

132. Roberts P A, Holland A J, Halliday R J et al 2002 Congenital lobar emphysema: like father, like son. Journal of Pediatric Surgery 37: 799–801

133. Roguin N, Peleg H, Lemer J et al 1980 The value of cardiac catheterization and cineangiography in infantile lobar emphysema. Pediatric Radiology 10: 71–74

134. Rothenberg S S 2000 Thoracoscopic lung resection in children. Journal of Pediatric Surgery 35: 271–274

135. Rotschild A, Ling E W, Wensley D F et al 1994 Unilateral cervical spinal cord lesion in a term newborn associated with ipsilateral diaphragmatic atrophy and pulmonary hypoplasia. Pediatric Pulmonology 18: 53–57

136. Rutledge J C, Jensen P 1986 Acinar dysplasia: a new form of pulmonary maldevelopment. Human Pathology 17: 1290–1293

137. Sapin E, Lejeune V, Barbet J P et al 1997 Congenital adenomatoid disease of the lung: prenatal diagnosis and perinatal management. Pediatric Surgery International 12: 126–129

138. Savic B, Birtel F J, Tholen W et al 1979 Lung sequestration: report of seven cases and review of 540 published cases. Thorax 34: 96–101

139. Senyuz O F, Danismend N, Erdogan E et al 1989 Congenital lobar emphysema – a report of 5 cases. Japanese Journal of Surgery 19: 764–767

140. Spranger J, Langen L O, Maroteaux P 1970 Increasing frequency of a syndrome of multiple osseous defects? Lancet 2: 716

141. Stigers K B, Woodring J H, Kanga J F 1992 The clinical and imaging spectrum of findings in patients with congenital lobar emphysema. Pediatric Pulmonology 14: 160–170

142. Stocker J T, Drake R M, Madewell J E 1978 Cystic and congenital lung disease in the newborn. Perspectives in Pediatric Pathology 4: 93–154

143. Sturgess J M, Thompson M W, Czegledy-Nady E et al 1986 Genetic aspects of immotile cilia syndrome. American Journal of Medical Genetics 25: 149–160

144. Szaflik K, Kozarzewski M, Adamczewski D 1998 Fetal bladder catheterization in severe obstructive uropathy before the 24th week of pregnancy. Fetal Diagnosis and Therapy 13: 133–135

145. Thakral C L, Maji D C, Sajwani M J 2001 Congenital lobar emphysema: experience with 21 cases. Pediatric Surgery International 17: 88–91

146. Thomas R J, Lathif H C, Sen S et al 1998 Varied presentations of unilateral lung hypoplasia and agenesis: a report of four cases. Pediatric Surgery International 14: 94–95

147. Thompson A J, Reid A J, Reid M 2000 Congenital lobar emphysema occurring in twins. Journal of Perinatal Medicine 28: 155–157

148. Thompson J, Forfar J O 1958 Regional obstructive emphysema in infancy. Archives of Disease in Childhood 33: 97–102

149. Thompson P J, Greenough A, Blott M et al 1990 Chronic respiratory morbidity following PROM. Archives of Disease in Childhood 65: 878–880

150. Thompson P J, Greenough A, Dykes E et al 1993 Impaired respiratory function in infants with anterior abdominal wall defects. Journal of Pediatric Surgery 28: 664–666

151. Thompson P J, Greenough A, Nicolaides K H 1992 Lung volume measured by functional residual capacity in infants following first trimester amniocentesis or chorion villus sampling. British Journal of Obstetrics and Gynaecology 99: 479–482

152. Thompson P J, Greenough A, Nicolaides K H 1993 Respiratory function in infancy following pleuro-amniotic shunting. Fetal Diagnosis and Therapy 8: 79–83

153. Thorpe-Beeston J G, Nicolaides K H 1994 Cystic adenomatoid malformation of the lung: prenatal diagnosis and outcome. Prenatal Diagnosis 14: 677–688

154. Todd D W, Tinguely S J, Norberg W J 1986 A thoracic expansion technique for Jeune's asphyxiating thoracic dystrophy. Journal of Pediatric Surgery 21: 161–163

155. van Leeuwen K, Teitelbaum D H, Hirschl R B et al 1999 Prenatal diagnosis of congenital cystic adenomatoid malformation and its postnatal presentation, surgical indications, and natural history. Journal of Pediatric Surgery 34: 794–798

156. Van Raemdonck D, De Boeck K, Devlieger H et al 2001 Pulmonary sequestration: a comparison between pediatric and adult patients. European Journal of Cardio-thoracic Surgery 19: 388–395

157. Vergani P, Locatelli A, Strobelt N 1997 Amnioinfusion for the prevention of pulmonary hypoplasia in second-trimester rupture of membranes. American Journal of Perinatology 14: 325–329

158. Vilos G A, McLeod W J, Carmichael L et al 1984 Absence or impaired response of fetal breathing to intravenous glucose is associated with pulmonary hypoplasia in congenital myotonic dystrophy. American Journal of Obstetrics and Gynecology 148: 558–562

159. Vyas H, Milner A D, Hopkin I E 1982 Amniocentesis and fetal lung development. Archives of Disease in Childhood 57: 627–628

160. Waszak P, Claris O, Lapillonne A et al 1999 Cystic adenomatoid malformation of the lung: neonatal management of 21 cases. Pediatric Surgery International 15: 326–331

161. Weinbaum P J, Bors-Koefoed R, Green K W et al 1989 Antenatal sonographic findings in a case of intra-abdominal pulmonary sequestration. Obstetrics and Gynecology 73: 860–862

162. Whitelaw A, Evans A, Corrin B 1981 Immotile cilia syndrome: a new cause of neonatal respiratory distress. Archives of Disease in Childhood 56: 432–435

163. Williams A J, Vawter G, Reid L M 1984 Lung structure in asphyxiating thoracic dystrophy. Archives of Pathology and Laboratory Medicine 108: 658–661

164. Winn H N, Chen M, Amon E et al 2000 Neonatal pulmonary hypoplasia and perinatal mortality in patients with midtrimester rupture of amniotic membranes – a critical analysis. American Journal of Obstetrics and Gynecology 182: 1638–1644

165. Yoshimura S, Masuzaki H, Miura K et al 1999 Diagnosis of fetal pulmonary hypoplasia by measurement of blood flow velocity waveforms of pulmonary arteries with Doppler ultrasonography. American Journal of Obstetrics and Gynecology 180: 441–446

PART 6

Diaphragmatic hernia

Mark Davenport

Introduction

A number of diaphragmatic abnormalities may present with respiratory problems during infancy, the most common being a posterolateral congenital diaphragmatic hernia (CDH). This is usually associated with severe lung hypoplasia, and, despite many advances in its management, still has a high mortality. Anterior diaphragmatic hernias are smaller and tend to present later in infancy, often with gastrointestinal symptoms alone. Eventration of the diaphragm is a condition in which the cupola becomes thinned, stretched and immobile but yet is still intact. Some degree of respiratory impairment is seen in most of these cases.

Congenital posterolateral diaphragmatic hernia

In 1848, the Czech anatomist Vincent Bochdalek described bowel herniation through the posterior part of the diaphragm, attributing it to the effects of an inverted fetus and rupture of the lumbocostal membrane.[10] Although such posterolateral hernias are still widely known by the eponym Bochdalek's hernia, he was certainly not the first to describe this type of diaphragmatic defect. Detailed reports of CDH in both children[47] and adults[13] had been published previously.

The embryological development of the diaphragm is complex (p. 594): its mesenchyme is derived from the septum transversum and the dorsal mesentery of the oesophagus, and its muscular component from the innermost muscle layer of the thoracic cage and descending cervical myoblasts.[57] The nerve supply to this muscle is via the phrenic nerve (C3–5). There is a communication between the pleural and the peritoneal cavities (the pleuroperitoneal canal) up to the 8th week of gestation.

The orthodox hypothesis of the aetiology of CDH ascribes intestinal herniation to a failure to close completely the initially patent pleuroperitoneal canal. There is then visceral migration into the hemithorax and interference with the developing lung bud. This herniation would therefore occur during the late embryonic period at 8–10 weeks' gestation.

An important alternative hypothesis has also been advanced more recently, which suggests that the primary defect is that of lung hypoplasia. Thus it has been suggested that the pleuroperitoneal canals are actually too small to accommodate even a single loop of bowel[56] and that the diaphragmatic defect occurs in the posterior mesenchymal part of the nascent diaphragm rather than the pleuroperitoneal canal.[48] Such studies also suggest that the defect therefore occurs earlier and equivalent to about 5 weeks' gestation, i.e. within the early embryonic period.

Most recent studies investigating causative factors in CDH have used animal models. These can be divided into surgically created diaphragmatic hernias in large animals (typically sheep) during the latter stages of gestation[51,75] and those resulting from exposure of small animals (typically rats and mice) to teratogens, such as the pesticide Nitrofen, during the early stages of gestation.[48,55,57,61]

Anatomy and pathophysiology (Fig. 27.56)

The diaphragmatic defect occurs in the posterolateral segment, although it may range from a simple muscular slit to complete agenesis.[90] Left-sided hernias account for about 80% of most series.[21,35,79,89] Bilateral CDHs occur rarely and are associated with an awful prognosis.[8,17] In left-sided hernias, the hemithorax contains herniated bowel, stomach, spleen, and often part of the left lobe of the liver. The herniated bowel is inevitably malrotated because of its abnormal development, although consequent duodenal obstruction is uncommon. A thin, almost translucent hernial sac

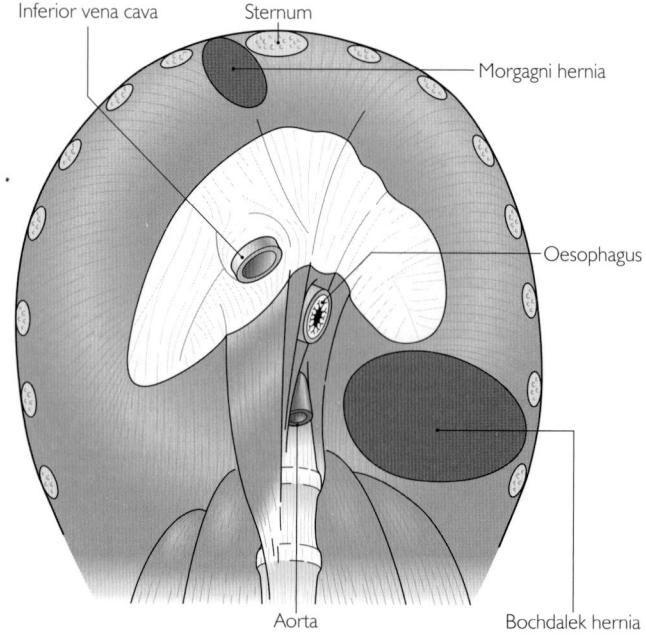

Fig. 27.56 Schematic illustration of the anatomy of congenital diaphragmatic hernia: posterolateral hernia of Bochdalek and anterior hernia of Morgagni.

occurs in about 20% of cases. Right-sided hernias usually contain the right lobe of the liver, and because of its volume, this tends to plug the defect and may minimise herniation of other viscera.

Some degree of lung hypoplasia occurs with virtually all diaphragmatic hernias[18] (pp. 583–4). This is most obvious on the ipsilateral side, where perhaps only a nubbin of tissue might remain, but is also seen on the contralateral side. Compared with normal term lungs, there is an absolute decrease in lung weight and volume and a decrease in compliance. The number of bronchial generations is reduced and true alveoli, which should start to be seen by 34 weeks' gestation, are uncommon. Most terminal air spaces are therefore still in the saccular phase of development. Along with an absolute decrease in lung tissue, there is a reduction in the total number of preacinar pulmonary vessels, although the ratio of capillaries per alveolus is retained. The pulmonary and intra-acinar arteries have an abnormally high smooth muscle content, although it is unclear why this should be so. There is increased expression of endothelin-1 (ET-1), a potent vasoconstrictor, and its receptors (ET_A and ET_B) in such arterioles and this may be one molecular explanation for the frequency of persistent pulmonary hypertension of the newborn (PPHN) in CDH.[72] There may be also changes in the developing cardiovascular system. For instance, the left ventricle and interventricular septum have been shown to be smaller both in CDH cases compared with age-matched human controls[86] and in the experimental CDH lamb model.[51] There is also some experimental evidence that the heart tissue is less mature in CDH, with a diminution of the proportion of cardiac extracellular matrix and hence greater myocardial 'stiffness' compared with controls.[37] However, cardiac anomalies may simply be due to direct compression by herniated viscera, as right-sided hernias have been shown to cause diminution of the right rather than the left ventricle.

The pathophysiological sequence that explains some of the clinical features of a CDH is illustrated in Fig. 27.57. There is also an exaggerated response of the abnormally muscularised arterial resistance vessels to hypoxia, acidosis and hypercarbia, which causes in turn pulmonary hypertension and shunting of blood at several different levels from the right to the left side of the heart – PPHN (pp. 496–502).

Demography

The prevalence of CDH at birth has been estimated to be from 1 in 2000 to 1 in 5000, and does not appear to have any predilection for race or geographical area.[17,78,93] The sex ratio is equal, although right-sided defects may be more common in males.[8] Although most CDHs are sporadic, with no known cause, there may be a genetic component in a small number, as there are reports of CDH in twins and families.[24,65]

Associations

Although CDH was once thought of as an isolated anomaly, more accurate studies (which include stillbirths and intrauterine deaths) and the advent of widespread prenatal ultrasound have shown this to be incorrect.[8,39,89,93] About 30–50% of diagnosed fetuses will have a further anomaly,[93] although, because of intrauterine deaths, terminations and stillbirths, this falls to about 20–30% in liveborn infants.

Various anomalies may be found, including chromosomal anomalies (e.g. Turner syndrome and trisomies 13, 18 and 21), major central nervous system malformations (e.g. anencephaly, neural tube defects) and most types of congenital cardiac defects (e.g. ventricular septal defect, aortic coarctation, tetralogy of Fallot, hypoplastic left heart and transposition of the great vessels).[8,39,93] Similarly, there is also a wide range of renal anomalies (e.g. agenesis and hydronephrosis) and, in males, undescended testes.[8] Other anomalies less easy to classify include foregut duplication cysts and pulmonary sequestrations.

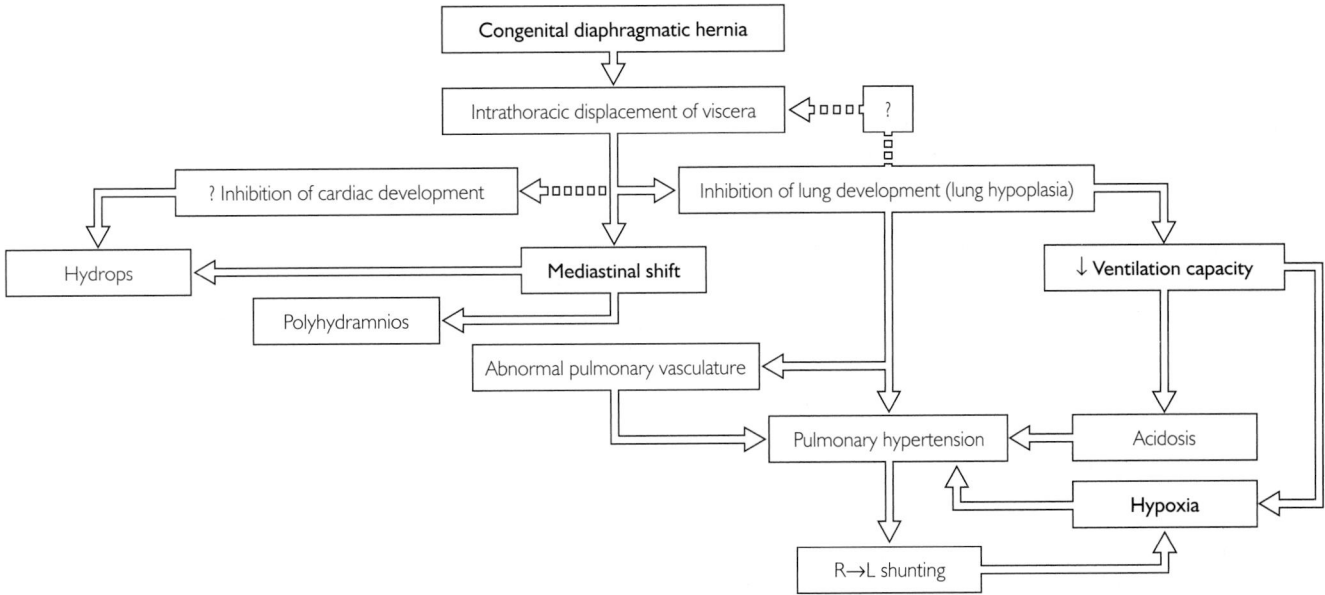

Fig. 27.57 Pathophysiology of congenital diaphragmatic hernia. Pulmonary hypertension, right–left shunting and hypoxia are the characteristic features of persistent pulmonary hypertension of the newborn.

Fryns syndrome is characterised by a diaphragmatic hernia in an infant with an abnormal facies, distal limb anomalies, undescended testes in males and various gut and genitourinary anomalies.[31,60]

Clinical features

Antenatal ultrasound diagnosis of a diaphragmatic hernia has been possible for well over two decades now.[24] The specific features include bowel loops, and liver or, more usually, stomach seen in the transverse four-chamber view within the thorax. Secondary features include mediastinal shift, hydrops fetalis and, most commonly, polyhydramnios. Right-sided defects are more difficult to diagnose, as the herniated fetal liver has a similar echogenicity to fetal lung.

The typical postnatal presentation is of increasing respiratory distress and cyanosis shortly after birth in a term infant. There are decreased breath sounds and air entry on the side of the hernia, with a shift of the trachea and cardiac impulse to the opposite side. The abdomen has a flat or even scaphoid appearance, as much of the viscera have already been displaced to the chest cavity.

A chest X-ray (CXR) is diagnostic in most infants and will show air-filled loops of bowel within the hemithorax, often with severe mediastinal displacement (Fig. 27.58). Occasionally there may be confusion with the radiographic appearance of a cystic adenomatoid malformation of the lung, which may also present with respiratory distress. This can be distinguished on the plain film by noting the normal abdominal gas pattern and diaphragmatic integrity, or more accurately by introducing radio-opaque contrast material into the stomach and proximal gastrointestinal tract (Fig. 27.59). An ultrasound scan can also differentiate these conditions. Occasionally, air does not enter the proximal bowel because of rapid intubation and resuscitation in the delivery room, especially if there has been an antenatal diagnosis. The usual radiographic appearance is then of complete opacification on the side of the hernia – a 'whiteout' (Fig. 27.60).

About 5% of infants with CDH will present beyond the first 24 hours of life, with failure to thrive, recurrent chest infections, a pleural effusion, or even as an incidental finding on a CXR.[63] It is important to note that a previously normal CXR does not exclude a CDH. There is an interesting association between the delayed presentation of a right-sided diaphragmatic hernia and group B streptococcal septicaemia.[5,77] Such infants present with respiratory distress and opacification of the right lung. Visceral herniation only occurs in the recovery phase of the illness, being diagnosed on a CXR or by computed tomography (CT).

Management

Antenatal

An increasing proportion of infants with CDH are diagnosed in utero by screening ultrasonography during the second trimester. An amniocentesis should be offered: if a chromosomal anomaly is found, most obstetricians would recommend termination, as this is an invariably lethal combination.

It is important that these infants are delivered in regional centres where there are the necessary obstetric, intensive care and neonatal surgical facilities. In our centre, we tend to induce vaginal delivery at about 38 weeks' gestation to minimise the risks of unintended early labour and delivery in a peripheral unit.

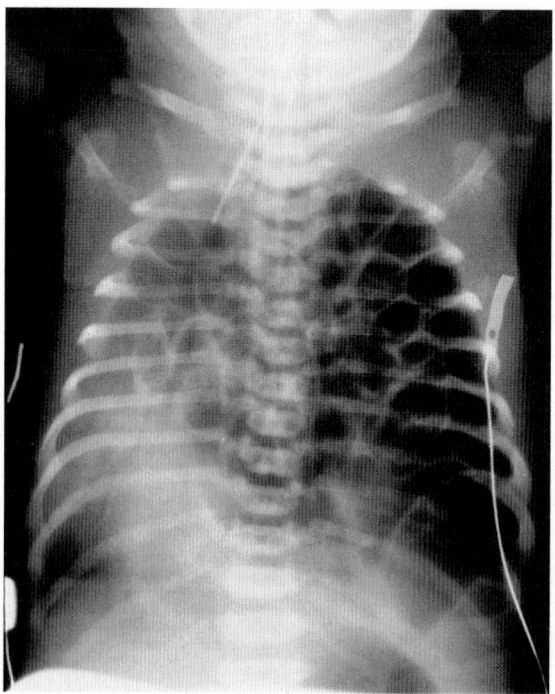

Fig. 27.58 Chest radiograph of infant at 1 hour of life, showing left diaphragmatic hernia, displacement of air-filled viscera into the hemithorax, and a marked shift of mediastinum and heart.

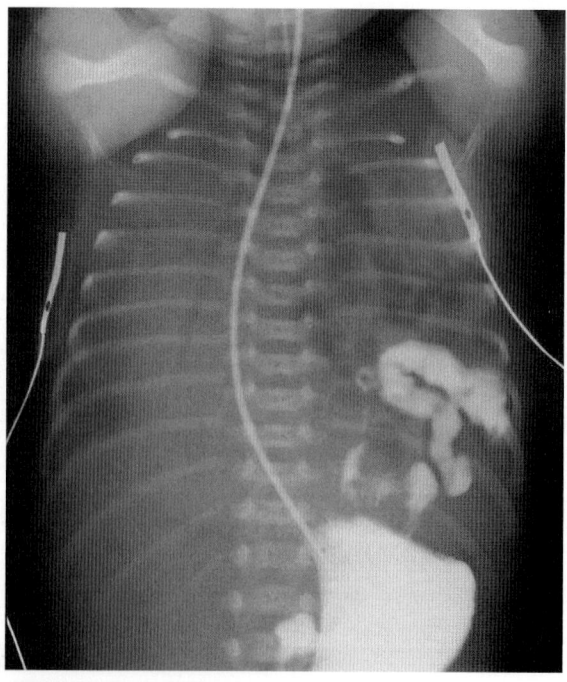

Fig. 27.59 Chest radiograph of infant with contrast medium in the stomach and small intestine, the latter lying within the left hemithorax.

In the UK and USA, innovative antenatal intervention techniques such as tracheal plugging or tracheal ligation are only offered as part of a research programme. Such techniques are discussed later.

Medical

Infants with CDH presenting within 24 hours of birth are at a considerable risk of death and should be endotracheally intubated, paralysed and ventilated. Prolonged attempts at bagging using a facemask can be dangerous and should be avoided, specifically because of the detrimental effects of intestinal distension. A large-bore nasogastric tube (e.g. 8 French gauge) should also be passed to decompress the stomach and small bowel. Neonatal resuscitation should then proceed on conventional lines. Initially, the main problem is hypoventilation due to lung hypoplasia, and there will be a proportion of infants in whom this is so extreme as to be incompatible with life, and who will die in the delivery room. Initial peak inflation pressures should be limited to 25 cmH$_2$O (to reduce barotrauma in small, stiff lungs), with rates of 60–80 per minute. Positive end-expiratory pressure is kept low to achieve maximum alveolar ventilation. In our institution, infants are paralysed (e.g. vecuronium 0.1–1.3 mg/kg/h) and have analgesia (e.g. fentanyl 2–8 mg/kg/h), although others

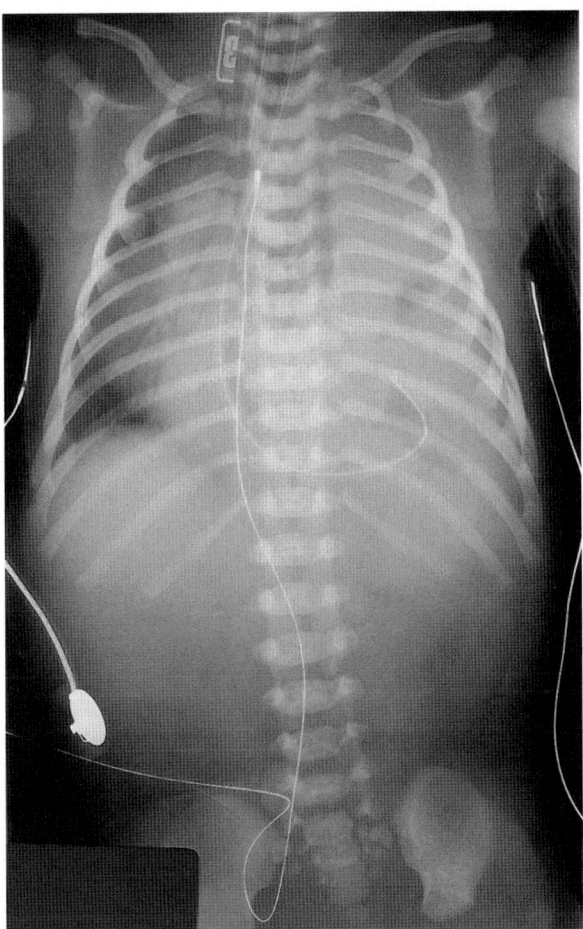

Fig. 27.60 Chest radiograph of early appearance of diaphragmatic hernia, with a 'whiteout' on the left side.

argue that spontaneous breathing without relaxants may be preferable.[12]

Most infants will respond to medical measures and achieve acceptable blood gases. This has been described as the 'honeymoon' phase, as these infants can be deceptively well for a period before becoming increasingly unstable, often with severe hypoxic episodes, hypercarbia and an uncorrectable acidosis. The dominant pathophysiological problem in this phase is pulmonary hypertension and right-to-left shunting. Such PPHN can be diagnosed clinically by the typical rapid swings in oxygenation, and confirmed by measuring pre- and postductal arterial oxygen levels. Echocardiography during this period will show an enlarged right heart with pulmonary and tricuspid regurgitation and a right – left shunt at the foramen ovale and ductus arteriosus.

Newer ventilation techniques, such as high-frequency oscillatory ventilation and high-frequency jet ventilation, have been used in infants with diaphragmatic hernia.[14,52] Although no particular type of ventilation or ventilator has been shown to be better than another, a consistent trend has been to apply 'gentle ventilation' to these infants[12] – that is, to avoid the risks of barotrauma by limiting use of high peak inspiratory pressures and accepting higher levels of CO$_2$ (permissive hypercapnea). There is also a range of pharmacological agents which have been used to treat the PPHN associated with a CDH, including tolazoline,[88] prostacyclin,[15] nitroprusside, diltiazem,[49] and, most recently, nitric oxide.[30,54] These options are discussed fully on pages 499–502. There is also a functional surfactant deficit in infants with CDH, and benefit has been shown from using exogenous surfactant both in experimental models and when administered to high-risk neonates prior to the first breath.[33,34]

Surgical

Nowadays there is no role for early (within 24 hours of birth) surgical repair. Abdominal replacement of the viscera and repair of the hernial defect causes a marked reduction in lung compliance and detrimental fluid shifts,[81] and should therefore be carried out only when the infant has achieved a period of cardiorespiratory stability (of at least 24 hours) with acceptable blood gases on conventional ventilation (e.g. F$_I$O$_2$ < 0.5, PO_2 > 8 kPa [60 mmHg]).[21]

European paediatric surgical centres were the first to delay surgical repair, during the early 1980s,[15,20,21,83] and this now seems to be prevalent in most other centres.[58,71] Although early reports did not show a clear survival advantage, probably because of the small numbers involved, they did show that the concept was not harmful. The largest single-centre experience with delayed surgery was reported from Manchester, where 86 high-risk infants had a survival rate of just over 70%.[21]

The surgical repair of a CDH is performed through a subcostal incision. The displaced viscera are removed from the hemithorax and returned to the abdomen. A hernial sac, if found, should be excised to allow a tension-free musculoaponeurotic closure. The posterior margin of the defect may not be apparent initially and most have to be developed from the posterior abdominal wall. Primary closure is possible in about 75% of cases, but in those where this is impossible because of excessive tension or agenesis, other techniques have to be used. A patch of artificial material or a rotation flap from an adjacent muscle group can be used to repair the defect.[9] A chest tube left in the empty hemithorax is not necessary, and may be dangerous if used with suction, as the hypoplastic lung may overexpand and rupture.

The role of extracorporeal membrane oxygenation

Extracorporeal membrane oxygenation (ECMO) is now an option for infants with CDH if conventional methods of medical therapy are failing. The concept behind this technique is simple: near-total cardiopulmonary support for a prolonged period of time (in practice, up to 10–14 days). ECMO was developed in the USA in the 1970s,[32] but has only recently become available in the UK because of the perceived lack of controlled data from its early trials.[6,73] Unfortunately, even the UK Collaborative ECMO trial[91] failed to recruit enough infants in the CDH subgroup for the differences in survival to be statistically significant. The North American ECMO experience suggests that a survival rate of about 40–60% will be found in infants with CDH, which is significantly worse than that achieved when ECMO is offered for other indications in neonates (e.g. meconium aspiration syndrome, pp. 502–8).[44,45,58,84]

The indications,[58,70] technique[6] and morbidity[68] associated with ECMO are fully discussed elsewhere (pp. 528–9, 781–2). Surgical repair of the hernia may be performed while on ECMO but should probably be deferred until the infant has improved enough to be almost ready for decannulation and cessation of heparinisation.[96]

Prediction of prognosis

It is logical to try and find specific or measurable features which will predict outcome in diaphragmatic hernia, because of the high mortality of this disease and the range of possible treatment options. A number of studies have assessed various factors as being of prognostic value, and can be divided into antenatal and postnatal.

Antenatal

Sebire et al reported a difference in outcome of CDH detectable as early as 10–14 weeks' gestation, on the basis of the ultrasound-measured nuchal translucency, with higher values predicting a poor prognosis. It seems that the earlier the diagnosis is made antenatally, the worse the outcome.[82] For instance, only 42% survived from a cohort of 83 fetuses with isolated CDH diagnosed before 24 weeks' gestation, compared with all of a cohort of 10 fetuses diagnosed after 24 weeks.[39] The development of polyhydramnios has also been a poor prognostic feature in some series,[3] although not in others.[25,85] The fetal stomach is found in the chest in most cases, but if it is found within the abdomen this seems to be a good prognostic feature.[25] The position of the fetal liver also seems to be important in that those with a significant (i.e. ultrasonically detectable) portion within the hemithorax have a poorer prognosis.[4] Various attempts have been made to estimate lung hypoplasia antenatally. Latterly, this has been refined into the calculation of a lung-to-head ratio (LHR), where

a ratio of <1 has an extremely poor prognosis,[62] and, by implication, requires antenatal intervention.

Associated congenital cardiac anomalies are, of course, indicative of a very poor outcome,[87,89] but a number of groups have also looked at echocardiographic features of the fetal heart as a measure of lung hypoplasia or pulmonary vascular anomalies. The ratio of left-to-right ventricular internal measurements[25,85] and the ratio of aortic-to-pulmonary artery diameters[25] have been put forward as valuable prognostic features in isolated diaphragmatic hernias. Both these indices reflect left ventricular underdevelopment.

Postnatal

For those infants who are not diagnosed antenatally, the age at presentation is important. The minority who present after 24 hours of life should have the prospect of a 100% survival. The earlier the symptoms, the worse the outcome. Survival is also worse in premature infants and those of low birthweight.[36,46]

Achieving normal blood gases is the final result of an effective pulmonary system, and the degree to which this is successful has been used as a prognostic factor. Initially, this is apparent clinically in the Apgar score. Skari et al recently reported on a multicentre cohort from Scandinavia (n = 157 high-risk early presenters), where there was significant association of mortality with low 1- and 5-minute Apgar scores.[87] Similarly, if a postductal $PaCO_2$ of <5.5 kPa (40 mmHg)[10] or a postductal PaO_2 of >13 kPa (100 mmHg)[74,98] can be achieved with conventional ventilation, this too suggests adequate lung tissue for survival and a good prognosis. In one series there was a survival of 91% in those infants who had achieved a postductal PaO_2 of >13 kPa (100 mmHg), compared with only 7% survival in those who did not.[98] The amount of ventilation required to achieve such blood gases can also be incorporated into a variety of ventilation indices (Table 27.16).[11,44,94,98]

At present it is not possible to measure the critical lung mass in neonates directly, although there have been attempts to measure some indirect indices of lung function (e.g. compliance and functional residual capacity [FRC]) early in the postnatal period in these infants.[28,29,53,81] Such studies have shown that day 1 compliance rather than FRC has a predictive relationship to outcome. Serial studies showed that, in survivors, only compliance increased over the first 2 weeks, FRC remaining constant.[53] Of course, measurement of lung volumes remains confined to specialist centres, but there has been some recent work on the predictive value of simply the CXR. Thus, Dimitriou et al have shown that there is a reasonable correlation (r = 0.51) between measured lung volume and computer-assisted measurement of lung area.[29] However, measured lung areas had predictive value

Table 27.16 Indices of ventilation

oxygenation index (OI) =

$$\frac{mean\ airway\ pressure\ (cmH_2O) \times F_IO_2 \times 100}{PaO_2\ (mmHg)}$$

ventilation index (VI) = respiratory rate (bpm)
× mean airway pressure (cmH_2O)

in postoperative infants only, not in preoperative infants, again similar to the findings for lung volumes.[53]

Echocardiography has been used to assess the degree of PPHN.[42,43] Some echocardiographic variables may also have value when performed sequentially, to show the improvement in pulmonary vascular stability and, perhaps, the most appropriate physiological time for surgery.[79]

The size of the diaphragm defect itself has been related to prognosis. Diaphragmatic agenesis[58,90] particularly, and all those where a patch is needed to repair the defect,[94] have been associated with a poorer outcome.

Outcome in congenital diaphragmatic hernia

No surgical series of diaphragmatic hernias has ever been able to emulate Robert Gross's first report of 100% survival in seven infants and children in 1946.[36] This paradox is, of course, entirely due to preselection, as only the less affected infants used to survive to reach paediatric surgical centres. Table 27.17 illustrates recent survival statistics from a number of different centres throughout the world.

Surviving infants have usually required a prolonged stay in intensive care, often with periods of hypoxia, hypercarbia and acidosis. Although early studies suggested that long-term complications in survivors were minimal, this was probably because of selection of a smaller but 'better-quality' cohort. Currently, more marginal survival is possible and the incidence of long-term problems is higher.[69]

Pulmonary function

Dramatic changes occur in lung structure after surgical repair, although not immediately. Lung weight and volumes do increase measurably after about 3 weeks. Sakai et al suggested that there was decrease in compliance in the early postoperative period,[81] although this has been disputed by more recent work,[53] perhaps because of variation in the timing of surgery. Histologically there is an increase in the number of alveoli, and a decrease in muscularisation of the interacinar arteries, although there is no actual change in bronchiolar airway generation.[7] The radiographic appearance of the chest does return to normal, although there are persisting anomalies in tested lung function (typically FEV_1 and FVC).[22] The progressive improvement in ventilation can be assessed using ventilation-perfusion scans, and such studies show particularly a long-term persistence of ipsilateral perfusion defects.[50]

Gastrointestinal function

The principal gastrointestinal problem is one of acid reflux caused by distortion of the gastro-oesophageal junction and crura; this may occur in up to 40% of survivors.[58] This may be manifest by vomiting and feeding difficulties, and can prolong respiratory morbidity, presumably due to recurrent aspiration. Twenty-four-hour intra-oesophageal pH measurement should be performed in all survivors where reflux is thought possible. Intensive medical treatment (e.g. antacids, H_2 receptor blockers, proton-pump blockers and prokinetic agents) should be tried, although, because of the anatomical basis for reflux, surgical correction (e.g. a Nissen antireflux procedure) may be necessary.

Neurological

There is a long-term worry of neurological impairment in survivors, which is presumed to be due to neonatal hypoxia and periods of cardiovascular instability. One study of selected high-risk long-term survivors found a major neurological handicap in two of 23 children, although there was no clear relationship

Table 27.17 Surgical outcome in infants with high-risk congenital diaphragmatic hernia

Series	n	Period	Treatment	Survival (%)
Heiss et al[44]	16	1974–1981	–	50
(Ann Arbor, USA)	34	1982–1987	ECMO	76
Charlton et al[21]	56	1976–1983	Immediate repair	55
(Manchester, UK)	86	1983–1989	Delayed repair	71
Goh et al[35]	69	1987–1990	Delayed repair	66
(London, UK)				
West et al[94]	65	1975–1987	–	43
(Indianapolis, USA)	46	1987–1992	ECMO & delayed repair	67
Bos et al[15]	46	1986–1989	Delayed repair	43
(Rotterdam, Holland)				
Skari et al[87]	157	1995–1998	Delayed repair & ECMO	65
(Scandinavian Multicentre)				
CDHSG*[23]	632	1995–1997	ECMO	53 (with ECMO)
(USA multicentre)				77 (no ECMO)
Boloker et al[12]	120	1992–2000	Delayed repair ECMO (13%)	76 overall
(New York, USA)			'gentle ventilation'	(62 with ECMO)

*Congenital Diaphragmatic Hernia Study Group

between poor outcome and measured indices of hypoxia and acidosis during the neonatal period.[26]

Innovations in therapy

Antenatal surgery

The realisation that most of the mortality associated with CDH is due to PPHN and lung hypoplasia and that these problems are ingrained by the time of birth has led to attempts to modify and, if possible, reverse the pulmonary pathology by various forms of antenatal manipulation.

The simplest concept is, of course, to repair the hernia completely in the fetus at some point following antenatal diagnosis and then return the fetus to complete its in-utero maturation. This approach was initiated and developed at the Fetal Treatment Center at the University of California, San Francisco.[1,40] In one report of its experience between 1989 and 1991, 61 antenatally diagnosed fetuses were referred for consideration of surgery.[40] Second-trimester surgery was attempted in 14 fetuses. Of these, five died during the operation; a further three died in utero shortly after closure of the hysterotomy, and two were born prematurely but died. Only four survived to term and eventually to leave hospital. The technical problems of intrauterine surgery and repair of a CDH are formidable and in humans there is a high risk of inducing preterm labour and obviating any pulmonary benefit from early intervention. Open fetal repair of CDH has now been discontinued in all centres.

A rather more elegant technique of antenatal therapy has been developed to achieve the same aim of in-utero reversal of pulmonary pathology. Thus, intrauterine tracheal occlusion, otherwise known by its acronym PLUG (plug the lung until it grows),[1,41,46] rose from the clinical observation that the lungs in congenital laryngeal atresia are grossly hyperplastic and even cause inversion of the domes of the diaphragm – the very opposite to the lungs in CDH.[95] Such pulmonary hyperplasia arises because fetal lungs are net fluid producers beyond the mid-gestational point, and occlusion therefore results in lung fluid retention and hence expansion. Experimental ligation of the trachea, mimicking laryngeal atresia, has been studied in a variety of animal models of diaphragmatic hernia[2,16,46,55,75] and lung hypoplasia.[97] There is reasonable experimental evidence to suggest that increase in lung mass, acceleration of lung growth and normalisation of abnormal pulmonary vasculature can occur, although it may be detrimental to the type II pneumocyte, causing a decrease in both their number and function.[75] There is, however, some evidence that a period of 'unplugging' towards the end of gestation might improve this aspect.

There are various methods of achieving such fetal tracheal occlusion in humans. Initially, this required a small hysterotomy and external dissection of the fetal trachea and then application of a clip. Subsequently, this has been modified by performing the tracheal clipping fetoscopically (four ports). Such external tracheal manipulations have been associated with tracheal or recurrent laryngeal nerve damage.[41] A joint Kings College Hospital/University of Leuven programme has recently been initiated using second-trimester minimally invasive intrauterine endoscopy

through a single uterine port. This technique allows intratracheal placement of a detachable balloon which effectively occludes lung fluid egress.[27,75] All such techniques invariably result in an obstructed trachea at the time of birth and therefore a further technique has had to be developed to secure the airway. Ex-utero intrapartum treatment (EXIT) is achieved by caesarian section on a relaxed uterus, partially delivering the fetus but leaving the placenta and cord intact to maintain a placental circulation.[67] Then, removal of the tracheal clip or balloon and tracheal intubation can occur within safe margins.

Lung transplantation

This is an obvious therapeutic concept for irreversible lung hypoplasia and has been reported in a ventilated infant with a right-sided CDH.[92] The upper and lower lobes of a right lung from a 6-week-old donor were successfully transplanted, resulting in successful weaning and survival.

Anterior diaphragmatic hernias

The Italian anatomist Giovanni Morgagni first described a hernia occurring between the costal and the sternal muscle origins of the diaphragm in a series published in 1769.[66] There is usually a hernial sac, and over 90% occur on the right side (Fig. 27.61). Compared with posterolateral defects, there is seldom any associated lung hypoplasia, and consequently, symptoms are mild. There may be other anomalies in a minority of cases, including

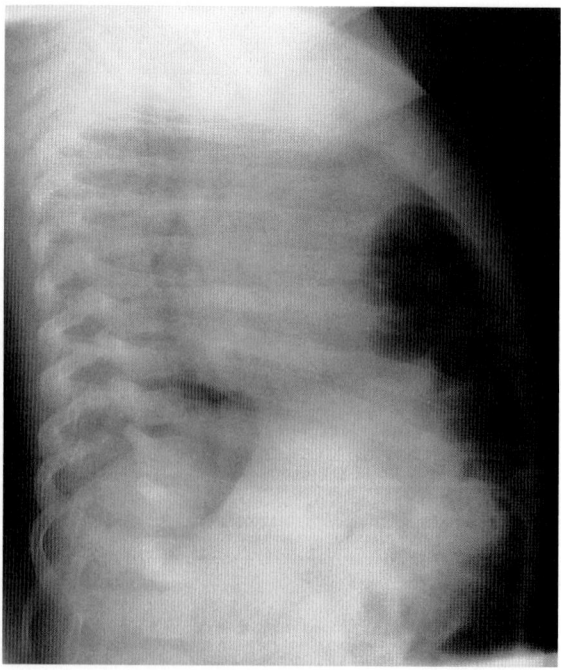

Fig. 27.61 Lateral chest radiograph of infant who presented with intermittent vomiting, showing anterior Morgagni hernia.

extralobar lung sequestrations and congenital cardiac defects. Morgagni hernias have also been described in Down syndrome.[38]

Most of the clinical features are due to incarceration of part of the bowel (commonly the transverse colon) and include vomiting, failure to thrive and intestinal obstruction. Some may be found incidentally on a CXR. Surgical repair is performed through an upper abdominal approach and is usually straightforward.

The pentalogy of Cantrell is a rare syndrome of an anterior diaphragmatic defect with pericardial defects, a short sternum, exomphalos and major intracardiac anomalies.[19,64] The defect itself differs anatomically from a Morgagni hernia and has been attributed to a defective septum transversum.

Diaphragmatic eventration

Eventration can be congenital or acquired. Congenital absence of anterior horn cells may be responsible (Werdnig–Hoffman disease), with others being due to intrauterine infection (e.g. rubella, cytomegalovirus) or as part of a more generalised chromosomal anomaly (e.g. trisomies 13–15 or 18). These anomalies are usually left-sided and may even be bilateral.[80] Diaphragmatic denervation due to phrenic nerve injury may be related to birth injury (when it is often associated with brachial plexus injury) or thoracic surgery (e.g. patent ductus arteriosus ligation).

Eventration may be asymptomatic, but most present in infancy with respiratory distress, recurrent chest infections or bronchiectasis. Paradoxical movement of the hemidiaphragm causes mediastinal shift, basal atelectasis and futile movement of air from the ipsilateral to the contralateral lung.

CXR (posteroanterior and lateral views) and fluoroscopic screening should establish the diagnosis, and radionuclide ventilation scans may allow assessment of the degree of ventilatory impairment. The management of eventration depends on the symptoms: if asymptomatic, an expectant course should be pursued; if there is respiratory distress, however, a more aggressive approach should be followed. Positive-pressure endotracheal ventilation overcomes any immediate problems, and once the infant is stable he should undergo definitive surgical correction. This is achieved by radial plication of the diaphragm by either an abdominal or a thoracic approach. The taut plicated diaphragm increases breathing capacity and tidal volume.

References

1. Adzick N S, Harrison M R 1994 Fetal surgical therapy. Lancet 343: 897–901
2. Adzick N S, Harrison M R, Glick P L 1984 Experimental pulmonary hypoplasia and oligohydramnios: relative contributions of lung fluid and breathing movements. Journal of Pediatric Surgery 19: 658–665
3. Adzick N S, Harrison M R, Glick P L, Nakayama D K, Manning F A, de Lorimier A A 1985 Diaphragmatic hernia in the fetus: prenatal diagnosis and outcome in 94 cases. Journal of Pediatric Surgery 20: 357–361
4. Albanese C T, Lopoo J, Goldstein R B et al 1998 Fetal liver position and perinatal outcome for congenital diaphragmatic hernia. Prenatal Diagnosis 18: 1138–1142
5. Banagale R C, Watters J H 1983 Delayed right-sided diaphragmatic hernia following group B streptococcal infection. Human Pathology 14: 67–69
6. Bartlett R H, Roloff D W, Cornell R G, Andrews A F, Dillon P W, Zwischenberger J B 1985 Extracorporeal circulation in neonatal respiratory failure: a prospective randomized study. Pediatrics 76: 479–487
7. Beals D A, Schloo B L, Vacanti J P, Reid L M, Wilson J M 1992 Pulmonary growth and remodelling in infants with high-risk congenital diaphragmatic hernia. Journal of Pediatric Surgery 27: 997–1002
8. Benjamin D R, Juul S, Siebert J R 1988 Congenital posterolateral diaphragmatic hernia: associated malformations. Journal of Pediatric Surgery 23: 899–903
9. Bianchi A, Doig C M, Cohen S J 1983 The reverse latissimus dorsi flap for congenital diaphragmatic hernia. Journal of Pediatric Surgery 18: 560–563
10. Bochdalek V A 1848 Einige Betrachtungen uber die Entstehung des angeborenen Zwerchfellbruches. Als Betrag zur pathologischen Anatomie der Hernien. Vierteljahrschrift fur die praktische Heilkunde 19: 89
11. Bohn D, Tamura M, Perrin D, Barker G, Rabinovitch M 1987 Ventilatory predictors of pulmonary hypoplasia in congenital diaphragmatic hernia, confirmed by morphological assessment. Journal of Pediatrics 111: 423–431
12. Boloker J, Bateman D A, Wung J-T, Stolar C J H 2002 Congenital diaphragmatic hernia in 120 infants treated consecutively with permissive hypercapnea/spontaneous respiration/elective repair. Journal of Pediatric Surgery 37: 357–366
13. Bonet T 1679 De Suffocatione Observatio XLI. Suffocatio excitata a tenium intestorum vulnus diaphragmatis, in thoracem ingrestu. Sepuhuchretum sive anatomia procteia et cadaveribus morbo denatus. Geneva
14. Boros S J, Mammel M C, Coleman J M et al 1985 Neonatal high frequency ventilation: four years' outcome. Pediatrics 75: 657–663
15. Bos A P, Tibboel D, Koot V C M, Hazebroek F W J, Molenaar J C 1993 Persistent pulmonary hypertension in high risk congenital diaphragmatic patients: incidence and vasodilator therapy. Journal of Pediatric Surgery 28: 1463–1465
16. Bratu I, Flageole H, Laberge J-M et al 2001 Pulmonary structural maturation and pulmonary artery remodeling after reversible fetal ovine tracheal occlusion in diaphragmatic hernia. Journal of Pediatric Surgery 36: 739–744
17. Butler N, Claireaux A E 1962 Congenital diaphragmatic hernia as a cause of perinatal mortality. Lancet i: 659–663
18. Campanale R P, Rowland R H 1955 Hypoplasia of the lung associated with congenital diaphragmatic hernia. Annals of Surgery 142: 176–189
19. Cantrell J R, Haller J A, Ravitch M M 1958 A syndrome of congenital defects involving the abdominal wall, sternum, diaphragm, pericardium and heart. Surgery, Gynecology and Obstetrics 107: 602–614
20. Cartlidge P H T, Mann N P, Kapilla L 1986 Preoperative stabilisation in congenital diaphragmatic hernia. Archives of Disease in Childhood 61: 1226–1228
21. Charlton A, Bruce J B, Davenport M 1991 Timing of surgery in congenital diaphragmatic hernia: low mortality after pre-operative stabilisation. Anaesthesia 46: 820–823
22. Chatrath R R, el-Shafie M, Jones R S 1971 Fate of hypoplastic lungs after repair of congenital diaphragmatic hernia. Archives of Disease in Childhood 46: 633–635
23. Congenital Diaphragmatic Hernia Study Group 1999 Does extracorporeal membrane oxygenation improve survival in neonates with congenital diaphragmatic hernia? Journal of Pediatric Surgery 34: 720–725
24. Crane J P 1979 Familial diaphragmatic hernia: prenatal diagnostic approach and analysis of twelve families. Clinical Genetics 16: 244–252
25. Crawford D C, Wright V M, Drake D P, Allan L D 1989 Fetal diaphragmatic hernia: the value of fetal echocardiography in the prediction of postnatal outcome. British Journal of Obstetrics and Gynaecology 96: 705–710
26. Davenport M, Rivlin E, D'Souza S W, Bianchi A 1992 Neurodevelopmental outcome following delayed surgery for congenital diaphragmatic hernia. Archives of Disease in Childhood 67: 1353–1356
27. Deprest J A, Evrard V A, Verbeken E K et al 2000 Tracheal side-effects of endoscopic balloon tracheal occlusion in the fetal lamb model. European Journal of Obstetrics, Gynecology and Reproductive Biology 92: 119–126
28. Dimitriou G, Greenough A, Chan V, Gamsu H R, Howard E R, Nicolaides K H 1995 Prognostic indicators in congenital diaphragmatic hernia. Journal of Pediatric Surgery 30: 1694–1697
29. Dimitriou G, Greenough A, Davenport M 2000 Prediction of outcome in infants with congenital diaphragmatic hernia from computer assisted analysis. Journal of Pediatric Surgery 35: 489–493
30. Finer N N, Etches P C, Kamstra B, Tierney A J, Peliowski A, Ryan C A 1994 Inhaled nitric oxide in infants referred for extracorporeal membrane oxygenation: dose response. Journal of Pediatrics 124: 302–308
31. Fryns J P, Moerman F, Goddeeris P et al 1979 A new lethal syndrome with cloudy corneae, diaphragmatic defects and distal limb deformities. Human Genetics 50: 65–70

32. German J C, Gazzaniga A B, Ragnar A 1977 Management of pulmonary insufficiency in diaphragmatic hernia using extracorporeal circulation with a membrane oxygenator. Journal of Pediatric Surgery 12: 905–912

33. Glick P L, Leach C L, Besner G E et al 1992 Pathophysiology of congenital diaphragmatic hernia. III: Exogenous surfactant therapy for the high-risk neonate with CDH. Journal of Pediatric Surgery 27: 866–869

34. Glick P L, Stannard V, Leach C L et al 1992 The fetal lamb CDH model is surfactant deficient. Journal of Pediatric Surgery 27: 382–388

35. Goh D W, Drake D P, Brereton R J, Kiely E M, Spitz L 1992 Delayed surgery for congenital diaphragmatic hernia. British Journal of Surgery 79: 644–646

36. Gross R E 1946 Congenital hernia of the diaphragm. American Journal of Diseases of Children 71: 580–592

37. Guarino N, Shima H, Puri P 2001 Structural immaturity of the heart in congenital diaphragmatic hernia in rats. Journal of Pediatric Surgery 36: 770–773

38. Harris G J, Soper R T, Kimura K K 1993 Foramen of Morgagni hernia in identical twins: is this an inheritable defect? Journal of Pediatric Surgery 28: 177–178

39. Harrison M R, Adzick N S, Estes J M, Howell L J 1994 A prospective study of the outcome for fetuses with diaphragmatic hernia. Journal of the American Medical Association 271: 382–384

40. Harrison M R, Adzick N S, Flake A W et al 1993 Correction of congenital diaphragmatic hernia in utero: VI. Hard-earned lessons. Journal of Pediatric Surgery 28: 1411–1418

41. Harrison M R, Mychaliska G B, Albanese C T et al 1998 Correction of congenital diaphragmatic hernia in utero. IX: Fetuses with poor prognosis (liver herniation and low lung-to-head ratio) can be saved by fetoscopic temporary tracheal occlusion. Journal of Pediatric Surgery 33: 1017–1022

42. Hasegawa S, Kohno S, Sugiyama T et al 1994 Usefulness of echocardiographic measurement of bilateral pulmonary artery dimensions in congenital diaphragmatic hernia. Journal of Pediatric Surgery 29: 622–624

43. Haugen S, Linker D, Eik-Nes S et al 1991 Congenital diaphragmatic hernia: determination of the optimal time for operation by echocardiographic monitoring of the pulmonary artery pressure. Journal of Pediatric Surgery 26: 560–562

44. Heiss K F, Clark R H 1995 Prediction of mortality in neonates with congenital diaphragmatic hernia treated with extracorporeal membrane oxygenation. Critical Care Medicine 23: 1915–1919

45. Heiss K, Manning P, Oldham K T et al 1989 Reversal of mortality for congenital diaphragmatic hernia. Annals of Surgery 209: 225–230

46. Hedrick M H, Estes K M, Sullivan K M et al 1994 Plug the Lung Until it Grows (PLUG): a new method to treat congenital diaphragmatic hernia in utero. Journal of Pediatric Surgery 29: 612–617

47. Holt C 1701 Child that lived two months with congenital diaphragmatic hernia. Philosophical Transactions 22: 992

48. Iritani I 1984 Experimental study on pathogenesis and embryogenesis of congenital diaphragmatic hernia. Anatomy and Embryology 169: 133–139

49. Islam S, Masiakos P, Schnitzer P et al 1999 Dilitiazem reduces pulmonary arterial pressures in recurrent pulmonary hypertension associated with pulmonary hypoplasia. Journal of Pediatric Surgery 34: 712–714

50. Jeandot R, Lambert B, Brendel A J, Guyot M, Demarquez J L 1989 Lung ventilation and perfusion scintigraphy in the follow up of repaired congenital diaphragmatic hernia. European Journal of Nuclear Medicine 15: 591–596

51. Karamanoukian H L, Glick P L, Wilcox D, O'Toole S J, Rosman J E, Azizkhan R G 1995 Pathophysiology of congenital diaphragmatic hernia XI: anatomic and biochemical characterisation of the heart in the fetal lamb CDH model. Journal of Pediatric Surgery 30: 925–929

52. Karl S R, Ballantine T V N, Snider M T 1983 High frequency ventilation at rates of 375 to 1800 cycles per minute in four neonates with congenital diaphragmatic hernia. Journal of Pediatric Surgery 18: 822–828

53. Kavvadia V, Greenough A, Laubscher B et al 1997 Perioperative assessment of respiratory compliance and lung volume in infants with congenital diaphragmatic hernia: prediction of outcome. Journal of Pediatric Surgery 32: 1665–1669

54. Kinsella J P, Neish S R, Ivy D, Shaffer E, Abman S H 1993 Clinical responses to prolonged treatment of persistent pulmonary hypertension of the newborn with low doses of inhaled nitric oxide. Journal of Pediatrics 123: 103–108

55. Kitano Y, Kanai M, von Allmen D et al 2001 Lung growth induced by prenatal tracheal occlusion and its modifying factors: a study in the rat model of congenital diaphragmatic hernia. Journal of Pediatric Surgery 36: 251–259

56. Kluth D, Keijzer R, Hertl M et al 1996 Embryology of congenital diaphragmatic hernia. Seminars in Pediatric Surgery 5: 224–233

57. Kluth D, Tenbrick R, Ekesparre M V et al 1993 The natural history of congenital diaphragmatic hernia and pulmonary hypoplasia in the embryo. Journal of Pediatric Surgery 28: 456–463

58. Lally K P, Paranka M S, Roden J et al 1992 Congenital diaphragmatic hernia, stabilisation and repair on ECMO. Annals of Surgery 216: 569–573

59. Langer J C, Filler R M, Bohn D J et al 1988 Timing of surgery for congenital diaphragmatic hernia: is emergency operation necessary? Journal of Pediatric Surgery 23: 731–734

60. Langer J C, Winthrop A L, Whelan D 1994 Fryns syndrome: a rare familial cause of congenital diaphragmatic hernia. Journal of Pediatric Surgery 29: 1266–1267

61. Leinwald M J, Tefft J D, Zhao J et al 2002 Nitrofen inhibition of pulmonary growth and development occurs in the early embryonic mouse. Journal of Pediatric Surgery 37: 1263–1268

62. Lipshutz G S, Albanese C T, Feldstein V et al 1997 Lung-to-head ratio predicts survival in fetal diaphragmatic hernia. Journal of Pediatric Surgery 32: 1634–1636

63. Malone P S, Brain A J, Kiely S M, Spitz L 1989 Congenital diaphragmatic defects that present late. Archives of Disease in Childhood 64: 1542–1544

64. Milne L W, Moroson A M, Campbell J R, Harrison M W 1984 Pars sternalis diaphragmatic hernia with omphalocele: a report of 2 cases. Journal of Pediatric Surgery 19: 394–397

65. Mishalany H, Gordo J 1986 Congenital diaphragmatic hernia in monozygotic twins. Journal of Pediatric Surgery 21: 372–374

66. Morgagni G B 1769 Seats and causes of disease investigated by anatomy, Vol 3. Translated by B Alexander. Millere and Cadell, London, p. 205

67. Mychaliska G B, Bealer J F, Graf J L et al 1996 Operating on placental support: the Ex-utero intrapartum treatment (EXIT) procedure. Journal of Pediatric Surgery 32: 227–231

68. Nagaraj H S, Mitchell K A, Fallat M E, Groff D B, Cook L N 1992 Surgical complications and procedures in neonates on extracorporeal membrane oxygenation. Journal of Pediatric Surgery 27: 1106–1109

69. Naik S, Greenough A, Zhang Y-X, Davenport M 1996 Prediction of morbidity following congenital diaphragmatic hernia repair. Journal of Pediatric Surgery 31: 1651–1654

70. Newman K D, Anderson K D, Meurs K V et al 1990 Extracorporeal membrane oxygenation and congenital diaphragmatic hernia: should any infant be excluded? Journal of Pediatric Surgery 25: 1048–1053

71. Nio M, Haase G, Kennaugh J, Bui K, Atkinson J B 1994 A prospective randomised trial of delayed versus immediate repair of congenital diaphragmatic hernia. Journal of Pediatric Surgery 29: 618–621

72. Okazaki T, Sharma H S, McCune S K et al 1998 Pulmonary vascular balance in congenital diaphragmatic hernia: enhanced endothelin-1 gene expression as a possible cause of pulmonary vasoconstriction. Journal of Pediatric Surgery 33: 81–84

73. O'Rourke P P, Crone R K, Vacanti J P et al 1989 Extracorporeal membrane oxygenation and conventional medical therapy in neonates with persistent pulmonary hypertension of the newborn: a prospective randomized study. Pediatrics 84: 957–963

74. O'Rourke P P, Vacanti J P, Crone R K, Fellows K, Lillehei C, Hougen T J 1989 Use of postductal PaO_2 as a predictor of pulmonary vascular hypoplasia in infants with congenital diaphragmatic hernia. Journal of Pediatric Surgery 23: 904–907

75. Papadakis K, De Paepe M E, Tackett L D et al 1998 Temporary tracheal occlusion causes catch-up lung maturation in a fetal model of diaphragmatic hernia. Journal of Pediatric Surgery 33: 1030–1037

76. Papadakis K, Luks F I, Deprest J A et al 1998 Single-port tracheoscopic surgery in the fetal lamb. Journal of Pediatric Surgery 33: 918–920

77. Philips A F, Bierny J-P, Crowe C P 1995 Perinatal/neonatal casebooks. Journal of Perinatology 15: 160–162

78. Puri P, Gorman W A 1987 Natural history of congenital diaphragmatic hernia. Implications for early intrauterine surgery. Pediatric Surgery International 2: 327–330

79. Reynolds M, Luck S R, Lappen R 1984 The 'critical' neonate with diaphragmatic hernia: a 21-year perspective. Journal of Pediatric Surgery 19: 364–369

80. Rodgers B M, Hawks P 1986 Bilateral congenital eventration of the diaphragm. Successful management. Journal of Pediatric Surgery 21: 858–864

81. Sakai H, Tamura M, Hosokawa Y, Bryan A C, Barker G A, Bohn D J 1987 The effect of surgical repair on respiratory mechanics in congenital diaphragmatic hernia. Journal of Pediatrics 111: 432–458

82. Sebire N J, Snijders R J, Davenport M, Greenough A, Nicolaides K H 1997 Fetal nuchal translucency thickness at 10–14 weeks' gestation and congenital diaphragmatic hernia. Obstetrics and Gynecology 90: 943–946

83. Shanbhogue L K R, Tam P K H, Ninan G, Lloyd D A 1990 Preoperative stabilisation in congenital diaphragmatic hernia. Archives of Disease in Childhood 65: 1043–1044

84. Shanley C J, Hirschl R B, Schumacher R E et al 1994 Extracorporeal life support for neonatal respiratory failure – a 20 year experience. Annals of Surgery 220: 269–282

85. Sharland G K, Lochhart S M, Heward A J, Allan L D 1992 Prognosis in fetal diaphragmatic hernia. American Journal of Obstetrics and Gynecology 166: 9–13

86. Siebert J R, Haas J E, Beckwith J B 1984 Left ventricular hypoplasia in congenital diaphragmatic hernia. Journal of Pediatric Surgery 19: 567–571

87. Skari H, Bjornland K, Frencker B et al 2002 Congenital diaphragmatic hernia in Scandinavia from 1995 to 1998: predictors of mortality. Journal of Pediatric Surgery 37: 1269–1275

88. Stevens D C, Screiner R L, Bull M J et al 1980 An analysis of tolazoline therapy in the critically ill neonate. Journal of Pediatric Surgery 15: 964–970

89. Sweed Y, Puri P 1993 Congenital diaphragmatic hernia: influence of associated malformations on survival. Archives of Disease in Childhood 69: 68–70

90. Tsang T M, Tam P K H, Dudley N E, Stevens J 1995 Diaphragmatic agenesis as a distinct clinical entity. Journal of Pediatric Surgery 30: 16–18

91. UK Collaborative ECMO Trial Group 1996 UK collaborative randomised trial of neonatal extracorporeal membrane oxygenation. Lancet 248: 75–82

92. Van Meurs K P, Rhine W D, Benitz W E et al 1994 Lobar lung transplantation as a treatment for congenital diaphragmatic hernia. Journal of Pediatric Surgery 29: 1557–1560

93. Wenstrom K D, Weiner C P, Hanson J W 1991 A five year statewide experience with congenital diaphragmatic hernia. American Journal of Obstetrics and Gynecology 165: 838–842

94. West K W, Bengstrom K, Rescorla F J, Engle W A, Grosfeld J L 1992 Delayed surgical repair and ECMO improves survival in congenital diaphragmatic hernia. Annals of Surgery 216: 454–462

95. Wigglesworth J, Hislop A 1987 Fetal lung growth in congenital larnygeal atresia. Pediatric Pathology 7: 515–525

96. Wilson J M, Bower L K, Lund D P 1994 Evolution of the technique of congenital diaphragmatic hernia repair on ECMO. Journal of Pediatric Surgery 29: 1109–1112

97. Wilson J M, DiFiore J W, Peters C A 1993 Experimental fetal tracheal ligation prevents the pulmonary hypoplasia associated with fetal nephrectomy: possible application for congenital diaphragmatic hernia. Journal of Pediatric Surgery 28: 1433–1440

98. Wilson J M, Lund D P, Lillehei C W, Vacanti J P 1991 Congenital diaphragmatic hernia: predictors of severity in the ECMO era. Journal of Pediatric Surgery 26: 1028–1034

PART 7

Airway problems

Gavin Morrison

Introduction

Continuing advances in neonatology present the paediatric otolaryngologist with an increasing range of baby and infant airway problems. This chapter attempts to review the causes, investigations and management of the compromised airway from the specialist paediatric airway surgeon's viewpoint. Investigation, management, and prognosis are discussed. Although this chapter is entitled Pulmonary Disease, airway obstruction in the newborn can involve any site from the nostrils to the alveoli. Higher upper airway obstruction (UAO), from the nose downwards, is therefore discussed, in addition to laryngotracheobronchial airway disease.

Tracheostomy, at one time the mainstay surgical procedure for airway obstruction, has seen changing trends over the years. Immunisation programmes against diphtheria, polio and *Haemophilus influenza* (acute epiglottitis) have dramatically reduced infective indications. The increased survival of very-low-birthweight (VLBW) babies and babies with multiple congenital abnormalities has led to a continued need for long-term tracheostomy in some infants and children. There is significant morbidity and mortality associated with tracheostomy, and newer developments now facilitate a trend away from tracheostomy, even for severe airway obstruction. Congenital and acquired subglottic stenosis (SGS) can often be successfully treated by single-stage laryngotracheal reconstruction (SS-LTR), thereby avoiding tracheostomy. The ex-utero intrapartum treatment (EXIT) procedure can also now be used in difficult cases with antenatally diagnosed airway obstruction. This chapter looks at assessment and management of the range of airway problems from a practical viewpoint.

Development of the nose, larynx and trachea, and lungs

At 4 weeks, a median laryngotracheal groove appears in the ventral wall of the developing primitive pharynx. This groove deepens and its edges fuse to create a tube, the laryngotracheal tube. At the cranial end of this tube, the lips do not fuse, remaining open into the pharynx with a slit-like aperture. This cranial end forms the larynx, the trachea lies below this, and caudally two lung buds arise and grow outward, forming the bronchi and bronchioles. The laryngotracheal tube is lined with endoderm, which becomes the respiratory epithelium. The epiglottis arises from the hypobranchial eminence at the tongue base and two arytenoid swellings appear, one on each side of the laryngotracheal groove. These develop from 6 weeks, into the epiglottis and arytenoids, creating a T-shaped laryngeal cleft. Soon after its formation, the epithelial walls of this cleft adhere to each other, and the aperture of the larynx remains occluded until the third month, when the lumen reappears. With further growth, this new definitive aperture forms above the initial primitive one and the detailed features of the larynx are created. The thyroid cartilage is developed from the ventral ends of the fourth and/or fifth branchial arches and appears as two lateral plates, while the cricoid cartilage develops from two sixth-arch cartilaginous centres, which fuse ventrally and gradually extend and fuse on the dorsal side as well.

The right and left lung buds commence before the laryngotracheal groove becomes a tube and develop out into the pleural passages. The lungs migrate caudally and at birth the bifurcation

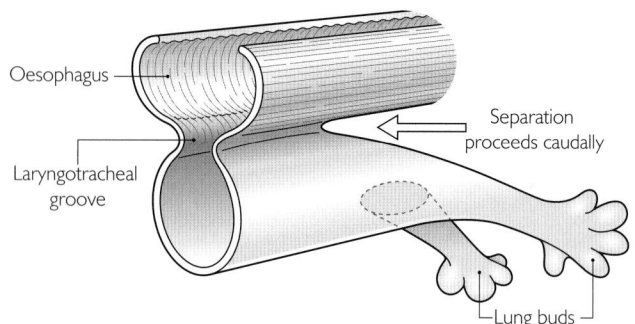

Fig. 27.62 The development of the trachea, bronchi and oesophagus.

of the trachea (carina) is at the level of the fourth thoracic vertebra.

The primitive foregut is in continuity with the pharynx and elongates to form the oesophagus. The continuity between the oesophagus and the laryngotracheal groove is not maintained and the separation between these structures proceeds cranially to achieve complete separation of the lung buds and trachea from the oesophagus (Fig. 27.62).

Laryngeal webs result from incomplete separation of the arytenoid regions. Laryngeal clefts are posteriorly sited and can result in notching of the posterior cricoid or complete failure of fusion of this ring. Incomplete fusion of the tracheo-esophageal wall can result in a laryngeal cleft superiorly and a tracheo-oesophageal fistula (TOF) more inferiorly. Congenital anomalies of the larynx and trachea are rare, estimated at between 1 in 10 000 and 1 in 50 000.[39] Laryngeal atresia results from failure of canalisation of the cricoid and/or separation of the arytenoids. If there is failure of development of the tracheoesophageal groove, then the lungs may arise from a common oesophagus or type 4 laryngeal cleft. Such infants can occasionally be resuscitated with oesophageal ventilation, but most will not survive the immediate neonatal period.

Higher upper airway obstruction

Choanal atresia

One in 7000 babies are born with choanal atresia.[26] It can be unilateral or bilateral. This congenital anomaly occurs where there has been failure of the opening at the back of the nose. The obstruction can be membranous or bony and membranous. It is most common to find a bony stenosis with a thin central bony atretic plate or membranous closure.

Choanal atresia can occur as an isolated anomaly or as part of the CHARGE association.[35] It is also sometimes found in association with other craniofacial conditions such as Treacher Collins syndrome. The atresia can be unilateral or bilateral in any of these conditions.

Diagnosis and management

The diagnosis of unilateral atresia may only become apparent when it proves impossible to pass a fine flexible catheter through each nostril into the pharynx, and there is a lack of mirror misting at the anterior nares. There is frequently no clinical airway obstruction, or just snuffly breathing. The diagnosis may therefore be delayed until later childhood. Bilateral choanal atresia, however, presents at birth, with severe UAO. This will usually require either intubation and ventilation, or maintenance of the upper airway by placing a Guedel airway orally, securely taped to prevent displacement, prior to definitive correction. Frequent oropharyngeal suctioning will then be required.

A high-resolution computed tomography (CT) scan in the axial plane, with bone and soft-tissue windows, should be undertaken. It is important for the paediatrician to attend the scan in order to decongest the nose with a few 0.5% ephedrine nose drops and then nasal suctioning to remove mucus immediately prior to imaging. Otherwise, mucus will be interpreted radiologically as a membranous atresia.

Surgery and postoperative care

Surgical correction of bilateral choanal atresia should be undertaken as soon as this is practicable, usually within the first 14 days of life. Unilateral atresia, unless there is unusually severe airway obstruction, is better corrected electively at any time from 6 months of age or even as a toddler. The surgical outcome will tend to be better in an older child. Either a transnasal or a transpalatal surgical approach is adopted. The bony atresia is drilled away under endoscopic control, and most surgeons then insert nasal stents fashioned from endotracheal tubing. These nasal tubes need to be kept clear by regular suctioning and irrigation with a few drops of saline or bicarbonate solution, as required. The baby's parent or guardian should be taught this process prior to discharge home. The nasal stents are usually removed after 2–6 weeks and subsequent anaesthetics for endoscopic examination, dilatation and sometimes laser treatments are required. There is a relatively high incidence of restenosis following this surgery, regardless of the technique employed. Samadi et al[35] reported that about five surgical procedures were required to achieve maintained patency. Holland & McGuirt[23] report improved outcomes using topical mitomycin C application at the time of surgery.

Oropharyngeal airway obstruction and stertor

Stertor describes the low-tone breathing noise resultant from turbulent airflow in an obstructed pharynx. It is almost a snoring, and typically arises from the level of the tonsils, adenoids or tongue base. It is usually quite easily distinguishable from the higher-pitched, almost musical, wheezy quality of stridor, which signifies airway obstruction at the laryngeal level or below. There will often be associated chest recession with stertor or stridor.

Table 27.18 Causes of high upper airway obstruction

- Nasal agenesis
- Congenital nasal septal deflection
- Nasal tumour (e.g. meningomyelocoele)
- Choanal stenosis
- Choanal atresia
- Craniofacial syndromes with midface hypoplasia
- Macroglossia
- Oropharyngeal lymphangioma or haemangiomata
- Micrognathia (e.g. Pierre Robin sequence)
- Glossoptosis, prolapsing tongue base
- Abnormally high or posterior larynx
- Vallecular or supraglottic cysts
- Pharyngeal hypotonia (neurological disease)
- Excessive oropharyngeal secretions
- Foreign bodies
- Adenotonsillar hypertrophy

In the neonate, stertor is unlikely to be caused by obstructive adenoid or tonsillar tissue which has yet to hypertrophy, but it will be seen in any condition in which there are rattley oropharyngeal secretions, or with altered muscular tone in the pharynx, associated with neurological disorders, and where the tongue base and epiglottic morphology is unusual or hypotonic, causing these structures to prolapse over the laryngeal opening on attempted respiration (glossoptosis). Pharyngeal UAO and stertor will be common therefore in infants with congenital abnormalities of the region, such as Treacher Collins syndrome, Pierre Robin sequence and in other conditions with an associated cleft palate. It will be seen with macroglossia (e.g. Beckwith–Weidermann syndrome). Other common conditions include lymphangioma (cystic hygroma) involving the tongue, pharynx, and neck.

Progressive UAO in the infant may indicate an enlarging mucus retention cyst, usually found in the vallecula, at the tongue base. It may be seen on a soft-tissue lateral X-ray of the neck and should be diagnosed at endoscopic laryngoscopy. Undiagnosed, this simple condition can be fatal. It requires drainage and excision or marsupialisation. Table 27.18 lists the causes of high UAO.

Management of oropharyngeal upper airway obstruction

Clinical assessment remains important, checking the patency of both nostrils, examining the oral cavity and oropharynx and studying the baby for dysmorphic features. The degree of stertor, recession and the pulse oximetry monitoring will give a good indication of the severity. A lateral soft-tissue X-ray of the neck can be helpful. Referral to a paediatric ENT surgeon should be made.

Initial treatment, with general supportive measures such as oxygen and perhaps humidification, will be helpful. Even inhaled or nebulised mixtures of helium and oxygen (Heliox, BOC Medical) can be considered. Continuous positive airway pressure (CPAP) delivered by nasal oxygen cannulae may stent the upper airway open and avoid the need for intubation. Sometimes the airway can be maintained by the insertion of a unilateral nasopharyngeal prong, which will bypass the airway obstruction and can also allow better delivery of CPAP, if required. The presence of the prong, however, stimulates increased secretions and causes feeding difficulty; regular suctioning will be required.

Where there is a removable obstructive cause, such as enlarged adenoids or tonsils or a retention cyst, ENT surgery will be corrective. Cystic hygroma in the airway may be reduced in a number of ways, such as surgical debulking, laser treatments or sclerosing agents (OK-432 or doxycycline).[19,27,42] If pharyngeal airway surgery and/or supportive measures are not successful in the long term, then tracheostomy surgery becomes indicated. Many causes of congenital UAO will slowly self-correct with growth, over a number of years, and allow much later decannulation of the tracheostomy.

Where the posterior tongue is bulky and prolapses, compressing the laryngeal inlet (glossoptosis), it may occasionally be possible to perform a posterior third midline wedge resection and lead to airway improvement. Maxillofacial techniques such as mandibular distraction surgery can also have a place in promoting earlier correction of the obstructed upper airway in association with the micrognathic mandible and even the hypoplastic midface in toddlers or children with craniofacial syndromes.

Prognosis of high upper airway obstruction

Acute inflammatory conditions associated with airway obstruction and surgically correctable conditions will hold a good prognosis. The baby requiring a tracheostomy because of congenitally compromised upper airway anatomy, however, may require a tracheostomy for 3 or 4 years of life, before there has been adequate resolution with growth.

Laryngotracheal airway obstruction

Assessment of airway obstruction and stridor

Stridor, a high-pitched audible noisy breathing, indicates airway obstruction within the larynx, trachea or bronchi. The history may help to diagnose the cause and localise the obstruction. Inspiratory stridor frequently arises from the supraglottis or the vocal cords. Laryngomalacia is the most common cause. Biphasic stridor usually indicates a vocal cord, or subglottic causes. A biphasic vocalisation noise is often found to be caused by bilateral congenital vocal cord paralysis in the newborn. Expiratory stridor progressing to wheeze indicates lower tracheal or bronchial obstruction. Exacerbating features and whether the stridor is constant or progressive, can be helpful. If the cry is absent or abnormal, there may be a congenital laryngeal lesion (e.g. web); a unilateral vocal cord paralysis can give a husky cry. An associated cough may indicate laryngitis and subglottic inflammation with laryngotracheobronchitis (LTB) or croup, while a harsh or barking cough is seen with tracheomalacia.

Stridor is frequently exacerbated by feeding. Stridor from laryngomalacia is often seen when the baby is asleep and lying supine. Stridor that is exacerbated by increased activity or upset tends to indicate a fixed, narrowed airway such as SGS.

Babies can adapt to slowly developing subglottic or tracheal stenosis, resulting in a prolonged expiratory phase which reduces recession and stridor, masking the severity of the obstruction. Acute-onset airway obstruction, in contrast, will tend to produce much more marked signs of obstruction, with tracheal tug, sub-costal and intercostal recession, use of accessory respiratory muscles, increased respiratory rate and sweating. It is note-worthy, however, that recession is not specifically a sign of air-way obstruction, but of airway effort, and is therefore also seen in babies with respiratory distress in the absence of significant obstruction (pp. 609, 1017).

Auscultation of the stridor over the sternum is helpful, espe-cially in a noisy ward, and can give a good indication of the vol-ume of airflow and severity of the obstruction.

The small newborn baby, even with airway obstruction, may initially show relatively little stridor, perhaps because of the small-volume, lower-speed airflow. With increasing age, stridor will tend to become more marked. Laryngomalacia, for example, will often develop only after the first few weeks of life, or even later.

The overall assessment of the baby with stridor should include oropharyngeal and chest examination and attention to the rest of the history, including an assessment of likely neuro-logical and cardiac status.

Pulse oximetry readings and capillary blood gases, taken in the context of other associated conditions, will be helpful. To rely solely on a pulse oximeter can be misleading (pp. 255–6). Clinical evaluation of the baby remains important.

Investigations for stridor

Investigation of the baby or infant with stridor should include a chest X-ray (CXR). A lateral X-ray of the neck may yield helpful information. Some institutions undertake the so-called Cincinnati view – a coned high-kilovolt anteroposterior X-ray of the medi-astinum, which can delineate the trachea and main bronchi. A barium swallow may demonstrate an abnormal swallowing reflex, aspiration or TOF, as well as compression from a vascular ring or sling. A pH study, CT scan and magnetic resonance imaging (MRI) scans, as well as an echocardiogram of the great vessels, are all additional investigations.

Investigations should be tailored to the individual baby, but the minimum investigations for a baby with stridor should include a CXR and referral to the paediatric ENT airway surgeons for diagnostic endoscopy.

Management of stridor and laryngotracheal airway obstruction

Universal supportive measures can be applied. Oxygen, humidi-fication and nebulisers or even heliox may be helpful. Adrenaline nebuliser (1 ml of 1:1000 adrenaline mixed with 2 ml of normal saline) can be administered every few hours to most babies. Nebulised steroids may be helpful,[13] and salbutamol is worth trying. Systemic steroids such as dexamethasone will reduce any acute inflammation, oedema or haemangioma. When there is respiratory failure despite these measures, CPAP or intubation and ventilation will be required.

Airway endoscopy

While the supportive measures and investigations described are helpful, almost all babies and infants with stridor and airway obstruction require endoscopy to confirm a diagnosis and, if pos-sible, to treat the condition endoscopically. Flexible laryngoscopy with a 2–4-mm diameter flexible rhinolaryngoscope (passed through the baby's mouth whilst awake on the ward) may allow a diagnosis of a supraglottic obstruction such as a vallecular cyst or laryngomalacia and might confirm vocal cord lesions or paralysis. The subglottic airway will not be readily assessed with a flexible endoscope. If the baby is intubated, the more distal tracheo-bronchial tree can be visualised with a very fine flexible fibre-optic endoscope passed down the endotracheal tube (ETT). Flexible endoscopes therefore have an increasing diagnostic role in the neonatal unit, but do not allow as accurate an assessment as rigid microlaryngoscopy and bronchoscopy (MLB) and generally do not allow correction of the problem (therapeutic endoscopy).

A formal MLB in the operating theatre, under light spontaneous-respiration general anaesthesia, will allow full assess-ment of airway obstruction and the possibility of endoscopic thera-peutic procedures. The technique requires no neuromuscular blockade and minimal sedation, so that spontaneous respiration allows a dynamic endoscopic assessment of the entire airway with-out the presence of an ETT. Oxygen and inhalational agents, such as isoflurane, can be delivered through a nasal prong. The technique relies heavily upon the use of lidocaine (lignocaine) spray to the lar-ynx (7 mg/kg stat.). Intravenous anaesthesia such as propofol is also employed. Views are obtained using the microscope and/or rigid endoscopes. Storz ventilating bronchoscopes do allow ventilation when assessing the tracheobronchial tree, if needed. These tech-niques allow coaxial instrumentation and laser treatments.

Care of the intubated baby

Airway obstruction and prematurity require babies to be intubated with speed and skill. Many factors appear to be associated with endotracheal airway damage leading to acquired SGS. Choice of an appropriately sized tube, movement, infection,[37] the length of time intubated and the number of reintubations are all factors. Downing & Kilbride[12] reported that variables more commonly found in patients with SGS included greater number of intub-ations, use of an inappropriately large ETT, and longer durations of intubation. Contencin & Narcy[8] believe the size of the ETT to be a major risk factor for acquired laryngotracheal stenosis in the neonate, recommending use of a size 2.5 ETT in babies under 2500 g weight. Supraglottic laryngeal damage from intu-bation, which will increase the likelihood of failed extubation, is significantly more common in active neonates than those who are quiescent.[1] Pashley[33] reviewed the risk factors and predictors of SGS, proposing a figure of the number of intubations × the number of days intubated × the number of days ventilated. A child with a risk factor figure of greater than 3000 was at high risk.

A small leak past the ETT is desirable. A tube smaller than size 3.0 will be more difficult to manage regarding patency and ventilation. Table 27.19 gives a guide to the expected diameter of the subglottis and trachea for age with appropriate endotracheal and tracheostomy tube sizes.

Tube design may be another important feature. The Cole shouldered tube provides easier and safer intubation because of the rigidity of the fatter oropharyngeal component, but positioning is important as the shoulder can prolapse through the glottis, and its increased diameter will then cause trauma or even malacia.[6] Tube fixation techniques and the preferences for oral or nasal intubation remain debated (pp. 1256–8). There is no strong evidence to support any particular method.

I feel strongly that an intubated baby who is allowed to be too active and mobile is at greatly increased risk of developing glottic laryngeal granulations and subglottic ulceration, leading to failed extubation and stenosis. Occult or overt acid reflux is considered to be a detrimental factor in laryngeal and subglottic trauma, leading to failed extubation.

Deep suctioning through an ETT will also cause mechanical trauma with ulcerations and granulations. Suction techniques should involve introducing the suction tip just beyond the end of the ETT and then applying the suction with rotation and a gradual withdrawal (Fig. 27.63).

Extubation

For the baby deemed fit for a trial of extubation, different weaning protocols have been studied. Randolph et al[34] found extubation failure rates are not significantly different from one another. Barrington et al[4] showed that nasal synchronised intermittent mandatory ventilation (nSIMV) was effective in preventing extubation failure compared with CPAP. The use of respiratory stimulants such as doxapram or methylxanthines to facilitate successful extubation has been studied, with mixed results. Most neonatal units use caffeine prior to extubation in babies of less than 32 weeks' gestation (p. 563).

When there is initial failure of extubation, and an airway obstructive cause seems probable, then reintubation for 48 hours with heavy sedation to reduce tube movement and the use of systemic steroids as well as ranitidine or a proton-pump inhibitor may allow subsequent successful extubation.

Failed extubation

Where there is repeated failure of extubation, referral should be made to a paediatric ENT surgeon. These babies tend to fall into three distinct categories: firstly, the premature neonate who has

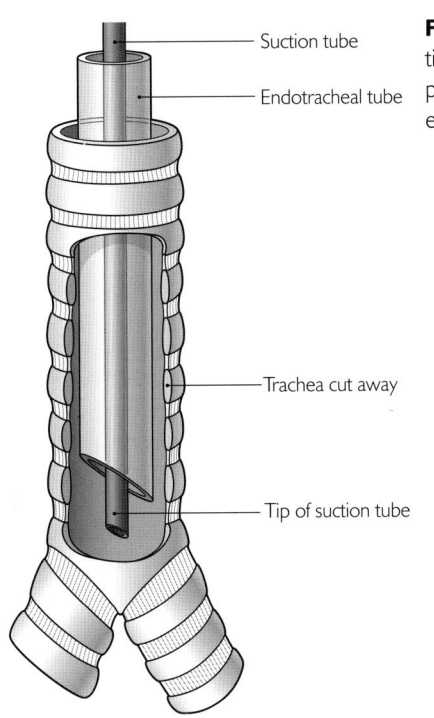

Suction tube
Endotracheal tube
Trachea cut away
Tip of suction tube

Fig. 27.63 The suction tip should usually be passed just beyond the endotracheal tube tip.

Table 27.19 Approximate neonatal and infant airway parameters

	Pre-30 weeks	30 weeks – term	1 month	6 months	12 months
Expected cricoid AP diameter	3.6 mm	4.4 mm	5.0 mm	5.8 mm	6.2 mm
Appropriate Portex blue line ETT size	2.5 (OD 3.4 mm)	3.0 (OD 4.3 mm)	3.0 (OD 4.3 mm)	3.5 (OD 4.8 mm)	4.0 (OD 5.4 mm)
ETT size without air leak indicating significant Cotton 1 subglottic stenosis	–	2.5	2.5	3.0	3.5
Expected transverse tracheal diameter	4.6 mm	4.75 mm	5.3 mm	6.0 mm	6.5 mm
Appropriate size of Shiley neonatal tracheostomy tube	3.0 (OD 4.5 mm)	3.0 (OD 4.5 mm)	3.0 (OD 4.5 mm)	3.5 (OD 5.2 mm)	4.0 (OD 5.9 mm)

AP, anteroposterior; ETT, endotracheal tube; OD, outer diameter.

Table 27.20 Causes of extubation failure

- **Central apnoea**
  Apnoea of prematurity
  Neurological disease
  Iatrogenic (opiates, sedatives)
  Hypocapnia

- **Peripheral apnoea**
  Neuromuscular blockade (vecuronium)

- **Cardiac causes**
  Congenital heart disease
  Heart failure (patent ductus arteriosis)

- **Lower respiratory tract**
  Infection
  Respiratory distress syndrome
  Chronic lung disease (BPD)
  Lung anomalies/hypoplasia

- **Airway obstruction**
  Any site

- **General sepsis**

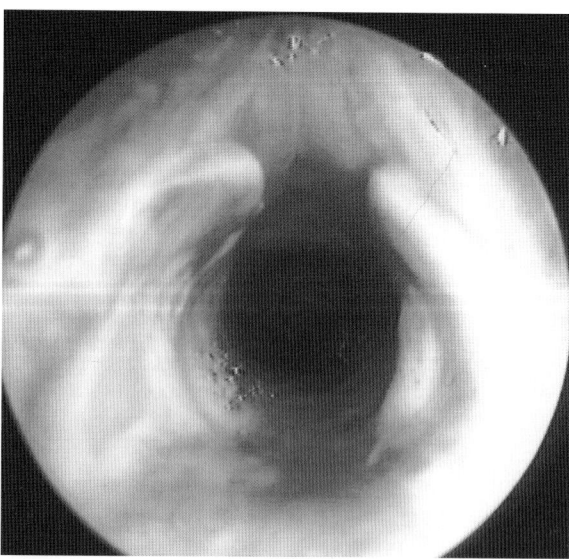

Fig. 27.64 Laryngeal granulomas and exposed cartilage following prolonged complicated intubation.

been ventilator dependent since birth and repeatedly fails attempts at extubation; secondly, the infant or baby who has breathed spontaneously but then fails extubation after a subsequent surgical procedure; lastly, the infant or older baby who has been readmitted and intubated for LTB or croup, pneumonia, epilepsy control or asthma, subsequently failing extubation. This latter category may include children with neurological impairment, such as children with cerebral palsy.

Extubation failure must imply that the baby is unable to maintain adequate arterial oxygenation and/or that the $PaCO_2$ has become unsustainably high. Table 27.20 lists possible causes for such failed extubation. Airway obstruction is only one of the important factors and each of the causes should be excluded. In simple terms, successful extubation requires:

- respiratory drive;
- neuromuscular function;
- adequate cardiac function and pulmonary gaseous exchange;
- clear unobstructed airways;
- no significant sepsis.

In our experience, the most common causes for neonatal intensive care extubation failure are chronic lung disease, apnoea of prematurity, sepsis, airway obstruction or multifactorial causes.

Assessing a preterm baby prior to his first extubation involves consideration of all these factors. As a broad guideline, a successful outcome is likely if the infant weighs over 1000 g, if there is an air leak around an age-appropriate ETT at less than 20 cmH$_2$O peak ventilator pressure, if oxygen saturations are being maintained in 35% oxygen or less and if the ventilator requirements have been weaned to satisfactory rates. A rate of 10–15 per minute with peak inspiratory pressure of 12 mmH$_2$O for a baby under 1 kg, and less than 18 mmH$_2$O for a baby over 1 kg, is a very rough guide.

Management of extubation failure

If extubation fails because of airway obstruction, a retrial after a period of 2–4 days on systemic dexamethasone, an acid-blocking agent, and heavy sedation or paralysis to reduce tube movement, may be successful.

Where there have been repeated failures of extubation, the paediatric ENT surgeon should assess the airway at MLB. The treatment of choice will depend upon the endoscopic findings. If there is relatively little airway trauma but some generalised oedema reducing the laryngeal or subglottic airway, then a further period of therapeutic reintubation may be successful. Sometimes the airway obstruction can be corrected endoscopically, for example by vapourising acquired subglottic cysts or prominent laryngeal granulations with a CO$_2$ laser. Extubation will then become possible 48–72 hours later. Where there is incipient or early SGS with oedema but a near-normal and clear airway at the level of the vocal cords and above, an anterior cricoid split operation can be undertaken. If the SGS is more severe and the fibrous tissue more mature, then an SS-LTR, employing a costochondral graft to augment the airway, is chosen. The reconstruction is supported by an ETT for 1–2 weeks, and, if successful, subsequent extubation allows avoidance of a tracheostomy.

Where there is severe transglottic inflammation with granulations or oedema in the supraglottis as well as the subglottis, then a tracheostomy is advised, as the entire larynx cannot settle with the continued presence of an ETT. Fig. 27.64 shows laryngeal granulations and exposed cartilage following prolonged complicated intubation. Very early reassessment of the larynx at endoscopy is advisable in such a situation. If after 3 weeks the inflammation has settled and the airway is adequate, tracheostomy decannulation should proceed. Unnecessary prolongation of the duration the tracheostomy is left in situ may otherwise exacerbate the development of progressive SGS.

Laryngotracheal airway obstruction – conditions and management

Laryngomalacia

Laryngomalacia is the most common cause of infant stridor. It results from laxity of the supraglottic structures: the epiglottis and the mucosa over the cuneiform and arytenoid cartilages can be sucked into the airway on inspiration. The epiglottis is usually curled and omega shaped and there are both short and tall aryepiglottic folds tethering the arytenoid mucosa to the epiglottis. Laryngomalacia is seen with associated reflux. The airway obstruction and increased intrathoracic negative pressure will increase acid reflux. Typically it presents with inspiratory stridor after the first few weeks (sometimes days) of life. It tends to increase in severity and is often worse on feeding and sleeping supine. The cry will be normal. It is twice as common in boys. The natural history is for self-correction with growth over a 12–24-month period, but it can persist. The diagnosis should usually be confirmed with endoscopy. Treatment is often expectant; however, when there is progressive or continuing stridor with marked recession and respiratory effort, the baby will fail to thrive. If the weight charts show a consistent fall-off down the percentiles, then surgical correction should be undertaken. The endoscopic operation of aryepiglottoplasty (or supraglottoplasty) involves trimming the redundant mucosa and cuneiform cartilages away, and freeing the tethered aryepiglottic folds with micro scissors. It is usually highly successful for posterior laryngomalacia, but there is a risk of supraglottic stenosis from scarring. When the laryngomalacia is of an anterior type, involving the epiglottis prolapsing back or into the laryngeal introitus, surgery may not be successful. Some paediatric ENT surgeons advocate an extended supraglottoplasty, resecting the lateral free edges of the curled epiglottis as well. Severe cases of laryngomalacia, not suitable for this endoscopic surgery, may require a tracheostomy, but this is rare.

Airway cysts and webs

Congenital laryngeal (mucous retention) cysts, laryngeal saccule cysts and supraglottic cysts can present in very early life or at a few months with stridor. A mucous cyst of the vallecula at the tongue base can present early with UAO and stridor or stertor. Lateral soft-tissue X-rays may be helpful, but these cysts are definitively diagnosed and treated endoscopically (Fig. 27.65).

Acquired subglottic cysts are commonly found in previously intubated infants, most frequently arising on the left-hand side. They will present with stridor sometimes at the time of a respiratory infection. They can be cured by laser vapourisation at endoscopy.[38]

Congenital webbing of the larynx, in which the vocal cords are fused together anteriorly, is rare, and will present with stridor and a posterior laryngeal airway. Open surgery and stenting with a keel is usually required.

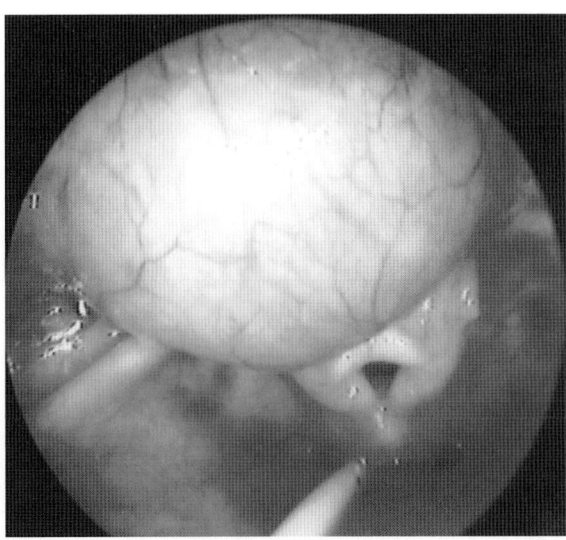

Fig. 27.65 Vallecular mucous retention cyst obstructing the airway at the tongue base.

Vocal cord paralysis

Vocal cord paralysis can be unilateral or bilateral, and congenital or acquired. Congenital causes include Arnold-Chiari malformation, other neurological disease and birth trauma, while acquired causes may be from neck trauma or open-heart surgery. Even congenital cases can show spontaneous recovery of movement with development and age. Unilateral cord palsy will present with a weak or husky cry and sometimes feeding difficulty. Stridor is present only if there is coexistent airway swelling. Bilateral cord paralyses, by comparison, will present with inspiratory or biphasic stridor with a vocal quality to the inspiratory noise. The cords lie very close to the midline, restricting the airway. Diagnosis is made at a dynamic microlaryngoscopy. Unilateral cases require no intervention, but bilateral cord paralysis often requires a tracheostomy.

Croup

LTB or croup is usually managed by paediatricians and only involves the ENT surgeons when there have been multiple failures of extubation (see above). Then, endoscopy (MLB) is indicated for diagnosis, and occasionally laser reduction of laryngeal granulations. The ex-premature baby requiring intubation for subsequent croup, however, is at increased risk of developing SGS.

Congenital posterior laryngeal cleft

A congenital laryngeal cleft occurs in the posterior larynx when there is failure of closure of the tracheo-oesophageal groove as high as the interarytenoid level, and a degree of failure of fusion of the posterior cricoid cartilage lamina. There are numerous classifications described,[31] but the most commonly accepted one is that of Benjamin & Inglis.[5] A type I cleft represents a failure of mucosal fusion in the posterior larynx, with the open

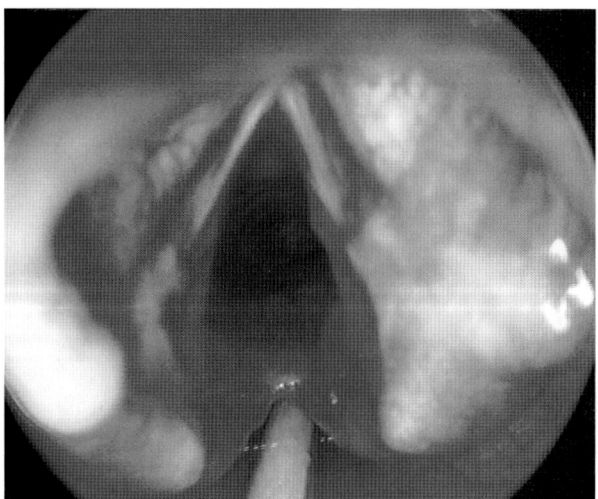

Fig. 27.66 Type I congenital posterior laryngeal cleft.

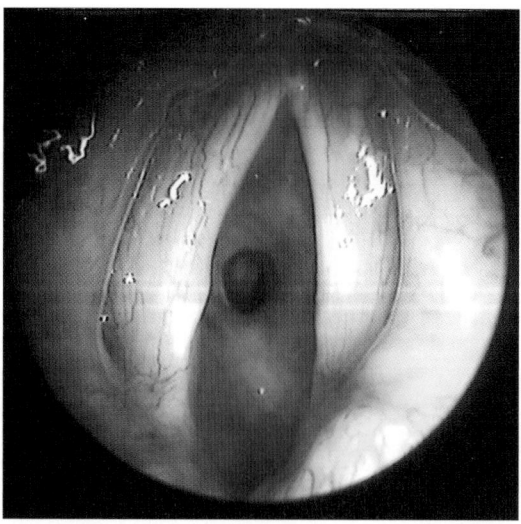

Fig. 27.67 Severe subglottic stenosis.

notch reaching the level of the vocal cords but not affecting the posterior cricoid plate (Fig. 27.66). A type 2 cleft notches into the cricoid cartilage below the cords. In a type 3 cleft there is complete cleft of the posterior cricoid cartilage and mucosa extending into the cervical trachea. The type 4 cleft extends down into the thoracic trachea (laryngotracheo-oesophageal cleft), even to the carina or beyond.

Type 1 clefts may present late, with repeated aspiration pneumonias and maybe inspiratory stridor similar to that of laryngomalacia. Type 2 and 3 clefts are more likely to present in early life, with airway embarrassment requiring ventilation and with failed extubations. The type 4 cleft may be an immediate neonatal emergency, with great difficulty maintaining an adequate ET tube position to ventilate the baby, as the tube tends to prolapse into the oesophagus. Such severe type 4 laryngeal clefts are often incompatible with long-term survival. The diagnosis is always confirmed by MLB.

Management of posterior laryngeal clefts

The type 1 clefts and some type 2 clefts can be repaired surgically from an endoscopic approach. Deeper type 2 clefts and worse will require an open neck or neck and median sternotomy approach. The cleft is repaired in layers, inserting a tibial periosteal graft in the trachealis region and perhaps a cartilage graft at the posterior cricoid level. The baby usually needs a tracheostomy as well. Tracheomalacia of the airway remains a significant problem in these challenging conditions.

Subglottic stenosis

In over 95% of babies, SGS is considered acquired,[9] following prolonged intubation of low-birthweight premature infants, who also develop chronic lung disease. The incidence varies but in our institution it occurs in approximately 2.5% of intubated, severely preterm babies. SGS can be congenital, when the unintubated baby is born with stridor. In these cases, endoscopy shows a narrowed, sometimes pear-shaped cricoid region or underriding of the first tracheal cartilage ring. If infants with a congenitally narrow subglottis do require intubation, the use of a standard-sized tube in this situation will cause trauma and may lead to a combined congenital and acquired SGS. The Cotton classification describes the severity of the stenosis, grade I representing up to 50% reduction in lumen cross-section, grade II between 50% and 70%, grade III 70–99%, and grade IV complete stenosis with no lumen. The percentage can be read off a chart according to the size of ET tube in relation to age.[32] Fig. 27.67 shows a mature severe SGS.

Factors influencing the development of SGS have been studied[36] and are similar to those for failed extubations. The duration of intubation, the number of ETTs inserted, the duration of mechanical ventilation, the presence of post-extubation stridor, and the size of the ETT in relation to gestational age are significantly correlated with the development of SGS.

The management of SGS will depend upon its severity and evolution. The mildest cases may be managed conservatively, and, with growth, the condition can improve. Early oedematous SGS may be treated by the cricoid split operation and more severe mature stenoses are likely to require laryngotracheal reconstruction (LTR) surgery or cricotracheal resection. A tracheostomy is frequently required for a number of years in these difficult cases.

Cricoid split

When there is failure of extubation caused by persistent isolated subglottic oedema, granulations or early soft or incipient SGS, then an open anterior cricoid split operation will often allow subsequent successful extubation. The neck is approached from a horizontal skin crease incision, the cricoid ring and adjacent airway divided vertically, preserving the vocal cords at the anterior commissure, and the baby is then reintubated with a large-sized ETT. This procedure allows oedema fluid to escape from the subglottic region, and the enlarged subglottis will usually heal quickly with an anterior fibrous union. Extubation is attempted, despite an absence of air leak, after 2 to 7 days following the use of systemic steroids and ranitidine. Tube movement should be kept to a minimum.

If there is accidental extubation, the risk of creating a false passage into the neck on reintubation can be reduced by rotating the ET tube through 180° as it is passed through the cords and asking an assistant to apply light digital pressure to the anterior neck wound. The use of a neck drain to avoid surgical emphysema is advised until well after successful extubation.

The reported success rate for cricoid split surgery is between 69% and 75%;[20] however, this procedure is not without potential complications, and failures will require a tracheostomy. In our own experience, the success rate was over 80%, but this was in a highly selected population.[30] VLBW neonates with a higher oxygen requirement are less likely to have a successful outcome.

Single-stage laryngotracheal reconstruction

Where the infant presents with failure of extubation or progressive stridor and is shown at endoscopy to have a definitive SGS, the problem can often be corrected by an SS-LTR. The SGS is usually a Cotton grade I or II. This procedure involves a vertical anterior split of the cricoid and adjacent tracheal rings with insertion of an anterior cartilage graft into the airway to enlarge its diameter. Every attempt is made to avoid disruption of the vocal cords at the anterior commissure, as blunting here will result in a poor-quality husky voice. If the SGS is more severe, or if there is posterior scarring, a posterior cricoid split or even posterior cricoid graft is also inserted. The graft is typically harvested from the costochondral cartilage from the lower ribcage anterolaterally.

After the grafts have been secured with resorbable monofilament sutures, the infant is reintubated for 5–14 days on a neonatal or paediatric intensive care unit (NICU, PICU). The postoperative protocols will be very similar to those for a cricoid split operation, except for a longer period of intubation. If extubation is successful, then the airway has been corrected without the need for a tracheostomy. Sometimes in the 'single-stage' operation an existing tracheostomy will be surgically reversed and closed at the same operation.

Post-extubation care will require close observation of the airway for a few weeks. There is usually the need for a further two or three MLB procedures in the first postoperative 6 weeks, to remove granulations from the airway as the graft becomes vascularised and epithelialised.

Hartnick et al[21] reported the Cincinnati experience of SS-LTR, finding first operation-specific extubation rates were between 67% and 82%, depending on the severity of stenosis. Almost all failures, however, were subsequently extubated or decannulated after a revision procedure. Morrison & Wareing[30] showed 80–90% success rates for SS-LTR.

Staged laryngotracheal reconstruction

Staged LTR for SGS is similar to the single-stage procedure, but with a tracheostomy in situ which is only removed later (Fig. 27.68). After the graft(s) have been inserted into the subglottis and upper trachea, the reconstructed lumen is stented for a period (typically 6 weeks), prior to stent removal at a second

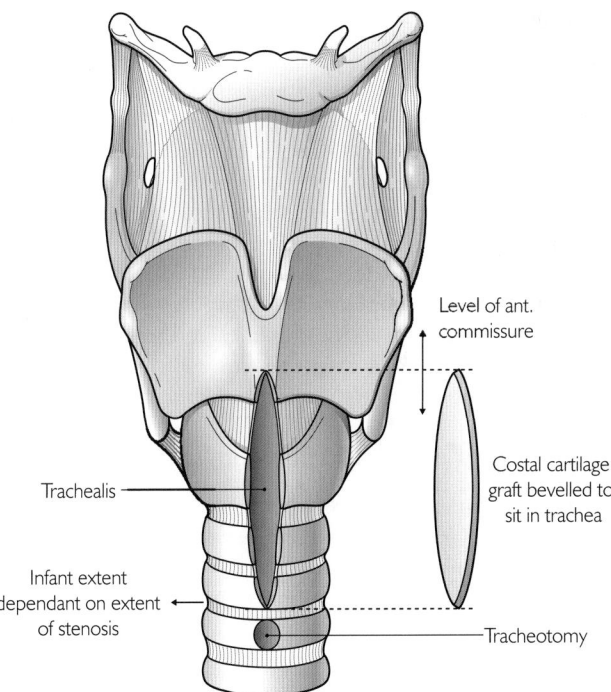

Fig. 27.68 Technique of laryngotracheal reconstruction.

Labels: Level of ant. commissure; Costal cartilage graft bevelled to sit in trachea; Trachealis; Infant extent dependant on extent of stenosis; Tracheotomy

stage. After removal of the stent, the airway requires a number of endoscopic procedures to keep it clear of granulations as the lumen and graft fully epithelialise. When healing is complete, the tracheostomy can be removed as a ward or surgical decannulation procedure. The airway usually takes time to stabilise and the time to decannulation of tracheostomy following successful staged LTR is often 3–6 months.

The surgery can distort the glottic anatomy, and cricoarytenoid joint movement is often impaired in these children as well. A long-term hoarse voice is therefore a common outcome following LTR surgery.

The staged LTR is usually reserved for more severe stenoses and revision procedures. For these multiple or double-staged LTRs, reported operation-specific decannulation rates for Myer–Cotton grades 2, 3, and 4 as 85% (18/21), 37% (23/61) and 50% (7/14), respectively, and the overall decannulation rates were between 74% and 95%.[21] Unfavourable results are encountered for the most severe stenoses, and because of this, the newer operation of cricotracheal resection evolved.

Cricotracheal resection

In recent years the operation of cricotracheal resection has gained popularity. First described by Philippe Monnier,[29] it is indicated for the more severe stenoses and involves resection of the narrowed or obliterated subglottic space including removal of most of the cricoid cartilage while preserving some of its posterior lamina. The trachea is mobilised and 'end-to-end' larynx-to-tracheal anastomosis is undertaken. The chin and neck may need to be secured in a flexed position with temporary external sutures during the postoperative healing period, to avoid tracheal separation. In a specialist centre,[28] 93% of patients were decannulated, over half had dysphonia.

Subglottic haemangioma

Subglottic haemangiomas usually present after 6 weeks of age, with progressive stridor and recession. They can be unilateral or bilateral and are seen as a soft smooth red swelling in the subglottis (Fig. 27.69). The haemangioma enlarges over the first year or so, and the airway may become compromised, requiring tracheostomy in about 60% of cases.[7] The presence of a cutaneous haemangioma may be a clue to the subglottic diagnosis. The natural history will be of spontaneous resolution over a few years.

MLB under general anaesthesia is required to make the diagnosis. The subglottis shows a smooth dark red swelling on one or both sides, more bulbous in the posterior airway.

Management of subglottic haemangioma

Small haemangiomata can be monitored endoscopically until they regress. If the airway is more significantly compromised, the choice is between a tracheostomy or an attempt to reduce the haemangioma and avoid or reverse a tracheostomy. Episodes on systemic steroids (prednisolone) or intralesional steroids can be beneficial and avoid a tracheostomy, but long-term systemic steroid therapy is not advised because of adverse side effects. Laser vaporisation of some of the haemangioma may improve the airway and allow avoidance of tracheostomy. Formerly, the CO_2 laser was employed, but results were disappointing. In one large series, the time to resolution of subglottic haemangiomas did not appear to be reduced by CO_2 laser therapy.[7] The physical characteristics of the KTP laser, with deeper penetration into the red spectrum of the haemangioma, may prove a better choice in the future.

For those patients who required a tracheostomy, the mean time from diagnosis to decannulation was 30 months.[7] More recently, in order to avoid a prolonged period with a tracheostomy, thereby reducing morbidity and enhancing language development, open single-stage excision of the haemangioma by a cricoid split approach and submucosal dissection, with or without a costal graft insertion, has achieved good results, with 80% successful extubation at the first open operation (G Morrison, unpublished data 2003).[16]

Vascular compression (rings and slings)

Investigation

The baby or infant with stridor always requires investigation. Particularly where there is evidence of a cardiac condition or associated swallowing difficulty (dysphagia lusoria), a barium swallow X-ray can be helpful. This may demonstrate a congenitally abnormal vascular ring or sling compressing the oesophagus, the trachea, or both structures.

Echocardiography can also demonstrate abnormal vessels in the chest, but as ultrasonography expertise is mostly focused on the heart itself, this investigation can miss some mediastinal vessels.

A diagnostic MLB remains the most important investigation and will visualise any pulsatile vascular compression with secondary tracheomalacia or bronchomalacia.

An MRI or CT scan of the thorax will allow clarification of the configuration of the great vessels and detect compression of the trachea or main bronchi by an aberrant vessel such as a double aortic arch (Fig. 27.70) or an aberrant left pulmonary artery.

Management of vascular anomalies

Once the diagnosis has been confirmed with MLB, echocardiography and scanning, the treatment of the condition is surgical correction by paediatric cardiac surgeons. Even after this, soft-tissue swelling will frequently compromise the tracheal or bronchial airway for many months. When necessary, a tracheostomy will treat this by stenting the distal trachea open until natural resolution occurs. If one main bronchus is occluded, then intraluminal bronchial stenting can be undertaken. This is not without complications, however. 'Palmaz' metal expandable mesh stents (Johnson & Johnson Interventional Systems Co, Warren, NJ) are

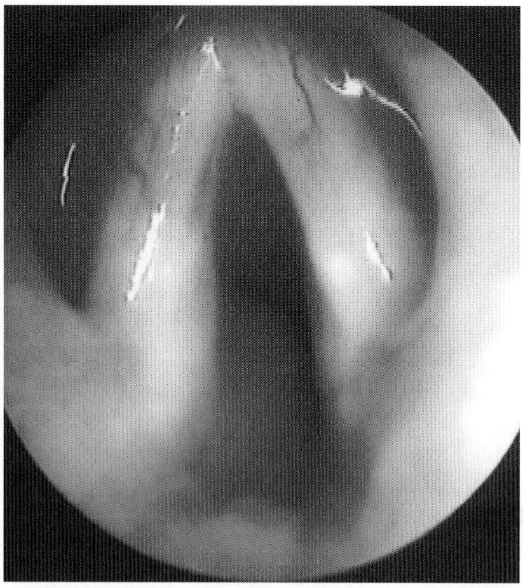

Fig. 27.69 Unilateral subglottic haemangioma.

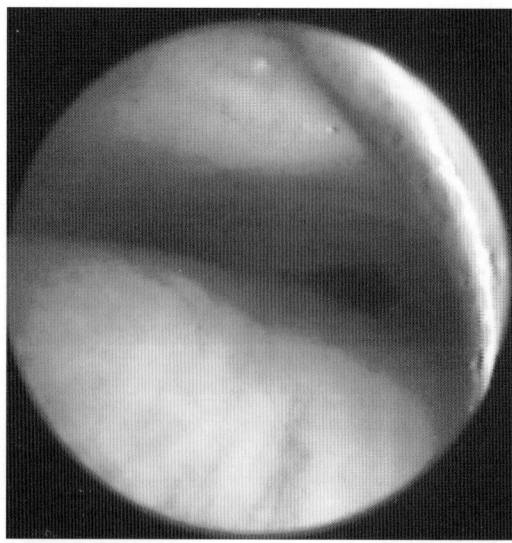

Fig. 27.70 Bronchoscopic view of double aortic arch, above the carina.

inserted at bronchoscopy or under radiological screening and are well accepted but become incorporated into the mucosal wall and cannot be easily removed at a future date. Silastic 'Hood' stents can be changed and removed, but may lead to more troublesome granulations in the airway. Stenting is advised only when the condition remains life threatening and other measures have failed.

Congenital microtrachea

This condition, also known as long-segment congenital tracheal stenosis and as stove-pipe trachea, occurs when some or all of the trachea forms with complete tracheal cartilage rings, rather than an open D configuration. There is a large range of severity, but, as the rings are smaller in diameter than normal and do not enlarge at a normal rate, stridor tends to become progressively worse, with increased oxygen needs, over early life. Presentation may be from birth for severe stenoses or only later in childhood for the less severe cases. The microtrachea can be an isolated anomaly, but it is commonly associated with a vascular anomaly, typically an aberrant left pulmonary artery, which passes to the right before looping around the back of the stenotic trachea to reach the left side of the mediastinum (Fig. 27.71).

Management of congenital tracheal stenosis

The mildest cases can be treated conservatively with serial endoscopy. Where there is an associated vascular anomaly, this

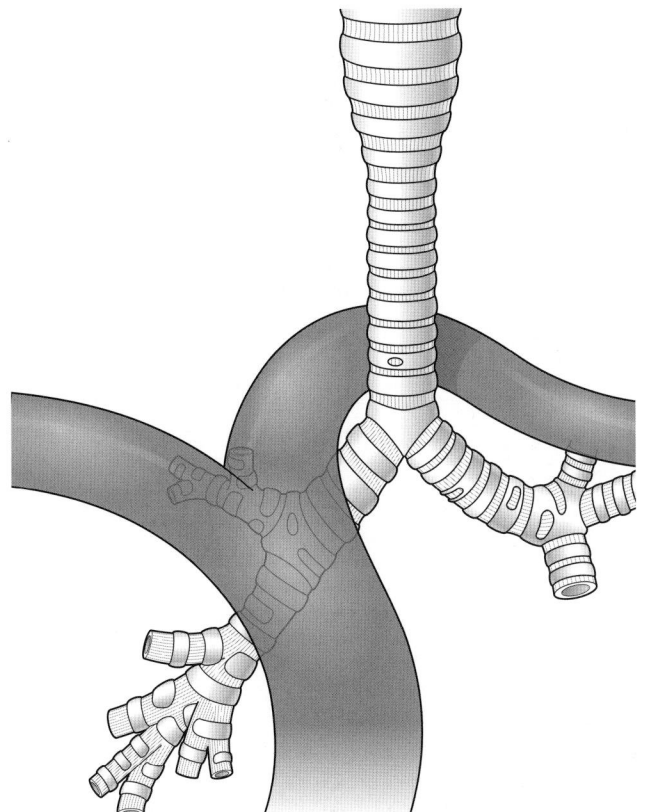

Fig. 27.71 Congenital long-segment tracheal stenosis with aberrant left pulmonary artery.

will require correction surgically. Numerous surgical techniques have been described to correct the microtrachea itself. Short-segment stenoses can be managed by resection and 'end-to-end' anastomosis of the trachea. Longer segments can be treated by a slide tracheoplasty operation, which widens the diameter at the same time as shortening it.[10,25] Pericardial patching to a split open trachea has also been employed, but collapse and lack of rigidity are problems with this technique.[3] All of these surgical treatments are carried out under cardiac bypass. Finally, the most severe stenoses have been treated by transplant of cadaveric tracheas.[22] This involves many months of intraluminal stenting with treatment of troublesome granulations.

Tracheomalacia, bronchomalacia

Tracheomalacia or bronchomalacia can be primary or secondary. When primary, there is generalised lack of support of the airway, with weak collapsing cartilage, causing a flattening of the normal D-shape cartilages on respiration and excessive collapse of the trachealis soft tissue into the lumen on respiration. This may involve one or both of the trachea and bronchi. The generalised tracheomalacia is likely to be self-correcting with growth. Secondary malacia occurs where there is extrinsic compression of the airway from an abnormal vessel, an unusually overriding aorta, or from a mediastinal tumour. It can also occur as localised tracheomalacia following cartilage resorption at the site of a tracheostomy or other airway surgery. Tracheomalacia will present with biphasic or primarily expiratory stridor, recession and a gruff barking cough. It is made worse by increased activity or respiratory effort, or concurrent infection.

Investigations for tracheobronchomalacia

Diagnostic MLB will confirm the tracheomalacia or bronchomalacia, so long as the study is dynamic, with the baby breathing spontaneously under a light general anaesthetic without CPAP from the anaesthetic circuit. Flexible bronchoscopy on a NICU, through an ETT, will also allow this assessment if there is no positive airway pressure. Such an assessment, however, can exaggerate the degree of malacia and in a flexible assessment of any normal infant making significant respiratory effort there will be some airway collapse and bulging in of the trachealis with respiration, because of the negative intrathoracic pressure. Radiology using a contrast bronchogram under screening or video recording will also demonstrate a malacic airway and help to localise the area of obstruction or image the tree distal to an endoscopically unpassable stenosis.

Management of tracheobronchomalacia

Primary malacia can be treated by positive pressure ventilation or CPAP until there is sufficient improvement. This conservative approach may not always be possible, however, in which case tracheostomy or intraluminal stenting are considered. Localised tracheomalacia, if severe, may require a tracheostomy, the tube stenting the airway open. Sometimes, customised longer tubes are required. Secondary tracheomalacia will tend to self-correct once the causative external compression is rectified, but airway stenting or tracheostomy can still be required for a period. Furman et al[17] reviewed six cases employing a Palmaz expandable stent, reporting two deaths and three long-term successes. Granulation formation within the airway was encountered. Aortic compression of the trachea can sometimes be improved by aortopexy surgery, in which the aorta is hitched anteriorly towards the sternum.

Cartilage malacia following localised surgery such as tracheostomy can require tracheal reconstruction with costal cartilage grafting or excision and 'end-to-end' anastomosis.

Bronchoscopy for atelectasis and air trapping

Infantile pneumonias are usually treated medically, with mechanical ventilation and with endotracheal suctioning and physiotherapy where necessary. Bronchoscopy is not generally considered as a first-line adjunctive treatment. However, on occasions, rigid bronchoscopy under light general anaesthesia will lead to an improvement in the condition. Firstly, if the segmental or main bronchi are obstinately plugged with mucus casts, it may be possible to clear these at bronchoscopy by bronchial saline lavage and aspiration. The topical irrigation at bronchoscopy of a mucolytic agent such as rhDNase therapy[14] has been highly effective in this regard in a small number of cases. Bronchoscopy can also allow accurate collection of a tenacious mucopurulent specimen for microbiology.

Finally, unilateral air trapping and emphysema with secondary mediastinal shift in neonates can be compromising; if the problem persists, a rigid bronchoscopy to clear the segmental bronchi and inflate the collapsed regions can restore a more symmetrical ventilation.

Tracheostomy

In the 19th century, indications for tracheostomy included inhaled foreign bodies, diphtheria and croup, but the mortality was very high. In recent years, indications have changed. Infective indications, especially bacterial, are much reduced, although intubation trauma to the laryngotracheal airway following ventilation for croup (LTB) remains a common problem. Increasing survival of VLBW babies and babies with multiple congenital abnormalities has led to a lowering of the average age of patients undergoing paediatric tracheostomy, more than half of which procedures are carried out in babies under 1 year old.[40] There is often continued need for long-term tracheostomy in these infants. Also, more paediatric tracheostomies are carried out for surviving babies with congenital UAOs as well as for those with neuromuscular diseases.

Broadly there are three categories of indication for a tracheostomy: (i) for airway obstruction, (ii) for assisted prolonged ventilation (especially if there is evidence of airway trauma), and (iii) to provide pulmonary toilet and/or non-ventilatory support. This last category will include infants with neurological impairment or immaturity who are ventilator dependent using an ETT but can be weaned to spontaneous respiration with a tracheostomy

and supportive airway toilet. This process allows rehabilitation away from an ICU setting.

In our institution, in a series of 65 cases over 3 years, almost half the paediatric tracheostomies performed were for airway obstruction; only 8.7% were for an acute airway infection and 12.3% were required for a congenital airway anomaly. The remainder of patients in this series required a tracheostomy for long-term ventilation, airway toilet or non-ventilatory respiratory support. Table 27.21 summarises the common causes of airway obstruction requiring tracheostomy.

Tracheostomy technique

Surgical tracheostomy technique in the baby or infant requires a vertical slit through the 2–5 tracheal rings. Removal of a window of cartilage is contraindicated, as it leads to tracheal wall collapse. Good practice either sutures the tracheal edge to the adjacent neck skin or employs two nylon tracheal 'rescue' stay sutures, one from each side of the trachea, taped to the chest. In the event of a tube displacement or obstruction, the attending staff can then facilitate reinsertion of a new tracheostomy tube by pulling the stay sutures up and outwards, making the tracheal opening pout forwards.

Post-tracheostomy ward care

Postoperatively, a CXR is routine to confirm the tracheostomy tube position and that there are no complications such as consolidation or pneumothorax. The tracheostomy tapes and the tube should not be changed or removed for the first week, except in airway distress, in order to allow a good tract to develop. A member of the medical staff should perform the first tube change; thereafter, weekly changes, or more frequently if there is a need, are advised. 'Velcro' tracheostomy tapes can be used after the first tube change. The tube must be kept patent at all times. Constant humidification of the ventilated or inspired air is recommended, to stop drying of obstructive secretions. If the baby is self-ventilating, formal humidification or the application of a 'Swedish nose' (Portex Thermovent T attachment) will achieve this.

Table 27.21 Airway indications for tracheostomy
■ Airway obstructed above larynx, (e.g. lymphangioma, Pierre Robin etc.)
■ Tongue base collapse, glossoptosis
■ Severe laryngomalacia
■ Laryngeal granulations and airway trauma (post intubation)
■ Subglottic stenosis
■ Subglottic haemangioma
■ Respiratory papillomatosis
■ Bilateral vocal cord palsy
■ Bilateral crico-arytenoid joint fixation
■ Vascular compression – aberrant pulmonary artery, double aortic arch
■ Primary tracheomalacia
■ Microtrachea and congenital bronchopulmonary deformities

Regular tracheostomy suctioning will be required to keep the airway free of mucus secretions. A flexible catheter is inserted just to the level of the tracheostomy tube tip, and then the suction is activated by occluding its vent with a thumb while the suction tube is gently swivelled between finger and thumb as it is withdrawn. Only occasionally is it necessary to run the suction tube significantly beyond the distal tube tip, to or beyond the carina. Overzealous suctioning of this type can lead to tracheal trauma with bleeding, and granulation formation.

When a tracheostomy is inserted for long-term airway ventilation in a neonate with chronic lung disease (bronchopulmonary dysplasia), initial ventilation may be unexpectedly difficult owing to there being a much larger air leak around the tracheostomy tube up through the larynx than was possible when the long snugger ETT was employed. Higher ventilator pressures may therefore be needed, and relatively larger tracheostomy tubes are often required, which may damage the trachea. This is one reason why tracheostomy is not necessarily a helpful procedure for the baby with severe lung disease who still requires long-term ventilatory support.

Types of tracheostomy tube

Different makes and patterns of tracheostomy tubes are available. In the neonatal and paediatric age group, plastic or Silastic tracheostomy tubes are most commonly employed, rather than the older rigid silver tubes such as the Negus or Alder Hey types. Of the Silastic tubes, the 'Shiley' tubes (manufactured by Mallincrodt) are popular, as they have a standard extension that accepts ventilator attachments and are available in a good range of sizes. The neonatal range of tubes are shorter than the equivalent paediatric tubes (size 3.0 neonatal is 32 mm long compared with 39 mm for paediatric, and the size 3.5 neonatal tube is 32 mm compared with 40 mm for the paediatric). These tubes are all non-cuffed, non-fenestrated tubes, without an inner tube. A preterm baby requiring ventilation through a tracheostomy tube would often require a 3 or 3.5 Shiley neonatal tracheostomy tube. Other makes of tracheotomy tube are Portex and the Great Ormond Street pattern. Occasionally, an extra-long tracheostomy tube is required to hold the carinal region open or bypass granulations. If a paediatric Shiley tube is insufficiently long, then a Mallincrodt Bivona adjustable flange tube can be used and customised to individual needs.

Complications and mortality of tracheostomy

Accidental decannulation and tube obstruction remain the most life-threatening complications. If the attempt to reinsert the tube results in a false passage, the attempts at ventilation will fail and can lead to pneumomediastinum and pneumothorax. Other complications include bleeding, surgical emphysema, wound infection, chest infection, airway trauma from overly vigorous suctioning, and cardiorespiratory arrest.

Late sequelae of tracheostomy include the frequent formation of a suprastomal granuloma within the trachea, tracheomalacia, deglutition difficulties, language delay, chest infections, and subsequent persistence of a tracheo-cutaneous fistula after decannulation. The most serious late complications remain tube obstruction and accidental displacement. Massive haemorrhage is rare, as is tracheal stenosis.

Mortality from tracheostomy is difficult to define. The range for paediatric published series is an overall raw mortality of 11% to 40%.[15] In our most recent series, the overall mortality is 19%. Tracheostomy tube-related deaths, however, are rare, ranging from 0.5% to 3.4% in different reported series.[15] Ward et al[40] reported a tracheostomy-related mortality rate of 2.9%, with mucous plugging of the tracheostomy being the most common cause of death.

There is a strong association between prematurity and mortality in infants with a tracheostomy, and higher comorbidity scores correlate with higher mortality rates. In one series,[18] 80% of deaths were in preterm infants, and among those who were under 3000 g weight at the time of tracheostomy, the mortality rate was 64%. The tube-related mortality rate, however, was low, at 1.6%. In our institution, the raw mortality rate among infants requiring a tracheostomy at under 1 year of (uncorrected) age was 25.6% and that among severe preterm infants requiring long-term ventilation was very much higher. Tracheostomy is not a cure-all treatment for these high-risk infants, and must be undertaken only after careful evaluation.

Home tracheostomy care

Home tracheostomy care will need to be arranged and will include local support services as well as guardians learning to care for the tracheostomy, change the tubes etc., and acquire appropriate resuscitation expertise. Special precautions are required for the baby with a tracheostomy, and include care with baths, refraining from swimming, and avoiding foreign bodies such as sand, dirt, talc or aerosols from entering the stoma. Care is also required with clothes and bibs and sleeping positions, to ensure that these items or the chin does not occlude the tracheostomy tube. A tube extension and 'Swedish nose' help avoid chin dipping as a cause of occlusion.

Decannulation from tracheostomy

The earliest possible decannulation is desirable. Prolonged placement of a tracheostomy tube, even in developmentally normal children, results in language delay.[24] The tracheostomy can be removed after definitive correction or spontaneous resolution of the underlying condition for which the tracheostomy was required and after the airway has been assessed at dynamic endoscopy. Prior to successful tracheostomy decannulation, there should be no serious aspiration or recurrent chest infections, no need for regular tracheal toilet, and no need for assisted ventilation. The upper airway must be adequate and assessed at MLB, which should include removal of any obstructing suprastomal granuloma, and assessment of vocal cord mobility and airway collapse on respiration.

Once the infant is considered fit for decannulation, the usual practice would be to try a ward decannulation procedure. The tracheostomy tube is downsized to the smallest available (usually a size 3 Shiley), and the tube is then occluded with a bung or tape for short periods, by day, with observation and saturation monitoring. The tube is then occluded for progressively longer periods if tolerated; when 24 hours of occlusion is achieved, the tube can be removed and an occlusive dressing applied to the fistula site. If this ward decannulation protocol fails, the airway will require reassessment. Sometimes a surgical decannulation is required. In this case, the tracheostomy is formally reversed and closed at surgery, usually with removal of an obstructive granuloma or repair of a suprastomal tracheal collapse. The baby is then managed on an ICU intubated and ventilated with relatively little tube movement for 2 to 7 days prior to elective extubation.[2]

Antenatal airway obstruction and EXIT

Increasing sophistication of antenatal diagnosis, initially with ultrasound, increasingly allows the detection of potential airway problems that will become apparent at birth or even beforehand. Fetal MRI is helpful to further define the pathology. When a prenatal diagnosis of airway obstruction is made, a multidisciplinary approach to the pregnancy and birth is important. If long-term survival seems possible, it is feasible to plan a special delivery by the EXIT procedure.[41] This procedure involves delivering the head and upper torso of the baby through a caesarian section approach while maintaining the utero-placental blood flow and maternofetal gas exchange. This allows time for the airway obstruction to be corrected and an airway secured, prior to full delivery and ligation of the umbilical cord.

Mass lesions obstructing the fetal airway will be detected on ultrasound. Cystic hygromas are common, but only those hygromas which seem to involve the pharynx or cause airway compression are likely to actually cause neonatal airway obstruction. Once an obstructing lesion is detected on ultrasound, rapid-sequence fetal MRI is recommended, where transverse, sagittal and coronal planes can be studied.

In a complete laryngeal atresia it may be difficult to see the larynx fully on fetal ultrasound, but the secondary changes in the trachea and lungs are apparent. Because there is total obstruction, the liquor produced in the lungs builds up, causing gross tracheal dilatation and hypoechogenic lungs. There is often polyhydramnios, an inverted diaphragm and ascites. This is described as CHAOS (congenital high airway obstruction syndrome) and it represents complete airway obstruction.[11] If the fetus can be brought to maturity, the EXIT procedure with tracheostomy is the management of choice.

References

1. Albert D M, Mills R P, Fysh J, Gamsu H, Thomas J N 1990 Endoscopic examination of the neonatal larynx at extubation: a prospective study of variables associated with laryngeal damage. International Journal of Pediatric Otorhinolaryngology 20: 203–212
2. Al-Saati A, Morrison G A J, Clary R A, Bailey C M 1993 Surgical decannulation of children with tracheostomy. Journal of Laryngology and Otology 107: 217–221
3. Backer C L, Mavroudis C, Gerber M E, Holinger L D 2001 Tracheal surgery in children: an 18-year review of four techniques. European Journal of Cardio-thoracic Surgery 19: 777–784
4. Barrington K J, Bull D, Finer N N 2001 Randomized trial of nasal synchronized intermittent mandatory ventilation compared with continuous positive airway pressure after extubation of very low birth weight infants. Pediatrics 107: 638–641
5. Benjamin B, Inglis A 1989 Minor congenital laryngeal clefts: diagnosis and classification. Annals of Otology, Rhinology and Laryngology 98: 417–420
6. Brewis C, Pracy J P, Albert D M 1999 Localized tracheomalacia as a complication of the Cole tracheal tube. Paediatric Anaesthesia 9: 531–533
7. Chatrath P, Black M, Jani P, Albert D M, Bailey C M 2002 A review of the current management of infantile subglottic haemangioma, including a comparison of CO$_2$ laser therapy versus tracheostomy. International Journal of Pediatric Otorhinolaryngology 64: 143–157
8. Contencin P, Narcy P 1993 Size of endotracheal tube and neonatal acquired subglottic stenosis. Study Group for Neonatology and Pediatric Emergencies in the Parisian Area. Archives of Otolaryngology – Head and Neck Surgery 119: 815–819
9. Cotton R T, Gray S D, Miller R P 1989 Update of the Cincinnati experience in pediatric laryngotracheal reconstruction. Laryngoscope 99: 1111–1116
10. Cunningham M J, Eavey R D, Vlahakes G J, Grillo H C 1998 Slide tracheoplasty for long-segment tracheal stenosis. Archives of Otolaryngology – Head and Neck Surgery 124: 98–103
11. DeCou J M, Jones D C, Jacobs H D, Touloukian R J 1998 Successful ex-utero intrapartum treatment (EXIT) procedure for congenital high airway obstruction syndrome (CHAOS) owing to laryngeal atresia. Journal of Pediatric Surgery 33: 1563–1565
12. Downing G J, Kilbride H W 1995 Evaluation of airway complications in high-risk preterm infants: application of flexible fiberoptic airway endoscopy. Pediatrics 95: 567–572
13. Durward A D, Nicoll S J, Oliver J, Tibby S M, Murdoch I A 1998 The outcome of patients with upper airway obstruction transported to a regional pediatric intensive care unit. European Journal of Pediatrics 157: 907–911
14. Durward A, Forte V, Shemie S 2000 Resolution of mucus plugging and atelectasis after intratracheal rhDNase therapy in a mechanically ventilated child with refractory status asthmaticus. Critical Care Medicine 28: 560–562
15. Dutton J M, Palmer P M, McCulloch T M, Smith R J 1995 Mortality in the pediatric patient with tracheotomy. Head and Neck 17: 403–408
16. Froehlich P, Stamm D, Floret D, Morgon A 1995 Management of subglottic haemangioma. Clinical Otolaryngology and Allied Sciences 20: 336–339
17. Furman R H, Backer C L, Dunham M E, Donaldson J, Mavroudis C, Holinger L D 1999 The use of balloon-expandable metallic stents in the treatment of pediatric tracheomalacia and bronchomalacia. Archives of Otolaryngology – Head and Neck Surgery 125: 203–207
18. Gianoli G J, Miller R H, Guarisco J L 1990 Tracheostomy in the first year of life. Annals of Otology, Rhinology and Laryngology 99: 896–901
19. Giguere C M, Bauman N M, Sato Y et al 2002 Treatment of lymphangiomas with OK-432 (Picibanil) sclerotherapy: a prospective multi-institutional trial. Archives of Otolaryngology – Head and Neck Surgery 128: 1137–1144
20. Grundfast K M, Coffman A C, Milmoe G 1985 Anterior cricoid split: a "simple" surgical procedure and a potentially complicated care problem. Annals of Otology, Rhinology and Laryngology 94: 445–449
21. Hartnick C J, Hartley B E, Lacy P D et al 2001 Surgery for pediatric subglottic stenosis: disease-specific outcomes. Annals of Otology, Rhinology and Laryngology 110: 1109–1113
22. Herberhold C, Stein M, von Falkenhausen M 1999 [Long-term results of homograft reconstruction of the trachea in childhood] (in German). Laryngo-Rhino-Otologie 78: 692–696
23. Holland B W, McGuirt W F Jr 2001 Surgical management of choanal atresia: improved outcome using mitomycin. Archives of Otolaryngology – Head and Neck Surgery 127: 1375–1380
24. Jiang D, Morrison G A J 2003 The influence of long-term tracheostomy on speech and language development in children. International Journal of Pediatric Otorhinolaryngology 67(suppl. 1): S217–S220
25. Lang F J, Hurni M, Monnier P 1999 Long-segment congenital tracheal stenosis: treatment by slide-tracheoplasty. Journal of Pediatric Surgery 34: 1216–1222
26. Lazar R H, Younis R T 1995 Transnasal repair of choanal atresia using telescopes. Archives of Otolaryngology – Head & Neck Surgery 121: 517–520
27. Molitch H I, Unger E C, Witte C L, vanSonnenberg E 1995 Percutaneous sclerotherapy of lymphangiomas. Radiology 194: 343–347
28. Monnier P, Lang F, Savary M 2001 [Treatment of subglottis stenosis in children by cricotracheal resection] (in French). Annales d'Oto-Laryngologie et de Chirurgie Cervico-Faciale 118: 299–305
29. Monnier P, Savary M, Chapuis G 1995 Cricotracheal resection for pediatric subglottic stenosis: update of the Lausanne experience. Acta Oto-Rhino-Laryngologica Belgica 49: 373–382

30. Morrison G A J, Wareing M 1999 Defining boundaries in cricoid split and single stage laryngotracheal reconstruction. Journal of Laryngology and Otology 113(suppl. 23): 49

31. Moungthong G, Holinger L D 1997 Laryngotracheoesophageal clefts. Annals of Otology, Rhinology and Laryngology 106: 1002–1011

32. Myer C M 3rd, O'Connor D M, Cotton R T 1994 Proposed grading system for subglottic stenosis based on endotracheal tube sizes. Annals of Otology, Rhinology and Laryngology 103: 319–323

33. Pashley N R T 1982 Risk factors and the prediction of outcome in acquired subglottic stenosis in children. International Journal of Pediatric Otorhinolaryngology 4: 1–6

34. Randolph A G, Wypij D, Venkataraman S T et al 2002 Effect of mechanical ventilator weaning protocols on respiratory outcomes in infants and children: a randomized controlled trial. Pediatric Acute Lung Injury and Sepsis Investigators (PALISI) Network. Journal of the American Medical Association 288: 2561–2568

35. Samadi D S, Shah U K, Handler S D 2003 Choanal atresia: a twenty-year review of medical comorbidities and surgical outcomes. Laryngoscope 113: 254–258

36. Sherman J M, Lowitt S, Stephenson C, Ironson G 1986 Factors influencing acquired subglottic stenosis in infants. Journal of Pediatrics 109: 322–327

37. Suzumura H, Nitta A, Tanaka G, Kuwashima S, Hirabayashi H 2000 Role of infection in the development of acquired subglottic stenosis in neonates with prolonged intubation. Pediatrics International 42: 508–513

38. Tierney P, Francis I, Morrison G A J 1997 Acquired subglottic cysts in low birth weight pre-term infants. Journal of Laryngology and Otology 111: 487–481

39. Van der Broek P, Brinkman W F B 1979 Congenital laryngeal defects. International Journal of Pediatric Otorhinolaryngology 1: 71–78

40. Ward R F, Jones J, Carew J F 1995 Current trends in pediatric tracheotomy International Journal of Pediatric Otorhinolaryngology 32: 233–239

41. Ward V M M, Langford K, Morrison G 2000 Prenatal diagnosis of airway compromise: EXIT (ex utero intra-partum treatment) and foetal airway surgery. International Journal of Pediatric Otorhinolaryngology 53: 137–141

42. Wimmershoff M B, Schreyer A, Glaessl A et al 2000 Mixed capillary/lymphatic malformation with coexisting port-wine stain: treatment utilizing 3D MRI and CT-guided sclerotherapy. Dermatologic Surgery 26: 584–587

CHAPTER 28

Cardiovascular disease

Nick Archer

Introduction

Neonatal cardiovascular disease can be primary or secondary, congenital or acquired, structural or functional. Whatever categories of abnormality are concerned, a similar systematic approach to history, examination and investigation is required to allow correct management. In many situations, an understanding of fetal as well as of neonatal cardiovascular physiology is necessary. In this chapter the approach is pathophysiological, with particular conditions being considered in the most appropriate category. A description of fetal and perinatal cardiovascular physiology is given and the growing practice of fetal cardiac diagnosis and therapy will be considered. Those seeking information on embryology of the heart are referred to reviews by Srivastava & Baldwin,[88] Mahony[63] and Pickoff.[78]

Fetal circulation

The basic differences between fetal and postnatal circulations are the presence of a low-resistance high-flow placental circulation in the fetus, and the fact that not more than 20% of total cardiac output enters the fetal pulmonary circulation at term and even less reaches the lungs in early gestation. Three vascular pathways which are an integral part of the different blood flow pattern in the fetus close soon after birth in a healthy term infant. These are the ductus venosus, the foramen ovale and the ductus arteriosus (DA). The first two allow oxygenated blood from the placenta to be channelled into the left atrium and thence via the left ventricle and ascending aorta to the coronary and cerebral circulations. The DA has pulmonary artery to aortic (right to left) flow because of high pulmonary vascular resistance (PVR). The DA is kept patent in utero by prostaglandins, both circulating and locally produced, and as gestation progresses, it becomes increasingly sensitive to the constricting influence of oxygen. The role of prostaglandins in maintaining fetal duct patency is important when considering the administration of prostaglandin synthetase inhibitors to pregnant women for any reason, such as to suppress premature labour or to treat polyhydramnios. In these circumstances, reversible fetal DA constriction has been documented.[66] However, there are reports of neonatal persistent pulmonary hypertension in association with maternal prostaglandin synthetase inhibitor ingestion.[65,115] This problem is probably related both to constriction of the DA and to changes in pulmonary vasculature induced by the drug. At birth, arterial oxygen tension rises and PVR begins to fall, allowing an increase in pulmonary blood flow. Also in response to higher oxygen tension, the DA starts to constrict; this process is functionally complete within 60 hours in 93% of term infants.[35] Increased lung blood flow causes increased pulmonary venous return, resulting in elevation of the left atrial pressure. This pushes the foramen ovale shut, although it may then exhibit left-to-right shunting, even into adult life. The ductus venosus closes as umbilical venous flow ceases, but it can provide vascular access to the right heart for a few days. Closure of all these structures may be delayed in pathological circumstances and may precipitate clinical deterioration in various structural cardiac conditions (Table 28.1). Continued patency of the DA and foramen ovale may contribute to clinical problems in some conditions (Table 28.2).

Table 28.1 Clinical problems associated with closure of the foramen ovale, ductus venosus and ductus arteriosus after birth

Foramen ovale	Poorer mixing in TGA Systemic/pulmonary venous obstruction in right/left heart obstructions
Ductus venosus	Worsening pulmonary venous obstruction in infradiaphragmatic TAPVC
Ductus arteriosus	Marked deterioration in duct-dependent pulmonary or systemic circulations

Table 28.2 Clinical problems associated with failure of closure of the foramen ovale, ductus venosus and ductus arteriosus after birth

Foramen ovale	Allows right-to-left shunting in PPHN and (probably less often) in respiratory causes of high right heart pressures
Ductus venosus	No definite problem identified
Ductus arteriosus	Associated with major respiratory and other problems in preterm infants Important left-to-right shunting only rarely seen in the newborn period in term infants with PDA

Table 28.3 Conditions with increased risk of fetal cardiac abnormalities, offer of fetal cardiac scan appropriate

- Autosomal dominant condition with cardiac implications in either parent
- Structural heart disease in parent or previous sibling
- Structural heart disease in two or more family members
- Maternal disease with increased risk of fetal cardiac problem, e.g. diabetes mellitus, collagen vascular disease
- Maternal teratogen exposure, e.g.
  - infection: rubella
  - medication: anticonvulsants, lithium
  - alcohol
- Abnormal nuchal translucency in first trimester with normal karyotype
- Abnormal four-chamber screening scan
- Non-cardiac abnormalities in fetus
- Suspected syndrome in fetus
- Maternal prostaglandin synthetase inhibitor therapy
- Abnormal heart rate/rhythm in fetus
- Hydropic fetus

Fetal cardiology

Diagnosis

Fetal cardiac anatomy, function and rhythm have been determined by transabdominal scanning from 18 weeks' gestation for the last two decades.[5] Transvaginal ultrasound has been used for detailed assessment of high-risk cases[46] but has also been used as a screening tool to detect cardiac abnormalities at 14 to 16 weeks.[13] Transabdominal scanning can now detect important abnormalities under 14 weeks of pregnancy.[19,91] An approach using both abdominal and (when necessary) transvaginal scanning in high-risk cases at 10–13 weeks allowed interpretable images in over 80% of cases,[51] with a probable low false-positive rate although verification was incomplete. Screening fetal cardiac anatomy with a four-chamber view at 18 weeks is part of general anomaly scanning in many regions, but this will pick up under 50% of cases of structural heart lesions, even in experienced hands.[101,117] Heart lesions picked up by a four-chamber screening scan are generally the more complex ones with a poorer outlook both prenatally and after delivery. If views of the outflow tracts are obtained in addition to the four-chamber view, the range of abnormalities detectable is increased.[18] In particular, transposition and tetralogy of Fallot and similar lesions should be recognised. Detailed evaluation of fetal cardiac anatomy by ultrasound is much more time consuming and is usually reserved for women with an increased risk of having a fetus with a cardiac problem (Table 28.3). However, when detailed echocardiography was used on all pregnancies, Stümpflen and colleagues reported an 86% sensitivity and 100% specificity.[101] The conditions missed were mainly atrial septal defects (ASDs) and small ventricular septal defects (VSDs). Other workers have pointed out the difficulty in diagnosing coarctation and total anomalous pulmonary venous return in the fetus.[3] Fetal heart rhythm can be determined by M-mode and Doppler studies. There are ethical aspects to fetal diagnosis and health workers need to be sensitive to parental views. Fetal cardiac scanning should be carried out in the context of expertise in all aspects of fetal medicine, including the provision of support to families. This is very important as the association with non-cardiac abnormalities is strong and these are often major influences in the natural history in utero and after birth, as well as in decisions about continuation of pregnancy. For example, in one study in which cardiac scans were performed for a variety of indications, 70% of fetuses with a cardiac anomaly had an underlying chromosome abnormality.[51]

Treatment

Accurate diagnosis of structural heart disease in a fetus allows information to be given to families. Some parents will opt for termination of pregnancy and about 5% of fetuses with structural cardiac abnormalities will die spontaneously in utero.[12] Cardiac diagnosis and prognosis must be viewed in the context of full fetal assessment, as non-cardiac abnormalities may well be more important in determining these. In pregnancies progressing to viability, a cardiac diagnosis will, in a minority of cases, influence place, time or mode of delivery, and non-cardiac factors also need to be taken into account. The most important specific point with respect to early postnatal management of heart disease is whether or not the lesion is likely to be duct dependent, thereby allowing prostaglandin to be used before symptoms develop. Progressive underdevelopment of the ventricle in the fetus with severe arterial valve stenosis is well recognised[92,106] and arterial valve balloon valvuloplasty can be successful.[57,106] Many structural lesions do not progress with advancing gestation to such an extent that in-utero interventions need to be considered. There is evidence that fetal diagnosis of severe duct-dependent congenital heart disease (CHD) results in babies reaching a cardiac centre in better condition than those not diagnosed until after delivery.[22] Benefit from fetal diagnosis in terms of improved survival and morbidity has been shown for coarctation,[40] and in improved mortality in transposition[10] and hypoplastic left heart,[108] although in the last two conditions benefit from prenatal diagnosis has not always been demonstrated.[58] Reassurance of normality or the chance to prepare for the arrival of an abnormal baby are valued by many parents but cannot easily be quantified.

Accurate diagnosis of fetal dysrhythmias is essential to avoid unnecessary intervention and to allow appropriate treatment which can improve outlook for the fetus with a haemodynamically compromising rhythm disturbance. Diagnosis and management of abnormal fetal rhythms are discussed in the section on neonatal rhythm disturbances (pp. 651–7).

Incidence and aetiology of fetal and neonatal heart disease

Structural CHD occurs in approximately 8 per 1000 live births.[50] In populations uninfluenced by fetal diagnosis, between 30% and 40% of these children will be symptomatic in early infancy and about two-thirds of them will have been diagnosed by the end of the first year of life. There are various studies on the prevalence of CHD: diagnostic methods and criteria vary, but Table 28.4 gives figures for those presenting in the first year of life. Fetal echocardiography has shown that some severe cardiac lesions result in death in utero[12] and the effect of prenatal

Table 28.4 Congenital heart disease diagnosed by any means, presenting in the first year of life, Alberta, 1981–1984 inclusive

Lesion/group	Rate/1000 live births	% of total
Ventricular septal defect	1.905	34.4
Left heart obstruction	0.716	12.9
Right heart obstruction	0.600	10.8
Atrial septal defect	0.580	10.5
Transposition of the great arteries	0.280	5.1
Patent ductus arteriosus	0.251	4.5
Atrioventricular septal defect	0.242	4.4
Tetralogy of Fallot	0.203	3.7
Complex	0.193	3.5
Double-outlet right ventricle	0.145	2.6
Total anomalous pulmonary venous drainage	0.087	1.6
Other	0.338	6.1
Total	5.541	100

Notes: (i) cases given a principal diagnosis and only counted once; (ii) excludes bicuspid aortic valve; (iii) patent ductus arteriosus only included if symptomatic after day 10; (iv) left heart obstruction includes coarctation, aortic stenosis, hypoplastic left heart, mitral stenosis or atresia; (v) right heart obstruction includes pulmonary stenosis or atresia, tricuspid atresia; (vi) complex includes absent pulmonary valve, transposition with atrioventricular septal defect and truncus arteriosus; (vii) other includes congenital complete heart block, heart muscle disease and symptomatic vascular rings.
Information obtained from Grabitz et al.[43]

diagnosis on postnatal prevalence and spectrum of disease may be considerable.[14] Acquired heart disease, such as endocarditis and myocarditis, may also present in the newborn period. Metabolic disorders which may involve heart muscle can produce symptoms in the newborn period. There are not reliable figures for the incidence of these problems nor for the incidence of fetal and neonatal arrhythmias. Aetiological factors and important associations of CHD are outlined in Table 28.5 and are discussed in more detail by Brennan,[11] Burn[17] and Clark.[23]

Clinical implications of adaption to birth

Normal adaptation

Normal adaptation may have adverse haemodynamic effects in certain cardiovascular conditions, and failure of normal changes to occur may be disadvantageous under certain circumstances. These two situations will be considered for each of the four structures concerned.

Foramen ovale

If exit of blood from the left atrium through the mitral valve is impaired, the presence of a foramen ovale is important in allowing decompression of the left atrium as it is forced open by the abnormally high pressure in the left atrium. Failure of this mechanism by virtue of a small foramen ovale results in pulmonary venous hypertension and respiratory distress. This problem is an important part of the pathophysiology of mitral atresia or hypoplasia. A restrictive foramen ovale is also important in obstructive lesions in the right heart, such as tricuspid atresia, pulmonary atresia with intact ventricular septum, and critical pulmonary stenosis. In such circumstances, right atrial enlargement and hydops fetalis may occur in utero, but even if it does not, there may be postnatal problems from systemic venous engorgement and poor cardiac output. In the context of transposition of the great arteries (TGA), a small foramen ovale results in poor mixing of oxygenated and deoxygenated blood. In many of these conditions, particularly TGA, enlargement of the foramen ovale by balloon septostomy is an important part of the initial management. In some circumstances, surgical septostomy or septectomy may be indicated, as in mitral atresia. Failure of the foramen ovale to close has the same consequences as the presence of an ASD; indeed, distinguishing between patent foramen ovale (PFO) and ASD in newborn infants can be difficult. The consequences are right-to-left shunting in the presence of structural or functional obstruction to right heart flow and left-to-right shunting otherwise. The balance between favourable and deleterious effects is different for different lesions. In general, left-to-right shunting at atrial level in early infancy is rarely a major disadvantage, whereas right-to-left shunting will worsen systemic arterial desaturation – but this may be less of a disadvantage than very high venous pressures or poor left ventricular filling resulting from poor forward flow through the right heart.

Table 28.5 Aetiological factors in congenital heart disease, with examples (not comprehensive) (See also Brennan[11], Burn[17])

Category	Example	Cardiac lesions include
Chromosome abnormality	Down syndrome (trisomy 21)	AVSD, VSD, tetralogy of Fallot
	Edwards' syndrome (trisomy 18)	VSD
	Patau syndrome (trisomy 13)	VSD
	Turner syndrome (XO)	Coarctation, AS, MS, PAPVC
	Catch 22 (22 q 11 del)	Truncus, IAA, tetralogy of Fallot, any
	Williams syndrome (7 q del)	Supravalvar AS, PABS
Non-specific genetic	Parent or sibling with CHD	Any
Teratogen exposure	Virus: rubella	Coarctation, PABS, VSD, PDA
	Drug:	
	Alcohol	VSD
	Phenytoin	ASD
	Lithium	Ebstein's anomaly
	Warfarin	VSD, tetralogy of Fallot
Syndromes	Autosomal dominant:	
	Noonan	PS, ASD, HCM
	Holt–Oram	ASD
	Autosomal recessive: TAR	ASD, tetralogy of Fallot
	Sporadic:	
	DiGeorge	(p. 128)
	Williams	(pp. 788, 798, 799)
	Cornelia de Lange	VSD
Maternal disease	Diabetes mellitus	VSD, HCM
	Collagen vascular diseases	CHB
Association with non-cardiac malformations	Oesophageal atresia	VSD, tetralogy of Fallot
	Diaphragmatic hernia	Any
	Exomphalos	Any
	Pierre Robin	VSD

Ductus venosus

Closure of the ductus venosus is of importance in that it removes the possibility of central venous access being obtained via the umbilical vein for monitoring, balloon septostomy or cardiac catheterisation. It will also result in marked deterioration in cases of total anomalous pulmonary venous connection (TAPVC) to the portal vein as it will cause severe pulmonary venous obstruction with pulmonary oedema (Fig. 28.1). In this condition, closure of the ductus venosus may not occur until some days after birth. Delay in or failure of closure of the ductus venosus is probably rare and never of significance.

Ductus arteriosus

Closure of the DA will cause marked deterioration in duct-dependent pulmonary and duct-dependent systemic circulations; in the first instance causing worsening cyanosis, and in the latter, shock and heart failure. Systemic arterial oxygenation in TGA will also deteriorate when the DA closes. These conditions are all discussed in more detail below (see cyanosis and collapse).

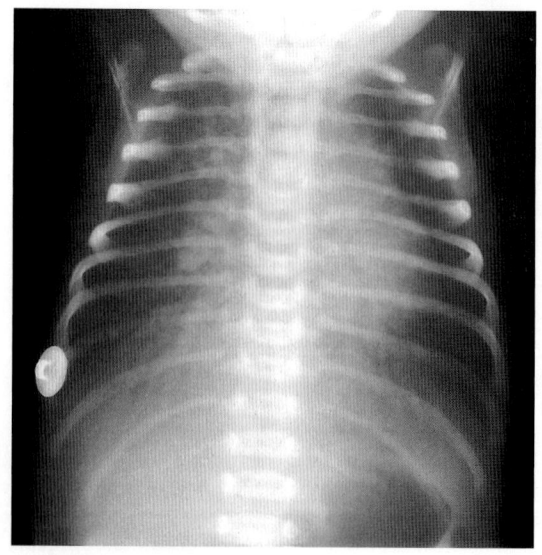

Fig. 28.1 CXR showing pulmonary venous engorgement and normal heart size in obstructed TAPVC.

Pulmonary vascular resistance

Pulmonary blood flow increases rapidly at birth as PVR falls. This normal process will have adverse effects if an increase in pulmonary venous return is disadvantageous as discussed above in the presence of pulmonary venous obstruction from any cause or if exit of blood from the left atrium is impeded. Increased pulmonary blood flow secondary to lesions allowing left-to-right shunting will cause respiratory distress and heart failure as PVR falls. This usually is not a problem in the early newborn phase and often is not apparent until 2 or 3 months of age. A common exception to this statement is patent ductus arteriosus (PDA) in the preterm infant (see below). Any shunt lesion may become symptomatic at an earlier postnatal age in preterm infants than in term ones; this is attributed to less well developed pulmonary vascular musculature in the premature infant.[49] Delay in the normal fall in PVR may quickly result in a clinical problem (persistent pulmonary hypertension of the newborn, PPHN, p. 496) or it may become important in the pathophysiology of chronic lung disease (CLD) and in the development of permanent pulmonary vascular changes in structural heart disease, with unrestricted transmission of systemic pressures into the pulmonary circulation, such as in large VSD and complete atrioventricular septal defect (AVSD). PPHN may also be seen when there has been underdevelopment of the pulmonary vascular tree in utero (such as in diaphragmatic hernia) or if there has been in-utero exposure to prostaglandin synthetase inhibitors as a result of maternal therapy. Hypoxaemia in PPHN is due to right-to-left shunting which can be either within the lungs or extrapulmonary, in which case it can be at ductal level or intracardiac through the foramen ovale. Detailed consideration of PPHN is given on pages 496–502.

History and examination

These are basic in the evaluation of a newborn infant with suspected cardiac disease. History taking involves details of the current symptom as well as obtaining pregnancy, perinatal, family and social information. Much of this will be available in maternity records, but clarification and expansion is often required when a particular clinical picture presents. Examination of the newborn is dealt with in Chapter 14; a number of points with specific reference to the cardiovascular system will be considered here.

Dysmorphic features and non-cardiac malformations

These must be carefully sought and described in detail in relation to all body systems. They are clearly important if a syndrome is to be diagnosed and may influence treatment plans and prognostic information given to families. It may be relevant to investigate other systems on the basis of certain cardiac diagnoses, for example chromosome analysis or immunological assessment. In some circumstances, recognition of an abnormality in an infant will result in a diagnosis being made in a parent, for example Noonan syndrome. When certain non-cardiac structural abnormalities are recognised, a detailed cardiac evaluation is appropriate, as in Down syndrome and many gastrointestinal abnormalities.[107]

Pulses

If femoral pulses cannot be felt easily because an infant is too active, a further attempt should be made when the baby is settled. Impalpable or weak femoral pulses in the presence of good volume upper limb pulses suggest coarctation of the aorta, in which case other signs may well be present and might include upper limb hypertension, systolic pressure difference of 20 mmHg or more between arms and legs, evidence of aortic valve abnormality (ejection click), a bruit between the scapulae and signs of heart failure. If all pulses are weak, then left ventricular outflow obstruction, hypovolaemia or left ventricular dysfunction should be considered. Hypoplastic left heart may be associated with stronger femoral than right brachial pulses before the DA closes. A preterm infant severely compromised by PDA may have very weak femoral pulses. A baby with interrupted aortic arch usually collapses in the first week of life; the diagnosis and the site of interruption can sometimes be deduced by comparing arm and neck pulses as they will be much stronger proximal to the interruption.

Blood pressure

Blood pressure (BP) should be measured in both arms and in one leg in any newborn infant with cardiac symptoms and in an asymptomatic infant if other signs raise the possibility of coarctation. A difference in systolic BP of 20 mmHg or more between arm and leg is strongly suggestive of coarctation, although smaller gradients in term babies can be normal and the absence of such a difference does not rule out the diagnosis of coarctation if the DA is still patent. BP should also be measured in any unwell baby, as well as in those with urinary tract abnormalities, those on steroids, in CLD and in the infants of drug-addicted mothers. It is essential that the baby is settled; results on crying (or recently crying) babies are misleading. Monitoring BP is part of the management of severely ill babies and this should be carried out invasively wherever possible. Obtaining a definitive non-invasive BP requires patience and attention to detail. The arterial pulse can be detected by palpation or with a Doppler probe. Both methods will only give a systolic value. Auscultation is very difficult and the flush method rarely used. Oscillometric monitors may be useful in sequential BP monitoring of immobile babies but even then are subject to error at low pressures infants with extremely low birthweight. Cuff size is important and for the arm it should cover 75% of the distance from axilla to elbow or have a width that is 40–50% of the arm circumference.[70] The bladder should virtually encircle the arm. Leg BP can be measured using the same cuff around the calf with detection of a dorsalis pedis or posterior tibial pulse. Normal BP values are given in Appendix 4.

Cyanosis

Peripheral cyanosis is very common in normal newborn babies. Central cyanosis can be mimicked by facial petechiae (traumatic cyanosis) and in markedly polycythaemic infants. Plethoric infants with a low normal oxygen saturation may have enough deoxygenated haemoglobin to give true central cyanosis. Pigmentation of the lips can also confuse the observer and it is important to look at the tongue to get the best possible assessment of saturation. Anaemia and desaturation make a baby look pale grey rather than really blue, and methaemoglobinaemia (p. 638) gives babies a slate black or grey colour which is often mistaken for cyanosis. Cyanotic, often termed 'dusky', episodes are very common and are only occasionally a presenting feature for structural heart disease; persistent cyanosis is far more likely to be cardiac, although it may vary in intensity. Cyanosis whilst crying is rarely pathological if colour and behaviour return to normal rapidly when the infant stops crying. Hypercyanotic episodes as seen in tetralogy of Fallot and related conditions are rare in the newborn period.

Heart failure

The signs of heart failure in the newborn are listed in Table 28.6. These features can be masked or caused by respiratory disease and by circulatory collapse from any cause. Most causes of heart failure will be associated with other cardiovascular signs and with cardiomegaly on chest X-ray (CXR).

Heart murmur

Heart murmurs in the newborn may be the presentation of both major and minor cardiac lesions[2] but also can be a normal physiological finding.[7] Many serious cardiac conditions have unimpressive or even no murmurs. Other auscultatory and general cardiovascular signs are very important in assessing the significance of a murmur. The absence of any other features of cardiac disease as well as the presence of certain positive murmur characteristics are required to diagnose innocent heart murmurs. The typical heart murmur in newborn babies comes from the pulmonary artery branches (Table 28.7) and disappears before 6 months of age in term infants.

Investigations

History and examination often allow cardiac disease to be suspected or ruled out. They sometimes allow a definite diagnosis to be made. Investigations consist of those readily available in any neonatal nursery (CXR, electrocardiogram [ECG], and hyperoxia test) and those only available at cardiac centres (cardiac catheterisation and magnetic resonance imaging [MRI]). Echocardiography is being increasingly used outside cardiac centres and with suitable equipment and trained operators is very valuable in the care of the newborn, particularly to confirm or rule out a cardiac abnormality in those cases where clinical assessment, ECG and CXR have been inconclusive. The value of ECG and CXR in differentiating normal from abnormal murmurs in the newborn has not been systematically examined, and they are less often used now. The main question is establishing which babies with murmurs should have echocardiography before being discharged from hospital (see below).[2] The role of pulse oximetry as a screening test is also discussed below (see hyperoxia test).

Electrocardiogram

The ECG provides useful information in a number of areas (Table 28.8) providing attention is paid to technical aspects of obtaining a good recording, which can be difficult in a neonatal nursery. Systematic reading of the ECG will optimise the information obtained and reference should be made to normal values (see Appendix 3) and to a standard text for detailed interpretation of ECGs.[75]

Table 28.6 Features of neonatal heart failure

- Poor feeding
- Excess or unexpected weight gain
- Poor peripheral perfusion, clammy mottled skin, cold sweatiness
- Oedema – usually late but characteristic of fetal heart failure (hydrops) often with pericardial, pleural and peritoneal fluid
- Tachycardia (unless cause of failure is heart block)
- Hepatomegaly
- Respiratory distress, added sounds in chest
- Gallop rhythm
- Specific signs of causative lesion

Table 28.7 Features of innocent neonatal heart murmurs

Source/type	Characteristics	Comment
Pulmonary arteries	Base of heart, chest bilaterally	Gone by 6 months
Ductus arteriosus	No definite evidence that it can be heard whilst closing normally	
Tricuspid regurgitation (without structural heart disease)	Sound like VSD	Often with perinatal stress and transient ST/T changes on ECG; resolves in days
Still's innocent murmur	Vibratory Mid-systolic Between LLSE AND apex	Rarely heard in newborn period; lasts years

LLSE, lower left sternal edge; ST/T, ST segment and T wave.

Table 28.8 Information obtainable from the electrocardiogram

- Rhythm
- Atrial:
  - Position
  - Enlargement
- Ventricular:
  - Position
  - Hypertrophy
  - Strain/ischaemia

Heart rhythm

Abnormal heart rate can be confirmed on the ECG and heart rhythm usually can be ascertained. Sinus rhythm is characterised by normal P waves (frontal plane axis 0° to +90°) preceding every QRS complex. Sinus rate varies between 70 and 180/min in healthy babies, reaching as much as 220/min in sick babies. In these circumstances, P waves can be hard to see but all leads should be examined and paper run at a faster speed (50 mm/s) if necessary. First-degree heart block (prolonged PR interval) is rarely of importance in its own right in the newborn but may be a marker for structural heart disease such as ASD or Ebstein's anomaly. A short PR interval is a marker for an increased tendency to supraventricular tachycardia (SVT), although delta waves in the QRS complex may easily be overlooked in neonates. A short PR interval also accompanies some structural heart lesions (Ebstein's anomaly) and may be seen in glycogen storage disease. Partial atrioventricular (AV) dissociation (second-degree heart block) and complete heart block are considered below, as are SVT and ventricular tachycardia (VT).

Information on the atria

Inverted P waves in lead 1 may be a sign of an incorrectly wired ECG (right arm/left arm reversed); this can be checked by looking at lead V_6. If I and V_6 look similar, the ECG is wired up correctly and negative P waves in I then suggest one of the following:

- not sinus rhythm (Fig. 28.2);
- heart in abnormal position;
- heart in normal position but atria in abnormal spatial relationship to each other.

Right atrial enlargement is indicated by tall (>2.5 mV) P waves and left atrial enlargement shown by broad (>3 mm) P waves at standard paper speed (25 mm/s).

Information on the ventricles

Abnormal ventricular positions within the chest, as in dextrocardia, or in relationship to each other, as in congenitally corrected transposition, can be suspected from abnormalities in QRS progression across the chest leads. In dextrocardia, complexes do not evolve between V_1 and V_6 but simply get progressively smaller. Q waves in V_1 mean one of the following:

- abnormal intraventricular conduction (as in left bundle branch block or some cases of pre-excitation);

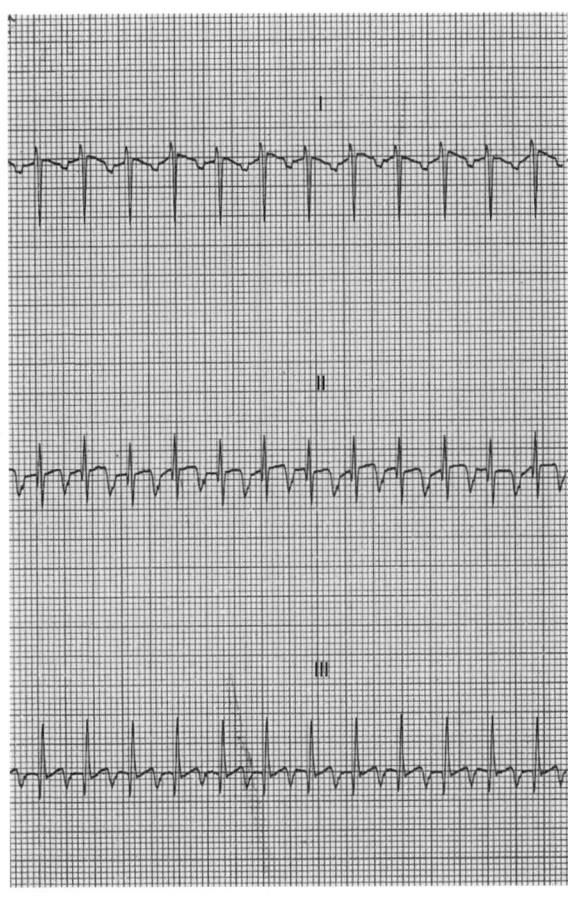

Fig. 28.2 ECG leads I, II and III, showing inverted P wave in I. SVT at 190/min.

- severe right ventricular hypertrophy (RVH);
- spatial relationship between right and left ventricles abnormal (as in congenitally corrected transposition).

RVH is suggested by one or more of the following:

- right axis deviation;
- Q in V_1;
- large RV_1 or SV_6 (see Appendix 3);
- upright T in V_1 after day 3 (Fig. 28.3).

It is important to note that conditions causing marked RVH in later infancy may cause no ECG abnormality in the immediate newborn period and only an upright T wave in V_1 in the later newborn period.

Left ventricular hypertrophy is suggested by one or more of the following:

- adult R/S progression V_1 to V_6 (dominant SV_1 dominant RV_6);
- large SV_1 or RV_6 (see Appendix 3).

Biventricular hypertrophy is indicated by a combination of these findings.

Ventricular strain or ischaemia is indicted by ST depression or T-wave inversion in left chest leads (II, aVL, V_{5-6}) and may point to a primary cardiac muscle disorder or be secondary to a severe

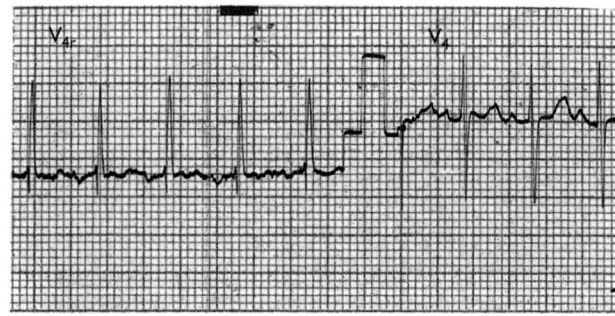

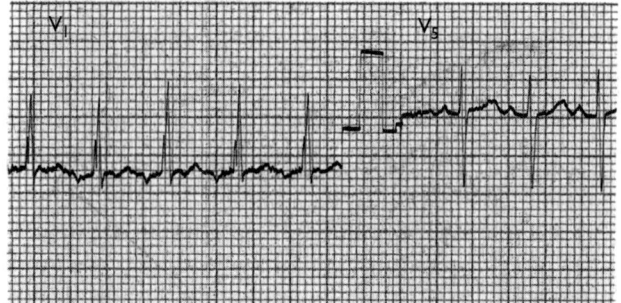

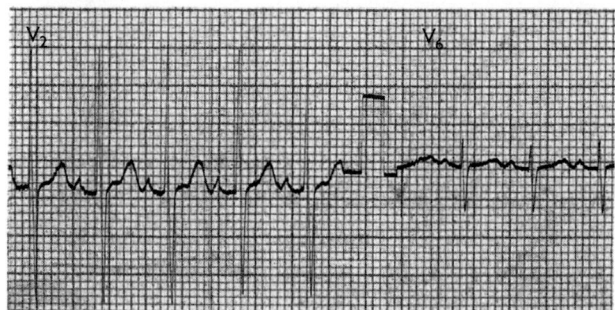

Fig. 28.3 ECG chest leads in a 6-day-old infant. Neonatal R/S progression (normal) but upright T wave V₁ indicating RVH.

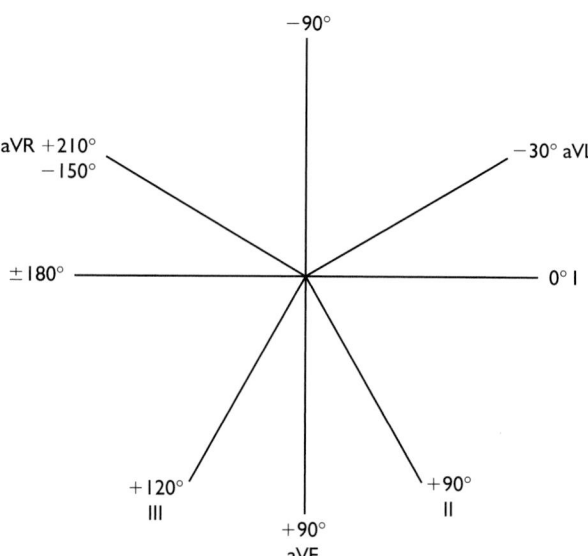

Fig. 28.4 Hexaxial reference system for calculating frontal plane axis of QRS complex (and of P and T waves if required). Frontal axis of QRS complex can be estimated from the diagram showing polarity of ECG leads I, II, III, aVL, aVF and aVR. To obtain the frontal axis of a QRS complex:

i. Identify the lead in which R and S waves are most nearly of equal size.
ii. Look at right angles (+90° and −90°) to the lead identified in step i.
iii. One of the leads identified in step ii will be predominantly positive, the other predominantly negative.
iv. The predominantly positive lead identified by step iii is approximately the QRS axis (depolarisation towards a lead produces a positive deflection).
v. The approximate QRS axis obtained from step iv can be made more accurate by estimating the equiphasic lead (step i) more accurately by 'imagining' it between actual leads.

If all leads appear equiphasic, the QRS axis is described as indeterminate; this is rarely normal.

structural abnormality causing pressure or volume load on the heart. T-wave changes are seen after perinatal stress and resolve in under a week. Pericarditis is rare in the newborn period but ST segment and T-wave changes are seen.

QRS axis

The frontal QRS axis can be calculated as shown in Figure 28.4. An abnormal QRS axis may be an important diagnostic clue in a number of conditions, including AVSD (Fig. 28.5) and tricuspid atresia (QRS usually −30°); in the former case it makes the ECG a valuable screening investigation in newborn infants with Down syndrome, in whom clinical features of AVSD may be absent or very subtle.

Chest X-ray

The plain CXR is widely used in the investigation of suspected cardiac disease. Features to look for in this context are listed in Table 28.9; examples are shown in Figures 28.6–28.9.

Hyperoxia test

The hyperoxia (or nitrogen washout) test was described in the era before echocardiography to help distinguish cardiac from respiratory cyanosis without resorting to cardiac catheterisation. Babies with cyanotic heart disease usually show little rise in arterial oxygen tension in response to increased inspired oxygen. A rise of PaO_2 to a value below 20 kPa after 10 minutes in 85% or more inspired oxygen makes heart disease likely, whereas an increase in PaO_2 above 20 kPa makes respiratory disease likely. There are exceptions to this pattern in that babies with desaturating cardiac disease with high lung blood flow (as in unobstructed TAPVC and double-inlet ventricle, for example) will pass, whereas those with very severe respiratory disease and with PPHN may fail. When it is essential to have an accurate measurement of arterial oxygen content, an arterial blood sample must be obtained, and further information of importance in the management of ill infants will also be available from a blood gas analysis.

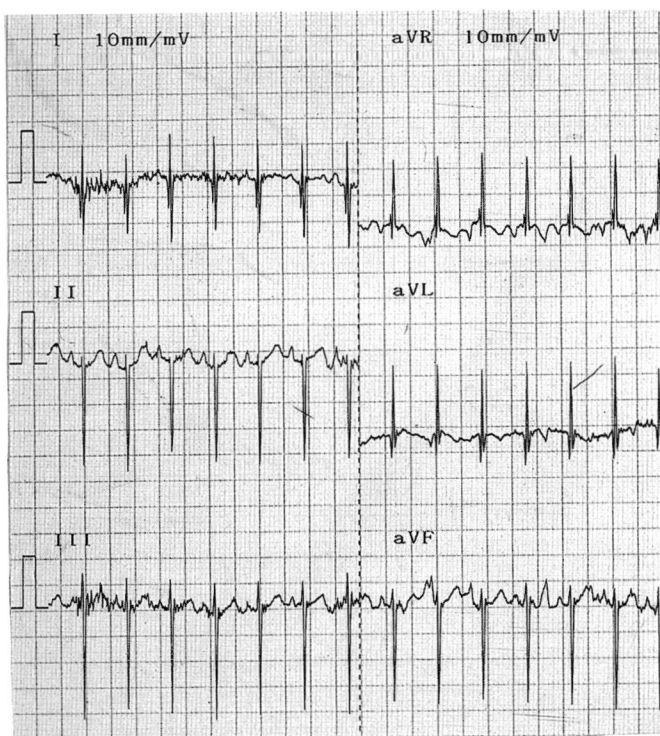

Fig. 28.5 ECG standard leads, superior QRS axis (−90°), newborn with complete AVSD.

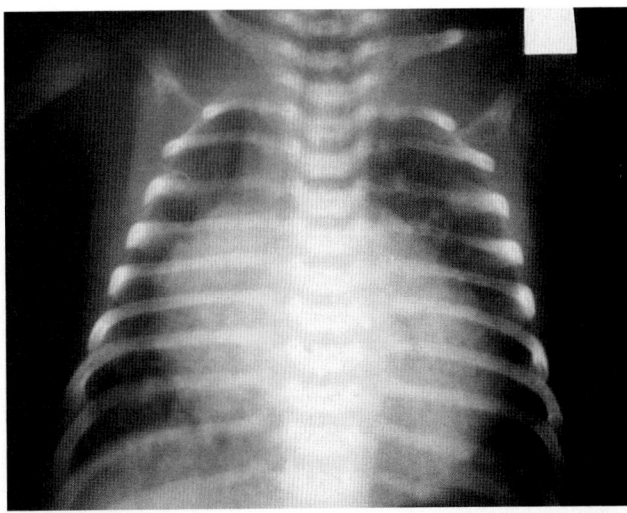

Fig. 28.6 CXR showing cardiomegaly and pulmonary plethora.

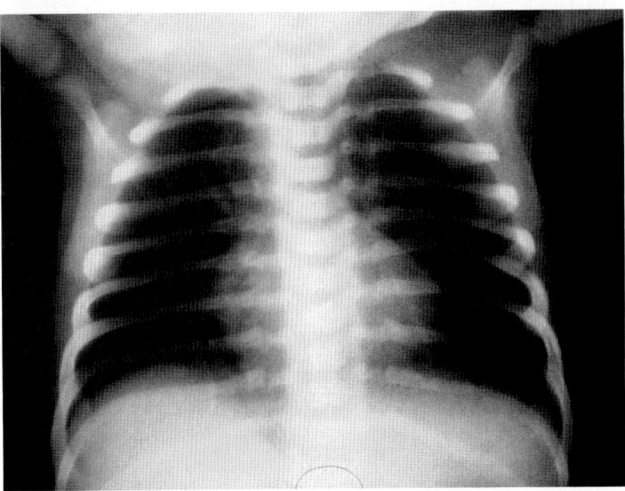

Fig. 28.7 CXR showing normal heart size and pulmonary oligaemia (tetralogy of Fallot).

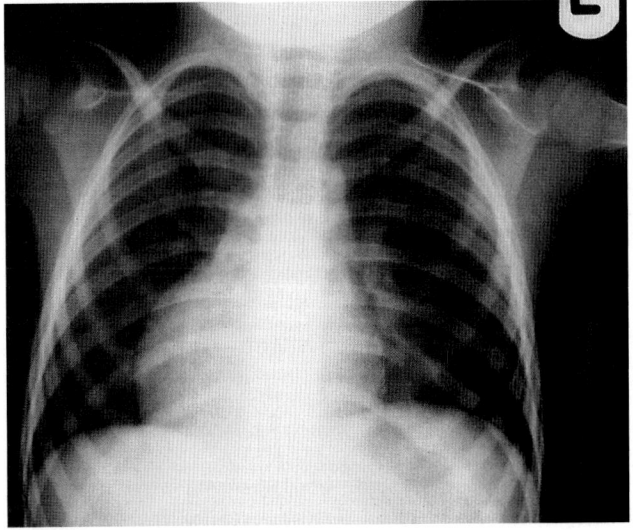

Fig. 28.8 CXR showing dextrocardia and apex to the right. Abdominal situs not seen (normal heart).

Table 28.9 Features to assess on chest X-ray in infant with suspected cardiac disease

Feature	Comment
Quality of film	Adequate inspiration Normal penetration Centred on mid chest Not rotated
Abdominal situs Bronchial situs	Normal/inverted/ambiguous
Aortic arch side	Left or right
Heart	Side Direction of apex Size Contour
Lung vasculature	Plethora Oligaemia Pulmonary venous engorgement
Diaphragm	Distinct Side of apex should be more caudal
Lung fields	Any pathology
Musculoskeletal	Vertebral/rib abnormalities Fractures

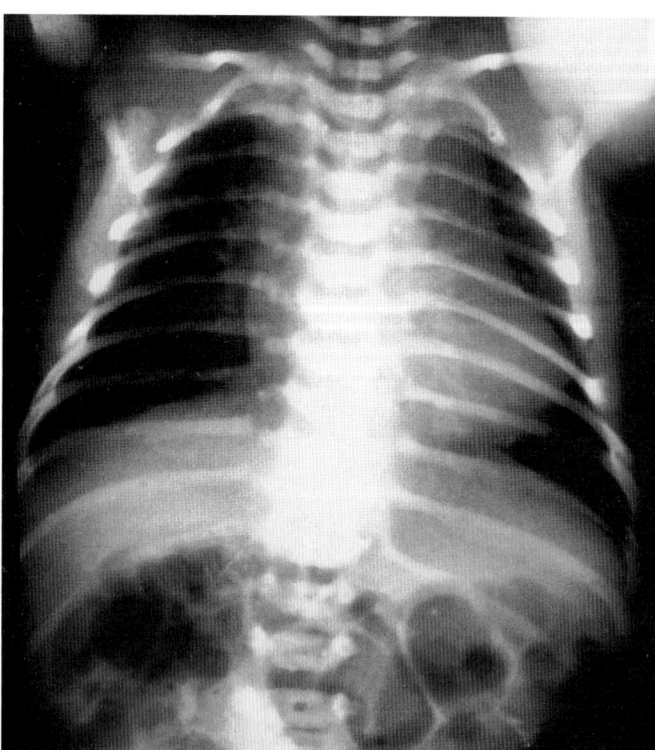

Fig. 28.9 CXR showing laevocardia, apex to the left, midline liver, stomach not clearly lateralised, pulmonary oligaemia (right isomerism, cardiac lesion with severe pulmonary outflow obstruction).

Table 28.10 Uses of different ultrasound modalities

Modality	Uses
2D imaging	Anatomical detail Chamber size, wall thickness Function
Doppler	Signals reflect direction and velocity of flow, turbulence and flow patterns.
Colour flow	Rapid identification of site of abnormal flow patterns Detection of regurgitation and small shunts
Pulsed wave	Sampling in a localised region May be inaccurate with high velocities
Continuous wave	Excellent for high velocities Not precisely localised
M mode	Dimensions and function

detected. This approach is time consuming and has not yet been widely applied nor compared directly with other screening strategies.

Echocardiography

Transthoracic echocardiography has a major role in diagnosis and management of neonatal heart disease. It has resulted in a dramatic reduction in the need for diagnostic cardiac catheterisation and can be used to guide interventions such as balloon atrial septostomy. All ultrasound modalities have a role in evaluating the cardiovascular system (Table 28.10). Imaging gives anatomical detail. Doppler identifies or clarifies shunt lesions and regions of turbulent flow and allows quantification of stenosis by measuring blood velocity, which allows a pressure difference across a valve or between ventricles through a VSD to be calculated by the modified Bernouilli equation ($P = 4V^2$, where P = instantaneous peak systolic pressure gradient in mmHg, V = velocity distal to the site of obstruction in m/s). Detailed consideration of the ultrasound features of different conditions is outside the scope of this chapter, but Skinner and colleagues[96] give a useful pragmatic approach for neonatal paediatricians, including further references. Standard echocardiographic windows and images of the heart are shown in Figure 28.10; examples of clinical scans are given in Figures 28.11–28.13. Transoesophageal echocardiography (TOE) can be used on term newborn infants and has a role in postoperative assessment when precordial or subcostal images can be hard to obtain. The group of babies from whom transthoracic echocardiograms are most difficult to get are those with severe respiratory disease receiving assisted ventilation. Many of these infants are of low birthweight and too small to allow a TOE probe to be passed. As echocardiographic skills become more widespread, telemedicine allows neonatal units to collaborate with cardiac centres to optimise the transfer arrangements of babies or to avoid transfer altogether.[20]

Transcutaneous oxygen tension monitors placed on the right upper chest (that is preductal) can be used instead of arterial sampling as a screening test if other information is not required. Oxygen pulse saturation monitors will not provide the same assurance of a pass, as an infant will show 100% saturation at a PaO_2 value well below 20 kPa. A well baby who is clearly blue does not need a hyperoxia test result; a sick baby on assisted ventilation in whom cardiac disease is suspected needs echocardiography irrespective of the result, and a look through the blood gas chart of such a baby is likely to serve the same purpose without a formal test. Babies for whom hyperoxia is potentially harmful (p. 359), even for a short period, should not be tested. The role of the hyperoxia test has therefore changed since its inception, but it is still helpful in two circumstances:

■ When a well baby seems dusky and there is uncertainty as to whether a cyanotic cardiac condition is present. A failed transcutaneous or pulse oximeter hyperoxia test strongly points to cyanotic heart disease.

■ A well baby with signs of heart disease who looks pink may fail the hyperoxia test, thus alerting the physician to the presence of a more complex lesion.

An additional use for pulse oximetry in screening for heart disease is to perform oximetry on the foot of a baby breathing air. A value of less than 95% is found in about 5% of apparently well infants.[83] If these infants are further evaluated (by repeating the test initially), few cases of important structural heart disease are overlooked and some other potentially unwell infants are also

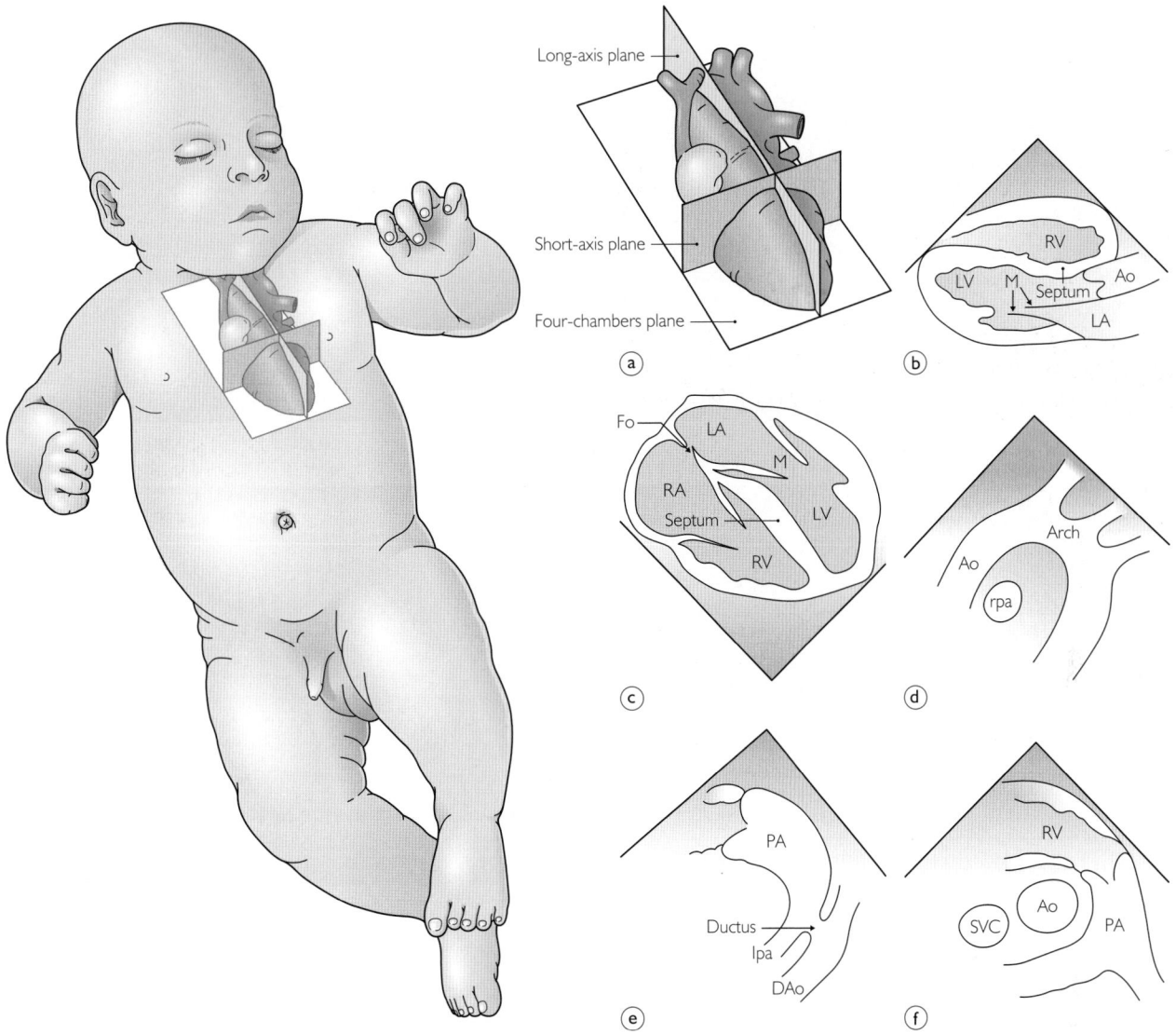

Fig. 28.10 (a) Diagram illustrating echocardiographic cross-sectional planes (two-dimensional). The long-axis plane is approximately sagittal; the four-chambers plane is approximately frontal; the short-axis plane is approximately transverse. (b–f) Diagrammatic representations of normal; cross-sectional views. (b) Long-axis cut as seen with transducer in parasternal position. (c) Four-chambers cut as seen from subxiphoid site. (d) Semi-long-axis cut of aortic arch as obtained from suprasternal view. (e) High long-axis cut (parasagittal) to show ductus arteriosus. (f) Short-axis cut through the great arteries just above the heart. Ao, aorta; Dao, descending aorta; Fo, foramen ovale; LA, left atrium; lpa, left pulmonary artery; LV, left ventricle; m, mitral valve leaflets; PA, pulmonary artery; RA, right atrium; rpa, right pulmonary artery; RV, right ventricle; svc, superior vena cava; t, tricuspid valve leaflets. (From Wilkinson & Cooke.[116])

Cardiac catheterisation

Cardiac catheterisation may be diagnostic for haemodynamic or anatomical data or therapeutic. Diagnostic catheterisation is rarely required in the newborn baby with present-day ultrasound capability, and when it is, there is usually only a small amount of information required in order to complement that already obtained by echocardiography. Therapeutic catheterisation can be performed under ultrasound control, such as for balloon septostomy, but more complex therapeutic interventions usually require X-ray screening in addition to or instead of ultrasound. Conditions treated in the newborn period by interventional cardiac

catheterisation are listed in Table 28.11. Vascular access is obtained via the umbilicus or percutaneously in the femoral region, and cut-down techniques are rarely needed. Babies must have general and specific resuscitation before and during the procedure, with particular reference to body temperature, blood glucose, circulating volume, acid/base balance and ventilation. If proper attention is paid to these things, as well as ensuring adequate sedation or anaesthesia, complications are rare, with vascular damage being the commonest. Mortality in diagnostic and interventional catheterisation in the newborn is less than 1%, but acute morbidity may occur in up to 25% of interventional procedures.[120]

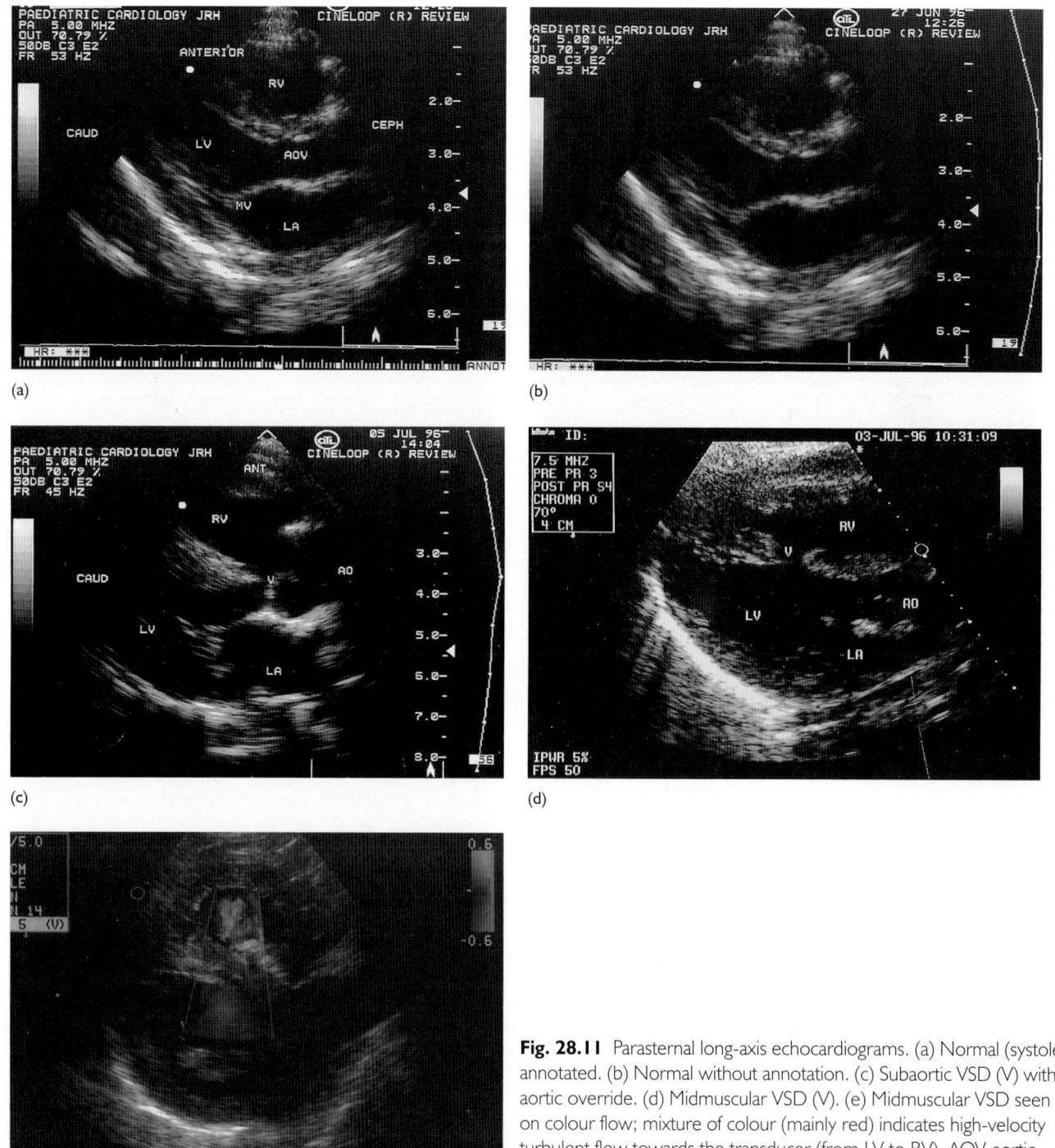

Fig. 28.11 Parasternal long-axis echocardiograms. (a) Normal (systole), annotated. (b) Normal without annotation. (c) Subaortic VSD (V) with aortic override. (d) Midmuscular VSD (V). (e) Midmuscular VSD seen on colour flow; mixture of colour (mainly red) indicates high-velocity turbulent flow towards the transducer (from LV to RV). AOV, aortic valve; caud, caudal; ceph, cephalad; LA, left atrium; LV, left ventricle; MV, mitral valve; RV, right ventricle.

Magnetic resonance imaging

MRI provides excellent anatomical images, but, in the newborn, echocardiography usually provides more than adequate information. MRI is useful in older children in evaluating aortic arch and pulmonary arterial abnormalities. Whereas MRI involves no radiation hazard, it does require heavy sedation or general anaesthesia in an environment where detailed monitoring is rather more complicated to achieve and where instant access to the baby can be difficult.

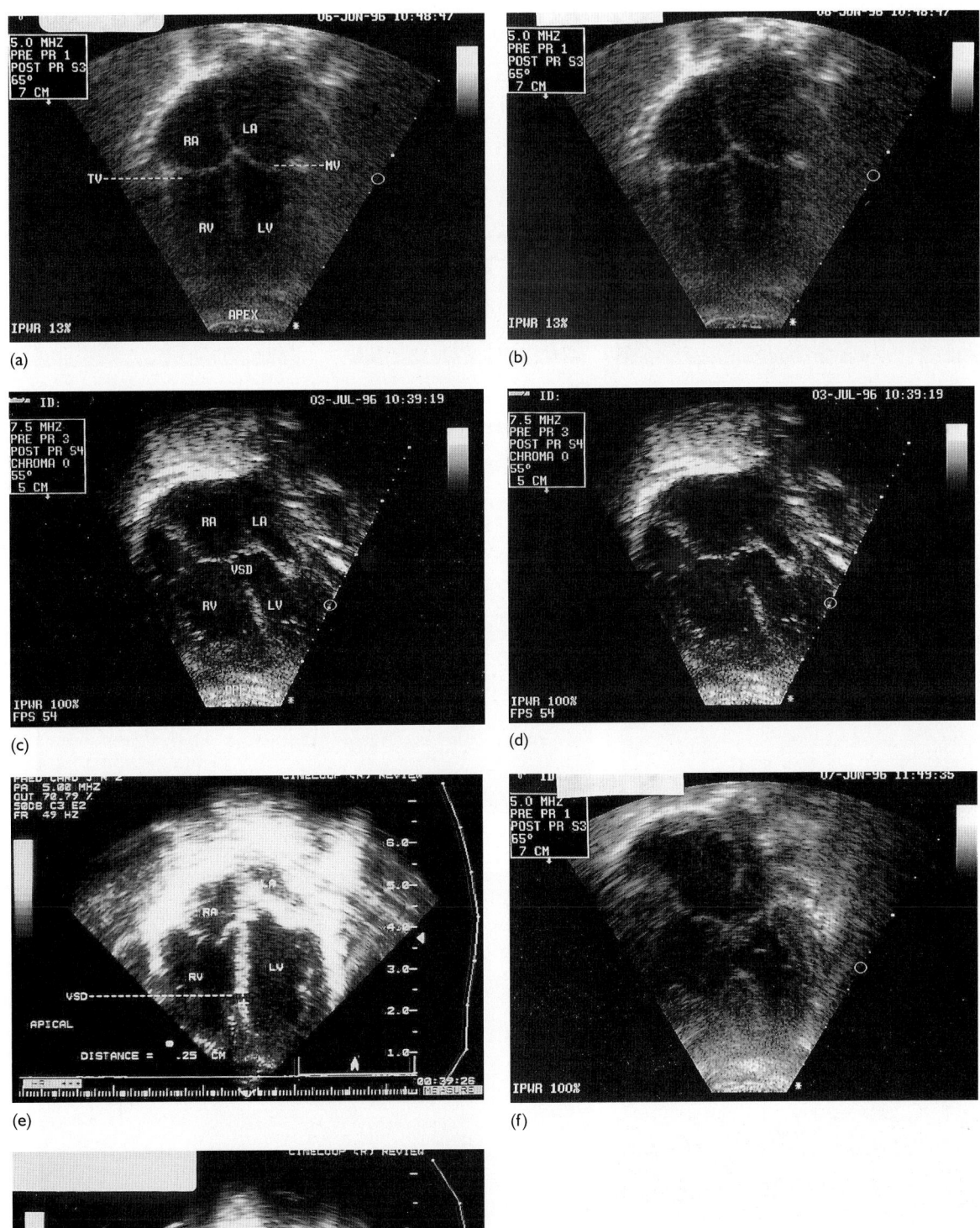

Fig. 28.12 Apical four-chamber echocardiograms. (a) Normal (systole), anno-
tated. (b) Normal without annotation. (c) Perimembranous VSD with annotation.
(d) Perimembranous VSD without annotation. (e) Midmuscular VSD.
(f) Complete AVSD (systole). Common AV valve closed with adjacent large
ASD and VSD. (g) Massively thickened ventricular muscle, especially septum and
LV (glycogen storage disease). AOV, aortic valve; caud, caudal; ceph, cephalad;
LA, left atrium; LV, left ventricle; MV, mitral valve; RA, right atrium; RV, right ventricle;
TV, tricuspid valve.

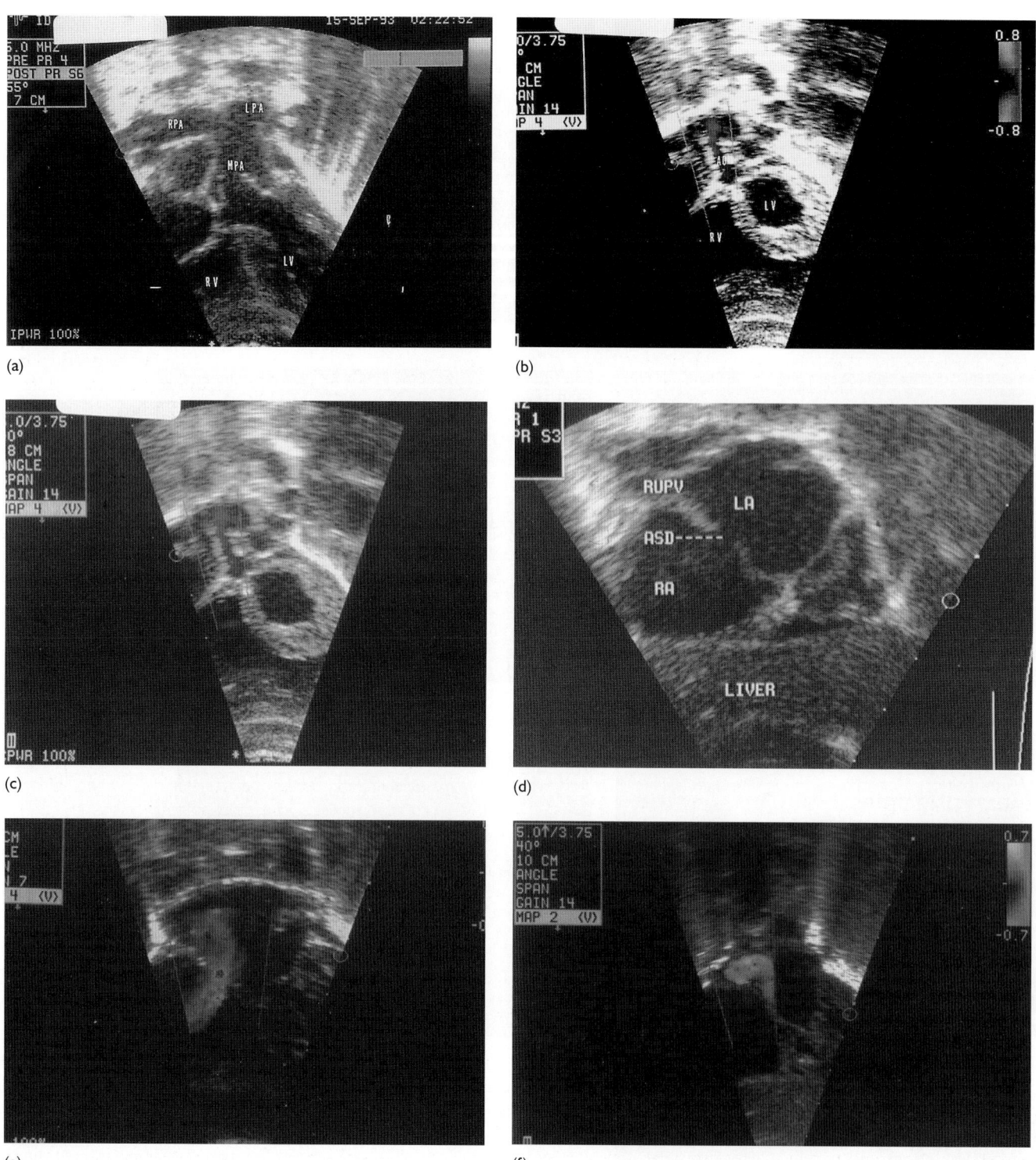

Fig. 28.13 Subcostal echocardiograms. (a) Transposition. Main pulmonary artery (MPA) arising from LV divides into right and left pulmonary arteries (RPA, LPA). (b) Hypoplastic left heart. Tiny ascending aorta (AO) separated from thick-walled LV with small cavity by atretic aortic valve. Hugely dilated RV. (c) Same image with colour Doppler showing red signal (flow towards transducer) in ascending aorta, which is filled retrogradely via DA rather than through aortic valve. (d) View of atria. (e) Same view showing red colour Doppler signal towards transducer, shunting LA to RA through ASD. (f) Similar view showing blue colour Doppler signal in ASD, indicating flow away from transducer (RA to LA).

Table 28.11 Interventional cardiac catheterisation in newborn infants

Technique	Comment
Balloon septostomy	TGA and restrictive PFO in mitral obstruction or hypoplastic right heart
Balloon dilatation	
Pulmonary valve	Widely used as first choice for stenosis
Aortic valve	First choice in some centres for stenosis
Coarctation	Lower success and higher complication rates than surgery
Infundibulum	Occasionally in TOF
Ductus arteriosus	Rarely, if prostaglandin fails
Pulmonary atresia	Becoming widespread if no VSD Occasionally used if VSD present Radiofrequency assisted valvuloplasty
Stent techniques	
Ductus arteriosus	Being explored as part of initial palliation of hypoplastic left heart
Embolisation techniques	
Cerebral AVM	Treatment of choice for neonates in heart failure
Scimitar syndrome	For aberrant arterial supply to right lung

Table 28.12 Prostaglandin (PG) dosage regimens

Drug and route	Dose	Comment
PGE$_1$ i.v.	0.005–0.1 micrograms/kg/min	For both drugs, start at low dose and increase at 15- to 30-minute intervals if no response. More than threefold increase in dose rarely needed. Side effects increase with higher doses
PGE$_2$ i.v.	0.005–0.05 micrograms/kg/min	
PGE$_2$ oral/nasogastric	25–40 micrograms/kg/h	Start hourly at lower dose. For long-term use, can go stepwise to 4- to 6-hourly

Table 28.13 Heart failure management

Acute	Restrict fluid to approximately two-thirds maintenance Furosemide (frusemide) i.v. 1 mg/kg 6- to 12-hourly Optimise oxygenation, avoid hyperoxia Treat anaemia Consider dopamine or dobutamine if myocardial dysfunction (do not use in hypertrophic cardiomyopathy)
Chronic	Avoid fluid restriction if possible, in order to maximise calorie intake Oral diuretic: furosemide (frusemide) 2–6 mg/kg/day (in two or three doses) and potassium-sparing diuretic or potassium supplement If heart muscle dysfunction, consider digoxin 4 micrograms/kg twice daily orally or ACE inhibitor (not in hypertrophic cardiomyopathy)

Treatment

General principles

Attention to general aspects of medical care to achieve stability prior to transfer and intervention of any kind is a very important aspect of minimising morbidity and mortality for any cardiac condition. Similarly expert neonatal care after intervention is required to ensure optimal outcomes. Specific cardiac interventions can be pharmacological, transcatheter or surgical and are considered in this section.

Ductal manipulation

Establishing and maintaining an open DA is a crucial part of the resuscitation of babies with duct-dependent pulmonary or systemic circulations and usually greatly improves oxygenation in TGA. Prostaglandin E1 and prostaglandin E2 will both dilate the DA. Dosage regimens for both drugs are given in Table 28.12. Acute side effects of prostaglandin include apnoea, jitteriness, convulsions, diarrhoea, flushing and fever. These are usually manageable without loss of therapeutic effect by stopping the infusion for a few minutes and restarting it at a lower dose. Long-term oral or nasogastric use[95] is sometimes of value, for example in a low-birthweight infant with duct-dependent pulmonary circulation in whom somatic growth is considered desirable before surgical intervention. Whether this approach allows useful increase in the size of pulmonary arteries in term infants is unclear.[62]

Important side effects with gastric administration are rare. Bone periosteal reaction during chronic administration of prostaglandin is very uncommon with the doses currently recommended. When increasing the dose to allow for less frequent administration, it is advisable to observe the infant for apnoea. Manipulation of the DA in order to close it is considered on page 636.

Heart failure

Management of heart failure is outlined in Table 28.13. In order to achieve as good a nutritional state as possible, it is desirable to minimise fluid restriction. In the long term it is usually possible to regulate fluid status with diuretics and allow a good volume intake. Additives to increase the calorific value of milk are often needed and nasogastric feeding may be required. Loop diuretics may cause hyponatraemia; a reduction of dose with modest fluid restriction if necessary often brings this under control. Increasing sodium supplements in this context is to be avoided if possible, as this will also cause fluid retention. There is considerable experience of angiotensin-converting enzyme (ACE) inhibitor usage in infancy[68,90] but far less in newborns, particularly in preterm newborns; the latter group appear to tolerate ACE inhibition poorly. If an ACE inhibitor is to be used, it is important not to have the patient dehydrated with diuretics before commencing the drug. Digoxin may be of value in chronic heart failure associated with poor muscle function, but neither it nor ACE inhibitors should be used when dynamic left ventricular outflow obstruction is present.

Persistent pulmonary hypertension of the newborn

Therapy is considered in Chapter 27, Part 2.

Antiarrhythmic drugs

Arrhymias and their management are considered on pages 651–7. Doses of commonly used antiarrhythmic agents are given in Table 28.30.

Interventional catheterisation

This is considered on page 629 and in Table 28.11. This area is changing all the time and choosing between surgical and catheter interventions for the same condition is influenced by many factors.[85]

Surgery

Cardiac surgery can be open (as in intracardiac repairs) or closed (as in coarctation repair, clipping of the DA, Blalock–Taussig systemic-to-pulmonary anastomoses and pulmonary artery banding). Open cardiac surgery is generally performed through a median sternotomy using either hypothermic cardiac arrest or cardiopulmonary bypass or both. Closed operations are frequently performed through a posterolateral thoracotomy. There is an overall trend toward operations at a younger age and toward attempts at physiological, if not necessarily anatomical, corrections rather than palliation. Many conditions do not need surgery in the newborn period and a significant proportion of neonatal surgery is still palliative. Practice will vary from centre to centre but neonatal primary correction is the treatment of choice in simple TGA and in those cases of TAPVC that present in the newborn period. Operative mortalities are given in the discussion of particular conditions. As surgical mortality rates improve, there is greater concern about morbidity, which may be a feature of an underlying or associated condition or a consequence of the cardiac intervention.[42,59]

Cardiovascular problems in the preterm infant

Patent ductus arteriosus

In the absence of respiratory distress syndrome (RDS), the DA closes in the same timescale after birth in preterm babies as it does in term-born babies, being closed in over 90% of infants by 60 hours of age.[35] Information on well, extremely preterm infants is obviously scarce. Closure of the DA in infants over 30 weeks' gestation with mild RDS takes place over a similar timescale, with 90% being closed by the fourth day of life.[81] Thus, failure of the DA to close in preterm infants is not an abnormality of the DA but rather due to abnormal stimuli such as acidosis and continuing high circulating prostaglandin levels or due to the absence of normal stimuli such as an increase in oxygen tension. Failure of the DA to close is associated with more severe RDS,[28,54] and interventions to close the DA are associated with short-term improvements in respiratory status.[28,118]

Causative factors for PDA

Prematurity and RDS are the two major causative factors. Fetal exposure to indometacin (indomethacin) increases the likelihood of symptomatic PDA (sPDA) and is associated with a lower closure rate in response to postnatal indometacin.[71]

Prevention of PDA

Antenatal steroid administration reduces the incidence and severity of RDS and one possible mechanism for this is steroid-induced reduction in ductal sensitivity to prostaglandin.[25,67] Maintaining good oxygen delivery and avoiding acidosis make good theoretical sense. It is very attractive to close the DA actively in babies with RDS before sPDA becomes apparent, and both surgery[21] and drug therapy[64] have been advocated, although surgery is not easy to arrange in many neonatal units. However, predicting which infants will develop sPDA has not been particularly reliable, although there is evidence that DA minimum diameter on colour flow Doppler of 1.5 mm or greater in babies less than 1500 g birthweight and postnatal age less than 10 days is strongly predictive of the development of sPDA (Fig. 28.14b).[56] A left atrial to aortic root ratio of greater than 1.5 after the first day of age also helps predict sPDA.[53] The Doppler waveform across the ductus (Fig. 28.14e–g) has been used to predict sPDA in a similar group of babies under 5 days old[103] and in managing drug treatment (see below).[102] Su and colleagues[103] identified low-velocity (not above 1.5 m/s) left-to-right shunting through the DA (termed a pulsatile pattern – Fig. 28.14f) in the first 4 days after birth in ventilated babies under 1500 g birthweight as indicating a high risk of developing sPDA (sensitivity 93.5%, specificity 100%). A rather lower sensitivity and specificity (64.5% and 81.1%, respectively) for sPDA was reported for babies in the same study[103] with low-velocity predominantly left-to-right shunting and very brief right-to-left shunting in

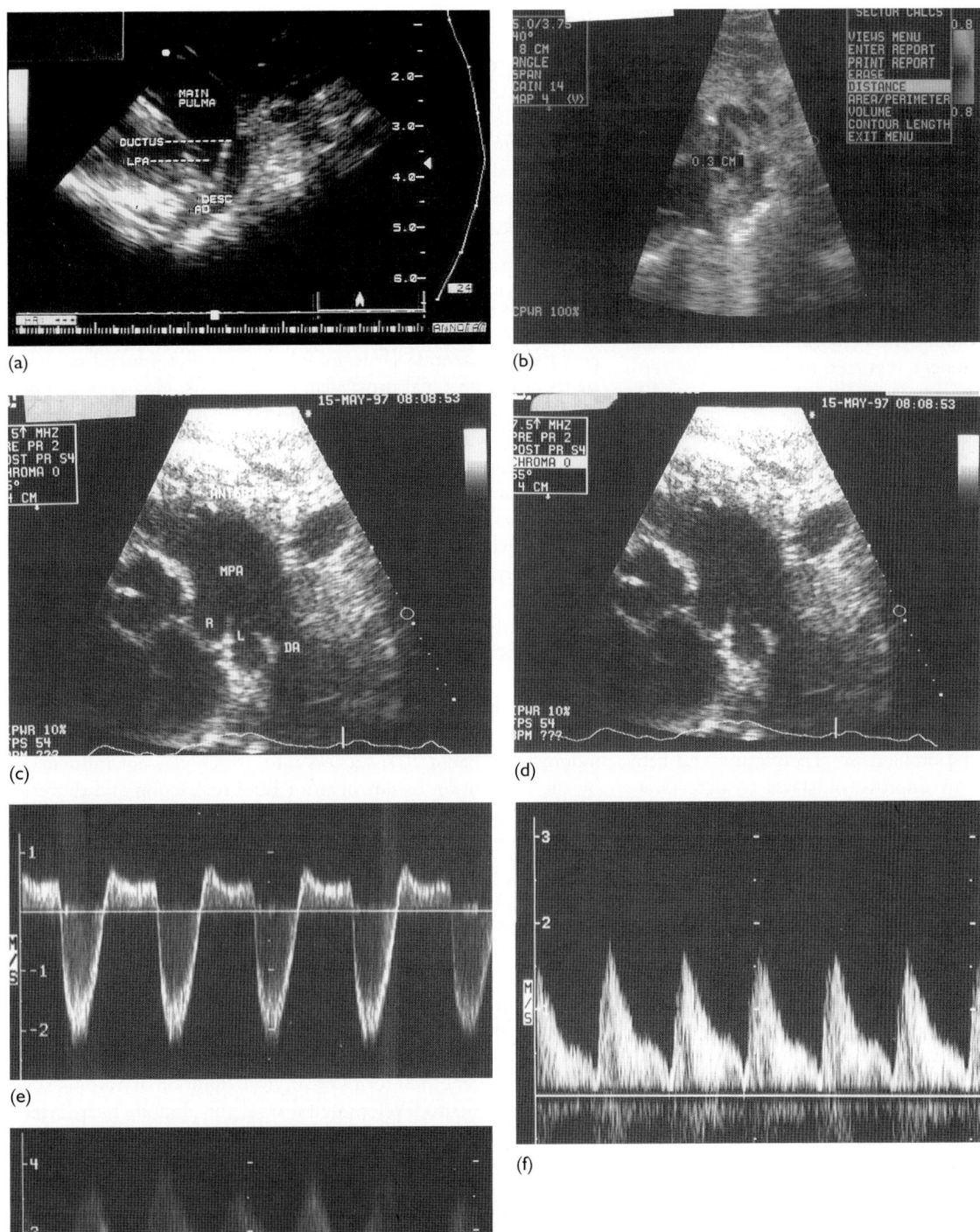

Fig. 28.14 (a) High parasternal ultrasound scan showing PDA. (b) Same view showing red colour Doppler signal toward transducer (descending aorta to pulmonary artery); width of signal indicates size of DA. (c) Parasternal short-axis view showing PDA (annotated). (d) Same view as (c), not annotated. (e) Pulsed-wave Doppler signal across DA showing low velocity bidirectional pattern of no predictive value. (f) Pulsed-wave signal showing pulsatile pattern – see text. (g) High velocity ductal left-to-right shunting, a closing pattern. DESC AO, descending aorta; LPA, left pulmonary artery; MAIN PULMA, main pulmonary artery.

early systole (termed a growing pattern). It may be that these developments will allow better selection of suitable infants for prophylactic intervention with resultant improvement in outcome, but, to date, long-term benefit has not been demonstrated following prophylactic indometacin.[39,86] However, there is considerable evidence that indometacin reduces the occurrence of all grades of germinal matrix/intraventricular haemorrhage, and what long-term evidence there is suggests favourable rather than unfavourable long-term neurological consequences following its use.[114] There is little evidence that prophylactic administration of indometacin is associated with less short-term morbidity than use of the drug as soon as sPDA is detected.[24] Use of another prostaglandin synthetase inhibitor, ibuprofen, within 3 hours of birth has been reported to reduce short-term mordidity and length of hospital stay.[110] Ethamsylate, used to prevent intraventricular haemorrhage, has been associated with a reduced incidence of sPDA[6] but there is insufficient evidence to support its widespread use for PDA prophylaxis. It has also been reported that prophylactic indometacin has a significant relapse rate for sPDA[28] from a unit with an overall low incidence of sPDA.

Incidence, clinical features and diagnosis

Definitions of sPDA vary widely and quoted incidences consequently also show much variation, but rates of up to 50% or more in infants under 800 g have been reported;[105] rates diminish as birthweight and gestation increase. The picture of a baby with RDS who is failing to improve or starts to deteriorate between 5 and 10 days of age, who has some or all of bounding pulses, an active precordium and a continuous murmur in the pulmonary area, is easy to recognise. Progressive cardiomegaly and worsening lung shadowing on X-ray may be seen. Less gross physical signs in the clinical context may still allow a diagnosis to be made even in the absence of a murmur. sPDA can occur well before 5 days of age, particularly in infants who have received exogenous surfactant;[29,80] indeed, PDA may be important in the pathogenesis of pulmonary haemorrhage occurring after surfactant administration. Apnoea in a non-ventilated baby is sometimes a manifestation of PDA and necrotising enterocolitis may be secondary to a widely patent duct. Echocardiography is more sensitive and specific than clinical signs[33] but is not always needed unless there is doubt about the diagnosis or other cardiac problems are suspected or surgery is intended. A continuous murmur in a preterm infant is far more likely to be due to PDA than to any structural lesion, but, if doubt exists, echocardiography must be performed. The little understood systemic-to-pulmonary collateral arteries detected in preterm infants appear to be a transitory finding[1] in most cases but cause a continuous murmur and can confuse in the diagnosis of PDA. The contribution of these vessels to CLD and the indications for intervention are unclear. Echocardiographic features of PDA include volume overloading of the left heart, visualisation of the ductus itself and Doppler evaluation of the pulmonary artery, the ductus and the descending aorta (Fig. 28.14).[33] Unless prophylactic drug therapy is intended, the significance of echocardiographic detection of PDA is evaluated in the light of the clinical picture.

Treatment of sPDA

The DA will close spontaneously in time in nearly all preterm infants without specific therapy but with considerable morbidity. It is therefore appropriate to recommend early and aggressive treatment for sPDA in the preterm infant, although, as discussed above, prophylactic pharmacological treatment cannot yet be advocated unreservedly.[24,39] First-line treatment involves optimising oxygen delivery by treating anaemia and achieving adequate arterial oxygen tension, as well as employing fluid restriction and diuretics. Loop diuretics such as furosemide (frusemide) are the most commonly used, although there are theoretical reasons as well as modest clinical evidence[44] to suggest that furosemide (frusemide) may promote ductal patency by its effect on renal prostaglandin synthesis. However, a short trial of fluid restriction and diuretic treatment is sometimes associated with clinical improvement, but, if there is no improvement after 24 hours, ductal closure should be attempted either pharmacologically or by surgery. Drug treatment should be tried first unless a contraindication to it exists. Indometacin is the most widely used drug. In a multicentre trial of babies under 1750 g birthweight,[41] 21% developed sPDA and indometacin closed the ductus within 48 hours of administration in 79% of the 135 infants who received it. Spontaneous closure occurred in only 28% of controls in the same timescale. One-third of responders relapsed but many of these did not require further intervention. Many of those who did have further intervention responded to additional indometacin administration. Overall, indometacin had a 70% success rate, which was not influenced by the application or not of prior fluid restriction and diuretic therapy. Many other studies have demonstrated similar results. Gestation under 28 weeks and postnatal age beyond 2 weeks are associated with lower success rates, as is antenatal indometacin exposure.[71]

Indometacin is usually given intravenously in a dose of 0.2 mg/kg on three occasions, with 8 to 12 hours between each dose. If a response is seen but with later relapse, it is reasonable to give a further course of indometacin. Indometacin used in this way has a beneficial effect on ventilatory requirements and also allows improved nutrition. However, there is little clear evidence of long-term benefit in terms of survival, duration of hospital stay or improved neurodevelopmental outcome. Indometacin interferes with platelet function and thrombocytopenia is a contraindication to its use, as are markedly elevated or rapidly rising blood urea or creatinine concentrations. As well as constricting the DA, indometacin causes renal vasoconstriction, resulting in oliguria, fluid retention, hyponatraemia and elevation of blood urea and creatinine concentrations. These effects are transitory and rarely serious if fluid restriction is applied during treatment; they may also be lessened by the use of dopamine during indometacin treatment, although this has not been a consistent finding.[37] Peripheral vasoconstriction during indometacin administration causes hypertension[32] and derangement of intestinal arterial haemodynamics.[27] The effect on gastrointestinal blood flow may be the explanation for gastrointestinal haemorrhage and perforation, which are seen in less than 10% of recipients of indometacin. Cranial Doppler ultrasound demonstrates significant falls in cerebral blood flow velocity after rapid intravenous administration of indometacin[32] but not if the drug is given over 30 minutes.[26] However, near-infrared spectroscopy shows marked and prolonged reduction in cerebral blood flow and volume, cerebral oxygen delivery and cerebral vascular responsiveness, regardless of the speed of administration of the drug.[31] The evidence that indometacin reduces cerebral blood flow is countered by clear evidence that it reduces the incidence of intraventricular haemorrhage[114] and that PDA has adverse effects on cerebral haemodynamics.[36,94] A 5-day course of indometacin[47] has been shown to reduce relapse rate, and a 6-day lower-dose (0.1 mg/kg/day) course[82] is associated with lower relapse rates and less biochemical disturbance. It is not known what cerebral haemodynamic disturbances accompany these longer courses of indometacin. Ductal Doppler waveforms referred to above[103] have been used to reduce the number of doses of indometacin used if evolution in the pattern from growing or pulsatile to closing (high-velocity left-to-right, Fig 28.14 g) is documented before a standard course of the drug is completed. Side effects would also appear to be reduced by this approach.[102] Ibuprofen has been shown to be as effective at closing the ductus in extremely preterm infants but without disturbances of cerebral haemodynamics as demonstrated by near-infrared spectroscopy[76,77] and also to cause less disturbance of renal function[109] than three doses of indometacin 0.2 mg/kg administered 12 hours apart. There are problems with availability of a suitable intravenous preparation of ibuprofen in many countries.

Surgery

Surgical occlusion of sPDA is indicated if a clear contraindication to indometacin administration exists, or if the drug is ineffective. Relapse after a second short course of indometacin or after a single 6-day course are also indications for surgery. Surgery can be performed in the neonatal intensive care nursery with acceptable morbidity and low short-term mortality, although this group of patients have been reported to have a 10% mortality before discharge from hospital.[84] If the above approaches are followed, most babies with sPDA should have had successful occlusion of it either pharmacologically or by surgery before 14 days of age, some even in the first week of life, and all well before they are 3 weeks old.

Chronic lung disease

The pathogenesis of CLD is complex (Chapter 27, Part 3) and a contribution from PDA seems likely, although early intervention to close PDA has not been shown to reduce its incidence. Other left-to-right shunt lesions may contribute to or be masked by chronic respiratory problems. Sustained or recurrent hypoxaemia secondary to CLD results in elevation of PVR with consequent pulmonary hypertension and right heart enlargement. Steroid administration may cause cardiac hypertrophy with or without systemic hypertension which may result in dynamic left ventricular outflow obstruction.[34] These changes are rarely of clinical significance and resolve with cessation of steroid therapy. Electrocardiographic and echocardiographic assessment of infants with CLD is appropriate to judge RVH and to get non-invasive

(Doppler) evaluation of right heart pressures. Diuretics are of value if pulmonary oedema occurs and are also indicated if systemic venous engorgement occurs secondary to elevated right heart pressures. Reduced ventricular function or atrial dysrhythmias are late and very serious findings.

Structural heart disease

Structural heart disease can be present in the preterm infant and may easily be overlooked because respiratory signs mask cardiac ones and CXR can be hard to interpret. Any possibility of structural heart disease warrants echocardiographic evaluation if intervention for sPDA is contemplated and such assessment is essential before surgery for PDA. Duct-dependent cardiac conditions can be particularly problematic in extreme preterm infants and long periods of intravenous or gastric prostaglandin administration can be used whilst growth to a size where corrective or palliative interventions are feasible occurs. It is not yet clear that this alters outcome, which is less good than for the equivalent conditions in term infants.[30,119]

Endocarditis

Infective and non-infective thrombotic endocarditis occur in critically ill newborn infants with structurally normal hearts, particularly the preterm.[73] Clinical features are non-specific, but recurrent or relapsing bacteraemia or the presence of multiple infected sites should raise suspicion of infective endocarditis. Splenomegaly and microscopic haematuria are often present, but these have many other possible causes. Indwelling arterial or central venous cannulae are risk factors for thromboembolic phenomena and infection. Echocardiography is helpful in diagnosis by recognition of intracardiac vegetations. Treatment involves removal of infected or potentially infected lines and culture-guided antibiotic therapy, which may need to be prolonged.

Persistent pulmonary hypertension may complicate respiratory disease in the preterm infant as well as being seen in term infants, and is considered on pages 496–502.

Structural heart disease in the newborn

Heart disease in the newborn presents in one of four main ways:

- cyanosis;
- respiratory distress (heart failure);
- collapse;
- asymptomatic.

Cyanosis

The causes of cyanosis are listed in Table 28.14. In practice, it is often possible to distinguish respiratory and cardiac causes on

Table 28.14 Conditions presenting with neonatal cyanosis

Category	Detail	Comment
Respiratory	Any respiratory disease	
Cardiac	*Common mixing:*	
	TAPVC	Especially if obstructed
	DIV $\}$ DOV	Degree of cyanosis reflects severity of PS
	Truncus arteriosus	Heart failure common
	Right-to-left shunt:	
	Pulmonary atresia, IVS	
	Pulmonary atresia, VSD	
	Tricuspid atresia	
	Tetralogy of Fallot	20% cyanosed as newborn
	Transposition	
Persistent pulmonary hypertension	See pp. 496–502	
Haematological	Methaemoglobinaemia	Grey/black rather than blue, arterial oxygen tension normal

Table 28.15 Clinical features helpful in distinguishing respiratory from cardiac cyanosis. Note all categories have overlap between respiratory and cardiac causes

	Respiratory cyanosis	Cardiac cyanosis
History	Prematurity, meconium liquor/below cords, risk of infection	Family history of congenital heart disease
Respiration	Marked respiratory distress	Little or no respiratory distress unless shocked or metabolic acidosis
Cardiovascular examination	Normal	May have clear signs
Response to oxygen	Cyanosis likely to improve	Cyanosis unlikely to improve
Chest X-ray	Obvious respiratory pathology	No respiratory pathology, abnormal heart shadow or lung vasculature may be seen
ECG	Normal	May be normal, may be helpful
Blood gases	Hypercapnia	Hypo- or normocapnia

Table 28.16 Management of newborn infant with suspected cyanotic congenital heart disease

1. General measures:
   - Maintain temperature
   - Avoid hypoglycaemia
   If well, proceed to 3
2. If ill:
   - Arterial blood gas
     - Treat respiratory failure; ventilate if necessary
     - Hypoxaemia alone not reason to ventilate
     - Treat metabolic acidosis
     - Consider hyperoxia test
   - Consider prostaglandin
3. Chest X-ray:
   - Diagnostic clues may be present
   - Aid in management
     - Oligaemia: start prostaglandin
     - Plethora: start prostaglandin if very hypoxaemic or metabolic acidosis
4. ECG: may point to specific diagnosis
5. Review:
   - Drugs
     - Prostaglandin as above
     - Alkali
     - Diuretic if heart failure/pulmonary congestion
   - Antibiotics if risk of serious infection
   - Need for hyperoxia test: it may help, see pages 626, 628
6. Echocardiography:
   - If infant requires transfer, stabilise first
   - Occasionally needed to confirm/rule out cardiac cause
   - Usually gives precise cardiac diagnosis

clinical grounds; Table 28.15 gives details of helpful discriminating features. If cardiac disease is thought definite or likely, an approach to management is given in Table 28.16. Clinical features, ECG and CXR often allow an approximate cardiac diagnosis to be made (Table 28.17). Echocardiography allows very precise diagnosis in the vast majority of cases. It is more important to stabilise an infant before transfer to a cardiac centre than to get a precise diagnosis by ultrasound. Differentiating cardiac disease from PPHN may require echocardiography and the two may coexist (Table 28.18). Specific cyanotic conditions are discussed below.

Transposition

TGA represents approximately 5% of cases of structural CHD; it is rarely found in preterm infants and is rarely associated with extracardiac abnormalities or syndromes. It is commoner in males by a factor of 3. Associated cardiac conditions include ASD, VSD, PDA, valvar and subvalvar pulmonary stenosis, and aortic coarctation. Clinical signs will be determined by the associated abnormalities; in particular, the fewer and smaller the shunt lesions, the more severe the cyanosis will be. Presentation is occasionally delayed beyond the first week of life but in those

Table 28.17 Clinical features of structural heart lesions presenting with cyanosis

Condition	Pulses	Respiratory distress	Precordium	Auscultation	ECG	CXR	Extracardiac abnormalities
Transposition	Normal	Mild	RV+	S2 single ± RVOT/LVOT systolic murmur	T↑V₁	RV+, lung fields normal or plethora Oligaemia if severe PS	Rare
Pulmonary atresia	Normal	Mild	Normal	S2 single ± TR	RA + LV + QRS 0° to 90°	Heart normal or large. Oligaemia	Rare
Pulmonary atresia with VSD (+MAPCAs)	Normal	Mild	Normal or RV+	S2 single ± continues murmur (MAPCAs)	T↑V₁	Heart normal or large Small PA Right arch Oligaemia (plethora if many MAPCAs)	Common (GI, GU chromosomes)
Tetralogy of Fallot	Normal	None	RV+	S2 single RVOT systolic murmur	T↑V₁	Heart normal Small PA Oligaemia Right arch	Common (GI, GU chromosomes)
Tricupsid atresia	Normal	None	Normal	VSD or PS systolic murmur	RA + LAD (0° to −90°)	Heart size normal RA+ Oligaemia	Rare
TAPVC (obstructed)	Normal or weak	Marked	RV+	S2 may be wide P2 loud No murmur	T↑V₁ RSRV₁	Heat normal if obstructed Pulmonary venous engorgement	Rare
Complex lesions	Normal, full or weak	Variable	Active	S2 often single Various murmurs	Abnormal P waves Abnormal QRS axis	Dextrocardia, situs inversus/ambiguus Oligaemia	Common including heterotaxy (p. 642)

Note: Any lesion may have ductal murmur in addition to signs listed.
Abbreviations: ↑ upright; ± – with or without; + – hypertrophied or enlarged.

Table 28.18 Features helpful in differentiating PPHN from cyanotic heart disease

	Persistent pulmonary hypertension	Cyanotic heart disease
History	Maternal prostaglandin synthetase inhibitor therapy	May have positive family history
Delivery	Fetal distress, birth asphyxia	Uneventful
Examination	Respiratory and/or neurological signs	May have clear cardiac signs
Chest X-ray	May have respiratory pathology	May have cardiac/pulmonary vascular signs. Often non-specific
ECG	May have RAH, ischaemic changes	May have clear abnormality
Hyperoxia test	Variable response, may pass, not if severe; fluctuating arterial oxygen tensions seen	Usually poor response
Upper/lower limb saturations	Lower limb often lower (if DA patent)	Occasionally marked discrepancy
Echocardiography	Usually can exclude heart abnormality but can be difficult	Usually diagnostic

Note: There can be marked overlap and both can coexist.

with no shunts is usually within a few hours of birth. Marked pulmonary outflow obstruction will result in worse cyanosis as well as a loud murmur with pulmonary oligaemia on CXR, whereas in the absence of pulmonary stenosis, pulmonary plethora is the more usual finding. Cases with large shunt lesions will not require immediate intervention to improve oxygenation; those without large shunt lesions will usually improve oxygenation enough to avoid metabolic acidosis if the DA is opened with prostaglandin. In most cases, enlargement of the foramen ovale by balloon septostomy will be necessary to obtain adequate entry of well-saturated blood into the right ventricle, even if the DA has been reopened. Balloon septostomy can be done in the neonatal nursery under ultrasound control if angiography is not needed. Coexistent coarctation must be repaired and the arterial switch operation is performed in the newborn period unless there is marked fixed pulmonary outflow obstruction, in which case the switch operation is not appropriate and a systemic-to-pulmonary anastomosis will be needed, with definitive surgery being deferred for some years. The arterial switch operation must be performed before left ventricular muscle has involuted in response to serving the lower resistance pulmonary circulation. The timescale in which this happens is unclear, but surgery under 3 weeks of age is within a safe margin. If there is a large VSD that does not reduce in size spontaneously, the timescale is not as pressing but there is no particular advantage in delaying surgery beyond 2 months. A baby with TGA who presents beyond the early newborn period needs careful assessment to be sure that the left ventricular pressure remains high. Coronary artery anatomy is clearly important to the surgeon and can often be delineated by echocardiography, but even if it cannot, few centres now perform angiography to clarify it. Neonatal arterial switch operative mortality is <5% for simple TGA. Repair of transposition by intra-atrial repair (Mustard or Senning operations) is uncommonly performed now because of long-term problems with arrhythmias and right ventricular failure.

Congenitally corrected transposition of the great arteries

This very rare abnormality (<1% of structural heart lesions) involves not only ventriculoarterial discordance (as in TGA) but also atrioventricular discordance. Thus, pulmonary venous blood passes from the left atrium through the tricuspid valve into the morphological right ventricle and then is ejected into the aorta. Desaturated systemic venous blood passes through the right atrium and morphological left ventricle into the pulmonary artery. There may be dextrocardia and sometimes situs inversus. If there are no associated defects, infants are pink and the condition is not suspected until long after the newborn period. VSDs occur in 75–80% of patients and will often cause heart failure in infancy unless important pulmonary stenosis coexists, in which case cyanosis will occur, sometimes in the newborn period. Systemic AV valve regurgitation develops in about 30% of cases in later life and arrhythmias can develop at any age from fetal life onwards, including all degrees of AV block and SVT. Cyanosis or heart failure may be present; there is RVH and P2 is single. Murmurs depend on associated lesions. The ECG may have heart block of any degree or a pre-excitation pattern. There are Q waves in V_1 and none in V_{5-6}. CXR will be affected by associated lesions; it may show an abnormal heart position and often has a prominent left upper heart border due to the ascending aorta. Palliative surgery in the form of pulmonary artery banding or systemic-to-pulmonary anastomosis is indicated in symptomatic infants.

Pulmonary atresia

In all forms of this condition, the pulmonary valve and sometimes the subvalvar ventricular outflow tract is completely blocked, so there can be no forward flow from the right ventricle into the pulmonary artery. Valve morphology varies and may consist of two or three thin cusps which are fused, or the cusps may be extremely thick, dysplastic and immobile. Whatever cusp morphology exists, the valve ring itself is usually small in addition. Hearts with pulmonary atresia can be further subdivided as follows:

- with intact ventricular septum – pulmonary circulation always duct dependent (includes neonates with critical pulmonary valve stenosis);
- with VSD – pulmonary circulation duct dependent or pulmonary blood supply from major aortopulmonary communicating arteries (MAPCAs);
- as part of complex cyanotic heart disease, for example as in asplenia with AVSD ± TGA.

Pulmonary atresia with intact ventricular septum

This condition always presents with severe cyanosis in the early newborn period, thereby making up 2.5% of symptomatic newborns with CHD but <1% of all lesions. The main pulmonary artery and its branches are usually confluent and of reasonable size, whereas the right ventricle and tricuspid valve are underdeveloped, sometimes severely so. The tricuspid valve is frequently malformed by displacement of its septal leaflet toward the apex (Ebstein's malformation). Anomalies of the coronary supply to the right ventricle are common and may affect outcome. There is total right-to-left shunting at atrial level. If the foramen ovale is or becomes restrictive, marked right atrial enlargement and systemic venous engorgement occur. Pulmonary blood flow is duct dependent, and extreme cyanosis with metabolic acidosis develops as duct closure progresses. Clinical features are given in Table 28.17. Resuscitation includes prostaglandin and sometimes balloon atrial septostomy. Interventional catheterisation can be used as initial treatment[48] but many centres use a surgical approach, the exact sequence depending on echocardiographic assessment of right ventricular cavity and tricuspid valve sizes. In what way coronary abnormalities should affect management is unclear. Primary opening up of the right ventricular outflow tract (RVOT) is desirable if at all possible; systemic-to-pulmonary arterial anastomosis may be required in addition. These approaches give survival to school age in the region of 80%. If right ventricular hypoplasia is so severe that a biventricular circulation cannot ultimately be established, a systemic-to-pulmonary shunt is performed in the newborn period with the eventual aim of achieving a Fontan-type circulation in which systemic veins are connected to the pulmonary arteries without passage of systemic venous blood through a ventricle. Critical pulmonary valve stenosis has many features in common with this situation except that there is forward flow through the pulmonary valve and the right heart is not markedly hypoplastic. Infants with critical pulmonary stenosis can be treated with either balloon dilatation or surgery with a good result, even if further intervention in the form of pulmonary balloon dilatation is needed in later infancy.

Pulmonary atresia with VSD (see Table 28.17)

These infants may have non-confluent and severely underdeveloped pulmonary arteries. Pulmonary blood supply may come entirely via the DA or it may come partly or entirely from other vessels arising from the aorta (MAPCAs) or head and neck branches. The degree of cyanosis and other physical signs will depend on the amount of flow into the pulmonary circulation. If MAPCAs are large or plentiful, cyanosis is milder, continuous murmurs are heard all over the chest and heart failure may develop. This group of conditions has a significant association with extracardiac malformations, syndromes and chromosomal abnormalities. DiGeorge syndrome and 22q11 deletions must be remembered as they have important implications for management, with increased risk of symptomatic hypocalcaemia, immunodeficiency and, if transfused cellular blood products, of graft-versus-host disease. If pulmonary blood flow is duct dependent, prostaglandin will be needed and early palliative surgery is indicated. If sources of lung blood supply are complex, detailed evaluation with angiography is required in early infancy in order to assess surgical options. Long-term outcome is variable, but a survival of 80% or more is likely, even if multiple surgical procedures are required.

Pulmonary atresia as part of a complex lesion

These infants usually have duct-dependent pulmonary blood flow and their condition will be improved by prostaglandin. Obstruction to the systemic arterial outflow of the heart exceedingly rarely coexists, just as complex lesions with systemic outflow obstruction very rarely have significant pulmonary outflow obstruction. However, almost any other cardiac structural abnormality can coexist. Thus, clinical features in addition to cyanosis vary, as do appropriate treatments. In the newborn period, surgical interventions, if indicated at all, are likely to be only palliative. Extracardiac abnormalities are common and long-term outcome is often poor for both cardiac and non-cardiac reasons, particularly in those with dextro-isomerism (pp. 590, 625, 627, 639, 640), in whom asplenia with an increased risk of serious bacterial infection is usually present.

Tetralogy of Fallot (see Table 28.17)

This constitutes 10% of all cases of structural heart disease, but only 20% of cases of tetralogy of Fallot are cyanotic in the newborn period. Right ventricular outflow obstruction is always subvalvar (infundibular) but may be valvar and supravalvar in addition. Right ventricular outflow obstruction and a large VSD cause RVH. The VSD is subaortic with the aorta arising in part from the right ventricle (overriding aorta); it is rarely restrictive and additional significant VSDs are occasionally found. PFO or ASD commonly coexist;

rarely the pulmonary valve is absent (see below) and the condition can coexist with complete AVSD. The cases presenting with cyanosis as newborns may have pulmonary atresia or a very narrow but patent RVOT. Those with pulmonary atresia will be duct dependent. Tetralogy of Fallot without cyanosis in the newborn period is associated with a pulmonary outflow murmur although it is frequently mistaken for a VSD murmur. Cyanosis is progressive during the first year of life as subvalvar muscular RVOT obstruction increases. Hypercyanotic spells due to infundibular constriction are rare in the newborn period but are an indication for palliative or corrective surgery. Emergency management of spells includes:

- intermittent knee/chest position if feasible;
- facial oxygen (although whilst the spell occurs it is unlikely to improve oxygenation);
- morphine (50–100 micrograms/kg s.c., i.m. or i.v.);
- phenylephrine 20 micrograms/kg i.v.;
- propranolol 20 micrograms/kg slowly i.v., may be repeated once;
- heavy sedation/anaesthesia and assisted ventilation.

It is rare to need to progress beyond morphine in this protocol. Intravenous drugs should only be used in a setting where ventilation and full cardiopulmonary resuscitation can be given. Spells are usually mild initially and get progressively more frequent, severe and prolonged. Oral propranolol (1–2 mg/kg) three times daily usually prevents recurrent spells in the short and medium term whilst surgical strategies are decided. Cardiac catheterisation may be carried out prior to corrective surgery for tetralogy of Fallot to assess coronary anatomy, to look for additional VSDs and to display pulmonary artery anatomy in detail. Cardiac catheterisation is not required prior to the creation of a systemic-to-pulmonary anastomosis.

Tetralogy of Fallot with absent pulmonary valve

This rare variant of tetralogy (<5% of cases) has small dysplastic pulmonary valve leaflets resulting in marked pulmonary regurgitation and dilatation, often massive, of the pulmonary arteries. The large pulmonary arteries compress the bronchi so that bronchomalacia develops in utero. Presentation in the newborn period is with airway obstruction causing pulmonary collapse or over-inflation. Cyanosis is not usually marked in early infancy. Impressive systolic and diastolic murmurs from the RVOT with a single S2 in the context of airway obstruction strongly suggest the diagnosis. The dilated pulmonary arteries are seen on CXR; RVH is apparent on ECG. Severe bronchomalacia and pulmonary hypoplasia often cause death even if technically satisfactory cardiac surgical repair is achieved. Surgical mortality in those with severe pulmonary problems may be as high as 50%.

Tricuspid atresia

Tricuspid atresia represents about 2% of structural heart lesions. Associated abnormalities include VSD and TGA. Those without TGA may have pulmonary stenosis; those with TGA may have coarctation. Blood leaves the right atrium via the foramen ovale or an ASD. If the VSD is large or there is TGA, pulmonary blood flow will be high and cyanosis mild, with the possibility of heart failure developing. A restrictive VSD and/or severe pulmonary

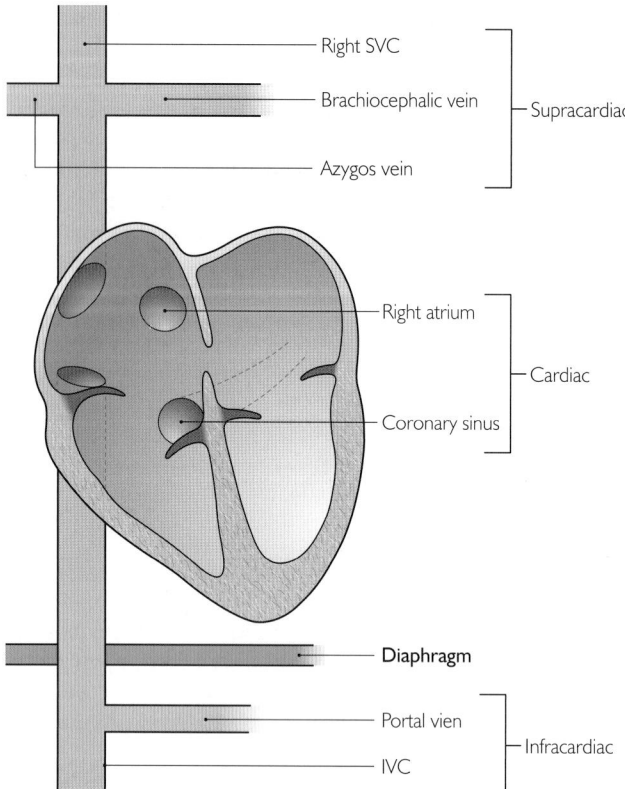

Right SVC ⎤
Brachiocephalic vein ⎬ Supracardiac
Azygos vein ⎦

Right atrium ⎤
⎬ Cardiac
Coronary sinus ⎦

Diaphragm

Portal vien ⎤
⎬ Infracardiac
IVC ⎦

Fig. 28.15 Possible sites of total anomalous pulmonary venous connection; mixed connections can occur.

stenosis will produce duct-dependent pulmonary circulation. Coarctation with TGA may result in collapse from duct-dependent systemic circulation. Clinical features are given in Table 28.17. Coarctation should be repaired at presentation. The long-term goal is a Fontan circulation, and either systemic-to-pulmonary anastomosis or pulmonary artery banding are usually required in infancy as palliation and, if the VSD is large, to ensure undamaged pulmonary vasculature. In the context of tricuspid atresia with TGA, an arterial switch operation may be performed; although in this circumstance the switch is only palliative, it does ensure that the systemic ventricle is the morphologically left ventricle, an advantage for long-term ventricular function. Tricuspid atresia is the lesion with the best long-term outlook with a Fontan circulation, with an operative mortality in childhood of under 10% and a 75% 15-year good-quality survival thereafter.

Total anomalous pulmonary venous connection

Entry of pulmonary veins into systemic venous pathways can be at one site or several (mixed TAPVC). Most commonly, the pulmonary veins all enter a confluence behind, but separate from, the left atrium. The confluence then drains directly or indirectly into the right atrium. Drainage can be classified as in Figure 28.15. Obstruction to the pulmonary venous return can occur at a number of sites, including the pulmonary vein orifices, on entry of the confluence to the systemic veins, on passage through the

diaphragm and on passage through the liver after the ductus venosus closes in infradiaphragmatic TAPVC. Obstruction to the pulmonary veins will cause worse cyanosis, marked respiratory distress and less cardiomegaly than unobstructed TAPVC and may prove difficult to distinguish from PPHN even with echocardiography. There is always a PFO and often an ASD, with entry of blood to the left heart only through these means; thus, varying degrees of left ventricular underdevelopment are common. Coarctation and even severe hypoplasia of the left heart are occasionally present. TAPVC forms part of the complex abnormalities associated with heterotaxy states (left and right isomerism). These are considered in more detail on pages 590, 625, 627, 639, 640. In general, the more severe the pulmonary venous obstruction, the earlier the infant is symptomatic. Infradiaphragmatic TAPVC to the portal vein is associated with marked cyanosis and respiratory distress which gets dramatically worse when the ductus venosus shuts. Infants with completely unobstructed TAPVC are sometimes not recognised until after the newborn period when recurrent or chronic chestiness and failure to thrive occur. As they sometimes present early and very blue, infants with obstructed TAPVC often receive prostaglandin, sometimes with benefit to their general state. This improvement is presumably due either to opening of the DA and decompression of the right heart or to opening the ductus venosus and ameliorating pulmonary venous hypertension in TAPVC to the portal vein. Management is by corrective surgery, with mortality below 10% and an excellent long-term outlook unless pulmonary vein stenosis is present.

Complex structural cyanotic congenital heart disease

These conditions often include more than one of the above abnormalities as well as shunt lesions and obstruction to either systemic or pulmonary arterial outflow tracts. Important pulmonary and systemic obstruction only very rarely coexist. Association with extracardiac abnormalities is common and in addition to specific system abnormalities the occurrence of heterotaxy states must be considered. Heterotaxy states, sometimes termed situs ambiguus, exist when abdominal, bronchial and atrial anatomy is neither the usual arrangement (situs solitus) nor a mirror image of the usual arrangement (situs inversus). The usual arrangement of viscera involves spleen and stomach being on the left-hand side and liver on the right, a morphologically left lung being on the left and a morphologically right lung (three-lobed) being on the right with a morphologically left atrium being to the left of the morphologically right atrium. Situs inversus is a mirror image of this arrangement and situs ambiguus exists when both lungs are of the same morphology (right or left) and both atria are of the same morphology (right or left). When this situation exists, the liver tends to be midline, stomach position is variable and there is either asplenia (in right isomerism) or polysplenia (in left isomerism). Very rarely the situation is less clear-cut and there are features of more than one arrangement of situs. Generally speaking, right isomerism is associated with severe cyanotic CHD comprising TAPVC, complete AVSD and pulmonary atresia or severe pulmonary stenosis with or without transposition. The cardiac abnormalities associated with left isomerism are more variable in range and severity, but abnormalities of the pulmonary venous drainage are invariable,

Table 28.19 Cardiac conditions presenting with neonatal respiratory distress

Category	Comments
Heart muscle disease	
Ischaemia	With birth asphyxia
Myocarditis	Any cause
Cardiomyopathy	Hypertrophic or dilated
Arrhythmias	
Arteriovenous malformation	Cranial or other with PPHN
Structural heart disease	
Week I	
Hypoplastic left heart	May also present with
Interrupted arch	collapse, see Tables 28.24
Aortic atresia/critical stenosis	and 28.25
Coarctation	
Week 2–3	
Truncus	May also present with
DOV, DIV, TAPVC	cyanosis, see Table 28.14
TGA + VSD	
Week 3	
Left-to-right shunt lesions	Any
Time Variable	
Tetralogy with absent pulmonary valve	Neonatal symptoms are due to airway obstruction

DIV, double-inlet ventricle; DOV, double-outlet ventricle; TAPVC, total anomalous pulmonary venous connection; TGA, transposition of the great arteries; VSD, ventricular septal defect.

although often only partially anomalous. Cardiac lesions with left isomerism are not always cyanotic. Clues to the presence of a complex abnormality include a midline liver and dextrocardia. Immediate management principles include deciding whether prostaglandin is indicated: the same criteria apply in these circumstances as in any other.

Conclusion

There are other structural lesions which may present with cyanosis in the newborn infant, such as truncus arteriosus and double-inlet or double-outlet ventricle, but frequently they are not diagnosed until beyond the newborn period. They are considered under respiratory distress (see below).

Respiratory distress

Cardiac conditions presenting with respiratory distress are listed in Table 28.19 and clinical details given in Tables 28.20 and 28.21. Some of these conditions may present with collapse and in retrospect a period of respiratory distress may have been present prior to collapse. Cardiac conditions causing respiratory distress usually do so through heart failure, the signs of which are given in Table 28.6. Cardiac disease will also cause respiratory distress if there is marked pulmonary venous engorgement or metabolic acidosis has developed; these two occurrences can be associated with cyanotic cardiac conditions. Some conditions characteristically cause both cyanosis and heart failure (Table 28.22). Signs of cardiac disease will be absent in respiratory causes of respiratory distress and a CXR usually allows the distinction to be made with confidence; in addition, cardiac causes of respiratory distress are likely to have signs related to the cardiac diagnosis.

Arrhythmias (see Table 28.20)

These are considered in detail on pages 651–7.

Heart muscle disease (see Table 28.20)

There is little information on the incidence of heart muscle disease in the newborn, but cardiomyopathy is much more frequent under 1 year of age (about 8 per 100 000 per year) than in childhood overall (about 1 per 100 000 per year).[60,72]

Myocardial ischaemia

Subclinical myocardial ischaemia in asphyxiated and otherwise stressed infants is quite common.[9] Involvement severe enough to cause hypotension is less common, although a transient murmur from tricuspid regurgitation in association with ST depression and T-wave inversion in the left chest leads is a common finding. Specific therapy for heart failure is sometimes required; such infants usually have neurological and renal impairment in addition. Myocardial infarction in neonates may cause heart failure or sudden collapse. ECG changes include deep and wide Q waves and initial elevation of the ST segment, followed by T-wave inversion some days later. Q waves persist indefinitely but ST segment changes resolve in a week or so and T waves return to normal over a much longer timescale. Enzyme studies can be difficult to interpret in the early newborn period as other tissues may be the source of the enzymes and cardiac-specific isoenzymes need to be measured. Myocardial infarction can occur as part of generalised perinatal asphyxia or secondary to thromboembolic events[104] and has a high mortality. Anomalous origin of the left coronary artery from the pulmonary artery (ALCAPA) is rarely symptomatic in the early weeks of life, as it is well tolerated whilst the pulmonary artery pressure remains high. It is a cause of pale sweating episodes (presumably angina), heart failure from dilated cardiomyopathy (DCM) and myocardial infarction after the newborn period. Ischaemia secondary to birth asphyxia usually recovers fully without any apparent long-term sequelae, even if intravenous inotrope support is required acutely. Long-term outlook after neonatal myocardial infarction is less well documented.

Myocarditis

Myocarditis is usually presumed rather than definitely proven to be viral in origin, although occasionally a virus is identified

Table 28.20 Clinical features of cardiovascular conditions not involving intracardiac structural abnormalities presenting with respiratory distress in the newborn

Condition	Pulses	Precordium	Auscultation	ECG	Extracardiac associations
Arrhythmia	Normal or weak	Normal	Gallop	Diagnostic	Rare
Heart muscle disease					
Myocarditis	Normal or weak	Normal	Gallop, MR murmur, rub	Small QRS ST↑, T↓	Common (hepatitis etc.)
Ischaemia	Normal or weak	Normal	Gallop, MR murmur, TR murmur	ST↑, T↓	Features of perinatal asphyxia
DCM	Normal or weak	Normal	Gallop, MR murmur	LV+, ST↓↓, T↓↓	Rare
EFE	Weak	Normal or active	Gallop, MR murmur	LV+, ST↓↓, T↓↓ V_{5-6}	Rare
HCM	Normal or jerky	Normal or active	Gallop, LVOT or RVOT	LV/RV + ST↑ or ↓T↓	Common (macrosomia, usually maternal diabetes)
AVM					
Cranial	Normal or weak femorals	Active	Gallop, MR murmur, cranial bruit	LV/RV+ ST↓, T↓	Neurological signs
Coronary	Full	Active	Gallop, continuous murmur	LV or RV+ ST↓, T↓	

Note: Cyanosis is not present in any condition unless PPHN occurs and all have cardiomegaly and pulmonary congestion on chest X-ray.

Table 28.21 Structural heart lesions presenting with respiratory distress (heart failure) after the first week of life

Condition	Pulses	Cyanosis	Precordium	Auscultation	ECG	Extracardiac associations
Truncus arteriosus	Normal or full	Mild	Active	S2 single, EC Systolic	RV+ ± LV+ ST↓, T↓ V_{5-6}	Common (DiGeorge)
TGA + VSD	Normal	Mild/moderate	RV+	S2 single ± VSD murmur	LV+ or RV+	Rare
TAPVC (unobstructed)	Normal or weak	Mild/moderate	RV+	S2 wide, P2 loud ± RVOT murmur	RV+ RsRV₁	Rare
DIV/DOV without PS	Normal	Mild	Active	P2 loud VSD murmur	Variable	Rare
PDA	Full	None	Active	Continuous murmur at base	LV+ ± RV+	Occasional
VSD	Normal	None	Active	P2 loud PSM LLSE	LV+ ± RV+	Occasional
Complete AVSD	Normal	None	Active	P2 loud VSD murmur LLSE MR murmur apex	RA+ RV+ Superior QRS axis	Very common (Down syndrome)
AP window	Normal or full	None	Active	P2 loud, continuous murmur at midsternal edge	LV+ RV+	Rare

Table 28.22 Structural cardiac conditions in which cyanosis and heart failure commonly coexist in the newborn

- Transposition
  - with coarctation
  - with large VSD
- Truncus arteriosus
- Tricuspid atresia
  - with large VSD
  - with TGA and coarctation
- Double-inlet ventricle
- Total anomalous pulmonary venous connection
  - with obstructed pulmonary veins
- Hypoplastic left heart syndrome
- Arteriovenous malformation – usually intracerebral, often have PPHN

If significant pulmonary stenosis coexists, heart failure is unlikely and cyanosis is more marked

Table 28.23 Blood and urine screening tests for hypertrophic and dilated cardiomyopathy in infants if no clinical diagnosis apparent. Abnormal findings need detailed investigation

Blood for:	Vacuolated lymphocytes
	Carnitine and acyl carnitine
	Lactate and pyruvate (fasting)
	Creatine kinase MM
	Thyroid function
	Autoimmune screen
	Amino acids
	Virology (especially entero-, adeno- and parvoviruses)
Urine for:	Amino and organic acids
	Glycosaminoglycans
	Virology
Nasopharyngeal aspirate for:	Virology

directly or by serology, often in the context of a generalised viraemic illness with hepatitis and meningo-encephalitis. Heart failure and either tachy- or bradyarrhythmias can occur. Detection of a pericardial rub is rare in the newborn; pericardial effusion and even tamponade can occur. There is no specific therapy: heart failure should be treated in the usual way, but digoxin used cautiously because of the risk of arrhythmias. Digoxin should not be used if tamponade is suspected as it will slow the heart rate and reduce cardiac output if venous return is already impaired. Symptomatic, large or increasing pericardial effusions should be drained. Usually this is possible percutaneously (pp. 1264–5). Precise outcome figures are scarce, but if death does not occur, there may be complete recovery or the development of chronic DCM.

Dilated cardiomyopathy

This usually presents after the newborn period but fetal and neonatal presentation with heart failure do occur. Tachyarrhythmia must be excluded as a cause, as must anomalous origin of the left coronary artery, which is unlikely to present this young (see above). Detailed investigations for infective and metabolic causes are appropriate[16] (Table 28.23) if ischaemia or infarction is not clearly responsible. If any of the screening investigations reveal possible aetiologies, enzyme studies on lymphocytes, fibroblasts or other tissue biopsies are indicated. If a metabolic cause is suspected from investigations or other clinical features such as skeletal myopathy, the question of blind treatment needs to be considered if the infant is critically ill. This may be appropriate if one of the carnitine deficiency states is suspected.[52] First-degree relatives of infants with DCM should be evaluated clinically, by ECG and echocardiography, as familial occurrence is recognised even when precise metabolic diagnoses are lacking.

Endocardial fibroelastosis

This can be primary, in which case it has close clinical similarities to DCM, with marked left ventricular hypertrophy on ECG. The endocardium is echogenic on ultrasound. Information on prognosis is difficult to interpret as diagnostic criteria differ, but complete recovery is described. Endocardial fibroelastosis is often secondary to obstructive left heart lesions, in which case the clinical picture and prognosis is influenced by the nature and severity of the accompanying pathology.

Hypertrophic cardiomyopathy (HCM)

This can be primary as a manifestation of an autosomal dominant genetic disease, or secondary – for example, in association with Noonan's syndrome (also autosomal dominant). Most common is HCM secondary to hyperinsulinism, usually maternal diabetes mellitus (or at least maternal glucose intolerance during pregnancy which may not have been recognised) but rarer causes of hyperinsulinism can also cause neonatal cardiac hypertrophy. Infants receiving corticosteroids for CLD may develop reversible cardiac hypertrophy out of proportion to the degree of hypertension; they rarely show symptoms.[34] The majority of infants born to mothers with diabetes or gestational diabetes have no clinical effects from HCM. Some have a left ventricular outflow murmur and a few develop respiratory distress attributed more often to impaired left ventricular filling than to outflow obstruction. Hypertrophy can be global or localised and this is reflected in the ECG and echocardiographic findings. Infants of diabetic mothers also have an increased incidence of structural heart disease (5%), making detailed assessment including echocardiography important if there are any cardiac symptoms or signs in such infants. If maternal glucose intolerance cannot be confirmed, a search for metabolic causes of cardiac hypertrophy is indicated (see Table 28.23).[15,45] Management of symptomatic cases should not usually include digoxin, inotropes or vasodilators as these all may exacerbate left ventricular outflow obstruction. Propranolol is occasionally indicated in severely symptomatic cases, although hypoglycaemia needs to be carefully guarded against if it is used. Cardiac hypertrophy in association with maternal diabetes resolves over 6 to 12 months.[113]

Isolated left ventricular non-compaction

This form of left ventricular abnormality[72] is now well recognised in children (about 10% of childhood cases of cardiomyopathy) and has recently been described in the fetus.[55]

Arteriovenous malformation (AVM) (see Table 28.20)

Arteriovenous fistulae may present in the newborn period with heart failure; there may be associated PPHN. Intracranial fistulae are the most common; intrahepatic fistulae are occasionally encountered and may coexist with intracranial shunts. As well as heart failure, signs include a bruit over the affected site. Management consists of medical support for the circulation and intervention to stop or at least reduce the shunt through the AVM. This involves catheter embolisation for intracranial abnormalities, which are most commonly vein of Galen aneurysms. The outcome is determined by the ability to achieve a marked reduction in or abolition of the arteriovenous shunt and by the severity of secondary hydrocephalus and cerebral ischaemic lesions. Babies with an in-utero diagnosis of AVM who have hydrops fare particularly badly.

Duct-dependent systemic circulation

This group of conditions comprises hypoplastic left heart syndrome (HLHS), interrupted aortic arch, coarctation, aortic atresia and critical aortic stenosis (AS), and is discussed in detail under Collapse (p. 648).

Truncus arteriosus (see Table 28.21)

This malformation constitutes <1% of congenital heart lesions; it is associated with DiGeorge syndrome in 30% of cases. A single artery arises from the heart giving rise to coronary and pulmonary circulations as well as to the aortic arch, which is right-sided in 30% of cases and interrupted in 5–10%, in which case the association with DiGeorge syndrome is very high. The VSD is usually large and the common arterial trunk overrides it; the truncal valve is abnormal and may be regurgitant or stenosed. Pulmonary arteries arise either laterally from the truncus, adjacent and posteriorly, or from a short main pulmonary artery. Absence of one pulmonary artery occasionally occurs. Stenosis at the origin of a pulmonary artery if present is rarely severe; thus, high pulmonary blood flow and pressure result in pulmonary vascular disease (PVD) if the baby survives infancy without surgery. Clinical presentation is with tachypnoea or heart failure in the later newborn period. Severity of cyanosis varies but is usually only mild; other features are listed in Table 28.21. The severity and haemodynamic effect of the truncal valve abnormality influence the signs detected, as does the PVR. Definitive diagnosis is by ultrasound, and, providing both pulmonary arteries can be demonstrated, further cardiac investigation is not normally required before surgery. Corrective surgery is indicated in early infancy to avoid irreversible progressive PVD. Chromosome 22q11 deletion and immune status should be investigated preoperatively. The long-term outlook is determined not only by the cardiac state but also by neurodevelopmental and immunological aspects of DiGeorge syndrome.

Corrective surgery in early infancy has a mortality of 10% or less and further surgery in the form of replacement of the right ventricular to pulmonary artery conduit will be required in later childhood. In addition, many cases will need truncal valve surgery at some stage, although not usually at initial intervention; if valve replacement is required in early infancy, surgical mortality can be up to 50%.

Transposition with ventriculoseptal defect (TGA+VSD)

Transposition is discussed in detail in the section on cyanosis (pp. 638–40). Clinical features of TGA + VSD are given in Table 28.21.

Total anomalous pulmonary venous connection

Unobstructed TAPVC presents with respiratory distress; it is discussed on page 642. Clinical features are given in Tables 28.17 and 28.21.

Double-inlet and double-outlet ventricle

These terms cover a wide spectrum of abnormalities. Double-inlet ventricle is one type of univentricular AV connection when both atria empty into one ventricle; this is sometimes termed single ventricle. The other form of single ventricle is when one AV valve is atretic, that is tricuspid or mitral atresia (absent right or absent left AV connection, respectively). A double-inlet ventricle may receive atrial blood through one common or two separate AV valves. If there are two AV valves draining into one ventricle, it is most usually the morphological left ventricle – double-inlet left ventricle (DILV). Double-outlet ventricle exists when both great arteries arise chiefly from the same ventricle. Double-outlet right ventricle (DORV) is the usual form. Details of AV valve anatomy and great arterial arrangements vary greatly. Thus, blood flow patterns and pathophysiology in DORV may resemble large VSD, TGA + VSD or tetralogy of Fallot, depending on the associated abnormalities. Single-ventricle arrangements and double-outlet ventricle anatomy each constitute 1% of structural heart lesions. The clinical features in common between double-inlet and double-outlet ventricle are that heart failure is likely to develop as PVR falls unless there is important pulmonary stenosis, in which case cyanosis will be the presenting feature. Coarctation may be present in cases without pulmonary stenosis.

Left-to-right shunt lesions (see Table 28.21)

These conditions have a lot of features in common. Some lesions may be small and asymptomatic, as is the case with many VSDs. Symptoms do not develop until PVR falls enough to permit excessive pulmonary blood flow; this may happen more quickly in preterm infants, related to the relative paucity of muscle in immature lung arterioles. In some circumstances when the defect is large, PVR may not fall sufficiently to result in excessive lung blood flow. These infants remain relatively well and pass into the phase of progressive vascular damage without heart failure occurring. Whether or not a period of heart failure occurs, the development of pulmonary vascular changes is universal and rapid in complete AVSD but unusual and not until adult life in secundum-type ASD. Other lesions lie between these extremes in both frequency and rapidity of progression to PVD. Extracardiac factors may influence the risk and hasten the development of PVD. These include extreme prematurity, CLD, airway obstruction, life at high altitude, and Down syndrome.

Patent ductus arteriosus

Prematurity and PDA are considered on pages 634–7. As an isolated lesion outside the context of RDS and prematurity, PDA accounts for nearly 10% of congenital heart lesions. Clinical features are given in Table 28.21; diagnosis is often clinical and confirmed by echocardiography. sPDA in term infants is an indication for surgical closure. If the infant is asymptomatic without evidence of pulmonary hypertension, intervention is often delayed until after infancy, when occlusion by catheter-delivered device or by surgery is performed. The size at which catheter closure can be performed is being reduced all the time. Surgery and transcatheter closure both have high success rates and excellent long-term prognosis. The factors influencing which method is chosen are many and are evolving.

Atrial septal defect

Isolated ostium secundum ASDs very rarely, if ever, cause symptoms in newborn infants, but are occasionally suspected on auscultation. Left-to-right shunting at atrial level is often found on echocardiography either as an isolated finding or in conjunction with physiological pulmonary artery branch stenosis, PDA or more complex lesions. It is not always clear whether the shunt is through an ASD or merely through a prolapsing PFO (see p. 619). Approximately 85–90% of atrial shunts detected by ultrasound in the newborn period disappear and defects sized ≤3 mm always do.[79]

Ventricular septal defect

VSDs without associated abnormalities account for at least 15% of structural heart lesions; up to 65% of them resolve spontaneously. They may be single or multiple and can occur in any part of the ventricular septum. The site is of importance with respect to associated lesions, likely natural history and surgical approaches. Symptoms may never occur and if heart failure does develop, it frequently does not do so until after the newborn period; indeed, there may be no murmur until several weeks of age. This is because there is little flow across a VSD whilst PVR is high. Diagnosis is usually clinical (see Table 28.21) with echocardiographic confirmation and identification of precise location. Heart failure is treated as necessary (see Table 28.13). Surgery is rarely needed in the newborn period unless there are associated lesions such as coarctation. Surgery is indicated for cases in which heart failure cannot be well enough controlled to permit satisfactory weight gain or if pulmonary artery pressure is over 50% of systemic; this can usually be assessed by Doppler echocardiography. Surgical repair of VSD has a low mortality (<3%) even in the newborn period. Palliative pulmonary artery banding is only considered when there are multiple VSDs or if surgery is indicated for another lesion such as coarctation. When VSD is part of a more complex lesion, strategies are different; in some circumstances a sizeable VSD is essential for satisfactory haemodynamics, for example in DILV with TGA.

Atrioventricular septal defect

The basic abnormality in this condition is in the AV septum, which in a normal heart separates the left ventricle from the right atrium. A defect here will always be associated with an abnormality of the AV valves. There may be an intra-atrial defect only (ostium primum ASD, termed partial AVSD), or additionally an intraventricular defect may also exist, in which case a complete AVSD is present and the AV valve has a single large orifice rather than two separate ones. In both forms there can be AV regurgitation including left ventricular to right atrial shunting. Partial AVSD constitutes <2% of CHD and complete AVSD accounts for 2% of CHD. Either lesion can be part of the complex cardiac abnormalities found in left isomerism (partial AVSD) or right isomerism (complete AVSD), as described above (p. 642). Partial AVSD is frequently undetected in the newborn period and may not cause heart failure in infancy, although surgical correction is required in childhood to prevent right heart failure or PVD in adult life; cases with heart failure in infancy often have left AV valve regurgitation as well as left-to-right shunting at atrial level and require valve repair as well as surgical closure of the shunt. Eighty percent of cases of complete AVSD are associated with Down syndrome; in the region of 35% of infants with Down syndrome and CHD have complete AVSD. Occasionally, tetralogy of Fallot coexists with AVSD, as may PDA or coarctation. In some cases of complete AVSD, one ventricle is much larger than the other; usually they are approximately equal sizes with volume overloading of the right ventricle. Clinical features of complete AVSD are given in Table 28.21. Heart failure may never develop and as PVD develops rapidly, particularly in Down syndrome, it is desirable to make the diagnosis in the newborn period. It is for this reason and because signs can be subtle that at least an ECG is desirable by way of cardiac investigation in newborn infants with Down syndrome; if this is done, complete AVSD will not be overlooked, as the QRS axis is superior ('north-west', +180° to +270°/−90°). Diagnosis is by echocardiography; angiography is not usually needed. Survival without surgery is not always beyond infancy, because of heart failure; however, of those alive at 1 year, survival into the late teens or twenties is common. Corrective surgery for cases detected in infancy improves outlook, with a surgical mortality of under 10%.

Aortopulmonary window

This rare abnormality involves a connection between the ascending aorta and the main pulmonary artery. It has haemodynamic and clinical features similar to large PDA and truncus arteriosus; it may coexist with PDA and with aortic arch interruption (see Table 28.21). It can be easily overlooked on echocardiography, especially if a coexistent lesion is recognised. Surgical treatment at diagnosis is appropriate and has a high success rate.

Coronary arteriovenous fistula

This is another rare shunting lesion which presents with systolic and diastolic murmurs with or without bounding pulses and heart failure depending on the size of the shunt. The coronary fistula can be into any heart chamber or to the pulmonary artery. Ultrasound usually delineates the anatomy but angiography may be needed. Surgery or transcatheter occlusion is indicated for cases causing symptoms or signs in the newborn period.

Conclusion

All the diseases and conditions discussed above may present in other ways such as asymptomatic murmurs and coincidental findings in investigations done for other reasons. In such circumstances, management will need to be tailored in the light of the clinical picture and likely natural history.

Collapse

Conditions that commonly present with collapse are listed in Table 28.24. Differentiating cardiac from non-cardiac causes is usually not difficult although conditions with duct-dependent circulation can, when the duct closes, mimic septicaemia and primary metabolic disorders.

Table 28.24 Cardiac conditions which may present with collapse

Arrhythmias – primary or secondary
Duct-dependent circulation
    Transposition – ASD, VSD, PDA
    Pulmonary
        Pulmonary atresia – without collaterals
        Tricuspid atresia – with restrictive VSD
    Systemic
        Hypoplastic left heart
        Aortic atresia
        Critical aortic stenosis
        Interrupted arch
        Coarctation

Duct-dependent cardiac conditions often present with other signs (cyanosis or respiratory distress) before collapse occurs.

Arrhythmias

These are discussed in a separate section (pp. 651–7). In the newborn period, arrhythmias that cause sudden unexpected collapse with no signs and a normal ECG between episodes are very rare.

Duct-dependent pulmonary circulation and transposition

These infants will normally be recognised as cyanosed and are discussed under that heading (p. 624). Duct-dependent pulmonary circulation will result in extreme cyanosis and metabolic acidosis when ductal closure occurs, as will TGA if there is no mixing between systemic and pulmonary circulations via a VSD or large ASD.

Duct-dependent systemic circulation

These lesions are listed in Table 28.24 with clinical features being given in Table 28.25. They are all likely to have at least mild respiratory distress and some physical signs prior to collapse, but those features may have been unrecognised, especially if early discharge home occurred. Resuscitation with prostaglandin (see Table 28.12) will usually be carried out before definitive diagnosis by ultrasound has been performed; resuscitation must not be delayed awaiting echocardiography if the clinical picture is at all suggestive of duct-dependent systemic circulation.

Hypoplastic left heart syndrome

This constitutes 1% of CHD but nearly 10% of symptomatic neonatal CHD in series dating from the era before fetal diagnosis. Extracardiac abnormalities are only occasionally encountered in live-born infants with HLHS. The condition consists of a small left atrium, atresia of mitral and aortic valves, and extreme hypoplasia of the left ventricle and aorta proximal to the DA. There is coarctation in 60–70% of cases. The right heart is dilated and hypertrophied with a large pulmonary artery. Head

Table 28.25 Structural heart lesions presenting with respiratory distress or collapse in the early newborn period. All may have cyanosis if PPHN or shocked; all have cardiomegaly with congested lung fields on chest X-ray

Condition	Pulses	Cyanosis	Precordium	Auscultation	ECG	Extracardiac associations
Hypoplastic left heart	Weak, femoral stronger if DA open	Mild	Active	Gallop	Small LV voltages	Uncommon
Aortic arch interruption	Strong proximal to lesion	None	Active	Gallop LVOT, systolic murmur	LV/RV+ T↓V$_{5-6}$	Common (DiGeorge)
Coarctation	Weak femoral	None	Active	Gallop, EC, LVOT, systolic murmur Murmur between scapulae	RA+ RV+ T↓V$_{5-6}$	Uncommon (Turner)
Critical aortic stenosis	Weak	None	Active	Gallop, EC, LVOT, systolic murmur	LV+ ST↓, T↓V$_{5-6}$	Uncommon

and coronary arterial flow is through retrograde filling of the transverse and ascending aorta via the DA. Clinical features are given in Table 28.25; before ductal closure occurs, femoral pulses may be stronger than upper limb pulses. Death occurs rapidly after ductal closure and usually between 5 and 10 days after birth; occasional survival to a few months can occur. The advent of prostaglandin and ultrasound and, more recently still, fetal diagnosis has meant that most live-born infants with HLHS can be stabilised whilst treatment options for this universally fatal condition are considered. The treatment options are:

- No active treatment.
- Heart transplantation. There are major problems with organ availability, and even if initially resuscitated and stabilised, infants may not be able to be kept in good condition long enough for a donor organ to become available. Long-term sequelae of transplantation need to be discussed with families before embarking on this pathway. Neonatal heart transplantation has up to 80% survival at 5 years.[8]
- Palliative measures in the form of surgery described by Norwood and subject to a number of variations.[100] This essentially consists of reconstruction of the systemic outflow of the heart using the native pulmonary artery with repair of coarctation if present and establishing another source of pulmonary blood flow in the newborn period. Second and third procedures are performed in infancy and the preschool years to establish a Fontan circulation with the right ventricle as the systemic ventricle, a far from ideal physiological situation. Operative mortality is falling and is highest for the first stage, but there is an ongoing attrition rate between operations also. Survival beyond stage 3 for 50% of cases is now achieved in many centres. Organ availability for children and teenagers is better than for neonates and so the Norwood approach can be considered palliative until heart transplant is possible if needed; it is not clear at present how many will require this. Quality of life long term is improving for these patients, but information remains scarce.

Aortic valve atresia

This lesion very occasionally occurs without hypoplasia of the remainder of the left heart. The ascending aorta is very small. Presentation and clinical features resemble HLHS but an attempt to establish a biventricular circulation may be considered.

Critical aortic stenosis

This lesion lies at the end of a spectrum of severity of aortic valve abnormalities, the mildest of which may cause no symptoms even in adult life. It is commoner in males and the possibility of Turner's syndrome must be considered in affected females. The aortic valve may have one, two or three cusps and there is often post-stenotic dilatation of the ascending aorta. AS of any degree may be associated with some aortic regurgitation, mitral stenosis, VSD and coarctation. Symptomatic AS at sub- or supravalvar levels is rare in the newborn, but subvalvar AS may develop in treated or untreated valvar AS and in association with VSD and aortic coarctation or interruption. Symptomatic aortic regurgitation in neonates and infants is rare and is usually due to an aorticoventricular tunnel rather than a valvar

abnormality. Progression of AS and its unfavourable effect on the left ventricle in fetal life has been documented by ultrasound.[89] Death may occur in utero. The postnatal clinical picture (see Table 28.25) may be of an asymptomatic murmur with heart failure developing in early infancy or of pulseless collapse when the DA shuts. Angiography is not required for diagnosis, but cardiac catheterisation may be performed for balloon dilatation, although many centres prefer surgical valvotomy. Survival is mainly determined by the state of the left ventricle, which may either be dilated or severely hypertrophied. It is a matter of debate as to whether the most severe forms should be subject to Norwood-type surgery (see HLHS above). Fetal intervention is theoretically attractive but has yet to establish a role. Surgery is successful in most symptomatic infants; in some centres, balloon dilatation is the treatment of choice with similarly a low mortality.[61] All infants requiring intervention in the newborn period will ultimately have further interventions either for residual or recurrent stenosis or for aortic regurgitation.

Aortic arch interruption

This abnormality is present in 1% of congenital heart lesions. The DA supplies the descending aorta distal to the site of interruption, which is distal to the left subclavian artery in 30% (type A), between the left carotid and left subclavian arteries in 45% (type B) and between the innominate and left carotid in the remainder (type C). Approximately 50% of type-A interruptions are associated with DiGeorge syndrome. Associated cardiac lesions always include VSD, often valvar or subvalvar AS, sometimes mitral valve abnormalities, and very occasionally truncus arteriosus or aortopulmonary window. Clinical features are given in Table 28.25. Diagnosis can be strongly suspected clinically by careful attention to the pulses and is confirmed with clarification of associated lesions by ultrasound. Corrective surgery is usually performed through a median sternotomy with concurrent repair of intracardiac abnormalities, with up to 90% survival. Left ventricular outflow obstruction may progress even after successful neonatal surgery and often requires surgery; further intervention to the repaired aortic arch may also be required.

Coarctation

This makes up 10% of CHD, being more common in males but having a strong association with Turner's syndrome, 15% or more of whom have the condition. The position of the discrete narrowing of the aorta is distal to the left subclavian artery, opposite the point of entry to the aorta of the DA. The exact position varies and may actually evolve in relation to ductal closure and postnatal growth. The terms pre-, juxta- and postductal are used to describe the site of coarctation and bear some relationship to the age of presentation and clinical picture. Not all cases of coarctation cause symptoms in the newborn period or infancy; some remain asymptomatic for years or occasionally decades. Other lesions in the left heart are very commonly associated, as are VSDs. Transposition and more complex cyanotic conditions may have accompanying coarctation. In the newborn with coarctation and PDA, there is systemic pressure in the right ventricle, although until the DA starts to close, shunting is predominately left to right at ductal and atrial levels. Thus, as heart failure develops, the infant is pink with RVH on ECG. When the duct shuts, some constriction of the descending aorta probably occurs, as well in those babies who collapse. In others, duct closure is tolerated, although heart failure and hypertension may occur in the early weeks of life. Those infants who remain asymptomatic in the newborn period may develop heart failure in later infancy with LVH on ECG. After infancy and before middle age, coarctation presents with asymptomatic abnormalities of the pulses, with a murmur or with hypertension and its complications. The time and mode of presentation of infants with associated intracardiac lesions is influenced by the nature of the associated lesion. If the coexistent lesion presents early, great care must be taken not to overlook coarctation. Coarctation can be difficult to diagnose clinically (see Table 28.25) in the newborn as pulses and upper/lower limb BPs may be normal while the ductus is open, and if collapse occurs, all pulses can be weak if left ventricular dysfunction is marked. Similarly, echocardiography imaging and Doppler assessment can sometimes be inconclusive whilst the ductus is wide open; even angiography and direct pressure measurements can be inconclusive. If there is doubt, careful observation and serial echocardiography over a period of a few days is required until the DA constricts and the characteristic features develop. Coarctation causing collapse is resuscitated with prostaglandin and heart failure is treated with diuretics. Inotrope support is needed in critically ill infants and renal function must be watched carefully as occasionally renal failure develops. Infants who collapse or who are in heart failure should undergo surgical repair when stabilised. Coarctation as part of a more complicated lesion must be repaired before or at the same time as the intracardiac abnormality. In some circumstances, pulmonary artery banding is performed with coarctation repair if there is a cardiac lesion which will cause pulmonary plethora and which is not to be corrected in the newborn period, for example multiple muscular VSDs or DILV with VSD and TGA. There are disadvantages to pulmonary artery banding which mean it is desirable to avoid it if possible. Coarctation in the newborn period may be repaired using the left subclavian artery (subclavian flap repair). This results in an absent brachial pulse in the left arm but very rarely leads to ischaemic problems there. Some surgeons prefer excision of the coarctation and end-to-end repair in newborns, as is the case after infancy. Mortality of coarctation repair without major intracardiac lesions is <5%. Asymptomatic infants or those with easily controlled heart failure can be operated on in later infancy with the intention of achieving a lower recurrence rate, which may be as high as 20% in those repaired in the newborn period.

Conclusion

Any of the causes of collapse considered above may present less dramatically, usually with evidence of heart failure, which often precedes collapse. The precise diagnosis of which duct-dependent condition exists is not important at the resuscitation stage and if a collapsed infant could have structural heart disease as the cause, prostaglandin should be given. This is likely to be rapidly therapeutic as well as helpful in confirming a cardiac cause for the collapse. Absence of response to prostaglandin at doses at the top of the range (see Table 28.12) makes duct-dependent

systemic circulation unlikely but not impossible. Risks of surgery are increased if renal or multi-organ failure is present.

Cardiac conditions likely to present in the asymptomatic newborn (Table 28.26)

The commonest asymptomatic presentation of heart disease in the newborn period is the detection of a heart murmur, which may be a feature at an early stage of the natural history of many of the conditions discussed above.

Innocent heart murmurs

Detailed history and other features on physical examination are an important part of the evaluation of a heart murmur. The features of innocent murmurs in the newborn are given in Table 28.7. It is important to note that innocent murmurs have positive characteristics as well as being associated with no other clinical evidence of cardiovascular disease. It is unclear whether ECG and CXR help the experienced or trained observer distinguish innocent from pathological murmurs, and they are less often used.[38] A practical approach following the detection of a heart murmur is given below.

Pathological asymptomatic heart murmurs

The likely causes for such murmurs detected in the newborn are given in Table 28.26. The conditions listed are considered elsewhere in the chapter. As a general rule, obstructive lesions cause a murmur from birth, although mild pulmonary stenosis, trivial AS or simple bicuspid aortic valve are frequently not heard. Pulmonary and particularly aortic stenosis may progress in severity. Lesions associated with left-to-right shunts frequently cause no murmur in the immediate newborn period and may not be detected until a 6- or 8-week routine check. If a pansystolic murmur suggesting VSD is heard in the newborn period, it may be due to tricuspid regurgitation, which will resolve over a matter of a few weeks. A VSD detected immediately after birth is likely to be small. If a structural abnormality is suspected as the cause of an asymptomatic murmur, an ECG and CXR should be performed. These investigations may have diagnostic features and are of some help in deciding the severity of the lesion and therefore timescale in which cardiology review and echocardiography are indicated.

Practical approach to neonatal heart murmurs

When a heart murmur is detected in the early newborn period, a number of options are open which will be influenced by local considerations, particularly availability of specialist cardiological services and echocardiography. The following are common approaches:

- If symptoms or other signs of cardiac disease exist, an ECG and CXR should be performed and cardiology referral made; this can involve the use of telemedicine to have the cardiac ultrasound assessed by a paediatric cardiologist prior to or instead of transferring the infant.[20]

Table 28.26 Cardiac disease presenting in an asymptomatic newborn infant

Category	Detail	Comments
Fetal diagnosis	Any cardiac condition	Diagnosis known/ suspected before birth can be confirmed before infant becomes symptomatic
Murmur	Causes include: VSD Tricuspid regurgitation Aortic stenosis Pulmonary stenosis Patent ductus arteriosus Atrial septal defect AV septal defect Tetralogy of Fallot Innocent	See Table 28.7
Weak femoral pulses	Coarctation	Many non-cardiac causes of weak pulses
Rhythm or rate abnormality	Fast/slow/irregular	Some are normal variants See arrhythmia section

Some cardiac conditions are diagnosed when cardiac assessment is requested following a non-cardiac diagnosis being made (e.g. neonatal surgical conditions or certain syndromes).

Table 28.27 Features in an infant with an asymptomatic murmur which suggest the possibility of a serious (duct-dependent) lesion

Feature	Comment
No weight loss after birth or excessive weight gain, especially if feeding poorly	May suggest incipient heart failure
Any suggestion of symptoms	If 'dusky', a transcutaneous hyper-oxia test may help (pp. 626, 628)
Any doubt about quality of femoral pulses	Suggests coarctation
Right arm systolic blood pressure > 20 mmHg above leg pressure	
Murmur loudest between scapulae	Suggests coarctation, innocent pulmonary murmur well heard front and sides
Cardiomegaly on CXR	
Ventricular hypertrophy on ECG	

- If no symptoms or other signs are present but the murmur has features suggesting a structural lesion, an ECG and CXR should be performed and cardiology referral made.
- If no symptoms or other signs of cardiac disease are present and the murmur has features compatible with an innocent one (see Table 28.7), discharge from hospital is reasonable. The family should be warned about important signs and follow-up arranged for 4 to 6 weeks. It has not been shown that ECG and CXR aid in this decision.
- In some centres, all babies with heart murmurs are referred for echocardiography.[2] This is not practicable in most UK services, and if the above approaches are adopted consistently, the likelihood of a baby with serious cardiac disease coming to harm through delayed diagnosis is small.[38]

A baby with an asymptomatic murmur should not be allowed home until it is clear that no form of duct-dependent CHD is present; this is usually apparent on clinical grounds (Table 28.27). If there is any doubt, either a further period of observation in hospital is indicated or, preferably, echocardiography should be arranged.

Arrhythmias

In the newborn, primary cardiac arrhythmias requiring treatment are uncommon. Tachy- or bradyarrhythmias are much more likely to be secondary to extracardiac pathology, which must be identified and treated.

Recognition of arrhythmias

Infants with an arrhythmia may be asymptomatic or present with heart failure or very rarely with collapse. Some will have been recognised in utero. An ECG will usually allow precise diagnosis although occasionally this will not be possible either because the abnormal rhythm is intermittent or because the ECG is difficult to interpret. Sinus rhythm exists if each QRS complex is preceded by a P wave with an axis of 0° to +90° and with a normal PR interval (90–120 ms). An approach to assessing the ECG in a possible arrhythmia involves answering the questions given in Table 28.28. Arrhythmias can be classified in a number of ways. They will now be considered under the headings either supraventricular or ventricular. There are important normal variations in rhythm and rate,[98] which are mentioned at appropriate points below.

Supraventricular arrhythmias

Supraventricular arrhythmias usually have narrow QRS complexes which resemble those seen when the patient is in sinus rhythm.

Sinus bradycardia

When asleep or when straining, the interval between QRS complexes can lengthen transiently up to 1.5 s, but sustained rates,

Table 28.28 Approach to ECG interpretation of an arrhythmia

QRS complexes	Rate	Slow/norm/fast
	Rhythm	Regular/irregular
		If irregular: premature/delayed
	Configuration	Normal/abnormal
P waves	Seen/not seen	
	Rate	Slow/normal/fast
	Rhythm	Regular/irregular
		If irregular: premature/delayed
	Axis	Normal/abnormal
	Relationship to QRS complexes	None/constant/variable
		If constant: before/within/after
		If before, PR interval: Normal/long Fixed/changing

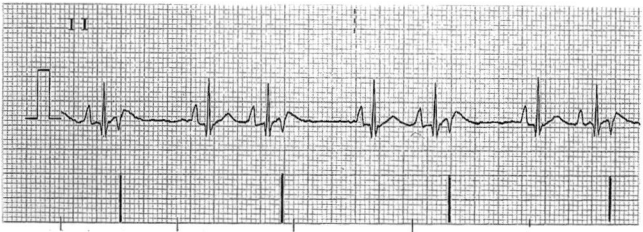

Fig. 28.16 ECG lead II, 25 mm/s. Blocked atrial ectopics on the upstroke of T wave of complexes 1, 3, 5 and 7.

even during sleep, below 80/min in term or 100/min in preterm infants are not normal. Sinus bradycardia is associated with normal P waves before every QRS complex; the complexes are normal unless the cause of the bradycardia has other effects on the myocardium. Sinus bradycardia is seen most commonly in association with apnoeic episodes. It may also be a manifestation of hypoxaemia, raised intracranial pressure of any cause, and hyperkalaemia. It is seen in association with stress from handling and interventions in critically ill infants. Drugs may cause sinus bradycardia, for example heavy sedation administered to the infant or before birth to the mother, digoxin and propranolol. Sustained sinus bradycardia in a relatively well infant is a feature of hypothyroidism.

Sinus arrhythmia and sinus arrest

These result in variable slowing of the heart rate. Neither is common in the newborn infant. Sinus arrhythmia is an increase in the heart rate during inspiration and results in a regular irregularity of heart rate in time with the respiratory cycle. Sinus arrest or pauses result in an occasional abnormally long pause (>1.6 s) between P waves, producing an irregular irregularity of the heart rate. These two variations of normal are of no significance of themselves. If they are very pronounced, they can be a marker of sinoatrial dysfunction which may be associated with symptomatic bradycardia or tachycardia.

Atrial ectopics

These are due to premature depolarisation of a site in an atrium earlier than the sinus node discharge so that either a premature QRS complex follows or, if the ectopic is so early as to occur whilst the ventricle is in its refractory period, there is no QRS complex (blocked atrial ectopics; Fig. 28.16). Intermediate between these two timings for the atrial ectopic, a QRS complex will be conducted aberrantly and be broad. If non-conducted

atrial ectopics occur regularly alternating with normally conducted sinus impulses, there will be bradycardia in the region of 60–80/min. If ectopics are frequent or non-conducted but not alternating with sinus beats, the heart rate will be irregular (Fig. 28.16). Atrial ectopics are harmless but may cause confusion when detected in the fetus causing bradycardia with or without an irregular rhythm. They can be correctly diagnosed by fetal ultrasound and thereby prevent unnecessary concern about fetal wellbeing being engendered. They are markers for an increased incidence of SVT, which may not necessarily be symptomatic.[97] Atrial ectopics resolve within 3 months in 90% of cases.

Sinus tachycardia

Sinus tachycardia is a heart rate above 160/min in term and above 180/min in preterm infants. P waves have a normal axis and precede every QRS complex. Sinus tachycardia is always secondary, usually to a non-cardiac cause. Causes to be considered include fever, hypovolaemia, pain, respiratory failure, anaemia, fluid overload, drugs (in particular, methylxanthines and inotropes) and septicaemia. Structural heart disease or heart muscle disease may cause sinus tachycardia. The cause should be identified and treated; therapy for sinus tachycardia itself is not indicated. In the newborn, sinus tachycardia can reach 230 beats/min, so that at its higher rates it can be difficult to distinguish from the pathological types of SVT.

Supraventricular tachycardia

A simple classification of SVT is given in Table 28.29.

Atrial flutter

This is a rare rhythm in the newborn. It may be diagnosed in utero, in which case maternal digoxin and/or flecainide therapy is indicated. There is an association with myocarditis, myocardial ischaemia and structural heart disease, although the heart is often structurally normal in neonates. Atrial rates usually exceed 300/min and ventricular rate and rhythm will vary with the degree and constancy of AV block. Consistent 2:1 AV block can make the rhythm hard to recognise as the characteristic flutter waves are hidden by QRS complexes, but they may become apparent when the degree of block varies spontaneously or with adenosine administration. Fetal or neonatal heart failure often develops. The rhythm can be well tolerated for short periods but attempts to restore sinus rhythm or at least to control ventricular

Table 28.29 Simple classification of SVT

Site	Rhythm	Comment
Sinus node	Sinus tachycardia	Always secondary
Atrium	Atrial flutter	Rare
	Atrial fibrillation	Very rare
	Atrial tachycardia	Very rare
AV junction	AV re-entry tachycardia	Common
	AV nodal re-entry tachycardia	Rare
Below AV node	His bundle tachycardia (junctional ectopic tachycardia)	Very rare Usually postoperative

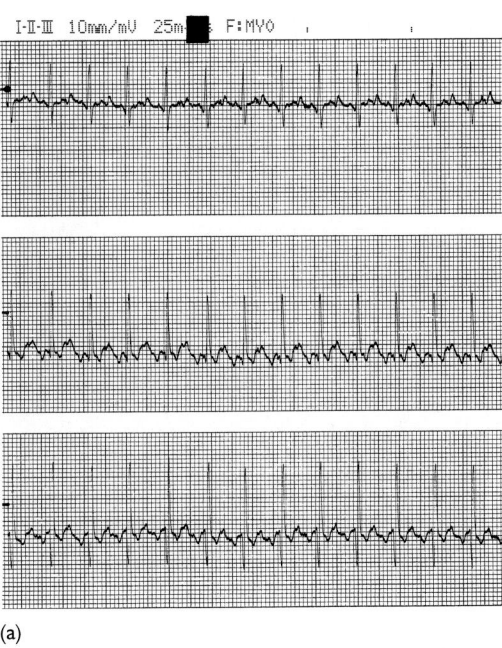

(a)

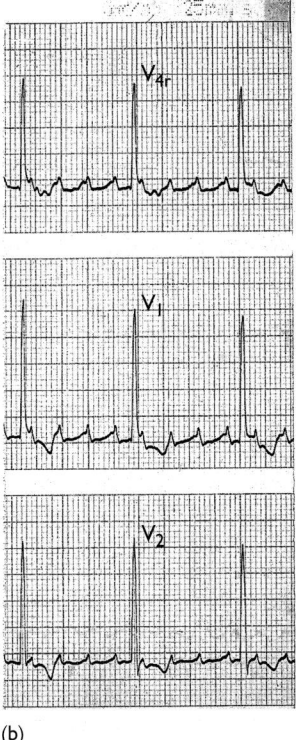

(b)

Fig. 28.17 (a) ECG leads I, II, III, 25 mm/s. Atrial flutter with 2:1 AV block. (b) ECG leads V_{4r}, V_1, V_2, 25 mm/s. Atrial flutter with 4:1 AV block. Flutter waves much easier to see than in (a).

rate are appropriate to prevent deterioration in heart muscle function. Adenosine will not restore sinus rhythm but may transiently increase AV block, allowing a diagnosis to be made if the rhythm has not been recognised prior to its use (Fig. 28.17). Shocked infants and those in heart failure warrant DC cardioversion or an attempt at oesophageal overpacing of the atria to establish sinus rhythm; neither of these therapies should be carried out without sedating the infant. Recurrence after cardioversion by either of these techniques may occur but is less likely in the newborn than in older children. Digoxin is used to slow ventricular rate and to help maintain sinus rhythm when achieved. Propranolol may be added to digoxin therapy to achieve further control of ventricular rate. If immediate restoration to and maintenance of sinus rhythm cannot be achieved, the outlook is still good, with spontaneous recovery, if ventricular rate and therefore symptoms can be controlled. Preventative antiarrhythmic therapy after early infancy is not required. A minority of patients have an underlying pre-excitation ECG and in many there is probably an underlying accessory pathway. The arrhythmia carries a small mortality in the newborn either from intractable heart failure or from progression to more malignant arrhythmias, spontaneously or in response to electrical or pharmacological intervention.

Atrioventricular re-entry tachycardia (AVRT)

This is the commonest form of SVT in the fetus and newborn and is associated with the presence of an accessory AV conduction pathway. Fetal SVT can be treated by administration of digoxin, flecainide or verapamil to the mother[4,93] in specialist centres. Administration of antiarrhythmics directly to the fetus is occasionally used. It is preferable to bring the arrhythmia under control before delivery, but in extreme circumstances this will not be possible. The ECG in sinus rhythm may have a pre-excitation pattern (short PR interval and delta wave on QRS upstroke) allowing Wolff–Parkinson–White syndrome to be diagnosed. Even if present, a pre-excitation pattern may be intermittent or disappear with age. The QRS complexes are narrow when SVT occurs unless aberrant conduction occurs, which is very unusual in the newborn. P waves may be visible between QRS complexes, but if they are, they have an abnormal axis. QRS rates vary from 180 to 300/min (see Fig. 28.2). Distinction from sinus tachycardia is occasionally difficult but the overall clinical picture usually allows this, as well as careful examination of the ECG for features mentioned above. Infants can be asymptomatic or have episodes of pallor and breathlessness or be in heart failure. Any form of structural heart disease, myocardial tumours, myocarditis, electrolyte disturbances or indwelling right atrial lines should be

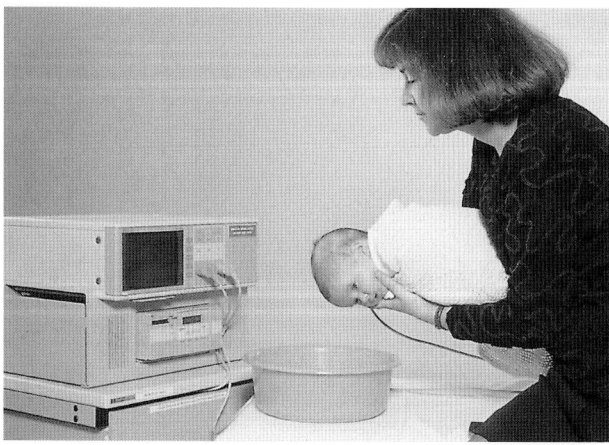

(a)

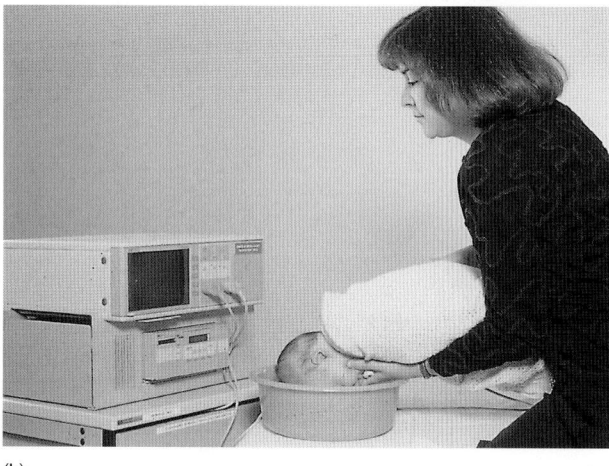

(b)

Fig. 28.18 (a,b) Simulated facial immersion in cold water for treatment of SVT. Note ECG monitor interfaced to paper printer.

considered as causes, but the heart is usually normal. Myocardial dysfunction and mitral regurgitation develop secondary to the arrhythmia and can be expected to resolve once control is achieved. If the clinical condition allows, facial immersion in cold water until conversion or for a maximum of 10 seconds (Fig. 28.18) is the treatment of choice, with an 85–90% success rate.[99] If this fails or is impracticable, application of ice to the face may be tried but has a lower success rate, and adenosine intravenously should be used. Adenosine also has an 85% success rate in restoring sinus rhythm and it may unmask atrial flutter if present. Contraindications to adenosine in the newborn are few. Dipyridamole will potentiate its effects. Side effects include transient profound bradycardia. If these measures fail and the baby is collapsed, synchronised DC shock should be given. Digoxin should be given if heart failure is marked; propranolol may be used instead if heart failure is not severe or in addition if it is. If these measures fail but DC shock is not indicated, a further trial of cold water or adenosine should take place before progressing to amiodarone or a type I antiarrhythmic (disopyramide, flecainide, quinidine), all of which should be discussed with a cardiology centre. Verapamil is

not recommended for intravenous administration in the newborn period or infancy because of the incidence of bradycardia and hypotension associated with its use. If the rhythm is well tolerated, it is acceptable to give digoxin at least 6–12 hours to work, even if loading doses have been used. In summary, acute treatment of SVT is as follows (drug doses are in Table 28.30):

- DC cardioversion if collapsed (sedate unless unconscious).
- Facial immersion/ice-bag.
- Intravenous adenosine if vagotonic manoeuvre fails.
- Intravenous propranolol if no heart failure and adenosine has failed.
- Start intravenous digitalisation if heart failure or if two doses of propranolol fail.
- Review need for cardioversion. Retry facial immersion and intravenous adenosine if DC cardioversion still not indicated.
- If baby stable without heart failure, continue digitalisation regimen and oral maintenance propranolol; infant may be watched for 6 to 12 hours. Further attempts at facial immersion and intravenous adenosine can be tried after 6 to 8 hours.
- If in heart failure, observation is not appropriate and amiodarone or a type I antiarrhythmic (flecanide) should be considered in conjunction with discussion with cardiology service.
- When sinus rhythm established, decide on appropriate maintenance preventative treatment (see text).

Once sinus rhythm is restored, maintenance therapy with whatever agent(s) restored it is usually given for about 6 months, although evidence for the efficacy of digoxin prophylaxis is weak.[74] Drug doses are given in Table 28.30.

Ventricular arrhythmias

Ventricular arrhythmias have QRS-T complexes which are always different in configuration and polarity from those in sinus rhythm; the QRS complexes are usually, but not necessarily, broad. Broad complexes can be hard to recognise in the newborn as the upper limit of normal for QRS duration is only 70 ms. Associated and causative conditions for ventricular arrhythmias include any type of cardiomyopathy, myocarditis, intracardiac tumours, electrolyte disturbances, hypoxaemia and acidosis, and only rarely structural CHD. Familial long QT syndromes[87] may be detected in the newborn if the family history is known or if ventricular arrhythmias occur.

Premature ventricular complexes

These are recognised by being abnormal premature QRS complexes without a preceding P wave. They are followed by a compensatory pause. Sometimes, complexes with features of both the ventricular ectopic and the normal QRS complex are seen (fusion complexes). Ventricular ectopics (VEs) have been found in up to 33% of healthy newborn infants.[98] They are rarely a sign of cardiac disease but conditions listed above must be considered. Occasional unifocal VEs with normal clinical examination and ECG require no action in the newborn period, merely

Table 28.30 Antiarrhythmic drug doses

Drug	Dose and route	Comment
Adenosine	0.05–0.25 mg/kg rapid i.v.	Start low and increase at 2-min intervals
Digoxin	10 micrograms/kg i.v. over 15 min, then 5 micrograms/kg i.v. after 6 h; repeat after a further 6 h After digitalisation regimen start maintenance at: 4 micrograms/kg/dose oral 12-hourly (give 60% of this if using i.v. route)	Acute loading doses. Ensure infant not hypokalaemic
Propranolol	0.05 mg/kg i.v. over 2 min 1–2 mg/kg/dose oral 8-hourly	Acute, may repeat once. Avoid in severe heart failure Beware hypoglycaemia Never use after verapamil
Verapamil		Better avoided in newborns Never use after propranolol
Lidocaine (lignocaine)	1 mg/kg i.v., then 1 mg/kg/h i.v.	
DC shock	SVT (synchronised) 0.5–1 J/kg VT/VF 1–2 J/kg	Sedation/anaesthesia required unless infant unconscious

Note: Other drugs used vary with local expertise. Advice should be sought.

review at 6–8 weeks. Very frequent VEs, the presence of a family history suggesting a long QT syndrome, cardiac physical signs or ECG abnormalities – particularly a long QT[111] or evidence for heart muscle disease – are an indication for echocardiography and 24-hour ECG monitoring (looking for VT). Isolated VEs with a normal heart require no treatment and will resolve within 2 months; if they do not, echocardiography and 24-hour ECG monitoring should be performed or repeated.

Ventricular tachycardia

This is rare in the newborn and consists of a series of VEs occurring sequentially with a rate of 150–250/min. Close examination reveals that there are minor irregularities in rate and that the P waves, if recognised, are either dissociated from the QRS complexes or conducted retrogradely. The rhythm may be paroxysmal or sustained; if paroxysmal, fusion beats may be seen. Neonates with VT may have underlying diseases as listed above but may have normal hearts. A well infant with no underlying disease may be asymptomatic; most cardiologists would still advocate preventative treatment in such cases initially. Collapsed infants should receive synchronised DC shock; less severely symptomatic infants should be treated with lidocaine (lignocaine) intravenously by bolus and then infusion. Pulseless VT should be treated with full cardiopulmonary resuscitation and DC shock (1–2 J/kg). Amiodarone is often advocated if pulseless VT does not respond to DC shock; local policy should be worked out in conjunction with paediatric cardiologists. If the rhythm reflects underlying electrolyte disturbance, this should be rapidly corrected. Propranolol is the traditional oral preventative; amiodarone may be used in certain cases (see Table 28.30).

Idioventricular rhythm

This has the morphology of VT but is slower (110–120/min), being around the same speed as sinus rhythm. It is rarely a sign of heart disease, is usually well tolerated and has a benign natural history.

Ventricular fibrillation

The QRS complexes are fast, bizarre and irregular. Full cardiopulmonary resuscitation should be instituted if the underlying pathology is unknown or considered remediable. Ventricular fibrillation is very rare in neonates and is usually terminal whatever the cause.

Atrioventricular conduction disturbances (heart block)

There are three degrees of AV conduction block.

First-degree heart block

This is present when the PR interval exceeds the upper limit of normal for age and heart rate; the maximum is 110 ms in the newborn. It is never symptomatic but may reflect underlying structural heart disease such as ASD, heart muscle disease or drug effect (for example, digoxin). It can occur in families and may progress to more severe degrees of block.

Second-degree heart block

This is present when not every P wave is followed by a QRS complex. There are two forms. Mobitz type I second-degree AV block shows the Wenckebach phenomenon in which the PR interval progressively increases until, after three to six cycles, the P wave is not conducted; the sequence then commences again. This phenomenon may be seen in sleep or under anaesthesia at any age and does not necessarily reflect underlying heart disease. Mobitz type II block has a fixed normal or long PR interval with intermittent non-conduction of the P wave. Failure to conduct the P wave is often at regular intervals such as 2:1, 3:1 and so on. Mobitz type II block is much more likely to reflect underlying cardiac disease and frequently progresses to complete heart block.

Third-degree heart block

This is also termed complete heart block (CHB). The P waves and QRS complexes in CHB are totally dissociated, with, most commonly, normal atrial rate and responsiveness and a ventricular rate between 40 and 80/min (Fig. 28.19). Fetal and neonatal CHB may be associated with a variety of usually complex structural heart lesions, in which case heart failure is the norm and outlook is frequently poor. Another group of patients with congenital CHB have structurally normal hearts. A high proportion of these infants have His bundle fibrosis secondary to maternal antibodies, termed anti Ro or SS Ro antibodies. Mothers with these antibodies may have connective tissue disorders but more usually are well with serological markers for connective tissue disease. Many neonates with normal hearts and CHB are asymptomatic. Heart failure may occur pre- or postnatally; Stokes Adams

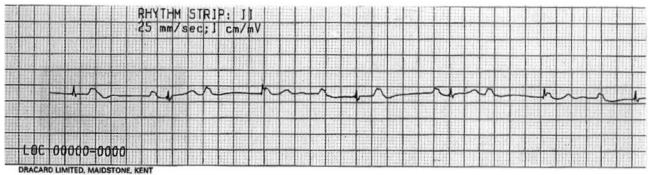

Fig. 28.19 ECG lead II, 25 mm/s. Complete heart block. Atrial rate 82/min (sleeping infant), ventricular rate 48/min.

Table 28.31 Causes of neonatal hypertension		
System	**Examples**	**Comment**
Renal	Renal artery emboli/thrombosis	May be UAC related (pp. 1240–6)
		May be acutely symptomatic
		Often improves over 12 months
	Renal vein thrombosis	Hypertension may be delayed-onset
	Dysplastic renal disease	
	Urinary tract obstruction	
	Renal infection	
	Renal failure	Any cause
Cardiovascular	Coarctation	
Endocrine	Congenital adrenal hyperplasia	
	Hyperaldosteronism	
	Hyperthyroidism	
	Phaeochromocytoma	
	Neuroblastoma	
Respiratory disease	Acute hypercapnia	Any cause
	Chronic lung disease	Often steroid-induced
Neurological disease	Raised intracranial pressure	Any cause
		Treating BP alone will reduce cerebral perfusion pressure
	Convulsions	Probably mediated via intracranial pressure, convulsion may be subtle or masked by drugs
Drugs	Neonatal exposure:	
	Corticosteroids	
	Methylxanthines	
	Phenylephrine	In eye drops
	Inotropes	Overdose
	Fetal exposure:	
	Maternal cocaine	

attacks are rare. A number of factors identify infants likely to have a poor outlook without intervention; these include structural heart disease, symptoms, resting heart rate below 55/min, little increase in heart rate in response to stress, and broad QRS complexes. If necessary, specific emergency management should include inotropes and diuretics and, if possible, temporary pacing through the oesophagus or transvenously. Permanent pacemaker insertion may be epicardial in newborn infants rather than endocardial. CHB in the fetus is usually well tolerated; if hydrops starts to develop, thought should be given to delivery. Evidence that the fetal heart rate can be significantly increased by drug administration to the mother is unclear; maternal steroid administration to prevent His bundle damage has been advocated but is not universally accepted. Fetal pacemaker insertion has yet to be successful.

Hypertension

Measurement of neonatal BP is discussed on page 623. Ill infants are likely to have direct invasive BP measurements. Normal BP increases with gestational and postnatal ages. Hypertension exists if BP is found above the upper limit of normal in a calm infant. Normal values are given in Appendix 4. Causes of hypertension are given in Table 28.31. Hypertension is rarely symptomatic but may cause heart failure, irritability and other neurological signs. Specific treatment is appropriate if there are symptoms; in their absence, therapy should be aimed at the underlying disease and hypotensive therapy only commenced if there is severe hypertension or evidence of progressive left ventricular hypertrophy. Some drugs commonly used to treat neonatal hypertension are listed in Table 28.32. In the rare circumstance of hypertensive encephalopathy or heart failure secondary to hypertension, rapid reduction of BP can be achieved by intravenous alpha blockade with phentolamine, oral ACE inhibitor (captopril) or oral nifedipine. Intravenous hydralazine, nitroprusside or diazoxide are rarely used. The prognosis in hypertension is that of the underlying cause, providing malignant hypertension is avoided or treated rapidly and effectively. Encephalopathic infants may need sedation or anticonvulsant medication as well as hypotensive therapy, but hypertensive encephalopathy is remarkably rare in the newborn.

Cardiac tumours

Symptomatic cardiac tumours are extremely rare in the newborn but are found more commonly since the widespread use of ultrasound scanning. So-called golf-ball tumours, usually in the left ventricle, are a fetal echocardiographic finding which have usually resolved by term and are of no functional significance. They may be a fetal marker for a syndrome if found in both ventricles. Cardiac tumours in the newborn may cause arrhythmias[69] or, less commonly, physical obstruction within the heart. Over 95% of intracardiac tumours in the newborn are benign and at least 75% of them are rhabdomyomata. Rhabdomyomata are often multiple and may resolve, which is a reason for being cautious about surgical intervention even if symptoms are present.[69] Multiple intracardiac tumours strongly suggest the possibility of tuberous sclerosis (TS); 50% of individuals with TS will have cardiac tumours detected by echocardiography if looked for in infancy.[112] Pericardial tumours may present with pericardial effusion and tamponade in the newborn period.

Table 28.32 Drugs for treating systemic hypertension

Drug	Dose and route	Comment
Vasodilators		
Phentolamine	0.1–0.5 micrograms/kg/min i.v.	Alpha blocker
Captopril	0.1–1.0 mg/kg/dose oral	ACE inhibitor Acute or chronic Start low and increase May cause severe hypotension, hyperkalaemia and elevated urea/creatinine
Nifedipine	0.2 mg/kg/dose oral	Acute
	0.1–0.5 mg/kg/dose oral	Chronic, 8-hourly
		Calcium channel blocker
Hydralazine	0.1–0.3 mg/kg/dose i.v.	Acute, can repeat after 20–30 min
	0.2–0.5 mg/kg/dose oral	Chronic, 8-hourly
Diuretics		
Furosemide	1 mg/kg/dose i.v.	Acute, 8-hourly
	1–2 mg/kg/dose oral	Chronic, 8–12-hourly
Chlorothiazide	25 mg/kg/dose oral	Chronic, 8–12-hourly
Beta-blocker		
Propranolol	1–2 mg/kg/dose oral	Chronic, 8-hourly

References

1. Acherman R J, Siassi B, Pratti-Madrid G et al 2000 Systemic to pulmonary collaterals in very low birth weight infants: color Doppler detection of systemic to pulmonary connections during neonatal and early infancy period. Pediatrics 105: 528–532

2. Ainsworth S B, Wyllie J P, Wren C 1999 Prevalence and clinical significance of cardiac murmurs in neonates. Archives of Disease in Childhood. Fetal and Neonatal Edition 80: F43–F45

3. Allan L D 1995 Echocardiographic detection of congenital heart disease in the fetus: present and future. British Heart Journal 74: 103–106

4. Allan L D, Chita S K, Sharland G K,Maxwell D, Priestley K 1991 Flecainide in the treatment of fetal tachycardias. British Heart Journal 65: 46–48

5. Allan L D, Crawford D C, Anderson R H, Tynan M 1985 Spectrum of congenital heart disease detected echocardiographically in prenatal life. British Heart Journal 54: 523–526

6. Amato M, Huppi P S, Markus D 1992 Prophylaxis of patent ductus arteriosus using ethamsylate in preterm infants treated with exogenous surfactant. Acta Paediatrica 81: 351–352

7. Arlettaz R, Archer N, Wilkinson A R 1998 Natural history of innocent heart murmurs in newborn babies: controlled echocardiographic study. Archives of Disease in Childhood. Fetal and Neonatal Edition 78: F166–F170

8. Bailey L I, Gundry S R, Razzook A J 1993 Bless the babies: one hundred fifteen late survivors of heart transplantation during the first year of life. Journal of Thoracic and Cardiovascular Surgery 105: 805–815

9. Barberi I, Calabro M P, Cordaro S et al 1999 Myocardial ischaemia in neonates with perinatal asphyxia. Electrocardiographic, echocardiographic and enzymatic correlations. European Journal of Pediatrics 158: 742–747

10. Bonnet D, Coltri A, Butera G et al 1999 Detection of transposition of the great arteries in fetuses reduces neonatal morbidity and mortality. Circulation 99: 916–918

11. Brennan P, Young I 2001 Congenital heart malformations: aetiology and associations. Seminars in Neonatology 6: 17–25

12. Brick D H, Allan L D 2002 Outcome of prenatally diagnosed congenital heart disease: an update. Pediatric Cardiology 23: 449–453

13. Bronshtein M, Zimmer E Z 2002 The sonographic approach to the detection of fetal cardiac anomalies in early pregnancy. Ultrasound in Obstetrics and Gynecology 19: 360–365

14. Bull C 1999 Current and potential impact of fetal diagnosis on prevalence and spectrum of serious congenital heart disease at term in the UK. Lancet 354: 1242–1247

15. Burch M 1994 Hypertrophic cardiomyopathy. Archives of Disease in Childhood 71: 488–489

16. Burch M, Runciman M 1996 Dilated cardiomyopathy. Archives of Disease in Childhood 74: 479–481

17. Burn J 2002 The aetiology of congenital heart disease. In: Anderson R H, Macartney F J, Shinebourne E A et al (eds) Paediatric cardiology (2nd edition). Churchill Livingstone, London, pp 141–213

18. Carvalho J S, Mavrides E, Shinebourne E et al 2002 Improving the effectiveness of routine prenatal screening for major congenital heart defects. Heart 88: 387–391

19. Carvalho J S, Moscoso G, Ville Y 1998 First trimester transabdominal fetal echocardiography. Lancet 351:1023–1027

20. Casey F A 1999 Telemedicine in paediatric cardiology. Archives of Disease in Childhood 80: 497–499

21. Cassady G, Crouse D T, Kirklin S W et al 1989 A randomised controlled trial of very early prophylactic ligation of the ductus arteriosus in babies who weighed 1000 g or less at birth. New England Journal of Medicine 320: 1511–1516

22. Chang A C, Huhta J C, Yoon G Y et al 1991 Diagnosis, transport and outcome in fetuses with left ventricular outflow obstruction. Journal of Thoracic and Cardiovascular Surgery 102: 841–848

23. Clark E B 2000 Etiology of congenital cardiovascular malformations: epidemiology and genetics. In: Allan H D, Gutgesell H P, Clarke E B et al (eds) Heart disease in infants, children and adolescents, 6th edition. Lippincott Williams and Wilkins, Philadelphia, pp 64–79

24. Clyman R I 1996 Recommendations for the postnatal use of indomethacin: an analysis of four separate treatment strategies. Journal of Pediatrics 128: 601–607

25. Clyman R I, Mauray F, Roman C, Rudolph A M, Heymann M A 1981 Glucocorticoids alter the sensitivity of the lamb ductus arteriosus to prostaglandin E2. Journal of Pediatrics 98: 126–128

26. Colditz P, Murphy D, Rolfe P, Wilkinson A R 1989 Effect of infusion rate of indomethacin on cerebrovascular responses in preterm neonates. Archives of Disease in Childhood 64: 8–12

27. Coombs R C, Morgan M E I, Durbin G M, Booth I W, McNeish A S 1990 Gut blood flow velocities in the newborn: effects of patent ductus arteriosus and parenteral indomethacin. Archives of Disease in Childhood 65: 1067–1071

28. Cotton R B, Haywood J L, Fitzgerald G A 1991 Symptomatic patent ductus arteriosus following prophylactic indomethacin. Biology of the Neonate 60: 273–282

29. Couser R J, Ferrata B, Wright G B et al 1996 Prophylactic indomethacin therapy in the first twenty-four hours of life for the prevention of patent ductus arteriosus in preterm infants treated prophylactically with surfactant in the delivery room. Journal of Pediatrics 128: 631–637

30. Dees E, Lin H, Cotton R B, Graham T P, Dodd D A 2000 Outcome of preterm infants with congenital heart disease. Journal of Pediatrics 137: 653–659

31. Edwards A D, Wyatt J S, Richardson C et al 1990 Effects of indomethacin on cerebral haemodynamics in very preterm infants. Lancet 335:1491–1495

32. Evans D H, Levene M I, Archer L N J 1987 The effect of indomethacin on cerebral blood flow velocity in premature infants. Developmental Medicine and Child Neurology 29: 776–782

33. Evans N 1993 Diagnosis of patent ductus arteriosus in the preterm newborn. Archives of Disease in Childhood 68: 58–61

34. Evans N 1994 Cardiovascular effects of dexamethasone in the preterm infant. Archives of Disease in Childhood. Fetal and Neonatal Edition 70: F25–F30

35. Evans N J, Archer L N J 1990 Postnatal circulatory adaptation in healthy term and preterm neonates. Archives of Disease in Childhood 65: 24–26

36. Evans N, Kluckow M 1996 Early ductal shunting and intraventricular haemorrhage in ventilated preterm infants. Archives of Disease in Childhood. Fetal and Neonatal Edition 75: F183–F186

37. Fajardo C A, Whyte R K, Steele B T 1992 Effect of dopamine on failure of indomethacin to close the patent ductus arteriosus. Journal of Pediatrics 121: 771–775

38. Farrer K F, Rennie J M 2003 Neonatal murmurs: are senior house officers good enough? Archive of Disease in Childhood. Fetal and Neonatal Edition 88: F147–F151

39. Fowlie P W 1996 Prophylactic indomethacin: systematic review and metaanalysis. Archives of Disease in Childhood. Fetal and Neonatal Edition 74: F81–F87

40. Franklin O, Burch M, Manning N et al 2002 Prenatal diagnosis of coarctation of the aorta improves survival and reduces morbidity. Heart 87: 67–69

41. Gersony W M, Peckham G J, Ellison R C, Miettinen O S, Nadas A S 1983 Effects of indomethacin in premature infants with patent ductus arteriosus: results of a national collaborative study. Journal of Pediatrics 102: 895–906

42. Goldberg C, Schwartz E M Brunberg J A et al 2000 Neurodevelopmental outcome of patients after the Fontan operation: a comparison between children with hypoplastic left heart syndrome and other functional single ventricle lesions. Journal of Pediatrics 137: 646–652

43. Grabitz R G, Joffres M R, Collins-Nakai R L 1988 Congenital heart disease: incidence in the first year of life. American Journal of Epidemiology 128: 381–383

44. Green T P, Thompson T R, Johnson D E, Lock D E 1983 Furosemide promotes patent ductus arteriosus in premature infants with respiratory distress syndrome. New England Journal of Medicine 308: 743–748

45. Guenthard J, Wylie F, Fowler B, Baumgartner R 1995 Cardiomyopathy in respiratory chain disorders. Archives of Disease in Childhood 72: 223–226

46. Haak M C, Bartelings M M, Gittenberger-de Groot A C et al 2002 Cardiac malformations in first trimester fetuses with increased nuchal translucency: ultrasound diagnosis and post mortem morphology. Ultrasound in Obstetrics and Gynecology 20: 14–21

47. Hammerman C, Aramburo M J 1990 Prolonged indomethacin therapy for the prevention of recurrences of patent ductus arteriosus. Journal of Pediatrics 117: 771–776

48. Hanley F L, Sade R M, Freedom R M, Blackstone E H, Kirklin J W 1993 Outcomes in critically ill neonates with pulmonary stenosis and intact ventricular septum: a multi-institutional study. Journal of the American College of Cardiology 22: 183–192

49. Heymann M A 1995 Fetal and postnatal circulations, pulmonary circulation. In: Emmanouilides E C, Riemens-Schneider T A, Allen H D, Gutgesell H P (eds) Heart disease in infants, children and adolescents, 5th edition. Williams & Wilkins, Baltimore, pp 41–47

50. Hoffman J I E, Christianson R 1978 Congenital heart disease in a cohort of 19,502 births with long-term follow up. American Journal of Cardiology 42: 641–647

51. Huggon I C, Ghi T, Cook A C et al 2002 Fetal cardiac abnormalities identified prior to 14 weeks' gestation. Ultrasound in Obstetrics and Gynecology 20: 22–29

52. Ino T, Sherwood G, Benson L N, Wilson G J, Freedom R M, Rowe R D 1988 Cardiac manifestations in disorders of fat and carnitine metabolism in infancy. Journal of the American College of Cardiology 11: 1301–1308

53. Iyer P, Evans N 1994 Re-evaluation of the left atrial to aortic root ratio as a marker of patent ductus arteriosus. Archives of Disease in Childhood. Fetal and Neonatal Edition 70: F112–F117

54. Jacob J, Gluck L, Di Sessa T et al 1980 The contribution of PDA in the neonate with severe RDS. Journal of Pediatrics 96: 79–87

55. Karatza A A, Holder S E, Gardiner H M 2003 Isolated non-compaction of the ventricular myocardium: prenatal diagnosis and natural history. Ultrasound in Obstetrics and Gynecology 21: 75–80

56. Kluckow M, Evans N 1995 Early echocardiographic prediction of symptomatic patent ductus arteriosus in preterm infants undergoing mechanical ventilation. Journal of Pediatrics 127: 174–179

57. Kohl T, Sharland G, Allan L et al 2000 World experience of percutaneous ultrasound-guided balloon valvuloplasty in human fetuses with severe aortic valve obstruction. American Journal of Cardiology 85: 1230–1233

58. Kumar R K, Newburger J W, Gauvreau K et al 1999 Comparison of outcome when hypoplastic left heart syndrome and transposition of the great arteries are diagnosed prenatally versus when diagnosis of these two conditions is made only postnatally. American Journal of Cardiology 83: 1649–1653

59. Limperopoulos C, Majnemer A, Shevell M I et al 2000 Neurodevelopmental status of newborns and infants with congenital heart defects before and after open heart surgery. Journal of Pediatrics 137: 638–645

60. Lipshultz S E, Sleeper L A, Towbin J A et al 2003 The incidence of pediatric cardiomyopathy in two regions of the United States. New England Journal of Medicine 348: 1647–1655

61. McCrindle B W, Blackstone E H, Williams W G et al 2001 Are outcomes of surgical versus transcatheter balloon valvotomy equivalent in neonatal critical aortic stenosis? Circulation 104(suppl. l): 152–158

62. Macmahon P, Gorham P R, Arnold R, Wilkinson J L, Hamilton D I 1983 Pulmonary artery growth during treatment with oral prostaglandin E2 in ductus dependent cyanotic congenital heart disease. Archives of Disease in Childhood 58: 187–189

63. Mahony L 2001 Development of myocardial structure and function. In: Allan H D, Gutgesell H P, Clarke E B et al (eds) Heart disease in infants, children and adolescents, 6th edition. Lippincott Williams and Wilkins, Philadelphia, pp 24–40

64. Mahony L, Carnero V, Brett C, Heymann M A, Clyman R I 1982 Prophylactic indomethacin therapy for patent ductus arteriosus in very low birth weight infants. New England Journal of Medicine 306: 506–510

65. Manchester D, Margolis H S, Sheldon R E 1976 Possible association between maternal indomethacin therapy and primary pulmonary hypertension in the newborn. American Journal of Obstetrics and Gynecology 126: 467–469

66. Moise K J, Huhta J C, Sharif D S et al 1988 Indomethacin in the treatment of premature labor. New England Journal of Medicine 319: 327–331

67. Momma K, Takao A 1989 Increased constriction of the ductus arteriosus with combined administration of indomethacin and betamethasone in fetal rats. Pediatric Research 25: 69–75

68. Montigny M, Biron P, Fournier A, Elie R, Davignon A, Fouron J-C 1989 Captopril in infants for congestive heart failure secondary to a large ventricular left to right shunt. American Journal of Cardiology 63: 631–633

69. Muhler E G, Kienas W, Turniski-Harder V, von Bernuth G 1994 Arrhythmias in infants and children with primary cardiac tumours. European Heart Journal 15: 915–921

70. National Institutes of Health 1987 Report of the Second Task Force on Blood Pressure Control in Children. Pediatrics 79: 1–25

71. Norton M E, Merrill J, Cooper B A B, Kuller J A, Clyman R I 1993 Neonatal complications after the administration of indomethacin for preterm labor. New England Journal of Medicine 329: 1602–1607

72. Nugent A W, Daubeney P E F, Chondros P et al 2003 The epidemiology of childhood cardiomyopathy in Australia. New England Journal of Medicine 348: 1639–1646

73. Opie G F, Fraser S H, Drew J H, Drew S 1999 Bacterial endocarditis in neonatal intensive care. Journal of Pediatrics and Child Health 35: 545–548

74. O'Sullivan J J, Gardiner H M, Wren C 1995 Digoxin or flecainide for prophylaxis of supraventriculr tachycardia in infants? Journal of American College of Cardiology 26: 991–994

75. Park M, Guntheroth W G 1992 How to read pediatric ECGs, 3rd edition. Year Book, Chicago

76. Patel J, Marks K A, Roberts I, Azzopardi O, Edwards A D 1995 Ibuprofen treatment for patent ductus arteriosus. Lancet 346: 255

77. Patel J, Roberts I, Azzopardi D, Hamilton P, Edwards A D 2000 Randomized double blind controlled trial comparing the effects of ibuprofen with indomethacin on cerebral hemodynamics in preterm infants with patent ductus arteriosus. Pediatric Research 47: 36–42

78. Pickoff A S 2001 Development and function of the cardiac conduction system. In: Allan H D, Gutgesell H P, Clarke E B et al (eds) Heart disease in infants, children and adolescents, 6th edition. Lippincott Williams and Wilkins, Philadelphia, pp 414–424

79. Radzik D, Davignon A, van Doesburg N, Fournier A, Marchand T, Ducharme G 1993 Predictive factors for spontaneous closure of atrial septal defect diagnosed in the first 3 months of life. Journal of the American College of Cardiology 22: 851–853

80. Raju T N K, Langenberg P 1993 Pulmonary hemorrhage and exogenous surfactant therapy: a meta analysis. Journal of Pediatrics 123: 606–610

81. Reller M D, Colasurdo M A, Rice M C, McDouall R W 1990 The timing of spontaneous closure of the ductus arteriosus in infants with respiratory distress syndrome. American Journal of Cardiology 66: 75–78

82. Rennie J M, Cooke R W I 1991 Prolonged low dose indomethacin for persistent ductus arteriosus of prematurity. Archives of Disease in Childhood 66: 55–58

83. Richmond S, Reay G, Abu Harb M 2002 Routine pulse oximetry in the asymptomatic newborn. Archives of Disease in Childhood. Fetal and Neonatal Edition 87: F83–F88

84. Robie D K, Waltrip T, Garcia-Prats J A, Pokorny WJ, Jaksic T 1996 Is surgical ligation of a patent ductus arteriosus the preferred initial approach for the neonate with extremely low birth weight? Journal of Pediatric Surgery 8: 1134–1137

85. Salmon A P, Keeton B R, Sethia B 1993 Developments in interventional catheterisation and progress in surgery for congenital heart disease: achieving a balance. British Heart Journal 69: 479–480

86. Schmidt B, Davis P, Moddemann D et al 2001 Long term effects of indomethacin prophylaxis in extremely low birth weight infants. New England Journal of Medicine 344: 1966–1972

87. Schwartz P J, Locati E H, Moss A J et al 1993 Diagnostic criteria for the long QT syndrome: an update. Circulation 88: 782–784

88. Srivastava D, Baldwin H S 2001 Molecular determinants of cardiac development. In: Allan H D, Gutgesell H P, Clarke E B et al (eds) Heart disease in infants, children and adolescents, 6th edition. Lippincott Williams and Wilkins, Philadelphia, pp 3–23

89. Sharland G K, Chita S K, Fagg N L K et al 1991 Left ventricular dysfunction in the fetus: relation to aortic valve anomalies and endocardial fibroelastosis. British Heart Journal 66: 419–424

90. Shaw N J, Wilson N, Dickinson D F 1988 Captopril in heart failure secondary to a left to right shunt. Archives of Disease in Childhood 63: 360–363

91. Simpson J M, Jones A, Callaghan N et al 2000 Accuracy and limitations of transabdominal fetal echocardiography at 12–15 weeks of gestation in a population at high risk for congenital heart disease. British Journal of Obstetrics and Gynaecology 107: 1492–1497

92. Simpson J M, Sharland G K 1997 Natural history and outcome of aortic stenosis diagnosed prenatally. Heart 77: 205–210

93. Simpson J M, Sharland G K 1998 Fetal tachycardias: management and outcome of 127 consecutive cases. Heart 79: 576–581

94. Shortland D B, Gibson N A, Levene M I, Archer L N, Evans D H, Shaw D E 1990 Patent ductus arteriosus and cerebral circulation in preterm infants. Developmental Medicine and Child Neurology 32: 386–393

95. Silove E D, Roberts D G U, De Giovanni J V 1985 Evaluation of oral and low dose intravenous prostaglandin E2 in management of ductus dependent congenital heart disease. Archives of Disease in Childhood 60: 1025–1030

96. Skinner J, Alverson D, Hunter S 2000 Echocardiography for the neonatologist. Churchill Livingstone, London

97. Southall D P, Johnson A M, Shinebourne E A, Johnstone P G B, Vulliamy D G 1981 Frequency and outcome of disorders of cardiac rhythm and conduction in a population of newborn infants. Pediatrics 68: 58–66

98. Southall D P, Richard J, Mitchell P, Brown D J, Johnston P G B, Shinebourne E A 1980 Study of cardiac rhythm in healthy newborn infants. British Heart Journal 43: 14–20

99. Sreeram N, Wren C 1990 Supraventricular tachycardia in infants: response to initial treatment. Archives of Disease in Childhood 65: 127–129

100. Starnes V A, Griffin M L, Pitlick P T et al 1992 Current approach to hypoplastic left heart syndrome. Journal of Thoracic and Cardiovascular Surgery 104: 189–195

101. Stümpflen I, Stümpflen A, Wimmer M, Bernaschek G 1996 Effect of detailed fetal echocardiography as part of routine prenatal ultrasonographic screening on detection of congenital heart disease. Lancet 348: 854–857

102. Su B-H, Peng C-T, Tsai C-H 1999 Echocardiographic flow pattern of patent ductus arteriosus: a guide to indomethacin treatment in premature infants. Archives of Disease in Childhood. Fetal and Neonatal Edition 81: F197–F200

103. Su B-H, Watanabe T, Shimizu M et al 1997 Echocardiographic assessment of patent ductus arteriosus shunt flow pattern in premature infants. Archives of Disease in Childhood. Fetal and Neonatal Edititon 77: F36–F40

104. Tillett A, Hartley B, Simpson J 2001 Paradoxical embolism causing fatal myocardial infarction in a newborn infant. Archives of Disease in Childhood. Fetal and Neonatal Edition 85: F137–F138

105. Trus T, Winthrop A L, Pyle S, Shah J, Langer J C, Lau G Y P 1993 Optimal management of patent ductus arteriosus in the neonate weighing less than 800 g. Journal of Pediatric Surgery 28: 1137–1139

106. Tulzer G, Artz W, Franklin R C G et al 2002 Fetal pulmonary valvuloplasty for critical pulmonary stenosis or atresia with intact ventricular septum. Lancet 360: 1567–1568

107. Tulloh R M R, Tansey S P, Parashar K, De Giovanni J V, Wright J G C, Silove E D 1994 Echocardiographic screening in neonates undergoing surgery for selected gastrointestinal malformations. Archives of Disease in Childhood. Fetal and Neonatal Edition 70: F206–F208

108. Tworetzky W, McElhinney D B, Reddy M et al 2001 Improved surgical outcome after fetal diagnosis of hypoplastic left heart syndrome. Circulation 103: 1269–1273

109. Van Overmeire B, Smets K, Lecouterie D et al 2000 A comparison of ibuprofen and indomethacin for closure of patent ductus arteriosus. New England Journal of Medicine 343: 674–681

110. Varvarigou A, Bardin C L, Beharry K et al 1996 Early ibuprofen administration to prevent patent ductus arteriosus in premature infants. Journal of the American Medical Association 275: 539–544

111. Villain E, Levy M, Kachaner J, Garson A 1992 Prolonged QT interval in neonates: benign, transient or prolonged risk of sudden death. American Heart Journal 124: 194–197

112. Wallace G, Smith H C, Watson G H, Rimmer S, D'Souza S W 1990 Tuberous sclerosis presenting with fetal and neonatal cardiac tumours. Archives of Disease in Childhood 65: 377–379

113. Way G L, Woolfe R R, Eshaghpour E, Bender R L, Jaffe R B, Ruttenberg H D 1979 The natural history of hypertrophic cardiomyopathy in infants of diabetic mothers. Journal of Pediatrics 95: 1020–1025

114. Wells J T, Ment L R 1995 Prevention of intraventricular hemorrhage in preterm infants. Early Human Development 42: 209–233

115. Wilkinson A R, Aynsley-Green A, Mitchell M D 1979 Persistent pulmonary hypertension and abnormal prostaglandin E levels in preterm infants after maternal treatment with naproxen. Archives of Disease in Childhood 54: 942–945

116. Wilkinson J L, Cooke R W I 1992 Cardiovascular disorders. In: Robertson's textbook of neonatology, 2nd edition. Churchill Livingstone, Edinburgh

117. Wyllie J, Wren C, Hunter S 1994 Screening for fetal cardiac malformations. British Heart Journal 71(suppl.): 20–27

118. Yeh T F, Luken J A, Thalji A, Raval D, Carr I, Pildes R S 1981 Intravenous indomethacin therapy in premature infants with persistent ductus arteriosus – a double-blind controlled study. Journal of Pediatrics 98: 137–145

119. Zecskes Z, Cartwright D W 2002 Poor outcome of very low birthweight babies with serious congenital heart disease. Archives of Disease in Childhood. Fetal and Neonatal Edition 87: F31–F33

120. Zeevi B, Berant M, Fogelman R et al 1999 Acute complications in the current era of therapeutic cardiac catheterisation for congenital heart disease. Cardiology in the Young 9: 266–272

CHAPTER 29

Gastroenterology

PART I

Neonatal jaundice

N Kevin Ives

Introduction

Jaundice is the most common clinical sign in neonatal medicine, but only rarely is it the harbinger of disease or associated with neurotoxicity. Some two-thirds of healthy term infants, and almost all premature infants, develop clinical jaundice in the first week of life. The majority of this jaundice is 'physiological', and results from an immaturity of the liver's excretory pathway for bilirubin at a time of its heightened production. It is the shared responsibility of all involved in the medical, nursing and midwifery care of the newborn to recognise the rare cases of 'exaggerated physiological jaundice' or truly 'pathological' jaundice that necessitate investigation and possible treatment. This is especially true in the current era of early postnatal discharge; jaundice is currently the most common reason for readmission to hospital in the first week of life.[85]

A 'kinder, gentler approach' to the management of jaundice in healthy full-term newborns has evolved over the past decade.[21,70] Undoubtedly, this has spared a large number of babies and their families the stress of blood tests, phototherapy, exchange transfusion and prolonged hospitalisation.[82] Inadvertently, however, a less vigilant approach to all forms of jaundice, including that of prematurity, may have been engendered. Earlier postnatal discharge, treatment guidelines with narrower margins for error, and the more relaxed approach to therapy may all be linked to the resurgence of kernicterus.[22,36,39,71]

Despite improved understanding of the mechanisms of bilirubin neurotoxicity, our ability to predict which babies are at greatest risk remains imprecise. Recent clinical research has focused on attempts to predict babies who are at risk of developing significant jaundice.[9,77,87]

Improvements in the delivery of phototherapy secure its place as the main treatment option for unconjugated hyperbilirubinaemia, and its role in reducing the requirement for exchange transfusion. Newer treatments, such as metalloporphyrins[101] and high-dose immunoglobulin in isoimmune haemolysis,[30] are gaining research credibility, but, as yet, have not entered widespread clinical practice.

Bilirubin biochemistry

Bilirubin is produced by a two-stage catabolism of haem in the reticuloendothelial system (Fig. 29.1). The majority of haem arises from the turnover of haemoglobin released from naturally decommissioned or pathologically destroyed erythrocytes. Haem (ferroprotoporphyrin IX) has a porphyrin ring structure which is opened preferentially at its α-methene bridge by haem oxygenase. The intermediate pigment, biliverdin IXα, is water-soluble, non-toxic and serves as the excretory product of haem in amphibians, reptiles and birds. In mammals, reduction of biliverdin IXα by biliverdin reductase results in the production of bilirubin IXα.

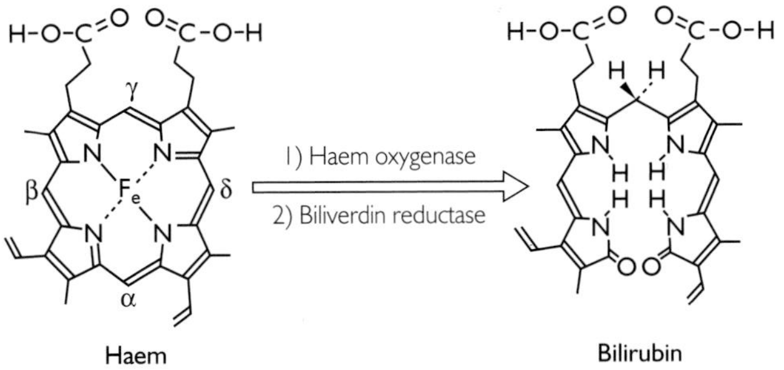

Fig. 29.1 Production of bilirubin from haem degradation. (Reproduced from McDonagh & Lightner.[56])

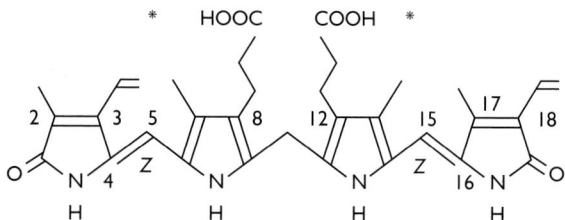

Fig. 29.2 Linear representation of bilirubin IXα with central proprionic acid groups [**]. (Reproduced from McDonagh & Lightner.[56]) Z – see text.

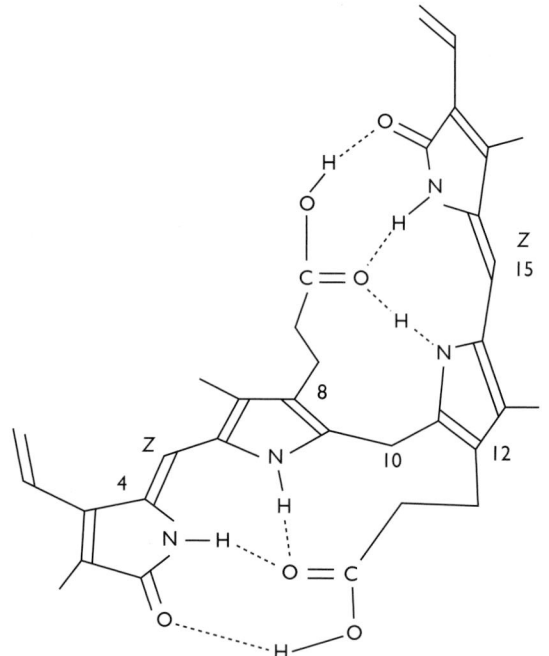

Fig. 29.3a Preferred conformation of bilirubin. (Reproduced from McDonagh & Lightner.[56])

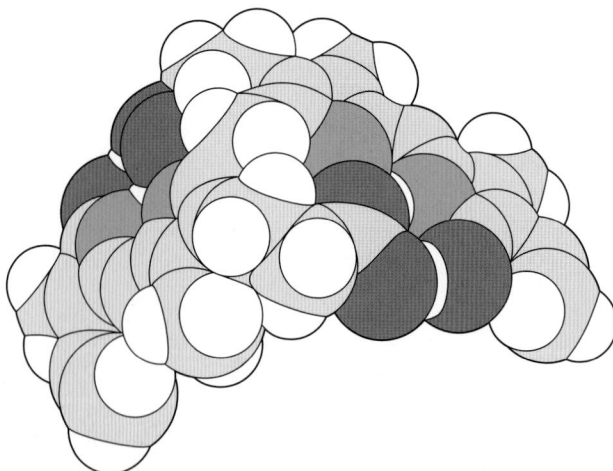

Fig. 29.3b Atomic representation of the bilirubin-IXa ZZ molecule (nitrogen mid grey; oxygen dark grey; carbon light grey and hydrogen white).

Bilirubin IXβ is the only toxic isomer of bilirubin. The small amounts of the IXα and IXδ isomers produced are non-toxic. Why mammalian species should expend energy producing and excreting a potentially neurotoxic haem byproduct remains unclear. One possible explanation stems from the discovery that bilirubin is an antioxidant, thus prompting the question: 'Is bilirubin good for you?'[55] Whatever the reason, we are left with the responsibility of ensuring that serum levels of free bilirubin IXα do not reach neurotoxic levels.

Diagrammatic representation of the bilirubin molecule conveys the impression of a tetrapyrrole aligned in a single plane (Fig. 29.2). The preferred conformation of the molecule is known to be partially folded at its mid methylene bridge (Fig. 29.3a,b). This shape facilitates intramolecular hydrogen bonding, which saturates the hydrophilic polar groupings, rendering bilirubin virtually insoluble in water at physiological pH. In this form, bilirubin has lipophilic properties which enable it to cross cell membranes and biological boundaries, such as the placenta and blood–brain barrier.

The proprionic acid groups attached to the inner two pyrrole rings of the bilirubin molecule are the site of conjugation with glucuronic acid. The mono- and diglucuronides of bilirubin so formed retain the more open, water-soluble conformation by reducing or preventing intramolecular hydrogen bonding. Polar groupings remain similarly exposed in the naturally occurring β and δ isomers of bilirubin and in the major products of phototherapy, enabling them to be freely excreted in bile.[24]

Bilirubin metabolism and excretion

The newborn bilirubin pool originates chiefly from the breakdown of red cells, but up to a quarter comes from ineffective erythropoiesis and other haem-containing compounds, such as myoglobin and cytochromes. Bilirubin is transported in the blood bound reversibly to serum albumin on high and low affinity sites, with a potential molar bilirubin to albumin ratio up to 3:1. Under normal circumstances, the proportion of free bilirubin circulating in the jaundiced newborn is very low (<5 nmol/l). Changes in serum pH do not affect the binding of bilirubin to albumin, but a fall in pH will increase the concentration of bilirubin acid and promote binding of bilirubin to cell membranes and organelles.[10]

A carrier assists transfer of bilirubin across the hepatocyte membrane, and specific binding proteins increase net uptake by reducing efflux of bilirubin from the hepatocyte.[14] Conjugation with glucuronic acid occurs in the smooth endoplasmic reticulum to form water-soluble mono- and diglucuronides of bilirubin. These reactions are catalysed by the microsomal enzyme hepatic uridine diphosphoglucuronosyl transferase (UDPGT). Conjugated bilirubin (chiefly the monoglucuronide in the newborn) is actively transported out of the liver cell and into the biliary canaliculi as a component of bile.

In adults, most of the conjugated bilirubin is converted by colonic flora to urobilinogen before elimination in the stool. In the newborn, a significant proportion is hydrolysed by β-glucuronidase in the small gut to yield glucuronic acid and unconjugated bilirubin, which can re-enter the circulating pool via the enterohepatic circulation.

Biochemical basis of phototherapy

Phototherapy detoxifies bilirubin and facilitates its excretion from the body via routes other than conjugation in the liver.[24,56] When bilirubin interacts with a photon of light energy, three photochemical reactions can occur. They are as follows:

- photo-oxidation;
- configurational isomerisation;
- structural isomerisation.

Photo-oxidation involves disruption of the bilirubin molecule to form colourless polar fragments that are readily excreted in urine. Although this process reminds us of the need to avoid exposure of serum samples to direct sunlight,[15] it is thought to play only a minor role in bilirubin excretion during phototherapy.

Configurational isomerisation results from molecular re-orientation around the double bonds between carbon atoms 4–5 and 15–16 (see Fig. 29.2). In the natural form, the arrangement of these double bonds, and hence the alignment of the end pyrrole rings, is classified as bilirubin-4Z,15Z (Z = *zusammen*, together). A photon of light striking the bilirubin molecule can temporarily disrupt the double bonds and initiate a 180° rotation of one or both end pyrrole rings to produce three isomeric forms, designated: 4Z,15E; 4E,15Z; and 4E,15E (E = *entgegen*, apart).

Formation of bilirubin-Z,E is favoured during phototherapy by the nature of the binding between bilirubin and albumin. Whilst bound to albumin, the configurational isomers remain stable for a number of hours. As shown in Figure 29.4, the conformation of bilirubin-Z,E maintains exposure of polar groups at one end of the molecule, enabling it to be excreted, unconjugated in bile. Once in bile, a rapid reversal of the reaction occurs, such that unconjugated bilirubin-Z,Z enters the gut and is available for uptake via the enterohepatic circulation.

Configurational isomerisation was originally thought to be the main excretory mechanism of phototherapy. It is now realised that, although rapidly produced, these isomers are slowly cleared in humans. The serum half-life of bilirubin-Z,E is about 15 hours, and after some 6–12 hours of phototherapy a steady state is achieved in which approximately 20% of the total serum bilirubin is in the form of the configurational isomer.[24] Importantly, this means that up to one-fifth of the circulating bilirubin is detoxified, despite not being in a form that is readily excreted.

Formation of the structural isomer, lumirubin, is now considered to be the chief mode of bilirubin excretion during phototherapy. Lumirubin is formed by 'cyclisation' of one end of the bilirubin molecule, as shown in Figure 29.5. This structural change is irreversible and allows the more polar product to be excreted in bile and urine. Lumirubin's more efficient elimination is reflected by its half-life of less than 2 hours and steady state concentration

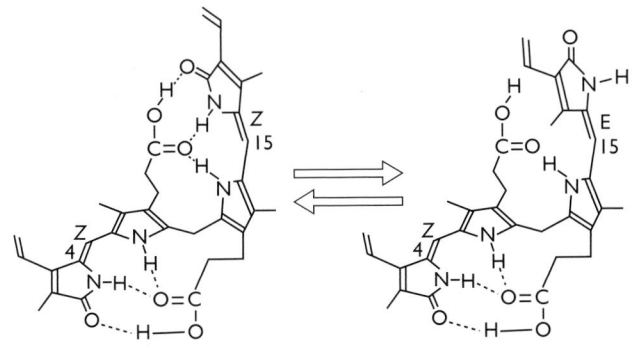

Fig. 29.4 Configurational photoisomerisation of bilirubin. (Reproduced from McDonagh & Lightner.[56])

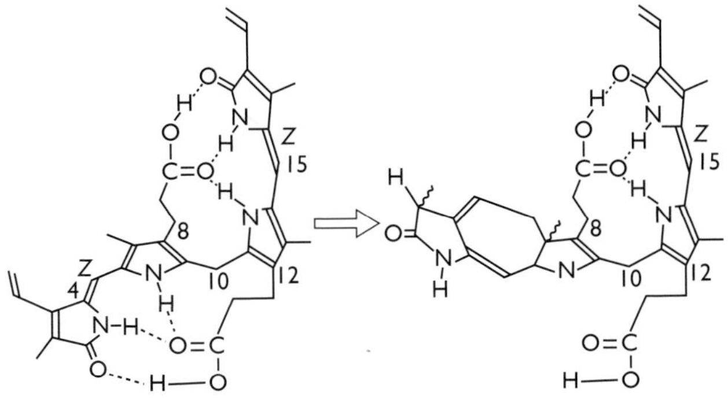

Fig. 29.5 Structural photoisomerisation of bilirubin to form lumirubin. (Reproduced from McDonagh & Lightner.[56])

during phototherapy of 2–6% of the total serum bilirubin.[24] Production of lumirubin follows a dose–response relationship with the irradiance of phototherapy applied and may be favoured by the use of light of a longer wavelength than that of conventional phototherapy.[23]

Physiological jaundice

The fetus excretes unconjugated bilirubin via the placenta and maternal liver. In the absence of pathological fetal hyperbilirubinaemia or maternal liver disease, the mean bilirubin level in cord blood at birth is in the region of 20–35 micromol/l.[49] Postnatally, most newborns exhibit a further elevation in serum bilirubin. In healthy term formula-fed babies, the serum bilirubin peaks on the third to fourth day of life, attaining clinically detectable levels (>80 micromol/l) in approximately two-thirds of the population. Following this phase I peak, serum bilirubin levels fall rapidly for 2–3 days and then more gradually, reaching normal adult values between 1 to 2 weeks of age (phase II). Exclusively breastfed babies may have a delayed serum bilirubin peak and a more prolonged pattern to their jaundice (see later, pp. 664–5). Physiological jaundice is the result of increased bilirubin

Table 29.1 Factors that exacerbate physiological jaundice in the newborn

Polycythaemia
  Delayed cord clamping
  Maternofetal transfusion
  Recipient of twin–twin transfusion
Extravasated blood
  Bruising (e.g. cephalhaematoma)
  Birth trauma
  Internal haemorrhage
Delayed passage of meconium
Swallowed blood
Hypocaloric feed intake
Dehydration
Breastfeeding
Prematurity

production at a time when the mechanisms for liver uptake, transport and conjugation of bilirubin are immature. At higher serum bilirubin levels, the carrier-mediated and saturable excretion of bilirubin into bile may also become rate limiting. The biphasic pattern of physiological jaundice results from a deficiency of UDPGT activity in the first phase[46] and low ligandin binding protein levels in the second.[29]

Premature babies exhibit a higher peak serum bilirubin level, occurring on days 5–7, and a longer phase II, persisting for 2–4 weeks. Even newborns bordering on prematurity are likely to exhibit heightened jaundice. A study population of babies of 37 weeks' gestation were four times as likely to attain bilirubin levels greater than 220 micromol/l than those of 40 weeks' gestation.[26]

Bilirubin production during the first weeks of life is more than double that of the adult. This excess bilirubin load in the newborn results from factors that include the higher haematocrit, increased red cell turnover, and a greater contribution from sources of haem other than senescent erythrocytes. In addition, a 10-fold higher level of β-glucuronidase in the small-bowel brush border of the newborn reverses the conjugation process,[27] liberating more unconjugated bilirubin to join the enterohepatic circulation. The high bilirubin content of meconium and the initial absence of gut bacteria are also thought to contribute. Other risk factors that heighten physiological jaundice are listed in Table 29.1.

Although the term 'physiological jaundice' is helpful in our understanding of the common pattern of newborn jaundice, it conveys the false impression of a benign status. Some clinicians prefer to ignore the term 'physiological jaundice' altogether. Others use the statistical limit of more than two standard deviations above the mean of a study population to denote 'pathological jaundice'. Attempts to define 'physiological' and 'pathological' jaundice using total serum bilirubin range is a futile exercise. It is more practical to be alerted to a pathological cause for jaundice in the following circumstances:

- jaundice on day one;
- total serum bilirubin level ⩾250 micromol/l by 48 hours;
- total serum bilirubin level ⩾275 micromol/l by 72 hours;
- total serum bilirubin level ⩾300 micromol/l by 96 hours.

That is not to say that all jaundice falling into one or other of these categories has a pathological cause. In the absence of an identifiable disease process, the term 'exaggerated physiological jaundice' may be more appropriate in such cases.[27] In using this term it must be remembered that 'exaggerated physiological jaundice' may attain unconjugated bilirubin levels capable of transient auditory derangement[90] and, rarely, permanent neurological damage.[39,62]

Epidemiology

The prevalence of breastfeeding and the incidence of preterm birth will influence the pattern of jaundice within a population. Why certain Greek, Chinese and Japanese babies develop a marked idiopathic hyperbilirubinaemia remains unclear. Developments in human genomics are destined to provide explanations for the epidemiological variation in neonatal hyperbilirubinaemia and susceptibility to bilirubin encephalopathy.[98] Gilbert's syndrome is being increasingly recognised as a contributory factor in pronounced and prolonged unconjugated jaundice.[67,98] In Gilbert's syndrome, a variant in the promoter for the gene encoding UDPGT results in a reduction of the enzyme's activity by as much as two-thirds. The syndrome is common in that it affects 5–10% of the population in the homozygous state. The heterozygous Gilbert's state, present in 42% of the population, has also been shown to have some contributory effect in hyperbilirubinaemia.[41] A genetic interaction between the Gilbert's genotype and that of glucose-6-phosphate dehydrogenase (G6PD) deficiency has been responsible for severe cases of hyperbilirubinaemia of greater severity than would be anticipated from their additive effect alone.[42]

Jaundice in the healthy breastfed infant

Breastfed babies develop more marked and prolonged jaundice than those who are purely formula-fed. They are more than three times as likely to develop serum bilirubin levels greater than 205 micromol/l, and over six times as likely to exceed levels of 256 micromol/l than formula-fed infants.[80] The peak bilirubin level in the formula-fed infant usually occurs on day 3 or 4, whereas in the breastfed baby it may not be reached until the end of the first week or into the second week of life.[28] The phenomenon of breast-milk jaundice also occurs in babies born prematurely.[54]

Up to one-third of breastfed babies remain clinically jaundiced beyond 2 weeks of age,[2] and they represent the majority of infants presenting for a prolonged jaundice screen. A reliable diagnosis of breast-milk jaundice can only be made on exclusion of pathological causes. Once the diagnosis is confirmed, parents should be warned that resolution of jaundice in the breastfed baby might take as long as 2–3 months. They should be advised to report back if the nature of the jaundice changes, there is failure to thrive or the jaundice persists beyond 3 months. Although interruption of breast milk feeds and supplementation with formula for 24 hours may be associated with a marked decline in serum bilirubin and lower rebound level on re-introduction, the practice is rarely justified. Also to be discouraged is the vogue for supplementing breastfed infants with water, regardless of their state of hydration. Newborns supplemented in this way have been shown to have higher maximum serum bilirubin levels.[17]

Several hypotheses have been put forward to explain the association between breastfeeding and heightened jaundice. There appears to be an early and late phase of such jaundice, and a valiant attempt to distinguish these phases as 'breastfeeding jaundice' (or more correctly 'breast-nonfeeding jaundice') and 'breast-milk jaundice' has been made.[28] However, the pathogenesis of this early and late jaundice is likely to be multifactorial with overlap between the two phases.

The exacerbated physiological jaundice commonly seen in the breastfed, as opposed to formula-fed, baby during the first week of life probably relates to lower calorie intake and slower passage of meconium. When marked, this pattern of jaundice in the breastfed newborn has been referred to as 'lack-of-breast milk jaundice'[34] or 'breast-nonfeeding jaundice'.[28] The importance of good caloric intake in the first days of life to prevent or ameliorate jaundice has been recently demonstrated by Bertini et al.[7] They looked at three groups of infants with differing feeds. The first group was exclusively breastfed; the second was breastfed but received formula supplementation for excessive weight loss; and the third was exclusively formula-fed. The infants who were successfully breastfed (without significant weight loss) were no more likely to develop jaundice than exclusively formula-fed babies. Those most likely to develop jaundice were the breastfed babies who received formula supplementation in response to excessive weight loss.

The prolonged form of jaundice seen in the breastfed baby beyond the second week of life is considered to be related to enhanced enterohepatic circulation of bilirubin. The presence in breast milk of β-glucuronidase – which unconjugates bilirubin in the infant gut, enabling it to re-enter the circulation – is thought to be contributory. Altered bacterial colonisation of the gut in the breastfed baby with a resultant decrease in the conversion of bilirubin glucuronides to urobilinoids may also play a role. Inhibition of hepatic conjugation of bilirubin has been postulated, but most of the mechanisms advanced, including the presence in breast milk of the steroid pregnane-3α,20β-diol, have been disproved.[31]

Pathophysiology of bilirubin encephalopathy

Kernicterus

Kernicterus is the name given to the characteristic pattern of yellow staining of parts of the brainstem, hippocampus, cerebellum and certain brainstem nuclei seen at autopsy in infants dying with acute bilirubin toxicity (see Fig. 29.8). The clinical manifestations of bilirubin encephalopathy arise from the susceptibility to damage of the basal ganglia, brainstem auditory pathways and oculomotor nuclei.[96] This anatomical preference for bilirubin deposition and

vulnerability to toxicity has not been fully explained, but may be a consequence of increased blood flow and metabolic activity in these areas.[11] Regional variation in bilirubin influx, detoxification and clearance may also play a part.

The blood–brain barrier is anatomically derived from tight junctions between the endothelial cells of cerebral blood vessels. This barrier remains permeable to lipid-soluble substances, but, whilst intact, excludes water-soluble substances and large molecules, such as proteins. Free bilirubin influxes and effluxes across the intact blood–brain barrier with a permeability in keeping with the behaviour of a lipid-soluble molecule. Disruption of the blood–brain barrier will allow an influx of albumin-bound bilirubin as well as free bilirubin into the brain. In terms of toxicity, the significance of albumin-bound bilirubin within the brain is uncertain. Of note is the lack of correlation between bilirubin staining and histological evidence of neuronal injury observed in the brains of premature infants dying in the so-called 'low bilirubin kernicterus' era.[91]

Bilirubin toxicity

What is known about the mechanisms of bilirubin brain toxicity has been reviewed recently.[35] Bilirubin's toxicity would appear to be that of a generalised cellular poison. Disruption of membrane function, lowering of action potentials, compromise of energy metabolism, and disturbance of neurotransmitter synthesis and neurotransmission, are some of the mechanisms implicated.[96] Neuronal vulnerability to bilirubin would appear to be both gestational and postnatal age dependent, possibly reflecting the functional status of specific brain areas at the time of the metabolic insult. Advances in human genomics are likely to identify factors that protect against or predispose to bilirubin encephalopathy. There is growing evidence to suggest that bilirubin is a substrate for P-glycoprotein, a plasma membrane efflux pump found on the luminal surface of brain capillary endothelial cells and considered responsible for limiting entry of certain lipophilic substrates into the central nervous system.[98] P-glycoprotein expression has been related to gestational maturity, and may be a factor contributing to the greater vulnerability of the premature brain to bilirubin neurotoxicity.

Attempts to reproduce bilirubin neurotoxicity experimentally point to the importance of coexisting risk factors, such as acidosis, hypoxia, hypercarbia and blood–brain barrier disruption, as being prerequisites for bilirubin's toxicity. Hypercarbia should not be underestimated as a risk factor. Respiratory acidosis will increase cerebral blood flow, and hypercarbia can open the blood–brain barrier.

Agents that interfere with the binding of bilirubin to serum albumin also promote neurotoxicity. The devastating effect of sulphisoxazole[86] in the 1960s serves as a reminder that all drugs used in neonatology should be assessed in terms of their potential to displace bilirubin from albumin.[74] Such testing has shown the antibiotics ceftriaxone, rifampicin and fusidic acid to be theoretically hazardous in this context. Also to be avoided in jaundiced infants are the diuretic chlorthiazide and large doses of radiographic contrast media. Free fatty acids, if they reach a molar ratio with albumin in excess of 4:1, interfere with bilirubin binding. Such ratios may be attained in sick immature newborns receiving high-dose intravenous lipid preparations. For this reason, lipid infusions should be reduced or stopped during the peak phase of jaundice in sick preterms. A cautious approach to the use of any preparation that has been shown experimentally to displace bilirubin from albumin would appear wise. However, apart from sulphisoxazole, no other drug or biochemical agent has been implicated as a cause of clinical kernicterus in humans.

Clinical bilirubin encephalopathy

The word kernicterus originated as a description of yellow nuclear staining of the brain, but has become synonymous with the acute and chronic neurological features of what are more correctly termed bilirubin encephalopathy and its sequelae. The terminology has been imprecise for some time, but a recent proposal to introduce the acronym BIND (bilirubin-induced neurologic dysfunction) and a BIND score adds little to our understanding of the condition or ability to prevent it.[40] Descriptions of 'classic kernicterus' arise from observations of markedly jaundiced infants with erythroblastosis fetalis before the advent of exchange transfusion. Three clinical phases have been identified.[13] The first day or so is characterised by lethargy, hypotonia, and poor suck. Towards the end of the first week, a second phase is heralded by hypertonia, which may include opisthotonus. At this stage, the baby commonly exhibits a high-pitched cry and fever and may have seizures. The third phase is entered as the hypertonia subsides to be replaced by hypotonia. Intervention during phase one with phototherapy and exchange transfusion may prevent evolution of long-term damage, but hypertonia during the second phase is a poor prognostic sign and is predictive of neurological sequelae.

The long-term features of bilirubin encephalopathy include extrapyramidal disturbances, auditory impairment, upward gaze palsies, and dental enamel dysplasia. The resulting cerebral palsy typically has an element of athetosis, which can develop as early as 18 months or be delayed for several years. High-frequency sensorineural deafness frequently accompanies the cerebral palsy, but may evolve in isolation. Cognitive impairment may result from bilirubin encephalopathy, but is commonly absent. A characteristic brain MRI pattern has been described in cases of kernicterus. The presence of high-intensity areas in the posteromedial border of the globus pallidus on T2-weighted imaging is considered the most sensitive finding.[103] Kernicteric brain MRI changes are illustrated in Figure 29.6.

Identifying the newborn at risk of bilirubin encephalopathy

Healthy term infants: total serum bilirubin concentration

A 'kinder, gentler approach'

Up until the last decade, treatment thresholds for phototherapy and exchange transfusion have reflected clinical experience gained with severe erythroblastosis fetalis half a century ago. Early exponents of exchange transfusion determined that kernicterus was unlikely to occur in affected infants if serum bilirubin levels were kept below 20 mg/dl (342 micromol/l). Kernicterus resulting from newborn haemolytic disease has been virtually eradicated wherever this threshold for treatment has been adopted. The impact was such that an 'irrational fear of 20 mg/dl' or 'vigintiphobia', as coined by Watchko and Oski,[99] led to the adoption of this exchange threshold for all infants, regardless of the cause of jaundice. A campaign for 'a kinder, gentler approach' to the treatment of jaundice in healthy, non-haemolysing term infants was started by Newman and Maisels,[70] who carried out an extensive review of the existing literature before proposing their less interventional management regimens. With respect to hearing, they could find no consistent association between sensorineural hearing loss and serum bilirubin levels in healthy term newborns. It should be noted, however, that the six studies reviewed reflected very little experience of bilirubin levels in excess of 440 micromol/l. On the question of bilirubin levels and IQ, Newman and Maisels[70] suggest that 'statistical significance has been mistaken for clinical significance'. From the results of the Collaborative Perinatal Project, which followed the progress of babies born to a cohort of more than 53 000 American women who became pregnant between 1959 and 1965, they estimate that the statistically significant correlation between IQ and bilirubin represents a deficit of only one IQ point per 85 micromol/l increase in serum bilirubin concentration. The relevance of this correlation to the healthy term infant is further undermined by the fact that the study population included babies with haemolysis and premature infants weighing more than 2.5 kg. In the case of studies of subtle neurological motor dysfunction secondary to hyperbilirubinaemia, it remains uncertain as to whether there are significant or long-term effects of moderate hyperbilirubinaemia.[63]

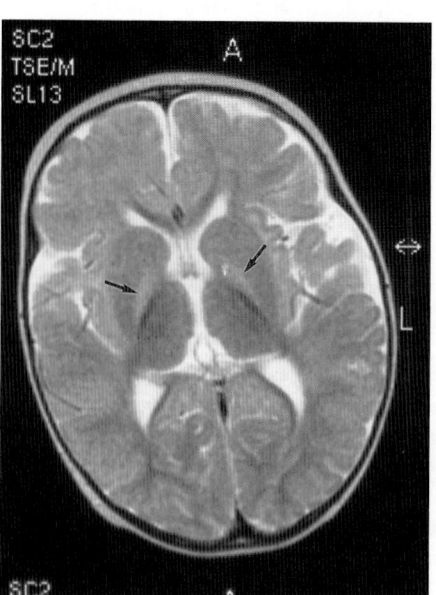

Fig. 29.6 T2-weighted axial section of the brain imaged with MRI, showing characteristic changes of kernicterus in the globus pallidus (arrowed).

Lessons from case reports of kernicterus in term infants

What is the evidence that an otherwise healthy, non-haemolysing term baby can develop kernicterus at any bilirubin level? Maisels and Newman[62] have reported six cases in which apparent 'exaggerated physiological jaundice' was associated with signs of acute bilirubin encephalopathy, and typical neurological sequelae. Peak recorded bilirubin levels with a range of 663–845 micromol/l occurred between days 4–10. Four of the babies were 37 weeks' gestation and four had significant weight loss. The possibility that these infants had a genetic predisposition to heightened jaundice, such as Gilbert's syndrome, has been raised.[98] Ebbesen[22] has reported experience of six cases of kernicterus in Denmark between 1994 and 1998. Spherocytosis was the cause of jaundice in one case and galactosaemia in another. ABO incompatibility is likely to have been implicated in a further two of the six cases. Of the remaining two cases, one had a gestational age of 36 weeks. All were breastfed and the range of maximum total serum bilirubin concentration was 531–745 micromol/l. Three of the infants were discharged within 24 hours (one at 12 hours), and it is not known whether they were clinically jaundiced at the time of discharge.

We may gain further insight into bilirubin encephalopathy by studying the case histories of infants who experience very high levels of bilirubin but escape neurological sequelae. Hanko et al[33] describe a baby with ABO incompatibility with a peak serum bilirubin at 19 hours of age of 636 micromol/l who appears to have escaped injury after the bilirubin level was reduced to <400 micromol/l by 35 hours of age. By contrast, they report two cases of apparently non-pathological jaundice with peak values of 650 and 717 micromol/l in which the bilirubin value was not reduced to <400 micromol/l until 60 and 68 hours, respectively. These babies went on to develop long-term neurological features consistent with bilirubin encephalopathy. The authors suggest that it may be the duration of hyperbilirubinaemia or 'area under the curve' that is important for neurotoxicity.

A large population-based case series in California[69] has identified 11 babies over 4 years (0.01% of the study population) who presented with bilirubin levels in excess of 510 micromol/l (range 525–778 micromol/l; mean 597 micromol/l). These cases arose despite the fact that there was a well-established follow-up policy and paediatric practice that adhered to the American Academy of Pediatrics (AAP) guidelines for phototherapy.[3] There were no neurodevelopmental sequelae in this small group, but the authors were correct to caution that 'additional studies are required to quantify the known, significant risk of kernicterus in infants with very high total serum bilirubin levels.'

Our clinical experience to date can be no more precise than to place the risk of bilirubin encephalopathy in healthy term newborns at a threshold of serum bilirubin somewhere between 425 micromol/l[70] and 650 micromol/l.[33,62] The anxiety previously engendered by a total serum bilirubin level >20 mg/dl (340 micromol/l) in such infants has been replaced by uncertainty as to the safety of levels of 25–30 mg/dl (425–510 micromol/l) in neonatal practice.

Predischarge prediction of the severity of jaundice

In the context of early postnatal discharge and a varying degree of community support, American authors[9] have recently proposed that all babies should have a predischarge serum bilirubin estimation in an attempt to categorise their risk of significant hyperbilirubinaemia based on an hour-specific bilirubin nomogram (Fig. 29.7). The nomogram was generated from measurements of total serum bilirubin in 2840 term and near-term (≤5 weeks) infants eligible for discharge between 24 and 72 hours of age. The predischarge bilirubin assay was performed with the routine metabolic screen at a mean age of 33.7 ± 14.6 SD hours. Postdischarge values were obtained to determine whether the initial measurement was predictive of the natural history of jaundice. This was a highly selected group that excluded many first-day discharges, babies with evidence of rhesus or ABO sensitisation, babies admitted to a SCBU/NICU, and newborns who required phototherapy before the age of 60 hours for a rapidly rising serum bilirubin. A little over 60% of the study population fell into a low-risk category and did not progress to significant jaundice. The remaining patients were in risk zones that were either high risk or they had the potential to move to the high-risk zone from an intermediate-risk zone. The authors suggest targeting these infants for individualised timing of paediatric follow-up. Some cases of kernicterus have been occurring in the USA as a result of a lapse in post-discharge follow-up for 1 to 2 weeks.[39]

In the UK we would like to think that the primary healthcare system provides a safety net for detecting significant post-discharge jaundice, but lessons with respect to good clinical practice can be gained from the hour-specific bilirubin nomogram. An accurate graphical plot of serum bilirubin against time is an essential guide to the rate of rise or fall. Alarm bells should ring in the following circumstances:

- jaundice on day one;
- total serum bilirubin level ≥250 micromol/l by 48 hours;

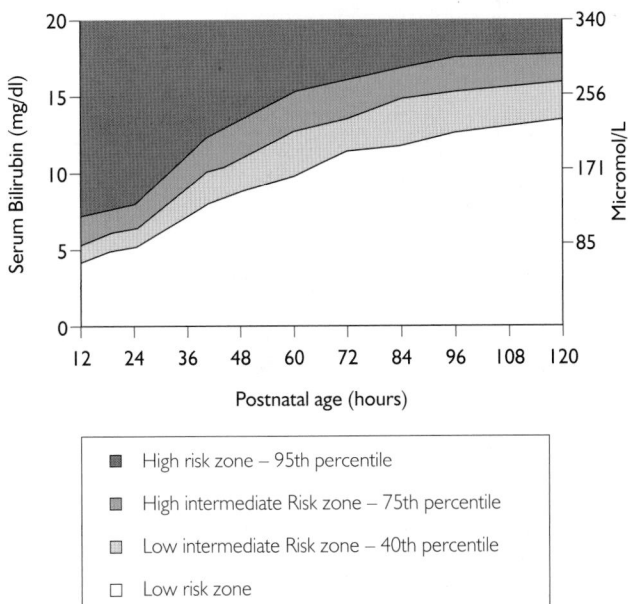

High risk zone – 95th percentile

High intermediate Risk zone – 75th percentile

Low intermediate Risk zone – 40th percentile

Low risk zone

Fig. 29.7 Hour-specific bilirubin values from a group of over 13 000 healthy babies. Note conversion of mg/dl to micromol/l requires multiplication by 17.1. (Adapted from Bhutani et al.[9])

- total serum bilirubin level ≥275 micromol/l by 72 hours;
- total serum bilirubin level ≥300 micromol/l by 96 hours.

No baby should be discharged home in the first week of life with a serum bilirubin level above 300 micromol/l. Moderately preterm babies of 35 and 36 weeks should not be discharged home with bilirubin levels above 275 micromol/l.

Premature infants: total serum bilirubin concentration

Premature infants are considered to be more prone to bilirubin encephalopathy than their full-term counterparts. The greater risk to the preterm brain was overstated in the past by false interpretation of autopsy findings in the so-called 'low-bilirubin kernicterus era' (1965–1982). This was a time when all yellow staining of the basal ganglia merited the description kernicterus, regardless of histological confirmation (Fig. 29.8). Agonal changes in blood–brain barrier permeability to albumin-bound as well as free bilirubin in infants dying from other causes have been implicated in this pattern of staining (Fig. 29.9).

Elevated serum bilirubin levels appear in some studies to be a risk factor for hearing loss in premature babies. The high incidence of bilateral sensorineural deafness in a population of sick very-low-birthweight (VLBW) infants with serum bilirubin levels >240 micromol/l was dramatically reduced when lower thresholds for intervention were adopted.[19,20] Deafness in this population was also shown to correlate with the mean duration of hyperbilirubinaemia. A comparison of clinical antecedents in 15 prematurely born babies (<33 weeks) with sensorineural hearing loss (SNHL) and 30 case-controls failed to identify peak serum bilirubin level or duration of jaundice as being individually associated with SNHL.[64] SNHL was more likely if acidosis occurred when peak bilirubin levels were >200 micromol/l, or if peak bilirubin levels coexisted with aminoglycoside use. The authors concluded that 'the coexistence of risk factors for hearing loss may be more important than the individual factors themselves.'

There have been calls to relax the more aggressive treatment regimens applied to the jaundiced preterm population.[100] The authors base their argument on experience gained in a pre-intensive care era (1950–1965) with relatively more mature (28–36 week gestation) infants, very few of whom were exposed to serum bilirubin levels in excess of 340 micromol/l. False reassurance is also gained from trials conducted against the backdrop of the more interventionalist therapeutic regimens of recent clinical practice. A study relating the neurodevelopmental outcome of preterm infants to their peak serum bilirubin levels failed to demonstrate any causal relationship with cerebral palsy or early developmental delay.[32] However, only three of the 249 preterm infants assessed had serum bilirubin levels greater than 250 micromol/l. The large National Institute of Child Health and Human Development (NICHHD) phototherapy trial failed to demonstrate an association between maximal serum bilirubin level and neurodevelopmental outcome in term or preterm infants.[79] However, the threshold criteria for exchange transfusion had meant that serum bilirubin levels were kept relatively low. A relationship between maximum total serum bilirubin level in the newborn period and cerebral palsy at 2 years of age was reported by van de Bor et al,[95] but the neurological picture was not characteristic of kernicterus and there was no correlation with auditory damage. By 5 years of age, the association between peak bilirubin level and neurological impairment was no longer apparent in the same study population.[94]

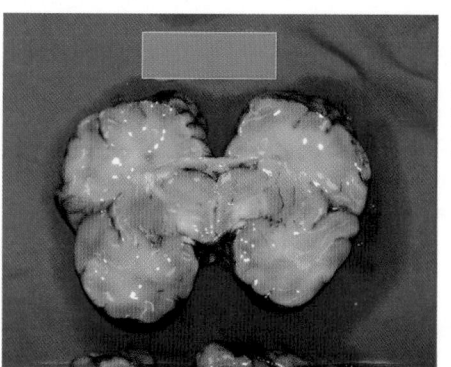

Fig. 29.8 Macroscopic appearance of brain in a term infant with kernicterus.

Markers of bilirubin toxicity

The imprecise relationship between total serum bilirubin levels and adverse neurological outcome has encouraged research seeking to identify more accurate markers of bilirubin toxicity. Assessment of free bilirubin levels, bilirubin binding capacity and brainstem auditory evoked responses has been proposed.[25] These markers may prove of value in research environments, but they are not all universally available, or indeed feasible, in the acute clinical situation. Although free bilirubin assay represents a scientifically more rigorous approach to the jaundiced infant, clinicians have traditionally focused on the total serum bilirubin as the arbiter of treatment thresholds. Correlation of abnormal auditory brainstem responses in infants of 28–32 weeks' gestation has been demonstrated with peak free bilirubin level but not the total bilirubin value in a range of moderate jaundice.[5]

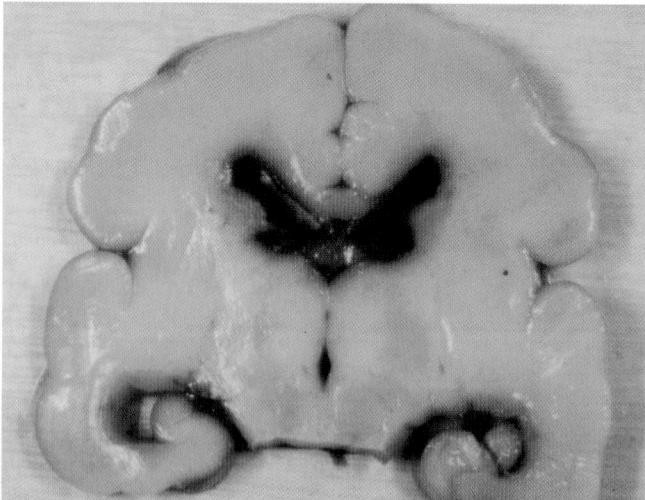

Fig. 29.9 Macroscopic appearance of brain in an ELBW infant with low-bilirubin 'kernicterus'.

More accessible than free bilirubin measurement is the bilirubin/albumin ratio, which acts as an indirect guide to the free bilirubin level. This has also been shown to correlate with abnormal auditory brainstem responses whereas total bilirubin did not.[5] On the basis of unbound bilirubin estimations, Ahlfors[1] has proposed an exchange transfusion threshold at a bilirubin/albumin ratio of 0.8 in the healthy term newborn, 0.72 in a sick term infant and 0.4 for the sick premature infant of <1250 g. Although this ratio has not gained wide clinical acceptance, it may help to inform the decision as to whether or not to perform an exchange transfusion in borderline cases. (Note that when calculating the bilirubin/albumin ratio, values for serum albumin concentration in g/l should be converted to micromol/l using the factor 15.15, as necessary.)

Clinical approach to the diagnosis of the jaundiced infant

Visual inspection

Clinical jaundice becomes apparent at serum bilirubin levels of 80–90 micromol/l, and is observed in the majority of newborns during the first week of life. Significant jaundice of the skin can be missed in black infants, in whom examination of the sclerae and gums may be more informative. Visual assessment is also unreliable under artificial light, and is meaningless once phototherapy has been commenced. If in doubt, measure the bilirubin level.

Newborns jaundiced within 24 hours of birth and all preterms with detectable jaundice, regardless of their postnatal age, should have their serum bilirubin determined. Clinical judgement should be exercised in assessing the need to investigate an otherwise healthy term infant, with no known risk factors, who develops jaundice from day 2 onwards. The cephalocaudal progression of dermal jaundice, which has long been observed,[50] has been validated by transcutaneous bilirubinometry.[48] The dermal zones of jaundice described by Kramer[50] can be used as a rough guide as to when formally to measure the serum bilirubin level in a term infant from day 2 onwards. From Kramer's observations, jaundice limited to the head and neck had an average value of 100 micromol/l with a range of 70 to 130 micromol/l. If dermal jaundice had reached beyond the elbows and knees, but not as far as the hands and feet, an average value of 250 micromol/l was found (range 190–310 micromol/l). Dermal jaundice of the hands and feet calls for formal serum bilirubin estimation, as a value >300 micromol/l is to be anticipated.

Transcutaneous bilirubinometry

Transcutaneous bilirubinometry has a role in screening otherwise healthy term and near-term newborns, provided that a safe threshold (e.g. total bilirubin level >300 micromol/l, or a value within 50 micromol/l of the chosen phototherapy cut-off) is established. Beyond such a value, blood sample assessment of the serum bilirubin level is mandatory. Bertini and Rubaltelli[8] have produced a recent review of the types of instrument available, and the characteristics of their use. A device that measures bilirubin in the skin as opposed to 'yellowness', and which is not confounded by differing racial skin pigmentation, appears to perform well in trial conditions.[76] Transcutaneous jaundice meters should eventually prove cost effective in terms of a reduction in the requirement for invasive measurement of serum bilirubin, and assist in the management of the otherwise healthy jaundiced term and near-term infant, both in hospital and at home. Phototherapy, through its bleaching effect on the skin, precludes the use of transcutaneous bilirubinometry to monitor the progress of treatment under the lights.[89]

Identifying pathological jaundice

Every jaundiced infant should be clinically evaluated to identify underlying pathology and to assess the risk potential for bilirubin encephalopathy. Family, maternal and infant history should be reviewed and the baby examined. Appropriate early investigation aims to identify treatable disease states, such as isoimmunisation, infection, hypothyroidism, biliary atresia and galactosaemia. Clinical features that suggest a pathological cause of jaundice and prompt further investigation are listed in Table 29.2. Many of the more commonly recognised causes of unconjugated hyperbilirubinaemia are listed in Table 29.3. Serum unconjugated bilirubin levels in excess of 300 micromol/l in an otherwise healthy newborn may reflect exaggerated physiological jaundice, but this is a diagnosis of exclusion and the peak bilirubin will still need to be monitored. Unless there are diagnostic pointers to the more rarely encountered causes of neonatal jaundice, stepwise investigation should aim to identify the more common ones first (Table 29.4).

Early-onset jaundice

Jaundice within the first 24 hours of life is likely to be the result of isoimmunisation or other cause of significant haemolysis. In the absence of haemolysis, the rare Crigler–Najjar syndromes should be considered. Urgent investigation is essential (see Table 29.4). Maternal rhesus status and blood group should be sought. The infants of known rhesus-negative mothers are likely to have had cord or postnatal blood sent for a direct antiglobulin test (DAT). The same approach to all infants born to blood group O mothers with the potential for the more frequently encountered ABO incompatibility has been suggested. Despite an ABO incompatibility set-up in 10–15% of pregnancies, the proportion that result in significant haemolysis is small. The finding of a positive DAT is not predictive of the severity of jaundice. A sixth-hour serum bilirubin measurement has been shown to help predict significant hyperbilirubinaemia (if ⩾68 micromol/l) and severe ABO haemolytic disease (if ⩾102 micromol/l) in a population of newborns with the set-up for ABO incompatibility.[77]

Other blood group incompatibilities will usually be known from the maternal history. The Kell group incompatibilities can cause severe haemolytic disease of the newborn, whereas complications of the Duffy, Kidd and other rare blood group systems are usually

Table 29.2 Clinical features that suggest a pathological cause of jaundice in the newborn

Jaundice appearing in the first 24 hours of life
Jaundice in a sick neonate
Total serum bilirubin level
    >250 micromol/l on day 2
    >300 micromol/l thereafter
Rapidly rising serum bilirubin >100 micromol/l/24 h
Prolonged jaundice
    >14 days in term infants
    >21 days in preterm infants
Conjugated serum bilirubin >25 micromol/l
Pale or acholuric stools and dark urine

Table 29.3 Causes of unconjugated jaundice in the newborn

Haemolysis
Isoimmunisation
    Rhesus
    ABO
    Minor blood groups
Other
    Spherocytosis*
    G6PD deficiency
    Pyruvate kinase deficiency†
    Sepsis‡
    Disseminated intravascular coagulation
    α-thalassaemia

Polycythaemia
Small for dates
Twin–twin transfusion
Delayed cord clamping
Maternofetal transfusion
Infant of diabetic mother

Extravasated blood
Bruising, e.g. cephalhaematoma
Pulmonary haemorrhage
Cerebral haemorrhage
Intra-abdominal haemorrhage

Increased enterohepatic circulation
Pyloric stenosis
Bowel obstruction
Swallowed blood

Endocrine/metabolic
Hypothyroidism
Hypopituitarism‡
Hypoadrenalism‡
Glucuronosyl transferase deficiency
Galactosaemia‡
Tyrosinaemia‡
Hypermethioninaemia‡

* and other red cell morphological abnormalities.
† and other red cell enzyme defects.
‡ conjugated jaundice often coexists.

Table 29.4 Investigation of jaundice in the newborn

Early-onset jaundice
Blood group and DCT
Haematocrit and FBC
Blood film and reticulocyte count
Infection screen if indicated
Serology for congenital infections
Urine for CMV culture
Stool for virology
G6PD screen
Red cell enzyme assays

Prolonged jaundice
Total and conjugated serum bilirubin
Thyroid function tests
Urine culture
Urine Clinitest for reducing substances
Liver function tests
α_1-antitrypsin assay and phenotype
Cystic fibrosis DNA screen
Immunoreactive trypsin
Plasma cortisol level
Serum aminoacid screen

less severe. A reticulocyte count of more than 6% after 3 days is suggestive of a haemolytic process, but reticulocyte counts and blood films carry a low sensitivity and specificity for diagnosing haemolysis in the newborn (Newman & Esterling 1994). Heightened carbon monoxide excretion serves as a useful marker of the rate of bilirubin production, being produced in equimolar quantities with bilirubin during haem catabolism. An automated end-tidal carbon monoxide analyser has been evaluated as an early warning device for significant haemolysis,[87] but this technology is yet to make the transition from research to widespread clinical use.

Applying a differential diagnosis to unconjugated jaundice

The maternal record should be checked for documentation of syphilis and hepatitis serology as well as any history suggesting congenital infection. Specific red cell morphological abnormalities, such as spherocytosis, or inborn errors of metabolism, such as galactosaemia or Crigler–Najjar syndrome types I and II, may be implicated from the family history. The jaundice associated with galactosaemia is likely to be predominantly unconjugated in the first week of life. Diagnostic pointers such as hepatomegaly, poor feeding and vomiting should prompt early screening for galactosaemia with urinalysis for non-glucose reducing substances (Clinitest). Urinalysis may provide false-negative and false-positive results in the first few weeks of life. Confirmation of the diagnosis of galactosaemia is made by assessment of erythrocyte galactose-1-phosphate uridyl transferase activity (p. 918).

The Crigler–Najjar syndromes characteristically present in the first few days of life with a rapidly evolving, non-haemolytic, unconjugated hyperbilirubinaemia. The type I disorder results from a complete absence of UDPGT within the hepatocyte, and is inherited in an autosomal recessive manner. Affected individuals frequently require exchange transfusions in the newborn period and nocturnal phototherapy in early childhood. Definitive treatment involves liver transplantation. Crigler–Najjar syndrome type II is a less severe condition in that there is partial UDPGT activity. Inheritance is thought to be autosomal dominant with variable expression, and serum bilirubin levels can be adequately controlled with a UDPGT inducer such as phenobarbital (phenobarbitone).

With parents of Mediterranean, Asian and African ethnicity, the increased likelihood of G6PD deficiency, especially in males, needs to be considered. Screening cord blood for evidence of G6PD deficiency may be appropriate in populations with a high incidence of this condition. It should be remembered that G6PD levels can be falsely elevated in the context of a high reticulocyte count. Marked jaundice may not present in affected babies until 3 to 5 days of age. The differing severity of jaundice probably reflects the variety of isoenzyme deficiencies involved. It is also suggested that the pronounced jaundice in neonates with G6PD deficiency may result from an associated partial defect in bilirubin conjugation.[43] This would be in keeping with end-tidal carbon monoxide measurements that have failed to demonstrate appreciable early haemolysis in such infants.[84] After the newborn period, an affected individual is at risk of haemolytic episodes triggered by a number of common drugs. Parents and family practitioners should be given a list of medications to be avoided (see Table 30.6).

Details of gestational age and evidence of birth asphyxia and trauma may explain heightened or prolonged jaundice. The mode and success of feeding should be noted and assessment made of the infant's state of hydration and weight trend since birth. Examination of the newborn should confirm gestational age and identify growth retardation. Polycythaemia, anaemia, hydrops, purpura and frank bruising should be looked for, along with signs of infection.

A low threshold for performing a full infection screen should be adopted. The set-up for a common blood group incompatibility should not delay consideration of coexisting infection. A full infection screen is not, however, an automatic requirement for cases of hyperbilirubinaemia in otherwise well newborns. No instance of bacterial septicaemia was identified from a study reporting the investigation of over 300 newborns readmitted with a mean peak serum bilirubin level of 316 micromol/l (range 217–498 micromol/l).[61] However, failure of unconjugated hyperbilirubinaemia to respond to phototherapy should alert the clinician to the possibility of infection.[53] A raised component of conjugated bilirubin may also suggest infection.

Prolonged jaundice

Visibly detectable jaundice beyond 2 weeks of age in the term infant and 3 weeks in the preterm is classified as 'prolonged jaundice'. The majority of term infants presenting with prolonged jaundice have an unconjugated hyperbilirubinaemia and will be breastfeeding. Providing there are no features in the history or on clinical examination that suggest a pathological cause (in particular, the urine and stool colour are normal and the baby is thriving),

screening investigations can be safely performed at 3 weeks of age. At that stage, the following first-phase tests are appropriate:

- total and conjugated serum bilirubin;
- full blood count;
- examination of blood film if haemolysis is suspected;
- thyroid function tests if result of heel-prick TSH screen is not known;
- urinalysis for reducing sugars (Clinitest);
- urinalysis for evidence of infection.

Further tests (see Table 29.4 and Chapter 29, Part 2) will be indicated according to the outcome of this initial screen. Greater urgency and a more direct approach to specific investigations are necessary in cases where a specific pathology, such as biliary atresia, is suspected.

Neonatal cholestasis (conjugated jaundice)

Definitions of conjugated hyperbilirubinaemia vary. Serum conjugated bilirubin levels of above 25 or 30 micromol/l are commonly adopted cut-offs; with an alternative being to allow a value of up 10% of the total serum bilirubin. Pale or acholuric stools and dark bile-stained urine are the clinical markers of established conjugated jaundice, but neither may be present in the first weeks of many hepatic disease states, including biliary atresia. The absence of bilirubin in the urine on early testing may also be falsely reassuring because the renal threshold for conjugated bilirubin may only be reached at 40 micromol/l.

Diagnosis of any associated clotting abnormality and its correction are urgent requirements in the infant with conjugated jaundice. Several conditions present with a mixture of raised unconjugated and conjugated bilirubin. Notable amongst these are the intrauterine infections, bacterial sepsis, galactosaemia, aminoacidaemias and congenital hypopituitarism. Some of the causes of conjugated hyperbilirubinaemia are listed in Table 29.5, and the initial investigations are found in Table 29.4.

If an obstructive aetiology is suspected, liver ultrasound and a hepatobiliary scan will be indicated. Visualisation of the gallbladder on ultrasound does not rule out biliary atresia. The importance of making an early diagnosis of biliary atresia and its prompt referral to a centre specialising in the medical and surgical management of childhood liver disorders cannot be overstated. McKiernan[59] has provided a recent practical approach to investigation and management of neonatal cholestasis, and conjugated hyperbilirubinaemia is further detailed in Chapter 29, Part 2.

Clinical management of the jaundiced infant

Invasive measurement of bilirubin

Laboratory measurement of bilirubin to determine the total and direct bilirubin is not a straightforward assay. Inter-laboratory variability in results from standard solutions have been disconcerting,

Table 29.5 Causes of conjugated jaundice in the newborn

Prolonged parenteral nutrition
Idiopathic neonatal cholestasis
Perinatal asphyxia
Severe haemolysis, e.g. erythroblastosis
Bacterial sepsis
Intrauterine infections
    Toxoplasmosis
    Rubella
    Cytomegalovirus
    Herpes simplex
    Coxsackie and other viruses
Biliary atresia
Choledochal cyst
Spontaneous bile duct perforation
Intrahepatic biliary hypoplasia (Alagille's)
α_1-antitrypsin deficiency
Cystic fibrosis
Progressive familial intrahepatic cholestasis
Inspissated bile plug syndrome
Galactosaemia
Tyrosinaemia

Table 29.6 Unconjugated jaundice: modes of treatment

Phototherapy
Exchange transfusion
Pharmacological agents
    Competitive inhibition of haem oxygenase
    Suppression of isoimmune haemolysis
    Induction of hepatic conjugation
    Inhibition of enterohepatic recirculation of bilirubin

but, more recently, assay precision has been improved by the use of commercial reagents and automated methodology.

For practical purposes, a bilirubinometer employing direct spectrometry is used in many neonatal units to provide rapid estimation of total serum bilirubin. It should be remembered that such instruments reflect the sum value of all species of bilirubin, conjugated and unconjugated, including photoisomers. Significant errors can arise from incorrect spectrometer use and poor maintenance. Failure by the operator to note that serum specimens are grossly lipaemic, or that the outside of the capillary tube or cuvette is dirty, will give misleading results. Instrument calibration and attention to regular quality control are necessary to provide early warning of machine drift. The bilirubinometer used should be accurate to within ±30 or ideally ±20 micromol/l, and the limitations of spectrometry should be known. Some devices are very inaccurate above values of bilirubin of 450 micromol/l, and show a 'flattening-off' with little incremental response for values >500 micromol/l. It is customary to confirm pre-exchange transfusion values of total serum bilirubin with a laboratory measurement, but transfusion should not be delayed if this service is not readily available.

Treatment

The different modes of treatment of unconjugated jaundice are shown in Table 29.6. The two established approaches are phototherapy and exchange transfusion. A number of drug therapies have been shown to modify neonatal jaundice, but have not entered routine clinical practice. It is essential that any infant undergoing treatment for jaundice should be adequately investigated for the cause. Unconjugated hyperbilirubinaemia that is judged to be above treatment thresholds, but below those that prompt immediate exchange transfusion, is most commonly controlled using phototherapy. A lack of response to adequate phototherapy may imply significant underlying haemolysis, necessitating exchange transfusion. An infant with a total serum bilirubin level that is rising towards or has already reached/exceeded an exchange transfusion threshold should have blood urgently cross-matched for the procedure. This is a neonatal emergency and an appropriate response time from the local transfusion service should be established and audited.

Phototherapy

Observation of the effect of sunlight on the serum bilirubin level of premature infants nursed outdoors prompted the first use of a 'cradle illumination machine' by Cremer et al.[15] It took a decade for phototherapy to gain clinical acceptance throughout the world, and a further 12 years before its mode of action started to be unravelled (see pp. 674–8).[57] Phototherapy of itself has not influenced neurodevelopmental outcome or cognitive performance in recipients,[78,83] but it remains a convenient and safe means of lowering serum bilirubin. Most importantly, phototherapy reduces the need for the more hazardous alternative, namely exchange transfusion. Optimal use of phototherapy in preterm physiological jaundice has made the need to resort to exchange transfusion in that context a rarity.

Phototherapy's ease of use has encouraged its overuse. Many infants are 'placed under the lights' unnecessarily or treated for too long. The vogue for 'prophylactic' phototherapy from birth in VLBW infants has been shown to neither reduce the peak nor shorten the duration of their jaundice.[16] Phototherapy would only appear to be effective as bilirubin enters the skin at serum levels >80 micromol/l.[88] Similarly, a small study randomising term infants with physiological jaundice to receive phototherapy at a threshold of either 250 or 320 micromol/l failed to demonstrate any significant difference in peak serum bilirubin levels between the two groups.[52]

The maximal effect of phototherapy is during the first 24–48 hours of its use. It is to be anticipated that, in the absence of haemolysis, phototherapy will reduce the serum bilirubin level by 25% to 50% during this initial phase. It has been suggested that the enterohepatic circulation of bilirubin-ZZ, reconstituted from configurational photoisomers in bile, causes the subsequent decay in response. Even without an impact on the serum bilirubin level, it is of reassurance that within a matter of hours of commencing phototherapy up to a fifth of the circulating bilirubin has been detoxified in the form of configurational photoisomers.[24]

Phototherapy has a benign reputation but it is not without side effects. The more commonly encountered are:

- diarrhoea;
- increased fluid loss via the skin;
- temperature instability;
- erythematous rashes;
- tanning;
- bronze baby syndrome.

The diarrhoea asssociated with phototherapy is thought to result from an irritant effect of photoisomers on the bowel. This and increased insensible water loss from the skin require attention to fluid balance. A general prescription of additional fluid is often used in these circumstances, but individualised assessment of fluid requirements, especially in the premature or sicker infant, is to be advised. Close attention to thermoregulation is also important, with the risks of cooling from surface exposure and overheating from standard phototherapy lamps. Nursing care should include regular monitoring of the infant's temperature, documentation of stool frequency and urine output, and a daily assessment of weight. The eyes of an infant receiving lamp phototherapy should be shielded to prevent potential retinal damage.[65] In-vitro evidence of light-induced DNA damage, particularly in the presence of bilirubin,[75] has not been mirrored by skin damage in clinical experience with newborns or from long-term phototherapy in children with Crigler–Najjar syndrome. The bronze baby syndrome results from an interaction between cholestatic jaundice and phototherapy.[72] The brown pigment produced (bilifuscin) stains the infant's skin and lingers for some weeks after phototherapy has been discontinued.

The recently developed fibreoptic systems for delivering phototherapy via a body pad or wrap have made its application more versatile. These devices are likely to gain greater acceptance in the context of healthy term infants nursed without eye pads and alongside their mothers. Trials have shown fibreoptic phototherapy to be as effective as conventional phototherapy in preterm infants, but less so in term infants.[66] A new generation of phototherapy unit has evolved using the technology of multiple light-emitting diodes (LEDs). These have the advantage of not emitting infrared or ultraviolet radiation, and so can be used closer to the infant's skin for maximal efficacy without the risk of burning.[81]

Optimal use of phototherapy

The efficacy of phototherapy depends on the dose and wavelength of light used and the proportion of the infant's surface area to which it is applied. The dose of phototherapy administered is expressed in terms of spectral irradiance ($\mu W/cm^2/nm$). Before the mode of action of phototherapy was better understood, it was thought that saturation of dose–response occurred within the blue light range at a spectral irradiance of $4 \mu W/cm^2/nm$. This is true of the configurational isomer bilirubin-Z,E. However, production of the most important photoisomer, lumirubin, has a dose–response relationship that does not attain saturation until a spectral irradiance of 25 to $30 \mu W/cm^2/nm$ is achieved.[24] Increasing the dose of phototherapy is most readily achieved by operating the light source at the minimum recommended safe distance from the infant.

Early phototherapy lights were designed to emit blue light at a wavelength of around 450 nm, in keeping with the maximal absorbance of bilirubin. Pure blue light is poorly tolerated by staff and can mask cyanosis in an infant. Combinations of broad-spectrum white light and blue light have proved more acceptable. There are theoretical reasons why green light delivered at high irradiance would be the most efficient choice. Compared with blue light, green preferentially favours formation of lumirubin, the main excretory photoisomer, and its longer wavelength enhances skin penetration.[23,24] The efficiency of treatment can also be improved by using more than one phototherapy lamp or by combining conventional lamps with a fibreoptic system. Double or multiple phototherapy applied to a greater proportion of the body surface area should be adopted in cases of severe jaundice, and especially in the instance of awaiting blood for an urgent exchange transfusion. With less severe jaundice, it may be safe to use intermittent phototherapy. Parents should be reassured that in taking their baby out of the lights for feeds and cuddles they are not jeopardising treatment. The fact that it takes up to 3 hours for bilirubin to return to the skin following removal of photoisomers has prompted intermittent phototherapy regimens based on 1 in 4 hours' exposure to lights. Claims that such regimens are equally effective as continuous phototherapy are based on experience with moderate physiological jaundice.[51] Jaundice that has reached a level that is within 50 micromol/l of the exchange transfusion threshold should be treated with continuous phototherapy.

Pharmacological agents

The use of synthetic metalloporphyrins to reduce bilirubin production through competitive inhibition of haem oxygenase has been an interesting development.[101] Tin protoporphyrin has been used to modify the course of hyperbilirubinaemia in ABO isoimmunisation.[45] Similarly, tin mesoporphyrin has been shown to supplant the need for phototherapy in term and near-term newborns with physiological jaundice,[44] and to significantly reduce phototherapy requirements in preterms.[93] These agents are likely to find a role in the treatment of forms of significant pathological jaundice, such as G6PD deficiency,[92] particularly in parts of the world where conventional management with phototherapy and exchange transfusion is less readily available. Whether they are destined to revolutionise our management of most forms of neonatal jaundice will depend on their safety profile over time.

Another preventative therapy that may be of benefit to newborns presenting with severe rhesus or ABO isoimmunisation is early administration of high-dose intravenous immunoglobulin (HDIVIG). Treatment of these conditions with HDIVIG has been shown to significantly reduce the need for exchange transfusion, the duration of phototherapy and the length of hospital stay.[30] A single 0.5 g/kg dose of IVIG on day 1, as soon as the diagnosis of haemolysis is made, appears to be beneficial. Patients treated with HDIVIG using current dosage regimens are more likely to require top-up red cell transfusions for late anaemia. One group advocates the use of recombinant erythropoietin in this context.[73] The optimum treatment dose of HDIVIG and whether or not further benefit is to be gained from repeat doses remain to be established. If HDIVIG attains a licence for such use, clinicians may need to consider the relative risks of transfusion-transmitted diseases and the complications of exchange transfusion in their practice.

Induction of hepatic conjugation and agents that decrease the enterohepatic recirculation of bilirubin have been studied, but are not currently recommended. These and other potential therapies and their side effects are covered in a recent review.[18]

Exchange transfusion

The practicalities of performing an exchange transfusion are covered elsewhere (Chapter 45). The indications for an exchange transfusion vary according to the underlying condition. In cases where there has been severe in-utero haemolysis, early exchange, irrespective of the bilirubin level, may be required to correct anaemia and to remove sensitised red cells. Previous guidelines based on cord blood values rarely apply, as most infants with severe erythroblastosis will have received in-utero transfusion. The timing of their last top-up and a Kleihauer estimation of the proportion of circulating fetal red cells are more likely to be predictive of the need for an early exchange. Many such infants respond to intensive phototherapy followed by a later top-up transfusion. If, despite double phototherapy, the serum bilirubin continues to rise by more than 10 micromol/l/h, exchange transfusion is to be anticipated. Whilst it would appear logical to keep the serum albumin level of a jaundiced infant within the normal range,[1] there is no agreement as to whether the practice of giving albumin before or during an exchange transfusion confers any benefit.[18]

In addition to a low risk of blood-borne infection, exchange transfusion carries a significant risk of morbidity and mortality from vascular accidents, cardiac complications and biochemical or haematological disturbance.[47] This is especially the case in sick premature newborns.[38] The mortality rate from the procedure is often quoted as being around 0.3%. This figure originates from a well-conducted trial[78] performed during an era when exchange transfusion was more commonly performed. Exchange transfusions are now rarely required, and so with dwindling practical expertise, the procedure is likely to have become more hazardous.

Exchange transfusion will remain necessary for infants who fail to respond to adequate phototherapy or who present late with bilirubin levels in excess of a given exchange value. In the latter case, the infant should be placed under multiple phototherapy, pending the availability of blood for the exchange. Attention should also be paid to correcting disturbances of hydration or acid–base balance, and to the treatment of any underlying infection. Signs and symptoms characteristic of acute bilirubin encephalopathy are an absolute indication for exchange transfusion.

Guidelines for the use of phototherapy and exchange transfusion

Infants with haemolysis or Crigler–Najjar syndrome

Kernicterus has been virtually eradicated by the adoption of thresholds for exchange transfusion taken from early experience

with severe erythroblastosis, and by the pre-emptive use of phototherapy to prevent, whenever possible, the exchange threshold being attained. Two groups of term-born infants would appear to remain at greater risk from bilirubin toxicity, i.e. newborns with haemolysis, and those born with Crigler–Najjar syndrome. It is prudent to maintain our respect for a total bilirubin level of 20 mg/dl (342 micromol/l) as being the indication for exchange transfusion in these patient groups, with phototherapy having been instituted at values of 200 micromol/l.

Premature infants

Formerly, no distinction was made between the thresholds for treatment of jaundiced term and preterm infants. Recognition that preterm newborns are at higher risk of bilirubin toxicity has given rise to sliding scales prompting earlier intervention on the basis of birthweight or gestational age. There are recommendations of a single treatment protocol for all preterms,[21] but it appears logical to have a greater margin for error in the lower gestation infant. Sick LBW newborns are more likely to have been exposed to a number of risk factors that increase their susceptibility to bilirubin toxicity, such as hypoxia, acidosis, hypercarbia, sepsis and hypoalbuminaemia. The counter argument holds that it may be beneficial to leave a premature infant with a moderate degree of jaundice to take advantage of bilirubin's antioxidant properties.[102]

An example of a sliding scale of bilirubin values for intervention in preterm newborns based on gestation is shown in Table 29.7. Phototherapy should be commenced in all preterm infants who become clinically jaundiced within the first 24 hours. Investigation of the cause of jaundice and assessment of the need for an early exchange transfusion are urgent considerations. From the second day onwards, it is recommended that phototherapy and exchange transfusion are considered if the serum bilirubin has reached the values shown in Table 29.7. Practice in the USA has tended to adopt birthweight categories for the sliding scale of treatment thresholds in the premature infant, and the guidelines are less interventional. An example is provided by Cashore,[12] reproduced as Table 29.8 after conversion of bilirubin values to micromol/l. The author provides a disclaimer to these guidelines by stating that 'these suggested levels for therapeutic intervention have not been validated by autopsy findings.' It is also suggested that 'exchange transfusion is preferred for rapid increases in bilirubin owing to haemolytic states.' On current evidence, calls to relax such an approach to the jaundiced preterm population any further[100] should be resisted.[37]

Term infants

Over the past 10–15 years, most paediatricians caring for healthy jaundiced newborns in the UK have been willing participants in a cautious relaxation of the threshold for phototherapy from 250 micromol/l to 300–350 micromol/l, and for exchange transfusion from 340 micromol/l to 400–450 micromol/l. How much further can this shift in practice be taken without placing such infants at greater risk of bilirubin toxicity? Newman and Maisels[70]

Table 29.7 Guidelines for treatment of preterms with phototherapy and exchange transfusion

Gestational age	Serum bilirubin concentration (micromol/l)		
	Phototherapy	Exchange transfusion	
		Sick*	Well
36 weeks	250	300	350
32 weeks	150	250	300
28 weeks	100	200	250
24 weeks	80	150	200

* Rhesus disease, perinatal asphyxia, hypoxia, acidosis, hypercapnia

Table 29.8 Phototherapy and exchange transfusion in VLBW and ELBW infants[12]

Weight (g)	Total bilirubin (micromol/l)	
	Start phototherapy	Consider exchange transfusion
500–750	85–135	205–255
750–1000	100–170	>255
1000–1250	135–170	255–305
1250–1500	170–205	290–340

Table 29.9 Newman & Maisels' treatment regimens for full-term infants[70]

Treatment	Total bilirubin level (micromol/l)	
	Well baby, no haemolysis	Haemolysis likely or sick
Phototherapy	300–375	225–300
Exchange transfusion	425–500	300–400

and Maisels,[70] was incorporated in a 'practice parameter' issued by a subcommittee of the American Academy of Pediatrics.[3] A summary of the AAP recommendations for the management of hyperbilirubinaemia in the healthy term newborn is shown in Table 29.10.

Most treatment guidelines rely on total bilirubin level, but, faced with the decision as to whether or not to perform an exchange transfusion, it is tempting (and may appear logical) to subtract the conjugated component. On the basis of unnerving case reports, others recommend the more cautious approach of not subtracting the direct bilirubin concentration from the total until it reaches 50%.[60] When considering an exchange transfusion in a baby receiving phototherapy, should allowance also be made for the fact that up to one-fifth of the circulating bilirubin pool may be in the form of non-toxic photoisomers? This practice could be hazardous, because the accuracy of such an assumption depends on the duration and efficiency of phototherapy provided.

In general, the best standard of care is to agree on a set of guidelines for phototherapy and exchange transfusion in healthy and sick, term and preterm infants in line with current-day practice, and to stick by them. As thresholds for exchange transfusion are relaxed, the margin for error is diminished. Failure to perform an exchange at a recommended or agreed therapy threshold will be difficult to defend if the infant goes on to develop bilirubin encephalopathy and kernictus.

carried out an extensive review of the topic and proposed new treatment regimens for full-term infants, as summarised in Table 29.9. The wide ranges of bilirubin values chosen were 'intended to encourage individualisation of treatment, taking preferences and biases of the parent and pediatrician into account'. When such 'preference' or 'bias' dictates that an infant's serum bilirubin level may be allowed to reach 500 micromol/l, it should be acknowledged that the evidence supporting the safety of such practice is sparse beyond bilirubin levels of 425 micromol/l. In the case of babies with proven or suspected haemolysis or who are otherwise sick, Newman and Maisels[70] maintain a more conventional range for exchange transfusion at bilirubin levels between 300 and 400 micromol/l. They suggest use of the lower end of this range for infants with severe haemolysis or who are sick for other reasons, and values closer to 400 micromol/l for equivocal cases, such as breastfeeding babies with ABO incompatibility and positive direct antiglobulin test but no anaemia.

The fact that healthy term babies appear to tolerate higher levels of bilirubin than their haemolysing or sick contemporaries has prompted calls for a more relaxed approach to the management of their jaundice from day 2 or 3 onwards. It should, however, be appreciated that in adopting the description 'healthy term infant' one is assuming that screening investigations (e.g. G6PD deficiency) are likely to prove negative. Similarly, at the time of presentation it is not known whether there is any contribution from Gilbert's syndrome or other genetic variable that may contribute to the severity of hyperbilirubinaemia.[98] The so-called 'kinder, gentler approach' to the jaundiced term infant, proposed by Newman

The benefits of a 'kinder, gentler approach' to jaundice treatment

The AAP 'practice parameter'[3] was considered too lax by some and too stringent by others, but applied to otherwise healthy full-term infants it has been associated in parts of the USA with a decrease in the use of phototherapy by more than 50% and of exchange transfusion by 87%.[82] The lessening of transfusion-associated morbidity and mortality is to be welcomed. It has been estimated that in the USA an increase in the exchange transfusion threshold from 340 micromol/l to 425 micromol/l in healthy term infants will have saved approximately 200 lives each year from procedural complications.[97] However, in terms of bilirubin neurotoxicity, the safety of this more relaxed approach to neonatal jaundice has yet to be verified. Some reassurance is gained from the fact that cases of kernicterus have not been reported in infant populations managed with strict adherence to the AAP 'practice parameter' or similar guidelines.[69,97]

Table 29.10 Management of jaundice in the healthy term newborn: American Academy of Pediatrics Guidelines 1994

Age (h)	Total serum bilirubin level (micromol/l)			
	Consider phototherapy	**Phototherapy**	**Exchange if intensive phototherapy fails***	**Exchange and intensive phototherapy**
25–48	⩾170	⩾260	⩾340	⩾430
49–72	⩾260	⩾310	⩾430	⩾510
>72	⩾290	⩾340	⩾430	⩾510

* Failure of intensive phototherapy to reduce serum bilirubin by 17 to 34 micromol/l within 4 to 6 h. (Reproduced from American Academy of Pediatrics Provisional Committee for Quality Improvement and Subcommittee on Hyperbilirubinemia.[3])

Why are we witnessing a resurgence of kernicterus?

One group of infants that the AAP 'practice parameter'[3] may fail to identify for investigation or early treatment are those infants discharged within 24 hours in whom day-1 jaundice was not apparent or had not been recognised.[22,39,62] Other cases of kernicterus that are occurring against the backdrop of the AAP 'practice parameter' are the result of failure to heed the exclusion criteria, such as clinical jaundice within 24 hours of life, prematurity, evidence of haemolysis or a sick infant. There is evidence that the guidelines are being 'stretched' to apply to treatment in near-term infants with gestational ages of 35 weeks and above[82] and amongst term infants the recommended phototherapy thresholds are not being adhered to.[6] The AAP Subcommittee on Hyperbilirubinaemia has revised its 'practice parameter' by issuing warnings on risk factors for severe jaundice and the clinical pitfalls that may result in kernicterus.[4]

Registering cases of kernicterus

A pilot kernicterus registry for term and near-term infants 'discharged as healthy from their place of birth' was established in the USA in 1992.[39] The level of case ascertainment and state coverage of this registry does not allow the authors to generate information on the national incidence of kernicterus. However, Johnson et al[39] are able to derive clinical pointers and have drawn some important lessons from the 61 infants who required medical intervention in the first week of life for hyperbilirubinaemia, with or without acute signs of kernicterus. All but two of the 61 infants were breastfed, and the two formula-fed infants turned out to be G6PD deficient. The median age at discharge was 1.5 days (range 12–72 hours), and 18 were discharged at ⩽1 day. The registry does not include cases of rhesus sensitisation. The cause of jaundice designated in the 61 infants was as follows: idiopathic (n = 19), G6PD deficiency (undiagnosed before hospital readmission; n = 19), haemolysis (n = 10), extensive bruising (n = 6), systemic infection (n = 4), Crigler–Najjar syndrome (n = 2) and galactosaemia (n = 1).

This work provides a valuable insight into some of the causes of kernicterus in the USA, and of the pitfalls of what appears to have been an unstructured system of paediatric follow-up. The infants were born between 1984 and 2001, and so the recommendation of a follow-up appointment within 2–3 days of early discharge (⩽48 hours of age) as advised by the 1994 AAP practice parameter only applies to the younger third of the cohort. The authors recommend a universal predischarge total serum bilirubin measurement plotted on an hour-specific bilirubin nomogram[9] to help customise the appropriate timing of follow-up appointments. They also call for a national (USA) registry reporting all infants with a total serum bilirubin value ⩾340 micromol/l at <72 hours of age and >425 micromol/l at >72 hours of age.

The British Paediatric Surveillance Unit (BPSU) is currently inviting case reporting throughout the UK and the Republic of Ireland of infants with an unconjugated serum bilirubin level ⩾510 micromol/l in the first month of life (D Manning, personal communication, 2003). The aims are to establish the incidence, causes and consequences of severe hyperbilirubinaemia. Lessons on clinical management are also likely to be generated by this study.

Current dilemmas in the management of jaundice

The potential danger of a move to a more relaxed attitude to jaundice in the healthy term infant, at the same time that the majority of newborns are at home by 24–48 hours of age, may be that of delaying the diagnosis in cases of more sinister jaundice. Heightened awareness of aspects of the history and clinical examination that suggest the likelihood of severe jaundice need to be maintained. Failure to do so may result in more infants being readmitted with bilirubin levels at or above exchange levels with conditions such as ABO incompatibility and G6PDH deficiency.[39,58]

There are inherent dangers in simply translating jaundice management protocols from one country to another without taking into account the differences in healthcare infrastructure.

This relates especially to arrangements for follow-up in the community. In the UK the responsibility for detecting significant post-discharge jaundice rests with the primary healthcare team of midwives, health visitors, general practitioners and, of course, informed parents. The BPSU survey may tell us whether this early warning system is sufficiently robust in the UK. If it proves not to be, we may need to consider the type of predictive testing being proposed in the USA,[9] and more objective community screening with one of the new generation of transcutaneous bilirubinometers.[76]

Useful resource

www.pickonline.org/parentsinfo.html

Parents of infants and children with kernicterus resource centre: has useful information and links, with videos of affected children.

References

1. Ahlfors C E 1994 Criteria for exchange transfusion in jaundiced newborns. Pediatrics 93: 488–494
2. Alonso E M, Whitington P F, Whitington S H et al 1991 Enterohepatic circulation of non-conjugated bilirubin in rats fed with human milk. Journal of Pediatrics 118: 425–430
3. American Academy of Pediatrics Provisional Committee for Quality Improvement and Subcommittee on Hyperbilirubinemia 1994 Practice parameter: management of hyperbilirubinemia in the healthy term newborn. Pediatrics 94: 558–565
4. American Academy of Pediatrics Subcommittee on Hyperbilirubinemia 2001 Neonatal jaundice and kernicterus. Pediatrics 108: 763–765
5. Amin S B, Ahlfors C, Orlando M S et al 2001 Auditory brainstem response and bilirubin binding in premature infants. Pediatrics 107: 664–670
6. Atkinson L R, Escobar G J, Takayama J I, Newman T B 2003 Phototherapy use in jaundiced newborns in a large managed care organization: do clinicians adhere to the guideline? Pediatrics 111(5 Pt 1): e555–e561
7. Bertini G, Dani C, Tronchin M et al 2001 Is breast-feeding really favoring early neonatal jaundice? Pediatrics 107(3): e41
8. Bertini G, Rubaltelli F F 2002 Non-invasive bilirubinometry in neonatal jaundice. Seminars in Neonatology 7: 129–133
9. Bhutani V K, Johnson L, Sivieri E M 1999 Predictive ability of a predischarge hour-specific serum bilirubin for subsequent significant hyperbilirubinaemia in healthy term and near-term newborns. Pediatrics 103: 6–14
10. Brodersen R, Stern L 1990 Deposition of bilirubin acid in the central nervous system: a hypothesis for the development of kernicterus. Acta Paediatrica Scandinavica 79: 12–19
11. Burgess G H, Oh W, Bratlid D et al 1985 The effects of brain blood flow on brain bilirubin deposition in newborn piglets. Pediatric Research 19: 691–696
12. Cashore W J 2000 Bilirubin and jaundice in the micropremie. Clinics in Perinatology 27: 171–179
13. Connolly A M, Volpe J J 1990 Clinical features of bilirubin encephalopathy. Clinics in Perinatology 17: 371–379
14. Crawford J M, Howsser S C, Gollan J L 1988 Formation, hepatic metabolism, and transport of bile pigments: a status report. Seminars in Liver Disease 8: 105–118
15. Cremer R J, Perryman P W, Richards D H 1958 Influence of light on the hyperbilirubinaemia of infants. Lancet i: 1094–1097
16. Curtis-Cohen M, Stahl G E, Costarino A T et al 1985 Randomized trial of prophylactic phototherapy in the infant with very low birth weight. Journal of Pediatrics 107: 121–124
17. De Carvalho M, Hall M, Harvey D 1981 Effects of water supplementation on physiological jaundice in breast-fed babies. Archives of Disease in Childhood 56: 568–569
18. Dennery P A 2002 Pharmacological interventions for the treatment of neonatal jaundice. Seminars in Neonatology 7: 111–119
19. DeVries L S, Lary S, Dubowitz L M S 1985 Relationship of serum bilirubin levels to ototoxicity and deafness in high-risk low birth-weight infants. Pediatrics 76: 351–354
20. DeVries L S, Lary S, Whitelaw A G et al 1987 Relationship of serum bilirubin levels and hearing impairment in newborn infants. Early Human Development 15: 269–277
21. Dodd K L 1993 Neonatal jaundice – a lighter touch. Archives of Disease in Childhood 68: 529–533
22. Ebbesen F 2000 Recurrence of kernicterus in term and near-term infants in Denmark. Acta Paediatrica 89: 1213–1217
23. Ennever J F 1990 Blue light, green light, white light, more light: treatment of neonatal jaundice. Clinics in Perinatology 17: 467–481
24. Ennever J F 1992 Phototherapy for neonatal jaundice. In: Polin R A, Fox W W (eds) Fetal and neonatal physiology. W B Saunders, Philadelphia, pp 1165–1173
25. Funato M, Tamai H, Shimada S et al 1994 Vigintiphobia, unbound bilirubin, and auditory brainstem responses. Pediatrics 93: 50–53
26. Gale R, Seidman D S, Dollberg S et al 1990 Epidemiology of neonatal jaundice in the Jerusalem population. Journal of Pediatric Gastroenterology and Nutrition 10: 82–86
27. Gartner L M 1994 Neonatal jaundice. Pediatrics in Review 15: 422–432
28. Gartner L M 2001 Breastfeeding and jaundice. Journal of Perinatology 21(suppl. 1): S25–S29
29. Gartner L M, Lee K-S, Vaisman S et al 1977 Development of bilirubin transport and metabolism in the newborn rhesus monkey. Journal of Pediatrics 90: 513–531
30. Gottstein R, Cooke R W I 2003 Systematic review of intravenous immunoglobulin in haemolytic disease of the newborn. Archives of Disease in Childhood. Fetal and Neonatal Edition 88: F6–F10
31. Gourley G R 2002 Breast-feeding, neonatal jaundice and kernicterus. Seminars in Neonatology 7: 135–141
32. Graziani L J, Mitchell D G, Kornhauser M et al 1992 Neurodevelopment of preterm infants: neonatal neurosonographic and serum bilirubin studies. Pediatrics 89: 229–234
33. Hanko E, Lindemann R, Hansen T W R 2001 Spectrum of outcome in infants with extreme neonatal jaundice. Acta Paediatrica 90: 782–785
34. Hansen T W R 1995 Kernicterus in a full-term infant: the need for increased vigilance (letter). Pediatrics 95: 798–799
35. Hansen T W R 2001 Bilirubin brain toxicity. Journal of Perinatology 21(suppl. 1): S48–S51
36. Hansen T W R 2002 Kernicterus: an international perspective. Seminars in Neonatology 7: 103–109
37. Ives N K 1992 Kernicterus in preterm infants: lest we forget (to turn on the lights). Pediatrics 90: 757–759
38. Jackson J C 1997 Adverse events associated with exchange transfusion in healthy and ill newborns. Pediatrics 99: E7
39. Johnson L H, Bhutani V K, Brown A K 2002 System-based approach to management of neonatal jaundice and prevention of kernicterus. Journal of Pediatrics 104: 396–403
40. Johnson L H, Brown A K, Bhutani V K 1999 BIND – a clinical score for bilirubin induced neurologic dysfunction in newborns. Pediatrics 104: 746–747
41. Kadakol A, Sappal B S, Ghosh S S et al 2001 Interaction of coding region mutations and the Gilbert-type promoter abnormality of the UGT1A1 gene causes moderate degrees of unconjugated hyperbilirubinaemia and may lead to neonatal kernicterus. Journal of Medical Genetics 38: 244–249
42. Kaplan M 2001 Genetic interactions in the pathogenesis of neonatal hyperbilirubinaemia: Gilbert's syndrome and glucose-6-phosphate dehydrogenase deficiency. Journal of Perinatology 21(suppl. 1): S30–S34
43. Kaplan M, Hammerman C 2002 Glucose-6-phosphate dehydrogense deficiency: a potential source of severe neonatal hyperbilirubinaemia and kernicterus. Seminars in Neonatology 7: 121–128
44. Kappas A, Drummond G S, Henschke C et al 1995 Direct comparison of Sn-mesoporphyrin, an inhibitor of bilirubin production, and phototherapy in controlling hyperbilirubinemia in term and near-term newborns. Pediatrics 95: 468–474
45. Kappas A, Drummond G S, Manola T et al 1988 Sn-protoporphyrin use in the management of hyperbilirubinemia in term newborns with direct Coombs'-positive ABO incompatibility. Pediatrics 81: 485–497
46. Kawade N, Onishi S 1981 The prenatal and postnatal development of UDP-glucuronyl transferase activity toward bilirubin and the effect of premature birth on this activity in the human liver. Biochemical Journal 196: 257–260
47. Keenan W J, Novak K K, Sutherland J M et al 1985 Morbidity and mortality associated with exchange transfusion. Pediatrics 75(suppl): 417–421

48. Knudsen A 1990 The cephalocaudal progression of jaundice in newborns in relation to the transfer of bilirubin from plasma to skin. Early Human Development 22: 23–28

49. Knudsen A, Lebech M 1989 Maternal bilirubin, cord bilirubin and placental function at delivery in the development of neonatal jaundice in mature newborns. Acta Obstetricia et Gynecologica Scandinavica 68: 719–724

50. Kramer L I 1969 Advancement of dermal icterus in the jaundiced newborn. American Journal of Diseases of Children 118: 454–458

51. Lau S P, Fung K P 1984 Serum bilirubin kinetics in intermittent phototherapy of physiological jaundice. Archives of Disease in Childhood 59: 892–894

52. Lewis H M, Campbell R H A, Hambleton G 1982 Abuse of phototherapy for physiological jaundice of newborn infants. Lancet ii: 408–410

53. Linder N, Yatsiv I, Tsur M et al 1988 Unexplained neonatal jaundice as an early diagnostic sign of septicemia in the newborn. Journal of Perinatology 8: 325–327

54. Lucas A, Baker B A 1986 Breast milk jaundice in premature infants. Archives of Disease in Childhood 61: 1063–1067

55. McDonagh A F 1990 Is bilirubin good for you? Clinics in Perinatology 17: 359–369

56. McDonagh A F, Lightner D A 1985 "Like a shrivelled blood orange": bilirubin, jaundice and phototherapy. Pediatrics 75: 443–455

57. McDonagh A F, Palma L A, Lightner D A 1980 Blue light and bilirubin excretion. Science 208: 145–1

58. MacDonald M G 1995 Hidden risks: early discharge and bilirubin toxicity due to glucose-6-phosphate dehydrogenase deficiency. Pediatrics 96: 734–738

59. McKiernan P J 2002 Neonatal cholestasis. Seminars in Neonatology 7: 153–165

60. Maisels M J 1994 Jaundice. In: Avery G B, Fletcher M A, MacDonald M G (eds) Neonatology: pathophysiology and management of the newborn, 4th edition. J B Lippincott, Philadelphia, pp 630–725

61. Maisels M J, Kring E 1992 Risk of sepsis in newborns with severe hyperbilirubinemia. Pediatrics 90: 741–743

62. Maisels M J, Newman T B 1995 Kernicterus occurs in otherwise healthy, breast-fed term newborns. Pediatrics 96: 730–733

63. Maisels M J, Newman T B 2001 Bilirubin and neurological dysfunction – do we need to change what we are doing? Pediatric Research 50: 677–678

64. Marlow E S, Hunt L P, Marlow N 2000 Sensorineural hearing loss and prematurity. Archives of Disease in Childhood. Fetal and Neonatal Edition 82: F141–F144

65. Messner K H, Maisels M J, Leure-DuPree A E 1978 Phototoxicity to the newborn primate retina. Investigative Ophthalmology and Visual Sciences 17: 178–182

66. Mills J F, Tudehope D 2003 Fibreoptic phototherapy for neonatal jaundice (Cochrane Review). The Cochrane Library, Issue 3. Oxford. Available: http://www.update-software.com/abstracts/ab002060.htm

67. Monaghan G, McLellan A, McGeehan A et al 1999 Gilbert's syndrome is a contributory factor in prolonged unconjugated hyperbilirubinaemia of the newborn. Journal of Pediatrics 134: 441–446

68. Newman T B, Easterling M J 1994 Yield of reticulocyte counts and blood smears in term infants. Clinical Pediatrics 33: 71–76

69. Newman T B, Liljestrand P, Escobar G J 2003 Infants with bilirubin levels of 30 mg/dL or more in a large managed care organization. Pediatrics 111: 1303–1311

70. Newman T B, Maisels M J 1992 Evaluation of jaundice in the term newborn: a kinder, gentler approach. Pediatrics 89: 809–818

71. Newman T B, Maisels M J 2000 Less aggressive treatment of neonatal jaundice and reports of kernicterus: lessons about practice guidelines. Pediatrics 105: 242–245

72. Onishi I, Itoh S, Isobe K et al 1982 Mechanism of development of the bronze baby syndrome in neonates treated with phototherapy. Pediatrics 69: 273–276

73. Ovaly F 2003 Late anaemia in Rh haemolytic disease. Archives of Disease in Childhood. Fetal and Neonatal Edition 88: F444

74. Robertson A, Carp W, Brodersen R 1991 Bilirubin displacing effect of drugs used in neonatology. Acta Paediatrica Scandinavica 80: 1119–1127

75. Rosenstein B S, Ducore J M 1984 Enhancement by bilirubin of DNA damage induced in human cells exposed to phototherapy light. Pediatric Research 18: 3–6

76. Rubaltelli F F, Gourley G R, Loskamp N et al 2001 Transcutaneous bilirubin measurement: a multicenter evaluation of a new device. Pediatrics 107: 1264–1271

77. Sarici S U, Yurdakok M, Serdar M A et al 2002 An early (sixth-hour) serum bilirubin measurement is useful in predicting the development of significant hyperbilirubinemia and severe ABO hemolytic disease in a selective high-risk population of newborns with ABO incompatibility. Pediatrics 109: e53

78. Scheidt P C, Bryla D A, Nelson K B et al 1990 Phototherapy for neonatal hyperbilirubinemia: six year follow-up of the NICHD clinical trial. Pediatrics 85: 455–463

79. Scheidt P C, Graubard B I, Nelson K B et al 1991 Intelligence at six years in relation to neonatal bilirubin level: follow-up of the National Institute of Child Health and Human Development Clinical Trial of Phototherapy. Pediatrics 87: 797–805

80. Schneider A P 1986 Breast milk jaundice in the newborn – a real entity. Journal of the American Medical Association 255: 3270–3274

81. Seidman D S, Moise J, Ergaz Z et al 2000 A new blue light-emitting phototherapy device: a prospective randomized controlled study. Journal of Pediatrics 136: 771–774

82. Seidman D S, Paz I, Armon Y et al 2001 The effect of the publication of the "Practice parameter for the management of hyperbilirubinaemia" on treatment of neonatal jaundice. Acta Paediatrica 190: 292–295

83. Seidman D S, Paz I, Stevenson D K et al 1994 Effects of phototherapy for neonatal jaundice on cognitive performance. Journal of Perinatology 14: 23–28

84. Seidman D S, Shiloh M, Stevenson D K et al 1995 Role of hemolysis in neonatal jaundice associated with glucose-6-phosphate dehydrogenase deficiency. Journal of Pediatrics 127: 804–806

85. Seidman D S, Stevenson D K, Zivanit E et al 1995 Hospital readmission due to neonatal hyperbilirubinemia. Pediatrics 96: 726–729

86. Silverman W A, Andersen D H, Blanc W A et al 1956 A difference in mortality rate and incidence of kernicterus among premature infants allotted to two prophylactic antibacterial regimens. Pediatrics 18: 614–625

87. Stevenson D K, Fanaroff A A, Maisels M J et al 2001 Prediction of hyperbilirubinemia in near-term and term infants. Pediatrics 108: 31–39

88. Tan K L 1982 The pattern of bilirubin response to phototherapy for neonatal hyperbilirubinemia. Pediatric Research 16: 670–674

89. Tan K L, Dong F 2003 Transcutaneous bilirubinometry during and after phototherapy. Acta Paediatrica 92: 327–331

90. Tan K L, Skurr B A, Yip Y Y 1992 Phototherapy and the brain-stem auditory evoked response in neonatal hyperbilirubinemia. Journal of Pediatrics 120: 306–308

91. Turkel S B, Miller C A, Guttenberg M E et al 1982 A clinical pathologic reappraisal of kernicterus. Pediatrics 69: 267–272

92. Valaes T, Drummond G S, Kappas A 1998 Control of hyperbilirubinemia in glucose-6-phosphate dehydrogenase-deficient newborns using an inhibitor of bilirubin production, Sn-mesoporphyrin. Pediatrics 101: 1–11

93. Valaes T, Petmezaki S, Henschke C et al 1994 Control of jaundice in preterm newborns by an inhibitor of bilirubin production: studies with tin mesoporphyrin. Pediatrics 93: 1–11

94. Van de Bor M, Ens-Dokkum M, Schreuder A et al 1992 Hyperbilirubinemia in low birthweight infants and outcome at five years of age. Pediatrics 89: 359–364

95. Van de Bor M, van Zeben-van der Aa T M, Verloove-Vanhorick S P et al 1989 Hyperbilirubinemia in very preterm infants and neurodevelopmental outcome at two years of age: results of a national collaborative survey. Pediatrics 83: 915–920

96. Volpe J J 1995 Neurology of the newborn, 3rd edition. W B Saunders, Philadelphia, pp 490–515

97. Watchko J F 2001 Recurrence of kernicterus in term and near-term infants in Denmark. Acta Paediatrica 90: 1080

98. Watchko J F, Daood M J, Biniwale M 2002 Understanding neonatal hyperbilirubinaemia in the era of genomics. Seminars in Neonatology 7: 143–152

99. Watchko J, Oski F 1983 Bilirubin 20 mg/dL = vigintiphobia. Pediatrics 71: 660–663

100. Watchko J F, Oski F A 1992 Kernicterus in preterm newborns: past, present, and future. Pediatrics 90: 707–715

101. Yao T C, Stevenson D K 1995 Advances in the diagnosis and treatment of neonatal hyperbilirubinemia. Clinics in Perinatology 22: 741–758

102. Yeo K L, Perlman M, Hao Y M P 1998 Outcomes of extremely premature infants related to their peak serum bilirubin concentrations and exposure to phototherapy. Pediatrics 102: 1426–1431

103. Yokochi K 1995 Magnetic resonance imaging in children with kernicterus. Acta Paediatrica 84: 937–939

PART 2

Liver disease

Giorgina Mieli-Vergani, Nedim Hadzic

Introduction

Liver disease in infancy is rare but is a serious cause of morbidity and mortality. A better awareness of the causes of liver disease in this age group and their mode of presentation have led to earlier diagnosis of treatable conditions, with considerable improvement in prognosis, and facilitated genetic counselling for those families with hereditary disorders.

Jaundice is usually the first sign of liver dysfunction, but its importance is often underestimated because of the frequent occurrence of physiological jaundice in the neonatal period (Chapter 29, Part 1). A raised serum bilirubin with a conjugated component of >20%, and urine which contains bile pigment, is always pathological even if the total bilirubin is as low as 85 micromol/l (5 mg/dl). The notion that jaundice could be due to liver disease should prompt health workers to assess the colour of the urine and the stools to ascertain whether the jaundice is due to cholestasis. A baby's urine is usually pale yellow and often colourless. Dark yellow urine (unless during phototherapy) and stools which are not yellow or green in an infant of any age, should suggest liver disease and trigger appropriate investigations. A persistently elevated unconjugated bilirubin, not explained by haemolysis or other neonatological problems, should suggest the possibility of liver-based inherited disorders of bilirubin metabolism.

Hepatitis syndrome of infancy

Hepatitis syndrome of infancy is characterised by clinical and laboratory features of liver dysfunction, of which the most distinct is conjugated hyperbilirubinaemia. Babies usually have inflammatory changes in the liver histology – hence the name hepatitis – but the cause is only rarely infective. In most cases the baby presents with conjugated jaundice, which follows physiological jaundice; the urine becomes dark and the stools pale. Less commonly, babies may present with complications of liver dysfunction such as a bleeding diathesis, hypoglycaemia or fluid retention. The bleeding diathesis is usually due to vitamin K deficiency associated with fat malabsorption, which may also cause failure to thrive. Unless parenteral vitamin K is given, these babies may bleed catastrophically. Hepatomegaly is almost universal. Palpable splenomegaly occurs in 40–60% of cases.

Hepatitis syndrome of infancy most commonly is due to intrahepatic disease, for which there are many associated disorders. It may be due to lesions of the biliary system. All babies require urgent investigation to identify disorders for which there is specific treatment and to prevent complications of cholestasis. If the stools contain no yellow or green pigment, cholestasis is complete and biliary atresia must be suspected. It is essential to arrange urgent referral to a specialist centre with the experience and skills to confirm the diagnosis and provide corrective surgery as early as possible.[54]

Pathology

Four main pathological entities cause the syndrome:

1. Hepatocellular disease (hepatitis).
2. Inflammation and bile duct reduplication in the portal tracts, leading in some instances to paucity of interlobular bile ducts.
3. Disorders of the main intrahepatic bile ducts, leading to sclerosing cholangitis.
4. Disorders of the extrahepatic bile ducts, most commonly biliary atresia.

Hepatocellular disease may be associated with a wide range of infective, genetic, endocrine, vascular, toxic, familial, genetic or chromosomal disorders.[57] Often there are no associated factors and the disorder is cryptogenic. Chronic liver disease rarely follows in infective or endocrine disorders, but occurs in at least 50% of genetic or familial disorders. Pathological categories 2, 3 and 4 are invariably associated with chronic liver disease unless surgery (category 4) is effective. Infants with a normal serum γ-glutamyl transpeptidase (GGT) activity or cholesterol concentration in the presence of jaundice and abnormal biochemical tests of liver function, are likely to have a form of progressive familial cholestasis or primary bile acid synthesis abnormality.[13,52,87] Together with babies with sclerosing cholangitis,[2,5] this group have a particularly poor prognosis.

For all pathological entities, in the acute stages, the intrahepatic pathology, as revealed by liver biopsy, is dominated by cholestasis, with varying degrees of giant-cell transformation of hepatocytes and inflammatory cell infiltrate in the portal tracts. In metabolic disorders, abnormal accumulation of microvesicular or macrovesicular fat, glycogen or other storage material may be found in hepatocytes or Kupffer cells. Portal tract widening with oedema, accumulation of fibrous tissue and bile duct proliferation is characteristic of disorders of the major bile ducts, the most common of which is biliary atresia. It may occur in genetic disorders such as α_1-antitrypsin deficiency (α_1ATD) and could be a harbinger of chronic liver disease.

Clinical features

The majority of babies with hepatitis syndrome present with conjugated hyperbilirubinaemia starting in the first 4 weeks of

Table 29.11 Clinical signs of diagnostic importance in conjugated hyperbilirubinaemia

Abnormal signs	Disorders
Skin lesions, purpura, chorioidoretinitis, myocarditis	Generalised viral infection (pp. 1053–61)
Cataract	Galactosaemia (p. 918) or intrauterine infection or hypoparathyroidism (pp. 882–3)
Multiple congenital anomalies	Trisomy 21, 13 or 18
Cystic mass below the liver	Choledochal cyst
Ascites and bile-stained herniae	Spontaneous perforation of the bile ducts
Systolic murmur, abnormal facies, posterior embryotoxon	Arteriohepatic dysplasia (Alagille syndrome)
Cutaneous haemangiomata	Hepatic or biliary haemangioma
Situs inversus with or without polysplenia	Extrahepatic biliary atresia
Optic nerve hypoplasia and/or micropenis	Septo-optic dysplasia

Table 29.12 Investigations in conjugated hyperbilirubinaemia

Immediate investigations in all cases
Bacterial culture of blood and urine
Urine microscopy and analysis for reducing substances
Prothrombin time
Full blood count and reticulocyte count
Blood sugar, creatinine and urea
Serum sodium, potassium, bicarbonate and calcium
Blood group and cross-match

Investigations when full laboratory service is available
Biochemical tests of liver function, including split bilirubin and γ-glutamyl transpeptidase
IgM/IgG to toxoplasma, listeria, cytomegalovirus, herpes virus, rubella, hepatitis A and C, HIV and syphilis serology
Hepatitis B surface antigen
α_1-antitrypsin phenotype or genotype
Red blood cell galactose-1-phosphate uridyl transferase
Sweat electrolytes and immunoreactive trypsin
Serum and urine amino acids
Serum lactate and pyruvate
Mass spectrometry for plasma or urine bile acids
Urine succinyl acetone and organic acids
Direct Coombs' test (if appropriate)
T4, TSH, cortisol
Chest X-ray/echocardiogram for cardiac lesions
Wrist X-ray for rickets
In the presence of ascites: tap for cytology, biochemical testing + culture
Ultrasound of liver to detect focal lesions and dilated bile ducts
Methyl-brom-IDA scan following phenobarbital (in selected cases)

Tissue diagnosis
Percutaneous liver biopsy
Skin biopsy for fibroblast culture and enzyme analysis (in selected cases)
Bone marrow aspirate for Niemann–Pick disease
Laparotomy, intraoperative cholangiography

life, but may occasionally present as late as 4 months of age. The second most common presentation is spontaneous bleeding, usually secondary to vitamin K malabsorption, the jaundice being mild or ignored because it is considered physiological by parents and their healthcare advisers. Rarely, babies present with features of hypoglycaemia or hypoalbuminaemia. Review of the perinatal case records and past medical history may reveal features suggesting intrauterine infection, exposure to toxins, drugs or intravenous nutrition, familial, genetic or metabolic disease or consanguinity.[57]

Clinical examination is likely to show hepatomegaly and splenomegaly. Babies with intrahepatic disease may show failure to thrive, but babies with biliary atresia typically are well nourished and have no stigmata of chronic liver disease in the first 2 months of life. Rarely, there are clinical signs of diagnostic importance (Table 29.11). If the stools are white or grey, there may be complete cholestasis, and conditions such as biliary atresia enter into the differential diagnosis. Standard tests of liver function, such as serum bilirubin, alkaline phosphatase, aspartate transaminase, GGT, albumin and prothrombin time, may be equally abnormal in each of the four main groups of disorders. Serum triglycerides and cholesterol are usually normal in the first 4 months of life but may increase thereafter, particularly in infants with bile duct hypoplasia. Serum α-fetoprotein values are high, particularly in tyrosinaemia, where the values may exceed 5000 ng/ml.[57]

Management (Table 29.12)

The first priority on admission to hospital is to identify the causes and complications for which urgent treatment is required. These are septicaemia, urinary tract infection, toxoplasmosis, syphilis, malaria, herpes simplex and the metabolic disorders – galactosaemia and fructosaemia. The most dangerous complication is spontaneous haemorrhage due to vitamin K malabsorption. Such

haemorrhage may well be intracranial. The initial investigations must include prothrombin time, full blood count, blood cultures, urine culture, and urine analysis for non-glucose reducing substances. Galactose and fructose must be excluded from the diet until it is shown that there is no metabolic abnormality primarily affecting their metabolism.[34] After these bloods have been taken, diagnostic investigations such as α_1-antitrypsin (α_1AT) phenotyping and galactose-1-phosphate uridyl transferase activity in red cells should be carried out. If the baby has received a blood transfusion, the parents need to be investigated for a possible heterozygote status.

If septicaemia is suspected, broad-spectrum antibiotic therapy is indicated. Even if septicaemia is confirmed, there may still be a serious underlying disease, such as galactosaemia, haemophagocytic lymphohistiocytosis (HLH), tyrosinaemia type 1, α_1ATD or biliary atresia. The finding of non-glucose reducing substances

Table 29.13 Surgically correctable disorders causing bile duct obstruction (see text)

Extrahepatic biliary atresia
Choledochal cyst
Spontaneous perforation of the bile ducts
Duodenal and low bile duct atresia
Gallstones
Haemangiomata
Extrinsic compression
Bile plugs in extrahepatic bile ducts

Table 29.14 Infections associated with conjugated hyperbilirubinaemia (see Chapter 40, Part 2)

Cytomegalovirus	Epstein–Barr virus
Rubella virus	Varicella-zoster virus
Hepatitis A	Psittacosis
Hepatitis B	Bacterial infections
Hepatitis C	Listeria
Non A–C hepatitis	*Treponema pallidum*
Herpes simplex virus 1 & 2	*Toxoplasma gondii*
Coxsackie A9, B	Malaria
Echovirus 9, 11, 14, 19	Tuberculosis
Adenovirus	HIV
Reo virus type III	

Table 29.15 Inherited metabolic disorders associated with hepatitis syndrome in infancy (see Chapter 35, Part 3)

Galactosaemia
Fructosaemia
Tyrosinaemia
α_1-antitrypsin deficiency
Progressive familial intrahepatic cholestasis
Mitochondrial cytopathies
Cystic fibrosis
Niemann–Pick type C
Gaucher disease
Wolman disease
Zellweger syndrome
Infantile polycystic disease (p. 776)
Haemophagocytic lymphohistiocytosis
Neonatal iron storage disease (perinatal haemochromatosis, p. 688)
Carbohydrate glycoprotein deficiency
Defects in synthesis of primary bile acids

Table 29.16 Endocrine disorders associated with hepatitis syndrome in infancy (see Chapter 35, Part 2)

Hypopituitarism
Diabetes insipidus
Hypoadrenalism
Hypothyroidism
Hypoparathyroidism

in the urine does not necessarily indicate galactosaemia, as they may occur in normal babies in the first 2 weeks of life and are common in all forms of liver damage.[57] Conversely, the absence of non-glucose reducing substances does not exclude galactosaemia, as very ill babies may feed poorly or vomit. If the prothrombin time is found to be prolonged, vitamin K (1 mg i.v.) should be given immediately and, if bleeding is still occurring, fresh-frozen plasma infused or exchange transfusion performed. The next priority is to identify those babies who require surgical correction of bile duct obstruction (Table 29.13). Ultrasound examination should be undertaken to exclude a choledochal cyst or focal intrahepatic lesions.

In all infants, infective (Table 29.14), metabolic (Table 29.15) and endocrine (Table 29.16) causes of liver damage affecting this age group must be excluded. With regard to infective conditions, it must be remembered that cytomegalovirus (CMV), rubella and hepatitis B virus have been found to occur in all types of hepatobiliary disease.[34] Seropositivity for these viruses should not preclude investigation of other causes of liver damage. Galactosaemia, fructosaemia and tyrosinaemia must be investigated promptly because dietary intervention in the first two conditions and treatment with 2-(2-nitro-4-trifluoro-methyl-benzoyl)-1-3-cyclohexanedione (NTBC)[47] in the last, need to be instituted urgently to avoid severe deterioration. α_1ATD, cystic fibrosis and Niemann–Pick disease type C need also to be sought in all infants because these are relatively common genetic conditions for which antenatal diagnosis is possible. α_1ATD must be excluded

in all cases by determining the α_1AT phenotype, rather than by means of the α_1AT concentration, which can be within the normal range in the presence of hepatitis or infection, as α_1AT is an acute-phase reactant.[78] This is perhaps the most important investigation in distinguishing severe hepatitis with complete cholestasis from extrahepatic biliary atresia, as the liver disease associated with phenotype PiZZ α_1ATD (see later) has many clinical and pathological similarities with biliary atresia.[22,69] Investigation for rarer metabolic diseases should be performed only if suggested by the family history or findings on percutaneous liver biopsy. The frequency with which infectious, genetic, pharmacological and toxic causes of hyperbilirubinaemia or structural biliary abnormalities can be identified depends not only on the prevalence of these in the community studied, but also on referral patterns and the sophistication of investigation facilities.[57]

In a study in south-east England of 54 infants who had conjugated hyperbilirubinaemia of at least 2 weeks' duration, it was found that idiopathic intrahepatic disorders were approximately three times more common than biliary atresia and four times as frequent as disease associated with α_1ATD or the combined incidence of all other specific disorders.[22] The relative frequency of the causes of conjugated hyperbilirubinaemia in infants referred to King's College Hospital, a tertiary referral centre, is shown in Table 29.17. A large number of infants defined as having

Table 29.17 Relative frequency of causes of conjugated hyperbilirubinaemia in infants referred to the Paediatric Liver Service, King's College Hospital, London

Disorder	Referred cases
Biliary atresia	337
Idiopathic hepatitis	331
α_1-antitrypsin deficiency	189
Alagille syndrome	41
Choledochal cyst	34
Spontaneous perforation of bile duct	6
Others	94

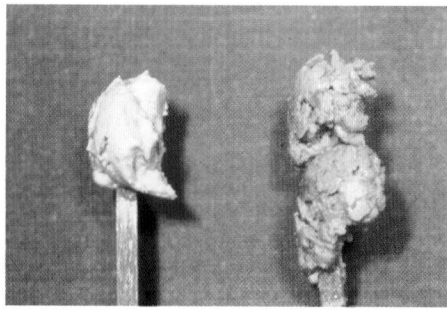

Fig. 29.10 Appearances of normal (right) and acholic baby stool (left) suggestive of biliary obstruction.

cryptogenic liver disease in this series, however, today would be diagnosed as having progressive familial intrahepatic syndromes or mitochondrial cytopathies, the clinical, biochemical and genetic characteristics of which have been described in recent years.[32,87]

Identifying bile duct obstruction

A most useful observation is the stool colour. Because of photosensitivity of bile pigments in the stool, all stools passed should be saved in the dark (e.g. in a black bag or in a container) and examined for yellow or green pigment; if absent, cholestasis is complete and biliary atresia must be excluded (Fig. 29.10). Referral to a specialist centre with experience in the identification of this condition and a reputation for its successful surgical correction is essential.[51,54] A skilfully interpreted percutaneous liver biopsy performed under local anaesthesia using the Menghini technique is diagnostic in up to 90% of cases. If all portal tracts show increased oedema, fibrosis and bile duct reduplication, this strongly suggests major bile duct disease, of which the most common is biliary atresia. This appearance can be found also in genetic disorders such as α_1ATD (PiZZ), cystic fibrosis, Alagille syndrome and endocrine disorders associated with septo-optic dysplasia. It occurs in some infants who will ultimately develop bile duct hypoplasia and in disorders of the intrahepatic bile ducts.[19,69] All of these disorders can cause complete cholestasis. It is essential that some of the material obtained is snap frozen at $-70°C$ for subsequent enzymatic analysis for inherited disorders (see Table 29.15) if indicated by the liver histology or other investigations.

If there are doubts as to whether there is pigment in the stools, a helpful investigation is radionucleotide demonstration of bile duct patency. This is only useful if isotope is demonstrated in the gut, thereby excluding biliary atresia and avoiding an unnecessary and potentially dangerous laparotomy. No excretion in the gut does not equate with biliary atresia. A ^{99m}Tc-tagged imminodiacetic acid derivative, such as methyl-brom-IDA, with good hepatic uptake and relatively poor renal uptake, must be used. Discrimination from intrahepatic cholestasis is enhanced if the infant is pretreated with phenobarbital (5 mg/kg/day for at least 3 days). Repeated imaging up to 24 hours after intravenous injection may be required to demonstrate isotope in the gut.

Equally effective discrimination may be achieved by computer analysis of distribution between the liver and heart within 10 minutes of intravenous injection.[25] Daily observation of the stool colour is essential even if patency of the bile ducts is demonstrated. If the stools remain acholic, the liver biopsy should be repeated, and further investigations may be necessary to identify the rare instances of late-onset biliary atresia.

The real difficulty arises if there is no excretion, the biopsy is not indicative of atresia and no genetic or endocrine disorder causing complete cholestasis has been identified. At specialised centres, endoscopic retrograde cholangiopancreatography (ERCP) is an important diagnostic tool in such ambiguous cases.[91] Unless filling of the intrahepatic ducts can be demonstrated by ERCP, such patients should have a laparotomy. It is essential that this be undertaken by an experienced surgeon who can correctly assess the changes in the porta hepatis and, being confident of the diagnosis, proceed to portoenterostomy.[50] Final confirmation of the diagnosis comes from histological examination of the excised biliary remnants, by which time an irreversible operation has been performed! Even with intraoperative cholangiography, extrahepatic ducts which are hypoplastic as a result of severe intrahepatic cholestasis may be considered atretic, leading to an unnecessary destructive operation.[53]

Surgically correctable disorders

Biliary atresia

Biliary atresia is the most frequent surgically correctable liver disorder in infancy, affecting 1:14 000 liveborns. It is unique to infancy and is characterised by complete obstruction of the bile flow owing to obliteration or destruction of part or all of the extrahepatic biliary tree. Study of bile duct remnants removed at surgery, and from macroserial sectioning and reconstruction of surgical and necropsy liver specimens, indicates that biliary atresia arises from a sclerosing inflammatory process affecting previously formed bile ducts (Fig. 29.11).[31] Recently, comparative anatomical studies have suggested that, in at least some cases, biliary atresia may be caused by failure of the intrauterine remodelling process at the hepatic hilum, with persistence of fetal bile ducts poorly supported by mesenchyme. As bile flow increases perinatally, bile leakage from these abnormal ducts may trigger an intense inflammatory reaction, with consequent obliteration of the biliary tree.[86] The extrahepatic ducts are

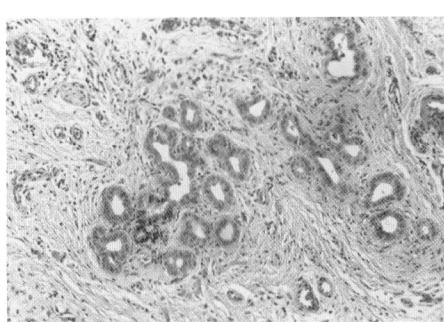

Fig. 29.11 Liver histology demonstrating expansion of the portal tract, bile duct proliferation and cholestasis, suggestive of extrahepatic biliary atresia (haematoxylin and eosin × 150).

Table 29.18 Requirements to improve the management of biliary atresia

- All babies jaundiced after 14 days of age should have urine analysis and total and direct serum bilirubin determination
- If conjugated bilirubin is present, the baby should be referred to a paediatrician for urgent investigation
- If the stools have no yellow or green pigment, the baby should be referred to a specialist centre to exclude or treat biliary atresia
- 'Well baby' clinics should be at 4 rather than 6 weeks of age to identify jaundice sufficiently early to increase the chances of successful treatment

primarily affected, whereas the intrahepatic bile ducts remain patent in early infancy but then also become affected, obliterated and eventually disappear. Cirrhosis with complications such as portal hypertension may appear at any time from 2 months of age, and death by 2 years of age is usual.

The cause of biliary atresia is unknown. Familial cases are extremely rare and, of 17 cases occurring in twins, in only two instances were both affected.[80] At our centre we have seen several twin pregnancies and one triplet pregnancy where only one infant was affected. HLA phenotype appears not to play a role.[23] Up to 25% of infants have minor or major abnormalities outside the biliary system, with a particularly high frequency of abnormalities of the vasculature below the diaphragm. Children with splenic malformations, including polysplenia and asplenia, with or without laterality defects (complete or partial situs inversus) may represent a separate aetiological subgroup – biliary atresia splenic malformation (BASM) syndrome.[18] It has also been suggested that the precarious blood supply to the biliary tree may be further jeopardised with such abnormalities. An increased incidence of maternal diabetes mellitus has been associated with the BASM syndrome.[18] Another suggested aetiological factor is a long common channel for the pancreatic and biliary ducts as they enter the duodenum, with the suggestion that pancreatic juice may reflux into the biliary system and initiate mucosal damage and subsequent inflammatory response. There have been many suggestions that perinatal infection may initiate biliary atresia, but all of the candidate viruses, e.g. Reovirus type III,[88] infect atresia patients no more frequently than other infants.[56] Other viruses suggested to be implicated in the aetiology of biliary atresia include CMV[27] and rotavirus.[73]

A specific problem in the diagnosis of biliary atresia is that, as mentioned above, in most cases it results from an obliterative disorder starting in formed extrahepatic ducts which eventually leads to their destruction.[31] The extrahepatic bile ducts and intrahepatic bile ducts may be patent in the first weeks of life, but become atretic later. Thus, in up to 30% of infants with atresia, stools are pigmented in the first weeks after birth, before bile flow is completely obstructed.[57] All too frequently the infant's apparent wellbeing causes paediatricians and other health workers to dismiss consideration of this disorder in early infancy, when the chances of successful surgery are high.[54] The longer biliary atresia has been present, the greater the likelihood

that the intrahepatic bile ducts will have been obliterated and that portoenterostomy will be less likely to be successful. It is essential to refer infants with acholic stools to units with experience in the interpretation of the diagnostic investigations outlined above, and in the surgical and postoperative management of biliary atresia (Table 29.18).[51]

At laparotomy, the surgeon must first confirm that the bile ducts are absent or atretic. This is not a simple task, and narrow but patent bile ducts in infants with intrahepatic disease and complete cholestasis have been removed by experienced surgeons.[53] In 5–10% of babies, the surgeon can identify a patent common bile duct containing bile and in continuity with intrahepatic bile ducts.[50] In these babies, a biliary–intestinal anastomosis via a long Roux-en-Y loop may allow bile to drain satisfactorily. In the majority of patients, however, the proximal common hepatic duct is completely obliterated or absent up to where it enters the liver, and at the porta hepatitis it is replaced by fibrous tissue. This tissue is transected flush with the liver and a Roux-en-Y loop of jejunum is anastomosed around the fibrous edges of the transected tissue, forming a porto-enterostomy (Kasai procedure). For surgery to be effective, the intrahepatic bile ducts must be patent to the porta hepatitis.[50] Modifications of the Kasai procedure undertaken to reduce the risks of cholangitis fail to do so and increase the risks of liver transplantation if this becomes subsequently necessary. Babies are started on phenobarbital preoperatively at a dose of 5–7 mg/kg/day to promote bile flow, and a dose of 45 mg/day is used postoperatively as maintenance in our unit.[18] If the jaundice reappears, the dose could be increased to 60–90 mg/day. With an experienced surgeon, good bile flow with normal serum bilirubin values can be achieved in more than 80% of children operated on by 60 days of age, but in only 20–30% with later surgery.[18,54,63] If bilirubin returns to normal, a 90% 15-year survival has been reported,[63] with a good quality of life into the fourth decade.[11] Up to 11% of children are free of clinical and biochemical signs of liver disease after 10-year follow-up.[33] If the bilirubin is not reduced, the rate of progression of cirrhosis is not slowed and survival beyond the second birthday is unusual. If bile drainage is partially effective, end-stage chronic liver disease may be delayed to 6 or 7 years of age.

An important postoperative complication is cholangitis. This is due to a wide range of microorganisms and occurs in over 50%

of cases in the first 2 years after surgery.[64] It is characterised by fever, recurrence or aggravation of jaundice, and frequently features of septicaemia. Blood culture, ascitic aspirate or liver biopsy to identify the organism responsible should precede intravenous antibiotic therapy, which is continued for 14 days if a pathogen is identified. Often, however, the diagnosis of cholangitis is not obvious and unexplained fever may be the only symptom. Antibiotics are then started empirically, after taking a blood culture and assessing liver function tests, C-reactive protein and full blood count. If the fever responds to antibiotics, these are continued for 5 days. Should the fever recur after stopping antibiotics, a liver biopsy is performed for histological examination and culture. Amoxicillin (amoxycillin) and cefuroxime are currently our initial choice pending in-vitro sensitivities. Long-term prophylaxis with rotating antibiotics may be indicated for recurrent cholangitis.[18]

Portal hypertension is present in almost all cases at the time of initial surgery. Approximately 50% of all survivors aged 5 years, even those with normal bilirubin levels, have oesophageal varices, but only 10–15% have gastrointestinal bleeding. For these, variceal banding or injection sclerotherapy are the treatments of choice. In approximately 10% of cases in whom the serum bilirubin returns to normal, intrahepatic cholangiopathy progresses and complications of biliary cirrhosis ultimately develop.[60] For these patients, and those for whom surgery has not been effective, liver transplantation should be considered.[59] With 1-year survival rates approaching 90%,[65] and 5-year survival rates over 80%,[59] liver transplantation is now a standard therapeutic option, but it still remains a formidable procedure. The recipient is likely to have one or more life-threatening complications in the perioperative or postoperative period. Lifelong immunosuppressive therapy is required, with a high risk of opportunistic and community-acquired infections, requiring close medical and surgical supervision. Most of the survivors have a good quality of life and attend school, although the long-term medical and psychological effects of liver transplantation in childhood are as yet unknown. The supply of donors of suitable size and blood group, even with an increased use of split grafts, where one donor liver is used for two recipients – usually one child and one adult – remains a major limiting factor in liver transplantation. Segmental graft transplant from living relatives has given survival rates of 90% in infants in whom Kasai portoenterostomy had been unsuccessful.[66] The results are better in children transplanted heavier than 10 kg (or after the age of 1 year) and if the procedure is done electively.[65] The precise indications and timing, and the optimum management of some of the intraoperative and postoperative problems, including the control of rejection, remain the subject of ongoing assessment and research. Although an important mode of management for end-stage liver disease, the role of liver transplantation in biliary atresia is complementary to that of portoenterostomy, except for infants in whom decompensated cirrhosis has developed because of delayed diagnosis.

Choledochal cysts

Choledochal cysts are dilatations of the biliary ducts which can be associated with intermittent biliary obstruction. If uncorrected,

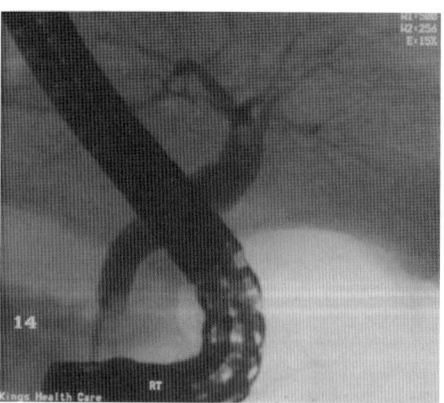

Fig. 29.12 Endoscopic retrograde cholangiopancreatography demonstrating a non-obstructive saccular dilatation of extrahepatic bile duct, strongly suggestive of a choledochal cyst.

they lead to increasing biliary fibrosis and ultimately cirrhosis. In the newborn period, the presentation is indistinguishable from neonatal hepatitis or biliary atresia. They may be diagnosed prenatally on routine ultrasound.[72,84] Children in whom a prenatal diagnosis of choledochal cyst is made should be referred promptly to a specialised paediatric hepatology centre, since this could also be the mode of presentation of biliary atresia.[72] Cholangitis, rupture, pancreatitis and gallstones are important complications of choledochal cyst which can occur even in early infancy, while chronic cholangitis and carcinoma of the cyst wall may be a long-term complication.

A cystic echo-free mass demonstrated in the biliary tree by ultrasound is strong evidence for this diagnosis. The intrahepatic bile ducts may be dilated due to the distal stasis. The cyst could be diagnosed by magnetic resonance cholangiopancreatography, but often ERCP or percutaneous transhepatic cholangiography (PTC) are needed (Fig. 29.12). The definitive treatment is surgical removal with biliary drainage via a Roux-en-Y loop.[36] With adequate surgery, the long-term prognosis is good.[84]

Spontaneous perforation of the bile duct

Spontaneous perforation of the bile duct at the junction of the cystic duct and common hepatic duct occurs when, for some unexplained reason, the common bile duct becomes blocked, usually at its distal end. Affected infants have mild jaundice, failure to gain weight, and abdominal distension due to ascites, which classically causes the development of bile-stained herniae. The stools are white or cream in colour, the urine is dark. Paracentesis confirms the presence of bile-stained ascites.[37]

If operative cholangiography shows free drainage of contrast into the duodenum, the ruptured duct may be sutured, but more commonly it is necessary to establish cholecysto-jejunostomy drainage via a Roux-en-Y loop. With effective surgery, the prognosis is excellent.[37] Delay in instituting surgery may lead to severe malnutrition, peritonitis and septicaemia.

Miscellaneous conditions

The remaining surgical conditions listed in Table 29.13 are very rare, and are usually dealt with either by flushing out the

Table 29.19 Causes of paucity of interlobular bile ducts

Syndromic
Alagille syndrome or arteriohepatic dysplasia

Non-syndromic
Idiopathic
α_1-antitrypsin deficiency
Biliary atresia after 6 months of age
Zellweger syndrome
Impaired cholic acid synthesis
Down syndrome
Intrauterine infection, e.g. rubella

Acquired
Graft-versus-host disease
Medications
Advanced chronic rejection after liver transplant

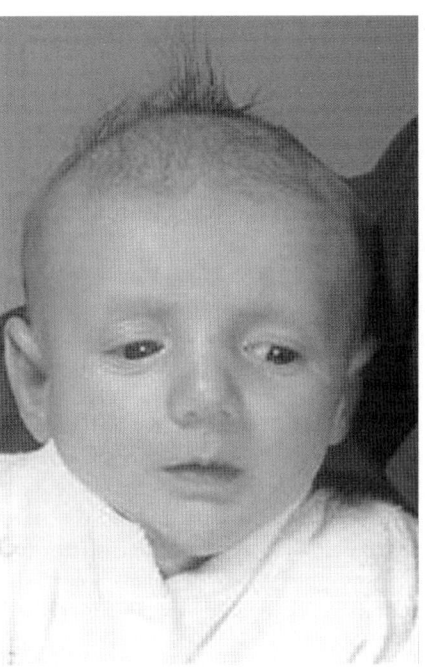

Fig. 29.13 Facial appearances of a baby with Alagille's syndrome. (Reproduced from Francavilla & Mieli-Vergani.[30])

obstruction with a percutaneous or operative cholangiogram or by a bypass procedure.

Conjugated hyperbilirubinaemia associated with erythroblastosis

The condition must be distinguished from the inspissated bile syndrome, a rare condition of unknown, but probably multifactorial, aetiology, in which the distal bile duct is obstructed by debris which can be flushed into the duodenum at percutaneous or operative cholangiography. The diagnosis of this disorder is made by ultrasonography and liver biopsy.

No specific treatment is available. No long-term hepatic sequelae such as cirrhosis or portal hypertension have been recorded.

Paucity of interlobular bile ducts (intrahepatic biliary hypoplasia)

This is a pathological diagnosis in which there is a decrease in the number of interlobular bile ducts seen in the portal tracts. It is found in many conditions causing hepatitis in infancy (Table 29.19). If it occurs with cardiovascular, skeletal and ocular anomalies, it is called Alagille syndrome (syndromic paucity of the intrahepatic bile ducts; arteriohepatic dysplasia)[1] and is inherited in an autosomal dominant fashion with variable expression. The estimated incidence is 1:100 000 livebirths. It is caused by mutations in the human *Jagged 1* gene on chromosome 20p12.[71] However, mutations in this gene can also be present in asymptomatic individuals and in other liver conditions, including biliary atresia.[45] There is a long-standing cholestasis causing jaundice, pruritus, hypercholesterolaemia and xanthomas. The severity of the cholestasis varies. Mild cases may have pruritus only. The majority have jaundice from the neonatal period, which in severe cases may persist but in others clears in late childhood or early adult life.

The long-term prognosis is uncertain, but some 15% may go on to develop cirrhosis and 5–10% die from liver disease.[49] In one series, 25% died from cardiac involvement, classically a peripheral pulmonary stenosis, or infection.[1] Diagnosis is supported by the finding of the typical facies: deep-set eyes, mild hypertelorism, overhanging forehead, a straight nose which in profile is in the same plane as the forehead, a small pointed chin, posterior embryotoxon (a remnant of an embryonic membrane between iris and cornea, seen by slit lamp), and vertebral arch defects on spinal radiographs (Fig. 29.13). A high serum cholesterol supports the diagnosis. The treatment is that of chronic cholestasis, with particular emphasis on adequacy of vitamin D, E, K and A supplements and the control of pruritus.[19]

Liver damage associated with parenteral nutrition

Prolonged intravenous nutrition, particularly in early infancy, causes cholestasis and hepatocellular damage, which may progress to cirrhosis if intravenous feeding continues with no enteral intake. Prevalence increases with the degree of prematurity, the duration of intravenous feeding and in the presence of associated medical and surgical conditions. Cholestatic jaundice, defined as a direct-reacting bilirubin concentration of greater than 34 micromol/l, occurred in 8.6% of 267 infants receiving intravenous nutrition.[67] The incidence was inversely proportional to the gestation, being 13.7% in babies of less than 32 weeks', 5.3% in babies of 32–36 weeks' and 1.4% in babies of greater than 36 weeks' gestation. In each gestational age group, the duration of parenteral therapy in babies with cholestasis was significantly longer than in those who remained free from this complication. The babies with cholestasis also tended to be without oral feeding for longer – 23 days as opposed to 15 days. Sepsis, hypoxia, shock, blood transfusion, intra-abdominal surgery and potentially hepatotoxic drugs may aggravate the liver damage.

Pathologically, there is a distinct cholestatic hepatitis, with bile stasis within the hepatocytes and in the bile canaliculi, and bile in the Kupffer cells. These cells also contain marked accumulation of periodic acid–Schiff (PAS)-positive pigment. The hepatocytes are oedematous and may have increased numbers of nuclei. There is a lobular disarray with distension of portal tracts by inflammatory cell infiltrate, bile duct proliferation and fibrosis. A fine panlobular sinusoidal or pericellular fibrosis may be noted in up to 50% of cases. Severe fibrosis and cirrhosis may develop if total intravenous feeding cannot be stopped. Acute acalculous cholecystitis, biliary sludge and cholelithiasis are frequent complications. Follow-up biopsies 5–9 months after the height of the illness still show mild hepatocellular cholestasis, lobular disarray with ballooning of hepatocytes, and increased fibrosis.

The aetiology of the hepatobiliary complications of total parenteral nutrition (TPN) is unknown.[70] Intravenous administration of amino acids, dextrose and protein hydrolysates can cause a rise in serum alkaline phosphatase concentrations above baseline levels during the first 3 weeks of administration. Intravenous amino acids, in addition, may cause hyperaminoacidaemia, metabolic acidosis or hyperammonaemia. Intravenous lipids cause a progressive rise in the concentration of lipoprotein X. How these abnormalities are associated with disturbances of intrahepatocyte metabolism is unknown at present. Other factors that have been suggested as possibly contributing to impaired hepatic function include a lack of essential nutrients, trace elements or an 'unbalanced' supply of amino acids. Other postulated causes include endotoxaemia, chronic hypoxia, toxins leached from central venous catheters and lack of intestinal stimulation of bile secretion because of lack of oral intake.[70] Hypersensitivity reactions to drugs must also be considered.

The first clinical indication of hepatic involvement is usually the appearance of conjugated hyperbilirubinaemia. Hepatomegaly may be noted. Biochemical tests of liver function are abnormal. It is important to consider other causes of cholestasis in this age group before concluding that the disorder is due to intravenous nutrition. If TPN can be withdrawn, the jaundice settles within 4–6 weeks, although liver function tests may remain abnormal for 5 months and liver biopsy changes persist for up to a year.

The prognosis of TPN-associated jaundice is more serious in children with anatomical anomalies or functional intestinal failure (necrotising enterocolitis, gastroschisis, microcolon, etc.), who are TPN-dependent for longer. They may progress to end-stage chronic liver disease, requiring isolated liver transplantation or combined liver and small bowel transplantation.[58]

There are no reported long-term follow-up studies. It is clearly important, therefore, to monitor closely liver function tests in babies who are receiving TPN, particularly if they are premature. Intravenous nutrition should be curtailed as much as possible if conjugated hyperbilirubinaemia or other signs of hepatocellular injury appear in infancy. Tests of liver function should be carried out at least weekly during intravenous feeding. Treatment of the liver dysfunction associated with parenteral nutrition aims at improving bile flow with the use of ursodeoxycholic acid (UDCA; 20–25 mg/kg/day) or phenobarbital (5 mg/kg/day). The most effective treatment, however, is the reintroduction of total or partial enteral nutrition, if tolerated.

Liver disease associated with α_1-antitrypsin deficiency

α_1ATs are glycoproteins synthesised largely in the liver. In vitro and probably in vivo they act as inhibitors of inflammatory response. Over 90 different alleles, controlled by a single gene, have been isolated and identified in alphabetical nomenclature as protease inhibitors (Pi). The predominant type is PiM. The alleles of α_1AT are inherited in an autosomal co-dominant fashion, the most common phenotype being PiMM. Liver disease is associated with the PiZZ, Pinulnul or PiZnul variants. These are among the most common single gene defects, occurring in about 1:2000–1:7000 newborns of European origin.[69,76] The plasma deficiency of the glycoprotein is associated with a defect in secretion from the endoplasmic reticulum rather than a defect in the synthesis of the Z polypeptide.[78]

The clinical features associated with the deficiency state are very variable, with some having no overt disease, up to 20% developing liver disease of variable severity, and up to 60% developing emphysema.[29,85] Cigarette smoking is closely associated with the development of emphysema, but the cause of the liver disease is still not fully elucidated.[48,76]

The putative pathogenic mechanism for the liver disease in PiZZ α_1ATD is abnormal 'loop sheet' polymerisation of the mutant α_1AT protein, leading to abnormal folding and inefficient export from the rough endoplasmic reticulum of the hepatocytes.[48,78] It is likely that genetic and environmental modifiers play a role in development of the liver disease and its severity. Suggested additional pathogenic factors include possession of HLA DR3, absence of breastfeeding and male sex, defects in chemotaxis, liver-specific autoimmune reactions, complement activation, and the increase in the synthesis of acute-phase reactants during febrile episodes in infection.[48,76]

Although over 50% of infants with the deficiency state have abnormal biochemical tests of liver function, and these remain abnormal in over 30% throughout the first 12 years of life, only 10–15% develop symptomatic liver disease.[85] In 90% this takes the form of a conjugated hyperbilirubinaemia with hepatosplenomegaly and disturbed biochemical tests of liver function presenting in the first 4 months of life. In 10% of these infants a serious bleeding diathesis due to vitamin K malabsorption is an important component of their illness, potentially leading to intracranial bleeding and permanent neurological abnormality; 1–2% present in later childhood or adult life with cirrhosis with no history of prior jaundice in infancy.[69] Emphysema usually has its onset in early adult life.

The identification of liver disease associated with α_1ATD in the individual baby is important for diagnostic, genetic and prognostic reasons. Such babies could be considered on clinical, biochemical and histological evidence to have extrahepatic biliary atresia and be subjected to the risks of unnecessary laparotomy. Infants with liver disease associated with α_1ATD have a significantly worse prognosis than those with hepatitis of unknown cause. In an epidemiological study in south-east England, seven cases of hepatitis in infants were associated with α_1ATD.[22] By 3 years of age, four had died of cirrhosis, and cirrhosis was present in one of two reviewed at 10 years of age. In contrast, only two of 28 with idiopathic hepatitis in this study died, and none at 10 years had cirrhosis. Our experience with 82 children with PiZ phenotype and liver disease was that approximately 25% died of cirrhosis by adolescence, a further 25% had histologically proven cirrhosis, 25% had persisting liver disease with possible cirrhosis, and 25% apparently recovered from liver disease showing no clinical or biochemical abnormality.[69]

The prognosis of the liver disease associated with PiZZ α_1ATD is correlated with the presence of fibrosis and the severity and duration of the acute hepatitis in early infancy.[29] In the individual baby, the liver biopsy is the most helpful guide to prognosis. In those who die or have persistent hepatic abnormality, there is a marked increase in portal tract oedema and fibrosis in the first 6 months of life. Unfortunately, there is no specific treatment for this form of liver disease, apart from liver transplantation.

Patients with α_1ATD may have renal involvement with a variety of glomerulonephropathies.[83] Renal involvement may cause haematuria and/or proteinuria and contribute to hypoalbuminaemia. The development of renal complications adds to the difficulties after liver transplantation, particularly severe hypertension.

Reliable methods of genotyping from chorionic villus sampling at 8–10 weeks of gestation are available. Genetic counselling is difficult because of the varying severity of the clinical associations and difficulties in predicting the prognosis. Such families should be carefully assessed and offered the option of prenatal diagnosis.

Cryptogenic (idiopathic) hepatitis in infancy

Despite an increasing number of specific disorders associated with hepatitis syndrome in infancy, in a high proportion of children the cause remains unidentified. These children are often born after an abnormal pregnancy and sometimes have a low birthweight. Frequently, they come to medical attention for complications of prematurity or intrauterine growth retardation, and then subsequently develop evidence of liver disease. Although the liver disease may be severe, the mortality in such cases is usually less than 15% and long-term hepatic problems occur in less than 10%. The histological features are often non-specific, with portal and lobular inflammation, giant-cell transformation of hepatocytes and variable degree of cholestasis. The indicators of poor prognosis are severe cholestasis with proliferation and/or damage of the intralobular bile ducts and presence of fibrosis, cholangiography showing

sclerosing cholangitis,[2] family history of liver disease in childhood, or consanguinity,[5,20] and normal serum GGT in the presence of abnormality of other liver function tests indicating persistent liver disease.[52] This latter finding suggests either a primary abnormality of bile acid formation, which must be promptly excluded, as treatment with oral primary bile salts reverses liver damage,[12] or a progressive familial intrahepatic cholestatic (PFIC) syndrome[14] due to FIC1 disease,[10] or bile salt export pump (BSEP) deficiency (see below), which typically present as non-specific neonatal hepatitis with normal or low GGT.[82] In this context it is important to remember that the normal values for GGT in premature infants, neonates and infants younger than 6 months are several-fold higher than in older children and adults.[9]

Progressive familial intrahepatic cholestasis syndromes

Over the last decade, different types of PFIC syndromes, associated with a low or a high GGT phenotype, have been characterised.[87] These autosomal recessive conditions can present in infancy with prolonged conjugated jaundice. GGT in the liver is normally bound to the canalicular membrane and to the cholangiocyte biliary epithelium. Under cholestatic conditions, the detergent effect of the bile acids liberates GGT from the membrane. When this is combined with a poor bile flow, GGT leaks back into the circulation, where elevated levels can be detected. In the absence of bile acids in the bile, even when there is poor bile flow, GGT is not released and the serum levels remain normal. Therefore, in the presence of cholestasis, a normal serum level of GGT correlates very well with low levels of biliary bile acids. These patients usually have low biliary but high serum levels of bile acids, in the absence of a defect in bile acid synthesis.

The original patients described with this phenotype were amongst the Old Order Amish.[14] One of the original families was called Byler, and this condition has become widely known as Byler disease. Byler disease, or FIC1, represents a third of the patients with low-GGT PFIC and maps to chromosome 18.[10] These patients may present with neonatal hepatitis of variable severity. The FIC1 gene is widely expressed, with only relatively low-level expression in the liver. Thus, some patients with FIC1 disease have extrahepatic manifestations. Expression of FIC1 is particularly high in the small intestine and pancreas. FIC1 patients may have pancreatitis and many have significant malabsorption, which is not improved by liver transplantation. A proportion of them will have abnormal sweat test.

A further third of patients with low-GGT PFIC have an isolated defect in bile acid transport due to deficiency of the BSEP. The condition maps to chromosome 2 and is due to mutations of the ABCB11 gene.[82] These patients mostly present in the first few months of life with a mild neonatal hepatitis. The disease progresses and pruritus usually becomes a prominent problem towards the end of the first year. The rate of progression is variable, resulting in end-stage liver disease between 2 and 10 years of age, or possibly even later. No treatment apart from transplantation has shown to be of benefit, and it is particularly noteworthy that these patients appear to be incapable of excreting UDCA.[39] Treatment with modest doses of UDCA, however, may have a beneficial effect by further suppressing endogenous bile acid production. As expression of the gene appears to be entirely limited to the liver, liver transplantation has proved to be curative.

The genetic basis of the remaining third of the low-GGT PFIC spectrum has not been clarified as yet.

A form of high-GGT PFIC is associated with MDR3 deficiency, due to mutations of the *ABCB4* gene.[21] It is believed that the MDR3 gene product plays a critical role in the excretion of phosphatidylcholine, the major lipid component of human bile. A defect in phosphatidylcholine excretion is likely to result in the production of highly detergent bile, which can cause considerable tissue damage. Indeed, children with MDR3 deficiency have marked portal inflammation and bile duct proliferation. Some patients, particularly those who have some residual protein function, show a clinical response to UDCA, which reduces the hydrophobicity of the bile. Preliminary data from a murine model show that transplanted hepatocytes are capable of ameliorating the phenotype, suggesting that such transport defects in humans are good candidates for hepatocyte transplantation or gene therapy.

Neonatal haemochromatosis

Neonatal haemochromatosis (NH), or neonatal iron storage disorder, is a rare and often fatal disorder which causes either death in utero or acute liver failure in the neonatal period. The pathogenesis is uncertain. It may represent a single phenotypic expression of different aetiologies. NH has been observed in siblings and it has been suggested to have an autosomal recessive mode of inheritance.[42] However, we[41] and others[89] have observed NH in neonates conceived by different fathers, suggesting a specific role for maternal factors, possibly mitochondrial[89] or related to pregnancy. Often the pregnancy is complicated by oligohydramnios and/or megaplacenta. Histologically, the condition is characterised by intense deposition of stainable iron in the liver, hepatocellular necrosis, and diffuse hepatic fibrosis with nodular regeneration. Other organs are also typically iron overloaded, including the pancreas, heart, thyroid and salivary glands, with a characteristic sparing of the reticuloendothelial system.[43] Serum ferritin is usually elevated, but its levels do not allow differentiation of neonatal liver failure due to haemochromatosis from that due to other causes.[46] The diagnosis should be confirmed by lip biopsy to demonstrate stainable iron in the salivary glands.[43]

Apart from rare cases of spontaneous recovery with supportive care,[15] the disease, if untreated, is fatal. The efficacy of antioxidant–chelating treatment is controversial. After reports of successful use of the cocktail including prostaglandin E_1, selenium, desferrioxamine, N-acetyl-cysteine and vitamin E,[75,77] further reports have failed to show its beneficial effects.[79] These discrepant results may be due to different aetiologies for the same clinical syndrome, variably responsive to antioxidant–chelating treatment, to a wrong diagnosis of NH, or to the different degree of severity of liver damage. The antioxidant cocktail was largely ineffective in our own series of 19 severe

cases. Nine of the 10 treated infants, in fact, required transplantation or died before transplantation could be carried out. Of two children who survived without transplantation, one received the cocktail and one did not, making it impossible to draw conclusions on the efficacy of the antioxidant–chelation therapy. Liver transplantation is at the moment the only procedure able to divert the natural course of the disease. In our group, of the seven survivors, five have received a liver transplant.[41] Liver transplantation therefore remains the only real therapeutic option in the presence of severe liver failure.[6]

Prevention of NH is important. Genetic counselling is useful when recessive inheritance is likely (e.g. should consanguinity exist). The recurrence of NH is high in subsequent pregnancies. Although placental abnormalities have been described in NH, they are not sufficiently specific for antenatal diagnosis. High-dose intravenous immunoglobulin therapy during gestation, on the assumption that the condition may be due to some immune dysregulation, has not prevented recurrence of NH, but appears to reduce its severity to permit survival without transplantation.[90]

Haemophagocytic lymphohistiocytosis

A primary (familial) form of HLH is an established, but probably still underdiagnosed, cause of liver and multi-organ failure in early infancy. It is thought that an underlying immune disorder, linked to perforin deficiency, is responsible for lack of NK-cell function and an uninhibited response of the immune system to infection.[44] Perforin is pivotal for translocation of granzyme B from cytotoxic cells into invading microorganisms to initiate apoptosis. Primary HLH or perforin deficiency has an autosomal recessive inheritance and mutations have been mapped to 10q22,[81] although other loci for primary HLH have also been suggested.[62] Clinically, the condition presents acutely with fever, hepatosplenomegaly, pancytopenia, skin rash, and renal and respiratory failure. Laboratory investigations demonstrate hypertriglyceridaemia, hypofibrinogenaemia and hyperferritinaemia. The diagnosis is confirmed by cytological demonstration of haemophagocytosis in the bone marrow, ascitic fluid or cerebrospinal fluid (CSF). Severe coagulopathy often precludes liver biopsy or lumbar puncture. Despite heroic supportive measures, the mortality in the presence of liver failure is more than 90%. Cytotoxic treatment with etoposide or lymphocyte ablation and cyclosporin A have been suggested for milder forms.[35] If remission is achieved, the condition can be corrected by stem-cell transplantation.[38]

Mitochondrial cytopathies

An increasing number of infants with hypoglycaemia, sepsis, biochemical signs of liver failure and lactic acidosis are diagnosed with various mitochondrial disorders. These include respiratory chain complex (I–V) deficiency, mitochondrial DNA depletion syndrome, Pearson marrow–pancreas syndrome and primary fatty acid oxidation defects. Most of them do not follow a Mendelian mode of inheritance since mitochondrial DNA is inherited maternally and does not recombine. More than 90% of mitochondrial cytopathies are caused by mutations in nuclear genes, only a few of which have been identified.[32]

Multi-organ involvement is often present since mitochondria provide energy for intracellular processes of oxidative phosphorylation throughout the body. The clinical suspicion of a mitochondrial disorder should be raised in the presence of hypoglycaemia, feeding difficulties, multi-organ and liver failure, neurological impairment, pancreatic insufficiency and failure to thrive. These children are usually not dysmorphic. Elevated serum and CSF lactate are frequently detected. MRI or CT imaging of the head could reveal various anatomical and myelinisation defects. Treatment is of a limited help and includes prevention of hypoglycaemia, ubiquinone (coenzyme Q10), thiamine, riboflavine and dichloroacetate. The major management difficulty is consideration for liver transplantation of those children who present with liver failure but have not developed, as yet, signs of neurological impairment or respiratory failure. Whether or not these children should be offered transplantation in view of the possibility of later neurological or respiratory complications is still under debate.[24]

Management of disorders causing hepatitis syndrome in infancy

The essence of management is to define the site of the main pathological involvement and to identify any associated disorder, particularly those for which there is specific therapy. Infections must be treated with appropriate anti-infective agents.

Fructose and galactose are omitted from the diet until fructosaemia and galactosaemia have been excluded by specific tests. Fat-soluble vitamin deficiencies must be prevented by oral or parenteral supplements.[57] The exact vitamin requirements depend on the degree of malabsorption and metabolic demands. It is mandatory to monitor the prothrombin time (vitamin K), serum calcium, phosphate and wrist X-rays (vitamin D), and serum vitamin E and A concentrations, to assess adequacy of supplementation. Vitamin K deficiency is an immediate risk.

If cholestasis persists for more than 3 months, laboratory or radiological signs of vitamin D deficiency are likely to appear, with pathological evidence of vitamin E deficiency occurring after 5 months. Clinical evidence of vitamin A deficiency develops after some years, but biochemical evidence may be present earlier.[3] Oral supplements are given in doses of three to five times normal requirements if cholestasis is incomplete. In complete cholestasis, doses of vitamin K 1 mg orally per day, vitamin D 30 000 units intramuscularly at 4-weekly intervals, and vitamin A 50 000 units intramuscularly at 4-weekly intervals will usually prevent laboratory evidence of deficiency. Vitamin E parenterally in a dose of 10 mg/kg at 2-weekly intervals is required to maintain the serum vitamin E level.[57] In infants with failure to thrive, dietary supplements of carbohydrate polymers and medium-chain triglycerides (if defects of fat oxidation have been excluded) are required.

Colestyramine (cholestyramine) with or without phenobarbital, UDCA or rifampicin may be required for pruritus. There is no medical treatment that influences the progression of idiopathic disorders.

Inherited disorders of bilirubin metabolism

Gilbert syndrome

A chronic, mild, variable unconjugated hyperbilirubinaemia, with serum bilirubin levels around 34–85 micromol/l (2–5 mg/dl), in the absence of significant haemolysis or abnormality of liver function, is the characteristic feature of this condition. The pathogenesis is undetermined. Impaired hepatic uptake of bilirubin, deficient uridine diphosphate glucuronyl transferase (UDPGT) activity and a mild excretory defect have been suggested.[55] An abnormality of the promotor region of the *UDPGT1* gene, inherited in an autosomal recessive fashion, has been demonstrated.[7] The frequency of the abnormal promotor among the normal population is 40%. Because clinically manifested Gilbert syndrome occurs in 3–10% of the population, other factors, such as an increased bilirubin production, must be present to bring this disease to expression. The diagnosis is rarely made with confidence before 10 years of age and is based on exclusion of other causes of unconjugated hyperbilirubinaemia. Treatment is unnecessary. Whether the condition contributes to hyperbilirubinaemia in the newborn is difficult to ascertain.

Crigler–Najjar disease

This rare disorder is characterised by elevated unconjugated hyperbilirubinaemia from birth. Crigler–Najjar disease type 1 results from a complete deficiency of UDPGT, and type 2 from a partial deficiency. In Crigler–Najjar disease type 1, serum bilirubin values are in excess of 350 micromol/l and the bile contains only traces of bilirubin conjugates. Crigler–Najjar disease type 2 is less severe, with serum bilirubin values not exceeding 350 micromol/l. The bile of these patients contains bilirubin mono- and diglucuronides in low concentration. Genetically, both diseases result from mutations of the *UDPGT1* gene.[4,74] Both Crigler–Najjar type 1 and type 2 are inherited in an autosomal recessive fashion.[40] The diagnosis is suspected on the basis of the clinical features and needs to be confirmed by mutation analysis, assessing bilirubin conjugates in the bile collected at endoscopy, or by measuring UDPGT activity in a percutaneous liver biopsy specimen. In Crigler–Najjar type 2, serum bilirubin levels decrease by at least 30% with phenobarbital treatment. Patients with Crigler–Najjar type 1 are at risk of developing neurological damage and kernicterus throughout their life. Most patients require exchange transfusions to control hyperbilirubinaemia in the newborn period, and thereafter require continuous phototherapy of sufficient intensity to keep the serum bilirubin below 340 micromol/l. This is most conveniently achieved by sleeping undressed for up to 12–15 hours under a specially built phototherapy device incorporating as many as 32 phototherapy tubes.[92] Oral colestyramine may reduce the phototherapy requirement by binding bilirubin in the gut. After 4 years of age, phototherapy gradually becomes less effective and liver transplantation becomes necessary to prevent kernicterus.[68] Auxiliary liver transplant, where the left lateral segment of the recipient is removed and substituted with the donor's left lateral segment, has proved successful in correcting the enzymatic defect. Hepatocyte transplantation is a therapeutic option which may offer non-surgical correction of the enzymatic defect.[28]

References

1. Alagille D, Estrada A, Hadchouel M et al 1987 Syndromic paucity of interlobular bile ducts (Alagille's syndrome or arteriohepatic dysplasia): review of eighty cases. Journal of Pediatrics 110: 195–200

2. Amedee-Manesme O, Bernard O, Brunelle F et al 1987 Sclerosing cholangitis with neonatal onset. Journal of Pediatrics 111: 225–229

3. Amedee-Manesme O, Mourey M S, Courturier M, et al 1988 Short- and long-term vitamin A treatment in children with cholestasis. American Journal of Clinical Nutrition 47: 690–693

4. Aono S, Yamada Y, Keino H et al 1993 Identification of defect in the genes for bilirubin UDP-glucuronosyl-transferase in a patient with Crigler-Najjar syndrome type II. Biochemical and Biophysical Research Communications 197: 1239–1244

5. Baker A, Portmann B, Westaby D et al 1993 Neonatal sclerosing cholangitis in two siblings: a category of progressive intrahepatic cholestasis. Journal of Pediatric Gastroenterology and Nutrition 17: 317–322

6. Bonatti H, Muiesan P, Connelly S et al 1997 Hepatic transplantation in children under 3 months of age: single centre's experience. Journal of Pediatric Surgery 32: 486–488

7. Bosma P J, Chowdhury J R, Bakker C et al 1995 The genetic basis of the reduced expression of bilirubin UDP-glucuronosyl-transferase 1 in Gilbert's syndrome. New England Journal of Medicine 333: 1171–1175

8. Brown W R, Sokol R J, Levin M J et al 1988 Lack of correlation between infection with reovirus 3 and extrahepatic biliary atresia or neonatal hepatitis. Journal of Pediatrics 113: 670–676

9. Cabrera-Abreu J C, Green A 2002 Gamma-glutamyl-transferase: value of its measurement in paediatrics. Annals of Clinical Biochemistry 39: 22–25

10. Carlton V E, Knisely A S, Freimer N B 1995 Mapping of a locus for progressive familial intrahepatic cholestasis (Byler disease) to 18q21-q22, the benign recurrent intrahepatic cholestasis region. Human Molecular Genetics 4: 1049–1053

11. Chiba T, Ohi R, Nio M, Ibrahim M 1992 Late complications in long term survivors of bilary atresia. European Journal of Pediatric Surgery 2: 22–25

12. Clayton P T, Casteels M, Mieli-Vergani G, Lawson A M 1995 Familial giant cell hepatitis associated with greatly increased urinary excretion of bile alcohols: a new inborn error of bile acid synthesis? Pediatric Research 37: 424–431

13. Clayton P T, Leonard J V, Lawson A M et al 1987 Familial giant cell hepatitis associated with synthesis of 3β,7α-dihydroxy- and 3β,7α,12α-trihydroxy-5-cholenoic acids. Journal of Clinical Investigation 79: 1031–1038

14. Clayton R J, Iber F L, Reubner B H, McKusick V A 1969 Fatal familial intrahepatic cholestasis in an Amish kindred. American Journal of Diseases of Children 117: 112–124

15. Colletti R B, Clemmons J J W 1988 Familial neonatal hemochromatosis with survival. Journal of Pediatric Gastroenterology and Nutrition 7: 29–45

16. Collins J, Goldfischer S 1990 Perinatal hemochromatosis: one disease, several diseases or a spectrum? Hepatology 12: 176–177

17. Davenport M, Kerkar N, Mieli-Vergani G, Mowat A P, Howard E R 1997 Biliary atresia: the King's College Hospital experience, 1974–1995. Journal of Pediatric Surgery 32: 479–485

18. Davenport M, Savage M, Mowat A P, Howard E R 1993 Biliary atresia splenic malformation syndrome: an etiological and prognostic subgroup. Surgery 113: 662–667

19. Deprettere A, Portmann B, Mowat A P 1987 Syndromic paucity of the intrahepatic bile ducts: diagnostic difficulty; severe morbidity throughout childhood. Journal of Pediatric Gastroenterology and Nutrition 6: 865–871

20. Deutsch J, Smith A L, Danks D, Campbell P E 1985 Long-term prognosis for babies with neonatal liver disease. Archives of Diseases in Childhood 60: 447–451

21. de Vree J M, Jacquemin E, Sturm E et al 1998 Mutations in the MDR3 gene cause progressive familial intrahepatic cholestasis. Proceedings of National Academy of Sciences of the United States of America 95: 282–287

22. Dick M C, Mowat A P 1985 Hepatitis syndrome in infancy – an epidemiological study with 10-year follow-up. Archives of Disease in Childhood 60: 512–515

23. Donaldson P T, Clare M, Constantini P K et al 2002 HLA and cytokine gene polymorphisms in biliary atresia. Liver 22: 213–219

24. Dubern B, Broue P, Dubuisson C et al 2001 Orthotopic liver transplantation for mitochondrial respiratory chain disorders: a study of 5 children. Transplantation 71: 633–637

25. El Tumi M A, Clark M D, Barrett J J, Mowat A P 1987 A ten minute radiopharmaceutical test in suspected biliary atresia. Archives of Disease in Childhood 62: 180–184

26. Emond J C, Whitington P F 1995 Selective surgical management of progressive familial intrahepatic cholestasis (Byler's disease). Journal of Pediatric Surgery 30: 1635–1641

27. Fishler B, Ehrnst A, Forsgren M, Orvell C, Nemeth A 1998 The viral association of neonatal cholestasis in Sweden: a possible link between cytomegalovirus infection and biliary atresia. Journal of Pediatric Gastroenterology and Nutrition 27: 57–64

28. Fox I J, Chowdhury J R, Kaufman S S et al 1998 Treatment of the Crigler-Najjar syndrome type I with hepatocyte transplantation. New England Journal of Medicine 338: 1463–1465

29. Francavilla R, Castellaneta S P, Hadzic N et al 2000 Prognosis of alpha-1-antitrypsin deficiency-related liver disease in the era of paediatric liver transplantation. Journal of Hepatology 32: 986–992

30. Francavilla R, Mieli-Vergani G 2002 Liver and biliary disease in infancy. Medicine 30: 45–47

31. Gautier M, Elliot N 1981 Extrahepatic biliary atresia: morphological study of 94 biliary remnants. Archives of Pathology and Laboratory Medicine 105: 397–402

32. Gillis L, Kaye E 2002 Diagnosis and management of mitochondrial diseases. Pediatric Clinics of North America 49: 203–219

33. Hadzic N, Davenport M, Tizzard S et al 2003 Long-term survival following Kasai portoenterostomy: is chronic liver disease inevitable? Journal of Pediatric Gastroenterology and Nutrition 37: 430–433

34. Henriksen N T, Drablos P A, Aagenaes O 1981 Cholestatic jaundice in infancy. The importance of familial and genetic factors in the aetiology and prognosis. Archives of Disease in Childhood 56: 622–627

35. Hirst W J, Layton D M, Singh S et al 1994 Haemophagocytic lymphohistiocytosis – experience at two UK centres. British Journal of Haematology 88: 731–739

36. Howard E R 1989 Choledochal cysts. In: Schwarz C, Ellis H (eds) Maingot's abdominal operations, 9th edn. Appleton-Century-Crofts, New York, p. 1366

37. Howard E R, Johnstone D I, Mowat A P 1976 Spontaneous perforation of the common bile duct in infants. Archives of Disease in Childhood 51: 883–886

38. Jabado N, de Graeff-Meeder E R, Cavazzana-Calvo M et al 1997 Treatment of familial hemophagocytic lymphohistiocytosis with bone marrow transplantation from HLA genetically nonidentical donors. Blood 90: 4743–4748

39. Jansen P L, Strautnieks S S, Jacquemin E et al 1999 Hepatocanalicular bile salt export pump deficiency in patients with progressive familial intrahepatic cholestasis. Gastroenterology 117: 1370–1379

40. Kadakol A, Ghosh S S, Sappal B S et al 2000 Genetic lesions of bilirubin uridine-diphosphoglucuronate glucuronosyl-transferase (UGT1A1) causing Crigler-Najjar and Gilbert syndromes: correlation of genotype to phenotype. Human Mutations 16: 297–306

41. Kallas M B E, Baker A, Nash R, Mieli-Vergani G 1997 Chelation/antioxidant treatment is unsuccessful in neonatal hemochromatosis presenting with acute liver failure. Hepatology 26: 534A

42. Kelly A L, Lunt P W, Rodrigues F et al 2001 Classification and genetic features of neonatal haemochromatosis: a study of twenty-seven affected pedigrees and molecular analysis of genes implicated in iron metabolism. Journal of Medical Genetics 38: 599–610

43. Knisely A S 1992 Neonatal hemochromatosis. Advances in Pediatrics 39: 383–403

44. Kogawa K, Lee S M, Villanueva J et al 2002 Perforin expression in cytotoxic lymphocytes from patients with hemophagocytic lymphohistiocytosis and their family members. Blood 99: 61–66

45. Kohsaka T, Yuan Z R, Guo S X et al 2002 The significance of human jagged 1 mutations detected in severe cases of extrahepatic biliary atresia. Hepatology 36: 904–912

46. Lee W S, McKiernan P J, Kelly D A 2001 Serum ferritin level in neonatal fulminant liver failure. Archives of Disease in Childhood. Fetal and Neonatal Edition 85: F226

47. Lindstedt S, Holme E, Lock E A et al 1992 Treatment of hereditary tyrosinaemia type I by inhibition of 4-hydroxyphenylpyruvate dioxygenase. Lancet 340: 813–817

48. Lomas D A, Evans D L, Finch J T, Carrell R W 1992 The mechanism of Z alpha₁-antitrypsin accumulation in the liver. Nature 357: 605–607

49. Lykavieris P, Hadchouel M, Chardot C, Bernard O 2001 Outcome of liver disease in children with Alagille syndrome: a study of 163 patients. Gut 49: 431–435

50. McClement J W, Howard E R, Mowat A P 1985 Results of surgical treatment of extrahepatic biliary atresia in the United Kingdom. British Medical Journal 290: 345–349

51. McKiernan P J, Baker A J, Kelly D A 2000 The frequency and outcome of biliary atresia in the UK and Ireland. Lancet 355: 4–5

52. Maggiore G, Bernard O, Riely C A et al 1987 Normal serum gamma-glutamyl-transpeptidase activity identifies groups of infants with idiopathic cholestasis with poor prognosis. Journal of Pediatrics 111: 251–252

53. Markowitz J, Daum F, Kahn E I et al 1983 Arteriohepatic dysplasia. I. Pitfalls in diagnosis and management. Hepatology 3: 74–76

54. Mieli-Vergani G, Howard E R, Portmann B, Mowat A P 1989 Late referral for biliary atresia: missed opportunities for effective surgery. Lancet I: 421–423

55. Monaghan G, Ryan M, Seddon R, Hume R, Burchell B 1996 Genetic variation in bilirubin-UDP-glucuronosyltransferase gene promotor and Gilbert's syndrome. Lancet 347: 578–581

56. Morecki R, Glaser J 1989 Reovirus 3 and neonatal biliary disease: discussion of divergent results. Hepatology 10: 515–517

57. Mowat A P 1994 Hepatitis and cholestasis in infancy: intrahepatic disorders. In: Liver disorders in childhood, 3rd edn. Butterworths, London, pp 43–78

58. Muiesan P, Dhawan A, Novelli M et al 2000 Isolated liver transplant and sequential small bowel transplantation for intestinal failure and related liver disease in children. Transplantation 69: 2323–2326

59. Nagral S, Muiesan P, Vilca-Melendez H et al 1997 Liver transplantation for extrahepatic biliary atresia. Tohoku Journal of Experimental Medicine 181: 117–127

60. Nietgen G W, Vacanti J P, Perez-Atayade A 1992 Intrahepatic bile duct loss in biliary atresia despite portoenterostomy: a consequence of ongoing obstruction. Gastroenterology 102: 2126–2133

61. Odievre M, Hadchouel M, Landrieu C, Alagille D, Elliot N 1981 Long-term prognosis for infants with intrahepatic cholestasis and patent extrahepatic biliary tract. Archives of Disease in Childhood 56: 373–376

62. Ohadi M, Lalloz M R, Sham P et al 1999 Localisation of a gene for familial hemophagocytic lymphohistiocytosis at chromosome 9q21.3-22 by homozygosity mapping. American Journal of Human Genetics 64: 165–171

63. Ohi R, Nio M, Chiba T et al 1990 Long-term follow-up after surgery for patients with biliary atresia. Journal of Pediatric Surgery 25: 442–445

64. Ohkohchi N, Chiba T, Ohi R, Mori S 1989 Long-term follow-up of patients with cholangitis after successful Kasai operation in biliary atresia: selection of recipients for liver transplantation. Journal of Pediatric Gastroenterology and Nutrition 9: 416–420

65. Otte J B, Yandza T, De Ville de Goyet J et al 1988 Pediatric liver transplantation: report on 52 patients with a 2-year survival of 86%. Journal of Pediatric Surgery 23: 250–253

66. Ozawa K, Uemoto S, Tanaka K et al 1992 An appraisal of pediatric liver transplantation from living relatives. Initial clinical experience in 20 pediatric liver transplantations from living relatives as donors. Annals of Surgery 216: 547–553

67. Pereira G R, Sherman M S, Digiacimo J 1981 Hyper-alimentation induced cholestasis. American Journal of Diseases of Children 135: 842–845

68. Pett S, Mowat A P 1987 Crigler-Najjar syndrome types I and II. Clinical experience – King's College Hospital 1972–1987. Phenobarbitone, phototherapy and liver transplantation Molecular Aspects of Medicine 9: 473–482

69. Psacharopoulos H T, Mowat A P, Cook P J L et al 1983 Outcome of liver disease associated with alpha 1-antitrypsin deficiency (PiZ); implications for genetic counselling and antenatal diagnosis. Archives of Disease in Childhood 58: 882–887

70. Quigley E M, Marsh M N, Shaffer J L, Markin R S 1993 Hepatobiliary complications of total parenteral nutrition. Gastroenterology 104: 1583–1584

71. Rand E B 1998 The genetic basis of the Alagille syndrome. Journal of Pediatric Gastroenterology and Nutrition 26: 234–236

72. Redkar R, Davenport M, Howard E R 1998 Antenatal diagnosis of congenital anomalies of the biliary tract. Journal of Pediatric Surgery 33: 700–704

73. Riepenhoff-Talty M, Gouvea V, Evans M J et al 1996 Detection of group C rotavirus in infants with extrahepatic biliary atresia. Journal of Infectious Diseases 174: 8–15

74. Ritter J K, Yeatman M T, Ferreira P, Owens I S 1992 Identification of a genetic alteration in the code for bilirubin UDP-glucuronosyltransferase in the UGT1 gene complex of a Crigler-Najjar type I patient. Journal of Clinical Investigation 90: 150–155

75. Roberts E A, James A, Chitayat D et al 1999 Prenatal surveillance, rapid diagnosis and prompt institution of medical treatment in perinatal hemochromatosis (abstract). Journal of Pediatric Gastroenterology and Nutrition 29: 511A

76. Schwarzenberg S J, Sharp H L 1990 Pathogenesis of alpha 1-antitrypsin deficiency-associated liver disease. Journal of Pediatric Gastroenterology and Nutrition 10: 5–12

77. Shamieh I, Kibort P K, Suchy F J, Freese D K 1993 Antioxidant therapy for neonatal iron storage disease. Pediatric Research 33: 109A

78. Sifers R N, Finegold M J, Woo S L C 1992 Molecular biology and genetics of alpha-1-antitrypsin deficiency. Seminars in Liver Diseases 12: 301–310

79. Sigurdsson L, Reyes J, Kocoshis S A et al 1998 Neonatal hemochromatosis; outcomes of pharmacological and surgical therapies. Journal of Pediatric Gastroenterology and Nutrition 26: 85–89

80. Silveira T R, Salzano F M, Howard E R, Mowat A P 1991 Extrahepatic biliary atresia and twinning. Brazilian Journal of Medical and Biological Research 24: 67–71

81. Stepp S E, Dufourcq-Lagelouse R, Le Deist F et al 1999 Perforin gene defects in familial hemophagocytic lymphohistiocytosis. Science 286:1957–1959

82. Strautnieks S S, Kagalwalla A F, Tanner M S et al 1997 Identification of a locus for progressive familial intrahepatic cholestasis PFIC2 on chromosome 2q24. American Journal of Human Genetics 61: 630–633

83. Strife C F, Hug G, Chuck G et al 1983 Membranoproliferative glomerulonephritis and alpha 1-antitrypsin deficiency in children. Pediatrics 71: 88–92

84. Stringer M D, Dhawan A, Davenport M et al 1995 Choledochal cysts: lessons from a 20-year experience. Archives of Disease in Childhood 73: 528–531

85. Sveger T, Eriksson S 1995 The liver in adolescents with alpha-1-antitrypsin deficiency. Hepatology 22: 514–517

86. Tan C E, Driver M, Howard E R, Moscoso G J 1994 Extrahepatic biliary atresia: a first trimester event? Clues from light microscopy and immunohistochemistry. Journal of Pediatric Surgery 29: 808–814

87. Thompson R J, Jansen P L 2000 Genetic defects in hepatocanalicular transport. Seminars in Liver Disease 20: 365–372

88. Tyler K L, Sokol R J, Oberhaus S M et al 1998 Detection of reovirus RNA in hepatobiliary tissues from patients with extrahepatic biliary atresia and choledochal cysts. Hepatology 27: 1475–1482

89. Verloes A, Temple I K, Hubert A F et al 1996 Recurrence of neonatal haemochromatosis in half sibs born of unaffected mothers. Journal of Medical Genetics 33: 444–449

90. Whitington P F 2002 Immunomodulatory therapy during pregnancy prevents recurrent lethal neonatal hemochromatosis (abstract). Hepatology 36: 336A

91. Wilkinson M L, Mieli-Vergani G, Ball C, Portmann B, Mowat A P 1991 Endoscopic retrograde cholangiopancreatography (ERCP) in infantile cholestasis. Archives of Disease in Childhood 66: 121–123

92. Yohannan M D, Perry M J, Littlewood J M 1983 Long-term phototherapy in Crigler-Najjar syndrome. Archives of Disease in Childhood 58: 460–462

PART 3

Gastrointestinal disorders

Simon J Newell

Structure and function of the developing gastrointestinal tract

Basic embryology

Embryological development is described in Chapter 9.

Neonatal gastrointestinal function

Digestion and absorption

This is dealt with in detail on page 737.

Motility

The ontogeny of motility lags behind digestive and absorptive function (Fig. 29.14). Disordered motor function presents clinically as 'poor tolerance of feeds'. Symptoms include vomiting, high gastric residual volume, bile staining of the gastric aspirate, abdominal distension and reduced stool frequency.

The oesophagus has two complementary functions: swallowing and the prevention of gastro-oesophageal reflux. Nutritive swallowing is seldom present in the infant of less than 34 weeks' gestation, and 75% of healthy preterm infants require tube feeding until this postconceptional age.[76] The fetus begins to swallow liquor at around 16 weeks gestation. Initially small volumes are

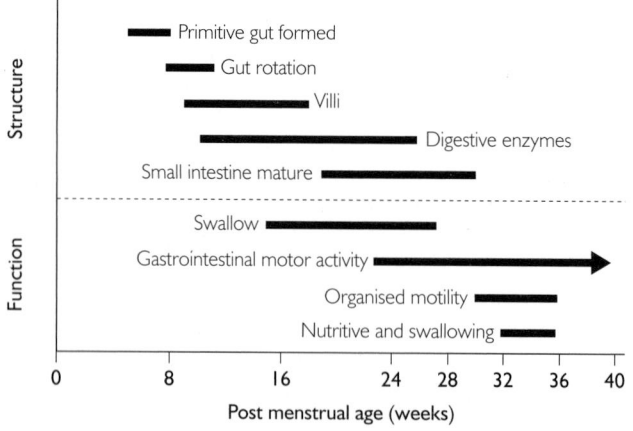

Fig. 29.14 Ontogenic timetable of gut structural and functional development. (Redrawn from Newell S J, Chapman S, Booth I W 1993 Ultrasonic assessment of gastric emptying in the preterm infant. Archives of Disease in Childhood 69: 32–36.)

swallowed, increasing to around 500 mL/day by term. Fetal swallowing is an important mechanism in the regulation of liquor volume, and reduced swallowing explains the polyhydramnios seen in oesophageal atresia or in fetuses with neuromuscular conditions.[144]

Swallowed liquor is important ontogenetically. Liquor contains protein, carbohydrate and triglyceride, which may be luminal nutrients. Amniotic fluid is rich in growth factors (epidermal growth factor, insulin-like growth factor, granulocyte-colony stimulating factor, erythropoietin) and fetal swallowing may stimulate enteric hormone secretion.[88,102,120,162,166] In the animal model, ligation of the fetal oesophagus results in gut hypoplasia, unless liquor or growth factors are infused into the intestine.[125,169] Artificial amniotic fluid in the preterm infant has been subjected to a phase 1 clinical trial of early feeding for in induction of gastrointestinal maturity.[166]

In the term infant, the complex mechanism of swallowing with movement of the bolus of milk into the stomach, protection of the airway, inhibition of respiration and appropriate relaxation of oesophageal sphincter and gastric fundus is achieved within a day or two of birth.[103] The mature suck-swallow pattern has bursts of sucks at a rate of 2 per second, with oesophageal transit on a few occasions during each burst.[141] In the preterm infant, uncoordinated motor activity[132] is similar to that seen in older children with reflux oesophagitis.[38]

Competent lower oesophageal sphincter (LOS) activity is essential to prevent reflux.[87] The high pressure in the sphincter is a function of the diaphragm, the intra-abdominal segment of the oesophagus and the muscular sphincter. Term infants have LOS pressure similar to that seen in older children[87] but in the preterm infant pressure is low and rises with postconceptional age.[135] Resting LOS pressure is reduced by caffeine[132] but function is not disrupted by nasogastric intubation.[1] Most gastro-oesophageal reflux occurs during transient relaxation of the sphincter.[139]

Gastric emptying can be observed in the fetus during the second trimester[49] but may be slow in the preterm infant, presenting as failure to tolerate milk feeds.[20] Half emptying time for breast milk has been estimated as 20–40 minutes.[23,57,133] Emptying is faster with breast milk than formula.[57] A number of other factors affect gastric emptying (Fig. 29.15). Breast milk fortifier does not affect gastric emptying during the introduction of milk feeds[110] although emptying is slower with full volume, 3 hourly feeds.[60]

In the preterm infant, propagative small intestinal motility is poorly organised, with short bursts of motor activity before 30 weeks' gestation, which subsequently become coordinated, coincident with the timing of nutritive sucking.[184] Small intestinal motility and tolerance of feeds is enhanced by previous exposure to enteral nutrition.[8,111]

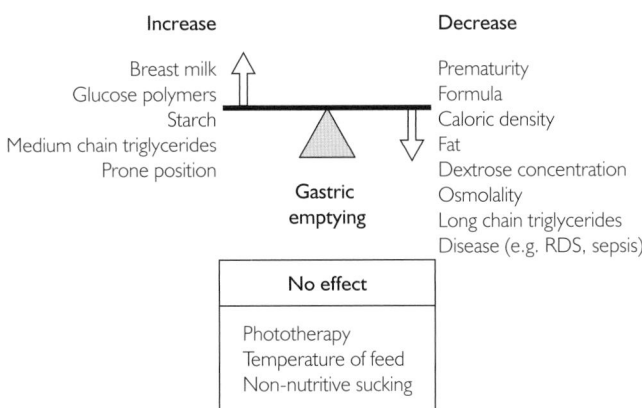

Fig. 29.15 Factors affecting gastric emptying. (Redrawn from Newell S J 1996 Gastrointestinal function and its ontogeny: how should we feed the preterm infant. In: Ryan S (ed) Seminars in neonatology 1. W B Saunders, London, pp 59–66.)

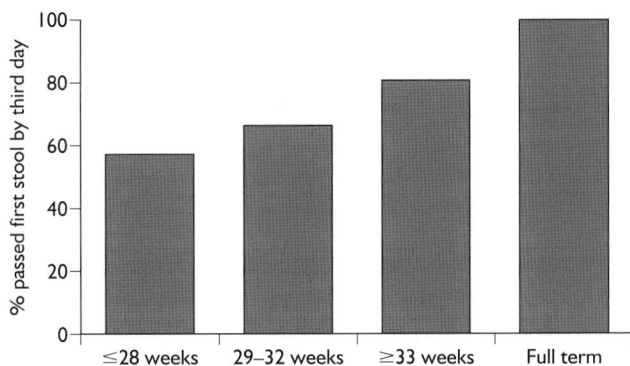

Fig. 29.16 Time of passage of first stool after birth.[29,157,179]

Table 29.20 The gastrointestinal barrier: factors that may protect against intestinal pathogens, toxins and antigens

Non-immune
Intraluminal
■ Gastric acid
■ Motility
■ Pancreaticobiliary secretions
■ Breast milk factors
  – Lysozyme
  – Lactoferrin
  – Oligosaccharides

Mucosal
■ Mucus, bicarbonate and glycocalyx
■ Microvillous membrane

Immune
■ Secretory IgA
■ Cellular immunity (GALT and milk)
  – Macrophages
  – Lymphocytes
  – Leukocytes
  – Complement

Total gut transit time varies between 1 and 5 days.[7,111] Passage of stool occurs within 24 hours of birth in 94–98% of healthy term infants. The passage of stools is slower in the preterm infant and frequency is inversely related to gestation (Fig. 29.16).[29,157,179] Around half of infants under 28 weeks gestation have not passed their first stool within the first 3 days.[179]

Barrier function

Mucosal protection is afforded by luminal, mucosal and systemic mechanisms (Table 29.20). Gastric acid, the first-line defence, reduces gastric pH below 4 within hours of birth, in all but the most immature infants in whom this occurs within the first week.[87] Enteral feeds buffer gastric acidity.[160]

Intact absorption of large molecules occurs across the neonatal gut. Macromolecular absorption is higher in preterm and small for gestational age infants[9] and diminishes over the first months of life. This process of gut closure may occur more rapidly if breast milk is given rather than cow's milk formula.[178] The biological and clinical significance of macromolecular absorption in the human is unclear.[83]

Signs of gastrointestinal disease

Vomiting

Vomiting is a common sign and assessment should take account of volume, frequency and content of the vomitus and associated symptoms. Effortless regurgitation may represent gastro-oesophageal reflux (see below). Vomiting is often a sign of disease outside the gastrointestinal tract, notably infection (meningitis, pyelonephritis, hepatitis; pp. 1011–75), disease of the central nervous system (intracranial haemorrhage, hydrocephalus; pp. 1194–6), metabolic disorders (galactosaemia, congenital adrenal hyperplasia, thyrotoxicosis; pp. 851–907) and heart disease (cardiac failure; p. 624).

Persistent vomiting may indicate obstruction. Upper gastrointestinal obstruction leads to vomiting shortly after birth while incomplete or lower obstruction presents later. Polyhydramnios during pregnancy or the 'mucusy' baby at delivery demands exclusion of oesophageal atresia before a feed is given. Fetal ultrasound reliably detects most cases of diaphragmatic hernia and duodenal atresia but malrotation, upper gut atresia, partial obstruction or web and duplications cysts are less often diagnosed antenatally. Most obstruction occurs distal to the ampulla of Vater, including the vast majority of duodenal atresias. Bile-stained vomiting indicates a surgical problem (p. 711). Herniae are an important site of obstruction at all ages (pp. 736–7).

Vomiting later in the neonatal period is less specific to obstruction. Functional obstruction occurs in necrotising enterocolitis (NEC) and ileus. Luminal obstruction may occur and is seen in meconium ileus (pp. 724–6), meconium plug syndrome (pp. 694, 732) and, rarely, lactobezoar. In malrotation, initial symptoms may be intermittent. Hirschsprung's disease may not present with typical features of abdominal distension and vomiting and this diagnosis should be considered following delayed passage of meconium (p. 751). Hypertrophic pyloric stenosis (pp. 693–4, 717–20) is a difficult diagnosis to make when signs begin – we have all been caught out by a preterm infant developing hypertrophic pyloric stenosis in front of our eyes!

Upper gastrointestinal bleeding

The appearance of small amounts of fresh blood or 'coffee grounds' in vomitus is not rare. In most infants a cause is not found and the prognosis is good. Swallowed maternal blood during birth or breastfeeding may lead to haematemesis or melaena. If blood is fresh, differentiation between adult and fetal haemoglobin is helpful.

Gastrointestinal bleeding may mark a bleeding diathesis. Classical haemorrhagic disease of the newborn (p. 262) still occurs if adequate vitamin K prophylaxis is not given.[148] Late vitamin K deficiency bleeding is more common in babies with liver disease (pp. 679–91). Disseminated intravascular coagulation (pp. 759–60) and inherited clotting disorders make assessment of coagulation status imperative if there is gastrointestinal bleeding.

Upper gastrointestinal ulceration occurs in the fetus,[3] the newborn after perinatal stress[43] and infants receiving intensive care.[119] At endoscopy, an oesophagogastritis of unknown aetiology occurs in a large proportion of infants presenting with haematemesis, frequent regurgitation or poor growth.[43] Rarely, haematemesis indicates congenital varices, true peptic ulcer, gastric or intestinal volvulus, duplications or haemangioma.[176] The administration of dexamethasone[136] or tolazoline may be associated with bleeding or perforation. We routinely use ranitidine as prophylaxis in infants receiving dexamethasone.[86] H_2 blockade or proton pump inhibition is used for stress bleeding and other upper gastrointestinal bleeding.[3] Routine inhibition of gastric acid secretion is not recommended, and predisposes to NEC.[171]

Rectal bleeding

Rapid intestinal transit may allow upper gastrointestinal bleeding to appear as fresh blood per rectum. A small amount of fresh rectal bleeding is commonly due to an anorectal fissure. This is usually obvious on inspection or can be seen by inserting a lubricated auriscope speculum into the anal canal. Rectal perforation is a very rare complication of use of a rectal thermometer.[185] A wide variety of intestinal conditions may lead to rectal bleeding, including malrotation (pp. 721–2), volvulus (p. 776), intussusception (p. 726) and Hirschsprung's disease (pp. 726–8). Meckel's diverticulum (p. 736), haemangiomata and bowel telangiectasia most commonly present after the neonatal period.[44] In the preterm infant, rectal bleeding may denote NEC (see below).

Dietary protein intolerance is an important cause of bleeding and colitis, with blood and mucus per rectum (see below).

Diarrhoea

The immediate and universal consequence of diarrhoea is loss of water and electrolytes. Dehydration may be rapid because of low body mass and the relative importance of colonic water and electrolyte conservation. Infective causes are common and a history of contact and stool culture is important (p. 1046). Loose, abnormal stools may indicate NEC (see below) or even Hirschsprung's disease. In persistent diarrhoea, rare disorders of mucosal function should be considered (see below). In some of these conditions, diarrhoea in utero may produce polyhydramnios and stool output may be enormous. Pancreatic malabsorption occurs in cystic fibrosis, Schwachmann's syndrome and pancreatic hypoplasia but does not usually present in the neonatal period.

Constipation

Delayed passage of meconium may indicate obstruction or Hirschsprung's disease (pp. 726–8). Meconium ileus, with thick, inspissated stools and abdominal distension often associated with palpable faecal masses, is almost pathognomonic of cystic fibrosis (see below). In meconium plug syndrome, symptoms usually resolve after the first passage of meconium (p. 502). Hypothyroidism, hypercalcaemia, diabetes insipidus and renal tubular acidosis may all present with constipation. Intestinal pseudo-obstruction may lead to symptoms in the neonatal period.[74]

In very-low-birthweight (VLBW) infants, infrequent or delayed passage of meconium or stool may be associated with poor tolerance of feeds, particularly in the preterm infant with intrauterine growth restriction.[59] Suppositories may be helpful in inducing defaecation or a small dose of lactulose may be justified.

Necrotising enterocolitis

Epidemiology

The incidence of NEC lies between 1 and 3 cases per 1000 live births. NEC occurs in 2–5% of VLBW infants, and in 1–8% of admissions to neonatal intensive care.[4,96,97] This equates with 500–1500 cases each year in England and Wales. The British Paediatric Surveillance Unit survey reported an overall mortality of 22%.[107] Median gestation was 29 weeks and 65% were under 1500 g, but 12% of infants with NEC are born at term (Fig. 29.17).[4,31,96] Onset of signs is most commonly in the second week (Fig. 29.18). There are no reliable, seasonal, sexual or geographical patterns with NEC. The National Institute of Child Health and Human Development made the startling observation of a variation in prevalence from 4% to over 20% of VLBW infants between centres across North America.[170] This variability in incidence between centres suggests an iatrogenic component, which has yet to be identified.

Necrotising enterocolitis is a common end point precipitated by a number of different circumstances (Table 29.21). Babies with NEC may be divided broadly into three groups.[4] In the term baby, NEC is almost universally associated with major risk factors for gut ischaemia, principally perinatal asphyxia, and often occurs in the first days. NEC may occur at term in Hirschsprung's

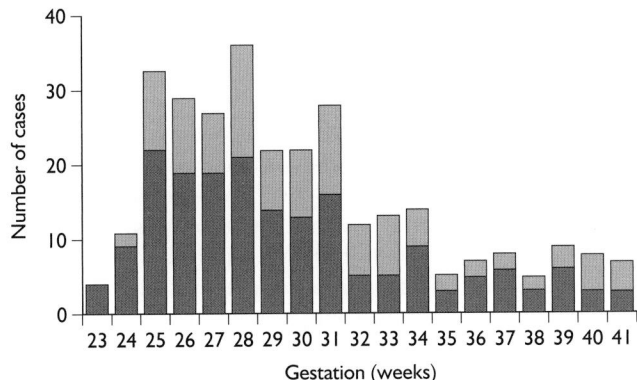

Fig. 29.17 Gestation at diagnosis of NEC: results of a survey in the UK over a period of 1 year. All cases are shown by the open bars. Cases confirmed at surgery, with gas in the portal tract, or free gas in the abdomen are shaded. (Redrawn from Lucas A, Abbott R in collaboration with the Royal College of Paediatrics and Child Health Research Unit.)

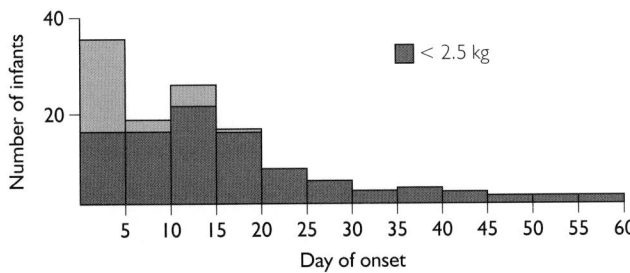

Fig. 29.18 Age at onset of NEC in 129 cases notified to the Communicable Diseases Surveillance Centre, July 1980 to June 1981. (Redrawn from Communicable Disease Report 1982 Neonatal necrotising enterocolitis surveillance. In: Communicable disease report 82/05. Communicable Disease Surveillance Centre, London.)

Table 29.21 'Risk' factors incriminated in the aetiology of necrotising enterocolitis

- Prematurity
- Intrauterine growth restriction
- Abruptio placentae
- Premature rupture of membranes
- Perinatal asphyxia
- Low Apgar score
- Umbilical catheterisation
- Hypoxia and shock
- Hypothermia
- Patent ductus arteriosus
- Non-human milk formula
- Hypertonic feeds
- Rapid introduction of enteral feeds
- Fluid overload
- Pathogenic bacteria
- Polycythaemia
- Thrombocytosis
- Anaemia
- Exchange transfusion
- Cyanotic congenital heart disease

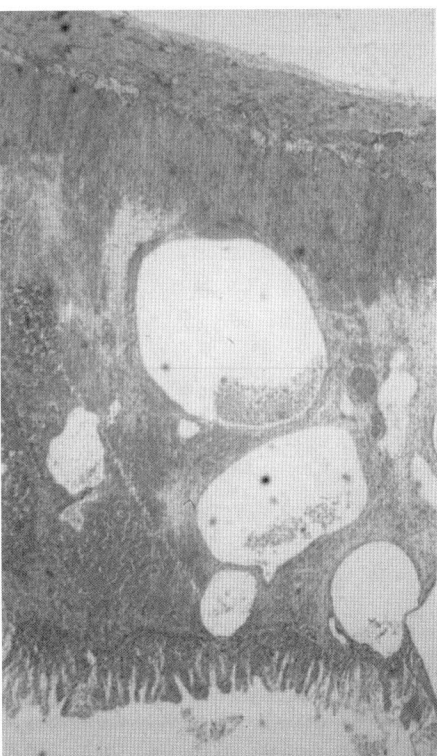

Fig. 29.19 Pathological specimen showing NEC. Pneumatosis is evident with gas bubbles within the bowel wall.

disease.[4] Preterm infants under 30 weeks gestation who develop NEC usually have no risk factors other than prematurity. In contrast, preterm infants of 30–36 weeks gestation have greater evidence of perinatal asphyxia than case controls and a higher rate of intrauterine growth restriction.[4] In most preterm infants, NEC develops in the second or third weeks, after the introduction of enteral feeds (Fig. 29.18).[33,120]

Pathology

Necrotising enterocolitis may affect any part of the gastrointestinal tract. In babies who come to surgery, or in those who die, the commonest sites of disease are the terminal ileum, caecum and ascending colon. NEC is a transmural disease. The bowel appears purple and discoloured, and is often distended with areas of serosal damage. Pneumatosis, the presence of submucosal and subserosal gas within the bowel wall, is the most characteristic appearance of the gut at laparotomy, histologically and radiographically (Fig. 29.19). This gas is largely nitrogen and hydrogen and is produced by gas forming bacteria.[55]

Histologically the earliest signs are a coagulative necrosis of the mucosa with microthrombus formation, leading to patchy mucosal ulceration, oedema and haemorrhage.[77] In focal intestinal perforation, haemorrhagic necrosis is a feature that distinguishes this condition from classical NEC.[145]

Cytokines have an important role in modulating intestinal inflammation and damage in NEC.[96] Raised levels of interleukins 1, 3 and 6, tumour necrosis factor (TNF)α, and platelet-activating factor (PAF) may predict the severity of the disease.[124] PAF, the lipid-derived, proinflammatory cytokine, has a central role.[56] Administration of PAF results in histological NEC in rats exposed to hypoxia, and pretreatment with PAF receptor antagonists reduces incidence and severity of NEC that has been induced by TNFα, lipopolysaccharide, hyperosmolar feeds and early exposure to non-pathogenic coliforms.[18,19] Human infants with NEC have high levels of PAF and low levels of PAF-acetylhydrolase, an enzyme important in PAF degradation.[96] PAF levels increase after enteral feeds in infants developing subsequently proven NEC.[116]

Aetiology

Numerous potential risk factors have been explored (Table 29.21). It is clear that none is in itself necessary or sufficient to produce NEC. The major candidate factors include hypoxia, prematurity and poor mucosal integrity, the bacterial flora and the presence of a metabolic substrate – milk – in the intestinal lumen (Fig. 29.20). These subjects will be discussed individually and have been reviewed extensively.[31,96,97]

Gut hypoxia

The pathology of NEC with vascular congestion, haemorrhage and ulceration accords with the importance of hypoxia. In the term infant with NEC, risk factors for gut hypoxia are almost invariably present. NEC may follow severe generalised hypoxia, maternal cocaine abuse and exchange transfusion.[4] In lambs, polycythaemia reduces oxygen delivery to the gut and produces NEC. In the infant, a high packed cell volume increases risk of NEC but an exchange transfusion is often the trigger.[182]

An adverse intrauterine environment leads to chronic fetal hypoxia and intrauterine growth restriction, and diversion of cardiac output away from the gut with reduced blood flow through the superior mesenteric artery.[71]

Studies have shown that abnormal fetal Doppler studies predispose to NEC.[71] Faced with poor oxygenation the fetus responds by redistributing blood flow, reducing splanchnic blood flow. In such infants reduction of gut blood flow is still evident after birth. A large multicentre European study showed increased perinatal mortality but no increase in NEC in infants with abnormal fetal umbilical Doppler studies.[85] The result is the consensus that infants with abnormal fetal Doppler studies, often associated with intrauterine growth restriction, are considered at high risk of NEC. In such fetuses, oligohydramnios and fetal echogenic bowel predict difficulties in the introduction of milk.[59] Intrauterine growth restriction is an important risk factor for NEC in infants over 29 weeks gestation.[4,168]

The preterm infant is at particular risk of intestinal hypoxia during intensive care. In the animal model, bacterial colonisation and excessive formula feeding do not precipitate NEC unless hypoxia is also present.[17] In the newborn, after feeds, intestinal oxygen use is increased but not blood flow, predisposing to tissue hypoxia.[37] Patent ductus arteriosus diminishes superior mesenteric artery blood flow and is more common in infants with NEC.[152] Indometacin (indomethacin), given for patent ductus arteriosus or to the mother in preterm labour for more than 2 days immediately before delivery, predisposes to NEC and focal intestinal perforation.[34,66]

Some of the earliest reports of NEC were in infants after exchange transfusion for rhesus haemolytic disease through a UVC. Umbilical arterial cannulation has been held to reduce gut blood supply and provoke embolisation or thrombus formation, predisposing to NEC. The studies confirming this relationship were all published prior to 1980.[97] In many centres this leads to avoidance of enteral feeding while an umbilical line is in place. More recently, prospective studies have shown no difference in the rate of NEC between high and low umbilical artery catheters,[30,89] or with early or late introduction of milk feeds while the arterial umbilical line is in place.[41] The umbilical venous catheter does not predispose to NEC.[147]

Mucosal integrity

Loss of mucosal integrity disrupts barrier function, allowing macromolecular absorption and bacterial translocation, and interferes with digestion. The preterm gut has an immature microvillous membrane with relative deficiency of mucus and secretory IgA, with increased permeability to small and large molecules. Further mucosal damage increases permeability to microorganisms and toxins.[79] This process may initiate NEC.[31,79,101] Antenatal corticosteroid administration induces intestinal maturation, decreases permeability and protects against NEC.[79]

Microbial infection

Most NEC is not infectious. In sporadic disease, the presence of bacteria is probably necessary for NEC to occur but is not

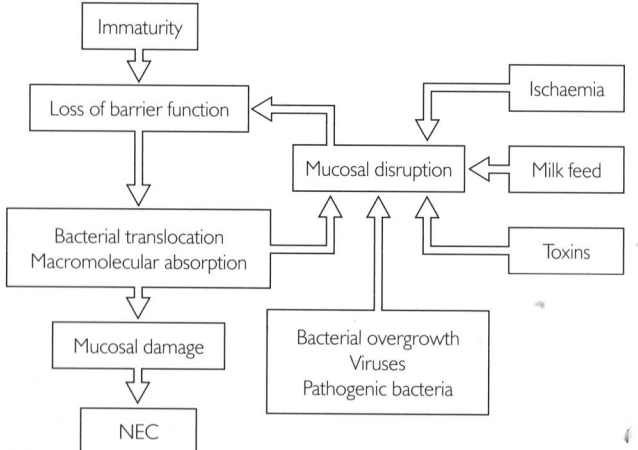

Fig. 29.20 Interaction of the main factors involved in the pathogenesis of NEC.

sufficient without other risk factors. In epidemic NEC there may be an identified infectious agent (Table 29.22).[31,151] Infection with clostridia, which produce a potent toxin, occurs in epidemics and in Hirschsprung's enterocolitis.[167] Infants with NEC during epidemics fare better than infants with sporadic disease, although this may be related to heightened awareness and earlier detection of NEC on the neonatal unit.[31]

In sporadic disease, a large variety of microorganisms are associated with the pathogenesis of NEC (Table 29.23).[31,33,101] Positive blood cultures are found in 10–50% and correlate with isolates from stool or peritoneal fluid.[4,25,117] Overall, the microbiological picture is dominated by *Escherichia coli*, *Klebsiella*, *Enterobacter* and coagulase negative staphylococci. Faecal Grampositive organisms may interact and increase pathogenicity of *E. coli*.[140] In surgical patients, peritoneal culture shows a wider variety of microorganisms in extremely low birthweight infants (under 1000 g), than in larger preterm infants.[152]

Unhindered proliferation of potentially pathogenic species may occur, promoting bacterial translocation and absorption toxic products,[101] explaining the increased risk of NEC in infants whose mothers were treated with co-amoxiclav after preterm rupture of membranes.[91] Among klebsiellas, rapid carbohydrate fermenters are more pathogenic.

Table 29.22 Organisms associated with epidemics of necrotising enterocolitis[31,151]

- *Klebsiella* spp.
- Non-pathogenic *Escherichia coli*
- Enterotoxigenic *Escherichia coli*
- *Enterobacter* spp.
- *Clostridium difficile*
- *Clostridium butyricum*
- *Clostridium perfringens*
- *Salmonella* spp.
- *Pseudomonas aeruginosa*
- Rotavirus
- Coronavirus

Table 29.23 Organisms isolated from blood cultures in infants with necrotising enterocolitis

Reference	94	33	4	117	25
Coagulase-negative staphylococci	–	10	6	11	2
Staphylococcus aureus	1	4	–	2	2
Escherichia coli	24	3	8	3	3
Klebsiella	6	1	7	5	–
Enterobacter spp.	–	–	1	4	4
Proteus mirabilis	1	1	–	1	–
Clostridium spp.	1	5	2	–	–
Streptococcus faecalis	2	1	1	–	–
Pseudomonas aeruginosa	2	–	–	–	1
Candida albicans	1	–	–	–	–
Miscellaneous	4	2	–	5	–

Reference numbers from reference list.

Enteral nutrition

The choice of milk and the management of enteral nutrition is crucial to the prevention of NEC. All studies have demonstrated that most infants with NEC have received milk.[4,94,152] In the British Paediatric Surveillance Unit survey, 90% of subjects had received enteral feeds prior to the onset of NEC.[107] In unfed infants with NEC, symptoms present early, often following an asphyxial insult.[31] Intraluminal milk may simply promote bacterial proliferation or increase bacterial endotoxin production by Gram-negative bacteria.[93] Bacterial action upon unabsorbed nutrients results in gas formation[55] and the production of short-chain fatty acids, which can be toxic to intestinal epithelium. Long-chain fats and undigested casein may contribute to inflammation and injury,[96] and the lipid in milk increases mucosal permeability. Immature patterns of motility and decreased digestive capacity predispose the preterm infant to NEC.[6,131] In healthy infants who do not develop NEC, milk induces a cellular and humoral inflammatory mucosal reaction with an increase in circulating cytokines.[96,116]

An early study showed reduction of NEC with a conservative enteral feeding regime[14] but prolonged delay of oral feeding is not recommended. The evidence that aggressive enteral feeding with rapid increase in feed volume is causative is more compelling,[117] although there is absence of good RCT data.[90] Hyperosmolar feeds produce mucosal damage[45] and in one study, NEC was seen in almost 90% of infants fed milk with twice the osmolality of breast milk.[10]

Breast milk protects against NEC.[106,115] Infants given breast milk are seven to ten times less likely to suffer from NEC, a benefit that is attenuated when breast milk is given with formula. Putative important factors in breast milk include immunoglobulins, lysozyme, complement, macrophages, growth factors, PAF-acetylhydrolase[96] and production of anti-inflammatory cytokines.[53] Polyunsaturated fatty acids in breast milk or added to formula modifies the cytokine and endotoxic response, avoiding NEC in the rat model.[19]

Trophic feeding – the use of minimal enteral feeds with parenteral nutrition – is of established value in preterm nutritional management and has not been shown to increase risk of NEC.[108,112] In infants of less than 32 weeks gestation, a recent trial of trophic feeding versus standard milk advancement was stopped because babies receiving the standard regimen had a higher rate of NEC (10% vs 1.4%).[7]

Clinical features

Presentation may vary from insidious deterioration with non-specific signs, lethargy, temperature instability and apnoeic episodes to a rapidly progressive illness with shock, peritonitis and death. In the infant without gastrointestinal symptoms, early recognition of NEC requires a high index of suspicion. The baby's general condition is similar to that seen in sepsis with pallor, skin mottling and jaundice. Bleeding may be due to disseminated intravascular coagulation (DIC). Some infants have initial mild feed intolerance and then demonstrate the classic triad of abdominal distension, bloody, mucusy stools and bile-stained vomit or aspirates.

The commonest abdominal sign is distension (Table 29.24). Careful assessment should be made for tenderness: often distended loops are palpable and an intra-abdominal mass may represent localised perforation. Blue abdominal discoloration suggests disease progression and occasionally the abdominal wall becomes indurated and red, a sign of underlying peritonitis. Proctoscopy with an auriscope may reveal friable haemorrhagic mucosa but should be performed with care. Equally important is a general assessment of cardiorespiratory function, blood pressure and perfusion.

Focal intestinal perforation is distinguished from NEC by pathology and clinical features. Focal intestinal perforation occurs earlier in life, characteristically in infants of low gestation who are receiving full intensive care, and is associated with blue discoloration of the abdomen.[120,145]

Investigation

Immediate investigations include haemoglobin, white cell and platelet counts, coagulation studies, urea, electrolytes and albumin and blood gas analysis. The platelet count initially rises, but falls with disease progression and DIC. Blood and fluid losses into the abdomen are often larger than appreciated and abnormalities of perfusion, anaemia and electrolyte balance are common. Metabolic acidosis is usually a marker of shock. Carbon dioxide retention or hypoxia may represent respiratory failure due to apnoea or diaphragmatic splinting and indicate the need for ventilatory support.

Abdominal radiography is mandatory. The bowel appearance varies from a gasless abdomen (Fig. 29.21) to dilated loops of thick-walled gut with fluid levels. The pathognomonic radiographic appearance is pneumatosis intestinalis due to bubbles of gas in the gut wall (Fig. 29.22). In severe disease gas collects within the portal venous system (see below).[97,152]

Radiological detection of perforation is not easy (Fig. 29.23). Free air may be seen in only two-thirds of infants in whom perforation is present. A lateral horizontal beam shoot-through

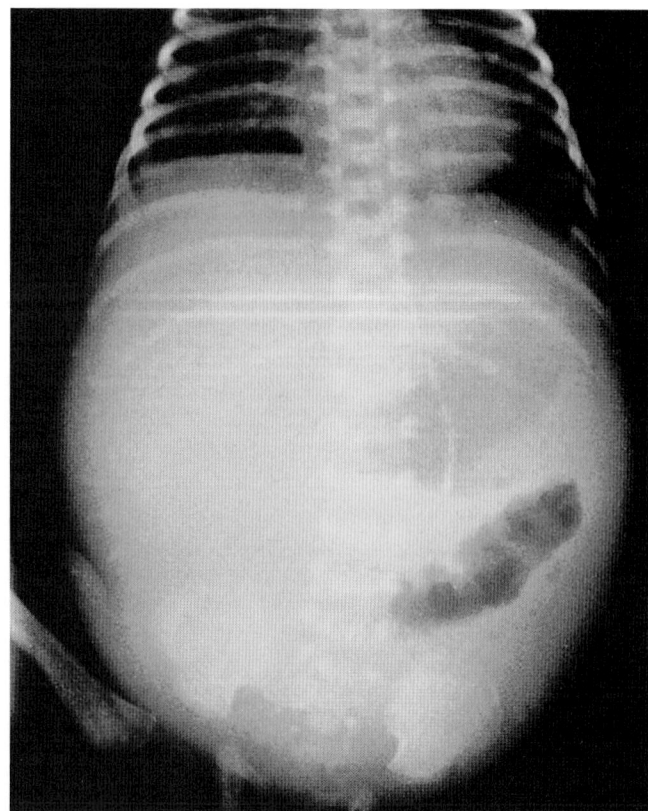

Fig. 29.21 Plain abdominal X-ray showing ascites in NEC.

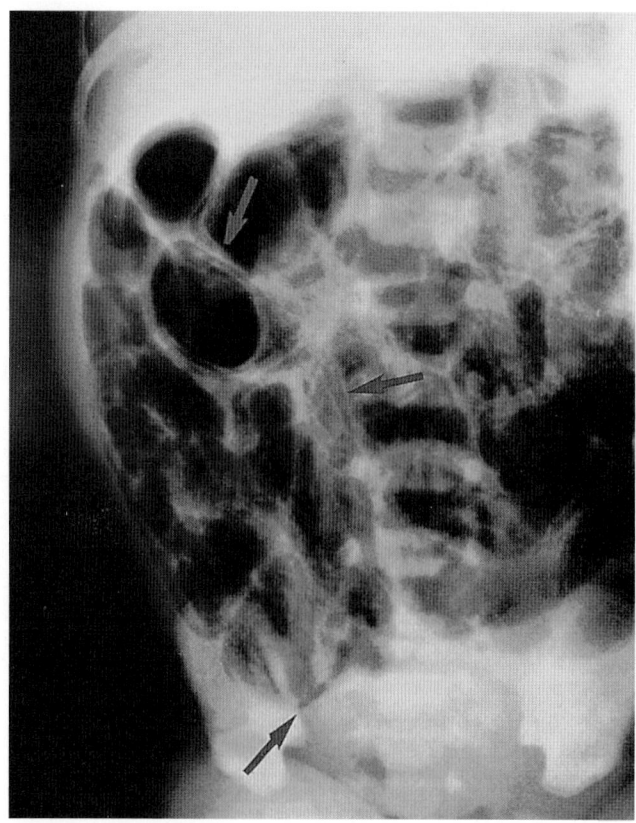

Fig. 29.22 Plain abdominal X-ray showing intraluminal gas (arrows) in NEC.

Table 29.24 Presenting features of necrotising enterocolitis (%)			
Reference	**94**	**33**	**107**
Abdominal distension	78	75	77
Lethargy	9	71	64
Visible blood in stool	28	70	39
Hypotonia	–	63	64
Vomiting/aspirates (±bile)	28	52	–
Abdominal tenderness	21	43	58
Apnoea	27	41	64
Bleeding diathesis	–	20	–
Abdominal wall oedema	–	19	–
Shock/sepsis	24	–	–

Reference numbers from reference list.

X-ray may allow easier detection of anterior collection of gas (Fig. 29.24) but, on a supine film, free gas is best seen between the liver and the diaphragm. Free gas in a generally gasless abdomen without pneumatosis favours focal intestinal perforation.[145]

Acute phase proteins (CRP) are helpful in monitoring progress. Stool contains raised levels of calprotectin, a marker of mucosal inflammation.[22] Exposure of the red cell T cryptantigen can occur in severe colitis, leading to massive haemolysis with blood product administration.[72] Screening for T antigen activation and use of low-titre anti-T blood products is now routine in some centres and currently this remains our practice. Recent data cast doubt upon the probable importance of T activation in NEC.[13] If there is doubt or reason to believe that T antigen related haemolysis is taking place, red blood cells reconstituted in SAG-M may be used. Abdominal ultrasound may allow detection of masses or ascites. Contrast studies are avoided during the acute phase and should not be done outside a centre capable of providing immediate surgery.

Differential diagnosis

In most cases, recognition of NEC is not difficult. Other causes of gut ischaemia, including malrotation, volvulus and hernia, should be considered. Isolated rectal bleeding has a differential diagnosis discussed above. Abdominal distension with regurgitation is common and, although NEC should be considered, it is reasonable to stop oral feeds for a few hours and observe the infant who has no other signs. 'NEC' may be the presenting feature of Hirschsprung's disease or cystic fibrosis.[167,183]

Treatment

The spectrum of clinical presentations makes it difficult and inappropriate to define a rigid regimen of management. Staging criteria may be helpful in tailoring treatment[5,177] (Table 29.25).

Prevention

Several preventive strategies are available but none have become standard practice (see pp. 702–3). They include:

- use of breast milk;
- minimal enteral feeding (0.5 ml/h) for 7 days before increasing feeds;
- slow feed advancement;

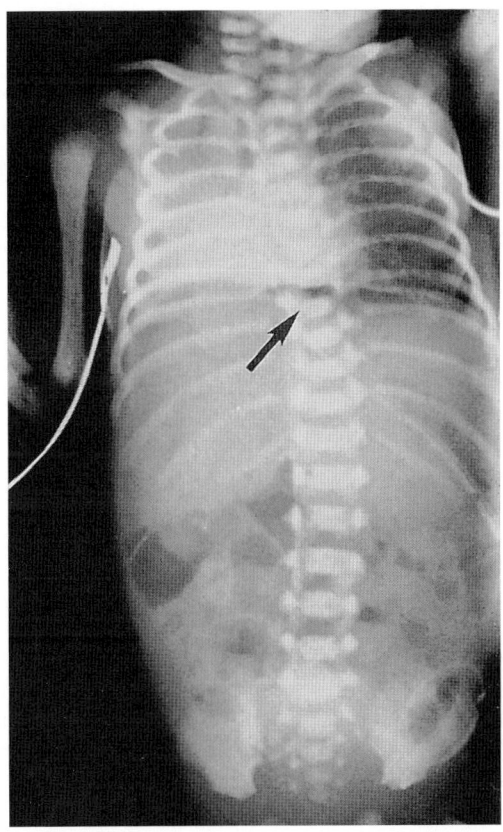

Fig. 29.23 Plain abdominal X-ray (anteroposterior supine) in the presence of a perforation: free gas is seen under the diaphragm (arrowed).

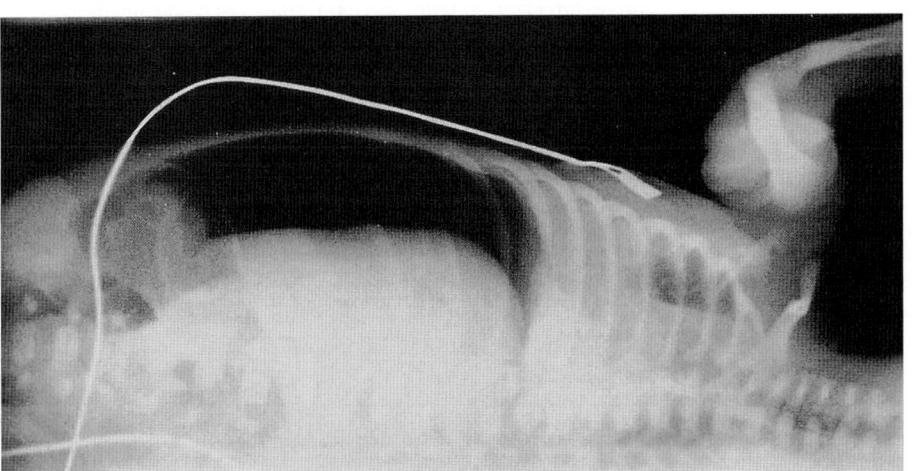

Fig. 29.24 Same infant as in Fig. 29.23 X-rayed lying on left side with a shoot-through horizontal beam film.

Table 29.25 Clinical staging system for necrotising enterocolitis[5]

Stage 1: suspected
- History of perinatal stress
- Systemic signs of ill health: temperature instability, lethargy, apnoea
- Gastrointestinal manifestations: poor feeding, increased volume of gastric aspirate, vomiting, mild abdominal distension, faecal occult blood (no fissure)

Stage 2: confirmed
Any of features of stage 1 *plus*:

- Persistent occult, or gross gastrointestinal bleeding, marked abdominal distension
- Abdominal radiograph: intestinal distension, bowel wall oedema, unchanging bowel loops, pneumatosis intestinalis, portal vein gas

Stage 3: advanced
Any of features of stages 1 or 2 *plus*:

- Deterioration in vital signs, evidence of shock or severe sepsis, or marked gastrointestinal haemorrhage
- Abdominal radiograph shows any of features of stage 2 *plus* pneumoperitoneum

- other specific interventions, such as lactobacilli, oral immunoglobulin (Ig)A, Doppler studies of blood flow velocity in the superior mesenteric axis before starting feeds.

Medical

The overall aim of treatment is to rest the gut, control infection, restore metabolic equilibrium and maintain the infant in an optimal condition until the bowel heals. The preterm infant is particularly vulnerable to undernutrition and, with the suspension of enteral feeding, parenteral nutrition should be provided. Surgery is indicated if intestinal perforation occurs, the infant's general condition deteriorates or intra-abdominal pathology persists beyond a few days.

The major components of medical management are:

- cessation of enteral feeding;
- nasogastric drainage with suction to minimise abdominal distension;
- monitoring of temperature, pulse, respiratory rate, blood pressure, fluid balance;
- plain abdominal radiography – if symptoms persist, radiographs should be repeated 6–12-hourly on the first day of NEC and while perforation remains likely;
- peripheral venous access for antibiotics, blood and plasma;
- blood cultures and septic screen; a lumbar puncture is not usually performed;
- intravenous antibiotics: a triple antibiotic regime is commonly used. *Gram-negative cover*: gentamicin or a third-generation cephalosporin (e.g. ceftazidime), although resistance to the latter is emerging. *Gram positive cover*: amoxicillin (amoxycillin) or vancomycin. The broad-spectrum regimen should

also include metronidazole. Second generation beta-lactamase-resistant cephalosporins (e.g. cefuroxime) are not effective against Gram-negative organisms, notably *Enterobacter*. The local regimen may take account of the dominant neonatal intensive care unit flora;

- volume replacement: fluid losses from the circulation into the gut or peritoneum are easily underestimated. Immediate management of suspected NEC in a baby infant who is ill includes appropriate volume replacement and circulatory support. Monitoring must include peripheral perfusion, peripheral-core temperature gradient, urine output and plasma bicarbonate or base excess;
- regular blood gas analysis and early recourse to assisted ventilation if there is evidence of respiratory distress, failure or apnoeic episodes;
- maintenance of normal urea, electrolytes, calcium and hydration by daily or twice-daily adjustments to rate and composition of intravenous fluids – prompt treatment of intercurrent problems such as hypoglycaemia (pp. 853–62), jaundice (pp. 661–78) and DIC (pp. 759–60);
- transfuse to maintain haemoglobin – the platelet count may fall and platelet transfusion will be necessary if the count is below 30×10^9/l or below 70×10^9/l before surgery;
- consider removal of umbilical cannulae – there is a balance of risks and if an umbilical artery catheter is the only arterial access in an ill baby of less than 1000 g birthweight the balance may be in favour of keeping the catheter in situ;
- insertion of a percutaneous central venous line for total parenteral nutrition if possible;
- total parenteral nutrition (Ch. 17) is always necessary in definite NEC, for which enteral starvation for at least 7–10 days is needed. During the first 24–48 hours, and when an infant is very ill, amino acid load is reduced and lipid infusion is avoided. In NEC is disproved, feeds may be recommenced after 48–72 h, and total; parenteral nutrition (TPN) may not be necessary;
- analgesics should be used liberally: infants with NEC suffer pain and considerable stress. An opiate infusion (e.g. morphine or diamorphine) is recommended. Opiate-induced apnoea is not a problem in a neonatal unit where intermittent positive pressure ventilation is available;
- barrier nursing: scrupulous hand washing will prevent most cross-infection – true barrier nursing may be needed in an outbreak of NEC.

The majority of babies with NEC who are managed medically recover steadily. Antibiotics, enteral starvation and TPN are usually prescribed for at least 7 days from the time of recovery from the initial severe illness. Perforation most often occurs in the first 48 hours but may become apparent at any time. By 7–14 days from diagnosis, most infants are free of signs of infection and have a soft abdomen, normal bowel sounds and a normal abdominal X-ray. Enteral feeding can then be restarted using 0.5–1.0 ml/h for the first 24 hours and thereafter increased cautiously. Expressed breast milk is the feed of choice; alternatively a preterm formula or donor expressed breast milk is used. Most infants who recover without surgery will tolerate one of these milks (see surgical management for alternative feeds).

Surgical

Twenty to 50% of infants with NEC require surgery.[4,107,161]

Indications

The cardinal indications for surgery in NEC are:

- perforation;
- formation of a mass;
- failure to respond to medical management.

The commonest indication for surgery is intestinal perforation, confirmed in 40–70% of infants who required surgery.[78,152] The commonest site of perforation is the terminal ileum, and multiple perforations are not unusual.[78,152] Perforation may occur without visible gas on the plain abdominal radiograph. Paracentesis showing at least 0.5 ml of brown-stained fluid, or bacteria on Gram stain, usually indicates perforation. Paracentesis is not widely used in the UK.[98,161]

Clinical deterioration despite medical treatment is more difficult to define. Abdominal signs, including a fixed dilated loop of intestine on serial radiographs, abdominal wall erythema or the development of an inflammatory mass, point to the need for surgery, as does general worsening in the infant's condition or a failure of intra-abdominal signs to resolve.[98,161]

Operation

At surgery, bowel necrosis is most commonly ileocaecal, and in around a third is limited to the colon, but it may occur at any point in the gut.[104] Extensive gut necrosis may be inoperable and lethal.[152] The choice of operation depends upon the extent of gut necrosis, the extent of NEC in non-necrotic gut and the general condition of the infant. Among the numerous surgical procedures described, four main options exist.[149]

The commonest procedure is laparotomy, resection of necrotic bowel, and creation of a proximal stoma and a distal mucous fistula.[78,149] This necessitates a second procedure to restore gut continuity. Large fluid, electrolyte and nutrient losses may occur through a small bowel stoma, especially when milk is reintroduced. This has led to earlier timing of the second procedure, which is often performed within 2 months of the initial surgery.[180] The possibility of stricture in the distal limb necessitates contrast study before the second operation, when a stricture can be resected.[68] Postoperative complications include systemic, wound and intra-abdominal sepsis, which, perhaps surprisingly, are unusual.[78] Stoma-related complications, such as dehiscence, are unusual and less likely with good nutritional status.[180]

Secondly, in the infant who is stable, with well-circumscribed disease, gut resection and primary anastomosis may be performed as one procedure. The anastomosis heals well, problems with losses from the stoma are avoided and hospital stay may be reduced.[161] In the two-stage procedure, strictures are nearly always in the distal loop of gut[155] and primary anastomosis may reduce the likelihood of stricture.[128]

An alternative strategy is peritoneal drainage, performed on the neonatal intensive care unit under local anaesthesia. One or two soft drains are inserted into the right lower quadrant, with broad-spectrum antibiotic cover and nasogastric aspiration. Initially used in babies who were too ill for surgery, it was found that some avoided surgery altogether. This technique has its proponents[46] and detractors.[16] In our practice, peritoneal drainage alone is usually reserved for small infants who are clinically unstable and unsuitable for laparotomy. After peritoneal drainage, laparotomy remains necessary in around 50%.[46]

Finally, in the group with a poor prognosis,[161] disease may be so extensive that resection cannot be performed or would entail extensive resection of intestine. Such extensive disease is usually lethal. A proximal jejunostomy can be used to defunction distal bowel. A 'second-look' laparotomy is performed if the baby survives, and necrotic gut is resected.

Postoperative management

Nutritional support and intensive care is usually needed for 2–3 weeks. Enteral feeds are reintroduced slowly using breast milk if available, as described above. If milk is not tolerated, a lactose-free formula containing hydrolysed protein and medium chain triglycerides is used and, in some centres, this is the feed of choice after NEC. If rapid gut transit and diarrhoea persists, loperamide may be used. In the infant who is tolerating feeds, but not gaining weight, salt and water depletion, malabsorption, and intestinal, systemic or urinary tract infection should be considered. Calories and protein may be added to breast milk using a commercial breast milk fortifier (pp. 316–17). Formula may be supplemented with a powdered carbohydrate/fat mixture in 2–5% solution, but this may provoke or exacerbate diarrhoea. Advice from a paediatric dietician is essential.

Late strictures due to submucosal thickening and fibrosis[155] may have become more common. In the baby who does not need surgery, strictures are less common and shorter.[100,104] Most strictures manifest within 6 weeks and almost all within 4 months.[104,155] Overall strictures occur in 10–40% and, although some narrowing seen on contrast studies may resolve spontaneously, most strictures need surgery. Most are colonic but strictures occur at the site of anastomosis and in the small bowel[82,104] (Fig. 29.25). Short bowel syndrome may require long-term management, especially if the ileocaecal valve has been resected (see below).

Outcome

In 5–10% of cases of NEC relapse occurs, usually within a month of initial presentation. Management is no different from that of the first attack. It is not clear if management of the first attack can alter risk of recurrence. Late complications are important (Table 29.26).[95]

Overall survival after NEC is 70–90%.[78,80,95,104,152] Mortality is higher in infants of less than 28 weeks gestation despite similar severity of disease. In babies with a birthweight of less than 1000 g the survival rate is poor compared with larger infants (around 60% vs over 90%).[26,46] Extensive disease, bacteraemia, DIC or persistent ascites are bad prognostic indicators.[78,94,104,152]

The nutrition, growth and gastrointestinal function of survivors depends upon the site and extent of disease and resection. In the absence of short bowel syndrome (see below), major nutritional problems are unusual, although short-term problems with rapid gut transit, diarrhoea and malabsorption are seen as gut adaptation occurs.[105] Specific nutritional deficiencies due to terminal ileal resection (particularly vitamin B$_{12}$) should not be forgotten.[32]

Long-term neurodevelopmental follow-up is essential in view of the high rate of disability in survivors of severe NEC.[80] Neurodevelopmental problems are more common among infants who need surgery compared with gestation- and birthweight-matched infants without NEC or those with NEC who only need medical treatment.[168] There is a link between NEC and PVL (pp. 1159–64), which may be due to common antenatal risk factors, or result from cause-and-effect via shock, cytokine release, hypotension or acidosis.

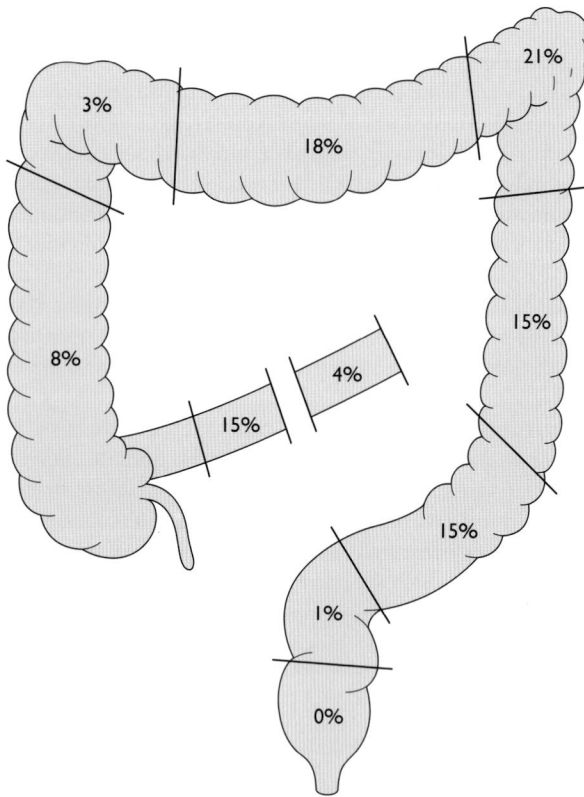

Fig. 29.25 Sites of intestinal stricture after NEC. (Redrawn from Janik J S, Ein S H, Mancer K 1981 Intestinal stricture after necrotising enterocolitis. Journal of Pediatric Surgery 16: 438–443.)

Table 29.26 Late complications of necrotising enterocolitis

- Recurrence
- Intestinal stricture
- Enterocyst
- Short gut syndrome
- Enterocolic fistula
- Anastomotic leak
- Cholestasis
- Malabsorption
- Atresias and aganglionosis
- Salt and water depletion
- Polyposis
- Treatment complications

Prevention

Future progress in NEC lies in its prevention. Despite many suggested preventive strategies,[175] the central difficulty of studying a relatively infrequent, sporadic disease thwarts attempts at good, prospective, randomised studies.

In the term infant, avoidance of perinatal asphyxia might reduce NEC.[4,31] In the infant with hypoxic ischaemic encephalopathy, our practice includes avoidance of feeds during the acute encephalopathy and low-volume feeds for 24 hours before full enteral feeding.

Maternal antenatal steroids reduce the risk of NEC by amelioration of preterm lung disease, or by a direct effect upon gut maturation and mucosal integrity.[79] Choice of antibiotic in preterm rupture of membranes is important, and co-amoxiclav should be avoided.[91] Surfactant replacement therapy in respiratory distress syndrome makes NEC less likely.[35] General measures including maintenance of good tissue perfusion, blood pressure, hydration and avoidance of hypotension, hypoxia and hypothermia are all likely to reduce NEC. In the preterm infant with hypotension resistant to volume expansion, inotropes improve gut perfusion.[75] Umbilical artery catheters should be removed if there is evidence of thrombosis or reduced blood flow to buttocks or lower limbs.

The timing, method and composition of enteral feeds in the face of immaturity of digestion, absorption, gut motility and barrier function has attracted most attention.[129] Breast milk should be given whenever possible.[106] Freezing breast milk for storage does not abolish benefit.[53] Meta-analysis suggests that donor breast milk will reduce risk of NEC fourfold compared with formula.[115] Hyperosmolar feeds should be avoided, and care should be taken when adding electrolytes to milk.

Prolonged delay in enteral feeding for the prevention of NEC cannot be recommended but rapid, incautious introduction and increase of enteral feeds in the face of poor feed tolerance is likely to lead to NEC.[6,117] In the VLBW infant, most advise introduction of milk feeds at 20–25 ml/kg/d, increased by the same amount daily.[7] In the UK, more units are giving milk feeds during neonatal intensive care.[109] Administration of small amounts of milk (minimal enteral feeding) is widely used to promote gut development.[108,112] Elective use of 10 days of minimal enteral feeding prior to feed increase may lead to a marked reduction in NEC so that a case of NEC is prevented for each ten infants managed in this way.[7] Special care is needed with the introduction of milk in the infant with intrauterine growth restriction.[59,114]

Control of infection is essential in the management of epidemic NEC[175] and is good practice in all cases. Prophylactic use of systemic antibiotics is not advised. Administration of enteral aminoglycosides is not without risk, as absorption may occur, but may reduce the risk of NEC.[175] Oral administration of immunoglobulins is used in a small number of centres.[54] Direct comparison of oral IgA–IgG and oral gentamicin suggests that the latter is more effective in a high-risk group.[62]

Future possibilities include non-antibody immune factors such as lactoferrin in formula milk, prostaglandin analogues, modification of cytokine activity, treatment with growth factors, supplementation with polyunsaturated fatty acids, prebiotics and probiotics.[21,31,40,79,175]

Short bowel syndrome

Short bowel syndrome (SBS) follows loss of a significant portion of the small intestine and comprises malabsorption, diarrhoea and growth failure due to loss of mucosal surface area and rapid gastrointestinal transit. Loss of bowel may follow pre- or postnatal damage to the gut[105,164] (Table 29.27). NEC is the commonest cause of SBS and intestinal failure[70] occurring at a time when, in fetal life, the small intestine is doubling in length. Among infants with NEC who require surgery and survive, 4–10% have SBS.[80,104]

Babies with less than 50% of their total bowel length, or less than 100 cm of small bowel, are at high risk of SBS.[24,105] Parenteral nutrition is usually needed when less than 40 cm of small intestine remains and is likely to be needed for longer if the ileocaecal valve is absent.[24,150]

The central tenet of management is nutritional support and maintenance of fluid and electrolyte balance, allowing a period of gradual intestinal adaptation during which growth in the length and diameter of the remaining bowel, and mucosal hypertrophy, occurs.[24,105,164,174] Most babies will achieve 90% absorption of carbohydrate and fats by 3 months.[105] This remarkable process of adaptation has allowed infants with less than 10 cm of small bowel to achieve full enteral feeds.[164] Preservation of the ileum is important as it has a greater ability to adapt than the jejunum, a longer transit time and the unique ability to absorb vitamin B_{12} and bile acids.

Most infants require initial TPN. If TPN is needed long-term, home administration has allowed these children good quality of life.[146] Enteral feeding is essential for adaptation but is often difficult. Most infants tolerate a protein hydrolysate, with medium-chain triglycerides and glucose polymers but no lactose (e.g. Pregestimil, Mead Johnson) and some require an amino acid formula (e.g. Neocate, SHS).[164] Caloric content may be increased by the addition of starch, glucose polymers or fats.

In some infants, a modular feed allows manipulation of individual nutrient components. Continuous feeds are usually tolerated well, although bolus feeds have the theoretical advantage of better promotion of gut development.[158] Specific nutrients may be used as primary therapy.[164] The diet must contain adequate calcium, magnesium, iron, fat- and water-soluble vitamins and trace elements. Vitamin B_{12} supplements may be necessary after terminal ileal resection.

Possible pharmacotherapy includes antibacterial drugs, antimotility drugs and hormonal therapies.[174] H_2 antagonists (ranitidine) or proton pump inhibitors may be required because of hypergastrinemia. Antimotility agents (loperamide) may be effective but should be used with care. Cholestyramine is indicated if there is evidence of bile acid diarrhoea after ileal resection. Close attention to dietary detail and follow-up requires multidisciplinary support.[164] Feeding and speech development should not be overlooked.

In a small proportion dependent upon TPN, and after at least a year to allow adaptation, surgery may be helpful. Procedures aim to slow intestinal transit time or increase absorptive surface area by the reconstruction of the ileocaecal valve, interposition of colon or antiperistaltic segments, recirculating loops or increasing intestinal length.[24,164] In children who cannot be maintained on TPN, small-bowel transplantation may be considered.[67]

The prognosis for SBS is now vastly better than it was 20 years ago, with survival rates exceeding 90%, even in those with less than 40 cm of small bowel. Linear growth may be impaired in the first year, although most climb back into the normal weight range by their third year, albeit on the lower centiles.[105]

Neonatal appendicitis

Appendicitis in the neonate is very rare, representing only 0.1–0.2% of childhood appendicitis.[48] The commonest presentation is with perforation and diffuse peritonitis, with signs like those of NEC[120] (Table 29.28). Neonatal appendicitis may complicate NEC, Hirschsprung's disease and cystic fibrosis.[163]

Table 29.27 Aetiology of short bowel

Prenatal
■ Vascular accidents
■ Intestinal atresia
■ Abdominal wall defects
■ Volvulus
■ Meconium peritonitis

Postnatal
■ Necrotising enterocolitis
■ Midgut or segmental volvulus
■ Inflammatory bowel disease
■ Abdominal trauma
■ Vascular thrombosis

Table 29.28 Signs of neonatal appendicitis ($n = 50$)[121]

Sign	% with finding
Abdominal distension	90
Fever	70
Vomiting	60
Refusal to feed	40
Pain (crying, restlessness)	30
Lethargy	30
Erythema/oedema of right lower quadrant	20
Mass in right lower quadrant	20
Diarrhoea	20
Bloody stools	20

The combination of physical signs in the right iliac fossa, abnormal gas pattern on plain abdominal X-ray and red and white cells in the urine point strongly to the diagnosis. Treatment is surgical, with intensive medical support and broad-spectrum antibiotic cover.

Intractable diarrhoea

Severe, protracted diarrhoea beginning soon after birth may be due to a congenital abnormality of gastrointestinal function. All are rare and investigation and management requires the support of a specialist centre. Intestinal mucosal biopsy is indicated, and fluid and electrolyte balance and support of nutrition are the central objectives of treatment.

Microvillous inclusion disease (congenital microvillous atrophy)

This is an autosomal recessive disorder of the cytoskeleton of the apical region of the enterocyte in which there is atrophy and involution of microvilli of the small and large bowel.[142] Massive diarrhoea is unresponsive to stopping feeds. To establish a diagnosis, mucosal biopsy is examined by electron microscopy. TPN is given but the prognosis is poor.[142] The future may lie in small intestinal transplantation.[15]

Congenital electrolyte transport defects

Congenital chloride diarrhoea is autosomal recessive due to a defect of the sodium-independent $[Cl^-\ HCO_3^-]$ exchanger in the ileum and colon.[118] Fetal diarrhoea produces polyhydramnios. Severe watery diarrhoea, which may be mistaken for urine in the nappy, abdominal distension, hypochloraemic alkalosis and rapid weight loss occur in the newborn period. Stool chloride is high. Congenital sodium diarrhoea, due to defective sodium/proton exchange, produces a similar picture but with high stool sodium losses.[11] Both conditions have been successfully managed with intravenous, and subsequently oral, mineral replacement.[47]

Congenital lactase deficiency

Symptoms immediately follow introduction of milk feeds, with acidic stools which contain lactose. Diagnosis is made by withdrawal of lactose-containing feeds and the demonstration of absent lactase activity on a jejunal mucosal biopsy.[154] It is very rare compared with secondary lactose intolerance.

Congenital glucose/galactose malabsorption

Watery acidic stools containing reducing substances, but possibly not lactose, are seen in the first days after birth. After rehydration, a fructose-based formula is given and the prognosis is good.[47]

Autoimmune enteropathy

Intractable diarrhoea, characteristically with a family history of autoimmune disease, may be due to an anti-enterocyte antibody and associated with a patchy enteropathy on biopsy.[123] A favourable response to cyclosporin has been reported.[126]

Gastro-oesophageal reflux

Clinical presentation

Gastro-oesophageal reflux (GOR) leads to vomiting, oesophagitis, recurrent apnoea, pulmonary aspiration, exacerbation of bronchopulmonary dysplasia and failure to thrive and prolongs stay in hospital.[65,130] Most episodes of reflux occur during transient relaxation of the lower oesophageal sphincter.[139] Reflux is more common in infancy than in childhood. The preterm infant is at high risk because of low resting LOS pressure (see above) and slow gastric emptying.[133,135] Reflux is often seen after repair of oesophageal atresia (pp. 715–17). Feeds, the supine position, nursing care and chest physiotherapy increase reflux.[58,132] Reflux is reduced by small volume tube feeds and during ventilation.[1,134,143]

Silent reflux, without the clinical clues of vomiting, should be suspected in infants with apnoea or respiratory problems resistant to usual therapy, or with unexplained deterioration.[12,99,132] Diagnosis is often made clinically. Contrast studies lack sensitivity but rule out anatomical abnormality. Prolonged oesophageal pH study is the gold standard for diagnosis in children but in newborns milk feeds lead to buffering of gastric acidity and reduce the diagnostic sensitivity.[181] Reference pH data vary according to prematurity and intensive care (Table 29.29).[132,137,172,173] The presence of acidic oro-pharyngeal secretions on litmus testing has a high positive predictive value for acid reflux.[81] Often a diagnostic trial of therapy is used. Oesophagitis may lead to bleeding, and endoscopy is feasible.[43]

Treatment

Changes in feed composition have little effect, although breast milk may be beneficial.[73] The prone, 30° head-up position reduces reflux but can only be recommended during inpatient monitoring. Left lateral positioning is effective.[58] Feed thickening reduces regurgitation and is widely used.[181] Infant Gaviscon contains approximately 1 mmol of sodium per dose. Cisapride is effective[2] but is no longer used because of potential cardiac dysrhythmia. Erythromycin in low, prokinetic dose may be used but efficacy is not established.[39] Metoclopramide is ineffective and risks unwanted extrapyramidal effects. In oesophagitis, Infant Gaviscon (Reckitt & Colman) or ranitidine may be used. Surgical fundoplication is rarely necessary in the neonatal period.[92] Antireflux surgery may be considered in recurrent aspiration, reflux-related life-threatening events or where severe reflux disease is unresponsive to medical therapy.

Table 29.29 Upper limits of reference range (median) for results of pH studies in infants without symptoms of gastroesophageal reflux

	NICU preterm infants[131] (n = 35)	Healthy preterm infants[137] (n = 21)	Infants[172] (n = 509)	Children 14–16 months[173] (n = 15)
Reflux index (%)	<11 (3)	<3 (1.1)	<10 (4)	<6.4 (2.7)
Episodes/24 h	<29 (9.5)	<30 (7.6)	<70 (27)	<46 (19)
Episodes >5 min/24 h	<7 (3)	<3 (1.1)	<9 (3)	<4.6 (2.2)
Longest episode (min)	<41 (8)	<16 (6.1)	<41 (12)	<22 (8.6)

The first study refers to preterm infants in neonatal intensive care units, the others to healthy infants. Almost all were receiving feeds.

The decision to start treatment is usually made on clinical grounds when reflux is thought to be the likely cause of feeding problems, recurrent apnoea or otherwise unexplained deterioration in chronic lung disease. A therapeutic trial of medical therapy is then reasonable but must be critically assessed. Successful treatment may lead to improved respiratory function or resolution of apnoea.[132] Prognosis is good and in most infants reflux resolves with maturation of the antireflux barrier. Persistent reflux is more common in those with neurodevelopmental problems.

Milk protein intolerance

Antigens provoking milk protein intolerance (MPI) include cow's milk whey proteins, β-lactoglobulin and α-lactalbumin, casein and soya proteins.[42] Immunogenic proteins may be absorbed and secreted in breast milk, explaining cow's milk colitis in exclusively breastfed infants.[159] In the newborn, gut barrier function is poor (see Table 29.20) and macromolecular absorption is high, although this does not fully account for allergic reactions.[83] MPI may follow any gastrointestinal insult, such as NEC or surgery.

Over 90% of MPI presents in the first months of life.[138] In a prospective study of healthy term infants, MPI was proven in 2.2%,[64] although over 50% with an atopic family history may develop MPI.[138] Infants with MPI often react to other antigens.

Clinical features

The commonest gastrointestinal symptoms are vomiting and diarrhoea (Table 29.30).[42,138,159] GOR is strongly linked with MPI.[153,159] MPI is the commonest cause of colitis in the young infant, with rectal bleeding with loose stools containing mucus. MPI enteropathy may result in weight loss, abdominal distension and steatorrhoea with patchy subtotal villous atrophy and crypt hyperplasia. MPI may be accompanied by lactose intolerance. Non-gastrointestinal symptoms of MPI range from acute reactions, including urticaria, to chronic atopic disease. Anaphylaxis is rare in the neonate.

Diagnosis rests upon remission of symptoms on exclusion diet and relapse on challenge. Intestinal biopsy, estimation of total IgE and specific antibodies (RAST), skin prick test and stool analysis may support the diagnosis. A hypoallergenic, lactose-free, milk-substitute-containing hydrolysed protein

Table 29.30 Gastrointestinal manifestations of milk protein intolerance

- Vomiting
- Gastro-oesophageal reflux
- Diarrhoea
- Failure to thrive
- Colic
- Colitis
- Villous atrophy and malabsorption
- Eosinophilic gastroenteropathy
- Occult blood loss

(Pregestimil, Nutramigen) is given. Infants with severe MPI, notably colitis, may be exquisitely sensitive to milk proteins and may require an amino-acid formula (Neocate). If breastfed, restriction of maternal diet, avoiding cow's milk and sometimes egg and soya, is recommended.[159] Goat's milk is only suitable for goats and is never a suitable food for babies (p. 311). Management demands close dietetic supervision. Challenge, to substantiate diagnosis and to demonstrate resolution of MPI, should be in hospital and is not usually in the neonatal period.[42] The vast majority of MPI resolves in the first 3 years.

Prevention

Prevention of MPI is contentious.[63] Early breastfeeding prevents atopic symptoms. Preventative strategies include exclusive breastfeeding for 6 months, late introduction of solid foods, restriction of maternal diet and hydrolysed formula. Immunomodulation may prove to be important and a recent trial of probiotic (*Lactobacillus*) indicates efficacy.[84]

Pancreatic disease

Cystic fibrosis

Cystic fibrosis (CF) is an autosomal recessive condition affecting 1/2400 live births in the UK.[50] The cystic fibrosis transmembrane conductance regulator (CFTR) regulates chloride and electrolyte transport across the cell membrane.[28] The commonest mutation is a single amino-acid substitution, ΔF508, which interferes with folding of the newly made CFTR so that it is held and degraded by the endoplasmic reticulum. Five classes of mutation are recognised and relate to prognosis and to potential therapy. In class I defects, where CFTR is not produced, for example, aminoglycosides inhibit the effect of a mutant stop codon so that full-length CFTR is made.[28,51] Around 1000 mutations are known and result in a wide range of severity and clinical phenotype. The carrier rate of CF mutations is about 1/25.

Table 29.31 Neonatal presentations of cystic fibrosis

- Antenatal mutation analysis
- Fetal hyperechogenic bowel
- Fetal gut dilatation
- Fetal intrabdominal calcification
- Neonatal screening
- Meconium ileus
- Cholestasis
- Meconium peritonitis
- Respiratory infection
- Exocrine pancreatic insufficiency
- Failure to thrive

Screening

Most neonatal screening uses the dried blood spot collected in the first week. Serum immune reactive trypsin (IRT) is elevated in almost all infants with CF in the neonatal period but over 90% of infants with a single positive result do not have CF. Combination of the IRT assay with DNA analysis provides a better screening method.[127] Neonatal screening is beneficial, and screening has been shown to reduce early respiratory morbidity[27] and improve growth on long-term follow-up.[61] Screening is now recommended by most authorities and is being introduced in Scotland with plans for introduction in the rest of the UK. Screening allows important choices about reproduction, which are taken up by about two-thirds of affected families.[52]

Clinical presentation

Most newborns with CF are asymptomatic. Neonatal diagnosis may follow screening or a variety of clinical presentations (Table 29.31). Most clinical presentation occurs in late infancy or childhood.[61] Some 10–15% of CF presents with meconium ileus resulting in intestinal obstruction within 48 hours of birth. It is associated with pre- or postnatal perforation, volvulus, chemical or bacterial peritonitis, intestinal atresia and microcolon. Conservative management with intravenous fluids, antibiotics and water-soluble, hyperosmolar contrast enema under fluoroscopic

Table 29.32 Nutritional management of cystic fibrosis[69,113]

Energy	
Routine	100–130 kcal/kg/d
Poor growth	150–200 kcal/kg/d
Milk	
Routine	Breast milk
	Standard infant formula
Poor growth	High energy infant formula
	OR supplement formula with: glucose polymer
	OR fat emulsion (e.g. Calogen) and glucose polymer
	OR mixed fat and carbohydrate (e.g. Duocal)
Post operative period, after meconium ileus or milk protein intolerance	Pregestimil, Peptijunior
Pancreatic enzymes (acid-resistant microspheres)	
Third to half capsule with feeds (e.g. Creon, Pancrease)	
Mix enteric coated granules with milk or water and give immediately from a spoon before a feed	
Vitamins	
Vitamin A	4000–5000 IU/d (e.g. Dalavit 0.6 ml)
Vitamin D	400 IU/d (e.g. Dalavit 0.6 ml)
Vitamin E	25–50 mg/d
Vitamin K	Routine neonatal prophylaxis, unless evidence of liver disease
	Repeat before surgery
(Monitor vitamin status and adjust)	

control should only be attempted in a specialised centre in collaboration with a paediatric surgeon (pp. 724–6). Neonatal mortality in meconium ileus is 10–20% but in survivors outcome is similar to that seen in other children with CF.[36] CF may be predicted by fetal ultrasound, although most fetal echogenic gut is not related to CF.[165]

Cystic fibrosis should not be forgotten as a cause for neonatal cholestasis.[156] Liver function tests are abnormal but liver biopsy may not be diagnostic. Ursodeoxycholic acid is used and jaundice usually clears in infancy.

Sweat testing is possible in the neonatal period but is not usually attempted before 4–6 weeks post term. A single sweat test is not diagnostic. Mutation analysis is usually diagnostic but can be misleading because of the large number of mutations that are implicated.

Management

The most important management step is referral to a specialised multidisciplinary team.[51,61] Early intervention, aggressive treatment of pathogens, chest physiotherapy and prophylactic anti-staphylococcal antibiotics should begin early.

Nutrition is vital. Increased energy requirements may relate to respiratory morbidity, fat malabsorption or the gene defect.[69] Breastfeeding should be encouraged.[69] Breast milk has lipolytic and anti-infective properties. Alternatively, a standard infant formula is used. Sodium supplements (2 mmol/kg/d) may be necessary. Energy supplements are provided if growth is suboptimal[113] (Table 29.32). A lactose-free hydrolysed protein feed containing medium-chain triglycerides may be better tolerated after meconium ileus. Pancreatic function is abnormal before birth[69] and malabsorption occurs in 60% by 8 weeks of age, rising to over 90% at 1 year. Pancreatic enzyme replacement therapy should be started when there are clinical features of steatorrhoea or laboratory evidence of pancreatic insufficiency, such as low levels of faecal elastase.

Schwachmann–Diamond syndrome

Pancreatic exocrine insufficiency is rare other than in CF. Pancreatic hypoplasia, isolated enzyme deficiencies, and a number of rare syndromes (e.g. Johanson Blizzard, Pearson's) may be associated with malabsorption.

Schwachmann's syndrome comprises pancreatic exocrine insufficiency, usually presenting in infancy, and variable or cyclical neutropenia, which may lead to clinical immunodeficiency. Short stature and metaphysial dysplasia are characteristic. Pancreatic enzyme replacement is needed in infancy.

References

1. Abe T, Hata Y, Sasaki F, Uchino J, Aoyama K, Nannbu H 1993 The effect of tube feeding on postprandial gastroesophageal reflux. Journal of Pediatric Surgery 28: 56–58

2. Ariagno R L, Kikkert M A, Mirmiran M, Conrad C, Baldwin R B 2001 Cisapride decreases gastroesophageal reflux in preterm infants. Pediatrics 107: E58

3. Bedu A, Faure C, Sibony O, Vuillard E, Mougenot J F, Aujard Y 1994 Prenatal gastrointestinal bleeding caused by esophagitis and gastritis. Journal of Pediatrics 125: 465–467

4. Beeby P J, Jeffrey H 1992 Risk factors for necrotising enterocolitis: the influence of gestational age. Archives of Disease in Childhood 67: 432–435

5. Bell M J, Ternberg J L, Feigin R D et al 1978 Neonatal necrotizing enterocolitis: therapeutic decisions based upon clinical staging. Annals of Surgery 187: 1–7

6. Berseth C L 1994 Gut motility and the pathogenesis of necrotizing enterocolitis. Clinics in Perinatology 21: 263–270

7. Berseth C L, Bisquera J A, Paje V U 2003 Prolonging small feeding volumes early in life decreases the incidence of necrotizing enterocolitis in very low birth weight infants. Pediatrics 111: 529–534

8. Berseth C L, Nordyke C 1993 Enteral nutrients promote postnatal maturation of intestinal motor activity in preterm infants. American Journal of Physiology 264: G1046–G1051

9. Boehm G, Jakobsson I, Mansson M, Raiha N C 1992 Macromolecular absorption in small-for-gestational-age infants. Acta Paediatrica 81: 864–867

10. Book L S, Herbst J J, Atherton S O, Jung A L 1975 Necrotizing enterocolitis in low birth weight infants fed an elemental formula. Journal of Pediatrics 87: 602–605

11. Booth I W 1985 Defective jejunal brush border Na$^+$/H$^+$ exchange: a cause of congenital secretory diarrhoea. Lancet 1: 1066–1069

12. Booth I W 1992 Silent gastro-oesophageal reflux: how much do we miss? Archives of Disease in Childhood 67: 1325–1327

13. Boralessa H, Modi N, Cockburn H et al 2002 RBC T activation and hemolysis in a neonatal intensive care population: implications for transfusion practice. Transfusion 42: 1428–1434

14. Brown E G, Sweet A Y 1978 Preventing necrotizing enterocolitis in neonates. JAMA 240: 2452–2454

15. Bunn S K, Beath S V, McKeirnan P J et al 2000 Treatment of microvillus inclusion disease by intestinal transplantation. Journal of Pediatric Gastroenterology and Nutrition 31: 176–180

16. Camberos A, Patel K, Applebaum H 2002 Laparotomy in very small premature infants with necrotizing enterocolitis or focal intestinal perforation: postoperative outcome. Journal of Pediatric Surgery 37: 1692–1695

17. Caplan M S, Hedlund E, Adler L, Hsueh W 1994 Role of asphyxia and feeding in a neonatal rat model of necrotizing enterocolitis. Pediatric Pathology 14: 1017–1028

18. Caplan M S, Hedlund E, Adler L, Lickerman M, Hsueh W 1997 The platelet activating factor receptor antagonist WEB 2170 prevents neonatal necrotizing enterocolitis in rats. Journal of Pediatric Gastroenterology and Nutrition 24: 296–301

19. Caplan M S, Russell T, Xiao Y, Amer M, Kaup S, Jilling T 2001 Effect of polyunsaturated fatty acid (PUFA) supplementation on intestinal inflammation and necrotizing enterocolitis (NEC) in a neonatal rat model. Pediatric Research 49: 647–652

20. Carlos M A, Babyn P S, Marcon M A, Moore A M 1997 Changes in gastric emptying in early postnatal life. Journal of Pediatrics 130: 931–937

21. Carlson S E, Montalto M B, Ponder D L, Werkman S H, Korones S B 1998 Lower incidence of necrotizing enterocolitis in infants fed a preterm formula with egg phospholipids. Pediatric Research 44: 491–498

22. Carroll D, Corfield A, Spicer R, Cairns P 2003 Faecal calprotectin concentrations and diagnosis of necrotizing enterocolitis. Lancet 361: 310–311

23. Cavell B 1982 Reservoir and emptying function of the stomach of the premature infant. Acta Paediatrica Scandinavica Supplement 296: 60–61

24. Chaet M S, Farrell M K, Ziegler M M, Warner B W 1994 Intensive nutritional support and remedial surgical intervention for extreme short bowel syndrome. Journal of Pediatric Gastroenterology and Nutrition 19: 295–298

25. Chan K L, Saing H, Yung R W H, Yeung Y P, Tsoi N S 1994 A study of pre-antibiotic bacteriology in 125 patients with necrotizing enterocolitis. Acta Paediatrica Supplement 396: 45–48

26. Chardot C, Rochet J S, Lezeau H et al 2003 Surgical necrotizing enterocolitis: are intestinal lesions more severe in infants with low birth weight?. Journal of Pediatric Surgery 38: 167–172

27. Chatfield S L, Owen G, Ryley H C et al 1991 Neonatal screening for cystic fibrosis in Wales and the West Midlands: clinical assessment after five years of screening. Archives of Disease in Childhood 66: 29–33

28. Choo-Kang L R, Zeitlin P L 2000 Type I, II, III, IV, and V cystic fibrosis transmembrane conductance regulator defects and opportunities for therapy. Current Opinion in Pulmonary Medicine 6: 521–529

29. Clark D A 1977 Times of first void and first stool in 500 newborns. Pediatrics 60: 457–459

30. Clark D A, Barkemeyer B M, Miller M J S 1993 Perinatal hypoxic-ischemic risk factors and necrotizing enterocolitis. Pediatric Research 32: 207

31. Clark D A, Miller M J S 1996 What causes neonatal necrotising enterocolitis and how can it be prevented? In: Hansen T N, McIntosh N (eds) Current topics in neonatology 1, W B Saunders, London, pp 160–176

32. Collins J E, Rolles C J, Sutton H, Ackery D 1984 Vitamin B$_{12}$ absorption after necrotizing enterocolitis. Archives of Disease in Childhood 59: 731–734

33. Communicable Disease Report 1982 Neonatal necrotising enterocolitis surveillance. In: Communicable disease report 82/05. Communicable Disease Surveillance Centre, London

34. Coombs R C, Morgan M E, Durbin G M, Booth I W, McNeish A S 1992 Abnormal gut blood flow velocities in neonates at risk of necrotising enterocolitis. Journal of Pediatric Gastroenterology and Nutrition 15: 13–18

35. Corbet A, Gerdes J, Long W et al 1995 Double-blind, randomized trial of one versus three prophylactic doses of synthetic surfactant in 826 neonates weighing 700 to 1100 grams: effects on mortality rate. American Exosurf Neonatal Study Groups I and IIa. Journal of Pediatrics 126: 969–978

36. Coutts J A, Docherty J G, Carachi R, Evans T J 1997 Clinical course of patients with cystic fibrosis presenting with meconium ileus. British Journal of Surgery 84: 555

37. Crissinger K D 1994 Regulation of hemodynamics and oxygenation in developing intestine: insight into the pathogenesis of necrotizing enterocolitis. Acta Paediatrica Supplement 396: 8–10

38. Cucchiara S, Staiano A, Di Lorenzo C et al 1986 Esophageal motor abnormalities in children with gastroesophageal reflux and peptic esophagitis. Journal of Pediatrics 108: 907–910

39. Curry J I, Lander T D, Stringer M D 2001 Review article: erythromycin as a pro-kinetic agent in infants and children. Alimentary Pharmacology and Therapeutics 15: 595–603

40. Dani C, Biadaioli R, Bertini G, Martelli E, Rubaltelli F F 2002 Probiotics feeding in prevention of urinary tract infection, bacterial sepsis and necrotizing enterocolitis in preterm infants. A prospective double-blind study. Biology of the Neonate 82: 103–108

41. Davey A M, Wagner C L, Cox C, Kendig J W 1994 Feeding premature infants while low umbilical artery catheters are in place: a prospective, randomized trial. Journal of Pediatrics 124: 795–799

42. David T J 1993 Cow's milk intolerance. in Food and food additive intolerance in children, Blackwell, Oxford, pp 25–84

43. De Boissieu D, Dupont C, Barbet J P, Bargaoui K, Badoual J 1994 Distinct features of upper gastrointestinal endoscopy in the newborn. Journal of Pediatric Gastroenterology and Nutrition 18: 334–338

44. De la Torre L, Carrasco D, Mora M A, Ramirez J, Lopez S 2002 Vascular malformations of the colon in children. Journal of Pediatric Surgery 37: 1754–1757

45. De Lemos R A, Rogers J H, McLaughlin W 1974 Experimental production of necrotizing enterocolitis in newborn goats. Pediatric Research 8: 380–387

46. Demestre X, Ginovart G, Figueras-Aloy J et al Peritoneal drainage as primary management in necrotizing enterocolitis: a prospective study. Journal of Pediatric Surgery 37: 1534–1539

47. Desjeux J-F 1996 Congenital transport defects. In : Walker W A et al (eds) Pediatric gastrointestinal disease, 2nd edn. B C Decker, Philadelphia, pp 792–816

48. Dessanti A, Porcu A, Scanu A, Dettori G 1995 Neonatal acute appendicitis in an inguinal hernia. Pediatric Surgery International 10: 561–562

49. Devane S P, Soothill P W, Candy D C A 1993 Temporal changes in gastric volume in human fetus in late pregnancy. Early Human Development 33: 109–116

50. Dodge J A, Morison S, Lewis P A et al 1997 Incidence, population, and survival of cystic fibrosis in the UK, 1968–95. UK Cystic Fibrosis Survey Management Committee. Archives of Disease in Childhood 77: 493–496

51. Doull I J 2001 Recent advances in cystic fibrosis. Archives of Disease in Childhood 85: 62–66

52. Dudding T, Wilcken B, Burgess B, Hambly J, Turner G 2000 Reproductive decisions after neonatal screening identifies cystic fibrosis. Archives of Disease in Childhood Fetal and Neonatal Edition 82: F124–F127

53. Dvorak B, Halpern M D, Holubec H et al 2003 Maternal milk reduces severity of necrotizing enterocolitis and increases intestinal IL-10 in a neonatal rat model. Pediatric Research 53: 426–433

54. Eibl M M, Wolf H M, Furnkranz H, Rosenkranz A 1988 Prevention of necrotizing enterocolitis in low birth weight infants by IgA-IgG feeding. New England Journal of Medicine 319: 1–7

55. Engel R R, Virnig N L, Hunt C E, Levitt M D 1973 Origin of mural gas in necrotizing enterocolitis. Pediatric Research 7: 292

56. Ewer A K 2002 Role of platelet-activating factor in the pathophysiology of necrotizing enterocolitis. Acta Paediatrica Supplement 91: 2–5

57. Ewer A K, Durbin G M, Morgan M E, Booth I W 1994 Gastric emptying in preterm infants. Archives of Disease in Childhood 71: F24–F27

58. Ewer A K, James M E, Tobin J M 1999 Prone and left lateral positioning reduce gastro-oesophageal reflux in preterm infants. Archives of Disease in Childhood Fetal and Neonatal Edition 81: F201–F205

59. Ewer A K, McHugo J M, Chapman S, Newell S J 1993 Fetal echogenic gut: a marker of intrauterine gut ischaemia. Archives of Disease in Childhood 69: 510–513

60. Ewer A K, Yu V Y 1996 Gastric emptying in pre-term infants: the effect of breast milk fortifier. Acta Paediatrica 85: 1112–1115

61. Farrell P M, Kosorok M R, Rock M J et al 2001 Early diagnosis of cystic fibrosis through neonatal screening prevents severe malnutrition and improves long-term growth. Wisconsin Cystic Fibrosis Neonatal Screening Study Group. Pediatrics 107: 1–13

62. Fast C, Rosegger H 1994 Necrotizing enterocolitis prophylaxis: oral antibiotics and lyophilized enterobacteria vs oral immunoglobulins. Acta Paediatrica (Supplement). 1994;396:86–90

63. Fiocchi A, Martelli A, De Chiara A, Moro G, Warm A, Terracciano L 2003 Primary dietary prevention of food allergy. Annals of Allergy Asthma and Immunology 91: 3–12

64. Ford R P, Schluter P J, Taylor B J, Mitchell E A, Scragg R 1996 Allergy and the risk of sudden infant death syndrome. The Members of the New Zealand Cot Death Study Group. Clinical and Experimental Allergy 26: 580–584

65. Frakaloss G, Burke G, Sanders M R 1998 Impact of gastroesophageal reflux on growth and hospital stay in premature infants. Journal of Pediatric Gastroenterology and Nutrition 26: 146–150

66. Fujii A M, Brown E, Mirochnick M, O'Brien S, Kaufman G 2002 Neonatal necrotizing enterocolitis with intestinal perforation in extremely premature infants receiving early indomethacin treatment for patent ductus arteriosus. Journal of Perinatology 22: 535–540

67. Ghanekar A, Grant D 2001 Small bowel transplantation. Current Opinion in Critical Care 7: 133–137

68. Gobet R, Sacher P, Schwobel M G 1994 Surgical procedures in colonic strictures after necrotizing enterocolitis. Acta Paediatrica Supplement 396: 77–79

69. Green M R, Buchanan E, Weaver L T 1995 Nutritional management of the infant with cystic fibrosis. Archives of Disease in Childhood 72: 452–456

70. Guarino A, De Marco G 2003 Natural history of intestinal failure, investigated through a national network-based approach. Journal of Pediatric Gastroenterology and Nutrition 37: 136–141

71. Hackett G A, Campbell S, Gamsu H, Cohen-Overbeek T, Pearce J M F 1987 Doppler studies in the growth retarded fetus and prediction of neonatal necrotising enterocolitis, haemorrhage, and neonatal morbidity. British Medical Journal 294: 13–16

72. Hall N, Ong E G, Ade-Ajayi N et al 2002 T cryptantigen activation is associated with advanced necrotizing enterocolitis. Journal of Pediatric Surgery 37: 791–793

73. Heacock H J, Jeffery H E, Baker J L, Page M 1992 Influence of breast versus formula milk on physiological gastroesophageal reflux in healthy, newborn infants. Journal of Pediatric Gastroenterology and Nutrition 14: 41–46

74. Heneyke S, Smith V V, Spitz L, Milla P J 1999 Chronic intestinal pseudo-obstruction: treatment and long term follow up of 44 patients. Archives of Disease in Childhood 81: 21–27

75. Hentschel R, Hensel D, Brune T, Rabe H, Jorch G 1995 Impact of blood pressure and intestinal perfusion of dobutamine or dopamine in hypotensive preterm infants. Biology of the Neonate 68: 318–324

76. Hey E N 1983 Special care nurseries: admitting to a policy. British Medical Journal 287: 1524–1527

77. Hopkins G B, Gould V E, Stevenson J K, Oliver T K 1970 Necrotizing enterocolitis in premature infants: a clinical and pathologic evaluation of autopsy material. American Journal of Diseases of Children 120: 229–232

78. Horwitz J R, Lally K P, Cheu H W, Vazquez W D, Grosfield J L, Ziegler M M 1995 Complications after surgical intervention in necrotizing enterocolitis: a multicenter review. Journal of Pediatric Surgery 30: 994–999

79. Israel E J 1994 Neonatal necrotizing enterocolitis, a disease of the immature intestinal mucosal barrier. Acta Paediatrica Supplement 396: 27–32

80. Jackman S, Brereton R J, Wright V M 1990 Results of surgical treatment of neonatal necrotising enterocolitis. British Journal of Surgery 77: 146–148

81. James M E, Ewer A K 1999 Acid oro-pharyngeal secretions can predict gastro-oesophageal reflux in preterm infants. European Journal of Pediatrics 158: 371–374

82. Janik J S, Ein S H, Mancer K 1981 Intestinal stricture after necrotizing enterocolitis. Journal of Pediatric Surgery 16: 438–443

83. Juvonen P, Mansson M, Andersson C, Jakobsson I 1996 Allergy development and macromolecular absorption in infants with different feeding regimens during the first three days of life. A three-year prospective follow-up. Acta Paediatrica 85: 1047–1052

84. Kalliomaki M, Salminen S, Poussa T, Arvilommi H, Isolauri E 2003 Probiotics and prevention of atopic disease: 4-year follow-up of a randomised placebo-controlled trial. Lancet 361: 1869–1871

85. Karsdorp V H M, Van-Vugt J M G, Van-Geijn H P et al 1994 Clinical significance of absent or reversed end diastolic velocity waveforms in umbilical artery. Lancet 344: 1664–1668

86. Kelly E J, Chatfield S L, Brownlee K G et al 1993 The effect of intravenous ranitidine on the intragastric pH of preterm infants receiving dexamethasone. Archives of Disease in Childhood 69: 37–39

87. Kelly E J, Newell S J 1994 Gastric ontogeny: clinical implications. Archives of Disease in Childhood 71: F136–F141

88. Kelly E J, Newell S J, Brownlee K G et al 1997 Role of epidermal growth factor and transforming growth factor α in the developing stomach. Archives of Disease in Childhood 76: F158–F162

89. Kempley S T, Bennett S, Loftus B G, Cooper D, Gamsu H R 1993 Randomised trial of umbilical arterial position: clinical outcome. Acta Paediatrica 83: 173–176

90. Kennedy K A, Tyson J E, Chamnanvanakij S 2000 Rapid versus slow rate of advancement of feedings for promoting growth and preventing necrotizing enterocolitis in parenterally fed low-birth-weight infants. Cochrane Database of Systematic Reviews 2: CD001241

91. Kenyon S L, Taylor D J, Tarnow-Mordi W 2001 Broad-spectrum antibiotics for preterm, prelabour rupture of fetal membranes: the ORACLE I randomised trial. ORACLE Collaborative Group. Lancet 357: 979–988

92. Kiely E M 1990 Surgery for gastro-oesophageal reflux. Archives of Disease in Childhood 65: 1291–1292

93. Kliegman R M 2003 The relationship of neonatal feeding practices and the pathogenesis and prevention of necrotizing enterocolitis. Pediatrics 111: 671–672

94. Kliegman R M, Fanaroff A A 1981 Neonatal necrotizing enterocolitis: a nine year experience. I. Epidemiology and uncommon observations. American Journal of Diseases of Children 135: 603–607

95. Kliegman R M, Fanaroff A A 1984 Necrotizing enterocolitis. New England Journal of Medicine 310: 1093–1103

96. Kliegman R M, Walker W A, Yolken R H 1993 Necrotizing enterocolitis: research agenda for a disease of unknown etiology and pathogenesis. Pediatric Research 34: 701–708

97. Kosloske A M 1994 Epidemiology of necrotizing enterocolitis. Acta Paediatrica Supplement 396: 2–7

98. Kosloske A M 1994 Indications for operation in necrotizing enterocolitis revisited. Journal of Pediatric Surgery 29: 663–666

99. Krishnamoorthy M, Mintz A, Liem T, Applebaum H 1994 Diagnosis and treatment of respiratory symptoms of initially unsuspected gastroesophageal reflux in infants. American Surgery 60: 783–785

100. Lamireau T, Llanas B, Chateil J F et al 1996 Frequence accrué et difficultés diagnostiques des stenose intestinales apres enterocolite ulceronecrosante. Archives de Pediatrie 3: 9–15

101. Lawrence G, Bates J, Gaul A 1982 Pathogenesis of neonatal necrotising enterocolitis. Lancet 1: 137–139

102. Lebenthal A, Lebenthal E 1999 The ontogeny of the small intestinal epithelium. Journal of Parenteral and Enteral Nutrition 23(Supple): S3–S6

103. Lebenthal E, Leung Y K 1988 Feeding the premature and compromised infant: gastrointestinal considerations. Pediatric Clinics of North America 35: 215–238

104. Lemelle J L, Schmitt M, de Miscault G, Vert P, Hascoet J M 1994 Neonatal necrotizing enterocolitis: a retrospective and multicentric review of 331 cases. Acta Paediatrica Supplement 396: 70–73

105. Liefaard G, Heineman E, Molenaar J C, Tibboel D 1995 Prospective evaluation of the absorptive capacity of the bowel after major and minor resections in the neonate. Journal of Pediatric Surgery 30: 388–391

106. Lucas, A., Cole, T. J. 1990 Breast milk and neonatal necrotising enterocolitis. Lancet 336: 1519–1523

107. Lucas A, Morley R 1998 Necrotising enterocolitis. British Paediatric Surveillance Unit, London

108. McClure R J 2001 Trophic feeding of the preterm infant. Acta Paediatrica Supplement 90: 19–21

109. McClure R J, Chatrath M K, Newell S J 1996 Changing trends in feeding policies for ventilated preterm infants. Acta Paediatrica 85: 1123–1125

110. McClure R J, Newell S J 1996 Effect of fortifying breast milk on gastric emptying. Archives of Disease in Childhood 74: F60–F62

111. McClure R J, Newell S J 1999 Randomised controlled trial of trophic feeding and gut motility. Archives of Disease in Childhood 80: F54–F58

112. McClure R J, Newell S J 2000 Randomised controlled trial of clinical outcome following trophic feeding. Archives of Disease in Childhood Fetal and Neonatal Edition 82: F29–F33

113. MacDonald A 1996 Nutritional management of cystic fibrosis. Archives of Disease in Childhood 74: 81–87

114. McDonnell M, Serra V, Gaffney G, Redman C W, Hope P L 1994 Neonatal outcome after pregnancy complicated by abnormal velocity waveforms in the umbilical artery. Archives of Disease in Childhood 70: F84–F89

115. McGuire W, Anthony M Y 2003 Donor human milk versus formula for preventing necrotising enterocolitis in preterm infants: systematic review. Archives of Disease in Childhood Fetal and Neonatal Edition 88: F11–F14

116. MacKendrick W, Hill N, Hsueh W, Caplan M S 1993 Increase in plasma platelet activating factor levels in enterally fed preterm infants. Biology of the Neonate 64: 89–95

117. McKeown R E, Marsh T D, Amarnath U, Garrison C Z, Addy C L, Thompson S J 1992 Role of delayed feeding and of feeding increments in necrotizing enterocolitis. Journal of Pediatrics 121: 764–770

118. Makela S, Kere J, Holmberg C, Hoglund P 2002 SLC26A3 mutations in congenital chloride diarrhea. Human Mutation 20: 425–438

119. Maki M, Ruuska T, Kuusela A-L 1993 High prevalence of asymptomatic esophageal and gastric lesions in preterm infants in intensive care. Critical Care Medicine 21: 1863–1867

120. Marchildon M B, Buck B E, Abdenour G 1982 Necrotizing enterocolitis in the unfed infant. Journal of Pediatric Surgery 17: 620–624

121. Marcy S M, Overturf G D 1997 Focal bacterial infections. In: Remington J S, Klein J O (eds) Infectious diseases of the fetus and newborn infant, 4th edn. WB Saunders, Philadelphia, pp 936–979

122. Marti U, Burwen S J, Jones A L 1989 Biological effects of epidermal growth factor, with emphasis on the gastrointestinal tract and liver: an update. Hepatology 9: 126–138

123. Mirakian R, Richardson A, Milla P J et al 1986 Protracted diarrhoea of infancy: evidence in support of an autoimmune variant. British Medical Journal 293: 1132–1136

124. Morecroft J A, Spitz L, Hamilton P A, Holmes S J K 1994 Plasma cytokine levels in necrotizing enterocolitis. Acta Paediatrica Supplement 396: 18–20

125. Mulvihill S J, Stone M M, Fonkalsrad E W, Debas H T 1986 Trophic effect of amniotic fluid on fetal gastrointestinal development. Journal of Surgical Research 40: 291–296

126. Murch S H 1997 The molecular basis of intractable diarrhoea of infancy. Baillières Clinical Gastroenterology 11: 413–440

127. Murray J, Cuckle H, Taylor G, Littlewood J, Hewison J 1999 Screening for cystic fibrosis. Health Technology Assessment 3: 1–104

128. Musemeche C A, Kosloske A M, Ricketts R R 1987 Enterostomy in necrotizing enterocolitis: an analysis of techniques and timing of closure. Journal of Pediatric Surgery 22: 479–483

129. Newell S J 1996 Gastrointestinal function and its ontogeny: how should we feed the preterm infant? In: Ryan S (ed). Seminars in neonatology 1. WB Saunders, London, pp 59–66

130. Newell S J 1999 GORD in infants and young children. International Journal of Gastroenterology 4: 9–12

131. Newell S J 2000 Enteral feeding in the micropremie. Clinical Perinatology 27: 221

132. Newell S J, Booth I W, Morgan M E, Durbin G M, McNeish A S 1989 Gastro-oesophageal reflux in preterm infants. Archives of Disease in Childhood 64: 780–786

133. Newell S J, Chapman S, Booth I W 1993 Ultrasonic assessment of gastric emptying in the preterm infant. Archives of Disease in Childhood 69: 32–36

134. Newell S J, Morgan M E, Durbin G M, Booth I W, McNeish A S 1989 Does mechanical ventilation precipitate gastro-oesophageal reflux during enteral feeding? Archives of Disease in Childhood 64: 1352–1355

135. Newell S J, Sarkar P K, Durbin G M, Booth I W, McNeish A S 1986 Maturation of the lower oesophageal sphincter in the preterm baby. Gut 29: 167–172

136. Ng P C, Brownlee K G, Dear P R F 1992 Gastroduodenal perforation in preterm babies treated with dexamethasone for bronchopulmonary dysplasia. Archives of Disease in Childhood 66: 1164–1166

137. Ng S C, Quak S H 1998 Gastroesophageal reflux in preterm infants: norms for extended distal esophageal pH monitoring. Journal of Pediatric Gastroenterology and Nutrition 27: 411–414

138. Oldaeus G, Anjou K, Bjorksten B, Moran J R, Kjellman N-I M 1997 Extensively and partially hydrolysed infant formulas for allergy prophylaxis. Archives of Disease in Childhood 77: 4–10

139. Omari T I, Barnett C P, Benninga M A et al 2002 Mechanisms of gastro-oesophageal reflux in preterm and term infants with reflux disease. Gut 51: 475–479

140. Panigrahi P, Gupta S, Gewolb I H, Morris J G 1994 Occurrence of necrotizing enterocolitis may be dependent on patterns of bacterial adherence and intestinal

colonisation: studies in Caco-2 tissue culture and weaning rabbit models. Pediatric Research 36: 115–121

141. Papaila J G, Wilmot D, Grosfeld J L, Rescorla F J, West K W, Vane D W 1989 Increased incidence of delayed gastric emptying in children with gastrosophageal reflux. A prospective evaluation. Archives of Surgery 124: 933–936

142. Phillips A D, Schmitz J 1992 Familial microvillous atrophy: a clinicopathological review of 23 cases. Journal of Pediatric Gastroenterology and Nutrition 14: 380–396

143. Pradeaux L, Boggio V, Gouyon J B 1991 Gastro-oesophageal reflux in mechanically ventilated preterm infants. Archives of Disease in Childhood 66: 793–796

144. Pritchard J A 1966 Fetal swallowing and amniotic fluid volume. Obstetrics and Gynaecology 28: 606–610

145. Pumberger W, Mayr M, Kohlhauser C, Weninger M 2002 Spontaneous localized intestinal perforation in very-low-birth-weight infants: a distinct clinical entity different from necrotizing enterocolitis. Journal of the American College of Surgeons 195: 796–803

146. Puntis J W L 1995 Home parenteral nutrition. Archives of Disease in Childhood 72: 186–190

147. Raval N C, Gonzalez E, Bhat A M, Pearlman S A, Stefano J L 1995 Umbilical venous catheters: evaluation of radiographs to determine position and associated complications of malpositioned umbilical venous catheters. American Journal of Perinatology 12: 201–204

148. Rennie J M, Kelsall A W 1994 Vitamin K prophylaxis in the newborn—again. Archives of Disease in Childhood 70: 248–251

149. Rescorla F J 1995 Surgical management of pediatric necrotizing enterocolitis. Current Opinions in Pediatrics 7: 335–341

150. Ricketts R R 1994 Surgical treatment of necrotizing enterocolitis and the short bowel syndrome. Clinics in Perinatology 21: 365–387

151. Rotbart H A, Levin M J 1983 How contagious is necrotizing enterocolitis?. Pediatric Infectious Disease Journal 2: 406–410

152. Rowe M I, Reblock K K, Kurkchubasche A G, Healey P J 1994 Necrotizing enterocolitis in the extremely low birth weight infant. Journal of Pediatric Surgery 29: 987–990

153. Salvatore S, Vandenplas Y 2002 Gastroesophageal reflux and cow milk allergy: is there a link? Pediatrics 110: 972–984

154. Savilathi E, Launiala K, Kuitunen P 1983 Congenital lactase deficiency: a clinical study of 16 patients. Archives of Disease in Childhood 58: 246–252

155. Schimpl G, Hollwarth M E, Fotter R, Becker H 1994 Late intestinal strictures following successful treatment of necrotizing enterocolitis. Acta Paediatrica Supplement 396: 80–83

156. Shapira R, Hadzic N, Francavilla R, Koukulis G, Price J F, Mieli-Vergani G 1999 Retrospective review of cystic fibrosis presenting as infantile liver disease. Archives of Disease in Childhood 81: 125–128

157. Sherry S N, Kramer I 1955 The time of passage of the first stool and first urine by the newborn infant. Journal of Pediatrics 46: 158–159

158. Shulman R J, Redel C A, Stathos T H 1994 Bolus versus continuous feedings stimulate small intestinal growth and development in the newborn pig. Journal of Pediatric Gastroenterology and Nutrition 18: 350–354

159. Sicherer S H 2003 Clinical aspects of gastrointestinal food allergy in childhood. Pediatrics 111: 1609–1616

160. Sondheimer J M, Clark D A, Gervaise E P 1985 Continuous gastric pH measurement in young and older healthy preterm infants receiving formula and clear liquid feedings. Journal of Pediatric Gastroenterology and Nutrition 4: 352–355

161. Spitz L, Stringer M D 1993 Surgical management of neonatal necrotising enterocolitis. Archives of Disease in Childhood 69: 269–271

162. Steeb C B, Trahair J F, Read L C 1995 Administration of insulin-like growth factor-I (IGF-I) peptides for three days stimulates proliferation of the small intestinal epithelium in rats. Gut 37: 630–638

163. Stiefel D, Stallmach T, Sacher P 1998 Acute appendicitis in neonates: complication or morbus sui generis?. Pediatric Surgery International 14: 122–123

164. Stringer M D, Puntis J W L 1995 Short bowel syndrome. Archives of Disease in Childhood 73: 170–173

165. Stringer M D, Thornton J G, Mason G C 1996 Hyperechoic bowel. Archives of Disease in Childhood 74: F1–F2

166. Sullivan S E, Calhoun D A, Maheshwari A et al 2002 Tolerance of simulated amniotic fluid in premature neonates. Annals of Pharmacotherapy 36: 1518–1524

167. Thomas D F M, Fernie D S, Bayston R, Spitz L 1984 Clostridial toxins in neonatal necrotising enterocolitis. Archives of Disease in Childhood 59: 270–272

168. Tobiansky R, Lui K, Roberts S, Veddovi M 1995 Neurodevelopmental outcome in very low birthweight infants with necrotizing enterocolitis requiring surgery. Journal of Paediatrics and Child Health 31: 233–236

169. Trahair J F, Harding R 1995 Restitution of swallowing in the fetal sheep restores intestinal growth after midgestation esophageal obstruction. Journal of Pediatric Gastroenterology and Nutrition 20: 156–161

170. Uauy R, Fanaroff A A, Korones S B, Phillips E A, Phillips J B, Wright L L 1991 Necrotizing enterocolitis in very low birth weight infants: biodemographic and clinical correlates. Journal of Pediatrics 119: 630–638

171. Udall J N 1990 Gastrointestinal host defence and necrotizing enterocolitis. Journal of Pediatrics 117: S33–S44

172. Vandenplas Y, Goyvaerts H, Helven R, Sacre L 1991 Gastroesophageal reflux, as measured by 24-hour pH monitoring, in 509 healthy infants screened for risk of sudden infant death syndrome. Pediatrics 88: 834–840

173. Vandenplas Y, Sacre Smits L 1987 Continuous 24-hour esophageal pH monitoring in 285 asymptomatic infants 0–15 months old. Journal of Pediatric Gastroenterology and Nutrition 6: 220–224

174. Vanderhoof J, Young R, Thompson J 2003 New and emerging therapies for short bowel syndrome in children. Paediatric Drugs 5: 525–531

175. Vasan U, Gotoff S P 1994 Prevention of neonatal necrotizing enterocolitis. Clinics in Perinatology 21: 425–435

176. Vinton N E 1994 Gastrointestinal bleeding in infancy and childhood. Gastroenterology Clinics of North America 23: 93–122

177. Walsh M C, Kliegman R M 1986 Necrotizing enterocolitis: treatment based on staging criteria. Pediatric Clinics of North America 33: 179–201

178. Weaver L T, Laker M F, Nelson R, Lucas A 1987 Milk feeding and changes in intestinal permeability and morphology in the newborn. Journal of Pediatric Gastroenterology and Nutrition 6: 351–358

179. Weaver L T, Lucas A 1990 Maturation of large bowel function in relation to gestational and postnatal age, feed volumes and composition in the newborn. Pediatric Reviews and Communications 4: 250

180. Weber T R, Tracy T F, Silen M L et al 1995 Enterostomy and its closure in newborns. Archives of Surgery 130: 534–537

181. Wenzl T G, Schneider S, Scheele F, Silny J, Heimann G, Skopnik H 2003 Effects of thickened feeding on gastroesophageal reflux in infants: a placebo-controlled crossover study using intraluminal impedance. Pediatrics 111: e355–e359

182. Wiswell T E, Cornish J D, Northam R S 1986 Neonatal polycythemia: frequency of clinical manifestations and other problems. Pediatrics 78: 26–28

183. Wood C M, Spicer R D, Beddis I R, Puntis J W L 1995 Pancreatic exocrine failure in cystic fibrosis presenting as necrotising enterocolitis. Journal of Pediatric Gastroenterology and Nutrition 20: 104–106

184. Wozniak E R, Fenton T R, Milla P J 1983 The development of fasting small intestinal motility in the human neonate. In: Roman C (ed) Gastrointestinal motility. MTP Press, Lancaster, pp 265–270

185. Young D G 1965 Spontaneous rupture of the rectum. Proceedings of the Royal Society of Medicine 58: 615–616

PART 4

Congenital defects and surgical problems

Mark D Stringer, Ian Sugarman, Alistair G Smyth

Introduction

This chapter discusses the management of major surgical conditions affecting the neonatal alimentary tract. Most are congenital malformations and, as such, are frequently multiple. Conditions are discussed in sequence down the gut, rather than in order of importance or severity. Some preliminary general comments about neonatal gastrointestinal surgery are necessary.

The survival of babies with congenital malformations has improved progressively as a result of advances in neonatal care and the concentration of these infants within specialist paediatric surgical units. An integrated multidisciplinary approach is essential in the management of premature surgical neonates and in those with complex congenital malformations.[6]

Prenatal ultrasound diagnosis of major structural gastrointestinal anomalies presents parents and clinicians with the opportunity to terminate the pregnancy or to deliver the baby in a centre with ready access to paediatric surgical expertise; in rare instances, fetal intervention may be appropriate. Prenatal diagnosis of gastrointestinal anomalies has had a major impact on the management of anterior abdominal wall defects in particular, not least because parents can be informed about management and prognosis. In other conditions, interpretation of ultrasound findings is less clear cut. For example, hyperechogenic fetal bowel (bowel of similar or greater echogenicity than surrounding bone; Fig. 29.26) may indicate the presence of meconium ileus or intestinal obstruction but it is a relatively soft marker of fetal pathology and most affected fetuses are normal after birth.[66]

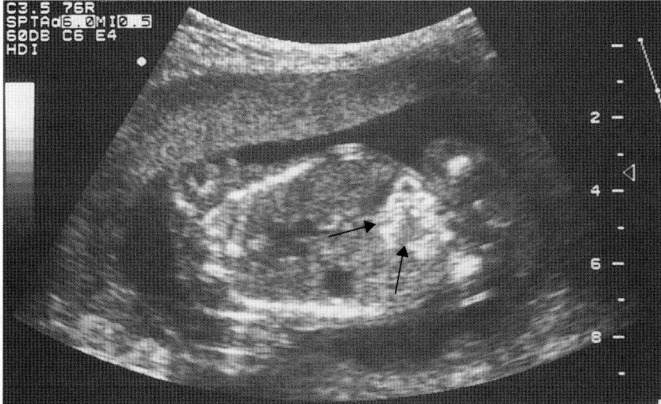

Fig. 29.26 Sonographic cross section of the fetal abdomen at 18 weeks' gestation showing hyperechogenic fetal bowel as bright as bone (arrows).

Similarly, intestinal dilatation is non-specific and may be seen in the fetus with midgut or hindgut atresia, meconium ileus, malrotation or Hirschsprung's disease.[52] A more complex picture with both dilated and hyperechogenic bowel, ascites and polyhydramnios may occur with meconium peritonitis. Duodenal atresia can often be diagnosed by prenatal ultrasound scan but the findings in oesophageal atresia are much less specific.

Many congenital gastrointestinal malformations present with symptoms and signs of intestinal obstruction in the newborn.

- **Vomiting**: this will be bile-stained if the obstruction is beyond the level of the ampulla of Vater. Bilious vomiting in the newborn should be attributed to intestinal obstruction until proven otherwise. In one prospective study of 63 consecutive neonates with bilious vomiting, a surgical cause was identified in 24 (38%): Hirschsprung's disease in nine, small bowel atresia in five, intestinal malrotation in four, meconium ileus in three, meconium plug in one, colonic atresia in one and milk inspissation in one.[29] Most of these babies had abdominal signs and an abnormal abdominal radiograph. No surgical cause for bilious vomiting was found in 39 (62%) infants whose symptoms resolved with conservative management. All neonates with bilious vomiting require investigation. Intestinal malrotation must be excluded. First-line investigations consist of a detailed clinical examination, a plain radiograph of the chest and abdomen, routine haematology and biochemistry, and blood and urine cultures. A more detailed septic screen may be indicated. Abdominal ultrasound and gastrointestinal contrast studies are often warranted and, in selected cases, a rectal biopsy may be necessary.
- **Abdominal distension**: an algorithm for assessing a baby who develops marked abdominal distension soon after birth is shown in Fig. 29.27. This must be interpreted in conjunction with the baby's gestational age and general condition.
- **Delay or failure to pass meconium**: over 95% of healthy term infants pass their first stool within 24 hours of birth.[58] Delayed passage of meconium after 48 hours in a term infant should always suggest the possibility of intestinal obstruction. However, such a delay is normal in premature infants.[71] In any baby who fails to pass meconium normally, the anus should be examined and its patency confirmed.

All babies with clinical features of intestinal obstruction should receive parenteral vitamin K. Bleeding is a rare manifestation of congenital gastrointestinal anomalies and more often indicates acquired disease. Upper gastrointestinal bleeding may be due to swallowed maternal blood, vitamin K deficiency bleeding or oesophagitis/gastritis. Peptic ulceration occurs occasionally and can be confirmed by endoscopy. Rectal bleeding in an otherwise well baby is most commonly due to an anal fissure or cow's milk

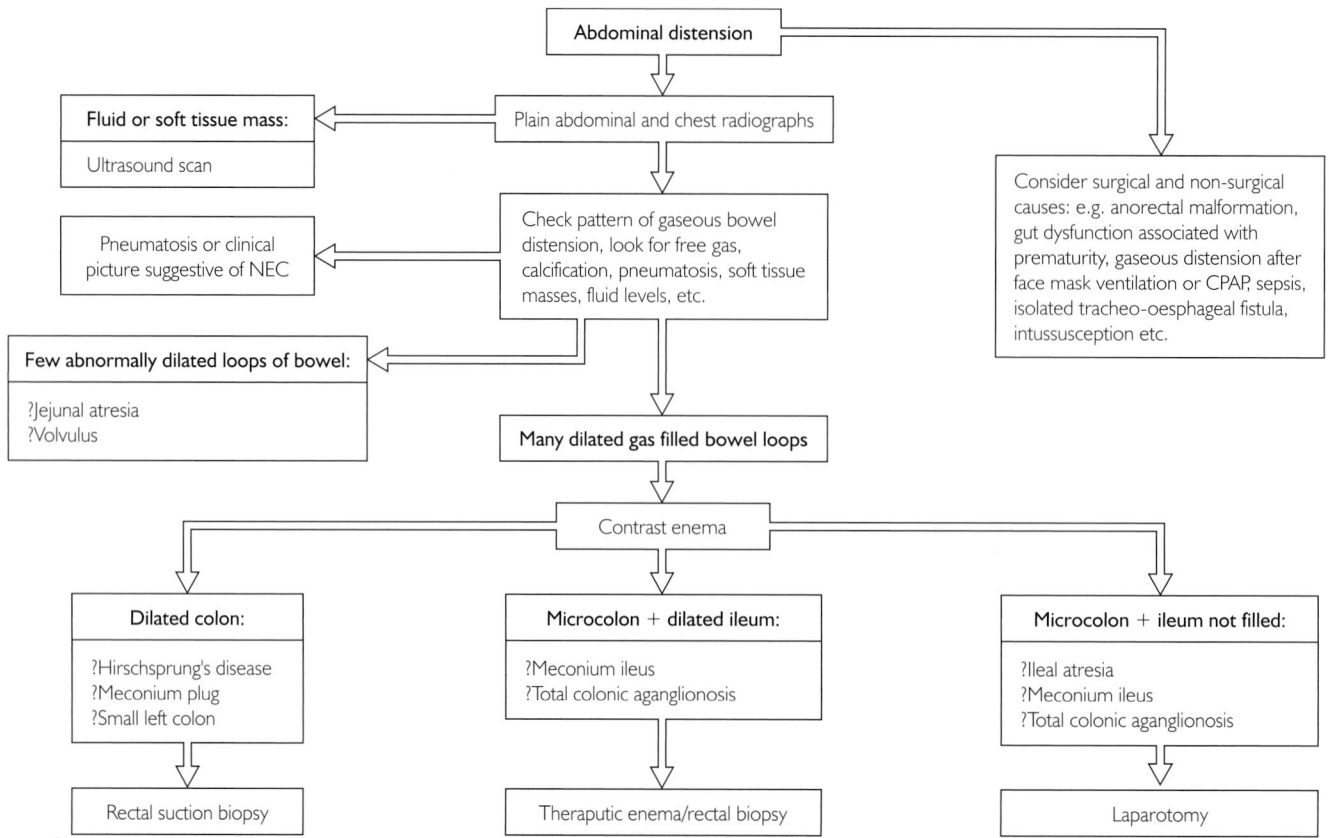

Fig. 29.27 An algorithm for investigating the neonate who develops abdominal distension soon after birth. This must be interpreted in conjunction with clinical and routine laboratory assessments.

protein intolerance. In a sick infant it may be from necrotising enterocolitis or malrotation with volvulus.

Mouth and nasopharynx

Cleft lip and palate

Cleft lip and palate is the commonest congenital anomaly in the craniofacial region, with an incidence in the UK of approximately 1/700 live births. Most clefts are diagnosed at birth but the diagnosis may be made by prenatal ultrasound scan. Cleft lip is twice as common on the left side than on the right but the reason for this remains obscure. Cleft lip with or without cleft palate is more than twice as common in males, whereas cleft palate alone is twice as common in females. In most patients the orofacial cleft will be the only defect. However, approximately 15% of all patients with cleft lip and/or palate will have other associated abnormalities, which together may form part of a recognised syndrome. Syndromal associations are more frequent in isolated cleft palate. With regard to non-syndromic cleft lip and palate, a family history of the condition may be present or a history of maternal exposure to drugs such as phenytoin. All babies presenting with cleft lip and/or palate should have a full examination and a standard karyotype investigation.

Isolated cleft palate accounts for about 50% of all clefts, the remaining groups consisting of unilateral cleft lip and palate (20%), cleft lip (20%) and bilateral cleft lip and palate (10%). This complex deformity can affect many aspects of development, including speech, hearing, facial appearance, dental development and facial growth. Treatment requires a multidisciplinary approach from birth to maturity. Outcomes can be remarkably good when this is provided in a skilled and co-ordinated manner, and remarkably bad when it is not.[57]

Cleft lip and palate services within the UK changed dramatically following the 1998 Clinical Standards Advisory Group report into cleft lip and palate services and treatment outcomes.[12] This document recommended a reduction in cleft units within the UK from the previous 57 units to eight to 15 specialist centres, allowing a concentration of expertise and resources. All patients should be cared for within a dedicated multidisciplinary cleft team with full access to the necessary specialist services.

Cleft lip

A cleft lip may result when fusion between the medial and lateral nasal processes with the maxillary process fails to occur. Cleft lip may occur in isolation or in conjunction with cleft palate. The lip cleft is usually to one side of the midline and may be incomplete (Fig. 29.28) or involve the full height of the lip (complete), extending into the floor of the nose. The cleft may be unilateral or bilateral and may extend on to the gum area

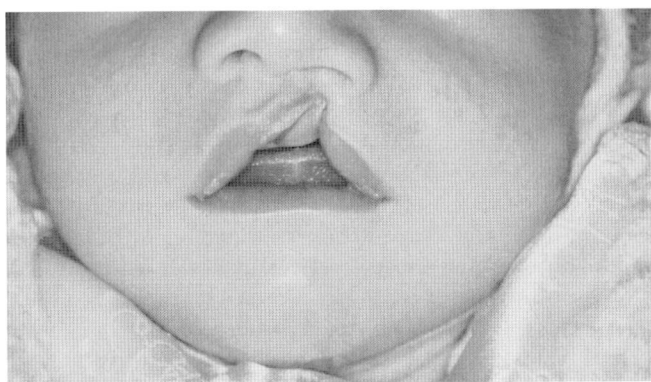

Fig. 29.28 Unilateral incomplete cleft lip.

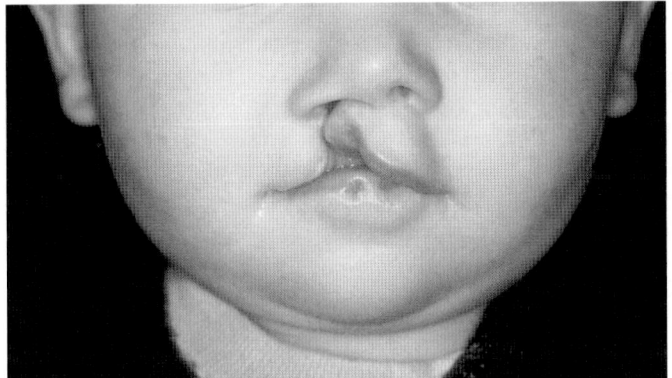

Fig. 29.29 Complete cleft lip and lower lip pits (Van der Woude syndrome).

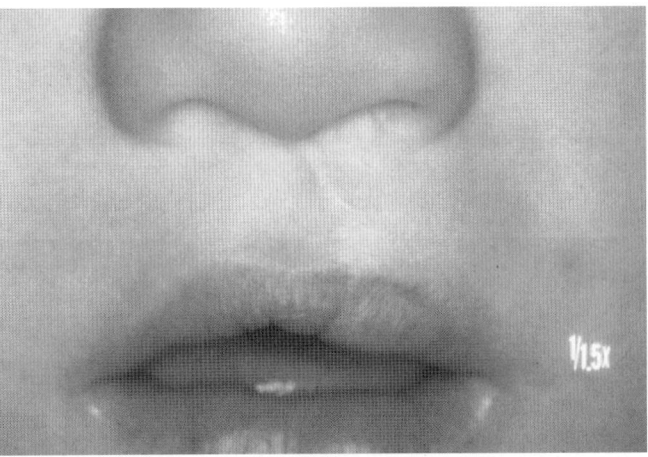

Fig. 29.30 Cleft lip and nose repair (same child as Fig. 29.28).

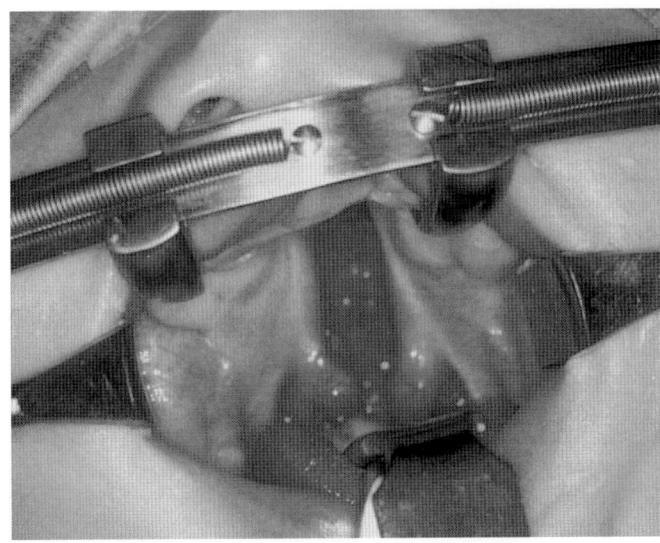

Fig. 29.31 Isolated cleft palate (seen at time of surgery).

(alveolus) of the upper jaw. Babies with isolated cleft lip usually manage to feed well from a soft bottle with teat and in many cases may also successfully breastfeed.

A rare midline cleft of the upper lip may occur as part of an oro-facial-digital syndrome (type I). Cleft lip can also occur in conjunction with lower lip pits – Van der Woude syndrome (Fig. 29.29) – an autosomal dominant condition with variable expressivity.

Outcomes from cleft lip treatment are often excellent and surgical repair is usually undertaken around 3 months of age. Primary nasal correction is carried out at the same time as lip repair (Fig. 29.30). If the alveolus is also involved then repair of the alveolar cleft with a bone graft may be required but this operation is usually performed in the mixed dentition around 9–11 years of age.

Cleft palate

Palatal fusion begins around the 6th week of intrauterine life and occurs from the front of the palate to the back. Interference with palatal shelf fusion from extrinsic factors such as phenytoin or intrinsic factors such as genetic predisposition or obstructing tongue position may result in a cleft palate. Cleft palate may occur in isolation or in combination with cleft lip. Isolated cleft palate may involve the posterior palate alone (soft palate) or may extend further forward into the hard palate up to the incisive

foramen just behind the front teeth (complete cleft palate). Cleft palate is a midline defect and may be incomplete or complete (Fig. 29.31).

Isolated cleft palate cannot be diagnosed antenatally and is noted after birth. Nasal regurgitation of milk is not pathognomonic of cleft palate and exclusion requires direct inspection of the full palate with a good light source with the tongue depressed. Digital palpation of the palate by itself is not sufficient, as incomplete clefts can be easily missed. Babies with cleft palate have difficulty with suction and are unlikely to breastfeed properly. Assisted bottlefeeding is often required using a soft bottle and teat. Midline clefts such as cleft palate are more likely to be associated with a chromosomal defect and therefore all babies born with cleft palate should have a fluorescent in-situ hybridisation (FISH) test for a chromosomal microdeletion on chromosome 22 (Catch-22, see p. 128) as well as a standard karyotype.

Pierre-Robin sequence (Fig. 29.32) is the association of an often wide U-shaped cleft palate (Fig. 29.33) with a small mandible (micrognathia) and a posteriorly placed tongue. Upper airway obstruction is a common association, which may require

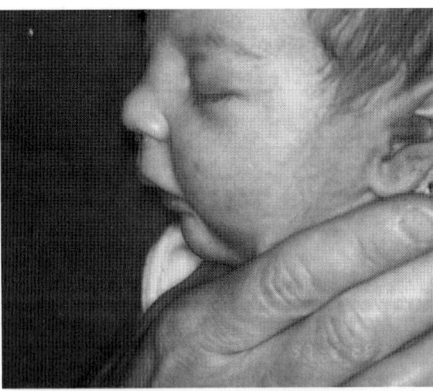

Fig. 29.32 Pierre-Robin sequence (note micrognathia).

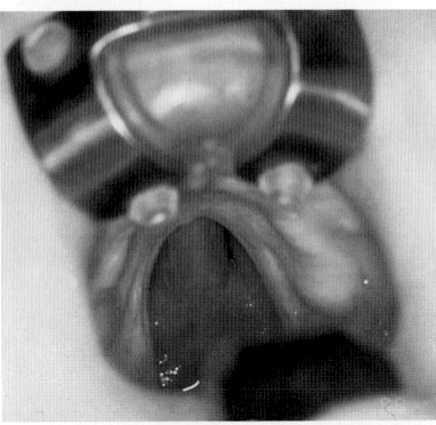

Fig. 29.33 Wide U-shaped cleft palate (Pierre-Robin sequence).

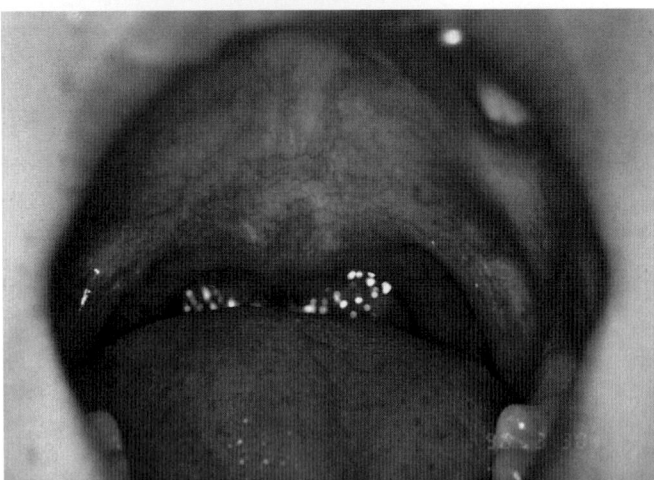

Fig. 29.34 Submucous cleft palate showing bifid uvula and midline groove/translucent line of soft palate.

intervention such as positioning the infant (side or prone) or insertion of a nasopharyngeal airway. Tracheostomy is rarely required. Pierre-Robin-associated syndromes should be considered, such as Stickler's syndrome and velo-cardio-facial syndrome (22q11 deletion).

Surgical repair of cleft palate is usually carried out around 8–9 months of age using local tissues and includes repair of the soft palate muscles. In Pierre-Robin-associated cleft palate, the repair may be further delayed to 1 year of age or older, depending on the degree of airway obstruction.

A subtype of cleft palate called a submucous cleft palate is often difficult to diagnose and typically may not present until the child is 4 or more years of age, often with accompanying speech problems. Indicators of a submucous cleft palate may include a bifid uvula, midline translucent zone of the soft palate and a palpable notch at the back of the hard palate (Fig. 29.34).

Children with a history of cleft palate require screening for chronic otitis media with effusion, which may require insertion of grommets or provision of a hearing aid. Speech and language monitoring is required for the possible development of cleft-type characteristics and velopharyngeal incompetence during speech.

Alveolar bone grafts

Clefts that involve the gum area (alveolus) of the upper jaw may benefit from the insertion of a bone graft to allow tooth eruption, provide bone support for the teeth and upper jaw and close off any remaining fistula. Secondary bone grafting just before the eruption of the permanent canine tooth produces the best outcome and is usually carried out between 9 and 11 years of age (Fig. 29.35).

Other facial clefts

Other, more extensive facial clefts are rare. The pathogenesis of these facial clefts such as the lateral and oblique facial cleft remains uncertain. The soft tissue clefts frequently involve the underlying facial bones and the orbit and a careful search is required for associated anomalies, including the central nervous system.

Multi-disciplinary management

Cleft lip and palate is a complex abnormality that demands coordinated care and treatment from a number of specialists and in the last 20 years there has been an increasing emphasis on the importance of the multidisciplinary team.[70] The core team often

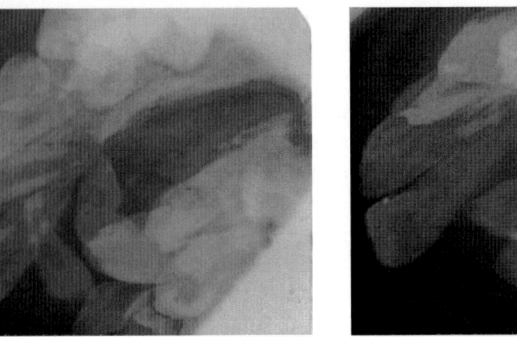

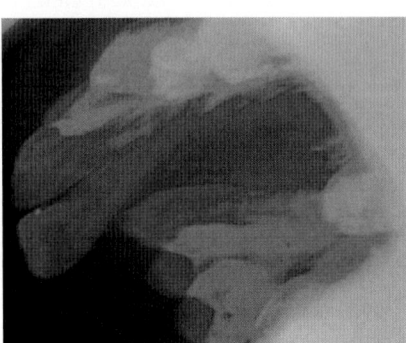

Fig. 29.35 Radiographs before (left) and 6 months after (right) alveolar bone graft operation.

consists of a cleft surgeon, orthodontist, speech and language therapist, paediatrician, clinical psychologist, clinical geneticist and specialist cleft nurses. While treatment interventions should be restricted to specific times to facilitate good outcomes and minimise the burden of care, follow-up by the cleft team is often required until growth has stopped (18–20 years of age). The Cleft Lip and Palate Association (CLAPA) is an active parent/patient support group within the UK providing essential feeding equipment and information.

The provision of high-quality primary surgery reduces the need for future interventions and evidence is accumulating in support of high-volume operators achieving better outcomes.[72] However, despite expert initial care including surgery, some patients may require further operative procedures to improve speech (pharyngoplasty) or benefit facial appearance and function.

Oesophagus and stomach

Oesophageal atresia

The commonest type of oesophageal atresia (OA), accounting for 85% of all cases, consists of a dilated, blind-ended upper oesophageal pouch and a narrow, distal tracheo-oesophageal fistula (TOF; Fig. 29.36a). Nearly 10% of infants with OA do not have a fistula but a long gap between the oesophageal segments (Fig. 29.36b). Rarely, there is a fistula between the upper oesophageal pouch and the trachea, with or without a distal fistula (Fig. 29.36d, e). An isolated TOF ('H' or 'N' fistula) is usually grouped with these anomalies although there is no atresia (Fig. 29.36c). More detailed classifications of oesophageal atresia have been reported.[33] The incidence of this spectrum of disorders is about 1/3500 births.

The trachea and oesophagus both develop from the primitive foregut but the pathogenesis of OA/TOF is uncertain. Some experimental studies have suggested that this malformation results from an abnormal separation of the primitive trachea and oesophagus while others have indicated that the fistula develops after these structures have separated. Oesophageal atresia is usually sporadic and rarely familial.

Maternal polyhydramnios and a small or absent fetal stomach bubble may suggest the possibility of OA prenatally but these sonographic findings are not specific.[64] Occasionally, a dilated upper oesophageal pouch may provide further evidence. Additional malformations suggestive of trisomy 13 or 18 or the VACTERL association (vertebral defects, anal atresia, TOF, radial and renal dysplasia with cardiac and limb defects) may be detected by prenatal ultrasound.

Postnatally, the baby typically dribbles frothy saliva and has episodes of choking, coughing and cyanosis, often precipitated by attempts to feed. This is caused by overflow of secretions into the larynx and trachea. Attempted passage of a 10–12 Fr radiopaque nasogastric tube will reveal a hold-up about 10 cm from the lips (a smaller tube tends to curl up in the upper pouch). The diagnosis is confirmed by anteroposterior and lateral radiographs of the chest with the tube in situ (Figs 29.37,

29.38). Air in the stomach indicates a TOF while a gasless abdomen usually signifies atresia without a fistula.

Associated congenital anomalies occur in 50% or more of infants.[11] Cardiovascular, genitourinary, skeletal and anorectal anomalies are found frequently. An echocardiogram, urinary tract ultrasound scan and radiographs of the chest, abdomen and spine will detect many of these additional malformations at an early stage. The VACTERL cluster includes vertebral, anorectal, cardiac, tracheo-oesophageal, renal and radial limb anomalies. Duodenal atresia is the commonest associated gastrointestinal anomaly. Rarely, OA may be associated with the CHARGE association (coloboma, heart defects, choanal atresia, retarded development and growth, genital hypoplasia and ear anomalies)[37] or with midline defects such as cleft lip and palate and exomphalos.

Initial management is aimed at keeping the airway free of secretions and excluding additional major malformations. It is rarely necessary to operate immediately. The infant should be placed slightly head-up, with a 10 Fr double-lumen Replogle tube in the proximal pouch on continuous low-pressure suction. Routine neonatal care will include regulation of temperature, fluid balance and blood glucose. As soon as the baby is stable, he should be transferred to a neonatal surgical unit.

The vast majority of neonates with OA/TOF can be treated successfully by surgical division of the fistula between the trachea and oesophagus and primary anastomosis of the oesophagus. This was first successfully accomplished in 1941.[31] The operation is usually performed through a small right thoracotomy but minimally invasive repair using a thoracoscope has recently been reported.[56] A preliminary tracheoscopy is often carried out to search for an upper pouch fistula and clarify the anatomy (Fig. 29.39). Postoperatively, after a straightforward operation, feeding is commenced enterally via a transanastomotic nasogastric tube or by mouth.

Two specific problems should be mentioned.

- The baby with OA/TOF and severe respiratory distress (associated with prematurity or secondary to acid aspiration via the fistula) is in danger. The fistula provides a low-resistance pathway for inspiratory gases, thus preventing efficient ventilation. Gastric distension (and subsequently rupture) further compromises ventilation. Various temporising measures may be helpful, such as positioning the tip of the endotracheal tube below the fistula, using low-pressure ventilation or attempting balloon catheter occlusion of the fistula, but the definitive treatment is emergency ligation of the fistula.[60] Gastrostomy is hazardous because it provides an even easier pathway for the escape of respiratory gases.
- The baby with long-gap oesophageal atresia may have OA without a fistula or a distal TOF but a wide gap between the oesophageal segments. In the former, surgery is typically delayed (delayed primary anastomosis). The upper and lower pouches are allowed to elongate and hypertrophy over a period of up to 3 months and can eventually be anastomosed. During this time the baby is fed through a gastrostomy and the upper pouch is kept clear of secretions. In wide-gap OA/TOF, the anastomosis is sometimes possible under tension. After the repair, disruptive forces at the anastomosis are minimised by electively paralysing and ventilating the baby for 5 days with

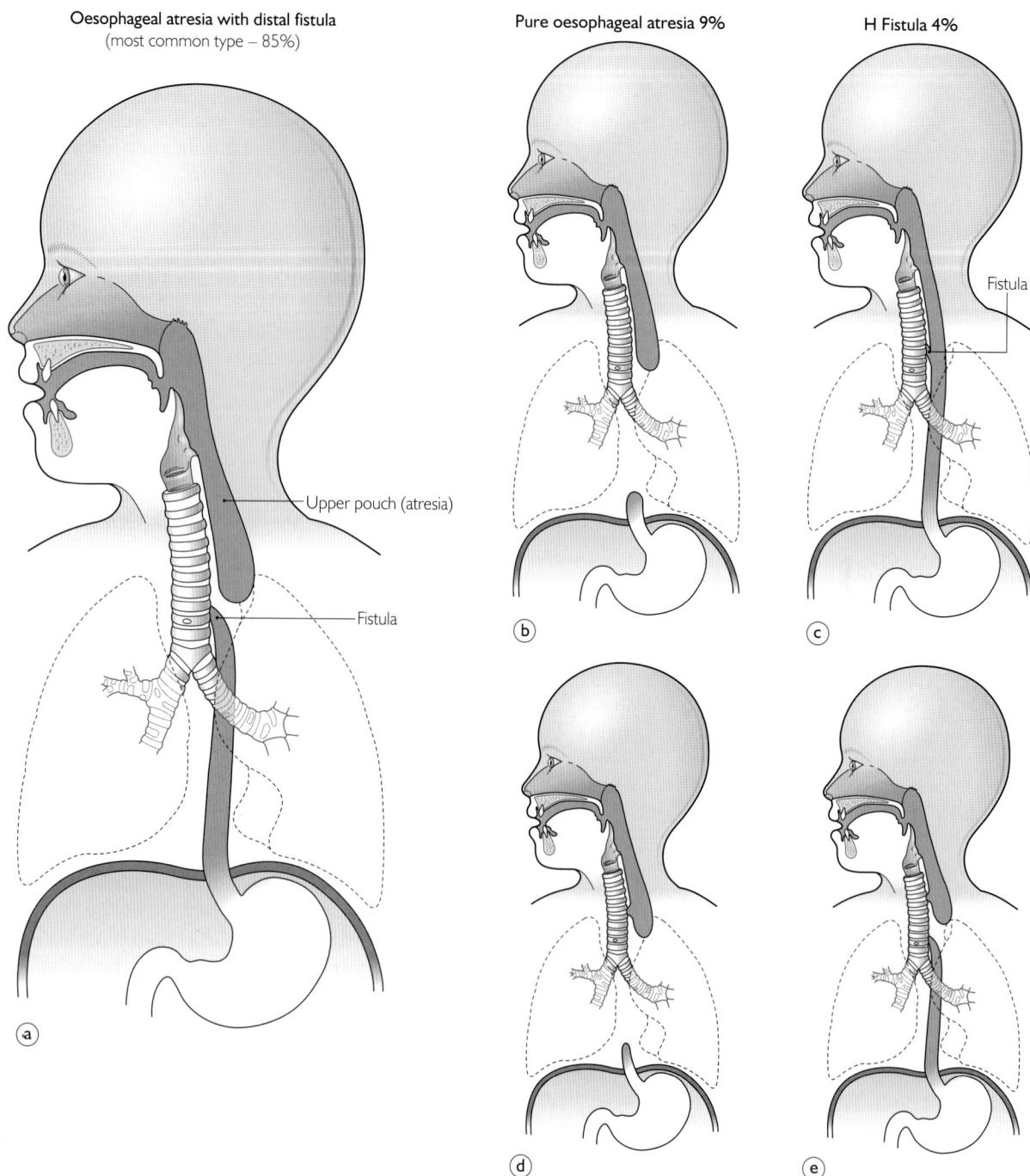

Oesophageal atresia with distal fistula
(most common type – 85%)

— Upper pouch (atresia)

— Fistula

(a)

Pure oesophageal atresia 9%

(b)

H Fistula 4%

Fistula

(c)

(d)

(e)

Fig. 29.36 Schematic representation of the spectrum of oesophageal atresia/tracheo-oesophageal fistula.

the neck flexed. Alternatively, the proximal oesophagus can be lengthened by dividing its outer muscle (myotomy) or by tubularising a proximal flap. In some cases, the oesophagus has to be abandoned – the TOF is divided and a cervical oesophagostomy and gastrostomy are fashioned (Fig. 29.40). The baby is sham fed and scheduled for oesophageal replacement (using the stomach or a segment of colon) when thriving.

Most infants can expect a good outcome after repair of OA/TOF but numerous complications may occur. An anastomotic leak is uncommon and typically manifests as a pneumothorax or sepsis;

conservative management with chest drainage, antibiotics and nutritional support is usually sufficient. In contrast, an anastomotic stricture is common but is easily treated by oesophageal dilatation. Gastro-oesophageal reflux is also common and requires antireflux medication. Intractable symptoms or reflux associated with a recalcitrant anastomotic stricture may merit fundoplication. A recurrent TOF is rare and presents with recurrent pneumonia, sometimes in the older child. In OA, the trachea is floppy and tends to collapse anteroposteriorly on expiration (tracheomalacia). Consequently, most children have a typical barking cough ('TOF cough'). In most, the tracheomalacia tends to improve during

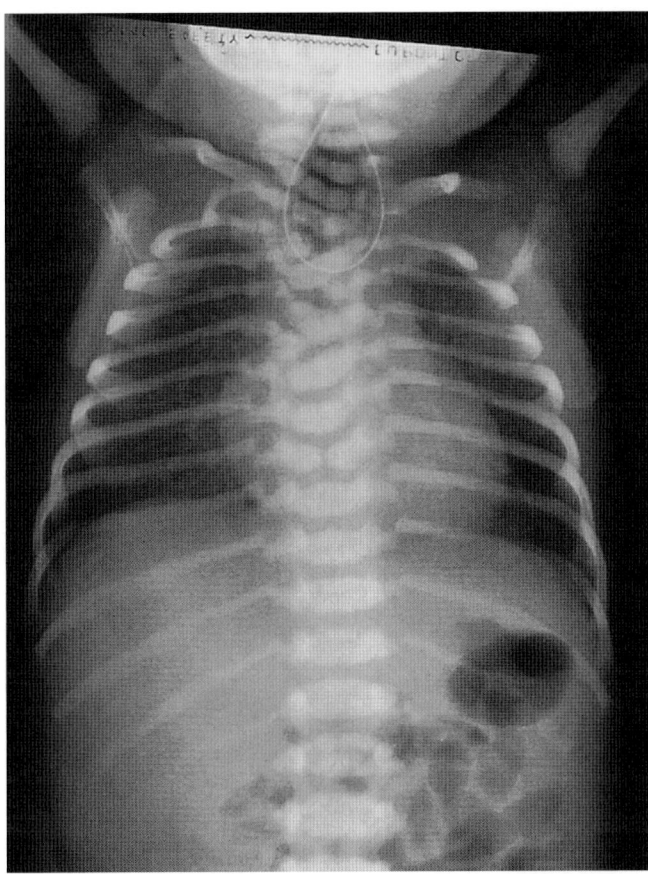

Fig. 29.37 Oesophageal atresia. Coiled feeding tube in proximal pouch. Note vertebral and rib abnormalities. Distal gas confirms a tracheo-oesophageal fistula.

infancy but, in some cases, life-threatening cyanotic episodes develop, requiring treatment by aortopexy and/or tracheopexy. All these complications can present with feeding difficulties and/or respiratory symptoms. Despite these problems, most children and adults enjoy a good quality of life after repair of OA/TOF.[10] In the UK, TOFS (Tracheo-Oesophageal Fistula Support Group) provides information for parents of affected children and a forum for sharing problems (www.tofs.org.uk).[41]

The two most important factors determining survival are very low birthweight and major congenital cardiac defects (those causing cardiac failure or requiring surgery). Without either factor, predicted survival is greater than 95%. With one factor present it is 60% and with both it is only 20%.[60]

Tracheo-oesophageal 'H' fistula

Congenital tracheo-oesophageal fistula without oesophageal atresia accounts for about 4% of all infants within the OA spectrum. It typically presents in the neonatal period with choking or cyanotic episodes associated with feeding. Some infants have marked gaseous abdominal distension from swallowed air. Right upper lobe pneumonia is common, especially when the fistula presents in older infants and children. In babies, a tube placed in the oesophagus with its external end under water may demonstrate

bubbles of air. The fistula can be visualised by a prone tube oesophagogram: with the infant lying prone and a tube positioned in the distal oesophagus contrast is gradually injected as the tube is withdrawn (Fig. 29.41). The fistula can be confirmed by bronchoscopy. Treatment is to divide the fistula, which is best approached through a low cervical incision rather than a thoracotomy.[17] Associated gastro-oesophageal reflux is common.

Laryngo-tracheo-oesophageal cleft

In this malformation, there is incomplete separation of the trachea and oesophagus. It can be associated with various other congenital anomalies, including oesophageal atresia and anorectal malformations. Clefts may be limited to the larynx and cricoid or involve the trachea. Recognising the disorder while intubating a baby with respiratory problems soon after birth is not easy. Difficulty in ventilating the infant may provide a clue. Any doubt about the anatomy of the posterior aspect of the larynx should prompt a detailed laryngoscopy, which will reveal whether it is cleft. Symptomatic or major clefts require surgical repair.[14] Treatment of the condition is often difficult and the longer-term problems of major clefts can be formidable.

Oesophageal perforation

Iatrogenic perforation of the upper oesophagus from the attempted passage of a nasogastric or endotracheal tube in a premature baby is rare.[35] It results in respiratory distress and feeding difficulties. A chest radiograph typically shows a right-sided pneumothorax or a pneumomediastinum (Fig. 29.42). A water-soluble contrast swallow helps to confirm the diagnosis, localise the perforation and direct treatment. Conservative management with chest tube drainage, antibiotics and parenteral nutrition is usually successful. Surgery is rarely required. Spontaneous rupture of the oesophagus in the neonate is extremely rare.

Hypertrophic pyloric stenosis

In hypertrophic pyloric stenosis (HPS) the pylorus is increased in length and diameter due to hypertrophy and hyperplasia of the circular muscle layer. This causes projectile vomiting, typically between 2 and 8 weeks of age. The incidence of HPS in the UK is approximately 3/1000 live births but regional and temporal variations are well recognised. Boys are affected four times more often than girls. Occasionally, HPS is seen in a premature neonate[67] and it has even been described in the fetus. However, HPS is fundamentally an acquired condition. One ultrasound study of asymptomatic newborns failed to show any pyloric abnormality in those babies who subsequently developed HPS.[55] Its exact cause remains uncertain. Various neural and histochemical changes have been described in the pylorus in HPS but whether these are cause or effect is not clear. Infants born with oesophageal atresia are at increased risk, as are premature babies fed through a transpyloric tube.[23] A genetic predisposition is apparent in some families.

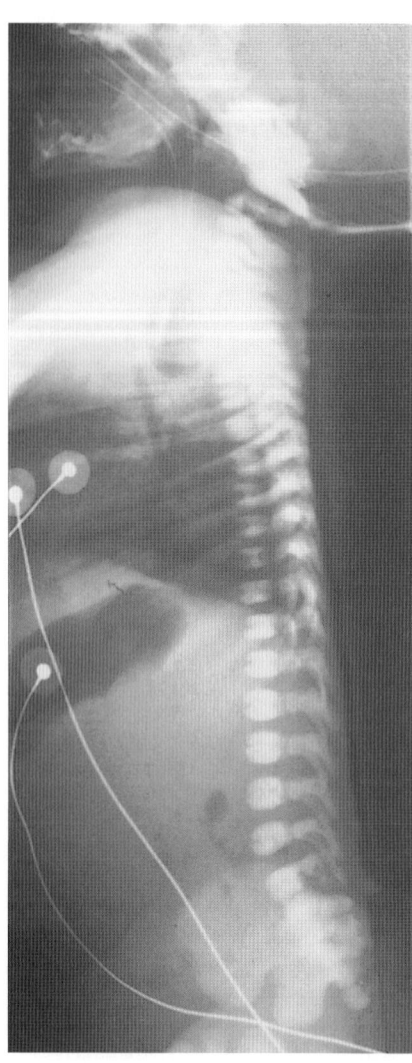

(a)

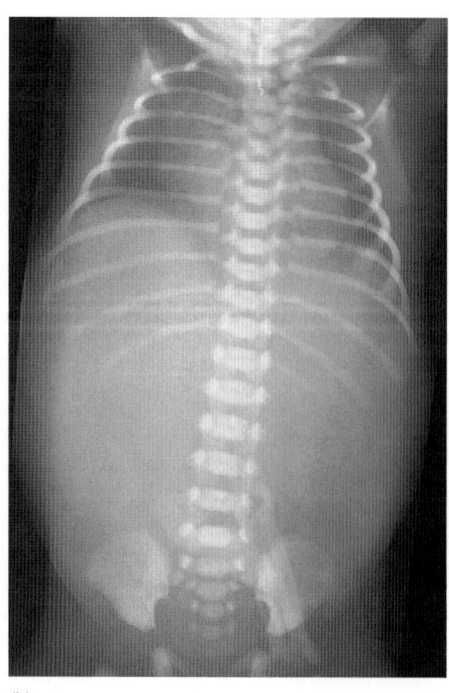

(b)

Fig. 29.38 (a) Lateral radiograph with radio-opaque tube in proximal pouch confirming the diagnosis of oesophageal atresia. Gas in the stomach confirms a tracheo-oesophageal fistula.
(b) Anteroposterior radiograph of oesophageal atresia with a tube in the upper pouch. A lack of gas in the abdomen usually indicates isolated oesophageal atresia with no distal tracheo-oesophageal fistula as in this case.

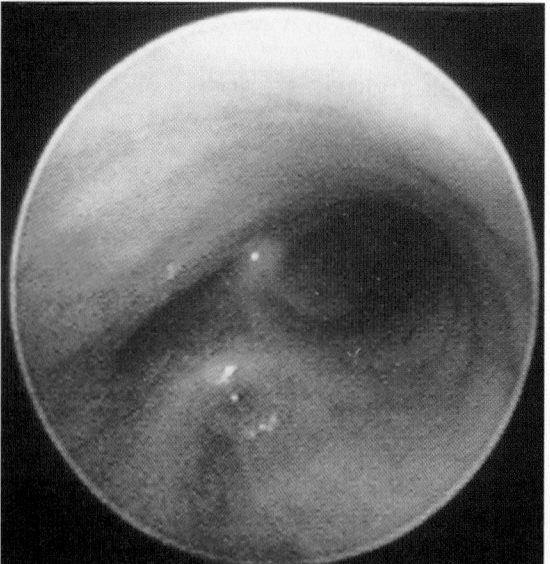

Fig. 29.39 Tracheoscopy in a baby with oesophageal atresia showing the site of a distal tracheo-oesophageal fistula just above the carina. The left main bronchus is partially collapsed from bronchomalacia.

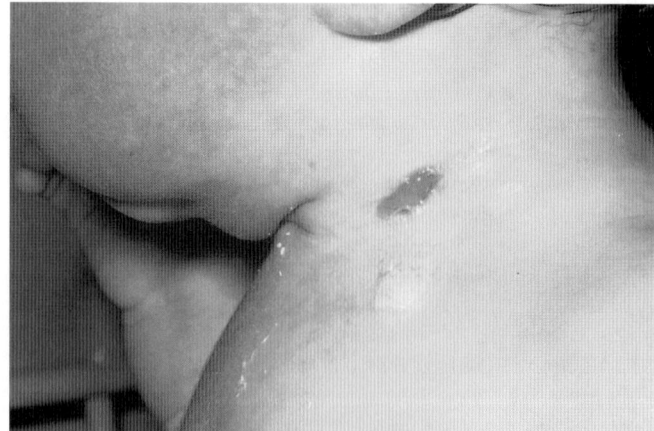

Fig. 29.40 Cervical oesophagostomy. This allows sham feeding.

Typically, the baby feeds hungrily and vomits toward the end of a feed. The vomit is non-bilious but may be bloodstained if there is an associated oesophagitis. Some affected infants are mildly jaundiced because of an unconjugated hyperbilirubinaemia. Electrolyte abnormalities are common, characteristically a

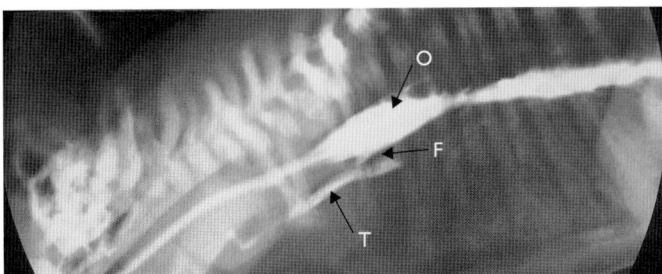

Fig. 29.41 An 'H' tracheo-oesophageal fistula outlined by contrast during a prone tube oesophagogram. A small amount of contrast has entered the trachea (T). O = oesophagus; F = fistula.

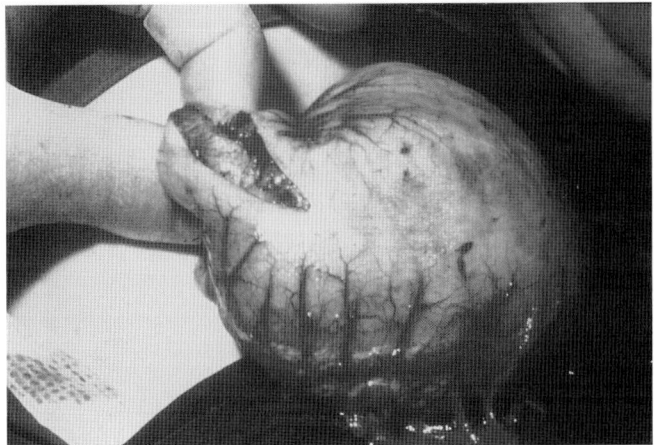

Fig. 29.43 Ultrasound appearance of hypertrophic pyloric stenosis. The arrows outline the hypertrophied pyloric muscle. 'S' is the stomach.

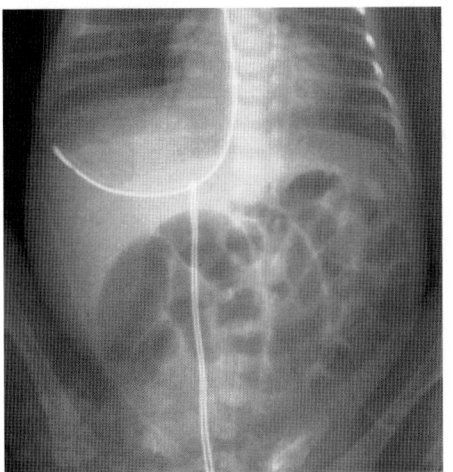

Fig. 29.42
(a) Abnormally positioned nasogastric tube in a premature baby following iatrogenic perforation of the upper oesophagus. (b) After the nasogastric tube was withdrawn and gently repassed into the stomach, a pneumomediastinum was evident. The baby recovered with conservative treatment.

(a)

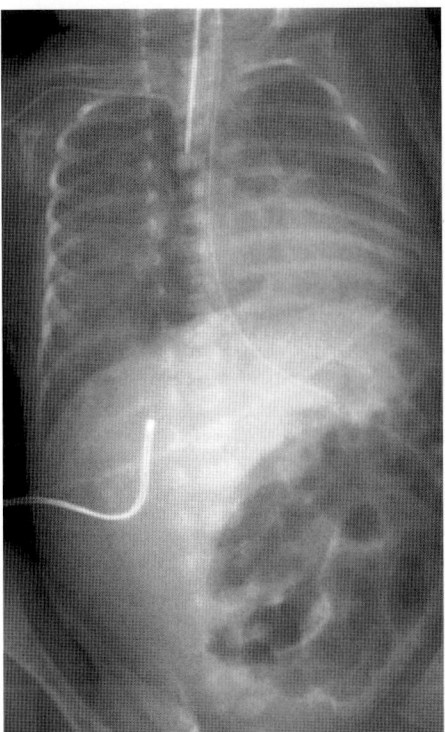

(b)

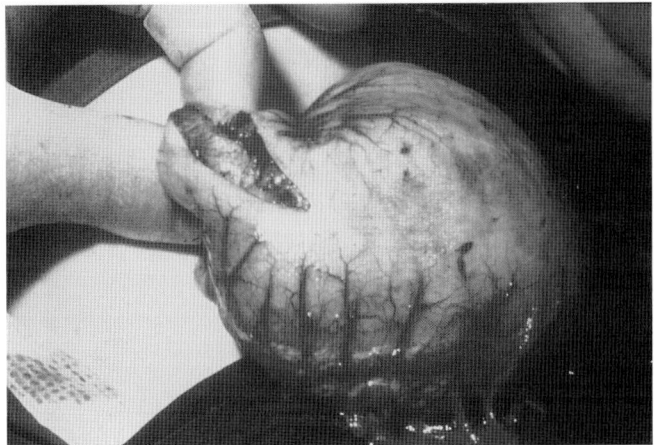

Fig. 29.44 Pyloromyotomy with mucosa projecting between the cut edges of the split hypertrophied muscle.

hypochloraemic alkalosis.[68] This disturbance may be severe and must be adequately corrected before surgery. Crystalloid solutions containing 0.45% saline and 5% dextrose with 20 mmol/l of potassium chloride are useful. Blood glucose should be monitored.

The diagnosis of HPS is made by feeling the hypertrophied pyloric muscle (similar to an olive) while the baby's abdominal muscles are relaxed, such as during a test feed. Gastric peristalsis is often visible. If doubt remains, an ultrasound scan by an experienced sonographer is helpful;[3] the pyloric muscle is usually 3–4 mm thick and the pyloric length and diameter are increased (Fig. 29.43). Contrast studies are rarely necessary.

The treatment of HPS is by Ramstedt's pyloromyotomy (Fig. 29.44). This can be performed through a transverse upper abdominal incision, a circum-umbilical incision (Fig. 29.45) or laparoscopically. Feeding can be reintroduced within 24 hours of surgery. Minor, transient postoperative vomiting is common. Persistent vomiting is unusual and most often due to associated gastro-oesophageal reflux. Complications of pyloromyotomy, which include duodenal perforation, haemorrhage, wound infection, wound dehiscence and incisional hernia, are rare.[73] There are almost no significant long-term sequelae after a successful pyloromyotomy.

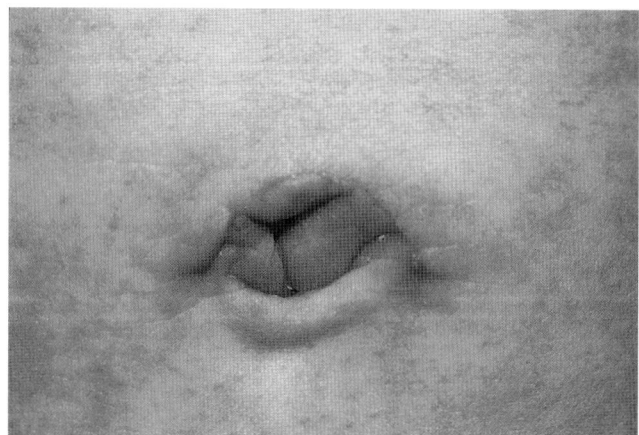

Fig. 29.45 Circum-umbilical wound a few weeks after surgery for hypertrophic pyloric stenosis.

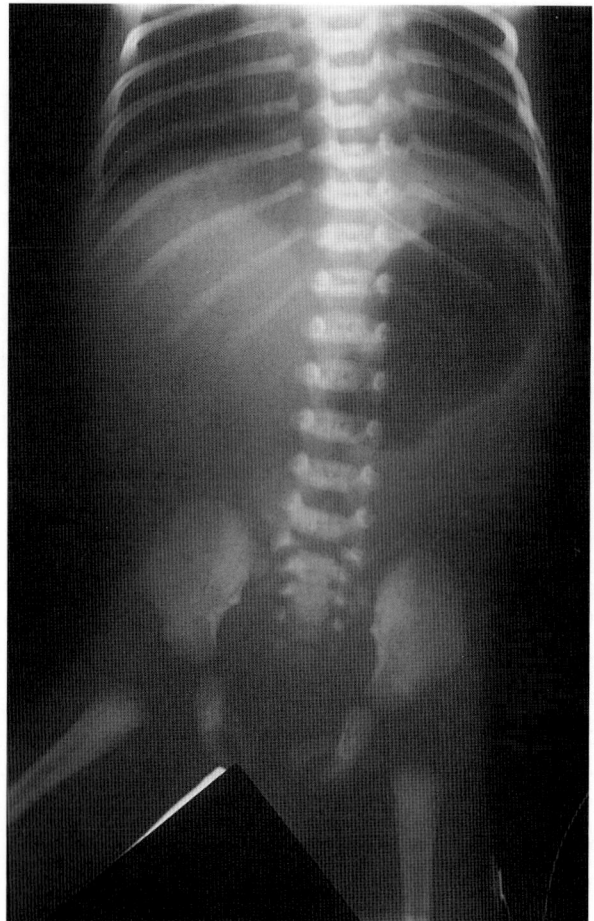

Fig. 29.46 Abdominal radiograph of a baby with pyloric atresia.

Pyloric atresia

Pyloric atresia is rare and causes congenital gastric outlet obstruction. The stomach is distended and an abdominal radiograph shows a gasless abdomen beyond the pylorus (Fig. 29.46). Treatment is surgical. The condition is familial in some cases.

Associations with epidermolysis bullosa and multiple intestinal atresias are well described.[45]

Gastric volvulus

Gastric volvulus is a rare, potentially life-threatening condition caused by abnormal rotation of the stomach about its axis resulting in a strangulating obstruction. Most instances of gastric volvulus in the newborn are associated with a diaphragmatic defect and/or deficient ligamentous attachments of the stomach.[63] Vomiting, haematemesis and respiratory distress are the dominant symptoms. A distended stomach in an abnormal position on a plain abdominal or chest radiograph should raise the possibility of gastric volvulus. Contrast studies clarify the anatomy. If possible, the stomach should be decompressed by the gentle passage of a nasogastric tube. At surgery, the volvulus is reduced, the stomach is fixed and any associated diaphragmatic defect is repaired.

Duodenum and small bowel

Duodenal obstruction in the neonate may be intrinsic or extrinsic or occasionally combined.

Duodenal atresia and stenosis

Intrinsic obstruction may be secondary to duodenal *atresia*, where there is either a gap between the duodenal segments (often with interposed pancreas) or an intact duodenal membrane with continuity of the duodenal wall, or duodenal *stenosis*, typically with a perforated duodenal web. Intrinsic duodenal obstruction affects approximately 1/6000 live births. Additional anomalies may include intestinal malrotation and, in one-third of patients, Down's syndrome. Whether the atresia is due to failure of recanalisation of the embryonic duodenum or to a later intrauterine event is not clear. The obstruction usually occurs in the region of the ampulla of Vater. Anomalies of the distal bile duct explain why, on rare occasions, an infant may have bile-stained vomiting and yet pass normal-coloured meconium.[1]

The frequent occurrence of polyhydramnios often results in duodenal atresia being detected by prenatal ultrasound.[27] The characteristic 'double bubble' may be seen only intermittently because of fetal vomiting. Prematurity is common.

Postnatally, duodenal atresia presents with bile-stained vomiting within hours of birth. In 20% of cases the obstruction is proximal to the common bile duct opening in the duodenum and the vomit is non-bilious. Duodenal stenosis causes partial obstruction and may not present during the neonatal period. Examination of the baby may show a distended stomach. A plain radiograph of the abdomen demonstrates the characteristic 'double bubble' sign of gas in the distended stomach and duodenum. This appearance is highlighted if the stomach is first aspirated via a nasogastric tube and 50 ml of air is instilled (Fig. 29.47). In most atresias there is no distal intestinal gas but occasionally a small amount of distal bowel gas may be seen if there is a Y-shaped termination of the common bile duct with limbs above and below

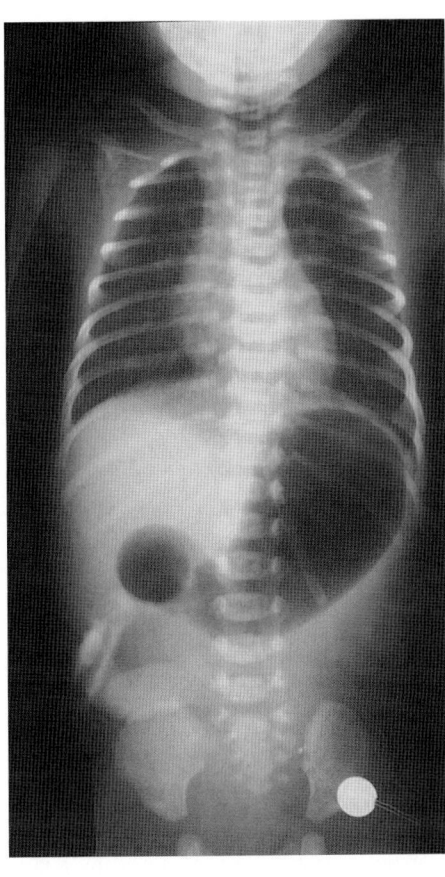

Fig. 29.47 Double bubble of duodenal atresia. Air has been injected through the nasogastric tube to highlight the anatomy.

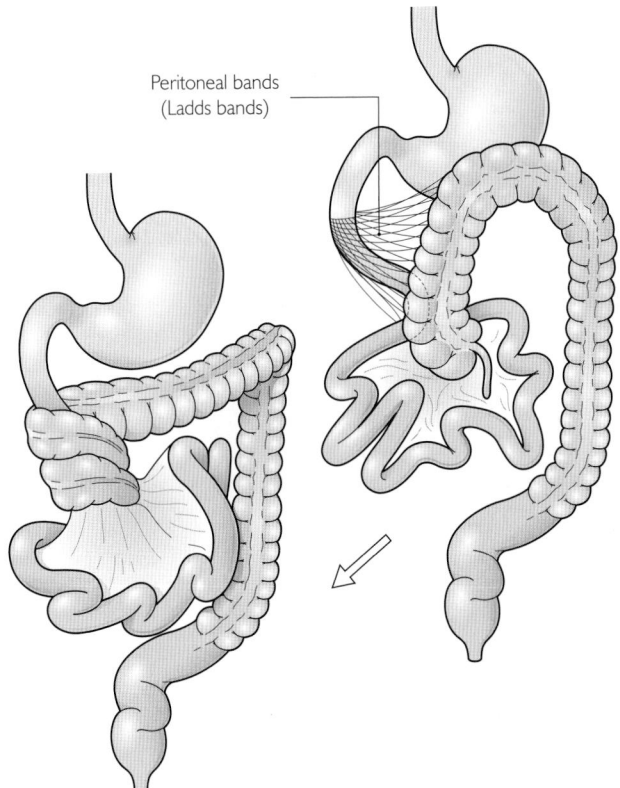

Peritoneal bands (Ladds bands)

Fig. 29.48 Intestinal malrotation. The classical type of intestinal malrotation predisposes to midgut volvulus.

the atresia. Significant amounts of distal gas with a distended stomach and duodenum should suggest the possibility of duodenal stenosis or intestinal malrotation and volvulus.

Management consists of nasogastric decompression, correction of any metabolic alkalosis or electrolyte imbalance, and early surgery. An echocardiogram should be performed in babies with Down's syndrome. At operation, the duodenum proximal to the site of atresia is anastomosed to the distal duodenum (duodeno-duodenostomy). Care must be taken not to damage the termination of the common bile duct. Because of the chronic nature of the obstruction, it may take a week or more before gastroduodenal function recovers sufficiently for the baby to tolerate full enteral feeding. Temporary parenteral nutrition is usually required. The outcome of intrinsic duodenal obstruction is related to associated anomalies, since the condition itself can be successfully corrected by surgery.

Intestinal malrotation

Unlike most cases of intrinsic duodenal obstruction, extrinsic obstruction due to intestinal malrotation with volvulus may be intermittent and incomplete and can present at any age. Boys are affected more often than girls. In classical intestinal malrotation, the midgut fails to complete its normal rotational development; the duodenojejunal flexure comes to lie on the right of the midline and the caecum is free-floating in the upper abdomen (Fig. 29.48). Consequently, the base of the small bowel mesentery, which extends between these two points, is a narrow pedicle. This predisposes to midgut volvulus around the superior mesenteric

vessels, which can lead to fatal midgut strangulation. Most patients with midgut volvulus present during the first month of life with bilious vomiting. Intestinal strangulation manifests as abdominal distension and rectal bleeding progressing to hypovolaemic shock.

Because the obstruction may be intermittent and incomplete the diagnosis may be delayed. While a plain abdominal radiograph may show an abnormal distribution of bowel gas, there is no single characteristic picture. The small bowel may be distributed more on the right and large bowel on the left of the abdomen. Alternatively, there may be a 'double bubble' of acute duodenal obstruction with a relatively gasless abdomen (Fig. 29.49). Any infant presenting with bile-stained vomiting should have an urgent upper gastrointestinal contrast study if malrotation cannot be excluded (Figs 29.50, 29.51). Colour Doppler imaging often demonstrates an abnormal relationship of the superior mesenteric artery and vein as a result of the malrotation.[48] A barium enema is less reliable in diagnosis but may confirm the abnormal position of the caecum.

Intestinal malrotation may be found in association with other congenital anomalies including congenital diaphragmatic hernia, abdominal wall defects, small bowel atresia, Hirschsprung's disease, situs inversus, polysplenia and biliary atresia.[26]

Surgery is mandatory for classical intestinal malrotation, even if the abnormality is diagnosed incidentally. This is because of the risk of midgut strangulation. Lesser degrees of intestinal malrotation rarely require surgery. The operation for classical intestinal malrotation is known as Ladd's procedure. It involves division of peritoneal bands extending from the caecum across the duodenum, broadening the base of the small bowel mesentery, placing the

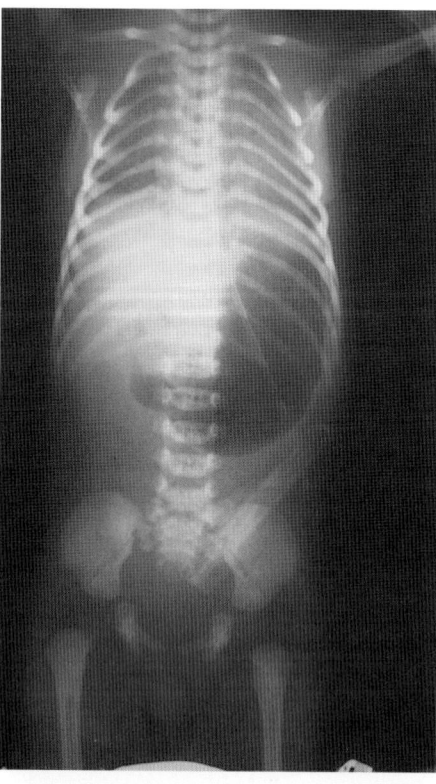

Fig. 29.49 Intestinal malrotation with neonatal midgut volvulus. The abdomen is virtually gasless beyond the distended stomach and duodenum.

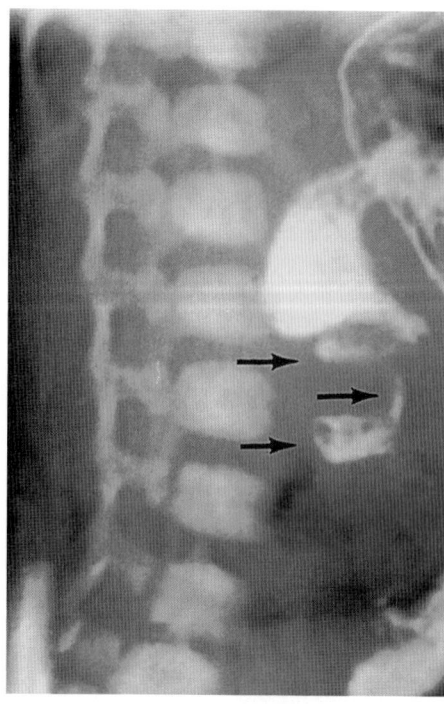

Fig. 29.51 Lateral radiograph showing barium passing down the duodenum and forming a cork-screw (arrows) configuration due to a midgut volvulus.

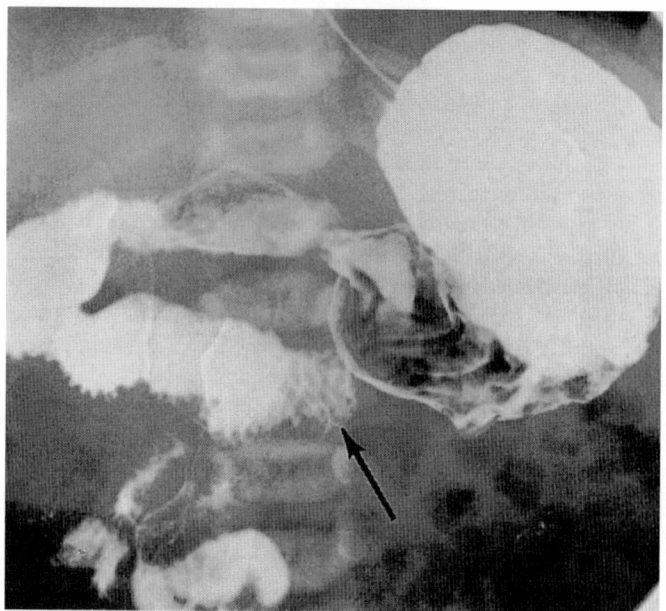

Fig. 29.50 Barium meal showing incomplete rotation of duodenum with the duodenojejunal flexure (arrow) in front of the vertebrae rather than to the left side of the abdomen.

small bowel on the right of the abdomen and the colon on the left, and appendicectomy. Subsequent peritoneal adhesions stabilise the gut in a position of non-rotation, thereby reducing the likelihood of volvulus. In cases where there is a volvulus at the time of surgery, this must be promptly untwisted and as much viable bowel as possible preserved. A repeat laparotomy performed 24 hours later may be helpful if bowel viability is initially uncertain.

Jejunal and ileal atresia

Atresia of the jejunum or ileum is most often caused by a late gestational interruption to the blood supply of the fetal gut. This was shown experimentally by Louw.[38] This intrauterine mesenteric vascular accident may arise from intestinal volvulus (associated with midgut malrotation, cystic fibrosis or a duplication cyst), intussusception, the action of vasoconstrictor drugs such as cocaine or constriction of the mesentery in a tight abdominal wall defect. A segment of small bowel is infarcted and reabsorbed, leaving a jejunal or ileal atresia. Multiple intestinal atresias are rare, may be familial and probably have a different pathogenesis.[49]

Jejunoileal atresias can be classified into four types[30] (Fig. 29.52). Type III is the commonest and is typically associated with a shorter bowel length. Type IIIb is known as an apple-peel deformity and consists of a proximal jejunal atresia, a wide mesenteric gap and a distal small bowel segment coiled around a marginal artery (Fig. 29.53). This classification is related more to the management and complications of intestinal atresia than to their presenting features.

Except for a lower mean birthweight, the baby with small bowel atresia often appears normal. There may be a history of maternal polyhydramnios or, rarely, dilated fetal bowel may have been detected by prenatal sonography.[52] Vomiting begins within a day or two of birth – the higher the atresia, the earlier the vomiting. Bilious vomiting is a typical feature of jejunal atresia and abdominal distension is often prominent with ileal atresia. The baby fails to pass normal meconium. Inspection of the baby's abdomen may show distended bowel loops. A plain abdominal radiograph demonstrates the characteristic picture of intestinal obstruction with dilated loops of bowel and multiple fluid levels (Figs 29.54, 29.55). The more distal the atresia, the greater the

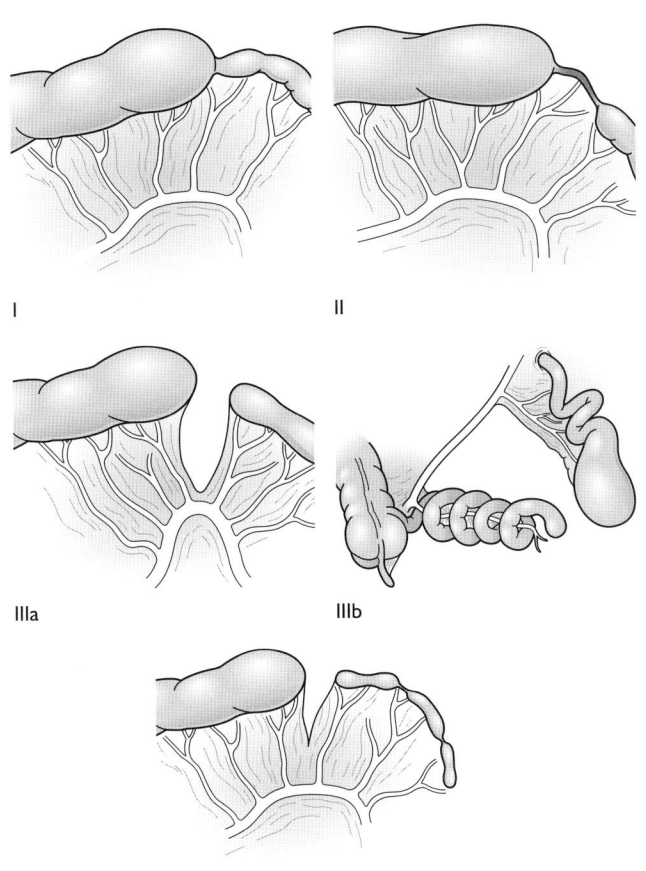

I   II

IIIa   IIIb

IV

Fig. 29.52 Classification of intestinal atresia: Type I – membranous atresia with intact bowel wall and mesentery; Type II – two atretic blind ends connected by a fibrous cord with an intact mesentery; Type III – two ends of atretic bowel separated by a V-shaped mesenteric defect; Type IIIb, 'apple-peel' deformity; Type IV – multiple atresias ('string of sausages'). (Reproduced with permission from Grosfeld J L, Ballantine T V N, Shoemaker R 1979 Operative management of intestinal atresia and stenosis based on pathologic findings. Journal of Pediatric Surgery 14:368–375.)

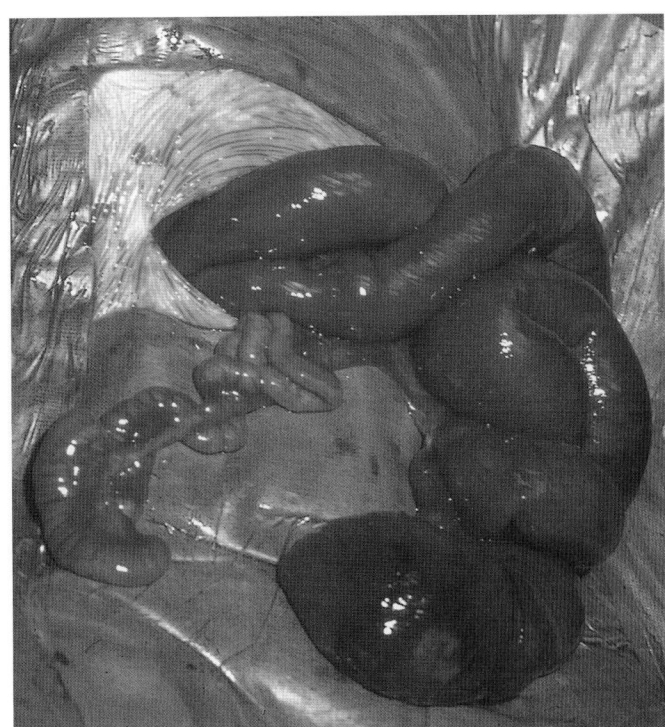

Fig. 29.53 Apple-peel atresia. The proximal bowel is dilated and congested.

number of distended bowel loops. Peritoneal calcification is a sign of intrauterine perforation. In a stable infant, a contrast enema may be required to clarify the cause of a distal bowel obstruction. Most infants with jejunoileal atresia have a microcolon.

After resuscitation, nasogastric decompression and any necessary urgent investigations, the baby should undergo surgery. At laparotomy the bowel distal to an obvious atresia must be examined carefully to exclude further atresias. Infants with type I and II atresias require resection of a short segment of dilated proximal bowel and an end-to-end anastomosis of the gut. Complications are infrequent and their long-term prognosis is good. Infants with type III defects require similar surgery but, because of the prenatal bowel loss, early postoperative digestive problems are common and parenteral nutrition is usually needed. Modified feeds may be necessary to optimise nutrition (see pp. 325–34). An anastomotic leak or stenosis is rare but episodes of functional intestinal obstruction are common during

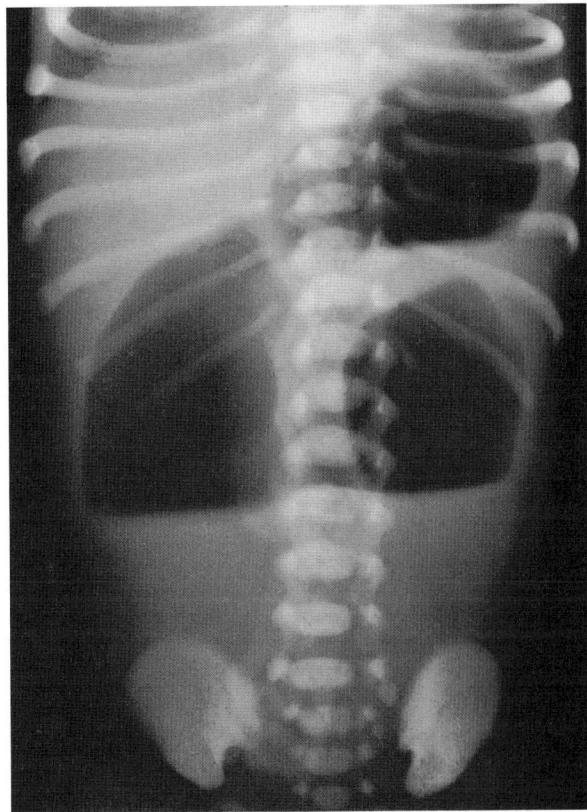

Fig. 29.54 Anteroposterior radiograph showing dilated bowel and fluid levels, indicating a proximal jejunal obstruction.

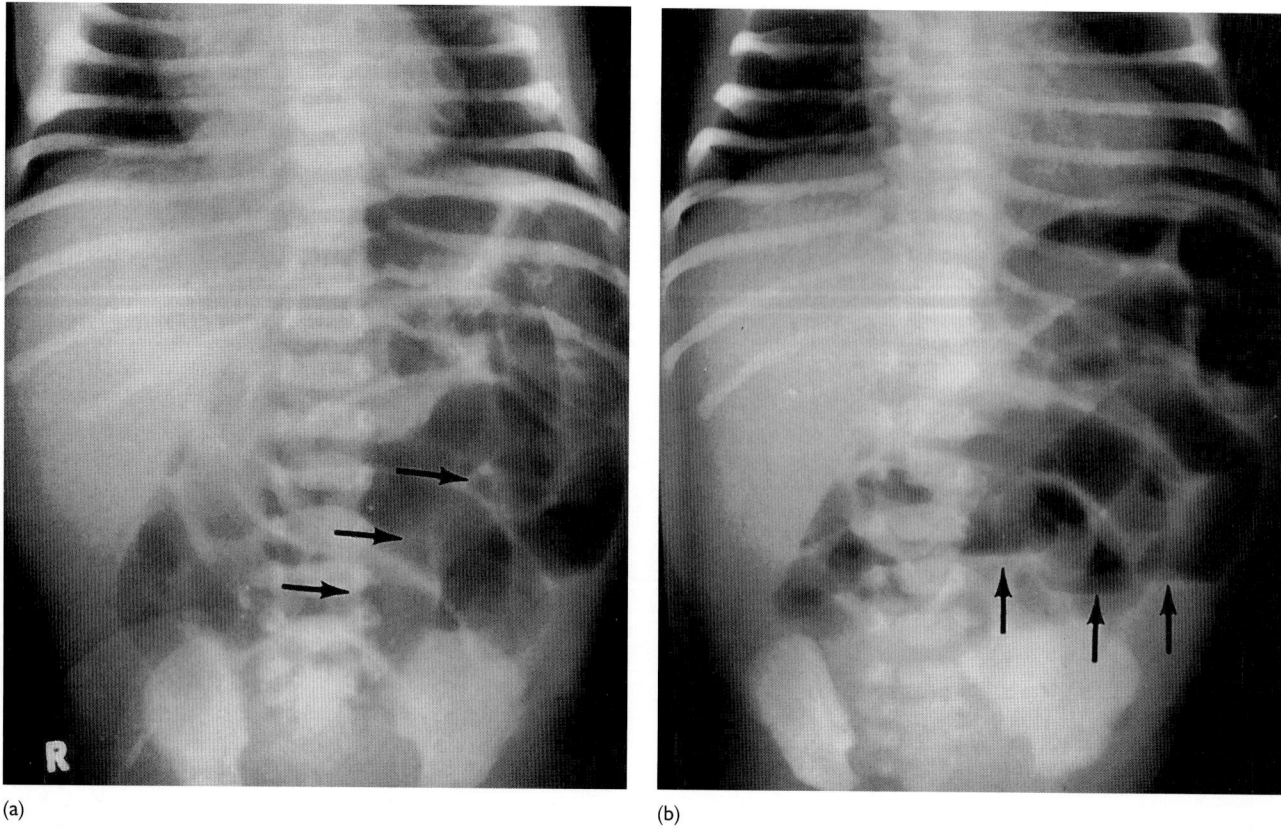

Fig. 29.55 (a) Supine radiograph showing ladder pattern of obstructed small bowel. (b) Erect film of same baby showing dilated bowel with fluid levels indicating ileal obstruction.

the early postoperative period. Despite this, adaptation occurs rapidly and long-term parenteral feeding is seldom required. In babies with multiple intestinal atresias, several anastomoses may be needed to preserve the maximum length of bowel. A sweat test and DNA mutational analysis are undertaken to exclude cystic fibrosis in infants with jujunoileal atresia.

Infants with a short gut require long-term follow-up to monitor their growth and development, address any nutritional deficiencies and detect and treat potential complications such as gallstones and late anastomotic ulceration.

Meconium ileus

In this condition, obstruction of the small bowel lumen is caused by highly viscid meconium containing excess protein. Cystic fibrosis (CF) is almost invariably the underlying cause, although exceptions do occur.[59] Approximately 10–15% of infants with CF present in this way.

Meconium ileus may be uncomplicated or complicated. In uncomplicated cases, there is small bowel obstruction, usually in the distal ileum. The proximal bowel is dilated and the distal small bowel is narrow and packed with grey-coloured meconium pellets. The unused colon is a narrow microcolon. Complicated meconium ileus is caused by a volvulus of meconium-laden bowel in the fetus. This may result in intestinal perforation, meconium peritonitis and meconium pseudocyst formation or an ileal atresia.

The neonate with meconium ileus usually has marked abdominal distension soon after birth, often accompanied by visible and palpable loops of bowel. There may be a palpable mobile abdominal mass.

The baby does not pass meconium, although small plugs or pellets of pale material may be passed. Vomiting becomes progressively worse and bile stained.

There may be a family history of CF and prenatal mutation analysis may already have been performed. Hyperechogenic fetal bowel (see above) or meconium peritonitis may have been identified by prenatal sonography. Postnatally, CF mutation analysis and sweat testing will confirm the aetiology. There is no clear-cut genotype correlation with meconium ileus but an association with delta F508 and G542X mutations has been reported.[25]

A plain abdominal radiograph shows marked bowel distension. Fluid levels are uncommon because of the viscid meconium. A 'soap bubble' appearance, caused by the admixture of air and viscid meconium may be noted (Fig. 29.56) but this is not pathognomonic for meconium ileus. In complicated cases intraperitoneal calcification or a cystic mass may be visible.

Neonates with complicated meconium ileus require surgery. In uncomplicated cases, an isotonic contrast enema is diagnostic, showing an unused microcolon (Fig. 29.57) and inspissated meconium in the terminal ileum. Prophylactic antibiotics are advisable prior to giving the enema. Occasionally, this same appearance is mimicked by total colonic aganglionosis. Passage of

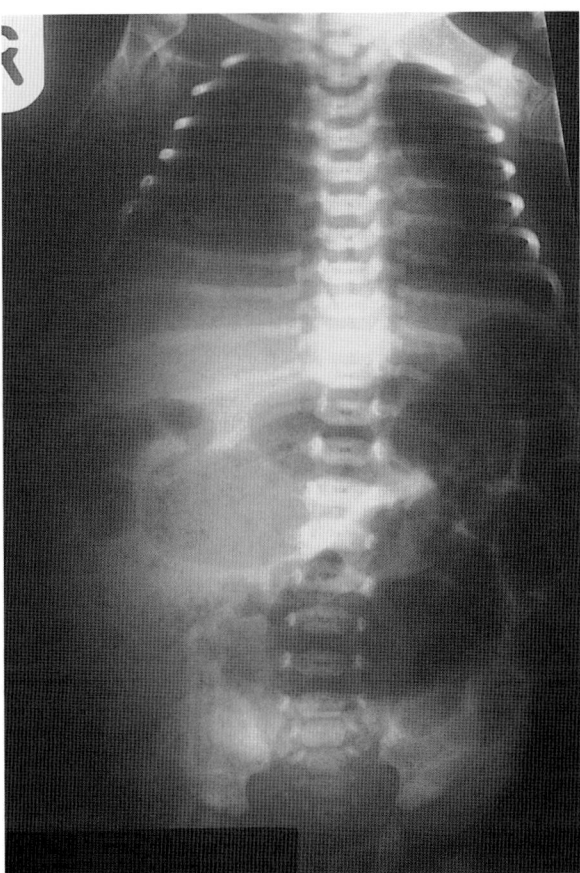

Fig. 29.56 Abdominal radiograph of a baby with meconium ileus. Note the lack of fluid levels and the soap bubble appearance in the right lower quadrant.

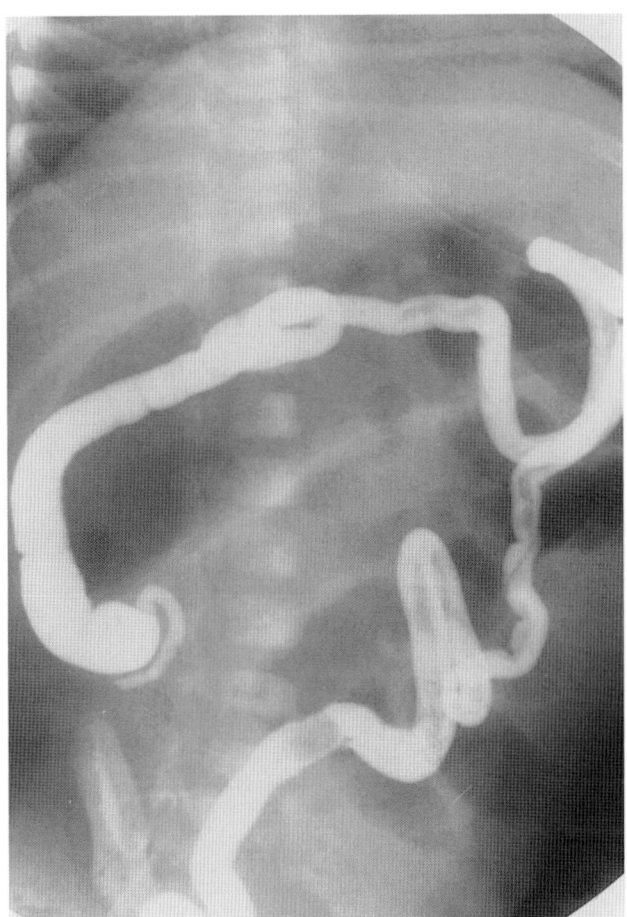

Fig. 29.57 Contrast enema showing a microcolon and dilated loops of proximal small bowel in meconium ileus.

contrast into dilated proximal bowel confirms its patency. Once this is determined, a therapeutic enema can be used (Fig. 29.58). Hyperosmolar solutions, such as dilute Gastrografin, draw fluid into the lumen of the gut, making the meconium less tenacious and encouraging its evacuation.[44] Additional intravenous fluids are required to compensate for this fluid loss. The enema may need to be repeated at daily intervals over the next few days before normal bowel movements are achieved.[5]

Non-operative management of uncomplicated meconium ileus is successful in about 50% of cases but it carries a risk of intestinal perforation. The presence of complicated meconium ileus precludes the use of a therapeutic enema and is an indication for surgery. Similarly, infants not responding to conservative management require operation. Various surgical procedures are used to treat meconium ileus, including intestinal resection and temporary stoma formation, resection and primary anastomosis and, in uncomplicated cases, enterotomy and irrigation of the bowel.

Survival rates for infants with meconium ileus have improved progressively. Recent reports document survival rates of 90% for complicated meconium ileus and a higher figure for uncomplicated cases.[43,51] Advances in the overall management of CF have contributed to this success. Infants with CF who present with meconium ileus have a relatively good long-term prognosis.[16]

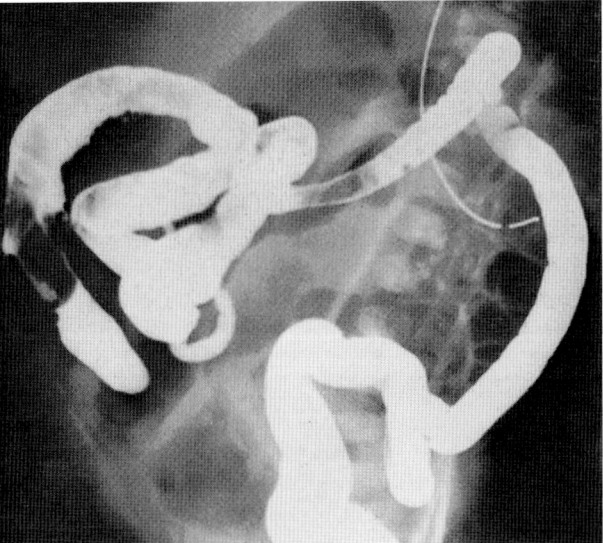

Fig. 29.58 Gastrografin enema filling the caecum and terminal ileum and outlining plugs of meconium in the distal ileum in a baby with meconium ileus.

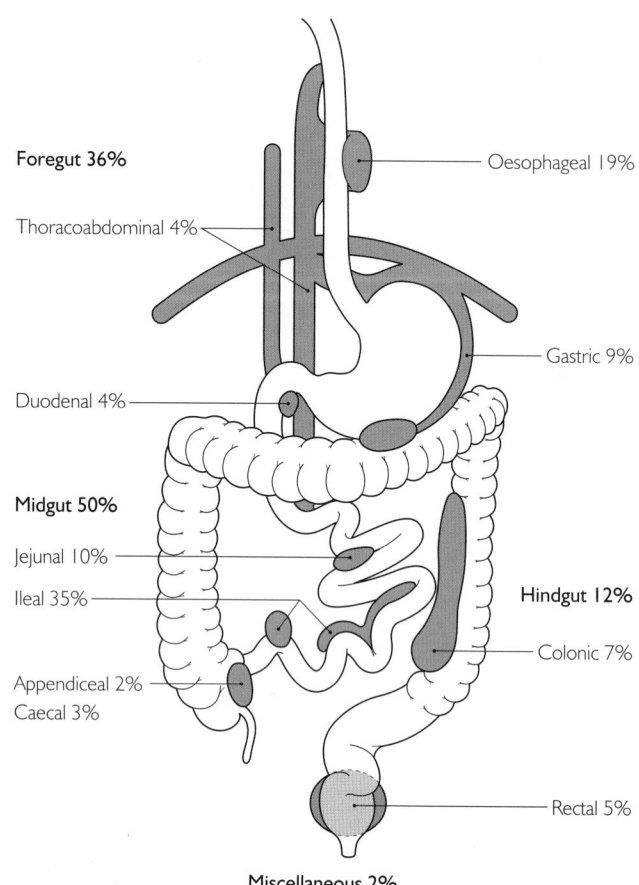

Fig. 29.59 Distribution of alimentary tract duplications. (Reproduced from Stringer et al 1995)

Alimentary tract duplications

Alimentary tract duplications are rare congenital malformations. Most are single, cystic lesions but some are tubular, running parallel to the gut. Typically, they are lined by alimentary tract mucosa and share a common smooth muscle wall and blood supply with the adjacent gut. Some communicate directly with the lumen of the native alimentary tract. About 50% of duplications occur in the midgut and 35% in the foregut (Fig. 29.59).[65]

One-third of duplication cysts present in the neonate with symptoms of obstruction, bleeding or inflammation. Some only become apparent during investigation of more severe congenital anomalies such as anorectal malformations, oesophageal atresia or bladder/cloacal exstrophy. Additional congenital abnormalities are common. Examples include exstrophy or myelomeningocele with hindgut duplication, intestinal malrotation with midgut lesions, and oesophageal atresia with foregut duplication. Some duplications, particularly foregut lesions, are associated with vertebral anomalies and even intraspinal pathology. Heterotopic gastric mucosa is found in one-third of duplications and may cause ulceration and bleeding.

Para-oesophageal cysts may present with respiratory symptoms or be noticed first on a chest radiograph (Fig. 29.60).

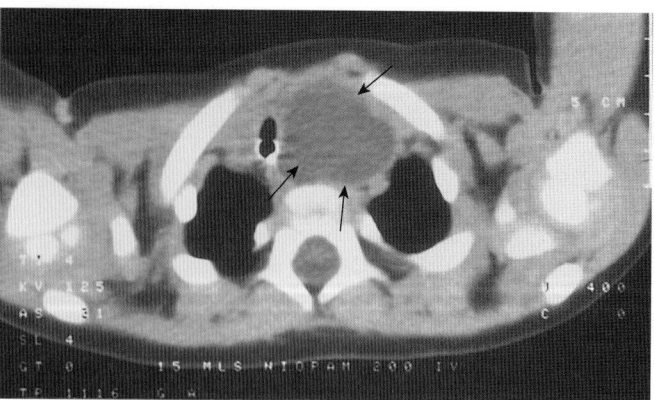

Fig. 29.60 Computed tomography scan of the thoracic inlet in an infant with a para-oesophageal duplication cyst causing tracheal deviation and respiratory symptoms.

Thoracoabdominal duplications have the greatest potential for complications; they usually lie to the right of the oesophagus in the posterior mediastinum and may communicate distally, through the diaphragm, with the upper gastrointestinal tract. Intestinal duplications most often present with bowel obstruction (from local compression, volvulus or intussusception). A small but increasing proportion of duplication cysts are discovered during prenatal ultrasound scans.

Duplications are best managed by early complete excision to avoid complications which include a small potential for malignant degeneration in adult life.

Other causes of neonatal small bowel obstruction

There are several other causes of intestinal obstruction in the newborn. Necrotising enterocolitis (see pp. 694–703) and an incarcerated inguinal hernia (see below) are relatively common causes. Rarer conditions include neonatal acute appendicitis, segmental small bowel volvulus (not due to midgut malrotation, CF or duplication cyst), an adhesion band connected to a vitellointestinal remnant, distal small bowel obstruction from inspissated formula milk curds[13] and pseudo-obstruction from intestinal neuropathy or myopathy. Neonatal intussusception may mimic necrotising enterocolitis.[69] An abdominal ultrasound scan and plain abdominal radiographs are often helpful in diagnosing these conditions.

Large bowel

Hirschsprung's disease

In a neonate with delayed passage of meconium, increasing abdominal distension and bilious vomiting, Hirschsprung's disease must be excluded.

Hirschsprung's disease is characterised by a congenital absence of intramural ganglion cells in the rectum. This aganglionosis and the presence of hypertrophied nerve trunks leads to a tonic contraction of the involved segment of gut, which causes a functional intestinal obstruction. The abnormalities of innervation extend into the proximal bowel to a variable degree. Harald Hirschsprung, a Danish paediatrician, provided the first comprehensive account of the disease in 1887, although he wrongly believed that the proximal dilated colon was the cause of the condition.[32]

The aganglionosis is restricted to the rectum and sigmoid colon in 75% of patients (*short-segment Hirschsprung's disease*), extends to the splenic flexure or transverse colon in 15% (*long-segment Hirschsprung's disease*) and along the entire colon and a variable length of terminal ileum in 8% (*total colonic aganglionosis*). Rarely, ganglion cells are absent as far proximally as the jejunum or duodenum.

Enteric ganglion cells are derived from vagal neural crest cells that migrate down the gut to the rectum in the embryo. Failure of this process is understood to be the cause of Hirschsprung's disease. The incidence of the condition is about 1/5000 live births, with a male to female ratio of 4:1; this sex difference is less marked in longer segment disease.

Numerous conditions are associated with Hirschsprung's disease. The most consistent association is with Down's syndrome but various other chromosomal abnormalities and syndromes are recognised.[62] Cardiac, genitourinary, central nervous system and gastrointestinal abnormalities are each recorded in about 5% of patients. Links with congenital central hypoventilation,[18] Waardenburg's syndrome,[42] multiple endocrine neoplasia and intestinal neuronal dysplasia are well described.

Advances in molecular genetics have confirmed that Hirschsprung's disease is a genetic disorder.[36] Most cases are sporadic but autosomal dominant, autosomal recessive and polygenic patterns of inheritance within families have been reported. Mutations in the *RET* proto-oncogene region of chromosome 10 are known to account for many cases. Other gene defects causing familial Hirschsprung's disease have been mapped to the endothelin-B receptor gene on chromosome 13. The association of Hirschsprung's disease with Down's syndrome, chromosomal anomalies and genetically determined syndromes emphasises the genetic nature of the condition.

Hirschsprung's disease typically presents during the neonatal period. Delayed passage of meconium is the cardinal clinical feature and is typically accompanied by progressive abdominal distension, reluctance to feed and vomiting, which is often bilious. Over 95% of healthy term infants pass their first stool within 24 hours of birth.[58] Delayed passage of meconium beyond 48 hours in a term infant should suggest the possibility of Hirschsprung's disease. Delayed passage of meconium is normal in premature infants[71] and this is therefore a less reliable feature of Hirschsprung's disease in this group.

Rectal examination typically reveals a tightly contracted anorectum and withdrawal of the finger may be followed by an explosive discharge of stool and gas. In some cases, this induces a temporary remission but the baby continues to have problems with constipation. If the obstruction is not relieved the infant is at risk of intestinal perforation, enterocolitis and death.

Hirschsprung's enterocolitis is a serious and potentially fatal complication. It is characterised by marked abdominal distension, explosive diarrhoea, vomiting and fever. The clinical and radiological picture may be indistinguishable from necrotising

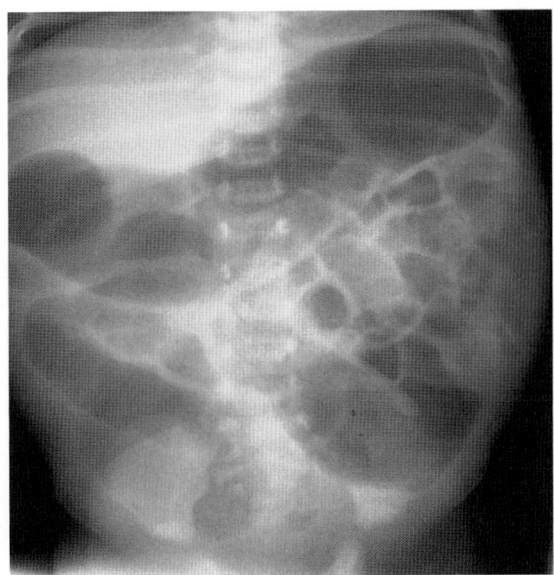

Fig. 29.61 Intestinal obstruction with an absence of gas in the rectum in a baby with Hirschsprung's disease.

enterocolitis. Obstruction, infection (e.g. *Clostridium difficile*) and impaired mucosal immunity are important predisposing factors. Bowel decompression by repeated rectal lavage with warm normal saline together with oral vancomycin or metronidazole is the usual first-line treatment. Intravenous broad spectrum antibiotics should be given in severe cases.

Histological examination of an adequate rectal biopsy by an experienced pathologist is the gold standard in the diagnosis of Hirschsprung's disease. The main diagnostic tools are:

- **Radiology**: plain abdominal radiographs characteristically show multiple dilated loops of bowel with an absent rectal gas shadow (Fig. 29.61) but the latter is not specific for Hirschsprung's disease. In infants with enterocolitis, thickening of the bowel wall, mucosal irregularity and/or a grossly dilated colon may be evident. A contrast enema performed by an experienced radiologist using an isotonic water-soluble contrast medium is often used to diagnose Hirschsprung's disease but the results are not always reliable. Typically, contrast outlines a narrow distal segment of rectum and colon, a cone-shaped transition zone and a proximal dilated colon (Fig. 29.62). However, the cone is not necessarily the site of the transition zone between abnormal and healthy bowel.

- **Anorectal manometry**: the resting pressure within the anal canal and lower rectum is raised and there is no anal relaxation in response to a distending stimulus in the rectum (absent rectoanal inhibitory reflex). Misleading results may occur and this technique is now used infrequently.

- **Rectal biopsy**: a suction rectal biopsy is taken from above the anal canal (usually 2–4 cm from the anal verge) and must contain adequate amounts of submucosa, be appropriately orientated and sectioned, and be examined by an experienced histopathologist. Diagnosis rests on the absence of ganglion cells, the presence of thickened nerve trunks and a marked increase in acetylcholinesterase activity in the hypertrophied nerve bundles.

Initial treatment of Hirschsprung's disease consists of decompressing the dilated proximal (ganglionic) bowel by rectal washouts using small volumes of warm saline (Fig. 29.63). Initially, this may be required twice daily but, with time, once a day is sufficient. If this fails to decompress the bowel then a stoma is necessary. The aim of definitive surgery for Hirschsprung's disease is to resect the aganglionic bowel and to join healthy ganglionic proximal bowel to the anorectal stump.

Various techniques are described (e.g. Duhamel's, Soave's and Swenson's operations) which implies that none is perfect. In the majority of infants, surgical correction is now performed as a single-stage procedure (primary pull-through) rather than the traditional approach of proximal stoma formation, definitive surgery and subsequent stoma closure. Recent developments include laparoscopically-assisted procedures and transanal operations, which obviate the need for an abdominal incision in short-segment disease. Primary pull-through procedures are best avoided if the colon cannot be adequately decompressed by rectal washouts (and this includes most cases with total colonic aganglionosis), if enterocolitis cannot be rapidly controlled by medical treatment or if intestinal perforation has occurred.

Most patients can expect good long-term bowel function after definitive surgery for Hirschsprung's disease. However, a significant proportion continue to have problems despite a technically adequate pull-through with fully ganglionic bowel. Potential long-term problems include enterocolitis, constipation and faecal incontinence. Long-term bowel function is influenced by early surgical complications, bowel training and the social background and intelligence of the child. In most series, about 75% of patients will achieve good bowel control as they reach adulthood.[22] Down's syndrome has a major adverse impact on the acquisition of faecal continence in Hirschsprung's disease.

The risk of disease in future offspring depends on the sex of the affected individual and the extent of the aganglionosis.[2]

Anorectal malformations

Anorectal malformations encompass a wide spectrum of congenital defects ranging from a minor malposition of the anus to complete agenesis of the anorectum. Classification of these anomalies

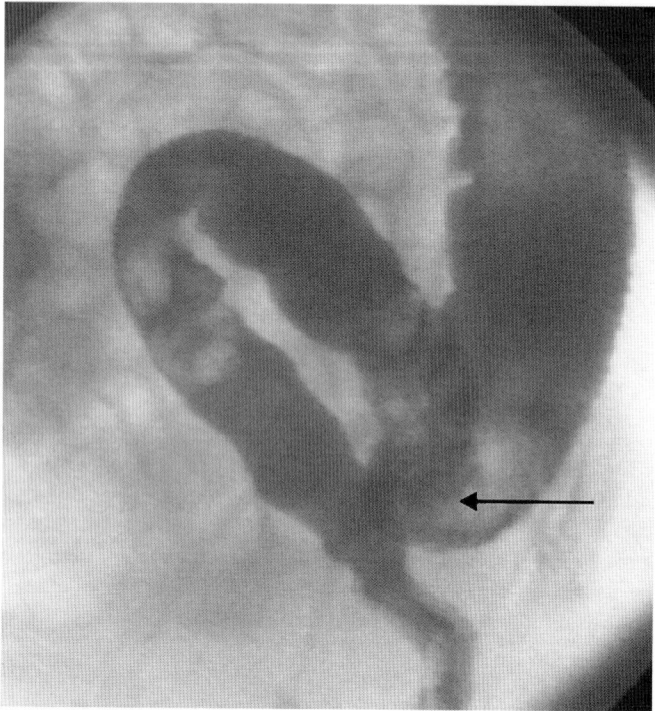

Fig. 29.62 Barium enema showing a 'transition zone' at the junction of the descending and sigmoid colon (arrow). The actual transition zone was found to be proximal to this site.

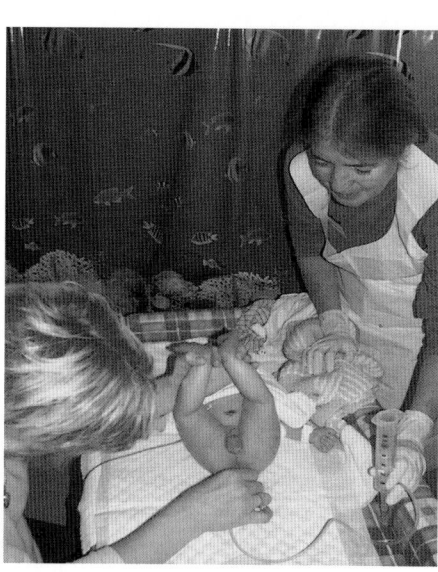

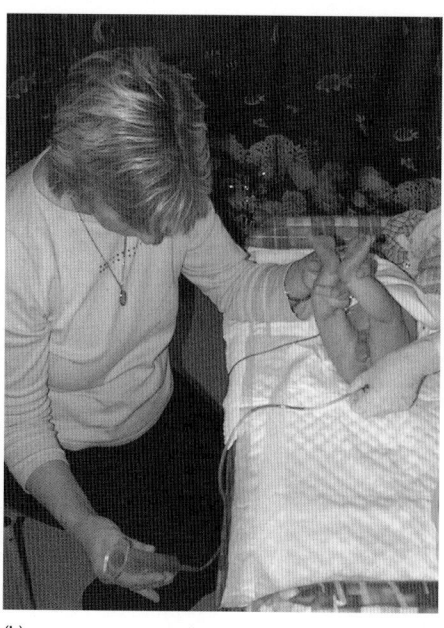

Fig. 29.63 Rectal washouts in Hirschsprung's disease. The mother is being supervised by a specialist nurse.

(a)   (b)

is difficult but Pena has suggested a practical approach based on gender and differences in treatment and prognosis.[46] The common types of malformation are listed in Table 29.33 and shown in Fig. 29.64.

Table 29.33 Types of anorectal malformation

Low defects	Higher lesions
Male	
Perineal fistula	Rectourethral fistula (bulbar or prostatic)
Anal membrane	Rectovesical fistula
Anal stenosis	Imperforate anus without fistula
	Rectal atresia and stenosis
	H-type fistula
Female	
Perineal fistula	Rectovestibular fistula
Anal membrane	Rectovaginal fistula (rare)
Anterior anus	Cloacal malformations
Anal stenosis	Imperforate anus without fistula
	Rectal atresia and stenosis
	H-type fistula

In low defects the rectum terminates close to the perineal skin while in high lesions it ends relatively higher in the pelvis.

In boys, an imperforate anus with the rectum terminating as a rectourethral fistula is the most frequent malformation. Next commonest is a low termination of the rectum and a perineal fistula. In girls, an anterior anus or perineal fistula or an imperforate anus with a rectovestibular fistula are the commonest lesions. Cloacal malformations account for about 10% of female defects.

The incidence of anorectal malformations is around 1/4–5000 live births. The cause of these defects is unknown. Most are sporadic. Traditionally, anorectal malformations have been understood to arise as a result of abnormal partitioning of the embryonic cloaca by the caudal descent of the urorectal septum but this view is almost certainly too simplistic.[34]

At least 40% of affected patients have additional congenital defects. This figure is higher in patients with high anorectal malformations.[53] Associated conditions include the following:

- **Genitourinary**: these are the commonest. Examples include absent, dysplastic, cross-fused or horseshoe kidneys, vesicoureteric reflux, hydronephrosis, hypospadias, bifid scrotum and cryptorchidism. Girls with cloacal anomalies may have vaginal and uterine malformations.
- **Skeletal**: lumbosacral vertebral anomalies are most common. Sacral defects are more frequent and more severe with high malformations. The absence of two or more sacral vertebrae is associated with a poor functional outcome.[46]

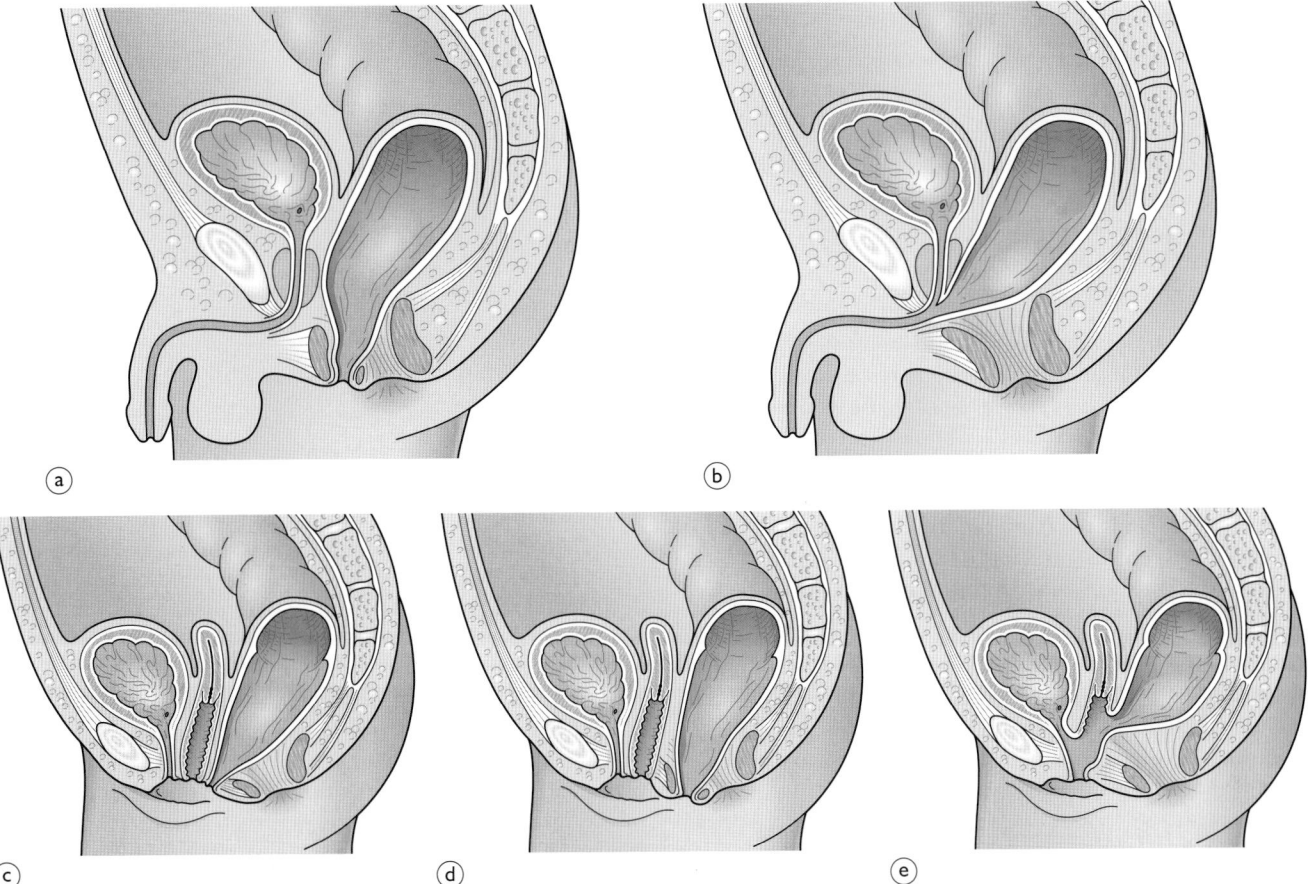

Fig. 29.64 Commoner varieties of anorectal malformations. (a) Perineal fistula in a boy, (b) Recto-urethral fistula in a boy, (c) Recto-vestibular fistula, (d) Anterior stenotic anus in a girl, and (e) Cloacal anomaly.

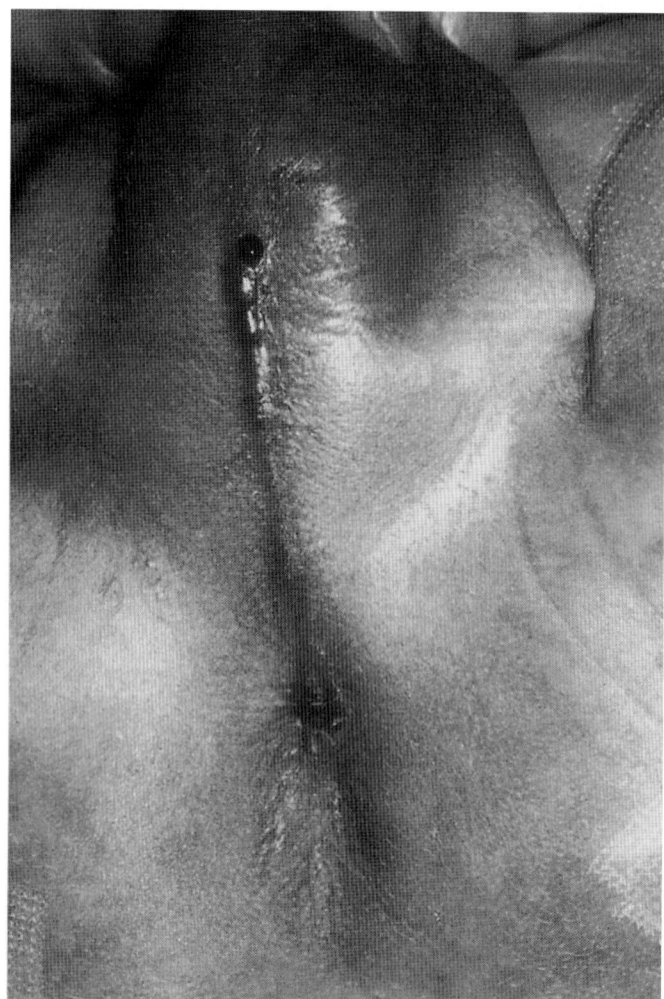

Fig. 29.65 Low anorectal anomaly. A subcutaneous track of meconium is visible within the midline raphe extending to the scrotum.

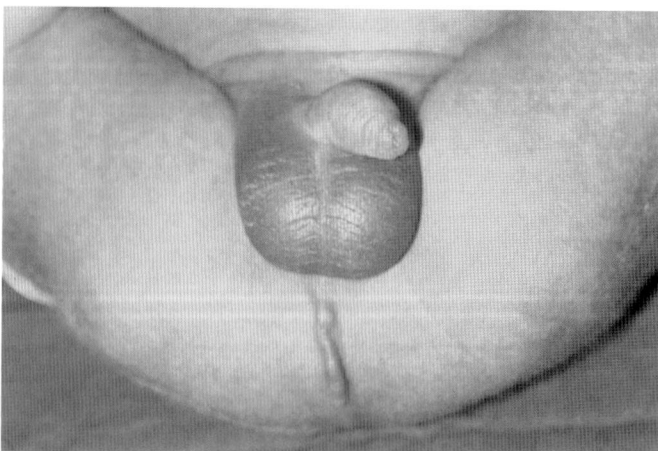

Fig. 29.66 Imperforate anus in a boy with a recto-urethral fistula.

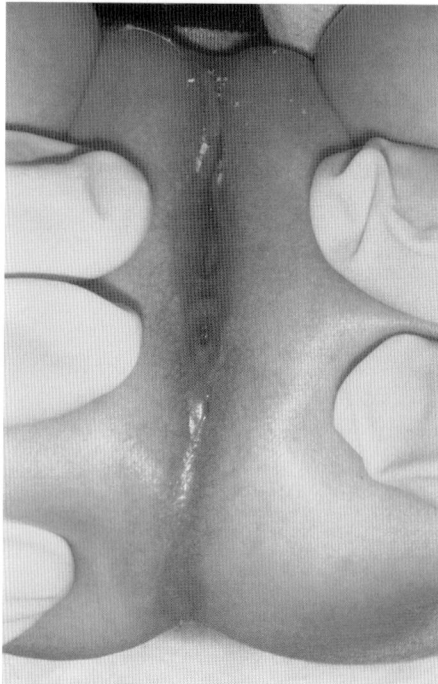

Fig. 29.67 An anterior stenotic anus in a girl.

- **Spinal cord**: a range of spinal cord anomalies have been described since the advent of magnetic resonance imaging.
- **Gastrointestinal**: the best known association is with oesophageal atresia as part of the VACTERL complex (see above).
- **Cardiovascular**: various abnormalities may coexist.
- **Syndromes**: the commonest is the VACTERL association. Another example is the Currarino triad due to an autosomal dominant gene on chromosome 7, manifesting as partial sacral agenesis, anal stenosis and a presacral mass (e.g. meningocele or sacrococcygeal teratoma).[19]

Early diagnosis is important to avoid complications such as intestinal perforation and urinary tract infection. All infants should be examined thoroughly, including the spine and genitalia. In most cases, a detailed inspection of the perineum can distinguish low and high malformations.

In boys with low lesions, the anus is imperforate or appears abnormal. There is a single abnormal opening on the perineum or a track may be seen running along the midline raphe to the scrotum (Fig. 29.65). Boys with low lesions have a well developed buttock cleft and anal dimple, good sphincter muscles and a normal sacrum. With higher lesions in boys, no perineal orifice is seen (Fig. 29.66) but meconium or bubbles may appear in the urine. In such cases, the pelvic and perineal muscles are less well developed and a sacral defect may be evident.

In normal girls, the anus is positioned midway between the posterior fourchette and the tip of the coccyx. A stenotic anterior anus (Fig. 29.67) is easily overlooked in the newborn and may not present until later, with severe constipation. In girls, it is important to count the number of perineal orifices. If only the vagina and urethra are visible, then the infant probably has a rectovestibular malformation in which the rectum opens immediately in front of the posterior fourchette (Fig. 29.68). Meconium is often passed through the fistula after birth. If there is only one perineal opening, then the baby has a cloacal malformation characterised by the confluence of rectum, vagina and urethra into a

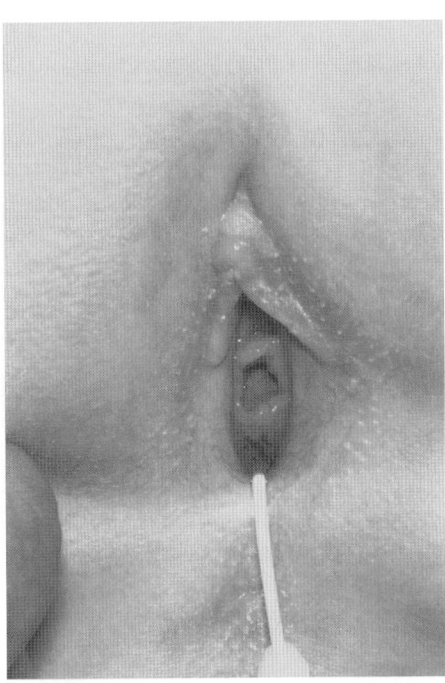

Fig. 29.68 A recto-vestibular fistula demonstrated with a cannula in the fistula.

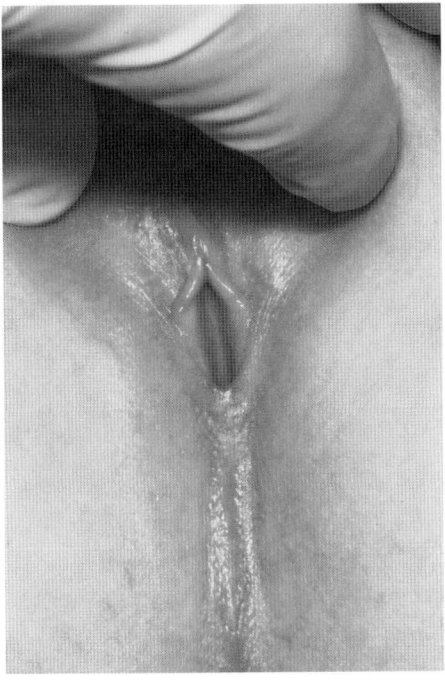

Fig. 29.69 A cloacal anomaly with a single perineal orifice only.

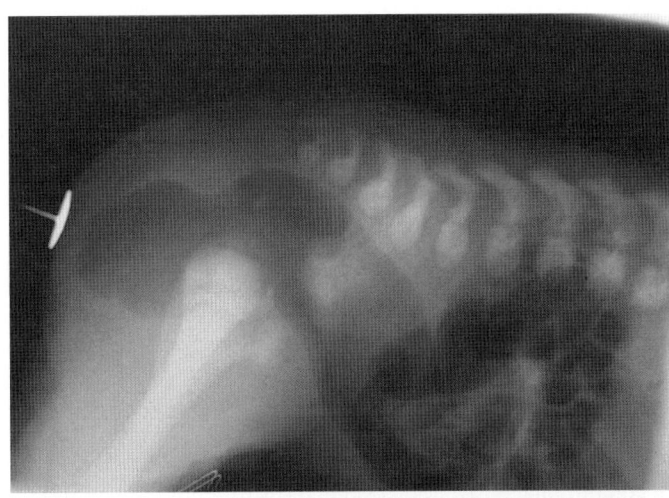

(a)

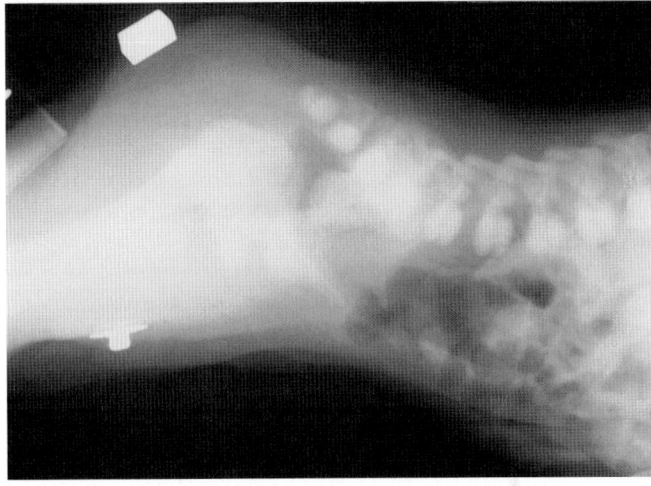

(b)

Fig. 29.70 Lateral prone radiograph with pelvic elevation at 24–36 hours of age in babies with (a) low and (b) high anorectal malformations. Note the distance between the rectal gas shadow and the anal marker in each case.

single common channel (Fig. 29.69). Neonatal hydrocolpos and urinary obstruction may complicate this anomaly.

If the clinical picture is unclear, a lateral prone radiograph at about 24 hours of age with the baby's pelvis elevated helps to distinguish high and low lesions. The anal dimple must be marked with a radiopaque marker (Fig. 29.70). The distance between the rectal termination and the anal skin can be measured. If this radiograph is performed too early, it may falsely suggest a high lesion because the gas has not yet reached the point of obstruction. The presence of air in the bladder is evidence of a rectourinary fistula.

Other useful investigations in a neonate with an anorectal malformation include lumbosacral and chest radiographs, a urinary tract ultrasound scan, echocardiography and, in selected cases, a karyotype.

Most low lesions can be successfully treated by an anoplasty soon after birth. Temporary use of an anal dilator is often needed. Constipation is a common problem but, provided this is managed aggressively, good bowel control can be achieved.[54] Higher malformations are usually treated by a diverting, proximal colostomy soon after birth and definitive repair of the malformation a few months later once the anatomy of the malformation has been defined and the infant is thriving. The posterior sagittal anorecto-plasty (PSARP) is the current standard reconstructive operative procedure.[46] Outcome in terms of constipation, soiling and faecal continence are affected by the type of anorectal malformation (many high lesions are associated with some faecal incontinence), the presence of a sacral defect and the method and timing of surgery. Many children require considerable help in achieving social continence and coping with psychosocial sequelae.[39]

Colonic atresia

This is a rare form of atresia, accounting for only 5% of intestinal atresias. It may be associated with limb anomalies, abdominal wall defects, Hirschsprung's disease or other atresias. Presentation is that of a low intestinal obstruction. The baby develops abdominal distension and progressive vomiting, and fails to pass meconium. An abdominal radiograph shows evidence of a distal bowel obstruction and a contrast enema demonstrates the level of the atresia. Staged surgery is often required, with initial relief of the obstruction by colostomy, followed later by large bowel anastomosis.

Meconium plug obstruction

Meconium plug obstruction occurs most often in the low-birth-weight baby who may also be compromised by other problems such as perinatal hypoxia, hypothermia and the effects of medication given to the mother in labour. It can be difficult to achieve a balance between subjecting the baby to potentially unnecessary investigations and overlooking genuine pathology. The main differential diagnosis is between meconium plug obstruction, Hirschsprung's disease and cystic fibrosis, all of which can occur in low-birthweight infants. Contrast enema studies in this situation may be misinterpreted as showing evidence of Hirschsprung's disease.

In preterm infants, expectant observation is usually the best approach. If abdominal distension is severe, gentle irrigation of the baby's rectum with warm saline usually relieves the obstruction and yields a pale plug of meconium (Fig. 29.71). Alternatively, warmed dilute Gastrografin may be instilled into the large bowel via a soft rectal catheter and a radiograph will demonstrate the meconium plug. This procedure often provokes passage of the plug and, once the infant has started passing motions, continuing difficulty is less marked. The infant with a meconium plug must be observed closely and followed up after discharge.

In full-term infants, delay in passage of meconium beyond 48 hours always merits investigation.

Megacystis–microcolon–intestinal hypoperistalsis syndrome

This rare entity, which is commoner in girls, is a form of visceral myopathy causing severe functional intestinal obstruction.[50] Intestinal and bladder motility are markedly impaired. Infants also have lax abdominal muscles and incomplete intestinal rotation. Most cases are reliant on long term parenteral nutrition for survival.

Small left colon syndrome

This term is used for a transient functional neonatal large bowel obstruction caused by a small-calibre left colon distal to the splenic flexure. It is associated with maternal insulin-dependent diabetes. The degree of obstruction is variable. A contrast enema is diagnostic and often therapeutic (Fig. 29.72). Hirschsprung's disease must be excluded.

Stomas

An intestinal stoma may be temporarily required in the management of various neonatal surgical conditions including necrotising enterocolitis, Hirschsprung's disease, anorectal malformations,

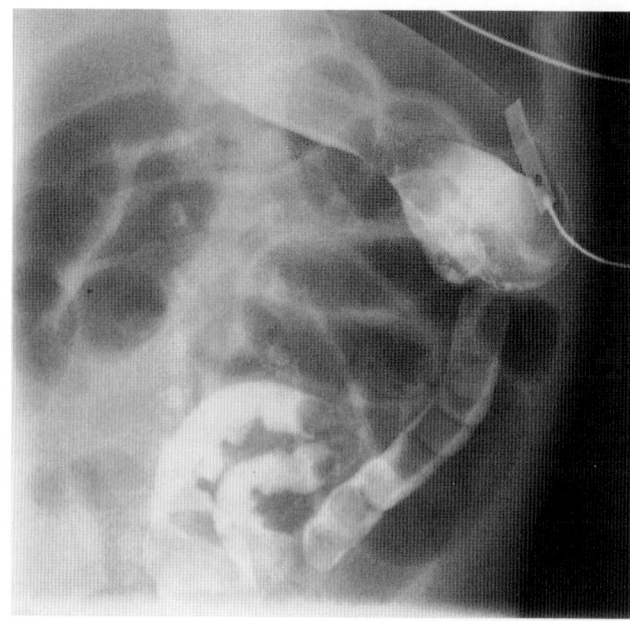

Fig. 29.72 Contrast enema in a baby with small left colon syndrome.

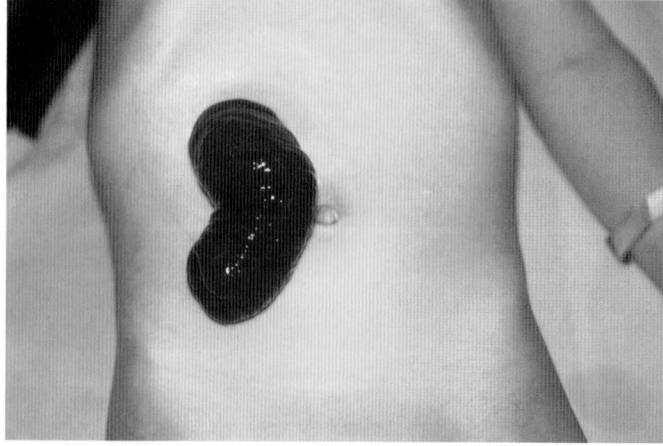

Fig. 29.73 Prolapse of a transverse loop colostomy.

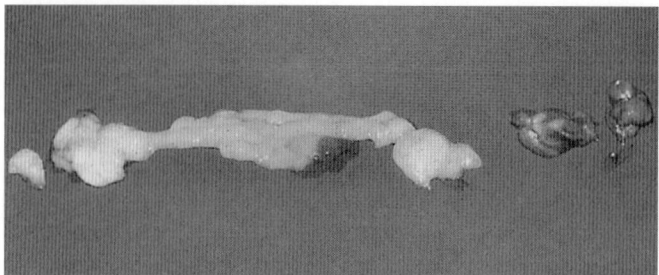

Fig. 29.71 Meconium plug.

intestinal atresia and complicated meconium ileus. Most are colostomies or ileostomies. Potential stoma complications include:

- mechanical, e.g. prolapse, stenosis, retraction – prolapse is more common with a loop stoma (Fig. 29.73);
- leakage and skin excoriation;
- fluid and electrolyte losses – especially with small bowel stomas;
- nutritional problems;
- wound infection, candidiasis.

Expert surgical nursing care and appropriate stoma appliances are paramount.

Sodium deficiency occurs frequently with neonatal ileostomies or proximal colostomies. Plasma sodium levels are usually normal but urinary sodium concentrations are consistently less than 10 mmol/l, indicating a total body sodium deficit.[4] A mild metabolic acidosis and growth failure ensue despite a good calorie intake. Before normal growth can be achieved, these babies must have their feeds supplemented with sodium chloride to restore normal urinary sodium excretion.

Anterior abdominal wall defects

Although gastroschisis was recognised as early as 1733,[7] only in the last 50 years has it been clearly differentiated from exomphalos. A distinction between these two anterior abdominal wall defects is clinically important but not all infants fall neatly into one or other category. The prevalence of gastroschisis is about 1/7000 total births[20] but there are significant regional variations within the UK and abroad.[21,61] Exomphalos is at least twice as common.[8,61] Gastroschisis has become more prevalent in the past 25 years while the frequency of exomphalos has remained much the same. Both sexes are similarly affected.

In simple terms, the anterior abdominal wall is formed by four separate embryological folds – cephalic, caudal, and lateral – each of which has a splanchnic and somatic component. Failure of union of the cephalic fold results in exomphalos with a sternal/diaphragmatic defect or the pentalogy of Cantrell.[9] Failure of the caudal fold to close results in exomphalos with bladder or cloacal exstrophy. Failure of the lateral folds to close results in exomphalos. The pathogenesis of gastroschisis is less clear. Suggested mechanisms include a local failure of differentiation of mesoderm forming the abdominal wall muscles, rupture of the membrane covering a hernia of the umbilical cord or a vascular insult interfering with the development of the somatopleure at the junction with the body stalk.[20]

Prenatal ultrasound is highly sensitive in the diagnosis of anterior abdominal wall defects. Most defects are detectable by 16–20 weeks' gestation and it is usually possible to differentiate between exomphalos and gastroschisis. This is important since exomphalos is frequently associated with chromosomal anomalies (e.g. trisomy 13, 18 and 21) and major congenital heart defects,[28] indicating the need for fetal karyotyping and echocardiography. Although exomphalos is seen more often than gastroschisis in utero, this relationship is reversed at birth because of fetal deaths and terminations in the exomphalos group. For the same reasons, the observed incidence of additional congenital anomalies in neonates with exomphalos is less than expected. Gastroschisis is rarely associated with aneuploidy.

Exomphalos

This term encompasses a spectrum of abnormalities ranging from a small umbilical defect with gut prolapsing into the cord (a *hernia into the cord*; Fig. 29.74), through umbilical defects less than 5 cm wide (*exomphalos minor*) to larger umbilical defects (*exomphalos major* or giant omphalocele; Fig. 29.75). Bowel and often liver are enclosed within the sac (unless it has

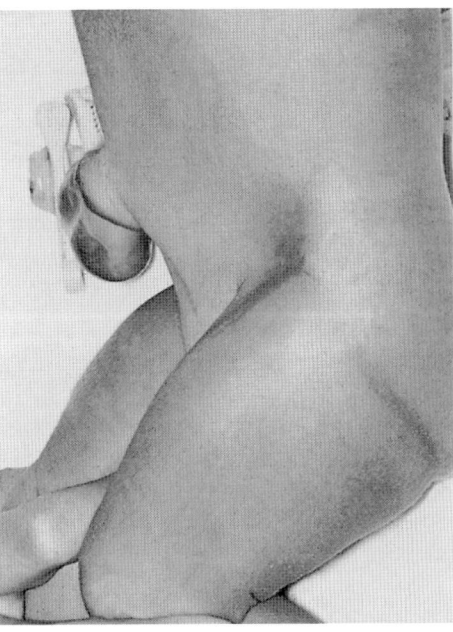

Fig. 29.74 A hernia into the cord. The infant had no other anomalies.

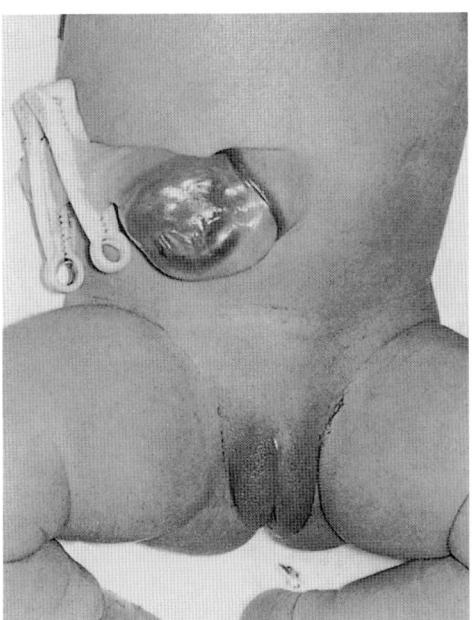

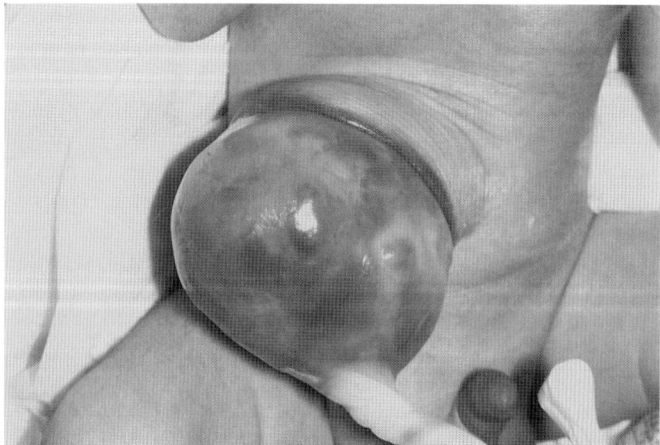

Fig. 29.75 Exomphalos major containing liver and bowel.

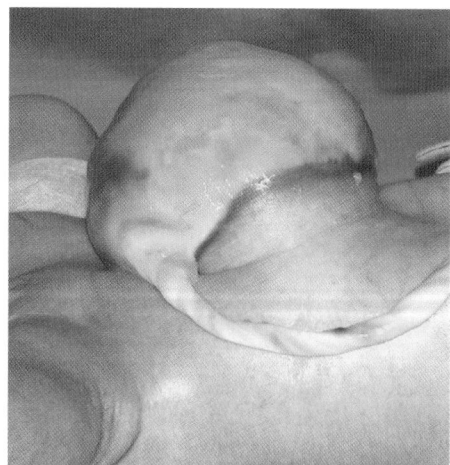

Fig. 29.77 Exomphalos major treated with flamazine. Note the epithelialisation of the sac at its edge.

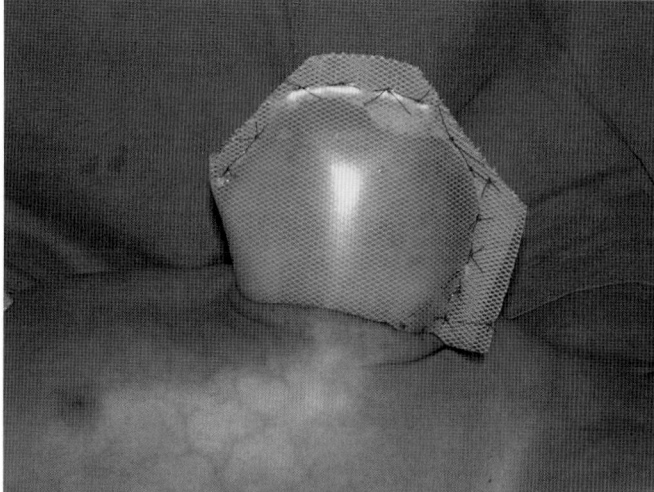

Fig. 29.76 Exomphalos treated with the application of a silo.

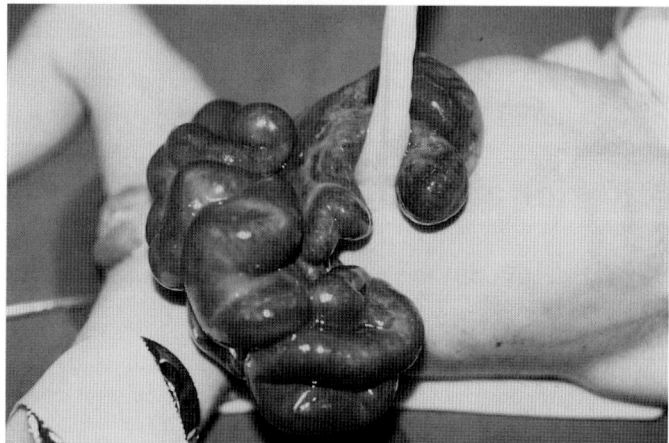

Fig. 29.78 Gastroschisis. The bowel is matted and has a fibrin peel. Note that the abdominal wall defect is just to the right of the umbilicus.

ruptured). Since the developing bowel has failed to complete its normal return to the abdominal cavity from the umbilical cord, disorders of intestinal rotation may be found with all these umbilical defects, but classical midgut malrotation is uncommon.

Urgent surgery is not indicated for the infant with an exomphalos and an intact amniotic sac. Echocardiography, karyotyping and, in selected cases, upper gastrointestinal contrast studies to assess gut rotation should be performed. Blood glucose must be monitored, particularly since Beckwith–Wiedemann syndrome (see p. 857) may present with exomphalos. Other associations include intestinal atresia or stenosis.

With a hernia into the cord or exomphalos minor, once the defect has been repaired the long-term outlook is good provided there is no associated syndrome or additional major congenital abnormality.

In exomphalos major, reduction of the herniated bowel and liver into the abdominal cavity can be difficult. It may require the surgical application of sterile prosthetic material to the rim of the abdominal wall defect and gradual reduction of the contents of this silo over a period of 7–10 days (staged silo repair; Fig. 29.76). The fascia and skin are repaired as the final procedure.

Temporary support with parenteral nutrition is often required. With this technique, potentially serious complications may occur. Consequently, a conservative approach is sometimes used. This involves treating the sac with desiccating antiseptic agents. Mercurochrome is potentially toxic[24] and has been replaced by silver sulfadiazine (silver sulphadiazine) ointment (Fig. 29.77) or povidone iodine spray. Thyroid function may be disturbed by prolonged use of the latter.[15] The sac gradually contracts, leaving a correctable abdominal wall defect.

Outcome is largely dictated by the severity of associated malformations. In some infants, both the abdominal and thoracic cavities are poorly developed and pulmonary hypoplasia may pose additional problems. A ruptured exomphalos requires urgent surgery.

Gastroschisis

In gastroschisis, the bowel prolapses through a defect that is typically just to the right of the umbilicus (Fig. 29.78). Unlike exomphalos, there is no covering membrane. The extent of evisceration is variable but may include stomach, small bowel, colon, and ovary and fallopian tube or testis. Only rarely is the liver involved.

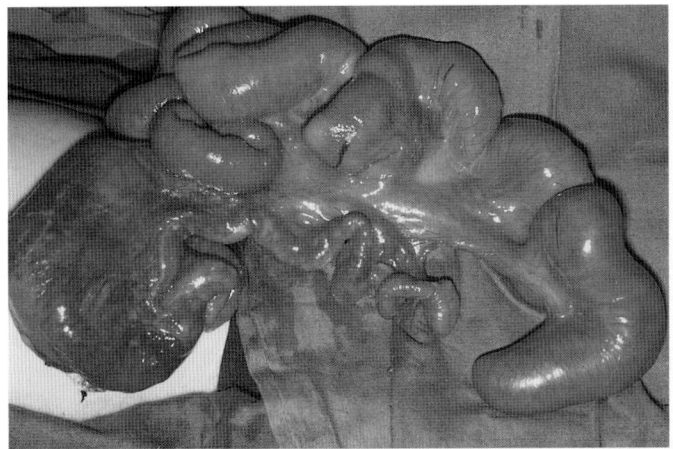

Fig. 29.79 Intestinal atresia associated with gastroschisis.

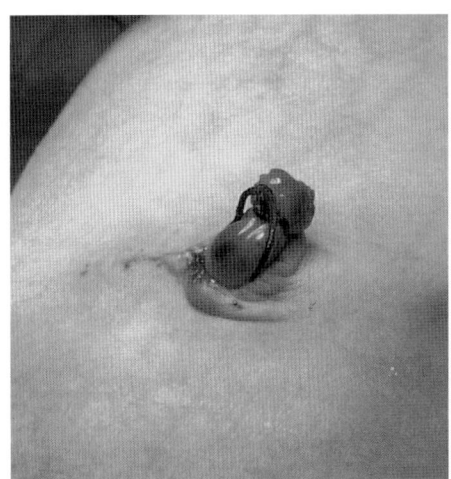

Fig. 29.81 Appearance of the umbilicus after primary repair of gastroschisis.

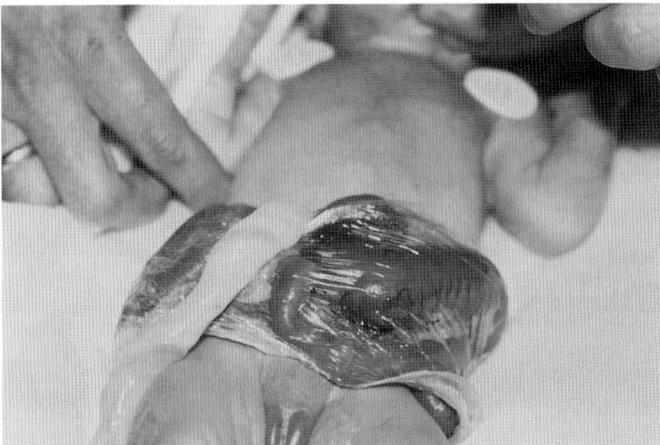

Fig. 29.80 The exposed gut can be temporarily insulated and stabilised with a 'cling-film' wrap.

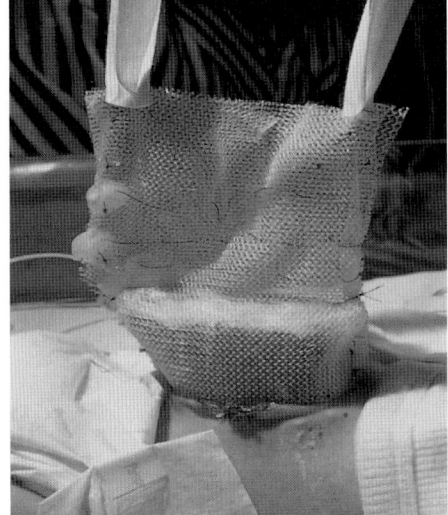

Fig. 29.82 Staged silo repair of gastroschisis. Repeated tucks have been taken in the silo to reduce the gut into the abdominal cavity.

Young maternal age (median 21 years) is consistently associated with the condition and other maternal risk factors have also been identified.[20] Infants with gastroschisis are typically of low birthweight (median 2.3 kg) and do not usually have other life-threatening anomalies. Intestinal atresia is found in about 10% of cases (Fig. 29.79) and the bowel in gastroschisis is non-rotated.

The postnatal appearance of the bowel varies from almost normal to a foreshortened, thickened mass covered in a dense fibrin 'peel'. The duration of exposure of the fetal gut to amniotic fluid may determine this appearance but clinical and experimental evidence suggests that it is related more to vascular compression of the mesentery of the gut by the edges of the abdominal wall defect.

Infants with gastroschisis lose fluid and heat readily from the exposed bowel. Immediately after delivery they require intravenous fluids, a nasogastric tube and measures to stabilise and insulate the bowel. Cellophane wrapping ('cling-film') allows the bowel to be inspected and prevents harmful traction on the mesentery (Fig. 29.80). In-utero transfer to a centre with obstetric and paediatric surgical services is preferable to postnatal transfer since it facilitates prompt postnatal surgical treatment and enables mother and baby to be together.

Under general anaesthesia, the bowel is reduced and the defect repaired (primary closure). This usually leaves a good cosmetic appearance (Fig. 29.81). In cases where the abdominal cavity is not large enough to accommodate the viscera, a staged silo repair (see above) is necessary (Fig. 29.82).

Although 90% or more of affected babies now survive, their postnatal course is often protracted. Full enteral feeding is usually not achieved for about 3 weeks after primary closure and during this period the infant requires total parenteral nutrition with its attendant risks and complications. Babies with gastroschisis often stay in hospital for several weeks. Those with atresias or severe short gut syndrome may have a more complicated course. Necrotising enterocolitis is an additional potential complication.

Cloacal exstrophy

This is an uncommon condition that affects both the alimentary and urinary tracts. Typically, there is an exstrophic central segment of bowel (ileocaecal region) flanked by two hemibladders but many variations are described (Fig. 29.83). Gender assignment

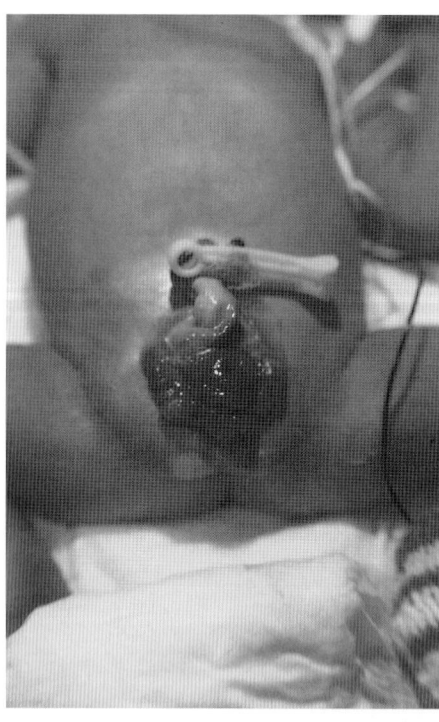

Fig. 29.83 Cloacal exstrophy. The gut is exposed between two hemibladders.

can be difficult and experienced multidisciplinary assessment is important. Major associated anomalies are common and reconstructive surgery is often complex.[40]

Hernias

Inguinal

Although girls may develop an inguinal hernia, boys are affected much more frequently because of failure of closure of the processus vaginalis after testicular descent. The prevalence of inguinal hernia is greatest during infancy, when at least 1% of boys are affected. In boys, 60% of inguinal hernias occur on the right, 30% on the left and 10% are bilateral. Inguinal hernias in general and bilateral hernias in particular are much more common in premature babies, as are associated undescended testes.

Inguinal hernias typically cause an intermittent swelling in the groin or scrotum when the baby cries or strains. If the hernia becomes obstructed (at the level of the external inguinal ring) it will manifest as a firm, tender lump in the groin or scrotum (Fig. 29.84). The baby may vomit and be irritable. Most incarcerated hernias in children can be successfully reduced by sustained gentle compression ('taxis') after analgesia. Surgery is delayed for 24–48 hours to allow resolution of oedema. If reduction is impossible, emergency surgery is required because of the risk of strangulation of bowel (or ovary) and damage to the testis.

The risk of incarceration/strangulation in an inguinal hernia is greatest in infancy and thus repair should generally be undertaken as soon as the infant is fit for surgery or prior to discharge from hospital in the case of a premature baby. Postoperative apnoea is a potential hazard in infants less than 44 weeks postconceptional

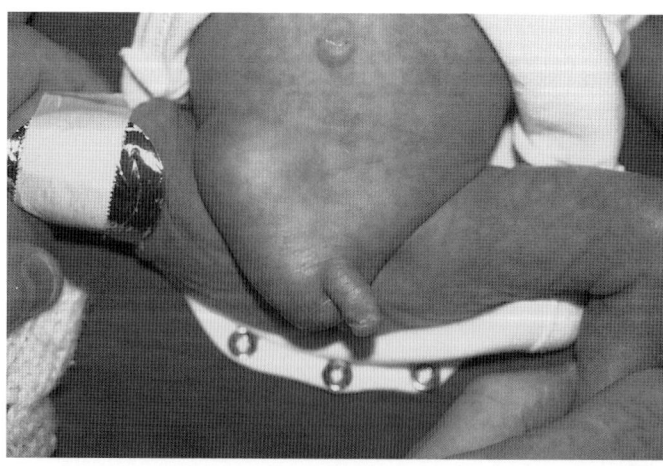

(a)

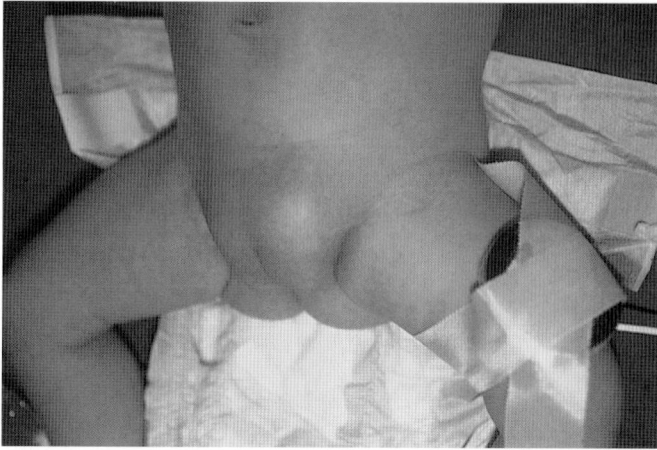

(b)

Fig. 29.84 Incarcerated inguinal hernias. (a) This boy's right inguinal hernia was reduced by taxis and subsequently repaired. (b) This baby girl had an ovary incarcerated in her irreducible inguinal hernia and required urgent surgery.

age. Inguinal herniotomy is usually performed under general anaesthesia but regional anaesthetic techniques are valuable for some infants with respiratory problems.[47] Most surgeons repair the hernia through an inguinal skin crease incision but laparoscopy has its advocates. Inguinal herniotomy is not a minor procedure in a neonate and demands anaesthetic and surgical expertise. Local complications are uncommon but may include recurrent hernia, interference with normal testicular descent, and injury to the vas or vessels.

Umbilical

Incomplete regression of the vitelline duct may result in a patent vitellointestinal duct (Fig. 29.85) or a Meckel's diverticulum. An umbilical hernia is caused by incomplete closure of the umbilical ring. Most resolve spontaneously within a year or two and surgical repair is rarely necessary. Incarceration in an umbilical hernia is rare in Western countries.

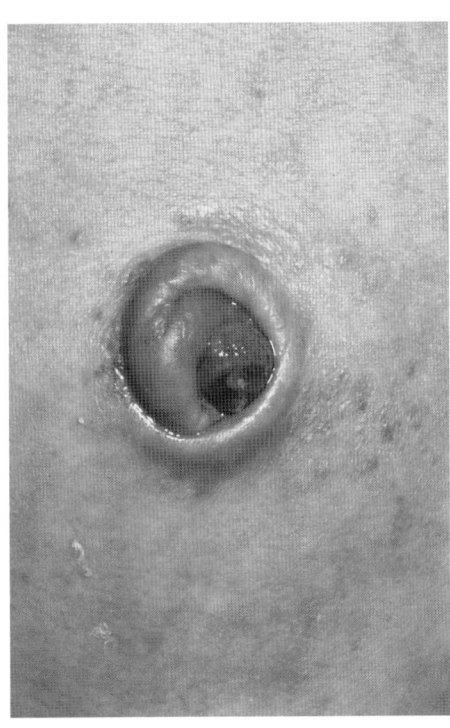

Fig. 29.85 A patent vitello-intestinal duct causing an intermittent umbilical discharge. Excision of the duct was curative.

Acknowledgements

We are grateful to Mr Carl F. Davis and Professor Dan G. Young from the Royal Hospital for Sick Children in Glasgow for some of the illustrations taken from the previous edition of this chapter.

References

1. Astley R 1969 Duodenal atresia with gas below the obstruction. British Journal of Radiology 42: 351–353
2. Badner J A, Sieber W K, Garver K L, Chakravarti A 1990 A genetic study of Hirschsprung's disease. American Journal of Human Genetics 46: 568–580
3. Blumhagen J D, Maclin L, Krauter D, Rosenbaum D M, Weinberger E 1988 Sonographic diagnosis of hypertrophic pyloric stenosis. American Journal of Roentgenology 150: 1367–1370
4. Bower T R, Pringle K C, Soper R T 1988 Sodium deficit causing decreased weight gain and metabolic acidosis in infants with ileostomy. Journal of Pediatric Surgery 23: 567–572
5. Boyd A, Carachi R, Azmy A, Raine P A M, Young D G 1988 Gastrografin enema in meconium ileus: the persistent approach. Pediatric Surgery International 3: 139–140
6. British Association of Paediatric Surgeons/Royal College of Surgeons of England 1999 Surgical Services for the Newborn. Joint publication by British Association of Paediatric Surgeons and the Royal College of Surgeons of England.
7. Calder J. Two examples of children with preternatural conformation of the guts. Medical Essays and observations, Vol 1. T and W Ruddimans, Medical Society of Edinburgh 1733; 1: 203
8. Calzolari E, Bianchi F, Dolk H, Milan M. Omphalocele and gastroschisis in Europe: a survey of 3 million births 1980–1990. EUROCAT Working Group. American Journal of Medical Genetics 1995; 58: 187–194
9. Cantrell J R, Haller J A Jr, Ravitch M M 1958 A syndrome of congenital defects involving the abdominal wall, sternum, diaphragm, pericardium and heart. Surgery of Gynecology and Obstetrics 197: 602–614
10. Chetcuti P, Myers N A, Phelan P D, Beasley S W 1988 Adults who survived repair of congenital oesophageal atresia and tracheo-oesophageal fistula. British Medical Journal 297: 344–346
11. Chittmittrapap S, Spitz L, Kiely E M, Brereton R I 1989 Oesophageal atresia and associated anomalies. Archives of Disease in Childhood 64: 364–368
12. Clinical Standards Advisory Group – Cleft Lip and/or Palate 1998; HMSO ISBN: 0 11 322 103 7.
13. Cook R C M, Rickham P P 1969 Neonatal intestinal obstruction due to milk curds. Journal of Pediatric Surgery 4: 599–605
14. Corbally M T 1993 Laryngo-tracheo-oesophageal cleft. Archives of Disease in Childhood 532–533
15. Cosman B C, Schullinger J N, Bell J J, Regan J A 1988 Hypothyroidism caused by topical povidone-iodine in a newborn with omphalocele. Journal of Pediatric Surgery 23: 356–358
16. Coutts J, Docherty J G, Carachi R, Evans T J 1997 Clinical course of cystic fibrosis presenting with meconium ileus. British Journal of Surgery 84: 555
17. Crabbe D C G, Kiely E M, Drake D P, Spitz L 1996 Management of the isolated congenital tracheo-oesophageal fistula. European Journal of Pediatric Surgery 6: 67–69
18. Croaker G D H, Shi E, Simpson E, Cartmill T, Cass D T 1998 Congenital central hypoventilation syndrome and Hirschsprung's disease. Archives of Disease in Childhood 78: 316–322
19. Currarino G, Coln D, Votteler T 1981 Triad of anorectal, sacral and presacral anomalies. American Journal of Roentgenology 137: 395–398
20. Curry J I, McKinney P, Thornton J G, Stringer M D 2000 The aetiology of gastroschisis. British Journal of Obstetrics & Gynaecology 107: 1339–1346
21. Di Tanna G L, Rosano A, Mastroiacovo P 2002 Prevalence of gastroschisis at birth: retrospective study. British Medical Journal 325: 1389–1390
22. Engum S A, Grosfeld J L 1998 Hirschsprung's disease: Duhamel pull-through. In: Stringer M D, Oldham K T, Mouriquand P D E, Howard E R (eds). Pediatric Surgery and Urology: long term outcomes. W B Saunders Co, 1998, London, pp. 329–339
23. Evans N J 1982 Pyloric stenosis in premature infants after transpyloric feeding. Lancet ii: 665
24. Fagan D G, Pritchard J S, Clarkson T W, Greenwood M R 1977 Organ mercury levels in infants with omphaloceles treated with organic mercurial antiseptic. Archives of Disease in Childhood 52: 962–964
25. Feingold J, Guilloud-Bataille M 1999 Genetic comparisons of patients with cystic fibrosis with or without meconium ileus. Clinical Centers of the French CF Registry. Annals of Genetics 42: 147–150
26. Filston H C, Kirks D R 1981 Malrotation – the ubiquitous anomaly. Journal of Pediatric Surgery 16: 614–620
27. Gee H, Abdulla U 1978 Antenatal diagnosis of fetal duodenal atresia by ultrasonic scan. British Medical Journal ii: 1265
28. Gilbert W M, Nicolaides K H 1987 Fetal omphalocele: associated malformations and chromosomal defects. Obstetrics and Gynecology 70: 633–635
29. Godbole P, Stringer M D 2002 Bilious vomiting in the newborn: How often is it pathologic? Journal of Pediatric Surgery 37: 909–911
30. Grosfeld J L, Ballantine T V N, Shoemaker R 1979 Operative management of intestinal atresia and stenosis based on pathologic findings. Journal of Pediatric Surgery 14: 368–375
31. Haight C, Towsley H A 1943 Congenital atresia of the esophagus with tracheo-esophageal fistula: extrapleural ligation of fistula and end-to-end anastomosis of esophageal segments. Surgery Gynecology and Obstetrics 76: 672–688
32. Hirschsprung H 1887 Stuhltragheit Neuegeborener in Folge von Dilatation und Hypertrophie des Colons. Jahrb Kinderheilk 27: 1–7
33. Kluth D 1976 Atlas of esophageal atresia. Journal of Pediatric Surgery 11: 901–919
34. Kluth D, Lambrecht W 1997 Current concepts in the embryology of anorectal malformations. Semin Pediatr Surg 6: 180–186
35. Krasna I H, Rosenfeld D, Benjamin B G, Klein G, Hiatt M, Hegyi T 1987 Esophageal perforation in the neonate: an emerging problem in the newborn nursery. Journal of Pediatric Surgery 22: 784–790
36. Kusafuka T, Puri P 1998 Genetic aspects of Hirshsprung's disease. Seminars in Pediatric Surgery 7: 148–155
37. Kutiyanawala M, Wyse R K H, Brereton R J et al 1992 CHARGE and esophageal atresia. Journal of Pediatric Surgery 27: 1136–1141
38. Louw J H 1959 Congenital intestinal atresia and stenosis in the newborn. Observations of pathogenesis and treatment. Annals of the Royal College of Surgeons of England 25: 209–234
39. Ludman L. Anorectal malformations: psychological aspects. In Stringer MD, Oldham KT, Mouriquand PDE, Howard ER (eds). Pediatric Surgery and Urology: Long Term Outcomes. 1998, pp386–392, W.B.Saunders, Philadelphia.
40. Lund DP, Hendren WH. 2001 Cloacal exstrophy: a 25-year experience with 50 cases. Journal of Pediatric Surgery 36:68–75
41. Martin V 1999 The TOF Child. Published by TOFS, Nottingham

42. Moore SW, Johnson AG 1998 Hirschsprung's disease: genetic and functional associations of Down's and Waardenburg syndromes. Seminars in Pediatric Surgery 7: 156–161

43. Mushtaq I, Wright V M, Drake D P, Mearns M B, Wood C B 1998 Meconium ileus secondary to cystic fibrosis. The East London experience. 1998 Pediatric Surgery International 13: 365–369

44. Noblett H 1969 Treatment of uncomplicated meconium ileus by gastrografin enema: a preliminary report. Journal of Pediatric Surgery 4: 190–197

45. Okoye B O, Parikh D H, Buick R G, Lander A D 2000 Pyloric atresia: five new cases, a new association and a review of the literature with guidelines. Journal of Pediatric Surgery 35: 1242–1245

46. Pena A 1995 Anorectal malformations. Seminars in Pediatric Surgery 4: 35–47

47. Peutrell J M, Hughes D G 1992 Epidural anaesthesia through caudal catheters for inguinal herniotomies in awake ex-premature babies. Anaesthesia 47: 128–131

48. Pracros J P, Sann L, Genin G, et al 1992 Ultrasound diagnosis of midgut volvulus: the 'whirlpool' sign. Pediatric Radiology 22: 18–20

49. Puri P, Fujimoto T 1988 New observations in the pathogenesis of multiple intestinal atresias. Journal of Pediatric Surgery 23: 221–225

50. Puri P, Tsuji M 1992 Megacystis-microcolon-intestinal hypoperistalsis syndrome (neonatal hollow visceral myopathy). Pediatric Surgery International 7: 18–23

51. Rescorla F J, Grosfeld J L 1993 Contemporary management of meconium ileus. World Journal of Surgery 17: 318–325

52. Richards C, Holmes S J 1995 Intestinal dilatation in the fetus. Archives of Disease in Childhood 72: F135–F138

53. Rintala R, Lindahl H, Louhimo I 1991 Anorectal malformations – results of treatment and long-term follow-up in 208 patients. Pediatric Surgery International 6: 36–41

54. Rintala R, Lindahl H, Rasanen M 1997 Do children with repaired low anorectal malformations have normal bowel function? Journal of Pediatric Surgery 32: 823–826

55. Rollins M D, Shields M D, Quinn R J M, Wooldridge M A 1989 Pyloric stenosis: congenital or acquired? Archives of Disease in Childhood 64: 138–140

56. Rothenberg S S 2002 Thoracoscopic repair of tracheoesophageal fistula in newborns. Journal of Pediatric Surgery 37: 869–872

57. Shaw W C, Sandy J R, Williams A C, Devlin H B 1996 Minimum standards for the management of cleft lip and palate: efforts to close the audit loop. Annals of the Royal College of Surgeons of England 78: 110–114

58. Sherry S N, Kramer I 1955 The time of passage of first stool and first urine by the newborn infant. Journal of Pediatrics 46: 158–159

59. Shigemoto H, Endo S, Isomoto T, Sano K, Taguchi K 1978 Neonatal meconium obstruction in the ileum without mucoviscidosis. Journal of Pediatric Surgery 13: 475–479

60. Spitz L 1996 Esophageal atresia: past, present, and future. Journal of Pediatric Surgery 31: 19–25

61. Stone D H, Rimaz S, Gilmour W H 1998 Prevalence of congenital anterior abdominal wall defects in the United Kingdom: comparison of regional registers. British Medical Journal 317: 1118–1119

62. Stringer M D 1999 Hirschsprung's Disease. In Surgery of the Anus, Rectum and Colon, 2(nd) edition, Keighley MRB, Williams NS (eds.). W.B Saunders, London, pp. 2635–2680

63. Stringer M D 2003. Gastric Volvulus. In: Newborn Surgery, 2(nd) edn. Puri P (ed.), Arnold, London, pp. 399–404

64. Stringer M D, McKenna K M, Goldstein R B, Filly R A, Adzick N S, Harrison M R 1995 Prenatal diagnosis of esophageal atresia. Journal of Pediatric Surgery 30: 1258–1263

65. Stringer M D, Spitz L, Abel R, Kiely E, Drake D P, Agrawal M, Stark Y, Brereton RJ 1995 Management of alimentary tract duplication in children. British Journal of Surgery 82: 74–78

66. Stringer M D, Thornton J G, Mason G C 1996 Hyperechogenic fetal bowel. Archives of Disease in Childhood 74: F1–F2

67. Tack E D, Perlman J M, Bower R J, McAlister WH 1988 Pyloric stenosis in the sick premature infant. Clinical and radiological findings. American Journal of Disease in Childhood 142: 68–70

68. Touloukian R J, Higgins E 1983 The spectrum of serum electrolytes in hypertrophic pyloric stenosis. Journal of Pediatric Surgery 18: 394–397

69. Wang N L, Yeh M L, Chang P Y, et al 1998 Prenatal and neonatal intussusception. Pediatric Surgery International 13: 232–236

70. Watson A C H, Sell D A & Grunwell P (eds) 2001 Management of cleft lip and palate. Whurr Publishers 2001. ISBN: 1 86156 158 X

71. Weaver L T, Lucas A 1993 Development of bowel habit in preterm infants. Archives of Disease in Childhood 68: 317–320

72. Williams A C, Sandy J R, Thomas S, Sell D, Sterne J 1999 Influence of surgeon's experience on speech outcome in cleft lip and palate. Lancet 354: 1697–1698

73. Zeidan B, Wyatt J, Mackersie A, Brereton R J 1988 Recent results of treatment of infantile hypertrophic pyloric stenosis. Archives of Disease in Childhood 63: 1060–1064

CHAPTER 30

Haematology

Irene A G Roberts, Neil A Murray

Developmental haemopoiesis

Introduction

The process which ensures lifelong production of cells of all the haemopoietic lineages is known as haemopoiesis. The principal cell lineages and organisation of this process (Fig. 30.1) are broadly similar in adults, children, neonates, the fetus and the embryo. However, there are fascinating differences in the regulation of haemopoiesis and its cellular components during ontogeny which contribute to the nature and management of many neonatal haematological problems.

Firstly, the sites of haemopoiesis vary during ontogeny. The first signs of haemopoiesis in humans occur in the yolk sac in the third week of gestation.[88] By 5 weeks' gestation, the main site of definitive haemopoiesis is a defined area of the embryonic dorsal aorta in the aorto-gonad-mesonephros (AGM) region.[121] Soon afterwards, AGM-derived haemopoietic stem cells migrate to the liver,

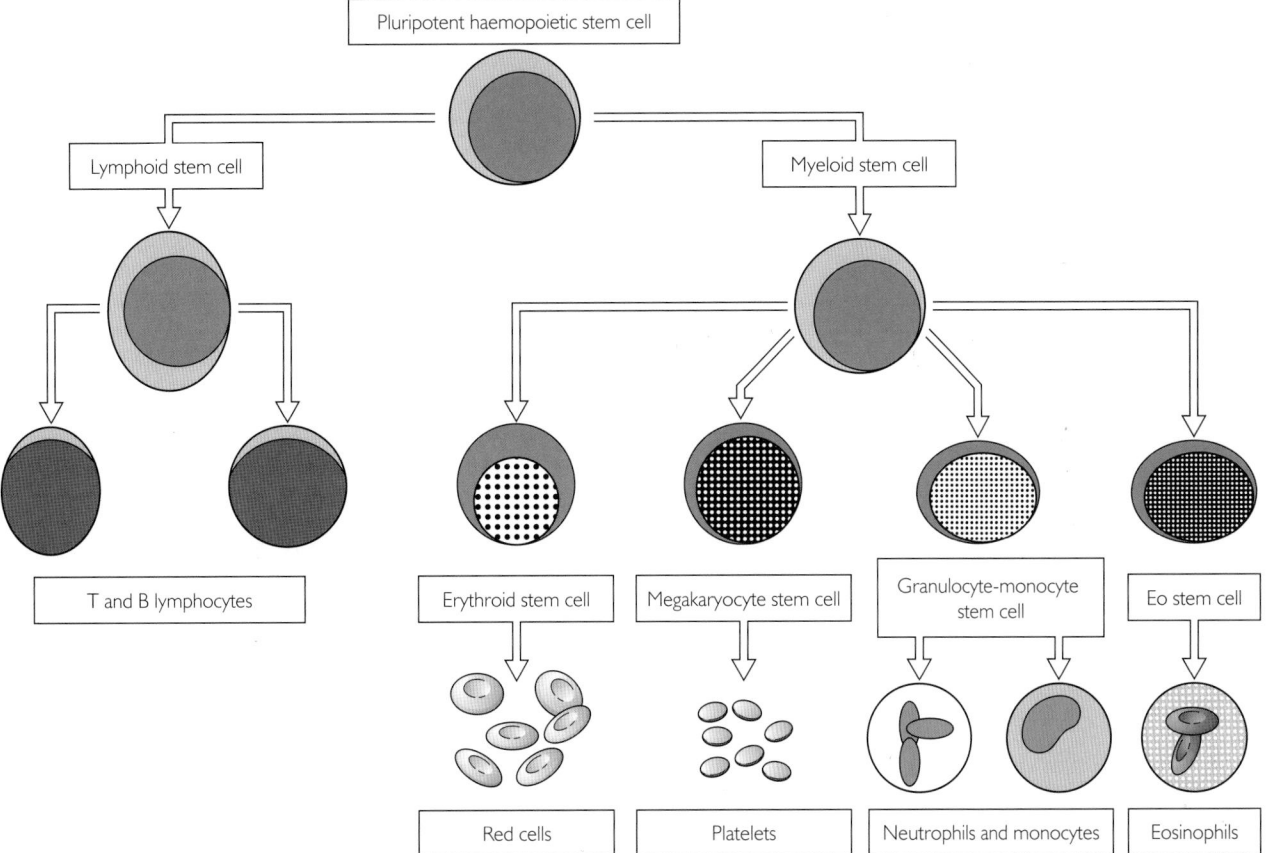

Fig. 30.1 Haemopoiesis in the newborn and adult. Simplified diagram of the process of haemopoiesis in term and preterm neonates and in adults.

which, by 6–8 weeks' gestation, becomes the primary site of blood cell production.[88] Even though signs of haemopoiesis begin in the bone marrow around the eleventh week of gestation, the fetal liver remains the principal site of haemopoiesis until the end of the third trimester.[176] Thus, for preterm infants, the liver is the main haemopoietic organ at and shortly after birth; this may be a contributory factor in a number of disorders, including the haematological abnormalities seen in neonates with intrauterine growth restriction (IUGR; see later sections).

Erythropoiesis in the fetus and neonate

Erythropoiesis is the first haemopoietic lineage to become established, with erythrocytes first being produced in the yolk sac at 3 weeks' gestation. There are a number of distinct characteristics of erythropoiesis in term and especially preterm neonates which are relevant both to our understanding of the normal changes in haemoglobin during this period and to identifying clinically significant acquired or inherited abnormalities of erythropoiesis:

■ **Rate of haemoglobin synthesis and red blood cell (RBC) production**: The rates of haemoglobin synthesis and of RBC production fall dramatically after birth and remain low for the first 2 weeks of life, probably in response to the sudden increase in tissue oxygenation at birth.[141] The physiological rise in red cell production begins several weeks later and by 3 months of age a healthy infant, whatever the gestation at birth, should be able to produce up to 2 ml of packed red cells per day.[141] Studies in preterm neonates have suggested that over the first 2 months of life the maximal rate of red cell production is about 1 ml/day since preterm babies receiving erythropoietin are unable to maintain their haemoglobin if >1 ml of blood per day is venesected for diagnostic purposes but can do so where sampling losses are less than this.[137]

■ **Reduced red cell lifespan**: Neonatal red cells, particularly from preterm babies, have a reduced lifespan compared with adult red cells. Calculated red cell lifespans for preterm infants are 35–50 days compared with 60–70 days for term infants and 120 days for healthy adults.[147] The reasons are unclear and are likely predominantly to reflect changes in the red cell membrane, including increased resistance to osmotic lysis, increased mechanical fragility, increased total lipid content and an altered lipid profile, increased insulin-binding sites and reduced expression of blood group antigens such as A, B and I.[141]

■ **Altered red cell metabolism**: There are numerous differences in the glycolytic and pentose phosphate pathways between neonatal and adult RBCs which lead to an increased susceptibility to oxidant-induced injury,[24,172] although the clinical implications of these differences are in many cases unclear. In addition, neonatal RBCs have reduced levels of NADH methaemoglobin reductase (about 60% of those in adult red cells). This makes them more likely to develop methaemoglobinaemia as they are more susceptible to the toxic effects of chemicals (e.g. nitric oxide) which oxidise haemoglobin iron more rapidly than the maximal rate of methaemoglobin reduction; methaemoglobin levels are, correspondingly, slightly higher in neonates than adults (mean 0.43 g/dl in preterm neonates, 0.22 g/dl in term neonates and 0.11 g/dl in adults).[141]

■ **Changes in globin chain synthesis in the fetus and newborn**: Knowledge of the normal evolution of embryonic, fetal and 'adult' haemoglobins during ontogeny is essential to our understanding of how haemoglobinopathies present in neonates (Table 30.1). The first globin chain produced is epsilon globin, followed almost immediately by α- and γ-globin chain production. HbF ($\alpha_2\gamma_2$) is therefore produced from early in gestation (4–5 weeks) and is the predominant haemoglobin until after birth. Adult haemoglobin (HbA: $\alpha_2\beta_2$) is also produced from an early stage (6–8 weeks' gestation) but remains at low levels (10–15%) until 30–32 weeks. After this time, the rate of HbA production increases at the same time as HbF production falls, resulting in an average HbF level at term birth of 70–80%, HbA of 25–30%, small amounts of HbA_2 and sometimes a trace of Hb Barts (β_4).[15] After birth, HbF falls to <2% at age 12 months with a corresponding increase in HbA. In term babies there is little change in HbF in the first 15 days after birth but it declines steeply thereafter as neonatal erythropoiesis starts. In preterm babies who are not transfused, HbF may remain at the same level for the first 6 weeks of life before HbA production starts to increase. It is this delay in HbA production (i.e. the switch from the γ-globin of HbF to the β-globin of HbA) which can make the diagnosis of β-globin disorders difficult in the neonatal period. By contrast, the fact that α-globin chains are absolutely essential for the production of both HbF and HbA means that α-thalassaemia major causes severe anaemia from early in fetal life.[81]

■ **Erythropoietin production in the fetus and newborn**: Erythropoietin is the principal cytokine regulating erythropoiesis in the fetus and newborn.[73,189] Since erythropoietin does not cross the placenta, erythropoietin-mediated regulation of fetal erythropoiesis is predominantly under fetal control.[189] The liver is the main site of erythropoietin production in the fetus[45] and the only stimulus to erythropoietin production under physiological conditions is hypoxia with or without anaemia. This explains the high erythropoietin levels in fetuses of mothers with diabetes or hypertension or those with IUGR or cyanotic congenital heart disease; erythropoietin is also increased in fetal anaemia of any cause, including haemolytic disease of the newborn (HDN).[195]

White cell production in the fetus and newborn

Neutrophils

There are few circulating neutrophils in first- and second-trimester blood ($0.1–0.2 \times 10^9$/l),[37] after which the numbers gradually rise to reach over 2×10^9/l by term, with slightly lower numbers in preterm neonates (Table 30.2). The principal difference between neutrophil production in the newborn and the adult is the diminished size of the neutrophil storage pool, particularly in preterm infants and most markedly so in those with IUGR or exposure to maternal hypertension.[41,102,139] The

Table 30.1 Composition of haemoglobins in the human embryo, fetus and neonate

Haemoglobin	Globin chains		Gestation
	α-globin gene cluster	β-globin gene cluster*	
Embryonic			
Hb Gower-1	ζ₂	ε₂	From 3–4 weeks
Hb Gower-2	α₂	ε₂	
Hb Portland	ζ₂	γ₂	From 4 weeks
Fetal			
HbF	α₂	γ₂	From 4 weeks
Adult			
HbA	α₂	β₂	From 6–8 weeks
HbA₂	α₂	δ₂	From 30 weeks

* The α-globin gene cluster is situated on chromosome 16 and the β-globin gene cluster on chromosome 11. Note that fetuses and neonates with α-thalassaemia major, who are unable to synthesise α-globin chains, will have Hb Portland as well as Hb Barts (β_4) detectable by haemoglobin electrophoresis or HPLC.

Table 30.2 Representative normal haematological values at birth and over the first 2 months of life in term babies*

	Birth	2 weeks	2 months
Hb (g/dl)	14.9–23.7	13.4–19.8	9.4–13
Haematocrit	0.47–75	0.41–0.65	0.28–0.42
MCV (fl)	100–125	88–110	77–98
Reticulocytes ($\times 10^9$/l)	110–450	10–85	35–200
WBC ($\times 10^9$/l)	10–26	6–21	5–15
Neutrophils ($\times 10^9$/l)	2.7–14.4	1.5–5.4	0.7–4.8
Monocytes ($\times 10^9$/l)	0–1.9	0.1–1.7	0.4–1.2
Lymphocytes ($\times 10^9$/l)	2.0–7.3	2.8–9.1	3.3–10.3
Eosinophils ($\times 10^9$/l)	0–0.85	0–0.85	0.05–0.9
Basophils ($\times 10^9$/l)	0–0.1	0–0.1	0.02–0.13
Nucleated RBC ($\times 10^9$/l)	<5	<0.1	<0.1
Platelets ($\times 10^9$/l)	150–450	150–450	150–450

These data are obtained from a number of sources and have been chosen to represent data most useful for interpreting the significance of haematological results.

neutrophil storage pool reflects the available reserve of neutrophils which the fetus or neonate can mobilize in response to infection. This may explain the frequency of bacterial infection in such infants. The neutrophil storage pool is defined as the numbers of segmented neutrophils, band neutrophils and metamyelocytes in the bone marrow and so is usually inferred (by the leukocyte response to bacterial sepsis) since bone marrow examination is rarely indicated in the newborn. Various cytokines stimulate neutrophil production in vitro and in vivo (e.g. granulocyte colony-stimulating factor [G-CSF] and granulocyte–macrophage colony-stimulating factor [GM-CSF])[41,139] but their exact physiological role is unclear.

Monocytes, eosinophils and lymphocytes

All types of leukocyte found in adult blood are also seen in the fetus and the newborn:[55] monocytes circulate from 4–5 weeks' gestation and eosinophils from 14–16 weeks' gestation, each cell type being present in low numbers and increasing slowly to the normal values at term (see Table 30.2). There are few studies of lymphopoiesis in the human fetus; both T lymphocytes and B lymphocytes are found in low numbers in the fetal liver at 7 and 8 weeks' gestation, respectively,[74] and T lymphocytes are detectable in fetal blood, marrow and thymus during the second trimester.[144] By term, T lymphocytes form 40–45% of circulating mononuclear cells, with a CD4:CD8 ratio of around 5:1, slightly higher than in adult blood (3.1:1). B lymphocytes are found in fetal blood and bone marrow from around 12 weeks' gestation and constitute 4–5% of circulating mononuclear cells by term.[74]

Megakaryocytopoiesis and platelet production in the fetus and newborn

Platelets first appear in the fetal circulation at 5–6 weeks post-conceptional age.[74] During the second trimester, the platelet count rises to normal adult values (175–250×10^9/l).[55] Thus, a platelet count of less than 150×10^9/l is abnormal even in the most preterm neonate. The principal cytokine regulating platelet production in the fetus and newborn is thrombopoietin, as in adults.[194] There are several differences between megakaryocytopoiesis and its regulation in the fetus and newborn compared with adults which may contribute to the frequent occurrence of thrombocytopenia in sick neonates. Fetal megakaryocytes are smaller and more immature than those in adult marrow;[48,77] the numbers of megakaryocyte progenitor cells, the precursor cells for maintaining megakaryocyte and platelet production, are reduced; and the ability to produce thrombopoietin is reduced, limiting the capacity to upregulate platelet production at times of increased demand, e.g. during thrombocytopenia in neonatal sepsis.[2,194]

Neonatal anaemia and other red cell disorders

Introduction and definition

Anaemia is the commonest haematological abnormality in the newborn. In the majority of neonates, the causes are straightforward, since they reflect a combination of well-recognised physiological changes and iatrogenic blood letting. However, it is important to identify those neonates with pathological anaemia who require additional investigations and more tailored management. In the neonatal period, the most frequent diseases associated with anaemia are immune haemolysis and genetic red cell disorders. A logical approach and appropriate use of straightforward investigations, as outlined below, reveals the cause in most babies. Treatment options for neonatal anaemia are limited and are based mainly on sensible use of blood transfusion (see pp. 764–8) and prevention of anaemia.

Table 30.3 Representative normal haematological values at birth in preterm babies

	24–25 weeks	26–27 weeks	28–29 weeks	30–31 weeks
Hb (g/dl)	19.4 ± 1.5	19.0 ± 2.5	19.3 ± 1.8	19.1 ± 2.1
Haematocrit	0.63 ± 0.04	0.62 ± 0.08	0.60 ± 0.07	60 ± 0.08
MCV (fl)	135 ± 0.02	132 ± 14.4	131 ± 13.5	127 ± 12.7
Reticulocytes ($\times 10^9$/l)	279 ± 23	454 ± 15	347 ± 12	278 ± 10
Platelets ($\times 10^9$/l)	150–450	150–450	150–450	150–450

Adapted from Oski.[141]

Normal values for red blood cells and blood volume

Normal values at birth for haemoglobin, haematocrit and mean corpuscular volume (MCV) for term and preterm babies are shown in Table 30.2 and Table 30.3, respectively, and in Appendix 1.

In term babies, the haemoglobin, haematocrit and red cell indices fall slowly over the first few weeks, reaching a mean haemoglobin of 13–14 g/dl at 4 weeks of age and 9.5–11 g/dl at 7–9 weeks of age, with a lower limit of normal for the MCV and mean corpuscular haemoglobin (MCH) of 77 fl and 26 pg, respectively. For preterm infants, these changes may be difficult to interpret, because of their variable clinical course and transfusion requirements. However, studies of well preterm infants carried out in the 1970s show a more rapid and steeper fall in haemoglobin, reaching a mean of 6.5–9 g/dl at 4–8 weeks postnatal age.[141] The reticulocyte count falls rapidly after birth as erythropoiesis is suppressed, and starts to increase in term babies at 7–8 weeks of age to reach 35–200 × 10^9/l (1–1.8%) at 2 months of age, and in preterm babies at 6–8 weeks of age.[32,122,141] Normal blood volume at birth varies with gestational age and the timing of clamping of the cord. In term infants, the average blood volume is 80 ml/kg (range 50–100 ml/kg), and in preterm infants is higher at 106 ml/kg (range 85–143 ml/kg).[166,183] Term and preterm babies have adequate stores of iron, folic acid and vitamin B_{12} at birth. However, stores of both iron and folic acid are lower in preterm infants and are depleted more quickly, leading to deficiency after 2–4 months if the recommended daily intakes are not maintained (see pp. 285, 293–4). In general, even term neonates with a normal haemoglobin at birth will have depleted their iron stores by the time they have doubled their birthweight.[152]

There are no useful published normal ranges for the numbers of circulating nucleated red cells, partly because it is only recently that automated blood counters have been able to distinguish nucleated red cells from white blood cells. Nevertheless, a useful 'rule of thumb' is that values of less than five nucleated RBCs per 100 white cells in a term baby and <20 nucleated red cells per 100 white blood cells in a preterm baby can be considered normal for the first 1–2 days of life. The commonest causes of increased numbers of circulating nucleated RBCs are:

- haemolysis (common in Rh haemolytic disease and α-thalassaemia major but uncommon in other types of haemolysis);
- haemorrhage (especially fetomaternal haemorrhage);
- chronic tissue hypoxia in utero (IUGR, maternal hypertension, maternal diabetes);
- perinatal asphyxia.

Definition of anaemia

Anaemia can be defined as a haemoglobin concentration below the normal range for a population of age- and sex-matched individuals. Normal values for term and preterm infants at birth are shown in Tables 30.2 and 30.3; from this it can be seen that, regardless of gestation, any neonate with a haemoglobin of <14 g/dl at birth in a properly taken blood sample should be considered anaemic. Not every neonate with a haemoglobin concentration at birth of <14 g/dl needs detailed further investigation, but thought should be given to the cause (Table 30.4) and appropriate investigations instituted. Where the reduced haemoglobin does not fit the clinical picture, the first step should be to repeat the sample, since in many cases the measured haemoglobin concentration is inaccurate because of the site of sampling (heel-prick versus venous blood) or the way in which the sample was collected. The haemoglobin concentration in venous samples is lower than in heel-prick samples collected simultaneously: in the first few hours of life this difference averages 2–4 g/dl and is greater at lower gestational ages.[141,178] The difference between the venous and capillary haemoglobin falls with increasing gestational age, and also with increasing postnatal age, such that by the fifth day of life there is almost no difference in haemoglobin concentration between a well taken heel-prick sample compared with a venous sample.[113,141]

The influence of cord clamping

The other major influence on haemoglobin concentration at birth is the timing of cord clamping and the position of the baby at the time of clamping. In term babies, the placental vessels contain around 100 ml of blood at birth. It has been estimated that 25% of the placental blood is transfused within the first 15 seconds and 50% (i.e. 50 ml in a term baby) by the end of the first minute.[112] The difference in haemoglobin concentration in the baby between early versus late cord clamping is around 3 g/dl.[204] Babies held below the level of the placenta continue to gain blood until the cord is clamped and have higher

Table 30.4 Causes of neonatal anaemia

A. Impaired red cell production
Diamond–Blackfan anaemia
Congenital infection, e.g. CMV, rubella
Congenital dyserythropoietic anaemia
Pearson's syndrome
Congenital leukaemia

B. Increased red cell destruction (haemolysis)
Alloimmune: haemolytic disease of the newborn (Rh, ABO, Kell, other)
Autoimmune, e.g. maternal autoimmune haemolysis
Red cell membrane disorders, e.g. hereditary spherocytosis
Red cell enzyme deficiencies, e.g. pyruvate kinase deficiency
Some haemoglobinopathies, e.g. α-thalassaemia major, HbH disease
Infection, e.g. bacterial, syphilis, malaria, CMV, toxoplasma, herpes simplex
Macro/microangiopathy, e.g. cavernous haemangioma, DIC
Galactosaemia

C. Blood loss
Occult haemorrhage before or around birth, e.g. twin-to-twin, fetomaternal
Internal haemorrhage, e.g. intracranial, cephalhaematoma
Iatrogenic: due to frequent blood sampling

D. Anaemia of prematurity
Impaired red cell production plus reduced red cell lifespan

haemo-globin levels than those held above the level of the placenta, who may lose blood into the placenta until the cord is clamped.[204]

Physiological impact of anaemia in the neonate

The clinical significance of anaemia in the newborn depends on whether or not the baby is able to maintain adequate tissue oxygenation. This does not depend solely upon the haemoglobin concentration. Tissue oxygenation is also influenced by the cardiopulmonary function of the baby and by the ability of the haemoglobin to unload the oxygen it is carrying. Fortunately, the oxygen unloading capacity of the blood has been shown to increase progressively from birth, reflecting the position of the haemoglobin–oxygen dissociation curve.

In neonates, the two most important factors determining the position of the haemoglobin–oxygen dissociation curve are the concentrations of HbF and of 2,3-diphosphoglycerate (2,3-DPG) within the RBCs: a high HbF and low 2,3-DPG both cause the curve to be shifted to the left, i.e. the affinity of haemoglobin for oxygen is increased, so less oxygen is released to the tissues. This is the situation just after birth both in term and preterm babies, as both have HbF concentrations above 50% at

birth. The high oxygen affinity may be more of a problem for preterm babies since the HbF levels are >90% in babies of 24–28 weeks' gestation, although this may not be significant in practice since very preterm neonates are more likely to require transfusion over the first few weeks of life. Over the first few months of life in term and preterm babies, 2,3-DPG levels rise and HbF levels fall, so the haemoglobin–oxygen dissociation curve gradually shifts to the right, i.e. the oxygen affinity of haemoglobin falls and oxygen delivery to the tissues increases, to some extent ameliorating the effects of the falling haemoglobin over the first months of life.

Pathogenesis and causes of neonatal anaemia

Anaemia in the neonatal period has distinct physiological features compared with that in older children and a distinct pathogenesis. Interpretation of diagnostic investigations has to be made on a background of these ontogeny-related changes that affect the red cell membrane, red cell enzyme concentrations, and the types and rate of haemoglobin production, which vary with gestational and postnatal age. Diagnostic tests are also often affected by whether the baby has been transfused and whether he is well or sick. Furthermore, anaemia in the neonate may be due to pregnancy-related or pre-existing disorders in the mother, such as the presence of red cell alloantibodies or genetic disorders. It is therefore important to remember that in many cases evaluating the blood count and blood film of the parents is the quickest way of identifying the underlying diagnosis in the neonate.

The principal causes of neonatal anaemia are shown in Table 30.4. In general, anaemia can result from one or more of the following mechanisms:

- inappropriately reduced red cell production;
- increased red cell destruction/reduced red cell lifespan;
- blood loss;
- a combination of these mechanisms (anaemia of prematurity).

Neonatal anaemia due to reduced red cell production

Anaemia due to reduced red cell production is not common in the neonatal period. Nevertheless, it is clinically important, because several of the disorders that present in this way are associated with severe, lifelong problems. The main diagnostic clues to reduced red cell production are the combination of a *low* reticulocyte count ($<20 \times 10^9$/l) together with a negative direct antiglobulin test (Coombs' test). The other useful diagnostic point is whether the disorder is confined to the red cell series (i.e. anaemia in the presence of a normal white cell and platelet count) or whether the blood count suggests that the white cells and/or platelets are also involved.

The most important causes are congenital infections (particularly due to parvovirus) and genetic disorders. Where failure of blood cell production is confined to the red cell series, as with Diamond–Blackfan anaemia (DBA) and most episodes of parvo-virus infection, the anaemia is said to be due to red cell aplasia. Reduced red cell production may also be part of a general failure of haemopoiesis and accompanied by leukopenia and/or thrombocytopenia, as seen in congenital infection due to cytomegalovirus (CMV), in congenital leukaemias (see p. 753 and Chapter 37) and in congenital bone marrow failure syndromes such as Pearson's syndrome (see p. 753).

Anaemia and congenital infection

Infections which cause anaemia due to reduced red cell production include parvovirus B19, CMV, toxoplasmosis, congenital syphilis, rubella and herpes simplex.[30,31] Identification of the causative organism is usually based on clinical suspicion prompted by well-recognised associated findings such as chorioretinitis, jaundice, pneumonitis, skin lesions, IUGR and hepatosplenomegaly, followed by specific diagnostic microbiological investigations. In infection due to CMV, toxoplasma or herpes simplex, the anaemia and reticulocytopenia are usually relatively mild.[30] In addition, the blood film often shows abnormal 'viral' lymphocytes, thrombocytopenia and/or neutropenia. Congenital parvovirus B19 can cause particular diagnostic difficulties and is discussed below.[31]

Parvovirus B19 and fetal/neonatal anaemia

Maternal infection with parvovirus B19 causes fetal anaemia which is severe enough to lead to intrauterine death in 9% of cases.[31,127,149] A diagnosis of fetal parvovirus B19 should be considered in every 'unexplained' case of fetal hydrops (Table 30.5) since it has been estimated that parvovirus B19 is responsible for 15% of cases of non-immune hydrops.[92,107,203] In addition to anaemia, parvovirus infection causes marked reticulocytopenia (usually $<10 \times 10^9$/l) and thrombocytopenia may also occur. The diagnosis of parvovirus B19 infection is primarily based on maternal serology together with the demonstration of B19 DNA in the fetus/neonate by dot blot hybridisation or polymerase chain reaction (PCR).[31,76] Where results are negative on blood samples but clinical suspicion of parvovirus is high, PCR for B19 should also be carried out on bone marrow.[31] Management

depends on the severity of the anaemia – severe cases diagnosed in utero may be treated by intrauterine transfusion; for those that survive, the majority have no long-term sequelae. However, a small number of neonates with chronic red cell aplasia, with or without evidence of persistent B19 DNA by PCR, have been reported, and for such cases intravenous immunoglobulin (IVIG) should be given to try and eradicate persistent viral infection.[31,54]

Failure of red cell production due to genetic disorders

Congenital or inherited disorders that usually or not infrequently present with neonatal anaemia due to reduced red cell production include DBA, congenital dyserythropoietic anaemia (CDA) and Pearson's syndrome. The other inherited bone marrow failure syndromes, such as Fanconi's anaemia, rarely present at birth.

Diamond–Blackfan anaemia

The principal cause of congenital red cell aplasia is DBA,[54] which has an incidence of 5–7 cases per million live births. There is a clear family history in 20% of cases (both autosomal dominant and autosomal recessive inheritance are reported); the remaining 80% are sporadic. Affected children nearly always present in the first year of life; most diagnoses are made around 2–3 months of age, but 25% of cases present at birth and rare cases present as mid-trimester fetal anaemia and hydrops.[14,58,188] The usual presentation is with anaemia in an otherwise healthy baby; 40% of infants have associated congenital anomalies, particularly craniofacial dysmorphism, IUGR, neck anomalies (Klippel–Feil syndrome) and thumb malformations (e.g. triphalangeal or bifid thumbs)[14,58,188] similar to those seen in Fanconi's anaemia. The important laboratory features are normochromic anaemia (which may be macrocytic), reticulocytopenia and absent erythroid precursors on the bone marrow aspirate. It is important to exclude parvovirus infection by appropriate serology and dot blot testing, and Fanconi's anaemia by diepoxybutane stress testing of peripheral blood lymphocytes.[63] If these tests are negative, the only other differential diagnosis of red cell aplasia with absent red cell precursors is transient erythroblastopenia of childhood, which, in contrast to DBA, resolves within a couple of months. Recent studies in DBA show that patients, and often one or more of their parents, have raised red cell levels of adenosine deaminase (ADA).[58] This may be useful to confirm the diagnosis, but normal red cell ADA levels do not exclude DBA. In addition, around 25% of cases (both familial and sporadic) have mutations of the ribosomal protein (RP) S19 gene on chromosome 19.[52] In the neonatal period, the treatment of DBA is red cell transfusion. Up to 75% of children with DBA respond to steroids and can often be weaned off transfusions, but this approach is not usually tried until after the first year of life.[58,188] DBA is a rather unpredictable disease: some cases resolve spontaneously; others wax and wane; but more than half of affected children have lifelong transfusion- or steroid-dependence and may be treated by bone marrow transplantation.[128]

Congenital dyserythropoietic anaemia

The CDAs are a rare group of disorders characterised by failure of red cell production due to ineffective erythropoiesis. Most

---

Table 30.5 Haematogical causes of hydrops fetalis (see Chapter 31 for other causes)

A. Reduced red cell production
Parvovirus B19
Diamond–Blackfan anaemia
Congenital dyserythropoietic anaemia
Congenital leukaemia

B. Increased red cell destruction (haemolysis)
Pyruvate kinase deficiency
α-thalassaemia major (or HbH hydrops)
Haemolytic disease of the newborn – Rhesus, Kell, ABO (rare)

C. Blood loss
Twin-to-twin transfusion
Fetomaternal haemorrhage

cases are autosomal recessive and a history of parental consanguinity is not uncommon. In contrast to DBA, the bone marrow has vastly increased numbers of erythroid precursors but they are grossly abnormal and do not properly differentiate into mature RBCs. CDA usually presents during childhood. However, a number of neonates with CDA presenting at birth or during fetal life have been reported and in severe cases the presentation may be with hydrops fetalis.[153] Most affected babies are normally grown with no dysmorphic features, have a normocytic anaemia with normal white cells and platelets but a low reticulocyte count and transfusion-dependent anaemia. CDA type 1 has recently been reported to be due to mutations in the codanin-1 gene[50] but the genetic basis of most cases of CDA is unknown. The prognosis of CDA is extremely variable. For transfusion-independent children with CDA, lifespan is usually normal and quality of life is good. For transfusion-dependent children, the treatment options are:

- splenectomy, which renders a small proportion of children transfusion-independent with a normal lifespan;
- bone marrow transplantation, the only curative treatment but one which carries a 10% risk of mortality or graft rejection;
- lifelong red cell transfusion with iron chelation therapy, which carries a similar prognosis to children with β-thalassaemia major (i.e. median survival of 30–40 years unless treatment compliance is very strictly enforced).

Pearson's syndrome

This rare disease is caused by mutations in mitochondrial DNA.[168] It often presents in neonates who are small for gestational age and thrive poorly in the first few weeks of life.[168] The anaemia is normocytic and associated thrombocytopenia and neutropenia are common; abnormal leukocyte vacuolation may be seen in the peripheral blood and highly characteristic vacuolation of early erythoid cells on the marrow aspirate should prompt blood to be sent for mitochondrial DNA analysis to establish the diagnosis. The prognosis of Pearson's syndrome is very poor, few children surviving beyond the second year of life.

Anaemia due to increased red cell destruction (haemolytic anaemia)

After anaemia of prematurity and anaemia due to blood letting, haemolysis is the commonest cause of neonatal anaemia. An understanding of the most likely causes and the diagnostic approach to their identification is therefore very useful in clinical practice. In addition, haemolysis should never be ignored even if the anaemia is mild and apparently trivial. This is because transient or mild haemolysis in the neonatal period may be the clue to an underlying problem with more serious manifestations later on in childhood (e.g. red cell enzymopathies) or to problems which might affect future siblings (e.g. alloimmune anaemia due to maternal red cell antibodies).

The principal clues which suggest a haemolytic anaemia are: increased numbers of reticulocytes and/or circulating nucleated RBCs, unconjugated hyperbilirubinaemia, a positive Coombs' test (if immune) and characteristic changes in the morphology of the red cells on a blood film (e.g. hereditary spherocytosis). The main types of neonatal haemolytic anaemia are listed in Table 30.4. It is usually straightforward to distinguish the cause, although rarer causes require specialist investigations which should be discussed with a haematologist once the basic investigations are to hand. The first step should be a Coombs' test, which will be positive only in the presence of immune haemolytic anaemia and not in non-immune haemolysis. The main cause of immune haemolytic anaemia is HDN (see below). The main causes of non-immune haemolysis in neonates are:

- red cell membrane disorders;
- red cell enzymopathies;
- haemoglobinopathies.

A number of congenital and primary infections can also cause haemolytic anaemia in the neonatal period, including CMV, toxoplasmosis, congenital syphilis, rubella, herpes simplex and, rarely, malaria.

Immune haemolytic anaemias including haemolytic disease of the newborn

The most common cause of Coombs'-positive haemolysis is HDN due to transplacental passage of maternal IgG alloantibodies to red cell antigens. Modern Coombs' reagents are so sensitive that a negative Coombs' test virtually excludes neonatal alloimmune haemolysis.[79] Maternal autoimmune haemolytic anaemia occasionally causes a positive Coombs' test in the neonate; however, both haemolysis and anaemia in the baby are extremely rare.

The principal alloantibodies that cause HDN are those against Rh antigens (anti-D, anti-c and anti-E), anti-Kell, anti-Kidd (J^k), anti-Duffy (F^y) and antibodies of the MNS blood group system, including anti-U. Anti-D remains the most frequent alloantibody to cause significant haemolytic anaemia, affecting 1 in 1200 pregnancies.[85,171,177] Anti-Kell antibodies are less common but can cause severe fetal and neonatal anaemia since they inhibit erythropoiesis as well as causing haemolysis.[186] Most babies with HDN present with jaundice and/or anaemia and are born to women with known antibodies. In neonates with severe anaemia, there is often evidence of extramedullary haemopoiesis, including hepatosplenomegaly and occasionally skin lesions producing the clinical appearance of 'blueberry muffin baby'.[23,190]

HDN due to ABO antibodies

ABO haemolytic disease occurs only in offspring of women of blood group O and is confined to the 1% of such women who have high-titre IgG antibodies. Haemolysis due to anti-A is more common (1 in 150 births) than anti-B. In contrast to anti-Rh antibodies, both anti-A and anti-B usually cause hyperbilirubinaemia without significant neonatal anaemia. This is mainly because there are relatively few group A or B antigenic sites on neonatal red cells, allowing the antibody-coated cells to persist for longer in the circulation.[141] As a reflection of this, the blood film in ABO haemolytic disease characteristically shows very large numbers of spherocytes with little or no increase in nucleated red cells; this contrasts to Rh HDN, where there are few spherocytes and vast numbers of circulating nucleated red cells. Management of ABO HDN usually just requires phototherapy; however, close monitoring is essential and exchange transfusion is occasionally required, particularly in cases of ABO HDN due to anti-B antibodies, which may cause severe anaemia as well as hyperbilirubinaemia.[190] Hydrops has occasionally been described.

Management of HDN

The antenatal diagnosis and management of pregnancies affected by red cell alloimmunisation requires co-operation between obstetric, paediatric and haematology teams.[68,171] All neonates at risk should have cord blood taken for measurement of haemoglobin, bilirubin and a Coombs' test and should remain in hospital until hyperbilirubinaemia and/or anaemia have been properly managed. Phototherapy should be given from birth to all Rh-alloimmunised infants with haemolysis, as the bilirubin can rise steeply after birth and this expectant approach will prevent the need for exchange transfusion in some infants. In HDN due to anti-Kell, anaemia is usually more prominent than jaundice and minimal phototherapy may be necessary despite severe anaemia.[68] Recent systematic reviews have found that treatment of neonates with alloimmune haemolysis with IVIG does reduce the need for exchange transfusion;[3,67] however, the number of studies and infants included is small and further well-designed studies are needed before IVIG can be recommended for the treatment of neonatal alloimmune haemolysis.[3]

Exchange transfusion in HDN is required for:

- severe anaemia: haemoglobin <10 g/dl at birth (with the possible exception of anti-Kell, as mentioned above); and/or
- severe or rapidly increasing hyperbilirubinaemia.

Details of the product to use for exchange transfusion are given on pages 765–7 and are summarised in the current British Committee for Standards in Haematology (BCSH) guidelines.[27]

'Late' anaemia presents at a few weeks of age in some babies with milder haemolytic disease who do not require exchange transfusion and in babies who have had earlier exchange transfusion. The blood film shows evidence of ongoing haemolysis and the anaemia is aggravated by the normal postnatal suppression of erythropoiesis. Such babies may require 'top-up' transfusion for symptomatic anaemia; conventional guidelines for neonatal transfusion can be followed (see p. 765) but irradiated blood must be used for infants previously receiving intrauterine transfusion, to prevent the risk of transfusion-associated graft-versus-host disease (TA-GVHD).[27,200] Thus, all babies found to have a positive Coombs' test at birth and all treated by intrauterine transfusion must be followed up to monitor the rate of haemoglobin fall. It is worth noting that babies with ABO HDN rarely require 'top-up' transfusion unless severe anaemia in the first few days of life (Hb <10 g/dl) has been a feature. Where the haemoglobin is falling more rapidly than normal, particularly in babies with unconjugated hyperbilirubinaemia, monitoring must be continued until the jaundice resolves and the haemoglobin reaches a plateau. This may take 8 weeks and it may be helpful to ask the haematologist to review the blood films each time, to look for evidence of ongoing haemolysis. Folic acid (500 micrograms/kg/day) should be given to all babies with haemolysis

until 3 months of age. Erythropoietin has been used to prevent the need for 'top-up' transfusion for late anaemia; both failures and successes of this approach have been reported and erythropoietin is unlikely to prevent the need for transfusion where ongoing haemolysis is brisk.[148,208]

Neonatal haemolytic anaemia due to red cell membrane disorders

A number of red cell membrane disorders may present in the neonatal period. The three most common types of presentation are:

- unexplained haemolysis with jaundice but usually only moderate anaemia (usually due to hereditary spherocytosis);
- as an incidental finding on a routine blood film in the absence of unusual jaundice or anaemia (usually hereditary elliptocytosis);
- severe, transfusion-dependent haemolytic anaemia with a characteristic very low MCV of 50–60 fl (usually due to hereditary pyropoikilocytosis).

The main clues that a neonate has a red cell membrane disorder are a family history, otherwise unexplained haemolysis and an abnormal blood film. Red cell membrane disorders can nearly always be recognised by the characteristic shape of red cells on a blood film. However, the identification of the exact type of membrane abnormality is more complex and requires specialised investigations on both the neonate and the parents and close liaison with a haematologist. The osmotic fragility test is of limited value in neonates and more often it is better to proceed to red cell membrane electrophoresis if the clinical pattern and appearance of the family blood films are suggestive of a membrane disorder. It is important to carry out these definitive diagnostic investigations (red cell membrane studies) on pre-transfusion blood samples to minimise diagnostic confusion due to transfused cells.[145]

A brief summary of the three main clinical disorders presenting in neonates is given below; for more detailed information, the reader is referred to recent reviews.[49,181]

Hereditary spherocytosis

This is the commonest red cell membrane defect. It occurs in 1 in 5000 live births to parents of Northern European extraction, but is less frequently seen in other ethnic groups.[49] It is autosomal dominant, but around 25% of cases are sporadic due to new mutations. Hereditary spherocytosis is genetically heterogeneous – mutations in spectrin, ankyrin, protein 4.1 and protein 3 have all been reported.[49,181] The usual presentation of hereditary spherocytosis in the neonate is with unconjugated hyperbilirubinaemia. Most affected neonates are not anaemic, but a small proportion have anaemia severe enough to require transfusion. The blood film in hereditary spherocytosis shows moderate numbers of spherocytes; the appearance is identical to that of ABO haemolytic disease, but the two disorders are distinguishable by the negative Coombs' test in hereditary spherocytosis. While some babies will require one or two transfusions during the first 1–2 months of life, very few remain transfusion-dependent after this time and it is important to stop transfusions to evaluate the nadir haemoglobin reached. All babies with hereditary spherocytosis should also receive folic acid supplementation (500 micrograms/kg/day or a total daily dose of 2.5 mg is sufficient in the first year of life).

Hereditary elliptocytosis
This is a more complex disorder. It is caused by different mutations in the genes for spectrin, ankyrin or protein 4.1.[49,181] In the common, autosomal dominant form of hereditary elliptocytosis, the heterozygotes have no clinical manifestations (i.e. no anaemia and no jaundice) apart from elliptocytes on the blood film. No treatment is required and folic acid prophylaxis is unnecessary, as folate deficiency is not a feature of this condition. Neonates who are homozygous or compound heterozygotes for hereditary elliptocytosis mutations have severe haemolytic anaemia; the most common form is hereditary pyropoikilocytosis (HPP).

Hereditary pyropoikilocytosis
Neonates with HPP have more than one mutation in a red cell membrane protein (they may be homozygous or compound heterozygotes).[49,181] HPP is uncommon but is important because it causes severe, transfusion-dependent haemolytic anaemia which does not improve with age. The diagnosis of HPP should easily be made by examining blood films from the baby (which shows lots of bizarre fragmented red cells and microspherocytes) and both parents (one or both often have red cell elliptocytosis); a useful diagnostic clue is the low MCV at birth (<60 fl). Red cell transfusion is usually necessary until the child is old enough to undergo splenectomy, to which there is an excellent response.

Neonatal haemolysis due to red cell enzymopathies

The principal red cell enzymopathies which present in the neonatal period are glucose-6-phosphate dehydrogenase (G6PD) deficiency and pyruvate kinase (PK) deficiency. They usually present with unconjugated hyperbilirubinaemia; clinically, they are indistinguishable from red cell membrane disorders, except that G6PD deficiency, being X-linked, is rare in female infants. Unlike with the membrane disorders, there are usually no diagnostic changes on the blood film.

Glucose-6-phosphate dehydrogenase deficiency
G6PD deficiency is seen in all ethnic groups but has a high prevalence in individuals from central Africa (20%) and the Mediterranean (10%). In neonatal G6PD deficiency, jaundice usually presents within the first few days of life and is often severe; anaemia is extremely rare and the blood film is completely normal, thus the diagnosis must be made by assaying G6PD on a peripheral blood sample.[115] It is not clear why some but not all G6PD-deficient neonates develop neonatal jaundice. In addition, the pathogenesis of the jaundice is also unclear, since most babies with G6PD deficiency have no evidence of haemolysis. The most important management issues in neonatal G6PD deficiency are close monitoring of the bilirubin, particularly

where interactions with other risk factors for neonatal hyperbilirubinaemia are present, such as Gilbert's syndrome or hereditary spherocytosis, since kernicterus has been reported in this setting,[94,95] and counselling parents of affected babies about which medicines, chemicals and foods may precipitate haemolysis (Table 30.6). If exchange transfusion is required for severe hyperbilirubinaemia, conventional guidelines for exchange transfusion can be followed (see p. 765). Certain uncommon variants of G6PD deficiency are associated with chronic haemolysis, and for these children folic acid supplements should be given.[115] However, for the vast majority of patients there is no chronic haemolysis and no anaemia and therefore folic acid supplements are not indicated.

Pyruvate kinase deficiency
PK deficiency is the second most common red cell enzymopathy in neonates. It is autosomal recessive and clinically heterogeneous, varying from anaemia severe enough to cause hydrops fetalis to a mild unconjugated hyperbilirubinaemia.[65,205] In severe cases, the jaundice has a rapid onset within 24 hours of birth and exchange transfusion may be required.[65] The diagnosis is made by measuring pre-transfusion red cell PK activity; in mild cases, the PK activity may be relatively modestly reduced, making the diagnosis difficult, and it is often useful to assay levels in the parents for confirmation. The blood film is sometimes distinctive but more often shows non-specific changes of non-spherocytic

Table 30.6 Drugs and chemicals associated with haemolysis in patients who are glucose-6-phosphate dehydrogenase (G6PD) deficient

A. Antimalarials
Primaquine
Pamaquine
(Quinine)*
(Chloroquine)*

B. Antibiotics
Nitrofurantoin
Sulphones, e.g. dapsone
Sulphonamides,† e.g. sulphamethoxazole (Septrin)
Quinolones, e.g. nalidixic acid, ciprofloxacin
(Chloramphenicol)‡

C. Analgesics
Aspirin (in high doses)
Phenacetin

D. Chemicals
Naphthalene (mothballs)
Divicine (fava beans – also known as broad beans)
Methylene blue

* Acceptable in acute malaria.
† Some sulphonamides do not cause haemolysis in most G6PD-deficient patients, e.g. sulfadiazine.
‡ To be avoided in some types of G6PD deficiency (can be taken by patients with the common, African A-form of G6PD deficiency).

haemolysis and therefore it is good practice to assay PK in all babies with unexplained haemolysis after the common causes have been excluded. Management in the neonatal period depends on the severity of the jaundice and anaemia; some but not all children are transfusion-dependent and folic acid supplements should be given to prevent deficiency due to chronic haemolysis.

Other red cell enzymopathies presenting in neonates

The other red cell enzymopathies are rare. The most important to be aware of in the neonatal period is triosephosphate isomerase deficiency, which is autosomal recessive.[163] One-third of cases present with neonatal haemolytic anaemia and this may be the only presenting feature at this age, the devastating neurological features of this disorder only becoming apparent 6–12 months later.[163] Persistent haemolysis should therefore always be investigated.

Neonatal haemolysis due to haemoglobinopathies

The haemoglobinopathies, with the exception of α-thalassaemia major, do not usually present in the neonatal period. Occasional non-thalassaemic, structural α-globin and γ-globin gene mutations, which are clinically completely silent in adults and children, cause transient haemolytic anaemia (and diagnostic confusion!) in the neonate (see below). Symptoms and signs of the major β-globin haemoglobinopathies (sickle cell disease and β-thalassaemia major) are rare in neonates, although modern techniques (e.g. HPLC, isoelectric focusing) allow the diagnosis to be made on neonatal blood samples where family studies indicate that both parents are carriers.[46] Many countries and regions with a high prevalence of haemoglobinopathies, including the UK, have neonatal screening programmes to facilitate early diagnosis, which is particularly important in sickle cell disease in order to start penicillin prophylaxis as soon as possible.[46,96,187]

Alpha-thalassaemia major

Alpha-thalassaemia major occurs when all four α-globin genes on chromosome 16 are deleted.[81] It predominantly affects families of south-east Asian origin and presents with mid-trimester fetal anaemia or hydrops fetalis which is fatal within hours of delivery (occasional babies have lived a few days). The only long-term survivors of α-thalassaemia major are those who received intrauterine transfusions.[44,165,169] In recent years there have been several reports of normal growth and development where intrauterine transfusion is commenced during the second trimester;[44,169] however, there is a high incidence of hypospadias in boys and other survivors have limb defects and/or severe neurological problems.[44,165] If intrauterine transfusions are delayed until the anaemia is severe, neonatal pulmonary hypoplasia is a cause of early mortality. The diagnosis of α-thalassaemia major should be suspected in any case of severe fetal anemia presenting in the second trimester and any case of hydrops fetalis with severe anaemia in which the parents come from south-east Asia (it is also seen occasionally in families who originate from India, the Middle East or the Mediterranean). Checking the blood counts of the parents will immediately identify whether they are at risk of having a child with α-thalassaemia major – both parents will be carriers of a chromosome 16 in which both of the two α-globin genes are deleted and so they will have hypochromic, microcytic red cell indices (MCV usually <74 fl and MCH usually <24 pg). The diagnosis of α-thalassaemia major is confirmed by haemoglobin electrophoresis or HPLC (which shows only Hb Barts and Hb Portland; HbF and HbA are absent); the blood film shows hypochromic, microcytic red cells with vast numbers of circulating nucleated red cells. Neonatal management of α-thalassaemia major has no impact on survival unless the baby has received intrauterine transfusions; for these transfused neonates, management is the same as for β-thalassaemia, i.e. lifelong red cell transfusions or bone marrow transplantation after the age of 2 years.[40,169]

Alpha- and gamma-globin chain structural abnormalities

Most α- and γ-globin gene variants are clinically silent. Occasional α-globin gene variants may cause haemolytic anaemia in the newborn because when the abnormal α-globin associates with γ-globin the resultant haemoglobin is unstable whereas when the variant α-globin associates with β-globin the resultant haemoglobin is stable. An example of this is Hb Hasharon: $\alpha^{214\text{Asp}\rightarrow\text{His}}$-$\gamma_2$ is unstable; but as γ-globin chain production is physiologically switched off and β-globin chain production predominates, the $\alpha^{214\text{Asp}\rightarrow\text{His}}$-$\beta_2$ produced is stable and the haemolytic anaemia completely resolves.[141] A similar principle occurs in the γ-globin variant HbF-Poole, which causes neonatal haemolytic anaemia that resolves as the switch from γ- to β-globin occurs.[110] These variants can be identified by haemoglobin HPLC and are worth considering when commoner causes of unexplained haemolysis have been excluded.

Beta-thalassaemias and sickle cell disease

Although these disorders are asymptomatic in neonates, if they are identified as a result of neonatal screening programmes, specialist advice should be sought as soon as possible. Babies with sickle cell disease (homozygous sickle cell disease, SC disease or S-β-thalassaemia) should be started on prophylactic penicillin V (62.5 mg twice daily) and folic acid (500 micrograms/kg/day).[187] Babies with β-thalassaemia major usually start to require transfusion around the age of 6 months but benefit from folic acid supplementation until regular transfusions begin.[140]

Anaemia due to blood loss

Blood loss causing neonatal anaemia may be very obvious, e.g. a cephalhaematoma or rupture of the cord, or be concealed and easy to miss unless specifically sought (e.g. fetomaternal bleeds). Conventionally, the causes of anaemia due to blood loss are classified according to the timing of the blood loss – during fetal life, at the time of delivery or postnatally (see Table 30.4). It is probably unnecessary to state that in neonates admitted to hospital the most common cause of anaemia is blood loss secondary to iatrogenic blood letting.

Blood loss prior to birth

Twin-to-twin transfusion

Twin-to-twin transfusion occurs in monochorionic twins with monochorial placentas (pp. 151–2).[197] Bleeding may be acute, particularly during the second stage of labour, or chronic.[197] Chronic twin-to-twin transfusion can cause a marked difference in birthweight between twins, although recent studies show that the majority of twin pairs have a discordance in haemoglobin of <5 g/dl.[197] The donor twin is smaller and may be pale and lethargic or have overt cardiac failure; the recipient twin may be plethoric, with hyperviscosity and hyperbilirubinaemia and may rarely have a haemoglobin as high as 30 g/dl. Where the haemoglobin/haematocrit are very high, disseminated intravascular coagulation (DIC) can occur. Management of DIC is described on pages 759–60, and that of polycythaemia on page 768.

Fetomaternal haemorrhage

This may occur spontaneously or secondary to trauma. Most spontaneous fetomaternal bleeds occur in the third trimester or during labour. Fetomaternal bleeds may also be increased by invasive procedures such as fetal blood sampling and caesarian section. The degree of anaemia is variable and the clinical presentation depends on the amount and rate of blood loss. Most episodes involve very small quantities of blood (0.5 ml or less) but acute loss of >20% of the blood volume may cause intrauterine death, circulatory shock or hydrops.[62] Diagnostic clues are anaemia at birth in an otherwise well term baby with no or minimal jaundice. The most useful diagnostic tests are a Coombs' test to exclude immune haemolysis, a reticulocyte count to exclude red cell aplasia, a Kleihauer test on maternal blood to quantitate the number of HbF-containing fetal RBCs in the maternal circulation, and a blood film.[84] Where the baby has bled acutely just prior to delivery, the blood film is normochromic/normocytic with large numbers of nucleated red cells. In this situation, the haemoglobin may be normal at delivery but fall rapidly as haemodilution occurs. Where there is chronic blood loss, the baby is often well but may present with cardiac failure; the blood film in this situation is hypochromic/microcytic, the nucleated red cells are less prominent and the Kleihauer result may be difficult to interpret. Another point of note is that where there is ABO incompatibility between the mother and baby, the fetal cells may be rapidly destroyed within the maternal circulation – a high index of suspicion of fetomaternal haemorrhage as a cause of neonatal anaemia is needed because it is important to perform the Kleihauer test as soon as possible, to increase the chance of detection of fetal cells. In many cases, an acute fetomaternal bleed supervenes upon chronic fetomaternal blood loss. In this situation, severe anaemia (Hb <5 g/dl) has been shown to confer a poor prognosis, as most survivors have evidence of brain injury.[62]

Blood loss at or after delivery

Blood loss around the time of delivery is usually due to obstetric complications, including placenta praevia, placental abruption or incision of the placenta during caesarean section. Such babies are often extremely ill with circulatory shock, anaemia worsening rapidly after birth, large numbers of circulating nucleated red cells and DIC. Similar haematological changes occur after massive internal bleeding in the baby, e.g. subaponeurotic or retroperitoneal bleeding, and may be particularly severe where there is damage to the liver. While most cases of internal bleeding will be associated with traumatic delivery, it is important to search for any underlying bleeding diathesis in such babies, particularly haemophilia A or B and vitamin K deficiency. Inherited and acquired coagulation disorders that may present with bleeding at birth or during the neonatal period are discussed on pages 756–60.

Anaemia of prematurity

Pathogenesis

The haemoglobin falls after birth in all newborns, regardless of gestational age. This normal physiological fall in haemoglobin is greater in preterm compared with term neonates and has been termed 'physiological anaemia of prematurity' since it does not appear to be associated with any abnormalities in the baby. The pathogenesis is not fully elucidated but contributory factors include the reduced red cell lifespan of fetal erythrocytes, the relatively low erythropoietin concentration and the rapid growth rate.[141] In practice, the routine supplementation of preterm neonates with folic acid and iron means that nutritional deficiency rarely plays a role.[57,70,152] On the other hand, for the majority of preterm infants in hospital, iatrogenic blood letting for diagnostic tests contributes to this physiological process. The clinical significance of anaemia of prematurity is mainly that the need for 'top-up' transfusion in preterm infants can be reduced if clinicians are aware of the normal nadir in erythropoiesis in neonates and the available measures to prevent the anaemia becoming severe.

Diagnosis

In a well term infant, the nadir in haemoglobin is as low as 9.4–11 g/dl and occurs at 8–12 weeks of age (see Table 30.2); for a preterm infant, the nadir in haemoglobin occurs earlier (4–8 weeks of age) and is lower (6.5–9 g/dl). The diagnosis is usually straightforward – a well preterm baby has a slowly falling haemoglobin with a completely unremarkable blood film showing normochromic/normocytic red cells, slightly low reticulocytes $(20 \times 10^9/l)$ and no nucleated red cells.

Management

There are three facets to the management of anaemia of prematurity. The first is to exclude other causes of anaemia using clinical features and diagnostic algorithm (see p. 750, Fig. 30.2). Secondly, a decision whether or not to transfuse should be made (the indications and principles of neonatal transfusion are discussed in detail on pp. 764–8). Thirdly, with increasing recognition of potential transfusion hazards, amelioration of neonatal anaemia to reduce the need for transfusion has become extremely important.

The role of erythropoietin and haematinics

The severity of anaemia of prematurity and thereby the need for red cell transfusion can be reduced by a combination of the

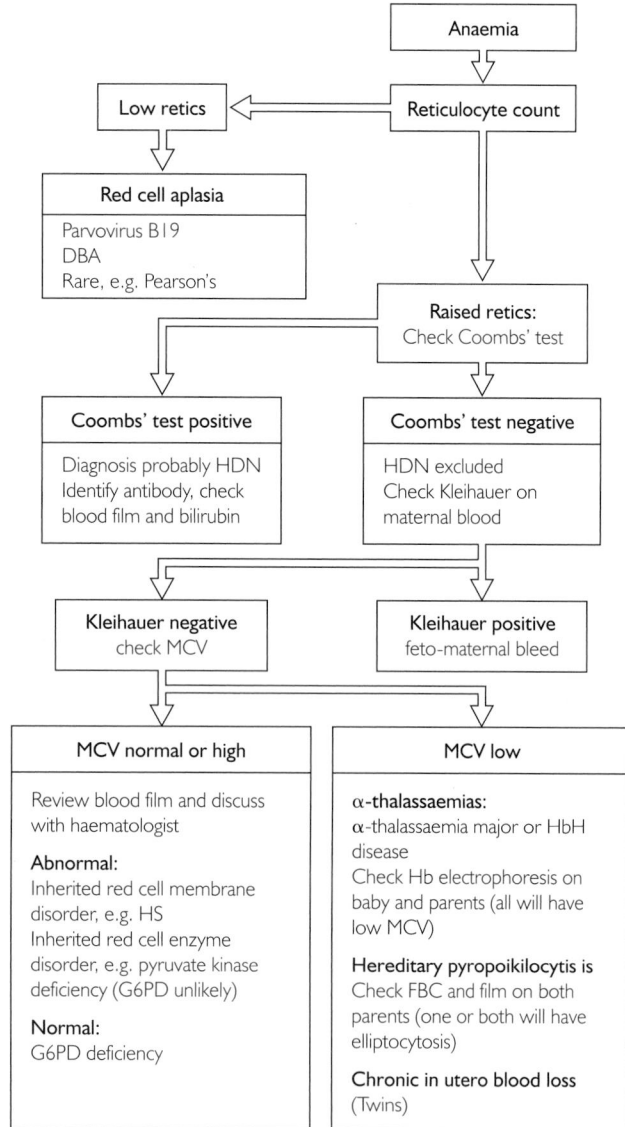

Fig. 30.2 A diagnostic algorithm for neonatal anaemia. The most useful screening tests for investigating unexplained neonatal anaemia are the reticulocyte (retic) count, the Coombs' test and the mean cell volume (MCV) of the red blood cells. DBA, Diamond–Blackfan anaemia; G6PD, glucose-6-phosphate dehydrogenase; HDN, haemolyic disease of the newborn; HS, hereditary spherocytosis.

following approaches:

- limiting iatrogenic blood loss by appropriate use of blood tests;[111,116]
- iron and folate supplementation for all preterm infants:
  - iron 3 mg/kg/day from 4–6 weeks of age (a pragmatic approach is to give 1 ml of sodium ironedetate – 'Sytron' – once daily) or iron-fortified formula with 0.5–0.9 mg/dl iron;[70,152]
  - folic acid 50 micrograms daily or 500 micrograms once weekly;[57]
- judicious use of erythropoietin.[61,136,185]

The many controlled trials of erythropoietin for prevention of neonatal anaemia have been extensively reviewed,[136] including two recent meta-analyses,[61,185] and are only briefly summarised here. Recombinant erythropoietin is biologically effective in that it stimulates erythropoiesis in all preterm infants and there is no evidence of erythropoietin insensitivity. Erythropoietin is also able to reduce red cell transfusion requirements in preterm infants.[61,118,125,136,185] However, in most studies there is no evidence to support the clinical effectiveness of erythropoietin, i.e. that it reduces the number of transfusions to an extent which demonstrably reduces the hazards of transfusion. At best, the studies show that erythropoietin reduces the number of transfusions in the relatively well infants with low transfusion requirements.[61,118,125,185] Unfortunately, even in high doses, the erythropoietin-mediated increase in red cell production is unable to increase sufficiently to cope with the need for frequent phlebotomy and multiple transfusions in sick preterm infants.[51,138] Despite its marginal role in reducing transfusion requirements, erythropoietin may become more important again if worries over the safety of blood transfusion lead to reduced availability and parental acceptance of red cell transfusion. At present, the main therapeutic roles for erythropoietin in neonates are:

- in preventing anaemia in infants who have received intrauterine transfusions for alloantibody-mediated anaemia;[208]
- in a non-emergency situation where red cell transfusions are against the parents' wishes and are not felt to be absolutely essential to save the life of the baby (e.g. preterm babies of Jehovah's witnesses).[83]

An effective dose of recombinant erythropoietin in this setting is 300 micrograms/kg as a single subcutaneous injection three times per week starting in the first week of life. Epoetin beta should be used in view of the potential risk of red cell aplasia described (in adults) with epoetin alpha, the alternative form of recombinant erythropoietin.[38] This is because the haemoglobin does not start to rise until about 10–14 days after erythropoietin has been commenced. In addition, iron supplements (Sytron, as above) should be started as soon as possible, to prevent the rapid development of iron deficiency in erythropoietin-treated infants (the dose may need to be increased up to a maximum of 9 mg/kg if iron deficiency develops on the standard dose of Sytron).[16]

A simple diagnostic approach to neonatal anaemia

Red cell disorders associated with neonatal or fetal anaemia present in three main ways: with a low haemoglobin (anaemia), with jaundice due to haemolysis or with hydrops. Table 30.4 lists the most common causes of anaemia, and the most common haematological causes of jaundice and hydrops are shown in Table 30.7 and Table 30.5, respectively. A diagnostic algorithm to help identify which of these causes is most likely, which can be excluded and what further investigations are most appropriate, is shown in Figure 30.2. This is based on simple observations and simple tests available in almost all haematology laboratories. Where in doubt about the best investigations to use and the interpretation of the results, discussion with a haematologist at an early stage should be helpful.

Table 30.7 Haematological causes of neonatal jaundice

A. *Immune*
   Haemolytic disease of the newborn
   Maternal autoimmune haemolytic anaemia

B. *Red cell membrane disorders*
   Hereditary spherocytosis
   Homozygous hereditary elliptocytosis
   Hereditary pyropoikilocytosis

C. *Red cell enzymopathies*
   G6PD deficiency
   Pyruvate kinase deficiency
   Other: e.g. glucose phosphate isomerase deficiency

D. *Haemoglobinopathies*
   α-thalassaemias (α-thalassaemia major; severe HbH disease)
   γ-thalassaemias (e.g. Hb Hasharon)
   Other: sickle cell syndromes (occasionally)

E. *Infection*
   Bacterial
   Viral, e.g. CMV, rubella, herpes simplex
   Protozoal, e.g. toxoplasma, malaria, syphilis

Table 30.8 Causes of neonatal polycythaemia

Intrauterine growth restriction
Maternal hypertension
Maternal diabetes
Chromosomal disorders: trisomy 21, 18 or 13
Twin–twin transfusion
Delayed clamping of the cord
Endocrine disorders: thyrotoxicosis, congenital adrenal
   hyperplasia

Polycythaemia

For both term and preterm infants, polycythaemia can be defined as a central venous haematocrit of >0.65. At haematocrits in excess of 0.65, there is an exponential rise in blood viscosity.[199] However, even at haematocrits >0.70, only a minority of neonates exhibit clinical signs of hyperviscosity. The clinical manifestations include lethargy, hypotonia, hyperbilirubinaemia and hypoglycaemia.[195] Polycythaemia may also be a contributory factor in neonatal seizures, stroke, renal vein thrombosis and necrotising enterocolitis (NEC).[71] Causes of polycythaemia are shown in Table 30.8. Treatment of neonatal polycythaemia is controversial and is probably not necessary in infants with very minor symptoms (e.g. borderline hypoglycaemia or poor peripheral perfusion). However, most of the evidence supports active management of infants with a haematocrit >0.65 in association with symptoms or signs indicative of an adverse long-term outcome (e.g. refractory hypoglycaemia, neurological signs). For these infants, partial exchange transfusion using a crystalloid solution such as normal saline should be performed to reduce the haematocrit to 0.55.[195] There is no evidence to support the use of fresh frozen plasma (FFP) or albumin[202] for this procedure, both of which carry the risk of transfusion-transmitted infection.

White cell disorders

Introduction and normal values

Apart from alterations in the numbers of white blood cells in response to infection, disorders of white cells are not common in neonates. Nevertheless, some diagnostic dilemmas do present in the neonatal period, in particular the causes and investigation of neutropenia and how to identify rare disorders such as congenital leukaemia (both described below). However, there is often a lot of very useful information that can be discovered just from looking carefully at the morphology of the white blood cells on a neonatal blood film. Not only can an early diagnosis of bacterial infection often be made in this way, but there may be indicators of the type of bacterial infection, of NEC, of congenital viral infections, or even of rare genetic and metabolic disorders, as discussed on page 753.

Normal values

Neutrophil and monocyte counts vary over the first few days of life even in healthy babies, increasing for the first 12 hours and then falling to a nadir at 4 days of age. Normal values for neutrophils at birth are also affected by other factors, including antenatal history, perinatal history and ethnic origin. The neutrophil count is higher in capillary samples and after vigorous crying; it is lower in neonates of African origin. All of the other types of white blood cell found in adult blood are also present in the newborn (see Table 30.2). Conversely, some cell types not found in healthy adults are seen in healthy preterm babies – these include blast cells, other early myeloid cells, nucleated red cells and even occasional megakaryocytes.

Neutropenia

Definition and causes of neonatal neutropenia

Transient neutropenia is fairly common in preterm neonates but is uncommon in term infants. The normal values for neutrophil counts vary both with gestational age and with postnatal age, particularly over the first few days of life. A pragmatic approach is to consider a neutrophil count at birth of $<2 \times 10^9$/l as abnormal and worth monitoring and a neutrophil count during the first month of life of $<0.7 \times 10^9$/l as significant enough to merit further investigation. The principal causes of neonatal neutropenia are shown in Table 30.9. The commonest cause in preterm neonates is neutropenia in association with IUGR and/or maternal hypertension,[102] while in term infants bacterial or viral infection is the usual explanation. Other important causes of

Table 30.9 Causes of neonatal neutropenia

1. Placental insufficiency
  Maternal hypertension
  Intrauterine growth restriction
  Maternal diabetes

2. Infection
  Acute, perinatal bacterial infection, e.g. group B streptococcus
  Congenital infections, e.g. CMV
  Postnatal bacterial infections
  Postnatal viral infections, e.g. CMV

3. Necrotising enterocolitis

4. Immune
  Alloimmune

5. Genetic
  Trisomies: 21, 13 and 18
  Kostmann's syndrome
  Schwachman's syndrome
  Pearson's syndrome
  Reticular dysgenesis
  Metabolic disorders, e.g. hyperglycinaemia, isovaleric,
    propionic and methylmalonic acidaemia

6. Marrow replacement
  Congenital leukaemia

neutropenia, as they may be the cause of severe neonatal infection, are alloimmune neutropenia and congenital neutropenia due to failure of neutrophil production (e.g. Kostmann's syndrome) (pp. 1006–7).

Neutropenia and infection

Any bacterial infection can cause acute neutropenia – where this is short-lived (6–12 hours) it is a normal response, but neutropenia lasting >12 hours in the setting of acute bacterial infection is usually a poor prognostic sign. Examination of the blood film is often helpful in differentiating neutropenia secondary to bacterial infection from that due to viral infection or IUGR. The classical signs of acute bacterial infection are the presence of an increased percentage of band neutrophils and toxic granulation of immature and mature neutrophils, followed after 1–2 days by a mature neutrophilia and after 3–5 days by eosinophilia. By contrast, there is no increase in band cells or toxic granulation in viral infections; instead, atypical 'viral' lymphocytes are seen, particularly in congenital CMV infection, where they may persist for several months.

Neutropenia and IUGR

The commonest cause of neutropenia in preterm infants is IUGR and/or maternal hypertension or maternal diabetes. In these disorders, neutrophil production is reduced because of inadequate numbers of neutrophil progenitors; most affected neonates also have thrombocytopenia and increased erythropoiesis (polycythaemia and/or increased circulating nucleated red cells).[195] The exact pathogenesis is unknown but evidence suggests that the haematological abnormalities are secondary to fetal tissue hypoxia.[195] The neutropenia resolves spontaneously, usually starting to recover 2–3 days after birth. However, both the duration and the severity of the neutropenia are directly related to the severity of the IUGR/maternal hypertension.[102,195] The main clinical significance of this form of neutropenia is firstly that recognition of its natural history prevents unnecessary treatment and investigations, and secondly that affected neonates do tend to have a 'blunted' neutrophil response to infection, i.e. the neutrophil response is both delayed and sometimes inadequate, which may lead to an increased frequency and duration of bacterial infections. There are no specific diagnostic tests for this form of neutropenia but clues that this is the explanation for the neutropenia are the clinical history, the concomitant presence of a platelet count $<150 \times 10^9/l$, an increased number of circulating nucleated RBCs (usually >20/100 white cells) and the severity (usually the neutrophil count is $>0.3 \times 10^9/l$). To date, neither of the recombinant haemopoietic growth factors available for therapeutic use in stimulating neutrophil production has been shown to be of clinical value in the treatment or prevention of IUGR-associated neutropenia, although both factors do increase the numbers of circulating neutrophils in such babies: within 24 hours in the case of G-CSF and slightly longer for GM-CSF.

Alloimmune neutropenia

Alloimmune neutropenia is the neutrophil equivalent of HDN and alloimmune thrombocytopenia. It occurs where fetal neutrophils express paternally derived neutrophil-specific antigens which are absent on maternal neutrophils and against which the mother produces IgG neutrophil alloantibodies.[117] The causative antibodies are usually anti-NA1 or anti-NA2.[173] It is widely quoted that alloimmune neutropenia affects 3% of all deliveries,[117] although relatively few cases are reported and in our experience this is a very uncommon clinical problem. This suggests that while the causative antibodies may be present in 3% of women, most neonatal cases are so mild that the signs do not merit medical attention. Therefore, from a practical perspective, the importance of neonatal alloimmune neutropenia is that it should be thought of as a possible cause of neutropenia in any neonate with a severe bacterial infection together with a neutropenia which persists for more than 3 days despite appropriate antibiotic treatment. Clinically significant neonatal alloimmune neutropenia presents in the first few days of life with fever and infections of the respiratory tract, urinary tract and skin, particularly due to *Staphylococcus aureus*. The diagnosis is made by demonstrating antineutrophil antibodies in the mother and baby which react against paternal, but not maternal, neutrophil antigens. The neutropenia is self-limiting, usually resolving within 1–2 months, and the mainstay of treatment is antibiotics. In severe cases, where there is clinical deterioration despite antibiotics, plasma exchange and/or G-CSF (10 micrograms/kg/day) may be helpful.[157]

Congenital and inherited neutropenias

All of the inherited and congenital neutrophil disorders are rare. The possible causes are listed in Table 30.9. These should be sought where the neutropenia is prolonged, if there is a relevant family history or consanguinity, or if the baby has typical dysmorphic features (e.g. thumb/radial abnormalities in Fanconi's anaemia). The most likely of these to present in the neonatal period is severe congenital neutropenia (Kostmann's syndrome; pp. 1006–7), in which neutrophil production is reduced due to an 'arrest' of differentiation at the myelocyte/promyelocyte stage. Infants with Kostmann's usually present with severe infections within a few weeks of birth.[206] Other clues to the diagnosis are that the neutropenia is marked (usually $<0.2 \times 10^9/l$) and there is often a marked compensatory monocytosis. The inheritance of Kostmann's can be either autosomal recessive or autosomal dominant. The diagnosis is made on the basis of the severity of the neutropenia, the bone marrow appearances, the clinical history and the absence of antineutrophil antibodies. Several cases of Kostmann's syndrome have recently been found to be due to mutations in the neutrophil elastase gene[12] and, where mutational analysis is available, this may prove useful for establishing the diagnosis and for prenatal diagnosis.

Congenital leukaemias and haematological abnormalities associated with Down syndrome

Congenital leukaemias

Congenital leukaemia is rare but the diagnosis is usually straightforward. The most common types are acute monoblastic leukaemia and acute megakaryoblastic leukaemia.[25] Around 25% of cases occur in babies with Down syndrome.[108] The usual presentation is with clinical signs of anaemia and skin lesions caused by focal infiltration by leukaemic cells. Rapid clinical deterioration due to severe anaemia and thrombocytopenia is common. Congenital leukaemia may also present as 'blueberry muffin' baby or hydrops fetalis.[23] Diagnostic clues to congenital leukaemia are the concomitant presence of severe and worsening anaemia and thrombocytopenia in a sick baby, usually with a very high white blood cell count. The diagnosis is established by examination of the blood film, which shows large numbers of primitive blast cells, and a bone marrow aspirate, bone marrow cytogenetics and immunophenotyping of the peripheral blood (or marrow) leukaemic cells. The prognosis is extremely poor; few are cured by chemotherapy, and bone marrow transplantation, which has been carried out successfully, may be the best option.[13]

Haematological abnormalities in neonates with Down syndrome and other trisomies

Haematological abnormalities are more common in neonates with chromosomal disorders, including Down syndrome, trisomy 13 and trisomy 18, all of which may be associated with pancytopenia. Most babies with Down syndrome have an apparently normal blood count, but at least 10% have one of the three following abnormalities:[108]

- acute leukaemia (discussed above);
- transient abnormal myelopoiesis (TAM);
- mild pancytopenia with subtle myelodysplastic changes.

TAM presents with leukocytosis and an abnormal blood film with circulating blast cells.[108] Mutations in GATA-1, a critical haemopoietic cell transcription factor, have recently been reported both in TAM and in the megakaryoblastic leukaemia associated with Down syndrome.[82,196] Usually, no treatment is indicated for TAM, which almost always resolves by the age of 2–3 months;[108] occasionally neonates die from fulminant hepatic involvement.

Abnormal leukocytes in neonatal systemic disease

Careful examination of the blood film often provides clues to other underlying disorders in the newborn. As well as classical features of acute bacterial and viral infections, characteristic changes can be seen in fungal infection, where vacuolation of the neutrophils and monocytes may be prominent and fungi may be seen within the phagocytic cells. In NEC, neutrophil and monocyte vacuolation are almost always present and is usually a very early feature. A number of metabolic and storage disorders also produce changes in the appearance of leukocytes:

- leukocyte vacuolation in Pearson's syndrome (see p. 743);
- giant neutrophil granules in Chediak–Higashi syndrome;
- Alder Reilly leukocyte granules in Hunter's syndrome, Hurler's syndrome and Sanfilippo's syndrome;
- lymphocyte vacuolation in Wolman's disease, α-mannosidosis, sialidosis and Sanfilippo's syndrome.

Haemostasis and thrombosis in the newborn

Introduction

Problems of disordered coagulation with or without obvious bleeding are relatively common in neonates, especially when they are sick. Thrombotic problems are also increasingly recognised in neonates, and the number of genetic and acquired causes of thrombophilia that can be identified in neonates and their families is rising. Therefore, in order to request and interpret the most useful laboratory tests, and to treat appropriately, it is important to have a basic understanding of normal haemostasis and how it differs in neonates compared with in older infants and children.

Haemostasis, the process of normal blood coagulation, takes place via a series of complex, tightly regulated interactions involving both activators and inhibitors of coagulation.[87] In general, defects in the coagulation proteins (such as the vitamin K-dependent factors), in platelet number or function, or in the fibrinolytic pathway are associated with an increased risk of bleeding. In contrast, defects in the naturally occurring anticoagulants (such as protein C) or in the vessel wall (such as damage from vascular catheters) are associated with thrombosis. However, in many cases, both pro- and anticoagulant abnormalities can occur at the same time, as seen, for example, in DIC.

The process can be summarised as follows. In the first stage, tissue factor (TF) binds to the coagulation factor VIIa, and the TF–VIIa complex, by converting factor X to Xa, leads to the generation of small amounts of thrombin (Fig. 30.3a). In the second stage, amplification of the coagulation cascade then occurs as the thrombin activates factor V and factor VIII, and the TF–VIIa activates factor IX, leading to the rapid generation of more thrombin. Thrombin also activates factor XI, further amplifying its own generation (see Fig. 30.3b). Finally, thrombin converts fibrinogen to fibrin with subsequent cross-linking by factor XIII to stabilise the clot. The role of TF has only relatively recently been recognised. It is of particular interest as it is produced not only by endothelial cells but also by monocytes.[123] TF is increased by endotoxin and proinflammatory cytokines and so is likely to play an important role in the pathogenesis of sepsis-associated DIC.[142]

Platelets

The role of platelets in coagulation is also critical, as shown by the risk of severe bleeding in patients with thrombocytopenia. Endothelial damage leads to exposure not only of TF but also of collagen, which binds von Willebrand's factor (vWF) produced by the endothelial cells. Platelets are first captured by the vWF via their glycoprotein Ib (Gp1b) receptors and are then 'tethered' by activation of their glycoprotein IIb/IIIa (GpIIb/IIIa) receptors, which bind to both vWF and fibrinogen. More and more platelets accumulate, followed by more vWF and fibrinogen, to form an occlusive platelet plug.

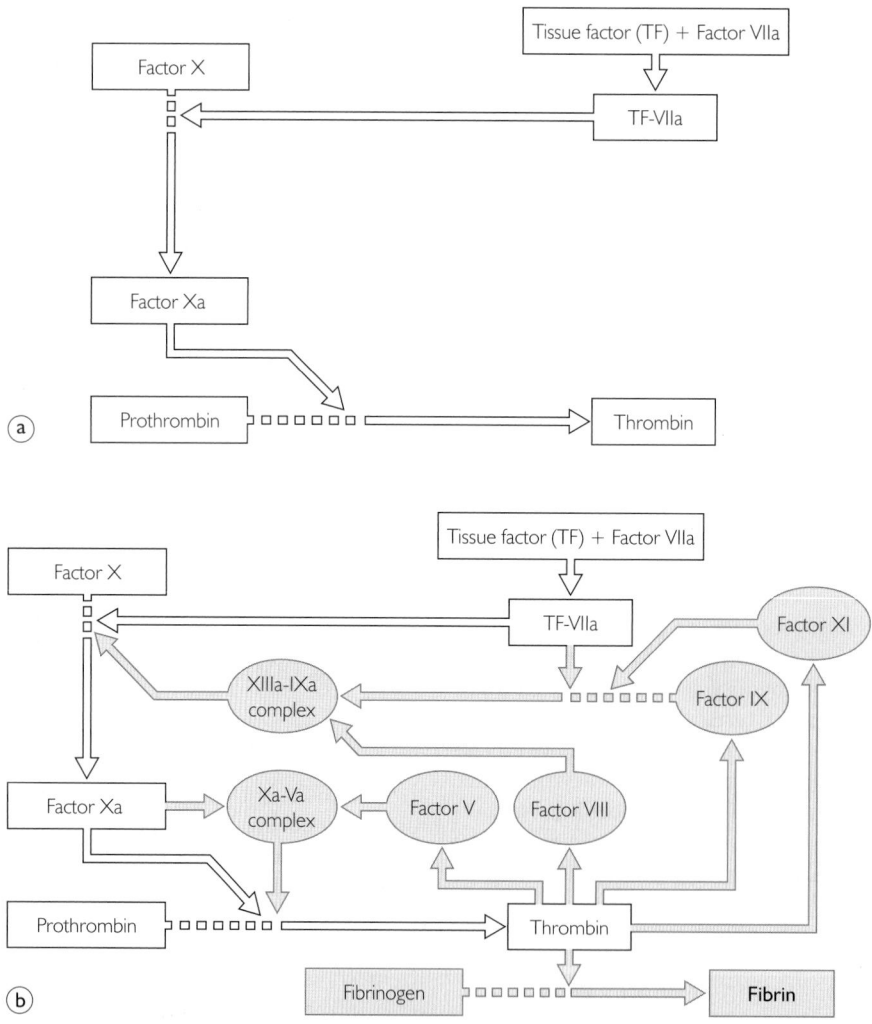

Fig. 30.3 A simplified scheme of the coagulation cascade. The first stage in the coagulation cascade is the binding of tissue factor (TF) to the coagulation factor VIIa. The TF–VIIa complex, by converting factor X to Xa, leads to the generation of small amounts of thrombin (a). In the second stage, amplification of the coagulation cascade then occurs as the thrombin activates factor V and factor VIII, and the TF–VIIa activates factor IX, leading to the rapid generation of more thrombin. Thrombin also activates factor XI, further amplifying its own generation (b). Finally, thrombin converts fibrinogen to fibrin with subsequent cross-linking by factor XIII to stabilise the clot.

Regulation of the procoagulant process by endogenous anticoagulants and fibrinolysis

The procoagulant process is regulated by a large number of mechanisms, some of which remain to be fully elucidated. These include the natural anticoagulants (antithrombin; protein C/protein S/thrombomodulin), TF pathway inhibitor (TFPI) and the fibrinolytic pathway.[53] The physiological importance of the natural anticoagulants is clear from the high propensity to thrombosis seen in patients with deficiency of one or more of these factors (see pp. 756–60). The main purpose of the natural anticoagulants is to limit the generation of thrombin and thereby prevent thrombosis. Antithrombin, heparin cofactor II and α_2-macroglobulin are direct inhibitors of thrombin. The protein C/protein S/thrombomodulin pathway is also activated by thrombin and does not function in the absence of thrombin. Current models (Fig. 30.4) indicate that activation of protein C requires binding of protein C to two receptors on the endothelial surface, thrombomodulin and the endothelial protein C receptor, which then act as a molecular switch to limit the procoagulant activity of thrombin.[103] The activated protein C then forms a complex with protein S and the protein C/S complex cleaves and inactivates factors Va and VIIIa, thus switching off thrombin generation. Consequently, vascular endothelium plays a key role in haemostasis not only by providing the principal initiator of coagulation (TF), but also by switching off the process via thrombomodulin. (It may also be relevant that intact endothelium secretes prostaglandin I_2 and nitric oxide, which promote vasodilatation and inhibit platelet aggregation, although the role of these compounds in preventing neonatal thrombosis is not clear.)

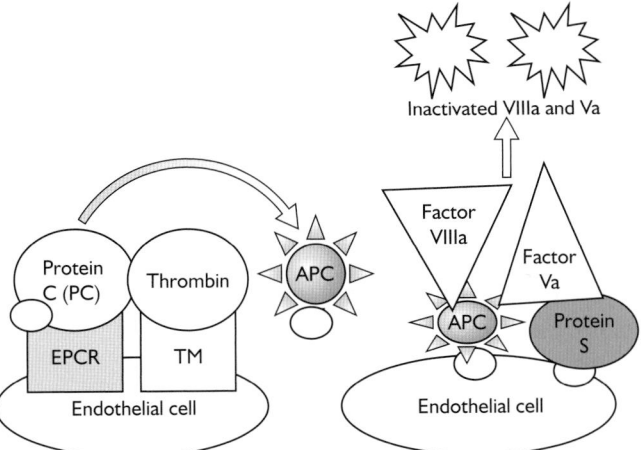

Fig. 30.4 Inactivation of activated factor VIII and factor V by the protein C/S pathway. The protein C/protein S/thrombomodulin pathway is activated by thrombin. The activation of protein C requires binding of protein C to two receptors on the endothelial surface, thrombomodulin (TM) and the endothelial protein C receptor (EPCR), which then act as a molecular switch to limit the procoagulant activity of thrombin. The activated protein C (APC) then forms a complex with protein S, and the protein C/S complex cleaves and inactivates factors Va and VIIIa, thus switching off thrombin generation.

A further mechanism preventing sustained activation of the procoagulant pathway is TFPI, which limits TF-induced initiation of coagulation, although its precise role remains to be defined, as deficiency states have not yet been characterised. Finally, the risks of uncontrolled thrombosis due to activation of the procoagulant process are limited by the fibrinolytic pathway. Fibrinolysis controls fibrin deposition at the site of injury via the activity of the serine protease plasmin and by thrombin-activated fibrinolysis inhibitor (TAFI).[22] Like other aspects of the haemostatic system, this pathway is subject to feedback control to provide a balance between coagulation and fibrinolysis. For example, fibrin itself stimulates release of tissue plasminogen activator (t-PA) and urokinase-type plasminogen activator (u-PA), which convert plasminogen into plasmin. Plasmin rapidly digests both fibrin and fibrinogen, leading to the production of fibrin degradation products (FDPs). Plasmin is also able to digest fibrin cross-linked by factor XIII, leading to the generation of D-dimers.

Developmental haemostasis

Coagulation proteins are synthesised by the fetus from the fifth week of gestation onwards and are present at measurable levels from the tenth week of gestation.[5] Levels gradually rise during fetal life but, with some exceptions (see below), do not reach adult values until several months after birth, even in term babies. Thus, 'normal values' in the neonate vary not only with gestational but also with postnatal age (Appendix 2). Coagulation proteins do not cross the placenta, or do so in very small amounts, and therefore need to be independently synthesised by the fetus. However, fetal coagulation factor synthesis can be affected by maternal factors (e.g. warfarin, severe maternal vitamin K deficiency).

There are relatively few data about the normal ranges of the coagulation factors at different gestational ages. In addition, the results can be difficult to interpret as there are differences between the levels measured in cord blood as compared with the levels collected from fetal blood by fetoscopy at the same gestational age, perhaps because of activation of coagulation during birth.[8] The published data for coagulation factor levels in preterm neonates are for those born between 30 and 36 weeks' gestation (Appendix 2).[7] Corresponding data are also available for term babies (Appendix 2).[8] Data for babies at <30 weeks' gestation derive from fetoscopy samples and show that the levels of the vitamin K-dependent factors (II, VII, IX and X) and of factors XI and XII are all low (<40% of adult values) and remain so during the first month of life.[154] By contrast, even in preterm babies (>30 weeks), levels of factor V, factor XIII and fibrinogen are normal at birth and levels of factor VIII and vWF are normal or increased.

Blood platelet counts at birth in term and preterm neonates are within the normal adult range.[155] Many studies have found impaired function of neonatal platelets in vitro in term and preterm infants; the most consistent abnormalities are reduced aggregation in response to adrenaline, ADP and thrombin. Their significance in clinical practice is unclear since the bleeding time tested with adult and neonatal devices is normal in term and preterm infants (<135 seconds)[174] and bleeding problems associated with abnormal platelet function are rare in neonates. There are also important gestational and postnatal age-related changes in the levels of the fibrinolytic and natural anticoagulant pathways (see p. 754).

Diagnostic approach to bleeding in neonates

Clinical presentation of bleeding disorders

The clinical presentation and likely cause(s) of bleeding in neonates depend on gestational age and whether the infant is sick or well. There are also particular patterns of bleeding which suggest the underlying diagnosis, such as bleeding from the umbilical cord stump in factor XIII deficiency and bleeding after circumcision in haemophilia. The most common sites of bleeding in preterm neonates are oozing from venepuncture sites, pulmonary haemorrhage, gastrointestinal bleeding and intracranial haemorrhage. In term neonates, cephalhaematomas are commonly seen following both normal and forceps deliveries. There is an increased incidence of cephalhaematoma and subarachnoid haemorrhage following vacuum extraction[198] but in otherwise healthy neonates these bleeding manifestations are unlikely to be markers of disordered haemostasis. However, a neonate with a large subaponeurotic or subdural haemorrhage should be screened for coagulation defects.[47] Germinal matrix/intraventricular haemorrhage (GMH-IVH) in term babies is also rare and should point to a possible coagulation defect. GMH-IVH and thalamic haemorrhage in term babies is often secondary to venous thrombosis (pp. 761–4) and a thrombophilia screen may be indicated. In any infant with abnormal bleeding, blood tests to identify the most likely cause should always be accompanied by a thorough clinical assessment, including sites of possible occult bleeding, and a careful history, including maternal/infant drugs (was vitamin K given?) and questions to elucidate a family history of bleeding disorders.

Screening tests for bleeding disorders

Nearly all significant bleeding disorders in neonates can be identified using simple screening tests as summarised below. Notable exceptions are factor XIII deficiency (which requires a specific assay) and platelet function disorders (which require specialised tests and are usually performed after the neonatal period, because of the difficulties of sample size and data interpretation in neonates). Where an inherited defect is suspected or where bleeding and coagulation assay derangement is severe, it is extremely important to test both parents for coagulation abnormalities. There are several reasons for this: there is considerable inter-individual variation in factor levels in neonates; there is also overlap between the deficiency states and the lower limit of normal, particularly in preterm neonates, when levels of many factors are physiologically low; and, finally, it is often difficult to obtain good-quality neonatal samples free from in-vitro activation or contamination with heparin.

The most useful screening tests in neonates are:

- *Prothrombin time* (PT) – this predominantly measures the activity of factors II, V, VII and X.
- *Activated partial thromboplastin time* (APTT) – this predominantly measures the activity of factors II, V, VIII, IX, X, XI and XII.
- *Thrombin time* (TT) – this tests for deficiency or dysfunction of fibrinogen.
- Quantitative fibrinogen assay.
- Platelet count.

The results of these tests along with the clinical history will guide subsequent investigation. A *Reptilase time* (so named because snake venom is used in the test) can also be very helpful; it assesses the same components as a TT but is unaffected by heparin and so is useful where heparin contamination from an indwelling line is suspected. Bleeding times are generally unhelpful in neonates and have been abandoned in most centres. Instead, platelet function is usually assessed by platelet aggregometry using a limited range of agonists and by a newly developed machine which measures platelet-dependent clot formation in whole blood (the platelet function analyser PFA-100™).[90]

Interpretation of coagulation screen results

Interpretation can often be difficult, particularly in preterm babies and in those who are sick, because the cause is usually multifactorial. Broadly there are two ways to approach this: firstly, by considering the causes for an abnormality in each individual test (Table 30.10), and secondly, by considering the pattern of results expected in the most common, clinically important conditions. These are discussed in more detail in the sections on inherited and acquired disorders (pp. 756–60).

Inherited coagulation disorders

While inherited coagulation disorders are rare, some of the most severe disorders may present in the neonatal period with life-threatening bleeding in otherwise healthy babies. The commonest are the X-linked disorders factor VIII deficiency (haemophilia A), which has a frequency of 1 in 5000 male births, and factor IX deficiency (haemophilia B), which occurs in 1 in 30 000 male births.[105] It is important to note that one-third of cases have no family history of haemophilia as they are due to new mutations. The other inherited coagulation disorders which may present with bleeding in the neonatal period are the severe forms of von Willebrand's disease (vWD; type 3 and occasionally type 2b), factor XIII deficiency, and deficiencies of factors II, V, VII, X and XI, which are all autosomal recessive and relatively rare.

Haemophilia A: factor VIII deficiency

Clinical presentation

The majority of cases of haemophilia A present in the second year of life and are diagnosed after presenting with a bleeding episode, which can be prolonged and life threatening. However, recent data show that almost 40% of cases present in the neonatal period.[105] In neonates, the most common sites of bleeding are intracranial haemorrhage (around 25% of cases), subgaleal or

Table 30.10 Causes of abnormal coagulation tests in the newborn

Prolonged APTT alone	Inherited deficiency of factor VIII, factor IX, factor XI, factor XII Heparin (therapeutic or heparin contamination*)
Prolonged PT alone	Inherited deficiency of factor VII Vitamin K deficiency (haemorrhagic disease of the newborn) Warfarin
Prolonged TT alone	Low fibrinogen Artefact: contamination with heparin from line or sample bottle*
Prolonged APTT + PT	Inherited deficiency of factor II, factor V, factor X Liver disease
Prolonged APTT, PT and TT	Inherited deficiency of fibrinogen DIC Severe liver disease
Normal APTT, PT and TT	Factor XIII deficiency Platelet defect: thrombocytopenia or rare platelet function abnormality (e.g. Bernard Soulier syndrome)

APTT, activated partial thromboplastin time; PT, prothrombin time; TT, thrombin time.

* The effect of heparin contamination can be distinguished by checking the Reptilase time on a coagulation sample; where a prolonged TT and/or a prolonged APTT is due to heparin contamination, the Reptilase time will be normal, but where a prolonged TT or APTT is due to a true coagulation defect, the Reptilase time will be abnormal.

cephalhaematomas (10–15% of cases), bleeding post circumcision (up to 30% of cases) and bleeding from venous or arterial puncture sites (10–20% of cases).[99,105,106] Prolonged bleeding from the umbilical cord is less common and haemarthroses are rare. Haemorrhage into major organs such as the liver, spleen or lungs is also uncommon but has been reported in up to 5% of published cases.[105]

Diagnosis

The diagnosis of haemophilia A in the neonatal period should be straightforward either on a cord blood or peripheral blood sample. The characteristic finding is a prolonged or very prolonged APTT together with a normal PT, TT, platelets and fibrinogen. The diagnosis is then established by measurement of factor VIII clotting activity, which is always reduced in haemophilia A (all other coagulation factors, including von Willebrand antigen, are normal). Clinically, the severity of the disease is classified according to the level of factor VIII activity: levels of <2% (i.e. < 0.02 IU/ml) are classified as severe disease, 2–10% (0.02–0.1 IU/ml) as moderate disease, and >10% (>0.1 IU/ml) as mild haemophilia. Where there is a family history of

haemophilia A, the diagnosis may be established prenatally by a variety of methods; most families choose early diagnosis by mutational analysis of the factor VIII gene on a chorionic villus biopsy in the first trimester.[93]

Neonatal management

Acute management of the bleeding neonate with haemophilia requires intravenous administration of recombinant factor VIII. If necessary, FFP or cryoprecipitate (15–20 ml/kg) may be used if there is any delay or doubt about the diagnosis. The usual treatment dose of factor VIII in neonates is 50–100 units/kg intravenously twice daily.[26,105] Since the half-life of factor VIII is shorter in children than in adults, more frequent dosing or a continuous factor VIII infusion may be required. The dose should be adjusted by monitoring plasma factor VIII activity to achieve factor VIII levels of 100% (1.0 IU/ml).[26,105] This is done by measuring plasma factor VIII activity and close liaison with a specialist haematologist. For neonates with intracranial bleeding, treatment with factor VIII should continue for at least 2 weeks. Note that venepuncture should be performed with great care in all haemophiliac neonates and arterial punctures should be avoided. In addition, lumbar punctures should be avoided unless essential for clinical management, and, if necessary, should be done by an experienced person in the presence of factor VIII cover. Fibrin glue may be useful in circumcision-associated bleeds.[98] Once the baby is ready for discharge it is vital to provide specialist family support and follow-up through a Haemophilia Centre. In the UK, all children are registered with such a centre and have access to clinical nurse specialists and haematologists with expertise in haemophilia. The UK Haemophilia Centres Doctors' Organization also publishes regularly updated guidelines on the recommended products for treatment of patients with hereditary coagulation disorders.[182] The Haemophilia Society provides very useful practical support and advice for families with affected children (http://www.haemophilia.org.uk).

Prenatal management and delivery

For patients diagnosed prenatally, the best mode of delivery is controversial and accurate data about the risks are very limited. It is clear that significant haemorrhage may occur whatever the mode of delivery; in particular, there is no evidence that elective caesarean section eliminates the risk of bleeding.[105,114] Vaginal delivery is regarded as safe provided there are no difficulties anticipated; however, vacuum extraction should be avoided because several studies have shown a high rate of subgaleal bleeds and cephalhaematomas in this situation.[105,179] In known or suspected haemophiliac newborns, cord blood should always be taken for a coagulation screen and factor VIII level to confirm the diagnosis. Oral vitamin K should be given at birth because the intramuscular route should be avoided in view of the risk of haematoma formation. The role of prophylactic factor VIII administration to haemophiliac newborns following difficult delivery to reduce the risk of intracranial bleeding is controversial.[33,105] The risk of intracranial haemorrhage at around the time of birth in baby boys with haemophilia is about 1–4%, and at least half have significant sequelae.[106] Any intervention that could reduce this morbidity deserves consideration. The main disadvantage of prophylactic factor VIII is that it may increase the risk of inhibitor formation leading to major problems with treatment later in childhood. Further, it has not been shown to work and may not prevent damage occurring from devastating perinatal intracranial bleeding. There is no current consensus view on the approach to the baby at risk and accurate data about the long-term risks of inhibitor formation after neonatal factor VIII administration are required before the best treatment option becomes clear. In the meantime, it may be reasonable to give prophylactic factor VIII to a newborn haemophiliac boy where a previous sibling has had a major intracranial bleed.

Haemophilia B: factor IX deficiency

Haemophilia B is clinically indistinguishable from haemophilia A. From the diagnostic point of view, both diseases cause an isolated prolonged APTT, but the diagnosis of factor IX deficiency is made by demonstrating a low factor IX level. Occasional diagnostic confusion may arise with mild factor IX deficiency, as factor IX levels also fall in liver disease and vitamin K deficiency. Although this is usually straightforward to resolve since there will be concomitant reductions in the other vitamin K-dependent factors in this situation, it is important to recheck factor IX levels at 6 weeks and 6 months of age if in doubt. Management of factor IX deficiency is similar to that of factor VIII deficiency. Treatment of bleeding is with recombinant factor IX concentrate once the diagnosis has been established (FFP can be used as an interim measure). The usual dose is 100 units/kg intravenously once daily, and treatment should be monitored to achieve a factor IX level of 80–100% (1.0 IU/ml).[26,105] As for haemophilia A, treatment for intracranial haemorrhage should be continued for at least 2 weeks.[105] Similarly, lumbar punctures should be avoided where possible and venepunctures kept to a minimum. Recommendations for prenatal management are as for haemophilia A.

von Willebrand's disease in neonates

vWD is caused by quantitative or qualitative defects in vWF. It is the commonest inherited bleeding disorder, affecting around 1% of the population.[39] There are several types of vWD, each of which have different clinical and genetic characteristics, but only two forms of the disease present in the neonatal period. Type 2b vWD is autosomal dominant and presents with thrombocytopenia; bleeding is uncommon. Type 3 vWD is the most severe form of the disease.[89] It is autosomal recessive and has a clinical phenotype similar to haemophilia, as levels of both vWF and factor VIII are low. The diagnosis is made by measuring vWF and factor VIII, and determining the pattern of vWF multimers; clinical clues are the presence of a haemophiliac pattern of bleeding in girls or families without X-linked inheritance and a poor response to factor VIII concentrates. Type 3 vWD is currently treated with intermediate-purity factor VIII (Haemate-P is the most commonly used product).[26]

Factor XIII deficiency

Factor XIII deficiency is a rare autosomal recessive disorder in which the routine diagnostic coagulation screen is normal. It usually presents clinically with delayed bleeding from the umbilical cord during the first 3 weeks of life.[10,11] Intracranial haemorrhage has been reported in up to 30% of neonates with homozygous factor XIII deficiency.[26] The diagnosis is made by measuring clot solubility in 5M urea solution as a screening test, followed by a specific factor XIII assay; molecular tests for the common mutations are also available.[167] The treatment of bleeding associated with factor XIII deficiency is factor XIII concentrate; cryoprecipitate (10 ml/kg) can be used prior to establishment of the diagnosis or where the specific concentrate is unavailable. Infants with homozygous factor XIII deficiency have a lifelong risk of intracranial haemorrhage, and current guidelines recommend monthly factor XIII to reduce this risk.[182]

Other inherited coagulation factor deficiencies

A number of rare coagulation deficiencies may present in neonates with bleeding or unexplained prolongation of coagulation tests. The majority are autosomal recessive and so a history of parental consanguinity is relatively common. Factor VII deficiency can produce a very severe bleeding disorder with a high incidence of intracranial haemorrhage. In some cases, factor VII has been shown to cross the placenta and in this way delay haemorrhage in severe factor VII deficiency until after birth. Recombinant factor VIIa is now available to treat this disorder but must be given at frequent intervals as it has a very short half-life.[42] Factor XI deficiency is most frequent in Ashkenazi Jews and presents in a similar way to haemophilia. There are a number of rare congenital fibrinogen disorders, including dysfibrinogenaemias and hypo/afibrinogenaemia. They may present with umbilical stump bleeding but other sites of haemorrhage are extremely unusual in neonates. Finally, one of the commonest inherited causes of an isolated prolonged APTT in a healthy baby with no signs of bleeding is factor XII deficiency; despite what is often a markedly prolonged APTT, affected individuals have no clinically apparent bleeding disorder throughout life!

Acquired disorders of coagulation

Vitamin K deficiency

Levels of the active forms of the vitamin K-dependent procoagulant factors (factors II, VII, IX and X), and of the natural anticoagulants protein C and protein S, are physiologically low at birth. There are many reasons for this. Vitamin K is essential for γ-carboxylation of these proteins, which converts them to their active form: placental transfer of vitamin K is insufficient to build up adequate stores in the neonate;[207] breast milk has a low vitamin K content; and bacterial vitamin K synthesis is lacking in the sterile neonatal gut. In neonates, vitamin K deficiency can lead to HDN, more recently referred to as vitamin K-deficiency bleeding (VKDB). It can be classified into early, classical and late disease according to the timing or presentation and the clinical features.

Early VKDB

This presents in the first 24 hours of life usually with severe haemorrhage, including gastrointestinal bleeding and intracranial haemorrhage. It is caused by severe vitamin K deficiency in utero, usually as a result of maternal medication that interferes with vitamin K, e.g. anticonvulsants (phenobarbital [phenobarbitone], phenytoin), antituberculous therapy and oral anticoagulants. Guidelines for prevention of early VKDB are discussed below.

Classical VKDB

This presents at 2–7 days old in babies who have not received prophylactic vitamin K at birth. The risk is increased in breastfed babies and in those with poor oral intake. The incidence in babies not receiving vitamin K supplementation has been estimated at 0.25–1.7%, depending on the study population,[180] although recent studies show that it may now be less common even in communities without routine prophylaxis.[80] Numerous studies have shown that classical VKDB is prevented by a single intramuscular dose of vitamin K at birth (reviewed by Puckett & Offringa[150]). Routine prophylactic vitamin K has been the subject of much controversy, which is briefly summarised below.

Late VKDB

This occurs after the first week of life, most often between 2 and 8 weeks after birth, although presentation after 15 weeks of age has been reported.[175] The characteristic presentation is of sudden intracranial haemorrhage in an otherwise well, breastfed term baby, or in babies with liver disease (e.g. biliary atresia, pp. 682–4) or malabsorptive states. Late VKDB in healthy breastfed babies can be prevented either by a single intramuscular dose of vitamin K or by repeated oral doses of vitamin K over the first 6 weeks of life. However, babies with chronic liver disease or malabsorption are likely to require prolonged vitamin K supplementation.

In all forms of VKDB, clotting studies show a prolonged PT with normal platelets and fibrinogen; in severe deficiency, the APTT may also be prolonged. In the presence of a typical clinical history, further diagnostic tests are usually unnecessary and correction of the PT following vitamin K administration provides additional confirmation. If doubt remains, factor assays of the vitamin K-dependent factors and of the inactive form of factor II (decarboxyprothrombin; PIVKA II) can be used to confirm the diagnosis.[26] Treatment of VKDB depends on the severity of the bleeding. In mild cases, vitamin K (1 mg), which should be given intravenously or subcutaneously (not intramuscularly due to risk of haematoma) should suffice, as this increases the levels of active vitamin K-dependent coagulation factors within a few hours; where there is significant bleeding, FFP may be given, in addition to vitamin K.[26]

Vitamin K prophylaxis

Guidelines for the prevention of early VKDB are to give a single intramuscular injection of vitamin K at birth together with antenatal administration of oral vitamin K to the mother during the last 4 weeks of pregnancy.[26] For classical and late VKDB, there are several options. This is because although vitamin K supplementation undoubtedly prevents classical and late VKDB, controversy surrounds the route of administration since the publication of studies by Golding et al,[66] which suggested a link between intramuscular vitamin K at birth and later childhood malignancies. These studies have been criticised on methodological grounds,[29] and at least nine further studies have since investigated this link (reviewed in references 150, 158 and 207). Although seven studies failed to confirm the link with malignancy, two produced equivocal results, and the controversy is unlikely to be resolved unequivocally in the short term. There is no link between oral vitamin K and malignancy.

The current situation is perhaps best summarised by the recent Cochrane Review,[150] which concludes that:

- Intramuscular vitamin K has been proven to prevent classical disease.
- Oral vitamin K has been proven to improve biochemical parameters of vitamin K deficiency in the first week of life.
- The efficacy of oral supplementation in preventing late disease is unproven. This probably reflects the unpredictable absorption and difficulties with compliance with repeated doses of oral vitamin K.

Both the American Academy of Paediatrics and the Royal College of Paediatrics and Child Health recommend vitamin K supplementation at birth. In healthy babies, the choice of administration route is increasingly being left to parents, who have to balance the remote risk of a borderline increase in leukaemia (odds ratio between 1.06 [CI 0.89–1.25] and 1.16 [CI 0.97–1.39]) against the slightly higher risk of VKDB (2.7/100 000) in infants given 1 mg of vitamin K orally at birth, 1 week and 1 month of age.[43]

Disseminated intravascular coagulation

The main precipitants of DIC in neonates are associated with severe hypoxia and/or acidosis and include peripartum haemorrhage, severe birth asphyxia, meconium aspiration and sepsis. The pathophysiology of DIC is complex and not fully understood. The process seems to be triggered by release of TF and cytokines from damaged endothelium and/or monocytes, which results in widespread activation of the coagulation cascade with subsequent consumption of clotting factors and a combination of thrombotic and haemorrhagic manifestations.[19] Clinically, DIC is seen in sick neonates and presents with generalised bleeding, including pulmonary haemorrhage and oozing from venepuncture sites. The usual pattern of coagulation abnormalities in DIC is prolongation of the PT, APTT and TT, together with low platelets and fibrinogen. D-dimers are increased but measurement is not necessary for diagnostic purposes and is often not done in neonates because of the need for an extra blood sample (results should also be interpreted with caution as D-dimers are not specific and can be found in healthy neonates with no evidence of coagulopathy).[97] The most important aspect of management of DIC is treatment of the underlying cause. Blood product replacement is indicated for the treatment of clinical bleeding: FFP is a good source of procoagulant proteins as well as protein C, protein S and antithrombin; cryoprecipitate contains higher concentrations of factor VIII and fibrinogen and is useful when the fibrinogen levels are low.[26] There are no recent randomised trials that address optimum management of bleeding associated with neonatal DIC. However, a pragmatic approach is to aim to maintain the platelet count above $30 \times 10^9/l$ and the fibrinogen >1 g/l.

Other acquired coagulation disorders

Other causes of acquired coagulopathy in neonates include liver disease, metabolic disorders (e.g. hyperammonemia), extracorporeal membrane oxygenation (ECMO) and the consumptive coagulopathy with thrombocytopenia secondary to giant haemangioendotheliomas (Kasabach–Merritt syndrome).[72]

Neonatal thrombocytopenia

Prevalence of neonatal thrombocytopenia

Thrombocytopenia (platelets $<150 \times 10^9/l$) is common in neonates. Several studies report a prevalence of thrombocytopenia of 1–5% of all newborns, around 10% of who will have severe thrombocytopenia (platelets $<50 \times 10^9/l$). In neonatal intensive care units (NICUs), thrombocytopenia develops in 22–35% of all admissions and in up to 50% of neonates who are preterm and sick.[155]

Causes of neonatal thrombocytopenia

Conventional lists of the causes of thrombocytopenia include a large number of possible diagnoses, most of which are very rare. However, in routine clinical practice, it is more useful to be aware of the common causes and patterns of thrombocytopenia. Thrombocytopenia usually presents in one of two clinical patterns which reflect the most common causes: early thrombocytopenia (within 72 hours of birth) and late thrombocytopenia (after 72 hours of life). The principal causes of early and late thrombocytopenia are shown in Table 30.11.

Early thrombocytopenia

The most frequent causes of early thrombocytopenia in preterm infants are conditions resulting in fetal hypoxia. This thrombocytopenia is self-limiting, usually resolving within 10 days.[131,195] It is seen in infants of mothers with pre-eclampsia, pregnancy-induced hypertension or diabetes; this form of thrombocyto-penia is also seen in infants with IUGR.[131,195] Thrombocytopenia is seen in virtually all such infants, although it is rarely severe (the platelet count usually remains above $50 \times 10^9/l$) except in neonates with severe IUGR. It is caused by reduced platelet production secondary to reduced megakaryocytopoiesis (this is discussed in more detail below). The most important cause of severe early neonatal thrombocytopenia is neonatal alloimmune thrombocytopenia (NAITP), which is also discussed below.

Late thrombocytopenia

The most common and clinically important causes of late thrombocytopenia are sepsis and NEC, which together account for $>80\%$ of cases.[130,155] This form of thrombocytopenia usually

Table 30.11 Causes of neonatal thrombocytopenia

Early (<72 hours)	Placental insufficiency (PET, IUGR, diabetes)
	NAITP
	Birth asphyxia
	Perinatal infection (group B streptococcus, *E. coli*, Listeria)
	Congenital infection (CMV, toxoplasmosis, rubella)
	Maternal autoimmune (ITP, SLE)
	Severe Rh HDN
	Thrombosis (renal vein, aortic)
	Aneuploidy (trisomy – 21, 18, 13)
	Congenital/Inherited (TAR, Wiskott–Aldrich)
Late (>72 hours)	Late-onset sepsis and necrotising enterocolitis
	Congenital infection (CMV, toxoplasmosis, rubella)
	Maternal autoimmune (ITP, SLE)
	Congenital/Inherited (TAR, Wiskott–Aldrich)

CMV, cytomegalovirus; HDN, haemolytic disease of the newborn; ITP, idiopathic thrombocytopenic purpura; IUGR: intrauterine growth restriction; NAITP, neonatal alloimmune thrombocytopenia; PET, pre-eclamptic toxaemia; SLE, systemic lupus erythematosus; TAR, thrombocytopenia with absent radii.

develops very rapidly over 1–2 days, is often very severe (platelets $<30 \times 10^9/l$) and takes 1–2 weeks to recover.[130] Such babies frequently require platelet transfusion.[130] The mechanism is likely to be a combination of increased platelet consumption, often but not always with evidence of DIC, and reduced platelet production.

Thrombocytopenia secondary to IUGR and maternal hypertension/diabetes

Neonates with IUGR have a number of distinctive haematological abnormalities which are present at birth, including neonatal thrombocytopenia, neutropenia, increased erythropoiesis (high numbers of circulating nucleated red cells with or without associated polycythemia) and evidence on the blood film of hyposplenism (spherocytes, target cells and Howell–Jolly bodies).[195] The underlying cause of the haematological abnormalities appears to be chronic fetal hypoxia since the same pattern of abnormalities occurs in several types of placental insufficiency, both maternal disorders such as pre-eclampsia, hypertension and diabetes mellitus, and fetal disorders manifest as 'idiopathic' IUGR. Erythropoietin levels are increased in affected fetuses and neonates.[160,195] In addition, the severity of the haematological abnormalities correlates both with serum erythropoietin levels and with the severity of the placental dysfunction.[160] We and others have shown that megakaryocytopoiesis is severely impaired at birth in such neonates, as shown by a marked reduction in circulating megakaryocytes and their precursor and progenitor cells, and that this is likely to be the principal reason for the neonatal thrombocytopenia since there is no evidence of increased platelet destruction/consumption.[131,194,195]

Immune neonatal thrombocytopenias

Neonatal alloimmune thrombocytopenia

This is the platelet equivalent of HDN and alloimmune neutropenia. NAITP affects around 1:1000 pregnancies.[34] In addition to the summary below, there are several useful recent reviews to which the reader is referred to for more detail about the diagnosis and treatment of this condition.[34,91,143,156] It is frequently severe and occurs in the first pregnancy in almost 50% of cases. Thrombocytopenia may present prenatally (as early as 20 weeks' gestation), in which case it is sometimes referred to as fetal alloimmune thrombocytopenia (FAITP), or at birth. The thrombocytopenia results from transplacental passage of maternal platelet-specific antibodies to human platelet antigens (HPA) which the mother lacks but which the fetus inherits from the father. In 80% of cases these are anti-HPA-1a antibodies and in 10–15% anti-HPA-5b; occasional cases are due to anti-HPA-3a.[34,143] Recent data indicate that the ability of an HPA-1a-negative woman to form anti-HPA-1a is controlled by the HLA DRB3*0101 allele such that HLA DRB3*0101-positive women are 140 times more likely to make anti-HPA-1a than are those who are HLA DRB3*0101-negative.[143] The main clinical problem in NAITP is intracranial haemorrhage; this occurs in 10% of cases, with long-term neurodevelopmental sequelae in 20% of survivors.[35] Affected neonates may present with seizures or other signs of intracranial haemorrhage, with petechiae or bruising, or with an incidental thrombocytopenia. The platelet count is usually $<30 \times 10^9/l$. The diagnosis of NAITP is made by demonstrating platelet antigen incompatibility between mother and baby (in 80% of cases of NAITP, the mother is HPA-1a-negative and the baby is HPA-1a-positive). This can usually be done within 1–2 days either serologically or by PCR, and is carried out in reference transfusion laboratories.[143] In addition, most mothers have detectable anti-HPA antibodies. The recommended management for neonates with NAITP is to transfuse 'severely affected' babies with HPA-compatible platelets (usually available 'off the shelf' from transfusion centres).[143] The definition of 'severely affected' varies in different studies but should be taken to include both asymptomatic neonates with severe thrombocytopenia (platelets $<30 \times 10^9/l$) and babies with evidence of haemorrhage despite less severe thrombocytopenia. If there is ongoing severe thrombocytopenia and/or haemorrhage despite HPA-compatible platelets, intravenous IgG (total dose 2 g/kg over 2–5 days) is often useful in ameliorating the thrombocytopenia until spontaneous recovery occurs 1–6 weeks after birth.[143] Prenatal management of NAITP remains controversial (reviewed in references 34, 91, 143 and 156). The principal options are an invasive approach using fetal blood sampling plus fetal transfusion with HPA-compatible platelets if thrombocytopenia is detected, or a non-invasive approach relying on maternal intravenous IgG therapy; each approach has evidence to support it.[34,91,143,156]

Neonatal autoimmune thrombocytopenia

This is secondary to transplacental passage of maternal platelet autoantibodies in maternal idiopathic thrombocytopenic purpura and systemic lupus erythematosus, which affects 1–5 in 10 000 pregnancies.[100] Around 10% of infants of affected mothers develop thrombocytopenia. However, the thrombocytopenia is usually mild and intracranial haemorrhage occurs in <1% of at-risk babies. In affected babies with severe thrombocytopenia, treatment with intravenous IgG is usually effective.[64]

Management of neonatal thrombocytopenia

Management of immune thrombocytopenias is described above. For other forms of neonatal thrombocytopenia, therapy depends upon the appropriate use of platelet transfusion. Evidence-based guidelines for neonatal platelet transfusion therapy are yet to be defined, although consensus guidelines are available.[27,155,156] Most recommend platelet transfusion for sick neonates where the platelet count is $<50 \times 10^9/l$; however, for stable, relatively well preterm and term infants, platelet counts of $30–50 \times 10^9/l$ are not associated with an increased risk of haemorrhage;[130] this approach conforms to the current UK guidelines.[27] Since platelet underproduction underlies the majority of neonatal thrombocytopenias, recombinant haemopoietic growth factors, including thrombopoietin and interkeukin-11, may be useful future therapies.[156]

Neonatal thrombosis: physiology and developmental aspects

Plasma concentrations of many of the inhibitors of coagulation are reduced in neonates. This, together with the frequent need for indwelling vascular catheters, is the main explanation for the increased risk of thrombosis in neonates (2.4 per 1000 hospital admissions) compared with in older infants and children. Of the direct inhibitors of thrombin, concentrations of antithrombin and heparin cofactor II are both decreased at birth while those of α_2-macroglobulin are increased and may partially compensate. In the protein C/S pathway, plasma concentrations of protein C are low at birth; total protein S levels are also low, but overall protein S activity is normal, as it exists mainly in its free active form due to the virtual absence of its binding protein (C4b-BP) in neonates.[5] Less is known about the third inhibitor pathway in neonates, TFPI, although neonates have slightly reduced TFPI levels in cord plasma compared with adult values. Finally, there are several age-related differences in the neonatal fibrinolytic system. Levels of plasminogen at birth are only 50% of adult values; since even homozygous plasminogen deficiency is not associated with thrombosis, the main clinical significance of this is that there is a reduced ability to generate plasmin in response to fibrinolytic agents. In contrast, the plasma levels of t-PA and its inhibitor (plasminogen activator inhibitor-1) are high, the clinical significance of which is unclear.[5]

Diagnostic approach to neonatal thrombosis: use of screening tests

The identification of an increasing number of risk factors for thrombosis in adults has led to increasing confusion about which of these factors are relevant to neonates and which neonates should be screened for congenital thrombophilia. Recent guidelines from the Haemostasis and Thrombosis Task Force of the BCSH[26] state that congenital thrombophilia should be considered and screened for in the following situations:

- any child with a clinically significant thrombosis, including spontaneous thrombotic events, unanticipated or extensive venous thrombosis, ischaemic skin lesions or purpura fulminans;
- a positive family history of neonatal purpura fulminans.

In fact, the only inherited deficiencies for which there is a proven causative role in neonatal thrombosis are homozygous/double heterozygote deficiencies in protein C and protein S which cause purpura fulminans (see below). For other types of thrombosis, such as neonatal stroke, in which the cause is almost certainly multifactorial, the contribution to the thrombotic process made by less severe thrombophilic defects (e.g. factor V Leiden or a mutation in the promoter of the prothrombin gene, prothrombin[20210A]) is difficult to assess. While uncertainty remains, it is probably reasonable to carry out the tests listed below. An important proviso is that all the data from such investigations should, where possible, be entered into national and/or international registries of paediatric thrombosis so that the role of inherited abnormalities can be determined.[162]

The screening tests that should be performed in all suspected cases of thrombophilia are:

- protein C activity;
- protein S;
- antithrombin;
- factor V Leiden;
- prothrombin[20210A].

These tests are all carried out on freshly collected anticoagulated blood samples (usually using the same type of sample bottle as employed for coagulation screen).

In addition, babies with thrombosis who are born to mothers with SLE and/or antiphospholipid syndrome should be tested for lupus anticoagulant, since antiphospholipid antibodies may cross the placenta and are a rare cause of neonatal thrombosis in such babies.[135] Tests for factor V Leiden and prothrombin[20210A] are carried out on DNA extracted from white blood cells in the coagulation sample (see above). Associations between neonatal thrombosis and increased serum lipoprotein a and the methylenetetrahydrofolate reductase (MTHFR) genotype C677T have recently been reported.[78] The relevance of serum lipoprotein a and the MTHFR genotype to neonatal management is unclear at present as there is no evidence that awareness of these laboratory abnormalities can be used to improve management. Therefore they are not currently listed as recommended screening tests for neonatal thrombophilia by the BCSH.[26] On the other hand, where these tests are performed, it is logical to include such data, together with clinical details, in one of the national or international thrombosis registries, in order to understand their relevance in the future.[162]

Inherited thrombotic disorders

Protein C deficiency

Babies who are homozygous or double heterozygotes for protein C deficiency have no normal protein C genes and undetectable or very low levels of plasma protein C. The condition is rare, occurring in 1 in 160 000 to 1 in 360 000 births.[120] Affected babies usually present within hours or days of birth with neonatal purpura fulminans in which there is DIC together with rapidly progressive, life-threatening, haemorrhagic necrosis due to dermal vessel thrombosis. Typically the lesions start as small ecchymoses, often in the extremities, buttocks or scalp and sometimes at sites of venepunctures. Neonates may also present with cerebral or renal vein thrombosis or with ophthalmic thrombosis, as suggested by vitreous and/or retinal haemorrhages and unreactive pupils.

The diagnosis of protein C deficiency is made by the characteristic clinical picture in conjunction with DIC and undetectable levels of protein C (<0.01 units/ml) in the patient, together with heterozygote levels in the parents.[26,103] Molecular analysis can be used to confirm the diagnosis retrospectively and for prenatal diagnosis in future pregnancies.[126] In contrast to homozygotes, patients who are heterozygous for protein C deficiency, and so have one normal protein C gene, rarely present as neonates unless there are additional prothrombotic factors; these individuals have low protein C levels which may overlap with the lower limit of normal in the first few months of life, delaying diagnosis until after the age of 6 months and sometimes until later in childhood. The treatment of neonatal purpura fulminans due to protein C deficiency is protein C concentrate starting at a dose of 40 units/kg and aiming to maintain a plasma level of >0.25 units/ml, which may require frequent dosing in the initial stages when DIC is ongoing.[26] FFP should be used until protein C concentrate is available, if any delay is likely. Heparin and antiplatelet agents are ineffective. In the long-term, lifelong protein C replacement and/or anticoagulation are necessary.[26]

Protein S deficiency

Homozygous or double heterozygosity for protein S deficiency is even rarer than protein C deficiency. It presents with features identical to those of protein C deficiency and the diagnosis is established by demonstrating undetectable levels of protein S (<0.01 units/ml). Treatment is with FFP (10–20 ml/kg) to maintain a plasma protein S level of >0.25 units/ml.[26] As for protein C deficiency, lifelong replacement therapy and/or anticoagulation is necessary.

Antithrombin deficiency

Homozygous antithrombin deficiency is extremely rare and is only seen where the mutation involves the heparin-binding site. It usually presents later in childhood but neonatal thrombosis has been reported, including deep venous thrombosis and inferior vena caval thrombosis.[78,104] Heterozygous antithrombin deficiency is more common (1 in 2000 to 1 in 5000 births); it usually presents in the second decade of life but neonatal presentation with venous and arterial thrombosis has been reported, including aortic thrombosis, myocardial infarction and cerebral dural sinus thrombosis. Neonatal purpura fulminans is not a feature. The diagnosis of both homozygous and hererozygous disease is made by measuring plasma antithrombin levels, although confirmation in heterozygotes may be delayed until 3–6 months of age because of the overlap with normal levels. The treatment of neonatal thrombosis due to antithrombin deficiency is replacement therapy with antithrombin concentrate together with heparin.[26]

Other inherited thrombotic disorders

The more recently discovered prothrombotic mutations such as factor V Leiden and the prothrombin 20210A promoter mutation (prothrombin[20210A])[78,135] have not yet been reported to cause neonatal thrombotic problems in isolation. Even in adults, heterozygosity for factor V Leiden or prothrombin[20210A] only increases the thrombotic risk by fourfold and twofold, respectively. Thus, these prothrombotic genotypes may play a role in the presence of other acquired risk factors, but since the majority of individuals with these mutations do not suffer thrombotic events even during adulthood, there is no evidence that management of neonates found to be harbouring these mutations should be any different from that of neonates without the mutations.

Acquired thrombotic problems

The most commonly identified risk factors for thrombosis are the presence of an intravascular catheter and shock in association with sepsis, hypoxaemia or hypovolaemia. The main sites, apart from catheters, of neonatal thrombosis are in the renal veins and, less commonly, in the aorta, aortic arch or cerebral vessels.[78,162]

Catheter-related thrombosis

This is the commonest cause of neonatal thrombosis; it is responsible for >80% of venous thrombosis and >90% of arterial thrombosis.[26,162] Symptomatic thrombosis occurs in 1% of neonates with indwelling vascular catheters, although postmortem studies suggest that asymptomatic thrombosis occurs in association with up to 20–30% of catheters. Arterial thrombosis can lead to peripheral gangrene or renal artery thrombosis with hypertension and heart failure (p. 624). Venous thrombosis can cause portal hypertension, varices and/or renal vein thrombosis with renal dysfunction (pp. 935–6). The diagnosis of catheter-related thrombosis is usually made by Doppler ultrasound[159,161] but this is notoriously unreliable, and may miss thrombosis in the aorta, right atrium or inferior vena cava, as well as in the upper limb. 'Linograms' (putting radio-opaque dye into the line) may also miss extensive thrombosis. For this reason, contrast angiography has been identified as the 'gold standard' for confirmation of thrombotic vessel occlusion.[161]

The treatment of catheter-related thrombosis depends on the severity and extent of thrombosis. The first step is prompt removal where possible;[4] although successful use of either t-PA or urokinase has been described, the risks of such an approach are likely to be much higher. If signs progress despite catheter removal, heparin should be started using a dosing regimen adapted for neonates.[6] Either unfractionated heparin or low-molecular-weight heparin (LMWH) can be used and suggestive dosage regimens developed by Maureen Andrew are summarised in Table 30.12. Thrombolytic therapy with urokinase or t-PA has been used successfully for catheter-related thrombosis in neonates but the number of reports in preterm neonates remains low. Where there is extensive thrombosis threatening limb viability or organ function, recent experience suggests that t-PA can be given with a reasonable safety profile if monitored very carefully. However, it seems better not to use thrombolytic therapy in milder cases, because of the known risk of life-threatening bleeding, including intracranial haemorrhage, and this risk may be higher in preterm infants.[75,109,124,191] There are very limited data about the best regimen to use but recent guidelines are

Table 30.12 Heparin schedules for neonates. (Modified from Andrew & de Veber G.[6])

A. Unfractionated heparin

	Dose (units/kg/h)	Check APTT
Loading dose	75	After 4 h
Maintenance	28	Daily or 4 h after dose change

Adjustment of maintenance by APTT:		
APTT <50 s	Increase by 20%	After 4 h
APTT 50–59 s	Increase by 10%	After 4 h
APTT 60–85 s	No change	24 h
APTT 86–120 s	Decrease by 10%	After 4 h
APTT >120 s	Stop for 1 h then decrease by 15%	After 4 h

B. Low-molecular-weight heparin	
Drug	Enoxaparin
Dose	1.5 mg/kg/dose twice daily
Monitoring	Measure anti-Factor Xa level (coagulation screen bottle)
	Therapeutic level is 0.5–1.0 units/ml anti-Factor Xa
	Check anti-Factor Xa 4–6 h after first dose
	If in therapeutic range, check once weekly
	If dose adjusted (see below), recheck 4 h after adjusted dose
	If <0.35 units/ml, increase by 25%
	If 0.35–0.49 units/ml, increase by 10%
	If 1.1–2 units/ml decrease by 20–30%
	If >2 units/ml, withold until anti-Factor Xa is <0.5 units/ml; restart at 40% of original dose

summarised in Table 30.12. In any neonates treated with thrombolytic therapy, it is important to maintain the fibrinogen >1 g/l and the platelet count $>50 \times 10^9$/l using cryoprecipitate and platelet transfusion, respectively. Heparin (starting dose 28 IU/kg/h) is often given to maintain vessel patency after thrombolytic therapy, although there is no evidence that this is beneficial. There is also no evidence that heparin prevents catheter-related thrombosis, although prophylactic low-dose heparin (0.5–5 units/h) has been shown to prolong umbilical artery catheter patency and is recommended.

Non-catheter-related thrombosis

The commonest non-catheter-related thrombosis is renal vein thrombosis, which presents in the neonatal period in nearly 80% of cases and may even develop in utero. Renal vein thrombosis is usually unilateral (75% of cases) and presents with a flank mass, haematuria, proteinuria, thrombocytopenia and reduced function of the involved kidney.[78] The most commonly identified risk factors which predispose to renal vein thrombosis are sepsis, maternal diabetes, polycythaemia, dehydration and prothrombotic mutations (therefore all such babies should have a thrombophilia screen performed). Management of renal vein thrombosis is controversial, as there are so few data. Treatment options include supportive treatment, anticoagulation with heparin, thrombolytic therapy or surgery. Recent guidelines recommend supportive therapy for small, clinically silent thromboses, with monitoring to detect extension of the original thrombus.[26] Anticoagulation with unfractionated heparin or LMWH is indicated for more extensive thrombosis, particularly where there is evidence of organ or limb dysfunction (see Table 30.12 for suggested regimens).[6,26] Thrombolysis should be reserved for extensive thrombosis where limb viability is threatened and should not be used within 10 days of surgery or where there are pre-existing bleeding problems.

Neonatal stroke

Neonatal stroke occurs in about 1 in 4000 births (pp. 183–4). An increased prevalence of thrombophilia in affected neonates, particularly factor V Leiden, is increasingly recognised and it is now considered that very few cases are due to hypoxia-ischaemia.[124] Factor V Leiden has also been shown to be associated with a poorer outcome in neonatal stroke compared with cases where factor V Leiden is absent.[124] Maternal or neonatal anticardiolipin antibodies have also been linked to neonatal stroke; these are often transient and their causal role is not yet established. However, it is important to note that all the evidence to date suggests that the aetiology of neonatal stroke is multifactorial and for the majority of thrombophilic mutations, including factor V Leiden, prothrombin[20210A] and the MTHFR genotype C677T, the presence of these genetic abnormalities alone has not been shown to be the direct cause of the stroke. For example, in the largest series reported, only five of the 24 children with neonatal stroke were factor V Leiden heterozygotes and in none of these children was there a family history of stroke.[124] This makes counselling extremely difficult, particularly when there are no series to suggest that stroke is more likely in siblings of a child

with neonatal stroke when the only family risk factor identified on thrombophilic screening is factor V Leiden, prothrombin[20210A] or MTHFR C677T. Thus, while it is likely that thrombophilia plays a role in neonatal stroke, additional risk factors may also be required and our current state of knowledge about the interactions between these factors does not allow any specific diagnostic or therapeutic guidelines to be established.

Transfusion of blood and blood products in the newborn

Introduction

Although sick neonates are one of the most heavily transfused groups of patients in modern medicine, neonatal transfusion remains opinion-based rather than evidence-based and there is a wide diversity of opinion and practice between different clinicians and institutions.[17,36,151] As blood products convey a risk of transmitting potentially serious infections and are increasingly costly, it is clearly important to define evidence-based and/or standardised protocols for blood product use in neonatal medicine.

Red cell transfusion

Aims of red cell transfusion

The principal aims of red cell transfusion in the newborn are to ensure adequate tissue oxygenation, particularly during intensive care, and to treat significant symptomatic anaemia. Indeed, given that cardiopulmonary function during intensive care will be optimised, the only way to increase tissue oxygenation is red cell transfusion. Unfortunately there are few data about using measures of tissue oxygenation to determine either the need for or the effects of red cell transfusion in neonates. Near-infrared spectroscopy has recently been used to measure peripheral fractional oxygen extraction (FOE) and thereby estimate oxygen delivery to the tissues and guide red cell transfusion in neonates.[192,193] In a study of 74 neonates of birthweight <1500 g, half of the babies were transfused on the basis only of a high peripheral FOE (>0.47) (suggesting inadequate tissue oxygen delivery) while the remaining babies were transfused according to a conventional protocol based on haemoglobin concentration. Neonates in the FOE group had lower median haemoglobin levels during the study, an increased time to first transfusion and no increase in major neonatal complications, suggesting that FOE may be a practical, as well as a more physiological, way of assessing trigger thresholds for red cell transfusion in preterm neonates and may reduce transfusions and donor exposure without adversely affecting outcome.

Capillary whole blood lactate concentration has also been used as an indicator of tissue oxygenation (in stable neonates, peripheral blood lactate levels decrease following red cell transfusions for 'symptomatic' anaemia).[59] However, during intensive care, lactate levels are of little use in deciding the need for red cell transfusion, since capillary lactate levels are highly variable because they reflect tissue perfusion rather than haemoglobin-limited oxygen unloading capacity to the tissues.[59]

Changing patterns of red cell transfusion in neonates

Numerous reports over the last 10–15 years show a trend towards increasingly conservative use of red cell transfusions, even in the most preterm neonates.[18,86] These changes have occurred without any significant increase in the need for respiratory support or oxygen therapy and without any increase in the incidence of intraventricular haemorrhage (IVH), NEC, sepsis or poor weight gain. These studies are well summarised in a number of reviews.[18,56,86,151] Similarly there is little evidence to suggest that maintaining a high haemoglobin improves outcome in preterm neonates; a recent study which aimed to ameliorate retinopathy of prematurity by maintaining a haematocrit greater than 40% showed not only no reduction in retinopathy of prematurity but also no change in IVH and NEC, which were recorded as secondary outcome measures.[28] This study only assessed preterm neonates over 28 days of life (i.e. outside the intensive care period). Since a low haemoglobin (as opposed to clinical signs of inadequate tissue oxygenation) is the sole trigger for transfusion in many intensive care situations, this suggests that haemoglobin-limited oxygen unloading capacity to the tissues is uncommon, even during intensive care.

Guidelines for transfusion of red cells in neonates

The BCSH recently revised their guidelines for transfusion of fetuses, neonates and older children.[27] Their recommendations about the products and indications for red cell transfusion in neonates are briefly summarised here (for a full discussion of recommendations for blood components for use in the newborn, see BCSH[27]).

Products for red cell transfusion in neonates

- Components for transfusion in utero or to children under 1 year of age must be prepared from donors who have given at least one donation within the previous 2 years which was negative for all mandatory microbiological markers.
- Dedicating aliquots from a single donation (multi-satellite packs) to allow sequential transfusions from the same donor for neonates who are likely to be repeatedly transfused is considered good practice.
- All cellular components should be leukocyte-depleted at the point of manufacture (to reduce the risk of transmission of infectious agents); this has been mandatory for all cellular components in the UK since 2001.
- Components transfused in the first year of life should be CMV-seronegative.
- Irradiation of red cells prior to transfusion is necessary in several situations (for detail, see BCSH[27]), including 'top-up' or exchange transfusion of neonates who have received an intrauterine transfusion, where a neonate has proven or suspected cellular immune deficiency and where the donated red cells are from a first- or second-degree relative.

- Blood group: samples from both the neonate and mother should be grouped to determine the ABO and Rhesus group and screened for atypical red cell alloantibodies; small volume 'top-up' transfusions can be given repeatedly over the first 4 months of life without further serological testing of the neonate provided that there are no atypical red cell antibodies in the neonate's or mother's serum and the baby's Coombs' test is negative (infants rarely produce atypical red cell antibodies unless they receive repeated large volume transfusions).[27]

Volume of red cell transfusion in preterm neonates

The few studies available suggest that large volume (20 ml/kg) red cell transfusions not only lead to larger rises in haemoglobin and fewer overall transfusions than small volume transfusions (10 ml/kg), but are also well tolerated in the majority of preterm neonates.[146]

Indications for RBC transfusion in preterm neonates

A number of groups have proposed RBC transfusion guidelines in preterm neonates, mostly in the setting of trials of erythropoietin to ameliorate neonatal anaemia.[119,164] These guidelines are based on combinations of ventilation requirements, oxygen requirements and haemoglobin/PCV levels. However, as improvements in both antenatal and neonatal care have led to a reduced incidence and severity of acute lung disease, the recommendations of these guidelines are being increasingly superseded by a similar but more conservative approach (Table 30.13). What is clear, however, is that adherence to strict neonatal transfusion guidelines (in whatever form) reduces both the number of transfusions and donor exposure.[1]

Whilst adverse transfusion reactions are rare in neonates, it should always be remembered that transfusion of all blood products is associated with finite risks[101] and that serious adverse reactions do occasionally occur.[201]

RBC T-antigen activation

The potential for transfusion-associated haemolysis in infants with T-activated RBCs has led to some centres screening infants and providing low-titre anti-T blood components. However, a recent study has shown that many 'T-activated' neonates are in fact expressing T antigen variants (Th and Tx) and Tk antigen.[21] This study also found no evidence of haemolysis in either T- or T-variant-activated neonates receiving standard blood components. The practice of providing low-titre anti-T blood components for neonates with sepsis or NEC cannot therefore be supported on current evidence.

Platelet transfusion

Studies of platelet transfusion to treat and prevent haemorrhage in neonates

Numerous studies suggest that neonatal thrombocytopenia is a risk factor for haemorrhage (particularly IVH), mortality and adverse neurodevelopmental outcome (reviewed by Roberts & Murray[156]).

Table 30.13 Guidelines for red cell transfusion for preterm neonates

Assisted ventilation				CPAP		Breathing spontaneously	
<28 days			≥28 days	<28 days	≥28 days	FiO₂ >0.21	Well in air
FiO₂ ≥0.3		FiO₂ <0.3					
Hb <12g/dl or PCV <0.40		Hb <11g/dl or PCV <0.35	Hb <10g/dl or PCV <0.30	Hb <10g/dl or PCV <0.30	Hb <8g/dl or PCV <0.25	Hb <8g/dl or PCV <0.25	Hb <7g/dl or PCV <0.20

RBC transfusion may be considered at higher thresholds than the above for neonates with:

- hypovolaemia (unresponsive to crystalloid infusion)
- septic shock
- necrotising enterocolitis
- undergoing/recovering from major surgery

However, whether these outcomes can be reduced by treating affected neonates with platelet transfusion is difficult to assess since there have been no neonatal trials which demonstrate reduced haemorrhage or improved outcome in neonates with non-immune-mediated thrombocytopenia treated with platelet transfusions. In the only randomised controlled trial in preterm neonates, Andrew et al[9] found no reduction in haemorrhage in neonates randomised to receive transfusions to maintain their platelet counts in the normal range ($>150 \times 10^9$/l) compared with control neonates with moderate thrombocytopenia (platelets $50-150 \times 10^9$/l) who were not transfused.

Studies of contemporary platelet transfusion practice in neonates

Three recent publications[60,130,170] retrospectively document platelet transfusion practice in three separate NICUs in the UK, US and Mexico. Despite the geographical differences, the findings of each study are similar:

- Platelet transfusion is fairly common in NICU patients, occurring in 2–9.4% of all admissions (more transfusions are given in NICUs with a high percentage of intensive care patients and in those units practising ECMO).
- The majority of platelet transfusions are given prophylactically to non-bleeding neonates with platelet counts below 50×10^9/l and most commonly in those with counts below 30×10^9/l, but a variety of platelet count triggers for transfusion are used.
- More than half of neonates given platelet transfusions receive more than one transfusion, with a significant proportion receiving more than four transfusions.
- Thrombocytopenic neonates who receive platelets are up to 10 times more likely to die than neonates who do not receive platelet transfusion (however, the severity of the clinical conditions causing the thrombocytopenia is stressed in all three reports as the major factor leading to mortality, as is the relative rarity of uncontrolled haemorrhage as a direct cause of death in such neonates).

Platelet transfusion guidelines

Until data from controlled trials become available, a number of countries have published consensus guidelines to help decide the indications for platelet transfusion in term and preterm neonates.[20,26,27,133] Our recent study has led us to modify these guidelines to fit the clinical problems we face within our unit (summarised in Table 30.14) and take into account what is already known about the incidence and natural history of haemorrhage in the newborn. Most neonates who bleed (particularly those with GMH-IVH) do so in the first days of life. However, with the exception of perinatal asphyxia, the conditions precipitating the majority of episodes of severe thrombocytopenia (e.g. late-onset sepsis and NEC) usually develop after the first few days of life and are rarely accompanied by major haemorrhage. We therefore believe that prophylactic platelet transfusions are not required for such patients until the platelet count falls to between 20×10^9/l and 30×10^9/l (see Table 30.14). However, we use a higher trigger level ($<50 \times 10^9$/l) for platelet transfusion for patients with the greatest risk of haemorrhage, especially ELBW neonates (<1000 g) in the first week of life and neonates with significant clinical instability, e.g. fluctuating ventilation requirements or blood pressure (Table 30.14). Platelet transfusions in neonates with platelet counts greater than 50×10^9/l should be reserved for patients with active bleeding, since there is no evidence that higher platelet counts are of any benefit.

Platelet transfusion: the products to use

Platelets for transfusion to neonates should be both ABO- and RhD-compatible since the plasma in the transfused product will contain anti-A and/or anti-B depending on the blood group and this may be sufficient amounts to cause haemolysis.[27] All blood products in the UK are leukocyte-depleted and are therefore highly unlikely to transmit CMV;[200] however, current guidelines recommend that platelets for transfusion to infants <12 months of age should be from CMV-seronegative donors.[27] There are no studies evaluating the volume of platelets which should be administered; in our practice we have found that a transfusion volume of 20 ml/kg is well tolerated even in VLBW babies and produces both a higher increment in platelet count and a more sustained increase than a transfusion volume of 10 ml/kg.

Granulocytes

A number of small trials (summarised by Vamvakas & Pineda[184]) have suggested that granulocyte transfusion may convey benefit

Table 30.14 Guidelines for platelet transfusion for neonates

Platelet count ($\times 10^9$/l)	Non-bleeding neonate	Bleeding neonate	NAITP (proven or suspected)
<30	Consider transfusion in all patients	Transfuse	Transfuse (with HPA-compatible platelets)
30–49	Do not transfuse if clinically stable Consider transfusion if: ■ <1000 g and <1 week of age ■ clinically unstable (e.g. fluctuating BP) ■ previous major bleeding complication (e.g. GMH-IVH) ■ current minor bleeding (e.g. petechiae, puncture site oozing) ■ concurrent coagulopathy ■ requires surgery or exchange transfusion ■ platelet count falling and likely to fall below 30	Transfuse	Transfuse (with HPA-compatible platelets)
50–99	Do not transfuse	Transfuse	Transfuse (with HPA-compatible platelets if major bleeding present)
>99	Do not transfuse	Do not transfuse	Do not transfuse

HPA, human platelet antigen; NAITP, neonatal alloimmune thrombocytopenia.

during neonatal sepsis. However, the practical difficulties of obtaining a sufficient dose of fresh granulocytes at the time of sepsis means that granulocyte transfusion has not entered routine practice in the UK for the treatment of neonatal sepsis.

Fresh frozen plasma and cryoprecipitate

Although FFP is widely used for a variety of indications in neonates, including prevention of IVH, volume replacement, as a source of 'opsonising factors' during sepsis and to 'support' haemostasis in neonates with thrombocytopenia, there is little or no evidence to support its use in any of these situations.[129] The only indications for FFP in neonates recommended in the recent BCSH guidelines and supported by evidence are: DIC, vitamin K-dependent bleeding and inherited deficiencies of coagulation factors.[26,27,129] The large study conducted by the Northern Neonatal Network clearly shows that prophylactic FFP administered to preterm neonates at birth does not prevent IVH or improve outcome at 2 years of life.[134] Similarly, FFP is not superior to other colloid or crystalloid solutions as a volume replacement solution in standard neonatal practice[132] and there is no evidence to support its use to 'correct' the results of abnormal coagulation screens.[26]

FFP: the product to use

The current BCSH guidelines state that FFP for transfusion to neonates should be group AB (since this contains neither anti-A nor anti-B) or the same ABO blood group as the neonate. Both 'standard' FFP and pathogen-inactivated FFP (either methylene blue treated or solvent-detergent treated) are available. In the UK, Department of Health recommendations state that single unit methylene blue-treated FFP (MB-FFP) should be used for neonates, as the 'standard' FFP carries a small risk of virus transmission (apart from CMV).[27] The residual levels of methylene blue have not been shown to be harmful in neonates.[27] The alternative to MB-FFP, solvent-detergent FFP (SD-FFP), is made from pooled plasma of several hundred donations and though shown to be generally safe in children in small studies, has been associated with transmission of parvovirus B19.[27] The dose of FFP is 10–20 ml/kg, with the larger dose given if possible in order to limit donor exposure where repeated dosing is likely.

Cryoprecipitate

Cryoprecipitate contains a higher concentration of fibrinogen and factor VIII per unit volume than FFP. It is useful in treating DIC associated with hypofibrinogenaemia, inherited afibrinogenaemia, or hypofibrinogenaemia and factor VIII deficiency (haemophilia A) if factor VIII concentrate is not immediately available.

Human albumin solution

The use of human albumin solution (HAS) has been reported to be associated with excess mortality in adults receiving intensive care. While data about the risks of HAS in neonates are not available, there are studies which clearly show that HAS is not superior to other colloid or crystalloid solutions for volume replacement in neonates.[202] In addition, there is no evidence from randomised trials that HAS is of any benefit in hypoalbuminaemic neonates with clinically significant peripheral oedema.[69] Together these data suggest that there is no good indication for the use of HAS in standard neonatal practice.

Exchange transfusion

As severe Rh HDN decreases in frequency, exchange transfusion is also becoming an increasingly rare procedure in neonatal medicine. Therefore, to ensure a high standard of practice, all neonatal units must adopt and maintain written practice guidelines for this procedure as outlined in the recent BCSH guidelines.[27]

Indications for exchange transfusion

Established indications for exchange transfusion of neonates are severe anaemia, particularly in the presence of heart failure, and/or hyperbilirubinaemia.[27] Controversial indications for exchange transfusion, for which there is insufficient evidence, include metabolic disease, septicaemia and DIC.[27]

Principles of exchange transfusion and the product to transfuse

The current BCSH guidelines state that blood for exchange transfusion should be group O, RhD-identical with the neonate, Kell-negative and <5 days old.[27] They also state that the blood should be CMV-negative, although universal leukocyte depletion of red cells in the UK means that CMV-untested blood is likely to be of equivalent safety to CMV-negative blood even in the newborn.[200] To prevent TA-GVHD, the blood should be irradiated *if the baby has received intrauterine transfusion;*[27] otherwise, irradiation of blood for exchange is recommended, but is not essential, and should only be requested where irradiation will not lead to a significant delay (the risks of severe hyperbilirubinaemia are greater than the remote risk of TA-GVHD).[27]

There is no consensus about whether whole blood or plasma-reduced red cells should be used for exchange transfusion in neonates; however, the current BCSH guidelines state that plasma-reduced red cells with a haematocrit of 0.50–0.60 should be suitable for both hyperbilirubinaemia and severe anaemia and this product is available from the National Blood Service in the UK.[27] It is important to note that packed red cells as supplied for 'top-up' transfusion may have a haematocrit of up to 0.75, leading to an unacceptably high post-exchange haematocrit, and, if used, will require dilution with colloid or saline. By contrast, whole blood, with a haematocrit of 0.35–0.45, may result in a post-exchange haemoglobin of <12 g/dl in a severely anaemic baby and thus increase the need for subsequent 'top-up' transfusion (whole blood is no longer widely available).[27] The pH of a unit of plasma-reduced red cells (and of whole blood) is around 7.0, which does not contribute to acidosis in the infant. Blood for exchange transfusion should be warmed to 37°C immediately prior to transfusion.

Dilutional exchange transfusion for polycythaemia

Dilutional exchange transfusion is undertaken to reduce whole blood viscosity in neonates with polycythaemia. There is no evidence to support the use of FFP or albumin for this procedure,[202] both of which carry the risk of transfusion-transmitted infection. In the assessment of such neonates it should always be remembered that umbilical venous catheterisation and dilutional exchange are not without complications. When considered clinically appropriate, a one-third whole blood volume exchange (80 ml/kg) is usually performed.

References

1. Alagappan A, Shattuck K E, Malloy M H 1998 Impact of transfusion guidelines on neonatal transfusions. Journal of Perinatology 18: 92–97
2. Albert T S E, Meng G, Simms P, Cohen R L, Phibbs R H 2000 Thrombopoietin in the thrombocytopenic term and preterm newborn. Pediatrics 105: 1286–1291
3. Alcock G S, Liley H 2002 Immunoglobulin infusion for isoimmune haemolytic jaundice in neonates (Cochrane Review). Cochrane Database of Systematic Reviews 3: CD003313
4. Alkalay A L, Mazkereth R, Santulli T, Pomerance J J 1993 Central venous line thrombosis in premature infants: a case management and literature review. American Journal of Perinatology 10: 323–326
5. Andrew M 1997 The relevance of developmental haemostasis to haemorrhagic disorders of newborns. Seminars in Perinatology 21: 70–85
6. Andrew M, de Veber G 1997 Paediatric thromboembolism and stroke protocols. B C Decker, Hamilton, Ontario
7. Andrew M, Paes B, Johnston M et al 1988 Development of the human coagulation system in the healthy premature infant. Blood 72: 1651–1657
8. Andrew M, Paes B, Milner R et al 1987 Development of the coagulation system in the full term infant. Blood 70: 165–172
9. Andrew M, Vegh P, Caco V C et al 1993 A randomized, controlled trial of platelet transfusions in thrombocytopenic premature infants. Journal of Pediatrics 123: 285–291
10. Anwar R, Miloszewski K J A 1999 Factor XIII deficiency. British Journal of Haematology 107: 468–484
11. Anwar R, Minford A, Gallivan L, Trinh C H, Markham A F 2002 Delayed umbilical bleeding – a presenting feature for factor XIII deficiency: clinical features, genetics, and management. Pediatrics 109: E32143
12. Aprikyan A A, Carlsson G, Stein S et al 2004 Neutrophil elastase mutations in severe congenital neutropenia patients of the original Kostmann family. Blood 103: 389
13. Bajwa R P, Skinner R, Windebank K P, Wariyar U K, Reid M M 2001 Chemotherapy and marrow transplantation for congenital leukaemia. Archives of Disease in Childhood. Fetal and Neonatal Edition 84: F47–F48
14. Ball S E, McGuckin C P, Jenkins G, Gordon-Smith E C 1996 Diamond-Blackfan anaemia in the UK: analysis of 80 cases from a 20-year birth cohort. British Journal of Haematology 94: 645–653
15. Bard H 1975 The postnatal decline in HbF synthesis in normal full-time infants. Journal of Clinical Investigation 55: 395–398
16. Bechensteen A G, Haga P, Halvorsen S et al 1993 Erythropoietin, protein, and iron supplementation and the prevention of the anaemia of prematurity. Archives of Disease in Childhood 69: 19–23
17. Bednarek F J, Weisberger S, Richardson D K et al 1998 Variations in blood transfusions among newborn intensive care units. SNAP II Study Group. Journal of Pediatrics 133: 601–607
18. Beeram M R, Krauss D R, Riggs M W 2001 Red blood cell transfusion practices in very low birth weight infants in 1990s postsurfactant era. Journal of the National Medical Association 93: 405–409
19. Bick R L 2002 Disseminated intravascular coagulation: a review of etiology, pathophysiology, diagnosis, and management: guidelines for care. Clinical and Applied Thrombosis/Hemostasis 8: 1–31
20. Blanchette V, Rand M L 1997 Platelet disorders in newborn infants: diagnosis and management. Seminars in Perinatology 21: 53–62
21. Boralessa H, Modi N, Cockburn H et al 2002 RBC T activation and hemolysis in a neonatal intensive care population: implications for transfusion practice. Transfusion. 42: 1428–1434

22. Bouma B N, Marx P F, Mosnier L O, Meijers J 2001 Thrombin-activatable fibrinolysis inhibitor (TAFI, plasma procarboxypeptidase B, procarboxypeptidase R, procarboxypeptidase U). Thrombosis Research 101: 329–354

23. Bowden J B, Hebert A A, Rapini R P 1989 Dermal hematopoiesis in neonates: report of five cases. Journal of the American Academy of Dermatology 20: 1104–1110

24. Bracci R, Martini G, Buonocore G et al 1988 Changes in erythrocyte properties during the first hours of life: electron spin resonance of reacting sulfhydryl groups. Pediatric Research 24: 391–395

25. Bresters D, Reus A C, Veerman A J, van Wering E R, van der Does-van den Berg A, Kaspers G J 2002 Congenital leukaemia: the Dutch experience and review of the literature. British Journal of Haematology 117: 513–524

26. British Committee for Standards in Haematology, Haemostasis and Thrombosis Task Force 2002 The investigation and management of neonatal haemostasis and thrombosis. British Journal of Haematology 119: 295–309

27. British Committee for Standards in Haematology, Transfusion Task Force. Transfusion guidelines for neonates and older children 24.2.03. *www.bcshguidelines.com/*

28. Brooks S E, Marcus D M, Gillis D et al 1999 The effect of blood transfusion protocol on retinopathy of prematurity: a prospective, randomized study. Pediatrics 104: 514–518

29. Brousson M A, Klein M C 1996 Controversies surrounding the administration of vitamin K to newborns: a review. Canadian Medical Association Journal 154: 307–315

30. Brown H L, Abernathy M P 1998 Cytomegalovirus infection. Seminars in Perinatology 22: 260–266

31. Brown K 2000 Haematological consequences of parvovirus B19 infection. Baillière's Best Practice & Research. Clinical Haematology 13: 245–259

32. Brown M S, Phibbs R H, Garcia J F, Dallman P R 1983 Postnatal changes in erythropoietin levels in untransfused premature infants. Journal of Pediatrics 103: 612–617

33. Buchanan G R 1999 Factor concentrate prophylaxis for neonates with hemophilia. Journal of Pediatric Hematology/Oncology 21: 254–256

34. Bussel J B 2001 Alloimmune thrombocytopenia in the fetus and newborn. Seminars in Thrombosis and Hemostasis 27: 245–252

35. Bussel J, Kaplan C 1998 The fetal and neonatal consequences of maternal alloimmune thrombocytopenia. Baillière's Clinical Haematology 11: 391–408

36. Calhoun D A, Christensen R D, Edstrom C S et al 2002 Consistent approaches to procedures and practices in neonatal hematology. Clinics in Perinatology 27: 733–753

37. Campagnoli C, Fisk N, Overton T, Bennett P, Watts T, Roberts I 2000 Circulating hematopoietic progenitor cells in first trimester fetal blood. Blood 95: 1967–1972

38. Casadevall N, Nataf J, Viron B et al 2002 Pure red-cell aplasia and antierythropoietin antibodies in patients treated with recombinant erythropoietin. New England Journal of Medicine 346: 469–475

39. Castaman G, Federici A B, Rodeghiero F, Mannucci P M 2003 von Willebrand's disease in the year 2003: towards the complete identification of gene defects for correct diagnosis and treatment. Haematologica 88: 94–108

40. Chik K W, Shing M M, Li C K et al 1998 Treatment of hemoglobin Bart's hydrops with bone marrow transplantation. Journal of Pediatrics 132: 1039–1042

41. Christensen R D, Calhoun D A, Rimsza L M 2000 A practical approach to evaluating and treating neutropenia in the neonatal intensive care unit. Clinics in Perinatology 27: 577–601

42. Chuansumrit A, Nuntnarumit P, Okascharoen C, Teeraratkul S, Suwansingh S, Supapannachart S 2002 The use of recombinant activated factor VII to control bleeding in a preterm infant undergoing exploratory laparotomy. Pediatrics 110: 169–171

43. Cornelissen M, von Kries R, Loughnan P, Schubiger G 1997 Prevention of vitamin K deficiency bleeding: efficacy of different multiple oral dose schedules of vitamin K. European Journal of Pediatrics 156: 126–130

44. Dame C, Albers N, Hasan C et al 1999 Homozygous alpha-thalassaemia and hypospadias – common aetiology or incidental association? Long-term survival of Hb Bart's hydrops syndrome leads to new aspects for counselling of alpha-thalassaemic traits. European Journal of Pediatrics 158: 217–220

45. Dame C, Fahnenstich H, Freitag P et al 1998 Erythropoietin mRNA expression in human fetal and neonatal tissue. Blood 92: 3218–3225

46. Davies S C, Cronin E, Gill M, Greengross P, Hickman M, Normand C 2000 Screening for sickle cell disease and thalassaemia: a systematic review with supplementary research. Health Technology Assessment 4: iii–v, 1–99

47. Davis D J 2000 Neonatal subgaleal hemorrhage: diagnosis and management. Canadian Medical Association Journal 164: 1452–1453

48. de Alarcon P A, Graeve J L 1996 Analysis of megakaryocyte ploidy in fetal bone marrow biopsies using a new adaptation of the feulgen technique to measure DNA content and estimate megakaryocyte ploidy from biopsy specimens. Pediatric Research 39: 166–170

49. Delaunay J 2002 Molecular basis of red cell membrane disorders. Acta Haematologica 108: 210–218

50. Dgany O, Avidan N, Delaunay J et al 2002 Congenital dyserythropoietic anemia type I is caused by mutations in codanin-1. American Journal of Human Genetics 71: 1467–1474

51. Donalto H, Vain N, Rendo P et al 2000 Effect of early versus late administration of human recombinant erythropoietin on transfusion requirements in premature infants: results of a randomized, placebo-controlled, multicenter trial. Pediatrics 105: 1066–1072

52. Draptchinskaia N, Gustavsson P, Andersson B et al 1999 The gene encoding ribosomal protein S19 is mutated in Diamond-Blackfan anaemia. Nature Genetics 21: 169–175

53. Edstrom C S, Calhoun D A, Christensen R D 2000 Expression of tissue factor pathway inhibitor in human fetal and placental tissues. Early Human Development 59: 77–84

54. Fisch P, Handgretinger R, Schaefer H 2000 Pure red cell aplasia. British Journal of Haematology 111: 1010–1022

55. Forestier F, Daffos F, Galacteros F 1986 Hematological values of 163 normal fetuses between 18 and 30 weeks of gestation. Pediatric Research 20: 342–346

56. Franz A R, Pohlandt F 2001 Red blood cell transfusions in very and extremely low birthweight infants under restrictive transfusion guidelines: is exogenous erythropoietin necessary? Archives of Disease in Childhood. Fetal and Neonatal Edition 84: F96–F100

57. Fuller N J, Bates C J, Cole T J, Lucas A 1992 Plasma folate levels in preterm infants, with and without a 1mg daily folate supplement. European Journal of Pediatrics 151: 48–50

58. Freedman M H 2000 Diamond-Blackfan anemia. Baillière's Clinical Haematology 13: 391–406

59. Frey B, Losa M 2001 The value of capillary whole blood lactate for blood transfusion requirements in anaemia of prematurity. Intensive Care Medicine 27: 222–227

60. Garcia M G, Duenas E, Sola M C et al 2001 Epidemiologic and outcome studies of patients who received platelet transfusions in the neonatal intensive care unit. Journal of Perinatology 21: 415–420

61. Garcia M G, Hutson A D, Christensen R D 2002 Effect of recombinant erythropoietin on 'late' transfusions in the neonatal intensive care unit: a meta analysis. Journal of Perinatology 22: 108–111

62. Giachoia G P 1997 Severe fetomaternal hemorrhage: a review. Obstetrical and Gynecological Survey 52: 372–380

63. Giampietro G F, Adler-Brecher B, Verlander P C, Pavlakis S G, Davis J G, Auerbach A D 1993 The need for more accurate and timely diagnosis in Fanconi anemia: a report from the International Fanconi Anemia Registry. Pediatrics 91: 1116–1120

64. Gill K K, Kelton J G 2000 Management of idiopathic thrombocytopenic purpura in pregnancy. Seminars in Hematology 37: 275–289

65. Gilsanz F, Vega M A, Gomez-Castillo E, Ruiz-Balda J A, Omenaca F 1993 Fetal anaemia due to pyruvate kinase deficiency. Archives of Disease in Childhood 69: 523–524

66. Golding J, Greenwood R, Birmingham K, Mott M 1992 Childhood cancer, intramuscular vitamin K, and pethidine given during labour. British Medical Journal 305: 341–346

67. Gottstein R, Cooke R W I 2003 Systematic review of intravenous immunoglobulin in haemolytic disease of the newborn. Archives of Disease in Childhood. Fetal and Neonatal Edition 88: F6–F10

68. Grant S R, Kilby M D, Meer L, Weaver J B, Gabra G S, Whittle M J 2000 The outcome of pregnancy in Kell alloimmunisation. BJOG 107: 481–485

69. Greenough A, Emery E, Hird M F, Gamsu H R 1993 Randomised controlled trial of albumin infusion in ill preterm infants. European Journal of Pediatrics 152: 157–159

70. Griffin I J, Cooke R J, Reid M M, McCormick K P B, Smith J S 1999 Iron nutritional status in preterm infants fed formulas fortified by iron. Archives of Disease in Childhood. Fetal and Neonatal Edition 81: F45–F49

71. Hakanson D O, Oh W 1977 Necrotizing enterocolitis and hyperviscosity in the newborn infant. Journal of Pediatrics 90: 458–461

72. Hall G W 2001 Kasabach-Merritt syndrome: pathogenesis and management. British Journal of Haematology 112: 851–862

73. Halvorsen S, Bechensteen A G 2002 Physiology of erythropoietin during mammalian development. Acta Paediatrica. Supplement 91: 17–26

74. Hann I M 1991 The normal blood picture in neonates. In: Hann I M, Gibson B E S, Letsky E A (eds) Fetal and neonatal haematology. Baillière Tindall, London

75. Hartmann J, Hussein A, Trowitzscha E, Beckerb J, Henneckeb K-H 2001 Treatment of neonatal thrombus formation with recombinant tissue plasminogen

activator: six years experience and review of the literature Archives of Disease in Childhood. Fetal and Neonatal Edition 85: F18–F22

76. Heegaard E D, Brown K E 2002 Human parvovirus B19. Clinical Microbiology Reviews 15: 485–505

77. Hegyi E, Nakazawa M, Debili N et al 1991 Developmental changes in human megakaryocyte ploidy. Experimental Hematology 19: 87–94

78. Heller C, Schobess R, Kurnik K et al 2000 Abdominal venous thrombosis in neonates and infants: role of prothrombotic risk factors – a multicentre case-control study. For the Childhood Thrombophilia Study Group. British Journal of Haematology 111: 534–539

79. Herschel M, Karrison T, Wen M, Caldarelli L, Baron B 2002 Isoimmunization is unlikely to be the cause of hemolysis in ABO-incompatible but direct antiglobulin test-negative neonates. Pediatrics 110: 127–130

80. Hey E 2003 Vitamin K – what, why, and when. Archives of Disease in Childhood. Fetal and Neonatal Edition 88: F80–F83

81. Higgs D R 1993 Alpha-thalassaemia. Baillière's Clinical Haematology 6: 117–150

82. Hitzler J K, Cheung J, Li Y, Scherer G W, Zipursky A 2003 GATA1 mutations in transient leukemia and acute megakaryoblastic leukemia of Down syndrome. Blood 101: 4301–4304

83. Horan M, Stutchfield P R 2001 Severe congenital myotonic dystrophy and severe anaemia of prematurity in an infant of Jehovah's Witness parents. Developmental Medicine and Child Neurology 43: 346–349

84. Howarth D J, Robinson F M, Williams M, Norfolk D R 2002 A modified Kleihauer technique for the quantitation of foetomaternal haemorrhage. Transfusion Medicine 12: 373–378

85. Howard H, Martlew V, McFadyen I et al 1998 Consequences for fetus and neonate of maternal red cell alloimmunisation. Archives of Disease in Childhood. Fetal and Neonatal Edition 78: F62–F66

86. Hume H 1997 Red blood cell transfusions for preterm infants: the role of evidence-based medicine. Seminars in Perinatology 21: 8–19

87. Hutton R A, Laffan M A, Tuddenham E G D 1999 Normal haemostasis. In: Hoffbrand A V, Lewis S M, Tuddenham E G D (eds) Postgraduate haematology, 4th edition. Butterworth-Heinemann, London, pp 550–580

88. Huynh A, Dommergues M, Izac B et al 1995 Characterization of hematopoietic progenitors from human yolk sacs and embryos. Blood 86: 4474–4485

89. Ikenboom J C 2001 Congenital von Willebrand disease type 3: clinical manifestations, pathophysiology and molecular biology. Best Practice & Research. Clinical Haematology 14: 365–379

90. Israels S J, Cheang T, McMillan-Ward E M, Cheang M 2001 Evaluation of primary hemostasis in neonates with a new in vitro platelet function analyzer. Journal of Pediatrics 138: 116–119

91. Jolly M C, Letsky E A, Fisk N M 2002 The management of fetal alloimmune thrombocytopenia. Prenatal Diagnosis 22: 96–98

92. Jordan J A 1996 Identification of human parvovirus B19 infection in non-immune hydrops fetalis. American Journal of Obstetrics and Gynecology 174: 37–42

93. Kadir RA 1999 Women and inherited bleeding disorders: pregnancy. Seminars in Hematology 36: 28–35

94. Kaplan M 2001 Genetic interactions in the pathogenesis of neonatal hyper-bilirubinemia: Gilbert's syndrome and glucose-6-phosphate dehydrogenase deficiency. Journal of Perinatology 21(suppl. 1): S35–S39

95. Kaplan M, Hammerman C 2002 Glucose-6-phosphate dehydrogenase deficiency: a potential source of severe neonatal hyperbilirubinaemia and kernicterus. Seminars in Neonatology 7: 121–128

96. Karnon J, Zeuner D, Ades A E, Efimba W, Brown J, Yardumian A 2000 The effects of neonatal screening for sickle cell disorders on lifetime treatment costs and early deaths avoided: a modelling approach. Journal of Public Health Medicine 22: 500–511

97. Karpatkin M 1999 Coagulation problems in the newborn. Seminars in Neonatology 4: 1–7

98. Kavakli K 1999 Fibrin glue and clinical impact on hemophilia care. Haemophilia 5: 392–396

99. Kavakli K, Aldecort LM 1998 Circumcision and haemophilia: a perspective. Haemophilia 4: 1–3

100. Kelton J G 2002 Idiopathic thrombocytopenic purpura complicating pregnancy. Blood Reviews 16: 43–46

101. Kleinman S, Chan P, Robillard P 2003 Risks associated with transfusion of cellular blood components in Canada. Transfusion Medicine Reviews 17: 120–162

102. Koenig J M, Christensen R D 1989 Incidence, neutrophil kinetics, and natural history of neonatal neutropenia associated with maternal hypertension. New England Journal of Medicine 321: 557–562

103. Kottke-Marchant K, Comp P 2002 Laboratory issues in diagnosing abnormalities of protein C, thrombomodulin, and endothelial cell protein C receptor. Archives of Pathology and Laboratory Medicine 126: 1337–1348

104. Kuhle S, Lane D A, Jochmanns K et al 2001 Homozygous antithrombin deficiency type II (99 Leu to Phe mutation) and childhood thromboembolism. Thrombosis and Haemostasis 86: 1007–1011

105. Kulkarni R, Lusher J 2001 Perinatal management of newborns with haemophilia. British Journal of Haematology 112: 264–274

106. Kulkarni R, Lusher J M 1999 Intracranial and extracranial hemorrhages in newborns with hemophilia: a review of the literature. Journal of Pediatric Hematology/Oncology 21: 289–295

107. Lallemand A V, Doco-Fenzy M, Gaillard D A 1999 Investigation of nonimmune hydrops fetalis: multidisciplinary studies are necessary for diagnosis – review of 94 cases. Pediatric and Developmental Pathology 2: 432–439

108. Lange B 2000 The management of neoplastic disorders of haematopoiesis in children with Down's syndrome. British Journal of Haematology 110: 512–524

109. Leaker M, Massicotte M P, Brooker L A, Andrew M 1996 Thrombolytic therapy in pediatric patients: a comprehensive review of the literature. Thrombosis and Haemostasis 76: 132–134

110. Lee-Potter J P, Deacon-Smith R A, Simpkiss M J, Kamuzora H, Lehmann H 1975 A new cause of hemolytic anemia in the newborn. Journal of Clinical Pathology 28: 317–320

111. Lin J C, Strauss R G, Kulhavy J C et al 2000 Phlebotomy overdraw in the neonatal intensive care nursery. Pediatrics 106: E19

112. Linderkamp O, Nelle M, Kraus M, Zilow E P 1992 The effect of early and late cord clamping on blood viscosity and other hemorheological parameters in full-term infants. Acta Paediatrica 81: 745–750

113. Linderkamp O, Versmold H T, Strohhacker I, Messow-Zahn K, Riegel K P, Betke K 1977 Capillary-venous hematocrit differences in newborn infants: I. Relationship to blood volume, peripheral blood flow and acid base parameters. European Journal of Pediatrics 127: 9–14

114. Ljung R, Lindgren A C, Petrini P, Tengborn L 1994 Normal vaginal delivery is to be recommended for haemophilia carrier gravidae. Acta Paediatrica 83: 6901–6911

115. Luzzatto L 1993 Glucose-6-phosphate dehydrogenase deficiency. In: Nathan A, Oski F A (eds) Hematology of infancy and childhood, 4th edition. W B Saunders, Philadelphia, pp 674–695

116. Madsen L P, Rasmussen M K, Bjerregaard L L, Nohr S B, Ebbesen F 2000 Impact of blood sampling in very preterm infants. Scandinavian Journal of Clinical and Laboratory Investigation 60: 125–132

117. Maheshwari A, Christensen R D, Calhoun D A 2002 Immune neutropenia in the neonate. Advances in Pediatrics 49: 317–339

118. Maier R F, Obladen M, Muller-Hansen I et al 2002 Early treatment with erythropoietin beta ameliorates anemia and reduces transfusion requirements in infants with birth weights below 1,000 g. Journal of Pediatrics 141: 8–15

119. Maier R F, Obladen M, Scigalla P et al 1994 The effect of epoetin beta (recombinant human erythropoietin) on the need for transfusion in very-low-birth-weight infants. European Multicentre Erythropoietin Study Group. New England Journal of Medicine 330: 1173–1178

120. Marlar R A, Montgomery R R, Broekmans A W 1989 Diagnosis and treatment of homozygous protein C deficiency. Report of the Working Party on Homozygous Protein C Deficiency. International Committee of Haemostasis and Thrombosis. Journal of Pediatrics 114: 528–534

121. Marshall C J, Thrasher A J 2001 The embryonic origins of human haematopoiesis. British Journal of Haematology 112: 838–850

122. Matoth Y, Zaizov R, Varsano I 1971 Postnatal changes in some red cell parameters. Acta Paediatrica Scandinavica 60: 317–320

123. Mattsson E, Herwald H, Bjorck L, Egesten A 2002 Peptidoglycan from Staphylococcus aureus induces tissue factor expression and procoagulant activity in human monocytes. Infection and Immunity 70: 3033–3039

124. Mercuri E, Cowan F, Gupte G et al 2001 Prothrombotic disorders and abnormal neurodevelopmental outcome in infants with neonatal cerebral infarction. Pediatrics 107: 1400–1404

125. Meyer M P, Sharma E, Carsons M 2003 Recombinant erythropoietin and blood transfusion in selected preterm infants. Archives of Disease in Childhood. Fetal and Neonatal Edition 88: F41–F45

126. Millar D S, Johansen B, Berntorp E et al 2000 Molecular genetic analysis of severe protein C deficiency. Human Genetics 106: 646–653

127. Miller E, Miller C K, Cohen B J, Seng C 1998 Immediate and long-term outcome of human parvovirus B19 infection in pregnancy. British Journal of Obstetrics and Gynaecology 105: 174–178

128. Mugishima H, Gale R P, Rowlings P A 1995 Bone marrow transplantation for Diamond-Blackfan anemia. Bone Marrow Transplantation 15: 55–58

129. Muntean W 2002 Fresh frozen plasma in the pediatric age group and in congenital coagulation factor deficiency. Thrombosis Research 107(suppl. 1): S29

130. Murray N A, Howarth L J, McMcloy M, Letsky E A, Roberts I A G 2002 Platelet transfusion in the management of severe thrombocytopenia in neonatal intensive care unit (NICU) patients. Transfusion Medicine 12: 35–41

131. Murray N A, Roberts I A G 1996 Circulating megakaryocytes and their progenitors in neonatal thrombocytopenia. Pediatric Research 40: 1–8

132. Niermeyer S, Kattwinkel J, Van Reempts P et al 2000 International Guidelines for Neonatal Resuscitation: an excerpt from the Guidelines 2000 for Cardiopulmonary Resuscitation and Emergency Cardiovascular Care: International Consensus on Science. Contributors and Reviewers for the Neonatal Resuscitation Guidelines. Pediatrics 106: E29

133. Norfolk D, Ancliffe P J, Contreras M et al 1998 Consensus Conference on Platelet Transfusion, Royal College of Physicians of Edinburgh, 27-28 November 1997. Synopsis of background papers. British Journal of Haematology 101: 609–617

134. Northern Neonatal Nursing Initiative Trial Group 1996 Randomised trial of prophylactic early fresh-frozen plasma or gelatin or glucose in preterm babies: outcome at 2 years. Lancet 348: 229–232

135. Nowak-Gottl U, Kosch A, Schlegel N 2001 Thromboembolism in newborns, infants and children. Thrombosis and Haemostasis 86: 464–474

136. Ohls R K 2000 The use of erythropoietin in neonates. Clinics in Perinatology 27: 681–696

137. Ohls R K 2002 Erythropoietin in extremely low birthweight infants: blood in versus blood out. Journal of Pediatrics 141: 3–6

138. Ohls R K, Ehrenkrantz R A, Wright L L et al 2001 Effects of early erythropoietin on the transfusion requirements of preterm infants below 1250 grams birth weight: a multicenter, randomized, controlled trial. Pediatrics 108: 934–942

139. Ohls R K, Li Y, Abdel-Mageed A, Buchanan G Jr, Mandell L, Christensen R D 1995 Neutrophil pool sizes and granulocyte colony-stimulating factor production in human mid-trimester fetuses. Pediatric Research 37: 806–811

140. Olivieri N F 1999 The beta-thalassemias. New England Journal of Medicine 341: 99–109

141. Oski F A 1993 The erythrocyte and its disorders. In: Nathan A, Oski F A (eds) Hematology of infancy and childhood. W B Saunders, Philadelphia, pp 18–43

142. Osterud B, Bjorklid E 2001 The tissue factor pathway in disseminated intravascular coagulation. Seminars in Thrombosis and Hemostasis 27: 605–617

143. Ouwehand W H, Smith G, Ranasinghe E 2000 Management of severe alloimmune thrombocytopenia in the newborn. Archives of Disease in Childhood. Fetal and Neonatal Edition 82: F173–F175

144. Pahal G, Jauniaux E, Kinnon C, Thrasher A J, Rodeck C H 2000 Normal development of human fetal hematopoiesis between eight and seventeen weeks' gestation. American Journal of Obstetrics and Gynecology 183: 1029–1034

145. Palek J, Jarolim P 1993 Clinical expression and laboratory detection of red blood cell membrane protein mutations. Seminars in Hematology 30: 249–283

146. Paul D A, Leef K H, Locke R G, Stefano J L 2002 Transfusion volume in infants with very low birth weight: a randomized trial of 10 versus 20 ml/kg. Journal of Pediatric Hematology/Oncology 24: 43–46

147. Pearson H A 1967 Life span of the fetal red blood cell. Journal of Pediatrics 70: 166–171

148. Pessler F, Hart D 2002 Hyporegenerative anemia associated with Rh hemolytic disease: treatment failure of recombinant erythropoietin. Journal of Pediatric Hematology/Oncology 24: 689–693

149. Public Health Laboratory Service Working Party on Fifth Disease 1990 Prospective study of human parvovirus (B19) infection in pregnancy. British Medical Journal 300: 1166–1170

150. Puckett R M, Offringa M 2000 Prophylactic vitamin K for vitamin K deficiency bleeding in neonates (Cochrane Review). Cochrane Database of Systematic Reviews 4: CD002776

151. Ramasethu J, Luban N L C 1999 Red blood cell transfusion in the newborn. Seminars in Neonatology 4: 5–16

152. Rao R, Georgieff M K 2002 Perinatal aspects of iron metabolism. Acta Paediatrica. Supplement 91: 124–129

153. Remacha A F, Badell I, Pujol-Moix N et al 2002 Hydrops fetalis-associated congenital dyserythropoietic anemia treated with intrauterine transfusions and bone marrow transplantation. Blood 100: 356–358

154. Reverdiau-Moalic P, Delahousse B, Body G, Bardos P, Leroy J, Gruel Y 1996 Evolution of blood coagulation activators and inhibitors in the healthy human fetus. Blood 88: 900–906

155. Roberts I A G, Murray N A 2001 Neonatal thrombocytopenia: new insights into pathogenesis and implications for clinical management. Current Opinion in Pediatrics 13: 16–21

156. Roberts I A G, Murray N A 2003 Thrombocytopenia in the newborn. Current Opinion in Pediatrics 15: 17–23

157. Rodwell R L, Gray P H, Taylor K M, Minchinton R 1996 Granulocyte colony stimulating factor treatment for alloimmune neonatal neutropenia. Archives of Disease in Childhood. Fetal and Neonatal Edition 75: F57–F58

158. Roman E, Flear N T, Ansell P et al 2002 Vitamin K and childhood cancer: analysis of individual patient data from six different case-control studies. British Journal of Cancer 86: 63–69

159. Roy M, Turner-Gomes S, Gill G, Mernagh J, Gillie P, Schmidt B 1997 Incidence and diagnosis of neonatal thrombosis associated with umbilical venous catheters. Thrombosis and Haemostasis 78: PS2953

160. Salvesen D R, Brudenell J M, Snijders R J, Ireland R M, Nicolaides K H 1993 Fetal plasma erythropoietin in pregnancies complicated by maternal diabetes mellitus. American Journal of Obstetrics and Gynecology 168: 88–94

161. Schmidt B, Andrew M 1992 Report of the Scientific and Standardization Subcommittee on Neonatal Hemostasis: diagnosis and treatment of neonatal thrombosis. Thrombosis and Haemostasis 67: 381–382

162. Schmidt B, Andrew M 1995 Neonatal thrombosis: report of a prospective Canadian and international registry. Pediatrics 96: 939–943

163. Schneider A S 2000 Triosephosphate isomerase deficiency: historical perspectives and molecular aspects. Baillière's Best Practice & Research. Clinical Haematology 13: 119–140

164. Shannon K M, Keith J F 3rd, Mentzer W C et al 1995 Recombinant human erythropoietin stimulates erythropoiesis and reduces erythrocyte transfusions in very low birth weight preterm infants. Pediatrics 95: 1–8

165. Singer S T, Styles L, Bojanowski J, Quirolo K, Foote D, Vichinsky E P 2000 Changing outcome of homozygous alpha-thalassemia: cautious optimism. Journal of Pediatric Hematology/Oncology 22: 539–542

166. Sisson T R C, Lund C J, Whalen L E, Telek A 1959 The blood volume of infants. I. The full term infant in the first year of life. Journal of Pediatrics 55: 163–179

167. Smith P 1990 Congenital coagulation protein deficiencies in the perinatal period. Seminars in Perinatology 14: 384–392

168. Smith O P, Hann I M, Woodward C E, Brockington M 1995 Pearson's marrow/pancreas syndrome: haematological features associated with deletion and duplication of mitochondrial DNA. British Journal of Haematology 90: 469–472

169. Sohan K, Billington M, Pamphilon D, Goulden N, Kyle P 2002 Normal growth and development following in utero diagnosis and treatment of homozygous alpha-thalassaemia. BJOG 109: 1308–1310

170. Sola M C, Del Vecchio A, Rimsza L M 2000 Evaluation and treatment of thrombocytopenia in the neonatal intensive care unit. Clinics in Perinatology 27: 655–679

171. Stockman J A, de Alarcon P A 2001 Overview of the state of the art of Rh disease: history, current clinical management, and recent progress. Journal of Pediatric Hematology/Oncology 23: 385–393

172. Stockman J A, Oski F A 1978 Erythrocytes of the human neonate. Current Topics in Hematology 1: 193–232

173. Stroncek D 2002 Neutrophil alloantigens. Transfusion Medicine Reviews 16: 67–75

174. Stuart M J, Graeber J E 1998 Normal hemostasis in the fetus and newborn: vessels and platelets. In: Polin R A, Fox W M (eds) Fetal and neonatal physiology. W B Saunders, Philadelphia, pp 1834–1848

175. Sutor A H, von Kries R, Cornelissen E A, McNinch A W, Andrew M 1999 Vitamin K deficiency bleeding (VKDB) in infancy. ISTH Pediatric/Perinatal Subcommittee. International Society on Thrombosis and Haemostasis. Thrombosis and Haemostasis 81: 456–461

176. Tavian M, Hallais M F, Peault B 1999 Emergence of intraembryonic hematopoietic precursors in the pre-liver human embryo. Development 126: 793–803

177. Thompson J 2002 Haemolytic disease of the newborn: the new NICE guidelines. Journal of Family Health Care 12: 133–136

178. Thurlbeck S M, McIntosh N 1987 Preterm blood counts vary with sampling site. Archives of Disease in Childhood 62: 74–87

179. Towner D, Castro M A, Eby-Wilkens E, Gilbert W 1999 Effect of mode of delivery in nulliparous women on neonatal intracranial injury. New England Journal of Medicine 341: 1709–1714

180. Tripp J H, Cornelissen M, Loughnan P et al 1995 Suggested protocol for the reporting of prospective studies of vitamin K deficiency bleeding (previously called hemorrhagic disease of the newborn). In: Sutor A H, Hathaway W E (eds) Vitamin K in infancy. Schattauer Verlag, Stuttgart, pp 395–401

181. Tse W T, Lux S E 1999 Red blood cell membrane disorders. British Journal of Haematology 104: 2–13

182. United Kingdom Haemophilia Centres Doctors' Organization Executive Committee 1997 Guidelines on therapeutic products to treat haemophilia and other hereditary coagulation disorders. Haemophilia 3: 63–77

183. Usher R, Lind J 1965 Blood volume of the newborn premature infant. Acta Paediatrica Scandinavica 54: 419

184. Vamvakas E C, Pineda A A 1996 Meta-analysis of clinical studies of the efficacy of granulocyte transfusions in the treatment of bacterial sepsis. Journal of Clinical Apheresis 11: 1–9

185. Vamvakas E C, Strauss R G 2001 Meta-analysis of controlled clinical trials studying the efficacy of rHuEPO in reducing blood transfusions in the anemia of prematurity. Transfusion 41: 406–415

186. Vaughan J I, Manning M, Warwick R M, Letsky E, Murray N A, Roberts I A G 1998 Inhibition of erythroid progenitor cell growth by anti-Kell (K): a mechanism for fetal anemia in K-immunized pregnancies. New England Journal of Medicine 338: 798–803

187. Vichinsky E, Hurst D, Earles A, Kleman K, Lubin B 1988 Newborn screening for sickle cell disease: effect on mortality. Pediatrics 81: 749–755

188. Vlachos A, Klein G W, Lipton J M 2001 The Diamond-Blackfan Anemia Registry: tool for investigating the epidemiology and biology of Diamond-Blackfan anemia. Journal of Pediatric Hematology/Oncology 23: 377–382

189. Vora M, Gruslin A 1998 Erythropoietin in obstetrics. Obstetrical and Gynecological Survey 53: 500–508

190. Waldron P, de Alarcon P 1999 ABO hemolytic disease of the newborn: a unique constellation of findings in siblings and review of protective mechanisms in the fetal-maternal system. American Journal of Perinatology 16: 391–398

191. Wang M, Hays T, Balasa V et al; Pediatric Coagulation Consortium 2003 Low-dose tissue plasminogen activator thrombolysis in children. Journal of Pediatric Hematology/Oncology 25: 379–386

192. Wardle S P, Garr R, Yoxall C W, Weindling A M 2002 A pilot randomised controlled trial of peripheral fractional oxygen extraction to guide blood transfusions in preterm infants. Archives of Disease in Childhood. Fetal and Neonatal Edition 86: F22–F27

193. Wardle S P, Weindling A M 2001 Peripheral fractional oxygen extraction and other measures of tissue oxygenation to guide blood transfusions in preterm infants. Seminars in Perinatology 25: 60–64

194. Watts T L, Murray N A, Roberts I A G 1999 Thrombopoietin has a primary role in the regulation of platelet production in preterm babies. Pediatric Research 46: 28–32

195. Watts T L, Roberts I A G 1999 Haematological abnormalities in the growth-restricted infant. Seminars in Neonatology 4: 41–54

196. Wechsler J, Greene M, McDevitt M A et al 2002 Acquired mutations in GATA1 in the megakaryoblastic leukaemia of Down syndrome. Nature Genetics 32: 148–152

197. Wee L Y, Fisk N M 2002 The twin-twin transfusion syndrome. Seminars in Neonatology 7: 187–202

198. Wen S W, Liu S, Kramer M S et al 2001 Comparison of maternal and infant outcomes between vacuum extraction and forceps deliveries. American Journal of Epidemiology 153: 103–107

199. Werner E J 1995 Neonatal polycythemia and hyperviscosity. Clinics in Perinatology 22: 693–710

200. Williamson L M Leucocyte depletion of the blood supply – how will patients benefit? British Journal of Haematology 110: 256–272

201. Williamson L, Cohen H, Love E, Jones H, Todd A, Soldan K 2000 The Serious Hazards of Transfusion (SHOT) initiative: the UK approach to haemovigilance. Vox Sanguinis 78(suppl. 2): 291–295

202. Wong W, Fok T F, Lee C H, Ng P C, So K W, Ou Y, Cheung K L 1997 Randomised controlled trial: comparison of colloid or crystalloid for partial exchange transfusion for treatment of neonatal polycythaemia. Archives of Disease in Childhood. Fetal and Neonatal Edition 77: F115–F118

203. Yaegashi N, Okamura K, Yajima A, Murai C, Sugamura K 1994 The frequency of human parvovirus B19 infection in non-immune hydrops fetalis. Journal of Perinatal Medicine 22: 159–163

204. Yao A C, Lin J, Tiisala R, Michelsson K 1969 Placental transfusion in the premature infant with observation on clinical course and outcome. Acta Paediatrica Scandinavica 58: 561–566

205. Zanella A, Bianchi P 2000 Red cell pyruvate kinase deficiency: from genetics to clinical manifestations. Baillière's Best Practice & Research. Clinical Haematology 13: 57–81

206. Zetterstrom R 2002 Kostmann disease – infantile genetic agranulocytosis: historical view and new aspects. Acta Paediatrica 91: 1279–1281

207. Zipursky A 1999 Prevention of vitamin K deficiency bleeding in newborns. British Journal of Haematology 104: 430–437

208. Zuppa A A, Maragliano G, Scapillati M E et al 1999 Recombinant erythropoietin in the prevention of late anaemia in intrauterine transfused neonates with Rh-haemolytic disease. Fetal Diagnosis and Therapy 14: 270–274

CHAPTER 31

Non-immune hydrops fetalis

Phillip Etches, Nestor Demianczuk, Radha Chari

Introduction

'Hydrops fetalis' describes a fetus or neonate with a pathological increase in total and interstitial body water, manifested as generalised subcutaneous oedema, accompanied by serous fluid collections within one or more of the pericardial, pleural, or peritoneal spaces. Associated antenatal ultrasound findings include polyhydramnios and placental oedema.[21] In-utero diagnosis of fetal hydrops identifies a clinical entity which has a myriad of underlying aetiologies and associations. This diagnosis also implies that the fetus is significantly compromised and at imminent risk for serious morbidity or mortality. However, the risks and prognosis are dependent upon the actual aetiology of the hydrops and any antenatal or postnatal therapy that may be available. Consequently, the antenatal detection of fetal hydrops requires an expeditious and diligent search for the underlying cause in order to direct appropriate pregnancy counselling and management.

Classification and epidemiology

There are two major categories of hydrops fetalis:

- immune hydrops secondary to erythroblastosis fetalis from Rhesus isoimmunisation or other maternal-fetal blood group incompatibilities;
- 'non-immune hydrops' (NIH), which includes all other causes.

Historically, Rh isoimmunisation was the leading cause of hydrops, accounting for 82% of cases in 1970.[62] However, with the institution of passive maternal immunisation and fetal intrauterine transfusion over the last few decades, NIH has become comparatively more prevalent. In 1992, Santolaya et al[87] reported a series of 76 hydropic fetuses, 87% of which were non-immune, and more recently, in a report from Taiwan, 78 out of 79 cases of hydrops were non-immune: of these, homozygous α-thalassaemia accounted for 31%.[102] The reported incidence of NIH at delivery varies from 1 in 830 to 1 in 3500.[43,62,96] From a pathological standpoint, an autopsy series from Northern France reported that 6% of fetal deaths were due to NIH, of which one-third had chromosomal abnormalities,[56] thus implying that many cases of fetal hydrops do not reach viability. This conclusion is supported by reports describing the early (10–17 weeks) ultrasound diagnosis of NIH, in which there was a high prevalence of chromosomal abnormalities (47–78%) and a very high fetal mortality (95–100%).[44,83] The prognosis for NIH, even if the pregnancy reaches viability, remains poor, with a perinatal mortality rate in excess of 50%.[14,43,98] Mortality remains high even in series reported in the 1990s.[70,100] Factors that contribute to this poor outcome are multiple, and include chromosomal anomalies, major malformations, pulmonary hypoplasia (pp. 583–4) and preterm delivery.

Pathophysiology

Interstitial fluid is produced at the level of the capillary, through the ultrafiltration of plasma. The normal transcapillary filtration rate is determined by the balance between the capillary and interstitial hydrostatic and colloid osmotic pressures, together with the capillary permeability.[91] Infection, fetal anaemia, cardiac failure, congenital anomalies and metabolic disorders may lead to increased central venous and/or lymphatic pressures, alteration in capillary permeability, and changes in colloid osmotic pressure, leading to interstitial fluid accumulation.[4,13] These processes are facilitated in the fetus by a relatively greater capillary filtration coefficient and greater interstitial compliance; in some cases, the fluid accumulation may be mediated by the renin–angiotension system causing placental fluid retention.[25,61]

Figure 31.1 summarises the possible interrelationships between the more common underlying aetiologies and the pathophysiological mechanisms that may lead to the development of hydrops. As illustrated, a single aetiology may lead to hydrops through

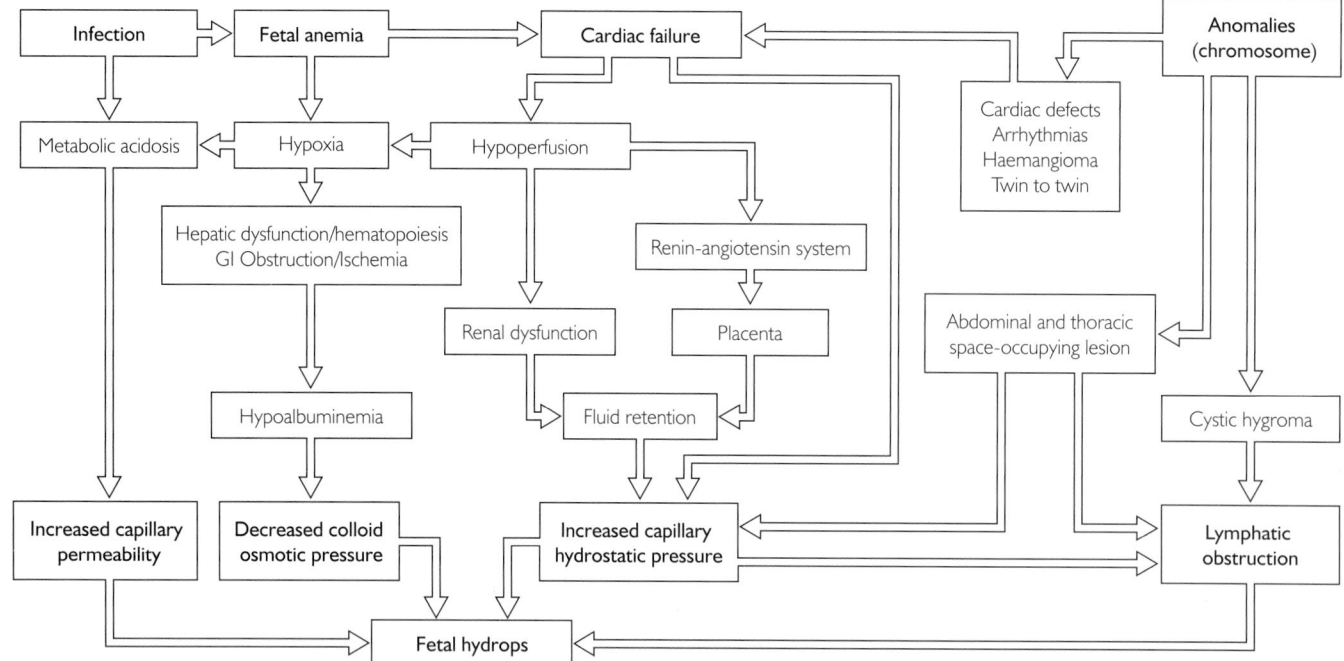

Fig. 31.1 Pathophysiological mechanisms whereby associated conditions may lead to fetal hydrops.

more than one pathophysiological mechanism.[6] In many cases, only by removing or correcting the underlying cause may the abnormal accumulation of interstitial fluid be reversed. This principle is important when in-utero shunting is being considered in order to drain body cavity fluid collections, for although one or two cavities may be decompressed, fluid accumulation in inaccessible vital areas of the fetus may still continue. Therefore, in generalised fetal NIH, the treatment of specific symptoms may neither alter the overall course of the disease nor improve the prognosis.

Diagnosis and antenatal management

Hydrops fetalis is not a diagnosis, but an ominous sign of underlying fetal abnormality or disease. Therefore, referral to a tertiary care unit for assessment, investigation, counselling and management is required.

History and physical examination

A family history of anaemia, a maternal history of consanguinity, Mediterranean or Asian ancestry, antepartum haemorrhage, infection during pregnancy, Graves' disease, polyhydramnios, or use of certain drugs may flag the pregnancy at risk for NIH. A clinical maternal status which mimics that of the hydropic fetus has also been described. This 'mirror syndrome' includes maternal peripheral oedema, hypertension, proteinuria, and a hyperdynamic circulation.[73] A maternal blood type and routine antibody screen will rule out virtually all *immune* causes of hydrops.

Ultrasound examination

Ultrasound allows the physician to determine the degree and extent of the fetal hydrops, assess fetal wellbeing, and search for fetal abnormalities. Polyhydramnios is commonly associated with hydrops fetalis.[39] The umbilical cord and placenta are scanned for evidence of masses such as cord cysts or chorioangiomas.[90] A thickened placenta may be associated with fetal anaemia,[86] which can also be assessed using the middle cerebral artery peak systolic velocity flow.[20] The earliest ultrasound finding may be increased nuchal translucency thickness at 10 to 15 weeks' gestation.[46]

Specific evaluation of the fetal anatomy is critical. A thorough fetal cardiac scan is indicated, as up to 26% of fetal hydrops cases are associated with cardiac disease.[64] Occasionally, visualisation of the heart is suboptimal secondary to compression from a pericardial or pleural effusion and some authors have found it helpful to drain this excess fluid in utero to obtain a transient improvement in visualisation of the fetal heart.[72] A search for cardiac arrhythmia is also required, as both tachyarrhythmias and bradyarrhythmias have been associated with the development of NIH. Evaluation of abnormal fetal posture and movement may suggest particular chromosomal or neuromuscular disorders.[94] The size and appearance of the liver and spleen should be also evaluated, as their enlargement may suggest congenital hepatitis or various inherited disorders of metabolism.[47]

Investigations

The maternal history and ultrasound assessment will direct further investigations. Fetal tissue can be obtained by amniocentesis, chorionic villus sampling, or cordocentesis, for genetic or infectious evaluation. For those cases where a definite cause is not evident, reference to Table 31.1 may help. Specific maternal

Table 31.1 Categorisation of conditions associated with NIH, a frequency estimate as a percentage of cases of NIH, and possible pathophysiological mechanisms. Most, if not all, of these conditions may occur without NIH. (Adapted from Holtzgreve et al,[41] Jones,[47] Cassady[13] and others.)

FETAL: FOCAL ABNORMALITY

Cardiac
Left-sided lesions
  Hypoplastic left heart
  Mitral stenosis
  Aortic valvular stenosis
  Coarctation of the aorta
Right-sided lesions
  Ebstein's anomaly of the tricuspid valve
  Atrioventricular canal defect
  Hypoplastic right heart
Central lesions
  Premature closure or restriction of the
    foramen ovale
  Premature closure or restriction of the ductus
    arteriosus
  Transposition of the great vessels
Rhythm abnormalities
  Supraventricular tachycardia
  Atrial flutter
  Atrial fibrillation
  Ventricular tachycardia
  Sinus bradycardia
  Heart block
Cardiac tumours
  Rhabdomyomas
  Haemangiomas
  Teratomas
  Hamartomas
Myocardial lesions and other
  Cardiomyopathy
  Myocarditis
  Myocardial infarction
  Idiopathic arterial calcification
  Endocardial fibroelastosis
Associated lesions, likely not causative
  Atrial septal defect
  Ventricular septal defect
  Tetralogy of Fallot
  Truncus arteriosus
	19–26%	Elevation of right atrial and central venous pressure is probably the common factor associated with the development of hydrops in structural cardiac disease. Cardiac tumours may cause hydrops by obstruction of blood flow and by their association with arrhythmia. Tachycardia-induced cardiac dysfunction results in elevation of right atrial and central venous pressure. Congenital heart block with bradycardia suggests a possible diagnosis of autoimmune disease in the mother. Myocardial disease may cause hydrops by inadequate myocardial contraction. Structural cardiac defects commonly are accompanied by cytogenetic and other anomalies

Intrathoracic lesions or masses Diaphragmatic hernia Cystic adenomatoid malformation Extralobar pulmonary sequestration Chylothorax Pulmonary lymphangiectasia Mediastinal teratoma Hamartomatous malformation of lung Mesenchymal malformation of lung Familial pulmonary lymphatic hypoplasia Pulmonary fibrosarcoma Laryngeal or tracheal atresia	8–10%	In the presence of a space-occupying lesion, hydrops develops because of abnormal lymphatic drainage or obstructed venous return resulting in increased central venous and/or lymphatic pressures. Upper airway atresia or stricture leads to pulmonary overdistension and thus to impaired cardiac filling

(Continued)

Table 31.1 (*Continued*)

Gastrointestinal Duodenal atresia Jejunoileal atresia Imperforate anus Volvulus Duodenal diverticulum Meconium peritonitis	1%	Hydrops may develop because of decreased intravascular colloid osmotic pressure. Protein may be lost as a transudate into the bowel or there may be abnormalities of lymphatic drainage in the splanchnic bed. Venous thrombosis may also play a role in obstructed venous return. Hydrops and meconium peritonitis may be related to fetal viral infection in many cases
Hepatic Hepatic fibrosis Polycystic disease of the liver Hepatic haemangioma Cholestasis Cirrhosis with portal hypertension Congenital portal dysplasia Giant cell hepatitis Neuroblastoma Hepatic adenoma Hepatic calcification	1%	Portal venous obstruction may lead to elevated central venous pressure. Hepatic dysfunction may occur when liver architecture is disrupted by haematopoietic tissue resulting in hypoproteinaemia. Viral infection may result in hepatic lesions causing alteration in organ blood flow
Renal Polycystic kidney Renal vein thrombosis Renal dysplasia Congenital nephrosis Hypoplastic kidney Pelvic kidney Mesoblastic nephroma	2–3%	Activation of the renin–angiotensin system may play a role in the pathogenesis of hydrops fetalis secondary to renal causes. Increased levels of plasma renin concentration secondary to asphyxia have been shown to be associated with the development of hydrops. Osmotic disturbances due to hypoalbuminaemia in nephrosis and lymphatic vessel overload by urinary ascites may also play a role in the progression to hydrops in some fetuses
Vascular/Tumours Vena cava thrombosis Absent ductus venosus Arteriovenous malformation Umbilical cord torsion or varix Arterial calcification Vein of Galen aneurysm Haemangioendothelioma Mesoblastic nephroma Neuroblastoma Fetal intracranial teratoma Sacrococcygeal teratoma	2–4%	Hydrops occurring in fetuses with tumours may be due to circulatory obstruction of blood or lymphatic fluid with resultant increased central venous pressure, or arteriovenous shunting resulting in high output cardiac failure. Vascular malformations may lead to high-output cardiac failure or hypoxia due to haemorrhage
FETAL: GENERALISED ABNORMALITY **Infectious causes** Cytomegalovirus Coxsackie virus Syphilis Toxoplasmosis Parvovirus B19 Rubella Herpes simplex Chagas disease Leptospirosis Respiratory syncytial virus Varicella	1–8%	Direct viral infection of the myocardium may lead to myocarditis and intrauterine congestive heart failure. Viraemia may also result in high-output congestive heart failure from severe anaemia by destruction of erythroid progenitor cells. Fetal infection can also cause alterations in organ blood flow and change microvascular hydrostatic pressures with escape of fluid through endothelial gaps and the basement membrane. Meconium peritonitis and hydrops is commonly associated with viral infection, particularly parvovirus B19

(*Continued*)

Table 31.1 (*Continued*)

Skeletal dysplasias Achondroplasia Achondrogenesis types I, IA and II Osteogenesis imperfecta type II Lethal osteoporosis Asphyxiating thoracic dysplasia Thanatophoric dwarfism	4%	Isolated case reports of various other osteochondrodysplasias have been reported to be associated with hydrops. The cause of hydrops in these cases is largely unknown. Hepatic enlargement with large vessel compression may occur secondary to proliferation of blood cell precursors to compensate for a small bone marrow volume. Thoracic abnormality secondary to various chondrodysplasias may cause increased intrathoracic pressure leading to obstructed venous return

Metabolic disorders
Lysosomal storage disorders
  Gaucher's disease
  GM$_1$ gangliosidosis
  Mucopolysaccharidosis I and IVb
  Mucolipidosis types I and II
  Niemann–Pick diseases types A and C
  Sialic acid storage disorder
  Galactosialidosis
Glucose phosphate isomerase deficiency
Pyruvate kinase deficiency
Carnitine deficiency
Hypothyroidism
	1%	Genetic metabolic diseases that cause hydrops may do so through myocardial involvement leading to congestive heart failure, or ascites secondary to hepatic sinusoidal infiltration resulting in disturbance of intrahepatic circulation. There may also be hypomobility secondary to muscle involvement. Erythrocyte enzymopathies can cause haemolytic anaemia with resultant hydrops

Chromosomal disorders Trisomy 21, 18, 13, 15, 16 45,XO (Turner syndrome) Partial duplication of chromosome 11, 15, 17, 18 Partial deletion of chromosome 13p Partial deletion of chromosome 18q Rearrangement of chromosome 22q 46,XX/XY mosaic Triploidy, tetraploidy	35%	There is no single clear pathogenesis for hydrops in chromosomally abnormal fetuses that have no cardiovascular abnormality or lymphatic drainage abnormality. In structurally normal fetuses, one theory for the hydrops involves fetal hypoxia from placental abnormalities. Hydrops and pericardial effusion may complicate trisomy 21 with myeloproliferative disorder
Fetal anaemia Alpha-thalassaemia Fetal closed-space haemorrhage Immune haemolysis Maternofetal haemorrhage Twin-to-twin transfusion Acardiac twin Diamond–Blackfan anaemia Leukaemia Methaemoglobinaemia Neonatal haemosiderosis	10–27%	Hydrops occurs due to severe anaemia and congestive heart failure. Usually there is extreme hepatic erythropoiesis in response to the anaemia, secondary portal hypertension, and hypoalbuminaemia/hypoproteinaemia
Syndromes *Autosomal dominant* Opitz–Frias syndrome (G syndrome) Myotonic dystrophy Cornelia de Lange syndrome Noonan syndrome Yellow nail syndrome Tuberous sclerosis Wiedemann–Beckwith syndrome	8–9%	It is not known how hydrops develops in these various syndromes. In syndromes characterised by immobility, fetal hydrops may result from a lack of respiratory movement of the chest wall leading to a secondary rise in intrathoracic pressure. This in turn causes a rise in the systemic venous pressure, leading to oedema. In cases associated with cystic hygroma, the explanation is that of an embryonal malformation of the lymphatic ducts leading to a hypoplasia of the main lymphatic trunk with resulting fluid accumulation

(*Continued*)

Table 31.1 (Continued)

Autosomal recessive Orofaciodigital syndrome type II Polysplenia Pena–Shokeir syndrome Lethal multiple pterygium syndrome Neu–Laxova syndrome Idiopathic recurrent hydrops Isolated recurrent cystic hygroma Elejalde syndrome Hypophosphatasia Prune belly syndrome Klippel–Trenaunay–Weber syndrome Massive cystic hygroma Fanconi syndrome type III		
Twinning Monozygotic twins with twin-to-twin transfusion syndrome (in recipient, donor, or both) Acardiac twins	4–8%	Hydrops in the recipient twin may be through reduced perfusion by hyperviscous blood. Hydrops in the donor is due to anaemia, cardiac failure, and hypoproteinaemia
PLACENTAL/UMBILICAL Chorioangioma True knots of the cord Angiomyxoma of the umbilical cord Aneurysm of the umbilical artery Haemorrhagic endovasculitis of the placenta Chorionic vein thrombosis Placental and umbilical vein thrombosis Umbilical cord torsion	2–6%	Chorioangioma acts as an arteriovenous shunt, bypassing normal placental tissue. The resultant physiological effects are increased pulse pressure, increased venous return to the heart, tachycardia, cardiac enlargement and hypervolaemia
MATERNAL Maternal indometacin (indomethacin) use Lupus erythematosus Hyperthyroidism Hypothyroidism	<1%	Hydrops may develop in these instances owing to premature closure or restriction of flow in the ductus arteriosus or because of fetal cardiac arrhythmia resulting in congestive heart failure

and fetal investigations are outlined in Table 31.2 and Table 31.3, respectively.

Involvement of a clinical geneticist often assists in directing prenatal diagnosis,[92] especially when single gene or metabolic disorders are suspected. The advent of fluorescent in-situ hybridisation (FISH) allows for interphase analysis of chromosome aberrations otherwise not detected by conventional cytogenetic techniques, such as familial Wiedemann–Beckwith syndrome.[22] Utilisation of FISH on amniocytes has also allowed for rapid screening for trisomies 13, 18 and 21, and Turner syndrome (45XO) within 48 to 72 hours. This facilitates clinical decision making after viability, and has reduced the need for the technically more challenging and hazardous cordocentesis.

An aetiology may be found in up to 85% of NIH when investigation is thorough.[64] After the birth, pathological investigation of the placenta and other tissues may be required to complete the work-up.[52]

Fetal therapy: general considerations

Only a limited number of causes of NIH are amenable to specific antenatal therapy, and of these, only some will be successful. Therefore, prior to viability, termination of pregnancy should be considered. If this choice is made, or if the pregnancy results in a stillbirth or neonatal death, then autopsy of the fetus is strongly recommended to verify aetiology (Table 31.4). This information plays a critical role in counselling the parents for future pregnancies.

At gestations after viability, the management should be individualised in each case. Delivery following steroid administration may be the simplest option, particularly if there is evidence of fetal compromise. A team approach, involving the perinatologist, neonatologist, obstetrician, geneticist, paediatric specialists and the parents, is required. The parents must be fully informed of the working diagnosis, prognosis, and the risks and benefits of available management options. Depending on the underlying

Table 31.2 Maternal investigation of fetal hydrops

Investigation	Underlying condition
Blood type, antibodies	Immune hydrops
Complete blood count and peripheral film Haemoglobin electrophoresis/ molecular analysis	Alpha-thalassaemia
Serology (IgG and IgM) Toxoplasma Rubella Cytomegalovirus Herpes Syphilis Parvovirus B19	Infectious cause
Kleihauer–Betke test	Fetomaternal haemorrhage
Autoimmune serology (fetal bradycardia)	Collagen vascular disease
Thyroid function	Thyroid dysfunction

Table 31.3 Fetal investigation of hydrops*

Investigation	Underlying condition
Chromosomes Single gene disorders	Fetal aneuploidy
Complete blood count, platelets, reticulocytes, film	Anaemia
Haemoglobin electrophoresis/ molecular analysis	Alpha thalassaemia
Blood type, antibodies	Immune hydrops
OD450	Haemolysis
Protein, albumin	Hypoproteinaemia
Serology (IgG and IgM): toxoplasma, rubella, cytomegalovirus, herpes, parvovirus, B19	Fetal infection
Fetal cell culture/blood	Inborn errors of metabolism
Amniotic fluid, fetal tissue/fluid culture	Viral infection
Pleural fluid analysis	Chylothorax
Muscle biopsy	Muscular dystrophy

* These investigations may be considered using samples of amniotic fluid, placental tissue, or fetal blood, fluid or tissue, obtained by amniocentesis, chorionic villus sampling, cordocentesis or paracentesis.
OD450, optical density at 450 nm.

aetiology, these management options could cover a wide spectrum and may range anywhere from non-intervention with compassionate neonatal care to antenatal fetal surgical interventions with aggressive neonatal support.

Table 31.4 Investigation of a stillbirth or neonatal death with hydrops fetalis*

Detailed placental examination
Detailed postmortem examination
Skin biopsy for fibroblast culture, karyotype
Liver biopsy for histopathology
Tissue (liver, kidney, spleen) for B19 DNA
X-rays
Photograph

* See Tables 31.2, 31.3, and 31.5 for maternal investigations and details of other tests which merit consideration.

Specific fetal therapies

Fetal anaemia

Fetal anaemia is a serious sign of multiple underlying aetiologies. Rhesus and other immune-mediated aetiologies are covered in Chapter 40.

Fetomaternal haemorrhage

Fetal anaemia may result from severe fetomaternal haemorrhage, which can be confirmed by a maternal Kleihauer–Betke test. Successful outcome utilising intrauterine transfusion has been reported, and multiple transfusions may be required in some cases to effect resolution of fetal hydrops and prolongation of pregnancy.[37]

Alpha-thalassaemia

This cause for fetal anaemia and hydrops has been reported in association with the maternal 'mirror syndrome'.[60] Cases of serial intrauterine transfusions improving fetal hydrops and maintaining fetal growth to viability have been described, although such neonatal survivors will also require lifelong blood transfusion therapy.[12] The mainstay of management remains antenatal screening of susceptible populations, combined with prenatal diagnosis utilising DNA hybridisation techniques from fetal cells.[71] Early ultrasound may be used to assess the fetal cardiothoracic ratio as a screening test in pregnancies at risk.[57] This approach may narrow the target population requiring invasive testing.

Fetal infections

Intrauterine vertical transmission of certain maternal infections to the fetus may result in NIH. More common specific infections include toxoplasmosis, parvovirus B19 and syphilis.

In maternal toxoplasmosis, large studies from France have shown 92% sensitivity in the diagnosis of fetal infection employing culture of fetal blood and amniotic fluid and fetal blood testing for toxoplasma-specific IgM, combined with ultrasound examination.[18] Maternal therapy with pyrimethamine and sulphonamides or with spiramycin, alone or in combination, may be effective.[40]

Parvovirus B19 is now well established as a cause for NIH by producing an aplastic crisis leading to severe anaemia and high-output cardiac failure, with possibly an additional direct cytopathic effect on the fetal myocardial cells.[69] About 10% of B19 infection in pregnancy leads to NIH and B19 may account for 15–20% of idiopathic NIH.[101] The particular association of B19 virus and isolated pleural or pericardial effusions has been described,[78] and ascites may be associated with meconium peritonitis.[104] Diagnosis is confirmed with positive maternal IgM serocoversion, and the detection of B19 DNA in amniotic fluid or fetal blood using the polymerase chain reaction. Although NIH due to this cause may resolve spontaneously, intrauterine transfusions to correct the anaemia have been shown to improve fetal survival.[26]

Syphilis has long been recognised as a cause for NIH. Appropriate diagnosis and maternal therapy with penicillin may allow the fetus to survive despite the presence of hydrops.[8]

Fetal thyroid abnormalities

Both fetal hyperthyroidism[95] and hypothyroidism[48] have been described in association with the development of NIH. Fetal hyperthyroidism may develop secondary to maternal autoantibodies in Graves' disease (p. 880), which cross the placenta and stimulate the fetal thyroid, even in the previously treated mother, who may be euthyroid or hypothyroid in pregnancy.

Fetal arrhythmias

Fetal tachycardia
Fetal tachyarrhythmia is thought to cause NIH through cardiac failure resulting in elevation in venous pressure and a reduction in fetal lymph flow. Tachyarrhythmias are usually supraventricular in origin, and include paroxysmal supraventricular tachycardia (SVT), Wolff–Parkinson–White syndrome, atrial fibrillation and atrial flutter. There are associated anatomical abnormalities in only 6–7% of cases.[84] The most commonly used therapy is maternal administration of digoxin, which appears to achieve adequate levels in the fetus,[88] unless there is severe hydrops.[103] Direct fetal therapy by intravenous,[28] intramuscular[35] and intraperitoneal[29] administration have also been used. Other drugs employed include verapamil[51] alone or in combination with digoxin,[77] quinidine,[33] propanolol,[84] amiodarone,[85] procainamide[51] and flecainide.[53] Of these therapies, flecainide may hold the most promise, according to a series from the Netherlands involving 49 fetuses with supraventricular tachycardia, 35 of which were treated transplacentally.[27] Flecainide was effective in all non-hydropic fetuses where digoxin failed, and was associated with reduced mortality in hydropic fetuses. Another recent innovation is the direct fetal intravenous injection of adenosine, which terminates the SVT.[54] This is of short duration, and therefore this approach should be combined with long-acting maintenance therapy, using digoxin or flecainide. Finally, recent work has suggested sotalol as an alternative first-line therapy in the treatment of fetal tachycardias,[76] with a successful conversion rate of 80% in fetuses with atrial flutter and 60% in fetuses with SVT. Of interest are recent reports of maternal digoxin therapy producing resolution of NIH in the absence of documented tachyarrhythmia.[15,82]

Fetal bradyarrhythmia
Fetal heart block is a less common cause of NIH, but is more difficult to treat antenatally. If it occurs with an associated structural cardiac abnormality, the prognosis is extremely poor.[30] In the presence of normal cardiac structure, NIH secondary to fetal bradyarrhythmia is unusual. The other well-known association of congenital heart block is with maternal autoantibodies due to connective tissue disorders, where therapy with maternal steroids may be of help.[17] Other therapeutic choices have included maternal administration of sympathomimetic drugs,[89] intra-abdominal fetal administration of sympathomimetics[67] and ventricular pacing.[19] If the fetus is near term, early delivery to allow for ventricular pacing may be considered. Some success with non-specific medical therapy (digoxin and diuretics) has been reported.[36]

Fetal tumours

Sacrococcygeal teratoma (p. 961)
This tumour has been associated with arteriovenous shunting leading to high-output cardiac failure, NIH, and death. Fetuses with a sacrococcygeal teratoma that is mainly solid in appearance and is highly vascularised have a higher risk of developing NIH.[99] There is at least one case report of a successful fetal sacrococcygeal teratoma resection in a hydropic fetus by the fetal surgery group in San Francisco.[31]

Intrathoracic space-occupying lesions
These include congenital cystic adenomatoid malformation of the lung (p. 156), pulmonary sequestration (pp. 587–8), congenital diaphragmatic hernia (Chapter 27, part 6) and other intrathoracic tumours. These mass lesions may produce pulmonary hypoplasia and reduce systemic venous return, leading to NIH.[10] Some of these lesions resolve,[63] and although association with hydrops often leads to fetal demise, spontaneous resolution of hydrops in utero has also been observed.[24] Current therapeutic options include shunting or aspiration of large intrathoracic cystic lesions.[74] Fetal lobectomy may be successful in expert hands.[1] Experimental radiofrequency thermal ablation in the sheep model has been assessed as a potential treatment for hydropic fetuses with a large chest mass.[68]

Twin-to-twin transfusion (pp. 151–2)

This syndrome occurs in multiple gestations where there are vascular anastomoses between monochorionic twins, with hydrops being more common in the recipient twin. This complication can occur at any time during pregnancy, but is most serious when it presents in the second trimester with fetal growth discordance and/or amniotic fluid volume discrepancy between the two sacs. The current recommendation is serial reduction amniocentesis. Although this may lead to complications such as abruption and preterm labour, several authors have shown success in improving survival with this method.[66] An experimental technique utilising fetoscopic laser coagulation has been described by some investigators, with a potential role for serious cases that present under 20 weeks' gestation.[32]

Fetal fluid accumulation

Fetal pleural effusions may either be associated with NIH of multiple origins, or may initiate the development of fetal hydrops by shifting the mediastinum and impeding venous return. An example of a primary pleural effusion is a chylothorax (pp. 518–19). Some pleural effusions may resolve spontaneously,[34] or after thoracocentesis (p. 517).[2] If this does not occur, therapy consists of placement of a thoraco-amniotic shunt under ultrasound guidance.[5] This treatment should be reserved for known primary pleural effusions in which genetic and infectious abnormalities have been excluded. Similar approaches have been used to drain fetal ascites.

Neonatal management of hydrops fetalis

Antenatal diagnosis should prompt transfer to a tertiary centre which allows for a planned delivery in a controlled setting, usually by caesarean section. This permits the neonatal team to assemble all the equipment and to make any appropriate surgical preparations. If anaemia is suspected, blood and exchange transfusion equipment should be prepared.[93]

Resuscitation

Hydropic infants tolerate labour poorly, and are usually depressed at birth.[23] Intubation is almost always required, which may be difficult because of oedema. Ventilation may require high pressures on account of pulmonary oedema and pulmonary hypoplasia secondary to pleural effusions and/or ascites. A prolonged initial breath at fairly high pressures (20–25 cmH$_2$O) for 1–4 seconds may help to establish a functional residual capacity, following which ventilation at rapid rates of 80–120 breaths/min is usually most effective.[80] Prophylactic surfactant may be given. Careful attention should be paid to temperature control. Preparations should be made for possible immediate abdominal paracentesis, thoracocentesis and, rarely, pericardiocentesis.

Subsequent management

Umbilical arterial and venous catheterisation will almost always be required, and these may be utilised to monitor arterial and central venous pressure. Although an intense vasoconstrictor response to asphyxia may produce elevated pressures, these babies are usually hypovolaemic.[81] Cautious correction of metabolic acidosis, volume replacement with blood or colloid depending on haematocrit, or exchange transfusion for severe anaemia is undertaken as indicated using central venous pressure as a guide. Fresh frozen plasma is preferable to albumin, both as a volume expander and to raise plasma protein concentration and oncotic pressure, and also to treat the frequently associated disseminated intravascular coagulation, for which platelets, cryoprecipitate or exchange transfusion may also be required.[23,80]

However, if severe hypoproteinaemia is present, 2 ml/kg of 25% albumin may be preferable, to avoid the risk of volume overload.[65]

Circulatory support with inotropic agents is often necessary to maintain blood pressure and urine output. We use dopamine early,[50] but usually find adrenaline is additionally required to increase systemic pressure,[7] likely mediated by increased systemic vascular resistance.[16] In the presence of reduced perfusion, dobutamine may be preferable.[75] Moderate fluid restriction (60–80 ml/kg per 24 h) and the use of diuretics such as furosemide (frusemide; 1 mg/kg/dose) help to promote a diuresis and the resolution of oedema.

Meticulous attention must be paid to evaluation of electrolytes, creatinine, liver function tests, and particularly glucose. Specific therapy for particular causative conditions as outlined in Table 31.1 may be necessary. Alternatively, if there are severe congenital abnormalities, discussion at this stage may take place with the parents regarding the withdrawal of active support. If this occurs, detailed pathological examination should be obtained with parental consent, as outlined in Table 31.4.

Investigation

Table 31.5 outlines tests which may be considered for the neonate with NIH, guided by the presenting features.

Ventilation

The baby's respiratory status may improve rapidly after a few hours of ventilation at high pressure, but more commonly there is ongoing respiratory insufficiency due to reaccumulation of pleural or peritoneal fluid, pulmonary oedema, hyaline membrane disease (HMD), pulmonary hypertension or pulmonary hypoplasia. It is usually very difficult or impossible to determine the relative contribution of the last four of these factors. Effective pleural and/or peritoneal and/or pericardial drainage is essential. Pulmonary oedema may improve with diuretics and increased levels of end-expiratory pressure, which will also be effective in HMD. Usually, antenatal steroids will have already been administered, and surfactant therapy should be considered in most cases. High-frequency ventilation may offer an advantage,[55] particularly when combined with surfactant therapy.[45] Inhaled nitric oxide (INO) reduces the need for extracorporeal membrane oxygenation (ECMO) in near-term infants with respiratory failure.[97] We have also found INO to improve oxygenation in preterm infants with 'pulmonary hypoplasia' from prolonged oligohydramnios,[79] although the overall benefits in preterm infants are marginal at best.[49]

Extracorporeal membrane oxygenation

If severe hypoxaemia persists, then it is probably due to pulmonary hypoplasia-associated pulmonary hypertension, which can be estimated echocardiographically. If the baby is at least 34 weeks' gestation, does not have any of the usual contraindications,

Table 31.5 Neonatal investigation of hydrops fetalis

Imaging	
X-rays	Chest, abdomen, skull, long bones (as appropriate)
Ultrasound	Heart, abdomen, brain
Pleural/ascitic fluid	Cytology, karyotype
	Total protein, albumin, triglyceride
	Viral and bacterial culture
Urine	Urinalysis, protein
	Virus and bacterial culture
	Inborn errors of metabolism
Blood	Complete blood count, platelets, reticulocytes, film
	PT, PTT, fibrinogen, fibrin split products
	Blood type, antibodies
	Haemoglobin electrophoresis/ molecular analysis
	Electrolytes, creatinine, glucose
	Total protein, albumin, bilirubin
	Liver function tests
	Thyroid function tests
	Serology (IgG and IgM) for toxoplasma, rubella, cytomegalovirus, herpes, syphilis, parvovirus B19
	Chromosomes
	Single gene disorders
	Inborn errors of metabolism
Electrocardiogram	
Placenta	Macroscopic examination
	Microscopic examination
	Cytogenetics
	Culture

and meets the local ECMO criteria for severe refractory respiratory failure, then ECMO may permit lung rest and resolution of pulmonary hypertension. Bealer et al[9] reported a survival rate of 54% for 'idiopathic' NIH treated with ECMO in a timely fashion (mean age of ECMO initiation 17.5 hours for survivors).

Outcome

Overall, the prognosis for neonates with NIH is very poor, with mortality rates ranging from 50% to 100%,[14,23,43,70,100] which is related to prematurity, chromosomal abnormalities, associated lethal malformations, and the presence of ascites or pleural effusions producing pulmonary hypoplasia, which is the most consistent postmortem finding.[3,14,43] Factors reported to be associated with survival, in the absence of underlying lethal congenital malformations or chromosomal anomalies, have been normal plasma proteins,[42] absence of proven infection,[100] not more than one fluid-filled cavity,[98,100] especially absence of

pleural effusion,[70] and a normal biventricular diastolic outer dimension measured on ultrasound.[11] Ayida et al[5] described six cases without structural and chromosomal anomalies, of which five survived to discharge following fetal therapy (four shunts, one transfusion).

The long-term outcome of survivors of NIH is difficult to predict, and will clearly be related to any associated problems. In a pathological series of 38 cases, 23 were found to exhibit hypoxic-ischaemic lesions, mostly in the white matter of the brain.[59] Similar findings were reported in the stillbirths and neonatal deaths described by Laneri et al;[58] of the 10 survivors in this report, six were neurologically abnormal at the time of discharge. In a series of 51 cases born between 1983 and 1994, there were 21 survivors (41%), two of whom died before 1 year of age.[70] Of the 19 evaluated subsequently, 13 (68%) showed normal development; three patients with severe psychomotor delay and cerebral palsy all had significant underlying conditions. Haverkamp et al[38] recently reported on the follow-up of 33 of 61 surviving infants with NIH; 24 of the 28 examined appeared normal. In many cases in this series the hydrops had resolved prior to delivery, either spontaneously or with antenatal therapy. The major therapeutic hope therefore lies in identifying those fetuses that may be amenable to antenatal intervention.

References

1. Adzick N S, Harrison M R, Crombleholme T M et al 1998 Fetal lung lesions: management and outcome. American Journal of Obstetrics and Gynecology 179: 884–889
2. Aguirre O A, Finley B E, Ridgway L E III et al 1995 Resolution of unilateral fetal hydrothorax with associated non-immune hydrops after intrauterine thoracocentesis. Ultrasound in Obstetrics and Gynecology 5: 346–348
3. Andersen H M, Drew J H, Beischer N A et al 1983 Non-immune hydrops fetalis: changing contribution to perinatal mortality. British Journal of Obstetrics and Gynaecology 90: 636–639
4. Apkon M 1995 Pathophysiology of hydrops fetalis. Seminars in Perinatology 19: 437–446
5. Ayida G A, Soothill P W, Rodeck C H 1995 Survival in non-immune hydrops fetalis without malformation or chromosomal abnormalities after invasive treatment. Fetal Diagnosis and Therapy 10: 101–105
6. Barnes S E, Bryan E M, Harris D A et al 1977 Oedema in the newborn. Molecular Aspects of Medicine 1: 187–282
7. Barrington K, Chan W 1993 The circulatory effects of epinephrine infusion in the anesthetized piglet. Pediatric Research 33: 190–194
8. Barton J R, Thorpe E M Jr, Shaver D C et al 1992 Nonimmune hydrops fetalis associated with maternal infection with syphilis. American Journal of Obstetrics and Gynecology 167: 56–58
9. Bealer J F, Mantor P C, Wehling L et al 1997 Extracorporeal life support for nonimmune hydrops fetalis. Journal of Pediatric Surgery 32: 1645–1647
10. Bullard K M, Harrison M R 1995 Before the horse is out of the barn: fetal surgery for hydrops. Seminars in Perinatology 19: 462–473
11. Carlson D E, Platt L D, Medearis A L et al 1990 Prognostic indicators of the resolution of nonimmune hydrops fetalis and survival of the fetus. American Journal of Obstetrics and Gynecology 163: 1785–1787
12. Carr S, Rubin L, Dixon D et al 1995 Intrauterine therapy for homozygous alpha-thalassemia. Obstetrics and Gynecology 85: 876–879
13. Cassady G 2001 Hydrops fetalis. Online. Available: http://www.emedicine.com/PED/topic1042.htm
14. Castillo R A, Devoe L D, Hadi H A et al 1986 Nonimmune hydrops fetalis: clinical experience and factors related to a poor outcome. American Journal of Obstetrics and Gynecology 155: 812–816
15. Chavkin Y, Kupfersztain C, Ergas Z et al 1996 Successful outcome of idiopathic nonimmune hydrops fetalis treated by maternal digoxin. Gynecologic and Obstetric Investigation 42: 137–139

16. Cheung P-Y, Barrington K J, Pearson J et al 1997 Systemic, pulmonary and mesenteric perfusion and oxygenation effects of dopamine and epinephrine. American Journal of Respiratory and Critical Care Medicine 155: 32–37

17. Copel J A, Buyon J P, Kleinman C S 1995 Successful in utero therapy of fetal heart block. American Journal of Obstetrics and Gynecology 173: 1384–1390

18. Daffos F, Forestier F, Capella-Pavlovsky M et al 1988 Prenatal management of 746 pregnancies at risk for congenital toxoplasmosis. New England Journal of Medicine 318: 271–275

19. Davison M B, Radford D J 1989 Fetal and neonatal congenital complete heart block. Medical Journal of Australia 150: 192–198

20. Detti L, Mari G, Akiyama M et al 2002 Longitudinal assessment of the middle cerebral artery peak systolic velocity in healthy fetuses and in fetuses at risk for anemia. American Journal of Obstetrics and Gynecology 187: 937–939

21. Driscoll S G 1966 Hydrops fetalis. New England Journal of Medicine 275: 1432–1434

22. Drut R M, Drut R 1996 Nonimmune fetal hydrops and placentomegaly: diagnosis of familial Widemann-Beckwith syndrome with trisomy 11p15 using FISH. American Journal of Medical Genetics 62: 145–149

23. Etches P C, Lemons J A 1979 Nonimmune hydrops fetalis: report of 22 cases including three siblings. Pediatrics 64: 326–332

24. Etches P C, Tierney A J, Demianczuk N 1994 Successful outcome in a case of cystic adenomatoid malformation of the lung complicated by fetal hydrops, using extracorporeal membrane oxygenation. Fetal Diagnosis and Therapy 9: 88–91

25. Faber J J, Anderson D F 1997 Angiotensin mediated interaction of fetal kidney and placenta in the control of fetal arterial pressure and its role in hydrops fetalis. Placenta 18: 313–326

26. Fairley C K, Smoleniec J S, Caul O E et al 1995 Observational study of the effect of intrauterine transfusions on outcome of fetal hydrops after parvovirus B19 infection. Lancet 346: 1335–1337

27. Frohnmulder I M, Stewart P A, Witsenburg M et al 1995 The efficacy of flecainide versus digoxin in the management of fetal supraventricular tachycardia. Prenatal Diagnosis 15: 1297–1302

28. Gembruch U, Hansmann M, Bald R 1988 Direct intrauterine fetal treatment of fetal tachyarrhythmia with severe hydrops fetalis by antiarrhythmic drugs. Fetal Therapy 3: 210–215

29. Gembruch U, Hansmann M, Redel D A et al 1988 Intrauterine therapy of fetal tachyarrhythmias: intraperitoneal administration of antiarrhythmic drugs to the fetus in fetal tachyarrhythmias with severe hydrops fetalis. Journal of Perinatal Medicine 16: 39–44

30. Gembruch U, Hansmann M, Redel D A et al 1989 Fetal complete heart block: antenatal diagnosis, significance and management. European Journal of Obstetrics and Gynecology and Reproductive Biology 31: 9–22

31. Graf J L, Albanese C T, Jennings R W et al 2000 Successful fetal sacrococcygeal teratoma resection in a hydropic fetus. Journal of Pediatric Surgery 35: 1489–1491

32. Gratacos E, van Schoubroeck D, Carreras E et al 2002 Impact of laser coagulation in severe twin-twin transfusion syndrome on fetal Doppler indices and venous blood flow volume. Ultrasound in Obstetrics and Gynecology 20: 125–130

33. Guntheroth W G, Cyr D R, Mack L A et al 1985 Hydrops from reciprocating atrioventricular tachycardia in a 27-week fetus requiring quinidine for conversion. Obstetrics and Gynecology 66: 29S–33S

34. Hagay Z, Reece E A, Roberts A et al 1993 Isolated fetal pleural effusion: a prenatal management dilemma. Obstetrics and Gynecology 81: 147–152

35. Hallak M, Neerhof M G, Perry R et al 1991 Fetal supraventricular tachycardia and hydrops fetalis: combined intensive, direct, and transplacental therapy. Obstetrics and Gynecology 78: 523–525

36. Harris J P, Alexson C G, Manning J A et al 1993 Medical therapy for the hydropic fetus with congenital complete atrioventricular block. American Journal of Perinatology 10: 217–219

37. Hartung J, Rabih C, Bollmann R 2000 Nonimmune hydrops from fetomaternal hemorrhage treated with serial fetal intravascular transfusion. Obstetrics and Gynecology 95: 844

38. Haverkamp F, Noeker M, Gerresheim G et al 2000 Good prognosis for psychomotor development in survivors with nonimmune hydrops fetalis. British Journal of Obstetrics and Gynaecology 107: 282–284

39. Hill L M, Breckle R, Thomas M L et al 1987 Polyhydramnios: ultrasonically detected prevalence and neonatal outcome. Obstetrics and Gynecology 69: 21–25

40. Hohlfeld P, Daffos F, Thulliez P et al 1989 Fetal toxoplasmosis: outcome of pregnancy and infant follow-up after in utero treatment. Journal of Pediatrics 115: 765–769

41. Holtzgreve W, Holtzgreve B, Curry C J R 1985 Nonimmune hydrops fetalis: diagnosis and management. Seminars in Perinatology 9: 52–67

42. Iliff P J, Nicholls J M, Keeling J W et al 1983 Non-immunologic hydrops fetalis: a review of 27 cases. Archives of Disease in Childhood 58: 979–982

43. Im S S, Rizos N, Joutsi P et al 1984 Nonimmunologic hydrops fetalis. American Journal of Obstetrics and Gynecology 148: 566–569

44. Iskaros J, Jauniaux E, Rodeck C 1997 Outcome of nonimmune hydrops fetalis diagnosed during the first half of pregnancy. Obstetrics and Gynecology 90: 321–325

45. Jackson J C, Truog W E, Standaert T A et al 1994 Reduction in lung injury after combined surfactant and high-frequency ventilation. American Journal of Respiratory and Critical Care Medicine 150: 534–539

46. Jauniaux E 1997 Diagnosis and management of early non-immune hydrops fetalis. Prenatal Diagnosis 17: 1261–1268

47. Jones D C 1995 Nonimmune fetal hydrops: diagnosis and obstetrical management. Seminars in Perinatology 19: 447–461

48. Kessel I, Makhoul I R, Sujov P 1999 Congenital hypothyroidism and nonimmune hydrops fetalis: associated? Pediatrics 103: E9

49. Kinsella J P, Walsh W F, Bose C L et al 1999 Inhaled nitric oxide in premature neonates with severe hypoxaemic respiratory failure: a randomised controlled trial. Lancet 354: 1061–1065

50. Klarr J M, Faix R G, Pryce C J E et al 1994 Randomized, blind trial of dopamine versus dobutamine for treatment of hypotension in preterm infants with respiratory distress syndrome. Journal of Pediatrics 125: 117–122

51. Kleinman C S, Copel J A, Weinstein E M et al 1985 In utero diagnosis and treatment of fetal supraventricular tachycardia. Seminars in Perinatology 9: 113–129

52. Knisely A S 1995 The pathologist and the hydropic placenta, fetus, or infant. Seminars in Perinatology 19: 525–531

53. Kofinas A D, Simon N V, Sagel H et al 1991 Treatment of fetal supraventricular tachycardia with flecainide acetate after digoxin failure. American Journal of Obstetrics and Gynecology 165: 630–631

54. Kohl T, Tercanli S, Kececioglu D et al 1995 Direct fetal administration of adenosine for the termination of incessant supraventricular tachycardia. Obstetrics and Gynecology 85: 873–874

55. Kugelman A, Gonen R, Bader D 2000 Potential role of high-frequency ventilation in the treatment of severe congenital pleural effusion. Pediatric Pulmonology 29: 404–408

56. Lallemand A V, Doco-Fenzy M, Gaillard D A 1999 Investigation of nonimmune hydrops fetalis: multidisciplinary studies are necessary for diagnosis – review of 94 cases. Pediatric and Developmental Pathology 2: 432–439

57. Lam Y H, Ghosh A, Tang M H Y et al 1997 Early ultrasound prediction of pregnancies affected by homozygous alpha-thalassaemia-1. Prenatal Diagnosis 17: 327–332

58. Laneri G G, Claassen D L, Scher M S 1994 Brain lesions of fetal onset in encephalopathic infants with nonimmune hydrops fetalis. Pediatric Neurology 11: 18–22

59. Larroche J C, Aubry M C, Narcy F 1992 Intrauterine brain damage in nonimmune hydrops fetalis. Biology of the Neonate 61: 273–280

60. Liang S T, Wong V C, So W W et al 1985 Homozygous alpha-thalassaemia: clinical presentation, diagnosis, and management. A review of 46 cases. British Journal of Obstetrics and Gynaecology 92: 680–684

61. Lumbers E R, Gunn A J, Zhang D Y et al 2001 Nonimmune hydrops fetalis and activation of the renin-angiotensin system after asphyxia in preterm fetal sheep. American Journal of Physiology – Regulatory, Integrative and Comparative Physiology 280: R1045–R1051

62. Macafee C A J, Fortune D W, Beischer N A 1970 Non-immunological hydrops fetalis. Journal of Obstetrics and Gynaecology of the British Commonwealth 77: 226–237

63. MacGillivray T E, Harrison M R, Goldstein R B et al 1993 Disappearing fetal lung lesions. Journal of Pediatric Surgery 28: 1321–1325

64. Machin G A 1989 Hydrops revisited: literature review of 1,414 cases published in the 1980s. American Journal of Medical Genetics 34: 366–390

65. McMahan M J, Donovan E F 1995 The delivery room resuscitation of the hydropic neonate. Seminars in Perinatology 19: 474–482

66. Mahoney B S, Petty C N, Nyberg D A et al 1990 The 'stuck twin' phenomenon: ultrasonographic findings, pregnancy outcome, and management with serial amniocentesis. American Journal of Obstetrics and Gynecology 163: 1513–1522

67. Martin T C, Arias F, Olander D S et al 1988 Successful management of congenital atrioventricular block associated with hydrops fetalis. Journal of Pediatrics 112: 984–986

68. Milner R, Kitano Y, Olutoye O et al 2000 Radiofrequency thermal ablation: a potential treatment for hydropic fetuses with a large chest mass. Journal of Pediatric Surgery 35: 386–389

69. Morey A L, Keeling J W, Porter H J et al 1992 Clinical and histopathological features of parvovirus B19 infection in the human fetus. British Journal of Obstetrics and Gynaecology 99: 566–574

70. Nakayama H, Kukita J, Hikino S et al 1999 Long-term outcome of 51 liveborn neonates with non-immune hydrops fetalis. Acta Paediatrica 88: 24–28

71. Nakayama R, Yamada D, Steinmiller V et al 1986 Hydrops fetalis secondary to Bart hemoglobinopathy. Obstetrics and Gynecology 67: 176–180

72. Nicolaides K H, Azar G B 1990 Thoraco-amniotic shunting. Fetal Diagnosis and Therapy 5: 153–164

73. Nicolay K S, Gainey H L 1964 Pseudotoxemic state associated with severe Rh immunization. American Journal of Obstetrics and Gynecology 89: 41–45

74. Nugent C E, Hayashi R H, Rubin J 1989 Prenatal treatment of type 1 congenital cystic adenomatoid malformation by intrauterine fetal thoracocentesis. Clinical Ultrasound 17: 675–677

75. Osborn D, Evans N, Kluckow M 2002 Randomized trial of dobutamine versus dopamine in preterm infants with low systemic blood flow. Journal of Pediatrics 140: 183–191

76. Oudijk M A, Maiike M, Michon M D et al 2000 Sotalol in the treatment of fetal dysrhythmias. Circulation 101: 2721–2726

77. Owen J, Colvin E V, Davis R O 1988 Fetal death after successful conversion of fetal supraventricular tachycardia with digoxin and verapamil. American Journal of Obstetrics and Gynecology 158: 1169–1170

78. Parilla B V, Tamura R K, Ginsberg N A 1997 Association of parvovirus infection with isolated fetal effusions. American Journal of Perinatology 14: 357–358

79. Peliowski A, Finer N N, Etches P C et al 1995 Inhaled nitric oxide for premature infants after prolonged rupture of the membranes. Journal of Pediatrics 126: 450–453

80. Phibbs R H 1985 Hydrops. In: Nelson N M (ed) Current therapy in neonatal-perinatal medicine 1985-1986. B C Decker, Toronto, pp 201–207

81. Phibbs R H, Johnson P, Kitterman J A et al 1976 Cardiorespiratory status of erythroblastotic newborn infants. III. Intravascular pressure during the first hours of life. Pediatrics 58: 484–493

82. Pinette M G, Pinette P Y, Blackstone J et al 1995 A new approach to the treatment of nonimmune hydrops associated with polyhydramnios using therapeutic amniocentesis and maternal digoxin. Journal of Maternal-Fetal Investigation 5: 254–259

83. Recep H 2001 Non-immune hydrops fetalis in the first trimester: a review of 30 cases. Clinical and Experimental Obstetrics and Gynecology 28: 187–190

84. Reed K L 1989 Fetal arrhythmias: etiology, diagnosis, pathophysiology, and treatment. Seminars in Perinatology 13: 294–304

85. Rey E, Duperron L, Gauthier R et al 1985 Transplacental treatment of tachycardia-induced fetal heart failure with verapamil and amiodarone: a case report. American Journal of Obstetrics and Gynecology 153: 311–312

86. Saltzman D H, Frigoletto F D, Harlow B L et al 1989 Sonographic evaluation of hydrops fetalis. Obstetrics and Gynecology 74: 106–111

87. Santolaya J, Alley D, Jaffe R et al 1992 Antenatal classification of hydrops fetalis. Obstetrics and Gynecology 79: 256–259

88. Schlebusch H, von Mende S, Grunn U et al 1991 Determination of digoxin in the blood of pregnant women, fetuses and neonates before and during anti-arrhythmic therapy, using four immunochemical methods. European Journal of Clinical Chemistry and Biochemistry 29: 57–66

89. Schmidt K G, Ulmer H E, Silverman N H et al 1991 Perinatal outcome of fetal complete atrioventricular block: a multicenter experience. Journal of the American College of Cardiology 91: 1360–1366

90. Seifer D B, Ferguson J E, Behrens C M et al 1985 Nonimmune hydrops fetalis in association with hemangioma of the umbilical cord. Obstetrics and Gynecology 66: 283–286

91. Starling E H 1896 On the absorption of fluids from the connective tissue spaces. Journal of Physiology 19: 312–326

92. Steiner R D 1995 Hydrops fetalis: role of the geneticist. Seminars in Perinatology 19: 516–524

93. Stephenson T, Zuccollo J, Mohajer M 1994 Diagnosis and management of non-immune hydrops in the newborn. Archives of Disease in Childhood. Fetal and Neonatal Edition 70: F151–F154

94. Stratton R F, Patterson R H 1993 DNA confirmation of congenital myotonic dystrophy in non-immune hydrops fetalis. Prenatal Diagnosis 13: 1027–1030

95. Stulberg R A, Davies G A L 2000 Maternal thyrotoxicosis and fetal nonimmune hydrops. Obstetrics and Gynecology 95: 1036

96. Swain S, Cameron A D, McNay M B et al 1999 Prenatal diagnosis and management of nonimmune hydrops fetalis. Australian and New Zealand Journal of Obstetrics and Gynaecology 39: 285–290

97. The Neonatal Inhaled Nitric Oxide Study Group 1997 Inhaled nitric oxide in full-term and nearly full-term infants with hypoxic respiratory failure. New England Journal of Medicine 336: 597–604

98. Wafelman L S, Pollock B H, Kreutzer J et al 1999 Nonimmune hydrops fetalis: fetal and neonatal outcome during 1983-1992. Biology of the Neonate 75: 73–81

99. Westerburg B, Feldstein V A, Sandberg P L et al 2000 Sonographic prognostic factors in fetuses with sacrococcygeal teratoma. Journal of Pediatric Surgery 35: 322–326

100. Wy C A W, Sajous C H, Loberiza F et al 1999 Outcome of infants with a diagnosis of hydrops fetalis in the 1990s. American Journal of Perinatology 16: 561–567

101. Yaegashi N, Niinuma T, Chisaka H et al 1998 The incidence of, and factors leading to, parvovirus B19-related hydrops fetalis following maternal infection; Report of 10 cases and meta-analysis. Journal of Infection 37: 28–35

102. Yang Y H, Teng R J, Tang J R et al 1998 Etiology and outcome of hydrops. Journal of the Formosan Medical Association 97: 16–20

103. Younis J S, Granat M 1987 Insufficient transplacental digoxin transfer in severe hydrops fetalis. American Journal of Obstetrics and Gynecology 157: 1268–1269

104. Zerbini M, Gentilomi G A, Gallinella G et al 1998 Intra-uterine parvovirus B19 infection and meconium peritonitis. Prenatal Diagnosis 18: 599–606

CHAPTER 32

Malformation syndromes

Michael Patton

Specific chromosomal abnormalities

Frequency of chromosomal abnormalities

At birth the frequency of sex chromosome abnormalities is about 3 per 1000, and that of autosomal abnormalities about 4 per 1000. Of the latter group, about 1.5 per 1000 represent autosomal trisomies (mainly Down syndrome), the remainder being translocations, mainly balanced. The frequency of chromosome abnormalities in miscarriages is much higher. Studies that include abortuses expelled up to the end of the second trimester show a frequency of 20–30%, whereas in those studies including only the early stages of pregnancy the figure is closer to 50%. A brief description of the more common chromosomal abnormalities recognisable at birth is given below. Fuller descriptions and photographs may be found in Jones.[100]

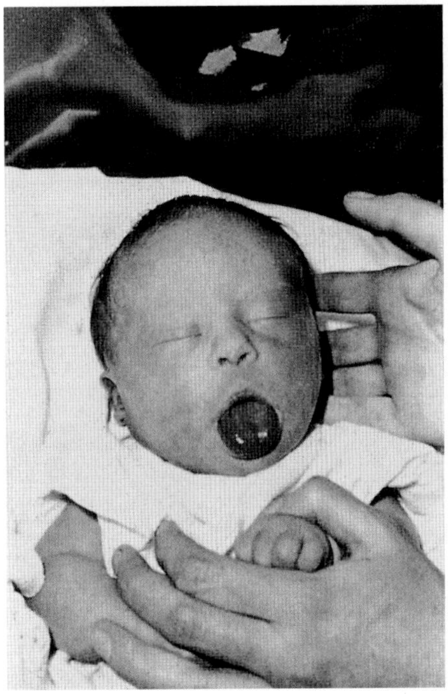

Fig. 32.1
Down syndrome (trisomy 21).

Down syndrome (Fig. 32.1)

The commonest autosomal anomaly is Down syndrome which is present in about 1 in 600–700 livebirths. In the majority of cases there are 47 chromosomes, the extra chromosome being number 21.

This syndrome is usually due to non-disjunction during oogenesis in the mother. The incidence of Down syndrome due to non-disjunction shows a marked association with maternal age. The overall prevalence of Down syndrome in children born to 18-year-old mothers is about 1 in 2300, whereas at 40 it is 1 in 100, and at a maternal age of 46 it is about 1 in 45.

The clinical diagnosis of Down syndrome is seldom a problem to the neonatologist. Recognition is based on the upward slant of the eyes, prominent epicanthic folds, Brushfield spots in the iris, a flat nasal bridge, protruding tongue, short neck and flat occiput. In the limbs, short broad hands, short incurved little fingers, single transverse palmar creases and a sandal gap between the first and second toes are typical. Congenital heart disease occurs in

about 40% of cases. Atrioventricular canal, atrial and ventricular septal defects are the commonest lesions.

Although 95% of babies with Down syndrome are of the usual trisomic type, in about 2.5% there is mosaicism, with a population of normal cells being present, and in the remainder of cases a chromosome translocation chromosome 21 is involved. The translocations mostly involve a number 14 and 21 chromosome. Of these, about three-quarters are de-novo events and one-quarter are inherited from a balanced translocation carrier parent. Very rarely, a parent carries a balanced Robertsonian translocation between two chromosomes 21. In this case, all offspring will have Down syndrome.

Management

Almost all are agreed that the suspected diagnosis should be disclosed early on, provided the clinician is confident of the clinical diagnosis. Confirmation, by means of a chromosome analysis,

Table 32.1 Recurrence risk figures in Down syndrome

	Risk
After one trisomic child (mother aged under 39 years)	1%
If mother aged over 39 years	Double maternal age risk
Mother is a 14/21 translocation carrier	10%
Father is a 14/21 translocation carrier	2%
One parent is a 21/21 translocation carrier	100%

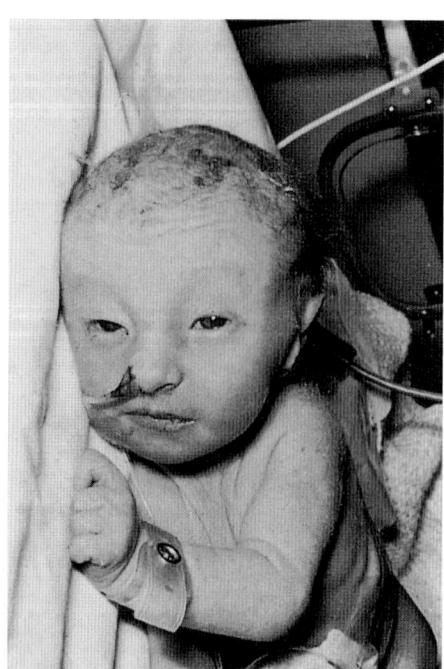

Fig. 32.3 Edward syndrome (trisomy 18).

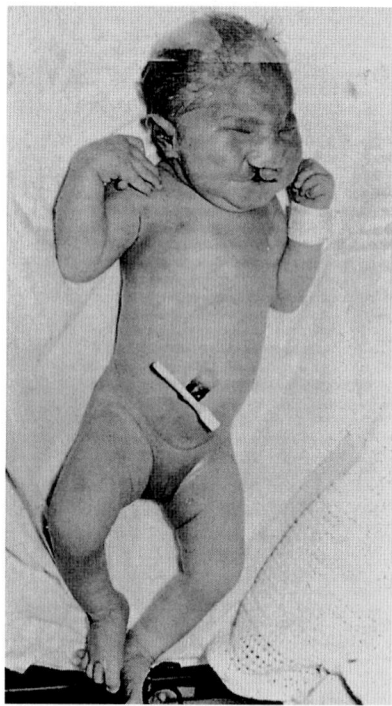

Fig. 32.2 Patau syndrome (trisomy 13).

ulnar side) and the overlapping of fingers are frequent features, as are rocker-bottom feet. Urogenital abnormalities and malrotation of the gut frequently occur.

Most complete trisomy 13s are spontaneous events with a slight maternal age effect, but where the extra number 13 is in the form of an unbalanced translocation, an examination of the parental chromosomes is mandatory. Recurrence risks for another child with trisomy 13 are small; however, there is about a 1% risk of a numerical chromosome abnormality in future pregnancies. The most common problem would be Down syndrome. Under these circumstances, most clinicians would offer an amniocentesis in subsequent pregnancies.

should be available within a week. As well as advice about the management and prognosis of the infant, the parents will need counselling about risks to future children. This is best carried out some months after the birth, and should include full explanation of prenatal diagnosis (amniocentesis or chorionic villus sampling) and the associated risk. A rough guide to the recurrence risk in Down syndrome is given in Table 32.1.

Trisomy 13 (Patau syndrome) (Fig. 32.2)

This aneuploidy has a frequency of 1 in 7000 livebirths. Survival after the first year of life is unusual, although survival until over the age of 5 years has been described. The head is small, triangular in shape (trigonocephaly), with a sloping forehead. The eyes are small and colobomata of the iris are common. Bilateral cleft lip and palate in the presence of the small head and jaw, in conjunction with the eye abnormalities, suggest the syndrome on inspection of the face alone. Congenital heart defects are present in more than 80% of cases, and in the limbs polydactyly (on the

Trisomy 18 (Figs 32.3 & 32.4)

Trisomy 18, or Edward syndrome, has a distinctive clinical picture. The incidence is about 1 in 5000. Those affected have a prominent occiput, a dolichocephalic (disproportionately long) head and a small chin. The ears are low-set and malformed (especially the auricles). The mouth opening is small, and ptosis and wide epicanthic folds are common. In the hands, the second finger overlaps the third, and occasionally the fifth overlaps the fourth. Dermatoglyphic examination of the finger pads reveals a preponderance of low arches, and the distal crease on the fifth finger might be absent. Cryptorchidism is common and the majority of cases have congenital heart defects, especially an atrial septal defect or patent ductus arteriosus. Renal defects are also common. Mental retardation in survivors is severe, however: only 10% of babies survive the first year of life.

The association of trisomy 18 with increasing maternal age is not as obvious as in trisomy 21. However, the mean maternal age (32 years) is well above the population mean. Recurrence risks are similar to those for trisomy 13.

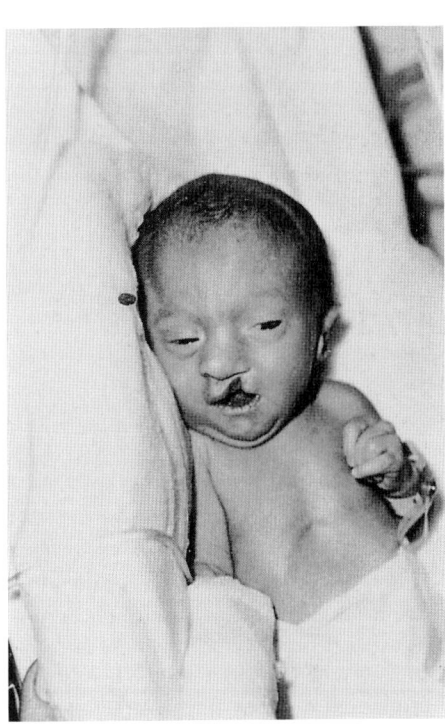

Fig. 32.4 Edward syndrome (trisomy 18).

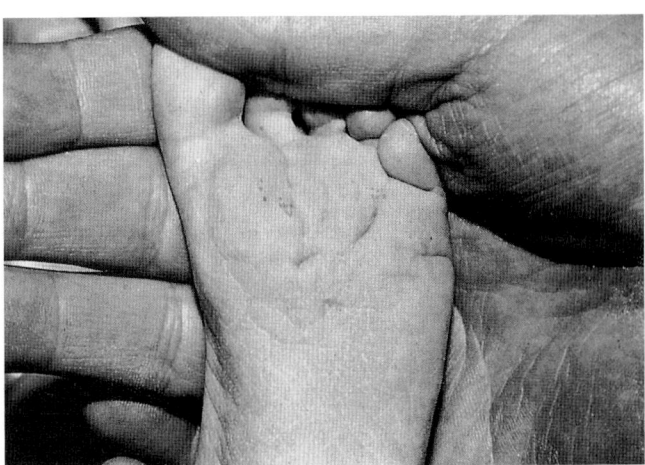

Fig. 32.5 Partial trisomy 8.

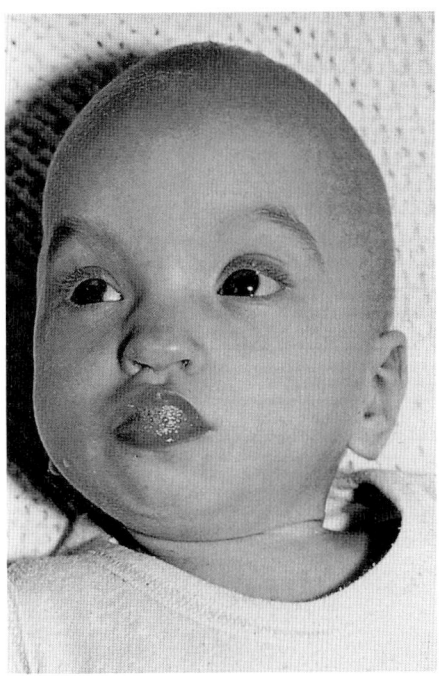

Fig. 32.6 Wolf–Hirschhorn syndrome (4p-syndrome).

Trisomy 8 (Fig. 32.5)

Most of these infants are mosaic for trisomy 8 cells and normal cells. The most characteristic neonatal abnormality is the presence of deep grooves on the soles and palms. Mild camptodactyly and limitation of elbow extension might also be present. The face may not be very unusual, but there is a tendency for rather 'coarse' features, consisting of a broad nasal root, thick lips, prominent forehead and protuberant ears. Eventual development reveals mild to severe retardation.

Deletion of the short arm of 4 (4p-) (Wolf–Hirschhorn syndrome) (Fig. 32.6)

Severe mental and growth retardation is invariably present. The head is small and midline scalp defects are common. Preauricular cutaneous pits and tags draw attention to the possible diagnosis, and colobomata of the iris, a fish mouth, cleft lip and palate, and simple low-set ears are frequently found. The prominent glabella, lack of an angle between the forehead and the broad nasal bridge, and hypertelorism give the face a 'Greek warrior helmet' appearance. Cardiac defects (atrial septal defects and ventricular septal defects) occur in one-third of cases. Grand mal epilepsy is common. It is associated with a high mortality rate.

Deletion of short arm of 5 (5p-) (cri du chat syndrome) (Fig. 32.7)

Even in the absence of the typical neonatal cry (not invariably present), the cri du chat syndrome is in most instances recognisable because of the presence of a round face, small head, widely spaced eyes, prominent epicanthus, antimongoloid eye slant and low-set ears. Cleft lip and palate, and cardiac and renal anomalies are sometimes present.

Partial trisomy of the short arm of 9

Trisomy 9p is now established as a definitive clinical entity. The facial appearance of this mental retardation syndrome is characterised by a large globulous nose, the effect of which is emphasised by deep-set, widely spaced eyes on a small head. Epicanthic folds, an antimongoloid obliquity of the eyes, down-turned mouth, protruding ears with abnormal antihelix, hypoplastic phalanges (especially the fifth finger middle phalanx) and extra skin folds in the neck are the other common features.

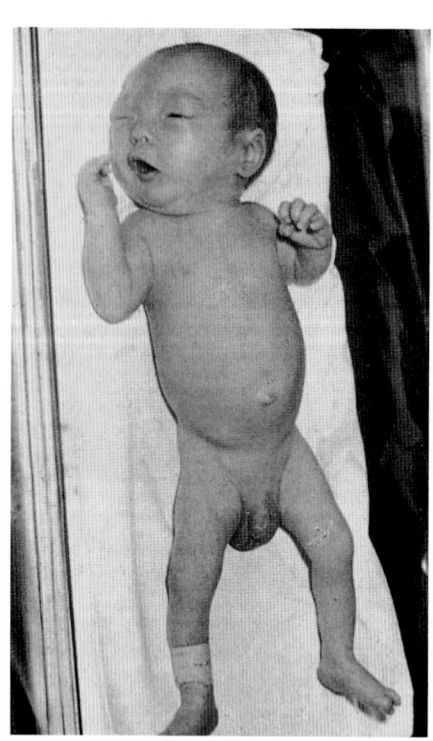

Fig. 32.7 Cri du chat syndrome (5p-syndrome).

Table 32.2 Microdeletion syndromes that may be diagnosed using laboratory probes

Condition	Main features	Locus
Williams	Supravalvular aortic stenosis, hypercalcaemia	7q11
Prader–Willi	Floppiness, hypogonadism in males	15q11
Miller–Dieker	Lissencephaly	17p13
DiGeorge	Hypocalcaemia, heart defects	22q11
Wolf–Hirschhorn	Facial abnormality (see Fig. 32.6)	4pter

Deletion of the long arm of 11 (11q-)

The craniofacial abnormalities are sometimes distinctive. The occiput is flared and the forehead is keel-shaped. The eyes are downslanting and ptosis is sometimes present. The jaw is small, the ears low-set, the mouth is characteristically carp-shaped and the philtrum long. Congenital heart defects, especially a ventricular septal defect, are common. Multiple joint contractures may be present.

Deletion of the long arm of 13 (13q-)

There is usually a broad, prominent nasal bridge and glabella on a small and often trigonocephalic head. Epicanthic folds are wide and colobomata of the iris may be present. Ears are commonly large, low-set and malformed.

There is evidence to suggest that there is a difference in the clinical features when the distal or proximal segment is implicated in the deletion. Protruding upper incisor teeth are, for instance, common in the distal deletion, as is the frontal bossing, whereas retinoblastoma and mild mental retardation are more often found with proximal or interstitial deletions. Like most of the chromosomal syndromes, abnormalities are widespread. Absent or hypoplastic thumbs, congenital heart defects, cryptorchidism, hypospadias and webbing of the neck have all been described on more than one occasion.

Deletion of the long arm of 18 (18q-)

A deletion of the long arm of a number 18 chromosome can be diagnosed on clinical grounds. The most characteristic feature is the mild facial flattening, with a prominent jutting jaw. The eyes are widely spaced and nystagmus, epicanthus and pale optic discs are found. The ears are prominent with large antihelices and antitragi, but the external canal is narrow and deafness is common. The mouth is downturned and 'carp-like'. In the hands, the thumbs are proximally implanted and the fingers are tapered. Dimples over the extensor surfaces of joints are a feature.

Trisomy 22

The head is small and the ears are low-set, malformed and angled forward. An unusual clinical feature is the frequent presence of preauricular skin tags, which, although not unique to the syndrome, are pointers to trisomy 22. A beaked nose, anteverted nostrils, long philtrum, cleft palate and downslanting eyes occur frequently. The neck is short and redundant skin folds accentuate the short-necked appearance. Cardiac anomalies are found in 50% of cases. In the hands, fingerised or broad thumbs are the more common manifestations.

The association of colobomata and anal atresia with an additional small acrocentric chromosome has long been recognised. Referred to as the cat-eye syndrome (distinct from cat cry), most cases were described during the pre-banding era. It now appears that the syndrome represents a partial trisomy or tetrasomy of the long arm of 22.

Microdeletion syndromes

All neonates who look unusual or have one or more malformations need a chromosome analysis. There are, however, a small but significant number of conditions that, despite being chromosomal in origin, have changes (mostly small deletions) that cannot be detected in this way. Over the past few years, new techniques have been developed to detect these submicroscopic deletions, the most commonly used being fluorescence in-situ hybridisation. The problem for the clinician is that a presumptive diagnosis needs to be made so that the laboratory can use the appropriate probes. Table 32.2 shows some of the more common conditions that may be diagnosed in this way.

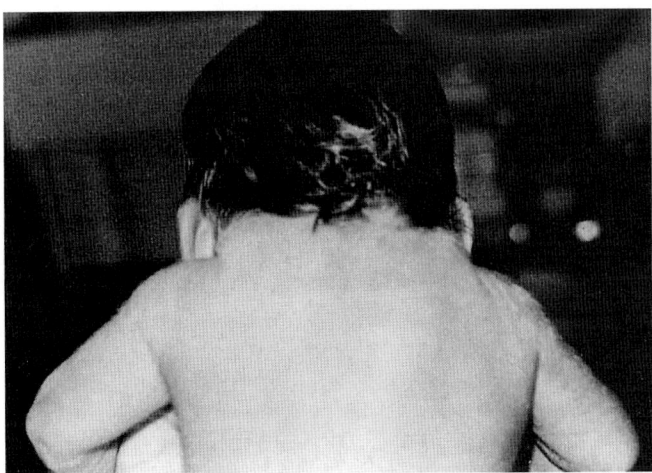

Fig. 32.8 Turner syndrome (45,XO).

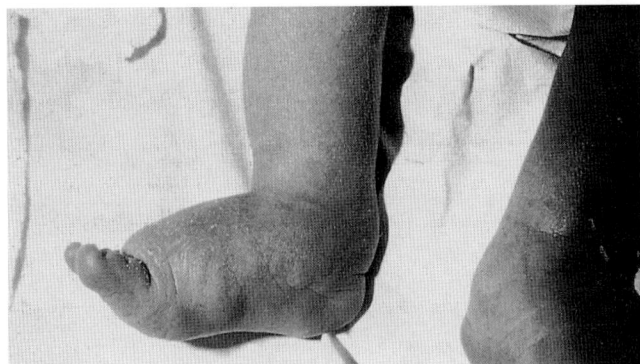

Fig. 32.9 Turner syndrome (45,XO).

Sex chromosome abnormalities

Of the common sex chromosome anomalies, fragile X mental retardation, Klinefelter syndrome (47,XXY), 47,XXX females and 47,XYY males show few phenotypic abnormalities in the neonatal period and are rarely diagnosed at this time. In general, all non-disjunction syndromes are maternal age-related, but not to the same extent as in Down syndrome.

Turner syndrome (45,XO)

The prevalence of this disorder is 1 in 5000 births. The most striking features may be a webbed skin fold at the neck (pterygium colli), with a low, trident posterior hairline (Fig. 32.8). Lymphoedema of the dorsum of the hands and feet is common (Fig. 32.9). The chest may be broad with widespread nipples, and cardiac defects, especially coarctation of the aorta, occur in about 20% of cases. Minor abnormalities that might be noted at birth include small, convex, deep-set nails, pigmented naevi on the skin and an increased carrying angle at the elbow. Short stature is the rule, with a mean final height of 4 feet 7 inches. Streak gonads are usually present, with the consequence that normal menstruation does not occur and infertility is the rule. Replacement

oestrogens are indicated at around the time of puberty. Outlook for final intelligence is good. Recurrence risks are small, probably less than those given for the autosomal trisomies.

Higher degrees of sex chromosome aneuploidy

With increasing numbers of sex chromosomes (e.g. 49,XXXXY; 48,XXXX; 49,XXXXX etc.), mental retardation becomes the rule. Pointers in the neonatal period include a tendency to mongoloid eye-slant, a short or webbed neck, and joint abnormalities, especially radioulnar synostosis.

An approach to the chromosomally normal malformed neonate

General considerations

One child in every 40 has a congenital malformation. Some of these are single; others are part of more complex dysmorphic syndromes. Single minor abnormalities are common (Table 32.3), but they also occur with an increased frequency in children with single or multiple major malformations. As pointed out by Marden et al,[126] multiple minor malformations occur alone in 0.8% of the population, whereas multiple minor malformations occur with single major malformations in 6.9% of affected infants. Multiple minor malformations occur in 56.2% of infants with multiple major malformations.

Syndrome recognition is an essential prerequisite for accurate genetic counselling, immediate management and prognosis. Syndrome identification in the neonate is based on an accurate evaluation of the dysmorphic features. For instance, hypertelorism (increased interpupillary distance) must be differentiated from telecanthus (increased distance between inner canthi).

Ideally this should be done with measurements and centile charts, and these do exist for certain modalities. Eventually photogrammetry might supersede clinical measurement, but at present a traditional clinical approach is used. Experience has shown that it is easier to make a syndrome diagnosis when a clearly delineated unusual feature or constellation of features is present. For example, cleft palate and polydactyly are more useful than those features that are common in normal neonates, such as inguinal hernia. Abnormal dysmorphic features might be thought of as 'handles', and there is a hierarchy of 'handles' in order of their usefulness for the syndromologist. Some malformations are minor and blend into normal variations; others are too frequent and therefore unhelpful. An approach to the diagnosis of the dysmorphic child will be discussed, using various 'handles' (Fig. 32.10).

Developmental considerations

In the assessment of the dysmorphic child it is necessary to decide whether there is (a) a malformation, (b) a deformation,

Table 32.3 Incidence of some common minor abnormalities

Minor abnormality	Frequency per 1000
Epicanthus	4.2
Small ears	1.4
Auricular sinus	1.2
Preauricular tags	2.3
Fifth finger clinodactyly	9.9
2/3 syndactyly (toes)	1.6
Single palmar crease	
Unilateral	40 (or 4% of pop.)
Bilateral	10 (or 1% of pop.)

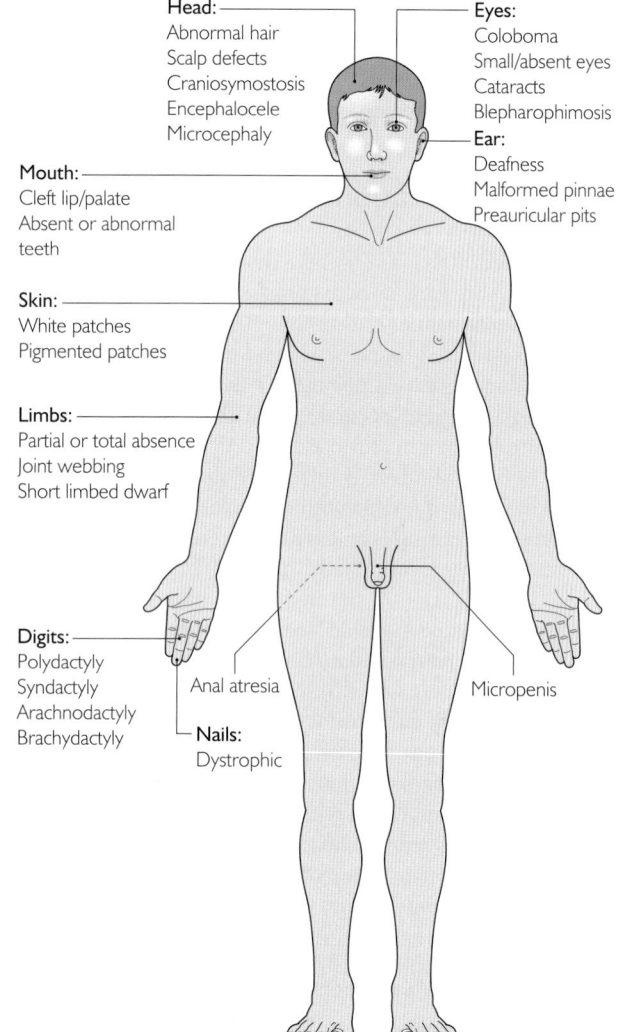

Head:
Abnormal hair
Scalp defects
Craniosymostosis
Encephalocele
Microcephaly

Eyes:
Coloboma
Small/absent eyes
Cataracts
Blepharophimosis

Ear:
Deafness
Malformed pinnae
Preauricular pits

Mouth:
Cleft lip/palate
Absent or abnormal teeth

Skin:
White patches
Pigmented patches

Limbs:
Partial or total absence
Joint webbing
Short limbed dwarf

Digits:
Polydactyly
Syndactyly
Arachnodactyly
Brachydactyly

Anal atresia

Micropenis

Nails:
Dystrophic

Fig. 32.10 An approach to the diagnosis of the dysmorphic child (see text).

or (c) a disruption. These can be defined as follows:[175]

a. A malformation results from an intrinsic abnormal developmental process. The developmental potential is abnormal (e.g. spina bifida).

Table 32.4 Important points in history taking

Question	Relevance
Personal/family history	
1. Elderly mother	? Chromosomal aneuploidy
2. Elderly father	? de novo AD mutation
3. Maternal disease, e.g. diabetes	Associated abnormalities, e.g. sacral agenesis and maternal diabetes
4. Poor social history	Possible alcohol/drug problems
5. Racial origin	Some genetic diseases confined to specific racial groups
6. Parental consanguinity	Autosomal recessive disorders
7. Multiple miscarriages	Chromosome rearrangements
Pregnancy history	
8. Maternal drug or alcohol ingestion	Teratogenic effects
9. Exposure to radiation	Possible teratogenic or mutation effects
10. Early rupture of membranes	Possible fetal compression
11. Oligohydramnios	? Renal agenesis
12. Polyhydramnios	? Oesophageal atresia
13. Poor fetal movements	? Neuromuscular disorder or fetal compression
14. Breech presentation	? Neuromuscular disorder

b. A deformation results from mechanical alteration to a developing part after a period of normal development (e.g. talipes equinovarus caused by fetal constraint).

c. A disruption – after an initially normal development, a breakdown of or an interference with organ development occurs, resulting in the destruction of that part (e.g. amniotic bands).

Having decided which of the three broad categories is appropriate, then, taking a malformation as an example, the designation to this category should be followed by the questions:

- Is it a single or multiple malformation?[100]
- If there are multiple malformations, are they part of a syndrome or a sequence?

If a single insult leads onto or initiates further defects, then it is a *malformation sequence*. This implies that there is a cascade of secondary consequences. For example, renal agenesis causes oligohydramnios, which in turn gives rise to 'Potter's facies' and pulmonary hypoplasia. If the initial insult causes multiple defects but these are not the consequence of one another, then the term *malformation syndrome* might be appropriate. It should be noted that a syndrome is a pattern of malformations thought to be pathogenically related. If the multiple malformation complex under consideration is not thought to be a syndrome or sequence, there could be a known association between the various components. An *association* is a non-random occurrence of multiple anomalies not

Table 32.5 Microcephaly

Syndrome	Features present at birth	Features developing later	Inheritance	Location	Gene	References
Bloom	IUGR, malar hypoplasia	Telangiectasia, low IgA and IgM, lymphoreticular tumours	AR	15q26	RecQ	53, 93
Cornelia de Lange (Fig. 32.11)	Synophrys, flared nostrils, thin upper lip, hirsutism	Growth delay and mental retardation	Usually sporadic	3q26		95, 100
Dubowitz	IUGR, ptosis, micrognathia	Short stature, eczema	AR			202
Fetal alcohol	IUGR, smooth philtrum, small finger nails	Mild to moderate mental retardation				
Fetal CMV	Hepatosplenomegaly, thrombocytopenia	Mental retardation, deafness				
Fetal rubella	IUGR, cataract, chorioretinitis, congenital heart disease	Deafness, mental retardation				
Lissencephaly	Wrinkled skin on forehead, jaundice, seizures	Mental handicap	AR, microdeletion	17p13	LIS1	48, 50
Maternal phenylketonuria	IUGR, cardiac defects	Mental retardation				185
Neu–Laxova (Fig. 32.12)	Absent eyelids, peripheral oedema, colloidion skin	Lethal	AR			187
Seckel	IUGR, beaked nose, dislocated elbows	Mental retardation, extreme short stature	AR	3q22		77, 122, 184
Smith–Lemli–Opitz	Anteverted nostrils, ptosis, hypospadias, 2–3 syndactyly of toes	Mental retardation	AR	7q32	SLOS	100, 145
True microcephaly	Sloping forehead, large ears	Mental retardation	AR	1q31 8p33	Microcephalin	186

known to be a sequence or a syndrome. It is a statistical concept. The importance of these distinctions is that deformations or disruptions are rarely genetically determined, whereas the malformation syndromes might be chromosomal, or inherited in a Mendelian way.

A clinical approach

History

Many important clues can be obtained by a careful history taken from the parents and detailed examination of the obstetric notes. A summary of important questions is given in Table 32.4.

Clinical examination

The malformed neonate with normal chromosomes might have a specific syndrome. Its recognition should be approached as follows:

Gestalt recognition

It might be that the individual malformation can easily be organised into a meaningful problem without consciously analysing the individual abnormalities. Recognition is immediate. For instance, diagnosis of the Cornelia de Lange syndrome (Fig. 32.11) is often possible from the examination of craniofacial features alone. Nevertheless, care should be taken not to overdiagnose syndromes on this basis, and a careful evaluation of other physical abnormalities which might help to confirm the initial diagnostic suspicion should be made. It is also better to diagnose a child as having an 'undiagnosed syndrome' rather than providing an inappropriate diagnosis which will be difficult to undo at a later date.

Identification of suitable handles

Where immediate recognition is not possible, it is necessary to identify one or more features (handles) which might lead the syndromologist to make a diagnosis. Useful handles are:

- Well-defined but unusual physical signs, e.g. polydactyly. These should be carefully evaluated and described. For example, polydactyly can be of different degrees, associated with syndactyly, and can be on the radial side (preaxial) or ulnar side (postaxial).
- Signs which are the subject of comprehensive reviews, e.g. anal atresia (see Pinsky[153]).

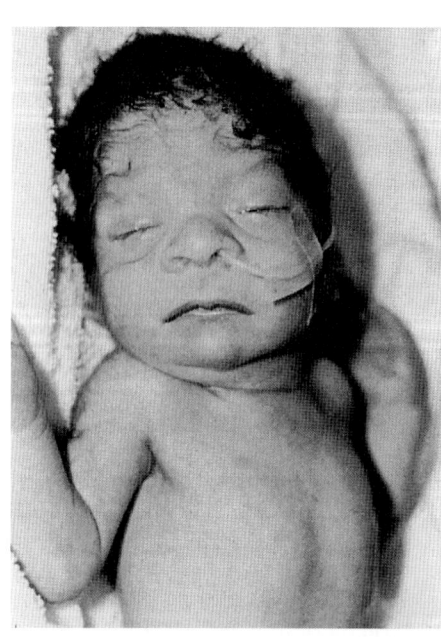

Fig. 32.11 De Lange syndrome.

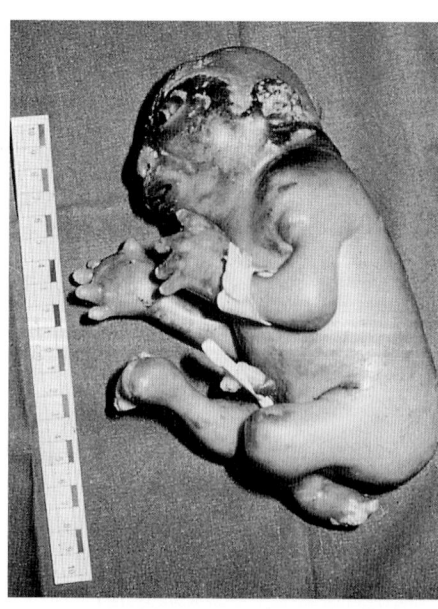

Fig. 32.12 Neu–Laxova syndrome.

Table 32.6 Macrocephaly

Syndrome	Features present at birth	Features developing later	Inheritance	Location	Gene	References
Achondroplasia	*see Short limbs – moderate (Table 32.27)*					
Albers–Schonberg	Osteopetrosis, pancytopenia		AR (severe type)	11q13 16p13	TCIRG1 CLCN7	64, 100
Bannayan–Zonana	Capillary haemangiomas	Lipomas	AD	10q22–23	PTEN	130
Grieg	*See Polydactyly (Table 32.28)*					
HARD + E	Hydrocephalus, small encephalocoele, retinal dysplasia, cataracts	Mental retardation	AR			48, 50
Neurofibromatosis	*see Skin abnormalities (Table 32.42)*					
Robinow	*see Hypertelorism (Table 32.13)*					
Russell Silver	Small for dates	Triangular facies	Sporadic	17		146
Sotos	Large birthweight, advanced bone age	Mild mental retardation	AD	5q35	NSD1	36, 109, 206
Sturge–Weber	*see Skin abnormalities (Table 32.42)*					
X-linked hydrocephalus	Adducted thumbs, aqueduct stenosis	Mental retardation	XLR	Xq28	L1CAM	65, 105

If one handle does not lead to a diagnosis, then other combinations should be tried. Computer databases are now available which will furnish a manageable list of syndromes, with references for all possible combinations.[203] Lists of good handles are contained in Tables 32.5–32.42, which follow. The lists are not exhaustive but they attempt to cover most of the useful signs present in the neonate.

New molecular tests

With the increasing identification of the genes responsible for the dysmorphic syndromes, there will be an increasing demand to use these tests in making a diagnosis. At present their role is mainly in confirming a diagnosis, and if a mutation is found, then early prenatal diagnosis can be offered in future pregnancies.

Table 32.7 Unusual-shaped skull

Syndrome	Features present at birth	Features developing later	Inheritance	Location	Gene	References
Apert syndrome (Figs 32.13 & 32.14)	Craniostenosis, beaked nose, cleft palate, mitten-shaped syndactyly in hands	Mild to moderate mental retardation	AD	10q25–26	FGFR2	100, 200
Baller–Gerold	see Radial defects (Table 32.35)					
Carpenter	see Polydactyly (Table 32.28)					
Crouzon	Craniostenosis, brachycephaly, prominent forehead, proptosis, hypoplastic mid face	Normal intelligence	AD	10q25–26	FGFR2	100, 158
Fetal compression	see Multiple joint contractures/ dislocations (Table 32.38)					
Hypophosphatasia	see Very short limbs (Table 32.36)					
Pfeiffer	Brachycephaly, craniostenosis, broad thumb and hallux	Normal intelligence	AD	8p11, 10q25–26	FGFR1, FGFR2	100, 166
Saethre–Chotzen	Ptosis, asymmetric facies, brachycephaly, prominent ear crus, mild syndactyly	Usually normal intelligence	AD	7p21	TWIST	91, 100, 157

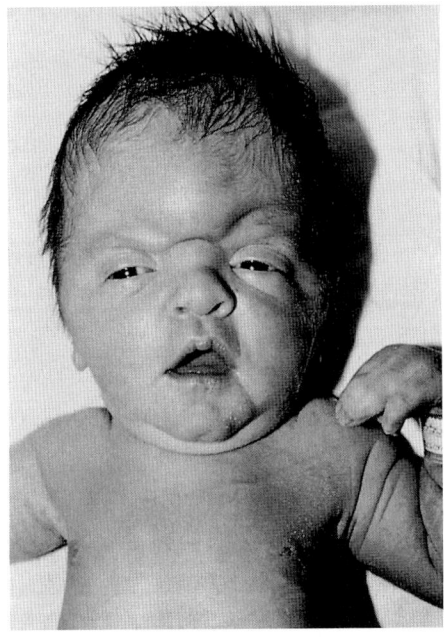

Fig. 32.13 Apert syndrome.

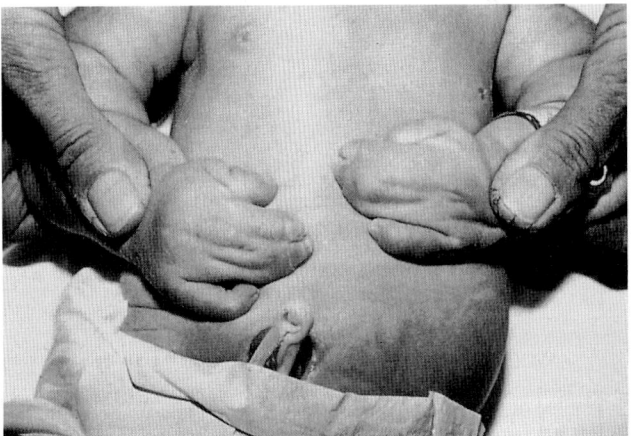

Fig. 32.14 Apert syndrome.

Unfortunately, at the moment the tests are very expensive and cannot pick up all the children affected by a syndrome, as the diagnostic testing cannot easily screen the entire sequence in the gene. With the development of increasing automation in gene diagnosis, the situation may change.

Abbreviations used in Tables 32.5–32.42
AD, autosomal dominant
AR, autosomal recessive
XLD, X-linked dominant
XLR, X-linked recessive

Table 32.8 Fontanelles – wide

Syndrome	Features present at birth	Features developing later	Inheritance	Location	Gene	References
Cleidocranial dysostosis	Prominent forehead, sloping shoulders, absent or hypoplastic clavicles	Wide-spaced carious teeth, hypoplasia of distal phalanges	AD	6p21	CBFA1	55, 100
Hallerman–Strieff	see Cataracts (Table 32.10)					
Hypophosphatasia	see Very short limbs (Table 32.36)					
Hypothyroidism	Prolonged jaundice, constipation, umbilical hernia	Coarse facial features, large tongue, dry skin, sparse hair, mental retardation if untreated	Usually sporadic but some metabolic			
Kenny	Hypocalcaemia, thin medullary cavities to long bones on X-ray	Short stature, myopia	AD	1q42		100
Osteogenesis imperfecta	see Very short limbs (Table 32.36)					
Pyknodysostosis	Beaked nose, small mandible, hypoplastic scapulae, short terminal phalanges, osteosclerosis	Fractures, short stature, crowded teeth	AR	1q21	Cathepsin K	13, 70
Russell Silver	see Macrocephaly (Table 32.6)					
Thanatophoric dysplasia	see Very short limbs (Table 32.36)					
Zellweger	see Cataracts (Table 32.10)					

Table 32.9 Coloboma

Syndrome	Features present at birth	Features developing later	Inheritance	Location	Gene	References
CHARGE association	Choanal atresia, external ear abnormality, hypogenitalism, congenital heart disease	Short stature, deafness	Mostly sporadic			144
Cohen	Antimongoloid slant to eyes	Obesity, prominent teeth, thin fingers, mental retardation	AR	8q22–23		141, 180
Goltz	see Skin abnormalities (Table 32.42)					
Linear sebaceous naevus	see Skin abnormalities (Table 32.42)					
Meckel Gruber	see Polydactyly (Table 32.28)					
Rieger	Aniridia, flat upper lip, prominent skin around umbilicus	Hypoplastic, widely spaced teeth	AD	4q25–27	RIEG	101, 169

An approach to the chromosomally normal malformed neonate

Table 32.10 Cataract

Syndrome	Features present at birth	Features developing later	Inheritance	Location	Gene	References
Cerebro-oculo-facio-skeletal (COFS)	see Multiple joint contractures/dislocations (Table 32.38)					
Hallermann–Streiff	Brachycephaly, prominent forehead, sparse hair, micrognathia, pinched nose, neonatal teeth	Short stature, usually normal intelligence	Usually sporadic			30, 100
Incontinentia pigmenti	see Skin abnormalities (Table 32.42)					
Lowe	Glaucoma, aminoaciduria, renal tubular acidosis	Mental retardation	XLR	Xq25	OCRL	1, 114
Fetal rubella	see Microcephaly (Table 32.5)					
Neu–Laxova	see Microcephaly (Table 32.5)					
Chondrodysplasia punctata	see Short limbs – moderate (Table 32.37)					
Rothmund Thomson	see Skin abnormalities (Table 32.42)					
Zellweger	Prominent forehead, stippled epiphyses, hypotonia	Mental retardation, lethal in childhood	AR	1p22–21, 7q11, 8q21	PXMP3 PMP70	128, 131

Table 32.11 Dislocated lens

Syndrome	Features present at birth	Features developing later	Inheritance	Location	Gene	References
Homocystinuria	Arachnodactyly, pes cavus, homocystine in urine	Sparse hair, malar flush, arterial and venous thrombosis	AR	21q22	CBS	125
Marfan	see Arachnoidactyly (Table 32.30)					
Sulphite oxidase deficiency	Sulphite and inorganic sulphate in urine	Mental retardation, lethal in childhood	AR			120
Weill–Marchesani	Brachydactyly, spherical lens	Short stature	AR	14q24, 6p21 19p13	MOCS1 MOCS2	205, 207

Table 32.12 Microphthalmia

Syndrome	Features present at birth	Features developing later	Inheritance	Location	Gene	References
Cerebro-oculo-facio-skeletal (COFS)	see Multiple joint contractures/dislocations (Table 32.38)					
Cross	Hypopigmentation of skin, seizures	Mental retardation	AR			40
Cohen	see Coloboma (Table 32.9)					
Cryptophthalmos (Fraser syndrome)	Fused eyelids, syndactyly, genital anomalies, laryngeal stenosis, renal anomalies	Stillbirth common	AR			69, 71
Goltz	see Skin abnormalities (Table 32.42)					
Hallermann–Streiff	see Cataracts (Table 34.10)					
Incontinentia pigmenti	see Skin abnormalities (Table 32.42)					
Lenz	Prominent ears, genital abnormalities	Sloping shoulders, crowded teeth	XLR		Xq27	11, 60, 190
Neu–Laxova	see Microcephaly (Table 32.5)					
Meckel Gruber	see Polydactyly (Table 32.28)					
Oculo-dento-digital (ODD)	Pinched nose, syndactyly	Enamel hypoplasia of teeth, osteopetrosis	AD	6q22–q24	GJA1	72, 149

Table 32.13 Hypertelorism

Syndrome	Features present at birth	Features developing later	Inheritance	Location	Gene	References
Aarskog	Ptosis, shawl scrotum	Short stature, mild mental retardation	XLR	Xp11	FGD1	14, 20, 155
Alagille	Deep-set eyes, pulmonary stenosis, liver disease		AD	20p11	Jagged1	132, 134
Frontonasal dysplasia	Bifid nasal tip, anterior encephalocoele, cleft palate		Sporadic			177
Greig	see Polydactyly (Table 32.28)					
Larsen	see Multiple contractures/dislocations (Table 32.38)					
Noonan	see Short neck (Table 32.27)					
Opitz G/BBB	Hypospadias, apnoeic episodes (cleft larynx)	Mental retardation	AD	22q11; Xp22	MID1	67, 129
Otopalato-digital	see Cleft palate (Table 32.21)					
Robinow	Short limbs (mesomelia), gingival hypertrophy, fetal facies, vertebral defects, micropenis	Short stature, scoliosis	AR/AD	9q22	ROR2	2, 3, 100
Waardenburg	Heterochromia	White forelock, deafness	AD	2q37; 3q12	PAX3 MITF	61, 100, 191

Table 32.14 Ptosis

Syndrome	Features present at birth	Features developing later	Inheritance	Location	Gene	References
Aarskog	see Hypertelorism (Table 32.13)					
Blepharophimosis ptosis epicanthus inversus (BPES)	Short palpebral fissures, prominent epicanthic folds, dysplastic ears	Occasionally female infertility	AD	3q22–23	FOXL2	143, 174
Dubowitz	see Microcephaly (Table 32.5)					
Fetal alcohol	see Microcephaly (Table 32.5)					
Moebius	Immobile face, limb defects, strabismus, syndactyly		Usually sporadic	13q12–13		8
Noonan	see Short neck (Table 32.27)					
Saethre Chotzen	see Unusual-shaped skull (Table 32.7)					
Schwartz–Jampel	Small mouth, myotonia, flexion deformities, cataracts	Mild mental retardation, short stature	AR	1p34–36	HSPG2 (perlecan)	12, 140

Table 32.15 Aplastic alae nasi (i.e. lack of flare in nostrils)

Syndrome	Features present at birth	Features developing later	Inheritance	Location	Gene	References
Fetal warfarin	see Flat or depressed nose (Table 32.17)					
Freeman–Sheldon	see Small mouth (Table 32.19)					
Hallermann Streiff	see Cataracts (Table 32.10)					
Johanson–Blizzard	Aplasia cutis of scalp, microcephaly, hypothyroidism, malabsorption, imperforate anus	Deafness, mental retardation, sparse hair	AR			92
Langer–Giedion	Microcephaly, bulbous nose, thin upper lip, prominent ears, cutis laxa	Sparse hair, cone-shaped epiphyses on X-ray of fingers	AD or sporadic	8q24	TRPS1, EXT1	89, 100
Oculo-dento-digital	see Microphthalmia (Table 32.12)					

Table 32.16 Beaked nose (i.e. convex outline)

Syndrome	Features present at birth	Features developing later	Inheritance	Location	Gene	References
Apert	see Unusual-shaped skull (Table 32.7)					
Crouzon	see Unusual shaped skull (Table 32.7)					
Rubinstein–Taybi	Microcephaly, antimongoloid eye slant, prominent nasal columella, hirsutism, broad thumbs	Microcephaly, mental retardation	Usually sporadic	16p13	CBP	100, 152
Seckel	see Microcephaly (Table 32.5)					

Table 32.17 Flat or depressed nasal bridge

Syndrome	Features present at birth	Features developing later	Inheritance	Location	Gene	References
Achondroplasia	see Short limbs – moderate (Table 32.37)					
Anhidrotic ectodermal dysplasia	Broad forehead, hyperthermia, lack of sweating, sticky eyes	Sparse fine hair, dry skin, hypodontia	Mostly XLR	Xq12–13	EDA	100, 209
Blepharophimosis	see Ptosis (Table 32.14)					
Cleidocranial dysostosis	see Fontanelle – wide (Table 32.8)					
Fetal alcohol	see Microcephaly (Table 32.5)					
Fetal hydantoin (phenytoin)	see Small or hypoplastic nails (Table 32.34)					
Fetal warfarin	Mid-face hypoplasia, stippled epiphyses, short proximal segments of limbs	Mental retardation in some				
Larsen	see Multiple joint contractures/dislocations (Table 32.38)					
Marshall Stickler	Cleft palate, anteverted nostrils, flat mid face, micrognathia	Epiphyseal dysplasia, cataract, joint stiffness, deafness	AD	12q13–14 6p21–22 1p21	COL2A1 COL11A2 COL11A2	9, 62
Williams (Fig. 32.15)	Supravalvular aortic stenosis, hypercalcaemia, stellate iris, thick lips, long philtrum	Mental retardation, short stature, nephrocalcinosis	Mostly sporadic	7q11	Elastin	41, 100

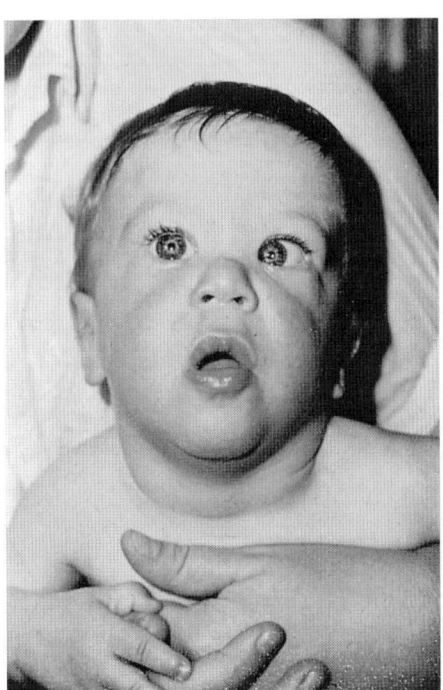

Fig. 32.15 Williams syndrome.

Table 32.18 Long philtrum

Syndrome	Features present at birth	Features developing later	Inheritance	Location	Gene	References
Cornelia de Lange	see Microcephaly (Table 32.5)					
Femoral hypoplasia, unusual facies	see Short limbs – moderate (Table 32.36)					
Langer–Giedion	see Aplastic alae nasi (Table 32.15)					
Robinow	see Hypertelorism (Table 32.13)					
Smith–Lemli–Opitz	see Microcephaly (Table 32.5)					
Williams	see Flat or depressed nasal bridge (Table 32.17)					

Table 32.19 Small mouth

Syndrome	Features present at birth	Features developing later	Inheritance	Location	Gene	References
Freeman–Sheldon	Broad forehead, blepharophimosis, long philtrum, puckered lips, talipes	Ulnar contraction of fingers, short stature	AD			100
Marden Walker	see Arachnoidactyly (Table 32.30)					
Schwartz–Jampel	see Ptosis (Table 32.14)					

Table 32.20 Cleft lip

Syndrome	Features present at birth	Features developing later	Inheritance	Location	Gene	References
Amniotic bands	see Split hands/reduction defects (Table 32.32)					
EEC	see Split hands/reduction defects (Table 32.32)					
Fetal hydantoin (phenytoin)	see Small or hypoplastic nails (Table 32.34)					
Mohr	Broad nasal tip, midline cleft lip and palate, aberrant frenulae, cleft tongue	Deafness, short stature	AR			127, 160
Oro-facio-digital (OFD)	see Syndactyly (Table 32.31)					
Popliteal web	Cleft lip and palate, web of the skin at the knees		AD	1q32–41	IRF6	66, 82
Rapp–Hodgkin	Dysplastic nails, pinched nose, cleft palate, hypospadias	Sparse hair	AD			19, 167
Roberts	see Radial defects (Table 32.35)					
Van der Woude	Cleft palate, lip pits on lower lip		AD	1q32–41	IRF6	99, 100, 136

Table 32.21 Cleft palate

Syndrome	Features present at birth	Features developing later	Inheritance	Location	Gene	References
Apert	see Unusual-shaped skull (Table 32.7)					
Camptomelic dysplasia	see Short limbs – moderate (Table 32.37)					
Cerebrocosto-mandibular	see Mandible – small (Table 32.25)					
CHARGE	see Coloboma (Table 32.9)					
Diastropic dysplasia	see Very short limbs (Table 32.36)					
Fetal hydantoin	see Small or hypoplastic nails (Table 32.34)					
Larsen	see Multiple joint contractures/dislocations (Table 32.38)					
Marshall Stickler	see Flat or depressed nasal bridge (Table 32.17)					
Mohr	see Cleft lip (Table 32.20)					
Otopalato-digital	Hypertelorism, flat mid face, broad tips to the fingers and toes	Prominent forehead and supraorbital ridges, deafness	XLR	Xq28		15, 150
Pierre Robin sequence	Small mandible, glossoptosis	Mental retardation in small proportion	Mostly sporadic			100
Popliteal web	see Cleft lip (Table 32.20)					
Spondyloepiphyseal dysplasia congenita	see short limbs – moderate (Table 32.37)					
Van der Woude	see Cleft lip (Table 32.20)					

Table 32.22 Oral frenulae

Syndrome	Features present at birth	Features developing later	Inheritance	Location	Gene	References
Ellis van Crevald	see Polydactyly (Table 32.28)					
Hypoglossia hypodactyly	see Mandible – small (Table 32.25)					
Mohr	see Cleft lip (Table 32.20)					
Oro-facio-digital (OFD)	see Syndactyly (Table 32.31)					
Popliteal web	see Cleft lip (Table 32.20)					

Table 32.23 Tongue abnormalities

Syndrome	Features present at birth	Features developing later	Inheritance	Location	Gene	References
Beckwith–Weideman	Large tongue, exomphalos, macrosomia, creases on ears	Mental retardation, renal tumours in 5%	Mostly sporadic	11p15		54, 87
GM$_1$ gangliosidosis	Large tongue, hypertrophied alveolar ridges, hepatomegaly	Coarse facial features, cloaking of long bones on X-ray	AR	3p21	GLB1	172
Hypothyroidism	Large tongue see Fontanelle – wide (Table 32.8)					
Mohr	Cleft tongue see Cleft lip (Table 32.20)					
Oor-facio-digital (OFD)	Tumours of the tongue see Syndactyly (Table 32.31)					

Table 32.24 Thick alveolar ridges

Syndrome	Features present at birth	Features developing later	Inheritance	Location	Gene	References
GM$_1$ gangliosidosis	see Tongue abnormalities (Table 32.23)					
I-cell disease	Coarse facial features, stiff skin, periosteal cloaking of long bones	Short stature, stiff joints, progressive coarsening of facial features, dysostosis multiplex	AR	4q21–23	GNPTA	116, 133
Robinow	see Hypertelorism (Table 32.13)					
Smith–Lemli–Opitz	see Microcephaly (Table 32.5)					

Table 32.25 Mandible – small

Syndrome	Features present at birth	Features developing later	Inheritance	Location	Gene	References
Bloom	see Microcephaly (Table 32.5)					
Cerebrocosto-mandibular	Cleft palate, defects in ribs, redundant skin	Mental retardation	AR			52, 115
Cerebro-oculo-facio-skeletal (COFS)	see Multiple joint contractures/dislocation (Table 32.38)					
Cornelia de Lange	see Microcephaly (Table 32.5)					
Dubowitz	see Microcephaly (Table 32.5)					
Femoral hypoplasia unusual facies	see Short limbs – moderate (Table 32.37)					
Goldenhar	see Ears – dysplastic (Table 32.26)					
Hypoglossia hypodactyly	Small tongue, transverse limb defects		Sporadic			
Marshall Stickler	see Flat or depressed nasal bridge (Table 32.17)					
Pierre Robin sequence	see Cleft palate (Table 32.21)					

Table 32.26 Ears – dysplastic or small

Syndrome	Features present at birth	Features developing later	Inheritance	Location	Gene	References
Beal's contractural arachnoidactyly	Crumpled ear see Arachnoidactyly (Table 32.30)					
Branchio-oto-renal (BOR)	Preauricular skin tags or pits; renal dysplasia	Deafness	AD with variable penetrance	8q13	EYA1	27, 33
CHARGE	see Coloboma (Table 32.9)					
Diastrophic dysplasia	Cystic deformed ears see Very short limbs (Table 32.36)					
Goldenhar	Preauricular skin tags, facial asymmetry, epibulbar dermoid, vertebral defects		Usually sporadic			34, 100
Roberts	see Radial defects (Table 32.35)					
Townes	see Anal atresia (Table 32.40)					
Treacher Collins	Antimongoloid slant to eyes, lower-lid coloboma, malar hypoplasia, small mandible	Deafness, normal intelligence	AD with variable penetrance	5q32	Treacle	47, 100

Table 32.27 Short neck (and/or webbing)

Syndrome	Features present at birth	Features developing later	Inheritance	Location	Gene	References
Goldenhar	see Ears – dysplastic (Table 32.26)					
Jarcho–Levin	Severe vertebral anomalies, broad forehead, short thorax, finger abnormalities	Early death from respiratory failure	AR	19q13	DLL3	24, 103
Klippel–Feil	Fusion of cervical vertebrae, low hairline, webbed neck, torticollis	Kyphoscoliosis, deafness	Sporadic	8q22–23		32
Multiple pterygium	see Multiple joint contractures/dislocations (Table 32.38)					
Noonan	Webbed neck, low hairline, antimongoloid slant to eyes, ptosis, hypertelorism, pulmonary stenosis	Short stature, bleeding problems, squints	AD	12q22	PTPN11	98, 170, 171, 181
Wildervanck	Cervical vertebral abnormalities, Duane anomaly, cleft palate	Deafness, occasional mental retardation	Uncertain			199

Table 32.28 Polydactyly

Syndrome	Features present at birth	Features developing later	Inheritance	Location	Gene	References
Opitz C	Trigonocephaly, oral frenulae, syndactyly	Mental retardation	AR			80, 165
Carpenter	Craniosynostosis, congenital heart defects, polydactyly	Mental retardation	AR			
Ellis van Creveld (Fig. 32.16)	Narrow thorax, atrial septal defect, oral frenulae, short limbs		AR	4p16	EVC	16, 154, 163
Greig	Syndactyly, frontal bossing, macrocephaly, hypertelorism		AD	7p13	GLI3	7, 75
Jeune	Narrow chest, short ribs, polydactyly	Renal dysfunction, cone-shaped epiphyses	AR	12p11–12		137
Kaufman–McKusick	see Anal atresia (Table 32.40)					
Laurence–Moon–Biedl		Obesity, retinitis pigmentosa, nephritis, mental retardation	AR	16q13, 3p11, 15p, 11q		100
Meckel–Gruber	Encephalocoele, polycystic kidneys,	May be stillborn or die in neonatal period	AR	17q22 11q, 8q		63, 164
Mohr	see Cleft lip (Table 32.20)					
Short rib polydactyly	Very small thorax, short limbs, usually lethal in utero		AR	Various types		

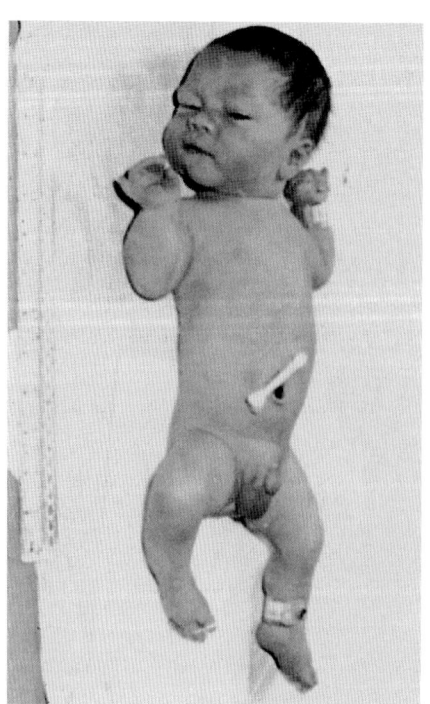

Fig. 32.16 Ellis van Creveld syndrome.

Table 32.29 Camptodactyly

Syndrome	Features present at birth	Features developing late	Inheritance	Location	Gene	References
Beal's contractural arachnoidactyly	*see* Arachnoidactyly (Table 32.30)					
Cerebro-oculo-facio-skeletal (COFS)	*see* Multiple joint contractures/dislocations (Table 32.38)					
Gordon	Talipes equinovarus, cleft palate		AD			57, 94, 161
Marden Walker	*see* Arachnoidactyly (Table 32.30)					
Multiple pterygium	*see* Multiple joint contractures/dislocations (Table 32.38)					

Table 32.30 Arachnodactyly

Syndrome	Features present at birth	Features developing later	Inheritance	Location	Gene	References
Beal's contractural arachnodactyly	Contractures of fingers and other joints; crumpled ears	Kyphoscoliosis, contractures improve	AD	5q23	FBN2	82, 121
Frontometaphyseal dysplasia	Prominent forehead	Frontal bossing, joint limitation, deafness, optic atrophy, metaphyseal flaring	Possible AD			59
Homocystinuria	see Dislocated lens (Table 32.11)					
Marden Walker	Blepharophimosis, cleft palate, talipes equinovarus, congenital heart disease	Mental retardation	AR			96, 201
Marfan	Dislocated lens, high arched palate, pectus excavatum, aortic and mitral incompetence	Dissection of aorta	AD	15q21	FBN1	44, 100

Table 32.31 Syndactyly

Syndrome	Features present at birth	Features developing later	Inheritance	Location	Gene	References
Apert	see Unusual-shaped skull (Table 32.7)					
Opitz C	see Polydactyly (Table 32.28)					
Cryptophthalmos	see Microphthalmia (Table 32.12)					
Goltz	see Skin abnormalities (Table 32.42)					
Greig	see Polydactyly (Table 32.28)					
Incontinentia pigmenti	see Skin abnormalities (Table 32.42)					
Moebius	see Ptosis (Table 32.14)					
Oro-facio-digital (OFD)	Midline cleft lip, oral frenulae, cleft palate, brachydactyly	Sparse hair	XLD, lethal in males	Xp22	CXORF5	10, 189
Pfeiffer	see Unusual-shaped skull (Table 32.7)					
Poland	Absence of pectoral muscle unilaterally	Poor breast development on affected side				43, 45
Saethre–Chotzen	see Unusual-shaped skull (Table 32.7)					

Table 32.32 Split hands/reduction defects

Syndrome	Features present at birth	Features developing later	Inheritance	Location	Gene	References
Amniotic bands	Facial clefts, ring constrictions					
Cornelia de Lange	see Microcephaly (Table 32.5)					
EEC	Ectodermal dysplasia, ectrodactyly, cleft lip and palate	Renal infections	AD	3q27 7q21	p63	22, 110
Hypoglossia–hypodactyly	see Mandible – small (Table 32.25)					
Isolated cleft hand (ectrodactyly)			AD			

Table 32.33 Abnormal thumbs

Syndrome	Features present at birth	Features developing later	Inheritance	Location	Gene	References
Aase	Triphalangeal thumbs, anaemia	Late closure of fontanelles Short stature	? XLR			74, 135
Cornelia de Lange	see Microcephaly (Table 32.5)					
Diastrophic dysplasia	'Hitchhiker' thumbs see Very short limbs (Table 32.36)					
DOOR (Deafness, Onycho-Osteodystrophy, Retardation)	Triphalangeal thumb see Small or hypoplastic nails (Table 32.34)					
Fanconi's anaemia	Hypoplastic thumbs, pigmented skin lesions, increased chromosome breakage, small penis	Pancytopenia, lymphoreticular malignancies	AR	3p22–26 9q22 16q24	FA(A) FA(C)	156
Fibrodysplasia ossificans progressiva	Hypoplastic thumbs and hallux	Soft tissue calcification	AD	4q27		38, 39
Holt–Oram	Hypoplastic thumbs and/or radius, ASD, VSD		AD variable expression	12q	TBX5	118, 138
Otopalato-digital	Broad thumbs see Cleft palate (Table 32.21)					
Pfeiffer	Broad thumbs see Unusual-shaped skull (Table 32.7)					
Rubenstein–Taybi	Broad thumbs see Beaked nose (Table 32.16)					
Townes	Triphalangeal thumbs see Anal abnormalities (Table 32.40)					
VATER	Hypoplastic thumbs see Vertebral anomalies (Table 32.41)					
X-linked hydrocephalus	Adducted thumbs see Macrocephaly (Table 32.6)					

Table 32.34 Small or hypoplastic nails

Syndrome	Features present at birth	Features developing later	Inheritance	Location	Gene	References
Coffin–Siris	Sparse scalp hair, microcephaly, coarse facial features, thick lips	Mental retardation, body hirsutism	AR			25, 100, 117
DOOR (Deafness, Onycho Osteodystrophy, Retardation)	Triphalangeal thumbs, small terminal phalanges	Deafness, mental retardation	AR			18, 148
Ellis van Crevald	see Polydactyly (Table 32.28)					
Fetal alcohol	see Microcephaly (Table 32.5)					
Fetal hydantoin (phenytoin)	Hirsuitism, cleft palate, midfacial hypoplasia	Developmental delay in some				68
Goltz	see Skin abnormalities (Table 32.42)					
Nail patella	Talipes equinovarus, joint contractures, ileal spur on pelvic X-ray	Nephritis, triangular lacunae on nails	AD	9q34	LMXIB	79, 100
Rapp–Hodgkin	see Cleft lip (Table 32.20)					

Table 32.35 Radial defects

Syndrome	Features present at birth	Features developing later	Inheritance	Location	Gene	References
Aase	see Abnormal thumbs (Table 32.33)					
Baller–Gerold	Craniosynostosis		AR			35, 151
Fanconi	see Abnormal thumbs (Table 32.33)					
Holt–Oram	Variable limb defects see Abnormal thumbs (Table 32.33)					
Juberg	Cleft lip and palate, microcephaly	Mental retardation	AR			102, 195
Roberts	Phocomelia, cleft lip and palate, facial dysmorphism Chromosome abnormality	Often stillborn or lethal in infancy	AR			5, 192, 208
Thrombocytopenia – absent radius (TAR)	Thrombocytopenia		AR			81, 111
VATER	see Vertebral abnormalities (Table 32.41)					

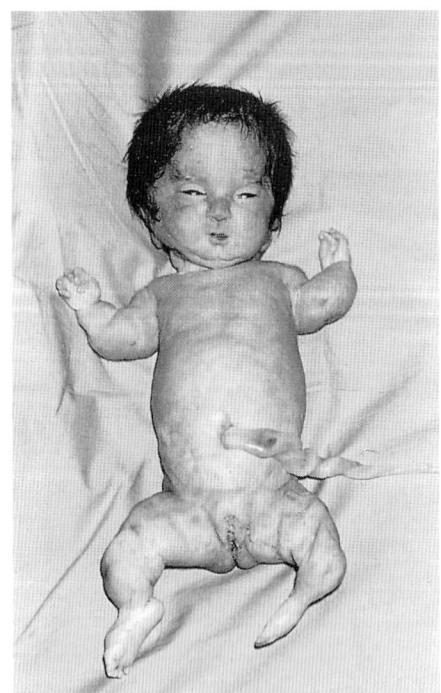

Fig. 32.17 Osteogenesis imperfecta congenita.

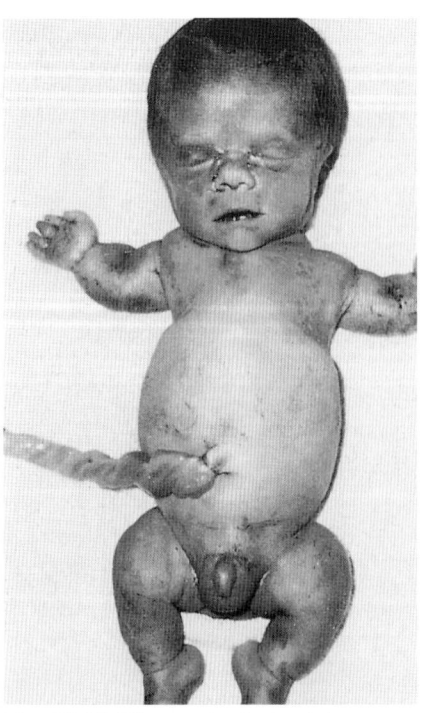

Fig. 32.18 Thanatophoric dysplasia.

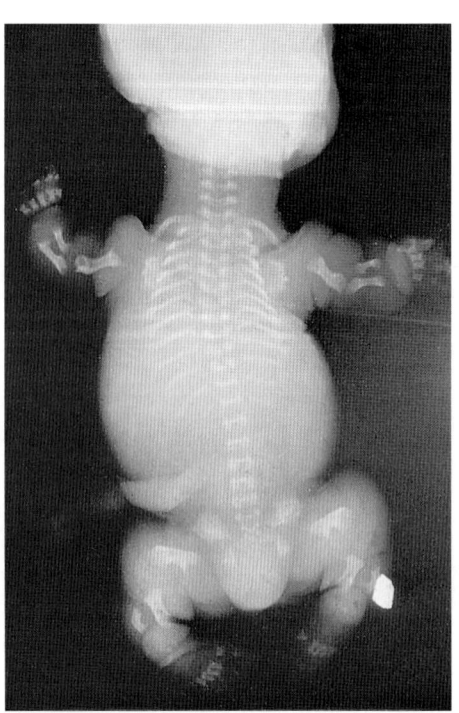

Fig. 32.19 Thanatophoric dysplasia.

Table 32.36 Very short limbs

Syndrome	Features present at birth	Features developing later	Inheritance	Location	Gene	References
Achondrogenesis	Large head, underossification	Lethal	Two types AR AR	5q31 12q13	DTDST COL2A1	179
Diastrophic dysplasia	'Hitchhiker' thumbs, talipes, cleft palate, respiratory difficulties	Kyphoscoliosis, cystic deformed ear	AR	5q21	DTDST	86
Hypophosphatasia	Underossification, low alkaline phosphatase	Two forms; severe form lethal	AR in severe form	1p34	ALPL	78
Kniest	Broad chest, cleft palate, flat mid face	Myopia, retinal detachment	Probably AD	12q13	COL2A1	17
Osteogenesis imperfecta (Fig. 32.17)	Blue sclera, poor ossification, multiple fractures	Severe forms lethal, mild form improves with age	AR and AD	7q21–22 17q21–22	COL1A1 COL1A2	37
Short ribbed polydactyly	see Polydactyly (Table 32.28)					
Thanatophoric dysplasia (Figs 32.18 & 32.19)	Large head, small thorax	Lethal	Sporadic	4p16	FGFR3	182

Table 32.37 Short limbs – moderate

Syndrome	Features present at birth	Features developing later	Inheritance	Location	Gene	References
Achondroplasia	Large head, trident hand, flat mid face	Lumbar lordosis, short stature	AD	4p16	FGFR3	194
Camptomelic dysplasia	Bowing of long bones, small thorax, sex reversal, cleft palate	Early demise, poor mental development	AR	17q24	SOX9	90, 123
Chondrodysplasia punctata (Conradi)	Flat mid face, ichthyosis, stippled epiphyses, cataract	Short stature	AD, AR, XLR	Xp11	EBP	83, 104
Ellis van Creveld	see Polydactyly (Table 32.28)					
Femoral hypoplasia Unusual facies	Hypoplastic femora/fibula Micrognathia		Rule out maternal diabetes			
Hypochondroplasia	Short limbs	Short stature	AD	4p16	FGFR3	139
Leri–Weill	Madelung's deformity	Mild short stature	XLD	Xp	SHOX	56, 119
Robinow	see Hypertelorism (Table 32.13)					
Spondyloepiphyseal dysplasia congenita	Cleft palate, short trunk, flat mid face, delayed epiphyses	Progressive scoliosis, myopia, retinal detachment	AD	12q13	COL2A1	6, 85

Table 32.38 Multiple joint contractures/dislocations

Syndrome	Features present at birth	Features developing later	Inheritance	Location	Gene	References
Arthrogryposis	Multiple joint contractures	Many different causes, neuromuscular disorders must be excluded				106
Beal's contractural arachnoidactyly	see Arachnoidactyly (Table 32.30)					
Cerebro-oculo-facio-skeletal (COFS)	Microcephaly, deep-set eyes, cataracts, rocker-bottom feet	Like trisomy 18, also lethal	AR	10q11	ERCC6	97, 204
Ehlers–Danlos	Dislocated joints see Skin abnormalities (Table 32.42)					
Fetal compression	Unusual skull shape micrognathia, facial compression	Lethal if due to renal agenesis (Potter's syndrome)				
Gordon	see Camptodactyly (Table 32.29)					
Larsen	Flat mid face, cleft palate	Accessory ossification centre in calcaneum	Mostly AD	3p14	FLNB	113, 188
Marden Walker	see Arachnoidactyly (Table 32.30)					
Multiple pterygium	Pterygia at elbows, neck, knees		AR			82
Nail patella	see Small or hypoplastic nails (Table 32.34)					
Schwartz–Jampel	see Ptosis (Table 32.14)					

Table 32.39 Hypogenitalism (male)/hypospadias

Syndrome	Features present at birth	Features developing later	Inheritance	Location	Gene	References
CHARGE	see Coloboma (Table 32.9)					
Cornelia de Lange	see Microcephaly (Table 32.5)					
Laurence–Moon–Biedl	see Polydactyly (Table 32.28)					
Meckel–Gruber	see Polydactyly (Table 32.28)					
Opitz G/BBB	see Hypertelorism (Table 32.13)					
Prader–Willi	Hypotonia, feeding difficulties	Obesity, almond-shaped eyes, small hands and feet, mental retardation	Mostly sporadic	15q11	SNRPN	23, 31
Robinow	see Hypertelorism (Table 32.13)					
Smith–Lemli–Opitz	see Microcephaly (Table 32.5)					

Table 32.40 Anal atresia (or abnormal placement)

Syndrome	Features present at birth	Features developing later	Inheritance	Location	Gene	References
Asymmetric crying facies	Congenital heart disease		Mostly sporadic			
Crytophthalmos	see Microphthalmia (Table 32.12)					
Johanson–Blizzard	see Aplastic alae nasi (Table 32.15)					
Kaufman–McKusick	Polydactyly, congenital heart disease, hydrometrocolpos		AR			29
Maternal diabetes	Congenital heart disease, sacral agenesis, limb defects					
Townes	Dysplastic ears, preauricular skin tags, abnormal thumbs		AD	16q12	SALL1	142, 159
VATER	see Vertebral abnormalities (Table 32.41)					

Table 32.41 Vertebral anomalies

Syndrome	Features present at birth	Features developing later	Inheritance	Location	Gene	References
Costovertebral dysplasia	Rib defects		AD or AR			
Goldenhar	see Ears – dysplastic (Table 32.26)					
Jarcho–Levin	see Short neck (Table 32.27)					
Klippel–Feil	see Short neck (Table 32.27)					
Robinow	see Hypertelorism (Table 32.13)					
SED congenita	see Short limbs – moderate (Table 32.37)					
VATER association	Vertebral defects, anal atresia, tracheo-oesophageal fistula, renal and radial limb defects	Congenital heart disease	Mostly sporadic			
Wildervanck	see Short neck (Table 32.27)					

Table 32.42 Skin abnormalities

Syndrome	Features present at birth	Features developing later	Inheritance	Location	Gene	References
Conradi	Ichthyosis *see* Short limbs – moderate (Table 32.37)					
Cutis laxa	Loose folds of skin	Emphysema, premature aged appearance	AD, AR, XLR	14q32 Xq12	FBLN5 Copper ATPase	4, 193
EEC	Ectodermal dysplasia *see* Split hand (Table 32.32)					
Ehlers–Danlos	Hyperextensible skin, loose joints, blue sclera	Abnormal scarring, vascular fragility, joint dislocation	At least 8 types		Mostly collagen genes	21, 28, 88, 107
Fetal alcohol	Haemangioma *see* Microcephaly (Table 32.5)					
Goltz	Focal dermal hypoplasia, syndactyly, microphthalmos	Abnormal teeth, alopecia, mental retardation	XLD – possibly lethal in males	Xp22		76, 183
Hypomelanosis of Ito	Hypopigmented streaks of skin	Seizures, possibly mental retardation				42, 162
Incontinentia pigmenti	Bullous eruptions of skin, cataract	Whorls of skin pigmentation, microcephaly, seizures	XLD, lethal in males	Xq28	NEMO	26, 112, 124, 173
Klippel–Trenaunay–Weber	Haemangiomata, overgrowth of limbs		Sporadic			198
Leopard	Lentigenes, pulmonary stenosis, hypertelorism	Deafness, short stature	AD	12q2 17q11	PTPN11 NF1	
Leprechaunism	Hirsutism, lack of subcutaneous tissue, hypoglycaemia	Growth deficiency	AR	19p13	INSR	46, 197
Limb reduction, ichthyosis	Unilateral ichthyosis with ipsilateral limb hypoplasia	Possible mental retardation	Possibly AR			100, 178
McCune–Albright	Café-au-lait patches	Fibrous dysplasia of bone	Sporadic	20q13	GNAS1	168
Rothmund–Thomson	Telangiectasia and atrophy	Cataract, premature ageing	AR	8q24	RECQL4	
Sturge–Weber	Port-wine stain on face	Intracerebral calcification, seizures	Sporadic			
Neurofibromatosis	Café-au-lait patches	Many complications	AD	17q11	NF1	196

References

1. Abbassi V, Lowe C U, Calcagno P L 1968 Oculo-cerebro-renal syndrome: a review. American Journal of Diseases of Children 115: 145–168
2. Afzal A R, Rajab A, Fenske C et al 2000 Linkage of recessive Robinow syndrome to a 4 cM interval on chromosome 9q22. Human Genetics 106: 351–354
3. Afzal A R, Rajab A, Fenske C D et al 2000 Recessive Robinow syndrome, allelic to dominant brachydactyly type B, is caused by mutation of ROR2. Nature Genetics 25: 419–422
4. Agha A, Sakati N O, Higginbottom M C et al 1978 Two forms of cutis laxa presenting in the newborn period. Acta Paediatrica Scandinavica 67: 775–780
5. Allingham-Hawkins D J, Tomkins D J 1991 Somatic cell hybridization of Roberts syndrome and normal lymphoblasts resulting in correction of both the cytogenetic and mutagen hypersensitivity cellular phenotypes. Somatic Cell and Molecular Genetics 17: 455–462
6. Anderson I J, Goldberg R B, Marion R W et al 1990 Spondyloepiphyseal dysplasia congenita: genetic linkage to type II collagen (COL2A1). American Journal of Human Genetics 46: 896–901
7. Ausems M G E M, Ippel P F, Renardel de Lavalette P A W A 1994 Greig cephalopolysyndactyly syndrome in a large family: a comparison of the clinical signs with those described in the literature. Clinical Dysmorphology 3: 21–30
8. Baraitser M 1977 Genetics of the Moebius syndrome. Journal of Medical Genetics 14: 415–417

9. Baraitser M 1982 Marshall/Stickler syndrome. Journal of Medical Genetics 19: 139–140

10. Baraitser M 1986 The orofaciodigital (OFD) syndromes. Journal of Medical Genetics 23: 116–119

11. Baraitser M, Winter R M, Taylor D S I 1982 Lenz microphthalmia – a case report. Clinical Genetics 22: 99–101

12. Beighton P 1973 The Schwartz syndrome in Southern Africa. Clinical Genetics 4: 548–555

13. Bennani-Smires C, El Alamy N R, Bouchareb N 1984 Pyknodysostosis, typical and atypical features and report on seven cases. Journal of Radiology 65: 689–695

14. Berry C, Cree J, Mann T 1980 Aarskog's syndrome. Archives of Disease in Childhood 55: 706–710

15. Biancalana V, Le Marec B, Odent S et al 1991 Oto-palato-digital syndrome type I: further evidence for assignment of the locus to Xq28. Human Genetics 88: 228–230

16. Blackburn M G, Belliveau R E 1971 Ellis van Creveld syndrome. A report of previously undescribed anomalies in two siblings. American Journal of Diseases of Children 122: 267–270

17. Bogaert R, Wilkin D, Wilcox W R et al 1994 Expression, in cartilage, of a 7-amino-acid deletion in type II collagen from two unrelated individuals with Kniest dysplasia. American Journal of Human Genetics 55: 1128–1136

18. Bos C J M, Ippel P F, Beemer F A 1994 DOOR syndrome: additional case and literature review. Clinical Dysmorphology 3: 15–20

19. Breslau-Siderius E J, Lavrijsen A P M, Otten F W A et al 1991 The Rapp-Hodgkin syndrome. American Journal of Medical Genetics 38: 107–110

20. Brondum-Nielsen K 1988 Aarskog syndrome in a Danish family: an illustration of the need for dysmorphology in paediatrics. Clinical Genetics 33: 315–317

21. Burrows N P, Nicholls A C, Yates J R W et al 1996 The gene encoding collagen alpha 1(V) (COL5A1) is linked to mixed Ehlers-Danlos syndrome type I/II. Journal of Investigative Dermatology 106: 1273–1276

22. Buss P W, Hughes H E, Clarke A 1995 Twenty-four cases of the EEC syndrome: clinical presentation and management. Journal of Medical Genetics 32: 716–723

23. Butler M G, Meaney F J, Palmer C G 1986 Clinical and cytogenetic survey of 39 individuals with Prader Labhart Willi syndrome. American Journal of Medical Genetics 23: 793–809

24. Cantu J M, Urrusti J, Rosales G, Rojas A 1971 Evidence for autosomal recessive inheritance of costovertebral dysplasia. Clinical Genetics 2: 149–154

25. Carey J C, Hall B D 1978 The Coffin-Siris syndrome. American Journal of Diseases of Children 132: 667–671

26. Carney R G 1976 Incontinentia pigmenti: a world statistical analysis. Archives of Dermatology 112: 535–542

27. Chen A, Francis M, Ni L et al 1995 Phenotypic manifestations of branchio-otorenal syndrome. American Journal of Medical Genetics 58: 365–370

28. Chiodo A A, Hockey A, Cole W G 1992 A base substitution at the splice acceptor site of intron 5 of the COL1A2 gene activates a cryptic splice site within exon 6 and generates abnormal type I procollagen in a patient with Ehlers-Danlos syndrome type VII. Journal of Biological Chemistry 267: 6361–6369

29. Chitayat D, Hahm S Y E, Marion R W et al 1987 Further delineation of the McKusick-Kaufman hydrometrocolpos-polydactyly syndrome. American Journal of Diseases of Children 141: 1133–1136

30. Christian C L, Lachman R S, Aylsworth A S et al 1991 Radiological findings in Hallermann-Streiff syndrome: report of five cases and a review of the literature. American Journal of Medical Genetics 41: 508–514

31. Chu C E, Cooke A, Stephenson J B P et al 1994 Diagnosis in Prader-Willi syndrome. Archives of Disease in Childhood 71: 441–442

32. Clarke R A, Singh S, McKenzie H, Kearsley J H, Yip M-Y 1995 Familial Klippel-Feil syndrome and paracentric inversion inv(9)(q22.2q23.3). American Journal of Human Genetics 57: 1364–1370

33. Clarke-Fraser F, Ling D, Clogg D, Nogrady B 1978 Genetic aspects of the Bor syndrome – branchial fistulas, ear pits, hearing loss, and renal anomalies. American Journal of Medical Genetics 2: 241–252

34. Cohen M M Jr, Rollnick B R, Kaye C I 1989 Oculoauriculovertebral spectrum: an updated critique. Cleft Palate Journal 26: 276–286

35. Cohen M M Jr, Toriello H V 1996 Is there a Baller-Gerold syndrome? American Journal of Medical Genetics 61: 63–64

36. Cole T R P, Hughes H E 1994 Sotos syndrome: a study of the diagnostic criteria and natural history. Journal of Medical Genetics 31: 20–32

37. Cole W G, Dalgleish R 1995 Syndrome of the month. Perinatal lethal osteogenesis imperfecta. Journal of Medical Genetics 32: 284–289

38. Connor J M, Evans D A P 1982 Genetic aspects of fibrodysplasia ossificans progressiva. Journal of Medical Genetics 19: 35–39

39. Connor J M, Skirton H, Lunt P W 1993 A three generation family with fibrodysplasia ossificans progressiva. Journal of Medical Genetics 30: 687–689

40. Cross H E, McKusick V A, Breen W 1967 A new oculocerebral syndrome with hypopigmentation. Journal of Pediatrics 70: 398–406

41. Curran M E, Atkinson D L, Ewart A K et al 1993 The elastin gene is disrupted by a translocation associated with supravalvular aortic stenosis. Cell 73: 159–168

42. David T J 1981 Hypomelanosis of Ito: a neurocutaneous syndrome. Archives of Disease in Childhood 56: 798–800

43. David T J 1982 Familial Poland anomaly. Journal of Medical Genetics 19: 293–296

44. De Paepe A, Devereux R B, Dietz H C, Hennekam R C M, Pyeritz R E 1996 Revised diagnostic criteria for the Marfan syndrome. American Journal of Medical Genetics 62: 417–426

45. Der Kaloustian V M, Hoyme H E, Hogg H et al 1991 Possible common pathogenetic mechanisms for Poland sequence and Adams-Oliver syndrome. American Journal of Medical Genetics 38: 69–73

46. Der Kaloustian V M, Kronfol N M, Takla R, Habash A, Khazin A, Najjar S S 1971 Leprechaunism: a report of two new cases. American Journal of Diseases of Children 122: 442–445

47. Dixon M J 1995 Syndrome of the month. Treacher-Collins syndrome. Journal of Medical Genetics 32: 806–808

48. Dobyns W B, Gilbert E F, Opitz J M 1985 Further comments on the lissencephaly syndromes. American Journal of Medical Genetics 22: 197–211

49. Dobyns W B, Kirkpatrick J B, Hittner H M et al 1985 Syndromes with lissencephaly. II: Walker-Warburg and cerebro-oculo-muscular syndromes and a new syndrome with type II lissencephaly. American Journal of Medical Genetics 22: 157–195

50. Dobyns W B, Truwit C L 1995 Lissencephaly and other malformations of cortical development: 1995 update (Review). Neuropediatrics 26: 132–147

51. Donnai D, Farndon P A 1986 Walker-Warburg syndrome (Warburg syndrome, HARD ± E syndrome). Journal of Medical Genetics 23: 200–203

52. Drossou-Agakidou V, Andreou A, Soubassi-Griva V, Pandouraki M 1991 Cerebrocostomandibular syndrome in four sibs, two pairs of twins. Journal of Medical Genetics 28: 704–707

53. Ellis N A, German J 1996 Molecular genetics of Bloom's syndrome. Human Molecular Genetics 5: 1457–1463

54. Engstrom W, Lindham S, Schofield P 1988 Wiedemann-Beckwith syndrome. European Journal of Pediatrics 147: 450–457

55. Feldman G J, Robin N H, Brueton L A et al 1995 A gene for cleidocranial dysplasia maps to the short arm of chromosome 6. American Journal of Human Genetics 56: 938–943

56. Felman A H, Kirkpatrick J A 1970 Dyschondrosteosis: mesomelic dwarfism of Leri and Weill. American Journal of Diseases of Children 120: 329–331

57. Ferrante M I, Giorgio G, Feather S A et al 2001 Identification of the gene for oro-facial-digital type I syndrome. American Journal of Human Genetics 68: 569–576

58. Finegold D N, Armitage M M, Galiani M et al 1994 Preliminary localization of a gene for autosomal dominant hypoparathyroidism to chromosome 3q13. Pediatric Research 36: 414–417

59. Fitzsimmons J S, Fitzsimmons E M, Barrow M, Gilbert G B 1982 Fronto-meta-physeal dysplasia. Further delineation of the clinical syndrome. Clinical Genetics 22: 195–205

60. Forrester S, Kovach M J, Reynolds N M et al 2001 Manifestations in four males with and an obligate carrier of Lenz microphthalmia syndrome. American Journal of Medical Genetics 98: 92–100

61. Foy C, Newton V, Wellesley D et al 1990 Assignment of the locus for Waardenburg syndrome type 1 to human chromosome 2q37 and possible homology to the splotch mouse. American Journal of Human Genetics 46: 1017–1023

62. Francomano C A, McIntosh I, Wilkin D J 1996 Bone dysplasias in man: molecular insights. Current Opinion in Genetic Development 6: 301–308

63. Fraser F C, Lytwyn A 1981 Spectrum of anomalies in the Meckel syndrome, 'or maybe there is a malformation syndrome with at least one constant anomaly'. American Journal of Medical Genetics 9: 67–73

64. Frattini A, Orchard P J, Sobacchi C et al 2000 Defects in TCIRG1 subunit of the vacuolar proton pump are responsible for a subset of human autosomal recessive osteopetrosis. Nature Genetics 25: 343–346

65. Fried K 1972 X-linked mental retardation and/or hydrocephalus. Clinical Genetics 3: 258–263

66. Froster-Iskenius U G 1990 Syndrome of the month. Popliteal pterygium syndrome. Journal of Medical Genetics 27: 320–326

67. Funderburk S J, Stewart R 1978 The G and BBB syndromes: case presentations, genetics and nosology. American Journal of Medical Genetics 2: 131–144

68. Gaily E 1990 Distal phalangeal hypoplasia in children with prenatal phenytoin exposure: results of a controlled anthropometric study. American Journal of Medical Genetics 35: 574–578

69. Gattuso J, Patton M A, Baraitser M 1987 The clinical spectrum of the Fraser syndrome: report of the three new cases and review. Journal of Medical Genetics 24: 549–555

70. Gelb B D, Edelson J G, Desnick R J 1995 Linkage of pycnodysostosis to chromosome 1q21 by homozygosity mapping (Letter). Nature Genetics 10: 235–237

71. Ghose S, Sihota R, Dayal Y 1988 Symmetrical partial lateral 'cryptophthalmos': a new concept of its embryological pathogenesis. Ophthalmic Paediatrics and Genetics 9: 67–76

72. Gladwin A, Donnai D, Metcalfe K et al 1997 Localization of a gene for oculodentodigital syndrome to human chromosome 6q22-q24. Human Molecular Genetics 6: 123–127

73. Glass R B J, Rosenbaum K N 1995 Frontometaphyseal dysplasia: neonatal radiographic diagnosis. American Journal of Medical Genetics 57: 1–5

74. Gojic V, van't Veer-Korthof E T, Bosch L J et al 1994 Congenital hypoplastic anemia: another example of autosomal dominant transmission. American Journal of Medical Genetics 50: 87–89

75. Gollop T R, Fontes L R 1985 The Greig cephalopolysyndactyly syndrome: report of a family and review of the literature. American Journal of Medical Genetics 22: 59–68

76. Goltz R W, Henderson R R, Hitch J M, Ott J E 1970 Focal dermal hypoplasia syndrome: a review of the literature and report of two cases. Archives of Dermatology 101: 1–11

77. Goodship J, Gill H, Carter J et al 2000 Autozygosity mapping of a seckel syndrome locus to chromosome 3q22 -24. American Journal of Human Genetics 67: 498–503

78. Greenberg C R, Evans J A, McKendry-Smith S et al 1990 Infantile hypophosphatasia: localization within chromosome region 1p36.1-34 and prenatal diagnosis using linked DNA markers. American Journal of Human Genetics 46: 286–292

79. Guidera K J, Satter-White Y, Ogden J A et al 1991 Nail patella syndrome: a review of 44 orthopedic patients. Journal of Pediatric Orthopedics 11: 737–742

80. Haaf T, Hofmann R, Schmid M 1991 Opitz trigonocephaly syndrome. American Journal of Medical Genetics 40: 444–446

81. Hall J G 1987 Thrombocytopenia and absent radius (TAR) syndrome. Journal of Medical Genetics 24: 79–83

82. Hall J G, Reed S D, Rosenbaum K N, Gershanik J, Chen H, Wilson K M 1982 Limb pterygium syndromes: a review and report of eleven patients. American Journal of Medical Genetics 12: 377–409

83. Happle R 1979 X-linked dominant chondrodysplasia punctata: review of literature and report of a case. Human Genetics 53: 65–73

84. Happle R, Effendy I, Megahed M, Orlow S J, Kuster W 1994 CHILD syndrome in a boy. American Journal of Medical Genetics 62: 192–194

85. Harrod M J E, Friedman J M, Currarino G et al 1984 Genetic heterogeneity in spondyloepiphyseal dysplasia congenita. American Journal of Medical Genetics 18: 311–320

86. Hastbacka J, Sistonen P, Kaitila I et al 1991 A linkage map spanning the locus for diastrophic dysplasia (DTD). Genomics 11: 968–973

87. Hatada I, Morisaki H, Nakayama M et al 1996 An imprinted gene p57KIP2 is mutated in Beckwith-Wiedemann syndrome. Nature Genetics 14: 171–173

88. Hautala T, Byers M G, Eddy R L et al 1992 Cloning of human lysyl hydroxylase: complete cDNA-derived amino acid sequence and assignment of the gene (PLOD) to chromosome 1p36.3→p36.2. Genomics 13: 62–69

89. Hou J, Parrish J, Ludecke H J et al 1995 A 4-megabase YAC contig that spans the Langer-Giedion syndrome region on human chromosome 8q24.1: use in refining the location of the trichorhinophalangeal syndrome and multiple exostoses genes (TRPS1 and EXT1). Genomics 29: 87–97

90. Houston C S, Opitz J M, Spranger J W et al 1983 The Camptomelic syndrome: review: report of 17 cases and follow-up on the currently 17 year old boy first reported by Maroteaux in 1971. American Journal of Medical Genetics 15: 3–28

91. Howard T D, Paznekas W A, Green E D 1997 Mutations in TWIST, a basic helix-loop-helix transcription factor, in Saethre-Chotzen syndrome. Nature Genetics 15: 36–41

92. Hurst J A, Baraitser M 1989 Johanson-Blizzard syndrome. Journal of Medical Genetics 26: 45–48

93. Hustinix T W J, Ter Haar B G A, Scheres J M J C et al 1977 Bloom's syndrome in two Dutch families. Clinical Genetics 12: 85–96

94. Ioan D M, Belengeanu V, Maximilian C, Fryns J-P 1993 Distal arthrogryposis with autosomal dominant inheritance and reduced penetrance in females: the Gordon syndrome. Clinical Genetics 43: 300–302

95. Ireland M, English C, Cross I et al 1995 Partial trisomy 3q and the mild Cornelia de Lange syndrome phenotype (Letter). Journal of Medical Genetics 32: 837–838

96. Jaatoul N Y, Haddad N E, Khoury L A, Afifi A K, Bahuth N B, Deeb M E 1982 Brief clinical report and review: the Marden-Walker syndrome. American Journal of Medical Genetics 11: 259–271

97. Jaeken J, Klocker H. Schwaiger H et al 1989 Clinical and biochemical studies in three patients with severe early infantile Cockayne syndrome. Human Genetics 83: 339–346

98. Jamieson C R, van der Burgt I, Brady A F et al 1994 Mapping a gene for Noonan syndrome to the long arm of chromosome 12. Nature Genetics 8: 357–360

99. Janku P, Robinow M, Kelly T et al 1980 The van der Woude syndrome in a large kindred: variability, penetrance, genetic risks. American Journal of Medical Genetics 5: 117–123

100. Jones K L 1988 Smith's recognizable patterns of human malformation, 4th edn. W B Saunders, London

101. Jorgenson R J, Levin L S, Cross H E, Yoder F, Kelly T E 1978 The Rieger syndrome. American Journal of Medical Genetics 2: 307–318

102. Juberg R C, Hayward J R 1969 A new familial syndrome of oral, cranial, and digital anomalies. Journal of Pediatrics 74: 755–762

103. Karnes P S, Day D, Berry S A, Pierpont M E M 1991 Jarcho-Levin syndrome: four new cases and classification of subtypes. American Journal of Medical Genetics 40: 264–270

104. Kelley R I, Wilcox W G, Smith M et al 1999 Abnormal sterol metabolism in patients with Conradi-Hunnerman-Happle syndrome and sporadic lethal chondrodysplasia punctata. American Journal of Medical Genetics 83: 213–219

105. Kenwrick S, Jouet M, Donnai D 1996 X linked hydrocephalus and MASA syndrome. Journal of Medical Genetics 33: 59–65

106. Kobayashi H, Baumbach L, Matise T C et al 1995 A gene for a severe lethal form of X-linked arthrogryposis (X-linked infantile spinal muscular atrophy) maps to human chromosome Xp11.3-q11.2. Human Molecular Genetics 4: 1213–1216

107. Kontusaari S, Tromp G, Kuivaniemi H et al 1992 Substitution of aspartate for glycine 1018 in type III procollagen (COL3A1) causes type IV Ehlers-Danlos syndrome: the mutated allele is present in most blood leukocytes of the asymptomatic and mosaic mother. American Journal of Human Genetics 51: 497–507

108. Kumar D 1990 Syndrome of the month. Moebius syndrome. Journal of Medical Genetics 27: 122–126

109. Kurotaki N, Imaizumi K, Harada N et al 2002 Haploinsufficiency of NSD1 causes Sotos syndrome. Nature Genetics 30: 365–366

110. Kuster W, Majewski F, Meinecke P 1985 EEC syndrome without ectrodactyly? Report on 8 cases. Clinical Genetics 28: 130–135

111. Labrune P, Pons J C, Khalil M et al 1993 Antenatal thrombocytopenia in three patients with TAR (thrombocytopenia with absent radii) syndrome. Prenatal Diagnosis 13: 463–466

112. Landy S J, Donnai D 1993 Syndrome of the month. Incontinentia pigmenti (Bloch-Sulzberger syndrome). Journal of Medical Genetics 30: 53–59

113. Latta R J, Graham C B, Aase J, Scham A M, Smith D W 1971 Larsen's syndrome: a skeletal dysplasia with multiple joint dislocations and unusual facies. Journal of Pediatrics 78: 291–298

114. Leahey A-M, Charnas L R, Nussbaum R L 1993 Nonsense mutations in the OCRL-1 gene in patients with the oculocerebrorenal syndrome of Lowe. Human Molecular Genetics 2: 461–464

115. Leroy J G, Devos E A, Bulcke V L J, Robbe N S 1981 Cerebro-costomandibular syndrome with autosomal dominant inheritance. Journal of Pediatrics 99: 441–443

116. Leroy J G, Spranger J W, Feingold M, Opitz J M, Crocker A C 1971 I-cell disease: a clinical picture. Journal of Pediatrics 79: 360–365

117. Levy P, Baraitser M 1991 Syndrome of the month. Coffin-Siris syndrome. Journal of Medical Genetics 28: 338–341

118. Li Q Y, Newbury-Ecob R A, Terrett J A et al 1997 Holt-Oram syndrome is caused by mutations in TBX5, a member of the brachyury (T) gene family. Nature Genetics 15: 21–29

119. Lichtenstein J R, Sundaram M, Burdge R 1980 Sex-influenced expression of Madelung's deformity in a family with dyschondrosteosis. Journal of Medical Genetics 17: 41–43

120. McKusick V A 1978 Mendelian inheritance in man, 5th edn. Johns Hopkins University Press, Baltimore, MD

121. MacNab A J, D'Orsogna L, Cole D E C et al 1991 Cardiac anomalies complicating congenital contractural arachnodactyly. Archives of Disease in Childhood 66: 1143–1146

122. Majewski F, Goecke T 1982 Studies of microcephalic primordial dwarfism. I: Approach to a delineation of the Seckel syndrome. American Journal of Medical Genetics 12: 7–21

123. Mansour S, Hall C M, Pembrey M E, Young I D 1995 A clinical and genetic study of camptomelic dysplasia. Journal of Medical Genetics 32: 415–420

124. Mansour S, Woffendin H, Mitton S et al 2001. Incontinentia pigmenti in a surviving male is accompanied by hypohirotic ectodermal dysplasia and recurrent infection. American Journal of Medical Genetics 99: 172–177

125. Marble M, Geraghty M T, de Franchis R et al 1994 Characterization of a cystathionine beta-synthase allele with three mutations in cis in a patient with B6 nonresponsive homocystinuria. Human Molecular Genetics 3: 1883–1886

126. Marden P M, Smith D W, McDonald M J 1964 Congenital anomalies in the newborn infant, including minor variations. Journal of Pediatrics 64: 357–371

127. Martinot V L, Manouvrier S, Anastassov Y et al 1994 Orodigitofacial syndromes type I and II: clinical and surgical studies. Cleft Palate-Craniofacial Journal 31: 401–408

128. Masuno M, Kuroki Y, Shimozawa N et al 1994 Assignment of the human peroxisome assembly factor-1 gene (PXMP3) responsible for Zellweger syndrome to chromosome 8q21.1 by fluorescence in situ hybridization. Genomics 20: 141–142

129. McDonald-McGinn D M, Driscoll D A, Bason L et al 1995 Autosomal dominant 'Opitz' GBBB syndrome due to a 22q11.2 deletion. American Journal of Medical Genetics 59: 103–113

130. Miles J H, Zonana J, McFarlane J et al 1984 Macrocephaly with hamartomas: Bannayan-Zonana syndrome. American Journal of Medical Genetics 19: 225–234

131. Monnens L, Heymans H 1987 Peroxisomal disorders: clinical characterisation. Journal of Inherited Metabolic Disease 10(suppl.): 23–32

132. Moog U, Engelen J, Albrechts J, Hoorntje T, Hendrikse F, Schrander-Stumpel C 1996 Alagille syndrome in a family with duplication 20p11. Clinical Dysmorphology 5: 279–288

133. Mueller O T, Wasmuth J J, Murray J C, Lozzio C B, Lovrien E W, Shows T B 1987 Chromosomal assignment of N-acetylglucosaminyl phosphotransferase, the lysosomal hydrolase targeting enzyme deficient in mucolipidosis II and III (abstract). Cytogenetics and Cell Genetics 46: 664

134. Mueller R F 1987 The Alagille syndrome (arteriohepatic dysplasia). Journal of Medical Genetics 64: 621–626

135. Muis N, Beemer F A, Van-Dijken P 1986 Aase syndrome. Case report and review of the literature. European Journal of Pediatrics 145: 153–157

136. Murray J C, Nishimura D Y, Buetow K H et al 1990 Linkage of an autosomal dominant clefting syndrome (Van der Woude) to loci on chromosome 1q. American Journal of Human Genetics 46: 486–491

137. Nagai T, Nishimura G, Kato R et al 1995 Del(12)(p11.21p12.2) associated with an asphyxiating thoracic dystrophy or chondroectodermal dysplasia-like syndrome. American Journal of Medical Genetics 55: 16–18

138. Najjar H, Mardini M 1988 Variability of the Holt-Oram syndrome in Saudi individuals. American Journal of Medical Genetics 29: 851–856

139. Naski M C, Wang Q, Xu J, Ornitz D M 1996 Graded activation of fibroblast growth factor receptor 3 by mutations causing achondroplasia and thanatophoric dysplasia. Nature Genetics 13: 233–237

140. Nicole S, Davione C S, Topaloglu H et al 2000 Perlecan, the major proteoglycan of basement membranes, is altered in patients with Schwartz-Jampel syndrome (chondrodysplasia myotonia). Nature Genetics 26: 480–483

141. North C, Patton M A, Baraitser M, Winter R M 1985 The clinical features of the Cohen syndrome: further case reports. Journal of Medical Genetics 22: 131–134

142. O'Callaghan M, Young I D 1990 Syndrome of the month. Townes-Brocks syndrome. Journal of Medical Genetics 27: 457–461

143. Oley C, Baraitser M 1988 Blepharophimosis, ptosis epicathus inversus syndrome (BPES syndrome). Journal of Medical Genetics 25: 47–51

144. Oley C A, Baraitser M, Grant D B 1988 A reappraisal of the Charge association. Journal of Medical Genetics 25: 147–157

145. Opitz J M, Penchaszadeh V B, Holt M C et al 1994 Smith-Lemli-Opitz (RSH) syndrome bibliography: 1964-1993. American Journal of Medical Genetics 50: 339–343

146. Patton M A 1988 Syndrome of the month. Russell-Silver syndrome. Journal of Medical Genetics 25: 557–560

147. Patton M A, Afzal A R 2002 Robinow syndrome – syndrome of the month. Journal of Medical Genetics 39: 305–310

148. Patton M A, Krywawych S, Winter R M et al 1987 Door syndrome (deafness, onycho-osteodystrophy, and mental retardation), elevated plasma and urinary 2-oxoglutarate in three unrelated patients. American Journal of Medical Genetics 26: 207–215

149. Patton M A, Laurence K M 1985 Three new cases of oculodentodigital (ODD) syndrome. Development of the facial phenotype. Journal of Medical Genetics 22: 386–389

150. Pazzaglia U E, Beluffi G 1986 Oto-palato-digital syndrome in four generations of large family. Clinical Genetics 30: 338–344

151. Pelias M Z, Superneau D W, Thurmon T F 1981. A sixth report (8th case) of craniosynostosis-radial aplasia (Baller-Gerold) syndrome. American Journal of Medical Genetics 10: 133–139

152. Petrij F, Peters D J M, Breuning M H et al 1995 Rubinstein-Taybi syndrome caused by mutations in the transcriptional co-activator CBP. Nature 76: 348–351

153. Pinsky L 1978 The syndromology of anorectal malformation (atresia, stenosis, ectopia). American Journal of Medical Genetics 1: 461–474

154. Polymeropoulos M H, Ide S E, Wright M et al 1996 The gene for the Ellis-van Creveld syndrome is located on chromosome 4p16. Genomics 35: 1–5

155. Porteous M E, Curtis A, Lindsay S et al 1992 The gene for Aarskog syndrome is located between DXS255 and DXS566 (Xp11.2-Xq13). Genomics 14: 298–301

156. Pronk J C, Gibson R A, Savoia A et al 1995 Localisation of the Fanconi anaemia complementation group A gene to chromosome 16q24.3 (Letter). Nature Genetics 11: 338–340

157. Reardon W, Winter R M 1994 Syndrome of the month. Saethre-Chotzen syndrome. Journal of Medical Genetics 31: 393–396

158. Reardon W, Winter R M, Rutland P et al 1994 Mutations in the fibroblast growth factor receptor 2 gene cause Crouzon syndrome. Nature Genetics 8: 98–103

159. Reid I S, Turner G 1976 Familial anal abnormality. Journal of Pediatrics 88: 992–994

160. Rimoin D L, Edgerton M T 1967 Genetic and clinical heterogeneity in the oral-facial-digital syndromes. Journal of Pediatrics 71: 94–102

161. Robinow M, Johnson G F 1981 The Gordon syndrome: autosomal dominant cleft palate, camptodactyly, and club feet. American Journal of Medical Genetics 9: 139–146

162. Ruiz-Maldonado R, Toussaint S, Tamayo L et al 1992 Hypomelanosis of Ito: diagnostic criteria and report of 41 cases. Pediatric Dermatology 9: 1–10

163. Ruiz-Perez V L, Ide S E, Strom T M et al 2000 Mutations in a new gene in Ellis-van-Crevald syndrome and Weyers acrodental dysostosis. Nature Genetics 24: 283–286

164. Salonen R 1984 The Meckel syndrome: clinicopathological findings in 67 patients. American Journal of Medical Genetics 18: 671–689

165. Sargent C, Burn J, Baraitser M et al 1985 Trigonocephaly and the Opitz C syndrome. Journal of Medical Genetics 22: 39–45

166. Schell U, Hehr A, Feldman G J et al 1995 Mutations in FGFR1 and FGFR2 cause familial and sporadic Pfeiffer syndrome. Human Molecular Genetics 4: 323–328

167. Schroeder H W, Sybert V P 1987 Rapp-Hodgkin ectodermal dysplasia. Journal of Pediatrics 110: 72–75

168. Schwindinger W F, Francomano C A, Levine M A 1992 Identification of a mutation in the gene encoding the alpha subunit of the stimulatory G protein of adenylyl cyclase in McCune-Albright syndrome. Proceedings of the National Academy of Sciences of the United States of America 89: 5152–5156

169. Semina E V, Zabel B U, Carey J C et al 1996 Cloning and characterization of a novel bicoid-related homeobox transcription factor gene, RIEG, involved in Rieger syndrome. Nature Genetics 14: 392–399

170. Sharland M, Burch M, McKenna W M, Patton M A 1992 A clinical study of Noonan syndrome. Archives of Disease in Childhood 67: 178–183

171. Sharland M, Patton M A, Talbot S et al 1992 Coagulation-factor deficiencies and abnormal bleeding in Noonan's syndrome. Lancet 339: 19–21

172. Shows T B, Scrafford-Wolff L, Brown J A, Meisler M 1978 Assignment of a beta-galactosidase gene (beta-GAL-alpha) to chromosome 3 in man. Cytogenetics and Cell Genetics 22: 219–222

173. Smahi A, Courtois G, Vabres P et al Genomic rearrangement in NEMO impairs NF-kappaB inactivation and is a cause of incontinentia pigmenti. The International Incontinentia Pigmenti (IP) Consortium. Nature 405: 466–472

174. Small K W, Stalvey M, Fisher L et al 1995 Blepharophimosis syndrome is linked to chromosome 3q. Human Molecular Genetics 4: 443–448

175. Spranger J, Benirschke K, Hall J G et al 1982 Errors of morphogenesis: concepts and terms. Journal of Pediatrics 100: 160–165

176. Spranger S, Spranger M, Meinck H-M, Tariverdian G 1995 Two sisters with Escobar syndrome. American Journal of Medical Genetics 57: 425–428

177. Stevens C A, Qumsiyeh M B 1995 Syndromal frontonasal dysostosis in a child with a complex translocation involving chromosomes 3, 7, and 11. American Journal of Medical Genetics 55: 494–497

178. Stosiek N, Ulmer R, von den Driesch P et al 1994 Chromosomal mosaicism in two patients with epidermal verrucous nevus. Demonstration of chromosomal breakpoint. Journal of the American Academy of Dermatology 30: 622–625

179. Superti-Furga A 1996 Achondrogenesis type 1B. Journal of Medical Genetics 33: 957–961

180. Tahvanainen E, Norio R, Karila E et al 1994 Cohen syndrome gene assigned to the long arm of chromosome 8 by linkage analysis. Nature Genetics 7: 201–204

181. Tartaglia M, Mehler E L, Goldberg R et al 2001 Mutations in the protein tyrosine phosphatase gene PTPN11 cause Noonan syndrome. Nature Genetics 29: 465–468

182. Tavormina P L, Shiang R, Thompson L M et al 1995 Thanatophoric dysplasia (types I and II) caused by distinct mutations in fibroblast growth factor receptor 3. Nature Genetics 9: 321–328

183. Temple I K, MacDowall P, Baraitser M, Atherton D J 1990 Syndrome of the month. Focal dermal hypoplasia (Goltz syndrome). Journal of Medical Genetics 27: 180–187

184. Thompson E, Pembrey M E 1985 Seckel syndrome: an overdiagnosed syndrome. Journal of Medical Genetics 22: 192–201

185. Tolmie J L, Harvie A, Cockburn F 1992 The teratogenic effects of undiagnosed maternal hyperphenylalaninaemia: a case for prevention? British Journal of Obstetrics and Gynaecology 99: 347–348

186. Tolmie J L, McNay M, Stephenson J B et al 1987 Microcephaly: genetic counselling and antenatal diagnosis after the birth of an affected child. American Journal of Medical Genetics 27: 583–594

187. Tolmie J L, Mortimer G, Doyle D et al 1987 The Neu-Laxova syndrome in female sibs: clinical and pathological features with prenatal diagnosis in the second sib. American Journal of Medical Genetics 27: 175–182

188. Topley J M, Varady E, Lestringant G G 1994 Larsen syndrome in siblings with consanguineous parents. Clinical Dysmorphology 3: 263–265

189. Toriello H V 1993 Review. Oral-facial-digital syndromes, 1992. Clinical Dysmorphology 2: 95–105

190. Traboulsi E I, Lenz W et al 1988 The Lenz microphthalmia syndrome. American Journal of Ophthalmology 105: 40–45

191. Van Camp G, Van Thienen M N, Handig I et al 1995 Chromosome 13q deletion with Waardenburg syndrome: further evidence for a gene involved in neural crest function on 13q. Journal of Medical Genetics 32: 531–536

192. Van Den Berg D J, Francke U 1993 Roberts syndrome: a review of 100 cases and a new rating system for severity. American Journal of Medical Genetics 47: 1104–1123

193. Van Maldergem L, Vamos E, Liebaers I et al 1988. Severe congenital cutis laxa with pulmonary emphysema: a family with three affected sibs. American Journal of Medical Genetics 31: 455–464

194. Velinov M. Slaugenhaupt S A, Stoilov I et al 1994 The gene for achondroplasia maps to the telomeric region of chromosome 4p. Nature Genetics 6: 314–317

195. Verloes A, Le Merrer M, Davin J-C et al 1992 The orocraniodigital syndrome of Juberg and Hayward. Journal of Medical Genetics 29: 262–265

196. Wallace M R, Marchuk D A, Andersen L B et al 1990 Type 1 neurofibromatosis gene: identification of a large transcript disrupted in three NF1 patients. Science 249: 181–186

197. Wertheimer E, Lu S-P, Backeljauw P F et al 1993 Homozygous deletion of the human insulin receptor gene results in leprechaunism. Nature Genetics 5: 71–73

198. Whelan A J, Watson M S, Porter F D, Steiner R D 1995 Klippel-Trenaunay-Weber syndrome associated with 5:11 balanced translocation. American Journal of Medical Genetics 59: 492–494

199. Wildervanck L S, Hoksema P E, Penning L 1966 Radiological examination of the inner ear of deaf-mutes presenting the cervico-oculo-acusticus syndrome. Acta Oto-Laryngologica 61: 445–453

200. Wilkie A O M, Slaney S F, Oldridge M et al 1995 Apert syndrome results from localized mutations of FGFR2 and is allelic with Crouzon syndrome. Nature Genetics 9: 165–172

201. Williams M S, Josephson K D, Wargowski D S 1993 Marden-Walker syndrome: a case report and a critical review of the literature. Clinical Dysmorphology 2: 211–219

202. Winter R M 1986 Dubowitz syndrome. Journal of Medical Genetics 23: 11–13

203. Winter R M, Baraitser M 1998 The London Dysmorphology Database. Oxford University Press, Oxford

204. Winter R M, Donnai D, Crawford M D'A 1981 Syndromes of microcephaly, microphthalmia, cataracts, and joint contractures. Journal of Medical Genetics 18: 129–133

205. Wirtz M K, Gorlin R J, Godfrey A et al 1996 Weill-Marchesani syndrome – possible linkage of the autosomal dominant form to 15q21.1 American Journal of Medical Genetics 65: 68–75

206. Wit J M, Beemer F A, Barth P G et al 1985 Cerebral gigantism (Sotos syndrome). Compiled data of 22 cases. Analysis of clinical features, growth and plasma somatomedin. European Journal of Paediatrics 144: 131–140

207. Young I D, Fielder A R, Casey T A 1986 The Weill-Marchesani syndrome in mother and son. Clinical Genetics 30: 475–480

208. Zergollern L, Hitrec V 1982 Four siblings with Robert's syndrome. Clinical Genetics 21: 1–6

209. Zonana J, Jones M, Browne D et al 1992 High-resolution mapping of the X-linked hypohidrotic ectodermal dysplasia (EDA) locus. American Journal of Human Genetics 51: 1036–1046

CHAPTER 33

Neonatal dermatology

Maureen Rogers

Introduction

There are important differences between the skin of the neonate, in particular the preterm neonate, and that of the child or adult, and understanding of their implications is vital to the appropriate care of the baby.

There are some skin disorders which are very specific to the neonatal period. These are mostly benign and transient and their main importance is the fact that they can imitate more serious disorders. Cutaneous infections in the neonate are almost all potentially serious and may have atypical presentations. Further, the first sign of certain systemic infections can also be cutaneous. Some important systemic disorders may present in the neonatal period with skin signs. Most naevi are present at birth and a number of skin tumours can be congenital or appear in the neonatal period. Finally, several important ongoing skin diseases may manifest in the first month of life. The recognition of these patterns of disease is important so that, if required, appropriate investigations and intervention can be instituted and so that the parents can be reassured or offered a realistic prognosis.

Structure and function of the neonatal skin

By 24 weeks' gestation, the anatomy of the skin is essentially similar to that of the older individual, but it is some years before functional maturity is achieved.

The epidermis of the baby is fragile,[25] especially in preterm neonates, with a susceptibility to fissuring and an increased risk of injury from adhesives, chemical burns from alcohol swabs and disinfectant solutions,[18] and thermal burns from transcutaneous oxygen monitors.[25]

Compared with that of the older child, there is an increased permeability of neonatal skin, again especially in the preterm baby.[55] This increases the risk of toxic effects of the application of such agents as iodine, hexachlorophene, gammabenzene hexachloride and phenol, and possibly some of the myriad over-the-counter preparations which are applied to the skin of babies. The absorption of topical steroid preparations is much increased, leading to potential side effects, both local and systemic. This tendency to complications from the use of applied agents is exaggerated by the large surface area to bodyweight ratio of the baby.

Vasomotor instability is characteristic in the neonate and is responsible for certain essentially benign and physiological, but clinically striking, entities. A rubor or generalised redness is often present in the early hours of life. Peripheral acrocyanosis presents as a bilaterally symmetrical, intermittent, blue discoloration of the hands and feet, which usually disappears after the early weeks. Harlequin colour change is a vascular phenomenon probably caused by an immature autonomic regulatory mechanism.[34,57] When the neonate is lying on one side, the lower half of the body is red and the upper half is pale, with a clear midline separation. This colour change reverses on altering the baby's position. It is a very transient phenomenon and does not indicate any significant neural or vascular abnormality. Physiological cutis marmorata or livedo reticularis is a benign transient blue or purple cutaneous mottling, most marked when the baby is cool, lasting minutes to hours but reversing quickly on warming.[34] The tendency to the condition lasts for weeks or months.

However, livedo is not always physiological (Table 33.1). A more persistent livedo may be seen in a number of syndromes, in congenital hypothyroidism and rarely in neonatal lupus. A very striking segmental livedo, associated with dilated veins and, sometimes, cutaneous atrophy, is a feature of cutis marmorata telangiectatica congenita, a rare vascular malformation.

Neonatal skin often manifests the same type of hyperpigmentation seen in pregnancy. This is believed to be due to the influence of maternal and placental hormones as part of the 'mini-puberty'

Table 33.1 Some causes of cutis marmorata (livedo reticularis) in the neonate

Physiological cutis marmorata
Down syndrome
Trisomy 18
Homocystinuria
Cornelia de Lange syndrome
Neonatal lupus erythematosus
Congenital hypothyroidism
Cutis marmorata telangiectatica congenita

Table 33.2 Some causes of hypertrichosis in the neonate

Physiological lanugo hair
Congenital hypertrichosis lanuginosa
Primary isolated hypertrichosis
Hypertrichosis as part of various syndromes
    Hypertrichosis with gingival fibromatosis
    Congenital erythropoietic porphyria
    Cornelia de Lange syndrome
    Coffin–Siris syndrome
    Leprechaunism
    Seip–Berardinelli syndrome
    Rubenstein–Taybi syndrome
Drug-induced hypertrichosis
    Diazoxide
    Fetal alcohol syndrome
    Maternal minoxidil

Table 33.3 Conditions which may present with pustules in the neonate

Toxic erythema of the newborn
Transient neonatal pustular dermatosis
Infantile acropustulosis
Eosinophilic pustulosis
Pustular miliaria
Neonatal cephalic pustulosis and neonatal acne
Varicella
Herpes simplex
Staphylococcal impetigo
Streptococcal impetigo
Candida
Scabies
Incontinentia pigmenti
Hyper-IgE syndrome
Myeloproliferative disorder in Down syndrome

Table 33.4 Conditions which may present with vesicles, blisters or erosions in the neonate

Sucking blisters
Herpes simplex
Varicella
Staphylococcal infections
    Impetigo
    Staphylococcal scalded-skin syndrome
Scabies
Aspergillus
Candida
Syphilis
Epidermolysis bullosa
Contact irritant dermatitis, chemical burn
Mastocytosis
Bullous ichthyosis
Incontinentia pigmenti
Neonatal pemphigus
Neonatal herpes gestationis
Congenital erosive and vesicular dermatosis
Zinc deficiency
Langerhans cell histiocytosis
Porphyrias
    Congenital erythropoietic porphyria
    Errythropoietic protoporphyria
    Transient porphyrinaemia in Rh incompatibility

of the newborn. It affects particularly the external genitalia, and the linea alba is instead a linea nigra.[34]

Lanugo is the fine silky hair found to cover neonates, especially preterm babies. It is most marked on the shoulders, back and cheeks. This is usually shed within 3 months. There is an extremely rare inherited disorder, congenital hypertrichosis lanuginosa, characterised by a very profuse and persistent, widespread covering of lanugo hair.[32] There are a number of causes of neonatal hypertrichosis featuring an excess of either vellus hair (normal childhood non-scalp hair) or terminal hair (adult or scalp-type hair). While this may occur alone, it is usually part of a syndrome with other diagnostic features. Certain drugs may cause a neonatal hypertrichosis. Some of these conditions are listed in Table 33.2.

Scalp hair may be sparse or abundant at birth. A well-defined patch of alopecia commonly develops in the occipital area. This is not, as is commonly believed, due to rubbing the back of the head on the bedding surface. It is explained by understanding the fetal and neonatal hair cycles.[51] By 20 weeks' gestation, there are well-developed hair follicles containing anagen (growing) hairs all over the scalp. Although the hair roots enter telogen (the resting stage, which lasts 10–12 weeks before the hairs inevitably fall) in a progressive manner from frontal to parietal areas at 26–28 weeks' gestation, those in the occipital area remain in anagen until birth, when they abruptly enter telogen. These hairs fall at 9–12 weeks of postnatal life. In some babies there are still large numbers of hairs in the parietal area still in telogen at birth and a more extensive postnatal alopecia occurs, with hair remaining only at the vertex.

Pustules, blisters and erosions in the neonate

There are a large number of conditions, some transient and benign and others serious, which present with pustules, blisters or erosions. Some of these are listed in Table 33.3 and Table 33.4.

Benign transient neonatal disorders presenting with sterile pustules

There are many benign conditions that may present in the neonatal period with sterile pustules[34,41] (see Table 33.3), which may mimic serious infections. Of course, it is vital to exclude infection in any pustular eruption in a neonate.

Toxic erythema of the newborn

This is a self-limiting, benign condition, of unknown aetiology, which occurs in about two-thirds of all neonates[34] but almost never in premature babies. The onset is usually between 24 and 48 hours, but may occur at any time from birth to 14 days. The characteristic lesions are poorly demarcated erythematous macules, often surmounted by central pale papules, but occasionally pustules develop. The lesions may occur anywhere on the body surface apart from palms and soles, particularly on the face and trunk. When cases present at birth, lesions are more sacrally distributed and are more often pustular. Smears taken from pustules and stained with Wright or Giemsa stain demonstrate numerous eosinophils and a peripheral blood eosinophilia is present. The disorder rarely lasts more than a few days.

Transient neonatal pustular dermatosis (transient neonatal pustular melanosis)

This condition presents at birth or in the first hours of life as lesions which quickly evolve from blisters to large flaccid pustules (Fig. 33.1).[34,39,48] These occur mainly on the trunk and buttocks, but may be widespread. Over the next 1–2 days, the pustules rupture, with the formation of a peripheral collarette of scale, which separates after a further day or so to leave either normal skin or, in dark-skinned individuals, a temporary post-inflammatory hyperpigmentation. Because the pigmentation depends on the skin colour, the term dermatosis is preferred to the earlier term melanosis. Occasionally, a few further crops of lesions appear. The pustules, which can closely simulate infective conditions, contain numerous neutrophils but are sterile on culture.

Infantile acropustulosis

This is another benign idiopathic condition which commences in the neonatal period or early infancy.[34,37] Recurrent crops of extremely pruritic 2–4-mm vesicopustules develop on the hands and feet, especially on palmar and plantar surfaces (Fig. 33.2).[21] Initially, each crop lasts 7–14 days and recurrences occur at 2- to 3-week intervals. As time goes on, the duration of each attack becomes shorter and the time between attacks longer, until the condition resolves spontaneously after many months. Cultures of the pustules are sterile. A clinically identical condition occurs as a post-scabetic reaction following successful treatment of severe neonatal or infantile scabies. When reports of infantile acropustulosis are studied, it becomes clear that almost all of the patients have been treated for scabies[37] and the existence of the condition as a distinct entity unrelated to scabies is in some doubt. The duration of the episode may be shortened with the use of strong topical steroids for a few days.

Eosinophilic pustulosis (eosinophilic pustular folliculitis)

This is a relatively rare condition in which recurrent groups of sterile pustules, centered around hair follicles, develop on the scalp in the first few months of life.[26,34] The lesions begin as small, closely grouped red papules which quickly develop into

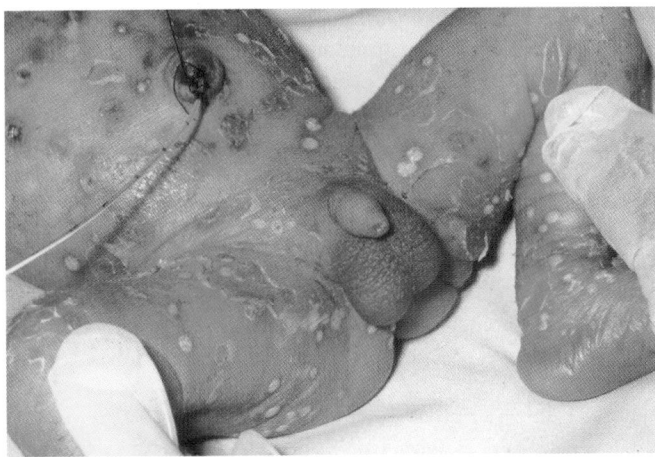

Fig. 33.1 Transient neonatal pustular dermatosis.

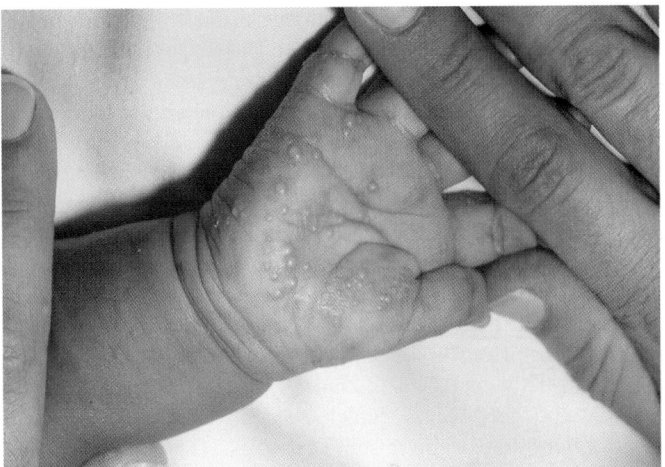

Fig. 33.2 Infantile acropustulosis.

pustules and then form crusted lesions which heal over several days. Several groups may occur at one time on the scalp. The lesions are characteristically very itchy. Occasionally there are a few follicular lesions at other sites, and in older infants, follicular and non-follicular lesions away from the scalp become more prominent. Cropping of lesions may continue for many months before eventual spontaneous resolution of the condition. Smears from the pustules show variable proportions of neutrophils and eosinophils and no evidence of infection on culture. There is often a peripheral blood eosinophilia present at the time of onset of new lesions. The use of fairly potent topical steroids may shorten the duration of each episode a little but has no effect on the overall course of the condition.

Miliaria

This is a sweat-retention condition common in young babies.[34] An obstruction, the nature of which is unknown, develops in the intraepidermal part of the sweat duct and sweat is trapped. The duct may rupture and sweat then leaks into the surrounding epidermis. Lesions begin as small red macules and are then surmounted by red papules (miliaria rubra) or pustules (pustular miliaria). Unlike miliaria in older individuals, the condition in infancy often occurs in the absence of fever or significant external occlusion of the skin. Lesions occur mainly on the face, scalp and upper trunk. There is often a mixture of red and pustular lesions, and the distribution and severity of the condition characteristically vary considerably from day to day or even within the same day. It is noted to be worse in areas of occlusion, such as where the face has been against the breast, and also at times of increased heat. It is important to stress to the parents that this is a benign phenomenon over which they have little control and which, if anything, will be worsened by the application of topical agents.

Neonatal cephalic pustulosis and neonatal acne

Both of these terms are used to describe a condition presenting within the first 3–4 weeks of life with erythematous papules and pustules but no comedones, occurring primarily on the cheeks (Fig. 33.3) but scattered elsewhere on the face and extending to the scalp and resolving after several more weeks.[1,34] The condition is quite separate from infantile acne, which is predominantly comedonal, occurs almost entirely in boys and rarely presents before 3 months of age. There is an opinion that the term neonatal acne should be abandoned in favour of neonatal cephalic pustulosis.[34] There is a suggestion that the lesions of cephalic pustulosis may be an inflammatory reaction to Malassezia species, but these are found as commensals on neonatal skin, so their pathogenic role is difficult to assess.[1] It is doubtful whether antifungal treatment significantly shortens the duration of this self-limiting condition. This condition is clinically very similar to pustular miliaria, and only biopsy, which clearly would be unjustified, could differentiate them in some cases.

Infective conditions presenting with pustules, blisters or erosions

A variety of infections can present in the neonatal period with pustules (see Table 33.3), blisters (see Table 33.4) or erosions. Some present predominantly with one or other type of lesion, but some infections can produce all types. Most of these conditions are described in more detail in Chapter 40 and only the cutaneous presentations are described here.

Varicella[2]

Because the infection in the neonate is usually severe, there may be many lesions in the same stage of development. Hence, the condition may present as a widespread vesicular or pustular disorder with a wide differential diagnosis. It may not be recognised clinically as varicella until the characteristic crusts form several days later. Congenital varicella may present as erosions but often stellate scarring is already present at birth.

Herpes simplex[20,50]

The skin lesions are grouped blisters, localised initially on the presenting part, usually the head, with the onset usually between the fourth and eighth days of life. Sometimes the lesions become pustular (Fig. 33.4), but they soon burst to form erosions, which may be deep and haemorrhagic. A characteristic pattern is individual lesions a few millimetres across coalescing to produce larger erosions with a geographical shape or scalloped border. On the thick skin of the palms or soles, the blisters or pustules may remain intact, producing a more confusing clinical picture.

Impetigo

This is usually a staphylococcal bullous impetigo, originating in an infected umbilical wound. The lesions first appear as intact vesicles, then become intact pustules, which eventually rupture

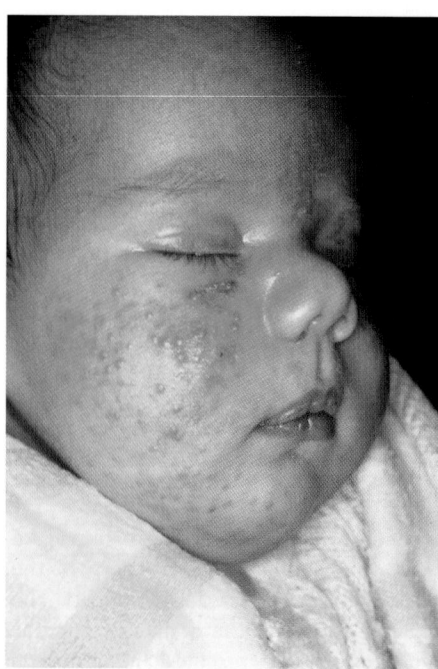

Fig. 33.3 Neonatal cephalic pustulosis.

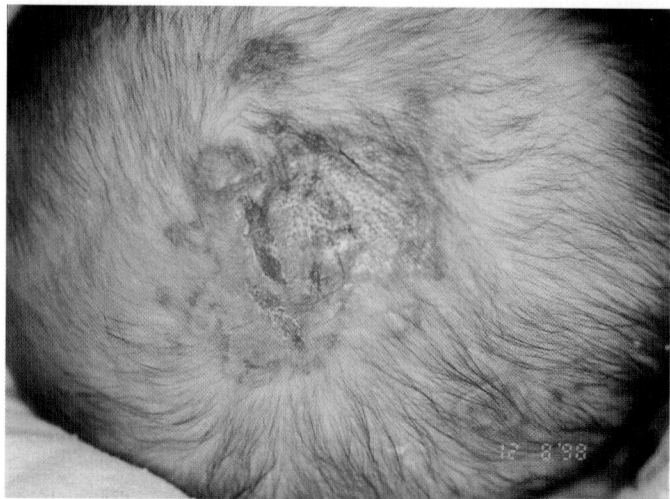

Fig. 33.4 Herpes simplex on the scalp.

to form fast-spreading erosions which, being very superficial, quickly dry out to form shiny crusts. Occasionally group A streptococcal infections present as pustules, but a non-specific omphalitis is more common. Systemic antibiotics are required, with oral administration usually adequate.

Staphylococcal scalded-skin syndrome

The condition commences with a macular erythema, initially on the face and in the major flexures and then becoming generalised. The skin is exquisitely tender. After 2 days, flaccid bullae develop and the skin wrinkles and shears off (Fig. 33.5). The exfoliation is most marked in the groin, neck fold and around the mouth and may involve the entire body surface, but mucosae remain uninvolved. The child is usually febrile but, because of the superficial level of the split, fluid loss is rarely significant. The erosions crust and dry and heal with desquamation over 4–8 days leaving no sequelae. Cultures from affected skin and blister fluid are usually negative. The usual source in a neonate is an infected umbilical stump. The condition responds quickly to intravenous anti-staphylococcal antibiotics.

Candida

In congenital candidiasis, the infection is acquired in utero and presents in the first 2 days of life with a diffuse eruption of papules, papulovesicles and pustules, often on an erythematous base (Fig. 33.6).[7] These usually settle in a few days with superficial desquamation.

In neonatal candidiasis, the infection is contracted during passage through an infected birth canal and there are several different presentations depending on the maturity and status of the neonate.

Localised neonatal candidiasis

This includes oral thrush and candida napkin dermatitis.[46] The latter demonstrates a beefy-red erythema extending a variable distance from the groin folds, with a thick white accumulation deep in the fold. There are often satellite pustules which rupture to form a peripheral scale.

Invasive fungal dermatitis

This is a term used to describe primary cutaneous, erosive, crusted, sometimes necrotic lesions occurring in very-low-birthweight (VLBW) infants.[54] A similar condition can occur with other fungal infections, including Aspergillus.

Cutaneous lesions of systemic candidiasis

VLBW infants with systemic candidiasis can present with an extensive burn-like dermatitis followed by peeling.[46]

Scabies

Clinical manifestations of scabies have been reported as early as the second week of life.[47] The lesions in neonatal scabies, which include papules, nodules, vesicles and pustules, tend to be very widespread, often with facial and scalp involvement, which is rare in older infants. Vesicles or pustules on the palms and soles are common features. Secondary eczematisation and secondary infection may complicate the clinical picture. Permethrin 5% cream is regarded as safe at any age, except possibly in the VLBW infant. Nodules frequently persist, and even become more numerous, for some weeks even after successful treatment. A common post-scabetic phenomenon is recurrent episodes of pustules on the palms and soles, clinically identical to the condition designated infantile acropustulosis.

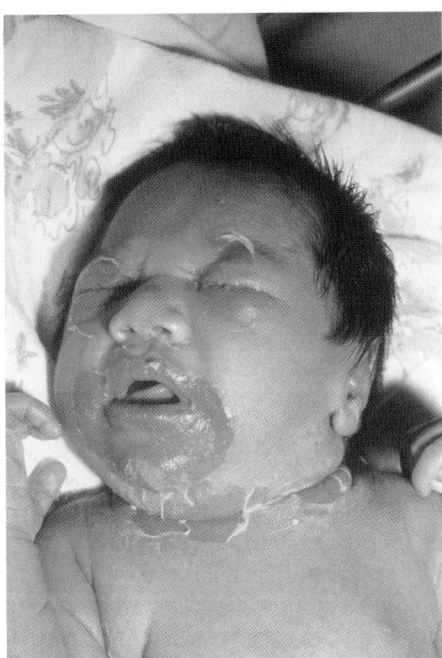

Fig. 33.5 Staphylococcal scalded-skin syndrome.

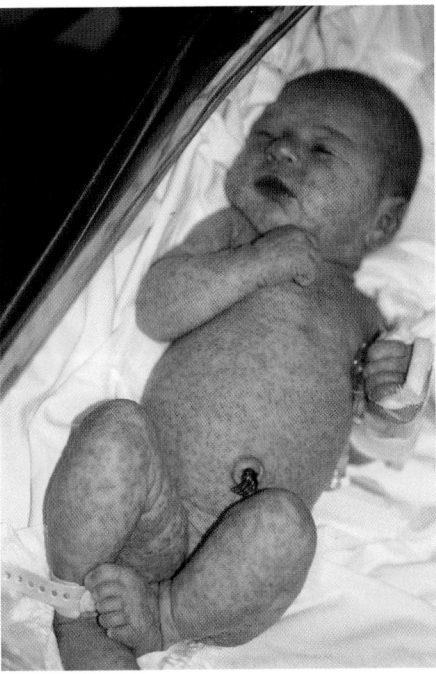

Fig. 33.6 Congenital candidiasis.

Syphilis[5,33]

While macular or maculopapular eruptions are more frequently seen, neonates with congenital syphilis may present with vesicles, bullae and erosions. Blisters form on an erythematous base and rupture easily, leaving a macerated area, sometimes with a peripheral annular scale. Haemorrhagic bullae on the palms and soles are particularly suggestive of syphilis.

Dermatological conditions presenting with pustules, blisters or erosions (see Tables 33.3 & 33.4)

Epidermolysis bullosa (EB)

This is a group of diseases characterised by trauma-induced blistering of skin (Fig. 33.7) and mucosae.[13,38] There are over 15 types now identified, separated on the basis of inheritance, clinical features and electron microscopic (EM) identification of the cleavage plane of the blister: within the epidermis, between the epidermis and dermis, or in the upper dermis. Blisters are clear or filled with serosanguinous material depending on their level. They may rupture or spontaneously subside. Secondary bacterial infection is common. Milia are small retention cysts resulting from a split through pilosebaceous or sweat ducts; these eventually extrude. Permanent scarring is mainly a feature of the forms with a deeper level of split and varies from mild, with minor cosmetic significance, to severe, with gross deformity and functional disability. Sometimes EB presents with extensive areas of denuded skin, particularly on the legs, as well as blistering; some of these cases may be associated with pyloric atresia.[23,29] A firm diagnosis should always be established as soon as possible by EM examination of a new blister. This enables a prognosis to be given and a management plan to be established for present and future.

In the severe forms with extensive neonatal blistering, the infant should initially be nursed naked in a humidicrib, lying on non-adherent material, with barrier nursing to prevent infection. Blisters should be drained and antibacterial creams such as silver sulfadiazine (sulphadiazine) applied to large erosions. Vaseline gauze or non-adherent plastic dressings should be used as required, secured with tubular gauze or by other means but never taped to the skin with adhesive. A squeeze bottle or dropper should be used for feeding when there is severe oral ulceration. Nasogastric tubes should be avoided. Tourniquets, adhesive urine collection bags, identification bands and pacifiers should all be avoided. The parents should be encouraged to hold the baby, but the need for extreme gentleness in handling must be explained and demonstrated. Secondary bacterial infection is treated with topical or oral antibiotics.

Mastocytosis

This is a condition in which the skin and sometimes other organs are infiltrated with benign mast cells. The cutaneous presentations vary from a single or a few isolated 1–5-cm lesions (mastocytoma),

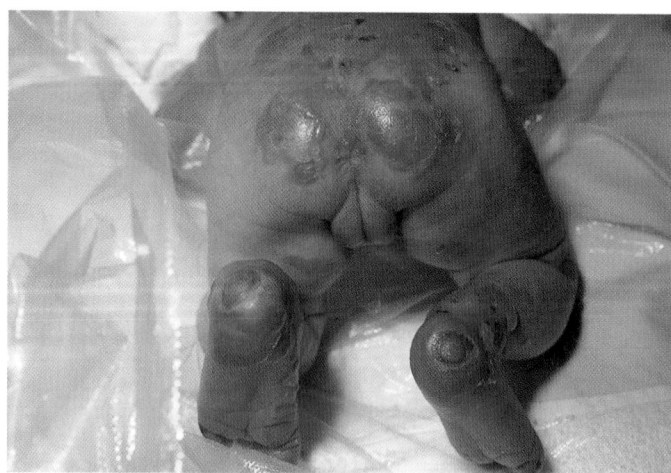
Fig. 33.7 Epidermolysis bullosa.

through multiple smaller often pigmented lesions (urticaria pigmentosa), to diffuse infiltration of the entire skin surface (diffuse cutaneous mastocytosis, bullous mastocytosis).[16] Mast cells contain various mediators of which the most important are histamine, prostaglandins and heparin, and the local and systemic effects of these account for many of the clinical features in this condition.

Urticaria pigmentosa is rarely present at birth but the other forms are usually congenital. Mastocytomas present as pink, pale-brown or yellowish nodules or plaques with a peau d'orange appearance on the surface. On rubbing, a red flush and oedema ('urtication') are seen on the lesion and beyond it. Spontaneous or friction-induced blistering is common, as a result of local histamine release. Systemic spread of the histamine may lead to a generalised flushing. In diffuse cutaneous mastocytosis, there is a generalised thickening and oedema of the skin, usually with widespread haemorrhagic blistering (Fig. 33.8). Flushing, hypotension, shock, gastrointestinal haemorrhage, bronchospasm and diarrhoea may occur from the systemic effects of the mediators. There may be hepatosplenomegaly and lymphadenopathy due to infiltration with mast cells. A number of drugs will cause degranulation of mast cells and release of mediators, and these should be avoided or used with caution; they include aspirin, opiates, tubocurarine, pilocarpine and iodine-containing radiographic agents.

All forms of mastocytosis improve with time, sometimes with complete resolution.

Bullous ichthyosis[9]

This is an autosomal dominant condition, now known to be due to mutations in keratin genes. At birth the skin is diffusely erythematous with widespread erosions and maceration, and, sometimes, intact bullae (Fig. 33.9). In just a few days, the redness and blistering settle and the skin begins to thicken and become verrucous, taking on the appearance which will persist through life.

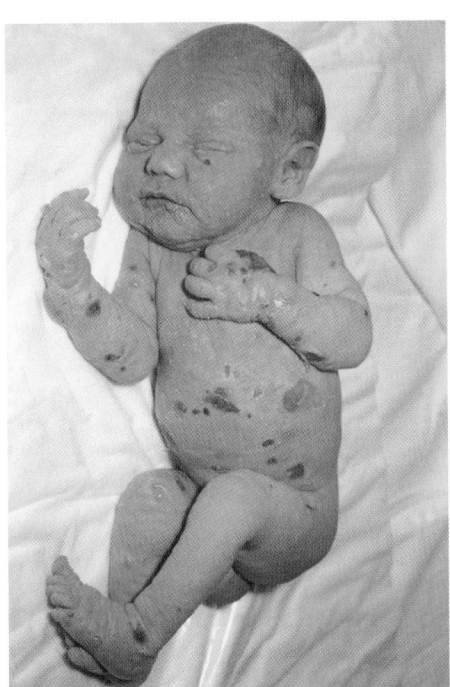

Fig. 33.8 Diffuse cutaneous mastocytosis.

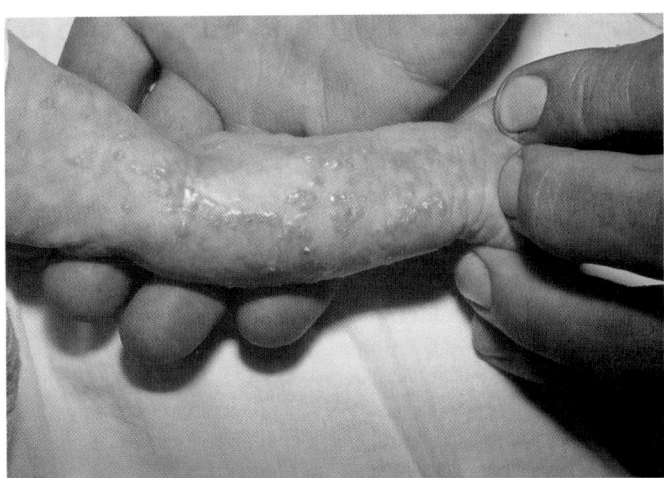

Fig. 33.10 Incontinentia pigmenti.

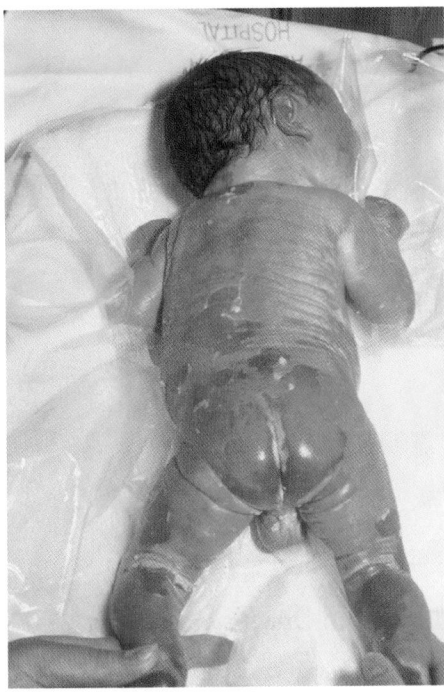

Fig. 33.9 Bullous ichthyosis.

seizures may be anticipated or explained. These comprise linear groups of vesicles (Fig. 33.10), which quickly become pustular, situated mainly on the limbs and appearing at birth or in the first days of life. They are accompanied by a peripheral blood eosinophilia and clear spontaneously over several weeks. The linear pattern is due to the fact that the lesions follow the lines of Blaschko, typical of mosaic disorders. Mosaicism in this X-linked condition occurs as a result of lyonisation.

Neonatal pemphigus

Blisters may occur in the newborn as a result of transplacental passage of IgG antibodies from mothers who have pemphigus vulgaris or pemphigus foliaceus. The lesions are usually present at birth and vary from tense or flaccid bullae to large erosions. It is rare for new blisters to develop after the early days of life and the condition quickly resolves.

Neonatal herpes gestationis

Babies born to mothers with herpes gestationis in pregnancy may develop cutaneous disease as a result of transplacental passage of immunoglobulins formed against the maternal basement membrane zone.[24] The disorder may be evident at birth or within several hours, and red macules or papules, often progressing to vesicles or bullae, can occur. Spontaneous resolution usually occurs by 1 month of age.

Incontinentia pigmenti

This is a multi-system disorder inherited as an X-linked dominant trait and usually lethal in males.[43] There are four cutaneous stages of the disease, vesiculopustular, verrucous, pigmented and hypopigmented, with stage one being present in the neonatal period. Abnormalities in other organ systems, especially neurological, ocular and skeletal, occur in about 70% of cases and seizures may occur in the neonatal period. It is therefore very important to recognise the stage 1 cutaneous lesions so that

Congenital erosive and vesicular dermatosis

The aetiology of this rare disorder is unknown. It presents at birth with extensive blisters, erosions and crusts over most of cutaneous surface.[56] Lesions heal in several weeks with a strange supple and reticulated scarring. The babies are usually premature and may have underlying neurological defects, including developmental delay and seizures. The face, palms, and soles are characteristically spared. Nails are absent or hypoplastic and patchy alopecia is seen on the scalp.

Disorders with systemic significance which can present with neonatal pustules, blisters or erosions

Zinc-deficiency dermatosis

This occasionally presents initially as a blistering rash. Acrodermatitis enteropathica is an autosomal recessive condition in which there is a defective absorption of zinc, possibly due to the absence of a specific carrier protein. The clinical features rarely appear in the early months of life. However, an identical condition occurs earlier in infants with nutritional zinc deficiency.[15] This may occur as a result of prematurity with low zinc stores, particularly in bottle-fed babies (as there is a lower bioavailability of zinc in bovine milk as compared with breast milk), or as a result of low breast-milk zinc. The condition usually presents with a very well-marginated eczematous or psoriasiform rash occurring in a horseshoe shape on the chin and cheeks and in the napkin area (Fig. 33.11). It also often occurs around the eyes and nose and may involve fingers and toes. There is usually a very characteristic dark-coloured scale at the periphery. Sometimes it presents with bullae, particularly in the acral areas, but these soon become erosions and subsequently crust. These children are very irritable and if the condition goes untreated may develop diarrhoea and alopecia and fail to thrive. Zinc deficiency also occurs in acquired immunodeficiency disease, cystic fibrosis and other causes of malabsorption, and in infants on parenteral nutrition solutions not containing adequate zinc. A clinically similar rash can occur with other metabolic conditions, including methylmalonicacidemia and propionicacidemia.

Langerhans cell histiocytosis (LCH)

This can present at birth, or very soon after, as a widespread vesicular or bullous disorder,[19] sometimes simulating staphylococcal scalded-skin syndrome. Usually some haemorrhagic changes point to the correct diagnosis. It may also present at birth as a small number of crusted nodules (Fig. 33.12) which often heal spontaneously after a few weeks. The most common presentation, however, is at several months of age, with a scaly and purpuric rash involving the major flexures, centrofacial area, scalp and ear canals. These children require a full assessment for systemic involvement, whether or not the lesions are apparently healing.

Hyper-IgE syndrome (Job syndrome)

This important immunodeficiency disorder (p. 827) may present in the neonatal period with inflammatory papules, vesicles and pustules, particularly on the face, scalp and upper trunk, but occasionally more widespread.[22] The appearance may be very reminiscent of a pustular miliaria, but the condition is much more persistent and the pustules may be large and tense. As the lesions resolve, they develop a characteristic dark crust. Histologically, the lesions show an intense eosinophilic infiltrate; a peripheral blood eosinophilia is present and the IgE level starts to rise after the early weeks of life. The infant soon begins to develop troublesome infections, particularly with *Staphylococcus aureus* and candida.

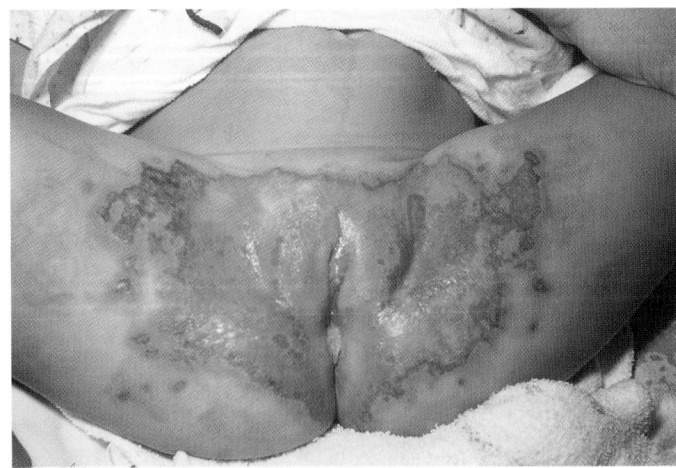

Fig. 33.11 Zinc-deficiency dermatosis.

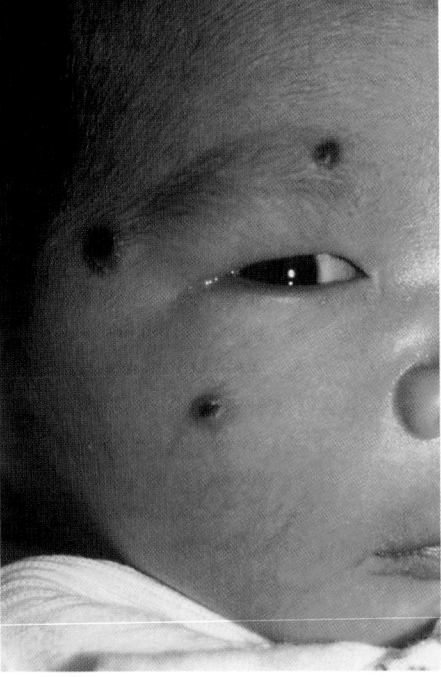

Fig. 33.12 Langerhans cell histiocytosis.

Myleoproliferative disorder in Down syndrome

Babies with Down syndrome are at increased risk of developing haematological abnormalities, including leukemoid reaction, transient myeloproliferative disorder and congenital leukaemia. These entities may be accompanied by a very striking vesiculopustular disorder starting in the early days of life, most marked on the face but sometimes widespread.[44] It spontaneously resolves after a few weeks. The cells identified on skin smear or biopsy reflect those found in the peripheral blood.

Porphyrias

These are a group of disorders of heme synthesis leading to the accumulation of heme precursors which, when present in the skin, produce a photosensitivity. The porphyrias are designated hepatic or erythropoietic depending on the organ predominantly expressing the defect. They can be further separated by the assessment of plasma and red cell porphyrins and the pattern of porphyrin excretion in urine and faeces. Some of these may become symptomatic in the neonatal period.

Congenital erythropoietic porphyria presents soon after birth with severe photosensitivity, with bullae on areas exposed to sun or phototherapy machines and red urine. A later feature is red discoloration of the teeth and their fluorescence on Wood's light examination.

Erythropoietic protoporphyria usually presents later in childhood but occasionally erythema and blistering occur during phototherapy in the neonate. This has been reported also in the homozygous variants of *coproporphyria* and *variegate porphyria*.

A *transient porphyrinemia*, of unclear aetiology, is described in haemolytic disease of the newborn.[36] This can produce marked erythema, purpura and blistering in areas exposed to phototherapy. There is a normalisation of the elevated plasma levels in a few weeks or months.

When photosensitivity occurs in the neonate, porphyrin levels in red cells, plasma, urine and faeces should be measured. The differential diagnosis of neonatal photosensitivity also includes neonatal lupus (see below), xeroderma pigmentosum (with early dark freckling) and drug-induced phototoxicity (e.g. frusemide [furosemide], fluorescin dye).

Other transient neonatal conditions

Sebaceous hyperplasia

This is a common neonatal condition, probably representing the effect of maternal androgens on the neonatal glands.[34] The hyperplastic sebaceous glands are seen as tiny yellow–white papules on the nose, especially at the tip. They disappear in several weeks.

Milia

These represent retention cysts of the pilosebaceous follicles.[34] They occur in approximately 50% of neonates, manifesting as firm pearly-white 1–2-mm papules, particularly on the face. They usually disappear by 4 weeks of age. Persistent milia occur in certain syndromes, including Bazex syndrome, oral-facial-digital syndrome type I and Marie Unna hypotrichosis.

Sucking blisters

These are present at birth and occur on the hands and forearms as a result of sucking in utero. The lesion is initially a tense fluid-filled blister, which ruptures to produce an erosion.[34]

Sucking calluses or sucking pads

These develop on the lips as localised or extensive thickenings of the vermilion border. They may be present at birth, but more commonly occur postnatally, and are due to vigorous sucking.[34]

Subcutaneous fat necrosis

This is a necrosis of subcutaneous fat in the newborn, probably induced by ischaemia. It occurs only in full-term infants. There is usually a history of a difficult labour and delivery, with such complications as prolonged labour, fetal distress and perinatal asphyxia. The lesions appear between the second and third weeks of life as tender, firm, skin-coloured or red–purple nodules or plaques occurring particularly on the buttocks, shoulders, upper back, proximal limbs and cheeks. New nodules may develop over several weeks. They usually disappear spontaneously without complication in several months, leaving no trace. However, sometimes they become fluctuant, ulcerate or calcify. In patients with calcified lesions, troublesome hypercalcaemia may develop.[31] Fluctuant lesions should be aspirated, secondary infection should be dealt with if it complicates ulcerated lesions, and serum calcium levels should be monitored in the presence of calcified lesions.

Neonatal lupus erythematosus (LE)

This occurs due to the passage of maternal SS-A or SS-B (anti-Ro, anti-La) antibodies through the placenta, where the mother suffers from clinical or subclinical LE or Sjögren syndrome.[60] The most important feature of neonatal LE is heart block, but there seems to be an inverse relationship between cutaneous and cardiac lesions. Other rare complications include autoimmune haemolytic anaemia, thrombocytopenia, hepatitis, pneumonitis and splenomegaly. Lesions appear soon after the first sun exposure. The most characteristic is a mauve erythema on the face with a clear lower border on the cheeks, extending up around the eyes into the hairline (Fig. 33.13). A similar erythema may occur on the arms. Occasionally lesions are annular, scaly or telangiectatic. The condition in the baby settles spontaneously in a few months, when the antibodies disappear. The finding of antibodies in either mother or child is adequate proof of the diagnosis and biopsy is unnecessary.

The red scaly baby

A number of important conditions can present with diffuse redness and variable scaliness (erythroderma) in the neonate or young baby (Table 33.5). These babies can have major problems with temperature regulation and fluid balance and may seriously fail to thrive.

Seborrhoeic dermatitis

There is a dull red erythema with a greasy yellow scale, involving particularly the scalp, centrofacial area and all the flexures but

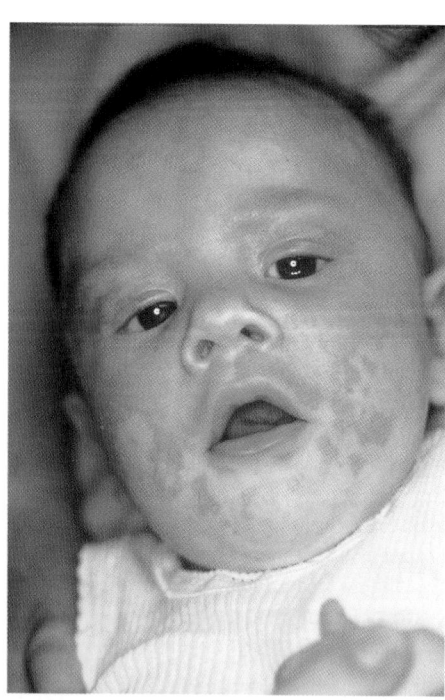

Fig. 33.13 Neonatal lupus erythematosus.

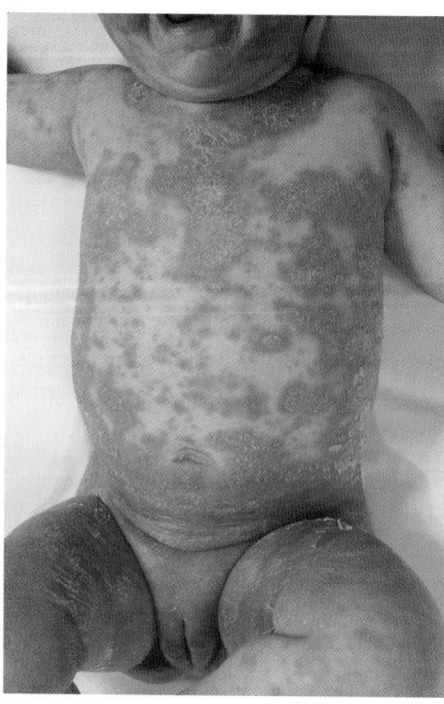

Fig. 33.14 Napkin psoriasis with dissemination.

Table 33.5 Conditions which may present with generalised erythema in the neonate
Seborrhoeic dermatitis
Atopic dermatitis
Psoriasis
Ichthyoses
Collodion baby phenotype
Netherton syndrome
Harlequin ichthyosis
Immunodeficiency disorders
Congenital mastocytosis
Staphylococcal scalded-skin syndrome
Cystic fibrosis

sometimes more widespread. The scale may be absent in the flexures and secondary candidiasis is common. It is usually asymptomatic and self-limiting after the early months of life. It responds to weak steroids and anti-candidal agents.

Atopic dermatitis

Very rarely this condition presents in the neonatal period with a widespread red scaly and itchy rash. These patients are likely to go on to difficult long-term disease. Management involves emollients and careful use of weak topical steroids, sometimes with wet dressings.

Psoriasis

A dramatic form of psoriasis seen in babies is napkin (diaper) psoriasis with dissemination.[40] A well-marginated, bright-red napkin rash develops initially and then small scaly patches spread beyond the margins. There is then an explosive spread of psoriatic lesions to the scalp and face and then all over the trunk (Fig. 33.14). The baby remains well and the condition is usually self-limiting in a few weeks. Weak topical steroids and wet dressings may speed the resolution a little. Very rarely, psoriasis may present in the neonatal period or even at birth as a generalised erythroderma, sometimes progressing to a pustular psoriasis. Infantile generalised pustular psoriasis may be associated with lytic bone lesions and the capillary leak syndrome.[30]

Ichthyoses

Collodion baby phenotype[3]

This is a descriptive term for the child who is encased at birth in a shiny tight membrane resembling collodion or plastic skin, producing ectropion and eclabium and fissuring (Fig. 33.15). The membrane peels off in days or weeks. This may be a presentation of various forms of ichthyosis, particularly congenital ichthyosiform erythroderma and lamellar ichthyosis, but also trichothiodystrophy, Gaucher disease, neutral lipid storage disease and Conradi–Hünermann syndrome. Rarely, the membrane peels off to leave normal skin; this condition is called lamellar exfoliation of the newborn. Collodion babies show temperature instability and excessive fluid loss. Corneal exposure may result if the eyes are not covered, and the eclabium may necessitate squeeze-bottle, tube or dropper feeding. As the fissures appear, secondary infection becomes a risk. The child should be nursed in a humidicrib with minimum handling. Emollients are best avoided in the early stages.

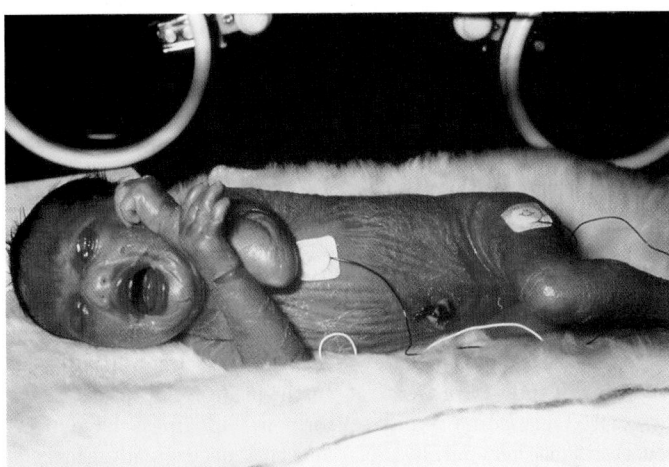

Fig. 33.15 Collodion baby.

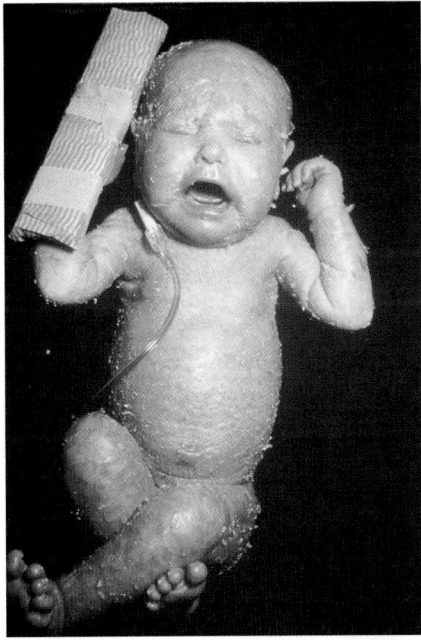

Fig. 33.16 Netherton syndrome.

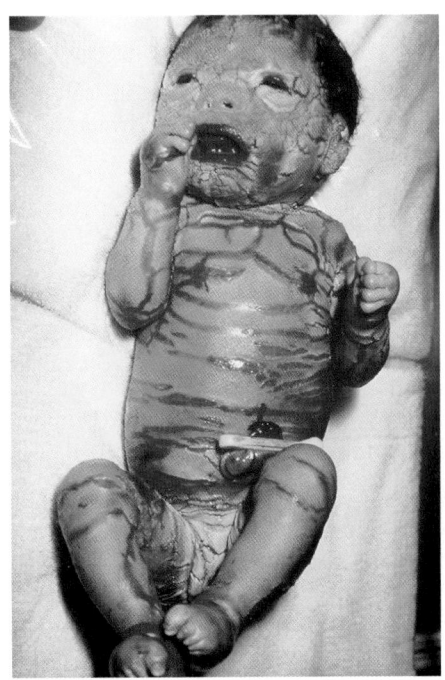

Fig. 33.17 Harlequin ichthyosis.

X-linked ichthyosis

This may present in the first month with pale shiny plates of scale, without redness, in a widespread distribution, lasting several days before exfoliating. It is only several months later that the typical dark scale of this condition appears.

Netherton syndrome[4]

This is a genetic disorder which may present as a congenital erythroderma with generalised redness and scale (Fig. 33.16). There is a severe failure to thrive and a risk of hypernatremic dehydration. These babies usually have no hair at all at birth. When hair develops, it is fragile and appears short, broken and sparse and histologically shows trichorrhexis invaginata (bamboo hair). Some infants with Netherton syndrome have a different cutaneous picture, presenting with multiple annular lesions with a double-edged scale, designated ichthyosis linearis circumflexa.

Harlequin ichthyosis

It is only in recent years that survivors with this condition have been reported.[27,53] In most cases, initial survival has been a result of retinoid therapy, but some cases have survived without specific therapy. These babies are at birth encased in a carapace of white hyperkeratotic skin, leading to severe distortion of facial features, ears, hands and feet. The skin soon splits, leaving bleeding fissures (Fig. 33.17), and then peels off, leaving red scaly skin beneath and a clinical picture similar to the severe end of the spectrum of congenital ichthyosiform erythroderma.[27] Death in these infants occurs as a result of infection or respiratory failure due to prenatal collection in the lungs of squamous material contaminating the amniotic fluid.

Immunodeficiencies

Patients with severe combined immunodeficiency, Omenn syndrome (T-cell deficiency, abnormal histiocytic cells and elevated IgE level; p. 824) and other immunodeficiencies may present with a widespread red scaly rash commencing in the neonatal period but not present at birth.[12,14,49] In some cases this represents a congenital graft-versus-host reaction. These babies usually demonstrate recurrent infections, diarrhoea and failure to thrive. What was described in the past as *Leiner disease* is now recognised as not a specific entity but a phenotype of non-congenital early-onset erythroderma, diarrhoea and failure to thrive. Some of the patients initially diagnosed as having Leiner disease have subsequently been recognised as having Netherton syndrome, while others have had a variety of immunodeficiencies. Skin biopsy and detailed study of immunological parameters is essential in any erythrodermic baby in whom another clear diagnosis has not been established. The terms Leiner disease and Leiner syndrome would be best abandoned.

Cystic fibrosis

Rarely, babies with cystic fibrosis develop widespread scaly red lesions and even a diffuse erythroderma in the early months of life as a manifestation of global malnutrition.

Birthmarks and other naevoid conditions

Pigmented birthmarks

Congenital melanocytic naevi

These occur at birth as raised verrucous or lobulated lesions of varying shades of brown to black, sometimes with blue or pink components, with an irregular margin and, often, growing long dark hairs. Giant-sized lesions may produce considerable redundancy of skin and often occur in a 'garment' distribution on the trunk and adjacent limbs. Malignancy in giant naevi can occur in childhood and the incidence over a lifetime is possibly of the order of 5%. In medium and small lesions, the risk is a lot lower and any development of malignancy is always post-pubertal. Lesions occurring over the spine, especially the upper part, may be associated with meningeal melanocytosis, which may be complicated by melanoma or obstructive hydrocephalus. Lesions over the lower spine may rarely be associated with spinal dysraphism and tethered cord. Large axial lesions or multiple scattered medium to large lesions may be associated with posterior cranial fossa malformations. All patients with these types of lesions should have imaging studies performed as soon as possible.

Naevoid pigmentary disorders

These are flat areas of hyperpigmented or hypopigmented skin which may be evident at birth. They occur in characteristic patterns – either segmental, or whirled and streaky following the lines of Blaschko.[42] Sometimes there is a combination of hypo- and hyperpigmented streaks. These distributions are now recognised as genetic mosaic patterns, indicating that, as a result of a post-zygotic mutation, the individual comprises more than one population of cells. They may have smooth or irregular edges and occur anywhere on the trunk, limbs or face. They usually occur as isolated phenomena but, particularly when extensive, may be associated, as part of certain mosaic phenotypes, with neurological, skeletal and other abnormalities.[42]

Important in the differential diagnosis are the café-au-lait spots of neurofibromatosis and the hypopigmented macules of tuberous sclerosis, both of which may occasionally be present at birth but which tend to be smaller, do not follow mosaic patterns and increase in number with time.

Mongolian spots

These are flat, blue or slate-grey lesions with poorly defined margins. They may be single or multiple and occur particularly on the lumbosacral area, although the shoulders, upper back and occasionally other areas may be involved. They are found in over 80% of Oriental and black infants and in up to 10% of white infants, particularly those of Mediterranean origin. They usually fade considerably by puberty, but may remain unaltered through life.

Naevus of Ota

This is a persistent patchy blue–grey discoloration of the skin of the face, particularly on the cheek, periorbital area and brow. It is usually unilateral and often there is a similar pigmentation of the sclera of the ipsilateral eye. It is most common in Oriental individuals and is present at birth in over 50% of cases. Associated glaucoma[35] and sensorineural deafness have been reported, and, very rarely, melanoma may occur in adult life.

Epidermal naevi

Epidermal naevi arise from the basal layer of the embryonic epidermis which gives rise to skin appendages as well as keratinocytes. These naevi have conventionally been classified according to the tissue of origin into keratinocytic, sebaceous and follicular types.[17] They can involve any area of skin. They may be present at birth or appear in the first few years of life and may extend well beyond their original distribution. On the scalp and face they have a yellowish colour due to prominent sebaceous glands and present as a hairless, often linear plaque, usually flat in infancy and childhood and becoming verrucous at puberty. Sometimes they are more papillomatous (Fig. 33.18). Lesions elsewhere are usually dark brown but occasionally are paler than the normal skin. They occur as single or multiple warty plaques or lines, often arranged in a linear or swirled

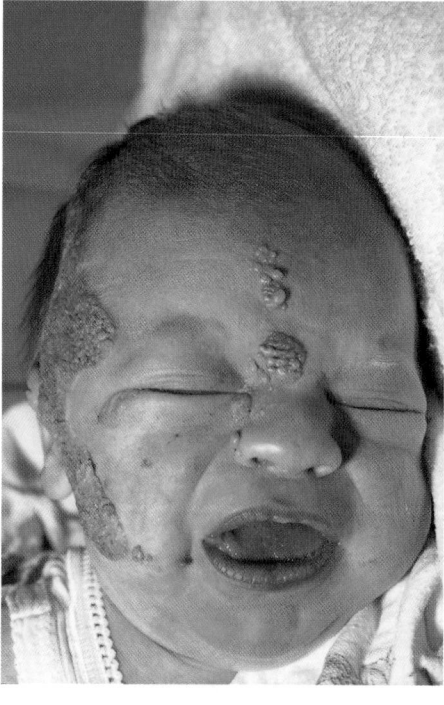

Fig. 33.18
Papillomatous sebaceous naevus.

pattern. It is now clear that the linear and swirled patterns taken by epidermal naevi follow the lines of Blaschko, and that all epidermal naevi can be explained on the basis of genetic mosaicism, with each type of naevus representing the cutaneous manifestation of a different mosaic phenotype. In most patients the naevus is the only detectable manifestation, but in some patients there are associated abnormalities in other organ systems, particularly skeletal, neurological and ocular. Skeletal abnormalities occur particularly with naevi of keratinocytic type on the limbs, and neurological and ocular abnormalities with naevi of sebaceous type on the head. These patients should have a careful physical examination, but imaging studies are generally not indicated in the absence of abnormal signs or symptoms.

Vascular birthmarks

These can be divided into haemangiomas, which are proliferative vascular tumours, and vascular malformations, which represent fixed collections of dilated abnormal vessels.

Haemangiomas

Haemangiomas usually appear just after birth, undergo a fast growth phase, and then, over a long period, tend to spontaneous resolution.[11] It is now clear that haemangiomas, whether superficially or deeply located in the skin, have the same structure, being composed in the early stage of proliferating masses of endothelial cells with occasional lumina and later, as they resolve, of large endothelial lined spaces. The terms capillary, cavernous and capillary–cavernous are misleading and should be abandoned in favour of the simple term haemangioma.

Superficial haemangiomas are usually not present at birth but appear in the first weeks of life as an area of pallor followed by a telangiectatic patch. They then grow rapidly into a lobulated, well-demarcated, bright-red tumour. Rapid growth continues over the first 6 months; the growth rate then slows and further growth after 10 months is unusual. After a stationary phase, signs of involution begin with the appearance of grey areas, which enlarge and coalesce. The lesions gradually fade and flatten, and, if uncomplicated, often resolve completely over several years. Deeper haemangiomas may occur alone or beneath a superficial lesion. They also usually appear after birth and undergo a growth phase. The overlying skin is normal or bluish in colour. As they resolve, they soften and shrink over, and complete disappearance occurs in many cases. Apparent deep haemangiomas which show no sign of resolution are now recognised as vascular malformations, usually of venous type, and are not haemangiomas at all.

Redundant tissue may remain in the place of large lesions, and residual telangiectasia may persist in the area of superficial lesions. Ulceration can occur during the rapid growth phase of superficial haemangiomas. If secondary infection is controlled, the ulcers usually heal in a few weeks, but some scarring is inevitable. Ulceration of lesions on eyelids, lips or ala nasae can lead to full-thickness tissue loss. Scarring following ulceration of lesions on or near the eyelids can result in a cicatricial ectropion, and alopecia may be permanent after scalp ulceration.

Haemangiomas may encroach on vital structures. A haemangioma closing the eye for as little as 4 weeks in infancy can produce amblyopia. However, even without occluding the pupil, an eyelid lesion, by pressing on the eye and producing astigmatism, can lead to failure of development of binocular vision and partial amblyopia. Large haemangiomas around the mouth may interfere with feeding and one blocking both nares can lead to respiratory difficulties while the child is being fed. A large deep haemangioma around the neck may displace the pharynx or trachea: also the upper respiratory tract may be directly involved with the haemangioma. The possibility of laryngeal involvement should be considered with an extensive lower face or neck haemangioma (Fig. 33.19), particularly when there is accompanying intraoral involvement, and a lateral airways X-ray should be arranged. If there is stridor, urgent laryngoscopy is mandatory. Even when traumatised, uncomplicated haemangiomas rarely bleed significantly.

Lesions over the lower spine may be associated with spinal fusion abnormalities and a tethered spinal cord; lesions involving the sacral area, with urogenital and rectal abnormalities; and large hemifacial lesions, with Dandy–Walker and other posterior cranial fossa abnormalities.[11] Early imaging studies should be undertaken when haemangiomas are in these positions.

Simple observation and reassurance while awaiting natural resolution is the ideal approach for most haemangiomas. Showing serial photographs of resolved lesions is encouraging. Indications for active intervention are an alarming growth rate, threatening ulceration in areas where serious complications could ensue, interference with vital structures, and severe bleeding. Oral corticosteroids will slow the growth of potentially dangerous or cosmetically serious lesions. They have no place once growth has ceased. Intralesional steroids may be used in very experienced hands to shrink periorbital haemangiomas that fail to respond to

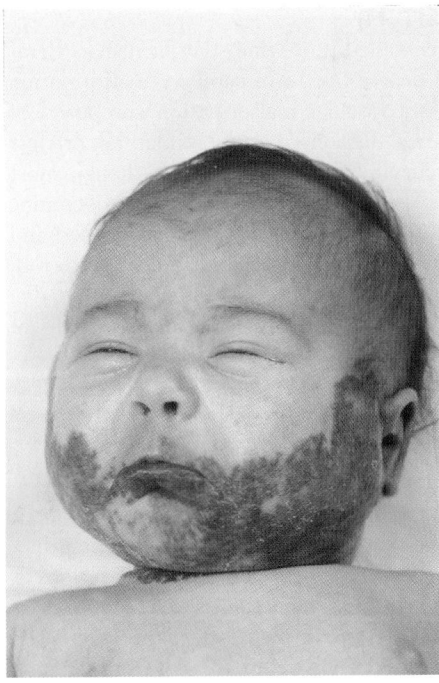

Fig. 33.19 Lower face haemangioma with laryngeal involvement.

oral steroids, and interferon-α (IFN-α) has been effective in some life-threatening cases. Cosmetic surgical procedures can improve the appearance when loose tissue remains. Laser therapy has a place for upper respiratory tract lesions and as an adjunct or alternative to surgery in some complicated lesions.

Diffuse infantile haemangiomatosis

This is a condition with multiple small haemangiomas in a widespread distribution.[11] There is a benign form, with lesions limited to the skin; however, in the potentially serious systemic form, lesions may occur in many organs, particularly the liver, gastrointestinal tract, lungs and central nervous system, with or, rarely, without cutaneous lesions. These patients should be carefully assessed, with full blood count, chest X-ray and examination for cardiac failure due to arteriovenous shunts, and for bleeding from the gastrointestinal tract. Ultrasound or abdominal CT scan should be performed to exclude hepatic involvement, and other organs should be further investigated as indicated. More sophisticated studies such as angiography and technetium-labelled red blood cell scans can delineate further the extent of internal involvement. With severe systemic involvement, high-dose corticosteroids are required along with management of cardiac failure and other complications.

Vascular malformations

Vascular malformations are structural abnormalities and, as such, are present at birth, grow in proportion to the patient's growth and have no tendency to resolution. They can be further divided according to their vessel of origin into capillary, arterial, venous, lymphatic and mixed types. Ultrasound is the most useful non-invasive investigation and, along with history and clinical examination, can identify the elements of most vascular malformations and separate them from hemangiomas.

Capillary malformation (CM)

This has previously been called port-wine stain or naevus flammeus but the accurate descriptive term capillary malformation should be used. This is a vascular malformation composed of dilated mature capillaries. Lesions may be unilateral or, less often, bilateral and occur anywhere on the body, though most commonly on the face. They are deep pink in infancy, becoming later more purple. After puberty, they may become raised and nodular. Until recently, only cosmetic cover could be offered, but good results are now being achieved with the pulsed dye laser and commencement of treatment in the early months of life gives the best results.

Sturge–Weber syndrome

This is the association of a facial CM and a vascular malformation of the ipsilateral meninges and cerebral cortex. The cutaneous lesion always involves the skin in the distribution of the first division of the trigeminal nerve.[59] The neurological manifestations of the syndrome include convulsions, hemiparesis and mental retardation. When the facial lesion involves the skin innervated by both the first and second divisions of the trigeminal nerve,

congenital glaucoma may occur:[59] this does not occur when only one division is involved. Patients presenting with a CM in the appropriate distribution should have early neurological and ophthalmological consultation and continued close follow-up. An MRI scan may demonstrate the intracranial malformations in the first few months of life.

Venous malformation (VM)

This appears as a bluish tumour, which empties with pressure and when elevated, and fills when dependent.

Lymphatic malformation (LM; lymphangioma, cystic hygroma)

Macrocystic deep lesions present as skin-coloured tumours, often with bruising (Fig. 33.20); superficial lesions present as groups of haemorrhagic vesicles or warty lesions.[8]

Arteriovenous malformation (AVM)

A localised AVM presents as a skin-coloured lump which may demonstrate a bruit on auscultation. More often, an AVM is part of a complex mixed malformation.

Mixed malformations

All combinations of malformation can occur, with two, three or even four elements being present. The eponym *Klippel–Trenaunay syndrome* refers to a CM, VM and sometimes LM associated with either overgrowth of a limb, with soft tissue hypertrophy and/or bony hypertrophy, or very rarely hypotrophy.[11] The eponym *Parkes–Weber syndrome* refers to a CM and AVM with limb hypertrophy.[11] These mixed vascular malformations are best described by their component parts rather than using the eponyms.

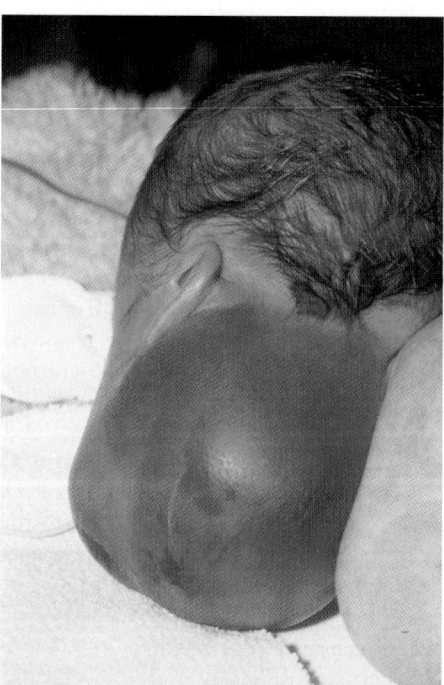

Fig. 33.20 Cervical lymphatic malformation with haemorrhage.

Some congenital tumours

Vascular tumours

Rare vascular tumours that may be present at birth include tufted angioma (TA), kaposiform haemangioendothelioma (KHE) and an entity presently designated rapidly involuting congenital haemangioma (RICH). All of these have typical histological features and RICH has a characteristic ultrasound appearance.

TA is a rare vascular proliferation which may be congenital.[11] It presents as a red to brown or violaceous plaque or nodule; some resolve, while others persist and spread. It is rarely associated with Kasabach–Merritt syndrome (KMS). KHE is a yellow, blue or red plaque-like lesion, usually present at birth and commonly associated with KMS.[11]

RICH is a vascular tumour which bears some clinical resemblance to a common hemangioma of infancy but is quite distinct from it and has a characteristic ultrasound appearance.[52] It proliferates in utero and is fully developed at birth. It presents as a raised plaque or tumour, bluish or violaceous in colour, sometimes studded with telangiectases and often surrounded by a characteristic pale halo. Unlike standard hemangiomas, it does not demonstrate an accelerated postnatal growth phase. Instead, involution commences promptly and progresses rapidly, often leaving an area of atrophy. The majority regress totally by 12 months of age.

Kasabach–Merritt syndrome

This was initially believed to be a complication of large haemangiomas, but it is now clear that the associated lesions are not haemangiomas but represent other vascular tumours, including TA and KHE (see above).[11] Thrombocytopenia is caused by entrapment of platelets within the lesion and is sometimes followed by disseminated intravascular coagulation (DIC). Initially there is bleeding into the lesion, which rapidly enlarges, and then widespread life-threatening haemorrhage may follow. When bleeding is confined to the tumour, the approach can be conservative. In severe cases, steroids, IFN-α and vincristine have been used to shrink the tumour, or removal can be considered if feasible. There is a definite concern about the use of IFN-α in the very young, with increasing numbers of reports of the later development of spastic diplegia. Management also involves resuscitation, transfusion, and dealing with the DIC, usually with heparinisation.

Langerhans cell histiocytosis (p. 824)

This may occasionally present with a single or small numbers of tumours. They are usually red nodules, often with an eroded surface, and often resolve spontaneously.

Congenital leukaemia (p. 753)

This may present with multiple, skin-coloured or, more often, purpuric nodules, or, occasionally, a single nodule which histologically demonstrates a leukaemic infiltrate.

Sarcomas (pp. 956–8)

Fibrosarcoma, rhabdomyosarcoma and undifferentiated sarcoma can all present as a deep red firm mass with a shiny surface and rapid growth.

Congenital neuroblastoma (pp. 958–60)

Cutaneous metastases present at birth or soon after, as multiple bluish firm nodules, which may demonstrate persistent blanching on pressure.

Infantile myofibromatosis

In most cases, this presents at birth or soon after; the lesions may be solitary or multicentric, with possible involvement of bones and multiple internal organs.[58] Solitary lesions are usually large red tumours on the skin or in the oral cavity. In the multicentric form, cutaneous lesions present as small nodules or indented areas of skin due to surface tethering. Extensive imaging studies are required in these patients to detect internal involvement.

Juvenile xanthogranuloma

These may be present at birth as yellow or red (the non-lipidised variant) nodules. They usually involute after many months. These patients are normolipaemic.

Dermoid cysts

These are congenital cysts occurring along embryonic fusion lines as asymptomatic, non-compressible nodules[45] with a typical ultrasound appearance. The commonest positions are over the anterior fontanelle, at the lateral end of the eyebrow and in the midline of the upper nose. Dermal sinuses are short tracks connecting the dermoid to the skin surface, where a punctum is seen.

Cephaloceles and heterotopic brain tissue

Cephaloceles (encephalocele, meningocele) represent herniation of intracranial structures through a scalp defect (pp. 1190–1).[10] Atretic encephaloceles and meningoceles have an intact skull underneath but are usually clinically indistinguishable from lesions with intracranial connections.[10] Local markers of these lesions include a capillary malformation and superimposed or surrounding hypertrichosis (the hair collar sign).[56] Heterotopic brain tissue occurs away from the scalp and includes the well-recognised 'nasal glioma' and nodules elsewhere on the face, again often marked by hypertrichosis.

Gluteal granulomas

These occur on top of a pre-existing napkin rash as impressive purplish nodules, histologically demonstrating a benign mixed inflammatory infiltrate, which tend to be oval in shape, following the lines of the skin folds. The cause is unclear but they settle slowly with standard treatment with weak steroid and barrier preparations.

Aplasia cutis

Aplasia cutis (AC) is a congenital absence of skin, usually localised but sometimes occurring as multiple lesions in a widespread distribution. The commonest form is membranous AC, which presents as single or multiple round or oval lesions, with an intact but atrophic surface on the scalp or side of the face, sometimes with a surrounding hair collar,[6] and probably representing incomplete closure of embryonic fusion lines.[10] Another form is as a large stellate erosion at or near the midline of the scalp, which crusts and finally, after some months, heals with a scar which is often hypertrophic.

Imaging to detect an underlying skull defect is essential in all cases of scalp AC.

Scalp AC occurs in a number of syndromes, including trisomy 13, Johanson–Blizzard syndrome and Adams–Oliver syndrome.

Extensive truncal and limb AC may be associated with a fetus papyraceus.[28]

References

1. Bergman J N, Eichenfield L F 2002 Neonatal acne and cephalic pustulosis: is malassezia the whole story? Archives of Dermatology 138: 255–257
2. Brunell P A 1992 Varicella in pregnancy, the fetus, and the newborn: problems in management. Journal of Infectious Diseases 166(suppl. 1): S42–S47
3. Buyse L, Graves C, Marks R et al 1993 Collodion baby dehydration: the danger of high transepidermal water loss. British Journal of Dermatology 129: 86–88
4. Chavanas S, Garner C, Bodemer C et al 2000 Localization of the Netherton syndrome gene to chromosome q32, by linkage analysis and homozygosity mapping. American Journal of Human Genetics 66: 914–921
5. Chawla V, Pandit P, Nkrumah F 1988 Congenital syphilis in the newborn. Archives of Diseases in Childhood 63: 1393–1394
6. Commens C, Rogers M 1989 Heterotropic brain tissue presenting as bald cysts with a collar of hypertrophic hair. Archives of Dermatology 125: 1253–1256
7. Darmstadt G L, Dinulos J G, Miller Z 2000 Congenital cutaneous candidiasis: Clinical presentation, pathogenesis, and management guidelines. Pediatrics 105: 438–444
8. Davies D, Rogers M 2000 Morphology of lymphatic malformations: a pictorial review. Australasian Journal of Dermatology 41: 1–7
9. Digiovanna J J, Bale S J 1994 Clinical heterogeneity in epidermolytic hyperkeratosis. Archives of Dermatology 130: 1026–1035
10. Drolet B A 2001 Developmental abnormalities. In: Eichenfield L F, Frieden I J, Esterly N B (eds) Textbook of neonatal dermatology. W B Saunders, Philadelphia, pp 126–130
11. Enjolras O, Garzon M 2001 Vascular stains, malformations and tumors. In: Eichenfield L F, Frieden I J, Esterly N B (eds) Textbook of neonatal dermatology. W B Saunders, Philadelphia, pp 324–352
12. Farrell A, Scerri L, Stevens A et al 1995 Acute graft-versus-host disease with unusual cutaneous intracellular vacuolation in an infant with severe combined immunodeficiency. Pediatric Dermatology 12: 311–313
13. Fine J D, Johnson L B, Suchindran C et al 1999 Cutaneous and skin associated musculoskeletal manifestations of inherited epidermolysis bullosa: the National Epidermolysis Bullosa Registry experience. In: Fine J, Bauer E, McGuire J et al (eds) Epidermolysis bullosa: clinical, epidemiologic, and laboratory advances and the findings of the National Epidermolysis Bullosa Registry. Johns Hopkins University Press, Baltimore, pp 114–146
14. Glover M T, Atherton D J, Levinsky RJ 1988 Syndrome of erythroderma, failure to thrive and diarrhea in infancy: a manifestation of immunodeficiency. Pediatrics 81: 66–72
15. Goskowicz M, Eichenfield L F 1993 Cutaneous findings of nutritional diseases in children. Current Opinion in Pediatrics 5: 441–445
16. Hannaford R, Rogers M 2001 Presentation of cutaneous mastocytosis in 173 children. Australasian Journal of Dermatology 42: 15–21
17. Happle R, Rogers M 2002 Epidermal nevi. Advances in Dermatology 18: 175–201
18. Harpin V A, Rutter N 1982 Percutaneous alcohol absorption and skin necrosis in a premature infant. Archives of Diseases in Childhood 57: 477–479
19. Herman L E, Rothman K F, Harawi S et al 1990 Congenital self-healing reticulo-histiocytosis. A new entity in the differential diagnosis of neonatal papulovesicular eruptions. Archives of Dermatology 126: 210–212
20. Jacobs R F 1998 Neonatal herpes simplex virus infections. Seminars in Perinatology 22: 64–71
21. Jennings J L, Burrows W M 1983 Infantile acropustulosis. Journal of the American Academy of Dermatology 9: 733–738
22. Kamei R, Honig P J 1988 Neonatal Job's syndrome featuring a vesicular eruption. Pediatric Dermatology 5: 75–82
23. Kanzler M H, Smoller B, Woodley D T 1992 Congenital localized absence of the skin as a manifestation of epidermolysis bullosa. Archives of Dermatology 128: 1087–1090
24. Karna P, Broecker AH 1991 Neonatal herpes gestationis. Journal of Pediatrics 119: 299–301
25. Lane A T 1987 Development and care of the premature infant's skin. Pediatric Dermatology 4: 1–5
26. Larralde M, Morales S, Munoz A S et al 1999 Eosinophilic pustular folliculitis in infancy: report of two new cases. Pediatric Dermatology 16: 118–120
27. Lawlor F 1989 Progress of a harlequin fetus to non-bullous ichthyosiform erythroderma. Pediatrics 82: 870–873
28. Leaute-Lebreze C, Depaire-Duclos F, Sarlangue J et al 1998 Congenital cutaneous defects as complications of surviving co-twins; aplasia cutis congenita and neonatal Volkmann ischemic contracture of the forearm. Archives of Dermatology 134: 1121–1124
29. Lestringant G G, Akel S R, Qayed K 1992 The pyloric atresia-junctional epidermolysis bullosa syndrome. Report of a case and review of the literature. Archives of Dermatology 128: 1083–1086
30. Levy M L, Spraker M K 2001 Erythrokeratodermas: the red scaly baby. In: Eichenfield L F, Frieden I J, Esterly N B (eds) Textbook of neonatal dermatology. W B Saunders, Philadelphia, pp 260–275
31. Lewis A, Cowen P, Rodda C et al 1992 Subcutaneous fat necrosis of the newborn complicated by hypercalcaemia and thrombocytopenia. Australasian Journal of Dermatology 33: 141–144
32. Littler C M 1997 Laser hair removal in a patient with hypertrichosis lanuginosa congenita. Dermatologic Surgery 23: 705–707
33. Lowy G 1992 Sexually transmitted diseases in children. Pediatric Dermatology 9: 329–334
34. Lucky A W 2001 Transient benign cutaneous lesions in the newborn. In: Eichenfield L F, Frieden I J, Esterly N B (eds) Textbook of neonatal dermatology. W B Saunders, Philadelphia, pp 88–102
35. Lui J C, Ball S F 1991 Nevus of Ota with glaucoma: report of three cases. Annals of Ophthalmology 23: 286–289
36. Mallon E, Wojnarowska F, Hope P et al 1995 Neonatal bullous erption as a result of transient porphyrinemia in a premature infant with hemolytic disease of the newborn. Journal of the American Academy of Dermatology 33: 333–336
37. Mancini A J, Frieden I J, Paller A S 1998 Infantile acropustulosis revisited: history of scabies and response to topical corticosteroids. Pediatric Dermatology 15: 337–341
38. Marinkovich M 1999 Update on inherited bullous dermatoses. Dermatologic Clinics 17: 473–485
39. Merlob P, Metzker A, Reisner S H 1982 Transient neonatal pustular melanosis. American Journal of Diseases of Children 136: 521–522
40. Morris A, Rogers M, Fischer G, Williams K 2001 Childhood psoriasis: a clinical review of 1262 cases. Pediatric Dermatology 18: 188–198
41. Nanda S, Reddy B S N, Ramji S et al 2002 Analytical study of pustular eruptions in neonates. Pediatric Dermatology 19: 210–215
42. Nehal K S, PeBenito R, Orlow S J 1996 Analysis of 54 cases of hypopigmentation and hyperpigmentation along the lines of Blaschko. Archives of Dermatology 132: 1167–1170
43. Nelson-Adesokan P, Mallory S B 1992 Incontinentia pigmenti. Pediatric Dermatology 9: 304–308
44. Nijhawan A, Baselga E, Gonzalez-Ensenat M A et al 2001 Vesiculopustular eruptions in Down syndrome neonates with myeloproliferative disorders. Archives of Dermatology 137: 760–764

45. Paller A S, Pensler J, Tomita T 1991 Nasal midline masses in infants and children. Dermoids, encephaloceles, and nasal gliomas. Archives of Dermatology 127: 362–366

46. Pong A L, McCuaig C C 2001 Fungal infections, infestations and parasitic infections in neonates. In: Eichenfield L F, Frieden I J, Esterly N B (eds) Textbook of neonatal dermatology. W B Saunders, Philadelphia, pp 223–240

47. Quarterman M J, Lesher J L1994 Neonatal scabies treated with permethrin 5% cream. Pediatric Dermatology 11: 264–266

48. Ramamurthy R S, Riveri M, Esterly N B et al 1976 Transient neonatal pustular melanosis. Journal of Pediatrics 88: 831–835

49. Ricci, G, Patrizi A, Specchia F 1997 Omenn syndrome. Pediatric Dermatology 14: 49–52

50. Riley L E 1998 Herpes simplex virus. Seminars in Perinatology 22: 284–292

51. Rogers M. 2001 Hair disorders. In: Eichenfield L F, Frieden I J, Esterly N B (eds) Textbook of neonatal dermatology. W B Saunders, Philadelphia, pp 487–503

52. Rogers M, Lam A, Fischer G 2002 Sonographic findings in a series of rapidly involuting congenital hemangiomas (RICH). Pediatric Dermatology 19: 5–11

53. Rogers M, Scarf C 1989 Harlequin baby treated with etretinate. Pediatric Dermatology 6: 216–221

54. Rowen J L, Atkins J T, Levy M L et al 1995 Invasive fungal dermatitis in the <1000-gram neonate. Pediatrics 95: 682–687

55. Rutter N 1987 Percutaneous drug absorption in the newborn: hazards and uses. Clinics in Perinatology 14: 911–930

56. Sadick N S, Shea C R, Schlessel J S 1995 Congenital erosive and vesicular dermatosis with reticulate, supple scarring: a neutrophilic dermatosis. Journal of the American Academy of Dermatology 32: 203–206

57. Selimoglu M A, Dilmen U, Karakelleoglu C et al 1995 Harlequin color change. Archives of Pediatric and Adolescent Medicine 149: 1171–1172

58. Stanford D, Rogers M 2000 Dermatological presentations of infantile myofibro-matosis: a review of 27 cases. Australasian Journal of Dermatology 41: 156–161

59. Tallman B 1991 Location of port-wine stain and the likelihood of ophthalmic and/or central nervous system complications. Pediatrics 87: 323–327

60. Weston W L, Morelli J, Lee L A 1999 The clinical spectrum of anti-Ro-positive cutaneous neonatal lupus erythematosus. Journal of the American Academy of Dermatology 40: 675–681

CHAPTER 34

Neonatal ophthalmology

Alistair R Fielder, Esther J Posner

The eye at birth and early visual development

At full term the eye is relatively well developed; the axial length is about 16–17 mm, compared with 24 mm for the average adult eye. Most of eye growth occurs in the first 3 years, although there is some increase in length of the eye over the first two decades. The front of the eye is relatively well developed at full term and reaches adult dimensions during early infancy. Similarly, the posterior section of the eye, the area including the optic disc and macula, grows little during childhood, so that most of eye growth takes place in the retinal periphery, just behind the lens. This arrangement permits growth to take place with minimal interruption to vision.

While the eye is growing the refractive state of the eye is changing and it is not surprising that during this period transient refractive aberrations occur. Most newborn infants are mildly hypermetropic, although premature infants tend to be transiently myopic. Astigmatism is common in infancy, but along with many other refractive errors at this time tends to reduce during early childhood.[12,91,117] Emmetropisation is the name given to this trend towards emmetropia (no refractive error). It is genetically and environmentally influenced and is fine-tuned by visual feedback. Emmetropisation may be disturbed by certain pathological conditions, such as congenital retinal dystrophies[178] and retinopathy of prematurity (ROP).[121]

The visual pathways are not fully developed at birth. While the peripheral retina is relatively well developed at this time, development of the macular region is not complete for about 4 years.[78,188] Maturational changes along the optic nerve[114] and posterior visual pathways[62] continue for several years after birth.

The immaturity of foveal cones and postreceptoral pathways is reflected by the low level of acuity in babies. At birth, babies can follow a coarse visual target. More sophisticated measures of visual acuity such as forced-choice preferential looking or neurophysiological techniques have shown that visual acuity develops rapidly, so that at 3 months it is about 6/60, reaching 6/18 by 1 year of age, with adult levels being achieved by 4–5 years.[44,168] Preterm birth neither hastens nor retards visual development, but it is critical that the clinician appreciates that visual acuity develops according to gestational age rather than postnatal age. Failure to appreciate this results in the ex-preterm infant being considered as being visually unresponsive: thus the visual acuity of a 28-week gestational age baby at 14 weeks postnatal age should be that of a baby 2 weeks post-term.[146,180] Other visual functions also mature during infancy, but colour vision is rather well developed by 3 months of age and binocular vision also appears around this time.

Abnormal visual development

Amblyopia

Amblyopia is defined as a reduction of visual acuity that results from an obstacle to visual development. The word 'development' is key because the developing visual system alone has a degree of plasticity, so that it is only during this period that blurred vision can cause amblyopia, and plasticity permits improvement if treated. Also included in the definition, and rather confusingly, the visual defect cannot be explained by physical examination of the eye itself and amblyopia persists after the obstacle to visual development has been removed. For instance, following surgery for congenital cataract, the vision will remain reduced despite optical correction. The deficit that remains after surgery is amblyopia, and will persist unless specific treatment is instituted. The neural basis of amblyopia lies in the striate visual cortex, although extrastriate areas may also be involved.[13]

Amblyopia is the commonest cause of visual loss in childhood, affecting 2–5% of children, and is classified according to its associations (Table 34.1). The causes of amblyopia are: refractive

Table 34.1 Classification of amblyopia

Amblyopia type	Proportion of all amblyopia in childhood (%)
Anisometropia	20
Strabismus	35
Mixed anisometropia and strabismus	40
Form deprivation	3–5

error (usually unilateral – anisometropia), strabismus and form (stimulus) deprivation (any lesion obstructing vision – cataract, ptosis, haemangioma of the eyelid, etc.). Amblyopia is usually unilateral but can affect both eyes.

Amblyopia types are listed in Table 34.1 (an approximate guide) and they refer to the childhood period as a whole. So, while form deprivation is the least frequent type of amblyopia in childhood, in infancy it is the most common and profound type of amblyopia. Ideally, complete unilateral ptosis, congenital cataracts and glaucoma should be detected and treated in early infancy. The routine neonatal examination includes assessment of the red reflex (p. 839), and screening for signs of visual problems should continue during infancy.[74] Parents should be questioned about their child's visual behaviour, and examination of babies should include their ability to fix and track (p. 847).

Broadly, the treatment of amblyopia has three phases:

1. removal of any obstacle to clear vision (e.g. cataract)
2. correction of any refractive error so that the retina receives a clear and focused image
3. patching of the preferred eye until vision is equal in the two eyes.

The visually unresponsive infant

The commonest cause of a visually unresponsive infant is delayed visual maturation (DVM). This is a diagnosis of exclusion.

Most (80–85%) childhood vision impairment has its origins before or at birth, and once the perinatal period has passed risk of a severe vision impairment has reduced significantly. The major cause of vision impairment in childhood in the UK is cortical (cerebral) vision impairment (CVI). Low birthweight contributes disproportionately to childhood visual impairment.[35,138] More than 65% of children with vision impairment have additional impairments.[35] These data refer to most high-income countries but do not reflect the pattern of childhood vision impairment in middle- and low-income countries.

The conditions that may cause the infant and child not to see well can be broadly subdivided into those conditions that are associated with an obvious ophthalmic abnormality and those that are not (Table 34.2). Such a simplistic approach has its limitations,

but two major points are worth emphasising. First, disorders of the front of the eye are relatively obvious. Second, many optic nerve and retinal disorders are either subtle and easily missed (are included in both categories) or do not have an ophthalmoscopic abnormality. So, the infant who cannot see but who does not have an obvious ocular abnormality may still have an optic nerve or retinal disorder.

Congenital ocular motor apraxia does not cause vision impairment, but is included because the absence of horizontal eye movements can be misinterpreted as visual unresponsiveness.

Delayed visual maturation

The term DVM describes the infant who is visually unresponsive in early infancy but who subsequently improves (Table 34.3).

Delayed visual maturation is not a single entity but a broad clinical spectrum.[52,54,148] So, while most babies who present as being blind are otherwise normal (type 1 DVM), some have major neurodevelopmental or ophthalmic disorders. This is important because, while infants with Type 1 DVM improve to develop normal vision, those with types 2–4 do not, the outcome being determined by the severity of the ocular or neurological condition.

The clinical features are as follows: all infants with DVM are behaviourally visually unresponsive and fail to smile or follow a visual stimulus. For infants in whom there are no neurological or ocular abnormalities (type 1 DVM) ophthalmic examination is

Table 34.3 Types of delayed visual maturation

Type 1	DVM as an isolated anomaly A. Normal perinatal period B. With perinatal problems
Type 2	DVM associated with obvious and persistent neurodevelopmental problems
Type 3	DVM associated with infantile nystagmus including albinism
Type 4	DVM associated with severe congenital, bilateral structural abnormalities (excluding albinism)

Table 34.2 The visually unresponsive infant – aetiology

'Obvious' ophthalmic abnormality	No 'obvious' ophthalmic abnormality
Anterior segment of the eye Maldevelopment (e.g. corneal opacity, aniridia) Cataract **Posterior segment of the eye** Coloboma Optic nerve hypoplasia Optic atrophy Cicatrical retinopathy of prematurity *And others* **Acute intracranial pathology**	**Posterior segment of the eye** Albinism Congenital achromatopsia Leber's amaurosis Optic nerve hypoplasia Optic atrophy **Neurological** Delayed visual maturation Cortical vision impairment 'Congenital ocular motor apraxia' **Acute intracranial pathology**

normal and there is no nystagmus. These (type 1) infants exhibit rapid visual improvement between 3 and 5 months of age, frequently over a very short time (a day or so), and from that time vision is normal and there are no developmental sequelae.[176] The term DVM was confined solely to this category until the broader spectrum became apparent. Transient oscillations may be seen in some infants but nystagmus is not a feature in type 1 DVM, although it appears around the time of improvement in type 3. Nystagmus is also a feature in type 4 DVM and is present even before vision improves.

The time and speed of visual improvement in infants with type 3 DVM (typically the infant with albinism) is similar to that which occurs in DVM type 1 but is differentiated by the development of nystagmus in type 3. For children with severe neurodevelopmental (type 2) or ocular problems (type 4) the improvement can take many months and is incomplete. For infants with type 1 DVM, the electroretinogram and pattern visually evoked potentials are normal compared to age matched controls.[105]

It is unlikely that a common underlying pathogenesis links all DVM types. In types 1 and 3, the retinogeniculostriate pathways are intact but deficits of subcortical and/or higher cortical functions[32,148] or a cortical maturational delay[86] have all been suggested. The mechanism of improvement in types 2 and 4 is unknown.

Delayed visual maturation is a complex clinical spectrum and the diagnosis can only be made with certainty once vision has improved.[161] However, DVM is the most common cause of vision impairment in early infancy and, if there are no ocular or systemic associations, the outlook is excellent.

Common eye problems in the neonate

Several transient ocular abnormalities may be found on routine examination of the neonate and are of no serious significance. Bruising of the face, including the lids, and subconjunctival and retinal haemorrhages are common immediately after birth and resolve spontaneously. Transient ocular motor abnormalities are also common in the first few weeks of life.

Premature babies may show additional abnormalities that are related to their low gestational age and immaturity of ocular development. In babies born at 26 weeks of gestation or less the lids are often fused but are easily separated. Similarly, in early extrauterine life the lens is vascularised, and this vascularisation (tunica vasculosa lentis) is frequently seen in premature babies and may be used to assess gestational age (p. 844). The vessels gradually regress and regression is usually complete by 34 weeks.[82] Other transient abnormalities seen in premature infants include lens vacuoles,[112] mild corneal clouding, vitreous haze and persistence of the hyaloid artery.

Conjunctivitis is common in the neonate and is considered in detail on page 797. Gonococcal ophthalmia remains rare in the UK, but *Chlamydia* is common and early and appropriate treatment is essential in order to prevent pneumonia.

Ocular motor abnormalities

Strabismus

The eyes of babies often appear to be divergent but this is probably a consequence of eye shape at this age.[172] Intermittent squints are common in the first few weeks of life.[87,120] Transient VIth nerve palsies,[15,143] which may be related to birth trauma, and transient disorders of vertical gaze may also be seen.[87] Any constant squint persisting after the age of 6 weeks should be referred to an ophthalmologist. Strabismus may also be the presenting sign of unilateral visual loss, for example in unilateral congenital cataract or retinoblastoma, hence the need for early referral.

Convergent strabismus (esotropia)

The commonest form of persistent strabismus in early infancy is infantile (congenital) esotropia with its onset around two to four months. In this disorder there is a large-angled convergent squint, which is often alternating. Other rare causes of esotropia in infancy include VIth nerve palsy, Duane's retraction syndrome or Moebius' syndrome, but in each case there is defective abduction of the affected eye.

Divergent strabismus

Far less common than convergent squints, but if persistent may indicate neurological or visual impairment.

Vertical strabismus

Vertical squints are only rarely evident in the neonatal period, except in the case of congenital IIIrd nerve palsy, when the marked ptosis is usually the presenting sign. Other causes, such as superior oblique palsy, Brown's syndrome and double elevator palsy, usually present with an abnormal head posture in later infancy or childhood.[49]

Nystagmus

Sustained nystagmus is rare in the first few weeks after birth, although a few beats are frequently seen. Nystagmus is classified as: physiological, associated with neurological conditions, sensory deprivation, infantile nystagmus, spasmus nutans and special types of nystagmus.

Central nervous system conditions – neurological nystagmus

Nystagmus can occur in many central nervous system conditions, such as cerebellar, brainstem and vestibular lesions, and may develop at any age. Roving eye movements have been reported in association with intraventricular haemorrhage.[45]

Sensory deprivation nystagmus

Bilaterally reduced vision in infancy and early childhood results in nystagmus, but only if the lesion involves the anterior visual pathway thus, nystagmus is not a feature of cortical blindness.[182] Conditions include: ocular and optic nerve pathology. Nystagmus due to reduced vision does not usually develop until about 3 months of age.

Infantile (congenital) nystagmus

The term 'infantile nystagmus' should be reserved for nystagmus presenting in infancy that is not associated with ocular or neurological pathology – a diagnosis of exclusion. Infantile nystagmus is sometimes referred to as motor nystagmus to avoid confusion with nystagmus due to sensory deprivation. The condition may be inherited as a dominant, recessive or X-linked disorder.

Spasmus nutans

This syndrome consists of the triad of nystagmus, head nodding and torticollis, commences between 4 and 18 months of age and usually resolves within 1–2 years. Not all features are present simultaneously. Although the nystagmus of spasmus nutans is usually bilateral, it can be asymmetrical and either horizontal or vertical. Infants with spasmus nutans can have intracranial tumours[5] and a full neurological assessment is mandatory.[70,71]

Special nystagmus types

Many other types of nystagmus not considered here may have important neurological implications – such as downbeat, upbeat, see-saw, dissociated (e.g. in internuclear ophthalmoplegia), ocular bobbing, and retraction nystagmus.

The investigation of nystagmus

Nystagmus may be the first sign of a serious neurological or ocular disorder. The pattern of eye movement must be carefully evaluated but accurate diagnosis is rarely possible from the observation of the nystagmus pattern alone. Because the incidence of neurological and visual pathway disorders is high and these cannot always be differentiated on a clinical basis, all infants with nystagmus should have a full ophthalmic and paediatric–neurological assessment, which includes electrophysiological investigations (electroretinogram and visual evoked potential) and frequently neuroimaging.

Ocular motor apraxia

In this disorder there is an inability to generate horizontal fast (saccadic) eye movements; vertical saccades are normal.[76] Infants with this disorder may be thought to have severe visual loss because they are unable to move their eyes to the left or right, although they can look up and down. After around 6 months the infant develops the characteristic head thrust, which is used to place the eyes so that they can view a new object of interest.[51]

Motor delay is a very frequent association and reduces throughout childhood but does not always fully resolve. Older children with this disorder show an absence of horizontal saccades and the typical head thrusts. Ocular motor apraxia may be associated with structural abnormalities of the central nervous system or, rarely, be seen in association with brain-stem tumour.[156]

Other eye movement disorders

Transient disorders of vertical gaze may be seen in healthy neonates but do not persist beyond a few weeks.[87] Vertical-gaze palsies may be seen in infantile hydrocephalus and preterm babies with intraventricular haemorrhage,[165] when the lids may be retracted and the eyes deviated downwards (the 'setting sun sign'). This disorder, which is thought to be caused by pressure on the vertical gaze centre by an enlarged third ventricle, usually resolves after shunt surgery but may recur with shunt blockage.

Ocular flutter, in which there are intermittent rapid bursts of horizontal saccades or opsoclonus, in which both horizontal and vertical saccadic abnormalities occur, may be seen in infants with encephalitis or, rarely, as a remote effect of neuroblastoma. Often chaotic eye movements are seen, which may be associated with tremor of the arms or legs. The eye movements usually resolve spontaneously or will respond to adrenocorticotrophic hormone.

Congenital abnormalities of the globe

A failure of the development of the optic vesicle in early embryonic life may give rise to anophthalmos, microphthalmos or ocular colobomata. Other developmental disorders of the globe, such as aniridia, congenital glaucoma and congenital cataract, may also present in early infancy.

Anophthalmos and microphthalmos

In anophthalmos there is complete absence of the globe; the orbit is usually small and the palpebral fissure narrow, often with partial fusion of the eyelids. A computed tomography or magnetic resonance scan of the orbit may be necessary to demonstrate that the globes are completely absent. Most cases are sporadic, although anophthalmos may be seen in chromosomal disorders, especially trisomy 13 (p. 786) and rarely may be inherited, when it is seen as the severe end of a spectrum of ocular malformation that includes microphthalmos and coloboma. Anophthalmos, like microphthalmos and coloboma, may be seen in association with a number of other congenital malformations.[75]

Microphthalmos, in which the globes are smaller than normal, is more common. Mild cases may have completely normal vision but in severe microphthalmos the eye may be effectively blind. Many cases have associated ocular colobomata and, in some cases, there are associated orbital cysts, which may cause proptosis or distend the lower lid. Most cases are sporadic but autosomal dominant, autosomal recessive and X-linked inheritance have been described, as have a variety of associated malformations.[179]

Ocular coloboma

Failure of closure of the fetal eye fissure in early development gives rise to ocular coloboma. This may affect the iris, lens, retina, choroid and optic nerve. Vision ranges from normal to blindness. There is considerable variation but the typical case shows absence of the iris inferiorly so that the pupil is keyhole-shaped. Chorioretinal defects are seen as white areas in the inferior fundus.

Ocular colobomata are usually sporadic but may be inherited as an autosomal dominant trait. They are also commonly seen in chromosomal abnormalities and in a variety of other genetic syndromes, including the CHARGE syndrome (p. 794), Aicardi's syndrome, focal dermal hypoplasia and Lenz's microphthalmos syndrome.[125]

Congenital cataract

Cataract is the commonest cause of treatable blindness in children worldwide.[60] Severe visual impairment from cataract in the industrialised world is becoming less common with earlier detection and more effective treatment, although congenital cataract remains difficult to detect with the current routine neonatal examination system.[137,139] The best results are achieved if surgery and visual rehabilitation are performed soon after birth, before form deprivation amblyopia becomes established. Thus, any abnormal red reflex needs urgent referral to an ophthalmologist.

Aetiology is diverse[103] and can be established in up to 50% with bilateral cataract but in a smaller number with unilateral cataract. The causes of congenital cataract include:

- idiopathic – accounting for more than 90% of unilateral and nearly 40% of bilateral congenital cataracts; some may represent new autosomal dominant mutations[140]
- hereditary – most are autosomal dominant, although X-linked and autosomal recessive cases have also been reported, which are usually bilateral[61]
- metabolic – e.g. galactosaemia (p. 911)
- congenital infections – e.g. rubella and toxoplasmosis (pp. 1067–9) (Fig. 34.1)
- associated with systemic syndromes – e.g. Conradi's syndrome, Hallermann–Streiff syndrome, Lowe's syndrome.[26]

Management depends on whether the cataract is felt to be visually significant, as this would then result in dense stimulus deprivation amblyopia.[109,167] If this is the case, early surgery is required, within the first few weeks after birth.[18] Early optical correction in babies is essential and is usually achieved by contact lenses, although intraocular lens implantation is increasingly used and is standard for cataract surgery in older children. There are benefits of this approach but also significant problems.[102,106,127] In the developing world, however, intraocular lenses may be the most suitable form of visual correction.[184,187] Following surgery,

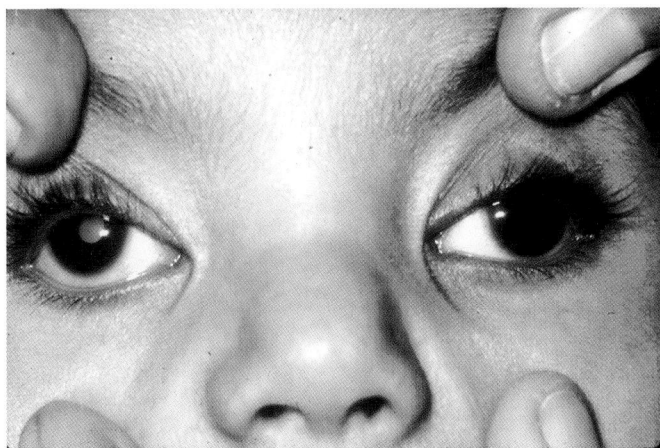

Fig. 34.1 Appearances of a cataract due to congenital rubella.

the greatest threat to vision is amblyopia and this requires very careful optical correction and ocular occlusion regimes (patching) for many years. The management of infantile cataract requires prolonged intensive effort by the parents, and this must be discussed before surgery.[167]

Congenital glaucoma

Congenital glaucoma is an infrequent condition but remains one of the major causes of preventable blindness in childhood.[162] Presenting at birth, or during early infancy, early recognition and treatment is essential, as the resulting optic disc cupping is reversible and visual prognosis good in the early stages. Most infantile glaucoma is caused by a developmental abnormality in the trabecular meshwork that prevents normal drainage of aqueous humour from the eye and results in raised intraocular pressure. The disease may be classified by aetiology:[177]

- Primary – an isolated anomaly of the iridocorneal angle; accounts for approximately 50% of infantile glaucoma. Most cases are sporadic. Approximately 10% are familial and may be autosomal recessive. Polygenic or multifactorial aetiologies have also been suggested, particularly as boys are preferentially affected.[150] Infantile glaucoma as an isolated abnormality is usually bilateral but can be asymmetrical (Fig. 34.2).
- Associated with ocular and/or systemic disease, including:
  - aphakia – usually following congenital cataract extraction
  - malformations of the anterior segment of the eye such as neural crest dysgenesis (Rieger's syndrome, Peters' anomaly), Marfan's syndrome, aniridia
  - metabolic disease – Lowe's syndrome
  - inflammatory – congenital rubella
  - syndromes associated with glaucoma – Rubinstein–Taybi and Down's syndromes, neurofibromatosis
  - secondary glaucoma – homocystinuria, Weill–Marchesani syndrome, persistent hyperplastic primary vitreous (PHPV), severe ROP.

The most severe cases usually present in the neonatal period. Raised intraocular pressure causes corneal oedema, manifest

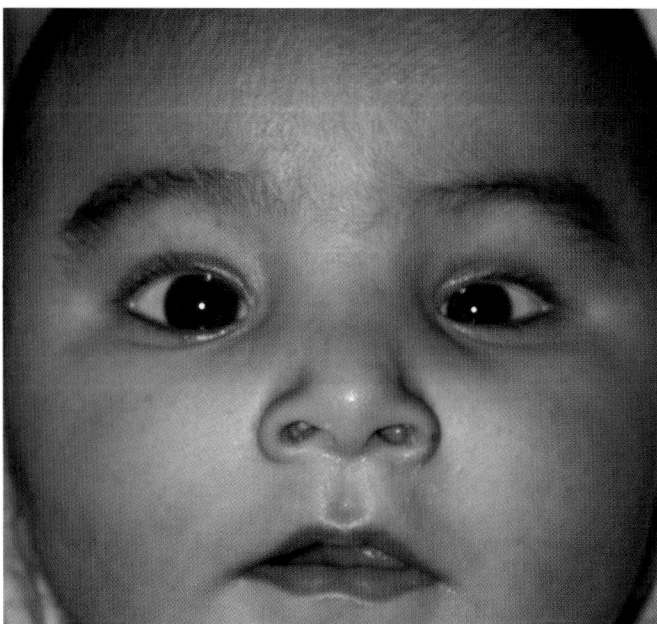

Fig. 34.2 Congenital glaucoma of the right eye.

as corneal clouding and progressive globe enlargement (buphthalmos), which are the most common presenting features (Fig. 34.2).[153] Corneal enlargement is a subtle sign, especially if bilateral. Optic disc cupping develops, with gradual loss of visual field and visual acuity. There is a classic triad of symptoms – photophobia, excess tearing and blepharospasm. It is clearly of critical importance that the symptoms are not confused with the much commoner and benign congenital nasolacrimal duct obstruction, which typically presents with watering eyes that are also sticky, but in which the eyes are not red and there is no photosensitivity or corneal enlargement.

Treatment is surgical and usually requires repeat examinations under anaesthesia for some years to assess intraocular pressure, corneal diameters and optic disc morphology. A major cause of visual loss in infantile glaucoma is amblyopia and this requires careful monitoring and treatment.[14]

Aniridia

This is a rare bilateral congenital anomaly in which the iris is either clinically absent or markedly underdeveloped. All affected infants have nystagmus and are visually disabled. Other ocular anomalies seen in aniridia include corneal changes, cataract, ectopia lentis, foveal and optic nerve hypoplasia.

Most cases of aniridia are inherited as an autosomal dominant trait with almost complete penetrance but variable expressivity. Approximately 20% of sporadic aniridia cases develop Wilms' tumour (nephroblastoma, p. 958) by 3 years of age. The PAX6 gene has been identified as the aniridia gene,[94] situated on the short arm of chromosome 11. This site encompasses a contiguous set of genes, including PAX6 and a Wilms' tumour gene, WT1, and a deletion at this locus appears to trigger tumour development.[72] Clinical and genetic analysis in these patients is

therefore of importance in assessing the risk of developing a Wilms' tumour.[36]

Other developmental abnormalities of the anterior segment

There are other rare malformations of the anterior segment of the eye.[48] In megalocornea the cornea is enlarged but the normal intraocular pressure differentiates this from congenital glaucoma. Bilateral corneal oedema without glaucoma is seen in a rare inherited ocular disorder, congenital hereditary endothelial dystrophy.

In Peters' anomaly there is a central corneal opacity with adhesions between the iris and posterior cornea; there may be associated glaucoma. Most cases are bilateral and are not associated with any systemic abnormalities. However, in Peters' plus syndrome the ocular abnormalities may be associated with a variety of systemic malformations, including cleft lip and palate, developmental delay and congenital heart disease. Some cases of Peters' anomaly are associated with mutations of the PAX6 gene.

Rieger's anomaly is a developmental abnormality of the eye in which there is hypoplasia of the iris stroma.[157] The pupil is often misshapen and eccentric, and there may be more than one pupil. Iridocorneal adhesions and peripheral corneal opacities are common. Glaucoma may complicate the disorder in infancy or childhood. Rieger's anomaly may be inherited as an autosomal dominant trait, but many cases have no family history. In Rieger's syndrome the ocular phenotype is accompanied by a number of systemic abnormalities, including facial and dental abnormalities, umbilical hernia and hypospadias. Rieger's syndrome is inherited as an autosomal dominant trait and exhibits very variable expression. Mutations have been identified in a novel homoeobox gene in some patients with Rieger's syndrome.[154] In sclerocornea there is peripheral corneal opacification and vascularisation which, if extensive, may involve the central cornea. It is usually seen as an isolated ocular abnormality.

Albinism

Melanin plays a vital role in ocular development. Albinism is a disorder resulting from a deficiency in melanin biosynthesis and results in characteristic ocular abnormalities (Fig. 34.3). Involvement of the skin, hair and eyes is termed oculocutaneous albinism[20] whereas involvement of the eye alone is called ocular albinism. Inheritance may be autosomal recessive or X-linked (ocular albinism). Progress in unravelling the underlying genetic and molecular pathways[123] will allow accurate prognostic information as well as genetic counselling. Babies with skin involvement need expert dermatological advice, and their skin must be protected with sunscreen.

There are two main types of oculocutaneous albinism: tyrosinase negative and positive. The latter children have slightly more pigment than tyrosinase-negative children and their skin and hair

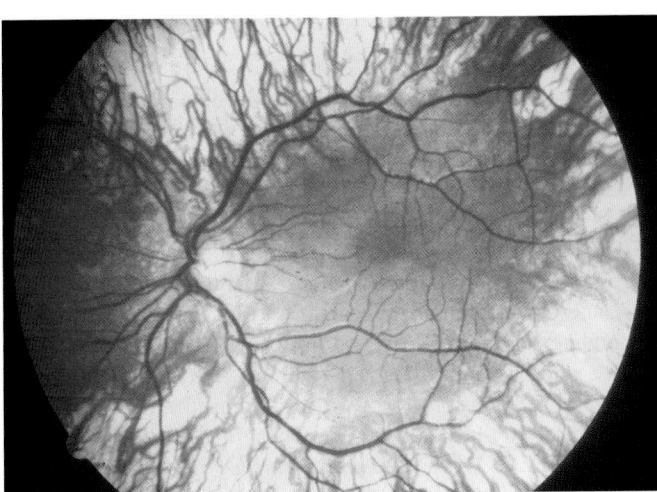

Fig. 34.3 The fundus in albinism.

darken to some extent with time. The clinical manifestations of albinism include: iris translucency, abnormally blond fundus and foveal hypoplasia which is the main cause of reduced visual acuity. Affected individuals develop nystagmus. The degree of hypopigmentation depends on the genetic subtype, race and age. In general visual acuity parallels the degree of pigmentation. Babies with albinism are frequently visually unresponsive in the first few weeks after birth, with vision improving around the time that there is visual improvement at 3–8 months of life – a form of DVM.[176] There is abnormal decussation of nerve fibres at the optic chiasm – essentially, all, instead of 50%, visual pathway fibres decussate which can be confirmed by visual evoked potential studies.[4]

There are two rare genetic disorders associated with albinism that are important to diagnose:

- Hermansky–Pudlak syndrome is associated with a bleeding disorder and the accumulation of ceroid-like material in different tissues including the lungs[163]
- Chédiak–Higashi syndrome is characterised by impaired immunity resulting in increased susceptibility to bacterial infection and malignancy and progressive neurologic abnormalities.[22]

Optic nerve anomalies

Optic nerve hypoplasia is a non-progressive developmental abnormality in which the affected optic nerve is smaller than normal with fewer axons. It is a significant cause of childhood vision impairment.[92,115] Vision ranges from good to complete blindness.

Optic nerve hypoplasia has also been reported in association with maternal intake of certain drugs, such as phenytoin, LSD, quinine, alcohol and crack cocaine[175] and may be more common in infants born to diabetic mothers and young primiparous parents.[135] Two genes have recently been implicated including the *PAX6* gene – which is expressed in many different ocular tissues and in the central nervous system during development.[10,164]

Optic nerve hypoplasia may be associated with midline brain abnormalities, especially absence of the septum pellucidum. Neuroendocrine dysfunction, particularly growth hormone deficiency of hypothyroidism, develops in up to 30% of children.[152] As this may not become apparent until 2–5 years of age, surveillance is required. While magnetic resonance imaging scanning in infants with optic nerve hypoplasia may help predict those who will develop later endocrine problems,[19,24] the absence of a septum pellucidum does not predict intellectual, behavioural or neurological deficits.[183]

Lid and orbital disorders

These are uncommon in the neonatal period.

Ptosis is the commonest disorder. The pathogenesis remains uncertain, although most agree that the primary defect is in the levator palpebrae superioris.[11] It is usually an isolated defect in a healthy child, although it may be associated with other anomalies and various chromosomal and inheritance patterns, for example congenital fibrosis of the extraocular muscles, the blepharophimosis syndrome, Marcus Gunn's jaw-winking syndrome.[11,149] Other neurogenic causes include congenital Horner's syndrome or IIIrd nerve palsy. Mechanical ptosis may result from lid masses. Treatment of primary congenital ptosis is surgical but this is rarely required before the age of 4–5 years unless the pupillary axis is obscured, in which case there is a risk of amblyopia developing and correction is required immediately.

Vascular lesions may affect the eyelids and orbit and can essentially be divided into haemangiomas and vascular malformations such as port-wine stains and lymphangiomas.[63] The vast majority of haemangiomas occur in isolation, although Sturge–Weber syndrome should be excluded when the ophthalmic division of the trigeminal nerve is involved (p. 830). Capillary haemangiomas may not be visible at birth, especially if this is preterm, but all are present within a few weeks. They undergo a phase of rapid growth in the first 3–6 months and regress slowly over the ensuing 7 years or so. Indications for treatment are usually for vision-threatening lesions or poor cosmesis, and treatment includes systemic and intralesional steroids, laser for superficial vascular malformations (port-wine stains), surgery, sclerotherapy and embolisation for malformations affecting the orbit and adnexa.[63,69,124,159]

Other lid conditions affecting babies include epiblepharon, an exuberant fold of skin that pushes the normal lower lid lashes against the cornea. This is relatively common, especially in Oriental babies, and usually resolves spontaneously.

Proptosis in the neonatal period may occur as the result either of shallow orbits in craniofacial disorders, e.g. Crouzon's syndrome, Apert's syndrome or vascular malformations, and rarely of a tumour such as retinoblastoma or neuroblastoma.

Nasolacrimal duct obstruction

This affects up to 20% of babies and results from failure of the nasolacrimal duct to open into the inferior meatus at the level of the valve of Hasner. It presents with persistent watery and sticky eye in the first few weeks after birth. Massage over the lacrimal sac area may accelerate opening of the lower end of the duct.[166] In most cases there is spontaneous resolution by 12–15 months of age but if symptoms persist probing and syringing of the lacrimal system may be indicated.

Congenital dacryocele or lacrimal sac mucocele is uncommon and appears within few days after birth as a tense bluish swelling of the lacrimal sac. It may disappear on compression, or become infected, in which case treatment by systemic antibiotics is required. Following this alarming infective episode, almost all cases resolve completely.

Retinal disorders

Leber's congenital amaurosis

This is one of the more common inherited causes of blindness in childhood[130] and is inherited by the autosomal recessive mode. Leber's amaurosis usually presents in early infancy with poor vision from birth and nystagmus. The pupillary responses are abnormal. The fundus is often normal early on, although later in life a variety of appearances may be seen, such as a pigmentary retinopathy or a retinitis pigmentosa-like appearance. The diagnosis has to be made by electrophysiological studies with a markedly diminished or absent electroretinogram. Several genes have been identified,[95] which are thought to account for about half of all cases.

Leber's amaurosis mostly occurs in otherwise normal children but it may be associated with systemic disorders, particularly neurodevelopmental conditions. On brain imaging, several different abnormalities have been seen – most consistently hypoplasia of the cerebellar vermis.[119] This can also be seen in other entities, such as Joubert's syndrome, in which Leber's amaurosis is also seen. Clinical appearances similar in many ways to Leber's amaurosis have also been reported in association with renal abnormalities particularly juvenile nephronophthisis,[80] and peroxisomal disorders (pp. 1170–2) such as infantile Refsum's disease, Zellweger's syndrome and infantile leukodystrophy.

As there are a number of other disorders that can present with similar ocular features to Leber's congenital amaurosis, thorough systemic evaluation and electrophysiological studies are usually necessary to differentiate them.

Retinoblastoma

This is the most common primary intraocular tumour of childhood, with an incidence of about 1 per 20 000 live births. The most common presenting features are leukocoria (white pupil), strabismus and glaucoma. The average age at diagnosis is 18 months but the diagnosis has been made prenatally. Retinoblastoma is described in more detail on pages 956–8. A gene therapy trial has started in the USA.[89]

There are a number of other conditions that may present with leukocoria (Table 34.4, Fig. 34.4).

Retinal dysplasia

This is caused by failure of the retina to develop normally during embryonic life. It is characterised by the presence at birth of a retrolental mass in a (usually) microphthalmic eye. Unilateral cases are usually solitary but bilateral involvement can occur in Norrie's disease, Patau's syndrome (p. 782), incontinentia pigmenti (Bloch–Sulzberger syndrome, pp. 1005–6),[84] Warburg's syndrome, osteoporosis-pseudoglioma–mental retardation syndrome and chromosomal abnormalities, especially trisomy 13.

The gene for Norrie's disease has been identified[16,21,28] and accurate genetic counselling is possible. A mutation in the gene may also be responsible for a separate clinical entity, X-linked (or very rarely dominantly inherited) familial exudative vitreoretinopathy (FEVR).[27,155] This resembles ROP in a larger and often

Table 34.4 Causes of leukocoria in the neonate

Retinoblastoma
Congenital cataract
Retinal dysplasia
Persistent hyperplastic primary vitreous (PHPV)
Retinopathy of prematurity – end stage (ROP)
Optic nerve coloboma

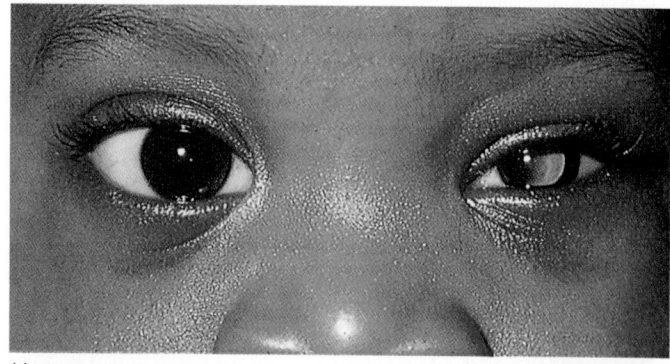
(a)

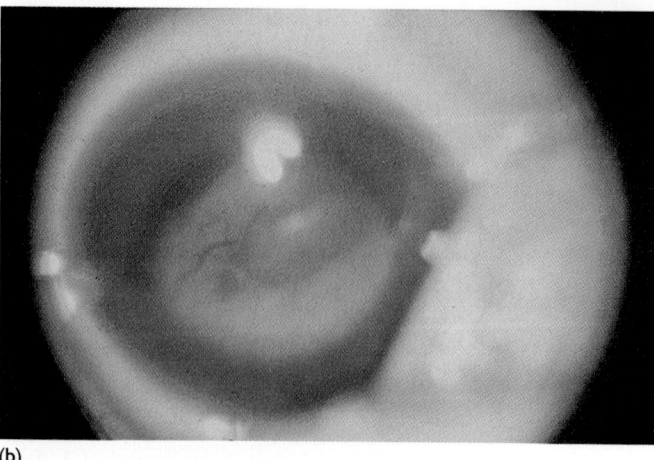
(b)

Fig. 34.4 (a) Infant with leukocoria of the left eye. (b) Infant with leukocoria due to a total retinal detachment.

full-term baby or infant. Both incontinentia pigmenti and FEVR have a acute proliferative phase rather similar to that seen in ROP and treatment by laser has been recommended.[185]

Persistent hyperplastic primary vitreous

This is caused by a failure of regression of the primary vitreous and can be divided into anterior and posterior types. Anterior persistent hyperplastic primary vitreous (PHPV) is much more common and is fortunately unilateral in 90% of cases. It is characterised by a retrolental mass. There may be associated microphthalmos, cataract and secondary glaucoma. The visual prognosis is very poor.

Retinopathy of prematurity

Retinopathy of prematurity was first described in 1942 by Terry.[171] Although potentially blinding, much sight-threatening ROP can be prevented by meticulous neonatal care, and blindness can largely be prevented by ophthalmic screening and treatment.

Table 34.5 Classification of retinopathy of prematurity

Stage 1	Demarcation line
Stage 2	Ridge
Stage 3	Ridge with extraretinal fibrovascular proliferation
Stage 4	Subtotal retinal detachment
	a) Extrafoveal
	b) Involving the fovea
Stage 5	Total retinal detachment

From Committee for the Classification of Retinopathy of Prematurity 1984 The international classification of retinopathy of prematurity. British Journal of Ophthalmology 68: 690–697.

Retinal vascular development

Retinal vascularisation commences at about 15 weeks' gestation and proceeds from the optic disc towards the retinal periphery.[134] The nasal retina is vascularised by about 32 weeks, and the temporal retina by about 37–40 weeks gestational age. It is at the advancing edge of retinal vascularisation that acute ROP develops.

Describing retinopathy of prematurity

Acute-phase ROP is described by the international classification[33,34] by four parameters: severity by stage, location, extent and plus disease, each of which should be recorded at every examination (Table 34.5).

There are five ROP stages (Table 34.5, Fig. 34.5). Stages 1 and 2 are referred to as mild ROP (Fig. 34.5a) and if they do not progress to stage 3 will resolve without sight-threatening sequelae. Stages 3 (Fig. 34.5c) to 5 therefore are referred to as severe ROP as stage 3 carries a risk, and stages 4 and 5 the certainty, of a visually disabling outcome.

The retina is divided into three zones, centred on the optic disc, with zone 1 most posterior, zone 3 peripheral and an intermediate zone 2 (Fig. 34.6). Location by zone is one of the most important predictors of outcome. Thus, for ROP in zone 1 over 50% of eyes require treatment[41] often with a poor outcome, whereas ROP in zone 3 hardly ever requires treatment and has a close to zero risk of visual impairment.[99] Disease extent is recorded as though the retinal circumference is divided like a clock face affected (Fig. 34.6).

Plus is the least well documented feature of acute-phase ROP yet it is a key prognostic indicator that ROP is, or may become, severe (Fig. 34.5b). Plus disease is constellation of signs: abnormal dilatation and tortuosity of the posterior retinal vessels, vascular engorgement of the iris blood vessels, pupillary rigidity and vitreous haze.

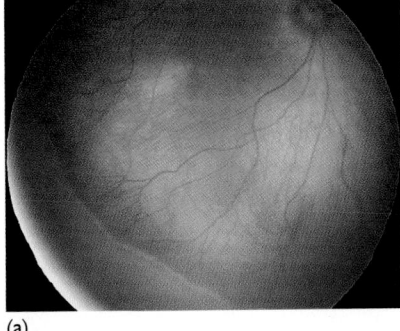 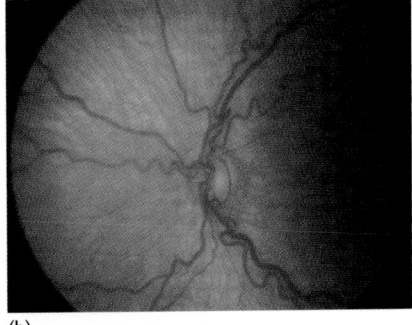 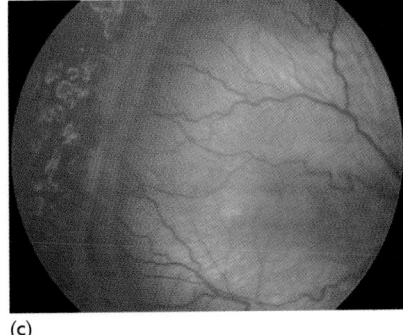

(a) (b) (c)

Fig. 34.5 (a) Stage 1 and 2 ROP. White ridge (stage 2) at the advancing edge of the retinal vessels and lying at the junction of the vascularised and non-vascularised retina. Towards to left, the ridge is flatter, a line of stage 1 ROP. (b) Plus disease. Grossly engorged retinal venules and tortuous retinal arterioles – compare with figure of stage 1 and 2. This baby had severe stage 3 ROP and this can be predicted from the plus disease alone without directly visualising the ROP lesion itself. (c) Stage 3 ROP and treatment. The retinal blood vessels are engorged and tortuous. Towards the left there is a raised neovascular lesion at the junction of the vascularised and non-vascularised retina. This is florid stage 3. Delta-like arborisation of vessels is seen running into the lesion, which is elevated above the retinal surface. This baby has been treated by laser – the pigmented laser lesions can be seen in the non-vascularised retina. The ROP lesion is not treated itself as the aim is to reduce VEGF production in the non-vascularised retina. Images obtained by wide-field digital imaging.

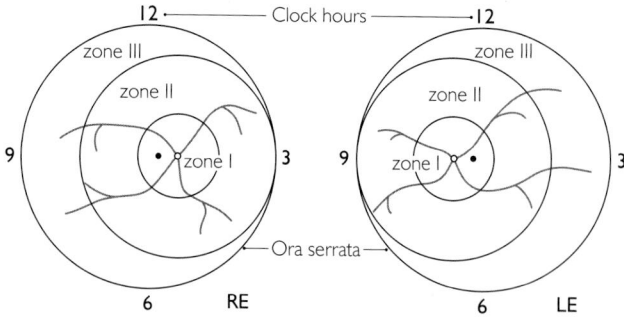

Fig. 34.6 Schematic representation of the retina of both eyes, showing the limits of each zone. The extent of disease may be described in clock hours as shown (the radius of zone I is twice the distance from the edge of the disc to the macula [shown as a black dot in the diagram]).

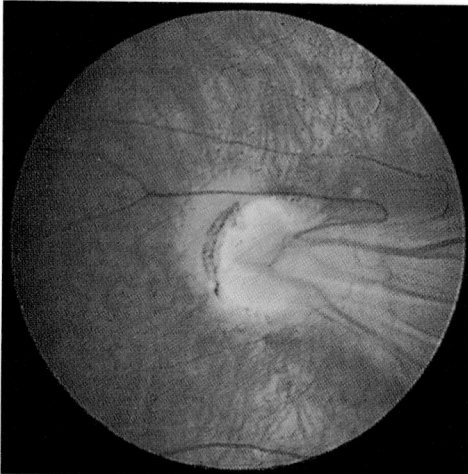

Fig. 34.7 Cicatricial ROP with dragging of the retinal vessels towards the retinal periphery.

All mild ROP undergoes complete regression, while severe ROP leaves retinovascular and cicatricial retinal changes (Fig. 34.7) which may be recorded separately.

Retinopathy of prematurity risk factors

Although the original epidemic of ROP in the 1950s was clearly related to the introduction of oxygen into nurseries, it is now evident ROP is multifactorial. There are several excellent reviews of the subject.[50,57,110,111,181]

Birthweight and gestational age

Retinopathy of prematurity incidence is inversely related to birthweight and gestational age.[58,97,118] About 70–80% of infants with birthweight less than 1000 g[58,118,142] show acute changes, for babies under 1251 g birthweight the incidence of stage 3 is around 18%, 6% of whom required treatment.[126] There is a suggestion[90] but not proven on a large scale, that the incidence of ROP is decreasing. While, in high income countries severe ROP is largely confined to babies under 1000 g birthweight, in middle income countries larger babies may be affected.[53,67]

Oxygen administration

The early studies in the 1950s[98,107] demonstrated that high levels of inspired oxygen was an ROP risk factor. Subsequent reduction of oxygen usage in clinical practice led to a fall in the incidence of severe ROP but was accompanied by increased neonatal mortality[8] and neurological morbidity.[113] It became necessary to attempt to define a safe level of oxygen usage for clinical practice. A multicentre study[97] designed to assess the relationship between arterial oxygen and ROP failed to find any significant difference between PaO_2 values in infants with and without ROP. More recently, a randomised controlled trial comparing continuous transcutaneous oxygen monitoring with standard neonatal care, although showing some benefit in larger infants (>1000 g), demonstrated no difference in the incidence or severity of ROP in infants of birthweight less than 1000 g.[58] A reanalysis of these data found a significant association between the duration of transcutaneous $PO_2 \geqslant 80$ mmHg and the incidence and severity of ROP.[59] Cunningham et al[37] and York et al[186] also confirmed that arterial oxygen levels are critical, particularly within the first few weeks (probably 4–6) after birth.

While no direct relationship has been demonstrated between arterial oxygen levels and ROP,[50] oxygen remains firmly centre stage in ROP pathogenesis. Current neonatal research is exploring the safe upper and lower limits of oxygen arterial saturation. A randomised controlled trial, comparing oxygen saturation ranges of 91–94% against 95–98%, reported no difference in infant growth, neurodevelopment or rates of ROP.[7] Exploring the lower safe limit; a recent study reported that babies with target saturation levels of 94–98% had a much higher incidence of ROP requiring treatment than those nursed with target oxygen levels of 70–90%, with no increase in neurological morbidity in the latter.[173,174] Chow et al[29] reported a fall in the incidence of ROP stage 3 associated with a strict oxygen management regimen that minimised fluctuations and avoided high saturation levels. It is evident that careful control of oxygen administration does reduce the incidence of ROP but it has proved impossible to define a safe level of oxygen.

Surfactant

Surfactant has reduced the severity of respiratory distress syndrome and chronic lung disease but studies have not demonstrated an influence of surfactant on the incidence of ROP.[9,96,129,170]

Exchange transfusions

Several studies[1,30,158] have shown an association between exchange transfusion and the incidence of ROP, but this is not confirmed by all[25] so it is still unclear whether exchange transfusion is an independent risk factor for the development of ROP or purely an indicator of the high-risk neonate.

Vitamin E

Kretzner and Hittner[101] suggested that vitamin E, a naturally occurring antioxidant, might play a role in ROP prophylaxis. Despite several trials of vitamin E supplementation[56,81,93,131] the protective effect of vitamin E has not been clearly demonstrated. Overall, high-dose vitamin E supplementation does not appear to reduce the incidence of ROP, although it may have an effect on the severity of disease. The possible side-effects of treatment, including sepsis, necrotising enterocolitis and intraventricular and retinal haemorrhage,[131] has meant that it is not in routine use. Following a meta-analysis Raju et al[141] reported a reduction in the incidence of stage 3 plus ROP and made a plea for the role of vitamin E in ROP to be re-evaluated.

Ethnic and genetic factors

All very-low-birthweight infants share common risk factors but only a small minority develop severe disease. The factors that underlie disease incidence and severity are ill-understood but significant ethnic differences have been reported.[67,118,151] The genetic basis for ROP susceptibility is poorly understood, but recently Shastry et al[155] have identified missense mutations in the Norrie's disease gene in some patients with advanced ROP. This finding was not confirmed in a recent study, although C597A polymorphisms of the Norrin gene were increased.[73]

Other factors

Other factors have been suggested to be associated with ROP. Acidosis is an ROP risk factor;[133] hypercarbia is not.[64] Prenatal steroids have been reported to be protective for ROP development[79] but postnatal steroids confer no such benefit.[43] Terry[171] suggested that exposure to light might be a causative factor but it took over 40 years for a prospective randomised clinical trial, the LIGHT-ROP study,[145] to demonstrate that light reduction had no effect on the incidence or severity of ROP. Other factors, including recurrent apnoea, hypercapnia, respiratory distress syndrome and blood viscosity, have been suggested as risk factors but none has been confirmed.[111,116]

Pathogenesis of retinopathy of prematurity

There are two largely historical theories of ROP pathogenesis. According to the first – 'classic' – theory developed by Ashton[6] and Patz,[128] ROP consists of two phases of equal importance. First, there is a hyperoxic phase, the phase in oxygen that causes retinal arteriolar constriction, irreversible vaso-obliteration and dissolution of the retinal capillary endothelial cells. This is followed by the second phase, on removal from the hyperoxic environment, the phase in air, which is characterised by a vasoproliferative response and is induced by the ischaemia consequent upon the capillary closure of the first phase.

The second – 'gap junction' – theory, proposed by Kretzer and Hittner[101] is based on the activity of the mesenchymal spindle cell precursors of the retinal capillaries that migrate centrifugally from the optic disc. These cells canalise to form capillaries just behind the advancing vanguard. Under normal in-utero-relative hyperoxic extrauterine conditions, gap junctions appear between adjacent spindle cells. Gap junctions interfere with normal migration and vessel formation and the angiogenic factors secreted by damaged spindle cells trigger the neovascular response.

Current concepts of ROP pathogenesis are a logical extension to both 'classic' and 'gap-junction' theories but with greater understanding of events at a cellular level. The increase of retinal thickness during development creates increased metabolic need and thus local 'physiological' hypoxia in advance of the developing retinal vessels. Astrocytes in this hypoxic region respond by secreting vascular endothelial growth factor (VEGF), which promotes vascular development to meet this increasing metabolic need by stimulating endothelial migration, differentiation and proliferation. Oxygen-dependent VEGF plays a part in all stages of vascular development and works in conjunction with other factors such as oxygen-independent insulin-like growth factor (IGF-1).

Thus, VEGF is secreted in response to physiological hypoxia in the maturing avascular retina, just anterior of the advancing retinal vessels. Neonatal hyperoxia causes shut-down of sections of the retinal vasculature, by apoptosis and excessive capillary regression, resulting in retinal ischaemia. This retinal ischaemia stimulates an overproduction of VEGF, resulting in the neovascularisation known as ROP.[2,132,160] IGF-1 has also been implicated in controlling VEGF activation: when IGF-1 is low, vessels do not grow. Fetal IGF-1, levels of which rise in the second and third trimester, is provided mainly by the placenta. Thus, oxygen-independent IGF-1 and oxygen-dependent VEGF are complementary and synergistic. A low serum IGF-1 is said to predict ROP[77] but IGF-1 is expressed by many tissues and a low serum level therefore could be a general marker of a sick baby at risk of ROP rather than a specific marker for retinal disease.

According to all three theories, there is an oxidative insult so normal vasculogenesis is impeded. Recent research explains why hyperoxia is important in the initial phase and how vascular shutdown is the consequence of oxygen-induced VEGF downregulation.

The epidemics of retinopathy of prematurity

There have been two ROP epidemics.[53,65,66] The first, in the 1940s, was due to high unrestricted, unmonitored oxygen and was brought to an end by oxygen restriction, which followed the discovery that oxygen supplementation was a factor in ROP causation. The second epidemic began in the late 1960s and is ongoing. During the first epidemic, the survival of neonates of less than 1000 g birthweight was around 5–8% and most of the babies blinded during this period were of heavier birthweight. Advances in neonatal care have largely eliminated the risk of severe ROP in babies of more than 1000 g birthweight. The second epidemic involves mainly the very immature neonate, who previously had a low survival rate. The first epidemic could now be considered to be largely preventable while the second currently is not.

The two epidemics are not discrete, historically separated, entities. In high-income countries such as the USA and much of Europe, ROP-induced disability accounts for 3–8% of childhood vision impairment.[138,169] In middle-income communities (e.g. Latin America, eastern Europe) technology permits the increased survival of the preterm baby but limited health resource limit the standard of care.[67] Consequently, babies with a wider range of birthweights and gestational ages are at risk of developing severe ROP and ROP-induced blindness contributes up to

39% of childhood vision impairment. In effect, the current epidemic occurring in middle-income countries contains elements from the first and second epidemics: increased survival, but associated with limited resources that do not permit high quality neonatal care. In contrast, in low-income countries such as Africa and Albania, very few babies survive to develop ROP.[67]

Screening for retinopathy of prematurity

The aim of screening is to ensure timeous identification of babies who require treatment for ROP,[53] mindful that the treatment criteria changed in 2003 (see below). Published clinical guidelines from the UK[147] and USA[3] do not differ greatly, although neither has yet incorporated the recently modified indications for intervention. In high-income communities, severe ROP (stage 3 or higher) is confined to infants of birthweight below 1501 g and less than 32 weeks gestational age, and only these babies need to be examined. The UK guidelines do not include a sickness criterion or recommend the screening of larger babies who have required prolonged oxygen therapy. In the USA screening is recommended for all babies less than 1501 g or with a gestational age of less than 29 weeks. Infants between 1500 g and 2000 g birthweight who had an unstable clinical course, and are considered to be at risk of ROP are examined in the USA but not the UK. In reality, the difference between UK and US criteria is small. In low- and middle-income countries, larger babies are also at risk of developing severe ROP. Thus the UK and US criteria will certainly *not* include all babies at risk.[67] It is essential in these communities, therefore, for the screening net to be cast wider, based on local data.

The onset and progression of ROP is governed predominantly by postconceptional age rather than postnatal age or neonatal events.[55,126] Most babies require treatment between 37 and 39 weeks gestation equivalent,[39,53] with a range from about 32 weeks to 10 weeks after term. Thus, while most current clinical guidelines recommend the commencement of screening between 4 and 7 weeks, Reynolds et al[144] devised an algorithm, based on postconceptional age, for examining the most immature baby later postnatally than the more mature baby.

Practical aspects

Each unit should have a clear protocol so that all infants at risk of severe ROP are identified and screened appropriately by an experienced ophthalmologist. When neonates are transferred between units it is important that the appropriate ROP information is communicated.

The pupils should be dilated with cyclopentolate 0.5% and phenylephrine 2.5%, repeated once, if necessary, 30 minutes before the examination. The use of a lid speculum, binocular indirect ophthalmoscopy and a scleral depressor permits complete examination of the peripheral retina. The results may then be recorded on a standardised form using the international classification. Wide-field digital imaging is increasingly used for ROP screening. (See Figs 34.5a,b,c)

Infants with acute ROP should be reviewed every 1–2 weeks until regression occurs or the threshold for treatment has been reached. Almost all examinations can be undertaken in hospital before the baby is discharged home, which is much more convenient for the family.

Treatment

Cryotherapy, at threshold stage (see below), has been shown to be effective in reducing the progression to blinding disease.[38–40,42] Laser delivery through the indirect ophthalmoscope has allowed the use of laser photocoagulation as an alternative to cryotherapy for the ablation of peripheral retina in ROP.[31] Diode laser therapy is as effective as cryotherapy and has now almost entirely superseded cryotherapy as the preferred treatment modality. While cryotherapy dramatically improved the outcome for severe ROP, it is no panacea, for at 10 years after treatment, 45% of eyes saw 6/60 or less.[42] The need to improve outcome generated the multicentre Early Treatment for Retinopathy of Prematurity Randomized Trial (ETROP), which reported a benefit of treating certain eyes at an earlier stage.[47]

The revised indications for treatment following the publication of ETROP are listed below:

- **Threshold ROP** (as defined by the CRYO-ROP study 1998):[38] At least 5 continuous or 8 cumulative clock hours of stage 3 ROP in zones I or II, in the presence of plus disease. Such eyes should be treated.
- **Prethreshold – type 1** (as defined by ETROP study[47]): Defined as: zone I, any stage of ROP with plus disease; zone I, stage 3 with or without plus disease, or zone II, stage 2 or 3 with plus disease. These eyes have highly active ROP and should be considered for early treatment.
- **Prethreshold – type 2** (as defined by ETROP study[47]): Defined as: zone I, stage 1 or 2 with no plus disease or zone II, stage 3 with no plus disease. These eyes may be followed conservatively unless they become type 1 prethreshold or reach threshold ROP.

The window for treatment is a maximum of 2 weeks and treatment should be undertaken as soon as possible – within 2–3 days of threshold identification. Clearly determining the urgency of treatment requires clinical judgement. Treatment should ideally be performed in the neonatal intensive care unit where there are full neonatal support facilities.

Outcome

Being born early can have many effects on the visual system. These range from the subtle and functionally insignificant to severe visual disability. Sequelae can be attributed to prematurity per se, ROP or neurological damage (see elsewhere).

Preterm birth alone has a mild effect on visual functions so that they are lower compared to control subjects while still falling within the normal range.[17,121] Mild ROP (stages 1 and 2) resolves spontaneously and has no additional adverse effect on visual function. Clearly severe ROP may impact vision.[42,83,121] The outcome following treatment of retinal detachment in advanced disease is poor.[100,136] Children who are born preterm have an increased prevalence of refractive errors, especially myopia.[41,108,121] Mild myopia is a sequela of low birthweight even in the absence of any ROP. Myopia that complicates severe ROP ranges from mild to severe. The prevalence of strabismus is increased by preterm birth and also by ROP stage (even mild ROP) and rises to about 30% for severe disease.[23,83,122] All infants who develop stage 3 ROP, whether or not they require treatment, should be reviewed during early childhood because of the high incidence of visual impairment, strabismus and refractive errors.

Cerebral visual impairment

Severe visual impairment in early infancy may be due to damage to the higher visual pathways. Referred to variously as cortical blindness and cortical visual impairment, the preferred term now is cerebral visual impairment (CVI).[46,68,85,88]

Affected infants have poor visual responses, with absence of normal fixation and following, but normal pupil reactions and usually a normal fundus examination or mild optic atrophy. Nystagmus is rarely present. Electrophysiological testing shows a normal electroretinogram but absent, normal or abnormal visual evoked responses. Computed tomography or magnetic resonance imaging may show abnormalities of the visual cortex or optic radiations but in some cases there is no evidence of structural change. The visual prognosis appears best in those infants with a normal scan.[104]

The causes of CVI include prenatal malformations, intrauterine infection and toxaemia. Perinatal causes include: hypoxic–ischaemic encephalopathy such as occurs in neonatal asphyxia and intracerebral haemorrhage, hypoglycaemia, meningitis and encephalitis. CVI acquired after the perinatal period may be caused by meningitis, encephalitis, cardiac arrest, neurodegenerative disorders, trauma, cortical vein thrombosis and shunt failure.

Children with CVI may have generalised brain damage, periventricular leukomalacia, damage to the occipital cortex with or without damage to the anterior visual pathway, etc., depending on the nature of the causative process.[104] It is rare that infants with CVI are totally blind and visual improvement may occur over a prolonged period (DVM type 2). In addition to DVM children later exhibit reduced acuity, visual field defects and visuoperceptual problems.[46]

References

1. Allegaert K, de Coen K, Devlieger H, on behalf of the EpiBel Study 2004 Threshold retinopathy at threshold of viability: the EpiBal study. British Journal of Ophthalmology 88: 239–242
2. Alon T, Hemo I, Itin A et al 1995 Vascular endothelial growth factor acts as a survival factor for newly formed retinal vessels and has implications for retinopathy of prematurity. Nature Medicine 1: 1024–1028
3. American Academy of Pediatrics, American Association for Pediatric Ophthalmology and Strabismus, American Academy of Ophthalmology 2001 Screening examination of premature infants for retinopathy of prematurity. Pediatrics 108: 809–811
4. Apkarian P, Tijssen R 1992 Detection and maturation of VEP albino asymmetry: an overview and a longitudinal study from birth to 54 weeks. Behavioural Brain Research 49: 57–67
5. Arnoldi K A, Tycheson L 1995 Prevalence of intracranial lesions in children initially diagnosed with disconjugate nystagmus (spasmus nutans). Journal of Pediatric Ophthalmology and Strabismus 32: 296–301
6. Ashton N 1980 Oxygen and retinal blood vessels. Transactions of the Ophthalmological Societies of the United Kingdom 100: 359–362
7. Askie L M, Henderson-Smart D J, Irwig L et al 2003 Oxygen-saturation targets and outcomes in extremely preterm infants. New England Journal of Medicine 349: 959–967
8. Avery M E, Oppenheimer E H 1960 Recent increase in mortality from hyaline membrane disease. Journal of Pediatrics 57: 553–559
9. Axer-Siegel R, Snir M, Ma'ayan A et al 1996 Retinopathy of prematurity and surfactant treatment. Journal of Pediatric Ophthalmology and Strabismus 33: 171–174
10. Azuma N, Yamaguchi Y, Handa H et al 2003 Mutations of the PAX6 gene detected in patients with a variety of optic-nerve malformations. American Journal of Human Genetics 72: 1565–1570
11. Baldwin H C, Manners R M 2002 Congenital blepharoptosis: a literature review of the histology of levator palpebrae superioris muscle. Ophthalmic Plastic and Reconstructive Surgery 18: 301–307
12. Banks M 1990 Infant refraction and accommodation. International Ophthalmology Clinics 20: 205–232
13. Barrett B T, Bradley A, McGraw P V 2004 Understanding the neural basis of amblyopia. Neuroscientist 10: 106–117
14. Beck A D 2001 Diagnosis and management of pediatric glaucoma. Ophthalmology Clinics of North America 14: 501–512
15. Benson P F 1962 Transient unilateral external rectus muscle palsy in newborn infants. British Medical Journal 1: 1055
16. Berger W, van der Pol D, Warburg M et al 1992 Mutations in the candidate gene for Norrie disease. Human Molecular Genetics 1: 461–465
17. Birch E E, O'Connor A R 2001 Preterm birth and visual development. Seminars in Neonatology 6: 467–497
18. Birch E E, Stager D R 1996 The critical period for surgical treatment of dense unilateral congenital cataract. Investigative Ophthalmology and Visual Science 37: 1532–1538
19. Birkebaek N H, Patel L, Wright N B et al 2003 Endocrine status in patients with optic nerve hypoplasia: relationship to midline central nervous system abnormalities and appearance of the hypothalamic-pituitary axis on magnetic resonance imaging. Journal of Clinical Endocrinology and Metabolism 88: 5281–5286
20. Biswas S, Lloyd I C 1999 Oculocutaneous albinism. Archives of Disease in Childhood 80: 565–569
21. Black G, Redmond R M 1994 The molecular biology of Norrie disease. Eye 8: 491–496
22. Blume R S, Wolff S M 1972 The Chédiak–Higashi syndrome: studies in four patients and a review of the literature. Medicine 51: 247–280
23. Bremer D L, Palmer E A, Fellows R R, et al for the Cryotherapy for Retinopathy of Prematurity Cooperative Group 1998 Strabismus in premature infants in the first year of life. Archives of Ophthalmology 116: 329–333
24. Brodsky M C, Glazier C M 1993 Optic nerve hypoplasia. Clinical significance of associated central nervous system abnormalities on magnetic resonance imaging. Archives of Ophthalmology 111: 66–74
25. Brooks S E, Marcus D M, Gillis R N et al 1999 The effect of blood transfusion protocol on retinopathy of prematurity: a prospective, randomized study. Pediatrics 104: 514–518
26. Cassidy L, Taylor D 1999 Congenital cataract and multisystem disorders. Eye 13: 464–473
27. Chen Z, Battinelli E M, Fielder A et al 1993 A mutation of the Norrie disease gene (NDP) associated with X-linked familial vitreoretinopathy. Nature Genetics 5: 180–183
28. Chen Z, Hendriks R W, Jobling A et al 1992 Isolation and characterisation of a candidate gene for Norrie disease. Nature Genetics 1: 203–208
29. Chow L C, Wright K W, Sola A and the CSMC Oxygen Administration Study Group 2003 Can changes in clinical practice decrease the incidence of severe retinopathy of prematurity in very low birth weight infants? Pediatrics 111: 339–345
30. Clark C, Gibbs J A H, Maniello R et al 1981 Blood transfusions: a possible risk factor in retrolental fibroplasia. Acta Paediatrica Scandinavica 70: 535–539
31. Clark D J, Hero M 1994 Indirect diode laser treatment for stage 3 retinopathy of prematurity. Eye 8: 423–426
32. Cocker K D, Moseley M J, Stirling H F et al 1998 Delayed visual maturation: pupillary responses implicate subcortical and cortical visual systems. Developmental Medicine and Child Neurology 40: 160–162
33. Committee for the Classification of Retinopathy of Prematurity 1984 The international classification of retinopathy of prematurity. British Journal of Ophthalmology 68: 690–697
34. Committee for the Classification of Retinopathy of Prematurity 1987 The classification of retinal detachment. Archives of Ophthalmology 105: 906–912

35. Crofts B J, King R, Johnson A. The contribution of low birth weight to severe vision loss in a geographically defined population. British Journal of Ophthalmology 1998; 82: 9–13

36. Crolla J A, Cawdery J E, Oley C A et al 1997 A FISH approach to defining the extent and possible clinical significance of deletions at the WAGR locus. Journal of Medical Genetics 34: 207–212

37. Cunningham S, Fleck B W, Elton R A et al 1995 Transcutaneous oxygen levels in retinopathy of prematurity. Lancet 346: 1464–1465

38. Cryotherapy for Retinopathy of Prematurity Cooperative Group 1988 Multicentre trial of cryotherapy for retinopathy of prematurity (preliminary results). Archives of Ophthalmology 106: 471–479

39. Cryotherapy for Retinopathy of Prematurity Cooperative Group 1990 Multicentre trial of cryotherapy for retinopathy of prematurity. Three month outcome. Archives of Ophthalmology 108: 195–204

40. Cryotherapy for Retinopathy of Prematurity Cooperative Group 1993 Multicentre trial of cryotherapy for retinopathy of prematurity. 3 year outcome – structure and function. Archives of Ophthalmology 111: 339–344

41. Cryotherapy for Retinopathy of Prematurity Cooperative Group 1994 The natural outcome of premature birth and retinopathy. Status at one year. Archives of Ophthalmology 112: 903–912

42. Cryotherapy for Retinopathy of Prematurity Cooperative Group 2001 Multicenter trial of cryotherapy for retinopathy of prematurity: ophthalmological outcome at 10 years. Archives of Ophthalmology 119: 1110–1118

43. Cuculich P S, DeLozier K A, Mellen B G et al 2001 Postnatal dexamethasone treatment and retinopathy of prematurity in very-low-birth-weight neonates. Biology of the Neonate 79: 9–14

44. Dobson V, Teller D Y 1978 Visual acuity in human infants: a review and comparisons of behavioural and electrophysiological studies. Vision Research 18: 1469–1483

45. Dubowitz L M S, Levene M I, Morante A, Palmer P, Dubowitz V 1981 Neurologic signs in neonatal intraventricular hemorrhage: a correlation with real-time ultrasound. Journal of Pediatrics 99: 127–133

46. Dutton G N, Jacobson L K 2001 Cerebral visual impairment in children. Seminars in Neonatology 6: 477–485

47. Early Treatment for Retinopathy of Prematurity Cooperative Group 2003 Revised indications for the treatment of retinopathy of prematurity. Archives of Ophthalmology 121: 1684–1696

48. Elston J 1997 Developmental abnormalities of the anterior segment. In: Taylor D S I (ed) Paediatric ophthalmology, 2nd edn. Blackwell Scientific, Oxford, pp 252–265

49. Elston J 1997 Incomitant strabismus and cranial nerve palsies. In: Taylor D S I (ed) Paediatric ophthalmology, 2nd edn. Blackwell Scientific, Oxford, pp 937–968

50. Fielder A R 1997 Retinopathy of prematurity. Clinical Risk 3: 47–51

51. Fielder A R, Gresty M A, Dodd K L, Mellor D H, Levene M I 1986 Congenital ocular motor apraxia. Transactions of the Ophthalmological Societies of the UK 105: 589–598

52. Fielder A R, Mayer D L Delayed visual maturation. Seminars in Ophthalmology 1991; 6: 182–193

53. Fielder A R, Reynolds J D 2001 Retinopathy of prematurity: clinical aspects. Seminars in Neonatology 6: 461–475

54. Fielder A R, Russell-Eggitt I R, Dodd K L, Mellor D H 1985 Delayed visual maturation. Transactions of the Ophthalmological Society of the United Kingdom 104: 653–661

55. Fielder A R, Shaw D E, Robinson J, Ng Y K 1992 Natural history of retinopathy of prematurity: a prospective study. Eye 6: 233–242

56. Finer N N, Grant G, Schindler R F et al 1982 Effect of intramuscular vitamin E on frequency and severity of retrolental fibroplasia: a controlled trial. Lancet 1: 1087–1091

57 Flynn J T 1987 Retinopathy of prematurity. Pediatric Clinics of North America 34: 1487–1516

58. Flynn J T, Bancalari E, Bawol R et al 1987 Retinopathy of prematurity. A randomised, prospective trial of transcutaneous oxygen monitoring. Ophthalmology 94: 630–638

59. Flynn J T, Bancalari E, Snyder E S et al 1992 A cohort study of transcutaneous oxygen monitoring and the incidence and severity of retinopathy of prematurity. New England Journal of Medicine 326: 1050–1054

60. Foster A, Gilbert C, Rahi J 1997 Epidemiology of cataract in childhood: a global perspective. Journal of Cataract and Refractive Surgery 23(Suppl): 601–604

61. Francis P J, Berry V, Bhattacharya S S, Moore A T 2000 The genetics of childhood cataract. Journal of Medical Genetics 37: 481–488

62. Garey L J, De Courten C 1983 Structural development of the lateral geniculate body and visual cortex in monkey and man. Behavioural Brain Research 10: 3–13

63. Garza G, Fay A, Rubin P A D 2001 Treatment of pediatric vascular lesions of the eyelid and orbit. International Ophthalmology Clinics 41: 43–55

64. Gellen B, McIntosh N, McColm J R et al 2001 Is the partial pressure of carbon dioxide in the blood related to the development of retinopathy of prematurity? British Journal of Ophthalmology 85: 1044–1045

65. Gibson D L, Sheps S B, Schechter M T, Wiggins S, McCormick A Q 1989 Retinopathy of prematurity: a new epidemic? Pediatrics 83: 486–492

66. Gibson D L, Sheps S B, Uh S H, Schechter M T, McCormick A Q 1990 Retinopathy of prematurity-induced blindness: birth weight-specific survival and the new epidemic. Pediatrics 86: 405–412

67. Gilbert C, Rahi J, Eckstein M, O'Sullivan J, Foster A 1997 Retinopathy of prematurity in middle income countries. Lancet 350: 12–14

68. Good W V, Jan J E, Burden S K, Skoczenski, Candy R. Recent advances in cortical visual impairment. Developmental Medicine and Child Neurology 2001; 43: 56-60

69. Gorst C M, Munnoch D A, Hancock K 2001 Combined treatment of a proliferative peri-orbital haemangioma with a tuneable dye laser and intra-lesional steroids to prevent deprivation amblyopia. Journal of the Royal College of Surgeons of Edinburgh 46: 234–236

70. Gottlob I, Zubcov A, Catalano R A et al 1990 Signs distinguishing spasmus nutans (with and without central nervous system lesions) from infantile nystagmus. Ophthalmology 97: 1166–1175

71. Gottlob I, Zubcov A A, Wizow S S, Reinecke R D 1992 Head nodding is compensatory in spasmus nutans. Ophthalmology 99: 1024–1031

72. Gronskov K, Olsen J H, Sand A et al 2001 Population-based risk estimates of Wilms tumor in sporadic aniridia. A comprehensive mutation screening procedure of PAX6 identifies 80% of mutations in aniridia. Human Genetics 109: 11–18

73. Haider M Z, Devarajan L V, Al-Essa M, Kumar H 2002 A C597-A polymorphism in the Norrie disease gene is associated with advanced retinopathy of prematurity. Journal of Biomedical Science 9: 365–370

74. Hall D M B, Elliman D (eds) 2003 Health for all children, 4th edn. Oxford University Press, Oxford

75. Handler L F, Heher K L, Katowitz J A 1994 Congenital and acquired anophthalmia. Current Opinion in Ophthalmology 5: 84–90

76. Harris C M, Shawkat F, Russel-Eggitt I et al 1996 Intermittent horizontal saccade failure (ocular motor apraxia) in children. British Journal of Ophthalmology 80: 151–158

77. Hellström A, Peruzzi C, Ju M et al 2001 Low IGF-1 suppresses VEGF-survival signalling in retinal endothelial cells: direct correlation with clinical retinopathy of prematurity. Proceedings of the National Academy of Sciences of the USA 98: 5804–5808

78. Hendrickson A E 1994 Primate foveal development: a microcosm of current questions in neurobiology. Investigative Ophthalmology and Visual Science 35: 3129–3133

79. Higgins R D, Mendelsohn A L, DeFeo M J et al 1998 Antenatal dexamethasone and decreased severity of retinopathy of prematurity. Archives of Ophthalmology 116: 236–137

80. Hildebrandt F, Omram H 2001 New insights: nephronophthisis-medullary cystic kidney disease. Pediatric Nephrology 16: 168–176

81. Hittner H M, Godio L B, Rudolph A J et al 1981 Retrolental fibroplasia: efficacy of vitamin E in double blind clinical study of preterm infants. New England Journal of Medicine 305: 1365–1371

82. Hittner H M, Hirsch N J, Rudolph A J et al 1977 Assessment of gestational age by examination of the anterior capsule of the lens. Journal of Pediatrics 91: 455–458

83. Holmström G, el Azzazi M, Kugelberg U 1999 Ophthalmological follow up of preterm infants: a population based, prospective study of visual acuity and strabismus. British Journal of Ophthalmology 83:143–150

84. Holmstrom G, Thoren K 2000 Ocular manifestations of incontinentia pigmenti. Acta Ophthalmologica 78: 348–353

85. Hoyt C S 2003 Visual function in the brain-damaged child. Eye 17: 369–384

86. Hoyt C S, Jastrzebski G, Marg R 1983 Delayed visual maturation in infancy. British Journal of Ophthalmology 67: 127–130

87. Hoyt C S, Mousel D K, Weber A A 1980 Transient supranuclear disturbances of gaze in healthy neonates. American Journal of Ophthalmology 89: 708–713

88. Huo R, Burden S K, Hoyt C S, Good W V 1999 Chronic cortical visual impairment in children: aetiology, prognosis, and associated neurological deficits. British Journal of Ophthalmology 83: 670–675

89. Hurwitz R L, Chevez-Barrios P, Chintagumpala M et al 2000 Gene therapy for retinoblastoma. Proceedings of the 4th Great Basin Visual Science Symposium 2000 vol 4. Available on line at: http://insight.med.utah.edu/gbs/gbs4/pdf/hurwitz_paper.pdf

90. Hussain N, Clive J, Bhandari V 1999 Current incidence of retinopathy of prematurity, 1989–1997. Pediatrics 104: 1–8

91. Ingram R M, Barr A 1979 Changes in refraction between the ages of 1 and 3 years. British Journal of Ophthalmology 63: 339–342

92. Jan J E, Robinson G C, Tinnis C et al 1977 Blindness due to optic nerve atrophy and hypoplasia in children. An epidemiological study (1944–1974). Developmental Medicine and Child Neurology 19: 353–363

93. Johnson L, Quinn G E, Abbasi S et al 1988 Vitamin E and retinopathy of prematurity. Pediatrics 81: 329–331

94. Jordan T, Hanson I, Zaletayev D et al 1992 The human *PAX6* gene is mutated in two patients with aniridia. Nature Genetics 1: 328–332

95. Keen T J, Mohamed M D, McKibbin M et al 2003 Identification of a locus (*LCA9*) for Leber's congenital amaurosis on chromosome 1p36. European Journal of Human Genetics 11: 420–423

96. Kennedy J, Todd D A, Watts J, John E 1997 Retinopathy of prematurity in infants less than 29 weeks gestation: 3 years pre- and postsurfactant. Journal of Pediatric Ophthalmology and Strabismus 34: 289–292

97. Kinsey V E, Arnold H J, Kalina R E et al 1977 PaO₂ levels and retrolental fibroplasia: a report of the co-operative study. Pediatrics 60: 655–668

98. Kinsey V E, Twomey J T, Hamphill F M 1956 Retrolental fibroplasia and the use of oxygen. Archives of Ophthalmology 56: 481–529

99. Kivlin J D, Biglan A W, Gordon R A et al 1996 for the Cryotherapy for Retinopathy of Prematurity (CRYO-ROP) Cooperative Group. Early retinal vessel development and iris vessel dilatation as factors in retinopathy of prematurity. Archives of Ophthalmology 114: 150–154

100. Knight-Nanan D M, Algawi K, Bowell R et al 1996 Advanced cicatricial retinopathy of prematurity – outcome and complications. British Journal of Ophthalmology 80: 343–345

101. Kretzer F L, Hittner H M 1988 Retinopathy of prematurity: clinical implications of retinal development. Archives of Disease in Childhood 63: 1151–1167

102. Lambert S R 1999 Management of monocular congenital cataracts. Eye 13: 474–479

103. Lambert S L, Drack A V 1996 Infantile cataract. Survey of Ophthalmology 40: 427–458

104. Lambert S, Hoyt C S, Han J E, Barkovich J, Fiddmark O 1987 Visual recovery from hypoxic cortical blindness during childhood. Computed tomograhic and magnetic resonance imaging predictors. Archives of Ophthalmology 105: 1371–1377

105. Lambert S R, Kriss A, Taylor D 1989 Delayed visual maturation. A longitudinal clinical and electrophysiological assessment. Ophthalmology 96: 524–529

106. Lambert S R, Lynn M, Drews-Botsch C et al 2001 A comparison of grating visual acuity, strabismus, and reoperation outcomes among children with aphakia and pseudophakia after unilateral cataract surgery during the first six months of life. Journal of the American Association for Pediatric Ophthalmology and Strabismus 5: 70–75

107. Lanman J T, Guy L P, Danus I 1954 Retrolental fibroplasia and oxygen therapy. Journal of the American Medical Association 55: 223–226

108. Larsson E K, Rydberg A C, Holmstrom G E 2003 A population-based study of the refractive outcome in 10-year old preterm and full-term children. Archives of Ophthalmology 121: 1430–1436

109. Lloyd C, Dowler J, Kriss A et al 1994 Preferential looking and the management of congenital cataract: new occlusion protocols. In: Cotlier E, Lambert S, Taylor D, eds. Congenital cataracts. RG Landes, Austin, TX, pp 93–101

110. Lucey J L, Dangman B 1984 A re-examination of the role of oxygen in retrolental fibroplasia. Pediatrics 73: 82–96

111. McColm J R, Fleck B W 2001 Retinopathy of prematurity: causation. Seminars in Neonatology 6: 453–460

112. McCormick A Q 1968 Transient cataracts in premature newborn infants – a new clinical entity. Canadian Journal of Ophthalmology 3: 202–205

113. McDonald A D 1963 Cerebral palsy in children of very low birth weight. Archives of Disease in Childhood 38: 579–588

114. Magoon E H, Robb R M 1981 Development of myelin in human optic nerve and tract. Archives of Ophthalmology 99: 655–659

115. Margalith D, Jan J E, McCormick A Q et al 1984 Clinical spectrum of optic nerve hypoplasia. Review of 51 patients. Developmental Medicine and Child Neurology 26: 311–322

116. Marlow N 1997 Clinical care and the prevention of retinopathy of prematurity. Clinical Risk 3: 37–41

117. Mohindra I, Held R, Gwiazda J, Brill S 1978 Astigmatism in infants. Science 202: 329–330

118. Ng Y K, Fielder A R, Shaw D E, Levene M I 1988 Epidemiology of retinopathy of prematurity. Lancet 2: 1235–1238

119. Nickel B, Hoyt C S 1982 Leber's congenital amaurosis. Is mental retardation a frequent associated defect? Archives of Ophthalmology 100: 1089–1092

120. Nixon R B, Helveston E M, Miller K et al 1985 Incidence of strabismus in neonates. American Journal of Ophthalmology 100: 798–801

121. O'Connor A R, Stephenson T, Johnson A et al 2002 Long-term ophthalmic outcome of low birth weight children with and without retinopathy of prematurity. Pediatrics 109: 12–18

122. O'Connor A R, Stephenson T J, Johnson A et al 2002 Strabismus in children of birth weight less than 1701 g. Arch Ophthalmol 120: 767–771

123. Oetting W S 1999 Albinism. Current Opinion in Pediatrics 11: 565–571

124. O'Keefe M, Lanigan B, Byrne S A 2003 Capillary haemangioma of the eyelids and orbit: a clinical review of the safety and efficacy of intralesional steroid. Acta Ophthalmologica Scandinavica 81: 294–298

125. Onwochei B C, Simon J W, Bateman J B et al 2000 Ocular colobomata. Survey of Ophthalmology 45: 175–194

126. Palmer E A, Flynn J T, Hardy R J 1991 The Cryotherapy for Retinopathy of Prematurity Cooperative Group. Incidence and early course of retinopathy of prematurity. Ophthalmology 98: 1628–1640

127. Pandey S K, Wilson M E, Trivedi R H et al 2001 Pediatric cataract surgery and intraocular lens implantation: current techniques, complication, and management. International Ophthalmology Clinics 41: 175–196

128. Patz A 1954 Oxygen studies in retrolental fibroplasia IV. Clinical and experimental observations. American Journal of Ophthalmology 38: 291–308

129. Pennefather P M, Tin W, Clarke M P et al 1996 Retinopathy of prematurity in a controlled trial of prophylactic surfactant treatment. British Journal of Ophthalmology 80: 420–424

130. Perrault I, Rozet J-M, Gerber S et al 1999 Leber congenital amaurosis. Molecular Genetics and Metabolism 68: 200–208

131. Phelps D L, Rosenbaum A, Isenberg S J, Leake R D, Davey F J 1987 Tocopherol efficacy and safety for preventing retinopathy of prematurity: a randomised controlled double masked trial. Pediatrics 79: 489–500

132. Pierce E A, Foley E D, Smith L E 1996 Regulation of vascular endothelial growth factor by oxygen in a model of retinopathy of prematurity. Archives of Ophthalmology 114: 1219–1228

133. Prendiville A, Schulenburg W E 1988 Clinical factors associated with retinopathy of prematurity. Eye 522–527

134. Provis J M 2001 Development of the primate retinal vasculature. Progress in Retinal and Eye Research 20: 799–821

135. Purvin V A 2002 Superior segmental optic nerve hypoplasia. Journal of Neuro-Ophthalmology 22: 116–117

136. 104. Quinn G E, Dobson V, Barr C C et al 1996 Visual acuity of eyes after vitrectomy for retinopathy of prematurity – follow up of 5 years. Ophthalmology 103: 595–600

137. Rahi J S, Botting B 2001 Ascertainment of children with congenital cataract through the National Congenital Anomaly System in England and Wales. British Journal of Ophthalmology 85: 1049–1051

138. Rahi J S, Cable N on behalf of the British Childhood Visual Impairment Study Group 2003 Severe visual impairment and blindness in children in the UK. Lancet 362: 1359–1365

139. Rahi J S, Dezateux C 1999 Capture-recapture analysis of ascertainment by active surveillance in the British Congenital Cataract Study. Investigative Ophthalmology and Visual Science 40: 236–239

140. Rahi J S, Dezateux C 2000 Congenital and infantile cataract in the United Kingdom: underlying or associated factors. British Congenital Cataract Interest Group. Investigative Ophthalmology and Visual Science 41: 2108–2114

141. Raju T N, Langenberg P, Bhutani V et al 1997 Vitamin E prophylaxis to reduce retinopathy of prematurity: a reappraisal of published trials. Journal of Pediatrics 131: 844–850

142. Reisner S H, Amir I, Shohat M et al 1985 Retinopathy of prematurity: incidence and treatment. Archives of Disease in Childhood 60: 698–701

143. Reisner S H, Perlman M, Ben Tovin N et al 1971 Transient lateral rectus muscle paresis in the newborn infant. Journal of Pediatrics 78: 461–465

144. Reynolds J D, Dobson V, Quinn G E, Fielder A R et al on behalf of the CRYO-ROP and LIGHT-ROP Cooperative Groups 2002 Evidence-based screening for retinopathy of prematurity: natural history data from CRYO-ROP and LIGHT-ROP Studies. Archives of Ophthalmology 120: 1470–1476

145. Reynolds J D, Hardy R J, Kennedy K A et al for the Light Reduction in Retinopathy of Prematurity (LIGHT-ROP) Cooperative Group 1988 Lack of efficacy of light reduction in preventing retinopathy of prematurity. New England Journal of Medicine 338: 1572–1576

146. Roy M S, Barsoum-Homsy M, Orquin J, Benoit J 1995 Maturation of binocular pattern visual evoked potentials in normal full-term and preterm infants from 1 to 6 months of age. Pediatric Research 37: 140–144

147. Royal College of Ophthalmologists and the British Association of Perinatal Medicine 1996 Retinopathy of prematurity: guidelines for screening and treatment. The report of a joint working party. Early Human Development 46: 239–258

148. Russell-Eggitt I, Harris CM, Kriss A 1998 Delayed visual maturation: an update. Developmental Medicine and Child Neurology 40: 130–136

149. Sakol P J, Mannor G, Massaro B M 1999 Congenital and acquired blepharoptosis. Current Opinion in Ophthalmology 10: 335–339

150. Sarfarazi M, Stoilov I, Schenkman J B 2003 Genetics and biochemistry of primary congenital glaucoma. Ophthalmology Clinics of North America 16: 543–554

151. Saunders R A, Donahue M, Christmann L M et al 1997 Racial variation in retinopathy of prematurity. Archives of Ophthalmology 115: 604–608

152. Scarf B, Hoyt C S 1984 Optic nerve hypoplasia in children. Archives of Ophthalmology 102: 62–67

153. Seidman D J, Nelson L B, Calhoun J H et al 1986 Signs and symptoms in the presentation of primary infantile glaucoma. Pediatrics 77: 399–404

154. Semina E V, Reiter R, Leyesens N J et al 1996 Cloning and characterization of a novel bicoid-related homeobox transcription factor gene, *RIEG*, involved in Rieger syndrome. Nature Genetics 14: 392–399

155. Shastry B S, Pendergast S D, Hartzer M K, Liu X, Trese M T 1997 Identification of missense mutations in the Norrie disease gene associated with advanced retinopathy of prematurity. Archives of Ophthalmology 115: 651–655

156. Shawkat F S, Kingsley D, Kendall B et al 1995 Neuroradiological and eye movement correlates in children with intermittent saccade failure ('ocular motor apraxia'). Neuropaediatrics 26: 298–305

157. Shields M B, Buckley E, Klintworth G K, Thresher R 1985 Axenfield–Rieger syndrome. A spectrum of developmental disorders. Survey of Ophthalmology 29: 387–409

158. Shohat M, Reisner S H, Krikler R et al 1983 Retinopathy of prematurity: incidence and risk factors. Pediatrics 72: 159–163

159. Sires B S, Goins C R, Anderson R L et al 2001 Systemic corticosteroid use in orbital lymphangioma. Ophthalmic Plastic and Reconstructive Surgery 17: 85–90

160. Smith L E H 2002 Pathogenesis of retinopathy of prematurity. Acta Paediatrica Supplement 437: 26–28

161. Snead M, Moore A T 1996 The investigation of the apparently blind infant. In: Jay B, Kirkness C M (eds) Recent advances in ophthalmology. Churchill Livingstone, Edinburgh, pp 155–178

162. Steinkuller P G, Du L, Gilbert C et al 1999 Childhood blindness. Journal of the American Association of Pediatric Ophthalmology and Strabismus 3: 26–32

163. Summers C G, Knobloch W H, Witkop C J Jr et al 1988 Hermansky–Pudlak syndrome: ophthalmic findings. Ophthalmology 95: 545–554

164. Tajima T, Hattorri T, Nakajima T et al 2003 Sporadic heterozygous frameshift mutation of *HESX1* causing pituitary and optic nerve hypoplasia and combined hormone deficiency in a Japanese patient. Journal of Clinical Endocrinology and Metabolism 88: 45–50

165. Tamura E E, Hoyt C S 1987 Oculomotor consequences of intraventricular hemorrhages in premature infants. Archives of Ophthalmology 105: 533–535

166. Tan A D, Rubin P A D, Sutula F C, Remulla H D 2001 Congenital nasolacrimal duct obstruction. International Ophthalmology Clinics 41: 57–69

167. Taylor D, Wright K W, Amaya L et al 2001 Should we aggressively treat unilateral congenital cataracts? British Journal of Ophthalmology 85: 1120–1126

168. Teller D Y, McDonald M A, Preston K, Sebris S L, Dobson V 1986 Assessment of visual acuity in infants and children: the acuity card procedure. Developmental Medicine and Child Neurology 28: 779–789

169. Termote J, Schalif-Delfos N E, Donders A R T et al 2003 The incidence of visually impaired children with retinopathy of prematurity and their concomitant disabilities. Journal of the American Association of Pediatric Ophthalmology and Strabismus 7: 131–136

170. Termote J U M, Schalij-Delfos N E, Wittebolpost D et al 1994 Surfactant replacement therapy: a new risk factor for developing retinopathy of prematurity. European Journal of Paediatrics 153: 113–116

171. Terry T L 1942 Extreme prematurity and fibroplastic overgrowth of persistent vascular sheath behind each crystalline lens. American Journal of Ophthalmology 25: 203–204

172. Thorn F, Gwiazda J, Cruz A A V, Bauer J A, Held R 1994 The development of eye alignment, convergence, and sensory binocularity in young infants. Investigative Ophthalmology and Visual Science 35: 544–553

173. Tin W, Milligan D W A, Pennefather P et al 2001 Pulse oximetry, severe retinopathy of prematurity, and outcome at one year in babies of less than 28 weeks gestation. Archives of Disease in Childhood Fetal and Neonatal Edition 84: F107–F110

174. Tin W, Wariyar U 2002 Giving small babies oxygen: 50 years of uncertainty. Seminars in Neonatology 7: 361–367

175. Tornqvist K, Ericsson A, Kallen B 2002 Optic nerve hypoplasia: risk factors and epidemiology. Acta Ophthalmologica Scandinavica 80: 300–304

176. Tresidder J, Fielder A R, Nicholson J 1990 Delayed visual maturation: ophthalmic and neurodevelopmental aspects. Developmental Medicine and Child Neurology 32: 872–881

177. Wagner R S 1993 Glaucoma in children. Pediatric Clinics of North America 40: 855–867

178. Wagner R S, Caputo A R, Nelson L, Zanoris D 1985 High hyperopia in Leber's congenital amaurosis. Archives of Ophthalmology 103: 1507–1509

179. Warburg M 1993 Classification of microphthalmos and coloboma. Journal of Medical Genetics 30: 664–669

180. Weinacht S, Kind C, Monting JS, Gottlob I 1999 Visual development in preterm and full-term infants: a prospective masked study. Investigative Ophthalmology and Visual Science 40: 346–353

181. Wheatley C M, Dickinson J L, Mackey D A, Craig J E, Sale M M 2002 Retinopathy of prematurity: recent advances in our understanding. Archives of Disease in Childhood 86: 696–700

182. Whiting S, Jan J E, Wong F K H, Flodmark O, Farrell K, McCormick A Q 1985 Permanent cortical visual impairment in children. Developmental Medicine and Child Neurology 27: 730–739

183. Williams J, Brodsky M C, Griebel C M, Caldwell D, Thomas P 1993 Septo-optic dysplasia: the clinical significance of an absent septum pellucidum. Developmental Medicine and Child Neurology 35: 490–501

184. Wilson M E, Pandey S K, Thakur J 2003 Paediatric cataract blindness in the developing world: surgical techniques and intraocular lenses in the new millennium. British Journal of Ophthalmology 87: 14–19

185. Wong G A E, Willoughby C E, Parslew R, Kaye S B 2004 The importance of screening for sight-threatening retinopathy in incontinentia pigmenti. Pediatric Dermatology 21: 242–245

186. York J R, Landers S, Kirby R S et al 2004 Arterial oxygen fluctuation and retinopathy of prematurity in very-low-birth-weight infants. Journal of Perinatology 24: 82–87

187. Yorston D, Wood M, Foster A 2001 Results of cataract surgery in young children in East Africa. British Journal of Ophthalmology 85: 267–271

188. Yuodelis C, Hendrickson A 1986 A qualitative and quantitative analysis of the human fovea during development. Vision Research 26: 847–855

CHAPTER 35

Metabolic disease

PART I

Disorders of blood glucose homeostasis in the neonate

Jane Hawdon

Introduction

Neonatal hypoglycaemia has been recognised for many years,[29,130,145] although with time there have been wide swings of opinion regarding the definition of the condition, its clinical significance and its optimal management. For example, in the era when routine postnatal management involved the withholding of feeds from healthy infants for up to 24 hours, and even longer in sick or small babies, many were found to have low blood glucose concentrations, and this became accepted as a normal finding.[35] However, to others it was apparent that some of these babies had clinical signs of hypoglycaemia, and the risk of reduced glucose availability to the brain was acknowledged. Neligan[117] summarised the level of anxiety: 'Certainly the risk of such complications forms a cogent incentive to all concerned to make the diagnosis as early as possible in every case.'

Such anxieties were later reawakened by the publication of papers by Koh et al[91] and Lucas et al[101] which suggested that there were significant neurological sequelae of hypoglycaemia. This resulted in a swing towards the treatment of large numbers of infants with intravenous (i.v.) glucose, which involved separation from their mothers and placed at risk the establishment of breastfeeding. Subsequent research has demonstrated that many infants may be protected from the neurological effects of hypoglycaemia by virtue of the availability of alternative cerebral fuels, so that this management may be overly intensive if applied to all babies.[33,49] Therefore, it is important to identify those infants most at risk of neurological sequelae and determine the most effective and least invasive regimens for prevention of hypoglycaemic brain injury.[33] To date, no controlled study has addressed either of these issues.

Hyperglycaemia was recognised as a neonatal complication over a century ago,[90] and until recent times was a rare phenomenon. However, it is now commonly seen in the increasing numbers of extremely-low-birthweight (ELBW) infants who are cared for in our neonatal units. As such, there is still some uncertainty as to its clinical significance and optimal management.

To manage these disorders of blood glucose homeostasis, it is essential to understand the metabolism of the fetus and neonate and the changes that occur at birth in the healthy infant. This chapter will summarise the current knowledge of the disorders of blood glucose homeostasis, and aims to provide a practical and pragmatic approach to the management of babies with hypoglycaemia and hyperglycaemia.

Glucose homeostasis in the healthy fetus and neonate

Fetal metabolism

During pregnancy the human fetus receives from its mother, via the placental circulation, a supply of substrates necessary for growth, for the deposition of fuel stores which are essential after birth (see below), and for energy to meet the basal metabolic rate and requirements for growth. Glucose is transported across the placenta by facilitated diffusion, but during maternal starvation or placental insufficiency the fetus is capable of endogenous glucose production.[75] Glucose metabolism accounts for 65% of fetal energy production, with lactate probably accounting for most of the remainder.[75] Glucose is not the only fuel utilised by the fetal brain. Studies of perfused human fetal brain have demonstrated that uptake of ketone bodies, the products of β oxidation of fatty acids, is greater than that of glucose and it is likely that the fate of ketone bodies is both incorporation into brain lipids and for use as a cerebral energy source.[1] Lactate may also be metabolised.

The fetus is usually capable of regulating its glucose concentrations independently of maternal hormones. This capacity is seen in some cases of placental insufficiency (see above), when gluconeogenesis is activated, and in the fetus of the diabetic mother (Chapter 22), who responds to the high placental transfer of glucose by secreting high concentrations of insulin. However, the healthy fetus differs from adults in that there is a blunted insulin response to high glucose concentrations, and that insulin secretion is more sensitive to amino acids than glucose.[110,118] In fact, it appears that insulin has a greater role in fetal growth than in fetal metabolic control. Similarly, the fetus is less sensitive than the neonate to the glucose-mobilising actions of glucagon, although sensitivity increases with gestational age.[146,147]

Under extreme circumstances, fetal blood glucose control fails. For example, in some cases of placental insufficiency leading to intrauterine growth retardation (IUGR), fetal hypoglycaemia may occur.[143] If prolonged periods of postnatal hypoglycaemia cause long-term neurological damage, it is possible that such profound and prolonged fetal hypoglycaemia may have the same effect and may explain some of the handicap following IUGR, even when there have been no postnatal complications.

Metabolic changes at birth

These changes are essential to preserve fuel supplies for vital organ function when the continuous flow of nutrients from the placenta is abruptly discontinued. As oxygen supply also temporarily fails during delivery, anaerobic metabolism must occur and this requires higher substrate availability than aerobic metabolism. In addition, the newborn infant must adapt to the fast-feed cycle and to the change in major energy source, from glucose from the placenta to fat from adipose tissue stores and in milk feeds. After birth, plasma insulin levels fall and there are rapid surges of catecholamine and pancreatic glucagon release.[62,147] These endocrine changes switch on the essential enzymes for glycogenolysis (the release of glucose stored as glycogen in liver, cardiac muscle and brain), for gluconeogenesis (glucose production from 3-carbon precursor molecules by the liver), lipolysis (release of fatty acids from adipose tissue stores), and ketogenesis (the β oxidation of fatty acids by the liver). Although glucose is the major metabolic fuel for most organs in the immediate postnatal period, there is evidence that lactate may be the preferred cerebral fuel over glucose and ketone bodies at this time.[106]

Neonatal metabolism

The metabolic processes of fetal life and at birth are repeated on a smaller scale during the milk-fed infant's fast-feed cycles. Immediately after a feed there is availability of metabolic fuels, namely fatty acids and, to a lesser extent, sugars from milk. Some tissues, for example the kidney, are obligate glucose users, but others burn fatty fuels and the respiratory quotient falls after birth, reflecting the fact that fat oxidation accounts for about 75% of oxygen consumption. Of the organs that utilise alternative fuels to glucose, the brain is the most important in that it takes up and oxidises ketone bodies at higher rates than seen in adults, and the neonatal brain uses ketone bodies more efficiently than glucose.[51]

Any excess glucose available after a feed is stored as glycogen in the liver or converted to fat for deposition in adipose tissue, along with fatty acids absorbed after milk feeds.

Between feeds, blood glucose levels start to fall and glycogenolysis and gluconeogenesis are again activated to ensure availability for organs which are obligate users (Fig. 35.1). Glycogenolysis is an exhaustible source of glucose whose capacity varies according to fetal growth and maturity,[135] and after approximately 2 hours gluconeogenesis must become the major glucose-providing process. Stable isotope turnover studies have shown that neonatal glucose production rates are 4–6 mg/kg/min.[21,23] Between feeds, lipolysis and ketogenesis provide alternative fuels to glucose for organs such as the brain, which are not obligate glucose utilisers.[72] The process of ketogenesis also provides energy and cofactors which are utilised in gluconeogenesis, again highlighting the importance of fatty fuels.

The control of neonatal metabolism is dependent first on the synthesis of key enzymes, such as hepatic phosphorylase for glycogenolysis, phosphoenolpyruvate carboxykinase (PEPCK) for gluconeogenesis, and carnitine acyltransferases for ketogenesis, and secondly, on the induction of enzyme activity by hormonal changes. Glucagon is the major neonatal glucoregulatory hormone.[147] Its concentration increases when blood glucose levels fall, and it induces activity of the enzymes of glycogenolysis, gluconeogenesis and ketogenesis in the liver. The glucoregulatory role of insulin in the neonate is less clear and may well differ from that in the adult (see below). In most neonates, insulin does not appear to have a major influence on normal blood glucose homeostasis, but in some extreme cases (see below) high insulin concentrations may result in hypoglycaemia. Finally, it is unlikely that other hormones, such as the catecholamines, cortisol, thyroid hormones and growth hormone, are important regulators in the fast-feed cycle of the healthy neonate, but rare cases of hypopituitarism or cortisol deficiency (see below) may present with neonatal hypoglycaemia, which suggests that minimum basal levels are needed to maintain normoglycaemia.

Finally, the change from fetal to neonatal metabolism must take into account the important role of gastrointestinal adaptation. It is possible that the introduction of enteral feeding triggers the secretion of gastrointestinal regulatory peptides and hormones, which in turn induce the features of gut adaptation, namely gut growth, mucosal differentiation, induction of motor activity and the development of digestion and absorption.[13,100]

Differences between neonatal and adult metabolism

It is apparent that neonates do not follow the same metabolic 'rules' as adults. Milk-fed neonates produce and utilise ketone bodies to the extent seen in adults only after a prolonged fast, and thus have the mechanisms to support this. Other fuels such as lactate may also be used, in addition to glucose and ketone bodies. Insulin plays a lesser role in glucoregulation in the neonate than in the adult, in that its release in response to glucose is blunted and delayed when compared with the adult, and that there may be end-organ insensitivities to its action.[83] In fact, healthy neonates have insulin–glucose relationships that differ markedly from those of older subjects.[67,69] Therefore, when interpreting studies of

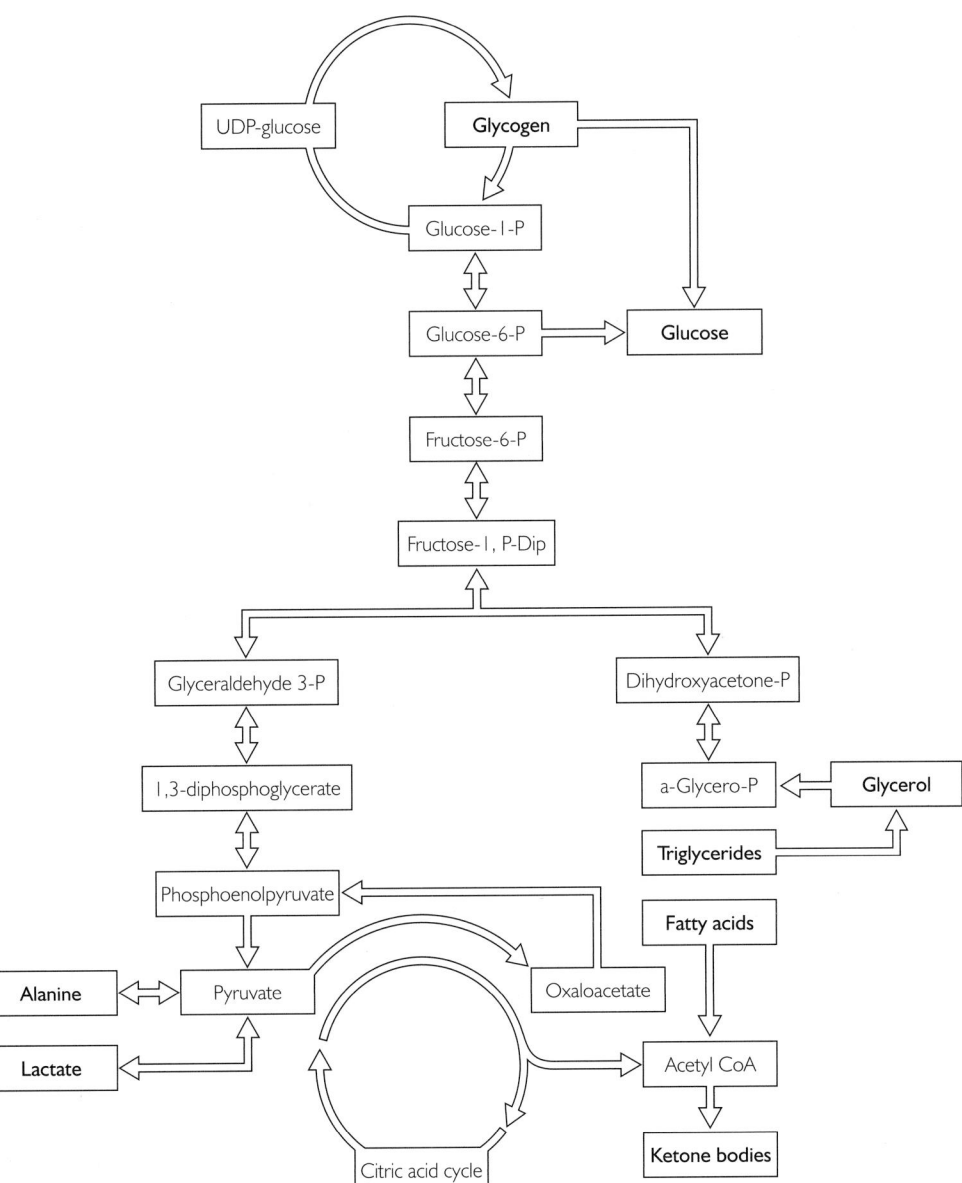

Fig. 35.1 Metabolic pathways involved in gluconeogenesis (pathways below glucose-6-P) and in glycogen synthesis (above glucose-6-P) and glycogenolysis. Galactose enters the pathways above glucose-6-P.

impaired neonatal glucoregulation it is essential to have reference data from healthy infants, rather than comparing the neonatal concentrations and interrelationships of fuels and hormones with those of adults. Also, it is impossible to consider glucose alone, and the availability of alternative fuels must be established.

Hypoglycaemia

Clinical significance

The controversy regarding the clinical significance of neonatal hypoglycaemia mirrors that surrounding its definition.[33] Blood glucose levels fall immediately after birth but rise after a few hours, either spontaneously or in response to feeding, in almost all healthy full-term infants.[72,124,149] This brief period when blood glucose level is low cannot be considered of clinical significance, and indeed, if it were so, would lead to the admission of large numbers of infants to neonatal units for treatment.

No study has yet addressed the duration of hypoglycaemia or of acute neurological dysfunction which is harmful to the human neonate, but a study of Rhesus monkeys has shown that a duration of neonatal hypoglycaemia (blood glucose less than 1.5 mmol/l) of 6.5 hours had no demonstrable long-term effects, whereas 10 hours of hypoglycaemia was associated with 'motivational and adaptability problems', but no motor or cognitive deficit, on testing at 8 months of age.[129]

In the light of the paucity of human neonatal data and the variability between babies with regard to exacerbating factors and protective mechanisms, it is impossible to state the duration of hypoglycaemia that is harmful to human neonates, but we suspect that prolonged periods (at least 12–24 hours) in the 'at-risk' groups of human neonates may lead to neurological sequelae, and that brief self-limiting episodes are of no neurological significance if not accompanied by clinical signs or coexisting clinical complications.[33]

Acute neurophysiological changes at low blood glucose levels have been demonstrated in human neonates and those of other species.[91,159] However, the long-term significance of these acute changes is not clear. There is no doubt that a number of infants have fits or a reduced level of consciousness when blood glucose levels are low, and some authors have described adverse long-term outcomes when neurological signs have been present.[60,131] Profound hypoglycaemia, usually the result of serious inborn errors of metabolism, may even result in 'cot death' or apparent life-threatening events. Other clinical signs have often been associated with hypoglycaemia, namely tremor, irritability, 'jitteriness', apnoea, hypotonia, abnormal cry, tachypnoea, pallor and feeding difficulties. However, these are as likely to be the result of coexisting clinical complications, such as perinatal asphyxia, or the cause of hypoglycaemia (e.g. poor feeding) than the specific effects of hypoglycaemia.

No study has clearly demonstrated the independent contribution of hypoglycaemia (with or without signs) to neurodevelopmental outcome, because all studies to date are of neonates who had other adverse clinical factors.[33,39,65] There is also a paucity of information regarding the histopathological and neuroradiological changes associated with neonatal hypoglycaemia, and the reports of past studies are conflicting. However, there is evidence that profound and prolonged hypoglycaemia is associated with both transient and permanent structural changes in the brain.[8,12,15,17,61,86,87,115,144] Grey matter damage is most commonly reported but there is no consistently described characteristic pattern of brain injury after neonatal hypoglycaemia.

Animal studies have shown that structural changes, when present, are in a distribution characteristic of dendritic loss secondary to a neurotoxic agent, and it is postulated that neuroexcitatory transmitters such as glutamate accumulate during hypoglycaemia and that their action on neuronal NMDA receptors causes depolarisation and cell damage.[12]

Hypoglycaemia is likely to be most significant when occurring shortly after or coincident with other insults, such as hypoxia-ischaemia. For infants with multisystem problems (for example the preterm or asphyxiated infant), all potential causes of neurological damage should be prevented and treated as far as possible, and in practice the prevention of hypoglycaemia is often the easiest of clinical issues.

It is likely that healthy full-term neonates, even some of those who are small for gestational age (SGA), are protected from the neurological sequelae of low blood glucose levels by metabolising ketone bodies.[45,49,65]

Finally, the impact of hypoglycaemia and its treatment on the mother and baby must be considered. The early neonatal period is an emotionally sensitive time, and the diagnosis of hypoglycaemia may create or add to anxiety for the parents. Treatment of the infant with i.v. glucose usually involves separation of the baby and mother, and may be perceived as invasive or painful. The implications for the establishment of breastfeeding must also not be forgotten, especially as there is evidence that breastfeeding and avoidance of formula supplementation augments ketogenesis.[49,53,64] Therefore, emphasis should be on the early prevention

of hypoglycaemia and strategies of management that do not involve the separation of mother and baby.[63]

Definition and diagnosis

Definition

Much controversy and confusion has surrounded the definition of hypoglycaemia.[33,92] For example, Koh et al[92] demonstrated that the definition varied widely not only among standard paediatric textbooks but also among neonatologists, with values given ranging from below 1 mmol/l to below 4 mmol/l.

Previous widely used definitions were based on cross-sectional samples from newborn babies, with the assumption that those with the lowest blood glucose levels were abnormal. This led to definitions of hypoglycaemia as follows: term infants less than 48 hours old – blood glucose level less than 1.7 mmol/l; term infants more than 48 hours old – less than 2.2 mmol/l; preterm infants – less than 1.1 mmol/l. However, these definitions were proposed at a time when, unlike the present, infants were starved for considerable periods after birth, and small and preterm infants received less milk than healthy term infants. Therefore, it is not surprising that so many infants on the first postnatal day had low blood glucose levels. The trend towards early feeding of infants has been associated with a more rapid increase in blood glucose concentration after the immediate postnatal fall (Fig. 35.2).[13,149] Fortunately, the long-standing belief that the brains of preterm infants were more able to withstand low blood glucose levels than those of term infants is now less widely accepted.[92]

Later, this statistical definition of hypoglycaemia was challenged and a 'functional' definition was proposed, which is 'at

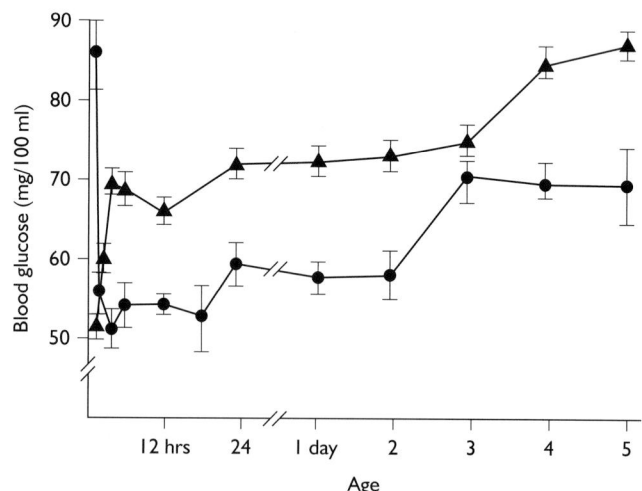

Fig. 35.2 Blood glucose levels (mean ± SE) in full-term infants, showing the changing pattern of development during the first postnatal days in 1965 compared with 1986 (circles, Cornblath & Reisner;[34] triangles, Srinivasan et al[149]). To convert mg/100 ml into mmol/l, divide by 18.

what level of blood glucose is the body's function, particularly that of the brain, compromised?' It is not possible to define hypoglycaemia from the blood glucose level at which symptoms occur, because, unlike adults and older children, babies cannot complain of symptoms and by the time blood glucose levels have fallen so low that clinical signs of cerebral dysfunction occur in neonates there is a risk that brain damage may have been sustained. There is no doubt that any low blood glucose concentration of any duration which causes clinical signs, such as fits or coma, is *too low*, regardless of its numerical value, and must be treated. In fact, the rapid clinical resolution of the signs after the i.v. administration of glucose confirms the diagnosis of acute cerebral dysfunction secondary to hypoglycaemia.

Only two studies have explored the 'safe level' for blood glucose concentrations in neonates without apparent clinical signs.[91,101] In a neurodevelopmental follow-up study of very-low-birthweight (VLBW) preterm infants, Lucas et al[101] found that neonatal blood glucose concentrations below 2.6 mmol/l on at least 3 days were associated with a poor neurodevelopmental outcome. The neurophysiological study of Koh et al[91] demonstrated that in a group of subjects which included five neonates of varying birthweights and gestations, no baby with a blood glucose level above 2.6 mmol/l had abnormal sensory-evoked brainstem potentials (SEPs). No differences were found in the blood glucose threshold for abnormal SEPs between subjects who had symptoms of hypoglycaemia and those who were asymptomatic. Thus, both studies suggested that blood glucose levels less than 2.6 mmol/l are associated with abnormal acute and prolonged neurological function, and that levels above this could be considered safe. However, the subjects of the studies were not representative of all neonates and the data cannot be extrapolated to other neonatal groups. There have been no prospective studies of the effects of neonatal hypoglycaemia in individual 'at-risk' groups which satisfactorily control for the effects of other neonatal complications.

Another factor not previously addressed is that babies vary in their ability to mount protective metabolic responses when blood glucose levels are low. Indeed, there is evidence that glucose utilisation by the neonatal brain is less than in subsequent months, and the role of alternative fuels must be considered.[88] For example, it has recently become apparent that neonates differ in terms of their ability to produce ketone bodies in response to hypoglycaemia. Low blood glucose concentrations (less than 2.6 mmol/l) are commonly found during the first 3 postnatal days in healthy appropriate-for-gestational-age (AGA) and SGA term neonates, particularly those who are breastfed. These infants have high ketone body levels when blood glucose concentrations are low, and it is likely that this protects them from neurological sequelae.[49,72,156] Therefore, it is inappropriate to consider low blood glucose levels in such infants as a pathological diagnosis. However, other groups, such as those who are preterm, IUGR, asphyxiated or hyperinsulinaemic, may have impaired ketogenesis; in these babies, circulating blood glucose concentrations acquire greater clinical significance and hypoglycaemia, if present, must be diagnosed and treated effectively.[33,70–72,74] The presence of additional neonatal complications which may add to neurological risks, such as asphyxia, acidosis, hyperbilirubinaemia and polycythaemia, must also be considered when deciding what level of blood glucose is acceptable.

The ideal definition of hypoglycaemia should include the blood glucose concentration considered to be the minimum safe level, the length of time beyond which the low blood glucose level is considered to be harmful, the presence of clinical signs, the group of infants studied, the consideration of alternative fuel availability, the conditions of sampling and the assay methods. Most of these criteria have never been adequately addressed by previous studies or publications. This paucity of data has resulted in a pragmatic approach proposed by a group of clinicians that is based on thresholds for intervention rather than attempts to define hypoglycaemia as a single numerical term.[33] This group suggested that, for infants who are at risk of neurological sequelae by virtue of their inability to mobilise ketone bodies at low blood glucose levels (Table 35.1), intervention to raise blood glucose should be considered if two consecutive blood glucose levels are below 2 mmol/l (measured using an accurate device) or a single blood glucose level is below 1 mmol/l. It would be prudent to apply this most rigorously to infants with coexisting clinical complications. Regardless of the blood glucose concentration, neurological signs in association with low blood glucose levels should prompt investigations to establish a firm diagnosis of hypoglycaemia and its underlying cause, and the institution of urgent treatment.

Diagnosis

The accurate measurement of blood glucose levels is essential in the diagnosis of hypoglycaemia. It is well known that glucose reagent strips, commonly used in neonatal and maternity units, are insufficiently reliable for the diagnosis.[33,89,105,127] Therefore, if these strips are used for neonatal screening, all low values should be confirmed by accurate measurement. These samples should be assayed promptly, as blood glucose levels diminish with time, even in fluoridated tubes.[84] Accurate determination may be conveniently performed using a blood glucose analyser sited in a neonatal unit laboratory. Usually, whole blood samples are taken, and it may be of relevance that glucose levels in plasma samples are 13–18% higher than in whole blood. In terms of safety, accurate blood glucose measurements in whole blood samples will not underestimate the severity of hypoglycaemia, except in polycythaemia.

Interesting new techniques of glucose monitoring by subcutaneous microdialysis should be noted, as they reduce the need for venepuncture and heelpricks.[19] However, the clinical significance and validity of glucose measurements using these techniques are not fully evaluated.

Table 35.1 Mechanisms of hypoglycaemia

Increased glucose utilisation
    Hyperinsulinism
Inadequate glucose supply
    Reduced availability of gluconeogenic precursors
    Inactivity of enzymes of glycogenolysis and gluconeogenesis
    Glucoregulatory hormone imbalance

Table 35.2 Infants who are at risk for the neurological sequelae of hypoglycaemia

At-risk group	Mechanisms	Management
Preterm ($\leq$ 36 weeks)	Low substrate stores Immature hormone and enzyme responses Fluid/energy restriction Feeding difficulties	Early, frequent and adequate feeds i.v. glucose (if necessary)
Intrauterine growth retardation (b.wt <3rd percentile or clinically wasted)	Low substrate stores Immature hormone and enzyme responses Feeding difficulties	Early, frequent and adequate feeds i.v. glucose (if necessary) i.m./i.v. glucagon
Infant of diabetic mother (poor antenatal control) Beckwith – Wiedemann syndrome Rhesus haemolytic disease	Hyperinsulinism	Early, frequent and adequate feeds i.v. glucose (if necessary) Diazoxide Somatostatin
Islet-cell dysregulation syndrome Islet-cell adenoma	Hyperinsulinism	Pancreatectomy/resection adenoma
Perinatal asphyxia (requiring admission to NNU)	Low substrate stores 'Exhausted' stress response Hyperinsulinism Fluid/energy restriction Feeding difficulties	Adequate energy provision
Maternal β-blocker administration	Suppressed catecholamine response	Early, frequent and adequate feeds i.v. glucose (if necessary)
Septicaemia	Inhibition of counter-regulatory enzymes Fluid/energy restriction Feeding difficulties	Adequate energy provision
Inborn errors of metabolism	Defects of enzymes of glycogenolysis, gluconeogenesis or fatty acid β oxidation	Investigate Adequate energy provision

In addition to diagnosing hypoglycaemia, the underlying cause must be determined. This is usually self-evident from the obstetric history or clinical examination, but if this is not the case and the hypoglycaemia is profound or persistent despite treatment, further investigations must be performed to identify rare but serious inborn errors of metabolism or hormone deficiencies (Table 35.2). As these tests are most informative when carried out at the time of hypoglycaemia, it is important to take the necessary blood and urine samples during such episodes and process and store them if necessary out of laboratory working hours. Each unit should devise an appropriate protocol for this in liaison with local and regional specialised laboratories.

Prevalence of neonatal hypoglycaemia

Because clinical practices have changed to such an extent since the risks of hypoglycaemia were first identified, and because of the controversy surrounding definition, it is difficult to ascertain the prevalence of hypoglycaemia in the at-risk groups. For example, using the definition proposed by Cornblath,[35] prevalences ranged from 5% to 7.9% for term infants and from 3.2% to 15% in preterm infants.[35,54,72,77] Using the more recently suggested level for blood glucose concentrations (2.6 mmol/l), Lucas et al[101] reported a prevalence of 67%, whereas a more recent study of

clinically stable, AGA, term and preterm neonates reported prevalences of 10% and 4%, respectively.[72] The lower incidence reported in preterm infants in the most recent study[72] may reflect the trend away from clinicians accepting the previous definitions of hypoglycaemia and thus aiming to maintain higher blood glucose levels in preterm infants. The prevalence of low blood glucose concentrations in the healthy, AGA, term population is unlikely to be of clinical concern in the light of the protective ketone body response, but early monitoring and the prevention of hypoglycaemia in at-risk groups should take place in order to minimise its occurrence therein.

Mechanisms and at-risk groups

Hypoglycaemia may be secondary to increased utilisation of glucose, to inadequate endogenous or exogenous supply of glucose, or to a combination of the two (see Table 35.1).

Increased glucose utilisation

The most common cause of excessive utilisation of glucose is neonatal hyperinsulinism. Hyperinsulinism should be confirmed by the use of a highly specific insulin assay for plasma insulin concentrations and its interpretation with reference to normal

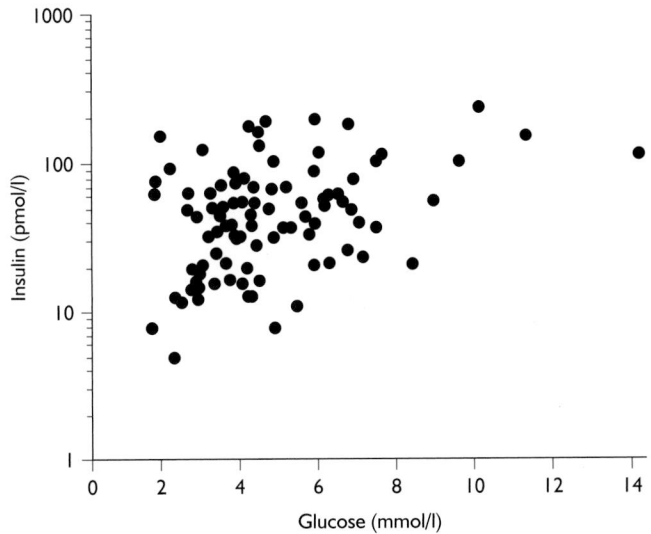

Fig. 35.3 Insulin–glucose relationship in preterm neonates, insulin concentrations measured using a highly specific immuno-radiometric assay. (Reproduced from Hawdon et al.[69])

neonatal insulin–glucose relationships (Fig. 35.3).[66,69] Clinical features are that glucose requirements to maintain normoglycaemia are high, in excess of the 4–6 mg/kg/min usually required by neonates, and the infant may be macrosomic (Fig. 35.4). Investigation of suspected hyperinsulinism will demonstrate low fatty acid and ketone body concentrations during hypoglycaemia, but this feature is not specific to hyperinsulinism as some infants who are not hyperinsulinaemic, such as some who are preterm or IUGR, also fail to mount lipolytic and ketogenic responses.

Self-limiting hyperinsulinism

Hyperinsulinism may be a temporary phenomenon when the fetus has been rendered hyperglycaemic by poorly controlled maternal diabetes (Chapter 22), antenatal administration of thiazide diuretics or the administration of glucose to the mother in labour, and in infants shortly after abrupt discontinuation of i.v. glucose infusions, after bolus doses of glucose, or if glucose has been infused through an umbilical arterial catheter whose tip is close to the coeliac axis.[99,132] Rhesus haemolytic disease and perinatal asphyxia have also been associated with transient fetal and neonatal hyperinsulinism, although the aetiological link is not known.[30,70,113] It has been suggested that hyperinsulinism contributes to hypoglycaemia after IUGR, but normal insulin–glucose relationships (using neonatal reference data) have been demonstrated in IUGR neonates.[31,66,67,74]

Beckwith–Wiedemann syndrome

This condition, described independently by Beckwith[20] and Wiedemann,[162] is characterised by exomphalos, macroglossia, visceromegaly, earlobe abnormalities and an increased later incidence of malignancies. Hyperinsulinism is a common but not invariable feature causing high glucose requirements in the early neonatal period, which usually resolves some time after birth. It is likely that the previously reported long-term developmental difficulties were related to undiagnosed and untreated hypoglycaemia, and it

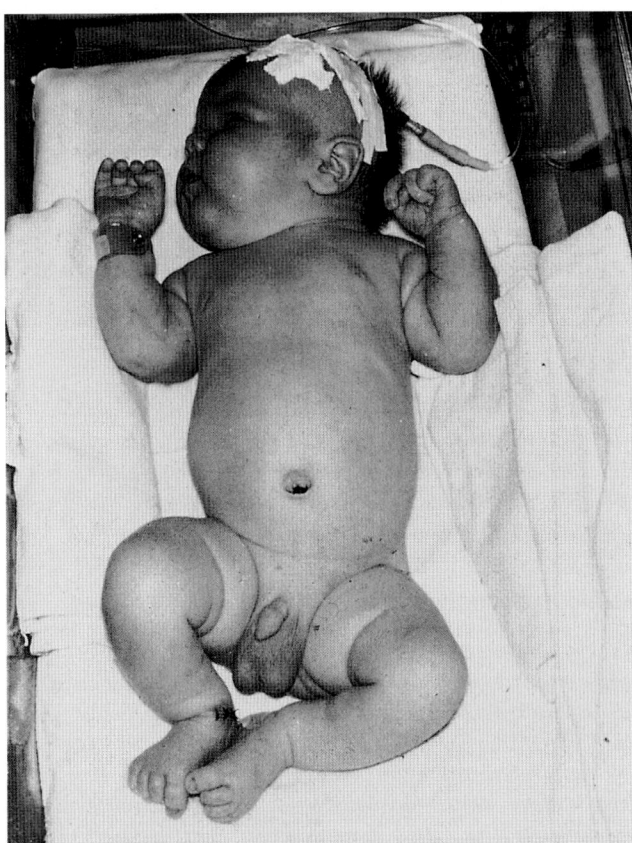

Fig. 35.4 Newborn infant with pancreatic islet-cell dysregulation syndrome (nesidioblastosis) showing increased adiposity and resemblance to an infant of a diabetic mother.

is anticipated that awareness of the condition and prevention of hypoglycaemia should result in improved outcome.

Hyperinsulinism in infancy (HI)

Although a rare condition, this is the most common cause of recurrent and persistent hypoglycaemia in infancy and childhood.[79] It is usually associated with macrosomia and always with extreme hyperinsulinism and high glucose requirements. The condition may be self-limiting in the neonatal period but more often extends beyond this time. As there is no protective ketone body response to hypoglycaemia, there are usually neurological signs and the risk of brain damage is high. Therefore, urgent treatment is required (see below). Many descriptive terms, such as 'nesidioblastosis', 'islet-cell dysregulation syndrome' or 'persistent hyperinsulinaemic hypoglycaemia of infancy', have been applied to the condition. Currently, histological classification is into diffuse and focal forms.[126]

Several underlying pathologies have been demonstrated.[51,136] In 30–40% of cases of persistent HI there are mutations in the genes encoding for SUR1 and KIR6.2, subunits of the K^+ATP channel. The functional loss of this channel results in dysregulation of calcium fluxes and thus unregulated insulin release.[57] Other forms of hyperinsulinism, which tend to be milder or present later, are linked to defects in genes encoding for glucokinase and glutamate dehydrogenase, enzymes essential for K^+ATP channel function. These forms are termed HI-GK and

HI-GLUD. The latter may be associated with hyperammon-aemia, necessitating measurement of ammonia levels whenever hyperinsulinism is suspected.[47,136] More recently, a mutation in the gene encoding the enzyme l-3-hydroxyacyl-CoA dehydrogenase (SCHAD) has been reported to cause HI.[28]

Rarely, an isolated islet-cell adenoma may present with neonatal hyperinsulinaemic hypoglycaemia.[141]

Recognition of hyperinsulinism and early prevention and treatment of hypoglycaemia, with referral to a specialist centre, is essential to reduce the incidence of permanent neurological damage which has been widely reported.[82,108,109,142]

'Leucine-sensitive hypoglycaemia'

This was previously described as a distinct entity, but it is more likely that hypoglycaemia in response to leucine administration represents underlying hyperinsulinism and should be investigated and treated as such.[169]

Insufficient supply of glucose

Hypoglycaemia is most often the result of reduced delivery of glucose into the blood. In the enterally fed infant, all the circulating glucose is provided either by the absorption and conversion of sugars or by glycogenolysis and gluconeogenesis, and in some babies there may be a contribution from i.v. glucose infusion. Thus, if the infant fails to switch on glycogenolysis or gluconeogenesis in response to falling blood glucose levels, or clinicians prescribe insufficient i.v. glucose, hypoglycaemia may occur. Three possible mechanisms may cause the failure of glucose production:

- *Reduced availability of gluconeogenic precursors.* Glycogenolysis and gluconeogenesis may be limited by availability of glycogen, gluconeogenic precursors or the energy provided by fatty acid oxidation. This may occur after preterm delivery, IUGR, maternal alcohol abuse or perinatal hypoxia-ischaemia, or as a consequence of inadequate substrate intake after birth.[119,120,134,139]
- *Reduced activity of enzymes of glycogenolysis and gluconeogenesis.* There may be failure of synthesis and activation of the key enzymes described above. This may be the result of a specific inherited metabolic disorder, in which case hypoglycaemia is usually severe, and recurrent or persistent, or there may be generalised immaturity of enzymes, as in preterm infants. In these cases the infant is resistant to the effects of the postnatal surges of counterregulatory hormones. Finally, enzyme activity may be suppressed by acquired conditions, such as perinatal bacterial infection. Defective gluconeogenesis may also be the cause of hypoglycaemia complicating cases of congenital heart disease and cold injury.[76,104]
- *Impaired counterregulatory hormone response.* This will result in failure to activate enzymes of glycogenolysis and gluconeogenesis. Hyperinsulinism has a dual mechanism in that glucose utilisation is increased (see above) but also counterregulatory hormone release is inhibited. In this way, hyperinsulinism inhibits glycogenolysis, gluconeogenesis, and lipolysis. Failure of release of counterregulatory hormones may play a role in hypoglycaemia in preterm and IUGR babies, and after maternal medication with β-blockers in pregnancy.[114,119] Finally, there may be rare permanent disorders which result in insufficiency of

counterregulatory hormones, for example low growth hormone and cortisol levels in septo-optic dysplasia and congenital hypopituitarism, and low glucocorticoid levels in adrenocortical deficiencies.[37,55,98]

In summary, mechanisms of hypoglycaemia vary among groups of infants, and for some there may be more than one aetiological mechanism (see Table 35.2). This is most applicable to neonates who have been subject to IUGR, which for many reasons may result in failure of glycogenolysis and gluconeogenesis after birth. Animal and clinical studies have demonstrated that IUGR may reduce the availability of alternative fuels for cerebral metabolism.[44,71,74] However, another clinical study has shown that many IUGR babies can mount a ketogenic response, and suggests that excessive formula milk supplementation to these babies may be the cause of the suppressed response.[49] It is important to note that not all IUGR infants will be SGA (Chapter 10), and clinical examination is important for the identification of the 'wasted' neonate. Conversely, not all SGA infants will have been subject to placental insufficiency: they may be constitutionally small and may not experience the postnatal problems in metabolic adaptation. The early identification of at-risk neonates and the understanding of underlying mechanisms of hypoglycaemia are important for the diagnosis and treatment of the disorder.

Prevention and management of neonatal hypoglycaemia (Table 35.3)

Normal babies

As described above, healthy full-term AGA neonates often have low blood glucose concentrations in the first 2–3 postnatal days, but are thought to be protected by the presence of ketone bodies and lactate as alternative fuels. Thus, it is now recognised in Europe and North America that for this group it is not appropriate to carry out routine blood glucose monitoring, to label low blood glucose as a pathological entity, or to initiate treatment which is invasive or which may interfere with the establishment of breastfeeding.[33,52,63,116] Because of the healthy infant's ability to counterregulate, problems with establishment of successful breastfeeding are equally likely to present with excessive weight loss (in excess of 10% birthweight), dehydration and jaundice as with clinically significant hypoglycaemia. Therefore, breastfeeding advice and intervention should not be based on blood glucose levels but on full assessment of the baby – proceeding to blood glucose measurement if there are clinical concerns. Midwives and doctors must be alert to the possibility that other conditions, such as infection or, more rarely, inborn errors of metabolism, may present with the neurological signs of hypoglycaemia, for which specific investigations should be performed (Table 35.4).

At-risk babies (see Table 35.2)

For practical purposes, the following discussion focuses only on the infants who are at risk of the neurological sequelae of

Table 35.3 Roberton Textbook of Neonatology, 4th Edition, in press

1. Identify at-risk infants (See Table 38.2)	

2. Early energy provision (within 1 hour of birth):

If enteral feeding planned:	*If enteral feeding contraindicated:*
Breastfeed if mother's wish	i.v. 10% glucose infusion of at least 3 ml/kg/h
Encourage kangaroo care and unlimited access to breast	
If not breast fed, formula feed of 12 ml/kg	
Minimum between-feed interval of 3 hours	

3. Blood glucose monitoring:
Pre-feed measurement
Before second feed, then frequency according to progress (at least 4–6-hourly in first 48 hours)
Accurate method or confirm reagent stick measurements <3.0 mmol/l with accurate method
Discontinue when 2 readings at least 2.0 mmol/l (3.0 mmol/l for hyperinsulinism)
Recommence if energy intake falls, e.g. vomiting or condition of baby changes
Measure blood glucose in any baby with abnormal clinical signs

4. Maintain energy provision:
Increase feed interval if BG ≥ 2.0 mmol/l (3.0 mmol/l for hyperinsulinism)

Mother plans to breastfeed:	*Mother plans to bottle feed:*
Encourage kangaroo care and unlimited access to breast	Start at 100 ml/kg/day
Encourage mother to express	Demand feed when BG ≥ 2.0 mmol/l
Offer breast before formula feeds	(3.0 mmol/l for hyperinsulinism)
Formula/EBM supplements by gavage, cup or bottle	
Volume and frequency as indicated by BG monitoring and clinical condition	
Discontinue when BG ≥ 2.0 mmol/l (3.0 mmol/l for hyperinsulinism)	
Continue milk feeds if tolerated even if i.v. therapy commenced	

i.v. therapy:
Make gradual reductions, e.g. by 1–2 ml/h if BG ≥ 2.0 mmol/l (3.0 mmol/l for hyperinsulinism)
Resite drips promptly

5. If blood glucose <2.0 mmol/l on at least 2 occasions, but no clinical signs:

If enterally fed:	*If i.v. 10% glucose already running:*
Increase feed volume and frequency	Increase infusion rate or concentration
Commence i.v. glucose if BG remains <2.0 mmol/l despite above	
If BG persistently low, trial of glucagon i.m./i.v. 100 micrograms/kg	

6. If BG < 1.0 mmol/l and/or major clinical signs e.g. fits/coma:
Take sample for accurate BG but don't wait for result
If possible take diagnostic hormone and metabolite samples
i.v. 10% glucose bolus of 3 ml/kg, repeated if signs do not resolve
Followed immediately by i.v. glucose infusion of at least 3 ml/kg/h, adjust according to signs and BG
If problems siting i.v. and diagnosis is hyperinsulinism, give glucagon i.m./i.v. 100 micrograms/kg
Investigate for other causes e.g. infection
Collect and freeze next urine sample
Hourly BG measurements until ≥2.0 mmol/l

7. If hypoglycaemia severe or persistent:
Investigate as in Table 35.4

8. Summary:
Milk feeds: to maximum volume tolerated
i.v. glucose: minimum necessary to maintain BG ≥ 2.0 mmol/l (3.0 mmol/l for hyperinsulinism)

hypoglycaemia (see Table 35.2). Early prevention of hypoglycaemia is optimal for these infants, so the first step in management must be to identify them. Although this is easy in some cases (such as the preterm baby), for others clinical observations are important (for example, to identify the wasted appearance of the growth-retarded neonate who may not necessarily have a low birthweight).

These at-risk infants should have regular pre-feed blood glucose monitoring (at least 4–6-hourly initially). In addition, it is imperative that any infant with neurological signs, even if not in an at-risk group, should have urgent, accurate blood glucose measurement. The monitoring schedule for at-risk infants will vary according to local protocols, but we suggest that monitoring

Table 35.4 Samples for the investigation of severe or persistent hypoglycaemia. NB: Each condition is a rare cause of neonatal hypoglycaemia

Sample	Assay	Diagnosis
Blood	Glucose*	Confirm diagnosis
Blood	pH* Lactate*	Lactic acidosis in: glucose-6-phosphatase deficiency fructose-1,6-diphosphatase deficiency pyruvate carboxylase deficiency phosphoenolpyruvate carboxykinase deficiency Acidosis in disorders of amino acid metabolism
Blood	Intermediary metabolites	Disorders of gluconeogenesis
Blood	Ketone bodies	Disorders of fatty acid β oxidation (NB: low ketone body levels in preterm, IUGR and hyperinsulinaemic infants)
Plasma	Fatty acids	Disorders of fatty acid β oxidation
Plasma	Insulin+	Hyperinsulinism
Plasma	Glucagon Catecholamines Corticosteroids Growth hormone	Isolated hormone deficiency or in association with others, e.g. septo-optic dysplasia
Plasma/urine	Amino acid profile	Disorders of amino acid metabolism
Urine	Organic acids	Disorders of fatty acid β oxidation
Fibroblasts/leukocytes	Enzyme activities	Selected inborn errors of metabolism

* Analysers available for use in neonatal unit laboratory.
+ Use specific assay and neonatal reference data.[66,75]

should be commenced before the first feed and that pre-feed monitoring be continued until the infant has had at least two satisfactory measurements. Monitoring should be recommenced if the infant's clinical condition worsens or energy intake decreases. If monitoring is by reagent strip, low levels must be confirmed by accurate measurement (see above).

The importance of early milk feeding has been appreciated for many years.[140] Both breast and formula milks provide important gluconeogenic precursors and fatty acids for β oxidation. As they contain sources of energy other than carbohydrate, they have a higher joule/ml content than 10% dextrose. In addition, enteral milk feeding stimulates the secretion of gut hormones, which may facilitate postnatal metabolic adaptation.[100] Therefore, all infants who are expected to tolerate enteral feeds should be fed with milk as soon as possible after birth, and at frequent intervals thereafter. Babies who are capable of sucking should be offered the breast at each feed (if this is the mother's wish). The need for formula supplementation will vary between babies, will diminish with the successful establishment of breastfeeding, and will be guided by regular pre-feed blood glucose monitoring, the clinical condition of the baby and assessment of breastfeeding. In the breastfed baby, formula intake should be kept to the minimum necessary, so as to enhance breastfeeding and avoid suppression of normal metabolic adaptation.[49]

When full enteral feeding is not anticipated, for example in the very preterm or sick infant, an i.v. glucose infusion should be commenced as soon as possible after birth. Usually, 10% dextrose at 3 ml/kg/h (5 mg glucose/kg/min) is sufficient to prevent hypoglycaemia, but in some cases (such as hyperinsulinism) more is required. If the amount of glucose administered is limited by fluid restriction, more concentrated dextrose solutions may be required and central venous lines should be used, because these solutions are sclerotic to peripheral veins and cause tissue damage if they leak.

If low blood glucose levels persist or are associated with clinical signs in the milk-fed infant despite the above measures, it may be possible to increase further the volumes and/or frequencies of feeds. If this is not possible, or if the hypoglycaemia is resistant to this strategy, i.v. glucose will be required. If the infant is tolerating milk feeds, these should be neither stopped nor reduced. The initial rate of 10% glucose infusion should be 3 ml/kg/h (5 mg/kg/min; Table 35.5), but adjusted according to frequent accurate blood glucose measurements. If the need for fluid restriction limits the amount of glucose that may be given, more concentrated solutions may need to be infused (see Table 35.5). If hypoglycaemia persists despite i.v. glucose, it is important to check the infusion site and the infusion apparatus to confirm glucose delivery. Leaking drips should be promptly resited. Boluses of concentrated glucose solution should be avoided because of the risk of rebound hypoglycaemia and cerebral oedema;[133] if boluses are required (for example, if there are neurological signs of hypoglycaemia), they should be of 10% dextrose (3–5 ml/kg),

Table 35.5 Chart for conversion of rate of glucose infusion from ml/kg/24 h to mg/kg/min depending on strength of dextrose solution

Rate of infusion		Strength dextrose solution mg/kg/min			
ml/kg/24 h	ml/kg/h	4%	10%	15%	20%
60	2.5	1.7	4.2	6.2	8.4
72	3.0	2.0	5.0	7.5	10.0
80	3.3	2.2	5.6	8.3	11.2
100	4.2	2.8	6.9	10.4	13.8
120	5.0	3.3	8.3	12.5	16.6
150	6.3	4.2	10.4	15.6	20.8
180	7.5	5.0	12.5	18.7	25.0
200	8.3	5.6	13.9	20.8	27.8

given slowly, and always followed by an infusion. All reductions in infusion rate should be gradual. In cases of hyperinsulinism, intramuscular (i.m.) glucagon will have a temporary glycaemic effect if there is delay in siting an i.v. infusion (see below).

Specific treatments

Hyperinsulinism

It should be stressed again that, when hyperinsulinism is not self-limiting and requires or is resistant to very high glucose infusion rates, referral to a specialist centre must be made.[14] The treatments outlined below should only be administered in non-specialist units on the advice of a specialist centre and as a holding measure pending transfer. The risk of precipitating heart failure, especially if there is a coexisting hypertrophic cardiomyopathy, must be considered.

Glucose delivery should be prescribed to maintain blood glucose levels above 3 mmol/l and early siting of an umbilical venous catheter or venous central line is essential to allow adequate delivery rates. If hypoglycaemia is still resistant to high glucose delivery rates, it is possible to administer diazoxide (10–20 mg/kg/day), which suppresses pancreatic insulin release. It may be given enterally (available through Idis World Medicines). The effect is optimal if a daily dose of chlorthiazide (7–10 mg/kg) is given to potentiate the hyperglycaemic effect and prevent the fluid-retentive effect of diazoxide. In cases of persistent hyperinsulinism, response to diazoxide is variable; patients with HI-GK and HI-GLUD tend to show the best response.

Work defining the molecular basis of hyperinsulinism has demonstrated that some cases respond to the calcium channel blocker nifedipine.[18,136]

Somatostatin analogue (octreotide, Sandostatin), administered i.v. or subcutaneously at a dose of 10 micrograms/kg/day, also suppresses insulin release.[14] However, tolerance may develop and there is concern about possible effects on the secretion of other hormones; because of the latter, glucagon is administered simultaneously at a dose of 1 microgram/kg/h.[73]

Glucagon (200 micrograms/kg bolus i.v. or i.m., or infusion 5–10 micrograms/kg/h), has a temporary glycaemic effect via its glycogenolytic action and given alone may be a useful holding measure, for example when resiting glucose infusions. However, its

prolonged use is limited because glucagon further stimulates insulin release.

In some cases of neonatal hyperinsulinism, 95% pancreatectomy is required, and for this, referral should be made to regional neonatal surgical centres. Some groups use pancreatic catheterisation to determine by intraoperative histological and biochemical studies the site of a focal islet-cell hyperplasia in the pancreas and to allow limited pancreatic resection.[46,48]

Intrauterine growth retardation

Of more interest is the potential role of glucagon when hypoglycaemia is secondary to IUGR. It appears that its mechanism of action when given in pharmacological doses (30–200 micrograms/kg) is to mimic the postnatal glucagon surge and the 'switching on' of the enzymes of gluconeogenesis.[68,107] Thus, it is a useful adjunct to i.v. glucose therapy and, after further evaluation, may prove an alternative treatment to i.v. glucose.

Adrenocortical insufficiency

Although parenteral hydrocortisone has been used for many years for the treatment of hypoglycaemia of various aetiologies, its place is solely as a replacement therapy for cortisol deficiency.

Inborn errors of metabolism

The management of the rare inborn errors of metabolism varies according to diagnosis and is beyond the scope of this chapter. In general, the aim is to provide adequate calories to prevent hypoglycaemia and catabolism.

Neonatal hypoglycaemia in developing countries

In developing countries, growth retardation, hypothermia, practices of late feeding and maternal nutritional factors are risk factors for hypoglycaemia.[165,166] However, there are few published data regarding the prevalence of hypoglycaemia in any developing country, and comparison of data with those from the developed world is hampered by differing definitions, populations, labour room practices, timing and technical methods. A study in Nepal using glucose test strips demonstrated that 38% of newborns during the first 3 days experienced a blood glucose of less than 2.6 mmol/l, compared with 18% of newborns of the same age in Newcastle-upon-Tyne, UK.[9,72] It is not known whether babies born in such circumstances are at risk of hypoketonaemia during hypoglycaemia, but if there is a high prevalence of IUGR, the vulnerability of these infants to the potential sequelae of hypoglycaemia should be considered. A recent study in Kathmandu, Nepal of 578 newborn infants showed that neonatal hypoglycaemia is more common in a developing country setting, but may not be a clinical problem unless all fuel availability is reduced.[36,123] Some 'textbook' risk factors, like hypothermia, disappeared after controlling for confounding variables. Early feeding reduced the risk of moderate hypoglycaemia in the second 12 hours of life. Some SGA and post-term infants increased counterregulatory ketogenesis with early neonatal hypoglycaemia, but hypothermia, male gender and low infant thyroxine (T_4) were associated with impaired counterregulation after birth. Hypoglycaemic infants generally had lower levels of alternative fuels through either reduced availability or increased consumption.

Therefore, it may not be appropriate to apply the guidelines described so far in this chapter to babies born in developing countries, and specific measures may be required to minimise the risk of neonatal hypoglycaemia. For example, the Baby Friendly Hospital initiative developed by UNICEF since 1992 has enjoyed considerable success in changing the culture of maternity hospitals, so that early breastfeeding is promoted, assisted by changes in facilities and procedures to ensure continual contact between mothers and their babies.[59] In addition, health education before and after childbirth, early suckling and promotion of breastfeeding, swaddling, and early breastfeeding or skin-to-skin contact should reduce the risk of hypothermia and hypoglycaemia.[157]

Neonatal mortality accounts for 50–60% of all infant deaths in developing countries.[11] It is possible that neonatal hypoglycaemia, arising as a consequence of fetal malnutrition, birth asphyxia, postnatal hypothermia or infection, could be responsible for some of the hitherto unexplained neonatal deaths.

Summary

The prevention and management of hypoglycaemia depends upon the administration of sufficient energy via either enteral or parenteral routes. In fact, many cases of hypoglycaemia are iatrogenic as a result of a failure to ensure adequate calorie intake for at-risk babies, or to prescribe sufficient glucose to fluid-restricted babies. Correcting these deficiencies is usually sufficient and only rarely are additional treatments required.

Neonatal hypoglycaemia is a common but usually preventable condition. Its prompt recognition, prevention and management are important to reduce the as yet unquantified but worrying risk of neurological sequelae.

Hyperglycaemia

Neonatal hyperglycaemia has been recognised for over a century,[90] and during this time it has become apparent that it represents several distinct clinical entities. As with hypoglycaemia, much uncertainty exists regarding definition, clinical significance and treatment.

Neonatal diabetes mellitus

Classic diabetes mellitus has been described as first presenting in the neonatal period. It was the subject of a British Paediatric Surveillance Unit study, whose results yielded exciting data regarding the genetics of the condition.[137,153,154] The condition is rare (1:500 000).[138] Early reports suggested that the condition was usually transient, characteristically occurring in SGA infants in the first 6 postnatal weeks and presenting with very high blood glucose levels, low plasma insulin concentrations, dehydration, fever and failure to thrive despite adequate feeding.[78,80,122] The mean duration of insulin therapy, if required, was 69 days for the transient form, and it was thought that very few infants developed permanent diabetes in later life.[35] More recent reviews of reported cases of neonatal diabetes mellitus have confirmed its occurrence predominantly in SGA infants. However, they demonstrated that 46% developed permanent diabetes in the neonatal period, 23% developed permanent diabetes in childhood or adolescence, and in 31%, diabetes resolved in the neonatal period. Ten cases had coexisting clinical conditions and six families had more than one affected individual (including two pairs of twins).[138,161]

Self-limiting neonatal hyperglycaemia

Neonatal hyperglycaemia is most often a transient disorder which resolves spontaneously and has few features in common with classic diabetes mellitus. The prevalence of transient hyperglycaemia appears to be increasing in parallel with the increased survival of ELBW infants and the early use of parenteral nutrition solutions and corticosteroid therapy in these babies.[96] The following sections refer to the most common condition, transient hyperglycaemia in small or sick infants.

Clinical significance

It is of the utmost importance to remember that neonatal hyperglycaemia may be a sign of a serious underlying disorder, such as infection. However, it is still not known whether the high glucose concentrations themselves place the infant at further risk. Unlike adults with insulin deficiency, hyperglycaemic neonates do not develop ketosis or metabolic acidosis.[56] There is a risk that glycosuria and osmotic diuresis may cause fluid and electrolyte imbalance with dehydration, and such disturbances are themselves common in the groups of infants who develop hyperglycaemia, but studies of large numbers of infants have reported that osmotic diuresis is not an invariable consequence of neonatal hyperglycaemia.[42,125,150] There is also concern that changes in blood osmolality and fluid shifts may result in cerebral damage. However, cerebral pathology and adverse neurodevelopmental outcome have never been demonstrated to occur as the direct result of hyperglycaemia, and it is thought that blood glucose levels above 20 mmol/l are required to exert significant osmolar effects.[10,38,50,112]

As described above, neonatal hyperglycaemia is clinically significant in that it may herald a serious underlying disorder. Once such disorders have been ruled out or treated, there is no evidence that self-limiting hyperglycaemia secondary to immaturity of glucoregulation or excessive glucose intakes and not associated with osmotic diuresis, has adverse effects at blood glucose levels below 20 mmol/l.

Definition and diagnosis

There is no established definition of neonatal hyperglycaemia, but blood glucose levels above 7 mmol/l are usually considered to be high. However, the upper 'safe' limit of blood glucose concentration in the neonate is entirely unknown (see below) and, as with hypoglycaemia, there is likely to be great variation among practising neonatologists in terms of the diagnosis and management of hyperglycaemia.

The use of glucose reagent strips is more useful in the diagnosis of hyperglycaemia than for hypoglycaemia because the strips are more reliable at high blood glucose levels, and inaccuracies of 0.5–1.0 mmol/l are of less clinical relevance in the context of hyperglycaemia. However, clinicians should be urged to confirm the diagnosis with a laboratory measurement. It may also be useful to monitor urine for glycosuria, but it should be remembered that neonates, particularly those who are preterm, have a low renal threshold for glucose and fractional excretion of glucose varies widely, so that glycosuria may be present even in normoglycaemia.[163]

Prevalence

Without a clear definition of hyperglycaemia, it is difficult to comment on its frequency. Studies of prevalence vary according to their subjects, with hyperglycaemia found most frequently in VLBW and preterm infants.[26,168] SGA infants who are preterm are more at risk for developing hyperglycaemia than hypoglycaemia when receiving standard i.v. infusions.[27] Reported prevalences vary from 29% to 86% in VLBW neonates.[50,97]

Mechanisms and at-risk groups

The mechanisms underlying neonatal hyperglycaemia vary and, as with hypoglycaemia, are best understood with reference to the expected metabolic changes at birth. In contrast to hypoglycaemia resulting from a low glucose production rate or a high glucose uptake rate, hyperglycaemia may be the result of a high glucose production or infusion rate or a low glucose uptake rate.

Neonatal hyperglycaemia is usually secondary to a high glucose appearance rate and it is often seen when glucose infusion rates are high.[67,97,112] To maintain control, the infant must be able to adapt to the exogenous administration of glucose by suppressing glucose production by the liver. The ability to glucoregulate in this way has been demonstrated in normoglycaemic neonates.[85,93] However, there is evidence from clinical and animal studies that some neonates do not suppress glucose production in response to glucose infusion and/or increased blood glucose levels.[40,41,43,67,158]

The inability to suppress gluconeogenesis may in turn be the result of disordered glucoregulatory hormone control. Although the glucoregulatory role of insulin in the neonate is unclear and may vary between infants, it has been suggested that hyperglycaemia results from decreased insulin secretion in immature subjects.[111,168] This is analogous to the adult insulin-dependent diabetic. Animal studies have also shown that after chronic hyperglycaemia, the fetal pancreas cannot mount an insulin response to a further glucose surge.[25] This may be analogous to the condition in preterm babies receiving constant high-rate glucose infusions, whose pancreatic response to hyperglycaemia may be 'exhausted'.

Alternatively, circulating insulin concentrations may be appropriate for the blood glucose concentration, but hyperglycaemia may result from end-organ insensitivity to insulin. This is analogous to 'maturity-onset diabetes', which is characterised by insulin resistance. Neonatal insulin resistance has been demonstrated by the persistence of hyperglycaemia in the presence of raised insulin concentrations, by the poor hypoglycaemic response to large exogenous doses of insulin, and by the high insulin concentrations needed to suppress gluconeogenesis.[58,81,94,125,152] Insulin resistance may be secondary to immaturity or downregulation of peripheral receptors, to the effect of high fatty acid levels resulting from infusion of fat emulsion, or to the peripheral actions of counterregulatory hormones.[167]

Clinical data demonstrate that some hyperglycaemic preterm infants have inappropriately low plasma insulin concentrations and high plasma catecholamine levels, whereas others have apparently appropriate insulin concentrations and may have insulin resistance (Fig. 35.5) (Hawdon et al, unpublished data). The former group were those who had other clinical complications such as infection, and the latter were either very preterm or preterm and SGA.

The excess secretion of counterregulatory hormones, which themselves stimulate glycogenolysis and gluconeogenesis, may in addition block the secretion of insulin and inhibit its peripheral action, thereby contributing to insulin resistance.[32] This is the

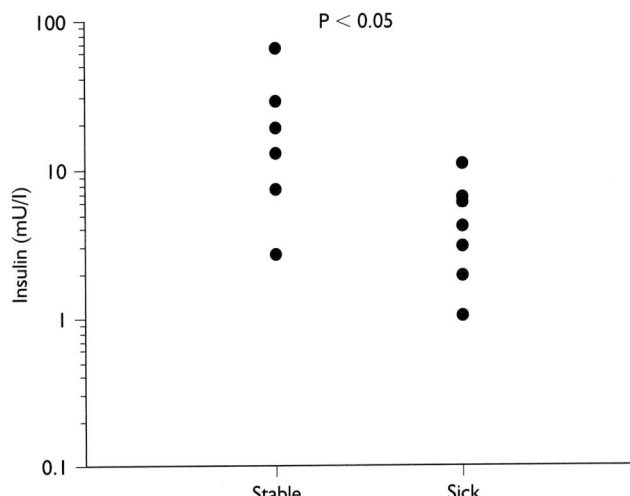

Fig. 35.5 Plasma insulin concentrations in preterm infants who were clinically stable or who had clinical complications such as infection or necrotising enterocolitis (sick infants).

mechanism of hyperglycaemia secondary to exogenous cortico-steroids, sometimes administered in large doses to neonates with lung disease.[155] It has even been suggested that antenatal cortico-steroid administration contributes to the failure to suppress post-natal gluconeogenesis.[158] Aminophylline, used for the prevention of apnoea of prematurity, mimics the action of catecholamines and induces glycogenolysis.[164] To date, growth hormone has not been implicated in the aetiology of neonatal hyperglycaemia.[168]

These hormonal disturbances may be the consequence of underlying clinical stresses such as infection, respiratory distress, pain or surgery.[3,5,24,95,97,148,151,168] Studies by Anand et al[2–7] demonstrated that with minimal anaesthesia for major surgical procedures in term and preterm neonates, high glucagon and catecholamine levels and inhibition of insulin secretion led to a number of metabolic abnormalities, including hyperglycaemia and hyperlactataemia. This response was in proportion to the severity of surgical stress and could be prevented by the addition of opioid analgesia or halothane to anaesthetic regimens. In some conditions associated with severe clinical stress, such as peri-natal asphyxia, hyperglycaemia may occur as the result of high counterregulatory hormone concentrations but hypoglycaemia is more often seen, probably because the latter represents the situation found after the stress response is exhausted.

Despite the frequency with which hyperglycaemia is now observed, the aetiology and optimal management of this metabolic disorder have not been established. Clinical, animal and laboratory studies suggest that glucose production is not suppressed in the face of hyperglycaemia, but there are conflicting data regarding the role of defective glucoregulatory hormone responses.

Prevention and management (Fig. 35.6)

As neonatal hyperglycaemia is usually self-limiting and not associated with adverse sequelae, many clinicians choose not to treat raised blood glucose concentrations aggressively. However, the first step in management, especially in a baby who has previously been normoglycaemic, must be to seek and treat serious underlying disorders. The second step is to prevent the occurrence of high blood glucose concentrations secondary to high glucose infusion rates by instituting careful management of i.v. fluid prescriptions. Clinicians often increase fluid infusion rates to counter renal and extrarenal losses in the immature neonate. It must be recognised that increasing the rate of administration of a glucose solution will result in a proportionate increase in glucose administration. For example, 200 ml/kg/day of 10% dextrose provides 14 mg/kg/min glucose, which is well in excess of the neonate's requirements. Thus it is not surprising that hyperglycaemia occurs and the extra glucose given is 'wasted'. Therefore, glucose infusion rates should be calculated, and if they are found to be excessive (for example, above 4–6 mg/kg/min), more dilute solutions should be used.

Hyperglycaemia may still occur in some neonates who are clinically stable and who are not receiving excessive glucose intakes. These infants are usually of extremely low birthweight and less than 1 week old. Often they have received early parenteral nutrition and thus fairly high rates of glucose infusion in combination with amino acids. At the same time, they may have high counterregulatory hormone levels, rendering them 'catabolic'

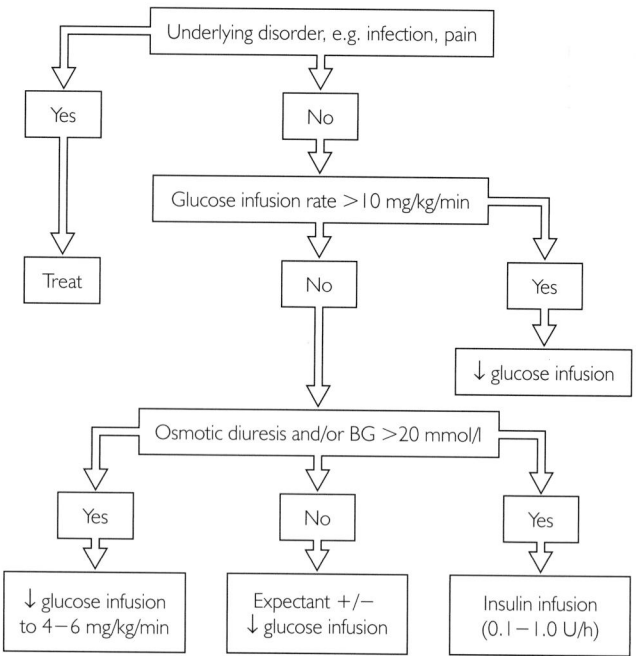

Fig. 35.6 Steps in the management of neonatal hyperglycaemia.

with or without peripheral insulin resistance, so that they cannot utilise the infused substrates. The condition is usually self-limiting and may be prevented by the more gradual introduction of parenteral nutrition solutions in those at risk.

There are three strategies for management of hyperglycaemia when it occurs in these circumstances.

First, moderate hyperglycaemia may be 'tolerated' if it does not appear to be causing osmotic diuresis. Our experience is that the condition resolves within a few days even if no action is taken.

Secondly, the rate of glucose infusion may be carefully reduced to the rate at which blood glucose levels become normal, and then gradually increased as tolerated. This carries the possible disadvantage of reducing the infant's energy intake, but it is likely that immature infants are unable to effectively utilise all the glucose offered, especially if at a rate in excess of 5 mg/kg/min.[158]

Thirdly, insulin may be administered in order to lower the blood glucose concentration without reducing the glucose infusion rate. Controlled studies of insulin administration to adult intensive care patients on i.v. nutrition have demonstrated that although there is a short-term improvement in nitrogen balance, there is no advantage in terms of either weight gain or body composition, and that a number of patients become hypoglycaemic.[102,128] Although there are a number of reports of this practice in the neonatal literature, there is no consistency regarding the clinical situations in which insulin has been given, only short-term outcome measures have been reported, and there are few prospective controlled trials.[22,121,160] They reported that the administration of insulin (20–400 mU/h, and 2–86 mU/kg/h) was associated with the ability to tolerate increased glucose infusion rates. However, as these studies were neither controlled nor randomised, and in the absence of long-term outcome measures, it is impossible to conclude that insulin therapy conferred a clinical advantage. All of these studies reported hypoglycaemia in some infants even after the discontinuation of insulin infusion.

One controlled trial of hyperglycaemic preterm neonates demonstrated that insulin administration (40–1000 mU/h) allowed glucose infusion rates of 20 mg/kg/min, compared with 13 mg/kg/min in infants who did not receive insulin (both are higher rates of glucose infusion than would be used in current clinical practice). There was more rapid early weight gain in the treated group, but this may have been related to higher rates of fluid infusion. Infected infants had extremely high insulin requirements and high circulating insulin concentrations, suggesting significant insulin resistance.[32]

There is marked variation between and within studies regarding the doses of insulin required, and some authors have raised the possibility of the development of tolerance in some babies, so that hyperglycaemia recurs despite large increases in insulin dosage.[22,32,58,121] This is surprising in the face of the clinical observation that without insulin treatment neonatal hyperglycaemia is usually a transient and self-limiting condition, and it may be that insulin administration in some way hinders spontaneous recovery.

Recent studies have suggested that intrauterine nutritional and endocrine status may influence adult metabolism and susceptibility to disease.[16] The long-term clinical significance of early high-energy intakes in association with large doses of exogenous insulin in the preterm neonate, and of possible up- or downregulation of insulin receptors, has not yet been considered.

Finally, the introduction of enteral feeding with small volumes of milk as soon as the infant's gastrointestinal tract will tolerate this may hasten the control of blood glucose homeostasis by inducing surges of gut hormones which may promote insulin secretion (the enteroinsular axis).[13]

The pathogenesis of neonatal hyperglycaemia and the mechanism of action of exogenous insulin administration are not clearly understood. Therefore, the increasing practice of prescribing insulin to neonates without understanding its mode of action is of concern. It is not known whether insulin administration promotes linear growth in neonates, or merely converts glucose into fat. A prospective randomised controlled trial of insulin therapy in preterm neonates who become glucose intolerant would assess the impact of insulin therapy on glucose tolerance, metabolism and growth in the short and long term. Until such a study is performed, it is impossible to judge whether insulin therapy does confer clinical advantage over expectant management of a condition which is usually self-limiting.

Summary

In this chapter, an approach to the controversy surrounding the definition, diagnosis and management of babies with neonatal hypoglycaemia has been presented. Much more information is needed before the same aspects of the present pragmatic approach, based on the safest possible practice, can be established on a more secure scientific basis. The following summarises the key questions that still need to be addressed.

First, the long-term effects of moderate and/or asymptomatic hypoglycaemia must be established. For example, we do not know whether the preterm infant's brain is more or less vulnerable to hypoglycaemia than that of the term infant, what duration of hypoglycaemia results in permanent disability, and whether the effects of hypoglycaemia are exacerbated by concurrent complications such as hyperbilirubinaemia or pre-existing hypoxia-ischaemia. We do not know whether the differences that we have demonstrated between preterm and term infants in metabolic adaptation persist beyond the first postnatal week, and whether there are implications for the preterm infant in terms of persistent impairment of metabolic responses.

Secondly, more information must be gathered relating to other factors regulating glucose availability to the brain – namely, cerebral blood flow, the ontogeny of glucose transporter proteins, and the role of the astrocyte in neuronal metabolic support.

Finally, as we realise the inadequacy of glucose reagent sticks for the diagnosis and monitoring of hypoglycaemia, improved accurate near-patient systems should be developed for the measurement of blood glucose concentrations, and the ability to measure blood ketone body concentrations in these circumstances would markedly enhance management.

In 1954, McQuarrie[103] urged the physician caring for children to be constantly aware of the risk of hypoglycaemia. This exhortation is still relevant in the 21st century, but much still needs to be learned and there are many challenging areas of research for the clinical investigator.

Acknowledgement

The author wishes to thank Dr A. M. de L. Costello for contributing to the section on neonatal hypoglycaemia in developing countries and Dr K. Hussain for contributing to the section on hyperinsulinism.

References

1. Adam P A J, Raiha N, Rahiala E C, Kekomahl M 1975 Oxidation of glucose and hydroxybutyrate by the early human fetal brain. Acta Paediatrica Scandinavica 64: 17–24
2. Anand K J S, Aynsley-Green A 1988 Measuring the severity of surgical stress in newborn infants. Journal of Pediatric Surgery 23: 297–305
3. Anand K J S, Brown M J, Causon R C, Christofides N D, Bloom S R, Aynsley-Green A 1985 Can the human neonate mount an endocrine and metabolic response to surgery? Journal of Pediatric Surgery 20: 41–48
4. Anand K J S, Hickey P R 1987 Pain and its effects on the human neonate and fetus. New England Journal of Medicine 317: 1321–1329
5. Anand K J S, Sippell W G, Aynsley-Green A 1985 Metabolic and endocrine effects of surgical ligation of patent ductus arteriosus in the human neonate: are there implications for further improvement of postoperative outcome? In: Falkner R, Kretchner N, Rossi E (eds) Modern problems in paediatrics. Karger, Basle, pp 145–157
6. Anand K J S, Sippell W G, Aynsley-Green A 1987 Randomised trial of fentanyl anaesthesia in preterm neonates undergoing surgery. Effects on the stress response. Lancet i: 62–66
7. Anand K J S, Sipell W G, Schofield N, Aynsley-Green A 1988 Does halothane anaesthesia decrease the metabolic and endocrine stress response of newborn infants undergoing surgery? British Medical Journal 296: 668–672
8. Anderson J M, Milner R D G, Strich S J 1967 Effects of neonatal hypoglycaemia on the nervous system: a pathological study. Journal of Neurology, Neurosurgery and Psychiatry 30: 295–310

9. Anderson S, Shakya K N, Shrestha L N, Costello A M de L 1993 Hypoglycaemia: a common problem among uncomplicated newborn infants in Nepal. Journal of Tropical Pediatrics 39: 273–277

10. Arant B S, Gorsh W M 1978 Effects of acute hyperglycemia on the central nervous system of neonatal puppies. Pediatric Research 12: 549

11. Ashworth A, Waterlow J C 1982 Infant mortality in developing countries. Archives of Disease in Childhood 57: 882–884

12. Auer R N, Siesjo B K 1993 Hypoglycaemia: brain neurochemistry and neuropathology. Baillières Clinical Endocrinology and Metabolism 7: 611–625

13. Aynsley-Green A 1988 Metabolic and endocrine interrelationships in the human fetus and neonate: an overview of the control of the adaptation to postnatal nutrition In: Lindblad B A (ed) Perinatal nutrition. Academic Press, New York, pp 162–191

14. Aynsley-Green A, Hussain K, Hall J et al 2000 Practical management of hyperinsulinism in infancy. Archives of Disease in Childhood. Fetal and Neonatal Edition 82: F98–F107

15. Banker B Q 1967 The neuropathological effects of anoxia and hypoglycaemia in the newborn. Developmental Medicine and Child Neurology 9: 544–550

16. Barker D J P 1990 The fetal and infant origins of adult disease. British Medical Journal 301: 1111

17. Barkovich A J, Ali F A, Rowley H A, Bass N 1998 Imaging patterns of neonatal hypoglycaemia. American Journal of Neuroradiology 19: 523–528

18. Bas F, Darendeliler F, Demirkol D, Bundak R, Saka N, Gunoz H 1999 Successful therapy with calcium channel blocker (nifedipine) in persistent neonatal hyperinsulinemic hypoglycemia of infancy. Journal of Pediatric Endocrinology and Metabolism 12: 873–878

19. Baumeister F A, Rolinski B, Busch R, Emmrich P 2001 Glucose monitoring with long-term subcutaneous microdialysis in neonates. Pediatrics 108: 1187–1192

20. Beckwith J B 1963 Extreme cytomegaly of the adrenal fetal cortex, omphalocele, hyperplasia of kidneys and pancreas and Leydig cell hyperplasia. Another syndrome? Proceedings of the Western Society for Pediatric Research, November 1963, Los Angeles

21. Bier D M, Leake R D, Haymond M W et al 1977 Measurement of 'true' glucose production rates in infancy and childhood with 6, 6-dideuteroglucose. Diabetes 26: 1016–1023

22. Binder N D, Raschko R K, Benda G I, Reynolds J W 1989 Insulin infusion with parenteral nutrition in extremely low birthweight infants with hyperglycemia. Journal of Pediatrics 114: 273–280

23. Bougneres P F 1987 Stable isotope tracers and the determination of fuel fluxes in newborn infants. Biology of the Neonate 52(suppl. 1): 87–96

24. Bryan M H, Wei P, Hamilton J R, Chance G W, Swyer P R 1973 Supplemental intravenous alimentation in low birthweight infants. Journal of Pediatrics 82: 940–944

25. Carver T D, Anderson S M, Aldoretta P A, Esler A L, Hay W W 1995 Glucose suppression of insulin secretion in chronically hyperglycemic fetal sheep. Pediatric Research 38: 754–762

26. Chaivorarat O, Dweck H S 1976 Effect of prolonged continuous glucose infusion in preterm neonates. Pediatric Research 10: 406

27. Chance G W, Bower B D 1966 Hypoglycaemia and temporary hyperglycaemia in infants of low birth weight for maturity. Archives of Disease in Childhood 41: 279–285

28. Clayton P T, Eaton S, Aynsley-Green A et al 2001 Hyperinsulinism in short-chain L-3-hydroxyacyl-CoA dehydrogenase deficiency reveals the importance of beta-oxidation in insulin secretion. Journal of Clinical Investigation 108: 457–465

29. Cobliner S 1911 Blutzuckeruntersuchungen bei Säuglingen. Zeitschrift für Kinderheilkunde 1: 207–216

30. Collins J E, Leonard J V 1984 Hyperinsulinism in asphyxiated and small for dates infants with hypoglycaemia. Lancet ii: 311–313

31. Collins J E, Leonard J V, Teale D et al 1990 Hyperinsulinaemic hypoglycaemia in small for dates babies. Archives of Disease in Childhood 65: 1118–1120

32. Collins J W Jr, Hoppe M, Brown K, Edidin D V, Padbury J, Ogata E S 1991 A controlled trial of insulin infusion and parenteral nutrition in extremely low birthweight infants with glucose intolerance. Journal of Pediatrics 118: 921–927

33. Cornblath M, Hawdon J M, Williams A F et al 2000 Controversies regarding definition of neonatal hypoglycemia: suggested operational thresholds. Pediatrics 105: 1141–1145

34. Cornblath M, Reisner S H 1965 Blood glucose in the neonate, clinical significance. New England Journal of Medicine 272: 378–381

35. Cornblath M, Schwartz R 1976 Disorders of carbohydrate metabolism in infancy, 2nd edn. W B Saunders, Philadelphia

36. Costello A M de L, Pal D K, Manandhar D S, Rajbhandari S, Land J M, Patel N 2000 Neonatal hypoglycaemia in Nepal. 2. The role of alternative fuels. Archives of Disease in Childhood. Fetal and Neonatal Edition 8: F52–F58

37. Costello J M, Gluckman P D 1988 Neonatal hypopituitarism: a neurological perspective. Developmental Medicine and Child Neurology 30: 190–199

38. Coulthard M G, Hey E N 1999 Renal processing of glucose in well and sick neonates. Archives of Disease in Childhood. Fetal and Neonatal Edition 81: F92–F98

39. Cowett R M 1999 Neonatal hypoglycaemia: a little goes a long way. Journal of Pediatrics 134: 389–391

40. Cowett R M, Andersen G E, Maguire C A, Oh W 1988 Ontogeny of glucose homeostasis in low birth weight infants. Journal of Pediatrics 112: 462–465

41. Cowett R M, Oh W, Schwartz R 1983 Persistent glucose production during glucose infusion in the neonate. Journal of Clinical Investigation 71: 467–475

42. Cowett R M, Schwartz R 1979 The role of hepatic control of glucose homeostasis in the aetiology of neonatal hypo and hyperglycemia. Seminars in Perinatology 3: 327

43. Cowett R M, Susa J B, Oh W, Schwartz R 1978 Endogenous glucose production during constant glucose infusion in the newborn lamb. Pediatric Research 12: 853–857

44. Dahlquist G 1976 Cerebral utilization of glucose, ketone bodies and oxygen in starving infant rats and the effect of intrauterine growth retardation. Acta Paediatrica Scandinavica 98: 237–247

45. De Boissieu D, Rocchiccioli F, Kalach N, Bougnere P F 1995 Ketone body turnover in term and in premature newborns in the first two weeks after birth. Biology of the Neonate 67: 84–93

46. De Lonlay P, Fournet J C, Rahier J et al 1997 Somatic deletion of the imprinted 11p15 region in sporadic persistent hyperinsulinaemic hypoglycaemia of infancy is specific of focal adenomatous hyperplasia and endorses partial pancreatectomy. Journal of Clinical Investigation 100: 802–807

47. De Lonlay P, Fournet J C, Touati G et al 2002 Heterogeneity of persistent hyperinsulinemic hypoglycemia. A series of 175 cases. European Journal of Pediatrics 161: 37–48

48. De Lonlay-Debeny P, Poggi-Travert F, Fournet J C et al 1999 Clinical features of 52 infants with hyperinsulinism. New England Journal of Medicine 340: 1169–1175

49. de Rooy L J, Hawdon J M 2002 Nutritional factors that affect the postnatal metabolic adaptation of full-term small- and large-for-gestational-age infants. Pediatrics 109: E42

50. Dweck H S, Cassady G 1974 Glucose tolerance in infants of very low birthweight. I. Incidence of hyperglycemia in infants of birthweights 1100 grams or less. Pediatrics 53: 189–195

51. Edmond J, Auestad N, Robbins R A, Bergstrom J D 1985 Ketone body metabolism in the neonate: development and effect of diet. Federal Proceedings 44: 2359–2364

52. Eidelman A I 2001 Hypoglycemia and the breastfed neonate. Pediatric Clinics of North America 48: 377–387

53. Elander G, Lindberg T 1984 Short mother-infant separation during first week of life influences the duration of breast feeding. Acta Paediatrica Scandinavica 73: 237–240

54. Fluge G 1974 Clinical aspects of neonatal hypoglycaemia. Acta Paediatrica Scandinavica 63: 826–832

55. Gemelli M, De Luca F, Barberio G 1979 Hypoglycaemia and congenital adrenal hyperplasia. Acta Paediatrica Scandinavica 68: 285–286

56. Gentz J C H, Cornblath M 1969 Transient diabetes of the newborn. Advances in Pediatrics 16: 345–363

57. Glaser B, Thornton P, Otonkoski T, Junien C 2000 Genetics of neonatal hyperinsulinism. Archives of Disease in Childhood. Fetal and Neonatal Edition 82: F79–F86

58. Goldman S L, Hirata T 1980 Attenuated response to insulin in very low birthweight infants. Pediatric Research 14: 50–53

59. Grant J 1995 UNICEF: State of the world's children. Oxford University Press, Oxford

60. Griffiths A D 1968 Association of hypoglycaemia with symptoms in the newborn. Archives of Disease in Childhood 43: 688–694

61. Griffiths A D, Lawrence K M 1974 The effects of hypoxia and hypoglycaemia on the brain of the newborn human infant. Developmental Medicine and Child Neurology 16: 308–319

62. Hägnevik K, Faxelius G, Irestedt L, Lagercrantz H, Lundell B, Persson B 1984 Catecholamine surge and metabolic adaptation in the newborn after vaginal delivery and caesarean section. Acta Paediatrica Scandinavica 73: 602–609

63. Haninger N C, Farley C L 2001 Screening for hypoglycemia in healthy term neonates: effects on breastfeeding. Journal of Midwifery and Womens Health 46: 292–301

64. Hawdon J M 1993 Neonatal hypoglycaemia: the consequences of admission to the special care nursery. Maternal and Child Health Feb: 48–51

65. Hawdon J M 1999 Hypoglycemia and the neonatal brain. European Journal of Pediatrics 158: S9–S12

66. Hawdon J M, Aynsley-Green A, Alberti K G M M, Ward Platt M P 1993 The role of pancreatic insulin secretion in neonatal glucoregulation. I. Healthy term and preterm infants. Archives of Disease in Childhood 68: 274–279

67. Hawdon J M, Aynsley-Green A, Bartlett K, Ward Platt M P 1993 The role of pancreatic insulin secretion in neonatal glucoregulation. II. Infants with disordered blood glucose homeostasis. Archives of Disease in Childhood 68: 280–285

68. Hawdon J M, Aynsley-Green A, Ward Platt M P 1993 Neonatal blood glucose concentrations: metabolic effects of intravenous glucagon and intragastric medium chain triglyceride. Archives of Disease in Childhood 68: 255–261

69. Hawdon J M, Hubbard M, Hales C N, Clark P 1995 Use of a specific immunoradiometric assay to determine preterm neonatal insulin-glucose relations. Archives of Disease in Childhood. Fetal and Neonatal Edition 73: F166–F169

70. Hawdon J M, Ward Platt M P 1992 Metabolic and hormonal interrelationships in perinatal asphyxia. Biology of the Neonate 62: 300

71. Hawdon J M, Ward Platt M P 1993 Metabolic adaptation in small for gestational age infants. Archives of Disease in Childhood 68: 262–268

72. Hawdon J M, Ward Platt M P, Aynsley-Green A 1992 Patterns of metabolic adaptation for preterm and term infants in the first neonatal week. Archives of Disease in Childhood 67: 357–365

73. Hawdon J M, Ward Platt M P, Lamb W H, Aynsley-Green A 1990 Tolerance to Sandostatin in neonatal hyperinsulinaemic hypoglycaemia. Archives of Disease in Childhood 65: 341–343

74. Hawdon J M, Weddell A, Aynsley-Green A, Ward Platt M P 1993 Hormonal and metabolic response to hypoglycaemia in small for gestational age infants. Archives of Disease in Childhood 68: 269–273

75. Hay W W Jr, Sparks J W 1985 Placental, fetal and neonatal carbohydrate metabolism. Clinical Obstetrics and Gynecology 28: 473–485

76. Haymond M W, Strauss A W, Arnold K J, Bier D M 1979 Glucose homeostasis in children with severe cyanotic congenital heart disease. Journal of Pediatrics 95: 220–227

77. Heck L J, Erenberg A 1987 Serum glucose levels in term neonates during the first 48 hours of life. Journal of Paediatrics 110: 119–122

78. Hoffman W H, Knoury C, Byrd H A 1980 Prevalence of permanent congenital diabetes mellitus. Diabetologia 19: 487–488

79. Hussain K, Aynsley-Green A 2000 Management of hyperinsulinism in infancy and childhood. Annals of Medicine 32: 544–551

80. Hutchinson J H, Keay A J, Kerr M N 1962 Congenital temporary diabetes mellitus. British Medical Journal ii: 436–440

81. Issad T, Pastor-Anglada M, Coupe C, Ferre P, Girard J 1990 Glucose metabolism and insulin sensitivity during suckling period in rats. In: Cuezva J M, Paseaud-Leone A M, Patel M S (eds) Endocrine development of the fetus and neonate. Plenum Press, New York, pp 61–66

82. Jacobs D G, Haka-Ikse K, Wesson D E, Filler R M, Sherwood G 1986 Growth and development in patients operated on for islet cell dysplasia. Journal of Pediatric Surgery 21: 1184–1189

83. Johnston V, Frazzini V, Davidheiser S, Przybylski R J, Kleigman R M 1991 Insulin receptor number and binding affinity in newborn dogs. Pediatric Research 29: 611–614

84. Joosten K J, Schellehens A P, Waellens J J, Wulffraat N M 1991 Erroneous diagnosis 'neonatal hypoglycaemia' due to incorrect preservation of blood samples. Nederlands Tijdschrift Geneeskunde 135: 1691–1694

85. Kalhan S C, Oliver A, King K C, Lucero C 1986 Role of glucose in the regulation of endogenous glucose production in the human newborn. Pediatric Research 20: 49–52

86. Kinnala A, Korvenranta H, Parkkola R 2000 Newer techniques to study neonatal hypoglycemia. Seminars in Perinatology 24: 116–119

87. Kinnala A, Rikalainen H, Lapinleimu H, Parkkola R, Kormano M, Kero P 1999 Cerebral magnetic resonance imaging and ultrasonography findings after neonatal hypoglycaemia. Pediatrics 103: 724–729

88. Kinnala A, Suhonen-Polvi H, Aarimaa T et al 1996 Cerebral metabolic rate for glucose during the first six months of life: an FDG positron emission tomography study. Archives of Disease in Childhood. Fetal and Neonatal Edition 74: F153–F157

89. Kirkham P, Watkins A 1995 Comparison of two reflectance photometers in the assessment of neonatal hypoglycaemia. Archives of Disease in Childhood. Fetal and Neonatal Edition 73: F170–F173

90. Kitselle J F 1852 Kinderh Leipsic XVIII 313

91. Koh T H H G, Eyre J A, Aynsley-Green A 1988 Neural dysfunction during hypoglycaemia. Archives of Disease in Childhood 63: 1353–1358

92. Koh T H H G, Eyre J A, Aynsley-Green A 1988 Neonatal hypoglycaemia – the controversy regarding definition. Archives of Disease in Childhood 63: 1386–1389

93. Lafeber H N, Sulkers E J, Chapman T E, Sauer P J J 1990 Glucose production and oxidation in preterm infants during total parenteral nutrition. Pediatric Research 28: 153–157

94. Le Dune M A 1971 Insulin studies in temporary neonatal hyperglycaemia. Archives of Disease in Childhood 46: 392–394

95. Lilien L D, Rosenfield R C, Pildes R S 1979 Hyperglycemia in small stressed neonates. Journal of Pediatrics 94: 454–459

96. Lindblad B S, Settegren G, Feychting H 1977 Total parenteral nutrition in infants. Blood levels of glucose, lactate, pyruvate, free fatty acids, glycerol, D β hydroxybutyrate, triglycerides, free amino acids and insulin. Acta Paediatrica Scandinavica 66: 409–419

97. Louik C, Mitchell A A, Epstein M F, Shapiro S 1985 Risk factors for neonatal hyperglycemia associated with 10% dextrose infusion. American Journal of Diseases of Children 139: 783–786

98. Lovinger R D, Kaplan S L, Grumbach M M 1975 Congenital hypopituitarism associated with neonatal hypoglycemia and microphallus. Journal of Pediatrics 87: 1171–1181

99. Lucas A, Adrian T E, Aynsley-Green A, Bloom S R 1980 Iatrogenic hyperinsulinism at birth. Lancet i: 144–145

100. Lucas A, Aynsley-Green A, Bloom S R 1981 Gut hormones and the first meals. Clinical Science 60: 349–353

101. Lucas A, Morley R, Cole T F 1988 Adverse neurodevelopmental outcome of moderate neonatal hypoglycaemia. British Medical Journal 297: 1304–1308

102. MacFie J, Yule A G, Hill G L 1981 Effect of added insulin on body composition of gastroenterologic patients receiving intravenous nutrition – a controlled clinical trial. Gastroenterology 81: 285–289

103. McQuarrie I 1954 Idiopathic spontaneously occurring hypoglycemia in infants. American Journal of Diseases of Children 87: 399–428

104. Mann T P, Elliot R I K 1957 Neonatal cold injury due to accidental exposure to cold. Lancet i: 229–231

105. Medical Devices Agency 1996 Extra-laboratory use of blood glucose meters and test strips: contraindications, training and advice to the users. Safety Notice MDA SN 9616

106. Medina J M, Fernandez E, Bolaros J P, Vicario C, Arizmendi L 1990 Fuel supply to the brain during the early postnatal period. In: Cueza J M, Pasaud-Leone A M, Patel M S (eds) Endocrine development of the fetus and neonate. Plenum Press, New York, pp 175–194

107. Mehta A, Wootton R, Cheng K N, Penfold P, Halliday D, Stacey T E 1987 Effect of diazoxide or glucagon on hepatic glucose production rate during extreme neonatal hypoglycaemia. Archives of Disease in Childhood 62: 924–930

108. Meissner T, Brune W, Mayatepak E 1997 Persistent hyperinsulinemic hypoglycemia of infancy: therapy, clinical outcome and mutational analysis. European Journal of Pediatrics 156: 754–757

109. Menni F, de Lonlay P, Sevin C et al 2001 Neurologic outcomes of 90 neonates and infants with persistent hyperinsulinemic hypoglycemia. Pediatrics 107: 476–479

110. Milner R D G, Fekete M, Assan R 1972 Glucagon, insulin and growth hormone response to exchange transfusion in premature and term infants. Archives of Disease in Childhood 17: 186–189

111. Milner R D G, Ferguson A W, Naidu S H 1971 Aetiology of transient neonatal diabetes. Archives of Disease in Childhood 46: 724–726

112. Miranda L, Dweck H S 1977 Perinatal glucose homeostasis: the unique character of hyperglycemia and hypoglycemia in infants of very low birthweight. Clinics in Perinatology 4: 351–365

113. Molsted-Pedersen L, Trautner H, Jorgensen K R 1973 Plasma insulin and K values during intravenous glucose tolerance test in newborn infants with erythroblastosis fetalis. Acta Paediatrica Scandinavica 62: 11–16

114. Munshi U K, Deorari A K, Paul V K, Singh M 1992 Effects of maternal labetalol on the newborn infant. Indian Pediatrics 29: 1507–1512

115. Murakami Y, Yamashita Y, Matsuishi T, Utsonomiya H, Okudera T, Hashimoto T. 1999 Cranial MRI of neurologically impaired children suffering from neonatal hypoglycaemia. Pediatric Radiology 29: 23–27

116. National Childbirth Trust 1997 Hypoglycaemia of the newborn. Modern Midwife 7: 31–33

117. Neligan G 1965 Idiopathic hypoglycaemia in the newborn. In: Gairdner D (ed) Recent advances in paediatrics III. Churchill, London

118. Obershain S S, Adam P A J, King K C et al 1970 Human fetal response to sustained maternal hyperglycemia. New England Journal of Medicine 283: 566–572

119. Ogata E S 1986 Carbohydrate metabolism in the fetus and neonate and altered neonatal glucoregulation. Pediatric Clinics of North America 33: 25–45

120. Ogata E S, Paul R I, Finley S L 1987 Limited maternal fuel availability due to hyperinsulinemia retards fetal growth and development in the rat. Pediatric Research 22: 432–437

121. Ostertag S G, Jovanovic L, Lewis B, Auld P A M 1986 Insulin pump therapy in the very low birthweight infant. Pediatrics 78: 625–630

122. Pagliara A S, Karl I E, Kipnis D B 1973 Transient neonatal diabetes: delayed maturation of the pancreatic beta cell. Journal of Pediatrics 82: 97–101

123. Pal D K, Manandhar D S, Rajbhandari S, Land J M, Patel N, Costello A M de L 2000 Neonatal hypoglycaemia in Nepal. 1. Prevalence and risk factors. Archives of Diseases of Childhood. Fetal and Neonatal Edition 82: F45–F51

124. Persson B, Gentz J 1966 The pattern of blood lipids, glycerol and ketone bodies during the neonatal period, infancy and childhood. Acta Paediatrica Scandinavica 55: 353–362

125. Pollack A, Cowett R M, Schwartz R, Oh M D 1978 Glucose disposal in low birthweight infants during steady state hyperglycemia: effects of exogenous insulin administration. Pediatrics 61: 546–549

126. Rahier J, Guiot Y, Sempoux C 2000 Persistent hyperinsulinaemic hypoglycaemia of infancy: a heterogeneous syndrome unrelated to nesidioblastosis. Archives of Disease in Childhood. Fetal and Neonatal Edition 82: F108–F112

127. Reynolds G J, Davies S 1993 A clinical audit of cotside blood glucose measurement in the detection of neonatal hypoglycaemia. Journal of Paediatrics and Child Health 29: 289–291

128. Ross R J M, Miell J P, Buchanan C R 1991 Avoiding autocannibalism. British Medical Journal 303: 1147–1148

129. Schrier A M, Wilhelm P B, Church R M et al 1990 Neonatal hypoglycaemia in the Rhesus monkey: effect on development and behaviour. Infant Behaviour and Development 13: 189–297

130. Sedgwick J P, Ziegler M R 1920 The nitrogenous and sugar content of the blood of the newborn. American Journal of Diseases of Children 19: 429–432

131. Senior B 1973 Current concepts. Neonatal hypoglycemia. New England Journal of Medicine 289: 790–793

132. Senior B, Slone D, Shapiro S 1976 Benzothiazides and neonatal hypoglycaemia. Lancet ii: 377

133. Shah A, Stanhope R, Matthew D 1992 Hazards of pharmacological tests of growth hormone secretion in childhood. British Medical Journal 304: 173–174

134. Shelley H J, Basset J M 1975 Control of carbohydrate metabolism in the fetus and newborn. British Medical Bulletin 31: 37–43

135. Shelley H J, Neligan G S 1966 Neonatal hypoglycaemia. British Medical Bulletin 22: 34–39

136. Shepherd R M, Cosgrove K E, O'Brien R E, Barnes P D, Ammala C, Dunne M J, on behalf of the EU funded European Network for Research into Hyperinsulinism in Infancy (ENRHI) 2000 Hyperinsulinism of infancy: towards a better understanding of unregulated insulin release. Archives of Disease in Childhood. Fetal and Neonatal Edition 82: F87–F97

137. Shield J P 2000 Neonatal diabetes: new insights into aetiology and implications. Hormone Research. 53(suppl. 1): 7–11

138. Shield J P H, Gardner R J, Wadsworth E J K et al 1996 Transient neonatal diabetes: a study of its aetiopathology and genetic basis. Archives of Disease in Childhood. Fetal and Neonatal Edition 76: F39–F42

139. Singh S P, Pullen G L, Snyder A K 1988 Effects of ethanol on fetal fuels and brain growth in rats. Journal of Laboratory and Clinical Medicine 112: 704–710

140. Smallpiece V, Davies P A 1964 Immediate feeding of premature infants with undiluted breast milk. Lancet ii: 1349–1356

141. Soltész G, Aynsley-Green A 1984 Hyperinsulinism in infancy and childhood In: Prader A (ed) Advances in internal medicine and paediatrics, Vol. 51. Springer, Berlin, pp 151–202

142. Soltész G, Jenkins P A, Anysley-Green A 1984 Hyperinsulinaemic hypoglycaemia in infancy and childhood: a practical approach to diagnosis and medical treatment based on experience of 18 cases. Acta Paediatrica Academiae Scientiarum Hungaricae 25: 319–322

143. Soothill P W, Nicolaides K H, Campbell S 1987 Prenatal asphyxia, hyperlacti-caemia, hypoglycaemia and erythroblastosis in growth retarded fetuses. British Medical Journal 294: 1051–1053

144. Spar J A, Levine J D, Orrison W W Jr 1994 Neonatal hypoglycemia: CT and MR findings. American Journal of Neuroradiology 15: 1477–1478

145. Spence J C 1921 Some observations on sugar tolerance, with special reference to variations found at different ages. Quarterly Journal of Medicine 14: 314–326

146. Sperling M A, Ganguli S, Leslie N, Landt K 1984 Fetal-perinatal catecholamine secretion: role in perinatal glucose homeostasis. American Journal of Physiology 247: E69–E74

147. Sperling M A, Grajwer L A, Leake R, Fisher D A 1976 Role of glucagon in perinatal glucose homeostasis. Metabolism 25(suppl. 1): 1385–1386

148. Srinivasan G, Jain R, Pildes R S, Kannon C R 1986 Glucose homeostasis during anaesthesia and surgery in infants. Journal of Pediatric Surgery 21: 718–721

149. Srinivasan G, Pildes R S, Cattamanchi G, Voora S, Lilien L D 1986 Plasma glucose values in normal neonates: a new look. Journal of Pediatric Surgery 21: 114–117

150. Stonestreet B S, Rubin L, Pollack A, Cowett R M, Oh W 1980 Renal function of low birthweight infants with hyperglycemia and glucosuria produced by glucose infusion. Pediatrics 66: 561–567

151. Stubbe P, Wolf H 1971 The effect of stress on growth hormone, glucose and glycerol levels in newborn infants. Hormone and Metabolic Research 3: 175–179

152. Susa J B, Cowett R M, Oh W 1979 Suppression of gluconeogenesis and endogenous glucose production by exogenous insulin administration in the newborn lamb. Pediatric Research 13: 594–599

153. Temple I K, Gardner R J, Robinson D O et al 1996 Further evidence for an imprinted gene for neonatal diabetes localised to chromosome 6q22-q23. Human Molecular Genetics 5: 1117–1121

154. Temple I K, James R S, Crolla J A et al 1995 An imprinted gene(s) for diabetes. Nature Genetics 9: 110–112

155. The Vermont Oxford Network Steroid Study Group 2001 Early postnatal dexamethasone therapy for the prevention of chronic lung disease. Pediatrics 108: 741–748

156. Thurston J H, Hawhart R E, Schiro J A 1986 β-hydroxybutyrate reverses insulin-induced hypoglycaemic coma in suckling-weanling mice despite low blood and brain glucose levels. Metabolism and Brain Research 1: 63–82

157. Van den Bosch C A, Bullough C H W 1990 The effect of suckling on term neonates' core body temperature. Annals of Tropical Paediatrics 10: 347–353

158. Van Goudoever J B, Sulkers E J, Chapman T E 1993 Glucose kinetics and glucoregulatory hormone levels in ventilated preterm infants on the first day of life. Pediatric Research 33: 583–589

159. Vannucci R C, Nardis E E, Vannucci J S, Campbell P A 1981 Cerebral carbohydrate and energy metabolism during hypoglycemia in newborn dogs. American Journal of Physiology 240: R192–R199

160. Vaucher Y E, Watson P D, Morrow G 1982 Continuous insulin infusion in hyperglycemic, very low birthweight infants. Journal of Pediatric Gastroenterology and Nutrition 1: 211–217

161. Von Muhlendahl K E, Herkenhoff H 1995 Long term outcome of neonatal diabetes. New England Journal of Medicine 333: 704–708

162. Wiedemann H R 1964 Complexe malformatif familial avec hernie umbilicale et macroglossie. Un 'syndrome nouveau'? Journal de Génétique Humaine 13: 223–232

163. Wilkins B H 1992 Renal function in sick very low birthweight infants: 4: Glucose excretion. Archives of Disease in Childhood 67: 1162–1165

164. Wilkinson A R, Fok T-F, Au-Yeung H 1984 High incidence of clinical problems in the newborn possibly attributable to theophylline therapy (abstract). Pediatric Research 18: 89

165. World Bank 1995 World Development Report. Oxford University Press, Oxford

166. World Health Organisation 1991 Child health and development: health of the newborn. Report of the Director General of the World Health Organisation EB89/26: 15–17

167. Yunis K A, Oh W, Kalhan S, Cowett R M 1989 Mechanisms of glucose perturbation following intravenous fat infusion in the low birthweight infant. Pediatric Research 25: 299A

168. Zarif M, Pildes R S, Vidyasagar D 1976 Insulin and growth hormone responses in neonatal hyperglycemia. Diabetes 25: 428–433

169. Zuppinger K A 1975 Hypoglycaemia in childhood. Monographs in paediatrics 4. S Karger, Basle

PART 2

Endocrine disorders

Tim Cheetham

An obvious physical abnormality, such as ambiguous genitalia, may indicate underlying endocrine pathology, but the signs are usually more subtle, and a low threshold for the suspicion of endocrine disease is required. This is particularly true of abnormalities of anterior and posterior pituitary function. Knowledge of the changes in hormone release and handling as the fetus undergoes the transition to independent life is helpful. Awareness of the impact of gestational and postnatal age on endocrine function is also important. Endocrine disorders in the newborn may be serious and potentially life threatening but are nearly always treatable. It is therefore particularly important that they are identified as soon as possible.

Advances in the field of molecular biology have now clarified the cellular basis of many endocrine disorders, but this chapter will focus on the presentation, differential diagnosis and management of these conditions. For fuller discussions of the clinical and molecular aspects of endocrine disease, the reader is referred to standard works on paediatric or general endocrinology, such as Sperling,[312] Brook & Hindmarsh[48] or Wilson & Foster.[364]

Hypothalamus and anterior pituitary

Normal function

The hypothalamus and anterior pituitary form a neuroendocrine unit that mediates between the central nervous system (CNS) and the peripheral tissues. The hypothalamic nerve fibres liberate humoral substances into the capillaries of the primary plexus in the median eminence, to be carried by the portal vessels to excite or inhibit the secretion of the cells of the anterior pituitary. The principal hypothalamic releasing hormones are corticotrophin-releasing hormone (CRH), thyrotrophin-releasing hormone (TRH), gonadotrophin-releasing hormone (GnRH) and growth hormone releasing hormone (GHRH), with two inhibitory hormones, somatostatin and dopamine. These factors regulate the secretion of the pituitary trophic hormones adrenocorticotrophic hormone (ACTH), thyroid-stimulating hormone (TSH), follicle-stimulating hormone (FSH), luteinising hormone (LH), growth hormone (GH) and prolactin into the circulation. They, in turn, stimulate the production of cortisol, thyroxine, sex steroids and insulin-like growth factor-I (IGF-I), which will then feed back and modulate hypothalamic and pituitary hormone release. Many other neurotransmitters and neuropeptides are involved in the regulation of pituitary hormone release and there is considerable interaction between the various axes; GH production is, for example, modulated by thyroxine, cortisol and sex steroids as well as by IGF-I.

Hypothalamic and anterior pituitary disease

Children with congenital pituitary hormone deficiency (PHD) have quantitative and qualitative abnormalities of the production of one or more pituitary hormones. The incidence of isolated GH deficiency is approximately 1 in 3500,[185,343] and that of multiple or combined pituitary hormone deficiency (CPHD) around 1 in 8000. Many children with 'hypopituitarism' have an abnormal hypothalamus which cannot manufacture and release the relevant hypothalamic hormones appropriately. There is an association between PHD and other midline CNS malformations[95] as well as midline malformations elsewhere in the body, such as cleft palate.[286,332] Chromosomal defects such as 18p- are also associated with PHD.[21] Many patients with PHD – more than 90% of those with CPHD – have midline CNS abnormalities on magnetic resonance imaging (MRI). These include an abnormal pituitary gland and/or hypothalamus as well as the absent septum pellucidum and optic nerve hypoplasia characteristic of septo-optic dysplasia (SOD).[27,124,333] Patients with PHD represent a spectrum of hormonal and associated midline abnormalities. At one end of the spectrum is the child with isolated GH deficiency and a structurally normal brain. At the other end of the spectrum is the patient with SOD and associated CPHD.[74,244,313]

The molecular basis of some cases of PHD has now been elucidated. A series of genes act in a sequential manner during the development of the hypothalamus, pituitary and other midline structures. A defect of one of these genes can impact on the normal developmental process and result in deficiencies of one or more hypothalamic and/or pituitary hormones. Defects of the transcription factor *Pit-1* are typically associated with a deficiency of GH, TSH and prolactin,[83,255,267,323] whilst the gene *Prop-1*, active at an earlier stage of pituitary gland development, is associated with deficiency of GH, TSH, prolactin, gonadotrophins[78,366] and sometimes ACTH deficiency, too.[335] The genes *Hes X1* and *Lhx 3*[225] appear to have an earlier and more fundamental role in CNS development. Homozygous and heterozygous mutations of *Hes X1* are a recognised cause of SOD, whilst heterozygous defects can also cause isolated GH deficiency.[73,321,328] All of these genetic defects can present with signs of PHD in the neonatal period, although deficiencies can also evolve with time.[341]

Isolated deficiencies of GH,[265,346] TSH,[89] ACTH[173] or gonadotrophins[178,179,257,356] may also arise from abnormalities of the respective genes. Mutations of the GH-1 gene can

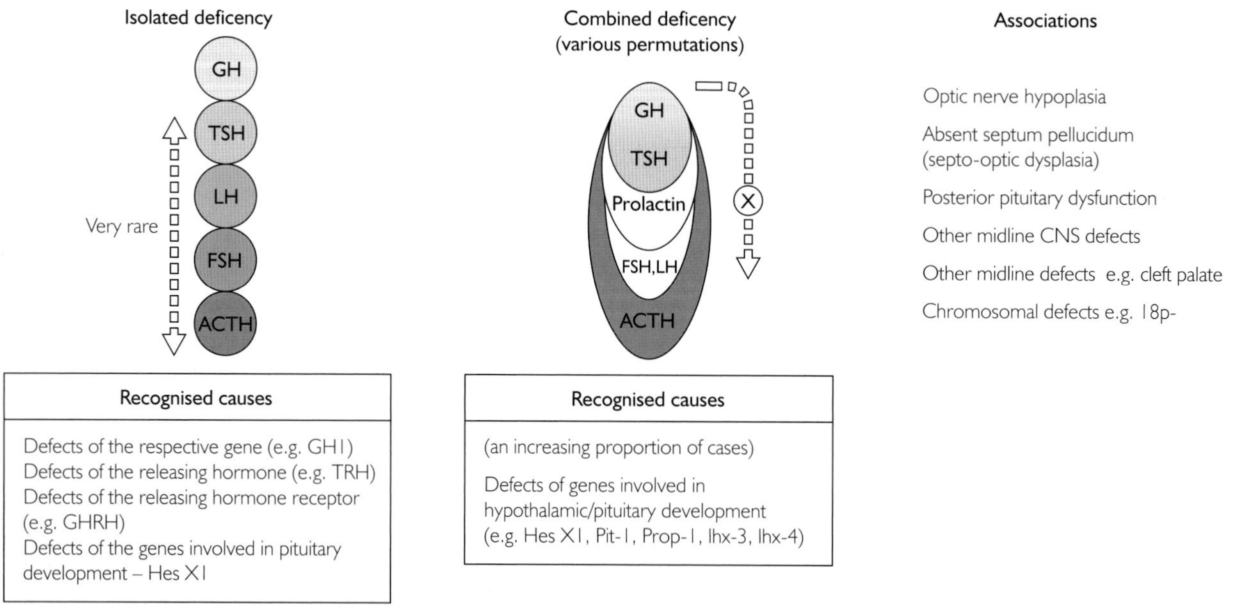

Fig. 35.7 Isolated pituitary hormone deficiency and the different combinations of combined pituitary hormone deficiency in the newborn. Endocrinopathies can evolve in later life as indicated by the broken arrow.

result in recessive and dominantly inherited isolated GH deficiency (Fig. 35.7).[35,65,148,258] Genetic defects of the GHRH receptor can also be associated with isolated GH deficiency (Fig. 35.7).[347]

Hypopituitarism has been linked to traumatic delivery in the past and there is a high incidence of breech and forceps delivery in some series.[68] Rona and Tanner[280] calculated that a male first-born delivered by breech has an 11-fold increased risk of GH deficiency. The fetus with isolated anterior pituitary aplasia[161] and most children with hypopituitarism still present in the cephalic position,[333] and altered movement in utero secondary to the underlying defect in brain development may be the common link between hypopituitarism and breech delivery.[82,260]

Holoprosencephaly is another extreme example of a midline brain malformation and is associated with anomalies that include aplasia of the olfactory bulbs and craniofacial abnormalities. Patients with holoprosencephaly can have anterior (and posterior) PHD. Patients may have an underlying chromosomal abnormality,[52] and a number of single gene defects have been identified in these babies.[224,348] The prevalence appears to be higher in young mothers[239] and in mothers with diabetes.[28] MRI may show an abnormal pituitary gland as well as the characteristic forebrain abnormalities seen in this disorder.

Clinical features (Table 35.6)

Clinical recognition of hypopituitarism in the newborn can be difficult. GH deficiency leads to relatively subtle changes in body form and whilst some authors report a reduction in length of about 1 SD with a normal birthweight[114] other studies indicate that birth length is unaffected.[250] Micropenis is a feature of GH deficiency and is also an important sign in the male with

Table 35.6 Clinical and biochemical assessment of the infant with suspected hypopituitarism

Clinical features
- Micropenis
- Hypoglycaemia – may be reflected by episodes of discoloration and fits
- Poor feeding
- Prolonged jaundice – typically conjugated hyperbilirubinaemia
- Associated defects – e.g. cleft palate

Investigations
1. Biochemistry at the time of hypoglycaemia
   - Cortisol (values greater than 560 nmol/l make ACTH deficiency unlikely)
   - GH
2. Other baseline investigations
   - Electrolytes – hyponatraemia may reflect cortisol deficiency
   - Thyroid function (TSH may be paradoxically raised)
   - Prolactin – usually high in the newborn period
   - LH/FSH – unrecordable levels, particularly at 2–3 months of age, suggest gonadotrophin deficiency
3. Dynamic testing (may not always be feasible)
   - Glucagon (to assess pituitary GH and ACTH/cortisol production)
   - TRH testing

   Other dynamic tests to assess the hypothalamo-pituitary axis
   - Synacthen
   - CRH test

gonadotrophin deficiency (pp. 896–7).[291] GH promotes longitudinal growth but it is also an insulin antagonist with lipolytic and ketogenic activity. Ketones are an important fuel in the newborn period and so hypoglycaemia can occur in the infant with isolated GH deficiency.[188] Hypoglycaemia is often severe in the infant with adrenocortical insufficiency and so both GH and ACTH status should be considered in these circumstances. Prolonged neonatal jaundice with a conjugated hyperbilirubinaemia is a further well-recognised feature of congenital hypopituitarism[132] and is closely linked to cortisol deficiency. Symptomatic hypothyroidism is not usually a prominent feature of hypopituitarism, reflecting the less profound effect on thyroid hormone production when the thyroid gland is intact but understimulated. All neonates with suspected PHD should have an opthalmological assessment because of the possiblility of underlying SOD.

Further investigations (Table 35.6)

Cortisol deficiency secondary to ACTH deficiency is associated with hyponatraemia because cortisol inhibits arginine vasopressin (AVP) production and is required to excrete a water load. Biochemical confirmation of hypopituitarism requires the measurement of pituitary and other hormones at the time of initial presentation with or without hypoglycaemia and after stimulation with hypothalamic and pituitary hormones such as TRH, CRH and ACTH. Biochemical testing can be extremely helpful but requires careful planning and is potentially misleading because, like all tests, there are false positives and negatives.

The synacthen test is still used by many clinicians to investigate possible secondary hypoadrenalism (ACTH deficiency) prior to commencing hydrocortisone in the infant with hypoglycaemia and suspected hypopituitarism (p. 870). The CRH test is increasing in popularity but both tests are hampered by concerns about sensitivity and specificity, a lack of reliable normative data, as well as the more complex and (in the case of the CRH test) limited availability of the ACTH assay. TSH levels can, paradoxically, be mildly elevated in secondary hypothyroidism and there may be an exaggerated response to TRH.[120] The increase in TSH levels and exaggerated response in hypothalamic hypothyroidism may reflect the presence of detectable but bioinactive TSH[253] or alternatively the abnormal production of TSH in the absence of hypothalamic hormones such as somatostatin.

GH levels are often elevated in the first days of life and a low or unrecordable GH concentration at the time of a documented hypoglycaemic episode raises the possiblity of hypothalamo-pituitary disease. Non-specific stimulation of GH release with glucagon may also be used in the older infant. GnRH administration with assessment of LH and FSH levels may be helpful but the assessment of other axes is more important if there is a limited amount of blood available. It should be remembered that drugs such as dopamine may interfere with endocrine investigations.[84]

It can be difficult to balance the desire to obtain comprehensive biochemical data with the need to treat the sick, hypoglycaemic neonate as soon as possible. If the clinical picture strongly suggests hypopituitarism, it is wise to treat and then reassess the neonate biochemically at a later stage.

It is now recognised that hormone deficiencies can evolve with time and a neonate who is ACTH sufficient can become ACTH, and hence cortisol, insufficient in later childhood.

MRI of the CNS can be difficult to arrange in the neonatal period but will provide extremely helpful information about pituitary/hypothalamic anatomy as well as information about the presence/absence of other midline structures and CNS development as a whole (see above).

Treatment

Hypopituitarism is treated by replacing the missing pituitary hormone (GH) or the product of their target organs (thyroxine or hydrocortisone). Although the cortisol production rate in the newborn is 6.6–8.8 mg/m^2/24 h,[205] the absorption and bioavailability of hydrocortisone can vary.[59] Adrenal replacement (secondary to ACTH deficiency) should be with hydrocortisone in a dose around 10 mg/m^2/24 h (in three or four divided doses). There are concerns about the bioavailability of some hydrocortisone suspensions which also needs to be borne in mind.[201] For thyroid replacement, thyroxine in a single dose of approximately 5–10 micrograms/kg/24 h in the newborn is suitable initially. The objective is to obtain thyroxine levels in the upper part of the normal range and the dose should be adjusted accordingly. TSH levels will be low in secondary hypothyroidism once therapy has commenced and so they cannot be used to guide replacement. GH replacement may be needed to control the hypoglycaemia of hypopituitarism if this proves intractable and therapy may also be warranted from an early stage if growth is to be optimised.

Resistance to the actions of anterior pituitary hormones

Endocrine disorders in which hormone action is impaired or absent due to abnormalities of the receptor or abnormal post-receptor events are well recognised. The phenotypic features of these rare conditions may suggest hypopituitarism, but the levels of pituitary hormones are usually normal or elevated. The best-described example is insensitivity to GH (Laron syndrome), which can present with hypoglycaemia and micropenis in the newborn period.[115,296]

Abnormalitites of the TSH receptor leading to hypothyroidism (see below), the ACTH receptor leading to glucocorticoid deficiency, and the LH receptor leading to genital ambiguity, are considered in more detail in the appropriate sections below.[172,318,354]

Posterior pituitary[276]

Normal function

From the end of the first trimester, oxytocin and vasopressin (AVP) are manufactured as part of larger protein precursor molecules in the hypothalamic supraoptic and paraventricular nuclei. The protein precursor is then modified and cleaved before being incorporated in neurosecretory granules. The prohormone is further cleaved to release AVP and its binding protein, neurophysin, as it is conveyed along the neurons of the neurohypophyseal tract to the posterior pituitary. The neurosecretory granules which include AVP bound to neurophysin are then stored in the nerve terminals until they are released under neural control. Secretion is primarily controlled by the osmoreceptors of the hypothalamus, although non-osmotic stimuli, notably blood volume and blood pressure, also influence vasopressin release via the stretch receptors of the left atrium and the baroreceptors in the carotid sinus. Vasopressin acts to conserve body water by altering the permeability of the distal convoluted and renal collecting tubules, thereby reducing urine output. The capacity to concentrate urine in the immediate newborn period is not as refined as in the older child.[18] This, coupled with the higher rate of insensible water loss in infancy, helps to explain susceptibility to hypernatraemia and dehydration when feeding is not established satisfactorily.[235]

Cranial diabetes inspidus[61]

In the absence of vasopressin, urine volume and tonicity are changed only minimally in the distal tubule and collecting ducts. Urine volume can reach nearly 10% of the glomerular filtrate, with an osmolality of 100 mmol/kgH$_2$O or less. The infant with AVP deficiency (cranial diabetes insipidus) will therefore tend to pass inappropriately large amounts of dilute urine for a given plasma osmolality.

The causes of diabetes insipidus in the newborn are shown in Table 35.7 and include congenital brain malformations such as SOD and holoprosencephaly.[332] Trauma can cause diabetes insipidus although the site of injury will determine whether or not this is permanent. Damage to the supraoptic nucleus or high stalk section causes permanent severe pituitary diabetes insipidus, with more distal lesions usually causing transient dysfunction.

Table 35.7 Causes of cranial (vasopressin-deficient) diabetes insipidus

I. Primary

Genetic
Autosomal dominant (vasopressin – neurophysin gene)
Autosomal recessive (vasopressin – neurophysin gene)
Autosomal recessive – Wolfram (DIDMOAD) syndrome
X-linked recessive

With congenital malformations (which may also have a genetic, single gene, basis)
Hypopituitarism
Septo-optic dysplasia
Holoprosencephaly
Midline defects

2. Secondary
Trauma
Infection/inflammation
Vascular, including haemorrhage
Hypoxic-ischaemic encephalopathy

Clinically the condition is characterised by excessive fluid output and intake. Diagnosis is difficult in the newborn because a high urine output is easily overlooked and persistent crying and weight loss can easily be attributed to a cause other than water loss. Infants may therefore present late, with non-specific symptoms such as anorexia, vomiting, poor weight gain, constipation or delayed development. Failure to thrive can occur[231] but is less pronounced than in children with nephrogenic diabetes insipidus, because the urine tends to be less dilute. The low osmolar load associated with breastfeeding may also help to maintain a normal serum osmolality and reduce symptoms.

The diagnosis is confirmed by a failure to concentrate the urine in spite of plasma hypertonicity, with reversal by administration of the vasopressin analogue desmopressin (DDAVP). Polyuria due to hypercalcaemia or potassium deficiency must be excluded, and allowance made for the lesser concentrating power of the neonatal kidney. Circulating vasopressin concentrations can be measured, although a relatively large amount of plasma is required. The principal differential diagnosis is nephrogenic diabetes insipidus, where there is an inherited resistance to the effects of circulating AVP (pp. 941–2).

Treatment

Treatment is with DDAVP, which is a vasopressin analogue. This compound is more potent than the native molecule and has a longer half-life.[277] The standard solution (100 micrograms/ml) may be diluted with 0.9% NaCl solution to create a more manageable volume (for example, 10 micrograms/ml – discuss with the hospital pharmacy) and can be instilled into the nose using a 1-ml syringe or with a graduated rhinyl catheter. A suitable starting dose in the newborn is 0.1–1.0 micrograms once or twice daily, although, when therapy with DDAVP is commenced, it is wise to administer the second dose only when the impact of the first has been established. The dose can be altered as necessary for adequate antidiuretic effect, since the absorption and therapeutic effects are variable in degree and duration. Experience with tablets and intravenous (i.v.) solution administered orally is increasing[61,316] and a suitable starting dose is around 1–5 micrograms daily, increased to twice a day once the impact of the first dose has been established. It is extremely important to be aware of the danger of water overload, which will develop in the presence of too much DDAVP for a given sodium and water load. Weight and serum sodium/osmolality should be checked regularly, particularly in the initial phase while the dose is being adjusted. It is safer in both the short and the long term for an infant with diabetes insipidus (and an intact sense of thirst) to be allowed to compensate for a relatively low dose of DDAVP by feeding or drinking more. Parents should be actively involved in management from an early stage and encouraged to gauge both fluid input and output. Daily weights in hospital and at home can provide useful information about water balance.

Excess vasopressin secretion (syndrome of inappropriate ADH secretion)

This is described on pages 340–1.

The hormonal regulation of appetite and feeding behaviour

An increasing number of hormones and receptors are known to be involved in the regulation of feeding behaviour and growth.

The hormone leptin is produced by the *ob* gene in the adipocyte and circulating levels provide the hypothalamus with information about nutritional status. This in turn will influence feeding behaviour, as vividly illustrated by rare examples of leptin deficiency or resistance.[97,214] Leptin levels are a reflection of fat mass and cord leptin levels are positively related to birthweight.[64,306] Feeding behaviour will influence growth, and leptin status has been shown to be related to weight gain in the first months of life.[240]

The MC4 receptor in the hypothalamus is a more distal component of the appetite and feeding regulatory pathway. The ligand for the MC4 receptor, alpha melanocyte-stimulating hormone (α-MSH), is produced together with ACTH by cleavage of the peptide preproopiomelanocortin (POMC). Leptin promotes MSH production and this then interacts with the MC4 receptor and reduces food intake. As many as 5% of children with severe, early-onset obesity may have defects of the MC4 receptor[98,99] and patients with rare abnormalities of the POMC gene can present with ACTH deficiency and demonstrate obesity with associated rapid growth in early life.[173]

The gut peptide PYY has been shown to inhibit food intake,[30] and another hormone with orexigenic effects, ghrelin, has also been described.[47] Ghrelin is a GH secretogogue produced by a number of tissues, including the gastrointestinal tract and the hypothalamus, where it appears to act as a 'hunger' hormone. Reduced insulin levels between feeds are associated with a rise in ghrelin release and GH production. This may prove to be an important link between feeding, fasting, hormone production and the regulation of intermediate metabolism and fuel supply in the newborn period.[58,127,151]

Thyroid

Disorders of thyroid gland development and/or function are relatively common, affecting approximately one newborn infant in 3000. Recent advances in this field reflect the development of more refined biochemical assays, the elucidation of genes involved in thyroid gland development and hormone synthesis, as well as information gained from screening programmes for congenital hypothyroidism.

Normal function

Thyroid function in utero

TSH, modulated by TRH, stimulates the synthesis and release of T_4 and T_3 from the thyroid into the plasma, where they circulate, strongly bound to proteins. Maternal T_4, but not TSH or T_3, can cross the placenta in physiologically significant amounts and this explains the relatively normal phenotype in hypothyroid infants at birth.[345] The importance of maternal thyroxine delivery to the fetus in early gestation, whilst the fetal thyroid axis is developing, is supported by studies of neurodevelopment in infants of mothers with relatively low thyroxine levels.[121] The significance of thyroxine transfer in the latter stages of pregnancy is illustrated by the life threatening illness seen in hypothyroid infants of hypothyroid mothers.[83,367]

The greater part of circulating T_3 is derived from peripheral monodeiodination of the outer ring of T_4, which therefore acts as a reservoir or prohormone for the more active T_3. An alternative monodeiodination affects the inner ring of T_4 and produces inactive reverse T_3 (rT_3). This mechanism permits a balance between production of the most and least active thyroid hormones. There are three deiodinases – type I (D1), which has inner and outer deiodination activity, type II deiodinase (D2), which catalyses outer-ring deiodination, and type III deiodinase (D3), which catalyses inner-ring deiodination.

Fetal thyroid hormone metabolism is characterised by a predominance of D3 activity outside the CNS in tissues such as the liver, kidney and placenta, which converts maternal and endogenous T_4 preferentially to rT_3. This presumably helps to reduce tissue thermogenesis and enhance tissue anabolism. Thyroxine (rather than T_3) is required by the developing brain, and the appropriate deiodinases (particularly D2) are expressed in a temporal and spatial manner in different brain regions. Sulphotransferase enzymes also have an important role in normal thyroid hormone metabolism. T_4 sulphation blocks outer-ring deiodination to T_3 whilst promoting inner-ring conversion to inactive rT_3. The activity of sulphotransferase enzymes in tissues like the liver will also, therefore, play a key role in determining thyroid hormone availability.[102]

Thyroid function in the neonatal period

After birth there is an acute discharge of TSH, provoked by cooling, which reaches a peak at 30 minutes, before falling towards basal levels within the first 3 days. There is an associated release of thyroid hormones and enhanced peripheral conversion of T_4 (closely linked to D2 activity), which results in a pronounced increase in T_3 in the first hours of life. There is a further increase in total T_3 and free T_3 levels for about 36 hours around the time of the postnatal peak in T_4 (Fig. 35.8), and free T_4 levels remain relatively high for the first weeks of life.[104] Preterm infants (>30 weeks) delivered before this maturational process is complete show similar but lesser changes in TSH and thyroid hormone concentrations (see below). By 1–2 months of age, thyroid hormone levels are comparable to those in term infants. In the case of infants under 30 weeks' gestation, the postnatal surge does not occur[36] and T_4 levels frequently fall to a nadir around 1–2 weeks of age, which is more pronounced with increasing prematurity.[200,338] Thyroxine levels remain below those of full-term infants through the first few weeks of life[108] and climb gradually to normal postnatal levels.

Congenital hypothyroidism

This is a heterogeneous group of patients, some of whom will have functioning tissue and some of whom will not. In those with functioning tissue, the gland may be normally sited and of

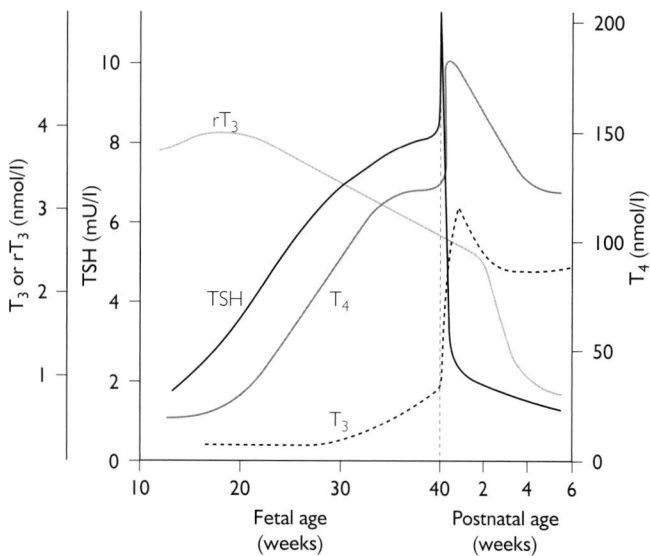

Fig. 35.8 The trend in fetal and neonatal plasma TSH/T$_4$/T$_3$ and reverse T$_3$ (rT$_3$) levels. (Adapted from Fisher.[100])

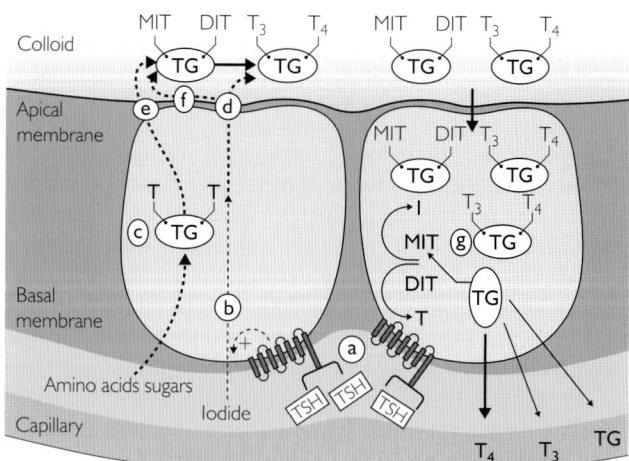

Fig. 35.9 Thyroid hormone production and disorders of thyroid hormone synthesis (dyshormonogeneses). *Thyroid hormone production:* Amino acids and glucose are used to produce thyroglobulin to which tyrosine residues are attached. Iodine is incorporated into these residues at the apical membrane to produce iodotyrosines. These are stored as extracellular colloid. *Thyroid hormone secretion:* Colloid droplets are invaginated to release thyroglobulin and the iodotyrosines including T$_4$ and T$_3$ which are released into the circulation. The other iodotyrosinases (DIT and MIT) are deiodinated and the iodine re-used. *Dyshormonogeneses:* a, TSH receptor defects; b, Abnormalities of iodide uptake (sodium iodide symporter); c, Defects of thyroglobulin synthesis; d, Abnormalities of iodine transport at the apical membrane (pendrin); e, Abnormalities of the enzyme system incorporating iodine into tyrosine (thyroid peroxidase); f, Abnormalities of the enzyme system involved in H$_2$O$_2$ generation (Thox); and g, Abnormalities of the deiodinase system.

normal size, hypoplastic or ectopic. There have been major developments in our understanding of the aetiology of congenital hypothyroidism in recent years, although the cause in most patients is still unknown.

Malformations besides defects of thyroid gland development and function are more common in infants with congenital hypothyroidism.[238] It is helpful to divide patients into those with thyroid dysgenesis and those patients with an abnormality of one of the enzymes or factors involved in thyroid hormone synthesis (dyshormonogenesis).

Thyroid dysgenesis

Embryological defects resulting in thyroid dysgenesis are the most common cause of congenital primary hypothyroidism, and range from thyroid agenesis to an ectopic and/or hypoplastic gland. Some thyroid tissue is demonstrable in approximately two-thirds of affected infants, and there is a spectrum of biochemical severity. The frequency is around 1 in 3500 and is twice as common in females as in males, with only minor racial and seasonal differences in incidence described. As genetic factors involved in thyroid development and thyroid-specific gene expression have been described, then so abnormalities of these same genes have been identified in a small number of patients with thyroid dysgenesis. Mutations in transcription factors such as TTF1 (NKX2-1), TTF2 and Pax-8 have been published, but a strict Mendelian inheritance pattern is uncommon[174,182,251] and the aetiology of thyroid dysgenesis in most patients is unknown.

Thyroid hormone replacement abolishes the physical manifestations of hypothyroidism but intellectual and neurological prognosis is poor unless treatment is started within the first few weeks of life.

Dyshormonogenesis (Fig. 35.9)

Recessively inherited biochemical defects of iodothyronine synthesis are the second most common cause of permanent congenital hypothyroidism, with a frequency in Europe and North America of

approximately 1 in 30 000–50 000, accounting for some 10–15% of patients identified by screening. The sex incidence is equal. A goitre may be present at birth but, unless large, may be difficult to detect and may not develop until later in life. The degree of clinical hypothyroidism is variable and some patients are euthyroid. Dyshormonogenesis may also be a cause of transient hypothyroidism when the extra demands in early life cannot be met. An isotope scan or ultrasound usually shows normal thyroid anatomy and site (a eutopic gland). In many dyshormonogeneses there is excessive discharge of iodide from the thyroid gland after administration of perchlorate (the perchlorate discharge test), due to an abnormality of iodide organification into thyroglobulin. Compensated primary hypothyroidism with normal isotope imaging due to abnormalities of the TSH receptor has also been described. Recognised abnormalities of thyroid hormone synthesis include abnormalities of the TSH receptor, which may be associated with a normally sized or hypoplastic gland,[32,318] and abnormalities of the thyroglobulin gene,[147,322] the sodium iodide symporter,[111,261] pendrin,[67,96] thyroid peroxidase[14,23,33,34] and THOX.[215] Delineation of the precise biochemical defect in these disorders does not alter the need for thyroxine replacement, but can be important when counselling families about the likelihood of recurrence.

Neonatal screening[1,94,331]

When radioimmunoassays were developed for measurement of T$_4$ and TSH in very small samples of serum or whole blood

Table 35.8 Clinical features of congenital hypothyroidism
At birth
Postmaturity, large size
Large posterior fontanelle
Umbilical hernia
Goitre
Early signs
Placid, sleepy
Poor feeding
Constipation, abdominal distension
Respiratory problems
Peripheral cyanosis
Oedema
Prolonged jaundice
'Cretinous' appearance
Later signs
Large tongue
Hoarse cry
Dry skin, hair
Slow responses
Delayed development
Growth failure

spotted onto filter paper, screening was rapidly adopted in many countries. Most programmes used a single blood sample taken between the fifth and tenth days of life, by which time relative stability has returned to the thyroid axis after the abrupt postnatal perturbation. T_4 screening alone proved inadequate because of the overlap between normal and hypothyroid values. The alternatives were therefore either to add a TSH assay in all cases or for the lower range of T_4 values, or to use TSH as the primary test and accept that the rare cases of secondary hypothyroidism may be missed. Programmes based on both systems were successful and both retain advocates. Many programmes in the USA measure T_4 levels, with TSH measurement in babies with the lowest 10% of T_4 values. Most European countries have adopted the primary TSH approach, although there are pitfalls in this, as in all forms of screening. In some parts of the world, a combined approach with measurement of both TSH and free T_4 has been implemented.[22] Guidelines for neonatal screening programmes have been published.[1,246,331]

The returns from screening proved even greater than had been expected: in both America and Europe, the frequency of congenital hypothyroidism was approximately 1 in 3500, almost double that suggested by retrospective surveys.[103] The early manifestations of congenital hypothyroidism are non-specific and development of the typical features usually occurs slowly (Table 35.8). Even in the most medically advanced countries, no more than half the affected infants could be diagnosed clinically by the age of 3 months.[13] With screening, treatment could be started by 4 weeks and ideally by 2 weeks of age.[1,331]

Diagnosis

The diagnosis of congenital hypothyroidism is confirmed by finding low serum thyroid hormone concentrations (free T_4) and a high TSH. The T_3 level is variable and is preserved in the normal range for longer. It remains essential to exclude hypothyroidism in any infant in whom there is clinical suspicion, because, first, errors inevitably occur in all screening programmes; secondly, mild hypothyroidism may escape detection by all screening methods (see below); and thirdly, there may be a late rise in TSH levels, particularly in the preterm infant.[142] The major clinical features are summarised in Table 35.8. Infants with low thyroxine values are more likely to have clinical signs such as feeding difficulties, lethargy, prolonged jaundice, umbilical hernia and macroglossia.[118] Such infants are more likely to have an aplastic rather than a hypoplastic or ectopic gland. A gestation over 40 weeks, induction of labour and a birthweight above 3500 g are all more common among infants with hypothyroidism.

Further investigation

The biochemistry primarily determines whether an infant requires thyroxine treatment. Further investigations do not have a major impact on the short-term management of the hypothyroid infant but imaging can, nevertheless, provide information about the nature and prognosis of the underlying defect.

Isotope scanning (technetium or ^{123}I) can be undertaken before or within a few days of starting thyroxine replacement treatment, when the TSH levels are still high. Thyroid ultrasonography is also performed in some centres,[252] and, whilst it is a highly operator-dependent technique, it can provide information about gland morphology. An ultrasound can be conducted on the neonatal unit and may be of particular value in the infant exposed to iodine-containing compounds whose isotope scan may be hard to interpret.

In thyroid dysgenesis, an isotope scan or ultrasound will reveal an absent, small or ectopic gland. This condition has a very low risk of recurrence in further children. The infant with thyroid aplasia or ectopia will need treatment for life and is unlikely to benefit from a trial of treatment in later childhood. If the gland is anatomically normal and the uptake is high, then hypothyroidism is probably due to a dyshormonogenesis and may be inherited in an autosomal recessive (AR) manner. Absent isotope uptake in a normally sited gland on ultrasonography also suggests a dyshormonogenesis.

A plain radiograph of the knee to assess epiphyseal maturity was frequently performed in the past; however, whilst it may reflect the degree of fetal hypothyroidism, it is of limited clinical value.

A TRH stimulation test is rarely indicated, but has been used in babies with mild thyroid dysfunction. An exaggerated and prolonged TSH response is observed if TSH levels are mildly elevated because of a compromised thyroid gland.[271]

Treatment

Thyroxine is used for replacement and there is no advantage in giving tri-iodothyronine (see above). It is a matter of some urgency to start treatment, and when the diagnosis is reasonably certain, it may be preferable to collect further specimens and start treatment without waiting for the results.

An appropriate starting dose of thyroxine in the newborn with low T_4 levels is 10–15 micrograms/kg/24 h given as a single daily dose.[42,92,290] Full-term infants should be commenced on 37.5–50 micrograms daily, which usually brings the TSH into the normal range quickly. Tablets of 25 micrograms are available and because of the long half-life of thyroxine the dose can be adjusted by giving a higher or lower dose on alternate days, such as 25 micrograms one day and 50 micrograms the next. Thyroxine suspensions are available, although there are concerns about the stability of these preparations.

The aim of therapy is rapidly to normalise T_4/freeT_4 levels as well as TSH concentrations. High T_4 levels may be seen after treatment is commenced but this picture does not usually suggest overtreatment if TSH levels are normal or elevated. TSH levels do not always normalise promptly and there may be a degree of pituitary thyroid hormone resistance in infancy in some patients.[105] The dose of thyroxine will fall with time when calculated on a weight basis and a suppressed TSH indicates overtreatment. The heterogeneity of congenital hypothyroidism has been highlighted earlier and babies with only mild or moderately elevated baseline TSH levels may require smaller doses of thyroxine than babies with agenesis, where the baseline TSH is typically very high.[126] Replacement is usually satisfactory if the serum total T_4 and free T_4 are in the upper part of the quoted laboratory normal range for age, but suboptimal compliance needs to be excluded if TSH values remain elevated despite a substantial thyroxine dose.

There is accumulating evidence to suggest that higher initial starting doses of thyroxine may have a beneficial impact on neurodevelopment,[42,290] although there has been concern that this might be at the expense of an increase in behavioural problems.[134,139,284] Severe overdosage may also cause accelerated growth and even craniosynostosis, but the danger of impaired neurological development from underdosage is probably greater.

Higher doses of thyroxine treatment in early life as well as a milder baseline biochemical picture have been associated with increased stature in mid-childhood and at final height[87,116,133] although this has not been a consistent observation.[289]

Follow-up and prognosis

Growth, clinical progress and thyroid function should be checked after 2 and then 4 weeks on treatment, and then at 1–2-monthly intervals through the first year and regularly thereafter.

If needed, definitive reassessment of thyroid status can be undertaken after the age of 2 years, when brief cessation of treatment will have no adverse effect. Most children with a permanent defect of thyroid hormone generation will develop abnormal biochemistry without any adverse symptoms if thyroxine is stopped for 4 weeks at this stage. In addition to a biochemical assessment of thyroid function, the opportunity can be taken to obtain or repeat an isotope thyroid scan.

Congenital hypothyroidism is associated with impaired motor development, a reduced intelligence quotient (IQ) and impaired hearing and language problems.[81,285] These features are related to the severity of hypothyroidism at birth.[283] In one study, total T_4 levels below 42 nmol/l in the neonatal period were associated with a 10-point deficit in IQ at school entry.[330] Individuals with T_4 values above 42 nmol/l were no different from controls, suggesting a 'threshold' effect. Thus it seems that the degree of pre- and perinatal hypothyroidism has implications for CNS function

in the long term. A formal hearing assessment is recommended in the hypothyroid infant because of the tenfold increase in hearing loss in these babies.[339]

Other abnormalities of thyroid function in early life

Secondary (pituitary/hypothalamic) hypothyroidism (see pages 873–4)

Secondary hypothyroidism (TSH deficiency) should be suspected if free T_4 and T_3 levels are low in the presence of a low, normal or paradoxically raised TSH. The differential diagnosis of this biochemical picture includes euthyroid illness and prematurity (see below). Isolated TSH deficiency is very rare and most infants with secondary hypothyroidism will have other pituitary hormone deficiencies with associated clinical and biochemical features. The TSH response to TRH in patients with secondary hypothyoidism may be normal, poor or even exaggerated.[120]

Abnormalities of binding proteins – thyroxine-binding globulin deficiency and familial dysalbuminaemic hyperthyroxinaemia

The major carrier protein of the thyroid hormones is thyroxine-binding globulin (TBG). Deficiency of TBG is usually inherited as an X-linked dominant trait and has an incidence in male infants of 1:2400 with an overall frequency around 1:4000–4300 in North America.[142,192] Affected patients are euthyroid. Total T_4 and T_3 levels are low, but the free fractions are normal and the resting and stimulated TSH values are also normal. TBG measurement is needed for a definitive diagnosis.

Familial dysalbuminemic hyperthyroxinemia is a relatively common disorder, affecting 1 in 100 people. It is characterised by increased thyroxine levels in clinically euthyroid individuals because of an abnormal albumin molecule that has an increased affinity for thyroid hormone. The abnormal albumin molecule will also interfere with some thyroid hormone assays, leading to spurious and potentially confusing results.[262] This condition underlines the importance of measuring TSH concentrations in infants with raised thyroid hormone concentrations.

Transient disorders of thyroid function

Transient hypothyroxinaemia[270]

All premature infants have some degree of hypothyroxinaemia because cord serum T_4 values increase with gestational age. Low thyroxine levels in the preterm infant reflect the loss of the normal maternal thyroxine supply, immaturity of the hypothalamo–pituitary–thyroid axis, as well as other factors such as the ongoing fetal tendency to convert thyroid hormone to inactive rT_3. Low thyroid hormone values persist in the first 1–2 weeks in association with low free T_4 and normal TSH levels. This biochemical picture tends to be more profound in the more preterm, lighter babies, and thyroid hormone levels also tend to be lower in those with illness such as respiratory distress syndrome.[338] This was thought to be of little consequence in the short term, but more recent evidence indicates that there is a relationship between thyroxine concentrations in preterm and low-birthweight (LBW) infants and subsequent neurodevelopmental outcome.[80,183,199,273] Although many of these studies have attempted to consider potential confounding variables, it is possible that in some infants thyroxine levels are simply a marker of fetal wellbeing. A low thyroxine concentration in the first weeks of life may therefore be an adaptation to illness in preterm infants, analogous to the sick-euthyroid syndrome or non-thyroidal illness seen in older children. A significant number of pregnant women may be iodine-deficient, and maternal iodine status and postnatal iodine supply are further potential confounding factors.

The impact of thyroid hormone administration on the short- and longer-term outcome following preterm delivery has yet to be established. Improvements in survival have been reported in some studies[298] but not others,[63] and early neurodevelopmental outcome does not appear to be affected by treatment.[338] A subgroup analysis in the study by van Wassenaer et al[338] suggested a potential benefit of thyroxine treatment (8 micrograms/kg/day) on the Bayley Mental Development Index in babies of 25–26 weeks' gestation. However, evidence from the same and other studies has suggested that increasing thyroxine delivery in babies born at 27–29 weeks may have an adverse effect on neurodevelopment. The most recent report from the same group, as the children reach school age, has confirmed the improved IQ with a reduction in behavioural problems in those receiving T_4 at <27 weeks, and the lower IQ with more behavioural problems in those receiving T_4 at >27 weeks.[46] The effects of thyroxine administration may therefore depend on the gestation and age of the infant treated, with protective mechanisms ensuring an adequate supply of tri-iodothyronine in all but the most preterm. At this moment in time, the routine supplementation of babies of any gestation in whom TSH levels are normal is not recommended.

It is important to remember that preterm infants with hypothyroxinaemia may have a permanent abnormality of thyroid function which will only become apparent with longer term follow-up.[142]

Transient hypothyroidism and hyperthyrotropinaemia

In this heterogeneous group of disorders, the TSH is raised and thyroid hormone concentrations are within the age-related reference range (hyperthyrotropinaemia) or low (hypothyroidism). Patients may have had a mild abnormality of thyroid function detected by the screening programme or the infant may have had thyroid function checked for other reasons. Although thyroid function may normalise within the first few months of life, some of these infants may have a permanent albeit subtle abnormality of thyroid function.[55,72] There are well-established causes of transient thyroid dysfunction, but overlap with congenital hypothyroidism is illustrated by the transient hyperthyrotropinaemia that can occur in infants with an underlying dyshormonogenesis.[215] These babies are presumably unable to meet the demand for thyroxine in the early neonatal period. A list of causes of hyperthyrotropinaemia/hypothyroidism is outlined in Table 35.9. Noteworthy causes include intrauterine exposure to antithyroid drugs,[62] iodine deficiency[19,166] and exposure to topical iodinated antiseptic agents. These are readily absorbed and should be avoided or carefully removed following

Table 35.9 Causes of transient hypothyroidism and hyperthyrotropinaemia

- Dyshormonogenesis
  e.g. Thox defects and TSH receptor mutations
- Thyroid dysgenesis
- Maternal antibodies
- Iodine deficiency
- Exposure to iodine-containing compounds
- Pseudohypoparathyroidism
- Down syndrome
- In association with prematurity

initial application.[51,184,308] Transient hypothyroidism may also be due to the transplacental passage of thyrotropin receptor-blocking antibodies in approximately 2% of cases of congenital hypothyroidism[50] and it is wise to check a mother's thyroid status in these circumstances. Transient hypothyroidism and hyperthyrotropinaemia appear to be more common in the preterm infant.[79,108,193] The late rise in TSH observed in some preterm and very-low-birthweight (VLBW) infants may reflect hypothalamopituitary immaturity, the negative iodine balance in early life, illness with a compensatory rise in TSH, as well as earlier exposure to drugs such as dopamine[84] which can suppress TSH levels. Causes of permanent hyperthyrotropinaemia include subtle abnormalities of the TSH receptor.[11]

Intervention is important in those patients with low thyroid hormone levels and increasingly there is a move towards treatment if the TSH is raised in the presence of thyroxine levels within the laboratory normal range, because even subtle abnormalities may suggest that the CNS is thyroid hormone deficient.[101,269] Therapy should be safe provided the infant is monitored appropriately, and can always be stopped at a later stage beyond the critical phase of brain growth.

The 'low T_3 syndrome' (non-thyroidal illness)

This term is used to describe thyroid function tests characterised by low serum T_3 concentrations, normal or raised rT_3, variable T_4 and normal TSH. Fetal T_3 levels are low throughout gestation because of enhanced conversion of T_4 to rT_3, and this picture is frequently observed in preterm infants. As in older patients, T_3 levels may be further reduced by intercurrent illness and by poor nutrition in infants of all gestational ages. Low T_3 levels, like T_4, have been linked to a reduction in IQ in later life.[189] Thyroxine administration to infants of less than 30 weeks' gestation does not increase T_3 levels.[339]

Hyperthyroidism

Neonatal thyrotoxicosis[236]

Neonatal thyrotoxicosis is a relatively rare but serious condition, usually caused by the transplacental passage of TSH receptor-stimulating antibodies from the serum of a mother with active, inactive or treated Graves' disease.[191,325] It may also occur when the mother has autoimmune thyroid disease other than Graves'.[137] The disease is usually transient, resolving within the timespan of the circulating antibodies. Neonatal hyperthyroidism is under-recognised but it can often be predicted and treated prenatally.

TSH receptor-stimulating antibodies may be demonstrated in the majority of patients with Graves' disease and they cross the placenta freely. Thyrotoxicosis in the fetus may lead to preterm labour, LBW, stillbirth and neonatal death. Approximately 1 in 70–100 babies of mothers with Graves' disease becomes overtly thyrotoxic, although the absolute risk is related to the concentration of TSH receptor-stimulating antibodies in the maternal serum[219,307,370] and some babies will be biochemically toxic but asymptomatic. Thyroid dysfunction has been detected in as many as 16.5% of babies born to women with Graves' disease.[212] TSH receptor-blocking antibodies may be present as well, and the clinical and biochemical picture will reflect a range of factors, including the impact of altered maternal and fetal thyroid hormone levels on fetal hypothalamopituitary function as well as the nature and concentration of prevailing antibody concentrations. Exposure to antithyroid drug treatment in utero will also influence the neonatal picture. Hence, an infant who is initially hyperthyroid can subsequently become hypothyroid (requiring thyroxine replacement) and an initially hypothyroid infant can become hyperthyroid.[62,128,196]

Although neonatal thyrotoxicosis is usually due to the transplacental passage of TSH receptor-stimulating antibodies, in some babies such antibodies are not present and yet the hyperthyroidism persists. These children suffer more complications and long-term morbidity, in particular growth failure in spite of early accelerated skeletal maturity, behaviour problems, and even mental retardation. It is likely that most of the reported cases are due to constitutively activating mutations of the TSH receptor.[93,168]

Clinical features (Table 35.10)

The signs of thyrotoxicosis in the fetus include tachycardia and intrauterine growth retardation (IUGR). Infants with perinatal thyrotoxicosis may show signs of hyperthyroidism immediately after birth, but symptoms may be delayed as long as 4–7 weeks.[307,369] This may be due to the effect of maternal antithyroid drugs or to the relative effects of both blocking and stimulating antibodies. Infants may have a palpable goitre, and although eye signs, especially proptosis and lid retraction, can be present at birth, they are often mild or absent throughout the course of the disease. Very rarely, a mother with euthyroid ophthalmic Graves' disease may produce an infant with eye involvement but no evidence of thyrotoxicosis. Signs of CNS stimulation, such as irritability, restlessness and 'jitteriness', usually predominate and there is tachycardia and occasionally arrhythmia, which may progress rapidly to severe and intractable heart failure. Other signs of hypermetabolism include an excessive appetite with weight loss or inadequate weight gain, diarrhoea, sweating and flushing. Less predictable clinical features include hepatosplenomegaly, jaundice and accelerated bone maturation, which can cause premature closure of the skull sutures and occasionally microcephaly. Mortality rates of 16–25% have been reported and the long-term outcome is uncertain.[307]

Management (Fig. 35.10)

Hyperthyroid pregnant women should be treated with the antithyroid thiourea derivatives carbimazole or propylthiouracil.[282] The use of radioactive iodine is absolutely contraindicated during pregnancy, and surgery may precipitate preterm delivery. The antithyroid drugs cross the placenta, and the lowest dose that controls the hyperthyroidism should be used. This is often lower in pregnancy than the dose normally required in adults. The 'block and replace' regimen, using higher doses of antithyroid drugs in combination with replacement thyroxine, should be avoided. If maternal antithyroid treatment causes goitre formation and bradycardia in the fetus, it is possible to give thyroxine by intramniotic injection. There may be biochemical evidence of transient hypothyroidism in clinically euthyroid babies of mothers treated with antithyroid drugs.[62] If fetal tachycardia suggests hyperthyroidism, treatment should be adjusted to maintain the fetal heart rate below 160 beats per minute and careful assessment of fetal growth is necessary. Cordocentesis may be used to confirm the diagnosis.

Severe hyperthyroidism carries a high mortality in the newborn. The key to successful management is, first, anticipation and prevention, then control of thyroid status until the disease runs its self-limited course. If the fetus was hyperthyroid and the mother received a thionamide during pregnancy, then the wisest course will usually be to continue the same preparation in a suitable neonatal dosage, which is propylthiouracil 5–10 mg/kg/24 h or carbimazole 0.5–1.5 mg/kg/24 h in divided doses by mouth every 6–8 hours. Regular assessment of thyroid function is necessary. As at other ages, it may be difficult to maintain a stable euthyroid state on treatment. Babies who are clinically euthyroid but subsequently show signs of hyperthyroidism will also need to be treated. Neonatal thyrotoxicosis usually remits after 2–5 months and so antithyroid medication can be cautiously withdrawn around this time. It is essential to maintain close observation until treatment has been successfully stopped and the infant is well, because fatal acute recurrent

Table 35.10 Clinical features of neonatal hyperthyroidism	
Thyroid	Goitre
Central nervous system	Irritability, restlessness, 'jitteriness'
Eyes	Stare, lid retraction, oedema, proptosis
Cardiovascular system	Tachycardia, cardiac failure, arrhythmia
Gastrointestinal tract	Excessive appetite, weight loss, emaciation, diarrhoea
Other	Sweating, flushing, acrocyanosis, hepatosplenomegaly, lymphadenopathy, thymic enlargement, thrombocytopenia, bruising, petechiae, hyperviscosity, advanced skeletal maturation, craniosynostosis, microcephaly

thyrotoxicosis has occurred at this stage. Administration of a generous dose of antithyroid drug and simultaneous replacement with thyroxine ('block and replace') has been used in thyrotoxic infants but the relatively short duration of the hyperthyroid phase makes this approach impractical in most babies. If a baby is thought to be at particular risk of hyperthyroidism, if a sibling was symptomatic or if there is a high titre of maternal antibodies, then close clinical and biochemical surveillance should be continued for the first weeks of life. Treatment with an antithyroid preparation should be started promptly if necessary.

If acute thyrotoxicosis does occur, then in addition to a thionamide, propranolol 2.0 mg/kg/24 h in divided doses by mouth 6–8-hourly can be used to control the peripheral stimulatory effects of thyroid hormones and/or potassium iodide, as aqueous iodine (Lugol's) solution (5% potassium iodide ~8 mg per drop) one drop 8-hourly can be administered to prevent synthesis and release of thyroid hormones from the gland. Saturated potassium iodide (48 mg iodine per drop) may also be used in a dose of one drop daily. Radiographic iodine-containing agents such as sodium ipodate (0.5 mg every 3 days) have also been used in the

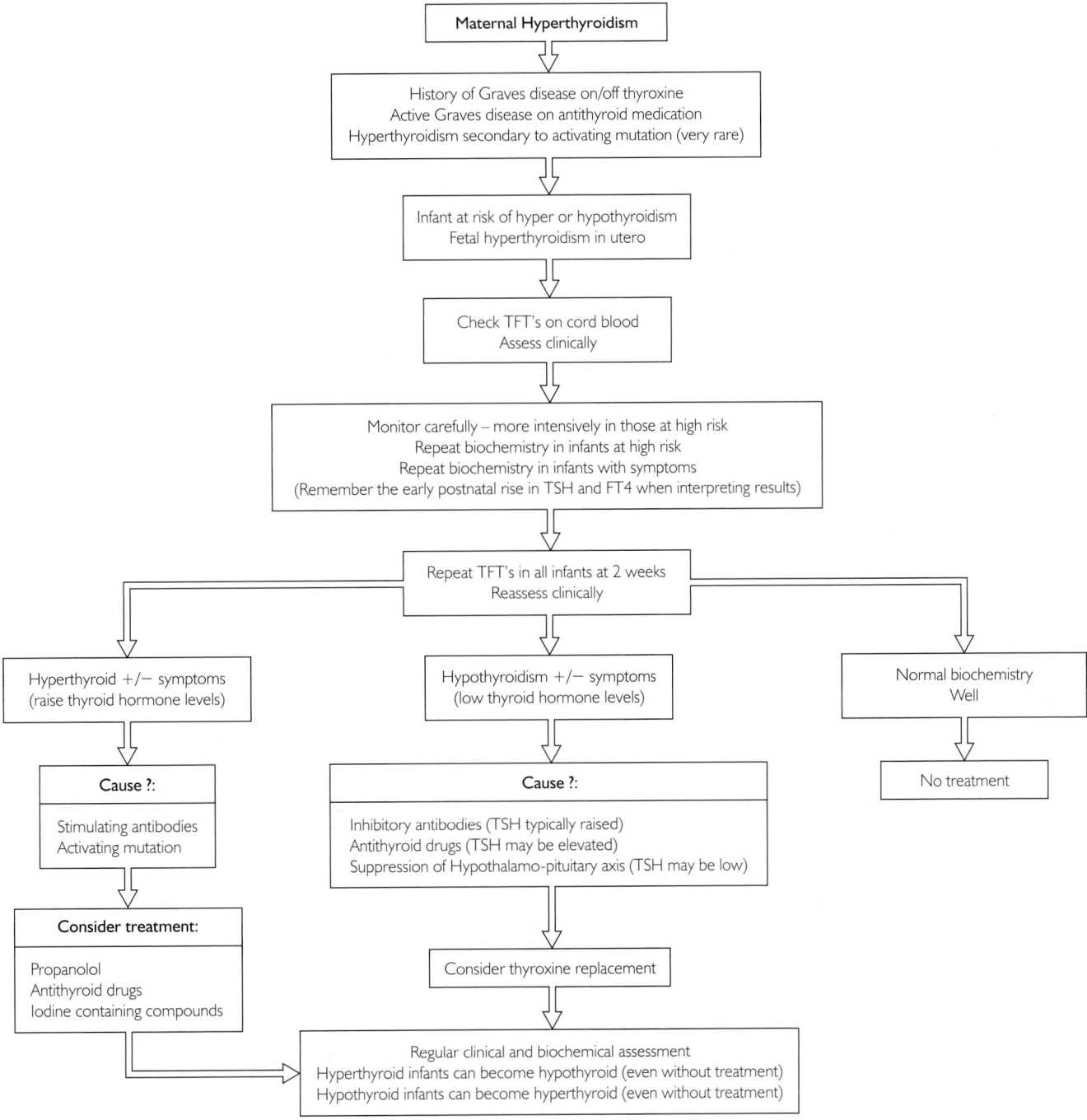

Fig. 35.10 An approach to the assessment and management of children with or at risk of neonatal hyper- or hypothyroidism.

treatment of neonatal Graves' disease, partly because of the relatively rapid response.[160] Severely ill babies can be treated with sedatives as well as a glucocorticoid such as prednisolone (2 mg/kg/day) which suppresses T_4 to T_3 conversion.

Occasionally an infant born to a mother with Graves' disease will be found to have a hypothyroid picture with low thyroid hormone levels and a raised or suppressed TSH. In some instances, a low TSH and low T_4 reflect suppression of the hypothalamus–pituitary–thyroid axis by the transplacental passage of thyroid hormone from a hyperthyroid mother, and these babies will need thyroxine replacement whilst the axis recovers.[181,196,212] The transplacental passage of blocking antibodies and exposure to antithyroid drug may also account for low thyroid hormone levels.

Thyroid hormone resistance[272,357]

Resistance to thyroid hormone (RTH) is caused by mutations in the thyroid hormone receptor (TR) (beta) gene. The clinical presentation of RTH is highly variable and the majority of individuals are completely asymptomatic. Occasionally neonates will be found to have this disorder because of a goitre or because of a raised TSH. A minority may have symptoms suggestive of hypothyroidism such as growth retardation and impaired cognitive ability, whilst others have signs of thyroid hormone excess such as tachycardia or hyperactivity.[37] The typical picture is of a healthy, clinically euthyroid infant with a raised TSH and raised T_4 and T_3. The disorder is usually inherited in an autosomal dominant (AD) manner and so one of the parents will have similar biochemistry.

Disorders of calcium metabolism

Normal physiology

Calcium has a central role in many physiological processes, including transmission across membranes, activation and inhibition of enzymes, the secretion and action of hormones, blood coagulation, muscle contraction and nerve transmission. In addition, calcium gives structural stability to the skeleton, which contains approximately 99% of total body calcium. Most of this large calcium pool is metabolically inactive and can be mobilised only slowly, but a small available fraction is under close regulation.

Calcium is present in serum in two major fractions, protein-bound (~50% of the total) and ionised calcium. There is also a small amount of diffusible non-ionised calcium present as complexes with phosphate and citrate. The ionised fraction is metabolically active and available for regulation. Of the protein-bound calcium, approximately 80% is attached to albumin and 20% to globulin, but this varies with the concentration of albumin and the pH. A rough 'correction' of the serum calcium concentration can be made by adding or subtracting 0.1 mmol/l for each 4 g/l of albumin above or below the mean serum albumin for age. Hydrogen ions compete with calcium for binding sites and so a decrease in pH causes a release of calcium from albumin

and an increase in ionised calcium, whilst alkalosis has the opposite effect.

There is active transport of calcium and phosphate by the placenta to the fetus, with a 1:1.4 mother/fetus gradient, so that the fetus is relatively hypercalcaemic compared with the mother.[170] Serum total and ionised calcium concentrations are high in cord blood but decrease rapidly in the first hours after birth, remaining relatively low for the first 2–4 days[197] before rising to adult levels in week 2 of life.

The maintenance of serum calcium levels in the physiological range is a complex process that reflects the function of, and interaction between, the calcium-sensing receptor, parathyroid hormone (PTH) and vitamin D (Fig. 35.11).

The calcium-sensing receptor

The extracellular calcium ion-sensing receptor is one of a group of 'G-protein coupled' receptors which responds to alterations in the concentration of calcium ion, thereby regulating PTH release and renal tubular calcium reabsorption.[247] A lowering of ionised calcium in extracellular fluid is detected by this receptor and leads to enhanced PTH secretion by the parathyroid chief cell. Gene defects that result in impaired or enhanced receptor activity can alter the 'set-point' and lead to hypo- or hypercalcaemia. AD familial benign hypocalciuric hypercalcaemia (impaired receptor function) and hypercalciuric hypocalcaemia (enhanced receptor function) may present in the neonatal period. These rare but important causes of neonatal hyper- and hypocalcaemia are described in more detail below.

Parathyroid hormone

PTH is secreted by the four parathyroid glands that lie behind the thyroid gland. It has 84 amino acid residues, of which the amino-terminal 34 have full biological activity. The primary stimulus for PTH synthesis and secretion is a low serum calcium level, but the secretion of PTH is also reduced by a low magnesium concentration. When PTH is released, it is rapidly degraded into a number of fragments, the more active of which include the amino-terminal sequence and have a half-life of only a few minutes. Some inactive fragments remain in the circulation much longer. The primary action of PTH is on the osteoclasts, where it promotes the release of calcium from bone. It also acts on the kidney, where it increases the excretion of phosphate (and sodium, potassium and bicarbonate) and decreases that of calcium (and magnesium and hydrogen ion). These are the primary actions that regulate calcium levels acutely, but PTH also increases the formation of 1,25-dihydroxyvitamin D, and so indirectly increases calcium absorption from the gut in the longer term.

Vitamin D

This term describes a number of compounds related to cholesterol. The two naturally occurring forms are ergocalciferol (D_2), which is derived from plants, and cholecalciferol (D_3), which is derived from 7-dehydrocholesterol by the effects of ultraviolet light on the skin. Cholecalciferol is also absorbed from animal

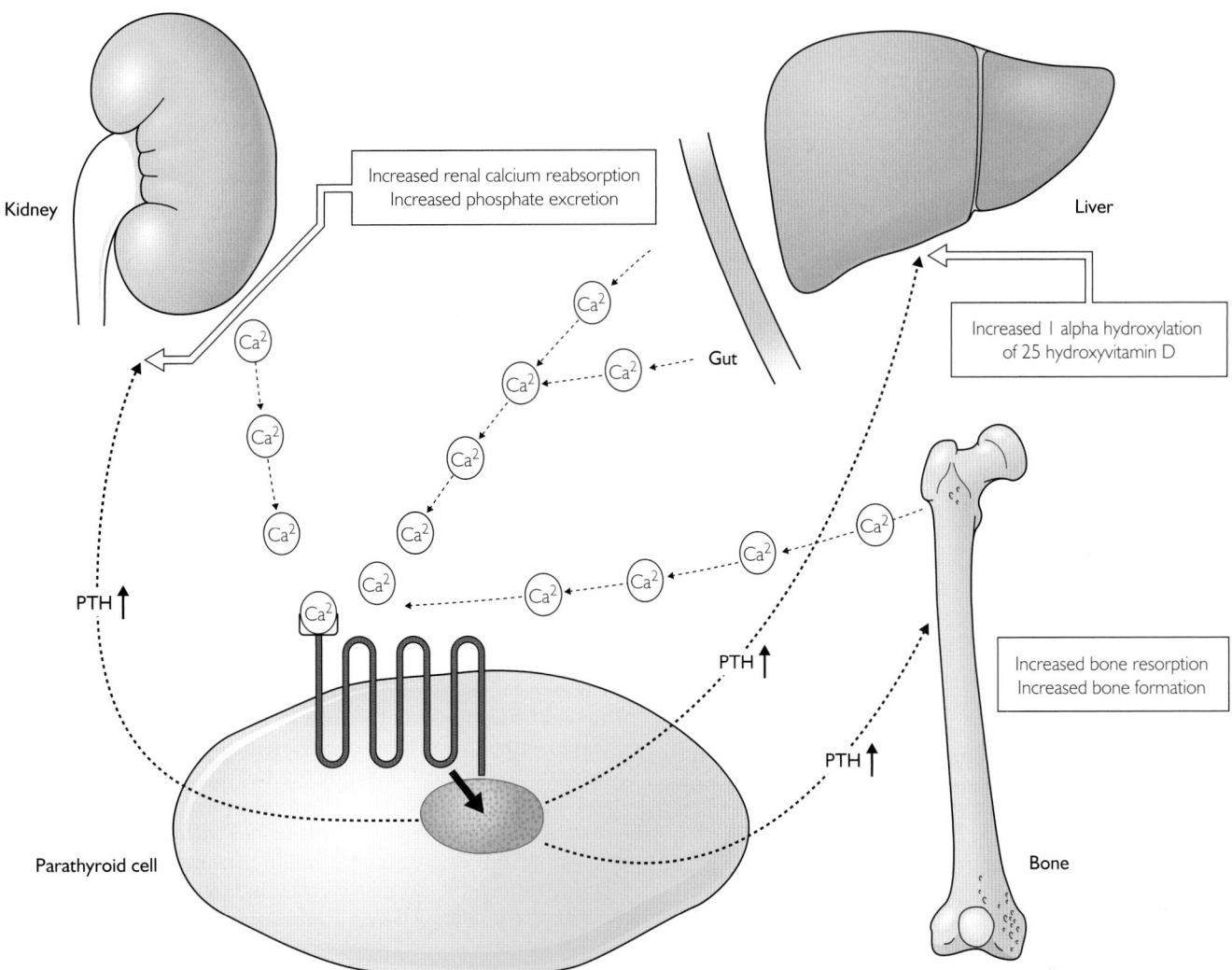

Fig. 35.11 The role of the calcium-sensing receptor and PTH production in calcium homeostasis. Calcium is detected by the calcium-sensing receptor on the surface of the parathyroid chief cell. Low calcium concentrations result in a rise in PTH release. The effects of PTH include enhanced calcium resorption by the kidney, increased 1α-hydroxylation of 25-hydroxyvitamin D by the liver, and increased bone resorption.

sources in the diet, from the upper part of the small intestine. Cholecalciferol and absorbed ergo-/cholecalciferol are hydroxylated, primarily by the liver, to 25-hydroxyvitamin D, which is the major circulating vitamin D metabolite. This undergoes 1-hydroxylation in the kidney to 1,25-dihydroxyvitamin D, the metabolically active form, or to 1,24,25-trihydroxyvitamin D or 24,25-dihydroxyvitamin D (see below). 1-hydroxylation is stimulated and 24-hydroxylation inhibited by hypocalcaemia, hypophosphataemia and PTH. Only 1–3% of circulating vitamin D is free, with most bound to vitamin D binding protein, an α₂-globulin.

The major effect of vitamin D is to increase serum levels of calcium and phosphate by facilitating their absorption from the gut. Vitamin D also enhances the mobilisation of calcium and phosphate from bone when dietary calcium is inadequate and promotes bone mineralisation by maintaining adequate concentrations of calcium and phosphate in the vicinity of unmineralised

osteoid. Fetal 1,25-dihydroxyvitamin D is probably the major stimulus for the placental transfer of calcium.

Other peptide hormones implicated in calcium homeostasis

PTH-related peptide (PTHrP)[317]
PTHrP has very similar actions to PTH. Circulating levels are low but it is found in breast milk and may have a role in calcium homeostasis in the fetus. Local production of PTHrP has been implicated in the development of tumour-related hypercalcaemia.

Calcitonin
This 32 amino acid peptide hormone is secreted by the parafollicular C cells of the thyroid in response to hypercalcaemia. It lowers serum calcium by inhibiting bone resorption, increasing urinary calcium and phosphate loss, and probably by decreasing

intestinal calcium absorption. Although it can produce hypocalcaemia in humans, neither removal of the thyroid gland nor massive hypersecretion in medullary thyroid carcinoma affects the serum calcium, and its physiological significance in man is unclear.

Hypocalcaemia[305]

The clinical features of hypocalcaemia infants, clinical features may include irritability, tremors, twitching and seizures, but some infants may in contrast be lethargic, feed poorly and vomit. The Chvostek and Trousseau signs are not reliable in the newborn but the QT interval of the ECG is increased.

Causes

The causes of hypocalcaemia are shown in Table 35.11.

Treatment

Severe symptoms of hypocalcaemia, such as seizures, may be treated with 10% calcium gluconate (9.4% calcium by weight) 2 ml/kg by slow i.v. injection over 5–10 minutes. If necessary, this may be followed by continuous infusion of diluted 10% calcium gluconate, 2.5 ml/kg/24 h, with careful monitoring of cardiac rate and rhythm and serum calcium concentration. A move to oral therapy at an early stage is advisable, and oral calcium supplements (e.g. Calcium Sandoz 4 ml/kg = 2.16 mmol Ca^{2+}/kg) and vitamin D or a vitamin D analogue may be needed for long-term management. This will depend on the cause of the hypocalcaemia and will be discussed under the appropriate diagnoses.

Table 35.11 Causes of hypocalcaemia

Neonatal hypocalcaemia
   Early (preterm, asphyxiated, infants of diabetic mothers)
   Late (inappropriate feeds)
Secondary to hypomagnesaemia
Hypoparathyroidism
   Microdeletions of chromosome 22q11 and 10p (including
      DiGeorge syndrome)
   X-linked
   Autosomal dominant, including HDR syndrome
   Autosomal recessive
   Mitochondrial DNA mutations
Maternal hypercalcaemia
Calcium-sensing receptor defects (activating – hypocalcaemic
   hypercalciuria)
Vitamin D deficiency
Vitamin D-dependent rickets (types I and II)
Pseudohypoparathyroidism (seldom presents in the newborn)
Alkalosis, bicarbonate therapy, citrate in blood transfusion
Renal failure
Malabsorption
Hypoalbuminaemia

Early hypocalcaemia

Symptomatic hypocalcaemia during the first 3 days of life occurs more commonly in preterm babies, infants of diabetic mothers and those who suffer birth asphyxia or other perinatal stress. This can be viewed as an exaggeration of the normal postnatal fall in calcium levels. Although the mechanisms leading to low calcium levels in preterm infants are not well defined, the levels of PTH are not usually low.[279,288] A degree of PTH resistance may be present, and a sudden interruption in calcium supply at a time of high demand may also account for the fall in calcium levels. Calcitonin secretion is high in the neonatal period, and, although it then falls rapidly during early infancy, it has been suggested that this increases susceptiblity to the development of early neonatal hypocalcaemia.[39,75] A low milk intake, or blood transfusions, which cause non-ionisable salt formation, can exacerbate hypocalcaemia still further. Many infants with early neonatal hypocalcaemia, especially those with diabetic mothers, also have low serum magnesium levels, which, like the hypocalcaemia, usually improve spontaneously. In some intances the cause of transient hypocalcaemia remains unclear.[110,211]

Late hypocalcaemia due to inappropriate feeds

This clinical picture is now much less common than it was when unmodified cow's milk formulas were widely used. It usually presented with seizures in apparently normal term infants on the fifth to tenth days of life. Classically this was due to the high phosphate and relatively low calcium content of cow's milk (pp. 284, 303). Increased absorption of phosphate caused hyperphosphataemia, which in turn depressed the serum calcium. An increased incidence during the winter months indicated that susceptibility might be compounded by a borderline maternal vitamin D status. The treatment needed was to control the fits and change the feed to breast milk or to a modified low-phosphate formula.

Other causes of hypocalcaemia

Hypomagnesaemia[85]
Hypomagnesaemia may cause hypocalcaemia both by inhibiting the secretion of PTH and by reducing PTH responsiveness. As many as 80% of infants with hypocalcaemic fits may be hypomagnesaemic, and hypocalcaemia may prove difficult to correct until the hypomagnesaemia has itself been corrected. This is most easily done by giving intramuscular (i.m.) magnesium sulphate in 50% solution, 0.2 ml/kg every 4–8 hours. The serum magnesium should therefore be measured in all infants with persistent hypocalcaemia.

There are other, rare, primary abnormalities of intestinal magnesium absorption (AR familial hypomagnesaemia with hypocalaemia) and renal magnesium handling (primary hypomagnesaemia) which need to be considered in the hypomagnesaemic, hypocalcaemic patient. Hypomagnesaemia may be a feature of Gitelman syndrome and Bartter syndrome, but these patients are not hypocalcaemic.

Hypoparathyroidism
Hypoparathyroidism is a rare cause of hypocalcaemia in the newborn period. It usually presents after 5 days of age with overt

signs of hypocalcaemia. Other biochemical findings include hyperphosphataemia, hypomagnesaemia and a normal or low alkaline phosphatase. The diagnosis is confirmed by the finding of low or absent immunoreactive PTH levels. This condition may be familial, with X-linked recessive, AD and AR patterns of inheritance described. Hypoparathyroidism, thymic aplasia, congenital abnormalities of the heart and great vessels, and other dysmorphic features may result from deletions within chromosome 22q11.[287] The DiGeorge syndrome links thymic hypoplasia with hypocalcaemia and forms part of a constellation of abnormalities which collectively has been termed the CATCH phenotype (cardiac abnormality, T-cell deficit, clefting, and hypocalcemia).[53,362] Some patients with 22q11 deletions have a preponderant cardiac presentation (Takao syndrome) and some have more prominent craniofacial and palatal abnormalities (Shprintzen syndrome). A small number of cases of DiGeorge syndrome have defects in other chromosomes, notably 10p.[76] The presence of hypocalcaemia with congenital abnormalities should prompt detailed genetic analysis, although it should be remembered that calcium levels may return to normal spontaneously.

Causes of hypoparathyroidism also include the HDR syndrome (hypoparathyroidism, deafness and renal dysplasia) due to defects in the GATA3 gene at 10p15.[337] This is an AD disorder which can present with hypocalcaemia in early life, although the diagnosis of hypoparathyroidism may be delayed by many years. Defects in the PTH gene are rare and can be associated with AD and AR isolated hypoparathyroidism.[20,243] Mutations of the GCMB gene on the short arm of chromosome 6 can also cause recessively inherited hypoparathyroidism.[88] Other rare causes of hypoparathyroidism include the Kenny–Caffey syndrome, where there is associated growth retardation and medullary stenosis of tubular bones, and mitochondrial disease such as Kearns–Sayre syndrome.

In the past high doses of vitamin D_2 were used to treat hypoparathyroidism, but the potent water-soluble analogues are preferable. A suitable dose in the newborn is α-calcidol (1α-hydroxycholecalciferol) or calcitriol (1,25-dihydroxycholecalciferol) 0.03–0.08 micrograms/kg/24 h up to a maximum of 1–2 micrograms. The maintenance dose needed varies not only between patients but also in the same patient at different times; frequent measurement of the serum calcium is therefore necessary, with dose adjustments to keep the level within the normal range. Supplementary oral calcium is not essential but may help to stabilise the serum calcium.

Maternal hypercalcaemia

In the presence of maternal hypercalcaemia, the fetus is exposed to chronic hypercalcaemia from excessive transplacental passage of calcium. Parathyroid suppression may result in hypocalcaemia after birth,[327] but this generally resolves spontaneously. Maternal calcium levels should be checked whenever there is unexplained hypocalcaemia in the newborn.

Hypercalciuric hypocalcaemia

Hypocalcaemia with hypercalciuria due to activating mutations of the calcium-sensing receptor may present in childhood with seizures. This rare condition should be suspected when hypocalcaemia is associated with hypercalciuria PTH levels that are within the normal range, in contrast to infants with hypoparathyroidism.[249] It is important to be aware of this condition because vitamin D administration may lead to nephrocalcinosis.

Vitamin D-deficient rickets

Hypocalcaemia and rickets may occur in association with maternal and infant vitamin D deficiency.[6,302] This is a well-recognised cause of neonatal seizures which will occur before a skeletal phenotype has evolved. Although some racial groups are more susceptible to hypocalcaemia and rickets than others, this remains a worldwide problem. The vitamin D status of an infant will reflect the mother's diet and her exposure to sunlight, as well as postnatal factors such as the type of feed. Most commercial milk preparations contain enough vitamin D to prevent rickets, but supplementation is advisable in breastfed babies. A dose of 400 IU of vitamin D per day is appropriate in most infants. Babies with vitamin D deficiency should be treated with vitamin D (ergo- or cholecalciferol) in a dose of 2000 IU for 6 months or 5000 IU for 2 months.

Vitamin D-dependent rickets (VDDR)

VDDR type I is due to defective renal hydroxylation of vitamin D,[165] whereas in VDDR type II there is cellular resistance to hormone action which is usually due to mutations in the steroid-binding domain or the DNA-binding domain of the vitamin D receptor.[141] Levels of 1,25-dihydroxyvitamin D are reduced in type I VDDR but elevated in type II. These rare conditions can present with rickets in infancy.

Pseudohypoparathyroidism

The term pseudohypoparathyroidism is used to describe several related disorders characterised by peripheral unresponsiveness to the action of PTH as a result of a receptor or postreceptor defect. This is an uncommon cause of hypocalcaemia in infancy which can, for similar reasons, result in TSH resistance and neonatal hyperthyrotropinaemia (see above). The characteristic biochemical findings are hypocalcaemia with hyperphosphataemia, raised levels of PTH and an absent or impaired response to exogenous PTH. These conditions are usually inherited as an AD trait with variable penetrance. Treatment of hypocalcaemia in this disorder requires calcium supplements and a vitamin D analogue.

Miscellaneous causes of neonatal hypocalcaemia

Hypocalcaemia may occur in alkalosis, with citrate administration in blood transfusion, and in hypoalbuminaemic states. It may also arise in infants with renal failure who have hyperphosphataemia.

Hypercalcaemia[278]

Hypercalcaemia is an uncommon problem in infancy and can be defined as a serum calcium above 2.75 mmol/l. The causes of hypercalcaemia are shown in Table 35.12 and are described in more detail below, but conceptually can be thought of as reflecting vitamin D or calcium excess, disease associated with reduced bone formation (hypophosphatasia) or increased bone resorption (e.g. some tumours). Occasionally a raised serum calcium can reflect an abnormality of the calcium-sensing receptor (hypocalciuric hypercalcaemia) with an associated altered 'set-point' and it may also be a manifestation of Williams syndrome. Primary hyperparathyroidism (as opposed to neonatal severe hyperparathyroidism resulting from a calcium-sensing receptor defect) probably does not occur in infancy. Clinical manifestations of hypercalcaemia include hypotonia, weakness and irritability, poor feeding, weight loss, constipation, vomiting, polydipsia and polyuria. Hypercalciuria can give rise to nephrocalcinosis.

Treatment

The primary cause must be corrected if possible but the key component of short-term treatment in many neonates with hypercalcaemia is a reduction in dietary calcium intake using low-calcium feed. Generous hydration and furosemide (frusemide) diuresis promote urinary calcium loss if a more acute reduction is needed. Glucocorticoids (e.g. hydrocortisone 1 mg/kg 6-hourly) reduce intestinal calcium absorption but the effect is slow and they should not be used if neoplasia is suspected. Calcitonin (10 U/kg i.v.) may be useful and has its maximum effect in 1 hour; infusions may be repeated 4-hourly. The hormone is antigenic and so the synthetic derivative salcatonin should be used in the longer term. Experience with the bisphosphonates is increasing and palmidronate in a dose of 0.5–1.0 mg/kg as an i.v. infusion is a useful medication. Long-term safety data following administration in infancy are not yet available.

Causes of hypercalcaemia (Table 35.12)

Hypercalcaemia in association with excess vitamin D

Infantile hypercalcaemia was common in the UK for some years when there was liberal vitamin D supplementation of foods. It generally presented with symptoms of hypercalcaemia in the early months of life, but was mild and self-limiting (Lightwood syndrome). The incidence fell when the use of vitamin D supplements was reduced, and it is thought to have affected infants with unusual sensitivity to vitamin D, when the cumulative daily dose could reach 2000–4000 IU or more. Hypercalcaemia due to excessive vitamin D intake has been reported in association with prolonged administration of preterm formula.[223]

Idiopathic infantile hypercalcaemia[177]

Idiopathic infantile hypercalcaemia remains a poorly defined entity seen by many as a diagnosis that is made only by the exclusion of other causes. Infants can present with the symptoms and signs of hypercalcaemia, including polyuria and polydipsia, and some have features in common with Williams syndrome such as facial dysmorphism and cardiac defects.[195] There is evidence to suggest that the hypercalcaemia is linked to abnormal vitamin D metabolism as well as abnormal PTHrP production. The hypercalcaemia can be more difficult to treat than in Williams syndrome and tends to persist for longer.

Williams syndrome (pp. 788, 798, 799)

This rare but serious condition is characterised by intermittent hypercalcaemia, a characteristic 'elfin' or 'pekinese' facial appearance, moderate mental retardation and vascular stenoses, most commonly supravalvular aortic stenosis. There is early failure to thrive, with severe anorexia, vomiting and constipation, hypotonia, polyuria and polydipsia. The hypercalcaemia and consequent symptoms tend to resolve spontaneously, but the other features persist. Radiologically there is sclerosis of the skull base, spine and long bones, and there may be metastatic calcification. Most children with Williams syndrome, and particularly those in whom there are cardiovascular manifestations, have deletions of the elastin gene on chromosome 7.[230] The condition is usually sporadic, although familial AD inheritance has also been observed.[217] In the hypercalcaemic phase, treatment is with a low-calcium milk/diet, with a cautious reintroduction of calcium once the biochemistry has been normalised. Controlling serum calcium does not affect the progression of the other features of the disease.

Hypercalcaemia due to phosphate depletion

Severe hypercalcaemia may occur in LBW preterm infants with hypophosphataemia due to a low phosphate intake from breast milk or parenteral feeding (pp. 284, 303, 328–9). The hypercalcaemia responds to phosphate repletion.[190,209]

Benign familial hypocalciuric hypercalcaemia and neonatal severe hyperparathyroidism[248]

These conditions are associated with mutations in the extracellular calcium ion-sensing receptor which lead to loss of function. The 'set-point' at which PTH is released is therefore altered. Benign familial hypercalcaemia is inherited as an AD trait (one abnormal allele), whereas the severe neonatal form is associated with both heterozygous and homozyous mutations of the calcium-sensing receptor gene.[263] Factors influencing the phenotype in this disorder include the number of mutant genes as well as the extent to which the calcium receptor is compromised.[130,264] The phenotype may also be influenced by the pattern of inheritance: if the infant inherits the mutant allele

Table 35.12 Causes of hypercalcaemia

Excess vitamin D
Idiopathic infantile hypercalcaemia
Williams' syndrome
Phosphate depletion in low-birthweight infants
Calcium-sensing receptor defects (inactivating)
  Benign familial hypercalcaemia with hypocalciuria
  Neonatal severe hyperparathyroidism
Maternal hypoparathyroidism
Subcutaneous fat necrosis
Hypophosphatasia
Malignancy
Vitamin A intoxication
Activating PTH receptor mutations (Jensen syndrome)

from the father, then PTH production will be more pronounced, because of the discrepancy between the maternal and fetal calcium-sensing receptor 'set-point' in utero. The neonatal form can lead to hypotonia, respiratory distress and failure to thrive, in association with hypercalcaemia and elevated PTH levels. There is skeletal undermineralisation, with rib fractures and subperiosteal erosions. The treatment of severe cases, usually homozygous for receptor mutations, may entail urgent parathyroidectomy, but some neonatal cases appear to run a milder, self-limiting course.[361] Some of these cases will be heterozygote infants with the abnormal allele inherited from the father. Earlier reports of primary hyperparathyroidism in neonatal life probably included children with calcium receptor abnormalities.

Hyperparathyroidism secondary to maternal hypoparathyroidism[187]

Secondary hyperparathyroidism may be due to untreated maternal hypoparathyroidism, which causes fetal hypocalcaemia and parathyroid hyperplasia; this condition is self-limiting but the hypercalcaemia may need treatment with hydration and calcitonin.

Subcutaneous fat necrosis

Hypercalcaemia may occur in association with extensive neonatal subcutaneous fat necrosis (p. 825), which is seen especially after traumatic delivery of large infants. This may be due to unregulated production of 1,25-dihydroxyvitamin D by the affected adipose tissue.[175]

Hypophosphatasia[359]

Hypophophatasia is an AR disorder that is due to defects in the gene for tissue non-specific (bone/liver/kidney) alkaline phosphatase. Hypophosphatasia is divided into perinatal, infantile, childhood and adult forms depending on the age at which skeletal lesions are discovered. The perinatal form is characterised by extreme skeletal hypomineralisation and babies die in utero or in early postnatal life. The infantile form is defined by a presentation before the age of 6 months. Clinical features include poor feeding, hypotonia, craniotabes, blue sclerae and a richetic deformity of the limbs. Hypercalcaemia and hypercalciuria reflect poor skeletal growth and mineralisation. Treatment options are limited[77] and the infantile form of the disease is fatal in approximately 50% of patients. There is a relationship between biochemistry and phenotype and so the severe perinatal and infantile forms are associated with lower alkaline phosphatase levels than are the milder childhood and adult forms.

Miscellaneous causes of hypercalcaemia

Vitamin A excess, adrenal failure, drugs such as thiazide diuretics, muscle disease with associated inactivity, and malignancy are rare causes of hypercalcaemia in early life. Constitutively activating PTH receptor mutations result in Jansen syndrome and a phenotype that includes hypercalcaemia and short-limbed dwarfism.[297]

Adrenal

Normal development and function

The adrenal gland has two embryologically and functionally distinct components. The medulla is formed from neural crest cells which enter the gland at about the seventh week of gestation and secrete catecholamines. Clinically significant abnormalities of function are not recognised in the newborn, although dysplasia and hypofunction is seen in patients with congenital adrenal hyperplasia.[202] The cortex is derived from mesodermal cells near the cephalic part of the mesonephros. It shares common primordial cells with the gonads, which also secrete steroids and may express similar enzyme deficiencies. The fetal adrenal is 20–30 times larger than the adult gland relative to body weight (twice as large in absolute terms) which reflects their contribution to oestrogen production in utero. At birth both glands together weigh 7–9 g. They are largely composed of the histologically distinct fetal cortex, which comprises 80% of the gland at birth and which then involutes rapidly, reducing to half its size by 2 weeks and disappearing by 6 months.

The enzyme activities of the fetal adrenal and the placenta are complementary; thus the placenta lacks the enzymatic activity necessary to generate adrenal androgens from the precursors, pregnenolone and progesterone (17α-hydroxylase and 17,20-desmolase; Fig. 35.12), whereas the fetal adrenal lacks the enzymatic activity to produce oestrogen from androgens, until the later stages of gestation. The adrenal androgens (primarily dehydroepiandrosterone and its sulphate) are therefore converted to oestrogen by the placenta, which expresses the necessary sulphatase and aromatase enzyme activity. Hence the fetal adrenal provides the precursors necessary for placental oestrogen production, and steroid production by the fetoplacental unit promotes maturation of organs such as the lungs. A deficiency of placental aromatase leads to virilisation of the mother and female infants during pregnancy.[304]

The adrenal cortex secretes three major groups of steroid hormones: glucocorticoids, mineralocorticoids and androgens. The gland has three histologically distinct zones. The outer zone, the zona glomerulosa, contains the enzymes for aldosterone biosynthesis but little 17α-hydroxylase, so it produces little cortisol or androgen. Aldosterone release is primarily controlled by the renin–angiotensin system and by the plasma concentrations of sodium and potassium, with ACTH playing a minor role. The two inner zones, fasciculata and reticularis, secrete cortisol and androgens, respectively, but no aldosterone. ACTH is the primary regulator of cortisol synthesis and also has a role in the regulation of androgen production.

Whilst umbilical cord cortisol concentrations are positively related to gestation,[157] cortisol concentrations subsequently fall with increasing postnatal and postconceptional age.[131,207,300] Cortisol levels reach a nadir in the first weeks of life in well term and preterm infants although the pattern will be influenced by general wellbeing.[300] Cortisol levels tend to be lower in the very sick, preterm infant[143] although the more mature preterm infant (greater than 30 weeks' gestation) may be able to mount a more appropriate stress response.[329] Hence, the postnatal trend in

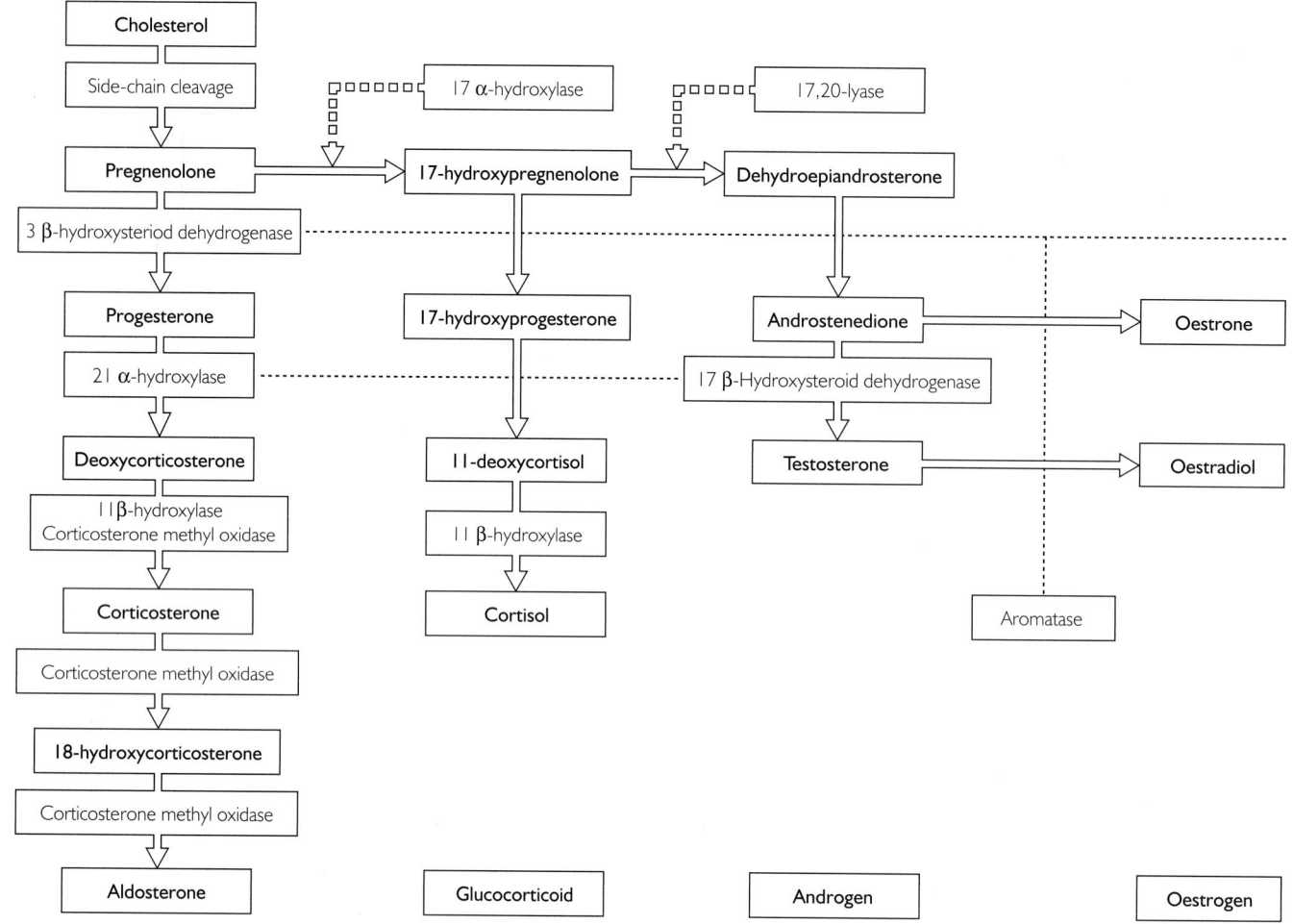

Fig. 35.12 Adrenal steroid biosynthesis. Steroids and steroid precursors are in bold.

cortisol concentrations pattern is linked to gestational age, post-natal age as well as other factors such as intrauterine growth and the presence of intercurrent illness.[300] The apparent inability of the more preterm infant to mount an appropriate stress response may be linked to enzymatic immaturity of the adrenal gland, with an associated inability to manufacture cortisol directly from cholesterol.[136,204,349] The ability of the adrenal gland to respond more appropriately to stress-related ACTH production has developed by 2 weeks of age.[227] The normal circadian pattern of cortisol release is usually established by 3 months of age, but has been identified as early as 2 weeks post delivery.[294]

Inherited disorders of steroidogenesis – the congenital adrenal hyperplasias (CAH)[210,311]

CAH is a generic term used to describe a series of AR disorders that prevent normal adrenal steroidogenesis. The phenotype of an affected infant is the result of steroid hormone deficiency coupled with the effects of excess steroidogenic precursors. CAH is the principle cause of ambiguous genitalia, and more than 95% of cases are due to 21α-hydroxylase deficiency. Some of the steroidogenic steps are common to the adrenal gland and gonad

and so impaired glucocorticoid and mineralocorticoid production can be associated with reduced gonadal sex steroid production.

Pathogenesis

A simplified schematic representation of adrenal steroid biosynthesis is shown in Fig. 35.12, and with this background, some of the consequences of a given enzyme defect can be determined. These are summarised in Table 35.13.

21α-hydroxylase deficiency

This condition classically presents as 'salt-losing', 'simple virilising' or 'late-onset' forms. There is a close link between residual enzyme activity and phenotype: the more severe gene defects result in the salt-losing form, whilst patients with significant residual enzyme activity will have the milder, late-onset form. Boys are under-represented in most series and some have presumably succumbed to adrenal insufficiency before the diagnosis was made. The prevalence in the UK and Europe is approximately 1 in 10 000[315] and worldwide approximately 1 in 14 000.[242] Population screening in an Italian region revealed a frequency of 1 in 8600.[54] The majority of affected individuals presenting in

Table 35.13 Major clinical and biochemical features of enzymatic blocks in adrenocortical steroid biosynthesis

Enzyme defect	Clinical features		
	Male	Female	Salt status
21α-Hydroxylase			
Simple virilising	N	Virilised	N
Salt-losing	N	Virilised	Loss
11β-Hydroxylase	N	Virilised	Retention (salt loss may occur in early life)
3β-Hydroxysteroid	Undervirilisation	N or mild virilisation	N or loss
17α-Hydroxylase	Female or inadequate virilisation	N	Retention with hypertension
Lipoid CAH (StAR and side-chain cleavage defects)	Female	N	Severe loss

N, normal.

early life have salt loss, but some produce enough mineralocorticoid to maintain sodium homeostasis; these children generate sufficient aldosterone while on appropriate glucocorticoid replacement, despite impaired enzyme activity. The genetics of 21α-hydroxylase deficiency have been extensively studied. There are two 21α-hydroxylase genes, one of which is inactive (*CYP21A*) and one active (*CYP21B*). They are both located on chromosome 6, interspersed between the genes encoding the C4 component of complement and in close proximity to the HLA complex (Fig. 35.13). Most affected individuals will be compound heterozygotes for a relatively small number of gene defects; the *CYP21B* locus (normally the active gene sequence) is affected by a gene conversion whereby part or all of this gene is converted to the inactive gene sequence of *CYP21A*. Alternatively, there may be a gene deletion extending from a point within the *CYP21A* gene to a corresponding part of the *CYP21B* gene. Most patients with salt loss have gene deletions or conversions that severely impair enzyme activity, whereas the 'late-onset' form is an allelic variant with higher enzyme levels that are sufficient to maintain health and a normal phenotype in the newborn period.

Clinical presentation

The clinical features reflect the combination of impaired cortisol/aldosterone production and androgen excess. Reduced cortisol generation leads to enhanced ACTH production with hyperplasia of the adrenal cortex and excess androgen release as the gland attempts to overcome the steroidogenic block. In the simple virilising form the steroidogenic defect is not as profound as in the salt-wasting form and residual enzyme activity can generate sufficient cortisol and aldosterone to survive but not enough to prevent excess androgen release. In male babies there may be some increase in pigmentation, especially of the scrotum, but there is no anatomical abnormality. If the infant with simple virilising CAH is not treated, then continued postnatal overproduction of androgen causes virilisation and rapid growth, although this does not usually become obvious until the second year of life and beyond.

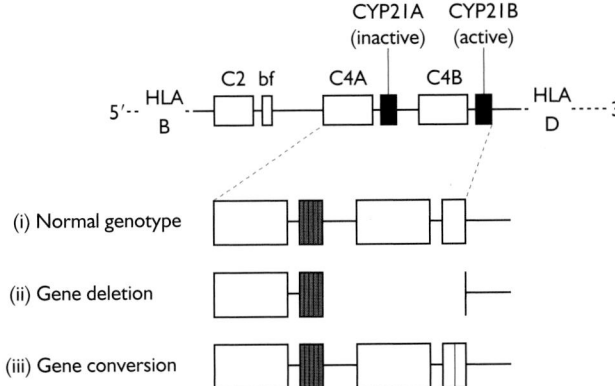

Fig. 35.13 Schematic diagram illustrating the proximity of the inactive (21A) and active (21B) 21α-hydroxylase genes to the HLA loci on chromosome 6. (i) The vertical lines in the 21A gene represent some of the mutations that lead to gene inactivity and that may be incorporated into the normally active 21B locus. (ii) The genotype of an affected infant will usually include 21B gene deletions and/or (iii) gene conversions, leading to impaired 21α-hydroxylase activity. C2, C4A, C4B – genes coding for complement components. HLA B, HLA D – genes for HLA antigens.

In females the prenatal androgen overproduction will virilise the external genitalia. In the least affected infants there may be only slight clitoral enlargement, whilst in the more severely virilised cases there is fusion of the labioscrotal folds and the clitoris becomes almost as large as a normal neonatal penis. These female babies can resemble a cryptorchid male and may be misdiagnosed as such (p. 786). A moderately severely virilised female with CAH is shown in Fig. 35.14 and the spectrum through from normal female to an apparently normal male is shown in Fig. 35.15.

In salt-losing CAH, inadequate production of aldosterone leads to renal salt loss. Affected neonates can become seriously unwell because of sodium depletion, with a median age at presentation of around 12 days.[90] The early signs are vomiting, anorexia and, sometimes, diarrhoea, which, if untreated, may develop into full Addisonian crisis (pp. 891–2). Further investigations reveal hyponatraemia, hyperkalaemia and acidosis and this picture should raise the possibility of CAH if it has not been suspected previously. Conditions that may be confused with salt-wasting CAH include renal tract malformations, urinary tract infection and pyloric stenosis. The cortisol deficiency can cause hypoglycaemia, but this occurs relatively infrequently, probably because the enzymatic block is often incomplete.

Diagnosis

A child presenting with a biochemical picture suggestive of a salt-wasting crisis requires resuscitation and an urgent renal and pelvic ultrasound. This can help to exclude renal malformations, and the identification of enlarged echogenic adrenals is a helpful pointer towards CAH at a time when 17-hydroxyprogesterone (17-OHP) levels are usually unavailable.[10] When the genitalia are ambiguous, establishing the genetic sex of the infant by examination of the karyotype is a priority. In 21α-hydroxylase deficiency, there is gross elevation of the plasma 17-OHP concentration. Levels are relatively high in healthy infants in the first hours of life and seriously ill preterm infants may also show moderate elevation of plasma 17-OHP in the absence of adrenal hyperplasia.[220] By 24 hours of age, the test is usually diagnostic of CAH. The plasma ACTH level is raised in all states of cortisol deficiency, so this is a non-specific test and it is also a less widely available assay. 11β-hydroxylase deficiency can be misdiagnosed as simple virilising 21α-hydroxylase deficiency and so it is wise to collect a sample of urine at presentation for urinary steroid profile analysis by gas chromatography. If this is collected before or in the very early stages of treatment, then the precise enzyme defect can usually be established for certain. It is possible to measure plasma 11-deoxycortisol (raised in 11β-hydroxylase deficiency) as well as 17-OHP, but poor assay specificity can lead to confusion. A case has been made for confirming the diagnosis of 21α-hydroxylase deficiency at the molecular level, partly because it can help to define the severity of 21α-hydroxylase deficiency.[233]

Prenatal diagnosis and treatment[153]

The prenatal administration of glucocorticoids to the mother of a female fetus with 21α-hydroxlase deficiency can reduce the degree of fetal virilisation and hence the need for postnatal surgery.[226] There are also behavioural implications of androgen exposure which may be influenced by glucocorticoid administration in utero.[232]

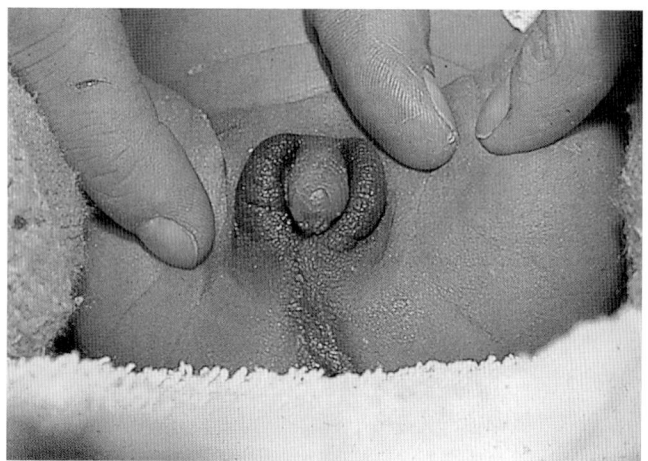

Fig. 35.14 Genitalia of a female infant with 21α-hydroxylase deficiency.

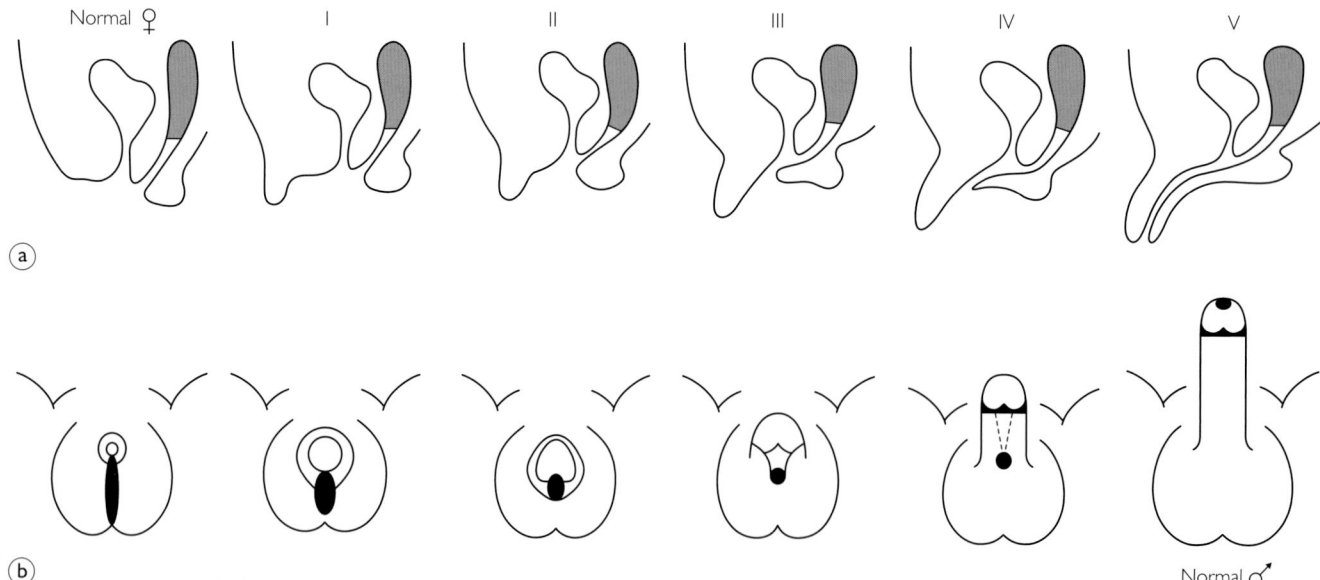

Fig. 35.15 Virilisation of the external genitalia based on the staging system of Prader and adapted from Miller.[210] A spectrum from normal female through to normal male is shown. Virilisation of a normal female (as in congenital adrenal hyperplasia) will result in any stage from I to V, and undervirilisation of a male (XY karyotype) will result in any appearance from IV through to normal female (as in partial or complete androgen insensitivity syndrome).

Before the pregnancy, the potential benefits and risks of prenatal treatment must be explained to the parents. Some will decline treatment, especially if a previous affected child was only mildly virilised. In some families the phenotype may vary, so it is not possible to state that subsequent children will not be more severely affected.[365]

In a pregnancy at risk, the mother can be given dexamethasone in a dose of 20 micrograms/kg/day in two or three divided doses as soon as the pregnancy is confirmed. Dexamethasone crosses the placenta and suppresses fetal ACTH secretion, and so the excess androgen production is curtailed. The treatment needs to be started as early as possible, and certainly before 8 weeks' gestation. It is then necessary to establish the sex of the fetus and whether or not it is affected. As the treatment is needed only for female fetuses with homozygous or compound heterozygous 21α-hydroxylase deficiency, glucocorticoid can be stopped in the seven out of eight pregnancies where the fetus is either male or an unaffected female.

The prenatal diagnosis of 21α-hydroxylase deficiency was originally made by finding raised 17-OHP levels in amniotic fluid. More recently, the likelihood of a pregnancy being affected has been established by HLA typing of the parents, index case and fetus, or by linkage analysis using markers in the region of the 21α-hydroxylase gene.[176] These techniques depend on the proximity of the locus for the 21α-hydroxylase gene to the HLA antigens on chromosome 6 or other 'adjacent' genes. It has also become possible to use specific DNA probes or allele-specific polymerase chain reaction (PCR) to screen for one of the relatively few number of mutations in family members, and then in the fetus, using tissue obtained by chorionic villus sampling at 10–12 weeks.[210]

Treatment of the mother with a potent steroid throughout pregnancy clearly carries some risk, and excessive weight gain, glucose intolerance, a rise in blood pressure, gastrointestinal upset and Cushingoid features have been recorded. No clear adverse effects on the fetus have been observed to date[226] although there are theoretical risks and careful follow-up studies are required.[49]

Population screening[138,326]

Measurement of 17-OHP in dried capillary blood samples (like those collected for screening for phenylketonuria and hypothyroidism) (p. 377) is possible and screening has been implemented in some parts of the world, including some states in North America. Screening programmes can operate effectively despite the need for a rapid turnaround[315] but there are currently no plans to include CAH in the UK national neonatal screening programme.

Treatment[153]

This entails replacing glucocorticoid and, if necessary, mineralocorticoid as well. The majority of affected girls will also require surgical correction of the virilisation.

A baby presenting in Addisonian crisis should be treated as detailed below. Thereafter the need to suppress ACTH, and hence androgen levels, means that a dose of hydrocortisone of 10–15 mg/m²/24 h administered as a thrice-daily (t.d.s.) regimen is appropriate in most infants. This should be trebled to cover significant acute illness and *must* be given parenterally if oral therapy cannot be tolerated. Liquid preparations can be unpredictable[201] but 2.5-mg tablets are available and an average dose for a full-term newborn infant, surface area 0.2 m², will therefore be around 1.25 mg t.d.s. Fludrocortisone can be given in an initial dose of 50–200 micrograms twice daily and then adjusted according to sodium levels, blood pressure and renin levels; divisible 100-microgram tablets are available. Salt supplements should also be provided to the salt-wasting infant and can be added to the milk: 2–8 mmol/kg/day of additional sodium chloride daily will ensure adequate intake until the diet contains more salt and until the infant's renal function becomes more refined (Fig. 35.16).

The long-term management consists of giving, first, enough glucocorticoid to maintain suppression of the excess androgen production but not enough to cause iatrogenic Cushing syndrome and growth retardation, and secondly, enough mineralocorticoid to ensure normal salt balance without excessive salt retention and hypertension. Although treatment in infancy requires close observation with careful measurement of growth, blood pressure, electrolytes, renin activity and plasma steroid measurement,[38] the skeleton is relatively resistant to the growth-promoting effects of sex steroids at this stage of life. The glucocorticoid dose will rise in infancy as the child grows, but the fludrocortisone dose will fall as the infant kidney becomes more sensitive to mineralocorticoid.[210] A profile of plasma 17-OHP (which can be estimated on fingerprick samples) probably gives the best simple estimate of biochemical control. Levels should be relatively low but not suppressed and later in infancy there should be evidence of diurnal variation.[259] The sodium dose can usually remain unchanged

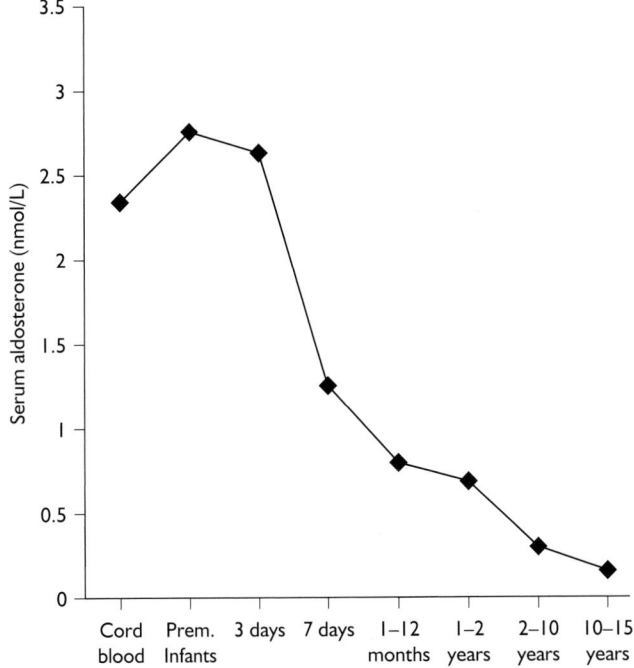

Fig. 35.16 Aldosterone levels as a function of age. This helps to explain why the neonate is more susceptible to salt wasting than are older children and why such a relatively large dose of aldosterone is required. (Adapted from Miller.[210])

beyond the neonatal period and the supplements stopped before the child's first birthday.

The management of 21α-hydroxylase deficiency in childhood and adolescence is not straightforward because of frequent difficulties achieving a balance between the need to suppress androgens on the one hand and yet avoid glucocorticoid toxicity on the other. Medical treatment with additional agents that block sex steroid effects may enable a more physiological replacement dose of glucocorticoid to be used.[203] The nature and timing of surgery in virilised girls remains a controversial issue and early assessment by a multidisciplinary team that includes an experienced paediatric urologist is important.[69] One possible approach to the surgical management of the virilised girl with CAH is to perform a clitoral reduction in early life, with reassessment and possible vaginoplasty in the teenage years, when tissues have grown and matured. The family and health professionals may also feel that it is appropriate to defer any decision regarding surgical management until a later date. A single-stage procedure in early life which involves both clitoral reduction and vaginoplasty has seemed an attractive option in the past but there are concerns about long-term outcome, including susceptibility to scarring and vaginal stenosis. Increased steroid cover is, of course, needed for surgery.

11β-hydroxylase deficiency[210,358]

This is the second most common cause of CAH, but accounts for less than 5% of cases in the UK. There is a relatively high incidence in the Middle East. Affected females are virilised but males have a normal phenotype at birth. Plasma 11-deoxycortisol, deoxycorticosterone (DOC) and their metabolites are increased and there is also an increase in 17-OHP. The increased intermediate compounds in the aldosterone pathway (notably DOC) can cause hypertension in later life but there may be salt-wasting in infancy because of a relative mineralocorticoid resistance at this stage.[210] It is important to be aware of the potential for confusing 11β-hydroxylase deficiency with 21α-hydroxylase deficiency because some assays for 11-deoxycortisol have had a suboptimal specificity and have been detecting 17-OHP. The antenatal treatment of affected pregnancies with dexamethasone in an attempt to reduce virilisation has been successful in some cases.[57]

Corticosterone methyloxidase (CMO) deficiency

This enzyme is responsible for the distal steps in aldosterone synthesis in the zona glomerulosa. It is very similar in sequence and structure to 11β-hydroxylase and is able to convert DOC to corticosterone in the zona glomerulosa (like 11β-hydroxylase), as well as corticosterone to aldosterone via 18-hydroxycorticosterone (see Fig. 35.12). Enzyme defects lead to salt wasting in early life and investigation demonstrates high plasma renin activity with low aldosterone levels. These patients will respond to treatment with fludrocortisone, although ongoing production of DOC by 11β-hydroxylase helps to explain why these patients may be able to manage off therapy in later life when the kidney becomes more sensitive to mineralocorticoid. CMO deficiency can be divided into CMOI and CMOII, depending upon the impact of mutations on enzyme function. CMOI deficiency

results from a loss of 18-hydroxylase and methyloxidase activity,[254] whilst CMOII deficiency is the consequence of a selective deficiency in the ability of the enzyme to convert 18-hydroxycorticosterone to aldosterone (18-methyloxidase activity).[245]

3β-Hydroxysteroid dehydrogenase deficiency

See p. 897

Congenital lipoid adrenal hyperplasia

See pp. 896–7

17α-Hydroxylase deficiency and 17,20-desmolase deficiency (see p. 897)

A single protein is responsible for these two separate enzyme activities. When this is deficient, there are varying degrees of cortisol deficiency with excessive mineralocorticoid production, driven primarily by ACTH feedback, sometimes causing hypertension and hypokalaemic alkalosis in infancy. The glucocorticoid activity of the excess mineralocorticoid may in part compensate for a lack of cortisol. In later life, affected females develop minimal secondary sexual characteristics and are amenorrhoeic, and males show absent or inadequate virilisation. This defect should be considered in the differential diagnosis of suspected androgen insensitivity in genetic males and primary hypogonadism in females.

Adrenocortical insufficiency[210]

There are a number of other disorders that can result in adrenal insufficiency in the newborn in addition to the congenital adrenal hyperplasias. A classification of the causes of adrenocortical insufficiency is shown in Table 35.14.

Smith–Lemli–Opitz syndrome

Although not stricly one of the adrenal hyperplasias, there are similarities between Smith–Lemli–Opitz syndrome (SLO) and other early abnormalities of steroidogenesis. The reduction in 7-dehydrocholesterol reductase activity with reduced generation of cholesterol from 7-dehydrocholesterol impairs steroidogenesis and can lead to adrenal insufficiency[16] as well as undervirilisation in genetic males (see below).

Wolman disease

In this disorder there is a failure to mobilise cholesterol from lipid droplets because of an abnormality of lysosomal acid lipase. Adrenal insufficiency is a consequence of the inadequate supply of cholesterol to facilitate normal steroidogenesis. The severe infantile-onset Wolman disease and the milder late-onset cholesteryl ester storage disease are caused by mutations in different parts of the lysosomal acid lipase gene.[15]

Congenital adrenal hypoplasia

Primary adrenocortical insufficiency due to congenital hypoplasia or atrophy of the glands has been estimated to have a frequency of 1 in 12 500 births. The X-linked recessive form is due to

Table 35.14 Causes of adrenocortical insufficiency

Primary
Congenital adrenal hyperplasia
    Deficiency of glucocorticoid and mineralocorticoid
        ■ 21α-hydroxylase deficiency, salt-losing
        ■ 11β-hydroxylase deficiency (in early life)
        ■ 3β-hydroxysteroid dehydrogenase deficiency
        ■ Lipoid CAH (steroidogenic acute regulatory
          protein and side-chain cleavage defects)
    Deficiency of glucocorticoid
        ■ 21α-hydroxylase deficiency, non-salt-losing
        ■ 11β-hydroxylase deficiency
        ■ 17α-hydroxylase deficiency
    Deficiency of mineralocorticoid
        ■ corticosterone methyl oxidase deficiency I
        ■ corticosterone methyl oxidase deficiency II

Early abnormalities of steroidogenesis
    Smith–Lemli–Opitz (7-dehydrocholesterol reductase
    deficiency)
    Lysosomal acid lipase deficiency (Wolman's syndrome)

Congenital adrenal hypoplasia
    X-linked (abnormalities of DAX-I/NROBI)
    Autosomal recessive
    IMAGE association

Adrenal hypoplasia in association with SF-1 mutations

Adrenoleukodystrophy

Adrenal necrosis or haemorrhage

Acute infection (Waterhouse–Friderichsen syndrome)

Isolated glucocorticoid deficiency
    Familial glucocorticoid deficiency
    Triple-A syndrome

Iatrogenic, post glucocorticoid therapy

Secondary
Hypopituitarism
Withdrawal from glucocorticoid therapy
Maternal Cushing's

---

mutations of the gene encoding a nuclear hormone receptor, *DAX-1*,[4,221] which resides in the region Xp21. The *DAX-1* gene product is expressed in the adrenal and testis, and also has a role in the normal production of gonadotrophins by the hypothalamopituitary axis. Hence, this form of adrenal hypoplasia is also associated with primary and secondary gonadal failure although gonadotrophin and gonadal function may appear normal in early life.

Congenital adrenal hypoplasia is a well-recognised cause of an adrenal 'Addisonian' crisis in the neonatal period and later childhood. Poor feeding, vomiting, poor weight gain and dehydration, apnoeas, fits and shock may all be manifestations of glucocorticoid and mineralocorticoid deficiency. The biochemical findings include hypoglycaemia, hyponatraemia, hyperkalaemia and a metabolic acidosis. Hyperpigmentation is rare until the third week of life, and cortisol deficiency may also present as prolonged jaundice.

Occasionally the picture has been confused with upper-intestinal obstruction, and renal tract malformations need to be excluded. The clinical and biochemical picture in the neonatal period is very similar to CAH but 17-OHP levels are not raised in congenital adrenal hypoplasia (see below). ACTH and renin levels are raised but cortisol and aldosterone reduced. Adrenal stimulation tests are not usually necessary but tetracosactrin stimulation shows an absent or greatly reduced cortisol response.

The diagnosis may be suspected antenatally if maternal oestriol values are very low, but adrenal hypoplasia cannot thus be differentiated from the more common – and also X-linked – placental sulphatase deficiency. It is important to remember that there is not always a close correlation between genotype and phenotype and so brothers with the same genetic defect can present at different ages.

Congenital adrenal hypoplasia has been described in association with IUGR, metaphyseal dysplasia and genital anomalies (IMAGe association). The three male children described had micropenis with cryptorchidism and developed adrenal insufficiency in the newborn period. All had a normal *DAX-1* coding sequence.[342]

Steroidogenic factor-1 (see below)

Steroidogenic factor-1 (SF-1) is a nuclear receptor which has a crucial role in the development of steroidogenic tissue. Defects of SF-1 can therefore lead to adrenal failure and abnormal gonadal development (see below).

Adrenal haemorrhage

The large hyperaemic fetal gland is vulnerable to vascular damage. Birth trauma presumably accounts for most adrenal haemorrhage seen at autopsy in the newborn although haemorrhage has also been detected antenatally. Bilateral haemorrhage has also been described in neonatal tuberculosis or syphilis. The incidence is increased in preterm infants and after prolonged or complicated labour. The bleeding may be sufficient to form a palpable mass, which may be mistaken for a tumour, especially if unilateral, or may rupture into the peritoneum and cause intestinal obstruction or a scrotal haematoma.[163,208] There may also be signs of acute blood loss or, at a later stage, anaemia and jaundice. If both glands are infarcted, the baby can present acutely with hypoglycaemia, shock and Addisonian features.

The diagnosis can be difficult to make unless there is scrotal/perineal bruising or a mass is palpable, but ultrasound is useful to confirm suspected haemorrhage. Adrenal calcification has been observed as early as the fifth day, but usually occurs much later. The presentation of adrenal insufficiency may be delayed but the regenerative capacity of the adrenal is great, and most adrenal haemorrhage is not associated with significantly impaired function.

Adrenal (Addisonian) crisis

Crisis may supervene in all forms of adrenal insufficiency pre- or post diagnosis. It may develop insidiously or be precipitated by acute illness or surgery. Hypoglycaemia can occur independently of salt and water loss. Features include poor feeding, poor weight gain and then vomiting, diarrhoea, vascular collapse, prostration and coma. Hypoglycaemia, hyponatraemia, hyperkalaemia and metabolic acidosis may all be present.

Treatment consists of i.v. fluid, glucose, and electrolyte replacement, steroid replacement, and treatment of any underlying disease. A bolus of i.v. glucose (0.5–1.0 g/kg over several minutes) and a rapid infusion of normal saline (20 ml/kg initially) may be needed. If the response is satisfactory, rehydration can be continued with i.v. normal saline and added glucose. Intravenous hydrocortisone 10 mg should be given *statim* in the neonate, then 100–200 mg/m^2/day as 4-hourly bolus therapy or, ideally, by continuous infusion.[60] When the baby's condition is stable, the dose can be reduced. Hydrocortisone may also be administered i.m. if venous access is difficult. The mineralocorticoid effect of hydrocortisone is adequate at these doses. (p. 1280).

Waterhouse–Friderichsen syndrome

Acute adrenal insufficiency from adrenal haemorrhage and infarction complicating septicaemic illness with disseminated intravascular coagulation is a rare event in the newborn, but can cause circulatory collapse and death.

Adrenoleukodystrophy

See pp. 1170–2

Isolated glucocorticoid deficiency

There are at least two AR causes of glucocorticoid deficiency characterised by high circulating ACTH levels: familial glucocorticoid deficiency and triple-A syndrome.[12,218] Familial glucocorticoid deficiency presents with signs of cortisol deficiency in infancy, or later in childhood, when hyperpigmentation may provide a diagnostic clue. Some, but not all, cases are due to abnormalities of the ACTH receptor.[292,353,354] The triple-A syndrome is the association of glucocorticoid deficiency with achalasia of the cardia and deficient tear production. It is caused by mutations of the *AAAS* gene on chromosome 12.[292,334]

Glucocorticoids and adrenal function in the neonate

There are a number of situations where the fetus or neonate may be exposed to or treated with exogenous glucocorticoid.

Maternal steroid administration, hyperadrenocorticism and fetal adrenal function

Short courses of dexamethasone or betamethasone are frequently given to mothers in preterm labour because of the beneficial impact on neonatal lung maturity, with an associated decreased incidence of hyaline membrane disease.[70] Transient biochemical changes in adrenal function have been identified in these infants.[24,91] The value of repeated courses of steroids, for example in infants with premature rupture of membranes, lacks a firm evidence-base but could have a detrimental effect on fetal and neonatal health. Adrenocortical insufficiency in the newborn may arise following maternal Cushing syndrome or the administration of large doses of steroid[45,171] and the potential for adrenal suppression must be considered in any infant exposed to exogenous glucocorticoid in pregnancy. Long-term dexamethasone administration during pregnancy to treat prenatally diagnosed fetal CAH usually leads to side effects in the mother, but has not been associated with overt abnormalities in the infant (see above).

Ventilator dependency and glucocorticoid administration

Oxygen- or ventilator-dependent neonates may be given an exogenous glucocorticoid such as dexamethasone to assist weaning, although concerns about safety have reduced this practice in the first weeks of postnatal life.[123] Glucocorticoid administration has numerous potential dose-related side effects such as hypertension, hyperglycaemia and glycosuria. Steroids also make the infant catabolic, impair growth and are associated with gastrointestinal perforation. However, it is the association with cerebral palsy and their detrimental effect on other aspects of long-term CNS function that are, perhaps, the major concern.[241,303,314]

Large doses of dexamethsone (500 micrograms/kg/day) have been shown to suppress the hypothalamo-pituitary-adrenal (HPA) axis,[157,229,363] but smaller doses, as well as inhaled steroids, can also influence HPA function. If an infant has received glucocorticoid for more than 1 week, it is wise to reduce the dose gradually and/or change to an alternate-day regimen prior to stopping treatment, bearing in mind that 50 micrograms of dexamethasone will probably suppress the adrenal gland completely.[135] It should also be remembered that an infant who has recently stopped glucocorticoid treatment may require steroid cover in association with subsequent illness or surgery.[229]

Hypotension, respiratory function and relative adrenal insufficiency

Sick preterm infants may have inappropriately low baseline and stimulated cortisol levels. This relative adrenal insufficiency may be linked to immaturity of the steroidogenic pathway[180] and has been associated with hypotension and the development of chronic lung disease.[143,351,352] There may be a role for a short course of hydrocortisone in the sick hypotensive infant (e.g. 0.25–2.5 mg/kg every 6 hours), although this is an area of neonatal practice that requires further study.[301,350]

Biochemical assessment of adrenal function in the neonate

The assessment of HPA integrity is not straightforward. The simple, non-invasive test of the HPA axis which can easily be interpreted with a reassuring test sensitivity and specificity remains an elusive goal. Differences in cortisol assay performance and the absence of appropriate reference data remain significant confounding factors when assessing adrenal function in babies (see below).

The cortisol response to i.v. synacthen administration is used by many units to assess the HPA axis. In some primary adrenal pathologies, cortisol production is compromised, and if secondary hypoadrenalism is suspected, the test is conducted on the basis that an understimulated adrenal will produce less cortisol than a normal, stimulated gland. Diagnosing secondary hypoadrenalism and avoiding 'false negative' tests is frequently a concern; this is reflected in the huge disparity in the synacthen doses used in babies, e.g. 0.1 micrograms/kg,[169] 0.5 micrograms,[143] 0.5 micrograms/1.73 m^2,[71] 1.0 microgram/1.73 m^2,[158] 15 micrograms/kg,[237] 36 micrograms/kg,[136] 62.5 micrograms,[125] and the various intervals between synacthen administration and cortisol sampling.[159] The higher synacthen doses represent a pharmacological rather than a physiological stimulus and it is well known that a normal response does not exclude a degree of adrenal suppression (suboptimal sensitivity).

As a general rule, a baseline or 20–30-minute post-synacthen cortisol response (any dose of synacthen) that is greater than 560 nmol/l makes adrenal insufficiency (primary or secondary) very unlikely. However, it needs to be recognised that some healthy infants will have a response that is below this threshold. Random plasma cortisol concentrations may be difficult to interpret, but adrenal suppression or insufficiency should be suspected if baseline cortisol values are below 140 nmol/l in stressed preterm infants[152] or when the response to synacthen stimulation is below 360 nmol/l in preterm infants.[363]

Data from children and adolescents that can be applied with caution to the infant population indicate that hypoadrenalism is also unlikely if the cortisol peak at 20 or 30 minutes is 500 nmol/l and/or the increment is >200 nmol/l following synacthen administration in a 'low' dose of 0.5 micrograms/1.73 m^2.[5]

Concern about the performance of the synacthen test has generated interest in other approaches to the assessment of HPA axis integrity. The ACTH response (typically measured at 20–30 minutes) and cortisol response (typically measured at 60 minutes) to CRH is a more logical approach to the assessment of the adrenal axis because it is examining pituitary function directly,[125,158,227,228,351] although there are still issues about the optimum CRH dose.[41] A cortisol response that is <360 nmol/l at 60 minutes post CRH administration (CRH 1.0 micrograms/kg) suggests adrenal insufficiency.

Adrenal hyperfunction

There are very few causes of adrenal hyperfunction in early life apart from CAH. Infants with adrenal hyperfunction usually have abnormal cell signalling (McCune–Albright syndrome) or an underlying neoplasia.

McCune–Albright syndrome is a well-recognised cause of endocrine gland hyperfunction in childhood. It results from activating mutations of the G protein component adjacent to the cell surface receptor. Hyperfunction of the gonadotrophin receptor/G protein complex explains the precocious puberty in this disorder (characterised by the triad of precocious puberty, café-au-lait lesions and polyostotic fibrous dysplasia), but activation of the ACTH receptor can also lead to glucocorticoid excess and Cushing's syndrome.[26,164]

Adrenal tumours have been reported in early life and when they occur the possiblity of an underlying tumor predisposition

syndrome such as Li-Fraumeni syndrome must be considered. The clinical picture will reflect the adrenal steroid produced in excess, with glucocorticoid leading to signs of Cushing's syndrome and androgens leading to signs of virilisation.[293]

Disorders of sexual development

Normal sexual differentiation

The physical basis of a person's sex reflects their genotype, gonads, the internal sexual organs, the external sexual organs and the development of secondary sexual characteristics at puberty. In the disorders of sexual development there is abnormal or discordant development of one or more of these factors.

The primary event in sexual determination is the fertilisation of an ovum by either an X- or a Y-bearing spermatozoon. Normally this initiates a cascade of events which culminates in female or male development. A 46,XX genotype results in the undifferentiated bipotential gonads developing into ovaries by the twelfth week of fetal life. Subsequent female development, as first shown in the classic studies of Jost,[155] proceeds normally in a castrated fetus irrespective of the genetic sex. There is persistence and development of the müllerian ducts, which form the fallopian tubes, uterus and upper vagina, and the external genitalia will take a female form. This is a rapidly expanding field and it is clear that a number of genes will contribute to the process of ovarian development (see below). In the individual with a normal 46,XY genotype, the sex-determining region of the Y chromosome (SRY) is the first of a series of genes that induce testicular differentiation.[167] SRY is a sequence of 14 kilobases adjacent to the pseudoautosomal region of the short arm of the Y chromosome that encodes for a DNA-binding regulatory protein. Other genes 'downstream' of this initial event are steadily being elucidated and include SOX9, abnormalities of which are associated with campomelic dysplasia with genital and gonadal malformations in XY individuals (see below). The presence of testicular tissue therefore indicates the presence of a Y chromosome except in rare instances such as XX males in whom SRY can usually be identified somewhere in the genome. In the presence of SRY the indifferent gonads transform into testes by the fifth to sixth week of intrauterine life and then play an active role in further development by secreting two hormones, testosterone and antimüllerian hormone (AMH).

Testosterone is secreted from the Leydig cells, initially under the stimulus of placental chorionic gonadotrophin, which is why gonadotrophin deficiency is associated with micropenis and/or cryptorchidism and not with ambiguous genitalia. It acts locally to stimulate development of the wolffian ducts into epididymis, vas deferens and seminal vesicles. It also reaches androgen-sensitive peripheral cells via the circulation, where it binds to the androgen receptor in the cell cytoplasm and nucleus. Testosterone is also converted to the potent androgen dihydrotestosterone (DHT) in peripheral tissues by the enzyme 5α-reductase. In the fetus, testosterone and DHT induce virilisation of the urogenital sinus and the external genitalia. This process is complete by 13 weeks of embryonic life. The

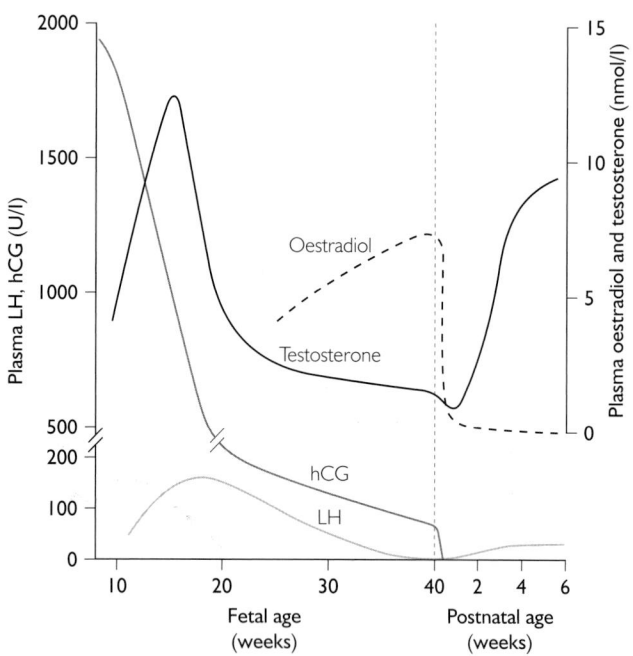

Fig. 35.17 The trend in fetal and neonatal plasma hCG, LH, testosterone and oestradiol concentrations in the male. (Adapted from Fisher.[100])

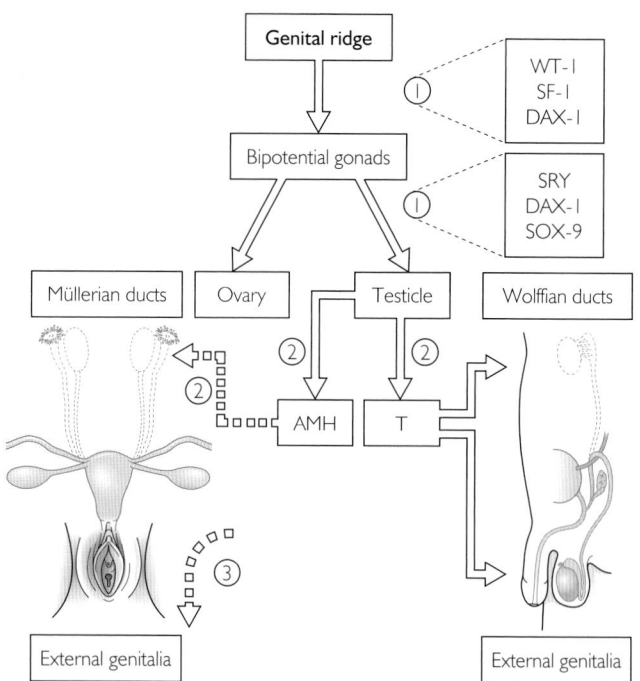

Fig. 35.18 Abnormal sexual development.
1. Disorders of urogenital and gonadal development.
2. Undervirilised males – XY individuals with abnormalities of steroidogenesis/AMH production or who are unable to respond to androgen or AMH in the normal way.
3. Virilised females – XX individuals exposed to excess androgen (see text for further details).

normal pattern of human chorionic gonadotrophin (hCG), gonadotrophin and androgen release in the male fetus is shown in Fig. 35.17.

The fetal testes also produce AMH, a high-molecular-weight glycoprotein secreted by the Sertoli cells, which causes regression of the müllerian ducts.

Abnormal sexual development

In the neonatal period the most common presentation of disorders of sexual development is with genital ambiguity. The abnormalities can vary from a minor degree of labial fusion in the female or hypospadias in the male to gross virilisation in a genetic female or what appear to be female external genitalia in a genetic male (see Fig. 35.15).

The major disorders of sexual development in this chapter will be classified into three major groups:

- Disorders of urogenital and gonadal development.
- Undervirilised males (male pseudohermaphroditism) – XY individuals with abnormalities of steroidogenesis/AMH production or who are unable to respond to androgen or AMH in the normal way.
- Virilised females (female pseudohermaphroditism) – XX individuals exposed to excess androgen.

The sexual organs may also be involved in a wide variety of dysmorphic syndromes which are not currently known to be related to specific disorders of sexual development but may sometimes closely mimic them.

Disorders of urogenital and gonadal development (Fig. 35.18 and Table 35.15)[8,295]

These disorders may be the consequence of a single gene defect affecting urogenital and/or gonadal development or may arise because of chromosomal mosaicism. There is the potential for both müllerian and wolffian duct development in one individual and variable potential for germ cell development and gonadal endocrine function as well as neoplasia. The renal tract may also be abnormal. Diagnosis in the newborn period usually depends on recognising an abnormality of the external genitalia, which is frequently present.

Genes involved in the formation of the bipotential gonad

A number of genes operating 'upstream' from *SRY* are important in the development of the bipotential gonad. These include *SF-1* and *WT-1*.

Steroidogenic factor-1

SF-1 is a nuclear receptor which has a crucial role in the development of steroidogenic tissue and so defects of *SF-1* can be associated with failure of adrenal and gonadal development.[3] Affected infants may present with adrenal failure, and XY

Table 35.15 Disorders of urogenital and gonadal development

Genes involved in development of the bipotential gonad
WT-1
SF-1

Genes involved in development of the testis
SRY
Sox-9

Genes involved in development of the ovary
DAX-1

Other causes of abnormal gonadal development
True hermaphroditism
XX males
Klinefelter
Mixed gonadal dysgenesis
Turner syndrome
Pure gonadal dysgenesis
Anorchia

individuals can have a female phenotype with persistent müllerian structures. The effects of SF-1 are complex and sensitive to a gene dosage effect as well as gene activity.

WT-1

The Denys–Drash syndrome and Frasier syndrome both result from abnormalities of the gene *WT-1* on chromosome 11. The nature of the underlying defect in the *WT-1* gene determines phenotype. The Denys–Drash syndrome is characterised by childhood renal cancer, glomerular nephropathy and abnormal gonadal and genital development. Gonadal abnomalities are also found in XX individuals.[186] The Frasier syndrome is a variant of Denys–Drash and is characterised by complete XY gonadal dysgenesis, nephropathy and increased susceptibility to gonadoblastomas.

Genes involved in normal testicular development

SRY and XY females

SRY encodes a protein that is highly conserved amongst mammalian species. SRY appears to bend DNA, thereby allowing other proteins access to genes along the DNA sequence. Defects in the *SRY* gene can be identified in some patients with XY sex reversal, streak gonads and müllerian structures.[129] However, most patients with this phenotype have a normal *SRY* gene, suggesting that many other genetic factors are involved in testicular development. This view has been reinforced by the recent report of an *SRY* gene mutation associated with XY sex reversal in one family member but not her father.[154]

SOX9

Heterozygous loss-of-function mutations of *SOX9* are associated with campomelic dysplasia, which is a skeletal abnormality associated with male-to-female sex reversal.[107,194,256] The skeletal features include micrognathia, cleft palate, eleven pairs of ribs, and bowing of the long bones, and most individuals die from respiratory failure in early life. The link between skeletal and

gonadal development is unclear but 75% of affected XY fetuses show female or ambiguous genitalia.

Factors involved in normal ovarian development

Duplication of the gene *DAX-1* is associated with male-to-female sex reversal,[25] which suggests that this gene may have an important role in normal ovarian development. However, isolated defects of *DAX-1* in XY individuals cause congenital adrenal hypoplasia with associated adrenal and testicular failure. *DAX-1* is expressed during ovarian development and the temporal effects of *DAX-1* and interactions with genes like *SF-1* may facilitate ovarian development in females whilst also contributing to normal testicular development and function in males following *SRY* expression.[198,319] Animal studies have shown that other genes (such as *Wnt-4*) may also be important in the process of ovarian development and increasingly this is viewed as an active rather than a passive process.

Other causes of abnormal gonadal development

True hermaphroditism

This diagnosis rests on the histological demonstration of ovarian and testicular tissue in a single individual, either in separate gonads or, more commonly, in ovotestes. There is nearly always some genital ambiguity and the internal sexual organs are variable. Most patients have an XX karyotype, although molecular analysis has identified Y sequences in some of these patients.[266] Pedigrees with XX true hermaphrodites and XX males have been described, which suggests varying penetrance of a mutated gene involved in sexual differentiation.[268] Many affected children have been raised as males in the past, but female gender assignment should be considered as there is good potential for sexual function and even fertility, and a high risk of tumour formation in dysgenetic testicular tissue.[122]

XX males

Individuals with this rare condition (1 in 20 000) have testes despite an XX karyotype. The genitalia are usually male, although there may be ambiguity, which can lead to presentation in infancy. Y-specific DNA sequences, sometimes including the *SRY* gene, can be identified in 80–90% of cases.[355]

Klinefelter syndrome

This relatively common condition (around 1–2 per 1000 live male births) is associated with a 47,XXY karyotype (p. 789). Many patients remain undiagnosed,[40] but when the diagnosis is made it is typically because the karyotype is checked antenatally or because of concerns about learning difficulties, a small phallus or small testes.[299] The diagnosis is sometimes made when a couple are investigated for infertility.

Mixed gonadal dysgenesis

Children with this condition have genetic mosaicism, including cell lines with and without Y-chromosome material. The phenotype is extremely varied, ranging from apparently normal male to apparently normal female, but is typified by a child with a testis and wolffian structures on one side of the body and a streak gonad with müllerian structures on the other. The karyotype in peripheral blood is usually 45,X/46,XY.[324] Stigmata of Turner syndrome are present in more than 50% of presenting children. There is a high risk of gonadoblastoma, which may even present in pre-puberty, and so most clinicians recommend laparoscopy with removal of dysgenetic gonads. Studies on prenatal diagnosis have shed new light on the condition, with 80% of 45,X/46,XY cases detected having an apparently male phenotype.[140]

Turner syndrome (p. 789)

A clinical diagnosis may be made in the newborn period because of the characteristic lymphoedema of the hands and feet, or suspected because of the presence of other associated abnormalities such as aortic coarctation (pp. 649–50). This permits early counselling and detection of problems such as growth failure and primary gonadal failure.

Pure gonadal dysgenesis

Affected infants are phenotypic females (usually with an XX karyotype, but they may also be XY) with normal external genitalia and bilateral streak gonads. This condition usually presents in adolescence with primary amenorrhoea, rather than in the neonatal period. It has now been shown that some XX individuals with hypergonadotrophic ovarian dysgenesis have abnormalities of the FSH receptor.[9]

Anorchia

The impact of anorchia on phenotype depends on the stage of development at which it occurs. Involution early in fetal life results in phenotypically normal or slightly virilised female genitalia with neither wolffian nor müllerian internal structures.[117] Later involution may cause the 'micropenis with rudimentary testes' syndrome[222] or absent testes in an otherwise normal male.[113] It has been suggested that testicular torsion in utero or in the perinatal period may be responsible for some cases[310] although familial cases suggests a genetic aetiology in some families.

Undervirilised male (male pseudohermaphroditism – incomplete virilisation in a genetic male) (see Fig. 35.18 and Table 35.16)[8]

This condition arises when a genetic male with well-differentiated testes fails to virilise normally because of an inability to manufacture androgen normally or a failure to respond to androgen appropriately. The phenotype can vary from that of a normal female through all degrees of ambiguity to normal male external genitalia.

Testosterone or dihydrotestosterone deficiency

The biosynthesis of testosterone can be affected at one of various stages, resulting in suboptimal testosterone production and fetal and usually postnatal undervirilisation. Steroid synthesis in the adrenal cortex as well as in the testis can be affected if the enzyme block occurs at a relatively early stage of steroidogenesis.

Table 35.16 Causes of male undervirilisation

Testosterone deficiency
Deficiency of
   7-dehydrocholesterol reductase
   (Smith–Lemli–Opitz syndrome)
   StAR or side-chain cleavage, causing lipoid CAH
   3β-hydroxysteroid dehydrogenase
   17α-hydroxylase/17,20-desmolase
   17β-hydroxysteroid dehydrogenase
   5α-reductase
Luteinising hormone receptor defects

Androgen insensitivity
Partial
Complete

AMH resistance and deficiency

Idiopathic
Including the association with IUGR and dysmorphic syndromes

These defects can produce severe undervirilisation, and associated cortisol/aldosterone deficiency can produce an adrenal crisis with hyponatraemia and hypoglycaemia.

Luteinising hormone receptor defects

Impaired androgen production by the testis may be due to end-organ insensitivity arising from molecular defects in the LH receptor.[172] The gonad is unable to respond normally to hCG in early pregnancy and then to LH in later gestation. Affected individuals may be described as having Leydig-cell hypoplasia because of the associated histological findings.

Smith–Lemli–Opitz syndrome

Patients with SLO are unable to manufacture cholesterol from dehydrocholesterol and so adrenal and gonadal steroidogenesis is compromised. The external genitalia in XY infants with SLO can vary from normal male to normal female depending on the extent to which testosterone synthesis is affected.[162]

Congenital lipoid adrenal hyperplasia

Congenital lipoid adrenal hyperplasia (lipoid CAH) is usually due to mutations in the steroidogenic regulatory protein (StAR) which promotes cholesterol transport into the mitochondria.[43] Impaired StAR activity leads to deficient synthesis of all steroid products, including aldosterone, cortisol and androgen. The synthesis of adrenal and gonadal steroids is impaired and so there is salt loss and hypoglycaemia in infancy and the genitalia will be female in appearance in the XY individual. At postmortem the adrenals are enlarged and full of accumulated cholesterol. Survival is possible with prompt recognition and appropriate treatment.

   Recently, an XY individual with female external genitalia was found to have lipoid CAH due to a mutation in cholesterol side-chain cleavage.[320] The relatively late development of adrenal failure in this patient and some patients with StAR defects probably reflects the gradual accumulation of cholesterol and associated cellular damage.

3β-Hydroxysteroid dehydrogenase deficiency (see Fig. 35.12)

In this condition, the variable degree of impaired enzyme activity can cause considerable phenotypic heterogeneity, including varying degrees of adrenal insufficiency. There are two 3β-hydroxysteroid dehydrogenase isoenzymes and it is type 2 (expressed in gonads and adrenals) rather than type 1 (expressed in placenta, prostate and skin) that is abnormal. Affected males may have perineal hypospadias. Females are either normal in appearance or are virilised, probably because of increased ACTH-stimulated production of the weak androgen dehydroepiandrosterone, which can be converted to more potent androgens. Some, but not all, affected children develop salt wasting or signs of glucocorticoid deficiency.[213,275]

17α-Hydroxylase deficiency and 17,20-desmolase deficiency (see Fig. 35.12)

A single protein is responsible for these two separate enzyme activities. Affected males are inadequately virilised, whereas females are phenotypically normal in early life.[368] Patients may subsequently present with delayed puberty or hypertension because of impaired sex steroid production and mineralocorticoid excess.

17β-Hydroxysteroid dehydrogenase deficiency (see Fig. 35.12)

This enzyme is responsible for the last step in testosterone production.[112] At birth, affected males are poorly virilised, and many have been reared as females before being investigated at puberty, when marked virilisation occurs.[344] Females are unaffected.[281] Presentation in infancy with herniae and palpable gonads has also been reported.[119]

5α-Reductase deficiency

Genetic males with 5α-reductase deficiency have external genitalia that are largely female in appearance. The defect was described in families living in an isolated community in the Dominican Republic, where affected individuals were raised as females but at puberty there was virilisation of the genitalia and body habitus and the development of male psychosexual orientation; most then converted to the male role.[150] The condition has now been recognised in many countries.[17] Clinically, there is normal fetal development of wolffian structures, which are testosterone dependent, but poor development of the external genitalia, which require DHT. Biochemically, the key finding is a high testosterone/DHT ratio in serum and analogous changes on urinary steroid analysis.[234]

Androgen insensitivity[7]

Partial androgen insensitivity

In this X-linked recessive condition, the genital abnormality arising from the insensitivity to androgen varies widely, ranging from a near-normal female appearance to normal male virilisation with azoospermia. This is an important cause of perineal hypospadias.[29] Many affected children have inherited defects of the androgen

Table 35.17 Causes of female virilisation

Virilising congenital adrenal hyperplasia
Deficiency of
21α-hydroxylase
11β-hydroxylase
3β-hydroxysteroid dehydrogenase
Aromatase deficiency
Maternal androgen excess
Endogenous
Exogenous

receptor (which maps to the long arm of the X-chromosome). The genetics of this disorder have been studied in detail.

Complete androgen insensitivity

Complete androgen insensitivity, also inherited as an X-linked recessive condition, is seldom diagnosed in the neonatal period unless there is a positive family history or gonads are palpable in the groin. Affected infants are otherwise indistinguishable from normal females. Müllerian regression occurs normally under the influence of AMH but the wolffian ducts fail to differentiate. The normal postnatal surge in LH and testosterone[106] is absent in complete androgen insensitivity syndrome, presumably because the hypothalamus and pituitary are unable to respond to androgen.[44] At puberty there is breast development but no virilisation.

AMH resistance and deficiency

In the persistent müllerian duct syndrome, the uterus and fallopian tubes fail to regress during development. Affected infants usually present when undergoing surgery for cryptorchidism or inguinal hernia repair, when the müllerian structures are identified. A number of mutations of the AMH gene, leading to AMH deficiency, or of the type II AMH receptor, resulting in AMH resistance, have been described in these patients.[31,149]

Virilised females (female pseudohermaphroditism) (see Fig. 35.18 and Table 35.17)

These conditions are characterised by a normal female karyotype, normal ovaries, and normal female internal genitalia but virilised external genitalia. Exposure of a female fetus to excess androgen can occur in four ways, although the commonest cause of this picture by far is CAH due to 21α-hydroxylase deficiency. The remaining three causes are very rare. The causes are shown in Table 35.17.

Congenital adrenal hyperplasia

The three virilising forms are discussed above (pp. 886–90).

Aromatase deficiency[261]

Normal conversion of fetal and maternal androgens to oestrogen by placental aromatase enzyme activity was thought to be essential for survival of the conceptus, but recently there have been reports of aromatase gene mutations leading to impaired placental enzyme activity and subsequent maternal and fetal virilisation.[66,304] It therefore appears that a pregnancy can be viable despite a marked reduction in oestrogen production, but that the associated rise in androgens in aromatase deficiency may lead to female pseudohermaphroditism.

Excess maternal androgens

Fetal virilisation may rarely occur in response to excess maternal androgen production from an adrenal or ovarian tumour. The degree of virilisation will depend on the timing and degree of androgen overproduction.[340]

Iatrogenic fetal virilisation

Fetal virilisation was formerly observed in female infants of mothers treated with androgens or androgenic progestins during pregnancy. These were administered in an attempt to prevent recurrent spontaneous abortion,[360] but such treatment is now rarely used.

IUGR and gonadal function

An association between small size at birth and hypospadias has been recognised for some time[56,109] and a link between SGA and altered gonadal (and adrenal) function in later life has now also been identified. Prenatal growth restriction is associated with a reduction in uterine and ovarian size[144] and an increase in FSH production in males and females, with oligo-ovulation and anovulation at adolescence.[145,146] This is likely to remain an area of intense research activity in the years ahead.

The clinical approach to problems of intersex[2,206]

Introduction

There is inevitable distress when parental questions about infant sex and wellbeing cannot be answered immediately. The initial discussions should emphasise that:

- Abnormalitites of sexual development are usually confined to the genital tract.
- The cause can be determined and treatment planned, usually with little delay.
- The prognosis for life and health and also for sexual function is good, but that for fertility must be guarded.

An early anxiety of the parents will be what to tell grandparents, siblings, friends and colleagues. It may be possible to delay announcing the birth, or, alternatively, to announce only that the baby has a problem requiring treatment and that the parents would prefer not to discuss progress for a few days. The birth should not be registered until the sex of rearing is decided. Choice of a name suitable for either sex is probably unwise at this early stage.

Whatever the genetic status and the anatomy of the internal sexual organs, successful integration in either sexual role depends on the configuration and function of the external genitalia, against the background of the prevailing social and religious attitudes. It is impossible, even with the most expert modern reconstructive surgery, to create an adequate erectile penis from inadequate tissue. Conversely, the impact of androgen exposure on the infant brain and the well-recognised instances of female-assigned XY patients requesting gender change must be considered. The prospects for fertility must also be borne in mind but are of secondary importance. There may be strong ethnic, social or religious pressures influencing the family's choice, and these clearly need to be respected.

Psychological adjustment to the sex of rearing does not usually cause problems as long as this is chosen early and accepted by those handling the child.[206] Experience with 5α-reductase deficiency and other conditions has shown that greater flexibility in sexual role is possible than was previously believed. Many physicians feel that the sex of rearing should be selected as early in infancy as possible and there is frequently a desire on the part of physician and parents to complete any genital surgery necessary to produce cosmetically acceptable external genitalia as early as is practicable. However, this is a contentious topic that is complicated by a dearth of long-term data and by the desire to involve the patient in the decision-making process.[69,86]

Initial assessment

The degree of virilisation should be determined and this will include an assessment of phallus dimensions, position of urethral opening and the extent of labioscrotal fold fusion. The calibre of the corpora and not merely the amount of shaft and preputial skin should be assessed. Attention should also be paid to the presence/absence and location of the gonads.

- Severe hypospadias with a small phallus and bilateral descended gonads is likely to be an undervirilised male irrespective of the position of the urethral opening.
- A neonate with any degree of virilisation and without palpable gonads may have CAH and the measurement of 17-OHP levels is a particularly crucial investigation in such circumstances.
- Genital ambiguity with asymmetry and unilateral gonadal descent increases the likelihood of gonadal dysgenesis.[156]

Most patients with ambiguous genitalia should be transferred to the local tertiary centre at an early stage because of the need for multidisciplinary input from individuals who manage these complex cases regularly. Urgent investigations in the neonate with ambiguous genitalia include a karyotype and pelvic and renal imaging. 17-OHP should also be measured and serum stored so that LH, FSH and androgens can be measured. It may also be appropriate to image the internal genitalia more precisely using contrast or by endoscopy. Virilised females and undervirilised males may have adrenal insufficiency and so electrolytes and glucose will need to be monitored in the neonatal period until a diagnosis has been reached or adrenal insufficiency excluded.

Subsequent assessment

Patients can usually be assigned to one of the three main categories of abnormal sexual development when the karyotype and imaging results are available. The more common scenarios are described first.

1. Virilised female. Karyotype 46,XX and probable ovaries and müllerian structures (uterus and fallopian tubes) on ultrasound.
This is one of the more common scenarios and the diagnosis is usually CAH. Salt-losing CAH will be manifest by a rising potassium and falling sodium. 17-OHP levels will typically be markedly elevated and the child will need glucocorticoid and mineralocorticoid replacement. Check that a urinary steroid profile has been taken and sent before therapy is commenced. Much rarer causes of androgen exposure in utero include placental aromatase deficiency and a maternal androgen-producing tumour. Girls with these defects have normal female internal genitalia and are potentially fertile, so most physicians feel that, whatever the degree of virilisation, they should be reared as females.

2. Undervirilised male. Karyotype XY with or without descended gonads and no evidence of müllerian structures (e.g. uterus) on ultrasound.
The cause of undervirilisation frequently remains unknown; however, it is important to look for dysmorphic features that may help to establish a diagnosis (e.g. SLO). Identifiable causes can usually be linked to insufficient androgen or impaired androgen action:

- testosterone biosynthetic or metabolism defect, e.g. 17β-hydroxysteroid dehydrogenase deficiency;
- partial androgen insensitivity syndrome.

Important investigations include measurement of:

- testosterone/DHT (abnormal ratio in 5α-reductase deficiency);
- androstenedione (raised relative to testosterone in 17β-hydroxysteroid dehydrogenase deficiency);
- urinary steroid profile (to exclude disorders such as 3β-hydroxysteroid dehydrogenase deficiency).

hCG stimulation with measurement of androstenedione, testosterone and DHT response may also be helpful. Serum should be stored for the subsequent measurement of factors such as AMH, which is a potentially useful marker of Sertoli cell function.[274] Levels tend to be low in patients with abnormal gonadal development, normal in conditions associated with impaired testosterone secretion, and high in androgen insensitivity syndrome. Imaging with contrast may help to delineate the internal anatomy (Fig. 35.19), and examination under anaesthetic and cystoscopy may also be helpful.

If surgery is required, a genital skin biopsy should be taken for androgen-binding studies and it may also be appropiate to discuss androgen receptor sequencing if the clinical and biochemical picture points towards this diagnosis.[7] The choice of sex of rearing will depend on the external genitalia. If the phallus is extremely small, then the prospects for further phallic growth may be poor and the female sex more appropriate. If there is remaining doubt, a course of depot testosterone, 25 mg i.m. monthly for 3 months can be given. Good phallic growth confirms the potential for virilisation at puberty.

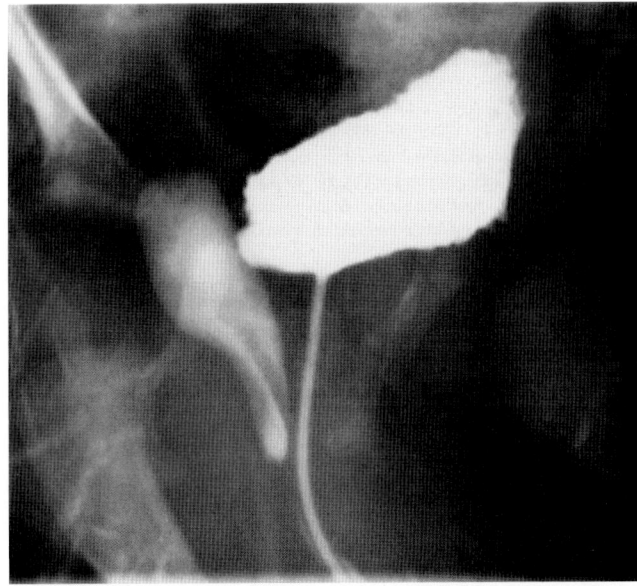

Fig. 35.19 The 'genitogram' of an infant with XY karyotype and ambiguous genitalia. Note the clearly defined blind-ending but adequately sized 'vaginal' cavity posterior to the urethra. This infant proved to have partial androgen unresponsiveness and was reared in the female sex.

3. Gonadal dysgenesis/abnormal gonadal differentiation.
4. Müllerian structures in an XY individual with no or abnormal gonadal tissue.
The differential includes:

- abnormal formation of the bipotential gonad;

5. Genital ambiguity in an individual with an abnormal karyotype, e.g. XO/XY or XX/XY.
The differential includes:

- a patient on the spectrum that runs from an undervirilised 'male' with dysgenetic gonads, through mixed gonadal dysgenesis to virilised 'Turner' syndrome with dysgenetic gonads;
- true hermaphroditism.

In the disorders of gonadal development there is considerable diversity and discordance between the genetic and anatomical findings. There is frequently asymmetry, and imaging, including a renal/pelvic ultrasound, MRI and a genitogram, may be particularly important to detail the nature and structure of internal genitalia and gonads. Laparoscopy and gonadal biopsy may also be necessary in order to obtain a comprehensive picture. The genitogram may reveal a 'vaginal' cavity, and if this is of reasonable size, the prospect of female rearing is made more acceptable. Even in the absence of such a cavity, however, it is possible surgically to construct a functional vagina later in life.

References

1. [Anonymous] 1999 Revised guidelines for neonatal screening programmes for primary congenital hypothyroidism. Working Group on Neonatal Screening of the European Society for Paediatric Endocrinology. Hormone Research 52: 49–52
2. [Anonymous] 2000 Evaluation of the newborn with developmental anomalies of the external genitalia. American Academy of Pediatrics. Committee on Genetics. Pediatrics 106: 138–142

3. Achermann J C, Ito M, Ito M, Hindmarsh P C, Jameson J L 1999 A mutation in the gene encoding steroidogenic factor-1 causes XY sex reversal and adrenal failure in humans. Nature Genetics 22:125–126

4. Achermann J C, Ito M, Silverman B L et al 2001 Missense mutations cluster within the carboxyl-terminal region of DAX-1 and impair transcriptional repression. Journal of Clinical Endocrinology and Metabolism 86: 3171–3175

5. Agwu J C, Spoudeas H, Hindmarsh P C, Pringle P J, Brook C G 1999 Tests of adrenal insufficiency. Archives of Disease in Childhood 80: 330–333

6. Ahmed I, Atiq M, Iqbal J, Khurshid M, Whittaker P 1995 Vitamin D deficiency rickets in breast-fed infants presenting with hypocalcaemic seizures. Acta Paediatrica 84: 941–942

7. Ahmed S F, Cheng A, Dovey L et al 2000 Phenotypic features, androgen receptor binding, and mutational analysis in 278 clinical cases reported as androgen insensitivity syndrome. Journal of Clinical Endocrinology and Metabolism 85: 658–665

8. Ahmed S F, Hughes I A 2002 The genetics of male undermasculinization. Clinical Endocrinology 56: 1–18

9. Aittomäki K, Lucena J L D, Pakarinen P et al 1995 Mutation in the follicle-stimulating hormone receptor gene causes hereditary hypergonadotropic ovarian failure. Cell 82: 959–968

10. Al-Alwan I, Navarro O, Daneman D, Daneman A 1999 Clinical utility of adrenal ultrasonography in the diagnosis of congenital adrenal hyperplasia. Journal of Pediatrics 135: 71–75

11. Alberti L, Proverbio M C, Costagliola S et al 2002 Germline mutations of TSH receptor gene as cause of nonautoimmune subclinical hypothyroidism. Journal of Clinical Endocrinology and Metabolism 87: 2549–2555

12. Allgrove J, Clayden G S, Grant D B, McCauley J C 1978 Familial glucocorticoid deficiency with achalasia of the cardia and deficient tear production. Lancet 1: 1284–1286

13. Alm J, Larsson A, Zetterstrom I R 1978 Congenital hypothyroidism in Sweden. Incidence and age at diagnosis. Acta Paediatrica Scandinavica 67: 1–3

14. Ambrugger P, Stoeva I, Biebermann H, Torresani T, Leitner C, Gruters A 2001 Novel mutations of the thyroid peroxidase gene in patients with permanent congenital hypothyroidism. European Journal of Endocrinology 145: 19–24

15. Anderson R A, Byrum R S, Coates P M, Sando G N 1994 Mutations at the lysosomal acid cholesteryl ester hydrolase gene locus in Wolman disease. Proceedings of the National Academy of Sciences of the United States of America 91: 2718–2722

16. Andersson H C, Frentz J, Martinez J E, Tuck-Muller C M, Bellizaire J 1999 Adrenal insufficiency in Smith-Lemli-Opitz syndrome. American Journal of Medical Genetics 82: 382–384

17. Andersson S, Berman D M, Jenkins E P, Russell D W 1991 Deletion of steroid 5 alpha-reductase 2 gene in male pseudohermaphroditism. Nature 354: 159–161

18. Aperia A, Zetterstrom R 1982 Renal control of fluid homeostasis in the newborn infant. Clinics in Perinatology 9: 523–533

19. Ares S, Escobar-Morreale H F, Quero J et al 1997 Neonatal hypothyroxinemia: effects of iodine intake and premature birth. Journal of Clinical Endocrinology and Metabolism 82: 1704–1712

20. Arnold A 1990 Mutation of the signal peptide-encoding region of the pre-proparathyroid hormone gene in familial isolated hypoparathyroidism. Journal of Clinical Investigation 86: 1084–1087

21. Artman H G, Morris C A, Stock A D 1992 18p- syndrome and hypopituitarism. Journal of Medical Genetics 29: 671–672

22. Asakura Y, Tachibana K, Adachi M, Suwa S, Yamagami Y 2002 Hypothalamo-pituitary hypothyroidism detected by neonatal screening for congenital hypothyroidism using measurement of thyroid-stimulating hormone and thyroxine. Acta Paediatrica 91: 172–177

23. Bakker B, Bikker H, Vulsma T, de Randamie J S, Wiedijk B M, De Vijlder J J 2000 Two decades of screening for congenital hypothyroidism in The Netherlands: TPO gene mutations in total iodide organification defects (an update). Journal of Clinical Endocrinology and Metabolism 85: 3708–3712

24. Ballard P L, Gluckman P D, Liggins G C, Kaplan S L, Grumbach M M 1980 Steroid and growth hormone levels in premature infants after prenatal betamethasone therapy to prevent respiratory distress syndrome. Pediatric Research 14: 122–127

25. Bardoni B, Zanaria E, Guioli S et al 1994 A dosage sensitive locus at chromosome Xp21 is involved in male to female sex reversal. Nature Genetics 7: 497–501

26. Bareille P, Azcona C, Stanhope R 1999 Multiple neonatal endocrinopathies in McCune-Albright syndrome. Journal of Paediatrics and Child Health 35: 315–318

27. Barkovich A J, Fram E K, Norman D 1989 Septo-optic dysplasia: MR imaging. Radiology 171: 189–192

28. Barr M Jr, Hanson J E, Currey K et al 1983 Holoprosencephaly in infants of diabetic mothers. Journal of Pediatrics 102: 565–568

29. Batch J A, Evans B A J, Hughes I A, Patterson M N 1993 Mutations of the androgen receptor gene identified in perineal hypospadias. Journal of Medical Genetics 30: 198–201

30. Batterham R L, Cowley M A, Small C J et al 2002 Gut hormone PYY(3-36) physiologically inhibits food intake. Nature 418: 650–654

31. Belville C, Josso N, Picard J Y 1999 Persistence of Mullerian derivatives in males. American Journal of Medical Genetics 89: 218–223

32. Biebermann H, Schoneberg T, Krude H, Schultz G, Gudermann T, Gruters A 1997 Mutations of the human thyrotropin receptor gene causing thyroid hypoplasia and persistent congenital hypothyroidism. Journal of Clinical Endocrinology and Metabolism 82: 3471–3480

33. Bikker H, den Hartog M T, Baas F, Gons M H, Vulsma T, de Vijlder J J 1994 A 20-basepair duplication in the human thyroid peroxidase gene results in a total iodide organification defect and congenital hypothyroidism. Journal of Clinical Endocrinology and Metabolism 79: 248–252

34. Bikker H, Vulsma T, Baas F, de Vijlder J J 1995 Identification of five novel inactivating mutations in the human thyroid peroxidase gene by denaturing gradient gel electrophoresis. Human Mutation 6: 9–16

35. Binder G, Ranke M B 1995 Screening for growth hormone (GH) gene splice-site mutations in sporadic cases with severe isolated GH deficiency using ectopic transcript analysis. Journal of Clinical Endocrinology and Metabolism 80: 1247–1252

36. Biswas S, Buffery J, Enoch H, Bland J M, Walters D, Markiewicz M 2002 A longitudinal assessment of thyroid hormone concentrations in preterm infants younger than 30 weeks' gestation during the first 2 weeks of life and their relationship to outcome. Pediatrics 109: 222–227

37. Blair J C, Mohan U, Larcher V F et al 2002 Neonatal thyrotoxicosis and maternal infertility in thyroid hormone resistance due to a mutation in the TRbeta gene (M313T). Clinical Endocrinology 57: 405–409

38. Bode H H, Rivkees S A, Cowley D M, Pardy K, Johnson S 1999 Home monitoring of 17-hydroxyprogesterone levels in congenital adrenal hyperplasia with filter paper blood samples. Journal of Pediatrics 134: 185–189

39. Body J J, Chanoine J P, Dumon J C, Delange F 1993 Circulating calcitonin levels in healthy children and subjects with congenital hypothyroidism from birth to adolescence. Journal of Clinical Endocrinology and Metabolism 77: 565–567

40. Bojesen A, Juul S, Gravholt C H 2003 Prenatal and postnatal prevalence of Klinefelter syndrome: a national registry study. Journal of Clinical Endocrinology and Metabolism 88: 622–626

41. Bolt R J, van Weissenbruch M M, Cranendonk A, Lafeber H N, Delemarre-Van De Waal H A 2002 The corticotrophin-releasing hormone test in preterm infants. Clinical Endocrinology 56: 207–213

42. Bongers-Schokking J J, Koot H M, Wiersma D, Verkerk P H, de Muinck Keizer-Schrama S M 2000 Influence of timing and dose of thyroid hormone replacement on development in infants with congenital hypothyroidism. Journal of Pediatrics 136: 292–297

43. Bose H S, Sugawara T, Strauss J F III, Miller W 1996 The pathophysiology and genetics of congenital lipoid adrenal hyperplasia. New England Journal of Medicine 335: 1870–1878

44. Bouvattier C, Carel J C, Lecointre C et al 2002 Postnatal changes of T, LH, and FSH in 46,XY infants with mutations in the AR gene. Journal of Clinical Endocrinology and Metabolism 87: 29–32

45. Bradley B S, Kumar S P, Mehta P N, Ezhuthachan S G 1994 Neonatal cushingoid syndrome resulting from serial courses of antenatal betamethasone. Obstetrics and Gynecology 83: 869–872

46. Briet J M, van Wassenaer A G, Dekker F W, de Vijlder J J, van Baar A, Kok J H 2001 Neonatal thyroxine supplementation in very preterm children: developmental outcome evaluated at early school age. Pediatrics 107: 712–718

47. Broglio F, Gottero C, Arvat E, Ghigo E 2003 Endocrine and non-endocrine actions of ghrelin. Hormone Research 59: 109–117

48. Brook C D G, Hindmarsh P C (eds) 2001 Clinical pediatric endocrinology. Blackwell Science, Oxford

49. Brook C G 2000 Antenatal treatment of a mother bearing a fetus with congenital adrenal hyperplasia. Archives of Disease in Childhood. Fetal and Neonatal Edition 82: F176–F181

50. Brown R S, Bellisario R L, Botero D et al 1996 Incidence of transient congenital hypothyroidism due to maternal thyrotropin receptor-blocking antibodies in over one million babies. Journal of Clinical Endocrinology and Metabolism 81: 1147–1151

51. Brown R S, Bloomfield S, Bednarek F J, Mitchell M L, Braverman L E 1997 Routine skin cleansing with povidone-iodine is not a common cause of transient neonatal hypothyroidism in North America: a prospective controlled study. Thyroid 7: 395–400

52. Bullen P J, Rankin J M, Robson S C 2001 Investigation of the epidemiology and prenatal diagnosis of holoprosencephaly in the North of England. American Journal of Obstetrics and Gynecology 184: 1256–1262

53. Burn J 1999 Closing time for CATCH22. Jourrnal of Medical Genetics 36: 737–738

54. Cacciari E, Balsamo A, Cassio A et al 1983 Neonatal screening for congenital adrenal hyperplasia. Archives of Disease in Childhood 58: 803–806

55. Calaciura F, Motta R M, Miscio G et al 2002 Subclinical hypothyroidism in early childhood: a frequent outcome of transient neonatal hyperthyrotropinemia. Journal of Clinical Endocrinology and Metabolism 87: 3209–3214

56. Calzolari E, Contiero M R, Roncarati E, Mattiuz P L, Volpato S 1986 Aetiological factors in hypospadias. Journal of Medical Genetics 23: 333

57. Cerame B I, Newfield R S, Pascoe L et al 1999 Prenatal diagnosis and treatment of 11beta-hydroxylase deficiency congenital adrenal hyperplasia resulting in normal female genitalia. Journal of Clinical Endocrinology and Metabolism 84: 3129–3134

58. Chanoine J P, Yeung L P, Wong A C, Birmingham C L 2002 Immunoreactive ghrelin in human cord blood: relation to anthropometry, leptin, and growth hormone. Journal of Pediatric Gastroenterology and Nutrition 35: 282–286

59. Charmandari E, Johnston A, Brook C G, Hindmarsh P C 2001 Bioavailability of oral hydrocortisone in patients with congenital adrenal hyperplasia due to 21-hydroxylase deficiency. Journal of Endocrinology 169: 65–70

60. Charmandari E, Lichtarowicz-Krynska E J, Hindmarsh P C, Johnston A, Aynsley-Green A, Brook C G 2001 Congenital adrenal hyperplasia: management during critical illness. Archives of Disease in Childhood 85: 26–28

61. Cheetham T D, Bayliss P B 2002 Diabetes insipidus in children. Pathophysiology, diagnosis and management. Pediatric Drugs 4: 785–796

62. Cheron R G, Kaplan M M, Larsen P R, Selenkow H A, Crigler J F 1981 Neonatal thyroid function after propylthiouracil therapy for maternal Graves' disease. New England Journal of Medicine 304: 525–528

63. Chowdhry P, Scanlon J W, Auerbach R, Abbassi V 1984 Results of controlled double blind study of thyroid replacement in very low birth weight premature infants with hypothyroxinaemia. Pediatrics 73: 301–305

64. Christou H, Connors J M, Ziotopoulou M et al 2001 Cord blood leptin and insulin-like growth factor levels are independent predictors of fetal growth. Journal of Clinical Endocrinology and Metabolism 86: 935–938

65. Cogan J D, Ramel B, Lehto M et al 1995 A recurring dominant negative mutation causes autosomal dominant growth hormone deficiency – a clinical research center study. Journal of Clinical Endocrinology and Metabolism 80: 3591–3595

66. Conte F A, Grumbach M M, Ito Y, Fisher C R, Simpson E R 1994 A syndrome of female pseudohermaphrodism, hypergonadotropic hypogonadism, and multi-cystic ovaries associated with missense mutations in the gene encoding aromatase (P450arom). Journal of Clinical Endocrinology and Metabolism 78: 1287–1292

67. Coyle B, Reardon W, Herbrick J A et al 1998 Molecular analysis of the PDS gene in Pendred syndrome. Human Molecular Genetics 7: 1105–1112

68. Craft W H, Underwood L E, Van Wyk J J 1980 High incidence of perinatal insult in children with idiopathic hypopituitarism. Journal of Pediatrics 96: 397–402

69. Creighton S M, Minto C L, Steele S J 2001 Objective cosmetic and anatomical outcomes at adolescence of feminising surgery for ambiguous genitalia done in childhood. Lancet 358: 124–125

70. Crowley P 2000 Prophylactic corticosteroids for preterm birth (Cochrane Review). Cochrane Database of Systematic Reviews (2): CD000065

71. Crowley S, Hindmarsh P C, Honour J W, Brook C G D 1993 Reproducibility of the cortisol responses to stimulation with a low dose of ACTH(1-24): the effect of basal cortisol levels and comparison of low-dose with high-dose secretory dynamics. Journal of Endocrinology 136: 167–172

72. Daliva A L, Linder B, DiMartino-Nardi J, Saenger P 2000 Three-year follow-up of borderline congenital hypothyroidism. Journal of Pediatrics 136: 53–56

73. Dattani M T, Martinez-Barbera J P, Thomas P Q et al 1998 Mutations in the homeobox gene HESX1/Hesx1 associated with septo-optic dysplasia in human and mouse. Nature Genetics 19: 125–133

74. Dattani M T, Robinson I C 2000 The molecular basis for developmental disorders of the pituitary gland in man. Clinical Genetics 57: 337–346

75. David L, Salle B, Putet G, Grafmeyer D 1981 Serum immunoreactive calcitonin in low birthweight infants. Description of early changes in serum calcium, phosphorus, magnesium, parathyroid hormone and gastrin levels. Pediatric Research 15: 803–808

76. Daw S C M, Taylor C, Kraman M et al 1996 A common region of 10p deleted in DiGeorge and velocardiofacial syndromes. Nature Genetics 13: 458–461

77. Deeb A A, Bruce S N, Morris A A, Cheetham T D 2000 Infantile hypophosphatasia: disappointing results of treatment. Acta Paediatrica 89: 730–733

78. Deladoey J, Fluck C, Buyukgebiz A et al 1999 "Hot spot" in the PROP1 gene responsible for combined pituitary hormone deficiency. Journal of Clinical Endocrinology and Metabolism 84: 1645–1650

79. Delange F, Henderson P, Bourdoux P et al 1986 Regional variations of iodine nutrition and thyroid function during the neonatal period in Europe. Biology of the Neonate 49: 322–330

80. Den Ouden A L, Kok J H, Verkerk P H, Brand R, Verloove-Vanhorick S P 1996 The relation between neonatal thyroxine levels and neurodevelopmental outcome at age 5 and 9 years in a national cohort of very preterm and/or very low birth weight infants. Pediatric Research 39: 142–145

81. Derksen-lubsen Verkerk P H 1996 Neuropsychologic development in early treated congenital hypothyroidism: analysis of literature data. Pediatric Research 39: 561–566

82. De Zegher F, Kaplan S L, Grumbach M M, Van den Berghe G, Francois I, Vanhole C 1995 The foetal pituitary, postmaturity and breech presentation. Acta Paediatrica 83: 1100–1102

83. De Zegher F, Pernasetti F, Vanhole C, Devlieger H, Van den Berghe G, Martial J A 1995 The prenatal role of thyroid hormone evidenced by fetomaternal Pit-1 deficiency. Journal of Clinical Endocrinology and Metabolism 80: 3127–3130

84. De Zegher F, Van den Berghe G, Devlieger H, Eggermont E, Veldhuis J D 1993 Dopamine inhibits growth hormone and prolactin secretion in the human newborn. Pediatric Research 34: 642–645

85. Diamond F B, Root AW 2002 Disorders of calcium metabolism in the newborn and infant. In: Sperling M A (ed) Pediatric endocrinology. WB Saunders, Philadelphia, pp 97–110

86. Diamond M, Sigmundson H K 1997 Management of intersexuality. Guidelines for dealing with persons with ambiguous genitalia. Archives of Pediatrics and Adolescent Medicine 151: 1046–1050

87. Dickerman Z, De Vries L 1997 Prepubertal and pubertal growth, timing and duration of puberty and attained adult height in patients with congenital hypothyroidism (CH) detected by the neonatal screening programme for CH – a longitudinal study. Clinical Endocrinology 47: 649–654

88. Ding D, Buckingham B, Levine M 2001 Familial isolated hypoparathyroidism caused by a mutation in the gene for the transcription factor GCMB. Journal of Clinical Investigation 108: 1215–1220

89. Doeker B M, Pfaffle R W, Pohlenz J, Andler W 1998 Congenital central hypothyroidism due to a homozygous mutation in the thyrotropin beta-subunit gene follows an autosomal recessive inheritance. Journal of Clinical Endocrinology and Metabolism 83: 1762–1765

90. Donaldson M D C, Thomas P H, Love J G, Murray G D, McNinch A W, Savage D C L 1994 Presentation, acute illness, and learning difficulties in salt-wasting 21-hydroxylase deficiency. Archives of Disease in Childhood 70: 214–218

91. Dorr H G, Versmold H T, Sippell W G, Bidlingmaier F, Knorr D 1986 Antenatal betamethasone therapy: effects on maternal, fetal, and neonatal mineralocorticoids, glucocorticoids, and progestins. Journal of Pediatrics 108: 990–993

92. Dubuis J-M, Glorieux J, Richer F, Deal C L, Dussault J H, van Vliet G 1996 Outcome of severe congenital hypothyroidism: closing the developmental gap with early high dose levothyroxine treatment. Journal of Clinical Endocrinology and Metabolism 81: 222–227

93. Duprez L, Parma J, Van Sande J et al 1994 Germline mutations in the thyrotropin receptor gene cause non-autoimmune autosomal dominant hyperthyroidism. Nature Genetics 7: 396–401

94. Dussault J H 1999 The anecdotal history of screening for congenital hypothyroidism. Journal of Clinical Endocrinology and Metabolism 84: 4332–4334

95. Ellyin F, Khatir A H, Singh S P 1980 Hypothalamic-pituitary function in patients with trans-sphenoidal encephalocele and mid-facial anomalies. Journal of Clinical Endocrinology and Metabolism 51: 854–856

96. Everett L A, Glaser B, Beck J C et al 1997 Pendred syndrome is caused by mutations in a putative sulphate transporter gene (PDS). Nature Genetics 17: 411–422

97. Farooqi I S, Jebb S A, Langmack G et al 1999 Effects of recombinant leptin therapy in a child with congenital leptin deficiency. New England Journal of Medicine 341: 879–884

98. Farooqi I S, Keogh J M, Yeo G S, Lank E J, Cheetham T, O'Rahilly S 2003 Clinical spectrum of obesity and mutations in the melanocortin 4 receptor gene. New England Journal of Medicine 348: 1085–1095

99. Farooqi I S, Yeo G S, Keogh J M et al 2000 Dominant and recessive inheritance of morbid obesity associated with melanocortin 4 receptor deficiency. Journal of Clinical Investigation 106: 271–279

100. Fisher D A 1992 Endocrinology and fetal development. In: Wilson J D, Foster D W (eds) Williams textbook of endocrinology. W B Saunders, Philadelphia, pp 1049–1077

101. Fisher D A 1999 Hypothyroxinemia in premature infants: is thyroxine treatment necessary? Thyroid 9: 715–720

102. Fisher D A 2002 Disorders of the thyroid in the newborn and infant. In: Sperling M (ed) Pediatric endocrinology. W B Saunders, Philadelphia, pp 161–185

103. Fisher D A, Dussault J H, Foley T P Jr et al 1979 Screening for congenital hypothyroidism: results of screening one million North American infants. Journal of Pediatrics 94: 700–705

104. Fisher D A, Nelson J C, Carlton E I, Wilcox R B 2000 Maturation of human hypothalamic-pituitary-thyroid function and control. Thyroid 10: 229–234

105. Fisher D A, Schoen E J, La Franchi S et al 2000 The hypothalamic-pituitary-thyroid negative feedback control axis in children with treated congenital hypothyroidism. Journal of Clinical Endocrinology and Metabolism 85: 2722–2727

106. Forest M G, Cathiard A M, Bertrand J A 1973 Total and unbound testosterone levels in the newborn and in normal and hypogonadal children: use of a sensitive radioimmunoassay for testosterone. Journal of Clinical Endocrinology and Metabolism 36:1132–1142

107. Foster J W, Dominguez-Steglich M A, Guioli S et al 1994 Campomelic dysplasia and autosomal sex reversal caused by mutations in an SRY-related gene. Nature 372: 525–530

108. Frank J E, Faix J E, Hermos R J et al 1996 Thyroid function in very low birth weight infants: effects on neonatal hypothyroidism screening. Journal of Pediatrics 128: 548–554

109. Fredell L, Kockum I, Hansson E et al 2002 Heredity of hypospadias and the significance of low birth weight. Journal of Urology 167: 1423–1427

110. Fujisawa Y, Yamashita K, Hirai N, Terada K, Kida K 1997 Transient late neonatal hypocalcemia with high serum parathyroid hormone. Journal of Pediatric Endocrinology and Metabolism 10: 433–436

111. Fujiwara H, Tatsumi K, Miki K et al 1997 Congenital hypothyroidism caused by a mutation in the Na$^+$/I$^-$ symporter. Nature Genetics 16: 124–125

112. Geissler W M, Davis D L, Wu L et al 1994 Male pseudohermaphroditism caused by mutations of testicular 17 beta-hydroxysteroid dehydrogenase 3. Nature Genetics 7: 34–39

113. Glenn, J F, McPherson H T 1971 Anorchism: definition of a clinical entity. Journal of Urology 105: 265–270

114. Gluckman P D, Gunn A J, Wray A et al 1992 Congenital idiopathic growth hormone deficiency is associated with prenatal and early postnatal growth failure. Journal of Pediatrics 121: 920–923

115. Godowski P J, Leung D W, Meacham L R et al 1989 Characterization of the human growth hormone receptor gene and demonstration of a partial gene deletion in two patients with Laron-type dwarfism. Proceedings of the National Academy of Sciences of the United States of America 86: 8083–8087

116. Grant D B 1994 Growth in early treated congenital hypothyroidism. Archives of Disease in Childhood 70: 464–468

117. Grant D B, Dillon M J 1975 Micropenis associated with testicular agenesis. Archives of Disease in Childhood 50: 247–249

118. Grant D B, Smith I, Fuggle P W, Tokar S, Chapple J 1992 Congenital hypothyroidism detected by neonatal screening: relationship between biochemical severity and early clinical features. Archives of Disease in Childhood 67: 87–90

119. Gregory J W, Aynsley-Green A, Evans B A, Hughes I A, Werder E A, Zachmann M 1993 Deficiency of 17-ketoreductase presenting before puberty. Hormone Research 40: 145–148

120. Gruneiro de Papendieck L, Iorcansky S, Rivarola M A, Heinrich J J, Bergada C 1982 Patterns of TSH response to TRH in children with hypopituitarism. Journal of Pediatrics 100: 387–392

121. Haddow J E, Palomaki G E, Allan W C et al 1999 Maternal thyroid deficiency during pregnancy and subsequent neuropsychological development of the child. New England Journal of Medicine 341: 549–555

122. Hadjiathanasiou C G, Brauner R, Lortat-Jacob S et al 1994 True hermaphroditism: genetic variants and clinical management. Journal of Pediatrics 125: 738–744

123. Halliday H 2001 Adverse effects of early dexamethasone treatment in extremely-low-birth-weight infants. Journal of Pediatrics 139: 163–164

124. Hamilton J, Blaser S, Daneman D 1998 MR imaging in idiopathic growth hormone deficiency. AJNR. American Journal of Neuroradiology 19: 1609–1615

125. Hanna C E, Keith L D, Colasurdo M A et al 1993 Hypothalamic pituitary adrenal function in the extremely low birth weight infant. Journal of Clinical Endocrinology and Metabolism 76: 384–387

126. Hanukoglu A, Perlman K, Shamis I, Brnjac L, Rovet J, Daneman D 2001 Relationship of etiology to treatment in congenital hypothyroidism. Journal of Clinical Endocrinology and Metabolism 86: 186–191

127. Haqq A M, Farooqi I S, O'Rahilly S et al 2003 Serum ghrelin levels are inversely correlated with body mass index, age, and insulin concentrations in normal children and are markedly increased in Prader-Willi syndrome. Journal of Clinical Endocrinology and Metabolism 88: 174–178

128. Hashimoto H, Maruyama H, Koshida R, Okuda N, Sato T 1995 Central hypothyroidism resulting from pituitary suppression and peripheral thyrotoxicosis in a premature infant born to a mother with Graves' disease. Journal of Pediatrics 127: 809–811

129. Hawkins J R, Taylor A, Goodfellow P N, Migeon C J, Smith K D, Berkovitz G D 1992 Evidence for increased prevalence of SRY mutations in XY females with complete rather than partial gonadal dysgenesis. American Journal of Human Genetics 51: 979–984

130. Heath H, Odelberg S, Jackson C E et al 1996 Clustered inactivating mutations and benign polymorphisms of the calcium receptor gene in familial benign hypocalciuric hypercalcemia suggest receptor functional domains. Journal of Clinical Endocrinology and Metabolism 81: 1312–1317

131. Heckmann M, Wudy S A, Haack D, Pohlandt F 1999 Reference range for serum cortisol in well preterm infants. Archives of Disease in Childhood. Fetal and Neonatal Edition 81: F171–F174

132. Herman S P, Baggenstoss A M, Cloutier M D 1975 Liver dysfunction and histologic abnormalities in neonatal hypopituitarism. Journal of Pediatrics 87: 892–895

133. Heyerdahl S, Ilicki A. Karlberg J, Kase B F, Larsson A 1997 Linear growth in early treated children with congenital hypothyroidism. Acta Paediatrica 86: 479–483

134. Hindmarsh P C 2002 Optimisation of thyroxine dose in congenital hypothyroidism. Archives of Disease in Childhood 86: 73–75

135. Hindmarsh P C, Brook C G D 1985 Single dose dexamethasone suppression test in children: dose relationship to body size. Clinical Endocrinology 23: 67–70

136. Hingre R V, Gross S J, Hingre K S, Mayes D M, Richman R A 1994 Adrenal steroidogenesis in very low birth weight preterm infants. Journal of Clinical Endocrinology and Metabolism 78: 266–270

137. Hoffman W H, Sahasrananan P, Ferandos S S, Burek C L, Rose N R 1982 Transient thyrotoxicosis in an infant delivered to a longacting thyroid stimulator (LATS) and LATS protector negative, thyroid stimulating antibody positive woman with Hashimoto's thyroiditis. Journal of Clinical Endocrinology and Metabolism 54: 354–356

138. Honour J W, Torresani T 2001 Evaluation of neonatal screening for congenital adrenal hyperplasia. Hormone Research 55: 206–211

139. Hopwood N J 2002 Treatment of the infant with congenital hypothyroidism. Journal of Pediatrics 141: 752–754

140. Hsu L Y F 1989 Prenatal diagnosis of 45X/46XY mosaicism – a review and update. Prenatal Diagnosis 9: 31–48

141. Hughes M R, Malloy P J, Kieback D G et al 1988 Point mutations in the human vitamin D receptor gene associated with hypocalcemic rickets. Science 242: 1702–1705

142. Hunter M K, Mandel S H, Sesser D E et al 1998 Follow-up of newborns with low thyroxine and nonelevated thyroid-stimulating hormone-screening concentrations: results of the 20-year experience in the Northwest Regional Newborn Screening Program. Journal of Pediatrics 132: 70–74

143. Huysman M W A, Hokken-Koelega A C S, De Ridder M A J, Sauer P J J 2000 Adrenal function in sick very preterm infants. Pediatric Research 48: 629–633

144. Ibanez L, Potau N, Enriquez G, de Zegher F 2000 Reduced uterine and ovarian size in adolescent girls born small for gestational age. Pediatric Research 47: 575–577

145. Ibanez L, Potau N, Ferrer A, Rodriguez-Hierro F, Marcos M V, de Zegher F 2002 Reduced ovulation rate in adolescent girls born small for gestational age. Journal of Clinical Endocrinology and Metabolism 87: 3391–3393

146. Ibanez L, Valls C, Cols M, Ferrer A, Marcos M V, De Zegher F 2002 Hypersecretion of FSH in infant boys and girls born small for gestational age. Journal of Clinical Endocrinology and Metabolism 87: 1986–1988

147. Ieiri T, Cochaux P, Targovnik H M et al 1991 A 3' splice site mutation in the thyroglobulin gene responsible for congenital goiter with hypothyroidism. Journal of Clinical Investigation 88: 1901–1905

148. Igarashi Y, Ogawa M, Kamijo T et al 1993 A new mutation causing inherited growth hormone deficiency: a compound heterozygote of a 6.7 kb deletion and a two base deletion in the third exon of the GH-1 gene. Human Molecular Genetics 2: 1073–1074

149. Imbeaud S, Carre-Eusebe D, Rey R, Belville C, Josso N, Picard J Y 1994 Molecular genetics of the persistent mullerian duct syndrome: a study of 19 families. Human Molecular Genetics 3: 125–131

150. Imperato-McGinley J, Peterson R E, Gautier T, Sturla E 1979 Androgens and the evolution of male-gender identity among pseudohermaphrodites with 5α-reductase deficiency. New England Journal of Medicine 300: 1233–1237

151. Iniguez G, Ong K, Pena V, Avila A, Dunger D, Mericq V 2002 Fasting and post-glucose ghrelin levels in SGA infants: relationships with size and weight gain at one year of age. Journal of Clinical Endocrinology and Metabolism 87: 5830–5833

152. Jett P L, Samuels M H, McDaniel P A et al 1997 Variability of plasma cortisol levels in extremely low birthweight infants. Journal of Clinical Endocrinology and Metabolism 82: 2921–2925

153. Joint LWPES/ESPE CAH Working Group 2002 Consensus statement on 21-hydroxylase deficiency from the Lawson Wilkins Pediatric Endocrine Society and the European Society for Paediatric Endocrinology. Journal of Clinical Endocrinology and Metabolism 87: 4048–4053

154. Jordan B K, Jain M, Natarajan S, Frasier S D, Vilain E 2002 Familial mutation in the testis-determining gene SRY shared by an XY female and her normal father. Journal of Clinical Endocrinology and Metabolism 87: 3428–3432

155. Jost A 1953 Problems of fetal endocrinology: the gonadal and hypophyseal hormones. Recent Progress in Hormone Research 8: 379–413

156. Kaefer M, Diamond D, Hendren W H et al 1999 The incidence of intersexuality in children with cryptorchidism and hypospadias: stratification based on gonadal palpability and meatal position. Journal of Urology 162: 1003–1006

157. Kari M A, Raivio K O, Stenman U H, Voutilainen R 1996 Serum cortisol, dehydroepiandrosterone sulfate, and steroid-binding globulins in preterm neonates: effect of gestational age and dexamethasone therapy. Pediatric Research 40: 319–324

158. Karlsson R, Kallio J, Irjala K, Ekblad S, Toppari J, Kero P 2000 Adrenocorticotropin and corticotropin-releasing hormone tests in preterm infants. Journal of Clinical Endocrinology and Metabolism 85: 4592–4595

159. Karlsson R, Kallio J, Toppari J, Kero P 1999 Timing of peak serum cortisol values in preterm infants in low-dose and the standard ACTH tests. Pediatric Research 45: 367–369

160. Karpman B A, Rapoport B, Filetti S, Fisher D A 1987 Treatment of neonatal hyperthyroidism due to Graves disease with sodium ipodate. Journal of Clinical Endocrinology and Metabolism 64: 119–123

161. Kato F, Kikudhi K, Miyamoto S, Ohie T, Yamaguchi S 1995 Congenital hypo-pituitarism with hypoplasia of the anterior pituitary gland. Acta Paediatrica 84: 1201–1203

162. Kelley R I, Hennekam R C 2000 The Smith-Lemli-Opitz syndrome. Journal of Medical Genetics 37: 321–335

163. Khuri F J, Alton D J, Hardy B E, Cook G T, Churchill B M 1980 Adrenal hemorrhage in neonates: report of 5 cases and review of the literature. Journal of Urology 124: 684–687

164. Kirk J M, Brain C E, Carson D J, Hyde J C, Grant D B 1999 Cushing's syndrome caused by nodular adrenal hyperplasia in children with McCune-Albright syndrome. Journal of Pediatrics 134: 789–792

165. Kitanaka S, Takeyama K, Murayama A et al 1998 Inactivating mutations in the 25-hydroxyvitamin D3 1alpha-hydroxylase gene in patients with pseudovitamin D-deficiency rickets. New England Journal of Medicine 338: 653–661

166. Köhler B, Schnabel D, Biebermann H, Grüters A 1996 Transient congenital hypothyroidism and hyperthyrotropinemia: normal thyroid function and phys-ical development at the ages of 6-14 years. Journal of Clinical Endocrinology and Metabolism 81: 1563–1567

167. Koopman P, Gubbay J, Vivian N, Goodfellow P, Lovell-Badge R 1991 Male development of chromosomally female mice transgenic for Sry. Nature 351: 117–121

168. Kopp P, van Sande J, Parma J et al 1995 Brief report: Congenital hyper-thyroidism caused by a mutation in the thyrotropin-receptor gene. New England Journal of Medicine 332: 183–185

169. Korte C, Styne D, Merritt T A, Mayes D, Wertz A, Helbock H J 1996 Adrenocortical function in the very low birth weight infant: improved testing sensitivity and association with neonatal outcome. Journal of Pediatrics 128: 257–263

170. Kovacs C S, Kronenberg H M 1997 Maternal-fetal calcium and bone metabolism during pregnancy, puerperium, and lactation. Endocrine Reviews 18: 832–872

171. Kreines K, DeVaux W D 1971 Neonatal adrenal insufficiency associated with maternal Cushing's syndrome. Pediatrics 47: 516–519

172. Kremer H, Kraaij R, Toledo S P A et al 1995 Male pseudohermaphroditism due to a homozygous missense mutation of the luteinizing hormone receptor gene. Nature Genetics 9: 160–164

173. Krude H, Biebermann H, Luck W, Horn R, Brabant G, Gruters A 1998 Severe early-onset obesity, adrenal insufficiency and red hair pigmentation caused by POMC mutations in humans. Nature Genetics 19: 155–157

174. Krude H, Schutz B, Biebermann H et al 2002 Choreoathetosis, hypothyroidism, and pulmonary alterations due to human NKX2-1 haploinsufficiency. Journal of Clinical Investigation 109: 475–480

175. Kruse K, Irle U, Uhlig R 1993 Elevated 1,25-dihydroxyvitamin D serum concentrations in infants with subcutaneous fat necrosis. Journal of Pediatrics 122: 460–463

176. Lako M, Ramsden S, Campbell R D, Strachan T 1999 Mutation screening in British 21-hydroxylase deficiency families and development of novel microsatellite based approaches to prenatal diagnosis. Journal of Medical Genetics 36: 119–124

177. Langman C B 1999 Hypercalcemic syndromes in infants and children. In: Favus M J (ed) Primer on the metabolic bone diseases and disorders of mineral metabolism. Lippincott Williams & Wilkins, Philadelphia, pp 219–223

178. Layman L C, Lee E J, Peak D B et al 1997 Delayed puberty and hypogonadism caused by mutations in the follicle-stimulating hormone beta-subunit gene. New England Journal of Medicine 337: 607–611

179. Layman L C, Porto A L, Xie J et al 2002 FSH beta gene mutations in a female with partial breast development and a male sibling with normal puberty and azoospermia. Journal of Clinical Endocrinology and Metabolism 87: 3702–3707

180. Lee M M, Rajagopalan L, Berg G J, Moshang T Jr 1989 Serum adrenal steroid concentrations in premature infants. Journal of Clinical Endocrinology and Metabolism 69: 1133–1136

181. Lee Y S, Loke K Y, Ng S C, Joseph R 2002 Maternal thyrotoxicosis causing central hypothyroidism in infants. Journal of Paediatrics and Child Health 38: 206–208

182. Leger J, Marinovic D, Garel C, Bonaiti-Pellie C, Polak M, Czernichow P 2002 Thyroid developmental anomalies in first degree relatives of children with congenital hypothyroidism. Journal of Clinical Endocrinology and Metabolism 87: 575–580

183. Leviton A, Paneth N, Reuss M L et al 1999 Hypothyroxinemia of prematurity and the risk of cerebral white matter damage. Journal of Pediatrics 134: 706–711

184. Linder N, Davidovitch N, Reichman B et al 1997 Topical iodine-containing antiseptics and subclinical hypothyroidism in preterm infants. Journal of Pediatrics 131: 434–439

185. Lindsay R, Feldkamp M, Harris D, Robertson J, Rallison M 1994 Utah Growth Study: growth standards and the prevalence of growth hormone deficiency. Journal of Pediatrics 125: 29–35

186. Little M, Wells C 1997 A clinical overview of WT1 gene mutations. Human Mutation 9: 209–225

187. Loughead J L, Mughal Z, Mimouni F, Tsang R C, Oestreich A E 1990 Spectrum and natural history of congenital hyperparathyroidism secondary to maternal hypocalcemia. American Journal of Perinatology 7: 350–355

188. Lovinger R D, Kaplan S L, Grumbach M M 1975 Congenital hypopituitarism associated with neonatal hypoglycaemia and microphallus. Four cases secondary to hypothalamic hormone deficiencies. Journal of Pediatrics 87: 1171–1181

189. Lucas A, Morley R, Fewtrell M S 1996 Low triiodothyronine concentration in preterm infants and subsequent intelligence quotient (IQ) at 8 year follow up. British Medical Journal 312: 1132–1133

190. Lyon A J, McIntosh N, Wheeler K, Brooke O G 1984 Hypercalcaemia in extremely low birthweight infants. Archives of Disease in Childhood 59: 1141–1144

191. McKenzie J M, Zakarija M 1978 Pathogenesis of neonatal Graves' disease. Journal of Endocrinological Investigation 1: 183–189

192. Mandel S, Hanna C, Boston B, Sesser D, LaFranchi S 1993 Thyroxine-binding globulin deficiency detected by newborn screening. Journal of Pediatrics 122: 227–230

193. Mandel S J, Hermos R J, Larson C A, Prigozhin A B, Rojas D A, Mitchell M L 2000 Atypical hypothyroidism and the very low birthweight infant. Thyroid 10: 693–695

194. Mansour S, Hall C M, Pembrey M E, Young I D 1995 A clinical and genetic study of campomelic dysplasia. Journal of Medical Genetics 32: 415–420

195. Martin N D, Snodgrass G J, Cohen R D 1984 Idiopathic infantile hypercalcaemia – a continuing enigma. Archives of Disease in Childhood 59: 605–613

196. Matsuura N, Harada S, Ohyama Y et al 1997 The mechanisms of transient hypothyroxinemia in infants born to mothers with Graves' disease. Pediatric Research 42: 214–218

197. Mayne P D, Kovar I Z 1991 Calcium and phosphorus metabolism in the premature infant. Annals of Clinical Biochemistry 28: 131–142

198. Meeks J J, Weiss J, Jameson J L 2003 Dax1 is required for testis determination. Nature Genetics 34: 32–33

199. Meijer W J, Verloove-Vanhorick S P, Brand R, van den Brande J L 1992 Transient hypothyroxinaemia associated with developmental delay in very preterm infants. Archives of Disease in Childhood 67: 944–947

200. Mercado M, Yu V V, Francis I, Szymonowicz W, Gold H 1988 Thyroid function in very preterm infants. Early Human Development 16: 131–141

201. Merke D P, Cho D, Calis K A, Keil M F, Chrousos G P 2001 Hydrocortisone suspension and hydrocortisone tablets are not bioequivalent in the treatment of children with congenital adrenal hyperplasia. Journal of Clinical Endocrinology and Metabolism 86: 441–445

202. Merke D P, Chrousos G P, Eisenhofer G et al 2000 Adrenomedullary dysplasia and hypofunction in patients with classic 21-hydroxylase deficiency. New England Journal of Medicine 343: 1362–1368

203. Merke D P, Keil M F, Jones J V, Fields J, Hill S, Cutler G B Jr 2000 Flutamide, testolactone, and reduced hydrocortisone dose maintain normal growth velocity and bone maturation despite elevated androgen levels in children with congenital adrenal hyperplasia. Journal of Clinical Endocrinology and Metabolism 85: 1114–1120

204. Mesiano S, Jaffe R B 1997 Developmental and functional biology of the primate fetal adrenal cortex. Endocrine Reviews 18: 378–403

205. Metzger D L, Wright N M, Veldhuis J D, Rogol A D, Kerrigan J R 1993 Characterization of pulsatile secretion and clearance of plasma cortisol in premature and term neonates using deconvolution analysis. Journal of Clinical Endocrinology and Metabolism 77: 458–463

206. Meyer-Bahlburg H F 1999 Gender assignment and reassignment in 46,XY pseudohermaphroditism and related conditions. Journal of Clinical Endocrinology and Metabolism 84: 3455–3458

207. Midgley P C, Holownia P, Smith J et al 2001 Plasma cortisol, cortisone and urinary glucocorticoid metabolites in preterm infants. Biology of the Neonate 79: 79–86

208. Miele V, Galluzzo M, Patti G, Mazzoni G, Calisti A, Valenti M 1997 Scrotal hematoma due to neonatal adrenal hemorrhage. Pediatric Radiology 27: 672–674

209. Miller R R, Menke J A, Menster M I 1984 Hypercalcaemia associated with phosphate depletion in the neonate. Journal of Pediatrics 105: 814–817

210. Miller W 2001 The adrenal cortex and its disorders. In: Brook C D G, Hindmarsh P C (eds) Clinical pediatric endocrinology. Blackwell Science, Oxford, pp 321–337

211. Minagawa M, Yasuda T, Kobayashi Y, Niimi H 1995 Transient pseudohypoparathyroidism of the neonate. European Journal of Endocrinology 133: 151–155

212. Mitsuda N, Tamaki H, Amino N, Hosono T, Miyai K, Tanizawa O 1992 Risk factors for developmental disorders in infants born to women with Graves disease. Obstetrics and Gynecology 80: 359–364

213. Moisan A M, Ricketts M L, Tardy V et al 1999 New insight into the molecular basis of 3beta-hydroxysteroid dehydrogenase deficiency: identification of eight mutations in the HSD3B2 gene in eleven patients from seven new families and comparison of the functional properties of twenty-five mutant enzymes. Journal of Clinical Endocrinology and Metabolism 84: 4410–4425

214. Montague C T, Farooqi I S, Whitehead J P et al 1997 Congenital leptin deficiency is associated with severe early-onset obesity in humans. Nature 387: 903–908

215. Moreno J C, Bikker H, Kempers M J et al 2002 Inactivating mutations in the gene for thyroid oxidase 2 (THOX2) and congenital hypothyroidism. New England Journal of Medicine 347: 95–102

216. Morishima A, Grumbach M M, Simpson E R, Fisher C, Qin K 1995 Aromatase deficiency in male and female siblings caused by a novel mutation and the physiological role of estrogens. Journal of Clinical Endocrinology and Metabolism 80: 3689–3698

217. Morris C A, Thomas I T, Greenberg F 1993 Williams syndrome: autosomal dominant inheritance. American Journal of Medical Genetics 47: 478–481

218. Moshang T, Rosenfield R L, Bongiovanni A M 1973 Familial glucocorticoid insufficiency. Journal of Pediatrics 82: 821–826

219. Munro D S, Dirmikis S M, Humphries H, Smith T, Broadhead G D 1978 The role of thyroid stimulating antibodies of Graves' disease in neonatal thyrotoxicosis. British Journal of Obstetrics and Gynaecology 85: 837–843

220. Murphy J F, Joyce B G, Dyas J, Hughes I A 1983 Plasma 17-hydroxyprogesterone concentration in ill newborn infants. Archives of Disease in Childhood 58: 532–534

221. Muscatelli F, Storm T M, Walker A P et al 1994 Mutations in the *Dax-1* gene give rise to both X-linked adrenal hypoplasia congenita and hypogonadotropic hypogonadism. Nature 372: 672–676

222. Najjar S S, Takla R J, Nasser V H 1974 The syndrome of rudimentary testes: occurrence in five siblings. Journal of Pediatrics 84: 119–122

223. Nako Y, Fukushima N, Tomomasa T, Nagashima K 1993 Hypervitaminosis D after prolonged feeding with a premature formula. Pediatrics 92: 862–864

224. Nanni L, Ming J E, Bocian M et al 1999 The mutational spectrum of the Sonic hedgehog gene in holoprosencephaly: SHH mutations cause a significant proportion of autosomal dominant holoprosencephaly. Human Molecular Genetics 8: 2479–2488

225. Netchine I, Sobrier M L, Krude H et al 2000 Mutations in LHX3 result in a new syndrome revealed by combined pituitary hormone deficiency. Nature Genetics 25: 182–186

226. New M I, Carlson A, Obeid J et al 2001 Prenatal diagnosis for congenital adrenal hyperplasia in 532 pregnancies. Journal of Clinical Endocrinology and Metabolism 86: 5651–5657

227. Ng P C, Lam C W, Lee C H et al 2002 Reference ranges and factors affecting the human corticotropin-releasing hormone test in preterm, very low birth weight infants. Journal of Clinical Endocrinology and Metabolism 87: 4621–4628

228. Ng P C, Wong G W K, Lam C W K et al 1997 The pituitary-adrenal responses to exogenous human corticotropin-releasing hormone in preterm, very low birth weight infants. Journal of Clinical Endocrinology and Metabolism 82: 797–799

229. Ng P C, Wong G W K, Lam C W K et al 1997 Pituitary-adrenal suppression and recovery in preterm very low birthweight infants after dexamethasone treatment for bronchopulmonary dysplasia. Journal of Clinical Endocrinology and Metabolism 82: 2429–2432

230. Nickerson E, Greenberg F, Keating M T, McCaskill C, Shaffer L G 1995 Deletions of the elastin gene at 7qII.23 occur in ~90% of patients with Williams' syndrome. American Journal of Medical Genetics 56: 1156–1161

231. Nijenhuis M, van den Akker E L T, Zalm R et al 2001 Familial neurohypophysial diabetes insipidus in a large Dutch kindred: effect of the onset of diabetes on growth in children and cell biological defects of the mutant vasopressin prohormone. Journal of Clinical Endocrinology and Metabolism 86: 3410–3420

232. Nordenstrom A, Servin A, Bohlin G, Larsson A, Wedell A 2002 Sex-typed toy play behavior correlates with the degree of prenatal androgen exposure assessed by CYP21 genotype in girls with congenital adrenal hyperplasia. Journal of Clinical Endocrinology and Metabolism 87: 5119–5124

233. Nordenstrom A, Thilen A, Hagenfeldt L, Larsson A, Wedell A 1999 Genotyping is a valuable diagnostic complement to neonatal screening for congenital adrenal hyperplasia due to steroid 21-hydroxylase deficiency. Journal of Clinical Endocrinology and Metabolism 84: 1505–1509

234. Odame I, Donaldson M D C, Wallace A M, Cochran W, Smith P J 1992 Early diagnosis and management of 5α-reductase deficiency. Archives of Disease in Childhood 67: 720–723

235. Oddie S, Richmond S, Coulthard M 2001 Hypernatraemic dehydration and breast feeding: a population study. Archives of Disease in Childhood 85: 318–320

236. Ogilvy-Stuart A L 2002 Neonatal thyroid disorders. Archives of Disease in Childhood. Fetal and Neonatal Edition 87: F165–F171

237. Ohrlander S, Gennser G, Nilsson K O, Eneroth P 1977 ACTH test to neonates after administration of corticosteroids during gestation. Obstetrics and Gynecology 49: 691–694

238. Olivieri A, Stazi M A, Mastroiacovo P et al 2002 The Study Group for Congenital Hypothyroidism. A population-based study on the frequency of additional congenital malformations in infants with congenital hypothyroidism: data from the Italian Registry for Congenital Hypothyroidism (1991–1998). Journal of Clinical Endocrinology and Metabolism 87: 557–562

239. Olsen C L, Hughes J P, Youngblood LG, Sharpe-Stimac M 1997 Epidemiology of holoprosencephaly and phenotypic characteristics of affected children: New York State, 1984-1989. American Journalof Medical Genetics 73: 217–226

240. Ong K K, Ahmed M L, Sherriff A et al 1999 Cord blood leptin is associated with size at birth and predicts infancy weight gain in humans. ALSPAC Study Team. Avon Longitudinal Study of Pregnancy and Childhood. Journal of Clinical Endocrinology and Metabolism 84: 1145–1148

241. O'Shea T M, Kothadia J M, Klinepeter K L et al 1999 Randomized placebo-controlled trial of a 42-day tapering course of dexamethasone to reduce the duration of ventilator dependency in very low birth weight infants: outcome of study participants at 1-year adjusted age. Pediatrics 104(1 Pt 1): 15–21

242. Pang S, Wallace M A, Hofman L et al 1988 Worldwide experience in newborn screening for classical congenital adrenal hyperplasia due to 21-hydroxylase deficiency. Pediatrics 81: 866–874

243. Parkinson D, Thakker R 1992 A donor splice mutation in the parathyroid hormone gene is associated with autosomal recessive hypoparathyroidism. Nature Genetics 1: 149–152

244. Parks J S, Brown M R, Hurley D L, Phelps C J, Wajnrajch M P 1999 Heritable disorders of pituitary development. Journal of Clinical Endocrinology and Metabolism 84: 4362–4370

245. Pascoe L, Curnow K M, Slutsker L, Rosler A, White P C 1992 Mutations in the human CYP11B2 (aldosterone synthase) gene causing corticosterone methyloxidase II deficiency. Proceedings of the National Academy of Sciences of the United States of America 89: 4996–5000

246. Pass K A, Lane P A, Fernhoff P M et al 2000 US newborn screening system guidelines II: follow-up of children, diagnosis, management, and evaluation. Statement of the Council of Regional Networks for Genetic Services (CORN). Journal of Pediatrics 137(4 suppl.): S1–S46

247. Pearce S H S, Brown E M 1996 The genetic basis of endocrine disease. Disorders of calcium ion sensing. Journal of Clinical Endocrinology and Metabolism 81: 2030–2035

248. Pearce S H S, Trump D, Wooding C et al 1995 Calcium-sensing receptor mutations in familial benign hypercalcaemia and neonatal hyperparathyroidism. Journal of Clinical Investigation 96: 2683–2692

249. Pearce S H S, Williamson C, Kifor O et al 1996 A familial syndrome of hypocalcemia with hypercalciuria due to mutations in the calcium-sensing receptor. New England Journal of Medicine 335: 1115–1122

250. Pena-Almazan S, Buchlis J, Miller S, Shine B, MacGillivray M 2001 Linear growth characteristics of congenitally GH-deficient infants from birth to one year of age. Journal of Clinical Endocrinology and Metabolism 86: 5691–5694

251. Perry R, Heinrichs C, Bourdoux P et al 2002 Discordance of monozygotic twins for thyroid dysgenesis: implications for screening and for molecular pathophysiology. Journal of Clinical Endocrinology and Metabolism 87: 4072–4077

252. Perry R J, Hollman A S, Wood A M, Donaldson M D 2002 Ultrasound of the thyroid gland in the newborn: normative data. Archives of Disease in Childhood. Fetal and Neonatal Edition 87: F209–F211

253. Persani L, Ferretti E, Borgato S, Faglia G, Beck-Peccoz P 2000 Circulating thyrotropin bioactivity in sporadic central hypothyroidism. Journal of Clinical Endocrinology and Metabolism 85: 3631–3635

254. Peter M, Fawaz L, Drop S L, Visser H K, Sippell W G 1997 Hereditary defect in biosynthesis of aldosterone: aldosterone synthase deficiency 1964–1997. Journal of Clinical Endocrinology and Metabolism 82: 3525–3528

255. Pfäffle R W, DiMattia G E, Parks J S et al 1992 Mutation of the POU-specific domain of Pit-1 and hypopituitarism without pituitary hypoplasia. Science 257: 1118–1121

256. Pfeifer D, Kist R, Dewar K et al 1999 Campomelic dysplasia translocation breakpoints are scattered over 1 Mb proximal to SOX9: evidence for an extended control region. American Journal of Human Genetics 65: 111–124

257. Phillip M, Arbelle J E, Segev Y, Parvari R 1998 Male hypogonadism due to a mutation in the gene for the beta-subunit of follicle-stimulating hormone. New England Journal of Medicine 338: 1729–1732

258. Phillips J A III, Hjelle B, Seeburg P H, Zachmann M 1981 Molecular basis for familial isolated growth hormone deficiency. Proceedings of the National Academy of Sciences of the United States of America 78: 6372–6375

259. Pincus D R, Kelnar C J H, Wallace A M 1993 17-hydroxyprogesterone rhythms and growth velocity in congenital adrenal hyperplasia. Journal of Paediatrics and Child Health 29: 302–304

260. Pinto G, Netchine I, Sobrier M L, Brunelle F, Souberbielle J C, Brauner R J 1999 Pituitary stalk interruption syndrome: a clinical-biological-genetic assessment of its pathogenesis. Journalof Clinical Endocrinology and Metabolism 82: 3450–3454

261. Pohlenz J, Rosenthal I M, Weiss R E, Jhiang S M, Burant C, Refetoff S 1998 Congenital hypothyroidism due to mutations in the sodium/iodide symporter. Identification of a nonsense mutation producing a downstream cryptic 3' splice site. Journal of Clinical Investigation 101: 1028–1035

262. Pohlenz J, Sadow P M, Koffler T, Schonberger W, Weiss R E, Refetoff S 2001 Congenital hypothyroidism in a child with unsuspected familial dysalbuminemic hyperthyroxinemia caused by a mutation (R218H) in the human albumin gene. Journal of Pediatrics 139: 887–891

263. Pollak M R, Brown E M, Wu Chou Y-H et al 1993 Mutations in the human Ca^{2+}-sensing receptor gene cause familial hypocalciuric hypercalcemia and neonatal severe hyperparathyroidism. Cell 75: 1297–1303

264. Pollak M R, Wu Chou Y-H, Marx S J et al 1994 Familial hypocalciuric hypercalcemia and neonatal severe hyperparathyroidism. Effects of mutant gene dosage on phenotype. Journal of Clinical Investigation 93: 1108–1112

265. Procter A M, Phillips J A 3rd, Cooper D N 1998 The molecular genetics of growth hormone deficiency. Human Genetics 103: 255–272

266. Queipo G, Zenteno J C, Pena R et al 2002 Molecular analysis in true hermaphroditism: demonstration of low-level hidden mosaicism for Y-derived sequences in 46,XX cases. Human Genetics 111: 278–283

267. Radovick S, Nations M, Du Y, Berg L A, Weintraub B D, Wondisford F E 1992 A mutation in the POU-homeodomain of Pit-1 responsible for combined pituitary hormone deficiency. Science 7: 1115–1118

268. Ramos E S, Moreira-Filho C A, Vicente Y A et al 1996 SRY-negative true hermaphrodites and an XX male in two generations of the same family. Human Genetics 97: 596–598

269. Rapaport R 2000 Congenital hypothyroidism: expanding the spectrum. Journal of Pediatrics 136: 10–12

270. Rapaport R, Rose S R, Freemark M 2001 Hypothyroxinemia in the preterm infant: the benefits and risks of thyroxine treatment. Journal of Pediatrics 139: 182–188

271. Rapaport R, Sills I, Patel U et al 1993 Thyrotropin-releasing hormone stimulation tests in infants. Journal of Clinical Endocrinology and Metabolism 77: 889–894

272. Refetoff S, Weiss R E 1997 Resistance to thyroid hormone. In: Thakker T V (ed) Molecular genetics of endocrine disorders. Chapman & Hill, London, pp 85–122

273. Reuss M L, Paneth N, Pinto-Martin J A, Lorenz J M, Susser M 1996 The relation of transient hypothyroxinemia in preterm infants to neurologic development at two years of age. New England Journal of Medicine 334: 821–827

274. Rey R A, Belville C, Nihoul-Fekete C et al 1999 Evaluation of gonadal function in 107 intersex patients by means of serum antimullerian hormone measurement. Journal of Clinical Endocrinology and Metabolism 84: 627–631

275. Rheaume E, Simard J, Morel Y et al 1992 Congenital adrenal hyperplasia due to point mutations in the type II 3 beta-hydroxysteroid dehydrogenase gene. Nature Genetics 1: 239–245

276. Robertson G L 2001 Disorders of water balance. In: Brook C G D, Hindmarsh P C (eds) Clinical pediatric endocrinology. Blackwell Scientific, Oxford, pp 193–221

277. Robinson A G 1976 DDAVP in the treatment of central diabetes insipidus. New England Journal of Medicine 294: 507–511

278. Rodd C, Goodyer P 1999 Hypercalcemia of the newborn: etiology, evaluation, and management. Pediatric Nephrology 13: 542–547

279. Romagnoli C, Zecca E, Tortorolo G, Diodato A, Fazzini G, Sorcini-Carta M 1987 Plasma thyrocalcitonin and parathyroid hormone concentrations in early neonatal hypocalcaemia. Archives of Disease in Childhood 62: 580–584

280. Rona R J, Tanner J M 1977 Aetiology of idiopathic growth hormone deficiency in England and Wales. Archives of Disease in Childhood 52: 197–208

281. Rosler A, Silverstein S, Abeliovich D 1996 A (R80Q) mutation in 17 beta-hydroxysteroid dehydrogenase type 3 gene among Arabs of Israel is associated with pseudohermaphroditism in males and normal asymptomatic females. Journal of Clinical Endocrinology and Metabolism 81: 1827–1831

282. Roti E, Minelli R, Salvi M 1996 Management of hyperthyoidism and hypothyroidism in the pregnant woman. Journal of Clinical Endocrinology and Metabolism 781: 1679–1682

283. Rovet J F 1999 Congenital hypothyroidism: long-term outcome. Thyroid 9: 741–748

284. Rovet J F, Ehrlich R M 1995 Long-term effects of L-thyroxine therapy for congenital hypothyroidism. Journal of Pediatrics 126: 380–386

285. Rovet J, Walker W, Bliss B, Buchanan L, Ehrich R 1996 Long-term sequelae of hearing impairment in congenital hypothyroidism. Journal of Pediatrics 128: 776–783

286. Rudman D, Davis T, Priest J H et al 1978 Prevalence of growth hormone deficiency in children with cleft lip and palate. Journal of Pediatrics 93: 378–382

287. Ryan A K, Goodship J A, Wilson D I et al 1997 Spectrum of clinical features associated with interstitial chromosome 22q11 deletions: a European collaborative study. Journal of Medical Genetics 34: 798–804

288. Saggese G, Baroncelli G I, Bertelloni S, Cipolloni C 1991 Intact parathyroid hormone levels during pregnancy, in healthy term neonates and in hypocalcemic preterm infants. Acta Paediatrica Scandinavica 80: 36–41

289. Salerno M, Micillo M, Di Maio S et al 2001 Longitudinal growth, sexual maturation and final height in patients with congenital hypothyroidism detected by neonatal screening. European Journal of Endocrinology 145: 377–383

290. Salerno M, Militerni R, Bravaccio C et al 2002 Effect of different starting doses of levothyroxine on growth and intellectual outcome at four years of age in congenital hypothyroidism. Thyroid 12: 45–52

291. Salisbury D M, Leonard J V, Dezateux C A, Savage M O 1984 Micropenis: an important early sign of congenital hypopituitarism. British Medical Journal 288: 621–622

292. Sandrini F, Farmakidis C, Kirschner L S et al 2001 Spectrum of mutations of the AAAS gene in Allgrove syndrome: lack of mutations in six kindreds with isolated resistance to corticotropin. Journal of Clinical Endocrinology and Metabolism 86: 5433–5437

293. Sandrini R, Ribeiro R C, DeLacerda L 1997 Childhood adrenocortical tumors. Journal of Clinical Endocrinology and Metabolism 82: 2027–2031

294. Santiago L B, Jorge S M, Moreira A C 1996 Longitudinal evaluation of the development of salivary cortisol circadian rhythm in infancy. Clinical Endocrinology 44: 157–161

295. Sarafoglou K, Ostrer H 2000 Clinical review 111: familial sex reversal: a review. Journal of Clinical Endocrinology and Metabolism 85: 483–493

296. Savage M O, Burren C P, Blair J C et al 2001 Growth hormone insensitivity: pathophysiology, diagnosis, clinical variation and future perspectives. Hormone Research 55(suppl. 2): 32–35

297. Schipani E, Langman C B, Parfitt A M et al 1996 Constitutively activated receptors for parathyroid hormone and parathyroid hormone-related peptide in Jansen's metaphyseal chondrodysplasia. New England Journal of Medicine 335: 708–714

298. Schonberger W, Grimm W, Emmrich P, Gempp W 1981 Reduction of mortality rate in premature infants by substitution of thyroid hormones. European Journal of Pediatrics 135: 245–253

299. Schwartz I D, Root A W 1991 The Klinefelter syndrome of testicular dysgenesis. Endocrinology and Metabolism Clinics of North America 20: 153–163

300. Scott S M, Watterberg K L 1995 Effect of gestational age, postnatal age, and illness on plasma cortisol concentrations in premature infants. Pediatric Research 37: 112–116

301. Seri I, Tan R, Evans J 2001 Cardiovascular effects of hydrocortisone in preterm infants with pressor-resistant hypotension. Pediatrics 107: 1070–1074

302. Shaw N J, Pal B R 2002 Vitamin D deficiency in UK Asian families: activating a new concern. Archives of Disease in Childhood 86: 147–149

303. Shinwell E S, Karplus M, Reich D et al 2000 Early postnatal dexamethasone treatment and increased incidence of cerebral palsy. Archives of Disease in Childhood. Fetal and Neonatal Edition 83: F177–F181

304. Shozu M, Akasofu K, Harada T, Kubota Y 1991 A new cause of female pseudo-hermaphroditism: placental aromatase deficiency. Journal of Clinical Endocrinology and Metabolism 72: 560–566

305. Singh J, Pearce S, Moghal N, Cheetham T D 2003 The investigation of hypocalcaemia and rickets. Archives of Disease in Childhood 88: 403–407

306. Sivan E, Lin W M, Homko C J, Reece E A, Boden G 1997 Leptin is present in human cord blood. Diabetes 46: 917–919

307. Skuza K A, Sills I N, Stene M, Rapaport R 1996 Prediction of neonatal hyperthyroidism in infants born to mothers with Graves disease. Journal of Pediatrics 128: 264–267

308. Smerdely P, Lim A, Boyages S C et al 1989 Topical iodine-containing antiseptics and neonatal hypothyroidism in very-low-birthweight infants. Lancet ii: 661–664

309. Smith C, Thomsett M, Choong C, Rodda C, McIntyre H D, Cotterill A M 2001 Congenital thyrotoxicosis in premature infants. Clinical Endocrinology 54: 371–376

310. Smith N M, Byard R W, Bourne A J 1991 Testicular regression syndrome – a pathological study of 77 cases. Histopathology 19: 269–272

311. Speiser P W 2001 Congenital adrenal hyperplasia owing to 21-hydroxylase deficiency. Endocrinology and Metabolism Clinics of North America 30: 31–59

312. Sperling M (ed) 2002 Pediatric endocrinology. W B Saunders, Philadelphia

313. Stanhope R, Preece M A, Brook C G D 1984 Hypoplastic optic nerves and pituitary dysfunction. Archives of Disease in Childhood 59: 111–114

314. Stark A R, Carlo W A, Tyson J E et al 2001 Adverse effects of early dexamethasone in extremely-low-birth-weight infants. National Institute of Child Health and Human Development Neonatal Research Network. New England Journal of Medicine 344: 95–101

315. Steigert M, Schoenle E J, Biason-Lauber A, Torresani T 2002 High reliability of neonatal screening for congenital adrenal hyperplasia in Switzerland. Journal of Clinical Endocrinology and Metabolism 87: 4106–4110

316. Stick S M, Betts P R 1987 Oral desmopressin in neonatal diabetes insipidus. Archives of Disease in Childhood 62: 1177–1178

317. Strewler G J 2000 The physiology of parathyroid hormone-related protein. New England Journal of Medicine 342: 177–185

318. Sunthornthepvarakul T, Gottschalk M E, Hayashi Y, Refetoff S 1995 Resistance to thyrotropin caused by mutations in the thyrotropin-receptor gene. New England Journal of Medicine 332: 155–160

319. Swain A, Narvaez V, Burgoyne P, Camerino G, Lovell-Badge R 1998 Dax1 antagonizes Sry action in mammalian sex determination. Nature 391: 761–767

320. Tajima T, Fujieda K, Kouda N, Nakae J, Miller W L 2001 Heterozygous mutation in the cholesterol side chain cleavage enzyme (p450scc) gene in a patient with 46,XY sex reversal and adrenal insufficiency. Journal of Clinical Endocrinology and Metabolism 86: 3820–3825

321. Tajima T, Hattorri T, Nakajima T et al 2003 Sporadic heterozygous frameshift mutation of HESX1 causing pituitary and optic nerve hypoplasia and combined pituitary hormone deficiency in a Japanese patient. Journal of Clinical Endocrinology and Metabolism 88: 45–50

322. Targovnik H M, Rivolta C M, Mendive F M, Moya C M, Vono J, Medeiros-Neto G 2001 Congenital goiter with hypothyroidism caused by a 5' splice site mutation in the thyroglobulin gene. Thyroid 11: 685–690

323. Tatsumi K-I, Miyai K, Notomi T et al 1992 Cretinism with combined hormone deficiency caused by a mutation in the PIT1 gene. Nature Genetics 1: 56–58

324. Telvi L, Lebbar A, Del Pino O, Barbet J P, Chaussain J L 1999 45,X/46,XY mosaicism: report of 27 cases. Pediatrics 104: 304–308

325. Teng C S, Tong T C, Hutchinson J H, Yeung R T T 1980 Thyroid stimulating immunoglobulins in neonatal Graves' disease. Archives of Disease in Childhood 55: 894–895

326. Therrell B L 2001 Newborn screening for congenital adrenal hyperplasia. Endocrinology and Metabolism Clinics of North America 30: 15–30

327. Thomas B R, Bennett J D 1995 Symptomatic hypocalcemia and hypoparathyroidism in two infants of mothers with hyperparathyroidism and familial benign hypercalcemia. Journal of Perinatology 15: 23–26

328. Thomas P Q, Dattani M T, Brickman J M et al 2001 Heterozygous HESX1 mutations associated with isolated congenital pituitary hypoplasia and septo-optic dysplasia. Human Molecular Genetics 10: 39–45

329. Thomas S, Murphy J F, Dyas J, Ryalls M, Hughes I A 1986 Response to ACTH in the newborn. Archives of Disease in Childhood 61: 57–60

330. Tillotson S L, Fuggle P W, Smith I, Ades A E, Grant D B 1994 Relation between biochemical severity and intelligence in early treated congenital hypothyroidism: a threshold effect. British Medical Journal 309: 440–445

331. Toublanc J E 1999 Guidelines for neonatal screening programs for congenital hypothyroidism. Working Group for Neonatal Screening in Paediatric Endocrinology of the European Society for Paediatric Endocrinology. Acta Paediatrica. Supplement 88: 13–14

332. Traggiai C, Stanhope R 2002 Endocrinopathies associated with midline cerebral and cranial malformations. Journal of Pediatrics 140: 252–255

333. Triulzi F, Scotti G, di Natale B et al 1994 Evidence of congenital midline brain anomaly in pituitary dwarfs: a magnetic resonance imaging study in 101 patients. Pediatrics 93: 409–416

334. Tullio-Pelet A, Salomon R, Hadj-Rabia S et al 2000 Mutant WD-repeat protein in triple-A syndrome. Nature Genetics. 26: 332–335

335. Vallette-Kasic S, Barlier A, Teinturier C et al 2001 PROP1 gene screening in patients with multiple pituitary hormone deficiency reveals two sites of hypermutability and a high incidence of corticotroph deficiency. Journal of Clinical Endocrinology and Metabolism 86: 4529–4535

336. Vanderschueren-Lodeweyckx M, Debruyne F, Dooms L, Eggermont E, Eeckels R 1983 Sensorineural hearing loss in sporadic congenital hypothyroidism. Archives of Disease in Childhood 58: 419–422

337. Van Esch H, Groenen P, Nesbit M et al 2000 GATA3 haplo-insufficiency causes human HDR syndrome. Nature 406: 419–422

338. Van Wassenaer A G, Kok J H, de Vijlder J J M et al 1997 Effects of thyroxine supplementation on neurologic development in infants born at less than 30 weeks' gestation. New England Journal of Medicine 336: 21–26

339. Van Wassenaer A G, Kok J H, Endert E, Vulsma T, de Vijlder J J 1993 Thyroxine administration to infants of less than 30 weeks' gestational age does not increase plasma triiodothyronine concentrations. Acta Endocrinologica (Copenhagen) 129: 139–146

340. Verhoeven A T M, Mostblum J L, Van Lousden H A I M 1973 Virilisation in pregnancy coexisting with an ovarian mucinous cystadenoma: a case report and review of virilising ovarian tumours in pregnancy. Obstetric and Gynecological Survey 28: 597–622

341. Vieira T C, Dias da Silva M R, Cerutti J M et al 2003 Familial combined pituitary hormone deficiency due to a novel mutation R99Q in the hot spot region of Prophet of Pit-1 presenting as constitutional growth delay. Journal of Clinical Endocrinology and Metabolism 88: 38–44

342. Vilain E, Le Merrer M, Lecointre C et al 1999 IMAGe, a new clinical association of intrauterine growth retardation, metaphyseal dysplasia, adrenal hypoplasia congenita, and genital anomalies. Journal of Clinical Endocrinology and Metabolism 84: 4335–4340

343. Vimpani G V, Vimpani A F, Lidgard G P, Cameron E H, Farquhar J W 1977 Prevalence of severe growth hormone deficiency. British Medical Journal 2: 427–430

344. Virdis R, Saenger P, Senior B 1978 Endocrine studies in a pubertal male pseudohermaphrodite with 17-ketosteroid reductase deficiency. Acta Endocrinologica 87: 212–224

345. Vulsma T, Gons M H, de Vijlder J J 1989 Maternal-fetal transfer of thyroxine in congenital hypothyroidism due to a total organification defect or thyroid agenesis. New England Journal of Medicine 321: 13–16

346. Wagner J K, Eble A, Hindmarsh P C, Mullis P E 1998 Prevalence of human GH-1 gene alterations in patients with isolated growth hormone deficiency. Pediatric Research 43: 105–110

347. Wajnrajch M P, Gertner J M, Harbison M D, Chua S C Jr, Leibel R L 1996 Nonsense mutation in the human growth hormone-releasing hormone receptor causes growth failure analogous to the little (lit) mouse. Nature Genetics 12: 88–90

348. Wallis D, Muenke M 2000 Mutations in holoprosencephaly. Human Mutation 16: 99–108

349. Watterberg K L, Gerdes J S, Cook K L 2001 Impaired glucocorticoid synthesis in premature infants developing chronic lung disease. Pediatric Research 50: 190–195

350. Watterberg K L, Gerdes J S, Gifford K L, Lin H M 1999 Prophylaxis against early adrenal insufficiency to prevent chronic lung disease in premature infants. Pediatrics. 104: 1258–1263

351. Watterberg K L, Scott S M 1995 Evidence of early adrenal insufficiency in babies who develop bronchopulmonary dysplasia. Pediatrics 95: 120–125

352. Watterberg K L, Scott S M, Backstrom C, Gifford K L, Cook K L 2000 Links between early adrenal function and respiratory outcome in preterm infants: airway inflammation and patent ductus arteriosus. Pediatrics 105: 320–324

353. Weber A, Clark A J 1994 Mutations of the ACTH receptor gene are only one cause of familial glucocorticoid deficiency. Human Molecular Genetics 3: 585–588

354. Weber A, Toppari J, Harvey R D et al 1995 Adrenocorticotropin receptor gene mutations in familial glucocorticoid deficiency: relationships with clinical features in four families. Journal of Clinical Endocrinology and Metabolism 80: 65–71

355. Weil D, Wang I, Dietrich A, Poustka A, Weissenbach J, Petit C 1994 Highly homologous loci on the X and Y chromosomes are hot-spots for ectopic recombinations leading to XX maleness. Nature Genetics 7: 414–419

356. Weiss J, Axelrod L, Whitcomb R W, Harris P E, Crowley W F, Jameson J L 1992 Hypogonadism caused by a single amino acid substitution in the beta subunit of luteinizing hormone. New England Journal of Medicine 326: 179–183

357. Weiss R E, Refetoff S 1999 Treatment of resistance to thyroid hormone – primum non nocere. Journal of Clinical Endocrinology and Metabolism 84: 401–404

358. White P C 2001 Steroid 11 beta-hydroxylase deficiency and related disorders. Endocrinology and Metabolism Clinics of North America 30: 61–79

359. Whyte M P 1994 Hypophosphatasia and the role of alkaline phosphatase in skeletal mineralization. Endocrine Reviews 15: 439–461

360. Wilkins L M 1960 Masculinisation of the female fetus due to the use of orally given progestagens. Journal of the American Medical Association 172: 1028–1032

361. Wilkinson H, James J 1993 Self limiting neonatal primary hyperparathyroidism associated with familial hypocalciuric hypercalcaemia. Archives of Disease in Childhood 69: 319–321

362. Wilson D, Burn J, Scrambler P, Goodship J 1993 DiGeorge syndrome: part of CATCH 22. Journal of Medical Genetics 30: 852–856

363. Wilson D M, Baldwin R B, Ariagno R L 1988 A randomized, placebo-controlled trial of effects of dexamethasone on hypothalamic-pituitary-adrenal axis in preterm infants. Journal of Pediatrics 113: 764–768

364. Wilson J D, Foster D W (eds) 2003 Williams textbook of endocrinology. W B Saunders, Philadelphia

365. Wilson R C, Mercado A B, Cheng K C, New M I 1995 Steroid 21-hydroxylase deficiency: genotype may not predict phenotype. Journal of Clinical Endocrinology and Metabolism 80: 2322–2329

366. Wu W, Cogan J D, Pfaffle R W et al 1998 Mutations in PROP1 cause familial combined pituitary hormone deficiency. Nature Genetics 18: 147–149

367. Yasuda T, Ohnishi H, Wataki K, Minagawa M, Minamitani K, Niimi H 1999 Outcome of a baby born from a mother with acquired juvenile hypothyroidism having undetectable thyroid hormone concentrations. Journal of Clinical Endocrinology and Metabolism 84: 2630–2632

368. Zachmann M 1996 Prismatic cases: 17,20-desmolase (17,20-lyase) deficiency. Journal of Clinical Endocrinology and Metabolism 81: 457–459

369. Zakarija M, McKenzie J M 1983 Immunoglobulin G inhibitor of thyroid-stimulating antibody is a cause of delay in the onset of neonatal Graves' disease. Journal of Clinical Investigation 72: 1352–1356

370. Zakarija M, McKenzie J M, Hoffman W H 1986 Prediction and therapy of intrauterine and late onset neonatal hyperthyroidism. Journal of Clinical Endocrinology and Metabolism 62: 368–371

PART 3

Inborn errors of metabolism in the neonate

James E Wraith

Introduction

All paediatricians have been presented with a desperately sick neonate for whom no diagnosis is readily available. It is in this group of patients that an inborn error of metabolism (IEM) is near the top of the differential diagnostic list. It is important to keep IEMs in mind as a possible cause of symptoms in the neonatal period, and to accept that it is worth investigating 10 babies to diagnose one. Most neonatologists find it easy to maintain this attitude towards bacterial infection, but difficult to sustain the same approach to IEMs. It is very important that a diagnosis of an IEM is established promptly, not only because many disorders are now amenable to effective treatment, but also because of the genetic implications for the families concerned. Even in disorders where treatment is unsatisfactory, prenatal diagnosis in subsequent pregnancies may allow parents to avoid the recurrence of a serious disease.

In most cases, an IEM will be diagnosed during the newborn period because of severe clinical symptoms (Table 35.18), and the bulk of this chapter will concentrate upon the recognition of IEMs in babies who become ill without any prior warning.

In some families, the neonatologist or preferably the obstetrician will be alerted to the risk of a particular IEM which has been present in a previous sibling (or other family members in the case of X-linked disorders). In other families, less specific but equally important clues may exist, such as previous unexplained neonatal deaths, particularly if there is a history of parental consanguinity. It is important always to take a very careful family history and examine the obstetric notes carefully.

The importance of being prewarned about the possibility of an IEM cannot be overemphasised. Most disorders are much easier to treat before the onset of symptoms, and the prognosis for a good neurological outcome is often directly related to the age at which effective treatment commences. This is particularly true for disorders associated with neonatal encephalopathy, such as maple syrup urine disease, organic acidaemias or urea cycle defects. *Remember: the outcome is directly related to the speed of diagnosis.*

IEMs can present in other ways, for instance as a result of mass screening of newborn babies, giving the clinician the opportunity of starting treatment before damage is done. Unfortunately, this approach is not really practicable for most of the disorders that cause neonatal illness. The potential expansion of the newborn

Table 35.18 Clues to the presence of an IEM

Antenatal
Consanguinity
Previous neonatal death
Recurrent non-immune hydrops fetalis
Siblings with known IEMS
Maternal HELLP syndrome or AFLP

Clinical
Unexplained clinical deterioration in an infant who was well
  at birth
Persistent vomiting with no anatomical cause
Persistent hiccups
Major organ failure, e.g. heart or liver
Cardiomyopathy
Dysmorphism or multiple congenital anomalies
Unusual odours
Cataracts
Encephalopathy/coma and/or seizures

Biochemical
Unexplained metabolic acidaemia
Ketosis
Unexpected hypoglycaemia
Hyperammonaemia

Haematological
Neutropenia and thrombocytopenia

Postmortem
Fatty liver and/or heart

Table 35.19 Investigations for diagnosis of an IEM

First-line investigations (available in all units providing neonatal care)
Full blood count
Urea and electrolytes
Blood gas and acid–base analysis
Blood ammonia
Urine-reducing substances
Urine ketones (dipstick)

Second-line investigation (available in each region)
Urine amino acids
Urine organic acids
Plasma amino acids
Blood and CSF lactate and/or pyruvate
Plasma carnitine and acylcarnitine analysis
Urine orotic acid
Beutler test (for galactosaemia)

Specialised investigations (available on a supraregional basis)
Specific enzyme assays on blood or skin fibroblasts, e.g. lysosomal
  enzyme studies etc.
DNA mutation analysis
Special metabolite studies, e.g. very-long-chain fatty acids, bile
  acid analysis etc.

screening programme by the use of tandem mass spectrometry is likely to make this group more important in the future.

Although the primary concern of this chapter is with those IEMs that cause signs in the newborn period, it is important to recognise that a number of disorders which normally present in older infants are capable of producing profound abnormalities in the neonate. The neonatologist needs to be alert to the possibility of encountering these conditions for the first time, or even of encountering a new IEM not previously described.

Finally, it is important to remember that infants with IEMs can be severely dysmorphic, and investigation of this latter group of patients can never be considered complete until one has considered the possibility of an IEM in the infant, or indeed in the mother.

Details of the long-term management of individual IEMs and the laboratory methods used for detection and follow-up are beyond the scope of this chapter. This information is available in the major reference work on IEMs.[31]

The organisation of clinical and laboratory services

A large number of IEMs present in the newborn period. A wide range of techniques are required for diagnosis, and the level of clinical and biochemical experience required for their effective treatment is substantial. Ideally, clinical and laboratory services for IEMs should be integrated, as prompt clinical interpretation of abnormal results is required if treatment is to proceed smoothly. Neonatologists must initiate appropriate investigations (Table 35.19), but they must recognise that rapid and correct diagnosis and treatment of these conditions is a highly specialised skill. A high index of suspicion of an IEM is a reason for referral to a paediatrician expert in the management of metabolic diseases, and not just a reason for sending blood and urine samples to a laboratory.

Some of the investigations performed in the laboratory are relatively simple and can be applied to every patient in whom there is the slightest suspicion of an IEM. Other tests are very complex and should be used only in carefully defined situations. Errors or delays in the use of the right tests or the best forms of therapy can prove very damaging – even fatal – to the affected neonate, especially those with a disorder of intermediary metabolism such as an organic acid defect or a urea cycle disorder. Close collaboration between clinician and laboratory is essential. Each health region within the UK should have the facilities to screen for the more common IEMs, as well as a clinician specialising in the clinical management of affected patients. Laboratory services for subacute and chronic disorders can be centralised for much larger populations and areas, giving rise to National Reference Laboratories for these groups of IEMs.

Before sending samples always:

- phone the laboratory to indicate urgency;
- give all details of drugs, diet and previous blood transfusions;
- arrange suitable transport for samples;

- discuss which tests are indicated with the metabolic consultant;
- freeze and save all urine passed by the infant.

Pathogenesis of IEMs

The majority of disorders are autosomal recessive, but a few are X-linked recessive, e.g. ornithine carbamyl transferase (OCT) deficiency. Deficiency of the E1 α-subunit of pyruvate dehydrogenase is X-linked dominant, with almost all cases, both male and female, due to new mutations.[7] In the X-linked recessive disorders, one occasionally sees partial manifestation in heterozygous females, e.g. OCT deficiency. The defective genotype is present from conception and in most cases the enzyme controlled by the gene in question is active during fetal life. Nonetheless, most IEMs have no effect on the health and development of the fetus, because placental perfusion can correct the disturbance in systemic metabolite levels caused by the enzyme defect. Consequently, most babies with IEMs are of normal birthweight and are in good general condition at birth.

This statement applies to those IEMs in which systemic accumulation of a toxic metabolite (or deficiency of an essential metabolite) damages cells of organs such as the brain. Hyperammonaemia can be taken as a classic example of this. Defective conversion of ammonia to urea in the liver leads to elevated levels of circulating ammonia and intoxicating effects on the brain. A readily dialysed compound such as ammonia is removed very effectively by the placenta before birth, and accumulation commences only after delivery.

There are some exceptions to this concept of 'placental protection'. Defects in cellular energy production (e.g. mitochondrial disorders) may have severe effects prenatally, including defects in embryonic development presenting as physical malformations at birth, or destructive processes later in fetal life (e.g. patchy brain destruction). In lysosomal storage disorders, intracellular accumulation of the substrate of the defective enzyme can be demonstrated early in fetal life, even though the serious symptoms may not develop until some years after birth.

In some IEMs the primary defect is in cerebral metabolism (e.g. glycine encephalopathy) and the abnormalities observed in blood and urine merely represent overflow from the brain. Placental perfusion may have a very small effect on this disease in utero, but not enough to prevent affected infants from being born with hypotonia, lethargy, seizures and often established structural brain damage.

Finally, symptoms of some IEMs develop after birth because the substrate of the defective enzyme becomes available in large amounts only after the baby begins to feed, as in galactosaemia and hereditary fructose intolerance.

Clinical presentation of IEMs

The affected child is likely to be normal at birth. The signs and symptoms produced by IEMs are non-specific and most are shared by many other more common neonatal disorders, especially serious generalised infections. The high frequency of bacterial infections in the newborn period makes it easy to forget the possibility of an IEM. To complicate the matter further, septicaemia is a frequent secondary event in some IEMs, e.g. galactosaemia.

A metabolic cause is particularly likely in babies who develop symptoms one or several days after birth, having been entirely normal for an initial period. Dramatic improvements during a period of intravenous fluid administration, followed by relapse when put back on milk feeding, is another strongly suggestive feature.

Although the range of possible symptoms is very wide indeed, there are two particularly frequent patterns of illness. The first begins with vomiting, acidosis and circulatory disturbance, followed by depressed consciousness and convulsions, and is particularly suggestive of one of the organic acidaemias. The second is dominated by neurological features, with lethargy, refusal to feed, drowsiness, unconsciousness and apnoea. Hypotonia may be a prominent feature. Primary defects of the urea cycle and glycine encephalopathy present in this way.

There are a few more specific symptoms of IEMs. Abnormal body odour is noted in some organic acidaemias, e.g. the smell of maple syrup in maple syrup urine disease, and of sweaty feet in isovaleric acidaemia or glutaric aciduria type II. *Most babies who have an unusual or powerful odour do not have an IEM, but there are exceptions.*

Jaundice and a haemorrhagic tendency occur in those diseases that damage the liver (galactosaemia and acute hereditary tyrosinaemia), but may also be seen as a very late sign in other IEMs, such as urea cycle defects. *The presence of cataracts in an infant with liver disease should lead to urgent investigation to exclude galactosaemia.*

Although convulsions may occur in many different IEMs, the pattern of convulsions in pyridoxine dependency is particularly characteristic and the onset is usually very early.[23] This classic pattern does not occur in every instance, and patients have been described whose convulsions began later than the first 24 hours or were of a very minor type, and some in whom there were considerable periods of freedom from convulsion without specific administration of pyridoxine.[2,13] Formal exclusion of this condition is desirable in all babies with persistent convulsions, regardless of the pattern of onset and progression and regardless of the existence of other apparent aetiological factors (e.g. birth asphyxia).

Hypoglycaemia is a very common finding in the newborn period and is only occasionally due to an IEM. However, this possibility must be borne in mind when hypoglycaemia occurs in atypical circumstances or recurs. To have the best chance of making a diagnosis in a hypoglycaemic infant, collect the samples whilst the sugar is low.

Some patients with IEMs present with prominent cardiac disease. Cardiac failure, particularly with an accompanying hypertrophic cardiomyopathy and hypotonia, is suggestive of a mitochondrial respiratory chain disorder or a defect in long-chain fatty acid oxidation. The multisystem congenital disorders of glycosylation (e.g. congenital disorder of glycosylation type I [CDG]) may also present soon after birth with pericardial effusion. In addition, affected patients fail to thrive and have a variable dysmorphic appearance, which often includes abnormal fat distribution ('fat pads'), large ears and inverted nipples.[18]

Dysmorphic features can also be produced by other metabolic disturbances in the embryo. The resulting infants have physical malformations at birth, including abnormal facies and cardiac, cerebral, renal and skeletal defects. The conditions responsible include those that affect mitochondrial energy production directly (glutaric aciduria type II, pyruvate dehydrogenase deficiency) or indirectly (3-hydroxy isobutyryl CoA deoxylase deficiency). Multiple morphogenic and congenital anomalies are also a feature of the inherited disorders of cholesterol biosynthesis.[37] *Always remember IEMs as a possible cause of multiple congenital anomalies.*

Hypothermia may suggest hypothyroidism or, less often, Menkes disease. The majority of infants with this X-linked recessive disorder have temperature instability which can be noted in the newborn period, although most are not diagnosed until other features of the disease appear in later infancy.

Microcephaly, hydranencephaly and porencephaly with severe neurological deficits are other important presenting features seen in some peroxisomal defects and in pyruvate dehydrogenase deficiency ('cerebral' lactic acidosis, seen generally in females). Rapidly progressive cerebral degeneration starting in the newborn period is seen in both molybdenum cofactor deficiency and isolated sulphite oxidase deficiency. Severe peripheral arteriospasm with marked pallor may occur in primary lactic acidosis. This causes a particularly difficult differential because poor perfusion may cause secondary lactic acidosis.

Finally, one group of disorders in the fetus has the potential to produce severe illness in the mother during pregnancy. Fetal long-chain L-3-hydroxyacyl-coenzyme A dehydrogenase deficiency (LCHAD) is associated with several pregnancy-specific disorders, including pre-eclampsia, HELLP syndrome (haemolysis, elevated liver enzymes, low platelets), hyperemesis gravidarum, acute fatty liver of pregnancy, and maternal floor infarct of the placenta.[29] A floor infarct is a lesion in which fibrin is deposited in the placenta, leading to necrosis of villi. Other mitochondrial fat oxidation disorders such as fetal trifunctional protein deficiency[8] and short-chain acyl coenzyme A dehydrogenase deficiency[22] have also been implicated in these severe maternal disorders.

A summary of some of the commoner presentations is given in Table 35.20. It should be recognised that this is not an exhaustive list and that some symptoms, such as poor feeding, lethargy and failure to thrive, are almost universal in infants with IEMs. Those who find algorithms useful are guided to Saudubray et al.[30]

Investigation of a baby who may have an IEM

General approach

The approach to diagnosis varies with the severity and nature of the symptoms. In some babies, one can make a very good guess at the diagnosis clinically and choose the test or tests most likely to give the answer – for example, a baby hypotonic at birth who

becomes more depressed within the first 24 hours and who develops seizures with a 'burst-suppression' pattern on EEG is very likely to have glycine encephalopathy. However, it is more usual to need to perform a group of tests to reach a diagnosis, as many different IEMs may cause very similar symptoms.

It is important to discuss investigations with the laboratory and also to give some indication of urgency. Many non-urgent samples for amino acid and organic acid analysis are received by metabolic laboratories, and it is often difficult from the clinical information (if any is provided!) on the sample cards to obtain any idea of the urgency of the situation. In addition, appropriate transportation to the laboratory must be arranged if an urgent analysis is requested. Full details of drugs and feeding history should be provided so that proper interpretation of results can be made. If an infant has received a blood transfusion prior to metabolic screening, this should be made known to the laboratory, as this will interfere with the commonly used screening test to exclude galactosaemia.

Some general tests are easily performed and should be used in all infants in whom there is even a slight possibility of an IEM (see Table 35.20). These will include 'routine' tests of electrolyte analysis, bilirubin, acid–base balance, blood glucose and calcium, as well as haematological assessment. Plasma ammonia should be measured in all infants with neurological depression. A simple bedside test for ketones can be very useful, as a heavy ketonuria in an infant with unexplained illness, especially if associated with metabolic acidosis, should be followed by urgent organic acid analysis. Urine testing for reducing substances should not be relied upon to make or refute a diagnosis of possible galactosaemia. Infants presenting with vomiting and acute liver disease, often with a secondary coagulopathy, must be screened urgently for galactosaemia using a specific screening test on blood. In patients with acidosis, calculation of the anion gap – the sum of the serum concentrations of sodium and potassium minus the sum of the serum concentrations of chloride and bicarbonate – can be helpful. Patients with an increased anion gap, and especially those with a value greater than 25 mmol/l (normal range 12–16 mmol/l), are likely to have a specific organic acidaemia. Patients with a normal anion gap and acidosis are most likely to have renal tubular acidosis or intestinal bicarbonate loss.[12] Never ignore a raised anion gap: if it is associated with ketosis, an organic acidaemia is very likely.

Specific tests: 'the metabolic screen'

Occasionally, experts are asked to give advice after a baby's death, and although it is possible to perform some investigations post mortem, early suspicion and collection of the appropriate tissues and samples from a living child permit a more comprehensive screen for metabolic disease.

Although techniques will vary, most metabolic laboratories will require a sample of blood (1–2 ml in a heparinised tube) and urine (5–10 ml in a sterile container with no preservatives) for a metabolic screen. It is now essential that these basic samples are supplemented by a sample of blood (3–5 ml in an EDTA bottle) for subsequent DNA extraction and storage. In addition, a capillary blood sample on filter paper should be collected for acylcarnitine

Table 35.20 Signs suggestive of an IEM

Sign or symptom	Disorder	Test(s)
Hydrops fetalis	Lysosomal storage disease	Urine MPS, WCEs
Coma/Encephalopathy	Organic acidaemias	UOAs, acylcarnitines
	Maple syrup urine disease	U/PPAs
	Urea cycle disorders	NH_4, orotic acid, U/PAAs
	Non-ketotic hyperglycinaemia	CSF/P glycine ratio
	Mitochondrial disease	P/CSF lactate
Coma + hypoglycaemia	GSD I	Enzyme assay
	Organic acidaemias	UOAs, acylcarnitines
	Fructose	Enzyme assay
	1,6-bisphosphatase	
	Fat oxidation defects	UOAs, acylcarnitines
	Hyperinsulinism	Insulin, c-peptide
	Other endocrine causes	GH, cortisol
Odours	Maple syrup urine disease	U/PAAs
	Isovaleric acidaemia	UOAs
	Glutaric aciduria type II	UOAs
Cataracts	Galactosaemia	Beutler test
Seizures	Pyridoxine dependency	Pyridoxine i.v
	Non-ketotic hyperglycinaemia	CSF/P glycine ratio
Liver disease	Galactosaemia	Beutler test
	Tyrosinaemia	UOAs, P/UAAs
	α_1-antitrypsin deficiency	α_1-AT level
	Niemann–Pick type C	Cholesterol esterification
	Fat oxidation defects	UOAs, acylcarnitines
	Mitochondrial disease	P/CSF lactate
Severe diarrhoea	Congenital chloride diarrhoea	Blood and stool chloride
	Glucose/galactose malabsorption	Faecal sugars
	CDG syndrome	Plasma transferrins
Cardiomyopathy	Fat oxidation defects	UOAs
	Primary carnitine deficiency	Acylcarnitine
	Mitochondrial disease	P/CSF lactate
Severe hypotonia	Zellweger syndrome	VLCFAs, DHAP-AT
	Mitochondrial disease	P/CSF lactate
Dysmorphism	Peroxisomal disorders	VLCFAs, DHAP-AT
	Glutaric acidura II	UOAs
	PDH deficiency	P/CSF lactate
	CDG syndrome	Plasma transferrins
	Smith–Lemli–Opitz	Plasma 7-dehydrocholesterol and fasting cholesterol

MPS, mucopolysaccharide
WCEs, white cell enzymes
UOAs, urine organic acids
UAAs, urine amino acids
PAAs, plasma amino acids
GH, growth hormone

VLCFAs, very-long-chain fatty acids
DHAP-AT, dihydroacetone phosphate acyl transferase
P/CSF, plasma/CSF ratio
GSD, glycogen storage disease
PDH, pyruvate dehydrogenase
CDG, congenital disorder of glycosylation

analysis by tandem mass spectrometry. This powerful technique is the easiest and quickest way of diagnosing most fat oxidation disorders. The technique can also be used to diagnosis amino acid disorders and some organic acidaemias.[15]

It is good practice to save and freeze all urine passed by the baby for future analysis and to save a heparinised sample of blood from all babies who require an exchange transfusion (in case galactosaemia screening is thought to be necessary).

In the laboratory, amino acid concentrations can be estimated in blood and urine by one-dimensional paper chromatography. Abnormal results are then characterised quantitatively. Gas–liquid chromatography with mass spectrometry should be used for urinary organic acid analysis. In infants who are hyperammonaemic, amino acid analysis should be performed, and the urinary orotic acid level is determined by high-performance liquid chromatography. Occasionally, more specialised investigations will be required, e.g. plasma carnitine or amino and organic acid analysis of cerebrospinal fluid (CSF). If this is the case, it is best to discuss the clinical problem with the laboratory to ensure that the appropriate samples are collected.

Babies with lactic acidosis present a difficult problem. It is often impossible to distinguish those with a primary defect in pyruvate metabolism from those with lactic acidosis secondary to hypoxia, cardiac disease, infection or convulsions. It is necessary to treat possible underlying causes aggressively while attempting to separate the two groups. Venous obstruction by tourniquet, crying or breath-holding may raise venous lactate and pyruvate levels as much as two- or threefold. Arterial samples are generally required, preferably from an arterial line that has been in place for some time. A persistent elevation of blood lactate greater than 2 mmol/l in a baby who was not asphyxiated and who was not hypoxic or suffering from other organ failure at the time of collection should lead to further mitochondrial investigations, especially if the clinical presentation is suggestive, e.g. prominent neuromuscular symptoms.

Urinary lactate (measured on the standard organic acid procedure) can be helpful. In those patients with secondary lactic acidosis, the urinary lactate falls (although this may take 2–3 days) as the underlying disorder improves, but babies with a primary defect in pyruvate metabolism presenting in the newborn period are generally unresponsive to treatment. Often the child dies before a clear distinction can be made, and one has to rely upon formal assay of the enzymes known to cause lactic acidosis. This is an unsatisfactory approach, as many patients with strong evidence of a primary defect have no biochemical abnormality detectable on enzyme testing. Lactic acidosis is a heterogeneous group of disorders, and it is likely that many defects have not been fully defined or are tissue specific, e.g. limited to muscle or the central nervous system (CNS). Babies with primary disorders of pyruvate metabolism are very difficult to diagnose; the lactic acidosis is usually persistent and severe (>6 mmol/l).

In many cases these investigations will provide a definitive diagnosis or a high suspicion of a known IEM, and appropriate treatment can be commenced. The complete characterisation of the particular condition involves more specific studies, such as enzyme assays, studies of in-vitro cofactor requirements, DNA mutation analysis and often further family studies. Most of the biochemical work-up can often be performed on cultured skin fibroblasts or transformed lymphoid lines.

Management while awaiting results

The severity of symptoms dictates the management. Very mild symptoms may occasion no change in management while awaiting results. It may be prudent to cease milk-containing feeds if symptoms are more than very mild, as protein catabolism is generally the source of the toxic metabolites. Glucose can be given orally or intravenously, but care must be taken to avoid inducing intestinal sugar intolerance by too large an oral glucose load.

In more severe cases, intravenous fluids will certainly be needed, and bicarbonate may be necessary to correct acidosis. Other additives should be dictated by laboratory results, the aim being to achieve glucose and electrolyte homeostasis. Dextrose 10% (with appropriate additives) should generally be used to try and inhibit catabolism, except when a primary lactic acidosis is possible, as some forms will be aggravated by a carbohydrate load.

If the patient is extremely ill, or is deteriorating rapidly, then very aggressive therapy may be warranted even before a diagnosis has been made.

Management of babies with severe acute IEMs

There can be no doubt that the greatest impact on the prognosis for infants with severe acute IEMs has been the improvement in neonatal intensive care that has occurred over the last 20 years or so. In particular, improvements in mechanical ventilation techniques, the use of central access and the ability to dialyse very small infants have been critical, but if treatment is to be successful, great emphasis must be placed on precision and attention to detail.

Appropriate intravenous fluids must be given, but care must be taken to avoid overhydration in the presence of impaired renal function.

Acid–base imbalance must be corrected promptly and adequately. This may require very large doses of sodium bicarbonate (e.g. 20–30 mmol/kg/day) in some of the organic acidaemias, and this will lead to hypernatraemia of a degree sufficient to necessitate dialysis or haemofiltration, especially in the presence of impaired renal function. Correction of acidosis may unmask hypokalaemia, which must be corrected quickly. It is always important to check the electrolyte levels frequently (e.g. 6-hourly) during correction of acidosis and liaise closely with the metabolic team and nephrologists who will be involved in the acute management of these patients.

Good tissue perfusion is essential if secondary lactic acidosis is to be avoided. Oxygen therapy may be needed as well as blood transfusion to correct anaemia (which may occur as an iatrogenic problem). The most common reason for poor tissue oxygenation is hypoventilation due to cerebral depression, and most babies with severe IEMs will require mechanical ventilation. Direct toxic effects of accumulating metabolites (e.g. ammonia) upon the brain may cause cerebral oedema, and this can be easily aggravated by hypercapnia due to inadequate ventilation. Ventilatory support should therefore be used early in order to treat carbon dioxide retention long before measurable hypoxia develops, and should be continued until the baby is breathing vigorously. If an IEM causes coma (as in hyperammonaemia) one usually has to wait at least 48 hours after metabolic correction before clinical recovery occurs to a degree sufficient to cease ventilator support. Hypoglycaemia or hypocalcaemia may require correction initially or during the recovery phase.

Nutrition in the acute phase requires careful attention, as most IEMs are aggravated by tissue catabolism, which is very difficult to reverse during the first 24 hours of severe illness. Intravenous glucose (with appropriate electrolyte additives) should be used initially and, when acid–base balance has been restored and tissue perfusion and oxygenation improved, one should attempt to encourage the development of an anabolic state. This may mean infusing 20% dextrose via a central venous catheter, the amount given being increased until a mild hyperglycaemia is induced (e.g. blood glucose 7–12 mmol/l). Small doses of insulin (0.05 U/kg/h as an infusion) may be used to help initiate anabolism, but this must be used with caution as some infants are exquisitely sensitive and become hypoglycaemic very rapidly. If tolerated, intravenous lipid emulsions can be used as a source of calories, and in some units, growth hormone is also being used as an anabolic agent.[21] Total parenteral nutrition (TPN) will be needed in those patients who are so severely affected that enteral feeding seems unlikely to be achieved quickly. Initially, protein should be added in an amount sufficient to meet minimal daily requirements, and then carefully titrated according to the results of biochemical monitoring.[27] Intravenous L-carnitine (100 mg/kg/day) is also given to compensate for urinary losses, and for some disorders, more specific therapies may be indicated.[9,36] *Oxygenation, good tissue perfusion, the correction of acidosis, and anabolism are the cornerstones of supportive therapy.*

Once the infant's catabolic state has been stabilised – often apparent as an increase in the amount of glucose tolerated, and accompanied by a diuresis (as well as improvement in general condition) – one should introduce oral protein into the diet fairly quickly. This should start at 0.5 g protein per kilogram bodyweight for the first 24 hours; this can then be increased (if tolerated) by 0.25–0.5 g/kg/day on successive days up to a maximum of around 1.5 g/kg/day. In addition, one should supply 120 kcal/kg, and this combination of protein and energy should be sufficient to promote and sustain anabolism. In some infants, especially those with urea cycle defects, protein may need to be maintained at slightly lower levels (1.2 g/kg/day), but in all cases, sufficient must be given to allow the infant to grow and gain weight. Usually the infant has recovered sufficiently to tolerate the protein as a formula given by nasogastric tube, but if not, parenteral feeding regimens can also be used.

Haemodialysis and haemofiltration, have replaced peritoneal dialysis and are important in the management of these patients. *Exchange transfusion is not a useful adjunct to therapy*, except in exceptional circumstances when access to dialysis is not immediately available. Often one will have to start one or other of these treatments while awaiting biochemical results, especially if the baby has a history strongly suggestive of an IEM and is unconscious or deteriorating rapidly despite supportive treatment. Peritoneal dialysis can be effective in infants with organic acid defects or hyperammonaemia due to a urea cycle defect, and it can be used with safety in infants in whom vascular access proves difficult, although haemodialysis or haemofiltration remains the method of choice. Dialysis or haemofiltration will generally be required for 5–7 days, and one should continue with therapy until the baby is established on enough protein to maintain anabolism.

A number of metabolic disorders are known to have vitamin-responsive forms, and it has become traditional to administer a combination of vitamins in pharmacological dosages to sick infants while awaiting results. It is difficult to justify this blind approach to therapy, as the ready availability of metabolic investigations in most regions should allow for diagnosis to proceed rapidly. This can be followed by the use of the appropriate vitamin cofactor (in a dose approximately 100 times the daily requirement) once diagnosis has been confirmed. *'Blunderbuss' vitamin therapy is never indicated.*

Long-term management after the acute phase has passed

The first problem is to achieve a form of treatment which can be continued in the long term and which is compatible with normal growth and development. This can be very difficult when the mainstay of treatment is protein restriction, as the amount of protein tolerated may be insufficient for growth.

The next step is to obtain some information about the margin of latitude available in the treatment of a particular patient. A patient who tolerates very little protein (e.g. <1.5 g/kg/day) will demonstrate metabolic imbalance very rapidly during the course of intercurrent infections, and will be at great risk if the parents or local paediatricians are not familiar with the child's illness. *An emergency regimen, giving clear, written instructions on how to deal with infections*, particularly those associated with anorexia, diarrhoea or vomiting, should be discussed with the parents before the baby is discharged from hospital. A copy should also be made available for the GP and referring paediatrician. We instruct the parents to be cautious and to bring the child early to hospital for assessment, particularly during the first two or three episodes of intercurrent illness. This allows the metabolic team as well as the parents to get some idea of how the individual child responds to different stresses. With experience, the parents become experts in judging how to respond to these intercurrent episodes. One must guard against undue complacency on the part of parents or of doctors in hospital emergency departments as well as in the community, who are not experienced with these conditions.

Management when no diagnosis can be made

As all metabolic disorders have genetic implications for the family, every effort must be made to keep the infant alive so that investigations can be completed. Even if the initial metabolic screen is normal, biochemical correction by dialysis or haemofiltration is still indicated in infants with hyperammonaemia, as severe *transient* hyperammonaemia is well recognised. These infants, often premature, may have very high plasma ammonia levels, but with aggressive treatment have a good prognosis and no long-term metabolic disturbance.

Further management when death is inevitable

If a baby cannot be kept alive, it is still important to think very carefully about the possibility of an underlying metabolic disorder. An autopsy is essential, and this must be performed quickly if metabolic studies are to be interpretable.[28] In this situation it is always best to discuss the infant's poor prognosis fully and frankly with the parents and obtain written permission for the autopsy or biopsies before the infant's demise. Tissues should be prepared for electron microscopy and portions of the relevant organs (usually liver, muscle and brain) snap-frozen in liquid nitrogen. Parallel samples should be taken for histology and histochemistry, and it is best to work in close liaison with the pathologist and metabolic specialist to ensure that the correct specimens are collected. It is important not to forget the appropriate viral and bacterial cultures. A careful examination for structural abnormalities of the brain, heart and other organs is also necessary, and it is therefore vital for the pathologist to be involved in the urgent autopsy irrespective of the time of day or night.

Special management when an IEM can be anticipated

Sometimes one knows in advance that a baby may be born with a particular IEM. This may be true when a sibling has the condition, or when the mother is a proven or suspected carrier of the gene for an X-linked IEM. The optimal treatment can be planned in advance and one can decide whether to treat the baby as affected from the time of delivery (or before), or to investigate promptly and treat only after a diagnosis has been established. The choice will vary from one disease to another.

In other circumstances, the birth of a child who may have an IEM is anticipated without any precise information about what IEM may be present, e.g. when one or two children in a family have died in circumstances that suggest an IEM but without adequate investigation or without achieving a diagnosis. In families like this, consideration should be given to transfer to the metabolic unit soon after delivery.[11] All the investigations listed above should be done immediately, and repeated after the infant has started protein-containing feeds if the initial set are negative.

By using this approach it is hoped to achieve a diagnosis before symptoms develop, and to initiate appropriate therapy. If symptoms develop without any diagnostic biochemical findings, the prognosis is very poor.

Potential hazards of aggressive treatment

Some paediatricians are concerned that an aggressive approach to management may keep alive a grossly brain-damaged infant, but in practice this is not a significant problem. If improvement does not occur within a few days and the prospects of near-normal cerebral function appear remote, one can merely refrain from employing extraordinary measures in the next acute episode of deterioration which will inevitably occur. This approach does carry the risk of producing a survivor with a mild-to-moderate degree of brain damage, but this is true in all acute neonatal illnesses and in all IEMs that can affect the brain.

Detection of IEMs by mass screening

Screening for hypothyroidism is considered on page 377. Phenylketonuria (PKU) is the only IEM which has received universal acceptance for mass newborn screening in the UK and this has been a source of frustration to metabolic paediatricians. It is worth reflecting on the characteristics of PKU, as it illustrates an almost ideal situation for mass screening and is serving as the yardstick against which other mass screening programmes for other IEMs in the newborn period are being measured. A pilot programme for screening for MCAD deficiency will be starting in the UK in April 2004 and will be judged against this yardstick.

Babies with PKU are born in good health, protected by the intrauterine environment. They begin to be affected by their metabolic disorder after birth, but these effects are gradual and probably take several weeks before leading to severe, irreversible change. The outcome of treatment is excellent if it is initiated within the first 2–3 weeks of life, but is not good if treatment is delayed until symptoms are apparent. In addition, there are a number of cheap and simple laboratory methods available, using microsamples of blood, which are very reliable in detecting the disorder. Finally, PKU occurs with a frequency (1 in 10 000–15 000 in the UK) sufficient to justify detection by screening.

Tests suitable for mass screening have been developed for a large number of IEMs but none of these has achieved universal acceptance within the UK.[1] Presymptomatic identification of the conditions that cause acute illness in the newborn period would obviously be an advantage and for many conditions this can now be achieved with introduction of tandem mass spectrometry techniques.[35] The sample used for PKU screening is collected between the fifth and seventh days of life by the visiting nurse (midwife or health visitor) in most regions of the UK, depending on the method used for analysis. This is too late for conditions that cause severe symptoms within the first day or so of life. Tandem mass spectrometry is a very sensitive technique and samples may be collected much earlier (at 48–72 hours), allowing for the diagnosis of many disorders before initial decompensation. If an earlier sample were collected (before discharge from the maternity hospital), it would be a challenge to organise a system that could handle the large number of samples concerned and get results back within the 24-hour period that might be available before decompensation in some disorders. Despite this many parts of the world have started expanded screening programmes using TMS to detect disorders of intermediary metabolism. Umbilical cord blood is probably unsuitable for the vast majority of disorders, as metabolite levels are too close to normal in the cord blood to be diagnostic in most diseases, although this approach may work for some disorders of intermediary metabolism and requires further study.

False negative results for PKU may occur if samples are taken too early or if the infant has not been established on a good protein intake,[34] and this would be a concern if an earlier age of screening was introduced. Premature or sick babies may be

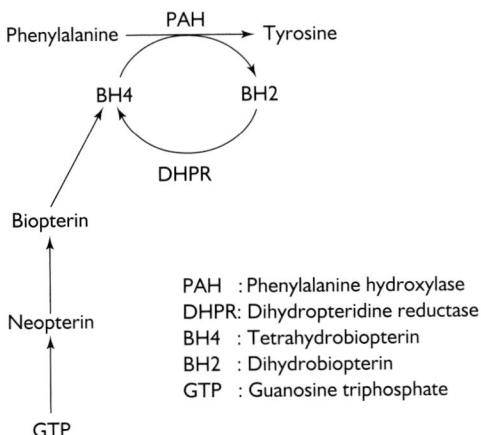

Fig. 35.20 Metabolic pathways for hyperphenylalaninaemia, which, in the classic form, is due to lack of phenylalanine hydroxylase. Rarer variants are due to defects in the tetrahydrobiopterin cofactor system.

PAH : Phenylalanine hydroxylase
DHPR: Dihydropteridine reductase
BH4 : Tetrahydrobiopterin
BH2 : Dihydrobiopterin
GTP : Guanosine triphosphate

receiving intravenous fluids at the time of the test. A false positive result may be obtained from a sick neonate on TPN. The elevation of phenylalanine will be accompanied by increases in the level of other amino acids, and in practice is not a diagnostic problem. Details of feeds should be recorded on the screening card and a further test performed when the infant has been established on a normal protein intake for 48–72 hours.

The PKU screening test identifies all babies with elevated levels of blood phenylalanine, but not all will have 'classic' PKU. Some will have mild hyperphenylalaninaemia (blood phe <500 micromol/l and will not require dietary therapy, but all should be seen in the metabolic unit for assessment. Infants with defects in the synthesis or recycling of the tetrahydrobiopterin cofactor for phenylalanine hydroxylase activity (Fig. 35.20) need to be distinguished from those with 'classic' PKU, as the low-phenylalanine diet has to be supplemented with neurotransmitter therapy in these patients. Specific enzyme assays for cofactor defects, combined with urine pterin analysis and/or tetrabiopterin loading tests, are necessary in all patients found to have raised phenylalanine on neonatal screening. It is important to remember that blood phenylalanine may only be marginally elevated in infants with cofactor disorders.

Each metabolic unit will have its own approach to the management of PKU. We recommend dietary treatment for all infants with a blood phenylalanine >400 micromol/l. The treatment of PKU (like other metabolic disorders) should be carried out only by those with substantial experience, and details of management are beyond the scope of this chapter. In principle, most of the infant's amino acid requirements are provided in synthetic form, and natural proteins are used in portions sufficient to supply the phenylalanine required for growth, leaving no excess to be broken down to tyrosine.

Screening for other IEMs now varies tremendously throughout the world. Many centres, including a number in Australasia, Japan, USA and Europe (not the UK), have introduced comprehensive metabolic screening programmes based on tandem mass spectometry. The simultaneous detection of more than 30 disorders affecting either fatty acid or amino acid metabolism is now possible. Concerns remain about this approach in the UK,

since many individuals will be detected who would have otherwise remained asymptomatic, as the natural history of a number of the conditions detected is not yet fully established.[17] A pilot screening programme for medium chain acyl-coA dehydrogenase deficiency.

Consideration of specific IEMs

Amino acid disorders (Fig. 35.21)

Maple syrup urine disease

This rare disorder usually presents towards the end of the first week of life, with vomiting and an encephalopathy characterised by drowsiness, seizures and dystonia. A maple syrup odour is often detectable and affected infants have severe ketoacidosis and are often hypoglycaemic.

Elevated levels of the branched-chain amino acids (leucine, isoleucine and valine) in blood and urine and of the corresponding 2-ketoacids in urine are characteristic. Deficiency of the branched-chain 2-ketoacid dehydrogenase complex can be demonstrated in cultured skin fibroblasts. The prognosis is directly related to the age at diagnosis[16] and recent reports suggest a very good outcome is possible with very careful treatment.[24] Very rarely the disorder occurs as a thiamine-responsive variant.

Acute hereditary tyrosinaemia (tyrosinaemia type I)

The acute neonatal form of this disorder presents with progressive liver disease (occasionally, acute hepatic necrosis) and renal tubular dysfunction. A diffuse hyperplasia of the pancreatic islet cells is seen in florid cases, and the subsequent hypoglycaemia can be resistant to treatment. Plasma tyrosine and methionine levels are raised, phosphate and potassium levels are low, and there is usually a gross generalised aminoaciduria, glycosuria and phosphaturia. The diagnosis is established by demonstrating increased urinary succinyl acetone excretion on urinary organic acid analysis. The enzyme fumarylacetoacetase is deficient when assayed in lymphocytes or fibroblasts.

The prognosis for affected infants has been revolutionised by the introduction of treatment with 2-(2-nitro-4-trifluoro-methylbenzoyl)-1,3-cyclohexanedione (NTBC). This chemical inhibits the enzyme 4-hydroxyphenylpyruvate dioxygenase and prevents the formation of maleylacetoacetate and fumarylacetoacetate, thus averting the risk of liver damage and normalising porphyrin synthesis in affected patients.[20]

Although there is a panethnic incidence, the disorder is particularly common in a French-Canadian isolate in Quebec, as well as in certain areas of Scandinavia.

Non-ketotic hyperglycinaemia (glycine encephalopathy)

This usually presents in the neonatal period, with drowsiness and lethargy, hypotonia and hypoventilation. Seizures are

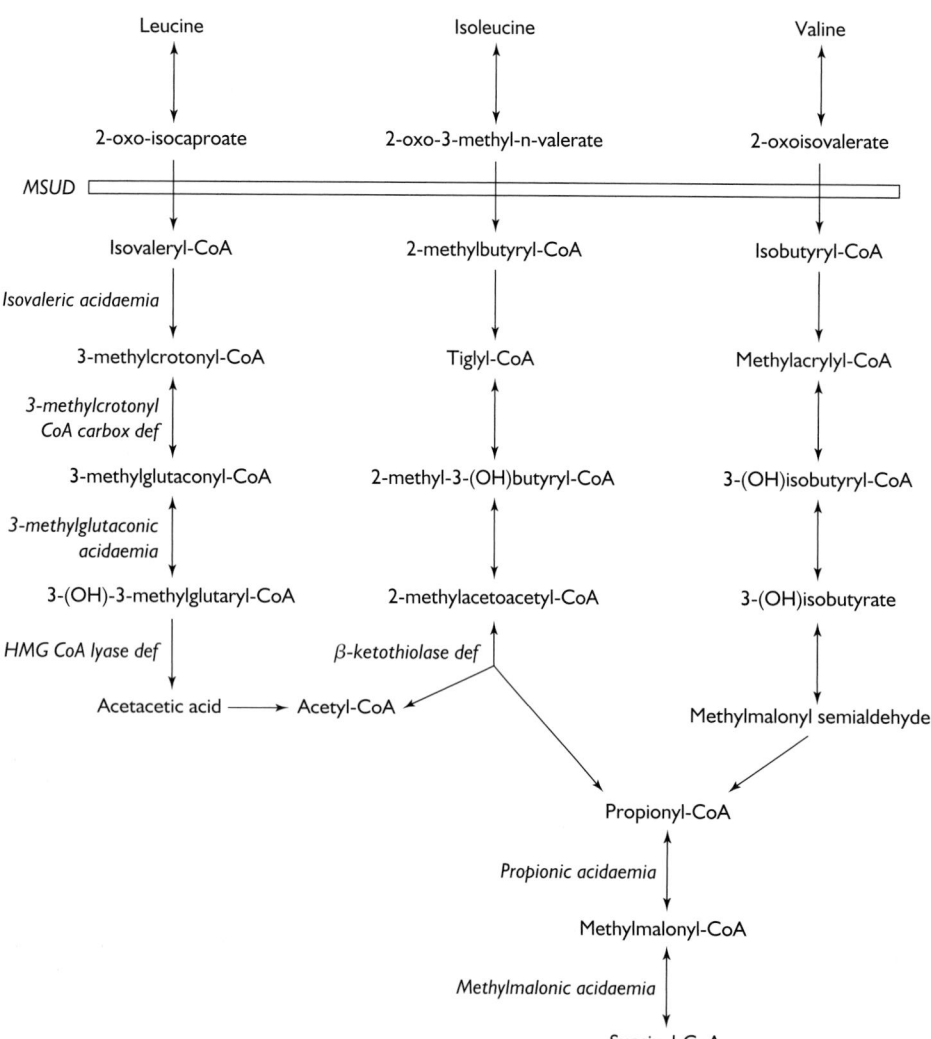

Fig. 35.21 Metabolic pathways in several important IEMs presenting in the neonatal period. The disorders (italics) are placed next to the metabolic step for which the enzyme (see text) is lacking.

prominent and are often myoclonic in nature. The EEG often shows a 'burst-suppression' pattern. Hiccuping and opisthotonus are common features. These may be present at birth and some mothers have reported reduced fetal movements in utero. In these latter cases, intracranial anomalies have been reported, and the disorder is one cause of agenesis of the corpus callosum.

Plasma glycine levels are very variable in affected patients, and can be normal. Large amounts of glycine are usually excreted in the urine, but the glycine elevation is much more marked in the CSF, reflecting the primary disturbance of neuronal glycine metabolism. Organic acids are not increased in the urine as they are in the various forms of ketotic hyperglycinaemia.

The effects of the disease are caused by the excitatory effects of glycine at the cortical NMDA receptor. Treatment that modifies the systemic levels of glycine have little effect on the disease, and specific inhibitors of glycine at the NMDA receptor, such as strychnine or tryptophan, may lead to an improvement in seizure control and hypotonia but do not usually affect the prognosis, which is very gloomy, death usually occurring in early childhood.

The basic defect is in the multicomplex glycine cleavage enzyme, and diagnosis can be confirmed on transformed lymphocytes or liver biopsy, but *not* cultured skin fibroblasts.[14]

Urea cycle disorders (Table 35.21)

The predominant clinical features of all of these conditions are similar and are a result of the accumulation of ammonia and glutamine. Presentation in the neonatal period is usually with episodes of vomiting and drowsiness, proceeding to unconsciousness and seizures. The absence of acidosis is an important point.

Once hyperammonaemia (levels above 200 micromol/l are usually due to an IEM) has been established by measurement of the blood ammonia level, the diagnosis of a primary urea cycle defect can usually be made after measuring plasma and urine amino acids and by screening the urine for organic acids and orotic acid. Hyperammonaemia secondary to an organic acidaemia will be excluded by a normal urinary organic acid profile and the absence of ketosis and metabolic acidosis.

Table 35.21 Urea cycle disorders

	CPS	OTC	ASAS	ASAL	ARG
Incidence	1:100 000	1:100 000	1:100 000	1:100 000	1:100 000
Inheritance	AR	XLR	AR	AR	AR
Enzyme deficiency	CPS	OTC	ASAS	ASAL	ARG
Mutations	2p	Xp21.1	9q34	7cen-p21	6q23
Prenatal	Fetal liver or DNA	Fetal liver or DNA	Enz-CVB	Enz-CVB	Fetal blood or DNA

CPS, carbamyl phosphate synthetase
OTC, ornithine transcarbamylase
ASAS, argininosuccinic acid synthetase (citrullinaemia)

ASAL, argininosuccinic acid lyase (argininosuccinic aciduria)
ARG, arginase (argininaemia)

In carbamyl phosphate synthetase (CPS) deficiency and ornithine transcarbamylase (OTC) deficiency, plasma ammonia levels are grossly elevated (2000–3000 micromol/l), but plasma amino acid levels are usually normal apart from elevation of glutamine. The two conditions can be differentiated by measuring urinary orotic acid, which is grossly elevated in OTC deficiency but not in CPS deficiency. Citrullinaemia, argininosuccinic aciduria and arginase deficiency all show characteristic elevations of the respective amino acids in plasma and urine.

Definitive diagnosis is obtained by measuring the individual enzymes in a liver biopsy (all defects), cultured skin fibroblasts (citrullinaemia, argininosuccinic aciduria and arginase deficiency) or erythrocytes (argininosuccinic aciduria).

Treatment of urea cycle disorders includes arginine (which becomes an essential amino acid in all but arginase deficiency) supplementation (2 ml/kg of 10% arginine HCl) and the use of alternative pathways to excrete nitrogen waste. Amino acid nitrogen may be excreted as hippuric acid if sodium benzoate (250–500 mg/kg/day) is administered, or as phenylglutamine after sodium phenylbutyrate (250–500 mg/kg/day) administration. These methods have made a great difference to the outcome of this group of patients.[3,4] Essential amino acid supplements can also be used to provide some of the nitrogen requirement.

It is important to remember that OTC deficiency is one of the X-linked IEMs. Female heterozygotes can be symptomatic in the newborn period and are often protein intolerant later in life. In this disorder, the neurological outcome is directly related to the plasma ammonia at diagnosis.[25] Carrier testing is possible by performing an allopurinol-loading test.[32] The OTC gene has been identified and a number of mutations characterised. Direct mutation analysis is playing an increasing role in both carrier detection and prenatal diagnosis in this disorder.

Transient neonatal hyperammonaemia

Plasma ammonia levels of over 1500 micromol/l have been described in a small number of comatose newborn infants who have recovered completely after very aggressive treatment, with no biochemical evidence of a specific enzyme defect in the urea cycle. These babies have subsequently tolerated a normal protein intake without any symptoms. The biochemical basis of the condition is unknown, but as it mainly occurs in preterm infants, immaturity of enzyme systems has been postulated.

Organic acid disorders (see Fig. 35.21)

Propionic acidaemia

In its acute form, this disorder presents early in the newborn period, with severe metabolic acidosis, poor feeding, vomiting and drowsiness which rapidly proceeds to coma. Hyperammonaemia and hypoglycaemia are often present. The blood ammonia may be elevated to levels similar to those seen in primary urea cycle defects.

In less severe forms, the features are poor feeding, failure to thrive and recurrent vomiting. Ketoacidosis and hyperglycinaemia are the main biochemical features, and some patients are neutropenic.

The urine contains large amounts of a wide variety of organic acids, including 3-hydroxypropionate, methylcitrate and triglycine, as well as some unusual ketone bodies. Diagnosis is suggested by a characteristic pattern of acylcarnitine metabolites on tandem mass spectrometry of a blood spot and confirmed by assay of propionyl-CoA carboxylase in white blood cells or cultured skin fibroblasts.

Long-term treatment relies upon protein restriction, alkali therapy, sodium benzoate and carnitine replacement. Because of the poor prognosis for neurological outcome in most patients on conventional therapy, liver transplantation may offer a better long-term prognosis although this is by no means certain.[19]

Methylmalonic acidaemia

The clinical features of this disorder are very similar to those of propionic acidaemia. However, it can be distinguished by the pattern of acylcarnitine metabolites, excretion of methylmalonic acid in the urine and by specific enzyme assay. Methylmalonic acidaemia can be subdivided into a number of different categories, depending on whether the defect is in the methylmalonyl-CoA mutase enzyme or in one of the steps in the formation of its cofactor adenosylcobalamin. They all present with vomiting, acidosis and neurological symptoms and they can be differentiated only by careful enzyme studies in cultured cells to distinguish defects of different steps in adenosylcobalamin synthesis as well as responsiveness to vitamin B_{12} therapy. The degree of response to vitamin B_{12} varies depending on the step in cofactor synthesis that is affected.

Hyperammonaemia can occur in any of the more severe forms of methylmalonic acidaemia, as in propionic acidaemia, although it is usually not so severe. Methylmalonic acidaemia plus homocystinuria may be seen in defects in the early steps of cobalamin cofactor biosynthesis. Long-term therapy is relatively simple and very effective in the vitamin B_{12}-responsive cases, but difficult in the remainder, in whom stringent protein restriction is required. Intercurrent infective illnesses frequently cause exacerbations of acidosis requiring intravenous therapy. Late complications such as progressive renal damage or acute infarction of the basal ganglia may occur, and liver transplantation may be a better long-term therapy.

Isovaleric acidaemia

This disorder, caused by a deficiency of the enzyme isovaleryl-CoA dehydrogenase, may present in the newborn period with vomiting and severe ketoacidosis. Affected infants are often neutropenic and thrombocytopenic during the acute episode, and the urine has a characteristic 'sweaty feet' odour owing to the excretion of isovaleric acid. Treatment with protein restriction, carnitine and glycine supplementation generally results in normal development in those infants who survive the newborn period unscathed.

Defects in carbohydrate metabolism

Galactosaemia

Infants with 'classical' galactosaemia due to deficiency of the enzyme galactose-1-phosphate uridyl transferase present towards the end of the first week of life with vomiting, failure to thrive and jaundice. Neurological symptoms are common and 30–40% develop a superadded septicaemia, usually due to *Escherichia coli* infection, which often starts as a urinary tract infection. This may be diagnosed and treated without recognising the underlying metabolic disease, especially as milk feeds are stopped during the treatment of this acute illness. Recurrence of symptoms when milk is reintroduced may alert the neonatologist to the principal diagnosis. Hepatomegaly is always present and the clinical course is dominated by the progressive liver damage. Cataracts may appear even in the first week, and there may be early evidence of renal damage, with proteinuria and aminoaciduria.

The diagnosis may be suspected by the urinary excretion of galactose and is readily confirmed by measurement of erythrocyte galactose-1-phosphate uridyl transferase. If the infant has had a prior blood transfusion, enzyme analysis is unreliable and diagnosis is achieved by measuring galactose-1-phosphate levels in blood.

Long-term treatment is with a milk-free diet. Cataracts regress and the liver heals, but the intellectual outcome remains poor, with most affected adults having IQ scores of 60–80. There is often a specific speech delay, and a cerebellar syndrome

with ataxia becomes prominent in some affected adults. Ovarian failure occurs in at least 80% of affected female patients and is not related to delays in postnatal treatment. An effect on fetal ovarian development has been postulated.

Fructose-1,6-bisphosphatase deficiency

This disorder may present in the newborn period with severe lactic acidosis. Affected infants hyperventilate, are often hypoglycaemic and can deteriorate rapidly with apnoea and death. Later episodes in survivors are often triggered by intercurrent fasting or infections. Gluconeogenesis is severely impaired and hypoglycaemia is prominent, with the accumulation of gluconeogenic precursors such as lactate, amino acids and ketones. Unlike hereditary fructose intolerance, patients do not vomit after the ingestion of fructose and an aversion to sweets does not develop. The diagnosis can be established on white blood cell enzyme assay. A fructose tolerance test is not necessary.

Glycogen storage disease (GSD) type I

All variants of GSD type I (e.g. GSD Ia and Ib) can present in the newborn period with profound hypoglycaemia. In addition there is lactic acidosis, hyperuricaemia and hyperlipidaemia. Hepatomegaly is usually obvious, but the very soft liver in GSD I may be difficult to define by palpation. The diagnosis is usually established by enzyme assay (glucose-6-phosphatase) performed on a liver biopsy sample and mutation analysis is also becoming more widely available. Treatment is aimed at maintaining normoglycaemia with frequent daytime feeds and continuous nocturnal intragastric infusion of glucose. Patients with type Ib disease also suffer from chronic neutropenia and functional deficiencies of neutrophils and monocytes, which requires therapy with granulocyte colony-stimulating factor to restore myeloid function.[10]

Primary disorders of pyruvate metabolism

All the primary disorders of pyruvate metabolism are associated with lactic acidosis and all have similar clinical features, with profound peripheral circulatory disturbance and severe neurological abnormalities. Pyruvate dehydrogenase deficiency deserves special mention.

Pyruvate dehydrogenase deficiency

Pyruvate dehydrogenase, a multienzyme complex, is a major metabolic control point in the aerobic oxidation of carbohydrates and some gluconeogenic amino acids. The action of pyruvate dehydrogenase is controlled by a specific kinase (inactivation) and phosphorylase (activation), which are tightly regulated in response to metabolite concentrations within the mitochondrion. The enzyme complex itself comprises three main enzymes, E1 or pyruvate decarboxylase (with α and β subunits), E2 or lipoyl transacetylase, and E3, a dihydrolipoyl-dehydrogenase. Defects in all three main components have been described, and early presentation is generally with severe acidosis or with profound neurological deficit in a baby with minimal or no acidosis (often with structural brain lesions, 'cerebral lactic acidosis'). Milder cases may present later, with intermittent ataxia or acidosis.

Deficiency of the E1 α-subunit (the subunit which is subject to most of the acute metabolic controls over enzyme activity) is the most frequent defect. The gene for this subunit is on the short arm of the X chromosome. Both hemizygous males and heterozygous females are affected, nearly all cases being the result of new mutations. The patients with the 'cerebral' form are females with severe enzyme lesions which destroy patches of the brain in which the mutant gene is active. Males predominate among those with early severe acidosis, and usually have an incomplete enzyme deficiency.

Patients with E3 deficiency may excrete large amounts of 2-ketoglutarate and branched-chain 2-ketoacids in addition to lactate, as this component appears to be common to all 2-ketoacid dehydrogenase complexes.

Patients with these defects deteriorate when given a high glucose intake, and prompt recognition is therefore important. It is very difficult to give the high-lipid, high-protein, low-carbohydrate regimens that in theory would be best for these patients. Occasional patients have been described who respond to large doses of thiamine, but there is no way of differentiating these patients clinically or biochemically from those with unresponsive forms.[38] Lactic acidosis presents a very complex set of problems. The first difficulty arises in diagnosis in an acutely ill newborn infant. Primary lactic acidosis can cause the very effects (vasoconstriction, convulsions, severe acidosis) that can cause secondary lactic acidosis when present for other reasons. The matter is further complicated by the existence of some disorders leading to lactic acidosis which require treatment with carbohydrate supplementation (e.g. fructose 1,6-bisphosphatase deficiency and some other gluconeogenic defects), and others which are made worse by this regimen (e.g. pyruvate dehydrogenase deficiency and some other mitochondrial disorders). The presence of structural CNS defects makes the latter group more likely, but often one has to gamble. As the gluconeogenic defects generally have the better prognosis, it is usually preferable to err on the side of carbohydrate supplementation in practice, especially as the profound hypoglycaemia which can occur in these disorders can cause severe brain damage.

In all forms of severe lactic acidosis, muscle paralysis and ventilatory support have a specific role in reducing muscle lactate production and, as with other IEMs that can affect the brain, ventilatory support should be considered early, especially in infants with significant (pH < 7.1) or persistent metabolic acidosis.

Fatty acid oxidation defects

A number of defects in fatty acid oxidation have been identified. Some prevent uptake of fatty acids into the mitochondria and others affect specific steps in the β-oxidation within the mitochondria. These enzymes have specificity based on the length of the fatty acid carbon chain. All can present in the newborn period and can commonly present with life-threatening or fatal illness. Deficiency of medium-chain fatty acyl-CoA dehydrogenase (MCAD) is the most frequently recognised. Diagnosis in this disorder has been considerably simplified by the finding of a common genetic mutation, which accounts for nearly 90% of mutant chromosomes in the Caucasian population. This disorder usually presents with hypoketotic hypoglycaemia between the ages of 3 and 18 months, although neonatal presentation is now well recognised.[39] Our ability to diagnose disorders of fat oxidation has been considerably enhanced by the introduction of acylcarnitine analysis by tandem mass spectrometry.

One other serious presentation of this group of disorders is with hypertrophic cardiomyopathy, which can cause heart failure or cardiorespiratory arrest in the newborn period. This occurs in multiple acyl-CoA dehydrogenase deficiency (glutaric aciduria type II), long-chain fatty acyl-CoA dehydrogenase deficiency, 3-hydroxyacyl-CoA dehydrogenase deficiency and the primary disorders of carnitine metabolism.[33] As mentioned earlier, these disorders, when present in the fetus, can be associated with severe maternal disease during pregnancy.

Diagnosis of defects in fatty acid metabolism relies on a combination of biochemical abnormalities, which may include evidence of liver disease (raised transaminases, hyperammonaemia) and muscle disease (raised CPK). A characteristic pattern of blood acylcarnitine metabolites and abnormal urinary organic acid profiles is usually enough to clinch the diagnosis. Specific enzyme assays on cultured skin fibroblasts are a difficult and specialised investigation and are not readily available. Decreased rates of catabolism of radiolabelled fatty acid substrates can be used to demonstrate a defect somewhere in the β-oxidation pathway, and can be helpful when interpreted with the clinical presentation and supporting biochemical abnormalities.

Disorders of subcellular organelles

Mitochondrial disease

Mitochondria are unique among cytoplasmic organelles as they contain their own genetic material. The mitochondrial genome is a circular DNA molecule of approximately 16 500 base pairs which encodes some (but not all) of the polypeptides of the respiratory transport chain and some other components of mitochondrial transcription and translation (22 transfer RNAs and two ribosomal RNAs). There are multiple copies of mitochondrial DNA (mtDNA) in each mitochondrion and many mitochondria in each cell, so that each cell contains several thousand mtDNA molecules. The phenotype and rate of progression of mitochondrial disorders appears to be determined by the proportion and segregation of abnormal mtDNA molecules at cell division, combined with a 'threshold effect' in various tissues, depending on energy requirements and functional reserve. Brain and muscle appear to be most sensitive to mitochondrial dysfunction.

The other major characteristic of mtDNA is that it is transmitted between generations only by the mother, probably because at fertilisation only the head of the sperm enters the egg and the mitochondria in the rest of the sperm are lost. Maternal inheritance patterns are seen in those disorders where there is a primary mtDNA mutation responsible for the disease.

Clinical features are extremely variable and the diagnosis should be suspected in infants where there is multiple organ involvement. Lactic acidosis is usual and there may be abnormalities on routine haematological and biochemical analyses, depending on the main target organs affected. Specific biochemical

Table 35.22 Peroxisomal disorders

	Zellweger	RCDP	NALD/INF.REF.
Incidence	1: 50 000	1:100 000	Very rare
Inheritance	AR	AR	AR
Enzyme deficiency	Membrane protein	Import protein	Membrane protein
Mutation data	8q21.1	?	?
Diagnosis	VLCFA/DHAP-AT	As Zellweger	As Zellweger
Initial treatment	None	None	None
Long-term treatment	None	None	None

RCDP, rhizomelic chondrodysplasia punctata; NALD, neonatal adrenoleukodystrophy; INF.REF., infantile Refsum's disease.

investigation will include assay of respiratory transport chain activity on muscle biopsy material. Histological changes in muscle tissue can be important, and the characteristic pathological finding in patients with many forms of mitochondrial disease is the 'ragged red fibre' on staining with Gomori trichrome. The clinical presentation of these disorders in childhood has recently been reviewed.[6]

In a number of mitochondrial disorders, underlying or associated genetic changes have been defined in mtDNA. These include large structural rearrangements (deletions and duplications) and point mutations. When present, these are a highly specific and sensitive addition to the biochemical investigations.

Peroxisomal disorders (Table 35.22)

These disorders present in the neonatal period and are all disorders of peroxisomal biogenesis or peroxisomal protein transportation. Not all defects have been fully categorised and there are a number of different complementation groups described. Single peroxisomal enzyme defects have been described and some can present neonatally.[5]

There are over 20 different peroxisomal disorders, caused by an impairment of one or more peroxisomal functions. The more profound and complex disorders of peroxisomal biogenesis or of multiple peroxisomal enzyme deficiency present in the newborn period with severe neurological abnormalities plus various other features, including abnormal facies and body build, cataracts, punctate epiphyseal calcification, liver fibrosis, renal cysts, and adrenal or hepatic failure. Increased levels of very-long-chain fatty acids (VLCFA, C26+) in plasma and/or deficiency of dihydroacetone phosphate acyl transferase (DHAP-AT) are useful biochemical markers. The absence of peroxisomes on liver histology is typical of Zellweger syndrome. There is no effective treatment, but prenatal diagnosis is possible.

Lysosomal disorders

The lysosomal disorders are conditions in which a defective lysosomal enzyme leads to the accumulation of specific substrates within the cell which eventually interfere with normal cellular function. The disorders are progressive and usually present in childhood or later, but some can produce dramatic neonatal presentation, usually in such cases with hydrops fetalis as a prominent feature. Diagnosis is established by enzyme assay on white blood cells or cultured skin fibroblasts. The neonatal presentation of these disorders has recently been reviewed.[40]

Miscellaneous disorders

Congenital disorders of glycosylation

This newly described group of metabolic disorders is characterised by a deficiency in the carbohydrate moiety of secretory glycoproteins, including a characteristic change in transferrin, which can be used as a diagnostic test. A number of variants have been described, including a type that can produce severe neonatal disease.[18]

During the first 24 hours of life, many infants with CDG feed poorly and are often floppy and hypothermic. Birthweight is usually normal, but a variable dysmorphism is often present, including abnormalities of the skin (*peau d'orange*) or subcutaneous tissue (fat pads). A number of serious complications can develop, including pericardial effusion and liver dysfunction. Failure to thrive and psychomotor delay are usual.

Menkes disease

Most babies with this X-linked recessive disease have difficulty in maintaining body temperature in the neonatal period, but few are diagnosed at this stage. Most are diagnosed at 2–4 months because of poor development, seizures and abnormal 'steely' hair. Low plasma levels of copper confirm the diagnosis.

The basic defect is in copper transport across the intestinal mucosa and in body cells. Parenteral copper therapy improves copper enzyme levels, but has little effect on development. Treatment after symptomatic diagnosis can only prolong existence with severe brain damage.

Inherited disorders of cholesterol biosynthesis

Cholesterol plays a crucial role in fetal development, and a number of inherited disorders of cholesterol biosynthesis show that low cholesterol levels may have severe consequences for human development. At least seven different defects linked to the cholesterol biosynthetic pathway have been described, the most common of which is the Smith–Lemli–Opitz syndrome (SLO).[37]

SLO had been recognised as a 'dysmorphic syndrome' for many years prior to the identification of the defect in cholesterol metabolism responsible for the clinical phenotype. Affected patients have characteristic craniofacial features, cleft palate, hypospadias, postaxial polydactyly and toe syndactyly. A number of biochemical abnormalities were known to be associated with the syndrome, including a very low plasma cholesterol level. Further investigation led to the finding of grossly elevated 7-dehydrocholesterol levels in the plasma of affected children, and this is now the basis of the biochemical confirmation of this disorder. This compound is the immediate precursor in the cholesterol biosynthetic pathway. A deficiency of the enzyme 3β-hydroxysterol Δ7-reductase has been shown to be the primary genetic lesion in affected infants. Treatment with bile acid supplementation and a high cholesterol diet has been attempted in a number of patients, but it is too early to say whether this will be of benefit.[26]

References

1. Bamforth F J 1994 Laboratory screening for genetic disorders and birth defects. Clinical Biochemistry 27: 333–342
2. Bankier A, Turner M, Hopkins I J 1983 Pyridoxine-dependent seizures – a wider clinical spectrum. Archives of Disease in Childhood 58: 415–418
3. Batshaw M L, Brusilow S W, Danney M et al 1984 Treatment of episodic hyperammonemia in children with inborn errors of urea synthesis. New England Journal of Medicine 310: 1630–1634
4. Batshaw M L Brusilow S, Waber L et al 1982 Treatment of inborn errors of urea synthesis. Activation of alternative pathways of waste nitrogen synthesis and excretion. New England Journal of Medicine 306: 1387–1392
5. Baumgartner M R, Saudubray J M 2002 Peroxisomal disorders. Seminars in Neonatology 7: 85–94
6. Borchert A, Wolf N I, Wilichowski E 2002 Current concepts of mitochondrial disorders in childhood. Seminars in Pediatric Neurology 9: 151–159
7. Brown R M, Dahl H H, Brown G K 1989 X-chromosome localization of the functional gene for the E1α subunit of the human pyruvate dehydrogenase complex. Genomics 4: 174–181
8. Chakrapani A, Olpin S, Cleary M, Walter J H, Wraith J E, Besley G T 2000 Trifunctional protein deficiency: three families with significant maternal hepatic dysfunction in pregnancy not associated with E474Q mutation. Journal of Inherited Metabolic Disease 23: 826–834
9. Chakrapani A, Wraith J E 2002 Principles of management of the more common metabolic disorders. Current Paediatrics 12: 117–124
10. Chou J Y, Matern D, Mansfield B C, Chen Y T 2002 Type I glycogen storage diseases: disorders of the glucose-6-phosphatase complex. Current Molecular Medicine 2: 121–143
11. Danks D M 1974 Management of newborn babies in whom serious metabolic disease is anticipated. Archives of Disease in Childhood 49: 576–578
12. Gabow P A, Kaeburg W D, Fennessey P V et al 1980 Diagnostic importance of an increased anion gap. New England Journal of Medicine 330: 854–858
13. Goutieres F, Aicardi J 1985 Atypical presentation of pyridoxine-dependent seizures: a treatable cause of intractable epilepsy in infants. Neurology 17: 117–120
14. Hayasaka K, Tada K, Fueki N et al 1987 Non-ketotic hyperglycinaemia: analysis of glycine cleavage system in typical and atypical cases. Journal of Pediatrics 110: 873–877
15. Jones P, Bennett M 2002 The changing face of newborn screening: diagnosis of inborn errors of metabolism by tandem mass spectrometry. Clinica Chimica Acta 324: 121–128
16. Kaplan P, Mazur A, Field M et al 1991 Intellectual outcome in children with maple syrup urine disease. Journal of Pediatrics 119: 46–50
17. Leonard J V, Dezateux C 2002 Screening for inherited metabolic disease in newborn infants using tandem mass spectrometry. British Medical Journal 324: 4–5
18. Leonard J, Grunewald S, Clayton P 2001 Diversity of congenital disorders of glycosylation. Lancet 357: 1382–1383
19. Leonard J V, Walter J H, McKiernan P J 2001 The management of organic acidaemias: the role of transplantation. Journal of Inherited Metabolic Disease 24: 309–311
20. Lindstedt S, Holme E, Lock E A et al 1992 Treatment of hereditary tyrosinaemia type I by inhibition of 4-hydroxyphenylpyruvate dioxygenase. Lancet 340: 813–817
21. Marsden D, Barshop B A, Capistrano-Estrada et al 1994 Anabolic effect of human growth hormone: management of inherited disorders of catabolic pathways. Biochemical Medicine, Metabolism and Biology 52: 145–154
22. Matern D, Hart P, Murtha A P et al 2001 Acute fatty liver of pregnancy associated with short chain acyl coenzyme A dehydrogenase deficiency. Journal of Pediatrics 138: 585–588
23. Minns R 1980 Vitamin B6 deficiency and dependency. Developmental Medicine and Child Neurology 22: 795–799
24. Morton D H, Strauss K A, Robinson D L, Puffenberger E G, Kelley R I 2002 Diagnosis and treatment of maple syrup urine disease. Pediatrics 109: 999–1008
25. Nicolaides P, Liebsch D, Dale N, Leonard J, Surtees R 2002 Neurological outcome of patients with ornithine carbamyltransferase deficiency. Archives of Disease in Childhood 86: 54–56
26. Nwokoro N A, Mulvihill J J 1997 Cholesterol and bile acid replacement therapy in children and adults with Smith-Lemli-Opitz (SLO/RSH) syndrome. American Journal of Medical Genetics 68: 315–321
27. Ogier de Baulny H 2002 Management and emergency treatments of neonates with a suspicion of inborn errors of metabolism. Seminars in Neonatology 7: 17–26
28. Perry T L 1981 Autopsy investigation of disorders of amino acid metabolism. In: Barson A J (ed) Laboratory investigation of fetal disease. Wright, Bristol, pp 429–451
29. Rakheja D, Bennett M J, Rogers B B 2002 Long chain L-3-hydroxyacyl-coenzyme A dehydrogenase deficiency: a molecular and biochemical review. Laboratory Investigation 82: 815–824
30. Saudubray J M, Nassogne M C, de Lonlay P, Touati G 2002 Clinical approach to inherited metabolic disorders in neonates: an overview. Seminars in Neonatology 7: 3–15
31. Scriver C R, Beaudet A L, Sly W S, Valle D (eds) 2001 The metabolic and molecular bases of inherited disease. McGraw-Hill, New York
32. Sebesta I, Fairbanks L D, Davies P M et al 1994 The allopurinol loading test for identification of carriers for ornithine carbamoyl transferase deficiency: studies in a healthy control population and females at risk. Clinica Chimica Acta 224: 45–54
33. Servidei S, Bertini E, DiMauro S 1994 Hereditary metabolic cardiomyopathies. Advances in Pediatrics 41: 1–32
34. Starfield B, Holtzman N A 1975 A comparison of screening for phenylketonuria in the United States, United Kingdom and Ireland. New England Journal of Medicine 293: 118–121
35. Sweetman L 1996 Newborn screening by tandem mass spectrometry (MS-MS). Clinical Chemistry 42: 345–346
36. Walter J H 2002 Investigation and initial management of suspected metabolic disease. Current Paediatrics 12: 110–116
37. Waterham H R 2002 Inherited disorders of cholesterol biosynthesis. Clinical Genetics 61: 393–403
38. Wick H, Schweizer K, Baumgartner R 1977 Thiamine dependency in a patient with congenital lactic acidaemia due to pyruvate dehydrogenase deficiency. Agents and Actions 7: 405–410
39. Wilcken B, Carpenter K H, Hammond J 1993 Neonatal symptoms in medium chain acyl coenzyme A dehydrogenase deficiency. Archives of Disease in Childhood 69: 292–294
40. Wraith J E 2002 Lysosomal disorders. Seminars in Neonatology 7: 75–83

PART 4

Metabolic bone disease

Nick Bishop

Background

The majority of neonatal metabolic bone disease is seen in infants born prematurely, and is due largely to substrate deficiency. Additional adverse effects on the skeleton may result from administration of steroids (suppression of bone turnover), diuretics and immobilisation. The effects on bone of inflammatory cytokines such as tumour necrosis factor-α and interleukin-6, which are produced during intercurrent illness and increase bone resorption in children and adults, have not been investigated in this population.

Diagnostic criteria vary considerably between centres, leading to estimates of incidence that range from 32% to 92%.[7,35,45]

Diagnosing metabolic bone disease in preterm infants

Bone disease in preterm infants is characterised in the short term by a sequence of events which begins with biochemical evidence of disturbed mineral metabolism,[1,8,9,34,42,44,60,65] continues with reduced bone mineralisation,[11,32,36,69,70,75] and results in abnormal bone remodelling[21] and reduced linear growth velocity.[42] In extreme forms, fractures of ribs and the distal ends of long bones[39] and craniotabes have been reported.[21,45] The progression of radiological changes is most clearly recorded in the literature prior to the introduction of formula and breast-milk supplementation, in particular in the work of Eek & Gabrielson.[21]

In the longer term, height may be reduced,[42] there is a trend towards earlier presentation with fracture (excluding non-accidental injury cases),[15] and bone mineral accretion,[4] bone turnover and height in later childhood may also be influenced.[23–25]

Aetiology

Disturbed mineral metabolism in the neonatal period

Calcium and phosphate

Whole blood ionised calcium falls within 18–24 hours of delivery. This is a physiological rather than pathological event, reflecting continued calcium accretion into bone in the face of reduced exogenous calcium input, and a postnatal surge in calcitonin production of unknown aetiology.[58] In term infants, symptomatic neonatal hypocalcaemia may reflect maternal vitamin D insufficiency.[16] The initial manifestation of disturbed mineral metabolism in the premature infant is hypophosphataemia.[8,60] Plasma phosphate falls below 1.0 mmol/l at between 7 and 14 days of age and is accompanied by hypophosphaturia, with tubular reabsorption of phosphorus, typically >90%.[1,65] Where persistent phosphate wasting is observed, investigations for renal tubular problems should be undertaken.

In phosphate-depleted infants, both hypercalcaemia (plasma calcium >2.7 mmol/l) and hypercalciuria are frequently observed.[9,44] These changes may also occur secondary to immobilisation.

Phosphate depletion can be monitored by serial urinary calcium:phosphate ratios.[64] This test can be performed on a spot sample (ideally immediately pre-feed) and should be <1 by age 3 weeks if the infant is phosphate-replete (calcium and phosphate both measured in mmol/l).

Lucas et al,[42] in a prospective study of 857 preterm infants fed different diets, could not demonstrate a relationship between initial or later linear growth and plasma phosphate, after adjusting for the effects of diet and plasma alkaline phosphatase activity. Ryan and colleagues[59] found a weak negative correlation of serum phosphate concentrations with forearm bone mineral content.

Bone turnover

There are now available a range of assays for assessing bone turnover (Table 35.23 and Table 35.24). It is important to remember that the values obtained reflect the summation of both bone modelling – bone formation from the calcified cartilage of the growth plate and the combined effects of periosteal apposition and endosteal resorption – and remodelling activity which results from the resorption of discrete packets of bone and new bone formation at the same site.

In general, the studies show a period of increased bone turnover in the initial weeks after birth, followed by a period of stability and then a subsequent decline.[13] Crofton et al also looked at the effects of steroids: dexamethasone suppressed bone activity (both formation and resorption) in a dose-dependent manner in keeping with results at later ages.[14] Further follow-up is required to examine whether there are any longer-term consequences of early steroid exposure (either pre- or postnatally) for bone growth or turnover.

Of the available markers, only plasma (tissue non-specific) alkaline phosphatase is routinely measured in neonatal units and so has been the subject of many reports of bone health in infants born prematurely, including long-term follow-up studies.

Table 35.23 Bone turnover markers

Formation	Measures	Resorption	Measures
Alkaline phosphatase (ALP)	New bone formation and/or rate of mineralisation	Cross-linked N-telopeptide of type I collagen (NTx)	Rate of bone type I collagen breakdown
N-terminal propeptide of type I collagen (PINP)	Rate of type I collagen incorporation into matrix	Cross-linked C-telopeptide of type I collagen (CTx)	Rate of bone type I collagen breakdown
C-terminal propeptide of type I collagen (PICP)	Rate of type I collagen incorporation into matrix	TRAP-5b	Number of osteoclasts
Osteocalcin	New bone formation	Type I collagen C-terminal telopeptide (ICTP)	Rate of type I collagen breakdown
		Pyridinoline	Rate of type I collagen breakdown (non-specific)
		Deoxypyridinoline	Rate of type I collagen breakdown
		Hydroxyproline	Rate of type I collagen breakdown (non-specific)

Table 35.24 Summary of change in markers over time in infants born prematurely

	0–4 weeks	4–10 weeks 'poor' diet	4–10 weeks 'good' diet	>10 weeks
Formation	↑*↓°	↑#	→/↑† then ↓	↓
Resorption	↑↓†	No data	→/↑ then ↓†	↓

* Seki et al.[63]
° Bhandari et al.[3]
Gross,[34] Lucas et al,[42] Michaelsen et al.[48]
† Crofton et al.[13]

Plasma alkaline phosphatase activity typically rises over the first 3 weeks of postnatal life to levels two- to threefold greater than the maximum of the adult normal range. Activity increases further (from age 5–6 weeks) in infants who receive diets low in mineral substrate compared with those who receive diets with increased mineral content.[34,42] In the short term, plasma alkaline phosphatase activity greater than five times the maximum of the adult normal range is associated with progressive slowing of linear growth velocity.[42] In the longer term (18 months and 9–12 years), such levels are associated with reduced height.[23]

Vitamin D and its metabolites

Where routine supplementation of door-step milk and cereals is practised, cord blood levels of 25-hydroxyvitamin D_3 are typically >20 nmol/l, indicating vitamin D sufficiency. In the UK, some yellow margarines and breakfast cereals are supplemented; dairy products are not. Maternal supplementation with vitamin D results in higher cord blood levels of 25-hydroxyvitamin D, but not 1,25-dihydroxyvitamin D.[16] Where maternal vitamin D intake during pregnancy has been poor, or where there is pre-existing maternal vitamin D deficiency, neonatal vitamin D stores may be low, and supplemental vitamin D of more than the normal 400 IU/day may be required. South Asian children living in the UK are at particular risk of vitamin D insufficiency.[41,53] Insufficiency tends to be familial, and parents and other siblings should be tested (plasma 25-hydroxyvitamin D, parathyroid hormone [PTH]) if a neonate presents with features of insufficiency.

A number of studies have identified low/borderline plasma 25-hydroxyvitamin D and elevated 1,25-dihydroxyvitamin D levels in plasma of preterm infants fed unsupplemented human milk,[33,62] suggesting an increased requirement for vitamin D during rapid bone turnover in phosphate-depleted infants. Many studies indicate that vitamin D supplementation does improve calcium absorption and retention, although the magnitude of this improvement is variable, possibly reflecting mineral as well as vitamin D status. There are no data indicating improved long-term outcome for infants receiving higher doses of vitamin D (>1000 IU/day). There is no good evidence suggesting frank vitamin D deficiency in the majority of preterm infants.

Reduced or static bone mineral accretion

Bone is composed of two elements, matrix and mineral. The commonly used methods of measuring bone mass utilise the attenuation of one or more X-ray beams. The values obtained reflect both total amount of bone material and the degree of its mineralisation.

Most of the published literature up to the early 1990s reported data obtained using single photon absorptiometry (SPA) measuring principally cortical bone at an appendicular site such as the distal forearm. Since the advent of dual energy X-ray absorptiometry (DXA), which measures total and regional body bone mineral and which can also estimate total body lean and fat mass, SPA has been less often used. Both SPA and DXA are 'areal' techniques that reduce a three-dimensional quantity to two dimensions (volume becomes area). Both therefore measure bone mass rather than bone density. The effects of body (and bone) size must be considered, since an areal technique gives a greater value for the same true volumetric density in larger bones. Neither technique gives any indication of cortical thickness (relevant when considering fracture risk, particularly post discharge).

The estimation of bone mineral content (BMC) in both term and premature infants has been reported from many centres but remains largely a research technique. The studies undertaken of mineralised bone mass accretion, irrespective of the technique used, have shown lower values than those expected had the infant remained in utero.[11,32,36,69,75] In general terms, healthy preterm infants who receive cow's milk-based diets supplemented with large amounts of calcium and phosphorus show improved mineral accretion that approaches the in-utero accretion rate.[11,32,36,69,75,77] However, many studies do not relate BMC to body size; it remains unclear whether low BMC reflects the infants' smaller body and bone size, or true under-mineralisation. Growth-retarded infants may have low BMC compared to appropriate-for-gestational-age (AGA infants), although the differences frequently disappear when BMC is related to body size rather than gestation.[50] There have been no reports of reduced mineral accretion during the period of initial hospitalisation being predictive of later outcomes such as growth, fracture risk, later mineral accretion or skeletal homeostasis.

Radiological changes

Radiological abnormalities are occasionally seen at birth in very growth-retarded infants, often in association with severe maternal malnutrition, including celiac disease.[40] The majority of infants developing radiological abnormalities (Fig. 35.22) (rachitic changes, cortical thinning, periosteal elevation, fractures) either weigh <1000 g at birth, or receive diets grossly deficient in mineral substrate (<1 mmol/kg/day of calcium and phosphate).

Koo et al, in 1982, described a scoring system based on single-view radiographs of the wrist or ankle at postnatal ages 5 and 10 weeks.[38] Lyon and colleagues found that over 70% of infants weighing less than 1000 g had evidence of abnormal remodelling using this system.[45] In older reports, metaphyseal cupping, splaying and fraying, and craniotabes were observed in half of all infants born before 33 weeks' gestation. Fractures of the ribs and long bones were also widely reported[21,73,76] along with periosteal double contours, presumably reflecting the periosteal deposition of unmineralised osteoid. A recent review of 262 cases of fractures in infancy referred for the exclusion of osteogenesis imperfecta

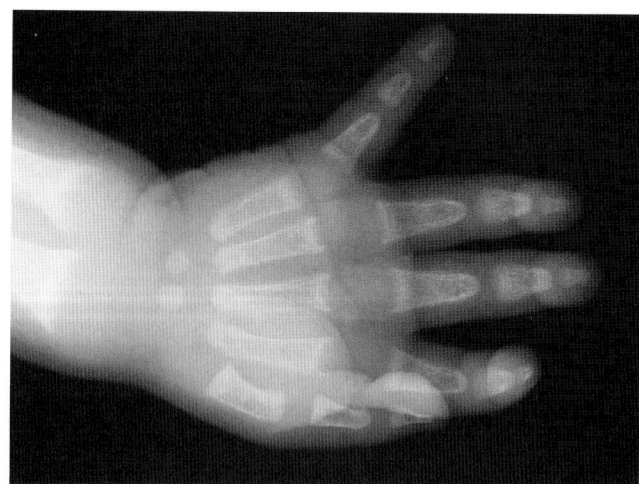

Fig. 35.22 X-ray of an ex-preterm infant showing rachitic changes.

(OI) to a centre in Seattle identified a higher than expected proportion of infants born prematurely amongst the referral population.[46]

Effects of drugs and immobilisation

Steroids reduce bone turnover (vide supra) and reduce linear growth. Oral steroid use clearly causes osteoporosis in adults but this effect has not been clearly shown in preterm infants; the difficulties of interpreting the confounding effects of steroids on growth, bone size and bone mass have prevented a clear picture emerging. Furosemide (frusemide) causes hypercalciuria, but without a clear effect on growth or mineral homeostasis. Steroids and furosemide (frusemide) together have been reported to cause nephrocalcinosis; immobilisation in infants receiving such treatment is likely to exacerbate this problem.[22]

Immobilisation leads to disuse osteoporosis in older children and adults. Moyer-Mileur et al showed a substantial gain in forearm BMC in infants undergoing up to 10 minutes of passive exercise per day over a 4-week period compared with matched controls.[51,52] A recent review by Rauch and Schönau explored the contribution of lack of mechanical stimulation to the changes observed in infants born prematurely.[57]

Treatment – prevention is better than cure

The objectives of treatment are:

- prevention of abnormal bone-remodelling activity during the period of hospitalisation;
- optimisation of growth potential, including effects on bone size and mass.

The principal aetiological factor remains inadequate mineral supply and therapeutic strategies are suggested with this in mind.

Organic phosphate solutions (sodium glycerophosphate, glucose-1-phosphate) are available. In combination with inorganic calcium solutions, these could provide adequate mineral substrate even before intravenous feeding is started.

All enterally fed preterm infants should receive 2 mmol/kg/day of phosphate. Phosphate retention is of the order of 90–95%. For the infant receiving human milk, with a typical phosphate content of 0.5 mmol/100 ml, this means a total daily supplement when on full feeds, of 1 mmol/kg/day of phosphate.

For infants receiving preterm formula, no further supplements should be necessary. Term formula is not an acceptable diet for preterm infants.[43] In practical terms it seems reasonable to start oral phosphate supplements when oral intake is ⩾ 2 ml/h.

Once phosphate supplementation is adequate, a relative deficiency of calcium may become evident.[64] Such a deficiency is evidenced by radiological osteopenia and high plasma alkaline phosphatase activity in the face of normal plasma phosphate (i.e. >1.8 mmol/l). Calcium supplementation is then warranted.

If both calcium and phosphate are being added to human milk, the phosphate should be added first and allowed to stand for at least 5 minutes, and then the calcium added subsequently; co-precipitation is kept to a minimum by this method.

There is no place for the use of active metabolites of vitamin D, other than the treatment of rare inherited disorders (see below).

All infants should receive 400 IU/day of vitamin D. It is not at all clear that supplements beyond this amount are associated with improved long-term outcome, but growth is certainly slower in unsupplemented term infants. Some authors believe that 1000 IU/day of vitamin D is needed for the more immature infants and there is no indication from the literature that this is an excessive or unsafe dose.

Passive physical exercise substantially improves weight gain and bone mineral accretion in preterm infants and should be considered a routine part of care in the prevention of immobilisation-induced bone loss.

Monitoring and adjusting treatment in affected infants

Most infants will have a weekly biochemical profile during their period in the NICU. Senterre & Salle[66] suggested the use of a random calcium:phosphate urine sample at age 3 weeks to identify infants who were becoming phosphate-depleted. Expressing both measurements as mmol, the ratio should be less than one in phosphate-replete infants. Later (from age 4 weeks onwards), persistently elevated serum alkaline phosphatase activity (more than three times the upper limit of the adult normal range) should lead the clinician to suspect metabolic bone disease. In each case, the remedy is the same – consider first the intake of mineral substrates and adjust the intake accordingly. In older infants, hypercalciuria has been reported in association with radiographic osteopenia. For these infants, an element of immobilisation may be contributing to their bone disease and gentle passive physiotherapy should be given if it is not already part of routine care.

There is no evidence for the use of vitamin D in high doses or by the intramuscular route being an effective intervention in any of these situations.

Inherited metabolic bone disease

Rachitic disorders

The three principal inherited types of rickets rarely present in the neonatal period, but clinical suspicion may indicate investigation where there is a relevant family history.

Familial hypophosphatemic rickets (XLH)

True familial hypophosphatemic rickets is an X-linked dominant condition characterised by renal phosphate wasting and a defective osteoblastic response to vitamin D metabolites.[17–19] There are a few reported cases with autosomal recessive inheritance. Clinical neonatal manifestations are unusual; investigations in affected infants show hypophosphataemia, elevated plasma calcitriol and hyperphosphaturia. Treatment with oral phosphate and calcitriol is not usually tolerated until age 3 months, at which stage the diagnosis can usually be substantiated; a fasting phosphate estimation is required to demonstrate hypophosphatemia.[49] The protein product of the affected gene (PHEX) is thought to act as an endopeptidase, cleaving phosphaturic substrates. FGF-23 has been identified as a putative substrate; in three separate phosphaturic disorders, FGF-23 is elevated.[5,67,79] FGF-23 may inhibit the conversion of 25-hydroxyvitamin D to 1,25-dihydroxyvitamin D in addition to this phosphaturic effect.

Hereditary vitamin D-resistant rickets (HVDRR)

This rare autosomal recessive disorder arises because of a non-functioning vitamin D receptor. Neonatal presentation is unusual. Clinical signs are persistent hypocalcaemia, elevated plasma 1,25-dihydroxyvitamin D_3, rachitic changes on X-ray and alopecia.[47] Treatment is difficult. Some cases have responded to regular intravenous infusions of calcium,[78] followed by large oral doses.[61] Similar strategies may be required in cases of severe infantile vitamin D-deficiency rickets complicated by fractures and respiratory compromise (own observations of two cases).

Pseudo-vitamin D deficiency rickets (PDDR)

This results from absence of the 25-hydroxyvitamin D 1-α hydroxylase enzyme. The clinical picture is of a rachitic, apathetic infant, typically 4–6 months old, with hypocalcaemia, who fails to thrive and may have fits.[2] The condition responds completely to treatment with calcitriol.[28]

Disorders of osteogenesis

A problem with osteogenesis may be suggested antenatally by ultrasound demonstration of shortened limbs.

Hypophosphatasia

Hypophosphatasia is the congenital absence of bone/liver/kidney-specific alkaline phosphatase in all tissues and serum.[81] Cases presenting early (infantile form) are characterised by severely defective osteogenesis. Chorionic villus sampling has been successfully applied in affected families.[6] Other biochemical abnormalities include elevated urinary excretion of inorganic pyrophosphate and phosphoethanolamine. There are case reports of successful treatment with frequent fresh plasma infusions,[80] and also with a combined bone marrow/stem cell transplantation approach, but at least 50% of affected infants perish.

Osteogenesis imperfecta

The diagnosis of OI remains difficult because of the extreme variability in phenotype,[68] the lack of a definitive biochemical test and the heterogeneity of the genetic alterations – more than 300 separate mutations in the type I collagen genes have been described to date. Genetic studies looking for the individual mutations typical in types III and IV can now be undertaken on genomic DNA (i.e. on 5 ml of blood) using exon-spanning primers on high-throughput DNA sequencing instruments, but the procedure remains labour intensive and costly. In those with a clear family history (frequent fractures and/or dislocations, hearing loss, hernias, fragile teeth, early-onset osteoporosis), 90% will have a mutation in the type I collagen genes.[71]

Fractures at birth may occur in any type of OI, but are more often seen in children with types II, III and IV.

OI type I (characterised by a 50% deficit in type I collagen production, autosomal dominant inheritance) rarely causes problems in the neonatal period. Types II–IV result from mutations in the collagen gene that affect the protein's ability to form the normal triple helices.

Type II is uniformly lethal. It is important to make the diagnosis, however, since parental germ-line mutations effectively create an autosomal dominant inheritance, engendering a significant risk (empirically approximately 7%) of a second affected child.[12]

Multiple early fractures leading to limb shortening are characteristic of OI III; affected infants typically have blue sclerae. In contrast to infants with OI II, there are few rib fractures and thus no thoracic dysplasia. Differentiating types III and IV is really only possible post-neonatally, although children with OI IV may have white rather than blue sclerae. Lax skin and ligaments are seen in all these types of OI.

Post-neonatally, the principal differential diagnosis is non-accidental injury; in such cases, the importance of family history and clinical examination is evident. As stated previously, genetic analysis can be undertaken by screening genomic DNA or by the older method of skin biopsy, culture of fibroblasts and analysis, either at the protein or mRNA level.

Recently, three more forms of relatively severe OI have been described, with most initially presenting outside the neonatal period.[30,31,56]

Treatment of severely affected infants with OI should be undertaken in a specialist centre that has a dedicated multidisciplinary team. Pamidronate given intravenously has been used to treat infants as young as 2 weeks old with type III OI.[55] The available data suggest that such treatment, in combination with occupational and physiotherapy, improves bone mass, reduces fracture rates, reduces bone pain and enables the reconstruction of previously crush-fractured vertebrae.[29,55] There is, as yet, no information on the long-term outcome of treated infants, and the ideal dose and preferred drug are still the subject of research endeavours.

Thanatophoric dwarfism

Both type I (cloverleaf skull, curved femora, marked platyspondyly) and type II (cloverleaf skull, short, straight long bones, mild platyspondyly) thanatophoric dwarfism result from mutations in fibroblast growth factor receptor 3 gene.[54,72] Mutations in other parts of the same gene are responsible for achondroplasia and hypochondroplasia.

Osteopetrosis

A large number of mutations in different genes involved in cellular processes such as ion transport and energy production within osteoclasts have been found.[10,26] Recently, one of the two 'adult' forms of the disease has been found to be due to activating mutations in the LDL receptor-related protein 5 (LRP5) gene, a regulator of bone formation.[74] Rarely, osteopetrosis may arise as a result of the absence of osteoclasts but the mechanisms underlying such cases have yet to be determined.[20] The clinical features of 'marble bones' and immunodeficiency in the autosomal recessive form arise from defective osteoclastic (bone-resorbing) activity and reduced leukocyte superoxide production.

Pancytopenia is common, and retinal degeneration reported from age 2 months.[27] Treatment with interferon gamma-1 b may be effective initially[37] but later bone marrow or stem cell transplantation is still likely to be needed and management in a specialist centre is recommended.

References

1. Atkinson S A, Radde I C, Anderson G H 1983 Macromineral balances in premature infants fed their own mothers' milk or formula. Journal of Pediatrics 102: 99–106
2. Balsan S 1991 Hereditary pseudo-deficiency rickets or vitamin D-dependency type I. In: Glorieux F H (ed) Rickets. Raven Press, New York
3. Bhandari V, Fall P, Raisz L, Rowe J 1999 Potential biochemical growth markers in premature infants. American Journal of Perinatology 16: 339–349
4. Bishop N J, Dahlenburg S L, Fewtrell M S, Morley R, Lucas A 1996 Early diet of preterm infants and bone mineralization at age five years. Acta Paediatrica 85: 230–236
5. Bowe A E, Finnegan R, Jan de Beur S M et al 2001 FGF-23 inhibits renal tubular phosphate transport and is a PHEX substrate. Biochemical and Biophysical Research Communications 284: 977–981
6. Brock D J, Barron L 1991 First-trimester prenatal diagnosis of hypophosphatasia: experience with 16 cases. Prenatal Diagnosis 11: 387–391
7. Callenbach J C, Sheehan M B, Abramson S J, Hall R T 1981 Etiologic factors in rickets of very low-birth-weight infants. Journal of Pediatrics 98: 800–805
8. Carey D E, Goetz C A, Horak E, Rowe J C 1985 Phosphorus wasting during phosphorus supplementation of human milk feedings in preterm infants. Journal of Pediatrics 107: 790–794

9. Carey D E, Hopfer S M 1987 Hypophosphatemic rickets with hypercalciuria and microglobulinuria. Journal of Pediatrics 111: 860–863

10. Chalhoub N, Benachenhou N, Rajapurohitam V et al 2003 Grey-lethal mutation induces severe malignant autosomal recessive osteopetrosis in mouse and human. Nature Medicine 9: 399–406

11. Chan G M, Mileur L, Hansen J W 1988 Calcium and phosphorus requirements in bone mineralization of preterm infants. Journal of Pediatrics 113: 225–229

12. Cole G C 1994 Osteogenesis imperfecta as a consequence of naturally occurring and induced mutations of type I collagen. Journal of Bone and Mineral Research 8: 167–204

13. Crofton P M, Shrivastava A, Wade J C et al 1999 Bone and collagen markers in preterm infants: relationship with growth and bone mineral content over the first 10 weeks of life. Pediatric Research 46: 581–587

14. Crofton P M, Shrivastava A, Wade J C et al 2000 Effects of dexamethasone treatment on bone and collagen turnover in preterm infants with chronic lung disease. Pediatric Research 48: 155–162

15. Dahlenburg S L, Bishop N J, Lucas A 1989 Are preterm infants at risk for subsequent fractures? Archives of Disease in Childhood 64: 1384–1385

16. Delvin E E, Salle B L, Glorieux F H, Adeleine P, David L S 1986 Vitamin D supplementation during pregnancy: effect on neonatal calcium homeostasis. Journal of Pediatrics 109: 328–334

17. Ecarot B, Caverzasio J, Desbarats M, Bonjour J P, Glorieux F H 1994 Phosphate transport by osteoblasts from X-linked hypophosphatemic mice. American Journal of Physiology 266: E33–E38

18. Ecarot B, Glorieux F H, Desbarats M, Travers R, Labelle L 1992 Defective bone formation by Hyp mouse bone cells transplanted into normal mice: evidence in favor of an intrinsic osteoblast defect. Journal of Bone and Mineral Research 7: 215–220

19. Ecarot B, Glorieux F H, Desbarats M, Travers R, Labelle L 1992 Effect of dietary phosphate deprivation and supplementation of recipient mice on bone formation by transplanted cells from normal and X-linked hypophosphatemic mice. Journal of Bone and Mineral Research 7: 523–530

20. Edwards T P B, Grabowski N J 2002 Failure of osteoclast induction from peripheral blood in a child with osteopetrosis. Bone 30: C62

21. Eek S, Gabrielson L H 1957 Prematurity and rickets. Pediatrics 20: 63–77

22. Ezzedeen F, Adelman R D, Ahlfors C E 1988 Renal calcification in preterm infants: pathophysiology and long-term sequelae. Journal of Pediatrics 113: 532–539

23. Fewtrell M S, Cole T J, Bishop N J, Lucas A 2000 Neonatal factors predicting childhood height in preterm infants: evidence for a persisting effect of early metabolic bone disease? Journal of Pediatrics 137: 668–673

24. Fewtrell M S, Prentice A, Cole T J, Lucas A 2000 Effects of growth during infancy and childhood on bone mineralization and turnover in preterm children aged 8–12 years. Acta Paediatrica 89: 148–153

25. Fewtrell M S, Prentice A, Jones S C et al 1999 Bone mineralization and turnover in preterm infants at 8–12 years of age: the effect of early diet. Journal of Bone and Mineral Research 14: 810–820

26. Frattini A, Orchard P J, Sobacchi C et al 2000. Defects in TCIRG1 subunit of the vacuolar proton pump are responsible for a subset of human autosomal recessive osteopetrosis. Nature Genetics 25: 343–346

27. Gerritsen E J, Vossen J M, van Loo I H et al 1994 Autosomal recessive osteopetrosis: variability of findings at diagnosis and during the natural course. Pediatrics 93: 247–253

28. Glorieux F H 1990 Calcitriol treatment in vitamin D-dependent and vitamin D-resistant rickets. Metabolism 39(4 suppl. 1): 10–12

29. Glorieux F H, Bishop N J, Plotkin H, Chabot G, Lanoue G, Travers R 1998 Cyclic administration of pamidronate in children with severe osteogenesis imperfecta. New England Journal of Medicine 339: 947–952

30. Glorieux F H, Rauch F, Plotkin H et al 2000 Type V osteogenesis imperfecta: a new form of brittle bone disease. Journal of Bone and Mineral Research 15: 1650–1658

31. Glorieux F H, Ward L M, Rauch F, Lalic L, Roughley P J, Travers R 2002 Osteogenesis imperfecta type VI: a form of brittle bone disease with a mineralization defect. Journal of Bone and Mineral Research 17: 30–38

32. Greer F R, McCormick A 1988 Improved bone mineralization and growth in premature infants fed fortified own mother's milk. Journal of Pediatrics 112: 961–969

33. Greer F R, Searcy J E, Levin R S, Steichen J J, Steichen-Asche P S, Tsang R C 1982 Bone mineral content and serum 25-hydroxyvitamin D concentrations in breast-fed infants with and without supplemental vitamin D: one-year follow-up. Journal of Pediatrics 100: 919–922

34. Gross S J 1983 Growth and biochemical response of preterm infants fed human milk or modified infant formula. New England Journal of Medicine 308: 237–241

35. Hillman L S, Hoff N, Salmons S, Martin L, McAlister W, Haddad J 1985 Mineral homeostasis in very premature infants: serial evaluation of serum 25-hydroxyvitamin D, serum minerals, and bone mineralization. Journal of Pediatrics 106: 970–980

36. James J R, Congdon P J, Truscott J, Horsman A, Arthur R 1986 Osteopenia of prematurity. Archives of Disease in Childhood 61: 871–876

37. Key L L Jr, Rodriguiz R M, Willi S M et al 1995 Long-term treatment of osteopetrosis with recombinant human interferon gamma. New England Journal of Medicine 332: 1594–1599

38. Koo W W, Gupta J M, Nayanar V V, Wilkinson M, Posen S 1982 Skeletal changes in preterm infants. Archives of Disease in Childhood 57: 447–452

39. Koo W W, Sherman R, Succop P et al 1988 Sequential bone mineral content in small preterm infants with and without fractures and rickets. Journal of Bone and Mineral Research 3: 193–197

40. Krishnamachari K A, Iyengar L 1975 Effect of maternal malnutrition on the bone density of the neonates. American Journal of Clinical Nutrition 28: 482–486

41. Lawson M, Thomas M 1999 Vitamin D concentrations in Asian children aged 2 years living in England: population survey. British Medical Journal 318: 28

42. Lucas A, Brooke O G, Baker B A, Bishop N, Morley R 1989 High alkaline phosphatase activity and growth in preterm neonates. Archives of Disease in Childhood 64: 902–909

43. Lucas A, Morley R, Cole T J et al 1990 Early diet in preterm babies and developmental status at 18 months. Lancet 335: 1477–1481

44. Lyon A J, McIntosh N, Wheeler K, Brooke O G 1984 Hypercalcaemia in extremely low birthweight infants. Archives of Disease in Childhood 59: 1141–1144

45. Lyon A J, McIntosh N, Wheeler K, Williams J E 1987 Radiological rickets in extremely low birthweight infants. Pediatric Radiology 17: 56–58

46. Marlowe A, Pepin M G, Byers P H 2002 Testing for osteogenesis imperfecta in cases of suspected non-accidental injury. Journal of Medical Genetics 39: 382–386

47. Marx S J 1991 1,25-dihydroxyvitamin D3 receptors and resistance: implications in rickets, osteomalacia, and other conditions. Rickets 21: 167–184

48. Michaelsen K F, Johansen J S, Samuelson G, Price P A, Christiansen C 1992 Serum bone gamma-carboxyglutamic acid protein in a longitudinal study of infants: lower values in formula-fed infants. Pediatric Research 31: 401–405

49. Minamitani K, Minagawa M, Yasuda T, Niimi H 1996 Early detection of infants with hypophosphatemic vitamin D resistant rickets (HDRR). Endocrine Journal 43: 339–343.

50. Minton S D, Steichen J J, Tsang R C 1983 Decreased bone mineral content in small-for-gestational-age infants compared with appropriate-for-gestational-age infants: normal serum 25-hydroxyvitamin D and decreasing parathyroid hormone. Pediatrics 71: 383–388

51. Moyer-Mileur L J, Brunstetter V, McNaught T P, Gill G, Chan G M 2000 Daily physical activity program increases bone mineralization and growth in preterm very low birth weight infants. Pediatrics 106: 1088–1092

52. Moyer-Mileur L, Luetkemeier M, Boomer L, Chan G M 1995 Effect of physical activity on bone mineralization in premature infants. Journal of Pediatrics 127: 620–625

53. Mughal M Z, Salama H, Greenaway T, Laing I, Mawer E B 1999 Lesson of the week: florid rickets associated with prolonged breast feeding without vitamin D supplementation. British Medical Journal 318: 39–40

54. Paterson C R 1997 Osteogenesis imperfecta and other heritable disorders of bone. Baillieres Clinical Endocrinology and Metabolism 11: 195–213

55. Plotkin H, Rauch F, Bishop N J et al 2000 Pamidronate treatment of severe osteogenesis imperfecta in children under 3 years of age. Journal of Clinical Endocrinology and Metabolism 85: 1846–1850

56. Primorac D, Rowe D W, Mottes M et al 2001 Osteogenesis imperfecta at the beginning of bone and joint decade. Croatian Medical Journal 42: 393–415

57. Rauch F, Schönau E 2002 Skeletal development in premature infants: a review of bone physiology beyond nutritional aspects. Archives of Disease in Childhood. Fetal and Neonatal Edition 86: F82–F85

58. Romagnoli C, Zecca E, Tortorolo G, Diodato A, Fazzini G, Sorcini-Carta M 1987 Plasma thyrocalcitonin and parathyroid hormone concentrations in early neonatal hypocalcaemia. Archives of Disease in Childhood 62: 580–584

59. Ryan S W, Truscott J, Simpson M, James J 1993 Phosphate, alkaline phosphatase and bone mineralization in preterm neonates. Acta Paediatrica 82: 518–521

60. Sagy M, Birenbaum E, Balin A, Orda S, Barzilay Z, Brish M 1980 Phosphate-depletion syndrome in a premature infant fed human milk. Journal of Pediatrics 96: 683–685

61. Sakati N, Woodhouse N J, Niles N, Harfi H, de Grange D A, Marx S 1986 Hereditary resistance to 1,25-dihydroxyvitamin D: clinical and radiological improvement during high-dose oral calcium therapy. Hormone Research 24: 280–287

62. Salle B L, Glorieux F H, Delvin E E 1988 Perinatal vitamin D metabolism. Biology of the Neonate 54: 181–187

63. Seki K, Furuya K, Makimura N, Mitsui C, Hirata J, Nagata I 1994 Cord blood levels of calcium-regulating hormones and osteocalcin in premature infants. Journal of Perinatal Medicine 22: 189–194

64. Senterre J 1991 Osteopenia versus rickets in premature infants. In: Glorieux F H (ed) Rickets. Raven Press, New York, pp 145–154

65. Senterre J, Salle B 1982 Calcium and phosphorus economy of the preterm infant and its interaction with vitamin D and its metabolites. Acta Paediatrica Scandinavica. Supplement 296: 85–92

66. Senterre J, Salle B 1988 Renal aspects of calcium and phosphorus metabolism in preterm infants. Biology of the Neonate 53: 220–229

67. Shimada T, Muto T, Urakawa I et al 2002 Mutant FGF-23 responsible for autosomal dominant hypophosphatemic rickets is resistant to proteolytic cleavage and causes hypophosphatemia in vivo. Endocrinology 143: 3179–3182

68. Sillence D O, Senn A, Danks D M 1979 Genetic heterogeneity in osteogenesis imperfecta. Journal of Medical Genetics 16: 101–116

69. Steichen J J, Asch P A, Tsang R C 1988 Bone mineral content measurement in small infants by single-photon absorptiometry: current methodologic issues. Journal of Pediatrics 113: 181–187

70. Steichen J J, Gratton T L, Tsang R C 1980 Osteopenia of prematurity: the cause and possible treatment. Journal of Pediatrics 96: 528–534

71. Sykes B, Ogilvie D, Wordsworth P et al 1990 Consistent linkage of dominantly inherited osteogenesis imperfecta to the type I collagen loci: COL1A1 and COL1A2. American Journal of Human Genetics 46: 293–307

72. Tavormina P L, Shiang R, Thompson L M et al 1995 Thanatophoric dysplasia (types I and II) caused by distinct mutations in fibroblast growth factor receptor 3. Nature Genetics 9: 321–328

73. Tulloch A L 1974 Rickets in the premature. Medical Journal of Australia 1: 137–140

74. Van Wesenbeeck L, Cleiren E, Gram J et al 2003 Six novel missense mutations in the LDL receptor-related protein 5 (LRP5) gene in different conditions with an increased bone density. American Journal of Human Genetics 72: 763–771

75. Venkataraman P S, Blick K E 1988 Effect of mineral supplementation of human milk on bone mineral content and trace element metabolism. Journal of Pediatrics 113: 220–224

76. Von Sydow G 1946 A study of the development of rickets in premature infants. Acta Paediatrica 22(2)

77. Wauben I P, Atkinson S A, Grad T L, Shah J K, Paes B 1998 Moderate nutrient supplementation of mother's milk for preterm infants supports adequate bone mass and short-term growth: a randomized, controlled trial. American Journal of Clinical Nutrition 67: 465–472

78. Weisman Y, Bab I, Gazit D, Spirer Z, Jaffe M, Hochberg Z 1987 Long-term intracaval calcium infusion therapy in end-organ resistance to 1,25-dihydroxyvitamin D. American Journal of Medicine 83: 984–990

79. White K E, Evans W E 2002 Circulating FGF-23 concentrations in oncogenic hypophosphatemic osteomalacia (OHO) patients pre- and post-surgery. Journal of Bone and Mineral Research 17: F398

80. Whyte M P, Magill H L, Fallon M D, Herrod H G 1986 Infantile hypophosphatasia: normalization of circulating bone alkaline phosphatase activity followed by skeletal remineralization. Evidence for an intact structural gene for tissue non-specific alkaline phosphatase. Journal of Pediatrics 108: 82–88

81. Whyte M P, McAlister W H, Patton L S et al 1984 Enzyme replacement therapy for infantile hypophosphatasia attempted by intravenous infusions of alkaline phosphatase-rich Paget plasma: results in three additional patients. Journal of Pediatrics 105: 926–933

CHAPTER 36

Disorders of the kidney and urinary tract

PART I

Renal function and renal disease in the newborn

George Haycock

Morphological development of the kidney

The kidney develops from the most caudal segment of the nephrogenic ridge, the *metanephros*, a specialised population of mesodermal cells which condenses around the tip of the ureteric bud from about 5 weeks' gestation. Normal growth and development of the ureteric bud is a precondition for the development of a normal kidney. As the ureteric bud branches and rebranches, forming first the major calices, then the minor calices, and finally the arborising system of collecting ducts, nephron formation is induced in relation to the successive divisions of the duct system. Nephrogenesis proceeds centrifugally: nephrons that eventually lie deepest in the cortex (the *juxtamedullary* nephrons) are the first to be formed, and those in the most superficial (*subcapsular*) cortex are the last. The first few generations of nephrons atrophy without having functioned. The first permanent nephrons, and the production of urine, date from 8–10 weeks' gestation; the last nephrons are formed by 36 weeks. Once nephrogenesis is complete, nephrons that die cannot be replaced. The number of nephrons per kidney in mammalian species is proportional to the size of the adult, from 10 000 in the mouse to more than 10 million in the pilot whale, with humans somewhere near the middle of the range at about 1 million. Intrauterine growth retardation is associated with a reduction in nephron number,[34] with probable adverse long-term consequences for blood pressure and renal function.[47] Although renal mass continues to increase rapidly after 36 weeks, this is due to growth of tubules, not the development of new nephrons.

Renal function in the term human newborn

Glomerular filtration rate

Glomerular filtration rate (GFR) is low in the newborn. GFR at the age of a week or so, after the transition from the fetal to the neonatal circulation has taken place, is about 2.5–5 ml/min in absolute terms, or 20–40 ml/min/1.73 m^2 body surface area. This increases to about 50 ml/min/1.73 m^2 at 1 month, 60 ml/min/ 1.73 m^2 at 3 months, 80 ml/min/1.73 m^2 at 6 months, and 100 ml/min/ 1.73 m^2 at 12 months. The adult value of about 120 ml/min/ 1.73 m^2 (range 80–150) is reached during the second year of life. Fig. 36.1 depicts GFR, measured by creatinine clearance, in neonates after the first 4 postnatal days, born at various gestational ages.

Formal measurement of GFR is not often done for clinical purposes, especially in infants. The most widely used proxy for GFR is the plasma creatinine concentration (Pcr), which in a steady state is inversely proportional to GFR. A baby's Pcr at birth (e.g. in cord blood) reflects the mother's, not the baby's, renal function. In term newborns, the Pcr at birth is typically 70–90 micromol/l (about 1 mg/dl), falling to about 30 micromol/l (0.3 mg/dl) with a range of 15–40 micromol/l (0.17–0.45 mg/dl) by 1 week of age and remaining at this level for the remainder of the first month.[77] It is important to note that some methods in routine use for estimating Pcr are unreliable at these low concentrations and will give a falsely high value due to interference by other chromogens in normal plasma. This should be discussed with the clinical chemistry staff of the relevant laboratory before reliance is placed on reported results.

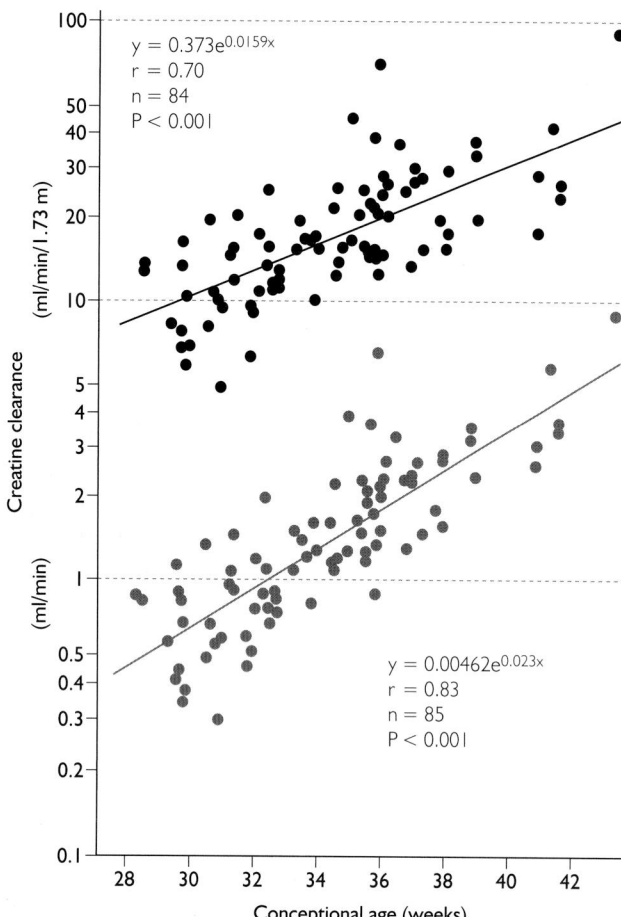

y = 0.373e^{0.0159x}
r = 0.70
n = 84
P < 0.001

y = 0.00462e^{0.023x}
r = 0.83
n = 85
P < 0.001

Fig. 36.1 Glomerular filtration rate (GFR), measured by creatinine clearance, in newborn preterm and term infants after the first 4 postnatal days. The open circles and lower regression line represent absolute values for GFR (ml/min); the closed circles and upper regression line represent GFR corrected to a notional body surface area of 1.73 m². (From Al-Dahhan et al.[2])

Following the introduction of formulae that relate GFR to body length (or height) and Pcr into paediatric practice in the 1970s,[63] attempts have been made to adapt these for use in the newborn, which involves recalculating the empirical constant *k* that relates these variables thus:

$$\text{GFR (ml/min/1.73 m}^2) = \frac{k \times \text{height}}{\text{Pcr}}$$

Note that this formula predicts GFR corrected for body surface area. If length is expressed in centimetres and Pcr in micromols per litre, approximate values for *k* are 50 for children, 40 for term infants and 30 for preterm infants.[29] Although there is a reasonable statistical correlation between measured GFR and the estimate obtained in this way, the scatter is so wide that it is doubtful if the method adds anything useful to simple comparison of Pcr with the age-related normal range.

Renal blood flow and filtration fraction

Early studies using the renal clearance of para-amino hippurate (PAH) gave results suggesting that renal plasma flow (RPF) was lower in newborns and young infants than would be expected from the GFR. However, PAH extraction is incomplete in newborns and underestimates RPF.[12] When correction is made for this, the filtration fraction (GFR/RPF) is similar to that in adults, about 0.2, i.e. 20% of the plasma entering the glomerular capillaries forms glomerular filtrate. RPF is regulated by changes in the vascular tone of the afferent and efferent glomerular arterioles. Drugs that cause constriction or dilatation of these vessels – angiotensin-converting enzyme (ACE) inhibitors, nonsteroidal anti-inflammatory drugs (NSAIDs) and powerful vasodilators such as tolazoline – can lead to acute renal failure if used incautiously.[76]

Proximal tubular function

Amino acid reabsorption

In adults and children, the fractional reabsorption of filtered amino acids is almost complete (>98% for all amino acids except histidine). In term neonates and young infants in the first few weeks, mild aminoaciduria is present, particularly affecting glycine, imino acids (proline and hydroxyproline), dibasic amino acids and taurine: fractional reabsorption of all the others is relatively complete.[10] This presumably reflects immaturity of the proximal tubular amino acid transporters for these particular classes of amino acids. However, if dietary intake is adequate (e.g. that provided by human milk), this has no significant adverse nutritional consequences.

Glucose reabsorption

The mean urinary glucose concentration in the term newborn is slightly higher than in older children and adults (mean values 0.83 mmol/l [15 mg/dl] vs 0.33 mmol/l [6 mg/dl]).[4] The results of early studies suggested that this was due to *glomerulotubular imbalance*, i.e. that the functional development of the glomeruli had outstripped the reabsorptive capacity of the proximal tubule. More careful studies using techniques that avoided volume expansion during manipulation of the blood glucose level showed this to be false: the capacity to reabsorb filtered glucose in the newborn actually equals or exceeds that in the adult when factored by GFR.[5] As with amino acids, the trivial degree of glycosuria seen in term newborns is of no nutritional significance. The finding of more marked glycosuria in a term infant cannot be attributed to physiological immaturity and should be investigated for the presence of pathological causes (hyperglycaemia, inherited tubulopathies).

Phosphate reabsorption

The normal plasma phosphate concentration is higher in the fetus and the healthy newborn infant than in older subjects. This is associated with a renal tubular phosphate threshold (the plasma phosphate concentration above which phosphate appears in the urine) that is higher than that in adults,[39] reflecting the need for phosphate retention in the rapidly growing infant, mainly to support skeletal growth. Since human milk contains little or no excess phosphate over the dietary needs of the infant, urinary phosphate excretion is normally low. Interestingly, if excess dietary phosphate is given (as used to be commonly the case when bottle-fed infants were given skimmed cows' milk as their main intake), phosphate retention may occur, leading to a form of transient neonatal tetany, confirming that the neonatal kidney is 'programmed' to retain, not to excrete, phosphate and other minerals.

Bicarbonate reabsorption

Filtered bicarbonate is completely reabsorbed in the proximal tubule provided the plasma bicarbonate is below the threshold value: the renal bicarbonate threshold, in fact, determines the plasma bicarbonate concentration in most circumstances. The plasma bicarbonate in healthy term neonates is 20–23 mmol/l, about 3 mmol/l lower than in adults.[1] This is physiological, reflecting a slightly lower renal bicarbonate threshold which may be due to the relatively expanded extracellular fluid (ECF) volume seen in the newborn period.

Distal tubular function

Urinary concentrating and diluting ability and urine flow rate

The adult kidney can produce urine with an osmolality of greater than 1000 (typically 1200–1400) mOsmol/kg water. A neonate can only achieve an osmolality of 500–700 mOsmol/kg. This value increases gradually during the first few months, and approximates to the adult value by about 1 year of age. However, in thirsted adults, about half of the solute contributing to urinary osmolality is urea, the remainder being electrolytes. Infants, being normally in a state of marked anabolism (growth), have a much lower urea production rate than adults and therefore have less need to produce highly concentrated urine in order to conserve water. If the urea production rate of infants is increased towards that of adults by means of high protein feeding or addition of urea to the diet, even young infants can concentrate their urine almost as well as adults, as shown in Fig. 36.2.[18] The capacity of the neonate to dilute urine, on the other hand, matches that of adults (minimum urine osmolality <50 mOsmol/kg H_2O).[61]

The factors determining urine flow rate (V) are solute excretion rate and the capacity of the kidney to concentrate and dilute the urine. The total potential solute content of the diet of a breastfed newborn is about 20 mOsmol/kg/day. However, most of this is retained and incorporated in new tissue: thus the actual solute load requiring excretion is 5–10 mOsmol/kg/day. A urine flow rate of approximately 0.5 ml/kg/h is needed to avoid solute retention (i.e. uraemia). This calculation agrees well with the clinical observation that when term neonates were thirsted for 2–3 days after birth, their urine output fell to 0.3–0.5 ml/kg/h.[25] Sick babies are catabolic and therefore generate more solute for excretion than healthy ones. In this setting, a urine flow rate

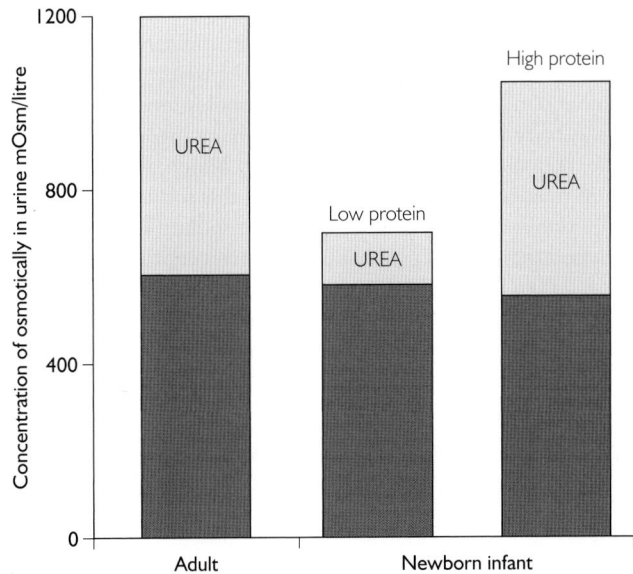

Fig. 36.2 The effect of increasing the blood urea concentration, and therefore the urinary urea excretion rate, on urinary concentrating ability in term neonates. The black bars represent non-urea urinary solute (mainly electrolytes). (From Edelmann et al.[18])

of <1 ml/kg/h suggests a degree of renal insufficiency. The maximum urine output at the same solute excretion rate is about 15 ml/kg/h, although this capacity is never needed in normal circumstances. Between the limiting values of 1 and 15 ml/kg/h, V is determined by water intake. Healthy infants, demand fed on their mothers' milk, usually produce urine approximately isotonic to plasma at about 3 ml/kg/h, demonstrating that the ratio of solute to water in mature human breast milk is close to the ideal for the needs of the infant.

Urinary acidifying capacity

Newborn infants can lower urinary pH to values similar to those of healthy adults.[19] The capacity to excrete an acid load depends on the presence of urinary buffers (mainly inorganic phosphate and ammonium). Maximal net acid excretion (NAE) rate in term newborns is comparable to the adult value if factored by GFR. Since GFR is lower than in adults, there is some reduction of maximal NAE standardised to 1.73 m^2. In normal circumstances this poses no problems for the infant, since the same strongly anabolic state that limits the urea production rate also leads to a relatively low production rate of non-volatile acid requiring excretion by the kidney.[45]

Sodium excretion

Healthy, term infants are able to produce virtually sodium-free urine (fractional sodium excretion, FE_{Na}, much less than 1%).[2] FE_{Na} describes the proportion of filtered sodium that is excreted in the final urine, and is calculated from simultaneous plasma and urine samples by the equation:

$$FE_{Na}(\%) = \frac{U_{Na} \times P_{cr}}{P_{Na} \times U_{cr}} \times 100$$

A timed urine collection is not necessary. A trap for the unwary: creatinine must be expressed in the same units in the numerator and the denominator of the equation, not in mmol/l in urine and micromol/l in plasma, as commonly reported by laboratories. A baby fed on his mother's milk has a low sodium intake, in the region of 1–1.5 mmol/kg daily, which is close to the amount needed for growth. Virtually all this sodium must therefore be retained. The ability to excrete a sodium load is less well developed than in older individuals.[3] However, it is unphysiological for a newborn baby to be exposed to such a challenge. In most circumstances, the prime requirement of the neonatal kidney is conservation, not excretion, of sodium.

Why is renal function so low in the newborn infant?

The low solute excretion rate of the growing (anabolic) baby places a proportionately low demand on the kidney: 'growth is the third kidney.'[45] If the GFR were similar to that of an adult (80–150 ml/min/1.73 m²), the resulting large increase in filtered sodium would have to be reabsorbed by the tubules. This is an energy-intensive process: maintaining this level of renal function in the newborn would increase total energy expenditure by about 3% (7 kcal/day/1.73 m²). It can be seen, therefore, that the optimal level of renal function in the newborn infant is the minimum that meets his limited excretory and homeostatic needs, while anything in excess of this would pose an unnecessary energy cost to the mother–baby dyad.

Renal function in the premature human infant

Glomerular filtration rate

GFR is typically 0.5–1 ml/min in babies of 28–32 weeks' gestation, measured during the first week of extrauterine life, rising in an approximately linear fashion from 32 weeks to achieve the value of 3–5 ml/min at 40 weeks.[2, 65] This corresponds to a rise from 10 to 30 ml/min/1.73 m² over the same period (Fig. 36.1). These figures refer to well babies. Sick babies have reduced renal function compared with healthy, equally premature controls, especially if they are hypoxic, hypotensive or if they are receiving mechanical ventilatory support.

Some have proposed that premature and term infants follow different patterns of postnatal development of GFR. However, if infants born at different stages of gestation are compared at the same absolute or postconceptional age, they follow similar tracks once they have passed the transitional period of adjustment to the change from intrauterine to extrauterine life (the first few postnatal days). For example, two groups of infants with identical postconceptional ages (245 ± 23 and 247 ± 19 days, respectively) had identical GFR, both corrected and uncorrected for surface area, even though the first

group were studied at 5–6 days postnatal age and the second at 26–68 days.[2]

Renal blood flow and filtration fraction

In animal studies, there is a progressive rise in renal blood flow (RBF) with development, in parallel with the increase in GFR. This rise is determined primarily by a fall in renal vascular resistance rather than by a rise in perfusion pressure.[23] Anatomical and physiological investigations in several species have shown that the deep (juxtamedullary) nephrons, which are the first to be formed, are preferentially perfused during early development and that more recently formed glomeruli are recruited centrifugally.[70] The most superficial (subcapsular) glomeruli, which are formed at 34–36 weeks in the human, are therefore the last to function. Although no data are available in humans, the pattern in other species, from rodents to non-human primates, is so consistent that it is overwhelmingly likely that the same sequence occurs in babies. The relatively low RBF and GFR characteristic of the very premature infant are therefore due to the fact that only the deepest and ontologically oldest glomeruli are perfused and filtering, the more superficial ones being vasoconstricted.

Proximal tubular function

Amino acid reabsorption

There is very little reliable published information concerning amino acid reabsorption and excretion in premature human infants, especially the very small infants who are now routinely surviving. Amino acid excretion is generally higher in preterm than in term infants, and relatively severe generalised aminoaciduria is occasionally seen in very preterm infants, although such descriptions are mainly anecdotal rather than systematic. It is not clear whether such cases represent simple immaturity of tubular function or secondary tubular dysfunction due to concomitant illness. In one study of 27 infants weighing <1500 g at birth, all had generalised, non-specific aminoaciduria, which persisted for at least 4 weeks in 56%.[33] The degree and persistence of aminoaciduria was not influenced by dietary protein intake, which varied between 2.2 and 3.0 g/100 kcal. Fractional excretion of taurine, in particular, is very high in low-birthweight (LBW) infants (38–68% in one study).[81] Since taurine is necessary, inter alia, for normal retinal development, it is important that taurine is provided in adequate amounts for infants receiving total parenteral nutrition (TPN).

Glucose reabsorption

The previously described increase in urinary glucose concentration observed in term infants is exaggerated in the preterm, typically to about 3.6 mmol/l (65 mg/dl).[4] This has not been adequately investigated, but if it is due to a low renal tubular glucose threshold it has important implications for control of the plasma glucose concentration: even moderate hyperglycaemia in the presence of a low threshold would lead to substantial glycosuria and the inevitable attendant osmotic diuresis. It is therefore essential that blood glucose levels are monitored in very-low-birthweight (VLBW) infants, especially those receiving TPN.

Phosphate reabsorption

The renal phosphate threshold, already higher in term infants than in adults and children, is higher still in preterm infants and falls with increasing postconceptional age. Since the tubular phosphate threshold (TmP/GFR) is the main determinant of plasma phosphate concentration, except in phosphate depletion, this indicates the importance of renal phosphate retention for normal growth and development. Premature infants on a low phosphate diet produce phosphate-free urine and frequently develop bone disease of prematurity, a form of phosphate-deficiency rickets. If a LBW infant is producing phosphate-free urine, the probability is that dietary intake (whether enteral or parenteral) is inadequate and should be increased. Phosphaturia in the presence of normal or low plasma phosphate concentrations is not seen as a consequence of immaturity alone, and should be investigated appropriately.

Bicarbonate reabsorption

The bicarbonate threshold is lower in preterm than in term infants, leading to an acid–base profile that is more acidotic.[64] This is probably due in part to volume expansion, and bicarbonate levels rise after the first few days. Fig. 36.3 shows the distribution of plasma bicarbonate concentrations (measured as tCO_2) in a group of healthy, newborn premature infants. An infant who has a low pH and bicarbonate (by adult standards), but who is (a) thriving and (b) not producing maximally acid urine, should be regarded as having physiological hypobasaemia of prematurity rather than pathological acidosis. The syndrome of late metabolic acidosis is due to imbalance between the non-volatile acid production rate and the capacity of the distal tubule to excrete the associated hydrogen ion load,[41] and is further discussed under *urinary acidifying capacity* (see below).

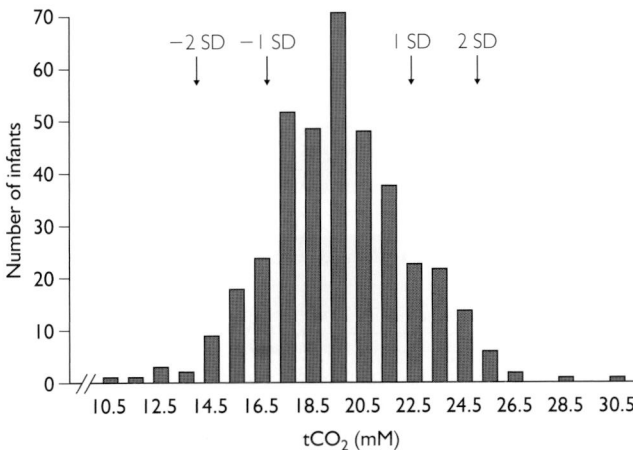

Fig. 36.3 Distribution of plasma total CO_2 concentration in well, pre-term neonates. (From Schwartz et al.[64])

Distal tubular function

Urinary concentrating and diluting ability and urine flow rate

Premature infants have an even more limited capacity to concentrate their urine than those born at term, with a maximum urine osmolality of about $500\,mOsmol/kg\,H_2O$. Also, the osmotic threshold for release of antidiuretic hormone (ADH) appears to be higher in preterm infants (plasma osmolality $290 \pm 4\,mOsmol/kg\,H_2O$) than in term infants (plasma osmolality $282 \pm 4\,mOsmol/kg\,H_2O$).[73] Therefore, premature infants do not begin to concentrate their urine until significantly more dehydrated than term infants, and at any degree of dehydration preterm infants produce less concentrated urine than term ones and are therefore more vulnerable to hypernatraemia and hyperosmolality. Preterm infants thirsted for up to 72 hours reduced urine flow rate to approximately 1 ml/kg/h, about twice that observed in term babies.[25] Diluting ability, by contrast, is well developed even in very premature infants, who can dilute their urine to $50–60\,mOsmol/kg\,H_2O$, a value only slightly less than term infants.[61] Well hydrated premature infants typically have a urine flow rate of 2–3 ml/kg/h with a range of about 1–10 ml/kg/h. Because of the limited capacity of newborn infants to reduce water excretion, especially if preterm, it is very important to ensure that their water intake is adequate to allow them to maintain normal body fluid tonicity. This applies especially in the case of sick infants, in whom the rate of addition of solute to the ECF may be increased because of interruption of growth and anabolism. Monitoring of urinary specific gravity or (better) osmolality is useful in this respect.

Urinary acidifying capacity

Even very preterm infants can lower urine pH to a level that would be adequate to prevent acidosis in older individuals in most circumstances (urine pH < 5.5). However, the defence against systemic acidosis depends on at least two other factors: GFR and an adequate supply of urinary buffers. As previously discussed, GFR is very low in premature newborns. Since phosphate is in high demand for bone mineralisation and may be in short dietary supply, there is very little available for urinary excretion (where it is an important buffer). The newborn renal tubule can synthesise ammonia, but this also is limited in supply because of small tubular mass. The main non-volatile acid needing urinary excretion is sulphuric acid derived from protein metabolism. If the infant is appropriately fed and growing, anabolism limits the production of sulphuric acid to a level at which even the kidneys of very premature infants can cope. If the baby is ill and catabolic, or fed protein much in excess of dietary need, metabolic acidosis can easily develop.[41] Borderline metabolic acidosis may be commoner than is recognised in very premature babies. It has been reported that babies who are excreting maximally acid urine, although not acidotic by standard, age-adjusted criteria, may thrive less well than those with higher urine pH, and that weight gain may be improved by alkali, suggesting that they are operating at the limit of their acid excretory capacity.[36,37] This possibility deserves exploration in preterm infants with poorer than expected weight gain in whom other explanations are lacking.

Sodium excretion

Neonates born at or after 32–33 weeks' gestation can produce virtually sodium-free urine, equivalent to $FE_{Na} \ll 1\%$ of the filtered load, from the first few days of life. Infants born before this time lose sodium in the urine, so that if dietary sodium intake is in the range 1.3–1.5 mmol/kg/day they are in negative sodium balance for up to 10–14 days.[2,75] Extremely premature babies (gestational age 28 weeks) may have FE_{Na} of 5% or more. This commonly leads to the development of hyponatraemia by the second or third week of life. It has been argued that this is due to excessive water intake and is therefore dilutional. The fact that unsupplemented premature infants have high plasma concentrations of aldosterone, noradrenaline and vasopressin, and that these are suppressed by sodium replacement,[74] suggests that ECF volume is contracted. Several groups have showed that salt supplementation, begun after the transitional period (the first 3–6 days of extrauterine life), improves early weight gain without apparent adverse effects[2,79] (for review, see Haycock & Aperia[30]).

Why is sodium reabsorption inefficient in the premature infant?

Sodium is actively reabsorbed in all tubular segments except the descending limb and the thin part of the ascending limb of Henle's loop. In the adult, about 65% of filtered sodium is reabsorbed in the proximal tubule, about 25% in the thick ascending limb of the loop (TAL), and the remaining 9–10% in the distal convoluted tubule and collecting duct. The proximal tubule accounts for a smaller fraction of total sodium reabsorption in newborns than in adults, and this fraction is even less in the premature than in the term baby.[61] An inevitable consequence of reduction of proximal tubular sodium absorption is an increase in the amount delivered to more distal parts of the tubule. Premature babies born after 32–33 weeks of gestation do not waste salt in the urine: it follows that they must compensate for reduced proximal sodium transport by a proportionate increase in distal tubular reabsorption. In extremely premature neonates, the distal tubule is incapable of the necessary compensation due to immaturity, and perhaps to an impaired response to circulating aldosterone: the result is natriuresis, negative salt balance and hyponatraemia.

Transition from the fetal to the neonatal kidney

That main function of the fetal kidney is production of amniotic fluid. It is therefore in a state of relative water and sodium diuresis, associated with an expanded ECF volume. This diuresis is sustainable because the water and electrolyte losses can be

replaced, partly by transplacental addition from the maternal circulation and partly by the fetus swallowing amniotic fluid. After birth, the diuresis is markedly attenuated, at least in part by activation of the renin–angiotensin–aldosterone system. For the first 2 or 3 days after birth, the infant is in a state of negative salt and water balance, resulting in a progressive contraction of the ECF volume, to a value of about 35% of bodyweight after a few days. This is necessary to prevent circulatory overload in the newborn baby, both in the term and the preterm infant. Although very preterm infants can develop hyponatraemia secondary to urinary sodium loss after the first few days of life, as mentioned above, it is not appropriate to attempt to prevent this by giving additional sodium or fluid in the first few days.[26–28] Data are available for sodium and water excretion, as well as GFR, in newborn babies.[2] Comparable direct measurements are not available for the human fetus, but reasonable estimates of GFR and FE_{Na} can be made on the basis of published values for urine flow rate,[56] urine[54] and plasma[52] sodium and creatinine concentrations. Fig. 36.4 shows that both GFR and

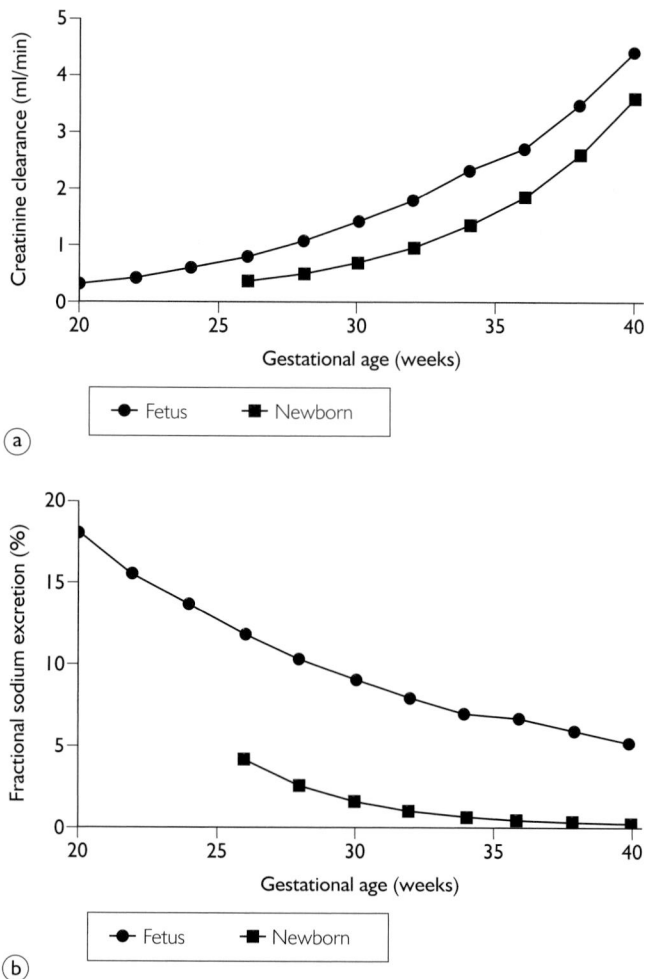

(a)

(b)

Fig. 36.4 Glomerular filtration rate and fractional sodium excretion in newborn premature infants (squares) and fetuses in utero (circles) at similar gestational ages. Values for infants taken from Al-Dahhan et al.[2] Values for fetuses calculated by the author from published data.[52,54,56]

FE_{Na} are much higher in the fetus than in the prematurely born infant at the same absolute gestational age.

Acute renal failure

Acute renal failure (ARF) is the syndrome that results from an abrupt, potentially reversible, reduction in GFR. The chief function of the kidneys is regulation of the volume and composition of the ECF; ARF is present when GFR is reduced sufficiently to cause adverse changes in either or both of these. There is no consensus as to what absolute or proportional change in GFR is necessary for the diagnosis of ARF in the neonate. A persistent rise in the Pcr concentration above 1.5 mg/dl (about 130 micromol/l), corresponding to a fall in GFR to <50% of normal, was suggested by Chevalier et al[13] and was later recommended by Stapleton et al;[71] both more and less stringent criteria have been proposed.

Incidence of acute renal failure in the newborn

The apparent incidence of ARF depends on the definition used. In a retrospective analysis of 2515 admissions to a single neonatal unit, Stapleton et al found that 75(3%) had been diagnosed as having ARF. However, in a prospective study in the same unit in which Pcr was monitored, values persistently >1.5 mg/dl occurred in 15 of 186 prospective admissions (8%).[71] This suggests that many cases of neonatal ARF will be missed if relevant investigations are not done in infants at risk from the condition. Over several years, ARF severe enough to need dialysis occurred in about 1% of admissions to the neonatal intensive care unit at Guy's Hospital, London, a figure similar to that seen in a much larger obstetric unit in Memphis, Tennessee (Arant B S, personal communication). This is an incidence of about 0.1% of all deliveries. These figures apply to modern experience in developed countries: in poor and developing countries where access to good obstetric care is limited, it may be much higher, as for example in Brazil (Zagury A, personal communication).

Clinical features of acute renal failure

There is often a clinical history of factors known to predispose to ARF (see below). Oliguria (urine flow < 1 ml/kg/h) is usually present but is not necessary to the diagnosis. Non-oliguric ARF occurs but is infrequently diagnosed except serendipitously or in prospective surveys; in fact, it is probably more frequent than oliguric ARF and represents the mild end of the spectrum of renal injury.[13] The commonest clinical sign in infants with ARF is oedema, due to continuation of normal fluid intake in the presence of unrecognised oliguria. Oedema is not a feature of non-oliguric ARF, and polyuria and natriuresis may lead to salt depletion and dehydration. ARF is commonly detected in the absence of specific physical signs by the finding of typical biochemical abnormalities during the investigation of an ill infant.

Biochemical features of acute renal failure

When renal function is normal, wide dietary variations are tolerated without measurable change in the chemical composition of the ECF. When renal function is absent or severely compromised, this freedom is lost and the composition of the ECF becomes dependent on dietary input, further modified by accumulation of products of metabolism (e.g. urea, creatinine, urate and non-volatile acid) and 'leakage' of constituents of intracellular fluid (e.g. potassium and inorganic phosphate) into the ECF. The fluid given to both well and sick infants is normally markedly hypotonic (e.g. breast milk with a sodium concentration of <10 mmol/l), and by the time ARF is suspected, hyponatraemia is present in most cases. The changes in ECF (i.e. plasma) biochemistry typical of ARF are listed in Table 36.1.

Classification and causes of acute renal failure

Renal function depends on:

- perfusion of the kidney with blood at sufficient pressure for filtration;
- functional integrity of the kidney;
- patency of the urinary passages.

ARF may therefore be caused by:

- failure of perfusion, due to either hypovolaemia or hypotension – prerenal failure;
- acute damage to the renal parenchyma – true or intrinsic renal failure;
- obstruction of the urinary tract – postrenal failure.

Intrinsic ARF due to acquired renal diseases, well recognised in older children, is virtually unknown in the neonatal period. For practical purposes, intrinsic renal failure in the newborn is

Table 36.1 Typical changes in plasma biochemical values in acute renal failure

Solute	Direction of change from normal
Creatinine	↑
Urea	↑
Uric acid	↑
Sodium	↓
Potassium	↑
Chloride	↑ or ↓
Hydrogen ion	↑
Bicarbonate	↓
Calcium	↓
Inorganic phosphate	↑

Hyponatraemia is dilutional, due to water retention, in oliguric renal failure, but may be exaggerated by urinary sodium loss in non-oliguric renal failure. The chloride concentration tends to be lowered by the same mechanisms as the sodium, but the fall may be attenuated by metabolic acidosis.

Table 36.2 Causes of prerenal and intrinsic renal failure in the newborn

Prerenal failure	Acute tubular necrosis
Hypovolaemia:	Anoxia/asphyxia
■ Haemorrhage	Sepsis
■ Dehydration	Nephrotoxic drugs:
■ Third-space losses	■ Aminoglycosides
Normovolaemic hypotension:	■ Non-steroidal anti-
■ Sepsis	inflammatory drugs
■ Vasodilator drugs	Disseminated intravascular
■ Low cardiac output	coagulation
– Congenital heart disease	
– Post-cardiopulmonary bypass	
– Post-asphyxial	

synonymous with acute tubular necrosis (ATN), with renal vein thrombosis a rare complication. Congenital chronic (i.e. irreversible) renal failure (CRF) commonly mimics ARF in its presentation. This is because the homeostatic and excretory needs of the fetus are met by the maternal, not the fetal, kidneys via the placenta, which acts as a highly efficient dialyser. Biochemical values measured in cord blood therefore reflect maternal, not fetal, renal function. The apparent postnatal deterioration in renal function that occurs in babies with severely reduced renal mass follows a similar time course to that observed in babies with true (i.e. acquired) ARF. Imaging studies serve to distinguish between congenital CRF and postrenal failure, on the one hand, and prerenal failure and ATN, on the other. Causes of ARF in the other two categories are given in Table 36.2. It should be noted that prerenal failure can progress to ATN if the predisposing cause or causes persist to the point where hypoxic-ischaemic injury occurs.

Factors predisposing to acute tubular necrosis

Hypoxia, sepsis and exposure to nephrotoxic drugs, separately or in combination, cause most episodes of ARF in the newborn. The use of aminoglycoside antibiotics in sick babies should always be monitored by serial measurement of trough levels of the drug and the plasma creatinine concentration. In fact, most infants who have suffered perinatal anoxia either do not develop ARF at all, or experience only a transient period of prerenal failure. The management of established ATN is much more difficult than that of prerenal failure. Moreover, if conventional fluid management is given to an infant with unrecognised ATN, marked biochemical abnormalities may occur before the diagnosis is made. It would be useful to identify prospectively a subgroup of infants at high risk of ATN, so that close monitoring of blood chemistry and modified fluid and electrolyte management could be instituted from the outset. Both myoglobinaemia and myoglobinuria are highly predictive of ATN, and in a study of asphyxiated infants Roberts et al found that myoglobinaemia, heavy myoglobinuria and increased urinary excretion of retinol-binding protein (RBP) discriminated with 100% specificity and sensitivity between those who developed ATN and those who

did not.[59] Hyperuricaemia has also been suggested as a marker of severity of tissue injury in infants and children subjected to cardiac surgery.[31] Further work is necessary to confirm these findings, which are based on rather small numbers of cases, but screening asphyxiated infants for urinary myoglobin and RBP is promising as a way of targeting at-risk babies for particularly close clinical and biochemical monitoring.

Diagnosis of acute renal failure

Evidence of reduced GFR is essential to the diagnosis, whether or not oliguria is present. Pcr is widely used as a rough marker for GFR, and a value of >1.5 mg/dl (130 micromol/l) persisting for more than 24 hours is a reasonable criterion. The plasma urea concentration is influenced by too many other factors to be a reliable index of GFR, although high levels indicate that the child's excretory needs are not being met and may be one factor pointing to the need for dialysis (see below). Other biochemical changes are summarised in Table 36.1.

Ultrasonography of the kidneys and urinary tract should be performed in infants with ARF, mainly to exclude CRF and postrenal failure. Renal vein thrombosis can also be confirmed or excluded by this investigation. If ultrasonography is normal, the diagnosis lies between prerenal failure and ATN. Radionuclide imaging studies are of little value in distinguishing between causes of ARF in the newborn.

Urinary indices in the diagnosis of acute renal failure

The oliguria of prerenal failure is a physiological response to renal underperfusion, leading to the production of urine of high osmolality, high urea and creatinine and low sodium concentrations. That of ATN is due to the passage of a small amount of 'poor quality' urine, i.e. urine similar in composition to glomerular filtrate because of the inability of the damaged tubules to modify it appropriately. Analysis of the urine therefore allows a degree of differentiation between prerenal failure and ATN (Table 36.3). The most discriminating test is measurement of FE_{Na}, the formula for which is given above. The so-called renal failure index (RFI) is sometimes used as an alternative to FE_{Na}:

$$RFI = \frac{U_{Na} \times Pcr}{Ucr}$$

However, inspection of this equation reveals that it is simply the formula for FE_{Na} with the number 100 substituted for measured P_{Na}. There is no good reason to prefer one over the other: both give essentially the same information. An FE_{Na} of >2.5–3% (equivalent to RFI > 4) is consistently present in oliguric ATN in term infants.[20] Very preterm babies (=32 weeks' gestation) have high urinary sodium concentrations and excretion rates even in health. In this subgroup, suitable 'cut-off' points for the diagnosis of ATN are an RFI of >8 or FE_{Na} >6%.[49]

The diagnosis of prerenal failure is confirmed by improvement in urine flow and renal function in response to fluid repletion. Provided there is no clinical evidence of circulatory

Table 36.3 Urinary biochemical indices in prerenal failure and acute tubular necrosis

Test	Prerenal failure	Acute tubular necrosis
Urine urea	High	Low
Urine creatinine	High	Low
Urine osmolality	High ($>500\,mOsmol/kg$)	Low ($\cong 300\,mOsmol/kg$)
Specific gravity	High (>1.025)	Low ($\cong 1010$)
Urine sodium	Low ($<10\,mmol/l$)	High ($>20\,mmol/l$)
U:P urea	High (>10)	Low
U:P creatinine	High (>40)	Low
U:P osmolality	High (>2)	Low ($\cong 1$)
FE_{Na}	Low ($<1\%$)	High ($>3\%$)
RFI	Low (<1)	High (>4)

FE_{Na}, fractional sodium excretion; RFI, renal failure index. See text for calculation of these, and for their interpretation in very-low-birthweight babies.

overload, a 'fluid challenge' of isotonic saline, 10 ml/kg, should be given intravenously over 1 hour. Failure to respond confirms ATN as the diagnosis.

Management of acute renal failure

Conservative management

Fluid balance

Meticulous attention to fluid balance is essential. Hypovolaemia should be corrected with isotonic fluid or colloid according to clinical assessment. Fluid losses, e.g. urine output and gastrointestinal losses, must be accurately measured and, providing the clinical condition allows it, the infant should be regularly weighed. Maintenance fluid is then calculated as insensible water loss (IWL) plus urine output and adjusted according to clinical assessment of the patient. In the term newborn, IWL is typically 180–$310\,ml/m^2$ surface area daily (15–$25\,ml/kg/day$), of which about 60% is transepidermal[24] and 40% respiratory.[57] Transepidermal water loss (TEWL) is greatly increased in very premature infants, according to the equation:

$$TEWL = 4.17 + 64.78e^{-\frac{G.A.-24.99}{2.73}}$$

where G.A. is gestational age in weeks.[24] TEWL is also increased in those nursed under radiant warmers; respiratory water loss is minimal in infants mechanically ventilated with humidified gases.

Nutrition

Nutrition is important in ARF and may be limited by the imposed fluid restriction. Provision of adequate energy is necessary in order to promote anabolism and prevent catabolism which potentiates hyperkalaemia, hyperphosphataemia and acidosis.

Enteral nutrition is preferred if the patient's condition allows, but parenteral nutrition may be necessary. Inability to meet the baby's nutritional needs because of limitation of the amount of fluid that can be given is an indication for dialysis.

Hyperphosphataemia

Hyperphosphataemia is managed by the addition of oral calcium carbonate to feeds. This binds phosphate, rendering it insoluble, thereby reducing intestinal absorption. Aluminium hydroxide should not be used as a phosphate binder in neonates, because of the risk of neurotoxicity. Although aluminium neurotoxicity in adults has only been described in patients on maintenance haemodialysis, it has been reported in infants who were not dialysed.[7] Hyperphosphataemia is usually accompanied by hypocalcaemia: additional calcium should not be given until the plasma phosphate has been reduced to normal, or ectopic calcification may occur. In babies who are not enterally fed, parenteral phosphate intake should be adjusted in response to changes in the plasma concentration.

Hyperkalaemia

Severe hyperkalaemia is a medical emergency since it may cause potentially lethal cardiac arrhythmias. Hypocalcaemia and hypomagnesaemia, both of which frequently occur in ARF, potentiate the toxic effect of hyperkalaemia on the heart. It is therefore important to maintain normocalcaemia using 10% calcium gluconate (0.1–$0.2\,ml/kg$) as necessary.

Short-term measures to control hyperkalaemia and to protect against its cardiotoxic effects include:

- Intravenous salbutamol ($4\,\mu g/kg$ over 5 minutes) – this has been shown to be a safe and highly effective treatment in hyperkalaemic infants and children.[53] Nebulised salbutamol is also effective in children and, although not formally evaluated in neonates, anecdotal experience suggests that this route is effective in this age group.[46]
- Intravenous glucose and insulin infusion (12 units soluble insulin in 100 ml 25% glucose – 5 ml/kg given over 30 minutes) – this is highly effective and has an additive effect with salbutamol. The blood glucose concentration must be closely monitored during and after treatment since fluctuations commonly occur.
- Intravenous sodium bicarbonate ($1\,mmol/kg$) – this is effective even in patients who are not acidotic.

These measures shift potassium from the extracellular to the intracellular compartment but do not eliminate it from the body. They are, therefore, only temporarily effective, allowing time to prepare for dialysis. Oral/rectal cation exchange resins, e.g. calcium polystyrene sulphate (Resonium), are effective in permanent removal of potassium from the body but may be complicated by bowel obstruction and perforation, and should preferably not be used in sick newborns who are already at risk of necrotising enterocolitis. Although it can be given rectally and then removed by gentle saline lavage, dialysis is probably a safer option if the measures listed above are insufficient to normalise the plasma potassium concentration.

Sodium intake

Dietary sodium intake should be about 1 mmol/kg/day in babies who are anuric or severely oliguric. Depending on acid–base status, it may be preferable to give this as bicarbonate rather than chloride. Babies with non-oliguric ARF may have very large urinary sodium losses, up to 10 mmol/kg/day, and these must be replaced. It is not possible to give a general formula for dietary sodium needs in this group of patients, and intake should be adjusted according to serial measurement of plasma sodium content and clinical assessment.

Acidosis

Metabolic acidosis should be treated with sodium bicarbonate in a dose sufficient to normalise the plasma pH and bicarbonate. Half correction of the base deficit should be followed by repeat estimation of acid–base status. If correction cannot be achieved within the infant's sodium and fluid allowance, dialysis should be considered.

Management by dialysis

Dialysis is now regarded as a routine therapy for ARF in the neonate. Both peritoneal and haemodialysis are possible in infants weighing <1 kg. The main indications for dialysis are given in Table 36.4.

Dialysis is the removal of small solutes across a semi-permeable membrane by diffusion down their concentration gradient. The membrane may be the peritoneum, separating blood in the splanchnic capillaries from dialysis fluid within the peritoneal cavity, or may be synthetic, as in haemodialysis, with blood and dialysis fluid pumped on opposite sides of the membrane. This process differs from ultrafiltration, in which there is convective removal of plasma water and small solutes as a result of a pressure gradient across a highly permeable membrane. Treatments can consist of pure dialysis, pure filtration or both.

Peritoneal dialysis

Peritoneal dialysis (PD) is the modality of choice in most neonates, the advantage being relative ease of access and technical simplicity in comparison with haemodialysis. The preferred means of access to the peritoneal cavity for dialysis is via a biologically inert, silastic Tenckhoff catheter inserted using sterile technique by a surgeon experienced in the procedure. Catheters can be inserted over a guidewire using the Seldinger technique, but these have a shorter functional life and are more prone to blockage, leakage and infection than those placed surgically. In VLBW infants, in whom insertion of this type of catheter is not feasible, PD can be carried out via an angiography catheter, intravenous cannula or thoracic drain. Infants as small as 380 g have been successfully dialysed using such techniques.[69,72] A relative contraindication to PD is major abdominal surgery, although there have been reports of success in some cases.[50]

The fill volume is calculated from the patient's weight. An initial fill volume of 10–20 ml/kg is usually used, increasing up to 30 ml/kg as tolerated. Larger fill volumes may splint the diaphragm and cause respiratory embarrassment. The dialysate is run into the abdomen by gravity. An automatic cycler, e.g. the 'Pac-X' machine, will perform this function, and with paediatric lines has a minimum cycle volume of 50 ml. Therefore, in LBW infants, where a smaller cycle volume is required, dialysis must be performed manually, usually using modified intravenous giving sets with suitably sized burettes.

It may be more difficult to achieve adequate ultrafiltration in neonates than in older children because their relatively larger functional peritoneal surface area, more permeable peritoneal membrane, and higher energy requirement all cause rapid absorption of glucose from the peritoneal cavity into the blood. This leads to loss of the osmotic gradient required to drive the convective transport of water from blood to the peritoneal cavity. Shorter dwell times, relatively larger volumes and higher dialysate glucose concentrations help to overcome this problem. However, prolonged exposure to high dialysate glucose concentrations may cause a peritoneal inflammatory reaction, reducing the permeability of the membrane and diminishing filtration. Table 36.5

Table 36.4 Indications for dialysis in acute renal failure

- Volume overload
- Hyperkalaemia
- Severe metabolic acidosis
- Hyperphosphataemia/hypocalcaemia
- To 'make space' for nutrition and drug administration
- Failure of conservative management

Table 36.5 Composition of some commonly used peritoneal dialysis fluids

Fluid	Glucose (%)	Sodium	Calcium	Magnesium	Chloride	Lactate	Osmolality
PD1 (1.36)	1.36	132	1.75	0.75	102	35	347
PD1 (2.27)	2.27	132	1.75	0.75	102	35	398
PD1 (3.86)	3.86	132	1.75	0.75	102	35	486

Concentrations are expressed as mmol/l except for glucose (g/100 ml) and osmolality (mOsmol/kg). The higher glucose concentrations are used to facilitate water removal by osmosis, but are less well tolerated than PD1 1.36 and their use should be kept to a minimum. Calcium-free solutions are available for use in hypercalcaemic patients. Potassium can be added in the uncommon patient with renal failure who is hypokalaemic. The fluids in the table are manufactured by Baxter Healthcare Ltd. GB, Thetford, Norfolk, UK.

gives the composition of three standard, widely used PD solutions. Special dialysate preparations are available which contain polymers (dextrins) in place of glucose, these being less prone to absorption because of their higher molecular weight. Common complications of PD include peritonitis, catheter exit-site infection, failure of drainage due to catheter blockage or occlusion by omentum, and hyperglycaemia due to absorption of glucose from the dialysate. To reduce the risk of blockage, some surgeons routinely perform an omentectomy when inserting a catheter.

Haemofiltration and haemodialysis

There are occasions when PD fails or is contraindicated, necessitating the use of haemofiltration and/or haemodialysis. While it is preferable to perform these techniques continuously in order to avoid swings in intravascular volume and biochemistry, intermittent haemodialysis has been used successfully in neonates.[62]

Continuous arteriovenous haemofiltration

The simplest technique is continuous arteriovenous haemofiltration (CAVH), in which an artery and a vein are cannulated and blood is driven across a suitable filter (e.g. 'Amicon minifilter') by the patient's own systemic blood pressure.[44]

Arterial access can be obtained via the umbilical or femoral vessels and venous access via the umbilical, femoral or jugular veins. A systemic blood pressure of at least 40 mmHg is required to maintain adequate flow across the filter and if necessary a volumetric infusion pump can be inserted into the circuit to improve this.[32] The ultrafiltration pressure can be increased by increasing the vertical height between the filter and the collection vessel and further adjusted by applying gentle suction with a pump across the filter. The pump also prevents excessive ultrafiltration. Using this system, ultrafiltration rates of up to 5 ml/kg/h have been achieved.[8] Replacement fluid can be infused into the venous port of the circuit if desired. Parenteral nutrition can be given by this route if indicated.

Most infants will tolerate a maximum extracorporeal volume of 10% of their blood volume. The smallest extracorporeal volume that can currently be achieved with CAVH is 12 ml (using an 'Amicon minifilter' and neonatal lines). LBW infants will therefore require blood priming of the circuit prior to initiation of treatment. Various combinations of whole blood, packed cells, plasma and albumin have been used for priming filtration and dialysis circuits in neonates. Banked blood may have a potassium

concentration of up to 20 mmol/l; therefore fresh whole blood is preferable. The citrate anticoagulant may cause sudden hypocalcaemia, leading to the recommendation that fresh whole blood anticoagulated with heparin should be used if possible.[17]

Heparin infusion is required to prevent clotting of the circuit. This is infused into the arterial port at a rate of 5–15 IU/kg/h following an initial bolus of 25–100 IU/kg. The infusion rate is adjusted, ideally according to the activated clotting time measured at the cot side, although laboratory-measured activated partial thromboplastin times can be used. In many neonates, the haematocrit is relatively high and the mean arterial pressure relatively low, resulting in sluggish flow across the filter and a requirement for increased heparinisation in order to prevent clotting. Where systemic heparinisation is contraindicated, heparin can be infused into the arterial port and protamine into the venous port.

Haemofiltration removes solute by convection but not diffusion. Occasionally this solute removal is inadequate, especially if the patient is catabolic with a raised urea generation rate. If so, diffusive clearance can be added by running dialysis fluid through the ultrafiltrate compartment of the filter in the opposite direction to blood flow, thereby converting the process to haemodiafiltration.[6,9] Fig. 36.5 illustrates the principles of haemofiltration and haemodiafiltration. A major disadvantage of CAVH in the neonate is the requirement for arterial access, which can be difficult to obtain, and in the case of brachial and femoral lines carries a risk of limb ischaemia and later reduced limb growth. CAVH may not be possible in patients who are hypotensive or have poor cardiac function.

Continuous venovenous haemofiltration

An alternative technique is continuous venovenous haemofiltration (CVVH), in which access is obtained either via two venous lines or a single double-lumen venous line, and a pump is used to control blood flow through the circuit. Unfortunately, systems specifically designed for CVVH in the neonate are not currently available. Yorgin et al first described CVVH in a neonate in 1990, using a standard dialysis unit to control blood flow.[80] Bunchman et al have successfully adapted a 'Gambro AK-10' haemodialysis machine for CVVH and, using an 'Amicon minifilter' and neonatal lines, have reduced the extracorporeal circuit volume to 38 ml.[11] Blood priming is therefore required in infants weighing <4.5 kg. Alternatively, a volumetric infusion pump can be used to regulate blood flow. This allows a lower blood flow and requires less technical support than does use of a standard dialysis machine. However, there is an increased risk of air embolus since the circuit does not contain a bubble trap and air detector.

More recently, a manual syringe-driven technique has been described which allows venovenous ultrafiltration and haemodialysis to be performed in infants weighing <1000 g, the smallest to whom the technique has been applied being 630 g.[16] The technique is very labour intensive, although automation may be possible in the future. As with CAVH, dialysis can be added to CVVH by running dialysate through the filter in the opposite direction to blood flow.

In virtually all cases, dialysis is possible in the neonate with ARF. PD remains the technique of first choice, although advances continue to be made in CAVH and CVVH. Ultimately, the

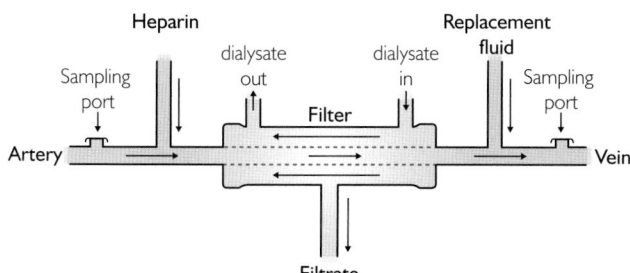

Fig. 36.5 Schematic representation of arteriovenous haemofiltration and haemodiafiltration (see text for details).

choice of dialysis modality depends upon the individual patient and the technical support available within the unit.

Chronic renal failure

Causes of chronic renal failure in the newborn

CRF presenting in the newborn period may be truly congenital, caused by irreversible renal damage already present before birth, or acquired due to perinatal renal injury so severe that the kidneys do not recover function. Bilateral renal agenesis and bilateral multicystic renal dysplasia are incompatible with survival, since the severe oligohydramnios caused by absence of fetal urine production leads to the Potter sequence and lethal pulmonary hypoplasia. Renal dysplasia, usually associated with gross bilateral vesico-ureteric reflux (VUR) or obstructive uropathy, is the commonest cause of 'true' congenital CRF. It is about twice as common in boys as girls because of the male predominance in posterior urethral valves and severe VUR. Acquired causes include bilateral renal arterial or venous thrombosis and severe ATN progressing to renal cortical necrosis. It is unusual for congenital renal dysplasia to be severe enough to require dialysis in the newborn period in a viable baby: if renal function is sufficient to prevent pulmonary hypoplasia, it is generally adequate for the baby to survive for at least a few weeks or months with supportive treatment alone. The recessive form of polycystic kidney disease (see below) occasionally causes renal failure in the neonatal period, but this is only in a small proportion of patients with an already rare disease.

Clinical features of chronic renal failure

The usual presentation is with failure to thrive in the newborn period, with the typical biochemical changes of renal failure (see above). Since the symptoms are non-specific, it is quite common for CRF to be missed for weeks or even months, with potentially irreversible adverse effects on growth and development: a simple test of renal function (urea, electrolytes and creatinine) is mandatory in any young infant with persistent, unexplained poor weight gain. Many babies with renal dysplasia have obligate high urinary sodium excretion, and are prone to become salt depleted if adequate replacement is not provided. Arterial hypertension may be present, but usually not in those with significant urinary salt loss. There are numerous rare, inherited syndromes with renal involvement that may lead to CRF, but it is exceptional for them to do so in the neonatal period and they will not be discussed further here.

Management of neonatal chronic renal failure

The biggest single problem in most babies with CRF is achieving an adequate energy intake: uraemia causes anorexia and sometimes nausea and vomiting. This nearly always requires tube feeding. Most units use nasogastric tubes, although some prefer elective gastrostomy.[14] The ideal feed is breast milk or a low-phosphate artificial formula. In order to achieve normal or near normal growth, an energy intake of 150–180 kcal/kg/day is the target, considerably more than in healthy infants. This will require the addition of energy supplements to the basic feed. The baby is encouraged to take as much feed as possible by sucking and swallowing, a necessary learned skill, but will have to be topped up by tube. A very successful stratagem is to administer intermittent feeds by day and continuous intragastric infusion by night using a Kangaroo or similar pump. Sodium bicarbonate is added to the feed in an amount sufficient to maintain the plasma bicarbonate at 22–24 mmol/l. If there is any tendency to hyponatraemia, or if weight gain is poor despite adequate energy intake, sodium chloride should also be added in a dose that maintains normal plasma sodium concentrations without inducing fluid overload or hypertension. Calcium carbonate is often necessary to maintain the plasma phosphate in the normal range (N.B. the normal range for plasma phosphate is higher in babies than in older individuals). When serum phosphate is adequately controlled, calcidiol or calcitriol should be added if the plasma calcium concentration is low. This is a difficult and demanding regimen and requires skilled and sympathetic coaching of the parents (or equivalent carers) by a team of experienced nurses, dieticians and nephrologists. Further details of management of CRF in infancy may be found in a comprehensive review.[58]

Polycystic kidney disease

Autosomal dominant polycystic kidney disease (ADPKD) is a fairly common condition (incidence about 1 in 500–600) which seldom causes clinical problems in the newborn period. However, cysts may be visible on ultrasonography in early childhood[38] and occasionally in the newborn or, rarely, the fetus.[51] The largest reported experience is that of a group in Denver, Colorado, who have sequentially followed 312 children from 131 affected families.[21, 22] They discovered that some children eventually found to be affected had hyperechoic kidneys in utero or in the neonatal period, and that cysts were identifiable in 60% of them by the age of 5 years. At any age, affected children had larger kidneys than those not affected and had a tendency to higher blood pressure, although few had blood pressures outside the age- and sex-related normal range. Of the two known loci for ADPKD, PKD-1 is more likely to present early than PKD-2. With very rare exceptions, GFR does not begin to decline measurably during infancy and childhood.

Autosomal recessive polycystic kidney disease (ARPKD) is rare (1 in 10 000–40 000 births) and very variable in expression. It is caused by mutations in a gene at 6p21, which codes for a protein recently identified and named fibrocystin.[82] The most severely affected cases have a version of Potter's syndrome and die of pulmonary insufficiency. Many are now detected antenatally by ultrasonography. All those who survive the neonatal period are destined to develop end-stage renal failure (ESRF), some in infancy but many not until later childhood or even adolescence or early adult life. Congenital hepatic fibrosis is a consistent associated finding. Those who develop ESRF in the newborn period or infancy should be managed as other infants of the same age with ESRF of other causes, with two exceptions. First, it may be necessary to remove both kidneys to make PD a practical proposition. Second, hypertension is a frequent feature of ARPKD and is often resistant to treatment. The combination of hypertension and renal salt loss is unusual, but certainly occurs in some babies with this disease and can be particularly difficult to manage.

Congenital nephrotic syndrome

The nephrotic syndrome is rare in the neonatal period in most populations. Acquired causes include congenital infection due to syphilis, toxoplasmosis, rubella, cytomegalovirus, human immunodeficiency virus and malaria. These should be sought in all cases where epidemiologically appropriate, because, although very rare, some of these are at least potentially treatable. Congenital nephrotic syndrome (CNS) of the Finnish type is the least rare cause. This is an autosomal recessive condition. It is due to mutations in a gene, *NPHS1*, at 19q13.1, that codes for nephrin, a protein that is an essential part of the glomerular ultrafilter, preventing leakage of albumin from the glomerular capillaries into Bowman's space.[40, 48] The name derives from the fact that the gene frequency is uniquely high in Finns, leading to an incidence of the disease of 1:8200 livebirths. It is much less common in other populations but has been described in most ethnic groups. Heavy albuminuria is invariably present from early in gestation, as shown by the consistent finding of very high amniotic fluid α-fetoprotein levels before 16–20 weeks' gestation.

Clinical features

Most affected babies are born prematurely, typically at about 36 weeks. The placenta is large, the mean ratio of placental to infant weight being 0.43 (average normal 0.18). Clinically evident oedema and abdominal distension is present in 25% of cases at birth and in 90% within the first week. The serum albumin concentration is <10 g/l unless artificially supported. Typical facies include wide sutures and fontanelle, small nose, wide-set eyes and low-set ears, although these may not be apparent at birth.[35]

Treatment

Conservative treatment is difficult and involves intensive intravenous albumin infusions, attempts to reduce proteinuria by altering glomerular filtration dynamics by means of ACE inhibitors and NSAIDS and, in some units, elective unilateral nephrectomy.[15] By these means, growth and nutrition can often be improved but not to normal standards. The definitive treatment is bilateral nephrectomy and renal transplantation. The unit in Helsinki, which has the greatest experience of the condition, interposes a period of several months on dialysis between nephrectomy and transplantation, to optimise nutrition and growth and to normalise the plasma albumin concentration and secondary metabolic abnormalities such as hyperlipidaemia. Newborns with CNS should be transferred on diagnosis to a regional paediatric nephrology unit with full dialysis and transplant facilities as well as an appropriate level of neonatal care.

Tubulopathies in the newborn

Bartter's syndrome(s)

Bartter's syndrome is due to mutations in one of three membrane transporters in the thick segment of the ascending limb of the loop of Henlé, resulting in failure of reabsorption of sodium, potassium and chloride.[66–68] The consequent large increase in salt delivery to the distal nephron results in the salt loss, volume depletion, hyperaldosteronism, hypokalaemia and metabolic alkalosis typical of the disease. The most severely affected cases may present in the neonatal period with failure to thrive, polyuria and polydipsia and the above biochemical features. In some cases, polyuria is of sufficient degree in utero to cause polyhydramnios.[55] All the features of Bartter's syndrome are perfectly mimicked by administration of loop diuretics (which block one of the transporters previously mentioned), an important point in differential diagnosis. Similar biochemical findings can occur due to non-renal electrolyte losses in cystic fibrosis (transcutaneous) and congenital chloride-losing diarrhoea (intestinal). The crucial diagnostic investigation is the urinary chloride concentration, which is high in Bartter's syndrome but low (virtually chloride-free urine) if the losses are non-renal. DNA analysis can now confirm the diagnosis but takes weeks or months. Treatment consists of potassium supplementation in all cases, salt supplementation in some and the use of indometacin (indomethacin) in a dose of up to 3 mg/kg/day in divided doses. The closely related syndrome of Gitelman is a much milder disease and seldom, if ever, presents in the neonatal period.

Nephrogenic diabetes insipidus

Nephrogenic diabetes insipidus (NDI) is due to renal resistance to ADH, which normally promotes osmotic water reabsorption in the collecting duct, enabling the production of concentrated urine. The main clinical features are polyuria and hypernatraemic dehydration: polydipsia only occurs in patients who can express thirst or gain independent access to drinks and is therefore not apparent in neonates. Unless there is a family history it is unusual for the diagnosis to be made in the newborn. The condition should be considered in any baby with persistent or recurrent hypernatraemia corrected by an increase in water intake. A formal water deprivation test is unnecessary in the newborn period and may be dangerous. If the plasma osmolality is above 300 mOsmol/kg H$_2$O and the sodium above 147–150 mmol/l, the urine should be maximally concentrated for age (see above). If it is not, and certainly if the urine is hypotonic to plasma, the diagnosis should be provisionally assumed and water supplementation given to maintain normonatraemia. The commonest variety of inherited

NDI is X-linked recessive, due to mutations in the tubular ADH receptor (V_2 receptor).[43] However, there is an even less common form that is inherited as an autosomal recessive condition. This is due to mutations in the gene for aquaporin 2, a tubular water channel that is inserted into the tubular cell membrane when V_2 receptors are occupied by ADH.[78] The two forms are clinically identical and it is important not to exclude the diagnosis of NDI merely because the baby is female.

Renal tubular acidosis

As previously mentioned, the proximal tubular bicarbonate threshold is lower in the newborn than in older infants and children, and lower in preterm than in term babies. The syndrome of late metabolic acidosis of prematurity was first described by Kildeberg[41] and occurs either when babies are fed inappropriately high protein intakes with consequent increase in the generation of non-volatile (mostly sulphuric) acid, and/or when normal growth is interrupted for any reason, when the 'third kidney' effect of growth is lost. This syndrome is seen much less often now than when first described, probably due to changes in infant feeding practices, but may still be seen in a subtle, 'incipient' form in infants who are thriving less well than expected: the hallmark is the finding of maximally acid urine, even if the blood profile is not frankly acidotic.[37] A comprehensive review of acid–base disturbances in newborn and young infants can be found in the classic monograph by Kildeberg.[42]

A form of primary proximal renal tubular acidosis (RTA) was described in newborn infants in the 1960s in New York.[60] These babies, who were carefully and rigorously investigated, had proximal tubular bicarbonate wasting and were able to acidify their urines normally but only at a blood pH lower than that at which healthy infants produce maximally acid urine. This condition was self-limiting and resolved spontaneously in all infants by 18 months of age. Mysteriously, this form of RTA seems to have disappeared since its original description: its cause is unknown. It is possible that it was due to exposure to some unknown dietary or other environmental factor that is no longer present, but it is unlikely that this little mystery will ever be solved. Proximal RTA is seen in infants with the renal Fanconi syndrome, of which the commonest cause in British children is cystinosis, but it is relatively unusual (although not unknown) for it to be apparent in the neonatal period. The presence of other features of the Fanconi syndrome (glycosuria, generalised aminoaciduria, phosphaturia) should lead to suspicion that this may be the case in any child with persistent, unexplained acidosis of the proximal type.

As in cases of unexplained metabolic (non-respiratory) acidosis at any age, it is important to measure the anion gap (AG), the difference between the sodium concentration and the sum of the chloride and bicarbonate:

$$AG = Na^+ - (Cl^- + HCO_3^-)$$

Calculated in this way, the normal value is 8–16 mmol/l. Confusingly, some authors include the potassium in the calculation, in which case the normal value is about 4 mmol/l higher. In reality, the total cations and total anions in a solution always balance exactly, and the apparent gap is due to unmeasured anions, mainly albumin, phosphate and small amounts of organic anions including lactate. If the anion gap is increased above the normal range, there must be present either an increase in the amount of one of the 'normal' unmeasured anions (e.g. lactate), or another organic anion normally present in no more than trace amounts (e.g. ketoacids, complex organic anions in various inborn errors of metabolism). Conversely, metabolic acidosis with a normal anion gap (hyperchloraemic metabolic acidosis) is generally due to renal or gastrointestinal loss of bicarbonate or failure of renal secretion of hydrogen ions (distal renal tubular acidosis).

References

1. Albert M S, Winters R W 1966 Acid-base equilibrium of blood in normal infants. Pediatrics 37: 728–732
2. Al-Dahhan J, Haycock G B, Chantler C, Stimmler L 1983 Sodium homeostasis in term and preterm neonates. I. Renal aspects. Archives of Disease in Childhood 58: 335–342
3. Aperia A, Broberger O, Thodenius K, Zetterstrom R 1975 Development of renal control of salt and fluid homeostasis during the first year of life. Acta Paediatrica Scandinavica 64: 393–398
4. Arant B S Jr 1973 Developmental patterns of renal functional maturation compared in the human neonate. Journal of Pediatrics 92: 705–712
5. Arant B S Jr, Edelmann C M Jr, Nash M A 1974 The renal reabsorption of glucose in the developing canine kidney: a study of glomerulotubular balance. Pediatric Research 8: 638–646
6. Assadi F K 1988 Treatment of acute renal failure in an infant by continuous arteriovenous hemodialysis. Pediatric Nephrology 2: 320–322
7. Baluarte H J, Gruskin A B, Hiner L B, Foley C M, Grover W D 1977 Encephalopathy in children with chronic renal failure. Proceedings of the Clinical Dialysis and Transplant Forum 1977; 7: 95–8
8. Bauer M, Stewart S 1988 Renal failure following cardiac surgery in a 2.8 kg infant managed with continuous arteriovenous hemofiltration. Annals of Thoracic Surgery 45: 225–226
9. Bishof N A, Welch T R, Strife F, Ryckman F C 1990 Continuous hemodiafiltration in children. Pediatrics 85: 819–823
10. Brodehl J, Gellissen K 1968 Endogenous renal transport of free amino acids in infancy and childhood. Pediatrics 42: 395–404
11. Bunchman T E, Maxvold N J, Kershaw D B, Sedman A B, Custer J R 1995 Continuous venovenous hemodiafiltration in infants and children. American Journal of Kidney Diseases 25: 17–21
12. Calcagno P L, Rubin M I 1963 Renal extraction of para-aminohippurate in infants and children. Journal of Clinical Investigation 42: 1632–1639
13. Chevalier R L, Campbell F, Brenbridge A N 1984 Prognostic factors in neonatal acute renal failure. Pediatrics 74: 265–272
14. Coleman J E, Watson A R, Rance C H, Moore E 1998 Gastrostomy buttons for nutritional support on chronic dialysis. Nephrology, Dialysis, Transplantation 13: 2041–2046
15. Coulthard M G 1989 Management of Finnish congenital nephrotic syndrome by unilateral nephrectomy. Pediatric Nephrology 3: 451–453
16. Coulthard M G, Sharp J 1995 Haemodialysis and ultrafiltration in babies weighing under 1000g. Archives of Disease in Childhood. Fetal and Neonatal Edition 73: F162–F165
17. Coulthard M G, Vernon B 1995 Managing acute renal failure in very low birthweight infants. Archives of Disease in Childhood. Fetal and Neonatal Edition 73: F187–F192
18. Edelmann C M Jr, Barnett H L, Troupkou V 1960 Renal concentrating mechanism in newborn infants. Effect of dietary protein and water content, role of urea and responsiveness to antidiuretic hormone. Journal of Clinical Investigation 39: 1062–1069
19. Edelmann C M Jr, Boichis H, Soriano J R, Stark H 1967 The renal response of children to acute ammonium chloride acidosis. Pediatric Research 1: 452–460
20. Ellis E N, Arnold W C 1982 Use of urinary indexes in renal failure in the newborn. American Journal of Diseases of Children 136: 615–617

21. Fick G M, Johnson A M, Strain J D et al 1993 Characteristics of very early onset autosomal dominant polycystic kidney disease. Journal of the American Society of Nephrology 3: 1863–1870

22. Fick-Brosnahan G M, Tran Z V, Johnson A M, Strain J D, Gabow P A 2001 Progression of autosomal-dominant polycystic kidney disease in children. Kidney International 59: 1654–1662

23. Gruskin A B, Edelmann C M Jr, Yuan S 1970 Maturational changes in renal blood flow in piglets. Pediatric Research 4: 7–13

24. Hammarlund K, Sedin G 1979 Transepidermal water loss in newborn infants. III. Relation to gestational age. Acta Paediatrica Scandinavica 68: 795–801

25. Hansen J D L, Smith C A 1953 Effects of withholding fluid in the immediate postnatal period. Pediatrics 12: 99–112

26. Hartnoll G, Betrémieux P, Modi N 2000 Randomised controlled trial of postnatal sodium supplementation on oxygen dependency and body weight in 25–30 weeks gestational age infants. Archives of Disease in Childhood. Fetal and Neonatal Edition 82: F19–F23

27. Hartnoll G, Betrémieux P, Modi N 2000 Randomised controlled trial of postnatal sodium supplementation on body composition in 25–30 weeks gestational age infants. Archives of Disease in Childhood. Fetal and Neonatal Edition 82: F24–F28

28. Hartnoll G, Betrémieux P, Modi N 2001 Randomised controlled trial of postnatal sodium supplementation in infants of 25–30 weeks gestational age: effects on cardiopulmonary adaptation. Archives of Disease in Childhood. Fetal and Neonatal Edition 85: F29–F32

29. Haycock G B 1989 Creatinine, body size and renal function. Pediatric Nephrology 3: 22–24

30. Haycock G B, Aperia A 1991 Salt and the newborn kidney. Pediatric Nephrology 5: 65–70

31. Hencz P, Deverall P B, Crew A D, Steel A E, Mearns A J 1979 Hyperuricemia of infants and children: a complication of open heart surgery. Journal of Pediatrics 94: 774–776

32. Heney D, Brocklebank J T, Wilson N 1989 Continuous arteriovenous haemofiltration in the newlyborn with acute renal failure and congenital heart disease. Nephrology, Dialysis, Transplantation 4: 870–876

33. Hillman L S, Salmons S S, Erickson M M, Hansen J W, Hillman R E, Chesney R 1994 Calciuria and aminoaciduria in very low birth weight infants fed a high-mineral premature formula with varying levels of protein. Journal of Pediatrics 125: 288–294

34. Hinchcliffe S A, Lynch M R J, Sargent P H, Howard C V, van Velzen D 1992 The effect of intrauterine growth retardation on the development of renal nephrons. British Journal of Obstetrics and Gynaecology 99: 296–301

35. Huttunen N P 1976 Congenital nephrotic syndrome of Finnish type. Study of 75 patients. Archives of Disease in Childhood 51: 344–348

36. Kalhoff H, Diekmann L, Kunz C, Stock G J, Manz F 1997 Alkali therapy versus sodium chloride supplement in low birthweight infants with incipient late metabolic acidosis. Acta Paediatrica 86: 96–101

37. Kalhoff H, Manz F, Diekmann L, Kunz C, Stock G J, Weisser F 1993 Decreased growth rate of low-birth-weight infants with prolonged maximum renal acid stimulation. Acta Paediatrica 82: 522–527

38. Kaplan B S, Rabin I, Nogrady M B, Drummond K N 1977 Autosomal dominant polycystic renal disease in children. Journal of Pediatrics 90: 782–783

39. Kaskel F J, Kumar A M, Feld L G, Spitzer A 1988 Renal reabsorption of phosphate during development: tubular events. Pediatric Nephrology 2: 129–134

40. Khoshnoodi J, Tryggvason K 2001 Congenital nephrotic syndromes. Current Opinion in Genetics and Development 11: 322–327

41. Kildeberg P 1964 Disturbances of hydrogen ion balance occurring in premature infants. II. Late metabolic acidosis. Acta Paediatrica 53: 517–526

42. Kildeberg P 1968 Clinical acid-base physiology. Studies in neonates, infants and young children. Munksgaard, Copenhagen, 1968

43. Knoers N V, van den Ouweland A M, Verdijk M, Monnens L A, van Oost B A 1994 Inheritance of mutations in the V2 receptor gene in 13 families with nephrogenic diabetes insipidus. Kidney International 46: 170–176

44. Lieberman K V, Nardi L, Bosch J P 1985 Treatment of acute renal failure in an infant using continuous arteriovenous hemofiltration. Journal of Pediatrics 106: 646–649

45. McCance R A 1959 The maintenance of stability in the newly born. 1. Chemical exchange. Archives of Disease in Childhood 34: 361–370

46. McClure R J, Prasad V K, Brocklebank J T 1994 Treatment of hyperkalaemia using intravenous and nebulised salbutamol. Archives of Disease in Childhood 70: 126–128

47. Mackenzie H S, Brenner B M 1995 Fewer nephrons at birth: a missing link in the etiology of essential hypertension? American Journal of Kidney Diseases 26: 91–98

48. Mannikko M, Kestaila M, Holmberg C et al 1995 Fine mapping and haplotype analysis of the locus for congenital nephrotic syndrome on chromosome 19q13.1. American Journal of Human Genetics 57: 1377–1383

49. Mathew O P, Jones A S, James E, Bland H, Groshong T 1980 Neonatal renal failure: usefulness of diagnostic indices. Pediatrics 65: 57–60

50. Mattoo T K, Ahmad G S 1994 Peritoneal dialysis in neonates after major abdominal surgery. American Journal of Nephrology 14: 6–8

51. Michaud J, Russo P, Grignon A et al 1994 Autosomal dominant polycystic kidney disease in the fetus. American Journal of Medical Genetics 51: 240–246

52. Moniz C F, Nicolaides K H, Bamforth F J, Rodeck C H 1985 Normal reference ranges for biochemical substances relating to renal, hepatic, and bone function in fetal and maternal plasma during pregnancy. Journal of Clinical Pathology 38: 468–472

53. Murdoch I A, Dos Anjos R, Haycock G B 1991 Treatment of hyperkalaemia with intravenous salbutamol. Archives of Disease in Childhood 66: 527–528

54. Nicolaides K H, Cheng H H, Snijders R J M, Moniz M D 1992 Fetal urine biochemistry in the assessment of obstructive uropathy. American Journal of Obstetrics and Gynecology 166: 932–937

55. Proesmans W 1997 Bartter syndrome and its neonatal variant. European Journal of Pediatrics 156: 669–679

56. Rabinowitz R, Peters M T, Vyas S, Campbell S, Nicolaides K H 1989 Measurement of fetal urine production in normal pregnancy by real-time ultrasonography. American Journal of Obstetrics and Gynecology 161: 1264–1266

57. Riesenfeld T, Hammarlund K, Sedin G 1995 Respiratory water loss in relation to gestational age in infants on their first day after birth. Acta Paediatrica 84: 1056–1059

58. Rigden S P, Start K M, Rees L 1987 Nutritional management of infants and toddlers with chronic renal failure. Nutrition and Health 5: 163–174

59. Roberts D S, Haycock G B, Dalton R N et al 1990 Prediction of acute renal failure after birth asphyxia. Archives of Disease in Childhood 65: 1021–1028

60. Rodriguez-Soriano J, Boichis H, Stark H, Edelmann C M Jr 1967 Proximal renal tubular acidosis. A defect in bicarbonate reabsorption with normal urinary acidification. Pediatric Research 1: 81–98

61. Rodríguez-Soriano J, Vallo A, Oliveros R, Castillo G 1983 Renal handling of sodium in premature and full-term neonates: a study using clearance methods during water diuresis. Pediatric Research 17: 1013–1016

62. Sadowski R H, Harmon W E, Jabs K 1994 Acute hemodialysis of infants weighing less than five kilograms. Kidney International 45: 903–906

63. Schwartz G J, Haycock G B, Edelmann C M Jr, Spitzer A 1976 A simple estimate of glomerular filtration rate in children derived from body length and plasma creatinine. Pediatrics 58: 259–263

64. Schwartz G J, Haycock G B, Edelmann C M Jr, Spitzer A 1979 Late metabolic acidosis: a reassessment of the definition. Journal of Pediatrics 95: 102–107

65. Siegel S R, Oh W 1976 Renal function as a marker of human fetal maturation. Acta Paediatrica Scandinavica 65: 481–485

66. Simon D B, Bindra R S, Mansfield T A et al 1997 Mutations in the chloride channel gene, CLCNKB, cause Bartter's syndrome type III. Nature Genetics 17: 171–178

67. Simon D B, Karet F E, Hamdan J M, Di Pietro A, Sanjad S A, Lifton R P 1996 Bartter's syndrome, hypokalemic alkalosis with hypercalciuria, is caused by mutations in the Na-K-2Cl transporter NKCC2. Nature Genetics 13: 183–188

68. Simon D B, Karet F E, Rodriguez-Soriano J 1996 Genetic heterogeneity of Bartter's syndrome revealed by mutations in the K+ channel, ROMK. Nature Genetics 14: 152–156

69. Sizun J, Giroux J-D, Rubio S, Guillois B, Alix D, De Parscau L 1993 Peritoneal dialysis in the very low-birth-weight neonate (less than 1000 g). Acta Paediatrica 82: 488–489

70. Spitzer A, Brandis M 1974 Functional and morphologic maturation of the superficial nephrons. Journal of Clinical Investigation 53: 279–287

71. Stapleton F B, Jones D P, Green R S 1987 Acute renal failure in neonates: incidence, etiology and outcome. Pediatric Nephrology 1: 314–320

72. Steele B T, Vigneux A, Blatz S, Flavin M, Paes B 1987 Acute peritoneal dialysis in infants weighing <1500 g. Journal of Pediatrics 110: 126–129

73. Sujov P, Kellerman L, Zeltzer M, Hochberg Z 1984 Plasma and urine osmolality in full-term and pre-term infants. Acta Paediatrica Scandinavica 73: 722–726

74. Sulyok E, Németh M, Tényi I, Csaba I F, Varga L, Varga F 1981 Relationship between the postnatal development of the renin-angiotensin-aldosterone system and the electrolyte and acid-base status in the sodium chloride supplemented premature infant. Acta Paediatrica Academiae Scientarum Hungaricae 22: 109–121

75. Sulyok E, Varga F, Györy E, Jobst K, Csaba I F 1979 Postnatal development of renal sodium handling in premature infants. Journal of Pediatrics 95: 787–792

76. Trompeter R S, Chantler C, Haycock G B 1981 Tolazoline and acute renal failure in the newborn [letter]. Lancet 1: 1219

77. Trompeter R S, Turner C, Haycock G B, Chik G, Chantler C 1983 Normal values for plasma creatinine concentration related to maturity in normal term and preterm infants. International Journal of Pediatric Nephrology 4: 145–148

78. van Lieburg A F, Verdijk M A, Knoers V V et al 1994 Patients with autosomal nephrogenic diabetes insipidus homozygous for mutations in the aquaporin 2 water-channel gene. American Journal of Human Genetics 55: 648–652

79. Vanpée M, Herin P, Broberger U, Aperia A 1995 Sodium supplementation optimizes weight gain in premature infants. Acta Paediatrica 84: 1312–1314

80. Yorgin P D, Krensky A M, Tune B M 1990 Continuous venovenous hemofiltration. Pediatric Nephrology 4: 640–642

81. Zelikovic I, Chesney R W, Friedman A L, Ahlfors C E 1990 Taurine depletion in very low birth weight infants receiving prolonged total parenteral nutrition: role of renal immaturity. Journal of Pediatrics 116: 301–306

82. Zerres K, Rudnik-Schoneborn S, Senderek J, Eggermann T, Bergmann C 2003 Autosomal recessive polycystic kidney disease (ARPKD). Journal of Nephrology 16: 453–458

PART 2

Urology

Duncan T Wilcox, Pierre Mouriquand

Urinary tract anomalies

Urinary tract abnormalities are increasingly detected by antenatal ultrasound, with 1:800 pregnancies having an antenatally diagnosed uropathy.[3,56,58] Despite improvements in technique, some children with an abnormal urinary tract still avoid detection and present during childhood with signs and symptoms of a urinary tract infection (UTI). Antenatally diagnosed dilatation of the urinary tract can occur either from impairment of urine flow or by retrograde reflux of urine, the pathological consequences of which are discussed below.

Pathology

Urine flow impairment (UFI) can occur at any level in the urinary tract, and may affect one or both sides. Dilatation of the pelvis and calyces is the first anatomical response to UFI and may lead to histological damage of the renal parenchyma and changes in renal function. Histological damage is related to the degree and level of UFI and its duration. Renal atrophy, as seen in patients with multicystic dysplastic kidney, is the ultimate response to UFI related to the onset of apoptosis.[26] When UFI is significant early in pregnancy, the renal parenchyma develops dysplasia,[25] and in severe cases there is a reduction of the ipsilateral glomerular filtration rate (GFR) and an increase in the contralateral GFR. When UFI becomes significant later in gestation or is partial, it generates dilatation of the excretory system[7,30] without affecting the parenchymal structure.

Before the advent of antenatal scanning all renal damage (scars) seen in patients with vesicoureteric reflux (VUR) was thought to be secondary to postnatal infection. Subsequently, early preinfection studies on neonates diagnosed antenatally with reflux have shown renal scars.[70] In these kidneys the scarring was global, compared with the segmental scarring seen following infection. This suggests that kidneys are damaged in utero, or that they develop abnormally. As with UFI, not all kidneys are affected: less than 50% of these infants had renal scarring. Mackie and Stephens postulated that an abnormal development of the ureteric bud would lead to anomalous development of the kidney, resulting in renal dysplasia.[41] This suggests that abnormal development leads to both reflux and renal scarring.

Investigation of a neonate with antenatally detected uropathy

When an antenatal uropathy is diagnosed, it is imperative to confirm the diagnosis postnatally. This should be done by ultrasound on day 3 or 4 of life;[14] ultrasonography earlier than this can lead to a false negative result, due to the relative oliguria of the newborn period. Structural anomalies of the renal parenchyma can be detected at this time. If no abnormality is detected, which with advances in antenatal ultrasound is unusual, a repeat ultrasound scan should be performed at 6 weeks of age. Until the diagnosis is made, all infants should be kept on prophylactic antibiotics, although the evidence for this is still limited.

If the postnatal ultrasound scan shows a unilateral dilatation, no further investigations need to be done until 6 weeks of age. Isotope renography (p. 1230) can then be performed at 6–12 weeks, when the kidneys have matured sufficiently for this to be reliable. Bilateral dilatation requires an early micturating cystourethrogram (MCUG) to exclude bladder outlet obstruction.

The role of the MCUG in neonates with unilateral dilatation is less well established, and there is still controversy. Initially it was felt that all babies required an MCUG in order to exclude reflux, which is present in approximately 15–20%.[63] More recent studies have questioned the clinical significance of this reflux and many centres now advocate performing an MCUG only in patients with bilateral dilatation, unilateral hydronephrosis with a dilated ureter or where there is a suspicion of an abnormal bladder.[69] These centres consider that MCUG is not necessary when there is unilateral hydronephrosis and a normal contralateral kidney. Other centres recommend that an MCUG is done in all cases of antenatally diagnosed dilatation.

Following the initial newborn and 6-week investigations, a diagnosis can be made in the majority of infants. Renal parenchymal anomalies occur in approximately 13% and dilatation in the remainder.[60] The renal anomalies include:

- multicystic dysplastic kidney;
- unilateral and bilateral renal agenesis.

The common causes of dilatation are listed in Table 36.6.[60] The routine postnatal management of these patients with dilatation is outlined in Fig. 36.6. The individual diagnoses are discussed below.

Pyeloureteric junction anomalies

Pyeloureteric junction (PUJ) anomalies are the most common antenatally diagnosed uropathy.[62,64] The diagnosis of unilateral or bilateral PUJ anomaly can be suspected antenatally when an ultrasound scan of the fetus shows a dilated renal pelvis without

---

Table 36.6 Common causes of antenatally diagnosed uropathy

- Pelvi-ureteric junction anomaly
- Vesicoureteric reflux
- Vesicoureteric junction anomaly
- Multicystic dysplastic kidney
- Duplex kidney
- Posterior uretheral valves

---

ureteric dilatation. Significant pathology may be suspected after 18 weeks' gestation if the pelvis is dilated, associated with changes in the parenchymal appearance[46] or with a reduction in the amount of amniotic fluid when the anomaly is bilateral, which is extremely rare. In that case, oligohydramnios is usually detected during the second half of pregnancy.

Although many PUJ anomalies are diagnosed antenatally, some may present as problems in infancy. Abdominal mass was one of the principal symptoms of PUJ anomaly in babies before the ultrasound era.[21] Loin pain reflects the intermittent distension of the renal pelvis. Haematuria, hypertension and UTIs are rare problems of PUJ anomalies.

Associated urological anomalies include ureteric hypoplasia,[1] VUR,[33,47] partial or complete ureteric duplication[36,43] and horseshoe kidney. PUJ anomalies also can be associated with anorectal anomalies, congenital heart disease and VATER syndrome (pp. 806, 807).[22]

The natural history of UFI located in the upper urinary tract is now better understood following the numerous randomised clinical studies[8,42,50] comparing non-operative with surgical management of antenatally diagnosed dilated upper tracts. These studies have shown that the majority of patients with antenatally diagnosed upper tract dilatation improve spontaneously; however, approximately 25% will require surgical intervention.[15] The difficulty is in identifying who needs an operation, and this can only be decided upon after a period of regular assessment.

Conservative management of PUJ anomalies is justified in most patients during the first year of life. Three conditions are

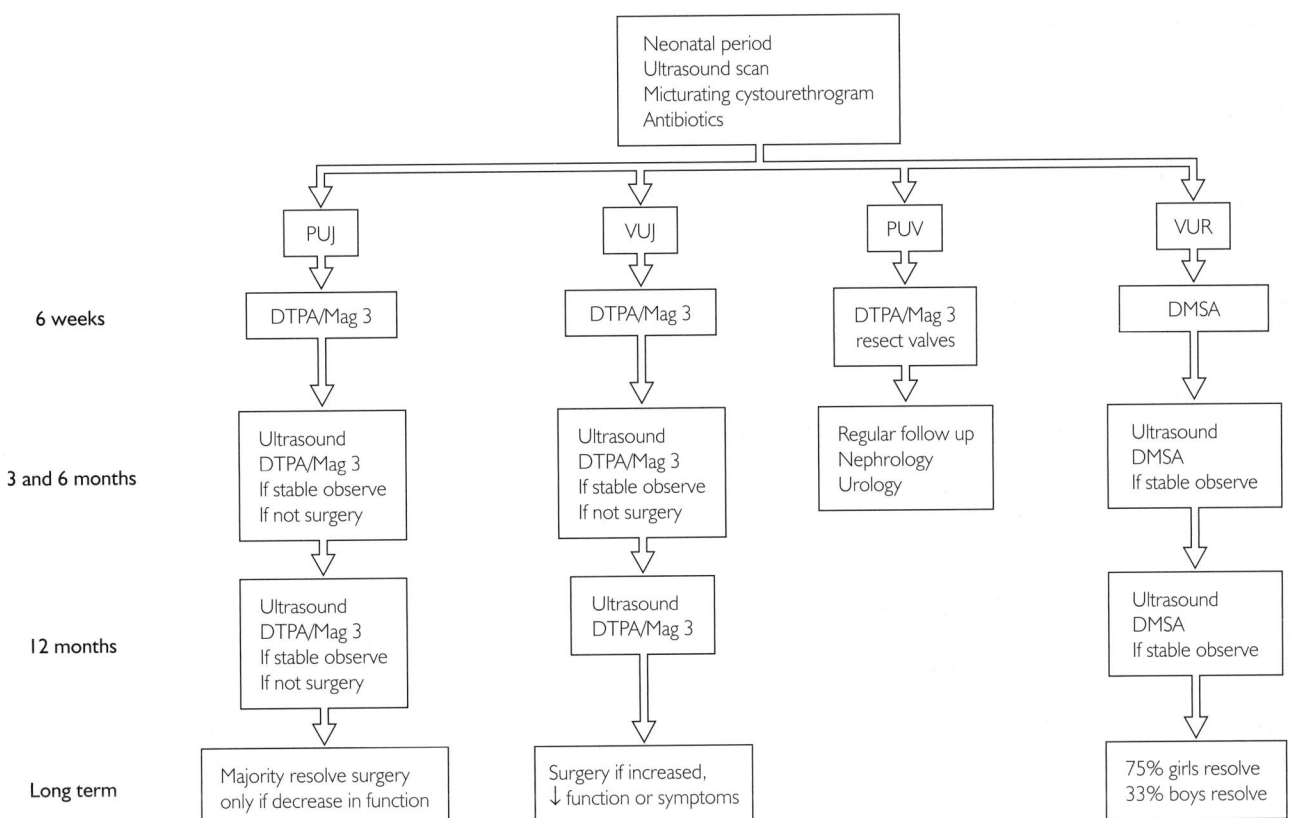

Fig. 36.6 Flow chart detailing the postnatal investigation pathways of a child born with a antenatally diagnosed dilatation.

required before it can be considered appropriate to follow a baby with unilateral PUJ anomaly medically:

■ The baby must be asymptomatic.
■ The degree of pelvic dilatation, measured with ultrasound, should be stable or decreasing.
■ The relative function of the affected kidney (measured with radioisotope studies) should be either stable or improving.

Antibiotic prophylactic cover is recommended, although no studies have to date proved that it prevents UTI. This conservative approach, initially proposed by Ransley et al,[50] is now adopted by many centres and requires 3-monthly ultrasound scans during the first year of life. The anterior–posterior diameter of the renal pelvis in the transverse plane should be measured with ultrasound, as this is a good predictor of significant UFI (Fig. 36.7).[16]

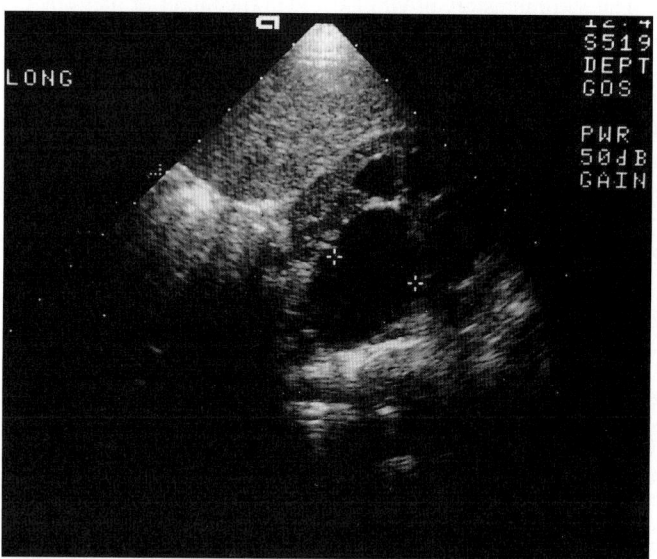

Fig. 36.7 Ultrasound scan showing a pyelouretric junction anomaly. The markers indicate the lateral margins of the dilated renal pelvis.

In addition, nuclear renography should be performed at 6–12 weeks and again at 1 year (Fig. 36.8).

Temporary diversion of the pelvic urine is indicated in infants with severe pelvic dilatation and poor relative function (<15%). The next question is whether or not to remove the poorly functioning kidney. To answer this, in our view it is necessary to place a percutaneous nephrostomy for 3–4 weeks, followed by reassessment of the relative function. Either the function will have improved and a pyeloplasty should be performed, or the function will remain poor and a nephrectomy should be discussed. Some paediatric urologists feel that a period of percutaneous drainage is unnecessary, arguing that DMSA scan can accurately predict the true function of the kidney when the obstruction is relieved.[65]

Surgical treatment of a PUJ anomaly is advocated by most urologists when the following conditions exist:

■ a symptomatic PUJ anomaly;
■ declining function in the dilated kidney;
■ moderate pelvic dilatation with dilatation of the calyces;
■ an increasing pelvic dilatation;
■ bilateral moderate-to-severe dilatation of the pelvis.[15]

These indications are not accepted by all: some operate on infants during the first year of life arguing that the outcome of pyeloplasty is usually excellent in terms of drainage and preserved renal function.[29] Conversely, others will follow a conservative approach even with an increased pelvic dilatation.[40] When surgery is performed, the most common operation is a pyeloplasty.

Vesicoureteric junction anomaly (megaureter)

Many classifications of megaureter have been reported[38] but practically there are only two: megaureter with or without reflux. However, distal anatomical obstruction of the ureter and VUR may occur together. Investigations include ultrasound scan of

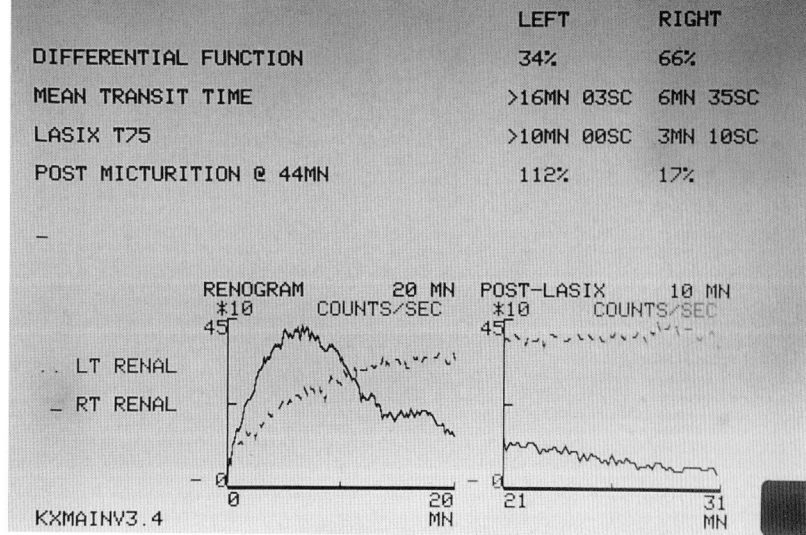

	LEFT	RIGHT
DIFFERENTIAL FUNCTION	34%	66%
MEAN TRANSIT TIME	>16MN 03SC	6MN 35SC
LASIX T75	>10MN 00SC	3MN 10SC
POST MICTURITION @ 44MN	112%	17%

RENOGRAM   20 MN   POST-LASIX   10 MN
*10   COUNTS/SEC   *10   COUNTS/SEC
45   45
.. LT RENAL
_ RT RENAL
0   0
0   20   21   31
MN   MN
KXMAINV3.4

Fig. 36.8 MAG 3 renogram showing a left unilateral pyelouretric junction anomaly. The dotted line represents the radioactivity in the left kidney; the plain line represents the radioactivity in the right kidney. The right kidney takes up the radioactive marker promptly and then within 20 minutes, as shown by the down-sloping line, has excreted the marker. This is a normal curve. The left kidney has poor uptake, indicating reduced function, confirmed by the differential function of 34%, and by 30 minutes the radioactivity remains high, showing impaired urinary excretion.

the urinary tract (Fig. 36.9) and an MCUG. Functional studies (diuresis renography) are useful to assess the degree of function. It is sometimes difficult to distinguish a PUJ from a vesicoureteric junction (VUJ) anomaly, as they can occur together. In these complicated cases, a contrast antegrade pyelogram may be the only way to differentiate the two conditions.

Spontaneous improvement of ureteric dilatation is a frequent event in megaureters related to a faulty VUJ. Conservative management of megaureters is recommended when renal function and dilatation of the upper tract remain stable (or improve), and when the child remains asymptomatic.[53] Antibiotic prophylaxis is recommended, especially in refluxing megaureters. Regular isotope assessments are required to follow these children.

When the conservative approach fails, i.e. when infections recur in spite of an adequate antibiotic prophylactic cover, or when renal function decreases on repeated isotope studies or when dilatation of the urinary tract increases, ureteric reimplantation is usually recommended, except where renal function is poor (<15%), when nephroureterectomy is indicated. The aim of the operation is to excise the distal obstructive segment of the ureter and reimplant the ureter with an antireflux mechanism.

Ureterocoeles

Ureterocoeles are a cystic dilatation of the intravesical portion of the ureter. They occur in approximately 1:500 people. In children they are almost always associated with a duplex kidney and occur in the ureter draining the upper pole, although rarely they can occur in a simplex system.[67] Ureterocoeles occur more frequently in girls and in the Caucasian population.[67] Ureterocoeles have been classified in many ways, but a simple classification is to divide them into those arising from a single or duplex kidney, and then further into intravesical and extravesical types.

Postnatally these babies need to be placed on prophylactic antibiotics and investigated with an ultrasound scan (Fig. 36.10); in addition, functional studies are required to assess the relative function in the upper and lower poles of the duplex kidney. As reflux occurs in 20–40% into the lower pole, many centres recommend an MCUG.

There is considerable controversy over the management of ureterocoeles, which varies from simple endoscopic puncture of the ureterocoele to upper-pole heminephrectomy and bladder reconstruction. Increasingly, a more conservative approach is being adopted. In patients who present in the neonatal period, the appropriate first procedure is endoscopic puncture: this was the only procedure required in 73% of babies, and resulted in drainage and preservation of the upper pole in over 90%.[8] In this and other studies, ureteric reflux was created in 20–40% of patients, and further surgery, including upper-pole heminephrectomy plus or minus bladder reconstruction, was required in 20–80%.[8,18]

Posterior urethral valves

A posterior urethral valve (PUV) is a congenital membrane obstructing or partially obstructing the posterior urethra. It is the most common cause of lower urinary obstruction in males, but has extremely rarely been described in females.[6] The incidence is between 1:4000 and 1:25 000.[5,37]

PUV should be suspected in a fetus with a thick-walled bladder and bilateral dilatation of the upper urinary tract, whether or not associated with renal dysplasia and oligohydramnios. Oligohydramnios is usually noticed during the second part of pregnancy, when most of the amniotic fluid is fetal urine. Despite modern ultrasonic equipment, only 16–55% of patients with PUV are detected before 24 weeks' gestation.[19] Children with antenatal diagnosis of PUV seem to have a worse renal prognosis than those with later diagnosis, and earlier diagnosis and treatment do not appear to improve the clinical prognosis.[52]

In the newborn, there can be symptoms of severe metabolic disorders related to renal failure, respiratory problems (spontaneous pneumothorax or pneumomediastinum) and UTI.[57] Palpation of the kidney(s) and the bladder is usually easy. In infants and young children, urinary symptoms are more common (dysuria, haematuria, UTI, septicaemia), sometimes accompanied by

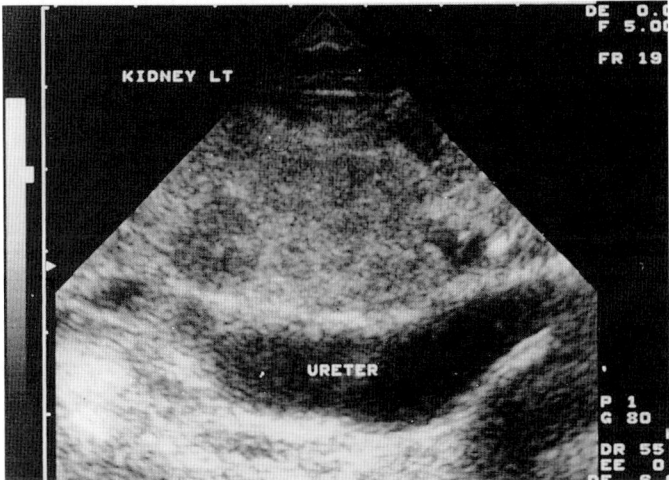

Fig. 36.9 Ultrasound scan showing a dilated megaureter which has a tortuous route.

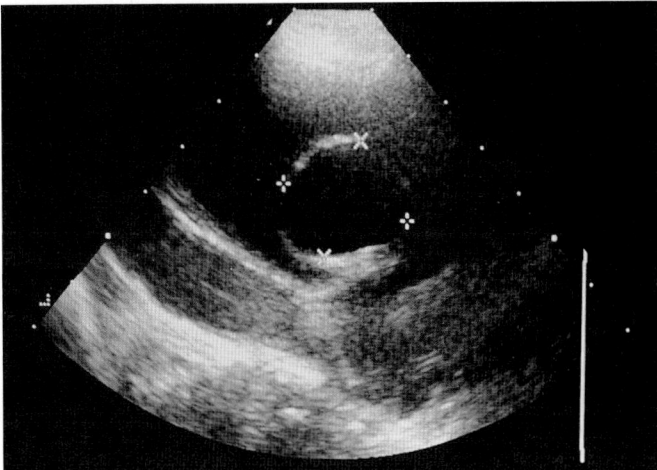

Fig. 36.10 Ultrasound scan. The cystic structure outlined by the markers is a ureterocoele situated within the bladder.

rectal prolapse. Renal failure may be present. In the older child, urinary incontinence, urgency and dysuria are also sometimes seen.

Ultrasound scan of the urinary tract is the first-line investigation. This shows the dilatation of the upper urinary tract, and, sometimes, abnormal echogenicity of the renal parenchyma is seen. There is usually a thick bladder wall associated (or not) with bladder diverticula, and a dilated posterior urethra. Perineal ultrasound is increasingly able to detect urethral anomalies. MCUG is still the gold-standard investigation to detect PUV (Fig. 36.11). Insertion of a transurethral catheter can damage the anatomy of the valve, and some paediatric urologists prefer to perform an MCUG via a suprapubic catheter. Isotope studies are essential to assess the renal consequences of PUV.[28,66]

Antenatal treatment is rarely indicated but may be justified when the liquor volume is reducing in a fetus with bilateral dilatation of the upper urinary tract.[32] Insertion of a double-J stent between the fetal bladder (or the dilated kidneys) and the amniotic cavity, under ultrasound guidance, allows decompression of the urinary tract, possible preservation of development of the fetal kidney, and maturation of the fetal lungs by restoration of an adequate volume of amniotic fluid. These antenatal diversions are usually done quite late in pregnancy and, once again, the benefit of such interventions in children with PUV has not been demonstrated.[32]

After birth, three main principles of treatment are to resuscitate the child, adequately drain the bladder and destroy the valves. Resuscitation implies hydration, electrolyte replacement and antibiotics. Urine drainage can usually be achieved by inserting either a transurethral or a suprapubic catheter. Occasionally, a surgical vesicostomy is required to drain the bladder. If the baby is severely ill and infected, drainage of the upper tract may be the best option (ureterostomy or, preferably, percutaneous nephrostomy). Destruction of the valve is performed when resuscitation is achieved, usually within a week of birth. Surgical destruction of the valve is performed endoscopically.

Renal failure is a common complication of PUV and is seen in 40–50% of cases at the time of diagnosis. The type of primary surgical treatment does not seem to influence the progression of renal failure or body growth in children with PUV. Regardless of the surgical or medical treatment, which can greatly influence mortality, renal failure develops in almost 50% of children with PUV.[52] Four factors have been identified as being associated with poor long-term outcome: presentation before the age of 1 year, bilateral VUR, proteinuria, and daytime incontinence at the age of 5 years.[48]

Incontinence is reported to occur in between 14% and 38%[12,35] of boys after treatment of PUV. The incontinence tends to improve at puberty, presumably as a result of further prostatic development. The association of poor renal outcome with urinary incontinence suggests that continuing bladder dysfunction plays a major role in secondary renal damage in these boys with PUVs.

Prune-belly syndrome

Prune-belly syndrome is an extremely rare condition in which the infant has three characteristic features: bilateral undescended testes, absence of the muscle of the anterior abdominal

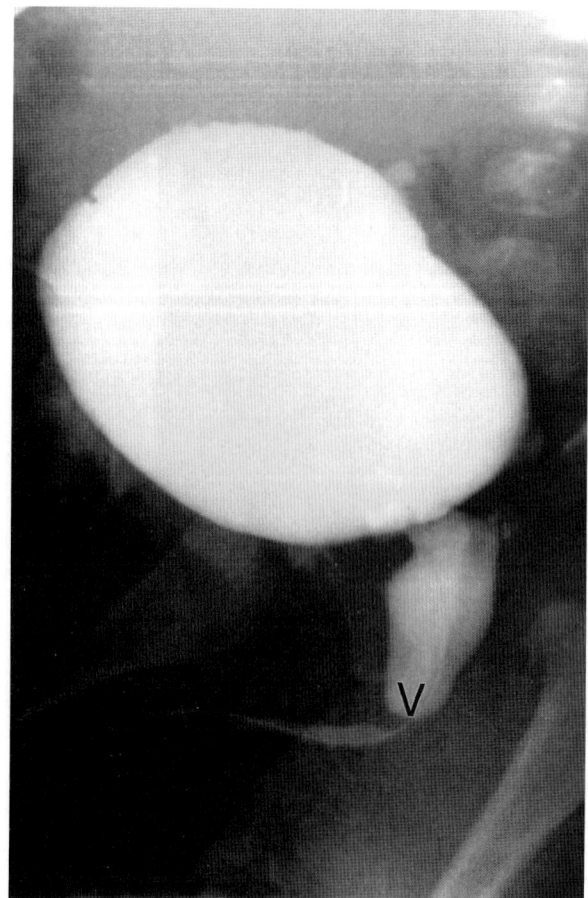

Fig. 36.11 Micturating cystogram showing a posterior urethral valve. Below the bladder is the dilated posterior urethra, from which runs a fine line of contrast. The posterior urethral valves are situated at the transition between the dilated posterior urethra and the thin urethra (V).

wall, and anomalies of the urinary tract. The incidence of this condition appears to be decreasing, probably associated with an increase in antenatal diagnosis and termination of the pregnancy. Because of the infrequency with which this condition is seen, management needs to be individualised. Prognosis is usually poor and dependent on the renal situation.[39]

Vesicoureteric reflux

VUR occurs when urine flows retrogradely from the bladder into the ureters. Previously, reflux was diagnosed in patients being investigated for UTIs; however, with improvements in antenatal scanning, pelvicalyceal dilatation can be identified during pregnancy, which subsequently is diagnosed as reflux and accounts for approximately 25% of all antenatally diagnosed dilatation.[2] Over 90% of those with antenatally diagnosed reflux are boys; this is in contrast to those with postnatally diagnosed reflux, who are mainly girls, and may be explained by the increased voiding pressure required in male fetuses.[2]

When reflux has been identified (Fig. 36.12), it is important to proceed to a DMSA isotope scan so that individual renal function and the presence of renal scarring can be assessed.

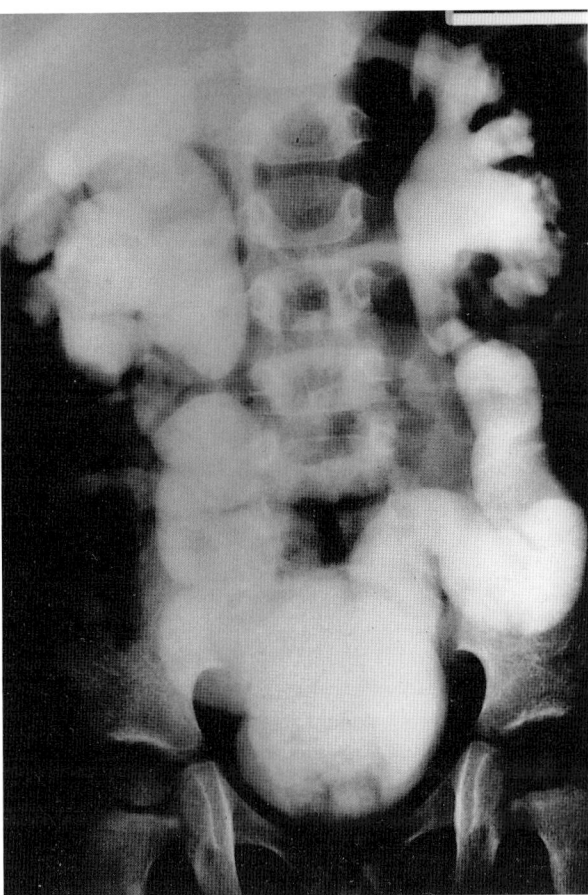

Fig. 36.12 Micturating cystogram showing bilateral vesicoureteric reflux. There is gross bilateral dilatation of the ureters and marked clubbing of the calyces and renal pelvis.

Approximately 60% of kidneys with reflux, within the first 4 weeks of life, have an abnormal renogram;[2] in the majority this was before a UTI had occurred. This suggests that abnormalities in renal development occur with reflux during intrauterine life.[2]

Treatment of reflux is initially non-operative, as reflux requires infected urine to further scar the kidneys.[51] All patients should be placed on prophylactic antibiotics in an attempt to avoid infection, in addition to general methods to reduce infections. Some centres suggest that circumcision can reduce the number of UTIs, but this has not been proved by a controlled trial despite being supported by considerable anecdotal evidence.[68] Following this, adequate and regular bladder emptying should be achieved. Only when these methods fail to prevent recurrent UTIs, or where there is a significant decrease in renal function associated with scarring, is reimplantation of the ureter required to surgically correct the reflux.

Abnormal formation, migration and fusion of the kidney

The absence of a kidney on ultrasound can be due to a congenital deficiency (unilateral or bilateral), involution of a multicystic dysplastic kidney or, alternatively, it could represent an ectopically placed kidney which has yet to be identified.

Renal agenesis

Renal agenesis can be unilateral or bilateral and probably results from a failure of the ureteral bud to induce development in the kidney. This may be due to a defect either in the ureteral bud or in the developing kidney.[44] The incidence of unilateral agenesis is between 1:1000 and 1:1500.[54] An ectopic kidney needs to be excluded by performing a renal isotope scan (DMSA) that visualises all functioning renal tissue. Associated urogenital anomalies are common. The ipsilateral ureter is absent or partially atretic in all cases. The contralateral kidney is either malrotated or ectopic in 15% of cases, and has associated VUR in 37%.[59]

The incidence of bilateral renal agenesis (Potter syndrome) is 1:4000 births. Bilateral renal agenesis is more common in males and within the same family, suggesting a genetic component.[55] Diagnosis is usually made antenatally by ultrasonography, which reveals oligohydramnios and absence of the kidneys. The ureters are usually absent or partially developed. Testicular absence has been found in approximately 10% of cases, but the vas deferens is often present, suggesting that renal agenesis is not due to a failure of the wolffian duct to develop.[4] Potter syndrome is, of course, fatal. The main differential diagnosis is bilateral involuted multicystic dysplastic kidneys.

Multicystic dysplastic kidney

Multicystic dysplastic kidney is increasingly being diagnosed during pregnancy. It is more commonly unilateral, although bilateral cases have been reported. Associated contralateral problems are frequently encountered. Postnatally, diagnosis is confirmed with an ultrasound showing multiple cysts that have completely replaced the kidney (Fig. 36.13). Nuclear renograms show that the multicystic dysplastic kidney is non-functioning. Anomalies in the contralateral kidney are seen in 25% of patients: these include PUJ anomalies and VUR.

Recently, the management of these patients has changed to a non-operative approach. Serial ultrasounds show that these kidneys frequently involute. The size of the kidney at initial presentation appears to predict involution, with few multicystic dysplastic kidneys greater than 6 cm disappearing spontaneously. If the kidney is not decreasing in size, many centres offer nephrectomy, as there have been reports of hypertension and malignant change associated with multicystic dysplastic kidneys, although these are extremly rare.[27,61]

Ectopic kidneys

Ectopic kidneys are caused by an abnormality in renal ascent and/or renal fusion. If an ectopic kidney is suspected, an ultrasound and DMSA scan should be performed for diagnostic reasons. Ectopic kidneys can be divided into simple, horseshoe, and crossed renal ectopia.

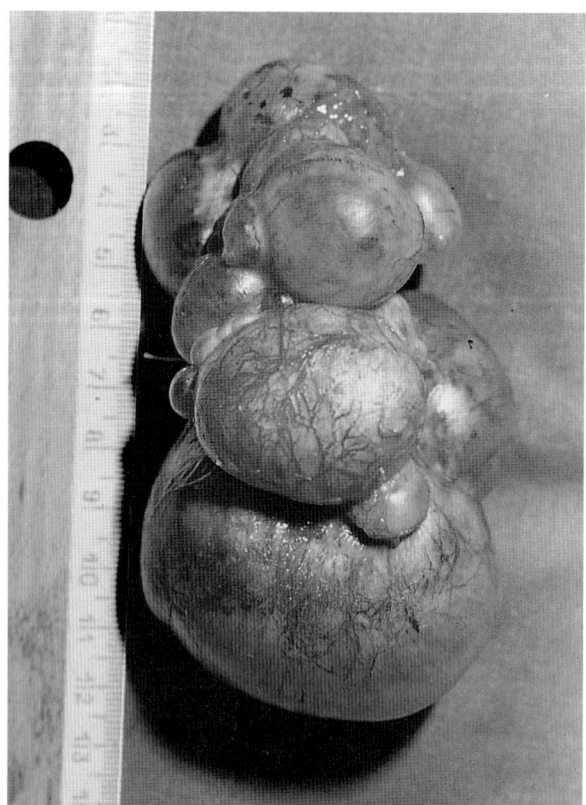

Fig. 36.13 Post-mortem specimen showing a multicystic dysplastic kidney.

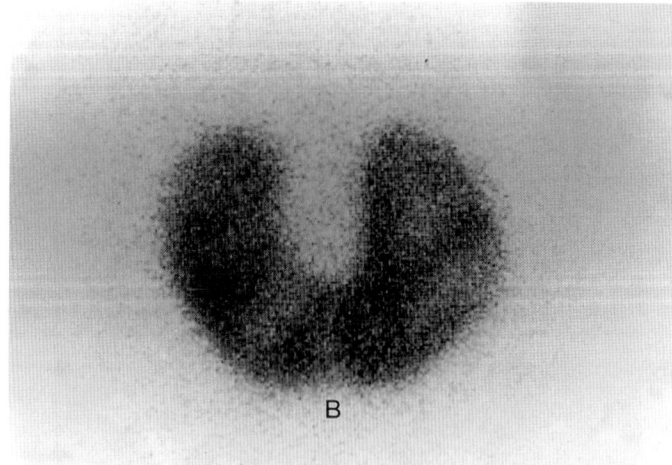

Fig. 36.14 MAG 3 renogram showing a horseshoe kidney; the bridge of renal tissue connecting the right and left kidneys can be seen (B).

Simple

The most common location for a simple ectopic kidney is pelvic, which occurs in 60% of cases. It is usually unilateral, with a slight predilection for the left side, but is found bilaterally in 10% of cases.[54] In addition to its abnormal location, a pelvic kidney is frequently small and irregular in shape. The remaining ectopic kidneys lie between the pelvis and the normal position. Very rarely, the kidney can be found within the thorax.

Ectopic kidneys are associated with genital and contralateral urinary abnormalities, such as absence of the vagina,[31] retrocaval ureter, bicornuate uterus, supernumerary kidney[23] and contralateral ectopic ureter.[9]

Horseshoe kidney

The incidence of horseshoe kidney varies between 1:400 and 1:1800[11] autopsies, and is more common in males. In 95% of cases, the lower poles of the two kidneys are joined by a bridge of renal tissue, which can be normal, dysplastic or fibrous (Fig. 36.14). In about 40% of cases, the isthmus lies at the level of L4, just beneath the origin of the inferior mesenteric artery. In 20% the isthmus is in the pelvis; in the rest it lies at the level of the lower poles of normally placed kidneys.[31] A small number of horseshoe kidneys have fusion at their upper poles. The ureters arch anteriorly to pass over the isthmus,[10] which may explain the relatively high incidence of pyeloureteric anomalies (20%) associated with horseshoe kidneys. Associated abnormalities are common: these can involve the central nervous system, gastrointestinal tract, and the skeletal and cardiovascular systems.

Crossed renal ectopia

Crossed renal ectopia can occur either with renal fusion (80%) or without fusion. It is slightly more common in boys and the left kidney usually crosses to the right side, where the upper pole of the crossed kidney fuses with the lower pole of the uncrossed kidney. As with all renal ectopia, treatment is only required for clinically significant consequences, which are fortunately rare, such as VUR or PUJ obstruction (Fig. 36.15).

Genitourinary tract anomalies

Hypospadias

Hypospadias occurs in 1 in 300 male births. This congenital abnormality consists of three features: an abnormally placed urethral meatus, which can be found anywhere from the glans to the penoscrotal junction; chordee of the penis, which forces the penis to point towards the scrotum when erect; and a foreskin which, instead of being wrapped around the penis, is present only on the dorsal side (Fig. 36.16).[45] The underlying pathology is not fully understood, but it is probably caused by an incomplete virilisation of the penis. The important consideration when examining a child with hypospadias is to be certain that this is not a virilised female or an XY/XO mosaic. This can be assessed by palpation of the testes: if there are two, the karyotype is XY; however, if one or both testes are undescended, then intersex problems must be excluded (see Chapter 35).[49] In the majority, the hypospadias is an isolated problem that necessitates appropriate referral and requires surgical reconstruction between 1 and 2 years of age.

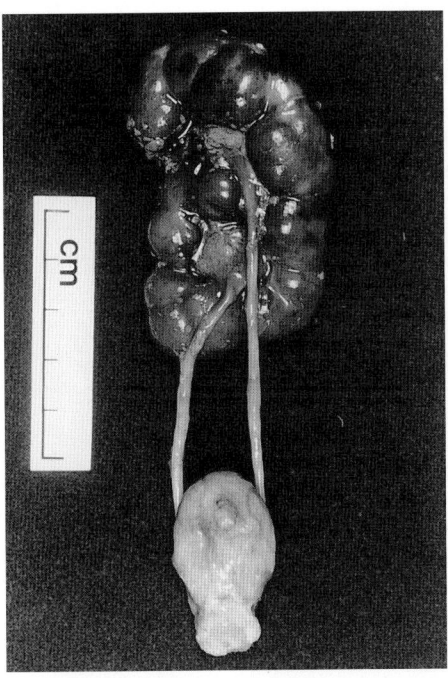

(a)

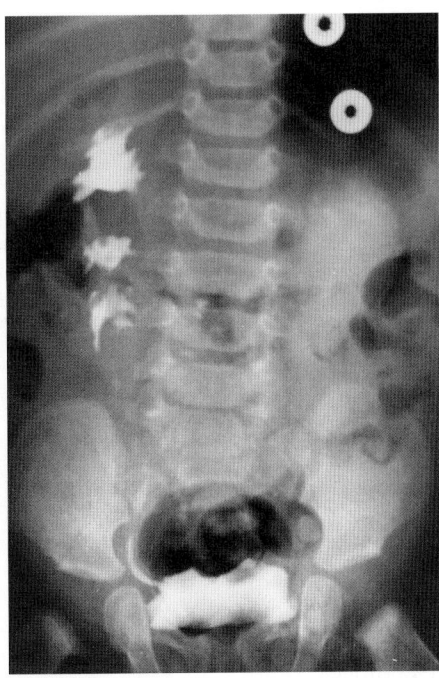

(b)

Fig. 36.15 (a) Post-mortem specimen showing a crossed fused ectopia. (b) Intravenous urogram showing a crossed fused ectopia, with both collecting systems visualised on the right side.

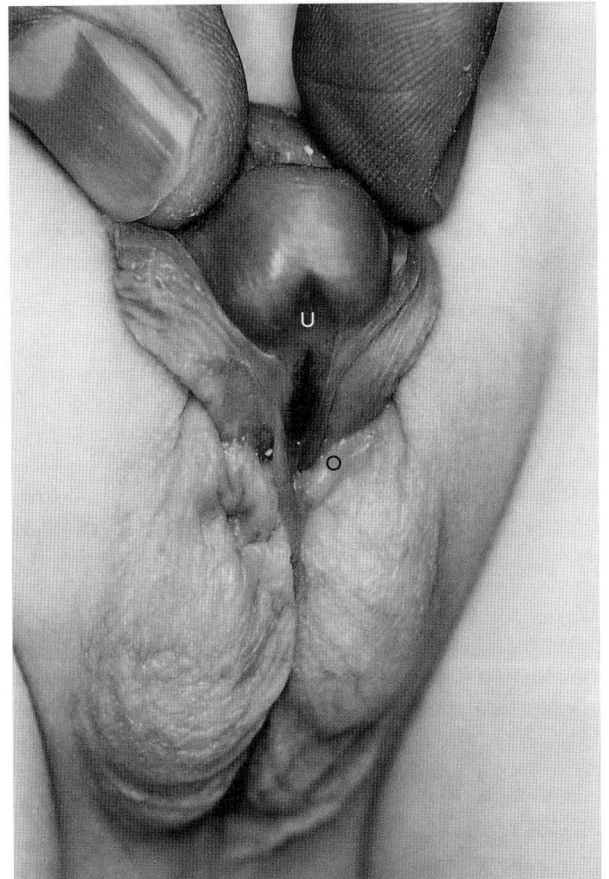

Fig. 36.16 Boy with hypospadias. This shows the urethral plate (U) with the urethral opening (O) on the scrotum and the hooded foreskin all behind the penis.

Undescended testicle

At birth, in term boys, both testicles have usually descended. The incidence of undescended testicles at term is 1:50 to 1:100; however, because the testicles descend from the fifth to the seventh months of gestation, premature boys have an increased risk of undescended testicles.[13] The left testicle descends first, therefore a right undescended testicle is slightly more common. Undescended testicles can be of two types: true undescended testicles (20%), which lie along the original line of descent but which have not reached the scrotum, and ectopic testes, which have deviated from the normal line of descent, the most common place being in the superficial pouch above the external inguinal ring. A retractile testis is often incorrectly diagnosed as an undescended testis. A retractile testis which has been milked into the scrotum may return into the inguinal canal due to the cremasteric reflex: these testes are normal and do not require further treatment, as they will become permanently situated in the scrotum with time.

Once the diagnosis of undescended testicle is made, it is important to keep the baby under review, because occasionally a previously undescended testis can complete descent, and there is a strong association between undescended testicle and a hernia sac. If a hernia occurs, it is necessary both to repair the hernia and to perform an orchidopexy soon in order to prevent a strangulated hernia. In most cases of undescended testicle, a definitive operation to bring the testicle down into the scrotum is performed between 1 and 2 years of age. The benefits of orchidopexy include the following:

■ Cosmetic and psychological benefits of having two testes in the scrotum.
■ The undescended testis has an increased risk of malignancy – placement in the scrotum enables easy palpation.

- It places the testis in a lower-temperature environment, which may improve the long-term chances of fertility.
- A malpositioned testis is more susceptible to damage from trauma.

Hydrocoeles

Congenital hydrocoele results from an incomplete obliteration of the patent processus vaginalis. Normally, the processus vaginalis, which accompanies the descending testicle into the scrotum, has been obliterated by the seventh month of pregnancy. If the processus remains patent around the testicle and there is a small lumen connecting it to the peritoneal cavity, fluid can enter and stay in the processus vaginalis, forming a hydrocoele. The only difference between a hydrocoele and hernia, therefore, in anatomical terms, is that in a hernia the lumen allows the bowel to enter the processus.

Hydrocoeles usually present with a scrotal swelling. The features which differentiate hydrocoele from hernia are that hydrocoeles transilluminate, and that it is possible to 'get above' a hydrocoele, whereas a hernia extends into the peritoneal cavity. It is vital that a hernia is excluded in the diagnosis, as the two conditions have very different treatments. Most hydrocoeles can be left alone, as the vast majority spontaneously resolve by 3 years of age. Surgical ligation of the processus vaginalis should be carried out if the hydrocoele remains, becomes symptomatic (very rare), or cannot be differentiated from a hernia.

Neonatal testicular torsion

Neonatal or intrauterine torsion of the testicle usually presents as a swollen testicle. The scrotum is often red, oedematous, and may be tender on examination. Often a black testicle can be identified within the scrotum. Occasionally the initial event is not identified and the torted testicle is only noticed when a fibrotic atrophied testicle is seen during exploration for an undescended testicle. The established treatment is early surgical exploration and fixation of the contralateral testis. However, in the neonatal period the testicle is always necrotic and it is now common practice to treat the boy with analgesia and antibiotics alone. Controversy exists about whether to fix the contralateral testis, but because asynchronous torsion has been described we believe it is prudent to perform surgical fixation. If at the time of presentation both testicles appear torted, then surgical exploration is recommended.[20]

Tight foreskin

At birth the prepuce and the glans of the penis are firmly adherent, gradually separating over the first 4 years. During this time, retraction of the foreskin is not possible – so-called 'physiological phimosis'. It is unusual to require circumcision during the neonatal period. The indications for circumcision are:

- religious reasons;
- a fibrous scarred foreskin;

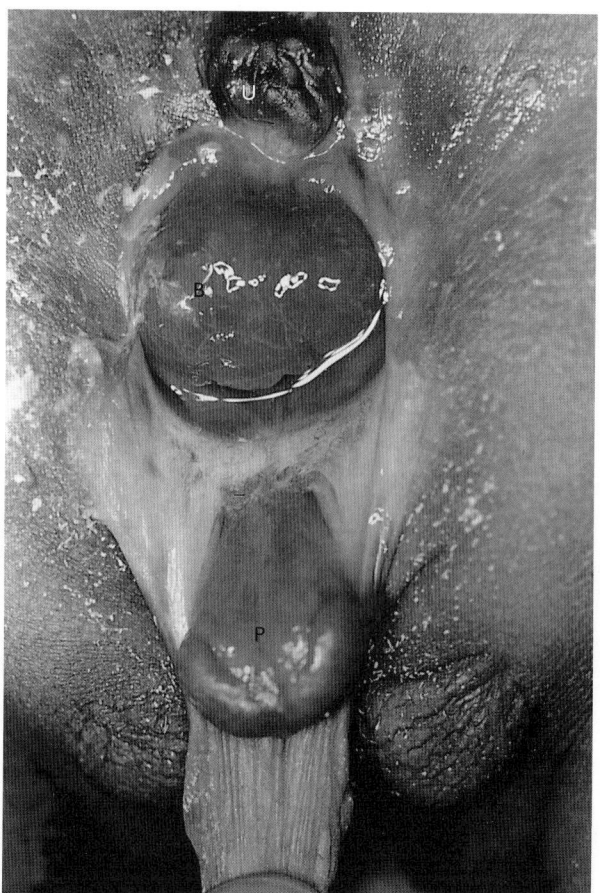

Fig. 36.17 A child with bladder exstrophy. The umbilicus is at the top of the photograph (U); below this is the bladder plate (B) with an open bladder neck and an epispadic penis (P).

- babies under a year with severe underlying uropathies who continue to present with recurrent UTIs despite prophylaxis.

All other indications are considerably less definite. Pathological tightness of the foreskin (pathological phimosis) does occur but is rare before 5 years of age, and even then can usually be successfully treated with gentle parental retraction of the foreskin and local steroid cream (after the age of 4). Many factors have been put forward in defence of circumcision, including a decreased incidence of penile and cervical cancer and a reduction in the incidence of UTIs.[68] However, once religion, social class and social activity are taken into consideration, many of these factors lose their significance. The one definite contraindication for circumcision is in boys with other penile anomalies, where the prepuce may be required to reconstruct the urethra; for religious reasons, parents can be reassured that once the hypospadias repair has been performed their child will be circumcised.

Epispadias and bladder exstrophy

Epispadias, bladder exstrophy and cloacal exstrophy represent a spectrum of congenital malformations in which there is an abnormal development of the cloacal membrane and consequently incomplete midline fusion of the cloacal structures.

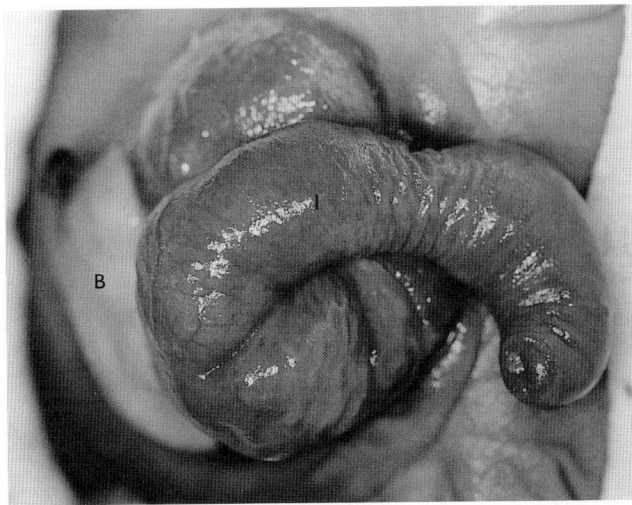

Fig. 36.18 Child with cloacal exstrophy. Prolapsed ileum (I) is seen coming from the exstrophied caecum; on the left side is an exstrophied hemibladder (B).

Epispadias is the mildest form: it is rare, with an incidence of 1 in 100 000, and can occur in both sexes, although it is more common in boys. In epispadias, the bladder is covered and the urethra opens onto the dorsal surface of the penis; in addition, the penis is often short and wide, with marked dorsal chordee. In girls the urethra is patulous and the clitoris has not fused in the midline. Treatment consists of reconstructing the genitalia; however, as the bladder neck and sphincter are often involved, further treatment to ensure urinary continence is often required.

Bladder exstrophy occurs in 1 in 30 000 livebirths. In this anomaly, the bladder opens onto the abdominal wall, there is marked separation of the pubic bones and epispadias of the genitalia (Fig. 36.17). Like epispadias, this is more common in boys. Treatment requires closure of the bladder and pubic ring within the first few days of life, then a staged approach to correct the epispadias and reconstruct the bladder neck. These patients will require lifelong follow-up, but despite the many problems the majority are socially continent and sexually active.

Cloacal exstrophy is the most severe and fortunately the rarest form of the exstrophy complex. It has an incidence of 1 in 250 000 and, unlike bladder exstrophy, is more common in girls.[17] In cloacal exstrophy, the bowel, usually at the ileocaecal valve, opens in the midline with two hemibladders lateral to it (Fig. 36.18). There is also epispadias of the genitalia and pubic bone separation.[34] Until 1960 this was uniformly fatal, but since 1980 the survival rate has been over 90%.[34]

References

1. Allen T D, Husmann D A 1989 Ureteropelvic junction obstruction associated with ureteral hypoplasia. Journal of Urology 142: 353–355
2. Anderson P A, Rickwood A M K 1991 Features of primary vesicoureteric reflux detected by prenatal sonography. British Journal of Urology 67: 267–271
3. Arthur R J, Irving H C, Thomas D F M 1989 Bilateral fetal uropathy; what is the outlook? British Medical Journal 298: 1419–1420
4. Ashley D J B, Mostofi F K 1960 Renal agenesis and dysgenesis. Journal of Urology 83: 211–230
5. Atwell J D 1983 Posterior urethral valves in the British Isles: a multicenter BAPS review. Journal of Pediatric Surgery 18: 70–74
6. Bakker N J 1958 Valves in the female urethra. Urologia Internationalis 6: 187–190
7. Beck A D 1971 The effect of intra-uterine urinary obstruction upon the development of the fetal kidney. Journal of Urology 105: 784–789
8. Blyth B, Snyder H M, Duckett J W 1993 Antenatal diagnosis and subsequent management of hydronephrosis. Journal of Urology 149: 693–698
9. Borer J G, Corgan F J, Krantz R, Gordon D H, Maiman M, Glassberg K I 1993 Unilateral single vaginal ectopic ureter with ipsilateral hypoplastic pelvic kidney and bicornuate uterus. Journal of Urology 149: 1124–1127
10. Boullier J, Chehval M J, Purcell M H 1992 Removal of a multicystic half of a horseshoe kidney: significance of preoperative evaluation in identifying abnormal surgical anatomy. Journal of Pediatric Surgery 27: 1244–1246
11. Campbell M F 1970 Anomalies of the kidney. In: Campbell M F, Harrison J H (eds) Urology, 3rd edn, vol 2. W B Saunders, Philadelphia, p. 1416
12. Cass A S, Stephens F D 1974 Posterior urethral valves: diagnosis and management. Journal of Urology 112: 519–525
13. Chilvers C, Dudley N E, Gough M H, Jackson M B, Pike M C 1986 Undescended testis: the effect of treatment on subsequent risk of subfertility and malignancy. Journal of Pediatric Surgery 21: 691–696
14. Dhillon H K 1995 Imaging and follow up of neonatal hydronephrosis. Current Opinion in Urology 5: 75–78
15. Dhillon H K 1998 Prenatally diagnosed hydronephrosis: the Great Ormond Street experience. British Journal of Urology 81(suppl. 2): 39–44
16. Dhillon H K 2002 Prenatally diagnosed hydronephrosis: selective postnatal intervention. Dialogues in Pediatric Urology 25: 5–7
17. Diamond D A 1990 Cloacal exstrophy: associated anomalies. Dialogues in Pediatric Urology 13: 6–8
18. Di Benedetto V, Meyrat B J, Sorrentino G, Monfort G 1995 Management of duplex ureteroceles detected by prenatal ultrasound. Pediatric Surgery International 10: 485–487
19. Dinneen M D, Dhillon H K, Word H C, Duffy P G, Ransley P G 1993 Antenatal diagnosis of PUV. British Journal of Urology 72: 364–369
20. Driver C D, Losty P D 1998 Neonatal testicular torsion. British Journal of Urology 82: 855–858
21. Flashner S C, Lower R K 1992 Ureteropelvic junction. In: Kelalis P P, King L R, Belman A B (eds) Clinical pediatric urology, 3rd edn. W B Saunders, Philadelphia, pp 693–725
22. Flashner S C, Mesrobian H G J, Flatt J A, Wilkinson R H, King L R 1993 Nonobstructive dilatation of upper urinary tract may later convert to obstruction. Urology 42: 569–573
23. Flyer M A, Haller J O, Feld M, Kantor A 1994 Ectopic supernumerary kidney: another cause of a pelvic mass. Abdominal Imaging 19: 374–375
24. Freedman A L, Johnson M P, Smith C A, Gonzalez R, Evans M I 1999 Long term outcome in children with antenatal intervention of obstructive uropathies. Lancet 354: 374–377
25. Glick P L, Harrison M R, Noall R A, Villa R L 1983 Correction of congenital hydronephrosis in utero. III. Early mid-trimester ureteral obstruction produces renal dysplasia. Journal of Pediatric Surgery 18: 681–687
26. Gobe G C, Axelsen R A 1987 Genesis of renal tubular atrophy in experimental hydronephrosis in the rat. Role of apoptosis. Laboratory Investigation 56: 273–281
27. Gough D C S, Postlethwaite R J, Lewis M A, Bruce J 1995 Multicystic renal dysplasia diagnosed in the antenatal period: a note of caution. British Journal of Urology 76: 244–248
28. Groshar D, Embdon O M, Sazbon A, Koritny E S, Frenkel A 1988 Radionuclide assessment of bladder outlet obstruction: a noninvasive (1-step) method for measurement of voiding time, urinary flow rates and residual urine. Journal of Urology 139: 266–269
29. Hanna H K 1991 The case for early operation. Dialogues in Pediatric Urology 14(2)
30. Harrison M R, Nakayama D K, Noall R, DeLorimier A A 1982 Correction of congenital hydronephrosis in utero; decompression reverses the effects of obstruction on the fetal lung and urinary tract. Journal of Pediatric Surgery 17: 965–974
31. Hendren W H, Donahoe P K 1986 Renal fusions and ectopia. In: Welch K J, Randolph J G, Ravitch M M, O'Neill J A Jr, Rowe M I (eds) Pediatric surgery, 4th edn. Year Book Medical Publishers, Chicago, pp 1134–1145
32. Hendron C D, Ferrer F A, Freedman A, McKeena P H 2000 Consensus on the prenatal management of antenatally detected urological abnormalities. Journal of Urology 164: 1052–1056
33. Hollowell J G, Altman H G, Snyder H M, Duckett J W 1989 Coexisting ureteropelvic junction obstruction and vesicoureteral reflux: diagnostic and therapeutic implications. Journal of Urology 142: 490–493

34. Hurwitz R S, Mansoni G A M, Ransley P G, Stephens F D 1988 Cloacal exstrophy: a report of 34 cases. Journal of Urology 138: 1065–1068

35. Johnson J H, Kulatilake A E 1971 The sequelae of posterior urethral valves: British Journal of Urology 43: 743–748

36. Joseph D B, Bauer S B, Colodny A H, Mandell J, Lebowitz R L, Retik A B 1989 Lower pole ureteropelvic junction obstruction and incomplete renal duplication. Journal of Urology 141: 896–899

37. Kaplan G W, Scherz H L 1992 Infravesical obstruction in clinical pediatric urology, 3rd edn. W B Saunders, Philadelphia, pp 821–864

38. Kass E J 1992 Megaureter. In: Kelalis P P, King L R, Belman A B (eds) Clinical pediatric urology. W B Saunders, Philadelphia, p. 782

39. Keating M A, Duckett J W 1993 Prune belly syndrome. In: Ashcraft K W, Holder T M (eds) Pediatric surgery. W B Saunders, Philadelphia, pp 721–739

40. Koff S A, Campbell K D 1994 The nonoperative management of unilateral neonatal hydronephrosis: natural history of poorly functioning kidneys. Journal of Urology 152(2 Pt 2): 593–595

41. Mackie G G, Stephens F D 1975 Duplex kidneys: a correlation of renal dysplasia with position of the ureteral orifice. Journal of Urology 114: 274–280

42. Madden N P, Thomas D F M, Gordon A C, Arthur R J, Irving H C, Smith S E W 1991 Antenatally detected pelviureteric junction obstruction. Is non-operation safe? British Journal of Urology 68: 305–310

43. Mesrobian H G J 1986 Ureteropelvic junction obstruction of the upper pole moiety in complete ureteral duplication. Journal of Urology 136: 452–453

44. Mesrobian H G J, Sulik K K 1992 Characterization of the upper urinary tract anatomy in the Danforth spontaneous murine mutation. Journal of Urology 148: 752–755

45. Mouriquand P D E, Mollard P 1995 Hypospadias repair: the paediatric urologist's point of view. European Urology Update Series 4: 106–111

46. Nicolini U, Fisk N M, Rodeck C H, Beacham J 1992 Fetal urine biochemistry: an index of renal maturation and dysfunction. British Journal of Obstetrics and Gynaecology 99: 46–50

47. Paltiel H J, Lebowitz R L 1989 Neonatal hydronephrosis due to primary vesico-ureteric reflux: trends in diagnosis and treatment. Radiology 170: 787–789

48. Parkhouse H F, Barratt T M, Dillon M J et al 1988 Long-term outcome of boys with posterior urethral valves. British Journal of Urology 62: 59–62

49. Rajfer J, Walsh P C 1976 The incidence of intersexuality in patients with hypospadias and cryptorchidism. Journal of Urology 116: 769–770

50. Ransley P G, Dhillon H K, Gordon I, Duffy P G, Dillon M J, Barratt T M 1990 The postnatal management of hydronephrosis diagnosed by prenatal ultrasound. Journal of Urology 144: 584–587

51. Ransley P G, Risdon R A 1979 The pathogenesis of reflux nephropathy. Contributions to Nephrology 16: 90–97

52. Reinberg Y, De Castano I, Gonzales R 1992 Prognosis for patients with prenatally diagnosed posterior urethral valves. Journal of Urology 148: 125–126

53. Rickwood A M K, Jee L D, Williams M P L, Anderson A P 1992 Natural history of obstructed and pseudo-obstructed megaureters detected by prenatal ultrasonography. British Journal of Urology 70: 322–325

54. Ritchey M 1992 Anomalies of the kidney. In: Kelalis P P, King L R, Belman A B (eds) Clinical pediatric urology, 3rd edn. W B Saunders, Philadelphia, pp 500–529

55. Rizza J M, Downing S E 1971 Bilateral renal agenesis in two female siblings. American Journal of Diseases of Children 121: 60–63

56. Scott J E S, Renwick M 1988 Antenatal diagnosis of congenital abnormalities in the urinary tract. Results from the northern region fetal abnormality survey. British Journal of Urology 62: 295–300

57. Sheldon C A 1995 Male external genitalia. In: Rowe M I, O'Neill J A, Grosfeld J L, Fonkalsrud E W, Coran A G (eds) Essentials of pediatric surgery. Mosby, St Louis, pp 775–776

58. Smith D, Egginton J A, Brookfield D S K 1987 Detection of abnormality of fetal urinary tract as a predictor of urinary tract disease. British Medical Journal 294: 27–28

59. Song J T, Ritchey M L, Zerin M, Bloom D A 1995 Incidence of vesicoureteral reflux in children with renal agenesis. Journal of Urology 153: 1249–1251

60. Thomas D F 1998 Prenatally detected uropathy: epidemiological considerations [review]. British Journal of Urology 81(suppl. 2): 8–12

61. Thomas D F 1996 Unilateral multicystic dysplastic kidney. Archives of Disease in Childhood 77: 368–369

62. Thomas D F, Irving H C, Arthur R J 1995 Prenatal diagnosis: how useful is it? British Journal of Urology 57: 784–787

63. Tibballs J M, De Bruyn R 1996 Primary vesicoureteric reflux – how useful is postnatal ultrasound? Archives of Disease in Childhood 75: 444–447

64. Turnock R R, Shawis R 1984 Management of fetal urinary tract anomalies detected by prenatal ultrasonography. Archives of Disease in Childhood 59: 962–965

65. Upsdell S M, Gupta S, Gough D C 1994 The radionuclide assessment of prenatally diagnosed hydronephrosis. British Journal of Urology 74: 31–34

66. van der Vis-Melsen M J E, Baert R J M, Rajnherc J R, Groen J M, Bemelmans L M M J, De Nef J J E M 1989 Scintigraphic assessment of lower urinary tract function in children with and without outflow tract obstruction. British Journal of Urology 64: 263–269

67. Whitten S M, Wilcox D T 2001 Duplex systems. Prenatal Diagnosis 21: 952–957

68. Wiswell T E, Smith F R, Bass J W 1985 Decreased incidence of urinary tract infections in circumcised male patients. Pediatrics 75: 901–903

69. Yerkes E B, Adams M C, Pope J C 4th, Brock J W 3rd 1999 Does every patient with prenatal hydronephrosis need voiding cystourethrography? Journal of Urology 162(3 Pt 2): 1218–1220

70. Yeung C K, Godley M L, Dhillon H K, Gordon I, Duffy P G, Ransley P G 1997 The characteristics of primary vesico-ureteric reflux in male and female infants with pre-natal hydronephrosis. British Journal of Urology 80: 319–327

CHAPTER 37

Neonatal malignancy

Roger Palmer, Denise Williams

Introduction

Neonatal cancer is rare, a surprising fact in view of the rapid cell division and growth occurring throughout fetal life. Our understanding of the factors affecting cell growth and the genetic events responsible for the development or progression of malignant disease continues to increase at a rapid rate. Genes controlling cell growth are termed proto-oncogenes. Research efforts have led to the identification of two major classes of genes associated with malignancy. Oncogenes are mutated proto-oncogenes and give rise to excessive cell growth and proliferation, whilst tumour-suppressor genes act in normal cells to suppress proliferation, but, if inactivated, remove the normal constraint to growth, and target cells are allowed to proliferate in an uncontrolled way.[23]

Knudson's 'two-hit' theory of carcinogenesis has been verified by this recent knowledge of the genetic factors that control cell growth.[36] The 'hits' could be a wide variety of agents – viral, chemical or radiation – and cause mutation of a proto-oncogene or inactivation or loss of a tumour-suppressor gene. This first 'hit' would allow all cells in the body, including the germ cells, to carry the defect, which could then be passed on to the next generation. The second 'hit' would be in the somatic cells of a target organ. The proto-oncogene would become an oncogene, or the loss of a homologous tumour-suppressor gene would allow uncontrolled cellular growth. The time during which the second 'hit' could occur is probably confined to the period when the cells of the target organ are undergoing mitotic activity, but ceases when they are fully mature. For example, retinoblasts differentiate to become photoreceptor cells by the age of 3 years, and this may explain why retinoblastoma is unusual in older children or adults.

Oncogenes exert their effect on cells through a variety of mechanisms. These include control of cellular growth factors or their receptors, or by modifying the signals sent from growth receptors to the nucleus of the cell. This may result in an effect on DNA repair, apoptosis or the cells' ability to metabolise toxins.

Neonatal malignancy presents many therapeutic challenges. Chemotherapy is poorly tolerated in young infants, and myelosuppression and life-threatening complications of therapy are common.[52] This may be because of altered pharmacokinetics in the neonatal age group.[52] The long-term effects of chemotherapy, surgery and radiation in terms of growth, development and second tumours[52] have been recognised for many years, and both short-term and long-term effects of treatment should be taken into account when planning therapy. Increasingly, cancer research is attempting to exploit the genetic mutations for therapeutic purposes. This, in the future, may provide more specific tumour-targeted therapies, increasing cure rates with a reduction in toxicity.

The routine use of antenatal ultrasound, and the improved quality of the images, have led to an increase in the diagnosis of congenital tumours, particularly teratomas and neuroblastomas, and an increase in the understanding of their natural history.[47] It allows close monitoring of affected pregnancies, and management planning with appropriate multidisciplinary team involvement.

Incidence and survival (Table 37.1A&B)

Neonatal malignancy is disproportionately represented within childhood, where the incidence of cancer is 11–15 per 100 000 population less than 15 years of age. Defining neonatal malignancy as malignant and central nervous system (CNS) tumours diagnosed in the first 6 weeks of life, the UK National Registry of Childhood Tumours (NRCT) incidence between 1981 and 2000, from 394 cancer registrations, was 2.74 per 100 000 live births, with 45.4% of these tumours presenting in the first week of life, 14.8% in the second and approximately 10% per week thereafter. This is similar to reports from other cancer registries (Table 37.1B). Suspected risk factors for the development of childhood cancer include certain congenital syndromes (Table 37.2), in-utero exposure to certain drugs (e.g. diethylstilbestrol), vaginal adenocarcinoma, and irradiation (all cancer types). There remains no convincing evidence that intramuscular vitamin K given at birth is associated with an increased risk of childhood leukaemia.[46]

Survival is dependent upon tumour type and site, and condition of the infant at diagnosis. Survival statistics, although improving,

Table 37.1 UK registration data and previously published series of neonatal tumours

Table 37.1A Single-centre experience

Institution	Toronto, Canada (Campbell et al[14])	Philadelphia, USA (Gale et al[25])	Los Angeles, USA (Isaacs[34])	Texas, USA (Xue et al[55])	Glasgow, UK (Davis et al[20])	Durham, USA (Halperin[29])	Memphis, USA (Crom et al[19])
Years	1922–1982	1952–1978	1958–1982	1941–1981	1955–1986	1930–1998	1962–1988
Percentage of all paediatric cancers	2%		2.6%			2%	3.2%
Male:female ratio	1.7:1	1:1.1			1:1.4	1:2.3	1:1
Survival	42%	2-year 45%	37%	78% (solid tumours only)	Approx. 50%[b] (solid only)[c]	Approx. 60%[d]	68%
Tumour numbers	102	22	49 (61[a])	45	16 (35)	15 (8)	34
Neuroblastoma	48	11	14	6	7	5	19
Retinoblastoma	17		2	3	3	4	3
Sarcoma	12	3	8 (16)	15	4 (4)	1	
Central nervous system	9		5	5		4	
Leukaemia	8	3	11	13			6
Wilms' tumour	4	1	3 (3 mesoblastic nephroma)	1	(9 mesoblastic nephroma)		2
Liver tumours	1 hepatoblastoma		1 hepatoblastoma (3 hamartoma)		(2 haemangioma, 1 hamartoma)		
Malignant teratoma	1	3	1 (39 other teratomas)		1 (18 SCT, 1 orbital teratoma)	1 retroperitoneal (6 other teratomas)	1 SCT, 1 oropharyngeal
Others	1 Schwannoma, 1 YST testis	1 parotid carcinoma	2 carcinoma, 2 LCH	2 melanoma	1 squamous cell carcinoma	1 (glossal glial choristoma, 1 haemangioma with Kasabach–Merritt)	2 melanoma

Abbreviations: YST – yolk sac tumour, LCH – Langerhans' cell histiocytosis, SCT – sacrococcygeal teratoma.

( ) – Number and type of benign neoplasms also reported.

[a] Haemangiomas (5 hepatic haemangiomas reported) and lymphangiomas excluded.

[b] 1 patient unaccounted for (malignant SCT).

[c] Central nervous system tumours and leukaemias excluded.

[d] 1 patient unaccounted for (rhabdomyosarcoma).

Table 37.1B Cancer registry experience

Cancer registry	Denmark (Borch et al[10])	West Midlands, UK (Parkes et al[41])	Third National Cancer Survey, USA (Bader & Miller[3])	National Registry of Childhood Tumours[g], UK
Years	1943–1985	1960–1989	1969–1971	1981–2000
Incidence per 100 000 live births	2.38 (up to 28 days old)	7.2 (up to 3 months old)	3.65 (up to 28 days old)	2.74 (up to 6 weeks old)
Male:female ratio	1:1.4	1:1.1	Not reported	1:1
Survival	5-year 25%	1-year 55%[e] 5-year 47%[e]	Not reported	1-year 57% 5-year 51%
Tumour numbers	76	98 (72)	39	394 (213[f])
Neuroblastoma	20	31	21	113
Retinoblastoma	2	14		37
Sarcoma	14	6 (11)	4	38
Central nervous system	8	14	1	61
Leukaemia	12	21	5	74
Wilms' tumour	4	1 (7 mesoblastic nephroma)	5 including mesoblastic nephromas	7
Liver tumours		2 hepatoblastoma, 1 rhabdoid tumour (5 unspecified)		9 hepatoblastoma
Malignant teratoma	4 (2 other teratomas), all retroperitoneal	(49 mature teratoma – 4 malignant recurrences)		40 MGCT, of which 2 gonadal
Others	8 unspecified	3 HLH, 3 LCH, 1 malignant thymoma, 1 malignant stromal cell tumour of testes	1 carcinoma, 1 lymphoma, 1 unspecified	5 extra-renal rhabdoid tumours, 4 peripheral PNET, 3 melanoma, 1 malignant histiocytosis, 1 pancreatoblastoma, 1 unspecified

Abbreviations: LCH – Langerhan's cell histiocytosis, MGCT – malignant germ cell tumour, HLH – haemophagocytic lymphohistiocytosis.

( ) – Number and type of benign neoplasms also reported.

[e] Includes benign tumours.

[f] Further 213 non-malignant tumours reported (not population based): 2 myelodysplasia/myeloproliferative disease, 26 mesoblastic nephroma, 12 LCH, 8 HLH, 10 fibromatosis, 9 haemangiopericytoma, 14 other non-malignant soft-tissue sarcoma, 5 neurofibromatosis, 120 non-malignant teratoma, 7 unspecified.

[g] Acknowledgement to Mr C Stiller, Childhood Cancer Research Group, University of Oxford, for providing data from the National Registry of Childhood Tumours.

Table 37.2 Tumours associated with specific malformations, syndromes and chromosomal abnormalities (After Berry[7])

Inherited syndrome	Childhood cancer
Hamartoses	
Tuberous sclerosis	Giant cell astrocytoma
Neurofibromatosis	Gliomas
Basal cell naevus (Gorlin's) syndrome	Medulloblastoma, basal cell carcinoma
Turcot syndrome	Medulloblastoma
Multiple mucosal neuroma syndrome	Medullary thyroid carcinoma, phaeochromocytoma
Neurocutaneous melanosis sequence	Melanoma
Aicardia syndrome	Germ cell tumour, hepatoblastoma
Metabolic disorders	
Glycogenosis type I, hereditary tyrosinaemia & α1-antitrypsin deficiency	Hepatocellular carcinoma
Chromosome breakage and repair defects	
Bloom syndrome	Leukaemia, Wilm's tumour & gastrointestinal tumours
Ataxia telangiectasia	Leukaemia, lymphoma
Fanconi's anaemia	Leukaemia, hepatoma, hepatoblastoma
Xeroderma pigmentosum	Skin cancers, melanoma
Werner syndrome	Sarcomas, meningioma
Immune deficiency disorders	
Wiscott–Aldrich syndrome	Leukaemia, lymphoma (often in the central nervous system)
X-linked lymphoproliferative disease (Duncan disease)	B-cell lymphoma
Severe combined immunodeficiency	Leukaemia, lymphoma
Bruton's agammaglobulinaemia	Leukaemia, lymphoma
Xeroderma pigmentosa	Non-melanomatous skin carcinomas
Chromosomal anomaly	
Down syndrome (trisomy 21)	Acute leukaemias
Turner syndrome (45XO)	Neurogenic tumours, germ cell tumours
13q syndrome	Retinoblastoma
11p syndrome	Wilms' tumour (nephroblastoma)
Monosomy 7	Pre-leukaemia & non-lymphoblastic leukaemia
XY gonadal dysgenesis, aniridia–Wilms' tumour association	Gonadoblastoma
Edwards syndrome (trisomy 18)	Wilms' tumour (nephroblastoma)
Klinefelter syndrome (XXY)	Leukaemia, teratoma, breast carcinoma
Congenital anomaly	
Hemihypertrophy & Beckwith–Wiedemann syndrome	Wilms' tumour, adrenal cortical carcinoma & hepatoblastoma
Sporadic aniridia, Denys–Drash syndrome, Fraser syndrome & Perlman syndrome, Sotos syndrome	Wilms' tumour (nephroblastoma)
Simpson–Golabi–Behmel syndrome	Germ cell tumour, Wilms' tumour
Poland anomaly	Leukaemia
Hirschsprung disease	Neuroblastoma
Pyloric stenosis	Germ cell tumour
Other	
Monozygotic twins	Sacrococcygeal teratoma

(Table 37.1A&B) are inherently unreliable due to the rarity of neonatal malignancy and advances in treatment over the decades. The NRCT reports a 1- and 5-year survival of 57% and 52%, respectively, for neonatal malignancy diagnosed between 1981 and 2000. This remains lower than for malignancy during childhood as a whole.

Neuroblastoma

Neuroblastoma is the commonest neonatal malignancy, accounting for 30–50% of all tumours in the newborn period. Approximately 30% of cases are diagnosed on the first day of life and a

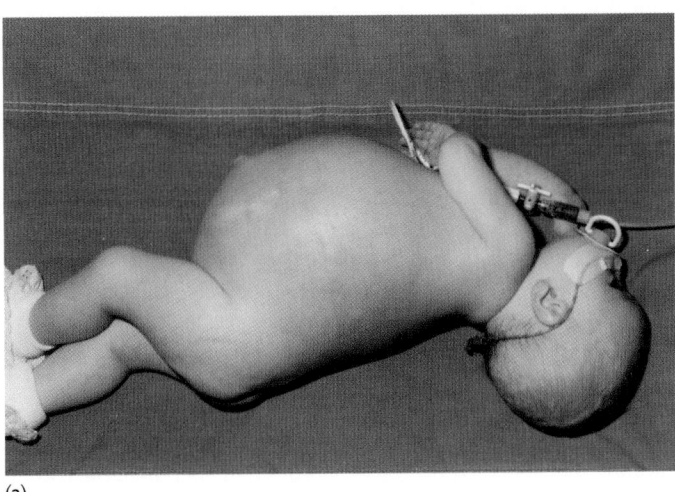

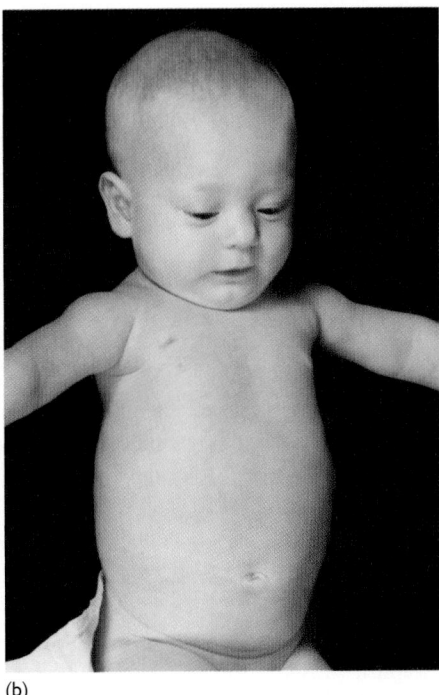

(a)   (b)

Fig. 37.1 (a) Enlarged abdomen in stage 4s neuroblastoma (left adrenal gland), presenting in the neonatal period with poor feeding, hepatomegaly and coagulopathy. (b) Same patient 5 months later, following a single course of low-dose OJEC chemotherapy (vincristine, cyclophosphamide, etoposide and carboplatin).

further 20% within the first week.[38] Neuroblastomas originate from neural crest cells, which give rise to the adrenal medulla and the sympathetic ganglia, but are also found in nearly all organs, including skin. Spontaneous differentiation and apoptosis may explain the 50-fold increase in frequency of small foci of neuroblastoma cells found at perinatal autopsies compared with documented cases of neuroblastoma.

Tumour genetics may be important in predicting rates of tumour progression and response to treatment and are important to determine at the time of diagnosis. Deletion of the short arm of chromosome 1, probably resulting in the loss of a tumour-suppressor gene, is associated with a poor prognosis.[13] Hyper-diploid tumours occur more commonly in infants and are associated with a good response to chemotherapy, while a diploid DNA index is associated with advanced and aggressive disease. Amplification of *MYCN*, the *c-myc*-related oncogene, found on chromosome 2, is an adverse prognostic biological marker associated with rapid disease progression and a poor outcome.[13]

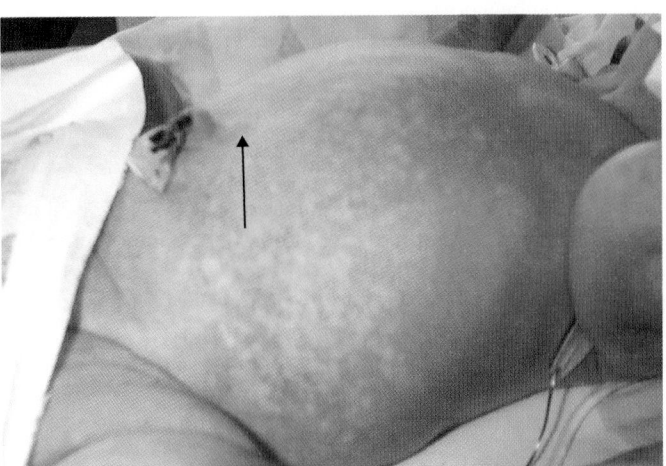

Fig. 37.2 Stage 4s neuroblastoma presenting on the first day of life with abdominal distension and marked hepatomegaly. 'Blueberry muffin' skin deposit adjacent to the umbilicus and intense cutaneous vasomotor reaction in response to handling.

Clinical features

A neuroblastoma arises anywhere in the neural crest tissues. Around 45% arise within the adrenal medulla, presenting as an abdominal mass (Fig. 37.1), while those arising in the posterior mediastinum may present with respiratory difficulties, swallowing problems or a unilateral Horner's syndrome. Approximately 60% of infants will have metastatic disease at presentation, common sites being bone, bone marrow, and skin. The so-called 'blueberry muffin' skin deposits (Fig. 37.2) are indistinguishable clinically from those seen in congenital leukaemia. Spinal cord compression due to intraspinal extension of tumour may give rise to paraplegia or neurological signs.

Hypertension secondary to circulating catecholamines is not uncommon. Rarely, neonatal neuroblastoma may metastasise to the placenta and lead to placental insufficiency or hydrops fetalis. Maternal pre-eclampsia secondary to catecholamine release has been reported.[50]

The use of antenatal ultrasound has led to an increase in prenatal diagnosis.[47]

Staging

The international staging system for neuroblastoma (INSS)[38] is based on the clinical and radiological features and the operability of the tumour. The clinical stage at diagnosis is a good predictor of overall survival, and, together with knowledge of biological factors, dictates treatment.

Stage 4s disease

Stage 4s denotes an infant with a localised primary lesion and dissemination restricted to skin, bone marrow and liver but excluding bone. Spontaneous regression usually occurs,[42] although close observation is necessary, as a grossly enlarging liver may result in respiratory compromise, hepatic dysfunction and coagulopathy, renal dysfunction or failure to thrive, any of which may be an indication for chemotherapy.

Diagnosis

A tissue diagnosis, although often confirming the diagnosis in a baby with a typical presentation and elevated catecholamines, vanillylmandelic acid (VMA) and homovanillic acid (HVA),[38] is important to provide additional biological and prognostic information. The presence of *MYCN* amplification will influence treatment. Staging involves a bone scan and bone marrow examination. Use of ^{131}I-labelled MIBG (meta-iodobenzyl guanidine), taken up by neurosecretory granules, will give a positive scan in about 90% of patients.

Treatment

Total surgical excision is usually curative in stages 1 and 2, and chemotherapy not indicated. A number of chemotherapeutic agents are active for higher-stage disease, and as numbers are small, in the UK such babies are treated as part of a European collaborative study. Spinal cord compression requires urgent treatment with dexamethasone and chemotherapy. Surgery may have a role in removing residual disease, although there is increasing evidence that complete resection is not necessary in those patients without poor-risk biological factors.[35]

Prognosis

At all stages, babies with neuroblastoma have a much better prognosis than older children. The overall survival with localised disease is in the region of 90% and with metastatic disease around 70%. Deaths in those with 4s disease may occur as a result of hepatic dysfunction or respiratory compromise. As in older children, the presence of adverse biological factors, particularly *MYCN* amplification, significantly affects the prognosis.

Screening

Approximately 90% of infants with neuroblastoma have raised urinary catecholamines and these can be measured quantitatively to screen for disease. Screening programmes for children under 1 year of age were introduced in Japan in 1985. However, a number of studies have now shown that infant screening is associated with a twofold increase in the documented incidence of neuroblastoma but no decrease in the incidence of advanced stage disease in older children[54] and no improvement in overall survival.

Teratoma and other germ cell tumours (GCTs)

Teratomas (the word being derived from the Greek *teras-atos*, meaning monster, and *-oma*, denoting tumour) are tumours derived from the three embryonic germ cell layers – ectoderm, mesoderm and endoderm. They are predominantly benign and arise in the gonads or in midline extragonadal sites. In the neonate, the commonest site is the sacrococcygeal region, occurring in 1:35 000–45 000 live births (the commonest tumour of the newborn) with a 3:1 female to male preponderance.[43] Tumours in this region may be postsacral (external), presacral (internal) or dumbbell shaped (external and internal portions). Sacrococcygeal teratomas (SCTs) are mature in 65–70% of cases, immature in 5–15% (both benign) and classified as mixed malignant GCTs in 15–30% of cases. The risk of malignancy, invariably yolk sac tumour, is greater in males and in cases with delayed surgery, and increases with the proportion of internal tumour (presacral). Of neonatal teratomas, 45% arise in the sacral area, 20% in the ovary, 20% in the testis, 10% intracranially, with the cervical region and the mediastinum accounting for 5%.

Clinical features

The most common presentation in the newborn is that of a SCT, with a readily recognisable tumour lying postanally between the buttocks. The tumour varies in size, from one that appears as a slight elevation or discoloration over the coccyx to one which equals the size of the baby and may cause hydrops or obstruction of labour. Diagnosis by antenatal ultrasound allows elective caesarean section, although the baby may still succumb if the tumour is in a site causing vital organ obstruction (cervical lesions) or heart failure. With the huge postsacral SCTs (Fig. 37.3) there is usually very little presacral extension. However, presacral tumours may not be as rare in this age group as supposed and only become apparent in the older child, by which time they have a greater chance of being malignant.

Investigations

A lateral X-ray of the abdomen may show anterior displacement of the rectum and possible calcification within the tumour. A chest X-ray including a lateral view is important to rule out pulmonary metastases. Computed tomography (CT) scan of the abdomen and pelvis with bowel contrast may determine whether primary surgery is feasible. Serum tumour markers, alpha-fetoprotein (AFP) and human chorionic gonadatrophin (hCG)

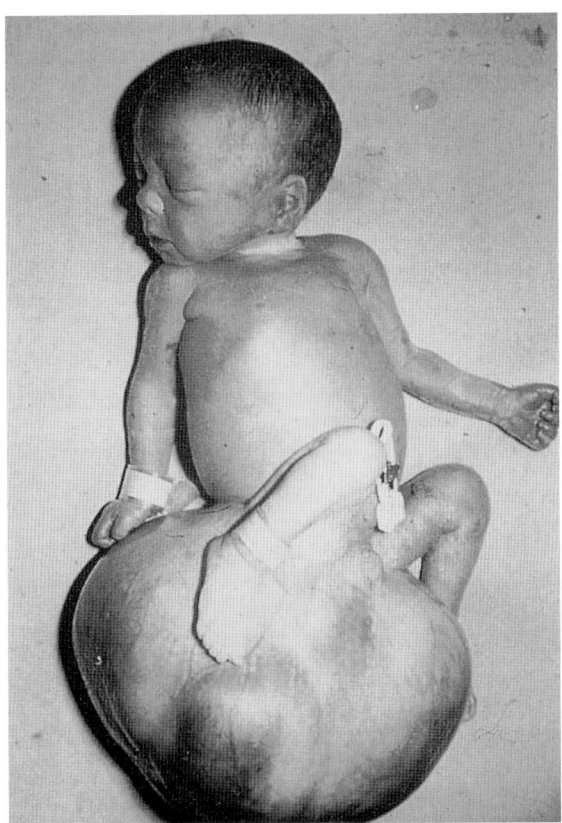

Fig. 37.3 Sacrococcygeal teratoma. (Courtesy of Dr J Berry.)

should be measured. High AFP levels are found in the normal newborn (mean 50 000 kU/l), which gradually fall to adult levels (less than 10 kU/l) over the first year of life (p. 1300).[8] This protein is produced by cells derived embryologically from either fetal yolk sac or liver, and the level is grossly elevated, often to several million kU/l, in malignant teratoma, where yolk sac tissue is the malignant element. High AFP readings, as found in the normal newborn, should fall sequentially at an expected rate based on the half-life of AFP (5–7 days) in the absence of a malignant yolk sac tumour and fall at a similar rate after surgery. Failure to fall at the expected rate after surgery, or a subsequent rise, would indicate residual malignant yolk sac elements or the development of metastases.

Choriocarcinomas are occasionally seen and may secrete hCG. In infancy, they probably result from migration of maternal or placental tissue, and are perhaps better termed 'gestational trophoblastic tumours', being less aggressive than the highly malignant pure choriocarcinoma of adolescence and adulthood. Testicular yolk sac tumours may also present in this period.

Treatment

The treatment of benign SCTs is surgical removal. Removal of the entire coccyx 'en bloc' is essential. Failure to do this will result in a local recurrence approaching 40%. Approximately 10% of neonatally detected SCTs recur as malignant GCTs up to 3 years of age.[43] Follow-up of neonates, with tumour markers,

for this period is therefore essential. Malignant recurrence usually requires chemotherapy, although the key prognostic intervention is the completeness of subsequent surgical resection. Surgery alone with long-term monitoring may be sufficient for small local relapses.

Where malignancy is suspected at the initial presentation (usually late diagnosis with raised AFP, bulky infiltrating lesion on imaging, or metastases identified), preoperative chemotherapy is preferable and significantly increases the chance of complete resection and long-term survival.[26]

Functional impairment after surgery, particularly for large tumours and those with intrapelvic extension, may be commoner than previously thought. Follow-up to detect bladder or bowel dysfunction, or lower limb weakness is mandatory.[43]

Other malignant GCTs are generally treated with chemotherapy until the tumour markers have returned to normal, although surgery may be required to remove residual disease. The exception is stage 1 gonadal tumours, where surgical excision alone suffices. With modern chemotherapy using platinum-based drug regimens, the few neonates with malignant GCTs have an excellent chance of cure.

Acute leukaemia

Congenital and neonatal leukaemia represents <1% of all childhood leukaemia,[12] but is the second most common neonatal malignancy, exceeded only by neuroblastoma. Acute leukaemia in the neonatal period is equally distributed between acute lymphoblastic (ALL) and acute myeloid (AML) subtypes, unlike older children, where ALL accounts for about 80% of cases of leukaemia.

Clinical features

Infants may present with a range of clinical symptoms. Hepatosplenomegaly is common, together with symptoms of anaemia and thrombocytopenia such as bruising, pallor and poor feeding. CNS involvement is common and may present as a bulging fontanelle or neurological signs. A high white cell count with hyperviscosity may be responsible for respiratory, cardiac or neurological compromise. Skin infiltration, seen in about 20% of cases,[21] presents as firm mobile nodules ranging in colour from blue to brown which typically wax and wane. Congenital leukaemia is a rare cause of hydrops and stillbirth.

Diagnosis

As congenital and infant leukaemia frequently presents with a high white count, diagnosis may be possible by morphology and the appropriate immunohistochemistry of the peripheral blood. If non-diagnostic, a bone marrow aspirate is necessary. Biopsy of the skin nodules will show immature blast cells.

Up to 75% of cases of neonatal leukaemia have chromosome rearrangements involving the mixed lineage leukaemia (MLL) gene, usually arising from the translocation t(4;11)(q21;q23).[27]

Other translocations found in infant leukaemia include t(1;11), t(11;19) in ALL and t(9;11), t(8;21) in AML.[27] Recent studies of twins with concordant leukaemia suggest that acute leukaemia in childhood may have a prenatal origin. This has been further supported by the finding of chromosomal fusion sequences in archived Guthrie blood spots matched to children who later developed leukaemia.[53]

Treatment/prognosis

ALL

The current treatment protocol is an intensive hybrid therapy consisting of both ALL and AML elements, as part of an international collaboration, the Interfant 99 study. In a recent report of UK ALL infant protocols,[16] the 4-year event-free survival was 33%, with an overall survival of 46%. Multivariate analysis of prognostic factors showed young age, CNS involvement and high presenting white count to be adverse prognostic factors.

AML

Despite the many poor prognostic factors found in neonatal AML, such as high presenting white count and extramedullary disease (CNS and skin involvement), the outcome after intensive chemotherapy is similar to that of older children with AML, with 60–65% overall survival.[15]

Transient myeloproliferative disorder and Down syndrome

A number of neonates with Down syndrome will have a leukaemia-like syndrome, or a transient myeloproliferative disorder (TMD) that resolves spontaneously within the first few months of life. TMD may present with marked organomegaly and be associated with hydrops and cardiac failure. Circulating blasts are myeloid and may range from a count of 5 to 384 000.[30] Cytogenetics of the blasts show trisomy 21 only, whereas cytogenetics in true AML is likely to show additional chromosomal abnormalities. It is estimated that approximately 30% of Down infants with TMD will go on to develop acute leukaemia, most commonly M7 AML. Leukopheresis and/or exchange transfusion may be necessary to treat signs or symptoms of hyperviscosity, or organ failure. Chemotherapy is rarely needed, although low-dose cytarabine has been used to treat leukocytosis refractory to leukopheresis.[49]

Renal tumours

Mesoblastic nephroma accounts for approximately 80% of solid renal masses in the neonate and for around 4% of early-infancy tumours. Although considered benign, they may rarely metastasise.[41] They are composed of immature stromal cells that infiltrate the kidney parenchyma, synonymous with leiomyomatous hamartoma. Wilms' tumour and rhabdoid tumour are malignant renal neoplasms, and although both are treated similarly, the latter has a considerably worse outcome.

Wilms' tumour, or nephroblastoma, is rare in the neonatal period, accounting for <1% of all Wilms' tumours, with an incidence of 0.49 per million live births. This represents 1.8% of tumours diagnosed in the first 6 weeks of life (NRCT data). Various congenital abnormalities are associated with an increased risk of developing Wilms' tumour, many involving chromosome 11p, where the tumour-suppressor gene *WT1* (11p13) is found.[11] Loss of *WT1* is seen in WAGR syndrome (*W*ilms' tumour, *A*niridia, *G*enitourinary tract abnormalities and mental *R*etardation), Denys–Drash syndrome (congenital nephrotic syndrome and ambiguous genitalia) and the related Fraser syndrome, along with 10–15% of sporadic Wilms' tumours. The *WT2* gene (11p15) is affected in Beckwith–Wiedemann syndrome.[11] Additionally, 40% of all Wilms' tumours show loss of heterozygosity for alleles on chromosome 11.[11] Other associated clinical conditions where 11p is not implicated include Edwards syndrome (trisomy 18), Sotos syndrome (5q35) and Bloom syndrome (15q26).

Clinical features

Most neonatal Wilms' tumours are discovered on clinical examination at a median age of 2 days, although more recently there has been an increase in antenatally detected masses.[45] Haematuria, unexplained anaemia and hypertension may be presenting features. Mesoblastic nephroma is typically diagnosed in the first week of life, uncommon beyond 3 months, and sometimes associated with hypercalcaemia. The resulting polyuria is potentially a cause of polyhydramnios, occasionally seen with the condition.[24]

Hydrocephalus, due to cerebral deposits of renal rhabdoid tumour, has also been reported.[9]

Investigations

Abdominal CT with intravenous contrast will delineate the primary tumour. Chest X-ray is required as a minimum to identify metastases. Hypercalcaemia responds to nephrectomy, but hypertension needs careful evaluation as it is associated with a high intraoperative morbidity.[31]

Treatment

Mesoblastic nephroma is treated by nephrectomy alone. Chemotherapy is only considered with incomplete excision or tumour rupture of the atypical/cellular histological type rather than the classical, leiomyomatous form.

For unilateral Wilms' tumours, current practice is surgery and postoperative chemotherapy according to surgical staging. Following biopsy, bilateral tumours receive chemotherapy first, in the hope that renal-sparing surgery may be possible later. Radiotherapy is avoided because of long-term sequelae.

Prognosis

The prognosis for mesoblastic nephroma is excellent (98% 2-year overall survival),[31] with the only death reported secondary to chemotherapy use predating the current recommendations. Wilms' tumours are invariably of favourable histology and predominantly stage 1. Their survival is excellent, >90%, with median follow-up of 31 months.[45]

Rhabdoid tumours are usually fatal irrespective of treatment.[45]

Screening

Routine radiological screening for at-risk groups has been debated for many years and some would advocate of dubious benefit, where simple clinical examination may suffice.[17] There is increasing support internationally for routine ultrasound for those with at least a 5% risk, 3-monthly and continuing until 7 years of age.[11] This generally includes those with Beckwith–Wiedemann syndrome (4–10% risk), WT1-associated syndromes, familial Wilms', or offspring of a parent previously treated for bilateral disease (if unilateral, risk <5%). Certain hemihypertrophy associations are likely to become included as more becomes known about the natural history.

Brain tumours

Whilst the most common solid malignancy in childhood, CNS malignancies are rare in the neonatal period, accounting for only 0.5–1.5% of all childhood CNS neoplasms.[51] Between 1981 and 2000, 15.5% of NRCT registrations in the first 6 weeks of life were CNS tumours, an incidence of 4.24 per million live births.

Neonatal brain tumours are predominantly supratentorial, and teratomas account for a third to a half of all cases. Teratomas frequently occur in the pineal or suprasellar region and may contain calcium visible on CT scan. Typically they are very large, rapidly growing and often histologically mature. Because of their size, they are rarely totally excised and there is a high operative mortality.[33]

Glial tumours such as astrocytomas account for 20–30% of neonatal tumours, with primitive neuroectodermal tumours (PNETs or medulloblastoma if infratentorial) the next most common. Choroid plexus papillomas are infrequent but overrepresented in this age group, whilst others such as craniopharyngiomas, ependymomas and meningiomas are rarely seen.[33]

Clinical features

The majority will present with macrocephaly, which may be diagnosed antenatally, or present with obstructed labour. Otherwise, a rapidly enlarging head circumference may become evident in the first week, frequently associated with hydrocephalus. Vomiting, listlessness, poor weight gain, neurological signs and seizures may occur but are less common, due to the ability of the skull to expand.[33,51]

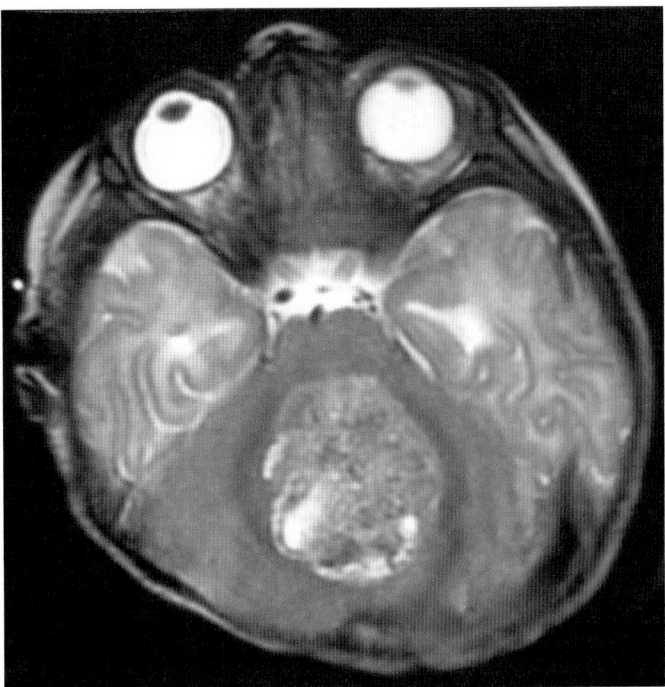

Fig. 37.4 Brain tumour.

Investigations

Neonatal brain tumours are often large, heterogeneous and rapidly growing. CT or magnetic resonance imaging (MRI) will delineate the tumour (Fig. 37.4), and determine operability and the presence of metastases. Extracranial metastases are seen in some cases of PNET.[33]

Low-grade gliomas, particularly of the optic tract, may be predictive of type 1 neurofibromatosis, whilst subependymal giant-cell astrocytomas are unique to tuberous sclerosis and are usually seen outside the neonatal period (see Table 40.2).

Treatment

Complete surgical resection is the treatment of choice for most tumours, although operability is dependent upon the site and size of the primary. Chemotherapy may be used as part of an aggressive treatment approach for PNET and ependymomas, although it is unclear whether this confers any survival advantage, due to the small numbers reported to date. Radiotherapy is avoided owing to the high incidence of cognitive, endocrine and neuropsychological sequelae.

Prognosis

A recent literature review of 250 published neonatal cases determined an overall survival of 28%.[33] Teratomas and PNETs generally had a very poor outcome, whilst survival was significantly better for astrocytomas and choroid plexus papillomas.

Retinoblastoma

Retinoblastoma is the commonest intraocular tumour of childhood and accounts for 3% of all childhood tumours. It produces progressive destruction of the retina, and occupies the globe, before spreading to the orbit and brain. Familial in up to 70% of cases and with a female preponderance 1.5:1,[1] the incidence in the neonatal period will depend on the local screening policy regarding those with a family history. The NRCT has recorded 37 cases of retinoblastoma over a 20-year period (1981–2000), accounting for 9% of malignancies in the first 6 weeks of life, with an incidence of 2.57 per million live births. A review of all neonatal retinoblastomas seen in New York[1] identified 46 cases diagnosed in the first 30 days of life (2.5% of all retinoblastomas), of which 56% were unilateral. Of these unilateral cases, 85% subsequently developed a tumour in the contralateral eye during follow-up (i.e. 91% had bilateral disease at some point).

The retinoblastoma gene was identified on chromosome 13q14, and is either partially or totally deleted in retinoblastoma.[22] As more becomes known about the retinoblastoma gene (*Rb1*) and there is further progress in molecular and cytogenetic techniques, it may be possible to predict the occurrence of these tumours by fetal chromosome analysis, especially in familial cases.

Clinical features

Those tumours not detected by elective screening are most likely to present with leukocoria (Fig. 37.5), heterochromia of the iris and strabismus.

Investigations

Staging by the Reese–Ellsworth classification[1] is based on the size and number of tumours, and their relationship to the globe's equator is by ophthalmoscopic examination under anaesthetic, together with CT scanning or MRI.

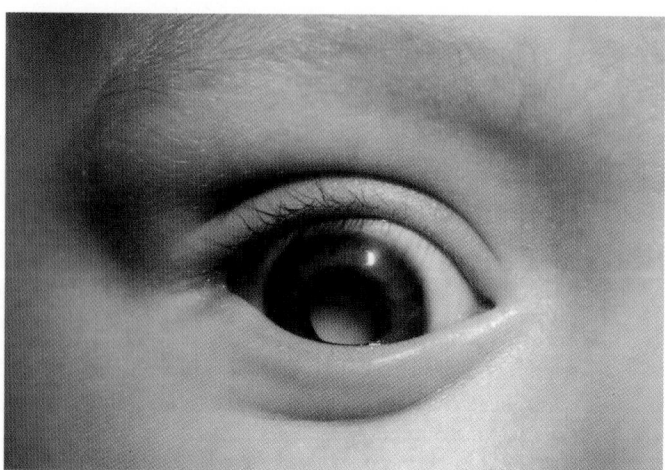

Fig. 37.5 Leukocoria.

Treatment

Treatment is dependent upon tumour extent and there has been a move towards eye-sparing therapy. The choice of therapy depends upon the location as well as the size of the tumour, and may include cryotherapy, laser or plaque therapy, or cyclical chemotherapy. In the New York series,[1] 79% of diseased eyes were salvaged. Stage 5 tumours usually require enucleation. If bilateral, conservative management is usually attempted first, in order to preserve the less severely affected eye. External-beam radiotherapy is avoided where possible because of the physical effects and a marked increase in secondary tumour risk.

Prognosis

For unilateral neonatal retinoblastoma, there is an 85% chance of retinoblastoma development in the contralateral eye,[1] hence regular ophthalmic follow-up is required. The prognosis is dependent upon the treatment modality employed, but generally 5-year survival exceeds 90%. The outcome in cases of metastatic disease is exceedingly poor.

There is an increased chance of developing a second tumour, most frequently an osteosarcoma, the locus for which is closely linked to that of the retinoblastoma gene. This usually follows local irradiation, with a cumulative risk of 1–2% per year for a secondary non-ocular malignancy.[1] Secondary malignancies are predominantly of high grade and carry a poor prognosis. Pineoblastoma is the second tumour most frequently seen in familial (bilateral) retinoblastoma. There is an increased risk of such tumours in the first 4 years of life, and, because of retinal differentiation seen on histology, these have been termed 'trilateral retinoblastomas'. They are thought to be muliticentric primaries rather than metastatic deposits and are usually fatal.

Risk to offspring

Germline mutations in familial disease are inherited in an autosomal dominant fashion with 90% penetrance. There is a 50% risk of carriage and a 45% risk of disease. Where neither parent is affected, the sibling risk for retinoblastoma is 1% in unilateral disease and 6% in bilateral or multifocal disease. This risk falls with every subsequent unaffected child.[39]

Sarcomas

Malignant soft-tissue tumours account for 11% of neonatal tumours, but only 2% of childhood sarcomas are diagnosed in the newborn period.[40]

Infantile fibrosarcoma is one of the commonest soft-tissue sarcomas. Although histologically similar to fibrosarcoma in adults, the biology is often not malignant and classification as a true sarcoma is questionable. It presents as a soft-tissue mass, most commonly in the head, neck or extremities. Cytogenetic abnormalities have been described.[48] The treatment of choice is surgical excision, although local recurrences have been reported. Metastases are rare. Because of the overall benign nature of the condition, the role of chemotherapy is limited to those where surgical resection would be disfiguring. The most commonly used agents are vincristine, actinomycin D and cyclophosphamide.[28]

Rhabdomyosarcomas rarely present at birth. Of the 3217 patients entered on the Intergroup Rhabdomyosarcoma Study (IRS), 14 were <30 days of age.[37] The most common primary sites are the genitourinary system, extremities or head and neck. Rhabdomyosarcoma has been classified histologically as alveolar, embryonal or botyroid. The latter two are the most common types in the neonatal period. Chromosomal abnormalities are commonly found and may be helpful both in diagnosis and in the understanding of tumourogenesis.[6] Treatment consists of chemotherapy and surgery. Radiotherapy is generally avoided, because of the effects on growth and function. Prognosis depends on the presence of metastases and, to a lesser extent, on the site of disease and the histological subtype. Approximately 20–25% of patients with metastatic disease are expected to be long-term survivors, as compared with 70% of those with localised disease.[18,40]

Rare neonatal sarcomas include Ewing's tumour, extraosseous Ewing's tumours, liposarcomas and leiomyosarcomas.[40]

Liver tumours

The only primary liver malignancy seen in the neonatal period is hepatoblastoma, which may be associated with hemihypertrophy or Beckwith–Wiedemann syndrome (see Table 40.2). The differential diagnosis of liver masses includes secondary deposits from neuroblastoma or choriocarcinoma, along with benign lesions such as haemangiomas, hamartomas, adenomas and cysts. Haemangioma and hepatoblastoma are the commonest lesions, often difficult to distinguish by imaging (angiogram or MRI), or by tumour markers, due to the normally high AFP seen at birth. They may require biopsy for diagnosis. Around 40 cases of neonatal hepatoblastoma have been reported in the literature, although few have received standard infant treatment (chemotherapy followed by surgery) and consequently the reported mortality rate is high.[2] Metastases are usually pulmonary in the older child, although this is rarely seen in the neonate, where 10–15% have metastases, usually at non-pulmonary sites. This is thought to be due to the fetal circulation bypassing the pulmonary vasculature. Bone scan and MRI of the brain are required for staging.

Histiocytosis

Histiocytosis includes a group of poorly understood conditions resulting from abnormal proliferation of histiocyte/mononuclear cells (including antigen-presenting cells). Predominantly benign conditions, they are frequently overseen by paediatric oncologists, as they may require intervention with chemotherapy or, rarely, irradiation, despite a strong immunological basis to the disease, with cytotoxic T-cell deficiency and excessive interleukin and PGE$_2$ production.

Langerhans' cell histiocytosis (LCH) is a clonal proliferation of Langerhans' cells distinguished by the presence of Birbeck granules on electron microscopy, and is usually benign (p. 831). It may present in the neonate with unifocal or, more typically, multiorgan disease.[32] Solitary lesions can present with painful swelling, isolated rash or be discovered incidentally on X-ray. Diagnosis is confirmed on biopsy. Although most spontaneously involute, local treatments may become necessary: topical corticosteroids for skin lesions, intralesional steroid or local low-dose radiotherapy for worrying bony disease such as spinal involvement.[32] Multifocal disease is less likely to spontaneously resolve, presenting with rash, auricular and oral lesions, lymphadenopathy, hepatosplenomegaly and lung involvement. Treatment with chemotherapy may be necessary for organ dysfunction. Response to chemotherapy is variable, with an overall mortality of 18%.[32]

Hashimoto–Pritzker disease[32] is a congenital self-healing reticulohistiocytosis and cutaneous form of LCH. Red–purple nodules, similar to healing chickenpox lesions, occur predominantly on the scalp, spontaneously regressing over a few weeks or months.

Haemophagocytic lymphohistiocytosis (HLH) is rarely seen in the neonatal period. This is usually the familial form and there may be a family history (autosomal recessive) or consanguinity. HLH is a non-clonal proliferation of histiocytes without Birbeck granules. This manifests with fever, splenomegaly, pancytopenia, hypofibrinogenaemia and hypertriglyceridaemia. Haemophagocytosis is seen in lymph node biopsy or bone marrow, and untreated, the median survival is 2 months.[32] Treatment involves chemotherapy and allogeneic bone marrow transplantation, with a 3-year event-free survival of 44%.[4] Secondary HLH is a consequence of infection or malignancy, for which supportive therapy and chemotherapy alone is preferred.

Other rare tumours

Many other rare malignancies may also occur in the neonatal period and appear as isolated cases within incidence series.[14,20,25,34]

Melanoma is the most frequent, and may arise in large congenital pigmented naevi or following transplacental spread. These lesions can regress spontaneously. Treatment is surgery and, rarely, chemotherapy, with less than 60% surviving 18 months.[44]

Throughout the chapter, histologically benign tumours have been included, as they are important in the differential diagnosis of malignant tumours (e.g. mature teratomas, mesoblastic nephroma) or may be fatal, often due to the site of disease (e.g. CNS tumours, hepatic haemangiomas).

Haemangiomas may occur at any site and be associated with high-output cardiac failure or thrombocytopenia, the Kasabach–Merritt syndrome (p. 831). They may respond to α-interferon, although spastic diplegia has been reported as a consequence of treatment.[5]

Cystic hygromas (congenital lymphatic malformation) are most frequently seen in the posterior neck (p. 830), often associated with Turner syndrome or the trisomies (pp. 895–6). Surgery is preferred, although inoperable or recurrent malformations may respond to intralesional bleomycin or OK-432.

Other benign lesions include rhabdomyomas (seen in tuberous sclerosis), myofibromatoses, xanthogranulomas, lipomas, ovarian cysts, and epidermal or dermal cysts. Many are excised, although some spontaneously regress or require no intervention.

References

1. Abramson D H, Du T T, Beaverson K L 2002 (Neonatal) retinoblastoma in the first month of life. Archives of Ophthalmology 120: 738–742
2. Ammann R A, Plaschkes J, Leibundgut K 1999 Congenital hepatoblastoma: a distinct entity. Medical and Pediatric Oncology 32: 466–468
3. Bader J L, Miller R W 1979 US cancer incidence and mortality in the first year of life. American Journal of Diseases of Children 133: 157–159
4. Baker K S, DeLaat C A, Steinbuch M et al 1997 Successful correction of hemophagocytic lymphohistiocytosis with related or unrelated bone marrow transplantation. Blood 89: 3857–3863
5. Barlow C F, Priebe C J, Mulliken J B et al 1998 Spastic diplegia as a complication of interferon alfa-2a treatment of hemangiomas of infancy. Journal of Pediatrics 132: 527–530
6. Barr F G 1997 Molecular genetics and pathogenesis of rhabdomyosarcoma. Journal of Pediatric Hematology and Oncology 19: 483–491
7. Berry P J 1987 In: Keeling J W (ed) Congenital tumours in foetal and neonatal pathology. Springer-Verlag, London, pp 229–247
8. Blair J I, Carachi R, Gupta R et al 1987 Plasma alpha fetoprotein reference ranges in infancy: effect of prematurity. Archives of Disease in Childhood 62: 362–369
9. Bonnin J M, Rubinstein L J, Palmer N F et al 1984 The association of embryonal tumors originating in the kidney and in the brain. A report of seven cases. Cancer 54: 2137–2146
10. Borch K, Jacobsen T, Olsen J H et al 1992 Neonatal cancer in Denmark 1943–1985. Pediatric Hematology and Oncology 9: 209–216
11. Bove K E 1999 Wilms' tumor and related abnormalities in the fetus and newborn. Seminars in Perinatology 23: 310–318
12. Bresters D, Reus A C, Veerman A J et al 2002 Congenital leukaemia: the Dutch experience and review of the literature. British Journal of Haematology 117: 513–524
13. Brodeur G M, Maris J M, Yamashiro D J et al 1997 Biology and genetics of human neuroblastomas. Journal of Pediatric Hematology and Oncology 19: 93–101
14. Campbell A N, Chan H S, O'Brien A et al 1987 Malignant tumours in the neonate. Archives of Disease in Childhood 62: 19–23
15. Chessells J M, Harrison C J, Kempski H et al 2002 Clinical features, cytogenetics and outcome in acute lymphoblastic and myeloid leukaemia of infancy: report from the MRC Childhood Leukaemia working party. Leukemia 16: 776–784
16. Chessells J M, Harrison C J, Watson S L et al 2002 Treatment of infants with lymphoblastic leukaemia: results of the UK Infant Protocols 1987–1999. British Journal of Haematology 117: 306–314
17. Craft A W, Parker L, Stiller C et al 1995 Screening for Wilms' tumour in patients with aniridia, Beckwith syndrome, or hemihypertrophy. Medical and Pediatric Oncology 24: 231–234
18. Crist W, Gehan E A, Ragab A H et al 1995 The Third Intergroup Rhabdomyosarcoma Study. Journal of Clinical Oncology 13: 610–630
19. Crom D B, Wilimas J A, Green A A et al 1989 Malignancy in the neonate. Medical and Pediatric Oncology 17: 101–104
20. Davis C F, Carachi R, Young D G 1988 Neonatal tumours: Glasgow 1955–86. Archives of Disease in Childhood 63: 1075–1078
21. Frangoul H A, Patterson K 1998 Complications of acute leukemia. Case one: congenital acute myelogenous leukemia with cutaneous involvement. Journal of Clinical Oncology 16: 3199–3200
22. Friend S H, Bernards R, Rogelj S et al 1986 A human DNA segment with properties of the gene that predisposes to retinoblastoma and osteosarcoma. Nature 323: 643–646
23. Friend S H, Dryja T P, Weinberg R A 1988 Oncogenes and tumor-suppressing genes. New England Journal of Medicine 318: 618–622
24. Fung T Y, Fung Y M, Ng P C et al 1995 Polyhydramnios and hypercalcemia associated with congenital mesoblastic nephroma: case report and a new appraisal. Obstetrics and Gynecology 85: 815–817
25. Gale G B, D'Angio G J, Uri A et al 1982 Cancer in neonates: the experience at the Children's Hospital of Philadelphia. Pediatrics 70: 409–413
26. Gobel U, Schneider D T, Calaminus G et al 2001 Multimodal treatment of malignant sacrococcygeal germ cell tumors: a prospective analysis of 66 patients of the German cooperative protocols MAKEI 83/86 and 89. Journal of Clinical Oncology 19: 1943–1950
27. Greaves M F 1996 Infant leukaemia biology, aetiology and treatment. Leukemia 10: 372–377
28. Grier H E, Perez-Atayde A R, Weinstein H J 1985 Chemotherapy for inoperable infantile fibrosarcoma. Cancer 56: 1507–1510
29. Halperin E C 2000 Neonatal neoplasms. International Journal of Radiation Oncology, Biology, Physics 47: 171–178
30. Homans A C, Verissimo A M, Vlacha V 1993 Transient abnormal myelopoiesis of infancy associated with trisomy 21. American Journal of Pediatric Hematology and Oncology 15: 392–399
31. Howell C G, Othersen H B, Kiviat N E et al 1982 Therapy and outcome in 51 children with mesoblastic nephroma: a report of the National Wilms' Tumor Study. Journal of Pediatric Surgery 17: 826–831
32. Huang F, Arceci R 1999 The histiocytoses of infancy. Seminars in Perinatology 23: 319–331
33. Isaacs H 2002 I. Perinatal brain tumors: a review of 250 cases. Pediatric Neurology 27: 249–261
34. Isaacs H Jr 1985 Perinatal (congenital and neonatal) neoplasms: a report of 110 cases. Pediatric Pathology 3: 165–216
35. Kaneko M, Iwakawa M, Ikebukuro K et al 1998 Complete resection is not required in patients with neuroblastoma under 1 year of age. Journal of Pediatric Surgery 33: 1690–1694
36. Knudson A G Jr 1985 Hereditary cancer, oncogenes, and antioncogenes. Cancer Research 45: 1437–1443
37. Lobe T E, Wiener E S, Hays D M et al 1994 Neonatal rhabdomyosarcoma: the IRS experience. Journal of Pediatric Surgery 29: 1167–1170
38. Lukens J N 1999 Neuroblastoma in the neonate. Seminars in Perinatology 23: 263–273
39. Margo C E, Harman L E, Mulla Z D 1998 Retinoblastoma. Cancer Control 5: 310–316
40. Palumbo J S, Zwerdling T 1999 Soft tissue sarcomas of infancy. Seminars in Perinatology 23: 299–309
41. Parkes S E, Muir K R, Southern L et al 1994 Neonatal tumours: a thirty-year population-based study. Medical and Pediatric Oncology 22: 309–317
42. Pritchard J, Hickman J A 1994 Why does stage 4s neuroblastoma regress spontaneously? Lancet 344: 869–870
43. Rescorla F J, Sawin R S, Coran A G et al 1998 Long-term outcome for infants and children with sacrococcygeal teratoma: a report from the Children's Cancer Group. Journal of Pediatric Surgery 33: 171–176
44. Richardson S K, Tannous Z S, Mihm M C Jr 2002 Congenital and infantile melanoma: review of the literature and report of an uncommon variant, pigment-synthesizing melanoma. Journal of the American Academy of Dermatology 47: 77–90
45. Ritchey M L, Azizkhan R G, Beckwith J B et al 1995 Neonatal Wilms tumor. Journal of Pediatric Surgery 30: 856–859
46. Roman E, Fear N T, Ansell P et al 2002 Vitamin K and childhood cancer: analysis of individual patient data from six case-control studies. British Journal of Cancer 86: 63–69
47. Sbragia L, Paek B W, Feldstein V A et al 2001 Outcome of prenatally diagnosed solid fetal tumors. Journal of Pediatric Surgery 36: 1244–1247
48. Schofield D E, Fletcher J A, Grier H E et al 1994 Fibrosarcoma in infants and children. Application of new techniques. American Journal of Surgical Pathology 18: 14–24
49. Tchernia G, Lejeune F, Boccara J F et al 1996 Erythroblastic and/or megakaryoblastic leukemia in Down syndrome: treatment with low-dose arabinosyl cytosine. Journal of Pediatric Hematology and Oncology 18: 59–62
50. Voute P A, Jr, Wadman S K, van Putten W J 1970 Congenital neuroblastoma. Symptoms in the mother during pregnancy. Clinical Pediatrics 9: 206–207
51. Wakai S, Arai T, Nagai M 1984 Congenital brain tumors. Surgical Neurology 21: 597–609
52. Weitzman S, Grant R 1997 Neonatal oncology: diagnostic and therapeutic dilemmas. Seminars in Perinatology 21: 102–111
53. Wiemels J L, Xiao Z, Buffler P A et al 2002 In utero origin of t(8;21) AML1-ETO translocations in childhood acute myeloid leukemia. Blood 99: 3801–3805
54. Woods W G, Tuchman M, Robison L L et al 1996 A population-based study of the usefulness of screening for neuroblastoma. Lancet 348: 1682–1687
55. Xue H, Horwitz J R, Smith M B et al 1995 Malignant solid tumors in neonates: a 40-year review. Journal of Pediatric Surgery 30: 543–545

CHAPTER 38

Orthopaedic problems in the neonate

Christopher J Dare, Nicholas M P Clarke

Introduction

With the advent of high-resolution ultrasound scanning (USS), orthopaedic problems are being increasingly detected during routine antenatal screening – for example, talipes equinovarus, limb deficiency and complex syndactyly. This is creating a need for neonatologists and those in fetal medicine to have a better knowledge of orthopaedic problems relevant to the newborn infant. Early diagnosis should facilitate appropriate referral and counselling, which should lead to an improvement in parent satisfaction and outcome for the child.

A whole range of factors can impact on the developing fetus, resulting in orthopaedic problems in the neonate. Some of these are well understood, such as genetic influences in achondroplasia and drug-related problems such as thalidomide; others are less well understood, such as congenital talipes equinovarus (CTEV) and developmental dysplasia of the hip. In this chapter we aim to give the reader some understanding and a working knowledge of the common and rarer orthopaedic problems affecting the neonate.

Lower limb abnormalities

Developmental dysplasia of the hip

Terminology

The nomenclature of this condition has been open to debate recently, as it encompasses a whole range of conditions other than frank dislocation of the hip. These include congenital subluxation of the hip, developmental dysplasia, and dislocatable hip. It is now accepted that hips are rarely truly dislocated at birth but are merely unstable and go on to develop problems at a later stage. Therefore, the condition formerly known as congenital dislocation of the hip (CDH) is more correctly referred to as developmental dysplasia of the hip (DDH).[33] DDH is the term used throughout this book.

Hips that are truly dislocated at birth are rare, and the cause usually involves teratologic factors. The aetiology is thus entirely different to DDH, and is usually secondary to neuromuscular conditions such as arthrogryposis multiplex congenita (AMC) and spina bifida.

Incidence of DDH

The incidence of DDH is approximately 1–2 per 1000 livebirths. The incidence of unstable hips at birth ranges from 5 to 20 per 1000 livebirths, but the majority (60%) of these go on spontaneously to stabilise.[7] The difference in incidence is thought to be due to transplacental passage of maternal relaxin causing temporary ligamentous instability in the early neonatal period, as well as to differences in diagnostic method and timing of evaluation. There are geographical variations thought to be genetic in Northern Italians and environmental in North American Indians.[27]

Risk factors

For 60% of neonates with DDH, no known risk factor(s) can be identified.[49] In 20% of cases, the condition is bilateral. There are, however, well-documented risk factors for DDH, such as positive family history, female sex, firstborn children, oligohydramnios, macrosomia and breech presentation. When there is a positive family history, there is a 6% risk for one affected child, a 12% risk with one affected parent and a 36% risk with one affected child and one affected parent. In monozygotic twins there is 43% concordance, with 3% concordance in dizygotic twins. Girls are affected more than boys at a ratio of 5:1. There is an increased incidence in firstborn Caucasian children.[27] Oligohydramnios and macrosomia increases the risk owing to the simple mechanics of a crowded intrauterine environment. The left hip is more often affected than the right, which is attributed to the right shoulder more often being anterior in breech presentation. With the right shoulder anterior, the left hip is compressed against the maternal sacral promontory, a position favouring dislocation. Breech presentation increases the risk particularly in breech with extended knees, which increases the incidence by a factor of 10.[11] Extrauterine factors that increase the risk of DDH include swaddling clothes and that now historic use of cradle boards to hold the hips in the extended position.

DDH is also associated with other congenital anomalies, including torticollis, metatarsus adductus, CTEV, congenital vertical talus (CVT) and calcaneovalgus (v.i.).[11]

Screening

Since 1966, as part of routine postnatal screening, the hips of newborn children are clinically examined by employing the Ortolani[43] and Barlow[7] tests (p. 260). Both these tests are subject to inter- and intra-observer variability and hence their sensitivity varies with the experience of the examiner. In some reported studies, as many as 50% of established cases of clinical hip abnormality are missed by clinical examination alone. They remain, however, the standard screening test for DDH in the newborn infant in the UK.

Prior to the advent of routine screening, the number of cases of DDH matched the number requiring surgery (1–2/1000). However, since the introduction of routine clinical screening, the number of identified cases of DDH has increased significantly (5–20/1000) along with the number undergoing abduction splinting (3–4/1000). Alongside this increase has been a significant decrease in the number undergoing surgery for DDH (0.2–0.7/1000). However, since the introduction of clinical screening, the number of late-presenting cases of DDH has changed very little and may have increased slightly. This may be because primary clinical examination fails to identify hip displacement or that no clinical abnormality was present or detectable at that stage. This questions the validity of clinical examination alone as a screening tool and it is now accepted that the clinical tests are not 100% specific or sensitive.

Clinical examination and findings

Ortolani's test is performed by flexing and abducting the hips. A dislocated hip will 'clunk' back into the normal acetabular position as the hip is abducted. The Barlow test, however, is a provocative test, which aims to displace a dysplastic hip from its normal acetabular position. This test is performed by adducting and flexing the hip to 90°, and applying downward force through the femur in a posterolateral direction while the pelvis is stabilised. A positive test is indicated by the hip displacing posteriorly when this force is applied. With older children, these tests become less appropriate, because secondary signs develop (restriction of abduction, shortening, and thigh crease asymmetry). Finally, a child with undiagnosed unilateral DDH will often be noted to have asymmetric limb lengths and will walk with a limp.

Investigations

The femoral head in the newborn is an entirely cartilaginous structure and only begins to ossify between 4 and 7 months of age. Radiological assessment of the hip in the first few months of life is difficult, and in most centres, ultrasound is employed.

USS has proved to be a very cost-effective, non-invasive, non-irradiating way of assessing hip stability (Fig. 38.1). Ultrasound visualises the cartilaginous and soft-tissue structures around the hip (Fig. 38.2) and is now the first-line investigation for DDH in neonates with clinical suspicion or when there are risk factors.[10,15]

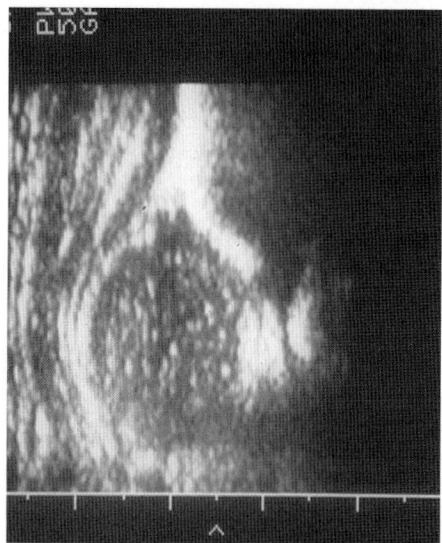

(a)

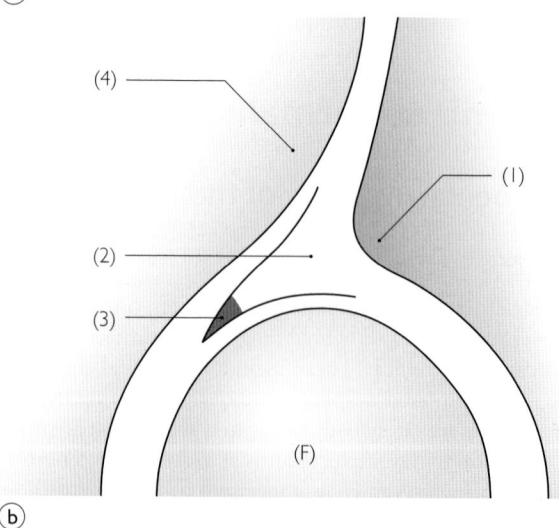

(b)

Fig. 38.2 (a) Ultrasound scan image of a normal neonatal hip. (b) The acetabular rim area of the right hip: (1) osseous rim; (2) cartilaginous rim; (3) fibrocartilaginous limbus; (4) joint capsule; (5) recess between the limbus and the periosteum; (F) femoral head (Reproduced from Graf.[24]).

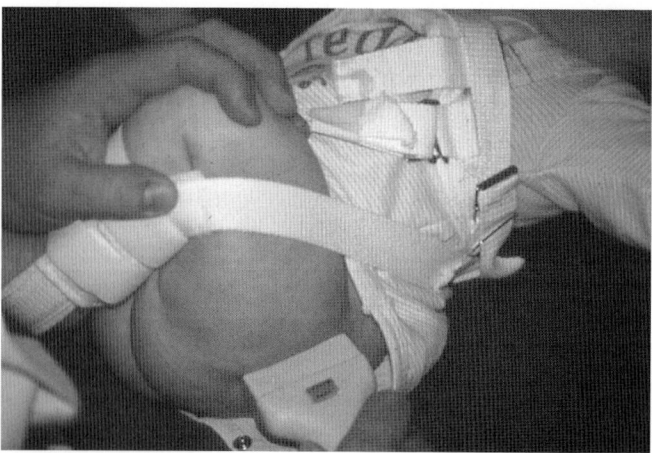

Fig. 38.1 Dynamic ultrasound of a left hip of a child in a Pavlik harness.

In some centres in the UK, both static and dynamic ultrasonography are now routinely used in the initial assessment and for the assessment of treatment of DDH.[52]

There currently exist no national set guidelines on the initial diagnosis and management of DDH. Some children will be splinted on clinical suspicion alone, while others will also undergo USS in addition to clinical assessment. The recent UK Hip Trial recommends the use of ultrasound assessment of clinically unstable hips but advocates caution with clinically stable hips in at-risk children.[20] This stance is taken because of the risk of exposing babies to unnecessary abduction splinting when the natural history of ultrasound-diagnosed hip dysplasia is not clearly understood.

Referral and treatment

Following detection of the at-risk neonate by either clinical assessment or risk factor identification, the baby is referred on for further assessment by ultrasonography. (The authors use treatment algorithms for subsequent management; Figs 38.3 & 38.4).[52] Those neonates with clinically unstable hips are referred and seen urgently within 2 weeks, and those with identified risk factors or 'clicky' hips are seen at 6 weeks.

There has been much debate about the role of ultrasound in the screening process, as some believe that ultrasonographic screening is too sensitive and therefore overdiagnoses DDH. As a result, a small percentage of babies are exposed to the risks of unnecessary splinting. As more information is gathered on the natural history of subtle ultrasound abnormalities of the neonatal hip, and abduction splintage is delayed in these cases until persistent ultrasonographic abnormalities are present at 6 weeks, this overdiagnosis of significant DDH is likely to decrease in the future.

Once assessed by ultrasound, subsequent management is dictated by the degree or otherwise of hip instability, with the mainstay of treatment being the abduction harness (Fig. 38.5).

The Pavlik[46] harness is the commonest abduction device which encourages dynamic hip relocation.[13] Other abduction devices do exist, such as the Von Rosen and Denis Browne splints, which are rigid in structure. Failure to respond to treatment or delay in presentation results in a more invasive surgical treatment which includes arthrography (Fig. 38.6).

Although it is now standard practice to apply abduction splintage when a diagnosis of DDH is made, concerns have been raised about how sound this treatment strategy is. Despite abduction splinting commencing before 8 weeks of age, a small percentage of babies will still have radiological evidence of hip dysplasia and 12% will have undergone surgery by the age of 2 years. It is clear that some babies will develop dysplasia despite splinting and these babies will be exposed to the risks of abduction splinting. Because the unaffected hip in unilateral DDH is also splinted, there is a small risk of iatrogenic complications. These include avascular necrosis (1–4% of cases), pressure sores, epiphysitis, femoral nerve palsy, inferior dislocation of the hip

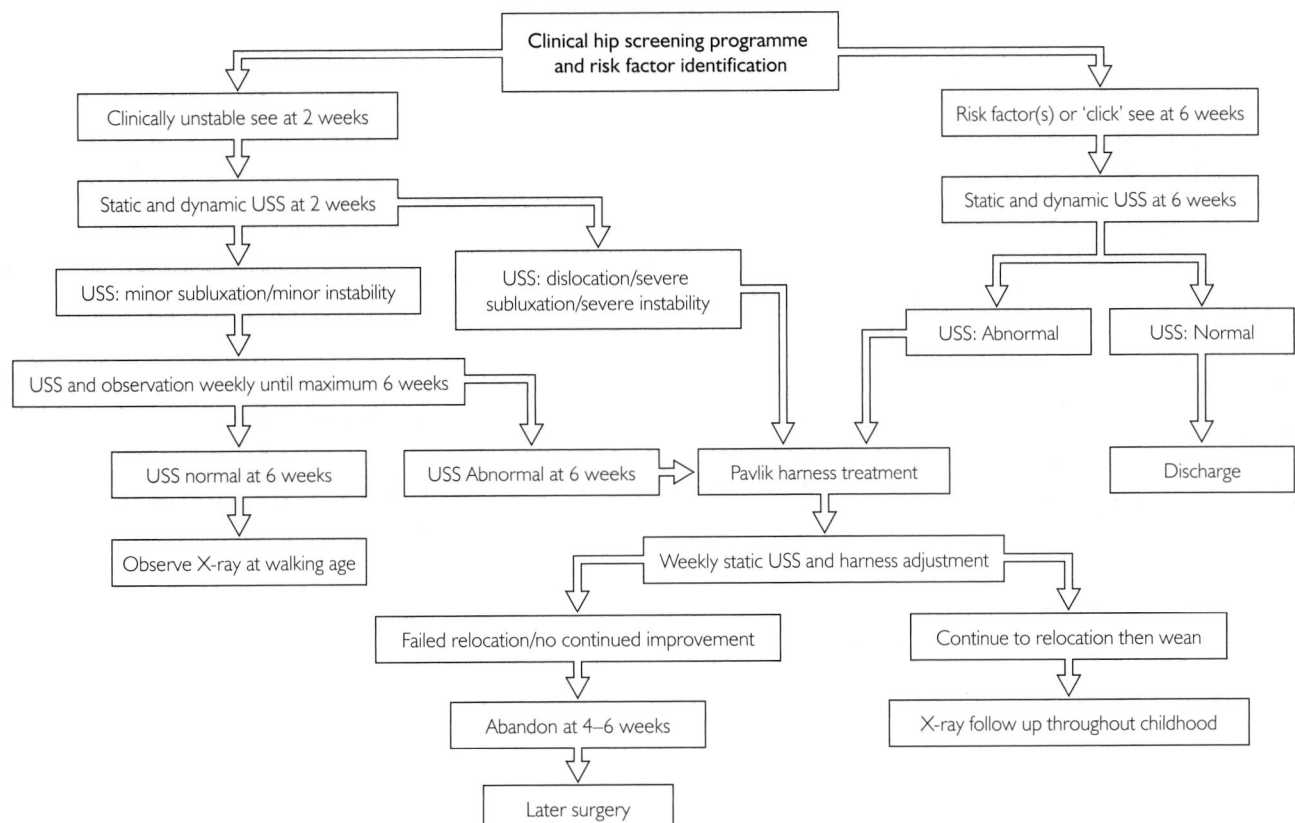

Fig. 38.3 Treatment algorithm for developmental dysplasia of the hip in the newborn.

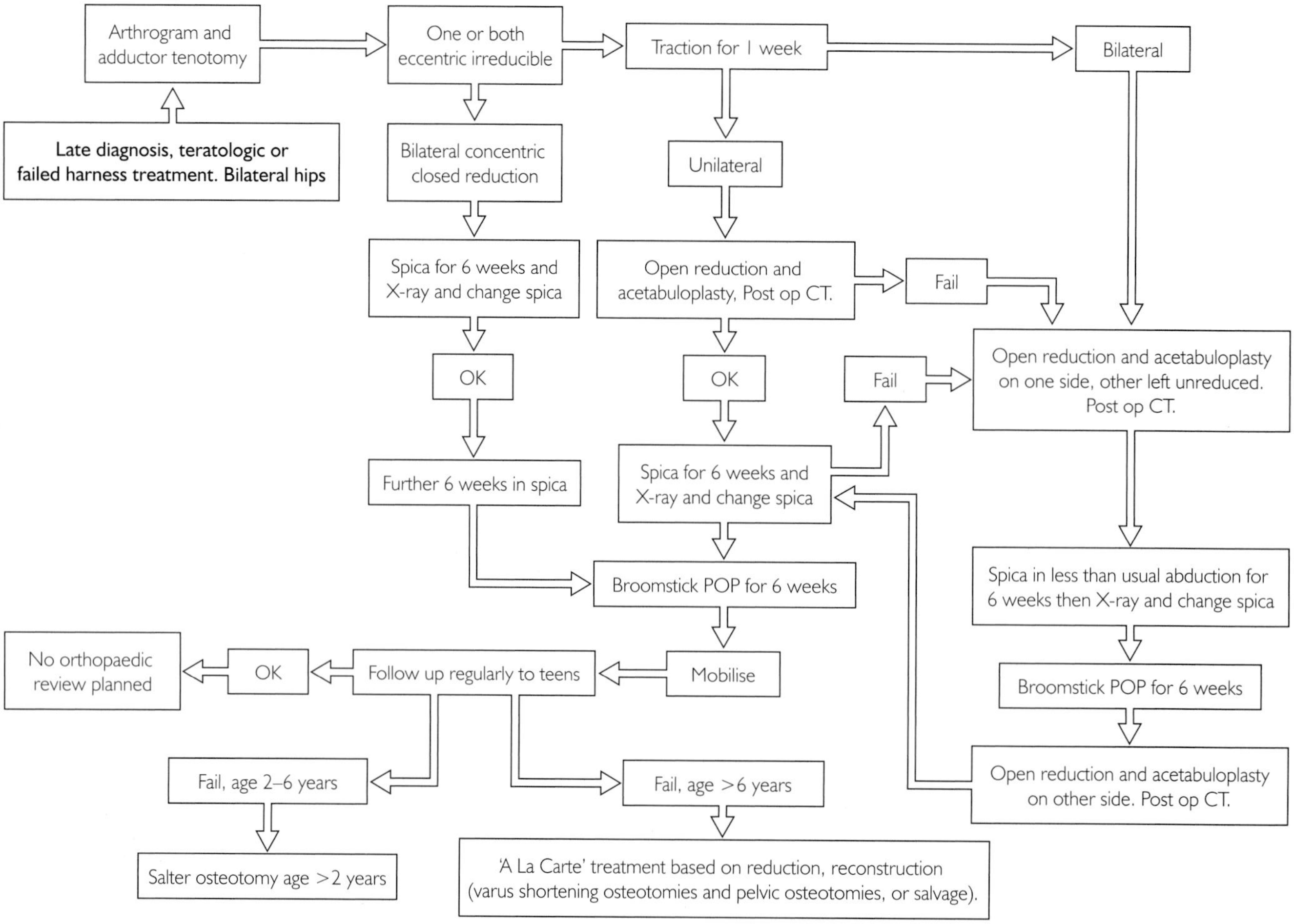

Arthrogram and adductor tenotomy → One or both eccentric irreducible → Traction for 1 week → Bilateral

Late diagnosis, teratologic or failed harness treatment. Bilateral hips

Bilateral concentric closed reduction

Unilateral

Spica for 6 weeks and X-ray and change spica

Open reduction and acetabuloplasty, Post op CT. → Fail

OK

OK

Fail → Open reduction and acetabuloplasty on one side, other left unreduced. Post op CT.

Further 6 weeks in spica

Spica for 6 weeks and X-ray and change spica

Spica in less than usual abduction for 6 weeks then X-ray and change spica

Broomstick POP for 6 weeks

No orthopaedic review planned ← OK ← Follow up regularly to teens ← Mobilise

Broomstick POP for 6 weeks

Fail, age 2–6 years

Fail, age >6 years

Open reduction and acetabuloplasty on other side. Post op CT.

Salter osteotomy age >2 years

'A La Carte' treatment based on reduction, reconstruction (varus shortening osteotomies and pelvic osteotomies, or salvage).

Fig. 38.4 Treatment algorithm for developmental dysplasia of the hip in children with delayed presentation or failed Pavlik treatment.

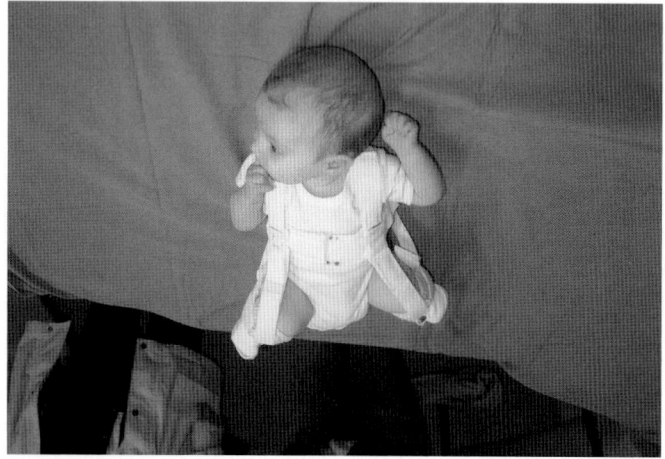

Fig. 38.5 Child in a Pavlik harness.

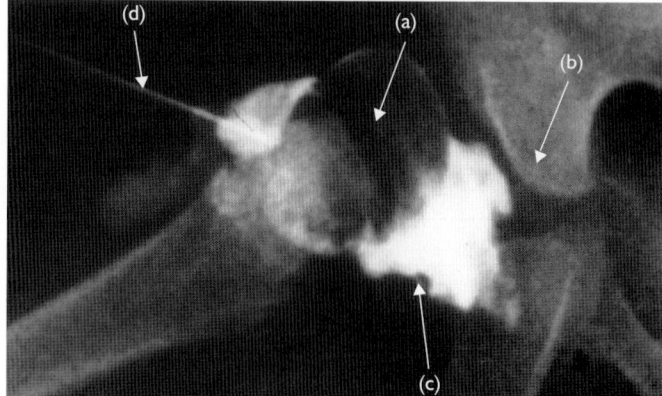

Fig. 38.6 Arthrogram of a dislocated right hip: (a) femoral head (dislocated); (b) dysplastic acetabulum; (c) medial pooling of contrast; (d) spinal needle to introduce contrast.

and medial instability of the knee joint. These risks are inevitable when treating an affected hip but may be unacceptable if they affect the 'normal' hip. Therefore, much of the current research on the management of DDH is focused on identifying those 'clicky' hips that will resolve spontaneously and those that will definitely require some form of intervention.

The efficacy of abduction splinting has been shown in prospective longitudinal trials but this method of treatment has not yet been subject to a randomised trial. It is now apparent that this will be necessary to develop treatment strategies for hips which are clinically stable but demonstrate borderline abnormalities on ultrasound.

As has been previously stated the current clinical screening tests are not the most reliable, and much debate has been generated about the inclusion of routine USS screening to identify those hips that require treatment and those that do not. This is an important issue, as there may be significant adverse long-term sequelae if DDH is not diagnosed and treated. Therefore, a dichotomy exists between overdiagnosing and overtreating DDH which may settle spontaneously, exposing the baby to unnecessary risk, and underdiagnosing DDH which may result in degenerative changes of the hip in early adult life.

This begs the question of whether there is a need for a national screening programme inclusive of ultrasound assessment, for all children, to identify all cases of DDH in the absence of clinical instability. However, until the use of abduction harnesses has been properly evaluated and further expertise in neonatal hip ultrasonography is developed nationally, this would be premature. A national screening programme incorporating USS, as seen in Germany and Norway, is unlikely to be instigated in the UK in the foreseeable future because of financial and personnel resource problems.

Congenital dislocation of the knee

Incidence

The incidence of congenital dislocation of the knee (CDK) is approximately 1 per 100 000 livebirths, which is about 100 times less than that of DDH, making it exceedingly rare. It is commonly associated with other congenital anomalies, DDH in 45% of cases and CTEV in 35% of cases, as well as torticollis and congenital dislocation of the elbow. It is a more frequent finding in children with AMC and myelodysplasia and those with Larsen's syndrome (a condition of ligamentous laxity). It is bilateral in approximately a third of cases and has a predilection for females at a ratio of 2:1.[5,17,41,42,50]

Aetiology

The underlying cause for CDK is poorly understood but several factors have been postulated. In an otherwise normal breech child, oligohydramnios has been proposed as a mechanical cause, with crowding in utero holding the legs in an extended position with the feet locked under the mandible or axillae. Other suggestions include congenital abnormalities of the quadriceps (fibrous contracture) and absent cruciate ligaments, although these may be secondary findings as a result of the dislocation.

It has also been described in children with Down syndrome and in children with other chromosomal defects.

Clinical findings and presentation

The abnormality is usually obvious at birth, with the knee(s) hyperextended (recurvatum) (Fig. 38.7a). In severe forms, the tibia may be in contact with the chest, with the feet tucked under the axilla or mandible.[50] X-ray evaluation (Fig. 38.7b) will reveal complete dislocation in the severe form, with the proximal tibia anterior and lateral to the distal femur. Clinically, the patella may

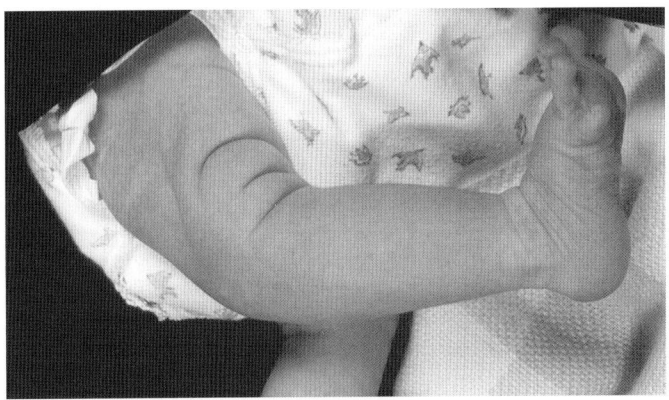

(a)

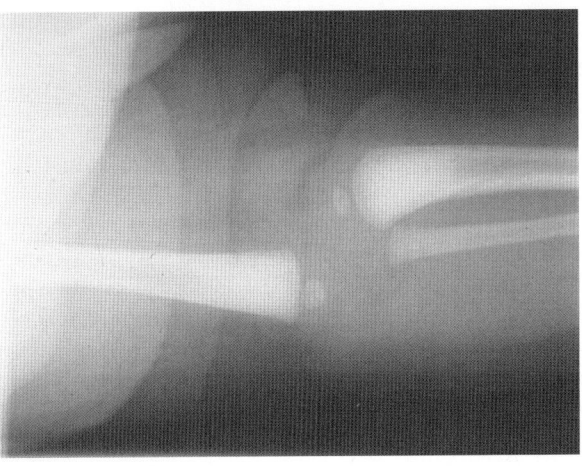

(b)

Fig. 38.7 (a) Clinical appearance of a right congenitally dislocated knee. (b) X-ray demonstrating the radiological appearance of a right congenitally dislocated knee.

be subluxed laterally and the femoral condyles are prominent posteriorly. In the first few hours after birth the knee is usually flexible but any delay in treatment can result in a fixed deformity.

Referral and treatment

CDK is an orthopaedic emergency and immediate orthopaedic referral is essential. The optimal treatment for CDK remains controversial, with some advocating early surgical intervention others conservative treatment.[5] Success of conservative treatment is dependent on early referral within the first 24 hours following delivery. The exception to this is when CDK is found in association with Larsen's syndrome and arthrogryposis. A variety of conservative treatments are available, including serial casting, Pavlik harness, skin traction and skeletal traction.

If it is possible, gentle traction and direct reduction should be attempted in the first 24 hours, followed by splinting or casting with the knee in 90° of flexion. If this is not possible, then passive stretching of the quadriceps and the anterior knee capsule, combined with splinting or serial casting of the knee in an increasingly flexed position, is an alternative method.

It has been suggested that the pathoanatomy of CDK resembles that of DDH in that failure to reduce the joint early results in soft-tissue contracture with a resultant fixed deformity, which requires surgical correction.[17,42,50]

Prognosis

When CDK is treated in the early stages, i.e. the first day of life, then conservative measures are most likely to produce a good functional range of movement of the knee with no further intervention required. In those cases of CDK associated with other musculoskeletal abnormalities, the prognosis remains good but conservative treatment tends to be more protracted. In older children with moderate to severe subluxation or with dislocation, surgical intervention is invariably required.

Congenital talipes equinovarus

This is a structural abnormality affecting the feet of children. It may be unilateral or bilateral, with the feet held in an adducted, supinated, plantar-flexed position (Fig. 38.8). This position is achieved by a combination of adduction and supination of the forefoot with a varus deformity of the heel and with the whole foot held in equinus at the ankle. The abnormal position is reflected in the bony architecture of the foot. The lateral malleolus is positioned posterolaterally and the head of the talus points anterolaterally (instead of anteromedially); the navicular is subluxed medially around the head of the talus and may even be in contact with the medial malleolus. With the talus lying obliquely in relation to the calcaneum, excess pressure on the anteromedial part of the calcaneum forces it into varus and equinus to compensate for the abnormally positioned talus.[12]

Incidence

In the UK, the incidence of CTEV is approximately 1 per 1000 livebirths, but geographical variations exist worldwide, with an incidence of 0.57 per 1000 for Orientals and 6.81 per 1000 in Polynesians. There is a sex difference, with a male preponderance of 2–3 to 1, and the condition is bilateral in 50% of cases.[6]

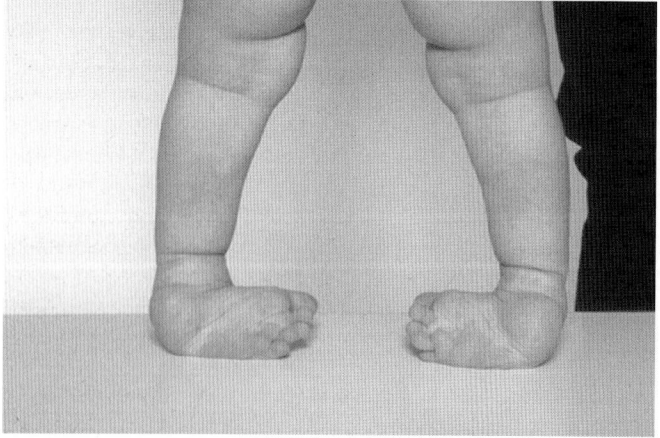

Fig. 38.8 Typical appearance of bilateral congenital talipes equinovarus.

Aetiology

The aetiology of CTEV is poorly understood but a variety of hypotheses have been put forward, including external compression in utero, abnormal tendon and ligament attachments, neuromuscular dysfunction and germ plasm defect.[12,51]

External compression in utero is thought to account for postural talipes, a variety of talipes deformity which is fully correctable at birth and resolves spontaneously with stretching. Abnormalities in the ligaments and tendons of CTEV feet have been well documented. Neurological dysfunction with abnormalities in muscle innervation and muscle imbalance and delayed muscle maturation have also been proposed as aetiological factors. However, the most widely accepted hypothesis is the germ plasm defect theory which suggests that the primary defect is in the development of the bones of the tarsus (principally the talus), and the other abnormalities are adaptive to this underlying defect.[6,11,12,51]

Clinical features and classification

The affected feet are held adducted, supinated and plantar-flexed (equinus) and classically have been graded as benign, moderate, severe and very severe. This classification is subjective and open to inter- and intra-observer errors. A variety of more objective grading systems do exist but the most widely adopted is the Dimeglio[18] classification.

Dimeglio grading system for CTEV

Dimeglio devised a scoring system based on the morphological characteristics and the stiffness of the foot, in an attempt to standardise the grading of CTEV and hence prognostic outlook and response to treatment. A score is attributed for morphological features, i.e. deep plantar crease and a deep heel crease. A second score is attributed for the suppleness of the foot. The sum of the scores attributes a Dimeglio grade to the feet. This is a complex and comprehensive system for producing a reproducible assessment of clubfeet, and should be employed at the first orthopaedic appointment. A simpler, easier, but less exact assessment, also described by Dimeglio, can be employed at the bedside to give a rough assessment of Dimeglio grade and hence prognosis.

A foot that is held in the classic position but is >90% correctable (20% of all clubfeet), and appears very similar to positional talipes, is said to be soft-soft (Dimeglio grade I). A foot that is reducible but partly resistant is said to be soft-stiff (Dimeglio grade II, 33% of all clubfeet). A foot that is resistant but partly reducible is said to be stiff-soft (Dimeglio grade III, 35% of all clubfeet). Feet that are almost irreducible are said to be stiff-stiff (Dimeglio grade IV, 12% of all clubfeet).

Radiological assessment of the feet plays no part in initial management of the feet in the neonate, as most of the bony structures of the foot remain cartilaginous anlages, making radiological assessment inaccurate. It is of more benefit in the older child, when ossification of the bony elements of the foot has occurred.

Referral and treatment

Antenatal diagnosis of CTEV is becoming increasingly common with the advent of high-resolution ultrasound, allowing time for appropriate antepartum counselling.

Early referral is important postnatally, even in the premature infant, as treatment should begin as soon as is practicable.

In the first instance, even before or simultaneously with orthopaedic referral, physiotherapy is required. Stretching exercises should be taught to the parent(s) and commenced as soon as possible, in order to stretch the tight ligaments and capsules at a time when they are likely to be most lax. Forceful correction of the deformity should, however, be avoided, as this may lead to harm.

Following orthopaedic assessment and grading, treatment will be either conservative or interventional. Conservative treatment is applied to Dimeglio grade I feet and consists of stretching exercises and regular orthopaedic review to assess progress and resolution.

Conservative treatment, proposed by Ponseti,[47] consists of application of serial above-knee plaster casts changed on a weekly basis for 5 weeks, gradually correcting the adductus and supination deformity by reducing the forefoot around the talus (Fig. 38.9). On the sixth week, a tendo Achillis tenotomy is undertaken to correct the equinus deformity and the plaster is applied for a further 4 weeks (Fig. 38.10). At the end of this period, the cast(s) are removed and the child placed in a splint – so-called 'boots-on-a-bar' (Fig. 38.11) – to maintain the correction until walking age.

Early relapse or failure to respond to treatment requires further intervention as outlined in the treatment algorithm for CTEV (Fig. 38.12).[54,55]

Prognosis

The prognosis for CTEV is difficult to quantify at present. On the whole, the long-term outlook is very good for all grades of feet, with only a very small number going on to require salvage surgery. But measures of outcome clearly differ between clinicians and parents. The principal aim of orthopaedic surgeons is to produce a functional pain-free foot, with cosmesis not being a clinical indication for intervention. With Dimeglio grade II–IV feet, in most cases the foot is never morphologically 'normal'. Parents, however, focus on the appearance of the child and look at appearance post treatment as a measure of outcome. Parents need to be made aware that the condition affects the whole of the lower limb as a unit and a small foot and calf are normal features,

particularly with Dimeglio grade IV feet. There may be significant variation in shoe size between affected and unaffected feet. A degree of forefoot adductus and dynamic supination may need to be accepted providing the foot is functional and pain-free, as to correct minor variations would involve major surgery for little gain.

Metatarsus adductus

This is a relatively common condition in the neonate, and parents should be reassured that it is usually self-correcting in 85% of cases.

It is important to note that approximately 5–10% of neonates with metatarsus adductus will have an associated DDH, and careful screening of the hips is therefore required.

The typical appearance is of a kidney-bean shape to the sole of the foot, with a curve on the lateral side beginning at the base of the fifth metatarsal and with the toes pointing inwards (Fig. 38.13). It is usually bilateral but not symmetrical and may

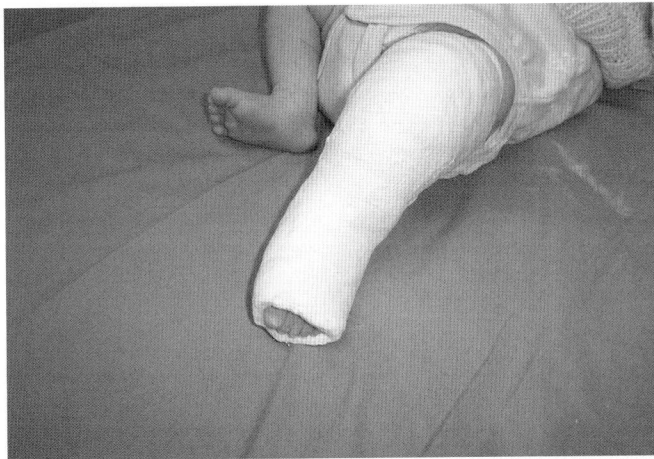

Fig. 38.10 The same foot as in Fig. 38.9, showing the cast in situ, demonstrating how the forefoot adductus, supination and equinus are held in a corrective position along with correction of the internal tibial torsion.

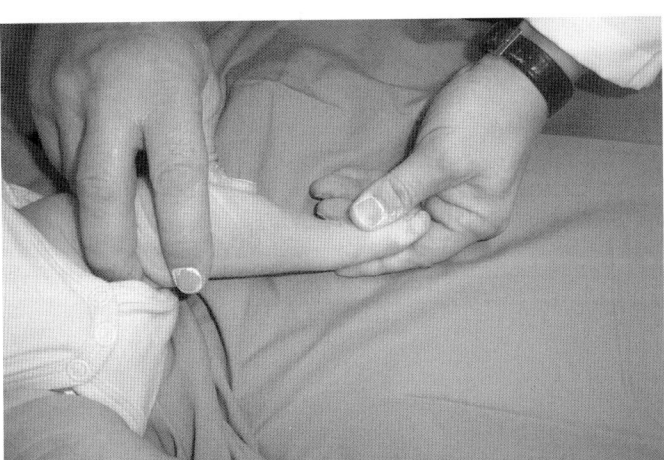

Fig. 38.9 Child undergoing the Ponseti regimen for CTEV, demonstrating the maximum amount of correction of the foot prior to application of the plaster cast.

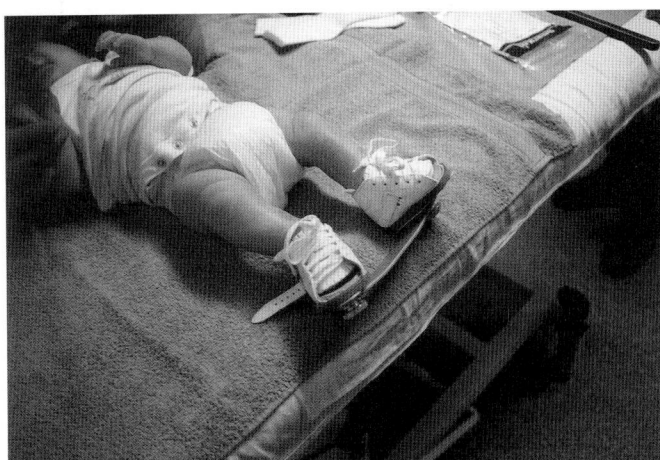

Fig. 38.11 Boots-on-a-bar, showing how the corrective position is maintained when the child is out of plaster following tendo Achillis tenotomy.

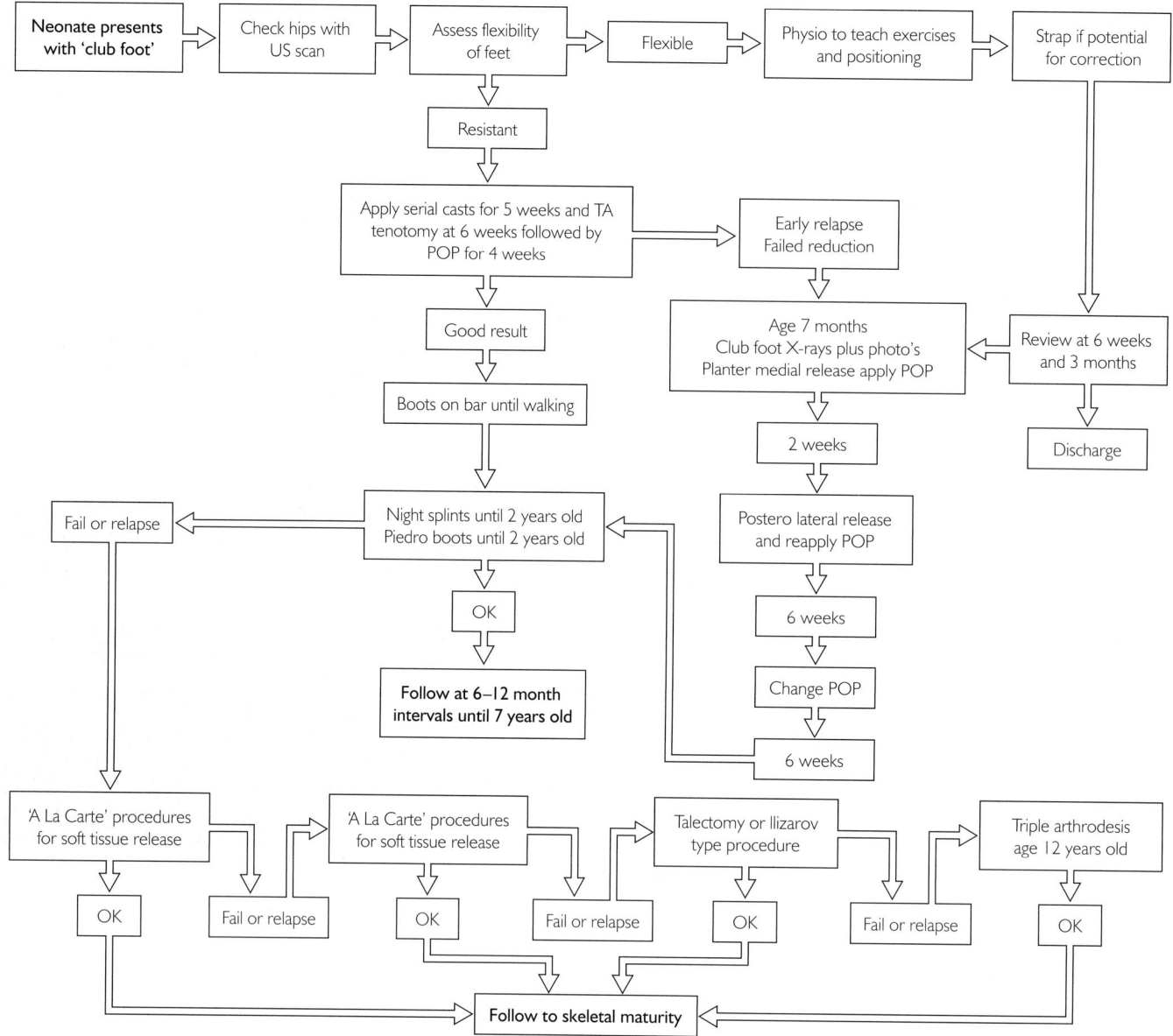

Fig. 38.12 Treatment algorithm for congenital talipes equinovarus.

have an associated internal tibial torsion. The abnormality is usually flexible and the forefoot can be corrected to the neutral position.

It is thought to occur in simple cases because of intrauterine moulding and can be compounded postnatally by neonates sleeping in the prone position, a sleeping position no longer advocated by paediatricians.

If there is still a significant problem at 12 months, serial casting or soft-tissue release may be indicated.[8,22]

In all but a very few children the deformity will be corrected by conservative measures alone.

Calcaneovalgus

This benign condition is not an infrequent neonatal finding. The ankle is unusually lax and the foot is noted to be excessively dorsiflexed – so much so, the forefoot touches the tibia (Fig. 38.14). The foot is also in valgus (away from the midline) and may even rest on the lateral side of the lower limb.

This condition is frequently associated with hip dysplasia, meaning that examination of the hips is required. We recommend USS of the hips in all babies with calcaneovalgus feet.

It is thought the aetiology of this condition is related to intrauterine moulding and hence it is a more frequent finding in oligohydramnios. Calcaneovalgus is also more common in first-born children.

Treatment is by passive stretching of the foot in the direction of neutrality. A paediatric physiotherapist should be involved early to educate the parent(s) and give instruction on stretching exercises. Occasionally the deformity is more rigid and serial casting may need to be employed, gradually to correct the deformity.

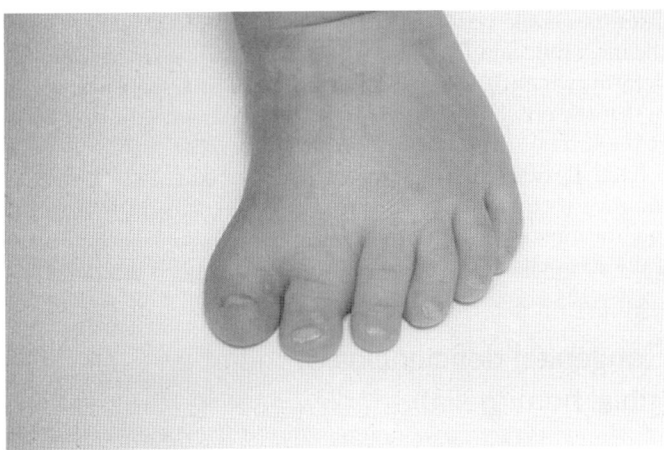

Fig. 38.13 Complex metatarsus adductus, demonstrating the curve of the lateral side of the foot beginning at the base of the fifth metatarsal. (In this case associated with duplication of the hallux.)

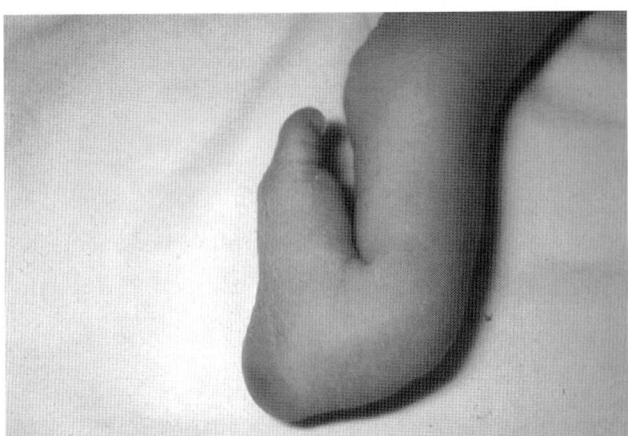

Fig. 38.14 Calcaneovalgus and tibial kyphoscoliosis in the same leg. The bow of the leg is directed posteromedially and the foot is in contact with the shin.

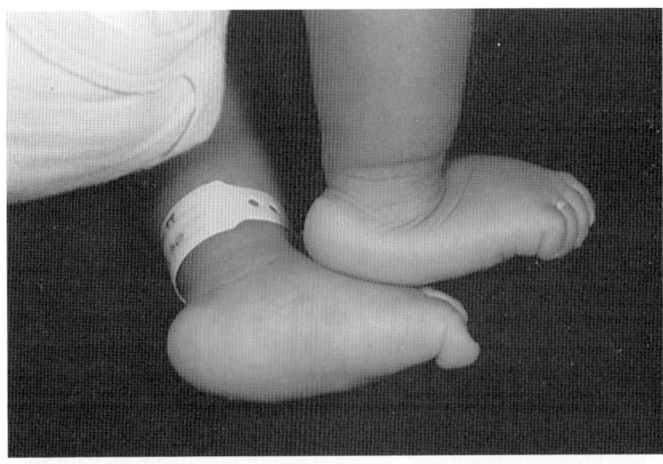

(a)

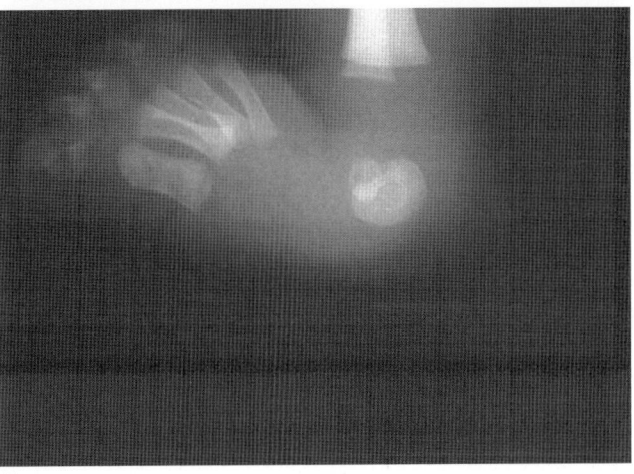

(b)

Fig. 38.15 (a) Clinical appearance of congenital vertical talus (CVT). (b) X-ray demonstrating the radiological appearance of CVT. The soft-tissue shadow clearly shows the rocker-bottom appearance of the sole of the foot.

The majority of cases resolve completely with these simple conservative measures.

Congenital vertical talus ('rocker-bottom' foot, congenital pes planus, congenital convex pes valgus)

This is a rare condition in the neonate and is characterised by a dysmorphic foot (Fig. 38.15a). The forefoot is dorsiflexed and abducted and the heel is in valgus and equinus. When viewed laterally, the plantar surface of the foot is curved, with the apex at the midtarsal joint. In contrast to calcaneovalgus, which may have a similar appearance, the deformity is fixed and non-flexible. If doubt exists about the diagnosis, X-rays are usually diagnostic (Fig. 38.15b). In 85% of cases there is an associated congenital anomaly such as AMC, myelomeningocoele, myelodysplasia, diastematomyelia, sacral agenesis, DDH, or Turner or Edward syndrome.[11,51]

Pathoanatomy

The talus is in a vertical position. There is lateral displacement of the calcaneum and hypoplasia of the sustentaculum tali, which results in subluxation of the talus medial to the calcaneum, making it palpable on the plantar surface of the foot. The talonavicular joint is dislocated, with the navicular lying on the dorsum and neck of the talus. The calcaneus is in an equinus position due to contracture of the tendo Achillis. The tibialis anterior, extensor hallucis longus and extensor digitorum tendons are shortened, as are the peroneal tendons, which are often subluxed anterior to the medial malleolus, causing the characteristic abduction and dorsiflexion.

Management

Early intervention is advocated, as late surgical correction has a poor outcome.

Initially treatment is conservative, with serial casting, which may be of benefit in stretching the soft tissues and aiding later surgical reduction. The optimum time for surgical intervention is at about 12 weeks. This involves lengthening the shortened tendons and open reduction of the navicular and talus, which are held in place with temporary wires and a well-moulded plaster. At 3 weeks postoperatively, the wires are removed and the plaster changed. A further 12 weeks is required in plaster, which is then replaced with an ankle foot orthosis until the child is walking.

Lower limb deficiencies[1,32]

In the developing fetus, the limb buds appear at the beginning of the fifth week. Specialised cells at the tip of the limb bud (apical ectodermal ridge [AER]) are instrumental in the normal development of the limbs, which develop in a longitudinal direction from proximal to distal. Any disruption in the intimate relationship between the AER and the underlying mesenchyme may result in a congenital limb deformity.[48]

These deformities can be classified according to the part of the limb affected. Arrest of longitudinal growth results in a transverse defect. Failure of development of the medial (postaxial) or lateral (preaxial) elements of the limb results in a longitudinal defect. Deficiencies of the central portion of the limb result in a central deficiency.

As with upper limb deficiencies, the deformity may be either transverse or longitudinal. Transverse abnormalities are usually obvious, with congenital absence of a whole or part of a limb.

Longitudinal deficiencies of the lower limb present with a shortened or abnormal-looking limb. Conditions that may be seen include hypolastic conditions of the femur, with shortening of the proximal limb and normally formed elements distally. Other conditions present with hypoplasia or absence of the fibula or tibia, with a variety of clinical deformities of the lower leg, knee and ankle joint.

Congenital femoral deficiencies

Abnormalities of the femur have been variously classified. Gillespie & Tarode[23] classified proximal deficiencies of the femur into group 1 (congenital short femur) and group 2 (true proximal focal femoral deficiencies).

Group 1

Group 1 conditions are truly hypoplastic and result in a leg-length discrepancy. The defect is obvious at birth, with asymmetric leg lengths and the foot on the affected side being at the mid-tibial level of the contralateral limb. The hip develops normally and there is a valgus deformity of the knee on the affected side. The femur is between 40% and 60% shorter than the normal femur. In the milder forms of congenital short femur, limb lengthening is a realistic treatment option at a later stage.

Group 2

Group 2 deficiencies have been further classified by Aitken[3] based on the radiological findings (Fig. 38.16). There are four categories in the classification, ranging from A to D, with A being the most mild and D the most severe deformity. Once again, the deformity is obvious at birth, but differs from hypoplastic femur in that the proximal leg is very much shorter, with the foot being at the level of the contralateral knee (Fig. 38.17). There is also a fixed flexion deformity of the hip and knee which fails to improve with growth. In group 2 children, surgery is aimed at modification of the limb to fit a suitably functional and cosmetically acceptable prosthesis, as limb lengthening is not possible.

Congenital deficiencies of the tibia (tibial hemimelia)

This is a rare condition, with an incidence of 1:1 000 000 live-births. It has been classified by Kalamchi & Dawe[32] (Fig. 38.18) into types I to III, with type I being the most severe. The classification is based on the radiological findings. In type I deformity there is complete absence of the tibia, which results in marked inversion and adduction of the foot, with or without absence of the medial rays. There is a fixed flexion contracture of the knee, with weak or absent quadriceps function. In type II, the distal tibia is absent, with the knee joint reasonably well preserved and a mild fixed flexion deformity. In the mildest form (type III), the distal tibia is dysplastic, with the foot in varus and a prominent lateral malleolus.

Management is aimed at producing a functional lower limb. In the milder forms, surgery is aimed at stabilisation of the ankle joint and correcting the leg-length discrepancy. In the more severe forms, surgery is aimed at fitting a prosthesis.

Congenital deficiency of the fibula (fibula hememelia)

Congenital deficiency of the fibula is a rare condition in which there is partial or complete absence of the fibula. It is seldom found in isolation but is frequently associated with anomalies of the foot, tibia and femur. The condition has been classified by Achterman & Kalamchi[1] and Coventry & Johnson,[16] the former classification being based on the radiological findings and the latter on the progressive severity of the deformity and the prognosis. In the most severe form (type III), there is complete absence of the fibula. This is frequently bilateral and associated with other limb deficiencies. The functional and cosmetic outlook is poor and treatment is usually by amputation and fitting of a prosthesis. In type II, the deficiency is unilateral, with complete absence of the fibula, marked hypoplasia of the entire lower limb and foot abnormalities. As with type I, the outlook is poor and management is usually with amputation. In the mildest form (type I), there is shortening or partial absence of the fibula, the foot is usually normal, with minimal leg-length inequality, and is associated with a good prognosis. With all types, there may be absence of the lateral rays of the foot.

As with any other skeletal anomaly, careful assessment of the neonate for other abnormalities should be undertaken along with referral to an orthopaedic surgeon with a specialist interest in paediatrics.

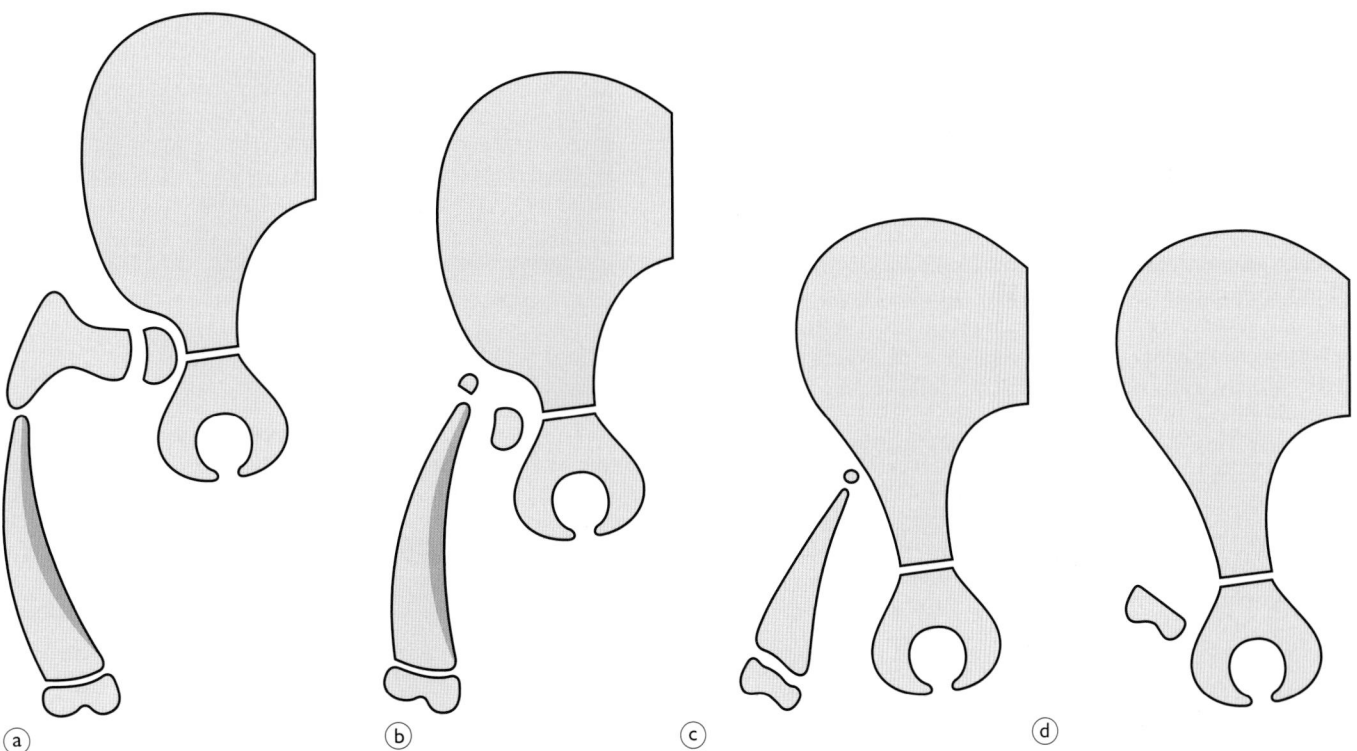

(a) (b) (c) (d)

Fig. 38.16 Aitken classification of proximal femoral focal deficiency.[3] (a) Type A – short femur with coxa vara and lateral bowing with thickening of the medial cortex. Adequate acetabulum with femoral head. (b) Type B – mildly dysplastic acetabulum with delayed ossification of the femoral head. Displacement of the proximal femur superiorly with a bony tuft connected to the femoral shaft by defective cartilage which will fail to ossify. (c) Type C – very dysplastic acetabulum and femoral head. No synchronous movement between the femoral shaft and head, with the proximal femoral shaft articulating with the iliac wing. (d) Type D – most severe deformity, with absent femoral head and acetabulum, and very short femoral shaft with no tufting. As is represented here, the femoral shaft may be represented by the femoral condyles only.

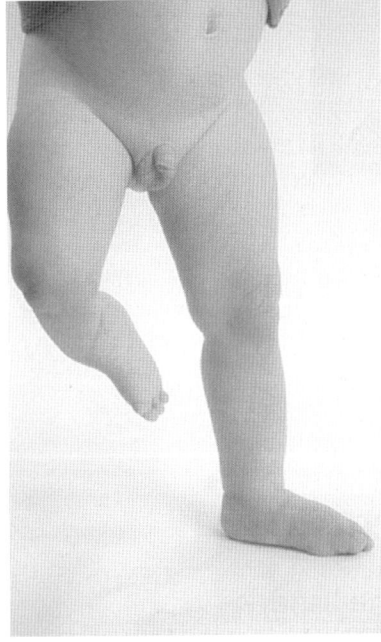

Fig. 38.17 Proximal femoral focal deficiency of the right leg in a boy, with the foot of the affected leg at the level of the knee of the unaffected contralateral leg.

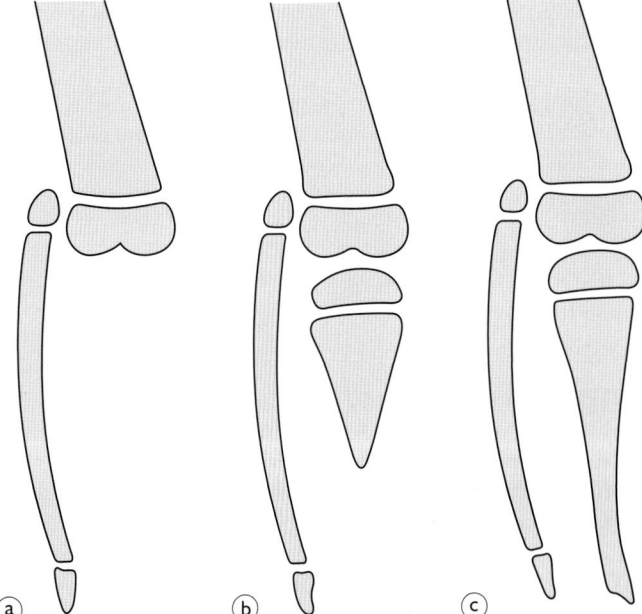

(a) (b) (c)

Fig. 38.18 Kalamchi & Dawe classification of congenital deficiencies of the tibia.[32] (a) Type I – complete absence of the tibia. (b) Type II – the distal tibia is absent, with presence of the proximal tibia to varying degrees. (c) Type III – dysplasia of the distal tibia with diastasis of the distal tibiofibular joint.

There is a whole spectrum of treatments available for congenital limb abnormalities, ranging from reconstruction to amputation. Those involved include orthopaedic and plastic surgeons, physiotherapists, occupational therapists and orthotists. The principle underlying any treatment is primarily to preserve or restore function, with cosmesis being a secondary issue.

Congenital constriction band syndrome (Simonart's bands, Streeter's dysplasia)

Congenital constriction band syndrome (CCBS) has a gamut of clinical presentations, ranging from simple bands around digits to limb amputation (Fig. 38.19). The aetiology is poorly understood and several theories have been proposed. The most popular aetiological theory is that a sequence of events occurs in utero: initially, early amniotic rupture, followed by temporary oligohydramnios, with resultant intrauterine compression and subsequent constriction of the fetal appendages by cords of torn amnion.[21,45,53]

The typical presentation of CCBS is that of limb reduction, constriction bands or syndactyly (especially acrosyndactyly). Other presentations include pseudoarthrosis, impending gangrene, peripheral nerve palsy and skin tube pedicles. Amniotic bands can also produce fetal death via a number of mechanisms.

Treatment is aimed at optimising early function and cosmesis, and should involve orthopaedic and plastic surgeons as well as physiotherapists.

Tibial kyphosis (posteromedial bowing of the tibia)

This is a dramatic-looking deformity of the lower limb (Fig. 38.14). Clinically, the foot is in extreme dorsiflexion and valgus, with the forefoot touching the anterolateral aspect of the shin (as seen in calcaneovalgus). In association with this is a posteromedial bow of the tibia, most marked distally. There is shortening of the lower leg on the affected side, with wasting of the muscles.

Fortunately, the condition is relatively benign, with rapid improvement in the foot position and the tibial bow in the first year of life.

Initial treatment consists of stretching exercises, as taught by a physiotherapist, which should begin as soon after birth as possible. For a marked deformity, serial casts may be applied. Residual deformity after the age of 3 years may require surgical intervention to correct the bow and leg-length discrepancy.

Congenital pseudoarthrosis of the tibia

This is a complex anomaly of the lower leg, of unknown aetiology, whose treatment and management is difficult and protracted. It is associated with neurofibromatosis type 1 in more than half of cases and has an incidence of approximately 1:200 000 livebirths. Other stigmata of neurofibromatosis may be present.

Rarely is there a fracture present at birth, but pathological fracture and pseudoarthrosis readily occur at some stage thereafter.

The deformity may be very slight or there may be mild or marked anterolateral bowing of the tibia. The condition is

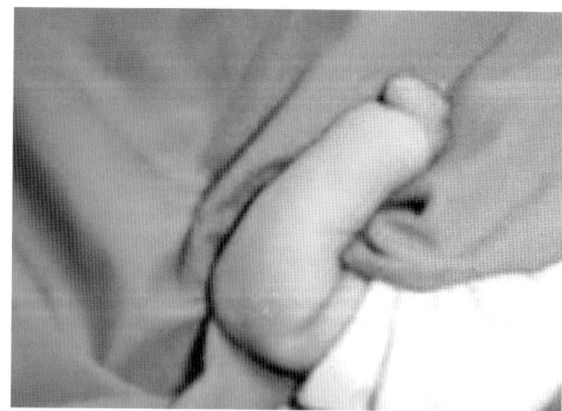

Fig. 38.19 Transverse deficiency of the upper limb secondary to congenital constriction band syndrome.

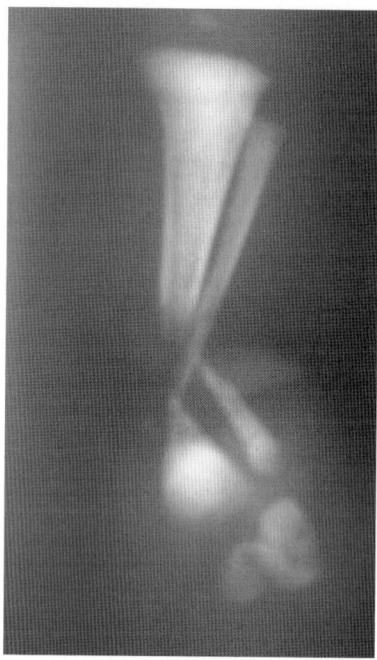

Fig. 38.20 Radiological appearance of congenital pseudoarthrosis of the tibia.

diagnosed by X-ray (Fig. 38.20) and attempts have been made to classify the condition radiologically. Initial treatment consists of protecting the tibia, which is at risk of fracture, until definitive treatment can be undertaken. There should be early involvement of an orthopaedic surgeon.

Upper limb abnormalities

Other anomalies of the hand

Syndactyly (congenital webbing of the hand, Fig. 38.21) occurs because of failure of apoptosis of the web spaces of the hand plate in utero. This is the most common congenital anomaly in the hand. The incidence is 1:2250 livebirths and the condition is

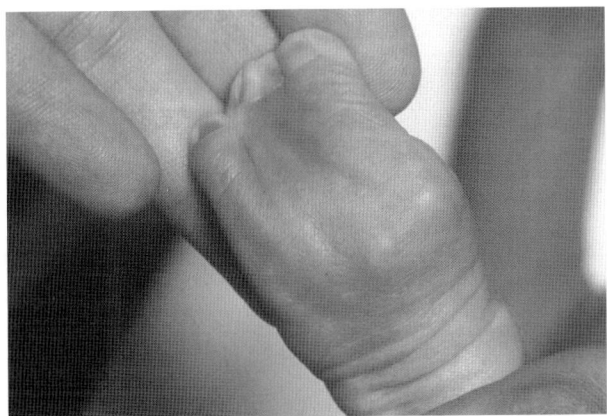

Fig. 38.21 Complex syndactyly in a neonate, showing fusion of all the web spaces in the right hand and bony union of the middle and ring fingers.

bilateral and symmetrical in 50% of cases. Boys are affected more than girls at a ratio of 2:1. Simple syndactyly involves simple skin bridges between the fingers, whereas complex syndactyly involves skin and bone. In acrosyndactyly, only the tips of the fingers are fused.

Varying degrees of complex syndactyly are seen in Apert's syndrome. Polydactyly and oligodactyly refer to excess or insufficient digits, respectively. Macrodactyly refers to overgrowth of a digit.

Trigger thumb is a common deformity, presenting with flexion of the interphalangeal joint of the thumb. Examination reveals a thickening of the flexor pollicis longus tendon. In 25% of cases the deformity is present at birth, with bilateral involvement in 50%. Left untreated, 30% will resolve spontaneously by 1 year.

Thumb-in-palm deformity (congenital clasped thumb) – characterised by marked flexion at the metocarpophalangeal joint with adduction of the thumb – is a rare anomaly which is familial. It affects males more than females at a ratio of 2:1 and is almost always bilateral. The deformity is caused by muscle imbalance in the thumb and may be seen in cerebral palsy and arthrogyposis but frequently has no other associated congenital anomalies. Treatment ranges from physiotherapy and splinting to tendon transfers, depending on the type and severity of the deformity.

Upper limb deficiencies

Transverse failure

Arrest of longitudinal growth of the arm can affect any part of the limb from the shoulder distally, with the most common being the proximal third of the forearm (Fig. 38.22a).

Longitudinal failure

Preaxial deficiencies present with hypoplasia or partial or complete absence of the radius and thumb, the 'radial club hand',

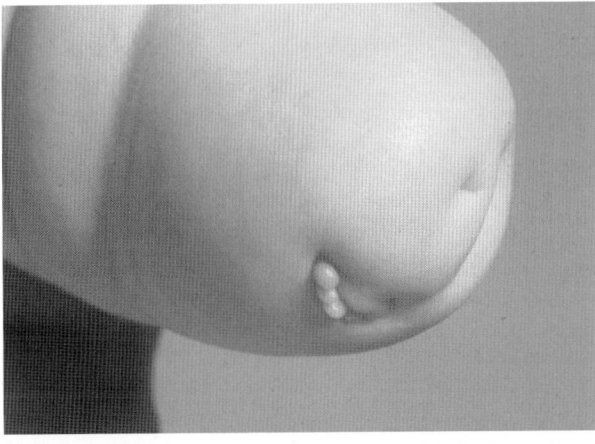

(a)

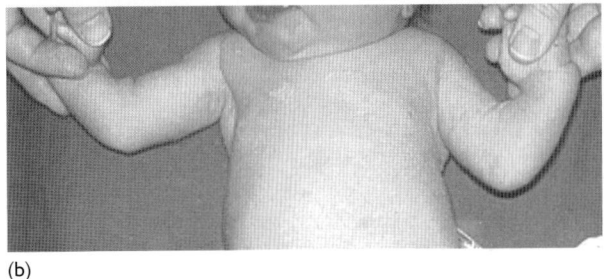

(b)

Fig. 38.22 (a) Transverse upper limb deficiency, showing absence of the arm just below the elbow. (b) Neonate with the thrombocytopenia–absent radius syndrome.

with marked deviation of the hand radially. The incidence is approximately 1:100 000 livebirths, with 50% being bilateral. In unilateral cases, the right arm is involved twice as often as the left. Males are affected more than females at a ratio of 1.5:1. Half the cases are found in association with congenital syndromes, including thrombocytopenia–absent radius (TAR) syndrome (Fig. 38.22b), Fanconi syndrome, Holt–Oram syndrome and Vater syndrome.[11,51]

Treatment is aimed at producing a functional hand. Initial treatment is passive stretching and splinting in the early phases. There are then a variety of surgical procedures aimed at centralising the carpus on the ulna and maintaining muscle balance in the forearm and creating a thumb. Functional outcome is usually good and in only a very few cases is a salvage wrist fusion required.

Postaxial longitudinal deficiencies of the arm present as absence of the ulna and a varying number of digits from the ulnar half of the hand. This condition is referred to as 'ulnar club hand'. It is one of the rarest upper limb anomalies and is associated with other skeletal anomalies rather than visceral defects.

Central longitudinal deficiency presents with absence of the second, third and fourth rays of the hand, with or without associated absence of the carpals. This results in a cleft or 'lobster claw' hand (Fig. 38.23). It accounts for approximately 2% of congenital hand anomalies. There is a male preponderance, with the condition usually being bilateral. In 50% of cases, cleft feet are also present. Associated anomalies include cleft lip and palate, cataracts, deafness, absence of nails, heart defects and imperforate anus.

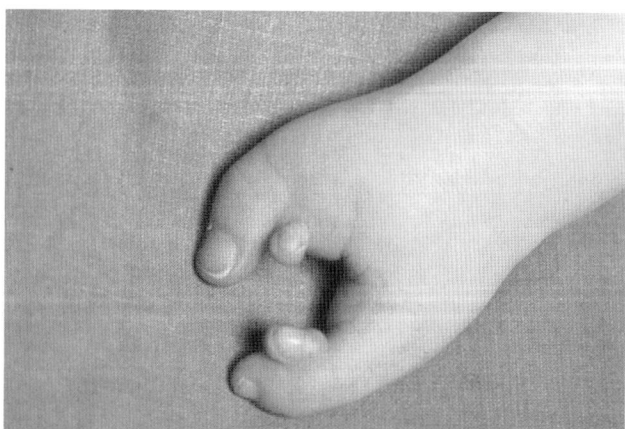

Fig. 38.23 Central longitudinal deficiency of the upper limb resulting in a 'lobster claw' hand.

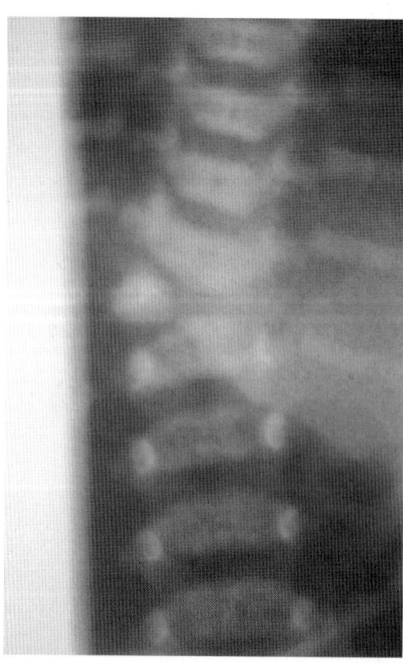

Fig. 38.24 X-ray showing a hemivertebra on the right in the thoracic region with an associated scoliosis.

Abnormalities of the spine and axial skeleton

Congenital spinal abnormalities (kyphosis and scoliosis)

During early embryonic life, at around the fourth week of gestation, the polymorphous mesenchyme of the segmented ventromedial somite, the sclerotome, surrounds the neural tube and notocord in development of the vertebral column. During further development, the cranial and caudal parts of the sclerotome proliferate and condense, ultimately uniting to form the pre-cartilaginous vertebral body.

The formation and subsequent rearrangement of the segmental sclerotomes into the definitive vertebrae is a complex process. It is not uncommon for adjacent vertebrae to fuse symmetrically or asymmetrically or for half the vertebrae to be missing (hemivertebra) (Fig. 38.24), or for the vertebrae to be wedged, resulting in congenital spinal anomalies.[48] With abnormalities of the spine, the overlying skin may contain angiomas, naevi, and patches of hair, dimples or a pad of fat (p. 258).

Osteopathic (congenital) scoliosis

Scoliosis refers to a lateral deviation of the spine. The most common cause of congenital scoliosis is failure of one side of a vertebra or adjacent vertebrae to segment, resulting in a unilateral unsegmented bar (an unbalanced anomaly). These are most commonly seen in the thoracic area. There is restricted growth of the unsegmented portion of the vertebra, with normal growth of the contralateral side, resulting in a curvature of the spine toward the bar. When there is one hemivertebra or two hemivertebrae on the same side, the curve will be severe. This deformity is progressive and carries the worst prognosis. The presence of hemivertebrae on opposite sides of the vertebral column, however, balance each other (balanced anomaly) and result in a relatively mild deformity.

Congenital scoliosis may be apparent at birth but may not manifest until later years. It is associated with a variety of congenital defects involving the spinal cord (diastematomyelia), cardiac system, renal system, gastrointestinal system (e.g. tracheo-oesophageal fistula) and limbs (e.g. congenital absence of the radius and hypoplasia of the thumb).[28,36] Careful and thorough clinical assessment is therefore required for any neonate presenting with a scoliosis.

Referral to an orthopaedic surgeon specialising in paediatric spines should be made. Surgical intervention is required for curves greater than 50° and for those children with a progressive curve that is likely to reach more than 50°. Initial treatment may consist of bracing, which does little to influence progression of the condition but may help in delaying surgery until the child is of a more appropriate age. Surgery is only undertaken following further assessment of the spinal cord with magnetic resonance imaging (MRI) to exclude a spinal cord abnormality. The surgical options consist of spinal fusion, correction with rods, hemivertebrae excision or osteotomy, depending on the age of the child and whether the deformity is fixed or flexible.[26,58] Corrective surgery usually results in permanent correction.

Congenital kyphosis

Kyphosis refers to an excessive outward curvature of the spine, causing forward bend of the back.

Congenital kyphosis is more often progressive than scoliosis, leading to a severe deformity in early life. It is categorised as type I or type II. In type I, there is failure of formation of the vertebrae; in type II, there is failure of segmentation of the vertebrae. Kyphosis may result from a combination of the two.

The common site for kyphosis is at the thoracolumbar junction between T10 and L2. Type I is the most common form and has a poorer prognosis than type II. Absence or hypoplasia of the anterior part of the vertebra results in progressive kyphosis and posterior displacement of the posterior hemivertebra, with a risk of cord compression.

Type II is characterised by an anterior unsegmented bar. As the posterior vertebrae grow, so there is progressive kyphosis.

Treatment is either surgical or conservative and is dictated by the type of kyphosis, the severity of the deformity and the age of the patient. If the curvature is greater than 50°, bracing with a Milwaukee brace is indicated. If the curvature is greater than 75°, corrective surgery is indicated. For less severe curves with no documented evidence of progression, careful follow-up is required.

The mainstay of treatment is spinal fusion, and for severe fixed deformities, osteotomies and correction with rods.[58]

Klippel–Feil syndrome (congenital synostosis of the cervical vertebrae, brevicollis, congenital short neck)

Klippel–Feil syndrome is a condition characterised by failure of vertebral segmentation in the neck, resulting in fusion of two (congenital block vertebrae) or more vertebrae, and may involve the whole neck. Other associated physical features, classically described but not always present, include a low posterior hairline and restricted head and neck movements.

This syndrome is associated with other congenital anomalies, the most common being a scoliosis. Other congenital anomalies include deafness, congenital heart disease and urological anomalies, particularly unilateral renal agenesis.[29] Any neonate with congenital cervical spine abnormalities should undergo USS of the renal tract.

The condition itself is relatively asymptomatic, except in a partial fusion there is a risk of non-traumatic spontaneous dislocation. Treatment is conservative with passive stretching exercises to obtain maximum range of movement, which should begin immediately after birth, initially under the guidance of a physiotherapist.

Spina bifida (dysraphism) (see also Chapter 41)

Spina bifida is a condition of the vertebral column with or without defects in the neural tube and has a spectrum ranging from a benign incidental finding to one causing significant disability.

During development of the vertebral column in utero, there is failure of the vertebral arch or arches to develop posteriorly and the lamina and spinous processes are absent at either one or multiple vertebral levels. In association with this, there may be a defect in the neural tube ranging from failure of separation of the skin from the neural tissue to complete exposure of the neural tissue to the surface.

Incidence

The incidence of spina bifida affecting the neural tube is approximately 2–4 per 1000 livebirths in the UK, and less than 1 per 1000 in the USA and Australia. There is a very slight sex difference, with girls more affected than boys, and a suggested polygenic mode of inheritance. There is a 10-fold increase in incidence with an affected sibling.

Aetiology

Environmental factors have been implicated, including folate and selenium deficiency, poor maternal nutrition, a high maternal alcohol intake, and maternal diabetes. Teratogens such as valproate have also been implicated. As yet, no single factor has been identified and therefore the aetiology is likely to be multifactorial.

The use of folic acid supplements preconceptually and during the first trimester of pregnancy is now advocated.

Screening

In the UK, antenatal ultrasound has replaced serum alpha fetoprotein as the screening method of choice (p. 1189).

Clinical presentation

Spina bifida occulta is one of the most common congenital anomalies, with approximately 25% of children showing some minor defect of the vertebral arches on X-ray. It may not manifest itself in the neonate but may be a serendipitous finding at a later stage. The skin overlying the defect is usually normal, but there may be failure of separation of the skin from the underlying neural tissue and it may contain pigmentation, dimples, pits, lipomas or hairy patches. The presence of these clinical findings should alert the examiner to the possibility of spina bifida, particularly if in association with neurological defects, which are rare in spina bifida occulta.

The remaining forms of spina bifida are collectively known as spina bifida cystica. The most benign form is a meningocoele, which is a cystic swelling overlying the bony defect with normal skin covering. The swelling is a bulge of CSF-filled meninges protruding through the underlying bony defect with the spinal cord remaining contained between the neural arches. This condition represents 5% of the spina bifidas and is rarely associated with neuromuscular deficiencies. In contrast, a myelomeningocoele, which is similar to a meningocoele, except the spinal cord is contained in the fundus of the sac (closed myelomeningocoele), is always associated with neuromuscular deficiencies. The most severe defect is a myelocoele (open myelomeningocoele), in which the primitive unfolded neural tube forms the roof of the cystic swelling and may be open to the air.

Associated lower limb deformities such as teratologic DDH, CTEV, claw toes and recurvatum are common with the myelomeningocoeles. In a third of neonates with myelomeningocoele there is complete lower motor neuron paralysis with loss of sensation and sphincter control below the affected level. In one-third there is a complete segmental lesion with preservation of a distal spinal segment, which results in a mixed neurological picture with intact reflexes and spastic muscle groups. In the final third the lesion is incomplete and there is some movement and sensation below the affected level.

Management

Management of spina bifida requires a multidisciplinary approach. The team is usually headed by a paediatrician, who coordinates the care. Others who input care include orthopaedic and neurosurgeons, urologists, physiotherapists and occupational therapists, and orthotists.

Congenital high scapula (Sprengel's deformity)

The scapula develops as a cervical appendage in the fifth week of gestation. It descends to the level of the posterior thorax by the end of the third month of gestation. Sprengel's deformity, described in 1863, occurs because of failure of separation and descent of the scapula at about 12 weeks' gestation. As a result, the scapula remains small and abnormally high and may remain tethered to the cervical spine by a tough fibrous band or by a cartilaginous or bony bar (the omovertebral bar).

The condition usually occurs sporadically but can be transmitted as an autosomal dominant trait. It is more common in female offspring, with the left shoulder being more affected than the right, and is occasionally bilateral.

It is frequently associated with other congenital abnormalities such as torticollis, scoliosis, kyphosis, diastematomyelia and Klippel–Feil syndrome.

Clinical presentation

The deformity is usually noticed at birth, with asymmetry of the shoulders. The elevation of the scapula is variable, depending on the severity of the condition. The clavicle is abnormally positioned and the pectoral girdle is hypoplastic due to wasting of the muscles. Abduction of the shoulder is limited owing to decreased scapulothoracic motion. With a bilateral deformity, there may be a low hairline and webbing of the neck.

Management

Management depends on the severity of the deformity and the degree of disability encountered. Mild cases are usually observed with no need for surgical intervention. Surgery is considered for cosmetic reasons and if the deformity is very fixed. Conjecture exists over the timing of surgery, some advocating early intervention in the first year and others before the age of 6.

Fractures in the newborn

Childbirth complicated by the necessity for rapid delivery, breech presentation or macrosomia may result in a birth fracture.[37] The site of fractures in descending order of frequency are: clavicle, humeral shaft, femoral shaft (Fig. 38.25),

epiphyseal separation at the upper and lower humerus, and, finally, separation of the upper and lower femoral epiphyses. Distal fractures below the elbow and the knee are rare.[11,37,51]

Long bone fractures are usually obvious and detected immediately by the obstetrician, as the bone can be heard and felt to break. There is usually associated pseudoparalysis of the affected limb. Long bone fractures are more likely when there is osteopenia, sometimes due to lack of fetal movements because of myopathy.

Clavicular fractures may go unnoticed, with the majority being relatively asymptomatic. All are unilateral, with most involving the anterior shoulder. The diagnosis may not come to light until callus formation creates the telltale lump seen in clavicular fractures. If suspected after birth, crepitus, tenderness and swelling are present on palpation of the clavicle and the diagnosis is confirmed by X-ray. There may be an associated brachial plexus injury. Treatment is conservative.

Long bone fractures of the humerus and femur are usually midshaft. Humeral shaft fractures may be associated with a radial nerve palsy. Such palsies are usually temporary and most have resolved by 6 weeks. Treatment is by immobilisation of the affected limb, with healing taking 2–3 weeks. Any residual angular deformity will invariably remodel with growth of the infant.

Physeal injuries are more difficult to diagnose and may go unnoticed if clinical suspicion is not present. However, if a birth is particularly difficult and there has been excess traction on a limb followed by swelling and immobility of the limb, then physeal injury should be considered. Immobility due to long bone fracture can easily be excluded by plain X-ray. Radiological findings in physeal injuries are initially difficult to interpret and a history of the clinical concern should be discussed with a paediatric musculoskeletal radiologist to aid interpretation. X-rays at a later stage of the injury reveal a florid periosteal reaction and callus formation.

If diagnosed early, treatment occasionally consists of manipulation, depending on the type of injury, and all early-diagnosed injuries should undergo a period of immobilisation of the affected limb for comfort. If diagnosis is delayed and healing has occurred, no treatment is necessary.

Multiple birth fractures are seen in AMC and osteogenesis imperfecta (p. 926).

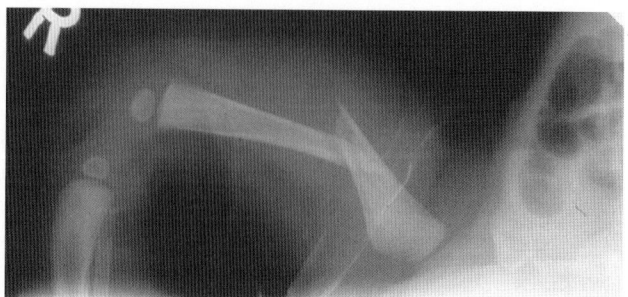

Fig. 38.25 X-ray demonstrating a birth fracture of the right femoral shaft.

Vascular conditions associated with orthopaedic problems in the newborn

Neonatal gangrene and amputation

Ischaemic gangrene of the extremity in the neonate has been recognised since 1828. It is a relatively uncommon condition, but failure to recognise the problem early can result in catastrophic sequelae, with loss of digits or limbs. It is important to make the distinction between ischaemic necrosis and necrotising fasciitis, a completely different entity requiring a different treatment.

There are four main causes of gangrene of the extremity in the neonate: following a complicated delivery, secondary to invasive monitoring, extravasation of intravenous fluids, and secondary to sepsis.

Any delivery complicated by a long second stage of labour with an abnormal fetal position resulting in compression of a limb for prolonged periods may result in thrombosis of the limb. There is an increased incidence in diabetic mothers because of macrosomia of the infant and increased blood viscosity. Twin delivery with twin-to-twin transfusion results in polycythaemia and hypercoagulability in one of the infants, increasing the risk of thrombosis of an extremity (Fig. 38.26).[34]

Peripheral arterial cannulation in the neonatal intensive care setting may compromise the circulation to the distal limb (pp. 1247–9). Cannulation of the femoral artery has been linked with ischaemia of the leg, as this site is an end artery. Also, failure to perform Allen's test prior to radial artery cannulation can compromise the circulation to the hand. Care also needs to be taken with repeated arterial blood sampling. With any insult of the peripheral arteries there is not only local trauma to the vessel but also possibly an associated intense vasospasm of the vessel proximally, with a risk of extensive gangrene.

Cannulation of the umbilical artery has been associated with aortic thrombosis and aortic branch occlusion, as well as digital thrombosis.

One of the most common procedures undertaken in the sick neonate is peripheral venous cannulation. Frequently, the cannula either erodes through the vessel wall or thromboses, with a risk of extravasation of fluid into the surrounding tissues. If the fluid being infused is hypertonic or irritant, such as total parenteral nutrition or calcium salts, there is blistering of the skin with local tissue necrosis (pp. 1252–5). Therefore, extreme vigilance is required when infusing such solutions through a peripheral cannula, and infusion pumps that alarm when the line is occluded are mandatory, as is regular observation of the infusion site.

Severe infections that cause disseminated intravascular coagulation can cause digital gangrene and skin necrosis.

It is important to look for peripheral ischaemia in at-risk neonates. Early clinical signs may be difficult to detect, but asymmetrically cool peripheries and absent pulses with skin mottling should alert the examiner. If there is a high index of clinical suspicion, there should be an aggressive search for the occlusion with Doppler ultrasound and angiography. If an occlusion is found, then either thrombolysis (p. 764) or thrombectomy should be considered and undertaken.

Despite best measures, it may not be possible to salvage a limb and the need for amputation arises. In the neonate, there is no urgency to amputate, as the early level of gangrene may be significantly lower than the final level. It is therefore important to wait for unequivocal demarcation of the gangrene prior to amputation.

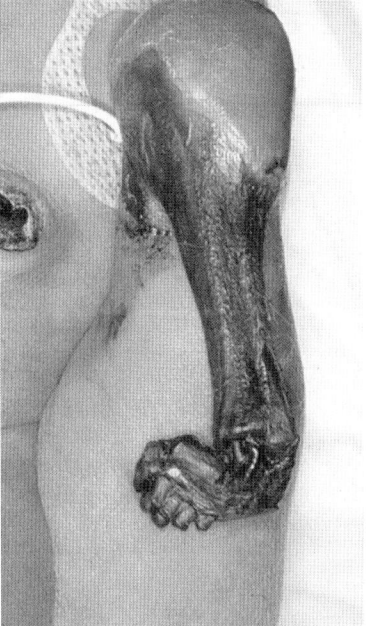

Fig. 38.26 Neonatal gangrene of the lower leg secondary to polycythaemia following twin-to-twin transfusion in utero.

Nerve and muscle conditions associated with orthopaedic problems in the newborn

Brachial plexus palsy

Damage to the brachial plexus during childbirth has long been recognised, first being reported in 1764.

Incidence

The reported incidence ranges from 0.4 to 2.5 cases per 1000 livebirths. There has been no reduction in incidence over the last few decades but much progress has been made in recovery rates. Recovery is dependent on the level and extent of the injury, which can range from a neuropraxic injury to complete neurotmesis.

Historically, recovery rates were bleak, with only 13% to 18% regaining full function. Today, rates of full recovery are in excess of 70% to 90% for upper plexus palsies.[2]

Risk factors

Brachial plexus injury is associated with gestational diabetes, grand multiparity, instrumental deliveries, shoulder dystocia, fetal macrosomia, prematurity and postmaturity, breech delivery and oxytocin use. More recent findings have associated obstetric brachial plexus palsy (OBPP) with the passage of meconium during delivery and neonatal hyperbilirubinaemia.[4,25,30]

Aetiology

The cause of many cases of upper OBPP (Erb's palsy), which involves the C5 and C6 nerve roots, is widening of the head–shoulder angle at delivery, and this is by far the most common brachial plexus injury. Klumpke's palsy, which involves the lower brachial plexus roots, C8 and T1, is a much less common finding, with an incidence of 0.6/1000 livebirths. The reduced incidence of lower OBPP is thought to be attributable to the decline in vaginal breech deliveries. These deliveries are associated with forced hyperabduction of the upper limb, with risk to the lower brachial plexus.[31]

Complete plexus palsies are more common than lower plexus palsies. The long-term outcome of complete brachial plexus palsy is very poor, with 66% having permanent dysfunction.[31]

Clinical presentation

The signs at birth are obvious. With an upper plexus palsy, the abductors and external rotators of the shoulder and the supinators are paralysed. Therefore, the arm is held to the side internally rotated and pronated and there may also be loss of finger extension, the classic 'waiter's tip' sign (Fig. 38.27). In an adult, one would expect to find sensory loss over the deltoid; however, tests of sensation are unreliable in a baby. Lower plexus palsies

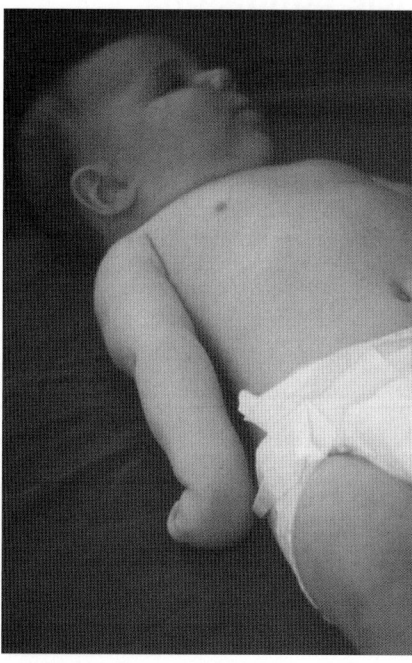

Fig. 38.27 The classic 'waiter's tip' posture of Erb's palsy following brachial plexus injury at birth.

result in clawing and wasting of the muscles of the hand. Complete plexus palsies result in a flail arm. The arm is pale with no motor function and there may be vasomotor impairment with a Horner's syndrome (meiosis, anhydrosis, ptosis and enopthalmos) on the affected side. Motor function of the arms can be tested in the neonate using the Moro reflex (p. 1099).

Referral and treatment

All babies with a suspected OBPP should be referred for an orthopaedic opinion. Occasionally, a birth fracture of the clavicle or the proximal humerus compounds the paralysis of the affected limb.

Prognosis

As most palsies are in the upper plexus with an excellent prognosis, the mainstay of treatment is to prevent stiffness and contractures, and early involvement of the paediatric physiotherapist is essential. The same applies for lower and complete plexus palsies, which have a higher risk of permanency. Regular orthopaedic review to monitor progress is essential. Absence of any motor function of the biceps at 3 months is an indication for further investigation with electrophysiological studies and possible surgical repair or grafting of the plexus.

Arthrogryposis multiplex congenita

Arthrogryposis is a generic term referring to a congenital, non-progressive fibrous ankylosis of joints resulting in reduced range of movement. It covers a heterogeneous group of syndromes, the most common being AMC.

AMC is an uncommon problem characterised by multiple joint contractures and absence of skin creases around joints, with occasional webbing on the flexor surface of immobile joints. It occurs sporadically with no known hereditary pattern.

Distal arthrogryposis causing clenched fists and foot deformities, however, is an autosomal dominant condition.[60]

Affected neonates with classic AMC have normal chromosomes and will generally develop normal intelligence.

Aetiology

As yet, no known cause for AMC has been found. Several aetiological theories have been postulated, including intrauterine infection (a similar condition is found in sheep, cows and horses secondary to Akabane virus), teratogens, environmental agents, or a metabolic cause.

AMC may be either neurogenic or myopathic. In the neurogenic form, there is depletion of motor neurons in the anterior horns of the spinal cord. In the myopathic form, there is depletion of muscle spindle fibres, although this may be secondary to neuropathic AMC.

It may be mimicked by other conditions which restrict fetal movements resulting in contracture deformities such as spina bifida, sacral agenesis and cerebral palsy.

Clinical presentation

The neonate presents with multiple rigid deformities which are usually bilateral and symmetrical. A characteristic posture is adopted in that the upper limb is adducted and internally rotated with the elbows extended and the wrists and fingers flexed **(Fig. 38.28a)**. The legs are held in a diamond shape, flexed and externally rotated at the hip with the knees partially flexed, with the feet invariably in the equinovarus position (Fig. 38.28b). There is marked muscle wasting proximal and distal to the joint contracture, with featureless skin and occasional webbing. In 92% of cases of AMC, all four limbs are affected; in 7%, lower limb only; and in 1%, upper limb only.[11] The condition is commonly associated with congenital vertical talus, CTEV and DDH of the teratologic variety.

Management

The deformities are at their worst at birth and, as the condition is non-progressive, are unlikely to advance with appropriate treatment. It is important that the baby is referred to an orthopaedic surgeon familiar with managing this condition.

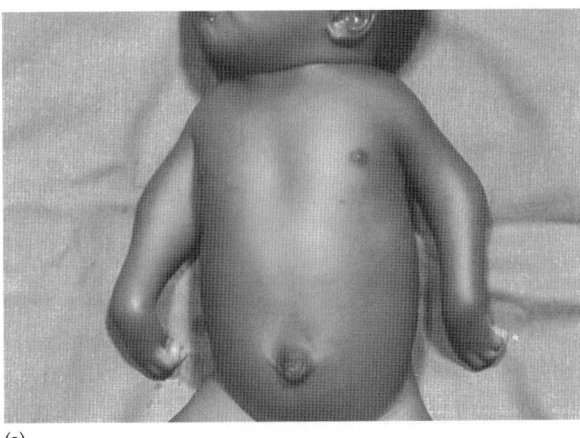

(a)

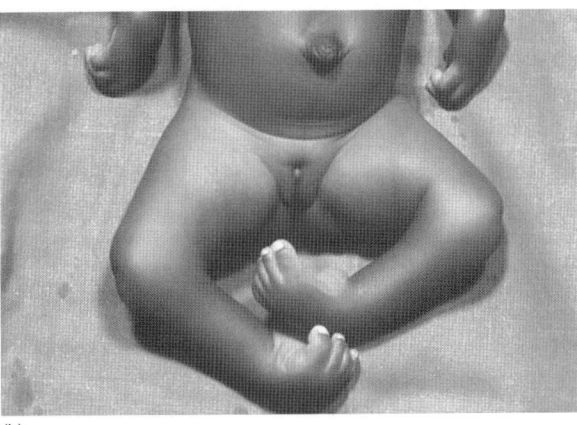

(b)

Fig. 38.28 (a) Clinical picture of the upper limbs in a baby with arthrogryposis. (b) The 'diamond' posture of the lower limbs in arthrogryposis

The mainstay of treatment in the initial phase is gentle stretching and splinting to correct the deformities and requires the input of specialist paediatric physiotherapists and occupational therapists. Care must be taken to avoid undue force when stretching, as the bones are thin and fracture easily. The therapists are closely involved with the family and provide invaluable support and advice, initially in the hospital setting and ultimately in the community.[44,57]

Invariably, affected children require some kind of surgical intervention in the form of soft-tissue release or tendon transfers, as well as management of DDH, CTEV or CVT if present.

On the whole, the outlook is good for genetically normal children with AMC, with 85% walking independently and having good wrist and hand function.[19]

Congenital muscular torticollis

The name torticollis is derived from Latin, *tortus* meaning twisted and *cullum* meaning neck. It presents with an abnormal head posture caused by shortening of one of the sternocleidomastoid (SCM) muscles in the neck. There is no information on incidence; it affects the right-hand side in 70% of cases and in 29% of cases is associated with DDH. This contracture prevents normal rotation of the head, pulling the chin away from the affected side when observed from the front and the ear towards the shoulder of the affected side when viewed from behind, the 'cock robin' posture (Fig. 38.29a).

The aetiology of congenital muscular torticollis (CMT) is poorly understood, but the condition is seen more commonly in traumatic births, leading to the suggestion that it is due to direct damage to the muscle resulting in a fibrous contracture following haematoma formation. CMT is seen in association with DDH and CTEV. Occasionally, the swelling of the muscle can be palpated in the affected SCM and is referred to as a 'tumour'. In other mature cases there is simply clinical thickening and tightness of the muscle and in some there is a torticollis posture with an absence of tightness or thickening of the SCM muscle.

Treatment initially is conservative with physiotherapy to increase range of movement. In most cases, the mass or thickening gradually disappears over the first year of life, and manual stretching is effective in 95% of cases referred before 1 year of age.[14]

Persistence of torticollis after 1 year (Fig 38.29b) requires further investigation and possible treatment. Occasionally, abnormal head posture may be due to an ocular or cerebral cause: in the absence of an obvious SCM tumour or tightening, ocular pathology should be excluded by ophthalomogical examination and cerebral pathology by MRI of the posterior fossae.[56]

Ultrasound assessment of the SCM muscle has been used to assess prognosis and need for surgical intervention. Ultrasound involvement of the distal third usually responds to conservative treatment, whereas involvement of the middle and distal thirds requires surgery in 6% of cases, and with whole muscle involvement, 35% of patients require surgery.[35] Failure to treat resistant CMT may result in facial moulding and asymmetry (plagiocephaly), and subsequent treatment is surgical, with release of the SCM muscle.

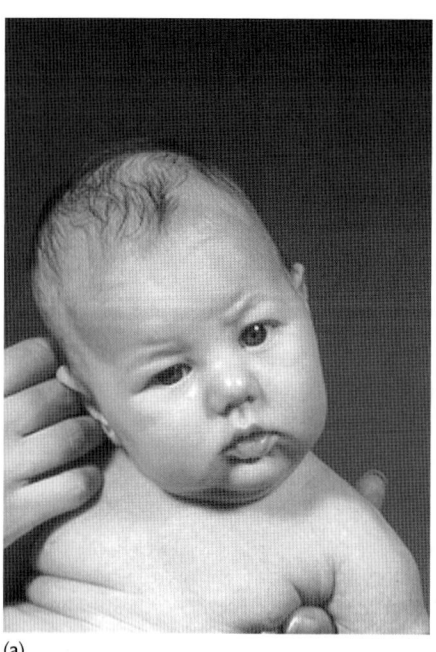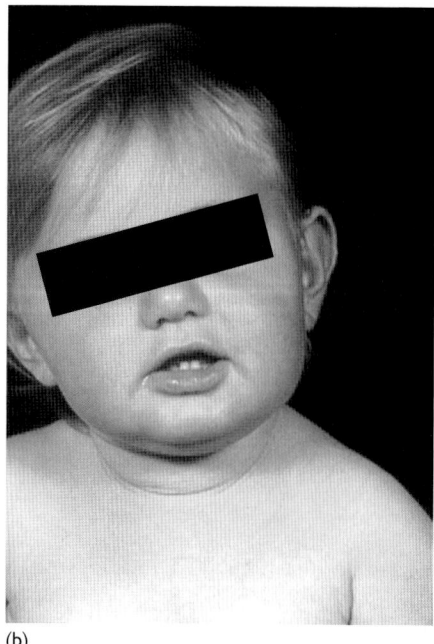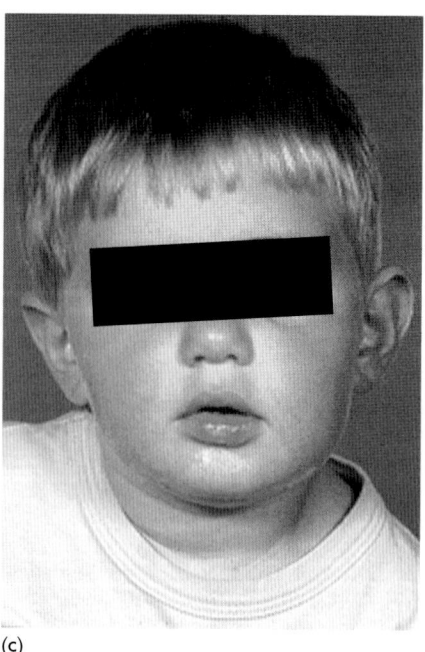

(a)   (b)   (c)

Fig. 38.29 (a) Congenital torticollis at birth. (b) The same child at the age of 1 year. (c) The same child at the age of 2 years.

Infectious disease associated with orthopaedic problems in the newborn

Septic arthritis[40]

Septic arthritis is an orthopaedic emergency and early involvement of an orthopaedic surgeon is mandatory. If there is any clinical suspicion of septic arthritis, an orthopaedic opinion should be sought urgently. It cannot be overemphasised that neonates may manifest very few systemic symptoms, making early diagnosis difficult, but if not considered in the differential of a child failing to thrive, the opportunity of early diagnosis and treatment will be missed.

Infection of a joint originates from three main sources: *haematogenous*, in which the synovium of the joint is inoculated from a distant source, i.e. the umbilicus; *direct extension* from an adjacent osteomyelitis; and *direct inoculation* from joint aspiration or arthrotomy. It must be remembered that taking blood from the femoral vein may lead to inadvertent joint puncture.

In order of frequency, the joints most often affected in the neonate are hip, knee and elbow, although any joint can be affected. The most common infecting organism is *Staphylococcus aureus* (60–80%), followed by *Streptococcus* and *Haemophilus* species. Unfortunately, only 50% of hip aspirates yield a positive culture.

As previously stated, clinical features may be slight and the characteristic high fever, systemic upset and immobility of the affected limb (pseudoparalysis) as seen in a child may be absent in the neonate. Failure to thrive may be the first clinical clue and careful clinical examination of the infant should be undertaken. Attention should be paid to any swelling, redness or tenderness of a joint, pain and stiffness on movement of a joint, pseudoparalysis, and observation of the position of the limbs. In septic arthritis of the hip, the limb is held in the position of most comfort, notably 40–60° of flexion, 10–20° of abduction and 10–15° of external rotation.

Markers of infection should be measured, including white cell count, C-reactive protein and a falling platelet count. These investigations are useful if the markers are raised, as they help to support the diagnosis. However, in the neonate these may be misleadingly normal, and if clinically suspected, further investigation is warranted.

Urgent ultrasound examination of the joint should be undertaken. This may simply identify a joint effusion, but the presence of echogenic debris may be more suggestive of infection. Bone scanning may be undertaken if the diagnosis is uncertain and may demonstrate increased activity around the joint. Plain X-rays in septic arthritis of the hip may be helpful, demonstrating lateral displacement of the hip or dislocation, but may also be entirely normal.

Delay in diagnosis and treatment results in joint destruction with secondary osteoarthritis or ankylosis, growth plate arrest, dislocation, and avascular necrosis.

Management

If there is clinical suspicion, the neonate should be prepared for surgery while investigations are taking place. Septic joints should be washed out and specimens sent for culture and sensitivity, and parenteral antibiotics commenced. The affected joint should be immobilised. Response to treatment can be monitored by the general wellbeing of the infant and, if raised initially, the restoration to normal values of inflammatory markers. Antibiotics must be continued for a minimum of 6 weeks, after which time

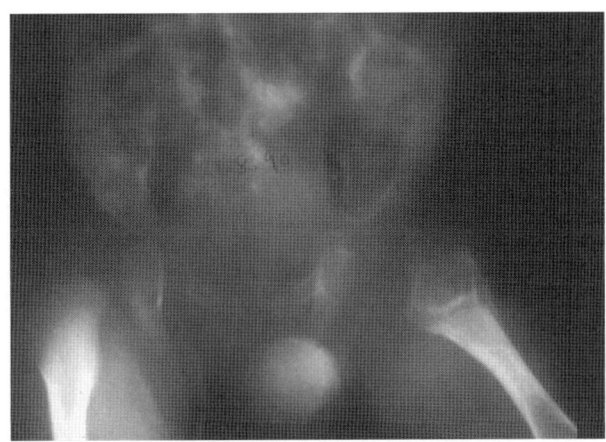

Fig. 38.30 Neonatal osteomyelitis of the left hip, showing lucency around the proximal femur and lifting of the periosteum.

splintage can be removed and clinical assessment of the joint made. After careful consideration, and only if the baby is doing well, it may be possible to convert parenteral antibiotics to enteral.

Osteomyelitis[38,39]

Neonatal osteomyelitis (Fig. 38.30) presents with swelling of the limb and septicaemia. Most commonly the infection is haematogenous in origin. The metaphyseal blood supply is sluggish, rendering this region of the bone susceptible to seeding of infection. In the neonate, the umbilicus is implicated as the portal for infection, particularly in the sick neonate who has undergone umbilical artery cannulation. In 70% of cases the adjacent joint becomes involved, because invariably the infected metaphysis is intracapsular.

Infecting organisms include group B beta-haemolytic streptococcus, *Streptococcus* species, *Staphylococcus aureus* and *Escherichia coli*.

In the newborn, there is often very little systemic response and, as with many childhood illnesses, there may simply be a failure to thrive. The most obvious clinical finding is absence of movement in the affected limb, 'pseudoparalysis'; other clues include instant crying when the affected limb is palpated or moved. There may also be local swelling and heat. There is spasm of the surrounding muscles that manifests as stiffness when the limb is moved.

Frequently, the signs of osteomyelitis are soft, and if it is clinically suspected, a bone scan should be organised. This may be helpful in determining all sites involved, as these may be multiple in the neonate. The scan may highlight a hotspot at the site of hyperaemia or a cold spot if bone infarction has occurred. A negative scan in the presence of high clinical suspicion should be followed by a gallium study, which is more sensitive in this age group.

Failure to make the diagnosis results in late sequelae of growth plate arrest, chondrolysis of the joint, early degenerative changes and avascular necrosis.

The mainstay of treatment is parenteral antibiotic therapy, ideally started after specimens and cultures have been obtained.

However, commencement of treatment should not be delayed. Antibiotic choice depends on local policy and advice should be sought from the microbiology department. As a guide, cefotaxime is a reasonable first-choice antibiotic, which should be continued until specific sensitivities are known. The affected limb should be splinted for comfort.

References

1. Achterman C, Kalamchi A 1979 Congenital absence of the fibula. Journal of Bone and Joint Surgery 61-B: 133–137
2. Adler J B, Patterson R L 1967 Erb's palsy: long term results of treatment in 88 cases. Journal of Bone and Joint Surgery 49-A: 1052–1064
3. Aitken G T 1969 Proximal focal femoral deficiency – definition, classification, and management. In: Aitken G T (ed) Proximal focal femoral deficiency: a congenital anomaly. National Academy of Sciences, Washington, DC, p. 1
4. Aston J W Jr 1977 Brachial plexus birth palsy. Orthopedics 2: 594–601
5. Austwick D H, Dandy D J 1983 Early operation for congenital subluxation of the knee. Journal of Pediatric Orthopedics 3: 85–87
6. Barlow I W, Clarke N M P 1994 Congenital talipes equinovarus. Surgery 12: 211–215
7. Barlow T G 1962 Early diagnosis and treatment of congenital dislocation of the hip. Journal of Bone and Joint Surgery 44-B: 292–301
8. Berg E E 1986 A reappraisal of metatarsus adductus and skewfoot. Journal of Bone and Joint Surgery 68-A: 1185–1196
9. Bialik V, Bialik G M, Blazer M, Sijov P, Weiner F, Berant M 1999 Developmental dysplasia of the hip: a new approach to incidence. Pediatrics 103: 93–99
10. Boeree N R, Clarke N M P 1994 Ultrasound imaging and secondary screening for congenital dislocation of the hip. Journal of Bone and Joint Surgery 76-B: 525–533
11. Broughton N S 1997 A textbook of paediatric orthopaedics. W B Saunders, Philadelphia
12. Carroll N C, McMurty R, Leete S F 1978 The pathoanatomy of congenital clubfoot. Orthopedic Clinics of North America 9: 225–231
13. Cashman J P, Round J, Taylor G, Clarke N M P 2002 The natural history of developmental dysplasia of the hip after early supervised treatment with a Pavlik harness. A prospective longitudinal follow up. Journal of Bone and Joint Surgery 84-B: 418–425
14. Cheng J C Y, Wong M W N, Tang S P et al 2001 Clinical determinants of the outcome of manual stretching in the treatment of congenital muscular torticollis in infants. A prospective study of eight hundred and twenty-one cases. Journal of Bone and Joint Surgery 83-A: 679–687
15. Clarke N M P, Harcke H T, McHugh P, Lee M S, Borns P F, MacEwen G D 1985 Real-time ultrasound in the diagnosis of congenital dislocation and dysplasia of the hip. Journal of Bone and Joint Surgery 67-B: 406–412
16. Coventry M B, Johnson E W J 1952 Congenital absence of the fibula. Journal of Bone and Joint Surgery 34-A: 941–945
17. Curtis B H, Fisher R L 1969 Congenital hyperextension with anterior subluxation of the knee. Journal of Bone and Joint Surgery 51-A: 255–269
18. Dimeglio A, Bensahel H, Souchet P, Mazeau P, Bonnet F 1995 Classification of clubfoot. Journal of Pediatric Orthopedics 4-B: 129–136
19. Drennan J C 1990 Neuromuscular disorders. In: Morrissy R T (ed) Lovell and Winter's pediatric orthopaedics, 3rd edn. J B Lippincott, Philadelphia, 381–463
20. Elbourne D, Dezateux C, Arthur R et al 2002 Ultrasonography in the diagnosis and management of developmental hip dysplasia (UK Hip Trial): clinical and economic results of a multicentre randomised controlled trial. Lancet 360: 2009–2017
21. Foulkes G D, Reinker K 1994 Congenital constriction band syndrome: a seventy year experience. Journal of Pediatric Orthopedics 14: 242–248
22. Ghali N N, Abberton M J, Silk F F 1984 The management of metatarsus adductus et supinatus. Journal of Bone and Joint Surgery 66-B: 376–380
23. Gillespie R, Torode I P 1983 Classification and management of congenital abnormalities of the femur. Journal of Bone and Joint Surgery 65-B: 557–568
24. Graf R 1984 New possibilities of the diagnosis of congenital hip joint dislocation by ultrasonography. Journal of Pediatric Orthopedics 3: 354–359
25. Hardy A E 1981 Birth injuries of the brachial plexus: incidence and prognosis. Journal of Bone and Joint Surgery 63-B: 98–101
26. Harrington P R 1960 Surgical instrumentation for management of scoliosis. Journal of Bone and Joint Surgery 42-A: 1448

27. Haynes R J 2001 Developmental dysplasia of the hip: etiology, pathogenesis, and examination and physical findings in the newborn. AAOS Instructional Course Lectures 50: 535–540

28. Hensinger R N, Jones E T 1981 Neonatal orthopaedics. Grune and Stratton, New York

29. Hensinger R N, Lang J R, MacEwen G D 1974 The Klippel-Feil syndrome: a constellation of related anomalies. Journal of Bone and Joint Surgery 56-A: 1246–1253

30. Jackson S T, Hoffer M M, Parrish N 1988 Brachial plexus palsy in the newborn. Journal of Bone and Joint Surgery 70-A: 1217–1220

31. Jennett R J, Tarby T J, Krauss R L 2002 Erb's palsy contrasted with Klumpke's and total palsy: different mechanisms are involved. American Journal of Obstetrics and Gynecology 186: 1216–1220

32. Kalamchi A, Dawe R V 1985 Congenital deficiency of the tibia. Journal of Bone and Joint Surgery 67-B: 581–584

33. Klisic P G 1989 Congenital dislocation of the hip – a misleading term. Journal of Bone and Joint Surgery 71-B: 136

34. Letts M, Blastorah B, Al-Azzam S 1997 Neonatal gangrene of the extremities. Journal of Pediatric Orthopedics 17: 397–401

35. Lin J N, Chou M L 1997 Ultrasonographic study of the sternocleidomastoid muscle in the management of congenital muscular torticollis. Journal of Pediatric Surgery 32: 1648–1651

36. MacEwen G D, Hardy J H 1972 Evaluation of kidney anomalies in congenital scoliosis. Journal of Bone and Joint Surgery 54-A: 1451–1454

37. Madsen E T 1955 Fractures of extremities in the newborn. Acta Obstetrica et Gynaecologia Scandinavica 34: 41–75

38. Mollan R A B, Piggot J 1977 Acute osteomyelitis in children. Journal of Bone and Joint Surgery 59-B: 2–7

39. Nade S 1983 Acute haematogenous osteomyelitis in infancy and childhood. Journal of Bone and Joint Surgery 65-B: 109–119

40. Nade S 1983 Acute septic arthritis in infancy and childhood. Journal of Bone and Joint Surgery 65-B: 234–241

41. Neibauer J J, King D E 1960 Congenital dislocation of the knee. Journal of Bone and Joint Surgery 42-A: 207–225

42. Nogi J MacEwen G D 1982 Congenital dislocation of the knee. Journal of Pediatric Orthopedics 2: 509–513

43. Ortolani M 1937 Un sengo poco noto e sua importanza per la diagnosi precoce di prelussazione congenital dell'anca. Pediatrica (Napoli) 45: 129–136

44. Palmer P M, MacEwen G D, Bowen J R, Matthews P A 1985 Passive motion therapy for infants with arthrogryposis multiplex congenita. Clinical Orthopaedics and Related Research 195: 53–59

45. Patterson T J S 1961 Congenital ring constrictions. British Journal of Plastic Surgery 14: 1–31

46. Pavlik A 1992 The functional method of treatment using a harness with stirrups as the primary method of conservative therapy for infants with congenital dislocation of the hip. 1957. Clinical Orthopaedics and Related Research 281: 4–10

47. Ponseti I V, Smoley E N 1963 Congenital clubfoot: the results of treatment. Journal of Bone and Joint Surgery 45-A: 261–275

48. Sadler T W 1990 Langman's medical embryology, 6th edn. Williams and Wilkins, Baltimore

49. Standing Medical Advisory Committee, Standing Nursing and Midwifery Advisory Committee Working Parties for the Secretary of State for Social Services and Wales 1986 Screening for the detection of congenital dislocation of the hip. Archives of Disease in Childhood 61: 921–926

50. Stern M B 1968 Congenital dislocation of the knee. Clinical Orthopaedics and Related Research 61: 261–268.

51. Tachdjian M O 1990 Pediatric orthopaedics, 2nd edn. W B Saunders, Philadelphia

52. Taylor G R, Clarke N M P 1997 Monitoring the treatment of developmental dysplasia of the hip with the Pavlik harness. The role of ultrasound. Journal of Bone and Joint Surgery 79-B: 719–723

53. Torpin R, Faulkner A 1966 Intrauterine amputation with the missing member found in the fetal membranes. Journal of the American Medical Association 198: 185–187

54. Uglow M G, Clarke N M P 2000 Relapse in staged surgery for congenital talipes equinovarus. Journal of Bone and Joint Surgery 82-B: 739–743

55. Uglow M G, Clarke N M P 2000 The functional outcome of staged surgery for the correction of talipes equinovarus. Journal of Pediatric Orthopedics 20: 517–523

56. Williams C R P, O'Flynn E, Clarke N M P, Morris R J 1996 Torticollis secondary to ocular pathology. Journal of Bone and Joint Surgery 78-B: 620–624

57. Williams P 1978 The management of arthrogryposis. Orthopedic Clinics of North America 9: 67–88

58. Winter R B 1981 Convex anterior and posterior hemiarthrodesis and hemiepiphysiodesis in young children with progressive congenital scoliosis. Journal of Pediatric Orthopedics 1: 361–366

59. Winter R B, Moe J H, Wang J F 1973 Congenital kyphosis. Its natural history and treatment as observed in a study of 130 patients. Journal of Bone and Joint Surgery 55-A: 223–256

60. Wynne-Davies R 1978 Heritable disorders in orthopedics. Orthopedic Clinics of North America 9: 1–14

CHAPTER 39

Neonatal gynaecology

D Keith Edmonds

Gynaecological problems in neonatal life are unusual and rare. Many conditions that are thought to be pathological are commonly physiological or anatomical variants, but these variants cause considerable anxiety amongst parents. A knowledge of the physiology and anatomy of the development of the genital tract during fetal life is therefore important, so that an explanation of these variations can be offered to parents in a reassuring manner.

The physiology of the fetal hypothalamo-pituitary axis

The early fetal brain undergoes rapid development, and by 5 weeks of gestation, gonadotrophin-releasing hormone (GnRH) can be detected in whole brain extract.[30] GnRH can be localised to the hypothalamus by 8–13 weeks' gestation,[2,15] and the hypothalamic GnRH content of female fetuses reaches a maximum at between 22 and 25 weeks' gestation and thereafter declines.[25] This is almost certainly in response to negative feedback of circulating oestradiol.

Luteinising hormones (LH) and follicle-stimulating hormone (FSH) can be identified within the pituitary gland by 9–11 weeks' gestation[7,12] and the portal circulation linking the hypothalamus with the pituitary is known to be intact by 12 weeks' gestation.[27] In response to GnRH release, FSH and LH reach their maximum between 16 and 24 weeks.[26] Subsequently, FSH levels decline, almost certainly owing to active secretion of inhibin from the granulosa cells in the ovary. During the latter part of fetal life, gonadotrophin levels are reduced and remain at low levels until birth.[26] Both inhibin and circulating oestradiol exhibit this negative feedback mechanism.

Following birth, the contribution of placental oestradiol to the fetal circulation is withdrawn, the fetal hypothalamo-pituitary axis becomes activated and both GnRH and gonadotrophin levels rise immediately.[29] FSH levels and LH levels remain elevated for several months after birth, but subsequent central suppression of GnRH leads to decline in gonadotrophin levels by around 6 months of age. The central suppression of the pulse generator in the arcuate nucleus of the hypothalamus may be brought about by several modulators, including noradrenaline, dopamine, central opiates, neuropeptide Y, glutamate or aspartate.[6,11,16,24] The cell receptors on the GnRH-secreting neurons are controlled by a gene encoding for transforming growth factor alpha,[18] and this gene may well itself be controlled by the secretion of leptin,[19] a hormone produced by adipose tissue; decreasing the body mass index towards later infancy and increasing body mass at puberty may be intimately involved in the activation of the gene.

Thus, throughout fetal and early neonatal life, the hypothalamo-pituitary ovarian uterine axis is fully developed and active, and capable of responding to all of the appropriate integrated mechanisms. It is only the genetic downregulation of central receptors that suppresses activity after birth.

Neonatal breast development

Breast development occurs during fetal life and is well described as proceeding in female infants for several months after birth. It is occasionally associated with secretions similar to lactation. Two studies suggest that, after birth, circulating levels of oestriol, which would be maternally derived, decline rapidly, and yet breast development continues for several months after birth.[1,21] Elevated levels of oestradiol and prolactin in the neonate are directly related to breast size, the relationship being particularly strong with prolactin. Therefore it would seem that the infant's own gonadal secretions are responsible for the control of the breast. Histological studies further support this theory.[20] Breast development in early neonatal life thus is a normal physiological process and ceases at 3–6 months of age; the breast bud may thereafter regress.

Supernumerary nipples are a common finding; they extend along the nipple line on either side of the chest wall, down the abdomen and may occur in the labia. Bilateral ectopic breast tissue has been described in the vulva.[17]

Vulval problems

Labial cysts in the newborn are rare, and occur in about 6 per 1000 female infants. These congenital cysts require no treatment whatsoever, and conservative management leads to complete resolution within 2–3 months of life. No surgical approach should be taken in these circumstances.[22]

Inguinal hernia in infants is very common and is encountered in approximately 1–3% of full-term newborns and 3–5% of premature babies.[8] Surgical management of this involves closure of the hernia when diagnosed. It is important to be aware that in female infants, a differential diagnosis of an irreducible inguinal mass must include the presence of either a prolapsed ovary or the uterus and ovary, and in female infants with ambiguous genitalia, the inguinal mass may be a testis. It is unusual for these to be seen in immediate infancy but they may result in the ensuing months after birth. Ultrasound of these masses can be extremely useful and may help to differentiate the presence of ovarian tissue in the hernia sac and also aid in differentiating the presence of an ovary or a testis. It is important than when these masses are detected, early treatment is embarked upon, as correction of this anatomical defect will reduce the risk of torsion and infarction and subsequent loss of the gonad. This is particularly important when the herniation is an ovary, as salvation of the ovary would be important in later life.

Abnormalities of the hymen

The hymen at birth is usually annular or fimbriated and commonly associated with external ridges. Hymenal tags are extremely common at birth,[23] and are often misdiagnosed as 'prolapse'. The hymen changes its characteristics during the first 3 years of life and becomes crescentic by age 3 years in the vast majority, with the external ridges disappearing.[4] Problems in neonatal life that are associated with peripheral oedema, often lead to oedema of the hymen, which may protrude beyond the vulval entrance and again be mistaken for a prolapse.

Failure of the hymen to perforate during embryological life may lead to retention of vaginal secretions which cannot escape and the vagina distends proximal to the hymen. Although these membranes are often referred to as imperforate hymen, it is likely that this is not strictly correct and that these membranes are transverse vaginal septae, resulting from failure of fusion of the urogenital sinus and the downgrowth of the vaginal plate from the müllerian structures. When a large quantity of fluid collects, there may be difficulty in emptying the bladder, as the distended vagina fills the pelvis, and the child may be very fretful and clearly in discomfort. The physical signs are of a lower abdominal cystic swelling and a bulging membrane at the introitus (Fig. 39.1). Diagnosis is extremely important, as misdiagnoses abound in which laparotomy has been performed, and even hysterectomy, and this is absolutely unnecessary. The most common misdiagnoses are to believe that this is either a swelling which is an ovarian cyst or, occasionally, a full bladder with urethral

prolapse. Ultrasound imaging may diagnose a hydrocolpos both antenatally and after delivery. It has been described as early as 25 weeks' gestation.[28] It is simple to demonstrate the uterus sitting above a distended vagina when the diagnosis of hydrocolpos can be made. Treatment is simple in most cases: the intact membrane is incised and the retained fluid released. Redundant portions of the membrane may be excised and the procedure completed. If the obstruction is more extensive owing to a wide transverse septum, great care is needed to avoid damage to the bladder and rectum, but an end-to-end anastomosis can be achieved to result in a normal vagina. One can only presume that these cases of hydrocolpos are exceptional, as most cases of transverse vaginal septum are not diagnosed until puberty.[9]

Vaginal bleeding problems

Bleeding from the genital tract in the newborn period is well described. A study from Huber in 1976[13] showed that vaginal bleeding occurs in 25% of newborn girls, although it is only macroscopically visible in 3.3%. Vaginal bleeding in the first week of life is extremely common. Persistent vaginal bleeding beyond the first year of life demands further investigation. The development of rhabdomyosarcoma, whilst extraordinarily rare in immediate

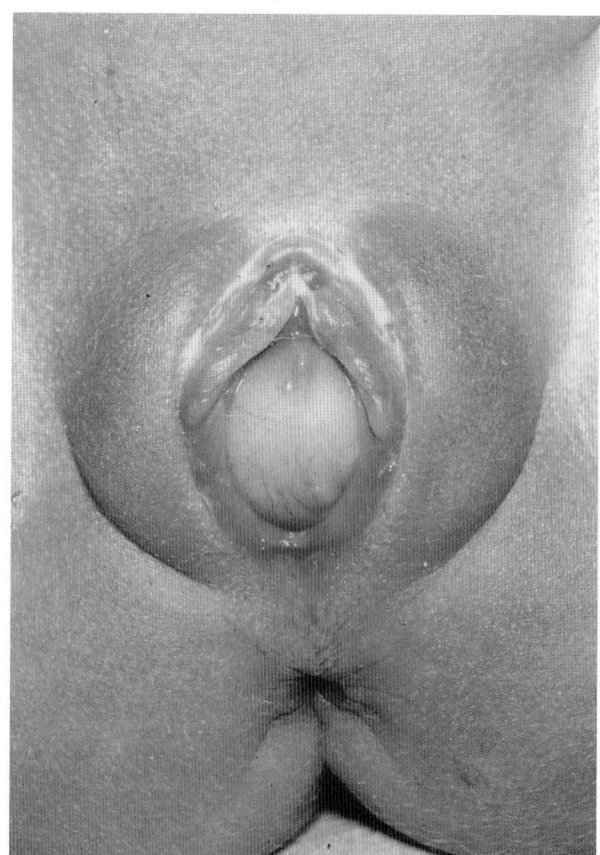

Fig. 39.1 Bulging membrane at the introitus in a case of transverse vaginal septum presenting in a newborn.

neonatal life, may present as bleeding at 2–3 months of age. Most of the genital lesions associated with rhabdomyosarcoma of the perineum, vulva and vagina occur in early childhood.

Uterine prolapse

Prolapse in the neonatal period is extremely rare, but may present with the cervix protruding through the vagina. A number of cases have been described and, although the aetiology of the problem remains obscure, some cases are associated with neurological abnormalities, e.g. spina bifida. Treatment is conservative and involves digital replacement of the prolapse into the vagina. This may have to be repeated on a number of occasions, but

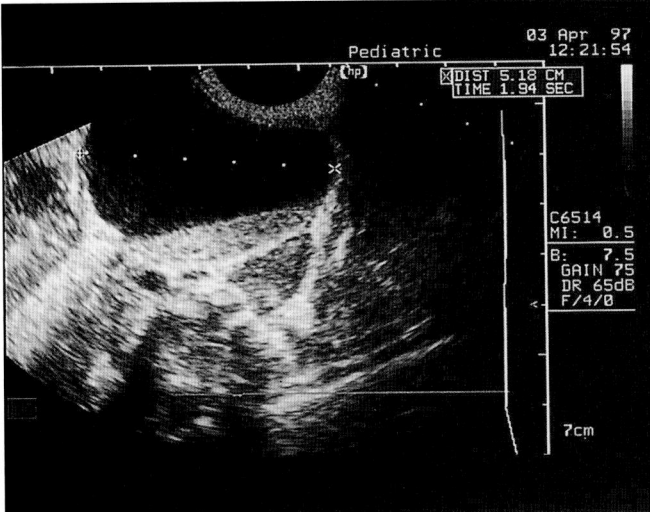

Fig. 39.2 Pelvic ultrasound scan showing an ovarian cyst 5 cm in diameter in a newborn girl.

eventually, by 3 months of age at the latest, all of these prolapses have resolved. Occasionally, pessaries may be required if the prolapse remains persistent, although these are very difficult to design for infants.[14] Recently, a surgical management using a ventrosuspension has been performed in an infant with a persisting problem.[3] No data exist to suggest whether or not these female infants will develop prolapse problems in a later stage of their lives, but it is likely that this will be the case, as the occurrence of prolapse in these circumstances may be associated with poor collagen development in the supporting tissue of the genital tract.

Urethral prolapse

Urethral prolapse in the neonatal period is extremely rare, but may present with vaginal bleeding. The urethral mucosa prolapses through the meatus and forms a sensitive vulval mass that bleeds on touch. The passage of urine may be unimpaired when the lesion is small, and in these circumstances the use of oestrogen cream may be beneficial. However, occasionally, urinary retention may be present, or the prolapse may recur following repeated oestrogen treatments and recurrence may require surgical excision if the lesion is large. This tends to be only rarely necessary and is usually only employed when urinary retention is present.

Ovarian cysts

Ultrasound of the fetus during pregnancy is now sophisticated enough to diagnose ovarian cysts in mid-pregnancy, and these may be detected as early as 16–18 weeks' gestation. The vast majority of these cysts are functional, benign follicular cysts and do not interfere with the course of pregnancy or birth. If these cysts are less than 5 cm in diameter as diagnosed during the

Fig. 39.3 Torted ovarian cyst at laparotomy in a young girl.

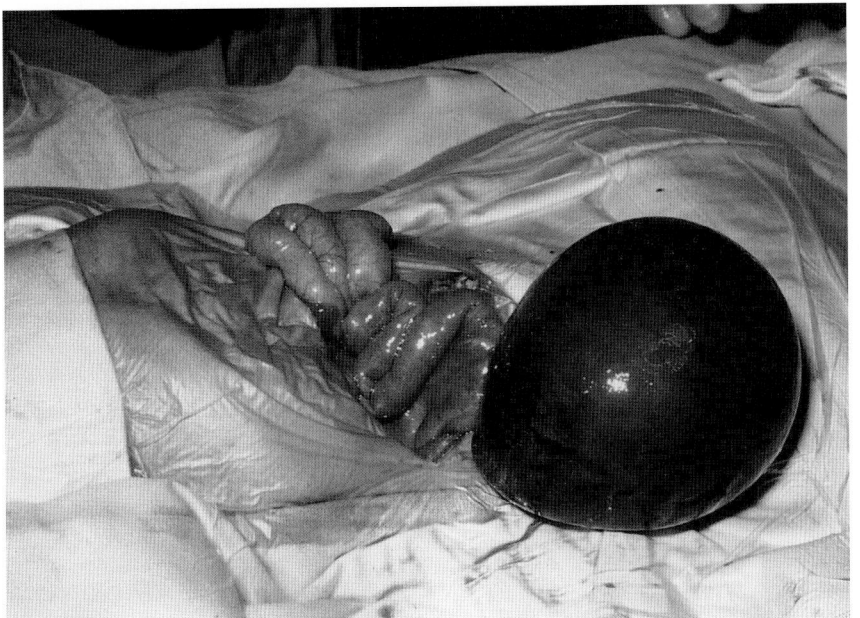

postnatal period, then they may be managed conservatively with serial ultrasound and the vast majority will resolve spontaneously.[5] This may take as long as 6 months to a year and this relates to stimulation of the ovary by elevated FSH levels which persist during this time. Cysts that are larger than 5 cm in diameter (Fig. 39.2) but do not contain any solid elements may be managed by percutaneous aspiration under local anaesthesia. Should this be performed, cytology should always be carried out for confirmation of a benign lesion. All cysts of 4 cm or more have the risk of torsion, and therefore care must be taken in their management and also in the advice that is given to parents. All larger cysts and complex cysts require more careful assessment and may require a surgical approach (Fig. 39.3) to ensure that the cyst is benign. This may be carried out laparoscopically.[10] Antenatal torsion of a cyst has been described in a pregnancy that resulted in premature birth, although the clinical course of the neonate was uneventful.

References

1. Anbazhagan R, Bartek J, Monaghan P, Gusterson B A 1991 Growth and development of the human infant breast. American Journal of Anatomy 192: 407–417

2. Aubert M L, Grumbach M M, Kaplan S L 1977 The autogenesis of human fetal hormones. IV. Somatostatin, luteinizing hormone releasing factor, and thyrotropin releasing factor in hypothalamus and cerebral cortex of human fetuses 10–22 weeks of age. Journal of Clinical Endocrinology and Metabolism 44: 1130–1141

3. Banieghbal B, Fonseca J 1998 Surgical management of uterine prolapse in an infant. European Journal of Pediatric Surgery 8: 119–120

4. Berenson A B 1995 A longitudinal study of hymenal morphology in the first 3 years of life. Pediatrics 95: 490–496

5. Brandt M L, Luks F I, Filiatrault D et al 1991 Surgical indications in antenatally diagnosed ovarian cysts. Journal of Pediatric Surgery 26: 276–281

6. Brann D W 1995 Glutamate: a major excitatory transmitter in neuroendocrine regulation. Neuroendocrinology 61: 213–225

7. Currie R W, Faiman C, Thliveris J A 1981 An immunocytochemical and routine electron microscopic study of LH and FSH cells in the human fetal pituitary. American Journal of Anatomy 161: 281–297

8. Dassonville M, Verstreken L, De Laet M H 1985 [Inguinal hernia in infants and children]. Acta Chirurgica Belgica 85: 341–347

9. Edmonds D K 1988 Practical paediatric and adolescent gynaecology. Butterworths, London, pp 86–95

10. Esposito C, Garipoli V, Di Matteo G, De Pasquale M 1998 Laparoscopic management of ovarian cysts in newborns. Surgical Endoscopy 12: 1152–1154

11. Gore A C, Mitsushima D, Terasawa E 1993 A possible role of neuropeptide Y in the control of the onset of puberty in female rhesus monkeys. Neuroendocrinology 58: 23–34

12. Hagen C, McNeilly A S 1977 The gonadotrophins and their subunits in foetal pituitary glands and circulation. Journal of Steroid Biochemistry 8: 537–544

13. Huber A 1976 [The frequency of physiologic vaginal bleeding of newborn infants]. Zentralblatt fur Gynakologie 98: 1017–1020

14. Johnson A, Unger S W, Rodgers B M 1984 Uterine prolapse in the neonate. Journal of Pediatric Surgery 19: 210–211

15. Kaplan S L, Grumbach M M, Aubert M L 1976 The ontogenesis of pituitary hormones and hypothalamic factors in the human fetus: maturation of central nervous system regulation of anterior pituitary function. Recent Progress in Hormone Research 32: 161–243

16. Lee P A 1988 The neuroendocrinology of puberty. Seminars in Reproductive Medicine 6: 13–20

17. Levin N, Diener R L 1968 Bilateral ectopic breast of the vulva. Report of a case. Obstetrics and Gynecology 32: 274–276

18. Ma Y J, Costa M E, Ojeda S R 1994 Developmental expression of the genes encoding transforming growth factor alpha and its receptor in the hypothalamus of female rhesus macaques. Neuroendocrinology 60: 346–359

19. MacDougald O A, Hwang C S, Fan H, Lane M D 1995 Regulated expression of the obese gene product (leptin) in white adipose tissue and 3T3-L1 adipocytes. Proceedings of the National Academy of Sciences of the United States of America 92: 9034–9037

20. McKiernan J, Coyne J, Cahalane S 1988 Histology of breast development in early life. Archives of Disease in Childhood 63: 136–139

21. McKiernan J F, Hull D 1981 Prolactin, maternal oestrogens, and breast development in the newborn. Archives of Disease in Childhood 56: 770–774

22. Merlob P, Bahari C, Liban E, Reisner S H 1978 Cysts of the female external genitalia in the newborn infant. American Journal of Obstetrics and Gynecology 132: 607–610

23. Mor N, Merlob P, Reisner S H 1983 Tags and bands of the female external genitalia in the newborn infant. Clinical Pediatrics 22: 122–124

24. Prasad B M, Conover C D, Sarkar D K et al 1993 Feed restriction in prepubertal lambs: effect on puberty onset and on in vivo release of luteinizing-hormone-releasing hormone, neuropeptide Y and beta-endorphin from the posterior-lateral median eminence. Neuroendocrinology 57: 1171–1181

25. Siler-Khodr T M, Khodr G S 1978 Studies in human fetal endocrinology. I. Luteinizing hormone-releasing factor content of the hypothalamus. American Journal of Obstetrics and Gynecology 130: 795–800

26. Takagi S, Yoshida T, Tsubata K et al 1977 Sex differences in fetal gonadotropins and androgens. Journal of Steroid Biochemistry 8: 609–620

27. Thliveris J A, Currie R W 1980 Observations on the hypothalamo-hypophyseal portal vasculature in the developing human fetus. American Journal of Anatomy 157: 441–444

28. Winderl L M, Silverman R K 1995 Prenatal diagnosis of congenital imperforate hymen. Obstetrics and Gynecology 85: 857–860

29. Winter J S, Faiman C, Hobson W C et al 1975 Pituitary-gonadal relations in infancy. I. Patterns of serum gonadotropin concentrations from birth to four years of age in man and chimpanzee. Journal of Clinical Endocrinology and Metabolism 40: 545–551

30. Winters A J, Eskay R L, Porter J C 1974 Concentration and distribution of TRH and LRH in the human fetal brain. Journal of Clinical Endocrinology and Metabolism 39: 960–963

CHAPTER 40

Neonatal infection

PART I

Immunodeficiency

Andrew J Cant, Andrew R Gennery

Introduction

The immune system distinguishes 'self' from 'non-self', destroying microorganisms but leaving other proteins unmolested. Immunological abnormalities result in an increased susceptibility to infection, as well as allergy and autoimmunity. The term neonate's immune system will generally respond appropriately, but failure occurs because of naïvete to an antigen or lack of fine-tuning (e.g. the antibody response to polysaccharide antigen). However, the preterm infant is immature in several respects, and in the neonatal unit, failure may also result from breaches of protective barriers by intravenous catheters and endotracheal tubes.

The immune system

Pathogen exclusion by physical and chemical barriers is very important. Epithelial surfaces and mucous membranes provide the first line of defence, augmented by cilia and respiratory tract mucus secretions, stomach acids and other mucous membrane secretions. Commensal intestinal and skin flora produce locally acting antibiotics, which exclude potential pathogens. These barriers are particularly important in the neonate, whose immunological immaturity renders him more susceptible to infections.

Specific and non-specific mechanisms of immunity

Pathogens that breach the barrier defences first encounter non-specific and then specific components of the immune system. These are interdependent; many specific immune mechanisms use non-specific elements to exert their effects and factors produced by the specific immune response can greatly potentiate non-specific functions.

Phagocytes such as neutrophils or monocytes, as well as the complement system, deliver highly effective non-antigen-specific immune responses using a limited number of receptors specific for conserved microbial structures.

The specific immune system responds to antigens by proliferation of antigen-specific T and B lymphocytes following antigen presentation to their receptor by cells of the non-specific (innate) system. These responses are then committed to 'immunological memory', resulting in more rapid and enhanced responses upon subsequent antigen exposure.

Non-specific immune mechanisms

Humoral

Complement is very important. When the central component, C3b, which can be activated by at least three pathways, is bound to an antigen, it interacts powerfully with C3b receptors on neutrophils and monocytes, enhancing phagocytosis. C3b also initiates a cascade activating further components such as C5–C9, which lyse cell membranes, a mechanism particularly important in the handling of systemic Neisserial infections.

Mannan-binding lectin (MBL), which binds to mannose on the surface of microorganisms, activates the classical complement pathway, which is important in the early stages of infection before antibody production, particularly in young children whose antibody-producing ability is immature.

Alpha- and beta-interferon (α-IFN, β-IFN) proteins are produced by virally infected cells. They render other cells immune to virus infection by producing an antiviral state. They also increase natural killer (NK) cell activity and increase HLA class I antigen expression on cells. IFN-γ, though having some antiviral effect, upregulates immune responses by enhancing intracellular killing of microorganisms such as mycobacteria.

Many bacteria require iron for growth, and decreasing its availability is one mechanism of defence used by the host. An avid iron-binding protein, lactoferrin, present in human milk, reduces the growth of *E. coli*. The removal of serum iron, which occurs during infections, increases the bacteriostatic effect of serum.

Lysozyme is found in neutrophil lysosomes and body secretions, including tears and saliva, and has antibacterial properties.

Cellular

Phagocytic cells such as neutrophils and monocyte/macrophages migrate to the site of infection attracted by products of the acute inflammatory response (chemotaxis), including cleaved complement fragments. Adherence to the bacterium and ingestion (phagocytosis) follows, aided by IgG and complement (C3b), which stick to bacteria and phagocyte cell surface receptors Fcγ and CR1/3, respectively (opsonisation). Following phagocytosis, lysosomes fuse with the bacterium-containing phagosome and release lysosomal enzymes (e.g. myeloperoxidase) and free oxygen radicals, which kill and digest microorganisms. Neutrophil numbers and function are enhanced by the inflammatory response.

Monocytes and macrophages kill extracellular bacteria more slowly and less efficiently than neutrophils but are important in defences against intracellular microorganisms, such as *Mycobacterium tuberculosis* and *Listeria monocytogenes*, because their activity is greatly enhanced by cytokines, particularly IFN-γ, produced by T lymphocytes.

NK cells are part of the non-T, non-B-cell lymphoid population and recognise and kill tumour and virus-infected cells.

Specific immune mechanisms

Specific responses are generated by T and B lymphocytes, whose receptors are antigen specific. Binding of antigen to receptor initiates antibody production or the generation of specific cytotoxic T lymphocytes (Fig. 40.1).

Antigen-presenting cells (APC), which include macrophages, dendritic cells and Langerhans cells as well as B lymphocytes, present antigens to T lymphocytes, degrade them to small peptide fragments and then express them on the cell surface in association with the major histocompatibility complex (MHC) molecules. The T-lymphocyte receptor (T-cell receptor, TCR) recognises the peptide in association with a self MHC molecule. CD4$^+$ helper T lymphocytes respond to antigen bound within the groove of class II MHC molecules (HLA-DR) whilst CD8$^+$ cytotoxic T lymphocytes respond to antigen bound within the groove of class I (HLA-AB) molecules. Other receptor–ligand interactions are also important for maximising T-lymphocyte stimulation.

There are two arms of the specific immune system – antibody-mediated and cell-mediated.

Antibodies

These are produced by B lymphocytes and their derivatives, plasma cells, in response to specific antigens such as microbial peptide or a vaccine.

The immunoglobulin class (isotype) is determined by the heavy chain. During B-lymphocyte development, genes coding for the variable and constant parts of the immunoglobulin chain are rearranged. One each of the variable (V), diversity (D) and joining (J) heavy-chain genes are rearranged to lie adjacent to the relevant heavy-chain constant-region gene, so that transcription produces a single protein with a constant and a variable portion (Fig. 40.2). Approximately 10^{16} different specific T-lymphocyte receptors (with a similar number of antibody receptors) are generated. Further rearrangement to bring a particular variable gene combination to lie adjacent to a different heavy-chain constant-region gene allows the B lymphocyte to switch to another antibody class (isotype) with the same antigen specificity. A μ chain is always produced first; class switching to other isotypes occurs later. Specific antibody diversity is created by the large number of possible combinations of variable-region genes that can be selected and is increased further by a very high mutation rate in V genes. A similar but slightly less complex process takes place with light chains, of which there are two types – kappa and lambda.

IgM is the first antibody class produced in primary immune responses. For most antigens, there is a subsequent switching to other classes. Its large pentameric structure confines it to the intravascular space, where it fixes complement.

IgG is the main class of antibody produced in secondary immune responses. Functions include opsonisation, complement fixation leading to C3 opsonisation and complement-mediated lysis, neutralisation of toxins or viruses, and participation in antibody-dependent cellular cytotoxicity. Though there is considerable overlap, the four subclasses of IgG tend to have different functions. Responses to protein antigens are mainly in the IgG1 and IgG3 subclasses. IgG2 binds polysaccharide such as group B streptococcal surface antigen. The role of IgG4 is, as yet, unclear.

IgA is the main antibody in secretions, where it forms a dimeric molecule. In addition to protecting mucous membranes and the gastrointestinal tract from infection, IgA may have a role in limiting food antigen uptake from the gut. Serum IgA is mainly in monomeric form, though dimeric and trimeric forms are also found. It is secreted in breast milk.

Mast cells and basophils have receptors for the Fc part of IgE. Antigen binding causes degranulation of the cells, triggering an immediate hypersensitivity response.

The final stages of B-lymphocyte differentiation require stimulation with the appropriate antigen, leading to maturation into plasma cells. The full process requires the co-operation of antigen-specific T helper (CD4$^+$) lymphocytes. Isotype switching from IgM production to the other antibody classes is critically dependent on T/B lymphocyte interaction via the B-lymphocyte CD40 antigen and the CD40 ligand expressed on activated T lymphocytes (CD40L, CD154).

Cell-mediated immunity

T (thymus-derived) lymphocytes kill intracellular microbes and regulate immune responses by secreting cytokines and growth factors.

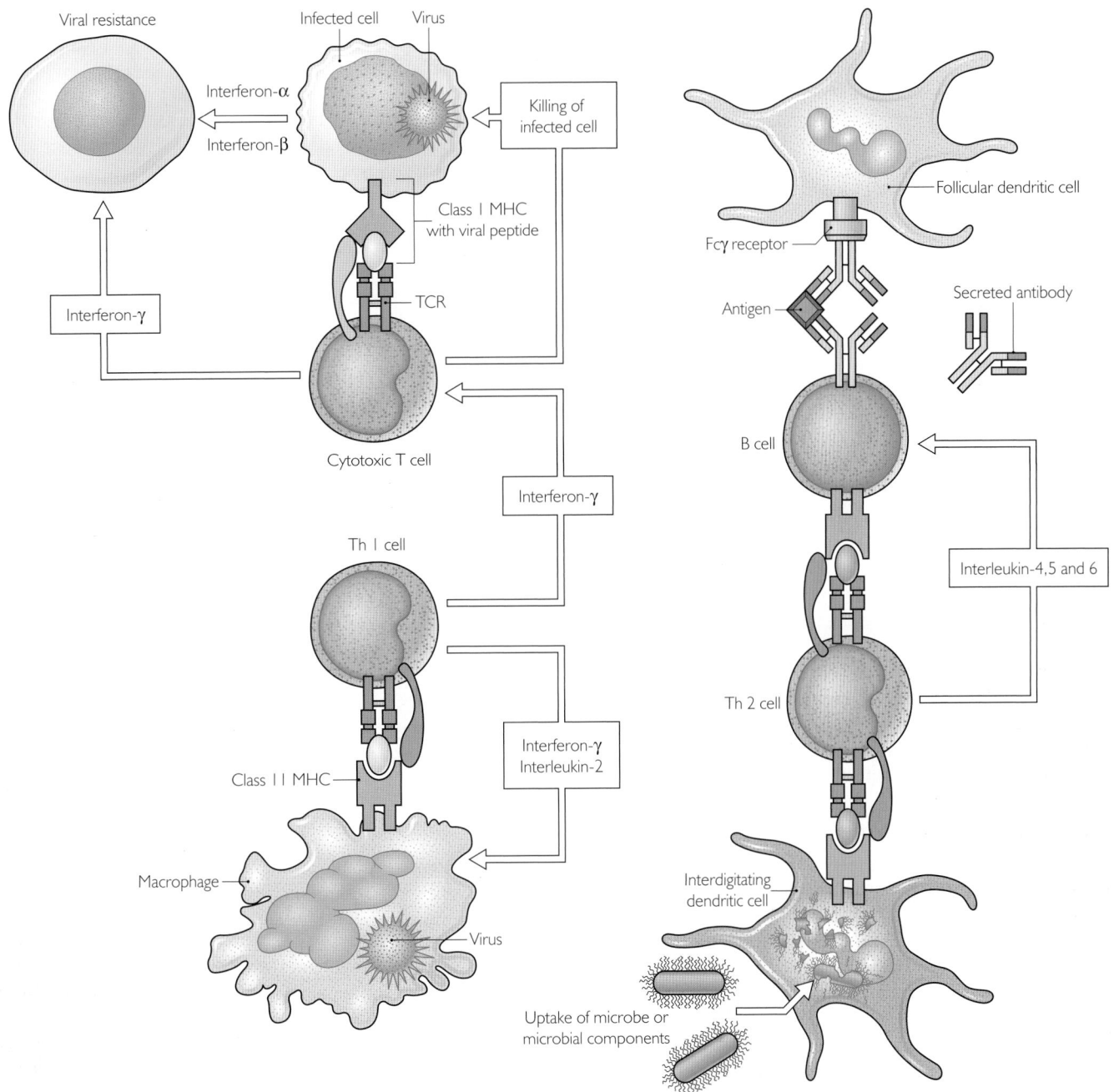

Fig. 40.1 Lymphocyte responses. T-lymphocyte receptors recognise specific processed antigen presented in association with MHC molecules by antigen-presenting cells. Cytotoxic (CD8+) T cells kill infected cells and prevent viral replication (left-hand diagram). Helper T cells (CD4+) either activate cytotoxic T cells and macrophages to kill intracellular organisms (TH1) or secrete cytokines to help B cells secrete antibody (TH2) (right-hand diagram). (Adapted with permission from Delves & Roitt IM.[17] Copyright © 2004 Massachusetts Medical Society. All Rights Reserved.)

T lymphocytes develop from bone marrow stem cells, but mature in the thymus, where their receptor genes (TCR) are rearranged to generate the diversity of lymphocyte receptors needed to counter every potential antigen. Self-reactive T lymphocytes are deleted and only those recognising antigen in association with self MHC are preserved and exit the thymus.

The TCR is similar to the immunoglobulin molecule, with constant and variable parts and the generation of diverse specificity achieved in a similar way. Recombinase activating genes 1 and 2 (RAG1,2) are critical for TCR gene rearrangement. During thymic maturation, T lymphocytes also acquire important functional surface molecules. CD3 is closely associated with the TCR. Initially, both CD4 and CD8 are expressed on the same cells; however, during thymic maturation, one of the molecules is lost. The CD4+ T-helper lymphocyte is the primary effector cell. Once switched on by antigen presentation,

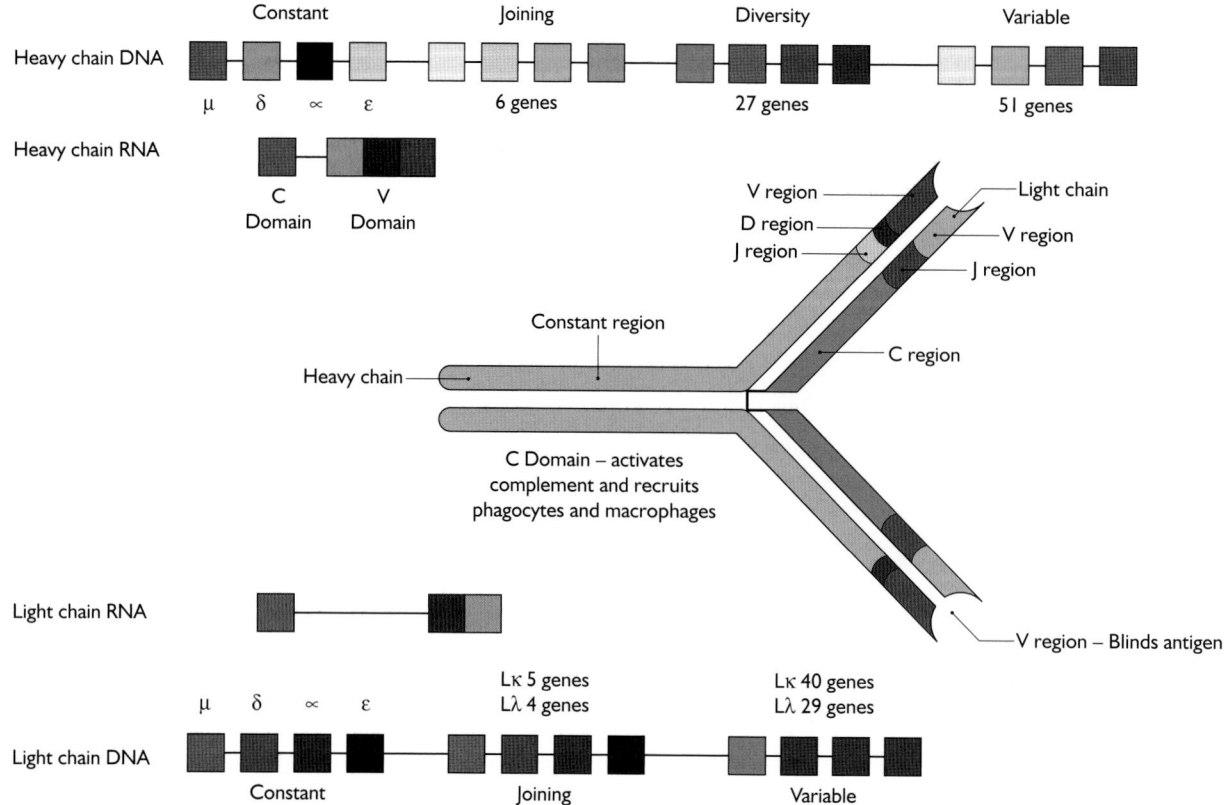

Fig. 40.2 Immunoglobulin heavy- and light-chain gene rearrangements. Discrete segments of the V, D and J heavy-chain genes are rearranged to lie adjacent to the relevant heavy-chain constant-region gene. Light-chain gene rearrangements using V and J segments from either kappa or lambda light chains complete the process. Transcription produces a single protein with a constant and a variable portion. (Adapted with permission from Gennery & Cant.[24])

these cells develop either by the TH1 route, with production of the cytokines interleukin-2 (IL-2) and IFN-γ, stimulating macrophage function, cell-mediated immunity and B lymphocyte class switching to IgG2 production, or to TH2 cells, which produce predominantly IL-4 and IL-10, which promote antibody responses and class switching, particularly towards IgG1, IgG4 and IgE. Allergic responses and those against parasites are of TH2 type. Antigen responses may follow a TH1 or TH2 route, depending on a complex set of circumstances. These responses are self-amplifying and production of IFN-γ or IL-4 promotes TH1 or TH2 responses, respectively, and inhibits the other.

The development of the immune system

Prenatal development

T and B lymphocyte development commences very early in human embryogenesis. Cells capable of responding in mixed lymphocyte culture or to mitogens, and recognisable NK cells are present in the fetal liver from 6 weeks. T- and B-lymphocyte precursors are identifiable from 7–8 weeks. T-lymphocyte precursors colonise the rudimentary thymus from the ninth week. By the second trimester, circulating lymphocytes with mature T-lymphocyte surface markers, including the CD3, CD4 and CD8, are present in fetal blood. Surface B-lymphocyte markers, including surface immunoglobulin, are also expressed at this stage. However, lymphocyte response to antigens, especially by making immunoglobulin, is limited until birth.

Absence of these lymphocyte markers can be used for the antenatal diagnosis of severe combined immunodeficiency (SCID) by fetal blood sampling.

The non-specific elements of immunity also develop early. Neutrophil precursors can be identified in the yolk sac; mature neutrophils appear in the circulation in the second trimester, but numbers are low until the onset of labour. Complement components are present by 6 weeks of gestation.

The immune system in the newborn

The full-term as well as preterm infant immune system exhibits a physiological immunodeficiency,[37] more marked in the premature and particularly sick or stressed infant. This accounts for the newborn's increased susceptibility to infection, whether overwhelming group B streptococcal sepsis, or disseminated herpes simplex infection. Placentally transferred IgG partially offsets the deficiency. However, transfer of immunoglobulin occurs late in gestation, and so preterm infants have significantly reduced levels; those at the limits of viability (23–24 weeks) have extremely low levels. The protective effect of maternal immunoglobulin depends on the mother having the appropriate antigen-specific IgG antibody, and in group B streptococcal sepsis, lack of specific maternal antibody is a major risk factor. The newborn infant shows particularly poor antibody responses to polysaccharide antigens, does not switch from making IgM to IgA and IgG so readily, and does not produce tightly sticking antibody. Diminished T lymphocyte expression of CD40 ligand reduces signalling to B lymphocytes via the CD40 receptor, and so depresses isotype switching.

Neonatal T lymphocytes differ in other ways. There is a high CD4:CD8 ratio, and there is usually less than 10% of the CD45RO (memory) isoform and predominant expression of the CD45RA (naïve) isoform. These proportions gradually reverse during childhood. Exposure to intrauterine infection often provokes a more 'mature' picture.

Naïve T lymphocytes are harder to stimulate, accounting for poorer responses in neonates. Furthermore, the overall balance of neonatal T-lymphocyte responsiveness is tilted towards a TH2 rather than a TH1 response. This may contribute to the susceptibility to intracellular bacterial pathogens, such as *Listeria monocytogenes* or *Salmonella* species, since defences to these pathogens rely on a TH1 pattern response.

Non-specific immune mechanisms are also immature at birth. Neutrophil bone marrow reserves are easily exhausted, leading to neutropenia; chemotaxis and cell deformability are also reduced,[30] whilst neutrophil numbers and function tend to deteriorate in the presence of infection. At term, complement levels and function are at approximately two-thirds of the adult value, and often below one-half in preterm babies, although it is not clear whether these findings significantly predispose to neonatal sepsis.

Whilst low immunoglobulin and complement levels are directly proportional to gestational age, depressed T-lymphocyte function may occur in babies who have suffered severe intrauterine growth restriction (IUGR). The latter has been demonstrated up to 5 years of age, though the clinical significance of such findings is unclear. The placental transfer of immunoglobulin in situations of severe intrauterine growth restriction is probably also compromised, though not all studies have confirmed this.[49]

Postnatal development

Following birth, exposure to a wide variety of antigenic stimuli triggers immunological maturation regardless of gestational age. Initially IgM is mostly produced, but gradually IgG responses develop, and by 2 months of age, infants are able to produce good IgG antibody responses to protein vaccines, such as tetanus toxoid. During this period, maternal IgG levels fall due to catabolism, and a physiological nadir in IgG level occurs at 3–6 months of age, before the infant's production picks up (Fig. 40.3). Thereafter, isotype levels rise at different rates; adult levels of IgM are achieved by 4–5 years, IgG by 7–8 years, whilst serum IgA levels (and secretory IgA) rise only very slowly, not achieving adult

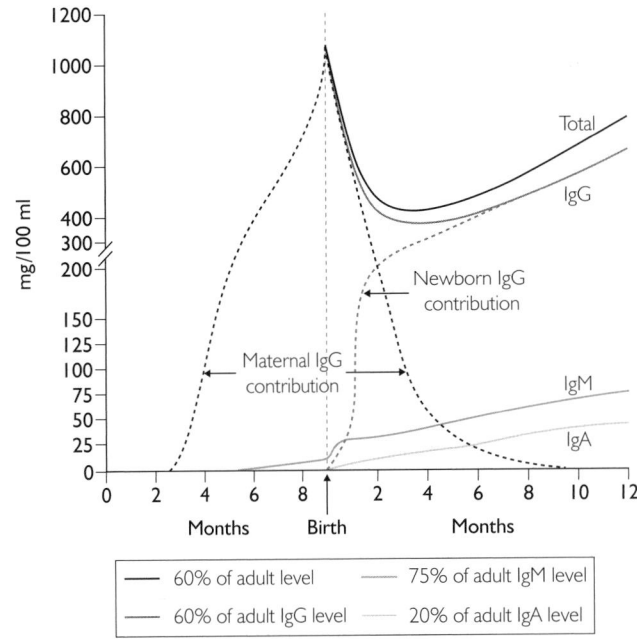

Fig. 40.3 Immunoglobulin levels in fetal life and the first year of postnatal life. (Adapted with permission from Braun & Steihm.[6])

values until teenage years. Most anti-polysaccharide IgG antibody in adults is found in the G2 subclass, and whilst young children make G1 polysaccharide responses, this immaturity probably explains infants' susceptibility to polysaccharide-encapsulated organisms, such as pneumococcus, and the lack of responsiveness of children under the age of 18–24 months to pure polysaccharide vaccines, such as pneumococcal vaccine. Conjugation of the polysaccharide to a protein or peptide facilitates early responsiveness to both components, as demonstrated by the high efficacy of Hib conjugate vaccine and the promising results with the new pneumococcal conjugate vaccines.[14]

T-lymphocyte immunity matures rapidly in the early weeks of life following antigen exposure. T-lymphocyte expression of CD40 ligand improves, as does cytokine production, with the TH1/TH2 balance shifting towards TH1. However, the differences in T-lymphocyte numbers and CD4:CD8 ratios between children and adults, and the unreliable responses of children to delayed hypersensitivity skin test antigens, such as Candida antigen, do suggest that maturation and development of the cell-mediated immune system continues through early childhood. Subtle immaturities in cell-mediated immunity probably account for the increased susceptibility of young children to tuberculosis, and of young infants to invasive salmonellosis and listeriosis.

The maternofetal immunological relationship

The close physiological contact at the placental interface of the fetus and mother has important effects on immunological development and disease. Maternal IgG is actively transferred across the placenta to the fetus from about 14 weeks' gestation, and by term, cord blood IgG levels are higher than those in maternal blood. IgG1 and IgG3 are principally transferred, but little IgG2 is transferred, compounding the poor neonatal response to encapsulated bacteria such as the group B streptococcus.

Placentally transferred maternal IgG occasionally causes fetal or neonatal disease. Most maternal anti-fetal immunoglobulins bind to fetal antigen expressed at the centre of the placental villus, and thus never cross to the fetus. However, some antigens expressed on highly differentiated fetal cells are not expressed at the placental villus, and so antibody can thus cross and cause disease such as Rhesus disease, neonatal thyrotoxicosis and myasthenia gravis. Maternal anti-Ro antibodies, found in systemic lupus erythematosus (SLE), can cause a transient neonatal SLE, but also damage the fetal cardiac conduction pathway, leading to permanent neonatal heart block (pp. 655–7), which may require cardiac pacing. Maternal medication can also cross the placental barrier, and maternally acquired immunosuppressive medication such as ciclosporin (cyclosporin) or azathioprine can lead to transient neonatal lymphopenia and hypogammaglobulinaemia. Viruses such as cytomegalovirus (CMV) can also cross the placenta and are not effectively excluded by fetal cell-mediated immunity, allowing progressive infection or persistent viral excretion.

Maternal breast milk is an important source of neonatal immunological protection. It contains secretory IgA, which acts locally in the neonatal gut to neutralise viral and bacterial pathogens. It may also modulate exposure to foreign milkprotein antigens, which may lessen the risk both of food intolerance and of atopy (e.g. eczema or asthma). Other protective factors in breast milk include soluble factors such as lactoferrin and lysozyme, as well as cells such as neutrophils and macrophages.

Immunodeficiency disorders: general principles

Classification and genetics

Immunodeficiency may be due to primary or secondary defects. The World Health Organisation (WHO) working party on immunodeficiency[46] has classified the primary disorders (Table 40.1). The incidence of any significant immune deficiency disorder (excluding selective IgA deficiency) is 1 in 10 000.

Many of the primary disorders have a genetic basis, and in many, the molecular basis is understood.[22] These discoveries have enhanced understanding of the immune response, and led to more focused treatment of primary immune deficiencies. Precise genetic diagnosis has also aided antenatal diagnosis.

Diagnosis and investigation of immunodeficiency

A careful history and examination should precede any laboratory tests as this will help determine which children should be investigated further and the nature and extent of investigations (Table 40.2).

History

Pregnancy and birth history may suggest possible congenital infection, intrauterine growth retardation or prematurity, all of which are associated with immune defects. Delayed separation of the umbilical cord, in the absence of local infection, may suggest a neutrophil defect. Risk factors for HIV in the parents should be sought. A family history may reveal other children with unusual or fatal infectious complications, suggesting an autosomal recessive (AR) or X-linked pattern of inheritance. A history of consanguinity is important. In some disorders, e.g. IgA deficiency, there may be a family history of collagen vascular or other immunopathological disease. Older relatives who are carriers of or who are affected by milder variants of primary immune defects may have autoimmune manifestations (e.g. mouth ulcers and SLE variant in chronic granulomatous disease [CGD]) or have a history of malignant disease (lymphoma in X-linked lymphoproliferative disease).

Examination

Examination should be directed towards potential sites of infection, including the throat, ears and mouth, and nappy area for candidiasis. The presence or absence of lymphoid tissue should be noted. In more severe antibody states such as SCID and X-linked agammaglobulinaemia, there is a lack of tonsils and lymphoid tissues, although visualising tonsillar tissue in neonates and small infants can be very difficult. Some diseases may have specific physical signs, such as oculocutaneous albinism in Chediak–Higashi syndrome (CHS), typical facies and/or cleft palate in DiGeorge syndrome, and disproportionate short stature in some forms of combined immune deficiency.

Radiological evaluation

Radiological evaluation, directed by findings from history and examination, may be useful. Bony abnormalities may be seen in adenosine deaminase (ADA) deficiency,[13] Shwachman–Diamond syndrome or other dysplasias associated with immune defects. Absence of a thymus on anterior-posterior and lateral chest radiographs is consistent with a combined immune defect in infants and young children, but thymic atrophy may also occur in response to stress (e.g. infection) and this finding is not diagnostic.

Laboratory investigation

There are little scientific data that help determine which infants should be investigated, but the following should trigger investigation: family history consistent with immune deficiency,

Table 40.1 Primary immunodeficiencies (Adapted from Rosen et al[46])

Immunodeficiency	Cells affected	Gene defect	Inheritance	Neonatal presentation
Cell mediated				
SCID				
$T^-B^+NK^-$	T, NK	CgC	XL	Yes
$T^-B^+NK^-$	T, NK	JAK3	AR	Yes
$T^-B^+NK^+$	T	IL7Ra	AR	Yes
$T^-B^-NK^+$	T, B	RAG 1,2	AR	Yes
$T^-B^-NK^+$	T, B	artemis	AR	Yes
$T^+B^-NK^+$		T-B-SCID with MFE or Omenn's syndrome	AR	Yes
ADA deficiency	T, B, NK	Adenosine deaminase	AR	Yes
PNP deficiency	T, B, NK	Purine nucleoside phosphorylase	AR	No
CID				
MHC II deficiency	Low T (CD4)	Defective MHCII expression	AR	No
MHC I deficiency	Low T (CD8)	Defective MHCI expression	AR	No
CD40L deficiency (XL hyper-IgM)	T	Defective CD40L	XL	No
Wiskott–Aldrich syndrome	T, B, platelet	WAS	XL	Yes
ZAP 70 kinase deficiency	T (low CD8)	ZAP 70 kinase	AR	No
XL lymphoproliferative disease	T, B	SAP	XL	No
DiGeorge syndrome	T, B	22q11 deletion	Sporadic, occasional AD	Yes
Cartilage hair hypolasia	T, B	RMRP gene	AR	Yes
Ataxia telangiectasia	T, B	ATM gene	AR	No
Nijmegen breakage syndrome	T, B	NBS1 gene	AR	Yes
Antibody deficiency				
X-linked agammaglobulinaemia	Absent B	Btk	XL	No
XL hyper-IgM (see CD40L deficiency)				
Autosomal recessive hyper-IgM syndrome	B	AID, CD40	AR	No
AR agammaglobulinaemia	Absent B	μ chain	AR	No
Transient hypogammaglobulinaemia of infancy		Unknown	Unknown	No
Phagocyte defects				
XL chronic granulomatous disease	Neutrophils	Killing gp91phox	XL	Yes
AR chronic granulomatous disease	Neutrophil killing	Killing gp22phox	AR	Unusual
		Killing gp47phox		
		Killing gp67phox		
LAD I	Neutrophil adherence	CD18	AR	Yes
Chediak–Higashi	Chemotaxis		AR	Yes
Griscelli	Chemotaxis		AR	Yes
Congenital neutropenia	Absent neutrophils	ELA gene – some	AR	Yes
		WAS	XL	
(Kostmann's syndrome)			Sporadic	
Shwachman syndrome	Chemotaxis	SBDS	AR	Yes

(Continued)

Table 40.1 (Continued)

Immunodeficiency	Cells affected	Gene defect	Inheritance	Neonatal presentation
Hyper-IgE syndrome	Unknown	Unknown	Sporadic, some AD	Yes
Mycobactericidal defect	Macrophages, T	IFNγ receptor 1,2	AR	Yes
		IL-12 receptor		
		IL-12		
Complement deficiencies				
C1–9		C1–9 gene defects	AR	No
Properdin		Properdin gene	XL	No
Factor H, I		Factor H, I gene	AR	No

Table 40.2 Neonatal immunodeficiency – diagnostic clues

History
Parental consanguinity
Family history of immunodeficiency
History of early infectious deaths
Autoimmune disease in the mother (e.g. SLE)
Immunosupressive drug therapy in the mother (e.g. azathioprine)
Infection during pregnancy (e.g. CMV)
Extreme IUGR with maternal hypertension
Risk factors for HIV
Persistent diarrhoea
Recurrent/chronic superficial candidiasis
Recurrent bacterial infections
Infection with unusual or opportunistic organism
Failure to thrive

Examination
Skin rash, eczema, pustulosis
Hepatosplenomegaly
Absence of lymphoid tissue
Axillary or inguinal lymphadenopathy
Cardiac disease especially truncus, Fallot, with reduced thymic
  shadow on X-ray
Oculocutaneous albinism
Unusual facies and cleft palate
Delayed separation of the umbilical cord
Sparse light hair and short length

Investigations
Lymphopenia ($<2.7 \times 10^9$/l)
Neutropenia
Abnormal blood film – leukocyte granules or Howell–Jolly bodies
Low immunoglobulins
Autoantibodies (may be maternal)
Thrombocytopenia with small platelets
Lack of thymic shadow on X-ray
ADA skeletal abnormalities (cupping deformities of the ends of
  the ribs, abnormal transverse vertebral processes, scapulae)

single infection with an unusual/opportunistic organism (e.g. *Pneumocystis carinii*), single infection which is atypically severe or has an atypical course, or more than one episode of serious bacterial infection.

Haematology

A full blood count and blood film examination is extremely useful. Neutropenia is readily detected. Bone marrow aspiration will distinguish between failure of production and increased peripheral destruction, and exclude a myelodysplastic or malignant process. Neutrophilia in the absence of overt infection may suggest a neutrophil adhesion defect or functional problem (e.g. CGD). Lymphopenia, using appropriate age-related ranges, is highly suggestive of a combined immune deficiency of primary or secondary aetiology,[28] but a normal lymphocyte count does not exclude SCID. A manual differential will differentiate nucleated red cells in infants and abnormal leukocyte morphology in sick children. Abnormal leukocyte granules are characteristic of CHS. Platelet volume is universally low in Wiskott–Aldrich syndrome.[41]

Tests of innate immunity

Complement function should be assayed by testing the ability of patient serum to lyse sensitised red blood cells, thus testing the whole pathway. Deficiency in any one component will result in a failure of lysis. Samples must be separated and frozen within 2 hours of venesection. If repeat testing shows a persistent abnormality, evaluation of individual complement components should be performed.

Neutrophil function tests are technically difficult, as neutrophils activate and then quickly die after venesection. The nitroblue tetrazolium (NBT) test is a rapid and sensitive test for CGD, but false normal results can be seen when the test is performed infrequently; it is now being superseded by the more reliable flow cytometric evaluation of the neutrophil oxidative burst.

Adaptive immune system

Test of humoral immunity
Immunoglobulins
IgG is the predominant circulating immunoglobulin, and in the neonate, most is maternal in origin. Smaller amounts of IgA, IgM, IgD and IgE are found in serum. IgG, IgA and IgM are routinely measured by nephelometry. Results must be compared with age-specific normal ranges (Appendix 6), as production of all five classes of immunoglobulin is low at birth and gradually matures over the first 5 years of life. Immunoglobulin can be lost via the gut or urinary tract. Low levels of immunoglobulin can only be attributed to a production defect if gut or renal losses have been excluded and the serum albumin is within the normal range. Measurement of IgE is indicated if hyper-IgE (Job's) syndrome is included in the differential diagnosis.

Measures of in-vivo antibody responses
Functional antibody is more important than the amount of circulating antibody. Functional tests of IgG production rely on measuring antibody titres to antigens to which the child is known to have been exposed either naturally or by vaccination. Responses to protein antigens such as tetanus and the conjugated Hib vaccine are widely available. If antibody titres are low, booster vaccinations should be given to assess the memory response.

Cell-mediated immunity
Cell-mediated defects are likely to result in poor antibody responses, as these depend on T-lymphocyte help in making an antibody response with memory.

Quantification of cell numbers
Lymphocytes can be enumerated using flow cytometry, characterised by their cell surface markers and expressed either as a percentage of the lymphocyte pool or as an absolute number. Proportions of different lymphocytes and absolute numbers vary with age, and age-related normal ranges should be consulted.[15]

In-vitro lymphocyte proliferation assays
Culturing lymphocytes for a defined time period with an appropriate non-specific stimulus and using the incorporation of tritiated thymidine or a non-radioactive marker such as bromodeoxyuridine into the DNA of dividing cells acts as a surrogate measure of cell proliferation.

Definition of molecular defects

The genetic basis of an increasing number of immune deficiencies is well defined. Usually, a gene defect coding for the protein results in no protein expression, expression of low amounts, or expression of abnormally sized protein, and can be detected by Western blotting and flow cytometry.[26] In the presence of an appropriate history or abnormal protein expression, genetic analysis may be undertaken.

Carrier testing

When a primary immunodeficiency is diagnosed, families should be offered genetic counselling. Parents can be tested for carrier status by mutation analysis if the mutation has been defined. Carrier status can also be determined by other tests such as the NBT, in which intermediate numbers of neutrophils will reduce NBT in mothers who carry the mutation, as will intermediate levels of ADA in carriers of ADA deficiency.

Antenatal diagnosis

Appropriate counselling by an individual conversant with the outcome of immune deficiencies in the modern era should be undertaken before antenatal diagnosis is offered. Due to the small risk of miscarriage, screening should be offered only to mothers in whom the result would determine whether the mother would terminate the pregnancy. The gestation at which antenatal diagnosis can be undertaken is influenced by the nature of the immune deficiency.

Specific primary immunodeficiencies

The complete spectrum of primary immunodeficiency is beyond the scope of this chapter, which will focus on those disorders that present very early in life. More comprehensive texts are recommended for those requiring more information.[42,52]

Disorders of cell-mediated immunity: severe combined immunodeficiencies

Failure to develop normal T and B lymphocytes is usually due to a specific gene defect affecting early lymphocyte development or subsequent signalling pathways, but as T lymphocytes are critical for the maturation and function of B lymphocytes, the more severe T-lymphocyte deficiencies are often accompanied by defective antibody responses and also result in combined deficiency. Combined immunodeficiency results from a large number of disorders with X-linked or AR inheritance, most of which are now molecularly defined (Fig. 40.4, Table 40.1).[8] The most severe phenotype is SCID (Fig. 40.5) associated with a profound T lymphopenia and panhypogammaglobulinaemia, with early death from infection. Whilst the usual clinical features of this group of diseases are well characterised, atypical presentations and 'leaky' forms with an attenuated phenotype are increasingly recognised. Circulating T-lymphocyte numbers are usually low or absent but may be normal. In the classic SCID presentation, lymphocyte responses to mitogen are absent. Patients usually have a limited diversity of T-lymphocyte receptor and immunoglobulin gene rearrangements. Identifying the molecular defect in specific patients with combined immunodeficiency

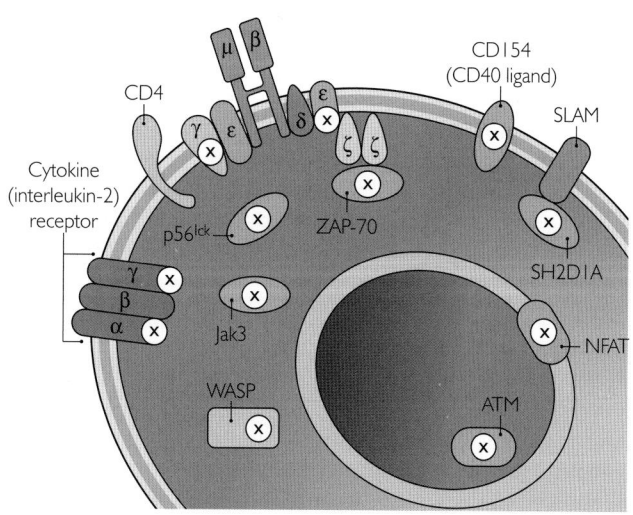

Fig. 40.4 Locations of mutant proteins in CD4$^+$ T cells identified in primary immunodeficiency diseases. Mutant proteins are marked with a red X. ZAP-70, zeta-associated protein; SLAM, signalling lymphocyte activation molecule; SH2D1A, SLAM-associated protein; ATM, ataxia telangiectasia mutation; NFAT, nuclear factor of activated T cells; Jak3, Janus kinase 3; WASP, Wiskott–Aldrich syndrome protein. (Adapted with permission from Buckley.[8] Copyright © 2004 Massachusetts Medical Society. All Rights Reserved.)

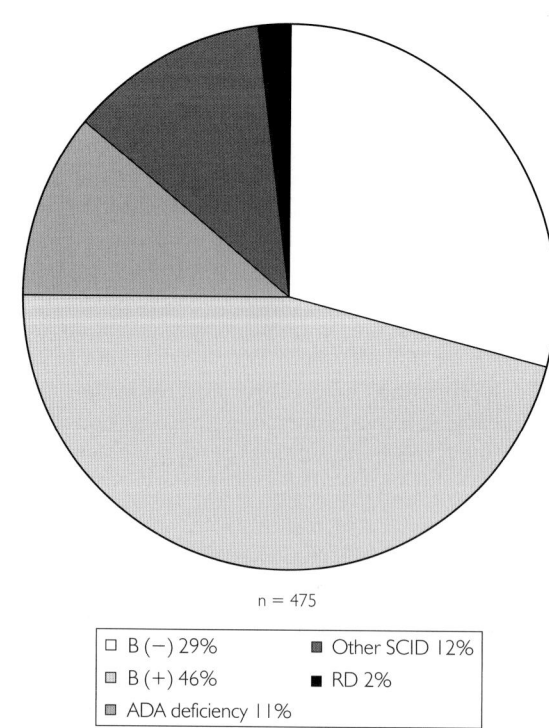

n = 475

☐ B (−) 29%	■ Other SCID 12%
▨ B (+) 46%	■ RD 2%
▥ ADA deficiency 11%	

Fig. 40.5 Relative frequencies of the various types of severe combined immunodeficiency among 475 European patients. (Adapted from Antoine et al.[1])

or SCID is important for prognosis, treatment and genetic counselling.

General features of severe combined immunodeficiency

Affected babies appear well at birth but within the first few months of life fail to clear infection and present with persistent respiratory tract or gut infection, failure to thrive and, sometimes, apparent food intolerance.[21] Persistent respiratory tract infection with respiratory syncytial virus or parainfluenza viruses is common, with failure to clear virus accompanying persistent bronchiolitic-like signs. An insidiously progressive persistent respiratory infection with radiological evidence of interstitial pneumonitis should raise the suspicion of *Pneumocystis carinii* infection, often a co-pathogen with respiratory viruses. Other presentations include prolonged otitis media and invasive bacterial infections, particularly staphylococcal or pseudomonas septicaemia and pneumonia, which may respond poorly to appropriate treatment. Severe invasive fungal infection is rare, but often fatal. Extensive persistent superficial candidiasis is more common. Occasionally babies present with disseminated BCG or vaccine-strain poliomyelitis virus. Epstein-Barr viral infection may lead to uncontrolled B lymphoproliferative disorders, similar to that seen in solid-organ transplant recipients.

Congenital graft-versus-host disease (GVHD) occurs because many infants with SCID are unable to reject foreign lymphocytes acquired either from the mother in utero or from an unirradiated blood transfusion. When clinically apparent, there is typically a mild reticular skin rash, sometimes with abnormal liver function tests. GVHD following transfusion with non-irradiated blood or white cell or platelet concentrates is generally more severe and can be fatal. In these cases, the skin rash is severe and lymphadenopathy and hepatosplenomegaly may be present. The clinical picture may be indistinguishable from Omenn's syndrome, but identification of maternal cells by karyotype or DNA fingerprinting will distinguish maternofetal GVHD from Omenn's syndrome.

Examination usually reveals a wasted child who has dropped through the growth centiles, with evidence of candidiasis and other infections. Skin rashes may indicate infection or GVHD. There is no clinically detectable lymphoid tissue. There may be hepatomegaly.

Investigation usually shows severe lymphopenia from birth. It should be remembered that in infancy a normal lymphocyte count is $>2.7 \times 10^9/l$ (unlike adults, where it is $>1.0 \times 10^9/l$). Lymphocytic phenotyping shows severely depleted T-lymphocyte numbers; B lymphocytes and NK cells may be present or absent, depending on the type of SCID. Occasional variants show unusual patterns of immature T-lymphocyte markers; in such cases, maternal engraftment should be excluded. Mitogen responses are usually absent. Immunoglobulin estimations show low levels of IgG, IgA and IgM but residual maternal IgG may give a falsely reassuring result and it can be difficult distinguishing IgA and IgM levels in SCID from the low levels seen in normal infants. Isohaemagglutinins are a useful measure of in-vitro IgM production, and absence is significant. If SCID is suspected, lymphocyte phenotyping is more reliable than immunoglobulin estimation.

Chest radiographs show an absent thymus and, if infection is present, hyperinflation and/or interstitial pneumonia.

In children who die, postmortem examination reveals severely depleted lymphoid tissue, with nodes and thymus showing no lymphoid follicles and absent Hassall's corpuscles in the thymus. Without treatment, patients die from infection by about 12 months of age. Currently, the only curative treatment is bone marrow transplantation (BMT), although clinical gene therapy trials for common gamma chain and ADA deficiency are in progress. Supportive interim treatments include antibiotic prophylaxis with co-trimoxazole as anti-pneumocystis treatment, antifungal prophylaxis and antibody replacement (intravenous immunoglobulin [IVIG]). Live vaccines, including BCG, must be avoided. The diagnosis of SCID is a paediatric emergency, and suspected cases should be urgently referred to a designated treatment centre for assessment and treatment.

Newborns suspected of having a severe immunodeficiency disorder should be protected using isolation techniques, including limitation of the numbers of persons involved with care; individuals with respiratory or gastrointestinal symptoms of infection should avoid contact. Breastfeeding should be encouraged. Wherever the child is managed, the importance of strict hand-washing procedures cannot be overemphasised. If BMT with conditioning chemotherapy is embarked upon, isolation in facilities with positive-pressure filtered air supply is necessary, mainly to reduce the risk of aspergillosis and droplet-borne viral infections. Blood products should be CMV negative and irradiated to avoid the risk of transfusion GVHD.

Types of severe combined and combined immunodeficiencies

T-negative B-positive SCID

Common gamma chain deficiency (X-linked SCID)
The most common form of SCID is characterised by severe lymphopenia, absence of mature T and NK lymphocytes, but normal numbers of circulating B lymphocytes (T⁻B⁺NK⁻). It is caused by a deficiency of the gamma chain common to the IL-2, IL-4, IL-7, IL-9 and IL-15 receptors.

JAK-3 deficiency
This AR form of SCID is phenotypically identical to X-linked SCID (T⁻B⁺NK⁻) but is due to mutations in the gene encoding Janus-associated-kinase 3, a signalling protein immediately downstream from the common gamma chain.

IL-7Ra deficiency
This rare AR form of SCID is characterised by a T⁻B⁺NK⁺ phenotype.

T-negative B-negative SCID
Two forms of this AR disorder have been described; in both, T and B lymphocytes are absent, but normal numbers of NK cells are present. The first is due to defects in the RAG genes, which code for enzymes that cut the DNA of the T- and B-cell receptor genes prior to gene rearrangement. In the second form, a

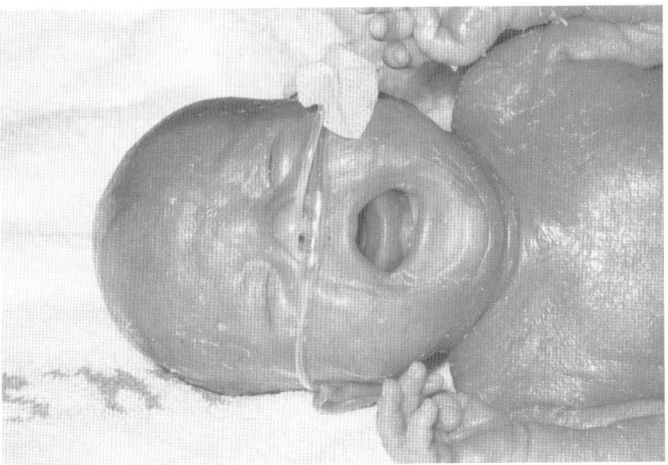

Fig. 40.6 Omenn's syndrome. Newborn infant with typical features of Omenn's syndrome, including generalised scaly erythroderma, alopecia, lymphadenopathy and hepatosplenomegaly. (Reproduced with permission from the Audiovisual Department, University of Newcastle.)

defect in the artemis genes prevents cells repairing DNA normally and so T- and B-cell receptor gene rearrangement is impaired and patients' fibroblasts show in-vitro radiosensitivity. 'Leaky' RAG defects have been shown in some patients with Omenn's syndrome.

Omenn's syndrome
Omenn's syndrome is characterised by a generalised erythematous rash, with scaling and erythroderma, lymphadenopathy, hepatosplenomegaly, increased serum IgE levels with a marked eosinophilia, and usual clinical features of SCID (Fig. 40.6).[40] Children usually present in early infancy, and may present at birth. There are high numbers of oligoclonal activated, poorly functional T lymphocytes of the TH2 phenotype but absent B lymphocytes and low levels of immunoglobulin. The syndrome is a 'leaky' form of SCID in that small numbers of very abnormal T lymphocytes 'leak' past the block in T-lymphocyte development. The underlying defect in some cases is a mutation in the RAG genes. In some families, one affected individual has presented with T⁻B⁻NK⁺ SCID whilst another has presented with Omenn's syndrome. The clinical picture may resemble SCID with maternofoetal engraftment, and molecular genetic studies to identify the origin of the dermal infiltrative T lymphocytes can differentiate the two disorders. BMT is the only curative treatment.

Netherton's syndrome
This triad of generalised infantile erythroderma, diarrhoea and failure to thrive may be associated with a variable immunodeficiency, including mild lymphopenia. The clinical features are similar to those seen in Omenn's syndrome and in SCID and maternofoetal engraftment. Distinguishing these entities is important, as the other conditions are treated by BMT, whereas Netherton's syndrome is not. Hair-shaft abnormalities are diagnostic (bamboo hairs).

Reticular dysgenesis

This rare AR-inherited form of SCID is characterised by defective lymphoid and myeloid differentiation. Bone marrow examination confirms the absence of myeloid precursors. Platelets and red cells are formed normally. The disorder may be due to other forms of SCID, complicated by severe maternal engraftment and bone marrow GVHD.[38] The absence of the non-specific cellular elements of the immune system makes the immune deficiency even more severe than in other forms of SCID. BMT is the only effective treatment.

Adenosine deaminase deficiency

This disorder due to a single gene defect results in absence of the purine salvage pathway enzyme ADA,[31] leading to accumulation of the toxic DNA breakdown products. Immature lymphocytes are particularly susceptible, with resulting cell death. Patients present early, with very low numbers of T, B and NK lymphocytes. Skeletal abnormalities, cupping deformities of rib ends, abnormal transverse vertebral processes and 'squaring off' of the scapulae, are seen in many cases.[13] Neurodevelopmental problems may also occur in some patients.[45] Very low erythrocyte ADA activity and high levels of dATP in the urine are diagnostic. First-trimester antenatal diagnosis can be made by assaying ADA activity in chorionic villus sampling. Treatment is by BMT or by use of replacement polyethelene glycol-coupled ADA (PEG-ADA).

Major histocompatibility complex class II deficiency

MHC class II antigens (HLA DR, DP, DQ) are expressed on a limited repertoire of cells and present antigen to CD4+ T lymphocytes, which, with the help of an appropriate second signal, leads to the activation of T-helper lymphocytes specific for that antigen and an effective immune response. Expression of MHC II in the thymus is also essential for positive selection of CD4+ T lymphocytes. Since HLA antigens are of vital importance for lymphocyte development and function, lack of MHC II expression results in a profound susceptibility to viral, bacterial, fungal and protozoal infections.[33]

Autosomal recessive MHC II deficiency is rare and can result from mutations in several different genes which code for a complex of regulatory factors controlling transcription of MHC II genes.

The clinical picture resembles SCID, although sometimes infections develop slightly later. Intestinal and hepatic complications due to cryptosporidial infections are more common than in other immune defects. Neurological manifestations due to a range of viral infections are also well described. Coxsackie virus, adenovirus and poliovirus are the most frequently reported causes of meningoencephalitis.

Most patients have a CD4 lymphopenia and hypogammaglobulinaemia; lymphocyte proliferation responses are normal. The diagnosis can be confirmed flow cytometrically by showing absent or significantly reduced levels of class II molecules on B lymphocytes and monocytes. Definitive treatment is BMT, although this has had limited success in comparison with in other types of SCID.

Combined immunodeficiency forming part of other syndromes

DiGeorge anomaly

This condition results from abnormal cephalic neural crest cell migration into the third and fourth pharyngeal arches in early embryological development. A microdeletion at chromosome 22q11.2 is present in 90% of cases, while the remainder are associated with other chromosomal anomalies, particularly 10p–. It is usually sporadic, though familial cases, some associated with 22q chromosomal deletions, have been reported, with a prevalence of 1 in 3000–4000 live births. Whilst classically recognised by the triad of congenital heart defects, immunodeficiency secondary to thymic hypoplasia, and hypocalcemia secondary to parathyroid gland hypoplasia, an expanded phenotype is increasingly recognised, with dysmorphic facies (low-set, abnormally formed ears, hypertelorism and antimongoloid slant, micrognathia, short philtrum to the upper lip and high arched palate), palatal abnormalities (cleft palate, velopharyngeal insufficiency), autoimmune phenomena, learning difficulties, (particularly speech delay), renal anomalies, neuropsychiatric disorders and short stature. Conotruncal heart defects are most often associated with the syndrome, but other defects seen include tetralogy of Fallot, septal defects, pulmonary atresia and aberrant subclavian vessels. Some patients have normal hearts.

Severe T-lymphocyte immunodeficiency presenting with a SCID phenotype of profound lymphopenia and poor lymphocyte proliferation is rare and accounts for <1.5% of cases.

However, all children suspected of having DiGeorge syndrome (with or without 22q11.2 deletion) should have an immunological evaluation including lymphocyte subset analysis, T-lymphocyte proliferative responses, immunoglobulin levels and specific antibody responses to vaccination antigens. Laboratory findings may show severe T-lymphocyte depletion with poor mitogen responses, or relatively normal findings. Immunoglobulin levels may be normal but hypogammaglobulinemia may develop, and minor humoral abnormalities are common. Chest X-ray shows lack of a thymic shadow.

Blood products should be irradiated if T-lymphocyte mitogen responses are poor. Patients with severe immune deficiency have been successfully treated with BMT. In the partial phenotype with normal T-lymphocyte function, the usual infant vaccination schedule can be followed. It is safe to give live vaccines such as oral polio vaccine, measles, mumps, rubella vaccine, or varicella zoster vaccine as long as the CD4 count exceeds 400/mm[3], and there are normal T-lymphocyte mitogen responses. Demonstration of good antibody responses to tetanus and *Haemophilus influenzae* type B vaccination give further reassurance that live vaccines can be safely administered.[20] Prophylactic antibiotics and, occasionally, IVIG can be helpful, particularly for young children with recurrent infection due to humoral deficiency.

Wiskott–Aldrich syndrome

Immunodeficiency, thrombocytopenia, eczema and an increased risk of autoimmune disorders and malignancy characterise this

X-linked recessive condition. Mutations in the same gene are found in patients with X-linked thrombocytopenia.

Clinical features of Wiskott–Aldrich syndrome can be surprisingly mild, especially in the newborn. Thrombocytopenia with a low mean platelet volume (<5 fl) is always present and should raise suspicion of the diagnosis even if bruising and bleeding are minimal.

Acute bleeding episodes may require platelet transfusions (irradiated to prevent GVHD). IVIG, with or without prophylactic antibiotics, reduces infections, and splenectomy may suppress autoimmune phenomena, but BMT is the only curative therapy. Without BMT, the prognosis is variable, but median life expectancy is 11 years.[53]

X-linked hyper-IgM syndrome (CD40 ligand deficiency)

X-linked hyper-IgM syndrome is a combined immunodeficiency caused by a T-lymphocyte defect and not an isolated antibody deficiency as was previously thought. The defect is in the gene encoding for the CD40 ligand (CD154) expressed on T lymphocytes which activate B lymphocytes and monocyte/macrophage-derived cells. Without CD40L binding, B lymphocytes cannot switch from IgM to IgA, IgG and IgE production. Pulmonary macrophages are not activated, resulting in *Pneumocytis carinii* pneumonia, and ineffective Kupffer cell function allows repeated infection with *Cryptosporidium parvum* and similar organisms, leading to sclerosing cholangitis, pancreatitis and malignancy. Absent IgA and IgG results in sinopulmonary and invasive bacterial infection. Neutropenia with oral ulceration is common and this together with low or absent IgA and IgG, and normal or raised IgM, should suggest the diagnosis.[39]

Patients should receive co-trimoxazole, as *Pneumocystis carinii* pneumonia (PCP) prophylaxis, and immunoglobulin replacement therapy. With adequate replacement, the rising IgM levels may normalise. The neutropenia sometimes responds to granulocyte colony-stimulating factor (G-CSF) and IVIG. All drinking water should be boiled. Azithromycin prophylaxis may lessen the risks of *Cryptosporidium parvum*. BMT is increasingly being recommended for this condition.

Immunodeficiency and short-limbed dwarfism

Cartilage hair hypoplasia is the best described form, inherited in an AR manner. Severe short-limbed short stature (−11.8 SD to −2.1 SD) with X-ray appearances of metaphyseal and spondyloepiphyseal dysplasia are always present, accompanied by sparse light hair in most patients. Severe anaemia and Hirschsprung disease are uncommon but well-recognised associations, as are malignancies, notably lymphoma and skin carcinoma. The immunodeficiency is surprisingly variable; most have T lymphopenia and impaired in-vitro mitogen proliferative responses, but only half suffer recurrent infection.[36] However, some have IgA and/or IgG subclass deficiencies, with frequent ear infections. Patients are excessively vulnerable to viral infections, particularly varicella-zoster virus, Epstein-Barr virus and other human herpesvirus infections, and the risk of infective death is 300 times greater than normal.[35] Severely affected patients should be assessed for BMT, which has been successful in correcting the immunodeficiency.

Abnormalities of T- and B-lymphocyte function are seen in a number of other osteochondrodysplasias, including Schwachmann syndrome, where there is neutropenia and pancreatic insufficiency and Schimke immuno-osseous dysplasia which features radiographic changes of spondyloepiphyseal dysplasia, nephrotic syndrome and cellular immunodeficiency.

DNA repair defects and immunodeficiency

The immune system uses cellular DNA repair mechanisms to generate the diversity of specific immune responses by rearrangement of the variable (V), diversity (D) and joining (J) gene segments that code for T- or B-lymphocyte receptor genes (VDJ recombination). Inability to repair DNA damage causes cellular apoptosis or malignant proliferation, and so individuals with defective DNA repair mechanisms have a predisposition to neurodegeneration, developmental anomalies and cancer, as well as defective immunity.[25] Single gene defects cause a number of distinct clinical entities of which ataxia telangiectasia is the best known, although the features are not apparent in the neonatal period. Nijmegen breakage syndrome (NBS), an AR disorder, is characterised by microcephaly, mental retardation, 'bird-like' facies, immunodeficiency, clinical radiation sensitivity and chromosomal instability.[29] It should be considered when investigating an infant with features of bird-headed dwarfism. Fanconi's anaemia presents with progressive bone marrow failure leading to pancytopenia. There may also be skeletal malformations, and immunodeficiency can occur.

Other immunodeficiencies

A number of syndromes that include primary immunodeficiency as part of the phenotype have been described. Although most lack clear definition, the syndrome is well described in some, and the underlying molecular defect has been elucidated in some.

Hoyeraal–Hreidarsson syndrome

This X-linked disorder is characterised by microcephaly, cerebellar hypoplasia, aplastic anaemia and growth retardation. A progressive combined immunodeficiency, with hypogammaglobulinaemia and lymphopenia, is a well-recognised association.

Anhydrotic ectodermal dysplasia, incontinentia pigmenti and defects in the NEMO gene

Until recently, incontinentia pigmenti and X-linked anhydrotic ectodermal dysplasia were thought to be unrelated disorders. Incontinentia pigmenti (p. 823) is a rare X-linked dominant condition characterised by developmental abnormalities of the skin, hair, teeth and central nervous system. Affected female infants present with a characteristic rash, occurring in four phases of erythema and vesicles, hyperkeratosis, hyperpigmentation and finally pallor and atrophy. Previously thought lethal in male fetuses carrying the affected X chromosome, rare male infants with a progressive combined immunodeficiency have been described. Patients with X-linked anhydrotic ectodermal dysplasia present with sparse scalp hair, conical teeth and absent sweat glands. Some suffer from recurrent sinopulmonary infection, often with encapsulated organisms, and have poor antibody responses to polysaccharide antigens, or frank hypogammaglobulinaemia. Recently, hypofunctional mutations in the NEMO gene encoding a protein required to activate the transcription factor NF-kB have been described in male patients with both incontinentia pigmenti and X-linked anhydrotic ectodermal dysplasia, suggesting that these conditions represent variants of the same disorder.[19]

IPEX syndrome

The IPEX (immune dysregulation, polyendocrinopathy, enteropathy, X-linked) syndrome is characterised by infantile ichthyosiform dermatitis, protracted diarrhoea, insulin-dependent diabetes mellitus and thyroiditis.[4] Mutations in the FOXP3 gene have recently been described in affected patients. BMT has been tried as a curative treatment.

ICF syndrome

The ICF (immunodeficiency, centromeric instability and facial anomalies) syndrome is an AR disorder characterised by structural chromosomal abnormalities in chromosomes 1, 9 and 16 in lymphocytes, easily seen on chromosome analysis. Other cells do not show these changes. Affected children develop severe recurrent infections and have immunoglobulin deficiency, often with agammaglobulinaemia but with normal numbers of T and B lymphocytes.[7] T-lymphocyte immunity is not normal and affected children can present with *Pneumocystis carinii* infection in infancy; severe viral warts and cutaneous fungal infection also occur.

Defects of antibody production

Isolated antibody deficiency does not usually present in the neonatal period because the presence of transplacentally acquired immunoglobulin obscures the affected child's inability to make antibody. Neonates can present with severe or recurrent bacterial infection and be found to have hypogammaglobulinaemia because of:

- failure of transfer of immunoglobulin due to prematurity;
- failure of transfer of immunoglobulin due to unrecognised maternal hypogammaglobulinaemia;
- immunoglobulin loss from the thoracic duct in chylothorax;
- immunoglobulin loss from gut in lymphangectasia.

Table 40.1 describes the main causes of primary hypogammaglobulinaemia which can often be screened for in the neonatal period when there is a positive family history.

Disorders of phagocytic cells

Chronic granulomatous disease

CGD results from inherited defects of the phagocyte nicotinamide adenine dinucleotide phosphate (NADPH) oxidase enzyme complex which generates free oxygen species needed to kill microorganisms ingested into phagosomes. The X-linked form is more common than the AR form.

The disease has protean clinical manifestations, but the hallmark is acute, and potentially fatal, bacterial or fungal infection.[23] In the neonatal period, a non-specific generalised pustulosis can be seen and the most common manifestation, acute suppurative lymphadenitis in the neck, axilla or groin, can sometimes be seen very early in life. Other frequent pyogenic infections include liver abscesses, osteomyelitis, arthritis, pneumonia, skin sepsis and perianal abscesses. Pathogens, such as *Staphylococcus aureus*, *Burkholderia cepacia*, *Aspergillus* species and *Serratia marcerens*, are common. Infections with catalase-negative organisms, such as *Streptococcus pneumoniae*, are rare. Fungal infection often manifests as pneumonia, but disseminated infection is frequently seen, with osteomyelitis and hepatic involvement. Once established, fungal infection is hard to treat and frequently fatal.

Diagnosis is suggested by failure of reduction of NBT or dihydrorhodamine by neutrophils. Prophylactic antibiotics – particularly co-trimoxazole, which is concentrated in neutrophils – significantly reduce morbidity and mortality from bacterial infections. Oral antifungal prophylaxis with an agent such as itraconazole probably reduces the incidence of fatal fungal disease.[11]

Infections or unexplained fevers should be treated aggressively. IFN-γ is a useful adjunctive treatment in severe bacterial or fungal infections. White cell infusions may also be used as adjunctive therapy in severe infection. Despite these therapeutic advances, considerable morbidity and mortality occurs and BMT should be considered.[48]

Other neutrophil disorders

Neutropenia (see also Chapter 30)

This may result from reduced production in the bone marrow or increased peripheral destruction, distinguished by the findings on bone marrow examination. Neutropenia most frequently follows decreased production induced by disease processes or drug treatments, as well as sepsis in preterm or stressed neonates. Increased consumption may occur in autoimmune states, including neonatal alloimmune neutropenia and those associated with immune deficiency. The degree of neutropenia will influence the clinical picture: neutrophil counts of less than $0.5 \times 10^9/l$ carry a major risk of infection, whilst counts below $0.2 \times 10^9/l$ are associated with a significant incidence of life-threatening sepsis.

Severe congenital neutropenia (Kostmann's syndrome)

This AR disease was originally described by Kostmann.[34] Onset is within the first year of life with recurrent and life-threatening infections. Symptoms include cellulitis, perirectal abscesses, peritonitis, stomatitis and meningitis. Bone marrow examination shows an arrest at the promyelocyte to myelocyte maturation stage. Recently a small number of patients with X-linked congenital neutropenia have been defined who have mutations that result in overactivity of WASP (Wiskott–Aldrich syndrome protein).[18]

Shwachman–Diamond syndrome

This rare AR disorder is characterised by exocrine pancreatic insufficiency, skeletal abnormalities, bone marrow dysfunction and recurrent infections. Neutropenia occurs in all patients, whilst 10–25% of patients also have pancytopenia. There is an increased incidence of malignancy.

Treatment of neutropenia with G-CSF results in increased counts and fewer infections in almost all patients with neutropenia not secondary to peripheral destruction. Concerns about the induction of leukaemias with prolonged use have not been realised, although pretreatment and annual bone marrow aspirates are recommended. BMT may be indicated in selected cases.

Chediak–Higashi syndrome

CHS is a rare AR disease with partial oculocutaneous albinism, recurrent bacterial infections and a high risk of developing macrophage activation syndrome (similar to that seen in haemophagocytic lymphohistiocytosis [HLH]), which is usually fatal. Variable neurological manifestations are also recognised. Characteristic giant lysosomal granules are seen in the cytoplasm of all cells containing these organelles, and are easily detected on a peripheral blood film. The gene for this disease codes for a regulator of lysosomal transport;[2] proteins normally transported through lysosomes enter these organelles but cannot exit, with subsequent lysosomal hypertrophy. In melanocytes, this is thought to result in abnormalities of melanin transport and consequent albinism. In neutrophils, degranulation of lysosomes cannot occur, with failure of release of bactericidal proteins into the phagosome and defective intracellular killing. Common pathogens in CHS include *Staphylococcus aureus*, streptococci and pneumococci. Prophylactic co-trimoxazole should prevent bacterial infection. The accelerated phase cannot be predicted, and patients should be closely monitored, particularly if febrile. The only definitive treatment is BMT. This should be considered early if there is a matched sibling donor. The effects of BMT on later neurological problems are not known.

Griscelli syndrome

Individuals with Griscelli syndrome resemble those with CHS in that they have variable hypopigmentation of the skin and hair and recurrent pyogenic infections associated with absent delayed-type cutaneous hypersensitivity and impaired NK cell function. Hypogammaglobulinaemia can be seen as a secondary phenomenon. In contrast to CHS, large lysosomal granules are not seen and examination of the hair by electron microscopy shows large clumps of pigment, with the accumulation of mature melanosomes in melanocytes. Neurological abnormalities are absent in these patients. They are also at high risk of developing macrophage activation syndrome unless treated by BMT.

Haemophagocytic lymphohistiocytosis (familial)

HLH is universally fatal without treatment (p. 688). Patients present with high swinging fevers, hepatosplenomegaly and pancytopenia, and may appear septic. Laboratory findings include an acute-phase response, elevated ferritin and elevated fasting triglycerides. Examination of bone marrow, cerebrospinal fluid, pleural effusions or ascitic fluid may demonstrate haemophagocytosis. This may be very difficult to find, and repeated sampling may be required. Haemophagocytosis may occur secondary to a number of infections, particularly viral infections, and careful exclusion of infections by serology/polymerase chain reaction should be undertaken. A clinical syndrome resembling HLH may also occur in a number of immunodeficient states, including Griscelli syndrome, CHS and X-linked lymphoproliferative disease. Diagnosis of familial HLH should be suspected in an infant with an appropriate clinical picture.

Between 20% and 30% of patients with familial HLH have a mutation in perforin, normally found in the granules of NK and cytotoxic T lymphocytes. Perforin may have a regulatory role, and absence leads to dysregulated immune activation.[51]

Treatment with a combination of chemotherapeutic agents, steroids, and monoclonal antibodies that deplete lymphocytes may induce remission, but only BMT is curative.

Leukocyte adhesion deficiency

Inherited defects in leukocyte cell surface molecules can prevent their egress into infected tissue, resulting in a characteristic clinical presentation. In leukocyte adhesion deficiency type I, deficiency of the 95 kD β chain (CD18), common to the β_2 integrin family of cell surface adhesive molecules, leads to a profound immunodeficiency affecting the function of neutrophils, monocytes and certain lymphocytes, including T and NK cytotoxic cells.[16] Inheritance is AR. Chemotaxis, adherence and phagocytosis are markedly depressed. The phenotype varies according to the severity of the mutation. Leukocytes are attracted to areas of infection and become fixed to the vessel walls at sites of inflammation in the usual way but cannot pass out into the tissues, causing infarction of small vessels and rapidly expanding necrotic lesions without pus.

Individuals with the most severe phenotype (<1% expression) present in the first weeks of life with delayed umbilical cord separation (the cord fails to shrink down and may not separate until 3–4 weeks of age) and rapidly progressive erosive perianal ulcers. Delayed umbilical cord separation does not occur in patients with some expression of the molecule (usually in the range 2–10% of normal expression). In all forms there is excessive susceptibility to bacterial and fungal infections. Gingivitis and periodontitis are common, and more deep-seated infections of bone, respiratory tract and gastrointestinal tract are often seen. Non-infective inflammatory lesions, particularly affecting the skin and resembling pyoderma gangrenosum, can occur in the partial forms of the deficiency and are often responsive to steroids.

There is almost always a neutrophilia (because of failure of the cells to migrate out of the circulation) and a profound neutrophil chemotactic defect. Diagnosis is confirmed by demonstrating the absence of the cell surface markers recognised by anti-CD11/CD18 monoclonal antibodies.

In the severe form, early death from infection occurs unless a successful BMT can be performed. In the partial forms, supportive and expectant management is pursued in the first instance, but BMT may become necessary.

Hyper-IgE syndrome (Job's syndrome)

This complex disorder is characterised by extreme elevation of the serum IgE level (usually in the range 2000–40 000 U/l), chronic dermatitis (p. 824), and repeated lung and skin infections.[27] Patients present in infancy with eczema, but in the neonatal period, a vesicular rash may be present in the first few days of life. *Staphylococcus aureus*, the predominant pathogen, can cause pneumatoceles and chronic lung damage. In addition to the high IgE level, there is a profound neutrophil chemotactic defect. Treatment is long-term anti-staphylococcal antibiotic prophylaxis, usually with flucloxacillin.

Secondary immunodeficiency

Congenital asplenia

Asplenia is seen when congenital cardiac defects are associated with right isomerism, and the presence of Howell–Jolly and Heinz bodies on a blood film should raise suspicion, asplenia being confirmed by abdominal ultrasound. Asplenic infants are at lifelong risk from invasive infection by organisms with polysaccharide coats, such as group B streptococcus and pneumococcus. Treatment is with lifelong prophylactic antibiotics. Penicillin is the antibiotic of choice, although in children less than 5 years of age we advocate using co-trimoxazole in order to prevent infection with the greater range of pathogens, including *Haemophilus influenzae* and Gram-negative organisms, to which younger children with asplenia are susceptible. Vaccination with conjugate pneumococcal vaccine is recommended before 2 years of age, and thereafter with polysaccharide pneumococcal vaccine.

Treatment of immunodeficiency

Vaccination of the child with a potentially impaired immune response

Immunocompromised children are more in need of the protection vaccination can offer because of their greater risk from infection, and yet are less likely to be vaccinated because of concerns about the underlying immunodeficiency. Children with primary immunodeficiency should be immunised. Live vaccines should be avoided in those with lymphocyte-mediated immunodeficiency; all other forms of immunodeficiency can safely have live vaccine administered, except BCG in patients with CGD. HIV-infected children should receive killed polio vaccine. Preterm infants should be vaccinated routinely, following the national immunisation programme. Children on pharmacological doses of steroids (an equivalent dose of prednisolone 2 mg/kg/day for >1 week, or 1 mg/kg/day for >1 month) or other immunosuppressive therapy should not be given live vaccines until 3 months after ceasing therapy.[50]

Supportive care

Children with immunodeficiency disorders often require the full spectrum of paediatric care. Particular attention needs to be paid to nutritional status and the management of dietary intolerances secondary to the gastrointestinal problems which frequently occur. Supporting the emotional needs of the family is also very important. Prevention and treatment of infections is the mainstay of supportive care.

Specific measures for prevention of infections

Co-trimoxazole as prophylaxis against *Pneumocystis carinii* should be given for defects involving cell-mediated immunity mechanisms. For PCP prophylaxis only, co-trimoxazole need only be given on 2 or 3 days a week. If this is not tolerated, alternatives include dapsone and atovaquone. Co-trimoxazole probably also reduces the incidence of pyogenic infections in these patients and those with phagocytic or humoral immune deficiencies, and for this purpose it is usually given daily (dose 30 mg/kg/day in one or two doses). In circumstances of poor nutrition, increased bone marrow turnover and in all cases after BMT, weekly folinic acid supplements are given to lessen the risk of bone marrow depression without compromising the antimicrobial efficacy. Antifungal prophylaxis should be used in combined immunodeficiencies or phagocytic cell defects. In CGD and other conditions where the risk of aspergillus infection is high, itraconazole is preferred. Otherwise, fluconazole or non-absorbed agents such as nystatin are used. Antiviral prophylaxis with aciclovir is used in patients with cell-mediated immunodeficiency and previous herpes simplex infection. It is also used in the context of BMT to prevent herpes simplex and CMV reactivation.

Treatment of infections

A policy of vigorous and early antimicrobial treatment of infections should be observed. Unusual agents may cause infection, and broader-spectrum antimicrobial cover may therefore be needed. In neutrophil disorders, it is particularly important to cover Pseudomonas and other Gram-negative bacilli. Early treatment of an infection may be life saving, but its initiation should not detract from full attempts at identification of the causative agent. Invasive diagnostic procedures, such as bronchoalveolar lavage or, if this fails to produce a diagnosis, open lung biopsy, can be fully justified on the basis that they will facilitate precise and optimal therapy. The mainstay of treatment for systemic fungal infection remains amphotericin B, mostly used in its liposomal form to reduce toxicity and enable larger doses to be given. Promising new agents for treating invasive aspergillosis include voriconazole and caspafungin.

Antivirals such as the broad-spectrum agent ribavirin and the anti-CMV agents ganciclovir and foscarnet are particularly useful in the immunocompromised infant. Newer antivirals include cidofovir (for resistant CMV, adenovirus and severe molluscum contagiosum) and pleconaril (for chronic enteroviral infections).

Intravenous immunoglobulin

IVIG is a blood product, and so its use is associated with all the risks of giving such products, such as hypersensitivity reactions (including anaphylaxis) during administration. Although modern manufacturing processes include steps which screen for and inactivate viruses such as hepatitis B and C, and HIV, transmission of infectious agents remains theoretically possible. Particular current concerns revolve around the issue of transmission of prion disease, although the risk of this is probably very small. Such factors mean that immunoglobulin treatment should be initiated only after due consideration of the risks and benefits. Before administration, liver function tests should be measured, and a sample of serum taken for long-term storage in case of future infective complications which may be attributable to the IVIG. Many studies have examined the role of immunoglobulin in either the prophylaxis or treatment of infection in preterm or low-birth-weight (LBW) infants. Taken overall, whilst IVIG prophylaxis gives a small (4–5%) reduction in the incidence of sepsis or serious infection, there is no difference in mortality, and only a trend towards shorter hospital stay. This has to be balanced against cost, risk of side effects (including potential transmission of infection), and recurrent venous access. There is currently no justification for the routine use of IVIG as prophylaxis against Gram-negative infection in preterm or LBW infants.[43]

IVIG has also been advocated as an adjunctive treatment to antibiotics in sepsis or suspected sepsis. A recent meta-analysis showed a borderline statistically significant reduction in mortality in cases of suspected sepsis given immunoglobulin, although the difference was more significant in cases that were proven sepsis.[44] Larger trials are needed to confirm this finding, but immunoglobulin treatment may have a role in the treatment of proven neonatal sepsis in specific cases.

Granulocyte colony-stimulating factor

Septic sick or preterm neonates become neutropenic because neutrophil stores are rapidly depleted, and granulopoiesis is depressed. G-CSF mobilises preformed neutrophils from the marrow into the circulation, and enhances neutrophil precursor proliferation. Several small studies have examined the effect of administering G-CSF to septic infants. Overall, no difference in mortality was found between placebo and treatment groups, although the treatment groups had higher neutrophil counts.[3,47] Other studies have addressed the issue of using G-CSF as prophylaxis by prospectively stimulating neutrophil production. Treated groups had less septic episodes and less sepsis-induced neutropenia, although there was no difference in mortality.[10,12] Further larger trials are necessary before G-CSF can be recommended routinely in prophylaxis or treatment of sepsis in preterm or growth-retarded neonates.

Blood product support

All blood products except IVIG and fresh frozen plasma contain viable leukocytes, and so before being given to patients with combined immunodeficiency or to those receiving intense immunosuppression, should be irradiated with 2000–3000 rad to prevent possible GVHD. In those with no evidence of previous exposure to CMV, blood products should be obtained from CMV antibody-negative donors. White cell infusions can benefit patients with CGD and other neutrophil disorders with invasive infections who respond poorly to antibiotic treatment, particularly if the leukocytes are harvested from G-CSF primed donors.

Bone marrow transplantation

Most primary T-lymphocyte and phagocyte immunodeficiency disorders can be corrected by BMT.[1] Best results are obtained using HLA-matched sibling donors, but these are available for only about 20% of patients. Since the early 1980s, techniques have been developed to allow HLA-mismatched parent-to-child (haploidentical) grafts, by removing mature T lymphocytes that would otherwise cause fatal GVHD. These are now the most common BMT procedure for patients with SCID.[5,9] Broadly matched volunteer-unrelated donor transplants are being increasingly used, particularly for non-SCID immunodeficiencies, and peripheral blood or umbilical cord stem cells are sometimes used instead of bone marrow.

Complications of bone marrow transplantation

The five main complications of BMT are toxicity from conditioning agents, graft failure, graft rejection, GVHD, and infection which may be pre-existing due to immunodeficiency or be acquired after BMT. Rejection is less likely following transplantation with whole rather than T-lymphocyte-depleted marrow, but the risk of GVHD after whole marrow is greater, particularly after unrelated-donor BMT. The risk of infectious complications is greatest in T-lymphocyte-depleted grafts where there is a prolonged period before functioning immunity develops.

Despite these problems, refinements of the technique over recent years have brought about continuing improvement in results, with success rates for SCID of around 78% for T-lymphocyte-depleted grafts, and >90% for matched sibling donors.[9] Success is dependent on type of SCID, with better results for B+ SCID than for the B− phenotype.[5] Age at presentation also influences outcome, with very good results for those transplanted in the neonatal period, before they have contracted infections.[32]

References

1. Antoine C, Muller S, Cant A et al 2003 Long-term survival and transplantation of haemopoietic stem cells for immunodeficiencies: a report of the European experience 1968–99. Lancet 361: 553–560

2. Barbosa M D F S, Barrat F J, Tchernev V T et al 1997 Identification of mutations in two major mRNA isoforms of the Chediak-Higashi syndrome gene in human and mouse. Human Molecular Genetics 6: 1091–1098

3. Bedford Russell A R, Emmerson A J B, Wilkinson N et al 2001 A trial of recombinant human granulocyte colony stimulating factor for the treatment of very low birthweight infants with presumed sepsis and neutropenia. Archives of Disease in Childhood. Fetal and Neonatal Edition 84: F172–F176

4. Bennet C L, Ochs H D 2001 IPEX is a unique X-linked syndrome characterised by immune dysfunction, polyendocrinopathy, enteropathy, and a variety of autoimmune phenomena. Current Opinion in Pediatrics 13: 533–538

5. Bertrand Y, Landais P, Friedrich W et al 1999 Influence of severe combined immunodeficiency phenotype on the outcome of HLA non-identical, T-cell-depleted bone marrow transplantation. Journal of Pediatrics 134: 740–748

6. Braun J, Steihm E R 1996 The B-lymphocyte system. In: Stiehm R E (ed) Immunological disorders in infants and children, 4th edn. W B Saunders, Philadelphia

7. Brown D C, Grace E, Sumner A T et al 1995 ICF syndrome (immunodeficiency, centromeric instability and facial anomalies): investigation of heterochromatin abnormalities and review of outcome. Human Genetics 96: 411–416

8. Buckley R H 2000 Primary immunodeficiency diseases due to defects in lymphocytes. New England Journal of Medicine 343: 1313–1324

9. Buckley R H, Schiff S E, Schiff R I et al 1999 Hematopoietic stem-cell transplantation for the treatment of severe combined immunodeficiency. New England Journal of Medicine 340: 508–516

10. Cairo M S, Agosti J, Ellis R et al 1999 A randomised, double-blind, placebo-controlled trial of prophylactic recombinant human granulocyte-macrophage colony-stimulating factor to reduce nosocomial infections in very low birthweight infants. Journal of Pediatrics 134: 64–70

11. Cale C M, Jones A M, Goldblatt D 2000 Follow up of patients with chronic granulomatous disease diagnosed since 1990. Clinical and Experimental Immunology 120: 351–355

12. Carr R, Modi N, Dore C J et al 1999 A randomised, controlled trial of prophylactic granulocyte-macrophage colony-stimulating factor in human newborns less than 32 weeks gestation. Pediatrics 103: 796–802

13. Cederbaum S D, Kartila I, Runoin D L et al 1976 The chondro-osseous dysplasia of adenosine deaminase deficiency with severe combined immunodeficiency. Journal of Pediatrics 89: 737–742

14. Choo S, Seymour L, Morris R et al 2000 Immunogenicity and reactogenicity of a pneumococcal conjugate vaccine administered combined with a Haemophilus influenzae type B conjugate vaccine in United Kingdom infants. Pediatric Infectious Diseases Journal 19: 854–862

15. Comans-Bitter W M, de Groot R, van den Beemd R et al. 1997 Immunophenotyping of blood lymphocytes in childhood. Reference values for lymphocyte subpopulations. Journal of Pediatrics 130: 388–393

16. Crowley C A, Curnutte J T, Rosin R E et al 1980 An inherited abnormality of neutrophil adhesion: its genetic transmission and its association with a missing protein. New England Journal of Medicine 302: 1163–1168

17. Delves P J, Roitt I M 2000 The immune system: second of two parts. New England Journal of Medicine 343: 108–117

18. Devrient K, Kim A S, Mathijs G et al 2001 Constitutively activating mutation in WASP causes X-linked severe congenital neutropenia. Nature Genetics 27: 313–317

19. Doffinger R, Smahi A, Bessia C et al 2001 X-linked anhidrotic ectodermal dysplasia with immunodeficiency is caused by impaired NF-kB signalling. Nature Genetics 27: 277–285

20. Driscoll D A, Sullivan K E 1999 DiGeorge syndrome: a chromosome 22q11.2 deletion syndrome. In: Ochs H D, Smith C I E, Puck J M (eds) Primary immunodeficiency diseases; a molecular and genetic approach. Oxford University Press, New York, pp 198–207

21. Fischer A 2000 Severe combined immunodeficiencies (SCID). Clinical and Experimental Immunology 122: 143–149

22. Fischer A 2001 Primary immunodeficiency diseases: an experimental model for molecular medicine. Lancet 357: 1863–1869

23. Fischer A, Segal A W, Seger R et al 1993 The management of chronic granulomatous disease. European Journal of Pediatrics 152: 896–899

24. Gennery A R, Cant A J 2001 Applied physiology: immune competence. Current Paediatrics 11: 458–464

25. Gennery A R, Cant A J, Jeggo PA 2000 Immunodeficiency associated with DNA repair defects. Clinical and Experimental Immunology 121: 1–7

26. Gilmour K C, Cranston T, Loughlin S et al 2001 Rapid protein-based assays for the diagnosis of T-B + severe combined immunodeficiency. British Journal of Haematology 112: 671–676

27. Grimbacher B, Holland S M, Gallin J I et al 1999 Hyper-IgE syndrome with recurrent infections – an autosomal dominant multisystem disorder. New England Journal of Medicine 340: 692–702

28. Hague R A, Rassam S, Morgan G et al 1994 Early diagnosis of severe combined immune deficiency syndrome. Archives of Disease in Childhood 70: 260–263

29. Hiel J A, Weemaes C M, van den Heuvel L P et al 2000 Nijmegen breakage syndrome. Archives of Disease in Childhood 82: 400–406

30. Hill H R, Joyner J L, Augustine N H 1999 The pathophysiology of neonatal neutrophil dysfunction. Pediatric Research 45: 761

31. Hirschhorn R, Vauter G F, Kirkpatrick J A Jr et al 1979 Adenosine deaminase deficiency frequency and comparative pathology in autosomally recessive severe combined immunodeficiency. Clinical Immunology and Immunopathology 14: 107–120

32. Kane L C, Gennery A R, Crooks B N A et al 2001 Neonatal bone marrow transplantation for severe combined immunodeficiency. Archives of Disease in Childhood. Fetal and Neonatal Edition 85: F110–F113

33. Klein C, Lisowska-Grospierre B, LeDeist F et al 1993 Major histocompatibility complex class II deficiency: clinical manifestations, immunologic features, and outcome. Journal of Pediatrics 123: 921–928

34. Kostmann R 1956 Infantile genetic agranulocytosis. A review with presentation of ten new cases. Acta Paediatrica Scandinavica 64: 362–366

35. Makitie O, Kaitla I 1993 Cartilage-hair hypoplasia – clinical manifestations in 108 Finnish patients. European Journal of Pediatrics 152: 211–217

36. Makitie O, Kaitla I, Savilahti E 1998 Susceptibility to infections and in vitro immune functions in cartilage-hair hypoplasia. European Journal of Pediatrics 157: 816–820

37. Marshall-Clarke S, Reen D, Tasker L et al 2000 Neonatal immunity: how well has it grown up? Immunology Today 21: 35–41

38. Muller S M, Ege M, Pottharst A et al 2001 Transplacentally acquired maternal T lymphocytes in severe combined immunodeficiency: a study of 121 patients. Blood 98: 1847–1851

39. Notarangelo L D, Hayward A R 2000 X-linked immunodeficiency with hyper-IgM (XHIM). Clinical and Experimental Immunology 120: 399–405

40. Notarangelo L D, Villa A, Schwarz K 1999 RAG and RAG defects. Current Opinion in Immunology 11: 435–442

41. Ochs H D, Slichter S J, Harker L A et al 1980 The Wiskott-Aldrich syndrome: studies of lymphocytes, granulocytes and platelets. Blood 55: 243–252

42. Ochs H D, Smith C I E, Puck J M (eds) 1999 Primary immunodeficiency diseases; a molecular and genetic approach. Oxford University Press, New York

43. Ohlsson A, Lacy J B 2002 Intravenous immunoglobulin for preventing infection in preterm and/or low-birth-weight infants (Cochrane Review). In: The Cochrane Library, Issue 4. Update Software, Oxford

44. Ohlsson A, Lacy J B 2002 Intravenous immunoglobulin for suspected or subsequently proven infection in neonates (Cochrane Review). In: The Cochrane Library, Issue 4. Update Software, Oxford

45. Rogers M, Lwin R, Fairbanks L et al 2001 Cognitive and behavioural abnormalities in adenosine deaminase deficient severe combined deficiency. Journal of Pediatrics 139: 44–50

46. Rosen F S, Eibl M, Roifman C et al 1999 Report of an IUIS Scientific Committee: primary immunodeficiency diseases. Clinical and Experimental Immunology 118 (suppl. 1): 1–28

47. Schibler K R, Osborne K A, Leung L Y et al 1998 A randomized, placebo-controlled trial of granulocyte colony-stimulating factor administration to newborn infants with neutropenia and clinical signs of early-onset sepsis. Pediatrics 102: 6–13

48. Seger R A, Gungor T, Belohradsky B H et al 2002 Treatment of chronic granulomatous disease with myeloablative conditioning and an unmodified hematopoietic allograft: a survey of the European experience 1985-2000. Blood 100: 4344–4350

49. Shapiro R, Beatty D W, Woods D L et al 1989 Serum complement and immunoglobulin values in small for gestational age infants. Journal of Pediatrics 99: 139–142

50. Skinner R, Cant A, Davies G et al 2002 Immunisation of the immunocompromised child. Best Practice Statement. Royal College of Paediatrics and Child Health, London

51. Stepp S E, Dufourcq-Lagelouse R, Le Deist F et al 1999 Perforin gene defects in familial hemophagocytic lymphohistiocytosis. Science 286: 1957–1959

52. Stiehm RE (ed) 1996 Immunological disorders in infants and children, 4th edn. W B Saunders, Philadelphia

53. Sullivan K E, Mullen C A, Blaese R M, Winkelstein J A 1994 A multi-institutional survey of the Wiskott-Aldrich syndrome. Journal of Pediatrics 125: 876–885

PART 2

Infection in the newborn

Peter Dear

Infection, as either prime pathology or a complication of other illness, is a major cause of neonatal mortality and morbidity throughout the world. The incidence of culture-confirmed neonatal sepsis in the USA is in the region of 0.7%.[652] Most infections occur in babies admitted to neonatal units, and a comprehensive study of systemic bacterial and fungal infections in neonatal units in Australia produced incidence figures of 0.22% for early-onset and 0.44% for late-onset sepsis.[407] The mortality rate for early-onset sepsis was 15% and for late-onset sepsis 9%. In a recent prospective study of bloodstream infections in three North American neonatal units, 11.2% of all babies had culture-proven sepsis.[64] Among infants requiring neonatal intensive care, the incidence of infection is twice as high,[561] with a mortality rate of about 16%.[303] Among very-low-birthweight (VLBW) infants undergoing prolonged intensive care, the rate of culture-proven sepsis may be as high as 30%, with a mortality rate of 30%.[652] In the developing world, neonatal sepsis is a greater problem. A recent study from Malaysia reported rates of neonatal sepsis of 5–10%, with case fatality rates of between 23% and 52%. Septicaemia accounted for between 11% and 30% of all neonatal deaths.[98]

The impact of infection can be reduced, as international comparisons show, but even in the most technologically advanced countries the contribution of sepsis to neonatal mortality and morbidity remains unacceptably high. The combination of a susceptible host, non-specific clinical presentation and an ever-changing population of pathogens makes for a great challenge. This chapter presents a systematic review of the pathogenesis, prevention, diagnosis and treatment of neonatal infection.

The pathogenesis of neonatal infection

The fetus normally encounters no microorganisms during development, and the newborn infant becomes harmlessly colonised by bacteria acquired from the birth canal and the environment. This happy state of affairs is evidence of the integrity of the barrier to infection provided by the placenta and membranes, the low pathogenicity of most colonising organisms, and the relative competence of the baby's defence mechanisms. It is usually when one or other of these factors is altered that fetal or neonatal infection occurs. These ideas provide a useful conceptual framework within which to discuss specific infections in detail.

Exposure to microorganisms

Transplacental

Certain infective agents have an inherent ability to penetrate the placental barrier, often damaging the placenta in the process, e.g. rubella virus (pp. 1064–6). The effects on the fetus are often devastating.

Ascending

Ascent of vaginal organisms into the uterine cavity prior to rupture of the membranes is rare but well recognised.[75] Once the membranes rupture, the risk increases progressively with time.

Intrapartum

Vaginal delivery inevitably results in contamination and the beginning of colonisation of the skin and the gut. The pattern of organisms and the heaviness of colonisation are usually closely similar between mother and baby (Fig. 40.7).[547] Vaginal flora

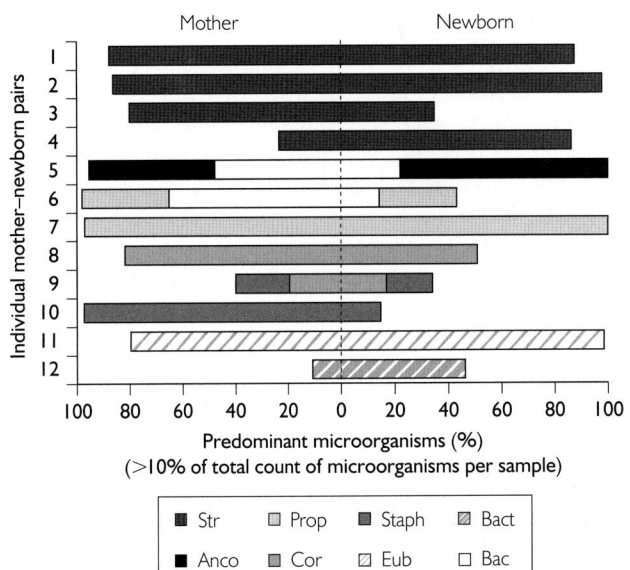

Fig. 40.7 Relationship between maternal and infant colonising flora. The figure shows the predominant species of microorganism grown from the baby's ear and the maternal vagina in 12 mother–infant pairs. Str, streptococci; Anco, anaerobic cocci; Prop, propionibacteria; Staph, staphylococci; Cor, corynebacteria; Bac, bacilli; Eub, eubacteria; Bact, bacteroides. (From Mandar & Mikelsaar.[547])

vary considerably from woman to woman,[547] and many cases of early-onset neonatal sepsis result from the vaginal carriage of opportunistic pathogens. Another potential source of intrapartum bacterial contamination is from the water used for 'water births'[358] and from repeated vaginal examinations.

Postnatal

In addition to the organisms acquired during birth, all babies are subject to further microbiological contamination from the environment. People are the main source of such contamination.

Colonisation

Bacterial colonisation is the inevitable lot of all creatures and it generally brings advantages. Competitive inhibition of potential pathogens is an important benefit, and as an example it can be shown that pharyngeal colonisation of the newborn with *Streptococcus viridans* reduces the risk of serious bacterial illness.[258]

Colonisation of normal infants

The nature of colonising organisms is determined by the pattern of flora in the birth canal and in the environment. Babies born at home are colonised by organisms derived primarily from the mother.[452] These organisms, and those acquired from other family members, tend to be community-derived antibiotic-sensitive organisms of limited pathogenicity, although even women choosing home delivery may harbour serious potential pathogens such as group B β-haemolytic streptococcus (GBS). On the postnatal ward the baby will acquire organisms from the ward environment, other babies and the clinical staff. The chance of encountering pathogens and their variety is considerably greater here than in the home environment.

The predominant intestinal organisms acquired by normal babies are enterobacteria (including *Escherichia coli*, *Klebsiella* species and *Citrobacter* species), *Bacteroides* species, enterococci, staphylococci, *Lactobacillus* species and *Bifidobacteria* species. Breastfeeding reduces the intensity of colonisation by the Enterobacteriaceae,[15,254] and *Bifidobacteria* species tend to predominate in breastfed infants.[53,860]

Colonisation of the upper respiratory tract occurs rapidly, and 90% of infants have positive pharyngeal cultures by the third day. Coagulase-negative staphylococci (CONS) are commonest, followed by *Str. viridans* and *Staphylococcus aureus*.[258] Exclusive breastfeeding does not influence the pattern of nasopharyngeal colonisation compared with exclusive formula feeding.[433]

Skin colonisation is very rapid, with the number of bacteria increasing 100-fold during the first week. CONS predominate, but *Staph. aureus* may be found in 65% of infants.[773] A host of other organisms can be found, including yeasts and a range of saprophytic bacteria. The umbilicus, perineum and axillae are most heavily colonised.

Colonisation of infants on a neonatal unit

These babies are at greatest risk of becoming colonised by pathogens, which often show resistance to antibiotics.[521] The pattern of bowel colonisation is very different among sick preterm infants. CONS and antibiotic-resistant Gram-negative organisms predominate.[235,236] Such organisms make a significant contribution to late-onset sepsis in these infants, and bacterial translocation through the gut wall is a likely mechanism in some cases.[812] The results of an attempt to replace this faecal reservoir of potential pathogens with virtually harmless *Lactobacillus* species have been reported.[568] Bowel colonisation with lactobacilli was achieved, but unfortunately the reservoir of potential nosocomial pathogens was not significantly reduced and no clinical benefit was found.

Skin colonisation on the neonatal intensive care unit (NICU) is mainly by CONS, which can be isolated from over 90% of all positive cultures.[454] *Staph. epidermidis* accounts for 80% and *Staph. haemolyticus* for almost all of the remainder.[90] These organisms show increasing resistance to antibiotics as the babies grow older (Fig. 40.8).[454] Interestingly, the skin of the preterm infant is much less heavily colonised than that of the adult, supports fewer species of bacteria and tends to have a transient rather than a stable resident population of organisms. Molecular biological techniques such as DNA fingerprinting, plasmid analysis and multilocus enzyme electrophoresis are increasingly being used to investigate the epidemiology of colonisation and infection with these and many other organisms.[509,783]

Colonisation and infection

Most babies become colonised without becoming infected, but in others, various host factors or the pathogenicity of the organisms result in tissue invasion and sepsis. It is useful to consider host and organism factors separately.

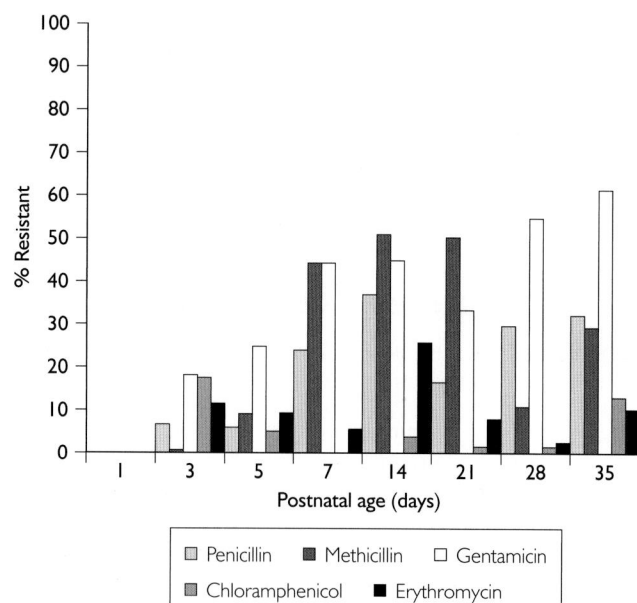

Fig. 40.8 Changes in percentage of cutaneous staphylococcus resistant to antibiotics with postnatal age. Measurements taken in all neonates at all sites. (From Keyworth et al.[454])

Features of the host

Portals of entry

Intact skin and mucous membranes present a formidable barrier to microorganisms. Abrasions and cuts, mucosal injury, cannulae, catheters and endotracheal tubes all open the way for bacterial invasion. Among inmates of a NICU, the risk of bacterial infection plummets as soon as intubation and vascular access are no longer required.[289]

Host immunity

Babies are less able than older children or adults to combat infection, an ability which is further compromised by prematurity. The local inflammatory response is particularly poor, so that infecting organisms easily enter the circulation. Accordingly, a much higher proportion of infections in babies have a septicaemic component than is the case with older children or adults.

Antibiotic exposure

Antibiotics are used freely in neonatology and increasingly so in obstetrics. The resulting obliteration of colonising flora predisposes to superinfection with pathogens such as yeasts, and antibiotic resistance becomes common.[189,521,526,569,747]

Prematurity

Premature babies have poorer immunity (pp. 996–7), less effective cutaneous and mucosal barriers, more portals of entry secondary to invasive procedures, and greater exposure to potential pathogens from their environment. There is a clear inverse relationship between birthweight and risk of sepsis.[205,446]

Features of the microorganisms

Pathogenicity

The following are notoriously pathogenic to babies: GBS, *Staph. aureus*, CONS, *Listeria monocytogenes*, *Haemophilus influenzae*, *E. coli*, *Pseudomonas aeruginosa*, *Klebsiella* species, *Serratia marcescens*, *Candida albicans* and herpes simplex (HSV).

Dose

The heavier the colonisation, the greater the risk of invasion and sepsis.[773] Efforts to reduce the level of colonisation by measures such as umbilical cord care, mouth care and bathing are important, even though complete eradication of the organisms is usually impossible.

Competition

Competition between bacteria is a controlling influence on the level of colonisation and risk of infection, for example the inhibition of yeasts by bacteria and the competitive inhibition of Gram-negative organisms by *Lactobacillus bifidus* in the gut of the breastfed infant.

Prevention of infection

If the newborn infant has little contact with anyone other than his mother and is breastfed from the outset, the risk of significant nosocomial infection is negligible. When babies are retained in a hospital environment with multiple carers, the risk is increased substantially. At the extreme end of the spectrum of risk is the tiny immature baby who spends weeks on a NICU, constantly invaded by tubes, needles and catheters and cared for by a multiplicity of staff, who are also caring for a large number of other similarly disadvantaged infants. Then, nosocomial infection is virtually inevitable and the emphasis is on early detection and treatment as much as on prevention. The principles of control of cross-infection in hospital are well established, and in the account that follows, those principles will be related mainly to the case of a baby on a neonatal unit.

Environmental factors

There are several important factors in the environment that can contribute, either by creating circumstances in which cross-infection is more likely to occur or by creating environmental reservoirs of potential pathogens.

Design of units

To minimise cross-infection, adequate space should be allowed around the cots. The Department of Health[192] recommends that the minimum space allocated to each incubator in a six-cot intensive care nursery should be $3\,m^2$ (100 sq feet). The ventilation to the rooms should deliver a maximum of $2.7\,m^3/s$, though in general there is no need to have special ventilation systems. Enough sinks must be provided so that handwashing protocols are easy to implement. There should be sufficient single rooms equipped for intensive care such that sick babies can be isolated if necessary. The floors, walls and all flat surfaces should be cleaned regularly, and ideally the unit should be sufficiently spacious for rooms to be vacated for cleaning on a regular rotational basis.

Equipment

Any medical equipment that comes into close contact with the baby is a potential source of infection, except for the moment when it is first removed from its sterile wrapping. Each baby in a normal nursery should have his own thermometer, and in the NICU he should have his own suction unit, stethoscope, laryngoscope, face mask etc. If the equipment has to be shared, either it should be wiped clean between patients (e.g. ultrasound transducers) or disposable devices should be used to connect the equipment to each patient (e.g. blood pressure cuffs). Equipment that comes into contact with potentially infective body fluids should be disposable. Three-way taps on intravenous (i.v.) or arterial lines should be changed every 24–48 hours and a meticulous regimen should be established for changing the drips and three-way taps connected to central lines used for total parenteral nutrition (TPN).

Humidified incubators are an infection hazard because Gram-negative bacilli, particularly *Pseudomonas* species, thrive in the wet and humid environment. Modern incubators are efficient when run dry, and many units only use humidification when they are having difficulty maintaining the temperature of particularly small babies. If incubator humidification is used, the humidifier should be drained daily and refilled with sterile distilled water. It should be swabbed regularly to look for Gram-negative colonisation. Incubators should be cleaned with conventional detergents and should be allowed to dry thoroughly before being reused. Incubators should be changed routinely every 2 to 3 weeks.

Ventilators pose an infection risk, as many parts of the circuit are inaccessible to sterilisation. Most ventilator circuits are now disposable, but the expense involved in changing them frequently is prohibitive. Changing them weekly seems a reasonable compromise between reducing infection risk and expense. As soon as the ventilator comes out of use, it is important to thoroughly clean the humidifier and all removable, cleanable items. The system should be allowed to dry thoroughly before being reused.

Admission policy

Babies should not be admitted to a neonatal unit if they can safely be managed at the mother's bedside. Any hospital can develop the concept of a transitional care ward (pp. 385–6), where babies can receive incubator care, tube feeding or a course of i.v. antibiotics at their mother's bedside.[191]

Cleanliness of the baby

Bacterial colonisation of the newborn is inevitable, but as the risk of invasive infection increases with the level of colonisation,[773] and as heavily colonised sites may cross-infect other sites on the same baby,[217] attempts to control the level of colonisation are warranted. Babies should be kept socially clean by the use of soap and water, but in the management of outbreaks of *Staph. aureus* infection, a limited period of use of an antibacterial agent for bathing babies is justified. An example of the effectiveness of such a regimen is the recently reported eradication of an outbreak of MRSA in a neonatal nursery brought about by bathing babies using a preparation containing 0.3% triclosan (Bacti-Stat).[863]

Cord care

The cord stump is generally the most heavily colonised area of the baby's surface and, traditionally, antiseptics have been applied in an attempt to reduce the risk of invasive infection, particularly with *Staph. aureus*. This is our current practice and we intend to continue it, as the evidence of the past is that the abandonment of such cord-care regimens is followed, sooner or later, by an increased prevalence of staphylococcal infection. A recent systematic review of 10 randomised or quasi-randomised trials, however, has concluded that, in developed countries at least, simply keeping the cord clean is as effective as using antibiotics or antiseptics.[869] In the developing world the situation is quite different, and improved attention to the care of the umbilical cord has a major impact on serious neonatal morbidity and on neonatal mortality.[39,286]

Invasive procedures

All invasive procedures can introduce colonising bacteria into the circulation. Areas of heavy colonisation, such as the groins, should be low down on the list of desirable sites for vascular access. The skin should be cleaned thoroughly, with either an iodine- or an alcohol-containing solution, which should be allowed to dry before the procedure is undertaken. A recent study[541] shows that more effective decontamination is obtained with a 30-second period of cleaning than with the conventional 5–10-second wipe. There is convincing evidence that catheter-related sepsis is more likely if the line is used frequently,[290,588] and every effort should be made to avoid doing so by the use of peripheral cannulae for blood transfusions and drug administration.

Other babies, staff and visitors

The greatest threat to an individual baby comes from bacteria colonising the skin, pharynx and gastrointestinal tract of other babies, visitors and staff, although the risk of acquiring infection from healthy visitors is trivial in relation to the social benefits of a reasonably open visiting policy (p. 374), as several studies have shown.[109,350,479] However, it should not be thought that visitors pose a zero risk, and epidemics of respiratory synctial virus (RSV) and rotavirus may be introduced by visiting siblings. Visitors must be shown how to wash their hands properly and must not touch babies other than their own.

Handwashing

The hands of the medical and nursing staff are the main potential route of cross-infection and, of all the measures for preventing nosocomial infection, handwashing is by far the most important. Hands should be washed before touching any baby and again immediately afterwards. Sleeves should be rolled up to the elbow and watches and jewellery removed. The highest bacterial kill rates are obtained with solutions or soaps containing iodine or alcohol. An effective approach is to use betadine- or chlorhexidine-containing solutions to thoroughly wash the hands and forearms occasionally during a stint of duty on the NICU, and then to simply rinse the hands in an alcohol-containing solution prior to and after touching each baby. Unfortunately, compliance with good handwashing practice is often poor. In a recent study conducted in a North American unit, handwashing immediately prior to patient contact was carried out by the medical staff on only 31.8% of occasions and by the nursing staff on only 24.7%.[127] Some improvement in staff compliance with good practice can be achieved by education and other measures.[353,748] Staff who only occasionally visit the neonatal unit, such as radiographers or physiotherapists, may have less opportunity to be educated in good handwashing habits.

Gowns, masks, caps and shoes

Routine use of gowns, masks, caps and shoes by staff or visitors is unnecessary on either the NICU or the postnatal wards.[168]

Overcrowding

Overcrowding and understaffing are associated with an increased incidence of nosocomial infection.[338]

Infectious disease in staff and parents

Medical and nursing staff with significant intercurrent infections should ideally stay away from work. Parents and siblings should take similar precautions, and be kept away from newborn babies. Staff with conditions such as gastroenteritis or skin infection should stay off duty, or stay away from babies. Infected parents, if they cover infected lesions and take appropriate precautions (masks, handwashing), can usually be allowed access to their baby (p. 386). HSV is a problem (pp. 1053–4) and staff with herpetic lesions should ideally stay off duty, certainly so if they have lesions on their hands. Herpetic lesions in parents should be treated with topical aciclovir and covered. Handwashing must be meticulous.

For serious infections in the mother and father, the routines outlined in Table 40.3 should be followed. Siblings and more distant family relatives should be kept away from the baby.

Use of antibiotics

Antibiotic use affects the pattern of nosocomial infection by influencing the colonising flora and by predisposing to antibiotic resistance.[434] In a study of antibiotic use in a North American NICU,[266] 75% of all infants, and 92% of VLBW babies, received antibiotics within 48 hours of birth. Five cross-sectional studies in the nursery showed point-prevalence rates of antibiotic use to be between 27% and 43% of the whole NICU population. These figures are almost certainly representative of most NICUs. It is difficult to know how, with the limitations of present investigational methods, the rate of initiating courses of antibiotics can safely be reduced, but there is a good deal that can be done in terms of stopping antibiotics sooner and rationalising the treatment once the infecting organisms have been identified (p. 1025).

Prophylactic antibiotic therapy is almost always undesirable, as, although it may protect the individual from infections by sensitive organisms, it predisposes to infection by resistant organisms and adds to the total amount of antibiotics prescribed, which over time encourages the emergence of resistant strains. Three randomised controlled trials (RCTs)[42,431,770] have demonstrated a convincing reduction in the incidence of CONS sepsis in infants who received parenteral nutrition fluids containing vancomycin. There may be a place for very limited use of this approach in selected high-risk cases but the practice will probably increase the risk of the emergence of strains of CONS and enterococci resistant to vancomycin,[542,814] and that would be a very serious problem.[483]

Human milk[633]

Human milk confers significant protection against infection, particularly in the developing world,[34] but also in affluent populations.[193] Apart from protection against necrotising enterocolitis (NEC), the evidence for human milk protection against systemic sepsis in preterm babies is less good, but there is a dearth of good literature on the subject.[400] Many units in the UK have abandoned milk banking since HIV came on the scene, but all presumably do (and certainly should) encourage the use of the baby's own mother's milk. Safe practice in running a breast-milk bank is described on page 1074. It is important to be aware, though, that human milk can be a vehicle for transmission of bacterial infection[93] and to culture milk when such an occurrence is suspected. Routine culture of milk is unnecessary.

Microbiological surveillance

The NICU and the microbiology department should collaborate in a microbiological surveillance programme, so that the pattern of infecting organisms and their antibiotic sensitivity is known at all times.[354] It is very helpful to have a microbiologist on the NICU ward round on a regular basis to discuss prevention measures and antibiotic policy.

Control of outbreaks of infection

When an outbreak of bacterial infection occurs within a NICU or on the postnatal wards, the following steps should be taken. How far down the list it is necessary to go will depend on many factors, and should be decided in discussion with a microbiologist and the control-of-infection officer. It will also depend on the available human resources.

1. Isolate the infected babies together, so far as is practical. They may need to be transferred to a satellite unit. Clean and disinfect vacated rooms before readmitting to them.
2. Increase attention to measures designed to minimise cross-infection, especially handwashing. The use of gowns by staff is also important, with a separate gown for each baby.[535] The use of gloves seems to have been useful in curtailing some outbreaks.[815]
3. Cohort the staff so that those caring for infected or colonised babies do not also care for non-colonised ones.
4. Culture all infants on the unit to identify asymptomatic carriers, and isolate them together if possible. Clean and disinfect vacated rooms before readmitting to them.
5. Change skin and cord care regimens, e.g. in a *Staph. aureus* outbreak.[863]
6. Culture equipment such as incubators, ventilators and blood gas analysers[315] and use settle plates to study the environment.
7. Where relevant, obtain surface cultures from all the unit staff to look for possible reservoirs and modes of transmission of infection.
8. Consider the use of prophylactic antibiotics for a short period, e.g. in an outbreak of streptococcal infection.
9. Restrict admissions or close the NICU until contacts are discharged or are known not to be carriers. This is a last resort and should only be done after discussion with the control-of-infection team. Very rarely, it will be necessary to close the maternity ward.

Table 40.3 Effect of perinatal maternal infections

Illness in mother	Access to normal baby	Treatment
Varicella	Access restricted until lesions crested: mother gowned, masked and gloved	Give 250 mg of zoster immune globulin i.m. to infant if maternal disease <7 days predelivery; consider prophylaxis with aciclovir (p. 1056)
Zoster	Access	None: baby immune because of transplacental maternal IgG
Measles	Access	Give 250 mg of human normal immunoglobulin i.m. to infant (hyperimmune if available)
Mumps	Access	Nil
Rubella	Access	No problem to neonate but keep mother away from antenatal patients
Herpes simplex (labial)	Access, but mother to wear face mask and treat lesion with aciclovir	None for baby
Herpes simplex (genital overt)	Access, but meticulous handwashing and gloves	Aciclovir orally to mother
Infectious hepatitis A (current)	Access	Give 250 mg of human normal immunoglobulin i.m. to baby
Recent acute hepatitis B or hepatitis B carrier	Access	Give 200 units of anti-hepatitis B immunoglobulin stat.; immunise baby with HBV vaccine stat. with booster at 1–6 months (p. 375)
HIV-positive (with or without AIDS)	Access	Nil. Breast-feeding probably contraindicated
TB open	Access	INAH to infant. BCG at 6 months if infant Mantoux negative: or give INAH-resistant BCG at once (pp. 375–6)
TB closed, on treatment or in the past	Access	BCG to infant
Brucella (active)	Access	Avoid breastfeeding[153]
Syphilis active	Access, meticulous handwashing, gloves for 24 hours	Penicillin to infant and mother (pp. 1070–2)
Gonorrhoea	Access	Treat mother and consort. Eye prophylaxis (p. 1049)
Malaria (active)	Access	Test infant's blood for parasites, especially if mother has falciparum malaria or if the infant develops symptoms. Treat congenital infection with chloroquine
Acute enteric infections (cholera, typhoid)	Nil during acute phase: mother too ill	Nil. Encourage breastfeeding if possible: immunise infant
Leprosy	Access	Continue maternal treatment
Other tropical diseases (i.e. trypanosomiasis, schistomiasis, filariasis)	Access	Nil, but consult local tropical disease hospital if infant symptomatic
Chlamydia	Access	Nil
Cytomegalovirus	Access	Nil
Acute respiratory infection (RSV, flu)	Access with masking and handwashing	Nil
Gastroenteritis	Access with meticulous handwashing	Nil
Listeria	Access if treated	Isolate and treat mother and baby
Streptococcal illness or carriage	Access, mask for group A streptococcal respiratory infection, handwashing for all	Nil
Skin infection (boils, impetigo)	Access. Meticulous handwashing. Antibiotic ointment to maternal lesions	Nil
Glandular fever	Access	Nil

INAH = Isonicotinic acid hydrazide.

Clinical presentation, investigation and management of neonatal sepsis

Neonatal infections can be caused by an extraordinary variety of microorganisms and can present many specific features. There are, though, many common principles relating to presentation, investigation and management which can usefully be considered before moving on to classify and deal with specific conditions.

Clinical presentation and assessment of the infant

Early recognition, diagnosis and treatment of serious infection in the neonate is essential because of the risk of permanent morbidity or mortality. Progression from mild symptoms to death can occur in less than 24 hours.[424] Most neonatal bacterial infections have an early bacteraemic phase preceding the development of a full-blown septicaemia or the localisation of infection in organs and tissues. During this phase the clinical signs are subtle, but this is when treatment must be started if there is to be intact survival. These factors dominate the clinician's approach to infants with apparently minor symptoms, and lead to an apparent, but totally justified, tendency to overinvestigate and overtreat. It is undoubtedly better to be proved wrong and to withdraw treatment after 48 hours from a well infant whose cultures are negative than to procrastinate for even a few hours with fatal consequences.

History

Ask about maternal, perinatal and neonatal events that put the baby at increased risk of infection.[765] If there is a possibility of congenital infection, take a detailed pregnancy history, enquiring about apparently trivial episodes of pyrexia or skin rash, as well as contact with known cases of infectious disease. Take the intrapartum history: was the mother unwell or febrile; did she have a tender uterus or a vaginal discharge; when did the membranes rupture (p. 198); were there any potentially infectious lesions on her cervix or vulva; was there a cervical suture; was there a fetal tachycardia: was there a raised C-reactive protein (CRP) or white cell count? If the mother has overt intrapartum infection, 15.2% of preterm babies and 4.1% of term babies will develop infection.[771] Maternal urinary tract infection (UTI) is an important risk factor for neonatal sepsis.[328,727] Are there factors predisposing to nosocomial infection, such as a history of possible contact with an infected person or environment? Has there been contact between the mother or other family members and patients with infectious disease? Do any of the staff have infections? What organisms are around the NICU at the time, and is there any evidence of an epidemic of infectious disease? Are there portals of entry for infection, such as a long line? If the baby presents with pyrexia, is this environmental in origin? If the baby is ventilated, have the requirements increased? Has jaundice or a bleeding tendency developed? Is there abdominal distension or blood in the stools?

Signs of neonatal sepsis

In the early stages, signs are subtle and often noted first by the nurses or the mother. Such concerns must always be taken seriously and should not be overridden by the findings of a single clinical examination, especially when risk factors for sepsis are present.

Early signs

- *'Going off'*. This is difficult to define, yet is often the earliest and most important sign. The mother or an experienced nurse thinks the baby is just not 'right'. He is slightly floppy, pale or mottled (cutis marmorata). He may be slightly irritable or unresponsive. He loses interest in feeding or sucks poorly.
- *Temperature change*. After excluding the effect of an abnormal environmental temperature (p. 576) and pyrexia in the first 1–2 hours of age in a baby of a pyrexial mother,[822] a temperature below 36°C or above 37.8°C sustained for more than an hour must be regarded as probably due to infection until proved otherwise.[228,822]
- *Jaundice*. Jaundice is far too common among newborn babies to have a useful positive predictive value for infection. However, infection enters into the differential list of causes of jaundice and should be considered if there is no other obvious explanation. Jaundice during sepsis is due to the effect of bacterial endotoxin on the liver, plus an increase in haemolysis.[690,753]
- *Apnoea*. In the preterm baby, apnoeic attacks are an early and significant sign of all types of infection.
- *Tachypnoea/recession*. Mild respiratory distress, as evidenced by a raised respiratory rate (sustained above 60 breaths per minute), and slight recession are among the first non-specific sign of sepsis.
- *Cardiovascular signs*. A tachycardia >160/min is often present early in sepsis.[316] In cases of myocarditis or endocarditis (p. 1032), cardiovascular signs will be more marked. Poor cutaneous circulation is common and is indicated by mottling and delayed capillary filling after the skin has been blanched by gentle pressure. The colour should normally return within 3 seconds.
- *Gastrointestinal*. The baby may vomit, have mild diarrhoea, or may develop an ileus with associated abdominal distension.
- *Irritability*. Infection may cause pain and may make the baby restless or whimper. Persistent moaning respiration is an ominous early sign.
- *Poor weight gain*. This may be a marker of chronic low-grade infection, such as UTI or an infected central line or shunt.
- *Skin*. Petechiae may be present (p. 1065) or there may be paronychia, septic spots or omphalitis.

Late signs of infection

The more obvious signs only appear with advanced infection, and if they occur, it usually means that the subtle signs have been present for some time beforehand, or the infecting organism was particularly virulent.

- *Respiratory*. Cyanosis, grunting and dyspnoea are the classic signs of neonatal lung disease (pp. 445–67). If present within the first 4–6 hours of life, pneumonia is a possibility, but many other diagnoses are possible (see Table 27.6). Beginning beyond 6–12 hours of age, these signs mean pneumonia until proved otherwise (pp. 1020–1).
- *Abdominal*. Signs of intestinal obstruction may be due to generalised sepsis as well as NEC (pp. 697–8) and structural malformations of the gastrointestinal tract (Chapter 29, Part 4). Bilious vomiting and abdominal distension are non-specific signs of obstruction, but flank lividity, abdominal redness and induration and periumbilical staining are late features of intraperitoneal sepsis.
- *Central nervous system* (CNS). A high-pitched cry, neck retraction, bulging fontanelle and convulsions are late features of neonatal meningitis, which has probably progressed to a cerebritis and cortical thrombophlebitis with a poor prognosis. In no other neonatal infection is it more important to consider the diagnosis as early as possible on the basis of the non-specific features.
- *Haemorrhagic diathesis*. Disseminated ontravascular coagulation (DIC) with petechiae and bleeding from puncture sites, the gut or the renal tract is a late sign of sepsis. Thrombocytopenia without evidence of DIC is also common with severe infection, especially fungal (p. 1061).
- *Sclerema* (p. 277). This is a non-specific feature of any serious neonatal illness. It may be seen in babies who have been septic for days, but is rarely found at presentation.
- *Pseudoparalysis*. The failure to move one limb, sometimes combined with the baby crying when moved, may be the only clue to septic arthritis or osteomyelitis.

Physical examination

Have the baby completely naked and look for:

- lesions of the skin or subcutaneous tissues;
- signs of respiratory distress, such as tachypnoea or expiratory grunting;
- signs of dehydration, suggesting fluid loss from vomiting or diarrhoea, or that the pyrexia is due to dehydration (p. 382);
- a red or discharging umbilicus or periumbilical flare.

In the formal examination, the following procedures should always be carried out:

- Examine the chest – is there tracheal shift, decreased air entry or added sounds?
- Check the heart rate and note the pulse volume – are there murmurs or a triple rhythm, suggesting myocarditis or endocarditis?
- Look for hepatosplenomegaly, which may accompany generalised septicaemia as well as hepatitis.
- Carefully palpate the kidneys – with pyelonephritis, a baby may have loin tenderness. Enlarged kidneys are a non-specific finding in early septicaemia.
- Is the abdomen tender, suggesting peritonitis? Is there redness or induration of the abdominal skin? Are there any underlying masses? Is peristalsis visible, and are bowel sounds present?
- Check the fontanelle tension, measure the head circumference, and check the spinal column and skull for pits or other skin defects, which might be the entry site for meningeal infections.
- Try to get an overall picture of the baby's neurological state. Is he obtunded or in a coma?
- Can osteomyelitis and septic arthritis be excluded by the presence of full and painless limb movements?
- Do not forget otitis media (p. 1032).
- Measure the blood pressure – always.

Investigation of neonatal sepsis[237,271]

Investigation and the value of tests

If the history and examination suggest infection, immediate investigation is indicated. The decision to treat will be determined mainly by the clinical assessment, but since septic infants deteriorate so rapidly, the threshold for a pre-emptive strike with antibiotics, pending further evaluation, should be very low, and the well-trained paediatrician will give antibiotics to a considerable number of non-infected infants.[294] To improve on this diagnostic accuracy, various tests have been developed and evaluated. Unfortunately, most evaluations have assessed the likelihood of a positive test in babies who have infection, and a negative test in babies shown not to have infection. This approach gives values for the sensitivity and specificity of the test. The question that the doctor wants the answer to, however, is 'What is the probability of this baby being infected, given the results of the test(s)?' The best approach to this question is a Bayesian one, through the use of likelihood ratios, which estimate the degree to which the result of a test alters the clinically assessed probability (prior probability) of infection being present. Unfortunately, few studies present their results in a form which allows likelihood ratios to be calculated and few tests for neonatal infection evaluated to date produce sufficiently large likelihood ratios to influence clinical decisions.[705]

Given the limited predictive power of existing tests, and the fact that few of them can produce results rapidly enough, decisions about antibiotic prescribing for unwell babies should continue to be made on clinical grounds. However, positive test results suggestive of infection may be sufficient reason to begin therapy even when the level of clinical suspicion is not high, for example a low white blood cell (WBC) count (say, $<5 \times 10^9/l$) in a slightly grunty term baby. The only test results that are more or less immediately available and sufficiently powerful to endorse a decision to go ahead with antibiotic therapy are cerebrospinal fluid (CSF) and urine microscopy, bacterial antigen tests, buffy coat microscopy and, possibly, the chest X-ray (CXR). The rest of the tests subserve one or both of the following functions:

- to provide retrospective evidence for or against the clinical diagnosis of infection;
- to establish the nature and antimicrobial sensitivity of the infecting organism.

The possible investigations are listed in Table 40.4.

Any baby who is suspected of being infected should have all of the routine tests performed immediately on presentation.

Table 40.4 Investigation of neonatal sepsis
Routine septic screen
Full blood count, including film
Blood culture
Swab from any site of inflammation
Throat and ear swab (in the case of suspected early-onset infection)
Urine microscopy and culture
Chest X-ray
C-reactive protein
Additional routine tests, indicated by the clinical situation/ availability
Lumbar puncture
Culture and Gram stain of gastric aspirate
Culture and Gram stain of a maternal high vaginal swab
Culture of endotracheal tube tip or tracheal aspirate
Culture of chest drain tip
Culture of removed vascular catheter
Quantitative blood cultures or multiple-site blood cultures
Organism-specific serial IgG concentrations
Organism-specific IgM concentration
Buffy coat microscopy
Non-routine or novel tests
Latex agglutination tests
Serum interleukin and TNFα
Immunoelectrophoresis
Acridine orange leukocyte cytospin test
NBT
DNA detection by PCR

The rest of the tests in Table 40.4 can be selected according to the circumstances. All are discussed below.

Microbiological investigation

Blood culture[140]

This is the definitive test, as the majority of neonatal infections are associated with bacteraemia. Continuous monitoring methods usually allow a positive blood culture to be reported within 12–24 hours, and virtually all cultures that are going to be positive have grown by 48 hours whatever the culture method.[558,696] Possible exceptions are *L. monocytogenes*, *H. influenzae* and yeasts, which may all take longer to grow. There are several pitfalls in collecting blood for culture and interpreting the findings.

Collecting blood for culture

Ideally, blood for culture should be taken from a peripheral vein after thoroughly cleaning the overlying skin with an antiseptic solution and allowing it to dry. Chlorhexidine with alcohol or an iodine-containing solution should be used. A better result can be obtained if the skin is cleansed for 30 seconds rather than the usual 5–10 seconds.[541] With good technique, skin contamination of blood cultures taken from peripheral veins can be reduced to an acceptable level. In a study of 677 paired cultures from blood and skin access sites, only nine of 58 positive blood cultures grew the same organism as was grown from the skin.[345] With modern laboratory techniques, 0.5 ml of blood may be sufficient for a successful culture,[449] but increasing the volume to 1 or 2 ml definitely increases the chance of a positive culture,[404,725] and to detect clinically significant low-level bacteraemia it has been suggested that up to 6 ml of blood may be necessary.[448] Taking two cultures from separate sites is a way to reduce false-positive diagnoses of infection.[784]

Cultures from freshly inserted long lines and umbilical artery catheters also give acceptable results. Capillary sampling can be adapted to give acceptable results if vascular access is a major problem, but contamination is more likely using this method.

Interpreting blood culture results

The problem lies in distinguishing septicaemia from skin contamination. A pure growth appearing within 24–48 hours is virtually always significant, but mixed organisms, bizarre organisms or growth that does not appear until after 72 hours of incubation should raise suspicion. However, in the case of the VLBW infant, it is unwise to ignore bizarre organisms (Table 40.5), or polymicrobial infection.

CONS present the greatest difficulty, because they colonise the skin of all babies and yet are the commonest pathogen among NICU inmates. Multiple-site blood cultures may improve the distinction between genuine septicaemia and skin contamination.[848] However, a recent study of multiple-site cultures, using plasmid typing and antibiotyping, has shown an incidence of unrelated strains of CONS from different sites of greater than 50%,[457] suggesting a high frequency of contamination. There is no easy answer to the problem of contamination in the case of CONS, and clinical assessment combined with the results of tests such as the blood count and CRP is often the only way to make a judgement about the likelihood of infection.

In septicaemia secondary to a long line, semiquantitative cultures on blood drawn from the line may be valuable in establishing the site of infection. The magnitude of the bacteraemia may also correlate with outcome, at least in the case of *Staph. aureus*.[730]

If conventional bacterial cultures are negative in a baby who has signs suggestive of septicaemia, it is important to exclude viral and fungal infection by sending appropriate samples after consultation with the clinical microbiologist.

Surface swabs

Swabbing sites of inflammation is important, but routine swabbing of sites such as the umbilicus, groin, ear, nose, throat, pharynx and rectum is much less so. Surface swabs are informative about colonisation, but all babies are soon colonised. Numerous studies have shown that the results of surface cultures are of limited value in diagnosis[670,867] and can probably be abandoned without detriment.[200] A study of the value of surveillance of pharyngeal colonisation in the detection of bacterial illness found concordance between pharyngeal isolates and blood-culture isolates in only 11% of cases.[258] In terms of producing likelihood ratios large enough to influence decision making, surface swabs perform poorly.[271]

Table 40.5 Organisms reported to cause neonatal sepsis (not specifically referred to in the main text). Most of these organisms cause a septicaemic type of illness and only focal features are referred to here

Organism	Focal and other features	References
Gram-positive cocci		
Group A streptococcus	Meningitis	Coulter et al 1984 Lancet ii:356
	Fasciitis	Nutman et al 1979 Arch. Dis. Child. 54:637
Group C streptococcus (*Streptococcus equisimilis*)	Meningitis	Hervas et al 1985 Ped. Inf. Dis. J. 4:694
Group D streptococcus		
1. α-haemolytic (viridans) (*Strep. sanguis, mitis*)	Meningitis	Freedman & Baltimore 1990 J. Perinatol. 10:272
		Heath et al 1980 Am. J. Obs. Gyn. 138:343
		Haftar et al 1983 J. Clin. Microb. 18:101
		Spigelblatt et al 1984 Ped. Inf. Dis. J. 4:56
2. *Strep. bovis*	Meningitis	Alexander & Giacoia 1978 J. Pediatr. 93:489
		Fikar & Levy 1979 Am. J. Dis. Child 133:1149
3. *Strep. faecalis*	Meningitis	Dobson & Baker 1990 Ped. Inf. Dis. J. 9:165
	Abscess	Jeffery et al 1977 Arch. Dis. Child. 52:683
		Luginbuhl et al 1987 Ped. Inf. Dis. J. 6:1022
α-haemolytic streptococcus (non-group D)	Meningitis	Broughton et al 1981 J. Pediatr. 99:450
Group F streptococcus		Well & Keeney 1980 Pediatrics 66:820
Group G streptococcus		Brans 1975 Pediatrics 55:745
		Dyson & Reld 1981 J. Pediatr. 99:944
Streptococcus milleri (usually group F, can be C, A, G)		Cox et al 1987 J. Clin. Pathol. 40:190
Streptococcus pneumoniae	Meningitis	Alzahawi et al 1988 Br. J. Obs. Gyn. 95:1198
		Geelen et al 1990 J. Perinat. Med. 18:125
		Jacobs et al 1990 Scand. J. Infect. Dis. 22:493
		Kaplan et al 1993 Am. J. Perinatol. 10:1
		Robinson 1990 Rev. Inf. Dis. 12:799
		Westh et al 1990 Rev. Inf. Dis. 12:416
		Wright et al 1990 J. Infect. 20:59
Leukonostoc	Meningitis	Friedland et al 1990 J. Clin. Microbiol. 28:2125
Peptostreptococcus (anaerobic)		Chow et al 1974 Pediatrics 54:736
		Noel et al 1988 Ped. Inf. Dis. J. 7:858
Gram-positive bacilli		
Bacillus anthracis	Septicaemia	Ozkaya et al 2000 Ped. Inf. Dis. J. 19:487
Bacillus fragilis	Osteomyelitis	Brock 1980 Clin. Pediat. 19:639
Bacillus licheniformis	Meningitis	Thompson et al 1990 Pediat. Rev. Comm. 4:147
Bacillus cereus	Meningitis	Feder et al 1988 Pediatrics 82:909
	Pneumonia	Jevon et al 1993 Ped. Inf. Dis. J. 12:251
Bifidobacterium		Noel et al 1988 Ped. Inf. Dis. J. 7:858
Clostridium perfringens (Welchii)	Congenital infection	Gallaher & Marks 1991 Am. J. Perinatol. 8:370
	Meningitis	Orzel et al 1983 Ped. Inf. Dis. J. 2:457
		Motz et al 1996 Ped. Inf. Dis. J. 15:708
	NEC	Long et al 1985 Ped. Inf. Dis J. 4:752
		Noel et al 1988 Ped. Inf. Dis J. 7:858
Lactobacillus	Meningitis	Broughton et al 1983 Ped. Inf. Dis. J. 2:382
Gram-negative cocci		
Moraxella catarrhalis	Meningitis	Daoud et al 1996 Ann. Trop. Paediatr. 16:199
	Pneumonia	Ohlsson & Bailey 1985 Scand. J. Inf. Dis. 17:225
	Cellulitis	Leighton et al 1982 Ped. Inf. Dis. J. 1:339

(Continued)

Table 40.5 (Continued)

Organism	Focal and other features	References
Neisseria gonorrhoea	Ventriculitis	Bland et al 1983 Am. J. Obs. Gyn. 147:1781
	Ophthalmia	Desenclos et al 1992 Sex. Transm. Dis. 19:105
	Vaginitis	Stark & Glade 1979 J. Pediatr. 94:298
Neisseria meningitidis	Intrauterine infection	Bhutta et al 1991 Ped. Inf. Dis. J. 10:868
	Abscess	Chugh et al 1988 Ped. Inf. Dis. J. 7:136
	Meningitis	Embree et al 1987 Ped. Inf. Dis. J. 6:299

Gram-negative bacilli

Organism	Focal and other features	References
Acinetobacter sp	Meningitis	Ibrahim 1995 West Afr. J. Med. 14:59
		Horrevorts et al 1995 J. Clin. Microb. 33:1567
		Morgan & Hart 1982 Arch. Dis. Child. 57:557
		Stone & Das 1985 J. Hosp. Inf. 6:42
		Vesikari et al 1985 Arch. Dis. Child. 60:542
Achromobacter xylosoxidans	Meningitis	Hearn & Gander 1991 Am. J. Clin. Pathol. 96:211
		Namuyak et al 1985 J. Clin. Microb. 22:470
Alkaligenes xylosoxidans	Meningitis	Boukadida et al 1993 Ped. Inf. Dis. J. 12:696
		Kishan et al 1987 Ind. J. Ped. 54:789
		Placzek & Whitelaw 1983 Arch. Dis. Child. 58:728
Bacteroides fragilis	Meningitis – metronidazole may be useful	Chow et al 1974 Pediatrics 54:736
		Ketter & Monif 1988 Obs & Gynecol 71:463
		Webber & Tuohy 1988 Ped. Inf. Dis. J. 7:886
		Noel et al 1988 Ped. Inf. Dis. J. 7:858
Brucella	Enterocolitis	Lubani et al 1988 Eur. J. Pediatr. 147:520
		Labrune et al 1990 Acta. Paed. Scand. 79:707
	Congenital infection	Chheda et al 1997 Ped. Inf. Dis. J. 16:81
		Shamo'on & Izzat 1999 Ped. Inf. Dis. J. 18:1110
	From blood tranfusion	al Kharfy 2001 Ann. Trop. Paediatr. 21:349
Campylobacter jejuni	Meningitis	Youngs et al 1985 Arch. Dis.Child. 60:480
	Gastroenteritis	Goosens et al 1986 Lancet ii: 146
		Forbes & Scheifele 1987 Ped. Inf. Dis. J. 6:494
Capnocytophaga		Feldman et al 1985 Ped. Inf. Dis. J. 4:415
Citrobacter (freundii, diversus)	Meningitis – abscesses common	Rae et al 1991 Drug Intell. Clin. Pharm. 25:27
		Kline et al 1988 J. Pediatr. 113:430
		Goering et al 1992 Ped. Inf. Dis. J. 11:99
		Saraswathi et al 1995 Ind Pediatr. 32:359
Corynebacterium amycolatum		Berner et al 1997 J. Clin. Microb. 35:1011
Edwardsiella tarda	Meningitis	Vohra et al 1988 Ped. Inf. Dis. J. 7:814
	Septicaemia	Mowbray et al 2003 Pediatrics 111:e296
Eikenella		Sporken et al 1985 Acta Obs. Gynecol. Scand. 64:683
Enterobacter cloacae	Meningitis	Acolet et al 1994 J. Hosp. Infect. 28:273
		Bannon et al 1988 Arch. Dis. Child. 64:1388
		Lacey & Want 1995 J. Infect. 30:223
		Modi et al 1987 Arch. Dis. Child. 62:148
		Verweij et al 1995 Infect. Control. Hosp. Epidemiol. 16:25
	NEC	Millar et al 1992 Arch. Dis. Child. 67:53
E. sakazakii	Meningitis	Muytjens et al 1983 J. Clin. Microb. 18:115
		Willis & Robinson 1988 Ped. Inf. Dis. J. 7:196
Flavobacterium meningosepticum	Meningitis – consider rifampicin	Thong et al 1981 J. Clin. Pathol. 34:429
		Linder et al 1984 Arch. Dis. Child. 59:582
		Tam et al 1989 Ped. Inf. Dis. J. 8:252
Fusobacterium	NEC	Noel et al 1988 Ped. Inf. Dis. J. 7:858
Haemophilus influenzae	Pneumonia and meningitis	al Mofada 1994 J. Infect. 29:283
		Bale & Watkins 1978 J. Pediatr. 92:233

(Continued)

Table 40.5 (*Continued*)

Organism	Focal and other features	References
		Berg et al 1981 Scand. J. Inf. Dis. 13:299
		Barton et al 1982 Am. J. Dis. Child. 136:463
		Kinney et al 1993 Ped. Inf. Dis. J. 12:739
		Lilien et al 1978 Pediatrics 62:299
		Meis et al 1991 Scand. J. Infect. Dis. 23:649
		Mendoza & Roberts 1991 J. Perinatol. 11:126
		Wong & Ng 1991 J. Paediatr. Child Health 27:113
		Webster et al 1995 Aust. N. Z. J. Obst. Gynecol. 35:102
		Milne et al 1988 Arch. Dis. Child. 63:83
	Osteomyelitis	Williams et al 1994 J. Infect. 29:203
H. parainfluenzae	Meningitis	Nakamura et al 1984 Am. J. Clin. Pathol. 81:388
Helicobacter cinaedi	Meningitis	Orlicek et al 1993 J. Clin. Microb. 31:569
Klebsiella oxytoca		Tullus et al 1992 Acta Pathol. Microb. Imm. Scand. 100:1008
Klebsiella pneumoniae	UTI	Reish et al 1993 J. Hosp. Inf. 25:287
		Coovadia et al 1992 J. Hosp. Infect. 22:197
	Meningitis	Cherubin et al 1982 Rev. Inf. Dis. 4, S:453
		McCracken et al 1980 Lancet i:187
		Morgan et al 1984 J. Hosp. Inf. 5:377
Mycobacterium cheloni		Speert et al 1980 J. Pediatr. 96:681
Pasteurella multocida	Meningitis – from animals	Thompson et al 1984 Ped. Inf. Dis. J. 3:559
Pasteurella pestis (plague)	Skin	White et al 1984 Am. J. Dis. Child. 135:418
Pleisomonas shigelloides	Meningitis	Waeker et al 1988 Ped. Inf. Dis. J. 7:877
		Billiet et al 1989 J. Inf. 19:267
Proteus mirabilis	Meningitis – abscesses common	Smith & Mellor 1980 Arch. Dis. Child. 55:308
		Velvis et al 1986 Ped. Inf. Dis. J. 5:591
Pseudomonas aeruginosa	Meningitis	Eisele et al 1990 Ear Nose Throat J. 69:119
		Gupta et al 1993 J. Trop. Pediatr. 39:32
		Jeffrey et al 1977 Arch. Dis. Child. 52:683
		Leigh et al 1995 Ped. Inf. Dis. J. 14:367
		Turkel et al 1986 Ped. Pathol. 6:131
		Ruderman et al 1983 Clin. Pediatr. 22:630
	Noma neonatorum	Juster Reicher et al 1993 Am. J. Perinatol. 10:409
		Freeman et al 2002 Ped. Inf. Dis. J. 21:83
Pseudomonas pseudomallei	Meningitis	Lumbiganon et al 1988 Ped. Inf. Dis. J. 7:634
Salmonella eimsbuettel	Gastroenteritis	McAlister et al 1986 Lancet i: 1262
Salmonella typhi	Gastroenteritis	Chin et al 1986 Arch. Dis. Child. 61:1228
	Typhoid fever	Reed & Klugman 1994 Ped. Inf. Dis. J. 13:774
Salmonella oranienburg	Gastroenteritis	Mehta et al 1987 Ind. J. Med. Res. 75:482
Salmonella sp. (heidelberg, typhimurium dublin, enteriditis, urbana, poona)	Meningitis	McCracken et al 1980 Lancet i: 787
		Davis 1981 Am. J. Dis. Child. 135:1096
		Gogate & Deodhar 1984 Ind. J. Pediat. 51:549
	Gastroenteritis	Kumar et al 1995 Indian Pediatr. 32:881
		Mahajan et al 1995 J. Commun. Dis. 27:10
		Umasankar et al 1996 J. Hosp. Inf. 34:117
		Sirinavin et al 1991 J. Hosp. Inf. 18:231
		Stone et al 1993 Am. J. Inf. Control. 21:270
Serratia marcescens	Meningitis	Lewis et al 1983 BMJ 287:1701
		Smith et al 1984 Lancet i: 151
Shigella sonnei	Late-onset gastroenteritis	Ruderman et al 1986 Ped. Inf. Dis. J. 6:379

(*Continued*)

Table 40.5 (Continued)

Organism	Focal and other features	References
Shigella flexneri	Gastroenteritis and bowel perforation	Starke & Baker 1985 Ped. Inf. Dis. J. 4:405
Vibrio cholera		Coovadia et al 1982 S. Afr. Med. J. 64:405
		Bose et al 2000 Ped. Inf. Dis. J. 19:166
Yersinia enterocolitica	Gastroenteritis	Paisley & Laver 1992 Ped. Inf. Dis. J. 11:331
Leptospira sp.		
Leptospirosis		Shaked et al 1993 Clin. Infect. Dis. 17:241
Legionella		
Legionella pneumophila	Pneumonia	Luck et al 1994 Eur. J. Clin. Microb. Inf. Dis. 13:565
		Holmberg et al 1993 Pediatrics 92:450
		Greene et al 1990 J. Perinatol. 10:183
Viruses		
Adenovirus	Systemic infection	Abzug & Levin 1991 Pediatrics 87:890
		Piedra et al 1992 Ped. Inf. Dis. J. 11:460
		Montone et al 1995 Diagn. Cytopathol. 12:341
		Chiou et al 1994 Ped. Inf. Dis. J. 13:664
Coronavirus	Pneumonia	Sizun et al 1995 Acta Paediatr. 84:617
Enteroviruses	Systemic infection	Abzug et al 1993 Ped. Inf. Dis. J. 12:820
	Respiratory illness	Pruekprasert et al 1995 J. Assoc. Acad. Minor. Phys. 6:134
Lymphocytic chroiomeningitis virus		Enders et al 1999 Ped. Inf. Dis. J. 18:652
Rhinovirus	In BPD	Chidekel et al 1997 Ped. Inf. Dis. J. 16:43
Parasites		
Blastocystis hominis	Diarrhoea	Galatowicz et al 1993 Ped. Inf. Dis. J. 12:345
Giardia lamblia	Gastroenteritis	Morrow et al 1992 J. Pediatr. 121:363
	Myiasis (blowfly larvae)	Amitay et al 1998 Ped. Inf. Dis. J. 17:1056

Gastric aspirate

This can be viewed as a sample of amniotic fluid, plus or minus some swallowed secretions from the birth canal. About one-third of gastric aspirates show bacteria on Gram stain (often potential pathogens, such as the Enterobacteriaceae, GBS and enterococci) and a similar proportion contain some polymorphs.[103] The great majority of these babies do not become septic, and the results of gastric aspirate microbiology cannot be considered an argument for antibiotic therapy. If a baby is thought to be infected on clinical grounds, however, it is important to choose antibiotic therapy that will cover any organisms seen in the gastric aspirate. The gastric aspirate can only contribute to the diagnosis of infection if taken immediately after birth and before the baby has been fed.

Maternal high vaginal swab

When babies present with signs of infection within the first 24–48 hours of birth, the source is likely to be the maternal vagina, and a high vaginal swab (HVS) may well grow the responsible organism. However, a low vaginal/perineal swab with enrichment media is more likely to yield a positive result for GBS. In common with the gastric aspirate and surface swabs, however, the HVS tells about possible exposure to pathogens and not about infection, and the results are available too late to influence initial decision-making

about therapy. They may help, though, to decide about the need to continue with therapy and on the choice of therapeutic agent.

Urine

There are two practical ways to obtain urine from babies for the purpose of diagnosing infection. One is to use a urine collection bag and the other is to perform a suprapubic aspiration (SPA) (pp. 1261–2). SPA overcomes the problem of contamination, and pus cells or organisms in a technically satisfactory SPA indicate urinary infection. To avoid delay and uncertainty, it may be worth performing an SPA in the initial assessment of the sick baby who is thought to be septicaemic.

As part of the routine septic screen it is usual to begin with a urine specimen collected in a bag applied to the perineum. The perineum should be cleaned carefully before the bag is applied, and the bag removed as soon as the urine is passed. It is not satisfactory to cover a urine bag with a nappy and remove it at the next nappy change! Urine should be microscoped as soon after voiding as possible. If bacteria and white cells are seen, this strongly suggests UTI. Because of the long-term implications of a diagnosis of UTI (p. 1047), the result of urinalysis must be interpreted with great care. The main value of bag urines is that if they are clear they exclude UTI. Positive bag urines should always be viewed with suspicion unless there are many white cells ($>150/mm^3$) and a pure growth of at least 10^8 organisms per litre of urine (10^5/ml). A mixed growth, or an organism other than *E. coli*, obtained from a bag urine should always be confirmed by performing an SPA.

It is also possible to screen for UTI in babies by means of dipsticks. These measure the concentrations of leukocyte esterase, nitrites and protein by a colour change which can be read using a photometer. One study has shown a negative predictive value for UTI of 99.4% in a cohort of newborn babies and infants.[498] Sticks have not yet been fully evaluated in the neonatal intensive care setting.

Tracheal secretions and endotracheal tube-tip culture

Undoubtedly, microorganisms recovered from the upper airway may be those causing septicaemia and lower respiratory tract infection, and this has been shown in the case of CONS, using ribotyping techniques,[87] and also with *Candida* species.[695] The results of cultures of respiratory secretions should therefore be used to inform the choice of antimicrobial agents for suspected pulmonary infection. However, it is naïve to base the diagnosis of pulmonary infection solely on the results of culture of respiratory secretions, as illustrated by a recent study comparing tracheal aspirate cultures from babies showing signs of respiratory deterioration with cultures from babies who were stable. No significant difference was found in the rate of positive cultures for bacteria, viruses, chlamydia or ureaplasmas. Cultures were positive in about one-third of the babies in each group.[798]

Vascular lines and thoracentesis tubes

The tips of umbilical cannulae, central lines and thoracentesis tubes should be sent for culture when removed. Central lines can be cultured using the 'Macki roll' technique, in which the line is rolled across the culture plate and a subsequent colony count performed. This can help to distinguish genuine line infection from skin contamination during removal of the line.

Lumbar puncture

Neonatal bacterial meningitis carries such a high morbidity and mortality (pp. 1040–2), especially if diagnosis and treatment are delayed, that a lumbar puncture (LP) should be performed as part of the infectious disease work-up of most ill babies before antibiotics are started. Exemptions can be made for babies with pulmonary infection complicating long-term intermittent positive-pressure ventilation (IPPV; pp. 521–4), babies with overt localised infection such as NEC or osteomyelitis, and babies who would not be able to tolerate the procedure.[343] However, these are rare and specific exemptions. Asymptomatic term babies merely at risk of sepsis do not require an LP.[426] As the LP is being used as a screening procedure, a large number of negative CSF results can be expected. In a recent survey, 99.05% of all CSF results were normal,[388] although it must be said that the threshold for performing an LP was extremely low, with 42% of all babies admitted to the neonatal unit concerned having their CSF examined. In keeping with this finding, the positive predictive value was low, at 46%. Whether or not babies presenting with respiratory distress syndrome (RDS) soon after birth should be added to the exemption list is debatable. Most clinicians do not

routinely LP preterm babies with RDS before starting antibiotics, and there is literature to support this stance.[365] However, there is a slight risk of missing or delaying the diagnosis of meningitis in preterm infants if the LP is omitted from the early sepsis screening.[847] In general, the LP is more likely to produce a positive result in late-onset than in early-onset sepsis.[738]

LP should be performed with strict sterile precautions (p. 1263). It is best performed with the baby sitting upright; however, if the baby is on his side, it is important to avoid excessive flexion of the trunk as this may cause respiratory embarrassment or apnoea. If it is essential to examine the CSF in an unstable baby, it may be safer to intubate and ventilate before proceeding. Babies with low platelet counts should be given platelets before the procedure is carried out.

CSF analysis

Although high WBC counts in CSF have sometimes been reported in babies without meningitis, a polymorphonuclear count higher than $20/mm^3$ should be regarded with suspicion,[16] and counts above $30/mm^3$ are strongly indicative of meningitis (Appendix 8). When bloodstained CSF is obtained, the ratio of red cells to white cells should be calculated. In uninfected CSF, this is usually $>500{:}1$.

Microscopy of the CSF is crucial and may, with caution, be used to direct the choice of initial antimicrobial therapy, although broad-spectrum antibiotics should be used until the results of the cultures are known. The isolation of *Candida* species from the CSF of infants in the absence of other CSF abnormality usually suggests contamination.[29]

The upper normal limit of CSF protein is 1.5–2.0 g/l in the term baby (Appendix 8). Preterm babies often have higher CSF protein concentrations but rarely greater than 3.0 g/l. The levels are usually raised in meningitis. CSF glucose levels should be related to a simultaneous measurement of blood glucose. The CSF glucose should be at least 50% of the blood glucose level, and a low level (<1.0 mmol/l or a value less than 30% of the blood glucose) suggests bacterial meningitis.

The CSF should be tested for the presence of group B streptococcal or *E. coli* K1 antigen, which gives accurate and prompt diagnostic information. A polymerase chain reaction (PCR) test for herpesvirus is available and should be requested when appropriate (see p. 131).

A new development in the diagnosis of meningitis in neonates and infants is the measurement of cytokines such as interleukin-6 (IL-6) and tumour necrosis factor alpha (TNFα) in the CSF. A recent study found IL-6 to be present in the CSF of each of 20 infants with bacterial meningitis and absent in all 20 infants without bacterial meningitis. In cases of aseptic meningitis, IL-6 was found in about half, but at only about 10% of the concentration found in bacterial meningitis. TNFα was found to be a less sensitive indicator of bacterial meningitis.[208] More research is needed to define the predictive value of tests for neonatal meningitis based on cytokine measurements.

Radiology

All babies with suspected sepsis should have a CXR. An abdominal X-ray and ultrasound are indicated if there are abdominal signs or suspicion of UTI. X-rays are not a good way to detect bone or joint infection in the early stages (pp. 1045–6).

Haematological investigation

Total white cell count

This is the least useful index, because the normal range is so wide (Appendix 1), varies with gestation and postnatal age, can be confused by machines including nucleated red blood cells in the count, and can be 30–40% lower in blood obtained from a central catheter than in a capillary sample. Furthermore, many non-infective catastrophes such as periventricular haemorrhage, convulsions and asphyxia can raise the total WBC count.

Neutrophil count

The neutrophil count is of more value. There are well-documented normal ranges in term and preterm infants at various postnatal ages (Appendix 1). Reference ranges for the total neutrophil count in the VLBW infant have recently been extended.[584] Within the first 48 hours of life, neutropenia (<2.0–$2.5 \times 10^9/l$) suggests bacterial infection, and at this cut-off value the sensitivity is around 20%.[331] Thereafter, both neutropenia and neutrophilia (>7.5–$8.0 \times 10^9/l$) have useful predictive power, although in neither case is the specificity or sensitivity greater than about 80%.

The appearance of the circulating neutrophils changes in infection, so that more immature forms are seen in the peripheral blood. These are commonly known as band forms. The absolute value for band forms is not of much use because it tends to rise late in infection, and in the most severely affected infants band cell production is limited as the marrow becomes exhausted. A slightly more useful indicator of infection is the ratio of immature to total neutrophils (I/T ratio). The maximum normal value is 0.16 during the first 24 hours, 0.14 by 48 hours, and 0.13 by 60 hours, where it remains until 5 days of age. Thereafter, the maximum normal I/T ratio is 0.12 until the end of the first month. Several studies have found that an I/T ratio >0.2 is a useful marker of infection and that a ratio <0.2 makes infection unlikely. Using a higher I/T ratio of 0.3 or 0.4 has been reported to marginally increase the positive predictive value of the tests.[336] An abnormal I/T ratio in the presence of a low absolute neutrophil count is more strongly suggestive of infection.

Another feature suggesting infection is the presence of toxic granulation in the neutrophils. Manroe et al[549] found this in only 11% of normal infants, compared with 63% of infants with confirmed sepsis.

It has been recommended that in neutropenic infected babies the WBC storage pool should be assessed by marrow puncture. However, as the test is invasive, the neutropenia usually transient and treatment by granulocyte transfusions still experimental,[143] there seems little purpose in doing this.

Lymphocyte count

Babies who have lymphocyte counts persistently below $2.8 \times 10^9/l$ should be investigated for severe combined immunodeficiency.[316,337]

Acridine orange test

Direct staining of microorganisms within WBCs using the acridine orange technique is a useful way of diagnosing septicaemia and fungaemia. In a study comparing diagnosis of central venous catheter sepsis, acridine orange was shown to be most accurate (87% sensitivity and 94% specificity).[700] Microscopy of a buffy-coat smear stained with methylene blue is also a useful test, with a high rate of concordance with blood culture results.[677]

Platelet count

In 50% of babies with bacterial infection, the platelet count will fall below $100 \times 10^9/l$, but this usually occurs after the baby is obviously septic. In a recent study, the sensitivity and specificity of thrombocytopenia for the diagnosis of septicaemia were reported as 65% and 47%, respectively.[81]

Viral infections, both congenital (e.g. rubella, CMV and herpes) and acquired (e.g. enterovirus, CMV, herpes), may cause a profound thrombocytopenia (p. 1066).

Acute-phase proteins

C-reactive protein

CRP is a better indicator of infection than the WBC indices,[81,331] especially if serial measurements are made[662] and a receiver operator characteristic curve is constructed to establish the best cut-off value. It takes several hours for the CRP concentration to rise in an infected baby, however, and so the CRP is not often of much value in deciding whether to treat with antibiotics. The greatest worth of the CRP is in the retrospective evaluation of a clinical diagnosis of sepsis after starting treatment. Culture-proven sepsis is unlikely if the CRP does not rise within 24–48 hours of the onset of the illness,[76,97,223] and the combination of a normal CRP and negative cultures at 48 hours is a generally safe basis for stopping antibiotic therapy which was started on clinical suspicion. Serial measurements of CRP are useful in monitoring the progress of infection and may help decide for how long to continue treatment. Persistently elevated CRP during antibiotic therapy for presumed bacterial infection should suggest the possibility of fungal infection, resistant organisms, or the development of a complication such as bacterial endocarditis or abscess formation. A raised CRP is often seen in association with meconium aspiration, even when there is no evidence of bacterial infection.

Other acute-phase proteins

Orosomucoids (α_1-acid glycoprotein), haptoglobin, α_1-antitrypsin and α_1-antichymotrypsin have all been used in assessing neonatal infection, but add little if anything to what is learnt from studying CRP. The same applies to fibronectin assays, although it is worth pointing out that many septic preterm infants develop significantly low plasma fibronectin concentrations, which may impair their ability to combat infection.[215,222]

Cytokines

TNFα and IL-6

Since TNFα is a principal initiator of systemic inflammation and together with IL-6 induces CRP, elevations of TNFα and IL-6 concentrations in plasma should provide an early indication of sepsis. IL-8 is also likely to be an early indicator of sepsis, as it is involved in neutrophil release from bone marrow and neutrophil activation. The value of these cytokines as markers of bacterial sepsis in newborn infants has recently been reviewed.[560] The authors concluded that wide methodological variations between the 31 studies evaluated, as well as small sample sizes, prevented meta-analysis or even any robust conclusions that would be valuable to clinicians – an all too familiar story! It is also the case that the cytokine assays used in research have turnover times that are too long to be of any use in practice. It appears that IL-6 is a better marker of early-onset sepsis than CRP and that combining cytokine and CRP measurements,[605] as well as serial testing,[636] improves the accuracy of the tests as markers of sepsis. Umbilical venous IL-6 (but not TNFα) concentrations have been shown to be elevated in very preterm babies with intrauterine or early-onset sepsis.[441]

Cellular antigens
Neutrophil CD64 and CD11b expression have been shown to be increased in neonatal sepsis[607,617] but the clinical utility of this type of test has not been established.

Serum procalcitonin[292]
Elevated serum concentrations of procalcitonin have recently been shown to predict neonatal sepsis with considerable accuracy,[538] but further studies are needed. Procalcitonin distinguishes between infection and inflammation (which CRP does not) and differentiates between bacterial and viral infection with high specificity.

Serum granulocyte colony-stimulating factor
Using a cut-off value of 120 pg/ml, the serum G-CSF concentration has been shown to have a sensitivity of 95%, a specificity of 73%, a positive predictive value of 40% and a negative predictive value of 99% in the diagnosis of culture-proven neonatal sepsis.[450]

Immunological studies
Antigen detection tests
Counterimmunoelectrophoresis has been used to detect the presence of bacterial antigens in blood, urine or CSF, but it is little used in neonatal practice. However, rapid screening for GBS using latex particle agglutination is in quite widespread use, for detecting both maternal and neonatal colonisation.[277,320,675] In screening neonates, it has been suggested that it may be best to concentrate the urine before testing.[65] However, a recent evaluation of the test on concentrated urine in screening for GBS within the first 24 hours of life found a sensitivity of 90%, a specificity of 70%, a positive predictive value of 12% and a negative predictive value of 99%.[846] These results suggest that the main value of the test may be in providing reassurance of the absence of GBS.

Antibody detection tests
These are of more value in viral infections, when a fourfold or greater rise in antibody titre in samples drawn 2 weeks apart is diagnostic. If there is suspicion of congenital infection, organism-specific IgM should be sought (p. 150), although this is not reliable for HIV (pp. 1073–5).

Genetic techniques[512]
It is now possible to amplify highly conserved DNA sequences from a variety of Gram-positive and Gram-negative organisms, as well as many viruses, using PCR, while avoiding the simultaneous amplification of associated human DNA.[520] This method has the potential to be automated and to provide rapid diagnosis of bacteraemia. Other DNA amplification techniques are also becoming available.

Treatment of neonatal sepsis

In this section the general principles of treatment of the septicaemic infant will be outlined. The overriding consideration is prompt and effective treatment, as infants with systemic sepsis deteriorate very rapidly because of poor host defences, and morbidity and mortality rates are high.

Antibiotics

The choice and administration of antibiotics for early-onset sepsis are discussed on pages 1028–33 and for late-onset sepsis on pages 1037–8. Other comments on antibiotics are linked to the discussion of focal infections.

Adjunctive therapies

Although antibiotics are the mainstay of treatment of neonatal bacterial infection, experience with immunodeficient patients shows that antibiotics alone are often unsuccessful in defeating bacteria if not supplemented by host defences. Because all neonates are to an extent immunodeficient, and preterm infants especially so, various attempts have been made to employ adjunctive therapies to improve host defences.

Immunoglobulin therapy

The prophylactic use of immunoglobulins is discussed on page 1038. The therapeutic use of immunoglobulin infusions in clinically suspected or proven sepsis has been less well studied. There is evidence of improved humoral immunity in babies after immunoglobulin infusion,[12] of enhanced opsonophagocytosis of CONS by neonatal blood after the addition of immunoglobulin,[175] and of enhanced production of TNFα by cord blood monocytes following incubation with IgG.[186] With regard to important clinical outcomes, the most recently published meta-analysis showed a statistically significant reduction in mortality (typical RR 0.55) when immunoglobulin was administered as part of treatment for proven infection (Fig. 40.9) but slightly less convincing evidence of a reduction in mortality in cases of suspected infection (Fig. 40.10).[626]

Fresh frozen plasma

Fresh frozen plasma (FFP) is commonly used as part of the treatment of the septic infant in an attempt to enhance humoral immunity.[782] Adult FFP enhances neonatal neutrophil chemotaxis in vitro.[224] However, when FFP was infused into infants, no effect on the serum concentrations of components of humoral

Review: Intravenous immunoglobulin for suspected or subsequently proven infection in neonates
Comparison: 02 IVIG vs placebo or no intervention for proved infection
Outcome: 01 Mortality from any cause

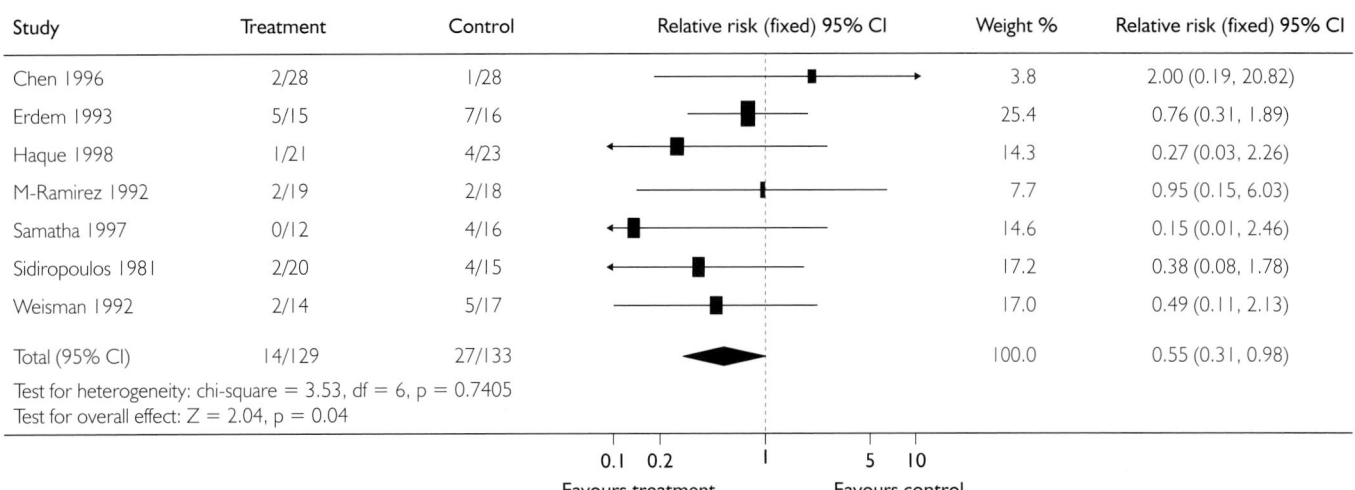

Study	Treatment	Control	Relative risk (fixed) 95% CI	Weight %	Relative risk (fixed) 95% CI
Chen 1996	2/28	1/28		3.8	2.00 (0.19, 20.82)
Erdem 1993	5/15	7/16		25.4	0.76 (0.31, 1.89)
Haque 1998	1/21	4/23		14.3	0.27 (0.03, 2.26)
M-Ramirez 1992	2/19	2/18		7.7	0.95 (0.15, 6.03)
Samatha 1997	0/12	4/16		14.6	0.15 (0.01, 2.46)
Sidiropoulos 1981	2/20	4/15		17.2	0.38 (0.08, 1.78)
Weisman 1992	2/14	5/17		17.0	0.49 (0.11, 2.13)
Total (95% CI)	14/129	27/133		100.0	0.55 (0.31, 0.98)

Test for heterogeneity: chi-square = 3.53, df = 6, p = 0.7405
Test for overall effect: Z = 2.04, p = 0.04

0.1 0.2   1   5   10
Favours treatment   Favours control

Fig. 40.9 Treatment with intravenous immunoglobulin versus either placebo or no intervention in cases of proven infection. Outcome measure is mortality from any cause. (From Ohlsson & Lacy.[626])

Review: Intravenous immunoglobulin for suspected or subsequently proven infection in neonates
Comparison: 01 IVIG vs placebo or no intervention for suspected infection
Outcome: 01 Mortality from any cause

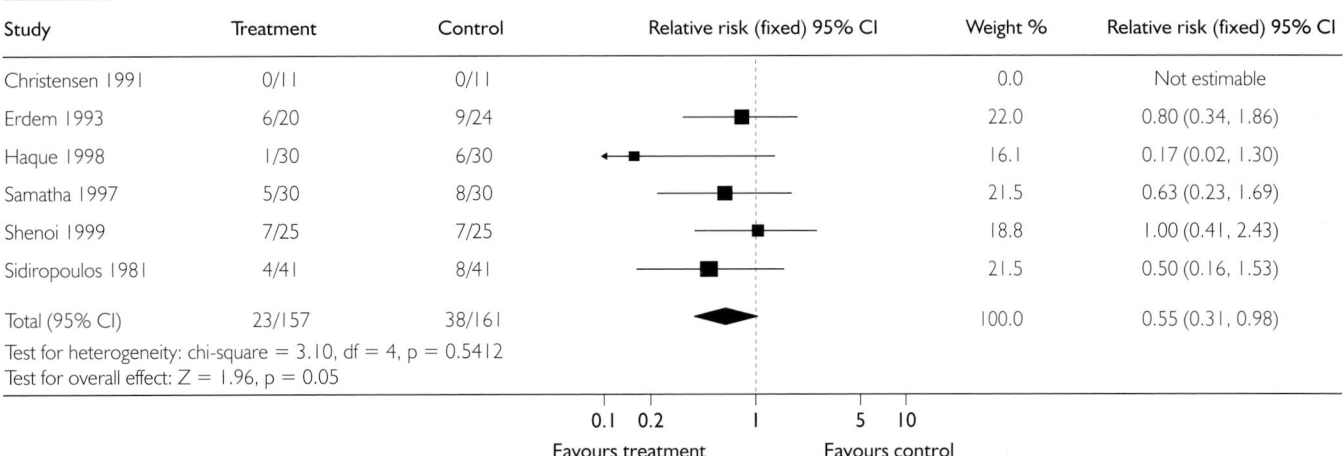

Study	Treatment	Control	Relative risk (fixed) 95% CI	Weight %	Relative risk (fixed) 95% CI
Christensen 1991	0/11	0/11		0.0	Not estimable
Erdem 1993	6/20	9/24		22.0	0.80 (0.34, 1.86)
Haque 1998	1/30	6/30		16.1	0.17 (0.02, 1.30)
Samatha 1997	5/30	8/30		21.5	0.63 (0.23, 1.69)
Shenoi 1999	7/25	7/25		18.8	1.00 (0.41, 2.43)
Sidiropoulos 1981	4/41	8/41		21.5	0.50 (0.16, 1.53)
Total (95% CI)	23/157	38/161		100.0	0.55 (0.31, 0.98)

Test for heterogeneity: chi-square = 3.10, df = 4, p = 0.5412
Test for overall effect: Z = 1.96, p = 0.05

0.1 0.2   1   5   10
Favours treatment   Favours control

Fig. 40.10 Treatment with intravenous immunoglobulin versus either placebo or no intervention in cases of suspected infection. Outcome measure is mortality from any cause. (From Ohlsson & Lacy.[626])

immunity was found.[12] There are also concerns about the safety of FFP (p. 767).[139] Unless evidence of the efficacy of FFP in treating neonatal sepsis is forthcoming from RCTs, there is little justification for its use in septic infants other than in treating associated DIC (pp. 759–60).

Exchange transfusion

Exchange transfusion provides humoral factors and removes some noxious products of septicaemia, such as bacterial toxins, fibrin degradation products and cytokines. Some studies have suggested that exchange transfusion with fresh whole blood is beneficial in neonatal sepsis,[807] but well-designed, prospective

RCTs are conspicuous by their absence. However, the improvement in some septicaemic babies after exchange with fresh blood is occasionally dramatic, and the technique should not necessarily be abandoned.

Granulocyte transfusion

Granulocytes obtained from donor blood, or by plasmapheresis, have been given to septic babies, in particular when their illness has been complicated by neutropenia and granulocyte storage pool depletion, as judged by bone marrow aspiration (p. 1264). Several efficacy studies have been published but are too flawed in their design to allow clear conclusions to be reached.[145,162,492]

The most recently published randomised trial has suggested a possible benefit,[147] but overall the literature is not convincing.

Granulocyte colony-stimulating factor and granulocyte–macrophage colony-stimulating factor[574]

G-CSF and GM-CSF are important in inducing granulocyte production and activation in the newborn during sepsis,[295,702] and may be a useful marker of infection.[436,450] The mononuclear cells of the newborn are less able to produce G-CSF than those from adults,[146] and this may be part of the explanation for the granulocytopenia that often accompanies severe neonatal sepsis. In human newborns, several trials of recombinant G-CSF and GM-CSF in suspected sepsis have shown an increase in neutrophil counts and enhanced functional activity, as judged by C3bi expression.[68,92,144,300,573,692,818] There are now several published studies on the influence of G-CSF and GM-CSF on outcome in neonatal sepsis when used either as treatment or prophylaxis.[67,92,471,573,726,818] An almost universal finding has been a sharp rise in the neutrophil count, and no acute toxicities have been identified. Evidence of efficacy in reducing mortality rates or other important outcome measures is not yet clearly established and almost all published reports state the necessity for larger and more definitive work, which is badly needed. In infants suffering from alloimmune neutropenia or congenital agranulocytosis, G-CSF and GM-CSF can be very effective,[686] and initial concerns about increased malignancy risk seem unfounded.[275]

Other innovations

Pentoxifylline (oxypentifylline)
Pentoxifylline (oxypentifylline) is an immunomodulating agent which can augment impaired neutrophil function in newborn infants. It has a wide range of effects, including altering neutrophil deformability and increasing nitoblue tetrazolium reduction and H_2O_2 production.[481] Its use in septic infants has not been evaluated.

Antilipid A monoclonal antibodies
Lipid A is responsible for the toxic effects of lipopolysaccharide in Gram-negative shock, and antilipid A monoclonal antibody decreases mortality in infected newborn rats.[313] Interestingly from a perinatal point of view, the antilipid antibody was administered to the pregnant female rat and passed transplacentally.

Supportive therapy

The septicaemic baby often requires full neonatal intensive care, as described in Chapter 19 and Chapter 27, Part 2. There are, though, one or two specific points that require special attention.

Arterial and venous lines
The preferred course of action is to remove any central lines that have been in place for more than 24 hours and to replace them with peripheral lines until the sepsis has been dealt with. This option may prove impossible to implement in tiny babies with difficult vascular access, in whom, despite the hazards, leaving the lines in place for both infusion and sampling in the early stages of the illness may be totally justified.

Bleeding diathesis
Thrombocytopenia and DIC are both common complications of neonatal septicaemia. Their management is discussed in detail on page 761.

Nutrition
Septicaemic babies are usually catabolic but rarely tolerate enteral feeds, because of a paralytic ileus, NEC or gastroenteritis. Intravenous feeding, particularly fat, is poorly tolerated during septicaemia. For this reason, dextrose and electrolytes alone should be used for the first 24–48 hours of infection. More complete parenteral or enteral nutrition should be established as soon as there is improvement in the baby's condition.

Classification of neonatal infections

Classification is useful in so far as it facilitates consideration of common principles of causation, presentation or treatment. The following is the most helpful to the practice of neonatal medicine.

- **Early-onset sepsis.** Definitions range from 24 hours to 7 days, but here the term means infections presenting within the first 48 hours of life and commonly caused by microorganisms acquired from the mother before or during birth. Other terms used for this pattern of infection are 'vertically transmitted' (meaning from mother to infant) and 'perinatally acquired'.
- **Late-onset sepsis.** This term means infection presenting after 48 hours of age and generally caused by microorganisms acquired from the environment rather than from the mother. The other terms used for this pattern of infection are 'nosocomial' and 'horizontally transmitted'. Nosocomial means literally 'of, or related to, a hospital'. In this sense many vertically transmitted infections are nosocomial, but it is more useful in studying epidemiology to separate infections acquired from the mother during birth from those acquired after birth.
- **Transplacental infection.** This is self-explanatory and is the usual term for infections such as congenital rubella, toxoplasmosis and CMV. It is also appropriate for many cases of HIV infection and hepatitis, and some cases of HSV infection.

Early-onset neonatal sepsis

Early-onset sepsis is usually a fulminating septicaemic illness, often complicated by meningitis or pneumonia. It is caused by pathogens acquired from the mother prior to, or during, birth. Important predisposing factors are prolonged rupture of the membranes, maternal UTI, prematurity, a particularly pathogenic microorganism, or a mother with no relevant antibody (as in GBS infection). It has also recently been reported that a significant proportion of the babies of mothers with severe pre-eclampsia are neutropenic and more than usually vulnerable to early-onset sepsis.[455,583] Although prematurity is an important risk factor, the mean birthweight of babies suffering from early-onset sepsis is significantly higher than that of babies suffering from late-onset sepsis. In two recent studies, the mean birthweight of babies with early-onset sepsis was 2472 g and 2213 g, and for babies with late-onset sepsis 1960 g and 1711 g, respectively.[205,407]

The incidence of early-onset sepsis (as defined here) is around 2–4 cases per 1000 livebirths.[407,735] The incidence may be falling in developed countries, especially among LBW infants, possibly owing to intrapartum antibiotic prophylaxis for group B streptococcal infection (pp. 1031–2).[652]

Most early-onset sepsis is probably still caused by *Str. agalactiae*, commonly known as GBS,[407] but there is recent evidence to suggest that Gram-negative organisms, such as *E. coli*, are taking over, probably the result of anti-GBS measures.[54,779] Other important organisms are streptococci other than GBS,[323] *H. influenzae*, *L. monocytogenes*, Gram-negative anaerobes,[123] fungi and *Chlamydia trachomatis*. The pattern of presentation is similar with most of the causative organisms, and early-onset sepsis with GBS will serve as the model for all.

Early-onset sepsis due to group B streptococcus

Epidemiology

The group B streptococcus is a commensal of the gastrointestinal tract and vagina, and colonises some 10% to 30% of pregnant women in the UK. There are numerous identifiable serotypes of GBS, based on capsular polysaccharide antigens: Ia, Ib, II, III, IV, V, VI, VII and VIII. All are implicated in early-onset disease, with national variations in prevalence,[554] but most neonatal infections are caused by types I, II and III.[355] Simultaneous infection with two distinct serotypes has been described.[255] In addition to the polysaccharide antigens there are surface-exposed protein antigens which may also contribute to the pathogenicity of particular strains,[165] although tissue invasiveness seems unrelated to known surface antigens.[810]

Recent publications have reported the prevalence of early-onset GBS sepsis in different countries as follows: in the USA, 1.8 per 1000 livebirths;[110] in Canada, 1.75 per 1000;[167] in Australia, 1.3 per 1000;[407] in Spain, 1.2 per 1000;[370] and in Finland, 0.76 per 1000.[435] In the UK, recently reported prevalences of either proven or proven/suspected GBS sepsis are 0.9 per 1000,[582] 0.6 per 1000,[359] 1.15 per 1000,[62] 2.6 per 1000,[66] and 0.57 per 1000.[622] From time to time, major outbreaks are reported during which the prevalence may be as high as 14 per 1000 livebirths.[13]

The two major factors influencing the prevalence of GBS sepsis are vaginal carriage rates among pregnant women and the effectiveness of strategies to prevent contamination of the baby at birth. During the last 10 years, vaginal and rectal carriage rates have been variously reported as 18.5%,[298] 12%,[423] 16.3%,[672] 23%,[30] 7.1%[370] and 17.8%.[781] Some of this variability relates to swabbing technique and the use of different culture media. The lowest rates are reported from European centres, and this is

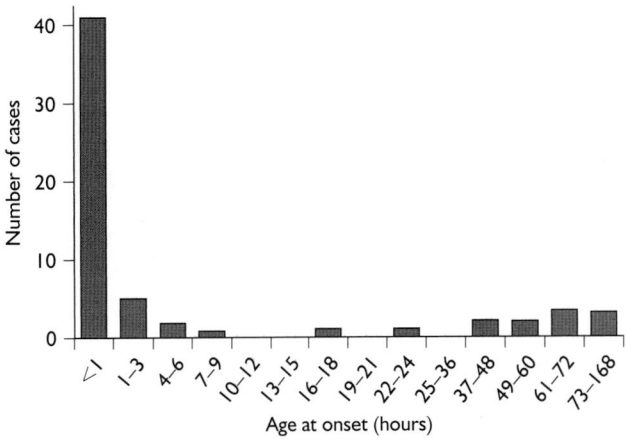

Fig. 40.11 Distribution of 61 cases of early-onset GBS infection. (Reproduced from Boyer & Gotoff.[112])

mirrored in the lower reported prevalence of early-onset GBS sepsis in Europe, certainly compared with the USA before preventive policies were instituted. Neonatal GBS infection can also occur as a result of infected breast milk but the presentation is later than with intrapartum transmission.[195,629]

Clinical picture

Most cases of GBS sepsis develop within the first 4–6 hours (Fig. 40.11) and almost 90% of cases present within 24 hours of birth,[285,856] even those cases that occur following the administration of intrapartum antibiotics.[122] GBS sepsis may masquerade as severe birth asphyxia or present immediately after resuscitation, with respiratory failure, cyanosis and shock. More often, the baby presents with the early signs of sepsis (pp. 1017–18), and this is when the condition **must be suspected**. Without prompt recognition and treatment, the baby's condition rapidly worsens and he requires intubation and IPPV for apnoea and severe hypoxaemia, often demonstrating the cardiorespiratory features of persistent pulmonary hypertension of the newborn (PPHN) (pp. 496–502). Hypotension, metabolic acidaemia, tachycardia and poor peripheral perfusion develop in severe cases, and then the prognosis is poor.

Pathophysiology

The hypotension, hypoxaemia, and lung and liver injury that characterise early-onset GBS sepsis in the newborn are very reminiscent of the systemic inflammatory release syndrome caused by the endotoxin of Gram-negative organisms. Gram-negative endotoxin exerts its effects mainly by stimulating the release of cytokines, such as TNFα, IL-1[811] and IL-6 from antigen-presenting cells, including macrophages and monocytes. TNFα causes progressive hypotension, decreased cardiac output, hypoxaemia and lung injury when infused directly into animals. TNFα can be detected in the serum and urine of babies with GBS sepsis (but not from healthy controls), and, in the laboratory, heat-killed washed GBS can induce the production of TNFα from monocytes and macrophages (Fig. 40.12).[844] Interestingly, mixed

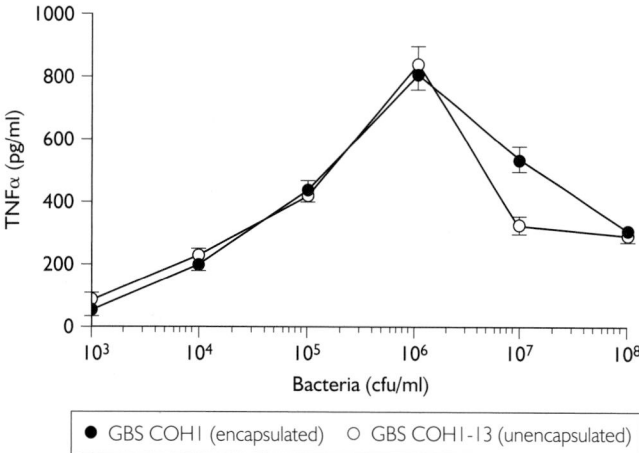

Fig. 40.12 Production of TNFα by monocytes and macrophages in response to encapsulated (COHI) and unencapsulated (COHI-13) type III GBS. (From Williams et al.[844])

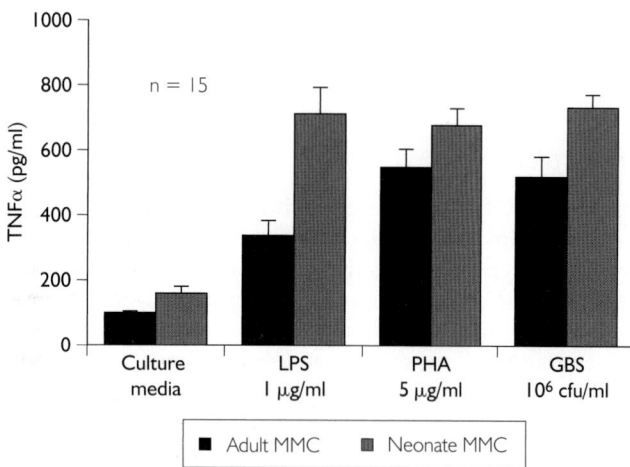

Fig. 40.13 Comparison of TNFα production by mixed mononuclear cells from adults and newborn infants in response to stimulation by GBS, phytohaemagglutinin (PHA) and *E. coli* endotoxin (LPS = lipopolysaccharide). (From Williams et al.[844])

mononuclear cells from neonates produced significantly more TNFα in response to GBS than did cells from adults (Fig. 40.13).[844] The cellular component of GBS responsible for causing septic shock is thought to be β-haemolysin.[684]

Another feature of the GBS is its ability to invade pulmonary endothelial cells,[234] especially the cells of the microvasculature, and lead to the release of the eicosanoids, such as prostacyclin and PGE$_2$.[299] In animals, injection of heat-killed GBS causes dose-dependent increases in pulmonary arterial pressure and pulmonary and systemic vascular resistance, and decreases in cardiac output and heart rate. The quantitative response of the pulmonary vascular resistance is strain dependent, with serotype Ib having a greater effect than serotype III.[177] Infection with different strains might go some way towards explaining different severities of illness.

Host defences against GBS include polymorphonuclear leukocytes, complement and type-specific antibodies directed against the polysaccharide and protein antigens. A baby is most susceptible to GBS when his mother, despite having GBS in her vagina, has little or no circulating anti-GBS IgG.[46] This is particularly likely if the baby is born prematurely. A concentration of IgG-specific antibody of >2 micrograms/ml in the serum of newborns seems protective.[46] Neonatal white cells find it difficult to kill the organism and, if antibody is present, GBS antigen causes neutrophil aggregation in the lung, with the consequent release of a multiplicity of cytokines which further contribute to tissue injury.[46]

Postmortem findings

There are no specific features, although many infants have alveolar hyaline membranes, as well as pneumonia.[5,642] In the preterm infant, surfactant-deficient hyaline membrane disease (HMD) may coexist,[417] but in term babies the hyaline membranes are a non-specific change caused by GBS toxicity.[688] The presence of hyaline membranes may in the past, in the absence of adequate bacteriological investigation, have resulted in many deaths due to GBS or other similar infections being attributed to surfactant-deficient RDS.

Investigation

On no account should the treatment of suspected early-onset sepsis be delayed pending the results of tests. The objective of performing tests is to provide retrospective confirmation of the diagnosis, to identify the responsible organism and to look for complications.

Microbiological

The blood culture will almost invariably be positive if the mother has not been treated with antibiotics. GBS will usually grow from most surface swabs and from the gastric aspirate (which often contains numerous Gram-positive cocci), although there is little benefit in investigating these sites in addition to blood. Meningitis is relatively unusual (circa 15%) in babies presenting in the first hours of life, but an LP should be performed in infants presenting with signs of early-onset sepsis (pp. 1028–33).[847] GBS antigen can be identified by latex particle agglutination tests on the infant's serum and concentrated urine (p. 1026).[277,675] However, in a recent multicentre study evaluating the latex particle agglutination test in the urine of babies with culture-proven GBS sepsis, only 53.5% of infected babies had a positive test.[65]

The organism is usually present in the mother's perineal swab, and new techniques may enable rapid detection of the organism on recto-vaginal swabs when the mother is admitted in labour.[776] The specificity of these tests appears to be good, but their sensitivity is relatively poor.[320]

Haematological/biochemical/clinical

Neutropenia and the presence of primitive cells in the peripheral blood are common[116,548] and neutropenia <1.5 × 10^9/l is an ominous sign.[642] However, the sensitivity, specificity and predictive values of haematological values in the diagnosis of early-onset sepsis are poor.[322,336] Anaemia and thrombocytopenia may develop in survivors. Acute-phase reactants such as CRP are generally highly elevated in GBS sepsis, but there may be a delay of 12 hours or so between the onset of signs and the rise in CRP.[651] Early acidosis and hypotension are bad signs.

Radiological

The CXR may be virtually normal or show widespread homogeneous opacity in those with coexisting RDS,[505] and is rarely helpful in differential diagnosis. Pleural effusions may occur.[642]

Treatment

Intravenous antibiotics, at the high end of the recommended dose range, must be started immediately the diagnosis is suspected. A combination of penicillin (or amoxicillin) and gentamicin is a good choice for blind treatment of early-onset sepsis in the newborn because of synergism between these antibiotics against GBS,[45,791] and because it is necessary to cover other organisms responsible for the syndrome (pp. 1032–3). A cephalosporin alone is unsatisfactory initial therapy for early-onset sepsis, as it will not treat *L. monocytogenes* or enterococci. Once the diagnosis of GBS sepsis is confirmed, therapy can be simplified to i.v. benzylpenicillin alone, continued for 10 days. GBS is very sensitive to penicillin, with most isolates having a minimal inhibitory concentration of less than 0.06 micrograms/ml. Surfactant should be given to GBS-infected infants in respiratory failure.[368]

Exchange transfusions using blood from a donor with anti-GBS antibodies have been considered helpful.[49,340] Use of immunoglobulin and GM-CSF is discussed on pages 1038–9.

Outcome

In the late 1970s, early-onset GBS sepsis had a mortality rate of around 50%,[43] rising to 100% for babies <1.50 kg.[671] The results have improved since then, and recent reports from European centres have reported overall mortality rates of 8%,[435] 11%[359] and 19.5%.[582] For mature babies, and those with late-onset disease, the mortality should now be <10%.[112,407,856] LBW babies still do less well and all of the deaths in the recently reported series from Oxford were all preterm.[582] A recent report from the North of England found that 0.8 neonatal deaths per 10 000 live-births were due to confirmed early-onset GBS sepsis.[230]

Preventing GBS sepsis

Maternal prophylaxis

Approximately 1% of babies born vaginally to mothers who carry GBS at the time of birth become infected. Important predisposing factors are chorioamnionitis, prolonged labour, prolonged rupture of the membranes, frequent pelvic examinations in labour, and low birthweight.[13,166,285,298,533,817] One or more of these predisposing factors is present in some 80% of cases of early-onset neonatal GBS sepsis.[285]

The main approach to preventing vertical transmission so far employed is intrapartum antibiotic prophylaxis, which appears to more than halve the risk of early-onset neonatal infection.[359,732]

Prophylaxis has been given to women known to carry GBS (a screening approach) and/or those who have obstetric risk factors (a risk-based approach).[82,653] A recent evaluation of these two approaches in the USA found that the risk of early-onset GBS sepsis was substantially lower among infants of women who had undergone screening between 35 and 37 weeks' gestation compared with those who were only treated on the basis of risk factors (relative risk 0.46; 95% CI 0.36–0.6).[731] In the same issue of *The New England Journal of Medicine* that reported this finding, however, was the report of an increase in the proportion of early-onset sepsis caused by Gram-negative bacteria,[779] suggesting that there may be a price to pay for widespread use of prophylactic intrapartum antibiotics. Intrapartum antibiotics are not effective in cases where intra-amniotic infection begins before labour, and this, coupled with concerns about widespread antibiotic prophylaxis, points to the need for other approaches to prevention.

In the UK there is much variation in practice regarding the prevention of vertical transmission of GBS. The pros and cons of various approaches have recently been reviewed,[113,406,581] and the RCOG/REPCH have produced guidelines. At present there is no support for a national screening policy in the UK, and the question has been addressed by the UK National Screening Committee and remains on the agenda (www.nsc.nhs.uk).

Immunisation against GBS is certainly possible and effective, although clinical trials are awaited;[46,442] however, international and secular changes in the distribution of GBS serotypes will be problematic.[187,355]

Management of premature rupture of the membranes and preterm, premature rupture of the membranes[309,312,564]

Once the amnion ruptures, the amniotic cavity and the fetus become accessible to microorganisms present in the vagina. The likelihood of such ascending infection increases with time. When the membranes rupture prior to the onset of labour – known simply as 'premature rupture of the membranes' (PROM) – the interval between membrane rupture and the birth of the baby may be prolonged. When the membranes rupture at less than 37 weeks' gestation – known as 'preterm, premature rupture of the membranes' (PPROM) – an even greater interval between membrane rupture and birth often occurs.

The evidence concerning the risk of neonatal sepsis following PROM at or near term is conflicting. Some studies suggest relatively little increased risk,[508] whereas others show a high risk and a high mortality.[17] Meconium staining of the liquor increases the risk of intra-amniotic infection.[837] A meta-analysis of RCTs of prophylactic antibiotics in the management of PROM at or near term has recently been concluded and shows no benefit in terms of neonatal sepsis.[263]

There is no doubt that PPROM carries a significant risk of sepsis,[37,371,508] although when membrane rupture occurs before 28 weeks of gestation, pulmonary hypoplasia is probably the greater threat to survival.[531] The risk of neonatal sepsis following PPROM has been reported to be about 3.5 times that without PPROM.[501] The risk can be reduced by prompt delivery following membrane rupture, but this has to be balanced against the risk of premature birth. A recently reported meta-analysis of trials of prophylactic antibiotics in PPROM showed some benefit

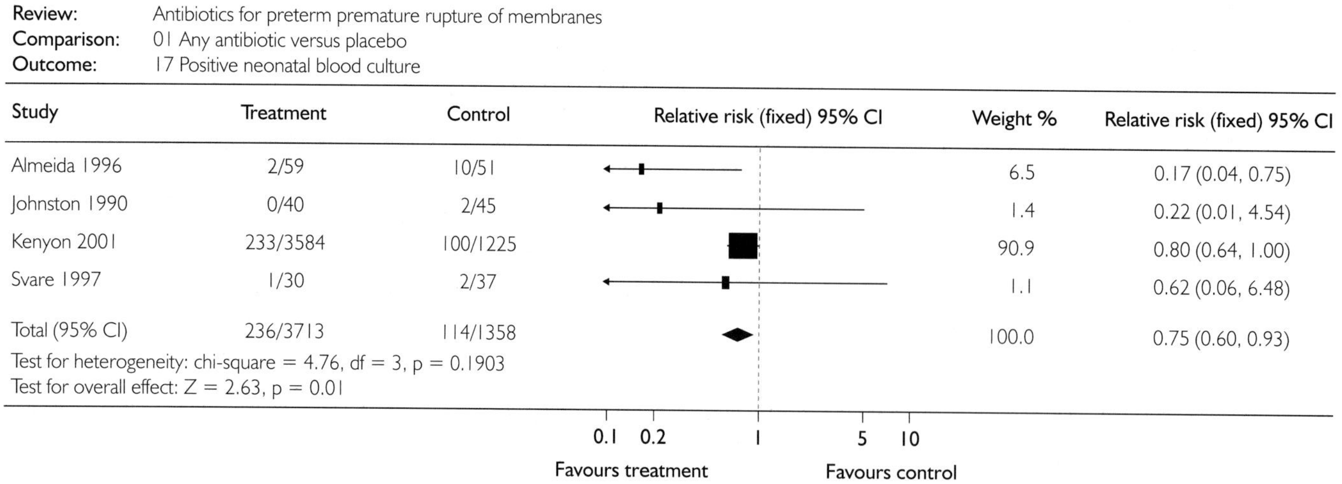

Review: Antibiotics for preterm premature rupture of membranes
Comparison: 01 Any antibiotic versus placebo
Outcome: 17 Positive neonatal blood culture

Study	Treatment	Control	Relative risk (fixed) 95% CI	Weight %	Relative risk (fixed) 95% CI
Almeida 1996	2/59	10/51		6.5	0.17 (0.04, 0.75)
Johnston 1990	0/40	2/45		1.4	0.22 (0.01, 4.54)
Kenyon 2001	233/3584	100/1225		90.9	0.80 (0.64, 1.00)
Svare 1997	1/30	2/37		1.1	0.62 (0.06, 6.48)
Total (95% CI)	236/3713	114/1358		100.0	0.75 (0.60, 0.93)

Test for heterogeneity: chi-square = 4.76, df = 3, p = 0.1903
Test for overall effect: Z = 2.63, p = 0.01

0.1 0.2   1   5   10
Favours treatment   Favours control

Fig. 40.14 Antibiotics for preterm premature rupture of membranes. Any antibiotic versus placebo. Outcome measure is positive blood culture from baby. (From Kenyon et al.[451])

in terms of both clinical evidence of neonatal sepsis and the frequency of positive blood cultures (Fig. 40.14).[451]

Neonatal prophylaxis

Whether or not to give prophylactic antibiotics to asymptomatic, term babies considered to be at risk of GBS sepsis is a controversial issue. Giving prophylactic penicillin to all babies cannot be justified given current evidence. Recommendations vary regarding management of asymptomatic babies born to known carrier mothers. The Royal College of Obstetrician and Gynaecologists (RCOG), the UK Government Health Protection Agency, and the Group B Strep Support (GBSS) group have all produced guidelines (www.rcog.org.uk; www.hpa.org.uk; www.gbss.org.uk). These range from the Health Protection Agency's statement that antibiotics should be 'considered' in this group, to those of the GBSS group, who think that treatment should be started in all babies whilst awaiting culture results. The RCOG discuss the risk factors, and point out that 'the argument for using prophylaxis is stronger in the presence of multiple risk factors but is still unproven'. Reasonable practice in the current state of flux is to observe asymptomatic babies of colonised mothers for 12 hours, but to screen and treat any who are asymptomatic but have any single risk factor (maternal pyrexia, fetal tachycardia, prolonged membrane rupture).

Recurrent GBS infection

Some unfortunate infants experience more than one distinct episode of GBS sepsis, although the risk of this is no more than about 1%. In a recently reported series of nine cases,[321] the mean age at the second infection was 42 days; six cases had septicaemia without a focus of infection and three had meningitis. In more than half of the cases, the organism causing the first and subsequent infection was shown by means of restriction enzyme digestion and pulsed-field gel electrophoresis to be the same. Whether these cases represent a relapse of the initial infection or a reinfection is unclear.

Table 40.6 Conditions caused by GBS (Reproduced from Baker & Edwards[44])

Early-onset septicaemia	Myocarditis
Asymptomatic bacteraemia	Ethmoiditis
Meningitis	Otitis media
Pneumonia	Conjunctivitis
Empyema	Endophthalmitis
Peritonitis	Breast abscess
Suprarenal abscess	Cellulitis
Arthritis	Fasciitis
Osteomyelitis	Impetigo
Brain abscess	Purpura fulminans
Subdural empyema	Omphalitis
Cerebritis	Dactylitis
Endocarditis	Superficial abscess
Pericarditis	Urinary infection

Other organisms causing early-onset neonatal sepsis

Many other organisms besides GBS can cause acute early-onset sepsis with a pattern of illness very similar to that described above (Table 40.5). These organisms can also cause late-onset septicaemia, as well as many of the specific infections listed in Table 40.6. It is because of this common presentation with such a diversity of pathogens that antibiotic therapy must be broad spectrum until the results of culture allow refinement. A few specific causes of early-onset sepsis warrant further discussion.

Haemophilus influenzae

H. influenzae, especially the non-capsulate non-serotypable strains, has an affinity for the female genital tract and is responsible for almost 10% of early-onset sepsis,[562] third only in importance to GBS and *E. coli*.[701] The prevalence of neonatal *H. influenzae* infection was recently reported to be 4.6 per 100 000 births in the Oxford region.[247] Risk factors operate as for GBS, and a recent study of early-onset *H. influenzae* sepsis reported preterm labour in 92%, PROM >12 hours in 63%, maternal fever in 64%, chorioamnionitis in 43% and vaginal discharge in 44%.[467] Most infants present immediately after birth with respiratory distress due to pneumonia. Meningitis and conjunctivitis are relatively common. The reported mortality is in the region of 50%.[850] Most *H. influenzae* causing early-onset sepsis in newborn infants in the UK are currently sensitive to ampicillin, and this is one of the reasons why ampicillin is preferable to benzylpenicillin as part of the blind initial treatment. However, ampicillin resistance is progressively emerging and cefotaxime should be added when there is reason to suspect *H. influenzae* sepsis.

Listeria monocytogenes (see also pp. 1047–8)

Early-onset neonatal sepsis with *L. monocytogenes* is far less common than it was in the late 1980s, presumably as a result of pregnant women heeding advice on the avoidance of potentially contaminated foods such as unpasteurised cheese. At present, fewer than 20 cases of neonatal listeria per annum are reported in England and Wales (http://www.phls.org.uk/topics_az/listeria/data_human.htm). Most vertically transmitted listeria infections present at ≤24 hours of birth as septicaemia, pneumonia or meningitis. Diarrhoea and an erythematous skin rash may occur. It is very important to realise that listeria is not effectively treated by third-generation cephalosporins, and high-dose ampicillin is the drug of choice.

Coagulase-negative staphylococci

Although a common cause of late-onset sepsis, CONS are also occasionally implicated in early-onset sepsis in preterm babies, and may cause pulmonary haemorrhage.[777]

Late-onset sepsis

Most neonatal infections which begin more than 48 hours after birth are caused by organisms acquired from the postnatal environment, rather than transplacentally or from the birth canal. The spectrum of late-onset sepsis ranges from minor skin infection to life-threatening septicaemia. In a prospective epidemiological study carried out in Australian neonatal units (using the 48-hour cut-off, as adopted here), the prevalence of late-onset systemic sepsis was 4.4 per 1000 livebirths, compared with 2.2 per 1000 for early-onset sepsis.[408] The mortality rate from late-onset sepsis was 9% as opposed to 15% for early-onset sepsis, and numerous studies have reported a much higher mortality rate from early-onset than from late-onset sepsis. The vast majority of episodes of serious late-onset sepsis occur in preterm infants on the NICU and babies of less than 750 g birthweight are reported to have almost 45 times the risk of late-onset

Table 40.7 Distribution of pathogens associated with episodes of late-onset sepsis treated with antibiotics for 5 or more days. (From Stoll et al[778])

Organism	No.	%
Gram-positive organisms		
Staphylococcus – coagulase-negative	1288	55
Staphylococcus aureus	209	9
Enterococcus/group D streptococcus	111	5
Group B streptococcus	53	2
Other	52	2
Gram-negative organisms		
Enterobacter	102	4
Escherichia coli	101	4
Klebsiella	85	4
Pseudomonas	53	2
Other	82	4
Fungi		
Candida albicans	111	5
Candida parapsilosis	57	2
Other	51	2
Total	**2355**	**100**

bacteraemia than those of more than 2000 g birthweight.[248] Rates of nosocomial infection among VLBW babies have been recently reported as 16%,[248] 19.1%[121] and 21%[780] in the USA, 15.6% in a group of units in Spain,[516] 30% in a national survey in Israel[540] and 50% in a Brazilian NICU.[593]

The commonest organisms causing late-onset systemic sepsis are CONS, Gram-negative bacilli (such as *Klebsiella* species, *E. coli*, *Serratia marcescens* and *Pseudomonas* species), *Staph. aureus* and various *Candida* species (Table 40.7). Numerous other species of microorganism are involved from time to time (see Table 40.5), most of which are normally commensals. Most minor superficial infections are caused by *Staph. aureus* and Gram-negative bacilli. GBS is quite often implicated in late-onset sepsis, and in this situation meningitis, osteomyelitis and cellulitis are seen more often than in early-onset disease.[359]

Epidemiology of nosocomial spread of infection

The important reservoirs of microorganisms involved in late-onset sepsis are people, including the subject's own skin and gastrointestinal tract, other babies, hospital staff and visitors. Rarely, the source is the physical environment. Occasionally, a specific contaminated source is discovered, for example mineral oil spreading *Listeria* species,[734] parenteral nutrition solutions containing *Acinetobacter* species,[606] or air-conditioners.[525] Modern methods of identifying specific strains of bacteria are proving useful in understanding the ecology of nosocomial pathogens, a step which is essential if the increasing rates of nosocomial infection and antibiotic resistance on the NICU are to be controlled.[265,287]

Predisposing factors to nosocomial infection

Any baby may acquire an infection from another person or from an environmental source, but certain babies and certain circumstances greatly increase this risk. Some of the more general predisposing factors relating to cross-infection were discussed in the section relating to preventative measures (pp. 1013–15), but there are two crucial factors over which there is little control.

Prematurity and low birthweight and the use of medical devices

There is a strong relationship between prematurity and LBW, and the risk of late-onset sepsis, especially that caused by CONS.[318,409,778] In recent studies of NICU inmates, rates of nosomial infection among babies weighing less than 1000 g have been reported as 44.4% and 22.6%, and among those weighing more than 2000 g as 10.1% and 0.6%.[205,408] This undoubtedly has something to do with the inherent susceptibility of such babies to infection,[141] but is also strongly influenced by factors in the NICU environment, such as the adverse microbiological ecology and the use of medical devices. Many studies have demonstrated a strong positive correlation between rate of nosocomial infection and the use – and duration of use – of ventilators, lines for central vascular access, i.v. fat emulsions and implanted shunts for hydrocephalus. The importance of exposure to these risk factors has been illustrated by the finding of a positive association between the rate of nosocomial infection and the overall average duration of stay on the NICU,[142,289] as well as the individual duration of stay on the NICU.[318] These findings show the importance of correcting for average duration of admission when making interhospital comparisons of nosocomial infection rates.

Specific examples of nosocomial infection

Coagulase-negative staphylococci

CONS currently account for the majority of late-onset sepsis in developed countries, followed by Gram-negative bacilli.[405,408,455] In developing countries, the organisms causing late-onset sepsis are quite different. In rural India, most cases are due to *Salmonella typhimurium* and *Pseudomonas* species,[678] whereas in Jordan, Gram-negative organisms predominate.[720] However, as countries implement modern neonatal medicine practices, CONS seem inevitably to emerge as the most important pathogens.[352]

Epidemiology

The CONS constitute a ubiquitous group of organisms found in abundance on human skin. They can be found on the skin of some premature infants from as early as 6 hours of age, and increase rapidly to colonise all infants during the first week of life (Fig. 40.15).[454] The most heavily colonised sites are the umbilicus and the nose.[90] CONS are found in the stools of 90% of preterm

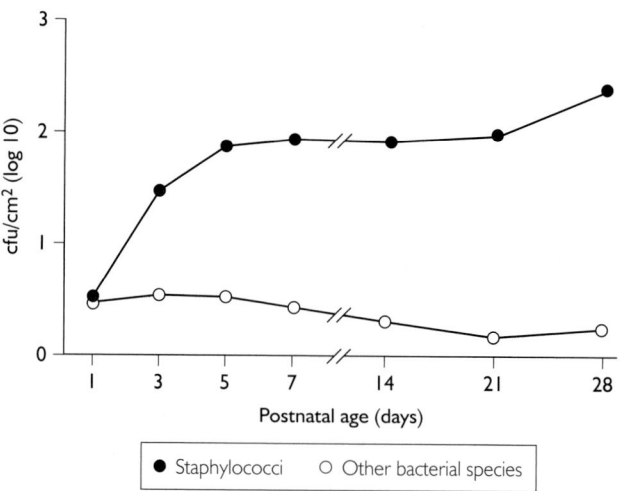

Fig. 40.15 Quantitative changes in cutaneous microflora with postnatal age. Measurements are logarithmically transformed and taken at eight sites in nine neonates. (From Keyworth et al.[454])

infants.[724] There are more than 20 species of CONS, but 60–80% of the isolates from babies are *Staph. epidermidis*, with *Staph. haemolyticus* making up most of the remainder and *Staph. warnerii* and *Staph. capitis* a long way behind.[90,454,602] Strains of CONS isolated from preterm infants exhibit low rates of susceptibility to penicillins and aminoglycosides.[602]

Infected infants are typically long-stay NICU patients on ventilators and with central venous access. Preterm infants seem particularly vulnerable to attack by CONS, and their deficiency of complement-mediated opsonic activity against *Staph. epidermidis* may be an important factor in this.[175] Infection is commonly with slime-producing strains.[329,391] Slime is a viscous extracellular polysaccharide substance which facilitates adherence to smooth surfaces such as the plastic or silicone used for vascular lines, shunts and endotracheal tubes.[161,649] Slime also inhibits neutrophil chemotaxis and phagocytosis and suppresses blastogenesis.[317,427] There is also some evidence that the slime can inhibit the action of glycopeptide antibiotics such as vancomycin.[249]

Clinical features

Most cases present between 7 and 14 days of age (Fig. 40.16). The clinical presentation of CONS sepsis is very variable. Ordinarily there is septicaemia without focal complication, although the longer the septicaemia persists the more likely is the infection to localise. Occasionally the baby is acutely ill and shows all the signs of fulminant sepsis described previously (pp. 1017–18), but more often the onset is subtle, even in those with endocarditis.[615] Transient apnoeic attacks, tachypnoea, mottled skin, abdominal distension, loose stools, the occasional vomit, a few spikes of fever up to 37.6°C or 38°C and the need for increased ventilatory support are typical.[248] More often the diagnosis is assumed when CONS, or another common skin commensal, grows in blood cultures from a baby who has a central line in place. The importance of intravascular catheters and shunts in CONS infection is such as to warrant a detailed discussion. A recent review article deals with catheter-related sepsis in detail.[376]

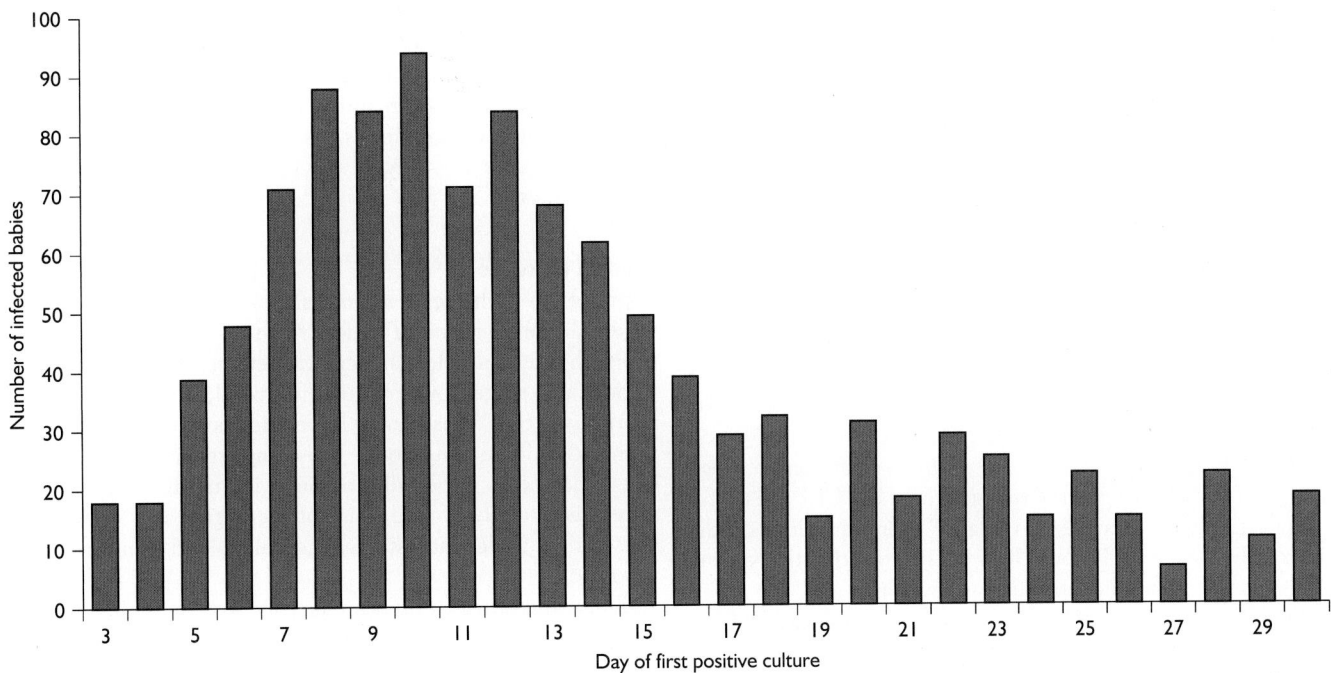

Fig. 40.16 Day of first positive culture of coagulase-negative staphylococci from blood or CSF. 160 babies whose first positive culture was at >30 days of age are not included. (From Isaacs.[405])

Catheter-related infections

The diagnosis of catheter-related sepsis can be established by one of the following criteria:

- a positive catheter-tip culture yielding the same organism as is grown from a peripheral blood sample;
- differential quantitative blood cultures with significantly greater colony counts from the catheter specimens than from peripheral blood cultures (p. 1019);
- clinical and culture-proven sepsis which is resistant to antibiotic therapy but which resolves when the catheter is removed.

More often the diagnosis is assumed when CONS, or another common skin commensal, grows in blood cultures from a baby who has a central line in place.

The emphasis is on central lines, which have a higher rate of bacterial colonisation than peripheral lines,[598] albeit that peripheral lines can sometimes act as portals of entry for CONS septicaemia.[284] Catheter-related sepsis rates among newborn infants have been variously reported as 10.3 per 1000 catheter days,[714] 10 per 1000 catheter days,[389] 3.7 per 1000 catheter days[468] and 13.1 per 1000 catheter days.[158] Most catheter-related infections occurring within a few days of insertion are probably caused by CONS migrating along the catheter from the skin around the insertion site. Infections of later onset, especially beyond 30 days, are probably due to colonisation of the catheter hub, followed by intraluminal migration into the bloodstream.[715] In a recent study of newborn infants with presumed catheter-related sepsis, 30% were found to have positive cultures for CONS from the entry site and 30% from the catheter hub.[795] Interestingly, molecular techniques showed that the isolates from blood and catheter hub were from identical clones in every case, but this was not so with the entry-site cultures, suggesting that the hub was the more likely source of infection. Further support for this is provided by a prospective study of catheter-hub contamination, in which 54% of episodes of catheter-related sepsis were preceded by, or associated with, contamination of the hub.[714]

There is a positive relationship between the length of time that a catheter is in place and the risk of infection.[142,290] Another important predisposing factor is the frequency with which the catheter is used for procedures such as giving drugs or blood transfusions.[290,588] The use of i.v. lipid preparations appears to have a major independent predisposing effect to catheter-related CONS sepsis.[38]

Catheter infections generally present with the low-grade clinical features outlined above, but occasionally may be complicated by blood vessel perforation,[57] central venous thrombosis,[699] bacterial endocarditis,[679] even when the heart is structurally normal,[559] and intestinal perforation.[565] The clinical presentation of vessel perforation is usually fairly dramatic, with peritonitis, respiratory distress or cardiac tamponade, depending on the location of the perforation. Endocarditis due to CONS is usually less dramatic, presenting as a persistent septicaemia despite appropriate antibiotics and catheter removal. Diagnosis is by echocardiography (pp. 629–33). The prognosis for endocarditis due to CONS is much better than for endocarditis due to Gram-negative organisms.

Ventricular shunt infections

The shunt infection rate for children under 6 months of age was recently reported as 15.7%, with 67% of these due to CONS.[660] High skin bacterial density prior to surgery and the presence of CONS with high adherence properties (a marker of pathogenicity) were found to be important risk factors.

Investigation

The problem of interpreting the results of blood cultures has already been discussed in some detail (p. 1019). In babies with shunts, as well as performing the blood culture, which is positive in almost all those with ventriculoatrial shunts but only in 25% of those with ventriculoperitoneal shunts, the shunt reservoir or tubing should also be aspirated and the CSF sent for culture. The LP may be negative in the presence of shunt infection.

Haematological changes are fairly common and include a rise in WBC and a fall in platelet count and haemoglobin concentration. The mean platelet volume often increases during CONS septicaemia, and this may be a useful adjunct to conventional tests.[621] The high specificity of the acridine orange leukocyte cytospin test for excluding line infection[700] (p. 1025) bears another mention here. Depression of the plasma fibronectin concentration has a usefully high specificity of 94% in suspected late-onset sepsis among VLBW babies.[222] Serial measurements of CRP are useful in monitoring the response to therapy,[640] and a failure of the CRP to fall as expected should lead to the consideration of line colonisation or a complication such as endocarditis.

Therapy is discussed below in the section on antibiotics for nosocomial infection. The question of whether to remove central venous catheters when there is CONS bacteraemia remains a vexed one. In about 50% of cases, the infection can be cleared without catheter removal, but when there is persisting bacteraemia, catheter removal must be considered.[440]

Staphylococcus aureus

Staph. aureus is inherently far more pathogenic than CONS, and epidemiological evidence suggests that some strains are more virulent than others. During the 1950s' heyday of perinatal *Staph. aureus* infection, phage type 80/81 showed itself to be particularly virulent.[252] This is partly explained by extracellular factors, especially the α-haemolysin, epidermolytic-toxin, enterotoxin, coagulase and leukocidin, and partly by surface components such as teichoic acid[23] which confers mucosal-binding properties. *Staph. aureus* was once the scourge of the newborn, but nowadays (in the developed world at least) it is a much rarer cause of systemic neonatal infection than either GBS, CONS or the Gram-negative bacilli. *Staph. aureus* remains, however, the commonest cause of infection in bones and joints,[79,197,412] skin and umbilical cord, and a common cause of eye infection. Systemic infections with *Staph. aureus* carry high morbidity and mortality rates. In the developing world, *Staph. aureus* is a common cause of neonatal sepsis, and in Nigeria it is the commonest pathogen causing neonatal meningitis[18] (interestingly, GBS was not encountered in this series, which is a common finding in developing countries). In Pakistan, *Staph. aureus* accounts for 15% of nosocomial infections, second only to *Salmonella typhi* and group A β-haemolytic streptococci (*Streptococcus pyogenes*).[89]

Epidemiology

Staph. aureus colonises the skin and upper gastrointestinal tract of many infants,[258] although is nowhere near as ubiquitous as CONS. In a recent study of *Staph. aureus* colonisation of the umbilicus, rates of 68% and 65% were found at 48 hours and 8/9 days respectively.[773] In that study, the rate of infection with *Staph. aureus* was

12% and there was a significant positive relationship between the level of colonisation and the risk of infection. *Staph. aureus* gains a foothold very easily, and quantitative studies have shown that fewer than 10 bacteria can initiate colonisation of the umbilicus in up to 50% of newborn infants. As with CONS, molecular methods are valuable in studying the epidemiology of outbreaks of *Staph. aureus*.[532,645,854]

Clinical features

Septicaemia with *Staph. aureus* is anything but subtle, and very urgent action is required if death or serious morbidity is to be avoided. There is a clear association between the severity of bacteraemia as judged by semiquantitative blood cultures, and the mortality rate.[730] Pustular or impetiginous skin lesions are common and provide a clue to the offending organism. Rapid seeding of organs occurs, especially to bones, joints and lungs.[597] *Staph. aureus* is a relatively rare cause of meningitis and an even rarer cause of UTI. Neonatal staphylococcal scalded skin syndrome is reported.[513,709]

Blood and other cultures are usually positive within 24 hours, and neutropenia and thrombocytopenia are common. Interpretation of a positive blood culture with *Staph. aureus* is less problematic than with CONS. The CRP usually soars and concentrations above 100 mg/l are often encountered within 12–24 hours of the onset of illness.

Therapy is discussed below in the section on antibiotics for nosocomial infection.

Gram-negative bacilli

These are a diverse group of organisms of widely differing genera. Most of those causing neonatal sepsis belong to the Enterobacteriaceae family, a large and heterogeneous group of Gram-negative rods whose natural habitat is the intestinal tract of humans and animals. Most of the species causing neonatal sepsis are part of the normal bowel flora, and only incidentally cause disease when they reach tissues outside the gut lumen. The most important Gram-negative bacilli causing neonatal sepsis in developed countries are *E. coli*, *Klebsiella pneumoniae*, *Ps. aeruginosa*, *Serratia marcescens*, *Citrobacter diversus*, *Proteus mirabilis* and *Enterobacter cloacae*. In the developing world these same organisms are prominent,[88] but, in addition, more overtly pathogenic members of the Enterobacteriaceae, such as the Salmonellae and Shigellae, are important causes of neonatal sepsis.[678] A recent study comparing intestinal organisms between babies born in Sweden and in Pakistan showed that the babies in Pakistan were more rapidly colonised by the Enterobacteriaceae, and that a much wider spectrum of organisms was present.[15] The Swedish babies harboured either *E. coli* or *Klebsiella* species, but the Pakistani babies often harboured *E. coli*, *Klebsiella* species, *Proteus* species, *Enterobacter* species and *Citrobacter* species simultaneously.

Epidemiology

Gram-negative bacilli currently account for around 20% of cases of late-onset sepsis, (Gladstone et al 1990) but this may be increasing.[369,743] In developing countries, Gram-negative organisms are more prominent, and in a recent study from Northern

Jordan, *Klebsiella* species accounted for 64% of culture-proven neonatal sepsis.[720] However, the Jordanian babies were totally spared infection by the GBS. In Kuala Lumpur, *Klebsiella* species are again the commonest cause of neonatal sepsis.[98] As with other organisms, molecular methods are proving useful in understanding the epidemiology of nosocomial infection.[94]

Clinical features

Systemic sepsis due to Gram-negative bacilli is usually fulminant and the mortality and morbidity are high, especially among VLBW infants.[439] A mortality rate of 50% was recently reported from the USA among a group of VLBW infants with *Ps. aeruginosa* septicaemia,[497] and from India a mortality rate of 23% for all babies with *Pseudomonas* sepsis.[332] In the United Arab Emirates, the mortality rates from *Ps. aeruginosa* and *Klebsiella* species sepsis have been reported as 71% and 59%, respectively.[477] Colonisation of the respiratory tract by Gram-negative bacilli is probably associated with increased severity of chronic lung disease (CLD).[173] Cholestatic liver disease is a common association with Gram-negative bacteraemia.[746]

Antibiotic therapy is discussed below in the section on antibiotics for nosocomial infection. Removal of central venous catheters is a necessary part of treatment in over half the cases, especially when bacteraemia has persisted for more than 1 day or when there is thrombocytopenia.[600]

Enterococci

These are mostly non-β-haemolytic. They are normal bowel organisms which only cause disease when they get out of their proper place. The organism causing most disease in babies is *Enterococcus faecalis*, with *Enterococcus faecium* a poor second.[163] Enterococci are a notorious cause of nosocomial infection in both adult and neonatal intensive care units. In the NICU, enterococci are an important cause of serious late-onset sepsis among VLBW infants.[199,534] Molecular methods are useful in establishing whether epidemic increases in enterococcal sepsis are due to the dissemination of a clonal strain or to multiple strains,[163] and this can be useful in planning antibiotic therapy for suspected cases. Enterococci are notoriously antibiotic resistant, especially *E. faecium*.[542] This resistance is partly intrinsic, but extrachromosomal resistance transferred by plasmid genes is also very important. Septicaemia with antibiotic-resistant enterococci carries a mortality rate of 75%.

Therapy is discussed below in the section on antibiotics for nosocomial infection.

Antibiotic therapy for late-onset bacterial infection

There should be a low threshold for starting antibiotic therapy pending the results of clinical observation, cultures and other tests. Antibiotics should be given i.v. in appropriate doses and at appropriate intervals for the age and gestation of the baby. The difficulty lies in the choice of antibiotics, given the wide range of potential pathogens and the propensity of some of the common bacteria responsible for late-onset infection to possess, or acquire, antibiotic resistance. The initial choice is guided by three considerations:

- Knowledge of the species of bacteria most likely to cause infection on the particular unit. This local knowledge is best acquired by the formal collection of data by the department of microbiology in the hospital.
- Knowledge of the antibiotic resistance patterns of the bacteria most likely to be responsible for the infection, from the information obtained from the point above. These vary from unit to unit and within a particular unit over time, mainly as a result of antibiotic use.[189]
- Knowledge of the patient's previous antibiotic therapy. This is important because previous antibiotic exposure predisposes to infection with multiply-resistant organisms. It is wise to choose different antibiotics from those used in a recently completed course.

Initial therapy

Unless there are local reasons to think otherwise, initial antibiotic therapy should be aimed at CONS and Gram-negative bacilli. If the locally endemic strains of CONS are sensitive to flucloxacillin, this should be the first choice. Commonly, though, CONS are flucloxacillin resistant and vancomycin should be used instead. Careful monitoring of serum drug concentration is required as the pharmacokinetics are very variable.[33]

The choice of an antibiotic for Gram-negative bacilli rests between an aminoglycoside and a third-generation cephalosporin, such as ceftazidime, and should be based on local knowledge of antibiotic resistance, the site of infection and the toxicity of particular combinations. For example, suspicion of Gram-negative meningitis might lead to cefotaxime being preferred over gentamicin (p. 1041), and concerns about impaired renal function might lead to vancomycin and a cephalosporin being preferred over vancomycin and gentamicin. If *Pseudomonas* species are suspected, ceftazidime should be used in preference to cefotaxime.

Although a combination of vancomycin and either a third-generation cephalosporin or an aminoglycoside will cover the majority of late-onset infections on the neonatal unit, neither combination is a panacea and a definitive choice can only be made if and when the organism responsible for the infection is identified and its antibiotic susceptibility established. Several newer antibiotics are finding a useful role in difficult cases. Aztreonam is valuable in the treatment of Gram-negative sepsis[569,758,786,805] in the newborn and may be used instead of a cephalosporin. Meropenem is proving to be a good second-line drug.[475,785]

Definitive antibiotic therapy

Once the infecting organism is identified, therapy is rationalised to maximise efficacy and to minimise the risk of inducing resistance. The following are suitable antibiotic choices for the common neonatal nosocomial pathogens.

- *CONS.* Vancomycin is the current drug of choice. The strains of CONS responsible for sepsis among babies on a NICU are commonly insensitive to penicillin, flucloxacillin and gentamicin. Routine susceptibility testing sometimes indicates that a CONS resistant to methicillin is sensitive to cephalosporins, but cross-resistance is common and all CONS that are resistant to penicillinase-resistant penicillins should be considered resistant to cephalosporins. Persistent infection with CONS despite vancomycin therapy has been treated successfully with a combination of vancomycin and rifampicin.[794]

For shunt infections, routine i.v. antibiotics should be given, and the CSF examined every other day to check that the infection is clearing. If not, it may be necessary to give intraventricular antibiotics, including vancomycin, either by direct infusion into the shunt or by inserting an Ommaya/Rickham reservoir. In general, however, the best results are obtained by removing the shunt and giving 10–14 days of antibiotics. The shunt can be reinserted once the infection has cleared.[733]

- *Staph. aureus.* An antistaphylococcal penicillin, such as flucloxacillin, should be used in preference to vancomycin if the organism is sensitive.
- *Methicillin-resistant Staph. aureus (MRSA).* Vancomycin is currently the drug of choice although there is evidence of a spectrum of decreased vancomycin susceptibilty among staphylococcal isolates.[395] Persistent infection with MRSA despite vancomycin therapy has been treated successfully with a combination of vancomycin and rifampicin.[794] An alternative treatment is with the recently introduced antibiotic known as linezolid, but only after discussion with a microbiologist. The usual dose for babies is 10 mg/kg 12-hourly, either i.v. or oral.
- *E. coli.* An aminoglycoside or a third-generation cephalosporin, depending on sensitivity pattern, should be used.
- *Klebsiella.* An aminoglycoside or a third-generation cephalosporin, depending on sensitivity pattern, should be used.
- *Enterobacter, Citrobacter, Serratia* and *Pseudomonas.* An aminoglycoside and a third-generation cephalosporin in combination should be used. Ceftazidime should be used if *Pseudomonas* is suspected.
- *Enterococci.* Ampicillin or vancomycin plus an aminoglycoside should be used.

Combination therapy is recommended partly to exploit synergistic antibiotic combinations and partly to prevent the emergence of antibiotic resistance.

Administering antibiotic therapy

Antibiotics should be given i.v., with careful attention to the recommended dosage, frequency, and the procedure for i.v. administration. If there is impaired renal or hepatic function, the antibiotic regimen will require modification if a safe course is to be steered between efficacy and toxicity. When gentamicin or vancomycin is used, serum concentrations should be monitored.

Duration of therapy
The duration of a course of antibiotic therapy will depend on whether or not infection is confirmed, the nature of the

infecting organism, and the location of infection. Little research exists to inform practice, but some guidelines can be given, as follows:

- If the clinical signs that led to treatment remit rapidly, and if after 48 hours there has been no rise in the CRP, no significant change in the WBC profile and the blood culture is negative, antibiotics can be stopped with minimal risk. A recent report has suggested that it may even be safe to stop antibiotics after 24 hours, by the application of a decision rule.[238] However, if the level of clinical suspicion at the time of starting treatment was high, then even in the absence of supportive or confirmatory tests, 5 days of treatment is easy to justify.
- In most cases where bacterial infection is confirmed by culture, or where there is strong clinical suspicion, supported by a CRP rise or a suggestive change in the WBC profile, but there is minimal or absent evidence of focal infection and a good clinical response to therapy, 7–10 days of antibiotic therapy is adequate. The duration of antibiotic therapy required to eradicate CONS infection is mainly determined by whether or not it is possible to remove indwelling vascular catheters or foreign bodies. Systemic infection with *Staph. aureus* should be treated for 3 weeks.
- In the case of focal infection, much depends on the location and the pathogen, and advice on these will be given in the sections that follow.

Prophylactic use of immunoglobulin

Preterm infants have lower serum IgG concentrations than their term counterparts and show a progressive fall in IgG concentration for many weeks after birth. Unsupplemented, about 15% of VLBW babies will develop IgG concentrations of less than 200 mg/dl by about 12 weeks of age.[172] There is evidence that VLBW babies who develop hospital-acquired infection have significantly lower serum IgG concentrations than those who do not.[491] It was found that if the serum IgG was less than 350 mg/dl during the first week, or less than 230 mg/dl in the second week, the risk of sepsis was five times greater than among babies with higher levels.

It is possible to maintain IgG concentrations in these infants by giving regular infusions of immunoglobulin. The question, though, is does this reduce the prevalence or severity of infection? Numerous studies have looked into this, and 19 of them have recently been the subject of an independent meta-analysis.[625] The main findings were that the prophylactic use of immunoglobulin resulted in a 3% reduction in sepsis (Fig. 40.17) and a 4% reduction in any serious infection (Fig. 40.18). There was no significant effect on mortality. One problem is the variation in antibody activity between different batches of immunoglobulin.[24,261,488,834] This may be improved by the development of immunoglobulin preparations with enhanced specific activity (p. 994). On balance, it seems reasonable to advocate immunoglobulin prophylaxis in the developing world, where infection plays such a large role in determining neonatal mortality and morbidity, but to regard the benefits as probably marginal in UK practice.

Review: Intravenous immunoglobulin for preventing infection in preterm and/or low-birth-weight infants
Comparison: 01 IVIG vs placebo or no treatment
Outcome: 01 Sepsis, one or more episodes

Study	Treatment	Control	Relative risk (fixed) 95% CI	Weight %	Relative risk (fixed) 95% CI
Bussei 1990a	20/61	23/65		6.5	0.93 (0.57, 1.51)
Chirico 1987	2/43	8/43		2.3	0.25 (0.06, 1.11)
Clapp 1989	0/56	5/59		1.6	0.10 (0.01, 1.69)
Conway 1990	8/34	14/32		4.2	0.54 (0.26, 1.11)
Fanaroff 1994	186/1204	209/1212		61.0	0.90 (0.75, 1.07)
Haque 1986	4/100	5/50		2.0	0.40 (0.11, 1.42)
Ratrisawadi 1991	10/68	13/34		5.1	0.38 (0.19, 0.79)
Sandberg 2000	19/40	13/41		3.8	1.50 (0.86, 2.61)
Tanzer 1997	3/40	8/40		2.3	0.38 (0.11, 1.31)
Weisman 1994a	40/372	39/381		11.3	1.05 (0.69, 1.59)
Total (95% CI)	292/2018	337/1957		100.0	0.85 (0.74, 0.98)

Test for heterogeneity: chi-square = 19.54, df = 9, p = 0.0210
Test for overall effect: Z = 2.30, p = 0.02

0.00 0.02 1 50 1000
Favours treatment   Favours control

Fig. 40.17 Intravenous immunoglobulin (IVIG) for preventing infection in preterm and/or low-birthweight infants. Treatment with IVIG versus either placebo or no treatment. Outcome measure is one or more episodes of sepsis. (From Ohlsson & Lacy.[625])

Review: Intravenous immunoglobulin for preventing infection in preterm and/or low-birth-weight infants
Comparison: 01 IVIG vs placebo or no treatment
Outcome: 02 Any serious infection, one or more episodes

Study	Treatment	Control	Relative risk (fixed) 95% CI	Weight %	Relative risk (fixed) 95% CI
Atici 1996	17/40	29/36		5.7	0.53 (0.36, 0.78)
Baker 1992	70/287	104/297		18.9	0.70 (0.54, 0.90)
Bussel 1990a	20/61	23/65		4.1	0.93 (0.57, 1.51)
Chirico 1987	6/43	12/43		2.2	0.50 (0.21, 1.21)
Chou Y-H 1998	6/31	5/30		0.9	1.16 (0.40, 3.40)
Clapp 1989	0/56	5/59		1.0	0.10 (0.01, 1.69)
Conway 1990	8/34	14/32		2.7	0.54 (0.26, 1.11)
Didato 1988	10/40	5/40		0.9	2.00 (0.75, 5.33)
Fanaroff 1994	208/1204	231/1212		42.7	0.91 (0.77, 1.07)
Haque 1986	4/100	7/50		1.7	0.29 (0.09, 0.93)
Ratrisawadi 1991	10/68	13/34		3.2	0.38 (0.19, 0.79)
Sandberg 2000	7/40	10/41		1.8	0.72 (0.30, 1.70)
Stabile 1988	4/46	3/48		0.5	1.39 (0.33, 5.88)
Tanzer 1997	3/40	8/40		1.5	0.38 (0.11, 1.31)
Van Overmire 1993	13/56	14/60		2.5	0.99 (0.51, 1.93)
Weisman 1994a	59/372	52/381		9.5	1.16 (0.82, 1.64)
Total (95% CI)	445/2518	535/2468		100.0	0.82 (0.74, 0.92)

Test for heterogeneity: chi-square = 29.96, df = 15, p = 0.0121
Test for overall effect: Z = 3.48, p = 0.00

0.1 0.2 1 5 10
Favours treatment   Favours control

Fig. 40.18 Intravenous immunoglobulin (IVIG) for preventing infection in preterm and/or low-birthweight infants. Treatment with IVIG versus either placebo or no treatment. Outcome measure is any serious infection, one or more episodes. (From Ohlsson & Lacy.[625])

Focal bacterial infections in the newborn

Meningitis

The prevalence of neonatal meningitis in the technologically developed world is falling according to some surveys,[751] but not according to others.[72,792] The current prevalence in England and Wales is reported as 0.39 cases per 1000 births, of which 0.21 cases were bacterial in origin.[382] In the developing world it is more like 2 per 1000.[18] Meningitis complicates 20% of cases of early-onset and 10% of cases of late-onset sepsis.[408] The risk increases with decreasing gestational age, and, as a group, preterm infants carry two or three times the risk that term infants do, and account for an even greater majority of the late-onset cases.[387]

Organisms

In the UK, GBS (mostly type III) and *E. coli* are responsible for just over 60% of all cases of neonatal bacterial meningitis, with *L. monocytogenes* a poor third (Table 40.8).[382] GBS is commoner in the early-onset cases, and *E. coli* and other Gram-negative organisms in the late-onset ones.[387] About 80% of *E. coli* causing neonatal meningitis carry the K1 capsular antigen,[586] and many show reduced interaction with host neutrophils[627] and aerobactin production.[803] In addition to the organisms mentioned, neonatal meningitis, like other forms of neonatal sepsis, can be caused by a host of bacteria (Table 40.5). The three organisms traditionally associated with meningitis in the older child, *H. influenzae*, *Str. pneumoniae* and *Neisseria meningitidis*, are usually only found in the late neonatal period or in the second month of life.[27,225,267,717]

Clinical features

Neonatal meningitis must be diagnosed on the basis of the 'softer' signs of early neonatal infection (pp. 1017–18), as by the time that signs such as a bulging fontanelle, high-pitched cry, altered consciousness or seizures occur, the disease has advanced to the stage at which permanent neurological sequelae are likely. In VLBW infants, recurrent apnoea, abdominal distension, hyponatraemia and loss of glucose homeostasis are common.[648]

During clinical examination, the head circumference should be measured and the skull and axial skeleton scrutinised for skin defects or pits that might have provided a portal of entry for infection.

Pathology

Inflammation, oedema and arachnoiditis are widespread in most cases of neonatal meningitis, as are vasculitis and superficial cortical thrombophlebitis, which cause superficial ischaemic damage to the brain. A useful rat model for neonatal meningitis has been developed.[462] Ventriculitis occurs in 70–90% of cases of neonatal meningitis, but is less common with GBS than with Gram-negative organisms. Severe encephalopathic changes often occur, probably as a result of direct penetration of the infection into the brain, and may result in widespread cerebral atrophy. The choroid plexus may be damaged, permanently compromising CSF production, and exudate may obstruct intraventricular foramina and arachnoid granulations, leading to hydrocephalus in around one-third of cases.[462] Abscess formation is commonly seen with meningitis caused by *Citrobacter* and *Proteus* species,[469] and occasionally with other coliforms. Abscess formation begins with a suppurative ventriculitis and progresses to periventricular abscess formation.[767]

Investigation

CSF analysis

The criteria for diagnosing meningitis are given on page 1024. Gram-negative meningitis generally produces a higher CSF white cell count than does GBS meningitis, in which the WBC count is often <100/mm³.[388] In most cases, bacteria can be identified when the CSF is stained by the Gram or acridine orange method; if no bacteria are seen, the possibility of a viral pathogen such as HSV should be considered. If the CSF cytology suggests meningitis but no organisms are seen, treatment with aciclovir should be started pending the results of further tests (p. 1055). Occasionally, in the early stages of fulminating infection, organisms may be seen without a significant pleocytosis. If no organisms are seen on Gram stain, latex agglutination testing on the CSF will identify GBS infection with a high degree of specificity.[675] Measurement of CSF β_2-microglobulin concentration provides a valuable distinction between babies with CNS infection and those without, at a cut-off level of 2.25 mg/l.[282]

The need for repeat LPs is debatable but we undertake a repeat after 48 hours of therapy. Failure of the lumbar CSF to improve is an indication for further investigation by ventricular puncture and ultrasound. An LP should be performed 48 hours after therapy is stopped. The last CSF may not show complete clearing of cells, but the sugar and protein values should be within the normal range, no organisms should be seen, the CRP should have fallen to a normal value, and the culture must, of course, be negative.

Table 40.8 Causative organisms in 274 cases of neonatal meningitis. Values in parentheses are percentages. CSF, cerebrospinal fluid. (From Holt et al[382])

	Number of cases	Died
Group B β-haemolytic streptococci	69 (25)	8 (12)
Escherichia coli	26 (10)	4 (15)
Listeria monocytogenes	7 (3)	1
Haemophilus influenzae	1 (<1)	0
Neisseria meningitidis	5 (2)	0
Streptococcus pneumoniae	8 (3)	1
Other Gram-positive bacteria	17 (6)	0
Other Gram-negative bacteria	11 (4)	0
Enteroviruses	18 (7)	0
Candida albicans	4 (2)	0
Sterile CSF	96 (35)	2 (2)
CSF sample not collected	12 (4)	2

Blood culture

Blood culture is commonly positive, because neonatal meningitis is usually secondary to a septicaemia. However, negative blood cultures may be found in around 15% of cases of neonatal meningitis with positive CSF culture.[387,820] The likelihood of a negative blood culture in meningitis is lowest in early-onset sepsis,[365,387] and this is when an LP may most safely be deferred if the baby is too ill to tolerate handling.[388]

Other tests

Cerebral ultrasonography will identify the cause of a rising occipito-frontal circumference (OFC). It can also be used to detect ventriculitis and to monitor the response to therapy. Parenchymal changes or ventriculomegaly identify babies at high risk of sequelae. If there is doubt about ultrasound findings, a CT or MRI scan is justified. In VLBW infants, progressive ventriculomegaly and the development of thalamic echodensities are quite common late findings, and suggest the need for serial brain ultrasound scanning.[648]

The EEG may be a useful guide to prognosis in neonatal meningitis and, when considered along with the presence or absence of seizures and alterations in conscious level, can predict outcome accurately in 93% of cases.[156]

Daily head circumference measurements are the simplest way of detecting the increasing cranial volume that occurs with cerebral oedema, hydrocephalus or subdural effusion (although this third complication is rare in neonatal meningitis).

Treatment

Antibiotics

Initial therapy

The safest initial blind treatment for suspected early-onset meningitis is still probably a combination of ampicillin and an aminoglycoside. This will effectively begin to treat meningitis caused by GBS, *L. monocytogenes*, enterococci, *H. influenzae* and many Gram-negative organisms. The alternative choice is a third-generation cephalosporin, such as cefotaxime or ceftriaxone, plus ampicillin. A combination of a third-generation cephalosporin and an aminoglycoside is sometimes used, but this will not effectively treat *L. monocytogenes* or enterococci. For late-onset cases, the blind choice is more difficult, but the combination of a third-generation cephalosporin and an aminoglycoside probably offers the best chance of immediately effective therapy.

When the Gram stain indicates the likely type of organism, prescribing is less speculative. For Gram-positive cocci, Gram-negative cocci or Gram-positive bacilli, ampicillin and an aminoglycoside should be used, and for Gram-negative bacilli, a combination of cefotaxime or ceftriaxone and an aminoglycoside. When the sensitivity pattern suggests that vancomycin is indicated, it is worth knowing that there is effective CSF penetration of vancomycin in preterm infants below about 32 weeks' gestation.[681]

Definitive therapy

GBS should be treated with benzylpenicillin, plus or minus gentamicin, with which there is some synergy. *L. monocytogenes* and enterococci are treated with ampicillin and gentamicin.[199]

Gram-negative bacilli vary so much in their sensitivity patterns that definitive therapy can only be decided after the microbiology department has carried out sensitivity testing. This is especially so in the case of nosocomial infections among the inmates of a NICU, who may acquire some very unusual and resistant pathogens. Combination therapy with cefotaxime or ceftriaxone and an aminoglycoside will be the most common choice. Aztreonam is emerging as a useful treatment for Gram-negative infections, including meningitis.[786] Antibiotic therapy for neonatal meningitis should be continued i.v. for at least 21 days.

Adjunctive treatment

Neonatal meningitis is such a potentially damaging condition, even with prompt and appropriate antibiotic therapy, that there is a need for additional interventions. In experimental animals, dexamethasone has been shown to prevent the brain injury associated with GBS meningitis almost completely.[462] There is no systematic study of steroid therapy in neonatal meningitis, and until such work is undertaken it is difficult to recommend steroids as part of routine treatment. It is likely that interventions aimed at the cytokines mediating inflammation and injury will eventually become routine. In experimental animals, the use of chemical agents to inhibit the binding of excitatory amino acids to neuronal receptors has been shown to lessen brain injury.[496]

Intraventricular antibiotic therapy

Ventriculitis is common in neonatal meningitis, especially when caused by Gram-negative bacilli. Before the introduction of the third-generation cephalosporins, ventriculitis with persistently positive CSF cultures was relatively common. The explanation for this is probably the poor CSF penetration of the aminoglycoside antibiotics that have so commonly been used to treat neonatal meningitis – with peak CSF concentrations often approximating to the minimal inhibitory concentration. Third-generation cephalosporins, such as cefotaxime and ceftriaxone, have very good CSF penetration and their introduction has led to a great reduction in the number of cases where ventriculitis has persisted. In a recently reported large study of neonatal meningitis in the UK, no baby required treatment with intraventricular antibiotics.[387] In the very unusual case of persistent ventriculitis despite adequate doses of appropriate antibiotics, recourse may still be made to CSF drainage procedures and direct instillation of antibiotics into the ventricles. However, controlled trials of both intrathecal[523] and intraventricular[524] aminoglycoside administration have failed to show significant benefit over systemic therapy.

Viral meningitis (p. 1057)

Mycoplasma meningitis

Fungal meningitis

Neurological complications

Cerebral abscess

This mainly occurs when meningitis is caused by *Citrobacter* or *Proteus* species, but may occasionally complicate meningitis caused by many other organisms, including *E. coli*, *Staph. aureus*, *Mycoplasma hominis*[260] and GBS.[43] Abscesses may present with signs of increased intracranial pressure in a baby who is responding poorly to treatment, but in some cases produce no obvious change in the clinical state.[772] Ultrasound or CT establishes the diagnosis. Multiple or small abscesses can be treated with high-dose i.v. antibiotics. If only one or two abscess cavities are present, or if abscesses fail to resolve with antibiotics, the cavities should be aspirated and an appropriate antibiotic instilled. Systemic antibiotic therapy should be maintained for at least 4 weeks.

Hydrocephalus

This may occur during the second week of the illness while the infant still has ventriculitis, or may present with increased head growth and CNS signs at almost any stage after bacteriological cure of the meningitis. If infection is still present, an intraventricular reservoir should be inserted and intraventricular and systemic antibiotics continued. External ventricular drainage is an alternative. In most cases, a permanent CSF shunt will be required after the infection is controlled.

Deafness

Bacterial meningitis is the single most important cause of acquired sensorineural hearing loss in childhood, and neonates are especially vulnerable.[268] All survivors of neonatal meningitis should routinely undergo audiological screening soon after recovery, and audiological follow-up.

Prognosis

Mortality

The mortality rate varies with the nature of the organism and the maturity of the patient, and there is limited value in quoting overall mortality rates for neonatal meningitis. For what it is worth, the overall mortality rate seems to have fallen during the last five decades, from around 60% in the 1950s and 1960s[517] to around 30% in the late 80s[522,586] down to 10% in the most recent series from England and Wales.[382]

In most reports, the mortality rate associated with Gram-negative meningitis is greater than that seen with meningitis caused by Gram-positive organisms.[272] In the recent England and Wales study, the mortality rate for neonatal *E. coli* meningitis was 15% and for GBS meningitis 12%.[382] Mortality is higher in preterm infants. Mulder et al[586] found a mortality in *E. coli* meningitis of 66% in babies of <31 weeks' gestation, 30% at 32–34 weeks', reducing to 19% in babies >35 weeks'.

Permanent CNS damage

In most series, adverse neurological sequelae occur in 30–50% of survivors.[522] It is commonly believed that babies with GBS meningitis do better than those with Gram-negative bacillary disease, with up to 70% of survivors being normal. However, some studies have found that only 50% of GBS meningitis survivors are intact.[221] The prognosis is worse in preterm babies. All forms of cerebral palsy, mental subnormality, epilepsy and cortical blindness may occur singly or in combination. In the most recently reported follow-up study, 38% of survivors were normal, 38% had mild disabilities and 24% had moderate to severe disabilities.[272]

Pneumonia

Neonatal pneumonia may be an isolated focal infection but is commonly part of a more widespread infective illness.[415] Definition and ascertainment of cause is generally more difficult with pneumonia than with other focal infections. This is partly because non-infective pulmonary pathology is so common in babies, and often impossible to distinguish radiologically, and partly because the isolation of bacteria from respiratory secretions is not synonymous with pneumonia in the same way that bacteria in the CSF are synonymous with meningitis. These uncertainties should be borne in mind when assessing the reported prevalence of neonatal pneumonia. Using a rigorous approach to diagnosis, in a prospective study the prevalence of neonatal pneumonia in an Oxford hospital was reported to be 3.7 per 1000 livebirths.[832] This was among a population of almost 20 000 babies born in a tertiary referral centre and included all cases of pneumonia occurring before discharge. This probably represents the best available estimate of the current prevalence of neonatal bacterial pneumonia.

There are several ways to classify neonatal pneumonia, but from a problem-orientated point of view, classification according to age of onset is most useful:

- congenital or intrauterine pneumonia;
- pneumonia presenting within the first 48 hours of life and commonly due to pathogens acquired from the birth canal;
- pneumonia occurring after 48 hours and usually acquired nosocomially.

Congenital or intrauterine pneumonia

This is rare and mainly occurs secondary to ascending infection and chorioamnionitis following PROM. The mortality rate is high and many affected infants appear asphyxiated at birth. Much of what is known about the pathogenesis has come from post-mortem histology, and this presents some paradoxes. Bacteria are by no means always to be seen and many of the histological changes usually associated with pneumonia are absent in congenital cases, particularly evidence of a pleural reaction and of infiltration and destruction of bronchopulmonary tissue.[188] This has led to the suggestion that many cases of so-called congenital pneumonia are predominantly cases of asphyxia. There is very little up-to-date literature to be found on the subject.

Early-onset pneumonia

The reported incidence of early-onset pneumonia is 1.79 per 1000 livebirths.[832] GBS accounts for 70% of cases, but *H. influenzae*,[467,701] *Str. pneumoniae*,[311,418,438,755,853] *L. monocytogenes*[373] and Gram-negative enteric bacilli contribute. Rarely, yeasts may be involved.[609] The same predisposing factors operate as for early-onset septicaemia (pp. 1028–33), and bronchoalveolar lavage fluid from ventilated babies, born following prolonged rupture of the membranes, contains increased numbers of WBCs and a high concentration of IL-6.[327] Numerous viruses may also cause early-onset pneumonia, e.g. adenovirus[9,159,579,655] and CMV.[737]

Clinical features

In term infants, early-onset pneumonia is comparatively easy to suspect, but in preterm infants, distinction from HMD is difficult and sometimes impossible (p. 476). Typically, in term infants, signs of respiratory distress accompanied by signs of systemic sepsis develop within a few hours of birth and progress rapidly. Pulmonary hypertension with hypoxaemia secondary to right-to-left shunting is a common complication, and in the case of GBS infection may be triggered by damage to the lung endothelium and the release of vasoconstrictor substances (p. 1030).[299]

Investigation

Blood culture is usually positive, and culture of nasopharyngeal aspirates grows the same organism as the blood culture in a high proportion.[832] If intubation is necessary, tracheal secretions should be obtained for microscopy and culture. Unfortunately, positive cultures from respiratory secretions do not prove pneumonia, but in rationalising the choice of antibiotics it is important to know what is grown. Cultures from other sites are less helpful. The radiological changes are quite variable and usually not of themselves diagnostic. They include nodular or coarse infiltrates, a diffuse picture with air bronchograms rather like HMD, perihilar streaking and well-defined areas of consolidation.

To make the diagnosis of pneumonia there should be evidence of an inflammatory process, such as a rise in the CRP or an abnormal WBC count, convincing CXR appearances, clinical findings and a positive blood culture. In many cases the evidence is less compelling. Babies with pneumonia have higher concentrations of IL-1 and TNFα in tracheal aspirates than do babies with uncomplicated RDS,[137] and tests based on recovered cytokines hold promise as discriminators in the future.

Differential diagnosis

The principal differential diagnosis in the preterm infant is HMD, and, as pneumonia can damage surfactant production and function, the two conditions may coexist (p. 1030).[494] Bacterial pneumonia should be suspected when there are features such as hypotension, poor tissue perfusion, metabolic acidosis and leukopenia. However, as it is impossible to exclude early pneumonia in preterm infants with apparent RDS, many neonatologists prescribe antibiotics for 48 hours until cultures are negative and the CRP has been seen not to rise.

If a previously well baby becomes dyspnoeic after 6 hours of age, pneumonia is the most likely diagnosis (see Table 27.6). Pulmonary oedema in infants with heart disease, and the very rare infant who presents late with a pneumothorax or an intrathoracic malformation, can usually be differentiated easily by a clinical examination, CXR and, if necessary, an echocardiograph. Care must also be taken to exclude other causes of tachypnoea, in particular that secondary to metabolic acidaemia.

Treatment

All babies showing signs of respiratory distress which does not have a clear non-infective cause must be treated with antibiotics, pending the results of further observations, cultures, CRP and other appropriate investigations. If the cultures are negative, the CRP does not rise and the baby makes a rapid recovery (as is often the case), treatment can be stopped. The safest 'blind' choice of antibiotic for presumed neonatal pneumonia is a combination of ampicillin and an aminoglycoside. A third-generation cephalosporin is an alternative if there is little likelihood of the pneumonia being due to *L. monocytogenes* or enterococci, and it does offer the benefit of reliable cover against *H. influenzae*, increasing numbers of which are now resistant to ampicillin. Antibiotic therapy for proven pneumonia should continue for 10 days, unless the pathogen is *Staph. aureus*, in which case at least 3 weeks should be employed.

Outcome

With modern neonatal intensive care, early-onset pneumonia in otherwise normal term babies carries a low mortality rate, but among preterm babies the mortality rate approaches 50%, especially when the CXR shows widespread atelectasis.[832] In infants with staphylococcal or coliform pneumonia, pneumatocoeles may develop, as, rarely, may lung abscess (p. 1045) and empyema. Abscesses and pneumatocoeles should be treated conservatively in the first place, using long-term i.v. antibiotics for the abscess. Empyema requires insertion of a thoracentesis tube for closed chest drainage, and i.v. antibiotics for several weeks.

Late-onset pneumonia

Pneumonia developing more than 48 hours after birth is commonest among preterm babies who are receiving IPPV. In the Oxford study referred to earlier, 92% of babies with late-onset pneumonia were preterm and 87% were on IPPV at the time of onset.[832] The mean postnatal age at onset was 35 days. The reported incidence of pneumonia in intubated babies varies from 10% to 35%. Halliday et al[344] reported an incidence of pneumonia of 35% among intubated babies with RDS. Using more stringent immunological criteria, Giacoia et al[296] diagnosed pneumonia in 24% of intubated babies, but in the Oxford study,[832] using strict radiological and laboratory criteria, only 10% of intubated babies had late-onset pneumonia.

Organisms and pathogenesis

The organisms implicated in late-onset pneumonia are in many respects similar to those already described as causing late-onset septicaemia (pp. 1033–9), except that Gram-negative bacilli are clear winners over CONS (Table 40.9). In long-stay patients with CLD, unusual organisms, including fungi, mycoplasma and chlamydia, as well as viruses such as RSV and CMV, must be considered.[148] Other unusual causes of nosocomial neonatal pneumonia are reported from time to time, e.g. *Legionella pneumophila*,[324,381,518] *Serratia marcescens*,[456] coronavirus[757] and rhinovirus.[157]

Pneumonia in ventilated babies can occur secondary to septicaemia or secondary to colonisation of the endotracheal tube. In contrast to early-onset cases, blood cultures are negative in most instances of late-onset pneumonia.

Clinical features

In an infant with primary lung disease already on IPPV, infection presents with deteriorating lung function (pp. 531–2) plus

Table 40.9 Bacterial isolates from nasopharyngeal or endotracheal secretions of 32 babies during 34 probable episodes of pneumonia of late onset. (From Webber et al[832])

Gram-negative bacilli:	30
Coliform sp.	15
P. aeruginosa	12
Escherichia coli	2
Proteus mirabilis	1
S. aureus	5
S. epidermidis	2
Group B streptococcus	1
H. influenzae	1
No organism identified	4

non-specific signs of infection (pp. 1017–18). An increase in endotracheal tube aspirate suggests infection, but can be confused with the bronchorrhoea seen in CLD. Localised and generalised crepitations may be heard.

Investigation

A method of surveillance for possible pneumonia in ventilated babies must be found, as it is a potentially serious cause of deterioration and additional lung injury. Our approach is to perform routine, twice-weekly CRP estimations on all ventilated babies, and to undertake a CXR, blood cultures and culture of respiratory secretions in any baby whose ventilatory requirement increases significantly or who develops a raised CRP. Interpretation of the results of tracheal secretion culture is discussed on pages 558 and 1024. In older babies, viral cultures and immunofluorescence studies for chlamydia (p. 1045) and RSV (p. 560) are indicated.

Treatment

The choice of initial antibiotic therapy for neonatal pneumonia is difficult because the list of potential pathogens is long and because it is more or less essential to cover CONS. Unless local knowledge suggests otherwise, a third-generation cephalosporin plus vancomycin is a good choice. Therapy should subsequently be modified to cover organisms grown from the blood or tracheal secretions, along the lines suggested for specific bacteria (p. 1015).

If the baby is already on antibiotics when deterioration from presumed pneumonia occurs, it is usually advisable to change the drugs and to broaden the spectrum of cover, often to include an antibiotic effective against *Pseudomonas* species. In babies on IPPV for several weeks, in whom *Chlamydia* species, *Mycoplasma* species, *Bordetella pertussis* or even *Pneumocystis carinii* are possible pathogens, antibiotics such as erythromycin and septrin should be considered.

Pneumonia in the baby with CLD (pp. 554–73)

In babies with long-term respiratory disease, pneumonia should always be at the top of the list of differential diagnosis if the lung disease deteriorates. Some of these babies are several months old and, in addition to the usual pathogens, the respiratory viral infections characteristic of that age group are common.[655] There is a suggestion from the literature that respiratory tract colonisation with Gram-negative organisms is associated with more severe CLD.[173] Babies with CLD who acquire added pulmonary infection often become extremely ill, and frequently require IPPV. Antibiotics should always be given. Viral respiratory infections in babies with CLD lead to a worsening of chronic respiratory morbidity, with signs of increased airway resistance, compared with those who avoid viral infection.[862]

Some specific neonatal lung infections

Ureaplasma urealyticum

U. urealyticum is a common vaginal commensal. It may be implicated in some cases of chorioamnionitis and premature delivery,[216,718] along with *Mycoplasma hominis*.[808] There is growing speculation that these organisms may cause acute neonatal pneumonia[628] and have a role in the pathogenesis of CLD, although the literature is confusing (p. 556).[108,152,179,216,281,361,634] Unfortunately, ureaplasmas require a special culture medium and may take several weeks to grow. However, a detection method for ureaplasma antibody has been described which should be useful in both clinical and research contexts.[673] Erythromycin is the antibiotic of choice for both ureaplasma and mycoplasma infections in the newborn.[824]

Respiratory syncytial virus

RSV infections are comparatively rare on the neonatal unit, but small epidemics occur from time to time and the effects on individual babies can be devastating, especially among those with severe CLD. Such babies may rapidly develop almost complete airway obstruction and become impossible to ventilate. Recurrent bradycardia is a common presenting feature, and the clinical course is occasionally complicated by atrial tachycardia.[31,203] RSV infection must always be considered when a baby with CLD experiences a deterioration in lung function, even if the typical physical signs of a bronchiolitis are absent. RSV is easily diagnosed by immunofluorescence on respiratory secretions. Stringent measures to limit cross-infection are required if a case of RSV infection occurs on a NICU.[535] Early institution of treatment with ribavirin has been recommended, although there is little evidence of efficacy in this group of patients. Extracorporeal membrane oxygenation (ECMO) should be considered early in deteriorating cases. Babies with CLD also remain very vulnerable to RSV infection for many months after discharge from the NICU[754] and hospital readmission is common.[149] There is growing evidence for the effectiveness of prophylaxis using the humanised RSV monoclonal antibody known as palivizumab.[623,768]

Other respiratory viruses

VLBW babies who remain on the NICU for many months may contract the usual viral respiratory infections of early childhood from their visitors and from nursing and medical staff. Symptoms are usually of a mild upper respiratory tract infection (URTI) accompanied by a low-grade pyrexia. More severe viral pneumonia, other than that caused by RSV, may also occur at any time in the neonatal period, and adenoviruses and coronaviruses are often responsible.[655,757]

Pertussis[384]

Severe pertussis can occur in the late neonatal period, presenting with paroxysmal cough, vomiting, apnoea and choking spells. Whooping is rare. Prolonged ventilatory support is often required.[348] Diagnosis is by culture of nasopharyngeal swabs or, in the case of babies who have started antibiotic therapy, by PCR.[220] Treatment is with erythromycin and sedation. In recent reports, the baby has acquired the infection from his unimmunised mother, who developed the disease perinatally.[70]

Chlamydia

Chlamydia trachomatis and *Chlamydia pneumoniae* can cause severe early-onset disease similar to that seen with GBS. Even birth by caesarean section with intact membranes does not preclude the possibility of vertical transmission,[74] and the organism can cross the intact membranes, causing fetal pneumonic stillbirth.[797] Chlamydial infection during pregnancy should be treated with either ampicillin or erythromycin in order to prevent perinatal transmission.[716] Chlamydial pneumonia in term infants is characteristically a disease in those over 4 weeks of age, but it can occur in the first week of life. The diagnosis is made by culture or immunofluorescence techniques in the presence of a suggestive clinical picture, which includes an afebrile pneumonia with tachypnoea and rales, diffuse CXR changes, an eosinophilia and previous neonatal conjunctivitis. Like other neonatal lung diseases, chlamydial pneumonia can cause long-term pulmonary damage. Treatment is with erythromycin.

Lung abscess

This is a rare occurrence in the newborn, presenting usually with dyspnoea and an area of opacification on CXR. It usually follows previous pneumonia and is usually caused by Gram-negative organisms, but can be caused by *Staph. aureus*. It should be treated initially with broad-spectrum antibiotics. If the lesion does not resolve, bronchoscopy or surgery may be indicated.

Cardiac infection

Endocarditis

Endocarditis is being recognised with increasing frequency in VLBW babies with structurally normal hearts. Virtually all of these babies have had central lines lying in the right atrium or right ventricle. The organisms responsible for most cases are CONS, but enterococci, *Staph. aureus* and *Candida* species are well-recognised causal agents.[559,679] Endocarditis in this group of infants usually presents with no more than persistent signs of sepsis and positive blood cultures despite appropriate antibiotic therapy, although in a few cases there are changing murmurs, heart failure, persisting haematuria or thrombocytopenia. A baby who presents any of these features and who has, or has recently

had, an intracardiac central line should have an echocardiogram performed. The demonstration of intracardiac vegetations, which are present in most patients, confirms the diagnosis.

Treatment and outcome

Remove the central line and check that the appropriate antibiotics are being given for the organism grown from the blood, at the correct dose and dose interval. If the signs of sepsis remit within a few days, and blood cultures become negative, antibiotic therapy should be continued for 10–14 days.[674] The prognosis for catheter-related endocarditis due to CONS is better than might be thought, with recovery rates of more than 60% reported from small series.[559,679] Endocarditis due to *Candida albicans* carries a poor prognosis. Rarely, vegetations persist or severe valve damage occurs, and then surgery may be indicated.

Pericarditis

This is extremely rare, and usually develops as a complication of pre-existing sepsis or an abscess near the mediastinum. Implicated organisms include *Staph. aureus*, *E. coli*, *H. influenzae*, *Klebsiella* species, *Pseudomonas* species and *Candida* species.[253,855] The CXR shows an increase in the size of the cardiac silhouette, but signs of tamponade are unusual. ECG changes are present, and the diagnosis can be confirmed by echocardiography and pericardial tap. The treatment is surgical drainage and long-term antibiotics.

Myocarditis (pp. 643, 645)

Bone and joint infection (see also pp. 986–7)

Septic arthritis and osteomyelitis are rare in the newborn, although their incidence does seem to vary quite a lot. Only five cases have occurred at St James's University Hospital in Leeds during the last 20 years (in over 90 000 births), whereas a recent report from an Australian tertiary centre describes an incidence of 9.6 cases per 1000 NICU admissions.[408] Osteomyelitis and septic arthritis are mainly caused by *Staph. aureus*,[197,412] but GBS is important[856] and several other organisms may be involved, including *H. influenzae*,[845,850] *U. urealyticum*,[302] *Candida* species,[305,835] *Neisseria gonorrhoea*[41,403] and *Str. pneumoniae*.[225] Osteomyelitis and septic arthritis often coexist, and are often indistinguishable clinically. There are two reasons for this. The infected metaphysis of the bone often lies within the capsule of the joint, and when the thin metaphyseal cortex collapses, infection enters the joint. In addition, blood vessels frequently pass through the thin epiphyseal plate of neonatal long bones, transmitting metaphyseal infection to the joint capsule.

Osteomyelitis/septic arthritis takes two forms. One is seen in acutely ill babies with complex problems, and often with indwelling cannulae, in whom multiple bone involvement may occur.[412] The other form is a more subtle presentation and usually only one site is affected. GBS is quite often responsible for this latter form. The sites most commonly affected are the pelvis, hip, knee and humerus, but any site may be involved. Skull osteomyelitis may occur following infection of a cephalhaematoma or a scalp puncture for fetal pH monitoring. Vertebral disease occasionally develops, and calcaneal disease may follow heel puncture. Isolated arthritis is rarely reported, but the organisms isolated are similar to those reported for osteomyelitis, except for the preponderance of coliform arthritis of the hip when this complicates femoral venepuncture.[375]

Clinical features

These disorders usually present in one of three ways:

■ with pseudoparalysis of the affected limb due to pain – the affected area may be warm and swollen;
■ following investigation of the baby with non-specific signs of sepsis;
■ incidentally on X-ray in a baby with multisystem disease.

Investigation and diagnosis

The affected bone or joint must be X-rayed as a baseline, although no changes are usually seen for 10–14 days, when bone rarefaction, lytic lesions, periosteal elevation and periosteal new bone formation are seen. Isotope scans are also useful in identifying 'hot spots' in joints or bones. MRI can be very valuable, especially to look at the spine and pelvis.[557] Aspiration of the affected joint or bone should usually be attempted, not only to achieve prompt bacteriological diagnosis by Gram stain and culture, but also because decompression is an important part of therapy.

Treatment

Vancomycin and a third-generation cephalosporin is a reasonable starting point until the results of blood cultures are available. Thereafter, the appropriate antibiotic(s) (pp. 986–7) should be given i.v. for at least 4–6 weeks. When pus is obtained at aspiration, orthopaedic advice should always be sought about surgical drainage of the bone or joint.

Prognosis

Mortality relates almost entirely to multisytem disease, but there is a high morbidity rate. Following staphylococcal and Gram-negative infections, permanent damage to the epiphyseal plate or the metaphysis is common. This may cause permanent arthritis, long-term growth problems or deformity, particularly in those with an acute onset or multiple sites of involvement, in whom up to 50% may have significant long-term orthopaedic problems.[650] Long-term clinical and radiological follow-up is essential, especially as impaired growth may not become evident for several years.[650] The prognosis for complete recovery from GBS infections is somewhat better.

Gastroenteritis

Neonatal gastroenteritis in Britain is commonly sporadic and usually mild. Infection may be acquired from the mother during birth, or subsequently by cross-infection or from contaminated feeds. Many nursery outbreaks are initiated by an asymptomatic infant who sheds the virus or bacterium. For some viral pathogens, such as rotavirus, nursery outbreaks often coincide with seasonal peaks of the disease in the community.[774] Breastfeeding is strongly protective, in the developing world at least.[515,859]

Organisms

Most neonatal gastroenteritis is due to rotavirus,[61,461,703,750] which may also be endemic in some nurseries without there being any evidence of it causing symptoms other than a mild increase in stool frequency. *E. coli, Salmonella* species and *Shigella* species all may cause neonatal gastroenteritis.[806] Neonatal campylobacter gastroenteritis has been described, often contracted from the baby's mother, as have infections with adenovirus, echovirus, coxsackievirus and astrovirus.

Symptoms and signs

Diarrhoea, rather than vomiting, is usually the predominant feature in neonatal gastroenteritis, and copious watery stools may be passed. Bloody stools are rare, except in infection with *Salmonella, Shigella* or *Campylobacter* species. Signs of dehydration soon appear and shock may develop, especially in preterm babies, who may rapidly lose more than 10% of their bodyweight. The infant is often pale and listless, with a distended abdomen and a metabolic acidosis.

Differential diagnosis and investigation

Healthy breastfed babies may pass up to 10 loosish yellow stools per day, but are thriving and otherwise completely asymptomatic. Frequent loose green stools are often seen in infants receiving phototherapy (pp. 672–3) and do not require further investigation. Severe diarrhoea can occasionally be caused by the inherited abnormalities of sugar absorption (p. 862), congenital chloride diarrhoea (p. 911) or cystic fibrosis (pp. 705–7). If these conditions are excluded, copious diarrhoea is almost always due to gastroenteritis. Stool culture is essential and, if appropriate, stools should also be examined by electron microscopy for virus particles.

Treatment

If the symptoms are mild and dehydration minimal, it may be worth persisting with breastfeeding or formula feeding, giving small frequent feeds. If the major problem is vomiting, this can usually be controlled with a glucose–electrolyte solution. In more severe cases, oral feeds should be stopped for 48 hours and i.v. fluids started. Infusions of sodium bicarbonate may need to be given to acidaemic preterm babies. After 48 hours, oral glucose–electrolyte solutions are usually well tolerated, and the baby can promptly restart milk feeds in the next 24–48 hours. There is no need to regrade the feeds from quarter to half to full strength. If diarrhoea returns, lactose intolerance (p. 705) or milk intolerance should be considered, and, if present, the baby should be started on an appropriate lactose-free hydrolysed milk such as Pregestimil.

Antibiotics should not be given routinely. However, if an epidemic of bacterial gastroenteritis develops, oral non-absorbable antibiotics such as neomycin or colomycin may be indicated.[806] If *Salmonella* species, *Shigella* species or campylobacter are grown, and particularly if the infant has systemic symptoms or is premature, parenteral antibiotics should be given using co-trimoxazole or a third-generation cephalosporin for *Salmonella*, ampicillin or co-trimoxazole for *Shigella*, and erythromycin or gentamicin for campylobacter. Antidiarrhoeal agents should not be used in the neonatal period.

Isolation

Term babies who develop mild symptoms on a postnatal ward can be isolated with their mothers. Sporadic cases on a neonatal unit should be isolated within the unit or, if appropriate facilities exist, transferred to the paediatric infectious disease unit. The management of epidemics is outlined on pages outlined above.

Urinary tract infection

The true incidence of UTI in the newborn is difficult to establish because the methods of urine collection employed in epidemiological surveys are all likely to lead to overdiagnosis, because of contamination. In term infants, the reported incidence is in the range 0.1–3%; among LBW infants, it is at least three times as high and possibly as much as 10 times as high.[219,314,838,849] If the higher quoted figures are true, most neonatal UTIs remain undiagnosed. There is a two- to threefold higher incidence in males at any gestation. Infants of cocaine users seem to be unusually susceptible to UTI.[314] UTI in the newborn is believed to occur mainly as a result of bloodstream spread of organisms to the kidney during a septicaemia, although no doubt the reverse situation can also apply. Breastfeeding offers a significant degree of protection.[658]

Organisms

The commonest pathogen by far is *E. coli*, and responsible strains are associated with P-fimbria, a limited number of serotypes, resistance to the bactericidal effects of serum, adhesion to epithelial cells and the production of haemolysins.[413,790] In addition, many Gram-negative enteric bacteria and some Gram-positive cocci, including CONS, *Staph. aureus* and enterococci, can cause neonatal UTI. *C. albicans* accounts for some 40% of UTIs in a neontal unit setting.[654] In the case of the VLBW baby, this is usually one component of a multisystem infection (pp. 1061–2).

Symptoms and signs

Neonatal UTI may present acutely with all the signs of septicaemia (pp. 1020, 1021), or insidiously with poor feeding, listlessness, poor weight gain and low-grade fever. Some infections only come to light if urinalysis is done as part of the routine investigation of a baby with, say, persisting jaundice, unexplained anaemia or poor weight gain. On examination, signs particularly relevant to the diagnosis of UTI include distress during renal palpation, renal enlargement due to hydronephrosis or some other congenital abnormality, and an enlarged bladder, suggesting outflow tract obstruction. The external genitalia must be examined to exclude stenoses or fistulae, and the blood pressure should be checked.

Investigation

If the UTI is part of a septicaemic illness, as it is in around a quarter of cases,[654] there will commonly be a positive blood culture in addition to a positive urine culture. The technique of urine collection and the diagnostic criteria for UTI are given on page 1218, and should be adhered to. All babies with a proven UTI must have their serum biochemistry checked.

Further investigation is essential, as between 35% and 50% will have an underlying abnormality, which in about two-thirds will be vesicoureteric reflux.[4,511] A renal ultrasound scan will demonstrate the presence, position and size of the kidneys, the size and thickness of the bladder, and dilatation of the collecting systems. Ultrasound may also show echogenic fungal material in the renal pelvis or ureter in around a third of cases of proven UTI due to *C. albicans*.[133,654] Ultrasound alone, however, cannot be relied upon to show scars or exclude vesicoureteric reflux,[759,760] and all children under the age of 1 year being investigated following proven UTI should have a micturating cysto-urethrogram (MCUG) and a dimercaptosuccinic acid (DMSA) scan in addition to ultrasound.[1,310] The MCUG will exclude bladder neck obstruction and urethral valves, but its most important role is to exclude vesicoureteric reflux. The DMSA scan can show scarring, which is probably commoner after renal infection than was once thought to be the case.[419] The intravenous urogram has fallen out of fashion but may be necessary on occasion to fully delineate an abnormality and plan further treatment. In children over 1 year of age, the diagnostic work-up is different.[304]

Treatment

If the baby presents with a systemic illness, the usual antibiotic combinations for either early- or late-onset sepsis should be used, and the treatment refined when the results of cultures are available. If UTI is confirmed, antibiotics should be continued for 10–14 days. Resolution of infection should be confirmed with further urine cultures. Once the infection has been treated, prophylaxis with low-dose trimethoprim, given in a single dose at night, should continue until radiological investigations have excluded underlying abnormalities. If the investigations are normal, prophylaxis can be discontinued, but the infant should be followed with urinalyses every 3 months for at least a year. If there is evidence of reflux, antibiotic prophylaxis should be continued. UTI due to *C. albicans* has traditionally been treated with amphotericin alone or in combination with one of the newer antimycotic drugs. A recent report has suggested that good results can also be obtained with a combination of fluconazole and flucytosine.[374]

Listeriosis

L. monocytogenes is a short Gram-positive rod which can be found both inside and outside cells. The most important reservoir for transmission to humans is probably food, especially dairy products, contaminated by infected farm animals.[262,291] Neonatal infection in the UK is now uncommon (see p. 1033). Women infected with HIV are considerably more susceptible to *L. monocytogenes* than are the general population.[243] Newborn infants are particularly susceptible for a variety of immunological reasons, including defects in macrophage response[414] and low opsonic activity.[106] Three main types of fetal and neonatal infection are found.

Transplacental infection

L. monocytogenes causes a non-specific influenzal or gastroenteritic illness in the pregnant woman, during which the organism may infect the fetus, either by haematogenous spread across the placenta or via infection of the amniotic fluid. First- or second-trimester infection may cause fetal death or miscarriage, and recurrent abortion due to listeria has been recorded in humans.[319] Later in pregnancy, infection may precipitate preterm labour,[291] with fetal distress and meconium staining of the liquor. Because meconium staining of the liquor is rare at gestations below 34 weeks, its presence should raise the suspicion of listeria. Liveborn babies are often extremely ill at birth. They may have a severe pneumonia, and hepatomegaly and meningitis may already be present. Blood and stool cultures are invariably positive. Characteristically, small (2–3 mm) pinkish-grey cutaneous granulomas are present and, at autopsy, similar small granulomatous lesions are widespread in the lung, liver, CNS and many other tissues and organs.

Early-onset infection, acquired intrapartum

Most cases of neonatal listeriosis are sporadic, but epidemics are described. At least two-thirds of infants who acquire listeria infection intrapartum are preterm, and almost all become ill within 24 hours of birth.[527] Most have disseminated infection, with pneumonia, meningitis, thrombocytopenia, anaemia and sometimes conjunctivitis. Small cutaneous granulomas may be found in some babies.

Late-onset infection, usually meningitis, probably due to nosocomial infection

Nosocomial spread of listeria is well documented and asymptomatic mothers of affected babies should be isolated.[250,528] Late-onset listeria infection is usually in the form of a meningitis (p. 1040) with or without concomitant septicaemia or colitis. The median age of onset is about 2 weeks. Associated brain abscess has been described.[55]

Investigation

The routine investigations of early-onset sepsis and meningitis reveal the diagnosis. However, listeria can pose problems for the microbiologist, as its uptake of the Gram stain can be variable and it may be slow-growing.

Therapy

The most effective antibiotic therapy is ampicillin plus gentamicin, and in units where listeria is a common pathogen there is much to be said for using this combination as the routine for early-onset sepsis. Listeria is resistant to all third-generation cephalosporins. Intrathecal treatment is not required for listerial meningitis. ECMO has recently been used successfully in the treatment of severe early-onset listeriosis.[373]

Outcome

The mortality for neonatal listeriosis is in the range 5–15%.[274,429] The prognosis for listerial meningitis is better than that for other neonatal bacterial meningitis.

Superficial infections

Umbilical cord infections

Devitalised tissue provides a good culture medium and the thrombosed cord vessels are a potential portal of entry into the circulation. In the days before effective prophylactic measures were introduced, staphylococcal infection of the cord and surrounding tissues, often leading to systemic infection, was commonplace. In the developing world, neonatal tetanus occurs mainly as a result of contamination of the umbilical cord stump by *Clostridium tetani*.[246,713]

Despite good cord care, minor umbilical infection still occurs in 2% of preterm and 0.5% of term neonates. Although *Staph. aureus* is still the most important pathogen, Gram-negative enteric bacilli, especially *E. coli* and *Klebsiella* species, are relatively common.[553] In most cases the clinical features are limited to periumbilical erythema, often with a small amount of discharge, but in other cases there is a spreading cellulitis of the abdominal wall, or even fasciitis.[553]

Investigation and treatment

Swab any exudate and take a blood culture. Usually, local treatment with an antiseptic such as chlorhexidine powder will suffice, but if there is evidence of invasion of the surrounding tissues or of systemic upset, a broad-spectrum antibiotic combination, effective against *Staph. aureus* and Gram-negative bacilli, should be given i.v. A combination of vancomycin or flucloxacillin and a third-generation cephalosporin, or flucloxacillin and gentamicin, would be a suitable initial treatment.

Skin infections

Staphylococcal

The commonest presentation is with a few flaccid intraepidermal bullae which are filled with a yellowish opalescent fluid, but occasionally larger bullae may be present, in which case the condition merges into bullous impetigo (pp. 820–1). Paronychia may also occur. The infant is usually well, with little or no local inflammation and no regional lymphadenitis. After taking swabs from the lesions, treatment should be with oral flucloxacillin. If there is any suggestion of a systemic illness, staphylococcal septicaemia should be suspected, appropriate investigations carried out, and parenteral antibiotics started.

Candida (thrush) (see pp. 1061–2)

Conjunctivitis

Up-to-date and useful epidemiological information on neonatal conjunctivitis is hard to come by. A recent study in Norway found an overall incidence of neonatal conjunctivitis of approximately 19%, of which 7% were classed as severe.[185] The incidence of conjunctivitis was approximately 15% among infants not receiving silver nitrate prophylaxis, and approximately 20% among those who did.

Organisms

Infective conjunctivitis can be caused by a wide variety of pathogens and the pattern varies considerably between reported series. In the UK, the top five would normally include *Staph. aureus*, *C. trachomatis*, *H. influenzae*, *Str. pneumoniae* and '*Streptococcus viridans*'. *N. gonorrhoeae* is rare in the UK at the present time. In all ill children with conjunctival discharge, in addition to the organisms mentioned, always consider HSV (pp. 1053–5), *L. monocytogenes* and *N. meningitidis*.

General considerations

Conjunctivitis can develop at any stage in the neonatal period. Late-onset and recurrent conjunctivitis is much more common if there is a blocked lacrimal duct with epiphora (pp. 841–2). The spectrum of severity ranges from mild crusting on the eyelids, through purulent discharge, conjunctival injection and eyelid oedema, to invasion of the eye and retro-orbital structures.

In infants with mild conjunctivitis, no treatment other than regular cleaning/bathing of the lids with a sterile saline swab 4–6-hourly for 2–3 days is required. However, if cultures are positive, discharge persists for more than 48 hours, or there is conjunctival or lid oedema, topical antibiotics should be started. Chloramphenicol, neomycin or gentamicin eye drops are common choices, administered 6-hourly. Because an important part of the therapy is irrigation, drops are preferable to ointment. Both eyes should be treated, even though infection is only apparent in one. In infants with epiphora, after instilling the antibiotics the lacrimal duct should be gently massaged towards the eye in an attempt to unblock it. Rarely, probing the lacrimal duct under anaesthesia may be necessary later in infancy (p. 842).

Gonococcal ophthalmia

This usually presents within 24 hours of delivery with a profuse, bilateral, purulent conjunctival discharge, but can present less dramatically at any time in the first month. Significant systemic upset is unusual, but because of the speed with which the infection can damage the cornea it is important that the diagnosis is made and treatment started immediately. A swab must be sent to the laboratory promptly for Gram stain and culture in an enriched medium. If Gram-negative intracellular diplococci are seen on microscopy, treatment must be started immediately, pending culture. Traditionally, treatment has been with systemic penicillin and penicillin eye drops and this is an effective regimen. Currently recommended treatment is with a single dose of ceftriaxone, 25–50 mg/kg i.v. or i.m. to a maximum dose of 125 mg. With this regimen, topical treament is not necessary.[154,383,486] The infected baby must be isolated with his mother from all other babies, and the mother and her contacts should be treated.

Chlamydial ophthalmia

This is now among the commonest causes of neonatal conjunctivitis, and some babies infected as neonates will develop chlamydial pneumonia later in infancy, which is often severe enough to require hospital admission. In Western Europe, chlamydial pneumonia is probably quite rare, and a recent study in Germany reported that only 1% of infants with pneumonia had evidence of chlamydia.[421] However, in areas of the world where chlamydial genital infection is much more common, 50% of all pneumonia in early infancy may be due to this organism.

The risk of vertical transmission of *C. trachomatis* has been variously reported. In some studies, 50% of babies delivered to mothers with genital chlamydia become infected, although only half of these are symptomatic with conjunctivitis or pneumonia.[74,763] However, a study in the UK reported that only 25% of infants of infected mothers were infected, with only 14% being symptomatic, and of those who did become symptomatic, only one-quarter developed pneumonia.[663]

Chlamydial conjunctivitis usually presents between 5 and 12 days' postnatal age. It may be unilateral initially, but often becomes bilateral. Rarely it can cause adhesions between the bulbar and tarsal conjunctiva, with some persisting pannus, but it almost never causes permanent visual impairment. Conventional cultures are negative and treatment with standard topical antibiotics is rarely successful: in many cases chlamydia is first suspected for these very reasons. Several tests are available for the identification of chlamydia from eye swabs, including enzyme immunoassay and immunofluorescence techniques,[210] the immune dot-blot test[95] and tissue culture. Now that PCR is available in routine laboratories, it is proving most useful.

Chlamydial eye infection is usually treated with tetracycline eye drops or ointment and oral erythromycin for 2 weeks. This should also prevent the baby developing chlamydial pneumonia in infancy.[95] There is evidence to suggest that a shorter course of azithromycin may be as effective.[347]

Attempts have been made to prevent both the neonatal conjunctivitis and pneumonia in infancy by some form of early neonatal prophylaxis. Silver nitrate eye drops and tetracycline or erythromycin eye ointment applied at delivery have all been used, with varying degrees of success.[190,346] It has recently been shown that a 2.5% ophthalmic solution of povidone-iodine is a more effective form of prophylaxis than either silver nitrate or erythromycin.[411] If maternal infection is detected antenatally, treatment with erythromycin for 1 week considerably reduces the risk of neonatal infection.[22,529,585] Alternatively, the mother can be treated with ampicillin.[22] The risk of perinatal transmission is reduced by caesarean section,[74] but few would consider this an indication for the operation.

Pseudomonal ophthalmia

Although a relatively rare cause of neonatal ophthalmia, *Ps. aeruginosa* has a remarkable ability to invade ocular tissue and to cause severe damage.[115] Most cases occur in preterm infants, usually as a result of cross-infection from an environmental source.[265] Many of these infants develop septicaemia as well as ophthalmia.[744] If pseudomonal ophthalmia is suspected, or if the organism is grown from an eye swab, parenteral therapy with a suitable antibiotic combination, such as gentamicin and ceftazidime, should be begun at once, in addition to locally applied gentamicin drops or ointment. Urgent ophthalmological opinion is required if invasive disease is suspected.

Dacrocystitis

This presents within the first week as a reddish-purple swelling over the course of the lacrimal duct and sac on the medial and inferior margin of the eye. Local pressure often results in a squirt of purulent material from the lacrimal punctum. The usual cause is *Staph. aureus*, but anaerobes may sometimes be involved.[124] Treatment is with systemic and topical antibiotics, usually in drops rather than ointment. Sequelae are rare.

Otitis media

This diagnosis is often ignored in the neonatal period, probably because of the great difficulty in visualising the oblique, downward-facing immobile tympanic membrane through the hairy, narrow neonatal external auditory meatus. However, otitis media has been reported to occur in two-thirds of infants ventilated through a nasotracheal tube, which compromises normal function at the lower end of the Eustachian tube, and infection may still be present at autopsy. However, in those who survive, the infection resolves. Otitis media is virtually universal in infants with cleft palate, in whom there is reflux of milk and secretions into the Eustachian tube. Finally, otitis media may occur in a previously healthy baby and in long-stay patients on a NICU who develop signs of an URTI.

Among the inmates of a NICU, the organisms responsible are often *E. coli* and *Staph. aureus*, but *H. influenzae* and *Str. pneumoniae* may be grown from previously asymptomatic babies who present later in the neonatal period. In many cases, fluid obtained by tympanocentesis is sterile.

Treatment of otitis media in the ill LBW baby on IPPV should be with the usual broad-spectrum antibiotic combination. In older infants with URTI and/or cleft palate, oral treatment with an antibiotic active against *Str. pneumoniae* and *H. influenzae*, such as amoxicillin or trimethoprim, is usually adequate.

Other neonatal bacterial infections

Localised abscesses

These may develop anywhere, but are most common at the site of heelpricks, i.v. infusions, or where the skin has been abraded by electrode adhesive or some other piece of monitoring equipment. There is localised swelling, redness and tenderness. The infection may spread to more important local tissues, such as bone, causing an osteomyelitis, or, rarely, septicaemia may develop. If a fluctuant area develops, incision or aspiration under local anaesthesia, using a wide-bore needle, is helpful. Broad-spectrum antibiotic cover should be given i.v., but if the baby is well this can be changed to an appropriate oral antibiotic once the culture and sensitivities are available. Treatment should usually be given for 7–10 days.

Breast abscess

Breast enlargement and redness in babies of either sex is not unusual and represents a transient hormonal stimulus, rather than infection. However, if tenderness and erythema are present with fluctuation, pyrexia or a purulent discharge from the nipple (not to be confused with neonatal breast milk/lactorrhoea, p. 380), then treatment with systemic antibiotics should be given.

Liver abscess

Postmortem examinations indicate that multiple microabscesses in the liver may occur in both preterm and term babies as a complication of generalised sepsis, vascular cannulae or abdominal surgery. In life there are few clues to their presence, although they may be associated with hepatomegaly and abnormal liver enzymes. Solitary liver abscesses have occasionally been reported in the newborn, mostly in preterm infants who have had umbilical vein catheterisation, but all of the references are quite old.[117] Most cases are caused by *Staph. aureus*. Ultrasound examination of the liver will discover an abscess quite reliably.[552] True bacterial hepatitis is very rare, but is a well-documented feature of congenital listeriosis. *C. albicans* can cause multiple liver abscesses in babies with immunodeficiency states.

Therapy for multiple microabscesses is that for septicaemia. Solitary abscesses may require drainage in addition, either percutaneously under ultrasound guidance[697] or by open operation.

Sialadenitis

The parotid or submandibular glands may become infected, with the latter more often involved in premature babies. Presentation is with a red indurated area over the gland, with pus draining from either Stensen's or Wharton's duct. *Staph. aureus* is the commonest pathogen, but *E. coli* and *Ps. aeruginosa* may also be implicated. Suppurative parotitis caused by anaerobic organisms has also been reported.[124,126] Treatment is with i.v. antibiotics, which should always include flucloxacillin.

Necrotising fasciitis

Bacterial infection of the subcutaneous tissues and fascia is a rare but potentially very serious condition in the newborn. The organisms most commonly implicated are streptococci of groups B, A and D, staphylococci, Gram-negative enterobacteria and various anaerobes.[125,390,482,553] Necrotising fasciitis can arise at any site, but the commonest is the abdominal wall, secondary to omphalitis. There is commonly marked tissue oedema and inflammation, which spreads rapidly. There are signs of systemic toxicity but blood cultures are positive in only about half the cases. The keys to a successful outcome are a high level of clinical suspicion, appropriate antibiotics, and prompt and aggressive surgical intervention.

Mycoplasma and ureaplasma infections[519]

If present in the mother's birth canal, these organisms may colonise as many as 50% of babies,[196,718] but their importance in causing infectious disease is incompletely understood.

Table 40.10 Neonatal infections caused by ureaplasmas and mycoplasmas

Organism	Infection	Reference
Mycoplasma hominis	Surgical wound infection	Brooker et al 1994 Ped. Inf. Dis. J. 13: 751
	Abscess	Sacker et al 1970 Pediatrics 46: 303
	Sialadenitis	Powell et al 1979 Pediatrics 63: 789
	Meningitis	Hjelm et al 1980 Acta Paed. Scand. 69: 415
		Waites et al 1988 Lancet i: 17
		McDonald & Moore 1988 Ped. Inf. Dis. J. 7: 795
	Septicaemia	Unsworth et al 1985 J. Inf. 10: 163
	Pericarditis	Miller et al 1982 Am. J. Dis. Child. 136: 271
Ureaplasma sp.	Meningitis	Waites et al 1988 Lancet I: 17
		Garland & Murton 1987 Ped. Inf. Dis. J. 6: 868

The probable role of *U. urealyticum* in neonatal pneumonia and CLD has been discussed (p. 1044). There is also little doubt that both *U. urealyticum* and *M. hominis* may occasionally cause focal infection[704] or septicaemia in ill LBW babies (Table 40.10). Some epidemiological studies, however, have found little evidence to suggest that babies colonised by either *U. urealyticum* or *M. hominis* are disadvantaged compared with those who are not.[362] Improved methods of detecting these organisms, such as PCR, should help to define their role further.[96]

Treatment

The most effective antibiotic against both mycoplasmas and ureaplasmas is erythromycin, and this should be given i.v.[825]

Tuberculosis

Tuberculosis is prevalent in almost all tropical developing countries and constitutes a special risk during pregnancy and lactation to mothers and babies.[257] In the UK, perinatal tuberculosis is currently extremely rare, although is probably set to increase. Transplacental infection usually occurs when the pregnant woman has clinical tuberculosis or a recent primary infection. In the former, but not in the latter, miliary lesions are present in the placenta. There is an absence of cellular response in the baby, and the primary focus and lymph nodes are caseous, with abundant tubercle bacilli. The peripheries of the lesions contain few lymphocytes and no giant cells. Co-infection with HIV is now recognised.[14,657]

Criteria for the diagnosis of congenital tuberculosis were first laid down by Beitzke,[71] and are rigorous enough for all time. There must be proof that the lesion is tuberculous, and in this regard a primary complex in the liver is almost certainly of intrauterine origin. If the liver primary complex is absent, the infection should be obvious in the fetus or in the neonate at birth or during the first week. Neonatal tuberculosis is the result either of intrauterine infection or of inhalation of tubercle bacilli during or soon after birth, through intimate contact with an adult with active pulmonary tuberculosis.

Clinical picture

The onset of symptoms is usually within the first month of life. The primary focus is often in the liver, and congenitally infected infants may present with hepatomegaly and jaundice caused by obstruction of bile drainage by enlarged lymph nodes at the porta hepatis. Sometimes a primary complex is found in the lung as a result of dissemination through the ductus venosus. The infant may then present with pneumonia, anaemia and hepatosplenomegaly, with radiological evidence of widespread pulmonary infection involving both lungs and mediastinal and hilar lymph nodes. There is usually no liver lesion in this clinical syndrome, the source of infection probably being the amniotic fluid or the maternal genital tract.[306] Examination of the gastric aspirate for acid-fast bacilli is the best diagnostic test. The infected neonate is not sensitive to tuberculin. Occasionally, localised infection is reported, such as otitis or cutaneous involvement,[766] and occasionally the presentation is as an acute sepsis syndrome.[556]

Management

Results are best when infected mothers have been detected by antenatal screening and antituberculous treatment instituted during pregnancy.[363] The management of an infant of a mother with the disease poses special problems. Isolation of the baby from the infected mother is usually not feasible and is in any case undesirable, because it would signal the end of breastfeeding and expose the infant to all the hazards of artificial feeding. Breastfeeding seems to be safe for the infant of a mother taking antituberculous drugs. The policy advocated here for asymptomatic infants of tuberculous mothers has been proved effective, and is as follows:

- Maintain breastfeeding (except where this is precluded by the gravity of the maternal illness).
- Treat the mother for tuberculosis.
- Give the infant prophylactic isoniazid in a single dose of 10 mg/kg daily, this to continue until the mother is confirmed to be sputum negative by repeated sputum examination.
- Carry out BCG immunisation in the infant using isoniazid-resistant BCG.

Treatment of proven neonatal infection is not well researched because of the relative rarity of the condition, although regimens that are effective in treating adults and children should be effective. One recommended regimen is isoniazid (20 mg/kg/day) plus rifampicin (20 mg/kg/day) and pyrazinamide (30 mg/kg/day) for 2 months, followed by 4 months of isoniazid and rifampicin. An alternative is a 9-month course of isoniazid and rifampicin. If isoniazid resistance is suspected, usually on the basis of the likely geographical source of the infection, at least one additional drug should be used until sensitivities are known. Streptomycin (20 mg/kg/day i.m.), ethambutol (20 mg/kg/day) or pyrazinamide (30 mg/kg/day) are suitable choices. Steroids have no place in treatment because of the lack of a host reaction. The infant with congenital tuberculosis should be vaccinated with isoniazid-resistant BCG to encourage active immunity. Breastfeeding should be encouraged, and if the mother is infected, she must also be treated with antituberculous drugs. Isoniazid prophylaxis for skin-test-negative neonatal contacts is appropriate and effective.[485,712]

Neonatal tetanus

Tetanus is an important cause of neonatal death (up to 60 per 1000 livebirths) worldwide because of local conditions and customs, rather than climate. Neonatal tetanus still accounts for between 25% and 65% of all neonatal deaths in some countries.[233,402] In rural India, the walls of the village houses are made of a mixture of earth and cowdung, and the ash of cowdung fires is used to dress the umbilical stump. Neonatal tetanus is known as the '8-day disease' in the Punjab, because so many babies die of tetanus on the eighth day of life. Infection of the umbilical stump caused by septic management of the cord and harmful cultural practices are the main reasons for the high frequency of neonatal tetanus in rural communities in the tropics.

The organism

Clostridium tetani is a Gram-positive rod and a strict anaerobe. It is present in animal faeces, though usually absent from human faeces. Spores of *Cl. tetani* are highly resistant to heat, chemicals and antibiotics, but can be destroyed if autoclaved. They can survive for many years in dry dust or earth. During germination and growth in anaerobic conditions, the organism produces two toxins, tetanospasmin and tetanolysin. Tetanospasmin is a potent exotoxin with high affinity for nervous tissue. It is produced by the vegetative form of *Cl. tetani* in conditions of reduced oxygen. Within the CNS, the toxin is bound to gangliosides, where it suppresses inhibitory influences on motor neurons and interneurons, directly enhancing excitatory synaptic action. Its action is similar to that of strychnine, inducing hypertonicity, spasms and seizures. The toxin also produces overactivity of the sympathetic nervous system, resulting in tachycardia, arrhythmias, labile hypertension, peripheral vasoconstriction, sweating, hypercarbia and increased urinary excretion of catecholamines. The site of absorption of tetanus toxin is at the peripheral motor and autonomic nerve endings. Toxin ascends the nerve fibres and crosses the synaptic cleft into the presynaptic endings of adjacent inhibitory spinal interneurons, where it is bound. Antitoxin

inhibits tetanospasmin only before it is fixed on to the presynaptic terminal.

Clinical features

The incubation period of neonatal tetanus varies from 3 to 14 days or more,[713] the severity of the disease being greater with a shorter incubation period. Both muscle rigidity and spasms are typical of tetanus.

Trismus, caused by spasm of the masseter muscles, a few days after birth is the presenting symptom in more than half of patients with neonatal tetanus. This is followed by stiffness of the neck muscles and difficulty in swallowing. The infant is irritable, restless and unable to feed. Spasm of the facial muscles produces risus sardonicus. Tonic contractions of the lumbar and abdominal musculature occur next, and result in opisthotonus. This is accompanied by flexion and adduction of the arms and clenching of the fists. Spasms which initially last a few seconds become more prolonged, and may persist for minutes as the disease progresses. The patient is conscious and crying because of intense pain from muscle spasms that become more powerful, and which are easily precipitated by any tactile, visual or auditory stimulus. Fever is a feature, probably because of overactivity of the muscles. Spasms of laryngeal and respiratory muscles may lead to obstruction, asphyxia and cyanosis. The natural history of tetanus is one of increasing severity during the first 7 days, followed by a plateau in the second week and gradual abatement over the next 2–6 weeks. Tetanus is often fatal in the neonate, with mortality as high as 50–90%.[484] Bronchopneumonia, aspiration pneumonia and atelectasis are common complications. When assisted ventilation and intensive care are available, the death rate can be substantially reduced.[713]

Management

The use of meagre resources to treat a serious infection with high mortality which can be eliminated by preventive measures raises some awkward ethical and administrative problems. The improved survival of patients with neonatal tetanus in centres where assisted ventilation, curarisation, i.v. nutrition and new spasmolytic drugs have been applied raises questions about the reasons for the disparity in medical services which on the one hand are insufficiently developed to prevent this dreadful disease but which on the other hand can employ expensive modern technology to treat it.

There is currently no agreed standard regimen of management of neonatal tetanus. The aims of treatment are to neutralise existing toxin before it enters the nervous system, to reduce further production of toxin, to control the neuromuscular and autonomic features, and to sustain the patient until the effects of toxin resolve.

General management includes skilful nursing care to prevent aspiration pneumonia and atelectasis, and the reduction to a minimum of stimuli that can precipitate a convulsion.

Penicillin 60 mg (100 000 units)/kg/day is given for 5 days to eliminate *Cl. tetani*. Concomitant infections should be treated with appropriate broad-spectrum antibiotics.

Tetanus antitoxin can only neutralise unbound circulating toxin and has no effect on toxin fixed in nerve cells. Although the

CNS is often affected by toxin before symptoms appear, patients given antitoxin have usually fared better than those not given antitoxin. Specific antitetanus human immunoglobulin is the preparation of choice. A single dose of 3000–5000 units given by i.m. injection is recommended. Equine antitetanus serum (ATS) remains the most widely used tetanus antitoxin. It should be used as early as possible in the course of the disease, as either a single i.m. injection of 5000 units or 750–1500 units daily for three doses. Massive doses of ATS have no significant advantage over smaller doses. There may be benefit in giving 1500 units of ATS intrathecally early in the disease. There is a significantly lower death rate in babies given intrathecal therapy (45%) compared with controls given i.m. ATS (82%). Infants who receive intrathecal ATS also have fewer complications than controls. There is no convincing evidence that periumbilical infiltration of ATS has a significant effect on the outcome of neonatal tetanus.

Paraldehyde for immediate control of spasms, followed by phenobarbital (phenobarbitone) and chlorpromazine or diazepam for continued sedation, is effective in the control of spasms. Combination therapy using phenobarbital, chlorpromazine and diazepam may help reduce mortality.[484] The mortality from neonatal tetanus has been strikingly reduced by the use of muscle relaxants and IPPV, and this approach should be used wherever the facilities to apply it exist.

Prevention

Tetanus in the newborn can be prevented by aseptic management of the umbilical cord at birth. The persistence of neonatal tetanus in many developing countries reflects the lack of rudimentary obstetric services for large sections of the population.[402] Education of traditional birth attendants in hygienic handling of the umbilical cord at birth has resulted in a sharp decline in the prevalence of neonatal tetanus. This provides a model which should be adopted with this disease in developing countries.

Active immunisation of pregnant women with tetanus toxoid reduces the risk of the disease by almost 90%,[333] but unfortunately those in greatest need of protection are not likely to attend antenatal clinics. Two doses of tetanus toxoid, 0.5 ml each, separated by 2 months, affords excellent immunity, but even one dose is very effective.[550] Passive immunisation of neonates at risk is the most frequently employed preventive measure in paediatric practice. The administration of 750 units of ATS to infants born in high-risk circumstances will provide protection.

Leprosy

Babies of mothers with leprosy

Babies of mothers with leprosy are of lower than average birthweight. Intrauterine growth retardation has been observed in babies of mothers with lepromatous leprosy as early as the 16th week of pregnancy. IgA antibodies to *M. leprae* have been found in 30% of cord sera of babies of mothers with active lepromatous leprosy. Specific IgA and IgM anti-*M. leprae* antibody production occurs during the first 6 months of life of these babies infected in utero. The prevalence of leprosy in children under

2 years of age whose mothers have active lepromatous leprosy is 5%. Diagnosis in these children has been made with positive skin tests to *M. leprae*, together with a marked increase in serum IgA and IgM anti-*M. leprae* antibody activity.

Management

The pregnant mother should receive multidrug therapy of dapsone 2 mg/kg daily, clofazimine 1 mg/kg daily and rifampicin 10 mg/kg monthly. Clofazimine will turn her milk pink, so mothers should be reassured that the colour change does not affect the quality of their milk. Folate supplements should be given. Women with leprosy should be encouraged to breastfeed their babies while they are receiving effective treatment. Heavy breast milk infection only occurs in advanced leprosy involving the nipple and milk ducts.

Newborn babies of mothers who were not treated during pregnancy should be treated with clofazimine 1 mg/kg daily, which may also be given to babies of treated women if indicated. Unlike dapsone, clofazimine will not induce haemolysis in children with glucose-6-phosphate dehydrogenase (G6PD) deficiency.

Perinatal viral infections

Several viral agents can cause serious neonatal illness with high mortality and morbidity rates. Most of these infections are acquired by vertical transmission, but some are the result of cross-infection postnatally.

Herpesviruses

Herpes simplex virus

HSV is a large virus containing double-stranded DNA, which encodes for some 70 polypeptides. It exists in two antigenically distinct forms: HSV-1, the cause of orolabial, ophthalmic and encephalitic herpes in older children and adults, and HSV-2, which until recently caused 80–85% of genital herpes and the majority of neonatal infections. The remaining 15–20% of cases of genital herpes, and up to 30% of neonatal infections, were due to HSV type 1. Lately, genital infection with HSV-1 has become commoner in the UK (probably as a result of the fear of HIV, leading to more oral sex) and the most recent incidence report has HSV-1 and HSV-2 accounting for equal proportions of neonatal infection.[800] The incidence of neonatal herpes in the UK is around 1 case per 50 000 births,[342,800] but 100-fold higher incidences are reported from North America.[840] Neonatal herpes is often fatal and neurological handicap is common in survivors. The preterm infant is most susceptible.

Modes of transmission
Transplacental infection
Transplacental transmission of HSV is rare and usually associated with primary maternal infection with HSV-2. This route accounts for around 5% of all cases of neonatal herpes[396] and some 70 cases

have been reported in the literature.[839] The infection may ascend through intact membranes.[399,646] The congenitally infected baby is usually profoundly damaged with microcephaly or hydranencephaly, chorioretinitis and skin lesions, but occasionally may just have mild eye involvement.[396] No treatment is available for these babies.

Vertical transmission

Neonatal HSV occurs as a result of maternal genital herpes in about 85% of cases[530] although most of the mothers are either asymptomatic at the time of birth or have no history of genital herpes.[546,858] Rarely, the virus may reach the fetus in utero following prolonged rupture of the membranes, in which case the baby may be born with skin and eye lesions. This form of infection is rare and carries a relatively good prognosis with effective antiviral treatment.[839] Usually, infection is acquired during passage down the birth canal. If the mother has an active, primary infection at the time of vaginal delivery, the risk of neonatal infection is about 50%,[130] but if the mother has a secondary recurrence of genital herpes, lower concentrations of virus are shed and the risk is reduced to around 3%.[129]

Nosocomial infection

HSV can be acquired from other neonatal cases, or from orolabial or cutaneous herpes in staff or family. Although this form of transmission is allegedly rare, the fact that the incidence of type 1 neonatal HSV is roughly double that of type 1 genital herpetic infections suggests that non-genital sources of neonatal infection may be more common than previously thought.[392]

Clinical features

Neonatal HSV infection occurs in three distinct forms, albeit with a degree of overlap.[229,546]

Localised to skin, mouth and eyes

Superficial infection ordinarily occurs during the second week of life and is a more common presentation if the mother has recurrent rather that primary infection.[543] The baby may develop a vesicular skin rash, keratoconjunctivitis or, rarely, intraoral vesicles. The disease can be localised to just one of these sites or may affect any combination of them. The skin vesicles are usually 1–2 mm in diameter, but may be much larger. They can be multiple or occur in clusters.

Babies who present with superficial infection generally do not develop disseminated disease, but a surprisingly high proportion (maybe up to 30%) show subsequent neurodevelopmental abnormalities.[840] Conversely, infants who present with disseminated disease may later develop cutaneous and eye lesions.

CNS disease

About one-third of babies with HSV infection present with isolated meningoencephalitis and symptoms similar to those seen in neonatal bacterial meningitis. The usual age of onset is around 10–14 days of age.[595] Many subsequently develop cutaneous or ocular herpes. This form of the disease may result either from haematogenous spread or from neural spread, with retrograde axonal transmission of the virus to the CNS.[326]

Disseminated disease

This most severe form of neonatal herpes presents during the first week of life,[543] and is probably a viraemia with secondary seeding of the CNS. About half of the cases will have only system disease and/or pneumonia, but the rest will have co-existing meningoencephalitis. Twenty per cent have no cutaneous manifestations, making diagnosis difficult.[829]

Infants with disseminated disease present like any critically ill septic baby (pp. 1017–18). They have respiratory distress as a result of pneumonitis, and usually require IPPV. They are often hypotensive, peripherally vasoconstricted, and have renal failure. Severe hepatitis[325] may occur with or without hepatosplenomegaly. DIC, causing petechiae and generalised bleeding, is common. Hypotonia, seizures and coma are common whether or not meningoencephalitis is present. Pneumonia and pleural effusions may occur.[80] Hydrops due to the intrauterine HSV has been reported.[25]

Diagnosis

Vesicular cutaneous, ocular or oral lesions strongly suggest herpes. Other vesicular lesions, such as staphylococcal skin infection or varicella, are usually easily differentiated by the history and their clinical appearance (pp. 820–1).[708]

The most rapid and useful diagnostic test that is widely available is immunofluorescence performed on vesicle fluid. DNA amplification tests are now well established and where available should be used on both serum and CSF, although negative results in a baby with clinically suspected HSV infection should not stop appropriate treatment being provided.[194,544] Viral culture should also be undertaken on vesicle fluid, conjunctival scrapings, nasopharyngeal swab and, where obtained, CSF. Cultures may show cytopathic changes within a few days. The virus may also grow from blood.[308] Serology is much less useful because of the difficulty in distinguishing between passively acquired maternal antibody and endogenously produced antibody.

In the absence of a maternal history of genital disease or of suspicious skin, eye or mouth lesions, disseminated HSV infection will only be diagnosed if viral cultures are a routine part of the investigation of all septic babies, with or without meningitis, from whom no bacterial pathogen is grown after 24–48 hours. Neonatal viral meningitis is usually a mild illness, so that if the CSF findings suggest it (p. 1040) but the baby is seriously ill, herpes is the most likely diagnosis. In some cases of herpetic meningoencephalitis, however, the CSF contains more than 1000 WBC/mm³, many of them polymorphs, together with many red cells, a markedly raised protein and a low glucose.[410] Differentiating these cases from bacterial meningitis depends on cultures.

If herpes is suspected, an EEG should be performed, as it may show characteristic temporoparietal high-voltage low-frequency activity. A CT scan should be performed to look for the characteristic necrosis and haemorrhage in the temporal lobes. These may only appear late in the disease, although MRI changes may occur earlier.[473] Visceral calcification has been reported with disseminated disease.[367]

If there is even a suspicion that systemic illness in a baby is due to herpes, treatment should be begun (see below) until a definite diagnosis is established. Nevertheless, some fulminating cases only come to light at postmortem, when widespread herpetic microabscesses are found, or the virus is grown or detected by

PCR.[610] Depressingly, there seems to have been little progress in decreasing the interval between onset of symptoms and the initiation of therapy.[464]

Treatment

Aciclovir is the current drug of choice, given i.v., 8-hourly, in a total daily dose of 30 mg/kg. As recurrences have occurred after a 10-day course, this should be continued i.v. for at least 14 days. An open-label evaluation of a higher-dose regimen (60 mg/kg/day for 21 days) has suggested improved outcome in disseminated disease but the incidence of significant neutropenia was high and there are no data from phase III trials.[465] Topical aciclovir should be applied to eye and skin lesions. Consideration should be given to prolonging therapy in babies with a positive PCR test for HSV DNA at the end of a normal course of treatment.[36] Alarmingly, aciclovir-resistant neonatal HSV infection is increasingly reported,[620] although there are some newer agents waiting in the wings.[630] In experimental animals, a combination of anti-HSV antibody and aciclovir is far superior to aciclovir alone in reducing mortality,[118] but there is no such study in newborn infants as yet.

Prognosis

The outcome of neonatal herpes before effective antiviral therapy was available was poor (Table 40.11). More recently the results have improved, partly because more cases are diagnosed early and have only localised disease. The mortality rate for disseminated disease is now between 35% and 60%, and for disease isolated to the CNS between 10% and 15%.[840] HSV-2 carries a much higher mortality rate than HSV-1.[543,841]

In terms of morbidity, the picture remains poor, with major adverse sequelae in some 85% of survivors of disseminated disease and in some 50–75% of survivors of meningoencephalitis.[379,410] HSV-2 infection has a worse prognosis than HSV-1;[545] in one study, only 25% of babies with HSV-2 infection were normal on follow-up compared to 100% of those with HSV-1.[174] An abnormal EEG in the neonatal period is a poor prognostic sign.[545]

Recurrent infection

Despite apparent complete resolution of the initial infection, there is a high incidence of recurrence in the following 6–12 months, owing to a defective immunological response to the virus.[472] In one series, relapses occurred in all congenital cases and 12 out of 25 neonatal cases.[787] Kohl[472] reports that most treated neonates will develop cutaneous recurrences in the first year of life. Encephalitic relapses may also occur,[787] and Gutman et al[335] have reported progressive neurological deterioration during the first year of life in a group of infants with neonatal encephalitis. The virus, however, is, still sensitive to, and may respond to, further courses of antiviral drugs. A phase I/II trial of oral aciclovir suppressive therapy has suggested a reduced incidence of cutaneous infection but there are no data on the effect of prophylaxis on neurological outcome and prophylaxis cannot be recommended at present.[466]

Prevention

The risk of transplacental infection is low,[130] only around 0.3% of women excreting the virus intrapartum.[129] The risk of neonatal infection is extremely small in babies born to the asymptomatic HSV excreter,[129] yet 60–80% of cases of neonatal herpes occur in babies whose mothers have neither a history of genital herpes nor any evidence of intrapartum infection.[631] These facts suggest that there is little point in routinely screening for HSV during pregnancy,[425,504] and that there is no need to deliver asymptomatic women with a history of herpes by caesarean section. The risk of neonatal herpes infection following vaginal delivery when the mother has overt primary genital herpes, however, is around 50%, and can be reduced to less than 20% if delivery is by caesarean section within 24 hours of membrane rupture. An apparently successful alternative approach is to treat women who have a primary herpes infection in pregnancy with aciclovir from 36 weeks' gestation until delivery[739] but the practice is of questionable merit.[664] Maternal immunisation in the mouse has shown reduced visceral dissemination but no reduction in CNS invasion.[242] There are no similar studies in humans. Arguably, the best strategy for the prevention of neonatal herpes, without greatly increasing the number of caesarean sections, is physical examination of the mother at the time of labour, with caesarean section for those who have lesions.[131]

Postnatally, the baby of the mother with covert genital herpes requires no treatment. Following vaginal delivery in the presence of overt genital herpes, the baby should stay with his mother and should be treated with i.v. aciclovir, although this is not always effective. If the mother has orolabial or cutaneous herpes, the baby should stay with her (p. 1016, Table 40.3) but her lesions should be covered, treated with topical aciclovir, and her handwashing technique should be meticulous. Other family members or staff with open herpes should stay away.

Table 40.11 Outcome of neonates with herpes infections. (Reproduced from Nahmias et al[594])

	No. of cases	Dead (%)	Alive but handicapped (%)	Alive and normal (%)
Disseminated herpes without CNS involvement	157	91	2	7
Disseminated herpes with CNS involvement	154	73	15	12
Localised CNS disease	116	41	42	17
Other localised disease	76	7	24	70

Varicella zoster virus

This is a member of the herpesvirus family. It causes varicella (chickenpox) as an acute primary infection, but when reactivated from its dormant site in the dorsal root ganglia it causes the cutaneous eruption known as zoster (shingles). Primary infection can occur in the fetus and newborn, sometimes with devastating effect. Reactivation of the virus to cause zoster is rare in the newborn period. Primary VZV infections can be classified as congenital, perinatal or postnatal. Congenital varicella is discussed on page 1069.

Perinatally acquired varicella

If a mother develops varicella during the 3 weeks prior to delivery, there is a 25% chance of her baby developing the illness.[591] Some babies may be born with the rash, in which case the prognosis is good, as it is if the baby develops a rash within 4 days of birth. The usual interval between the onset of the rash in the mother and the onset of rash in the fetus or infant is between 9 and 15 days.[596] The timing of birth in relation to the maternal infection is critical to outcome. Babies born 5 or more days after the mother develops the rash receive some transplacental immunity, have an excellent prognosis, and all reported cases have survived. Babies born less than 5 days after the mother develops the rash develop the disease some 5–10 days after delivery and experience a high mortality (Table 40.12).

Postnatally acquired varicella

Varicella acquired later in the neonatal period is usually a benign disease, although occasional fatalities occur.

Clinical features of neonatal varicella

The disease in the newborn can range from a few vesicles in a relatively well baby to severe disseminated infection complicated by pneumonitis. When pneumonitis occurs, the mortality is high.

Treatment

Babies born to mothers who develop varicella between 7 days antenatally and 7 days postnatally should receive a dose of zoster immume globulin (ZIG), 100 mg, as soon after delivery as possible, or as soon as possible after the mother becomes symptomatic. This will reduce the severity of the disease in the baby but will usually not prevent it. Miller et al[570] reported that 78 of 125 such babies developed varicella – 15 severely – but none died. This is a much better prognosis than suggested by Table 40.12. However, there are reports of neonatal deaths[379] in the high-risk group born within 7 days of the maternal presentation, despite the use of ZIG. For this group, therefore, in addition to giving ZIG, consider giving aciclovir 60 mg/kg/day, 8-hourly, if vesicles appear. Babies born to mothers with perinatal varicella should be isolated from other babies from birth.

If a baby is exposed to varicella postnatally, whether or not treatment is required depends on his immune status. All exposed infants should have their immune status checked using the varicella zoster ELISA test in order to avoid unnecessary treatment with a blood product.[608] If the baby is seronegative, ZIG should be administered, especially if he is less than 32 weeks' gestation or in some other high-risk category. If the baby has antibody, there is no need to give ZIG, unless he is more than 2 months old and still in a NICU.[276]

Zoster infection

Zoster has been reported in the neonate,[119] but the accuracy of the diagnosis must be questioned in the absence of confirmation by culture.[132] In babies who have congenital varicella (p. 1069), zoster may appear shortly after the first month of life, and may also occur in early infancy in babies who develop perinatal varicella.[570] Maternal zoster does not usually affect the baby,[231] although there are occasional reports of fetal damage.

Human herpesviruses type 6 & 7[463]

Human herpesvirus type 6 may be transmitted perinatally[624] but does not cause serious neonatal disease.[339,493]

Enteroviruses[721]

These are small spherical viruses containing a single strand of RNA. There are traditionally three main subgroups – namely, polioviruses, echoviruses and coxsackieviruses – but newly classified enteroviruses are now being numbered outside this classification, e.g. enterovirus 72 is hepatitis A virus.

Most neonatal enterovirus infections are mild and occur after the first week, often coinciding with epidemics in the community. Poliovirus infections are rare in developed countries, and becoming rarer in developing countries, but both echoviruses and coxsackieviruses regularly cause serious neonatal infection.[10] Enterovirus infection in the newborn can be acquired by both vertical and horizontal transmission. Infection due to vertical transmission tends to be more severe[409,410] and earlier in onset.[10] Horizontal spread is mainly via the faecal-oral route, but respiratory secretions may also be infectious.

Table 40.12 Outcome of neonates with varicella. (Reproduced from Hanshaw & Dudgeon[351])

	Total	Survived	Died (%)
Maternal varicella >5 days from delivery, neonatal varicella 0–4 days	27	27	0
Maternal varicella <4 days from delivery, neonatal varicella 5–10 days	23	16	7 (30%)

Echovirus

Many neonatal echovirus infections are asymptomatic, but some antigenic types, e.g. 6, 7, 11, 12, 14 and 17, can cause serious disease. Echovirus 11 has been responsible for the most severe cases[575] but severe nursery outbreaks with echovirus 17 have been reported.[420] Echovirus infection tends to follow one of three patterns.

Mild malaise

This is the commonest pattern. There is fever, malaise and mild gastrointestinal upset lasting for 3 or 4 days, and a full recovery is made. These cases are most often diagnosed during epidemiological surveys of outbreaks of serious disease. Investigation, apart from isolating the virus, is usually negative except for a few atypical mononuclear white cells on the differential white cell count. Recently it has become possible to detect enteroviruses in the serum and urine of infected babies using PCR.[11,722]

Viral meningitis

This is usually mild, and seizures and other major neurological signs are rare.[480] CSF analysis will show features typical of viral meningitis with up to 100–200 WBC/mm^3, mainly lymphocytes, and comparatively normal protein and sugar concentrations. No organisms are seen on Gram stain. The virus will grow from the CSF, and also usually from a throat swab and the stools. Atypical mononuclear cells may be seen on the blood film. Recovery is the rule, although evidence of focal encephalitis is increasingly recognised using modern imaging techniques.[693]

Severe viraemic illness

This is commonly caused by serotypes 6, 7 and 11, and is often acquired vertically. It is a serious infection, usually associated with hepatitis and often with meningoencephalitis, pneumonitis, myocarditis, gastroenteritis and DIC.[575,666] There is often rapid deterioration, with acidaemia, jaundice, apnoea, internal and external haemorrhage, and profound hypotension resistant to volume expansion and inotropic drugs. Renal failure often develops and bone marrow failure has been reported.[796] High mortality rates are reported, although a recent large survey found an overall mortality rate of 31%.[7] The autopsy findings are very characteristic, with massive hepatic necrosis and haemorrhagic necrosis of adrenals, renal tubules and myocardium.

Coxsackievirus

Coxsackievirus infections can be acquired by both vertical and horizontal transmission, but, unlike with the echovirus, the mode of transmission has little effect on the severity of illness. Most neonatal infections are due to type B. The spectrum ranges from a mild febrile illness, with or without diarrhoea, to meningoencephalitis,[575] myocarditis (pp. 643, 645) and a severe viraemic illness similar to that seen with the echoviruses.[851] The non-specific illnesses may progress to the more severe illnesses over several days and sometimes a biphasic illness is seen, with apparent recovery in between a mild illness and a fatal myocarditis.[207] Coxsackievirus infections are often accompanied by a rash, which is sometimes petechial.

Coxsackievirus B myocarditis may present gradually with tachycardia, breathlessness and poor feeding, or acutely with circulatory collapse. There is invariably cardiomegaly, often a murmur, and the ECG shows ST-segment depression and sometimes a supraventricular tachycardia. Viral RNA can be demonstrated in the myocardium using PCR.[372] This illness carries a high mortality rate and is often associated with signs of encephalitis or hepatitis.[437]

Meningoencephalitis usually occurs in small epidemics, and outbreaks due to many group A and B serotypes have been reported. The CSF shows a typical picture of viral meningitis and the virus can be grown from a throat swab, stools or CSF. The infant is rarely severely ill and usually recovers completely within 7–10 days. Neurological sequelae are extremely unusual.

It has recently been suggested that the children of women whose serum contained IgM to coxsackievirus B at delivery are at significantly increased risk of childhood-onset diabetes.[181]

Poliomyelitis

Neonatal polio typically presents with fever, listlessness, poor feeding, diarrhoea and flaccid paralysis of one or more limbs. There is often a CSF pleocytosis, and virus can usually be grown from the stools and CSF. Neonatal polio may occur following contact with an older patient known to have polio, or following birth to a mother who herself develops polio around the time of delivery.

Treatment of enterovirus infections

The only antiviral agent that has been used with apparent success in severe neonatal enteroviral hepatitis/disseminated infection is pleconaril, given enterally at a dose of 5 mg/kg 8-hourly.[26] Injections of pooled IVIG have been advocated to reduce the severity of illness as well as prevent transmission of an epidemic within a NICU,[638] although some studies have shown little benefit once the infection is established.[410] It has been suggested that higher doses of IVIG, or IVIG selected for its high titres of antibody to virulent enterovirus serotypes, may be beneficial.[8] Clinical trials are needed. Successful treatment of fulminant neonatal echovirus 11 infection by means of orthotopic liver transplantation has been recorded.[164]

Measles

Measles in pregnancy is even rarer than varicella. There is a substantial complication rate among pregnant women with measles, with high hospitalisation rates and pneumonia in around a quarter of cases. The measles virus is probably not teratogenic, but measles in pregnancy may lead to high rates of fetal loss and prematurity, mostly occurring within 2 weeks of the appearance of the rash. If the mother has measles around the time of delivery, the baby may be infected transplacentally and either be born with the rash or develop it within the first 10 days of life. Perinatal measles is often a mild illness, but may be severe and complicated by a fatal pneumonitis.[599] The older literature reports a high mortality rate but it is doubtful if this still applies in an era of broad-spectrum antibiotics and neonatal intensive care. The effect of hyperimmune antimeasles globulin in this situation has not been adequately evaluated, but it could be beneficial. There is a putative link between perinatal measles and the subsequent occurrence of Crohn's disease.[226]

Mumps

There is an unresolved controversy over whether congenital mumps infection can cause endocardial fibroelastosis in the neonate. Apart from this, prenatal mumps infection is apparently benign. Neonatal mumps seems to be extremely rare and is a mild disease.

Rubella

With a high level of maternal immunity in the community and a 3-week incubation period, primary rubella is highly unlikely to occur in the neonate, and when it does, it is usually mild.

Neonatal hepatitis

Neonatal hepatitis can be due to congenital, perinatal or postnatal infections. The main congenital causes are rubella (pp. 1064–6), CMV (pp. 1066–7), HSV (pp. 1053–5), toxoplasmosis (pp. 1067–9) and syphilis (pp. 1070–1). Perinatal infections, following intrapartum contact with infected maternal blood or secretions, include HSV (pp. 1053–4), CMV (pp. 1066–7), enteroviruses (pp. 1056–7),[10] varicella (p. 1056), adenovirus,[9] hepatitis A, B and C, and non-A, B or C hepatitis (see below). CMV is the only common postnatal cause of viral hepatitis.

Clinical presentation

Infants with congenital infective hepatitis are usually jaundiced within 24 hours of birth. Of the perinatally acquired causes of hepatitis, only HSV is likely to present within the first week of the neonatal period.[631] Hepatitis A, B and C usually present towards, or beyond, the end of the neonatal period, because of their long incubation times. Acquired CMV usually comes from blood transfusion (p. 481) and often presents in the postneonatal period in VLBW survivors who have had to stay in a neonatal unit for many weeks (p. 1059).

Babies with hepatitis are jaundiced and unwell. They usually have hepatosplenomegaly and often have dark urine and pale stools. A considerable proportion of the total bilirubin is conjugated and the liver enzymes are elevated. The commonest differential diagnosis is from conditions such as the inspissated bile syndrome following haemolytic jaundice, TPN-related cholestasis (p. 686) and α_1-antitrypsin deficiency. The more complex metabolic possibilities and whether or not the infant has biliary atresia are outlined on pages 682–4.

Hepatitis A

Transplacental hepatitis A infection has been reported extremely rarely,[244] and perinatal infection, even if the mother has active hepatitis at delivery, is very unusual.[507] Epidemics of hepatitis A in neonatal units have been reported, some associated with transfusion from an infected donor[495,691] and others with postnatal transmission from mother to baby.[830] No treatment for hepatitis A is available, but it is prudent to give 0.5–1.0 ml of pooled immunoglobulin to all infants delivered to women who have active hepatitis A within 2 weeks of delivery.

Hepatitis B

Epidemiology and vertical transmission

The majority of the 300 million asymptomatic carriers of hepatitis B virus (HBV) live in developing countries. Two-fifths of children with persistent infection who survive to adulthood die as a result of chronic liver disease and carcinoma. The prevalence of hepatitis B surface antigen, HBsAg, the marker for the carrier state of HBV in apparently healthy adults, varies from 0.1% in parts of Europe and North America to between 15% and 20% in parts of West Africa and East Asia. Transplacental passage of HBV is uncommon. Perinatal infection is caused by percutaneous or permucosal exposure to HBV-containing maternal blood, amniotic fluid or vaginal secretions during labour or at birth. Premature rupture of the membranes in a woman with chronic HBV infection probably merits no change in obstetric management.[259]

The risk of infection is high for babies born to carrier mothers in countries with high carrier rates, e.g. Taiwan, where the perinatal transmission rate is about 40%. Ethnic group susceptibility to infection is significant. Chinese HBsAg carrier mothers transmit infection more frequently to their infants than carriers among Africans, Asians or Caucasians in the UK. The presence of 'e' antigen, HBeAg, in the mother's blood greatly increases the risk of infection in the baby. This 'e' antigen is associated with a defective immune response to HBV, which permits continued replication of virus in liver cells.[804] The expression of 'e' antigen appears to be genetically determined. More Chinese women carriers (40%) of HBV are HBeAg-positive than are African carrier mothers (15%). Of children born to Chinese carrier mothers, between 40% and 70% become carriers; to African mothers, about 30%; to Indian mothers, 6–8%; and to European mothers, almost none.

Clinical picture

The majority of infected infants do not develop neonatal jaundice and remain asymptomatic. HBsAg appears in their blood between 6 weeks and 4 months after birth, and usually persists. Most of these infants become chronic carriers of HBV. A small number of infants with hepatitis B develop a fulminant illness and die with massive liver necrosis. The reasons for this are not understood. Although the clinical course for infected infants is usually mild, the long-term prognosis is blighted by their increased risk of chronic liver disease and primary hepatic carcinoma in adulthood. Convincing evidence of an association between HBsAg and hepatoma has emerged from a prospective study of 22 707 Chinese men in Taiwan, 15% of whom were HBsAg positive. Forty of the 41 cases of hepatocellular carcinoma detected in the 5-year study had HBsAg in their blood.[63]

Management and prevention

Once the carrier state has developed, it cannot be terminated by any therapeutic agent currently available. Prevention is therefore extremely important, and regimens based on a combination of active and passive immunisation are most effective.[614,740]

Current recommendations for preventing perinatal transmission of hepatitis B in the UK are shown in Table 40.13. If properly implemented, they are 85–95% effective in preventing perinatal transmission of the virus. The initial dose of vaccine should be given within 12 hours of birth. The hepatitis B vaccines employed are prepared using recombinant DNA technology and the active immunogen is the S-protein component of the HBsAg. Two licensed products are Energix B (SmithKline Beecham) and H-B-VaxII (Pasteur Merieux). These contain different concentrations of antigen, and manufacturer's guidelines should be followed. Immunisation is very effective and serious adverse effects are extremely rare.[503,741,843] Preterm infants develop lower titres of antibody than term infants and it has been suggested that revaccination after about 3 years might be indicated.[453] Further doses of vaccine are given at 1 and 6 months of age and a good deal of effort is required to ensure a complete and effective programme.[474,689] Serological testing should be undertaken at 9 to 15 months of age. Babies in whom immunoglobulin as well as vaccine is indicated should receive 200 IU (one vial) of human hepatitis B immunoglobulin (HBIG) by i.m. injection, within 12 hours of birth if possible.

It is worth noting that a lot of countries, including the USA and many in Western Europe, have followed the 1992 WHO recommendation that universal hepatitis B vaccination be introduced rather than vaccination of designated at-risk groups. Although the current prevalence of hepatitis B in the UK is lower than in countries that have adopted a universal approach, there have been appeals for change.[307]

Breastfeeding should not be discouraged, because transmission of the virus through breast milk or by ingestion of blood from excoriated nipples is negligible compared with the infant's exposure to contaminated maternal blood at delivery. Furthermore, the dangers of not breastfeeding in developing countries outweigh the very small chance of the baby becoming infected exclusively by the breast milk of the carrier mother. If given hepatitis B vaccine at birth, these babies will not even be exposed to this small risk of infection from breast milk.

Hepatitis C

Hepatitis C (HCV) can undoubtedly be transmitted vertically,[793] especially when the mother is coinfected with HIV.[698] In a recent report of 182 HCV-infected children in the UK and Ireland, vertical transmission accounted for 40 cases.[297] Breastfeeding, however, seems relatively safe.[506] This infection can also be acquired from transfusion, but in the UK all blood and blood products are now screened for HCV. Diagnosis is by means of antibody and antigen detection,[211] but cord blood is too often contaminated to be reliable. The incubation period is long and cases are unlikely to present within the neonatal period. The evidence so far is that vertically acquired HCV infection is usually benign,[868] although more follow-up data are needed and a case of aggressive liver disease presenting at 11½ years of age has been reported.[576]

Hepatitis non-A, B or C

Other hepatitis viruses are uncommon in the UK, but vertical transmission of hepatitis E causing serious neonatal hepatitis is well documented in developing countries.[458]

Cytomegalovirus

Serious illness, including hepatitis and pneumonia, is described in babies given CMV-positive blood during exchange transfusion, and following multiple top-up transfusions in VLBW babies. The pneumonitis can cause marked deterioration in lung function, especially among those with CLD.[665] Acquiring CMV may also predispose the VLBW baby to other serious infections. It is important to use only CMV-negative donors for transfusion of VLBW babies, even those of seropositive mothers, or to treat donor blood to remove the lymphocytes, which are the vectors of CMV (pp. 1066–7).

Babies may also acquire CMV from staff or infected babies. Recently, there has been a lot of interest in the transmission of CMV in breast milk,[134,349,749,821] which carries a risk of serious disease in very premature babies. There is as yet no solution to this problem and more research is required. Neonatal CMV is more likely to occur in babies of CMV-seronegative mothers, but also occurs in babies born to seropositive mothers after the titre of maternal antibody has declined postnatally.

Treatment is supportive. The use of high-titre CMV immunoglobulin and drugs such as ganciclovir, which have met with limited success in older immunosuppressed patients, has not been evaluated in neonates. VLBW babies who acquire CMV perinatally may have an increased incidence of handicap on follow-up, though more data are required.[637]

Influenza and parainfluenza viruses

Outbreaks of influenza A virus infection are rare but well described in the literature.[589,707] Respiratory and gastrointestinal symptoms

Table 40.13 Recommended scheme for use of hepatitis B vaccine and HBIG in relation to maternal disease status

	Baby should receive Hepatitis B vaccine	HBIG
Mother is HBsAg positive and HBeAg positive	+	+
Mother is HBsAg positive without e markers (or where they have not been determined)	+	+
Mother had acute hepatitis B during pregnancy	+	+
Mother is HBaAg positive and anti-HBe positive	+	−

Table 40.14 Reported fungal infections in the neonate

Organism	Symptoms	Treatment and comment	References
Alcaligenes xylosoxidans	Meningitis		Boukadida et al 1993 Ped. Inf. Dis. J. 12: 696
Aspergillus fumigatus	Sepsis	None diagnosed in life All fatal	Schwartz et al 1988 Ped. Inf. Dis. J. 7: 349
Aspergillus sp.	Cutaneous Cutaneous/systemic Pulmonary in myeloperoxidase deficiency	Amphotericin and flucytosine	Gupta et al 1996 Ped. Inf. Dis. J. 15: 464 Amod et al 2000 Ped. Inf. Dis. J. 19: 482 Chiang et al 2000 Ped. Inf. Dis. J. 19: 1027
Blastomycosis	Presented as SIDS	Presumed transplacental infection	Watts et al 1983 Ped. Inf. Dis. J. 2: 308
Candida parapsilosis	NICU outbreak of septicaemia		Welbel et al 1996 Ped. Inf. Dis. J. 15: 998
Candida glabrata		Case series	Fairchild et al 2002 Ped. Inf. Dis. J. 21: 39
Coccidioides	Pneumonia Vertically transmitted and nosocomial Congenital	Present in maternal cervical swab. Proved fatal	Bernstein et al 1981 J. Pediatr. 99: 752 Linsangan & Ross 1999 Ped. Inf. Dis. J. 18: 171 Charlton et al 1999 Ped. Inf. Dis. J. 18: 561
Curvularia lunata	Wound infection	Surgical excision	Yau et al 1994 Clin. Infect. Dis. 19: 735
Hansenula anomala	Sepsis, meningitis	Amphotericin and flucytosine Epidemic ceased with oral nystatin and betadine to venepuncture sites	Murphy et al 1986 Lancet i: 291
Malassezia furfur	Facial pustules confused with neonatal acne or miliaria	Ketoconazole cream. Remove lines and stop i.v. fat	Rapelanoro et al 1996 Arch. Dermatol. 132: 190 Powell et al 1984 J. Pediatr. 105: 987 Aschner et al 1987 Pediatrics 80: 535
Malassezia pachydermatis	Sepsis: common skin commensal	Amphotericin. Remove lines stop i.v. fat. Outlook good	Nickelsen et al 1988 J. Inf. Dis. 157: 1163 Larocco et al 1988 Ped. Inf. Dis. J. 7: 398
Pichia anomala			Aragao et al 2001 Ped. Inf. Dis. J. 20: 843
Rhizopus	Disseminated infection in a preterm infant Skin abscess	Surgery and amphotericin, but proved fatal Amphotericin. Resolved	Craig et al 1994 Pediatr. Dermatol. 11: 346 Ng & Dear 1989 Arch. Dis. Child. 64: 862
Torulopsis glabrata	Systemic infection in 2 preterm infants	Amphotericin. Successful outcome	Reich et al 1997 South. Med. J. 90: 246
Trichophyton rubrum	Systemic infection		Singal et al 1996 Pediatr. Dermatol. 13: 488
Trichosporon asahii	Cysto-peritoneal shunt infection Outbreak of systemic infection in a NICU Systemic illness ?NEC and sepsis Septicaemia	Shunt removal and antifungal agents Resistant to amphotericin Amphotericin and flucytosine Amphotericin	Ashpole et al 1991 Br. J. Neurosurg. 5: 515 Fisher et al 1993 Ped. Inf. Dis. J. 12: 149 Giacoia 1992 South. Med. J. 85: 1247 Rowen et al 1995 Pediatrics 95: 682 del Palacio et al 1990 Ped. Inf. Dis. J. 9: 520 Salazar & Campbell 2002 Ped. Inf. Dis. J. 21: 161 Panagopoulou et al 2002 Ped. Inf. Dis. J. 21: 169
Zygomyosis	Disseminated or necrotising cellulitis	Severe forms fatal	Grim et al 1984 Ped. Inf. Dis. J. 3: 61 White et al 1986 Pediatrics 78: 100 Robertson et al 1997

predominate, and low birthweight and mechanical ventilation are risk factors for more severe symptoms. The outlook is almost always favourable, although a fatal case of influenza B infection of the newborn has been described.[813] Parainfluenza virus type 3 can also cause nursery outbreaks of pulmonary infection.[577]

Fungal infections

Newborn infants are susceptible to invasive fungal infection because of their relative immunodeficiency. Particular factors are the 'naïve' state of neonatal T cells, mainly CD45RA type, and reduced T-cell cytotoxicity.[551] The prevalence of systemic candidiasis is increasing among inmates of neonatal units, probably because of increased survival of very immature babies and greater use of broad-spectrum antibiotics such as third-generation cephalosporins.[77,476,539,710] Among babies weighing more than 2500 g, the incidence is about 0.6%,[676] but among VLBW infants, prevalences of 5% and more are reported.[539,711] C. albicans accounts for most neonatal fungal infections, but C. parapsilosis is fast rising in prominence.[476,502] Several other species of fungi have been known to cause neonatal infection from time to time (Table 40.14).

Candida albicans

Cutaneous candidiasis is described on page 821.

Congenital candidiasis

Vaginal candidiasis is common in pregnancy and ascending fetal infection occasionally occurs, especially if an intrauterine contraceptive device is left in situ or a cervical suture is inserted. It is associated with preterm labour.[816] The infection spreads over the external and internal body surface rather than invading the bloodstream, and congenitally infected babies characteristically have skin and mucosal involvement and often a pneumonia.[393,609] Candida species can be cultured from gastric aspirates, superficial lesions and the lung, but rarely from the blood or CSF. Treatment is with amphotericin and flucytosine (see below), but, as with postnatally acquired systemic candidiasis, the mortality is high. C. albicans amnionitis has been successfully treated by amnioinfusion with amphotericin.[745]

Acquired systemic candidiasis[604]

This is an increasing problem in VLBW survivors of neonatal intensive care. The majority have been colonised by C. albicans from birth,[50] although around 15% acquire the organism nosocomially. As risk factors such as the presence of central lines,[711] ventriculoperitoneal shunts,[160] tracheal tubes[695] and extensive antibiotic use accumulate, the probability of invasive infection grows.[539] The use of i.v. hydrocortisone for the treatment of hypotension soon after birth may predispose to systemic candidiasis.[107]

Disseminated candidiasis presents like bacterial sepsis, and the spectrum of illness includes pneumonia, septicaemia with or without endocarditis, septic arthritis, osteomyelitis, endophthalmitis, intraperitoneal infection, liver abscesses, meningitis and renal tract infection. Preceding mucocutaneous candidiasis is common[107] and skin lesions are almost universal. Baley & Silverman[52] described mucocutaneous candidiasis in about half their cases of systemic disease, and the other half had a characteristic bright, erythematous, macular patchy dermatitis, usually on the trunk, often presenting within the first 72 hours. Localised cutaneous abscesses may also occur.

Neonatal sepsis caused by other Candida species, such as C. parapsilosis[227,762] and C. lusitaniae, presents a clinical picture indistinguishable from that caused by C. albicans. The profile of Candida species causing candidaemia in a NICU is illustrated in Fig. 40.19.[476] Recently there have been reports of invasive fungal dermatitis occurring during the first week or so of life in very immature infants,[694] and, as larger numbers of such babies are now surviving, this is something to watch out for.

Investigation

It is harder to diagnose fungal infection than bacterial infection, because positive blood cultures are less common. Even when the organisms are in the blood, it takes several days longer for cultures to become positive than is the case with most bacteria. In one study, the average time between the onset of symptoms and the initiation of antifungal therapy was 11 days.[51] When there is no typical mucocutaneous rash or some other clue to suggest fungal infection, the diagnosis is usually made during the routine investigation of an infant with suspected sepsis. In addition to culturing blood, urine and CSF where indicated, endotracheal tube aspirate and tubes removed from the baby, including chest drains and intravascular cannulae, can be examined microscopically for budding yeasts or fungal hyphae. A useful additional test is to examine a buffy-coat smear for the characteristic intracellular inclusions. Thrombocytopenia is common and should raise the level of suspicion. Serological tests to demonstrate the presence of both candida antigen and antibody have been developed, but have not as yet shown sufficient sensitivity or specificity to be of much use. Acute-phase proteins are usually very elevated in systemic candida infection.

In all cases of suspected or proven candidiasis, the following investigations should be undertaken. The renal tract should be examined with ultrasound to look for evidence of fungal and cellular debris, which may cause obstruction. If there is, or has recently been, a central line in situ, echocardiography should be performed to look for evidence of fungal endocarditis.[559] The CSF should be examined and ophthalmological examination should be performed to look for endophthalmitis. In the case of NICU outbreaks of candida infection, DNA fingerprinting may help to understand the mechanism of spread.[86]

Prevention

Limiting exposure to broad-spectrum antibiotics is important, and is anyhow sound practice. The early introduction of enteral feeding allows risk factors such as central lines and i.v. fat emulsions to be dispensed with. Attempts to prevent systemic candida infection by oral prophylaxis with antifungals have generally not been successful, although one report suggests some benefit in controlling an outbreak of infection.[182] Fluconazole given i.v. as

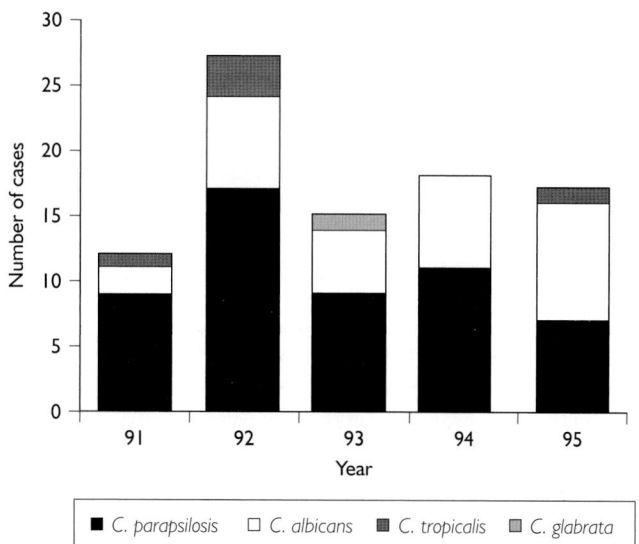

Fig. 40.19 Candida species causing candidaemia in the NICU from 1991 to 1995. (From Kossoff et al.[476])

prophylaxis has been shown to reduce the risk of invasive fungal infection quite dramatically in ELBW babies.[444]

Treatment

Immediately the diagnosis has been made, or even when there is a high level of suspicion in a sick infant, treatment with i.v. amphotericin B should be started. Because of the toxicity of amphotericin, it is probably preferable to use the liposomal form of the drug, ambisome.[723] Flucytosine acts synergistically with amphotericin, and many authorities advocate their combined use in the initial treatment of fungal infection in the newborn. Flucytosine may depress the marrow and damage the liver, so plasma levels should be monitored and weekly blood counts checked.

Fluconazole is being used increasingly and seems both safe and effective.[206,397,823] Fluconazole has good urinary tract penetration, including tubular excretion, and is recommended for treatment of renal candidiasis[374] and for fungal infection resistant to conventional treatment.[251,685] It is useful to remember that cultures often remain positive for more than 24 hours after effective therapy is begun, even in the absence of focal complications.[155] Intrathecal treatment is not usually required for candidal meningitis, as amphotericin has good CSF penetration. Several newer antifungal agents are undergoing evaluation.[836] Central vascular catheters should be removed if systemic candidiasis is diagnosed or strongly suspected.[706,715] Fungal material in the renal tract, demonstrated by ultrasound, usually disappears with medical treatment, although surgery is sometimes required.

Malsezzia species seem to be lipid dependent, and only occur if Intralipid is being given. Although amphotericin has been used in such patients, most cases resolve if the catheter is withdrawn and i.v. fat discontinued.

Prognosis

The reported mortality rate associated with systemic candidiasis in the newborn period ranges from 20% to 50%.[51,245] A significant proportion of cases are first diagnosed at postmortem. Adverse neurological outcome among ELBW babies with systemic candidiasis is about three times greater than among control infants.[278] The prognosis for candidal meningitis is very bleak.

Other neonatal fungal infections

Data on other fungi that have become opportunistic pathogens in ill VLBW babies are summarised in Table 40.14.

Parasitic infections

Pneumocystis carinii

Cases of *Pneumocystis carinii* pneumonia (PCP) were common, mainly in premature babies, in postwar Europe.[280] They usually presented just outside the neonatal period with progressive dyspnoea and increasing oxygen requirements, and, with symptomatic treatment, the mortality rate was around 50%. *Pneumocystis carinii* infection in the developed world now occurs almost exclusively among babies with an underlying immunodeficiency state,[386] often in combination with CMV infection. Prenatal or perinatal transmission of HIV infection has not been reported to cause *Pneumocystis carinii* infection in the neonate (p. 1002). The presentation is usually insidious, with progressive respiratory distress and a diffusely hazy CXR. The diagnosis requires a high level of clinical suspicion and acumen, and may be confirmed by direct microscopy of bronchial lavage material, although lung biopsy is much more likely to be successful. A PCR-based test is now a possibility.[756] Treatment is with high-dose co-trimoxazole or, if this is not successful, with pentamidine.

Trichomonas vaginalis

This protozoon has occasionally been reported to cause vaginitis and UTI in the neonate.[183] Case reports suggest that rarely it might cause pneumonia. If the organism is found on direct microscopy of a tracheal aspirate, or is isolated from any other infected site, treatment with metronidazole should be started.

Malaria

Pregnancy is associated with an increased susceptibility to malaria and with more severe infection. Primigravidae in Africa and Papua New Guinea have a peak prevalence of parasitaemia between 9 and 16 weeks of pregnancy. Parasitaemia and parasite density are higher in primigravidae than in multigravidae, and both decline progressively with parity. Involvement of the placental tissue is common, but fetal infection is relatively uncommon in endemic areas where there are high rates of maternal immunity. The risk of fetal infection increases with both the density of maternal parasitaemia and the severity of involvement of the placenta.[680] Simultaneous maternal HIV infection also increases the risk of fetal infection.[775]

Congenital malaria

In endemic areas it is difficult to distinguish congenital malaria from malaria acquired soon after birth, because the lifecycle of the protozoon means that symptoms from congenital malaria may be delayed for weeks or even months. However, a recent study in Nigeria estimated that 75% of neonatal malaria was of congenital origin.[401] Infection may occur with *Plasmodium falciparum*, *P. vivax* and *P. malariae*, and there is no evidence that one of these organisms is more likely to cause a congenital infection than any of the others. Congenital malaria is much more likely to occur when the mother has a clinical attack of malaria during pregnancy than when she has a chronic subclinical infection. This is mainly due to protection from maternally derived IgG antibody, which may protect the fetus even when there is major placental invasion.

Malarial parasites find it harder to thrive in erythrocytes containing fetal haemoglobin. This may explain the high gene frequencies of the thalassaemias and sickle cell anaemias in malaria-endemic areas.

The prevalence of malaria in pregnancy has recently been reported as 63% in Zambia in the rainy season[490] and 21% in Zaire,[619] despite some use of prophylaxis (see below) in both countries. The overall incidence of fetal parasitaemia in Zambia was 29%, and in Zaire 9%. A recent study in southwestern Nigeria reported a 23.7% prevalence of parasitaemia among newborn infants.[20]

Congenital malaria usually presents between 10 and 26 days of age, with the same symptoms as the acquired disease, namely, fever, jaundice, severe anaemia and massive splenomegaly.[514] Non-specific findings include poor feeding and failure to thrive, loose stools and diarrhoea. In the tropics, many infants with congenital malaria also suffer from other infections such as septicaemia and pneumonia.

An exclusive breast-milk diet has been shown to suppress malarial infection in infants and experimental animals by depriving the parasite of para-aminobenzoic acid, which is required for its growth in the erythrocyte.

Treatment

Chloroquine is the drug of choice in the treatment of congenital malaria, particularly in regions of stable malaria. Quinine is preferred for treatment in regions of chloroquine-resistant *P. falciparum* malaria, such as in Papua New Guinea, East Africa, and some areas of Central and West Africa, and in most regions of unstable (epidemic) malaria, but care is needed as cardiac arrythmias (prolonged QT interval and T-wave flattening), hypotension and hypoglycaemia may follow rapid i.v. infusion.

Chloroquine will eliminate sensitive strains of *P. falciparum*, *P. vivax*, *P. malariae* and *P. ovale*, but it will not prevent relapses of *P. vivax* and *P. ovale* infection. To ensure eradication of the exoerythrocytic forms of *P. vivax* and *P. ovale*, a 14-day course of primaquine is given following the chloroquine. Primaquine should not be administered to infants with G6PD deficiency, because of the danger of haemolysis.

Babies who require blood transfusions or exchange transfusion in malaria-endemic areas might be at risk of transfusion-acquired malaria. It is recommended that these infants receive a curative course of chloroquine following their transfusion. In areas now known to have chloroquine-resistant malaria, the treatment described above should be prescribed.

Trypanosomiasis

Trypanosomes are protozoa and produce two distinct diseases in man. African sleeping sickness is caused by *Trypanosoma (brucei) gambiense* and *T. (brucei) rhodesiense* and is transmitted by *Glossina* (tsetse) flies. Chagas' disease, found in Latin America, is caused by *T. cruzi* and transmitted by large Triatomidae bugs.

African trypanosomiasis

Trypanosomiasis during pregnancy often leads to abortion, hydramnios and preterm delivery. Congenital African trypanosomiasis has been reported with both *T. gambiense* and *T. rhodesiense*, although most cases involve *T. gambiense*. Fever and anaemia, with trypanosomes in the blood and/or CSF of the infant in the first weeks of life, is the usual presentation of congenital infection. In congenital infection in endemic areas, trypanosomes are found in the CSF by the end of the first week even before they are detected in the blood. Increased rouleau formation in the blood should raise the suspicion of trypanosomiasis. IgM is usually high in the blood and low in the CSF during the neonatal period in infected infants. Lymphadenopathy is not a feature of the congenital disease, although it is characteristic of infection acquired after birth.

Management

Treatment is hazardous because highly toxic drugs such as suramin, an organic urea, and melarsoprol, an arsenical compound, have to be used.

Congenital Chagas' disease

Chagas' disease is a major public health problem in South and Central America, where more than 65 million people living in rural areas are exposed to infection by *T. cruzi*. The frequency of congenital Chagas' disease is higher than suggested by the number of cases reported. Studies in Chile, Argentina and Brazil have shown that between 0.5% and 2% of LBW infants have congenital Chagas' disease.[334]

T. cruzi enters the fetal circulation through the placental trophoblast in acute, latent or chronic maternal disease. In most cases of transplacental infection the mother is asymptomatic. The diseased placenta is large, and in cases in which the fetus is hydropic it is indistinguishable from the placentitis of syphilis or toxoplasmosis. Abortions occur when the placenta is massively diseased. Congenital Chagas' disease has been observed to recur in subsequent pregnancies.

Most newborn infants with Chagas' disease are of low birthweight and may be either preterm or small for dates (SFD). Clinical manifestations of congenital infection may be obvious at birth or occur after a few months. Anaemia, jaundice, oedema, petechiae, hepatosplenomegaly, tremor and convulsions are common features. Anaemia may be so severe as to require blood transfusion. Dysphagia, with inflammatory infiltration of the oesophagus and absence of nerve cells of the myenteric plexus, interferes with feeding and has been described in a few cases. Prognosis of congenital infection depends upon the intensity of parasitaemia. Several organs, including the heart, oesophagus, brain, skin and skeletal muscle, show pathological changes, with inflammation, giant cells (a distinctive feature) and granulomas. Parasites have been found either in the muscle fibres or in the reticuloendothelial system. Long-term follow-up has shown a high frequency of neurological sequelae, such as mental retardation or behavioural and learning disabilities.

Diagnosis

Diagnosis of congenital Chagas' disease in the newborn is made on the presence of *T. cruzi* amastigotes in the blood using a fresh thin blood smear or a thick drop preparation. An indirect immunofluorescence reaction detects IgM of fetal origin specific for *T. cruzi*. High levels of fetal IgM and IgA have been observed on the first and 15th days after birth. A direct agglutination test using sera treated with 2-mercaptoethanol has also been introduced as a simple method of diagnosing congenital Chagas' disease. Recently, ELISA has been used with success.[613]

Management

No satisfactory treatment for Chagas' disease is currently available. Symptomatic treatment for heart failure may give temporary relief, but the prognosis remains gloomy because *T. cruzi* invades many organs and there is no satisfactory drug to eradicate it. Nifurtimox, a nitrofuran derivative, has been used in the acute phase of the disease, with the elimination of parasitaemia and remission of clinical symptoms, but it is very toxic.

Amoebiasis

Entamoeba histolytica, a unicellular protozoal parasite, has a global distribution and frequently causes intestinal disease in warm climates in communities with poor sanitation. Pregnant women may transmit the parasite to their newborn infants through faecal contamination at birth. The infant will usually present with bloody diarrhoea within a few days of birth.[683] Amoebic proctocolitis and liver abscess have been reported. Treatment is with metronidazole.

Strongyloides

A syndrome of respiratory distress, generalised pitting oedema and abdominal distension with ascites has been described in young infants from the age of 2 weeks in the Gulf Province of Papua New Guinea. Other prominent features of this syndrome include severe hypoproteinaemia with low serum albumin and heavy infestation of the stool with a *Strongyloides* species similar to *S. fulleborni*. The infection responds readily to thiabendazole.

Congenital infections

Congenital rubella

The incidence of congenital rubella is now less than 2 cases per 100 000 births in countries with high rates of immunisation, and a recent report from Western Australia reported an incidence of less than 2 cases per 10 000 births.[170] In Britain, 20–30 cases per annum were being notified to the Congenital Rubella Surveillance Programme in the mid-1980s. This had approximately halved by the mid-1990s;[571] a majority of the mothers of affected babies were from the immigrant population.[752]

Pathogenesis

The embryo or fetus becomes infected with rubella virus transplacentally during maternal viraemia. The placenta often sustains cellular and tissue damage in the process, and this may result in abortion, stillbirth or impaired fetal nutrition and oxygenation. In the embryo, the virus can cause widespread tissue injury and, despite evoking a vigorous antibody response, persists in the tissues until delivery and for some time thereafter. The timing of maternal infection has a major influence on outcome. When it occurs in the first 12–16 weeks of pregnancy, even within days of conception, there is virtually always embryonal or

Table 40.15 Rubella-associated defects following maternal rubella (without laboratory confirmation) by time of infection. (Reproduced from Munro et al[590])

| Gestational week | 1–2 | 3–4 | 5–6 | 7–8 | 9–10 | 11–12 | 13–14 | 15–16 | 17–18 | 19–20 | >20 | Total | % |
Number of cases	4	27	30	60	44	45	40	20	15	8	23	316	
Heart defects	–	15	13	22	6	4	2	1	1	1	1	66	21
CNS defects	3	12	13	15	11	8	5	4	2	1	3	77	24
Eye defects	2	18	20	26	15	5	6	3	1	–	1	97	31
Deafness	2	21	22	48	38	35	31	16	9	5	6	233	74
No defects	–	1	1	5	2	9	6	3	5	3	16	51	16

fetal infection. By the end of the second trimester, only a third of infected women transfer infection to their fetus. The risk of rubella-induced congenital abnormality also falls with advancing gestation. Malformations occur in 90% of infected infants whose mothers are infected in the first 2 months of pregnancy, but in only 50% of those infected in the third month and 20% of those infected in the fourth and fifth months. Congenital rubella is rare after 20 weeks of gestation because of maturation of fetal immune mechanisms. The type of defect caused by congenital infection at different stages of pregnancy is shown in Table 40.15.

Secondary infection with rubella in pregnancy

The risk of reinfection with rubella after the natural illness is around 5%, but after immunisation may be as high as 50%, as judged by serology.[385] The risk of fetal damage from reinfection is less than 5%.[138] There are, though, well-documented instances of fetal damage following secondary rubella infection in pregnancy.[447]

Clinical features (Fig. 40.20)[232]

The extended rubella syndrome presents as a sick baby with jaundice, petechiae and hepatosplenomegaly. On detailed examination, eye and bone abnormalities may be found and a murmur heard. About one-third of affected babies are below the third centile for birthweight. A long-term follow-up of cases from the 1963–1965 epidemic reported ocular disease in 78%, sensorineural hearing loss in 66%, psychomotor retardation in 62%, cardiac abnormalities in 58% and mental retardation in 42%.[301]

Eye defects

Cataracts may be detected at birth and may affect the whole of the lens or be central. Glaucoma also occurs, and requires urgent treatment (pp. 839–40). Microphthalmia is common. A fine pigmentary retinopathy (pepper-and-salt retinopathy) may be seen.

Deafness

This is usually sensorineural and bilateral. It is caused by inflammatory changes within the cochlea or the organ of Corti and, as its incidence increases throughout childhood, damage to these tissues is progressive. All babies suspected of congenital rubella should have auditory evoked responses checked as soon after delivery as possible.[842]

Central nervous system

Microcephaly, delayed motor development, various types of cerebral palsy and mental retardation, which in some cases can be profound, are common in isolation or in combination.

Cardiovascular

Viral damage to the endothelium of large blood vessels results in a high incidence of patent ductus arteriosus and peripheral pulmonary artery stenosis.

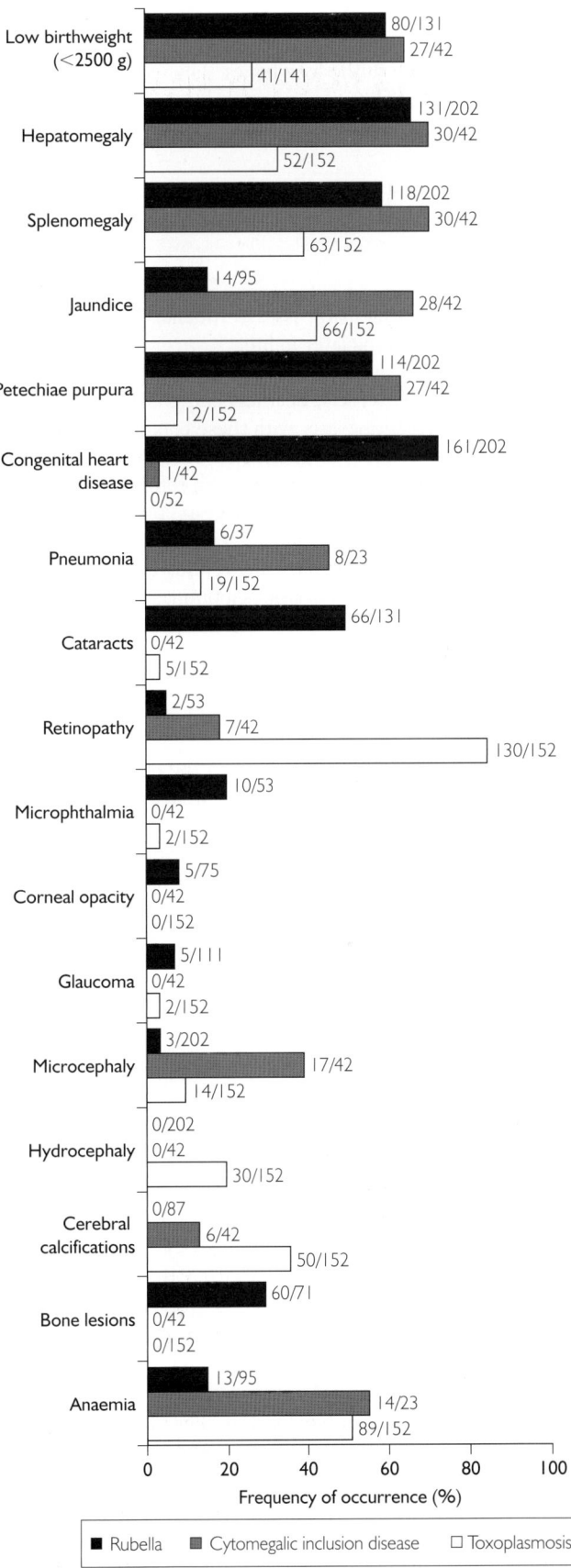

Fig. 40.20 Manifestations of symptomatic congenital rubella, CMV and toxoplasmosis. (Reproduced from Overall & Glasgow.[632])

Bone

In rubella osteitis there are irregular translucencies and an irregular trabecular pattern in the long bones. The radiological appearance is of a 'celery stick'.

Liver

Hepatitis causing prolonged jaundice is common in the extended rubella syndrome (pp. 1064–5).

Thrombocytopenia

This is found in most neonatal cases of rubella, though it is rarely found in cases presenting later in life.

Affected infants may present outside the neonatal period with neurological and eye defects, deafness and congenital heart disease. In infants presenting later with these conditions, it may not be possible to establish the diagnosis of congenital rubella by antibody studies, but culturing the virus from, for example, the lens at a cataract operation, strongly suggests prenatal infection. Infants presenting in the neonatal period, and those with a delayed presentation, may in later life develop a rubelliform rash, interstitial pneumonitis, hypogammaglobulinaemia, reduced cellular immunity, thyroid autoantibodies, thymic hypoplasia and diabetes mellitus.

Diagnosis

Congenital rubella is differentiated from the other organisms in Fig. 40.20 by culturing the virus from a throat swab or urine, and by demonstrating rubella-specific IgM in plasma. There is no value in screening otherwise normal SFD babies for congenital rubella.[537] Whenever the diagnosis is established in Britain, the baby must be notified to the Congenital Rubella Surveillance Programme.

Treatment

No specific treatment is available. Some babies with the extended rubella syndrome are quite ill and need intensive care. Platelet transfusion is often required, as is phototherapy or exchange transfusion. Cataracts and glaucoma must be treated early, and hearing aids fitted if there is any evidence of deafness.

The infants are highly infectious during the first few months of life and are a hazard to female members of the nursing and medical staff. Appropriate precautions should be taken, the most important of which is to ensure that these personnel are rubella immune.

Prevention

In Britain in 1988, the immunisation policy was changed from one in which only schoolgirls were given monovalent rubella vaccine, to one of giving children of both sexes the rubella vaccine as part of the MMR vaccine. Such a policy has virtually eliminated rubella in the USA. However, because of the risk to the fetus from secondary infection, pregnant women should avoid people with rubella. Immunisation during pregnancy is also best avoided, although there is no convincing evidence that it is teratogenic.

Any woman who has a rubella contact or who develops a febrile, exanthematous illness in the first few months of pregnancy should have rubella serology checked as soon as possible, and again 2–3 weeks later. If both rubella IgM and IgG are present in the first sample, recent infection is very likely and termination of pregnancy should be offered. If there is a rising titre between the two samples, the same applies. If the IgG level shows no rise and the IgM level is low, the diagnosis of recent infection remains in doubt and decision-making should reflect this uncertainty. Rubella RNA may be detected by PCR on tissue obtained by chorionic villus sampling early in the second trimester if further confirmation of fetal infection is required, although there is still limited experience with this technique.[809] The measurement of IgM in fetal cord blood has been described.[398]

Congenital cytomegalovirus

Epidemiology and incidence

CMV is the commonest cause of congenital infection, affecting 1–2% of infants worldwide, and probably the commonest cause of infection-related congenital abnormality.[47] The annual cost of treating the complications of congenital CMV in the USA has been put at $2 billion.[184] There are large international differences in incidence, and the estimated frequency in the UK is 0.3–0.4%. In the UK, just over half of all women presenting at antenatal clinics are seropositive for CMV.[799]

Transmission

Unlike rubella and toxoplasmosis, congenital acquisition of CMV occurs as a consequence of both recurrent and primary infection. The risk of transplacental transmission during reactivated infection is around 2%[857] (as opposed to as high as 25% during primary infection), but the high incidence of CMV seropositivity among pregnant women worldwide means that transplacental transmission during reactivated infection accounts for a high proportion of all congenitally acquired CMV infection. It has been estimated that 30–50% of congenital infections are due to reactivation of maternal virus, and there are well-documented cases of women having two affected infants.[611,737]

Of pregnant women who develop a primary infection, 10–25% will transmit the virus to the fetus, as assessed by the presence of CMV-specific IgM in cord blood, or positive cultures from throat swab or urine.[256] Women who fail to produce adequate amounts of CMV-neutralising antibody are more likely to transmit the virus transplacentally.[99] Other factors increasing the risk of transmission include maternal age less than 20 years, a weak response to CMV antigen in the lymphocyte transformation test, and the presence of CMV in the urine.[256,269]

Primary infection is much more likely to cause symptomatic congenital CMV and long-term sequelae than reactivation of infection.[270] In one study of 125 infants acquiring CMV as a result of primary maternal infection, 18% were symptomatic at birth and 25% had long-term sequelae.[270] Primary infection may also increase the risk of abortion, stillbirth and fetal hydrops.

Congenital acquisition of the virus during reactivated maternal infection is much less likely to lead to problems, although occasional fatalities are reported.[661] In one study,[270] none of 64 infants acquiring congenital CMV as a result of reactivated maternal infection was symptomatic at birth, and only 8% developed later sequelae. Women from poor socioeconomic backgrounds, who have a high incidence of seropositivity to CMV, are, therefore, less likely to have babies with serious congenital CMV infection. Women with AIDS may be more likely to transmit CMV to the fetus during a reactivation of infection.[737]

The observation that symptomatic congenital CMV is associated with lower maternal IgM levels at term than is asymptomatic infection suggests that early congenital infection is more likely to cause symptomatic disease.[101] Surprisingly, only one member of a twin pair may be severely affected, and there is even a report of variable outcome among infected quads.[728] An emerging mechanism of congenital CMV infection is that seen in the offspring of liver transplant patients.[487]

Clinical signs

Over 90% of infants with congenital CMV (culture and IgM positive) are asymptomatic in the neonatal period, though of slightly reduced birthweight. In the minority who are symptomatic, severe multisystem disease may be present which is clinically similar to congenital rubella or toxoplasmosis (Fig. 40.20). CMV hepatitis can lead to intrahepatic and extrahepatic bile duct destruction[356] as well as haemochromatosis. Oesophagitis is described.[40,833] CMV infection of the fetal brain causes microcephaly, with calcification in periventricular areas where the infection has caused brain necrosis. These lesions are clearly seen on ultrasound scanning. The pattern of CNS damage probably varies with the timing of injury, so that lissencephaly is a feature of early injury, and polymicrogyria of slightly later injury. When the gyral pattern is normal, the injury has probably occurred in the third trimester of pregnancy.[59] Hydrocephalus has been reported.[273] Eye involvement, with chorioretinitis, cataract and blindness, occurs in 10–20% of cases presenting in the neonatal period. Pneumonitis may develop in the first few months after birth, even in infants who were initially asymptomatic. There is a case report of aortic arch thrombosis secondary to CMV infection.[489]

Diagnosis

Fetal infection can be confirmed by cordocentesis or amniocentesis (fetal urine) in the mid-second trimester. In the absence of screening, most cases of congenital CMV will go unrecognised. Screening on saliva has been reported.[48] If the baby develops the severe form of the disease with jaundice and purpura, the diagnosis is best confirmed by rapid culture methods, staining for the presence of immediate-early nuclear CMV protein after 24 or 48 hours incubation, antigen assay to detect the CMV pp65 protein, or DNA detection by PCR or DNA hybrid capture.[864] Antibody tests are generally less accurate and more difficult to interpret in certain situations There is no need to screen asymptomatic SFD babies for congenital CMV.[537]

Treatment

CMV-infected infants excrete the virus for months or years, and should be segregated from potentially pregnant female members of staff. Whether there is a place for using anti-CMV chemotherapy in the neonatal period remains uncertain,[861] although there are some encouraging case reports on the use of ganciclovir.[279] One recent report showed benefit from a regimen of ganciclovir 7.5 mg/kg twice daily for 2 weeks followed by 10 mg/kg three times weekly for 3 months.[612]

Prognosis

Most infants with congenital CMV who are asymptomatic in the neonatal period develop normally and have a normal IQ,[416] and this includes the majority of cases caused by reactivation of maternal infection. About 10% of asymptomatic infants become deaf later in life, and constitute a major group of children with congenital deafness.[58] A small percentage may have other neurological defects, but this seems to be very rare except in those who are deaf.

The mortality from symptomatic neonatal CMV infection is between 10%[102] and 30%,[428] although much higher if the baby is premature.[647] Of those without signs of CNS involvement in the neonatal period, 30% will have neurological sequelae. If there is evidence of neurological involvement, including evidence of chorioretinitis, some 75% will have permanent neurological disability. Intracerebral calcification shown by CT imaging is associated with a bad neurological outcome, as are pseudocysts seen on ultrasound.[100] The duration of urinary CMV excretion has no bearing on the likelihood of adverse long-term cognitive outcome but shorter durations of urinary excretion may be associated with a greater risk of sensoineural hearing loss.[616]

Prevention

There is no successful CMV vaccine but there is a need to develop one,[659] as reactivation of CMV in immune women rarely causes sequelae in the baby (see above). If primary CMV infection is suspected in pregnancy, prenatal diagnosis may be attempted by examination of amniotic fluid, fetal blood or chorionic tissue for specific IgM and the presence of the virus, by culture or PCR.[201] As yet, though, the diagnostic accuracy of available tests is relatively poor in early pregnancy.[202]

Congenital toxoplasmosis

Toxoplasmosis is caused by the intracellular coccidian protozoan parasite *Toxoplasma gondii*. The definitive host, in which the organism completes its sexual cycle, is the cat. Toxoplasma organisms exist in three forms: the oocyst, which is excreted by the million in cat faeces; the tachyzoite, which is the active form and can migrate in tissues; and the cyst, which is a dormant form. There are three main genotypes of *Toxoplasma gondii* and most human disease is caused by type II.[19]

Incidence

In North America, Scandinavia and the UK, the number of women developing toxoplasmosis during pregnancy is in the range 1–6 per 1000. If only 5–10% of the babies of infected women develop symptomatic disease (see below) the incidence of significant congenital infection would be about 1:10 000, which was the incidence reported in Britain by Hall.[341] There are large differences in the prevalence of congenital toxoplasmosis between different racial and cultural groups.[422] The risk may be increased in infants of HIV-positive mothers, who are themselves at risk from toxoplasmosis, but there is controversy concerning this.[213]

Pathogenesis

Humans become infected either by direct contamination from infected cats or their excreta, or as a result of toxoplasma entering the human food chain through the intermediate host of the domestic farm animal. If meat is not adequately cooked, toxoplasma cysts are not destroyed and the organism is liberated during digestion. Contaminated vegetables used in salads are another important source. The world's largest reported outbreak of toxoplasmosis was in Canada in 1995, as a result of water contamination.[587]

Infected adults may remain asymptomatic or develop an influenza or glandular fever type of illness. Infection can reach the fetus at any stage of gestation, but whereas the risk of transplacental infection is greatest during the third trimester, first- and second-trimester infection is more likely to damage the fetus (Table 40.16). Fetal infection occurs almost exclusively during primary maternal infection but the odd case of infection from an immune mother is described.[366] During primary infection in pregnancy, the overall risk of fetal infection is about 25%.[827] However, the proportion of pregnant women who are seropositive for toxoplasmosis varies widely between populations, and is the major influence on the incidence of the congenital form of the disease. In the UK, about 30% of women are seropositive, and congenital infection occurs in fewer than 1 per 1000 infants. Of those fetuses infected, approximately 25% have subclinical disease affecting only the eyes, and only 5–10% develop widespread infection.[180,378]

Clinical features

The classic tetrad of congenital toxoplasmosis is hydrocephalus, epilepsy, cerebral calcification and chorioretinitis. Congenital toxoplasmosis may also involve the reticuloendothelial system, liver, lungs and muscles, including the myocardium (Fig. 40.20). CNS infection causes extensive cortical and periventricular necrosis. This necrotic tissue may become calcified, and can then be seen as diffuse intrahemispheric calcification on ultrasound. Periventricular damage around the aqueduct of the midbrain may obstruct CSF flow and lead to congenital hydrocephalus. Patchy myelitis with ascending paralysis has been reported.[21]

About a third of congenitally infected infants, i.e. around 5–10% of all babies born to mothers infected during pregnancy (Table 40.16), have neonatal symptoms and about 25% of these die as a result. These babies are often small for dates and can present with the classic tetrad. Hydrocephalus may obstruct delivery or be noted at birth. Eye abnormalities may occur, including microphthalmia and cataract. Congenital toxoplasmosis can also present with the typical congenital infection syndrome of jaundice, hepatosplenomegaly and petechiae (Fig. 40.20).

Diagnosis[111]

Diagnosing subclinical congenital toxoplasmosis is very important in order that treatment can be given early. Diagnosis is mainly by antibody assay, although, for reasons that are not fully understood, tests for toxoplasma-specific IgM are initially negative in some 25% of infected infants.[641] If there is doubt about the serological diagnosis, a repeat test can be performed 4 weeks later. Other approaches to distinguishing between active and passive antibody include measurement of IgG avidity[380] and measurement of specific IgE[852] and specific IgA.[85] CSF analysis may show a lymphocytosis, raised protein and tachizoites in centrifuged CSF. Positive serological or PCR tests for toxoplasmosis on CSF confirm the diagnosis. A test based on CD25 expression after incubation with soluble *T. gondii* antigen looks promising.[432] The pattern of intracerebral calcification is very specific for toxoplasmosis, and is different from the periventricular calcification seen with congenital CMV. Ophthalmological examination can be strongly suggestive.

Treatment

Unlike rubella and CMV, toxoplasmosis is a potentially treatable condition. If infection is diagnosed in pregnancy, the woman should be treated with spiramycin to reduce the risk of fetal infection. The diagnosis of fetal infection can be established by PCR for toxoplasma DNA in amniotic fluid[377] at 20 weeks' gestation. If the diagnosis is confirmed at that stage, termination of

Table 40.16 Incidence of congenital toxoplasmosis by gestational age at maternal infection. (Reproduced from Remington & Desmonts[682])

	Trimester of infection		
	1	**2**	**3**
Total women infected	126	246	128
SB or NND	6	5	0
Congenital toxoplasmosis			
Severe	7	6	0
Mild	1	13	8
Subclinical	3	49	68
No congenital infection	109 (86%)	173 (71%)	52 (41%)

Severe = overt clinical disease in neonatal period or subsequently.
Mild = no clinical sequelae except chorioretinitis, IQ normal.
Subclinical = serological evidence of infection only.
These data may underestimate the incidence since about two-thirds of these women were treated during pregnancy.

the pregnancy should be considered, although if antiparasitic therapy is given and serial fetal ultrasound scans are normal, this may not be necessary.[83,555] Fetal infection occurring after the first trimester can be treated with pyrimethamine and sulfadiazine, but these drugs are contraindicated in the first trimester.

Whether or not there are clinical signs, the congenitally infected baby should be given spiramycin (100 mg/kg/day) for 4–6 weeks, alternating with 3 weeks of pyrimethamine (1 mg/kg/day) plus sulfadiazine (50 mg/kg/day). The drugs in this regimen are synergistic against toxoplasma and should be continued for 1 year.[460] Serological rebounds are common after stopping treatment but are not currently considered to be a reason to restart treatment.[198] Worryingly, sulfonamide resistance has been recently reported,[35] but several novel and less toxic drugs are under evaluation.[293]

Prognosis

For seropositive infants with no intracranial calcification and, at most, chorioretinitis in the neonatal period (subclinical and mild cases in Table 40.16), the long-term prognosis is relatively good, although new areas of chorioretinitis may appear in untreated patients until early adult life. For those with neurological features or systemic disease, the outlook without treatment is bleak. About a quarter die and most of the survivors are handicapped. With treatment as outlined above, the outlook may be improved,[687] but there has been no controlled trial.

Prevention

Antenatal diagnosis can be achieved by regular serological testing of pregnant women. If this is combined with PCR to confirm fetal infection in mothers who seroconvert, antenatal treatment of the mother can be given or the pregnancy can be terminated (see above). In these ways, Daffos et al[180] suggest that symptomatic congenital toxoplasmosis can be eliminated. Whether or not antenatal screening is justifiable in the UK is debatable,[643] but it is not currently recommended. The other purpose of screening would be to educate those at risk about avoidance measures. Women who have high-avidity specific IgG during the first trimester are most unlikely to have a primary infection and their fetuses are at low risk.

Screening of newborn infants has been evaluated in both New England and Denmark, and there is no doubt that it can identify infected babies without overt clinical signs.[218,330] Infected infants were treated and appeared to have a better long-term outcome than expected, but there were no untreated controls, for obvious reasons.

Congenital varicella

Ninety-five per cent of women of childbearing age in the UK have had varicella in childhood and are immune. Varicella in pregnancy is therefore rare and prospective studies have shown it to be no more severe than at other times of life. The incidence of varicella in pregnancy is around 5 cases per 10 000,[742] and among those who develop varicella in early pregnancy, the risk of fetal damage is around 2%.[430,639]

VZV is teratogenic and infection during early pregnancy can cause chromosomal aberrations as well as a host of congenital structural defects, affecting the brain, eye, skeleton, gastrointestinal tract and renal tract.[430,536] Vocal cord paralysis has been reported.[678] A particular feature of congenital varicella is cutaneous scarring in a dermatomal distribution, which probably represents reactivation of the virus to cause zoster. Limb defects may be associated with severe cutaneous scarring.

Prevention

Pregnant women who are exposed to varicella but are uncertain of their immune status should have their antibody levels checked. Most will be found to be immune. Infection after 20 weeks of gestation will not cause congenital varicella (see above). With modern techniques of fetal imaging and blood sampling, it is now possible to assess the fetus for congenital infection in time to terminate the pregnancy if indicated.

Congenital Epstein–Barr virus infection

Maternal infection with the Epstein–Barr virus (EBV) is uncommon, as most women of childbearing age are immune. Whether or not maternal EBV infection can cause fetal malformations is still unclear, but rare cases have been described with LBW, abnormal facies, eye defects and congenital heart disease.

Congenital herpes (see pp. 1053–6)

Congenital parvovirus B19 infection

Human parvovirus B19 is best known as the cause of erythema infectiosum (fifth disease) in children. The virus has a predilection for rapidly dividing cells, including erythrocyte precursors, and can cause a haemolytic anaemia in the fetus.[828] The incidence of parvovirus infection in pregnancy is in the range 0.3–3.7%.[288] In almost 50% of these cases there is serological evidence of fetal infection,[470] and in 1–2% of these, the infection results in abortion, stillbirth or hydrops.[667] Between 10% and 25% of cases of non-immune hydrops are thought to be related to parvovirus.[580] In a significant proportion of cases the hydrops resolves as the infection subsides,[669,801] but in the remainder the prognosis seems to be very poor, with many infants dying. In some survivors the anaemia persists into childhood,[128] but in others lasts only for a few weeks.[802] In light of the significant spontaneous remission rate, the benefits of prenatal diagnosis and fetal transfusion at cordocentesis are difficult to evaluate, although some reports are encouraging.[360] Newer diagnostic techniques using PCR or ELISA may allow the prenatal diagnosis of parvovirus infection. It has been suggested that fetal parvovirus B19 infection can cause congenital structural abnormalities, by disrupting cell lines other than those involved in erythropoesis,[443] but more data are required to evaluate this possibility. Parvovirus can cause myocarditis, cardiomyopathy[769] and liver disease, and possible neonatal meningitis due to parvovirus has been reported.[789]

Congenital infections in the developing world

The intrauterine infections described in industrialised countries also occur in developing countries. Congenital rubella probably occurs more frequently in the absence of routine immunisation, but congenital CMV infection is relatively uncommon because most women of childbearing age in the developing world possess antibodies to CMV. *Toxoplasma gondii* infects the fetus in the pregnant mother who eats inadequately cooked infected meat. Syphilis and tuberculosis are rife in many cities in the developing world. Malaria is endemic throughout the tropics, HBV infection is a major public health problem in southeast Asia, and trypanosomiasis is endemic in tropical Africa. Congenital infections caused by these agents are encountered, but in the cases of tuberculosis, malaria and trypanosomiasis, congenital infections occur much less frequently than might be anticipated from the prevalence of these diseases in the population at large. As a cause of congenital abnormality, the intrauterine infections are important,[47] as shown by Table 40.17.

The clinical manifestations of congenital rubella, CMV, herpes simplex and toxoplasmosis in the tropics show no essential differences from those described in industrial countries, and will not be further considered in this section.

Syphilis

The classic sequence of events in untreated syphilis in a woman of childbearing age is one or more abortions followed by stillbirth or the livebirth of an affected infant. Fetal infection occurs in 40–50% of women with primary syphilis. Reactive syphilis serology is a significant risk factor for perinatal mortality in developing countries, where the prevalence of seropositivity among pregnant women may be as high as 10%.

In the UK, in the period 1994 to 1997, 139 women were treated for syphilis in pregnancy, 31 had congenitally transmissible disease and nine presumptive cases of congenital syphilis were reported.[394]

Treatment of syphilis in pregnancy

Penicillin is effective in preventing congenital infection.[826] In the USA it is now thought that eradication of congenital syphilis is feasible.[2]

Table 40.17 Incidences of congenital infection among 1688 Malaysian infants with congenital abnormalities. (From Balasubramaniam et al[47])

Type of infection	Proportion of children affected (%)
CMV	11.4
Syphilis	4.0
Rubella	3.7
Toxoplasmosis	1.0

Clinical manifestations of congenital syphilis

Many infants appear normal at birth and only develop signs of the disease weeks, months or, occasionally, years later. Early manifestations of congenital syphilis resemble the lesions of secondary syphilis in adults, and later manifestations correspond more to tertiary syphilis. Prematurity and LBW are commonly associated.

Early-onset congenital syphilis is a serious life-threatening disease, often presenting with general constitutional disturbance such as anaemia, oedema, jaundice, failure to thrive and pyrexia, in the absence of the more typical mucocutaneous lesions and other local signs of the disease. Conversely, the infant may initially show quite florid mucocutaneous lesions in the absence of significant constitutional disturbance.[78] Hepatomegaly is usual and splenomegaly and lymphadenopathy are common. Pulmonary abscesses may occur.[73]

Skin eruptions are common but vary considerably both in character and in distribution.[708] Usually the rash is maculopapular, but circinate lesions occur and are among the most characteristic eruptions encountered. Involvement of the skin of the palms and the soles is usual and provides one of the typical localising features of the rash of congenital syphilis. The palms and soles may become red, mottled and swollen, with superficial desquamation. A characteristic early sign is rhinitis, and ulceration of the nasal mucosa produces a profuse mucopurulent discharge which may be bloodstained and frequently causes excoriation around the nose and on the upper lip. Destruction of the nasal cartilage and bone will in time produce the flattened nasal bridge and 'saddle-nose' of congenital syphilis. Lesions at the mucocutaneous junctions of the mouth, nose, anus and vulva are common and produce moist fissuring and bleeding. Healing of deep fissures around the mouth leads to radiating scars called rhagades, one of the typical stigmata of congenital syphilis. Flat raised plaques with moist surfaces, called condylomata, may occur around the anus and female genitalia. Osteochondritis is a frequent and typical manifestation of the disease and may present as dactylitis, fracture or pseudoparalysis. Radiological examination of the bones is a most useful adjunct to the clinical diagnosis of congenital syphilis.[500] Radiological changes are usually multiple and widespread, and most easily evident around the wrists, elbows and knees. Osteochondritis is manifest by widening and alteration in the density of the epiphyseal line and by irregular destructive lesions in the epiphyseal end of the metaphyses. Periostitis can be widespread in the bones of the limbs and may also involve the skull. The radiological signs of congenital syphilis may not be very evident in the immediate neonatal period, but become more obvious during the early months of life. They may show spontaneous regression after the sixth month.

Signs of meningitis may occur with congenital syphilis, as may evidence of hydrocephalus. Even when there is no clinical evidence of CNS involvement, the CSF may be abnormal, although probably not often enough to justify routine LP in asymptomatic at-risk infants.[69] The classic changes in the CSF are a moderate increase in cells, mainly lymphocytes, an increased protein, normal sugar levels and positive serological tests for syphilis.

Investigation and diagnosis

The diagnosis of congenital syphilis relies on awareness of the condition and a high index of clinical suspicion. Syphilis has a justifiable reputation as a great imitator, and this is certainly true of the congenital form of the disease. Diagnosis is based on the following approaches.

Making the diagnosis in the mother

All pregnant women in the UK undergo routine serological testing for syphilis at booking. In the tropics, there might also be a case for screening by colposcopy.[499] False-positive results may occur in women previously infected with yaws (*Treponema pertenue*). Women who are seropositive for syphilis are twice as likely to be HIV-positive than are those who are seronegative.[459]

Demonstrating spirochaetes in samples from suspicious lesions

Spirochaetes can sometimes be demonstrated in the placenta or umbilical cord, or in material aspirated from bullae or papules. In a recent study, spirochaetes were identified in 89% of cords from babies born to mothers with untreated syphilis, using a combination of silver stains and immunofluorescence.[736]

Serological testing[719]

Despite continuing improvements, serological tests for syphilis still lack suffcient diagnostic precision to give a confident answer to the question: Is this possibly infected but asymptomatic infant infected or not? Serological tests for syphilis are traditionally of two kinds, those aimed at detecting non-treponemal antibodies, such as those to cardiolipin (VDRL test), and those aimed at detecting antitreponemal antibodies (FTA and TPHA tests). Serological testing for syphilis in the newborn is problematic because IgG antibody is transferred across the placenta. In non-infected babies, the VDRL test usually reverts to negative within 6 months, and the TPHA and FTA-ABS tests, based on IgG, within 1 year. Persistence of positive tests beyond these times is usually considered diagnostic. Tests based on specific IgM antibodies are considered unreliable. PCR tests to detect DNA from *T. pallidum* show promise, especially in detecting CNS disease.[566] At the present time, an approach to diagnosis which combines epidemiological, clinical and serological information is advisable.

Treatment

An algorithm to guide the investigation and treatment of the baby at risk of congenital syphilis has been produced by the Centres for Disease Control in the USA. This is illustrated in Fig. 40.21. Penicillin is the drug of choice in treatment, preferably aqueous penicillin G (benzylpenicillin) 50 000 units/kg (i.e. 30 mg/kg) i.v., twice daily for 10 days. In circumstances where follow-up is unlikely or doubtful, and meningeal involvement has been excluded, long-acting benzathine penicillin 10 0000 units/kg may be given in a single i.m. dose, although published evidence on the efficacy of this approach is lacking.

HIV infection and AIDS

At the time of writing, it is estimated that there are 42 million HIV-positive people in the world. Most new infections in children occur through vertical transmission. In the last edition of this book it was reported that, as of September 1996, a total of 7472 cases of AIDS in children had been reported in the USA, and that the number of children infected annually (the vast majority in the perinatal period) was between 1000 and 2000. Since the introduction of antiretroviral prophylaxis in the mid-1990s, the rate of vertical transmission has fallen sharply and currently it is estimated that fewer than 200 children acquire HIV infection each year.[788] Sadly, these advances are not yet universal.

In the UK, the prevalence of HIV positivity in the childbearing population remains relatively low, but is rising. Table 40.18 shows the numbers of children born to HIV-infected mothers in the UK up until June 2002.[3] Table 40.19 indicates the modes of acquisition of HIV by children.

Transmission

Mother to infant

The exact mechanisms of vertical transmission of HIV remain unclear but recent evidence suggests that approximately one-third of vertically transmitted infections occur transplacentally and the other two-thirds during delivery.[135] An important mechanism of transmission may be materno-fetal transfusion during placental separation.[135] Co-infection of twins is common when maternal virus load is high.[91]

The transmission rate varies between populations and is changing rapidly in some parts of the world as a result of the introduction of intervention with antiretroviral agents. In the UK in 1993, the vertical transmission rate was almost 20%, but this had fallen to just over 2% in 1998, by which time antiretroviral treatment was used in 97% of affected pregnancies (Fig. 40.22).[214] The risk of transmission is heightened if the mother is severely immuno-deficient, as evidenced by a low CD4 lymphocyte count and the presence of immune complex-dissociated p24 antigenaemia, which may in turn be reflections of a high maternal viral load.[6,114] Preterm birth is associated with a higher transmission rate, and in a European Collaborative Study[240] babies of less than 34 weeks' gestation were three times more likely to be infected than mature babies. How much of this effect is directly due to HIV status and how much to confounding factors, such as intravenous drug abuse, is unclear. Membrane rupture more than 4 hours before delivery is associated with an increased rate of mother–infant transmission.

Breastfeeding is an established mechanism for vertical transmission of HIV, increasing the risk by some 14% overall.[212] In women infected with HIV during lactation the risk of mother–infant transmission may be almost 30%.[635]

Blood transfusion

Hopefully this method of transmission has been virtually eliminated. The estimated risk in the USA is 1 in 153 000 transfusions and in the UK 1 in 1 million.

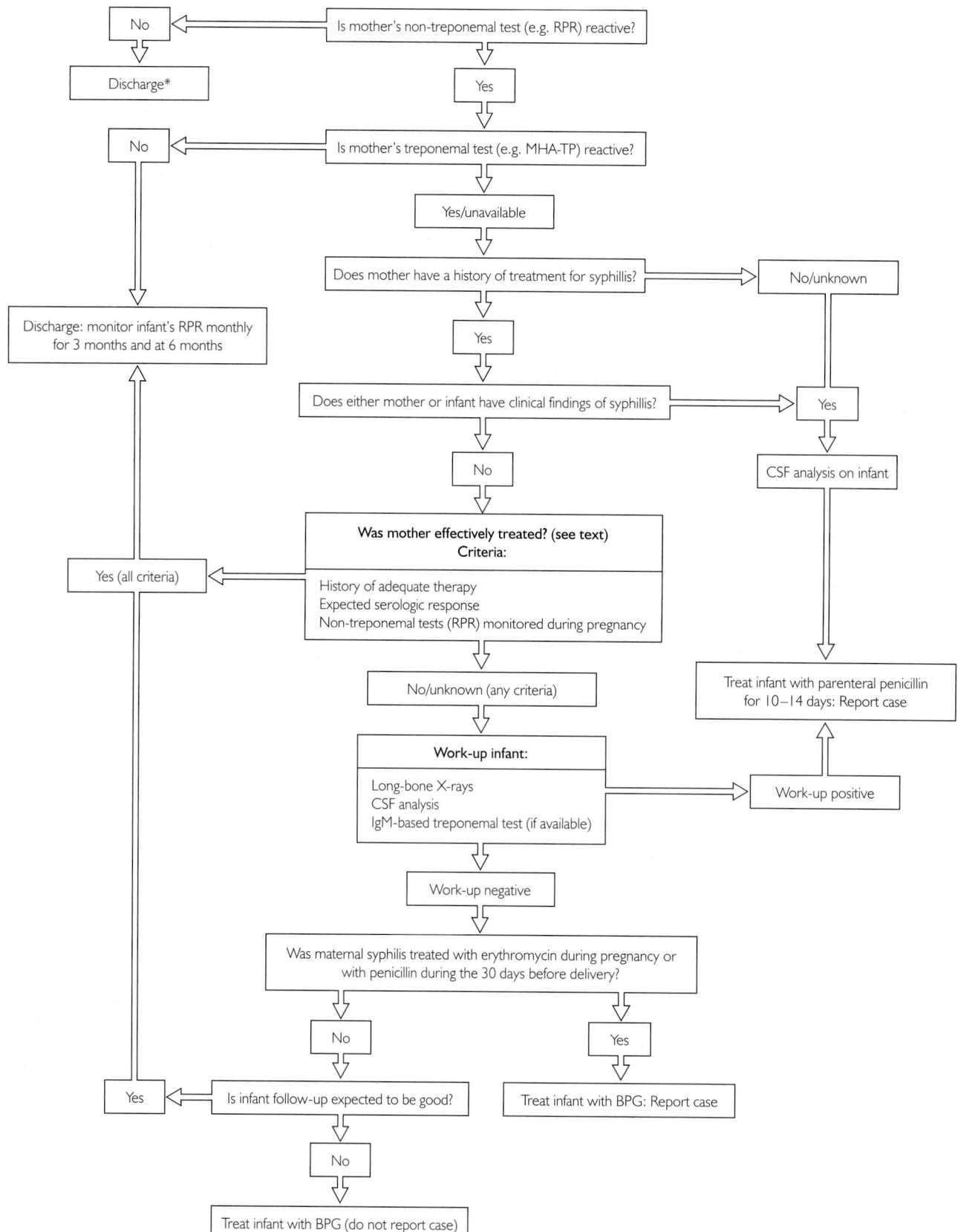

Fig. 40.21 Algorithm to aid the management of an infant at risk of congenital syphilis. The RPR non-treponemal test is equivalent to the VDRL test. Effective treatment of the mother is penicillin therapy, appropriate for the stage of syphilis in the mother, started at least 30 days before delivery. Reporting criteria are for the USA. BPG, benzathine penicillin. (From Zenker & Berman.[865])

Table 40.18 Children born to HIV-infected mothers*: year of birth and infection status

Year of birth	Infected		Indeterminate**	Not infected	Total	(Deaths)
	AIDS	Not AIDS	AIDS	Not AIDS		
1979–83	10	6	0	0	16	5
1984–85	23	16	4	15	58	12
1986–87	29	23	14	49	115	12
1988–89	51	31	14	52	148	25
1990–91	65	71	29	73	238	37
1992–93	76	63	38	89	266	41
1994–95	64	63	40	111	278	24
1996–97	63	69	35	172	339	22
1998–99	46	44	44	313	447	12
2000–01	29	19	387	384	819	8
2002	0	0	92	12	104	0
Total	456	405	697	1270	2828	198

* Due to ascertainment bias, the rate of vertical transmission cannot be estimated from these data.

** Aged less than 18 months when last tested positive for HIV antibody and without other evidence of HIV infection. Includes 95 children who were lost to follow-up.

Table 40.19 HIV infection and deaths in children by exposure category and sex: UK cases reported to the end of June 2002

How children probably acquired the virus	UK			Total	(Deaths)
	Male	Female	NS		
Mother to infant	438	420	2	860	179
Blood factor (e.g. for haemophilia)	285	0	0	285	123
Blood/tissue transfer (e.g. transfusion)	20	18	3	41	14
Other/undetermined	25	18	3	46	2
Total	768	456	8	1232	318

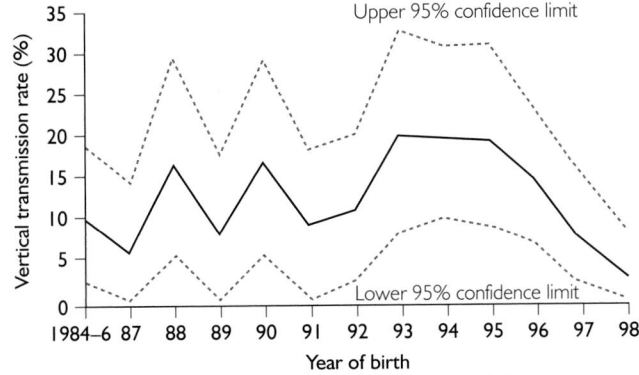

Fig. 40.22 Year-on-year estimates of vertical transmission rates (with 95% confidence intervals) for HIV among children born to mothers known to be infected with HIV and who did not breastfeed. (From Duong et al.[214])

Nosocomial spread

Casual household transmission of HIV has been documented on very few occasions and spread within a family is rare. The risk of a non-breastfeeding HIV-positive mother infecting her baby during the activities of normal care must be extremely slight.

Prevention of vertical transmission

The prevention of AIDS in children depends crucially on preventing perinatal transmission. There are many possible approaches to this, including health education, prevention of pregnancy and a combination of antenatal screening and termination of pregnancy. Once pregnancy in an HIV-positive woman has occurred and is to continue, however, there is now every possibility of successful intervention with antiretroviral drugs. The first RCT using a single antiretroviral (zidovudine) showed a reduction in the risk of perinatal transmission from 25.5% (in the placebo group) to 8.3% (in the treated group).[171] In the treatment group, zidovudine was given during late pregnancy, during labour and to the baby for 6 weeks after birth. The women enrolled in the trial were all in an early stage of HIV infection and would not normally have been receiving antiviral therapy, but subsequent studies have shown equivalent benefit in mothers with more advanced disease. Voluntary prenatal testing programmes have a reasonably high take-up rate but fail to identify a significant number of cases.[364,729] Implementing prevention strategies to full effect remains problematic.[28] Zidovudine prophylaxis is being superseded by prophylaxis with a combination of antiretroviral drugs.[644] The effect on the fetus of drugs other than zidovudine is much less well studied at present but there is reason to believe that there may be some serious risks and caution is required.[572,831] The development of drug resistance also needs careful evaluation.[178]

The British HIV Association has recently published detailed guidelines for managing HIV infection in pregnancy and preventing mother-to-child transmission.[120] Management of the baby depends on the circumstances. If it was a planned delivery to a known HIV-positive mother, the baby should receive antiretroviral monotherapy for a period of 4 weeks. If the mother was on zidovudine, this should be used for the baby also, but if the mother was on other monotherapy, specialist advice should be sought. In cases such as this, the risk of HIV transmission is very small and PCP prophylaxis with co-trimoxazole is not recommended. In the case of unplanned delivery before the mother has received antiretroviral therapy, the baby should be given zidovudine as for planned delivery plus combination therapy based on urgent specialist advice. Prophylaxis with co-trimoxazole is recommended. If mother's HIV positivity is only discovered after delivery, the baby should be given zidovudine within 48 hours of birth plus combination therapy based on urgent specialist advice. Prophylaxis with co-trimoxazole is recommended. The role of caesarean section in reducing perinatal transmission is still not completely clear, although evidence for benefit is mounting.[239,241]

Identifying the congenitally infected baby

Very occasionally, an HIV-infected baby presents with features such as hepatosplenomegaly, lymphadenopathy or thrombocytopenia, but as a rule they are indistinguishable from normal babies on clinical grounds. Recently, a pattern of early, aggressive disease has been described in developing countries.[656] These babies were growth-retarded and often premature and most were infected perinatally with tuberculosis, CMV or syphilis. Earlier reports of an associated dysmorphic syndrome have not been substantiated.

Because maternal IgG to HIV crosses the placenta, all babies born to HIV-positive women are initially seropositive. Most non-infected children become seronegative by about 9 months of age, although some may remain so for up to twice as long.[578] A small number of at-risk but seronegative infants have evidence of infection on clinical or virological grounds.[105] Because of the prolonged persistence of maternal antibody, an infant can only be declared free from HIV if there are no stigmata of disease and he is free of antigen and antibody after 18 months of age. Conversely, if antibody persists beyond this age, it strongly suggests that the child is infected. Neonatal screening has been argued for in certain populations, and the pros and cons of this have been discussed.[209]

The best approach to the definitive diagnosis of neonatal HIV infection is by means of serial PCR testing for HIV proviral DNA.[567] PCR tests should be performed on day 1 (but not from cord blood, because of the risk of contamination by maternal blood) and at 1 and 3 months. If all of these tests are negative and the baby is not being breastfed, he can be declared free of infection with a high level of confidence, although not with absolute certainty. The validity of current PCR tests for the detection of non-subtype B viruses, such as those most commonly found in Africa, is yet to be established.[668] Feasibility studies have shown the potential for screening newborn populations using the 'Guthrie card' (p. 1220).[169]

Cross-infection

HIV is not a highly contagious disease, unless there is direct contact with the patient's body fluids. The number of hospital staff infected by contact with HIV-positive patients worldwide is in the region of 100 cases, and the estimated risk of acquiring infection from a single cutaneous exposure is 0.3% (95% CI 0.18–0.46%). The labour ward, though, is one of the most bloody places in the hospital, and until all pregnant women are screened (and the pros and cons of this are much debated) labour ward staff are only likely to know the HIV status of women who have voluntarily agreed to testing, or who have already developed AIDS. For untested women in labour, a somewhat pejorative assessment of the risk can be made on the basis of their lifestyle and social circumstances, although a recent study has cast significant doubt on the validity of this approach.[357] In all situations, however, much greater care needs to be taken now than formerly, by all personnel, in dealing with blood or fomites potentially contaminated by HIV.

For the baby of the known HIV-positive mother, more stringent precautions should be instituted, including the use of full protective clothing.[510] Measures to reduce the risk of contaminating the baby with his mother's blood are also probably worth undertaking, such as avoiding airway suction where possible and avoiding crushing the umbilical cord with a clamp in the presence of maternal blood.[819]

Breastfeeding and breast-milk banking

The advice from both the American Academy of Pediatrics and the Department of Health is that HIV-positive mothers should not breastfeed. It is difficult to quibble with this advice in a western context. In the developing world, breastfeeding should not be discouraged, as the decrease in mortality it affords outweighs the risk of acquiring HIV infection in this way. Interestingly, a recent study in South Africa found that exclusive breastfeeding up to 6 months posed no additional risk over non-breastfeeding, whereas mixed breast/formula feeding posed a substantially increased risk of transmission.[176] However, beyond about 6 months of age, this risk/benefit balance of breastfeeding may reverse,[601] and there is a significant late-postnatal rate of acquisition of HIV by babies of infected mothers of around 4%.

Immunisation

Infants of HIV-positive mothers should be immunised at the normal times using DPT vaccine and substituting the Salk killed-polio vaccine for the Sabin oral polio vaccine. MMR should also be given, as the severity of these illnesses, especially measles, is increased in infants with AIDS. For measles immunisation to be maximally effective in HIV-infected children it should be given between 6 and 12 months of age. BCG can safely be given in the

Table 40.20 Congenital infections

Organism/disease	Symptoms	Treatment	Reference
Babesia microti	Fever, haemolytic anaemia	Clindamycin	Esernio Jenssen et al 1987 J. Pediatr. 110: 570 Lee 2001 Ped. Inf. Dis. J. 20: 816
Borrelia burgdorferi (Lyme disease)	Early neonatal death following birth asphyxia	Penicillin	Weber et al 1988 Ped. Inf. Dis. J. 7: 286
Respiratory papillomatosis	Presents with loss of voice or airways obstruction post extubation Condylomata not always present in the mother	Laser coagulation if severe	Sedlacek et al 1989 Am. J. Obs. Gyn. 161: 55 Chipps et al 1990 Ped. Pulmonol. 9: 125

neonatal period to babies from at-risk groups, but should not be given beyond the neonatal period, for fear of disseminated infection if immunodeficiency has developed.[84] Hepatitis B vaccination is relatively unsuccessful in babies who subsequently progress to AIDS, and failure to seroconvert may be a marker for a poor prognosis.[866] Similarly, a single dose of polyvalent polysaccharide pneumococcal vaccine does not seem to confer lasting immunity in children with perinatally acquired HIV infection.[32]

Prognosis

A few babies with undoubted HIV infection seem to recover completely and become seronegative.[136,603] For the rest, the prognosis is grim. In a recent large outcome study involving 2148 perinatally HIV-infected children, there was a 50% chance of developing AIDS, and a 25% chance of dying, by 5 years of age. The mean time from birth to developing AIDS was 4.8 years and the mean survival time was 9.4 years.[60] In a recent report from Australia, the median duration of survival was 8 years.[150] The prognosis is worse in those born with hepatosplenomegaly or adenopathy, in those with a low proportion of $CD4^+$ cells at birth, and in those who are culture or PCR positive.[764] HIV-infected infants also exhibit impaired physical growth and development relative to controls. Respiratory infection and cor pulmonale are common findings even in the first year of life.[56] Early treatment, especially of PCP, may improve the outlook.[592] In general, those who present early or are born prematurely do less well. The rapidity of virus growth in culture at 3 months of age has recently been shown to have considerable predictive value for outcome at 1 year.[283] Co-infection with CMV is associated with a more rapid disease progression.[104,204,478,563]

Congenital HTLV I/II infection

These viruses, the cause of T-cell lymphoma and adult T-cell leukaemia, are carried by a large number of women from Japan and the Caribbean. In Britain, up to 5% of women in London of African-Caribbean descent are antibody positive.

Although congenital infection with this virus is thought not to occur, some 40% of babies of infected women become infected, probably by breast milk.[618] Seropositive women should therefore be counselled not to breastfeed their babies, with the intention of significantly reducing the incidence of lymphatic malignancy in their babies 50 years later.

Human papillomavirus

Perinatal transmission of human papillomavirus and the persistence of viral DNA in infants is well described.[151,264,445,669,761] The risk of vertical transmission is in the region of 70%. Infected infants may present with minor hyperplastic growths of the oral mucosa or, rarely, with laryngeal papillomatosis. The human papillomavirus is associated with anogenital carcinoma in adults, although the potential seriousness of perinatal transmission has yet to be established.

Other congenital infections

Various other organisms have been shown to cause congenital infection by direct transplacental or intrapartum spread. Some of these are listed in Table 40.20.

References

1. [Anonymous] 1991 Guidelines for the management of acute urinary tract infection in childhood. Report of a Working Group of the Research Unit, Royal College of Physicians. Journal of the Royal College of Physicians of London 25: 36–42
2. [Anonymous] 2001 Congenital syphilis – United States, 2000. MMWR. Morbidity and Mortality Weekly Report 50: 573–577
3. [Anonymous] 2002 HIV and AIDS in the UK in 2001. London. An update November 2002. PHLS Communicable Disease Surveillance Centre, ICH (London), SCIEH
4. Abbott G D 1972 Neonatal bacteriuria: a prospective study of 1460 infants. British Medical Journal 1: 267–269
5. Ablow R C, Driscoll S G, Effmann E L et al 1976 A comparison of early-onset group B steptococcal neonatal infection and the respiratory-distress syndrome of the newborn. New England Journal of Medicine 294: 65–70

6. Abrams E J, Matheson P B, Thomas P A et al 1995 Neonatal predictors of infection status and early death among 332 infants at risk of HIV-1 infection monitored prospectively from birth. New York City Perinatal HIV Transmission Collaborative Study Group. Pediatrics 96: 451–458

7. Abzug M J 2001 Prognosis for neonates with enterovirus hepatitis and coagulopathy. Pediatric Infectious Disease Journal 20: 758–763

8. Abzug M J, Keyserling H L, Lee M L, Levin M J, Rotbart H A 1995 Neonatal enterovirus infection: virology, serology, and effects of intravenous immune globulin. Clinical Infectious Diseases 20: 1201–1206

9. Abzug M J, Levin M J 1991 Neonatal adenovirus infection: four patients and review of the literature. Pediatrics 87: 890–896

10. Abzug M J, Levin M J, Rotbart H A 1993 Profile of enterovirus disease in the first two weeks of life. Pediatric Infectious Disease Journal 12: 820–824

11. Abzug M J, Loeffelholz M, Rotbart H A 1995 Diagnosis of neonatal enterovirus infection by polymerase chain reaction. Journal of Pediatrics 126: 447–450

12. Acunas B A, Peakman M, Liossis G et al 1994 Effect of fresh frozen plasma and gammaglobulin on humoral immunity in neonatal sepsis. Archives of Disease in Childhood. Fetal and Neonatal Edition 70: F182–F187

13. Adams W G, Kinney J S, Schuchat A et al 1993 Outbreak of early onset group B streptococcal sepsis. Pediatric Infectious Disease Journal 12: 565–570

14. Adhikari M, Pillay T, Pillay D G 1997 Tuberculosis in the newborn: an emerging disease. Pediatric Infectious Disease Journal 16: 1108–1112

15. Adlerberth I, Carlsson B, de Man P et al 1991 Intestinal colonization with Enterobacteriaceae in Pakistani and Swedish hospital-delivered infants. Acta Paediatrica Scandinavica 80: 602–610

16. Ahmed A, Hickey S M, Ehrett S et al 1996 Cerebrospinal fluid values in the term neonate. Pediatric Infectious Disease Journal 15: 298–303

17. Airede A I 1992 Prolonged rupture of membranes and neonatal outcome in a developing country. Annals of Tropical Paediatrics 12: 283–288

18. Airede A I 1993 Neonatal bacterial meningitis in the middle belt of Nigeria. Developmental Medicine and Child Neurology 35: 424–430

19. Ajzenberg D, Cogne N, Paris L et al 2002 Genotype of 86 Toxoplasma gondii isolates associated with human congenital toxoplasmosis, and correlation with clinical findings. Journal of Infectious Diseases 186: 684–689

20. Akindele J A, Sowunmi A, Abohweyere A E 1993 Congenital malaria in a hyper-endemic area: a preliminary study. Annals of Tropical Paediatrics 13: 273–276

21. al Shahwan S, Rossi M L, al Thagafi M A 1996 Ascending paralysis due to myelitis in a newborn with congenital toxoplasmosis. Journal of the Neurological Sciences 139: 156–159

22. Alary M, Joly J R, Moutquin J M et al 1994 Randomised comparison of amoxycillin and erythromycin in treatment of genital chlamydial infection in pregnancy. Lancet 344: 1461–1465

23. Aly R, Shinefield H R, Litz C 1980 Teichoic acid in the binding of Staphylococcus aureus to nasal epithelial cells. Journal of Infectious Diseases 141: 463–467

24. Amato M, Huppi P, Imbach P, Llauto A, Burgi W 1995 Immunoglobulin subclass concentration in preterm infants treated prophylactically with different intravenous immunoglobins. American Journal of Perinatology 12: 306–309

25. Anderson M S, Abzug M J 1999 Hydrops fetalis: an unusual presentation of intrauterine herpes simplex virus infection. Pediatric Infectious Disease Journal 18: 837–839

26. Aradottir E, Alonso E M, Shulman S T 2001 Severe neonatal enteroviral hepatitis treated with pleconaril. Pediatric Infectious Disease Journal 20: 457–459

27. Arango C A, Rathore M H 1996 Neonatal meningococcal meningitis: case reports and review of literature. Pediatric Infectious Disease Journal 15: 1134–1136

28. Arbona S I, Melville S K, Hanson I C et al 2001 Mother-to-child transmission of the human immunodeficiency virus in Texas. Pediatric Infectious Disease Journal 20: 602–606

29. Arisoy E S, Arisoy A E, Dunne W M J 1994 Clinical significance of fungi isolated from cerebrospinal fluid in children. Pediatric Infectious Disease Journal 13: 128–133

30. Armer T, Clark P, Duff P, Saravanos K 1993 Rapid intrapartum detection of group B streptococcal colonization with an enzyme immunoassay. American Journal of Obstetrics and Gynecology 168: 39–43

31. Armstrong D S, Menahem S 1993 Cardiac arrhythmias as a manifestation of acquired heart disease in association with paediatric respiratory syncitial virus infection. Journal of Paediatrics and Child Health 29: 309–311

32. Arpadi S M, Back S, O'Brien J, Janoff E N 1994 Antibodies to pneumococcal capsular polysaccharides in children with human immunodeficiency virus infection given polyvalent pneumococcal vaccine. Journal of Pediatrics 125: 77–79

33. Asbury W H, Darsey E H, Rose W B, Murphy J E, Buffington D E, Capers C C 1993 Vancomycin pharmacokinetics in neonates and infants: a retrospective evaluation. Annals of Pharmacotherapy 27: 490–496

34. Ashraf R N, Jalil F, Zaman S et al 1991 Breast feeding and protection against neonatal sepsis in a high risk population. Archives of Disease in Childhood 66: 488–490

35. Aspinall T V, Joynson D H, Guy E, Hyde J E, Sims P F 2002 The molecular basis of sulfonamide resistance in Toxoplasma gondii and implications for the clinical management of toxoplasmosis. Journal of Infectious Diseases 185: 1637–1643

36. Atkins J T 1999 HSV PCR for CNS infections: pearls and pitfalls. Pediatric Infectious Disease Journal 18: 823–824

37. Averbuch B, Mazor M, Shoham Vardi I et al 1995 Intra-uterine infection in women with preterm premature rupture of membranes: maternal and neonatal characteristics. European Journal of Obstetrics, Gynecology and Reproductive Biology 62: 25–29

38. Avila-Figueroa C, Goldmann D A, Richardson D K, Gray J E, Ferrari A, Freeman J 1998 Intravenous lipid emulsions are the major determinant of coagulase-negative staphylococcal bacteremia in very low birth weight newborns. Pediatric Infectious Disease Journal 17: 10–17

39. Axelsson I 2002 [A Cochrane review on the umbilical cord care and prevention of infections. Antiseptic solutions are not necessary in developed countries but life-saving in developing countries.] Lakartidningen 99: 1563–1566

40. Azimi P H, Willert J, Petru A 1996 Severe esophagitis in a newborn infant. Pediatric Infectious Disease Journal 15: 385

41. Babl F E, Ram S, Barnett E D, Rhein L, Carr E, Cooper E R 2000 Neonatal gonococcal arthritis after negative prenatal screening and despite conjunctival prophylaxis. Pediatric Infectious Disease Journal 19: 346–349

42. Baier R J, Bocchini J A Jr, Brown E G 1998 Selective use of vancomycin to prevent coagulase-negative staphylococcal nosocomial bacteremia in high risk very low birth weight infants. Pediatric Infectious Disease Journal 17: 179–183

43. Baker C J, Edwards M S 1983 Group B streptococcal infections. In: Remington J S, Klein J O (eds) Infectious diseases of the fetus and newborn infant, 2nd edn. W B Saunders, Philadelphia, pp 820–881

44. Baker C J, Edwards M S 1990 Group B streptococcal infections. In: Remington J S, Klein J O (eds) Infectious diseases of the fetus and newborn infant, 3rd edn. W B Saunders, Philadelphia, pp 742–811

45. Baker C J, Melish M E, Hall R T, Casto D T, Vasan U, Givner L B 1992 Intravenous immune globulin for the prevention of nosocomial infection in low-birth-weight neonates. The Multicenter Group for the Study of Immune Globulin in Neonates [see comments]. New England Journal of Medicine 327: 213–219

46. Baker C J, Paoletti L C, Wessels M R et al 1999 Safety and immunogenicity of capsular polysaccharide-tetanus toxoid conjugate vaccines for group B streptococcal types Ia and Ib. Journal of Infectious Diseases 179: 142–150

47. Balasubramaniam V, Sinniah M, Tan D S, Redzwan G, Lo'man S G 1994 The role of cytomegalovirus (CMV) infection in congenital diseases in Malaysia. Medical Journal of Malaysia 49: 113–116

48. Balcarek K B, Warren W, Smith R J, Lyon M D, Pass R F 1993 Neonatal screening for congenital cytomegalovirus infection by detection of virus in saliva. Journal of Infectious Diseases 167: 1433–1436

49. Baley J E 1988 Neonatal sepsis: the potential for immunotherapy. Clinics in Perinatology 15: 755–771

50. Baley J E, Kliegman R M, Boxerbaum B, Fanaroff A 1986 Fungal colonisation in the very low birthweight infant. Pediatrics 78: 225–232

51. Baley J E, Kliegman R M, Fanaroff A A 1984 Disseminated fungal infections in very low birthweight infants: clinical manifestations and epidemiology. Pediatrics 73: 144–152

52. Baley J E, Silverman R A 1988 Systemic candidiasis: cutaneous manifestations in low birthweight infants. Pediatrics 82: 211–215

53. Balmer S E, Wharton B A 1989 Diet and faecal flora in the newborn: breast milk and infant formula. Archives of Disease in Childhood 64: 1672–1677

54. Baltimore R S, Huie S M, Meek J I, Schuchat A, O'Brien K L 2001 Early-onset neonatal sepsis in the era of group B streptococcal prevention. Pediatrics 108: 1094–1098

55. Banerji A, Noya F J 1999 Brain abscess associated with neonatal listeriosis. Pediatric Infectious Disease Journal 18: 305–307

56. Bannerman C, Chitsike I 1995 Cor pulmonale in children with human immunodeficiency virus infection. Annals of Tropical Paediatrics 15: 129–134

57. Bansal V, Strauss A, Gyepes M, Kanchanapoom V 1993 Central line perforation associated with Staphylococcus epidermidis infection. Journal of Pediatric Surgery 28: 894–897

58. Barbi M, Binda S, Caroppo S, Ambrosetti U, Corbetta C, Sergi P 2003 A wider role for congenital cytomegalovirus infection in sensorineural hearing loss. Pediatric Infectious Disease Journal 22: 39–42

59. Barkovich A J, Lindan C E 1994 Congenital cytomegalovirus infection of the brain: imaging analysis and embryologic considerations. AJNR. American Journal of Neuroradiology 15: 703–715

60. Barnhart H X, Caldwell M B, Thomas P et al 1996 Natural history of human immunodeficiency virus disease in perinatally infected children: an analysis from the Pediatric Spectrum of Disease Project. Pediatrics 97: 710–716

61. Bates P R, Bailey A S, Wood D J 1993 Comparative epidemiology of rotavirus, subgenus F (types 40 and 41) adenovirus, and astrovirus in children. Journal of Medical Virology 39: 224–230

62. Beardsall K, Thompson M H, Mulla R J 2000 Neonatal group B streptococcal infection in South Bedfordshire, 1993–1998. Archives of Disease in Childhood. Fetal and Neonatal Edition 82: F205–F207

63. Beasley R P, Hwang L Y, Lin C C, Chien C S 1981 Hepatocellular carcinoma and hepatitis B virus; a prospective study of 22707 men in Taiwan. Lancet 2: 1129–1132

64. Beck Sague C M, Azimi P, Fonseca S N et al 1994 Bloodstream infections in neonatal intensive care unit patients: results of a multicenter study. Pediatric Infectious Disease Journal 13: 1110–1116

65. Becker J A, Ascher D P, Mendiola J et al 1993 False-negative urine latex particle agglutination testing in neonates with group B streptococcal bacteremia. A function of improper test implementation? Clinical Pediatrics 32: 467–471

66. Bedford Russell A R, Breathnach A, Sender P 2001 Confirmed group B streptococcus infection: the tip of the iceberg. Archives of Disease in Childhood. Fetal and Neonatal Edition 84: F140

67. Bedford Russell A R, Emmerson A J, Wilkinson N et al 2001 A trial of recombinant human granulocyte colony stimulating factor for the treatment of very low birthweight infants with presumed sepsis and neutropenia. Archives of Disease in Childhood. Fetal and Neonatal Edition 84: F172–F176

68. Bedford Russell A R, Graham Davies E, Ball S E, Gordon-Smith E 1995 Granulocyte colony stimulating factor treatment for neonatal neutropenia. Archives of Disease in Childhood 72: 53–54

69. Beeram M R, Chopde N, Dawood Y, Siriboe S, Abedin M 1996 Lumbar puncture in the evaluation of possible asymptomatic congenital syphilis in neonates. Journal of Pediatrics 128: 125–129

70. Beiter A, Lewis K, Pineda E F, Cherry J D 1993 Unrecognized maternal peripartum pertussis with subsequent fatal neonatal pertussis. Obstetrics and Gynecology 82: 691–693

71. Beitzke H 1935 Uber die angeborne tuberculose infektion Ergebnisse der Gesamten. Tuberkulose-Forschung 7: 1–30

72. Bell A H, Brown D, Halliday H L, McClure G, McReid M 1989 Meningitis in the newborn – a 14 year review. Archives of Disease in Childhood 64: 873–874

73. Bell C, Taxy J 2002 Pulmonary abscesses in congenital syphilis. Archives of Pathology and Laboratory Medicine 126: 484–486

74. Bell T A, Stamm W E, Kuo C C, Wang S P, Holmes K K, Grayston J T 1994 Risk of perinatal transmission of Chlamydia trachomatis by mode of delivery. Journal of Infection 29: 165–169

75. Ben David Y, Hallak M, Evans M I, Abramovici H 1995 Amnionitis and premature delivery with intact amniotic membranes involving Staphylococcus aureus. A case report. Journal of Reproductive Medicine 40: 485–486

76. Benitz W E, Han M Y, Madan A, Ramachandra P 1998 Serial serum C-reactive protein levels in the diagnosis of neonatal infection. Pediatrics 102: e41

77. Benjamin J, Ross K, McKinney J, Benjamin D K, Auten R, Fisher R G 2000 When to suspect fungal infection in neonates: a clinical comparison of Candida albicans and Candida parapsilosis fungemia with coagulase-negative staphylococcal bacteremia. Pediatrics 106: 712–718

78. Bennett M L, Lynn A W, Klein L E, Balkowiec K S 1997 Congenital syphilis: subtle presentation of fulminant disease. Journal of the American Academy of Dermatology 36: 351–354

79. Bennett O M, Namnyak S S 1992 Acute septic arthritis of the hip joint in infancy and childhood. Clinical Orthopaedics and Related Research Aug: 123–132

80. Bennett R E Jr, Barnett D W 2001 Perinatal herpes simplex infection presenting with pneumonia and pleural effusions. Pediatric Infectious Disease Journal 20: 228–230

81. Berger C, Uehlinger J, Ghelfi D, Blau N, Fanconi S 1995 Comparison of C-reactive protein and white blood cell count with differential in neonates at risk for septicaemia. European Journal of Pediatrics 154: 138–144

82. Beri R, Lourwood D L 1997 Chemoprophylaxis for group B streptococcus transmission in neonates. Annals of Pharmacotherapy 31: 110–112

83. Berrebi A, Kobuch W E, Bessieres M H et al 1994 Termination of pregnancy for maternal toxoplasmosis. Lancet 344: 36–39

84. Besnard M, Sauvion S, Offredo C 1993 Bacillus Calmette-Guerin infection after vaccination of human immunodeficiency virus-infected children. Pediatric Infectious Disease Journal 12: 993–997

85. Bessieres M H, Roques C, Berreb, A, Barre V, Cazaux M, Seguela, J P 1992 IgA antibody response during acquired and congenital toxoplasmosis. Journal of Clinical Pathology 45: 605–608

86. Betremieux P, Chevrier S, Quindos G, Sullivan D, Polonelli L, Guiguen C 1994 Use of DNA fingerprinting and biotyping methods to study a Candida albicans outbreak in a neonatal intensive care unit. Pediatric Infectious Disease Journal 13: 899–905

87. Betremieux P, Donnio P Y, Pladys P 1995 Use of ribotyping to investigate tracheal colonisation by Staphylococcus epidermidis as a source of bacteremia in ventilated newborns. European Journal of Clinical Microbiology and Infectious Diseases 14: 342–346

88. Bhutta Z A 1996 Enterobacter sepsis in the newborn – a growing problem in Karachi. Journal of Hospital Infection 34: 211–216

89. Bhutta Z A, Naqvi S H, Muzaffar T, Farooqui B J 1991 Neonatal sepsis in Pakistan. Presentation and pathogens. Acta Paediatrica Scandinavica 80: 596–601

90. Bialkowska Hobrzanska H, Jaskot D, Hammerberg O 1993 Molecular characterization of the coagulase-negative staphylococcal surface flora of premature neonates. Journal of General Microbiology 139: 2939–2944

91. Biggar R J, Janes M, Pilon R et al 2002 Human immunodeficiency virus type 1 infection in twin pairs infected at birth. Journal of Infectious Diseases 186: 281–285

92. Bilgin K, Yaramis A, Haspolat K, Tas M A, Gunbey S, Derman O 2001 A randomized trial of granulocyte-macrophage colony-stimulating factor in neonates with sepsis and neutropenia. Pediatrics 107: 36–41

93. Bingen E, Denamur E, Lambert Zechovsky N et al 1992 Mother-to-infant vertical transmission and cross-colonization of Streptococcus pyogenes confirmed by DNA restriction fragment length polymorphism analysis, Journal of Infectious Diseases 165: 147–150

94. Bingen E H, Mariani Kurkdjian P, Lambert Zechovsky N Y et al 1992 Ribotyping provides efficient differentiation of nosocomial Serratia marcescens isolates in a pediatric hospital. Journal of Clinical Microbiology 30: 2088–2091

95. Bishop P N, Tullo A B, Killough R, Richmond S J 1991 An immune dot-blot test for the diagnosis of ocular infection with Chlamydia trachomatis. Eye 5: 305–308

96. Blanchard A, Hentschel J, Duffy L, Baldus K, Cassell G H 1993 Detection of Ureaplasma urealyticum by polymerase chain reaction in the urogenital tract of adults, in amniotic fluid, and in the respiratory tract of newborns. Clinical Infectious Diseases 17(suppl. 1): S148–S153

97. Bomela H N, Ballot D E, Cory B J, Cooper P A 2000 Use of C-reactive protein to guide duration of empiric antibiotic therapy in suspected early neonatal sepsis. Pediatric Infectious Disease Journal 19: 531–535

98. Boo N Y, Chor C Y 1994 Six year trend of neonatal septicaemia in a large Malaysian maternity hospital. Journal of Paediatrics and Child Health 30: 23–27

99. Boppana S B, Britt W J 1995 Antiviral antibody responses and intrauterine transmission after primary maternal cytomegalovirus infection. Journal of Infectious Diseases 171: 1115–1121

100. Boppana S B, Fowler K B, Vaid Y et al 1997 Neuroradiographic findings in the newborn period and long-term outcome in children with symptomatic congenital cytomegalovirus infection. Pediatrics 99: 409–414

101. Boppana S B, Pass R F, Britt W J 1993 Virus-specific antibody responses in mothers and their newborn infants with asymptomatic congenital cytomegalovirus infections. Journal of Infectious Diseases 167: 72–77

102. Boppana S B, Pass R F, Britt W J, Stagno S, Alford C A 1992 Symptomatic congenital cytomegalovirus infection: neonatal morbidity and mortality. Pediatric Infectious Disease Journal 11: 93–99

103. Borderon E, Desroches A, Tescher M, Bondeux D, Chillou C, Borderon J C 1994 Value of examination of the gastric aspirate for the diagnosis of neonatal infection. Biology of the Neonate 65: 353–366

104. Boriskin Y S, Sharland M, Dalton R, duMont G, Booth J C 1999 Viral loads in dual infection with HIV-1 and cytomegalovirus. Archives of Disease in Childhood 80: 132–136

105. Borkowsky W, Paul D, Bebenroth D 1987 Human immunodeficiency virus in infants negative for anti-HIV by enzyme-linked immunoassay. Lancet I: 1168–1171

106. Bortolussi R, Issekutz T B, Faulkner A 1986 Opsonization of Listeria monocytogenes type 4b by human adult and newborn sera. Infection and Immunity 52: 493–495

107. Botas C M, Kurlat I, Young S M, Sola A 1995 Disseminated candidal infections and intravenous hydrocortisone in preterm infants. Pediatrics 95: 883–887

108. Bowman E D, Dharmalingam A, Fan W Q, Brown F, Garland S M 1998 Impact of erythromycin on respiratory colonization of Ureaplasma urealyticum and the development of chronic lung disease in extremely low birth weight infants. Pediatric Infectious Disease Journal 17: 615–620

109. Boxall J, Orme R L, Cruickshank J G 1982 Shared care and infection in a special care baby unit. Nursing Times 78: 1848–1850

110. Boyer K M 1995 Neonatal group B streptococcal infections. Current Opinion in Pediatrics 7: 13–18

111. Boyer K M 2001 Diagnostic testing for congenital toxoplasmosis. Pediatric Infectious Disease Journal 20: 59–60

112. Boyer K M, Gotoff S P 1988 Antimicrobial prophylaxis of neonatal group B streptococcal sepsis. Clinics in Perinatology 15: 831–850

113. Boyer K M, Gotoff S P 1998 Alternative algorithms for prevention of perinatal group B streptococcal infections. Pediatric Infectious Disease Journal 17: 973–979

114. Boyer P J, Dillon M, Navaie M et al 1994 Factors predictive of maternal-fetal transmission of HIV-1. Preliminary analysis of zidovudine given during pregnancy and/or delivery. Journal of the American Medical Association 271: 1925–1930

115. Boyle E M, Ainsworth J R, Levin A V, Campbell A N, Watkinson M 2001 Ophthalmic Pseudomonas infection in infancy. Archives of Disease in Childhood. Fetal and Neonatal Edition 85: F139–F140

116. Boyle R J, Chandler B D, Stonestreet B S, Oh W 1978 Early identification of sepsis in infants with RDS. Pediatrics 62: 744–750

117. Brans Y W, Ceballos R, Cassady G 1974 Umbilical catheters and hepatic abscesses. Pediatrics 53: 264–267

118. Bravo F J, Bourne N, Harrison C J et al 1996 Effect of antibody alone and combined with acyclovir on neonatal herpes simplex virus infection in guinea pigs. Journal of Infectious Diseases 173: 1–6

119. Brazin S A, Simkovich J W, Johnson W T 1979 Herpes zoster during pregnancy. Obstetrics and Gynecology 53: 175–181

120. British HIV Association 2001 Guidelines for the management of HIV infection in pregnant women and the prevention of mother-to-child transmission. HIV Medicine 2: 314–334

121. Brodie S B, Sands K E, Gray J E et al 2000 Occurrence of nosocomial bloodstream infections in six neonatal intensive care units. Pediatric Infectious Disease Journal 19: 56–65

122. Bromberger P, Lawrence J M, Braun,D, Saunders B, Contreras R, Petitti D B 2000 The influence of intrapartum antibiotics on the clinical spectrum of early-onset group B streptococcal infection in term infants. Pediatrics 106: 244–250

123. Brook I 1995 Bacteroides infections in children. Journal of Medical Microbiology 43: 92–98

124. Brook I 1998 Dacryocystitis caused by anaerobic bacteria in the newborn. Pediatric Infectious Disease Journal 17: 172–173

125. Brook I 2002 Cutaneous and subcutaneous infections in newborns due to anaerobic bacteria. Journal of Perinatal Medicine 30: 197–208

126. Brook I 2002 Suppurative parotitis caused by anaerobic bacteria in newborns. Pediatric Infectious Disease Journal 21: 81–82

127. Brown J, Froese-Fretz A, Luckey D, Todd J K 1996 High rate of hand contamination and low rate of hand washing before infant contact in a neonatal intensive care unit. Pediatric Infectious Disease Journal 15: 908–910

128. Brown K E, Green S W, Antunez de Mayolo J et al 1994 Congenital anaemia after transplacental B19 parvovirus infection. Lancet 343: 895–896

129. Brown Z A, Benedetti J, Ashley R et al 1991 Neonatal herpes simplex virus infection in relation to asymptomatic maternal infection at the time of labor [see comments]. New England Journal of Medicine 324: 1247–1252

130. Brown Z A, Vontver L A, Benedetti J 1987 Effects on infants of a first episode of genital herpes during pregnancy. New England Journal of Medicine 317: 1246–1251

131. Brown Z A, Wald A, Morrow R A, Selke S, Zeh J, Corey L 2003 Effect of serologic status and cesarean delivery on transmission rates of herpes simplex virus from mother to infant. Journal of the American Medical Association 289: 203–209

132. Brunell P A 1992 Varicella in pregnancy, the fetus, and the newborn: problems in management [see comments]. Journal of Infectious Diseases 166(suppl. 1): S42–S47

133. Bryant K, Maxfield C, Rabalais G 1999 Renal candidiasis in neonates with candiduria. Pediatric Infectious Disease Journal 18: 959–963

134. Bryant P, Morley C J, Garland J S, Curtis N 2002 Cytomegalovirus transmission from breast milk in premature babies: does it matter? Archives of Disease in Childhood. Fetal and Neonatal Edition 87: F75–F77

135. Bryson Y J, Lazuriaga K, Wara D W 1993 Proposed definition for in utero versus intrapartum transmission of HIV-1. New England Journal of Medicine 327: 1246–1247

136. Bryson Y J, Pang S, Wei M S 1995 Clearance of HIV infection in a perinatally infected infant. New England Journal of Medicine 332: 833–838

137. Buck C, Gallati H, Pohlandt F, Bartmann P 1994 Increased levels of tumor necrosis factor alpha (TNF-alpha) and interleukin 1 beta (IL-1 beta) in tracheal aspirates of newborns with pneumonia. Infection 22: 238–241

138. Burgess M A 1992 Rubella reinfection – what risk to the fetus? Medical Journal of Australia 156: 824–825

139. Burgner D 1994 Fresh frozen plasma and neonatal sepsis [letter]. Archives of Disease in Childhood. Fetal and Neonatal Edition 71: F233

140. Buttery J P 2002 Blood cultures in newborns and children: optimising an everyday test. Archives of Disease in Childhood. Fetal and Neonatal Edition 87: F25–F28

141. Cadnapaphornchai M, Faix R G 1992 Increased nosocomial infection in neutropenic low birth weight (2000 grams or less) infants of hypertensive mothers. Journal of Pediatrics 121: 956–961

142. Cairns P A, Wilson D C, McClure B G, Halliday H L, McReid M 1995 Percutaneous central venous catheter use in the very low birth weight neonate. European Journal of Pediatrics 154: 145–147

143. Cairo M S 1990 The use of granulocyte transfusion in neonatal sepsis. Transfusion Medicine Reviews 4: 14–22

144. Cairo M S, Christensen R, Sender L S et al 1995 Results of a phase I/II trial of recombinant human granulocyte-macrophage colony-stimulating factor in very low birthweight neonates: significant induction of circulatory neutrophils, monocytes, platelets, and bone marrow neutrophils. Blood 86: 2509–2515

145. Cairo M S, Rucker R, Bennetts G A 1984 Improved survival of newborns receiving leukocyte transfusions for sepsis. Pediatrics 74: 887–892

146. Cairo M S, Suen Y, Knoppel E et al 1992 Decreased G-CSF and IL-3 production and gene expression from mononuclear cells of newborn infants. Pediatric Research 31: 574–578

147. Cairo M S, Worcester C C, Rucker R W et al 1992 Randomized trial of granulocyte transfusions versus intravenous immune globulin therapy for neonatal neutropenia and sepsis [see comments]. Journal of Pediatrics 120: 281–285

148. Campbell J R 1996 Neonatal pneumonia. Seminars in Respiratory Infections 11: 155–162

149. Carbonell-Estrany X, Quero J, Bustos G et al 2000 Rehospitalization because of respiratory syncytial virus infection in premature infants younger than 33 weeks of gestation: a prospective study. IRIS Study Group. Pediatric Infectious Disease Journal 19: 592–597

150. Carlin J B, Langdon P, Hurley S F et al 1996 Health care and its costs for children with perinatally acquired HIV infection. Journal of Paediatrics and Child Health 32: 42–47

151. Cason J, Kaye J N, Jewers R J et al 1995 Perinatal infection and persistence of human papillomavirus types 16 and 18 in infants. Journal of Medical Virology 47: 209–218

152. Cassell G H, Waites K B, Watson H L, Crouse D T, Harasawa R 1993 Ureaplasma urealyticum intrauterine infection: role in prematurity and disease in newborns. Clinical Microbiology Reviews 6: 69–87

153. Cataldo F, Scotto E, De Gregorio T 1983 Brucellosis in a five month old infant infected by mother. Acta Mediterranea Patologica Infettia et Tropica 62: 302–304

154. Centers for Disease Control and Prevention 2002 Sexually transmitted diseases treatment guidelines 2002. MMWR Recommendations and Reports 51: 1–78

155. Chapman R L, Faix R G 2000 Persistently positive cultures and outcome in invasive neonatal candidiasis. Pediatric Infectious Disease Journal 19: 822–827

156. Chequer R S, Tharp B R, Dreimane D, Hahn J S, Clancy R R, Coen R W 1992 Prognostic value of EEG in neonatal meningitis: retrospective study of 29 infants. Pediatric Neurology 8: 417–422

157. Chidekel A S, Rosen C L, Bazzy A R 1997 Rhinovirus infection associated with serious lower respiratory illness in patients with bronchopulmonary dysplasia. Pediatric Infectious Disease Journal 16: 43–47

158. Chien L Y, Macnab Y, Aziz K, Andrews W, McMillan D D, Lee S K 2002 Variations in central venous catheter-related infection risks among Canadian neonatal intensive care units. Pediatric Infectious Disease Journal 21: 505–511

159. Chiou C C, Soong W J, Hwang B, Wu K G, Lee B H, Wang H C 1994 Congenital adenoviral infection. Pediatric Infectious Disease Journal 13: 664–665

160. Chiou C C, Wong T T, Lin H H et al 1994 Fungal infection of ventriculoperitoneal shunts in children. Clinical Infectious Diseases 19: 1049–1053

161. Christensen G D, Simpson W A, Bisno A L 1982 Adherence of slime-producing strains of Staphylococcus epidermidis to smooth surfaces. Infection and Immunity 37: 318–322

162. Christensen R D, Rothstein G, Anstall H B 1982 Granulocyte transfusions in neonates with bacterial infection, neutropenia and depletion of mature marrow neutrophils. Pediatrics 70: 1–6

163. Christie C, Hammond J, Reising S, Evans Patterson J 1994 Clinical and molecular epidemiology of enterococcal bacteremia in a pediatric teaching hospital. Journal of Pediatrics 125: 392–399

164. Chuang E, Maller E S, Hoffman M A, Hodinka R L, Altschuler S M 1993 Successful treatment of fulminant echovirus 11 infection in a neonate by

orthotopic liver transplantation. Journal of Pediatric Gastroenterology and Nutrition 17: 211–214

165. Chun C S, Brady L J, Boyle M D, Dillon H C, Ayoub E M 1991 Group B streptococcal C protein-associated antigens: association with neonatal sepsis. Journal of Infectious Diseases 163: 786–791

166. Churgay C A, Smith M A, Blok B 1994 Maternal fever during labor – what does it mean? Journal of the American Board of Family Practice 7: 14–24

167. Cimolai N, Roscoe D L 1995 Contemporary context for early-onset group B streptococcal sepsis of the newborn. American Journal of Perinatology 12: 46–49

168. Cloney D L, Donowitz L G 1986 Overgown use for infection control in nurseries and neonatal intensive care units. American Journal of Diseases of Children 140: 680–683

169. Comeau A M, Hsu H W, Schwerzler M et al 1993 Identifying human immuno-deficiency virus infection at birth: application of polymerase chain reaction to Guthrie cards. Journal of Pediatrics 123: 252–258

170. Condon R J, Bower C 1993 Rubella vaccination and congenital rubella syndrome in Western Australia [see comments]. Medical Journal of Australia 158: 379–382

171. Connor E M, Sperling R S, Gelber R 1994 Reduction of maternal-infant transmission of human immunodeficiency virus type 1 with zidovudine treatment. New England Journal of Medicine 331: 1173–1180

172. Conway S P, Dear P R F, Smith I 1985 Immunoglobulin profile of the preterm baby. Archives of Disease in Childhood 60: 208–212

173. Cordero L, Ayers L W, Davis K 1997 Neonatal airway colonization with gram-negative bacilli: association with severity of bronchopulmonary dysplasia. Pediatric Infectious Disease Journal 16: 18–23

174. Corey L, Whitley R J, Stone E F, Mohan K 1988 Difference between herpes simplex type I and type II neonatal encephalitis in neurological outcome. Lancet i: 1–4

175. Correa A G, Baker C J, Schutze G E, Edwards M S 1994 Immunoglobulin G enhances C3 degradation on coagulase-negative staphylococci. Infection and Immunity 62: 2362–2366

176. Coutsoudis A, Pillay K, Kuhn L, Spooner E, Tsai W, Coovadia H 2001 Method of feeding and transmission of HIV-1 from mothers to children by 15 months of age: prospective cohort study from Durban, South Africa. AIDS 15: 379–387

177. Covert R F, Schreiber M D 1993 Three different strains of heat-killed group B beta-hemolytic streptococcus cause different pulmonary and systemic hemodynamic responses in conscious neonatal lambs. Pediatric Research 33: 373–379

178. Cunningham C K, Chaix M L, Rekacewicz C et al 2002 Development of resistance mutations in women receiving standard antiretroviral therapy who received intrapartum nevirapine to prevent perinatal human immunodeficiency virus type 1 transmission: a substudy of pediatric AIDS clinical trials group protocol 316. Journal of Infectious Diseases 186: 181–188

179. Da Silva O, Gregson D, Hammerberg O 1997 Role of Ureaplasma urealyticum and Chlamydia trachomatis in development of bronchopulmonary dysplasia in very low birth weight infants. Pediatric Infectious Disease Journal 16: 364–369

180. Daffos F, Forestier F, Capella-Pavlovsky M et al 1988 Prenatal management of 746 pregnancies at risk for congenital toxoplasmosis. New England Journal of Medicine 318: 271–275

181. Dahlquist G, Frisk G, Ivarsson S A, Svanberg L, Forsgren M, Diderholm H 1995 Indications that maternal coxsackie B virus infection during pregnancy is a risk factor for childhood-onset IDDM. Diabetologia 38: 1371–1373

182. Damjanovic V, Connolly C M, van Saene H K et al 1993 Selective decontamin-ation with nystatin for control of a Candida outbreak in a neonatal intensive care unit. Journal of Hospital Infection 24: 245–259

183. Danesh I S, Stephen J M, Gorbach J 1995 Neonatal Trichomonas vaginalis infection. Journal of Emergency Medicine 13: 51–54

184. Daniel Y, Gull I, Peyser M R, Lessing J B 1995 Congenital cytomegalovirus infection. European Journal of Obstetrics, Gynecology and Reproductive Biology 63: 7–16

185. Dannevig L, Straume B, Melby K 1992 Ophthalmia neonatorum in northern Norway. I: Epidemiology and risk factors. Acta Ophthalmologica 70: 14–18

186. Darville T, Tabor D, Simpson K, Jacobs R F 1994 Intravenous immunoglobulin modulates human mononuclear phagocyte tumor necrosis factor-alpha production in vitro. Pediatric Research 35: 397–403

187. Davies H D, Raj S, Adair C, Robinson J, McGeer A 2001 Population-based active surveillance for neonatal group B streptococcal infections in Alberta, Canada: implications for vaccine formulation. Pediatric Infectious Disease Journal 20: 879–884

188. Davies P A, Aherne W 1962 Congenital pneumonia. Archives of Disease in Childhood 37: 598–602

189. de Champs C, Franchineau P, Gourgand J M, Loriette Y, Gaulme J, Sirot J 1994 Clinical and bacteriological survey after change in aminoglycoside treatment to control an epidemic of Enterobacter cloacae. Journal of Hospital Infection 28: 219–229

190. de Toledo A R, Chandler J W 1992 Conjunctivitis of the newborn. Infectious Disease Clinics of North America 6: 807–813

191. Dear P R F, McLain B I 1987 Establishment of an intermediate care ward for babies and mothers. Archives of Disease in Childhood 62: 597–601

192. Department of Health 1989 Health building note No. 21. Maternity department. HMSO, London

193. Dewey K G, Heinig M J, Nommsen Rivers L A 1995 Differences in morbidity between breast-fed and formula-fed infants. Journal of Pediatrics 126: 696–702

194. Diamond C, Mohan K, Hobson A, Frenkel L, Corey L 1999 Viremia in neonatal herpes simplex virus infections. Pediatric Infectious Disease Journal 18: 487–489

195. Dinger J, Muller D, Pargac N, Schwarze R 2002 Breast milk transmission of group B streptococcal infection. Pediatric Infectious Disease Journal 21: 567–568

196. Dinsmoor M J, Ramamurthy R S, Gibbs R S 1989 Transmission of genital mycoplasmas from mother to neonate in women with prolonged membrane rupture. Pediatric Infectious Disease Journal 8: 483–487

197. Dirschl D R 1994 Acute pyogenic osteomyelitis in children. Orthopedic Reviews 23: 305–312

198. Djurkovic-Djakovic O, Romand S, Nobre R, Couvreur J, Thulliez P 2000 Serologic rebounds after one-year-long treatment for congenital toxoplasmosis. Pediatric Infectious Disease Journal 19: 81–83

199. Dobson S R, Baker C J 1990 Enterococcal sepsis in neonates: features by age at onset and occurrence of focal infection. Pediatrics 85: 165–171

200. Dobson S R, Isaacs D, Wilkinson A R, Hope P L 1992 Reduced use of surface cultures for suspected neonatal sepsis and surveillance. Archives of Disease in Childhood 67: 44–47

201. Dong Z W, Yan C, Yi W, Cui Y Q 1994 Detection of congenital cytomegalovirus infection by using chorionic villi of the early pregnancy and polymerase chain reaction. International Journal of Gynecology and Obstetrics 44: 229–231

202. Donner C, Liesnard C, Brancart F, Rodesch F 1994 Accuracy of amniotic fluid testing before 21 weeks' gestation in prenatal diagnosis of congenital cytomegalovirus infection. Prenatal Diagnosis 14: 1055–1059

203. Donnerstein R L, Berg R A, Shehab Z, Ovadia M 1994 Complex atrial tachycardias and respiratory syncytial virus infections in infants. Journal of Pediatrics 125: 23–28

204. Doyle M, Atkins J T, Rivera-Matos I R 1996 Congenital cytomegalovirus infection in infants infected with human immunodeficiency virus type 1. Pediatric Infectious Disease Journal 15: 1102–1106

205. Drews M B, Ludwig A C, Leititis J U, Daschner F D 1995 Low birth weight and nosocomial infection of neonates in a neonatal intensive care unit. Journal of Hospital Infection 30: 65–72

206. Driessen M, Ellis J B, Cooper P A et al 1996 Fluconazole vs. amphotericin B for the treatment of neonatal fungal septicemia: a prospective randomized trial. Pediatric Infectious Disease Journal 15: 1107–1112

207. Druyts Voets E, Van Renterghem L, Gerniers S 1993 Coxsackie B virus epidemiology and neonatal infection in Belgium. Journal of Infection 27: 311–316

208. Dulkerian S, Kilpatrick L, Costarino A T J et al 1995 Cytokine elevations in infants with bacterial and aseptic meningitis. Journal of Pediatrics 126: 872–876

209. Dumois A O 1995 The case against mandatory newborn screening for HIV antibodies. Journal of Community Health 20: 143–159

210. Dumornay W, Roblin P M, Gelling M, Hammerschlag M R, Worku M 1992 Comparison of a chemiluminometric immunoassay with culture for diagnosis of chlamydial infections in infants. Journal of Clinical Microbiology 30: 1867–1869

211. Dunn D T, Gibb D M, Healy M et al 2001 Timing and interpretation of tests for diagnosing perinatally acquired hepatitis C virus infection. Pediatric Infectious Disease Journal 20: 715–716

212. Dunn D T, Newell M L, Ades A E, Peckham C 1992 Risk of human immunodeficiency virus type 1 transmission through breastfeeding. Lancet 340: 585–588

213. Dunn D, Newell M L, Gilbert R 1997 Low risk of congenital toxoplasmosis in children born to women infected with human immunodeficiency virus. Pediatric Infectious Disease Journal 16: 84

214. Duong T, Ades A E, Gibb D M, Tookey P A, Masters J 1999 Vertical transmis-sion rates for HIV in the British Isles: estimates based on surveillance data. British Medical Journal 319: 1227–1229

215. Dyke M P, Forsyth K D 1993 Decreased plasma fibronectin concentrations in preterm infants with septicaemia. Archives of Disease in Childhood 68: 557–560

216. Dyke M P, Grauaug A, Kohan R, Ott K, Andrews R 1993 Ureaplasma urealyticum in a neonatal intensive care population. Journal of Paediatrics and Child Health 29: 295–297

217. Eastick K, Leeming J P, Bennett D, Millar M R 1996 Reservoirs of coagulase negative staphylococci in preterm infants. Archives of Disease in Childhood. Fetal and Neonatal Edition 74: F99–F104

218. Eaton R B, Petersen E, Seppanen H, Tuuminen T 1996 Multicenter evaluation of a fluorometric enzyme immunocapture assay to detect toxoplasma-specific immunoglobulin M in dried blood filter paper specimens from newborns. Journal of Clinical Microbiology 34: 3147–3150

219. Edelman C M, Ogwo J E, Fine B P 1973 The prevalence of bacteruria in full-term and premature newborn infants. Journal of Pediatrics 82: 125–129

220. Edelman K, Nikkari S, Ruuskanen O, He Q, Viljanen M, Mertsola J 1996 Detection of Bordetella pertussis by polymerase chain reaction and culture in the nasopharynx of erythromycin-treated infants with pertussis. Pediatric Infectious Disease Journal 15: 54–57

221. Edwards M S, Rench M A, Haffar A M, Murphy M A, Demond M M, Baker C J 1985 Long term sequelae of group B streptococcal meningitis in infancy. Journal of Pediatrics 106: 717–722

222. Edwards M S, Rench M A, Hall M A, Baker C J 1993 Fibronectin levels in premature infants with late-onset sepsis. Journal of Perinatology 13: 8–13

223. Ehl S, Gering B, Bartmann P, Hogel J, Pohlandt F 1997 C-reactive protein is a useful marker for guiding duration of antibiotic therapy in suspected neonatal bacterial infection. Pediatrics 99: 216–221

224. Eisenfeld L, Krause P J, Herson V C, Block C, Schick J B, Maderazo E 1992 Enhancement of neonatal neutrophil motility (chemotaxis) with adult fresh frozen plasma. American Journal of Perinatology 9: 5–8

225. Eisenstein E M, Gesundheit B 1998 Neonatal hand abscess, osteomyelitis and meningitis caused by Streptococcus pneumoniae. Pediatric Infectious Disease Journal 17: 760–761

226. Ekbom A, Wakefield A J, Zack M, Adami H O 1994 Perinatal measles infection and subsequent Crohn's disease. Lancet 344: 508–510

227. el Mohandes A E, Johnson Robbins L, Keiser J F, Simmens S J, Aure M V 1994 Incidence of Candida parapsilosis colonization in an intensive care nursery population and its association with invasive fungal disease. Pediatric Infectious Disease Journal 13: 520–524

228. El Radhi A S, Jawad M H, Mansor N, Ibrahim N, Jamil I I 1983 Infection in neonatal hypothermia. Archives of Disease in Childhood 58: 143–145

229. Elder D E, Minutillo C, Pemberton P J 1995 Neonatal herpes simplex infection: keys to early diagnosis. Journal of Paediatrics and Child Health 31: 307–311

230. Embleton N, Wariyar U, Hey E 1999 Mortality from early onset group B streptococcal infection in the United Kingdom. Archives of Disease in Childhood. Fetal and Neonatal Edition 80: F139–F141

231. Enders G, Miller E, Cradock Watson J, Bolley I, Ridehalgh M 1994 Consequences of varicella and herpes zoster in pregnancy: prospective study of 1739 cases. Lancet 343: 1548–1551

232. Epps R E, Pittelkow M R, Su W P 1995 TORCH syndrome. Seminars in Dermatology 14: 179–186

233. Eregie C O, Ofovwe G 1995 Factors associated with neonatal tetanus mortality in northern Nigeria. East African Medical Journal 72: 507–509

234. Eriksen N L, Blanco J D 1993 Group B streptococcal infection in pregnancy. Seminars in Perinatology 17: 432–442

235. Eriksson M, Bennett R, Nord C E, Zetterstrom R 1986 Fecal bacterial microflora of newborn infants during intensive care management and treatment with five antibiotic regimes. Pediatric Infectious Disease Journal 5: 533–539

236. Eriksson M, Melen B, Myrback K E, Winbladh B, Zetterstrom R 1982 Bacterial colonization of newborn infants in a neonatal intensive care unit. Acta Paediatrica Scandinavica 71: 779–783

237. Escobar G J 1999 The neonatal "sepsis work-up": personal reflections on the development of an evidence-based approach toward newborn infections in a managed care organization. Pediatrics 103: e360

238. Escobar G J, Zukin T, Usatin M S et al 1994 Early discontinuation of antibiotic treatment in newborns admitted to rule out sepsis: a decision rule. Pediatric Infectious Disease Journal 13: 860–866

239. European Centre for the Epidemiological Monitoring of AIDS 1994 AIDS surveillance in Europe. Quarterly Report No 44: 41–53

240. European Collaborative Study 1992 Risk factors for mother-to-child transmission of HIV-1. Lancet 339: 1007–1012

241. European Collaborative Study 1994 Caesarean section and risk of vertical transmission of HIV-1 infection. Lancet 343: 1464–1467

242. Evans I A, Jones C A 2002 Maternal immunization with a herpes simplex virus type 2 replication-defective virus reduces visceral dissemination but not lethal encephalitis in newborn mice after oral challenge. Journal of Infectious Diseases 185: 1550–1560

243. Ewert D P, Lieb L, Hayes P S, Reeves M W, Mascola L 1995 Listeria monocytogenes infection and serotype distribution among HIV-infected persons in Los Angeles County, 1985–1992. Journal of Acquired Immune Deficiency Syndromes and Human Retrovirology 8: 461–465

244. Fagan E A, Hadzic N, Saxena R, Mieli-Vergani G 1999 Symptomatic neonatal hepatitis A disease from a virus variant acquired in utero. Pediatric Infectious Disease Journal 18: 389–391

245. Faix R G 1992 Invasive neonatal candidiasis: comparison of albicans and parapsilosis infection. Pediatric Infectious Disease Journal 11: 88–93

246. Fajemilehin B R 1995 Neonatal tetanus among rural-born Nigerian infants. Maternal-Child Nursing Journal 23: 39–43

247. Falla T J, Dobson S R, Crook D W et al 1993 Population-based study of non-typable Haemophilus influenzae invasive disease in children and neonates. Lancet 341: 851–854

248. Fanaroff A A, Korones S B, Wright L L et al 1998 Incidence, presenting features, risk factors and significance of late onset septicemia in very low birth weight infants. The National Institute of Child Health and Human Development Neonatal Research Network. Pediatric Infectious Disease Journal 17: 593–598

249. Farber B F, Kaplan M H, Clogston A G 1990 Staphylococcus epidermidis extracted slime inhibits the antimicrobial action of glycopeptide antibiotics. Journal of Infectious Diseases 161: 37–41

250. Farber J M, Peterkin P I, Carter A O, Varughese P V, Ashton F E, Ewan E P 1991 Neonatal listeriosis due to cross-infection confirmed by isoenzyme typing and DNA fingerprinting [letter]. Journal of Infectious Diseases 163: 927–928

251. Fasano C, O'Keeffe J, Gibbs D 1994 Fluconazole treatment of neonates and infants with severe fungal infections not treatable with conventional agents. European Journal of Clinical Microbiology and Infectious Diseases 13: 351–354

252. Fekety F R, Buchbinder L, Shaffer E L 1958 Control of an outbreak of staphylo-coccal infections among mothers and infants in a suburban hospital. American Journal of Public Health 48: 298–303

253. Feldman W E 1979 Bacterial etiology and mortality of purulent pericarditis in paediatric patients. Review of 162 cases. American Journal of Diseases of Children 133: 641–647

254. Fernandes R M, Carbonare S B, Carneiro-Sampaio M M, Trabulsi L R 2001 Inhibition of enteroaggregative Escherichia coli adhesion to HEp-2 cells by secretory immunoglobulin A from human colostrum. Pediatric Infectious Disease Journal 20: 672–678

255. Fernandez M, Rench M A, Baker C J 1999 Neonatal sepsis caused simultan-eously by two serotypes of group B Streptococcus. Pediatric Infectious Disease Journal 18: 391–393

256. Fernando S, Pearce J M, Booth J C 1993 Lymphocyte responses and virus excretion as risk factors for intrauterine infection with cytomegalovirus. Journal of Medical Virology 41: 108–113

257. Figueroa-Damian R, Arredondo-Garcia J L 2001 Neonatal outcome of children born to women with tuberculosis. Archives of Medical Research 32: 66–69

258. Finelli L, Livengood J R, Saiman L 1994 Surveillance of pharyngeal coloniza-tion: detection and control of serious bacterial illness in low birth weight infants. Pediatric Infectious Disease Journal 13: 854–859

259. Fiore A E 2002 Chronic maternal hepatitis B infection and premature rupture of membranes. Pediatric Infectious Disease Journal 21: 357–358

260. Fischer E G, McLennan J E, Suzuki Y 1981 Cerebral abcess in children. American Journal of Diseases of Children 135: 746–749

261. Fischer G W 1994 Use of intravenous immune globulin in newborn infants. Clinical and Experimental Immunology 97(suppl. 1): 73–77

262. Fleming D W, Cochi S L, MacDonald K L 1985 Pasteurised milk as a vehicle of infection in an outbreak of listeriosis. New England Journal of Medicine 312: 404–407

263. Flenady V, King J 2002 Antibiotics for prelabour rupture of membranes at or near term (Cochrane Review). Cochrane Database of Systematic Reviews (3): CD001807

264. Fletcher J L J 1991 Perinatal transmission of human papillomavirus. American Family Physician 43: 143–148

265. Foca M, Jakob K, Whittier S et al 2000 Endemic Pseudomonas aeruginosa infection in a neonatal intensive care unit. New England Journal of Medicine 343: 695–700

266. Fonseca S N, Ehrenkranz R A, Baltimore R S 1994 Epidemiology of antibiotic use in a neonatal intensive care unit. Infection Control and Hospital Epidemiology 15: 156–162

267. Fortnum H, Davis A 1993 Hearing impairment in children after bacterial meningitis: incidence and resource implications. British Journal of Audiology 27: 43–52

268. Fortnum H M, Davis A C 1993 Epidemiology of bacterial meningitis. Archives of Disease in Childhood 68: 763–767

269. Fowler K B, Stagno S, Pass R F 1993 Maternal age and congenital cytomegalovirus infection: screening of two diverse newborn populations, 1980–1990. Journal of Infectious Diseases 168: 552–556

270. Fowler K B, Stagno S, Pass R F, Britt W J, Boll T J, Alford C A 1992 The outcome of congenital cytomegalovirus infection in relation to maternal antibody status. New England Journal of Medicine 326: 663–667

271. Fowlie P W, Schmidt B 1998 Diagnostic tests for bacterial infection from birth to 90 days – a systematic review. Archives of Disease in Childhood. Fetal and Neonatal Edition 78: F92–F98

272. Franco S M, Cornelius V E, Andrews B F 1992 Long-term outcome of neonatal meningitis. American Journal of Diseases of Children 146: 567–571

273. Fraser S H, O'Keefe R J, Scurry J P, Watkins A M, Drew J H, Chow C W 1994 Hydrocephalus ex vacuo and clasp thumb deformity due to congenital cytomegalovirus infection. Journal of Paediatrics and Child Health 30: 450–452

274. Frederiksen B, Samuelsson S 1992 Feto-maternal listeriosis in Denmark 1981–1988. Journal of Infection 24: 277–287

275. Freedman M H, Bonilla M A, Fier C 1999 Improved survival from granulocyte-colony stimulating factor therapy for congenital neutropenia unmasks predisposition to myelodysplasia and acute myeloid leukaemia. Pediatric Research 45: 747–752

276. Friedman C A, Temple D M, Robbins K K, Rawson J E, Wilson J P, Feldman S 1994 Outbreak and control of varicella in a neonatal intensive care unit. Pediatric Infectious Disease Journal 13: 152–154

277. Friedman C A, Wende D F, Rawson J E 1984 Rapid diagnosis of group B streptococcal infection utilizing a commercially available latex agglutination assay. Pediatrics 73: 27–30

278. Friedman S, Richardson S E, Jacobs S E, O'Brien K 2000 Systemic Candida infection in extremely low birth weight infants: short term morbidity and long term neurodevelopmental outcome. Pediatric Infectious Disease Journal 19: 499–504

279. Fukuda S, Miyachi M, Sugimoto S, Goshima A, Futamura M, Morishima T 1995 A female infant successfully treated by ganciclovir for congenital cytomegalovirus infection. Acta Paediatrica Japonica 37: 206–210

280. Gajdusek D C 1957 Pneumocystis carinii – etiologic agent of interstitial plasma cell pneumonia of perinatal and young infants. Pediatrics 19: 543–565

281. Gannon H 1993 Ureaplasma urealyticum and its role in neonatal lung disease. Neonatal Network 12: 13–18

282. Garcia Alix A, Martin Ancel A, Ramos M T et al 1995 Cerebrospinal fluid beta 2-microglobulin in neonates with central nervous system infections. European Journal of Pediatrics 154: 309–313

283. Garcia Rodriguez M C, Bates I, de Jose I et al 1995 Prognostic value of immunological data, in vitro antibody production, and virus culture in vertical infection with HIV-1. Archives of Disease in Childhood 72: 498–501

284. Garland J S, Dunne W M J, Havens P et al 1992 Peripheral intravenous catheter complications in critically ill children: a prospective study. Pediatrics 89: 1145–1150

285. Garland S M 1991 Early onset neonatal group B streptococcus (GBS) infection: associated obstetric risk factors. Australian and New Zealand Journal of Obstetrics and Gynaecology 31: 117–118

286. Garner P, Lai D, Baea M, Edwards K, Heywood P 1994 Avoiding neonatal death: an intervention study of umbilical cord care. Journal of Tropical Pediatrics 40: 24–28

287. Garrett D O, McDonald L C, Wanderley A et al 2002 An outbreak of neonatal deaths in Brazil associated with contaminated intravenous fluids. Journal of Infectious Diseases 186: 81–86

288. Gay N J, Hesketh L M, Cohen B J et al 1994 Age specific antibody prevalence to parvovirus B19: how many women are infected in pregnancy? Commicable Disease Report. CDR Review 4: 104–107

289. Gaynes R P, Martone W J, Culver D H et al 1991 Comparison of rates of nosocomial infections in neonatal intensive care units in the United States. National Nosocomial Infections Surveillance System. American Journal of Medicine 91: 192S–196S

290. Gellert G A, Ewert D P, Bendana N et al 1993 A cluster of coagulase-negative staphylococcal bacteremias associated with peripheral vascular catheter colonization in a neonatal intensive care unit. American Journal of Infection Control 21: 16–20

291. Gellin B G, Broome C V 1989 Listeriosis. Journal of the American Medical Association 261: 1313–1319

292. Gendrel D, Bohuon C 2000 Procalcitonin as a marker of bacterial infection. Pediatric Infectious Disease Journal 19: 679–687

293. Georgiev V S 1994 Management of toxoplasmosis. Drugs 48: 179–188

294. Gerdes J S 1991 Clinicopathologic approach to the diagnosis of neonatal sepsis. Clinics in Perinatology 18: 361–381

295. Gessler P, Kirchmann N, Kientsch Engel R, Haas N, Lasch P, Kachel W 1993 Serum concentrations of granulocyte colony-stimulating factor in healthy term and preterm neonates and in those with various diseases including bacterial infections. Blood 82: 3177–3182

296. Giacoia G P, Neter E, Ogra P 1981 Respiratory infections in infants on mechanical ventilators. The immune response as a diagnostic aid. Journal of Pediatrics 98: 691–695

297. Gibb D M, Neave P, Tookey P A et al 2000 Active surveillance of hepatitis C infection in the UK and Ireland. Archives of Disease in Childhood 82: 286–291

298. Gibbs R S, McDuffie R S J, McNabb F, Fryer G E, Miyoshi T, Merenstein G 1994 Neonatal group B streptococcal sepsis during 2 years of a universal screening program. Obstetrics and Gynecology 84: 496–500

299. Gibson R L, Soderland C, Henderson W R J, Chi E Y, Rubens C E 1995 Group B streptococci (GBS) injure lung endothelium in vitro: GBS invasion and GBS-induced eicosanoid production is greater with microvascular than with pulmonary artery cells. Infection and Immunity 63: 271–279

300. Gillan E R, Christensen R D, Suen Y, Ellis R, van de Ven C, Cairo M S 1994 A randomized, placebo-controlled trial of recombinant human granulocyte colony-stimulating factor administration in newborn infants with presumed sepsis: significant induction of peripheral and bone marrow neutrophilia. Blood 84: 1427–1433

301. Givens K T, Lee D A, Jones T, Ilstrup D M 1993 Congenital rubella syndrome: ophthalmic manifestations and associated systemic disorders [see comments]. British Journal of Ophthalmology 77: 358–363

302. Gjuric G, Prislin Muskic M, Nikolic E, Zurga B 1994 Ureaplasma urealyticum osteomyelitis in a very low birth weight infant. Journal of Perinatal Medicine 22: 79–81

303. Gladstone I M, Ehrenkranz R A, Edberg S C, Baltimore R S 1990 A ten-year review of neonatal sepsis and comparison with the previous fifty-year experience. Pediatric Infectious Disease Journal 9: 819–825

304. Gleeson F V, Gordon I 1991 Imaging in urinary tract infection. Archives of Disease in Childhood 66: 1282–1283

305. Glick C, Graves G R, Feldman S 1993 Neonatal fungemia and amphotericin B. Southern Medical Journal 86: 1368–1371

306. Gogus S, Umer H, Akcoren Z, Sanal O, Osmanlioglu G, Cimbis M 1993 Neonatal tuberculosis. Pediatric Pathology 13: 299–304

307. Goldberg D, McMenamin J 1998 The United Kingdom's hepatitis B immunisation strategy. Communicable Disease and Public Health 1: 79–83

308. Golden S E 1988 Neonatal herpes simplex viremia. Pediatric Infectious Disease Journal 7: 425–426

309. Goldenberg R L, Hauth J C, Andrews W W 2000 Intrauterine infection and preterm delivery. New England Journal of Medicine 342: 1500–1507

310. Goldman M, Lahat E, Strauss S et al 2000 Imaging after urinary tract infection in male neonates. Pediatrics 105: 1232–1235

311. Gomez M, Alter S, Kumar M L, Murphy S, Rathore M H 1999 Neonatal Streptococcus pneumoniae infection: case reports and review of the literature. Pediatric Infectious Disease Journal 18: 1014–1018

312. Gomez R, Ghezzi F, Romero R, Munoz H, Tolosa J E, Rojas I 1995 Premature labor and intra-amniotic infection. Clinical aspects and role of the cytokines in diagnosis and pathophysiology. Clinics in Perinatology 22: 281–342

313. Goto M, Zeller W P, Hurley R M, Jong J S, Lee C H 1991 Prophylaxis and treatment of newborn endotoxic shock with anti-lipid A monoclonal antibodies. Circulatory Shock 35: 60–64

314. Gottbrath Flaherty E K, Agrawal R, Thaker V, Patel D, Ghai K 1995 Urinary tract infections in cocaine-exposed infants. Journal of Perinatology 15: 203–207

315. Gravel Tropper D, Sample M L, Oxley C, Toye B, Woods D E, Garber G E 1996 Three-year outbreak of pseudobacteremia with Burkholderia cepacia traced to a contaminated blood gas analyzer [see comments]. Infection Control and Hospital Epidemiology 17: 737–740

316. Graves G G, Rhodes P G 1984 Tachycardia as a sign of early-onset neonatal sepsis. Pediatric Infectious Disease Journal 3: 404–406

317. Gray E S, Peters G, Verstegen M 1984 Effect of extracellular slime substance from Staphylococcus epidermidis on the human cellular immune response. Lancet i: 365–367

318. Gray J E, Richardson D K, McCormick M C, Goldmann D A 1995 Coagulase-negative staphylococcal bacteremia among very low birth weight infants: relation to admission illness severity, resource use, and outcome. Pediatrics 95: 225–230

319. Gray M L 1960 Genital Listeriosis as a cause of repeated abortion. Lancet 2: 296–297

320. Green M, Dashefsky B, Wald E R, Laifer S, Harge, J, Guthrie R 1993 Comparison of two antigen assays for rapid intrapartum detection of vaginal group B streptococcal colonization. Journal of Clinical Microbiology 31: 78–82

321. Green P A, Singh K V, Murray B E, Baker C J 1994 Recurrent group B streptococcal infections in infants: clinical and microbiologic aspects. Journal of Pediatrics 125: 931–938

322. Greenberg D N, Yoder B A 1990 Changes in the differential white blood cell count in screening for group B streptococcal sepsis. Pediatric Infectious Disease Journal 9: 886–889

323. Greenberg D, Leibovitz E, Shinnwell E S, Yagupsky P, Dagan R 1999 Neonatal sepsis caused by Streptococcus pyogenes: resurgence of an old etiology? Pediatric Infectious Disease Journal 18: 479–481

324. Greene K A, Rhine W D, Starnes V A, Ariagno R L 1990 Fatal postoperative Legionella pneumonia in a newborn. Journal of Perinatology 10: 183–184

325. Greenes D S, Rowitch D, Thorne G M, Perez Atayde A, Lee F S, Goldmann D 1995 Neonatal herpes simplex virus infection presenting as fulminant liver failure. Pediatric Infectious Disease Journal 14: 242–244

326. Gressens P, Langston C, Martin J R 1994 In situ PCR localization of herpes simplex virus DNA sequences in disseminated neonatal herpes encephalitis. Journal of Neuropathology and Experimental Neurology 53: 469–482

327. Grigg J M, Barber A, Silverman M 1992 Increased levels of bronchoalveolar lavage fluid interleukin-6 in preterm ventilated infants after prolonged rupture of membranes. American Review of Respiratory Disease 145: 782–786

328. Grio R, Porpiglia M, Vetro E et al 1994 Asymptomatic bacteriuria in pregnancy: maternal and fetal complications. Panminerva Medicine 36: 198–200

329. Gruskay J A, Nachamkin I, Baumgart S 1986 Predicting the pathogenicity of coagulase negative staphylococci in the neonate: slime production, antibiotic resistance and predominance of S. epidermidis species. Pediatric Research 20: 397A

330. Guerina N G, Hsu H W, Meissner H C et al 1994 Neonatal serologic screening and early treatment for congenital Toxoplasma gondii infection. The New England Regional Toxoplasma Working Group. New England Journal of Medicine 330: 1858–1863

331. Guillois B, Donnou M D, Sizun J, Bendaoud B, Youinou P 1994 Comparative study of four tests of bacterial infection in the neonate. Total neutrophil count, CRP, fibrinogen and C3d. Biology of the Neonate 66: 175–181

332. Gupta A K, Shashi S, Mohan M, lamba I M, Gupta R 1993 Epidemiology of Pseudomonas aeruginosa infections in a neonatal intensive care unit. Journal of Tropical Pediatrics 39: 32–36

333. Gupta S D, Keyl P M 1998 Effectiveness of prenatal tetanus toxoid immunization against neonatal tetanus in a rural area in India. Pediatric Infectious Disease Journal 17: 316–321

334. Gurtler R E, Segura E L, Cohen J E 2003 Congenital transmission of Trypanosoma cruzi infection in Argentina. Emerging Infectious Diseases 9: 29–32

335. Gutman L T, Wilfert C M, Eppes S 1986 Herpes simplex virus encephalitis in children: analysis of cerebrospinal fluid and progressive neurodevelopmental deterioration. Journal of Infectious Diseases 154: 415–421

336. Hachey W E, Wiswell T E 1992 Limitations in the usefulness of urine latex particle agglutination tests and hematologic measurements in diagnosing neonatal sepsis during the first week of life. Journal of Perinatology 12: 240–245

337. Hague R A, Rassam S, Morgan G, Cant A J 1994 Early diagnosis of severe combined immunodeficiency syndrome. Archives of Disease in Childhood 70: 260–263

338. Haley R W, Cushion N B, Tenover F C et al 1995 Eradication of endemic methicillin-resistant Staphylococcus aureus infections from a neonatal intensive care unit. Journal of Infectious Diseases 171: 614–624

339. Hall C B, Long C E, Schnabel K C et al 1994 Human herpesvirus-6 infection in children. A prospective study of complications and reactivation. New England Journal of Medicine 331: 432–438

340. Hall R T, Shigeoka A O, Hill H R 1983 Serum opsonic activity and peripheral neutrophil counts before and after exchange transfusion in infants with early onset group B streptococcal septicemia. Pediatric Infectious Disease 2: 356–358

341. Hall S M 1983 Congenital toxoplasmosis in England, Wales and Northern Ireland: some epidemiological problems. British Medical Journal 287: 453–455

342. Hall S, Glickman B 1991 The British Paediatric Surveillance Unit. New England Journal of Medicine 63: 344–346

343. Halliday H L 1989 When to do a lumbar puncture in a neonate [see comments]. Archives of Disease in Childhood 64: 313–316

344. Halliday H L, McClure B G, Reid D, Lappin T R, Meban C, Thomas P S 1984 Controlled trial of artificial surfactant to prevent respiratory distress syndrome. Lancet 1: 476–478

345. Hammerberg O, Bialkowska Hobrzanska H, Gregson D, Potters H, Gopal J, Reid D 1992 Comparison of blood cultures with corresponding venipuncture site cultures of specimens from hospitalised premature neonates. Journal of Pediatrics 120: 120–124

346. Hammerschlag M R, Cummings C, Roblin P M, Williams T H, Delke I 1989 Efficacy of neonatal ocular prophylaxis for the prevention of chlamydial and gonococcal conjunctivitis. New England Journal of Medicine 320: 769–772

347. Hammerschlag M R, Gelling M, Roblin P M, Kutlin A, Jule J E 1998 Treatment of neonatal chlamydial conjunctivitis with azithromycin. Pediatric Infectious Disease Journal 17: 1049–1050

348. Hampl S D, Olson L C 1995 Pertussis in the young infant. Seminars in Respiratory Infections 10: 58–62

349. Hamprecht K, Maschmann J, Vochem M, Dietz K, Speer C P, Jahn G 2001 Epidemiology of transmission of cytomegalovirus from mother to preterm infant by breastfeeding. Lancet 357: 513–518

350. Hamrick W B, Reilly L 1992 A comparison of infection rates in a newborn intensive care unit before and after adoption of open visitation. Neonatal Network 11: 15–18

351. Hanshaw J B, Dudgeon J A 1978 Viral disease of the fetus and newborn. W B Saunders, Philadelphia, p. 198

352. Haque K N, Chagia A H, Shaheed M M 1990 Half a decade of neonatal sepsis, Riyadh, Saudi Arabia. Journal of Tropical Pediatrics 36: 20–23

353. Harbarth S, Pittet D, Grady L et al 2002 Interventional study to evaluate the impact of an alcohol-based hand gel in improving hand hygiene compliance. Pediatric Infectious Disease Journal 21: 489–495

354. Harris J A 1998 Infection control for neonatal gram-negative bacterial infections. Pediatric Infectious Disease Journal 17: 532–533

355. Harrison L H, Elliot J A, Dwyer D M et al 1998 Serotype distribution of invasive group B streptococcal isolates in Maryland: implications for vaccine formulation. Maryland Emerging Infections Program. Journal of Infectious Diseases 177: 998–1002

356. Hart M H, Kaufman S S, Vanderhoof J A et al 1991 Neonatal hepatitis and extrahepatic biliary atresia associated with cytomegalovirus infection in twins. American Journal of Diseases of Children 145: 302–305

357. Hawken J, Chard T, Costeloe K, Jeffries D J, Hudson C N 1995 Risk factors for HIV infection overlooked in routine antenatal care. Journal of the Royal Society of Medicine 88: 634–636

358. Hawkins S 1995 Water vs conventional births: infection rates compared. Nursing Times 91: 38–40

359. Heath P, Nicoll A, Efstratiou A 2001 Group B streptococcal disease. In: Lynn R, Kirkbride H, Rahi J, Verity C (eds) British Paediatric Surveillance Unit 15th Annual Report 2000–2001. BPSU, London, pp 17–19

360. Heegaard E D, Hasle H, Skibsted L, Bock J, Brown K E 2000 Congenital anemia caused by parvovirus B19 infection. Pediatric Infectious Disease Journal 19: 1216–1218

361. Heggie A D, Bar-Shain D, Boxerbaum B, Fanaroff A A, O'Riordan M A, Robertson J A 2001 Identification and quantification of ureaplasmas colonizing the respiratory tract and assessment of their role in the development of chronic lung disease in preterm infants. Pediatric Infectious Disease Journal 20: 854–859

362. Heggie A D, Jacobs M R, Butler V T, Baley J E, Boxerbaum B 1994 Frequency and significance of isolation of Ureaplasma urealyticum and Mycoplasma hominis from cerebrospinal fluid and tracheal aspirate specimens from low birth weight infants. Journal of Pediatrics 124: 956–961

363. Henderson C E 1995 Management of tuberculosis in pregnancy. Journal of the Association for Academic Minority Physicians 6: 38–42

364. Henderson S L, Lindsay M K, Higgins J E, Clark W S, Bulterys M, Nesheim S R 2001 Experience with routine voluntary perinatal human immunodeficiency virus testing in an inner city hospital. Pediatric Infectious Disease Journal 20: 1090–1094

365. Hendricks Munoz K D, Shapiro D L 1990 The role of the lumbar puncture in the admission sepsis evaluation of the premature infant. Journal of Perinatology 10: 60–64

366. Hennequin C, Dureau P, N'Guyen L, Thulliez P, Gagelin B, Dufier J L 1997 Congenital toxoplasmosis acquired from an immune woman. Pediatric Infectious Disease Journal 16: 75–77

367. Herman T E, Siegel M J 1994 Special imaging casebook. Congenital disseminated herpes simplex infection with visceral calcifications. Journal of Perinatology 14: 80–82

368. Herting E, Gefeller O, Land M, van Sonderen L, Harms K, Robertson B & Members of the Collaborative European Multicenter Study Group 2000

Surfactant treatment of neonates with respiratory failure and group B strepto-coccal infection. Pediatrics 106: 957–964

369. Hervas J A, Ballesteros F, Alomar A, Gil J, Benedi V J, Alberti S 2001 Increase of Enterobacter in neonatal sepsis: a twenty-two-year study. Pediatric Infectious Disease Journal 20: 134–140

370. Hervas J A, Gonzalez L, Gil J, Paoletti L C, Madoff L C, Benedi V J 1993 Neonatal group B streptococcal infection in Mallorca, Spain. Clinical Infectious Diseases 16: 714–718

371. Hibbard J U, Hibbard M C, Ismail M, Arendt E 1993 Pregnancy outcome after expectant management of premature rupture of the membranes in the second trimester. Journal of Reproductive Medicine 38: 945–951

372. Hilton D A, Variend S, Pringle J H 1993 Demonstration of Coxsackie virus RNA in formalin-fixed tissue sections from childhood myocarditis cases by in situ hybridization and the polymerase chain reaction. Journal of Pathology 170: 45–51

373. Hirschl R B, Butler M, Coburn C E, Bartlett R H, Baumgart S 1994 Listeria monocytogenes and severe newborn respiratory failure supported with extracorporeal membrane oxygenation. Archives of Pediatrics and Adolescent Medicine 148: 513–517

374. Hitchcock R J, Pallett A, Hall M A, Malone P S 1995 Urinary tract candidiasis in neonates and infants. British Journal of Urology 76: 252–256

375. Ho N K, Low Y P, See H F 1989 Septic arthritis in the newborn – a 17 years' clinical experience. Singapore Medical Journal 30: 356–358

376. Hodge D, Puntis J W L 2002 Diagnosis, prevention, and management of catheter related bloodstream infection during long term parenteral nutrition. Archives of Disease in Childhood. Fetal and Neonatal Edition 87: F21–F24

377. Hohlfeld P, Daffos F, Costa J M, Thulliez P, Forestier F, Vidaud M 1994 Prenatal diagnosis of congenital toxoplasmosis with a polymerase-chain-reaction test on amniotic fluid. New England Journal of Medicine 331: 695–699

378. Hohlfeld P, Daffos F, Thulliez P et al 1989 Fetal toxoplasmosis: outcome of pregnancy and infant follow-up after in utero treatment [see comments]. Journal of Pediatrics 115: 765–769

379. Holland P, Isaacs D, Moxon E R 1986 Fatal neonatal varicella infection. Lancet ii: 1156

380. Holliman R E, Raymond R, Renton N, Johnson J D 1994 The diagnosis of toxoplasmosis using IgG avidity. Epidemiology and Infection 112: 399–408

381. Holmberg R E J, Pavia A T, Montgomery D, Clark J M, Eggert L D 1993 Nosocomial Legionella pneumonia in the neonate. Pediatrics 92: 450–453

382. Holt D E, Halket S, de Louvois J, Harvey D 2001 Neonatal meningitis in England and Wales: 10 years on, Archives of Disease in Childhood. Fetal and Neonatal Edition 84: 85–89

383. Hoosen A A, Kharsany A B, Ison C A 2002 Single low-dose ceftriaxone for the treatment of gonococcal ophthalmia – implications for the national programme for the syndromic management of sexually transmitted diseases. South African Medical Journal 92: 238–240

384. Hoppe J E 2000 Neonatal pertussis. Pediatric Infectious Disease Journal 19: 244–247

385. Horstmann D M, Schlueuderberg A, Emmons J E, Evans B K, Randolph M F, Andiman W A 1985 Persistence of vaccine-induced immune response to rubella: comparison with natural infection. Reviews of Infectious Diseases 7(suppl.): 80–85

386. Hostoffer R W, Litman A, Smith P G, Jacobs H S, Tosi M F 1993 Pneumocystis carinii pneumonia in a term newborn infant with a transiently depressed T lymphocyte count, primarily of cells carrying the CD4 antigen. Journal of Pediatrics 122: 792–794

387. Hristeva L, Booy R, Bowle I, Wilkinson A R 1993 Prospective surveillance of neonatal meningitis [see comments]. Archives of Disease in Childhood 69: 14–18

388. Hristeva L, Bowle I, Booy R, King A T, Wilkinson A R 1993 Value of cere-brospinal fluid examination in the diagnosis of meningitis in the newborn. Archives of Disease in Childhood 69: 514–517

389. Hruszkewycz V, Holtrop P C, Batton D G, Morden R S, Gibson P, Band J D 1991 Complications associated with central venous catheters inserted in criti-cally ill neonates. Infection Control and Hospital Epidemiology 12: 544–548

390. Hsieh W S, Yang P H, Chao H C, Lai J Y 1999 Neonatal necrotizing fasciitis: a report of three cases and review of the literature. Pediatrics 103: e53

391. Huebner J, Pier G B, Maslow J N et al 1994 Endemic nosocomial transmission of Staphylococcus epidermidis bacteremia isolates in a neonatal intensive care unit over 10 years. Journal of Infectious Diseases 169: 526–531

392. Hufert F T, Diebold T, Ermisch B, Von Laer D, Meyer Konig U, Neumann Haefelin D 1995 Liver failure due to disseminated HSV-1 infection in a new-born twin. Scandinavian Journal of Infectious Diseases 27: 627–629

393. Hung F C, Huang C B, Huang S C, Liu S T 1994 Congenital cutaneous candidiasis – report of two cases. Changgeng Yi Xue Za Zhi 17: 63–67

394. Hurtig A K, Nicoll A, Carne C, Lissauer T, Connor N, Webster J P, Ratcliffe L 1998 Syphilis in pregnant women and their children in the United Kingdom: results from national clinician reporting surveys 1994–7. British Medical Journal 317: 1617–1619

395. Hussain F M, Boyle-Vavra S, Shete P B, Daum R S 2002 Evidence for a contin-uum of decreased vancomycin susceptibility in unselected Staphylococcus aureus clinical isolates. Journal of Infectious Diseases 186: 661–667

396. Hutto C, Arvin A, Jacobs R 1987 Intrauterine herpes simplex virus infections. Journal of Pediatrics 110: 97–101

397. Huttova M, Hartmanova I, Kralinsky K et al 1998 Candida fungemia in neonates treated with fluconazole: report of forty cases, including eight with meningitis. Pediatric Infectious Disease Journal 17: 1012–1015

398. Hwa H L, Shyu M K, Lee C N, Wu C C, Kao C L, Hsieh F J 1994 Prenatal diagnosis of congenital rubella infection from maternal rubella in Taiwan. Obstetrics and Gynecology 84: 415–419

399. Hyde S R, Giacoia G P 1993 Congenital herpes infection: placental and umbilical cord findings. Obstetrics and Gynecology 81: 852–855

400. Hylander M A, Strobino D M, Dhanireddy R 1998 Human milk feedings and infection among very low birth weight infants. Pediatrics 102: e38

401. Ibhanesebhor S E 1995 Clinical characteristics of neonatal malaria. Journal of Tropical Pediatrics 41: 330–333

402. Idema C D, Harris B N, Ogunbanjo G A, Durrheim D N 2002 Neonatal tetanus elimination in Mpumalanga Province, South Africa. Tropical Medicine and International Health 7: 622–624

403. Ingram D L 1994 Neisseria gonorrhoeae in children. Pediatric Annals 23: 341–345

404. Isaacman D J, Karasic R B, Reynolds E A, Kost S I 1996 Effect of number of blood cultures and volume of blood on detection of bacteremia in children. Journal of Pediatrics 128: 190–195

405. Isaacs D 2003 A ten-year, multicentre study of coagulase negative staphylococ-cal infections in Australian neonatal units. Archives of Disease in Childhood. Fetal and Neonatal Edition 88: F89–F93

406. Isaacs D A V I 1998 Prevention of early onset group B streptococcal infection: screen, treat, or observe? Archives of Disease in Childhood. Fetal and Neonatal Edition 79: F81–F82

407. Isaacs D, Barfield C P, Grimwood K, McPhee A J, Minutillo C, Tudehope D I 1995 Systemic bacterial and fungal infections in infants in Australian neonatal units. Australian Study Group for Neonatal Infections. Medical Journal of Australia 162: 198–201

408. Isaacs D, Barfield C, Clothier T et al 1996 Late-onset infections of infants in neonatal units. Journal of Paediatrics and Child Health 32: 158–161

409. Isaacs D, Dobson S R, Wilkinson A R, Hope P L, Eglin R, Moxon E R 1989 Conservative management of an Echovirus 11 outbreak in a neonatal unit. Lancet 1: 543–545

410. Isaacs D, Moxon E R 1991 Neonatal infections. Butterworth Heinemann, Oxford, pp 149–166

411. Isenberg S J, Apt L, Wood M 1995 A controlled trial of povidone-iodine as prophylaxis against opthalmia neonatorum. New England Journal of Medicine 332: 562–566

412. Ish Horowicz M R, McIntyre P, Nade S 1992 Bone and joint infections caused by multiply resistant Staphylococcus aureus in a neonatal intensive care unit. Pediatric Infectious Disease Journal 11: 82–87

413. Israele V, Darabi A, McCracken G H 1987 The role of bacterial virulence factors and Tamm-Horsfall protein in the pathogenesis of Escherichia coli urinary tract infection in infants. American Journal of Diseases of Children 141: 1230–1234

414. Issekutz T B, Evans J, Bortolussi R 1984 The immune response of human neonates to Listeria monocytogenes infection. Clinical and Investigative Medicine 7: 263–266

415. Itoh K, Aihara H, Takada S et al 1990 Clinicopathological differences between early-onset and late-onset sepsis and pneumonia in very low birth weight infants. Pediatric Pathology 10: 757–768

416. Ivarsson S A, Lernmark B, Svanberg L 1997 Ten-year clinical, developmental, and intellectual follow-up of children with congenital cytomegalovirus infection without neurologic symptoms at one year of age. Pediatrics 99: 800–803

417. Jacob J, Edwards D, Gluck L 1980 Early-onset sepsis and pneumonia observed as respiratory distress syndrome: assessment of lung maturity. American Journal of Diseases of Children 134: 766–768

418. Jacobs J, Garmyn K, Verhaegen J, Devlieger H, Eggermont E 1990 Neonatal sepsis due to Streptococcus pneumoniae. Scandinavian Journal of Infectious Diseases 22: 493–497

419. Jakobsson B, Berg U, Svensson L 1994 Renal scarring after acute pyelonephri-tis. Archives of Disease in Childhood 70: 111–115

420. Jankovic B, Pasic S, Kanjuh B, Bukumirovic K, Cvetanovic G, Todorovic N, Djuricic S 1999 Severe neonatal echovirus 17 infection during a nursery outbreak. Pediatric Infectious Disease Journal 18: 393–394

421. Jantos C A, Wienpahl B, Schiefer H G, Wagner F, Hegemann J H 1995 Infection with Chlamydia pneumoniae in infants and children with acute lower respiratory tract disease. Pediatric Infectious Disease Journal 14: 117–122

422. Jara M, Hsu H W, Eaton R B, Demaria A Jr 2001 Epidemiology of congenital toxoplasmosis identified by population-based newborn screening in Massachusetts. Pediatric Infectious Disease Journal 20: 1132–1135

423. Jeffery H E, McIntosh E D 1994 Antepartum screening and non-selective intrapartum chemoprophylaxis for group B streptococcus. Australian and New Zealand Journal of Obstetrics and Gynaecology 34: 14–19

424. Jeffery H E, Mitchison R, Wigglesworth J S, Davies P A 1977 Early neonatal bacteraemia: comparison of group B streptococcal, other gram-positive and gram-negative infections. Archives of Disease in Childhood 52: 683–686

425. Jeffries D J 1991 Intra-uterine and neonatal herpes simplex virus infection. Scandinavian Journal of Infectious Diseases. Supplementum 80: 21–26

426. Johnson C E, Whitwell J K, Pethe K, Saxena K, Super D M 1997 Term newborns who are at risk for sepsis: are lumbar punctures necessary? Pediatrics 99: e10

427. Johnson G M, Lee D A, Regelmann W E 1986 Interference with granulocyte function by Staphylococcus epidermidis slime. Infection and Immunity 54: 13–16

428. Jones C A, Isaacs D 1995 Predicting the outcome of symptomatic congenital cytomegalovirus infection. Journal of Paediatrics and Child Health 31: 70–71

429. Jones E M, McCulloch S Y, Reeves D S, MacGowan A P 1994 A 10 year survey of the epidemiology and clinical aspects of listeriosis in a provincial English city. Journal of Infection 29: 91–103

430. Jones K L, Johnson K A, Chambers C D 1994 Offspring of women infected with varicella during pregnancy: a prospective study. Teratology 49: 29–32

431. Kacica M A, Horgan M J, Ochoa L, Sandler R, Lepow M L, Venezia R A 1994 Prevention of gram-positive sepsis in neonates weighing less than 1500 grams. Journal of Pediatrics 125: 253–258

432. Kahi S, Cozon G J, Peyron F 1999 Early detection of cellular immunity in congenitally Toxoplasma gondii-infected children. Pediatric Infectious Disease Journal 18: 846–847

433. Kaleida P H, Nativio D G, Chao H P, Cowden S N 1993 Prevalence of bacterial respiratory pathogens in the nasopharynx in breast-fed versus formula-fed infants. Journal of Clinical Microbiology 31: 2674–2678

434. Kalenic S, Francetic I, Polak J, Zele Starcevic L, Bencic Z 1993 Impact of ampicillin and cefuroxime on bacterial colonization and infection in patients on a neonatal intensive care unit. Journal of Hospital Infection 23: 35–41

435. Kalliola S, Vuopio-Varkila J, Takala A K, Eskola J 1999 Neonatal group B streptococcal disease in Finland: a ten-year nationwide study. Pediatric Infectious Disease Journal 18: 806–810

436. Kantar M, Kultursay N, Kutukculer N, Akisu M, Cetingul N, Caglayan S 2000 Plasma concentrations of granulocyte-macrophage colony-stimulating factor and interleukin-6 in septic and healthy preterms. European Journal of Pediatrics 159: 156–157

437. Kaplan M, Klein S W, McPhee J 1983 Group B coxsackievirus infections in infants younger than 3 months of age: a serious childhood illness. Reviews of Infectious Diseases 5: 1019–1032

438. Kaplan M, Rudensky B, Beck A 1993 Perinatal infections with Streptococcus pneumoniae. American Journal of Perinatology 10: 1–4

439. Karlowicz M G, Buescher E S, Surka A E 2000 Fulminant late-onset sepsis in a neonatal intensive care unit, 1988–1997, and the impact of avoiding empiric vancomycin therapy. Pediatrics 106: 1387–1390

440. Karlowicz M G, Furigay P J, Croitoru D P, Buescher E S 2002 Central venous catheter removal versus in situ treatment in neonates with coagulase-negative staphylococcal bacteremia. Pediatric Infectious Disease Journal 21: 22–27

441. Kashlan F, Smulian J, Shen-Schwarz S, Anwar M, Hiatt M, Hegyi T 2000 Umbilical vein interleukin 6 and tumor necrosis factor alpha plasma concentrations in the very preterm infant. Pediatric Infectious Disease Journal 19: 238–243

442. Kasper D L 1995 Designer vaccines to prevent infections due to group B streptococcus. Proceedings of the Association of American Physicians 107: 369–373

443. Katz V L, McCoy M C, Kuller J A, Hansen W F 1996 An association between fetal parvovirus B19 infection and fetal anomalies: a report of two cases. American Journal of Perinatology 13: 43–45

444. Kaufman D, Boyle R, Hazen K C, Patrie J T, Robinson M, Donowitz L G 2001 Fluconazole prophylaxis against fungal colonization and infection in preterm infants. New England Journal of Medicine 345: 1660–1666

445. Kaye J N, Starkey W G, Kell B et al 1996 Human papillomavirus type 16 in infants: use of DNA sequence analyses to determine the source of infection. Journal of General Virology 77: 1139–1143

446. Kazembe P, Simor A E, Swarney A E, Yap L G, Kreiswirth B, Ng J, Low D E 1993 A study of the epidemiology of an endemic strain of staphylococcus haemolyticus (TOR-35) in a neonatal intensive care unit. Scandinavian Journal of Infectious Diseases 25: 507–513

447. Keith C G 1991 Congenital rubella infection from reinfection of previously immunised mothers [see comments]. Australian and New Zealand Journal of Ophthalmology 19: 291–293

448. Kellogg J A, Ferrentino F L, Goodstein M H, Liss J, Shapiro S L, Bankert D A 1997 Frequency of low level bacteremia in infants from birth to two months of age. Pediatric Infectious Disease Journal 16: 381–385

449. Kennaugh J K, Gregory W W, Powell K R, Hendley J O 1984 The effect of dilution during culture on detection of low concentrations of bacteria in blood. Pediatric Infectious Disease Journal 3: 317–322

450. Kennon C, Overturf G, Bessman S, Sierra E, Smith K J, Brann B 1996 Granulocyte colony-stimulating factor as a marker for bacterial infection in neonates. Journal of Pediatrics 128: 765–769

451. Kenyon S, Boulvain M, Neilson J 2001 Antibiotics for preterm premature rupture of membranes (Cochrane Review). Cochrane Database of Systematic Reviews (4): CD001058

452. Kerr M M, Hutchison J H, McVicar J, Givan J, McAllister T A 1976 The natural history of bacterial colonization of the newborn in a maternity hospital. Scottish Medical Journal 21: 111–117

453. Kesler K, Nasenbeny J, Wainwright R, McMahon B, Bulkow L 1998 Immune responses of prematurely born infants to hepatitis B vaccination: results through three years of age. Pediatric Infectious Disease Journal 17: 116–119

454. Keyworth N, Millar M R, Holland K T 1992 Development of cutaneous microflora in premature neonates. Archives of Disease in Childhood 67: 797–801

455. Khadilkar V, Tudehope D, Fraser S 1995 A prospective study of nosocomial infection in a neonatal intensive care unit. Journal of Paediatrics and Child Health 31: 387–391

456. Khan E A, Wafelman L S, Garcia-Prats J A, Taber L H 1997 Serratia marcescens pneumonia, empyema and pneumatocele in a preterm neonate. Pediatric Infectious Disease Journal 16: 1003–1005

457. Khatib R, Riederer K M, Clark J A, Khatib S, Brisk L E, Wilson F M 1995 Coagulase-negative staphylococci in multiple blood cultures: strain relatedness and determinants of same-strain bacteremia. Journal of Clinical Microbiology 33: 816–820

458. Khuroo M S, Kamili S, Jameel S 1995 Vertical transmission of hepatitis E virus. Lancet 345: 1025–1026

459. Kidan K G, Fantahun M, Azeze B 1995 Seroprevalence of human immunodeficiency virus infection and its association with syphilis seropositivity among antenatal clinic attenders at Debretabor Rural Hospital, Ethiopia. East African Medical Journal 72: 579–583

460. Kieffer F, Thulliez P, Brezin A et al 2002 [Treatment of subclinical congenital toxoplasmosis by sulfadiazine and pyrimethamine continuously during 1 year: apropos of 46 cases.] Archives de Pediatrie 9: 7–13

461. Kilgore P E, Unicomb L E, Gentsch J R et al 1996 Neonatal rotavirus infection in Bangladesh: strain characterization and risk factors for nosocomial infection. Pediatric Infectious Disease Journal 15: 672–677

462. Kim Y S, Sheldon R A, Elliott B R, Liu Q, Ferriero D M, Tauber M G 1995 Brain injury in experimental neonatal meningitis due to group B streptococci. Journal of Neuropathology and Experimental Neurology 54: 531–539

463. Kimberlin D W 1998 Human herpesviruses 6 and 7: identification of newly recognized viral pathogens and their association with human disease. Pediatric Infectious Disease Journal 17: 59–67

464. Kimberlin D W, Lin C Y, Jacobs R F et al 2001 Natural history of neonatal herpes simplex virus infections in the acyclovir era. Pediatrics 108: 223–229

465. Kimberlin D W, Lin C Y, Jacobs R F et al 2001 Safety and efficacy of high-dose intravenous acyclovir in the management of neonatal herpes simplex virus infections. Pediatrics 108: 230–238

466. Kimberlin D, Powell D, Gruber W et al 1996 Administration of oral acyclovir suppressive therapy after neonatal herpes simplex virus disease limited to the skin, eyes and mouth: results of a phase I/II trial. Pediatric Infectious Disease Journal 15: 247–254

467. Kinney J S, Johnson K, Papasian C, Hall R T, Kurth C G, Jackson M A 1993 Early onset Haemophilus influenzae sepsis in the newborn infant [see comments]. Pediatric Infectious Disease Journal 12: 739–743

468. Klein J F, Shahrivar F 1992 Use of percutaneous silastic central venous catheters in neonates and the management of infectious complications. American Journal of Perinatology 9: 261–264

469. Kline A, Strickler J, Kempf J 1995 Factors associated with pregnancy and pregnancy resolution in HIV seropositive women. Social Science and Medicine 40: 1539–1547

470. Koch W C, Harger J H, Barnstein B, Adler S P 1998 Serologic and virologic evidence for frequent intrauterine transmission of human parvovirus B19 with a primary maternal infection during pregnancy. Pediatric Infectious Disease Journal 17: 489–494

471. Kocherlakota P, Gamma E F 1997 Human granulocyte colony-stimulating factor may improve outcome attributable to neonatal sepsis complicated by neutropenia. Pediatrics 100: e6

472. Kohl S 1989 The neonatal human's immune response to herpes simplex virus infection: a critical review. Pediatric Infectious Disease Journal 8: 67–74

473. Kohl S 1994 Herpes simplex virus infection – the neonate to the adolescent. Israel Journal of Medical Sciences 30: 392–398

474. Kohn M A, Farley T A, Scott C 1996 The need for more aggressive follow-up of children born to hepatitis B surface antigen-positive mothers: lessons from the Louisiana Perinatal Hepatitis B Immunization Program. Pediatric Infectious Disease Journal 15: 535–540

475. Koksal N, Hacimustafaoglu M, Bagci S, Celebi S 2001 Meropenem in neonatal severe infections due to multiresistant gram-negative bacteria. Indian Journal of Pediatrics 68: 15–19

476. Kossoff E H, Buescher E S, Karlowicz M G 1998 Candidemia in a neonatal intensive care unit: trends during fifteen years and clinical features of 111 cases. Pediatric Infectious Disease Journal 17: 504–508

477. Koutouby A, Habibullah J 1995 Neonatal sepsis in Dubai, United Arab Emirates. Journal of Tropical Pediatrics 41: 177–180

478. Kovacs A, Schluchter M, Easley K et al & The Pediatric Pulmonary and Cardiovascular Complications of Vertically Transmitted HIV Infection Study Group 1999 Cytomegalovirus infection and HIV-1 disease progression in infants born to HIV-1-infected women. New England Journal of Medicine 341: 77–84

479. Kowba M D, Schwirian P M 1985 Direct sibling contact and bacterial colonisation of newborns. Journal of Obstetric, Gynecologic, and Neonatal Nursing 14: 412–417

480. Krajden S, Middleton P J 1983 Enterovirus infections in the neonate. Clinics in Pediatrics 22: 87–92

481. Krause P J, Maderazo E G, Contrino J et al 1991 Modulation of neonatal neutrophil function by pentoxifylline. Pediatric Research 29: 123–127

482. Krebs V L, Koga K M, Diniz E M, Ceccon M E, Vaz F A 2001 Necrotizing fasciitis in a newborn infant: a case report. Revista do Hospital das Clinicas; Faculdade de Medicina da Universidade de Sao Paulo 56: 59–62

483. Krediet T G, Fleer A 1998 Should we use vancomycin as prophylaxis to prevent neonatal nosocomial coagulase-negative staphylococcal septicemia? Pediatric Infectious Disease Journal 17: 763–764

484. Kurtoglu S, Caksen H, Ozturk A, Cetin N, Poyrazoglu H 1998 A review of 207 newborn with tetanus. Journal of the Pakistan Medical Association 48: 93–98

485. Laartz B W, Narvarte H J, Holt D, Larkin J A, Pomputius W F III 2002 Congenital tuberculosis and management of exposures in a neonatal intensive care unit. Infection Control and Hospital Epidemiology 23: 573–579

486. Laga M, Naamara W, Brunham R C et al 1986 Single-dose therapy of gonococcal ophthalmia neonatorum with ceftriaxone. New England Journal of Medicine 315: 1382–1385

487. Laifer S A, Ehrlich G D, Huff D S, Balsan M J, Scantlebury V P 1995 Congenital cytomegalovirus infection in offspring of liver transplant recipients. Clinical Infectious Diseases 20: 52–55

488. Lamari F, Anastassiou E D, Stamokosta E et al 2000 Determination of slime-producing S. epidermidis specific antibodies in human immunoglobulin preparations and blood sera by an enzyme immunoassay: correlation of antibody titers with opsonic activity and application to preterm neonates. Journal of Pharmaceutical and Biomedical Analysis 23: 363–374

489. Lanari M, Lazzarotto T, Papa I et al 2001 Neonatal aortic arch thrombosis as a result of congenital cytomegalovirus infection. Pediatrics 108: E114

490. Larkin G L, Thuma P E 1991 Congenital malaria in a hyperendemic area. American Journal of Tropical Medicine and Hygiene 45: 587–592

491. Lassiter H A, Tanner J E, Cost K M, Steger S, Vogel R L 1991 Diminished IgG, but not complement C3 or C4 or factor B, precedes nosocomial bacterial sepsis in very low birth weight neonates. Pediatric Infectious Disease Journal 10: 663–668

492. Laurenti F, Ferro R, Isacchi G 1981 Polymorphonuclear transfusion for the treatment of sepsis in the newborn infant. Journal of Pediatrics 98: 118–123

493. Leach C T, Newton E R, McParlin S, Jenson H B 1994 Human herpesvirus 6 infection of the female genital tract. Journal of Infectious Diseases 169: 1281–1283

494. Lee D R, Moore G W, Hutchins G M 1991 Lattice theory analysis of the relationship of hyaline membrane disease and fetal pneumonia in 96 perinatal autopsies. Pediatric Pathology 11: 223–233

495. Lee K K, Vargo L R, Le C T, Fernando L 1992 Transfusion-acquired hepatitis A outbreak from fresh frozen plasma in a neonatal intensive care unit. Pediatric Infectious Disease Journal 11: 122–123

496. Leib S L, Kim Y S, Ferriero D M, Tuber M G 1996 Neuroprotective effect of excitatory amino acid antagonist kynurenic acid in experimental bacterial meningitis. Journal of Infectious Diseases 173: 166–171

497. Leigh L, Stoll B J, Rahman M, McGowan J J 1995 Pseudomonas aeruginosa infection in very low birth weight infants: a case-control study. Pediatric Infectious Disease Journal 14: 367–371

498. Lejeune B, Baron R, Guillois B, Mayeux, D 1991 Evaluation of a screening test for detecting urinary tract infection in newborns and infants. Journal of Clinical Pathology 44: 1029–1030

499. Leroy V, De Clercq A, Ladner J, Bogaerts J, Van de Perre P, Dabis F 1995 Should screening of genital infections be part of antenatal care in areas of high HIV prevalence? A prospective cohort study from Kigali, Rwanda, 1992–1993. The Pregnancy and HIV (EGE) Group. Genitourinary Medicine 71: 207–211

500. Levin T L, Schulman M, Zieba P, Goldman H S 1994 Absence of lower extremity ossification centers in term infants with congenital syphilis. Journal of Perinatology 14: 106–109

501. Levine C D 1991 Premature rupture of the membranes and sepsis in preterm neonates. Nursing Research 40: 36–41

502. Levy I, Rubin L G, Vasishtha S, Tucci V, Sood S K 1998 Emergence of Candida parapsilosis as the predominant species causing candidemia in children. Clinical Infectious Diseases 26: 1086–1088

503. Lewis E, Shinefield H R, Woodruff B A et al 2001 Safety of neonatal hepatitis B vaccine administration. Pediatric Infectious Disease Journal 20: 1049–1054

504. Libman M D, Dascal A, Kramer M S, Mendelson J 1991 Strategies for the prevention of neonatal infection with herpes simplex virus: a decision analysis [see comments]. Reviews of Infectious Diseases 13: 1093–1104

505. Lilien L D, Harris V J, Pildes R S 1977 Significance of radiographic findings in early-onset group B streptococcal infection. Pediatrics 60: 360–363

506. Lin H H, Kao J H, Hsu H Y et al 1995 Absence of infection in breast-fed infants born to hepatitis C virus-infected mothers. Journal of Pediatrics 126: 589–591

507. Linder N, Karetnyi Y, Gidony Y et al 1997 Placental transfer of hepatitis A antibodies in full term and preterm infants. Pediatric Infectious Disease Journal 16: 245–247

508. Linder N, Ohel G, Gazit G, Keidar D, Tamir I, Reichman B 1995 Neonatal sepsis after prolonged premature rupture of membranes. Journal of Perinatology 15: 36–38

509. Lipuma J J 1998 Molecular tools for epidemiologic study of infectious diseases. Pediatric Infectious Disease Journal 17: 667–67

510. Lissauer T 1989 Impact of AIDS on neonatal care [see comments]. Archives of Disease in Childhood 64(1 Spec No): 4–7

511. Littlewood J M L, Kite P, Kite B A 1969 Incidence of neonatal urinary tract infection. Archives of Disease in Childhood 44: 617–620

512. Litwin C M, Hill H R 1997 Serologic and DNA-based testing for congenital and perinatal infections. Pediatric Infectious Disease Journal 16: 1166–1175

513. Lo W T, Wang C C, Chu M L 2000 Intrauterine staphylococcal scalded skin syndrome: report of a case. Pediatric Infectious Disease Journal 19: 481–482

514. Loeffler A M, Milstein J M, Kosh D L 1996 Fever, hepatosplenomegaly and rash in a newborn. Pediatric Infectious Disease Journal 15: 721–722, 724

515. Lopez Alarcon M, Villalpando S, Fajardo A 1997 Breast-feeding lowers the frequency and duration of acute respiratory infection and diarrhea in infants under six months of age. Journal of Nutrition 127: 436–443

516. Lopez Sastre J B, Coto C D, Fernandez C B 2002 Neonatal sepsis of nosocomial origin: an epidemiological study from the 'Grupo de Hospitales Castrillo'. Journal of Perinatal Medicine 30: 149–157

517. Lorber J 1974 Neonatal bacterial meningitis. Medicine 27: 1579–1582

518. Luck P C, Dinger E, Helbig J H et al 1994 Analysis of Legionella pneumophila strains associated with nosocomial pneumonia in a neonatal intensive care unit. European Journal of Clinical Microbiology and Infectious Diseases 13: 565–571

519. Lyon A J 1996 Genital mycoplasmas and infection in the neonate. In: Hansen T N, McIntosh N (eds) Current topic in neonatology. W B Saunders, Philadelphia, pp 1–20

520. McCabe K M, Khan G, Zhang Y H, Mason E O, McCabe E R 1995 Amplification of bacterial DNA using highly conserved sequences: automated analysis and potential for molecular triage of sepsis. Pediatrics 95: 165–169

521. McCarthy A E, Victor G, Ramotar K, Toye B 1994 Risk factors for acquiring ampicillin-resistant enterococci and clinical outcomes at a Canadian tertiary-care hospital. Journal of Clinical Microbiology 32: 2671–2676

522. McCracken G H 1984 Management of bacterial meningitis; current status and future prospects. American Journal of Medicine 76: 215–223

523. McCracken G H, Mize S G 1976 A controlled study of intrathecal antibiotic therapy in gram-negative enteric meningits in infancy. Report of the Neonatal Meningitis Cooperative Study Group. Journal of Pediatrics 89: 66–72

524. McCracken G H, Mize S G, Threkeld N 1980 Intraventricular gentamicin therapy for gram-negative bacillary meningitis in infancy. Lancet 1: 787–791

525. McDonald L C, Walker M, Carson L A et al 1998 Outbreak of Acinetobacter spp. bloodstream infections in a nursery associated with contaminated aerosols and air conditioners. Pediatric Infectious Disease Journal 17: 716–722

526. McDuffie R S J, McGregor J A, Gibbs R S 1993 Adverse perinatal outcome and resistant Enterobacteriaceae after antibiotic usage for premature rupture of the membranes and group B streptococcus carriage. Obstetrics and Gynecology 82: 487–489

527. MacGowan A P, Cartlidge P H, MacLeod F, McLaughlin J 1991 Maternal listeriosis in pregnancy without fetal or neonatal infection. Journal of Infection 22: 53–57

528. MacGowan A P, O'Donoghue K, Nicholls S, McLauchlin J, Bennett P M, Reeves D S 1993 Typing of Listeria spp. by random amplified polymorphic DNA (RAPD) analysis. Journal of Medical Microbiology 38: 322–327

529. McGregor J A, French J I 1991 Chlamydia trachomatis infection during pregnancy. American Journal of Obstetrics and Gynecology 164: 1782–1789

530. McIntosh D, Isaacs D 1992 Herpes simplex virus infection in pregnancy. Archives of Disease in Childhood 67: 1137–1138

531. McIntosh N, Harrison A 1994 Prolonged premature rupture of membranes in the preterm infant: a 7 year study. European Journal of Obstetrics, Gynecology, and Reproductive Biology 57: 1–6

532. Mackenzie A, Johnson W, Heyes B, Norrish B, Jamieson F 1995 A prolonged outbreak of exfoliative toxin A-producing Staphylococcus aureus in a newborn nursery. Diagnostic Microbiology and Infectious Disease 21: 69–75

533. McLaren R A, Chauhan S P, Gross T L 1996 Intrapartum factors in early-onset group B streptococcal sepsis in term neonates: a case-control study. American Journal of Obstetrics and Gynecology 174: 1934–1937

534. McNeeley D F, Saint-Louis F, Noel G J 1996 Neonatal enterococcal bacteremia: an increasingly frequent event with potentially untreatable pathogens. Pediatric Infectious Disease Journal 15: 800–805

535. Madge P, Paton J Y, McColl J H, Mackie P L 1992 Prospective controlled study of four infection-control procedures to prevent nosocomial infection with respiratory syncytial virus [see comments]. Lancet 340: 1079–1083

536. Magliocco A M, Demetrick D J, Sarnat H B, Hwang W S 1992 Varicella embryopathy. Archives of Pathology and Laboratory Medicine 116: 181–186

537. Mahon B E, Yamada E G, Newman T B 1994 Problems with serum IgM as a screening test for congenital infection. Clinical Pediatrics 33: 142–146

538. Maire F, Heraud M C, Loriette Y, Normand B, Begue R J, Labbe A 1999 The value of procalcitonin in neonatal infections. Archives de Pediatrie 6: 503–509

539. Makhoul I R, Kassis I, Smolkin T, Tamir A, Sujov P 2001 Review of 49 neonates with acquired fungal sepsis: further characterization. Pediatrics 107: 61–66

540. Makhoul I R, Sujov P, Smolkin T, Lusky A, Reichman B 2002 Epidemiological, clinical, and microbiological characteristics of late-onset sepsis among very low birth weight infants in Israel: a national survey. Pediatrics 109: 34–39

541. Malathi I, Millar M R, Leeming J P, Hedges A, Marlow N 1993 Skin disinfection in preterm infants. Archives of Disease in Childhood 69: 312–316

542. Malik R K, Montecalvo M A, Reale M R et al 1999 Epidemiology and control of vancomycin-resistant enterococci in a regional neonatal intensive care unit. Pediatric Infectious Disease Journal 18: 352–356

543. Malm G, Berg U, Forsgren M 1995 Neonatal herpes simplex: clinical findings and outcome in relation to type of maternal infection. Acta Paediatrica 84: 256–260

544. Malm G, Forsgren M 1999 Neonatal herpes simplex virus infections: HSV DNA in cerebrospinal fluid and serum. Archives of Disease in Childhood. Fetal and Neonatal Edition 81: F24–F29

545. Malm G, Forsgren M, el Azazi M, Persson A 1991 A follow-up study of children with neonatal herpes simplex virus infections with particular regard to late nervous disturbances. Acta Paediatrica Scandinavica 80: 226–234

546. Malouf D J, Oates R K 1995 Herpes simplex virus infections in the neonate. Journal of Paediatrics and Child Health 31: 332–335

547. Mandar R, Mikelsaar M 1996 Transmission of mother's microflora to the newborn at birth. Biology of the Neonate 69: 30–35

548. Manroe B L, Rosenfeld C R, Weinberg A G, Browne R 1977 The differential leukocyte count in the assessment and outcome of early-onset group B streptococcal disease. Journal of Pediatrics 91: 632–637

549. Manroe B L, Weinberg A, Rosenfeld C R, Browne R 1979 The neonatal blood count in health and disease. I. Reference values for neutrophilic cells. Journal of Pediatrics 95: 89–98

550. Maral I, Cirak M, Aksakal F N, Baykan Z, Kayikcioglu F, Bumin M A 2001 Tetanus immunization in pregnant women. Serum levels of antitetanus antibodies at time of delivery. European Journal of Epidemiology 17: 661–665

551. Marodi L 1997 Local and systemic host defense mechanisms against Candida: immunopathology of candidal infections. Pediatric Infectious Disease Journal 16: 795–801

552. Martin D J 1985 Neonatal disorders diagnosed with ultrasound. Clinics in Perinatology 12: 219–231

553. Mason W H, Andrews R, Ross L A, Wright H T Jr 1989 Omphalitis in the newborn infant. Pediatric Infectious Disease Journal 8: 521–525

554. Matsubara K, Sugiyama M, Hoshina K, Mikamo H, Baba K 2000 Early onset neonatal sepsis caused by serotype VIII group B streptococci. Pediatric Infectious Disease Journal 19: 359–360

555. Matsui D 1994 Prevention, diagnosis, and treatment of fetal toxoplasmosis. Clinics in Perinatology 21: 675–689

556. Mazade M A, Evans E M, Starke J R, Correa A G 2001 Congenital tuberculosis presenting as sepsis syndrome: case report and review of the literature. Pediatric Infectious Disease Journal 20: 439–442

557. Mazur J M, Ross G, Cummings J, Hahn G A J, McCluskey W P 1995 Usefulness of magnetic resonance imaging for the diagnosis of acute musculoskeletal infections in children. Journal of Pediatric Orthopedics 15: 144–147

558. Meadow W L, Schwartz I K 1986 Time course of detection of positive blood cultures in childhood. Pediatric Infectious Disease Journal 5: 333–336

559. Mecrow I K, Ladusans E J 1994 Infective endocarditis in newborn infants with structurally normal hearts. Acta Paediatrica 83: 35–39

560. Mehr S, Doyle L W 2000 Cytokines as markers of bacterial sepsis in newborn infants: a review. Pediatric Infectious Disease Journal 19: 879–887

561. Mehr S S, Sadowsky J L, Doyle L W, Carr J 2002 Sepsis in neonatal intensive care in the late 1990s. Journal of Paediatrics and Child Health 38: 246–251

562. Mendoza J C, Roberts J L 1991 Early-onset Hemophilus influenzae sepsis in the neonate. Journal of Perinatology 11: 126–129

563. Mentzer D, Kreuz W 1999 CMV coinfection and disease progression in vertically acquired HIV infection. Archives of Disease in Childhood 81: 189

564. Merenstein G B, Weisman L E 1996 Premature rupture of the membranes: neonatal consequences. Seminars in Perinatology 20: 375–380

565. Meyer C L, Payne N R, Roback S A 1991 Spontaneous, isolated intestinal perforations in neonates with birth weight less than 1,000 g not associated with necrotizing enterocolitis. Journal of Pediatric Surgery 26: 714–717

566. Michelow I C, Wendel G D Jr, Norgard M V et al 2002 Central nervous system infection in congenital syphilis. New England Journal of Medicine 346: 1792–1798

567. Midani S, Rathore M H 1997 Polymerase chain reaction testing for early detection of HIV infection in children. Southern Medical Journal 90: 294–295

568. Millar M R, Bacon C, Smith S L, Walker V, Hall M A 1993 Enteral feeding of premature infants with Lactobacillus GG. Archives of Disease in Childhood 69: 483–487

569. Millar M R, MacKay P, Levene M, Langdale V, Martin C 1992 Enterobacteriaceae and neonatal necrotising enterocolitis. Archives of Diseases in Childhood 67: 53–56

570. Miller E, Craddock-Watson J E, Ridehalgh M K 1989 Outcome in newborn babies given anti-varicella-zoster immunoglobulin after perinatal maternal infection with varicella-zoster virus. Lancet 2: 371–373

571. Miller E, Tookey P, Morgan Capner P et al 1994 Rubella surveillance to June 1994: third joint report from the PHLS and the National Congenital Rubella Surveillance Programme. Communicable Disease Report. CDR Review 4: R146–R152

572. Mirochnick M, Siminski S, Fenton T, Lugo M, Sullivan J L 2001 Nevirapine pharmacokinetics in pregnant women and in their infants after in utero exposure. Pediatric Infectious Disease Journal 20: 803–805

573. Miura E, Procianoy R S, Bittar C et al 2001 A randomized, double-masked, placebo-controlled trial of recombinant granulocyte colony-stimulating factor administration to preterm infants with the clinical diagnosis of early-onset sepsis. Pediatrics 107: 30–35

574. Modi N, Carr R 2000 Promising stratagems for reducing the burden of neonatal sepsis. Archives of Disease in Childhood. Fetal and Neonatal Edition 83: F150–F153

575. Modlin J F 1986 Perinatal echovirus infection: insights from a literature review of 61 cases of serious infection and 16 outbreaks in nurseries. Reviews of Infectious Diseases 8: 918–925

576. Mohan P, Chandra R S, Kleiner D E, Luban N L C 2003 An unusual presentation of perinatally transmitted hepatitis C. Archives of Disease in Childhood 88: 160–161

577. Moisiuk S E, Robson D, Klass L et al 1998 Outbreak of parainfluenza virus type 3 in an intermediate care neonatal nursery. Pediatric Infectious Disease Journal 17: 49–53

578. Mok J 1991 HIV infection in children: millions will suffer. British Medical Journal 302: 921–922

579. Montone K T, Furth E E, Pietra G G, Gupta P K 1995 Neonatal adenovirus infection: a case report with in situ hybridization confirmation of ascending intrauterine infection. Diagnostic Cytopathology 12: 341–344

580. Morey A L, Porter H J, Keeling J W, Fleming K A 1992 Non-isotopic in situ hybridisation and immunophenotyping of infected cells in the investigation of human fetal parvovirus infection. Journal of Clinical Pathology 45: 673–678

581. Morita J Y, O'Brien K L, Schuchat A 1999 Prevention of perinatal group B streptococcal infections. Pediatric Infectious Disease Journal 18: 279–280

582. Moses L M, Heath P T, Wilkinson A R, Jeffery H E, Isaacs D 1998 Early onset group B streptococcal neonatal infection in Oxford 1985–96. Archives of Disease in Childhood. Fetal and Neonatal Edition 79: F148–F149

583. Mouzinho A, Rosenfeld C R, Sanchez P J, Risser R 1992 Effect of maternal hypertension on neonatal neutropenia and risk of nosocomial infection. Pediatrics 90: 430–435

584. Mouzinho A, Rosenfeld C R, Sanchez P J, Risser R 1994 Revised reference ranges for circulating neutrophils in very-low- birth-weight neonates. Pediatrics 94: 76–82

585. Much D H, Yeh S Y 1991 Prevalence of Chlamydia trachomatis infection in pregnant patients. Public Health Reports 106: 490–493

586. Mulder C J J, Zanen H C 1984 A study of 280 cases of neonatal meningitis in the Netherlands. Journal of Infection 9: 177–184

587. Mullens A 1996 "I think we have a problem in Victoria": MDs respond quickly to toxoplasmosis outbreak in BC. Canadian Medical Association Journal 154: 1721–1724

588. Mulloy R H, Jadavji T, Russell M L 1991 Tunneled central venous catheter sepsis: risk factors in a pediatric hospital. JPEN. Journal of Parenteral and Enteral Nutrition 15: 460–463

589. Munoz F M, Campbell J R, Atmar R L et al 1999 Influenza A virus outbreak in a neonatal intensive care unit. Pediatric Infectious Disease Journal 18: 811–815

590. Munro N D, Sheppard S, Smithells R W, Holzel H, Jones G 1987 Temporal relations between maternal rubella and congenital defects. Lancet ii: 201–204

591. Myers J D 1974 Congenital varicella in term infants: risk reconsidered. Journal of Infectious Diseases 129: 215–216

592. Nadal D, Hunziker U A, Schupbach J et al 1989 Immunological evaluation in the early diagnosis of prenatal or perinatal HIV infection. Archives of Disease in Childhood 64: 662–669

593. Nagata E, Brito A S, Matsuo T 2002 Nosocomial infections in a neonatal intensive care unit: incidence and risk factors. American Journal of Infection Control 30: 26–31

594. Nahmias A J, Keyserling H L, Kerrick G M 1983 Herpes simplex. In: Remington J S, Klein J O (eds) Infectious diseases of the fetus and newborn infant, 2nd edn. W B Saunders, Philadelphia, pp 636–678

595. Nahmias A, Whitley R, Vistine A M 1982 Herpes simplex virus encephalitis: laboratory evaluations and their diagnostic significance. Journal of Infectious Diseases 145: 829–836

596. Nankervis G A, Gold E 1973 Varicella-zoster viruses. In: Kaplan A S (ed) The herpesviruses. Academic Press, New York, pp 327–333

597. Narchi H, Gammoh S 1999 Multiple nodular pneumonitis in a three-week-old female infant. Pediatric Infectious Disease Journal 18: 471, 485–486

598. Narendran V, Gupta G, Todd D A, John E 1996 Bacterial colonization of indwelling vascular catheters in newborn infants. Journal of Paediatrics and Child Health 32: 391–396

599. Narita M, Togashi T, Kikuta H 1997 Neonatal measles in Hokkaido, Japan. Pediatric Infectious Disease Journal 16: 908–909

600. Nazemi K J, Buescher E S, Kelly R E, Karlowicz M G 2003 Central venous catheter removal versus in situ treatment in neonates with enterobacteriaceae bacteraemia. Pediatrics 111: e269–e274

601. Nduati R W, John G C, Richardson B A et al 1995 Human immunodeficiency virus type 1-infected cells in breast milk: association with immunosuppression and vitamin A deficiency. Journal of Infectious Diseases 172: 1461–1468

602. Neumeister B, Kastner S, Conrad S, Klotz G, Bartmann P 1995 Characterization of coagulase-negative staphylococci causing nosocomial infections in preterm infants. European Journal of Clinical Microbiology and Infectious Diseases 14: 856–863

603. Newell M L, Dunn D T, De Maria A 1996 Detection of virus in vertically exposed HIV antibody negative children. Lancet 347: 213–215

604. Ng P C 1994 Systemic fungal infections in neonates. Archives of Disease in Childhood. Fetal and Neonatal Edition 71: F130–F135

605. Ng P C, Cheng S H, Chui K M et al 1997 Diagnosis of late onset neonatal sepsis with cytokines, adhesion molecule, and C-reactive protein in preterm very low birthweight infants. Archives of Disease in Childhood. Fetal and Neonatal Edition 77: F221–F227

606. Ng P C, Herrington R A, Beane C A, Ghonheim A T M, Dear P R F 1989 An outbreak of acinetobacter septicaemia in a neonatal intensive care unit. Journal of Hospital Infection 14: 363–368

607. Ng P C, Li K, Wong R P, Chui K M, Wong E, Fok T F 2002 Neutrophil CD64 expression: a sensitive diagnostic marker for late-onset nosocomial infection in very low birthweight infants. Pediatric Research 51: 296–303

608. Ng P C, Lyon D J, Wong M Y et al 1996 Varicella exposure in a neonatal intensive care unit: emergency management and control measures. Journal of Hospital Infection 32: 229–236

609. Ng P C, Siu Y K, Lewindon P J, Wong W, Cheung K L, Dawkins R 1994 Congenital Candida pneumonia in a preterm infant. Journal of Paediatrics and Child Health 30: 552–554

610. Nicoll J A, Love S, Burton P A, Berry P J 1994 Autopsy findings in two cases of neonatal herpes simplex virus infection: detection of virus by immuno-histochemistry, in situ hybridization and the polymerase chain reaction. Histopathology 24: 257–264

611. Nigro G, Clerico A, Mondaini C 1993 Symptomatic congenital cytomegalovirus infection in two consecutive sisters. Archives of Disease in Childhood 69: 527–528

612. Nigro G, Scholz H, Bartmann U 1994 Ganciclovir therapy for symptomatic congenital cytomegalovirus infection in infants: a two-regimen experience. Journal of Pediatrics 124: 318–322

613. Nisida I V, Amato N V, Braz L M, Duarte M I, Umezawa E S 1999 A survey of congenital Chagas' disease, carried out at three health institutions in Sao Paulo City, Brazil. Revista do Instituto de Medicina Tropical de Sao Paulo 41: 305–311

614. Niu M, Targonski P V, Stoll B J, Albert G P, Margolis H S 1992 Prevention of perinatal transmission of the hepatitis B virus. Outcome of infants in a community prevention program [see comments]. American Journal of Diseases of Children 146: 793–796

615. Noel G J, Kreiswirth B N, Edelson P J et al 1992 Multiple methicillin-resistant Staphylococcus aureus strains as a cause for a single outbreak of severe disease in hospitalized neonates. Pediatric Infectious Disease Journal 11: 184–188

616. Noyola D E, Demmler G J, Williamson W D et al 2000 Cytomegalovirus urinary excretion and long-term outcome in children with congenital cytomegalovirus infection. Congenital CMV Longitudinal Study Group. Pediatric Infectious Disease Journal 19: 505–510

617. Nupponen I, Andersson S, Jarvenpaa A L, Kautiainen H, Repo H 2001 Neutrophil CD11b expression and circulating interleukin-8 as diagnostic markers for early-onset neonatal sepsis. Pediatrics 108: e12

618. Nyambi P N, Ville Y, Louwagie J et al 1996 Mother-to-child transmission of human T-cell lymphotropic virus types I and II (HTLV-I/II) in Gabon: a prospective follow-up of 4 years. Journal of Acquired Immune Deficiency Syndromes and Human Retrovirology 12: 187–192

619. Nyirjesy P, Kavasya T, Axelrod P, Fischer P R 1993 Malaria during pregnancy: neonatal morbidity and mortality and the efficacy of chloroquine chemo-prophylaxis. Clinical Infectious Diseases 16: 127–132

620. Nyquist A C, Rotbart H A, Cotton M et al 1994 Acyclovir-resistant neonatal herpes simplex virus infection of the larynx. Journal of Pediatrics 124: 967–971

621. O'Connor T A, Ringer K M, Gaddis M L 1993 Mean platelet volume during coagulase-negative staphylococcal sepsis in neonates. American Journal of Clinical Pathology 99: 69–71

622. Oddie S, Embleton N D 2002 Risk factors for early onset neonatal group B streptococcal sepsis: case-control study. British Medical Journal 325: 308

623. Oh P H, Lanctot K L, Yoon A et al 2002 Palivizumab prophylaxis for respiratory syncytial virus in Canada: utilization and outcomes. Pediatric Infectious Disease Journal 21: 512–518

624. Ohashi M, Ihira M, Suzuki K et al 2001 Transfer of human herpesvirus 6 and 7 antibodies from mothers to their offspring. Pediatric Infectious Disease Journal 20: 449–450

625. Ohlsson A, Lacy J B 2000 Intravenous immunoglobulin for preventing infection in preterm and/or low-birth-weight infants (Cochrane Review). Cochrane Database of Systematic Reviews (2): CD000361

626. Ohlsson A, Lacy J B 2000 Intravenous immunoglobulin for suspected or subsequently proven infection in neonates (Cochrane Review). Cochrane Database of Systematic Reviews (2): CD001239

627. Ohman L, Tullus K, Katouli M, Burman L G, Stendahl O 1995 Correlation between susceptibility of infants to infections and interaction with neutrophils of Escherichia coli strains causing neonatal and infantile septicemia. Journal of Infectious Diseases 171: 128–133

628. Ollikainen J, Hiekkaniemi H, Korppi M, Sarkkinen H, Heinonen K 1993 Ureaplasma urealyticum infection associated with acute respiratory insufficiency and death in premature infants [see comments]. Journal of Pediatrics 122: 756–760

629. Olver W J, Bond D W, Boswell T C, Watkin S L 2000 Neonatal group B streptococcal disease associated with infected breast milk. Archives of Disease in Childhood. Fetal and Neonatal Edition 83: F48–F49

630. Oram R J, Herold B C 1998 Antiviral agents for herpes viruses. Pediatric Infectious Disease Journal 17: 652–653

631. Overall J C J 1994 Herpes simplex virus infection of the fetus and newborn. Pediatric Annals 23: 131–136

632. Overall J C, Glasgow L A 1970 Virus infections of the fetus and newborn infant. Journal of Pediatrics 77: 315–333

633. Pabst H F 1997 Immunomodulation by breast-feeding. Pediatric Infectious Disease Journal 16: 991–995

634. Pacifico L, Panero A, Roggini M, Rossi N, Bucci G, Chiesa C 1997 Ureaplasma urealyticum and pulmonary outcome in a neonatal intensive care population. Pediatric Infectious Disease Journal 16: 579–586

635. Palasanthiran P, Ziegler J B, Stewart G J et al 1993 Breast-feeding during primary maternal human immunodeficiency virus infection and risk of transmission from mother to infant. Journal of Infectious Diseases 167: 441–444

636. Panero A, Pacifico L, Rossi N, Mancuso G, Stegagno M, Chiesa C 1997 Interleukin 6 in neonates with early and late onset infection. Pediatric Infectious Disease Journal 16: 370–375

637. Paryani S G, Yeager A S, Horsford-Dunn H et al 1985 Sequelae of acquired cytomegalovirus infection in premature and sick term infants. Journal of Pediatrics 107: 451–456

638. Pasic S, Jankovic B, Abinun M, Kanjuh B 1997 Intravenous immunoglobulin prophylaxis in an echovirus 6 and echovirus 4 nursery outbreak. Pediatric Infectious Disease Journal 16: 718–720

639. Pastuszak A L, Levy M, Schick B et al 1994 Outcome after maternal varicella infection in the first 20 weeks of pregnancy. New England Journal of Medicine 330: 901–905

640. Patrick C C, Kaplan S L, Baker C J, Parisi J T, Mason E O Jr 1989 Persistent bacteremia due to coagulase-negative staphylococci in low birth weight neonates [see comments]. Pediatrics 84: 977–985

641. Paul M, Petersen E, Pawlowski Z S, Szczapa J 2000 Neonatal screening for congenital toxoplasmosis in the Poznan region of Poland by analysis of Toxoplasma gondii-specific IgM antibodies eluted from filter paper blood spots. Pediatric Infectious Disease Journal 19: 30–36

642. Payne N R, Burke B A, Day D L, Christenson P D, Thompson T R, Ferrieri P 1988 Correlation of clinical and pathologic findings in early onset neonatal group B streptococcal infection with disease severity and prediction of outcome. Pediatric Infectious Disease Journal 7: 836–847

643. Peckham C, Logan S 1993 Screening for toxoplasmosis during pregnancy. Archives of Disease in Childhood 68: 3–5

644. Peckham C, Newell M L 2000 Preventing vertical transmission of HIV infection. New England Journal of Medicine 343: 1036–1037

645. Pekkala D H, Low D E, Wyper P A et al 1992 The utility of restriction endonuclease analysis and phage typing in the epidemiologic investigation of a Staphylococcus aureus outbreak in a neonatal nursery. Diagnostic Microbiology and Infectious Disease 15: 307–311

646. Peng J, Krause P J, Kresch M 1996 Neonatal herpes simplex virus infection after cesarean section with intact amniotic membranes. Journal of Perinatology 16: 397–399

647. Perlman J M, Argyle C 1992 Lethal cytomegalovirus infection in preterm infants: clinical, radiological, and neuropathological findings. Annals of Neurology 31: 64–68

648. Perlman J M, Rollins N, Sanchez P J 1992 Late-onset meningitis in sick, very-low-birth-weight infants. Clinical and sonographic observations. American Journal of Diseases of Children 146: 1297–1301

649. Peters G, Loscci R, Pulverer, G 1982 Adherence and growth of coagulase-negative staphylococci on surfaces of intravenous catheters. Journal of Infectious Diseases 146: 479–482

650. Peters W, Irving J, Letts M 1992 Long-term effects of neonatal bone and joint infection on adjacent growth plates. Journal of Pediatric Orthopedics 12: 806–810

651. Philip A G 1985 Response of C-reactive protein in neonatal group B streptococcal infection. Pediatric Infectious Disease 4: 145–148

652. Philip A G 1994 The changing face of neonatal infection: experience at a regional medical center. Pediatric Infectious Disease Journal 13: 1098–1102

653. Philipson E H, Herson V C 1996 Intrapartum chemoprophylaxis for group B streptococcus infection to prevent neonatal disease: who should be treated? American Journal of Perinatology 13: 487–490

654. Phillips J R, Karlowicz M G 1997 Prevalence of Candida species in hospital-acquired urinary tract infections in a neonatal intensive care unit. Pediatric Infectious Disease Journal 16: 190–194

655. Piedra P A, Kasel J A, Norton H J et al 1992 Description of an adenovirus type 8 outbreak in hospitalized neonates born prematurely. Pediatric Infectious Disease Journal 11: 460–465

656. Pillay T, Adhikari M, Mokili J et al 2001 Severe, rapidly progressive human immunodeficiency virus type 1 disease in newborns with coinfections. Pediatric Infectious Disease Journal 20: 404–410

657. Pillay T, Pillay D G, Pillay M, Adhikari M, Sturm A W 1999 Are specific strains of mycobacterium tuberculosis responsible for disease in newborns? Pediatric Infectious Disease Journal 18: 844–845

658. Pisacane A, Graziano L, Mazzarella G, Scarpellino B, Zona G 1992 Breast-feeding and urinary tract infection. Journal of Pediatrics 120: 87–89

659. Plotkin S A 1999 Vaccination against cytomegalovirus, the changeling demon. Pediatric Infectious Disease Journal 18: 313–325

660. Pople I K, Bayston R, Hayward R D 1992 Infection of cerebrospinal fluid shunts in infants: a study of etiological factors. Journal of Neurosurgery 77: 29–36

661. Portolani M, Cermelli C, Sabbatini A M et al 1995 A fatal case of congenital cytomegalic inclusion disease following recurrent maternal infection. New Microbiologica 18: 427–428

662. Pourcyrous M, Bada H S, Korones S B, Baselski V, Wong S P 1993 Significance of serial C-reactive protein responses in neonatal infection and other disorders [see comments]. Pediatrics 92: 431–435

663. Preece P M, Anderson J M, Thompson R G 1989 Chlamydia trachomatis infection in infants: a prospective study [see comments]. Archives of Disease in Childhood 64: 525–529

664. Prober C G 2001 Management of the neonate whose mother received suppressive acyclovir therapy during late pregnancy. Pediatric Infectious Disease Journal 20: 90–91

665. Prosch S, Lienicke U, Priemer C et al 2002 Human adenovirus and human cytomegalovirus infections in preterm newborns: no association with bronchopulmonary dysplasia. Pediatric Research 52: 219–224

666. Pruekprasert P, Stout C, Patamasucon P 1995 Neonatal enterovirus infection. Journal of the Association for Academic Minority Physicians 6: 134–138

667. Public Health Laboratory Service Working Party on Fifth Disease 1990 Prospective study of human parvovirus B19 infection in pregnancy. British Medical Journal 300: 1166–1170

668. Pugatch D 2002 Testing infants for human immunodeficiency virus infection. Pediatric Infectious Disease Journal 21: 711–712

669. Puranen M, Yliskoski M, Saarikoski S, Syrjanen K, Syrjanen S 1996 Vertical transmission of human papillomavirus from infected mothers to their newborn babies and persistence of the virus in childhood. American Journal of Obstetrics and Gynecology 174: 694–699

670. Puri J, Revathi G, Faridi M M, Talwar V, Kumar A, Parkash B 1995 Role of body surface cultures in prediction of sepsis in a neonatal intensive care unit. Annals of Tropical Paediatrics 15: 307–311

671. Pyati S P, Pildes R S, Ramamurthy R S, Jacobs N 1981 Decreasing mortality in neonates with early-onset group B streptococcal infection: reality or artifact. Journal of Pediatrics 98: 625–627

672. Pylipow M, Gaddis M, Kinney J S 1994 Selective intrapartum prophylaxis for group B streptococcus colonization: management and outcome of newborns. Pediatrics 93: 631–635

673. Quinn P A, Li H C, Th'ng C, Dunn M, Butany J 1993 Serological response to Ureaplasma urealyticum in the neonate. Clinical Infectious Diseases 179(suppl. 1): S136–S143

674. Raad I I, Sabbagh M F 1992 Optimal duration of therapy for catheter-related Staphylococcus aureus bacteremia: a study of 55 cases and review [see comments]. Clinical Infectious Diseases 14: 75–82

675. Rabalais G P, Bronfin D R, Daum R S 1987 Evaluation of a commercially available latex agglutination test for rapid diagnosis of group B streptococcal infection. Pediatric Infectious Disease Journal 6: 177–181

676. Rabalais G P, Samiec T D, Bryant K K, Lewis J J 1996 Invasive candidiasis in infants weighing more than 2500 grams at birth admitted to a neonatal intensive care unit. Pediatric Infectious Disease Journal 15: 348–352

677. Rabasa A I, Okolo A A 1996 Early diagnosis of septicaemia in infants with respiratory distress in the tropics. Tropical Doctor 26: 62–64

678. Rao P S, Baliga M, Shivananda P G 1993 Bacteriology of neonatal septicaemia in a rural referral hospital in south India. Journal of Tropical Pediatrics 39: 230–233

679. Rastogi A, Luken J A, Pildes R S, Chrystof D, LaBranche F 1993 Endocarditis in neonatal intensive care unit. Pediatric Cardiology 14: 183–186

680. Redd S C, Wirima J J, Steketee R W, Breman J G, Heymann D L 1996 Transplacental transmission of Plasmodium falciparum in rural Malawi. American Journal of Tropical Medicine and Hygiene 55(suppl.): 57–60

681. Reiter P D, Doron M W 1996 Vancomycin cerebrospinal fluid concentrations after intravenous administration in premature infants. Journal of Perinatology 16: 331–335

682. Remington J S, Desmonts G 1990 Toxoplasmosis. In: Remington J S, Klein J O (eds) Infectious diseases of the fetus and newborn infant, 3rd edn. W B Saunders, Philadelphia, pp 89–195

683. Rennert W, Ray C 2000 Fulminant amebic colitis in a ten-day-old infant. Pediatric Infectious Disease Journal 19: 1111–1112

684. Ring A, Braun J S, Pohl J, Nizet V, Stremmel W, Shenep J L 2002 Group B streptococcal beta-hemolysin induces mortality and liver injury in experimental sepsis. Journal of Infectious Diseases 185: 1745–1753

685. Robinson L G, Jain L, Kourtis A P 1999 Persistent candidemia in a premature infant treated with fluconazole. Pediatric Infectious Disease Journal 18: 735–737

686. Rodwell R L, Gray P H, Taylor K M, Minchinton R 1996 Granulocyte colony stimulating factor treatment for alloimmune neonatal thrombocytopenia. Archives of Disease in Childhood 75: 57–58

687. Roizen N, Swisher C N, Stein M A et al 1995 Neurologic and developmental outcome in treated congenital toxoplasmosis. Pediatrics 95: 11–20

688. Rojas J, Stahlman M 1984 The effects of group B streptococcus and other organisms on the pulmonary vasculature. Clinics in Perinatology 11: 591–599

689. Roome A, Rak M, Hadler J 2000 Follow-up of infants of hepatitis B-infected women after hepatitis B vaccination, Connecticut, 1994 to 1997. Pediatric Infectious Disease Journal 19: 573–575

690. Rooney J C, Hill D J, Danks D M 1971 Jaundice associated with bacterial infection in the newborn. American Journal of Diseases of Children 122: 39–41

691. Rosenblum L S, Villarino M E, Nainan O V et al 1991 Hepatitis A outbreak in a neonatal intensive care unit: risk factors for transmission and evidence of prolonged viral excretion among preterm infants. Journal of Infectious Diseases 164: 476–482

692. Rosenthal J, Healey T, Ellis R, Gillan E, Cairo M S 1996 A two-year follow-up of neonates with presumed sepsis treated with recombinant human granulocyte colony-stimulating factor during the first week of life. Journal of Pediatrics 128: 135–137

693. Rotbart H A 1995 Enteroviral infections of the central nervous system. Clinical Infectious Diseases 20: 971–981

694. Rowen J L, Atkins J T, Levy M L, Baer S C, Baker C J 1995 Invasive fungal dermatitis in the ≤1000-gram neonate. Pediatrics 95: 682–687

695. Rowen J L, Rench M A, Kozinetz C A, Adams J M J, Baker C J 1994 Endotracheal colonization with Candida enhances risk of systemic candidiasis in very low birth weight neonates. Journal of Pediatrics 124: 789–794

696. Rowley A H, Wald E R 1986 Incubation period necessary to detect bacteraemia in neonates. Pediatric Infectious Disease Journal 5: 590–591

697. Rubinstein, Z, Heyman Z, Morag B 1983 Ultrasound and computed tomography in the diagnosis and drainage of abscesses and other fluid collections. Israel Journal of Medical Sciences 19: 1050–1060

698. Ruiz-Extremera A, Salmeron J, Torres C et al 2000 Follow-up of transmission of hepatitis C to babies of human immunodeficiency virus-negative women: the role of breast-feeding in transmission. Pediatric Infectious Disease Journal 19: 511–516

699. Rupar D G, Herzog K D, Fisher M C 1990 Prolonged bacteraemia with catheter-related central venous thrombosis. American Journal of Diseases of Children 144: 879–882

700. Rushforth J A, Hoy C M, Kite P, Puntis J W 1993 Rapid diagnosis of central venous catheter sepsis. Lancet 342: 402–403

701. Rusin P, Adam R D, Peterson E A, Ryan K J, Sinclair N A, Weinstein L 1991 Haemophilus influenzae: an important cause of maternal and neonatal infections. Obstetrics and Gynecology 77: 92–96

702. Russell A R, Davies E G, McGuigan S, Scopes G J, Daly S, Gordon Smith E C 1994 Plasma granulocyte-colony stimulating factor concentrations ([G-CSF]) in the early neonatal period. British Journal of Haematology 86: 642–644

703. Ruuska T, Veskari T 1991 A prospective study of acute diarrhoea in Finnish children from birth to 2{1/2} years of age. Acta Paediatrica Scandinavica 80: 500–504

704. Sacker I, Brunell P A 1970 Abscess in newborn infants caused by mycoplasma. Pediatrics 46: 303–304

705. Sackett D, Haynes R B, Tugwell P, Guyatt G (eds) 1991 Clinical epidemiology. A basic science for clinical medicine. Lippincott Williams and Wilkins, Philadelphia

706. Sadiq H F, Devaskar S, Keenan W J, Weber T R 1987 Broviac catheterisation in low birthweight infants: incidence and treatment of associated complications. Critical Care Medicine 15: 47–50

707. Sagrera X, Ginovart G, Raspall F et al 2002 Outbreaks of influenza A virus infection in neonatal intensive care units. Pediatric Infectious Disease Journal 21: 196–200

708. Sahn E E 1994 Vesiculopustular diseases of neonates and infants. Current Opinion in Pediatrics 6: 442–446

709. Saiman L, Jakob K, Holmes K W et al 1998 Molecular epidemiology of staphylococcal scalded skin syndrome in premature infants. Pediatric Infectious Disease Journal 17: 329–334

710. Saiman L, Ludington E, Dawson J D et al 2001 Risk factors for Candida species colonization of neonatal intensive care unit patients. Pediatric Infectious Disease Journal 20: 1119–1124

711. Saiman L, Ludington E, Pfaller M et al 2000 Risk factors for candidemia in neonatal intensive care unit patients. The National Epidemiology of Mycosis Survey Study Group. Pediatric Infectious Disease Journal 19: 319–324

712. Saitoh M, Ichiba H, Fujioka H, Shintaku H, Yamano T 2001 Connatal tuberculosis in an extremely low birth weight infant: case report and management of exposure to tuberculosis in a neonatal intensive care unit. European Journal of Pediatrics 160: 88–90

713. Saltigeral Simental P, Macias Parra M, Mejia Valdez J, Sosa Vazquez M, Castilla Serna L, Gonzalez Saldana N 1993 Neonatal tetanus experience at the National Institute of Pediatrics in Mexico City. Pediatric Infectious Disease Journal 12: 722–725

714. Salzman M B, Isenberg H D, Shapiro J F, Lipsitz P J, Rubin L G 1993 A prospective study of the catheter hub as the portal of entry for microorganisms causing catheter-related sepsis in neonates. Journal of Infectious Diseases 167: 487–490

715. Salzman M B, Rubin L G 1995 Intravenous catheter-related infections. Advances in Pediatric Infectious Diseases 10: 337–368

716. Samson L, MacDonald N E 1995 Management of infants born to mothers who have Chlamydia infection. Pediatric Infectious Disease Journal 14: 407–408

717. Sanataella I O, Garcia M J M 1997 Neonatal meningococcal meningitis. Pediatric Infectious Disease Journal 16: 634

718. Sanchez P J 1993 Perinatal transmission of Ureaplasma urealyticum: current concepts based on review of the literature. Clinical Infectious Diseases 17(suppl. 1): S107–S111

719. Sanchez P J 1998 Laboratory tests for congenital syphilis. Pediatric Infectious Disease Journal 17: 70–71

720. Saoud A S, Abuekteish F, Obeidat A, el Nassir Z, al Rimawi H 1995 The changing face of neonatal septicaemia. Annals of Tropical Paediatrics 15: 93–96

721. Sawyer M H 1999 Enterovirus infections: diagnosis and treatment. Pediatric Infectious Disease Journal 18: 1033–1039

722. Sawyer M H, Holland D, Aintablian N, Connor J D, Keyser E F, Waecker N J J 1994 Diagnosis of enteroviral central nervous system infection by polymerase chain reaction during a large community outbreak. Pediatric Infectious Disease Journal 13: 177–182

723. Scarcella A, Pasquariello M B, Giugliano B, Vendemmia M, de Lucia A 1998 Liposomal amphotericin B treatment for neonatal fungal infections. Pediatric Infectious Disease Journal 17: 146–148

724. Scheifele D W, Bjornson G L, Dyer R A 1987 Delta-like toxin produced by coagulase-negative staphylococci is associated with neonatal necrotising enterocolitis. Infection and Immunity 55: 2268–2271

725. Schelonka R L, Chai M K, Yoder B A, Hensley D, Brockett R M, Ascher D P 1996 Volume of blood required to detect common neonatal pathogens. Journal of Pediatrics 129: 275–278

726. Schibler K R, Osborne K A, Leung L Y, Le T V, Baker S I, Thompson D D 1998 A randomized, placebo-controlled trial of granulocyte colony-stimulating factor administration to newborn infants with neutropenia and clinical signs of early-onset sepsis. Pediatrics 102: 6–13

727. Schieve L A, Handler A, Hershow R, Persky V, Davis F 1994 Urinary tract infection during pregnancy: its association with maternal morbidity and perinatal outcome. American Journal of Public Health 84: 405–410

728. Schneeberger P M, Groenendaal F, De Vries L S, van Loon A M, Vroom T M 1994 Variable outcome of a congenital cytomegalovirus infection in a quadruplet after primary infection of the mother during pregnancy. Acta Paediatrica 83: 986–989

729. Schoen E J, Limata C, Black S B 2001 Unsuccessful voluntary prenatal testing for human immunodeficiency virus infection. Pediatric Infectious Disease Journal 20: 79–81

730. Schonheyder H C, Gottschau A, Friland A, Rosdahl V T 1995 Mortality rate and magnitude of Staphylococcus aureus bacteremia as assessed by a semiquantitative blood culture system. Scandinavian Journal of Infectious Diseases 27: 19–21

731. Schrag S J, Zell E R, Lynfield R et al 2002 A population-based comparison of strategies to prevent early-onset group B streptococcal disease in neonates. New England Journal of Medicine 347: 233–239

732. Schrag S J, Zywicki S, Farley M M et al 2000 Group B streptococcal disease in the era of intrapartum antibiotic prophylaxis. New England Journal of Medicine 342: 15–20

733. Schreffler R T, Schreffler A J, Wittler R R 2002 Treatment of cerebrospinal fluid shunt infections: a decision analysis. Pediatric Infectious Disease Journal 21: 632–636

734. Schuchat A, Lizano C, Broome C V, Swaminathan B, Kim C, Winn K 1991 Outbreak of neonatal listeriosis associated with mineral oil. Pediatric Infectious Disease Journal 10: 183–189

735. Schuchat A, Zywicki S S, Dinsmoor M J et al 2000 Risk factors and opportunities for prevention of early-onset neonatal sepsis: a multicenter case-control study. Pediatrics 105: 21–26

736. Schwartz D A, Larsen S A, Beck Sague C, Fears M, Rice R J 1995 Pathology of the umbilical cord in congenital syphilis: analysis of 25 specimens using histochemistry and immunofluorescent antibody to Treponema pallidum. Human Pathology 26: 784–791

737. Schwebke K, Henry K, Balfour H H J, Olson D, Crane R T, Jordan M C 1995 Congenital cytomegalovirus infection as a result of nonprimary cytomegalovirus disease in a mother with acquired immunodeficiency syndrome. Journal of Pediatrics 126: 293–295

738. Schwersenski J, McIntyre L, Bauer C R 1991 Lumbar puncture frequency and cerebrospinal fluid analysis in the neonate. American Journal of Diseases of Children 145: 54–58

739. Scott L L, Sanchez P J, Jackson G L, Zeray F, Wendel G D Jr 1996 Acyclovir suppression to prevent cesarean delivery after first-episode genital herpes. Obstetrics and Gynecology 87: 69–73

740. Sehgal A, Sehgal R, Gupta I, Bhakoo O N, Ganguly N K 1992 Use of hepatitis B vaccine alone or in combination with hepatitis B immunoglobulin for immunoprophylaxis of perinatal hepatitis B infection. Journal of Tropical Pediatrics 38: 247–251

741. Seto D, West D J, Gilliam R R, Ioli V A, Ferrara D K, Rich B 1999 Antibody responses of healthy neonates of two mixed regimens of hepatitis B vaccine. Pediatric Infectious Disease Journal 18: 840–842

742. Sever J A, White L R 1969 Intrauterine viral infections. Annual Review of Medicine 19: 471–486

743. Shah S S, Ehrenkranz R A, Gallagher P G 1999 Increasing incidence of gram-negative rod bacteremia in a newborn intensive care unit. Pediatric Infectious Disease Journal 18: 591–595

744. Shah S S, Gallagher P G 1998 Complications of conjunctivitis caused by Pseudomonas aeruginosa in a newborn intensive care unit. Pediatric Infectious Disease Journal 17: 97–102

745. Shalev E, Battino S, Romano S, Blondhaim O, Ben Ami M 1994 Intraamniotic infection with Candida albicans successfully treated with transcervical amnioinfusion of amphotericin. American Journal of Obstetrics and Gynecology 170: 1271–1272

746. Shamir R, Maayan-Metzger A, Bujanover Y, Ashkenazi S, Dinari G, Sirota L 2000 Liver enzyme abnormalities in gram-negative bacteremia of premature infants. Pediatric Infectious Disease Journal 19: 495–498

747. Shamseldin el Shafie S, Smith W, Donnelly G 1995 An outbreak of gentamicin-resistant Klebsiella pneumoniae in a neonatal ward. Central European Journal of Public Health 3: 129–131

748. Sharek P J, Benitz W E, Abel N J, Freeburn M J, Mayer M L, Bergman D A 2002 Effect of an evidence-based hand washing policy on hand washing rates and false-positive coagulase negative staphylococcus blood and cerebrospinal fluid culture rates in a level III NICU. Journal of Perinatology 22: 137–143

749. Sharland M, Khare M, Bedford-Russell A 2002 Prevention of postnatal cytomegalovirus infection in preterm infants. Archives of Disease in Childhood. Fetal and Neonatal Edition 86: F140

750. Sharma R, Hudak M, Premachandra B et al 2002 Clinical manifestations of rotavirus infection in the neonatal intensive care unit. Pediatric Infectious Disease Journal 21: 1099–1015

751. Shattuck K E, Chonmaitree T 1992 The changing spectrum of neonatal meningitis over a fifteen-year period. Clinical Pediatrics 31: 130–136

752. Sheridan E, Aitken C, Jeffries D, Hird M, Thayalasekaran P 2002 Congenital rubella syndrome: a risk in immigrant populations. Lancet 359: 674–675

753. Sikuler E, Guetta V, Keynan A, Neumann L, Schlaeffer F 1989 Abnormalities in bilirubin and liver enzyme levels in adult patients with bacteremia. A prospective study [see comments]. Archives of Internal Medicine 149: 2246–2248

754. Simoes E A, King S J, Lehr M V, Groothuis J R 1993 Preterm twins and triplets. A high-risk group for severe respiratory syncytial virus infection. American Journal of Diseases of Children 147: 303–306

755. Singh J, Dick J, Santosham, M 2000 Colonization of the female urogenital tract with Streptococcus pneumoniae and implications for neonatal disease. Pediatric Infectious Disease Journal 19: 260–262

756. Sison A V 1992 Maternal and fetal infections. Current Opinion in Obstetrics and Gynecology 4: 48–54

757. Sizun J, Soupre D, Legrand M C et al 1995 Neonatal nosocomial respiratory infection with coronavirus: a prospective study in a neonatal intensive care unit. Acta Paediatrica 84: 617–620

758. Sklavunu Tsurutsoglu S, Gatzola Karaveli M, Hatziioannidis K, Tsurutsoglu G 1991 Efficacy of aztreonam in the treatment of neonatal sepsis. Reviews of Infectious Diseases 13(suppl. 7): S591–S593

759. Smellie J M, Rigden S P A 1995 Pitfalls in the investigation of children with urinary tract infection. Archives of Disease in Childhood 72: 251–258

760. Smellie J M, Rigden S P A, Prescod N P 1995 Urinary tract infection: a comparison of four methods of investigation. Archives of Disease in Childhood 72: 247–250

761. Smith E M, Johnson S R, Cripe T et al 1995 Perinatal transmission and maternal risks of human papillomavirus infection. Cancer Detection and Prevention 19: 196–205

762. Smith H, Congdon P 1985 Neonatal systemic candidiasis. Archives of Disease in Childhood 60: 365–369

763. Smith J R, Taylor Robinson D 1993 Infection due to Chlamydia trachomatis in pregnancy and the newborn. Baillieres Clinical Obstetrics and Gynaecology 7: 237–255

764. Smith R, Malee K, Charurat M et al 2000 Timing of perinatal human immunodeficiency virus type 1 infection and rate of neurodevelopment. The Women and Infant Transmission Study Group. Pediatric Infectious Disease Journal 19: 862–871

765. Soman M, Green B, Daling J 1985 Risk factors for early neonatal sepsis. American Journal of Epidemiology 121: 712–719

766. Sood M, Trehan A, Arora S, Jayashanker K, Marwaha R K 2000 Congenital tuberculosis manifesting as cutaneous disease. Pediatric Infectious Disease Journal 19: 1109–1111

767. Soriano A L, Russell R G, Johnson D, Lagos R, Sechter I, Morris J G J 1991 Pathophysiology of Citrobacter diversus neonatal meningitis: comparative studies in an infant mouse model. Infection and Immunity 59: 1352–1358

768. Sorrentino M, Powers T 2000 Effectiveness of palivizumab: evaluation of outcomes form the 1998 to 1999 respiratory syncytial virus season. Pediatric Infectious Disease Journal 19: 1068–1071

769. Soulie J C 1995 [Cardiac involvement in fetal parvovirus B19 infection.] Pathologie Biologie 43: 416–419

770. Spafford P S, Sinkin R A, Cox C, Reubens L, Powell K R 1994 Prevention of central venous catheter-related coagulase-negative staphylococcal sepsis in neonates. Journal of Pediatrics 125: 259–263

771. Sperling R S, Newton E R, Gibbs R S 1988 Intra-amniotic infection in low-birth-weight infants. Journal of Infectious Diseases 157: 113–117

772. Spirer Z, Jurgenson U, Lazewnick R, Reider-Grossvasser I 1982 Complete recovery from an apparent brain abcess treated without neurosurgery: the importance of early CT scanning. Clinical Pediatrics 21: 106–109

773. Stark V, Harrisson S P 1992 Staphylococcus aureus colonization of the newborn in a Darlington hospital. Journal of Hospital Infection 21: 205–211

774. Steele A D, Sears J F 1996 Characterisation of rotaviruses recovered from neonates with symptomatic infection. South African Medical Journal 86: 1546–1549

775. Steketee R W, Wirima J J, Bloland P B et al 1996 Impairment of a pregnant woman's acquired ability to limit Plasmodium falciparum by infection with human immunodeficiency virus type-1. American Journal of Tropical Medicine and Hygiene 55(suppl.): 42–49

776. Stiller R J, Blair E, Clark P, Tinghitella T 1989 Rapid detection of vaginal colonization with group B streptococci by means of latex agglutination. American Journal of Obstetrics and Gynecology 160: 566–568

777. Stoll B J, Fanaroff A 1995 Early-onset coagulase-negative staphylococcal sepsis in preterm neonate. National Institute of Child Health and Human Development (NICHD) Neonatal Research Network [letter]. Lancet 345: 1236–1237

778. Stoll B, Gordon T, Korones S B et al 1996 Late-onset sepsis in very low birthweight neonates: a report from the National Institute of Child Health and Human Development Neonatal Research Network. Journal of Pediatrics 129: 63–71

779. Stoll B J, Hansen N, Fanaroff A A et al 2002 Changes in pathogens causing early-onset sepsis in very-low-birth-weight infants. New England Journal of Medicine 347: 240–247

780. Stoll B J, Hansen N, Fanaroff A A et al 2002 Late-onset sepsis in very low birth weight neonates: the experience of the NICHD Neonatal Research Network. Pediatrics 110: 285–291

781. Stoll B J, Schuchat A 1998 Maternal carriage of group B streptococci in developing countries. Pediatric Infectious Disease Journal 17: 499–503

782. Strauss R G, Levy G J, Sotelo-Avila C 1993 National survey of neonatal transfusion practices: II. Blood component therapy. Pediatrics 91: 530–536

783. Struelens M 2002 Molecular typing: a key tool for the surveillance and control of nosocomial infection. Current Opinion in Infectious Diseases 15: 383–385

784. Struthers S, Underhill H, Albersheim S, Greenberg D, Dobson S 2002 A comparison of two versus one blood culture in the diagnosis and treatment of coagulase-negative staphylococcus in the neonatal intensive care unit. Journal of Perinatology 22: 547–549

785. Stuart R L, Turnidge J, Grayson M L 1995 Safety of imipenem in neonates. Pediatric Infectious Disease Journal 14: 804–805

786. Stutman H R 1991 Clinical experience with aztreonam for treatment of infections in children. Reviews of Infectious Diseases 13(suppl. 7): S582–S585

787. Sullender W M, Miller J L, Yasukawa L L et al 1987 Humoral and cell-mediated immunity in neonates with herpes simplex virus infection. Journal of Infectious Diseases 155: 28–37

788. Sullivan J L, Luzuriaga K 2001 The changing face of pediatric HIV-1 infection. New England Journal of Medicine 345: 1568–1569

789. Suzuki, N, Terada S, Inoue M 1995 Neonatal meningitis with human parvovirus B19 infection [letter]. Archives of Disease in Childhood. Fetal and Neonatal Edition 73: F196–F197

790. Svanborg C, Hausson S, Jodal U 1988 Host-parasite interaction in the urinary tract. Journal of Infectious Diseases 157: 421–425

791. Swingle H M, Bucciarelli R L, Ayoub E M 1985 Synergy between penicillins and low concentrations of gentamicin in the killing of group B streptococci. Journal of Infectious Diseases 152: 515–520

792. Synnott M B, Morse D L, Hall S M 1994 Neonatal meningitis in England & Wales: a review of routine national data. Archives of Disease in Childhood 71: 75–80

793. Tajiri H, Miyoshi Y, Funada S et al 2001 Prospective study of mother-to-infant transmission of hepatitis C virus. Pediatric Infectious Disease Journal 20: 10–14

794. Tan T Q, Mason E O J, Ou C N, Kaplan S L 1993 Use of intravenous rifampin in neonates with persistent staphylococcal bacteremia. Antimicrobial Agents and Chemotherapy 37: 2401–2406

795. Tan T Q, Musser J M, Shulman R J, Mason E O J, Mahoney D H J, Kaplan S L 1994 Molecular epidemiology of coagulase-negative Staphylococcus blood isolates from neonates with persistent bacteremia and children with central venous catheter infections. Journal of Infectious Diseases 169: 1393–1397

796. Tarcan A, Ozbek N, Gurakan B 2001 Bone marrow failure with concurrent enteroviral infection in a newborn. Pediatric Infectious Disease Journal 20: 719–721

797. Thorp J M Jr, Katz V L, Fowler L J, Kurtzman J T, Bowes W A Jr 1989 Fetal death from chlamydial infection across intact amniotic membranes. American Journal of Obstetrics and Gynecology 161: 1245–1246

798. Thureen P J, Moreland S, Rodden D J, Merenstein G B, Levin M, Rosenberg A A 1993 Failure of tracheal aspirate cultures to define the cause of respiratory deteriorations in neonates. Pediatric Infectious Disease Journal 12: 560–564

799. Tookey P A, Ades A E, Peckham C S 1992 Cytomegalovirus prevalence in pregnant women: the influence of parity. Archives of Disease in Childhood 67: 779–783

800. Tookey P, Peckham C S 1996 Neonatal herpes simplex virus infection in the British Isles. Paediatric and Perinatal Epidemiology 10: 432–442

801. Torok T J, Wang Q Y, Gary G W, Yang C F, Finch T M, Anderson L J 1992 Prenatal diagnosis of intrauterine infection with parvovirus B19 by the polymerase chain reaction technique. Clinical Infectious Diseases 14: 149–155

802. Tugal O, Pallant B, Shebarek N, Jayabose S 1994 Transient erythroblastopenia of the newborn caused by human parvovirus. American Journal of Pediatric Hematology and Oncology 16: 352–355

803. Tullus K, Brauner A, Fryklund B, Munkhammar T, Rabsch W, Reissbrodt R, Burman L G 1992 Host factors versus virulence-associated bacterial characteristics in neonatal and infantile bacteraemia and meningitis caused by Escherichia coli. Journal of Medical Microbiology 36: 203–208

804. Turner G C, Green H T, Blundell V T 1978 e-Antigen: a link between immune response and infectivity in hepatitis B? Journal of Hygiene 81: 405–414

805. Umana M A, Odio C M, Castro E, Salas J L, McCracken G H J 1990 Evaluation of aztreonam and ampicillin vs. amikacin and ampicillin for treatment of neonatal bacterial infections. Pediatric Infectious Disease Journal 9: 175–180

806. Umasankar S, Mridha E U, Hannan M M, Fry C M, Azadian B S 1996 An outbreak of Salmonella enteritidis in a maternity and neonatal intensive care unit. Journal of Hospital Infection 34: 117–122

807. Vain N E, Mazlumian J R, Swarner W 1980 Role of exchange transfusion in the treatment of severe septicaemia. Pediatrics 66: 693–698

808. Valencia G B, Banzon F, Cummings M, McCormack W M, Glass L, Hammerschlag M R 1993 Mycoplasma hominis and Ureaplasma urealyticum in neonates with suspected infection. Pediatric Infectious Disease Journal 12: 571–573

809. Valente P, Sever J L 1994 In utero diagnosis of congenital infections by direct fetal sampling. Israel Journal of Medical Sciences 30: 414–420

810. Valentin-Weigand P, Chhatwal G S 1995 Correlation of epithelial cell invasiveness of group B streptococci with clinical source of isolation. Microbial Pathogenesis 19: 83–91

811. Vallette J D Jr, Goldberg R N, Suguihara C et al 1995 Effect of an interleukin-1 receptor antagonist on the hemodynamic manifestations of group B streptococcal sepsis. Pediatric Research 38: 704–708

812. Van Camp J M, Tomaselli V, Coran A G 1994 Bacterial translocation in the neonate. Current Opinion in Pediatrics 6: 327–333

813. van den Dungen F A, Van Furth A M, Fetter W P, Zaaijer H L, Van Elburg R M 2001 Fatal case of influenza B virus pneumonia in a preterm neonate. Pediatric Infectious Disease Journal 20: 82–84

814. Van Houten M A, Uiterwaal C S, Heesen G J, Arends J P, Kimpen J L 2001 Does the empiric use of vancomycin in pediatrics increase the risk for Gram-negative bacteremia? Pediatric Infectious Disease Journal 20: 171–177

815. van Ogtrop M L, van Zoeren-Grobben D, Verbakel-Salomans E M A, van Boven C P A 1997 Serratia marcescens infections in neonatal departments: description of an outbreak and review of the literature. Journal of Hospital Infection 36: 95–103

816. Van Winter J T, Ney J A, Ogburn P L J, Johnson R V 1994 Preterm labor and congenital candidiasis. A case report. Journal of Reproductive Medicine 39: 987–990

817. Velaphi S, Siegel J D, Wendel G D Jr, Cushion N, Eid W M, Sanchez P J 2003 Early-onset group B streptococcal infection after a combined maternal and neonatal group B streptococcal chemoprophylaxis strategy. Pediatrics 111: 541–547

818. Venkateswaran L, Wilimas J A, Dancy R, Wang W C, Korones S, Hayden J, Hayes F A 2000 Granulocyte-macrophage colony-stimulating factor in the treatment of neonates with neutropenia and sepsis. Pediatric Hematology and Oncology 17: 469–473

819. Verkuyl D A A 1995 Practising obstetrics and gynaecology in areas with a high prevalence of HIV infection. Lancet 346: 293–296

820. Visser V H, Hall R T 1980 Lumbar puncture in the evaluation of neonatal sepsis. Journal of Pediatrics 96: 1063–1067

821. Vochem M, Hamprecht K, Jahn G, Speer C P 1998 Transmission of cytomegalovirus to preterm infants through breast milk. Pediatric Infectious Disease Journal 17: 53–58

822. Voora S, Srinivasan G, Lilien L D, Yeh T F, Pildes R S 1982 Fever in full term newborns in the first 4 days of life. Pediatrics 69: 40–44

823. Wainer S, Cooper P A, Gouws H, Akierman A 1997 Prospective study of fluconazole therapy in systemic neonatal fungal infection. Pediatric Infectious Disease Journal 16: 763–767

824. Waites K B, Crouse D T, Cassell G H 1993 Therapeutic considerations for Ureaplasma urealyticum infections in neonates. Clinical Infectious Diseases 17(suppl. 1): S208–S214

825. Waites K B, Sims P J, Crouse D T et al 1994 Serum concentrations of erythromycin after intravenous infusion in preterm neonates treated for Ureaplasma urealyticum infection. Pediatric Infectious Disease Journal 13: 287–293

826. Walker G J 2001 Antibiotics for syphilis diagnosed during pregnancy (Cochrane Review). Cochrane Database of Systematic Reviews (3): CD001143

827. Walpole I R, Hodgen N, Bower C 1991 Congenital toxoplasmosis: a large survey in western Australia. Medical Journal of Australia 154: 720–724

828. Ware R 1989 Human parvovirus infection [see comments]. Journal of Pediatrics 114: 343–348

829. Wareham J, Harris H, Whitman I 1995 Herpes simplex type II infection in monozygotic twins. American Journal of Perinatology 12: 75–77

830. Watson J C, Fleming D W, Borella A J, Olcott E S, Conrad R E, Baron R C 1993 Vertical transmission of hepatitis A resulting in an outbreak in a neonatal intensive care unit. Journal of Infectious Diseases 167: 567–571

831. Watson W J, Stevens T P, Weinberg G A 1998 Profound anemia in a newborn infant of a mother receiving antiretroviral therapy. Pediatric Infectious Disease Journal 17: 435–436

832. Webber S, Wilkinson A R, Lindsell D, Hope P L, Dobson S R M, Isaacs D 1990 Neonatal pneumonia. Archives of Disease in Childhood 65: 207–211

833. Weinstein M. Ford-Jones E, Cutz E 2001 Esophagitis and perinatal cytomegalovirus infection. Pediatric Infectious Disease Journal 20: 545–546

834. Weisman L E, Cruess D F, Fischer G W 1993 Standard versus hyperimmune intravenous immunoglobulin in preventing or treating neonatal bacterial infections. Clinics in Perinatology 20: 211–224

835. Weisse M E, Person D A, Berkenbaugh J T J 1993 Treatment of Candida arthritis with flucytosine and amphotericin. Journal of Perinatology 13: 402–404

836. Wellington M, Gigliotti F 2001 Update on antifungal agents. Pediatric Infectious Disease Journal 20: 993–995

837. Wen T S, Eriksen N L, Blanco J D, Graham J M, Oshiro B T, Prieto J A 1993 Association of clinical intra-amniotic infection and meconium. American Journal of Perinatology 10: 438–440

838. Wettergren B, Jodal U, Jonasson G 1985 Epidemiology of bacteriuria during the first year of life. Acta Paediatrica Scandinavica 74: 925–930

839. Whitley R J 1988 Neonatal herpes simplex virus infections. Clinics in Perinatology 15: 903–916

840. Whitley R J 1993 Neonatal herpes simplex virus infections. Journal of Medical Virology suppl. 1: 13–21

841. Whitley R, Arvin A, Prober C et al 1991 Predictors of morbidity and mortality in neonates with herpes simplex virus infections. The National Institute of Allergy and Infectious Diseases Collaborative Antiviral Study Group. New England Journal of Medicine 324: 450–454

842. Wild N J, Sheppard S, Smithells R W, Holzel H, Jones G 1989 Onset and severity of hearing loss due to congenital rubella infection. Archives of Disease in Childhood 64: 1280–1283

843. Williams I, Goldstein S, Tufa J, Tauillii S, Margolis H, Mahoney F 2003 Long term antibody response to hepatitis B vaccination beginning at birth and to subsequent booster vaccination. Pediatric Infectious Disease Journal 22: 157–163

844. Williams P A, Bohnsack J F, Augustine N H, Drummond W K, Rubens C E, Hill H R 1993 Production of tumor necrosis factor by human cells in vitro and in vivo, induced by group B streptococci. Journal of Pediatrics 123: 292–300

845. Williams R, Kirkbride V, Corcoran G D 1994 Neonatal osteomyelitis in Down's syndrome due to non-encapsulated Haemophilus influenzae. Journal of Infection 29: 203–205

846. Williamson M, Fraser S H, Tilse M 1995 Failure of the urinary group B streptococcal antigen test as a screen for neonatal sepsis. Archives of Disease in Childhood 73: 109–111

847. Wiswell T E, Baumgart S, Gannon C M, Spitzer A R 1995 No lumbar puncture in the evaluation for early neonatal sepsis: will meningitis be missed? Pediatrics 95: 803–806

848. Wiswell T E, Hachey W E 1991 Multiple site blood cultures in the initial evaluation for neonatal sepsis during the first week of life. Pediatric Infectious Disease Journal 10: 365–369

849. Wiswell T E, Roscelli J D 1986 Corroborative evidence for the decreased incidence of urinary tract infections in circumcised male infants. Pediatrics 78: 96–99

850. Wong S N, Ng T L 1991 Haemophilus influenzae septicaemia in the neonate: report of two cases and review of the English literature. Journal of Paediatrics and Child Health 27: 113–115

851. Wong S N, Tam A Y, Ng T H, Ng W F, Tong C Y, Tang T S 1989 Fatal Coxsackie B1 virus infection in neonates. Pediatric Infectious Disease Journal 8: 638–641

852. Wong S Y, Hajdu M P, Ramirez R, Thulliez P, McLeod R, Remington J S 1993 Role of specific immunoglobulin E in diagnosis of acute toxoplasma infection and toxoplasmosis. Journal of Clinical Microbiology 31: 2952–2959

853. Wright E D, Lortan J E, Perinpanayagam R M 1990 Early-onset neonatal pneumococcal sepsis in siblings. Journal of Infection 20: 59–63

854. Wu S, Shen L 1993 Plasmid analysis and phage typing in the study of staphylococcal colonization and disease in newborn infants. Chinese Medical Sciences Journal 8: 157–161

855. Wynn R J 1979 Neonatal E. coli pericarditis. Journal of Perinatal Medicine 7: 23–24

856. Yagupsky P, Menegus M A, Powell K R 1991 The changing spectrum of group B streptococcal disease in infants: an eleven-year experience in a tertiary care hospital. Pediatric Infectious Disease Journal 10: 801–808

857. Yamamoto A Y, Mussi-Pinhata M M, Cristina P, Pinto G, Moraes Figueiredo L T, Jorge S M 2001 Congenital cytomegalovirus infection in preterm and full-term newborn infants from a population with a high seroprevalence rate. Pediatric Infectious Disease Journal 20: 188–192

858. Yeager A S, Arvin A M 1984 Reasons for the absence of a history of recurrent genital infections in mothers of neonates infected with herpes simplex virus. Pediatrics 73: 188–193

859. Yoon P W, Black R E, Moulton L H, Becker S 1996 Effect of not breastfeeding on the risk of diarrheal and respiratory mortality in children under 2 years of age in Metro Cebu, The Philippines. American Journal of Epidemiology 143: 1142–1148

860. Yoshioka H, Iseki K-I, Fujita K 1983 Development and differences of intestinal flora in the neonatal period in breast-fed and bottle-fed infants. Pediatrics 72: 317–321

861. Yow M D 1989 Congenital cytomegalovirus disease: a NOW problem [see comments]. Journal of Infectious Diseases 159: 163–167

862. Yuksel B, Greenough A 1994 Viral infections acquired during neonatal intensive care and lung function of preterm infants at follow-up. Acta Paediatrica 83: 117–118

863. Zafar A B, Butler R C, Reese D J, Gaydos L A, Mennonna P A 1995 Use of 0.3% triclosan (Bacti-Stat) to eradicate an outbreak of methicillin-resistant Staphylococcus aureus in a neonatal nursery. American Journal of Infection Control 23: 200–208

864. Zaia J A 1999 Diagnosis of CMV. Pediatric Infectious Disease Journal 18: 153–154

865. Zenker P N, Berman S M 1991 Congenital syphilis: trends and recommendations for evaluation and management. Pediatric Infectious Disease Journal 10: 516–522

866. Zuccotti G V, Riva E, Flumine P et al 1994 Hepatitis B vaccination in infants of mothers infected with human immunodeficiency virus. Journal of Pediatrics 125: 70–72

867. Zuerlein T J, Butler J C, Yeager T D 1990 Superficial cultures in neonatal sepsis evaluations. Impact on antibiotic decision making. Clinical Pediatrics 29: 445–447

868. Zuin G, Saccani B, Di Giacomo S, Tanzi E, Zanetti A R, Principi N 1999 Outcome of mother to infant acquired GBV-C/HGV infection, Archives of Disease in Childhood. Fetal and Neonatal Edition 80: F72–F73

869. Zupan J, Garner P 2000 Topical umbilical cord care at birth (Cochrane Review). Cochrane Database of Systematic Reviews (2): CD001057

CHAPTER 41

Neurological problems in the newborn

PART 1

Assessment of the neonatal nervous system

Janet M Rennie

Introduction

Suspicion of neurological illness in the neonatal period is always important. As in any organ system disease, diagnosis and prognosis must be based on the findings of a full examination together with the results of appropriate investigation. Neonatal neurological assessment should include repeated careful examinations, which of necessity are dominated by examination of the baby's state of alertness and the motor system. Neurological examination of a baby receiving intensive care is difficult, but not impossible, and can be supplemented by a wide range of diagnostic tests. Cranial ultrasound scanning is now standard in neonatal units, and atlases have been published that can help clinicians interpret the findings.[18,39] Much valuable experience has been gained with magnetic resonance imaging (MRI) scanning of the neonatal brain.[6,43] Normal ranges exist for somatosensory, auditory and visual evoked potentials, and recording the electroencephalogram (EEG) can prove extremely helpful. The information in this short chapter can be supplemented by further reading from more detailed texts.[1,2,12,51] Much of the modern work on examination of the neonatal nervous system has built on the earlier teaching of Andre-Thomas,[5] Saint-Anne Dargassies,[44] Prechtl[33] and Illingworth.[24,25] For advice on general examination of the newborn see Chapter 14.

Examination systems

The endless fascination that observing babies provides is reflected in the number of schemes that have been developed for assessment of the neonatal nervous system. Majnemer and Mazer reviewed nine different systems,[28] many of which require special training and take up to an hour to carry out. This is not practical in clinical practice, or possible in sick babies. The recommendations vary from a 'cut down' version of an adult-style neurological examination to a totally unstructured approach involving observation of general spontaneous movement.[9] I agree with Amiel-Tison[1] that the allocation of a numbered score implies a degree of standardisation and accuracy which does not exist.

My current personal system is illustrated in Fig. 41.1 and can be carried out quickly and adapted for babies in intensive care. This scheme includes many of the items from the original and updated Dubowitz system, which has been developed after a great deal of careful research and was designed to be taught to junior resident staff and to be reproducible and quick to carry out. The updated scheme takes into account the newer emphasis on the importance of hand posture and presence or absence of individual finger movements, and has reduced duplication.[12,14] In addition to completing a suitable pro forma, there is no substitute for a short and pithy narrative note. For example:

At the start of the examination, Tom was lying prone in his incubator in a flexed posture with his knees tucked up under his abdomen, eyes closed and breathing regularly. His head circumference was 35 cm and his fontanelle felt normal.

When stroked lightly on his back he awoke and began fussing, with normal facial and body movements and a normal cry, but he soon calmed when stroked again. He sucked vigorously on a finger with a stripping action of his tongue, made eye contact readily and followed a target horizontally through 90° in each direction with ease. When observed lying on his back he kicked with both legs, and his truncal and limb tone and reflexes were normal. His hands were relaxed and open and he made individual movements of his fingers. He could not be taken out of the incubator to test stepping or ventral suspension today but his Moro response appeared full and symmetrical, although it was not possible to test head lag. As far as I can assess, Tom's neurological state was normal today.

Alice's head circumference is small for a term baby at 32 cm, and her ears appear prominent – they are not low-set. Her skull is a normal shape and although her fontanelle was small (little fingertip size) the tension felt

Neonatal CNS examination

Name: _____   Date of Exam: ___/___/___

DOB: ___/___/___   Examiner: _____

GA: _____ weeks

modified from Dubowitz 1981 and other sources © JMR 2004

States:
0. Coma: no/little response to pain
1. Deep sleep, no movement, regular breathing
2. Light sleep, eyes shut, some movement
3. Dozing, eyes opening and closing
4. Awake, eyes open, minimal movement
5. Wide awake, vigorous movement
6. Crying

* Do not examine starred items * in ventilated or very ill babies

Orientation and behaviour; note any adverse circumstances e.g. excessive noise

State at start	0	1 or 2	3 or 4	5 or 6
and end of exam	0	1 or 2	3 or 4	5 or 6
Level of consciousness	Comatose	Lethargic	Hyperalert, stary-eyed	Normal, easily aroused
Consolability	High pitched cry, continuous	Cries, difficult to console	Cries, easy to console	Not crying, consoling not needed
Irritability	Cries when not handled	Cries often and easily	Cries sometimes when handled, not irritable	Quiet all the time – too quiet
Visual orientation	Doesn't fix or follow, or roving eye movements	Fixes and follows but loses interest	Fixes and follows up to 90° horizontally	Fixes and follows reliably horizontally
Social interaction	Cannot engage at all	Tries to engage but does not succeed	Brief interest in stimuli or face of examiner	Easy to engage and makes eye contact

Posture and movement (normal and abnormal)

Posture: draw here	Opistotonus, or flexed arms extended legs 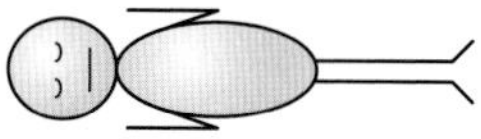	Arms + legs extended 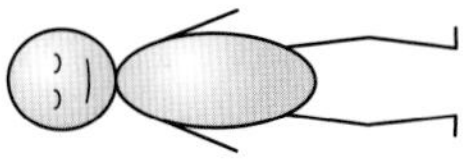	Legs flexed but not adducted 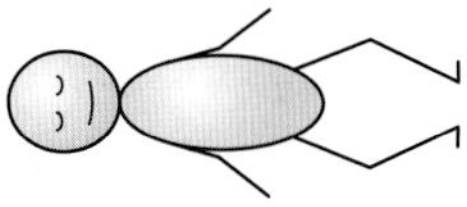	Normal, legs flexed. Legs well flexed near abdomen 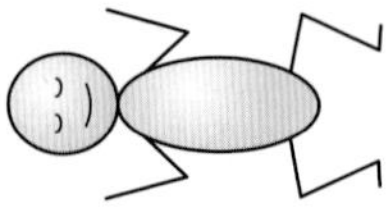

Spontaneous movements Observe quality and quantity	No spontaneous movement	Paucity of movement, occasional random jerky movement, only stretching	Stereotyped or monotonous	Rich variety, smooth, fluent, good variability and range
Hand movements	Thumb fixed in palm, hand fisted all the time	No finger movements, intermittent fisting	Some occasional finger movements	Fine elegant finger movements, hands open
Tremours/startles	None, no reaction to loud noise or stimuli	Continuous tremours and startles	Frequent spontaneous startles and tremours when awake	Tremour after Moro. occasional spontaneous startle
Clinical seizures – describe	More than 6/day	3–6/day	<3/day	None

Fig. 41.1 A system for neonatal neurological examination, adapted from Dubowitz, Prechtl, Amiel-Tison and others.

Trunk and limb tone

Head control/head lag* draw here	No attempt to raise head, complete lag 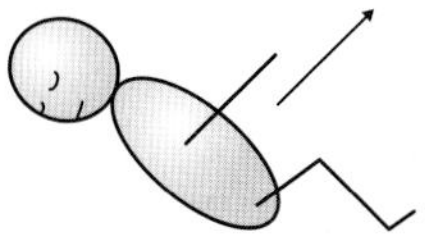	Tries to lift head but effort better felt than seen, head drops back 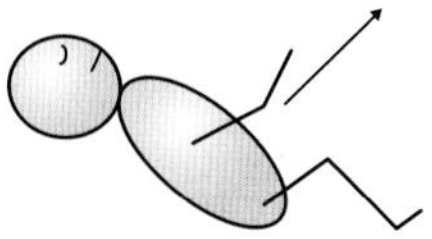	Raises head very briefly, in line with body 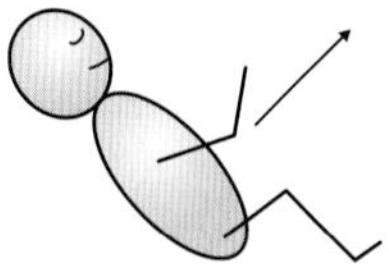	Raises head – remains vertical and in front of body for brief time 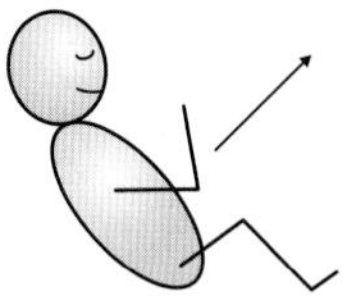
Ventral suspension* draw here	Back curved head and limbs hang straight 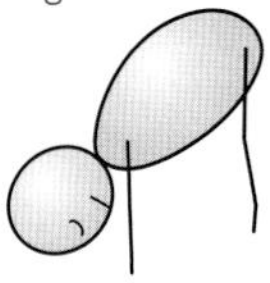	Back curved limbs slightly flexed 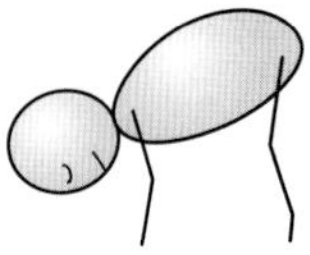	Back straight head in line limbs flexed 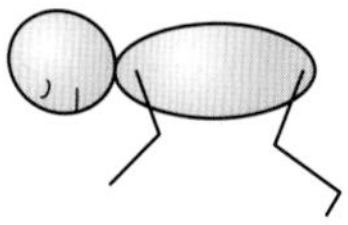	Back straight head above body 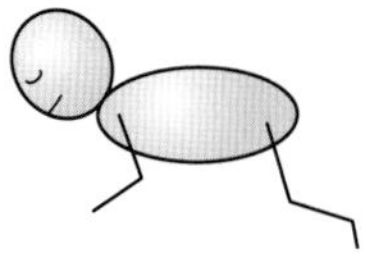
Leg recoil	No flexion	Incomplete	Complete, but slow	Complete and fast
Take both ankles with one hand, flex hips and knees, quickly extend, let go. Repeat × 3				
Truncal tone	Flaccid	Hyotonic	Hypertonic	Normal
Limb tone	Flaccid	Hyotonic	Hypertonic	Normal

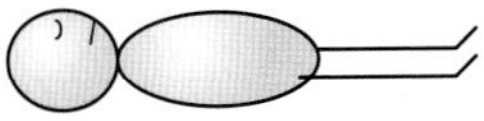

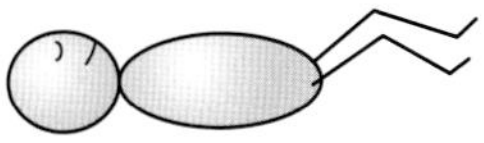

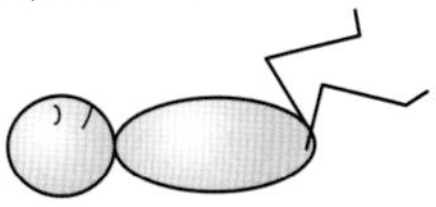

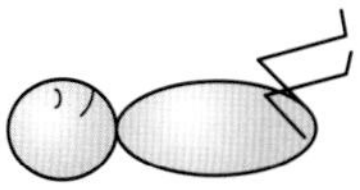

Reflexes

Tendon reflexes	Absent	Exaggerated	Clonus	Normal
Stepping*	No attempt to lift leg over the edge of the couch	Dorsiflexion of ankle	Flexes hip and knee and places sole on couch	Automatic walking easy to obtain
Moro*	Absent	Incomplete	Asymmetrical	Normal
Root*	Absent	Weak	Some head turning and mouth opening	Searches and localises
Asymmetric tonic neck	Absent			Present
Sucking	Absent	Bites, clenches	Weak irregular suck	Strong suck, strips

General observations

Fontanelle/OFC	OFC: cm	Tense	Full	Normal
Skull	Caput	Subgaleal haematoma	Sutures overriding	Cephalhaematoma
Respiration	IPPV for apnoea	Brief apnoeas	Hyperventilation	Normal
Stability during exam	Unstable	Abnormal state throughout, no change	Little transition of state, slow transition	Rapid transition of state, well tolerated

Comments:

Fig. 41.1 (Continued)

normal. When observed at the start, Alice was lying on her back, with outstretched arms and extended legs; she had a high pitched scream and was arching her back at times, digging her heels into the cot mattress. Her hands were fisted with the thumbs in both palms all the time and I did not observe her to open them. She could be consoled by swaddling and rocking but this took patience, and when she was handled her tone was high both in the trunk and the limbs. After some persuasion Alice fixed on a red woolly ball but did not track it consistently or through a wide range of arc. Alice did not make eye contact with me; she chomped on my finger and I note that the nurses are tube feeding her at the moment. Tendon reflexes were easy to obtain but I could not elicit a stepping or root reflex and her Moro was incomplete with a brisk adduction phase. I am concerned about Alice, whose neurological assessment was not normal today, and in my view a re-examination should be carried out before she is discharged home.

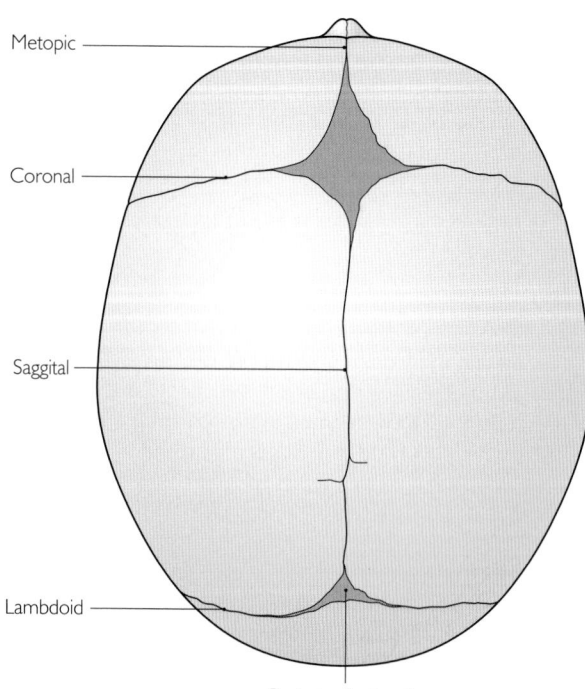

Fig. 41.2 Diagram to show the position of the cranial sutures and the fontanelles.

Labels: Metopic, Coronal, Saggital, Lambdoid, Posterior fontanelle

Scheme of neonatal neurological examination

General observations

Head size and shape

The head circumference should be measured as part of routine examination of the newborn (Ch 14), but the importance of documenting head size and head growth as part of neurological assessment cannot be overstressed. Fontanelle size and tension must be recorded.

The newborn skull is not fused and it is possible to palpate the cranial sutures, which should not be ridged or separated too far (Fig. 41.2). Observe any superficial swellings such as cephalhaematoma (p. 253) or subgaleal collections (pp. 1122–6). Fused sutures (craniosynostosis) may need treatment, or may be a clue to an underlying disorder such as Apert's syndrome (p. 793). Advice from a neurosurgeon may be needed.

Orientation and behaviour

Behavioural states

The initial assessment of the baby's nervous system should involve evaluation of behavioural state, a sensitive indicator of neural integrity. Behavioural states can be described on the basis of four features (Table 41.1, Fig. 41.1).[32,37,7]

Term babies spend about 50 minutes of each hour asleep, about 50% of the time in quiet sleep (state 1). Babies usually cycle between states, and failure to do so is abnormal; examples of conditions that cause this are drug withdrawal and hypoxic ischaemic encephalopathy.

Table 41.1 Features of neonatal behavioural states[37]

	Eyes open	Respiration regular	Gross movements	Vocalisation
State 1	−1	+1	−1	−1
State 2	−1	−1	0	−1
State 3	+1	+1	−1	−1
State 4	+1	−1	+1	−1
State 5	0	−1	+1	+1

Key: +1 = present; −1 = absent; 0 = present or absent

State 1 (deep or quiet sleep)
Quiet sleep begins when a baby who keeps his eyes closed begins to breathe regularly. Eye movements under the closed eyelids are not present. The baby is generally still and not moving. Rhythmical mouthing movements can appear, lasting a few seconds up to a maximum of a few minutes. Although gross motor movements are rare, startles do occur in this phase of sleep.

State 2 (light or rapid eye movement sleep)
In this phase of sleep respirations are irregular. The transition from state 1 into state 2 is frequently marked with a startle, gross movements or a sigh. Under the closed eyelids, slow eye movements can be observed. Small twitches are common in state 2 and are visible in the face, hands and feet. Grimaces, smiles and rhythmical mouthing are observable at times. The many movements result in frequently changing postures.

State 3 (awake; drowsy; dozing)

In state 3, the baby lies still and keeps his eyes open, although they may be heavy-lidded. Although there may be moments of staring, most of the time the baby seems to scan the environment with rapid eye movements. A stable posture and regular respiration are usual. Babies have a dazed look in this half-awake state. The longest such periods occur after a feed.

State 5 (alert)

The baby has his eyes open and moves his arms, legs and head around. Postures change frequently, and large and small movements are common. Movements have a writhing quality in newborn babies, which evolve to the fidgety movements characteristic of early infancy.

State 6 (crying)

Cry is a communication signal, and it is clear that parents and nurses can often discriminate between cries of discomfort, hunger and pain.

Behavioural state of the neonate less mature than 36 weeks gestation

Babies born before 36 weeks gestation spend a great deal of time asleep but their sleep states cannot be classified so easily as quiet and active sleep. Prechtl et al,[35] on the basis of a longitudinal study of very low-risk preterm infants, came to the following conclusion: 'Cycles of rest and activity, regular and irregular breathing, and epochs with and without eye movements may alternate independently and may accidentally overlap, but often do not coincide at all before 35–37 weeks'.

Abnormal states, abnormal state cycling and coma

Nearly every disorder that affects the central nervous system disturbs the level of alertness at some time. Babies are usually arousable, that is they will awaken to the sound of a bell or a bright light. Failure to arouse means that a baby is stuporose or comatose. Both in utero[36] and after birth, stereotyped movements are an indicator of disease and a rich variety of movement is an indicator of health.

In conclusion, in healthy newborns, both full-term and preterm, cycles of activity should be present: after 36 weeks these are recognised as distinct behavioural state cycles as described above; before 36 weeks these consist of more or less independently occurring cycles of activity and quiescence, of regular and irregular breathing, and of periods with and without rapid eye movements. Recognition of these cycles can be helped by looking at the electrocardiogram, respiratory pattern and transcutaneous PCO_2. Attention to assessment of behavioural state and behavioural state cycling may be the single most sensitive way to assess the integrity of the neonatal central nervous system, and should be the starting point for examination of the nervous system.

Consolability/cuddliness

During an examination, or when they are cold or hungry, babies often cry but are usually consolable. Brazelton and Nugent[7] stress that normal babies are 'cuddly' and will mould into the crook of an arm or nestle in the examiner's neck. Persistent, high-pitched crying is abnormal, as is the stiff 'uncuddly' behaviour of a baby with encephalopathy.

Posture, spontaneous movement and tone

Normal muscle offers a resistance to stretch which is felt by the examiner as tone. Passive flexor tone appears between 28 and 34 weeks and matures from the feet and legs upwards.[1] This is clear from the posture adopted by term babies, who lie with their limbs flexed and adducted, unlike preterm babies, who adopt an extended posture. Asymmetrical tone does not always indicate asymmetrical pathology in the newborn period. A pattern of mixed change in tone, with hypertonia in the limbs and hypotonia in the trunk, is abnormal, as is arching of the trunk at any age. When the whole body is arched, the term *opisthotonos* is used. Tone can alter considerably in relation to feeds and sleep state and repeated examinations are required to confirm physical signs.

A term newborn makes smooth, varied, spontaneous and symmetrical limb movements that stop when the baby's attention is diverted.[34] Finger movements are elegant and varied, involving the thumb, which can be abducted away from the palm by term.[17] A persistently adducted thumb (cortical thumb) in a tightly fisted hand is abnormal[25,12] and babies with brain injury often have this sign, with a paucity of fine finger movements.

Facial expression

Spontaneous facial movements are frequently seen in the normal newborn, although bilateral facial paralysis (as in Moebius' syndrome) is much more difficult to diagnose than the more common unilateral facial palsy. Normal facial expression in an otherwise hypotonic and flaccid newborn baby suggests a spinal cord problem. Babies of just a few days old will often imitate facial gestures, for example putting out their tongues.

Limb movement, tone and power

Before passive movements are used to assess tone it may be possible to observe spontaneous movements of the limbs against gravity. Failure to move part or the whole of a limb may be due to pain or paralysis. Limb tone is influenced by the tonic neck reflex in newborns, which means that it is important to have the head in the midline before beginning to elicit passive movements. These involve gentle flexion of the upper and lower limbs, then rapid extension and observation of recoil. A summary is contained within the protocol suggested by Dubowitz.[12] This examination system, like that of Amiel-Tison,[1] involves assessing angles made by bending and manipulating the limbs and trunk

(Fig. 41.3). These include the popliteal angle, the foot dorsiflexion angle and the scarf sign. A reduced popliteal angle and clusters of abnormal signs are sensitive indicators of later outcome.[13]

Jitteriness

The normal term newborn is in a state of relative hypertonicity, with brisk reflexes tending to clonus. This high tone can lead to the clinical sign of jittering. Jittering is a high frequency, generalised, symmetrical tremor of the limbs that is stilled by flexion or by inducing the baby to suck on a finger. Jittering is common in the first 2–3 days in term babies but if it is excessive or persistent it deserves investigation (see seizures, pp. 1105–19). Repetitive chewing movements or tongue thrusting are not part of jitteriness and imply seizures. Jitteriness is stimulus-sensitive, whereas seizures are not. In seizure the movement has a fast and slow component whereas in jittering the tremor is symmetrical. Jittering is never accompanied by physiological changes due to the activation of the autonomic nervous system such as tachycardia, hypertension or apnoea.

Trunk and neck tone and power

Normal term babies have sufficient power in their neck muscles to lift their heads slightly when prone or supine. Preterm babies can manage to turn their heads from side to side but have much less power, with complete head lag when pulled to sit. In order to judge tone in the neck and trunk, babies should be pulled to sit by holding them at the shoulders (Fig. 41.4). The pull-to-sit manoeuvre elicits an attempt to raise the head in a normal term newborn (Fig. 41.4a). If the head is unsupported it will gradually fall forwards or backwards: normal term babies will be able to raise their heads to the vertical again from either direction (Fig. 41.4b), but it is normal for the head of a term baby to wobble. Truncal tone can be assessed by placing the baby on his side, with one hand on the back and the other manipulating the legs. It is normally easier to flex a baby's trunk than to extend it.

Reflexes

Tendon and Babinski reflexes

Eliciting tendon reflexes is of less value in the newborn period than later in childhood. Knee and biceps jerks can usually be obtained. Reflexes at term are very brisk, because of the high tone, and a few beats of clonus at the ankle are usual. Very brisk reflexes and clonus are not reliable indicators of an upper motor neurone lesion until about 6 months of age.[4] A crossed adductor response to the knee jerk (see below) is also usual in the first months of life, whereas the sign is abnormal later on. The plantar reflex of Babinski is always extensor in babies, and this test is best omitted as the stimulus is painful and often results in a withdrawal response.

Primary neonatal reflexes

While these responses are intriguing to doctors and parents alike it is necessary to have a working knowledge of only a few. Primitive reflexes normally habituate after repeated performance.

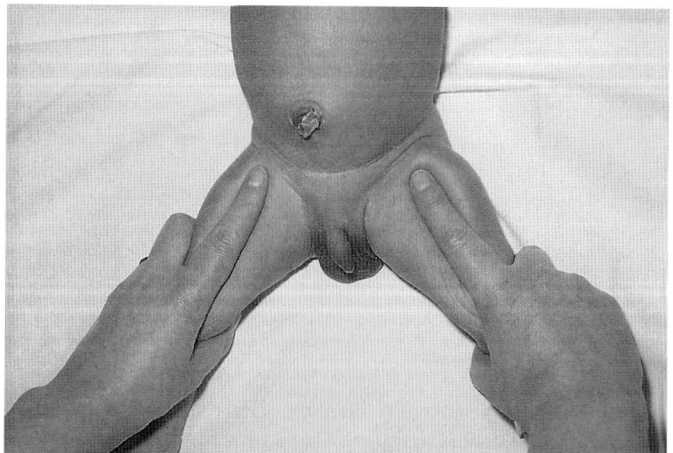

Fig. 41.3 Assessment of the adductor angle of the legs.

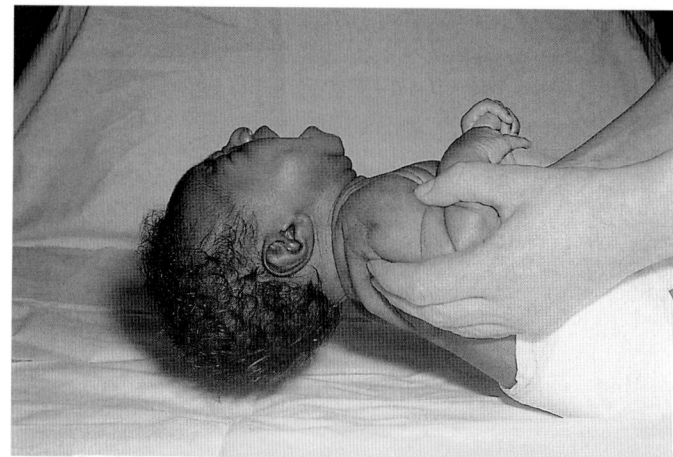

(a)

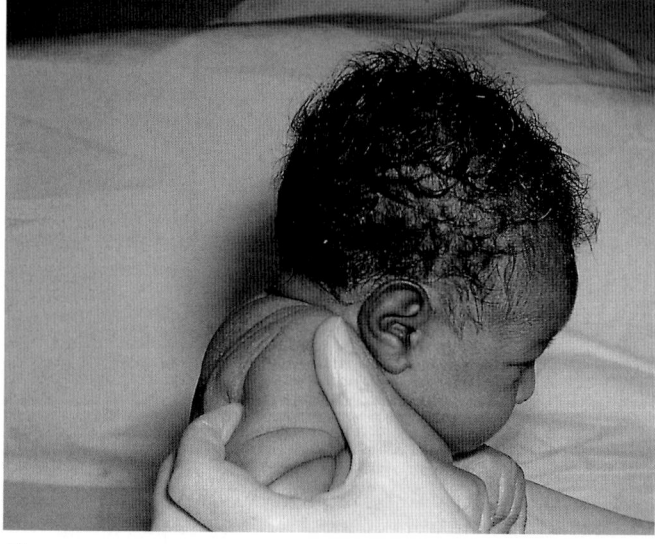

(b)

Fig. 41.4 (a) Pull-to-sit manoeuvre: this full-term baby is attempting to raise his head (b) After being pulled to sit the baby has raised his head to the vertical position, having let it fall forward.

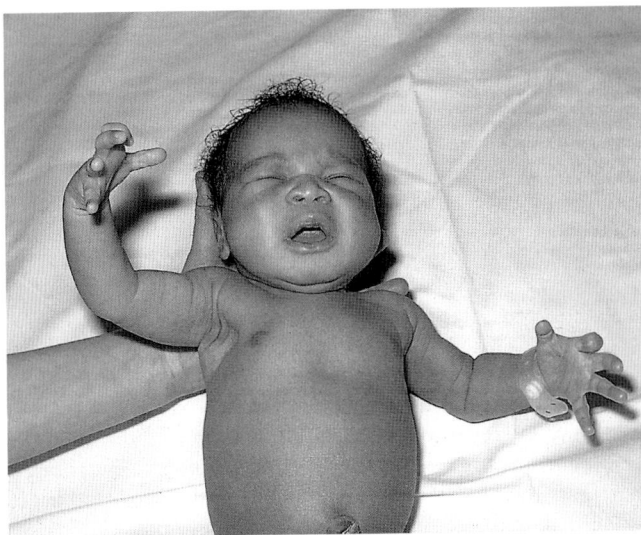

Fig. 41.5 The abduction phase of the Moro response; the baby's head has been allowed to fall back slightly but is then supported by the examiner's hand.

Persistence of primitive reflexes can inhibit normal movement in children with cerebral palsy.

Moro reflex

This reflex is usually elicited by allowing the previously supported head of a baby to fall backwards slightly, whereupon the baby extends and adducts both upper limbs, opening the hands (Fig. 41.5). Babies of more than 33 weeks' gestation subsequently adduct their arms. The Moro response is present from 28 weeks of gestation and usually disappears by 4 months. Persistence beyond 6 months is always abnormal.

Asymmetric tonic neck reflex

Starting with the baby supine and the head in the midline the head is slowly turned to one side. This results in increased extensor tone in the arm on the side to which the head is turned and increased flexor tone in the arm on the opposite side (fencing posture). The reflex appears by 35 weeks gestation, is very prominent by about 1 month of age and disappears by about 7 months.

Crossed extension (adduction) reflex

One leg is held in extension and the sole of the foot is rubbed. The other leg first withdraws and then extends with fanning of the toes. The third and final component of the fully developed reflex brings the other foot towards the side that was stimulated. Eliciting the knee jerk often produces this reflex in the neonatal period, which should not persist after 8 months of age.

Placing and stepping

By stimulating the dorsum of the foot, usually by bringing it into contact with the edge of the couch, a mature baby can be induced to 'step' over the edge (Fig. 41.6). The baby's toes fan out and he lifts his foot up and then places it on the surface. Babies will extend their legs on to a flat surface and 'support' their weight when held under the arms. With the feet in contact with a solid surface and the body tilted forwards the baby will 'walk'.

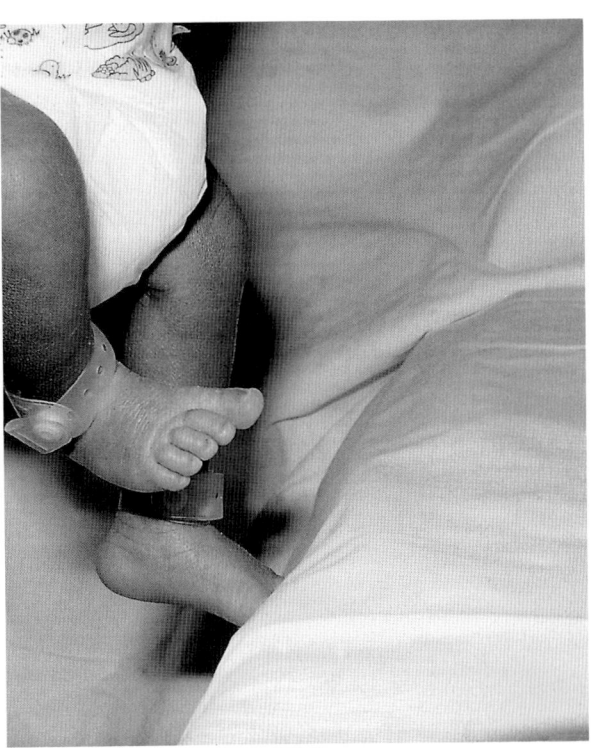

Fig. 41.6 The stepping reflex, elicited by bringing the dorsum of the baby's foot into contact with the couch.

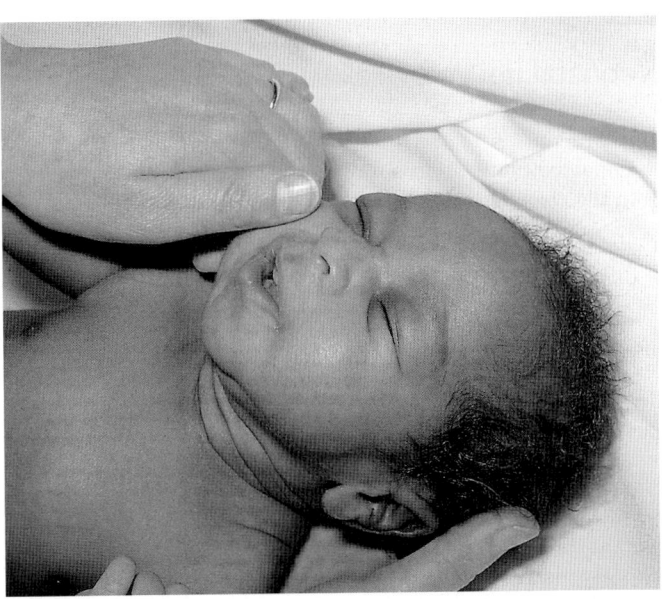

Fig. 41.7 The rooting reflex.

Rooting, sucking and swallowing

Stroking the upper lip of a baby of 28 weeks' gestation and above results in the baby searching for the nipple and opening the mouth. This reflex tests the sensation in the distribution of the Vth cranial nerve and the motor pathways of cranial nerves V, VII and XII (Fig. 41.7). Swallowing also involves cranial nerves IX and X. The sensory input for the sucking reflex comes from the hard palate, not the tongue or cheek. Sucking begins during the 11th week of intrauterine life. Co-ordination between sucking and swallowing exists from 28 weeks' gestation but the strength to sustain it and to synchronise the process with breathing is only adequate after 32–34 weeks' gestation. Sucking gradually builds up from bursts of three sucks at a time to eight or more, with a reduction in the interburst interval. If sucking is absent, test the gag reflex by gently stroking the soft palate with a cotton bud.

Palmar and plantar

The palmar reflex results from stroking the palmar surface of the hand, eliciting a grasp that is often strong enough to lift the baby from the crib (Fig. 41.8). It is present from 26 weeks' gestation and persists up to 4 months. Stroking the ball of the foot results in curling of the toes in a similar manner to the palmar response.

Pupillary reflex

The pupils respond to light only after 30 weeks gestation, and the response was present in all infants after 35 weeks.[40] Babies of less than 30 weeks gestation do respond to a bright light, by blinking or averting their eyes. The size of the pupil gradually decreases after the development of the light reflex. The amplitude of the response, that is the difference in size of the pupil before and after the light exposure, increases up to term. A small pupil on the side of an Erb's palsy suggests Horner's syndrome due to involvement of C8 and T1 nerve roots. A large pupil can indicate a congenital or acquired IIIrd nerve palsy.

Neonatal neurological alarm signals

Certain neonatal neurological signs are generally recognised as potential indicators of serious disease. These 'alarm signs', derived from the work of many authors,[2,3,8,12,26,44,48,51] are:

- persistent irritability;
- difficulty in feeding;
- persistent deviation of head and/or eyes;
- persistent asymmetry in posture and movements;
- persistently adducted thumbs in a fisted hand;
- opisthotonus;
- persistent posture of flexed arms and extended legs;
- apathy and immobility;
- floppiness, severe generalised hypotonia;
- convulsions;
- abnormal cry;
- the combination of setting-sun sign, vomiting, wide sutures and/or abnormal increase in skull circumference.

Respiratory difficulties and apnoea can be signs of neurological dysfunction although apnoea of prematurity is the commonest cause on a modern neonatal unit (Chapter 27). In one large study, recurrent apnoea (i.e. three or more episodes of apnoea of longer than 20 seconds' duration) occurred in 1% of 25 154 babies evaluated between 1974 and 1979.[21] Of the affected babies, apnoea commenced in the first 2 days of life in 77% and was unlikely to commence after 7 days.[21] The gestational age at birth had a major impact with respect to the postnatal age when the last apnoea was detected.

Special senses

Examination of vision, visual evoked potentials

The 26-week gestation preterm baby blinks in response to light; by 32 weeks there is eye closure; by 34 weeks a baby is able to fix and track a bright object briefly. By 37 weeks a baby will turn to soft light, and can track reliably (Fig. 41.9). Optokinetic nystagmus is present when a term baby looks at a striped rotating drum or a striped tape is moved in front of the baby's eyes. Changing the width of the stripes or forced-choice preferential looking at striped grids can be used to test visual acuity, which is equivalent to 20/150 vision at term.

The interpretation of deficient neonatal visual responses, however, is much more difficult. Dubowitz stresses the importance of the loss of previously good visual performance as a disturbing sign. Babies' eyes are usually in alignment, although a slight horizontal divergence is normal until 6 weeks of age, particularly in preterm

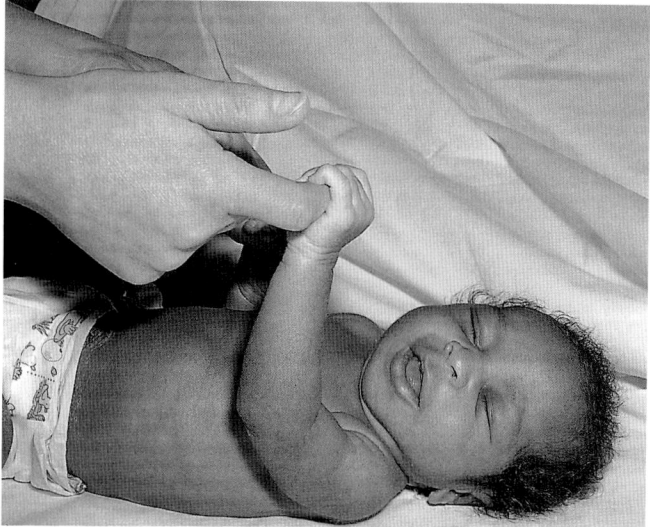

Fig. 41.8 The grasp reflex.

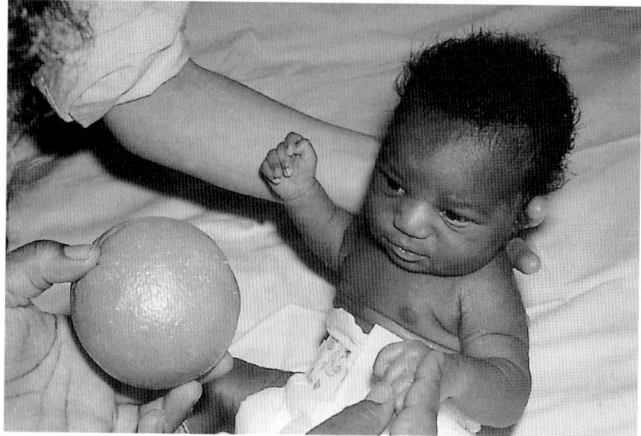

Fig. 41.9 Fixing and tracking an orange at term.

babies. Vertical or skew deviation is always abnormal and has been seen in association with germinal matrix/intraventricular haemorrhage (GMH-IVH).[51] For more information on abnormal and delayed visual development, and squint, see Chapter 34.

Visual evoked potentials (VEP) are produced within the occipital cortex as a result of repeatedly applying an appropriate visual stimulus so that the minute electrical response to it, which will be identical each time, can be extracted from the random background electrical noise (EEG) by computerised averaging. Stroboscopic or flashing red lights are used, which can penetrate closed eyelids. The electrical response 'matures' with advancing gestation and can be detected from 25 weeks. Study of VEPs has been found to be of value in predicting outcome after birth asphyxia[45] and is a sensitive test for the integrity of the visual pathway. Absent VEPs predicted cortical blindness in preterm infants with extensive cystic leukomalacia.[11]

Auditory testing in the neonatal period

The fetus responds to sound from 19 weeks of gestation.[22] Babies from 28 weeks of gestation respond to noise by turning their heads, arousing from sleep or increasing their body movements. Bilateral sensorineural deafness occurs in about 1.5 per 1000 children. Successful universal neonatal screening programmes developed for use in the UK[53,54] have been rolled out gradually since 2000. Universal neonatal hearing screening is now established in over 60 areas of England (about half the total) and in 32 states of the USA. Most of these programmes use transient otoacoustic emissions as the primary method, with automated brainstem evoked potential testing reserved for those who fail the initial screen (http://www.nhsp.info/). Universal neonatal hearing screening is more cost effective than the infant distraction test and children treated early have better speech and language skills, although debate continues about the strength of the evidence.[46]

Oto-acoustic emissions

Oto-acoustic emissions were discovered in 1978. Oto-acoustic emissions are low amplitude sound waves that are produced by the inner ear; they occur spontaneously as well as in response to a click stimulus. The automated method depends on the fact that a click stimulus, when presented to an intact hearing ear, evokes an oto-acoustic emission, which can be detected by a probe lying in the ear canal. Testing with oto-acoustic emissions is quicker than testing using an automated evoked brainstem response method but there are more false-positive results.

Brain-stem auditory evoked potential

These indicate electrical events generated in the brainstem auditory pathway in response to sound (usually a click) presented at the ear. The electrical signals are recorded with EEG electrodes on the scalp. The results of many click stimulations are summed by a computer, which uses coherent averaging to eliminate the background noise generated by the local EEG signal. The mature pattern consists of seven waves but these are poorly developed with increased latency and require a larger stimulus in order to elicit them in babies, in whom the response is present from 24 weeks.

Automated brainstem response equipment eliminates the need for extensive operator training and is a widely used method of hearing screening.

Imaging

For advice on the best imaging modality to choose when investigating the central nervous system see **Chapter 44**.

Examination of cerebrospinal fluid, intracranial pressure

Lumbar puncture is often done in babies because the signs of meningitis are subtle. For practical advice on how to perform the procedure see Chapter 45. In the neonatal period cerebrospinal fluid may be xanthochromic because of jaundice or old GMH-IVH. The cell count is higher than later in childhood. In preterm neonates the red and white cell counts can each be up to $30/mm^3$ (Appendix 8). In term babies after the first week of life more than 10 cells of each type per cubic millimetre is abnormal. A white cell count of more than $30/mm^3$ with neutrophils more than 66% of the total is suspicious, although in cases of meningitis the white cell count is usually more than $100/mm^3$. Seizures do not influence the results. Red cell counts of more than $1000/mm^3$ make the interpretation of cerebrospinal fluid results impossible: applying correction factors using the ratio of white cells to red cells has been shown to be inaccurate.[31,42] The only course of action is to repeat the lumbar puncture after 12 hours.

Measured accurately with pressure transducers at lumbar puncture the intracranial pressure was 0–5.5 mmHg[27] and 2 mmHg.[29]

Electroencephalography

Conventional multichannel EEG recordings are difficult to obtain in newborn babies but the results can provide very valuable information.[10,38] The montage of electrodes is hard to apply and maintain and many babies requiring investigation are in intensive care units, which are electrically noisy. Short recordings are of less value than prolonged ones as the EEG shows wide variability and changes not only with sleep state but also with the length of the preceding sleep epoch and the degree of maturity of the baby (pp. 1108–11).[16,38,41] Continuous monitoring is possible with a cerebral function monitor, which displays the amplitude of one or more channels of processed EEG, and modern equipment offers the opportunity to obtain multiple channels of raw EEG and a digital video signal in addition to a compressed and filtered amplitude integrated EEG (Fig. 41.10). Cerebral function monitoring has drawbacks but the advantages include continuous monitoring and relative ease of interpretation.[19]

Maturation of the electroencephalogram

The EEG of very preterm babies is markedly discontinuous, with a pattern of high-voltage slow activity with suppressed EEG activity termed *tracé discontinu* (p. 1108). Preterm babies also exhibit a pattern, called *delta brush* of fast waves superimposed on delta waves, which can be misinterpreted as convulsive activity. Delta brush is most abundant at 32 weeks gestation and is very rarely seen after term. With increasing gestation the interburst intervals decrease and the record becomes more continuous (Fig. 41.11). Abnormal background EEG activity, such as severe amplitude depression or burst suppression, correlates well with later adverse outcome in both preterm and asphyxiated term babies.[15,20,23,52]

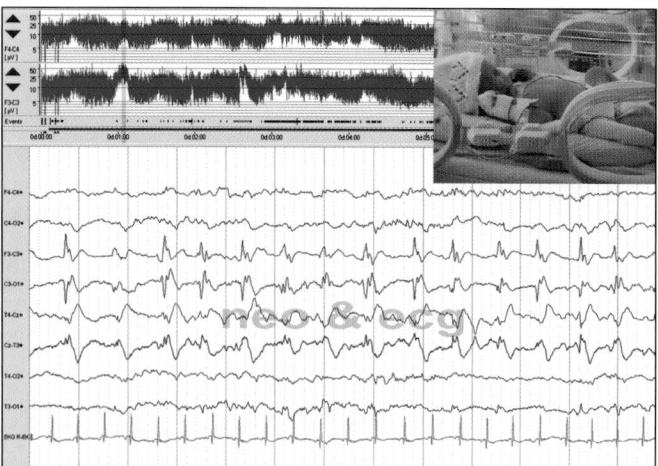

Fig. 41.10 Monitoring cerebral function with raw EEG, compressed and filtered EEG, and digital video monitoring.

Neurological examination before discharge, and follow-up

When assessing the predictive value of the neurological examinations before discharge, a distinction should be made between studies of low-risk and high-risk newborns. In low-risk full-term infants, there is a low but significant correlation between the neonatal neurological evaluation and follow-up evaluations to school age.[47,50] In high-risk preterm infants Touwen[49] found a much higher correlation between the neonatal and follow-up examinations during infancy. The neonatal hemisyndrome and hypertonia syndrome have distinct prognostic value, whereas hypotonia does not. With asphyxia, however, hypotonia that evolves to hypertonia correlates significantly with subsequent neurological disorders.[8] The neonatal hyperexcitability syndrome appears to correlate with subsequent developmental difficulties only when it persists for more than 6 weeks. If, upon discharge from the neonatal unit, it is concluded that the baby is definitely neurologically abnormal, on the basis of such established abnormalities as microcephaly or seizures, a nearly 100-fold increased risk of cerebral palsy does exist.[30]

Follow up of high-risk infants is an important part of neonatal intensive care provision (Ch. 19). Monitoring of head growth and neurodevelopment over the first months can give early warning of neurodevelopmental problems. A failure to achieve a normal pattern of head growth is an ominous sign.

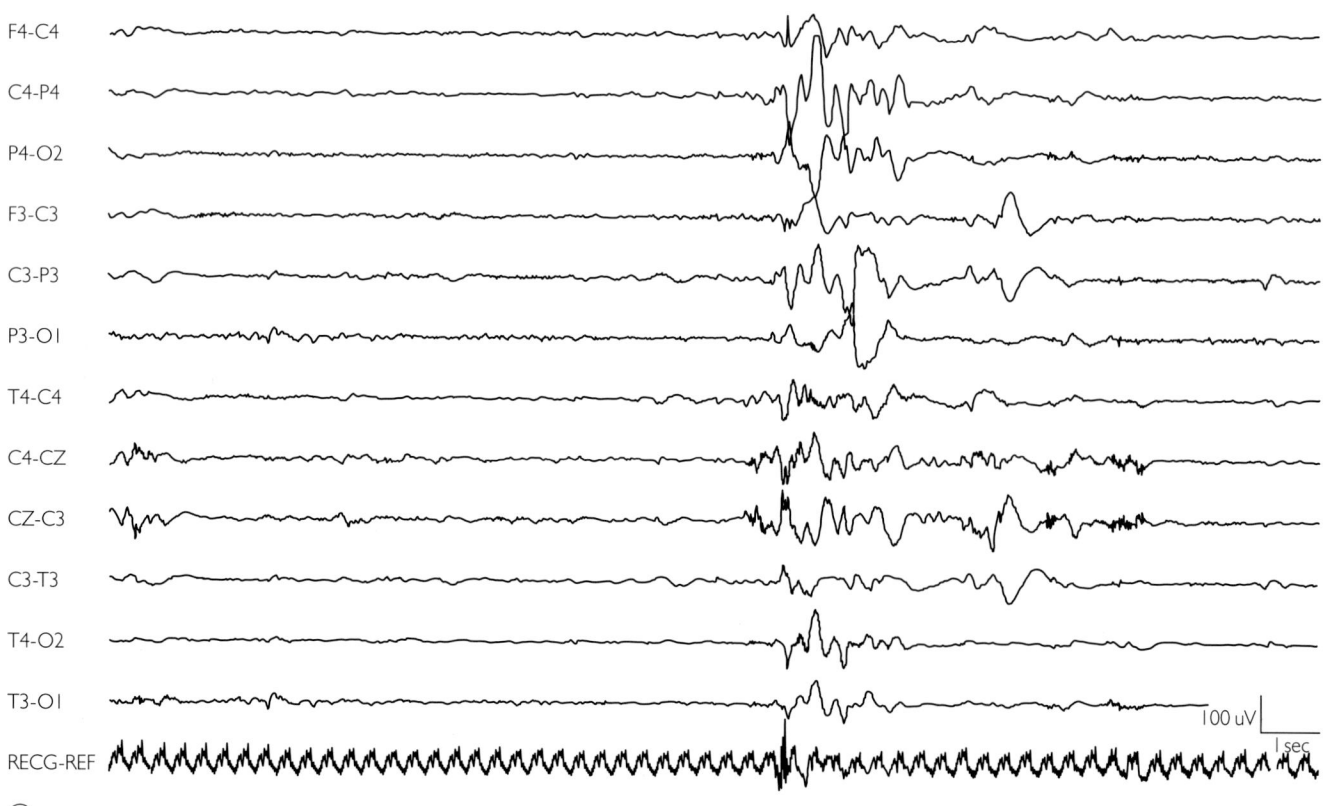

(a)

Fig. 41.11 Maturation of the EEG (a) 25 weeks; (b) 29 weeks; (c) 35 weeks; (d) 40 weeks.

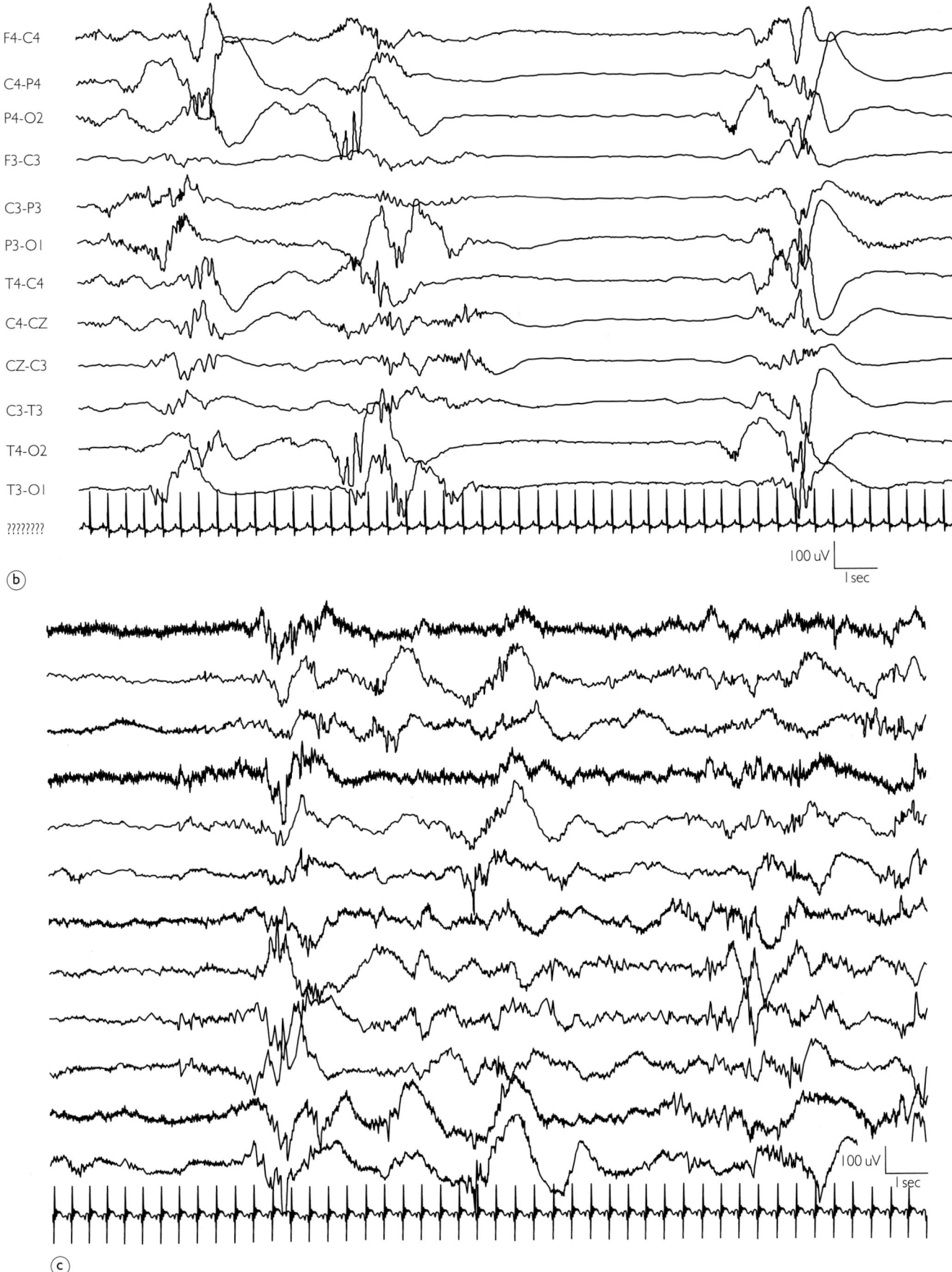

F4-C4

C4-P4

P4-O2

F3-C3

C3-P3

P3-O1

T4-C4

C4-CZ

CZ-C3

C3-T3

T4-O2

T3-O1

????????

100 uV

1 sec

(b)

100 uV

1 sec

(c)

Fig. 41.11 (Continued)

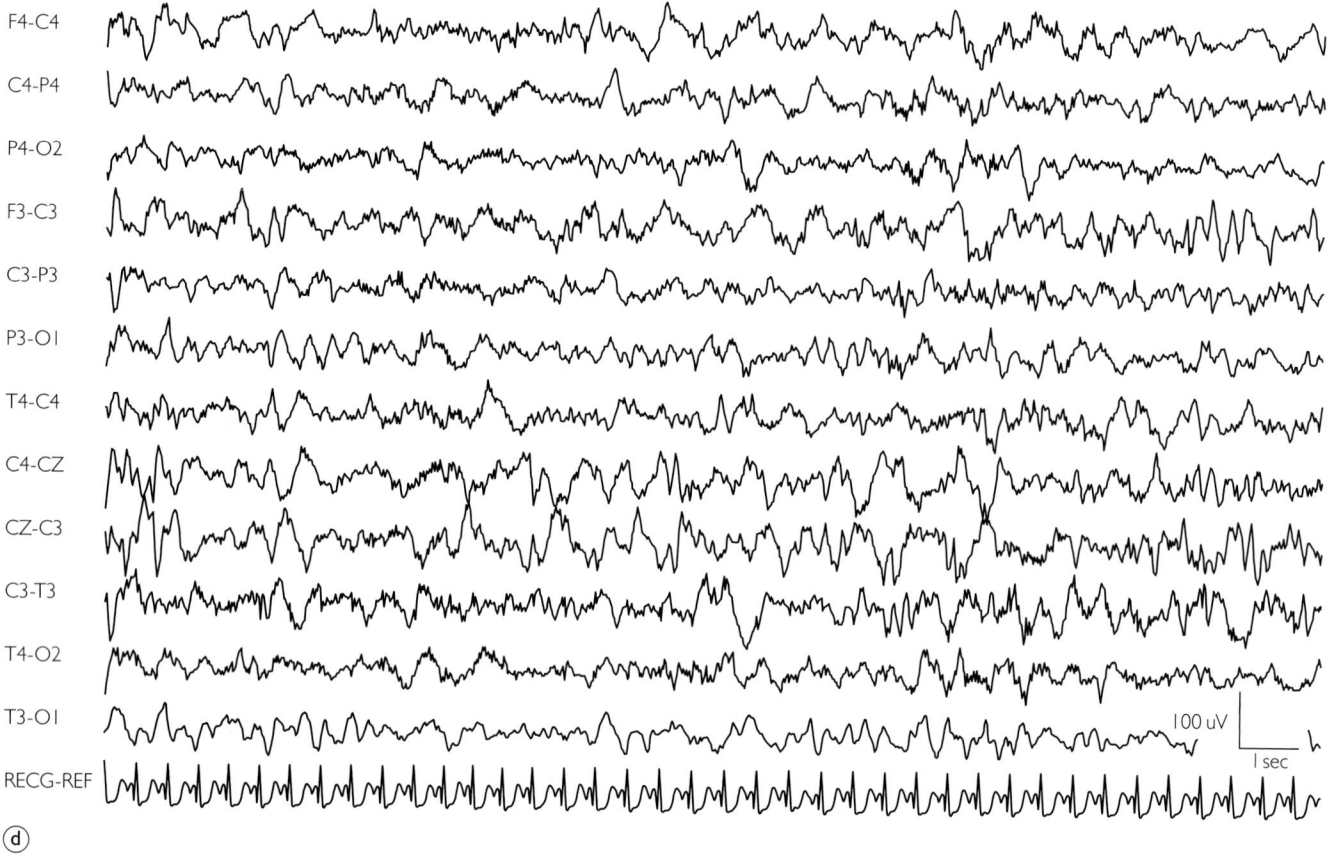

(d)

Fig. 41.11 (Continued)

References

1. Amiel-Tison C 2001 Clinical assessment of the infant nervous system. In: Levene M I, Chervenak F A, Whitte M (eds) Fetal and neonatal neurology and neurosurgery, 3rd edn. Churchill Livingstone, Edinburgh, pp 99–120

2. Amiel-Tison C 2002 Update of the Amiel-Tison neurologic assessment for the term neonate or at 40 weeks corrected age. Pediatric Neurology 27: 196–212

3. Amiel-Tison C, Grenier A 1980 Evaluation neurologique du nouveau-né et du nourrisson. Masson, Paris

4. Amiel-Tison C, Stewart A 1994 Apparently normal survivors: neuromotor and cognitive function as they grow older. In: Amiel-Tison C, Stewart A (eds) The newborn infant: one brain for life. INSERM-Doin, Paris, pp 227–237

5. Andre-Thomas Chesni Y, Saint-Anne Dargassies S 1960 The neurological examination of the infant. Clinics in Developmental Medicine no 1. McKeith Press, Cambridge

6. Barkovich J A 1999 Pediatric neuroimaging. Lippincott Williams & Wilkins, Philadelphia

7. Brazelton T B, Nugent J K 1995 Neonatal behavioural assessment scale, 3rd edn. Clinics in Developmental Medicine no 137. MacKeith Press, London

8. Brown J K, Purvis R J, Forfar J O, Cockburn F 1974 Neurological aspects of perinatal asphyxia. Developmental Medicine and Child Neurology 16: 567–580

9. Cioni G, Ferrari F , Einspieler C, Paolicelli P B, Barbani M T, Prechtl H F R 1997 Comparison between observation of spontaneous movements and neurologic examination in preterm infants. Journal of Pediatrics 139: 704–711

10. D'Allest A M, Andre M 2002 Electroencephalography. In: Lagercrantz H, Hanson M, Evrard P, Rodeck C (eds) The newborn brain: neuroscience and clinical applications. Cambridge University Press, Cambridge, pp 339–367

11. De Vries L S, Connell J, Dubowitz L M S, Oozeer R C, Dubowitz V, Pennock J M 1987 Neurological, electrophysiological and MRI abnormalities in infants with extensive cystic leukomalacia. Neuropediatrics 18: 61–66

12. Dubowitz L, Dubowitz V, Mercuri E 1999 The neurological assessment of the preterm and full term newborn infant, 2nd edn. Clinics in Developmental Medicine no.148. MacKeith Press, Cambridge

13. Dubowitz L M S, Dubowitz V, Palmer P G, Miller G, Fawer C-L, Levene M I 1984 Correlation of neurological assessment in the preterm newborn infant with outcome at 1 year. Journal of Pediatrics 105: 452–456

14. Dubowitz L, Mercuri E, Dubowitz V 1998 An optimality score for the neurological examination of the term newborn. Journal of Pediatrics 133: 406–416

15. Eken P, Toet M C, Groenendaal F, De Vries L S 1995 Predictive value of early neuroimaging, pulsed Doppler and neurophysiology in full term infants with hypoxic-ischaemic encephalopathy. Archives of Disease in Childhood 73: F75–F80

16. Eyre J A, Nanei S, Wilkinson A R 1988 Quantification of changes in normal neonatal EEGs with gestation from continuous 5 day recordings. Developmental Medicine and Child Neurology 30: 599–607

17. Ferrari F, Cioni G, Prechtl H F R 1990 Qualitative changes of general movements in preterm infants with brain lesions. Early Human Development 23: 193–231

18. Govaert P, de Vries L S 1997 An atlas of neonatal brain sonography. Clinics in Developmental Medicine no. 141–142. MacKeith Press, London

19. Hellstrom-Westas L 2002 Cerebral function monitoring. In: Lagercrantz H, Hanson M, Evrard P, Rodeck C (eds) The newborn brain: neuroscience and clinical applications. Cambridge University Press, Cambridge, pp 368–384

20. Hellstrom-Westas L, Rosen I, Svenningsen N W 1995 Predictive value of early continuous amplitude integrated EEG recordings on outcome after severe birth asphyxia in full term infants. Archives of Disease in Childhood 72: F34–F38

21. Henderson-Smart D J 1981 The effect of gestational age on the incidence and duration of recurrent apnoea in newborn babies. Australian Paediatric Journal 17: 273–276

22. Hepper P G, Shahidullah B S 1994 Development of fetal hearing. Archives of Disease in Childhood 71: F81–F87

23. Holmes G, Rowe J, Hafford J, Schmidt R, Testa M, Zimmerman A 1982 Prognostic value of the electroencephalogram in neonatal seizures. Electroencephalography and Clinical Neurophysiology 53: 60–72

24. Illingworth R S 1960 The development of the infant and young child. E & S Livingstone, Edinburgh

25. Illingworth R S 1980 The development of the infant and young child, 7th edn. Churchill Livingstone, Edinburgh

26. Joppich G, Schulte F J 1968 Neurologie des Neugeborenen. Springer, Berlin

27. Kaiser A M, Whitelaw A G L 1986 Normal cerebrospinal fluid pressure in the newborn. Neuropaediatrics 17: 100–102

28. Majnemer A Mazer B 1998 Neurologic evaluation of the newborn infant: definition and psychometric properties. Developmental Medicine and Child Neurology 40: 708–715

29. Minns R A 1984 Intracranial pressure monitoring. Archives of Disease in Childhood 59: 486–488

30. Nelson K B, Ellenberg J H 1979 Neonatal signs as predictors of cerebral palsy. Pediatrics 64: 225–232

31. Novak R W 1984 Lack of validity of standard corrections for white blood cell counts of blood-contaminated cerebrospinal fluid in infants. American Journal of Clinical Pathology 82: 95–97

32. Prechtl H F R 1974 The behavioural states of the newborn infant. Brain Research 76: 185–212

33. Prechtl H F R 1977 The neurological examination of the full term newborn infant, 2nd edn. Clinics in Developmental Medicine no. 63. MacKeith Press, London

34. Prechtl H F R 1990 Qualitative changes of spontaneous movements in fetus and preterm infant as a marker of neurological dysfunction. Early Human Development 23: 151–158

35. Prechtl H F R, Fargel VW, Weinaman HM, Bakker HH 1979 Postures, motility and respiration of low risk preterm infants. Developmental Medicine and Child Neurology 21: 3–7

36. Prechtl H F R, Nolte R 1984 Motor behaviour of preterm infants. In: Prechtl H F R (ed) Continuity of neural functions from prenatal to postnatal life. Clinics in Developmental Medicine no. 84. MacKeith Press, London

37. Prechtl H F R, O'Brien M J 1982 Behavioural states of the full term newborn. The emergence of a concept. In: Stratton P (ed) Psychobiology of the human newborn. John Wiley, New York, pp 53–73

38. Pressler R, Bady B, Binnie C D et al 2003 Neurophysiology of the neonatal period. In: Binnie C D, Cooper R, Mauguiere F, Osselton J, Prior P, Tedman B (eds) Clinical neurophysiology, vol 2. Elsevier, London

39. Rennie J M 1997 Neonatal cranial ultrasound. Cambridge University Press, Cambridge

40. Robinson J, Fielder A R 1990 Pupillary diameter and reaction to light in preterm neonates. Archives of Disease in Childhood 65: 35–38

41. Roffwarg H P, Muzio J N, Dement W C 1966 Ontogenetic development of human sleep dream cycles. Science 152: 604–619

42. Rubenstein J S, Yogev R 1985 What represents pleocytosis in blood contaminated ('traumatic tap') cerebrospinal fluid in children? Journal of Pediatrics 107: 249–252

43. Rutherford M A 2002 MRI of the neonatal brain. W B Saunders, London

44. Saint-Anne Dargassies S 1977 Neurological development in the full term and premature neonate. Elsevier-North Holland, Amsterdam

45. Taylor M J, Murphy W J, Whyte H E 1992 Prognostic reliability of SEPs and VEPs in asphyxiated newborn infants. Developmental Medicine and Child Neurology 34: 507–515

46. Thompson D C, McPhillips H, Davis R L, Lieu T A, Homer C J, Hefland M 2001 Universal newborn hearing screening: summary of evidence. Journal of the American Medical Association 286: 2000–2010

47. Touwen B C L 1972 The relationship between neonatal and follow up findings. In: Saling E, Schulte FJ (eds) Perinatale Medizin, vol II. Georg Thieme, Stuttgart, pp 303–306

48. Touwen B C L 1976 Neurological development in infancy. Clinics in developmental medicine no. 58. Spastics International Medical Publications/ Heinemann, London

49. Touwen B C L 1978 Early detection of developmental neurological disorders. In: Jonxis J H P (ed) Growth and development of the full term and premature infant. The Jonxis Lectures. Exerpta Medica, Amsterdam, pp 244–261

50. Touwen B C L, Lok-Mejjer T Y, Huisjes H J, Olinga A A 1982 The recovery rate of neurologically deviant newborns. Early Human Development 7: 131–148

51. Volpe J J 2001 The neurological examination: normal and abnormal features. In: Volpe J J (ed) Neonatal neurology, 4th edn. W B Saunders, Philadelphia, pp 103–133

52. Watanabe K, Miyazaki S, Hara K, Hakamanda A 1980 Behavioural state cycles, background EEGs and prognosis of newborns with perinatal hypoxia. Electroencephalography and Clinical Neurophysiology 49: 618–625

53. Watkin P M 1996 Neonatal otoacoustic emission screening and the identification of deafness. Archives of Disease in Childhood: F16–F25

54. Wessex Universal Neonatal Hearing Screening Trial Group 1998 Controlled trial of universal neonatal screening for early identification of permanent childhood hearing impairment Lancet 352: 1957–1964

PART 2

Seizures

Janet M Rennie

Introduction

Careful study of the unique biochemical properties of neonatal neurones has at last begun to clarify the reasons why seizures are so common in early life. In the adult brain, glutamate is the primary excitatory neurotransmitter, and there are three glutamate subreceptor types: *N*-methyl-D-aspartate (NMDA), alpha-amino-3-hydroxy-5-methyl-4-isoxazoleproprionate (AMPA) and kainic acid. Gamma-aminobutyric acid (GABA) is the main inhibitory transmitter. However, in the neonatal period opening the chloride-permeable GABA channels leads to depolarisation rather than hyperpolarisation (Fig. 41.12), with the result that GABA is excitatory.[40] There is an excess of excitatory synapses in the newborn brain compared with the adult, and immature neurones have a high chloride content. In due course, the significant advances in fundamental neuroscience research should lead to improved anticonvulsant treatment for the newborn.

All those who care for the newborn need a working knowledge of the likely causes and a management plan for this important emergency. Prompt diagnosis, investigation and treatment are vital as delayed recognition of a treatable cause can have a significant impact on the child's subsequent neurological outcome. In neonates, seizures are associated with conditions such as periventricular haemorrhage, cerebral infarction (stroke), hypoglycaemia, infection, cerebral malformations and hypoxic ischaemic encephalopathy.

There is increasing evidence that neonatal seizures have an adverse effect on neurodevelopmental outcome and predispose

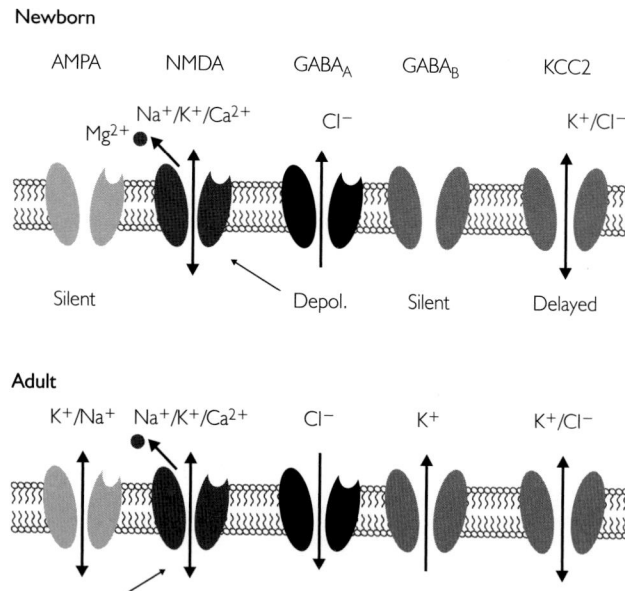

Newborn

AMPA NMDA GABA$_A$ GABA$_B$ KCC2

Mg^{2+} $Na^+/K^+/Ca^{2+}$ Cl^- K^+/Cl^-

Silent Depol. Silent Delayed

Adult

K^+/Na^+ $Na^+/K^+/Ca^{2+}$ Cl^- K^+ K^+/Cl^-

Depol. Hyperpol. Active

Fig. 41.12 Comparison of excitatory and inhibitory channels in neonate and adult. In the adult, AMPA responds to glutamate by opening and allowing Na^+ to enter cell. With depolarisation Mg^{2+} is displaced from the NMDA channel and Na^+ and Ca^{2+} enters the cell. GABA-A and GABA-B, through Cl^- and K^+ ionic flow, serve to hyperpolarize the cell. In the neonate, AMPA receptors, while present, are not functional (silent). NMDA channels, because of the block with Mg^{2+}, do not function at normal membrane resting potentials. Because of the higher Cl^- content of the immature brain, GABA activation results in an efflux of Cl^-, which serves to depolarise the cell. With depolarisation, the NMDA and voltage-gated channels can open. GABA-B, like AMPA, develops later and provides little postsynaptic inhibition in the neonate. The K^+/Cl^- co-transporter (KCC2), which is responsible for controlling intracellular Cl^-, is delayed in maturing, resulting in an increase in intracellular Cl^- in immature animals Depol = depolarisation; Hyperpol = hyperpolarisation. (Redrawn from Holmes G L, Khazipov R, Ben-Ari Y 2002 New concepts in neonatal seizures. Neuroreport 3: A3–A8.)

to cognitive, behavioural or epileptic complications in later life.[53] Seizures cause synaptic reorganisation with aberrant growth (mossy fibres), and may interfere with the normal synaptic pruning that takes place during development.[58] If seizures are not controlled the electrical activity can continue to circulate, a phenomenon known as kindling. Prolonged seizures cause progressive cerebral hypoxia, changes in cerebral blood flow, cerebral oedema and lactic acidosis; changes have been shown in human babies with Doppler ultrasound and using magnetic resonance spectroscopy.[9,62] Status epilepticus worsened the outcome for neonatal rats with hypoxic ischaemia.[101] Some clinical studies have shown a correlation between the number of seizures and outcome but others have not, although very few neonatal studies have been done using electroencephalographic (EEG) quantification of the seizure burden.[57]

Incidence

Seizures occur in 5–13% of very-low-birthweight infants and in 1–2 per 1000 of infants born at term.[18,47,48,50,55,81,83,90,98] Many of the cases in older studies were due to late-onset hypocalcaemia, which probably explains the higher incidence. The incidence of early (<48 hours) seizures in term infants has been proposed as an indicator of the quality of perinatal care because the most common cause in this group is hypoxic ischaemic encephalopathy. The incidence of early seizures varies, being 0.87 per 1000 in Dublin between 1980 and 1984,[18] 1.3 per 1000 in Cardiff during 1970–79[63] and 2.8 per 1000 in Fayette County, Kentucky in 1985–89.[48] The incidence of early seizures at term seems likely to become a core item in a minimum dataset requested from UK maternity units, but there are many problems in definition, which will become apparent to the reader. Subtle seizures are the most common type, particularly in premature infants, being present in 75% of the cases described by Sher et al.[84]

Time of onset

Most neonatal seizures start between 12 and 48 hours after birth; babies rarely present with seizures in the delivery room. In our experience, babies who are thought to be seizing on admission to the neonatal unit often have abnormal jittery movements without electrographic seizures. Animal work shows that seizures emerge 7–13 hours after a hypoxic–ischaemic insult[100] and this fits with what is known about glutamate release and damage during the secondary, reperfusion phase in this situation (p. 1111). The same sequence may occur in babies.[24] Late-onset seizures suggest meningitis, benign familial seizures or hypocalcaemia. Figure 41.13 shows the time of onset recorded in 277 neonatal cases.[39] A more recent study shows a very similar pattern.[83]

Diagnosis and classification

In 1870, J. Hughlings Jackson described a seizure as 'an excessive discharge of nerve tissue on muscle'. Today this definition is expanded to include the effects on the sensory and autonomic nervous systems, including paroxysmal alterations in behavioural state. Four main seizure types are recognised (Table 41.2) and within each type the seizures can be unifocal, multifocal or generalised. Classic 'tonic–clonic' seizures are very rare in babies, in whom there is the additional problem of electroclinical dissociation.[99]

Subtle

The clinical manifestations of seizures in infants can be extremely subtle. They can be divided into orofacial manifestations, including eye deviation, eyelid blinking, sucking, chewing and lip macking,

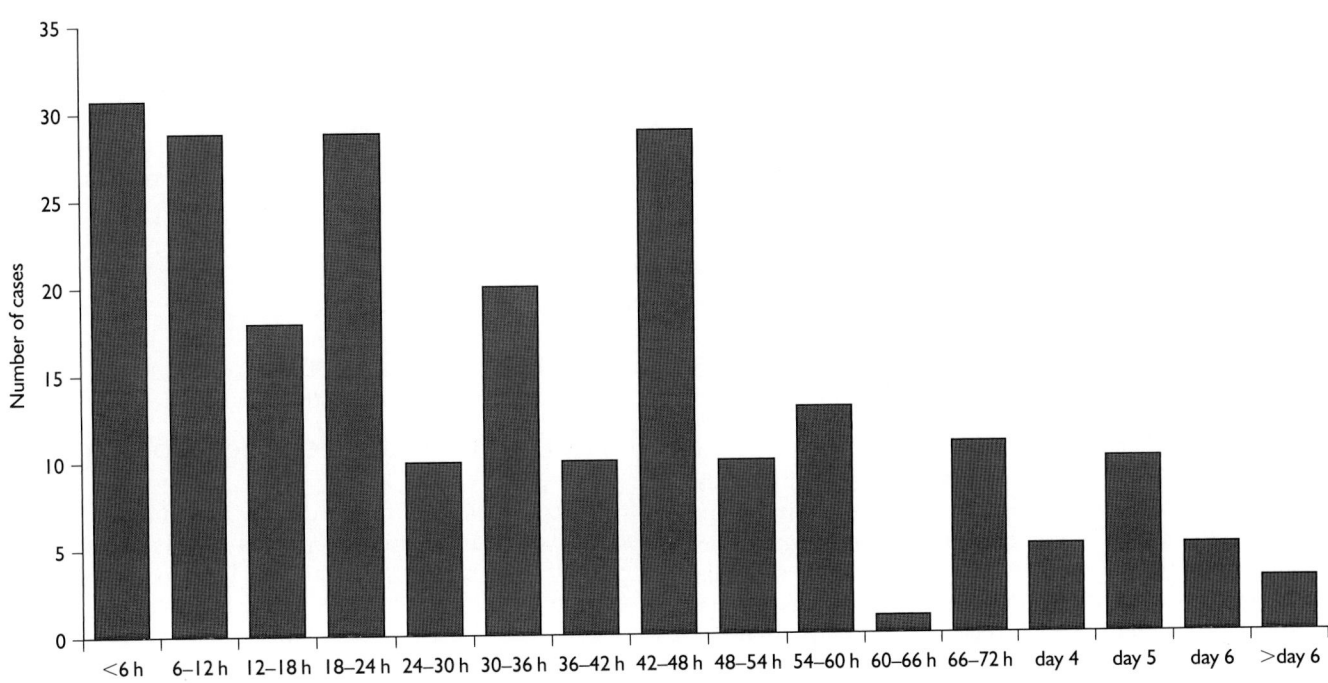

Fig. 41.13 Time of onset of seizures in 277 neonatal cases. Data from the National Collaborative Perinatal Project.[39] Note that the scale on the x axis starts as 6-hourly periods and is then grouped by days.

Table 41.2 Types of seizure in the newborn

Type	Clinical manifestation	Frequency and EEG correlate
Subtle	Eye signs – eyelid fluttering, eye deviation, fixed open stare, blinking. Apnoea. Cycling, boxing, stepping, swimming movements of limbs. Mouthing, chewing, lip smacking, smiling	About 50% of neonatal seizures; EEG correlation variable. EEG changes most likely with ocular manifestations
Tonic	Stiffening, decerebrate posturing	About 5% of neonatal seizures. EEG correlation variable
Clonic	Repetitive jerking, distinct from jittering. Can be unifocal or multifocal	25–30% of neonatal seizures. EEG correlation highly likely, especially if focal
Myoclonic	Myoclonic jerks; sleep myoclonus can be benign	15–20% of neonatal seizures. EEG normal if focal, or sleep myoclonus

and limb movements (often described as swimming, boxing or cycling). In addition, apnoeic episodes can be due to seizure and this diagnosis should be considered if there is slow response to bag and mask ventilation, particularly in a preterm neonate with an intracranial lesion. Another clue may be associated movements such as eyelid or mouth opening and a bradycardia that starts soon after the collapse. Autonomic changes, such as a change in blood pressure or increased salivation, often accompany subtle seizures and these may provide a clue to the correct diagnosis in the absence of EEG confirmation.

Clonic

Clonic seizures usually involve one limb or one side of the face or body jerking rhythmically at a frequency of 1–4 times per second.

This type of seizure is associated with a characteristic EEG discharge consisting of runs of sharp–slow-wave complexes that spread ipsilaterally from the hemisphere in which they originate. Clonic seizures in the neonate can have more than one focus or migrate in a non-Jacksonian fashion; for example jerking of one leg can be followed by similar movements in the opposite hand. Clonic seizures are often a clue to an underlying focal lesion such as a cortical infarction but they can be due to a metabolic cause. Infants are not usually unconscious during clonic seizures.

Tonic

Sustained posturing of the limbs or trunk, or deviation of the head or eyes are the usual manifestations of tonic seizures in the newborn.

Myoclonic

Myoclonic jerks tend to occur in the flexor muscle groups. Generalised myoclonic seizures resemble salaam spasms and are the type most likely to be associated with EEG change. Any type of myoclonic seizure (focal, multifocal or generalised) can occur in benign neonatal sleep myoclonus.[17]

Jitteriness

Jitteriness is an extremely common phenomenon amongst normal newborns, being observed in 44% of a sample of 936 babies.[72] Jittering is more common among infants born to mothers who use marijuana, and can be a sign of neonatal abstinence syndrome (Ch. 26). Jittering is a symmetrical tremor, without the fast and slow component of a clonic or myoclonic seizure, and occurs at a faster rate of 5–6 times per second. Jittering does not involve the face (unlike subtle seizures), is markedly stimulus-sensitive and ceases when the limb is held. The autonomic nervous system changes of a seizure, such as tachycardia or hypertension, are never seen in jittering.

Hyperekplexia

Hyperekplexia is a rare disorder characterised by hypertonia, especially in infancy, and a very exaggerated startle response.[94] The startles can look like myoclonic jerks and the high tone, hyperreflexia and jitteriness can lead to an erroneous diagnosis of seizure.[32] Hyperekplexia is probably the same condition previously known as hereditary stiff-baby syndrome.[56] Although the EEG is normal, the tonic spasms can be dangerous and treatment is warranted. Treatment with clonazepam (0.05–0.2 mg/kg/d) or low-dose clobazam (0.25–0.3 mg/kg/d) usually results in marked improvement, and the episodes usually disappear by the age of 2 years.[92] The disorder is caused by mutations in the alpha subunit of the inhibitory glycine receptor[91] and has been mapped to chromosome 5; it can be inherited in an autosomal dominant fashion, although some forms are autosomal recessive.[49]

Physiological changes during seizures

Blood glucose remains normal or rises during seizure but brain glucose falls markedly, with a rise in lactate. This implies that brain transport mechanisms are unable to keep up with the increased demand. The demand for oxygen is also increased, and cerebral blood flow rises to try to meet the need for oxygen and glucose. That metabolic demand outstrips supply in the newborn is supported by magnetic resonance spectroscopic data showing a shift in spectra from the high energy phosphate compounds towards inorganic phosphate.[103] The changes in the brain are similar to those seen in hypoxic–ischaemic injury. Glucose pretreatment is effective in reducing the high mortality of status epilepticus in rats, a benefit that is not seen with ketone body supplementation, although the neonatal brain is known to be able to utilise alternative fuels. Lactate accumulates during seizure, and the arterial pH falls. Systemic blood pressure increases, and cerebral blood flow rises. These dramatic short term effects are followed by the changes in cell structure and synaptic linkages referred to earlier.

Electroencephalographic diagnosis of seizures

The normal neonatal electroencephalogram

The EEG of the normal full-term baby is continuous, contains moderate voltage-mixed frequency activity, shows fully developed sleep cycles and is reactive to stimuli. The type of continuous activity present depends on whether the baby is awake, in active sleep or in quiet sleep (Ch. 28). During quiet sleep the EEG may show a pattern called high-voltage, slow-wave sleep (HVSW) that consists of continuous medium–high-voltage delta waves. As quiet sleep continues this pattern may become somewhat discontinuous, with periods of low-amplitude beta and theta activity, alternating with 3–5-second bursts of higher-voltage 1–3 Hz activity occurring at 3–10-second intervals. This pattern is called *tracé alternant*. In active sleep, the EEG is continuous, of lower voltage and contains mixed-frequency activity. In wakefulness the EEG also shows a lower-voltage mixed frequency pattern referred to as *activité moyenne*. The EEG of a full term baby is illustrated in Figure 41.14a. Specific normal maturational features that may be present in the full-term EEG are anterior slow dysrhythmia (first apparent from approximately 35 weeks) and frontal sharp transients.

The most striking feature of the very preterm EEG is long periods of quiescence interrupted only by bursts of high-voltage mixed-frequency waves (Fig. 41.14b). The lengths of quiescent periods (also referred to as interburst intervals) are directly proportional to the degree of prematurity and this normal background pattern is referred to as *tracé discontinu* or discontinuous pattern. This pattern is different from the tracé alternant pattern seen in full-term babies because the periods of quiescence can be completely flat. True quiescence is always less than 15 μV. In tracé alternant the discontinuous pattern is characterised by periods of high amplitude mixed frequency activity alternating with periods of lower amplitude activity at 25–50 μV (it is never completely flat). The degree of discontinuity seen in the preterm EEG would be very abnormal at term.[16]

Recent data suggests that the maximum interburst interval falls from 60 seconds at 24–26 weeks to 40 seconds at 27–29 weeks and 20 seconds at 30–32 weeks.[2,8,75,102] After 33–34 weeks and up to 37 weeks the EEG is discontinuous only in quiet sleep and the interburst interval should be no longer than 10 seconds.[75] After 37 weeks, the EEG is continuous in wakefulness and active sleep, and tracé alternant replaces tracé discontinu in quiet sleep. Specific normal maturational features of the preterm EEG include premature temporal theta activity, which is sharp activity

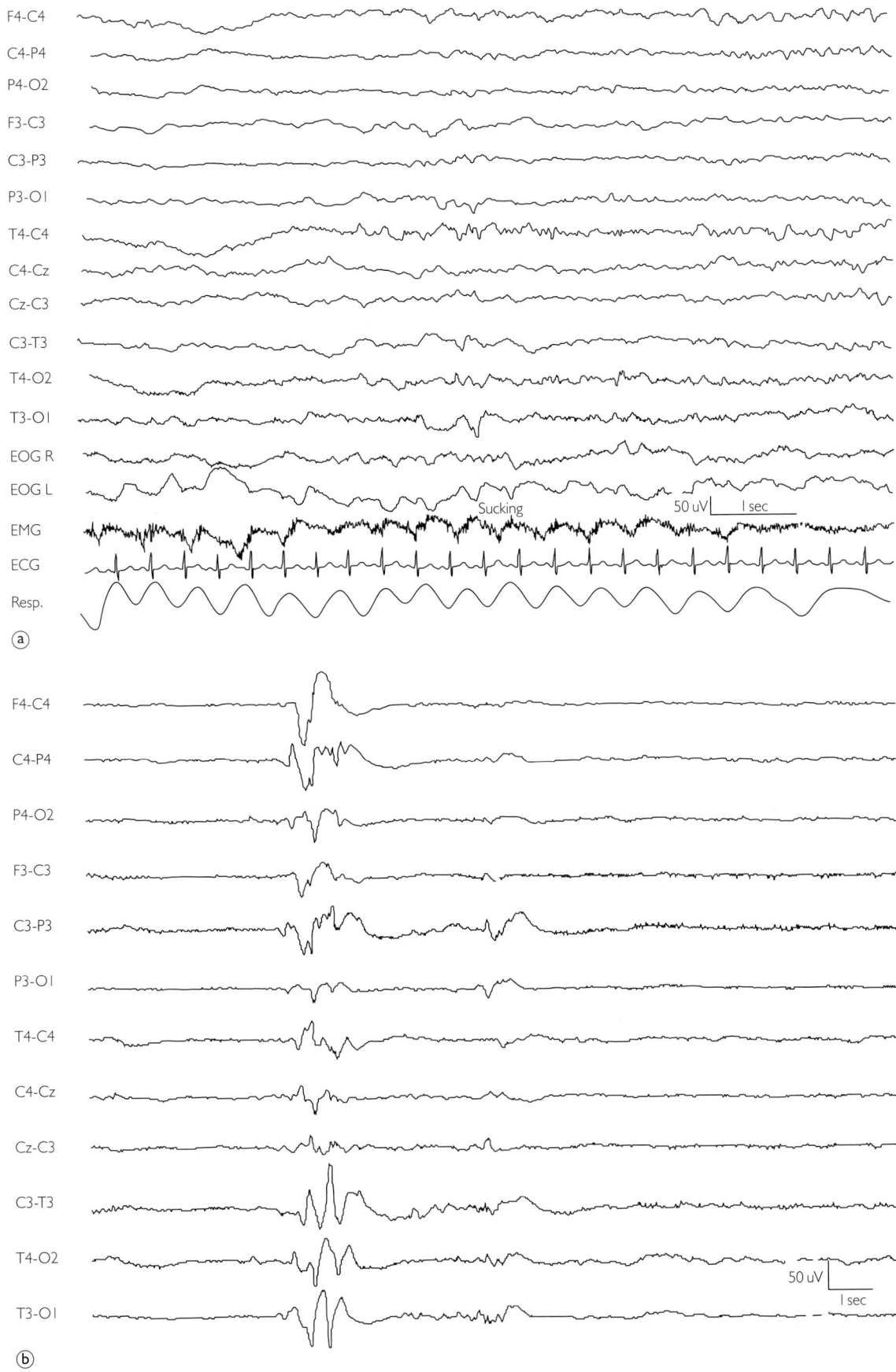

Fig. 41.14 EEG recordings showing normal term activity (a) normal preterm activity (b) and a seizure in a term baby (c) and a preterm baby (d).

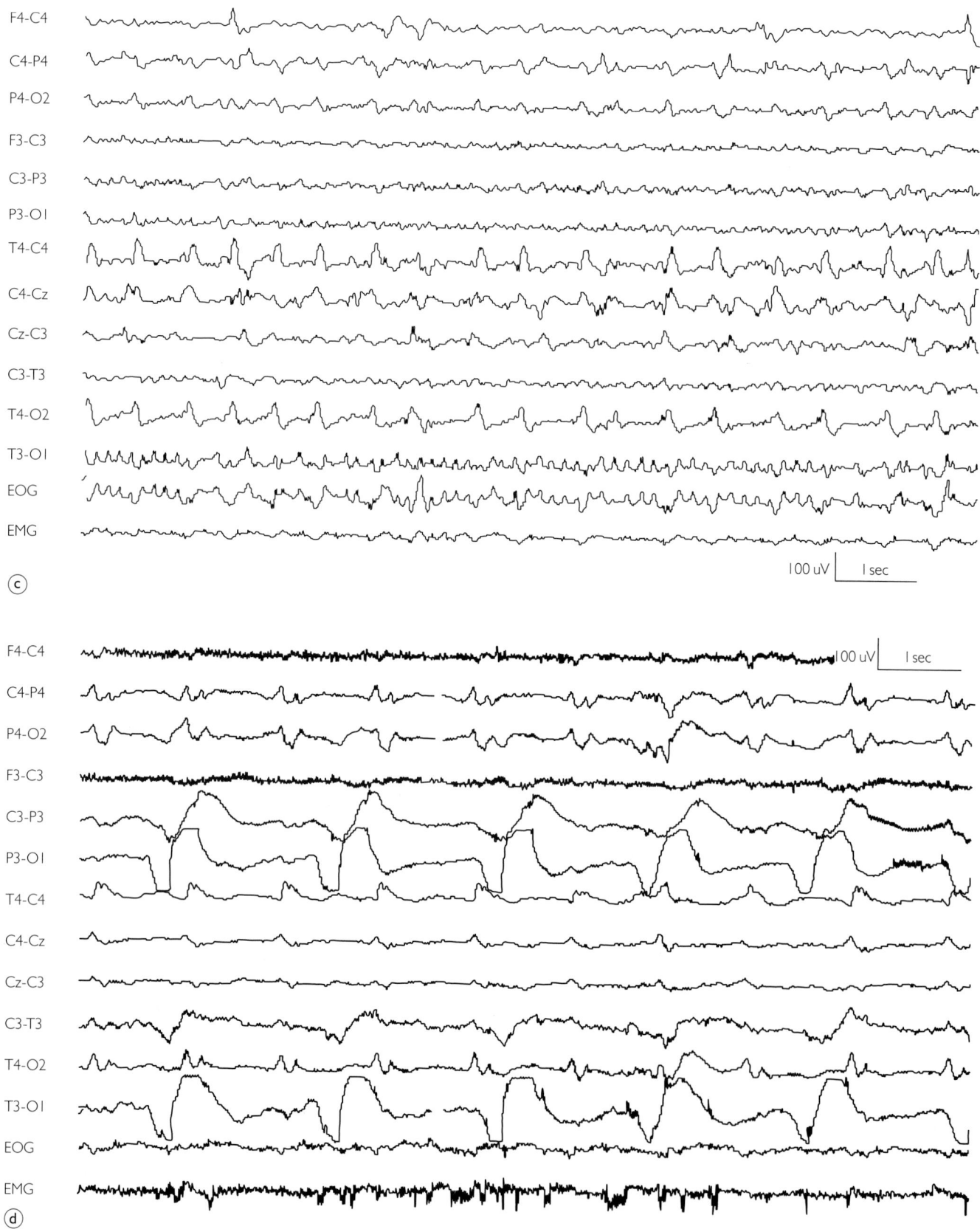

Fig. 41.14 (Continued)

with a characteristic 'saw-toothed' appearance seen from approximately 27 weeks, and delta brush activity, which is a combination of very slow delta activity with superimposed fast components, present from approximately 30 weeks.

The abnormal neonatal electroencephalogram

The neonatal EEG may be abnormal in a number of ways:

- disturbances of continuity, amplitude or frequency;
- interhemispheric asymmetry or asynchrony;
- abnormal waveforms may be present;
- disturbances of sleep state;
- seizure activity may be present.

Any periods of true quiescence in the term newborn are abnormal. However anticonvulsants and sedation may induce some periods of quiescence in the term newborn and prolong periods in the preterm baby. Ellison et al characterised the neonatal EEG mainly on the basis of the interburst interval, categorising the EEG of infants of less than 30 weeks gestation as abnormal if the interval was more than 60 seconds, using a figure of 30 seconds at term.[22] More recently, Menache and colleagues confirmed that an interburst interval of more than 30 seconds was abnormal at term, and presaged a poor outcome.[61]

Electrographic seizures

Neonatal seizure activity is quite variable in type and location of onset, morphology, and propagation.[73] Both term and preterm infants have the ability to generate a rich variety of ictal events, the most common site of seizure origin being the temporal lobe.

Few studies have quantified seizure duration in the newborn.[14,15,85] Clancy and Ledigo used an arbitrary cut-off of 10 seconds as a minimum duration and this definition was also adopted by Scher et al.[15,85] Others have used 5 seconds.[86] Very short bursts of abnormal electrical activity have also been termed BIRDs – brief intermittent rhythmic discharges. Electrographic seizures characteristically consist of monophasic repetitive discharges or spike and wave activity (Fig. 41.14c,d)[73] but there is a rich variety in the onset, morphology and propagation patterns of neonatal seizures, which do not always correlate with the underlying pathology. An electrographic seizure should have a clear onset and conclusion but these can be difficult to identify. Electrographic seizures may or may not be accompanied by stereotyped movements (see next section).

Electroclinical dissociation

There is asynchrony between the clinical and electrical diagnosis of neonatal seizures: in only one-third of cases studied with video surveillance were the clinical and electrical manifestations simultaneous.[64,99] Subtle stereotyped behaviour may or may not be associated with characteristic EEG changes, and continuous electrical monitoring detects many clinically silent seizures. One explanation is that the motor manifestations arise because of discharges from the brainstem and spinal cord which are 'released' because of lack of inhibition from higher centres. An alternative explanation is that scalp electrodes are incapable of recording from every part of the brain; depth electrodes reveal an otherwise unsuspected electrical focus in 10% of adult patients. The neurological effects of clinically silent (electrographic) seizures are not known, nor is it certain that treatment of clinically manifest seizures to electrical quiescence is required. This is an important question because phenobarbital (phenobarbitone) treatment frequently abolishes the clinical manifestations while the electrical paroxysms continue.[12] Our video-EEG studies have shown that there is a group of babies who only ever manifest 'clinical' seizures ('clinical-only'). These babies had not been treated with anticonvulsants, so this was not the reason for the lack of electrographic seizures. The babies had normal background EEG, normal neuroimaging and did well at follow-up, indicating that the phenomenon was benign.[10,12] The motor manifestations did not involve oro-facial movements.

Current clinical practice is to commence anticonvulsant treatment without obtaining an EEG in the newborn, and our experiences with this small group serve to underline the importance of attempting EEG confirmation if at all possible. Cerebral function monitoring is more widely available but this method fails to detect short seizures, low voltage seizures and seizures that remain localised.[77] There is as yet no information regarding any clinical benefits of treating to electrical quiescence, and in the current state of knowledge it is acceptable practice to aim to control clinically apparent seizures. In any case, it is virtually impossible to achieve electrical control in all cases with the anticonvulsants currently available for newborn use.

Aetiology

Causes of neonatal seizures in current order of importance are shown in Table 41.3.

Hypoxic ischaemic encephalopathy

This remains the most common cause of neonatal seizures at term, contributing over half the cases to most series. The characteristic time of onset is within 24 hours of birth, and seizures often begin in the first 12 hours (see Fig. 41.13). For more information on management and prognosis of this condition, see pages 1128–48.

Intracranial haemorrhage

Germinal matrix or intraventricular haemorrhage is the most frequent cause of seizures in preterm infants (Ch. 41).[44] Scher found that 45% of preterm infants with seizures had germinal matrix/intraventricular haemorrhage (GMH-IVH).[84]

Table 41.3 Causes of neonatal seizure

Study	Levene & Trounce 1986[54] (%)	Goldberg 1983[30] (%)	Andre et al 1988[3] (%)	Bergman et al 1983[7] (%)	Estan & Hope 1997[23] (%)	Lien et al 1995[55] (%)	Ronen & Penney 1995[80] (%)	Ortibus et al 1996[70] (%)
Number of cases			71	131	100	40	90	81
Hypoxic ischaemic encephalopathy	53	16	49	30	49	37	40	37
Cerebral infarction (stroke)					12	17	1	11
Intracranial haemorrhage (includes IVH and subdural haematomas)	17		14		7	12	15	9
Meningitis	8	3	2	7	5	5	20	9
Maternal drug withdrawal			4					
Hypoglycaemia	3	2	0.1	5	3		3	
Hypocalcaemia, hypomagnesaemia				22			5	
Rapidly changing serum sodium								
Congenitally abnormal brain		8		4	3	17	10	6
Fifth day fits (benign non-familial)		52						
Benign familial neonatal seizures							6	1
Pyridoxine-dependent seizures								
Hypertension			1.4					
Kernicterus					1			
Inborn errors of metabolism					3			

IVH = Intraventricular haemorrhage

Focal cerebral infarction

Preterm infants with GMH-IVH often have an associated haemorrhagic venous infarction, which acts as a focus for seizure (Ch. 41). Seizures in term infants with normal Apgar scores who remain alert between spasms are likely to be due to focal lesions, most commonly middle cerebral artery infarction (p. 1123). These often require magnetic resonance imaging (MRI) for identification, and the prognosis is better than when the underlying cause is hypoxic ischaemic encephalopathy. Diagnosis of stroke in the newborn period should trigger investigations to rule out an underlying thrombotic tendency (pp. 762–3).

Meningitis

Intracranial infections, both bacterial (pp. 1040–2), non-bacterial and congenital, cause neonatal seizures, usually after the first week of life. Lumbar puncture remains a mandatory investigation in babies with seizures.

Drug withdrawal (Ch. 26)

Maternal methadone addiction is more likely to be associated with neonatal withdrawal seizures than addiction to heroin.[38] Withdrawal seizures can occur for the first time at any age up to 3 weeks, with a median time of onset of 10 days. They can persist for several months. EEG abnormalities are present in 50% of cocaine-exposed neonates, persist up to 1 year and are associated with an adverse neurodevelopmental outcome. Tremors have been noted in children who received prolonged infusions of narcotics for analgesia[26] and there has been concern about the effects of midazolam for sedation in preterm babies (see below).[65]

Metabolic causes

Hypoglycaemia

Hypoglycaemia can be the sole cause of neonatal seizures and other neurological signs such as apnoea, lethargy and jitteriness. Often hypoglycaemia complicates hypoxic ischaemic encephalopathy or infection, and hypoglycaemia is also common in infants who are small for gestational age (Ch. 10). The adverse outcome associated with the underlying cause makes it difficult to determine the prognosis of uncomplicated hypoglycaemia. There is no doubt that the finding of a low glucose level in a baby who is seizing is an indication for urgent intravenous treatment, and every effort should be made to normalise the glucose level as soon as possible (Ch. 35).

Hypocalcaemia

Half the babies in the series of Brown et al[13] were hypocalcaemic (total serum calcium less than 1.75 mmol/l. Similarly high incidences of late hypocalcaemic seizures were reported prior to the introduction of modern low-phosphate milks; in the late 1960s infants were consuming doorstep cow's milk or a high phosphate formula. Hypocalcaemic seizures occasionally occur secondary to maternal hypercalcaemia (prolonged intrauterine exposure to high levels) or maternal vitamin D deficiency, and the neonatal diagnosis should prompt estimation of the maternal serum calcium. Low magnesium levels frequently accompany hypocalcaemia and require correction before the seizures will respond. Hypocalcaemia is common in ill very-low-birthweight babies and in babies with hypoxic ischaemic encephalopathy and is probably not causally related to the seizures in these cases.

Hyponatraemia

A very high, very low or rapidly changing serum sodium occurring in conditions such as the syndrome of inappropriate antidiuretic hormone secretion (pp. 340–1), Bartter's syndrome or severe dehydration can cause seizures.

Congenital malformations of the brain

Disorders of neuronal migration such as lissencephaly or schizencephaly can present with neonatal seizures. Diagnosis has been facilitated with the advent of MRI but is sometimes possible with ultrasound (p. 1137).

Inborn errors of metabolism

Pyridoxine-dependent seizures

The first case of an infant with intractable seizures controlled by pyridoxine was reported by Hunt et al in 1954.[41] These seizures can begin during intrauterine life (mothers describe 'hammering' movements lasting 15–20 minutes several times a day) and are very resistant to conventional anticonvulsant treatment, yet cease within minutes of parenteral pyridoxine (50–100 mg) and return within days of withdrawal. This therapeutic trial can cause hypotonia requiring ventilatory support and should be carried out in an intensive care unit.[46] There is no other way to make the diagnosis, although characteristic EEG abnormalities have been recognised.[66] Atypical cases who respond more slowly and who have late-onset seizures requiring unusually high doses of pyridoxine (up to 500 mg) have been described,[6,33] and yet others respond to very small doses. Gospe suggests that a trial of pyridoxine

should involve 100 mg intravenously every 10 minutes until the seizures stop or a total of 500 mg is reached.

The underlying defect is thought to be defective binding of the pyridoxal phosphate co-enzyme with glutamic acid decarboxylase (GAD), a step that is necessary for GABA synthesis.[34] The condition is autosomal recessive. Supplementation of the diet with pyridoxine (vitamin B_6) 20–100 mg twice daily is required for life, and the dose may need to be increased with age.[6] Unfortunately, many of these children are retarded despite early diagnosis and treatment. Recently, a better outcome has been achieved with bigger doses of pyridoxine, leading to the suggestion that sufficient pyridoxine should be given to restore the glutamate levels in the cerebrospinal fluid (CSF) to normal.

Glycine encephalopathy

Nonketotic hyperglycinemia is a rare inborn error of metabolism in which large amounts of glycine accumulate, causing intractable seizures (p. 909). Hiccups can be troublesome. Levels of glycine in blood, urine and cerebrospinal fluid are very high. Dextromethorphan monotherapy (35 mg/kg/d) was associated with cessation of seizures and normalisation of the EEG in a single case, but this regimen is not always successful.[87]

De Vivo's syndrome/GLUT-1 deficiency syndrome

Glucose transport across the blood–brain barrier is mediated by the facilitative glucose transporter isoform 1 (GLUT-1). A deficiency of this transporter results in impaired energy supply to the brain, and was recognised by De Vivo in 1991.[19] This rare disorder is important because treatment can lead to normal neurological outcome.[25] Babies have a strikingly low CSF glucose concentration, with low CSF lactate levels despite normal blood glucose concentrations. Treatment is with a ketogenic diet. There may be a transient form of the disorder that does not require long-term treatment, but the three cases so far described may have had alternative explanations for the low CSF glucose levels, such as low-grade meningitis or subarachnoid haemorrhage.[42]

Benign familial neonatal convulsions

This fascinating autosomal dominant condition was first recognised in 1964.[78] The seizures are dramatic and usually clonic, 80% beginning on the second or third day of life, usually ceasing by the age of 6 months. Genetic markers have shown a mutation on chromosome 20 leading to mutations in the potassium channel genes.[51,52] Seizure characteristics have been described.[82] In contrast to pyridoxine-dependent seizures these fits can be controlled by conventional medication and the prognosis for development is excellent.

Benign non-familial neonatal seizures (fifth day fits)

This benign self-limiting condition reached epidemic proportions in some Australian maternity units in the late 1970s.[76] Reports also came from France, but only two cases have been seen in Nancy since 1985 and the diagnosis has not been made in Camperdown since 1989.[4,68] The seizures began between days 3 and 5 and lasted for up to 2 weeks. The cause remains a mystery, although low CSF zinc was found in a few cases.[29] Recently we cared for a baby with this condition who had marked tonic-clonic seizures, which are otherwise very unusual in the newborn period; she has thrived.[35]

Benign neonatal sleep myoclonus

In this condition the myoclonic jerks only occur during sleep, when the EEG is normal. The myoclonus is present in all sleep states although its frequency is state-dependent and greatest during quiet sleep. The movements disappear by 6 months of age. No treatment is required and parents should be reassured that the jerks will cease eventually.

Hypertension

Rapid lowering of the blood pressure with captopril was accompanied by a seizure in one case,[74] and two cases of hypertensive seizure were reported in 1988.[3] True hypertensive encephalopathy causing neonatal seizures is extremely rare in the newborn, perhaps because of the compliance of the skull, and most neonatologists have never seen a case.[59]

Investigation

Essential laboratory investigations include:

- blood glucose;
- serum calcium, ionised calcium if possible;
- serum magnesium;
- arterial pH;
- serum sodium;
- serum urea and creatinine;
- lumbar puncture;
- blood culture;
- cranial ultrasound scan.

If the cause is not revealed, second-line investigations include specimens for virology and a congenital infection screen, MRI, samples such as hair or urine to look for maternal 'street' drugs, urinary and blood amino acid estimation, chromosomal analysis, blood ammonia and measurement of urinary organic acids. Consideration should be given to a trial of pyridoxine in resistant cases. The value of an EEG examination has already been discussed and an EEG should be obtained if at all possible, and certainly be done in difficult cases. MRI is superior to computed tomography for most purposes, and should be considered in all cases, and certainly if the cause is not revealed by first line investigations. Even if the cause is found, the information obtained from MRI can give valuable information about the prognosis.

Treatment

Indications for treatment

Most babies are treated on the basis of a clinical diagnosis alone, and treatment is also monitored this way. Continuous EEG studies show that a considerable electrographic seizure burden often remains after anticonvulsant treatment is begun, due to electro-clinical dissociation.[12] Whether or not treating to electrical quiescence can improve the outcome is not known, and as yet there is no anticonvulsant regimen that will achieve this in all cases. In the current state of knowledge most neonatologists would treat a baby who had more than three clinical seizures in an hour, or a single clinical seizure lasting more than 3 minutes; this remains reasonable practice, although every attempt should be made to obtain an EEG. Newer cerebral function monitors are available that allow access to the raw EEG signal and these should improve access to this important investigation.

General guidelines

Treatment is best started intravenously as absorption is erratic from intramuscular or enteral administration and the neonate has little muscle mass. Facilities to site and maintain intravenous lines and to institute artificial ventilation are necessary before treating seizures, as most of the available drugs depress respiration and ventilation can become inadequate due to frequent convulsions or the effects of treatment. The high total body water of the neonate means there is a large volume of distribution, hence the relatively large loading doses suggested in Table 41.4. Many of the drugs are protein-bound and can interact with other drugs and bilirubin.

Initiating treatment

Phenobarbital (phenobarbitone) remains the first-choice treatment for seizures in the newborn. There is a vast body of experience with this drug, and it will achieve clinical and electrographic control in one-third to half of babies within a few hours.[11,71] In our experience, phenobarbital is more likely to be effective when the background EEG is normal, and the seizure burden is low.

Phenytoin is our current second line, although this drug needs to be used with caution (and given slowly intravenously) in babies with cardiac depression secondary to perinatal hypoxic ischaemia. About a third of babies fail to respond to a combination of phenobarbital and phenytoin; they are usually suffering from severe hypoxic ischaemic encephalopathy and their prognosis is poor.[11] Very often these babies are given a vast range of anticonvulsants, resulting in a prolongation of their intensive care course and difficulty in assessing their neurological state. This temptation should be avoided, not least because there is as yet no evidence that the outcome can be improved even with thiopentone coma.[31]

Benzodiazepines have proved disappointing, although clonazepam remains a popular third-line choice. Lidocaine (lignocaine) should not be used if phenytoin has already been given, and sodium

Table 41.4 Anticonvulsant drug use in the newborn

Drug	Initial dose	Route	Maintenance dose	Route	Half life	Mode of excretion	Notes	Therapeutic level
Phenobarbital	20–40 mg/kg	IV	4–5 mg/kg/24 h	O	100–200 h	Hepatic P_{450} cytochrome oxidase	Slow oral absorption: liver enzyme inducer; vitamin K antagonist; risk of extravasation, cardiac toxicity and purple glove syndrome	20–40 mg/l 90–180 micromol/l
Phenytoin	20 mg/kg SLOWLY (1 mg/kg/min)	IV	5 mg/kg/24 h in 2 doses	IV/O	20 h (75 prems)	Liver glucuronidation	Protect from light and plastic	10–20 mg/l 40–80 micromol/l
Paraldehyde	0.3 ml/kg (0.6 ml/kg of mixture) PR	Rectal	For rectal use dilute 1:1 with arachis oil, give no more than t.d.s.	Rectal	7–27 h	Mainly liver, some lungs		
Diazepam	0.3 mg/kg	IV	0.3 mg/kg	IV	20–60 h	Liver glucuronidation	Flumazenil is an antidote to diazepam and midazolam; rapid clearance from the brain limits value	
Clonazepam	100 microg/kg	IV	4 microg/kg/h	IV	30 h	Liver glucuronidation	Tends to increase salivation and bronchial secretions	30–100 mg/l
Midazolam	60 microg/kg	IV	150 microg/kg/h	IV	6–12 h	Liver glucuronidation	Reports of myoclonic jerks in preterm babies	
Valproate	20 mg/kg	IV	10 mg/kg/12-hourly	O	26–47 h	Hepatic	GABA modifier. Increased ammonia levels. Hepatotoxicity may be a problem but not yet described in babies	40–50 mg/l 275–350 micromol/l
Lidocaine	2–4 mg/kg	IV	2 mg/kg/h maximum 6 mg/kg/h and for no more than 48 h	IV	200 min	Liver and kidney	Toxic metabolites accumulate in 24 hour	2.4–6 mg/l in adults – little known about therapeutic levels in babies

valproate remains virtually unevaluated. The newer anticonvulsants have yet to be tried in the newborn, and very few are available as an intravenous preparation.

Phenobarbital (phenobarbitone)

Give a large loading dose; it is reasonable to give 40 mg/kg if the patient is already ventilated, otherwise use 20 mg/kg initially. Gilman et al[28] achieved seizure control with phenobarbital alone in 77% of cases using a rapid sequential method in which they gave 15–20 mg/kg initially then further doses of 5–10 mg/kg every 30 minutes up to a maximum of 40 mg/kg to achieve a serum level of over 40 milligrams per litre (20–40 mg/l = 90–180 μmol/l). The half-life is very long and there have been concerns about toxic effects on the developing brain. Nevertheless, the drug has other actions, reducing cerebral metabolic rate and acting as a free radical scavenger, which make it a good choice as the first-line anticonvulsant. As discussed, the response to phenobarbital treatment is variable, but control is achieved in a third to a half of babies within a few hours.[11,71] A response is more likely in babies with a small seizure burden and normal or mildly abnormal background EEG.

Phenytoin

Phenytoin is probably the best choice as second-line treatment in babies who fail to respond to phenobarbital (phenobarbitone), and achieves control in about a further third of the total number of cases.[71] Intravenous phenytoin can cause arrhythmias if given too quickly, and this (and hypotension) may be a particular problem in babies with hypoxic ischaemic encephalopathy who have cardiac depression. The rate of administration should be no faster than 1 mg/kg/min and full monitoring must be in place (Table 41.4). The 'purple glove' syndrome that is recognised in older children and adults has been reported in babies, and there is a concern about the high rate of complications after intravenous phenytoin in children.[5,69,88] Some units use fosphenytoin as an alternative for this reason.[79]

Paraldehyde

Rectal administration of paraldehyde has been used for many years with safety and the drug is a useful second-line anticonvulsant. There is some experience with intravenous infusions, which can be inconvenient as the drug must be light-protected. Concern has been raised regarding pulmonary oedema and hepatic necrosis. Intramuscular administration often leads to sterile abscess formation and should be abandoned.

Benzodiazepines

Benzodiazepines increase GABA-mediated inhibition through activation of the GABA-A receptor. They are effective anticonvulsants in older children and adults but may be less so in the newborn because GABA is excitatory at this time. Benzodiazepines do have a good safety profile.

Midazolam

Midazolam is a water-soluble, short-acting benzodiazepine that has proved effective in treating status epilepticus in the paediatric population. There is very little experience with midazolam in babies.[89] We recently evaluated midazolam in an open comparison with lidocaine (lignocaine) as second-line treatment in babies whose seizures failed to respond to phenobarbital (phenobarbitone); seizures were monitored with continuous video-EEG.[11] Six babies received either clonazepam or midazolam but none responded.

We and others have seen clusters of abnormal movements in preterm babies receiving midazolam infusions, although the EEG usually remains normal.[67,96] The neurodevelopmental outcome was better in a group of babies sedated with morphine than it was when midazolam was used, and these results have led to concern about midazolam use in preterm babies.[1]

Clonazepam

Clonazepam is sometimes used as an infusion in babies with intractable neonatal seizures, although the half-life is such that intermittent dosing is probably just as good. Hypersalivation and increased bronchial secretions are a frequent problem when clonazepam is used.

Diazepam

Diazepam has a rapid onset of action but there is also very rapid clearance from the brain, which means that any anticonvulsant effect is short-lived. Cardiorespiratory instability can result when the drug is used in combination with phenobarbital (phenobarbitone), and the long half-life of the main metabolite, N-desmethyldiazepam, can contribute to sedation without achieving seizure control. For this reason, diazepam is not the benzodiazepine of choice in the newborn.

Lorazepam

Lorazepam is popular in the USA, where intravenous clonazepam is not available. There is little experience with this benzodiazepine in Europe.

Lidocaine (lignocaine)

Lidocaine (lignocaine) has a very narrow therapeutic range and accumulates in the blood, so that it can only be given as an infusion for 48 hours. There are reports of success with this agent, mainly from Scandinavia.[37,43] Three of the five babies who received lidocaine as second-line in our open study responded, but much more information is required before this drug can be recommended for routine use.[11] A baby who has been given phenytoin already should not receive lidocaine because of the risk of cardiac toxicity.

Table 41.5 Outcome of neonatal seizures by cause

	Dead (%)	Handicap (%)	Normal (%)	Reference
HIE grade II, III	50	25	25	
Preterm	58	23	18	Scher et al 1993,[84] Watkins et al 1988,[98] van Zeben-van der Aa et al 1990[95]
Meningitis	20	40	40	
Malformations	60	40		
Late-onset Hypocalcaemia			100	
Hypoglycaemia		50	50	Koivisto et al 1972[45]

Sodium valproate

Concern about the hepatotoxic effects, hyperammonaemia and hyperglycinaemia may limit the use of sodium valproate (valproic acid) in the newborn. Valproate proved effective in six intractable cases of neonatal seizure.[27]

Duration of treatment

Concern about the effects of anticonvulsant treatment on the developing brain means that most British neonatologists would only discharge a baby on maintenance phenobarbital (phenobarbitone) if the neurological examination was abnormal, although only 3% of US neonatologists discontinued treatment prior to discharge.[60] Only two of 55 Swedish infants discharged without medication relapsed.[36] Some perform an EEG at a month, or prior to discharge, and discontinue anticonvulsants if the EEG is normal. If babies are discharged on anticonvulsants, consider discontinuation of treatment if they remain seizure-free at 9 months. Babies can be allowed to 'grow out of' their dose, gradually reducing drug levels.

Maintenance anticonvulsants

Phenobarbital (phenobarbitone) in a dose of 5 mg/kg/day is the usual maintenance anticonvulsant chosen for the newborn. There is very little experience with alternative maintenance therapy at the present time and combinations are best avoided. Phenytoin is not a good choice for long-term therapy. Resistant cases should be treated with a combination of phenobarbital and carbamazepine, although sodium valproate can be successful in some cases.

Prognosis

This is mainly related to the cause of the seizures (Table 41.5). Following hypoxic ischaemic encephalopathy at term, 25% of those who develop grade II Sarnat and Sarnat encephalopathy will suffer sequelae. The combination of a 5-minute Apgar score of less than 5, fits and signs of encephalopathy was a poor one, with 33% dead and 55% with handicap.[21] Of 70 cases of clinical seizure in very-low-birthweight infants followed in Cambridge, 43 (59%) died, 16 (22%) had a major handicap and 11 (15%) were normal at 18 months (personal observations). These data are remarkably similar to those of Watkins et al,[98] van Zeben et al[95] and Scher et al.[84] The prognosis after hypocalcaemic seizure and in familial neonatal seizure is excellent. A normal background interictal EEG in a term baby with seizures is a good prognostic factor, with fewer than 10% of such infants experiencing sequelae.[97] The value of a normal neurological examination at discharge in providing early reassurance should not be underestimated; 11 of 14 infants with seizures who were normal at 4 years were assessed as normal at this stage.[20] However, this apparently normal group of Oxford children then had problems with spelling and memory in adolescence.[93]

Acknowledgement

Dr Geraldine Boylan, Department of Paediatrics, Cork University Hospital, Republic of Ireland contributed to the section on the EEG and provided the EEG figures.

References

1. Anand K J S, McIntosh N, Lagercrantz H, Young T E, Vasa R, Barton B A 1999 Analgesia and sedation in preterm neonates who require ventilatory support. Archives of Pediatric and Adolescent Medicine 153: 331–338
2. Anderson C M, Torres F, Faoro A 1985 The EEG of the early premature. Electroencephalography and Clinical Neurophysiology 60: 95–105
3. Andre M, Matisse M, Vert P, Debruille C 1988 Neonatal seizures – recent aspects. Neuropediatrics 19: 201–207
4. Andre M, Selton D 1993 Convulsions in the fifth day of life. A critical study. Archives of French Pediatrics 50: 197–200
5. Appleton R E, Gill A 2003 Adverse events associated with intravenous phenytoin in children: a prospective study. Seizure 12: 369–372
6. Baxter P 2001 Pyridoxine-dependent and pyridoxine-responsive seizures. Developmental Medicine and Child Neurology 43: 416–420

7. Bergman I, Painter M J, Hirsch R P, Crumin P K, David R 1983 Outcome in neonates with convulsions treated in ICU. Annals of Neurology 14: 642–647

8. Biagioni E, Mercuri E, Rutherford M et al 2001 Combined use of electroencephalogram and magnetic resonance imaging in full-term neonates with acute encephalopathy. Pediatrics 107: 461–468

9. Boylan G B, Panerai R B, Rennie J M, Evans D H, Rabe-Hesketh S, Binnie C D 1999 Cerebral blood flow velocity during neonatal seizures. Archives of Disease in Childhood 80: F105–F110

10. Boylan G B, Pressler R M, Rennie J M et al 1999 Outcome of electroclinical, electrographic, and clinical seizures in the newborn infant. Developmental Medicine and Child Neurology 41: 819–825

11. Boylan G B, Rennie J M, Chorley G et al 2004 Second line anticonvulsant treatment of neonatal seizures: a video-EEG monitoring study. Neurology 62: 486–488

12. Boylan G B, Rennie J M, Pressler R M, Wilson G, Morton M, Binnie C D 2002 Phenobarbitone, neonatal seizures, and video-EEG. Archives of Disease in Childhood 86: 165–170

13. Brown J K, Cockburn F, Forfar J O 1972 Clinical and chemical correlates in convulsions of the newborn. Lancet 1: 135

14. Bye A M E, Flanagan D 1995 Spatial and temporal characteristics of neonatal seizures. Epilepsia 36: 1009–1016

15. Clancy R R, Ledigo A 1987 The exact ictal and interictal duration of electroencephalographic neonatal seizures. Epilepsia 28: 537–541

16. Connell J A, Oozeer R C, Dubowitz V 1987 Continuous 4-channel EEG monitoring: a guide to interpretation, with normal values, in preterm infants. Neuropaediatrics 18: 138–145

17. Coulter D L, Allen R J 1982 Benign neonatal sleep myoclonus. Archives of Neurology 39: 191–192

18. Curtis P D, Matthews T G, Clarke T A et al 1988 Neonatal seizures. Archives of Disease in Childhood 63: 1065–1067

19. De Vivo D, Garcia-Alvarez M, Ronen G, Trifiletti R 1991 Defective glucose transport across the blood–brain barrier as a cause of persistent hypoglycorrhachia, seizures and developmental delay. New England Journal of Medicine 325: 703–709

20. Dennis J 1978 Neonatal convulsions: aetiology, late neonatal status and long term outcome. Developmental Medicine and Child Neurology 20: 143–158

21. Ellenberg J H, Nelson K B 1988 Cluster of perinatal events identifying children at high risk for death and disability. Journal of Pediatrics 113: 546–552

22. Ellison P, Franklin S, Brown P, Jones M G 1989 The evolution of a simplified method for interpretation of EEG in the preterm neonate. Acta Paediatrica Scandinavica 78: 210–216

23. Estan J, Hope P L 1997 Unilateral neonatal cerebral infarction in full term infants. Archives of Disease in Childhood 76: F88–F93

24. Filan P, Boylan G, Chorley G et al 2004 The relationship between the onset of electrographic seizure activity after birth and the time of cerebral injury in utero. British Journal of Obstetrics and Gynaecology 111: 1–4

25. Fishman R A 1991 The glucose transporter protein and gluconeogenic brain injury. New England Journal of Medicine 325: 731–732

26. French J P, Nocera M 1994 Drug withdrawal symptoms in children after continuous infusions of fentanyl. Journal of Pediatric Nursing 9: 107–113

27. Gal P, Oles K S, Gilman J T, Weaver R 1988 Valproic acid efficacy, toxicity, and pharmacokinetics in neonates with intractable seizures. Neurology 38: 467–471

28. Gilman J T, Gal P, Duchowny M S, Weaver R L, Ransom J L 1989 Rapid sequential phenobarbital treatment of neonatal seizures. Pediatrics 83: 674–678

29. Goldberg H J 1982 Fifth day fits – an acute zinc deficiency syndrome? Archives of Disease in Childhood 57: 633–635

30. Goldberg H J 1983 Neonatal convulsions – a ten year review. Archives of Disease in Childhood 57: 633–635

31. Goldberg P N, Moscoso P, Bauer C R 1986 Use of barbiturate therapy in severe perinatal asphyxia. Journal of Pediatrics 109: 851–856

32. Gordon N 1993 Startle disease or hyperexplexia. Developmental Medicine and Child Neurology 35: 1015–1024

33. Gospe S M 1998 Current perspectives on pyridoxine-dependent seizures. Journal of Pediatrics 132: 919–923

34. Gospe S M 2002 Pyridoxine-dependent seizures: findings from recent studies pose new questions. Pediatric Neurology 26: 181–185

35. Guerra M P, Wilson G A, Boylan G B, Rennie J M 2002 An unusual presentation of fifth-day fits in the newborn. Pediatric Neurology 26: 398–401

36. Hellstrom-Westas L, Blennow G, Lindroth M, Rosen I, Svenningsen N 1995 Low risk of seizure recurrence after early withdrawal of antiepileptic treatment in the neonatal period. Archives of Disease in Childhood 72: F97–F101

37. Hellstrom-Westas L, Westgren U, Rosen I, Svenningsen N W 1988 Lidocaine for treatment of severe seizures in newborn infants. Acta Paediatrica Scandinavica 77: 79–84

38. Herzlinger R A, Kandall S R, Vaugham H G Jr 1977 Neonatal seizures associated with narcotic withdrawal. Journal of Pediatrics 91: 638–641

39. Holden K R, Mellits E D, Freeman J M 1982 Neonatal seizures 1: correlation of prenatal and perinatal events with outcomes. Pediatrics 70: 165–176

40. Holmes G L, Khazipov R, Ben-Ari Y 2002 New concepts in neonatal seizures. Neuroreport 13: A3–A8

41. Hunt A D, Stokes J, McCrory W W, Stroud H H 1954 Pyridoxine dependency: report of a case of intractable convulsions in an infant controlled by pyridoxine. Pediatrics 13: 140–145

42. Klepper J, De Vivo D, Webb D W, Klinge L, Voit T 2003 Reversible infantile hypoglycorrhachia: possible transient disturbance in glucose transport? Pediatric Neurology 29: 321–325

43. Kobayashi K, Ito M, Miyajima T, Fujii T, Okuno T 1999 Successful management of intractable epilepsy with intravenous lidocaine and lidocaine tapes. Pediatric Neurology 21: 476–480

44. Kohelet D, Shochat R, Lusky A, Reichman B 2004 Risk factors for neonatal seizures in very low birthweight infants: population-based survey. Journal of Child Neurology 19: 1–9

45. Koivisto M, Blanco-Sequeiros M, Krause U 1972 Neonatal symptomatic and asymptomatic hypoglycaemia: a follow up study of 151 children. Developmental Medicine and Child Neurology 14: 603–614

46. Kroll J 1985 Pyridoxine for neonatal seizures: an unexpected hazard. Developmental Medicine and Child Neurology 27: 369–382

47. Lanska M J, Lanska D J 1996 Neonatal seizures in the United States: results of the National Hospital Discharge Survey, 1980–1991. Neuroepidemiology 15: 117–125

48. Lanska M J, Lanska D J, Baumann R J, Kryscio R J 1995 A population-based study of neonatal seizures in Fayette county, Kentucky. Neurology 45: 724–732

49. Lapunzina P, Sanchex J M, Cabrera M et al 2003 Hyperekplexia (startle disease): a novel mutation (S270T) in the M2 domain of the *GLRA1* gene and a molecular review of the disorder. Molecular Diagnosis 7: 125–128

50. Legido A, Clancy R R, Berman P H 1991 Neurological outcome after electroencephalographically proven neonatal seizures. Pediatrics 88: 583–595

51. Leppert M, Anderson V E, Quattlebaum T et al 1989 Benign familial neonatal convulsions linked to genetic markers on chromosome 20. Nature 337: 647–648

52. Leppert M, Singh N 1999 Benign familial neonatal epilepsy with mutations in two potassium channel genes. Current Opinion in Neurology 12: 143–147

53. Levene M 2002 The clinical conundrum of neonatal seizures. Archives of Disease in Childhood 86: 75–77

54. Levene M I, Trounce J Q 1986 Cause of neonatal convulsions: towards more precise diagnosis. Archives of Disease in Childhood 61: 78–79

55. Lien J M, Towers C V, Quilligan E J, de Veciana M, Toohey J S, Morgan M A 1995 Term early-onset neonatal seizures: obstetric characteristics, etiologic classifications and perinatal care. Obstetrics and Gynecology 85: 163–169

56. Lingham S, Wilson J, Hart E W 1981 Hereditary stiff baby syndrome. American Journal of Diseases of Children 135: 909–911

57. McBride M C, Laroia N, Guillet R 2000 Electrographic seizures in neonates correlate with poor neurodevelopmental outcome. Neurology 55: 506–513

58. McCabe B K, Silveira D C, Cilio M R et al 2001 Reduced neurogenesis after neonatal seizures. Journal of Neuroscience 6: 2094–2103

59. Mace S, Hirschfield S 1983 Hypertensive encephalopathy. American Journal of Diseases of Children 137: 32–33

60. Massingale T W, Boutross S 1993 Survey of treatment practices for neonatal seizures. Journal of Perinatology 13: 107–110

61. Menache C C, Bourgeois B F D, Volpe J J 2002 Prognostic value of the neonatal discontinuous EEG. Paediatric Neurology 27: 93–101

62. Miller S P, Weiss J, Barnwell A et al 2002 Seizure-associated brain injury in term newborns with perinatal asphyxia. Neurology 58: 542–548

63. Minchom P, Niswander K, Chalmers I et al 1987 Antecedents and outcome of very early neonatal seizures. British Journal of Obstetrics and Gynaecology 94: 431–439

64. Mizrahi E M, Kellaway P 1998 Diagnosis and management of neonatal seizures, 1st edn. Lippincott-Raven, Philadelphia

65. Montenegro M A, Guerreiro M M, Caldas J P S, Moura-Ribeiro M V L, Guerreiro C A M 2001 Epileptic manifestations induced by midazolam in the neonatal period. Arquivos de Neuro-psiquiatria 59: 242–243

66. Nabbout R, Soufflet C, Plouin P, Dulac O 1999 Pyridoxine dependent epilepsy: a suggestive electroclinical pattern. Archives of Disease in Childhood 81: F125–F129

67. Ng E, Klinger G, Shah V, Taddio A 2002 Safety of benzodiazepines in newborns. Annals of Pharmacotherapy 36: 1150–1155

68. North K N, Storey G N, Henderson-Smart D J 1989 Fifth day fits in the newborn. Australian Journal of Paediatrics and Child Health 25: 284–287

69. O'Brien T J, Cascino E L S, Hanna D R 1998 Incidence and clinical consequences of the purple glove syndrome in patients receiving intravenous phenytoin. Neurology 51: 1034–1039

70. Ortibus E L, Sum J M, Hahn J S 1996 Predictive value of EEG for outcome and epilepsy following neonatal seizures. Electroencephalography and Clinical Neurophysiology 98: 175–185

71. Painter M J, Scher M S, Stein A D et al 1999 Phenobarbital compared with phenytoin for the treatment of neonatal seizures. New England Journal of Medicine 341: 485–489

72. Parker S, Zuckerman B, Bauchner H, Frank D, Vinci R, Cabral H 1990 Jitteriness in full term neonates: prevalence and correlates. Pediatrics 85: 17–23

73. Patrizi S, Holmes G L, Orzalesi M, Allemand F 2003 Neonatal seizures: characteristics of EEG ictal activity in preterm and fullterm infants. Brain and Development 25: 427–437

74. Perlman J M, Volpe J J 1989 Neurologic complications of captopril treatment of neonatal hypertension. Pediatrics 83: 47–52

75. Pressler R, Bady B, Binnie C D, Boylan G B, Connell J A 2003 Neurophysiology of the neonatal period. In: Binnie C B et al (eds) Clinical neurophysiology, vol. 2: EEG, paediatric neurophysiology, special techniques and applications, 2nd edn. Elsevier, London

76. Pryor D S, Don B, Macourt D C 1981 Fifth day fits: a syndrome of neonatal convulsions. Archives of Disease in Childhood 56: 753–758

77. Rennie J M, Chorley G, Boylan G B, Pressler R, Nguyen Y, Hooper R 2004 Non-expert use of the cerebral function monitor for neonatal seizure detection. Archives of Disease in Childhood 89: 37–40

78. Rett A, Tuebel R 1964 Neugeborenen Krampfe im Rohmen einer epileptisch belasten Familie. Wiener Klinische Wochenschrift 76: 609–613

79. Riviello J J J 2004 Drug therapy for neonatal seizures: part 1. Neoreviews 5: e215–e220

80. Ronen G M, Penney S 1995 The epidemiology of clinical neonatal seizures in Newfoundland, Canada: a five-year cohort. Annals of Neurology 38: 518–519

81. Ronen G M, Penney S, Andrews W 1999 The epidemiology of clinical neonatal seizures in Newfoundland: a population based study. Journal of Pediatrics 134: 71–75

82. Ronen G M, Rosales T O, Connolly M, Anderson V E, Leppert M 1993 Seizure characteristics in chromosome 20 benign familial neonatal convulsions. Neurology 43: 1355–1360

83. Saliba R M, Annegers J F, Waller D K, Tyson J E, Mizrahi E M 1999 Incidence of neonatal seizures in Harris County, Texas, 1992–1994. American Journal of Epidemiology 150: 763–769

84. Scher M S, Aso K, Beggarly M E, Hamid M Y, Steppe D A, Painter M J 1993 Electrographic seizures in preterm and full-term neonates: clinical correlates, associated brain lesions, and risk for neurologic sequelae. Pediatrics 91: 128–134

85. Scher M S, Hamid M Y, Steppe D A, Beggarly M E, Painter M J 1993 Ictal and interictal electrographic seizure durations in preterm and term neonates. Epilepsia 34: 284–288

86. Schewman D A 1990 What is a neonatal seizure? Problems in definition and quantification for investigative and clinical purposes. Journal of Clinical Neurophysiology 7: 315–368

87. Schmitt B, Steinmann B, Gitzelman R, Thun-Hohenstein L, Mascher H, Dumermuth G 1993 Non-ketotic hyperglycinaemia: clinical and electrical effects of dextromethorphan, an antagonist of the NMDA receptor. Neurology 43: 421–424

88. Sharief N, Goonasekera C 1994 Soft tissue injury associated with intravenous phenytoin in a neonate. Acta Paediatrica 83: 1218–1219

89. Sheth R D, Buckley D J, Gutierrez A R, Gingold M, Bodensteiner J B, Penney S 1996 Midazolam in the treatment of refractory neonatal seizures. Clinical Neuropharmacology 19: 165–170

90. Sheth R D, Hobbs G R, Mullett M 1999 Neonatal seizures: incidence, onset, and etiology by gestational age. Journal of Perinatology 19: 40–43

91. Shiang R, Ryan S G, Fielder T J et al 1995 Mutational analysis of familial and sporadic hyperekplexia. Annals of Neurology 38: 85–91

92. Stewart W A, Wood E P, Gordon K E, Camfield P R 2002 Successful treatment of severe infantile hyperekplexia with low dose clobazam. Journal of Child Neurology 17: 154–156

93. Temple C M, Dennis J, Carney R, Sharich J 1995 Neonatal seizures: long term outcome and cognitive development among normal survivors. Developmental Medicine and Child Neurology 37: 108–118

94. Tohier C, Roze J C, David A, Veccierini M F, Renaud P, Mouzard A 1991 Hyperexplexia or stiff baby syndrome. Archives of Disease in Childhood 66: 460–461

95. Van Zeben-van der Aa D M, Veerlove-Vanhorick S P, den Ouden A L, Brand R, Ruhy J H 1990 Neonatal seizures in very preterm and low birthweight infants: mortality and handicaps at two years in a nationwide cohort. Neuropediatrics 21: 62–65

96. Waisman D, Weintraub Z, Rotschild A, Bental Y 1999 Myoclonic movements in very low birthweight premature infants associated with midazolam intravenous bolus administration. Pediatrics 104: 579

97. Watanabe K, Miyazaki S, Hara K, Hakamanda A 1980 Behavioral state cycles, background EEGs and prognosis of newborn with perinatal hypoxia. Electroencephalography and Clinical Neurophysiology 49: 618–625

98. Watkins A, Szymonowicz W, Jin X, Yu V Y H 1988 Significance of seizures in very low birthweight infants. Developmental Medicine and Child Neurology 30: 162–169

99. Weiner S P, Painter M J, Geva D, Guthrie R D, Scher M S 1991 Neonatal seizures: electroclinical dissociation. Pediatric Neurology 7: 363–368

100. Williams C E, Gunn A, Gluckman P D 1991 Time course of intracellular oedema and epileptiform activity following prenatal cerebral ischaemia in sheep. Stroke 22: 516–521

101. Wirrell E C, Armstrong E A, Osman L D, Yager J Y 2001 Prolonged seizures exacerbate perinatal hypoxic-ischemic brain damage. Pediatric Research 50: 445–454

102. Young G B, Da Silva O P 2000 Effects of morphine on the electroencephalograms of neonates: a prospective, observational study. Clinical Neurophysiology 111: 1955–1960

103. Younkin D P, Delivoria-Papadopoulos M, Maris J, Donlon E, Clancy R, Chance B 1986 Cerebral metabolic effects of neonatal seizures measured with in vivo ^{31}P NMR spectroscopy. Annals of Neurology 20: 513–519

PART 3

Intracranial haemorrhage at term

Malcolm Levene

Introduction

Bleeding into the brain and related structures is a very common neonatal event and is most frequently recognised in premature infants. Intracranial haemorrhage (ICH) involving the term baby occurs less commonly than in the preterm, and the affected sites and pathogenesis of the bleeding are far more heterogeneous. The pattern of ICH in the term baby has changed over the last 40 years. Subdural haemorrhage (SDH) was a common cause of death following traumatic delivery, but its incidence has fallen with improved obstetric management. In recent years, SDH has again become more frequently recognised, mainly owing to improved imaging techniques, which allows identification of smaller (and sometimes asymptomatic) lesions.

ICH in the term infant may occur at many sites (Fig. 41.15). In addition, it is important to consider other forms of intracranial pathology which predispose to bleeding or haemorrhagic infarction and which may be mistaken for primary haemorrhage. In particular, infarction of a cerebral artery and venous sinus thrombosis are two important causes that need to be considered.

ICH detected by imaging studies in apparently healthy term infants is relatively common. Studies have reported an overall incidence of 3.1–5.5%.[24] A study of 1000 unselected low-risk apparently healthy asymptomatic term babies showed that ICH was present in 3.5%, and all were periventricular in origin.[24] Before discussing in detail the various sites of intracranial bleeding in mature infants, this chapter will initially review the presentation and investigation of ICH in this group of infants.

Presentation

ICH in the term neonate usually presents with neurological symptoms and signs, but these are often non-specific in that they do not point to a focal site of cerebral pathology. Signs may be very general and not point directly to the brain as the source of the problem, and in some cases, clues to the cause of the haemorrhage may be obtained by general examination.

Neurological signs

The major neurological feature of intracranial pathology is seizures. Seizures occur commonly and are a feature of many different

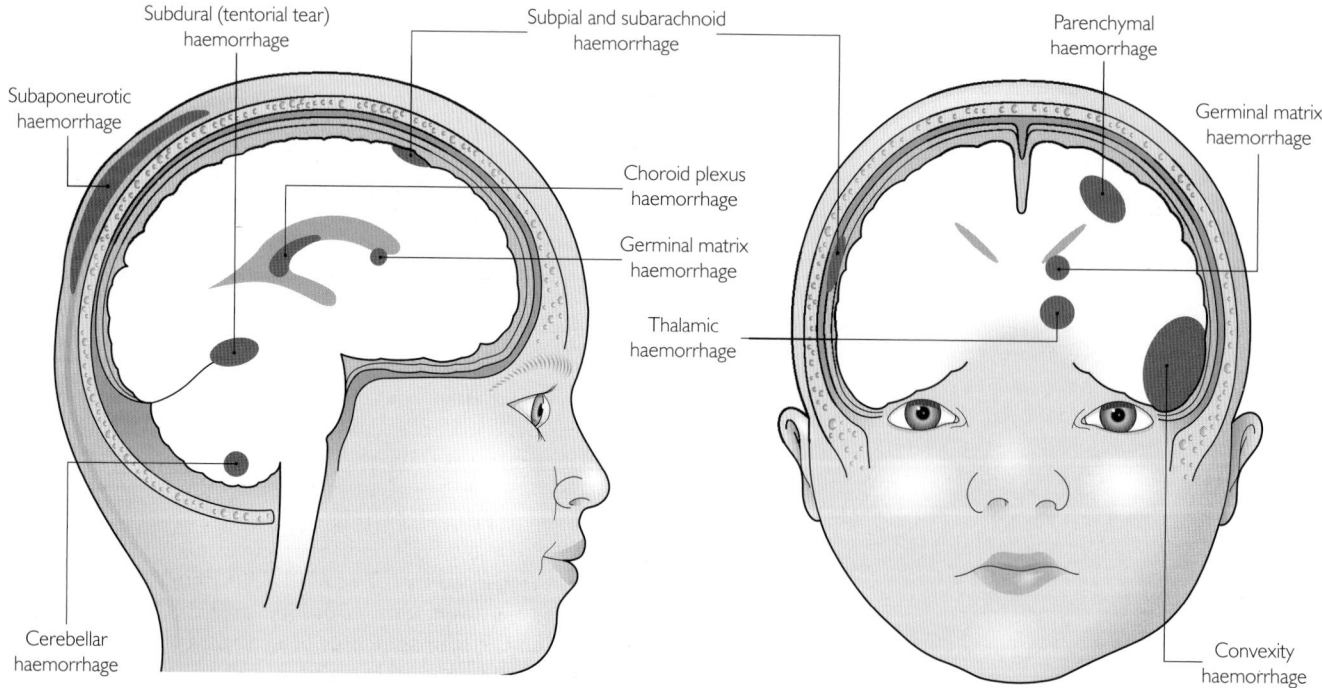

Fig. 41.15 Sites of intracranial haemorrhage.

forms of brain pathology (pp. 1105–19), but in the mature brain overt seizures occur as a result of ICH more frequently than in the premature infant.

A complicating factor in evaluating the significance of abnormal neurological signs is that they may be present as the result of underlying pathology that is the cause of the haemorrhage rather than the effect. Severe intrapartum asphyxia is an example of this sequence: the baby may develop seizures and other abnormal signs from shortly after birth and the development of ICH may not be considered because the abnormal signs are thought to be due to the more obvious pathology. Imaging must be carried out in all term babies with abnormal neurology. Ultrasound is a useful first-line investigation but is not as sensitive as magnetic resonance imaging (MRI), which should be considered if the cranial ultrasound scan is normal and no other obvious cause is found.

A common clinical course is for a baby to be born in good condition and show normal neurological behaviour for a number of days before developing an acute and major encephalopathic illness. This focuses the clinician's attention to the brain as the site of pathology, and appropriate imaging is likely to diagnose the precise cause if haemorrhage is present.

It is well recognised that 'silent' haemorrhages occur with little or no neurological abnormality. This is particularly common in premature infants with germinal matrix/intraventricular haemorrhage (GMH-IVH), but it is now well accepted to occur also in term infants with brain haemorrhage. This is usually the case with minor bleeding, particularly subarachnoid and small subdural haemorrhages.

Non-specific signs

Fever is relatively common with ICH. Meningitis must always be considered in a baby with fever and abnormal neurology, and lumbar puncture may reveal leukocytes and low cerebrospinal fluid (CSF) glucose levels, together with bloodstained CSF. This is a common finding following GMH-IVH and may make the distinction between meningitis and IVH very difficult.

Associated signs

Intracranial bleeding can occur as the result of a coagulopathy, and petechial or purpuric skin lesions may be widespread. Thrombocytopenia (pp. 760–1) or a congenital clotting factor abnormality (pp. 756–60) must be considered as the cause. Multiple cutaneous haemangiomata may rarely be associated with rupture of an intracranial haemangioma. A neurologically abnormal infant with extensive bruises also suggests the possibility of intracranial birth trauma, and this should be considered.

Investigations

Imaging is the most important method for confirming or excluding the diagnosis of ICH.

Ultrasound is widely used in neonatal intensive care units for brain imaging and is valuable in term neonates as a screening technique when ICH is suspected. However, its limitations must be recognised. It is very poor at diagnosing subarachnoid and/or subdural haemorrhages unless they are large. In addition, ultrasound may miss important associated pathology which predisposes to haemorrhage, such as cerebral artery infarction and venous sinus thrombosis.

I recommend that all infants in whom ICH is clinically suspected should undergo either computed tomography (CT) or MRI. MRI is the most versatile and sensitive imaging modality currently available. Pathology not detected on CT scan may be recognised on MRI, but the requirement for the infant to remain still is more critical than with CT. The decision as to whether to undertake CT or MRI depends on the type of pathology under consideration, the availability of techniques, and the local expertise and experience in interpreting the scans.

Intracranial haemorrhages

Subarachnoid haemorrhage

Bleeding into the subarachnoid space may be either primary or secondary. Primary subarachnoid haemorrhage (SAH) arises as the result of two separate mechanisms:

- rupture of veins bridging the subarachnoid space;
- rupture of vessels within the leptomeningeal plexus, which may represent ruptured subpial haemorrhage with consequent SAH.

Secondary SAH occurs as the result of haemorrhage from another site, usually intraventricular, draining into the subarachnoid space. SAH may also occur overlying an area of arterial infarction.

SAH is a very common finding at autopsy and does not necessarily indicate the presence of underlying brain injury. Many of these small lesions may actually represent subpial haemorrhages,[16] which are most commonly seen over the temporal or parietal lobes.[11,13] Larger lesions appear as a reddish-yellow layer of jelly-like consistency over the surface of the brain.[8] Large SAH is particularly likely in babies with coagulopathy.[6,16] Traumatic delivery has been reported to cause SAH in surviving infants.[47]

Diagnosis

Convulsions are the most common sign associated with SAH in the term infant and are usually present within the first 24 hours of life. Characteristically, the baby is said to be neurologically normal between seizures, but the larger the SAH, the more neurologically abnormal the baby is likely to be. Blood is always present in the subarachnoid fluid on lumbar puncture.

Diagnosis is made by CT or MRI. Ultrasound is an unreliable method for diagnosing this condition. A small SAH is most likely to appear on CT scan as an area of increased attenuation within the posterior interhemispheric fissure. It may be impossible to distinguish a large convexity SAH from SDH.

The prognosis for primary SAH is good unless there is massive convexity bleeding.

Convexity haemorrhage

In this condition, a large collection of clotted subarachnoid blood causes a convex space-occupying lesion, usually over the temporal or occipital region.[40] The convexity haemorrhage commonly causes compression of cortical and subcortical structures, with localised venous infarction adjacent to the lesion. Histologically it may be difficult to identify the origin of the bleeding, which in some cases has been reported to be subpial.[13]

Convexity haemorrhage is particularly associated with neonatal coagulopathy (see below), and Larroche[28] has reported its association with exchange transfusion. The lesion is usually well seen with ultrasound imaging (Fig. 41.16).

The prognosis for a large convexity haemorrhage is poor and is dependent on the degree of infarction of normal brain immediately adjacent to the lesion.

Subdural haemorrhage

Massive SDH causing death is now a rare occurrence; however, with the increased availability of modern imaging techniques, a second type of less severe SDH is recognised more frequently in surviving infants.

SDH arises as the result of three different mechanisms:

- rupture of bridging veins;
- tearing of the dural membranes owing to distorting forces;
- laceration of the dura from skull displacement (osteodiastasis); this latter variant is commonly associated with associated cerebellar haemorrhage (see below).

The cause of SDH is basically trauma to the head. This may be direct, which is now rare, or as a result of abnormal forces associated with instrumental delivery, particularly vacuum extraction.

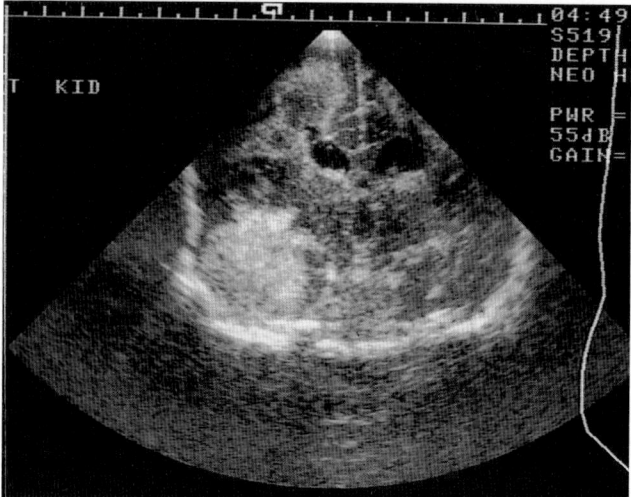

Fig. 41.16 Convexity haemorrhage. Ultrasound scan showing echodense haemorrhage in right temporal area.

The dura is a thick membrane which compartmentalises the brain. Folds of dura form the sagittally lying falx, which separates the two cerebral hemispheres. The posterior dural reflection forms the axially lying tentorium, which separates the cerebellum from the cerebral hemispheres. The venous sinuses lie within the folds of the dura and a tear to the dural membrane is likely to be associated with rupture of a venous sinus, causing extensive intradural and subdural haemorrhage. Bridging veins run from the dural membranes to the superior sagittal sinus, and these too may rupture, resulting in SDH.

SDHs occur equally frequently in the sub- or supraratentorial areas or may occur at multiple sites.[5] Blood may be visible either between the superior surface of the cerebellum and the tentorium or between the convexity of the cerebellar hemisphere and the occipital bone.[46] This type of SDH is often associated with severe hypoxic-ischaemic encephalopathy (HIE) and a tear of the tentorium.

Aetiology

Trauma is the underlying cause of SDH in almost all cases. Fetal SDH has been described as the result of direct trauma to the maternal abdomen at term.[29] The commonest cause of SDH is maldistribution of compressive forces on the head during delivery. If the head is distorted, excessive stress is applied to the tentorium and falx, causing a tear to the free edge of the tentorium (Fig. 41.17) with associated rupture of the vein of Galen or straight sinus. This is likely to occur as the result of prolonged labour, uncontrolled delivery of the fetal head where the compressive forces rapidly change, or to traction from forceps or vacuum extraction. SDH is increasingly being recognised as a complication

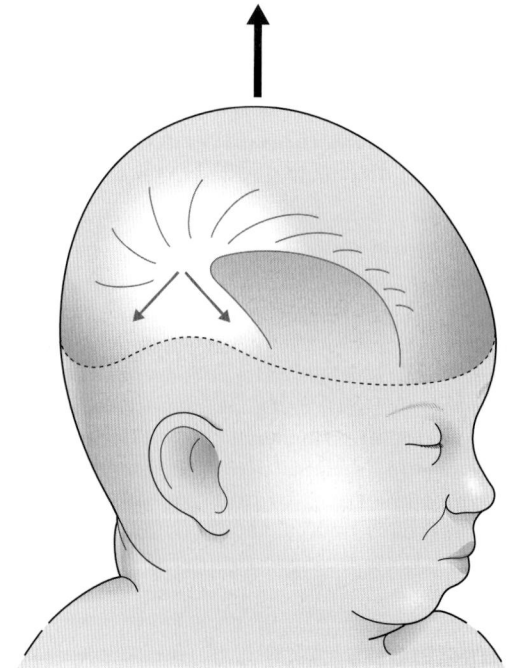

Fig. 41.17 Forces on the tentorium (small arrows) as the result of traction on the vertex, as occurs in vacuum extraction delivery (large arrow).

of vacuum extraction.[4,23] Elongation of the head by traction causes a particular strain on the apex of the tentorium, with rupture of bridging veins or venous sinuses. In one study, 10 unselected asymptomatic infants delivered by vacuum extraction showed evidence of intracranial bleeding, of which intradural or subdural haemorrhage was most common, although no baby appears to have sustained adverse neurodevelopmental outcome as a result.[1]

SDH is well recognised to occur in infants with severe HIE. Rebleeding up to 4 days after the first bleed has been described following primary non-fatal SDH.[8] The delayed bleed may occur as the result of restoration of blood pressure or as a result of falling intracranial pressure in the few days after the original bleed.[53] SDH may also occur secondary to maternal or fetal/neonatal coagulopathy.

Diagnosis

Govaert et al[17] reviewed 78 cases of SDH diagnosed during life. A recognisable symptom complex has been described, including tense fontanelle, hypotonia, lethargy with reduced primitive reflexes, and facial palsy. Symptoms related to posterior fossa injury include apnoea, irregular sighing respiration, fixed bradycardia, opisthotonos and skew deviation of the eyes. Seizures may not be prominent in subtentorial bleeding. In infants with smaller SDH, clinical signs may not become apparent until 12–14 hours after birth and are usually respiratory in nature.[5]

Imaging

SDHs are most reliably detected on CT or MRI scanning (Fig. 41.18). Autopsy studies have shown that a small intradural haemorrhage may be missed on CT.[32]

Management

Most children with SDH do not require active management of the haematoma. Review of reported cases suggests that there is some benefit to surgery,[17] but this may represent case selection

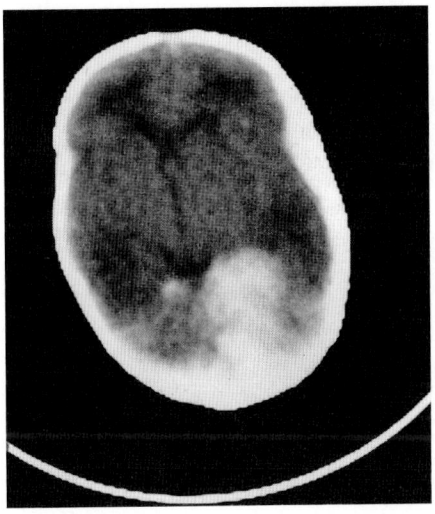

Fig. 41.18 CT scan of subdural haemorrhage associated with tentorial tear.

for surgery in that only those thought to have the best prognosis were operated on. Neurosurgical intervention depends on the size and position of the lesion and whether the baby shows clinical signs of brainstem compression (apnoea, severe bradycardia or hypotension) or obstruction to CSF outflow pathways.[41]

Complications

SDH can cause acute obstruction to the fourth ventricle, with impairment of CSF flow and brainstem compression. Infarction of the middle or posterior cerebral artery is a recognised complication following supratentorial SDH.[20] This occurs as the result of supratentorial subdural clot, with uncal herniation and occlusion of the ipsilateral posterior and middle cerebral artery. A convexity subdural or subarachnoid haemorrhage may cause obstruction to more peripheral branches of the middle cerebral artery.

Germinal matrix and intraventricular haemorrhage

GMH-IVH is a generic term which does not indicate the origin of the bleeding. In term babies, there are three major sites of origin:

- germinal matrix;
- choroid plexus;
- extension of an intraparenchymal haemorrhage.

In premature infants, the germinal matrix is the most likely origin of GMH-IVH, and this becomes progressively less common as the baby matures (Chapter 41, Part 5). GMH is well recognised to occur at term,[34,45] and is reported to occur in 2% of asymptomatic, unselected and apparently normal term infants.[24] Others have reported an incidence for symptomatic IVH of 0.036%.[27]

Haemorrhage from the choroid plexus is the commonest cause of large GMH-IVH in term infants, and was reported to occur in 1.1% of unselected healthy term infants.[24] Choroid plexus haemorrhage is discussed in detail below.

Rupture of an intraparenchymal haemorrhage (see below) into the ventricle is a relatively uncommon cause of GMH-IVH. These babies are usually symptomatic, with major signs of neurological disturbances. GMH-IVH has been reported in conjunction with deep venous thrombosis.[38] Massive GMH-IVH occurring prenatally in mature fetuses is well described[30] and may be associated with fetal or maternal coagulopathy.

GMH-IVH has also been reported to occur as the result of abdominal compression in a term infant[52] and following gentle aspiration of CSF from a ventricular reservoir in babies with hydrocephalus.[35] GMH-IVH is seen in infants who have survived extracorporeal membrane oxygenation (ECMO) treatment.[7,48]

Diagnosis

Small GMH-IVH may be asymptomatic. Larger haemorrhages present with severe neurological abnormalities, including convulsions, signs of raised intracranial pressure, and feeding difficulties. Hyperpyrexia has been reported as a frequent finding.[27,38] Diagnosis is suspected on the basis of abnormal neurological signs. Lumbar puncture reveals frankly bloodstained CSF.

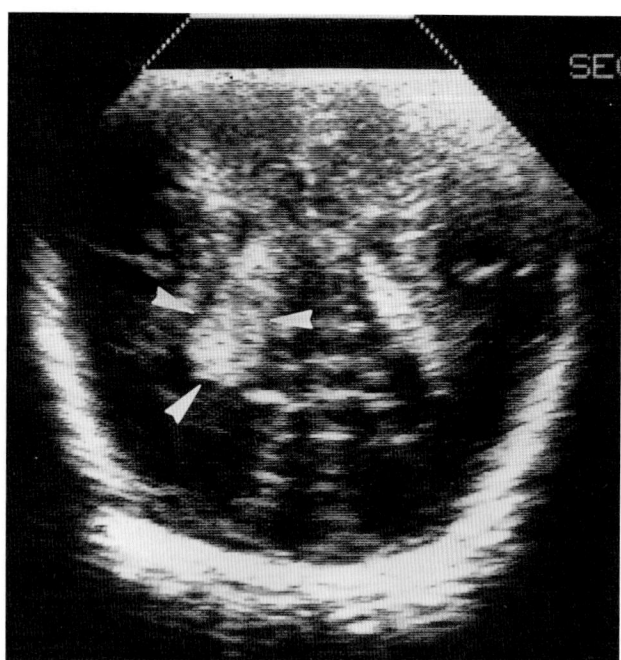

Fig. 41.19 Choroid plexus haemorrhage. Ultrasound scan showing echogenic clot adherent to one choroid plexus. (Reproduced from Spastics International Medical Publications.)

Prognosis

Jocelyn & Casiro[27] reported the outcome of 15 term infants with symptomatic GMH-IVH. One died, and of the survivors followed up for a mean age of 35 months, 36% had severe handicaps. They reported a correlation between severity of GMH-IVH and adverse outcome, but others have reported much better outcome even in babies with extensive GMH-IVH.[45] Posthaemorrhagic hydrocephalus is an important complication of GMH-IVH at term. The incidence of hydrocephalus requiring shunt placement is 35%.[27,45]

Choroid plexus haemorrhage

Haemorrhage from the veins of the choroid plexus is well described as a cause of IVH occurring in term neonates. The most frequent site of bleeding is into the posterior tufts at the level of the glomus. Choroid plexus haemorrhage was diagnosed by ultrasound in 1.1% of asymptomatic, non-selected term infants.[24]

Diagnosis is made by detection of thrombus adherent to the choroid plexus (Fig. 41.19). In infants with clot filling the major part of a lateral ventricle, it may not be possible to determine the origin of the bleed. The presence of IVH with no pathology in the germinal matrix is strongly suggestive of the choroid plexus as its site of origin. Clinical presentation is as for any cause of GMH-IVH.

Intraparenchymal lesions

Intraparenchymal lesions (IPLs) in the term infant represent a heterogeneous group of conditions. For a discussion of IPLs in preterm infants, see page 1149.

Table 41.6 Causes of intraparenchymal lesions at term

Coagulopathy
Trauma
Arterial infarction
Venous thrombosis
Hypoxia-ischaemia
Extracorporeal membrane oxygenation therapy
Arteriovenous malformation
Aneurysm
Tumour
Secondary thrombosis
    Protein C deficiency
    Protein S deficiency
    Factor V Leiden

Aetiology

Table 41.6 lists the causes of IPLs in term neonates. Birth trauma has been implicated as the cause for supratentorial intraparenchymal haemorrhage[47] and intrapartum asphyxia causes haemorrhage within both grey (the thalamic nuclei are particularly vulnerable) and white matter,[10] although this may represent bleeding into a previously infarcted area. In some cases it may be difficult to distinguish primary haemorrhage from haemorrhagic infarction. The distribution of the lesion may be the best clue to whether thrombosis was the primary cause (see below).

Infarction

Infarction may be either arterial or venous. The haemorrhage may be multifocal, which is suggestive of intrapartum asphyxia, an underlying coagulopathy or, rarely, an embolic cause. Arterial infarcts occur most commonly in the middle cerebral artery and may be due to a thrombophilic disorder (pp. 756–60). Infarction at multiple arterial sites may occur involving both intra- and extracranial vessels.

Increasingly recognised is haemorrhage secondary to venous infarction. Govaert and colleagues have described two different patterns of infarction involving neonatal venous drainage.[18,19] Seven infants (term and preterm) were identified with a unilateral focal haemorrhagic lesion in the region of the temporal lobe (Fig. 41.20), thought to be due to venous thrombosis in the region drained by the inferior ventricular vein.[18] In another case, bilateral haemorrhage in the temporal and parieto-occipital region was thought to be due to thrombosis in the basal veins of Rosenthal, which drain into the vein of Galen.[19] Sinus thrombosis is an important, but often unrecognised, cause of parenchymal haemorrhage.[2]

Coagulopathy

Coagulopathy due to clotting factor abnormality, α_1-antitrypsin deficiency or vitamin K deficiency is one of the most common causes of IPL at term. Rarely, spontaneous haemorrhage may occur as a result of thrombolytic therapy used in the neonatal period.[56]

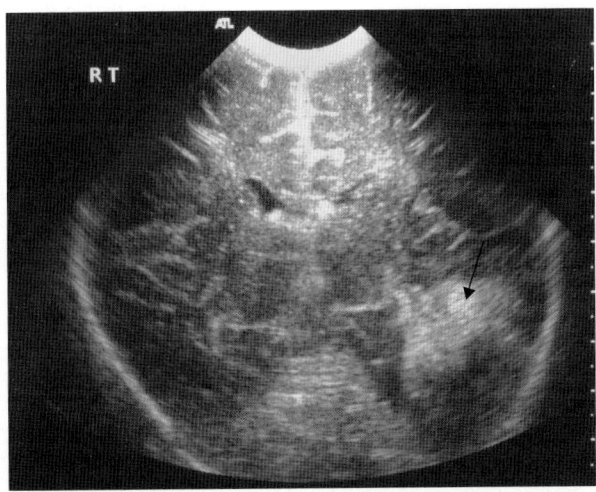

Fig. 41.20 Focal haemorrhage in the left temporal lobe (arrowed).

ECMO

IPL is a well-recognised complication of ECMO. This may be due to the underlying cardiorespiratory instability for which ECMO was given, anticoagulation necessary during the course of ECMO, or ischaemia induced by impairment of carotid artery blood flow. All forms of ICH are common in babies requiring ECMO, and intraparenchymal haemorrhage has been reported in 3–18%.[7,22,48] Sinus thrombosis is reported to be an important sequela of ECMO[55] and this may predispose to IPL. Sepsis as the primary indication for ECMO is a particular risk factor for ICH[3] and IPL occurred within 48 hours of the start of ECMO in 75% of cases.[3]

Structural anomalies

Arterial aneurysm,[33] arteriovenous malformation[51] and tumours[49] are rare causes of IPL at term.

Diagnosis

The baby usually shows acute onset of neurological signs at 1–5 days of age after a period of apparent normality. At presentation the baby is usually severely neurologically abnormal, but convulsions are not always a major feature of the clinical course. Focal signs rarely occur but if present may give a clue to the site of the lesion.

Investigations

The diagnosis may be suspected on ultrasound examination, but CT or MRI is much more reliable in accurately defining the position and possible aetiology of the lesion. If an aneurysm or venous thrombosis is suspected to be the underlying cause, magnetic resonance angiography is the investigation of choice; carotid or vertebral angiograms should be avoided. Repeated imaging in the weeks after the acute insult usually shows resolution of the lesion to a porencephalic cavity in the majority of cases.

Prognosis

This depends on the underlying cause of the lesion. It is reported that approximately one-third of infants die, one-third are handicapped and one-third are subsequently neurologically normal.

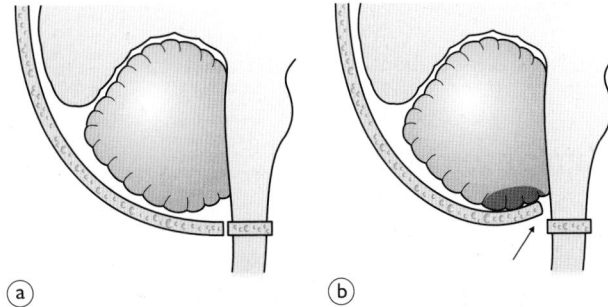

Fig. 41.21 Occipital diastasis. (a) Normal. (b) Diastasis with the occipital bone subluxing into the cerebellum.

Cerebellar haemorrhage

Bleeding into the posterior fossa is a well-recognised complication of breech delivery in a term infant. Haemorrhage may be due to subdural rupture, with bleeding from the venous sinus or from haemorrhage within the cerebellum. It is not uncommon for both types of bleeding to occur together. Although not all causes of cerebellar haemorrhages in term infants are related to trauma, this accounts for the majority of cases.

Cerebellar haemorrhage occurs as the result of:

- germinal matrix bleeding from the roof of the fourth ventricle;
- trauma to the cerebellum, of which occipital osteodiastasis with breech delivery is the most common cause.

As well as the cerebellar germinal matrix adjacent to the fourth ventricle, there is an area of poorly formed vascular tissue just below the pial layer of the cerebellum. These vessels are easily damaged, with ensuing haemorrhage into the cerebellar cortex. This appears to occur in both premature and term infants, but is not usually severe.

More severe bleeding into the cerebellum occurs as the result of trauma, usually sustained during breech delivery (Fig. 41.21). Overextension of the neck during delivery causes separation of the squamous and lateral portions of the occipital bone, with direct trauma to the cerebellum.[54] This is termed occipital osteodiastasis and is commonly associated with subdural tears.

A tight-fitting band around the head to maintain the position of a facemask has also been implicated in occipital diastasis with cerebellar infarction or haemorrhage.[39]

Diagnosis

Seizures are a less frequent presenting sign associated with cerebellar haemorrhage. The baby is usually lethargic, has episodes of apnoea or irregular ventilation, and bradycardia. He does not suck well and may show signs of raised intracranial pressure. Nystagmus and facial nerve palsy may be seen on examination.

Management

The role of craniotomy and evacuation of the clot is not certain (see Management of subdural haemorrhage). Successful conservative management of cerebellar haematomas has been described.[12]

Prognosis

There is little known about the long-term outcome.

Thalamic haemorrhage

This is now a well-recognised form of haemorrhage in the term baby.[9,44,50] Extension into the thalamus from GMH-IVH in the premature infant is a different condition (pp. 1150–9). It is almost always unilateral and must be distinguished from bilaterally bright basal ganglia, which are seen in severely asphyxiated infants (Chapter 41, Part 4). These babies are severely neurologically abnormal from birth, whereas primary thalamic haemorrhage arises de novo in an otherwise normal infant.

The cause of thalamic haemorrhage is unknown in most cases, but, rarely, haemorrhagic infarction, meningitis, coagulation disorders and sinus thrombosis have been associated factors.

Diagnosis

The baby is usually normal at birth and causes no concern until the development of dramatic and severe neurological abnormality 2–14 days later. This not uncommonly occurs after discharge from hospital. A particular feature of the neurological presentation is dramatic ocular signs, with sunsetting and eye deviation downward and outwards to the side of the thalamic lesion.[50] The abnormal eye posture is due to proximity of the haemorrhagic lesion to the frontomesencephalic pathway of the optic tract.

The haemorrhage is easily recognised on ultrasound imaging as well as on CT and MRI. Evidence of associated venous thrombosis has been reported on CT[44] and MRI.[15] A vascular malformation causing the haemorrhage is very rare, and if MRI does not suggest such a lesion, further invasive procedures are not warranted.

Prognosis

Initial reports of outcome were optimistic but this has not been borne out on longer-term follow-up. Roland et al[44] reported that less than 29% of term babies with primary thalamic haemorrhage were normal at follow-up. Cerebral palsy is a common sequel, but is often not severe. Cognitive deficit is common and may be severe. A particular form of epilepsy (continuous spike-wave during sleep) has been described.[36]

Subaponeurotic (subgaleal) haemorrhage

Bleeding into the loose connective tissue below the aponeurotic membrane is referred to as subaponeurotic or subgaleal haemorrhage. It is not an intracranial form of bleeding, but may be life threatening and deserves consideration here. A considerable volume of blood may be extravasated into this potential space before the extent of the bleeding has been realised, leading to hypovolaemia and possibly death.

The overall incidence of subaponeurotic haemorrhage is approximately 1:1250 deliveries,[37] but is particularly common following

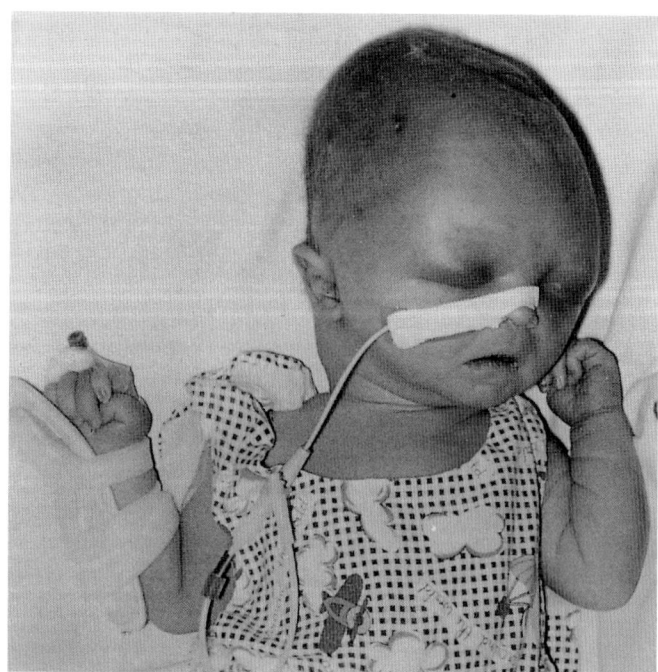

Fig. 41.22 Massive scalp enlargement caused by subaponeurotic haemorrhage.

vacuum extraction, with an incidence of 1:150.[37] It may be due to vitamin K deficiency and appears to be more common in babies of Afro-Caribbean descent.

Diagnosis

A history of fetal distress is noted in half of cases, and the infant may show abnormal neurological signs secondary to shock. This may make the distinction between fetal distress and bleeding as the primary cause of the encephalopathy a difficult clinical problem. A large volume of blood may extravasate into the subaponeurotic space before signs of haemorrhage are obvious. The first indication of abnormality may be anaemia, a rapid drop in haematocrit, or shock. The head size increases rapidly and may become enormous owing to the accumulation of blood (Fig. 41.22). The soft-tissue swelling crosses suture lines. Each centimetre enlargement has been said to correspond to a blood loss of 40 ml.

Management

Rapid diagnosis and blood replacement is the key to management, which may need to be directed towards supporting organs such as the kidneys and brain if shock has occurred.

Prognosis

Mortality from subaponeurotic haemorrhage is reported to be 17–25%.[21,37,42] In general, the prognosis for neurodevelopmental outcome in the survivors is good, providing there is no associated HIE.

Cerebral sinus and venous thrombosis

Thrombosis of the cerebral veins or sinuses is rarely diagnosed in life, but probably occurs more frequently than initially thought. It may occur in association with ICH or be mistaken for haemorrhage on imaging of the brain.

Thrombosis of the cerebral veins may occur spontaneously, but has been found in association with sepsis, trauma to the skull and underlying structures, dehydration with reduction in venous flow, and thrombophilic disorders. A recent study of eight neonates with this condition reported a high incidence of maternal pre-eclampsia.[26] ECMO and congenital heart disease have been recognised as additional risk factors.[55]

Diagnosis

There are no specific neurological signs that suggest neonatal cerebral venous thrombosis, but it should be suspected in infants with dehydration or those with pre-existing neurological disease if exacerbation of neurological features occurs. General signs include features of intracranial hypertension, convulsions, hypertonia and opisthotonus. Unexplained lethargy has been reported to be a consistent feature.[43]

Cerebral ultrasound and colour flow Doppler do not appear to offer diagnostic benefit. CT and MRI are the only methods for diagnosing this condition in life. On CT, the diagnosis is suspected by increased density of the vein of Galen and straight sinus or a high-density thrombus in a cerebral cortical vein. CT enhancement and MRI may reveal specific abnormalities.[31]

Management

Few case reports exist on the management of sinus thrombosis with urokinase.[14,25] The role of thrombolysis in this condition is uncertain, but may be appropriate in symptomatic cases.

Prognosis

Good follow-up data from survivors are scant, but the general view is that outcome is favourable. A recent report, however, suggests a more guarded prognosis, with adverse neurodevelopmental outcome in the majority of survivors.[26]

References

1. Avrahami E, Frishman E, Minz M 1993 CT demonstration of intracranial haemorrhage in term newborn following vacuum extractor delivery. Neuroradiology 35: 107–108
2. Bergman I, Bauer R E, Barmada M A et al 1985 Intracerebral hemorrhage in the full term neonatal infant. Pediatrics 75: 488–496
3. Biehl D A, Stewart D L, Forti N H et al 1996 Timing of intracranial hemorrhage during extracorporeal life support. ASAIO Journal 42: 938–941
4. Castillo M, Fordham L A 1995 MR of neurologically symptomatic newborns after vacuum extraction delivery. American Journal of Neuroradiology 16: 816–818
5. Chamnanvanakij S, Rollins N, Perlman J M 2002 Subdural hematoma in term infants. Pediatric Neurology 26: 301–304
6. Chaou W-T, Chou M-L, Eitzman D V 1984 Intracranial hemorrhage and vitamin K deficiency in early infancy. Journal of Pediatrics 105: 880–884
7. Cilley R E, Zwischernburger J B, Andrews A F, Bowerman R A, Roloff D W, Bartlett R H 1986 Intracranial haemorrhage during extracorporeal membrane oxygenation in neonates. Pediatrics 78: 699–704
8. Craig W S 1938 Intracranial haemorrhage in the newborn. Archives of Disease in Childhood 13: 89–124
9. De Vries L S, Smet M, Goemans N, Wilms G, Devlieger H, Caesar P 1992 Unilateral thalamic haemorrhage in the pre-term and full-term newborn. Neuropediatrics 23: 153–156
10. Eken P, Jansen G H, Groenendaal F, Rademaker K J, de Vries L S 1994 Intracranial lesions in the full-term infant with hypoxic ischaemic encephalopathy: ultrasound and autopsy correlation. Neuropediatrics 25: 301–307
11. Fenichel G M, Webster D L, Wong W K T 1984 Intracranial hemorrhage in the term newborn. Archives of Neurology 41: 30–34
12. Fishman M A, Percy A K, Cheek W R, Speer M E 1981 Successful conservative management of cerebellar hematomas in term neonates. Journal of Pediatrics 98: 466–468
13. Freide R L 1972 Subpial hemorrhage in infants. Journal of Neuropathology and Experimental Neurology 31: 548–556
14. Gebara B M, Goetting M G, Wang A-M 1995 Dural sinus thrombosis complicating subclavian vein catheterisation: treatment with local thrombolysis. Pediatrics 95: 138–140
15. Govaert P, Acten E, Vanhaesebrouck, P de Praeter C, van Damme J 1992 Deep cerebral venous thrombosis in thalamo-ventricular hemorrhage of the term newborn. Pediatric Radiology 22: 123–127
16. Govaert P, Bridger J, Wigglesworth J 1995 Nature of the brain lesion in fetal allo-immune thrombocytopenia. Developmental Medicine and Child Neurology 37: 485–495
17. Govaert P, Calliauw L, Vanhaesebrouck P, Martens F, Barrilari A 1990 On the management of neonatal tentorial damage. Eight case reports and a review of the literature. Acta Neurochirurgica 106: 52–64
18. Govaert P, Smets K, Matthys E et al 1999 Neonatal focal temporal lobe or atrial wall haemorrhagic infarction. Archives of Disease in Childhood. Fetal and Neonatal Edition 81: F211–F216
19. Govaert P, Swarte R, Oostra A et al 2001 Neonatal infarction within basal cerebral vein territory. Development Medicine and Child Neurology 43: 559–562
20. Govaert P, Vanhaesebrock P, de Praeter C 1992 Traumatic neonatal intracranial bleeding and stroke. Archives of Disease in Childhood 67: 840–845
21. Govaert P, Vanhaesebrock P, de Praeter C, Moens K, Leroy J 1992 Vacuum extraction, bone injury and neonatal subgaleal bleeding. European Journal of Pediatrics 151: 532–535
22. Grayck E N, Meliones N J, Kern F H, Hansell D R, Ungerleider R M, Greeley W J 1995 Elevated serum lactate correlates with intracranial hemorrhage in neonates treated with extracorporeal life support. Pediatrics 96: 914–917
23. Hanigan W C, Morgan A M, Stahlberg L K, Hiller J L 1990 Tentorial hemorrhage associated with vacuum extraction. Pediatrics 85: 534–539
24. Heibel M, Heber R, Bechinger D, Kornhuber H H 1993 Early diagnosis of perinatal cerebral lesions in apparently normal full-term newborns by ultrasound of the brain. Neuroradiology 35: 85–91
25. Higashida R T, Helmer E, Helbach V V 1989 Direct thrombolytic therapy for superior sagittal sinus thrombosis. American Journal of Neuroradiology 10: 54–56
26. Hunt R W, Badawi N, Laing S et al 2001 Pre-eclampsia: a predisposing factor for neonatal venous sinus thrombosis? Pediatric Neurology 25: 242–246
27. Jocelyn L J, Casiro O G 1992 Neurodevelopmental outcome of term infants with intraventricular hemorrhage. American Journal of Diseases of Children 146: 194–197
28. Larroche J-C 1977 Developmental pathology in the neonate. Excerpta Medica, Amsterdam
29. Larroche J-C 1986 Fetal encephalopathies of circulatory origin. Biology of the Neonate 50: 61–74
30. Larroche J-C 1995 Fetal cerebral pathology of circulatory origin. In: Levene M I, Lilford R J, Bennett M J, Punt J (eds) Fetal and neonatal neurology and neurosurgery, 2nd edn. Churchill Livingstone, Edinburgh, pp. 321–331
31. Levene M I, de Vries L S 1995 Neonatal intracranial haemorrhage. In: Levene M I, Lilford R J, Bennett M J, Punt J (eds) Fetal and neonatal neurology and neurosurgery, 2nd edn. Churchill Livingstone, Edinburgh, pp. 335–359
32. Ludwig B, Brand M, Brockerhoff P 1980 Postpartum CT examination of the heads of full term infants. Neuroradiology 20: 145–154
33. McLellan N J, Prasad R, Punt J 1986 Spontaneous subhyaloid and retinal haemorrhages in an infant. Archives of Disease in Childhood 61: 1130–1132

34. Mitchell W, Tuama L 1980 Cerebral intraventricular hemorrhages in infants: a widening age spectrum. Pediatrics 65: 35–39
35. Moghal N E, Quinn M W, Levene M I, Puntis J W L 1992 Intraventricular haemorrhage after aspiration of ventricular reservoirs. Archives of Disease in Childhood 67: 448–449
36. Monteiro J P, Roulet-Perez E, Davidoff V et al 2001 Primary neonatal thalamic haemorrhage and epilepsy with continuous spike-wave during sleep: a longitudinal follow-up of a possible significant relation. European Journal of Paediatric Neurology 5: 41–47
37. Ng P C, Siu Y K, Lewindon P J 1995 Subaponeurotic haemorrhage in the 1990s: a 3-year surveillance. Acta Paediatrica 84: 1065–1069
38. Palma P A, Miner M E, Morriss F H, Adcock E W, Denson S E 1979 Intraventricular hemorrhage in the neonate born at term. American Journal of Diseases of Children 133: 941–944
39. Pape K E, Armstrong D L, Fitzhardinge P M 1976 Central nervous system pathology associated with mask ventilation in the very low birthweight infant: a new etiology for intracerebellar hemorrhage. Pediatrics 58: 473–483
40. Pape K E, Wigglesworth J S 1979 Haemorrhage, ischaemia and the perinatal brain. Clinics in Developmental Medicine 69/70, London
41. Perrin R G, Rutka J T, Drake J M et al 1997 Management and outcomes of posterior fossa subdural hematomas in neonates. Neurosurgery 40: 1190–1200
42. Plauche W C 1980 Subgaleal hematoma. A complication of instrumental delivery. Journal of the American Medical Association 244: 1597–1598
43. Rivkin M J, Anderson M L, Kaye E M 1992 Neonatal idiopathic cerebral venous thrombosis: an unrecognised cause of transient seizures or lethargy. Annals of Neurology 32: 51–56
44. Roland E H, Flodmark O F, Hill A 1990 Thalamic hemorrhage with intraventricular hemorrhage in the full-term newborn. Pediatrics 85: 737–742
45. Scher M S, Wright F S, Lockman L A, Thompson T R 1982 Intraventricular hemorrhage in the full-term neonate. Archives of Neurology 39: 769–772
46. Scotti G, Flodmark O, Harwood-Nash D C, Humphries R P 1981 Posterior fossa hemorrhages in the newborn. Journal of Computer Assisted Tomography 5: 68–72
47. Strand R 1986 Traumatic parturitional intracranial haemorrhage. Developmental Medicine and Child Neurology 28: 156–164
48. Taylor G A, Fitz C R, Glass P, Short B L 1989 CT of cerebrovascular injury after neonatal extracorporeal membrane oxygenation: implications for neurodevelopmental outcome. American Journal of Roentgenology 153: 121–126
49. Tekkok I H, Ventureyra E C 1997 Spontaneous intracranial hemorrhage of structural origin during the first year of life. Child's Nervous System 13: 154–165
50. Trounce J Q, Dodd K L, Fawer C-L, Fielder A R, Punt J, Levene M I 1985 Primary thalamic haemorrhage in the newborn: a new clinical entity. Lancet i: 190–192
51. Wakai S, Andoh Y, Ngai M, Teremoto C, Tanaka G 1990 Choroid plexus arteriovenous malformation in a full-term neonate. Journal of Neurosurgery 72: 127–129
52. Wehberg K, Vincent M, Garrison B, Dilustro J F, Frank L M 1992 Intraventricular hemorrhage in the full-term neonate associated with abdominal compression. Pediatrics 89: 327–329
53. Welch K 1980 The intracranial pressure in infants. Journal of Neurosurgery 52: 693–699
54. Wigglesworth J S, Husemeyer R P 1977 Intracranial birth trauma in vaginal breech delivery: the continued importance of injury to the occipital bone. British Journal of Obstetrics and Gynaecology 84: 684–691
55. Wu Y W, Miller S P, Chin K et al 2002 Multiple risk factors in neonatal sinovenous thrombosis. Neurology 59: 438–440
56. Zenz W, Arlt F, Sodia S et al 1997 Intracerebral hemorrhage during fibrinolytic therapy in children: a review of the literature of the last thirty years. Seminars in Thrombosis and Hemostasis 23: 321–332

PART 4

Hypoxic–ischaemic brain injury

Malcolm Levene, David J Evans

Introduction

Definition

Understanding of hypoxic–ischaemic injury is handicapped by the lack of a generally accepted definition. The term asphyxia is defined as impairment of placental or pulmonary gas exchange resulting in hypoxaemia, hypercapnia and a mixed respiratory and metabolic acidosis. The essence of this is the simultaneous occurrence of hypoxia and ischaemia and the term hypoxic–ischaemic insult is now preferred. This may lead to injury to a variety of organ systems as a result of the hypoxic–ischaemic process.

Hypoxic–ischaemic injury may occur acutely or chronically and is most commonly due to impairment of placental blood flow associated with maternal factors (hypotension, severe hypoxia), cord factors (prolapse, occlusion) or placental factors (insufficiency, abruption). Hypoxic–ischaemic insult may occur less frequently as the result of neonatal events such as severe respiratory disease, shock and cardiac arrest.

There has been considerable debate regarding the contribution that hypoxia–ischaemia at birth contributes to the totality of brain injury. It has been suggested that the brain may have been significantly impaired by events during pregnancy and birth asphyxia is just the final insult making a relatively small contribution to the burden of damage. Cowan and colleagues[29] have recently shown in a magnetic resonance imaging and autopsy study that 80% of babies with neonatal encephalopathy showed only evidence of an acute lesion without evident earlier pathology.

The variable cause of the insult, the uncertainty of its duration and the distribution of injury to different organs varies widely and consequently there is no clinical entity for the effects of hypoxic–ischaemic insult. Each case must be carefully evaluated for each of these features and management directed towards the affected organs.

Incidence

Throughout the world intrapartum hypoxic–ischaemic insults remain an important cause of perinatally acquired brain injury in

Table 41.7 Incidence of neonatal encephalopathy and death or severe neurological impairment following intrapartum hypoxia–ischaemia

Place	Year	Total births	Criteria	Incidence per 1000 live births		Ref.
				Intrapartum hypoxia–ischaemia	Death and/or severe neurological disability	
Edinburgh, Scotland	1969–73	14 020	Encephalopathy	6.7	2.3	22
Edmonton, Canada	1974–78	20 155	Sarnat HIE	4.7	0.9	40
Leicester, England	1980–84	20 975	Levene HIE	6.0	1.1	66
Gothenburg, Sweden	1985–91	42 203	Apgar <7 at 5 min + HIE	1.8	0.5	129
Brussels, Belgium	1990s	10 065	Encephalopathy	5.9		143

full-term infants. The incidence varies depending upon the clinical definition used. Table 41.7 gives incidence figures from studies in term infants using neonatal encephalopathy as a main diagnostic criterion. The risk of death or severe neurological impairment following hypoxia–ischaemia is 0.5–1.0 per 1000 live births in this era of modern perinatal care, representing approximately up to 750 infants per year in the UK alone.

In developing countries intrapartum hypoxic–ischaemic injury appears to be more common, although studies in such countries often include preterm as well as full-term infants. Countries reporting high incidences include Kuwait[4] (9.4 per 1000), Malaysia[20] (18.7 per 1000), Nigeria[3] (26.5 per 1000, and 143 per 1000 in rural areas[38]), India[120] (New Delhi 59 per 1000) and Tanzania[58] (229 per 1000). Neonatal mortality in the first 24 hours following hypoxic–ischaemic injury in normal-birthweight infants was 18 per 1000 live births in the Tanzanian study.[58] Follow-up programmes are not well developed in these countries and the numbers of survivors with severe neurological impairment are unknown, but it is likely that hypoxic–ischaemic injury produces a huge burden of disability worldwide.

Having established that hypoxia–ischaemia is an important cause of death and disability, it is disappointing to note that the management of these infants is still largely empirical and until recently virtually no treatment regimen has been the subject of a randomised controlled trial.

Term versus preterm

It is unclear to what extent preterm babies can manifest similar clinical features following hypoxic–ischaemic injury compared to term babies. The immature central nervous system may respond differently to such insults, although clinical features of hypoxic–ischaemic encephalopathy have been described in an infant of 31 weeks' gestation.[90] Preterm infants are also at risk from additional insults outside the intrapartum period. Antenatal insults, including infection, may be more common than previously thought, and could be responsible for the onset of preterm labour. Postnatal problems such as respiratory illness, germinal matrix/intraventricular haemorrhage (GMH-IVH) and leukomalacia may cause further injury that leads to neurological morbidity. These additional insults can mask the significance of intrapartum hypoxia–ischaemia and can confound the study of preterm hypoxia–ischaemia. Therefore, the majority of information discussed in this chapter will refer to hypoxic–ischaemic injury in

the term infant, occurring most commonly as the result of an intrapartum insult.

Pathophysiology of hypoxia–ischaemia

As the intrauterine pressure exceeds 30 mmHg during contractions in active labour, the perfusion of the intervillous space is impaired, transiently interrupting placental gas exchange. This can be accommodated by the healthy fetoplacental unit, provided the contractions are of less than 60 seconds' duration, with sufficient respite (2–3 minutes) in between.[94]

Several additional stresses may occur; some represent acute hypoxic–ischaemic insults, others chronic or acute-on-chronic insults:

- interruption of the umbilical circulation (e.g. cord compression or cord prolapse);
- altered placental gas exchange (e.g. abruption, placental insufficiency);
- reduced maternal placental perfusion (e.g. maternal hypotension or hypertension);
- impaired maternal oxygenation;
- failure to establish adequate cardiopulmonary circulation after birth.

Fetal responses to hypoxia–ischaemia

The healthy fetus is able to use a variety of adaptive responses in order to help it overcome the hypoxic–ischaemic insult. These include:

- reduction in body movements, breathing movements and rapid eye movement sleep, thus reducing energy consumption and oxygen demand;
- increased oxygen extraction from the blood: the maternofetal circulation represents a high-output oxygen supply such that almost twice the amount of oxygen can be extracted by fetal haemoglobin before cardiac output needs to increase.[19] Erythropoietin concentrations are increased, stimulating fetal erythrocyte production;

- redistribution of blood supply to the central nervous system, myocardium and adrenals at the expense of the kidneys, gastrointestinal tract, liver and muscle;[25]
- within the brain, preferential oxygenation is maintained by diverting blood flow to the brainstem, midbrain and cerebellum;[99]
- sympathetic response: the high catecholamine levels seen during hypoxia–ischaemia increase peripheral vascular resistance and myocardial contractility in order to maintain perfusion, despite the fetal bradycardic response; the sympathetic stimulation also accelerates anaerobic glycolysis, with mobilisation of liver glycogen stores, thus maintaining the central nervous system (CNS) and myocardial energy substrate;
- the immature CNS can more readily utilise the lactate, pyruvate and ketones generated by anaerobic glycolysis as an alternative to glucose.[149] Babies with hyperinsulinaemia (e.g. those born to mothers with diabetes) are less able to generate these alternative energy sources and are therefore at greater risk from hypoxic–ischaemic injury.

Mechanisms of brain injury

The causes of neuronal death after a hypoxic–ischaemic insult are becoming gradually understood, although our knowledge to date is far from complete and further important information will emerge in this rapidly developing field. The earlier understanding of asphyxial brain insult was that the majority of neuronal death occurred during the hypoxic–ischaemic insult and, although clinical manifestations were noted to change after resuscitation, these changes were considered to be secondary to the effects of the insult and management might not influence outcome.

The modern view is that the majority of injury leading to neuronal death occurs after recovery from the initial hypoxic–ischaemic insult. The concept of at least two stages of neuronal compromise arising from numerous processes developing as the result a hypoxic–ischaemic insult has been formulated. These stages are summarised in Fig. 41.23.

Primary neuronal injury

During the hypoxic–ischaemic insult intracellular energy depletion occurs, and this has a major effect on cell membrane function. Ionic fluxes become deranged as a result of failure to gate neuroreceptors, with the effect of excess sodium, calcium and water entering the cell and leading to cytotoxic neuronal injury and primary neuronal death.[56] Although this mechanism is an important factor in neuronal death, it is now recognised that the majority of cell death occurs some hours, or even days, after resuscitation from the insult. The biochemical processes that influence this progression towards late cell death are referred to as secondary neuronal injury, and the major factors thought to be important in this process are described below. With increasing understanding of the pathways to neuronal death, strategies are now being developed to intervene and prevent neurons from dying.

Secondary neuronal injury

Reperfusion injury

Resuscitation after a hypoxic–ischaemic insult allows reperfusion and oxygenation of compromised tissues, with the initiation of a large number of abnormal biochemical processes. Immediately following resuscitation, a period of hyperperfusion of the brain will occur. This may be in response to accumulation of metabolites, including lactic acid and carbon dioxide, which causes vasodilatation.[57] Following this, vascular tone may increase with increasing reduction of cerebral blood flow, resulting in the so-called 'no reflow phenomenon'.[8] The cause of this phenomenon is not well understood but a number of factors are implicated, and mediated through injury to the vascular endothelial cell. Some of these mechanisms include the following.

Reactive oxygen metabolites (free radicals)

With reperfusion, reactive oxygen metabolites are produced, including oxygen free radicals and the more aggressive hydroxyl radicals, and these are generated by the action of the enzyme xanthine oxidase.[74] The vast majority of brain xanthine oxidase is derived from the endothelial cell. The generation of reactive oxygen metabolites further damage the arteriolar endothelium fuelling further generation of reactive oxygen metabolites (for review see Saugstad[113]).

It has been known for some time that, in animal experiments, where the organ is reperfused by blood-depleted in neutrophils there is a reduction in secondary hypoperfusion[35] and this may be mediated by cytokines expressed by neutrophils or microglia within the brain (see below). Intracellular adhesion molecule (ICAM)-1 and selectins are up-regulated as a result of hypoxic–ischaemic insult in the endothelial cell, which cause adherence of neutrophils to the vessel wall causing mechanical blockage to the vessel. These white cells migrate through the vessel wall and cause further reactive oxygen metabolites to be produced following activation by cytokines, with resultant damage to the neuron.

During ischaemic injury, platelet activating factor (PAF) is synthesised from the action of phospholipase A_2 on lipid membranes. PAF activates neutrophils, promotes platelet aggregation, increases vascular permeability resulting in vasogenic cerebral oedema and stimulates the release of vasoactive eicosanoids (thromboxanes, prostaglandins and leukotrienes).[151]

In summary, following an asphyxial insult blood flow is reduced to the brain as a result of a number of factors, including insult to the endothelial cell wall with resulting accumulation of white cells and platelets, which infiltrate into the cerebral interstitium, thereby setting off intracellular triggers which may further damage the cell. The clinical effect of this is to cause loss of cerebral autoregulation, reduction in cerebral blood flow and vasogenic oedema.

Intraneuronal compromise

Neuronal necrosis may occur as a result of a number of different processes which are currently being elucidated. These include:

Generation of reactive oxygen metabolites
As well as causing vascular damage these substances, generated as a result of endothelial damage in the extracellular space, attack the lipid components of the cell wall.

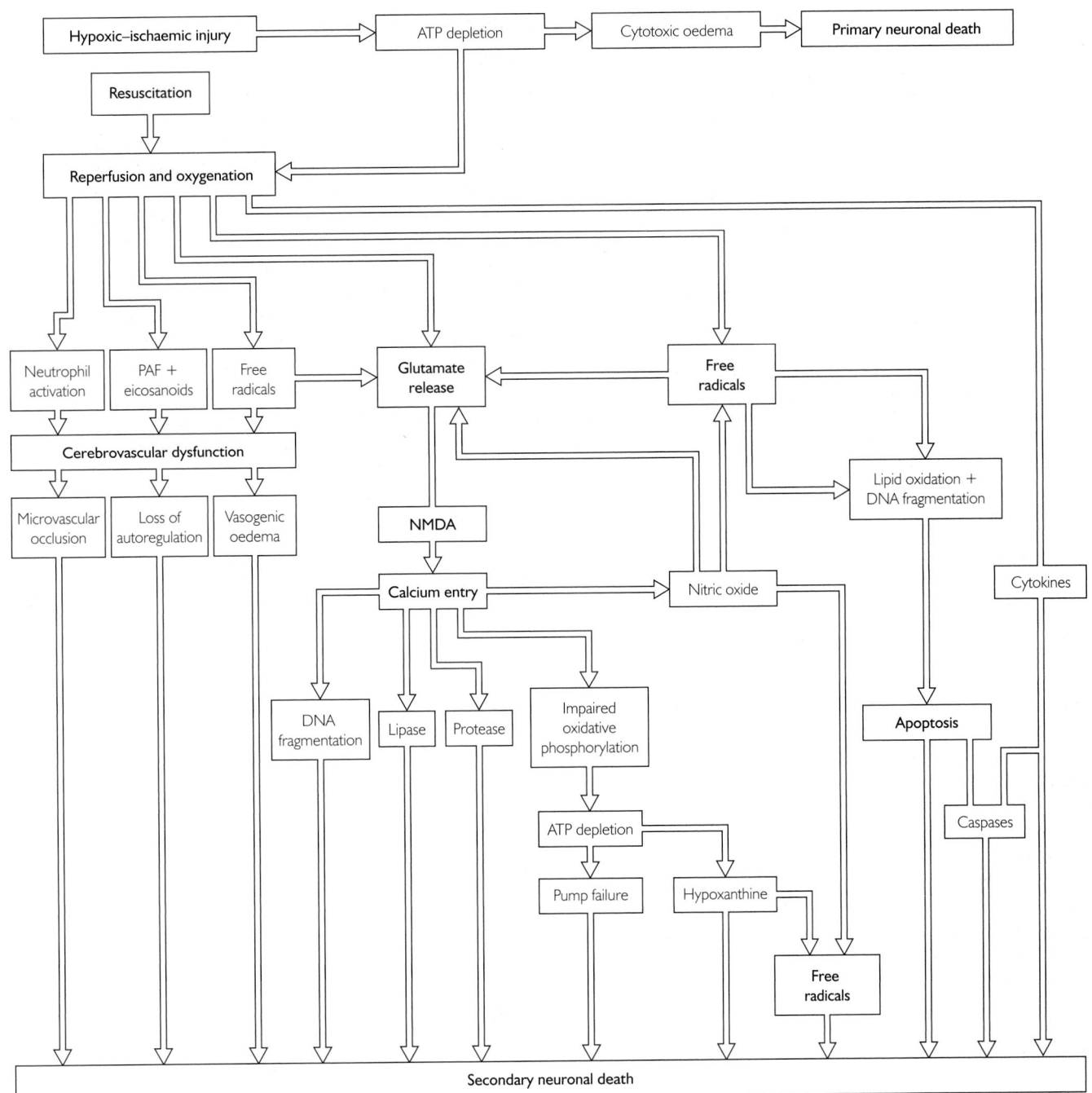

Fig. 41.23 Simplified schematic representation of the mechanisms involved in secondary neuronal injury following hypoxia–ischaemia.

Nitric oxide

Nitric oxide is generated in the cell as the result of stimulation of nitric oxide synthase (NOS). This has the effect of generating another reactive metabolite, peroxynitrite, causing lipid peroxidation of intracellular membranes with consequent loss of function. DNA degradation within the nucleus has also been described. Inhibition of NOS has given conflicting results in terms of reducing neuronal injury when given after the asphyxial event in animal models. In turn, DNA damage stimulates poly(ADP-ribose) polymerase (PARP), which further impairs mitochondrial regeneration of adenosine triphosphate, causing additional impairment to

membrane function. NO can diffuse through membranes and act as a retrograde messenger, further stimulating glutamate release.[61]

Excitotoxic injury

Hypoxic–ischaemic insult causes excessive release of the excitatory neurotransmitter glutamate. Glutamate acts on the N-methyl-D-aspartate (NMDA) receptor, a postsynaptic ion channel, permitting excessive calcium influx. An increase in intraneuronal calcium initiates activation of lipases, proteases, endonucleases and NOS. This generates further reactive oxygen metabolites, which may in turn increase glutamate release and exacerbate further entry of calcium into the cell, thereby setting up a vicious cycle culminating in neuronal necrosis.[71]

Certain regions of the brain appear to be particularly sensitive to NMDA-related injury, especially the basal ganglia and peri-rolandic cortex, which are particularly vulnerable in neonates following severe hypoxic–ischaemic insult. Elevated intramitochondrial calcium interfere with function of the structure and may stimulate further reactive oxygen metabolites to be produced.

Apoptosis

It is now recognised that neuronal death may occur as a result of necrosis, probably initiated through excessive calcium entry, or apoptosis in which the cell appears to initiate its own demise. Neuropathological studies can distinguish whether a cell dies as a result of necrosis or apoptosis.

Cell death following hypoxic–ischaemic insult is often due to both necrotic and apoptotic processes with interrelated pathogenesis. Necrosis is initiated by external factors, mitochondrial injury and disruption of the cell. Apoptosis is regulated by genetic factors with little loss of cellular membrane integrity, leading to contraction of the cells, which are subsequently consumed by macrophages. This is a highly conserved process with little inflammatory response. Neuronal apoptosis may be induced by genetic signals, including immediate early genes (e.g. c-*jun*, c-*fos*); other triggers of apoptosis include cytokines (tumour necrosis factor α) reactive oxygen metabolites and NO.

The final apoptotic signal, which causes cell death, appears to be the caspase mechanism. A variety of insults leading to disruption of the mitochondrial membrane active caspase-9, which in turn stimulates caspase-3. This undertakes cell execution to complete apoptosis.

Pathology

There is no single distinct or uniform pathological appearance of the brain following hypoxia–ischaemia. Cell death will occur when the metabolic demand fails to be met by substrate delivery via the blood. The pattern of injury depends upon the severity of asphyxial insult (total versus partial), its timing and duration (acute versus chronic), the developmental maturity of the brain and regional variations in vulnerability (due to local vascular factors, distribution of NMDA receptor etc.).

Observed patterns of injury following hypoxia–ischaemia

Cerebral oedema

Within 24–48 hours gross swelling of the cerebral tissue may occur, with marked flattening and widening of the gyri plus obliteration of the sulci, seen on imaging or at post mortem. It arises through two mechanisms: cytotoxic, when membrane pump failure leads to intracellular fluid accumulation, and vasogenic, when the impaired blood–brain barrier permits capillary leak and interstitial fluid accumulation.

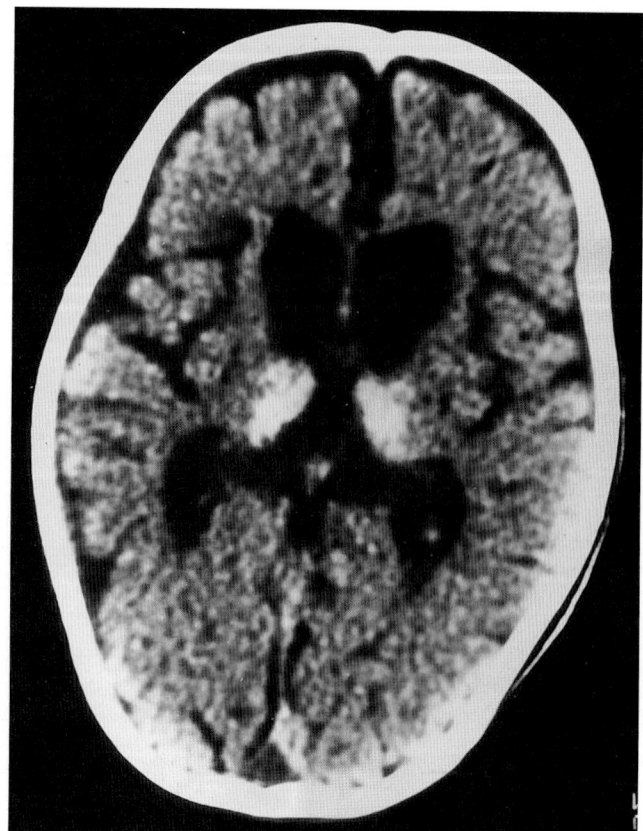

Fig. 41.24 CT scan of the brain of an asphyxiated neonate aged 18 months. Note the bilateral bright thalami and generalised cortical atrophy.

Selective neuronal necrosis

This is the most commonly observed pathology following hypoxia–ischaemia in term infants, affecting neurons in a scattered fashion and often widely distributed throughout the grey matter. The cerebral cortex layers III and IV and the hippocampus appear particularly vulnerable.[121] This may reflect differing metabolic rates of the various cortical structures.[60] Light-microscopy changes are apparent 24–36 hours following the insult, with cytoplasmic eosinophilia and nuclear fragmentation. Overt necrosis follows within a few days.

Basal ganglia and brainstem

In animal models this pattern of injury is seen following acute total asphyxia rather than chronic partial asphyxia.[82] Basal ganglion injury is thought to be responsible for the dyskinetic type of cerebral palsy seen in survivors of hypoxia–ischaemia, and abnormal signal intensity in the basal ganglia is a common finding on magnetic resonance imaging (MRI).[108] Within the first weeks, abnormal capillary proliferation and microcalcification can be seen on histology.[117] Abnormalities detected at this stage by ultrasound or computed tomography (CT) are thought to represent these pathological processes (Fig. 41.24).[137] If the infant survives for several months, an abnormal myelination pattern occurs that is detectable on MRI. This is responsible for the marble-like

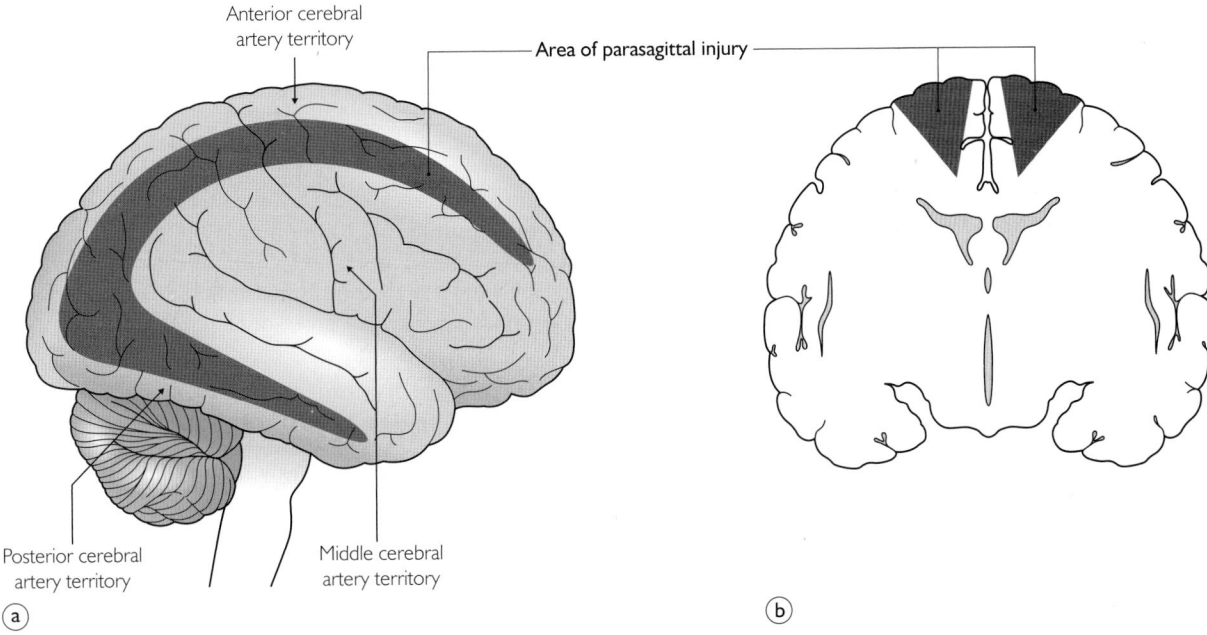

Fig. 41.25 Parasagittal injury. (a) Lateral view of the cerebral cortex. (b) Coronal section.

appearance of the basal ganglia seen at post mortem, known as status marmoratus.

Haemorrhage and haemorrhagic infarction affecting the thalami following hypoxia–ischaemia are also well recognised phenomena.

Parasagittal injury

This is an ischaemic injury affecting the cerebral cortex and subcortical white matter in vascular watersheds between the anterior, middle and posterior cerebral arteries, giving rise to a parasagittal distribution, and is often symmetrical (Fig. 41.25).[139]

White matter injury

Ischaemic insults in preterm infants produce periventricular leukomalacia. Periventricular glia are vulnerable to ischaemia in preterm infants. When ischaemic white matter injury occurs at term, it usually results in subcortical leukomalacia. The survivors of the most severe insults usually show a mixed pattern of injury, referred to as multicystic leukoencephalopathy (Fig. 41.26).

Focal cerebral infarction

Infarction of a major cerebral artery, most commonly the left middle cerebral artery, has in the past been reported in association with asphyxia,[141] but it is now realised that this lesion occurs much more commonly in infants with no evidence of intrapartum asphyxia (67%).[138] Further, thrombophilia screening is currently recommended in babies with a diagnosis of neonatal stroke, because a significant number will have disorders such as the factor V Leiden mutation. Early studies of stroke were reported before thrombophilia screening was available. For more information on thrombophilia screens see p. 762.

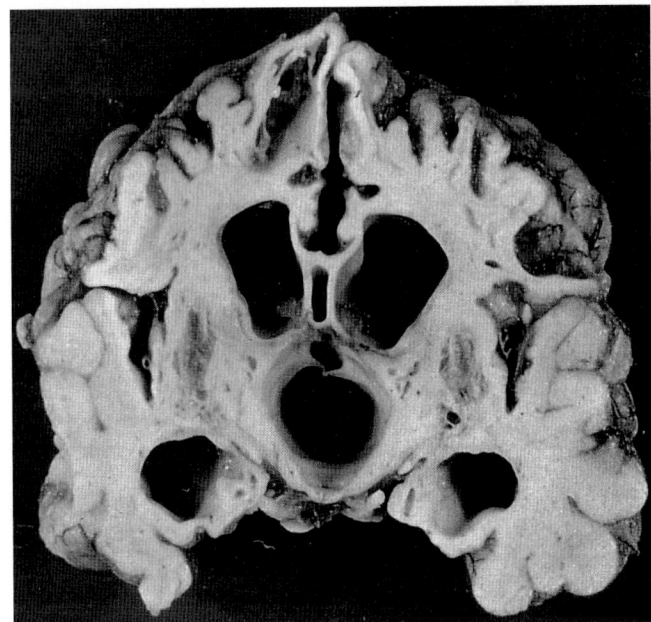

Fig. 41.26 Multicystic encephalopathy. Coronal section of a pathological specimen with areas of cystic degeneration throughout the periventricular white matter, subcortical white matter and basal ganglia. Also note the generalised cortical atrophy with ventricular enlargement.

Clinical definition: 'the asphyxia syndrome'

Despite the increasing knowledge of the pathophysiology of perinatal asphyxia, there is little agreement over its clinical definition.

This is reflected in the multitude of differing definitions used in studies of incidence, treatment and outcome. There are many clinical and biochemical features that are used as possible markers but, as with the definition of many other syndromes, no single feature alone should be taken as defining perinatal asphyxia. One problem in evaluating the relative importance of such features (or a combination of features) has been the lack of a 'gold standard' by which to weight their value. We cannot yet clinically define the nature, timing or severity of the asphyxial insult, and in many cases the observed outcome may not necessarily be a consequence of that insult. To diagnose 'asphyxia syndrome' it is necessary to ascertain positive features (Table 41.8), together with excluding alternative conditions that may mimic some of these features (Table 41.9).

Table 41.8 Evidence for intrapartum hypoxic–ischaemic injury causing cerebral palsy

Evidence for intrapartum asphyxia	Fetal distress
	Fetal acidosis
	Depressed Apgar scores
	Delayed onset of respiration
	Hypoxic–ischaemic encephalopathy
	Multiorgan involvement
Exclusion of alternative causes of neonatal encephalopathy (Table 41.9)	
Supporting evidence	Normal fetal brain growth until birth, followed by failure of normal brain growth
	Pattern of MRI abnormality suggestive of intrapartum hypoxia–ischaemia
Pattern of disability	Spastic quadriplegia
	Dyskinetic cerebral palsy

Table 41.9 Aetiology of early neonatal encephalopathy

Hypoxia–ischaemia	
Infection	Neonatal meningitis
Drug-related	Maternal anaesthesia /analgesia
	Maternal drug abuse
	Neonatal sedatives/anticonvulsants
CNS malformations	
Intracranial haemorrhage	
Metabolic	Hypoglycaemia
	Hyponatraemia /hypocalcaemia
	Bilirubin encephalopathy
	Amino acidaemias (e.g. non-ketotic hyperglycinaemia)
	Organic acidaemias
	Pyridoxine dependency
	Lactate acidaemias
	Urea cycle disorders

Fetal distress

The fetus is well adapted to cope with the physiological stress normally imposed by labour. The aim of intrapartum monitoring is to detect fetal 'distress' rather than 'stress', which is normal. If fetal distress is detected it cannot be assumed that the insult has occurred during labour. A fetus that has sustained a hypoxic–ischaemic insult before labour may not be able to mount the normal physiological coping responses during labour. Therefore, evidence of 'fetal distress' may in some cases be a marker of compromise prior to the onset of labour.

Intrapartum fetal monitoring

Electronic fetal monitoring

See pp. 203–7 for more information on cardiotocograph (CTG) interpretation.

In the 1970s electronic fetal monitoring (EFM) was introduced and it was assumed that more precise information about fetal heart rates would lead to improved outcomes.[146] Unfortunately, there is little evidence that this has resulted in a reduction of morbidity. Interpretation of the EFM trace has been variably applied and misinterpretation is reported to be the most frequently recorded clinical error associated with intrapartum death.[26] More recently, clinical guidelines have been published categorising features of the fetal heart rate (see Tables 12.1 and 12.2) to allow interpretation of the trace into normal, suspicious or pathological.[84] When considering the need to deliver the baby on the basis of an abnormal trace, it is recommended that fetal blood sampling (FBS) should be undertaken where possible.[88] A pH of less than 7.20 indicates that delivery should be carried out as rapidly as possible. However, meta-analyses of randomised controlled trials comparing EFM ± FBS versus intermittent auscultation do not show a reduction in intrapartum deaths or cerebral palsy, despite an increase in caesarean section rates.[85,126] None of the randomised controlled trials published to date, which compared EFM ± FBS with intermittent auscultation, had sufficient statistical power to demonstrate a reduction in the incidence of perinatal death or subsequent neurological impairment secondary to hypoxia–ischaemia.

The only benefit in neonatal outcome seen after electronic fetal monitoring was a reduction in the incidence of early neonatal seizures. The prevalence of cerebral palsy in the two randomised controlled trials with follow-up data was not significantly altered by EFM + FBS.[45,72] One meta-analysis reported a reduction in perinatal mortality due to fetal hypoxia.[136] However, this study did not show a reduction in overall perinatal mortality rate and, as there is no specific marker for hypoxic death, it is difficult to reliably ascertain the mortality due to fetal hypoxia.[11]

In conclusion, it appears that a normal heart rate pattern may be reassuring (negative predictive value of adverse outcome >96% in most studies) but an abnormal pattern is poorly predictive of fetal compromise. It appears that abnormal fetal heart rate patterns are unreliable markers of intrapartum antecedents of neurological damage, leading to obstetric intervention without proven benefit. It remains to be seen whether better markers can be developed from future work on the newer techniques of intrapartum monitoring.

Fetal ECG analysis

During myocardial ischaemia, anaerobic glycolysis changes the ion gradients across the myocardial cell membranes, resulting in a raised ST segment and a raised T/QRS ratio.[104] Randomised controlled trials of this technique have shown a reduction in operative intervention without worsening outcome.[145,38] A recent study also showed that CTG monitoring with automatic ST-waveform analysis resulted in a significantly lower rate of acidotic umbilical artery pH values compared with standard CTG monitoring.[7]

Systolic time intervals

Fetal ECG analysis in combination with Doppler analysis of the cardiac cycle has been used to assess myocardial function. The pre-ejection period (an electromechanical interval from initial deflection of the QRS complex to aortic valve opening) and the ventricular ejection time (duration of aortic valve opening) are thought to be sensitive indicators of myocardial contractility and have been used to detect deteriorating function during asphyxia.[68]

Fetal pulse oximetry

Continuous fetal oxygen saturation monitoring is possible and corresponds to results from fetal blood analysis.[73] However, signal quality is limited and the technique has not been tested in large-scale clinical practice.

Near-infrared spectroscopy

Light of near-infrared wavelengths can penetrate brain tissue for distances up to 8 cm. It is possible to obtain continuous quantification of changes in cerebral haemoglobin oxygen saturation and total cerebral haemoglobin concentration (representing cerebral blood volume) by analysis of the absorption spectra. During labour, an optical probe is inserted through the dilated cervix and on to the fetal head. A study of 41 fetuses during labour demonstrated good correlation between the mean cerebral oxygen saturation shortly before delivery and the umbilical arterial acid-base status immediately after birth.[5] This technique has not been applied in a large series or trial.

Passage of meconium

This occurs in 10–20% of all term deliveries but it is often taken as a marker of fetal distress. However, only 0.4% of term infants

with meconium-stained liquor during labour subsequently developed cerebral palsy.[88] Richey et al found no correlation between the passage of meconium and markers of acute asphyxia (umbilical arterial pH, lactate and hypoxanthine).[100]

Condition at birth

Apgar scores

A method of assessing an infant's condition at birth was first described by Virginia Apgar.[9] Originally scored at 1 minute of life by summation of five scored signs (p. 225), this was later extended to 5-minute intervals. A hypoxic–ischaemic insult can cause depression of the Apgar score but this is not invariable unless the insult occurs immediately prior to birth. Many non-asphyxial factors can cause depression, for example prematurity, maternal analgesia or anaesthetic. Nevertheless, prolonged depression of the Apgar score is related to death or major neurological disability[87] (Table 41.10). It is notable that almost 75% of children with cerebral palsy had Apgar scores of 7–10 at 5 minutes of life.

Acidosis

Metabolic acidosis is an index of anaerobic metabolism and is widely used as retrospective evidence of tissue hypoxia and 'fetal distress'. However, umbilical arterial acidaemia at delivery, considered on its own, is not associated with a poor outcome:[32,107] it is associated with a poor outcome only when in combination with abnormal fetal heart rate patterns, depressed Apgar scores and significant neonatal encephalopathy.[150] Severe fetal acidosis occurs in the moribund fetus but may also occur in the fetus who has compensated by preserving function in vital organs. Thus there is only a very loose association between fetal acidosis and severe fetal distress.

Clinical features after birth

Neonatal encephalopathy

Neonatal encephalopathy refers to abnormal neurological behaviour in the neonatal period and may be caused by a wide range of

Table 41.10 The outcome associated with latest* very low Apgar score (0–3)[87]

| Time (min) | Number liveborn | Death by 1 year (%) | <2501 | | >2500 | | | |
			Number known to 7 years	Cerebral palsy (%)	Number liveborn	Death by 1 year (%)	Number known to 7 years	Cerebral palsy (%)
1	428	25.5	257	1.9	1729	3.1	1330	0.7
5	163	55.2	56	7.1	286	7.7	217	0.9
10	67	67.2	15	6.7	66	18.2	43	4.7
15	51	84.3	8	0.0	23	47.8	11	9.1
20	139	95.7	7	0.0	39	59.0	14	57.1

* Counts at each time include only those children with very low Apgar scores at the time and no later very low Apgar score.

Table 41.11 A clinical grading system for hypoxic–ischaemic encephalopathy[66]

Grade I	Grade II	Grade III
Irritability		
Hyperalert	Lethargy	Comatose
Mild hypotonia	Marked abnormalities in tone	Severe hypotonia
Poor sucking	Requires tube feeds	Failure to maintain spontaneous respiration
No seizures	Seizures	Prolonged seizures

Table 41.12 Risk of death or severe handicap in remaining survivors associated with grade of hypoxic–ischaemic encephalopathy[95]

HIE grade	Risk of death or severe handicap in remaining survivors		
	Percentage	Likelihood ratio	(95% CI)
Mild (I)	1.6	0.05	0.02–0.15
Moderate (II)	24	0.94	0.71–1.23
Severe (III)	78	10.71	6.71–17.1

conditions. Very young infants recovering from a near-miss sudden infant death syndrome (SIDS) often show a predictable progression of neurological symptoms.[28] Initially there is a period of near normality, followed by the onset of seizures and a gradual deterioration in their consciousness level. Similar behaviour is seen in severely asphyxiated term infants. Sarnat and Sarnat introduced a grading system to describe the neurological abnormality, which they referred to as hypoxic–ischaemic encephalopathy (HIE)[112] and which has been modified by Levene et al (Table 41.11).[66] An important feature of HIE is the pattern of evolving neurological signs over the first few days of life, which contrasts with many other causes of neonatal encephalopathy where the baby shows an unremitting clinical course. It is important to consider alternative causes for a neonatal encephalopathy (see Table 41.9). Meningitis and severe hypoglycaemia are the most common treatable conditions that can produce encephalopathic features, and may coexist with hypoxia–ischaemia.

Mild (grade I) encephalopathy

This stage is characterised by hyperalertness, staring (decreased frequency of blinking), normal or decreased spontaneous motor activity and a lower threshold for all stimuli, including the easily elicited Moro reflex. Seizures are not a feature.

Moderate (grade II) encephalopathy

Seizures occur commonly. There is lethargy, hypotonia with reduced spontaneous movements, a higher threshold for primitive reflexes, and mainly parasympathetic responses. A consistent feature is differential tone between the upper and lower limbs, with the arms being relatively hypotonic compared to the legs.

Severe (grade III) encephalopathy

These neonates are comatose, with hypotonia and no spontaneous movements. Primitive reflexes and the suck reflex are often absent. Seizures may be frequent and prolonged, although in the most severe cases there may be no seizure activity and an isoelectric electroencephalogram (EEG).

Outcome

In a meta-analysis of studies examining the outcome of neonates with different HIE grades, it appears that stage I (mild HIE)

Table 41.13 Multiorgan dysfunction following hypoxia–ischaemia

Renal	Acute renal failure
	Myoglobinuria
	Haematuria
Gastrointestinal	Abnormal motility and feed intolerance
	Necrotizing enterocolitis
Cardiovascular	Reduced ventricular function
	Myocardial ischaemia (ECG)
	Papillary muscle necrosis
Pulmonary	Meconium aspiration
	Persistent pulmonary hypertension
	Apnoea
Haematological	Disseminated intravascular coagulation
Metabolic	Hyponatraemia/inappropriate ADH
	Hypoglycaemia
	Hypocalcaemia
	Elevated liver enzymes
	Elevated ammonia
	Metabolic acidosis

does not confer an increased risk of death or disability. Table 41.12 shows the risks of death and neurological abnormalities in survivors associated with HIE grade from this analysis.[95] A significant reduction in IQ at 8 years has been reported in children who had suffered from grade II HIE but who were neurologically normal, compared to children with grade I HIE.[102]

In a comparison of depression of Apgar scores with HIE grading in predicting outcome, an Apgar score of 5 or less at 10 minutes was found to be a more specific predictor of death or major neurological sequelae than HIE grades II and III (95% versus 78%), although it was less sensitive (57% versus 96%).[67]

Multiorgan dysfunction

During hypoxia–ischaemia, blood flow is redistributed in order to preserve circulation to the most vital organs – the brain, heart and adrenals. This is at the expense of the kidneys, liver and gastrointestinal tract, which are therefore vulnerable to hypoxic–ischaemic damage. Such damage to these and other organs serves as a further marker of hypoxia–ischaemia (Table 41.13).

Investigations

Many advances have been made in imaging techniques, enabling a greater understanding of the pathophysiology of perinatal asphyxia and allowing a more accurate prognosis. This is particularly important because accurate early detection is required in assessing the efficacy of potential neuroprotective therapies. However, some of the newer imaging techniques have not been fully evaluated because accurate neurodevelopmental follow-up is still awaited.

Cranial ultrasound

Ultrasound has proved most useful in the detection of GMH-IVH and ischaemic lesions in preterm infants, and it can also be of use in asphyxiated term infants. Initially, cerebral oedema can be recognised by a generalised increase in echodensity, a loss of anatomical landmarks, indistinct sulci and compression of the ventricles. 'Slit-like' ventricles are seen normally in the first 24 hours in term infants, and are only abnormal if persisting for more than 36 hours. The presence of oedema is not a useful prognostic sign, but later ultrasound scan findings associated with a poor neurodevelopmental outcome include bilateral, uniformly echogenic thalami, which represents severe basal ganglia hypoxic–ischaemic injury;[27] diffuse parenchymal echodensities (thought to represent neuronal necrosis); multifocal cystic changes; periventricular echodensities; and ventriculomegaly with cortical atrophy.[118] One of the major limitations of ultrasound in asphyxia has been its inability to assess peripheral cortical damage but, with the recent use of higher-resolution probes (10 MHz), increased cortical echogenicity associated with hypoxic–ischaemic damage can be detected.[36]

Cerebral blood flow velocities

Using pulsed-wave duplex Doppler with real-time spectral analysis of the back-scattered Doppler signal from a major cerebral artery (often the anterior), the cerebral blood flow velocities in that vessel can be determined. A relative increase in the end-diastolic blood flow velocity compared to the peak systolic blood flow velocity (Pourcelot's resistivity index <0.55) is associated with a poor outcome in asphyxiated infants.[10] It was later demonstrated that, if the anterior cerebral artery blood flow velocity rose to above three standard deviations from the mean, this was also associated with an adverse outcome (positive predictive value 94%).[79] This increased velocity lacked the normal variation with changing $PaCO_2$ and was thought to represent vasoparalysis of the cerebral vasculature. The cerebral blood flow velocities can take 24 hours to become abnormal following hypoxia–ischaemia, and have been found to be of little prognostic value if performed at 6 hours.[37]

Cerebral blood flow

In studies of infants with HIE using near-infrared spectroscopy, the cerebral blood volume was found to be increased, the normal response to changing CO_2 tension was markedly attenuated, and cerebral autoregulation to changing arterial pressure was also impaired.[148] Studies using the xenon clearance method for measuring cerebral blood flow have found that high flow and loss of autoregulation to changes in $PaCO_2$ are associated with a poor prognosis following hypoxia–ischaemia.[98]

Computed tomography

In a study of 43 asphyxiated term infants, cerebral CT scans were performed in the first 2 weeks and the appearances classified as normal or decreased density (subdivided into patchy, diffuse or global).[1] Diffuse or global decreased density indicates a poor prognosis (sensitivity 93%, specificity 80%). Other studies have shown little correlation unless the scans are performed after the first week.[69]

Magnetic resonance

Magnetic resonance imaging

Magnetic resonance imaging is now the imaging modality of choice following a significant asphyxial insult at term because of its excellent resolution and ability to predict outcome. The timing of early MR abnormalities has been reported by Martin and Barkovitch.[79] In the first 2–3 days after the acute event the first abnormalities are a low signal on T1-weighted images and a high signal on T2-weighted images. Following acute near-total asphyxia these abnormalities are seen in the lentiform nucleus as well as other parts of the basal ganglia. By day 4–5 T1-shortening appears in the affected areas and becomes most prominent by day 7. Abnormal T1-weighted signal may persist for 4 weeks or more. Low T2-weighted signal develops slowly over the first month and may persist for 2–3 months. Diffusion-weighted imaging appears to detect abnormalities earlier than those seen on T1- or T2-weighted scans and correlates well with areas of cytotoxic oedema.[103]

Magnetic resonance has been shown to be one of the best modalities for predicting outcome. Early changes that are associated with disability include abnormalities in the basal ganglia[2,12,109,111] and cortical highlighting in the perirolandic area (Fig. 41.27). The best predictor of bad outcome in the first 10 days of life is abnormality in signal intensity in the posterior limb of the internal capsule (PLIC), most obvious on inversion recovery sequences.[2] An abnormal or equivocal signal intensity within the PLIC predicted abnormal outcome (sensitivity 90%, specificity 100%, PPV 100%).

Late MRI findings associated with a poor neurodevelopmental outcome are delayed myelination, which is a marker of neuronal destruction, and other abnormalities, including cortical atrophy with thinning of the corpus callosum, persisting abnormal signal intensity in the basal ganglia, ventricular dilatation and extensive white matter changes (Fig. 41.28).[23,110] Patchy white matter changes, most obvious posteriorly, have been demonstrated in late MR scans of asphyxiated infants who presented with mild HIE and were apparently normal at 1 year.[110] These children may have any minor neurological dysfunction at school age.[13]

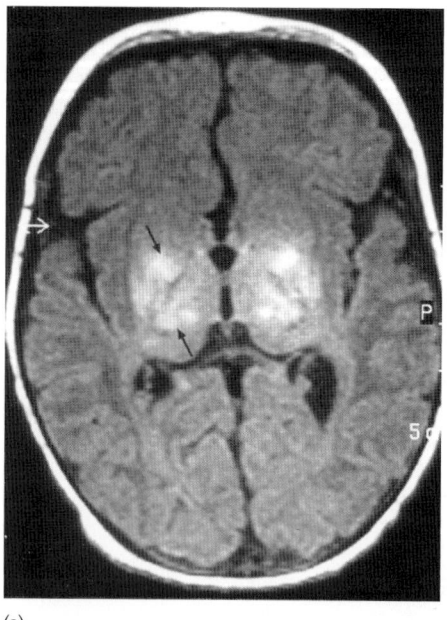

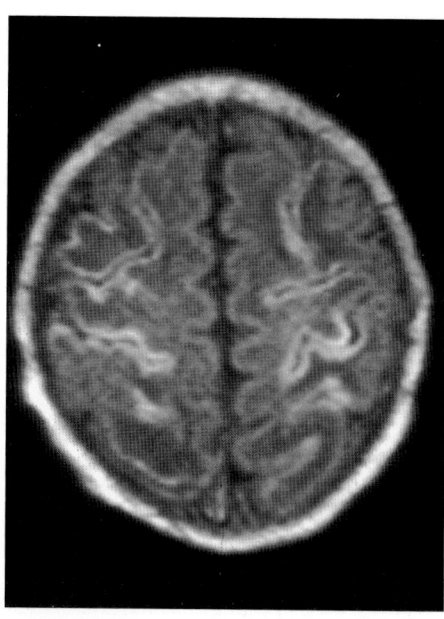

(a)

(b)

Fig. 41.27 Early MR changes predicting adverse outcome. (a) High signal on T1 axial section in the basal ganglia (arrowed). (b) Cortical highlighting in high axial T1 section.

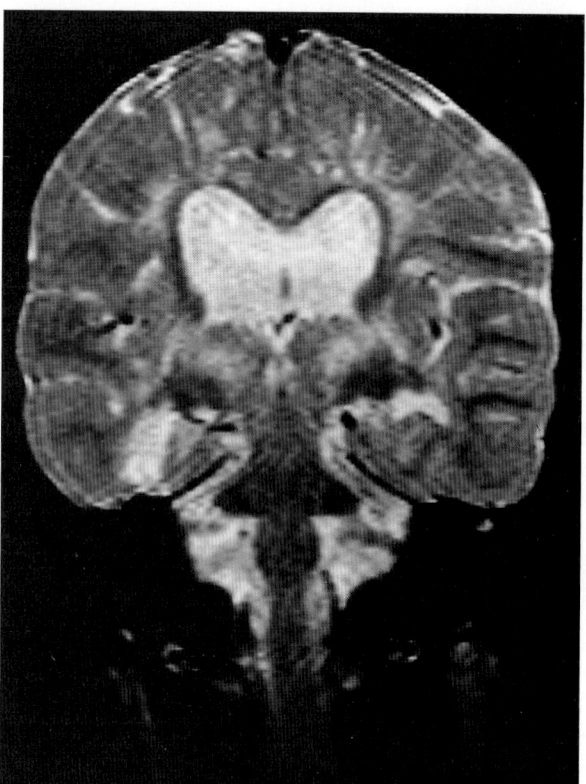

Fig. 41.28 MRI of the brain (T2-weighted coronal image) performed 2 years following an hypoxic–ischaemic insult. There is extensive abnormal high signal intensity in the periventricular white matter, basal ganglia plus ventricular enlargement.

Magnetic resonance spectroscopy

Intracerebral energy states can be measured in vivo by magnetic resonance spectroscopy (MRS) techniques using phosphorus-31 and hydrogen-1. Phosphocreatinine (PCr) and inorganic phosphate

(Pi) can be measured from the phosphorus-31 spectra. The PCr/Pi ratio represents the phosphorylated energy status within the brain, and a low PCr/Pi ratio in asphyxiated neonates is associated with later neurodevelopmental impairment,[80] with a sensitivity of 88% and specificity of 83%. Proton MRS detects a rise in lactate and a fall in N-acetyl-aspartate (Naa) following hypoxic–ischaemic injury. Prolonged high levels of lactate peaks predict a bad outcome.[96] A low Naa/creatinine or Naa/choline ratio has also been shown to be associated with a poor prognosis.[46,93] It appears that information from the proton resonance spectra occur before changes in the phosphorus-3 spectra, i.e. before cellular energy levels have been depleted.

Electrophysiology

Electroencephalography

Studies of neonatal EEGs in term infants with evidence of perinatal asphyxia have shown that background activity is an important prognostic indicator.[125] Continuous computer EEG analysis, allowing quantification and grading of the background activity, demonstrates that the more discontinuous the background, the worse the associated outcome.[144] An overview of the prediction of outcome based on four EEG studies of asphyxiated infants showed that severe EEG abnormalities (burst suppression, low-voltage, isoelectric) were associated with 95% risk of death or severe disability.[95]

There are many practical difficulties in obtaining extended EEG monitoring, thus limiting its use. Cerebral function monitors record amplitude-integrated EEG on a compressed timescale, providing a continuous trend of cerebral activity using just three electrodes. Hellström-Westas et al applied this technique in the first 6 hours and predicted the outcome correctly in 92% of infants[52] and others have reported similar findings.[6,130] Quantification of the abnormality following severe hypoxic–ischaemic insult has been reported by Naqeeb et al[6] based on measurement of the maximum and minimum voltage envelope. Moderate abnormality (upper margin $>10\,\mu V$, lower margin $<5\,\mu V$) relate to a poor outcome in most cases and severe abnormality (upper margin $<10\,\mu V$, lower edge $<5\,\mu V$) resulted in a uniformly poor outcome.

Evoked potentials

Persistently absent auditory brain-stem evoked responses (ABRs) and visual evoked potentials (VEPs) are predictive of sensorineural deafness and visual impairment respectively.[81,124] Somatosensory evoked potentials (SEPs) are technically the most difficult to perform but are useful in predicting neurological outcome because of the close proximity of sensory and motor axons within the deep periventricular white matter. In a study of term infants following hypoxic–ischaemic insult, a normal median nerve SEP within the first 24 hours accurately predicted normal outcome (sensitivity 94%), whereas an absent response was predictive of death or major handicap (specificity 59%).[34]

Markers of tissue injury

A number of biochemical markers have been proposed as indicators of hypoxic–ischaemic injury and as possible predictors of outcome. These include plasma lactate, CSF lactate dehydrogenase (LDH) and hydroxybutyrate dehydrogenase (HBDH),[30] plasma hypoxanthine, vasopressin and erythropoietin.[106] Many of the studies are in mixed preterm and term populations and the precise sensitivity and specificity of each assay requires further study. Of particular recent interest is the brain-specific isoenzyme of creatine kinase (CK-BB). In an analysis of three reports measuring CK-BB in term infants following hypoxic–ischaemia, those who died or were subsequently handicapped had a higher weighted mean CK-BB level in the first 6 hours than those without subsequent neurological impairment.[111] CSF CK-BB may be a more specific marker for adverse outcome.[33] Other CSF markers of recent interest include neuron-specific enolase,[44] glial fibrillary acidic protein (GFAP)[18] and excitatory amino acids.[48]

Management following hypoxia–ischaemia

Neonatal resuscitation

- It is important to establish adequate oxygenation and restore circulation by rapid and effective resuscitation.
- Newborn babies can be resuscitated as effectively in air as in 100% oxygen.[114] Babies resuscitated in 100% oxygen have increased oxidative stress levels for at least 1 month after birth compared with infants resuscitated in air.[135]
- If effective resuscitation fails to establish spontaneous cardiac output by 10 minutes, or respiratory activity by 30 minutes, the outlook for preterm and term infants alike is very poor.

Systemic management

The cornerstone of management following hypoxia–ischaemia is still supportive care and the careful maintenance of systemic homeostasis.

Respiratory support

Following resuscitation, respiratory support may be required for those patients with severe encephalopathy, co-existing lung disease (e.g. meconium aspiration syndrome, respiratory distress syndrome) or frequent and prolonged convulsions. Hypoxia should be avoided. Hyperoxia may promote oxygen free radical formation and may also be detrimental. Spontaneously breathing infants should be electively ventilated if their $PaCO_2$ rises above $7\,kPa$ (53 mmHg). The relationship between $PaCO_2$, cerebral blood flow and cerebral oedema is discussed later.

Cardiovascular support

Continuous intra-arterial monitoring and the prompt treatment of hypotension is recommended because systemic blood pressure needs to be adequate to maintain cerebral perfusion. Hypotension following hypoxia–ischaemia is common, owing to myocardial compromise rather than hypovolaemia. Therefore, caution must be used when using volume infusions in order not to further impair cardiac function. If there is not a rapid response to 10 ml/kg of crystalloid or colloid, or the central venous pressure is elevated, the early use of inotropes is recommended. Dopamine at doses of 7 microg/kg/min and above reduces cerebral blood flow through alpha-mediated vasoconstriction in beagle dogs.[140] Therefore, dobutamine (which lacks alpha effect), in combination with dopamine at a low dose (2–5 microg/kg/min), should be used. Although echocardiography may demonstrate poor myocardial contractility, it may not reliably exclude hypovolaemia.

Fluid and electrolyte therapy

Fluid restriction is commonly practised as a method of limiting cerebral oedema, although there is little evidence that fluid intake contributes to cerebral oedema. However, renal impairment and inappropriate antidiuretic hormone (ADH) are common sequelae of hypoxic–ischaemia, and therefore water overload can occur. The infant should be given only the volume of fluid necessary for adequate hydration, and a reasonable starting point is restricting to 20% less than the normal maintenance rate for the first 48 hours. Regular assessment of hydration, serum electrolytes, urine output and specific gravity or osmolality is required, aiming to maintain the serum osmolality in the region of 290 mmol/l and the urine specific gravity at 1010.

Infection

Early neonatal meningitis may have a similar presentation to hypoxic–ischaemic encephalopathy, and if there is any doubt a lumbar puncture must be performed. The routine use of antibiotics, without clinical indication, is not recommended.

Table 41.14 Suggested standard treatment of a term infant following intrapartum hypoxia–ischaemia

Respiratory	**Indications for ventilation**: frequent apnoea, $PaCO_2$ >7 kPa, hypoventilation secondary to anticonvulsants, meconium aspiration syndrome/pulmonary hypertension Maintain $PaCO_2$ 4.0–6.5 kPa
Blood pressure	Maintain mean arterial pressure >40 mmHg in term infants Cautious use of volume expansion (10 ml/kg colloid) Use dopamine (2–5 microg/kg/min) and dobutamine (5–15 microg/kg/min) if no response within 30 minutes
Fluids and electrolytes	Restrict to 20% less than maintenance for first 48 hours (anticipating SIADH or renal failure) Monitor fluid balance, infant's weight, serum electrolytes and osmolality, urine specific gravity and urinalysis Aim for neutral fluid balance (i.e. replacement of losses) Mannitol (1 g/kg) can be used if clinical signs of raised intracranial pressure (renally excreted) Treat hypocalcaemia if Ca <1.7 mmol
Seizures	Treat if frequent (≥1 per hour), prolonged (1 or more minutes), or interfering with respiration or ventilation
Glucose	Treat hypoglycaemia (<2.6 mmol) and hyperglycaemia (>8.0 mmol/l)
Infection	Blood cultures, consider lumbar puncture Antibiotics if clinically indicated
Haematology	Check clotting, give parenteral vitamin K Treat DIC with plasma, clotting factors, platelet transfusions, as necessary
Nutrition	Observe for NEC. Aspirate gastric contents Caution and patience with enteral feeds
Temperature	If pyrexial (>37°C), lower environmental temperature, use antipyretics Maintain environmental temperature in thermoneutral range
No indications for	Hyperventilation Corticosteroids Prophylactic anticonvulsants

Haemostasis

Disseminated intravascular coagulation (DIC) can occur, and therefore tests of clotting function must be performed following hypoxia–ischaemia. Treatment is with additional vitamin K, plasma or clotting factors and platelet transfusions, in sufficient quantity to restore clotting function.

Nutrition

Asphyxiated infants are at risk of developing necrotising enterocolitis, and also of aspiration if there is pharyngeal incoordination. A transient intolerance to enteral feeds is common because of the reduced small intestinal motility.[16] Enteral feeds should be introduced cautiously and it may take some time for the infant to breast-feed or feed from a bottle. In some cases the infant may be discharged with tube feeds continuing at home.

Traditional brain-oriented management

Much of the clinical management following hypoxia–ischaemia is largely empirical and has not been the subject of large randomised controlled clinical trials. When assessing the effectiveness of a particular treatment, problems arise because extrapolation from animal studies is difficult and comparison between clinical studies may not be possible if different definitions of hypoxia–ischaemia are used. Testing treatments in clinical trials with meaningful numbers of infants is, however, logistically difficult given the relatively low incidence of hypoxia–ischaemia for any individual centre. Table 41.14 summarises a pragmatic approach to the management of an asphyxiated term infant.

Cerebral oedema and intracranial hypertension

If cerebral oedema leads to reduced cerebral perfusion and cerebrovascular dysfunction, it is argued that treatment directed at reducing the oedema may be protective against further compromise. It is questionable whether cerebral oedema has a significant role in the development of further cerebral injury. Where intracranial pressure (ICP) has been measured with a subarachnoid catheter, raised ICP was found in 14 out of 23 asphyxiated infants and in only five cases could the raised ICP be medically controlled. Treatment of intracranial hypertension appears to have little influence on final outcome.[64]

Hyperventilation

Hypocapnia due to hyperventilation leads to an increase in cerebrovascular resistance, which reduces cerebral perfusion and may potentially compound an ischaemic insult. Hyperventilation appears to increase the risk of ischaemic lesions in preterm infants.[42] If vasoparalysis occurs following hypoxia–ischaemia,[98] the relationship between $PaCO_2$ and cerebrovascular resistance no longer holds. This vasoparalysis may result in increased perfusion to damaged areas at the expense of the less damaged areas with intact autoregulation (a 'reverse steal' effect). Mildly elevated $PaCO_2$ levels have been found to be more neuroprotective than normal $PaCO_2$ levels (both associated with less severe brain damage than hypocapnia) in the 7-day postnatal rat model.[133] Therefore, hyperventilation cannot be recommended and the $PaCO_2$ should be maintained at 5.0–6.5 kPa.

Steroids

These are only of benefit in treating cerebral oedema associated with cerebral mass lesions. Studies in adults following stroke, head trauma or hypoxic events have failed to show any benefit, and there are no data from perinatal animal models of hypoxia–ischaemia demonstrating that steroids improve outcome. In a case series of seven asphyxiated neonates, dexamethasone treatment reduced ICP but was accompanied by a fall in systemic blood pressure and no improvement in cerebral perfusion pressure.[63] Therefore, there is no evidence supporting the use of steroids following hypoxia–ischaemia and worries about high-dose steroids on long-term brain function further restrict their use in this context.

Osmotic agents

Mannitol has been used in a number of uncontrolled case series. In a heterogeneous group of 225 asphyxiated infants 1 g/kg of mannitol was given either early (before 2 hours) or late following hypoxic–ischaemia in a non-randomised fashion; the early-treatment group had a better outcome.[77] In a small study, four infants with raised ICP (measured by subarachnoid catheter) were given 1 g/kg mannitol over 20 minutes. This produced a transient fall in ICP and an improvement in cerebral perfusion pressure for around 4 hours.[63] Mannitol is also a free radical scavenger and has been shown to reduce brain injury following hypoxia–ischaemia, when given with another free radical scavenger and magnesium, in the rat model.[127] Although there is no good evidence for a beneficial effect, in practice mannitol can be used when there are clinical signs of raised intracranial pressure (e.g. bulging anterior fontanelle), provided renal function is adequate for its excretion.

Anticonvulsants

See also Chapter 41, Part 2.

Seizure control

Hypoxic–ischaemic encephalopathy is the most common cause of neonatal seizures at term. Seizures can substantially increase CNS metabolic demand, cause the release of excitatory neurotransmitters such as glutamate, lead to fluctuations in systemic arterial pressure, and cause hypoxia and hypercapnia. A variety of anticonvulsants have been employed to control seizures, and most experience relates to the use of barbiturates. In addition to their anticonvulsant activity, they are known to decrease CNS metabolic rate in high dose and reduce calcium entry post-ischaemia, and are free radical scavengers. However, long-term use leads to inhibition in brain growth and development in animal models.

There is now increasing evidence from animal studies that neonatal seizures have an adverse effect on neurodevelopmental progression and may predispose to cognitive, behavioural or epileptic complications later in life (see Levene[62] for review). Equally, anticonvulsants commonly used in the neonatal period have been shown to have adverse effects, so a balance must be struck between effective pharmacological management to avoid repeated or prolonged seizures and the use of multiple anticonvulsants in high doses. Our practice is to treat seizures when frequent (more than two in 1 hour) or prolonged (longer than 1 minute), particularly if they are interfering with respiration or ventilation. Initially a 20 mg/kg loading dose of phenobarbital (phenobarbitone) is used (a further 10 mg/kg loading may be given), followed by a maintenance dose of 3 mg/kg every 12 hours. Phenobarbital, however, is often ineffective as a first-line anticonvulsant particularly when the interseizure EEG is very abnormal.[21]

A one-off loading dose of phenytoin (20 mg/kg) given slowly over 30 minutes intravenously may be used as second line, followed by a continuous infusion of midazolam. Alternative drugs include clonazepam, lidocaine (lignocaine) and sodium valproate. The anticonvulsants can be discontinued once seizure control has been attained and the infant is neurologically normal. In the majority of cases anticonvulsants can be stopped prior to discharge.

Prophylaxis

Administration of barbiturates following hypoxia–ischaemia for neuroprotection has been attempted. An overview of five randomised studies of anticonvulsants given early to infants with hypoxia–ischaemia did not show any benefit from this form of treatment[39] and in particular no reduction in the incidence of seizures. The largest single study[50] demonstrated a significant reduction in the relative risk of severe neurodevelopmental disability or death, but there were methodological difficulties with this study.

Glucose

Hypoglycaemia

Animals rendered hypoglycaemic by insulin administration have a greatly reduced capacity to survive hypoxia–ischaemia.[134] However, 7-day postnatal rats that have been rendered hypoglycaemic through fasting prior to induced hypoxia–ischaemia show a reduction in brain damage compared to insulin-treated or normoglycaemic controls.[149] This neuroprotective effect may be due to the increased capacity of the immature brain to utilise lactate, pyruvate and ketones as an alternative energy source to glucose. The immature blood–brain barrier is more able to transport ketones, and the enzymes involved in ketone metabolism are induced rapidly after birth, in contrast to glycolytic enzymes. However, there is no evidence that depriving infants of glucose after hypoxia–ischaemia is neuroprotective, and the administration of ketones has not been tested. Best clinical practice is to maintain normoglycaemia.

Hyperglycaemia

In mature animals hyperglycaemia prior to the insult accentuates hypoxic–ischaemic injury.[83] The excessive accumulation of lactate appears responsible for this detrimental effect, possibly by causing endothelial damage. The converse occurs in the immature CNS: 7-day postnatal rats rendered hyperglycaemic prior to induced hypoxia–ischaemia survived twice as long as normoglycaemic counterparts.[142] The immature CNS has a lower capacity for glucose uptake and lactate production, and is more able to utilise lactate as an energy substrate, thus preventing harmful lactate accumulation. These differences in carbohydrate metabolism may account for the apparent paradox seen when comparing studies of hypoxic–ischaemic damage following hyperglycaemia in both adults and neonates. The evidence that inducing hyperglycaemia in immature animals following hypoxia–ischaemia is beneficial remains controversial, with conflicting results in the 7-day postnatal rat model.[51,116]

At present there is insufficient evidence to justify any other course of clinical management than the maintenance of normoglycaemia following hypoxia–ischaemia.

New neuroprotective approaches

Many neuroprotective approaches designed to be administered after hypoxic–ischaemic insult and calculated to protect the central nervous system from secondary neuronal injury are emerging from animal models, but few have been tested clinically. It seems unlikely that a single agent will confer complete neuroprotection, and therefore a combination of such agents may eventually be required.

Human studies

Allopurinol

This is a xanthine oxidase inhibitor. When given in high dosage (135 mg/kg) 15 minutes after hypoxic–ischaemic injury in 7-day-old rats it has been shown to reduce brain injury.[92] It appears to be effective at higher doses than simple enzyme inhibition; other effects include inhibition of neutrophil lysosomal enzyme release and scavenging of hydroxyl free radicals. When used to prevent free-radical-mediated injury in preterm infants it was found to be ineffective, although a relatively low oral dose was used (20 mg/kg).[105]

Allopurinol was given to 11 asphyxiated mature infants without apparent toxic effect.[132] The treated group showed a reduction in free radical formation, a reduction in cerebral blood volume and less inhibition of electrical brain activity compared with 11 untreated controls. No further reports on the surviving babies has been published and allopurinol as rescue treatment cannot be recommended.

Magnesium

This has been found to block the NMDA ion channel under resting conditions, occupying a binding site within the ion channel.[91] This block is voltage-dependent and is overcome during the axonal depolarisation that occurs with hypoxia–ischaemia.[55] If the extracellular magnesium concentrations are raised, this blockade can be restored.[53] The systemic administration of magnesium after a simulated hypoxic–ischaemic insult limits neurological damage in several animal models, including rat,[75,76,147] piglet[54] and mouse.[78] Magnesium has also been effective when used in combination with oxygen free radical scavengers, L-methionine and mannitol,[127]

and has the advantage of being less toxic than MK-801. It has been used in obstetric practice for over 60 years, and readily crosses the placenta without apparent harm to the fetus or neonate. Indeed, from epidemiological studies, the use of antenatal maternal magnesium therapy is associated with a lower incidence of intracranial haemorrhage (GMH-IVH and/or intraparenchymal lesion)[97] and cerebral palsy in the preterm population.[89] The efficacy of magnesium given postnatally or antenatally in providing neuroprotection has not been established in controlled clinical trials.

Hypothermia

Animal models suggest that hypothermia may be neuroprotective and have renewed interest in its potential role following hypoxia–ischaemia. These studies using a variety of immature animal models (rats, piglets and lambs) showed evidence of neuroprotection after the asphyxial insult with hypothermia (reduction of temperature by 4–6°C) for 3–72 hours (see Thoresen[128] for review).

In recent years a number of randomised controlled trials have been initiated to evaluate the role of therapeutic hypothermia in brain protection following human neonatal asphyxia. The largest of these to date is the Olympus Medical regional brain cooling study undertaken primarily in the USA. This study has completed patient recruitment (over 250 babies) and used a cooling cap to reduce brain temperature. No details of outcome are currently available but these are expected in 2004. A pilot study of regional hypothermia showed no adverse effects of this treatment in 21 babies compared with 15 historic controls.[119]

In a separate group of 13 babies submitted to head cooling in New Zealand the procedure was well tolerated by the babies.[14] Another report on tolerance of 19 asphyxiated babies treated with total body cooling of 34.5°C showed that this technique was well tolerated.[115] In a French study,[31] 25 newborn infants with moderate or severe HIE were cooled to 33–34°C for 72 hours and again no serious complications of the technique were recognised. Sinus bradycardia (70–80 bpm) with mild hypotension, thrombocytopenia without the need for platelet transfusion and mild hypoglycaemia were seen relatively commonly in the cooled group but these were not considered to be severe.

It appears that therapeutic hypothermia is a relatively safe technique but no evidence yet exists from studies in human babies that it improves outcome. To date there are at least five studies enrolling babies worldwide into randomised controlled trials, but this technique cannot be recommended until evidence for its efficacy and further evidence of safety is available.

Outcome

Interpreting clinical studies

The risk of death or major neurological sequelae following hypoxic–ischaemic insult is one of the foremost concerns of parents and clinicians alike. Many of the studies described in this chapter examine the outcome associated with a particular predictive factor. Table 41.15 gives the relative efficacy of methods

Table 41.15 Prognostic abilities of various techniques following hypoxic–ischaemia

Test	Result	Time assessed	No. in study	Sensitivity	Specificity	Predictive value of positive result for adverse outcome (%)	Predictive value of negative result for good outcome (%)	Prevalence of adverse outcome in study (%)	Ref.
Apgar score	5 or less	10 minutes	122	57	95	72	90	19	67
Encephalopathy	Sarnat grade III		200	50	10	100	84	28	101
	Sarnat grades II + III		200	100	52	43	100	28	101
Doppler ultrasound	PRI <0.55	24 hours	43	100	81	67	100	29	7
CT	Diffuse/global decreased density	7–14 days	43	93	80	90	86	65	1
MRI	Diffuse hyperintensity of cerebral hemispheres or basal ganglia changes (moderate–severe)	2–14 days	43	100	92	70	100	16	59
MRS	PCr/Pi below normal	1–5 days	32	88	83	64	95	25	80
	Naa/choline <0.80	1–20 days	21	90	73	75	89	48	46
Amplitude integrated EEG (cerebral function monitor)	Burst suppression, low voltage or flat	1–6 hours	47	95	89	86	96	40	52
Standard EEG	Burst suppression, low voltage or flat	1–4 days	44	84	88	84	88	41	52
Median nerve SSEP	Absent or delayed	24 hours	40	94	59	65	93	45	34

Sensitivity = proportion of infants with an adverse outcome correctly predicted by the investigation; Specificity = proportion of infants with a normal outcome correctly predicted by the investigation; Predictive values = positives: proportion of infants with positive or abnormal result that have an adverse outcome; negative: proportion of infants with negative or normal result that are normal on follow-up; Adverse outcome = death or major neurological impairment.

for predicting outcome following severe hypoxic–ischaemic injury. However, comparison between studies is difficult because of potential confounding variables:

- variation in the clinical definition of asphyxia;
- gestational age: factors associated with an adverse outcome identified by studies on a preterm population may not be applicable to the term infant;
- variation in the technique and timing of investigations, and definition of an abnormal result;
- variation in outcome variable assessed (e.g. mortality, cognitive, motor, neurological, behavioural) and definition of severe disability;
- age at assessment: early assessment allows for better inference as to the relationship between perinatal event and later outcome; later follow-up enables a more detailed assessment of higher-order cognitive functioning but is more likely to be confounded by environmental influences.

Withdrawal of ventilatory support

Following severe hypoxia–ischaemia many neonatologists consider that discontinuation of artificial ventilation is justified if the prognosis is poor. Early accurate information about prognosis is required in this situation. Unfortunately, the maximal degree of HIE may not be determined for a few days. The best early predictors of poor outcome are sustained low-voltage states or burst-suppression on the EEG, persisting beyond 6 hours, and abnormal Doppler cerebral blood flow velocities, appearing by 24 hours. Our personal practice is to perform these tests and, if the results of these investigations are unequivocally abnormal on two separate occasions after the first 24 hours, to explain the results and the poor prognosis to the parents. We offer to consider withdrawal of ventilatory support. If the parents choose this option care continues but is redirected towards supporting the parents and ensuring that the infant does not suffer distress. The parents are warned that the baby may not die if artificial ventilation is withdrawn.

Follow-up

The following general points can be made with some confidence.

- Condition at birth is a poor predictor of subsequent adverse outcome. Casalaz et al[24] reported 29 babies born at 36 weeks gestation or above with an Apgar score of zero who were successfully resuscitated; 45% of these babies were subsequently described as normal.
- Term infants with mild HIE are unlikely to have any subsequent neurodevelopmental problems and their parents should be strongly reassured.
- The best predictors of adverse outcome in the order in the sequence after birth in which they show abnormality are EEG (cerebral function monitoring), cerebral Doppler waveforms and MRI.
- The majority of infants admitted to a neonatal unit following hypoxia–ischaemia show signs of moderate HIE, making it

difficult for the clinician to accurately counsel the parents. A cluster of abnormal perinatal signs, including fetal heart rate pattern, acid–base status, depressed Apgar scores and multi-organ dysfunction, with an encephalopathy, is associated with later impairment.[150] Encouraging clinical features are the early establishment of breast or bottle feeds and the absence of neurological abnormalities on discharge.

- Severe HIE is clearly associated with a poor outcome. The classic disability suffered by survivors of severe HIE is cerebral palsy, in particular spastic quadriplegia or dyskinetic cerebral palsy. There may be associated intellectual impairment, blindness or epilepsy. Mental retardation alone is not a recognised sequel.
- The statement that the outcome of severe asphyxia is 'all or nothing' (if the baby does not have a severely adverse outcome – death or severe disability – then the outcome will be normal) can no longer be sustained in light of accumulating data (see below). Long-term follow-up is necessary to assess more subtle adverse outcomes.

'Late' neurological disability associated with hypoxia–ischaemia

There are relatively few follow-up data on long-term outcome of asphyxiated infants. In Canada a follow-up programme has tracked a group of asphyxiated babies through to 8 years of age.[101,102] They showed that there is a gradation of effect on the IQ for different degrees of severity of the asphyxial insult. At 3.5 years, the children with moderate HIE had a median Stanford Binet IQ of 92.3 compared with 101.5 in babies with mild HIE.[101] At 8 years there was a difference in IQ of 11 points when children with moderate HIE were compared with those sustaining mild HIE. The difference was 17 points between those with moderate HIE and an unasphyxiated control group.[102] There appears to be a continuum of cognitive deficit related to the severity of the asphyxial insult.

In another study assessing outcome at 5.5–6.5 years in 34 children without cerebral palsy but who had shown neonatal encephalopathy with Apgar scores of less than 5 at 1 minute, various tests of neurological function were performed.[13] All these survivors also had neonatal MR examination. It was found that 23.5% of the cohort had minor neurological dysfunction and/or perceptual motor difficulties. Of those with minor neurological dysfunction, 80% had mild or moderate basal ganglia abnormality or more marked white matter abnormalities on neonatal MR imaging. The authors comment that these children would be regarded as normal on short-term follow-up.

Medicolegal implications (Chapter 6)

In the 19th century, work by Little[70] suggested that the major cause of cerebral palsy and mental retardation was intrapartum 'brain damage', later translated into terms such as 'birth asphyxia' or 'hypoxic–ischaemic injury'. This resulted in undue emphasis being placed on the causative role of intrapartum events in cerebral palsy by the medical profession, lawyers and lay people. However, the incidence of cerebral palsy is largely unchanged despite increasing obstetric intervention.[47,123] In a case note analysis of the 183 cases of spastic cerebral palsy from the Western Australia Cerebral Palsy Register 1975–1980, 14.1% were judged to have suffered perinatal asphyxia. However, only 8.2% of cerebral palsy was judged to have been caused by asphyxia, as there were many cases of perinatal asphyxia in the control population without cerebral palsy.[17] Similar figures have been derived from other epidemiological studies.[86] Some MRI studies also suggest that the majority of cerebral palsy is due to prenatal brain injury.[131] Intrapartum asphyxia may be the first presentation of cerebral palsy if this prenatal insult impairs the ability of the fetus to cope with the physiological stress of labour.[49] Gaffney et al found that there had been a suboptimal clinical response to fetal distress (judged by case note review) in only 6.8% of children with cerebral palsy born to residents in the Oxford Region 1984–1987.[43] Lawyers and expert witnesses need to be aware that only a small proportion of cerebral palsy can be prevented by improvements in intrapartum care.[41,122]

Terminology

In this increasingly litigious world medical note-keeping following the birth of an infant in poor condition needs to be accurate and non-judgemental. Terms such as 'birth asphyxia' may be valid, but only if there is evidence to support the diagnosis (which should be documented). However, depressed Apgar scores alone do not make the diagnosis and the infant should be described as being born 'in poor condition' or 'with low Apgar scores', not 'asphyxiated'. Likewise, neonatal encephalopathy may not be asphyxial in origin, and therefore the term 'hypoxic–ischaemic encephalopathy' should be avoided until specific evidence for its origin becomes available.[15]

Evidence for medicolegal cases

When giving evidence in medicolegal cases the neonatal paediatrician will be required to consider whether the adverse outcome (e.g. cerebral palsy) resulted from intrapartum hypoxia–ischaemia. Table 41.8 gives the information required from the case notes for the paediatrician to be confident of causation. The obstetrician will need to consider liability when commenting upon the obstetric management. In order for a court to make a decision in such cases, three separate issues need to be addressed in light of the evidence presented by the paediatrician and obstetrician:

- was the adverse outcome a consequence of intra-partum hypoxia–ischaemia?
- was negligence demonstrated by the medical team responsible for management of the patient in labour?
- would a reasonable alternative management have resulted in a more favourable outcome?

References

1. Adsett D B, Fitz C R, Hill A 1985 Hypoxic-ischaemic cerebral injury in the term newborn: correlation of CT findings with neurological outcome. Developmental Medicine and Child Neurology 27: 155–160
2. Aida N, Nishimura G, Hachiya Y. MR imaging of perinatal brain damage: comparison of clinical outcome with initial and follow-up MR findings. American Journal of Neuroradiology 1998; 19: 1909–1921.
3. Airede A I 1991 Birth asphyxia and hypoxic–ischaemic encephalopathy: incidence and severity. Annals of Tropical Paediatrics 11: 331–335
4. Al-Alfry A, Carroll J E, Devarajan L V, Moussa M A 1990 Term infant asphyxia in Kuwait. Annals of Tropical Paediatrics 10: 355–361
5. Aldrich C J, D'Antona D, Wyatt J S, Spencer J A, Peebles D M, Reynolds E O R 1994 Fetal cerebral oxygenation measured by near-infrared spectroscopy shortly before birth and acid-base status at birth. Obstetrics and Gynecology 84: 861–865
6. Al Naqeeb N, Edwards A D, Cowan F M, Azzopardi D 1999 Assessment of neonatal encephalopathy by amplitude-integrated electroencephalography. Pediatrics 103: 1263–1271.
7. Amer-Wahlin I, Hellsten C. Noren H, Hagberg H 2001 Cardiotocography only versus cardiotocography plus ST analysis of fetal electrocardiogram for intrapartum fetal monitoring: a Swedish randomised controlled trial. The Lancet 358(9281): 534–538.
8. Ames A, Wright R L, Kowada M 1968 Cerebral insult: II. The no reflow phenomenon. American Journal of Pathology 52: 437–453
9. Apgar V 1953 A proposal for a new method of evaluation of the newborn infant. Anesthesia and Analgesia 32: 260–267
10. Archer L N J, Levene M I, Evans D H 1986 Cerebral artery Doppler ultrasonography for prediction of outcome after perinatal asphyxia. Lancet ii: 1116–1118
11. Bader T J, Morgan M A 1995 Intrapartum electronic fetal heart rate monitoring versus intermittent auscultation: a meta-analysis (letter). Obstetrics and Gynecology 85: 643
12. Barkovich A J, Hajnal B L, Vigneron D 1998 Prediction of neuromotor outcome in perinatal asphyxia: evaluation of MR scoring systems. American Journal of Neuroradiology 19: 143–149.
13. Barnett A, Mercuri E, Rutherford M, Haataja L, Frisone M F, Henderson S, Cowan F, Dubowitz L 2002 Neurological and perceptual-motor outcome at 5–6 years of age in children with neonatal encephalopathy: relationship with neonatal brain MRI. Neuropediatrics 33: 242–248.
14. Battin M R, Penrice J, Gunn T R, Gunn A J 2003 Treatment of term infants with head cooling and mild systemic hypothermia (35°C and 34.5°C) after perinatal asphyxia. Pediatrics 111: 244–251.
15. Bax M, Nelson K B 1993 Birth asphyxia: a statement. World Federation of Neurology Group. Developmental Medicine and Child Neurology 35: 1022–1024
16. Berseth C L, McCoy H H 1992 Birth asphyxia alters neonatal intestinal motility in term neonates. Pediatrics 90: 669–673
17. Blair E, Stanley F J 1988 Intrapartum asphyxia: a rare cause of cerebral palsy. Journal of Pediatrics 112: 515–519
18. Blennow M, Hagberg H, Rosengren L 1995 Glial fibrillary acidic protein in the cerebrospinal fluid: a possible indicator of prognosis in full-term asphyxiated newborn infants? Pediatric Research 37: 260–264
19. Bocking A D, White S E, Homan J, Richardson B S 1992 Oxygen consumption is maintained in fetal sheep during prolonged hypoxaemia and hypercapnia in sheep. Journal of Developmental Physiology 17: 169–174
20. Boo N Y, Lye M S 1991 Factors associated with clinically significant perinatal asphyxia in the Malaysian neonates: a case-control study. Journal of Tropical Pediatrics 38: 284–289
21. Boylan G B, Rennie J M, Pressler R M, Wilson G, Morton M, Binnie CD 2002 Phenobarbitone, neonatal seizures, and video-EEG. Archives of Disease in Childhood, Fetal & Neonatal Ed 86: F165-F170.
22. Brown J K, Purvis R J, Forfar J O, Cockburn F 1974 Neurological aspects of perinatal asphyxia. Developmental Medicine and Child Neurology 16: 567–580
23. Byrne P, Welch R, Johnson M A, Darrah J, Piper M 1990 Serial magnetic resonance imaging in neonatal hypoxic–ischaemic encephalopathy. Journal of Pediatrics 117: 694–700
24. Casalaz D M, Marlow N & Speidel B D 1998 Outcome of resuscitation following unexpected apparent stillbirth. Archives of Disease in Childhood, Fetal & Neonatal Ed. 78: F112-F115.

25. Cohn H E, Sachs E J, Heyman M A, Rudolph A M 1974 Cardiovascular responses to hypoxemia and acidaemia in fetal lambs. American Journal of Obstetrics and Gynecology 120: 817–824

26. Confidential Enquiry into Stillbirths and Deaths in Infancy 1997 Executive summary of the Fourth Annual Report. Maternal and Child Health Research Consortium, London

27. Connolly B, Kelehan P, O'Brien N et al 1994 The echogenic thalamus in hypoxic–ischaemic encephalopathy. Pediatric Radiology 24: 268–271

28. Constantinou J E C, Gillis J, Ouvrier R A, Rahilly P M 1989 Hypoxic-ischaemic encephalopathy after near miss sudden infant death syndrome. Archives of Disease in Childhood 64: 703–708

29. Cowan F, Rutherford M, Groenendaal F, Eken P, Mercuri E, Bydder G M, Meiners L C, Dubowitz L M S, de Vries L S 2003 Origin and timing of brain lesions in term infants with neonatal encephalopathy. Lancet 361: 736–742.

30. Dalens B, Viallard J-L, Raynaud E-J, Dastugue B 1981 CSF levels of lactate and hydroxybutyrate dehydrogenase as indicators of neurological sequelae after neonatal brain damage. Developmental Medicine and Child Neurology 23: 228–233

31. Debillon T, Daoud P, Durand P, Cantagrel S, Jouvet P, Saizou C, Zupan V 2003 Whole-body cooling after perinatal asphyxia: a pilot study in term neonates. Developmental Medicine & Child Neurology 45: 17–23.

32. Dennis J, Johnson A, Mutch L, Yudkin P, Johnson P 1989 Acid-base status at birth and neurodevelopmental outcome at four and one-half years. American Journal of Obstetrics and Gynecology 161: 213–220

33. De Praeter C, Vanhaesebrouck P, Govaert P, Delanghe J, Leroy J 1991 Creatine kinase concentrations in the cerebrospinal fluid of newborns: relationship to short-term outcome. Pediatrics 88: 1204–1210

34. De Vries L S 1993 Somatosensory evoked potential in term neonates with postasphyxial encephalopathy. Clinics in Perinatology 20: 463–482

35. Dukta A J, Kochanek P M, Hallenbeck J M 1989 Influence of granulocytopenia on canine cerebral ischaemia induced by air embolism. Stroke 20: 390–395

36. Eken P, Jansen G H, Groenendaal F, Rademaker K J, de Vries L S 1994 Intracranial lesions in the fullterm infant with hypoxic–ischaemic encephalopathy: ultrasound and autopsy correlation. Neuropediatrics 25: 301–307

37. Eken P, Toet M C, Groenendaal F, de Vries L S 1995 Predictive value of early neuroimaging, pulsed Doppler and neurophysiology in full term infants with hypoxic–ischaemic encephalopathy. Archives of Disease in Childhood 73: F75-F80

38. Etuk S J, Etuk I S 2001 Relative risk of birth asphyxia in babies of booked women who deliver in unorthodox health facilities in Calabar, Nigeria. Acta Tropica 79(2): 143–147

39. Evans D J, Levene M I 2001 Anticonvulsants for preventing mortality and morbidity in full term newborns with perinatal asphyxia (Cochrane Review). The Cochrane Library, Issue 1

40. Finer N N, Robertson C M, Richards R T, Pinnell L E, Peters K L 1981 Hypoxic-ischemic encephalopathy in term neonates: perinatal factors and outcome. Journal of Pediatrics 98: 112–117

41. Freeman J M, Nelson K B 1988 Intrapartum asphyxia and cerebral palsy. Pediatrics 82: 240–249

42. Fujimoto S, Togari H, Yamaguchi N, Mizutani F, Suzuki S, Sobajima H 1994 Hypocarbia and cystic periventricular leukomalacia in premature infants. Archives of Disease in Childhood 71: F107-F110

43. Gaffney G, Sellers S, Flavell V, Squier M, Johnson A 1994 Case-controlled study of intrapartum care, cerebral palsy, and perinatal death. British Medical Journal 308: 743–750

44. Garcia-Alix A, Cabanas F, Pellicer A, Hernanz A, Stiris T, Quero J 1994 Neuron-specific enolase and myelin basic protein: relationship of cerebrospinal fluid concentrations to the neurologic condition of asphyxiated full-term infants. Pediatrics 93: 234–240

45. Grant A, O'Brien N, Joy M, Hennessy E, MacDonald D 1989 Cerebral palsy among children born during the Dublin randomised trial of intrapartum monitoring. Lancet ii: 1233–1236

46. Groenendaal F, Veenhoven R H, van der Grond J, Jansen G H, Witkamp T D, de Vries L S 1994 Cerebral lactate and N-acetyl-aspartate/choline ratios in asphyxiated full-term neonates demonstrated in vivo using proton magnetic resonance spectroscopy. Pediatric Research 35: 148–151

47. Hagberg B, Hagberg G, Olow I 1993 The changing panorama of cerebral palsy in Sweden VI. Prevalence and origin during the birth year period 1983–1986. Acta Paediatrica 82: 387–393

48. Hagberg H, Thornberg E, Blennow M et al 1993 Excitatory amino acids in the cerebrospinal fluid of asphyxiated infants: relationship to hypoxic–ischemic encephalopathy. Acta Paediatrica 82: 925–929

49. Hall D M 1994 Intrapartum events and cerebral palsy. British Journal of Obstetrics and Gynaecology 101: 745–747

50. Hall R T, Hall F K, Daily D K 1998 High-dose phenobarbital therapy in term newborn infants with severe perinatal asphyxia: A randomized, prospective study with three-year follow-up. Journal of Pediatrics 132: 345–348

51. Hattori H, Wasterlain C G 1990 Posthypoxic glucose supplement reduces hypoxic–ischemic brain damage in the neonatal rat. Annals of Neurology 28: 122–128

52. Hellstrom-Westas L, Rosen I, Svenningsen N W 1995 Predictive value of early continuous amplitude integrated EEG recordings on outcome after severe birth asphyxia in full term infants. Archives of Disease in Childhood 72: F34–F38

53. Henneberry R C, Novelli A, Cox J A, Lysko P G 1989 Neurotoxicity at the N-methyl-D-aspartate receptor in energy-compromised neurons. An hypothesis for cell death in aging and disease. Annals of the New York Academy of Science 568: 225–233

54. Hoffman D J, Marro P J, McGowan J E, Mishra O P, Delivoria-Papadopoulos M 1994 Protective effect of $MgSO_4$ infusion on NMDA receptor binding characteristics during cerebral cortical hypoxia in the newborn piglet. Brain Research 644: 144–149

55. Hori N, Carpenter D O 1994 Transient ischaemia causes a reduction of Mg^{2+} blockade of NMDA receptors. Neuroscience Letters 173: 75–78

56. Hossman K A 1983 Neuronal survival and revival during and after cerebral ischaemia. American Journal of Emergency Medicine 1: 191–197

57. Hossman K A, Kleihues P 1973 Reversibility of ischaemic brain damage. Archives of Neurology 29: 375–385

58. Kinoti S N 1993 Asphyxia of the newborn in east, central and southern Africa. East African Medical Journal 70: 422–433

59. Kuenzle C, Baenziger O, Martin E et al 1994 Prognostic value of early MR imaging in term infants with severe perinatal asphyxia. Neuropediatrics 25: 191–200

60. Laroche J-C 1984 Perinatal brain damage. In: Adams J H, Corsellis J A N, Duchen L W (eds) Greenfield's neuropathology. Edward Arnold, London

61. Lawrence A J, Jarrott B 1993 Nitric oxide increases interstitial excitatory amino acid release in the rat dorsomedial medulla oblongata. Neuroscience Letters 151: 126–129

62. Levene M I 2002 The clinical conundrum of neonatal seizures. Archives of Disease in Childhood, Fetal & Neonatal Ed 86: F75–F77

63. Levene M I, Evans D H 1985 Medical management of raised intracranial pressure after severe birth asphyxia. Archives of Disease in Childhood 60: 12–16

64. Levene M I, Evans D H, Forde A, Archer L N 1987 Value of intracranial pressure monitoring of asphyxiated newborn infants. Developmental Medicine and Child Neurology 29: 311–319

65. Levene M I, Fenton A C, Evans D H, Archer L N J, Shortland D B, Gibson N A 1989 Severe birth asphyxia and abnormal cerebral blood flow velocity. Developmental Medicine and Child Neurology 31: 427–434

66. Levene M I, Kornberg J, Williams T H C 1985 The incidence and severity of post-asphyxial encephalopathy in full-term infants. Early Human Development 11: 21–26

67. Levene M I, Sands C, Grindulis H, Moore J R 1986 Comparison of two methods of predicting outcome in perinatal asphyxia. Lancet i: 67–69

68. Lewinsky R M 1994 Cardiac systolic time intervals and other parameters of myocardial contractility as indices of fetal acid-base status. Baillières Clinical Obstetrics and Gynecology 8: 663–681

69. Lipp-Zwahlen A E, Deonna T, Chrzanowski R, Micheli J L, Calame A 1985 Temporal evolution of hypoxic–ischaemic brain lesions in the asphyxiated full-term newborn assessed by computerized tomography. Neuroradiology 27: 138–144

70. Little W J 1862 On the influence of abnormal parturition, difficult labours, premature birth, and asphyxia neonatorum, on the mental and physical condition of the child, especially in relation to deformities. Transactions of the Obstetrical Society of London 3: 293–344

71. Loreck A, Takei Y, Cady E B et al 1994 Delayed ('secondary') cerebral energy failure after acute hypoxia–ischaemia in the newborn piglet: continuous 48-hour studies by phosphorus magnetic resonance spectroscopy. Pediatric Research 36: 699–706

72. Luthy D A, Shy K K, van Belle G et al 1987. A randomised trial of electronic fetal monitoring in preterm labour. Obstetrics and Gynecology 69: 687–695

73. Luttkus A, Fengler T W, Friedmann W, Dudenhausen J W 1995 Continuous monitoring of fetal oxygen saturation by pulse oximetry. Obstetrics and Gynaecology 85: 183–186

74. McCord J M 1985 Oxygen-derived free radicals in postischemic tissue injury. New England Journal of Medicine 312: 159–163

75. McDonald J W, Silverstein F S, Johnston M V 1990 Magnesium reduces N-methyl-D-aspartate (NMDA)-mediated brain injury in perinatal rats. Neuroscience Letters 109: 234–238

76. McIntosh T K, Vink R, Yamakami I, Faden A I 1989 Magnesium protects against neurological deficit after brain injury. Brain Research 482: 252–260

77. Marchal C, Costagliola P, Leveau P, Dulucq P, Steckler R, Rouquier F 1974 Traitement de la souffrance cérébrale néonatale d'origine anoxique par le mannitol. Revue de Pediatrie 9: 581–589

78. Marret S, Gressens P, Gadisseux J-F, Evrard P 1995 Prevention by magnesium of excitotoxic neuronal death in the developing brain: an animal model for clinical intervention studies. Developmental Medicine and Child Neurology 37: 473–484

79. Martin E, Barkovich A J 1995 Magnetic resonance imaging in perinatal asphyxia. Archives of Disease in Childhood 72: F62–F70.

80. Moorcraft J, Bolas N M, Ives N K et al 1991 Global and depth resolved phosphorus magnetic resonance spectroscopy to predict outcome after birth asphyxia. Archives of Disease in Childhood 66: 1119–112343

81. Muttitt S C, Taylor M J, Kobyashi J S, MacMillan L, Whyte H E 1991 Serial evoked visual potentials and outcome in full term birth asphyxia. Pediatric Neurology 7: 86–90

82. Myers R E 1972 Two patterns of perinatal brain damage and their conditions of occurrence. American Journal of Obstetrics and Gynecology 112: 246–276

83. Myers R E, Yamaguchi S 1977 Nervous effects of cardiac arrest in monkeys. Preservation of vision. Archives of Neurology 34: 65–74

84. National Institute for Clinical Excellence 2003 The use of electronic fetal monitoring: the use and interpretation of cardiotocography in intrapartum fetal surveillance 3, 5–6.

85. Neilson J P 1994 EFM + scalp sampling vs intermittent auscultation in labour: In: Enkin M W, Keirse M J N C, Renfew M J, Neilson J P (eds) Pregnancy Database of Systematic Reviews': Review No. 03297, 4 May 1994. Published through 'Cochrane Updates on Disk', Oxford: Update Software, 1994, Disk Issue 1

86. Nelson K B 1988 What proportion of cerebral palsy is related to birth asphyxia? Journal of Pediatrics 112: 572–573

87. Nelson K B, Ellenberg J H 1981 Apgar scores as predictors of chronic neurologic disability. Pediatrics 68: 36–44

88. Nelson K B, Ellenberg J H 1984 Obstetric complications as risk factors for cerebral or seizure disorder. Journal of the American Medical Association 251: 1843–1848

89. Nelson K B, Grether J K 1995 Can magnesium sulfate reduce the risk of cerebral palsy in very low birthweight infants? Pediatrics 95: 263–269

90. Niijima S, Levene M I 1989 Post-asphyxial encephalopathy in a preterm infant. Developmental Medicine and Child Neurology 31: 391–397

91. Nowak L, Bregestovski P, Ascher P, Herbet A, Prochiantz A 1984 Magnesium gates glutamate-activated channels in mouse central neurones. Nature 307: 462–465

92. Palmer C, Towfighi J, Roberts R L, Heitjan D F 1993 Allopurinol administered after inducing hypoxic–ischemia reduces brain injury in 7 day old rats. Pediatric Research 33: 405–411

93. Peden C J, Rutherford M A, Sargentoni J, Cox I J, Bryant D J, Dubowitz L M S 1993. Proton spectroscopy of the neonatal brain following hypoxic–ischaemic injury. Developmental Medicine and Child Neurology 35: 502–510

94. Peebles D M, Spencer J A, Edwards A D et al 1994 Relation between frequency of uterine contractions and human fetal cerebral oxygen saturation studied during labour by near infrared spectroscopy. British Journal of Obstetrics and Gynaecology 101: 44–48

95. Peliowski A, Finer N N 1992 Birth asphyxia in the term infant. In: Sinclair J C, Bracken M B (eds) Effective care of the newborn infant. Oxford University Press, Oxford, pp 249–279

96. Penrice J, Cady E B, Lorek A 1996 Proton magnetic resonance spectroscopy of the brain in normal preterm and term infants, and early changes after perinatal hypoxia–ischemia. Pediatric Research 40: 6.

97. Perlman J, Fernandez C, Gee J, Leveno K, Risser R 1995 Magnesium sulphate (Mg) administered to mothers with pregnancy-induced hypertension (PIH) is associated with a reduction in periventricular-intraventricular hemorrhage (PV-IVH). Pediatric Research 37: 231A

98. Pryds O, Greisen G, Lou H, Friis-Hansen B 1990 Vasoparalysis associated with brain damage in asphyxiated term infants. Journal of Pediatrics 117: 119–125

99. Richardson B S, Rurak D, Patrick J E, Homan J 1989 Cerebral oxidative metabolism during sustained hypoxaemia in fetal sheep. Journal of Developmental Physiology 11: 37–43

100. Richey S D, Ramin S M, Bawdon R E et al 1995 Markers of acute and chronic asphyxia in infants with meconium-stained amniotic fluid. American Journal of Obstetrics and Gynecology 172: 1212–1215

101. Robertson C, Finer N 1985 Term infants with hypoxic–ischemic encephalopathy: outcome at 3.5 years. Developmental Medicine and Child Neurology 27: 473–484

102. Robertson C M T, Finer N N, Grace M G A 1989 School performance of survivors of neonatal encephalopathy associated with birth asphyxia at term. Journal of Pediatrics 114: 753–760

103. Roelants-van Rijn A M, Nikkels P G J, Groenendaal F, van der Grond J, Barth P G, Snoeck I, Beek F J A, de Vries L S 2001 Neonatal diffusion-weighted MR imaging: relation with histopathology or follow-up MR examination. Neuropediatrics 32: 286–294.

104. Rosén K G 1986 Alterations in the fetal electrocardiogram as a sign of fetal asphyxia – experimental data with a clinical implimentation. Journal of Perinatology 14: 355–364

105. Russell G A B, Cooke R W I 1995 Randomised controlled trial of allopurinol prohylaxis in very preterm infants. Archives of Disease in Childhood 73: F27–F31

106. Ruth V, Autti-Ramo I, Granstrom M-L, Korkman M, Raivio K O 1988 Prediction of perinatal brain damage by cord plasma vasopressin, erythropoietin, and hypoxanthine values. Journal of Pediatrics 113: 800–815

107. Ruth V J, Raivio K O 1988 Perinatal brain damage: predictive value of metabolic acidosis and the Apgar score. British Medical Journal 297: 24–27

108. Rutherford M A, Pennock J M, Dubowitz L M S 1994 Cranial ultrasound and magnetic resonance imaging in hypoxic–ischaemic encephalopathy: a comparison with outcome. Developmental Medicine and Child Neurology 36: 813–825

109. Rutherford M A, Pennock J, Schwieso J 1996 Hypoxic-ischaemic encephalopathy: early and late magnetic resonance imaging finds in relation to outcome. Archives of Disease in Childhood 75: F145–F151.

110. Rutherford M, Pennock J, Schwieso J, Cowan F, Dubowitz L 1996 Hypoxic-ischaemic encephalopathy: early and late magnetic resonance imaging findings in relation to outcome. Archives of Disease in Childhood 75: F145–F151

111. Rutherford M A, Pennock J M, Counsell S J 1998 Abnormal magnetic resonance signal in the internal capsule predicts poor neurodevelopmental outcome in infants with hypoxic ischemic encephalopathy. Pediatrics 102: 323–329.

112. Sarnat H B, Sarnat M S 1976 Neonatal encephalopathy following fetal distress. Archives of Neurology 33: 696–705

113. Saugstad O D 2002 Free radical-mediated processes. In: Birth Asphyxia and the brain: basic science and clinical implications. Donn S M, Sinha S K, Chiswick M L (eds) 189–212.

114. Saugstad O D, Rootwelt T, Aalen A O 1998 Resuscitation of asphyxiated newborn infants with room air or oxygen: an international trial: the Resair 2 study. Pediatrics 102: e1.

115. Shankaran S, Laptook A, Wright L L, Ehrenkranz R A, Donovan E F, Fanaroff A A, Stark A R, Tyson J E, Poole K, Carlo W A, Lemons J A, Oh W, Stoll B J, Papile L U, Bauer C R, Stevenson D K, Korones S B, McDonald S 2002 Whole-body hypothermia for neonatal encephalopathy: animal observations as a basis for a randomized, controlled pilot study in term infants. Pediatrics 110: 377–385.

116. Sheldon R A, Partridge J C, Ferriero D M 1992 Postischemic hyperglycemia is not protective to the neonatal rat brain. Pediatric Research 32: 489–493

117. Shewmon D A, Fine M, Masdeu J C, Palacios E 1981 Postischemic hypervascularity of infancy: a stage in the evolution of ischemic brain damage with characteristic CT scan. Annals of Neurology 9: 358–365

118. Siegel M J, Shackelford G D, Perlman G M, Fulling K H 1984 Hypoxic-ischaemic encephalopathy in term infants: diagnosis and prognosis evaluated by ultrasound. Radiology 152: 395–399

119. Simbruner G, Haberl C, Harrison V, Linley L, Willeitner A E 1999 Induced brain hypothermia in asphyxiated human newborn infants: a retrospective chart analysis of physiological and adverse effects. Intensive Care Medicine 25: 1111–1117.

120. Singh M, Deorari A K, Khajuria R C, Paul V K 1991 A four year study on neonatal morbidity in a New Delhi hospital. Indian Journal of Medical Research 94: 186–192

121. Smith M L, Auer R N, Siesjo B K 1984 The density and distribution of ischemic brain injury in the rat following 2–10 min of forebrain ischemia. Acta Neuropathologica 64: 319–332

122. Stanley F 1994 Cerebral palsy. The courts catch up with the sad realities. Medical Journal of Australia 161: 236

123. Stanley F J 1994 Cerebral palsy trends. Implications for perinatal care. Acta Obstetrica et Gynecologica Scandinavia 73: 5–9

124. Stockard J E, Stockard J J, Kleinberg F, Westmoreland B F 1983 Prognostic value of brainstem auditory evoked potentials in neonates. Archives of Neurology 40: 360–365

125. Takeuchi T, Watanabe K 1988 The EEG evolution and neurological prognosis of perinatal hypoxia in neonates. Brain Development 11: 115–120
126. Thacker S B, Stroup D F, Peterson H B 1995 Efficacy and safety of intrapartum electronic fetal monitoring: an update. Obstetrics and Gynecology 86: 613–620
127. Thordstein M, Bagenholm R, Thiringer K, Kjellmer I 1993 Scavengers of free oxygen radicals in combination with magnesium ameliorate perinatal hypoxic–ischaemic brain damage in the rat. Pediatric Research 34: 23–26
128. Thoresen M 2002 Thermal influence on the asphyxiated newborn. In: Birth Asphyxia and the brain: basic science and clinical implications. Donn SM, Sinha SK, Chiswick ML (eds) 357–368
129. Thornberg E, Thiringer K, Odeback A, Milson I 1995 Birth asphyxia: incidence, clinical course and outcome in a Swedish population. Acta Paediatrica 84: 927–932
130. Toet M C, Hellstrom-Vestas L, Groenendaal F 1999 Amplitude integrated EEG 3 and 6 hours after birth in full-term neonates with hypoxic–ischaemic encephalopathy. Archives of Disease in Childhood, Fetal & Neonatal Edition 81: F19–F23
131. Truwit C L, Barkovich A J, Koch T K, Ferriero D M 1992 Cerebral palsy: MR findings in 40 patients. American Journal of Neuroradiology 13: 67–78
132. Van Bel F, Shadid M, Moison R M, Dorrepaal C A, Fontijn J, Monteiro L, Van de Bor M, Berger H M 1988 Effect of allopurinol on postasphyxial free radical formation, cerebral hemodynamics, and electrical brain activity. Pediatrics 101: 185–193
133. Vannucci R C, Towfighi J, Heitjan D F, Brucklacher R M 1995 Carbon dioxide protects the perinatal brain from hypoxic–ischemic damage: an experimental study in the immature rat. Pediatrics 95: 868–874
134. Vannucci R C, Vannucci S J 1978 Cerebral carbohydrate metabolism during hypoglycaemia and anoxia in newborn rats. Annals of Neurology 4: 73–79
135. Vento M, Asensi M, Sastre J 2001 Resuscitation with room air instead of 100% oxygen prevents oxidative stress in moderately asphyxiated term neonates. Pediatrics 107: 642–647
136. Vintzileos A M, Nochimson D J, Guzman E R, Knuppel R A, Lake M, Schifrin B S 1995 Intrapartum electronic fetal heart rate monitoring versus intermittent auscultation: A meta-analysis. Obstetrics and Gynecology 85: 149–155
137. Voit T, Lemburg P, Neuen E, Lumenta C, Stork W 1987 Damage of thalamus and basal ganglia in asphyxiated full-term neonates. Neuropediatrics 18: 176
138. Volpe J J 1995 Hypoxic-ischemic encephalopathy: neuropathology and pathogenesis. In: Volpe J J. Neurology of the newborn, 3rd edn. WB Saunders, Philadelphia, pp 279–313
139. Volpe J J, Herscovitch P, Perlman J M, Kreusser K L, Raiche M E 1985 Positron emission tomography in the asphyxiated term newborn: parasagittal impairment of cerebral blood flow. Annals of Neurology 17: 287–296
140. Von Essen C, Zervas N T, Brown D R, Koltun W A, Pickren K S 1980 Local cerebral blood flow in the dog during intravenous infusion of dopamine. Surgical Neurology 13: 181–188
141. Voorhies T M, Ehrlich M E, Frayer W, Lee B, Vannucci R C 1983 Occlusive vascular disease in perinatal cerebral hypoxia–ischaemia. American Journal of Perinatology 1: 1–5
142. Voorhies T M, Rawlinson D, Vannucci R C 1988 Glucose and perinatal hypoxic–ischemic brain damage in the rat. Annals of Neurology 24: 638–646
143. Wayenberg J L, Vermeylen D, Damis E 1998 Definition of asphyxia neonatorum and incidence of neurologic and systemic complications in the full-term newborn. Archives de Pediatrie 5(10): 1065–1071.
144. Wertheim D, Mercuri E, Faundez J C, Rutherford M, Acolet D, Dubowitz L 1994 Prognostic value of continuous electroencephalographic recording in full term infants with hypoxic ischaemic encephalopathy. Archives of Disease in Childhood 71: F97–F102
145. Westgate J, Harris M, Curnow J S H, Greene K R 1993 Plymouth randomised trial of cardiotocogram only versus ST waveform plus cardiotocogram for intrapartum monitoring in 2400 cases. American Journal of Obstetrics and Gynecology 169: 1151–1160
146. Wheble A M, Gillmer M D G, Spencer J A D, Sykes G S 1989 Changes in fetal monitoring practice in the UK: 1977–1984. British Journal of Obstetrics and Gynaecology 96: 1140–1147
147. Wolf G, Keilhoff G, Fischer S, Hass P 1990 Subcutaneously applied magnesium protects reliably against quinolinate-induced N-methyl-D-aspartate (NMDA)-mediated neurodegeneration and convulsions in rats: are there therapeutical implications? Neuroscience Letters 117: 207–211
148. Wyatt J S, Edwards A D, Azzopardi D et al Cerebral haemodynamics during failure of oxidative phosphorylation following birth asphyxia. Pediatric Research 26: 511A
149. Yager J Y, Heitjan D F, Towfighi J, Vannucci R C 1991 Effect of insulin induced and fasting hypoglycaemia on perinatal hypoxic–ischemic brain damage. Pediatric Research 31: 138–142
150. Yudkin P L, Johnson A, Clover L M, Murphy K W 1994 Clustering of perinatal markers of birth asphyxia and outcome at age five years. British Journal of Obstetrics and Gynaecology 101: 774–781
151. Yue T L, Feuerstein G Z 1994 Platelet activating factor. A putative neuromodulator and mediator in the pathophysiology of brain injury. Critical Reviews in Neurobiology 8: 11–24

PART 5

Preterm brain injury: preterm cerebral haemorrhage

Linda S de Vries, Janet M Rennie

Introduction

Despite the welcome decline in the incidence of bleeding into the brain of preterm infants reported in the 1990s, the condition remains the most common type of neonatal intracranial lesion. Cohort screening with ultrasound has provided information about the incidence, timing and evolution of neonatal cerebral lesions for over 20 years now. As yet, there have been very few cohorts of preterm babies who have been screened with MR imaging, but it is likely that this powerful technique will reveal that subtle intracerebral lesions are even more common than was previously suspected in this high risk group.

Terminology

In the past the term 'periventricular haemorrhage', abbreviated to PVH, was widely used in the generic sense to embrace germinal matrix haemorrhage, intraventricular haemorrhage and haemorrhage into the brain parenchyma. In our view, the term PVH

Table 41.16 Description of neonatal intracranial lesions seen early in life with ultrasound

Description	Generic term
Germinal matrix haemorrhage	Germinal matrix/intraventricular haemorrhage (GMH-IVH)
Intraventricular haemorrhage without ventricular dilatation	GMH-IVH
Intraventricular haemorrhage with acute ventricular dilatation (measure the ventricle)	GMH-IVH and ventriculomegaly
Intraparenchymal lesion – describe size, location, degree of echogenicity (see Table 41.17) and permanently record the image	Intraparenchymal lesion (IPL)

should be abandoned; it is now realised that neither are all parenchymal lesions haemorrhagic nor are they all periventricular. The Papile classification,[154] which was based on computed tomography (CT) scan appearances, is outmoded. The Papile classification was designed to grade a single CT 'snapshot' taken during the first week of life. In the Papile system grade I described a haemorrhage confined to the subependymal region, grade II was used for bleeding into the ventricular cavity but not distending it, grade III for an intraventricular bleed with ventricular enlargement and grade IV for any parenchymal lesion. There are several disadvantages to this system, including the fact that grade IV 'lumps' all parenchymal lesions together, whereas modern neuroimaging can distinguish many different types. Further, the system suggests that the types of intracranial lesion are linked in a hierarchical way, which is not the case.

The evolution of a parenchymal lesion often provides the best clue to which type of lesion it is. However, any system of classification must be applicable to the early ultrasound appearances because some babies will die before the evolving lesion can be studied, and very few babies undergo magnetic resonance imaging (MRI). In our view, the term germinal matrix/intraventricular haemorrhage (GMH-IVH) remains the most appropriate generic term for the common form of intracranial haemorrhage seen in preterm infants that does not involve the brain parenchyma. We prefer the term intraparenchymal lesion (IPL) to describe the early appearances of parenchymal lesions. Ultrasound cannot reliably distinguish between infarction and haemorrhage so we prefer not to use the term haemorrhagic periventricular infarction (HPI). Others have suggested the generic term 'white matter disease of prematurity'.[104]

It has been realised for some time now that direct extension into the parenchyma from pressure of blood in the ventricle is unlikely. Most authorities now agree that a unilateral parenchymal lesion accompanying GMH-IVH is usually caused by the presence of the GMH leading to impaired venous drainage and venous infarction.[67] Ischaemic white matter damage can be associated with secondary haemorrhage.

Intraparenchymal lesions seen early in life using ultrasound should be carefully described as to size, laterality, echogenicity and location. A permanent image should be made together with a

Table 41.17 Description of neonatal intraparenchymal lesions using ultrasound

Classification	Description
Flare or echodensity	Periventricular echodense area. Loss of the normal pattern of alternating echoreflectant and echopoor lines. Record size, side and position. Monitor duration of abnormal ultrasound appearance for at least a month and describe duration in days
Frontoparietal cystic periventricular leukomalacia (PVL)	Localised small frontoparietal cysts; lesions not involving the occipital cortex
Parieto-occipital cystic PVL	Multiple cysts in the parieto-occipital white matter
Subcortical cystic PVL	Multiple subcortical cysts in the deep white matter (multicystic leukoencephalomalacia – MCLE)
Porencephalic cyst	Single large cavity adjoining a ventricle and in communication with it

written description, which can be invaluable if the image degrades or is lost. The evolution of the parenchymal lesion should then be followed. When first seen with ultrasound most parenchymal lesions are echoreflectant, or 'bright'. Over the next weeks some resolve, many evolve into multiple small cysts and others evolve into single large cysts. Using ultrasound it is not possible to make a certain pathological diagnosis so the terms 'grade IV intraventricular haemorrhage' and 'parenchymal extension of intraventricular haemorrhage' should be abandoned. As yet there is no universal agreement on how to classify GMH-IVH or intraparenchymal lesions. A classification system suitable for describing early and late ultrasound appearances and based on that suggested by Volpe[208] and de Vries[39] is given in Tables 41.16–41.18. An attempt has been made to give equivalents (Table 41.18) so that alternative classification systems, which still exist in the literature, can be re-interpreted.

Table 41.18 Table of ultrasound descriptions with equivalent terms and pictorial examples

Description of ultrasound appearances, equivalent terms	Nomenclature used in this chapter	Examples of ultrasound appearances		
		Early	Mid	Late
Germinal matrix haemorrhage that forms a subependymal cyst Subependymal haemorrhage Uncomplicated periventricular haemorrhage Grade I PVH **NB.** Not equivalent to subependymal pseudocyst, which forms in a different place	Uncomplicated GMH-IVH			
Intraventricular haemorrhage that resolves without ventricular enlargement IVH Intraventricular haemorrhage, grade II PVH Uncomplicated periventricular haemorrhage	Uncomplicated GMH-IVH			
Intraventricular haemorrhage that at some stage is associated with enlarged ventricles (>97th centile of Levene,[14]) which does not progress to hydrocephalus Ventricular dilatation, grade III PVH	Complicated GMH-IVH GMH-IVH with non-progressive ventriculomegaly			
Intraventricular haemorrhage associated with enlarged ventricles that progresses to hydrocephalus with symptomatic raised intracranial pressure or excessive head growth Posthaemorrhagic hydrocephalus	Complicated GMH-IVH GMH-IVH with progressive hydrocephalus Posthaemorrhagic hydrocephalus			
Enlarged ventricles (usually with irregular margins) without preceding GMH-IVH Ventriculomegaly; cerebral atrophy	Enlarged ventricles without GMH-IVH Non-haemorrhagic ventriculomegaly Cerebral atrophy			
IPL (usually globular and unilateral, and usually associated with GMH-IVH) evolving to a single large porencephalic cyst Haemorrhagic periventricular infarction associated with PVH Grade IV PVH	Globular IPL with GMH-IVH evolving into porencephalic cyst			

IPL, usually unilateral, fan-shaped and associated with GMH-IVH but partially separate from the ventricle, evolving into multiple cysts Periventricular flare evolving into PVL	Fan-shaped IPL, with GMH-IVH, evolving into multiple cysts – describe anatomical location
IPL (usually bilateral) persisting for at least 48 hours without cystic evolution; can be associated with GMH-IVH, usually not Transient flare Periventricular flare	IPL persisting for 48 hours Transient flare
IPL (usually bilateral) persisting for at least 7 days without cystic evolution; can be associated with GMH-IVH, usually not Persistent flare Mild PVL Grade I PVL	IPL persisting for 7 days Prolonged flare
IPL persisting for 7 days and evolving into localised small frontoparietal cysts; lesions not involving the occipital cortex Cystic PVL Grade II PVL	IPL persisting for 7 days and evolving into localised small frontoparietal cysts Fronto-parietal cystic PVL
IPL persisting for days and evolving into multiple cysts in the parieto-occipital white matter Cystic PVL Grade III PVL	IPL persisting for days and evolving into multiple cysts in the parieto-occipital white matter Parieto-occipital cystic PVL
IPL persisting for days and evolving into multiple subcortical cysts in the deep white matter Cystic PVL Grade IV PVL	IPL persisting and evolving into multicystic leukoencephalomalacia Subcortical cystic PVL

Germinal matrix/intraventricular haemorrhage

Incidence

The first studies, using CT and ultrasound, were performed between 1978 and 1983 and showed the incidence of all forms of intracranial haemorrhage (encompassing GMH-IVH and IPL) to be 40–50% in infants with a birthweight of less than 1500 g. In the 1990s many groups noted a decline in the incidence of GMH-IVH and IPL together to about 20–30% of very-low-birthweight (VLBW) infants.[9,86,112,162] The rate of IPL alone in VLBW babies is about 8–11%.[86] The incidence and severity of GMH-IVH remains tightly related to gestational age (Fig. 41.29a). About a quarter of the cases are bilateral.

The Australian and New Zealand neonatal network reported that their IPL rate had fallen to 24% (in babies of 24–30 weeks gestation) by 1997 but that large interunit variation existed.[81] Variation in incidence between centres has also been reported from the Vermont-Oxford and National Institute of Health neonatal networks in the USA, in Canada[188] and in the Pacific Rim[129] (Fig. 41.29b). In the Canadian study, 40% of the variance was explained by differences in illness severity measured with SNAP-II. The UK and Europe have lagged behind the rest of the developed world in benchmarking, and as yet there are no similar comparative studies.

Timing

Although GMH-IVH occasionally occurs antenatally, the vast majority of preterm infants develop the lesion after birth. Sequential ultrasound studies enabled accurate timing of the onset after birth.[64] These studies showed that the majority of lesions occurred within 72 hours, with more than half occurring during the first 24 hours.[49,120,126,132,150] In 10–20% of cases extension occurs over the next 24–48 hours[113] (Fig. 41.30). GMH-IVH has been reported to occur very soon after birth in the least mature infants.[118,161] Only about 10% of GMH-IVH occurs beyond the end of the first week, in contrast to periventricular leukomalacia (PVL), where late onset is not uncommon.[2,44]

Pathogenesis

Anatomy and pathology of the preterm brain

Ruckensteiner and Zollner were the first to point out that GMH-IVH developed following haemorrhage in the subependymal germinal matrix, a structure that is most prominent between 24 and 34 weeks of gestation and has almost completely regressed by term.[174] Germinal matrix tissue is abundant over the head of the caudate nucleus and can also be found in the periventricular zone. Recently, MRI has confirmed just how extensive this tissue is in preterm infants. The germinal matrix contains neuroblasts and glioblasts, which undergo mitotic activity before the cells migrate

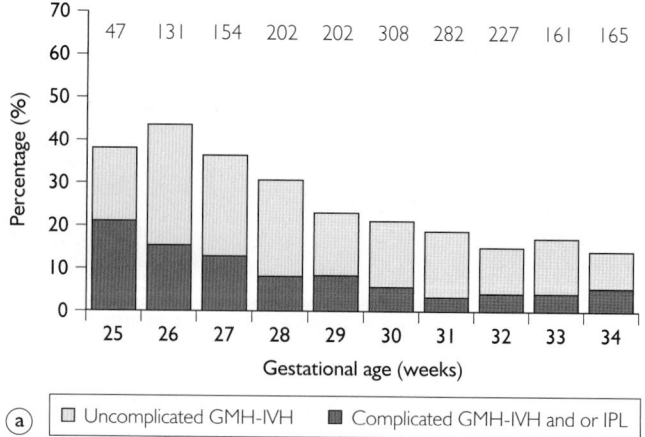

(a)

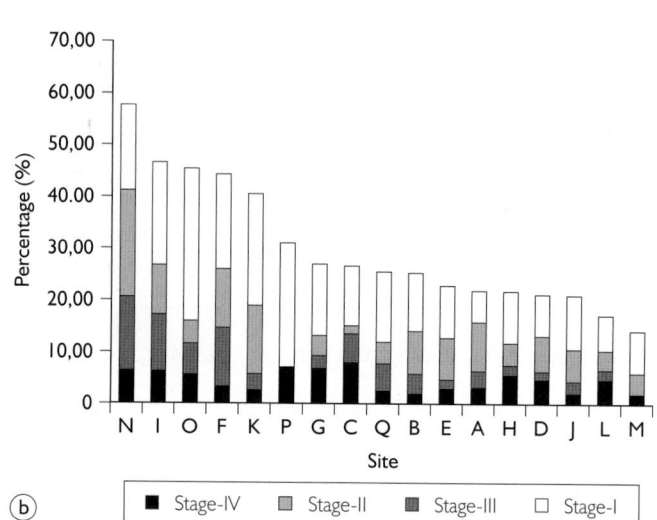

(b)

Fig. 41.29 (a) Incidence of GMH-IVH in premature infants in relation to gestational age. The number at the top of each column refers to the number of infants in each group. Data are from WKZ Hospital, the Netherlands, Sept 93–Sept 01. (b) Variation in incidence of GMH-IVH and IPL between centres. With permission from Synnes A R, Chien, L-Y, Peliowski A, Baboolal R, Lee S K 2001 Variations in intraventricular hemorrhage incidence rates among Canadian neonatal intensive care units. Journal of Pediatrics 138: 525–531.

to other parts of the cerebrum. Bleeding into the caudothalamic part of the germinal matrix was predominant in the large autopsy series from New Jersey but more than a third of cases also had bleeding into the temporal or occipital germinal matrix outer zones.[149] Choroid plexus bleeding was also common, particularly in more mature babies.

The germinal matrix receives its blood supply from a branch of the anterior cerebral artery known as Heubner's artery. The rest of the blood supply is derived from the anterior choroidal artery and the terminal branches of the lateral striate arteries.[76] Venous drainage of the deep white matter occurs through a fan-shaped leash of short and long medullary veins through which blood flows into the germinal matrix and subsequently into the terminal vein which lies below the germinal matrix.[191] The anatomical distribution of parenchymal lesions associated with GMH-IVH suggested venous infarction due to obstruction of this vein.[67] The

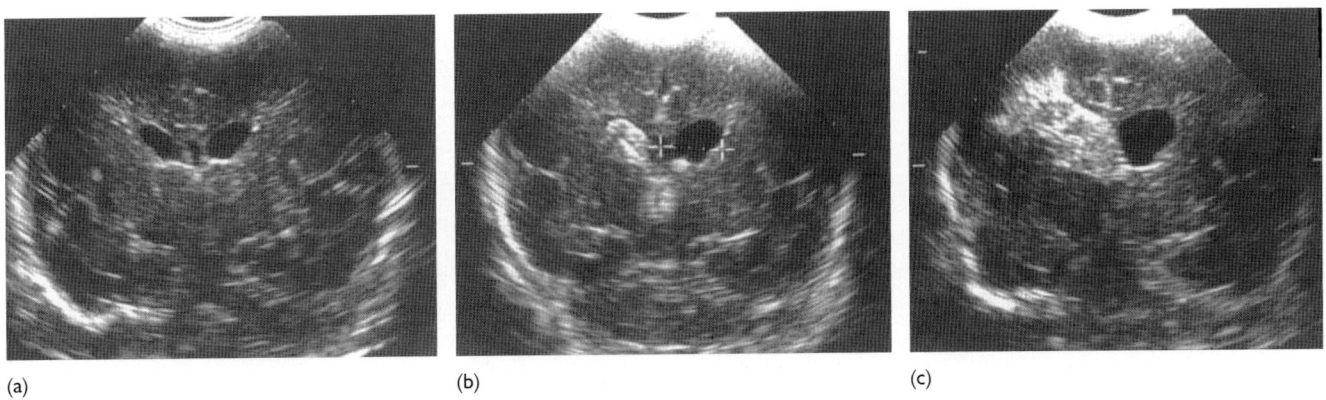

(a)   (b)   (c)

Fig. 41.30 Coronal view at 3, 12 and 36 hours. Mild ventricular dilation is seen on the first scan, a right sided IVH on the second and parenchymal involvement on the third.

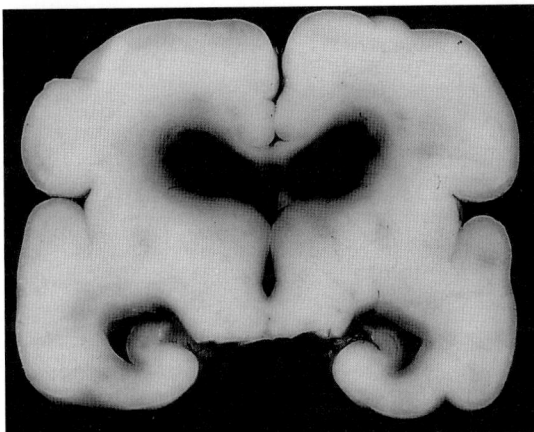

Fig. 41.31 Germinal matrix-intraventricular haemorrhage in an infant, with a gestational age of 26 weeks. Coronal section of brain.

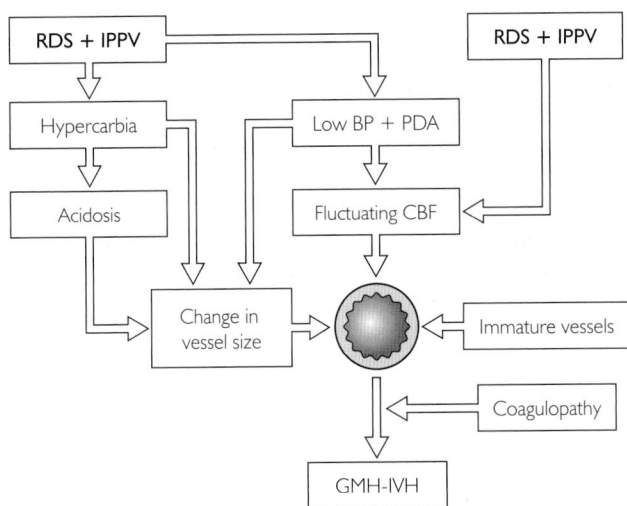

Fig. 41.32 Interaction of factors involved in the genesis of GMH-IVH.

blood can fill part of, or the entire ventricular system (Fig. 41.31), spreading through the foramen of Monro, the third ventricle, the aqueduct of Sylvius, the fourth ventricle and the foramina of Luschka and Magendie to eventually collect around the brainstem in the posterior fossa.

Cerebral blood flow and vascular factors

Prematurity and the presence of respiratory distress syndrome are the main risk factors for GMH-IVH. The best unifying hypothesis (Fig. 41.32) is that GMH-IVH occurs as a result of a combination of vulnerable immature anatomy, haemodynamic instability and the propensity to bleeding which is intrinsic to the newborn.[153] The neonatal platelet has a storage pool defect and the substances released by the neonatal endothelium tend to be vasodilators. The newborn of most species have low cerebral blood flow, and autoregulation is easily disturbed by insults such as hypoxia or acidosis, which are more likely to be present if there is respiratory disease. Impaired autoregulation renders the cerebral circulation 'pressure-passive' and hence unprotected against any wide swings or changes in blood pressure. All these factors combine to increase the risk of intracranial haemorrhage. Changes in cerebral blood flow have been documented with pneumothorax, handling and endotracheal suction,[84,160,220] all of which

have been implicated in the genesis of GMH-IVH. Carbon dioxide retention, artificial ventilation, hypoxia, hypoglycaemia, anaemia and seizures also alter cerebral blood flow.[84,168] Various prenatal and postnatal factors have been found to be associated with GMH-IVH in preterm infants (Table 41.19).[83,137,189,196,210,211]

The precise nature and origin of GMH-IVH remains uncertain. While some groups have suggested that the capillaries in the germinal matrix do not rupture easily, others have suggested that they can, because of the fact that the vessels are immature in structure with little evidence of basement membrane protein, and are of relatively large diameter.[74] Most now accept the concept that IPLs are due to venous infarction[67,191] or to a reperfusion injury following an ischaemic insult.[103,131] Ultrasound cannot reliably distinguish between haemorrhage and infarction in the early stages, hence the classification system proposed in Table 41.16.

Cerebral blood flow measurements in the newborn

There is no method that can accurately and repeatedly measure cerebral blood flow in life that is suitable for repeated use in sick preterm infants, so the pressure–passive circulation/ischaemia theories remain hypotheses. Using radioactive xenon, Lou et al

Table 41.19 Factors associated with an increased risk of GMH-IVH in preterm infants

Factor	Reference
Prenatal	
Failure to give antenatal steroids	pp. 473–4
	Crowley 1997,[32] Kari et al 1994,[99] Rennie et al 1996,[171] Shankaran et al 1995,[181] Cooke 1999,[27] Heuchan et al 2002,[81] Synnes et al 2001,[188] Linder et al 2003[120]
Maternal aspirin therapy	Rumak et al 1981[175]
Maternal smoking	Bada et al 1990,[6] Spinillo et al 1995[186]
Reason for prematurity other than pre-eclamptic toxaemia	Kuban et al 1992[106]
Male sex	Rennie et al 1996,[171] Heuchan et al 2002,[81] Synnes et al 2001[188]
Breech vaginal delivery (some studies)	Ment et al 1992[134]
Very preterm delivery	Most studies
At delivery	
Birth depression; asphyxia	Ment et al 1992,[134] Heuchan et al 2002,[81] Synnes et al 2001[188]
Birth trauma; bruising	Szymonowicz et al 1984[189]
Postnatal	
Respiratory distress syndrome, particularly if complicated by pneumothorax	Hill et al 1982,[82] Szymonowicz et al 1984,[189] Wallin et al 1990,[210] Tzogalis et al 1988,[197] Lipscomb et al 1981,[121] Linder et al 2003[120]
Hypercarbia	Wallin et al 1990,[210] Szymonowicz et al 1984,[189] Cooke 1981[26]
Acidosis	Bada et al 1990,[6] Synnes et al 2001,[188] Thorburn et al 1982[192]
Hypoxia	Bada et al 1990,[6] Weindling et al 1985[213]
Hypotension, low right ventricular output, low superior vena cava flow	Bada et al 1990,[7] Evans and Kluckow 1996,[52] Miall-Allen et al 1987,[137] Watkins et al 1989,[211] Synnes et al 2001,[188] Kluckow and Evans 2000,[103] D'Souza et al 1995,[33] Osborn et al 2002[147]
Fluctuating cerebral blood flow	Perlman et al 1983,[158] Van Bel et al 1987[198]
Low cerebral blood flow	Meek et al 1999[131]
Bruising and associated hyperkalaemia	Shortland et al 1987[183]
Coagulation disturbance (prematurity/ bruising/sepsis/low platelets)	McDonald et al 1984,[126] Thorburn et al 1982,[192] Khan et al 2002
Tolazoline therapy	Thorburn et al 1982[192]
Increased illness severity as measured by CRIB, SNAP-II	Synnes et al 2001[188], Martinez et al 2002,[129] de Courcy-Wheeler et al 1995,[36] Fowlie et al 1998[61]
Patent ductus arteriosus (low blood pressure, cerebral steal)	Evans and Kluckow 1996[52]
Postnatal transfer	Heuchan et al 2002,[81] Synnes et al 2001[188]

showed a direct linear relationship between blood pressure and cerebral blood flow in a small number of babies.[123] A fluctuating cerebral blood flow, mirroring changes in arterial blood pressure was demonstrated using Doppler ultrasound and this pattern was associated with an increased risk of GMH-IVH.[158] Muscle paralysis stabilised the fluctuating blood flow pattern and was followed by a reduction in GMH-IVH.[157] The importance of the fluctuating pattern was subsequently confirmed by some[7,198] but not by others.[136] The origin of the fluctuating pattern is almost certainly the infant fighting the ventilator and may be exaggerated in hypovolaemia.[71,167] Administration of surfactant has also been noted to cause a transient increase in cerebral blood flow by some[199] but not by others.[31] The benefits of surfactant therapy in ameliorating the severity of respiratory distress syndrome

hence reducing hypoxia, hypotension and hypercarbia clearly outweigh these theoretical risks, and surfactant therapy has generally been associated with fewer cases of GMH-IVH.[87,122]

Hypotension and cerebral ischaemia

Hypotension is a common complication of severe respiratory distress syndrome, and in the presence of a pressure passive cerebral circulation may lead to hypoxia–ischaemia of the germinal matrix and parenchyma. The brain may be damaged in the ischaemic phase or during subsequent reperfusion. Several groups have shown that arterial hypotension precedes the development of both GMH-IVH and IPL.[137,211] It has been suggested that the protective effect of antenatal steroids is due to a reduction in the

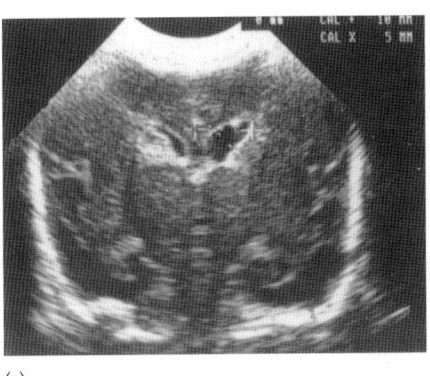
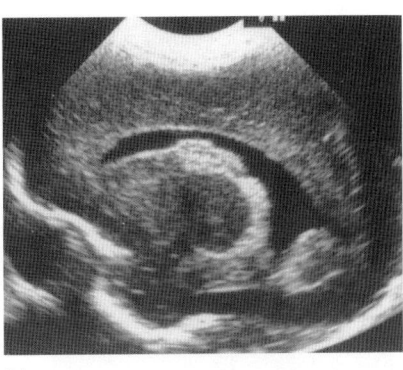

(a)　　　　　　　　　　(b)

Fig. 41.33 Coronal (a) and parasagittal (b) view showing a small GMH. Also note a small clot on the floor of the occipital horn.

need for blood pressure support, or by direct stabilisation of the capillary endothelium.[140] Early administration of gelofusin or fresh frozen plasma did not prevent either GMH-IVH or later handicap,[143] perhaps because hypotension can be due to either cardiac dysfunction or hypovolaemia.[66] Neither dopamine or dobutamine reduced the incidence of GMH-IVH.[147] Nevertheless, a reduction in GMH-IVH has been seen during an era of closer attention to blood pressure, gentle handling, synchronous ventilation and less severe respiratory distress syndrome due to antenatal steroid and postnatal surfactant therapy, rather than to any specific drug used as prophylaxis.[162,214]

Diagnosis

Clinical diagnosis

Volpe describes three clinical syndromes, the first one being *catastrophic deterioration*.[208] A sudden deterioration is noted in the baby's clinical state; examples include an increase in oxygen or ventilatory requirement, a fall in blood pressure and/or peripheral mottling, pallor, feed intolerance and acidosis. This change in condition is non-specific but, if accompanied by a drop in haematocrit, the occurrence of clinical seizures and a full fontanelle is very suggestive of GMH-IVH. The *saltatory syndrome* is more common and gradual in onset, presenting with a change in spontaneous general movements. The quality of the infant's movements may change from fluid and elegant to a paucity of cramped or stylised movements; there may be subtle seizures with eye deviation or lip-smacking (p. 1123). The third and most frequent presentation is *asymptomatic*; 25–50% of infants with GMH-IVH have no obvious clinical signs. Dubowitz et al were also able to recognise three phases on careful neurological assessment.[50] With the current ready availability of ultrasound in most neonatal units around the world, any abnormal central nervous system signs or a sudden unexplained deterioration in the general condition of a preterm neonate are indications for cranial imaging.

Ultrasound diagnosis

Cranial ultrasound is a reliable, portable and cheap non-invasive technique with which to diagnose GMH-IVH and IPL and to study their evolution over time. Good correlations with autopsy findings have been reported.[20,152,193] Most neonatal units routinely screen all VLBW admissions, partly as a form of audit and partly in order to provide an early warning of problems and to inform counselling about prognosis. The ideal protocol would include an admission scan, together with daily scans for the first week, reducing to twice weekly or weekly thereafter. Frequent scans enable accurate timing of the onset of lesions and monitoring of their evolution to assist in the final classification (Table 41.18). The records can be very helpful for audit and for medicolegal purposes, as lesions may have been evident before a given clinical event. If the available manpower or equipment allows for only a single scan then the optimal time is at the end of the first week, but repeated imaging is required to detect all lesions reliably. For more information on normal cranial ultrasound appearances see Chapter 3. Several atlases exist.[68,170]

A germinal matrix haemorrhage can be recognised as an echogenic area between the caudate nucleus and the ventricle, which evolves over a 2–4-week period into a cystic lesion that will eventually disappear (Fig. 41.33). An intraventricular bleed can be recognised as an echogenic structure within the normally echolucent ventricle (Fig. 41.34). When the amount of blood in the lateral ventricle is small, it is often difficult to make a distinction between a GMH and a GMH associated with a small IVH. A large IVH is easy to recognise and distends the ventricle in the acute stage (Fig. 41.34). Infants with GMH-IVH that is sufficiently large to form a cast of the entire ventricle are almost certain to develop posthaemorrhagic ventricular dilatation (see next section). A very large GMH-IVH that balloons the ventricle can be confused with an IPL.

Unilateral IPL associated with GMH-IVH is usually due to venous infarction. This type of lesion is classically triangular, or fan-shaped with the apex at the outer border of the lateral ventricle (Fig. 41.35). In some cases the lesion is globular with the apex of the triangle at the midline and a smooth outer border (Figure 41.35c,d) This globular type of lesion (usually unilateral) evolves over 2–3 weeks into a porencephalic cyst (Fig. 41.36) whereas those IPLs that are clearly separate from the ventricle at the start often form multiple small cysts[169] (Fig. 41.37). Porencephalic cysts do not disappear with time like those of PVL.

Magnetic resonance imaging diagnosis

Diagnosis of GMH-IVH with MRI has now been described by several groups, and the appearances of an IPL diagnosed with this method are shown in Fig. 41.38.

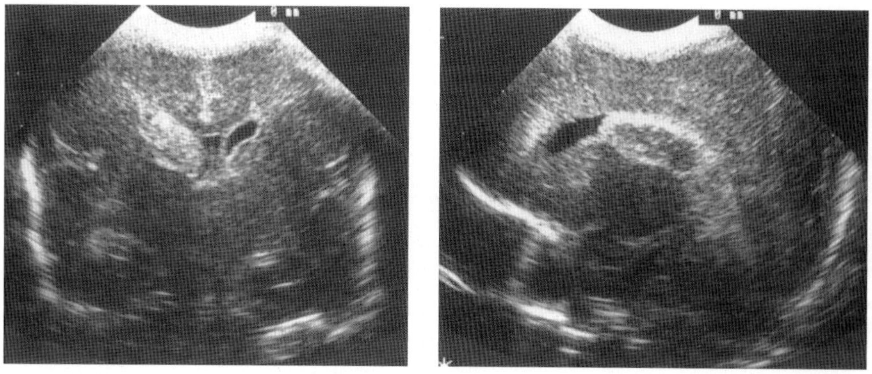

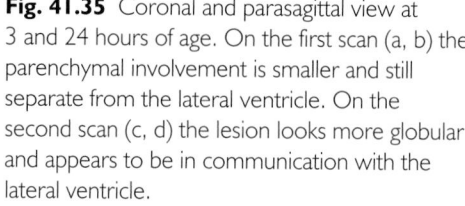

Fig. 41.34 Coronal (a) and parasagittal (b) view, showing an IVH, with a clot filling more than 50% of the right ventricle.

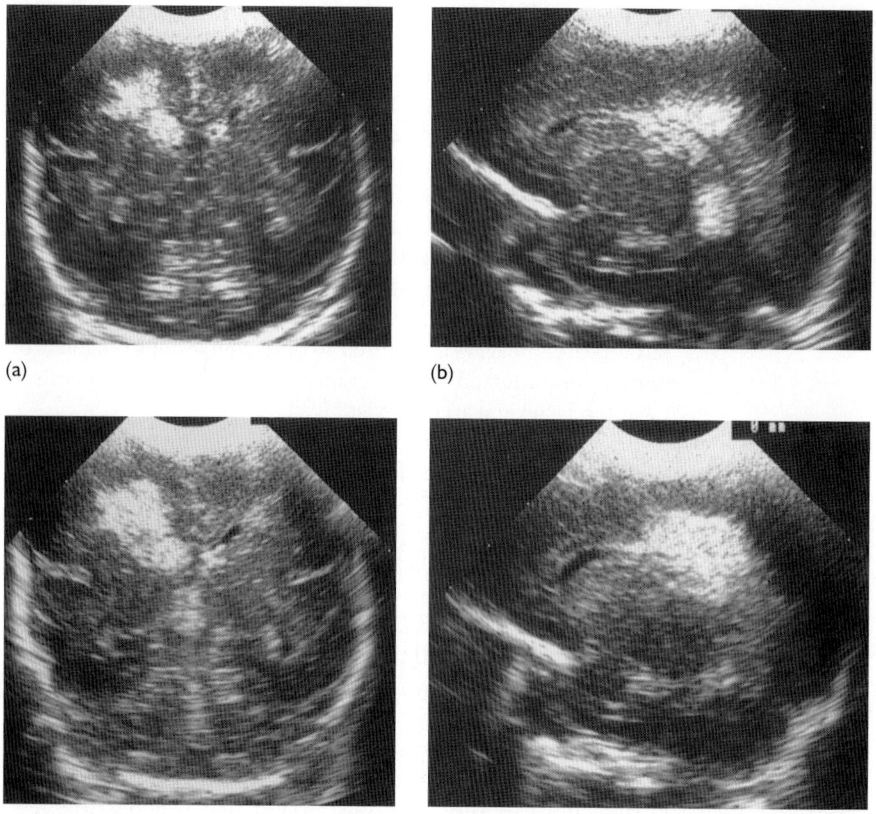

(a)

(b)

Fig. 41.35 Coronal and parasagittal view at 3 and 24 hours of age. On the first scan (a, b) the parenchymal involvement is smaller and still separate from the lateral ventricle. On the second scan (c, d) the lesion looks more globular and appears to be in communication with the lateral ventricle.

(a)

(b)

(c)

(d)

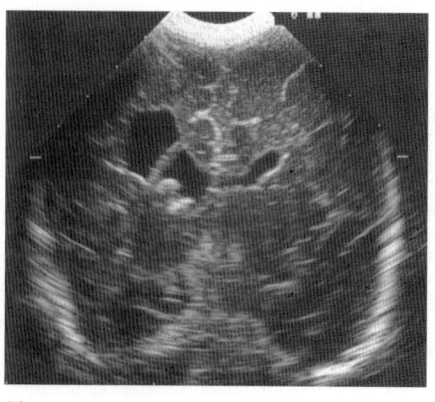

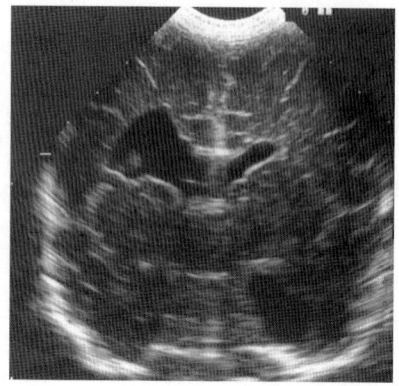

(a)

(b)

Fig. 41.36 Cranial ultrasound at 4 weeks of age; same infant as in Figure 41.30, showing the development of a porencephalic cyst, which is partially separate and partially in communication with the lateral ventricle.

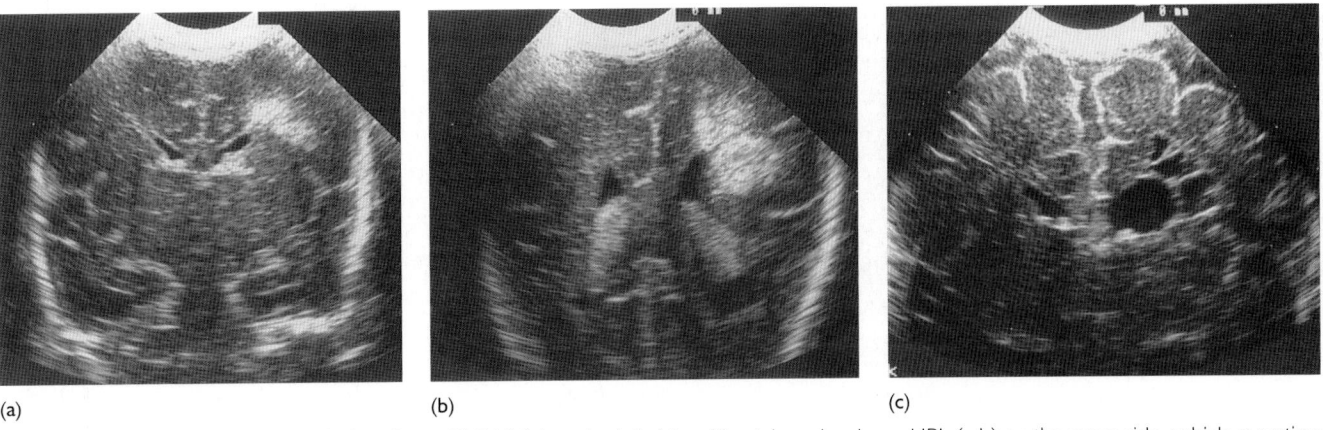

(a)   (b)   (c)

Fig. 41.37 Coronal views on day 3 showing a GMH-IVH on the left side with a triangular shaped IPL (a,b) on the same side, which over time evolves into multiple cystic lesions associated with mild ventricular dilatation on the affected side (c).

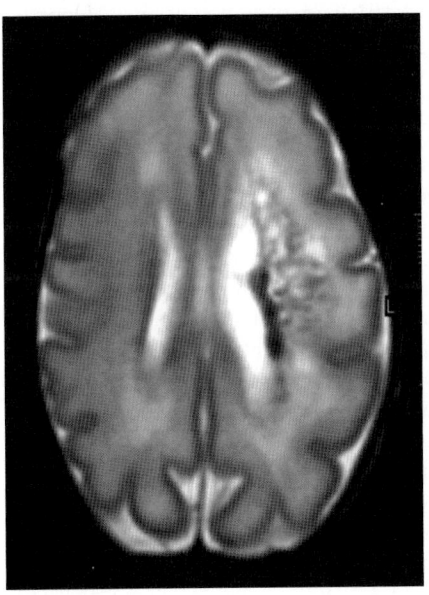

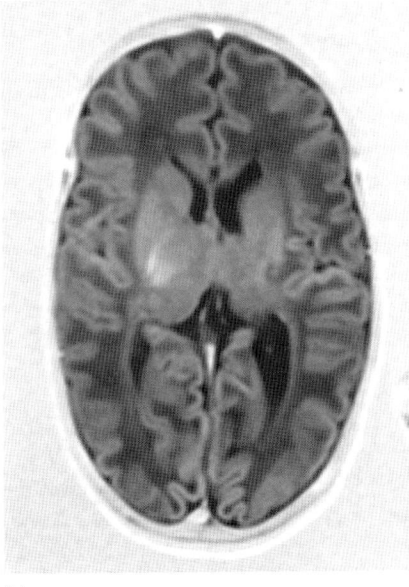

(a)   (b)

Fig. 41.38 (a) MRI, axial view, T2 TSE sequence performed at 2 weeks of age, showing the IPL with a triangular shape. The low signal is compatible with haemorrhage. (b) A repeat MRI, inversion recovery sequence, performed at 41 weeks postmenstrual age, shows asymmetry of the signal of the posterior limb of the internal capsule (PLIC), which is absent on the affected side.

Complications

Posthaemorrhagic ventricular dilatation

About 30% of infants with GMH-IVH go on to develop posthaemorrhagic ventricular dilatation (PHVD);[114] the more severe the GMH-IVH the higher the risk of developing PHVD. This condition is considered to be due to an obliterative arachnoiditis.[109] In this condition the arachnoid villi, situated over the vault of the brain, are damaged and cease to reabsorb cerebrospinal fluid (CSF), causing a communicating form of hydrocephalus. Some CSF is thought to be reabsorbed across the ependyma into small blood vessels, which become blocked with clot. Over time, transforming growth factor beta-1 may stimulate the production of extracellular matrix protein, which deposits and further blocks CSF pathways.[219]

Hydrocephalus usually develops between 10 and 20 days following the onset of the GMH-IVH. Ventricular dilatation seen using cranial ultrasound precedes the development of clinical symptoms by days or even weeks. The clinical signs are a full fontanelle, diastasis of the sutures and an increase in head size. Sunsetting of the eyes is a late sign. PHVD is transient in about half of the infants and is persistent or rapidly progressive in the remaining cases. Once it has been recognised that the ventricles are enlarged, the baseline size should be measured using ultrasound. The most widely adopted measurement system is that of Levene and Starte.[114] This 'ventricular index' is the distance between the midline and the lateral border of the ventricle measured in a coronal view in the plane of the third ventricle (Fig. 41.39). The measurement made from the scan image can then be compared to the chart of normal ranges (Fig. 41.40). There are many other reported measurement systems, including area and volume estimation, but this simple linear index has proved repeatable and robust and has a well established normal range. Another common measurement is the depth of the frontal horn taken just in front of the thalamic notch, a height of more than 3 mm being used to define ventriculomegaly and one of more than 8 mm to suggest hydrocephalus.

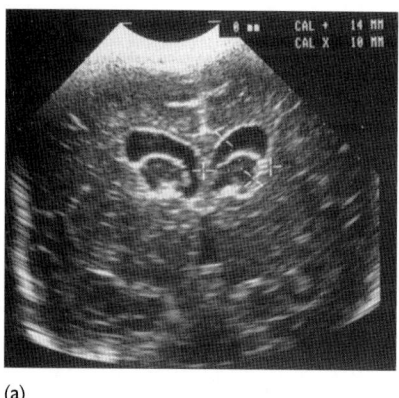
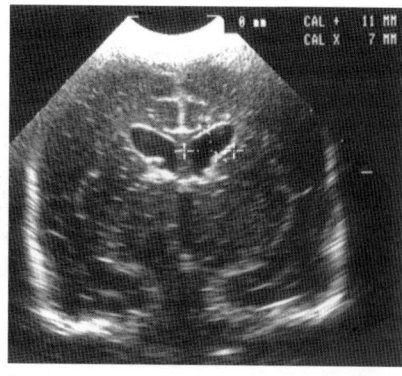

(a)   (b)

Fig. 41.39 Coronal views, showing posthaemorrhagic ventricular dilatation before and after repeated punctures from a reservoir. Both the width (the 'ventricular index') and the diagonal size are measured.

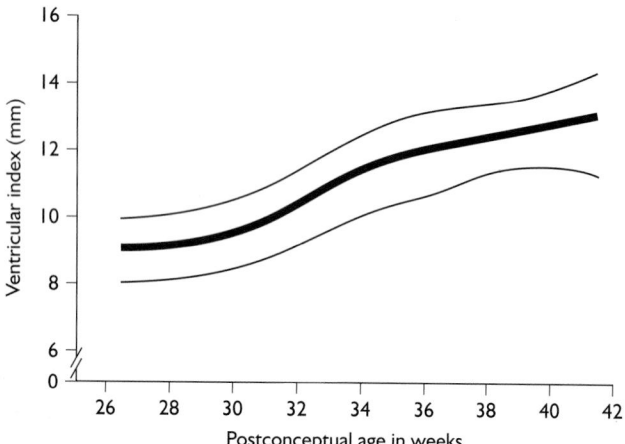

Fig. 41.40 Normal range for the ventricular index (Redrawn from Levene M I, Starte D R 1981 A longitudinal study of post haemorrhagic ventricular dilatation in the newborn. Archives of Disease in Childhood 56: 905–910.)

The key to management of PHVD is to distinguish between those cases who will require surgical treatment for progressive hydrocephalus (i.e. those with raised intracranial pressure) and those in whom the dilatation is due to cerebral atrophy (low pressure), who will not require surgery. Accurate measurement of pressure is a vital part of this assessment; the size of the ventricles cannot indicate the pressure. Progressive hydrocephalus is very likely if the CSF pressure, measured via the lumbar route in communicating hydrocephalus or via the ventricle in non-communicating cases, is more than 1.6 kPa (12 mmHg or 15.6 cm of CSF).[200,201] The upper limit of normal CSF pressure for newborns is 0.7 kPa (5.25 mmHg or 6.8 cmCSF).[97,98] Late progression has been described[156] and serial monitoring of head circumference is required for up to a year, with further ultrasound examinations if there is any concern about the pattern of head growth.

In the early stages PHVD should be monitored with serial ultrasound scans and head circumference measurements at least thrice weekly. Raised CSF pressure can cause symptoms. These include visual disturbance, seizure, feed intolerance and apnoea. In the long term, pressure-induced destruction of neuronal tissue causes motor handicap and mental retardation. Short-term adverse effects on the nervous system have been confirmed using somatosensory and visual evoked potentials,[37] Doppler estimates of cerebral blood flow velocity[179] and near infrared spectroscopy.[17]

Despite these findings there is no evidence that early drainage of CSF alters the natural history or outcome of PHVD, which is that about half of the infants will develop progressive hydrocephalus.[200,201] Once the diagnosis of ventriculomegaly has been made, a single lumbar puncture is indicated in order to measure the CSF pressure, assess whether there is communication between the lumbar and ventricular CSF, and exclude a low-grade meningitis as a cause for the ventriculomegaly. If the pressure is low at lumbar puncture but the hydrocephalus is rapidly progressive, the cause is likely to be non-communicating hydrocephalus, and ventricular drainage through an external drain or via a surgically inserted subcutaneous reservoir should be considered. Repeated ventricular taps are not recommended as they can result in multiple needle tracks through the brain, and the need for a shunt will not be prevented by this treatment.[200,201] In a large retrospective multicentre study from the Netherlands, 95 babies with large GMH-IVH and ventriculomegaly who received early or late treatment were compared.[43] The early-treated babies received treatment before their ventricular index reached 4 mm above the 97th centile of Levene and Starte; the late-treated babies were treated after their ventricles enlarged beyond this cut-off. There was a significantly reduced requirement for shunt insertion in the early intervention group, who also did better at follow-up, although this finding was not statistically significant.

Acetazolamide cannot be recommended. Results of a European randomised trial of diuretic therapy with acetazolamide in PHVD has shown no benefit from this combination of treatment; in fact the treated group did worse, with 81% disabled at a year.[94,100] A few babies have been treated with intraventricular fibrinolytic therapy which remains experimental.[217,218] Endoscopic third ventriculostomy is unlikely to be an option for many babies in view of their small size and the communicating nature of the hydrocephalus, and has not so far been successful in this group.

There is no absolute consensus regarding the point at which drainage is indicated. Some would argue that the following indications, derived from the collaborative ventriculomegaly trials, let the situation deteriorate too far and that earlier treatment leads to better results. However there can be no doubt that absolute indications for CSF drainage include:

- symptoms such as apnoea, seizure, irritability or vomiting (visual deterioration in older infants) associated with an intracranial pressure of more than 10 cmCSF;
- head circumference crossing two centile lines, or enlarging at twice the normal rate for more than 2 weeks.

Clues that the ventriculomegaly is likely to become progressive and that the child may need surgical drainage are a CSF pressure greater than 1.6 kPa at any stage (12 mmHg: 15.6 cmCSF), and a rapid progression of the ventricular index measurement. This knowledge may allow early transfer of an infant to a centre with a paediatric neurosurgeon before symptoms develop. Once it is established that treatment is required, the timing of the insertion of a suitable ventriculoperitoneal shunt can be discussed. Many neurosurgeons will insert such devices straight away, even in very small infants, but some advocate temporary external drainage or drainage via a surgically implanted subcutaneous reservoir in order to allow the infant to gain weight.[87a]

Temporary external drainage systems are prone to infection in this group and are less preferable to an indwelling device if shunt surgery has to be delayed. Some neurosurgeons regard a high CSF protein level of more than 1.5 or 2 g/l as a contraindication for permanent shunt insertion and use repeated intermittent drainage until the protein level has reduced.[65,215]

Prevention of GMH-IVH

A reduction in the incidence of GMH-IVH has been reported in many large neonatal units without any specific pharmacological prophylaxis, which is now largely historical. Details can be found in earlier editions of this book. The importance of good general care, with attention to careful control of blood pressure, coagulation defects, temperature and blood gases, gentle handling, gentle ventilation and the appropriate use of antenatal steroids and postnatal surfactant cannot be overemphasised.[207] With the low incidence of parenchymal lesions seen in most neonatal units nowadays, the use of prophylaxis against GMH-IVH, which will benefit only a few infants while exposing many to potentially serious side effects, is not recommended. The most promising specific prophylactic drug, excluding antenatal steroids, was indometacin (indomethacin).[60,133] Unfortunately the long-term outcome study[135] showed that no protection against neurodevelopmental handicap was gained from the early reduction in GMH-IVH, and this agent is not in widespread use for this purpose.

Prognosis: neurodevelopmental outcome

Uncomplicated GMH-IVH has a good prognosis. The risk of handicap in VLBW survivors with uncomplicated GMH-IVH or normal cranial ultrasound scans at discharge is 4%.[124,187,206] PHVD carries a high risk of adverse neurodevelopmental outcome, about 50%, and this increases to 75% if a shunt procedure is required.[57,148,182155,201] Only 11 of 112 infants enrolled in the

multicentre ventriculomegaly trial were normal at follow-up, underlining the poor prognosis for this group.[201] Babies were enrolled into the International PHVD drug trial 8 years later, and fewer of the control group required shunting when compared to the control arm of the early tapping trial (44% versus 62%), while more of the survivors were normal at a year (34% versus 11%). It is possible that the degree of associated white matter damage has reduced over time, but more studies are needed.

Prognosis after diagnosis of parenchymal involvement has become more difficult since the realisation that not all these lesions are haemorrhagic, and this will be discussed in the next section. Many older studies did not clearly distinguish between parenchymal involvement, ventriculomegaly and progressive hydrocephalus.[21] What is clear is that there is the occasional child with a large porencephalic cyst who is entirely normal. This is also true for a child with a few isolated cysts of PVL isolated to the anterior frontoparietal region. However, the mortality in series reporting the outcome of large IPL is high, 59% in one study,[75] with 86% of the survivors suffering hemiplegia or spastic quadriplegia. Single large porencephalic cysts are now less common, in our experience. Smaller IPLs that are only partly communicating with the lateral ventricle are more often seen nowadays and the outcome appears to be better. Of 45 babies found to have a unilateral IPL more than 1 cm in diameter, 38% did not have any motor sequelae at all at follow-up.[46] Early prediction of hemiplegia is now possible, using MRI at 40–42 weeks (Fig. 41.38). At term, myelination should be present in the posterior limb of the internal capsule; babies who have asymmetry or lack of myelination in the posterior limb of the internal capsule at term (Fig. 41.38b) went on to develop hemiplegia.[42] Diffusion tensor MR imaging can be used to visualise the tracts at an even earlier stage, but studies of preterm infants are in the very early stages.[88,138] Bilateral cystic PVL has a dismal prognosis (see next section).

Periventricular leukomalacia

History and terminology

Damage to the deep white matter in the centrum semiovale is the main reason for spastic diplegia, the most common adverse neurodevelopmental sequel of prematurity. The characteristic pattern of late white matter loss, particularly marked in the posterior trigone, is best demonstrated with MRI. Ultrasound remains important in the early evaluation of PVL despite its limitations. Myelination is actively proceeding in infants and damage to the myelin producing cells (oligodendroglia) leads to lipid accumulation, necrotic foci and cellular reaction. White matter damage in babies was observed by pathologists as early as 1867, when Virchow first described abnormal areas in the periventricular zone.[205] The term periventricular leukomalacia was coined in 1962 by Banker and Larroche, who described changes on histology in 51 infants.[8] The name was chosen as white (*leukos*) spots and softening (*malacia*) were seen in the periventricular white matter. Most of the infants in the study of Banker and Larroche were born at more than 28 weeks gestation (74% were preterm) and were several weeks old at the time of death. Anoxic events were recorded in all the cases; jaundice, sepsis and surgery were also mentioned as possible risk factors.

More recently Paneth et al[151] reported on autopsy findings in 22 very preterm infants, who died after 5 days. Although 15 of them had white matter necrosis, only three had the classical changes of PVL. Further observations were made by the same authors in their excellent monograph.[149] A total of 25 infants with white matter damage were autopsied. Only one had 'classic' PVL but the pathological changes of PVL were associated with GMH-IVH in 20 babies. Thirteen had been noted to have an increase in echogenicity in the periventricular white matter on ultrasound, and nine had ventriculomegaly apparently without GMH-IVH. We should be aware of these very important pathological studies when we are tempted to use the term PVL to describe a bright area in the brain parenchyma in a 26-week gestation infant on the first day of life. Classifying the ultrasound appearance as an IPL at this stage, as suggested by us, avoids a number of assumptions.

Pathology and vascular factors

Pathological changes include coagulation necrosis at 3–6 hours, followed by microglial activation at 6–8 hours. Several days later there is astrocytic degeneration and karyorrhexis with macrophage infiltration. Precisely when the earliest changes can be seen with ultrasound is not known; certainly a 'flare' can be seen 24–48 hours after a hypoxic–ischaemic insult in many cases. Less severe injury may not ever be detectable with ultrasound, although some babies develop late ventriculomegaly, and in others earlier imaging may show changes. Microcavities appear in the brain between 8 and 12 days with macroscopic cavities by 2 weeks, and these can be imaged with ultrasound. The pathological hallmark of PVL is coagulation necrosis. Liquefaction of the centre of the necrotic area can occur after 10–20 days and these small cavities are usually not in communication with the lateral ventricle when imaged with ultrasound (Fig. 41.41). The abnormalities reflect a response to tissue injury that is specific to highly metabolically active white matter that is undergoing rapid myelination.

Periventricular leukomalacia has long been thought to be vascular in origin and due to hypoperfusion of the boundary zones between ventriculofugal and ventriculopetal arteries.[8,190] The major arteries of the brain encircle the cerebrum and send off penetrating branches oriented towards the lateral ventricles. The discovery of a further radially arranged set of vessels travelling out from the ventricles (ventriculofugal) was thought to create a 'boundary zone' or 'watershed' susceptible to a reduction in blood supply[209] (Fig. 41.42). More recently, the existence of ventriculofugal and ventriculopetal arteries has been questioned.[105,130,142] This work used high-power stereomicroscopic instruments and the results suggested that ventriculofugal and ventriculopetal arteries are in fact transcerebral venous channels. These recent studies, suggesting that there is no ventriculofugal circulation and that the vessels previously thought to be arteries are in fact veins, have dealt a blow to the

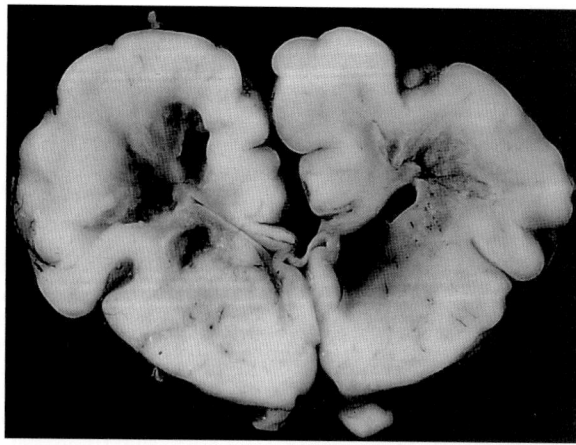

Fig. 41.41 Germinal matrix haemorrhage on the left and bilateral extensive cystic leukomalacia.

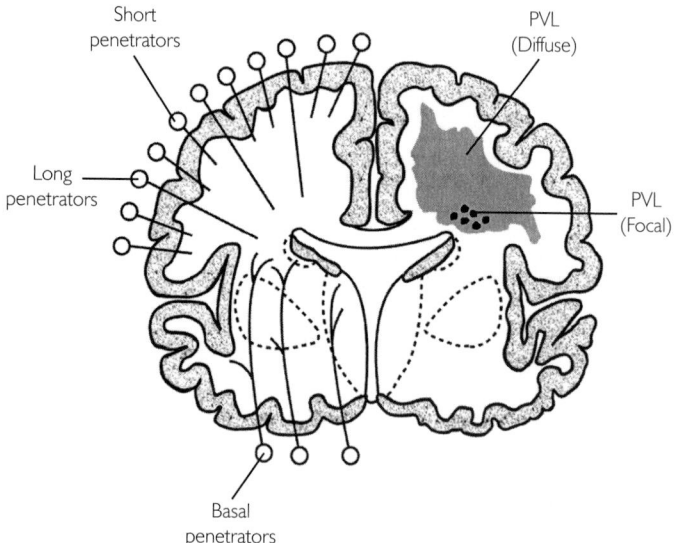

Fig. 41.42 Diagram showing coronal section with focal and diffuse components of PVL shown in one hemisphere and the cerebral vascular supply in the other hemisphere, with the long and short penetrators shown diagrammatically. Redrawn from Volpe J J 2001 Neurobiology of periventricular leukomalacia in the premature infant. Pediatric Research 50: 553–562.

ischaemia theory. However no better alternative explanation has been offered and the pathological findings clearly suggest hypoxia–ischaemia.

Incidence and timing

It is difficult to get a good idea about the incidence of PVL, as different research groups have used different classification systems in different cohorts. Often only infants with extensive cystic lesions are included, and sometimes globular unilateral IPL, usually due to haemorrhage into an area of venous infarction, is lumped together with cases of bilateral cystic PVL. Most

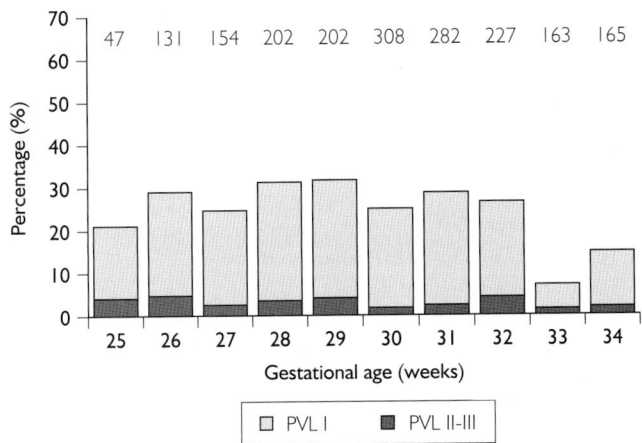

Fig. 41.43 Incidence of PVL in premature infants in relation to gestational age. The number at the top of each column refers to the number of infants in each group. Data are from WKZ Hospital, Netherlands, Sept 93–Sept 01.

large studies report an incidence of 3–10% for bilateral cystic leukomalacia.[45,54,111,112,194] When non-cystic PVL (bilateral IPL that does not progress to cystic change ('flare') is included, an incidence of 26% has been found,[111,194] which is comparable to our own experience (Fig. 41.43). A national survey in Japan, where many units have access to MRI, revealed an incidence of 5% (in babies of less than 33 weeks gestation) using ultrasound, and 8% when MRI was used to make the diagnosis.[62] There was a peak incidence at 27–28 weeks, and more PVL was seen in twins in this study.

The time of onset of PVL is much more variable than that of GMH-IVH. Occasionally the injury is of antenatal onset, for example following twin–twin transfusion syndrome with or without the death of one twin, chorioamnionitis, prolonged rupture of membranes or antepartum haemorrhage.[13,48,40,73,78,110,141,159] In these situations, fully developed cysts can be seen on the first image made shortly after birth. The time taken for an IPL of the 'flare' category (Table 41.17) to develop into cystic PVL is usually 2 weeks, although one recent Japanese study suggested that it might take longer: the median date of cyst formation was 18 days but the range was 10–39 days.[107] There is a clear relation between the severity of cystic PVL and the time it takes for the cysts to develop: i.e. the more localised the cysts the longer it takes for the cysts to develop.[164] Sometimes the initial IPL develops several weeks after birth following an acute clinical deterioration like septicaemia or necrotising enterocolitis.[2,44,176]

Pathogenesis

The pathogenesis of PVL is multifactorial and less well understood than for GMH-IVH. Hypoxic–ischaemic or toxic injury to the metabolically active oligodendroglia (OL) is thought to be important.[145] Using surface markers to identify the precise type of OL, it has been shown that the late oligodendrocyte precursor is the predominant type present at the time of peak incidence of

PVL, 32 weeks.[5] Steven Back and his colleagues describe finding the late progenitor OL in human brains between 23 and 32 weeks of gestation and believe that there is a 'developmental window of vulnerability' in the OL lineage. In tissue culture late progenitor OLs are exquisitely vulnerable to toxic effects,[4] far more vulnerable than the early OL progenitors and the more mature OLs, which are resistant to damage. It was recently shown in a culture model that glutamate is highly toxic to differentiating oligodendroglia.[145]

Several groups have found an association between ascending intrauterine infection, production of proinflammatory cytokines and white matter injury.[14,117,139,141,159,202] Leviton[116] has suggested that there may be release of tumour necrosis factor (TNF) in response to endotoxins, producing hypotension, disseminated intravascular coagulation and the production of platelet-activating factor. TNF promotes destruction of oligodendrocytes and the proliferation of astrocytes. Several groups have measured proinflammatory cytokines in the amniotic fluid, fetal plasma and cord blood. TNFα, interleukin (IL)-1 beta and interleukin-6 have been shown to be raised in the amniotic fluid of pregnant women with chorioamnionitis.[225] Others studied the in-situ expression of proinflammatory cytokines and found a high expression of TNFα, a myelinotoxic factor, in the brains of newborns with PVL.[96] The relationship between chorioamnionitis and cerebral palsy was evaluated in a recent meta-analysis and chorioamnionitis was found to be a risk factor for both cerebral palsy (RR 1.9; 95% CI 1.5–2.5) and cystic PVL (RR 2.6; 95% CI 1.7–3.9).[223] Others have shown that chorioamnionitis is associated not only with raised IL-1β and IL-6 but also with a decrease in mean and diastolic blood pressure after birth.[224] It is possible that haemodynamic disturbances make the newborn more susceptible to perinatal brain injury. In addition to antenatal cytokine exposure, postnatal infection may also be an independent risk factor for PVL.[203,216]

Like GMH-IVH, changes in blood pressure are more likely to matter if there is a pressure-passive cerebral circulation because autoregulation is lost. Studies using continuous blood pressure measurements have so far been unable to identify hypotension as an independent risk factor for white matter injury.[34,195,211] Near infrared spectroscopy (NIRS) was used in 32 preterm infants to evaluate the role of cerebral autoregulation.[196] Impaired autoregulation was confirmed in 53% using this technique and 47% of these infants developed severe intracranial abnormalities, compared to only 13% of the group with intact autoregulation. Cerebral 'steal' occurs when there is a large PDA. When this occurs there is an abnormal reversal of cerebral blood flow in diastole, rather than the normal situation of continuous forward flow, and this flow pattern has been linked to PVL.[184] Severe hypocarbia, which causes a decrease in cerebral blood flow, has been identified as an independent risk factor for PVL.[18,63,70,72,89,119,146,221] Both cerebral blood flow as well as cerebral oxygen delivery were found to be significantly reduced in infants who went on to develop PVL.[166]

The pathogenesis of bilateral IPLs that evolve into cystic PVL appears to be very different from a globular unilateral IPL that evolves into a porencephalic cyst. Bilateral cystic PVL occurs with or without GMH-IVH, the age of onset is much more variable and the lesion is much less tightly linked to gestational age.

More subtle white matter damage also occurs in the neonatal period and gives rise later to loss of white matter but goes undetected with ultrasound. These cases form the 'ultrasound-negative' group of ex-preterm children who develop cerebral palsy with an apparently normal neonatal cranial ultrasound scan, who are shown to have loss of myelin volume on MRI in later childhood.

Diagnosis and evolution

Clinical diagnosis

Compared with large GMH-IVH, the clinical signs occurring in infants who develop cystic PVL are less obvious and may easily go unnoticed, and often this devastating damage is remarkably silent from the clinical point of view. In the acute phase hypotonia and some degree of lethargy can be observed. Some 6–10 weeks later a characteristic clinical picture emerges. The infants become very irritable and are hard to pacify. They are hypertonic and show increased flexion of the arms and extension of the legs. Frequent tremors and startles can be noted and the Moro reaction is usually abnormal. General movement studies have reported these infants to have a 'cramped synchronised' movement pattern.[24] In spite of the cortical visual impairment that is often noted in later infancy in this group, visual tracking still appears normal at this stage.[51]

Electrographic diagnosis

Positive rolandic sharp waves on the EEG are an abnormal finding. These transient sharp waves are specifically associated with PVL in preterm infants and may assist in distinguishing those with a poor prognosis.[128] According to one study, the sensitivity is higher in the more mature babies (>28 weeks).[10] Others were able to make a distinction between acute and non-acute EEG changes, which was helpful in timing the onset of PVL to the antenatal or perinatal period.[79] EEG has proved a useful tool in the hands of other groups too.[25,108] One group has described a lower spectral edge frequency in the EEG of preterm babies who went on to develop white matter injury.[90]

Ultrasound diagnosis

Since 1983 many groups have shown that cystic PVL can be diagnosed using cranial ultrasound scans.[16,82,115] The angle of insonation should be wide enough to visualise the periventricular white matter and the resolution of the transducer should be high (7.5 MHz) in order to detect small cystic lesions.[39] Serial ultrasound scans, at least weekly, until discharge are essential for case ascertainment.[46a]

The recommendation made by the Committee of Child Neurology Society to perform one ultrasound examination between day 7 and day 14 would lead to many undiagnosed PVL cases, as cysts can take 10–14 days to develop. In babies with small and localised cysts, evolution takes more than 4 weeks in more than half the cases.[164] Correlation with autopsy findings has shown that ultrasound is less sensitive for the detection of PVL than for GMH-IVH.[47,54,193] The sensitivity was very high in infants who

died with cystic lesions diagnosed using ultrasound.[144] However, there have been many missed diagnoses in infants with non-cavitating PVL. Small areas of diffuse gliosis have often been seen at autopsy that had gone unnoticed with cranial ultrasound.[85,151] In the series described by Paneth most of the cases with haemorrhagic PVL were correctly diagnosed with ultrasound but those with focal non-haemorrhagic PVL were frequently missed.

Eventually the cystic lesions disappear and ventricular dilatation is often seen. The ventricular cavity typically has a scalloped inner wall and/or a square, straight-edged appearance of the trigone when imaged with MR, even years later. These findings can appear without preceding cysts or flare, probably because the damage to the oligodendroglia is too subtle to be detected with ultrasound. A glial scar can be left.

There is no generally accepted classification system for PVL. Table 41.17 gives a suggested classification.[39] Others[35] have suggested a subclassification of 'flare' into those of brief duration (1–6 days) intermediate (7–13 days) and prolonged (14 or more).

Diagnosis of periventricular flare

The main difficulty with ultrasound diagnosis of early PVL occurs with the requirement for a distinction between a genuinely echogenic patch and the normal peritrigonal 'blush' which is often seen in the brain of the very preterm infant. Ultrasound interpretation is prone to artefact due to poor transducer–skin contact and excessive gain settings and requires experience for accurate recognition. Interpretation is still subjective. Any abnormality of white matter will increase echogenicity so that the ultrasound findings are not specific.

A truly abnormal echogenic area is as bright as the choroid plexus, and the abnormality can be confirmed in more than one scan plane on more than one occasion. The genuinely abnormal area of confluent high intensity echoes completely obliterates the normal pattern of finely interlaced echogenic and echopoor lines that fan out from the periventricular zone. These gracile lines, which can normally be seen in the periventricular region, are thought to represent interfaces between the neural and vascular bundles. This abnormal ultrasound appearance, when present for more than 48 hours, is classified as a transient flare and when present for more than 7 days as a persistent flare (Tables 41.17, 41.18). A flare can coexist with GMH-IVH; if the echogenic area is globular and unilateral then it may represent a parenchymal venous infarction, as already discussed.

Areas of increased echogenicity (IPL) are usually seen 24–48 hours after the insult, whether it be a venous infarction with the globular type of IPL or the fan-shaped 'flare' that usually precedes bilateral cystic PVL. Bilateral flare can resolve within days. If areas of increased echodensity persist beyond day 7, but do not become cystic, they can be considered to represent mild leukomalacia. Mild ventricular dilatation with widening of the interhemispheric fissure is often seen with ultrasound studies later in infancy in these cases, suggesting cerebral atrophy. Gliosis has indeed been found in a few cases who died after neonatal cranial ultrasound appearances of flare evolving into mild ventriculomegaly.[47,54,127,193]

In other cases the echobright area evolves into localised small cysts a few millimetres in diameter over 2–3 weeks (Fig. 41.44, Fig. 41.45a,b).[164] These are often located in the frontoparietal

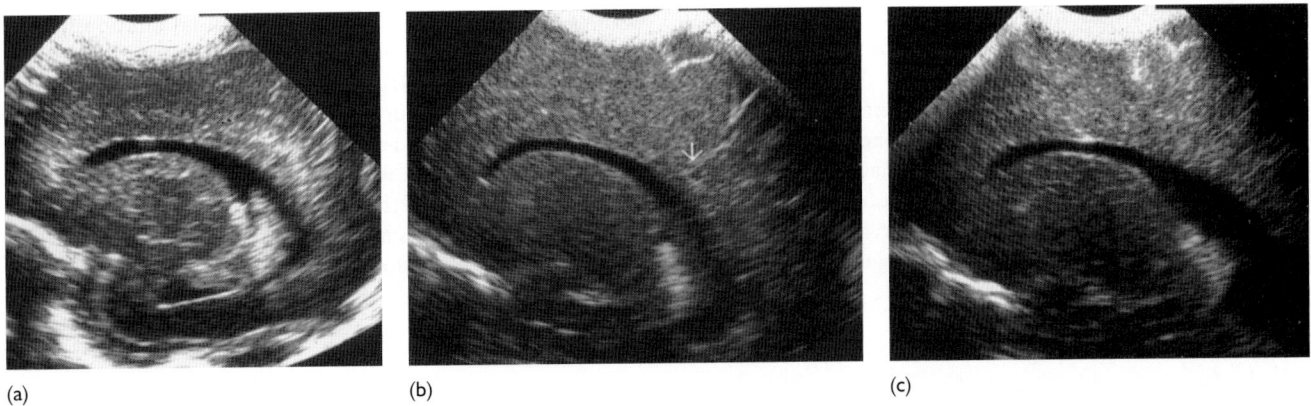

(a)   (b)   (c)

Fig. 41.44 Parasagittal views taken on day 2, 16 and 45, showing increased echogenicity in the periventricular white matter, posterior to the occipital horn, evolving into small cystic lesions (arrow) and subsequently into dilatation of the occipital horn of the lateral ventricle.

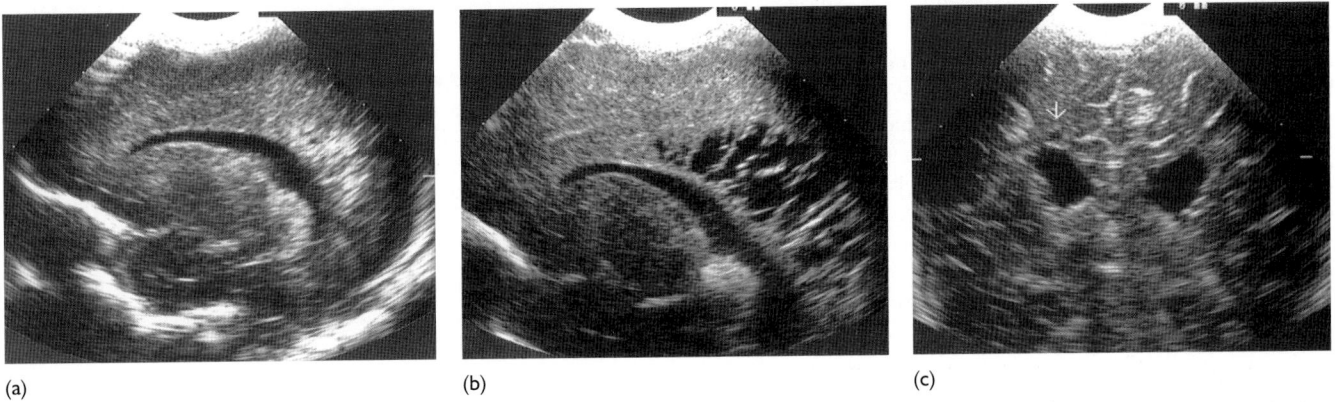

(a)   (b)   (c)

Fig. 41.45 Parasagittal views on days 2 and 21 and at 3 months, showing evolution from increased echogenicity into extensive cysts and finally dilatation ex vacuo.

periventricular white matter. In a minority of the infants extensive cystic lesions develop. These are often especially prominent in the parieto-occipital periventricular white matter (Fig. 41.45b). The cysts do not communicate with the lateral ventricle. They collapse after several weeks and are no longer visible with cranial ultrasound once the child is 2–3 months old. At this stage, irregular ventricular dilatation can be noted due to atrophy of the periventricular white matter (Fig. 41.45c). MRI performed in the second year of life confirms the irregular dilatation of the lateral ventricle and can also show white matter loss, particularly marked in the trigone, with extensive gliosis in the areas where the cysts were initially seen.[41,59]

Magnetic resonance imaging diagnosis

Ultrasonography has limitations in the diagnosis of non-cystic PVL. Even for babies with cystic PVL, MRI is superior to ultrasound: the cysts are detected earlier and often more cysts are seen with MR compared to ultrasonography.[172,185] Diffusion-weighted imaging (DWI) enables us to identify areas with cytotoxic oedema within hours of an insult. The use of DWI for early prediction of cystic evolution of areas of abnormal signal was reported by Inder.[92] The additional value of MRI is especially appreciated in

babies with non-cystic PVL. Focal areas of abnormal signal intensity are often present, referred to as punctate white matter lesions; these have signal intensity changes compatible with petechial haemorrhages.[22,125] More diffuse changes of the white matter can also be seen and are often referred to as diffuse excessive high signal intensity.[29,30,125]

The correlation of abnormalities in echogenicity with ultrasound and white matter abnormalities on MRI improves when ultrasound abnormalities persist for more than 7 days (positive predictive value 0.72 with 95% CI 0.58–0.87). Recent quantitative volumetric three-dimensional MRI techniques have been used in preterm babies with PVL. A reduction in cerebral cortical grey volume was found at term compared with either premature babies without PVL or normal term babies.[91]

Prevention

In contrast to GMH-IVH, where many intervention studies have been performed both before and after delivery, hardly any data are available with regard to the prevention of PVL. Prevention of systemic hypotension is considered to be important, in spite of the lack of convincing evidence that it is implicated. Normal blood pressure data continue to accrue (Appendix 4), but an arterial pressure of 30 mmHg is generally considered to represent a threshold for most preterm infants.[80,204,211]

Antenatal steroids are probably effective in helping to reduce the incidence of postnatal PVL, although one important study showed that it was only betamethasone that had a beneficial effect.[1,11,19] The lack of benefit for dexamethasone has been attributed to the presence of sulphite as a preservative.[12] Given the wealth of evidence that maternal chorioamnionitis is important, it is perhaps surprising that there is so little evidence (as yet) than antibiotics given antenatally are protective.[101]

Adjusting ventilatory settings in order to avoid severe hypocarbia can also be recommended on the basis of both animal studies and risk factor data in humans.[18,56,70,72,146,221,222] This may be especially important in infants ventilated with high frequency oscillation.[222]

High hypoxanthine and protein carbonyl levels were present at birth in infants who went on to develop PVL, suggesting that free radical damage might be important.[93,178] One randomised double-blind study used allopurinol, an inhibitor of xanthine oxidase, but no protective effect could be shown.[177] Another retrospective case control study showed that infants who were exposed to magnesium sulphate in utero were less likely to develop cystic PVL.[58] A prospective study is needed to support these findings.

Prognosis: neurodevelopmental outcome

There is no doubt that bilateral occipitoparietal cystic PVL is the most powerful predictor of cerebral palsy (usually spastic diplegia) among the neonatal cranial ultrasound lesions so far described.[16,77,212] In many preterm cohort follow-up studies almost all the cases of cerebral palsy had bilateral occipital leukomalacia in the neonatal period.[15,56,69,163,165,173] Earlier studies, reporting an association between ventricular dilatation and adverse outcome,[21,187] probably included some undiagnosed cases of PVL due to poor resolution of the older ultrasound scanners. Single cysts and cysts confined to the frontal region appear to have a better outcome than multiple bilateral occipital cysts, where the outlook is universally dismal.[21] Cerebral visual impairment is another important sequel and attempts should be made to recognise this early in infancy, for example using visual acuity cards.[23,51,180] Bilateral occipital cystic white matter damage carries a significantly higher risk of developing a major handicap than a large unilateral parenchymal haemorrhage.[38] As leukomalacia is almost always bilateral there is little scope for compensation by the contralateral hemisphere.

While transient densities were not taken very seriously to start with, they are now generally considered to be a mild form of leukomalacia provided they persist for at least 7–14 days. Both short- and long-term follow-up studies have shown an adverse effect on neurodevelopmental outcome, with a risk of developing spastic diplegia of 5–10%.[3,47,55,127] In the early follow-up studies almost half of infants surviving with persistent echodensity without cystic change were found to have transient abnormalities in tone. When these children were assessed again at the age of 6 years and compared with preterm infants with normal ultrasound scans, no difference was found in cognitive

abilities. However, the results of standardised motor assessment showed that performance decreased significantly if there had been prolonged periventricular echodensity.[95] Other groups have also noted abnormal neuromotor signs as well as lower cognitive abilities.[53] As yet, there is very little information on the outcome of babies with punctate white matter lesions.[28] Only one of our 10 preterm babies with this MRI finding had a delay in language development, while the others were considered normal at 2 years. No follow-up information is available for babies with diffuse excessive high signal intensity on their MRI.

Conclusion

For over 20 years the use of cranial ultrasound imaging has allowed documentation of a changing pattern of brain injury in preterm infants. In particular, the realisation that not all parenchymal lesions are of uniform aetiology has been an important finding. In view of the fact that the prognosis for bilateral occipital cystic white matter damage is so poor, the challenge for the next decade is to increase understanding of this condition. Neonatology would achieve much if a reduction in incidence could be obtained of similar magnitude to that which has been accomplished in GMH-IVH.

References

1. Agarwal R, Chiswick M L, Rimmer S et al 2002 Antenatal steroids are associated with a reduction in the incidence of cerebral white matter lesions in very low birthweight infants. Archives of Disease in Childhood Fetal and Neonatal Edition 86: F96–F101
2. Andre P, Thebaud B, Delavaucoupet J et al 2001 Late-onset cystic periventricular leukomalacia in premature infants: a threat until term. American Journal of Perinatology 18: 79–86
3. Appleton R E, Lee R E J, Hey E N 1990 Neurodevelopmental outcome of transient neonatal echodensities. Archives of Disease in Childhood 65: 27–29
4. Back S A, Han B H, Luo N L et al 2002 Selective vulnerability of late oligodendrocyte progenitors to hypoxia-ischaemia. Journal of Neuroscience 22: 455–463
5. Back S A, Luo N L, Borenstein N S, Levine J M, Volpe J J, Kinney H C 2001 Late oligodendrocyte progenitors coincide with the developmental window of vulnerability for human perinatal white matter injury. Journal of Neuroscience 21: 1302–1312
6. Bada H S, Korones S B, Perry E H et al 1990 Frequent handling in the neonatal intensive care unit and intraventricular hemorrhage. Journal of Pediatrics 117: 126–131
7. Bada H S, Krones S B, Perry E H et al 1990 Mean arterial blood pressure changes in premature infants and those at risk for periventricular hemorrhage. Journal of Pediatrics 117: 607–614
8. Banker B Q, Larroche J C 1962 Periventricular leukomalacia of infancy. A form of neonatal anoxic encephalopathy. Archives of Neurology 7: 386–410
9. Batton D G, Holtrop P, DeWitte D, Pryce C, Roberts C 1994 Current gestational age-related incidence of major intraventricular hemorrhage. Journal of Pediatrics 125: 623–625
10. Baud O, d'Allest, A-M, Lacaze-Masmonteio T et al 1998 The early diagnosis of periventricular leukomalacia in premature infants with positive rolandic sharp waves on serial electroencephalography. Journal of Pediatrics 132: 813–817
11. Baud O, Foix-L'Helias L, Kaminski M et al 1999 Antenatal glucocorticoid treatment and cystic periventricular leukomalacia in very premature infants. New England Journal of Medicine 341: 1190–1196

12. Baud O, Laudenbach V, Evrard P, Gressens P 2001 Neurotoxic effects of fluorinated glucocorticoid preparations on the developing mouse brain: role of preservatives. Pediatric Research 50: 706–711

13. Bejar R, Vigliocco G, Gramajo H, Solana C, Benirschke K, Berry C 1990 Antenatal origins of neurologic damage in newborns II. multiple gestations. American Journal of Obstetrics and Gynecology 162: 1230–1236

14. Bejar R, Wozniak P, Allard M et al 1988 Antenatal origin of neurologic damage in newborn infants I preterm infants. American Journal of Obstetrics and Gynecology 159: 357–363

15. Bennett F C, Silver G, Leung E J, Mack L A 1990 Periventricular echodensities detected by cranial ultrasound: usefulness in predicting neurodevelopmental outcome in low birthweight:preterm infants. Pediatrics 85: 400–404

16. Bozynski M E A, Nelson M N, Matalon T A S et al 1985 Cavitary periventricular leukomalacia: incidence and short-term outcome in infants weighing less than 1,200 grams at birth. Developmental Medicine and Child Neurology 27: 572–577

17. Caesar P, von Siebenthal K, van der Vlugt A 1993 Cytochrome aa3 and intracranial pressure in newborn infants: a near infrared spectroscopy study (letter). Neuropediatrics 23: 111

18. Calvert S A, Hoskins E M, Fong K W, Forsyth S C 1987 Etiological factors associated with periventricular leukomalacia. Acta Paediatrica Scandinavica 75: 254–259

19. Canterino J C, Verma U, Visintainer P F, Elimian A, Klein S A, Tejani H 2001 Antenatal steroids and neonatal periventricular leukomalacia. Obstetrics and Gynecology 97: 135–139

20. Carson S C, Hertzberg B S, Bowie J D, Burger P C 1990 Value of sonography in the diagnosis of intracranial hemorrhage and periventricular leukomalacia: a post mortem study of 35 cases. American Journal of Radiology 155: 595–601

21. Catto-Smith A G, Yu V Y H, Bajuk B, Orgill A A, Astbury J 1985 Effect of neonatal periventricular haemorrhage on neurodevelopmental outcome. Archives of Disease in Childhood 60: 8–11

22. Childs A-M, Cornette L, Ramenghi L A et al 2001 Magnetic resonance and cranial ultrasound characteristics of periventricular white matter abnormalities in newborn infants. Clinical Radiology 56: 647–655

23. Cioni G, Bertuccelli B, Boldrini A et al 2000 Correlation between visual function, neurodevelopmental outcome, and magnetic resonance imaging findings in infants with periventricular leucomalacia. Archives of Disease in Childhood 82: F134–F140

24. Cioni G, Prechtl H F R 1990 Preterm and early post-term motor behaviour in low-risk premature infants. Early Human Development 23 120–132

25. Connell J A, Oozeer R C, Regev R, de Vries L S, Dubowitz L M S, Dubowitz V 1987 Continuous 4 channel EEG in the evaluation of echodense ultrasound lesions. Archives of Disease in Childhood 62: 1019–1024

26. Cooke R W I 1981 Factors associated with periventricular haemorrhage in very low birthweight infants. Archives of Disease in Childhood 56: 425–431

27. Cooke R W I 1999 Trends in incidence of cranial ultrasound lesions and cerebral palsy in very low birthweight infants 1982–1993. Archives of Disease in Childhood 80: F115–F117

28. Cornette L G, Tanner S F, Ramenghi L A et al 2002 Magnetic resonance imaging of the infant brain: anatomical characteristics and clinical significance of punctate lesions. Archives of Disease in Childhood 86: 171–177

29. Counsell S J, Allsop J M, Harrison M C et al 2003 Diffusion-weighted imaging of the brain in preterm infants with focal and diffuse white matter abnormality. Pediatrics 112: 1–7

30. Counsell S J, Rutherford M A, Cowan F M, Edwards A D 2003 Magnetic resonance imaging of preterm brain injury. Archives of Diseases in Childhood 88: 269–274

31. Cowan F, Whitelaw A, Wertheim D, Silverman M 1991 Cerebral blood flow velocity after surfactant administration. Archives of Disease in Childhood 66: 1105–1109

32. Crowley P 1997 Corticosteroids prior to preterm delivery. In Neilson J P et al (eds) Pregnancy and childbirth module of the Cochrane Collaboration, 3rd edn. Update Software, Oxford

33. D'Souza S W, Janakova H, Minors D et al 1995 Blood pressure, heart rate, and skin temperature in preterm infants: association with periventricular haemorrhage. Archives of Disease in Childhood 72: F162–F167

34. Dammann O, Allred E N, Kuban K C K et al 2002 Systemic hypotension and white-matter damage in preterm infants. Developmental Medicine and Child Neurology 44: 82–90

35. Dammann O, Leviton A 1997 Duration of transient hyperechoic images of white matter in very-low-birthweight infants: a proposed classification. Developmental Medicine and Child Neurology 39: 2–5

36. De Courcy-Wheeler R, Wolfe C, Fitzgerald A, Spencer M, Goodman J, Gamsu H 1995 The use of the CRIB score in prediction of neonatal mortality and morbidity. Archives of Disease in Childhood 73: F32–F36

37. De Vries L S 1990 Short latency cortical SEP in infants with hydrocephalus. Neuropediatrics 21: 136–139

38. De Vries L S, Dubowitz L M S, Dubowitz V 1985 Predictive value of cranial ultrasound in the newborn baby : a reappraisal. Lancet 2: 137–140

39. De Vries L S, Eken P, Dubowitz L M S 1992 The spectrum of leukomalacia using cranial ultrasound. Behavioural Brain Research 49: 1–6

40. De Vries L S, Eken P, Groenendaal F, Rademaker K J, Hoogervorst B, Bruinse H W 1998 Antenatal onset of haemorrhagic and/or ischaemic lesions in preterm infants: prevalence and associated obstetric variables. Archives of Disease in Childhood 78: F51–F56

41. De Vries L S, Eken P, Groenendaal F, van Haastert I C, Meiners L C 1993 Correlation between the degree of periventricular leukomalacia diagnosed using cranial ultrasound and MRI later in infancy of children with cerebral palsy. Neuropediatrics 24: 263–268

42. De Vries L S, Groenendaal F, van Haastert I C, Eken P, Rademaker K J, Meiners L C 1999 Asymmetrical myelination of the posterior limb of the internal capsule in infants with periventricular haemorrhagic infarction: an early predictor of hemiplegia. Neuropediatrics 30: 314–319

43. De Vries L S, Liem K D, van Dijk K, Smit B J, Rademaker K J, Gavilanes A W D 2003 Early versus late treatment of posthaemorrhagic ventricular dilatation: results of a retrospective study from five neonatal intensive care units in the Netherlands. Acta Paediatrica 91: 212–217

44. De Vries L S, Regev R, Dubowitz L M S 1986 Late onset cystic leukomalacia. Archives of Disease in Childhood 61: 298–299

45. De Vries L S, Regev R, Pennock J M, Wigglesworth J S, Dubowitz L M S 1988 Ultrasound evolution and later outcome of infants with periventricular densities. Early Human Development 16: 225–233

46. De Vries L S, Roelants-van Rijn A M, Rademaker K J, van Haastert I C, Beek F J A, Groenendaal F 2001 Unilateral parenchymal haemorrhagic infarction in the preterm infant. European Journal of Paediatric Neurology 5: 139–149

46a. De Vries L S, Van Haastert I L, Rademaker K J, Koopman C, Groenendaal F 2004 Ultrasound abnormalities preceding cerebral palsy in high-risk preterm infants. J Pediatr 144: 815–820

47. De Vries L S, Wigglesworth J S, Regev R, Dubowitz L M S 1988 Evolution of periventricular leukomalacia during the neonatal period and infancy: correlation of imaging and post mortem findings. Early Human Development 17: 205–219

48. Denbow M L, Battin M R, Cowan F, Azzopardi D, Edwards A D, Fisk N M 1998 Neonatal cranial ultrasonographic findings in preterm twins complicated by severe fetofetal transfusion syndrome. American Journal of Obstetrics and Gynecology 178: 479–483

49. Dolfin T, Skidmore M B, Fong K W, Hoskins E M, Shennan A T 1983 Incidence, severity, and timing of subependymal and intraventricular hemorrhages in preterm infants born in a perinatal unit as detected by serial real-time ultrasound. Pediatrics 71: 541–546

50. Dubowitz L M S, Levene M I, Morante A, Palmer P, Dubowitz V 1981 Neurological signs in neonatal intraventricular hemorrhage: correlation with real time ultrasound. Journal of Pediatrics 99: 127–133

51. Eken P, van Nieuwenhuizen O, van der Graag Y, Schalij-Delfos N E, de Vries L S 1994 Relation between neonatal cranial ultrasound abnormalities and cerebral visual impairment in infancy. Developmental Medicine and Child Neurology 36: 3–15

52. Evans N, Kluckow M 1996 Early ductal shunting and intraventricular haemorrhage in ventilated preterm infants. Archives of Disease in Childhood 75: F183–F186

53. Fawer C-L, Calame A 1991 Significance of ultrasound appearances in the neurological development and cognitive abilities of preterm infants at 5 years. European Journal of Pediatrics 556: 515–520

54. Fawer C-L, Calame A, Perentes E, Anderegg A 1985 Periventricular leukomalacia: a correlation study between real time ultrasound and autopsy findings. Neuroradiology 27: 292–230

55. Fawer C-L, Diebold P, Calame A 1987 Periventricular leukomalacia and neurodevelopmental outcome in preterm infants. Archives of Disease in Childhood 62: 30–36

56. Fazzi E, Orcesi S, Caffi L, Ometto A, Rondini G, Telesca C 1994 Neurodevelopmental outcome at 5–7 years in preterm infants with periventricular leukomalacia. Neuropediatrics 25: 134–139

57. Fernell E, Hagberg G, Hagberg B 1993 Infantile hydrocephalus in preterm, low birthweight infants: a nationwide Swedish cohort 1979–1988. Acta Paediatrica 82: 45–48

58. Finesmith R B, Roche K, Yellin P B et al 1997 Effect of magnesium sulfate on the development of cystic periventricular leukomalacia in preterm infants. Americal Journal of Perinatology 14: 303–307

59. Flodmark O, Lupton B, Li D et al 1989 MR imaging of periventricular leukomalacia in childhood. American Journal of Neuroradiology 10: 111–118

60. Fowlie P W 1996 Prophylactic indomethacin: systematic review and a meta-analysis. Archives of Disease in Childhood 74: F81–F86

61. Fowlie P W, Tarnow-Mordi W, Gould C R, Strang D 1998 Predicting outcome in very low birthweight infants using an objective measure of illness severity and cranial ultrasound scanning. Archives of Disease in Childhood 78: F175–F178

62. Fujimoto S, Togari H, Takashima S et al 1998 National survey of periventricular leukomalacia in Japan. Acta Paediatrica Japonica 40: 239–243

63. Fujimoto S, Togari H, Yamaguchi N, Mizutami F, Suzuki S, Sobajima H 1994 Hypocarbia and cystic periventricular leukomalacia in preterm infants. Archives of Disease in Childhood 71: F107–F110

64. Funato M, Tamai H, Noma K et al 1992 Clinical events in association with timing of intraventricular hemorrhage in preterm infants. Journal of Pediatrics 121: 614–619

65. Gaskill S J, Marlin A E, Rivera S 1988 The subcutaneous ventricular reservoir: an effective treatment for posthaemorrhagic hydrocephalus. Childs Nervous System 4: 291–295

66. Gill A B, Weindling A M 1993 Randomised controlled trial of plasma protein fraction versus dopamine in hypotensive very low birthweight infants. Archives of Disease in Childhood 69: 284–287

67. Gould S J, Howard S, Hope P L, Reynolds E O R 1987 Periventricular intraparenchymal cerebral haemorrhage in preterm infants: the role of venous infarction. Journal of Pathology 151: 197–202

68. Govaert P, de Vries L S 1997 An atlas of neonatal brain sonography. Mackeith Press, London

69. Graham M, Levene M I, Trounce J Q, Rutter N 1987 Prediction of cerebral palsy in very low birthweight infants: prospective ultrasound study. Lancet 2: 593–594

70. Graziani L J, Spitzer A R, Mitchell D G et al 1992 Mechanical ventilation in preterm infants: neurosonographic and developmental studies. Pediatrics 90: 515–522

71. Greenough A, Wood S, Morley C J, Davis J 1984 Pancuronium prevents pneumothorax in ventilated preterm babies who actively expire against positive pressure inflation. Lancet 1: 1–3

72. Greisen G, Munck H, Lou H 1987 Severe hypocarbia in preterm infants and neurodevelopmental deficit. Acta Paediatrica Scandinavica 76: 401–404

73. Grether J K, Nelson K B, Emery E S, Cummins S K 1996 Prenatal and perinatal factors and cerebral palsy in very low birthweight infants. Journal of Pediatrics 128: 407–414

74. Grunnet M R L 1989 Morphometry of blood vessels in the cortex and germinal plate of premature neonates. Pediatric Neurology 5: 12–16

75. Guzzetta F, Shackleford G D, Volpe S, Perlman J M, Volpe J J 1986 Periventricular echodensities in the newborn period: critical determinant of neurologic outcome. Pediatrics 78: 955–1006

76. Hambleton G, Wigglesworth J S 1976 Origin of intraventricular haemorrhage in the preterm infant. Archives of Disease in Childhood 51: 651–659

77. Han T R, Bang M S, Lim J Y, Yoon B H, Kim I W 2002 Risk factors of cerebral palsy in preterm infants. American Journal of Physical Medicine and Rehabilitation 81: 297–303

78. Haverkamp F, Lex C, Hanisch C, Fahnenstich H, Zerres K 2001 Neurodevelopmental risks in twin-to-twin transfusion syndrome: preliminary findings. European Journal of Paediatric Neurology 5: 221–227

79. Hayakawa F, Okumura A, Kato T, Kuno K, Watanabe K 1999 Determination of timing of brain injury in preterm infants with periventricular leukomalacia with serial neonatal electroencephalography. Pediatrics 104: 1077–1088

80. Hegyi T, Carbone M T, Anwar M 1994 Blood pressure ranges in preterm infants: I – the first hours of life. Journal of Pediatrics 124: 627–633

81. Heuchan A M, Evans N, Henderson-Smart D J, Simpson J M 2002 Perinatal risk factors for major intraventricular haemorrhage in the Australian and New Zealand neonatal network, 1995–1997. Archives of Disease in Childhood 86: F86–F90

82. Hill A, Melson G L, Clark H B, Volpe J J 1982 Haemorrhagic periventricular leukomalacia: diagnosis by real time ultrasound and correlation with autopsy findings. Pediatrics 69: 282–284

83. Hill A, Perlman J M, Volpe J J 1982 Relationship of pneumothorax to occurence of intraventricular hemorrhage in the premature newborn. Pediatrics 69: 144–145

84. Hill A, Volpe J J 1981 Seizures, hypoxic-ischemic brain injury, and intraventricular hemorrhage in the newborn. Annals of Neurology 10: 109–121

85. Hope P L, Gould S J, Howard S, Hamilton P A, Costello A M, Reynolds E O R 1988 Precision of ultrasound diagnosis of pathologically verified lesions in the brains of very preterm infants. Developmental Medicine and Child Neurology 30: 457–471

86. Horbar J D, Badger G J, Carpenter J H et al 2002 Trends in mortality and morbidity for very low birthweight infants, 1991–1999. Pediatrics 110: 143–151

87. Horbar J D, Soll R F, Schaginger H 1990 A European multicentre randomized controlled trial of single dose surfactant therapy for idiopathic respiratory distress syndrome. European Journal of Pediatrics 149: 416–423

87a. Hudgins R J, Boydston W R, Gilreath C L 1998 Treatment of posthemorrhagic hydrocephalus in the preterm infant with a ventricular access device. Pediatric Neurosurgery 29: 309–313

88. Huppi P S, Murphy B, Maier S E et al 2001 Microstructural brain development after perinatal cerebral white matter injury assessed by diffusion tensor magnetic resonance imaging. Pediatrics 107: 455–460

89. Ikonen R S, Janas M O, Koivikko M J, Laippala P, Kuusinen E J 1991 Hyperbilirubinaemia, hypocarbia and periventricular leukomalacia in preterm infants. Acta Paediatrica Scandinavica 81: 802–807

90. Inder T E, Buckland L, Williams C E et al 2003 Lowered electroencephalographic spectral edge frequency predicts the presence of cerebral white matter injury in premature infants. Pediatrics 111: 27–33

91. Inder T E, Huppi P S, Warfield S et al 1999 Periventricular white matter injury in the premature infant is followed by reduced cerebral cortical gray matter volume at term. Annals of Neurology 46: 755–760

92. Inder T E, Huppi P S, Zientara G P et al 1999 Early detection of periventricular leukomalacia by diffusion-weighted magnetic resonance imaging techniques. Journal of Pediatrics 134: 631–634

93. Inder T E, Mocatta T, Darlow B, Spencer C, Volpe J J, Winterbourn C 2002 Elevated free radical products in the cerebrospinal fluid of VLBW infants with cerebral white matter injury. Pediatric Research 52: 213–218

94. International PHVD Drug Trial Group 1998 International randomised controlled trial of acetazolamide and furosemide in posthaemorrhagic ventricular dilatation in infancy. Lancet 352: 433–440

95. Jongmans M, Henderson S, de Vries L S, Dubowitz L 1993 Duration of periventricular densities in preterm infants and neurologic outcome at 6 years of age. Archives of Disease in Childhood 69: 9–13

96. Kadhim H, Tabarki B, Verellen G, De Prez C, Rona A-M, Sebire G 2001 Inflammatory cytokines in the pathogenesis of periventricular leukomalacia. Neurology 56: 1278–1284

97. Kaiser A M, Whitelaw A 1986 Cerebrospinal fluid pressure during post haemorrhagic ventricular dilatation in newborn infants. Archives of Disease in Childhood 60: 920–924

98. Kaiser A M, Whitelaw A G L 1986 Normal cerebrospinal fluid pressure in the newborn. Neuropediatrics 17: 100–102

99. Kari M A, Hallman M, Eronen M, Teramo K, Virtanen M, Koivisto M 1994 Prenatal dexamethasone treatment in conjunction with rescue therapy of human surfactant: a randomized placebo-controlled multicentre study. Pediatrics 93: 730–736

100. Kennedy C R, Ayers S, Campbell M J, Elbourne D, Hope P, Johnson A 2001 Randomized, controlled trial of acetazolamide and furosemide in posthemorrhagic ventricular dilation in infancy: follow-up at 1 year. Pediatrics 108: 597–607

101. Kenyon S L, Taylor D J, Tarnow-Mordi W 2001 Broad-spectrum antibiotics for preterm:relabour rupture of fetal membranes: the ORACLE 1 randomised trial. Lancet 357: 979–988

102. Khan D J, Richardson D K, Billett H H 2002 Association of thrombocytopenia and delivery method with intraventricular hemorrhage among very low birthweight infants. American Journal of Obstetrics and Gynecology 186: 109–116

103. Kluckow M, Evans N 2000 Low superior vena cava flow and intraventricular haemorrhage in preterm infants. Archives of Disease in Childhood 82: F188–F194

104. Kuban K C K, Allred E N, Dammann O et al 2001 Topography of cerebral white-matter disease of prematurity studied prospectively in 1607 very-low-birthweight infants. Journal of Child Neurology 16: 401–408

105. Kuban K C K, Gilles F 1985 Human telencephalic angiogenesis. Annals of Neurology 17: 539–548

106. Kuban K C K, Leviton A, Pagano M, Fenton T, Strassfield R, Wolff M 1992 Maternal toxemia is associated with reduced incidence of germinal matrix hemorrhage in premature babies. Journal of Child Neurology 7: 70–76

107. Kubota T, Okumura A, Hayakawa F et al 2001 Relation between the date of cyst formation observable on ultrasonography and the timing of injury determined by serial electroencephalography in preterm infants with periventricular leukomalacia. Brain and Development 23: 390–394

108. Kubota T, Okumura A, Hayakawa F et al 2002 Combination of neonatal electroencephalography and ultrasonography; sensitive means of early diagnosis of periventricular leukomalacia. Brain and Development 24: 698–702

109. Larroche J-C 1972 Post haemorrhagic hydrocephalus in infancy. Biology of the Neonate 20: 287–299

110. Larroche J-C 1986 Fetal encephalopathies of circulatory origin. Biology of the Neonate 50: 61–74

111. Larroque B, Marret S, Ancel P Y et al 2003 White matter damage and intraventricular hemorrhage in very preterm infants: the epipage study. Journal of Paediatrics 143: 477–483

112. Lemons J A, Bauer C R, Oh W et al 2001 Very low birthweight outcomes of the national institute of child health and human development neonatal research network, January 1995 through December 1996. Pediatrics 107: e1–e8

113. Levene M I, de Vries L S 1984 Extension of neonatal intraventricular haemorrhage. Archives of Disease in Childhood 59: 631–636

114. Levene M I, Starte D R 1981 A longitudinal study of post haemorrhagic ventricular dilatation in the newborn. Archives of Disease in Childhood 56: 905–910

115. Levene M I, Wigglesworth J S, Dubowitz V 1983 Haemorrhagic periventricular leukomalacia in the neonate: a real time ultrasound study. Pediatrics 71: 794–797

116. Leviton A 1993 Preterm birth and cerebral palsy : is tumour necrosis factor the missing link? Developmental Medicine and Child Neurology 35: 549–558

117. Leviton A, Gilles F H 1984 Aquired perinatal leukoencephalopathy. Annals of Neurology 16: 1–8

118. Leviton A, Pagano M, Kuban K C K, Krishnamoorthy K S, Sullivan K F, Alfred E N 1991 The epidemiology of germinal matrix haemorrhage during the first half day of life. Developmental Medicine and Child Neurology 33: 138–145

119. Liao S-L, Lai S-H, Chou Y-H, Kuo C-Y 2001 Effect of hypocapnia in the first three days of life on the subsequent development of periventricular leukomalacia in premature infants. Acta Paediatrica Taiwanica 42: 90–93

120. Linder N, Haskin O, Levit O et al 2003 Risk factors for intraventricular hemorrhage in very low birthweight premature infants: a retrospective case-control study. Pediatrics 111: e590–e595

121. Lipscomb A P, Thorburn R J, Reynolds E O R et al 1981 Pneumothorax and cerebral haemorrhage in preterm infants. Lancet 1: 414–416

122. Long W, Corbet A, Cotton R 1991 A controlled trial of synthetic surfactant (Exosurf) in infants weighing 1250 g or more with respiratory distress syndrome. New England Journal of Medicine 325: 1696–1703

123. Lou H C, Lassen N A, Friis-Hansen B 1979 Impaired ability of autoregulation of cerebral blood flow in the distressed newborn infant. Journal of Pediatrics 94: 118–121

124. Lowe J, Papile J A 1990 Neurodevelopmental performance of very low birthweight infants with mild periventricular, intraventricular haemorrhage. American Journal of Diseases of Children 144: 1242–1245

125. Maalouf E F, Duggan P J, Counsell S J et al 2001 Comparison of findings on cranial ultrasound and magnetic resonance imaging in preterm infants. Pediatrics 107: 719–727

126. McDonald M M, Koops B L, Johnson M L et al 1984 Timing and antecedents of intracranial hemorrhage in the newborn. Pediatrics 74: 32–36

127. McMenamin J B, Shackleford D G, Volpe J J 1984 Outcome of neonatal intraventricular hemorrhage with periventricular echodense lesions. Annals of Neurology 15: 285–290

128. Marret S, Parain D, Jeannot E, Eurin D, Fessard D 1992 Positive rolandic sharp waves in the EEG of the premature newborn: a five year prospective study. Archives of Disease in Childhood 67: 948–951

129. Martinez A, Taeusch H W, Yu V et al 2002 Variation in mortality and intraventricular haemorrhage in occupants of Pacific Rim nurseries. Journal of Paediatrics and Child Health 38: 235–240

130. Mayer, P L, Kier E L 1991 The controversy of the periventricular white matter circulation: a review of the anatomic literature. American Journal of Neuroradiology 12: 223–228

131. Meek J H, Tyszczuk L, Elwell C E, Wyatt J S 1999 Low cerebral blood flow is a risk factor for severe intraventricular haemorrhage. Archives of Disease in Childhood 81: F15–F18

132. Ment L R, Duncan C C, Ehrenkrantz R A et al 1984 Intraventricular haemorrhage in the neonate : timing and cerebral blood flow changes. Journal of Pediatrics 104: 419–425

133. Ment L R, Oh W, Ehrenkranz R A et al 1994 Low-dose indomethacin and prevention of intraventricular hemorrhage: a multicentre randomised trial. Pediatrics 93: 543–550

134. Ment L R, Oh W, Philip A G S et al 1992 Risk factors for early intraventricular hemorrhage in low birthweight infants. Journal of Pediatrics 121: 776–783

135. Ment L R, Vohr B, Oh W et al 1996 Neurodevelopmental outcome at 36 months corrected age of preterm infant in the multicenter indomethacin intraventricular hemorrhage prevention trial. Pediatrics 98: 714–718

136. Miall-Allen V M, de Vries L S, Dubowitz L M S, Whitelaw A G L 1989 Blood pressure fluctuation and intraventricular hemorrhage in the preterm infants of less than 31 weeks gestation. Pediatrics 83: 657–661

137. Miall-Allen V M, de Vries L S, Whitelaw A G 1987 Mean arterial blood pressure and neonatal cerebral lesions. Archives of Disease in Childhood 62: 1068–1069

138. Miller S P, Vigneron D B, Henry R G et al 2002 Serial quanitative diffusion tensor MRI of the premature brain: development in newborns with and without injury. Journal of Magnetic Resonance Imaging 16: 621–632

139. Minagawa K, Tsuji Y, Ueda H, Koyama K, Okumura H, Hashimoto-Tamaoki T 2002 Possible correlation between high levels of IL-18 in the cord blood of preterm infants and neonatal development of periventricular leukomalacia and cerebral palsy. Cytokine 17: 164–170

140. Moise A A, Wearden M E, Kozinetz C A, Gest A L, Welty S E, Hansen T E 1995 Antenatal steroids are associated with less need for blood pressure support in extremely premature infants. Pediatrics 95: 845–850

141. Murphy D J, Sellers S, MacKenzie I Z, Yudkin P L, Johnson A M 1995 Case-control study of antenatal and intrapartum risk factors for cerebral palsy in very preterm singleton babies. Lancet 346: 1449–1454

142. Nelson M D, Gonzalez-Gomez I, Gilles F H 1991 The search for human telencephalic ventriculofugal arteries. American Journal of Neuroradiology 12: 223–228

143. Northern Neonatal Nursing Initiative 1996 Randomised trial of prophylactic early fresh-frozen plasma or gelatin or glucose in preterm babies: outcome at 2 years. Lancet 348: 229–232

144. Nwaesei C G, Pape K E, Martin D J, Becker L E, Fitz C R 1984 Periventricular infarction diagnosed by ultrasound: a post mortem correlation. Journal of Pediatrics 105: 106–110

145. Oka A, Belliveau M J, Rosenberg P A, Volpe J J 1993 Vulnerability of oligodendroglia to glutamate: pharmacology, mechanisms and prevention. Journal of Neuroscience 13: 1441–1453

146. Okumura A, Hayakawa F, Itomi K et al 2001 Hypocarbia in preterm infants with periventricular leukomalacia: the relation between hypocarbia and mechanical ventilation. Pediatrics 107: 469–475

147. Osborn D, Evans N, Kluckow M 2002 Randomized trial of dobutamine versus dopamine in preterm infants with low systemic blood flow. Journal of Pediatrics 140: 183–191

148. Palmer P, Dubowitz L M S, Levene M I, Dubowitz V 1982 Developmental and neurological progress of preterm infants with intraventricular haemorrhage and ventricular dilatation. Archives of Disease in Childhood 57: 748–752

149. Paneth N, Kazam E, Monte W 1994 Brain damage in the preterm infant. MacKeith Press, London

150. Paneth N, Pinto-Martin J, Gardiner J et al 1993 Incidence and timing of germinal matrix/intraventricular hemorrhage in low birthweight infants. American Journal of Epidemiology 137: 1167–1176

151. Paneth N, Rudelli R, Monte W et al 1990 White matter necrosis in very low birthweight infants: neuropathologic and ultrasonographic findings in infants surviving six days or longer. Journal of Pediatrics 116: 975–984

152. Pape K E, Bennett-Button S, Szymonowicz W, Martin D J, Fitz C R, Becker L 1983 Diagnostic accuracy of neonatal brain imaging : a post mortem correlation of computed tomography and ultrasound scans. Journal of Pediatrics 102: 275–280

153. Pape K E, Wiglesworth J S 1979 Haemorrhage, ischaemia and the perinatal brain. MacKeith Press, London

154. Papile L-A, Burstein J, Burstein R, Koffler H 1978 Incidence and evolution of subependymal and intraventricular haemorrhage: a study of infants with birthweights less than 1500 g. Journal of Pediatrics 92: 529–534

155. Pellicer A, Cabanas F, Garcia-Alix A, Rodriguez J P, Quero J 1993 Natural history of ventricular dilatation in preterm infants: prognostic significance. Pediatric Neurology 9: 108–114

156. Perlman J M 1990 Late hydrocephalus after arrest and resolution of neonatal post haemorrhagic hydrocephalus. Developmental Medicine and Child Neurology 32: 725–742

157. Perlman J M, Goodman S, Kreusser K L, Volpe J J 1985 Reduction in intraventricular hemorrhage by elimination of fluctuating cerebral blood flow velocity in preterm infants with respiratory distress syndrome. New England Journal of Medicine 312: 1353–1357

158. Perlman J M, McMenamin J B, Volpe J J 1983 Fluctuating cerebral blood flow velocity in respiratory distress syndrome: relation to the development of intraventricular hemorrhage. New England Journal of Medicine 309: 204–209

159. Perlman J M, Risser R, Broyles R S 1996 Bilateral cystic periventricular leukomalacia in the premature infant: associated risk factors. Pediatrics 97: 822–827

160. Perlman J M, Volpe J J 1983 Suctioning the preterm infant : effects on cerebral blood flow velocity, intracranial pressure and arterial blood pressure. Pediatrics 72: 329–334

161. Perlman J M, Volpe J J 1986 Intraventricular haemorrhage in extremely small preterm infants. American Journal of Disease in Children 140: 1112–1114

162. Philip A G S, Allan W C, Tito A M, Wheeler L R 1989 Intraventricular hemorrhage in preterm infants: declining incidence in the 1980s. Pediatrics 84: 797–801

163. Pidcock F S, Graziani L J, Stanley C, Mitchell D G, Merton D 1990 Neurosonographic features of periventricular echodensities associated with cerebral palsy in preterm infants. Journal of Pediatrics 116: 417–422

164. Pierrat V, Duquennoy C, van Haastertt I C, Ernst M, Guilley N, de Vries L S 2001 Ultrasound diagnosis and neurodevelopmental outcome of localised and extensive cystic periventricular leucomalacia. Archives of Disease in Childhood 84: F151–F156

165. Pinto-Martin J A, Riolo S, Cnaan A, Holzman C, Susser M W, Paneth N 1995 Cranial ultrasound prediction of disabling and nondisabling cerebral palsy at age two in a low birthweight population. Pediatrics 95: 249–254

166. Pryds O 1994 Low neonatal cerebral oxygen delivery is associated with brain injury in preterm infants. Acta Paediatrica 83: 1233–1236

167. Pryds O, Greisen G, Lou H, Friis-Hansen B 1989 Heterogeneity of cerebral vasoreactivity in preterm infants supported by mechanical ventilation. Journal of Pediatrics 115: 638–645

168. Pryds O, Greisen G, Lou H, Friis-Hansen H B 1990 Increased cerebral blood flow and plasma epinephrine in hypoglycaemic preterm neonates. Pediatrics 85: 172–176

169. Rademakers K J 1994 Unilateral haemorrhagic parenchymal lesions in the preterm infant: shape, site and prognosis. Acta Paediatrica Scandinavica 83: 602–608

170. Rennie J M 1997 Neonatal cerebral ultrasound. Cambridge University Press, Cambridge

171. Rennie J M, Wheater M, Cole T J 1996 Antenatal steroid administration is associated with an improved chance of intact survival in preterm infants. European Journal of Pediatrics 155: 576–579

172. Roelants-van Rijn A M, Croenendaal F, Beek F J A, Eken P, van Haastert I C, de Vries L S 2001 Parenchymal brain injury in the preterm infant: comparison of cranial ultrasound, MRI and neurodevelopmental outcome. Neuropediatrics 32: 80–89

173. Rogers B, Msall M, Owens T et al 1994 Cystic periventricular leukomalacia and type of cerebral palsy in preterm infants. Journal of Pediatrics 125: S1–S8

174. Ruckensteiner E, Zollner F 1929 Uber die Blutungen im Gebiete der Vena terminalis bei Neugeborenen. Frankfurt Zeitschrift für Pathologie 37: 568–578

175. Rumak C M, Guggenheim M A, Peterson R G, Johnson M L, Braithwaite W R 1981 Neonatal IVH and maternal use of aspirin. Obstetrics and Gynecology 58: 52S–55S

176. Rushton D I, Preston P R, Durbin G M 1985 Structure and evolution of echodense lesions in the neonatal brain. Archives of Disease in Childhood 60: 798–808

177. Russell G A B, Cooke R W I 1995 Randomised controlled trial of allpurinol prophylaxis in very preterm infants. Archives of Disease in Childhood 73: F27–F31

178. Russell G A B, Jeffers G, Cooke R W I 1992 Plasma hypoxanthine: a marker for hypoxic ischaemic induced periventricular leukomalacia. Archives of Disease in Childhood 67: 388–392

179. Saliba E, Santini J J, Arbeille P 1985 Mesure non invasive du flux sanguin cerebral chez le nourisson hydrocephale. Archives françaises de pediatrie 42: 97–102

180. Scher M S, Dobson V, Carpenter N A, Guthrie R D 1989 Visual and neurological outcome of infants with periventricular leukomalacia. Developmental Medicine and Child Neurology 31: 353–365

181. Shankaran S, Bauer C R, Bain R, Wright L L, Zachary J 1995 Relationship between antenatal steroid administration and grade III and IV intracranial hemorrhage in low birthweight infants. American Journal of Obstetrics and Gynecology 173: 305–311

182. Shankaran S, Koepke T, Woldt E 1989 Outcome after posthemorrhagic ventriculomegaly in comparison with mild hemorrhage without ventriculomegaly. Journal of Pediatrics 114: 109–114

183. Shortland D B, Trounce J Q, Levene M I 1987 Hyperkalaemic cardiac arrhythmias and cerebral lesions in high risk infants. Archives of Disease in Childhood 62: 1139–1143

184. Shortland D B, Trounce J Q, Levene M I, Archer L N J, Evans D H, Shaw D E 1990 Patent ductus arteriosus and cerebral circulation in preterm circulation in preterm infants. Developmental Medicine and Child Neurology 32: 386–393

185. Sie L T, van der Knaap M S, van Wezel-Meijler G, Taets van Amerongen A H M, Lafeber H N, Valk J 2000 Early MR features of hypoxic-ischemic brain injury in neonates with periventricular densities on sonograms. American Journal of Neuroradiology 21: 852–861

186. Spinillo A, Ometto A, Bottino R, Piazzi G, Iasci A, Rondini G 1995 Antenatal risk factors for germinal matrix hemorrhage and intraventricular hemorrhage in preterm infants. European Journal of Obstetrics, Gynecology, and Reproductive Biology 60: 13–19

187. Stewart A L, Thorburn R J, Hope P L, Goldsmith M, Lipscomb A P, Reynolds E O R 1983 Ultrasound appearance of the brain in very preterm infants and neurodevelopmental outcome at 18 months of age. Archives of Disease in Childhood 58: 598–604

188. Synnes A R, Chien, L-Y, Peliowski A, Baboolal R, Lee S K 2001 Variations in intraventricular hemorrhage incidence rates among Canadian neonatal intensive care units. Journal of Pediatrics 138: 525–531

189. Szymonowicz W, Yu V Y H, Wilson F E 1984 Antecedents of periventricular haemorrhage in infants weighing 1250 g or less at birth. Archives of Disease in Childhood 59: 13–17

190. Takashima J, Tanaka K 1978 Development of cerebral architecture and its relationship to periventricular leukomalacia. Archives of Neurology 35: 11–16

191. Takashima S, Takashi M, Ando Y 1986 Pathogenesis of periventricular white matter haemorrhage in preterm infants. Brain Development 8: 25–30

192. Thorburn R J, Lipscomb A P, Stewart A, Reynolds E O, Hope P L 1982 Timing and antecedents of periventricular haemorrhage and of cerebral atrophy in very preterm infants. Early Human Development 7: 221–238

193. Trounce J Q, Fagan D, Levene M I 1986 Intraventricular haemorrhage and periventricular leucomalacia: ultrasound and autopsy correlation. Archives of Disease in Childhood 61: 1203–1207

194. Trounce J Q, Rutter N, Levene M I 1986 Periventricular leucomalacia and intraventricular haemorrhage in the preterm neonate. Archives of Disease in Childhood 61: 1196–1202

195. Trounce J Q, Shaw D E, Levene M I, Rutter N 1988 Clinical risk factors and periventricular leucomalacia. Archives of Disease in Childhood 63: 17–22

196. Tsuji M, Saul P, du Plessis A et al 2000 Cerebral intravascular oxygenation correlates with mean arterial pressure in critically ill premature infants. Pediatrics 108: 625–632

197. Tzogalis D, Fawer C L, Wong Y, Calame A 1988 Risk factors associated with the development of peri-intraventricular haemorrhage and periventricular leukomalacia. Helvetica Paediatrica Acta 43: 363–376

198. Van Bel F, Van de Bor M, Stijnen T, Baan J, Ruys J H 1987 Aetiological role of cerebral blood flow alterations in development and extension of per-intraventricular haemorrhage. Developmental Medicine and Child Neurology 29: 601–614

199. Van de Bor M, Ma E J, Walther F J 1991 Cerebral blood flow velocity after surfactant instillation in preterm infants. Journal of Pediatrics 118: 285–287

200. Ventriculomegaly Trial Group 1990 Randomised trial of early tapping in neonatal posthaemorrhagic ventricular dilatation. Archives of Disease in Childhood 65: 3–10

201. Ventriculomegaly Trial Group 1994 Randomised trial of early tapping in neonatal posthaemorrhagic periventricular dilatation: results at 30 months. Archives of Disease in Childhood 70: F129–F136

202. Verma U, Tejani N, Klein S et al 1997 Obstetric antecedents of intraventricular hemorrhage and periventricular leukomalacia in the low birthweight neonate. American Journal of Obstetrics and Gynecology 176: 275–281

203. Vermeulen G M, Bruinse H W, Gerards L J, de Vries L S 2001 Perinatal risk factors for cranial ultrasound abnormalities in neonates born after spontaneous labour before 34 weeks. Obstetrics and Gynaecology 94: 290–295

204. Versmold H T, Kitterman J A, Phibbs R H, Gregory G, Tooley W 1981 Aortic blood pressure during the first 12 hours of life in infants with birthweight 610 to 4220 grams. Pediatrics 67: 607–612

205. Virchow R 1867 Zur pathologischen Anatomie des Gehirns. I: congenitale Encephalitis und Myelitis. Virchows Archiv 38: 129–142

206. Vohr B, Garcia-Coll C, Flanagan P, Oh W 1992 Effects of intraventricular hemorrhage and socioeconomic status on perceptual, cognitive, and neurologic status of low birthweight infants at 5 years. Journal of Pediatrics 121: 280–285

207. Volpe J J 1990 Brain injury in the premature infant – is it preventable? Pediatric Research 27: 28–33

208. Volpe J J 2001 Intracranial haemorrhage: germinal matrix–intraventricular hemorrhage of the premature infant. In: Volpe J J (ed) Neurology of the Newborn, 4th edn. W B Saunders, Philadelphia, pp 429–493

209. Volpe J J 2001 Neurobiology of periventricular leukomalacia in the premature infant. Pediatric Research 50: 553–562

210. Wallin L A, Rosenfeld C R, Laptook A R et al 1990 Neonatal intracranial haemorrhage. II: Risk factor analysis in an inborn population. Early Human Development 23: 129–137

211. Watkins A M C, West C R, Cooke R W I 1989 Blood pressure and cerebral haemorrhage and ischaemia in very low birthweight infants. Early Human Development 19: 103–110

212. Weindling A M, Rochefort M J, Calvert S A, Fok, T-F, Wilkinson A 1985 Development of cerebral palsy after sonographic detection of periventricular cysts in the newborn. Developmental Medicine and Child Neurology 27: 800–806

213. Weindling A M, Wilkinson A R, Cook J, Calvert S A, Fok T-F, Rochefort M J 1985 Perinatal events which precede periventricular haemorrhage and leucomalacia in newborn. British Journal of Obstetrics and Gynaecology 92: 1218–1223

214. Wells J T, Ment L R 1995 Prevention of intraventricular haemorrhage in preterm infants. Early Human Development 42: 209–233

215. Weninger M, Salzer H R, Pollak A 1992 External ventricular drainage for treatment of rapidly progressive posthaemorrhagic hydrocephalus. Neurosurgery 31: 103–110

216. Wheater M, Rennie J M 2000 Perinatal infection is an important risk factor for cerebral palsy in very low birthweight infants. Developmental Medicine and Child Neurology 42: 364–367

217. Whitelaw A 1996 Phase i study of intraventricular recombinant tissue plasminogen activator for treatment of posthaemorrhagic hydrocephalus. Archives of Disease in Childhood 75: F20–F26

218. Whitelaw A, Pople I, Cherian S, Evans D, Thoresen M 2003 Phase 1 trial of prevention of hydrocephalus after intraventricular hemorrhage in newborn infants by drainage, irrigation, and fibrinolytic therapy. Pediatrics 111: 759–765

219. Whitelaw A, Thoresen M, Pople I 2002 Posthaemorrhagic ventricular dilatation. Archives of Disease in Childhood 86: 72–74

220. Wimberley P D, Lou H C, Pedersen H 1982 Hypertensive peaks in pathogenesis of IVH in newborn: abolition by phenobarbitone sedation. Acta Paediatrica Scandinavica 71: 537–542

221. Wiswell T E, Graziani L J, Kornhauser M S T et al 1996 Effects of hypocarbia on the development of cystic periventricular leukomalacia in premature infants treated with high frequency jet ventilation. Pediatrics 98: 918–924

222. Wiswell T E, Graziani L J, Kornhauser M S et al 1996 High-frequency jet ventilation in the early management of respiratory distress syndrome is associated with a greater risk for adverse outcomes. Pediatrics 98: 1035–1043

223. Wu Y W, Colford J M 2000 Chorioamnionitis as a risk factor for cerebral palsy. Journal of the American Medical Association 284: 1417–1424

224. Yanowitz T D, Jordan J A, Gilmour C H et al 2002 Hemodynamic disturbances in premature infants born after chorioamnionitis: association with cord blood cytokine concentrations. Pediatric Research 51: 310–316

225. Yoon B Y, Jun J K, Romero R et al 1997 Amniotic fluid inflammatory cytokines (interleukin-6, interleukin-1beta, and tumor necrosis factor-alpha), neonatal brain white matter lesions, and cerebral palsy. American Journal of Obstetrics and Gynecology 177: 19–26

PART 6

Hereditary and degenerative central nervous system disease

Peter G Barth

Introduction

Neurodegenerative diseases may start to affect the central nervous system during the fetal period. Their cause is usually a genetic defect. Signs at the time of birth include disturbed swallowing, stridor, abnormal posturing, nystagmus, seizures and arthrogryposis. External dysmorphic signs may be present or absent. Results of routine neuroimaging by ultrasound or magnetic resonance imaging (MRI) of the brain may cause some confusion with more common disorders. For example, intracranial calcification found on neuroimaging might suggest congenital viral infection (pp. 1053–61). The finding of an 'empty' space in the posterior fossa may invite a diagnosis of Dandy–Walker syndrome (p. 1196) unless more thorough evaluation corrects this to pontocerebellar hypoplasia (PCH). Absence of gyration suggestive of lissencephaly (pp. 1199–200) may result from massive neuronal death that starts after neuronal migration but before completion of the gyration process. Included in this chapter are some disorders that usually present during infancy, because they may start at birth.

A proper diagnosis is essential in each case of an inherited neurodegenerative disease. It will not help the neonate with a progressive and untreatable disorder but it is necessary to provide a guide to the paediatrician directing management, as well as to help the parents to cope with the situation. Coping includes taking rational decisions about life-prolonging therapies, including respiratory support. Since these disorders are usually genetically determined, an accurate diagnosis allows appropriate genetic counselling.

Many of the disorders that are described here are still not defined at the molecular level and for practical purposes their classification is morphological. An inventory of inherited disorders with prenatal brain degeneration encompasses:

- disorders of myelin and myelination;
- neuroaxonal dystrophies;
- neuronal degeneration;
- pontocerebellar hypoplasia;
- intracerebral calcification;
- cerebral vasculopathies.

Disorders of myelin and myelination

Myelination of the brain in the full-term newborn is largely limited to the brainstem and has hardly proceeded to the supratentorial structures. Myelination in the newborn brain can be studied by

MRI, preferably making use of transverse and sagittal T1-weighted inversion recovery images. This will show myelin in the cerebellar white matter, the dorsal (tegmental) part of the pons, the mesencephalon, the posterior limbs of the internal capsules and the postcentral parasagittal areas. The optic radiation is visible by the end of the first month.[59]

Disorders of myelination are generally divided in three groups: delayed myelination, dysmyelination and demyelination. Delayed myelination as observed by MRI is a non-specific finding due to a variety of causes, including axonal loss in perinatal hypoxic ischemic encephalopathies, some defined metabolic disorders, including disorders of serine biosynthesis and cholesterol biosynthesis, and also chromosome disorders. Dysmyelination refers to the formation of a biochemically and ultrastructurally unstable kind of myelin, appearing on MRI or in neuropathological sections as delayed myelination. This is to be followed in later stages of the disease by active demyelination.

Dysmyelinating and demyelinating disorders affect the synthesis or catabolism of myelin lipids in some peroxisomal and lysosomal disorders. The paradigm of inherited dysmyelination is Pelizaeus–Merzbacher disease, an X-linked genetic disorder that causes deficiency of proteolipid protein (PLP), an important constituent of myelin.

Various genetic disorders cause a process of myelin breakdown known as leukodystrophy. Leukodystrophy refers to myelin loss and severe structural changes including loss of the axons, and often an inflammatory reaction. Well identified leukodystrophies include genetic lysosomal and peroxisomal disorders such as sphingolipidoses and peroxisome biogenesis disorders. Most of these make their appearance past the newborn period. In some of these disorders, such as neonatal adrenoleukodystrophy (NALD) or Krabbe's disease, presentation may be at the time of birth or shortly thereafter. In one defined leukodystrophy, Alexander's disease, presentation may be within the first month after birth.

Pelizaeus–Merzbacher disease

Pelizaeus–Merzbacher disease is the best known form of dysmyelination. It is an X-linked disease. The gene encoding PLP, localised at Xq22, is organised in seven exons. Mutations to the *PLP* gene are of two types: intragenic mutations, including missense mutations, insertions and deletions, and gene duplications. The latter type is the most common.[54]

Proteolipid protein is a transmembrane protein that spans the thickness of the myelin lipid bilayer and has both extracytoplasmic and cytoplasmic domains. It is assumed to provide stability to the layered myelin structure by connecting the myelin layers and causing compaction as they become wrapped around the axon during the myelination process. Absence of PLP does not lead to absence of myelin but to impairment of the compaction process, causing instability, to be followed at a later stage by disintegration. This explains the sequence of delayed myelination to be followed later by demyelination.[11]

Symptoms may start at birth or in the first months of life, following a latent asymptomatic period. Typical nystagmoid eye movements may be present in the first weeks after birth and are often the presenting sign. Another early symptom, often encountered, is stridor. At this stage other findings are normal, including feeding behaviour and neonatal motor patterns.[46,51,57] At a later stage, lack of proper head control and delayed motor milestones become prominent, followed by spastic pareses. Suspicion may be aided by a positive family history suggestive of X-linked inheritance. Even in the absence of this the diagnosis may be suspected on the basis of the early symptoms. MRI documentation is scanty at this stage because of the physiological lack of myelin in the cerebral hemispheres at the time of birth. A useful diagnostic instrument is the brainstem acoustic evoked responses (BAER), by which decreased or absent responses past wave II may be found in Pelizaeus–Merzbacher disease, even in the newborn period.[24] Because the PLP protein is only expressed in brain, definite diagnosis requires mutation analysis of the *PLP* gene.

Wiedemann–Rautenstrauch syndrome

The neonatal progeroid or Wiedemann–Rautenstrauch syndrome is a rare autosomal recessive disorder. It presents with generalised lipoatrophy, except for fat pads in the suprabuttock areas; hypotrichosis of the scalp hair, eyebrows and eyelashes; relative macrocephaly; triangular face; natal teeth; and micrognathia.[43] No metabolic or molecular genetic cause has yet been found. Some studies have shown dysmyelination. No MRI studies are currently available. Differential diagnosis should include congenital defect of glycosylation 1A and Cockayne's syndrome type B or cerebro-oculo-facio-skeletal syndrome (COFS; see below).

Krabbe's disease

Krabbe's disease is an autosomal recessive deficiency of lysosomal galactosylceramidase. It typically presents in the first half year, usually in the first months of life, with cerebral and peripheral nerve demyelination. The first signs are irritability and spasticity with diminished tendon reflexes. While the usual onset is after the first months of life, some babies present as early as the first few days.[15,29,52] The main signs are irritability and feeding difficulty. No MRI findings of the early-onset form have been published. Absence of or diminished tendon reflexes should lead to determination of motor nerve conduction velocities, because Krabbe's disease features both central and peripheral demyelination. This may provide a useful clue to differential diagnosis. The ultimate diagnostic tool is determination of lysosomal galactosylceramidase in leukocytes or cultured skin fibroblasts.

Peroxisomal disorders

Neonatal adrenoleukodystrophy (NALD) and Zellweger's syndrome belong to the peroxisome biogenesis disorders, formerly known as generalised peroxisomal disorders.[62] Peroxisome biogenesis disorders are caused by impairment of targeted import of peroxisomal enzymes into the peroxisome, after their synthesis outside the peroxisomal environment on free ribosomes. This import failure results in catabolism of these enzymes in the cytosol and consequently in multiple peroxisomal enzyme defects occurring together. Normal peroxisomal assembly and targeted protein import require at least 12 PEX genes.[62]

The difference between NALD and Zellweger's syndrome is mainly phenotypical. For reasons not yet fully understood, deficiency of certain PEX genes may either result in NALD or in Zellweger's syndrome. These two disorders have phenotypical differences and similarities. Whereas in Zellweger's syndrome facial dysmorphic signs and neuronal migration disorder are prominent, these signs are less obvious or absent in NALD. Very large fontanelles and periarticular calcifications surrounding the large joints, especially the knees, are typical of Zellweger's syndrome but are not found in NALD. Liver enlargement and liver dysfunction are seen in both. Prolonged jaundice is usual in Zellweger's syndrome but uncommon in NALD. A frequent presenting sign in NALD is neonatal seizures, which may be difficult to manage.[55] Hypotonia is usually found in both disorders, and may lead to the need for gavage feeding. Although lipid storage is present in the adrenals at autopsy, overt adrenocortical deficiency does not occur in either condition. Meticulous examination of the eyes may reveal dot-like peripheral retinal pigmentary deposits in both disorders and these are very typical. Electroretinography is usually diagnostic of retinopathy in both disorders. Cataracts occur in a minority of cases in NALD, and may also be present in Zellweger's syndrome.

Neuroimaging provides helpful information leading to diagnosis, especially in Zellweger's syndrome. Neocortical polymicrogyria is typically found in Zellweger's syndrome (Fig. 41.46) but is not an obligatory finding in NALD. Zellweger's syndrome patients have delayed myelination; NALD patients have early demyelination. Demyelination in NALD affects the cerebral hemispheres and is also prominent in the cerebellar white matter.[5,34] No neonatal MRI studies are available on NALD yet. On the basis of neuropathological studies and previous computed tomography (CT) studies, signal changes of the white matter would be expected in NALD. MRI of the brain in Zellweger's syndrome will reveal impaired myelination, moderate enlargement of the ventricular system, especially the posterior horns, polymicrogyria and pachymicrogyria, a vertical upsweep of the sylvian fissure and often subependymal germinolytic cysts[7] (Fig. 41.47). Proton magnetic resonance spectroscopy may give additional clues leading to the diagnosis of a progressive neurodegenerative disorder.[27]

Confirmation of the diagnosis of NALD or Zellweger's syndrome requires the finding in plasma of increased levels of very-long-chain fatty acids, the bile acid precursors trihydroxycholestanoic acid and dihydroxycholestanoic acid, pristanic acid, phytanic acid and pipecolic acid. Etherphospholipids (plasmalogens) are decreased in blood cells but less in NALD than in Zellweger's syndrome, and plasmalogens may even be normal in NALD.[62] Because at least 12 proteins are involved in peroxisomal assembly, the defective gene has to be identified first by complementation studies, to be followed by mutation analysis.

Life expectation in Zellweger's syndrome patients is limited. Most babies die before the age of 6 months and survival beyond

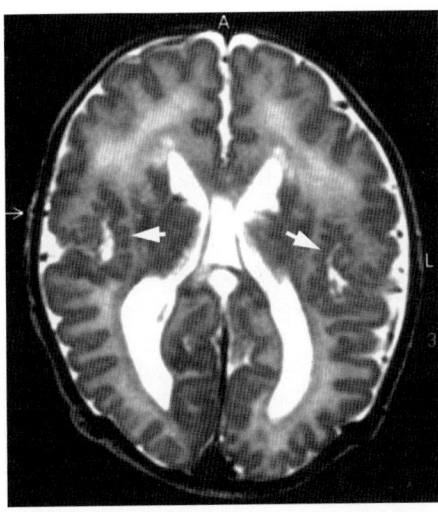

Fig. 41.46 Zellweger's syndrome. Transverse T2-weighted MR image. The sylvian fissure extends to a higher level than normal and is bordered by an abnormally structured cortex composed of minuscule gyri with absence of intervening sulci: polymicrogyria (arrows). The ventricular system is moderately enlarged. (Courtesy of Professor L S de Vries.)

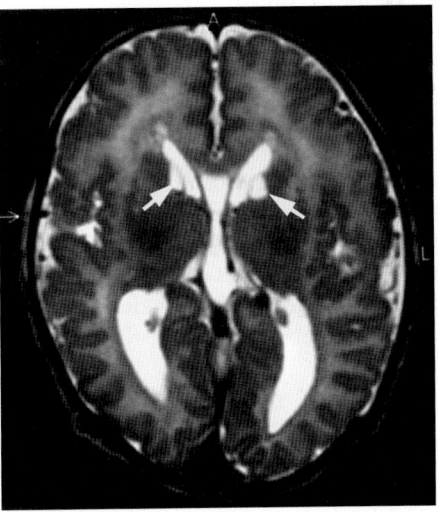

Fig. 41.47 Zellweger's syndrome. Transverse T2-weighted MR image. Germinolytic cysts are present, in the caudate–thalamic angles (arrows). (Courtesy of Professor L S de Vries.)

a year is rare. NALD patients have a slightly better prognosis but usually die in infancy or early childhood.

Acyl-co-enzyme A (CoA) oxidase-1 deficiency is a single peroxisomal enzyme deficiency that clinically mimics NALD with early signs of demyelination.[44,63] D-bifunctional protein is another peroxisomal beta-oxidation enzyme. The role of D-bifunctional protein deficiency in peroxisomal pathology (rather than that of L-bifunctional protein, as previously assumed) was established recently.[60] Deficiency of D-bifunctional protein leads to a neuronal migration disorder similar to Zellweger's syndrome.[63] In acyl-CoA oxidase-1 deficiency, as well as in D-bifunctional protein deficiency, peroxisomal import is normal but these single enzyme deficiencies retain many of the characteristics of NALD and Zellweger's syndrome. A detailed biochemical and molecular-genetic workup is necessary in each case presenting pheno-typical features of either NALD or Zellweger's syndrome to differentiate peroxisome biogenesis disorders from the mentioned single-enzyme disorders.

Alexander's disease

This disease, which has MRI features of a leukodystrophy, is a disease of astrocytes and represents a de novo dominant mutation of the gene encoding glial fibrillary acidic protein (GFAP),[14] resulting in abnormal thick glial filaments and proliferation of astrocytes. This progressive disease has its clinical onset in the first months of life, sometimes at the time of birth. Hydrocephalus, probably due to aqueductal stenosis, megalencephaly and cystic disintegration of affected brain tissue, especially in the frontal lobes, are common findings. Seizures are common and their treatment difficult. This affection leads to white matter involvement on MRI with frontal lobe predominance.[58]

Vanishing white matter disease

Demyelination accompanied by rarefaction and cavitation results from vanishing white matter disease, a group of autosomal recessive disorders associated with mutations in any of five genes encoding subunits of the translation initiation factor IF2B, which is necessary for protein synthesis and the regulation of this protein synthesis under different stress conditions. Newborn patients with the disease may have additional symptoms such as oligohydramnios, intrauterine growth retardation, cataracts, pancreatitis, hepatosplenomegaly, hypoplasia of the kidneys, and ovarian dysgenesis (Boltshauser et al 2002, van der Knaap et al 2003).[12a,59a]

Neuro-axonal dystrophies

Axonal swellings ('spheroids') with stored tubular and filamentous structures, usually at their distal endings, are the morphological marker of a heterogenous group of progressive inherited disorders of central and peripheral axons. Spheroids (Fig. 41.48) are found in the brain and spinal cord and may also be found in peripheral nerve endings, allowing diagnosis by biopsy (skin, conjunctiva, peripheral nerve, motor endplates) in the absence of a biochemical or genetic marker. The most common representative of this group is infantile neuroaxonal dystrophy, which becomes symptomatic around the first birthday. Several axonopathies with spheroids, probably unrelated to infantile neuroaxonal dystrophy, have their onset around or before birth as part of a multisystem disorder with extracerebral involvement. These include combinations with osteopetrosis,[21] cutis laxa[53] and cardiomyopathy and ophthalmic disease.[37] Some reported patients had mineralisation (calcification) of the thalamus

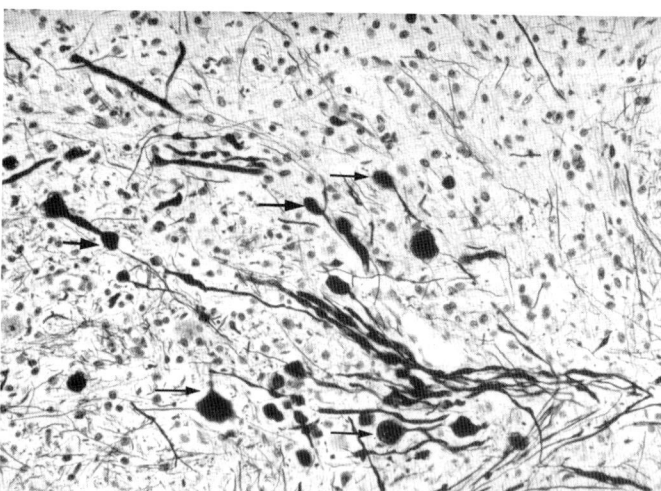

Fig. 41.48 Axonal spheroids present as solid round structures (arrows) on silver staining. Lumbar anterior horn. Autopsy of a newborn with atypical neuroaxonal dystrophy. Glees–Marsland stain.

and brainstem or basal ganglia combined with axonal neuropathy.[33,61] Diagnosis in this category may be difficult to establish by clinical means and eventually require neuropathological confirmation.

Neuronal degeneration

Progressive cortical atrophy due to massive loss of cortical neurons, together with spongiform changes and involvement of the basal ganglia, is characteristic of Alpers' syndrome, an inherited disorder that usually starts in the first months of life and is rapidly progressive with acquired microcephaly and intractable epileptic seizures. This disease may start at birth. It was first described as a neuropathological entity.[3] Accompanying liver cirrhosis is found in a significant proportion.[12,32] Later studies have revealed lactic acidosis and variable abnormalities on studies of the respiratory chain in muscle or liver biopsies.[6,45,56] It is doubtful whether all families stated to have prenatal onset of Alpers' syndrome represent variants of the postnatal-onset type. One reported family with progressive cortical degeneration starting before birth and presenting at birth with fetal akinesia sequence had a thorough biochemical study that did not reveal mitochondrial involvement.[23]

Cortical degeneration of neurons during the period of cerebral growth spurt will lead to microcephaly at birth and sometimes to a 'walnut' brain with huge cranio-cerebral disproportion. When such loss precedes cortical folding the process can be expected to result in a smooth brain surface, resembling lissencephaly but differing in pathogenesis from classic four layered (type I) or cobblestone (type II) lissencephalies because neuronal migration is not involved in the pathogenesis and the smooth cortical surface is the result of a degenerative (disruptive) process rather than malformation. Some authors propose calling this type of cortical pathology lissencephaly type III.[4,20] The cause of this type of cortical degeneration is heterogenous and no specific molecular causes have been defined yet.

Pontocerebellar hypoplasias

Pontocerebellar hypoplasia describes a heterogenous condition in which the cerebellum and pons are small. The cerebellar hemispheres are reduced in size and flattened in anteroposterior direction, giving the appearance of a butterfly (Fig. 41.49). The ventral pons, usually the larger part of the pons, is reduced in comparison to the pontine tegmentum (Fig. 41.50). Importantly, the size of the posterior fossa is not enlarged, excluding Dandy – Walker syndrome.

These features are best revealed by sagittal and coronal MRI sections. They are not specific for a particular diagnosis or subtype. They may be encountered in defined genetic disorders with neocortical dysplasia, which includes lissencephalies (Walker–Warburg syndrome, lissencephaly with cerebellar hypoplasia and *RELN* mutation)[48] and occasionally in merosin-deficient congenital muscular dystrophy.[42] They have been described also in the context of congenital disorders of glycosylation,[31] although the usual MRI pattern of congenital defect of glycosylation type 1A is cerebellar hypoplasia rather than PCH. PCH has also been described in the context of a mitochondrial disorder.[17] The disorders known as PCH types I and II have a different pathomechanism. Basically, these two disorders represent autosomal recessive neurodegenerative disorders with fetal onset.[8]

The name olivo-ponto-cerebellar atrophy/hypoplasia, which is used by some authors to describe the same group of disorders, suggests relationship to a group of mainly adult onset autosomal-dominant disorders traditionally known as olivo-ponto-cerebellar atrophies, more recently renamed spinocerebellar atrophies. While it is true that the olivary nucleus may be involved in PCH, this cannot be confirmed by MRI. For these reasons most paediatric neurologists prefer the name PCH to emphasise its unique genetic and pathologic features and to avoid confusion with spinocerebellar atrophies.

Pontocerebellar hypoplasia type I (PCH-1)

A detailed description of both clinical and pathological findings dates from 1977.[26] Affected babies had contractures at birth and poor respiration as a result of generalised muscle weakness. Mental and motor milestones were almost absent, and they died in infancy. Neuropathology showed PCH as well as spinal anterior horn degeneration morphologically similar to spinal muscular atrophy type I.

Microscopic findings in the brainstem and cerebellum showed that this disease is a progressive neurodegenerative process with the onset prenatally, rather than a malformation. Neurons in the pons were severely diminished in numbers with gliosis in the brainstem and cerebellar white matter, loss of dentate neurons, cerebellar granule cells and Purkinje cells. In a single case, contractures as well as pulmonary hypoplasia were found, together with PCH and neurogenic muscular atrophy.[39] Later

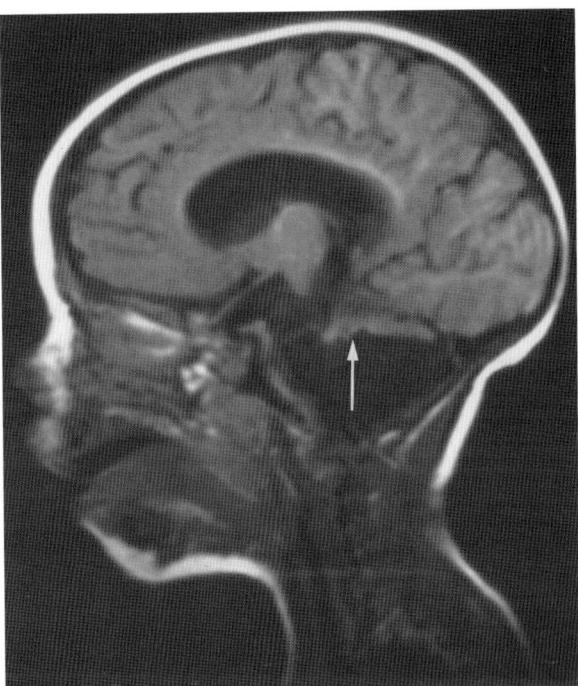

Fig. 41.49 Pontocerebellar hypoplasia. Sagittal T1-weighted MR image showing the hypoplastic cerebellar hemisphere lying under the tentorium (arrow) and leaving an empty space in the posterior fossa.

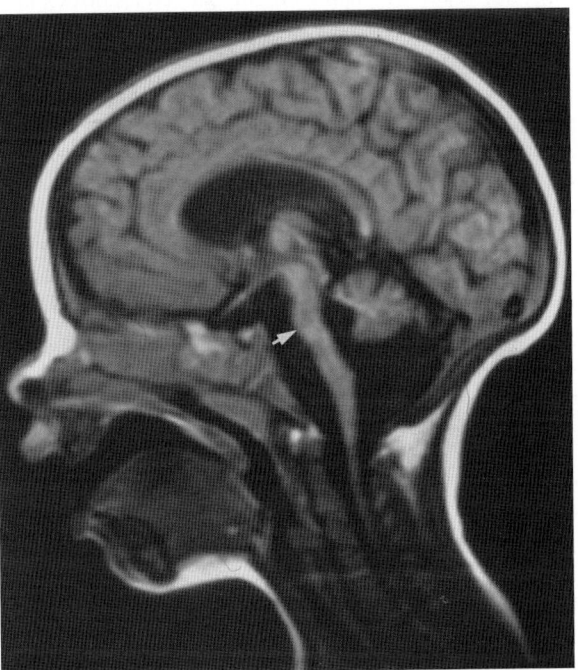

Fig. 41.50 Pontocerebellar hypoplasia. Midsagittal T1-weighted MR image showing the hypoplastic vermis and the flattening of the ventral pons (arrow).

investigations have excluded PCH-1 from the *SMA* gene on chromosome 5.[19,40]

There appears to be variability in the expression of this disease, with an overlapping spectrum from prenatal onset to onset within the first postnatal months.[49] This focuses discussion on whether to call the cerebellar anomalies 'hypoplasia' or 'atrophy'. Hypoplasia refers to small size and poor folial branching, while atrophy refers to shrinkage of folia with (retained) normal branching. Postnatal onset would lead to atrophy rather than hypoplasia. Apparently both phenomena are involved in longstanding cases with prenatal onset. PCH-1 is inherited in an autosomal recessive pattern, but so far the gene has not been identified. Because of the progressive nature of the cerebellar changes, antenatal ultrasonography cannot be regarded as a safe tool for prenatal diagnosis during the first half of pregnancy.

Pontocerebellar hypoplasia type I should be suspected in any newborn who presents with muscle contractures, especially of the lower limbs, due to intrauterine muscle weakness. Findings include functional disturbance of bulbar muscles, involving facial, tongue, palatal and laryngeal muscles. Respiratory movements are weak or absent. Impaired swallowing during pregnancy may lead to polyhydramnios.[8] Intrauterine growth, including head circumference, is normal.

Neuroimaging by ultrasound may show dilatation of the ventricular system but no other abnormalities above the tentorium. Images of the posterior fossa may reveal an enlarged fourth ventricle and disproportion between the size of the posterior fossa and its contents. Adequate neuroimaging requires the use of MRI, preferably sagittal and coronal images, and standard inversion recovery and spin-echo sequences. The latter may be helpful in defining the relative proportions of the tegmentum and the ventral part of the pons.

Pontocerebellar hypoplasia type II (PCH-2)

Progressive microcephaly from birth, severely impaired mental and motor development and chorea/dystonia together with MR or neuropathological features of PCH characterise PCH-2.[9,10] The absence of neurogenic muscular atrophy distinguishes this disorder from PCH-1. Survival in PCH-2 is better than in PCH-1 and patients may even reach young adulthood. However, increased liability to cot death and malignant hyperthermia restrict chances of survival.[9]

Newborns with PCH-2 have a normal size, including head circumference. Their presenting signs are restlessness and jitteriness, and poor swallowing. The latter is due to inadequate coordination of sucking and swallowing, rather than weakness, which is the predominant problem in PCH-1. Seizures are a problem in the majority of PCH-2 patients but rarely occur in the first month of life. Some reports refer to neonates with PCH with polyhydramnios and myoclonus not having spinal anterior horn involvement. This may be a variant of PCH-2 or a completely separate type.[2,28]

Intracerebral calcification

Cerebral calcification in the neonate is usually associated with perinatal infections, especially cytomegalovirus or toxoplasmosis, or with hypoxic–ischaemic damage. Some cases are due to genetic disorders.

Aicardi–Goutières syndrome

Aicardi–Goutières syndrome is an autosomal recessive disorder[1,25] with the following main features:

- progressive microcephaly, but normal head circumference at birth;
- developmental delay and regression, dystonia and mental handicap;
- cerebral and brainstem atrophy, loss of white matter and progressive calcification affecting the cerebral white matter, basal ganglia, thalamus and dentate nuclei;
- cerebrospinal fluid lymphocytosis and increase of alpha-interferon in cerebrospinal fluid and plasma.

One gene for this disease localises to 3p21.[16] The usual age at onset is the first months of life. Goutières et al described 27 patients: four had symptoms at birth consisting of irritability and feeding difficulties. In another case deceleration of head growth was documented before birth. Early in the course of the disease calcifications may not be conspicuous. Cerebrospinal fluid findings (lymphocytosis), together with cerebral calcifications, may closely mimic an intrauterine infectious disease (Fig. 41.51).

Cerebro-oculo-facio-skeletal syndrome/ Cockayne's syndrome type B

Cerebro-oculo-facio-skeletal syndrome was originally described in 1971[36] and later defined as an autosomal recessive disorder with multiple dysmorphia that included abnormalities of the brain (microcephaly) and eyes (microphthalmia, cataracts, blepharophimosis), facial dysmorphia (large ears, prominent root of the nose, micrognathia) and abnormalities of the skeletal system (flexion contractures at the elbows and knees).[41] In addition, these patients have generalised osteoporosis, severe failure to thrive and die early.

A detailed neuropathological study revealed the degenerative nature of this disease.[18] Findings in the brain besides microencephaly and widened ventricles are: dysmyelination; pericapillary and parenchymal mineralisation in the globus pallidus, putamen and cerebral cortex; and degenerative changes to the cerebellar internal granular layer and Purkinje cells. These findings are similar to Cockayne's syndrome.[35]

Cockayne's syndrome belongs to a group of nucleotide excision repair disorders together with xeroderma pigmentosum and the photosensitive form of trichothiodystrophy. Nucleotide excision repair is the mechanism by which DNA is repaired following the formation of so-called adducts, compounds that bind adjacent pyrimidines under influence of ultraviolet light and carcinogens and distort the helical structure.[13] Repair must precede transcription/translation of an active gene. A mechanism to effect this is known as transcription-coupled repair. Absence of this mechanism leads, among other effects, to hypersensitivity to sunlight, a typical finding in Cockayne's syndrome. Cockayne's syndrome patients are defective in the preferential

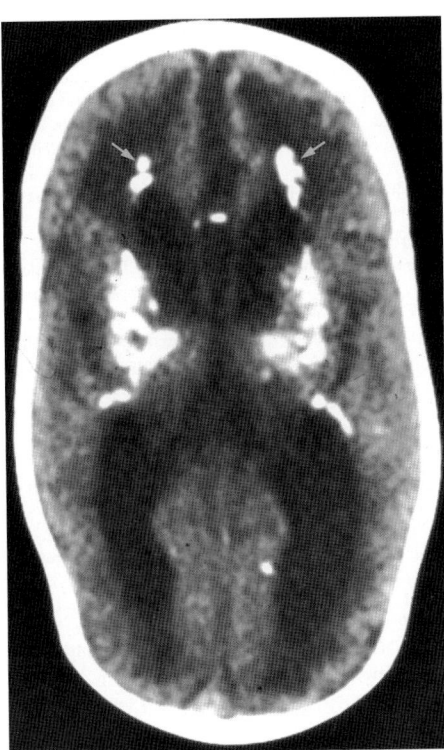

Fig. 41.51 Aicardi–Goutières syndrome. CT scan at 3 months of age showing characteristic distribution of calcifications. Arrows point to calcifications in the frontal white matter. Decreased density in this area is close to the density of cerebrospinal fluid because of tissue damage.

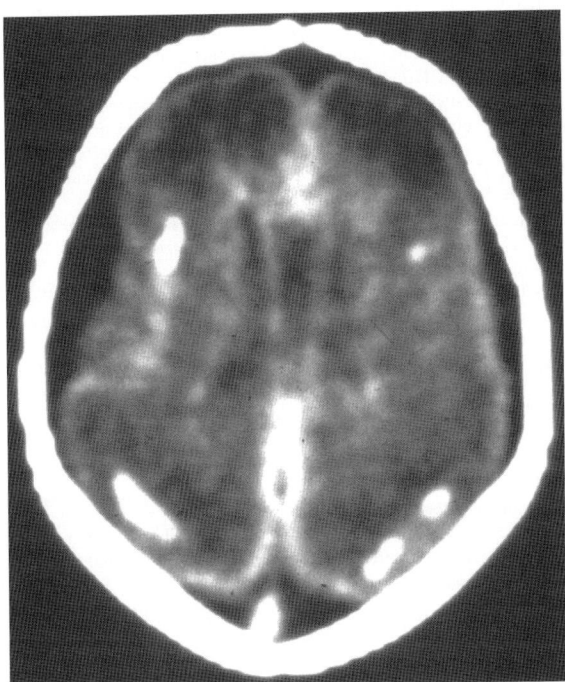

Fig. 41.52 Cerebro-oculo-facio-skeletal syndrome in a preterm newborn (32 weeks gestational age). CT scan shows subcortical calcification.

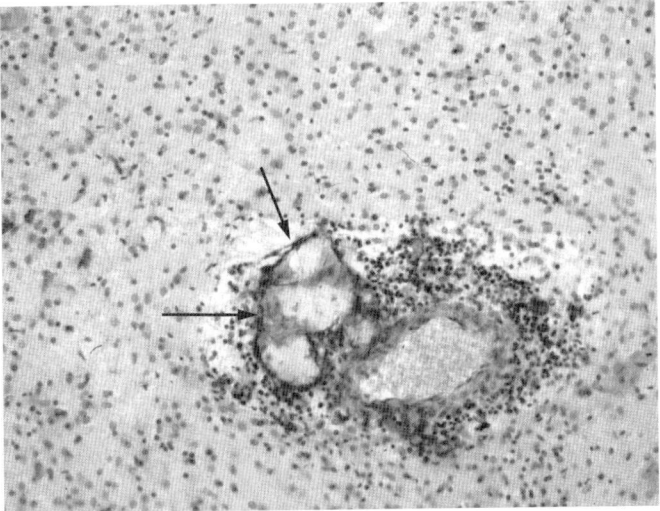

Fig. 41.53 Cerebro-oculo-facio-skeletal syndrome. Autopsy of the patient shown in Figure 41.52. Microscopic section of cerebral white matter. Two blood vessels are seen, with periadventitial calcification (arrow). Haematoxylin & eosin stain.

removal of oxidative damage from the transcribed strand of active genes by RA polymerase II. Two complementation groups exist in Cockayne's syndrome: CS A and CS B. COFS and CS B share mutations in the *ERCC6* gene,[38] proving their identity.

Cerebral pathology to be found on MRI or CT in COFS includes subcortical calcifications (Fig. 41.52) due to perivascular accumulation of calcium (Fig. 41.53). Definite diagnosis requires mutation analysis of the *ERCC6* gene.

Differential diagnosis of COFS/CS B includes Raine's syndrome,[47] a rare, probably autosomal recessive syndrome with microcephaly from birth; calcified brain lesions, often surrounding smaller blood vessels and located in the periventricular white matter, putamen and pallidum; together with osteosclerosis, proptosis and cataracts. Differential diagnosis also includes a rare syndrome with cerebral calcifications, neuronal migration disorder, severe neonatal lactic acidosis, and combined deficiency of respiratory chain complexes I and IV and pyruvate dehydrogenase complex.[50]

Vasculopathies

Fowler's disease

Fowler's disease is an autosomal recessive disorder presenting as fetal akinesia sequence and pterygia possibly due to a severe prenatal brain degeneration resulting in hydrocephaly, hydranencephaly and cerebral calcifications. Microscopic tufts of abnormal blood vessels, called 'glomeruli' are an important marker of this disease, allowing neuropathological differentiation from acquired fetal disorders.[22,30]

References

1. Aicardi J, Goutières F 1984 A progressive familial encephalopathy in infancy with calcifications of the basal ganglia and chronic cerebrospinal fluid lymphocytosis. Annals of Neurology 15: 49–54

2. Albrecht S, Schneider M C, Belmont J 1993 Fatal infantile encephalopathy with olivopontocerebellar hypoplasia and micrencephaly. Acta Neuropathologica 85: 394–399

3. Alpers B J 1931 Diffuse progressive degeneration of the gray matter of the cerebrum. Archives of Neurology and Psychiatry 25: 469–505

4. Attia-Sobol J, Encha-Razavi F, Hermier M et al 2001 Lissencephaly type III, stippled epiphyses and loose, thick skin: A new recessively inherited syndrome. American Journal of Medical Genetics 99: 14–20

5. Aubourg P, Scotto J, Rocchiccioli F et al 1986 Neonatal adrenoleukodystrophy. Journal of Neurology Neurosurgery and Psychiatry 49: 77–86

6. Bakker H D, Van den Bogert C, Drewes J G et al 1996 Progressive generalized brain atrophy and infantile spasms associated with cytochrome c oxidase deficiency. Journal of Inherited Metabolic Disease 19: 153–156

7. Barkovich A J, Peck W W 1997 MR of Zellweger syndrome. American Journal of Neuroradiology 18: 1163–1170

8. Barth PG 1993 Pontocerebellar hypoplasias. An overview of a group of inherited neurodegenerative disorders with fetal onset. Brain and Development 15: 411–422

9. Barth P G, Blennow G, Lenard H-G 1995 The syndrome of autosomal recessive pontocerebellar hypoplasia, microcephaly and extrapyramidal dyskinesia (pontocerebellar hypoplasia type 2): compiled data from ten pedigrees. Neurology 45: 311–317

10. Barth P G, Vrensen G F J M, Uylings H B M et al 1990 Inherited syndrome of microcephaly, dyskinesia and pontocerebellar hypoplasia: A systemic atrophy with early onset. Journal of the Neurological Sciences 97: 25–42

11. Baumann N, Pham-Dinh D 2001 Biology of oligodendrocyte and myelin in the mammalian central nervous system. Physiological Reviews 81: 871–927

12. Blackwood W, Buxton P H, Cumings J N et al 1963 Diffuse cerebral degeneration in infancy (Alpers' disease). Archives of Disease in Childhood 38: 193–204

12a. Boltshauser E, Barth P G, Troost D, Martin E, Stallmach T. "Vanishing White Matter" and ovarian dysgenesis in an infant with cerebro-oculo-facio-skeletal phenotype. Neuropediatrics 2002; 33(2): 57–62

13. Bootsma D, Kraemer K H, Cleaver J E et al 2001 Nucleotide excision repair syndromes: xeroderma pigmentosum, Cockayne syndrome, and trichothiodystrophy. In: Scriver C R, Beaudet A L, Sly W S, Valle D (eds) The metabolic and molecular bases of inherited disease, 8th edn. McGraw-Hill, New York, pp 677–703

14. Brenner M, Johnson A B, Boespflug-Tanguy O et al 2001 Mutations in GFAP, encoding glial fibrillary acidic protein, are associated with Alexander disease. Nature Genetics 27: 117–120

15. Clarke J T R, Ozere R L, Krause V W. Early infantile variant of Krabbe globoid cell leucodystrophy with lung involvement. Archives of Disease in Childhood 1981; 56: 640–642

16. Crow Y J, Jackson A P, Roberts E et al 2000 Aicardi–Goutières syndrome displays genetic heterogeneity with one locus (AGS1) on chromosome 3p21. American Journal of Human Genetics 67: 213–221

17. De Koning T J, de Vries L S, Groenendaal F et al 1999 Pontocerebellar hypoplasia associated with respiratory-chain defects. Neuropediatrics 30: 93–95

18. Del Bigio M R, Greenberg C R, Rorke L B et al Neuropathological findings in eight children with cerebro-oculo-facio-skeletal (COFS) syndrome. Journal of Neuropathology and Experimental Neurology 1997; 56: 1147–1157

19. Dubowitz V, Daniels R J, Davies K E 1995 Olivopontocerebellar hypoplasia with anterior horn cell involvement (SMA) does not localize to chromosome 5q. Neuromuscular Disorders 5: 25–29

20. Encha Razavi F, Larroche J C, Roume J et al 1996 Lethal familial fetal akinesia sequence (FAS) with distinct neuropathological pattern: type III lissencephaly syndrome. American Journal of Medical Genetics 62: 16–22

21. Fitch N, Carpenter S, Lachance R C 1973 Prenatal axonal dystrophy and osteopetrosis. Archives of Pathology 95: 298–301

22. Fowler M, Dow R, White T A et al 1972 Congenital hydrocephalus–hydrencephaly in five siblings, with autopsy studies: a new disease. Developmental Medicine and Child Neurology 14: 173–188

23. Frydman M, Jager-Roman E, deVries L et al 1993 Alpers progressive infantile neuronal poliodystrophy: an acute neonatal form with findings of the fetal akinesia syndrome. American Journal of Medical Genetics 47: 31–36

24. Garg B P, Markand O N, DeMyer W E 1983 Usefulness of BAER studies in the early diagnosis of Pelizaeus–Merzbacher disease. Neurology 33: 955–956

25. Goutières F, Aicardi J, Barth P G et al 1998 Aicardi–Goutières syndrome: an update end results of interferon-α studies. Annals of Neurology 44: 900–907

26. Goutières F, Aicardi J, Farkas E 1977 Anterior horn cell disease associated with pontocerebellar hypoplasia in infants. Journal of Neurology Neurosurgery and Psychiatry 40: 370–378

27. Groenendaal F, Bianchi M C, Battini R et al 2001 Proton magnetic resonance spectroscopy (^{1}H-MRS) of the cerebrum in two young infants with Zellweger syndrome. Neuropediatrics 32: 23–27

28. Grosso S, Mostadini R, Cioni M 2002 Pontocerebellar hypoplasia type 2: further clinical characterization and evidence of positive response of dyskinesia to levodopa. Journal of Neurology 249: 596–600

29. Hagberg B, Sourander P, Svennerholm L 1963 Diagnosis of Krabbe's infantile leucodystrophy. Journal of Neurology Neurosurgery and Psychiatry 26: 195–198

30. Harding B N, Ramani P, Thurley P 1995 The familial syndrome of proliferative vasculopathy and hydranencephaly–hydrocephaly: immunocytochemical and ultrastructural evidence for endothelial proliferation. Neuropathology and Applied Neurobiology 21: 61–67

31. Horslen S P, Clayton P T, Harding B N et al 1991 Olivopontocerebellar atrophy of neonatal onset and disialotransferrin developmental deficiency syndrome. Archives of Disease in Childhood 66: 1027–1032

32. Huttenlocher P R, Solitare G B, Adams G 1976 Infantile diffuse cerebral degeneration with hepatic cirrhosis. Archives of Neurology 33: 186–192

33. Jennekens F G I, Barth P G, Fleury P et al 1984 Axonal dystrophy in a case of connatal thalamic and brain stem degeneration. Acta Neuropathologica 64: 68–71

34. Kelley R I, Datta N S, Dobyns W B et al 1986 Neonatal adrenoleukodystrophy: new cases, biochemical studies, and differentiation from Zellweger and related peroxisomal polydystrophy syndromes. American Journal of Medical Genetics 23: 869–890

35. Lowry R B 1982 Early onset of Cockayne syndrome. American Journal of Medical Genetics 13: 209–210

36. Lowry R B, MacLean R, McLean D M et al 1971 Cataracts, microcephaly, kyphosis, and limited joint movement in two siblings: a new syndrome. Journal of Pediatrics 79: 282–284

37. Lyon G, Arita F, Le Galloudec E et al 1990 A disorder of axonal development, necrotizing myopathy, cardiomyopathy and cataracts: a new familial disease. Annals of Neurology 27: 193–199

38. Meira, L B, Graham J M Jr, Greenberg C R et al 2000 Manitoba aboriginal kindred with original cerebro-oculo-facio-skeletal syndrome has a mutation in the Cockayne syndrome group B (CSB) gene. American Journal of Human Genetics 66: 1221–1228

39. Moerman P, Barth P G 1987 Olivo-ponto-cerebellar atrophy with muscular atrophy, joint contractures and pulmonary hypoplasia of prenatal onset. Virchows Archiv A 410: 339–345

40. Muntoni F, Goodwin F, Sewry C et al 1999 Clinical spectrum and diagnostic difficulties of infantile ponto-cerebellar hypoplasia type 1. Neuropediatrics 30: 243–248

41. Peña S D J, Shokeir M H K 1974 Autosomal recessive cerebro-oculo-facio-skeletal syndrome. Clinical Genetics 5: 285–293

42. Philpot J, Cowan F, Pennock J et al 1999 Merosin-deficient congenital muscular dystrophy: the spectrum of brain involvement on magnetic resonance imaging. Neuromuscular Disorders 9: 81–85

43. Pivnick E K, Angle B, Kaufman R A et al 2000 Neonatal progeroid (Wiedemann-Rautenstrauch) syndrome: report of five new cases and review. American Journal of Medical Genetics 90: 131–140

44. Poll-Thé B T, Roels F, Ogier H et al 1988 A new peroxisomal disorder with enlarged peroxisomes and a specific deficiency of acyl-CoA oxidase (pseudo-neonatal adrenoleukodystrophy). American Journal of Human Genetics 42: 422–434

45. Prick M J J, Gabreëls F J M, Renier W O et al 1981 Progressive infantile poliodystrophy. Association with disturbed pyruvate oxidation in muscle and liver. Archives of Neurology 38: 767–772

46. Renier W O, Gabreëls F J M, Hustinx T W J et al 1981 Connatal Pelizaeus–Merzbacher disease with congenital stridor in two maternal cousins. Acta Neuropathologica (Berlin) 54: 11–17

47. Rickert C H, Rieder H, Rehder H et al 2002 Neuropathology of Raine syndrome. Acta Neuropathologica (Berlin) 103: 281–287

48. Ross M E, Swanson K, Dobyns W B 2001 Lissencephaly with cerebellar hypoplasia (LCH): a heterogeneous group of cortical malformations. Neuropediatrics 32: 256–263

49. Rudnik-Schöneborn S, Sztriha L, Aithala G R et al 2003 Extended phenotype of pontocerebellar hypoplasia with infantile spinal muscular atrophy. American Journal of Medical Genetics 117A: 10–17

50. Samsom J F, Barth P G, de Vries J I P et al 1994 Familial mitochondrial encephalopathy with fetal ultrasonographic ventriculomegaly and intracerebral calcifications. European Journal of Paediatrics 153: 510–516

51. Scheffer I E, Baraitser M, Wilson J et al 1991 Pelizaeus–Merzbacher disease: classical or connatal? Neuropediatrics 22: 71–78

52. Schochet S S Jr, Hardman J M, Lampert P W et al 1969 Krabbe's disease (globoid leukodystophy): electron microscopic observations. Archives of Pathology 88: 305–313

53. Shintaku M, Uemura Y, Fujii I et al 2000 Neuroaxonal leukodystrophy associated with congenital cutis laxa: report of an autopsy case. Acta Neuropathologica 99: 420–424

54. Sistermans E A, de Coo R F, De Wijs I J et al 1998 Duplication of the proteolipid protein gene is the major cause of Pelizaeus–Merzbacher disease. Neurology 50: 1749–1754

55. Takahashi Y, Suzuki Y, Kumazaki K et al 1997 Epilepsy in peroxisomal diseases. Epilepsia 38: 182–188

56. Tulinius M H, Holme E, Kristinasson B et al 1991 Mitochondrial encephalomyelopathies in childhood. II. Clinical manifestations and syndromes. Journal of Pediatrics 119: 251–259

57. Ulrich J, Herschkowitz N 1977 Seitelberger's connatal form of Pelizaeus–Merzbacher disease. Case report, clinical, pathological and biochemical findings. Acta Neuropathologica (Berlin) 40: 129–136

58. Van der Knaap M S, Naidu S, Breiter S N et al 2001 Alexander disease: diagnosis with MR imaging. American Journal of Neuroradiology 22: 541–552

59. Van der Knaap M S, Valk J 1995 Magnetic resonance of myelin, myelination, and myelin disorders,. 2nd edn. Springer Verlag, Berlin: pp 31–52.

59a. Van der Knaap M S, Van Berkel C G, Herms J, Van Coster R, Baethmann M, Naidu S, Boltshauser E, Willemsen M A, Plecko B, Hoffmann G F, Proud C G, Scheper G C, Pronk J C. eIF2B-Related Disorders: Antenatal Onset and Involvement of Multiple Organs. Am J Hum Genet 2003; 73(6): 1199–1207

60. Van Grunsven E G, van Berkel E, Mooijer P A W et al 1999 Peroxisomal bifunctional protein deficiency revisited: resolution of its true enzymatic and molecular basis. American Journal of Human Genetics 64: 99–107

61. Venkatesh S, Coulter D, Kemper T D 1994 Neuroaxonal dystrophy at birth with hypertonicity and basal ganglia mineralization. Journal of Child Neurology 9: 74–76

62. Wanders R J A, Barth P G, Heymans H S A 2002 Peroxisomal disorders. In: Rimoin D L et al (eds) Principals and practice of medical genetics, 4th edn. Churchill Livingstone, Edinburgh: vol 2, pp 2752–2787

63. Watkins P A, McGuinness M C, Raymond G V et al 1995 Distinction between peroxisomal bifunctional enzyme and acyl-CoA oxidase deficiencies. Annals of Neurology 38: 472–477

PART 7

Muscle disease

Francesco Muntoni, Adnan Manzur, Eugenio Mercuri

Introduction

Neuromuscular disorders is one of the fastest growing fields in medicine. This mainly reflects the impact of our improved understanding of the genetic basis of these disorders, with more than 200 responsible loci having been identified so far (for an extensive list of all neuromuscular disorders identified, visit http://www.elsevier.com/homepage/sah/nmd/menu.html). This has allowed a much better definition of the clinical phenotypes associated to the various forms and, to some extent, has also changed the diagnostic approach to these disorders. In this chapter we will review the current state of knowledge of the neuromuscular disorders with clinical onset in the neonatal period, focusing on their clinical presentation and giving an update on the rational approach to the diagnosis for each form.

Clinical presentation

Hypotonia is the most typical and common symptom of neuro-muscular involvement in the newborn infant.[7] There are, how-ever, many non-neuromuscular disorders that can also present with profound hypotonia and, in some cases, the differential diagnosis can be quite difficult. A detailed clinical examination and a good clinical and obstetric history provide in many cases the foundation to distinguish infants with peripheral involvement from those with central nervous system (CNS) involvement and, in some cases, provide important clues for a more specific diagnosis. Other presentations of neuromuscular disorders include arthrogryposis, feeding difficulties, sudden episodes of 'collapse' and unexplained respiratory failure.

Obstetric history

Reduced fetal movements throughout the pregnancy or normal movements initially followed by later reduction are frequently observed in infants with neuromuscular disorders and suggest weakness with onset in utero. The presence of polyhydramnios is also commonly associated with some conditions and indicates antenatal involvement of the swallowing muscles. A breech presentation is also a common feature and suggests failure of change in posture during the end of pregnancy.

Birth history

Breech presentation is relatively common. Profound osteopenia predisposing to spontaneous and sometimes multiple fractures is not a specific feature of individual neuromuscular disorder but can be observed in all conditions characterised by severe lack of movements in utero. It can be seen particularly frequently in nemaline myopathy and centronuclear myopathy, and in patients at the severe end of the spinal muscular atrophy spectrum.

Poor respiration at birth requiring intubation and mechanical ventilation is also a feature of children with severe congenital neuromuscular disorders; at times rigidity of the cervical spine, micrognathia and limited mandibulotemporal joint movement can complicate the intubation process.

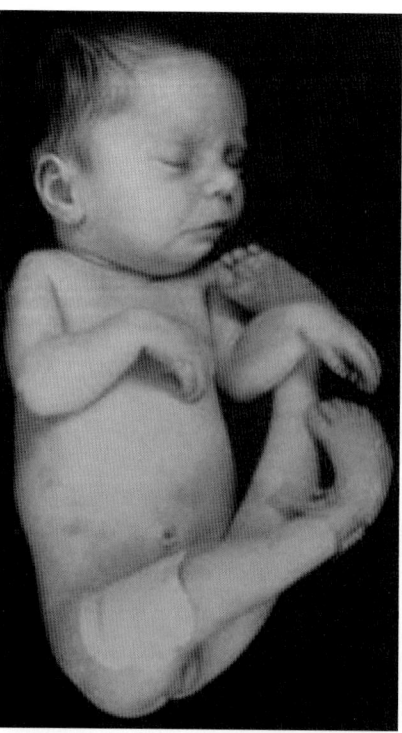

Fig. 41.54 Elbow, wrist and hip flexion contractures with extended knees in arthrogryposis.

Clinical examination

Fixed joint contractures can be observed in patients with intrauterine immobility and marked disease. Common patterns include flexion contractures at the elbows, knees, ankles and hips, or adducted thumbs, finger flexion contractures with poorly developed digits, or extended talipes, extended knee deformity with knee dislocation and hip dislocation (pp. 259–61) (Fig. 41.54). Scoliosis and rigidity of the spine can also be present. When movement in two or more joints is present at birth due to immobility in utero, the term arthrogryposis (pp. 984–5) is often used.[14] This is not a diagnosis but a description of symptoms that could potentially result from several different types of pathological process. Electromyography (EMG) and muscle biopsy are essential for the diagnosis, allowing myopathic or neurogenic patterns to be identified.[35] Bilateral talipes equinovarus (pp. 972–4) (Fig. 41.55) is classically described in infants with congenital myotonic dystrophy but can also be found in congenital myopathies and in some forms of congenital muscular dystrophy. Extended talipes is more rarely observed and is found in central core disease and in Ullrich's congenital muscular dystrophy.

Skin dimpling (Fig. 41.56) and poor dermatoglyphic pattern formation (Fig. 41.57) suggest immobility already in the first trimester of pregnancy and are also indicators of reduced fetal movements. Thin ribs on the chest radiograph (Fig. 41.58) is another indicator of poor respiratory muscle movements in utero. These signs are usually found in patients with neuromuscular disorders and are only rarely observed in infants in whom CNS insults occurred in the first trimester of pregnancy, such as neuronal migration disorders.

The presence or absence of antigravity movements is one of the key elements for detecting *weakness*. It is important to observe the baby for a while and judge movement at the peak of activity, such as when crying or stimulated. Weak babies, such as those with neuromuscular involvement, will show little movement, even in response to stimulation. Babies with CNS lesions, who may be equally hypotonic, will show occasional antigravity movements or 'unexpectedly good' resistance and antigravity movement to painful stimuli or, for example, during a seizure. Fluctuations of weakness and the relationship with the sleep–wake cycle should be noted, as this might be significant in myasthenia.

Facial weakness is often observed in infants with muscle diseases, such as myotonic dystrophy, congenital myopathies and congenital muscular dystrophy, while babies with the severe type of spinal muscular atrophy, despite being very weak, typically do

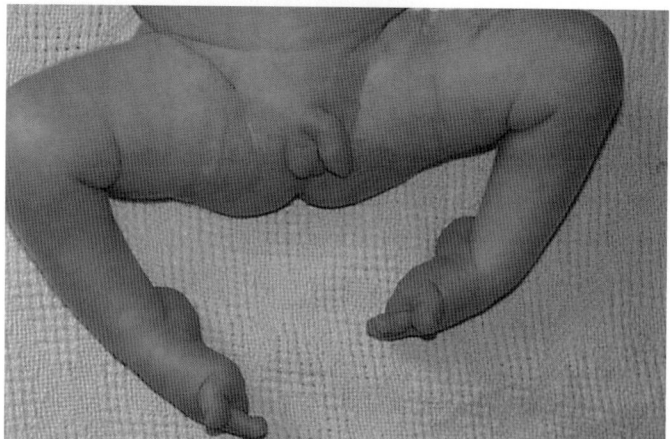

Fig. 41.55 Bilateral talipes equinovarus.

not show facial significant weakness and on the contrary appear to be alert and bright.

Swallowing difficulties are often observed. Babies with severe weakness may be totally unable to swallow their own secretions and require multiple suctioning each hour; feeding difficulties are also common and generally in keeping with the swallowing difficulties observed. Infants with non-neuromuscular conditions, such as Prader–Willi syndrome, can show poor feeding and sucking but are invariably able to manage their salivary secretions as swallowing is not affected.

Stridor can also be present in a few conditions, suggesting poor laryngeal muscle tone. Conditions in which bulbar function is more severely affected than other muscles include pontocerebellar hypoplasia type I and diaphragmatic spinal muscular atrophy (SMA).

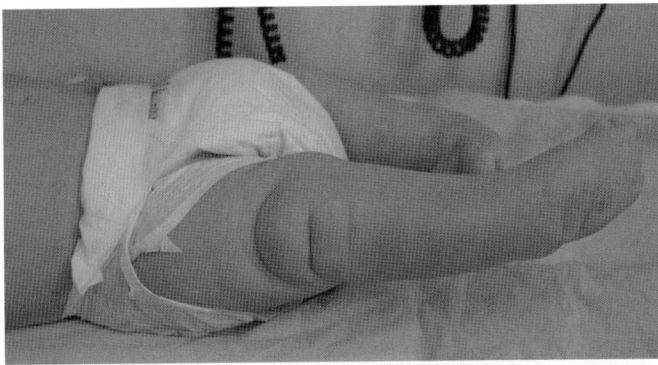

(a)

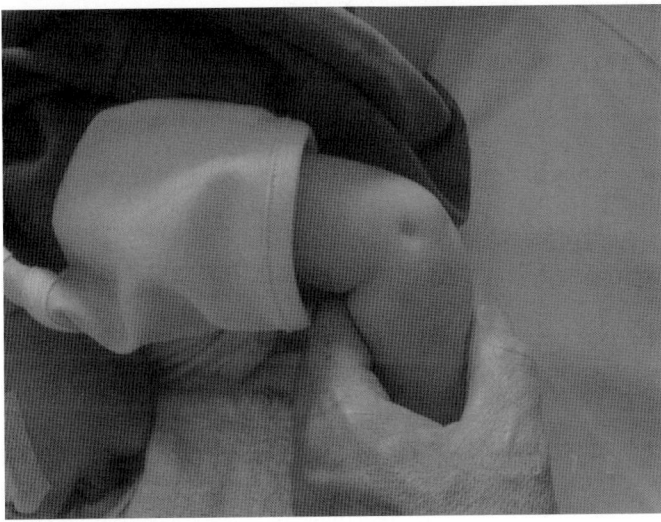

(b)

Fig. 41.56 Skin dimpling in arthrogryposis. (a) Knees. (b) Elbow.

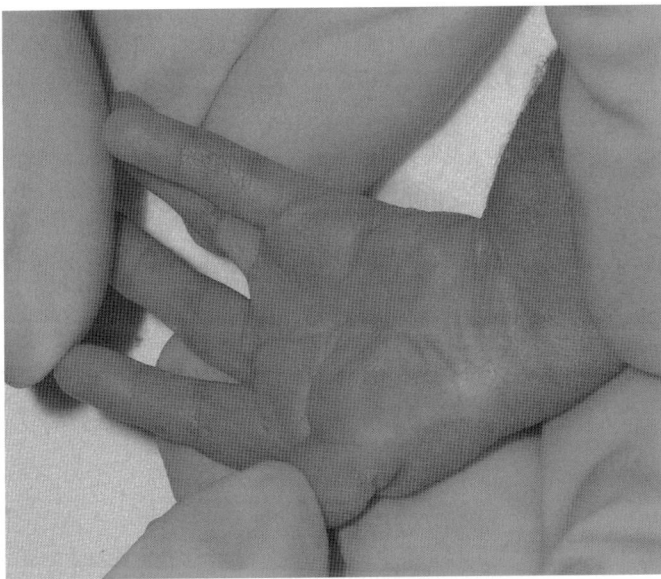

Fig. 41.57 Poor hand dermatoglyphic pattern secondary to immobility.

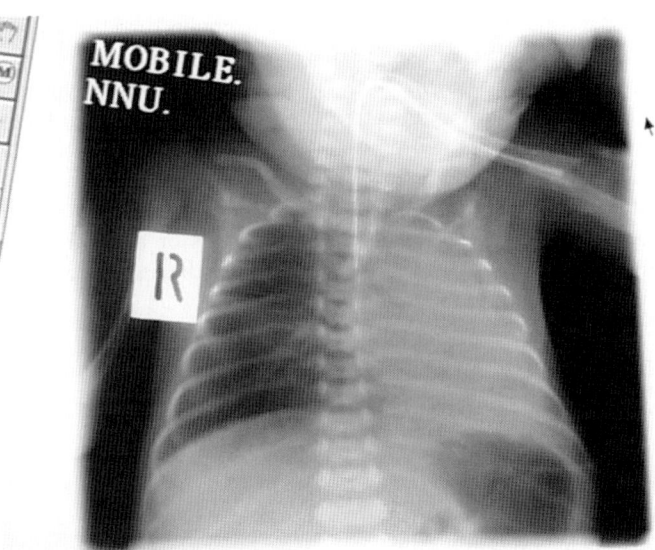

Fig. 41.58 Thin ribs and collapsed left lung in a ventilated infant with congenital myotonic dystrophy.

The assessment of the *respiratory muscle movement* is also important. In most muscle disorders there is diaphragmatic weakness with abdominal paradox (inward abdominal wall movement during inspiration). In some conditions, such as diaphragmatic SMA, this muscle is selectively affected. In spinal muscular atrophy, the weakness mainly affects intercostal muscles and the breathing pattern is abdominal, with the rib cage indrawing paradoxically during inspiration.

Deep tendon reflexes are usually absent or reduced in neuromuscular disorders. Normal tendon reflexes in a floppy infant can almost exclude spinal muscular atrophy or severe peripheral neuropathy but their absence does not necessarily suggest a muscle disorder. Brisk reflexes can be observed in myasthenia, in addition to conditions affecting the upper motor neuron.

Visual and auditory attention and level of alertness are generally preserved in babies with neuromuscular disorders, although very sick babies with severe respiratory compromise will often have reduced level of consciousness. If encephalopathy is present in a weak baby, the possibility of the association of CNS involvement with a neuromuscular disorder (for example in mitochondrial disorders or muscle–eye–brain disorders) should be considered, in addition to the possibility of a coincidental CNS involvement related to birth asphyxia.

Family history and examination

As most neonatal neuromuscular disorders are genetic, it is important to draw a pedigree going back three generations and to inquire about family history of neuromuscular diseases, stillbirth and neonatal death. When a dominant or an X-linked disorder is suspected, it is important to assess possible subclinical manifestations in the family. For example, myotonic dystrophy is inherited as an autosomal dominant trait. In many cases the mother and other affected family members may be mildly affected and unaware they have the disease. In these cases the examination of family members might detect abnormal physical signs, such as facial weakness (which may only consist of inability to bury the eyelashes), wasting of the facial muscles, percussion myotonia of the tongue and hands, and relaxation myotonia of the hands. A history of cataracts and early diabetes might also be present. Another neuromuscular disorder that should be considered is myasthenia gravis, which may lead to transient neonatal myasthenia due to passive transfer of antibody across the placenta. A previous history of miscarriages or arthrogryposis might further point towards maternal myasthenia, especially if there has not been a normal pregnancy in between.

Clinical investigations

The determination of serum creatine phosphokinase (CK) levels can be an important marker of possible muscle involvement. Serum CK levels are normally increased in cord blood up to five times the normal levels for adults, as a reflection of muscle damage during labour, and reach normal values by 5–10 days of age. Measurement of serum CK activity is likely to be of most value in some forms of muscular dystrophy, such as merosin-negative congenital muscular dystrophy, or in the variants of congenital muscular dystrophy associated with brain malformation, such as Walker–Warburg syndrome. However in congenital myopathies or other forms of congenital muscular dystrophy and in motor neurone disorders the levels can be normal or mildly elevated.

Electromyography is generally not as useful as in older children, as in the neonatal period interpretation can be difficult. EMG in experienced hands can, however, be used to assess the presence of myotonic discharges. Repetitive stimulation might help in the assessment of a baby with suspected myasthenia. Peripheral motor nerve conduction studies are easier to perform and to interpret. Slow nerve conduction velocity may point to a hereditary motor neuropathy, which may rarely present in early infancy, or to a neurometabolic disorder.

Ultrasound imaging of muscle can help to demonstrate the presence of muscle involvement and, in some cases, the selective involvement or sparing of muscles, which can be of considerable practical importance when taking a biopsy.

Muscle biopsy can be done either using an open technique or a needle. A needle technique in our experience is well tolerated and has an excellent success rate. An open technique, however, is necessary when dealing with infants in whom a suspected metabolic myopathy is suspected, as, for example, in mitochondrial encephalomyopathies. An open technique might also be the technique of choice in babies with severe contractures and bone fractures. While a muscle biopsy is indicated every time the clinical examination suggests a peripheral involvement, in a few conditions such as myotonic dystrophy and spinal muscular atrophy the diagnosis can be reached rapidly and reliably using molecular genetic techniques. When these conditions are suspected it is therefore important to proceed first with the non-invasive genetic testing before obtaining a muscle biopsy.

Brain imaging (cranial ultrasound and/or brain magnetic resonance imaging, MRI) can help to identify structural brain lesions, such as cerebellar hypoplasia or cortical dysplasia, which are features of some conditions such as Walker–Warburg syndrome, muscle–eye–brain disease, mitochondrial disorders or pontocerebellar hypoplasia type I, with both central and peripheral involvement. Brain imaging can also help to identify brain haemorrhage and/or ischaemic lesions or ventricular dilatation, which commonly complicate the clinical picture of congenital myotonic dystrophy and other severe congenital myopathies such as centronuclear myopathy.

Congenital myotonic dystrophy

This is the commonest neuromuscular disorder occurring in the neonatal period.

Classically, infants with congenital myotonic dystrophy are born following a pregnancy complicated by reduced fetal movements and polyhydramnios. If the polyhydramnios is severe, premature delivery can further complicate the picture. Affected infants typically have hypotonia, bilateral talipes equinovarus (see Fig. 41.55) and other contractures, mostly affecting the legs (flexion deformity of the knees and hips), in association with marked difficulty in sucking and swallowing. Other features invariably present are facial weakness, characterised by a striking facial diplegia, with a triangular-shaped open mouth. The severity of the weakness is variable and, while children at the severe end of the spectrum can be totally paralysed, children at the milder end of the spectrum can show partial antigravity power in the limbs. Respiratory muscle weakness is frequent and ventilation is often required to sustain these infants in the first weeks of life.

The severity of the respiratory involvement is the most important determinant of survival and previous studies have indicated that ventilation for more than 4 weeks in a term infant is a negative prognostic factor.[32] Prematurity should also be taken into account and additional time should be allowed before considering whether or not to discontinue care. The overall figures indicate a mortality of approximately 40% in the more severely affected patients.[20]

Severe neonatal feeding difficulties are also almost invariably present and require nasogastric tube feeding for several months, even in infants who breathe spontaneously. These feeding difficulties tend, however, to improve over the first months of life in the survivors, and gastrostomy feeding is very rarely needed.

Mental retardation is a very frequent feature of children with congenital myotonic dystrophy and this is one of the most important complications determining the difficulty of leading an independent life. Recent studies suggest that the mean IQ of patients with this form varies between 50 and 65 and less than 10% of the survivors achieve normal education and employment.[27]

It is important to realise that clinically evident myotonia is invariably absent in the neonatal period but can start to appear later on in childhood, when the progressive symptoms typical of the adult form of the disease become apparent. Children affected by the congenital variant of myotonic dystrophy who survive the first few months generally improve in the first 10 years of life. This is followed by a period of plateau and eventually by slow progression of weakness from the late teens onwards. Myotonia will usually appear in the first decade of life. Cardiac involvement, invariably present in older individuals with myotonic dystrophy, is rare in the neonatal period. A few cases of severe hypertrophic cardiomyopathy in infancy have, however, been reported.[16]

Neuroimaging in the neonatal period often shows non specific abnormalities such as ventricular dilatation, small haemorrhages or, in some cases, periventricular leukomalacia.[15,22,31]

A detailed pedigree, specifically asking both for other children born with similar problems and for individuals with hand weakness and myotonia, cataracts and diabetes, is helpful but it is often the examination of the mother that indicates the diagnosis, as the transmission of the disease is virtually always through the mother. There is no direct correlation between the severity of the condition in the mother and the infant, so that it is not unusual to deal with pauci–symptomatic mothers unaware of being affected. On detailed examination the mother might show either subtle facial weakness (inability to bury the eyelashes) or grip myotonia (better evaluated not by shaking hands but by asking the mother to tighten her fists for a few seconds and observing the delay in fist-releasing). Percussion myotonia can also be demonstrated in the thenar eminence or the tongue. The EMG will invariably demonstrate myotonic discharge in the mother and the diagnosis is confirmed by molecular genetic testing, which reveals expansion (increase in the number of CTG trinucleotide repeats) in the *DMPK* gene on chromosome 19.

The genetic diagnosis is essential for counselling, as prenatal diagnosis on chorionic villus biopsy is available.[1] A negative expansion study in the mother and the baby excludes the diagnosis of myotonic dystrophy. The muscle biopsy is not necessary in children with the congenital form of myotonic dystrophy. It is important to be aware that there is a very significant pathological overlap between congenital myotonic dystrophy and myotubular myopathy, and this has led to diagnostic confusion in several cases in the past.

Congenital muscular dystrophy

The term 'congenital muscular dystrophy' includes a heterogeneous group of muscle disorders characterised by weakness, usually from birth, and dystrophic changes on muscle biopsy. The classification of congenital muscular dystrophy (CMD) has become increasingly complicated because of the ever-growing number of genes and proteins identified.[21]

Until recently the classification of CMD was mainly based on the involvement of the CNS and on the presence or absence of merosin, an extracellular matrix protein found to be missing in approximately 35–45% of cases of CMD. The classification into merosin-deficient and merosin-positive CMD, however, is inadequate, as the group with normal merosin is a heterogeneous one including various forms that have been recently identified as genetically distinct entities. We can now recognise nine forms of CMD for which the genetic defect is known. On the basis of the clinical and immunohistopathological evidence, it is anticipated that several additional forms exist. Table 41.20 shows the classification of the CMD forms identified so far.

From a practical point of view, it is useful for the clinician to be able to separate forms with CNS involvement from those in which CNS involvement is absent or rare. We will describe the most frequent forms of CMD observable in the neonatal period, separating the three forms associated with structural brain changes and eye abnormalities (Fukuyama congenital muscular dystrophy, muscle–eye–brain disease, Walker–Warburg syndrome) from other forms of CMD that can be observed in the neonatal period, providing clinical, pathological and imaging details to help their identification.

Forms of congenital muscular dystrophy with structural brain changes and eye involvement

Although brain changes can be observed in a variety of forms of CMD, there are three forms in which CMD is associated with structural brain changes and ocular abnormalities. Despite their similarities, these three forms have been found to be genetically separate conditions.

Walker–Warburg syndrome

This is a relatively common form that occurs worldwide. This is the most severe of the conditions with CNS involvement. Severe neonatal hypotonia and weakness, poor visual attention and decreased alertness are invariably present, accompanied by ocular abnormalities that include retinal dysgenesis, microphthalmia, buphthalmos and anterior chamber malformations.

Brain MRI shows a type II lissencephaly with the typical micropolygyric cobblestone cortex; the white matter is also severely abnormal, showing dysmyelination or cystic changes.[5] Cerebellar hypoplasia is also always present, often associated with brainstem hypoplasia, Dandy–Walker syndrome or encephalocele. Progressive hydrocephalus often develops. Often, infants are considered only to have a CNS malformation until a markedly elevated serum CK suggests the presence of skeletal muscle involvement as well. The presence of a muscular dystrophy is confirmed by pathological studies. In a few cases, normal CK in the neonatal period has been documented, followed by progressive and marked subsequent elevation with time.

The gene responsible for approximately a quarter of all cases of WWS is *POMT1*, which codes for a glycosyltransferase.[26]

Muscle–eye–brain disease

This is a rare form of CMD initially believed to be confined to Finland and Turkey but more recently demonstrated to occur worldwide. Clinical signs are usually present at birth or in the first months of life, with hypotonia and weakness. Ocular abnormalities may become evident only after the first years of life. These children invariably develop severe mental retardation and, often, epilepsy;[33] approximately a quarter of them eventually learn to walk.

Table 41.20 Forms of congenital muscular dystrophy

Name	Abbreviation	Gene symbol	Location	Protein
Merosin deficient CMD	MDC1A	LAMA2	6q2	Laminin α2
Fukuyama CMD	FCMD	FKT1	9q3	Fukutin
Integrin-α7 deficiency	ITGA7	ITGA7	12q	Integrin α7
Muscle–eye–brain disease	MEB	POMGnT1	1p3	O-mann-CH_3-glucose-NH_2-transferase
CMD/rigid spine syndrome	RSMD1	SEPN1	1p36	SEPN1
CMD/muscle hypertrophy	MDC1B	?	1q4	?
CMD/muscle hypertrophy 2	MDC1C	FKRP	19q	FKRP
Ullrich's disease	UCMD	COL6A1, 2 and 3	2q–21q	Collagen 6
Walker–Warburg syndrome	WWS	POMT1	9q	O-mannosyltransferase

Brain MRI shows extensive abnormalities of neuronal migration, such as pachygyria and polymicrogyria and often brainstem and cerebellar hypoplasia and periventricular white matter changes. Recessive mutations in the POMGTn1, another glycosyltransferase are also responsible for this form of CMD.[14]

Fukuyama congenital muscular dystrophy

This form is exceptional outside Japan. The gene responsible codes for another glycosyltransferase named fukutin.[28] The clinical features of Fukuyama congenital muscular dystrophy are mild to moderate hypotonia at birth and a progressive course with increasing weakness, joint contractures, high CK levels, moderate to severe mental retardation and frequent association with epilepsy. Ocular abnormalities occur in approximately 70% of these children but are rarely severe.

Brain MRI shows structural changes consisting of pachygyria and polymicrogyria and low-density white-matter areas.

Other forms of congenital muscular dystrophy

Merosin-negative congenital muscular dystrophy

This form, classified as MDC1A, is an autosomal recessive form due to mutations in the LAMA2 gene on chromosome 6, encoding merosin (laminin-α2), an extracellular matrix protein.[37]

Children with merosin deficiency are usually symptomatic at birth or in the first few weeks of life with hypotonia and muscle weakness, weak cry and, in 10–30% of cases, contractures. Weakness often affects upper limbs more than lower limbs. These infants may present with feeding and respiratory problems, although these tend to recover in the first months. CK levels in these children are always grossly elevated (10 times the normal values). These children will show severe motor delay and never acquire independent ambulation.[30]

Brain MRI shows diffuse white matter changes on MRI, which are a typical feature of merosin-deficient CMD. These changes, however, become evident around 6 months, and are not obvious on the conventional scans performed in the first months of life,[23] although they can be suspected using more T2-weighted images.[24]

Recent studies have demonstrated that other patterns of brain lesions, such as cerebellar hypoplasia and/or cortical dysplasia,[36] can be observed in approximately one-tenth of children with merosin-deficient congenital muscular dystrophy.

Forms of congenital muscular dystrophy with normal merosin

Until recently the diagnosis of merosin-positive CMD was usually made after having excluded all the known forms of CMD.[9] It is now obvious, however, that this group is very heterogenous and a number of forms have been mapped to specific genes. In addition to these, a number of syndromes have been described on the basis of clinical, imaging and pathological findings. Table 41.20 provides a list of the forms more often observed in the neonatal period, together with clinical and imaging details and some relevant references.

Although many of these forms will develop specific features that will help their recognition later in life, the presenting signs in the neonatal period are often common and not specific. These are hypotonia, weakness and often contractures, which may or not be associated with feeding and respiratory involvement. Torticollis and hip dislocation are often reported in cases with Ullrich CMD, one of the most frequent forms of CMD due to mutations in one of the genes encoding collagen VI.[4,25]

Muscle biopsy will help in arriving at a more specific diagnosis, which is very important for counselling about both the short-term and long-term prognosis. The short-term prognosis mainly depends on the severity of respiratory involvement, while the long-term prognosis should be only discussed when the form of CMD has been identified.

Motor neurone disorders

Spinal muscular atrophy

Spinal muscular atrophy is the most common disease of the motoneuron in the newborn. The form affecting the newborn is the most severe of the subtypes of SMA and is classified as SMA type 1 or Werdnig–Hoffmann disease. Infants affected by this form are very weak, never acquire the ability to sit, have severe respiratory muscle weakness and die usually before the age of 1 year of an intercurrent respiratory infection.

The posture of the upper limbs in these babies is described as 'jug-handle', with a characteristic internal rotation of the shoulders and pronation of the forearms. There is a clear discordance between the weakness in the limbs, with little spontaneous activity, mainly limited to the feet and hands, and the sparing of the facial muscles, as infants with SMA generally show a bright expression and are very alert. Bulbar involvement can be present but is generally mild. Tongue fasciculations are frequent.

The intercostal muscles are always affected, while the diaphragm is relatively spared. The combination of very severe hypotonia with bright and alert face, tongue fasciculations and the respiratory pattern are generally strongly suggestive of the diagnosis. EMG showing fibrillation potentials at rest will further support the diagnosis, which will be confirmed by genetic analysis. Indeed, homozygous deletion of *SMN1* (motor neuron survival factor) exon 7 is found in more than 98% of SMA patients.

Spinal muscular atrophy type 0

A few cases of prenatal-onset spinal muscular atrophy with reduced fetal movements, severe weakness and asphyxia at birth have recently been reported.[18] These babies also show signs of CNS involvement due to birth asphyxia, which can be associated with non-specific signs of asphyxia on brain MRI. The survival time in these babies is short and, because they appear to be more severely affected than the typical SMA type I, the condition has been described as type 0. This form, which has also been confirmed by gene deletion studies, suggests that the phenotype of SMA is still expanding.[8]

Other forms of motor neurone disease

Motor neuron involvement can also be present in other forms not linked to chromosome 5. Many of these forms have onset after the neonatal period and in some cases, only in adulthood. Three of these however have onset at birth and should be taken in account. These include diaphragmatic SMA,[13,19] a form predominantly affecting the lower limbs and the form with pontocerebellar hypoplasia.[38]

Pontocerebellar hypoplasia type 1

In this form, spinal muscular atrophy is associated with pontocerebellar hypoplasia.[3] These babies have most of the motor features of typical SMA 1 but in addition have reduced alertness and poor visual behaviour. The clinical course is progressive, and respiratory and feeding difficulties, already present at birth or in early infancy, become more severe.

This form is not allelic to SMA[10] and the gene responsible for this form has not yet been identified. The diagnosis is mainly based on the association of clinical signs and MRI findings, showing hypoplasia of the cerebellar vermis and, often, of the cerebellar hemispheres, and a thin brainstem and pons.

Congenital myopathies

Four conditions, classified as 'structural congenital myopathies', can present in the neonatal period.[6] In order of frequency, these are nemaline myopathy, central core disease, myotubular myopathy and minicore disease, whose names derive from the typical muscle histopathological changes. Both minicore and central core disease present more frequently in early infancy as opposed to the neonatal period, although earlier presentation is possible.

Nemaline myopathy

The clinical spectrum of nemaline myopathy is wide and, in the neonatal period, the two most common forms are the severe congenital form, in which affected babies present with the classical fetal akinesia sequence (polyhydramnios/arthrogryposis/respiratory failure/complete immobility) to the so called 'classical' congenital form, characterised by hypotonia, general weakness predominantly affecting facial and axial muscles, and disproportionate bulbar and feeding difficulties, requiring frequent suctioning, tube feeding and gastrostomy. In our clinical experience the frequency of these two conditions is quite similar; rare cases might present with intermediate clinical features (for example only mild contractures at birth, and significant weakness, with transient respiratory failure).

The serum CK levels are usually normal, the EMG myopathic and the nerve conduction studies normal. The muscle biopsy shows an abundance of rod-like structures in muscle that stain red with the modified Gomori trichrome technique (Fig. 41.59).[17]

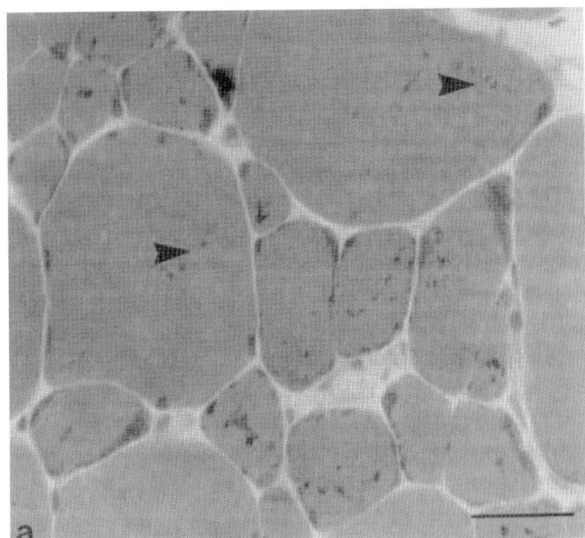

Fig. 41.59 Muscle biopsy showing nemaline rods (arrow).

The prognosis is invariably grim for children belonging to the 'severe congenital' category, as these infants do not appear to make any significant improvement of their limb, axial, bulbar and respiratory function, even after several months. On the other hand, the prognosis for babies with the classical form is much better, with most affected children acquiring independent ambulation. Frequent later complications are failure to thrive, scoliosis and nocturnal hypoventilation, even in ambulant cases.

The condition is genetically heterogeneous with at least five genes implicated in its pathogenesis. However, regarding the neonatal forms, de-novo dominant mutations in the *ACTA1* gene account for a significant proportion of the severe form (while the rest are due to mutations in an as yet unidentified gene). Most of the classical milder congenital forms are due to recessive mutations in the *NEB* gene.[17] Prenatal diagnosis is therefore available for the genetically defined variants.

Central core disease

Central core disease is characterised by a variable degree of hypotonia and axial and proximal muscle weakness, predominantly affecting the hip girdle. Presentation with weakness is usually in infancy or early childhood, although contractures at birth (equinovarus foot deformity; hip dislocation) are frequently found. Some patients at the severe end of the spectrum may present with severe arthrogryposis and scoliosis. Severe facial and respiratory muscle weakness and bulbar dysfunction are not a feature. Serum CK activity is usually normal or only moderately elevated. Most affected individuals achieve the ability to walk. The natural course is static or only slowly progressive. Malignant hyperthermia susceptibility is a common complication and all cases should be considered to be at risk.

The biopsy typically shows predominantly central, core-like areas on oxidative stains (Fig. 41.60); however, these striking abnormalities can be absent in the infantile period and only develop later on in life.[34] As the condition is usually inherited in an autosomal dominant way, careful examination of the parents (and if necessary the pathological study of the one likely to be affected) might help to clarify the diagnosis in these cases in whom the pathological changes are not clear. Central core disease is commonly transmitted as an autosomal dominant trait with variable penetrance but many sporadic cases have also been reported. Dominant missense mutations in the skeletal muscle ryanodine receptor gene (*RYR1*) are found in most affected cases. De novo dominant mutations are common and account for the majority of sporadic cases. A few recessive pedigrees have, however, been reported very recently and the affected children in these families are severely affected, often in the neonatal period.

Myotubular (centronuclear) myopathy

This term derives from the numerous centrally placed nuclei (Fig. 41.61) with a surrounding central zone devoid of oxidative enzyme activity seen on the histological and histochemical reactions. A similar histological picture can be found in patients with

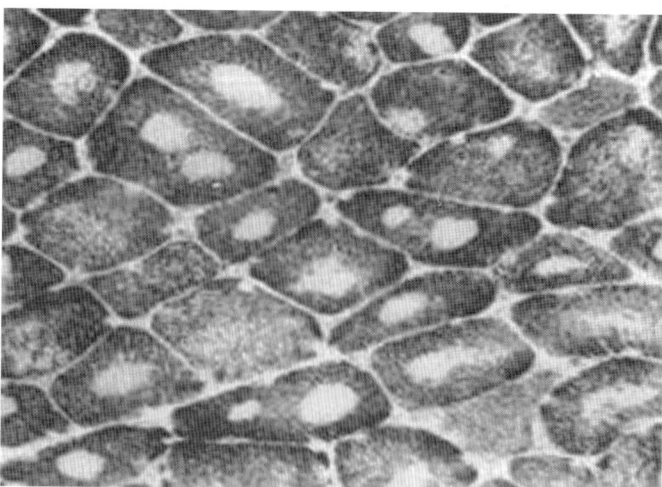

Fig. 41.60 Muscle biopsy showing central cores due to absent oxidative enzyme staining of the centre of the fibres (NADH).

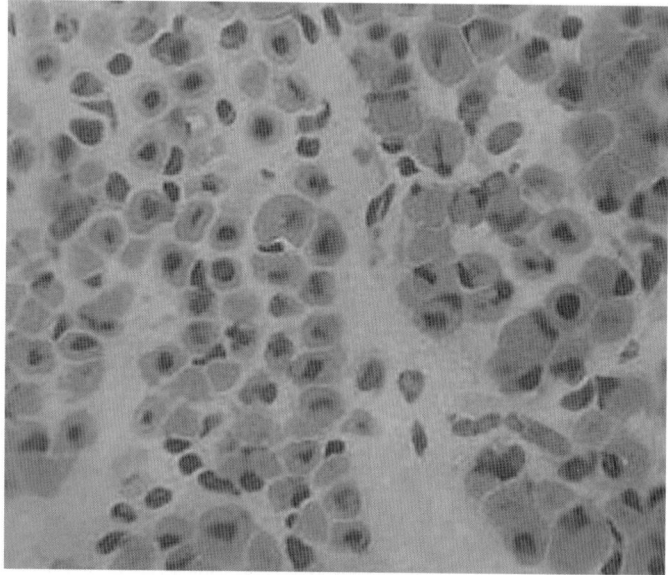

Fig. 41.61 Muscle biopsy showing multiple centrally placed nuclei in an infant with myotubular myopathy.

congenital myotonic dystrophy, and this may lead to diagnostic confusion if muscle biopsy is interpreted independently of the pedigree and clinical features in the affected infant and his/her mother.

The clinical phenotype of myotubular (centronuclear) myopathy is highly variable, depending on the mode of inheritance. The more common X-linked form results in a severe phenotype in males presenting with polyhydramnios, reduced fetal movements, marked hypotonia, a variable degree of external ophthalmoplegia, respiratory failure at birth and an often fatal course. Severely affected infants who are ventilator-dependent in the neonatal period may survive if receiving continuous invasive ventilation but show almost complete lack of motor developmental progress. The phenotype in the autosomal recessive forms can range from early presentation with marked proximal weakness and inability to walk to milder variants characterised by generalised weakness and a variable degree of external ophthalmoplegia.

The gene for the X-linked variant is the myotubularin gene (*MTM1*) on chromosome Xq28.

Minicore myopathy (multicore disease)

This is a rare condition, not usually presenting in the neonatal period. The most common phenotype features marked axial weakness with spinal rigidity, scoliosis and respiratory failure in late childhood. Another group of patients have associated partial or complete external ophthalmoplegia, and this is the variant that in our experience can present in the neonatal period. The name of the condition derives from the multifocal areas of myofibrillar disruption on oxidative enzyme staining. At least two genes are responsible for minicore disease: the *SEPN1* gene (the same one that when disrupted can give rise to rigid spine syndrome, suggesting that the two conditions are allelic) and recessive *RYR1* gene mutations.

Myasthenia gravis

Transient neonatal myasthenia

This self-limiting but potentially life-threatening immune-mediated form occurs in approximately 20% of infants born to mothers with acquired myasthenia gravis and is due to transplacental transfer of maternal antibodies directed against the acetylcholine receptor (AchR). The diagnosis in mothers is often known, with the myasthenia active or in remission. Transient myasthenia may rarely occur in infants born to undiagnosed mothers with subclinical disease but positive AchR antibody.[29] There is no direct relation between the severity of maternal myasthenia and symptoms in the infant.

Onset is within a few hours of birth and always within the first 3 days. Typical features include poor sucking/swallowing, generalised hypotonia, facial weakness and weak cry. Fatigability, especially during feeds, may be present. Respiratory difficulties may require mechanical ventilation. Ptosis and ophthalmoparesis are less common but diagnostically helpful, especially if variable. Recovery is anticipated by 2 months in 90% and by 4 months in all infants. Atypical presentation, in addition to the above symptoms, includes antenatal onset with polyhydramnios, decreased fetal movements and multiple joint contractures. Recurrent stillbirths with severe arthrogryposis secondary to maternal myasthenia have been described.[2]

Infants born to mothers with acquired myasthenia, either active or in remission, with or without AchR antibodies, should be considered at risk of developing neonatal myasthenia. Prenatal care includes surveillance for polyhydramnios, decreased fetal movements and consideration of maternal plasmaphaeresis to prevent fetal arthrogryposis. Infants should be observed for 3 days for development of symptoms. Once the first signs appear, diagnosis can be confirmed by anticholinesterase administration. Intramuscular neostigmine (single dose 0.15 mg/kg bodyweight) results in improvement in 15–30 minutes and lasts for 1–3 hours, allowing ample observation of the infant's feeding, crying, antigravity limb movements and respiration. This test should always be performed on the neonatal intensive care unit and a prior dose of atropine is helpful in reducing muscarinic side effects. Positive AchR antibodies, in the infant or the mother, are further evidence, but their absence does not rule out the diagnosis. In case of doubt, repetitive nerve stimulation at 3 Hz results in an electrodecremental response.

Management aims at supporting feeding and maintaining adequate ventilation until spontaneous recovery occurs. In symptomatic infants, neostigmine (or pyridostigmine) is given orally or by nasogastric tube 30 minutes before 4-hourly feeds. Gavage feeding and mechanical ventilation may be required in more severely affected infants. Anticholinesterases are gradually weaned off when the infant is no longer symptomatic, between 1 and 4 months of age.

Congenital myasthenic syndromes

Congenital myasthenic syndromes are inherited disorders resulting in neuromuscular transmission dysfunction. Inheritance is autosomal recessive, except for slow-channel syndrome, which is autosomal dominant. Depending on the site and mechanism of the neuromuscular transmission defect, they are classified into presynaptic, synaptic and postsynaptic categories, and the molecular basis of many of the congenital myasthenic syndromes has been described in the last decade.[12]

Symptomatic presentation at birth or in the early neonatal period is less common and only about half of the cases present in the first 2 years of life. Key features are fatigable weakness affecting ocular, bulbar, limb and respiratory muscles, apnoea and negative AchR antibodies. There may be a family history of similar illness or deaths during infancy. Although diagnostic algorithms are available,[11] the precise diagnosis of congenital myasthenic syndromes requires detailed neurophysiology. Molecular genetic analysis and patch clamping of muscle endplates confirm the diagnosis but are available only in specialised laboratories. The following are congenital myasthenic syndromes with neonatal presentation.

- **Congenital myasthenic syndrome with episodic apnoea (familial infantile myasthenia)**: Some babies present at birth with hypotonia and bulbar and respiratory muscle weakness, which gradually improves. Sudden apnoea and respiratory arrest in the course of intercurrent infection or fever in infancy is characteristic. In between these attacks, the infant may appear asymptomatic. Electrodecremental response is seen on 2 Hz repetitive stimulation and there is a good response to treatment with anticholinesterases. Recessive mutations in the choline acetyl transferase gene have been documented.
- **Endplate acetylcholinesterase deficiency**: Absence of acetylcholinesterase in the synaptic cleft results in a depolarisation block and, in the longer term, endplate myopathy. The pupillary light response may be slow and a repetitive compound action potential on motor nerve stimulation is present. Demonstration of mutations in the *COLQ* gene confirms the diagnosis. There is no response or worsening on anticholinesterase administration.

References

1. Aslanidis C, Jansen G, Amemiya C et al 1992 Cloning of the essential myotonic dystrophy region and mapping the putative defect. Nature 355: 1253–1255

2. Barnes P R, Kanabar D J, Brueton L et al 1995 Recurrent congenital arthrogryposis leading to a diagnosis of myasthenia gravis in an asymptomatic mother. Neuromuscular Disorders 5: 59–65

3. Barth P G 1993 Pontocerebellar hypoplasia. An overview of a group of inherited neurodegenerative disorders with fetal onset. Brain Development 15: 411–422

4. Camacho-Vanegas O, Bertini E, Zhang R Z et al 2001 Ullrich scleroatonic muscular dystrophy is caused by recessive mutations in collagen type VI. Proceedings of the National Academy of Sciences of the USA 98: 7516–7521

5. Dobyns W B, Pagon R A, Armstrong D et al 1989 Diagnostic criteria for Walker-Warburg syndrome. American Journal of Medical Genetics 32: 195–210

6. Dubowitz V 1995 Muscle disorders in childhood, 2nd edn. W B Saunders, London

7. Dubowitz V 1969 The floppy infant. Clinics in Developmental Medicine 31. Spastics International/Heinemann, London

8. Dubowitz V 1999 Very severe spinal muscular atrophy (SMA type 0): an expanding clinical phenotype. European Journal of Paediatric Neurology 3: 49–52

9. Dubowitz V 1994 Workshop report on 22nd ENMC-sponsored meeting on congenital muscular dystrophy held in Baarn, The Netherlands, 14–16 May 1993. Neuromuscular Disorders 4: 75–81

10. Dubowitz V, Daniels R J, Davies K E 1995 Olivopontocerebellar hypoplasia with anterior horn cell involvement (SMA) does not localize to chromosome 5q. Neuromuscular Disorders 5: 25–29

11. Engel A E 2001 Workshop report. 73rd ENMC international workshop: congenital myasthenic syndromes. Neuromuscular Disorders 11: 315–321

12. Engel A E, Ohno K, Sine S M 2003 Congenital myasthenic syndromes: Progress over the past decade. Muscle and Nerve 27: 4–25

13. Grohmann K, Schuelke M, Diers A et al 2001 Mutations in the gene encoding immunoglobulin mu-binding protein 2 cause spinal muscular atrophy with respiratory distress type 1. Nature Genetics 29: 75–77

14. Hageman G, Willemse J 1983 Arthrogryposis multiplex congenita. Neuropediatrics 14: 6–11

15. Hashimoto T, Tayama M, Myazaki M et al 1995 Neuroimaging study of myotonic dystrophy I. Magnetic resonance imaging of the brain. Brain Development 17: 24–27

16. Igarashi H, Momoi M Y, Yamagata T et al 1998 Hypertrophic cardiomyopathy in congenital myotonic dystrophy. Pediatric Neurology 18: 366–369

17. Jungbluth H, Sewry C A, Muntoni F 2003 What's new in neuromuscular disorders? The congenital myopathies. European Journal of Paediatric Neurology 7: 23–30

18. MacLeod M J, Taylor J E, Lunt P W et al 1999 Prenatal onset spinal muscular atrophy. European Journal of Paediatric Neurology 3: 65–72

19. Mercuri E, Goodwin F, Sewry C et al 2000 Diaphragmatic spinal muscular atrophy with bulbar weakness. European Journal of Paediatric Neurology 4: 69–72

20. Mercuri E, Heckmatt J, Dubowitz V 2001 The newborn with neuromuscular disorders. In: Levene M, Chervenak F A, Whittle M (eds) Fetal and neonatal neurology and neurosurgery. Churchill Livingstone, London

21. Mercuri E, Muntoni F 2001 Congenital muscular dystrophy. In: Emery A (ed) Muscular dystrophies. Oxford University Press, Oxford

22. Mercuri E, Muntoni F 2001 The neonate with neuromuscular disorder. In: Rutherford M, Bydder G (eds) Magnetic resonance imaging of the neonatal brain. W B Saunders, London

23. Mercuri E, Pennock J, Goodwin F et al 1996 Sequential study of central and peripheral nervous system involvement in an infant with merosin-deficient CMD. Neuromuscular Disorders 6: 425–429

24. Mercuri E, Rutherford M, DeVile C et al 2000 Early white matter changes on brain Magnetic Resonance Imaging in a newborn affected by merosin-deficient congenital muscular dystrophy. Neuromuscular Disorders 11: 297–299

25. Mercuri E, Yuva Y, Brown S C et al 2002 Collagen VI involvement in Ullrich syndrome: a clinical, genetic and immunohistochemical study. Neurology 58: 1354–1359

26. Muntoni F, Brockington M, Blake D J et al 2002 Defective glycosylation in muscular dystrophy. Review. Lancet 360; 360: 1419–1421

27. O'Brien J A, Harper P S 1984 Course prognosis and complications of childhood onset myotonic dystrophy. Developmental Medicine and Child Neurology 26: 62–67

28. Osawa M, Sumida S, Suzuki N et al 1997 Fukuyama type congenital progressive muscular dystrophy. In: Fukuyama Y, Osawa M, Saito K (eds) Congenital muscular dystrophies. Elsevier Science, London

29. Papazian O 1992 Transient neonatal myasthenia gravis. Journal of Child Neurology 7: 135–141

30. Philpot J, Sewry C, Pennock J et al 1995 Clinical phenotype in congenital muscular dystrophy: correlation with expression of merosin in skeletal muscle. Neuromuscular Disorders 5: 301–305

31. Regev R, de Vries L S, Heckmatt J Z et al 1987 Cerebral ventricular dilation in congenital myotonic dystrophy. Journal of Pediatrics 111: 372–376

32. Rutherford M A, Heckmatt J Z, Dubowitz V 1989 Congenital myotonic dystrophy: respiratory function at birth determines survival. Archives of Disease in Childhood 64: 191–195

33. Santavuori P, Somer H, Saino K et al 1989 Muscle eye brain disease (MEB). Brain Development 11: 147–153

34. Sewry C A, Muller C, Davis M et al 2002 The spectrum of pathology in central core disease. Neuromuscular Disorders 12: 930–938

35. Strehl E, Vanasse M 1985 EMG and needle muscle biopsy studies in arthrogryposis multiplex congenita. Neuropediatrics 16: 225–227

36. Sunada Y, Edgar T S, Lotz B P et al 1995 Merosin-negative congenital muscular dystrophy associated with extensive brain abnormalities. Neurology 45: 2084–2089

37. Tome F M, Evangelista T, Leclerc A et al 1994 Congenital muscular dystrophy with merosin deficiency. Comptes rendus de l'Academie des sciences. Serie III, Sciences de la vie 317–351

38. Van der Vleuten A J W, van Ravenswaaij-Arts C M A, Frijns C J M et al 1998 Localisation of the gene for a dominant congenital spinal muscular atrophy predominantly affecting the lower limbs to chromosome 12q23–q24. European Journal of Human Genetics 6: 376–382

PART 8

Central nervous system malformations

A Michael Weindling, Janet M Rennie

Epidemiological aspects

Incidence at birth

Congenital malformations of the central nervous system (CNS), consisting principally of spina bifida, anencephalus and hydrocephalus, form a large but progressively diminishing proportion of all major congenital malformations (Table 41.21, Fig. 41.62). Since the first edition of this book, there has been a sustained reduction in the prevalence of neural tube defects (NTDs) at birth. This has been due only in part to antenatal diagnosis and termination of pregnancy. At the same time, the use of magnetic resonance imaging (MRI) has resulted in an

Table 41.21 Number of babies (live and stillborn) with central nervous system defects born in England and Wales, and terminations of pregnancy for central nervous system defects

Year	Terminations of pregnancy	Anencephalus births	Spina bifida births	Congenital hydrocephalus births	Other CNS malformation births	Total CNS malformation births	Total CNS malformation
1974	34	849	1185	313	105	2452	4938
1976	81	644	880	267	124	1915	3911
1979	285	455	845	227	110	1637	3559
1983	511	114	422	194	187	917	2345
1987	529	31	202	117	161	511	1551
1990	452	26	120	92	122	360	1172
1993	536	14	81	71	88	255	1045
1996	N/A	27	61	76	90	254	N/A
1999	449	12	46	47	90	204	797
2001	411	12	47	65	109	233	726

Source: Office of National Statistics 1993, 2003 (www.statistics.gov.uk/statbase).

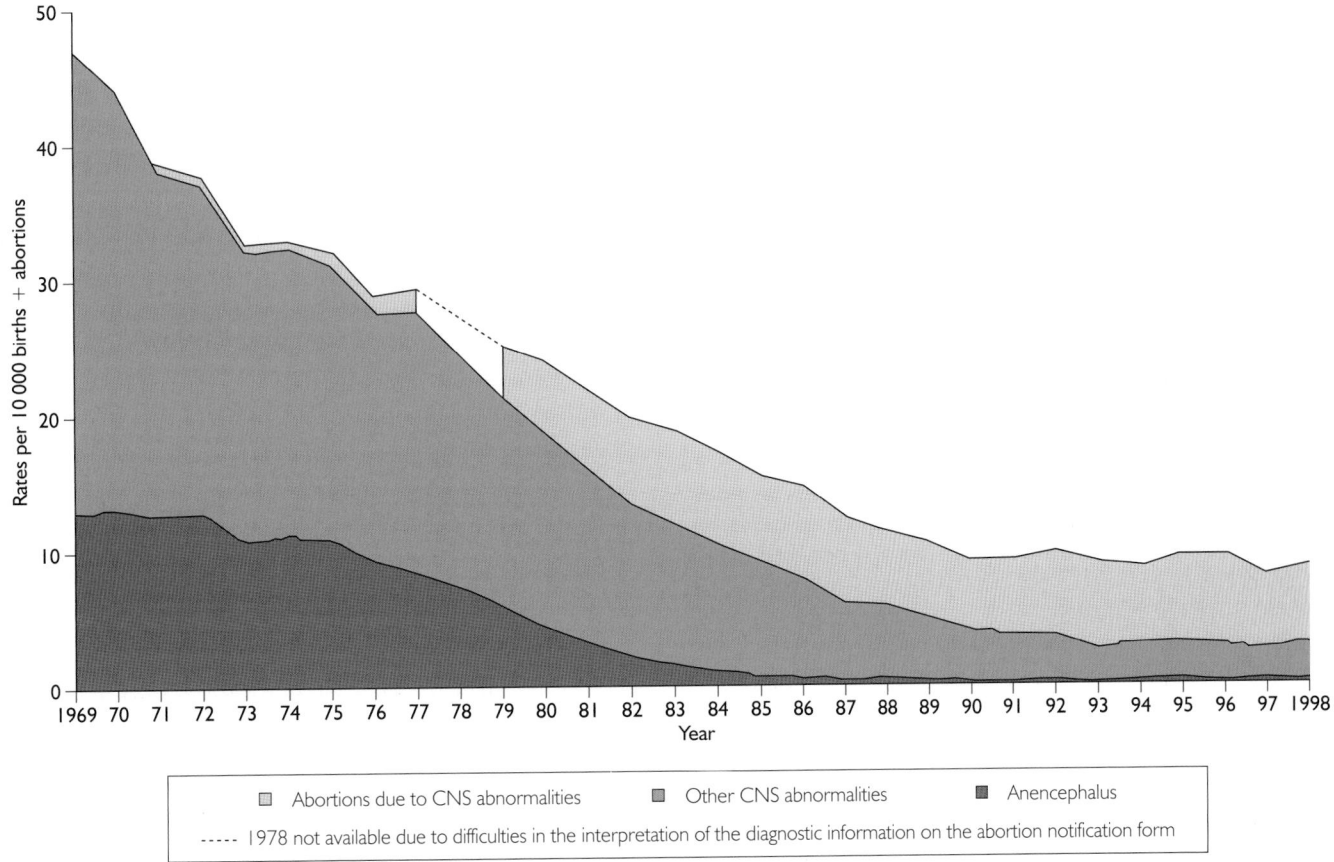

Fig. 41.62 Notification rates of anencephalus, other CNS anomalies and legal abortions for CNS anomalies in England and Wales 1968–1998. (With permission from Office for National Statistics 2002 Health statistics quarterly 16. ONS, London.)

increased diagnosis during life of cerebral malformations such as lissencephaly (meaning 'smooth brain', where gyral formation is reduced).

Antenatal diagnosis by ultrasound has also created new dilemmas, particularly for parents whose fetus has a condition for which the prognosis is uncertain, such as mild unilateral ventriculomegaly, isolated agenesis of the corpus callosum, hemimegalencephaly or a middle cranial fossa arachnoid cyst. In addition, a great deal of parental anxiety is engendered by the antenatal finding of a minor CNS malformation such as a choroid plexus cyst or an enlarged cisterna magna. This evolution in clinical practice has required a change of emphasis from earlier editions,

Table 41.22 Rates of central nervous system abnormalities per 10 000 total births, England and Wales 1991–2001

Malformation	Year of birth									
	1988	1990	1992	1994	1996	1997	1998	1999	2000	2001
All CNS	7.3	5.1	4.6	4.0	3.9	3.5	4.5	4.8	6.1	5.3
Anencephalus	0.6	0.4	0.5	0.4	0.4	0.5	0.3	0.4	0.4	0.5
Spina bifida	2.3	1.7	1.2	0.7	0.9	0.8	1.0	1.0	1.4	1.0
Hydrocephalus	2.0	1.3	1.4	1.2	1.2	1.0	1.2	1.0	1.6	1.4

Source: Office for National Statistics 2002 Health statistics quarterly 16. ONS, London: p 67.

and the reader is referred to the second edition in particular for an excellent and detailed account of NTDs.

In 1974, almost 5000 babies were conceived with CNS defects of all types. By 1993, this figure had reduced to just over 1000, and among live births CNS defects had reduced tenfold. During the same period, other malformations increased from 159 to 191 per 10 000 deliveries.[83,85] Anencephalic births fell from 13.1 to 0.2 per 10 000 between 1974 and 1993; spina bifida from 18.3 to 1.2 and hydrocephalus from 4.8 to 1.0 per 10 000. The rates of CNS abnormalities per 10 000 total births between 1988 and 2001 are shown in Table 41.22. The most recent data available (Summer 2004) showed no change in the rates of developmental abnormalities of the central nervous system between 1992 and 2002. The rates per 10,000 total births in England and Wales were 1.3 for anencephalus, 1.2 for spina bifida and 1.3 for hydrocephalus. These data add to the previous incidence figures contained in Table 41.22.

Interestingly, a nuclear accident in Chernobyl in the Ukraine in 1986 had no effect on the incidence of NTDs, or indeed any other congenital anomalies.[34]

Regional variations

There are large variations in the incidence of CNS defects in different parts of the world[38,108] and at different periods. In 1986, the incidence of NTDs in the USA was estimated at 1 per 1000 deliveries, anencephaly at 0.6–0.8 per 1000 deliveries and open spina bifida as 0.5–0.8 per 1000 deliveries.[4] In the British Isles, the highest incidence is in Ireland, where the incidence of anencephaly was 6.7 per 1000 deliveries in Belfast,[72] followed by Wales. In England, the highest incidence was in the north-west and the lowest in the south-east but these differences have been almost eliminated by antenatal diagnosis and terminations of pregnancies. The incidence in Thailand in a study undertaken between 1989 and 2000 was, by contrast, low: although the incidence of NTDs was similar to Western countries (0.66 per 1000 births), spina bifida occurred in only 0.06 per 1000 births.[59] Nevertheless, low socioeconomic status increases the risk of an NTD-affected pregnancy, with risk increasing across a gradient of socioeconomic indicators.[118]

Sex incidence

In anencephalus and in encephalocele, the sex ratio of females to males is 7:3 and in spina bifida it is 55:45, but in congenital hydrocephalus it is 4:6. An explanation of these differences might provide one possible clue to the causation of CNS defects.

Twins

Both twins are rarely affected by NTD. Furthermore, if both twins are affected by a CNS malformation, the site may be different. Analysis of a series of 887 pairs in which at least one twin had either anencephalus or spina bifida showed that the concordance rate was only 4.9%. In twin pairs with spina bifida alone, the concordance in like-sexed twins was 9% and in unlike-sexed twins 1%. In monozygous twins, the concordance was 12% of pairs.[70]

The family history and recurrence risks of spina bifida, anencephalus and congenital hydrocephalus

The risk of recurrence in siblings following the birth of a fetus or baby with an NTD is around 5%[19,20,65] and may be related to the incidence in the area at a given time. For example, in the British Isles the highest recurrence rate recorded was 8.8% in the high-incidence area of Belfast in the 1960s[80] and the lowest 3.4% in the south-east of England during the 1970s.[100] The risk is increased when the interval between the end of the previous pregnancy and the beginning of the current pregnancy is short. For example, when the interpregnancy interval is less than 6 months and the previous pregnancy resulted in a livebirth (as opposed to spontaneous abortion or elective termination), the risk of NTD is doubled (odds ratio, OR, 2.0, 95% confidence interval, CI, 1.0–3.8).[111] These observations are likely to be due to nutritional effects (see below).

The recurrence risk of an NTD is approximately 10% if the mother has already had two or more affected cases.[22,65,103] The risk to children of a parent who had spina bifida is of the same order as to siblings after a single affected case.[21] The risk to more distant relations is far less.

There is a considerably increased risk of CNS malformations to siblings of a child who has congenital hydrocephalus unassociated with spina bifida. In Sheffield, 187 patients with congenital hydrocephalus had 338 siblings: 13 (3.8%) had CNS defects, of which five had hydrocephalus and eight had spina bifida or anencephalus. It seems, therefore, that at least a part of the 'congenital hydrocephalus' group is of similar or identical aetiology to spina bifida and anencephalus.[66,68] In a smaller group in Belfast, there was a recurrence rate of 1.9% for congenital hydrocephalus, which was 26 times higher than the rate in the local population.[1] Cohen et al[27] collected data from various parts of the world to show that following the birth of a baby with isolated hydrocephalus the risk of anencephalus in subsequent pregnancies was 1%, of spina bifida 0.6% and of isolated hydrocephalus 1.5%.

Prevention of central nervous system defects

Antenatal diagnosis followed by termination of pregnancy

There is an elevated alpha-fetoprotein level in the maternal blood and amniotic fluid in the presence of an open NTD in the fetus.[12,13,116] Alpha-fetoprotein is widely offered as a serum screening test for the detection of NTDs in pregnancy (Ch. 9), in addition to a careful examination of the fetal brain and spine with ultrasound during an anomaly scan at 18–20 weeks gestation. Interpretation of the result is highly dependent on accurate dating of the pregnancy: high serum alpha-fetoprotein concentrations may also be obtained in cases of twin pregnancy, exomphalos and urinary tract abnormalities, as well as in cases of fetal death in utero. The predictive value can be improved by the analysis of the blood acetylcholinesterase concentration, which is also high in NTD pregnancies.[116]

Routine anomaly scanning during pregnancy can now detect many CNS malformations such as the Dandy–Walker malformation, enlarged ventricles, cerebral asymmetry and agenesis of the corpus callosum (Table 41.23). The accuracy of antenatal diagnosis of anencephaly and spina bifida is good, whereas for other malformations there is less precision. For many of these diagnoses the natural history is uncertain. For others, such as the Dandy–Walker malformation, the generally poor prognosis (see below) is sufficiently established for it to be reasonable to recommend termination of the pregnancy.

Vitamin supplementation

True prevention of NTDs is possible by periconceptional folate supplementation.[104,105] Furthermore, periconceptional exposure to folic acid antagonists, including carbamazepine, phenobarbital (phenobarbitone), phenytoin and trimethoprim, during the first or second month after the last menstrual period increases the risk of NTD almost threefold (OR 2.8, 95% CI 1.7–4.6).[47] Current UK recommendations are that all women who plan to become pregnant should take folate supplementation, in the form of 4 mg daily, from before conception to the 12th week of pregnancy.[39] A generally better diet has probably contributed to the fall in CNS malformations at conception, in spite of the fact that few women in antenatal clinics have heard of the government's

Table 41.23 Major central nervous system malformations that can be diagnosed antenatally by ultrasound

Diagnosis	Reference
Anencephaly	Campbell et al 1972[18]
	Goldstein et al 1989[43]
Spina bifida	Nicolaides et al 1986[81]
Lipomyelomeningocele	Seeds and Jones 1986[99]
Diastematomyelia	Anderson et al 1994[5]
Encephalocele	Chatterjee et al 1985[23]
Hydrocephalus	Chervenak et al 1983[24]
Holoprosencephaly	Chervenak et al 1985[25]
Hydranencephaly	Hadi et al 1986[46]
Callosal agenesis	Comstock et al 1985[28]
	Meizner et al 1987[74]
Schizencephaly	Kligensmith and Cioffi-Ragan 1986[60]
	Kormarniski et al 1990[61]
Lissencephaly	Saltzman et al 1991[94]
Hemimegalencephaly	Sandri et al 1991[95]
Microcephaly	Chervenak et al 1987[26]
	Den Hollander et al 2000[32]
Septo-optic dysplasia	Pilu et al 1990[90]
Vein of Galen malformation	Vintzileos et al 1986[113]
	Dan et al 1992[31]
Agenesis of the cerebellar vermis	Campbell et al 1984[18]
Dandy–Walker malformation	Russ et al 1989[93]
Arachnoid cyst	Chervenak et al 1983[24]
Porencephalic cyst	Vintzileos et al 1987[114]

advice about folate.[109] Maternal periconceptional multivitamin use has been suggested to reduce the incidence of fetal cleft palate[102] and childhood neuroectodermal tumours, particularly medulloblastoma (p. 958), but to increase the risk of twinning.[16,30]

Clinical aspects

Anencephalus

In anencephalus, the posterior parts of the skull bones fail to develop and fuse and a malformed rudimentary brain with absent cerebral hemispheres (or even more gross defects) is exposed and is covered with congested meninges (Fig. 41.63). There is often an associated spina bifida as well as other malformations. It is frequently associated with hydramnios.

All babies with anencephalus die. Although one case survived for several years because of artificial ventilation she did not develop any useful independent function.[6] The clinical importance of the condition lies in the increased probability of CNS defects, including spina bifida, in subsequent siblings. The parents should know the reason for the stillbirth or neonatal death and should be given genetic counselling.

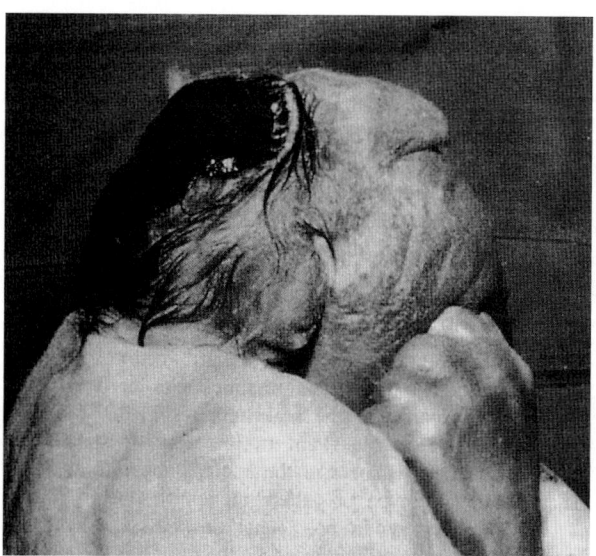

Fig. 41.63 Anencephaly. (From Forfar & Arneil's Textbook of Paediatrics, 5th edn. Churchill Livingstone, Edinburgh.)

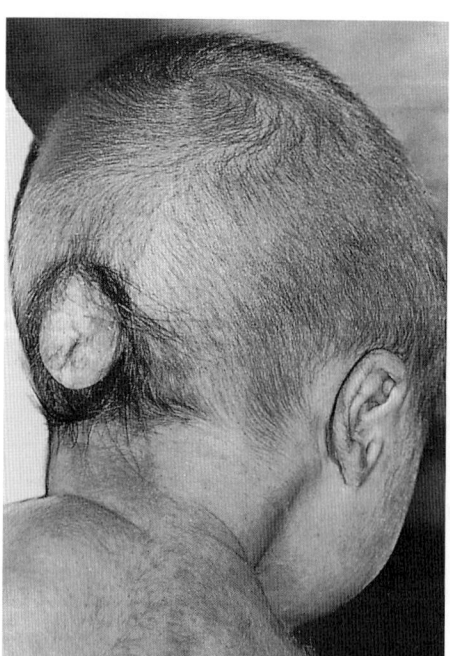

Fig. 41.64 Cranium bifidum: meningocele.

Cranial encephalocele and meningocele

The incidence of these conditions is about 1–3 per 10 000 in Western countries, but more in south-east Asia. Cranial encephalocele occurs in about four-fifths of all cases. In both conditions, the skull bone is deficient and a cystic swelling arises through the defect, usually in the occipital region. In cranial meningocele, the swelling is covered with skin or membrane and contains only cerebrospinal fluid (CSF) (Fig. 41.64) but in cranial encephalocele abnormal brain tissue is also present in the sac.

The rest of the brain is often also grossly abnormal. In about half the patients the swelling is over 6 cm in diameter and may be larger than the skull itself (Fig. 41.65). Microcephalus, where there is a decreased volume of brain substance, is very common. Hydrocephalus, where the ventricular volume is increased, occurs in about half.

Encephaloceles are usually occipital but can be parietal, frontal or protrude into the upper nasal cavity, causing considerable diagnostic difficulties. Frontal encephaloceles are commoner in south-east Asia. Frequently there are associated malformations, including myelomeningocele, cleft palate, the Klippel–Feil syndrome and a variety of other conditions. The Meckel–Gruber syndrome (MKS) is the most common monogenic cause of NTD. It is an autosomal recessive disorder. Other (variable) abnormalities, include: encephalocele, polycystic kidneys, hepatic ductal dysplasia and cysts, polydactyly and hydrocephalus. There is heterogeneity of the gene locus, which has been mapped to chromosome 17q21–24 in Finnish families (*MKS1*), to 11q13 in north African and Middle Eastern families (*MKS2*), and 8q24 in Indian families (*MKS3*), in whom polydactyly and possibly encephalocele seems to be less common.[78]

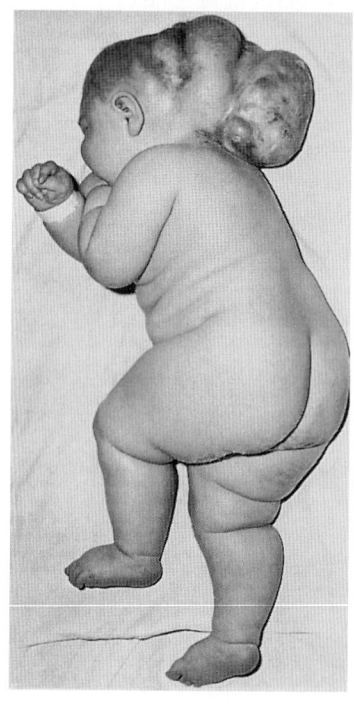

Fig. 41.65 Encephalocele.

Investigation and treatment

All infants with an encephalocele, even small ones, should be investigated with neuroimaging to investigate any intra-cranial malformations and to uncover incipient hydrocephalus. The lesion should be surgically treated, and the excision may need be followed by treatment of associated hydrocephalus. Babies with large lesions often die quickly. Nevertheless, surgical treatment is indicated for those who survive the first weeks, because a large unoperated lesion creates immense nursing problems.

Prognosis

The prognosis in occipital meningocele is good but in most with true encephaloceles it is poor. In a series of 147 cases followed

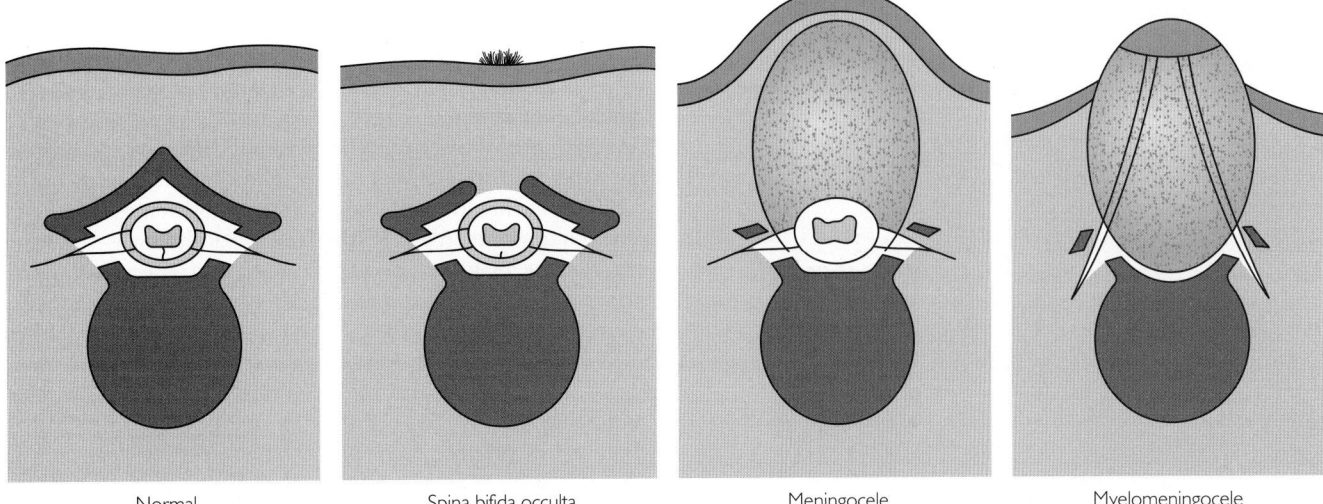

| Normal | Spina bifida occulta | Meningocele | Myelomeningocele |

Fig. 41.66 Classification of spina bifida. (Redrawn from Forfar & Arneil's Textbook of Paediatrics, 4th edn. Churchill Livingstone, Edinburgh.)

over 20 years, 90% of the 32 with meningocele survived, compared with 40% among the 115 with true encephalocele. Of the survivors with occipital meningocele, 48% were fully normal in contrast with only 4% of those with encephalocele, while 15% and 26% respectively were physically and mentally handicapped. The main physical handicaps in encephalocele are cortical blindness or partial sight, spastic quadriplegia, cerebellar ataxia and epilepsy. Very large lesions or microcephalus associated with the encephalocele carry the worst prognosis.[71]

Spina bifida

Spina bifida is due to failure of neural tube closure by days 26–28 after conception.[77] The term 'spina bifida', meaning disruption of the vertebral arches, encompasses several types of lesion. *Spina bifida aperta* refers to an open lesion where the skin is completely deficient. *Spina bifida cystica* refers to a lesion covered with a membrane that later epithelialises. Spina bifida cystica can be a meningocele or a myelomeningocele (Fig. 41.66). *Spina bifida occulta* refers to a failure of the vertebral arches to fuse, and this is always a completely skin-covered lesion. This group includes babies with dermal sinuses, lipomyelomeningocele and diastematomyelia. In diastematomyelia the spinal cord is split into two parts, sometimes by a bony bar.

The importance of recognising these latter conditions is because of the risk of cord tethering, with resultant neurological disability. It is possible to have neurological complications from tethered cord without any surface clues, but midline skin dimples or sinuses over the vertebral column should always be regarded with suspicion (pp. 1194, 1195). Blind-ending dimples and pits within an inch of the natal cleft can safely be ignored (see Chapter 38)[42] but any midline skin lesion on the back that is higher than this deserves further investigation. Ultrasound in experienced hands can provide sufficient reassurance but if there is doubt MRI of the spine is recommended.[42,62]

Meningocele

Between 5% and 10% of all spina bifida cystica lesions are cases of meningocele, a benign condition of mostly mesodermal origin. One or two spinous processes are absent and protruding through the gap is a small midline sac, which is covered either by membrane or by skin, contains only CSF and freely transilluminates (Fig. 41.66).

The frequency of hydrocephalus associated with meningocele is about 10%, which is far less than in myelomeningocele, and usually the hydrocephalus is less severe. Most infants would survive without operation but operative closure is advisable at a convenient time, either because the cystic lesion may burst, leading to meningitis, or for cosmetic reasons. The prognosis is excellent and most survive without handicap.

Meningocele is not always detected antenatally because it is a closed lesion; the amniotic fluid does not contain excess alphafetoprotein. In any case, termination of pregnancy is not indicated.

Myelomeningocele

A myelomeningocele has abnormalities in the spinal cord or cauda equina in addition to a cystic dilatation of the meninges, skin and a vertebral defect (Fig. 41.66). Affected infants show neurologic abnormalities below the level of the lesion. Myelomeningoceles are usually thoracolumbar (Fig. 41.67), which carry the worst prognosis, or lumbar, lumbosacral (Fig. 41.68) or, less commonly, purely sacral. Multiple lesions can occur. The lesion is usually symmetrical. A small proportion have hemimyelocele: only half of the affected segment is abnormal and forms the neural plaque.[36]

The lesions are often large, affecting several segments of the spinal cord with defects in the vertebrae including the splaying out and deformity of the spinal laminae with deformities of the vertebral bodies. In a minority, there is kyphosis at birth, which makes the prognosis much worse. Frequently, there are abnormalities of the vertebrae well above the lesion itself, which can only be detected by X-ray of the whole vertebral column and the

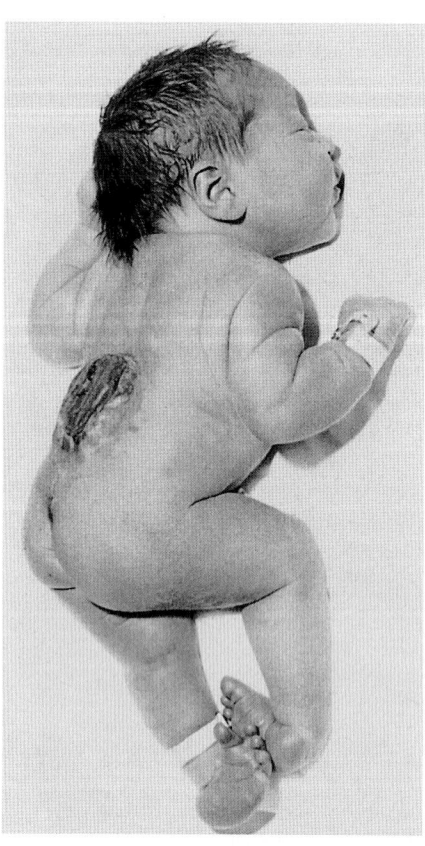

Fig. 41.67
Thoracolumbar
myelomeningocele.

chest: wedge-shaped vertebrae or hemivertebrae occur often associated with defects, fusion or absence of some ribs. These will invariably lead to severe scoliosis.

Clinical assessment

Examination of the newborn baby should be performed by a clinician with appropriate experience. The width and length of the spinal lesion should be measured and its position relative to the spinal column recorded. Within the cystic lesion is the neural plaque – the maldeveloped spinal cord that is exposed on the surface (Fig. 41.69). Immediately after birth, the nerve roots can be clearly seen through the CSF within the sac: they usually run horizontally or even upward because the physiological cranial migration of the cord was impeded during fetal life. The neural plaque may occupy the centre, or the upper or lower part of the whole lesion. A large plaque with a high upper level carries a bad prognosis, with extensive paralysis and analgesia.

Paralysis

There is a wide range of paralysis possible in the legs, from none to complete. Typically, the paralysis is of lower motor neurone type (flaccid). Knowledge (and a chart) of the segmental innervation of the leg muscles (Table 41.24[101]) is helpful and the neurological level of paralysis may be ascertained in each leg separately and charted. The neurological level does not necessarily coincide with the vertebral level. All muscles below the uppermost affected segment may be paralysed. Another pattern

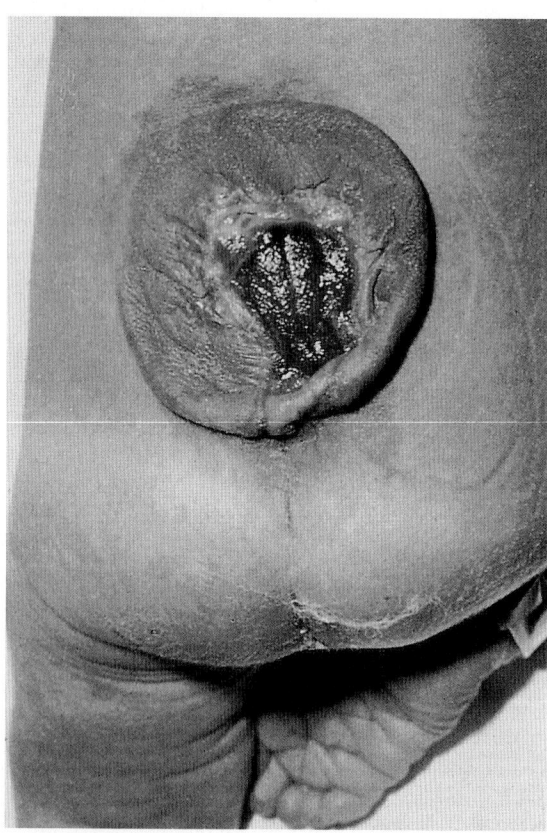

Fig. 41.68 Lumbosacral myelomeningocele with typical central neural plaque and patulous anus.

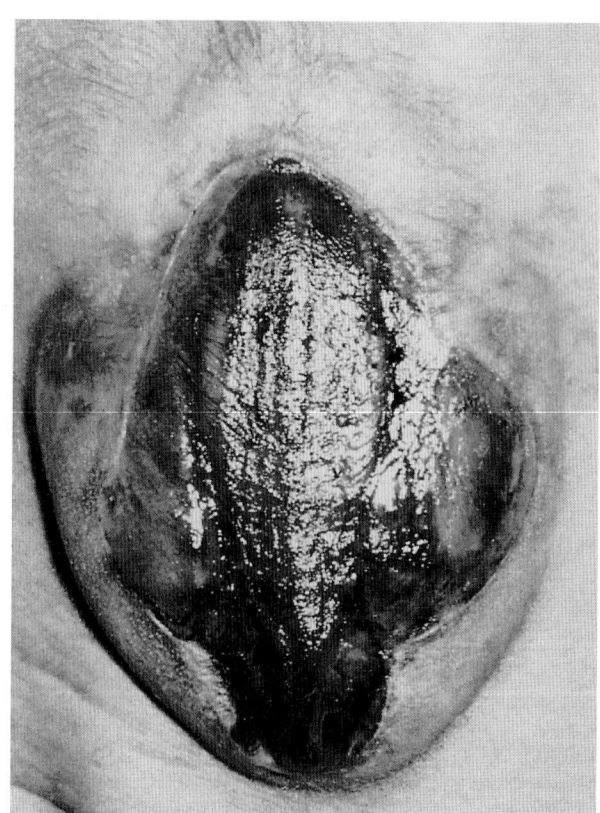

Fig. 41.69 Large open myelomeningocele showing the typical 'filleted' appearance of the central plaque.

also occurs, especially in thoracolumbar lesions, with flaccid paralysis of muscles deriving their innervation from the affected segments followed by reflex movements in muscles below the affected segments. Reflex activity, which later disappears and may be followed by spasticity,[106] should not be mistaken for useful voluntary movement. Stimulation of the legs may provoke reflex movements and mislead the examiner; it is better to stimulate the upper half of the body to elicit active movement in unaffected muscle groups.

The sphincters and the urinary tract

Almost all babies with myelomeningocele have paralysed urethral sphincters. Watching the baby may identify dribbling incontinence and inability to pass a stream of urine, although a moderate stream can be achieved when the baby is crying, due to contraction of the abdominal muscles. In the absence of normal sphincter control, urine can be expressed.

An intravenous urethrogram or a renal ultrasound and a micturating cysto-urethrogram will show whether there is hydronephrosis, retention of urine, trabeculation or diverticulae in the bladder and/or ureteric reflux. The expressibility of the bladder and the residual urine can also be demonstrated. Other renal defects, such as single kidney, horseshoe kidneys, pelvic kidney and double pelvis and ureters are some ten times commoner than in infants without NTDs. The anus is not visible in normal babies without separating the buttocks, but when the muscles of the perineum and of the rectal sphincters are paralysed it is on the surface and patulous. Perianal rugae may still be present. The anal sphincter cannot contract on perianal stimulation or grip a small finger inserted into the rectum.

Hydrocephalus

The maximum head circumference must be measured and charted and related to the baby's weight and gestational age. Cranial ultrasound is an essential early investigation in myelomeningocele and can reveal dilated ventricles before the head circumference enlarges. Ultrasound, computed tomography (CT) or MR imaging can also reveal the associated Chiari malformation, which can cause bulbar paresis. Treatment is by insertion of a ventricular shunt.

Treatment and prognosis

Emergency active treatment of all babies, irrespective of irreversible major neurological handicaps, led to the survival of

Table 41.24 Root innervation responsible for flexion and extension in regions of the lower limbs

	Flexion	Extension
Hip	L1–L2	S1–S2
Knee	L5–S1	L3–L4
Ankle	L4–L5	S1–S2
Toes	S2–S3	L4–S1

Adapted from Sharrard W J W 1964 The segmental innervation of the lower limb muscles in man. Annals of the Royal College of Surgeons 35: 106–122.

many severely handicapped children.[67,107] A selective approach was advocated by Lorber (see below) and adopted by many clinicians in the 1980s. Now far fewer babies are born with spina bifida. In those that are there has very often been an antenatal diagnosis, allowing early counselling.

Most infants are offered surgical repair. The survival rate has improved from that reported 25 years ago. There are North American studies that claim that almost all the children become ambulatory, although longer follow-up reveals that many become wheelchair-bound in adulthood.[50,51,63] Infants whose spina bifida lesion is surgically closed will usually develop progressive hydrocephalus and require insertion of a ventricular shunt, usually ventriculo-peritoneal.

The prognosis for mobility and continence depends on the level of the lesion, while the prognosis for intelligence mainly depends on the presence of hydrocephalus and the associated volume of brain parenchyma. When there is a Chiari malformation, there may be progressive further neurological deficit in later childhood, and syringomyelia can develop. Progressive spinal deformity can also produce severe problems. Cord tethering due to diastematomyelia is another cause of later progressive neurological deterioration in children with myelomeningocele.

The sensory level is the best guide to prognosis: by the age of 35 years all adults with a sensory level above L3 were wheelchair-bound (although some had been able to walk as teenagers), whereas half of those with a sensory level below L4 were community walkers.[50,51] Of this cohort, operated between 1963 and 1971, 70% were of normal intelligence (Fig. 41.70) but only 13/54 survivors were employed on the open market. Only 26% were fully continent; most of those who were successfully managing incontinence were using intermittent catheterisation. A sensory level above T11 was indicative of a poor prognosis, with a high mortality and severe disability probable in the survivors.

Fetal surgery for myelomeningocele

Fetal surgery has been the subject of limited investigation. A multicentre randomised controlled trial to compare the results of intrauterine repair of myelomeningocele at 19–25 weeks postconception with postnatal repair started in March 2003.[117] The overall conclusion, based on existing evidence, is that intrauterine repair of myelomeningocele decreases the incidence of hindbrain herniation and hydrocephalus but increases the risk of premature delivery.[15,110]

The arguments for prenatal surgery have been summarised by Walsh and Adzick:[117] in essence, they are that neural tissue, unprotected by its covering of skin and muscle, may be vulnerable to secondary destruction. It has been suggested that this may be due to chemical injury by amniotic fluid, direct trauma or trauma because of increased CSF pressure in the subarachnoid space, for example when the baby's head is compressed during labour, leading to damage to the spinal roots.[117] Some evidence for direct trauma to the cord comes from the observation that neural tissue is mainly lost where the uncovered cord protrudes dorsally.[35,52,76]

Spina bifida occulta

This affects some 5–10% of the population. Some have outward signs: a naevus, cutis aplasia, dimple, fatty pad or hairy tuft over

Neurological deficit in infancy in 117 consecutive cases of open spina bifida and outcome in 54 people who survived to mean age 35 years

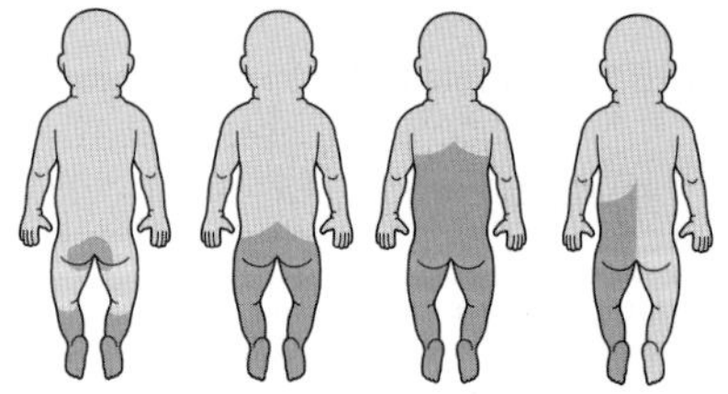

Sensory level in infancy

Below L3   L3–T11   Above T11   Asymmetrical

	Below L3	L3–T11	Above T11	Asymmetrical	P value for trend*
Whole cohort	38	32	42	5	
Those who died (n = 63)	14	17	30	2	<0.01

Disability and lifestyle in survivors (mean age 35):

	Below L3	L3–T11	Above T11	Asymmetrical	
Survivors	24	15	12	3	
No CSF shunt (n = 8)	7	0	1	0	<0.05
IQ ≥ 80 (n = 39)ℑ	21	11	6	1	0.05
Community walker (n = 16)#	16	0	0	0	<0.0001
Continent (n = 11)ξ	8	2	0	1	<0.05
Live independently (n = 22)λ	14	5	2	1	<0.05
Drive cars (n = 20)	14	4	2	0	<0.05
Open employment (n = 13)	9	2	2	0	0.18

* X² test. Asymmetrical sensory level excluded from analysis.
ℑ IQ recorded at age 5–15 years.
\# Able to walk ≥50 metres with aids if required.
ξ Continent without catheters or appliances.
λ Living in the community without help or supervision.

Fig. 41.70 Neurological deficit in infancy in 117 consecutive cases of open spina bifida and outcome in 54 people who survived to mean age 35 years. (With permission from Hunt G Oakeshott P 2003 Outcome in people with open spina bifida at age 35: prospective community based cohort study. British Medical Journal 326: 1365–1366.)

the lumbosacral region. Figure 41.71a shows a skin lesion that was associated with spina bifida occulta in the underlying vertebrae. A dermal sinus and evidence of cord tethering requiring surgery was revealed on MRI (Fig. 41.71b). Failure of the vertebral arches to fuse is not of itself significant but it may indicate more extensive involvement of the spinal cord. The finding of a cutaneous stigma on the back, other than a pit in or just above the natal cleft (p. 1195), is an indication for investigation with ultrasound and/or MRI. The entire length of the spine should be examined, as multiple lesions can exist.

Ultrasound appearances suggestive of spinal dysraphism include a low conus (below L3), a non-tapered conus and a thick filum terminale.[62] The median position of the conus was

midway between L1/L2 disc and L2 body in 105 infants studied at Northwick Park Hospital;[92] the range was from T12 to L3 with only 3% at L3. Infants with a conus below L3 should have MRI to exclude tethering. A normal spinal ultrasound, provided it has been performed by an experienced paediatric sonographer, can exclude spinal dysraphism.[42,62] Spinal lesions that can cause neurological complications later can exist without any cutaneous clues: two abnormal infants were found in the Northwick Park series.[92] Patients with spina bifida occulta do not have an increased risk of the Chiari malformation or hydrocephalus.

Investigation of cases of spina bifida occulta frequently uncovers lesions such as lipomyelomeningocele, diastematomyelia, dermoid cysts and sinuses. Most paediatric neurosurgeons recommend early surgery for these conditions in order to preserve urologic sphincter function.[58] Early surgery is particularly important in cases of dermoid sinus that predispose to meningitis.

Lipomyelomeningocele

Lipomyelomeningocele was once regarded as a purely cosmetic defect. It is now realised that the majority of children acquire disability in early childhood due to cord tethering or compression of neural elements by the mass. Bruce and Schut[14] reported that 88% of unoperated patients with lipomyelomeningocele lost neurologic function in the first few years of life, so that early surgery is recommended.[58,97] Malignant transformation has not been described. Some 11% of children followed up at around 7 years after surgery showed deterioration in mobility, 82% remained static (the others were non-ambulatory at the time of the operation); late deterioration was only seen in children with lipomyelomeningocele and was associated with obesity and re-tethering of the cord.[98]

Hydrocephalus

Congenital hydrocephalus

Congenital hydrocephalus unassociated with spina bifida may be a single abnormality or may be associated with other congenital CNS malformations such as agenesis of the corpus callosum, Dandy–Walker cyst or the Arnold–Chiari malformation. Hydrocephalus is also associated with non-CNS malformations such as congenital heart disease, intestinal atresia, chromosome abnormalities or anophthalmia. There is a rare, genetic, sex-linked form of aqueduct stenosis confined to males,[37] often associated with flexion and adduction defects of the thumbs. The commonest cause of hydrocephalus due to a congenital malformation but unassociated with spina bifida is aqueduct stenosis (Table 41.25). In preterm infants, the most common cause is following intraventricular haemorrhage, which may occur prenatally.

Clinical diagnosis of hydrocephalus in the newborn
Hydrocephalus may be evident at birth and the diagnosis is almost certain if a baby's maximal head circumference exceeds

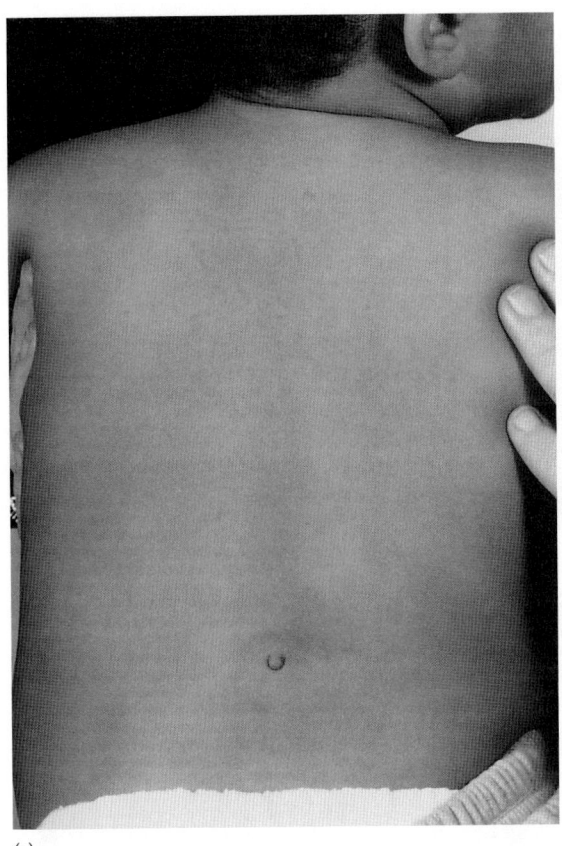

(a)

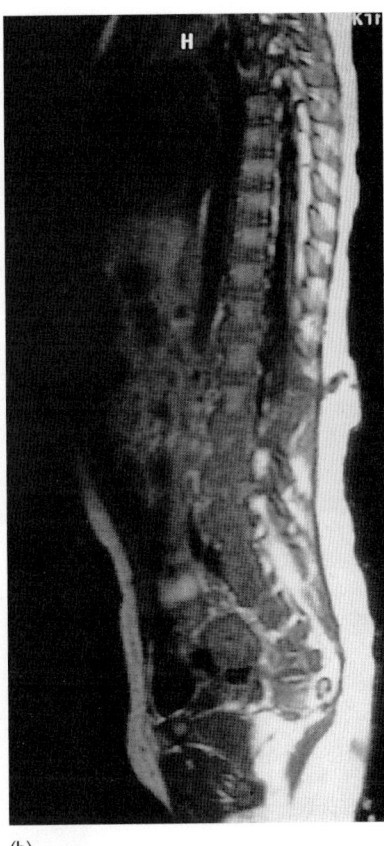

(b)

Fig. 41.71 (a) A midline skin lesion over the lumbar spine in an asymptomatic infant (Picture reproduced with permission from the child's parents, with thanks). (b) MRI scan of the same child revealed a tethered cord and a dermal sinus.

Table 41.25 Causes of neonatal hydrocephalus

Congenital malformations	Aqueduct stenosis
	Chiari malformation
	X-linked aqueduct stenosis
	Dandy–Walker malformation
Posthaemorrhagic	Intraventricular haemorrhage; preterm
	Intraventricular haemorrhage secondary to a bleeding disorder or asphyxia at term
	Subarachnoid haemorrhage
	Birth trauma
	Vitamin K deficiency bleeding
Postinfective	Neonatal meningitis
	Intrauterine viral infection
Neoplastic lesions	
Vascular malformations	Aneurysm of the vein of Galen, arteriovenous malformations
Choroid plexus papilloma	
Skull defects	Osteogenesis imperfecta
	Craniosynostosis

the 97th centile by 2 cm or more (corrected for gestational age and birthweight), the anterior fontanelle is large or bulging, the cranial sutures are widely separated and the posterior fontanelle is still open at term.

Many hydrocephalic babies have no suspicious signs at birth but their head grows abnormally fast: cranial growth is largely passive with the cranium increasing in size in response to the growth of its contents, normally brain but, if there is hydrocephaly, ventricular volume. Good practice includes measuring every baby's occipitofrontal head circumference at birth and plotting the measurement on a growth chart. The rate of increase in head size can then be assessed by subsequent measurements. Excessive cranial growth is an indication for early investigation, so that early treatment can be initiated to achieve the best possible result. Cranial ultrasound is the first investigation (Fig. 41.72), and can be particularly helpful in reassuring parents whose small baby is merely exhibiting catch-up growth of the head.

Benign enlargement of the subarachnoid space ('external' hydrocephalus)

Neuroimaging investigation of infants with large heads has revealed that a proportion have an enlarged subarachnoid space, without dilatation of the lateral ventricles or a subdural haematoma.[75] The infants, some of whom are ex-preterm infants, exhibit a pattern of head growth that is above and parallel to the 97th centile. Recognition of this diagnostic entity can save an accusation of non-accidental injury being made, based on the incorrect assumption that all enlargements of this type are subdural haematomas. Open opercula, wide CSF spaces and a rapidly increasing head circumference can be an early clue to glutaric acidemia.[11]

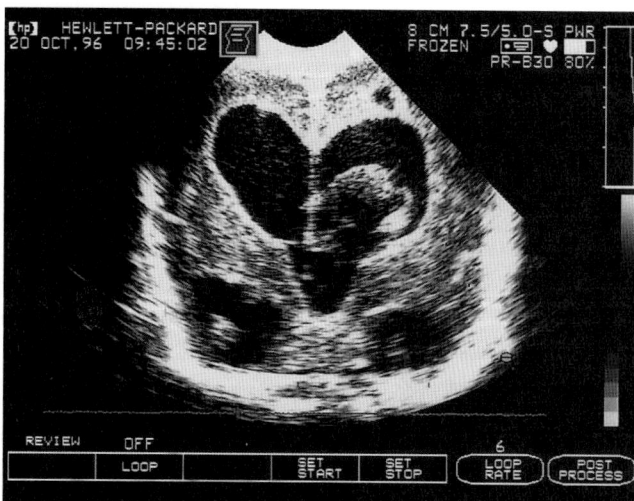

Fig. 41.72 Cranial ultrasound, coronal view, showing enlarged ventricles with a clot in the left ventricular cavity.

Other malformations

Dandy–Walker malformation

This is thought to be due to defective development of the roof of the neural tube at its cranial end, which is to occupy the posterior fossa (Fig. 41.73). It is usually defined as the association of three components:

- partial or complete agenesis of the cerebellar vermis;
- a cystic expansion in the posterior fossa communicating with the fourth ventricle, of which it is a diverticular expansion;
- hydrocephalus (this may not develop until adult life).

Males outnumber females by 3:1. There are often associated cerebral malformations such as agenesis of the corpus callosum or occipital encephaloceles and heterotopia of the lower olivary body.[2] The treatment is that of congenital hydrocephalus, although occasionally the cyst itself has to be removed.

The Dandy–Walker malformation is generally considered a sporadic condition, with a recurrence rate of less than 2%. The prognosis is guarded, with 27% dead in a summary of several published series and only half the survivors with a normal IQ.[48] Osenbach and Menezes[86] reported a personal series of 37 cases treated over 30 years; 91% had hydrocephalus at presentation. A third had developmental delay at follow-up. Only two children among a cohort of 38 with Dandy–Walker syndrome were completely normal in a series from Spain[88] and two-thirds of the survivors in Dublin were mentally retarded.[57] Aicardi points out that, since the Dandy–Walker syndrome is not invariably associated with neurodevelopmental dysfunction, its prenatal diagnosis raises ethical issues.[2]

Hypoplasia and agenesis of the corpus callosum

This is a congenital defect in which either the whole or part of the corpus callosum is missing. The abnormality may be quite common and was noted in 33 of 1447 cerebral scans carried out for various reasons, corresponding to an incidence of 1:20 000.

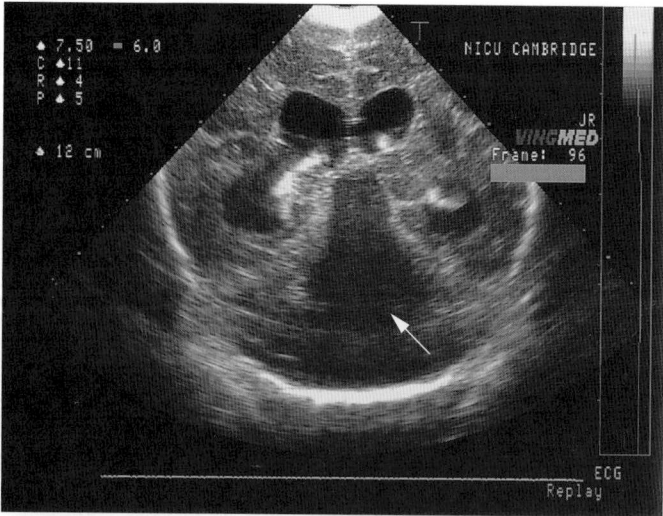

Fig. 41.73 (a) Cranial ultrasound scan in a case of Dandy–Walker syndrome, coronal view, showing a large cystic space in the posterior fossa (arrowed) and large lateral ventricles. (b) CT scan of the same case confirming the diagnosis of Dandy–Walker syndrome.

Post-mortem data suggests an incidence of 1:19 000.[45] There is a failure of the association fibres to traverse the midline, and the fibres form aberrant bundles (of Probst), which can be seen displacing the lateral ventricles to one side. There is often an associated colpocephaly, a term used to describe persistence of the fetal appearance of both posterior horns of the lateral ventricle which appear large, a part of the primary malformation of the brain in this disorder. Ultrasound, CT or MRI reveals a radial gyral pattern (sunburst gyri), colpocephaly and loss of the usually easily visualised callosal sulcus from the midline view (Fig. 41.74).

There are multiple causes for failure of development of the corpus callosum, which should be considered as a non-specific finding. It is often a feature of disorders of neuronal migration, with which development of the corpus callosum is coincident.[115] The condition is associated with several syndromes, such as trisomy 8, 13 or 18, Goldenhar's syndrome, Rubinstein–Taybi syndrome and orofacial digital syndrome. Acquired causes include exposure to excessive alcohol during pregnancy (the 'fetal alcohol syndrome')[55] and hyperglycinaemia.[33] Indeed, up to 2% of cases may be associated with a metabolic disorder.[2] Aicardi described a constellation of callosal agenesis, infantile myoclonic epilepsy, retinal lacunae and mental retardation in females in a syndrome that now bears his name.

Agenesis of the corpus callosum is unlikely to be recognised in the newborn unless the baby has a large head with hypertelorism, but is increasingly diagnosed antenatally. In one such series, 6/12 were normal at follow-up.[19] Those who did badly had other malformations, such as the CHARGE anomaly or the Dandy–Walker malformation, whereas those who did well were children with partial agenesis unassociated with another condition. CHARGE is an acronym referring to children with coloboma, heart defects, atresia choanae, retardation of growth and development, genitourinary problems and ear abnormalities. North et al[82] have suggested that the locus for the gene causing some of the CHARGE anomalies is at 14q22–14q24.3.

Hydranencephalus

This term is used when there has been massive bilateral brain damage, resulting in the destruction of both cerebral hemispheres and their replacement by CSF. Although this condition may rarely arise postnatally, its cause is generally prenatal; the cerebral hemispheres are thought to have been destroyed by a vascular event during early fetal life. It has been described in association with fetal exposure to cocaine.[115] The cavities are smooth-walled, in contrast to those of multicystic encephalomalacia, which is the result of an insult later in fetal life when the brain is capable of mounting a glial response. In the newborn, it can be difficult clinically to distinguish hydranencephalus from extreme degrees of hydrocephalus. If the intracranial pressure is high and the baby's head is enlarging rapidly, then it is worth treating the baby surgically with a shunt for cosmetic reasons and to ease nursing. In general, the outlook is grim and few survive beyond a year.

Megalencephaly

A large head without a bulging fontanelle or separated sutures and growing at a normal rate usually indicates a harmless, familial megalencephaly.[69] In such cases, it is only necessary to measure the parents' and the siblings' head circumference. In the newborn period, it is important to exclude pericerebral collections of blood or CSF by appropriate brain imaging. Megalencephaly may, however, be a manifestation of a cerebral abnormality (such as neuronal migration disorders[41] or neurofibromatosis[29]) and be associated with impaired intelligence, although benign enlargement of

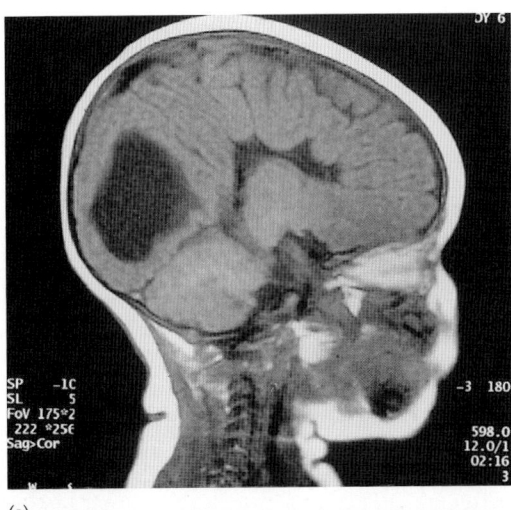

(a)

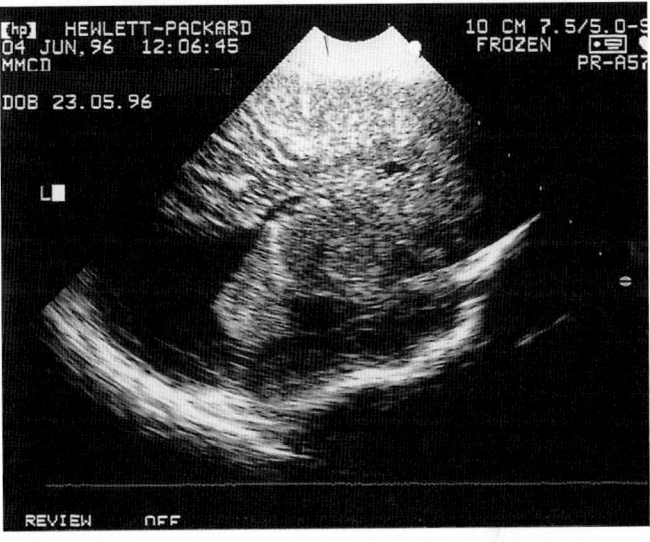

(b)

Fig. 41.74 (a) MRI scan in agenesis of the corpus callosum; there is a sunburst arrangement of the gyri, loss of the callosal sulcus, and an enlarged posterior horn of the lateral ventricle (colpocephaly). (b) Ultrasound scan of the brain in the same case. The sunburst gyri and the absence of the callosal sulcus, together with the colpocephaly, can be seen.

the subarachnoid space is the diagnosis in some of these cases. Megalencephaly may also be a feature when there is intra- or extra-cerebral venous anomalies, achondroplasia, cerebral gigantism (Sotos' syndrome), tuberose sclerosis and mucopolysaccharidoses. Megalencephaly can be the presenting feature in a wide variety of organic acid disorders, and an unexplained large head should prompt a screen including determination of amino acids, purines, pyrimidines and markers of peroxisomal function.[49] (see Chapter 35).

Hemimegalencephaly

Asymmetric enlargement of one side of the brain is often due to an underlying dysplastic hemisphere with a migration disorder of the cortical neurones.[7] There may be hemihypertrophy of the entire body. Intelligence is usually impaired and intractable epilepsy can be a problem.

Microcephalus

The term refers to a small brain. In clinical practice, this is most easily determined by the routine measurement of the occipito-frontal circumference, which increases passively in response to the increasing size of the contents of the cranium. The cut-off point, as with all measurements, is arbitrary, but most clinicians will accept the 3rd centile. The forehead is shallow and slopes backwards, and the ears appear large.

There are various causes of microcephaly. If prenatal cranial growth has been shown by ultrasound measurements made during the pregnancy to have been normal and a baby is born microcephalic, the chances are that abnormal brain growth occurred because of an intrauterine insult. Similarly, if a baby's head size is normal at birth but then becomes microcephalic, the likelihood is that serious cerebral damage occurred during the weeks or days just before birth, at birth or just afterwards. This acquired and non-genetic form of microcephaly may be of multiple aetiology: serious disturbance of the utero-placental blood supply, drugs, other chemicals, X-rays and hypoxic ischaemia prenatally or at birth may all cause microcephaly. Microcephaly may also be the result of transplacental infection during pregnancy (e.g. rubella, toxoplasmosis – p. 1065) or form part of the rarer chromosome defect syndromes (Ch. 32). Microcephalia vera, the genetic type of microcephaly, is rare. It is usually autosomal recessive, but dominant and X-linked forms have also been described and are even rarer.[2]

Holoprosencephaly

Holoprosencephaly is a rare major abnormality of the CNS. It occurs before the sixth week of embryogenesis and is characterised by midline defects. The cardinal abnormality of holoprosencephaly is an absence of the olfactory bulbs and tracts and failure of cleavage of the forebrain. Because sagittal cleavage of the prosencephalon to form the cerebral hemispheres occurs at about 35 days postconception and the olfactory bulbs and tracts only develop at 42 days, holoprosencephaly is frequently associated with absence of the olfactory structures.[115] A third of cases have trisomy 13 but the syndrome has also been linked with trisomy 9, translocations affecting chromosomes 9 and 13 and sonic hedgehog mutation.[112] The condition is rare, affecting between 1 in 15 000 and 1 in 20 000 births, but occurs much more often when there is spontaneous abortion, indicating that the condition is generally lethal. Cyclopia is the term used to describe a single fused orbit with a proboscis above it; cebocephaly means a normally placed nose with a single nostril. Ethmocephaly is the least common anomaly, in which there are two separate orbits with a proboscis between them. Hypotelorism with a midline facial cleft, and milder midline facial dysplasias, also signal the presence of holoprosencephaly.

Usually the brain is small and there are fewer than normal gyri, which are broad and often flat. There is a large monoventricle,

which may be associated with agenesis of the corpus callosum. There are often other midline disturbances, with midfacial hypoplasia, cleft lip and hypertelorism. Holoprosencephaly may occur on its own but more usually it is associated with other major somatic malformations, in which case there is also a demonstrable chromosome defect.

The disorder can be categorised into three subtypes: alobar holoprosencephaly, when the ventricles are fused throughout; lobar holoprosencephaly, when there is fusion of the frontal poles only; and semilobar holoprosencephaly, which is an intermediate form. The prognosis is poor and there is no effective treatment. The diagnosis can be made prenatally by either ultrasound or fetal MRI.

Septo-optic dysplasia

In this condition, the septum pellucidum is unformed and the optic nerves are hypoplastic. There may also be absence of the cerebellar vermis and/or the pituitary gland. The condition is not genetically determined. The children can have hypopituitarism, seizures, ataxia and mental deficiency.

Agenesis of the cerebellar vermis (including Joubert's syndrome)

Joubert's syndrome is an autosomal recessive disorder in which there is absence of the cerebellar vermis, and retinopathy often with optic disc colobomata and renal cysts.[56] Newborn babies can present with an effortless panting tachypnoea of 120–200 per minute and apnoeic pauses. Sarnat and Alcalá[96] reported a series of seven children with cerebellar hypoplasia. They observed hypotonia, which is also a feature of the Dandy–Walker malformation where there is also hypoplasia of the cerebellar vermis, delayed development, truncal titubation and intention tremor. Most had fixation nystagmus and three had seizures.

Arachnoid cysts

Congenital arachnoid cysts are another important cause of a CSF collection in the posterior and middle fossa, although they can occur anywhere within the brain or spinal cord. They are increasingly discovered in fetal life or during the first few years after birth by ultrasound scanning (Fig. 41.75). They have been observed as an incidental finding in about 5% of cases at autopsy.[79] The cysts are thought to form because of splitting of the arachnoid during embryogenesis with subsequent secretion of cerebrospinal fluid into the cavity. There is no continuity between such cysts and the fourth ventricle or the subarachnoid space.

Arachnoid cysts are generally asymptomatic but, if they enlarge, they may cause hydrocephalus by obstructing CSF flow in the posterior fossa or at the outflow of the fourth ventricle.[115] This is particularly likely if the cyst is in the suprasellar or quadrigeminal region, and these babies require careful follow-up with repeat neuroimaging (Fig. 41.75b). The cysts may be treated by fenestration of the wall or by a cysto-peritoneal shunt. Small asymptomatic cysts do not require any treatment. The prognosis is generally good, although sometimes there is epilepsy in childhood and bleeding can occur into the cysts at any time.

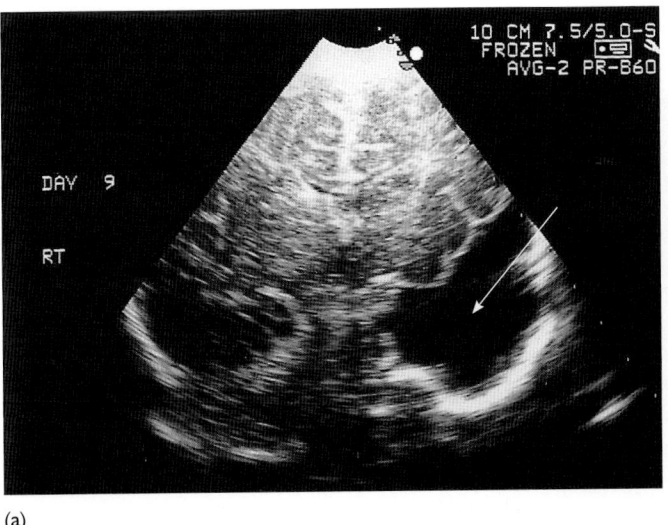

(a)

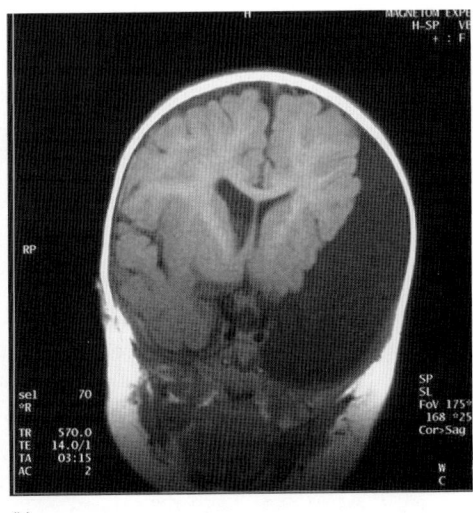

(b)

Fig. 41.75 (a) Arachnoid cyst on ultrasound. (b) Middle cranial fossa arachnoid cyst seen with MRI in the coronal plane.

Disorders of cortical development (neuronal migration disorders)

Ectoderm, mesoderm and endoderm are formed during the second embryonic week. The midline ectoderm develops into the neural plate, which then forms a groove. This develops into the neural tube, which closes during the fourth week, starting at the middle and proceeding to the extremities. At about day 33 the prosencephalon is cleaved to form the cerebral vesicles and the forebrain and face develop from the cranial neural crest at 5–6 weeks. The proliferation of the primitive cells that will form neurons and glia occurs mainly around the lumen of the neural tube and starts at about 30 days. Nerve cells originate in the ventricular and subventricular zones, sometimes called the germinative zone. An excess of cells are produced and the number is reduced by programmed cell death or apoptosis. (For a more detailed review, see Gressens.[44]) The first neurons migrate to form a subpial preplate, also known as the primitive plexiform zone or layer, at about 45–50 days postconception. Later neurons, which will form the cortical plate, move to their final position by following the processes of a specialised glial cell, the radial glial cell. As each wave of migrating cells moves to its final position, it 'leapfrogs' previous layers, i.e. the most superficial layer, the neocortex, is made up of the youngest cells. This process, by which neurons reach their final positions in the cortex, is known as neuronal migration. Migration to the cortex starts at about 10 weeks and is generally considered to be complete by 20 weeks.

Abnormalities of this complex process are caused by genetic or environmental effects. The resulting disorders depend on the timing and nature of the disturbance. There are disorders with absent or abnormal sulcation, such as lissencephaly ('smooth brain'), agyria ('no gyri'), pachygyria ('large gyri') and schizencephaly ('split brain') and cortical heterotopias.

Aicardi[2] usefully considers disorders of cortical development as:

- disorders of proliferation and differentiation;
- disorders of migration; and
- disorders of cortical organisation (Table 41.26).

Table 41.26 Main disorders of cortical development (after Aicardi 1998[2])

(a) Disordered proliferation and differentiation	Microcephaly
	Megalencephaly
	Hemimegalencephaly
	Schizencephaly
	Tuberose sclerosis
(b) Disordered migration	Periventricular heterotopias
	Subcortical heterotopias
	Lissencephaly and agyria
	Pachygyria
	Polymicrogyria
(c) Disordered cortical organisation	Cortical dysplasia
	Microdysgenesis

Lissencephaly and pachygyria

These disorders are becoming more frequently recognised with the advent of MRI scanning (Fig. 41.76). They cannot be diagnosed readily in early uterine life because the brain is not convoluted until 28 weeks and secondary gyri do not appear until 32 weeks. Early-onset seizures are frequent, but not invariable. The brain can be completely smooth – lissencephaly. More commonly there are a few thick gyri – pachygyria. There is often an agenesis of the septum pellucidum. Imaging with ultrasound can reveal the diagnosis, which is more easily made with CT or MRI.[89] Type I lissencephaly has areas that are agyric and others that are pachygyric.[8] The cerebral surface is said to resemble that of a 12-week fetus[115] (Fig. 41.76). There is also dilatation of the lateral ventricles and hypoplasia of the corpus callosum. Migration is thought to be affected at between 12 and 16 weeks. Affected children show bitemporal hollowing, micrognathia and occipital prominence.[44]

Miller–Dieker syndrome is a specific disorder in which there is a four-layer cortex resulting in lissencephaly or pachygyria, a

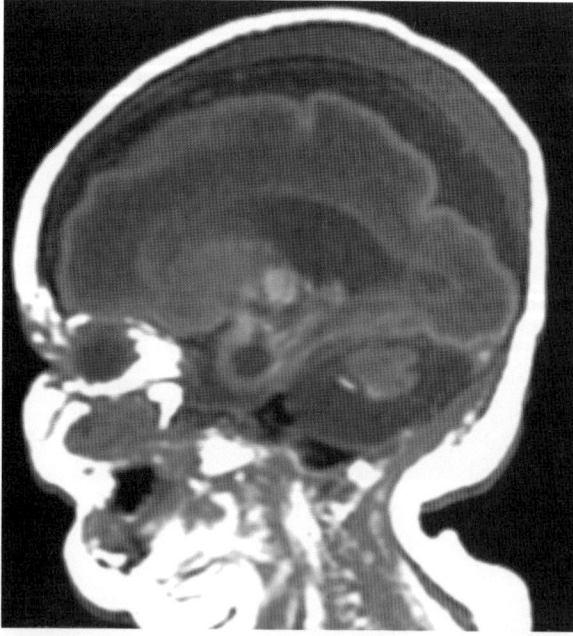

(a)

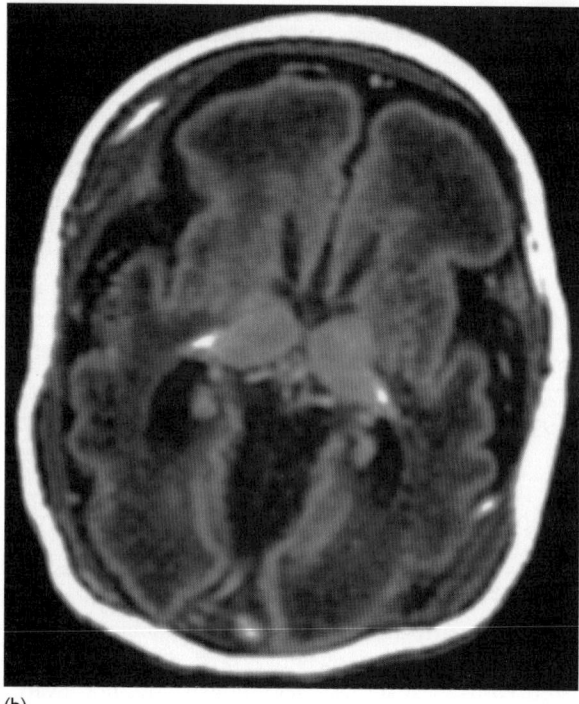

(b)

Fig. 41.76 (a) MRI scan in lissencephaly seen in the sagittal plane in a term baby. The normal pattern of sulci and gyri is absent. (b) MRI lissencephaly seen in the axial plane from the same case.

characteristic facies with bitemporal hollowing, an upturned nose and a thin vermilion border to the upper lip. Chromosomal analysis in the Miller–Dieker syndrome reveals a microdeletion of 17p. Cases of Miller–Dieker syndrome and about 40% of cases of isolated lissencephaly – it is probably not useful to distinguish the disorders clinically – have a hemideletion of the *LIS1* gene, which encodes the beta subunit of acetylhydrolase,

responsible for degrading platelet activating factor (PAF).[64,91] Neuronal migration in vitro is disrupted by stimulation of the PAF receptor.[9] Other males with isolated lissencephaly have abnormalities of the X-chromosome at the Xq24-q24 locus, where the gene for doublecortin is situated. Double cortin and PAF appear to be important in the regulation of migrating neurones.[115,44]

In Type II lissencephaly, there is a thickened and seriously disorganised cortex, which is disrupted by vascular and fibro-glial septa.[8,115,44] Notably, there are subcortical heterotopias. The meninges are thickened and adhere tightly to the cortex, obliterating the subarachnoid space and causing hydrocephalus. These patients present a similar picture to the Walker–Warburg syndrome (see below) with ophthalmic malformations, posterior encephaloceles, hydrocephalus and often hypotonia.[44] The cause is still unknown

In the Walker–Warburg syndrome there is lissencephaly, retinal dysplasia and congenital muscular dystrophy. The disorder is autosomal recessive and the same chromosomal deletion is not present. This disorder has also been termed the HARD(E) syndrome; *h*ydrocephalus, cerebral and cerebellar *a*gyria, *r*etinal *d*ysplasia, ±*e*ncephalocele.[87] There is no treatment for lissencephaly. Lissencephaly has also been found in association with metabolic disorders such as Zellweger's syndrome (pp. 1170–2), Menkes' syndrome (p. 920) and inherited amino-acid disorders. Focal areas of pachygyria can be seen after insults to the fetus in the first trimester. The neurodevelopmental outcome is generally poor but varies with the degree to which normal brain development has been disrupted.

Schizencephaly

There is a deep cleft in the brain, usually in the region of the sylvian fissure. The lips of the fissure can be open or closed. There is often an agenesis of the septum pellucidum and there may be hydrocephalus. The condition can be a primary malformation or can result from an insult in early fetal life, for example due to maternal cocaine abuse.

Cerebrovascular malformations

There are a number of rare congenital cerebrovascular malformations, but few are recognisable in the newborn. These include the Sturge–Weber syndrome and arteriovenous aneurysms, including aneurysm of the vein of Galen, which is characterised by heart failure and an intracranial murmur.

Vein of Galen malformation

Aneurysms of the vein of Galen are dilatations of the vein, which range from a large single malformation to multiple smaller communications. Antenatal diagnosis is possible, giving forewarning and allowing counselling and delivery in a centre with interventional radiology. Fetuses with hydrops and babies requiring ventilation for heart failure in the neonatal period usually die, although some groups report success with very aggressive management.[40] In the neonatal period, ultrasound and MRI confirm

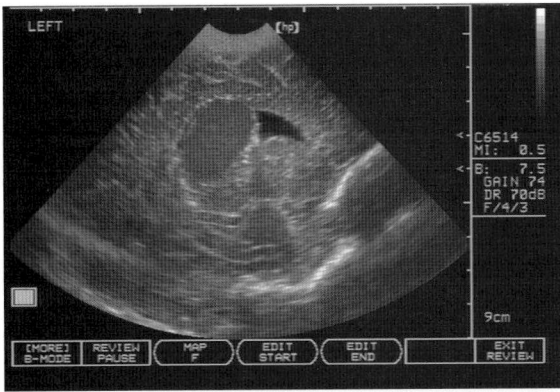

(a)

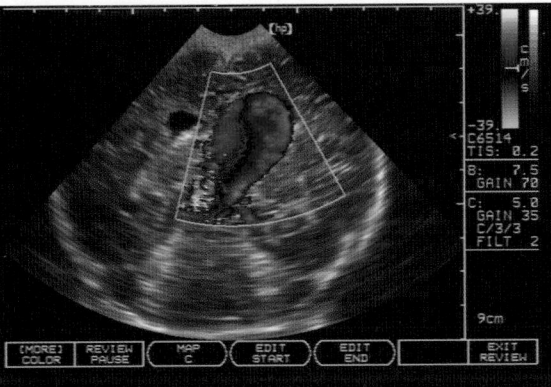

(b)

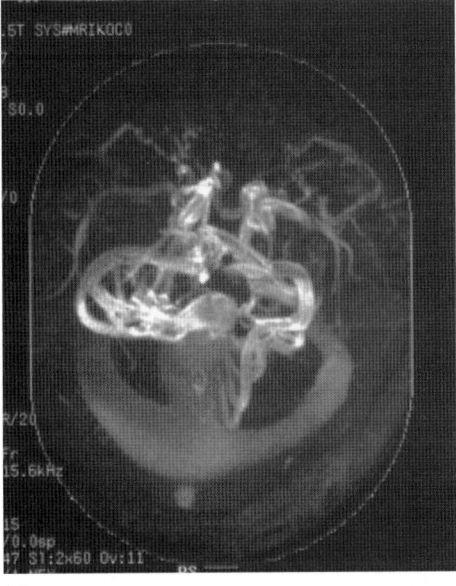

(c)

Fig. 41.77 (a) Ultrasound appearance of vein of Galen malformation – black and white picture in the sagittal plane, with the malformation appearing as an ovoid shape filling the posterior part of the lateral ventricle. (b) Ultrasound appearance of vein of Galen malformation – colour Doppler image in the coronal plane. The abnormal flow within the malformation is clearly seen. (c) MR angiogram of a large vein of Galen malformation.

the diagnosis and allow assessment of the feeder vessels (Fig. 41.77a,b,c). Previously the results of treatment of vein of Galen vascular malformations were poor but therapeutic options now include the transarterial insertion of coils in the abnormal vessels. Lylyk et al[73] treated 28 children this way, 11 of whom were neonates; 17 had a good long-term outcome.

Congenital brain tumours

These are very rare but sometimes come to attention because of associated hydrocephalus. Occasionally they can cause obstructed labour. Over half are supratentorial, the most common histological type in the newborn being an astrocytoma (p. 963).

Malformations of the skull

Craniosynostosis

Abnormal development or premature closure of one or more of the cranial sutures of the skull results in craniosynostosis, usually producing an abnormal head shape. The incidence of craniosynostosis is about 1 in 2000; the most common form is isolated sagittal synostosis (1 in 1000). Craniosynostosis can be a manifestation of a syndrome such as Apert's (p. 793) Crouzon's (p. 793) Pfeiffer's (p. 793) or Carpenter's (p. 793). About 140 syndromes have been identified in which craniosynostosis is a part. Many of these are autosomal dominant with a good prognosis.

Babies with single or multiple suture craniosynostosis can present in the neonatal period with suture ridging or an unusual shape of the head. Sometimes they present later in infancy because their heads deform during the rapid phase of skull growth during the first 6 months. The diagnosis can be confirmed with X-ray or three-dimensional CT. Surgery is only indicated if there is significant cosmetic deformity or raised intracranial pressure, which is obviously much more likely when more than one suture is involved. Some claim success with skull caps alone, or a combination of minimally invasive early surgery and postoperative helmet moulding for up to a year.[53]

The 'back to sleep' campaign has led to an increase in babies with flattening of the occiput. Genuine bilateral lambdoid synostosis is very rare, and the vast majority of these babies have a postural deformity that does not require treatment.[54]

References

1. Adams C, Johnston W P, Nevin N C 1982 Family study of congenital hydrocephalus. Developmental Medicine and Child Neurology 24: 493–498
2. Aicardi J 1998 Diseases of the nervous system in childhood, 2nd edition. McKeith Press, Cambridge
3. Aicardi J, Lefebvre J, Lerique-Koechlin A 1965 A new syndrome: spasm in flexion, callosal agenesis, ocular abnormalities. Electroencephalography and Clinical Neurophysiology 19: 609–610
4. American College of Obstetricians and Gynecologists 1986 Prenatal detection of neural tube defects. Technical Bulletin no. 99. ACOG, Washington, DC

5. Anderson N G, Jordan S, MacFarlane M R, Lovell-Smith M 1994 Diastomyelia: diagnosis by prenatal sonography. American Journal of Roentgenology 163: 911–914

6. Annas G J 1994 Asking the courts to set the standard of care – the case of baby K. New England Journal of Medicine 330: 1542–1545

7. Barkovich A J, Chuang S H 1990 Unilateral megalencephaly: correlation of MR imaging and pathologic characteristics. American Journal of Neuroradiology 11; 523–531

8. Barkovich A J, Gressens P, Evrard P 1992 Formation, maturation and disorders of neocortex. Americal Journal of Neuroradiology 13: 423–446

9. Bix G J, Clarke G D 1998 Platelet activating factor receptor stimulation disrupts neuronal migration in vitro. Journal of Neuroscience 18: 307–318

10. Blum A, André M, Droullé P, Husson S, Leheup B 1990 Prenatal echographic diagnosis of corpus callosum agenesis. The Nancy experience. Genetic Counselling 38: 115–126

11. Brismar J, Ozand P T 1995 CT and MR of the brain in glutaric acidemia type I: a review of 59 published cases and a report of 5 new patients. American Journal of Neuroradiology 16: 675–683

12. Brock D J H, Bolton A E, Scrimgeour J B 1974 Prenatal diagnosis of spina bifida and anencephaly through maternal plasma alpha-fetoprotein measurement. Lancet 1: 767–769

13. Brock D J H, Sutcliffe R G 1972 Alpha-fetoprotein in the antenatal diagnosis of anencephaly and spina bifida. Lancet 2: 197–199

14. Bruce D A, Schut L 1979 Spinal lipomas in infancy and childhood. Child's Brain 5: 192–203

15. Bruner J P, Tulipan N, Paschall R L et al Fetal surgery for myelomeningocele and the incidence of shunt-dependent hydrocephalus. Journal of the American Medical Association 1999; 282: 1819–1825

16. Bunin G R, Kuijten R R, Buckley J D, Rorke L B, Meadows A T 1993 Relation between maternal diet and subsequent primitive neuroectodermal brain tumours in young children. New England Journal of Medicine 329: 536–541

17. Campbell S, Johnstone F D, Holt E M, May P 1972 Anencephaly: early ultrasound diagnosis and active management. Lancet 2: 1226

18. Campbell S, Tsannatos C, Pearce J M 1984 The prenatal diagnosis of Joubert's syndrome of familial agenesis of the cerebellar vermis. Prenatal Diagnosis 4: 391–395

19. Carter C O, David P A, Laurence K M 1968 A family study of major central nervous system malformations in South Wales. Journal of Medical Genetics 16: 14–16

20. Carter C O, Evans K 1973 Spina bifida and anencephalus in Greater London. Journal of Medical Genetics 10: 209–234

21. Carter C O, Evans K 1973 Children of adult survivors with spina bifida cystica. Lancet 2: 924–926

22. Carter C O, Roberts J F 1967 The risk of recurrence after two children with central nervous system malformations. Lancet 1: 306–308

23. Chatterjee M S, Bondoz B, Adhate A 1985 Prenatal diagnosis of occipital encephalocele. Americal Journal of Obstetrics and Gynecology 153: 646–647

24. Chervenak F A, Berkowitz R L, Romero R et al 1983 The diagnosis of fetal hydrocephalus. American Journal of Obstetrics and Gynecology 147: 703–716

25. Chervenak F A, Isaacson G, Hobbins J C, Chitkara U, Tortora M, Berkowitz R L 1985 Diagnosis and management of fetal holoprosencephaly. Obstetrics and Gynecology 66: 322–326

26. Chervenak F A, Rosenberg J, Brightman R D et al 1987 A prospective study of ultrasound in predicting fetal microcephaly. Obstetrics Gynecology 69: 908–910

27. Cohen T, Stern E, Rosemann A 1979 Sib risk of neural tube defect: is prenatal diagnosis indicated in pregnancies following the birth of a hydrocephalic child? Journal of Medical Genetics 16: 14–16

28. Comstock C H, Culp, D, Gonzalez J, Boal D B 1985 Agenesis of the corpus callosum in the fetus: its evolution and significance. Journal of Ultrasound in Medicine 4: 613–616

29. Cutting L E, Cooper K L, Koth C W et al 2002 Megalencephaly in NF1: predominantly white matter contribution and mitigation by ADHD. Neurology 59: 1388–1394

30. Czeizel A E, Metneki J, Dudas I 1994 Higher rate of multiple births after peri-conceptional vitamin supplementation (letter). New England Journal of Medicine 330: 1687–1688

31. Dan V, Shalev E, Greif M, Weiner E 1992 Prenatal diagnosis of fetal brain arteriovenous malformation; the use of color Doppler imaging. Journal of Clinical Ultrasound 20: 149–151

32. Den Hollander N S, Wessels M W, Los F J et al 2000 Congenital microcephaly detected by prenatal ultrasound: genetic aspects and clinical significance. Ultrasound in Obstetrics and Gynecology 15: 282–287

33. Dobyns W B 1989 Agenesis of the corpus callosum and gyral malformations are frequent manifestations of non-ketotic hyperglycinaemia. Neurology 39: 817–820

34. Dolk H, Nichols and a EUROCAT working group 1999 Evaluation of the impact of Chernobyl on the prevalence of congenital anomalies in 16 regions of Europe. International Journal of Epidemiology 28: 941–948

35. Drewek M J, Bruner J P, Whetsell W O et al 1997 Quantitative analysis of the toxicity of human amniotic fluid to cultured rat spinal cord. Pediatric Neurosurgery 27: 190–193

36. Duckworth T, Sharrard W J W, Lister J, Seymour N 1968 Hemimyelocele. Developmental Medicine and Child Neurology (Suppl) 16: 69–75

37. Edwards J H 1961 The syndrome of sex linked hydrocephalus. Archives of Disease in Childhood 36: 486–493

38. Elwood J M, Elwood J H 1980 Epidemiology of anencephalus and spina bifida. Oxford University Press, Oxford

39. Expert Advisory Group 1992 Folic acid and the prevention of neural tube defects. Department of Health, Scottish Office Home and Health Department, Welsh Office, Department of Health and Social Security Northern Ireland. HMSO, London

40. Frawley G P, Dargaville P A, Mitchell P J, Tress B M, Loughnan P 2002 Clinical course and medical management of neonates with severe cardiac failure related to vein of Galen malformation. Archives of Disease in Childhood 87: F144–F149

41. Friede R L 1989 Developmental neuropathology, 2nd edition. Springer Verlag, Berlin

42. Gibson P J, Britton J, Hall D M B, Hill C R 1995 Lumbosacral skin markers and identification of occult spinal dysraphism in neonates. Acta Paediatrica Scandinavica 84: 208–209

43. Goldstein R B, Filly R A, Callen P W 1989 Sonography of anencephaly: pitfalls in early diagnosis. Journal of Clinical Ultrasound 17: 397–402

44. Gressens P 2002 Neuronal migration. In: Lagercrantz H, Hanson M, Evrard P, Rodeck C H (eds) The newborn brain – neuroscience and clinical applications. Cambridge University Press, Cambridge

45. Grogono J L 1968 Children with agenesis of the corpus callosum. Developmental Medicine and Child Neurology 10: 613–616

46. Hadi H A, Mashini I S, Devoe L D et al 1986 Ultrasonographic prenatal diagnosis of hydranencephaly. A case report. Journal of Reproductive Medicine 31: 254–256

47. Hernandez-Diaz S, Werler M M, Walker A M, Mitchell A A. Neural tube defects in relation to use of folic acid antagonists during pregnancy. American Journal of Epidemiology 2001; 153: 961–968

48. Hirsch J F, Pierre-Kahn A, Renier D, Sainte-Rose C, Hoppe-Hirsche E 1984 The Dandy–Walker malformation. A review of 40 cases. Journal of Neurosurgery 61: 515–522

49. Hoffman G F, Gibson K M, Trefz F K, Nyhan W L, Bremer H J, Rating D 1994 Neurological manifestations of organic acid disorders. European Journal of Pediatrics 153: S94–S100

50. Hunt G, Oakeshott P 2003 Outcome in people with open spina bifida at age 35: prospective community based cohort study. British Medical Journal 326: 1365–1366

51. Hunt G, Poulton A 1995 Open spina bifida: a complete cohort reviewed 25 years after closure. Developmental Medicine and Child Neurology 37: 19–29

52. Hutchins G M, Meuli M, Meuli-Simmen C et al 1996 Acquired spinal cord injury in human fetuses with myelomeningocele. Pediatric Pathology and Laboratory Medicine 16: 801–812

53. Jimenez D F, Barone C M, Cartwright C C, Baker L 2002 Early management of craniosynostosis using endoscopic assisted strip craniectomies and cranial orthotic moulding therapy. Pediatrics 110: 97–104

54. Jones B M, Hayward R, Evans R, Britto J 1997 Occipital plagiocephaly: an epidemic of craniosynostosis British Medical Journal 315: 693–694

55. Jones K, Smith D W, Ulleland C, Streissguth A P 1973 Pattern of malformations in offspring of chronic alcoholic mothers. Lancet 1: 1267–1271

56. Joubert M, Eisenring J-J, Robb J P, Andermann F 1969 Familial agenesis of the cerebellar vermis. Neurology 19: 813–825

57. Kalidasan V, Carroll T, Alcutt D, Fitzgerald R J 1995 The Dandy–Walker syndrome – a 10 year experience of its management and outcome. European Journal of Pediatric Surgery 5(Suppl 1): 16–18

58. Kanev P M, Bierbrauer K S 1995 Reflections on the natural history of lipomyelomeningocele. Pediatric Neurosurgery 22: 137–140

59. Kitisomprayoonul N, Tongsong T 2001 Neural tube defects: a different pattern in Northern Thai population. Journal of the Medical Association of Thailand 84: 483–488

60. Kligensmith W C, Cioffi-Ragan D T 1986 Schizencephaly: diagnosis and progression in utero. Radiology 159: 617–618

61. Kormarniski C A, Cyr D R, Mack L A, Weinberger E 1990 Prenatal diagnosis of schizencephaly. Journal of Ultrasound in Medicine 8: 337–339

62. Korsvik H E, Keller M S 1992 Sonography of occult dysraphism in neonates and infants with MR imaging correlation. Radiographics 12: 297–306

63. Kupka J, Geddes N, Carroll N C 1978 Comprehensive management in the child with spina bifida. Orthopedic Clinics of North America 9: 97–113

64. Lo Nigro C, Chong C S, Smith A C, Dobyns W B, Carrozzo R, Ledbetter D H 1997 Point mutations and an intragenic deletion of *LIS1*, the lissencephaly causative gene in isolated lissencephaly sequence and Miller–Dieker syndrome. Human Molecular Genetics 6: 157–164

65. Lorber J 1965 The family history of spina bifida cystica. Pediatrics 35: 589–595

66. Lorber J, De N C 1970 Family history of congenital hydrocephalus Developmental Medicine and Child Neurology (Suppl) 22: 94–100

67. Lorber J 1971 Results of treatment of myelomeningocele. An analysis of 524 unselected cases with special reference to possible selection for treatment. Developmental Medicine and Child Neurology 13: 279–303

68. Lorber J 1984 The family history of congenital hydrocephalus – an epidemiological study based on 250 index cases. British Medical Journal 289: 281–284

69. Lorber J, Priestley B L 1981 Children with large heads: a practical approach to diagnosis in 557 children, with special reference to 101 children with megalencephaly. Developmental Medicine and Child Neurology 23: 494–504

70. Lorber J, Rogers S C 1977 Spina bifida and anencephalus in twins. Zeitschrift für Kinderchirurgie 22: 565–571

71. Lorber J, Schofield J K 1979 Prognosis of occipital encephalocele. Zeitschrift für Kinderchirurgie 28: 347–352

72. Lorber J, Ward A M 1985 Spina bifida – a vanishing nightmare? Archives of Disease in Childhood 60: 1086–1091

73. Lylyk P, Vineula F, Dion J E et al 1993 Therapeutic alternatives for vein of Galen vascular malformations. Journal of Neurosurgery 78: 438–445

74. Meizner I, Barki Y, Hertzanu Y 1987 Prenatal sonographic diagnosis of agenesis of corpus callosum. Journal of Clinical Ultrasound 15: 262–264

75. Ment L R, Duncan C C, Geehr R 1981 Benign enlargement of the subarachnoid space in children. Journal of Neurosurgery 54: 504–508

76. Meuli M, Meuli-Simmen C, Hutchins G M et al 1997 The spinal cord lesion in human fetuses with myelomeningocele: implications for fetal surgery. Journal of Pediatric Surgery 32: 448–452

77. Moore K L 1998 The developing human: clinically oriented embryology, 6th edn. W B Saunders, Philadelphia: pp 455

78. Morgan N V, Gissen P, Sharif S M et al 2002 A novel locus for Meckel-Gruber syndrome, MKS3, maps to chromosome 8q24. Human Genetics 111: 456–461

79. Naidich T P, McLone D G, Radkowski M A 1985–86 Intracranial arachnoid cysts. Pediatric Neuroscience 12: 112–122

80. Nevin N C, Johnston W P 1980 A family study of spina bifida and anencephalus in Belfast, Northern Ireland (1964–1968). Journal of Medical Genetics 17: 203–211

81. Nicolaides K H, Campbell S, Gabbe S G, Guidetti R 1986 Ultrasound screening for spina bifida: cranial and cerebellar signs. Lancet 2: 72–74

82. North K N, Wu B I, Cao B N, Whiteman D A, Korf B R 1995 CHARGE association in a child with de novo duplication[14](q22?q24.3). American Journal of Medical Genetics 57: 610–614

83. Office of National Statistics 1990, 1993, 1999, 2002 Congenital malformations. Government Statistical Service, London

84. Office for National Statistics 2002 Health Statistics Quarterly 16. ONS, London; available on line at www.statistics.gov.uk

85. Office of Population Censuses and Surveys 1982, 1983, 1984, 1985, 1986, 1987 Monitor, congenital malformations. Government Statistical Service, London

86. Osenbach R K, Menezes A H 1992 Diagnosis and management of the Dandy–Walker malformation: 30 years of experience. Pediatric Neurosurgery 18: 179–189

87. Pagon R A, Chandler J W, Collie W R et al 1978 Hydrocephalus, agyria, retinal dysplasia, encephalocele (HARD +/− E) syndrome: an autosomal recessive condition. Birth Defects Original Articles Series 14: 233–241

88. Pascual-Castroviejo I, Velez A, Pascual-Pascual S I, Roche M C, Villarejo F 1991 Dandy–Walker malformation: analysis of 38 cases. Childs Nervous System 7: 88–97

89. Pellicer A, Cabanas F, Perez-Higueras A, Garcia-Alix A, Quero J 1995 Neural migration disorders studied by cerebral ultrasound and colour Doppler flow imaging. Archives of Disease in Childhood 73: F55–F61

90. Pilu G, Sandri F, Cerisoli M, Alvisi C, Salvioli G P, Boricelli L 1990 Sonographic findings in septo-optic dysplasia in the fetus and newborn. American Journal of Perinatology 7: 337–339

91. Pilz D T, Matsumoto N, Minnerath S et al *LIS1* and *XLS* (*DCX*) mutations cause most classical lissencephaly but different patterns of malformation. Human Molecular Genetics 1998; 7: 2029–2037

92. Rowland-Hill C A, Gibson P J 1995 Ultrasound determination of the normal location of the conus medullaris in neonates. American Journal of Neuroradiology 16: 469–472

93. Russ P D, Pretorius P M, Johnson M J 1989 Dandy–Walker syndrome: a review of fifteen cases evaluated by prenatal sonography. American Journal of Obstetrics and Gynecology 161: 401–406

94. Saltzman D H, Krauss C M, Goldman J M, Benacerraf B R 1991 Prenatal diagnosis of lissencephaly. Prenatal Diagnosis 11: 139–143

95. Sandri F, Pilu G, Dallacasa P, Foschi F, Salvioli G P, Bonecelli L 1991 Sonography of unilateral megalencephaly in the fetus and newborn infant. American Journal of Perinatology 8: 18–20

96. Sarnat H B, Alcalá H 1980 Human cerebellar hypoplasia: a syndrome of diverse causes. Archives of Neurology 37: 300–305

97. Sathi S, Madsen J R, Bauer S, Scott R M 1993 Effect of surgical repair on the neurologic function in infants with lipomeningocele. Pediatric Neurosurgery 19: 256–259

98. Schoenmakers M A, Gooskens R H, Gulmans V A et al 2003 Long-term outcome of neurosurgical untethering on neurosegmental motor and ambulation levels. Developmental Medicine and Child Neurology 45: 551–555

99. Seeds J W, Jones F D 1986 Lipomyelomeningocele: prenatal diagnosis and management. Obstetrics and Gynecology 67: 345–375

100. Seller M J 1981 Recurrence risks for neural tube defects in a genetic counselling clinic population. Journal of Medical Genetics 18: 245–248

101. Sharrard W J W 1964 The segmental innervation of the lower limb muscles in man. Annals of the Royal College of Surgeons of England 35: 106–122

102. Shaw G M, Lammer E J, Wasserman C R, O'Malley C D, Tolarova M M 1995 Risks of orofacial clefts in children born to women using multivitamins containing folic acid periconceptionally. Lancet 346: 393–396

103. Smithells R W, D'Arcy E E, McAllister E F 1968 The outcome of pregnancies before and after the birth of infants with nervous system malformations. Developmental Medicine and Child Neurology 15: 6–10

104. Smithells R W, Seller M J, Harris R et al 1983 Further experience of vitamin supplementation for prevention of neural tube defects. Lancet 1: 1027–1031

105. Smithells R W, Sheppard S, Scorah C J et al 1981 Apparent prevention of neural tube defects by periconceptional vitamin supplementation. Archives of Disease in Childhood 56: 911–918

106. Stark G D, Baker G C W 1967 The neurological involvement of the lower limbs in myelomeningocele. Developmental Medicine and Child Neurology 9: 732–744

107. Stein S C, Schut L, Ames M D 1974 Selection for early treatment in myelomeningocele: a retrospective analysis of various selection procedures. Pediatrics 54: 553–557

108. Stevenson A C, Johnston H A, Stewart M I P, Golding D R 1966 Congenital malformations. Bulletin of the World Health Organization 34(Suppl): 9–127

109. Sutcliffe M, Wild J, Perry A, Schorah C J 1994 Prevention of neural tube defects (letter). Lancet 344: 1578

110. Sutton L N, Scott Adzick N, Bilaniuk L T, Johnson M P, Crombleholme T M, Flake A W 1999 Improvement in hindbrain herniation demonstrated by serial fetal magnetic resonance imaging following fetal surgery for myelomeningocele. Journal of the American Medical Association 282: 1826–1831

111. Todoroff K, Shaw G M 2000 Prior spontaneous abortion, prior elective termination, interpregnancy interval and risk of neural tube defects. American Journal of Epidemiology 151: 505–511

112. Verlinsky Y, Rechitsky S, Verlinsky O et al 2003 Preimplantation diagnosis for sonic hedgehog mutation causing familial holoprosencephaly. New England Journal of Medicine 348: 1449–1454

113. Vintzileos A M, Eisenfeld L I, Campbell W A et al 1986 Prenatal ultrasonic diagnosis of arterio-venous malformation of the vein of Galen. American Journal of Perinatology 3: 209–211

114. Vintzileos A M, Havoc T J, Escat D T et al 1987 Congenital midline porencephaly: prenatal sonographic findings and review of the literature. American Journal of Perinatology 4: 125–128

115. Volpe J J 2001 Neurology of the newborn, 4th edition. WB Saunders, Philadelphia

116. Wald N J, Cuckle H S 1981 Amniotic fluid acetylcholinesterase electrophoresis as a secondary test in the diagnosis of anencephaly and open spina bifida in early pregnancy. Collaborative Acetylcholinesterase Study. Lancet 2: 321–324

117. Walsh D S, Adzick N S 2003 Foetal surgery for spina bifida. Seminars in Neonatology 8: 197–205

118. Wasserman C R, Shaw G M, Seldin S, Gould J B, Syme L S 1998 Socioeconomic status, neighborhood social conditions, and neural tube defects. American Journal of Public Health 88: 1674–1680

Section Six

Pathology, Radiology and Biochemistry

CHAPTER 42

Perinatal post mortem

Adrian K Charles, Nicholas M Smith

Introduction

Two recent public inquiries, Kennedy[8] and Redfern[1], and the subsequent retained organ reviews have thrown a spotlight onto the practice of the paediatric autopsy, with bereaved parents in particular expressing concern about organ retention, consent, the use of post-mortem tissue, and return of the tissue to the body. The effect on paediatric pathology in the UK and around the world has been profound.[15,23,52] The inquiries have demonstrated that families and the public expect more information and detailed autopsy consent procedures. The clinician requesting an autopsy must be informed about the autopsy procedure and the potential benefits. Perhaps most of all, the clinician needs to ensure that the counselling is compassionate, yet open and detailed, and tailored to the needs of the parents, both before and after the procedure. It is clear that many professionals and parents have little idea of what happens during the autopsy examination, and of the contribution the autopsy has made to medical progress.

The autopsy rate in stillbirths and neonatal deaths has declined over the last few years to around 50%,[9,22,25] well below the 75% rate suggested by the Joint Working Party of the Royal Colleges of Obstetricians and Gynaecologists and Pathologists.[20] This is contrary to the increased requirement for audit in medicine, risk management[28] and the scientific investigation of disease at the molecular level. Autopsies have a key role in the Confidential Enquiry into Stillbirths and Deaths in Infancy (CESDI) and similar epidemiological healthcare reviews.

The perinatal post-mortem examination remains an important part of clinical practice,[21] and the pathologist should be regarded as part of the perinatal/neonatal team. This requires good communication and regular multidisciplinary meetings.

Every parent has the right to be offered a post-mortem examination of their child, although it is equally their right (in most circumstances) to refuse. The parents and the children should form the focus of our care. Many parents request detailed information on what contributed to the death,[5] and some find solace in the fact that the knowledge gained from the examination may benefit others. Others have expressed a desire to be approached to donate tissue or organs.[36] Parental support of societies related to research into fatal childhood disease illustrates this interest. A recent review suggested that over 80% of parents, if asked, would agree to a post-mortem examination on their child[34] and many have found it beneficial.[27]

The autopsy has implicit tensions associated with it. Parents are confronted by a process that appears intrusive, and are required to understand detailed consent procedures while in a state of grief. Clinicians fear that the autopsy may reveal unexpected findings, which on occasion might result in litigation. The pathologist has one chance to obtain the data needed to provide answers to questions posed at the time and later, in the face of increasing constraints.

The request for autopsy is usually the responsibility of the treating clinician, and this chapter reflects the international changes that have been made in the practice of post mortems, with increasing complexity of consent forms, and new conditions and codes of conduct, and is aimed at providing the clinician with information on the hospital and coronial post-mortem examination.

The purpose of the perinatal post-mortem examination

Reasons for the performance of the autopsy extend beyond mere diagnostic purposes, and consent should take these purposes into account.[3,39,43]

Accurate cause of death

Despite the increasing complexity of diagnostic procedures in life, there is a consistent level of discrepancy between clinically recorded causes of death and findings at autopsy, of 24–45%.[9,12,17,25,32,40] In a significant number of these discrepant results, management is likely to have been different had the diagnosis been known.

Identification of disorders with implications for future pregnancies

A major benefit of the perinatal autopsy is identifying (and excluding) factors relating to future pregnancies, due to the high number of congenital anomalies, some unexpected congenital infections, and the occasional metabolic disorder found in this group. Subtle syndromic external features and internal anomalies may not be detected at delivery, or on the neonatal ward. Future pregnancies may need detailed monitoring, and counselling on recurrent disorders may be required.

Research

Diseases of neonates are often related to development and are different to diseases of children or adults. Post-mortem examination findings have led to a better understanding of neonatal diseases such as bronchopulmonary dysplasia, intracranial haemorrhages and leukomalacia. Post-mortem studies have demonstrated the neuropathological basis of abnormal ultrasound and MRI scans,[14,37] led to recognition of new disease entities, and allowed the identification of novel infectious diseases. The development of tissue banks of post-mortem material for research (with consent) needs wider acceptance and implementation if advances in technology are to be applied retrospectively to autopsy cases.

Quality control/audit

Audit is an essential part of a perinatal service, and post-mortem results provide vital information for this. The autopsy itself should be audited.[10,16,17,45,49,53] Rates of unexplained stillbirth may reflect the expertise of the pathologist, although pathologists differ on their interpretation of the significance of some autopsy findings. National studies such as CESDI can identify areas of healthcare needing guidelines or investigation. Post-mortem evidence of cardiac tamponade from long intravenous cannulas has led to changes in practice.[13] The few studies correlating antemortem MRI scans with the neuropathological findings are mentioned above. Full, frank and confidential discussion should occur at audit meetings, to maximise learning and benefit to future patients.[51]

Teaching

Use of the body for procedural practice such as insertion of long lines, or intubation, would now require specific consent. Cardiac surgeons and cardiologists have learnt the anatomy of rare cardiac malformations from museum cases, which are to a large extent no longer collected. Junior pathologists have traditionally learnt their normal histology from tissues obtained at autopsy.

Medicolegal

Most of the adult autopsies in the UK are performed as part of a coroner's investigation. Relatively few perinatal deaths are investigated by the coroner but reasons for referral to the coroner are discussed below. Any case may become a matter for litigation, and information from the autopsy is often important.

Alternatives to the full post-mortem examination

Post-mortem MRI scans, post-mortem needle biopsies, laparoscopic autopsies, and small incision access have been used as alternatives to a full post-mortem examination. MRI may be valuable in detection of subtle brain changes, but a final definite pathological cause of death can not be given, and there is no means to obtain tissue for diagnostic tests. The post-mortem examination, if performed to an acceptable standard, remains the gold standard in ascertaining cause of death. The value of a 'verbal post mortem', i.e. a review of events leading up to death, while considerable, cannot satisfy the requirements for a specific histopathological diagnosis. The Royal College working party found little evidence for valid alternatives to the paediatric post-mortem examination.[52]

In the perinatal period, a limited post mortem, or a thorough external examination, with measurements, weight, photographs and X-rays, and placental examination, may identify useful features such as chorioamnionitis, growth restriction or dysmorphism, but without a full internal examination, important features are likely to be undetected.

Coroner's versus hospital post mortems

In most jurisdictions, there are two types of post mortem, the coronial and the consented hospital post mortem. The same pathologist may perform them at the same location, but there are fundamental differences between the two in law, with different purposes for the examination, and this has important ramifications.[39]

Coroner's post mortem

The purpose of the coroner's post mortem is to determine the cause of death, and specifically whether it is natural or unnatural. Any other uses or benefits beyond those required for this investigation usually require specific next-of-kin consent. Examples of neonatal cases that should be referred to the coroner are:

- babies dead on arrival at hospital, or within 24 hours of admission;
- unattended stillbirth;
- deaths within 24 hours of an operation, anaesthetic or invasive procedure;
- deaths as a result of accident;
- unnatural, criminal or suspicious deaths, e.g. neglect, abuse, poisoning;

- deaths caused by drugs, prescribed or not;
- deaths as a result of medical mishap;
- deaths in which the doctor is uncertain of the cause of death, and unable to confidently complete the death certificate;
- unexpected death on the ward.

In doubt, discussion with an experienced coronial officer or the coroner himself is advised. The above list is a guideline only, which the coroner may choose to disregard in a specific case. For example, the coroner may choose not to investigate the unsuspicious death following pneumothorax of a 24-week gestation neonate on a ventilator. The wishes of the next of kin do not override the coroner's duty to order a post-mortem examination if he wishes, though some jurisdictions allow a legal challenge.

Ideally, coroners should arrange for paediatric pathologists rather than general or forensic pathologists to perform the post mortem,[52] and provide results to relevant clinicians.

The coroner's post mortem may result in an inquest. The coroner and his officer will be present, and usually the family. If you are asked to attend, you should report clearly what you did, observed, and deduced. You may be asked for an opinion, but unless you are present as an expert witness you should relay only what you know, and be clear to say when you do not know the answer to a question.

Hospital post mortem

The hospital post mortem has a much broader purpose than mere confirmation of the cause of death (the clinicians must complete a death certificate prior to this type of post mortem). The purpose is to document other contributing and non-contributing factors, audit, and answer questions related to the case.

Consent

Fully informed consent is the ideal goal, but there are considerable difficulties in the concept at this time of emotional distress.[26] Fortunately, post mortems rarely require immediate consent and a day or so can be spent discussing the options. Provision of a leaflet, a copy of the consent form, and use of a bereavement counsellor may be helpful.

Acquiring consent involves discussion of whether the post mortem is to be full, limited or stepwise, and whether there is specific permission to retain whole organs. The time or method of return or disposal of any whole organs retained must be clarified and documented. The fact that histological blocks are taken routinely should be made clear. Consent for use of tissues or whole organs for teaching should be discussed. Hospital consent forms should be regularly reviewed to ensure they address current ethical issues.

The pathologist should be consulted about any restrictions imposed. For example, consent that does not allow for the brain to be fixed may result in an inadequate post-mortem examination, and the pathologist may have reservations about an examination that cannot address significant questions. Any restrictions and the subsequent reduction of the information obtained need to be discussed with the parents and documented. Parents have the right to decline the post mortem, or impose strict limitations as to what is done. Pathologists vary in their opportunity and tendency for interaction with parents, but most are happy to meet parents together with the treating clinician, before and/or after the procedure, to explain what is done and why, and the significance of any findings. Having given consent, the majority of parents do not later regret their decision;[26] however, some parents who decline, later regret doing so.[33]

Cultural issues

Most religious leaders have accepted that the post mortem may be performed, subject to their codes. Hospitals should ensure that there is access to relevant religious authorities for advice.

Post-mortem procedure

The post-mortem examination requires a well-equipped mortuary, appropriately staffed, funded and accredited, with paediatric instruments, good photographic facilities, and access to a full range of histology techniques and genetic and metabolic services.[39]

Pathologist

The post-mortem examination of an infant is very different to that performed on an adult,[7,20,21,39,52] and ideally should be performed by a paediatric pathologist. Pathologists with paediatric training find a higher incidence of causes of death in infants,[11] provide a much higher proportion of adequate reports,[45,49] and their causes of death were infrequently revised by the CESDI review panel.[16]

The pathologist should know the main questions posed, the likely causes of death (registered in hospital cases), and the relevant neonatal history and be prepared to adapt technique accordingly before starting the autopsy. For example, difficult deliveries call for careful examination of the cervical spine,[50] and a similar approach may be needed for confirming cerebellar anomalies such as a Dandy Walker cyst.

Placenta

The placenta is an integral part of the perinatal post-mortem examination, and ideally all placentas should be retained for a few days after birth, to allow subsequent retrieval should an infant deteriorate, such as may happen with sepsis or a metabolic disorder. Chorioamnionitis is a common cause of premature labour and neonatal distress, and usually arises as a result of an ascending bacterial infection. Neutrophils marginating in the fetal vessels of the chorionic plate or in the umbilical cord are indicative of a fetal response, and are associated with cerebral white matter changes.[29] CMV, syphilis, and toxoplasma may also be

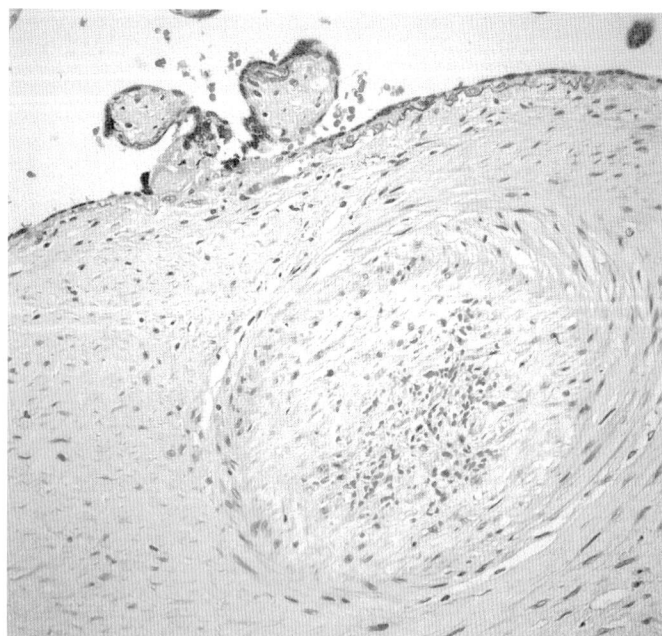

Fig. 42.1 Fetal stem vessel thrombus. Large villus with organising thrombus, and, above, small terminal avascular villi.

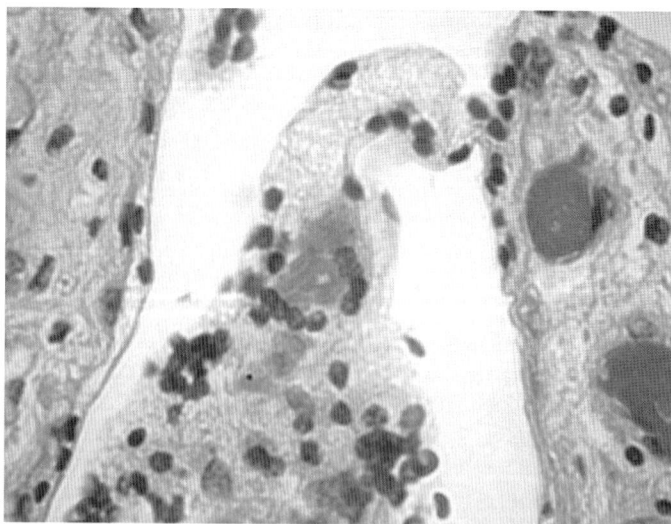

Fig. 42.2 GM1 gangliosidosis. Term infant. The cytotrophoblast at the periphery of the villi is pale and vacuolated.

diagnosed by the placental examination. 'Villitis of unknown aetiology' (VUE), appears to be due to an immunological response, and is associated with recurrent fetal compromise.[35]

The placenta may show evidence of pre-eclampsia, even when this has not been clinically apparent, with placental infarcts, ischaemic changes of the villi, maternal vessels unreconstructed by trophoblast, and atherosis. These lesions may be associated with maternal thrombotic disorders, which should also be considered if extensive fibrin deposition is seen. Fetal thrombotic disorders presenting with thrombi in the stem vessels of the placenta are associated with neurological deficits (Fig. 42.1).[24] Occasionally, an unrecognised twin pregnancy is seen, with a fetus papyraceous, and twin pregnancy has been associated with increased risk of neurological damage, some due to twin–twin transfusion syndrome.[31] A coexisting molar pregnancy or metastatic maternal or neonatal malignancy (neuroblastoma or leukaemia) is also a rare finding. Amniotic strands are associated with limb defects, or clefts, and some metabolic conditions may be first recognised from changes in the chorionic villi (Fig. 42.2).

In the mortuary

Many paediatric mortuaries provide parents with mementos such as photographs, hand- and footprints, and locks of hair.

Radiology should be completed before the body is opened.

The **full** post mortem starts with acquisition of a range of standardised photographs and measurements. The body is then examined externally, noting any dysmorphic features. Most pathologists use an incision from the sternum to the pubis, and a posterior vertex-to-neck or ear-to-ear head incision through the hair. The face and limb are not incised unless there is a specific indication and suitable consent has been obtained. Pneumothorax

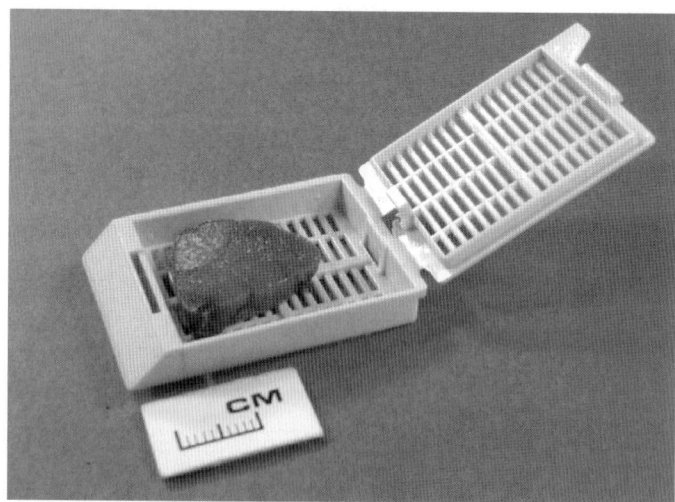

Fig. 42.3 Tissue processing block with typical tissue sample with 1-cm scale.

may be excluded by aspiration through the intercostal muscles. The sternum is removed by dividing lateral or medial to the costochondral junctions. A small piece of lung may be removed using aseptic technique for microbiology. The organs are examined in situ, and their connections established prior to their removal for weighing. Abnormalities are photographed. A small sample of each of the major organs is kept for histology, as many diseases can only be identified microscopically (Fig. 42.3). No whole major organ (brain, heart, liver, lung, kidney) is routinely retained, but these are returned to the body cavities after examination. The brain is usually very soft, and requires fixation in formalin for proper examination. This can be expedited, and brains fixed for 2–3 days are usually firm enough to be examined using normal neuropathological techniques. This allows the brain to be returned prior to burial or cremation. Hearts with difficult congenital anomalies are also easier to examine after fixation, allowing time for discussion with the cardiologists or cardiac surgeon.

Cytogenetic samples for chromosomal analysis or fibroblast culture are ideally taken shortly after death, but can be taken up to several days later. Microbiological samples (usually blood, urine and lung, but others including CSF, liver, heart and brain for viral illnesses) are often taken. A small piece of tissue (often muscle or spleen) may be snap frozen for later DNA extraction.

The **limited post mortem** will usually allow examination of a single body cavity or restrict the length of incision. An **external only examination** would include measurements, photographs and usually radiology, but no examination of the internal organs.

Following the post mortem, if the infant is dressed in age-appropriate attire, little evidence of the procedure is apparent.

Post-mortem report

The post-mortem report will usually comprise demographic details; a summary of the history as provided; the external examination findings, including weight and measurements; the internal examination findings, including organ weights; microscopic findings; results of ancillary examinations such as cytogenetics, microbiology, radiology etc.; a summary of findings; a commentary to suggest the most likely pathophysiological pathway; and a cause of death if appropriate.[38]

Other details ideally recorded are mode of identification, a list of samples taken, a record of X-rays and photographs taken, and details of the consent and any limitations imposed.

The post-mortem report is usually provided in two stages. The preliminary report is usually completed within 2 days of the examination, and covers the clinical history, samples taken, and macroscopic findings. Little interpretation may be given at this stage. The final report may take up to 6 weeks, allowing time for review of 30–40 slides, additional special stains, cytogenetic results, and neuropathology. Some complex genetic or metabolic work-ups require samples to be sent to national and international centres, and delays of 6–12 months are not uncommon for a final diagnosis in these cases.

Interpretation

The role of the pathologist is to document the findings and interpret these findings in the context of the clinical history, to put together the most likely pathophysiological processes leading to the death. The external measurements and weights of the organs give some clues about growth and gestational age (Table 42.1 and Table 42.2). The gestational age can be assessed microscopically.[21] Lung weights are helpful in assessing pulmonary hypoplasia. Assymetric growth restriction can be suggested by an abnormal brain:liver weight ratio.

Establishing the pathophysiological sequence leading up to death may require a team discussion. The identification of the various disease processes present may explain the clinical features, suggest alterations in prophylactic therapy, antibiotic protocols, or feeding protocols as part of an audit of unit practice, and also

Table 42.1 Foot length of the fetus (Modified from Streeter[44])

End of week	Mean foot length (mm)	Minimum foot length (mm)	Maximum foot length (mm)
14	14.0	12.5	15.5
15	16.8	15.2	18.5
16	19.9	18.2	21.6
17	23.0	21.0	25.0
18	26.8	24.8	28.8
19	30.7	28.5	33.0
20	33.3	31.0	35.7
21	35.2	32.5	38.0
22	39.5	36.0	43.0
23	42.2	39.0	45.5
24	45.2	42.0	48.5
25	47.7	44.5	51.0
26	50.2	47.0	53.5
27	52.7	49.0	56.5
28	55.2	51.5	59.0
29	57.0	53.0	61.0
30	59.2	55.5	63.0
31	61.2	57.5	65.0
32	63.0	59.0	67.0
33	65.0	61.0	69.0
34	68.2	64.0	72.5
35	70.5	66.0	75.0
36	73.5	69.0	78.0
37	76.5	72.0	81.0
38	78.5	74.0	83.0
39	81.0	76.0	86.0
40	82.5	77.5	87.5

aid the parents in coming to terms with the death, by showing that no easily remediable factor that would have prevented the death was missed.

The negative post mortem

Some causes of death leave no pathologically identifiable evidence, such as cardiac arrhythmias, epilepsy, gentle suffocation, and some metabolic conditions. Infections following antibiotic treatment are also difficult to identify. Accidental toxicity such as due to magnesium used for tocolysis,[19] or drug overdose may need to be excluded. The possibility of deliberate harm by staff, a parent or others should be considered; if the circumstances of the death warrant it, samples should be kept for toxicology.

Classification systems

Several systems of classification of perinatal death exist. Systematic classification is important for epidemiological studies,

Table 42.2 Organ weights of newborn infants by body weight (From Gruenwald & Minh[18])

Body weight (g)	Number of cases	Body length (cm)	Heart (g)	Lungs combined (g)	Spleen (g)	Liver (g)	Adrenals combined (g)	Kidneys combined (g)	Thymus (g)	Brain (g)	Gestational age Weeks	Days
500	317	29.4 ±2.5	5.0 ±1.6	12 ±5	1.3 ±0.8	26 ±10	2.6 ±1.7	5.4 ±2.1	2.2 ±0.8	70 ±18	23 ±2	5 3
750	311	32.9 ±3.0	6.3 ±1.8	19 ±6	2.0 ±1.2	39 ±12	3.2 ±1.5	7.8 ±2.6	2.8 ±1.3	107 ±27	26 ±2	0 6
1000	295	35.6 ±3.1	7.7 ±2.0	24 ±8	2.6 ±1.5	47 ±12	3.5 ±1.6	10.4 ±3.4	3.7 ±2.0	143 ±34	27 ±3	5 1
1250	217	38.4 ±3.0	9.6 ±3.3	30 ±9	3.4 ±1.8	56 ±21	4.0 ±1.7	12.9 ±3.9	4.9 ±12.1	174 ±38	29 ±3	0 0
1500	167	41.0 ±2.7	11.5 ±3.3	34 ±11	4.3 ±2.0	65 ±18	4.5 ±1.8	14.9 ±4.2	6.1 ±2.7	219 ±52	31 ±2	3 3
1750	148	42.6 ±3.1	12.8 ±3.2	40 ±13	5.0 ±2.5	74 ±20	5.3 ±2.0	17.4 ±4.7	6.8 ±3.0	247 ±51	32 ±2	4 6
2000	140	44.9 ±2.8	14.9 ±4.2	44 ±13	6.0 ±2.7	82 ±23	5.3 ±2.0	18.8 ±5.0	7.9 ±3.4	281 ±56	34 ±3	6 2
2250	124	46.3 ±2.9	16.0 ±4.3	48 ±15	7.0 ±3.3	88 ±24	6.0 ±2.3	20.2 ±4.9	8.2 ±3.4	308 ±49	36 ±13	4 0
2500	120	47.3 ±2.3	17.7 ±4.2	48 ±14	8.5 ±3.5	105 ±21	7.1 ±2.8	22.6 ±5.5	8.3 ±4.4	339 ±50	38 ±3	0 2
2750	138	48.7 ±2.9	19.1 ±3.8	51 ±15	9.1 ±3.6	117 ±26	7.5 ±2.7	24.0 ±5.4	9.6 ±3.8	362 ±48	39 ±2	2 2
3000	144	50.0 ±2.9	20.7 ±5.3	53 ±13	10.1 ±3.3	127 ±30	8.3 ±2.9	24.7 ±5.3	10.2 ±4.3	380 ±55	40 ±2	0 1
3250	133	50.7 ±2.6	21.5 ±4.3	59 ±18	11.0 ±4.0	145 ±33	9.2 ±3.4	27.3 ±6.6	11.6 ±4.4	395 ±53	40 ±1	4 6
3500	106	51.8 ±3.0	22.8 ±5.9	63 ±17	11.3 ±3.6	153 ±33	9.8 ±3.5	28.0 ±6.5	12.8 ±5.1	411 ±55	40 ±1	4 5
3750	57	52.1 ±2.3	23.8 ±5.1	65 ±15	12.5 ±4.1	159 ±40	10.2 ±3.3	29.5 ±6.8	13.0 ±4.8	413 ±55	40 ±2	6 3
4000	31	52.4 ±2.7	25.8 ±5.3	67 ±20	14.1 ±4.0	180 ±39	10.8 ±3.4	30.2 ±6.2	11.4 ±3.2	420 ±62	41 ±1	4 3
4250	15	53.2 ±2.5	26.5 ±5.3	68 ±16	13.0 ±2.5	197 ±42	12.0 ±3.7	30.7 ±15.8	11.7 ±3.7	415 ±38	41 ±2	2 1

and identification of factors in need of addressing in the local population. The assignment of the classification category is best decided by a group of clinicians, paediatricians, obstetricians, fetal medicine specialists, nurses, and midwives. The same classification system should be used within a region to allow meaningful comparisons, and there is a wide choice (see appendices in the CESDI reports).

Clinicopathological correlation and audit

The neonatologist must take the lead in correlating the post-mortem findings with the clinical history, and ensuring that parents get feedback. The pathologist also requires feedback for his own education and audit purposes.

It is important that the hospital supports grieving parents, and provides a forum whereby the parents can, if desired, meet clinical staff a few weeks after the death. Consideration should be made for how and when parents are seen, and who is present. Many of these parents have clinical depression,[48] need social and/or spiritual support, require advice for future pregnancies, and have specific questions. This process may involve a team of a neonatologist, obstetrician, fetal medicine specialist, midwife, counsellor, chaplain, pathologist and others. A bereavement counsellor can coordinate this and also be a neutral person for the parents to contact, particularly where the parents have concerns about their baby's treatment.

Specific post-mortem conditions

Cases of death due to an inborn error of metabolism (Chapter 35, Part 3) usually have a prodromal illness, and should be considered when there is unexpected liver failure, acidosis or hypoglycaemia.[4] Urine and blood should be taken before death, ideally before transfusions, and the laboratory notified to retain these samples. Liver and skeletal muscle are taken for histology and electron microscopy, and samples deep frozen ideally within an hour of death. The full autopsy can take place later, and a full neuropathological study is indicated, as subtle cerebral anomalies may be diagnostically useful. Some metabolic conditions may present with a specific pathology such as pulmonary alveolar proteinosis and lysinuric aciduria. Unfortunately, the metabolic changes relating to collapse or dying may make identification of the disease more difficult than in samples taken from a stable infant. Discussion between the clinician, paediatric biochemist and the paediatric pathologist is crucial to optimise the work-up of these difficult cases.

There are several pathological findings that may be identified **after a difficult delivery**. Small haemorrhages are commonly found in the meninges. Trauma to the brain with identification of cerebellar tissue in the pulmonary arteries may be seen after an instrumental delivery.[6] In breech deliveries and after difficult or instrumental deliveries, the pathologist should take special care to obtain cervical X-rays, to check for occipital osteodiastasis, and to carefully examine the posterior part of the cervical spine, the occipital bone, the posterior and inferior cerebellum and brainstem in situ.[50] The falx, dura, and tentorium should be carefully inspected to exclude tears. It should be noted that in many cases of apparent perinatal hypoxia there is evidence of previous ischaemic cerebral damage.[42]

Most **cardiac** lesions do not present immediately at birth or with sudden death, but histiocytoid cardiomyopathy[41] (which can be recognised at post mortem as yellow nodules in the myocardium) and left ventricular outlet obstruction by a rhabdomyoma may be identified. Antenatal ultrasound screening detects many cardiac lesions, but some, such as hypoplastic left heart, may develop and evolve during pregnancy. Anomalous pulmonary drainage may be missed on scans, and at post mortem the pulmonary venous anatomy needs to be clearly identified.

Identification of mild-to-moderate **pulmonary hypoplasia** can be very difficult, particularly when the infant has been ventilated. Criteria based on size of the thorax, combined lung weight (as a proportion of the bodyweight, normally <0.012 over 28 weeks' gestation[2]), or techniques based on DNA content are not easy to interpret. The airspaces and airways are also affected by ventilation, and assessment of development can be difficult. The radial alveolar count needs to allow for the gestational age. **Alveolar capillary dysplasia** usually presents as intractable pulmonary hypertension in infants a few days or weeks old. The vascular architecture of the lungs is disorganised, with increased capillaries, thickened alveolar walls, and pulmonary veins not in the normal position between lung lobules, but with the pulmonary arteries and bronchi in the centre of lobules (Fig. 42.4). This condition is not as rare as the published literature suggests, and should be considered in all cases of neonatal or early infantile onset of pulmonary hypertension for which there appears to be no cause.[46]

Renal tubular dysgenesis, with failure of the normal development of the proximal renal tubules, is seen in conditions where the kidneys are poorly perfused during pregnancy, such as in the

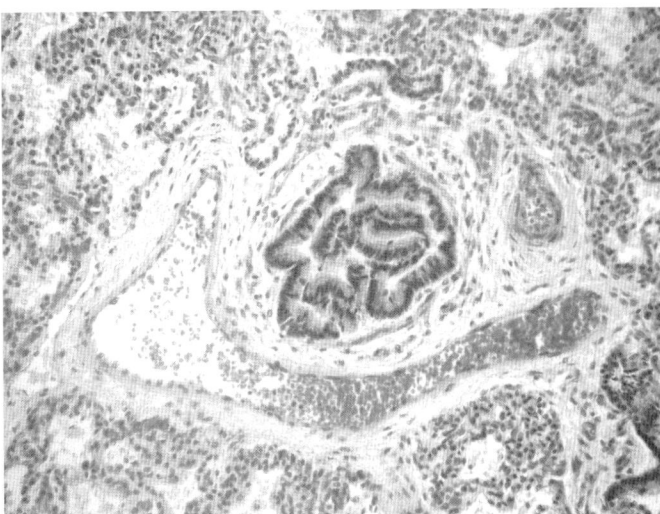

Fig. 42.4 Alveolar capillary dysplasia. Central bronchus with artery to the right, and anomalously sited vein. The adjacent alveoli are abnormal with increased capillaries.

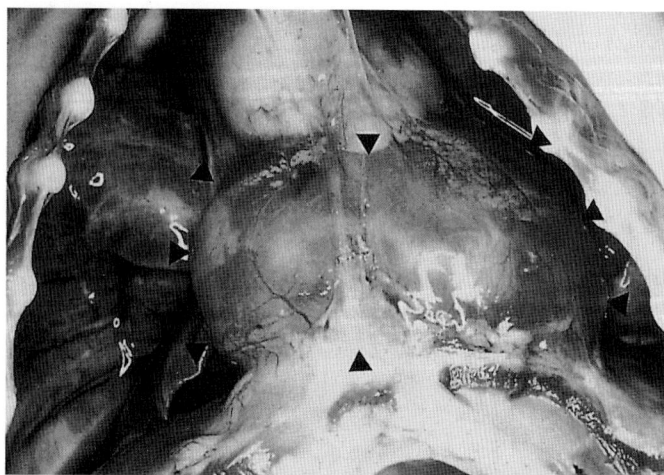

Fig. 42.5 Cardiac tamponade.

donor of twin-to-twin perfusion,[30] and with maternal use of angiotensin-converting enzyme inhibitors. It also can occur as a familial genetic condition.

Skeletal dysplasia diagnosis requires good-quality X-rays of the body and limbs, establishment of a fibroblast culture, and an analysis of the bones (by routine histology, electron microscopy and frozen samples), including femoral head, rib and vertebral body, usually obtained through the standard incisions. Bones may be replaced by a firm prosthesis to give a good cosmetic result.

In some genetic disorders, removal of the **eye** for examination may be required, but this needs specific consent. Glass eyes or special plastic moulds designed to maintain the socket shape and keep the eyelids closed are available.

Some degree of **iatrogenic disease** is commonly seen in neonatal autopsies:[47]

- Bronchopulmonary dysplasia.
- Necrotising tracheobronchitis may be seen, particularly with high-frequency ventilation.
- Chest drain damage to the lungs is now unusual but there may be intrapleural haemorrhage due to trauma to an intercostal artery.
- Myocardial damage due to adrenaline/noradrenaline may be present, though pressor lesions may be seen in any stressed neonate.
- Cardiac tamponade is a recognised complication of long lines situated in the right atrium (pp. 106, 491, 1208, 1223) (Fig. 42.5).
- Total parenteral nutrition (TPN) liver damage with cholestasis is a frequent finding.

The unexpected finding

Occasionally, a lesion is found at post mortem which has major implications for the family, such as tuberous sclerosis, cystic fibrosis, or some other familial disorder. There is a need to ensure genetic counselling is available if such a finding is made. Samples may be retained for DNA confirmation after discussion with the family. The requirement for specific consent for DNA testing or confirmation for a suspected genetic disease in this situation is unclear to most paediatric pathologists, as the diagnosis of some genetic diseases may be more firmly made by macroscopic or microscopic examination than by a DNA test.

Summary

Neonatalogists have traditionally been advocates of the post-mortem examination, a procedure which has recently been under much public scrutiny, with resultant distress to parents, pathologists and others. The wide range of benefits arising from the examination means that until other forms of examination can truly take over the myriad of its functions, the post-mortem examination will continue to have a crucial role in neonatal practice. Many parents wish to understand the reasons for their tragedy and it is crucial that government and regulatory bodies take on the responsibility of establishing clear guidelines, and continue to work to balance some of the conflicting pressures. Attending an infant autopsy and helping to explain the procedure to parents should be part of the training of every neonatologist.

Acknowledgement

We express our gratitude to all those parents who have consented to the examinations from which we have learned so much.

References

1. Alder Hey Inquiry 2001 The Royal Liverpool Children's Hospital Inquiry Report (Alder Hey). The Stationery Office, London. Available online: http://www.rlcinquiry.org.uk/ 7 Oct 2002
2. Askin F B 1998 Respiratory tract disorders in the fetus and neonate. In: Wigglesworth J S, Singer D B (eds) Textbook of fetal and perinatal pathology. Blackwell Science, Massachusetts, pp 555–592
3. Beckwith J B 1989 The value of the pediatric postmortem examination. Pediatric Clinics of North America 36: 29–36
4. Bennett M J, Rinaldo P 2001 The metabolic autopsy comes of age. Clinical Chemistry 47: 1145–1146
5. Berger L R 1985 Requesting the autopsy: a pediatric perspective. Clinical Pediatrics 17: 445–452
6. Bohm N, Keller K M, Kloke W D 1982 Pulmonary and systemic cerebellar tissue embolism due to birth injury. Virchows Archiv. A, Pathological Anatomy and Histopathology 398: 229–235
7. Bove K E 1997 Practice guidelines for autopsy pathology: the perinatal and pediatric autopsy. Autopsy Committee of the College of American Pathologists. Archives of Pathology and Laboratory Medicine 121: 368–376
8. Bristol Royal Infirmary Inquiry 2000 The Inquiry into the management of care of children receiving complex heart surgery at The Bristol Royal Infirmary. Interim Report, May 2002. Removal and retention of human material. Bristol Royal Infirmary Inquiry, Bristol. Available online: http://www.bristol-inquiry.org.uk/ 7 Oct 2002
9. Brodlie M, Laing I A, Keeling J W, McKenzie K J 2002 Ten years of neonatal autopsies in tertiary referral centre: retrospective study. British Medical Journal 324: 761–763
10. CESDI 1997 Management after fetal and infant death and pathology. In: CESDI 4th Annual Report. Maternal and Child Health Research Consortium, London, pp 50–54
11. Cote A, Russo P, Michaud J 1999 Sudden unexpected deaths in infancy: what are the causes? Journal of Pediatrics 135: 437–443
12. Craft H, Brazy J E 1986 Autopsy high yield in neonatal population. American Journal of Diseases of Children 140: 1260–1262

13. Department of Health 2001 Review of the deaths of four babies due to cardiac tamponade associated with the presence of a central venous catheter. Department of Health, London. Available online: http://www.doh.gov.uk/manchesterbabies/manchreport.pdf 7 Oct 2002

14. Felderhoff-Mueser U, Rutherford M A, Squier W V et al 1999 Relationship between MR imaging and histopathologic findings of the brain in extremely sick preterm infants. AJNR. American Journal of Neuroradiology 20: 1349–1357

15. Gould S 2001 Update on issues surrounding the post mortem. In: CESDI 8th Annual Report. Maternal and Child Health Research Consortium, London, pp 63–71

16. Gould S, Keeling J 2000 Sudden unexpected deaths in infancy – pathology. In: CESDI 7th Annual Report. Maternal and Child Health Research Consortium, London, pp 65–74

17. Gould S, Keeling J, Thornton C M 1999 Perinatal pathology. In: CESDI 6th Annual Report. Maternal and Child Health Research Consortium, London, pp 51–58

18. Gruenwald P, Minh H N 1960 Evaluation of body and organ weights in perinatal pathology. 1. Normal standards derived from autopsies. American Journal of Clinical Pathology 34: 247–253

19. Herschel M, Mittendorf R 2001 Tocolytic magnesium sulfate toxicity and unexpected neonatal death. Journal of Perinatology 21: 261–262

20. Joint Working Party of the Royal College of Obstetricians and Gynaecologists and the Royal College of Pathologists 1988 Report on fetal and perinatal pathology. Royal College of Pathologists, London

21. Keeling J 2001 The perinatal necropsy. In: Keeling J (ed) Fetal and neonatal pathology. Springer, London, pp 1–46

22. Khong T Y 2002 Falling neonatal autopsy rates: neonatologists, pathologists, and relatives need to boost neonatal pathology. British Medical Journal 324: 749–750

23. Khong T Y, Arbuckle S M 2002 Perinatal pathology in Australia after Alder Hey. Journal of Paediatrics and Child Health 38: 409–411

24. Khong T Y, Hague W M 2001 Biparental contribution to fetal thrombophilia in discordant twin intrauterine growth restriction. American Journal of Obstetrics and Gynecology 185: 244–245

25. Kumar P, Angst D B, Taxy J, Mangurten H H 2000 Neonatal autopsies: a 10-year experience. Archives of Pediatrics and Adolescent Medicine 154: 38–42

26. McHaffie H E, Fowlie P W, Hume R et al 2001 Consent to autopsy for neonates. Archives of Disease in Childhood. Fetal and Neonatal Edition 85: F4–F7

27. McPhee S J, Bottles K, Lo B et al 1986. To redeem them from death. Reactions of family members to autopsy. American Journal of Medicine 80: 665–671

28. Macpherson T 1996 The perinatal autopsy and risk management: the value of a 'standardised' approach. In: Donn S M, Fisher C W (eds) Risk management techniques in perinatal and neonatal practice. Futura, New York, pp 361–387

29. Nelson K B, Willoughby R E 2000 Infection, inflammation and the risk of cerebral palsy. Current Opinion in Neurology 13: 133–139

30. Oberg K C, Pestaner J P, Bielamowicz L, Hawkins E P 1999 Renal tubular dysgenesis in twin-twin transfusion syndrome. Pediatric and Developmental Pathology 2: 25–32

31. Pharoah P O D, Price T S, Plomin R 2002 Cerebral palsy in twins: a national study. Archives of Disease in Childhood. Fetal and Neonatal Edition 87: F122–F124

32. Porter H J, Keeling J W 1987 Value of perinatal necropsy examination. Journal of Clinical Pathology 40: 180–184

33. Rahman H A, Khong T Y 1995 Perinatal and infant postmortem examination. Survey of women's reactions to perinatal necropsy. British Medical Journal 310: 870–871

34. Rankin J, Wright C, Lind T 2002 Cross sectional survey of parents' experience and views of the postmortem examination. British Medical Journal 324: 816–818

35. Redline R W 1999 Disorders of the placental parenchyma. In: Lewis S H, Perrin E (eds) Pathology of the placenta. Churchill Livingstone, New York, pp 161–184

36. Rickard H, Willis M 2001 After AlderHey … can we survive? ACP News Summer: 11–13

37. Roelants-van Rijn A M, Nikkels P G J, Groenendaal F et al 2001 Neonatal diffusion-weighted MR imaging: relation with histopathology or follow-up MR examination. Neuropediatrics 32: 286–294

38. Royal College of Pathologists 2000 Guidelines for post mortem reports. Royal College of Pathologists, London. Available online: http://www.rcpath.org/activities/publications/pmrbook.html 7 Oct 2002

39. Royal College of Pathologists 2002 Guidelines on autopsy practice. Report of a working group of the Royal College of Pathologists. Royal College of Pathologists, London. Available online: http://www.rcpath.org/activities/publications/autopsy_practise_sept2002.html 7 Oct 2002

40. Saller D N, Lesser K B, Harrel U et al 1995 The clinical utility of the perinatal autopsy. Journal of the American Medical Association 273: 663–665

41. Shehata B H, Patterson K, Thomas J E et al 1998 Histiocytoid cardiomyopathy: three cases and a review of the literature. Pediatric and Developmental Pathology 1: 56–69

42. Squier W 2002 Pathology of fetal and neonatal brain damage: identifying the timing. In: Squier W (ed) Acquired damage to the developing brain. Timing and causation. Arnold, London, pp 110–127

43. Start R D, Cotton D W K 1997 The current status of the autopsy. In: Progress in pathology, volume 3. Churchill Livingstone, New York, pp 179–188

44. Streeter G L 1921 Weight, sitting height, head size, foot length and menstrual age of the human embryo. Contributions to Embryology, Carnegie Institute 55: 143–170

45. Thornton C, O'Hara M D 1998 A regional audit of perinatal and infant autopsies in Northern Ireland. British Journal of Obstetrics and Gynaecology 105: 18–23

46. Tibballs J, Chow C W 2002 Incidence of alveolar capillary dysplasia in severe idiopathic persistent pulmonary hypertension of the newborn. Journal of Paediatrics and Child Health 38: 397–400

47. Valdes-Dapena M 1989 Iatrogenic disease in the perinatal period. Pediatric Clinics of North America 36: 67–93

48. Vance J C, Boyle F M, Najman J M et al 2002 Couple distress after sudden death or perinatal death: a 30-month follow up. Journal of Paediatrics and Child Health 38: 368–372

49. Vujanic G M, Cartlidge P H T, Stewart J H 1998 Improving the quality of perinatal and infant necropsy examinations: a follow up study. Journal of Clinical Pathology 51: 850–853

50. Winter C, Savage P, Lawrence J et al 2000 Focus group – breech presentation at onset of labour. In: CESDI 7th Annual Report. Maternal and Child Health Research Consortium, London, pp 25–39

51. Womack C, Roger S, Lavin M 1997 Disclosure of clinical audit records in law: risks and possible defences. British Medical Journal 315: 1369–1370

52. Working Group 2002 The future of paediatric pathology services. Report of a Working Group to restore and develop specialist paediatric pathology. Royal College of Paediatrics and Child Health, London

53. Wright C, Cameron H, Lamb W 1998 A study of the quality of perinatal autopsy in the former Northern Region. British Journal of Obstetrics and Gynaecology 105: 24–28

CHAPTER 43

The clinical biochemistry laboratory

Ruth M Ayling

Introduction

Clinical biochemistry is involved, in varying amounts, in all medical specialities. In neonatology, biochemical tests are used for screening, diagnosis and monitoring the effect of treatment, and the laboratory may already have been involved in antenatal testing of maternal and fetal samples.

Successful working relationships between neonatologists and the staff of clinical biochemistry departments requires a mutual understanding of clinical and laboratory problems, which is often best achieved by the nomination of a designated clinical biochemist with a responsibility for the neonatal unit.

Specimen collection

Before requesting a biochemical investigation, the neonatologist should define the question to which the analysis would help provide an answer. The laboratory must be provided with the correct specimen and sufficient clinical information to ensure that the correct tests are performed and the results communicated with minimal delay. Tests should only be requested urgently if the results are required for immediate patient management. Various specimens can be used for biochemical tests (Table 43.1), although the majority of requests are for analysis of blood.

Table 43.1 Specimens used for biochemical analysis	
Blood	Other fluids, e.g.
capillary	synovial
venous	pleural
arterial	ascitic
Urine	Calculi
Faeces	Biopsy specimens, e.g.
Saliva	skin
Cerebrospinal fluid	liver
	muscle

Blood

It is essential to ensure that the correct sample is taken for the test required. There is often confusion as to the difference between plasma and serum samples. Plasma refers to the aqueous phase of the blood in vivo and to the supernatant obtained after centrifugation of a blood sample collected into a tube containing an anticoagulant, most commonly lithium heparin. Blood collected into a plain tube clots, and after centrifugation, serum is obtained. Whilst certain tests require plasma samples (e.g. ammonia, amino acids), the majority can be performed on either plasma or serum. There are some differences between the results obtained from plasma and serum samples; for example, the potassium concentration is higher in serum owing to release from platelets during clotting. If results are required with particular urgency, it is preferable to send a plasma sample, as it can be centrifuged and analysed immediately, without having to wait for the blood to clot in order to obtain the serum. Examples of tests requiring whole blood, i.e. blood collected into anticoagulant and not centrifuged, are genetic studies and investigations of white or red cell enzymes.

Blood samples from neonates are usually obtained by heel puncture (capillary samples), venepuncture or from indwelling catheters, usually situated in arteries. Whilst capillary sampling is widely used, venepuncture has been assessed to be less painful and more effective.[4] Capillary samples are not adequate for all tests – for example, they result in an increased potassium concentration, and contamination from sweat can cause spurious elevation of ammonia concentration. Capillary samples should not be used to provide meaningful estimates of pO_2. Prior to taking blood from an indwelling catheter, to prevent contamination from infusate, three to five times the dead-space volume should be withdrawn prior to sampling and this volume re-infused afterwards.

Sampling errors

Sampling errors may prevent the laboratory from producing meaningful results; examples of those arising most often are shown in Table 43.2.

Table 43.2 Examples of sampling errors which may cause spurious results

Error	Mechanism	Result
Blood sampling site	Dilution of sample by i.v. fluid	
Blood sampling technique	Difficulty in obtaining sample leads to haemolysis, resulting in release of red cell components	↑ Potassium ↑ Phosphate & AST
Stasis during venepuncture	Diffusion of plasma water from intravascular compartment and concentration of plasma	↑ Protein, albumin & protein-bound components, e.g. calcium
Incorrect specimen container	Glycolysis will not be inhibited unless a fluoride/oxalate preservative is used	↓ Glucose
	Effect of even a slight amount of potassium EDTA (the anti-coagulant in a 'full-blood count bottle')	↑ Potassium ↓ Calcium, ALP ↓ Magnesium
Delay in transit to laboratory	Metabolism of glucose Leakage of cellular components	↓ Glucose ↑ Potassium ↑ Phosphate

ALP, alkaline phosphatase; AST, aspartate transaminase.

Sample volume

A disadvantage of biochemical investigations in the neonate is that the volume of blood withdrawn may necessitate blood transfusion. Assuming a blood volume of 10 ml/kg and that transfusion may be required after loss of 10% of this, sending a total of 7.5 ml of blood to the laboratory from a 750 g infant over a short period (less than the usual volume received to perform one full biochemistry profile in an adult patient) may reach this threshold. It may be helpful for the laboratory to provide an indication of sample volume requirements and for clinicians and clinical biochemists to work together to provide guidelines for the frequency of biochemical monitoring.

Non-invasive techniques are obviously an attractive alternative to blood sampling and pulse oximetry and transcutaneous pO$_2$ monitors are important management tools. Transcutaneous glucose monitoring and bilirubinometry are under development but are not yet sufficiently reliable to be incorporated into routine practice.

Urine

Urine can be collected from babies by using plastic urine bags secured to the perineal area, but the adhesive used can cause irritation. An alternative method is to place a plastic glove containing several cotton-wool balls around the genital area, attached to the skin with plastic tape if necessary. The urine passed can be aspirated from the cotton wool and sent for analysis. This method is not suitable for samples for protein analysis owing to absorption of protein by the cotton wool. Timed urine

collections should be performed accurately in neonates as, owing to the small volumes passed, any losses are highly significant.

If a small sample of urine or other fluid is obtained, it may be preferable to send it to the laboratory in a bottle intended for serum collection, as all the available sample can be amalgamated by centrifugation. The same amount of fluid arriving in small drops on the sides of a Universal (urine) container that is too large to centrifuge may be deemed insufficient for analysis.

Cerebrospinal fluid

Cerebrospinal fluid for glucose analysis should be sent in a bottle containing fluoride/oxalate to prevent a result that is spuriously low. Samples for protein analysis should be sent in a plain container.

Faeces

Samples of faeces can generally be obtained from a nappy.

Reference ranges

Biochemical tests are interpreted in the light of a quoted reference range or, more correctly, reference interval. The reference range is usually determined as the interval into which the central 95% of apparently healthy individuals fall. If the distribution is

Gaussian, this is the range two standard deviations above and below the mean. With non-Gaussian distributions, this range is obtained by deleting the 2.5% at the upper and lower ends of ranked values. One in 20 (i.e. 5%) of apparently healthy babies will therefore have a value outside this range. The finding of a value outside the quoted reference range does not necessarily indicate the presence of a pathological cause, and the more tests performed which are independent variables, the greater the probability of finding a result outside the reference range. Similarly, the presence of abnormality is not excluded by a result within the reference range. It is difficult to obtain a sufficiently large population of healthy neonates for studies to define reference ranges, or to obtain the necessary informed consent to enable them to be carried out. Determining reference ranges in hospitalised, sick patients has advantages in neonatal practice, particularly for those analytes that are known to change in 'sick' patients.[2] When monitoring trends, it should be remembered that a difference in results could be due to a genuine change in biochemical status, itself the result of biological variation or pathological change, or to laboratory imprecision. A significant change is likely to have occurred when two results differ by more than 2.8 times the analytical standard deviation. Reference ranges may vary between laboratories, and reference ranges from other institutions and the literature should not be used to interpret a result without prior consultation with the clinical biochemist from the laboratory that performed the analysis.

Historically, laboratory testing for the newborn was performed in specialised laboratories using procedures and instruments suitable for the small volume of available samples. Different reference ranges were often necessitated by the differences in methodology. Technological advances have led to more widespread ability to use small sample volumes, and different reference intervals for neonates now tend to reflect their physiological differences from adult populations.

Near-patient testing

Near-patient, or point-of-care, testing refers to testing which is not performed in a central hospital laboratory but is carried out in a satellite laboratory or on the ward. Bedside monitoring of blood glucose using dry chemistry 'sticks' has been routine practice in neonatal units for many years, although often with a greater analytical error than is recommended.

Electrochemical biosensors (analytical devices that use biodetectors such as an enzyme or antibody to recognise the analyte without the need for specimen processing) for glucose are now in use, as are other systems that employ single-use disposable cartridges to perform a battery of tests on a drop of blood. Their use may have distinct advantages in the setting of a neonatal unit. Hospital laboratories run internal quality control such that standards with known values are measured by the staff using the equipment at regular intervals throughout the day. To attain accreditation it is compulsory to participate in external quality-assessment schemes whereby samples containing unknown amounts of substance must be measured and the values reported to external assessors. Laboratories that fail to reach satisfactory standards have their practice reviewed. Neonatologists embarking upon near-patient testing should do so in collaboration with the hospital laboratory and should consider quality control together with issues such as data handling, troubleshooting, staff training and competency evaluation.[3]

Inherited metabolic disease

The clinical biochemistry laboratory has a pivotal role in the investigation of suspected inherited metabolic disease, and neonatologists and clinical biochemists should work together to agree protocols for their investigation. If an inherited metabolic disease is suspected, it can be helpful to review the results of first-line biochemical investigations. Hypoglycaemia, hypocalcaemia, or renal or hepatic failure may be signs of underlying metabolic abnormality. If a metabolic acidosis is present, calculation of the anion gap ($[Na^+] + [K^+] - [Cl^-] + [HCO_3^-]$) may be helpful, a gap >20 mmol/l suggesting an organic acidaemia, whereas acidosis and a normal gap is more likely to be due to a renal tubular acidosis or bicarbonate loss from the gastrointestinal tract. More specific tests may then be appropriate, including measurement of ammonia, lactate, galactose-1-phosphate uridyl-transferase, amino acids and acyl carnitines in plasma, and amino and organic acids in urine. To enable full interpretation of the results, it is important to provide, with the specimens, accurate details regarding the date and time of sampling, and feeding and treatment regimens. If a dying infant is suspected of having a metabolic disorder, it may be helpful to obtain tissue specimens to facilitate diagnosis and therefore provide the opportunity for genetic counselling during future pregnancies. It is preferable to take such samples before death, although skin biopsies for fibroblast culture can be obtained up to 24 hours and liver and muscle samples up to 2 hours after death. Skin samples should be placed in a sterile container in transport media and stored at 4°C. Culture medium should be available from virology or cytogenetics departments; if not, isotonic (N/saline) can be used. Liver and muscle biopsies should be placed in a plastic tube, snap frozen in liquid nitrogen, and stored as cold as possible.

Particularly in non-specialist centres, investigations of patients with metabolic disorders are carried out infrequently. Some of the tests requested may be performed in specialised laboratories, which stipulate complex sample-handling processes prior to arrival. It is essential for both neonatologists and all laboratory personnel to ensure that robust mechanisms are in place, for example on-call and when the designated liaison individual is on leave, to ensure that these valuable specimens are dealt with correctly.

Sudden unexplained death in infancy

The clinical biochemistry laboratory also has a place in the investigation of sudden, unexplained death in infancy. A blood sample should be taken by cardiac puncture within 4 hours of death,

Table 43.3 Biochemical investigation of sudden unexplained death in infancy

	Investigation	Type of specimen required
Blood	Urea and electrolytes	Serum/lithium heparin
	Acyl carnitine	Blood spot card
	Metabolic studies	Lithium heparin
	Toxicology	Serum
	Chromosomes	Lithium heparin (*if infant is dysmorphic*)
Urine	Toxicology	
	Organic acids	
	Amino acids	

preferably within the first 30 minutes, and a sample of urine obtained if possible (Table 43.3). Care should be taken that erroneous diagnoses are not made on samples of blood showing postmortem changes, as results may reveal hypoglycaemia as well as spurious increases in serum potassium, phosphate, aspartate transaminase, lactate, ammonia and amino acids, due to protein autolysis and cellular breakdown. Other biochemical investigations should be carried out if indicated by the history and clinical findings.

Neonatal screening

Clinical biochemists are involved in testing all babies in the UK via the national neonatal screening programme. Screening is carried out in the first week of life using a sample of capillary blood placed onto a blood spot (Guthrie) card. This is usually performed by a community midwife in the child's home and it is important for hospital staff to remember to perform the test on babies who remain in-patients. Screening for phenylketonuria was introduced in the early 1960s and that for congenital hypothyroidism was added in the mid-1970s. The majority of centres use only an increased thyroid-stimulating hormone (TSH) concentration as their screening test for congenital hypothyroidism and do not measure thyroxine, so will fail to detect hypothyroidism secondary to hypothalamopituitary disease. In some areas, although not nationwide at present, screening for cystic fibrosis and sickle cell disease is performed. Clinical biochemists now have the capability to use molecular genetics and tandem mass spectrometry to screen for a number of other inherited metabolic disorders.[1] The neonatal screening programme is carried out at regional centres and the blood spot cards are retained there for some time, so can be obtained for later use, for example for metabolic or genetic studies in cases of neonatal death when no other samples are available.

Conclusion

The neonatal unit provides unique challenges for the clinical biochemistry laboratory, and mutual understanding of each other's resources and limitations should lead to the best possible diagnostic service. To achieve this, it may be helpful for neonatologists and clinical biochemists to work together to draw up practical guidelines and investigative approaches applicable to local circumstances – for example:

- standard test protocols and sample requirements;
- repertoire of tests offered and acceptable turnaround times (within and outside routine working hours);
- laboratory test values requiring telephoning directly to the ward;
- biochemical monitoring of fluid and electrolyte status;
- biochemical monitoring of patients receiving parenteral nutrition;
- investigation of persistent jaundice;
- investigation of hypoglycaemia;
- investigation of hypocalcaemia;
- investigation of sudden unexplained infant death.

As changes occur in neonatal practice and the management of currently untreatable inherited metabolic diseases, close contact with the clinical biochemistry laboratory will ensure that appropriate arrangements are made for service provision to take account of developments in neonatal screening, diagnosis and monitoring.

References

1. Clague A, Thomas A 2002 Neonatal biochemical screening for disease. Clinica Chimica Acta 315: 99–110
2. Hoffmann R G 1963 Statistics in the practice of medicine. Journal of the American Medical Association 185: 864–873
3. Lee-Lewandrowski E, Lewandrowski K 2001 Point of care testing. An overview and a look to the future. Clinics in Laboratory Medicine 21: 217–239
4. Shah V, Ohlsson A 2001 Venepuncture versus heel lance for blood sampling in term neonates (Cochrane Review). Cochrane Database of Systematic Reviews (2): CD001452

Further reading

Green A, Morgan I, Gray J 2003 Neonatology and laboratory medicine. ACB Venture Publications, London

CHAPTER 44

Neonatal imaging

David W Pilling

Introduction

Imaging in the neonate includes the whole range of imaging investigations available in the older child and adult. The cornerstone of imaging is still conventional radiography, but ultrasound also plays an important part. Computed tomography (CT), magnetic resonance imaging (MRI) and nuclear medicine play a much smaller part. Most neonatal imaging is undertaken on very sick and usually very small neonates in the intensive care unit and requires portable X-ray equipment of a very high specification that will give very short exposure times. Whilst in most departments conventional X-ray film is still used, there is a rapid advance towards using computerised radiography which enables digital images to be produced, aiming towards a filmless environment. Images are then available for viewing on monitors within the intensive care unit and can be transmitted electronically over large distances if a further opinion is required. Interpretation of intensive care radiology is often done on the spot by clinicians, who must receive appropriate training. Regular review meetings between clinical and radiology staff are essential for audit, training, and maintenance of skills.

Radiation safety

All involved in the management of neonates should sign up to the ALARA principle (as low as reasonably achievable) with regard to radiation dose. In the European Union, legislation has been enacted, which in the UK has led to the Ionising Radiation Medical Exposure Regulations 2000 – IRMER 2000[2] – governing both the justification (i.e. clinical needs for an examination) and optimisation (obtaining the best images with the lowest possible radiation dose).

Chest imaging

Chest radiography

Almost every baby admitted to a neonatal intensive care unit (NICU) will have one or more chest radiographs. It is most important that these answer the clinical question posed by the requesting doctor and that all those requesting such radiographs are able to interpret them. It is important that the film is technically satisfactory with the appropriate radiation exposure so that the lungs, soft tissues and bones can be adequately visualised on the radiograph produced. It is vital that the highest quality radiograph possible is obtained. The chest should be straight so that the hemithoraces in the normal situation would appear the same density. It is also important that the film is taken in full inspiration (Fig. 44.1). This is relatively easy to judge in a ventilated baby from the timing of the ventilator but requires a great degree of skill and judgment on the part of the radiographer if the baby is breathing spontaneously.

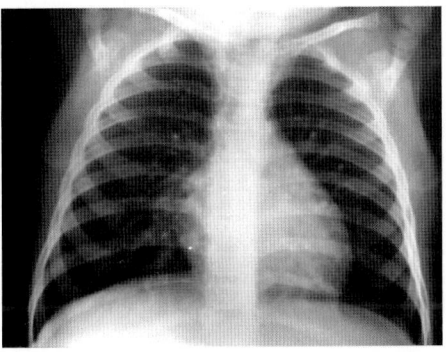
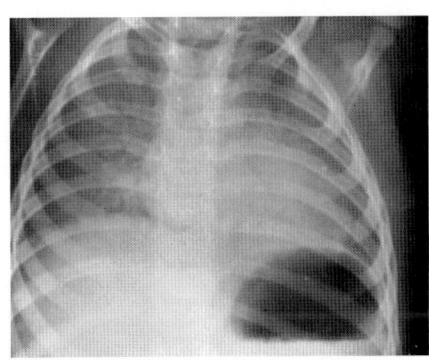

(a)

(b)

Fig. 44.1 Same-day films of the same patient with normal chest: (a) is in inspiration and (b) is in expiration.

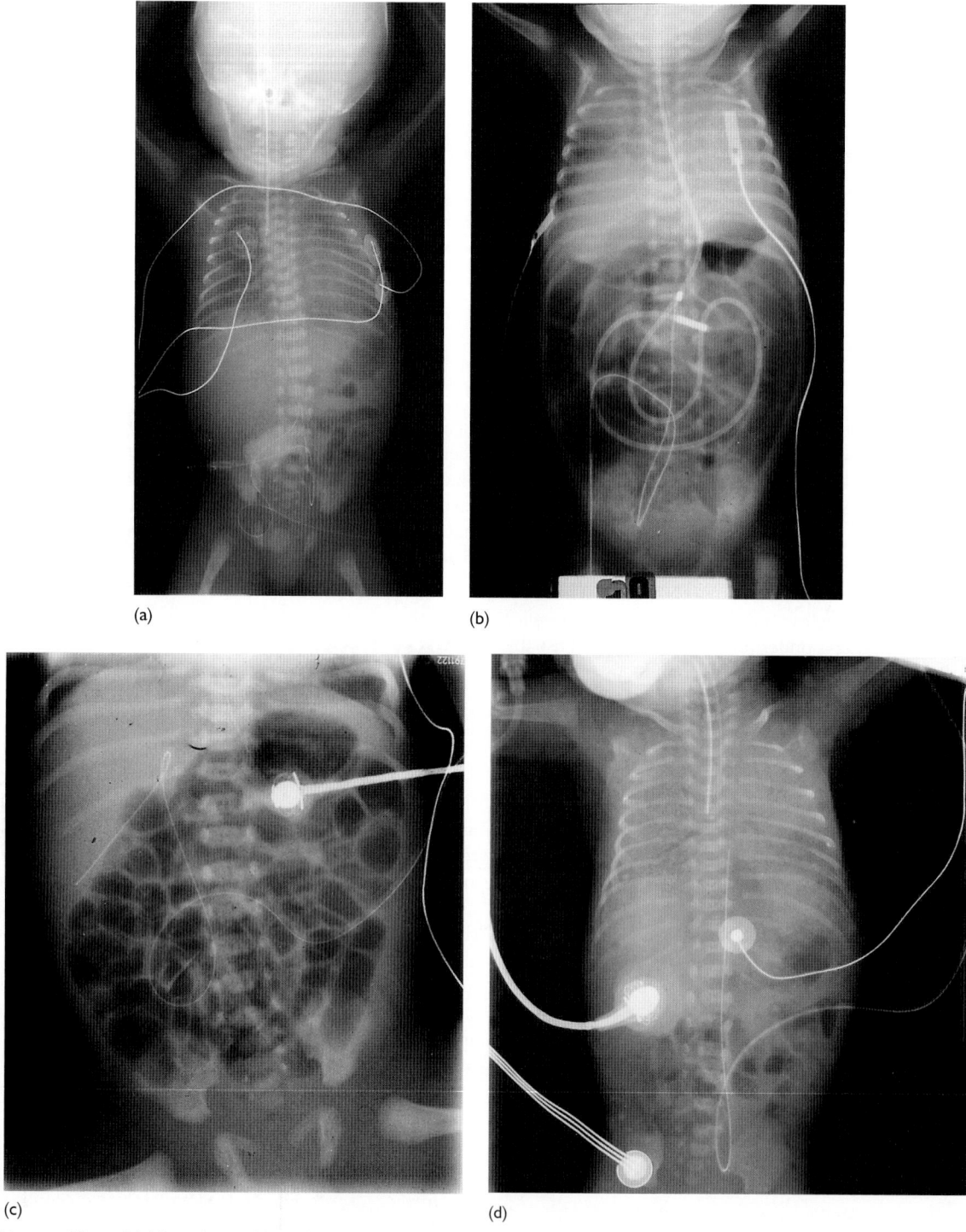

(a)　(b)

(c)　(d)

Fig. 44.2 Tubes and lines. (a) Note the position of the tips of the umbilical venous and arterial lines and endotracheal (ET) tube. The tip of the ET tube is too low. The ECG leads are badly placed over the lung fields. (b) The umbilical arterial catheter tip is at the level of T12. This is too near the origins of the mesenteric and renal arteries for safety. The tip of the feeding tube is well placed in the jejunum. (c) The tip of the umbilical venous catheter lies in the liver in the portal vein and should be moved. (d) Severe respiratory distress syndrome with an air bronchogram. The tip of the ET tube is too low but the tip of the umbilical arterial catheter is satisfactory.

There is considerable variability in the normal appearances of the mediastinum. In the neonate this consists largely of the heart and a prominent thymic shadow. The thymus can fill the whole of the upper mediastinum or be prominent on the right or the left. In case of difficulty and when considering a mediastinal mass, ultrasound can be very helpful. A normal thymus has an even texture similar to the liver, whereas an abnormal mass will almost certainly have a mixed echogenic pattern.

Tubes and lines

Whilst most chest radiographs are taken to assess lung or intrapleural pathology or cardiac shape and size, a significant number are taken either solely for or additionally to demonstrate the positions of various lines and tubes inserted in the treatment of the baby. It is most important that all those managing such neonates are aware of the appearances of these.

The most frequently used is the endotracheal tube, which usually has an opaque line in the side of it, making it clearly visible on a plain X-ray. The tip of the tube should lie between the level of the seventh cervical vertebra (C7) (just below the larynx) and the level of the carina, which is usually around about the level of the fourth thoracic vertebra (T4). Umbilical arterial lines (pp. 1240–6) are often used and can be identified by their opaque marker line. Position is confirmed by the course of the catheter which descends into the pelvis to enter the internal iliac artery on either side and then via the common iliac artery into the aorta. The tip of the line should lie between T4 and T10 when ideally positioned. Umbilical venous catheters are more difficult to position (pp. 1246–7). They enter through the umbilical vein and pass through the liver, entering the portal venous system, before passing through the ductus venosus to lie with their tip in the inferior vena cava. The ideal position is between the ductus venosus and the right atrium, a very small distance, which makes accurate positioning extremely difficult. Again, these lines have an opaque wall which makes their identification fairly simple (Fig. 44.2).

Small peripheral venous catheters are frequently used for venous access and these may be inserted in any of the four limbs or sometimes via a scalp vein (pp. 1252–5). The tip of such catheters should be in a large central vein but outside the heart. The tip of one of these catheters should not lie more centrally than the inferior limit of the superior vena cava or the superior limit of the inferior vena cava. There is some evidence that intracardiac placement of these catheters is associated with cardiac tamponade and death,[4] and these catheters should only be positioned within the heart when no other position is feasible.[3] These catheters are very fine and usually do not have an opaque line in them. Their position must be confirmed by radiography after insertion, either by radiographing with the introducer, which is often radiopaque, still in situ or by injecting 0.5 ml of intravenous contrast medium (such as Omnipaque or Niopam) to confirm the position of the tip of the catheter (Fig. 44.3). The question of how often the catheter position should be checked after insertion is a difficult one, about which there is no consensus, but all clinicians must be aware that catheter migration both distally and proximally can occur. The tip of the catheter can be extremely difficult to identify without contrast medium, particularly over the chest or abdomen, when overlying mediastinal structures or bowel can be extremely confusing. The positions of lines within the abdomen can also be determined by ultrasound, and whilst this is potentially an attractive option, it has not found favour, owing to difficulties with overlying bowel gas.

Common difficulties with X-ray interpretation

Pneumothorax

The majority of pneumothoraces are easily diagnosed on plain radiography as an area within the chest containing no lung markings

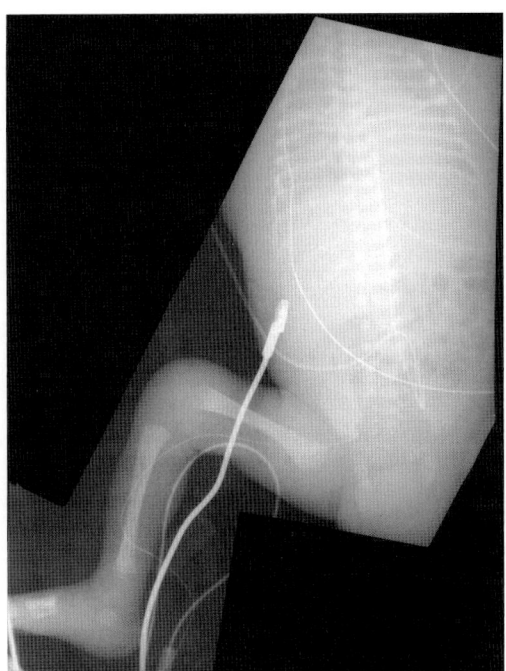

Fig. 44.3 Anteroposterior radiograph of the right lower limb and abdomen, a fine peripheral venous catheter enters the right leg. It is seen traversing the pelvis and its tip lies low in the inferior vena cava. Note how difficult it is to identify these catheters even with contrast medium within them.

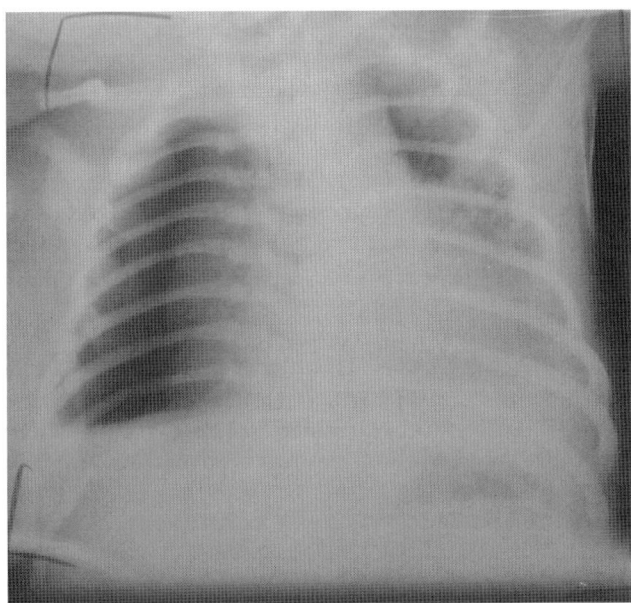

Fig. 44.4 Anteroposterior radiograph of the chest showing absence of lung markings peripherally in the right hemithorax due to a large right pneumothorax.

and with the edge of the lung clearly seen separating this from the lungs (Fig. 44.4). However, in neonates, frequently a small pneumothorax lies anteriorly and cannot be identified by these signs. There is usually a hyper-transradiancy of the chest on the affected side, which can only easily be identified with a high-quality film that is not rotated.[10] The appearance of the heart border or

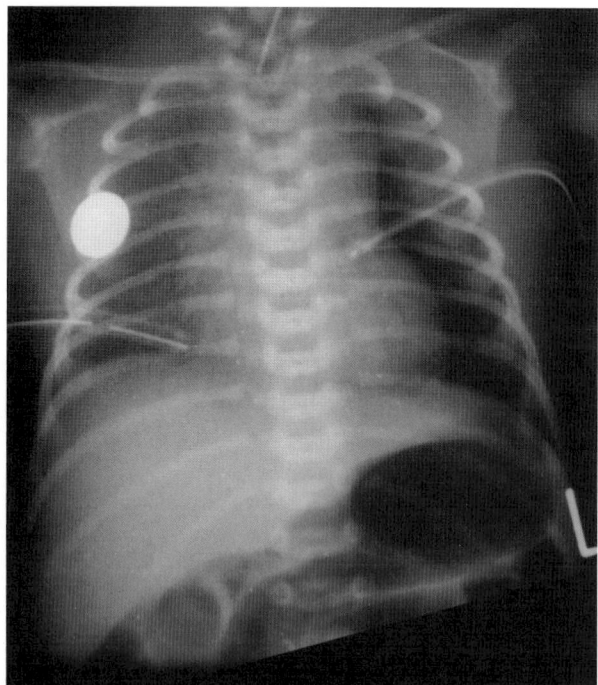

Fig. 44.5 Anteroposterior chest radiograph with bilateral chest drains. Notice how much clearer the left heart border is than the right, the so-called 'etched heart border' sign.

mediastinum appears clearer than in the usual situation where lung abuts the mediastinum, giving the so-called 'etched heart border' sign. It requires some experience to recognise this, but the importance of diagnosing a small pneumothorax in a sick neonate cannot be overstated (Fig. 44.5). Air adjacent to the mediastinum, a pneumomediastinum, also gives the 'etched heart border' sign and it can be extremely difficult to differentiate between a pneumomediastinum and a small anterior pneumothorax (Fig. 44.6). Pneumopericardium is usually easily recognised as an air shadow giving the same sign but confined to the cardiac contour.

Fluid or consolidation?

Opacity of the chest when uniform can be very difficult to evaluate. If there is an air bronchogram appearance (that is with air in the bronchi and consolidation in the lung) the abnormality must lie within the lung and be a form of consolidation, either hyaline membrane disease pneumonic consolidation or pulmonary oedema. If the shadowing has no particular characteristics, then it can either be fluid within the lung, such as pulmonary oedema infection haemorrhage, or fluid in the pleural space. It is not possible to differentiate on a plain film between a simple pleural effusion, a chylothorax or a haemothorax. Sometimes a pleural effusion can be differentiated from consolidation by seeing the lung edge separated from the chest wall either towards the apices or in the lower zone, but occasionally ultrasound is required to differentiate between these two conditions (Figs 44.7 & 44.8).

Rib fractures

These are uncommon but still seen in babies with extreme prematurity and marked osteopenia. They tend to be seen when the baby is recovering from the worst of his illness, as it is at this

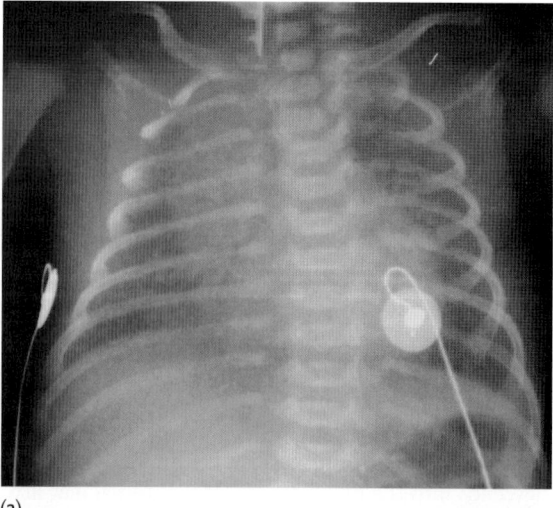

(a)

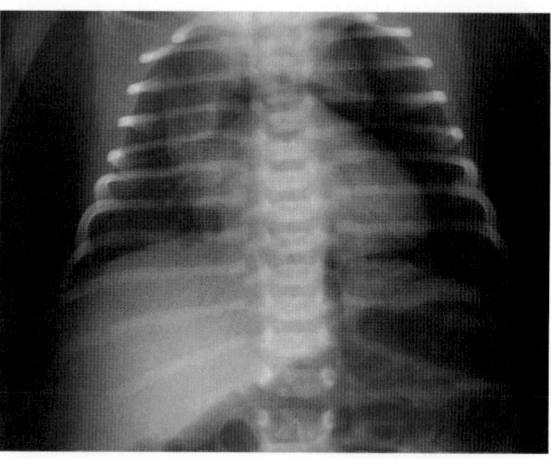

(b)

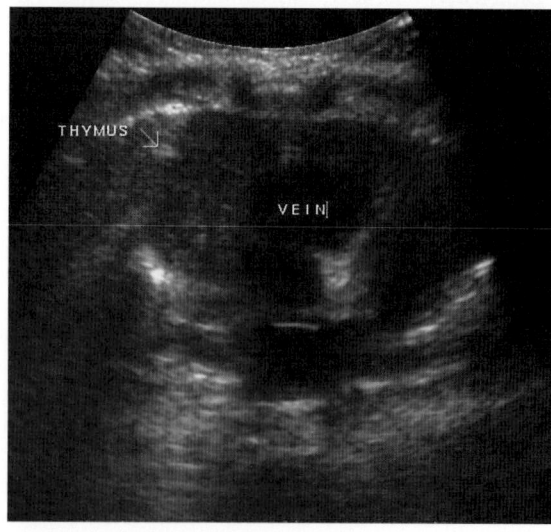

(c)

Fig. 44.6 (a) The whole of the mediastinum is widened almost down to the diaphragm by right-sided thymus. (b) A pneumomediastinum with air around the anterior-lying thymus. Note 'wave' sign of thymus where anterior end of right 4th rib presses on it. (c) Ultrasound of the thymus shows it to be homogeneous and lying in front of the great vessels in the upper mediastinum.

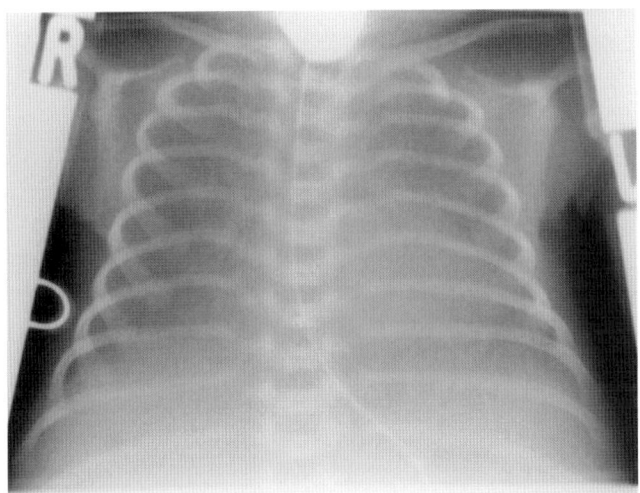

Fig. 44.7 Anteroposterior chest radiograph showing general hazy shadowing throughout the chest. Note the heart shadow is not clearly defined. This is widespread pulmonary oedema.

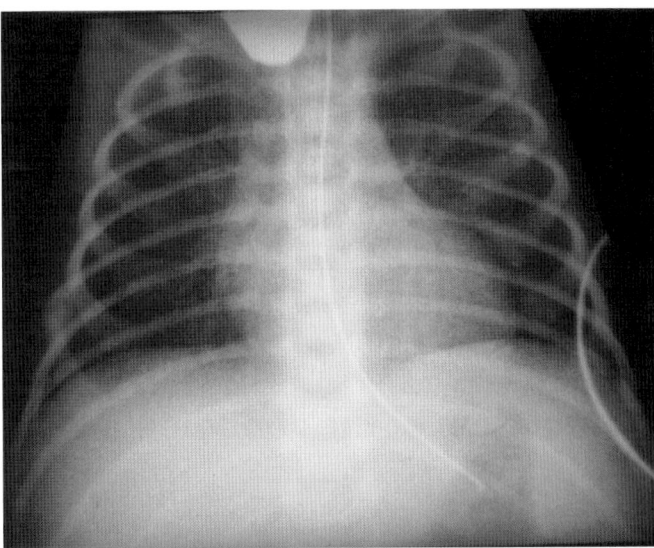

Fig. 44.9 Note the change in contour of the right 6th rib laterally due to a healing rib fracture.

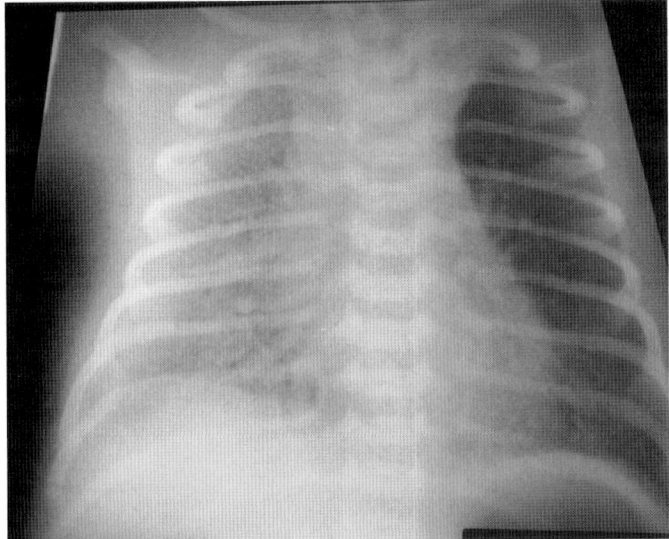

Fig. 44.8 As well as the bilateral pulmonary consolidation, note the separation of the right lung edge from the rib margin in the right upper zone due to a small right pleural effusion.

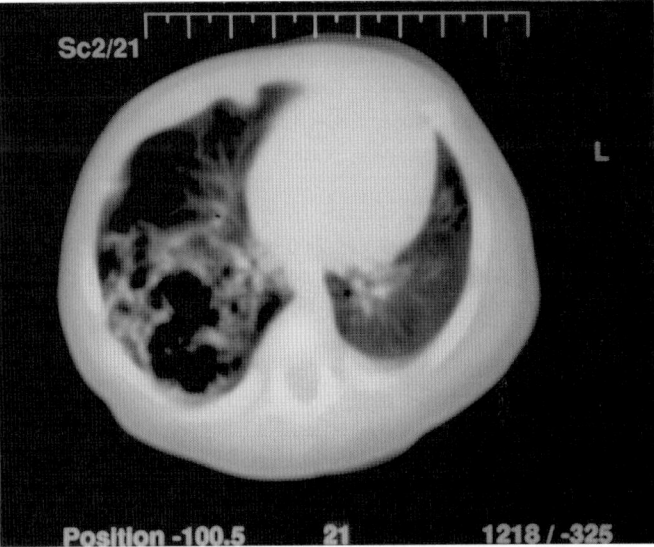

Fig. 44.10 Axial CT section of chest in lung window showing a right lower lobe lesion consisting of air-filled cysts and some solid tissue. This lesion was proven histologically to be a congenital cystic adenomatoid malformation.

stage that ossification occurs and can be identified as callus along the ribs. Recognition of these fractures and their likely aetiology is important so that other causes of rib fractures such as non-accidental injury can be excluded (Fig. 44.9).

Computed tomography of the chest

CT of the chest in the neonate is not often required. As it needs the baby to be moved from the NICU to the CT scanner, it is only appropriate for very specific problems. These are usually related either to mediastinal masses, differentiating the thymus from a pathological mass, or for evaluating a congenital lung mass. Many congenital lung lesions are now suspected antenatally and confirmation of the diagnosis (or resolution) is required in the neonatal period. In the acute situation, some of these lesions, such as congenital cystic adenomatoid malformations (pp. 584–5) or congenital lobar emphysema (pp. 589–90), may require urgent surgery, in which case cross-sectional imaging with CT may not be possible. In the majority of cases, respiratory symptoms are relatively minor and CT can be obtained. With modern helical CT or multislice CT, these examinations take only a few seconds to obtain high-quality images of the mediastinum, and on separate window settings, detail of the lungs can be obtained. Contrast injection is not usually necessary, although if there is concern about the vascular supply of a lung segment, contrast injections can be undertaken and appropriate images obtained. With multislice CT, multiplanar reconstructions are possible from a single cross-sectional series of images, although again, these are not often required (Fig. 44.10).

Magnetic resonance imaging of the chest

As with CT, these examinations are very limited. MRI of the lungs is not currently the modality of choice, but MRI of the mediastinum, and particularly of the heart and vascular structures, is often very helpful in assessing the cardiovascular anatomy. Echocardiography, however, should always be the first examination of the cardiovascular system, supplemented by MRI where there are particular issues that require further evaluation, such as vascular rings.

Examination of the abdomen

Plain radiography

Abdominal radiographs are often required for abdominal symptoms such as distension, bile-stained vomiting or palpable abdominal masses. Usually only a supine abdominal radiograph is required. On the plain radiograph there are only three common X-ray densities: soft tissue/fluid, gas and calcification.

Calcification is relatively rare and suggests a meconium perforation if it is within the peritoneum (Fig. 44.11). Intraluminal colonic calcifications suggest bowel/urinary tract communication.

Within the renal tract, calcification is much less common but suggests nephrocalcinosis.

Commonly in the sick neonate there may be very little gas in the bowel. Accurate diagnosis is then impossible on a plain X-ray. The more gas that is present, the easier it is to make a diagnosis.

The commonly asked questions are:

■ *What sort of bowel is it?*
  The stomach is usually easily recognised by its shape and position. In the neonate, gas-filled bowel has very much the same appearance whether it is small or large bowel. The large bowel usually appears round the periphery of the abdomen but it is often otherwise very difficult to tell large from small bowel. The rectum can usually be identified by its position (Fig. 44.12).
■ *Is there any free air?*
  Significant volumes of free air can usually be identified on a supine radiograph but this requires a certain amount of experience. The signs to look for are:
  – diffuse radiolucency over the upper abdomen, particularly towards the liver;
  – visibility of both sides of the bowel wall (Fig. 44.13).
  In the normal situation, the air in the lumen of the bowel shows one side of the bowel wall, the other side not being visible. When there is free air in the peritoneum, both sides of the bowel wall can be seen. The danger of this sign is that if there are multiple distended loops of bowel adjacent to one another, it is difficult sometimes to tell between free air outlining the outer wall of one loop of bowel and gas in two adjacent loops of bowel walls abutting one another giving a similar appearance. A decubitus or erect film will sometimes be necessary to confirm the presence of free air which will then move towards the non-dependent surface. In the presence of multiple

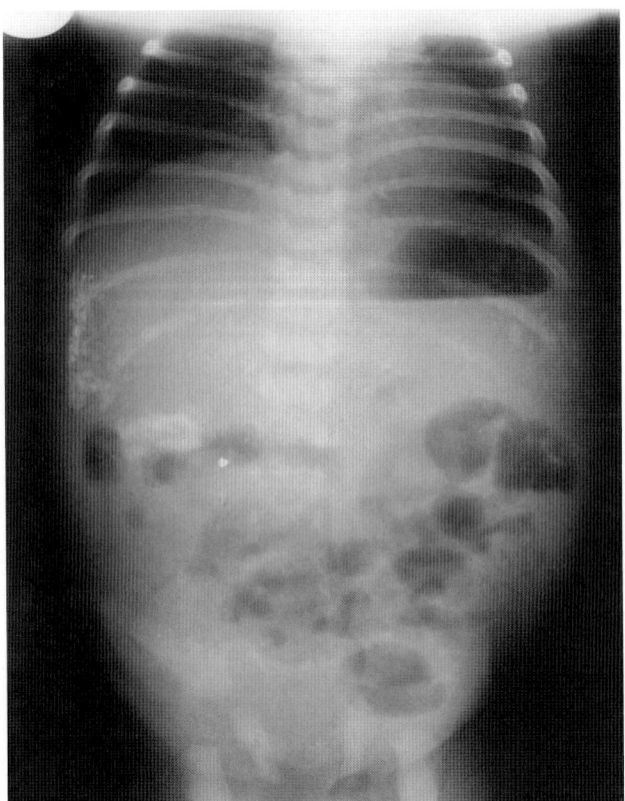

Fig. 44.11 Abdominal radiograph showing extensive plaques of calcification throughout the abdomen. Note how these are mainly peripherally situated consistent with peritoneal calcification. This is usually the end stage of meconium peritonitis secondary to a perforation in utero.

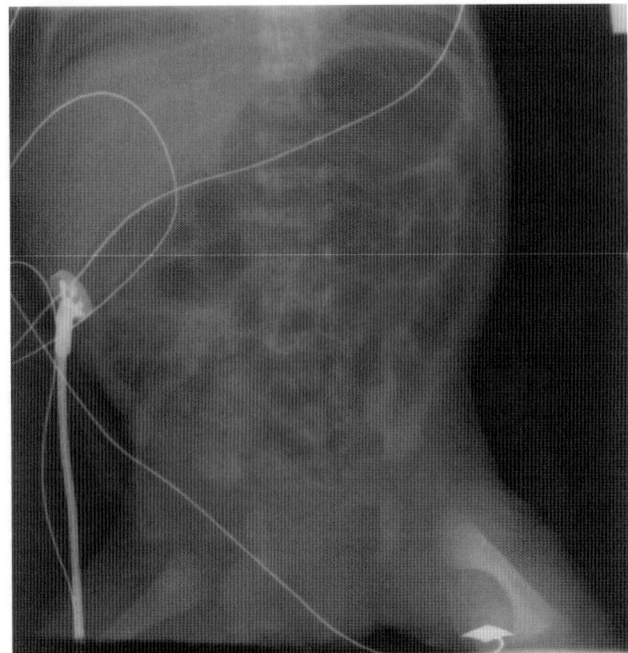

Fig. 44.12 Gas seen throughout the small and large bowel. The large bowel is peripherally situated and the small bowel more centrally so. This appearance is normal.

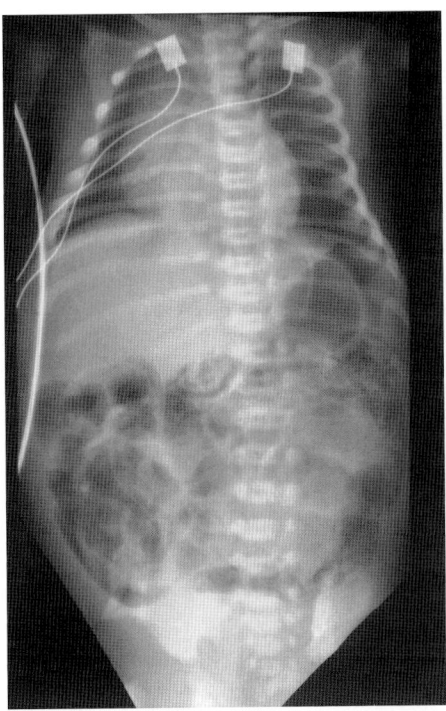

Fig. 44.13 Abdominal radiograph with a pneumoperitoneum. Note the diffuse haziness over the left lobe of the liver and in particular outlining the falciform ligament. In the right hypochondrium note both sides of the bowel wall can be identified, further confirming the presence of a pneumoperitoneum.

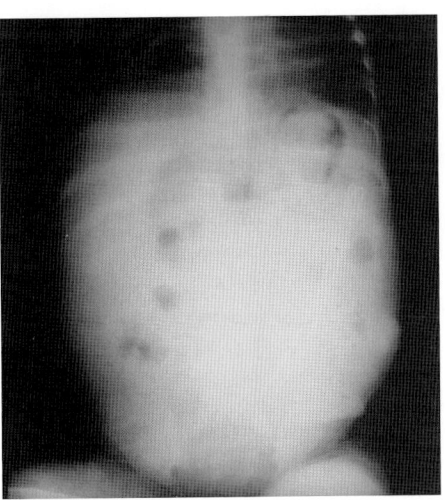

Fig. 44.14 Abdominal radiograph showing loops of bowel mainly centrally situated. The loops of air-filled bowel are floating towards the central abdomen within the ascitic fluid.

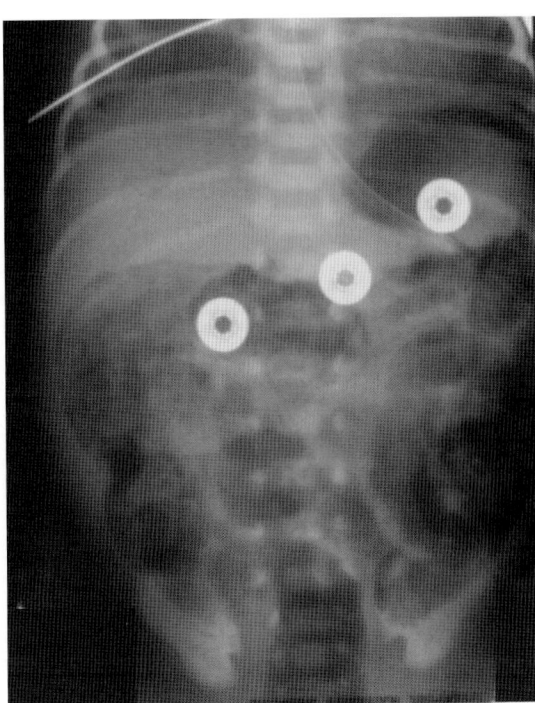

Fig. 44.15 Gas in the small and large bowel with intramural gas in the right side of the abdomen in particular. The baby had necrotising enterocolitis.

dilated loops of bowel, it can sometimes be quite difficult to differentiate free air from dilated loops.[7,9] There is no value whatsoever in a decubitus film looking for free air if there is no visible air on a supine film.

■ *Is there any free fluid?*
The presence of free fluid is suggested if air-filled loops of bowel remain centrally in the abdomen. The sick neonate, however, often has little bowel gas, and free fluid is therefore difficult to determine by plain radiography (Fig. 44.14). If the abdomen is distended but there is very little bowel gas, the hypothesis that free fluid is present can be confirmed using ultrasound.

■ *Is there any evidence of necrotising enterocolitis?*
This often is a very difficult question in the small premature neonate. The classical appearance of necrotising enterocolitis (NEC), with gas in the bowel wall appearing as linear streaks

or 'bubbles', is not often seen in the premature neonate (Fig. 44.15).[1] The condition is suggested on plain radiographs by some dilated loops of bowel (paralytic ileus). If these appear fixed from one radiograph to another, this is very suggestive of NEC (Fig. 44.16). Sometimes the bowel loops have an unusual contour to them, suggesting oedema, which can be a sign of NEC. This diagnosis is, however, usually a clinical one and radiology is of limited value, often only confirming the diagnosis on those uncommon occasions when there is a pneumoperitoneum due to perforation.

■ *Is it obstruction or ileus?*
This is often a difficult decision to make on a single film. If there is uniform dilatation of the bowel, it is more likely to be paralytic ileus. If there is more dilatation of distal than of proximal, then obstruction is more likely. If, over a period of time, the dilatation becomes progressive, then obstruction is more likely.

Uses of contrast studies

Bowel contrast studies have a relatively limited value in the neonate.

Oral contrast studies

The contrast medium used usually is one of the contrast media employed in adults and older children for intravenous use. These water-soluble contrast media are not absorbed from the bowel and have the advantage that radiographs over a period sometimes of several days can be obtained using the same contrast bolus.

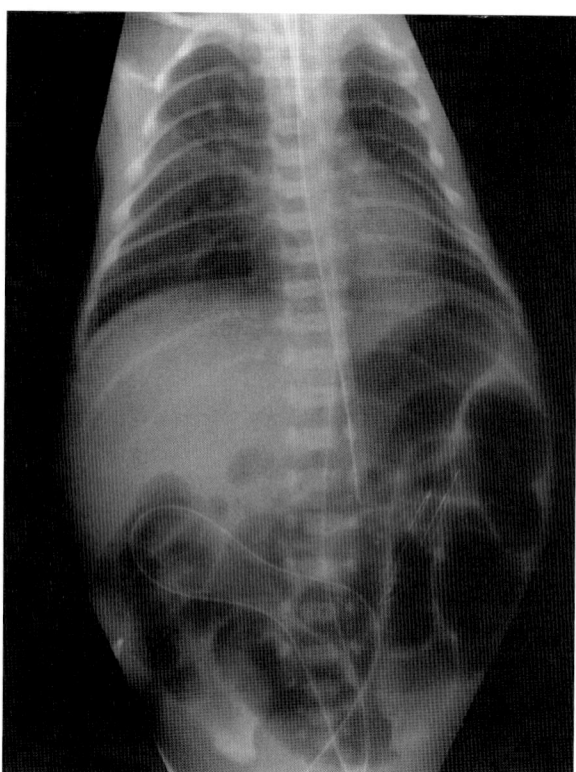

Fig. 44.16 Dilated loops of small and large bowel due to paralytic ileus. These loops did not change configuration over a period of several days. The clinical diagnosis was necrotising enterocolitis.

It is, however, still quite appropriate for upper GI studies to use barium, providing distal obstruction is not suspected.

Commonly asked questions are:

■ *Is there gastro-oesophageal reflux?*
Either barium or water-soluble contrast can be used for this. The baby is usually given this medium in a bottle to suck and swallow, with observation by fluoroscopy of the swallowing mechanism, and oesophageal and stomach anatomy. It is usual to assess for gastric emptying and obtain pictures of the duodenum. Gastro-oesophageal reflux can usually be demonstrated when the baby stops swallowing and either cries or is tilted gently with his head down, but often occurs spontaneously. It is important to exclude the presence of hiatus hernia at this stage also.

■ *Is there upper gastrointestinal obstruction?*
In this circumstance, it is usual to use water-soluble contrast media. This should be preceded by a plain X-ray of the abdomen, which is quite accurate at assessing the level of suspected obstruction. The examination should usually be undertaken using fluoroscopy so that the dynamic aspects of the examination can be followed as far as the duodenum. The stomach is examined and gastric emptying into the duodenum noted. It is important to obtain an anteroposterior view of the duodeno-jejunal flexure, which should be to the left of the midline and at the level of the pylorus, to exclude malrotation (Fig. 44.17). Follow-through films to look at the remainder of the GI tract can be taken on the intensive care unit at intervals. It is often helpful to obtain films at half an

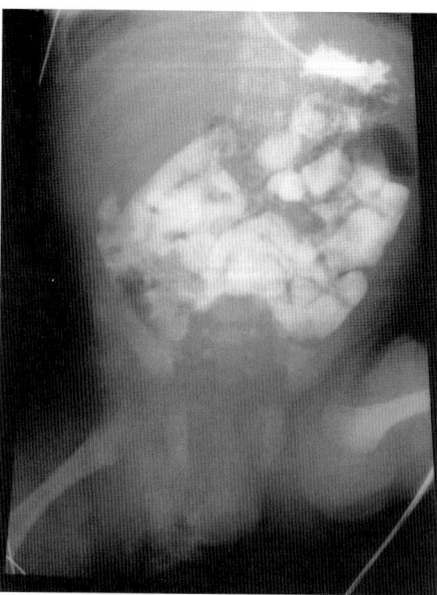

Fig. 44.17
Anteroposterior view of the abdomen in a neonate 30 minutes after the administration of 6 ml of Omnipaque. Note most of the contrast has left the stomach and is in the small bowel. The duodenojejunal (DJ) flexure was identified at an earlier stage to the left of the midline above the level of the pylorus. The remainder of the proximal small bowel appears normal.

hour, 1 hour, 2 hours and 4 hours, following the contrast through the bowel. It is often necessary then to take more delayed films at 8 and 24 hours until the obstruction has been identified or the rectum has been reached.

Lower gastrointestinal studies

These are almost always undertaken for suspected large-bowel obstruction, and need to be performed under fluoroscopic guidance. A small catheter (about 8F) can be inserted into the rectum and contrast instilled using a syringe until the large bowel has been demonstrated with reflux into the terminal ileum. The level of obstruction can usually easily be identified and appropriate films obtained (Fig. 44.18). This technique can also be used to instil dilute Gastrografin as a means of treating meconium ileus.

Loopogram

This is a special examination used to determine the patency of the distal loop of bowel following previous defunctioning bowel surgery. Contrast is introduced into the distal stoma, again using a small 8F catheter, and instilled using a syringe until the entire bowel has been identified and strictures excluded.

Micturating cystourethrography

Micturating cystourethrography is used for the following clinical indications:

■ hydronephrosis – antenatally or postnatally diagnosed;
■ large bladder on palpation or ultrasound;
■ urinary tract infection.

Catheterisation using a small (5F or 6F) feeding tube can usually be simply achieved. Use of water-soluble contrast, such as Urografin 150, is usually appropriate, with spontaneous micturition taking place when the bladder is full. It is recommended to obtain film of the male urethra in all cases, only removing the catheter during micturition when films of the full urethra with

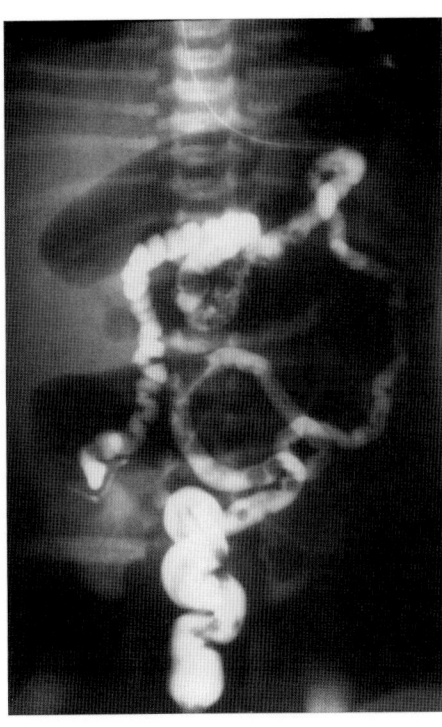

Fig. 44.18 Water-soluble contrast enema using Omnipaque is seen outlining the entire colon from rectum to caecum and appendix. This baby has meconium ileus and a micro colon.

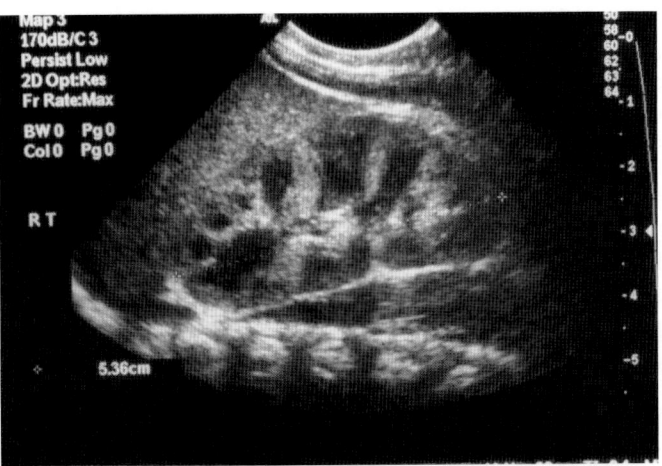

Fig. 44.19 Longitudinal ultrasound scan of the right kidney. Note the renal cortex is of similar echogenicity to the liver. This is normal in the neonate but the cortex would usually be of lower echogenicity in the older child and adult. Note the particularly obvious corticomedullary differentiation, again a normal feature.

catheter in situ have been obtained. Spot films to demonstrate vesicoureteric reflux when it occurs are necessary.

Ultrasound

Whilst ultrasound is easy to undertake within an incubator in even the sickest baby, the investigation should be focused on a specific clinical problem wherever possible, rather than reviewing the entire abdomen. This is because handling of these babies should be kept to the minimum.

Liver and spleen

Many neonates, particularly after long-term total parenteral nutrition (TPN), develop enlargement of the liver and spleen. Ultrasound is not good at measuring either liver or splenic volume, as these are organs with an irregular shape. There are accepted measurements for spleen length but these are of very limited value. More commonly ultrasound of the liver is undertaken when the bilirubin is elevated, in order to exclude an obstructive cause for hyperbilirubinaemia (p. 1237). In most cases the liver texture appears normal and the bile ducts are not dilated. The gall bladder can usually be identified with certainty and in TPN jaundice is often thick walled and smaller than average but should be considered normal if more than 15 mm long. The rare occurrence of a choledochal cyst can also be excluded confidently by ultrasound. Ultrasound, as well as demonstrating a normal gallbladder, can be used to assess the porta hepatis, and absence of the 'triangular cord sign' makes biliary atresia very unlikely.[6] The combination with ^{99m}Tc-labelled trimethyl bromo HIDA scanning further refines the differential diagnosis between neonatal hepatitis and biliary atresia, although biopsy is the ultimate arbiter. It is important to exclude the diagnosis of biliary atresia before 6 weeks of life.

Urinary tract

Ultrasound scanning of the urinary tract is often required for the following indications:

- anuria/oliguria;
- haematuria;
- antenatally diagnosed renal pelvic dilatation or hydronephrosis;
- urinary tract infection;
- associated congenital abnormalities, especially VATER association, exomphalos;
- palpable renal mass;
- distended bladder.

The renal cortex is often brighter in the neonate than in the older child and this exaggerates the normal corticomedullary differentiation (Fig. 44.19). Hyperechogenicity of the renal pyramids can be a transient phenomenon in the neonate and should not be presumed to be pathological in the first few days of life. As a rule of thumb, the renal length is approximately 1 mm per week of gestational age. Such a measurement at all gestations lies between the 5th and 95th centile.

Pylorus

Ultrasound is the definitive means of diagnosing pyloric stenosis. The hypertrophied pyloric muscle is clearly demonstrated in the right hypochondrium. A canal length of more than 15 mm and muscle thickness of more than 3 mm is diagnostic of pyloric stenosis in a term neonate. In the preterm infant, allowance has to be made for the smaller size, and repeat scanning is sometimes necessary a day or so after initial presentation, to confirm the diagnosis.

Peritoneal cavity

Ultrasound to evaluate palpable abdominal mass is a useful adjunct to clinical examination. Differentiating an abscess (most often related to NEC) from matted bowel loops can be difficult, but is worth trying. Assessing volumes of free fluid within the abdomen is not easy, but the confirmation of free fluid as a cause of abdominal distension may be helpful.

Nuclear medicine

Nuclear medicine has a very small part to play in neonatology.

Biliary scanning

99mTc-labelled trimethyl bromo HIDA is currently the most valuable biliary pharmaceutical. The neonate should be prepared by giving phenobarbital (phenobarbitone) at a dose rate of 5 mg/kg/day for 3 days before the scan is undertaken. This maximises biliary excretion of the pharmaceutical. The radiolabelled pharmaceutical is given by intravenous injection and scans obtained from 5 minutes onwards. A film after a feed is usually obtained about 1 hour post injection. Delayed films the following day are often necessary to confirm isotope in the bowel, which makes the diagnosis of biliary atresia unlikely.

Renal scanning

Renal scanning is not often required in the neonatal period. Owing to evolving renal function, renography using mercaptoacetyl-triglycine (MAG 3) or diethylenetriamine penta-acetic acid (DTPA) labelled with 99mTc is not usually reliable; indeed, values obtained by computer from renography need to be interpreted with extreme caution in the neonate. Renal cortical imaging with dimercaptosuccinic acid (DMSA) is also more effective after 2 months of age and rarely influences management in the early stage.

Head imaging

Ultrasound

Neonatal cranial ultrasound has developed dramatically in the last 20 years. A standard examination is undertaken with a small footprint probe of 5 or 7.5 MHz, the higher frequency being preferable, but in the term neonate, sometimes the penetration obtainable with 7.5 MHz is not adequate. The anterior fontanelle

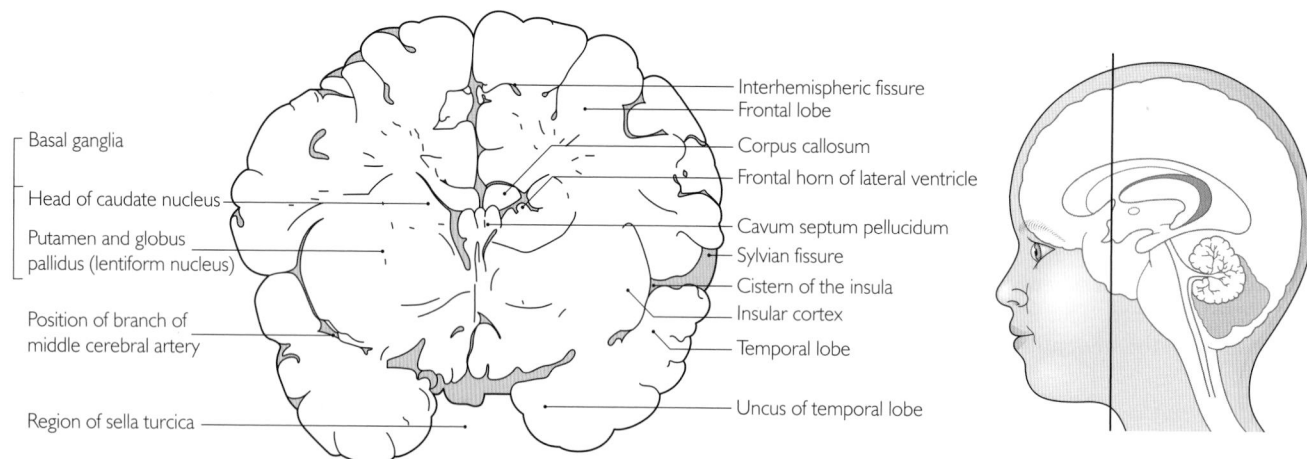

(a)

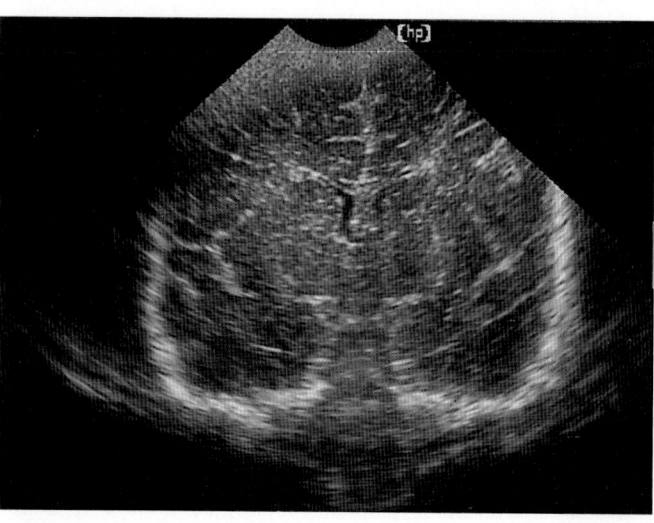

(b)

Fig. 44.20 (a) Labelled diagram of standard coronal section of the neonatal head imaged with ultrasound, with the corresponding scan picture in (b). (Reproduced from Rennie.[8])

is used almost exclusively as the portal of entry of ultrasound, giving enhanced resolution compared with scanning through the skull vault, where most of the ultrasound is absorbed. The standard views are coronal (Fig. 44.20) and it must be remembered that most views are coronal oblique, angled from the anterior fontanelle anteriorly or posteriorly and not true coronal. The midline sagittal scan (Fig. 44.21) can also be obtained, with oblique parasagittal views completing the examination. Whilst the concept of standard views is often used for the purpose of documentation, the examination is a dynamic one, with the probe sweeping from anterior to posterior and from side to side to obtain as full a view of the head as possible. Obviously the areas under the parietal convexities are not as well demonstrated as other areas using this approach and it must be appreciated that small subdural collections in this site will not be excluded by ultrasound.

Computed tomography

With modern helical and multislice CT scanners, the quality of resolution of the neonatal brain is exceptional. Obviously the examination has the disadvantage of the requirement to move the baby from his more controlled environment to the CT scanner and this is therefore somewhat restricted. The length of time of the examination has been reduced to a few seconds so that movement is considerably reduced and sedation is not usually needed. It is usual just to obtain axial sections of the brain as these give most of the relevant information with the lowest radiation dose. CT is the only diagnostic modality that confidently diagnoses calcification. However, changes relating to bleeding and particularly extra-axial bleeds are best assessed by CT, much better than ultrasound and at least equal to MRI.

Magnetic resonance imaging

The length of time taken for MR examinations and poor availability of scanning time restrict the use of MRI to a very small number of neonates. The lack of radiation, multiplanar capabilities and exquisite demonstration of differences in tissue density make this the gold standard for brain imaging. As well as being

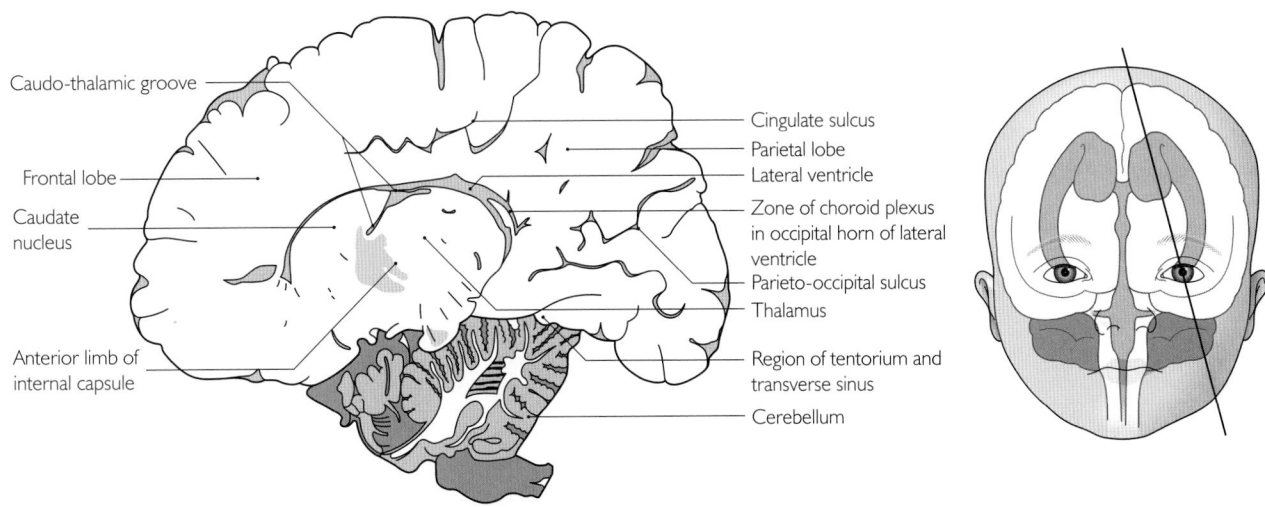

(a)

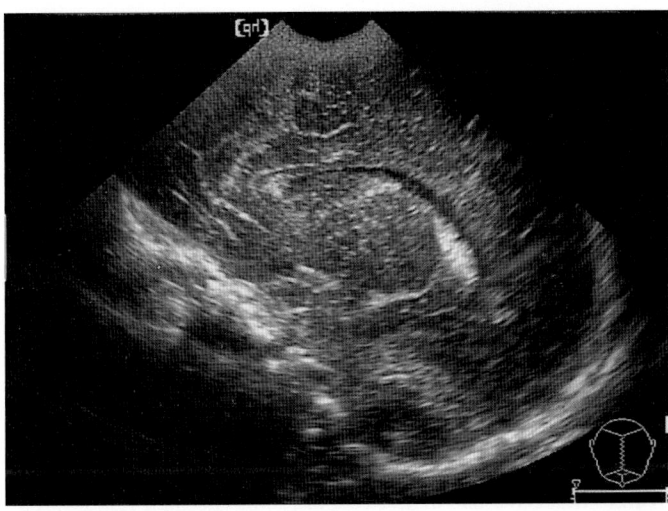

(b)

Fig. 44.21 Parasagittal section of the neonatal brain imaged with ultrasound. (a) Labelled diagram with the picture taken in the same plane in (b) (Reproduced from Rennie.[8])

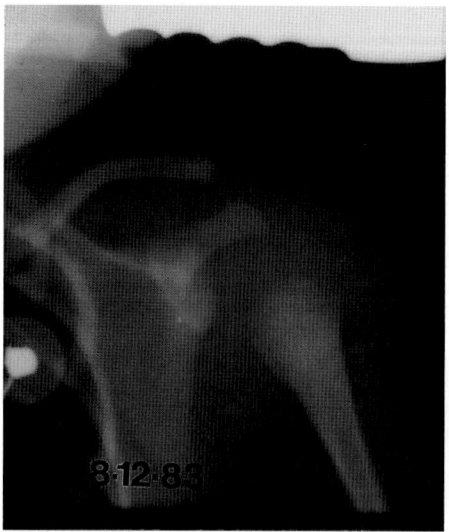

(a)

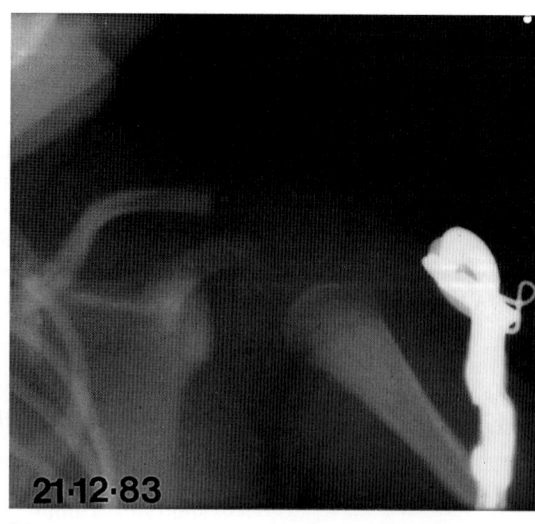

(b)

Fig. 44.22 Metabolic bone disease in a premature baby postoperatively following a congenital diaphragmatic hernia repair. (a) Normal proximal humerus; (b) 13 days later lucency in the humeral metaphysis indicates metabolic bone disease secondary to low calcium stores.

very efficient at assessing haemorrhage, hypoxia/ischaemia and maturation of the neonatal brain can be most accurately assessed using MRI and this will continue to evolve with more sophisticated software. The fact that the neonatal brain has a high water content means that specific sequences have been devised to maximise the information from MRI scans, especially using long T2 relaxation times.

Imaging the skeleton

Skeletal radiology

Most of the indications for skeletal radiographs in neonates are related to birth trauma. Although all fractures are uncommon in neonates, indications for skeletal radiography in the neonate are:

- birth trauma;
- clinical deformity;
- suspected skeletal dysplasia;
- suspected osteomyelitis;
- suspected metabolic bone disease of prematurity;
- other congenital abnormalities, e.g. VATER association.

Metabolic bone disease of prematurity has become less frequent in recent years (pp. 922–8) but isolated rib fractures are still quite often seen in babies surviving months of neonatal intensive care (Fig. 44.22). It is important that they are recognised for what they are and that the mechanism is also recognised. Osteomyelitis is an infrequent complication of neonatal intensive care (p. 987). It is often clinically asymptomatic and may only be recognised when the plain X-ray findings are fairly advanced. Isotope bone scans using ^{99m}Tc methylene diphosphonate (MDP) may be positive but a normal or negative isotope bone scan does not exclude the diagnosis. The late changes will

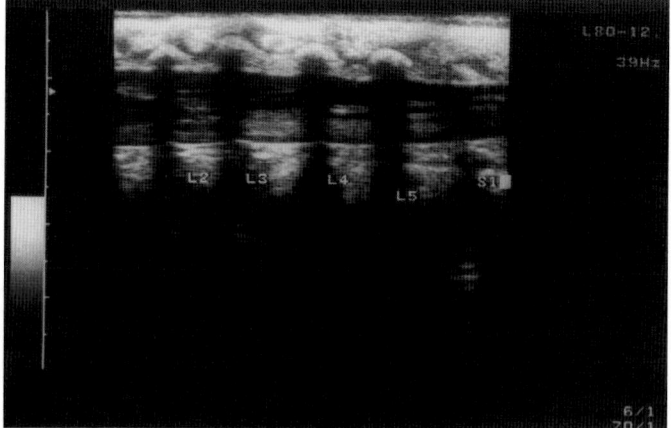

Fig. 44.23 Longitudinal section of the spinal canal showing the cord finishing at the L2 level. The nerve roots are seen lying against the anterior wall of the spinal canal. These are normal appearances.

be seen on plain X-ray, usually undertaken for unexplained limb swelling.

Hip ultrasound

Following upon the work of Graf[5] and others, the technique of ultrasound of the neonatal hip has been developed. The aim is to detect developmental dysplasia of the hip and to guide management (pp. 967–71). Normal measurements of the angles of the acetabulum, both bony and the cartilagenous labrum, are well documented. The technique requires considerable attention to detail. Applying ultrasound as a screening test to a whole population has been tried in Europe and in Coventry, UK, with some success. Selective use of the technique in the high-risk population is the usual current UK strategy (p. 968).

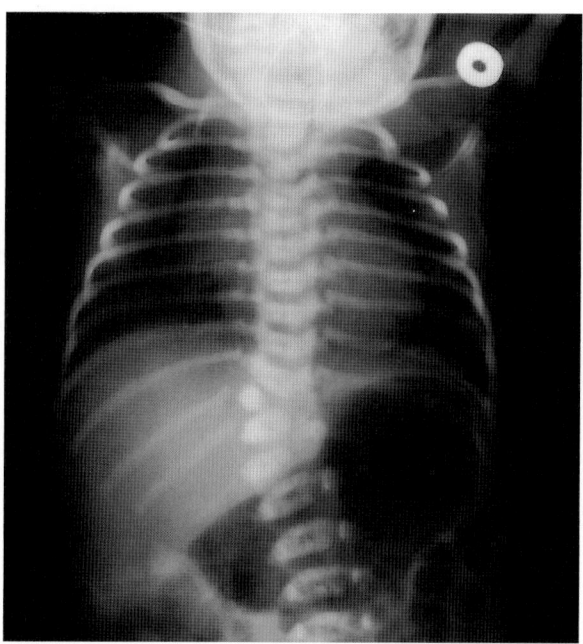

Fig. 44.24 VATER anomaly. Note thoracic and lumbar vertebral anomalies. Gas-filled stomach due to associated tracheo-oesophageal fistula.

Spinal imaging

In the neonate, ultrasound of the spine is a very effective way of demonstrating the cord and spinal canal contents. It is efficient because the vertebral arches are not ossified at this age and good access of ultrasound to the spine is therefore possible (Fig. 44.23). This can be used to demonstrate the cord, nerve roots and spinal contents very effectively. MRI, which is considered the gold standard, often does not give pictures that are as detailed as the ultrasound ones at this age and is a second-line investigation. Plain X-rays of the spine are unhelpful except for documenting segmentation defects (Fig. 44.24).

References

1. Daneman A, Woodward S, De Silva M 1978 The radiology of neonatal necro-enterocolitis (NEC). A review of 47 cases and the literature. Pediatric Radiology 7: 70–77
2. Department of Health 2000 Ionising radiation (medical exposure) regulations 2000. London: HMSO
3. Department of Health 2001 New guidance issued to the NHS on intravenous feeding of sick new born babies. HMSO, London
4. Department of Health 2001 Review of the deaths of four babies due to cardiac tamponade associated with the presence of a central venous catheter. HMSO, London
5. Graf R, Schule P 1986 Sonography of the infant hip: an atlas. VCH Publishers
6. Kim M J, Park Y N, Han S J et al 2000 Biliary atresia in neonates and infants: triangular area of high signal intensity in the portahepatis on T2 weighted magnetic resonance cholangiography with US and histopathologic correlation. Radiology 215: 395–401
7. Miller R E 1960 Perforated viscus in infants: a new Rontgen sign. Radiology 74: 65–67
8. Rennie J M 1997 Neonatal cranial ultrasound. Cambridge University Press, Cambridge
9. Rigler L G 1941 Spontaneous pneumoperitoneum. Rontgenologic sign found in the supine position. Radiology 37: 604–607
10. Swischuk L E 1976 Two lesser known but useful signs of neonatal pneumothorax. American Journal of Rontgenology 127: 623–627

Further reading

Armpilia C I, Fife I A, Crosdale P L 2002 Radiation dose quantities and risk in neonates in a special care baby unit. British Journal of Radiology 75: 590–595

Arthur R 2001 The neonatal chest X-ray. Paediatric Respiratory Reviews 2: 311–323

Barnes N, Pilling D W 1999 Interpretation of the neonatal chest X-ray. Hospital Medicine 60: 781–787

Carty H, Shaw D, Brunelle F, Kendall B 1994 Imaging children. Churchill Livingstone, Edinburgh

Kuhn J P, Slovis T, Haller J 2000 Caffeys pediatric diagnostic imaging, 10th edition. Mosby, St Louis

Siegel M J 2002 Pediatric sonography, 3rd edition. Lippincott Williams and Wilkins, Philadelphia

Swischuk L E 1997 Imaging of the newborn, infant, and young child, 4th edition. Lippincott Williams and Wilkins, Baltimore

Section Seven

Practical Procedures

CHAPTER 45

Procedures and iatrogenic disorders

Jagjit S Ahluwalia, Jeffrey L Brain, Anthony W Kelsall

Introduction

Many conditions in the newborn have an iatrogenic component (Tables 45.1 & 45.2): these are dealt with in other sections of this book and are well reviewed by Macpherson et al.[119]

Newborn intensive care necessarily involves the undertaking of multiple procedures on extremely sick and premature babies. All procedures carry some risk of a complication, no matter how small the risk or how insignificant the complication. This chapter describes, in practical detail, both common and less frequently undertaken procedures within a newborn intensive care setting. For each procedure, indications for its use are followed by detailed descriptions of how to undertake the procedure, with typical equipment requirements listed and common variations in how to undertake the procedure discussed. Recognised complications of each procedure together with the frequency of such complications are discussed and, where relevant, the appropriate management of these complications is highlighted.

In a climate of a changing workforce, with rising numbers of junior medical staff working on shift systems, the time available to acquire experience in practical procedures is ever reducing. The importance of adequate training in undertaking procedures has never been more critical. Doctors and nurses involved in undertaking practical procedures should receive specific training and supervision in the relevant procedures until such a time that they

Table 45.1 Neonatal disorders with an iatrogenic component

Condition	Damaging agent	Page no.
Retinopathy of prematurity	Oxygen	843–7
Necrotising enterocolitis	Hypotension	694–703
	Enteral feeding, formula	
Discrete intestinal perforation	Emboli from UAC, indometacin	562
Airleaks, e.g. pneumothorax	High PIP, high MAP, inadequate humidity during IPPV	487–91
Chronic lung disease	As for airleak	554–73
	Fluid overload	
	Infection, oxygen	
GMH-IVH	Hypotension, hypoxia, hypercarbia	1123–4
PVL	Sepsis, hypotension, hypocarbia	1159–64
Lung puncture	Treatment of pneumothorax	1260
Gastric rupture	Mask/nasal IPPV	519
	Nasogastric tube erosion	
Airway damage	ETT, oscillatory and jet ventilation	606
	Poor ETT fixation	
Nasal septum injury	Secondary to nasal CPAP fixation	521
Obstructive jaundice	TPN	671
Complex metabolic upsets	TPN	330
Intestinal obstruction	High calorie density milks	311

CPAP, continuous positive airways pressure; ETT, endotracheal tube; GMH-IVH, germinal matrix/intraventricular haemorrhage; IPPV, intermittent positive pressure ventilation; MAP, mean airway pressure; PIP, peak inflating pressure; PVL, periventricular leukomalacia; TPN, total parenteral nutrition; UAC, umbilical artery catheter.

Table 45.2 Drug-induced iatrogenic complications

Drug	Complication	Page no. Reference
General	Incorrect dosage	
	Incorrect drug	
	Incorrect concentration	
Specific		
Chloramphenicol	Grey baby syndrome	
Diuretics (especially frusemide)	Nephrocalcinosis	181, 231
Sulphisoxazole	Kernicterus	192
Tetracyclines	Stained teeth	100
Vitamin K analogues (menadione)	Jaundice	116
Vitamin E (Eferol)	Liver failure, haematuria	10
Tolazoline	Hypotension, haematuria, GI tract haemorrhage	218
Indometacin	Fluid retention, GI tract haemorrhage, decreased cerebral blood flow velocity	4
Dexamethasone	GI tract haemorrhage & perforation, hypertension, sepsis, cardiomyopathy, glycosuria, adrenal suppression	177
Hexachlorophane	Vacuolative encephalopathy	191
Glycol in i.v. multivitamin preparation	Fits, GMH-IVH	118
Benzyl alcohol in i.v. saline	Acidaemia & collapse, kernicterus	88, 114
Heparin	GMH-IVH	110
Phenylephrine (mydriatic)	Hypertension	86
Transcutaneous		
Tribiotic (neomycin)	Deafness	138
Iodine-containing antiseptics		
Transient hypothyroidism		199

are deemed competent as an independent practitioner for a given procedure. Such training should include the need to assess the risks versus the benefits of a given procedure, the role of parental consent for procedures, the importance of clear and contemporaneous documentation of any procedures performed (successfully or otherwise), specific instruction on undertaking the procedure itself, the use of relevant equipment, and guidance on recognition and management of potential complications. Patient identification should also be emphasised in such training, as should the need for universal infection precautions, the importance of aseptic technique, and the need to handle any sharps safely. Imaginative use of cotside teaching, use of skills laboratories, mannequins and other approaches are required to provide this training. Training episodes need to be recorded and procedural logbooks for individual trainees may soon form part of such a record. Induction training for new staff needs to ensure that they are made aware of the existence of local unit guidance for given procedures.

The role of parental consent for procedures on neonatal units remains the subject of ongoing debate (pp. 90–1), with no clear agreement on which procedures require explicit consent and for which procedures implied consent is acceptable. It is important to emphasise the basic principle that gaining consent is essential. A clinician who carries out a non-lifesaving procedure without consent will leave himself open to criticism, at the very least. However, it is also important to recognise the real practical difficulty which is involved if consent is sought for every possible procedure during a prolonged intensive care stay. Further, this will cause 'information overload' for parents already burdened with stress. Parent groups such as BLISS are producing literature describing common events in neonatal intensive care, and this is a welcome development.

Critical incident reporting (CIR) has to be established for complications of procedures. A robust CIR process will help in identifying problems such as an increase in the rate of unplanned extubations following a change in fixation device. Clinical audit can also play a role in the identification of iatrogenic procedure-related complications.

Percutaneous blood sampling

Modern laboratory analysers can perform increasing numbers of measurements on small samples. The choice and site of sampling depends on the volume of blood required. These procedures are painful and some form of analgesia, either a topical local anaesthetic cream, oral sucrose solution, suckling or swaddling, should be considered if possible. Appropriate volumes of blood should be collected and specimens labelled properly to avoid re-sampling.

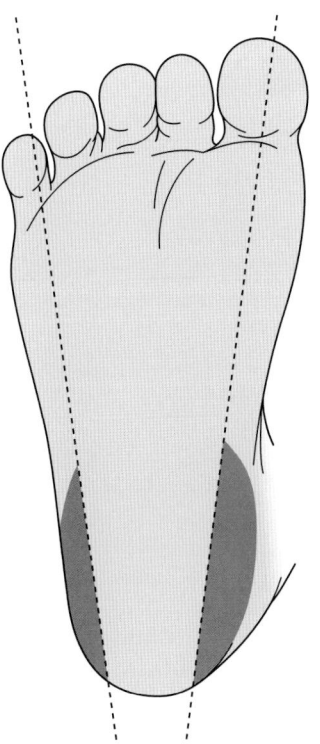

Fig. 45.1 Heel pricks for capillary sample; the shaded areas indicate the sites from which this type of blood should be collected, i.e. beyond the lateral and medial limits of the foot.

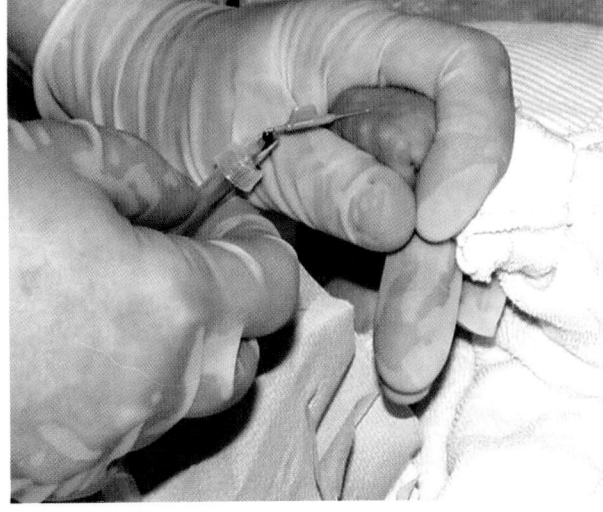

Fig. 45.2 Venous blood sampling from a flanged collection needle.

Capillary heel pricks

Indications

- Small volumes of blood for routine haematological, biochemical analyses
- Capillary blood gas analysis
- Blood glucose measurement.

Equipment

- Automated heel incision device, Minilet or Glucolet lancets
- Heparinised capillary tubes, appropriate sample bottles.

Procedure

1. The foot must be warm and well perfused. The heel should be cleaned with an antibacterial swab. Alcohol-containing swabs will interfere with blood glucose measurements. Petroleum jelly should also be avoided.
2. With the foot dorsiflexed, the skin of the lateral or medial margins of the heel should be punctured using an appropriately sized incision device.[26] The area over the calcaneus must be avoided (Fig. 45.1).
3. Gentle pressure produces blood.
4. Bleeding should be controlled using a cotton-wool ball.

Venepuncture blood samples

Indications

- Larger volumes of blood for laboratory analyses
- Samples for coagulation or microbiological studies.

Equipment

- G24 cannula or G25 butterfly
- G21 or G23 flanged collection needle
- Assay bottles, capillary tubes.

Procedure

1. Peripheral veins should be used initially, with proximal veins saved for central vascular access.
2. Clean skin with an antibacterial Steret and the vein stabilised.
3. The needle or butterfly is inserted at an angle of 30–45°.
4. Blood should be collected via a butterfly and attached syringe or dripped directly into bottles and capillary tubes from collection needles (Fig. 45.2).
5. After needle removal, gentle pressure with a cotton-wool ball prevents bruising/haematoma formation.

Complications from capillary and venous blood sampling

- Destabilisation of the baby
- Scars from skin punctures[49]
- Osteomyelitis or osteochondritis of the os calcis[112]
- Development of painful calcified heel nodules.[188]

Arterial 'stabs'

Indications

- Large volumes of uncontaminated blood for laboratory analysis
- Blood gas analysis.

Equipment

- G25 needle or butterfly
- Heparinised blood gas syringes, capillary tubes, sample bottles.

Procedure

1. The radial, posterior tibial and dorsalis pedis arteries are the most frequently used.
2. Sampling from the ulnar artery should only be considered when collateral circulation to the hand via the radial artery has been demonstrated (Allen's test).
3. The artery should be identified by palpation and transillumination with a *cold* light. Excessive extension or flexion at the wrist or ankle may impede blood flow.
4. Clean skin with an antibacterial swab.
5. The artery is entered at an angle of 30–45°; blood should flow freely into the needle.
6. After withdrawal of the needle, apply firm pressure with a cotton-wool ball for at least 5 minutes.

Complications

- Peripheral ischaemia[94]
- Aneurysm formation from repeated stabs[148,170]
- Destabilisation during handling.

Umbilical artery catheterisation

An umbilical artery catheter (UAC) provides secure long-term access. There is a wide range of catheters available; the most advanced provide continuous cotside display of arterial pH, oxygen and carbon dioxide levels, reducing the need for frequent blood sampling.[136] UACs have been positioned 'high' above the diaphragm at a level between the 6th and 10th thoracic vertebrae or 'low' below the 3rd lumbar vertebra, to avoid the coeliac, renal and mesenteric arteries. Recent reviews suggest the high position is safest (see below).

Indications

- Repeated intermittent sampling for blood gases and laboratory assays
- Monitoring of blood gas parameters via indwelling electrodes
- Monitoring of blood pressure
- Exchange transfusion
- Fluid infusions.

Equipment

- Catheterisation pack containing sterile gown, drapes, artery clamps, fine forceps, dilating probes.
- Umbilical catheters, typically 3.5 Fr for babies <1500 g and 5.0 Fr for those >1500 g. Catheters should have Luer-lock attachments. In emergencies, nasogastric tubes have been inserted, but there is greater risk of accidental disconnection and blood loss.
- Sterile cord ligature, three-way tap, Luer-lock extension sets, syringes, sutures.

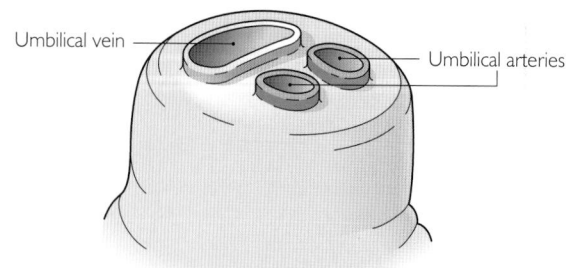

Fig. 45.3 The appearance of the cut surface of the umbilical cord.

- Heparinised saline or dextrose (1 U/ml).
- Blood pressure transducer (if required).

Procedure

1. Catheters must be inserted with aseptic technique with the infant draped and closely monitored.
2. The umbilical cord and skin surrounding the stump must be cleaned with antibacterial solution. Alcohol-based solutions can burn the skin; spillage around the flanks, buttocks and back must be avoided. The solution should be allowed to dry and then wiped off with sterile water.
3. The catheter and three-way tap must be flushed with saline. The insertion distance (in centimetres) for catheter placement above the diaphragm is calculated by the formula $(3 \times weight [in kg]) + 9 + stump length (in cm)$. Shoulder tip to umbilicus measurement can also be used.
4. The cord should be cut horizontally with a scalpel 1–2 cm above the abdominal wall; a cord ligature placed around the base of the stump minimises blood loss. The cut cord is held with artery forceps gripping the Wharton's jelly, and the two thick-walled arteries and a single thin-walled gaping umbilical vein identified (Fig. 45.3).
5. The artery should be gently dilated with a probe or fine non-toothed forceps which are introduced into the artery and allowed to open. Once the artery is gaping, the catheter should be introduced and advanced with gentle pressure to overcome resistance to the calculated depth. Passage into the artery will be confirmed by aspiration of pulsating blood. Prodding back and forth with the dilator or catheter may result in a false passage.
6. Catheters can be secured using a zinc oxide tape flag fitted around the catheter and two sutures carefully inserted into the stump avoiding occlusion of the vein if a venous catheter is intended (Fig. 45.4). Once catheters have been inserted, a purse-string suture should be placed around the top of the stump to prevent bleeding. H-tape bridges or commercial devices can be attached to the abdominal wall. The application of hydrocolloid dressing to the skin reduces epidermal damage (Fig. 45.5). The UAC site and lower limbs must not be covered. Careful observation is required to detect problems with the catheter or lower limb perfusion; remember to check the buttocks.
7. Correct placement must be confirmed with chest/abdominal X-ray showing the catheter looping through the iliac arteries

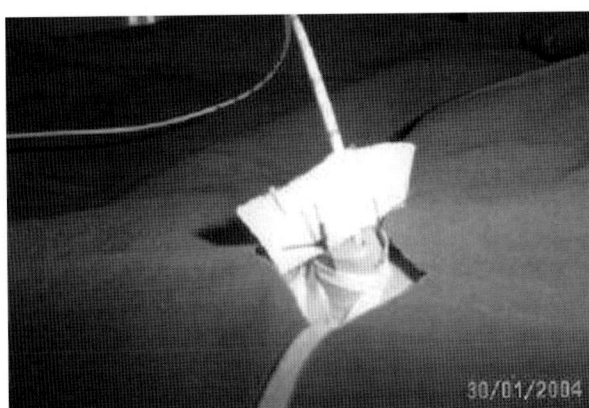

Fig. 45.4 Sutured flag fixation of umbilical catheter.

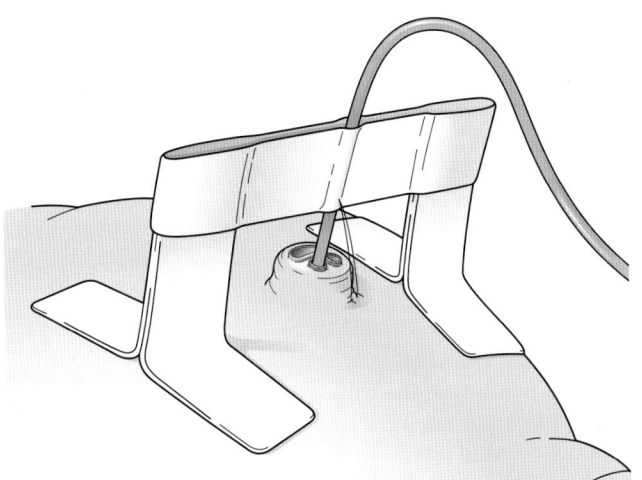

Fig. 45.5 'H' technique for immobilisation of the umbilical catheter.

into the aorta (p. 357). The UAC can be repositioned using a sterile technique. If perfusion to the perineum and lower limbs is suboptimal, volume expansion may improve matters.

8. Saline, dextrose, drug infusions and blood products can in theory be administered via UACs. Heparinised saline is the infusion of choice.[166]

9. In extremely premature infants, a functioning UAC may be critical for survival. In these circumstances, the benefits of repositioning or replacing blocked catheters may outweigh the risks of such procedures.

10. The procedure must be documented in the case notes, detailing blood loss, state of peripheral perfusion, presence of femoral pulses, position of UAC tip on X-ray and ease of sampling and flushing. The operator should ensure appropriate labels have been or will be applied. As with all indwelling intravascular catheters, there should be a clear record of regular nursing observations relating to the UAC and its use.

11. UACs must be removed if perfusion problems persist or if the UAC is no longer clinically required. Wharton's jelly needs to be carefully eased away from the catheter. Heparinised fluids are stopped 30 minutes before removal, the line is withdrawn with gentle traction, the last 5 cm removed over

Table 45.3 Complications of umbilical artery catheterisation

Complication	Reference
Aortic thrombosis	213
Thromboses affecting	
legs/toes/buttocks	72
kidneys	126
gut	77
Urachal damage and urinary leak	53
Hypoglycaemia	212
Aortic aneurysm	56
Gluteal skin necrosis	123
Sciatic nerve damage	164
Hypertension	34, 154
Paraplegia	79
Haemorrhage	77
Fracture of catheter with embolism	194, 200

several minutes, allowing arterial spasm which minimises bleeding. Pressure on the stump and suture insertion will control bleeding. The site must not be covered for a few hours after line removal.

Complications

Complications and problems associated with UACs can be broadly related to:

- insertion procedure – occurring at or during insertion;
- presence of the catheter;
- infusate.

Barrington has comprehensively reviewed the literature with respect to UACs[13–16] and concludes that:

- UACs should be sited in the thoracic (high) rather than in the lumbar (low) position.
- End-hole rather than side-hole catheters should be used.
- Heparinisation of infusates with at least 0.25 units of heparin per millilitre decreases catheter occlusion rates.
- Catheter material makes no difference to complication rates.

Table 45.3 lists the common complications associated with UACs.

Complications and problems during insertion

False passage

The rupture of the catheter either into a false passage within the arterial wall or through the wall into connective tissue is common but rarely causes any damage. There is usually an increased resistance to passage of the catheter and the attempt should be abandoned.

Haematoma

When a false passage is created, an asymptomatic haematoma may occasionally form. Occasionally the blood loss may be large and even fatal.[126,130] Such a lesion will present with signs of hypovolaemia and should be identified on ultrasound. Treatment involves transfusion, when appropriate, and correction of any coagulation disorder; surgery is occasionally required to ligate the bleeding site.[130]

Entry into the peritoneum

This occurs with deep dissection, either in a cord cut flush with the abdominal wall or after initially creating a false passage. It may also occur if there is a very small omphalocoele in the base of the cord, in which case small intestine[196] or just the appendix may appear.[24] No harm is done; the hole should be closed with a suture, taking care that a loop of bowel is not trapped.

Entry into the urachus

This arises while probing too deeply for the umbilical artery, invariably in a baby with a large urachal remnant. The sudden appearance of clear yellow fluid (urine) suggests that the renal tract has been entered. Surgical help should be sought, but the fistula usually closes spontaneously if the bladder is emptied via a urethral catheter.[93] The urinary leak may be intraperitoneal[53] and not recognised initially. Open surgery to repair the tear may then be required.

Catheterisation of the wrong vessel

Occasionally the catheter tip passes into a branch of the internal iliac, including the superior and inferior gluteal arteries,[44] and may be responsible for damage to the pelvic bones and gluteal skin (superior gluteal artery) and the sciatic nerves (inferior gluteal arteries; see below) (Table 45.3). Malposition of the UAC is the main reason for always confirming catheter tip position by X-ray immediately after insertion. Schreiber et al[183] have described a technique of passing another small (3.5 Fr) UAC alongside the malpositioned one. This second catheter then enters the aorta and the original one can be removed. Disturbance of flow down these branches is also responsible for peripheral ischaemic change, which can be seen following 'blind' injection of drugs inadvertently into the umbilical artery in the cord during resuscitation at birth – usually in mistake for the umbilical vein[47] (pp. 1242–4).

Haemorrhage from the umbilical vessels

During insertion there may be haemorrhage from the other umbilical artery or the vein. This can be prevented by placing a ligature loosely around the base of the cord before it is cut for the procedure (p. 1240).

Complications related to the presence of the catheter

Peripheral ischaemia and thrombosis

Ischaemic and thrombotic complications may occur as a result of the catheter or the infusate and are discussed below under complications related to the infusate.

Haemorrhage

This is an ever-present risk and is one of the commonest complications of UACs.[77,203] It can be prevented by meticulous nursing observation of all connections to the catheter. Luer-locks should be used for all connections, which must be visible at all times. Nursing the baby supine must remain the default position when a UAC is in situ, with prone nursing used only in exceptional circumstances, where the benefits of improved gas exchange are considered greater than the risk of UAC-related haemorrhage. In practice, the UAC will have been in situ for a day or more with good evidence of haemostasis before prone nursing is considered. If significant haemorrhage does occur, the treatment is immediate transfusion.

Air emboli

UAC are invariably maintained patent by a continuous infusion of heparinised saline, leading to risk of air being entrained in the line, creating systemic air embolism. However, because of the arterial pressure, leaks in the system are more likely to result in haemorrhage than in air being injected.

Severed catheter tip

During removal, a catheter may fracture or be severed when the retaining suture is cut. This can lead to haemorrhage, the catheter tip being retained within the umbilical artery or even floating free and embolising in the arterial tree.[200] These problems should be avoided by careful technique when removing the catheter; if they do occur, the catheter remnant should be retrieved by an interventional radiologist or cardiologist whenever possible.

Infection from the UAC

UACs will predispose the baby to sepsis, in particular *Staphylococcus epidermidis* (p. 1251).[107,215,220] The use of prophylactic antibiotics to avoid infection with prolonged UAC insertion cannot be justified. Scrupulous attention to handling technique and minimising the time the UAC is in situ is required.

Mycotic aneurysm

These usually occur around the tip of an indwelling UAC and are most common with thoracic placement. Most occur in babies with coexisting staphylococcal septicaemia. Although true aneurysms do occur,[40,113] in many cases there is a false aneurysm, with the aorta communicating through its wall with a sac that does not contain the normal tissues of the aortic wall[56] or is composed of an organising para-aortic haematoma.[167] In many reported cases, as well as the aneurysm there is associated thrombus of the aorta and its major branches.[61,113] Rarely the aneurysm may rupture, with fatal results.[147] In some cases it has been an incidental postmortem finding,[113] but in others, after treatment of the septicaemia with antibiotics and removal of the arterial catheter, surgical repair has given good results.[61] Aneurysms have also been detected incidentally in infants over 1 year of age, and have been successfully resected.[32,61]

Complications related to the infusate

Peripheral ischaemia and thrombosis

This is the second most common complication after haemorrhage. Initially, the features of peripheral ischaemia may be due to a large catheter partially occluding the aorta and iliac vessels,

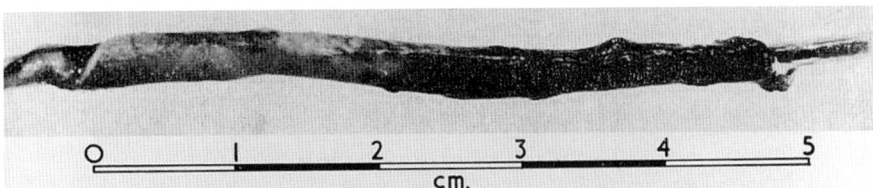

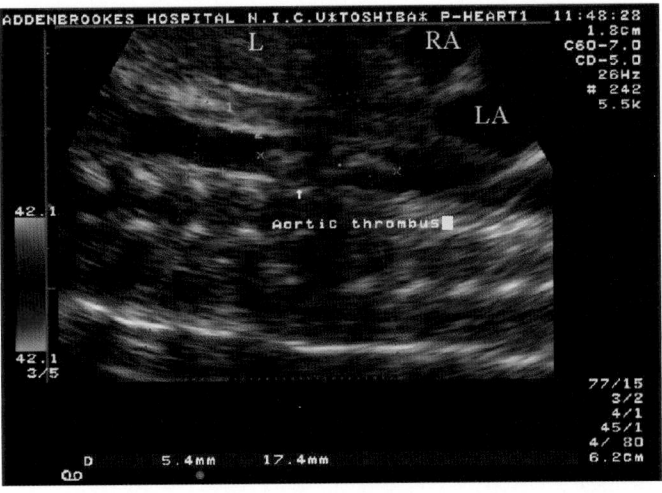

(a)

(b)

Fig. 45.6 (a) Sheaths of thrombus surrounding an umbilical artery catheter found at post mortem. (From Gupta et al.[77]) (b) Abdominal echocardiogram showing aortic thrombus (L, liver; RA, right atrium; LA left atrium).

or to arterial spasm following infusion of (hypertonic) solutions or vasoconstricting drugs such as catecholamines. It is to prevent the latter problem that the tip of the UAC is positioned well away from the major branches of the aorta. Hypertonic drugs must infuse slowly so that they are instantaneously diluted in rapidly flowing blood.

The serious consequence is that thrombosis develops. The incidence of this complication varies widely in reported series, from as little as 1.5%[77] (where only clinically detected or autopsy-proven cases were reported) to as high as 95%[141] (where aortography was used prior to removing the catheter). The literature[72] suggests that thombosis occurs soon after UAC insertion and rarely thereafter. Normally grown term babies suffering from hypoxic-ischaemic encephalopathy seem to be significantly over-represented in studies of thrombosis.[83,146,154,182,205,213]

Thrombus forms as a result of damage to the endothelial wall of the artery[36] and is likely to start near the hole in the catheter tip. Side-hole catheters, where the infusate impinges directly onto the endothelium of the artery, have been thought to create more problems than end-hole catheters, where the infusate is instantly diluted in the rapidly flowing arterial blood,[13–16,221] although there are conflicting reports.[38] Once thrombosis has formed, it may propagate down the aorta alongside the catheter, down branches of the aorta such as the renal and lumbar arteries, and, once formed on the aortic wall, may propagate up the aorta, obstructing branches proximal to the tip of the catheter. Thrombus may also disintegrate, with embolisation to any vessel distal to it. It is not clear how often conditions such as necrotising enterocolitis (NEC), haematuria or limb pallor, are due to emboli rather than to direct extension of the thrombus.

Clinical features

Many thrombi remain asymptomatic and are incidental findings on ultrasound scan or at post mortem (Fig. 45.6a, b).[126,141,149] Thrombi can present in various ways. Rarely, there may be heart failure due to total aortic obstruction.[83] Much more common is evidence of ischaemia to a limb or organ (Table 45.4, Figs 45.7–45.9). These signs and symptoms may appear when the catheter is in situ, but may also occur just after its removal, presumably due to dislodgement of thrombus on the aortic wall or to a sleeve of thrombus being left behind. Occasionally, signs develop days after a UAC has been removed, presumably as a result of thrombus developing on the previously damaged intima.[2,104]

In babies with obstruction to the renal or iliac arteries, the diagnosis is usually made promptly within minutes or hours of the obstruction, as the baby develops haematuria, reduced urine output, poor peripheral perfusion, ischaemia and reduced pulses in the distribution of one artery (Figs 45.7–45.10). However infants, who develop paraplegia, are often critically ill, hypotonic and may be paralysed on intermittent positive pressure ventilation (IPPV), so it is several days or even weeks before the paraplegia is recognised.

The role of UAC in the aetiology of NEC remains controversial, and most large epidemiological studies of this disorder do not show that the risk of NEC is greater in those babies who have a UAC. However, in the separate entity of focal or discrete intestinal perforation, emboli from a UAC are likely to be of importance.[145,176]

In addition to clinically obvious thrombotic or embolic lesions, autopsy studies have shown infarction secondary to UAC in the liver, adrenals, stomach, spleen and pancreas.[211]

Table 45.4 Clinical features of thrombotic or embolic obstruction secondary to umbilical artery catheterisation

Artery	Clinical features	Reference
Renal	Haematuria	213
	Oliguria	154
	Renal failure	34
	Hypertension	
Superior/inferior mesenteric	Abdominal distension	
	Melaena	
	NEC	145
	Discrete intestinal perforation	
Common/external iliac	Leg pallor, ischaemia, gangrene	77, 135
		(Figs 45.7 & 45.8)
Internal iliac, superior and inferior gluteal	Buttock necrosis	123 (Fig. 45.9)
	Pelvic bone necrosis	44
	Sciatic nerve damage	164
Lumbar	Paraplegia	79, 104

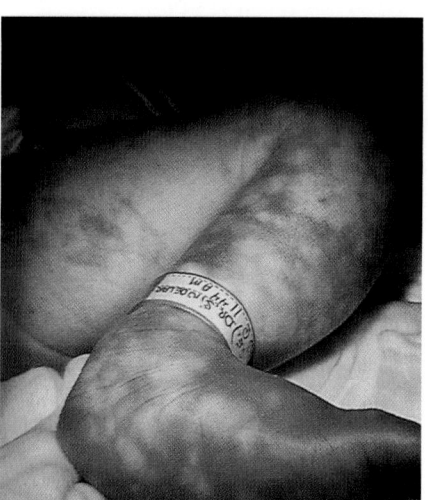

Fig. 45.7 Mottling of lower extremity in infant with umbilical artery catheter.

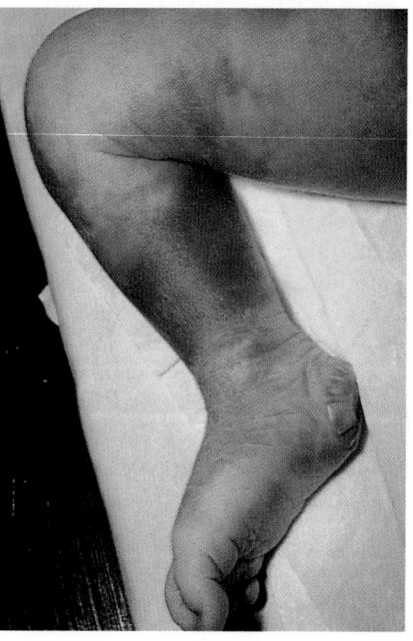

Fig. 45.8 Blanching and cyanosis in lower extremity in infant with umbilical artery catheter.

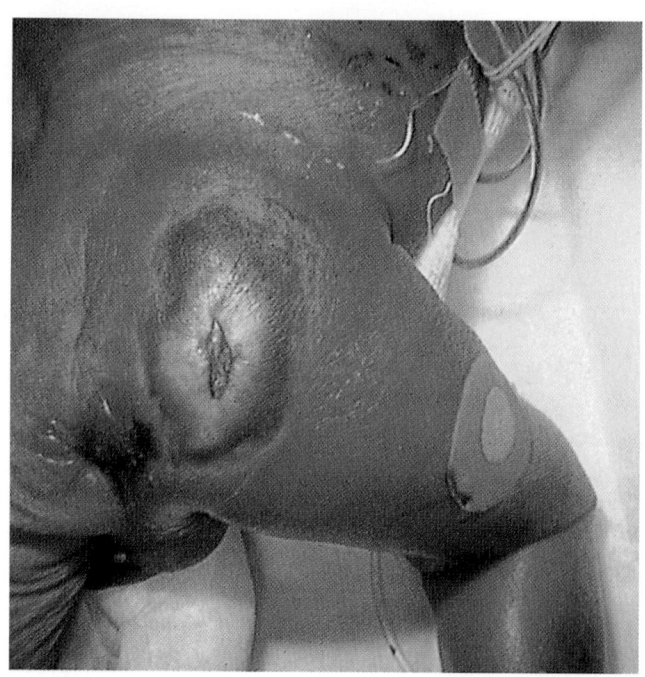

Fig. 45.9 Ischaemic injury in gluteal area.

Treatment

As soon as there is evidence of compromised circulation, the catheter should be removed unless hypovolaemia is contributing and volume infusion rapidly corrects the situation. In cases where there was simply obstruction of a blood vessel, UAC removal, together with treatment to improve systemic pressure with volume expansion or inotropes, will usually result in prompt reversal of the ischaemia with no sequelae. In the case occurring shortly after catheter insertion, the ischaemic changes are usually due to arterial spasm, in addition to simple vessel obstruction. The application or infusion of vasodilators such as nitroglycerine or tolazoline[82,227] may be useful to reverse the peripheral ischaemia. If there is clinical, radiological or ultrasound evidence of persistent ischaemia, thrombosis or arterial obstruction, careful assessment of

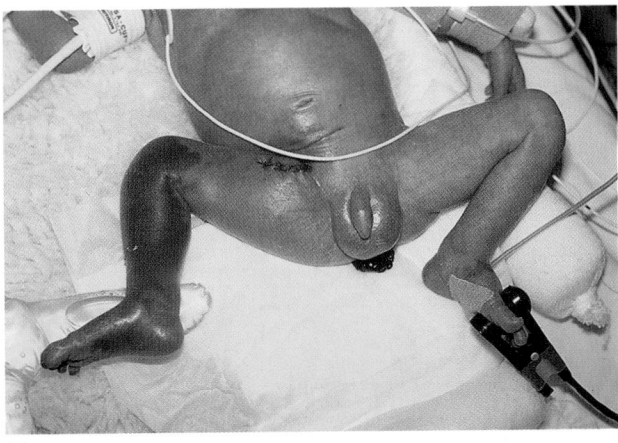

(a)

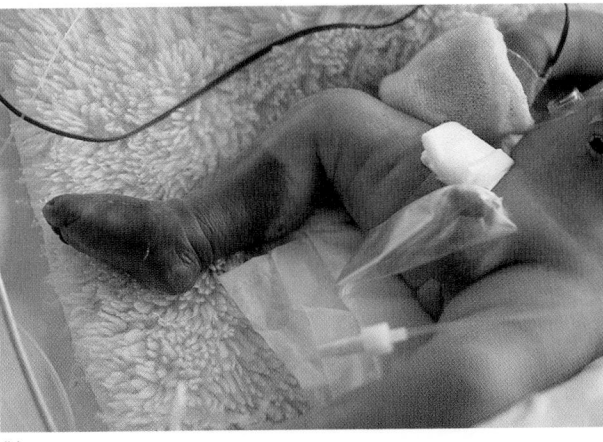

(b)

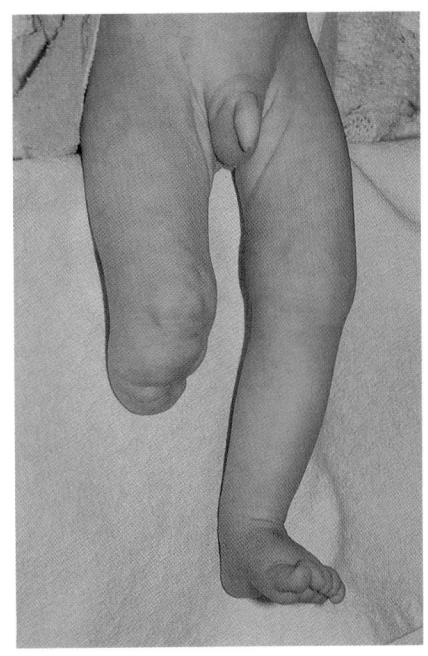

(c)

Fig. 45.10 (a) Acute ischaemia to the right leg following insertion of a femoral artery line. The level of injury appears to be above the knee. (b) Marked recovery with the line of demarcation below the knee. This resulted in below-knee amputation. (c) Immediately following the injury, the artery had been explored, but this was unsuccessful in saving the limb.

the extent of the thrombus should be carried out by ultrasound or angiography. Renal involvement should be assessed with radionuclide imaging.[34,213]

The treatment algorithm of Colburn et al[39] provides a good guide to subsequent treatment (Fig. 45.11). In most cases of aortic mural thrombosis, conservative therapy is appropriate; the clot will clear, and this has been confirmed with ultrasound imaging.[2,186] Investigation for a thrombophilic disorder such as protein C or protein S deficiency (p. 762) may be appropriate. However, if there are signs of persisting peripheral ischaemia or damage to other organs, the baby should be heparinised and thrombolytic therapy commenced.[69] Heparinisation may improve the outcome,[85,122,146] and should be given in the doses shown in Table 45.5. Rather more success has been reported with streptokinase or urokinase[122,172,205] (Table 45.5), although this is not always the case.[59] More recently there have been reports of success with tissue plasminogen activator[2,97,146] (Table 45.5). Full intensive care should be continued as appropriate during attempts to dissolve the clot, in particular treating hypertension (see below) and renal failure.[34,121,154]

If these medical procedures do not result in a rapid improvement in perfusion, particularly to a leg, operation and thrombectomy or embolectomy can be extremely successful.[69,105,154]

Amputation for irreversibly ischaemic limbs
It is important to wait for a clear line of demarcation between viable and non-viable tissue to properly determine the level of

amputation. Too early surgery may result in a higher level of amputation, as there may be some proximal recovery (Fig. 45.10a–c).

Hypertension
This is a frequently reported complication of UAC, almost always in association with aortic thrombosis, which involves the renal arteries. At the time of the thrombosis, the babies may have a high serum renin, and the cornerstone of early neonatal management is control of the hypertension with drugs[34,121] (p. 657).

Follow-up
The overall prognosis for aortic thrombosis and renal damage is surprisingly good. Hypertension in surviving babies resolves in the majority or is easily controlled.[34,121,213] In some cases, hypertension persists[154,161] and, if due to unilateral renal disease, may be cured by nephrectomy.[9,19]

Some babies do develop renal failure and ultimately require transplants. Damage to the sciatic nerve is usually permanent, as is paraplegia. Skin grafting may be required for severe cases of peripheral ischaemia.

For limb ischaemia, if gangrene does not develop, the prognosis is excellent. Leg growth is usually normal,[28] but one study reported that affected legs may be slightly wasted.[187] If gangrene

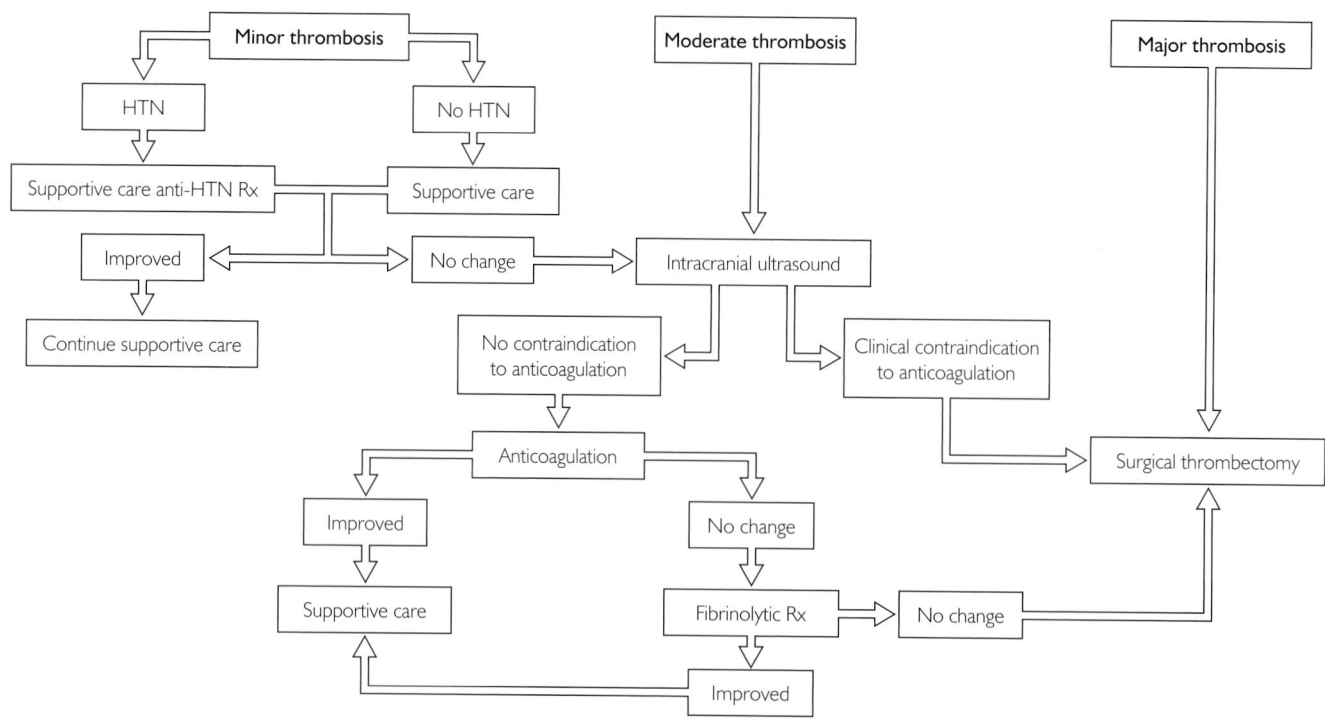

Fig. 45.11 Algorithm for management of neonatal aortic thrombosis. (From Colburn et al.[39]) HTN, hypertension; Rx, therapy.

Table 45.5 Anticoagulants, thrombolytics in the neonate

Drug	i.v. bolus dose	i.v. maintenance dose	Reference
Heparin			
<28 weeks' gestation	25 units/kg	15 units/kg/h	122
28–36 weeks' gestation	50 units/kg	20 units/kg/h	122
>36 weeks' gestation	100 units/kg	25 units/kg/h	122
Streptokinase	1000 units/kg	1000 units/kg/h*	122
Urokinase	–	200 units/kg/h for 24 h	7
Tissue plasminogen activator	0.5 mg/kg over 10 min	0.5 mg/kg/h	2

*Monitor fibrinogen levels, stop treatment if less than 1 g/l.

does develop, it may be very minor, involving the loss of just the pulp of one or two toes.[77]

Hypoglycaemia

If glucose is infused through a UAC whose tip is sited at the level of the coeliac axis, the pancreas is exposed to a constant high concentration of glucose, and hyperinsulinaemia and hence hypoglycaemia results.[212] This complication can be prevented by keeping the tip of the UAC away from the coeliac axis.

Umbilical venous catheterisation

A correctly positioned umbilical venous catheter (UVC) passes through the ductus venosus to lie at the junction of inferior vena cava/right atrium. A UVC provides secure vascular access during the first week of life, preserving peripheral veins.

Indications

- Emergency vascular access in delivery room during resuscitation
- Vascular access for administration of drugs, parenteral nutrition, vasoactive and hyper-osmolar infusions and blood products
- Exchange transfusion.

Equipment

- As for UAC insertion
- Single-, double- or triple-lumen catheters.

Procedure

1. Monitoring, catheter and cord preparation as for UAC catheterisation.

Table 45.6 Complications of umbilical venous catheterisation

Complication	Site of UVC tip (intended or after migration)	Reference
Air embolism	Supradiaphragmatic	99
Cardiac arrhythmias	Intracardiac	58
Sepsis	Any site	8, 22, 37, 89, 107, 208
Biliary-venous fistula	Hepatic venous tree	137
Hepatic abscess	Hepatic venous tree	31, 132, 225
Hepatic vein thrombosis and portal hypertension	Hepatic venous tree	92, 108, 151, 184, 208
Hepatic infarction and necrosis	Hepatic venous tree	179, 222
NEC	IVC, portal venous system	42, 84, 150, 210
Peritoneal perforation and ascites	Any site (during insertion)	134
Pericardial tamponade	Right atrium	87
Pulmonary haemorrhage, hydrothorax	Left atrium	25

2. The insertion distance (in centimetres) for catheter placement in the inferior vena cava is calculated by the formula ($2 \times$ weight [in kg]) $+ 5 +$ stump length (in cm). Shoulder tip to umbilicus measurement can also be used.

3. The vein is identified and may need little or no dilatation. The catheter should be inserted into the vein and advanced the required distance. Blood cannot always be aspirated.

4. Catheter dislodgement and bleeding around the catheter is more common with a UVC than a UAC. The catheter should be secured using a zinc oxide tape flag with sutures that pull the surrounding vein and jelly snugly onto the line, whilst avoiding artery damage if a UAC is intended (Fig. 45.4). It is usually easiest to insert the UAC first, followed by the UVC.

5. UVC placement should be confirmed with chest/abdominal X-ray showing the catheter running directly to, but not in, the right atrium. Catheters deviating from this course should be withdrawn or removed.

6. Documentation detailing line labelling, blood loss and state of haemostasis is important.

7. Fluids are infused at higher rates through UVCs and routine heparinisation is not universally used.

8. UVCs should be removed when not required, with care taken to achieve haemostasis.

Complications

UVCs have been in use since the 1950s and, like UACs, are associated with a large range of complications (Table 45.6). Again, complications arise at or during insertion, secondary to the presence of the catheter itself or due to the infusate. The site of the line tip will influence the nature of any complication (Table 45.6), with no ideal site available.

One of the principal complications remains sepsis, with infection rates of the order of 3% or 7 per 1000 catheter-days reported.[37,107] Use of antibiotics, duration of catheterisation and infusate type all are likely to influence catheter-related infection rates. Catheter removal in the face of sepsis is not always an option in the central venous line-dependent preterm, but serially positive blood cultures with coagulase-negative staphylococci or growth of Gram-negative organisms or *Staph. aureus* are indications for catheter removal.[22]

The risk of thrombosis can be reduced by heparinisation of the infusate, and if hepatic vein thrombosis does occur, it can be relieved with streptokinase.[169]

Hepatic abscesses can be managed conservatively or with percutaneous drainage.[132]

Peripheral arterial cannulation

Indications

- Continuous blood pressure monitoring
- Frequent blood sampling.

Equipment

- G24 cannula
- Steri-strips, blenderm or micropore tape, transparent dresssing, splints
- Three-way tap and Luer-lock extension sets
- Heparinised 0.9N saline or 0.45N saline
- Blood pressure transducer, if indicated.

Procedure

The peripheral artery should be identified, usually radial, posterior tibial or dorsalis pedis. When these vessels are no longer suitable, the axillary, femoral, brachial and ulnar arteries can be considered but there may be increased risk of compromising distal circulation. Allen's test should be performed before the ulnar artery is cannulated, to confirm perfusion. The hand blanches when both the radial and ulnar arteries are compressed; when

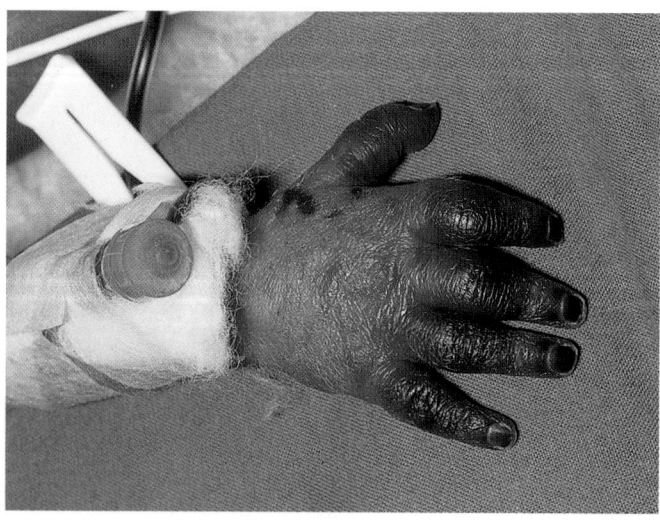
(a)

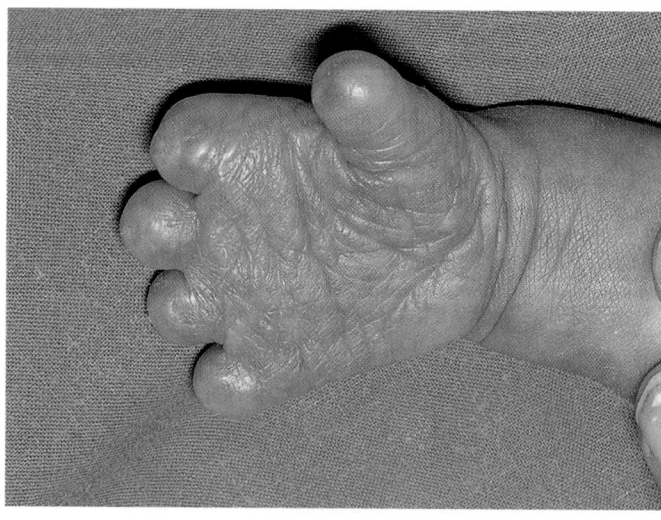
(b)

Fig. 45.12 (a) Gangrenous fingers following radial artery catheterisation. (b) Subsequent loss of fingers and thumbs.

Table 45.7 Peripheral arterial cannulation in the neonate

Artery	Comment	Reference
Superficial temporal	Not used now due to parietal lobe ischaemia	163
Axillary		160
Brachial	High risk of ischaemia (end artery)	171
Radial	Use Allen's test	78, 155, 209
Ulnar	Use Allen's test	12, 78, 217
Femoral		174
Posterior tibial		1, 12, 202
Dorsalis pedis		217

pressure is released alternately from each artery, normal perfusion should return, and if so, it is safe to proceed. Failure to perform this simple test may result in ischaemia with loss of fingers or part of the hand (Fig. 45.12).

1. Successful insertion and fixation usually requires two people.
2. The cannula should be inserted into the artery at an angle of 30–45°; as blood flushes into the chamber, advance the catheter into the artery. Sometimes the cannula may pierce the posterior wall of the artery. In this situation, withdrawing the cannula slightly may result in a flash-back of blood, indicating the cannula is now within the lumen of the artery. The catheter can then be fully advanced into position.
3. Pressure should be applied proximal to the cannula as the stylet is removed and during attachment of the extension set and three-way tap, to minimise blood loss.
4. The line must be secured with Steri-strips or tape; an overlying transparent dressing provides extra security whilst allowing visualisation of the entry site. Ensuring that the catheter is not kinked and the limb appropriately positioned with a splint will maximise the life of the line.
5. The line should sample easily, with no or only minimal and transient blanching around the site of insertion and distally during flushing.

6. A heparinised saline infusion should be commenced.
7. If the process fails, prompt removal of the cannula and adequate pressure over the artery is needed to prevent bruising and haematoma.
8. Documentation as for UAC insertion and use should be followed.

Complications

Cannulae have been placed in most accessible arteries (Table 45.7).
Complications, reportedly occurring in the minority of babies,[168] depend upon the site of cannulation and include:

- distal ischaemia from thrombi or emboli[33,35,193,198] (Figs 45.10a–c, 45.12, 45.13);
- proximal ischaemia from spasm proximal to the site of cannulation;[94]
- carpal tunnel syndrome in forearm artery cannulation;[101]
- damage to extensor muscles and tendons in forearm artery cannulation;[197]
- aneurysms;[170]
- adjacent nerve damage;[153]
- parietal lobe ischaemia.[33,193]

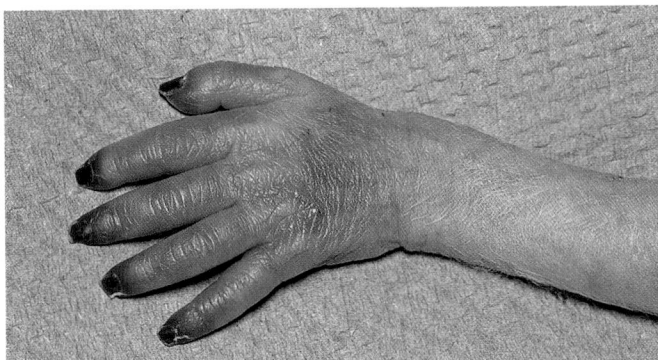

Fig. 45.13 Terminal digital ischaemia following accidental cannulation of the brachial artery while inserting a peripheral long line.

Complications may be reduced by:

- use of these cannulae for sampling and blood pressure monitoring only;
- continuous infusion of heparinised saline;
- avoidance of excessive or rapid bolus flushes;[115]
- clear labelling, to avoid inadvertent intravenous (i.v.) injection – if this does occur, administration of a systemic vasodilator drug may be useful.[82,227]

Immediate removal of the catheter in the presence of persistent ischaemic signs must remain the default, although there may be a role – as yet unproven – for infusion of vasodilator or thrombolytic agents via the peripheral arterial cannula itself.

Percutaneously inserted central venous lines

These catheters are usually inserted via proximal veins; the 27G lines can be inserted through standard 24G cannulae, allowing smaller veins to be used. The line tip should lie outside the right atrium in the superior vena cava if inserted above the diaphragm or in the inferior vena cava if inserted from the lower limb. Although these lines are said to be radio-opaque, they are so fine that X-ray with contrast should be undertaken to accurately identify tip position.

Indications

- Long-term administration of parentral nutrition and drug infusions
- Prolonged courses of bolus drugs. e.g. antibiotics.

Equipment

- Catheterisation pack containing sterile gown, drapes, fine forceps
- Long line with insertion butterfly, splitting needle or cannula
- Steri-strips, transparent dressing

- Luer-locked connectors and extension sets
- Injectable X-ray contrast.

Procedure

1. Using aseptic technique, percutaneous long lines can be threaded into position from the cephalic vein, brachial veins at the elbow, saphenous vein at the ankle or knee, superficial scalp veins and, occasionally, axillary or external jugular veins. Measurement from the site of insertion to the vena cava must be performed.
2. The surrounding skin must be cleaned with antibacterial solution and drapes positioned. Assistance may be required to stabilise the limb and vein.
3. Blood flows from the introducer needle after successful insertion into the vein. The saline-flushed catheter should then be threaded into position with non-toothed fine forceps. The arm or leg may need repositioning to allow the line to pass around the shoulder or through the groin (Fig. 45.14a).
4. The butterfly introducer needle or splitting needle should be taken off the catheter. If a cannula was used for venous cannulation, this should be withdrawn from the vein and positioned on the limb. The line, compression hub (if required) and extension set should be fixed to the skin with Steri-strips, avoiding kinking, and a transparent dressing applied (Fig. 45.14b).
5. The line should be flushed with 0.5–1.0 ml of contrast material prior to the X-ray, avoiding flushing during the X-ray itself. Lines with the tip within the heart must be withdrawn to the vena cava. Lines with the tip at the shoulder or groin may be used but there is more risk of extravasation. Line repositioning and fixation must be performed with sterile technique.
6. Documentation regarding insertion, X-ray findings and observations during use are required. Fluids are infused at higher rates and heparinisation is not needed. Pressure-sensitive pumps should be used, as the fine 27G lines often require high pressures to deliver the required infusion rates.

Femoral, jugular and subclavian venous lines

Cannulation of the femoral, subclavian and jugular veins should usually only be considered when all other vascular access has been exhausted. The femoral vein is the safest route for percutaneous line insertion by an experienced practitioner and is the approach described here. The pulsating femoral artery at the inguinal ligament is the landmark for all femoral vessel insertions. The procedural techniques are identical for both arterial and venous catheterisation, although smaller, usually single-lumen, catheters are used for arterial access. These lines may be inserted by a cut-down procedure.

Indications

- Vascular access for administration of drugs, parenteral nutrition, vasoactive and hyper-osmolar infusions and blood products.

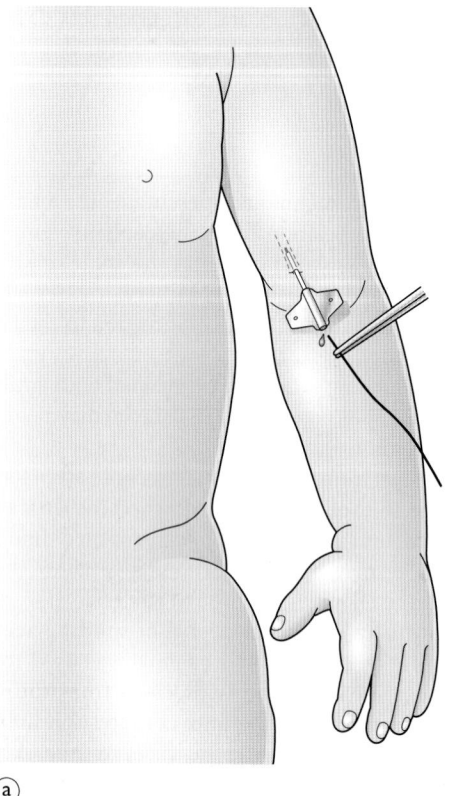

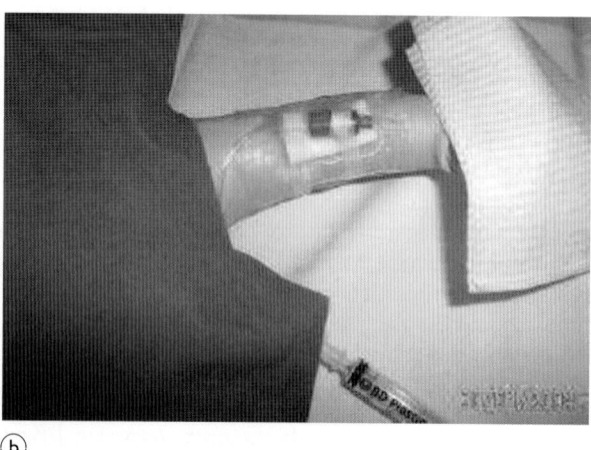

Fig. 45.14 (a) Central venous catheter insertion through a needle used as an introducer. (b) Fixation of central venous line to limb.

Equipment

- Catheterisation pack containing sterile gown, drapes, fine forceps
- Seldinger central line insertion pack with catheter.

Procedure

1. Aseptic technique.
2. Successful cannulation is unlikely if the baby is moving. Where possible, the baby should be ventilated, sedated and possibly paralysed for the procedure.

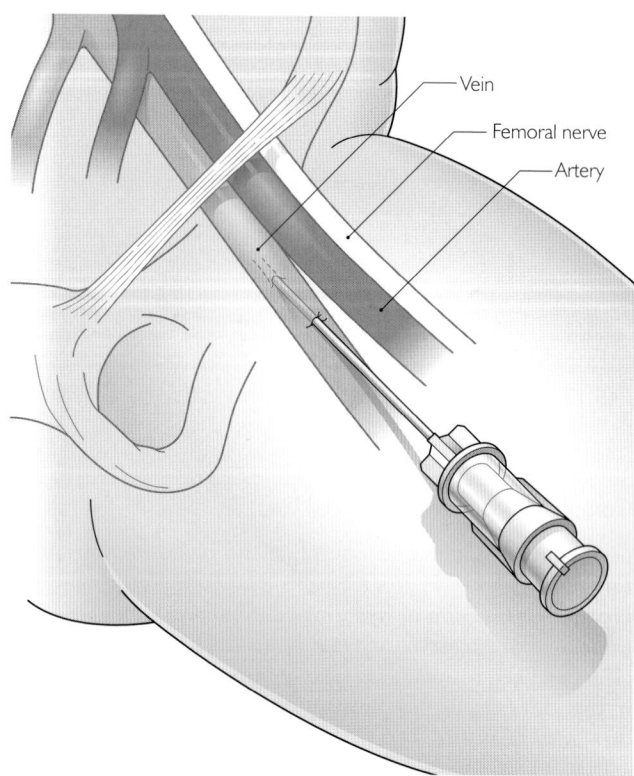

Fig. 45.15 Central line introducer inserted into the femoral vein, awaiting guidewire insertion.

3. Using the Seldinger technique, a venous catheter is threaded over a guidewire into place. The operator should be familiar with the equipment, ensuring that the guidewire passes through the introducer needle or 24G cannula.
4. The femoral vein lying medial to the artery is entered at an angle of 30–45°, aiming for the umbilicus; blood should flow or be aspirated freely (Fig. 45.15). Taking care not to dislodge the introducer, the guidewire is threaded into the vein. The introducing needle/cannula is then withdrawn over the guidewire. The operator has the choice of which catheter to insert over the wire. A standard cannula could be temporarily inserted, through which a standard fine long line can be positioned. Alternatively, larger multi-lumen central venous catheters (4.5 Fr, 20 G) can be inserted. A dilator will need to be passed over the guidewire to allow these larger lines to be inserted. The guidewire must be withdrawn as the catheter is advanced into place.
5. Successful cannulation will be confirmed by aspiration of blood from all of the catheter lumen. Pulsatile blood indicates that an artery has been cannulated. If so, this line can either be left in place as a guide or removed: pressure will need to be applied for several minutes to control blood loss. Following confirmation of correct placement, the line should be sutured in place and a transparent dressing applied to prevent it being dislodged (Fig. 45.16).
6. An X-ray should be taken to confirm position, with contrast unless a wide-bore catheter has been used.
7. Standard procedure documentation and observations during use are required.
8. Fluids are infused at higher rates, therefore heparinisation is not required.

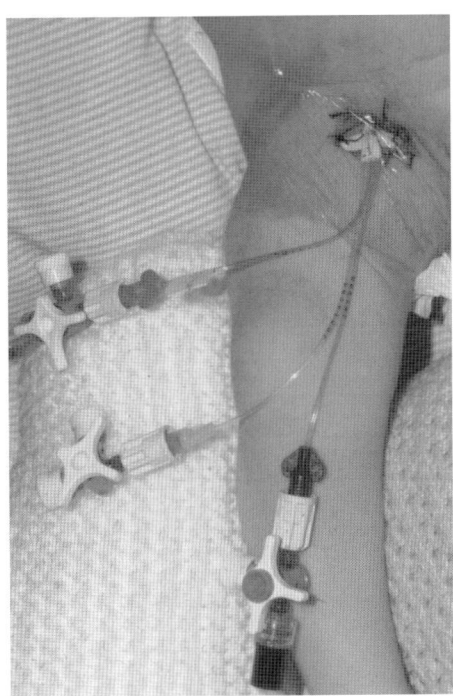

Fig. 45.16 Fixation of triple-lumen right femoral venous line.

Complications of central venous lines (all types)

Percutaneously inserted fine catheters or surgically inserted catheters (Broviac or Hickman) have been associated with five major groups of problems:

- infections, including endocarditis, particularly with *Staph. epidermidis* and fungi;
- thrombosis;
- ectopic placement or line migration, with extravasation;
- retention;
- air embolism.

The treatment of the first three is usually removal of the catheter, although attempts at sterilisation are often attempted, particularly when vascular access is difficult. Thrombosis is relatively rare, occurring in less than 5% of catheterised neonates, and is more common with the larger Broviac or Hickman type of catheter,[125,127] which take up more space in the blood vessel and are more rigid than fine silastic lines. Placement of Hickman or Broviac catheters with the tip outside the right atrium leads to a high incidence of thrombosis, possibly due to intimal damage. Caution should be exercised when these larger lines are left in situ for long periods: the baby's growth will result in the tip leaving the right atrium, and thrombosis can follow. Thrombosis may occur in the great veins or, more characteristically, within the right atrium, where the thrombus can be seen bobbing about on a cardiac ultrasound image.[125,128] Such thrombi are frequently accompanied by a positive blood culture for *Staph. epidermidis* or candida, and may result in pulmonary or systemic embolisation. They can resolve spontaneously,[128] but if infected should be treated with antibiotics, and thrombolytic therapy (Table 45.5)

Table 45.8 Sites of extravascular infusions with TPN catheters

Site	Reference
Pericardial	95, 206
Pleural, direct	95, 185
Pleural, secondary to SVC obstruction	52
With permanent phrenic nerve injury	224
Intra-abdominal	144
Subdural	178, 230
Intrapulmonary	175 (Fig. 45.17)
Hydrocephalus secondary to vena caval obstruction	204
Lumbar vein/intrathecal	96 (Fig. 45.18)

(urokinase, streptokinase, tissue plasminogen activator) should be considered.[3]

Unlike Broviac and Hickman catheters, percutaneously inserted fine silastic or polyurethane catheters should be sited outside of the heart, in line with recent UK Department of Health recommendations,[50] in order to reduce the risk of pericardial extravasation and cardiac tamponade. It is important to remember, however, that these fine catheters may migrate after insertion and continued vigilance with regard to potential complications is essential.

Where extravasation accompanies location of the tip in an inappropriate position (Table 45.8, Fig. 45.17), the situation must be handled accordingly. This includes removal of the line, aspiration of the extravasated material if clinically indicated, plus appropriate treatment for any accompanying respiratory failure (pleural fluid) or hypotension (pericardial fluid) that frequently coexists. Certainly the sudden cardiorespiratory compromise of an infant with an indwelling central venous line should lead to the immediate consideration and exclusion of pericardial effusion and cardiac tamponade. Where the clinical situation allows, a cardiac echo should be undertaken to exclude an effusion, but, *if in extremis*, pericardial aspiration should be attempted without echocardiographic evidence. One striking feature of this type of complication is that although a major vessel, or even the right atrium, is punctured for the extravasation to occur, haemorrhage is rare.

There are reports of the catheter becoming stuck by thrombus formation,[20,98] and we know of cases where the catheter has been severed and floated free, usually within the heart,[142] eventually becoming fixed to the endocardium. When tethered, catheters can be removed surgically.[20]

Catheters in the atria may provoke arrhythmias[45] and even cardiac arrest;[180] an air embolism has been reported in adults[157] and is a theoretical risk in neonates when infusion pumps are being used.

It is legitimate to leave a line in situ where the catheter tip lies, for example, in the subclavian or femoral vein, in particular if achieving vascular access has proved difficult. The major complication here is venous obstruction, in some cases complicated by thrombosis, with the limb becoming oedematous. Removal is indicated, with oedema resolution likely.

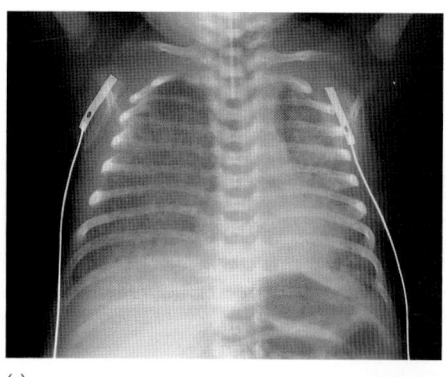

(a)

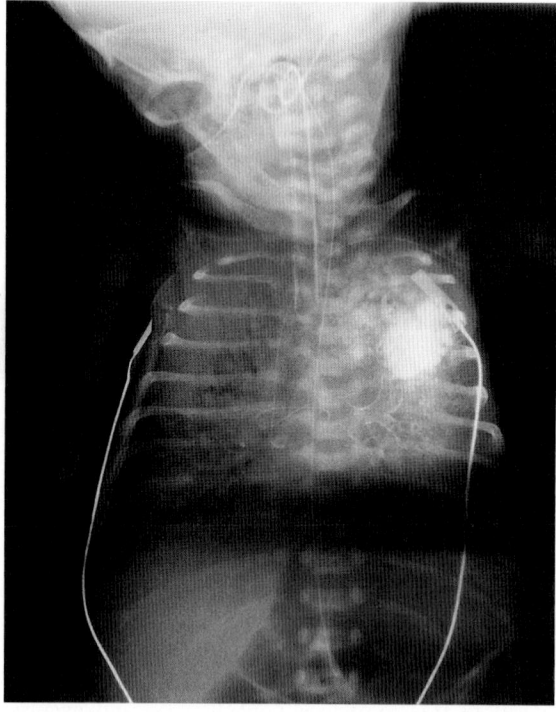

(b)

Fig. 45.17 Chest X-ray of a low-birthweight baby suffering from chronic lung disease. (a) Before, (b) after intrapulmonary infusion of total parenteral nutrition (TPN) solution when the TPN catheter had slipped from the right atrium into the left atrium and out into a pulmonary vein. The blob of interstitial TPN solution can be seen in the upper left zone. (From Rubin et al.[175])

Peripheral venous cannnulation

Peripheral venous cannulae should be inserted into veins in the hands, feet or scalp. More proximal veins should be reserved for central line insertion.

Indications

- Administration of antibiotics, fluids, drug infusions and blood products.

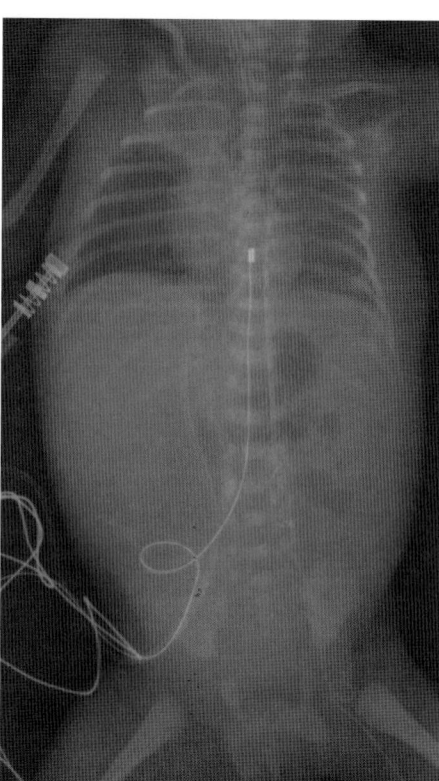

Fig. 45.18 Long line contrast injection into the vertebral venous plexus.

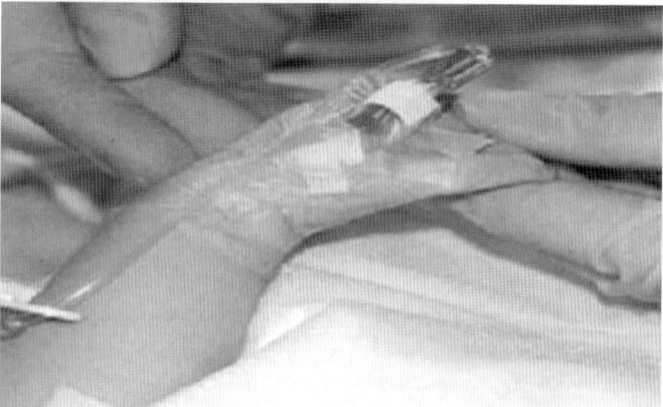

Fig. 45.19 Fixation of a peripheral venous cannula.

Equipment

- As for peripheral arterial cannulation
- G24 cannulae.

Procedure

1. The vein is identified and prepared as described in venous blood sampling.
2. The cannula, held at an angle of 30–45°, is inserted into the vein. As blood flushes into the chamber, the catheter is advanced along the vein. Blood may be aspirated if needed.
3. The catheter is secured with Steri-strips or tape; an overlying transparent dressing provides extra security, allowing visualisation of the entry site (Fig. 45.19).

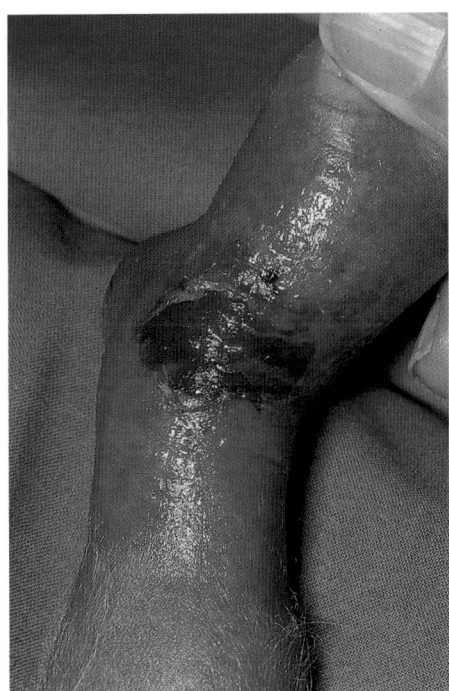

Fig. 45.20 Skin slough following infiltration of intravenous fluids.

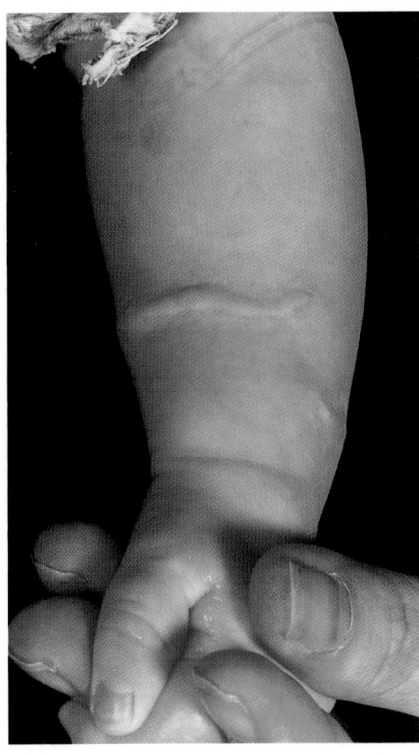

Fig. 45.22 Linear scar where an intravenous infusion had tissued proximal to a tightly occluded dressing.

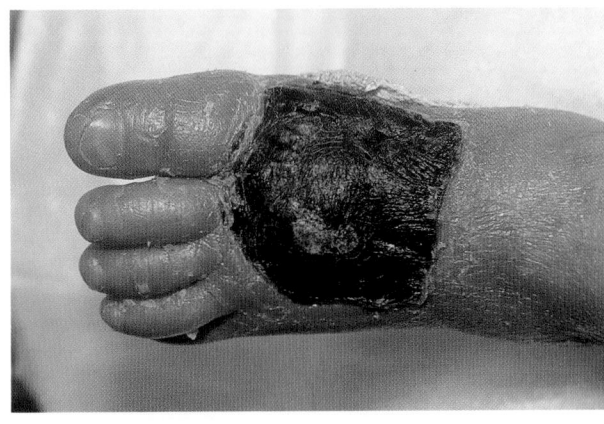

(a)

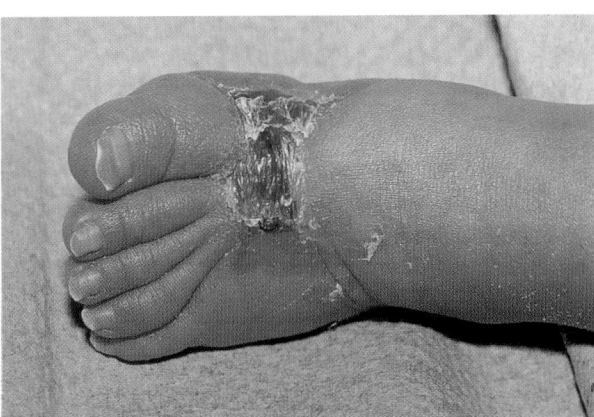

(b)

Fig. 45.21 Severe tissue damage to the dorsum of the foot following extravasation of total parenteral nutrition. This healed causing an extensor contracture. The time interval between (a) and (b) is 5 weeks.

4. Luer-locked connectors and valved connectors allow the use of syringes without needles, reducing the risk of injury to staff and the baby.
5. Fluids should infused with pressure-sensitive pumps.

Complications (intravenous drips)

Peripheral i.v. cannulae are associated with a high incidence of potential complications, including those detailed below.

Subcutaneous extravasation of infusate

This occurs in up to 90% of infusions,[66,131,158] due to spontaneous vessel rupture or thrombosis or if the cannula tip ruptures the vessel wall. Minor extravasation may be unavoidable and causes few problems unless the extravasated volume is large or the infusate hypertonic or an irritant. Some drugs, total parenteral nutrition (TPN) and calcium salts, which precipitate in the tissues, cause particular problem, resulting in skin blistering, ischaemia and necrosis. Large areas of skin and subcutaneous tissue can be damaged (Fig. 45.20), with deformity from the subsequent scarring (Fig. 45.21a, b).

To minimise serious sequelae of this complication:

■ The infusion site should be clearly visible.
■ The vessel should not be obstructed by tightly binding the limb to a splint proximal to the infusion (Fig. 45.22). Not only may this aggravate the tissue ischaemia by localising the subcutaneous infusion to a 'tight blister' if the drip does extravasate, but also the tightness may damage adjacent nerves.[63]
■ The site of an i.v. should always be checked hourly.

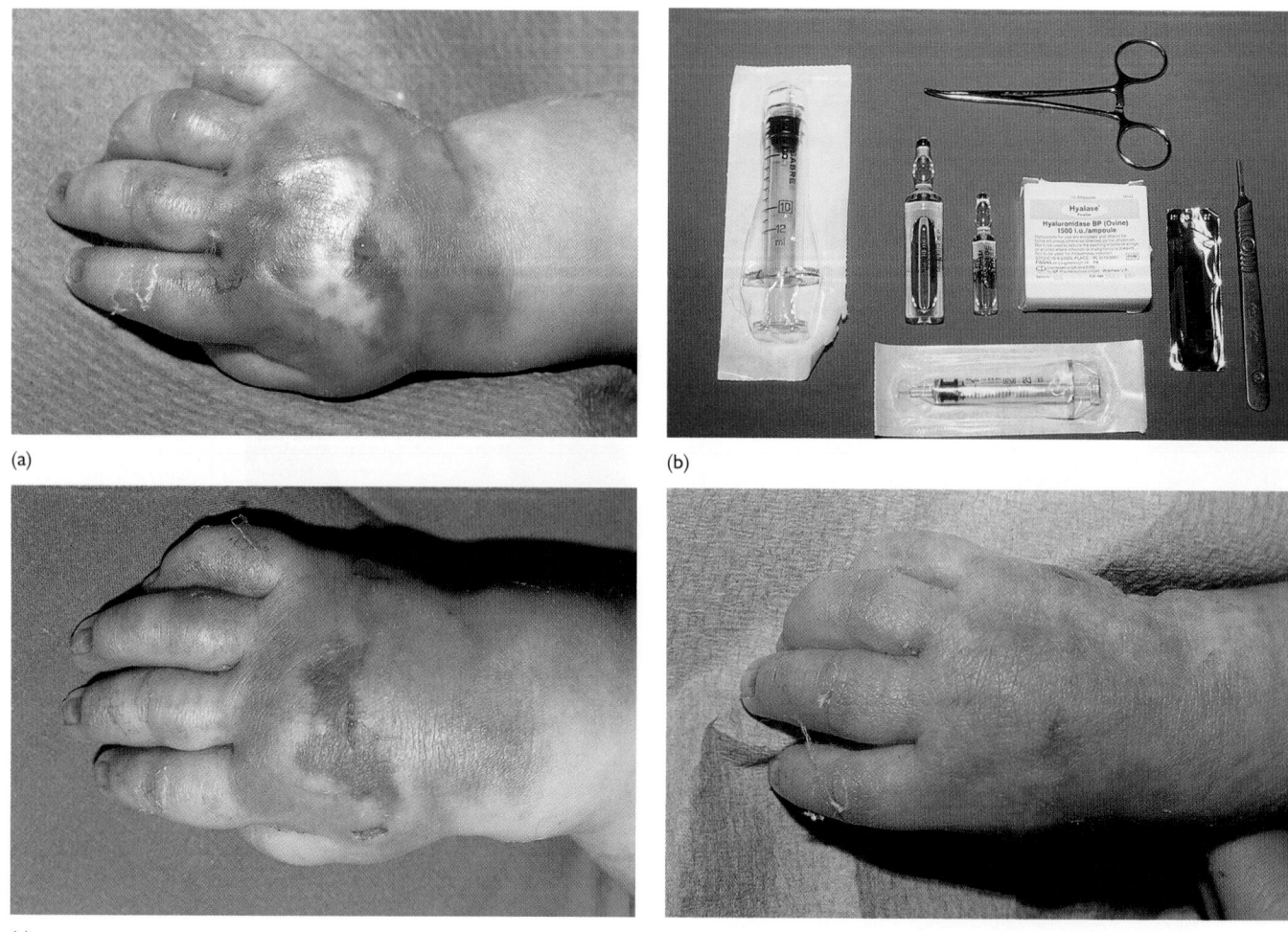

(a)

(b)

(c)

(d)

Fig. 45.23 (a) An acute TPN extravasation injury to the dorsum of the hand. (b) The simple kit needed to treat the problem by irrigation with hyaluronidase and saline. (c) Two small incisions are made on the medial and lateral aspects of the dorsum of the hand using local anaesthesia. The tissue planes are opened with artery forceps. Hyaluronidase and saline are then introduced via one of the incisions, irrigating the subcutaneous tissue on the back of the hand. The fluid exits from the incision on the other side. A marked improvement (c) can be seen immediately following this irrigation. (d) The result 24 hours after irrigation, with well vascularised skin and no sign of skin loss. Compare this with Fig. 45.21.

■ The risk of extravasation is less with Teflon i.v. cannulae than with steel scalp vein needles,[18,158] and if 0.5 U/ml of heparin is added to the infusion.[131]

Once extravasation occurs, the drip must be removed and the limb, if oedematous, should be elevated and kept dry. If there is impending or even established ischaemia or necrosis of the overlying skin, the tissues should be urgently flushed with hyaluronidase solution (500–1000 units of hyaluronidase, followed by free irrigation of up to 500 ml normal saline) to remove all irritant infusate (Fig. 45.23).[46]

Modern pressure-sensitive infusion devices which alarm when the drip is obstructed reduce (but do not eliminate) the risk of extravasation.

Infection

Local phlebitis may occur in about 10% of babies with a peripheral i.v. infusion. Bacteria, in particular *Staph. epidermidis*, may be grown from the site and the cannula. Septicaemia from peripheral i.v. sites is uncommon.[66,207]

Ischaemic change

Subcutaneous i.v. infusions may compromise the arterial supply, causing digital ischaemia[219] (Fig. 45.24). They may also damage adjacent nerves.[103]

Air embolism

This is a constant risk with any infusion.[111] Nursing vigilance is essential for prevention. Small air emboli (the occasional bubble) are common and seem to be without effect, but if more than 5–10 ml of air is infused, death or permanent CNS sequelae are likely.

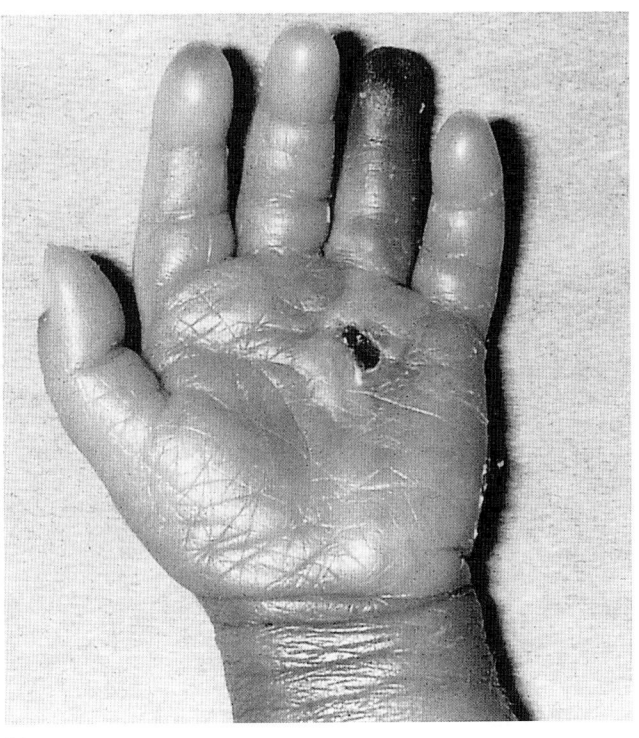

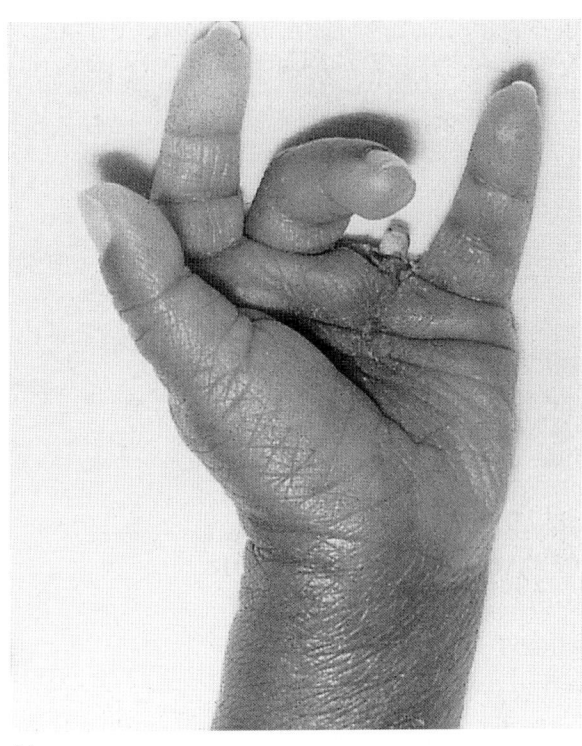

(a)   (b)

Fig. 45.24 (a) Ischaemic change in a finger following subcutaneous infusion and deep infection at a drip site on the dorsum of the hand. (b) Subsequent tissue loss; the remnant of the proximal phalanx was easily removed with forceps.

Limb fractures

Osteopenic babies have developed fractures in association with insertion and fixation of i.v. lines (Fig. 45.25).[159]

Intraosseous lines

Indications

- Collapsed infant, all other routes vascular access having failed
- Administration of resuscitation drugs, fluids, blood products and sampling.

Equipment

- G22, 1.5 inch spinal needle
- G18 intraosseous needle
- Luer-lock extension sets.

Procedure

1. Aseptic technique.
2. Intraosseous needles inserted into the anteromedial tibia 1–2 cm below the tuberosity.

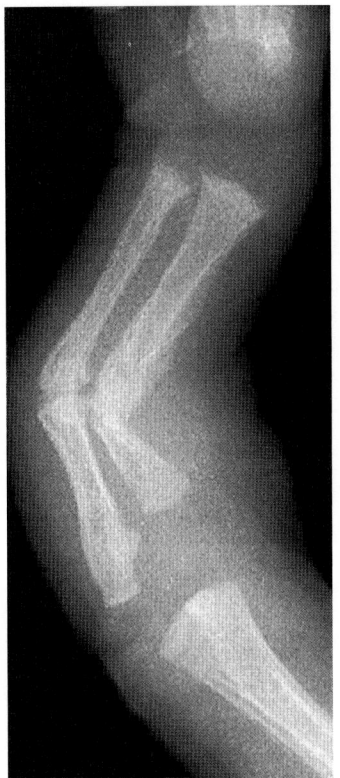

Fig. 45.25 X-ray showing fracture of the radius and ulna sustained during handling for intravenous line insertion in a baby with osteopenia of prematurity.

3. Needle with trochar should be screwed through the bone into the marrow cavity. In small infants, the spinal needle will be easier to use. Once in situ, the trochar should be removed; the needle will be securely held in place by surrounding bone.
4. Bone marrow may be aspirated and fluids infused without resistance. Soft-tissue swelling on the lateral aspect of the leg indicates the needle is incorrectly positioned.
5. Remove the needle when alternative vascular access has been established.

Complications

- Infection
- Fractures, especially in the preterm, osteopenic baby.

Endotracheal intubation

Indications

- Prolonged artificial mechanical ventilation
- Instillation of exogenous surfactant
- Removal of meconium or other secretions from the airway
- Transfer between neonatal units when a baby has poor respiratory drive or airway control.

Equipment

- Straight-blade laryngoscopes, Miller sizes 0 and 1; disposable blades are recommended
- Endotracheal tubes (ETT), straight and shouldered tubes size 2.0 to 4.0
- Resuscitation platform with oxygen, suction, light, heater and timer
- Magills forceps and lubricating jelly for nasal intubation
- Fixation devices, cord ligature, hydrocolloid dressing for the cheek and tape
- Introducer.

Procedure

1. Intubation requires coordination, the ability to visualise the airway holding the laryngoscope in the left hand and manipulate the ETT with the right hand.
2. Shouldered ETT are suitable for oral intubation, straight-sided ETT can be used for oral or nasal intubation. ETT size depends on the infant's birthweight and gestation, as a guide:

Birthweight	Gestation	ETT size
>3000 g	Term	3.5 mm
1000–3000 g	>28 weeks	3.0 mm
<1000 g	<28 weeks	2.5 mm

3. The baby should be positioned on the resuscitaire with the head in the neutral position and the neck slightly extended.

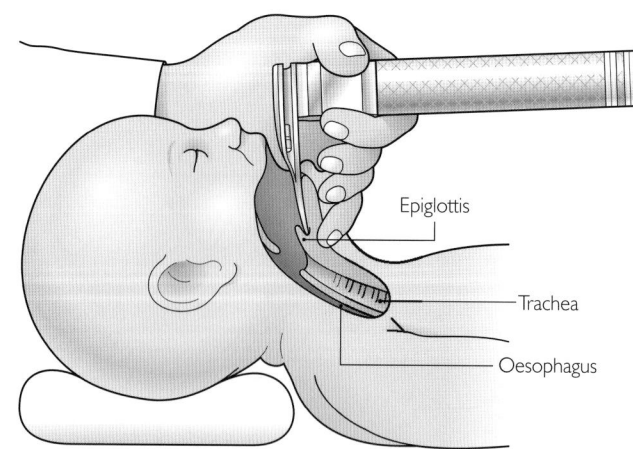

Fig. 45.26 Laryngoscopy. Laryngoscope blade positioned in the vallecula, lifting the epiglottis. Note cricoid pressure can be applied with the little finger.

Avoid over-extension, as the cords will be difficult to visualise. The oro- and nasopharynx should be suctioned to remove secretions. Holding the laryngoscope handle in the left hand, the blade is introduced into the right side of the mouth; the tongue is moved over to the left as the blade is advanced into the vallecula (Fig. 45.26). Gentle vertical traction with the laryngoscope and cricoid pressure with the little finger of the left hand will bring the epiglottis with vocal cords behind into view (Fig. 45.27).

4. An oral ETT should be introduced into the right side of the mouth and positioned over the cords. For nasal intubation, a lubricated straight-sided ETT should be passed vertically in to the nose and rotated horizontally to pass under the turbinates. Gentle pressure should be applied to pass the tube through the choanae into the oropharynx; excessive pressure may damage the cribriform plate, creating a false passage.
5. The ETT can be manipulated through the cords using a finger as a guide, by gripping with Magills forceps, or using an introducer in an oral tube. Introducers must be used with care – if they protrude beyond the tip of the ETT, the trachea may be perforated.
6. Under direct vision, the ETT tip should be positioned about 1 cm below the cords. When positive pressure ventilation is commenced, there should be equal air entry and chest wall movement bilaterally and improvement in heart rate and colour. The ETT should be firmly held at the nares or lip to prevent accidental extubation or migration into the bronchus.
7. The upper lip and cheek should be cleaned to remove vernix and secretions. A hydrocolloid dressing should be applied to the cheeks.
8. Nasal ETT should be secured with the assistance of nursing staff. A cord ligature is knotted above and below the tube; the ends are stuck down to the hydrocolloid with H-shaped zinc oxide tape which is partly wrapped around the tube for additional security (Fig. 45.28).
9. Oral tubes can be fixed with adhesive devices that are positioned along the top lip and cheeks. These devices incorporate a toothed clamp in velcro which securely grips the tube, avoiding distortion of the lips and mouth (Fig. 45.29).

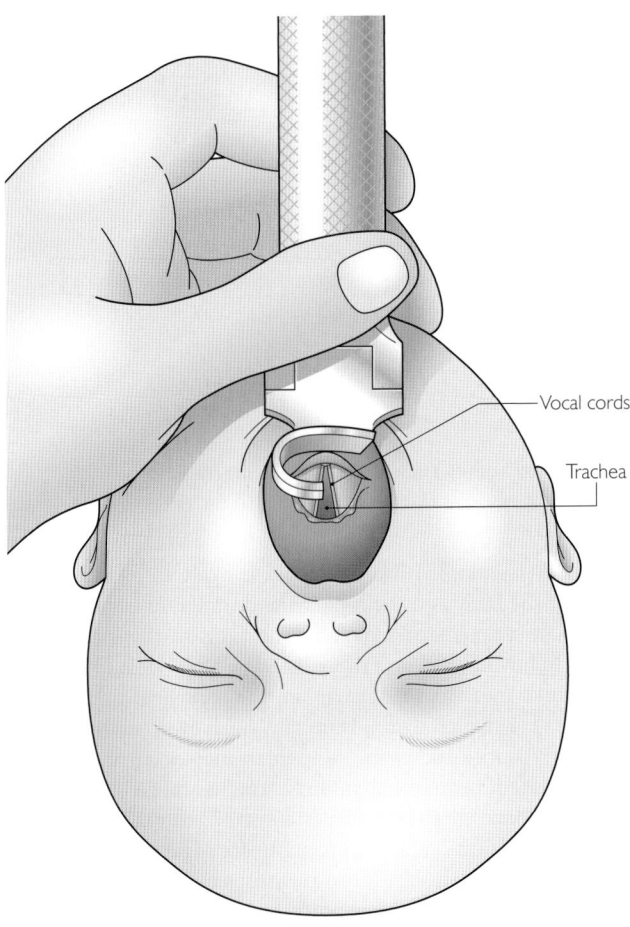

Fig. 45.27 Laryngoscopy. Visualisation of the vocal cords.

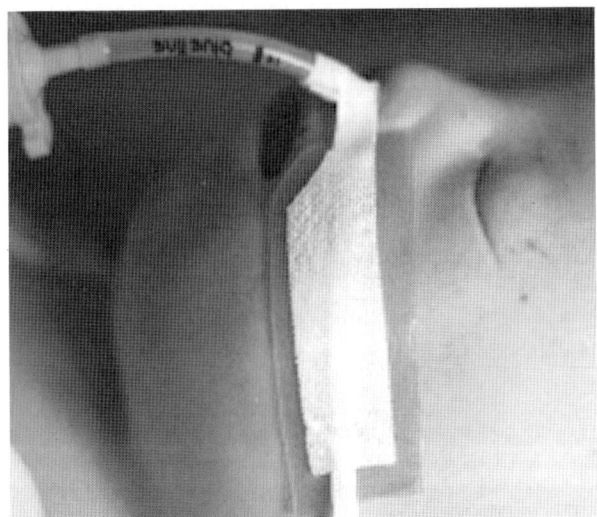

Fig. 45.28 Fixation of nasal endotracheal tube.

10. After fixation, air entry and chest wall movement should be checked; the ETT is cut down to reduce dead space and, if appropriate, surfactant administered via a fine catheter passed down the tube.

11. ETT position must be confirmed with a chest X-ray (CXR), noting the position at the lips or nose. Documentation must

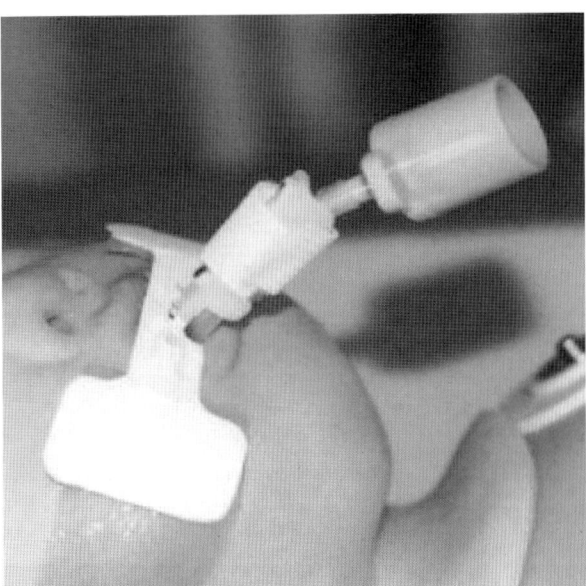

Fig. 45.29 Fixation device for oral endotracheal tube.

be completed. The tube must be carefully observed to ensure that it remains in place.

Elective reintubation

For elective intubations or reintubations, it is appropriate to sedate the baby with morphine (100 microgram/kg). Muscle relaxation with, for example, suxamethonium (3 mg/kg/dose) is more controversial, and experienced personnel must be available. If replacing an oral tube, a new nasal ETT can be positioned and gripped with Magill forceps to be advanced through the cords as the old tube is removed by an assistant. This can be accomplished within seconds with virtually no disturbance to the baby. Sometimes there is difficulty passing an ETT through the nose. In these cases, a fine feeding tube should be passed through the nose and visualised in the oropharynx; the nasal ETT can be threaded over the feeding tube with confidence that a false passage will not be created. Once through the nose, the feeding tube should be removed and the ETT manipulated through the cords.

Complications

These are wide-ranging and may be severe. The majority are dealt with elsewhere in this book. Complications related to fixation of the ventilatory devices are listed in Table 45.9.

A wide variety of local injuries can occur from acute and chronic trauma to the nose, mouth, pharynx, larynx (Fig. 45.30) and trachea (Fig. 45.31). Although some of these local complications are rare, others, such as the development of a palatal groove with an oral ETT, may occur in 50% of neonates so treated,[60] although only a small proportion of these progress to perforation, causing iatrogenic cleft palate.[57] Nasal damage is more likely with ETT (Fig. 45.32) than continuous positive airways pressure (CPAP) tubes, though it can still occur with double-prong

Table 45.9 Injury from application of ventilation devices

Injury	Comment	Reference
Local trauma to mouth, fauces with laryngoscope/ETT		
Subglottic stenosis		
Nasal damage and stenosis		21, 75, 173
Palatal grooves from oral ETT		60, 71
Acquired cleft palate		57
Defective dentition*		139
Perforation of airway with ETT		119, 190
Intracerebellar haemorrhage	From tight fixation	152
Corneal ulceration	Inappropriate size face mask	41

* This can be caused by pressure from the laryngoscope during intubation or from the indwelling oral endotracheal tube (ETT).

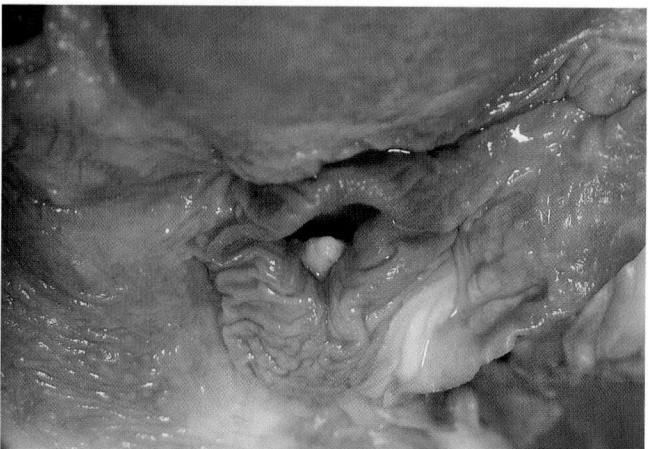

Fig. 45.30 Granuloma on interarytenoid fold in a baby of 30 weeks' gestation who had been on IPPV for 2 weeks.

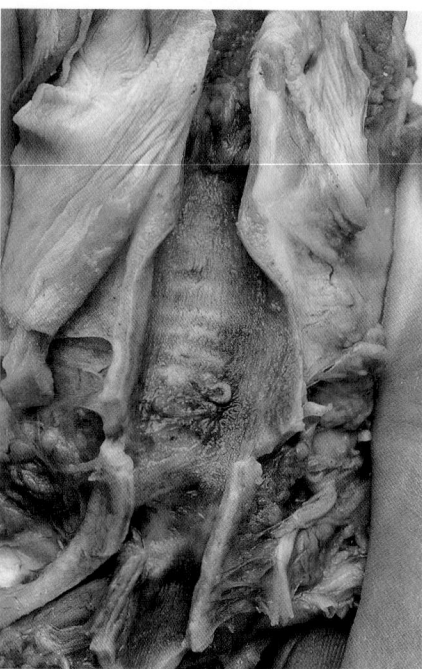

Fig. 45.31 Severe ulceration in distal trachea in a baby who had been on IPPV for several months.

nasal CPAP (Fig. 45.33). Nasal damage is likely to be more severe the smaller the baby and the longer the duration of intubation.

The most serious iatrogenic complications to the local airways and lungs following IPPV are those listed in Table 45.1. Other problems include metaplastic change in the laryngeal and tracheal mucosa,[68,91,226] which will eventually heal even with the ETT still in situ;[74] subglottic cysts,[43,55] which may occur in up to 7% of ex-intubated premature infants; tracheomegaly;[23] tracheobronchomalacia;[54] and bronchial stenosis,[140] though the latter is probably a complication of inappropriate and vigorous ETT suction.

The presence of the ETT compromises eustachian tube function, leading to otitis media.[51] Necrotising tracheobronchitis[27] is an often fatal complication which is almost specific to high-frequency jet ventilation (pp. 525–6).

Endotracheal suctioning may also cause local trauma to the mucosa, as shown by the frequent presence of flecks of blood in the aspirate. Granulomata may form at the carina or in the more peripheral airways[140] and the airways may be perforated by the suction catheter, resulting in pneumothorax and a bronchopleural fistula.[76,216]

Aspiration of the chest

Indications

- Drainage of a tension pneumothorax
- Drainage of a pleural effusion.

Equipment

- G21–G25 needle, three-way tap, syringe
- G21G–G25 butterfly, universal container, sterile water.

Procedure

1. Clinical, cold light, X-ray diagnosis of tension pneumothorax.
2. Aseptic technique, skin cleaned.

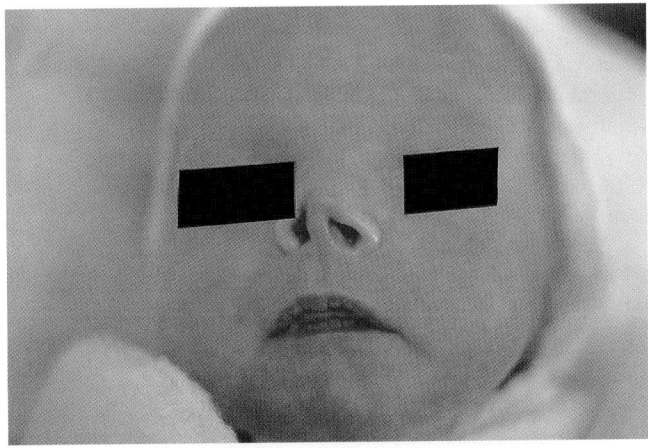

(a)

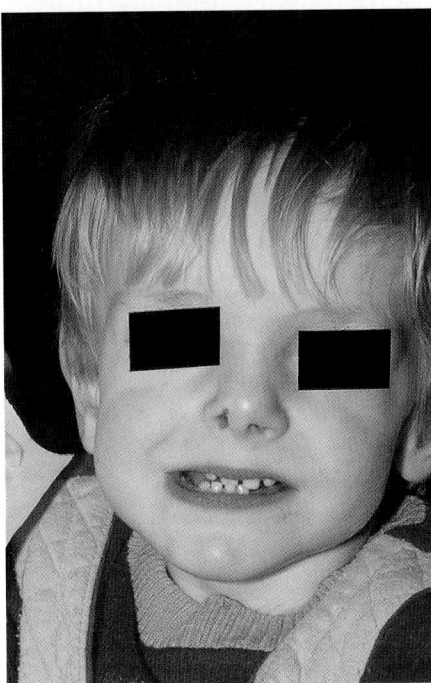

(b)

Fig. 45.32 (a) A notch in the nose cased by a nasoendotracheal tube during the neonatal period. (b) The same child more than 1 year later.

3. Pleural cavity entered through second intercostal space in mid-clavicular line.
4. Butterfly tubing should be placed under water and the air will bubble out. Needles should be connected to a short extension set which is placed under water. The tubing can also be attached to a three-way tap and air aspirated by syringe.
5. When no more air can be obtained, remove needle and cover entry site. Perform a CXR and consider formal chest drain insertion.
6. Document procedure.

Complications

See below, under chest drains.

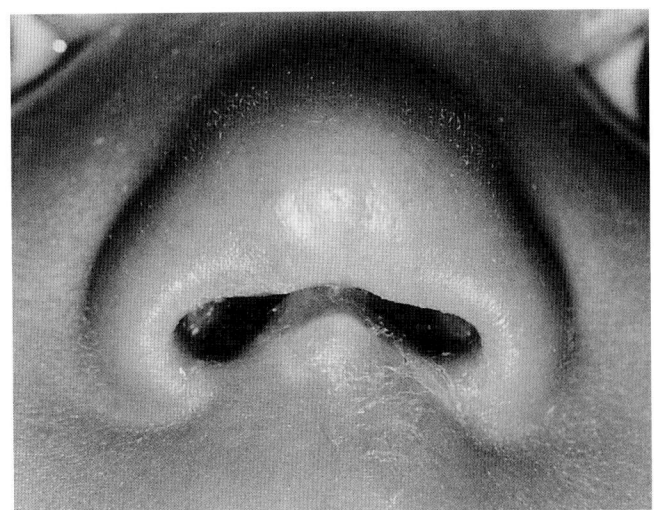

Fig. 45.33

Chest drain insertion

Indications

- Drainage of pneumothorax
- Drainage of pleural fluid.

Equipment

- Chest drain insertion pack containing drapes, intercostal drains, scalpel, sutures, Steri-strips, adhesive dressings
- Underwater drain, collection system.

Procedure

1. Aseptic technique. Confirm correct side of chest for insertion.
2. The infant should be positioned with the affected side elevated 45° to the horizontal, with a towel under the back. The baby should be held with the ipsilateral arm above the head.
3. The skin in the axilla should be cleaned with antibacterial solution. If time allows, 1% lidocaine (lignocaine) should be instilled in to the tissues of the fourth intercostal space in the mid-axillary line.
4. A small incision (1–2 cm) is made in the intercostal space, parallel to the ribs. The tissues down to the pleura should be bluntly dissected with artery forceps. The pleura should be nicked with the scalpel and the drain advanced 2–3 cm into the pleural cavity with the aid of artery forceps, not the introducer.
5. Chest drains may be inserted atraumatically using the Seldinger technique. An introducer is inserted through the intercostal chest wall and a guidewire passed into the pleural cavity. A track for insertion is created by threading a dilator over the guide and then the chest drain is threaded into position.
6. Drains inserted for the management of pneumothoraces should be directed anteriorly and apically.

7. Drains placed for the removal of pleural fluid should be directed posteriorly and towards the base of the lung.

8. When the drain is connected to the underwater system, bubbles should appear. Resolution of the pneumothorax will be aided by the application of negative pressure, 5–10 cm H_2O, via a pump connected to the underwater system. Fluid should flow freely if a pleural effusion is being drained.

9. A zinc oxide flag is placed around the drain close to the chest wall; two sutures are positioned through the wound and the skin pulled snugly around the drain to prevent air entry. A transparent dressing should be applied (Fig. 45.34). Purse-string sutures are not necessary and should not be used.

10. A CXR must be performed to confirm that the drain has been correctly placed and that the pneumothorax or pleural effusion is resolving.

Complications

- Haemorrhage may occur if the vascular bundle in the intercostal groove below each rib is damaged
- Distortion of breast growth – avoid the breast bud area
- Amazia – avoid the breast bud area
- Diaphragmatic eventration[124]
- Lung perforation[133]
- Lung puncture by the pneumothorax drain – this occurs in up to 25% of cases
- Pericardium damage[165]
- Thoracic duct damage[106]
- Phrenic nerve injury.[6]

Chest drain removal

Once the pneumothorax or pleural effusion has resolved, the drain should be removed. When bubbling ceases, suction should be discontinued, the drain can be clamped, and a repeat CXR performed to check that there has been no reaccumulation of the pneumothorax before the drain is removed.

Equipment

- Dressing pack, stitch cutter, Steri-strips.

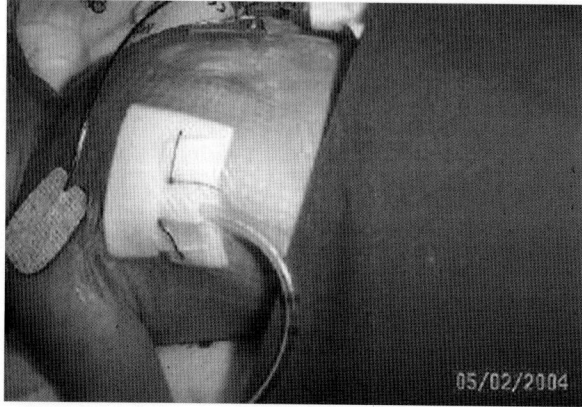

Fig. 45.34 Sutured tape fixation of chest drain.

Procedure

1. Remove dressings and cut anchoring sutures.
2. The chest drain should then be withdrawn rapidly from the pleural cavity while pinching the skin on either side of the drain site to close the incision.
3. Steri-strips should be applied across the incision and covered with a transparent dressing, providing an airtight seal. Purse-string sutures produce unsightly scars.
4. CXR to ensure that the pneumothorax has not reaccumulated.

Feeding tubes

Nasogastric/orogastric feeding tubes

Indications

- Facilitate enteral nutrition in preterm, ventilated infants
- Decompress distended stomach or bowel.

Equipment

- Feeding tubes (4 Fr <1000 g, 6 Fr other babies, 8–10 Fr for decompression)
- pH paper
- Hydrocolloid dressing and tape.

Procedure

1. Measurement of length for insertion: nasogastric (NG) tube, xiphisternum to ear tip + ear tip to nares; orogastric (OG) tube, xiphisternum to nares + 1 cm.
2. The baby should be supine with the head in the midline. NG tubes should be lightly lubricated and passed downwards through the nostril, and OG over the tongue and into the oropharynx to the predetermined length. Tubes should be passed in a few seconds. The baby must be closely observed for apnoea and bradycardia.
3. Correct placement is confirmed by the aspiration of acidic fluid on pH testing or auscultation over the stomach as air is injected; X-rays are not routinely required but should be performed if there is doubt about the tube position.
4. NG tubes are fixed to the cheek and OG tubes to the chin. The tube should be taped to the hydrocolloid dressing on the skin.
5. Tube position must be checked regularly. Bile-stained aspirates may indicate that the tube has slipped into the duodenum (yellow bile) or, more importantly, intra-abdominal pathology (green bile).
6. When a tube has been passed to decompress the bowel, an accurate record of fluid losses must be maintained, to ensure appropriate fluid replacement. When babies are on CPAP, feeding tubes should be left on free drainage to vent the stomach.[67]
7. Tubes should be changed every 7 days to prevent bacterial contamination.

Nasojejunal feeding tubes

Indications

- Facilitate enteral nutrition in infants with delayed gastric emptying.

Equipment

- Nasojejunal (NJ) feeding tube
- As for NG/OG tubes.

Procedure

1. Measurement of length for insertion: orogastric length + 8 cm or nares to ankle, and mark the NJ tube with length to stomach and jejunum.
2. With a separate gastric tube in situ, the NJ tube should be advanced to the stomach. Fluid injected into the NJ should be aspirated from the OG/NG tube. Turning the baby right side down encourages migration through the pylorus. With time, the jejunal marker should reach the tip of the nares, and the NJ position confirmed by X-ray. Secure the tube as described for NG tubes.
3. Continuous milk feeds should be commenced. Milk aspirates from the stomach indicate that the tube has slipped back.

Complications from nasogastric and nasojejunal tubes

Bleeding gastric erosions and ulcers occur frequently in ill very-low-birthweight neonates.[120] Indwelling NG tubes inevitably cause trauma to the mucosa of the stomach and oesophagus and so aggravate this problem. Coffee-ground aspirate is common, but frank haematemesis is rare. The tendency to haematemesis is aggravated by drugs, especially tolazoline, steroids and indometacin (indomethacin) (Table 45.2), and treatment with ranitidine is indicated (p. 1283).

The gut may be perforated at any level by NG and NJ tubes or during difficult endotracheal intubation. The pharynx and oesophagus are the most common sites.[90,102,109] Excessive force may not necessarily be the cause, as rupture may occur through an area of congenital weakness.

Babies present with oesophageal obstruction if the leak is limited to the mediastinum. However, if the pleural cavity is breached, they present with a pleural effusion, pneumothorax and respiratory distress. Treatment is conservative, with i.v. nutrition, drainage of the pleural fluid and antibiotics.[90]

Perforation of the upper small intestine presents with clinical deterioration and signs of peritonitis. Abdominal X-ray may show the tube to be incorrectly placed, together with a pneumoperitoneum.[102,129] PVC tubes, previously used for NJ feeding, become hard and rigid after being in situ for some time[29,81] and so should not be used. Silicone tubes are preferable, but even these can perforate the bowel.[156]

Perforation of the cribiform plate of the ethmoid bone by an NG tube seems an unlikely complication but this has been

reported.[214] A gentle technique and a knowledge of anatomy should be used whenever any sort of tube is passed.

Suprapubic aspiration

Indications

- Obtain uncontaminated urine for microbiological culture.

Equipment

- Sterile dressing pack
- Syringes (2.5, 5 ml), G25 needle.

Procedure

1. If possible, undertake abdominal ultrasound immediately before the procedure, to confirm full bladder (Fig. 45.35).
2. Spontaneous urination may occur, allowing a clean catch sample.
3. Aseptic technique. The skin between the umbilicus and symphysis pubis should be cleaned with antibacterial solution or swab.
4. With the baby supine, an assistant holds the lower limbs with hips abducted. The abdominal wall is punctured in the midline 1 cm above the symphysis and the needle (with syringe attached) advanced perpendicularly, aspirating continuously until urine is aspirated (Fig. 45.36). Send sample to the laboratory and cover puncture site.

Complications

These are rare.[162]

- Haematuria
- Viscus damage.[65]

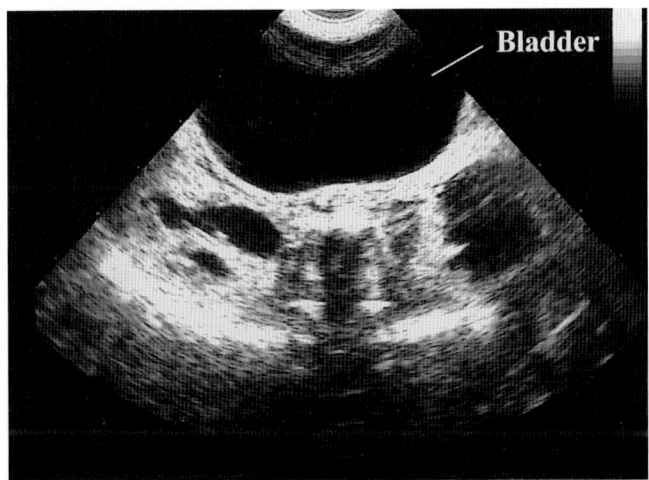

Fig. 45.35 Abdominal ultrasound scan confirming a full bladder.

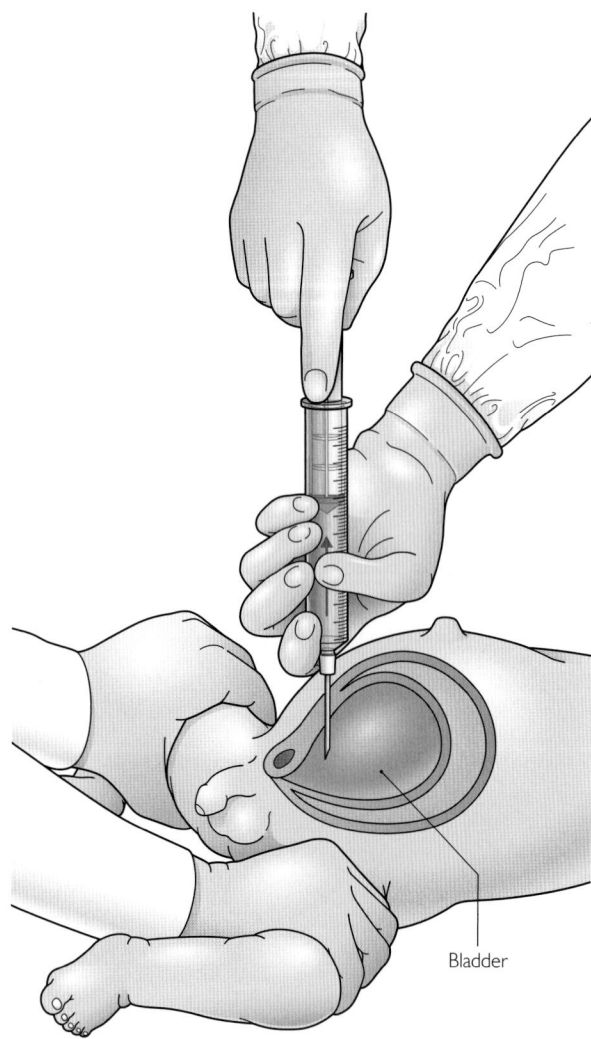

Fig. 45.36 Technique for suprapubic bladder aspiration.

Suprapubic catheterisation

Indications

- Suspected posterior urethral valves
- Urethral trauma
- Following urethral surgery.

Equipment

- Sterile dressing pack, local anaesthetic
- Suprapubic catheterisation pack and collection system.

Procedure

Ideally, this should be performed by or following consultation with paediatric urologist.

1. Abdominal ultrasound to confirm diagnosis.
2. Preparation and positioning as for suprapubic aspiration. Local anaesthetic instilled into the abdominal wall.
3. The bladder is entered with an introducer and urine obtained exactly as described for suprapubic aspiration. The guidewire is threaded into the bladder and the suprapubic catheter is positioned using the Seldinger technique or use 'Cystofix' kit.
4. The anchoring flange system is fitted and the system secured to the abdominal wall and collecting system attached.

Complications

- Infection
- Haematuria
- Viscus injury[65]
- Extravasation of urine.

Transurethral catheterisation

Indications

- To obtain uncontaminated urine specimen for culture, in/out catheterisation
- Close monitoring of urine output when nappy weighing is inaccurate or urinary retention is not responding to bladder expression.

Equipment

- Sterile dressing pack, Steri-strips
- Fine feeding tube.

Procedure

1. Aseptic technique. Clean the vulva/penis with antibacterial solution.
2. Lubricated feeding tube is gently advanced through the urethral meatus into the bladder. Free-flowing or aspirated urine indicates correct placement.
3. The catheter should be fixed to the abdominal wall with a sandwich of adhesive tape and connected to a collecting system. Catheters should be removed as soon as possible, to minimise infection.

Complications

- Septicaemia may result from instrumentation of the urinary tract in the presence of infection
- Creation of a false passage with the risk of a urethral stricture can result from traumatic catheterisation. If the catheter does not pass into the bladder with ease, specialist advice should be sought

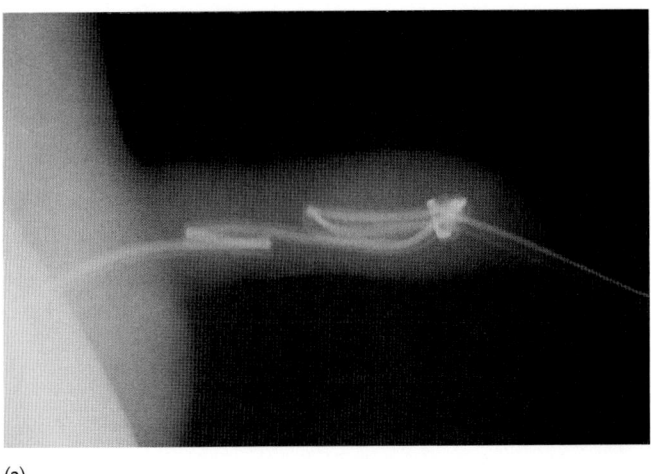
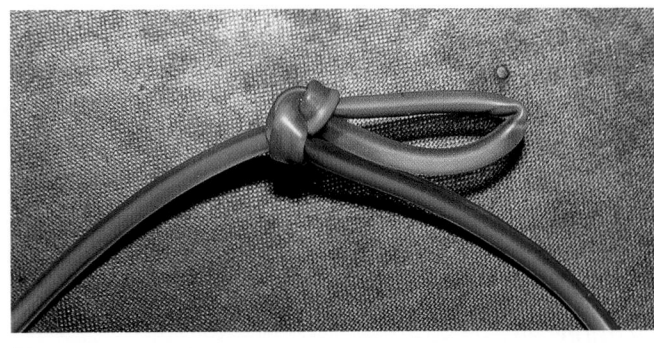

Fig. 45.37 The hazards of excessive length of bladder catheters. (a) The knotted catheter impacted in the penile urethra during attempted removal. (b) The knot after removal.

- Kinking of the catheter as the bladder empties, obstructing the lumen, leads to urine bypassing the catheter. This may occur with an excessive length of catheter in the bladder
- The catheter may tie itself into a knot, making removal very difficult (Fig. 45.37a, b).

Cerebrospinal fluid collection

Lumbar puncture

Indications

- Septic screen to diagnose meningitis
- Investigation of neonatal seizures
- Relief of raised intracranial pressure in communicating hydrocephalus.

Equipment

- Dressing pack, universal containers
- G22, 1.5 inch spinal needle with stylet.

Procedure

1. Contraindications include lumbosacral abnormalities, bleeding diathesis and thrombocytopenia.
2. An experienced assistant is vital to the success of the procedure. The infant is held left side down; the back must be vertical and gently flexed, opening the intervertebral spaces. Some infants may not tolerate this position and the investigation may need to be delayed or a lumbar puncture attempted with the infant in sitting position.
3. The L4 spinous process is identified on a line joining the iliac crests. The back is cleaned with antibacterial solution and the needle inserted though the L3/L4 intervertebral space. At a depth of 1–1.5 cm there will be a change of resistance as the dura is penetrated. Cerebrospinal fluid (CSF) should be obtained when the stylet is removed; flow may be facilitated by carefully rotating the needle. Bloodstained fluid indicates that the venous plexus on the posterior surface of the vertebral bodies has been damaged by inserting the needle too far; rarely, bloody taps are due to subarachnoid haemorrhages.
4. Three serial CSF samples are collected in universal containers for microscopy, culture and protein analysis. Two to three drops of CSF are collected in a fluoride tube for glucose measurement (for normal values, see Appendix 6).
5. In hydrocephalus, an opening pressure can be determined by attaching a manonometer to the spinal needle via a three-way tap.
6. After collection of sufficient fluid, the stylet should be replaced and the needle withdrawn. Adhesive dressing spray should be applied.

Ventricular tap

Indications

- Diagnosis of ventriculitis
- Drainage of CSF in non-communicating hydrocephalus
- Instillation of intrathecal antibiotics.

Equipment

- As for lumbar puncture.

Procedure

1. Cranial ultrasound is performed to confirm ventriculomegaly and determine the depth for needle insertion.
2. Hair is shaved from the lateral angle of the anterior fontanelle and the skin cleaned with antibacterial solution. Strict aseptic technique is required.

3. With the baby supine, an assistant holds the head in the midline. The spinal needle is inserted at the angle of the fontanelle and advanced smoothly in a medial direction to the required depth. The stylet is removed and an extension set carefully attached to the needle; opening pressure can be recorded with a manometer. Diagnostic samples for laboratory analysis can be obtained or therapeutic drainage undertaken with slow aspiration by syringe.
4. After needle removal, the area must be carefully sprayed with adhesive dressing.

Subdural taps

Indications

■ Diagnostic/therapeutic drainage of collections causing raised intracranial pressure.

Equipment

■ As for ventricular tap.

Procedure

1. Perform cranial imaging to confirm collection.
2. As for ventricular puncture: a short spinal needle, G22 butterfly, is inserted into the collection from the lateral angle of the anterior fontanelle, and aspirated.

Aspiration from Rickham reservoirs

Rickham reservoirs are surgically inserted for administration of intrathecal antibiotics or repeated CSF aspiration.

Procedure

1. Strict aseptic technique. The overlying skin is cleaned with antibacterial solution.
2. The reservoir is gently gripped and a G25 butterfly inserted perpendicularly through the skin and reservoir membrane. CSF (10–15 ml/kg) should be aspirated slowly over several minutes.
3. After removal of the needle, the site should be sprayed with adhesive dressing.

Complications of CSF drainage

■ Infection – there is a risk of introducing microorganisms during CSF sampling
■ Trauma – parenchymal cysts may develop along the needle track with venticular taps
■ Haemorrhage – usually local and settles spontaneously
■ Haematoma around spine – rare, but may cause permanent nerve damage. Coagulopathies and thrombocytopenia need excluding prior to the procedure.

Bone marrow aspiration

Indications

■ Investigation of marrow dysfunction
■ Diagnosis of marrow involvement in malignancies.

Equipment

■ Dressing pack
■ G22, 1.5 inch spinal needle, bone marrow aspiration needle
■ Appropriate slides and assay bottles.

Procedure

1. Aseptic technique. Local anaesthetic is infiltrated at the aspiration site.
2. The tibial tuberosity is the preferred site in the neonate; anterior iliac spine or posterior iliac crests can also be used.
3. The needle is held perpendicular to the bone, and carefully screwed into the bone marrow cavity.
4. Marrow should be aspirated and prepared as directed by the haematologist.

Complications

■ See intraosseous line insertion.

Drainage of pericardial effusion

Pericardial effusions should be suspected if an infant collapses with any form of central venous line in situ. More discrete clinical signs include tachycardia, poor perfusion, soft heart sounds and increasing cardiomegaly on CXR.

Indications

■ Cardiac tamponade confirmed by echocardiogram (Fig. 45.38)
■ Cardiac arrest in the presence of a central venous catheter.

Equipment

■ G22–G24 cannula, syringe.

Procedure

1. Echocardiographic confirmation only if time allows.
2. In an unresponsive arrest setting, a 'blind' pericardial tap must be performed using the subxiphisternal approach.

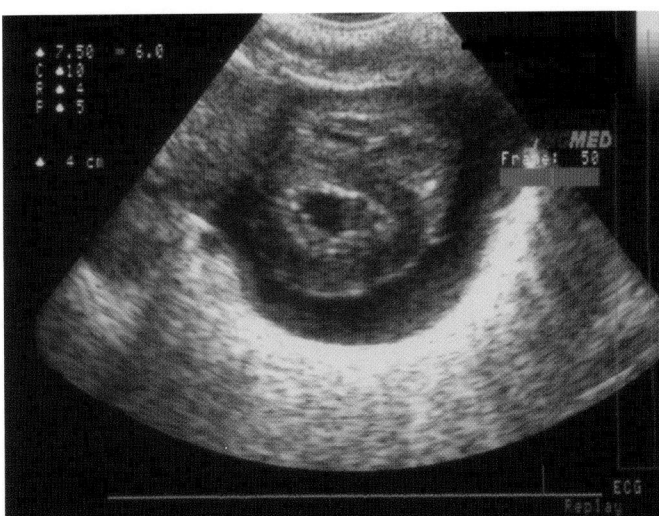

Fig. 45.38 Transthoracic echocardiogram showing large pericardial effusion.

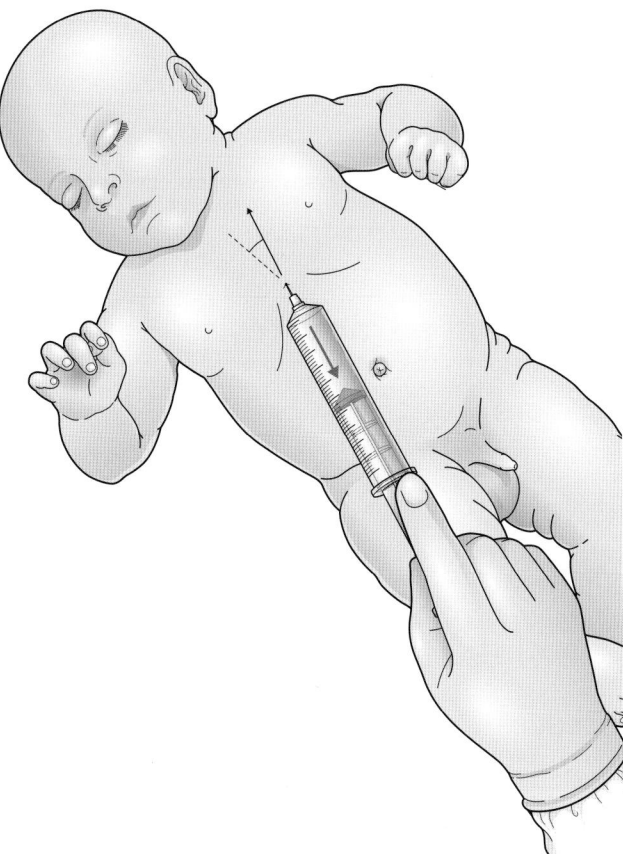

Fig. 45.39 The subxiphisternal approach to drain a pericardial effusion; note the cannula is directed toward the left shoulder.

3. After cleaning the skin, a 22G/24G cannula should slowly be inserted at an angle of 30° to the skin, directed towards the left shoulder, to a depth of between 1–2 cm, maintaining suction (Fig. 45.39). If blood is aspirated, the needle has been inserted into the heart. The withdrawal of a small volume of fluid (5–10 ml) can be lifesaving. Rarely, a cannula or drain is needed to be left in situ. Bleeding is not a problem when the cannula is withdrawn.

4. Careful cardiac observations are required following the procedure.

Complications

- Cardiac puncture
- Arrthymias.

Drainage of pneumopericardium/ pneumomediastinuem

Indications

- Consider this if there is sudden collapse in the presence of airleaks with no response to standard resuscitation.

Equipment

- As for pericardial effusion.

Procedure

1. X-ray confirmation if time allows; echocardiography will be unhelpful.
2. Approach and procedure as for drainage of pericardial effusion. Drainage of a pneumomediastinum will require superficial cannula insertion.
3. Drainage of a small volume of air may produce a dramatic improvement.
4. CXR following procedure.

Complications

- As for pericardial aspiration.

Exchange transfusion

Indications

- Hyperbilirubinaemia due to haemolytic disease or other causes
- Severe sepsis or disseminated intravascular coagulation.

Equipment

- Functioning arterial and/or central venous catheters
- Cross-matched fresh blood for either single or double volume exchange
- Blood administration sets, warming coils
- Three-way or four-way taps, depending on the method chosen.

Procedure

1. Careful cardiovascular, biochemical and haematological monitoring.
2. Secure vascular access must be established before this specialised blood is run through the warming coils, to avoid waste. Central lines are less likely to fail during this long procedure and offer the most secure route. An exchange transfusion can be performed as either an 'in and out' exchange via a single central umbilical venous (or arterial) line with a four-way tap, or a peripheral arterial catheter, UAC or UVC can be used to withdraw blood and a second large venous line used to infuse the fresh blood.
3. The administration set and blood-warming coil should be primed.
4. The volume of the aliquots is determined by the size of the baby; usually 5–20 ml of blood can be withdrawn over 5 minutes. A closed system should be employed; withdrawn blood must be discarded into a waste bag.
5. A 2.5 kg infant will require 400 ml of blood in a double volume exchange (80 ml/kg/exchange) withdrawing 20 ml aliquots over 5 minutes at a time. The whole procedure will last about 100 minutes. Acid–base status, electrolytes, calcium, coagulation, glucose and haematology should be measured at the midpoint and end of the exchange.
6. The catheters should be left in situ until no further exchanges are required.

Complications

- Infection
- Thromboembolic events
- Acid–base, electrolyte, glucose, coagulation and platelet disturbance
- Haemodynamic disturbance
- Hypothermia if blood not warmed
- Transfusion reactions
- Complications from intravascular lines used.

Dilutional exchange transfusion

Indications

- Polycythemia, central venous packed cell volume (PCV) >75% in asymptomatic infants

- PCV >65% in symptomatic, hypoglycaemic, jittery, growth-restricted infants.

Equipment

- Vascular access as for exchange transfusion; usually a peripheral arterial line with a venous line for return of saline
- Saline.

Procedure

1. PCV confirmed with free-flowing venous blood.
2. Calculate volume of blood to be removed and replaced using the formula:

$$\text{Volume (ml)} = \text{Total blood volume} \times \frac{(\text{Observed PCV} - \text{Desired PCV})}{\text{Observed PCV}}$$

3. Withdraw blood as for exchange transfusion; replace with saline.
4. Repeat free-flowing PCV.

Complications

- Potentially as for exchange transfusion, except for transfusion reactions.

Abdominal paracentesis

Indications

- Diagnostic tap
- Therapeutic tap, to reduce intra-abdominal pressure.

Equipment

- Dressing pack, G20/22/24 i.v. catheters.

Procedure

1. Aseptic technique. Local anaesthesia to incision site.
2. Fluid should be aspirated from the left iliac fossa to avoid the liver and spleen. The cannula is inserted through the abdominal wall into the peritoneal cavity and the soft catheter advanced as the trochar is withdrawn, minimising risk of bowel perforation.

Complications

- Infection
- Trauma to bowel or solid viscus
- Haemorrhage.

Peritoneal dialysis

The management of renal failure should be discussed with a paediatric nephrologist. Peritoneal dialysis (PD) will not be possible if there is intra-abdominal pathology nor when there is respiratory compromise which will deteriorate with a splinted diaphragm.

Indications

- Renal failure with significant hyperkalaemia, metabolic acidosis, oliguria.

Equipment

- Dressing pack, Luer-lock extension sets
- PD catheter, PD fluids
- Urinometer.

Procedure

1. Aseptic technique, local anaesthesia.
2. PD catheters can be inserted surgically or percutaneously using the Seldinger technique either in the left iliac fossa or midway between the umbilicus and symphysis pubis.
3. An introducer is inserted through the abdominal wall, the abdomen is filled with 20 ml/kg of warm dialysate and the PD catheter inserted over a guidewire.
4. Dialysis cycles should usually be 60 minutes: 20 ml/kg of dialysate is infused, dwell time 40 minutes, drainage time 20 minutes. The volumes and duration of cycles should be altered depending on the clinical response and after discussion with a nephrologist.
5. Discontinue PD when an adequate urine output and normalising biochemistry has returned.

Complications

- As for paracentesis
- Respiratory compromise from diaphragmatic splinting
- Fluid and electrolyte balance may be over-corrected.

Haemofiltration

Arteriovenous haemofiltration is technically more difficult than peritoneal dialysis, but it is the method of choice in the fluid-overloaded hydropic infant with respiratory difficulties. Successful haemofiltration can be carried out via large umbilical arterial and venous catheters, provided the infant has an adequate blood pressure to drive blood through the filter. This specialist procedure should be conducted in an intensive care unit under the supervision of paediatric nephrologists.

Miscellaneous skin, musculoskeletal and soft tissue injuries

Apart from the procedures discussed above, the baby's skin, soft tissues or indeed musculoskeletal system may be damaged by:

- cuts during caesarean section;
- clothing acting as tourniquets;[17]
- scalp clips[5] during labour;
- intramuscular injections;[11,70,143,189]
- cut-downs for vascular access;
- chest physiotherapy;[228]
- incubator-related injuries;[48]
- adhesive materials used for fixation – this may be reduced by the use of Opsite;[62]

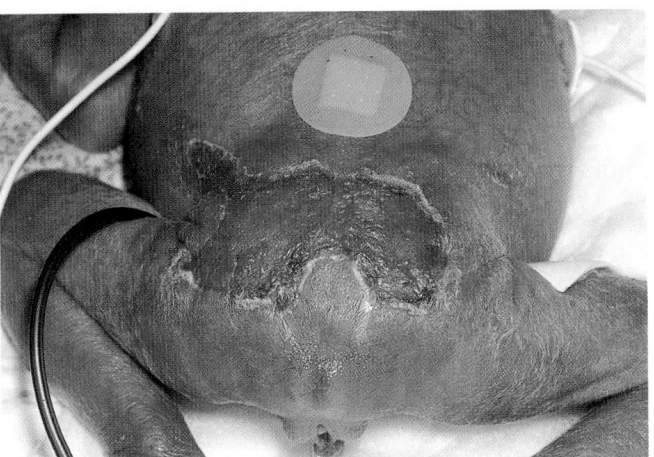

(a)

(b)

Fig. 45.40 (a) Burn; black area and surrounding erythema on the buttocks of a 1200 g baby who had lain in a pool of antiseptic during umbilical artery catheterisation. (b) Subsequent improvement in the lesion with clean exposed tissue which healed with minimal scarring.

- Iodine and alcohol, used as neonatal antiseptic solutions, can damage the preterm baby's skin – the baby's back and buttocks are particularly vulnerable, as these agents may trickle down following such procedures as umbilical catheterisation (Fig. 45.40a, b);[80,223]
- radiant heaters;[64,195]
- transcutaneous monitors, especially if used at 44°C;[30,73]
- pulse oximeters;[201,229]
- transilluminators.[117]

Awareness of the potential for such damage is perhaps the only unifying preventative measure.

References

1. Abrahamson E L, Scott R C, Jurges E, Al-Jawad S, Madden N 1993 Catheterization of posterior tibial artery leading to limb amputation. Acta Paediatrica 82: 618–619

2. Ahluwalia J S, Kelsall A W R, Diederich S, Rennie J M 1994 Successful treatment of aortic thrombosis after umbilical catheterization with tissue plasminogen activator. Acta Paediatrica 83: 1215–1217

3. Alkalay A L, Mazereth R, Santuili T, Pomerance J J 1993 Central venous line thrombosis in premature infants. A case management and literature review. American Journal of Perinatology 10: 323–326

4. Archer N 1993 Patent ductus arteriosus in the newborn. Archives of Disease in Childhood 69: 529–532

5. Ashkenazi S, Metzker A, Merlob P, Ovadia J, Reisner S H 1985 Scalp changes after fetal monitoring. Archives of Disease in Childhood 60: 267–269

6. Ayra H, Williams J, Ponsford S N, Bissenden J G 1991 Neonatal diaphragmatic paralysis caused by chest drains. Archives of Disease in Childhood 66: 441–442

7. Bagnall H A, Gomperts E, Atkinson J B 1989 Continuous infusion of low dose urokinase in the treatment of central venous catheter thrombosis in infants and children. Pediatrics 83: 963–966

8. Balagatas R C, Bell C E, Edwards L D, Levin S 1971 Risk of local and systemic infections associated with umbilical vein catheterization: a prospective study in 86 newborn patients. Pediatrics 48: 359–367

9. Baldwin C E, Holder T M, Asheraft K W, Amoury R A 1981 Neonatal renovascular hypertension. A complication of aortic monitoring catheters. Journal of Pediatric Surgery 16: 820–821

10. Balistreri W F, Farrell M K, Bove K E 1986 Lessons from the E-ferol tragedy. Pediatrics 78: 503–506

11. Barak M, Herschkowitz S, Montag J 1986 Soft tissue calcification: a complication of the vitamin E injection. Pediatrics 77: 382–385

12. Barr P A, Sumners J, Wirtschafter D, Porter R C, Cassidy G 1977 Percutaneous peripheral arterial cannulation in the neonate. Pediatrics 59: 1058–1062

13. Barrington K J 2000 Umbilical artery catheters in the newborn: effects of position of the catheter tip (Cochrane Review). Cochrane Database of Systematic Reviews (2): CD000505

14. Barrington K J 2000 Umbilical artery catheters in the newborn: effects of heparin (Cochrane Review). Cochrane Database of Systematic Reviews (2): CD000507

15. Barrington K J 2000 Umbilical artery catheters in the newborn: effects of catheter design (end vs side hole) (Cochrane Review). Cochrane Database of Systematic Reviews (2): CD000508

16. Barrington K J 2000 Umbilical artery catheters in the newborn: effects of catheter materials (Cochrane Review). Cochrane Database of Systematic Reviews (2): CD000949

17. Barton D J, Sloan G M, Nichter L S, Reinisch J F 1988 Hair-thread tourniquet syndrome. Pediatrics 82: 925–928

18. Batton D G, Maisels M J, Appelbaum P 1982 Use of peripheral intravenous cannulas in premature infants. A controlled study. Pediatrics 70: 487–490

19. Bauer S B, Feldman S M, Gellis S S, Retik A B 1975 Neonatal hypertension: a complication of umbilical artery catheterization. New England Journal of Medicine 293: 1032–1033

20. Bautista A B, Ko S H, Sun S C 1995 Retention of percutaneous venous catheter in the newborn. A report of three cases. American Journal of Perinatology 12: 53–54

21. Baxter R J, Johnson J D, Guetsman B W, Hackel A 1975 Cosmetic nasal deformities complicating prolonged nasal tracheal intubation in critically ill newborn infants. Pediatrics 55: 884–886

22. Benjamin D K, Miller W, Garges H et al 2001 Bacteremia, central catheters and neonates: when to pull the line. Pediatrics 107: 1272–1276

23. Bhutani V K, Ritchie W G, Shaffer T G 1986 Acquired tracheomegaly in very preterm neonates. American Journal of Diseases of Children 140: 449–452

24. Biagtan J, Rosenfeld W, Salazar D, Velcek F 1980 Herniation of the appendix through the umbilical ring following umbilical artery catheterization. Journal of Pediatric Surgery 15: 672–673

25. Biorklund L J, Mahngren N, Lindroth M 1995 Pulmonary complications of umbilical venous catheters. Pediatric Radiology 25: 149–152

26. Blumenfeld T A, Turi G, Blanc W A 1979 Recommended site and depth of newborn heel stick punctures based on anatomical measurements and histopathology. Lancet i: 230–233

27. Boros S J, Mammel M C, Lewallen P K, Coleman J M, Gordon M J, Ophoven J 1986 Necrotizing tracheobronchitis: a complication of high-frequency ventilation. Journal of Pediatrics 109: 95–100

28. Boros S J, Nystrom J F, Thompson T R, Reynolds J W, Williams H J 1975 Leg growth following umbilical catheter associated thrombus formation: a 4 year follow-up. Journal of Pediatrics 87: 973–976

29. Boros S J, Reynolds J W 1974 Duodenal perforation: a complication of neonatal nasojejunal feeding. Journal of Pediatrics 85: 107–108

30. Boyle R J, Oh W 1980 Erythema following transcutaneous PO_2 monitoring. Pediatrics 65: 333–334

31. Brans Y W, Ceballos R, Cassady G 1974 Umbilical catheters and hepatic abscesses. Pediatrics 53: 264–266

32. Brill P W, Winchester P, Levin A R, Griffith A Y, Kazam E, Zirinsky K 1985 Aortic aneurysm secondary to umbilical artery catheterization. Journal of Pediatric Surgery 15: 199–201

33. Bull M J, Schreiner R L, Garg B P, Hutton N M, Lemons J A, Gresham E L 1980 Neurological complications following temporal artery catheterization. Journal of Pediatrics 96: 1071–1073

34. Caplan M S, Cohn R A, Langman C B, Conway J A, Shkolnik A, Brouillette R T 1989 Favourable outcome of neonatal aortic thrombosis and renovascular hypertension. Journal of Pediatrics 115: 291–295

35. Cartwright G W, Schreiner R L 1980 Major complication secondary to percutaneous radial artery catheterization in the neonate. Pediatrics 65: 139–141

36. Chidi C C, King D R, Boles E T 1983 An ultrastructural study of the intimal injury induced by an indwelling umbilical artery catheter. Journal of Pediatric Surgery 18: 109–115

37. Chien L Y, Macnab Y, Aziz K, Andrews W, McMillan D D, Lee S K 2002 Variations in central venous catheter-related infection risks among Canadian neonatal intensive care units. Pediatric Infectious Diseases Journal 21: 505–511

38. Cohen R S, Ramachandran P, Kim E H, Glasscock G F 1995 Retrospective analysis of risks associated with an umbilical artery catheter system for continuous monitoring of arterial oxygen tension. Journal of Perinatology 15: 195–198

39. Colburn M D, Gelabert H A, Quinones-Baldrich W 1992 Neonatal aortic thrombosis. Surgery 111: 21–28

40. Colclough A B, Barson A J 1981 Infantile aortic aneurysm complicating umbilical arterial catheterization. Archives of Disease in Childhood 56: 795–797

41. Cole G F, Chaudhuri P R, Carroll L P 1982 Mask for continuous positive airways pressure: does it cause corneal abrasions? British Medical Journal 284: 19

42. Corkery J J, Dubowitz V, Lister J, Moosa A 1968 Colonic perforation after exchange transfusion. British Medical Journal iv: 345–349

43. Couriel J, Phelan P D 1981 Subglottic cysts: a complication of neonatal endotracheal intubation. Pediatrics 68: 103–105

44. Cumming W A, Burchfield D J 1994 Accidental catheterization of internal iliac branches: a serious complication of umbilical artery catheterization. Journal of Perinatology 14: 304–309

45. Daniels S R, Hannon D W, Meyer R A, Kaplan S 1984 Paroxysmal supraventricular tachycardia: a complication of jugular central venous catheters in neonates. American Journal of Diseases of Children 138: 474–475

46. Davies J, Gault D, Buchdahl R 1994 Preventing the scars of neonatal intensive care. Archives of Disease in Childhood. Fetal and Neonatal Edition 70: F50–F51

47. de Curtis M, Mastropasqua S, Paludetto R, Orzalesi M 1985 Gangrene of the buttock: a devastating complication of the infusion of hyperosmolar solutions in the umbilical artery at birth. European Journal of Pediatrics 144: 261–262

48. Dellagrammaticas H D, Papageorgeou A 1994 Unfriendly incubators. Archives of Disease in Childhood. Fetal and Neonatal Edition 71: F148

49. den Guden A L, Berger H M, Ruys J H 1986 Scarring of the hands after venepunctures in babies. European Journal of Pediatrics 145: 58–59

50. Department of Health 2001 Review of four neonatal deaths due to cardiac tamponade associated with the presence of a central venous line. HMSO, London

51. de Sa D J 1983 Mucosal metaplasia and chronic inflammation in the middle ear of infants receiving intensive care in the neonatal period. Archives of Disease in Childhood 58: 24–28

52. Dhande V, Kattwinkel J, Alford B 1983 Recurrent bilateral pleural effusions secondary to superior vena cava obstruction as a complication of central venous catheterization. Pediatrics 72: 109–113

53. Dmochowski R R, Crandell S S, Corrieri V N 1986 Bladder injury and uroascites from umbilical artery catheterization. Pediatrics 77: 421–422

54. Doull I J M, Mok Q, Tasker R C 1997 Tracheobronchomalacia in preterm infants with chronic lung disease. Archives of Disease in Childhood. Fetal and Neonatal Edition 76: F203–F205

55. Downing G J, Hayen L K, Kilbride H W 1993 Acquired subglottic cysts in the low birthweight infant. American Journal of Diseases of Children 147: 971–974

56. Drucker D E M, Greenfield L J, Ehrich F, Salzberg A M 1986 Aorto-iliac aneurysms following umbilical artery catheterization. Journal of Pediatric Surgery 21: 725–730

57. Duke P M, Coulson J D, Santos J I, Johnson J D 1976 Cleft palate associated with prolonged orotracheal intubation in infancy. Journal of Pediatrics 89: 990–991

58. Egan E A, Eitzman D V 1971 Umbilical vessel catheterization. American Journal of Diseases of Children 121: 213–218

59. Emami A, Saldanha R, Knupp C, Kodroff M 1987 Failure of systemic thrombolytic and heparin therapy in the treatment of neonatal aortic thrombosis. Pediatrics 79: 773–777

60. Erenberg A, Nowak A J 1984 Palatal groove formation in neonates and infants with orotracheal tubes. American Journal of Diseases of Children 138: 974–975

61. Esper E, Krabill K A, St Cyr J A, Patton C, Foker J E 1993 Repair of multiple mycotic aneurysms in a newborn. Journal of Pediatric Surgery 28: 1553–1556

62. Evans N J, Rutter N 1986 Reduction of skin damage from transcutaneous oxygen electrodes using a spray-on dressing. Archives of Disease in Childhood 61: 881–884

63. Fischer A Q, Strasburger J 1982 Foot drop in the neonate secondary to use of foot boards. Journal of Pediatrics 101: 1003–1004

64. Fleischman A R 1977 Another potential hazard of radiant warmers [letter]. Journal of Pediatrics 91: 984

65. Garcia Munoz M T, Cerezo Pancorbo J M, Martinez Bastida G, Sanchez Badia J L 1996 [Suprapubic bladder aspiration. Utility and complication.] Anales Espanoles de Pediatria 45: 377–379

66. Garland J S, Dunne W M, Havens P et al 1992 Peripheral intravenous catheter complications in critically ill children: a prospective study. Pediatrics 89: 1145–1150

67. Garland J S, Nelson D B, Rice T, Neu J 1985 Increased risk of gastrointestinal perforations in neonates mechanically ventilated with either face mask or nasal prongs. Pediatrics 76: 406–410

68. Gau G S, Ryder T A, Mobberley M A 1987 Iatrogenic epithelial change caused by endotracheal intubation of neonates. Early Human Development 15: 221–229

69. Gault D T 1992 Vascular compromise in newborn infants. Archives of Disease in Childhood 67: 463–467

70. Gilles F H, Matson D D 1970 Sciatic nerve injury following misplaced gluteal injection. Journal of Pediatrics 76: 247–254

71. Ginoza G, Cortez S, Modanlou H D 1989 Prevention of palatal groove formation in premature neonates requiring intubation. Journal of Pediatrics 115: 133–135

72. Goetzman B W, Stradalnik R C, Bogren H G, Blankenship W J, Ikeda R M, Thayer J 1975 Thrombotic complications of umbilical artery catheters. A clinical and radiographic study. Pediatrics 56: 374–379

73. Golden S M 1981 Skin craters: a complication of transcutaneous oxygen monitoring. Pediatrics 67: 514–516

74. Gould S J, Howard S 1985 The histopathology of the larynx in the neonate following endotracheal intubation. Journal of Pathology 146: 301–311

75. Gowdar K, Bull M J, Schreiner R L, Lemons J A, Gresham E L 1980 Nasal deformities in neonates. American Journal of Diseases of Children 134: 954–957

76. Grosfield J L, Lemons J L, Ballantine T V N, Schreiner R L 1980 Emergency thoracotomy for acquired bronchopleural fistula in the premature infant with respiratory distress. Journal of Pediatric Surgery 15: 416–421

77. Gupta J M, Roberton N R C, Wigglesworth J S 1968 Umbilical artery catheterization of the newborn. Archives of Disease in Childhood 43: 382–387

78. Hack W W M, Van der Lei J, Okken A 1990 Incidence and duration of total occlusion of the radial artery in newborn infants after catheter withdrawal. European Journal of Pediatrics 149: 275–277

79. Haldeman S, Fowler G W, Ashwal S, Schneider S 1983 Acute flaccid neonatal paraplegia: a case report. Neurology 33: 93–95

80. Harpin V, Rutter N 1982 Percutaneous alcohol absorption and skin necrosis in a preterm infant. Archives of Disease in Childhood 57: 477–479

81. Hayhurst E G, Wyman M 1975 Morbidity associated with prolonged use of polyvinyl feeding tubes. American Journal of Diseases of Children 129: 72–74

82. Heath R E 1986 Vasospasm in the neonate: response to tolazoline. Pediatrics 77: 405–408

83. Henry C G, Gutierrez F, Lee J T et al 1981 Aortic thrombosis presenting as congestive heart failure: an umbilical artery complication. Journal of Pediatrics 98: 820–822

84. Hillman L S, Goodwin S L, Sherman W R 1975 Identification and measurement of plasticizers in neonatal tissues after umbilical catheters and blood products. New England Journal of Medicine 292: 381–386

85. Horgan M J, Bartoletti A, Polansky S, Peters J C, Manning T J, Lamont B M 1987 Effect of heparin infusates in umbilical artery catheters on frequency of thrombotic complications. Journal of Pediatrics 111: 774–778

86. Isenberg S, Everett S 1984 Cardiovascular effects of mydriatics in low-birth-weight infants. Journal of Pediatrics 105: 111–112

87. Jacobson Z, Strom J 1999 Pericardial tamponade complicating central venous catheterisation in an infant with very low birth weight: role of echocardiography in diagnosis and treatment. Heart Disease 1: 133–135

88. Jardine D S, Rogers K 1989 Relationship of benzyl alcohol to kernicterus, intraventricular hemorrhage and mortality in preterm infants. Pediatrics 83: 153–160

89. Johnson D E, Base J L, Thompson T R et al 1981 Candida septicemia and right atrial mass secondary to umbilical vein catheterization. American Journal of Diseases of Children 135: 275–277

90. Johnson D E, Foker J, Munson D P, Nelson A, Athinarayanan P, Thompson T R 1982 Management of esophageal and pharyngeal perforation in the newborn infant. Pediatrics 70: 592–596

91. Joshi V V, Mandavia S G, Stern L, Wigglesworth F W 1972 Acute lesions induced by endotracheal intubation. American Journal of Diseases of Children 124: 646–649

92. Junker P, Egeblad M, Nielson O, Kamper J 1976 Umbilical vein catherization and portal hypertension. Acta Paediatrica Scandinavica 65: 499–504

93. Kaufman J M, Sharada P, Austin T L et al 1983 Neonatal bladder injury occurring after umbilical artery catheterization by cut down. Journal of the American Medical Association 250: 2968–2970

94. Keeling J W 1993 Fetal and neonatal pathology, 2nd edn. Springer-Verlag, London, p. 333

95. Keeney S E, Richardson C J 1995 Extravascular extravasation of fluid as a complication of central venous lines in the neonate. Journal of Perinatology 15: 284–288

96. Kelly M A, Finer N N, Dunbar L G 1984 Fatal neurological complication of parenteral feeding through a central vein catheter. American Journal of Diseases of Children 138: 352–353

97. Kennedy L A, Drummond W H, Knight M E, Millsaps M M, Wilhams J L 1990 Successful treatment of neonatal aortic thrombosis with tissue plasminogen activator. Journal of Pediatrics 116: 798–801

98. Khilnani P, Toce S, Reddy R 1990 Mechanical complications from very small percutaneous central venous silastic catheters. Critical Care Medicine 18: 1477–1478

99. Kitterman J A 1979 Fatal air embolism through an umbilical venous catheter. European Journal of Pediatrics 131: 71–73

100. Kline A H, Blattner R J, Lunin M 1964 Transplacental effect of tetracyclines on teeth. Journal of the American Medical Association 188: 178–182

101. Koenigsberger M R, Moessinger A C 1977 Iatrogenic carpal tunnel syndrome in the newborn infant. Journal of Pediatrics 91: 443–445

102. Krasna I H, Rosenfeld D, Benjamin B G, Klein G, Hiatt M, Hegyi T 1987 Esophageal perforation in the neonate: an emerging problem in the newborn nursery. Journal of Pediatric Surgery 22: 784–790

103. Kreusser K L, Volpe J J 1984 Peroneal palsy produced by intravenous fluid administration in a newborn. Developmental Medicine and Child Neurology 26: 522–524

104. Krishnamoorthy K S, Fernandex M D, Todres I D, DeLong G R 1976 Paraplegia associated with umbilical artery catheterization in the newborn. Pediatrics 58: 443–445

105. Krueger T C, Neblett W W, O'Neill J A, MacDonnell R C, Dean R H, Thiema G A 1985 Management of aortic thrombosis secondary to umbilical artery catheters in neonates. Journal of Pediatric Surgery 20: 328–332

106. Kumar S P, Belik J 1984 Chylothorax – a complication of tube placement in the neonate. Critical Care Medicine 12: 411–412

107. Landers S, Moise A A, Fraley J K, Smith E O'B, Baker C J 1991 Factors associated with umbilical catheter related sepsis in neonates. American Journal of Diseases of Children 145: 675–680

108. Larroche J C 1970 Umbilical catheterization: its complications. Biology of the Neonate 16: 101–116

109. Lee S B, Kahn J P 1976 Esophageal perforation in the neonate. American Journal of Diseases of Children 130: 325–329

110. Lesko S M, Mitchell A A, Epstein M F et al 1986 Heparin use as a risk factor for intraventricular hemorrhage in low birthweight infants. New England Journal of Medicine 314: 1156–1160

111. Levy I, Mosseri R, Garty B 1996 Peripheral intravenous infusion – another cause of air embolism. Acta Paediatrica 85: 385–386

112. Lilien L D, Harris V J, Ramamurthy R S, Pildes R D 1976 Neonatal osteomyelitis of the calcaneus: complication of heel puncture. Journal of Pediatrics 88: 478–480

113. Lobe T E, Richardson C J, Boulden T F, Swischuk L E, Hayden K E, Oldham K T 1992 Mycotic thromboaneurysm of the abdominal aorta in preterm infants: its natural history and its management. Journal of Pediatric Surgery 27: 1054–1060

114. Lovejoy F H 1982 Fatal benzyl alcohol poisoning in neonatal intensive care units. American Journal of Diseases of Children 136: 974–976

115. Lowenstein E, Little J W, Lo, H H 1971 Prevention of cerebral embolization from flushing radial artery cannulae. New England Journal of Medicine 285: 1414–1415

116. Lucey J F, Dolan R G 1959 Hyperbilirubinemia of newborn infants associated with the parenteral administration of a vitamin K analogue to the mothers. Pediatrics 23: 553–560

117. McArtor R D, Saunders B S 1979 Iatrogenic second degree burns caused by a transilluminator. Pediatrics 63: 422–424

118. MacDonald M G, Getson P R, Glasgow A M, Miller M K, Boeckx R L, Johnson E L 1987 Propylene glycol: increased incidence of seizures in low birthweight infants. Pediatrics 79: 622–625

119. Macpherson T A, Shen-Schwarz S, Valdes-Dapena M 1988 Prevention and reduction of iatrogenic disorders in the newborn. In: Guthrie R D (ed) Neonatal intensive care: Clinics in Critical Care Medicine No. 13. Churchill Livingstone, New York, pp 271–312

120. Maki M, Ruuska J, Kuusela A L, Karikoski-Leo R 1993 High prevalence of asymptomatic esophageal and gastric lesions in preterm infants in intensive care. Critical Care Medicine 21: 1863–1867

121. Malin S W, Baumgart S, Rosenberg H K, Foreman J 1985 Non-surgical management of obstructive aortic thrombosis complicated by renovascular hypertension in the neonate. Journal of Pediatrics 106: 630–634

122. Manco-Johnson M J 1990 Diagnosis and management of thromboses in the perinatal period. Seminars in Perinatology 14: 393–402

123. Mann N P 1980 Gluteal skin necrosis after umbilical artery catheterization. Archives of Disease in Childhood 55: 815–817

124. Marinelli P V, Ortiz A, Alden E R 1981 Acquired eventration of the diaphragm: a complication of chest tube placement in neonatal pneumothorax. Pediatrics 67: 552–554

125. Marsh D, Wilkerson S A, Cook L M, Pietsch J B 1988 Right atrial thrombus formation screening using two dimensional echocardiograms in neonates with central venous catheters. Pediatrics 81: 284–287

126. Marsh J L, King W, Barrett C, Fonkalsrud E W 1975 Serious complications after umbilical artery catheterization for neonatal monitoring. Archives of Surgery 110: 1203–1205

127. Mehta S, Connors A F, Danish E H, Grisoni E 1992 Incidence of thrombosis during central venous catheterization of newborns: a prospective study. Journal of Pediatric Surgery 27: 18–22

128. Mendoza G J B, Soto A, Brown E G, Dolgin S E, Steinfeld L, Sweet A W 1986 Intracardiac thrombi complicating central total parenteral nutrition: resolution without surgery or thrombolysis. Journal of Pediatrics 108: 610–613

129. Merton D F, Mumford L, Filstron H C, Brumley G W, Offman E L, Grossman H 1980 Radiological observations during transpyloric tube feeding in infants of low birthweight. Radiology 136: 67–75

130. Miller D, Kirkpatrick B V, Kodroff M, Ehrlich F E, Salzberg A M 1979 Pelvic exsanguination following umbilical artery catheterization in neonates. Journal of Pediatric Surgery 14: 264–269

131. Moclair A, Bates I 1995 The efficacy of heparin in maintaining peripheral infusions in neonates. European Journal of Pediatrics 154: 567–570

132. Moens E, Dooy J D, Jansens H, Lammens C, Op de Beeck B, Mahieu L 2003 Hepatic abscesses associated with umbilical catheterisation in two neonates. European Journal of Pediatrics 162: 406–409

133. Moessinger A C, Driscoll J M, Wigger H J 1978 High incidence of lung perforation by chest tube in neonatal pneumothorax. Journal of Pediatrics 92: 635–637

134. Mohan M S, Patole S K 2002 Neonatal ascites and hyponatraemia following umbilical venous catheterisation. Journal of Paediatrics and Child Health 38: 612–614

135. Mokrohisky S T, Levine R L, Blumhagen J D, Wesenberg R L, Simmons M A 1978 Low positioning of umbilical artery catheters increases associated complications in newborn infants. New England Journal of Medicine 299: 561–564

136. Morgan C, Newell S J, Ducker D A et al 1999 Continuous neonatal blood gas monitoring using a multiparametric-arterial sensor. Archives of Disease in Childhood. Fetal and Neonatal Edition 80: F93–F98

137. Mgobo K I, Wang D C 1997 Biliary venous fistula from umbilical catheter placement. Pediatric Radiology 27: 333–335

138. Morrell P, Hey E, Mackee I W, Rutter N, Lewis M 1985 Deafness in preterm baby associated with topical antibiotic spray containing neomycin. Lancet i: 1167–1168

139. Moylan F M B, Seldin E B, Shannon D C, Todres I D 1980 Defective primary dentition in survivors of neonatal mechanical ventilation. Journal of Pediatrics 96: 106–108

140. Nagaraj H S, Shott R, Fellows R, Yacoub U 1980 Recurrent lobar atelectasis due to acquired bronchial stenosis in neonates. Journal of Pediatric Surgery 15: 411–415

141. Neal W A, Reynolds J W, Jarvis C W, Williams H J 1972 Umbilical artery catheterization: demonstration of arterial thrombosis by aortography. Pediatrics 50: 6–13

142. Neubauer A-P 1995 Percutaneous central i.v. access in the neonate: experience with 535 silastic catheters. Acta Paediatrica 84: 756–760

143. Norman M G, Temple A R, Murphy J V 1970 Infantile quadriceps femoris contracture resulting from intramuscular injections. New England Journal of Medicine 282: 964–966

144. Nour S, Puntis J W L, Stringer M D 1995 Intra-abdominal extravasation complicating parenteral nutrition in infants. Archives of Disease in Childhood. Fetal and Neonatal Edition 72: F207–F208

145. Nowak C M, Waffarn F, Sills J H, Pousti T M, Warden M J, Cuningham M D 1994 Focal intestinal perforation in the extremely low birthweight infant. Journal of Perinatology 14: 450–453

146. Nowak-Gottl U, von Kries R, Gobel U 1997 Neonatal symptomatic thromboembolism in Germany: two year survey. Archives of Disease in Childhood. Fetal and Neonatal Edition 76: F163–F167

147. O'Neill J A, Neblett W W, Born M L 1981 Management of major thromboembolic complications of umbilical artery catheters. Journal of Pediatric Surgery 16: 972–978

148. Ontell S J, Gauderer M W L 1985 Iatrogenic arteriovenous fistula after multiple arterial punctures. Pediatrics 76: 97–98

149. Oppenheimer D A, Carroll B A, Garth K E 1982 Ultrasonic detection of complications following umbilical artery catheterization in the neonate. Radiology 145: 667–672

150. Orme R L'E, Eades S M 1968 Perforation of the bowel in the newborn as a complication of exchange transfusion. British Medical Journal iv: 349–351

151. Oski F A, Allen D M, Diamond L K 1963 Portal hypertension – a complication of umbilical vein catheterization. Pediatrics 31: 297–302

152. Pape K E, Armstrong D L, Fitzhardinge P M 1976 Central nervous system pathology associated with mask ventilation in the very low birthweight infant. A new etiology for intracerebellar hemorrhages. Pediatrics 58: 473–483

153. Pape K E, Armstrong D L, Fitzhardinge P M 1978 Peripheral median nerve damage secondary to brachial artery blood gas sampling. Journal of Pediatrics 93: 852–856

154. Payne R M, Martin T C, Bower R J, Canter C E 1989 Management and follow-up of arterial thrombosis in the neonatal period. Journal of Pediatrics 114: 853–858

155. Pearse R G 1978 Percutaneous catheterization of the radial artery in newborn babies using transillumination. Archives of Disease in Childhood 53: 549–554

156. Perez-Rodriguez J, Quero J, Frias E G, Omenaca F 1978 Duodenal perforation in a neonate by a tube of silicon rubber during transpyloric feeding. Journal of Pediatrics 92: 113–114

157. Peters J L, Armstrong R 1977 Air embolism as a complication of central venous catheterization. Annals of Surgery 187: 375–378

158. Phelps S J, Helms R A, 1987 Risk factors affecting infiltration of peripheral venous lines in infants. Journal of Pediatrics 111: 384–389

159. Phillips R R, Lee S H 1990 Fractures of long bones occurring in neonatal intensive therapy units. British Medical Journal 301: 225–226

160. Piotrowski A, Kawczynski P 1995 Cannulation of the axillary artery in critically ill newborn infants. European Journal of Pediatrics 154: 57–59

161. Plumer L B, Kaplan G W, Mendoza S A 1976 Hypertension in infants – a complication of umbilical arterial catheterization. Journal of Pediatrics 89: 802–805

162. Pollack C V, Pollack E S, Andrew M E 1994 Suprapubic bladder aspiration versus urethral catheterisation in ill infants: success, efficiency and complication rates. Annals of Emergency Medicine 23: 225–230

163. Prian G W 1977 Complications and sequelae of temporal artery catheterization in the high risk newborn. Journal of Pediatric Surgery 12: 829–835

164. Purohit P M, Levkoff A H, de Vito P C 1978 Gluteal necrosis with foot drop. Complications associated with umbilical artery catheterization. American Journal of Diseases of Children 132: 897–899

165. Quak J M E, Szatmari A, van den Anker J N 1993 Cardiac tamponade in a preterm neonate secondary to a chest tube. Acta Paediatrica 82: 490–491

166. Rajani K, Goetzman B W, Wemberg R P, Tumer E, Abildgaard C 1979 Effect of heparinization of fluids infused through an umbilical artery catheter on catheter patency and frequency of complications. Pediatrics 63: 552–556

167. Rajs J, Finnstrom O, Wesstrom G 1976 Aortic aneurysm developing after umbilical artery catheterization. Acta Paediatrica Scandinavica 65: 495–498

168. Randel S N, Tsang B H, Wung J T, Driscoll J M, James L S 1987 Experience with percutaneous indwelling peripheral arterial catheterization in neonates. American Journal of Diseases of Children 141: 848–851

169. Rehan V K, Cronin C M G, Bowman J M 1994 Neonatal portal vein thrombosis successfully treated by regional streptokinase infusion. European Journal of Pediatrics 153: 456–459

170. Rey C, Marache P, Watel A, Francart C 1987 Iatrogenic false aneurysm of the brachial artery in an infant. European Journal of Pediatrics 146: 438–439

171. Reynolds E O R 1963 Arterial blood gas tensions in acute disease of lower respiratory tract in infancy. British Medical Journal i: 1192–1195

172. Richardson R, Applebaum H, Touran T et al 1988 Effective thrombolytic therapy of aortic thrombosis in the small premature infant. Journal of Pediatric Surgery 12: 1198–1200

173. Robertson N J, McCarthy L S, Hamilton P A, Moss A L H 1996 Nasal deformities resulting from flow driver continuous positive airway pressure. Archives of Disease in Childhood. Fetal and Neonatal Edition 75: F209–F212

174. Rosenthal A, Anderson M, Thomson S J, Pappas A M, Fyler D C 1972 Superficial femoral artery catheterization. American Journal of Diseases of Children 124: 240–242

175. Rubin S P, Hewson P, Roberton N R C 1986 Pulmonary complications of total parenteral nutrition in a neonate. Journal of the Royal Society of Medicine 79: 545–547

176. Rubin S P, Roberton N R C 1991 Intestinal perforation without necrotizing enterocolitis in very low birthweight infants with umbilical arterial catheters. Pediatric Reviews and Communications 6: 51–54

177. Rush M G, Hazinski T A 1992 Current therapy of bronchopulmonary dysplasia. Clinics in Perinatology 19: 563–590

178. Rushforth A, Green M A, Levene M I, Puntis J W L 1991 Subdural fat effusion complicating parenteral nutrition. Archives of Disease in Childhood 66: 1350–1351

179. Sarrut S, Alain J, Alison F 1969 Les complications précoces de la perfusion par la veine ombilicale chez le prématuré. Archives Français de Pédiatrie 26: 651–667

180. Sasidharan P, Bilhnan D, Heimler R, Nelin L 1996 Cardiac arrest in an extremely low birthweight infant: complication of percutaneous central venous catheter placement. Journal of Perinatology 16: 123–126

181. Schell-Feith E A, Kist-van Holthe J E, Conneman N et al 2000 Etiology of nephrocalcinosis in preterm neonates: association of nutritional intake and urinary parameters. Kidney International 58: 2102–2110

182. Schmidt B, Andrew M 1995 Neonatal thrombosis: report of a prospective Canadian and international registry. Pediatrics 96: 939–943

183. Schreiber M D, Perez C A, Kitterman J A 1984 A double-catheter technique for caudally misdirected umbilical artery catheters. Journal of Pediatrics 104: 768–769

184. Scott J M 1965 Iatrogenic lesions in babies following umbilical vein catheterization Archives of Disease in Childhood 40: 426–429

185. Seguin J H 1992 Right sided hydrothorax and central venous catheters in extremely low birthweight infants. American Journal of Perinatology 9: 154–158

186. Seibert J J, Lindley S G, Sutterfield S L, Seibert R W, Mollitt D L 1986 Umbilical artery clot in the neonate: spontaneous resolution. Journal of Pediatric Surgery 11: 973–974

187. Seibert J J, Northington F J, Miers J F, Taylor B J 1991 Aortic thrombosis after umbilical artery catheterization in neonates. Prevalence of complications on long term follow-up. American Journal of Roentgenology 156: 567–569

188. Sell E J, Hansen R C, Struck-Pierce S 1980 Calcified nodules on the heel: a complication of neonatal intensive care. Journal of Pediatrics 96: 473–475

189. Sengupta S 1985 Pathogenesis of infantile quadriceps fibrosis and its correction by proximal release. Journal of Pediatric Orthopedics 5: 187–191

190. Serlin S P, Dally W J R 1975 Tracheal perforation in the neonate: a complication of endotracheal intubation. Journal of Pediatrics 86: 596–597

191. Shuman R M, Leech R W, Alvord E C 1974 Neurotoxicity of hexachlorophene in the human. 1. A clinical pathological study of 248 children. Pediatrics 54: 689–695

192. Silverman W A, Andersen D H, Blanc W A, Rozier D N 1956 A difference in mortality rate and incidence of kernicterus among premature infants allotted to two antibacterial regimes. Pediatrics 18: 614–625

193. Simmons M A, Levine R L, Lubchenko L O, Guggenheim M A 1978 Warning: serious sequelae of temporal artery catheterization. Journal of Pediatrics 92: 284

194. Sirnon-Fayard E E, Kroncke R S, Solarte D, Peverini R 1997 Non-surgical retrieval of embolised umbilical catheters in premature infants. Journal of Perinatology 17: 143–147

195. Simonsen K, Graem N, Rothman L P, Degn H 1995 Iatrogenic radiant heat burns in severely asphyxic newborn. Acta Paediatrica 84: 1438–1440

196. Simpson J S 1975 Misdiagnosis, complicating umbilical vessel catheterization. Clinical Pediatrics 14: 727–729

197. Skoglund R R, Giles E E 1986 The false cortical thumb. American Journal of Diseases of Children 140: 375–376

198. Slogoff S, Keats A S, Arlund C 1983 On the safety of radial artery cannulation. Anesthesiology 59: 42–47

199. Smerdely P, Boyages S C, Wu D et al 1989 Topical iodine-containing antiseptics and neonatal hypothyroidism in very low birthweight infants. Lancet ii: 661

200. Smith P L 1978 Umbilical catheter retrieval in the premature infant. Journal of Pediatrics 93: 499–502

201. Sobel D B 1992 Burning of a neonate due to a pulse oximeter: arterial saturation monitoring. Pediatrics 89: 154–155

202. Spahr R C, MacDonald H M, Holzrnan I R 1979 Catheterization of the posterior tibial artery in the neonate. American Journal of Diseases of Children 133: 945–946

203. Stavis R L, Krauss A N 1980 Complications of neonatal intensive care. Clinics in Perinatology 7: 107–124

204. Stewart D R, Johnson D G, Myers G G 1975 Hydrocephalus as a complication of jugular catheterization during total parenteral nutrition. Journal of Pediatric Surgery 10: 771–777

205. Strife J L, Ball W S, Towbin R, Keller M S, Dillon T 1988 Arterial occlusions of neonates. Use of fibrinolytic therapy. Radiology 166: 395–400

206. Sutcliffe A G 1995 Total parenteral nutrition tamponade. Journal of the Royal Society of Medicine 88: 173–174

207. Tager I B, Ginsberg M B, Ellis S E et al 1983 An epidemiological study of the risks associated with intravenous catheters. American Journal of Epidemiology 118: 839–851

208. Thompson E N, Sherlock S 1964 The aetiology of portal vein thrombosis with particular reference to the role of infection and exchange transfusion. Quarterly Journal of Medicine 33: 465–480

209. Todres L D, Rogers M C, Shannon D C, Moylan F C, Ryan J F 1975 Percutaneous catheterization of the radial artery in the critically ill neonate. Journal of Pediatrics 87: 273–275

210. Touloukian R J, Kadar A, Spencer R P 1973 The gastrointestinal complications of neonatal umbilical venous exchange transfusion. A clinical and experimental study. Pediatrics 51: 36–43

211. Tyson J E, de Sa D J, Moore S 1976 Thromboatheromatous complications of umbilical arterial catheterization in the newborn period: clinical pathological study. Archives of Disease in Childhood 51: 744–754

212. Urbach J, Kaplan M, Blondheim O, Hersch H J 1985 Neonatal hypoglycemia related to umbilical artery catheter malfunction. Journal of Pediatrics 106: 825–826

213. Vailas G N, Brouillette R T, Scott J P, Shkolnik A, Conway J, Wiringa K 1986 Neonatal aortic thrombosis: recent experience. Journal of Pediatrics 109: 101–108

214. van den Anker J N, Baerts W, Quak J M et al 1992 Iatrogenic perforation of the lamina cribrosa by nasogastric tube in an infant. Pediatric Radiology 22: 545–546

215. van Vliet P J K, Gupta J M 1973 Prophylactic antibiotics in umbilical catheterization in the newborn. Archives of Disease in Childhood 48: 296–300

216. Vaughan R S, Menke J A, Giacoia G P 1978 Pneumothorax: a complication of endotracheal tube suctioning. Journal of Pediatrics 92: 633–634

217. Wall P M, Kuhns L R 1977 Percutaneous arterial sampling using transillumination. Pediatrics 59: 1032–1035

218. Ward R M 1984 Pharmacology of tolazoline. Clinics in Perinatology 11: 703–713

219. Wehbe M A, Moore J H 1985 Digital ischemia following intravenous therapy. Pediatrics 76: 99–103

220. Wesstrom G, Finnstrom O 1979 Umbilical artery catheterization in newborns. II. Infections in relation to catheterization. Acta Paediatrica Scandinavica 68: 713–718

221. Wesstrom G, Finnstrom O, Stenport G 1979 Umbilical artery catheterization in newborns. 1. Thrombosis in relation to catheter type and position. Acta Paediatrica Scandinavica 68: 575–581

222. Wiedersberg H, Pawlowski P 1974 Anaemic necrosis of the liver after umbilical vein catheterization. Helvetica Paediatrica Acta 34: 53–62

223. Wilkinson A R, Baum J D, Keeling J W 1981 Superficial skin necrosis in babies prepared for umbilical arterial catheterization. Archives of Disease in Childhood 56: 237–238

224. Williams J H, Hunter J E, Kanto W P, Bhatia J 1995 Hemidiaphragmatic paralysis as a complication of central venous catheterization in a neonate. Journal of Perinatology 15: 386–388

225. Williams J W, Rittenberry A, Dillard R, Allen R G 1973 Liver abscess in newborn: complication of umbilical vein catheterization. American Journal of Diseases of Children 125: 111–113

226. Wiswell T E, Turner B S, Bley J A, Fritz D L, Hunt R E 1989 Determinants of tracheobronchial histologic alterations during conventional mechanical ventilation. Pediatrics 84: 304–311

227. Wong A F, McCulloch L M, Sola A 1992 Treatment of peripheral tissue ischemia with topical nitroglycerine ointment in neonates. Journal of Pediatrics 121: 980–983

228. Wood B P 1987 Infant ribs: generalized periosteal reaction resulting from vibrator chest physiotherapy. Radiology 162: 811–812

229. Wright I M R, Puntis J W L 1993 A case of skin necrosis related to a pulse oximeter probe. British Journal of Intensive Care 3: 394–398

230. Young S, MacMahon P, Kovar I Z 1989 Subdural intravenous fat collection – an unusual complication of central intravenous feeding in the neonate. Journal of Parenteral and Enteral Nutrition 13: 661–662

231. Whitelaw A, Kennedy C R, Brion L P 2001 Diuretic therapy for newborn infants with posthemorrhagic ventricular dilatation (Cochrane Review). Cochrane Database of Systematic Reviews (2): CD002270

Section Eight

Pharmacopoeia

CHAPTER 46

Pharmacopoeia

Sam Richmond

Table 46.1 Neonatal dosage of the more commonly used drugs. See also the Neonatal Formulary 4th edition. BMJ Books: London, 2003 (www.neonatalformulary.com)

Drug	Indication, mode of action and comments	Route	Dose	Post menstrual/ Chronological age	Frequency (times/24 hours)
Aciclovir	For Herpes Simplex and Varicella Treat HS for at least 2 weeks (3 weeks if disseminated or intracranial infection). Use with zoster immune globulin in Varicella. Increase dose interval in renal failure (Creatinine >150).	iv	20 mg/kg per dose* (*give over one hour) half this dose may be sufficient in the absence of disseminated or intracranial infection		3
Adenosine	Used to stop supraventricular tachycardia. An ECG record of the transition is invaluable.	iv by rapid bolus	200–400 microg/kg per dose		repeatable (half life less than one minute)
Adrenaline	Cardiac arrest. Usually given iv but can also be given by direct intracardiac injection or by the intraosseous or intratracheal routes.	iv	10–100 microg/kg per dose		repeatable
	For severe hypotension it can be given by infusion. (1/1000 = 1 mg/ml and 1/10 000 = 100 microg/ml)	iv infusion	0.1–0.3 microg/kg per minute (Up to 2 microg/kg per minute)		infusion
Amikacin	Semi-synthetic aminoglycoside antibiotic used for treating infection with gentamicin-resistant gram negative organisms.	iv, im	15 mg/kg per dose aim to keep trough level below 5 mg/l		1
Amiodarone	Class III anti-arrhythmic. *Should not be used except under direct supervision of a paediatric cardiologist.* Continuous infusion no longer advised as the drug leaches a toxic plasticiser from giving sets.	iv	5 mg/kg loading dose* 5 mg/kg maintenance dose* *give over at least 30 minutes		Can be repeated once 1 or 2
	IV preparation contains benzyl alcohol. Do NOT dilute with 0.9% saline.	oral	10 mg/kg for 10–14 days then 7.5 mg/kg thereafter		1
Amoxicillin	Broad spectrum semi-synthetic aminopenicillin. Better absorbed by mouth than ampicillin. Drug of choice for Listeria infection.	oral iv, im	50 mg/kg per dose (100 mg/kg in meningitis)	0–1 week 1–3 weeks 4 weeks or more	2 3 4
Amphotericin B	Polyene antifungal for systemic fungal infections. (see also flucytosine and fluconazole)	iv	1 mg/kg per dose (give over 4–6 hours) – standard preparation 2 mg/kg per dose (give over 30 minutes) – liposomal preparation		1 (reduce to every 48 hours after 7 days if using the standard preparation)
Ampicillin	Drug of choice for Listeria infection.	iv, im, oral	as amoxicillin	as amoxicillin	as amoxicillin
Atracurium	Competitive non depolarising muscle relaxant. Duration of action 15–30 minutes.	iv bolus	500 microg/kg		single dose
Atropine	Muscarinic blocker (not a resuscitation drug) – to treat bradycardia – for premedication	iv subcut, im	10 microg/kg		single dose
Azlocillin	Acylureidopenicillin used for pseudomonas infections (normally with an aminoglycoside for synergistic effect).	iv, im	50 mg/kg per dose 100 mg/kg per dose	0–3 weeks more than 3 weeks	3 (<37 wks–2) 3 (<37 wks–2)

Drug	Notes	Route	Dose	Age	Frequency
Aztreonam	Narrow spectrum beta lactam antibiotic active against aerobic gram negative bacteria only. Penetrates inflamed CSF. Increase dose interval in renal failure (Creatinine >150).	iv	30 mg/kg per dose	0–1 weeks 1–3 weeks 4 weeks or more	2 3 4
Caffeine citrate	Increases respiratory drive. Both the loading dose and the maintenance dose may be safely doubled. (1 mg of caffeine citrate = 0.5 mg of caffeine base.)	iv, oral	loading dose 20 mg/kg maintenance 5 mg/kg per dose		once only 1
Calcium gluconate	For temporary rapid control of cardiac effects of hyperkalemia; see also salbutamol. Precipitates with bicarbonate, sulphates or phosphates. For correction of hypocalcaemia (see also Mag. Sulph.)	iv oral	2 ml of 10% solution/kg slowly (i.e. 200 mg/kg per dose) 1.5 ml of 10% soln/kg per dose (or 1 ml/kg Ca Sandoz syrup)		once only 6 – in feeds (4 – in feeds)
Captopril	Angiotensin converting enzyme (ACE) inhibitor. Vasodilator, reduces afterload in heart failure, may cause hypotension. Unwise with renal impairment, hyponatraemia or hypovolaemia. Labetalol is a safer option for acute control of hypertension.	oral	start at 10 microg/kg increasing progressively to no more than 100 microg/kg per dose		3
Carbamazepine	Anticonvulsant. Build up to full dose over several days. Optimum plasma level 4–12 mg/l; 1 mg = 4.23 micromol.	oral	5–15 mg/kg per dose		2
Carbimazole	Thioamide antithyroid for thyrotoxicosis, alternative to propylthiouracil. (also see Iodine)	oral	0.5–1.5 mg/kg		1
Cefotaxime	Third generation cephalosporin especially useful in meningitis. Increase dosage interval in renal failure. (Creatinine >150 micromol/l).	iv, im	50 mg/kg per dose	0–1 week 1–3 weeks 4 weeks or more	2 3 4
Ceftazidime	Third generation cephalosporin especially useful for Pseudomonas. Increase dosage interval in renal failure. (Creatinine >150 micromol/l).	iv, im	25 mg/kg per dose (50 mg/kg in meningitis)	up to 4 weeks 4 weeks and over	2 3
Chloral hydrate	Hypnotic – for short term sedation – for sustained sedation.	oral	45 mg/kg single dose 30 mg/kg per dose		once only max 4 in 24 hours
Chloramphenicol	Drug levels should be checked if possible. Aim for a peak level of 15–20 mg/l in serum. (1 mg = 3.09 micromol). Good CSF penetration.	iv, oral	loading dose 20 mg/kg maintenance 12 mg/kg per dose	0–2 weeks 3 weeks or more	once only 2 3
Chlorothiazide	Thiazide diuretic usually combined with spironolactone.	oral	10 or 20 mg/kg per dose		2
Chlorpromazine	Tranquilliser.	oral	1 mg/kg per dose (max 6 mg/kg per day)		3
Cimetidine	Histamine H_2 receptor blocker used for reducing gastric acid secretion in the face of stress ulceration. Benefit remains unproven. Prolongs the half-life of theophylline.	oral	5 mg/kg per dose if active problem, half this if used prophylactically		4
Ciprofloxacin	Reserve broad spectrum quinolone antibiotic. Best avoided unless absolutely necessary. Prolongs half-life of theophylline and caffeine.	iv, oral	10 mg/kg per dose (lactate)		2 (under 4 wks of age)

(Continued)

Table 46.1 (Continued)

Drug	Indication, mode of action and comments	Route	Dose	Post menstrual/ Chronological age	Frequency (times/24 hours)
Clonazepam	Benzodiazepine anticonvulsant. Aim for a plasma level of 30–100 mg/l. (1 mg = 3.16 micromol). Increases bronchial secretions. No proven advantage over phenobarbitone in a randomised trial.	iv (oral)	100 microg/kg per dose		1
Dexamethasone	Start 4 hours before extubation in a baby with a traumatised or oedematous larynx. 4 mg of base = 4.8 mg of dex phosphate = 5 mg of dex sodium phosphate. Has been used for established ventilator dependent BPD but there are major concerns about neurological damage associated with treatment in survivors.	iv	200 microg of *base*/kg per dose		3 doses at 8 hourly intervals
Diamorphine	Analgesia in *ventilated* babies. Respiratory suppression may interfere with trigger ventilation. Half this dose will suffice for sedation. *Has no advantages over morphine.*	iv / iv infusion	loading dose 180 microg/kg / maintenance 15 microg/kg/hour		once only (over 30 mins) / infusion
Diazepam	Benzodiazepine anxiolytic. There are many better anticonvulsants. *Dosage required is very variable.*	iv	start with 300 microg/kg		once only
Diazoxide	Thiazide derivative – reduces insulin release, used to control refractory hypoglycaemia in hyperinsulinism. Oral administration preferred.	(iv), oral	5 mg/kg per dose		2
Digoxin	May improve myocardial contractility and sometimes used in supraventricular tachycardia with variable results. Narrow therapeutic range causing partial AV block and prolonged PR interval (>0.16 sec) in excess. Toxicity appears above 2–3 micrograms/l especially if hypokalaemic. For AV block use atropine: for severe toxicity – Digibind.	loading dose oral (very rarely iv) oral	10 microg/kg (over 15 mins) then 5 microg/kg after 6 hours then 5 microg/kg after a further 6 hours (p. 655) 2–4 microg/kg per dose		loading regime only 2
Dobutamine	Synthetic inotrope, improves ventricular function.	iv infusion	5–15 microg/kg per minute		infusion
Dopamine	Causes vasoconstriction and thus raises blood pressure. It is best to use a central vein. Very variable response. Correct any acidosis before use.	iv infusion	Start at 3 microg/kg per minute increasing as needed (monitor with cardiac echo if possible) max dose ~6–15 microg/kg/min		infusion
Doxapram	Central respiratory stimulant but also stimulates all levels of the cerebrospinal axis. Can cause fits in high doses. High doses should not be used for more than 2–3 days.	iv / iv infusion / oral	loading dose 2.5 mg/kg maintenance 0.3 mg/kg per hour *(max 1.5 mg/kg/hour)* 6 mg/kg per dose (best after iv loading dose)		once only infusion 4

Drug	Notes	Route	Dose	Frequency
Edrophonium	Cholinesterase inhibitor with rapid onset but brief duration of action. Sometimes used to diagnose myasthenia gravis ('Tensilon' test) but many prefer to use neostigmine both for diagnosis and treatment.	iv	100 microg/kg give the first 20% very slowly and have atropine available to control hypersalivation	once only
Enoximone	Selective phosphodiesterase inhibitor can be used with dobutamine to support cardiac output in sepsis. Contains 41.3% w/v of propylene glycol – sustained infusion can cause hyperosmolality esp in renal failure.	iv	600 microg/kg loading dose over 15 minutes then 10–20 microg/kg per minute	infusion
Epoprostenol (PGI₂ Prostacyclin)	Inhibits platelet aggregation. Short acting vasodilator. Can be used for pulmonary vasodilatation but causes systemic vasodilation as well.	iv infusion	10–15 nanograms/kg per minute (20 nanograms/kg per minute has been used)	infusion
Erythromycin	Drug of choice for Chlamydia. Well absorbed orally. Also a motilin agonist. Risk of arrythmia with cisapride.	iv, oral	10 mg/kg per dose (give over one hour if iv) for motility start with 3 mg/kg per dose orally	4; 4
Erythropoeitin	Stimulates marrow red cell production (supplemental iron may be needed) – reduces the need for transfusions (but not as effectively as limiting blood letting).	subcut injection	400 units/kg per dose	three times per week
Fentanyl	Synthetic opioid analgesic (for ventilated babies only). Infusion is not recommended as tolerance develops rapidly and withdrawal symptoms are common.	iv	5–15 microg/kg	repeatable
Flecainide	Class I antiarrhythmic for supraventricular arrhythmias. Should not be used except under the direct supervision of a paediatric cardiologist. Causes fatal arrhythmias in overdose. Monitoring of plasma levels is essential (therapeutic range 250–750 microg/l).	oral	start with 2.5 mg/kg per dose and adjust dosage based on clinical response and plasma levels.	3
Flucloxacillin	Beta lactamase resistant penicillin. Moderately well absorbed orally.	iv, oral, im	50 mg/kg per dose (for meningitis or osteitis use 100 mg/kg per dose)	0–1 week: 2; 1–3 weeks: 3; 4 weeks or more: 4
Fluconazole	Triazole antifungal agent. Increase dosage interval where renal function is poor. Do not use if the baby is on cisapride (risk of ventricular arrhythmias).	iv, oral	6 mg/kg per dose	0–2 weeks: once every 3 days; 2–4 weeks: once every 2 days; 4 weeks or more: 1
Flucytosine	Fluorinated pyrimidine often used with amphotericin for some systemic fungal infections. Increase dosage interval in renal failure. Aim for a serum level of 50–75 mg/l. (1 mg = 7.74 micromol)	iv, oral	50 mg/kg per dose	2
Furosemide	Powerful loop diuretic, increases urinary loss of Na⁺, K⁺ and Ca⁺⁺.	iv, im, oral	1–2 mg/kg per dose	1 or 2

(Continued)

Table 46.1 (Continued)

Drug	Indication, mode of action and comments	Route	Dose	Post menstrual/ Chronological age	Frequency (times/24 hours)
Fucidin (sodium fusidate, fusidic acid)	Narrow spectrum anti-staphylococcal antibiotic, moderately well absorbed orally and well distributed (except CSF). The dose may need to be reduced for administration for more than 5 days. Watch liver function tests for a rapid rise in enzyme levels.	iv oral	10 mg/kg per dose sodium fusidate over 6 hours 15 mg/kg fusidic acid		2 3
Gentamicin	Aminoglycoside antibiotic. Aim for a trough level of 1 mg/l or less. Extend dosage interval to 36 hours if level is 2 mg/l or greater just before the fourth dose.	iv, im	5 mg/kg check trough level with fourth dose		1
Glucagon	For immediate treatment of hypoglycaemia. Mobilises hepatic gycogen, increases hepatic glucose production. Half life <10 minutes.	im, iv iv infusion	200 microg/kg 0.3 microg/kg per minute		once only infusion
Heparin	Activates antithrombin III causing anticoagulation. Has some thrombolytic action. Used for anticoagulation. (Using 0.5 to 2 units per hour can increase the effective life of intravascular cannulae.)	iv loading iv infusion	50–75 units/kg 25 units/kg per hour Monitor Activated Partial Thromboplastin Time (APTT)	use lower loading dose under 36 wks	once only infusion
Hydralazine	Vasodilator – for maintenance control of hypertension. A beta blocker may be needed to control tachycardia. (Labetalol is better than hydralazine for urgent iv use)	oral (iv)	start with 0.5 mg/kg max 2–3 mg/kg (iv dose about half oral)		3
Hydrocortisone	For treatment of adrenal insufficiency in congenital adrenal hyperplasia (with fludrocortisone). Maintenance usually 25 mg/M². Can increase neonatal blood pressure.	iv oral iv	25 mg (with dextrose) in Addisonian crisis 2.5 mg 2 mg/kg stat then 1 mg 8 hourly		once only 3
Ibuprofen	For closure of patent ductus arteriosus. Much less effective after 2 weeks of age.	iv	10 mg/kg loading 5 mg/kg daily for 2 days		once 1
Immunoglobulin	May reduce mortality in severe infection and reduces thrombocytopenia in autoimmune thrombocytopenia due to maternal ITP or SLE.	iv	400 mg/kg over several hours		once (repeatable)
Indometacin	For closure of patent ductus arteriosus. Much less effective after 2 weeks of age. (Oral absorption variable)	iv (oral)	loading dose 200 microg/kg then 100 microg/kg for 5 days		once only 1
Insulin	Occasionally used to increase glucose uptake with parenteral nutrition. To reduce hyperkalaemia (with glucose). To control neonatal diabetes (v rare).	iv iv iv later subcut	0.05–0.5 (1.0) units/kg per hour 0.3–0.6 units/kg per hour 0.5–3 units/kg per day		infusion infusion infusion/1–2

Drug	Notes	Route	Dose	Age	Frequency
Iodine	Helpful in thyrotoxicosis; acts by suppressing thyroxine synthesis and inhibiting thyroxine release.	oral	Saturated potassium iodide (~48 mg per drop) Lugol's iodine (~8 mg per drop)		1 drop daily / 1–3 drops daily
Isoniazid	For TB prophylaxis and treatment in the neonate. Seek expert advice.	oral	5 mg/kg	0–2 weeks	1
Isoprenaline	Sympathomimetic for management of significant bradycardia or heart block.	iv infusion	0.02 microg/kg per minute (max 0.2 microg/kg per minute)		infusion
Labetalol	Non cardioselective alpha blocker with beta blocking effects. The best iv drug for controlling hypertension. Adult half life of 3–4 hours.	iv infusion	start with 0.5 mg/kg per hour double the dose every 3 hours until a satisfactory BP level is reached. (max 4 mg/kg per hour)		infusion
Levothyroxine	Thyroid hormone, for replacement therapy in congenital hypothyroidism. Monitor TSH and T4 levels. Aim for a T4 level more than 20 picograms/L within 2 wks and a fall in TSH to 10 milliunits/L within 4 wks of starting. Keep T4 levels in the upper part of the normal range.	Oral (iv)	Start at 10–15 micrograms/kg per day and monitor effect on T4 and TSH levels		1
Lidocaine (Lignocaine)	Local anaesthetic. Membrane stabiliser for cardiac arrythmias and fits. Third line anticonvulsant. Toxic levels (& fits) can occur if the higher doses are used for more than 12 hours.	subcut / iv / iv infusion	up to 0.3 ml/kg of 1% soln loading dose 4 mg/kg maintenance 2 mg/kg per hour. (max 6 mg/kg per hour)		once only / once only over 1 hour / infusion
Magnesium Sulphate	For control of hypocalcaemia. For vasodilatation in persistent pulmonary hypertension try to keep plasma Mg between 3.5 and 5.5 mmol/l.	im (deep) / iv / iv infusion	100 mg/kg per dose loading dose 250 mg/kg maintenance 20–75 mg/kg/hour		2 / once only over 15 min / infusion
Mannitol	Reduces damage after cerebral trauma probably by reducing blood viscosity rather than by setting up an osmotic gradient to reduce cerebral cell swelling.	iv	1.4 gram/kg over 10–20 minutes (7 ml/kg of a 20% solution)		repeat once after 6 hours if needed
Meropenem	Carbapenem β-lactam broad spectrum antibiotic. Increase dose interval in renal failure (Creatinine >150).	iv	try 20 mg/kg per dose (no neonatal data)	0–3 weeks / 4 weeks or more	2 / 3
Metronidazole	Used to treat anaerobic bacterial infections, especially in necrotising enterocolitis	iv (oral)	15 mg/kg loading dose 7.5 mg/kg	0–3 weeks / 4 weeks or more	once only / 2 / 3
Miconazole	Imidazole antifungal agent. Do not use orally if the baby is taking cisapride as it affects the metabolism of cisapride making ventricular arrhythmias possible.	oral / topical	apply 1–2 ml of 2.5% gel apply 2% cream		2 after feeds / 2
Milrinone	Selective phosphodiesterase inhibitor can be used with dobutamine to support cardiac output in sepsis. Precipitates with furosemide.	iv	60 microg/kg over 15 minutes, (repeated once in severe cases) then 30–60 microg/kg per hour		infusion

(Continued)

Table 46.1 (Continued)

Drug	Indication, mode of action and comments	Route	Dose	Post menstrual/ Chronological age	Frequency (times/24 hours)
Morphine	Opioid sedative and analgesic given by iv bolus or (best) by infusion. Can also be given im, orally or rectally but larger doses will be needed for oral administration. The *infusion* dose quoted will only sedate, serious pain requires double this loading and maintenance dose.	iv boluses / iv / iv infusion	100 microg/kg per dose (can be doubled *if ventilated*) / loading dose 120 microg/kg maintenance 10 microg/kg/hour		2 or 3 / once only infusion
Naloxone	Opioid antagonist – to reverse effect of maternal opioids – use the ADULT (400 microg/ml) preparation. To diagnose opioid sedation	im / iv	100 microg/kg (effect lasts up to 24 hours) / 40 microg (effect lasts 30 mins)		once only / repeatable
Neostigmine	Cholinesterase inhibitor prolongs muscarinic and nicotinic effects of acetylcholine. Used for the diagnosis & treatment of neonatal myasthenia, and to reverse the effect of non-depolarising muscle relaxants (e.g. pancuronium).	iv / im / iv	for diagnosis 50 microg/kg / for treatment 150–300 microg/kg per dose / for reversal 80 microg/kg (after 20 microg/kg of atropine)		once only / 3–6 / once only
Netilmicin	Aminoglycoside antibiotic. Said to be less ototoxic than gentamicin. Aim for a trough level of 1 mg/l or less. Extend dosage interval to 36 hours if level is 2 mg/l or greater just before fourth dose. (1 mg = 2.1 micromol)	iv, im	5 mg/kg check trough level with fourth dose		1
Noradrenaline (Norepinephrine)	Postganglionic sympathetic neurotransmitter, a potent vasoconstrictor sometimes used to maintain blood pressure in septic shock. Use a central vein. 1 mg noradrenaline acid tartrate = 0.5 mg of noradrenaline base	via central vein	start with 0.1 microg/kg per minute of noradrenaline base (max 1.5 microg/kg base per minute)		infusion
Nystatin	Polyene antifungal for candida infection.	oral, topical	100 000 units per dose		4 (after feeds)
Octreotide	Synthetic analogue of the hypothalamic hormone somatostatin.	subcut inj / iv	5 microg/kg per dose / 25 microg/kg per dose		3–4
Pancuronium	Competitive non depolarising muscle relaxant used to induce paralysis in ventilated babies.	iv, (im)	initial dose 100 microg/kg repeat doses 50 microg/kg		once only usually 4–6
Paracetamol	A useful analgesic. This drug has a large volume of distribution – if a loading dose is not given then a therapeutic level is not reached for four or more doses. Check the blood level if using high dose treatment for more than 24 hours in a baby less than 3 months old.	oral / rectal	24 mg/kg loading dose then 12 mg/kg thereafter / 36 mg/kg then 24 mg/kg	(less than 32 wks) / (less than 32 wks)	6 (3) / 6 (3)
Paraldehyde	Emergency anticonvulsant. Best given rectally mixed 1:1 by volume with olive oil.	deep im / rectal	0.2 ml/kg / 0.4 ml/kg of paraldehyde (0.8 ml/kg of mixture)		repeatable once / once

				0–1 week	1–3 weeks	4 weeks or more
Penicillin G (Benzylpenicillin)	Drug of choice for group B streptococcal infection.	iv, im	30 mg/kg per dose (60 mg/kg in meningitis)	2	3	4
Pethidine	A synthetic opioid that can be used for pain relief in ventilated babies but morphine is preferable.	iv, im	1 mg/kg	1 or 2		
Phenobarbitone	First line anticonvulsant. Aim for a serum level of 20–40 mg/l; 1 mg = 4.42 micromol. Where the standard loading dose does not suffice a further 10 mg/kg can be given but may well cause significant sedation.	iv, im iv, oral	loading dose 20 mg/kg maintenance 4 mg/kg (increase to 5 mg/kg after 2 weeks)	once only 1		
Phenytoin	Second line anticonvulsant. Plasma levels must be monitored if used for more than 48 hours. Aim for levels of 10–20 mg/l. 1 mg = 3.96 micromol	iv only	loading dose 20 mg/kg (give over 20 minutes with ECG) maintenance usually 2.5 mg/kg per dose	once only 2		
Propranolol	β blocker, antiarrythmic, used to control cyanotic spells in Fallots tetralogy and for neonatal thyrotoxicosis.	oral	250–750 microg/kg per dose initially, up to 2 mg/kg per dose.	3		
Propylthiouracil	Thioamide antithyroid for symptomatic hyperthroidism. (also see Iodine)	oral	1.5–3.5 mg/kg per dose	3		
Prostaglandin E_2	Used to keep the ductus arteriosus open in duct dependent cardiac malformations. Takes about 3 hours to reach maximal effect. Respiratory depression and apnoea can occur. E_2 is just as effective as E_1 and much cheaper.	iv infusion	0.6 microg/kg per hour (i.e. 10 nanog/kg/min) higher doses have been used but they are no more effective and cause more side effects, especially apnoea.	infusion		
Prostaglandin I_2 (Prostacyclin)	See Epoprostenol					
Pyridoxine	Used to diagnose pyridoxine dependency as a cause of seizures (watch for apnoea) – and for their treatment.	iv oral	100 mg bolus (with EEG monitoring) start with 30 mg/kg per dose	once only 1		
Ranitidine	H_2 histamine receptor blocker that inhibits gastric acid secretion (best avoided in renal failure). Or as a continuous infusion (which may be safer).	iv iv iv infusion	500 microg/kg per dose slowly to avoid arryhthmias loading dose 250 microg/kg maintenance 50 microg/kg/hour	4 (2 if less than 32 wks gestation) once only infusion		
Rifampicin	Antituberculous agent (seek expert advice) and potent (reserve) antistaphylococcal antibiotic usually used together with teicoplanin or vancomycin.	iv oral	10 mg/kg per dose over 60 minutes (20 mg/kg in TB meningitis) 20 mg/kg	2 1		
Salbutamol	Betamimetic and bronchodilator. Can rapidly reduce plasma potassium to buy time in an emergency.	nebulised iv	2.5 mg nebulised 4 microg/kg over 10 minutes	repeatable once		

(Continued)

Table 46.1 (*Continued*)

Drug	Indication, mode of action and comments	Route	Dose	Post menstrual/ Chronological age	Frequency (times/24 hours)
Sodium Bicarbonate	For correction of metabolic acidosis. 1 ml of 8.4% solution contains 1 mmol of bicarbonate. Can be given orally to correct late metabolic acidosis. Consider THAM if concerned about sodium loading.	iv	0.5 mmol/kg for each mmol of desired correction of base deficit give slowly (*max rate 0.5 mmol/kg per minute*)		repeatable
Spironolactone	Aldosterone antagonist, potassium sparing diuretic. Usually combined with chlorothiazide.	oral	1 or 2 mg/kg per dose		2
Streptokinase	Activates plasmin which causes lysis of clots. Can be used to dissolve arterial clots.	iv infusion	3000 units/kg loading dose then 500–1000 units/kg per hour		once only
Suxamethonium	Short acting depolarising muscle relaxant used to facilitate intubation. Effect lasts 5–10 mins.	iv	2–3 mg/kg		single dose
Teicoplanin	Reserve antibiotic for coagulase negative staphylococci. Double dosage interval in renal failure.	iv, im	loading dose 16 mg/kg maintenance 8 mg/kg		once only 1
THAM	Organic buffer used to treat metabolic acidosis, a sodium free alternative to sodium bicarbonate.	iv	0.6 mmol/kg for each mmol of desired correction of base deficit.		repeatable
Theophylline	Respiratory stimulant for neonatal apnoea (*but caffeine is both easier to use and safer*). By weight aminophylline is 85% theophylline and choline theophyllinate is 64% theophylline. Optimum levels 8–12 mg/l, side effects above 14 mg/l. (1 mg = 5.55 micromol)	iv oral	loading dose 8 mg/kg aminophylline maintenance 2.5 mg/kg per dose loading dose 9 mg/kg choline theophyllinate maintenance 4 mg/kg per dose		once only 2 once only 2
Thyroxine	See Lerothyroxine				
Tobramycin	Aminoglycoside antibiotic. Check level and adjust dosage interval around fourth dose. Aim for a trough level of 1 mg/l or less. Extend dosage interval to 36 hours if trough is 2 mg/l or greater. (1 mg = 2.14 mmol)	iv, im	5 mg/kg check trough level with fourth dose		1
Tolazoline	Alpha adrenergic antagonist used to produce pulmonary vasodilatation but also causes systemic vasodilatation and may cause hypotension. Works best if any significant acidosis is corrected first.	iv iv infusion	1 mg/kg bolus 0.2 mg/kg per hour		once only infusion
Trimethoprim	Antibiotic particularly valuable in urinary tract infection for both treatment and prophylaxis	oral (iv)	3–4 mg/kg per dose 2 mg/kg		2 (3 if other than urinary infection) once at night

Drug	Description	Route	Dose	
Vancomycin	Reserve antibiotic for gram positive organisms especially coagulase negative staphylococci. Monitoring levels is usually not necessary. [If monitoring then a trough level of (1 mg = 0.69 micromol)]	iv	15 mg/kg per dose (give over one hour) 5–10 mg/l is thought to be appropriate	less than 29 weeks 1 29–35 weeks 2 36 weeks or more 3
Vitamin D	Most term and preterm formulae are appropriately supplemented.	oral	300 units (7.5 microg) per dose	1
Vitamin K (Phytomenadione)	Prophylaxis against vitamin K deficiency bleeding. There is some concern that intramuscular dosage is associated with an increased risk of childhood cancer. The risk does not seem to extend to oral dosage.	im oral	1 mg at birth either 25 microg per day or 1 mg once per weeks	once only for 3 months if breast fed

Post menstrual age is the age in completed weeks from the mothers LMP. A baby born at 26 weeks gestation 4 weeks ago has a post menstrual age today of 30 weeks.
Chronological age is the age in completed weeks from birth.

Units

1 kilogram (kg) = 1000 grams
1 gram (g) = 1000 milligrams
1 milligram (mg) = 1000 micrograms
1 microgram (microg) = 1000 nanograms
1 nanogram (nanog) = 1000 picograms

Solutions

A 1:100 (1%) weight for volume (w/v) solution contains 1 g of substance in 100 ml of solution or 10 milligrams in 1 ml
A 1:1000 solution contains 1 milligram in 1 ml
A 1:10 000 solution contains 100 micrograms in 1 ml

APPENDIX 1

Haematological values in the newborn

Irene A G Roberts

Table A1.1 Red cell parameters in the fetus

Age (weeks)	Hb (g/dl)	PCV	RBC ($\times 10^{12}$/l)	MCV (fl)	MCH (pg)	MCHC (g/dl)	Nucleated RBC (% of WBC)	Reticulocytes (%)
12	8.0–10.0	0.33	1.5	180	60	34	5.0–8.0	40
16	10.0	0.35	2.0	140	45	33	2.0–4.0	10–25
20	11.0	0.37	2.5	135	44	33	1.0	10–20
24	14.0	0.40	3.5	123	38	31	1.0	5–10
28	14.5	0.45	4.0	120	40	31	0.5	5–20
34	15.0	0.47	4.4	118	38	32	0.2	3–10
Term 40 cord	16.8	0.53	5.25	107	34	31.7	0.01	3–7

Hb, haemoglobin; MCH = mean corpuscular haemoglobin; MCHC = mean corpuscular haemoglobin concentration; MCV = mean cell volume; PCV = packed cell volume; RBC = red blood cells; WBC = white blood cells.
Adapted from Oski F A, Naiman J L 1982 Hematologic problems in the newborn, 3rd edn. W B Saunders, New York.

Table A1.2 Normal leukocyte counts ($\times 10^9$/l) in the first month of life

Age	Total leukocytes Mean (range)	Neutrophils Mean (range)	%	Lymphocytes Mean (range)	%	Monocytes Mean	%	Eosinophils Mean	%
Birth	18.1 (9.0–30.0)	11.1 (6.0–26.0)	61	5.5 (2.0–11.0)	31	1.1	6	0.4	2
12 hrs	22.8 (13.0–38.0)	15.5 (6.0–28.0)	68	5.5 (2.0–11.0)	24	1.2	5	0.5	2
24 hrs	18.9 (9.4–34.0)	11.5 (5.0–21.0)	61	5.8 (2.0–11.5)	31	1.1	6	0.5	2
1 week	12.2 (5.0–21.0)	5.5 (1.5–10.0)	45	5.0 (2.0–17.0)	41	1.1	9	0.5	4
2 weeks	11.4 (5.0–20.0)	4.5 (1.0–9.5)	40	5.5 (2.0–17.0)	48	1.0	9	0.4	3
1 month	10.8 (5.0–19.5)	3.8 (1.0–9.0)	35	6.0 (2.5–16.5)	56	0.7	7	0.3	3

Neutrophils include band forms and a small number of metamyelocytes and myelocytes in the first few days of life.
With permission from Dallman P R 1977 In: Rudolph A M (ed) Pediatrics, 16th edn. Appleton-Century-Crofts, New York, p 1178.

APPENDIX 2

Coagulation values in term and preterm infants

Irene A G Roberts

Table A2.1 Reference values for coagulation tests in healthy term infants and in the adult (means and standard deviations)

Test	Day 1	Day 5	Day 30	Adult
PT (s)	13 ± 1.43	12.4 ± 1.46	11.8 ± 1.25	12.4 ± 0.78
APPT (s)	42.9 ± 5.8	42.6 ± 8.62	40.4 ± 7.42	33.5 ± 3.44
TCT (s)	23.5 ± 2.38	23.1 ± 3.07	24.3 ± 2.44	25 ± 2.66
Fibrinogen (g/l)	2.83 ± 0.58	3.12 ± 0.75	2.7 ± 0.54	2.78 ± 0.61
II (U/ml)	0.48 ± 0.11	0.63 ± 0.15	0.68 ± 0.17	1.08 ± 0.19
V (U/ml)	0.72 ± 0.18	0.95 ± 0.25	0.98 ± 0.18	1.06 ± 0.22
VII (U/ml)	0.66 ± 0.19	0.89 ± 0.27	0.9 ± 0.24	1.05 ± 0.19
VIII (U/ml)	1.00 ± 0.39	0.88 ± 0.33	0.91 ± 0.33	0.99 ± 0.25
vWF (U/ml)	1.53 ± 0.67	1.40 ± 0.57	1.28 ± 0.59	0.92 ± 0.33
IX (U/ml)	0.53 ± 0.19	0.53 ± 0.19	0.51 ± 0.15	1.09 ± 0.27
X (U/ml)	0.40 ± 0.14	0.49 ± 0.15	0.59 ± 0.14	1.06 ± 0.23
XI (U/ml)	0.38 ± 0.14	0.55 ± 0.16	0.53 ± 0.13	0.97 ± 0.15
XII (U/ml)	0.53 ± 0.20	0.47 ± 0.18	0.49 ± 0.16	1.08 ± 0.28
Plasminogen (U/ml)	1.95 ± 0.35	2.17 ± 0.38	1.98 ± 0.36	3.36 ± 0.44

All factors except fibrinogen and plasminogen are expressed as units per millilitre where pooled plasma contains 1.0 U/ml. Plasminogen units are those recommended by the Committee on Thrombolytic Agents.
APPT = activated partial thromboplastin time; PT = prothrombin time; TCT = thrombin clotting time; vWF = von Willebrand factor.
From Andrew M, Paes B, Milner R et al 1987 Development of the human coagulation system in the full term infant. Blood 70: 165–172.

Table A2.2 Reference values for coagulation tests in preterm infants (means and boundaries given, where the boundaries encompass 95% of the observations)

Test	Day 1	Day 5	Day 30	Adult
PT (s)	13 (10.6–16.2)	12.5 (10.0–15.3)	11.8 (10.0–13.6)	12.4 (10.8–13.9)
APPT (s)	53.6 (27.5–79.4)	50.5 (26.9–74.1)	44.7 (26.9–62.5)	33.5 (26.6–40.3)
TCT (s)	24.8 (19.2–30.4)	24.1 (18.8–29.4)	24.4 (18.8–29.9)	25.0 (19.7–30.3)
Fibrinogen (g/l)	2.43 (1.5–3.73)	2.8 (1.6–4.2)	2.54 (1.5–4.14)	2.78 (1.56–4.0)
II (U/ml)	0.45 (0.41–1.44)	0.57 (0.29–0.85)	0.57 (0.36–0.95)	1.08 (0.71–1.46)
V (U/ml)	0.88 (0.41–1.44)	1.0 (0.46–1.54)	1.02 (0.48–1.56)	1.06 (0.62–1.50)
VII (U/ml)	0.67 (0.21–1.13)	0.84 (0.3–1.38)	0.83 (0.21–1.45)	1.05 (0.67–1.43)
VIII (U/ml)	1.11 (0.50–2.13)	1.15 (0.53–2.05)	1.11 (0.5–1.99)	0.99 (0.5–1.49)
vWF (U/ml)	1.36 (0.78–2.1)	1.33 (0.72–2.19)	1.36 (0.66–2.16)	0.92 (0.5–1.58)
IX (U/ml)	0.35 (0.19–0.65)	0.42 (0.14–0.74)	0.44 (0.13–0.8)	1.09 (0.55–1.63)
X (U/ml)	0.41 (0.11–0.71)	0.51 (0.19–0.83)	0.56 (0.20–0.92)	1.06 (0.7–1.52)
XI (U/ml)	0.30 (0.08–0.52)	0.41 (0.13–0.69)	0.43 (0.15–0.71)	0.97 (0.67–1.27)
XII (U/ml)	0.38 (0.10–0.66)	0.39 (0.09–0.69)	0.43 (0.11–0.75)	1.08 (0.52–1.64)
Plasminogen (U/ml)	1.70 (1.12–2.48)	1.91 (1.21–2.61)	1.81 (1.09–2.53)	3.36 (2.48–4.24)

APPT = activated partial thromboplastin time; PT = prothrombin time; TCT = thrombin clotting time; vWF = von Willebrand factor. From Andrew M, Paes B, Milner R et al 1988 Development of the coagulation system in the healthy premature infant. Blood 72: 1651–1657.

Table A2.3 Reference values for the inhibitors of coagulation in healthy full-term infants (means $\pm$ standard deviations)

Coagulation inhibitor (U/ml)	Day 1	Day 5	Day 30	Adult
AT III	0.63 ± 0.12	0.67 ± 0.13	0.78 ± 0.15	1.05 ± 0.13
α_2 M	1.39 ± 0.22	1.48 ± 0.25	1.50 ± 0.22	0.86 ± 0.17
α_2 AP	0.85 ± 0.15	1.0 ± 0.15	1.0 ± 0.12	1.02 ± 0.17
C_1-INH	0.72 ± 0.18	0.9 ± 0.15	0.89 ± 0.21	1.01 ± 0.15
α_1 AT	0.83 ± 0.22	0.89 ± 0.20	0.62 ± 0.13	0.93 ± 0.19
Protein C	0.35 ± 0.09	0.42 ± 0.11	0.43 ± 0.11	0.96 ± 0.16
Protein S	0.36 ± 0.12	0.50 ± 0.14	0.63 ± 0.15	0.92 ± 0.16

α_1 AT = α_1 antitrypsin; α_2 AP = α_2 antiplasmin; α_2 M = α_2 macroglobulin; AT III = antithrombin III; C_1-INH = C_1 esterase inhibitor. From Andrew M, Paes B, Milner R et al 1987 Development of the human coagulation system in the full term infant. Blood 70: 165–172.

Table A2.4 Reference values for the inhibitors of coagulation in preterm infants (means and boundaries given, where the boundaries encompass 95% of the observations)

Coagulation inhibitor (U/ml)	Day 1	Day 5	Day 30	Adult
AT III	0.38 (0.14–0.62)	0.56 (0.30–0.82)	0.59 (0.37–0.81)	1.05 (0.79–1.31)
α_2 M	1.10 (0.56–1.82)	1.25 (0.71–0.77)	1.38 (0.72–2.04)	0.86 (0.52–1.2)
α_2 AP	0.78 (0.40–1.16)	0.81 (0.49–1.13)	0.89 (0.55–1.23)	1.02 (0.68–1.36)
C_1-INH	0.65 (0.31–0.99)	0.83 (0.45–1.21)	0.74 (0.40–1.24)	1.01 (0.71–1.31)
α_1 AT	0.90 (0.36–1.44)	0.94 (0.42–1.46)	0.76 (0.38–1.12)	0.93 (0.55–1.31)
Protein C	0.28 (0.12–0.44)	0.31 (0.11–0.51)	0.37 (0.15–0.59)	0.96 (0.64–1.28)
Protein S	0.26 (0.14–0.38)	0.37 (0.13–0.61)	0.56 (0.22–0.90)	0.92 (0.60–1.24)

α_1 AT = α_1 antitrypsin; α_2 AP = α_2 antiplasmin; α_2 M = α_2 macroglobulin; AT III = antithrombin III; C_1-INH = C_1 esterase inhibitor. From Andrew M, Paes B, Milner R et al 1988 Development of the coagulation system in the healthy premature infant. Blood 72: 1651–1657.

APPENDIX 3

Normal ranges for commonly assessed ECG values in the newborn

Nick Archer

	<1 day	1–3 days	4–7 days	8–10 days
Heart rate (beats/min)	94–155	92–158	90–166	106–182
PR lead II (ms)	80–100	81–139	74–136	72–138
QRS duration V5 (ms)	21–75	22–67	21–68	22–79
Frontal QRS axis (degrees)	+60 to +190	+62 to +196	+75 to +190	+65 to +160
QRS size (mV)				
V1				
Q	0	0	0	0
R	0.5–2.6	0.5–2.6	0.3–2.4	0.3–2.1
S	0–2.3	0–2.1	0–1.7	0–1.1
T	−0.3 to 4	−0.4 to 4	−0.45 to 2.5	−5 to −1
V6				
Q	0–0.17	0–0.21	0–0.28	0–0.28
R	0–1.1	0–1.2	0–1.2	0.25–1.6
S	0–1.0	0–0.9	0–1.0	0–1.0
R/S V1	0.2–9.8	0.2–6	0.2–9.8	1–7
R/S V6	0.2–10	0.2–11	0.2–10	0.2–12

Ranges given are approximately 2nd and 98th centiles, derived from Davignon A et al[1] Qtc = $QT/\sqrt{RR}$, using lead II and where the RR interval is the one preceding the QRS complex in which the QT interval is measured. Qtc 98th centile figure from Davignon and colleagues is <0.48, except in the first few days of life, when higher values may transiently be found. Other authors consider persistent values above 0.46 to be abnormal.[2]

References

1. Davignon A, Rautaharju P, Boisselle E, Soumis F, Megelas M, Choquette A
   1979/80 Normal ECG standards for infants and children. Pediatric Cardiology
   1: 123–131
2. Garson A 1990 Ventricular arrhythmias. In: Gillette P C, Garson A (eds)
   Pediatric arrhythmias: electrophysiology and pacing. W B Saunders, Philadelphia,
   pp 427–500

APPENDIX 4

Neonatal blood pressure: normal values

Nick Archer

Table A4.1 Day 1, healthy low-birthweight infants (not receiving inotropes or intermittent positive pressure ventilation)

Birthweight (g)	n	Systolic range (mmHg)	Diastolic range (mmHg)
501–750	18	50–62	26–36
751–1000	39	48–59	23–36
1001–1250	30	49–61	26–35
1251–1500	45	46–56	23–33
1501–1750	51	46–58	23–33
1751–2000	61	48–61	24–35

Some infants in added inspired oxygen, some receiving continuous positive airway pressure. Some recordings direct intra-arterial, some oscillometric.
From Hegyi T, Carbone M T, Anwar M et al 1994 Blood pressure ranges in premature infants: 1. The first hours of life. Journal of Pediatrics 124: 627–633.

Table A4.2 Day 1, healthy preterm infants

Gestation (weeks)	n	Systolic range (mmHg)	Diastolic range (mmHg)
<24	11	48–63	24–39
24–28	55	48–58	22–36
29–32	110	47–59	24–34
>32	68	48–60	24–34

Same infant characteristics and measurement methods as in Table A4.1.
From Hegyi T, Carbone M T, Anwar M et al 1994 Blood pressure ranges in premature infants: 1. The first hours of life. Journal of Pediatrics 124: 627–633.

Table A4.3 Week 1, healthy low-birthweight infants (<2000 g)

Day	n	Systolic range (mmHg)	Diastolic range (mmHg)
1	183	48–63	25–35
2	121	54–63	30–39
3	117	53–67	31–43
4	85	57–71	32–45
5	76	56–72	33–47
6	59	57–71	32–47
7	48	61–74	34–46

Same infant characteristics and measurement methods as in Tables A4.1 and A4.2.
From Hegyi T, Anwar M, Carbone M T et al 1996 Blood pressure ranges in premature infants: 2. The first week of life. Pediatrics 97: 336–342.

Table A4.4 Non-invasive (indirect) arm systolic blood pressures (mmHg) with pulse detected by Doppler probe

Age (days)	3	4	5	6	7	8–10
Awake						
Mean systolic BP (mmHg) ± SD	72 ± 6	74 ± 9	77 ± 10	77 ± 10	82 ± 9	88 ± 17
No. of infants	4	71	44	42	9	4
Asleep						
Mean systolic BP (mmHg) ± SD	68 ± 7	70 ± 8	72 ± 8	72 ± 9	72 ± 9	75 ± 9
No. of infants	72	681	426	322	47	18

All infants 38 weeks' gestation or more.
Derived from de Swiet M, Fayers P, Shinebourne E A 1980 Systolic blood pressure in a population of infants in the first year of life: the Brompton study. Pediatrics 65: 1028–1035.

APPENDIX 5

Birthweight and head circumference centiles

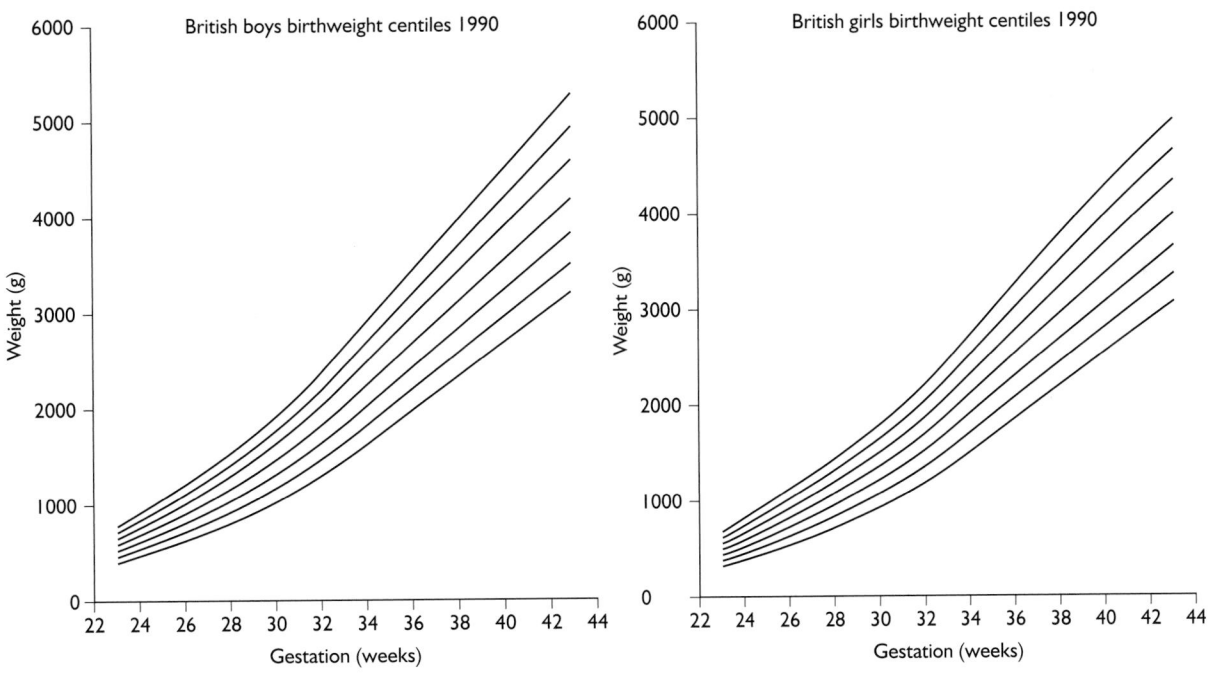

British 1990 growth reference birthweight centiles (g)

	Boys								Girls					
Weeks	3rd	10th	25th	50th	75th	90th	97th	Weeks	3rd	10th	25th	50th	75th	90th	97th
23	386	451	515	585	653	713	771	23	346	407	469	535	601	660	717
24	463	539	614	696	776	846	915	24	421	493	565	644	722	792	860
25	541	628	714	807	899	981	1060	25	497	576	662	753	843	924	1004
26	623	720	817	922	1026	1118	1208	26	576	669	762	864	967	1059	1149
27	710	817	924	1042	4458	1261	1362	27	660	762	866	980	1095	1198	1299
28	803	921	1040	1170	1299	1414	1527	28	750	863	977	1004	1231	1345	1458
29	906	1035	1166	1309	1452	1580	1705	29	849	972	1097	1237	1377	1504	1629
30	1020	1162	1305	1463	1620	1762	1901	30	961	1095	1232	1385	1540	1680	1819
31	1148	1303	1460	1634	1807	1964	2117	31	1086	1232	1382	1551	1721	1876	2029
32	1291	1459	1631	1822	2013	2185	2355	32	1226	1385	1548	1733	1920	2090	2259
33	1446	1630	1816	2025	2235	2424	2611	33	1378	1550	1728	1929	2134	2320	2506
34	1612	1811	2013	2240	2469	2676	2881	34	1541	1727	1919	2137	2359	2562	2765
35	1786	1999	2218	2463	2711	2935	3159	35	1712	1912	2118	2353	2593	2812	3032
36	1965	2192	2426	2689	2955	3197	3439	36	1889	2101	2321	2572	2828	3064	3301
37	2145	2385	2633	2913	3198	3457	3716	37	2066	2290	2523	2789	3062	3314	3567
38	2323	2576	2837	3133	3434	3709	3985	38	2243	2477	2722	3002	3290	3556	3824
39	2497	2761	3035	3345	3662	3952	4243	39	2461	2660	2915	3208	3509	3788	4070
40	2669	2944	3229	3553	3884	4189	4494	40	2584	2836	3101	3405	3720	4011	4305
41	2842	3127	3423	3760	4100	4424	4744	41	2748	3009	3282	3597	3923	4225	4531
42	3019	3313	3620	3970	4330	4662	4996	42	2914	3183	3465	3790	4127	4440	4759
43	3201	3505	3822	4186	4560	4906	5255	43	3086	3362	3653	3989	4338	4662	4993

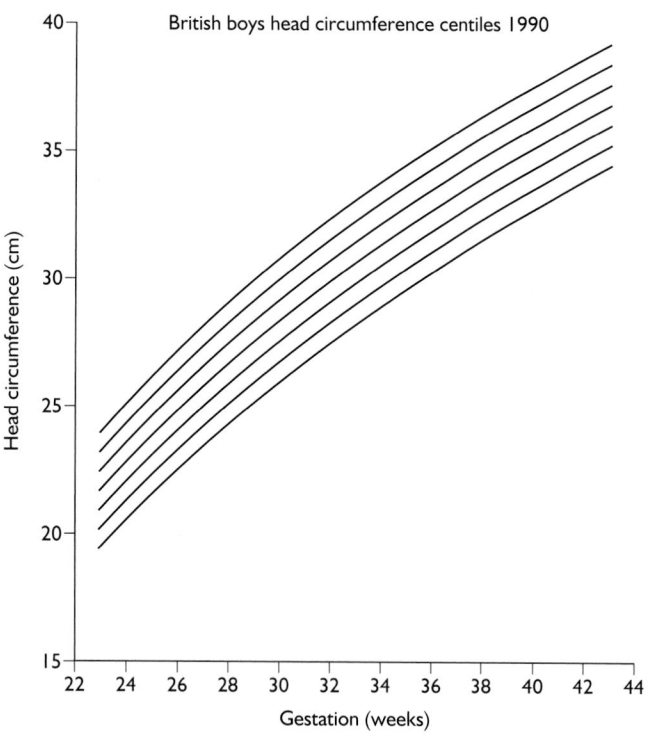

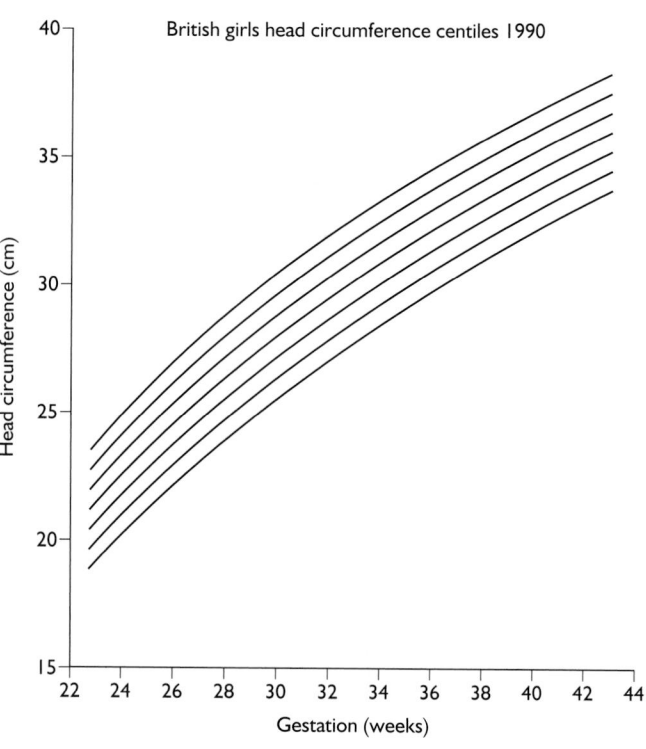

British 1990 growth reference head circumference centiles (cm)

	Boys								Girls					
Weeks	3rd	10th	25th	50th	75th	90th	97th	Weeks	3rd	10th	25th	50th	75th	90th	97th
23	19.3	20	20.8	21.6	22.4	23.1	23.8	23	18.9	19.6	20.4	21.2	22	22.8	23.5
24	20.4	21.2	21.9	22.7	23.6	24.3	25	24	20	20.8	21.5	22.4	23	24	24.7
25	21.4	22.2	22.9	23.8	24.6	25.4	26.1	25	21	21.8	22.5	23.5	24.3	25	25.8
26	22.4	23.2	24	24.8	25.7	26.4	27.2	26	22	22.8	23.6	24.4	25.3	26.1	26.8
27	23.4	24.2	24.9	25.8	26.6	27.4	28.2	27	23	23.7	24.5	25.4	26.3	27.1	27.8
28	24.3	25.1	25.9	26.7	27.6	28.4	29.1	28	23.9	24.7	25.5	26.3	27.2	28	28.8
29	25.2	25.9	26.7	27.6	28.5	29.3	30	29	24.8	25.5	26.3	27.2	28.1	28.9	29.7
30	26	26.8	27.6	28.4	29.3	30.1	30.9	30	25.6	26.4	27.2	28	28.9	29.7	30.5
31	26.8	27.5	28.3	29.2	30.1	30.9	31.6	31	26.3	27.1	27.9	28.8	29.7	30.4	31.2
32	27.5	28.3	29.1	29.9	30.8	31.6	32.4	32	27.1	27.9	28.6	29.5	30.4	31.2	31.9
33	28.3	29	29.8	30.7	31.6	32.4	33.1	33	27.8	28.6	29.4	30.2	31.1	31.9	32.7
34	29	29.7	30.5	31.4	32.3	33.0	33.8	34	28.5	29.3	30.1	30.9	31.8	32.6	33.3
35	29.7	30.4	31.2	32.1	33	33.7	34.5	35	29.2	29.9	30.7	31.6	32.4	33.2	34
36	30.3	31.1	31.9	32.7	33.6	34.4	35.2	36	29.8	30.6	31.4	32.2	33.1	33.8	34.6
37	30.9	31.7	32.5	33.4	34.2	35	35.8	37	30.4	31.2	31.9	32.8	33.6	34.4	35.2
38	31.6	32.3	33.1	34	34.9	35.6	36.4	38	31	31.8	32.6	33.4	34.2	35	35.7
39	32.2	33	33.7	34.6	35.5	36.2	37	39	31.6	32.4	33.1	34	34.8	35.6	36.3
40	32.8	33.6	34.3	35.2	36.1	36.8	37.6	40	32.2	33	33.7	34.5	35.4	36.1	36.9
41	33.4	34.1	34.9	35.8	36.6	37.4	38.2	41	32.8	33.5	34.3	35.1	35.9	36.7	37.4
42	34	34.7	35.5	36.3	37.2	38	38.7	42	33.3	34	34.8	35.6	36.4	37.2	37.9
43	34.5	35.3	36	36.9	37.7	38.5	39.3	43	33.9	34.6	35.3	36.1	37	37.7	38.4

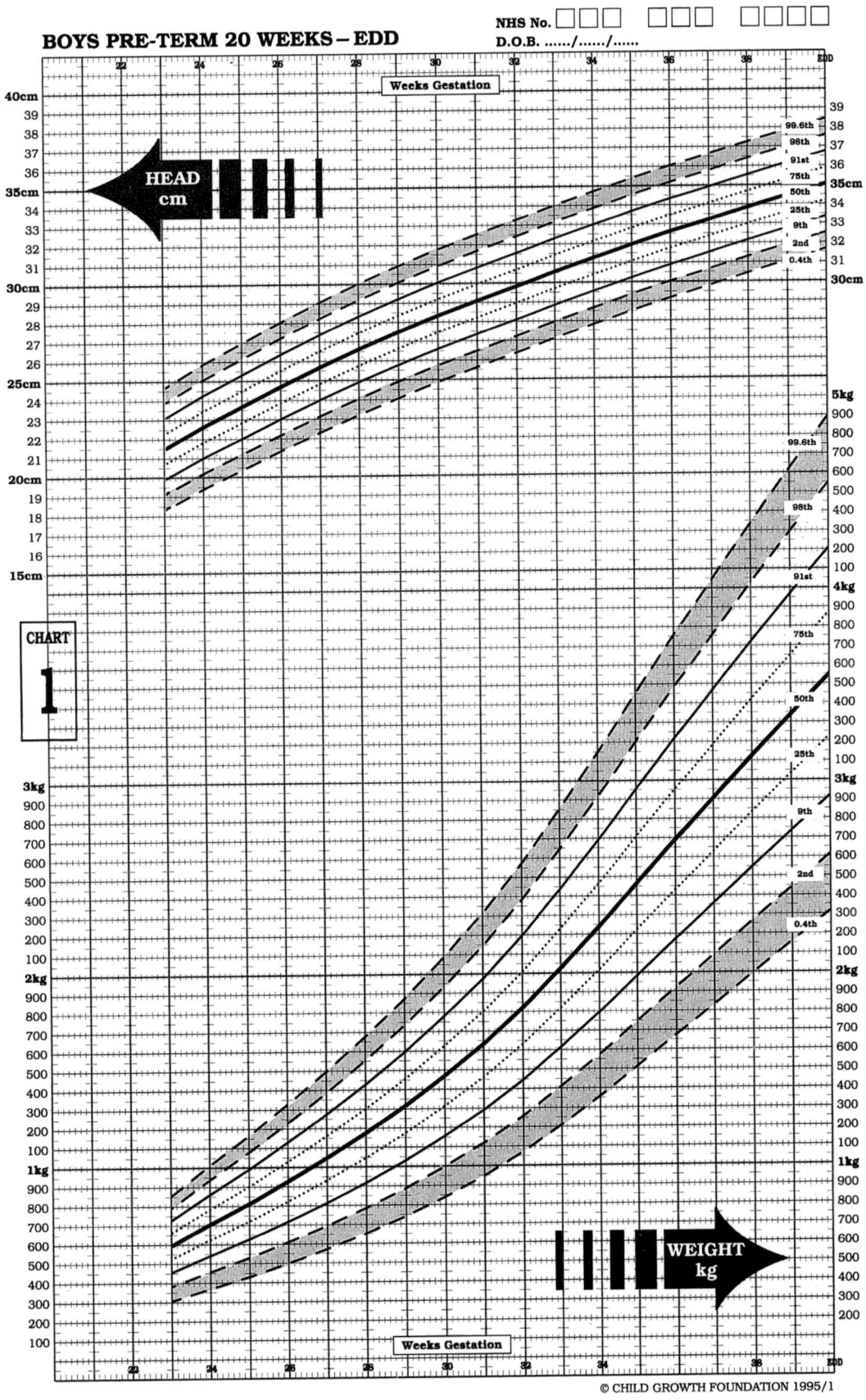

BOYS PRE-TERM 20 WEEKS — EDD

NHS No.

D.O.B. ....../....../......

Weeks Gestation

HEAD cm

CHART 1

WEIGHT kg

Weeks Gestation

© CHILD GROWTH FOUNDATION 1995/1

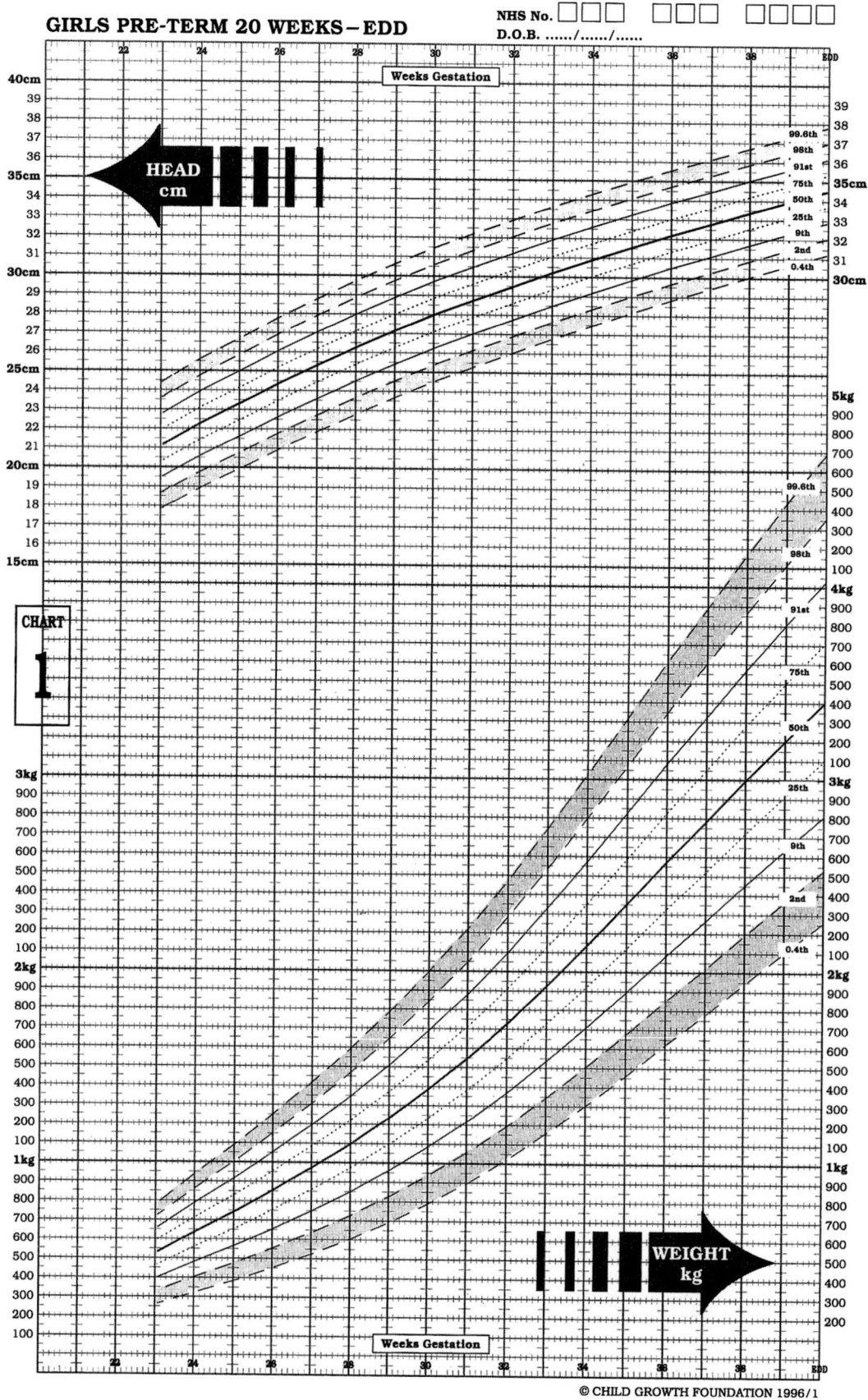

GIRLS PRE-TERM 20 WEEKS—EDD

NHS No.

D.O.B. ....../....../......

Weeks Gestation

HEAD cm

CHART 1

WEIGHT kg

Weeks Gestation

© CHILD GROWTH FOUNDATION 1996/1

APPENDIX 6

Neonatal biochemical reference ranges

Ruth M Ayling, Fiona Carragher

Analyte	Unit	Reference range					Comment
		Preterm			Term		
		Gestational age (weeks)	Age	Reference range	Age	Reference range	
Plasma/serum							
Alanine aminotransferase[50] (ALT)	IU/l				1–30 days	6–40	Range dependent on methodology
Albumin[59]	g/l	27		21–33	0–7 days	28–43	
		29		23–34	7–14 days	30–43	
		31		22–35	14–21 days	27–44	
		33		22–35	21–28 days	32–44	
		35		22–36			
Alkaline phosphatase[14] (ALP)	IU/l	26–27	5–10 days	319 ± 142	1–30 days	48–406	Range dependent on methodology. Higher activity in first week due to placental ALP
		28–29	5–10 days	291 ± 86			
		30–31	5–10 days	281 ± 84			
		32–33	5–10 days	253 ± 61			
		34–35	5–10 days	236 ± 61			
		36	5–10 days	207 ± 59			
Alpha$_1$-antitrypsin[10]	g/l				0–30 days	1.24–3.48	'Adult' concentrations at birth, falling after 2 weeks. To assess possible deficiency; phenotype should be determined if concentration <1.6 g/l
Alpha-fetoprotein[3] (AFP)	kU/l				Birth	7533–157 390	Higher in premature babies
					1 day	6561–137 082	
					2 days	5741–119 393	
					3 days	4977–103 988	
					4 days	4375–90 569	Half-life 5.1 days
					5 days	3819–79 796	
					6 days	3335–69 660	
					7 days	2911–60 811	
					8–14 days	1222–48 640	
					15–21 days	475–18 924	
					22–28 days	261–5212	
Aluminium[36]	micromol/l					0.07–0.80	
Ammonia[11]	micromol/l				0–30 days	17–91	Preterm and/or sick babies may have concentrations up to 200 micromol/l
Amylase[47]	IU/l				0–30 days	<30	Range dependent on methodology

Analyte	Units				Comments
Aspartate transaminase[50] (AST)	IU/l				Range dependent on methodology
Bilirubin[43]					
total	micromol/l			1-7 days 24-100 8-30 days 20-72 Birth-1 day <100 1-2 days <140 3-5 days <200 >14 days <20	Refer to neonatal treatment charts for further details
conjugated				0-30 days <4	
Caeruloplasmin[44]	g/l			1-30 days m 0.07-0.23 f 0.03-025	Increases from birth throughout first year
Calcium					
total[30,50,56]	mmol/l	21-28	2.14-2.65	1-2 days 2.18-2.48 2-3 days 2.14-2.64 3-4 days 2.22-2.55 4-6 days 2.25-2.68 6-12 days 2.26-2.69	Results should be interpreted in conjunction with serum albumin concentration
ionised[35]	mmol/l	25-36	1 day 0.81-1.41 2 days 0.72-1.44 3 days 1.04-1.52	1 day 1.05-1.37 3 days 1.10-1.44 5 days 1.20-1.48	
Chloride[15]	mmol/l			96-110	
Cholesterol[20]	mmol/l			1-30 days 1.4-4.01	Gradual increase from birth
Copper[29]	micromol/l	28-34	3.0-8.3	0-5 days 1.4-7.2 5-28 days 4.0-11.0	Rapid increase during first week
Cortisol[18,25]	mmol/l	24 25 26 27 28 29	0-14 days 73-562	1-7 days 204-1380 8-15 days 190-579	If there is doubt about the integrity of the hypothalamopituitary adrenal axis, a short synacthen test should be performed
C-reactive protein[5] (CRP)	mg/l			<5	
Creatine kinase[23] (CK)	IU/l			Cord blood 70-380 5-8h 214-1175 24-33h 130-1200 72-100h 87-725	% of total CK activity

% of total CK activity

	CKMB	CKBB
Cord	1.4	5.5
5-8h	4.6	9.1
24-33h	3.4	5.9
72-100h	3.4	10.3

Range dependent on methodology

(Continued)

Analyte	Unit	Reference range					Comment
		Preterm			Term		
		Gestational age (weeks)	Age	Reference range	Age	Reference range	
Creatinine[13,38,53]	micromol/l	24–28	1 day	35–136	2 days	37–113	Creatinine rises in the first 48 h, especially in infants <30 weeks' gestation[32]
		29–36	1 day	27–175	7 days	14–86	
		26–34	1 wk	69–141	14 days	18–58	
			2 wk	45–99	21 days	15–55	
			3–4 wk	39–71	28 days	12–48	
			5–6 wk	42–62			
			7–9 wk	39–48			
Cystatin C[13]	mg/l	24–28		0.65–3.37	0–28 days	0.81–2.32	
		29–36		0.62–4.42			
Ferritin[34]	microg/l				1–30 days	36–483	
Glucose (fasting)[16,54]	mmol/l				12–24 h	2.4–5.4	
					1–2 days	2.9–5.2	
					2–3 days	2.8–5.6	
					3–4 days	3.4–6.1	
					4–7 days	3.2–5.9	
					>7 days	3.9–7.0	
γ-Glutamyltransferase[53] (GGT)	IU/l				1–7 days	23–153	
					8–30 days	17–131	
17α-Hydroxyprogesterone[41] (17-OHP)	nmol/l				0–1 days	5–75	Premature and/or sick infants may have concentrations 2–3-fold higher
					1–7 days	1–10	
					7–28 days	0–8	
Immunoglobulins[2,12]							Lower in premature infants
Ig G	g/l	29–32	7 days	1.86–7.28	0–2 wk	5.0–17.0	
			14 days	1.19–6.37	2–4 wk	3.9–13.0	
			28 days	0.9–4			
Ig A	g/l	29–32	7 days	0–0.01	0–2 wk	0.01–0.08	
			14 days	0–0.08	2–4 wk	0.02–0.15	
			28 days	0–0.12			
IgM	g/l	29–32	7 days	0.02–0.39	0–2 wk	0.05–0.20	
			14 days	0.04–0.41	2–4 wk	0.08–0.40	
			28 days	0.06–0.3			
IgE	U/ml				0–30 days	<35	
Immunoreactive trypsin[19]	microg/l					<60	Blood spot

Analyte	Units	Gestation	Age	Reference range	Age	Reference range	Comments
Insulin[16]							Should be measured during documented hypoglycaemia. There may be cross-reactivity with proinsulins and values may be higher in premature infants, hence results should always be interpreted in light of clinical features and intravenous glucose requirements
Insulin-like growth factor-1[46] (IGF-1)	nmol/l		1–30 days	0.2–11.9			
Insulin-like growth factor binding protein-3[4] (IGFBP-3)	mg/l		0–1 wk 1–4 wk	0.42–1.39 0.77–2.09			
Iron[42]	micromol/l		1–30 days	5.2–22.7			May be higher at birth
Ketone bodies[17]	mmol/l	26–36	3 days	0.01–0.51	3 days	0.01–2.06	Low concentrations of ketone bodies and non-esterified fatty acids associated with hypoglycaemia are suggestive of hyperinsulinism
Lactate[28] (fasting)	mmol/l		Cord blood 1 h 24 h 7 days	1.5–4.5 0.9–2.7 0.8–1.2 0.5–1.4			
Lactate dehydrogenase[51] (LDH)	U/l		1–30 days	125–765			
Magnesium[31,35]	mmol/l	25–36	1 day 3 days 5 days 7–28 days	0.62–1.02 0.66–1.10 0.68–1.24 0.75–1.00	1 day 3 days 5 days 7–28 days	0.72–1.00 0.81–1.05 0.78–1.02 0.65–1.00	
Manganese[36]	nmol/l					<360	Risk of toxicity
Non-esterified fatty acids[17]	mmol/l	26–36	3 days	0.01–1.04	3 days	0.04–1.34	
Osmolality[9]	mosmol/kg		Birth 7 days 28 days	275–300 276–305 274–305		275–295	
Phenylalanine[22]	micromol/l			98–213		38–137	
Phosphate[55]	mmol/l		2–3 days 3–4 days 4–6 days 6–12 days 21 days	1.81–3.00 1.74–2.76 1.64–2.70 1.39–3.03 1.74–2.66			Tends to be higher in babies fed formula milk

(Continued)

Analyte	Unit	Reference range					Comment
		Preterm			Term		
		Gestational age (weeks)	Age	Reference range	Age	Reference range	
Potassium[15]	mmol/l		7 days	4.6–6.7	0–7 days	3.2–5.5	Results from capillary blood tend to be higher. Serum potassium concentrations are higher than those of plasma due to potassium released form platelets during clotting
					8–28 days	3.4–6.0	
Prolactin[7]	mU/l				0–30 days	9–2850	May be considerably higher in the first 2 weeks
Protein[21,59] (total)	g/l	22–36		36–63	1–30 days	41–63	
Pyruvate[43]	micromol/l				1–30 days	80–150	
Selenium[33]	micromol/l				0–4 wk	0.19–1.35	
Sodium[15]	mmol/l				0–30 days	133–146	
Thyroid-stimulating hormone[6] (TSH)	mU/l				1 day	3.0–120	Rapid increase during the first 24 h
					2 days	3.0–30	
					7 days	0.3–10	
					>7 days	0.3–5.0	
Thyroxine[1,8,24,48] free (FT$_4$)	pmol/l	25–30	0–7 days	6.4–42.5	1–3 days	25.7–68.2	
		31–36	0–7 days	16.7–60.6			
total (TT$_4$)	nmol/l	30–31	0–3 days	94–203	1–4 wk	142–277	
			3–10 days	53–146		106–214	
Triiodothyronine[1,8,24,48] free (FT$_3$)	pmol/l	29–36	1–3 days	1.2–7.3	1–3 days	2.5–9.3	Lower in small sick infants
			4–10 days	1.2–4.9	4–10 days	2.8–5.7	
total (TT$_3$)	nmol/l	<1850 g	0–3 days	0.28–0.63	1–30 days	0.2–3.2	
			21–28 days	0.63–1.17			
Triglyceride[49] (non-fasting)	mmol/l				0–7 days	0.24–2.06	
					8–30 days	0.34–2.08	
Urate[57]	micromol/l				0–1 days	300–505	
					1–2 days	200–490	
					2–3 days	190–395	
					3–7 days	150–290	
Urea[52]	mmol/l		7 days	0.5–4.2	1–7 days	0.7–4.6	May be higher in infants fed formula milk
					8–30 days	0.7–5.7	

Analyte	Units	Value	Age	Value	Age	Value	Age	Comments
Vitamin D[45]	microg/l					6–55	1–30 days	May show seasonal variation
Zinc[29,39]	micromol/l	28–34		10–24		9.9–21.4	0–5 days	Higher in preterms. Concentration decreases during first week
Urine								
Calcium[26]	mmol/l			0.2–1.6	0–7 days	<0.6	0–1 wk	
Calcium:creatinine ratio[40]	mmol/mmol					<2.4	1–4 wk	
Creatinine clearance[53]	ml/min/1.73m²			7–22 10–28 11–34 15–36 17–36	1 wk 2 wk 2–4 wk 5–6 wk 7–9 wk			
Fractional sodium excretion[37]	%					<0.72	0–3 days	$\dfrac{\text{Urinary [Sodium]} \times \text{Plasma [Creatinine]}}{\text{Plasma [Sodium]} \times \text{Urinary [Creatinine]}}$
Phosphate[58]	mmol/24h			<0.5–9.9 0.5–12	1–2 wk 3–4 wk	<18	0–7 days	
Potassium[58]	mmol/l mmol/kg/24h			2–28 0.2–1.2	0–30 days	<5		Dependent upon intake
Sodium[58]	mmol/l			1–15	0–30 days	<1		Dependent upon intake
Tubular phosphate reabsorption[37]	micromol/ml					1.89–2.37	0–30 days	Tubular phosphate reabsorption/ml GFR: $P[\text{phos}] - \dfrac{U[\text{phos}] \times P[\text{creat}]}{Ur[\text{creat}]}$
Urate:creatinine ratio[27]	mmol/mmol					0.1–2.0		The ratio is generally elevated in Lesch-Nyhan syndrome and <0.03mmol/m mol in sulphite oxidase deficiency

References

1. Adams L M, Emery J R, Clark S J et al 1995 Reference ranges for newer thyroid function tests in premature infants. Journal of Pediatrics 126: 122–127
2. Ballow M, Cates K L, Rowe J C et al 1986 Development of the immune system in very low birthweight (less than 1500 g) premature infants. Concentrations of plasma immunoglobulins and patterns of infections. Pediatric Research 20: 899–904
3. Blohm M E, Vesterling-Horner D, Calaminua G et al 1998 Alpha 1-fetoprotein (AFP) reference range values in infants up to 2 years of age. Paediatric Hematology and Oncology 15: 135–142
4. Blum W F, Ranke M B, Kietzmann K et al 1990 A specific radio-immunoassay for the growth hormone (GH)-dependent somatomedin-binding protein: its use for diagnosis of GH deficiency. Journal of Clinical Endocrinology and Metabolism 70: 1292–1298
5. Chiesa C, Signore F, Assumma M et al 2001 Serial measurements of C-reactive protein and interleukin-6 in the immediate postnatal period: reference intervals and analysis of maternal and perinatal confounders. Clinical Chemistry 47: 1016–1022
6. Clayton B E, Jenkins P, Round J M (eds) 1980 Paediatric chemical pathology. Blackwell Scientific, Oxford
7. Cook J F, Hicks J M, Godwin I D et al 1992 Pediatric reference ranges for prolactin. Clinical Chemistry 38: 959
8. Cuestas R A 1978 Thyroid function in preterm infants. Journal of Pediatrics 92: 963–967
9. Davies D P 1973 Plasma osmolality and protein intake in preterm infants. Archives of Disease in Childhood 48: 575–579
10. Davis M L, Austin C, Messmer B L et al 1996 IFCC-standardized pediatric reference intervals for 10 serum proteins using Beckman Array 360 system. Clinical Biochemistry 29: 489–492
11. Diaz J, Tornel P L, Martinez P 1995 Reference intervals for blood ammonia in healthy subjects determined by microdiffusion. Clinical Chemistry 41:1048
12. Drossou M, Cates K L, Rowe J C et al 1995 Concentrations of the main serum opsonins in early infancy. Archives of Disease in Childhood. Fetal and neonatal Edition 72: F172–F175
13. Finney H, Newman D J, Thakkar H et al 2000 Reference ranges for plasma cystatin C and creatinine measurements in premature infants, neonates and older children. Archives of Disease in Childhood 82: 71–75
14. Glass E J, Hume R, Hendry G M et al 1982 Plasma alkaline phosphatase activity in rickets of prematurity. Archives of Disease in Childhood 57: 373–376
15. Greeley C, Snell J, Colaco A et al 1993 Pediatric reference ranges for electrolytes and creatinine. Clinical Chemistry 39: 1172
16. Hawdon J M, Aynsley-Green A, Alberti K G M M et al 1993 The role of pancreatic insulin secretion in neonatal glucoregulation. I. Healthy term and preterm infants. Archives of Disease in Childhood 68: 274–279
17. Hawdon J M, Ward Platt M P, Aynsley-Green A 1992 Patterns of metabolic adaptation for preterm and term infants in the first week of life. Archives of Disease in Childhood 68: 274–279
18. Heckmann M, Wudy S A, Haack D et al 1991 Reference range for serum cortisol in well preterm infants. Archives of Disease in Childhood. Fetal and neonatal Edition 81: F171–F174
19. Heeley A F, Bangert S K 1992 The neonatal detection of cystic fibrosis by measurement of immunoreactive trypsin in blood. Annals of Clinical Biochemistry 29: 464–467
20. Hicks J M, Bailey J, Beatey J et al 1996 Pediatric reference ranges for cholesterol. Clinical Chemistry 42: S307
21. Hicks J M, Bjorn S, Beatey J et al 1995 Pediatric reference ranges for albumin, globulin and total protein on the Hitachi 747. Clinical Chemistry 41: S93
22. Hommes FA (ed) 1991 Techniques in diagnostic human biochemical genetics – a laboratory manual. Wiley Liss, New York
23. Jedeikin R, Makela S K, Shennan A T et al 1982 Creatine kinase isoenzymes in serum from cord blood and the blood of healthy full term infants during the first three postnatal days. Clinical Chemistry 28: 317–322
24. John R, Bamforth F J 1987 Serum free thyroxine and free triiodothyronine concentrations in healthy full term, pre-term and sick pre-term neonates. Annals of Clinical Biochemistry 24: 461–465
25. Jonetz-Mentzel L, Weidemann G 1993 Establishment of reference ranges for cortisol in neonates, infants, children and adolescents. European Journal of Clinical Chemistry 31: 525–529
26. Karlen J, Aperia A, Zetterstrom R 1995 Renal excretion of calcium and phosphate in preterm and term infants. Journal of Pediatrics 106: 814–819
27. Kaufman J M, Greene M I, Seegmiller J E 1968 Urine uric acid:creatinine ratio – a screening test for inherited disorders of purine metabolism. Journal of Pediatrics 73: 583–592
28. Koch G, Wendel H 1968 Adjustment of arterial blood gases and acid base balance in the normal newborn infant during the first week of life. Biologia Neonatorum 12: 136–161
29. Lockitch G, Halstead A, Wadsworth L et al 1988 Age and sex specific pediatric reference intervals and correlations for zinc, copper, selenium, iron, vitamins A and E and related proteins. Clinical Chemistry 34: 1625–1628
30. Mayne P D, Kovar I Z 1991 Calcium and phosphorus metabolism in the premature infant. Annals of Clinical Biochemistry 28: 131–142
31. Meites S (ed) 1989 Pediatric clinical chemistry, 3rd edition. AACC Press, Washington, p. 191
32. Miall L S, Henderson M J, Turner A J et al 1999 Plasma creatinine rises dramatically in the first 48 hours of life in preterm infants. Pediatrics 104: e76
33. Muntau A C, Steiter M, Kapple R 2002 Age-related reference ranges for serum selenium concentrations in infants and children. Clinical Chemistry 48: 555–560
34. Murthy J N, Hicks J N, Soldin S J 1995 Evaluation of the Technicon Immuno I random access immunoassay analyser and calculation of pediatric reference ranges for endocrine tests, T-uptake and ferritin. Clinical Biochemistry 28: 181–185
35. Nelson N, Finnstrom O, Larsson L 1989 Plasma ionised calcium, phosphate and magnesium in pre-term and small for gestational age infants. Acta Paediatrica Scandinavica 78: 351–357
36. NHS 1998 Supraregional assay service handbook, 3rd edn
37. Rossi R, Danzebrink S, Linnenburger K et al 1994 Assessment of tubular reabsorption on sodium, glucose, phosphate and amino acids based on spot urine samples. Acta Paediatrica 83: 1282–1286
38. Rudd P T, Hughes E A, Placzek M M et al 1983 Reference ranges for plasma creatinine during the first month of life. Archives of Disease in Childhood 58: 212–215
39. Rükgauer M, Klein J, Kruse-Jarres J D 1997 Reference values for the trace elements copper, manganese, selenium and zinc in the serum/plasma of children, adolescents and adults. Journal of Trace Elements in Medicine and Biology 1: 92–98
40. Sargent J D, Strubel T A, Kresel J et al 1993 Normal values for random urinary calcium to creatinine ratios in infancy. Journal of Paediatrics 123: 393–397
41. Soldin S J, Bailey J, Beatey J et al 1995 Pediatric reference ranges for 17α-hydroxyprogesterone. Clinical Chemistry 41: S92
42. Soldin S J, Bailey J, Bjorn J et al 1999 Pediatric reference ranges for iron on the Hitachi 747 with Boehringer Mannheim reagents. Clinical Chemistry 45: A22
43. Soldin S J, Brugnara C, Hichs J M (eds) 1999 Pediatric reference ranges, 3rd edn. AACC Press, Washington
44. Soldin S J, Hicks J M, Bailey J et al 1997 Pediatric reference ranges for β2-microglobulin and ceruloplasmin. Clinical Chemistry 43: S199
45. Soldin S J, Hicks J M, Bailey J et al 1997 Pediatric reference ranges for 25 hydroxy vitamin D during the summer and winter. Clinical Chemistry 43: S200
46. Soldin S J, Hicks J M, Bailey J et al 1997 Pediatric reference ranges for creatinine kinase and insulin-like growth factor I. Clinical Chemistry 43: S199
47. Soldin S J, Hickson J M, Bailey J et al 1995 Pediatric reference ranges for amylase. Clinical Chemistry 41: S94
48. Soldin S J, Morales A, Albalos F et al 1995 Pediatric reference ranges on the Abbott Imx for FSH, LH, prolactin, TSH, T4, T3, free T4, free T3, T-uptake, IgE and ferritin. Clinical Biochemistry 28: 603–606
49. Soldin S J, Morse A S 1998 Pediatric reference ranges for calcium and triglycerides in children <1 year old using the Vitros 500 analyser. Clinical Chemistry 44: A16
50. Soldin S J, Savwoir T V, Guo Y 1997 Pediatric reference ranges for alkaline phosphatase, aspartate aminotransferase, and alanine aminotransferase in children less than 1 year old on the Vitros 500. Clinical Chemistry 43: S199
51. Soldin S J, Savwoir T V, Guo Y 1997 Pediatric reference ranges for lactate dehydrogenase and uric acid during the first year of life on the Vitros 500 analyzer. Clinical Chemistry 43: S199
52. Soldin S J, Savwoir T V, Guo Y 1997. Pediatric reference ranges for gamma-glutamyltransferase and urea nitrogen during the first year of life on the Vitros 500 analyser. Clinical Chemistry 43: S199
53. Sonntag J, Prankel B, Waltz S 1996 Serum creatinine concentration, urinary creatinine excretion and creatinine clearance during the first 9 weeks in preterm infants with a birth weight below 1500 g. European Journal of Pediatrics 155: 815–819

54. Srinvason G, Pildes R S, Cattamanchi G et al 1986 Plasma glucose values in normal neonates: a new look. Journal of Pediatrics 109: 114–117

55. Thalme B 1962 Calcium, chloride, cholesterol, inorganic phosphorus and total protein in blood plasma during the early neonatal period studied with ultra-microchemical methods. Acta Paediatrica Scandinavica 51: 649–660

56. Wandrup J, Kroner J, Pryds O et al 1988 Age related reference values for ionized calcium in the first week of life in premature and full term newborns. Scandinavian Journal of Clinical Laboratory Investigation 48: 255–260

57. Wharton B A, Bassi U, Gough G et al 1971 Clinical value of plasma creatine kinase and uric acid levels during the first week of life. Archives of Disease in Childhood 46: 356–362

58. Wilkins BH 1992 Renal function in sick, very low birthweight infants. 3. Sodium, potassium and water excretion. Archives of Disease in Childhood 67: 1154–1161

59. Zlotkin S H, Casselman C W 1987 Percentile estimates of reference values for total protein and albumin in sera of premature infants (<37 weeks of gestation). Clinical Chemistry 33: 411–413

Normal blood gas values

N R C Roberton, Janet M Rennie

	PaO$_2$				PaCO$_2$				H$^+$			
	kPa	mmHg	kPa	mmHg	kPa	mmHg	kPa	mmHg	nmol/l	pH	nmol/l	pH
15 min	11.6	87			3.7	28			48	7.32		
30 min	11.4	86			4.3	32			43	7.37		
60 min	10.8	81			4.1	31			40	7.40		
1–6 h	8.0–10.6	60–80	*8.0–9.3*	*60–70*	4.7–6.0	35–45	*4.7–6.0*	*35–45*	46–49	7.31–7.34	*42–48*	*7.32–7.38*
6–24 h	9.3–10	70–75	*8.0–9.3*	*60–70*	4.4–4.8	33–36	*3.6–5.3*	*27–40*	37–43	7.37–7.43	*35–45*	*7.36–7.45*
48 h–1 week	9.3–11.3	70–85	*10.0–10.6*	*75–80*	4.4–4.8	33–36	*4.3–4.5*	*32–36*	42–44	7.36–7.38	*40–48*	*7.32–7.40*
2 weeks					4.8–5.2	36–39	*5.1*	*38*	43	7.37	*48*	*7.32*
3 weeks					5.3	40	*5.1*	*38*	42	7.38	*49*	*7.31*
1 month					5.2	39	*4.9*	*37*	41	7.39	*49*	*7.31*

The values at 15, 30 and 60 minutes are from our own unpublished observations on full-term infants. Data from 1 hour to 1 week are drawn from the literature on arterial samples. Data beyond 1 week are on capillary samples. Values in the table which are in *italics* are those for premature infants; those not in italics are for full-term infants.
Reproduced from Rennie J M & Roberton N R C 2002 Manual of neonatal intensive care 4e. Edward Arnold, London.

APPENDIX 8

Normal cerebrospinal fluid values

Janet M Rennie

All values are given as mean and range.

Type of infant	Red cell count (mm³)	White cell count (mm³)	Protein (g/l)	Glucose (mmol/l)
Preterm <7 days	30 (0–333)	9 (0–30)*	1 (0.5–2.9, but mostly <2 g/l)	3 (1.5–5.5)[†]
Preterm >7 days	30	12 (2–70)	0.9 (0.5–2.6, mostly <1.5)	3 (1.5–5.5)[†]
Term <7 days	9 (0–50)	5 (0–30)*	0.6 (0.3–2.5)	3 (1.5–5.5)[†]
Term >7 days	<10	3 (0–10)	0.5 (0.2–0.8)	3 (1.5–5.5)[†]

Sources: see reference list.[1,3,5,7,9,11,12,14–16]

* Gyllensward & Malmstrom[6] give values of up to 112 white cells per mm³ in preterm and 90 in term babies, but the study included babies with over 1000 red cells per mm³ and was done before routine ultrasound was available. The results are so much higher than other studies that I have not extended the range to include these values.

[†] CSF glucose usually 70–80% of plasma glucose, and at least 50%. Take plasma glucose sample *before* doing lumbar puncture (stress). Low CSF glucose levels can persist for weeks after intraventricular haemorrhage.[4]

Traumatic lumbar puncture

It has been suggested that it is possible to apply a formula to compare observed (O) to predicted (P) white cell counts in CSF samples with high red cell counts thought to be due to a 'traumatic tap'. The predicted white cell count P in the CSF is calculated from:

$$P = CSF \text{ red cell count} \times \frac{\text{Blood WCC}}{\text{Blood RBC}}$$

The O:P ratio was greater than 1 in all cases of meningitis in infants over the age of 1 month.[2] The ratio is less well evaluated in the newborn, who can have paradoxically low white cell counts in the CSF even when the culture is positive. Several authors have pointed out that this ratio 'overcorrects' the CSF white cell count in newborn infants.[8,10,13] Osborne & Pizer[9] suggested that contamination with fewer than 10 000 red cells per mm³ did not influence the white cell count. In suspicious clinical cases, the only course is to repeat the lumbar puncture after 12–24 hours.

References

1. Ahmed A, Hickey S M, Ehrett S et al 1996 Cerebrospinal fluid values in the term neonate. Pediatric Infectious Disease Journal 15: 298–303
2. Bonadio W A, Smith D S, Goddard S, Boroughs J, Khaja G 1990 Distinguishing cerebrospinal fluid abnormalities in children with bacterial meningitis and traumatic lumbar puncture. Journal of Infectious Diseases 162: 251–254
3. Bonadio W A, Stanco L, Bruce R, Barry D, Smith D 1992 Reference values of normal cerebrospinal fluid composition in infants ages 0 to 8 weeks. Pediatric Infectious Disease Journal 11: 589–591

4. Deonna T, Calame A, van Melle G, Prod'hom L S 1977 Hypoglycorrhachia in neonatal intracranial haemorrhage. Relationship to posthaemorrhagic hydrocephalus. Helvetica Paediatrica Acta 32: 351–361

5. Escobedo M, Barton L L, Volpe J J 1975 Cerebrospinal fluid studies in an intensive care nursery. Journal of Perinatal Medicine 3: 204–210

6. Gyllensward A, Malmstrom S 1962 The cerebrospinal fluid in immature infants. Acta Paediatrica Scandinavica 51(suppl. 135): 54–62

7. Naidoo B T 1968 The cerebrospinal fluid in the healthy newborn infant. South African Medical Journal 42: 933–935

8. Novak R W 1984 Lack of validity of standard corrections for white blood cell counts of blood-contaminated cerebrospinal fluid in infants. American Journal of Clinical Pathology 82: 95–97

9. Osborne J P, Pizer B 1981 Effect on the white cell count of contaminating cerebrospinal fluid with blood. Archives of Disease in Childhood 56: 400–401

10. Otila E 1948 Studies on the cerebrospinal fluid in premature infants. Acta Paediatrica Scandinavica 35(suppl. 9): 7–97

11. Portnoy J M, Olson L C 1985 Normal cerebrospinal fluid values in children: another look. Pediatrics 75: 484–487

12. Rodriguez A F, Kaplan S L, Mason E O 1990 Cerebrospinal fluid values in the very low birthweight infant. Journal of Pediatrics 116: 971–974

13. Rubenstein J S, Yogev R 1985 What represents pleocytosis in blood contaminated ('traumatic tap') cerebrospinal fluid in children? Journal of Pediatrics 107: 249–252

14. Sarff L D, Platt L H, McCracken G H Jr 1976 Cerebrospinal fluid evaluation in neonates: comparison of high risk infants with and without meningitis. Journal of Pediatrics 88: 473–477

15. Widell S 1958 On the cerebrospinal fluid in normal children and in patients with acute abacterial meningoencephalitis. Acta Paediatrica Scandinavica 47(suppl. 115): 1–102

16. Wolf H, Hoepffner L 1961 The cerebrospinal fluid in the newborn and premature infant. World Neurology 2: 871–877

APPENDIX 9

Oxyhaemoglobin dissociation curve

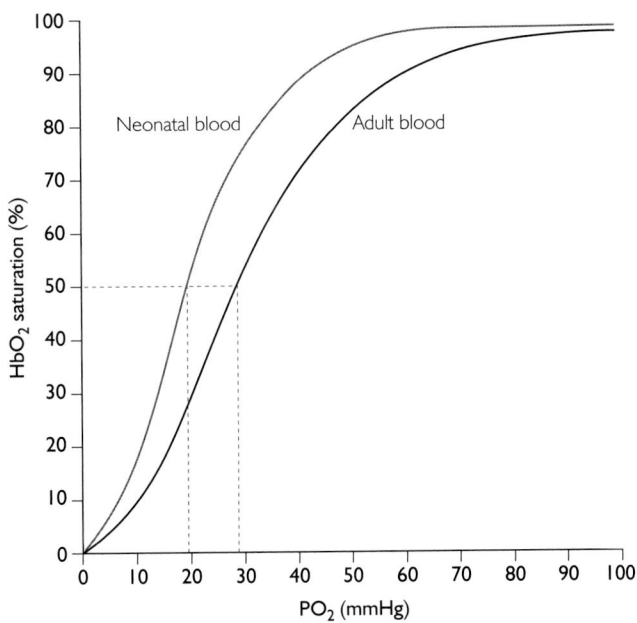

Oxyhaemoglobin dissociation curves for adult blood and neonatal blood. The dotted lines dropping from 50% saturation give the p50 values for neonatal blood (19 mmHg) and of adult blood (28 mmHg).

APPENDIX 10

The Siggaard-Andersen nomogram

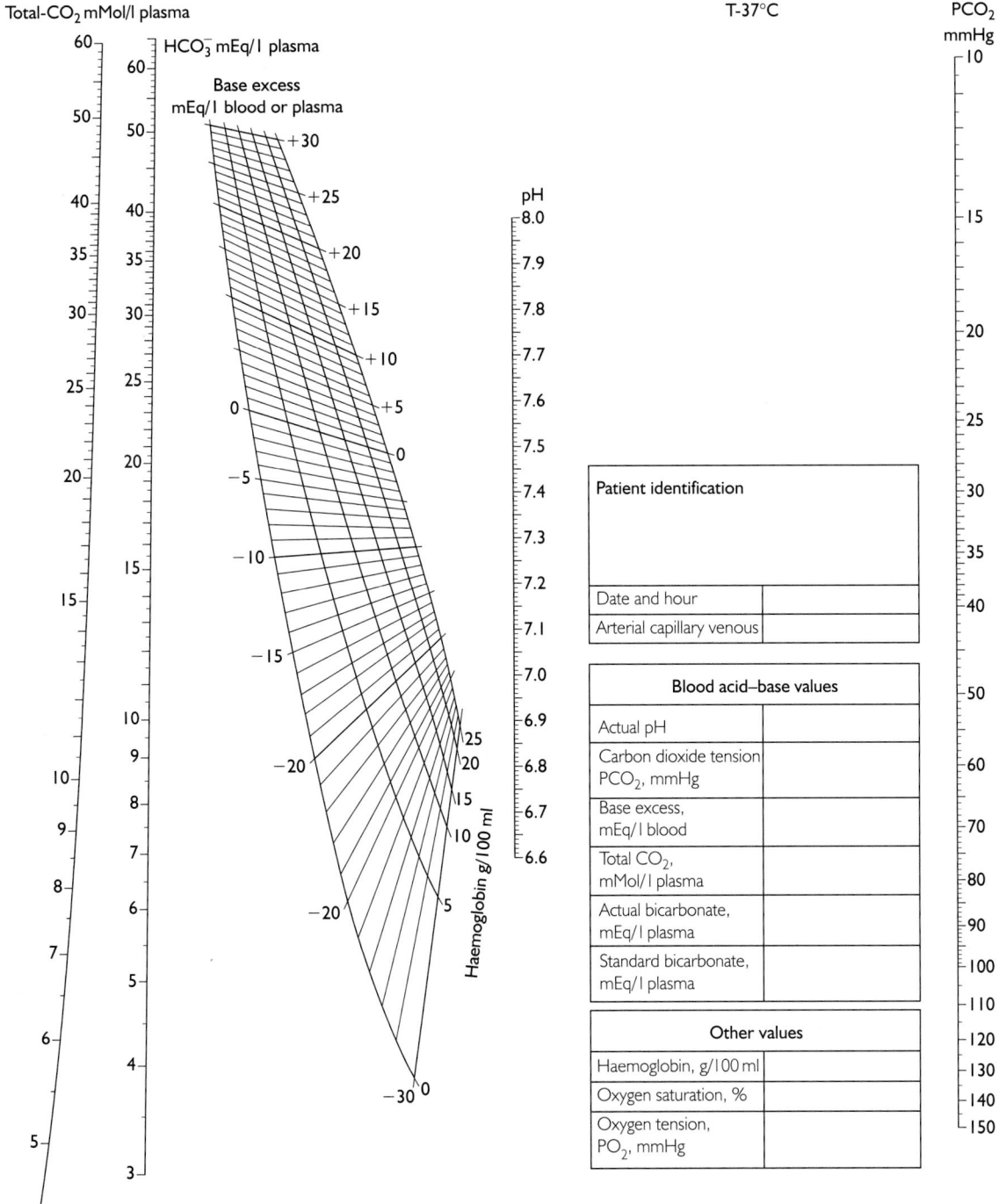

By knowing any two values of an acid–base measurement, the other values can be derived by connecting the two known points on this nomogram. For newborn babies, the haemoglobin can be assumed to be 15 g/100 ml. Reproduced from Siggaard-Andersen O 1963 Blood acid-base alignment nomogram. Scandinavian Journal of Clinical and Laboratory Investigation 15: 211–217.

Index